Miranda A. Farage • Kenneth W. Miller
Howard I. Maibach
Editors

Textbook of Aging Skin

Second Edition

Volume 1

With 574 Figures and 224 Tables

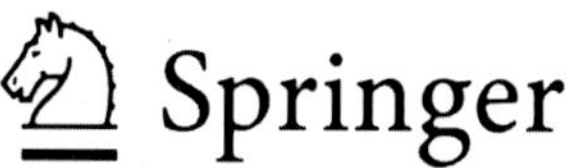

Editors
Miranda A. Farage
Winton Hill Business Center
The Procter and Gamble Company
Cincinnati, OH, USA

Kenneth W. Miller
Margoshes-Miller
Consulting, LLC
Cincinnati, OH, USA

Howard I. Maibach
Department of Dermatology
University of California
San Francisco, CA, USA

ISBN 978-3-662-47397-9 ISBN 978-3-662-47398-6 (eBook)
ISBN 978-3-662-47399-3 (print and electronic bundle)
DOI 10.1007/978-3-662-47398-6

Library of Congress Control Number: 2009938632

Printed on acid-free paper

This Springer imprint is published by Springer Nature
The registered company is Springer-Verlag GmbH Germany
The registered company address is: Heidelberger Platz 3, 14197 Berlin, Germany

Textbook of Aging Skin

Dedication
To a forgotten and sometimes lonely and scary aging journey – Much more dignity and respect are deserved for all of you. MAF, KWM, and *HIM*

When things go wrong as they sometimes will,
When the road you're trudging seems all uphill,
When the funds are low and the debts are high,
And you want to smile but you have to sigh,
When care is pressing you down a bit
Rest if you must, but don't you quit.
Success is failure turned inside out,
The silver tint on the clouds of doubt,
And you can never tell how close you are,
It may be near when it seems afar.
So, stick to the fight when you're hardest hit
It's when things go wrong that you mustn't quit.

—*Unknown*

Foreword

We mourn the loss of Professor Albert Kligman – a man whose energy, enthusiasm and intelligence benefited the specialty and many of us. His remarks below are as cogent today – as when written for the first Edition in December 2009.

Editors
MAF, KWM and HIM

The population is aging rapidly. Centenarians are no longer a rarity. The fastest growing segment of the population in the United States is people over 80. In the next 25 years, half of the population in the United States will be aged over 50.

These shifts will have a tremendous impact on the delivery of healthcare to the elderly and will require a new awareness of how cutaneous disorders affect the quality of life, comprising a heavy burden on health and wellbeing.

Physicians and healthcare workers are woefully ignorant of the distress, discomfort, and anxieties of people afflicted by disorders of the skin. There exists a widespread misconception that skin disorders are simply cosmetic nuisances that can be self-treated by a great assortment of anti-aging creams and lotions available at the local drug store. Most of these include high-sounding ingredients such as antioxidants, vitamins, nutrients, botanicals, and ancient folkloristic remedies, the efficacy and safety of which have never been tested. They offer little more than hope in a bottle. The fact is that common skin diseases may not often be lethal but can ruin enjoyment of life. Chronic itchy rashes can be maddening, lowering one's self-esteem, embarrassing, interfering with sleep, and often accompanied by depression, social isolation, and deterioration of appearance; they can also be uncomfortable, and, not least, costly to treat.

The elderly commonly take 15–20 oral supplements daily to fight the ailments of old age. These are generally useless and may be harmful, often interacting adversely with prescription drugs. The elderly often resort to alternative medicines instead of seeing their doctor to obtain FDA-approved drugs, and also often skip their daily doses to save money. Noncompliance is common. Misdiagnosis and mistreatment of the elderly by health-care workers are common. National surveys show that skin diseases increase steadily throughout our life-span. Old people may have as many as 5–10 coexistent cutaneous problems that are worthy of medical attention. Moreover, the clinical manifestations of skin diseases in the aged often have different

appearances than in the young, confounding diagnosis. Importantly, healing of chronic lesions, especially ulcers, is impaired in the elderly. Immunity is weakened, increasing susceptibility to infections. Response to treatment is slower, leading to noncompliance. Adverse drug reactions are common and too commonly not suspected. Management of chronic conditions is difficult and frustrating.

The above litany of problems makes this textbook edited by Farage, Miller, and Maibach a welcome addition to the literature. It is invaluable as a reference resource covering exhaustively an enormous number of clinical conditions. No topic is neglected including cosmetic treatments. The numerous contributions are by highly qualified experts who have a published record of expertise.

This comprehensive volume is also practical and relevant to the everyday world of clinical practice. The information will be useful to physicians, manufacturers of drugs and skincare products, educators, investigators, nursing home personnel, estheticians, and federal regulators.

This first edition is up to date, including much new material that belongs to the shelves of every library, which deals with geriatric problems. Dermatologists especially will be remiss if they do not put this volume within easy reach for consultation as they encounter a swelling clientele of aging patients.

University of Pennsylvania
Philadelphia, PA, USA

Albert M. Kligman M.D., Ph.D.
Professor Emeritus

Preface

The skin is a portal of knowledge on aging. From its softness and smoothness in infancy, through its suppleness in youth, to its wrinkled texture in elders, the skin displays the most visible and accessible manifestations of aging.

Due to falling birth rates and rising life expectancies in industrialized countries, the average age of the population is increasing. People are more preoccupied with looking and "staying" young, and research into the process of aging has expanded.

Although excellent compendia exist on the subject of aging skin, the body of knowledge is burgeoning and we still have more to learn. The purposes of this textbook are: (1) to compile the most current information into one comprehensive reference (it covers a range of topics, from the basics of skin structure and function to the cellular and molecular mechanisms of aging, to the latest bioengineering instruments used to assess age-related changes in the skin); (2) to guide on how to utilize skin as a tool for insights into the remainder of organs; and (3) to encourage the rapidly expanding universe of aging research in a more holistic aspect (heart, lung, brain, etc., as well as laboratories and investigators/foundations/government agencies) to utilize the readily available skin as an entry/surrogate for research on other organs.

Contributors are internationally recognized experts from multiple disciplines germane to this topic. We gratefully acknowledge all contributors for sharing their time and expertise.

We expect this second edition of the textbook to be valuable to researchers and students with an interest in aging skin, and the aging process in general. Because research progress in this area is rapid, we hope to update this compendium periodically as advances in the field dictate.

The editors welcome suggestions for the third edition.

Miranda A. Farage
Kenneth W. Miller
Howard I. Maibach

Acknowledgments

Deep appreciation and grateful thank yous are extended to the many experts who contributed both knowingly and indirectly to this book.

A special thank you to Drs. N. Enane-Anderson, G. Collier, P. Schofield, R. Leboeuf, Mr. Ron Visscher, and Mr. John Cooper, who generously offered their time and expertise to peer-review relevant chapters and for their support of this book. No praise is excessive for their efforts, and they have our heartfelt gratitude.

Many thanks go to the significant efforts of all the contributors of this book and the valuable time they dedicated preparing their chapters. This book represents the fruits of a jointly conceived and executed venture and has benefited from global and diverse partners.

We would also like to single out Ms. Sunali Mull (Springer Editorial-India) for a special recognition. Her great efforts, time, discipline, and dedication helped moved this book forward on a timely and organized manner. In addition, we would like to thank Mr. S. Klemp, Mr. A. Baroi, Ms. R. Amos, Ms. A. Singh, Ms. S. Friedrichsen, and Ms. S. Westendorf (Springer Office) for their help in moving this book forward. We acknowledge the usefulness of the new "SpringerMeteor" system which helped contributors and editors get the first glance of the future of electronic information/submission/editing.

In addition, Dr. D. A. Hutchins, Ms. Z. Schwen, Ms. W. Wippel, Ms. G. Entrup, Dr. T. L. Nusair, and Ms. P. Fifth (Rest in Peace our dear friend; your memories will always be with us) have all assisted with this book.

Above all, our everlasting gratitude, thanks, and love go to our parents who inspired us and to our families and children who supported, helped, and encouraged us all the way with their incredible patience. Your continuous care, unconditional love, and sacrifice made all this possible and easier to achieve.

MAF, *KWM*, and *HIM*

Contents

Volume 1

About the Editors

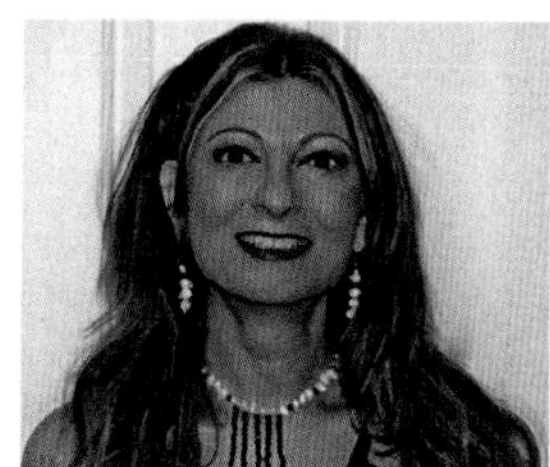

Miranda A. Farage is a Research Fellow in the Global Clinical Sciences Innovation at the Procter & Gamble Company, Cincinnati, Ohio. Dr. Farage leads global research on genital health, dermatological testing and claims, new clinical methods development, sensitive skin, physiology, clinical toxicology, women's health, quality of life, and related fields. Dr. Farage has invented novel state-of-the-art clinical test methods that have resulted in efficient ways of assessing new technologies and products as well as the filing of 15 patent applications. She has published more than 200 manuscripts and chapters in peer-reviewed journals and medical books. She is the Editor-in-Chief of several books such as *The Vulva*; *Textbook of Aging Skin*, first edition; *Topical Application and the Mucosa*; and *Skin, Mucosa and Menopause: Management of Clinical Issues*.

Dr. Farage is a member of many scientific societies including the American Academy of Dermatology, the European College of Society of Vulva Diseases, the National Vulvodynia Association, the American Society for Testing and Materials (ASTM) International, and the Science Advisory Board. Currently, she is serving on the editorial boards of more than a dozen scientific, dermatology, and medical journals. She received a Ph.D. in Medical Sciences and a master degree (MS) in Biology from the University of Illinois, Urbana-Champaign. Before joining Procter & Gamble, she was a faculty member at the Virginia Polytechnic Institute and State University (Virginia Tech).

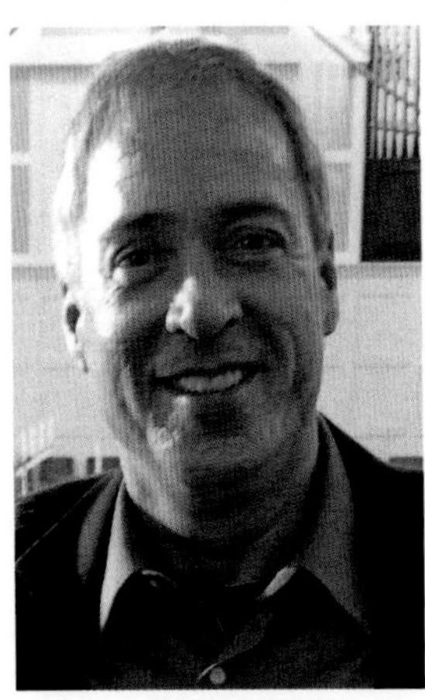

Kenneth W. Miller

- Principal Consultant, Margoshes Miller Consulting LLC, for Product Safety, Toxicology, and Regulatory Strategy (June 2015 to present).
- Associate Director, The Procter & Gamble Company (July 1984–June 2015), with global safety and regulatory experience in medical devices, OTC health care products, and food products.
- Diplomate, American Board of Toxicology (1986–2006).
- Postdoctoral Fellow, University of Medicine and Dentistry of New Jersey (June 1982–July 1984), Nutritional Biochemistry.
- Doctoral degree (Ph.D.): Cornell University, 1982, Toxicology and Food Chemistry.
- Master's degree (M.S.): Cornell University, 1979, Toxicology and Food Chemistry.
- Bachelor's degree (B.S.): Iowa State University, 1977, Biology.
- Dr. Miller has published over 50 manuscripts in the area of toxicology in peer-reviewed journals plus numerous abstracts, book chapters, and presentations at meetings of scientific societies. He is a member of several scientific and professional societies.

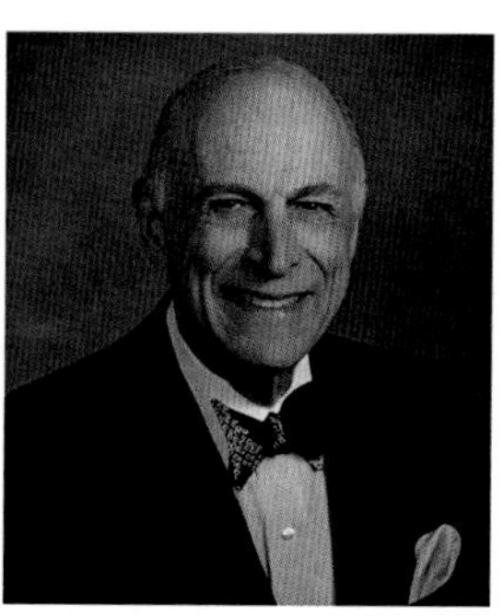

Howard I. Maibach
Present Title: Professor

Education	Degree
Tulane University, New Orleans, LA	A.B.
Tulane University, New Orleans, LA	M.D.
USPHS, Hospital of the University of Pennsylvania	Resident/Fellow

Honorary degrees	Degree	Year
L'Universite de Paris-Sud, France	Ph.D.	1985
Université Claude Bernard Lyon 1, France	Ph.D.	2008
University of Southern Denmark	M.D.	2010

Dr. Howard Maibach joined the University of California Faculty as Assistant Professor and is currently Professor of Dermatology.

Dr. Maibach, an expert in contact and occupational dermatitis, sees patients at the Environmental Dermatoses Clinic, which is part of the Dermatology Clinic at UCSF. His most active fields of research are in dermatopharmacology, dermatotoxicology, and environmental dermatoses. He has been doing human subject research for 45 years.

He has been on the editorial board of more than 30 scientific journals. His bibliography includes more than 2790 publications and 100 books.

He is member of 19 professional societies including the American Academy of Dermatology (AAD), San Francisco Dermatological Society (SFDS), North American Contact Dermatitis Group (NACDG), American Contact Dermatitis Society (ACDS), International Contact Dermatitis Research Group (ICDRG), Society of Toxicology (SOT), European Environmental and Contact Dermatitis Research Group (EECDRG), and the Internal Commission on Occupational Health. He is a consultant to government, academia, and industry worldwide.

Dr. Howard Maibach was honored as the 2013 recipient of The Master Dermatologist Award by The American Academy of Dermatology's 71st Annual Conference held in Miami, Florida. This prestigious award recognizes an Academy member's significant contributions to the field of dermatology and to the American Academy of Dermatology.

In March 2015, The International League of Dermatological Societies (ILDS) awarded Dr. Maibach their 2014 ILDS Certificate of Appreciation in recognition of his outstanding contribution to dermatology, both nationally and internationally, through his work, research, publications, and teaching in the USA and over 60 countries.

Contributors

Rami Abadi Department of Dermatology, American University of Beirut Medical Center, Beirut, Lebanon

Ossama Abbas Department of Dermatology, American University of Beirut Medical Center, Beirut, Lebanon

Jihane Abou Rahal Department of Dermatology, American University of Beirut Medical Center, Beirut, Lebanon

Jean Adamus Unilever Research and Development, Trumbull, CT, USA

Mohamed A. Adly Department of Zoology, Faculty of Science, Sohag University, Sohag, Egypt

Avani Ahuja Department of Biotechnology, Jaypee Institute of Information Technology, Noida, UP, India

Denize Ainbinder Institute of Drug Research, School of Pharmacy, The Hebrew University of Jerusalem, Jerusalem, Israel

A. Deniz Akkaya Department of Dermatology, Koç University Hospital, Istanbul, Turkey

Department of Dermatology, V.K. Foundation, American Hospital of Istanbul, Istanbul, Turkey

Ali Alikhan Department of Dermatology, University of Cincinnati, Cincinnati, OH, USA

Satoshi Amano Shiseido Research Center, Yokohama, Japan

Marco Ardigò Clinical Dermatology, IFO San Gallicano Dermatological Institute, Rome, Italy

Melina C. Armenaka Department of Dermatology and Venereology, University of Athens, A. Sygros Hospital, Athens, Greece

Hanan Assaf Department of Dermatology, Saudi German Hospital, Jeddah, Saudi Arabia

Daniel Asselineau L'Oreal, Research and Innovation, Aulnay-sous-bois, France

Carmela Rita Balistreri Department of Pathobiology and Medical Biotechnologies, University of Palermo, Immunosenescence Unit, Palermo, Italy

Elma Baron Department of Dermatology, Case Western Reserve University, Cleveland, OH, USA

Leslie S. Baumann Baumann Cosmetic and Research Institute, Miami, FL, USA

Enzo Berardesca San Gallicano Dermatological Institute, Rome, Italy

Françoise Bernerd L'Oreal Research and Innovation, Aulnay-sous-bois, France

Christiane Bertin SkinCare R&D, Johnson & Johnson Santé Beauté France, Issy-les-Moulineaux, France

Marianne Berwick Internal Medicine, Division of Epidemiology, University of New Mexico, Albuquerque, NM, USA

Tapan K. Bhattacharyya Otolaryngology-Head and Neck Surgery, University of Illinois, Chicago, IL, USA

Emil Bisaccia Columbia University College of Physicians and Surgeons, New York, NY, USA

Johannes Bischof Department of Cell Biology, Division of Genetics, University of Salzburg, Salzburg, Austria

Donald L. Bissett Beauty Technology Division, The Procter & Gamble Company, Sharon Woods Innovation Center, Cincinnati, OH, USA

Donald L. Bjerke The Procter & Gamble Company, Central Product Safety, Cincinnati, OH, USA

Thomas Blatt The Beiersdorf Research Center, Hamburg, Germany

Miroslav Blumenberg The R.O. Perelman Department of Dermatology, NYU Langone Medical Center, New York, NY, USA

Department of Biochemistry and Molecular Pharmacology, NYU Langone Medical Center, New York, NY, USA

Ulrike Blume-Peytavi Department of Dermatology and Allergy, Clinical Research Center for Hair and Skin Science, Charité-Universitätsmedizin Berlin, Berlin, Germany

Markus Böhm Department of Dermatology, Laboratory for Neuroendocrinology of the Skin and Interdisciplinary Endocrinology, University of Münster, Münster, Germany

Carol Bosko Unilever Research and Development, Trumbull, CT, USA

Mario Bramante Product Safety and Regulatory Affairs, Procter & Gamble Service GmbH, Schwalbach am Taunus, Germany

Douglas E. Brash Departments of Therapeutic Radiology, Genetics, and Dermatology, Yale School of Medicine, New Haven, CT, USA

Stéphane Brézillon Laboratoire de Biochimie, CNRS UMR 7369, Faculté de Médecine, Université de Reims-Champagne-Ardenne, Reims, France

Centre National de la Recherche Scientifique, CNRS UMR 7369, Reims, France

Carla Abdo Brohem R&D Department, Grupo Boticário, São José dos Pinhais, PR, Brazil

Robert L. Bronaugh Office of Cosmetics and Colors, Center for Food Safety and Applied Nutrition, Food and Drug Administration, College Park, MD, USA

John Jay P. Cadavona Department of Dermatology, University of California, San Francisco, CA, USA

Fernanda Camozzato Department of Dermatology, Brazilian Center for Studies in Dermatology, Porto Alegre, RS, Brazil

Giuseppina Candore Department of Pathobiology and Medical Biotechnologies, University of Palermo, Immunosenescence Unit, Palermo, Italy

Calogero Caruso Department of Pathobiology and Medical Biotechnologies, University of Palermo, Immunosenescence Unit, Palermo, Italy

Anne Lynn S. Chang Department of Dermatology, Stanford University School of Medicine, Redwood City, CA, USA

Duane L. Charbonneau The Procter & Gamble Company, Cincinnati, OH, USA

Alexandra Charruyer Department of Dermatology and Eli and Edythe Broad, Center of Regeneration Medicine and Stem Cell Research, University of California, Veterans Affairs Medical Center, San Francisco, CA, USA

Adele Chedraoui Department of Dermatology, Lebanese American University, Beirut, Lebanon

Ying Chen Global R&D, Equity and Claims, Reckitt Benckiser, Montvale, NJ, USA

Shujiang (Suzie) Cheng Colgate-Palmolive Company, Piscataway, NJ, USA

Raymond J. Cho Department of Dermatology, University of California, San Francisco, CA, USA

Yun-Hee Choi Anti-aging Research Institute of BIO-FD&C Co. Ltd., Incheon, Republic of Korea

Departments of Pharmacology and Global Medical Science, Institute of Lifestyle Medicine and Nuclear Receptor Research Consortium, Wonju College of Medicine, Yonsei University, Wonju, Republic of Korea

Kaare Christensen The Danish Twin Registry and The Danish Aging Research Center, Department of Public Health, University of Southern Denmark, Odense C, Denmark

Jin Ho Chung Department of Dermatology, Seoul National University College of Medicine, Seoul, Korea

Maria Grazia Cifone Life, Health and Environmental Sciences, University of L'Aquila, L'Aquila, Italy

Benedetta Cinque Life, Health and Environmental Sciences, University of L'Aquila, L'Aquila, Italy

Daniele Corridoni Division of Gastroenterology and Liver Disease, Department of Medicine, Case Western Reserve University School of Medicine, Cleveland, OH, USA

Giovanni Corsetti Department of Clinical and Experimental Sciences, Division of Human Anatomy and Physiopathology, University of Brescia, Brescia, Italy

Gertrude-Emilia Costin The Institute for In Vitro Sciences, Inc. (IIVS), Gaithersburg, MD, USA

Justine Courtois Laboratory of Skin Bioengineering and Imaging, Department of Dermatopathology, University Hospital of Liège, Liège, Belgium

Jonathan M. Crowther JMC Scientific Consulting Ltd, Surrey, UK

Shweta Dang Department of Biotechnology, Jaypee Institute of Information Technology, Noida, UP, India

Razvigor Darlenski Department of Dermatology and Venereology, Tokuda Hospital Sofia, Sofia, Bulgaria

Nancy C. Dawes The Procter and Gamble Company, Cincinnati, OH, USA

Philippe Delvenne Department of Dermatopathology, University Hospital of Liège, Liège, Belgium

Céline Deneuville L'Oreal, Research and Innovation, Aulnay-sous-bois, France

Luisa Di Marzio Department of Pharmacy, University of Chieti - Pescara "G d'Annunzio", Chieti - Pescara, Italy

Francesco S. Dioguardi Department of Internal Medicine and Community Health, University of Milan, Milan, Italy

Luisa A. DiPietro Center for Wound Healing and Tissue Regeneration, College of Dentistry, University of Illinois at Chicago, Chicago, IL, USA

Department of Biology, DePaul University, Chicago, IL, USA

Alexander S. Donath Cincinnati Facial Plastic Surgery, Cincinnati, OH, USA

Frank Dreher MERZ North America, Inc., San Mateo, CA, USA

Laurence Du-Thumm Colgate-Palmolive Company, Piscataway, NJ, USA

Christine Duval L'Oreal Research and Innovation, Aulnay-sous-bois, France

Kimberly M. Eickhorst Dermatology Associates Of W CT, Danbury, CT, USA

Moetaz El-Domyati Department of Dermatology, Al-Minya University, Al-Minya, Egypt

Akram Elmahdy Department of Dermatology, University of California, San Francisco, CA, USA

Peter Elsner Department of Dermatology and Dermatological Allergology, Universitätsklinikum Jena, Jena, Germany

Alex Eshaghian AE Skin, Encino, CA, USA

Khaled Ezzedine Department of Dermatology, CHU Saint-André, Bordeaux, France

Miranda A. Farage Winton Hill Business Center, The Procter & Gamble Company, Cincinnati, OH, USA

Susan P. Felter The Procter & Gamble Company, Cincinnati, OH, USA

Vincenzo Flati Department of Biotechnological and Applied Clinical Sciences, University of L'Aquila, L'Aquila, Italy

Sara Flores Department of Dermatology, University of Cincinnati, Cincinnati, OH, USA

Joachim W. Fluhr Department of Dermatology, Charité University Clinic, Berlin, Germany

Reema Gabrani Department of Biotechnology, Jaypee Institute of Information Technology, Noida, UP, India

Mary Carmen Gasco-Buisson P&G Brand Creation and Innovation, Procter & Gamble, Cincinnati, OH, USA

Licia Genovese Minerva Research Labs Ltd, London, UK

G. Frank Gerberick Human Safety Department, Procter and Gamble Company, Cincinnati, OH, USA

Ruby Ghadially Department of Dermatology and Eli and Edythe Broad, Center of Regeneration Medicine and Stem Cell Research, University of California, Veterans Affairs Medical Center, San Francisco, CA, USA

Paolo U. Giacomoni Elan Rose Int., Tustin, CA, USA

Sarah Girardeau-Hubert L'Oreal, Research and Innovation, Aulnay-sous-bois, France

Maurizio Giuliani Life, Health and Environmental Sciences, University of L'Aquila, L'Aquila, Italy

Francesca Giusti Department of Dermatology, University of Modena and Reggio Emilia, Modena, Italy

Paraskevi Gkogkolou Department of Dermatology, Laboratory for Neuro-endocrinology of the Skin and Interdisciplinary Endocrinology, University of Münster, Münster, Germany

Farzam Gorouhi Department of Dermatology, University of California, Davis, CA, USA

James C. Grotting Department of Plastic Surgery, University of Alabama, Birmingham, AL, USA

Linna Guan Department of Dermatology, Case Western Reserve University, Cleveland, OH, USA

Christiane Guinot Biometrics and Epidemiology Unit, CE.R.I.E.S., Neuilly-sur-Seine, France

David A. Gunn Unilever Research and Development, Colworth Science Park, Sharnbrook, Bedfordshire, UK

Madhulika A. Gupta Department of Psychiatry, Schulich School of Medicine and Dentistry, University of Western Ontario, London, ON, Canada

Prashant Gupta Department of Biotechnology, Jaypee Institute of Information Technology, Noida, UP, India

Sanjay Gupta Department of Biotechnology, Jaypee Institute of Information Technology, Noida, UP, India

Varun Gupta Department of Plastic Surgery, Vanderbilt University, Nashville, TN, USA

Bahman Guyuron Department of Plastic Surgery, University Hospitals of Cleveland, Case Western Reserve University, Cleveland, OH, USA

Elisabeth Hahnel Department of Dermatology and Allergy, Clinical Research Center for Hair and Skin Science, Charité-Universitätsmedizin Berlin, Berlin, Germany

Tomohiro Hakozaki Beauty Technology Division, The Procter & Gamble Company, Mason Business Center, Mason, OH, USA

Stacy S. Hawkins Unilever Research and Development, Trumbull, CT, USA

Valerie Haydont L'Oreal, Research and Innovation, Aulnay-sous-bois, France

Timothy P. Heffernan Departments of Therapeutic Radiology, Genetics, and Dermatology, Yale School of Medicine, New Haven, CT, USA

Peter Helmbold Department of Dermatology, University of Heidelberg, Heidelberg, Germany

Trinh Hermanns-Lê Laboratory of Skin Bioengineering and Imaging, Department of Dermatopathology, University Hospital of Liège, Liège, Belgium

Electron Microscopy Unit, Department of Dermatopathology, Unilab Lg, University Hospital of Liège, Liège, Belgium

Doris Hexsel Department of Dermatology, Brazilian Center for Studies in Dermatology, Porto Alegre, RS, Brazil

Department of Dermatology, Pontificia Universidade Católica do Rio Grande do Sul (PUC-RS), Porto Alegre, RS, Brazil

K. Kye Higdon Department of Plastic Surgery, Vanderbilt University, Nashville, TN, USA

Greg Hillebrand Amway Corporation, Ada, MI, USA

Tetsuji Hirao Faculty of Pharmacy, Chiba Institute of Science, Choshi, Japan

Regina Hourigan Colgate-Palmolive Company, Piscataway, NJ, USA

Christopher R. Hughes Internal Medicine, Division of Epidemiology, University of New Mexico, Albuquerque, NM, USA

Michael F. Hughes U.S. Environmental Protection Agency, Office of Research and Development, National Health and Environmental Effects Research Laboratory, Research Triangle Park, NC, USA

Young Hui University of California, San Diego, CA, USA

Mahmoud R. Hussein Department of Pathology, Assir Central Hospital, and Assuit University, Assuit, Egypt

Qunshan Jia The Procter & Gamble Company, Central Product Safety, Cincinnati, OH, USA

Mary B. Johnson Beauty Technology Division, The Procter & Gamble Company, Sharon Woods Innovation Center, Cincinnati, OH, USA

Nancy Karapasha The Procter & Gamble Company, Cincinnati, OH, USA

Alexandra Katsarou Department of Dermatology and Venereology, University of Athens, A. Sygros Hospital, Athens, Greece

Linda M. Katz Office of Cosmetics and Colors, Center for Food Safety and Applied Nutrition, Food and Drug Administration, College Park, MD, USA

Abdul Ghani Kibbi Department of Dermatology, American University of Beirut Medical Center, Beirut, Lebanon

Christine C. Kim Dermatology Institute and Skin Care Center, Santa Monica, CA, USA

Hyeong-Sik Kim Anti-aging Research Institute of BIO-FD&C Co. Ltd., Incheon, Republic of Korea

Ki Woo Kim Departments of Pharmacology and Global Medical Science, Wonju College of Medicine, Yonsei University, Wonju, Republic of Korea

Institute of Lifestyle Medicine and Nuclear Receptor Research Consortium, Wonju College of Medicine, Yonsei University, Wonju, Republic of Korea

Won-Serk Kim Department of Dermatology, Kangbuk Samsung Hospital, Sungkyunkwan University College of Medicine, Seoul, South Korea

Mayumi Komine Department of Dermatology, Jichi Medical University, Shimotsuke, Tochigi, Japan

Jan Kottner Department of Dermatology and Allergy, Clinical Research Center for Hair and Skin Science, Charité-Universitätsmedizin Berlin, Berlin, Germany

Aleksandar Krbanjevic Department of Dermatology, Indiana University School of Medicine, Indianapolis, IN, USA

Shalini Krishnasamy University of California, Los Angeles, CA, USA

Nils Krueger Rosenpark Research, Darmstadt, Germany

Jean Krutmann Environmental Health Research Institute (IUF), Heinrich-Heine-University, Duesseldorf, Germany

Atul Kulkarni Anti-aging Research Institute of BIO-FD&C Co. Ltd., Incheon, Republic of Korea

School of Mechanical Engineering, Sungkyunkwan University, Suwon, South Korea

Mazen Kurban Department of Dermatology, American University of Beirut Medical Center, Beirut, Lebanon

Department of Biochemistry and Molecular Genetics, American University of Beirut Medical Center, Beirut, Lebanon

Department of Dermatology, Columbia University, New York, NY, USA

Cristina La Torre Life, Health and Environmental Sciences, University of L'Aquila, L'Aquila, Italy

S. Lahtinen Active Nutrition, DuPont Nutrition and Health, Kantvik, Finland

Samuel M. Lam Willow Bend Wellness Center, Lam Facial Plastic Surgery Center and Hair Restoration Institute, Plano, TX, USA

William J. Ledger Department of Obstetrics and Gynecology, The New York-Presbyterian Hospital, Weill Medical College of Cornell University, New York, NY, USA

Jeong Hun Lee Anti-aging Research Institute of BIO-FD&C Co. Ltd., Incheon, Republic of Korea

Marianne Lesuisse Department of Dermatology, Unilab Lg, Regional Hospital Citadelle, Liège, Belgium

Department of Dermatology, Regional Hospital of Huy, Huy, Belgium

Jacquelyn Levin West Dermatology, Rancho Santa Margarita, CA, USA

Davina A. Lewis Department of Anatomic Pathology and Histology, Covance CLS, Indianapolis, IN, USA

Aikaterini I. Liakou Departments of Dermatology, Venereology, Allergology and Immunology, Dessau Medical Center, Dessau, Germany

University of Athens Medical School, Athens, Greece

Andrea Lichterfeld Department of Dermatology and Allergy, Clinical Research Center for Hair and Skin Science, Charité-Universitätsmedizin Berlin, Berlin, Germany

Low Chai Ling The Sloane Clinic, Singapore, Singapore

Chengxu Liu The Procter & Gamble Company, Cincinnati, OH, USA

Jane Y. Liu Department of Dermatology, University of California, School of Medicine, San Francisco, CA, USA

Márcio Lorencini R&D Department, Grupo Boticário, São José dos Pinhais, PR, Brazil

Isabelle Lorthois Centre LOEX de l'Université Laval, Québec, QC, Canada

Stefanie Luebberding Rosenpark Research, Darmstadt, Germany

Judit Lukács Klinik für Hautkrankheiten, Universitätsklinikum Jena, Jena, Germany

John Lyga Avon Global R&D, Suffern, NY, USA

Howard I. Maibach Department of Dermatology, University of California, San Francisco, CA, USA

Robert Maidof Avon Global R&D, Suffern, NY, USA

Evgenia Makrantonaki Departments of Dermatology, Venereology, Allergology and Immunology, Dessau Medical Center, Dessau, Germany

Geriatry Research Group, Charité Universitaetsmedizin Berlin, Berlin, Germany

Department of Dermatology and Allergology, University Medical Center Ulm, Ulm, Germany

Denis Malvy EA 3677 and Centre René-Labusquière, Université Victor Segalen, Bordeaux, France

Department of Internal Medicine and Tropical Diseases, University Hospital Center, Bordeaux, France

Valéria Maria Di Mambro R&D Department, Grupo Boticário, São José dos Pinhais, PR, Brazil

François-Xavier Maquart Laboratoire de Biochimie, CNRS UMR 7369, Faculté de Médecine, Université de Reims-Champagne-Ardenne, Reims, France

Centre National de la Recherche Scientifique, CNRS UMR 7369, Reims, France

Centre Hospitalier et Universitaire (CHU) de Reims, Reims, France

Anna Margolina Research and Development, Skin Biology, Bellevue, WA, USA

Claire Marionnet L'Oreal Research and Innovation, Aulnay-sous-bois, France

Slaheddine Marrakchi Department of Dermatology, Hedi Chaker Hospital, Sfax, Tunisia

Daniel S. Marsman The Procter & Gamble Company, Cincinnati, OH, USA

Jean-Yves Mary INSERM U717, Biostatistics and Clinical Epidemiology, DBIM, Saint-Louis Hospital, University Paris 7, Paris, France

Paul J. Matts Procter & Gamble, Greater London Innovation Centre, Egham, Surrey, UK

Walid Medhat Department of Dermatology, Al-Minya University, Al-Minya, Egypt

Reena Mehra Sleep Medicine Center, The Cleveland Clinic, Cleveland, OH, USA

Esterina Melchiorre Life, Health and Environmental Sciences, University of L'Aquila, L'Aquila, Italy

Helen Meldrum Unilever Research and Development, Trumbull, CT, USA

Joseph Merregaert Laboratory of Molecular Biotechnology, Department of Biomedical Sciences, University of Antwerp, Antwerp, Belgium

Afton Metkowski Department of Dermatology and Itch Center, Temple University School of Medicine, Philadelphia, PA, USA

Thomas A. Meyer Bayer Healthcare, Memphis, TN, USA

Gianfranca Miconi Life, Health and Environmental Sciences, University of L'Aquila, L'Aquila, Italy

Kenneth W. Miller Margoshes-Miller Consulting, LLC, Cincinnati, OH, USA

Jillian Wong Millsop Department of Dermatology, University of California, Davis, Sacramento, CA, USA

Shivangi Mishra Department of Biotechnology, Jaypee Institute of Information Technology, Noida, UP, India

Sang Hyun Moh Anti-aging Research Institute of BIO-FD&C Co. Ltd., Incheon, Republic of Korea

Akimichi Morita Department of Geriatric and Environmental Dermatology, Nagoya City University Graduate School of Medical Sciences, Nagoya, Japan

D. James Morré MorNuCo, Inc, West Lafayette, IN, USA

Dorothy M. Morré MorNuCo, Inc, West Lafayette, IN, USA

Zeenat Nabi Colgate-Palmolive Company, Piscataway, NJ, USA

Kouichi Nakagawa Department of Radiological Life Sciences, Graduate School of Health Sciences, Hirosaki University, Hirosaki, Aomori, Japan

J. Frank Nash The Procter & Gamble Company, Central Product Safety, Cincinnati, OH, USA

Dany Nassar Department of Dermatology, American University of Beirut Medical Center, Beirut, Lebanon

Department of Anatomy, Cell Biology and Physiological Sciences, American University of Beirut Medical Center, Beirut, Lebanon

Véronique Neiveyans L'Oreal, Research and Innovation, Aulnay-sous-bois, France

Isaac M. Neuhaus Department of Dermatology, University of California, San Francisco, CA, USA

Paul Nghiem Departments of Therapeutic Radiology, Genetics, and Dermatology, Yale School of Medicine, New Haven, CT, USA

Kasra Soltani Nia Department of Dermatology, University of California, School of Medicine, San Francisco, CA, USA

Georgios Nikolakis Departments of Dermatology, Venereology, Allergology and Immunology, Dessau Medical Center, Dessau, Germany

John Nip Unilever Research and Development, Trumbull, CT, USA

Jean-Luc Nizet Department of Plastic Surgery, University Hospital of Liège, Liège, Belgium

Alex Nkengne Clarins Laboratories, Pontoise, France

Kimberly G. Norman Institute for In Vitro Sciences, Gaithersburg, MD, USA

John Oblong Beauty Technology Division, The Procter & Gamble Company, Sharon Woods Innovation Center, Cincinnati, OH, USA

Mutsumi Okazaki Department of Plastic and Reconstructive Surgery, Graduate School of Science, Tokyo Medical and Dental University, Bunkyo-ku, Tokyo, Japan

Yasemin Oram Department of Dermatology, V.K. Foundation, American Hospital of Istanbul, Istanbul, Turkey

A. C. Ouwehand Active Nutrition, DuPont Nutrition and Health, Kantvik, Finland

Noritaka Oyama Dermatology and Dermato-Allergology, Matsuda General Hospital, Ohno, Fukui, Japan

Department of Dermatology, Fukui University, Fukui, Japan

Herve Pageon L'Oreal, Research and Innovation, Aulnay-sous-bois, France

Paola Palumbo Life, Health and Environmental Sciences, University of L'Aquila, L'Aquila, Italy

Apostolos Pappas The Johnson & Johnson Skin Research Center, CPPW, a Division of Johnson & Johnson Consumer Companies, Inc, Skillman, NJ, USA

Byung-Soon Park Cellpark Dermatology Clinic, Seoul, South Korea

Evasio Pasini "S. Maugeri Foundation", IRCCS, Cardiology Rehabilitative Division, Medical Centre of Lumezzane, Brescia, Italy

Paula C. Pennacchi Department of Clinical Chemistry and Toxicology, School of Pharmaceutical Sciences, University of Sao Paulo, Sao Paulo, Brazil

Jerrold Scott Petrofsky Department of Physical Therapy, Loma Linda University, Loma Linda, CA, USA

School of Allied Health, Loma Linda University, Loma Linda, CA, USA

Christina Phuong Department of Dermatology, University of California San Francisco, San Francisco, CA, USA

Loren Pickart Research and Development, Skin Biology, Bellevue, WA, USA

Gérald E. Piérard Laboratory of Skin Bioengineering and Imaging, Department of Dermatopathology, University Hospital of Liège, Liège, Belgium

Sébastien L. Piérard Telecommunication and Imaging Laboratory, INTELSIG, Montefiore Institute, University of Liège, Liège, Belgium

Claudine Piérard-Franchimont Laboratory of Skin Bioengineering and Imaging, Department of Dermatopathology, University Hospital of Liège, Liège, Belgium

Department of Dermatology, Regional Hospital of Huy, Huy, Belgium

Raimondo Pinna Plastic and Reconstructive Surgery and Burns Centre, Brotzu Hospital, Cagliari, Italy

Thomas G. Polefka Life Science Solutions, LLC, Somerset, NJ, USA

S. Brian Potterf Unilever Research and Development, Trumbull, CT, USA

Tarl W. Prow Dermatology Research Centre, School of Medicine, The University of Queensland, Princess Alexandra Hospital, Translational Research Institute, Brisbane, QLD, Australia

Prashant Rai L'Oreal China, Shanghai, China

Utkrishta L. Raj Department of Biotechnology, Jaypee Institute of Information Technology, Noida, UP, India

Vibha Rani Department of Biotechnology, Jaypee Institute of Information Technology, Noida, UP, India

Matthew J. Ranzer Center for Wound Healing and Tissue Regeneration, College of Dentistry, University of Illinois at Chicago, Chicago, IL, USA

Department of Biology, DePaul University, Chicago, IL, USA

Anthony P. Raphael Dermatology Research Centre, School of Medicine, The University of Queensland, Princess Alexandra Hospital, Translational Research Institute, Brisbane, QLD, Australia

Wellman Center for Photomedicine, Massachusetts General Hospital, Harvard Medical School, Boston, MA, USA

Christina Raschke Department of Dermatology, University Hospital Jena, Jena, Germany

Suresh I. S. Rattan Laboratory of Cellular Ageing, Department of Molecular Biology and Genetics, Aarhus University, Aarhus C, Denmark

Anthony V. Rawlings AVR Consulting Ltd, Cheshire, UK

Glen Rein Innovative Biophysical Technologies, Ridgway, CO, USA

Klaus Richter Department of Cell Biology, Division of Genetics, University of Salzburg, Salzburg, Austria

Sylvie Ricois L'Oreal, Research and Innovation, Aulnay-sous-bois, France

Mark Rinnerthaler Department of Cell Biology, Division of Genetics, University of Salzburg, Salzburg, Austria

Caroline Ritacco Laboratory of Skin Bioengineering and Imaging, Department of Dermatopathology, University Hospital of Liège, Liège, Belgium

Diana Alyce Rivers The Department of Basic Biomedical Sciences, Touro College of Osteopathic Medicine, New York, NY, USA

Michael K. Robinson Global Biotechnology and Life Sciences Technology Platform, The Procter & Gamble Company, Mason Business Center, Mason, OH, USA

Sheila Rocha Unilever Research and Development, Trumbull, CT, USA

Igor Roganin DAO Clinic, Moscow, Russia

Claudia Romano Department of Clinical and Experimental Sciences, Division of Human Anatomy and Physiopathology, University of Brescia, Brescia, Italy

David J. Rowe University Hospitals, Case Western Reserve University, Cleveland, OH, USA

Nelly Rubeiz Department of Dermatology, American University of Beirut Medical Center, Beirut, Lebanon

Anna Rufo Department of Biotechnological and Applied Clinical Sciences, University of L'Aquila, L'Aquila, Italy

Cindy A. Ryan The Procter and Gamble Company, Cincinnati, OH, USA

Shingo Sakai Basic Research Laboratory, Kanebo Cosmetics Inc., Kanagawa, Japan

Salah Salman Department of Dermatology, American University of Beirut Medical Center, Beirut, Lebanon

Preamjit Saonanon Department of Ophthalmology, King Chulalongkorn Memorial Hospital, The Thai Red Cross Society, Chulalongkorn University, Bangkok, Thailand

Giovanni Scapagnini Department of Health Sciences, University of Molise, Campobasso, Italy

Richard Scarborough University Hospitals Case Medical Center, Cleveland, OH, USA

Dwight Scarborough Clinical Assistant Professor of Medicine, Division of Dermatology, The Ohio State University Wexner Medical Center, Columbus, OH, USA

Megan E. Schrementi Center for Wound Healing and Tissue Regeneration, College of Dentistry, University of Illinois at Chicago, Chicago, IL, USA

Department of Biology, DePaul University, Chicago, IL, USA

Peter Schroeder Environmental Health Research Institute (IUF), Heinrich-Heine-University, Duesseldorf, Germany

Miri Seiberg Seiberg Consulting, LLC, Princeton, NJ, USA

Stefania Seidenari Department of Dermatology, University of Modena and Reggio Emilia, Modena, Italy

Hyo Hyun Seo Anti-aging Research Institute of BIO-FD&C Co. Ltd., Incheon, Republic of Korea

Garima Sharma Department of Biotechnology, Jaypee Institute of Information Technology, Noida, UP, India

Susan N. Sherman SNS Research, Cincinnati, OH, USA

Shuichi Shibuya Department of Advanced Aging Medicine, Chiba University Graduate School of Medicine, Chiba, Japan

Takahiko Shimizu Department of Advanced Aging Medicine, Chiba University Graduate School of Medicine, Chiba, Japan

William Shingleton General Electric Company, Cardiff, UK

Sara Sibilla Minerva Research Labs Ltd, London, UK

Neha Singh Department of Biotechnology, Jaypee Institute of Information Technology, Noida, UP, India

James E. Sligh Medicine, Dermatology, The University of Arizona, Tucson, AZ, USA

Jack Sobel Infectious Diseases, Wayne State University, Detroit, MI, USA

Mi Young Song Anti-aging Research Institute of BIO-FD&C Co. Ltd., Incheon, Republic of Korea

Yuli Song The Procter & Gamble Company, Mason Business Center, Mason, OH, USA

Dan F. Spandau Departments of Dermatology and Biochemistry and Molecular Biology, Indiana University School of Medicine, Indianapolis, IN, USA

Georgios N. Stamatas SkinCare R&D, Johnson & Johnson Santé Beauté France, Issy-les-Moulineaux, France

Robert Stern The Department of Basic Biomedical Sciences, Touro College of Osteopathic Medicine, New York, NY, USA

Maria Karolin Streubel Department of Cell Biology, Division of Genetics, University of Salzburg, Salzburg, Austria

Paul R. Summers University of Utah School of Medicine, Salt Lake City, UT, USA

Cheri L. Swanson The Procter & Gamble Company, Sharon Woods Innovation Center, Cincinnati, OH, USA

Hachiro Tagami Department of Dermatology, Tohoku University School of Medicine, Sendai, Japan

Haw-Yueh Thong Department of Dermatology, University of California, San Francisco, CA, USA

Kirsti Tiihonen Active Nutrition, DuPont Nutrition and Health, Kantvik, Finland

Danielle Tokarz Wellman Center for Photomedicine, Massachusetts General Hospital, Harvard Medical School, Boston, MA, USA

Princess Margaret Cancer Centre, University Health Network, Toronto, ON, Canada

Marjana Tomic-Canic Wound Healing and Regenerative Medicine Research Program, Department of Dermatology and Cutaneous Surgery and Hussman Institute of Human Genomics, University of Miami Miller Medical School, Miami, FL, USA

Salina M. Torres Department of Pathology, Center for HPV Prevention, University of New Mexico, Albuquerque, NM, USA

Elka Touitou Institute of Drug Research, School of Pharmacy, The Hebrew University of Jerusalem, Jerusalem, Israel

Jeffrey B. Travers Departments of Pharmacology and Toxicology and Dermatology, Boonshoft School of Medicine at Wright State University, Dayton, OH, USA

Joel Tsevat Division of General Internal Medicine, Department of Internal Medicine, University of Cincinnati College of Medicine and Cincinnati VA Medical Center, Cincinnati, OH, USA

Katsuhiko Tsuchida Research and Development Department, Naris Cosmetics Co. Ltd., Osaka, Japan

Gabe Tzeghai Wyoming, OH, USA

Efstratios Vakirlis Department of Dermatology and Venereology, Aristotle University of Thessaloniki, Thessaloniki, Greece

Giuseppe Valacchi Department of Life Sciences and Biotechnology, University of Ferrara, Ferrara (FE), Italy

Department of Food and Nutrition, Kyung Hee University, Seoul, South Korea

Rodrigo Valdes-Rodriguez Department of Dermatology and Itch Center, Temple University School of Medicine, Philadelphia, PA, USA

Fabien Valet Biostatistics Department, Institut Curie, Paris, France

Jessica Michelle Vasquez-Soltero Research and Development, Skin Biology, Bellevue, WA, USA

Annika Vogt Clinical Research Center for Hair and Skin Science, Department of Dermatology and Allergy, Charité-Universitätsmedizin Berlin, Berlin, Germany

Shilpa Vora Unilever Research and Development, Bangalore, India

Kenji Watanabe Department of Advanced Aging Medicine, Chiba University Graduate School of Medicine, Chiba, Japan

Yanusz Wegrowski Laboratoire de Biochimie, CNRS UMR 7369, Faculté de Médecine, Université de Reims-Champagne-Ardenne, Reims, France

Centre National de la Recherche Scientifique, CNRS UMR 7369, Reims, France

Horst Wenck The Beiersdorf Research Center, Hamburg, Germany

Katherine M. Whipple Envision Eye and Aesthetics, Fairport, NY, USA

Cornelia Wiegand Department of Dermatology, University Hospital Jena, Jena, Germany

Julian Winocour Department of Plastic Surgery, Vanderbilt University, Nashville, TN, USA

Klaus-Peter Wittern The Beiersdorf Research Center, Hamburg, Germany

Hidekazu Yamada Department of Dermatology of Kinki University, Faculty of Medicine Nara Hospital, Kinki University Antiaging Center, Higashiosaka, Osaka Prefecture, Japan

Paul S. Yamauchi Dermatology Institute and Skin Care Center, Santa Monica, CA, USA

David Geffen School of School of Medicine at UCLA, Los Angeles, CA, USA

Daniel B. Yarosh The Estee Lauder Companies, Inc., Melville, NY, USA

Max Yeslev Department of Plastic Surgery, Vanderbilt University, Nashville, TN, USA

Koutaro Yokote Department of Clinical Cell Biology and Medicine, Chiba University Graduate School of Medicine, Chiba, Japan

Hyun Sun Yoon Department of Dermatology, Seoul National University Boramae Hospital, Seoul, Korea

Gil Yosipovitch Department of Dermatology and Itch Center, Temple University School of Medicine, Philadelphia, PA, USA

Sidra Younis The R.O. Perelman Department of Dermatology, and Department of Biochemistry and Molecular Pharmacology, NYU Langone Medical Center, New York, NY, USA

Department of Biochemistry, Quaid-i-Azam University, Islamabad, Pakistan

Efterpi Zafiriou Department of Dermatology and Venereology, University of Thessaly, Larissa, Greece

Hanjiang Zhu Department of Dermatology, UC San Francisco, San Francisco, CA, USA

Ying Zou Department of Dermatology, UC San Francisco, San Francisco, CA, USA

Christos C. Zouboulis Departments of Dermatology, Venereology, Allergology and Immunology, Dessau Medical Center, Dessau, Germany

Helene Zucchi L'Oreal, Research and Innovation, Aulnay-sous-bois, France

Part I

Basic Sciences/Physiology/Histology

Histology of Microvascular Aging of Human Skin

1

Peter Helmbold

Contents

Abstract

Histological studies regarding the role of pericytes (PC) in the dermis with emphasis on dermal microvascular aging are summarized in this chapter. Aging of the dermis happens under special conditions. In addition to *chronological aging*, a powerful extrinsic factor – chronic UV light – leads to *photoaging*. Some known facultative intrinsic or extrinsic factors that influence dermal aging include diabetes mellitus, alcohol, cigarette smoking, and genodermatoses like progeria.

Introduction

In this chapter, various histological studies regarding the role of pericytes (PC) in the dermis will be summarized, focusing on dermal microvascular aging [1–4]. Aging of the dermis proceeds under special conditions. In addition to *chronological aging*, a powerful extrinsic factor – chronic UV light – leads to *photoaging* (actinic or solar aging). Some known facultative intrinsic or extrinsic factors that influence dermal aging include diabetes mellitus, alcohol, cigarette smoking, and genodermatoses like progeria [5–8]. Previous studies have shown that human dermal microvessel densities depend on age with reduction of functioning reserve capillaries, and there are typical ultrastructural changes in the microvasculature of elderly individuals [5, 6, 9].

P. Helmbold (✉)
Department of Dermatology, University of Heidelberg, Heidelberg, Germany
e-mail: peter.helmbold@med.uni-heidelberg.de

M.A. Farage et al. (eds.), *Textbook of Aging Skin*,
DOI 10.1007/978-3-662-47398-6_2

Most efforts in microvascular research focus on endothelial cells (EC). By contrast, progress in knowledge on PC which cover microvascular capillaries and venules on their abluminal surfaces has been slow. In the microvasculature, EC and PC are anatomical and functional neighbors. They are separated from each other by the EC basal lamina, which allows punctate direct contact and interdigitation [10]. Endothelin-1 [11] and vascular endothelial growth factors are thought to be the most important cytokines responsible for the interaction of the two cell types [11–13]. Pericytes have contractile function, and they are thought to regulate local blood flow [14]. Moreover, they are essential for microvessel stability and control of angioneogenesis [15, 16]. Pericytes are involved in the pathogenesis of diabetic microangiopathy [17, 18], hypertension [19], tumor growth [20], and retinopathy of prematurity [21]. In the skin, PC hyperplasia has been reported in chronic venous insufficiency and in scleroderma [3, 22]. Because of methodological difficulties, most of the dermatological research performed on PC was restricted to ultrastructural or unspecific identification of this cell type by their smooth muscle actin expression [10, 18, 23–25].

One of the most striking methodological problems in this field was identification and counting of a sufficient number of PC and EC in dermal microvessels. Ultrastructurally, 90–130 ultrathin sections are required for the reconstruction of one vessel segment with one to four PC [26]. Thus, two methods for identification of cutaneous PC and EC were recently developed: a direct but relatively expensive technique that allows identification of PC and EC nuclei in cryosections by 3G5 antigen and von Willebrand factor expression, and an indirect method that uses identification of PC and EC nuclei according to their anatomical relationship with the collagen IV-positive microvascular basal lamina [2, 3]. The indirect technique in particular allows rapid identification of all key microvascular parameters that were used in this study. From these studies, it can be concluded that the PC/EC ratio is a crucial "functional-morphological" parameter in the dermal microvasculature [3].

In the first study, 120 biopsies from normal skin of 87 patients were obtained from surplus areas (i.e., Burow's triangle) of routinely excised and histologically controlled benign nevus cell nevi of normal skin (it was previously verified that PC numbers or total microvascular counts were not influenced by noninflammatory nevus cell nevi, unpublished results). Biopsies with inflammatory cells (infiltrated nevus cell nevi) or histological conditions other than normal skin and biopsies from patients with known vasculopathies were strictly excluded from the study. To eliminate the influence of latent venous insufficiency, skin samples from the lower legs of patients older than 14 years were generally excluded. Known vascular diseases and diabetes mellitus were additional exclusion criteria. Each specimen was characterized by a set of clinical data: age, sex of the patient, and body location of the biopsy. Further methods are stated in [1]. The relative number of capillaries and venules as well as PC/EC ratios were counted in the upper horizontal dermal plexus, including papillar and the upper reticular dermis in collagen IV stained paraffin sections (hematoxylin counterstained) as reported previously [3] (Fig. 1a, b). In short, intraluminal nuclei (within the lumen that is surrounded by the inner layer of the microvascular basal lamina) were ascribed to EC. By contrast, nuclei found between the two layers of microvascular basal lamina were ascribed to PC. Segmented nuclei or nuclei without contact with the basal lamina were excluded. *Only clearly recognizable cross or longitudinal sections with unequivocal assignment of the nuclei* to the cell types to be determined were selected for examination (Fig. 1a, b). The mean coefficient of variation of this method was 5.7 ± 3.9 % [3].

In another experimental study, the PC/EC ratio was studied in clearly cross- or longitudinal-sectioned capillaries by colocalization analysis of 3G5 or vWF binding sites with nuclei in crysoctions by triple-staining with anti-3G5 (a pericyte marker), anti-von Willebrand factor (endothelial marker), and DNA fluorochrome (Hoechst 33258, Sigma) as reported before (Fig. 1c, d) [2, 3]. In a third study part, different TGFs, VEGFs, and PDGF-receptors in the upper dermal plexus were studied in paraffin sections (Fig. 1e, f).

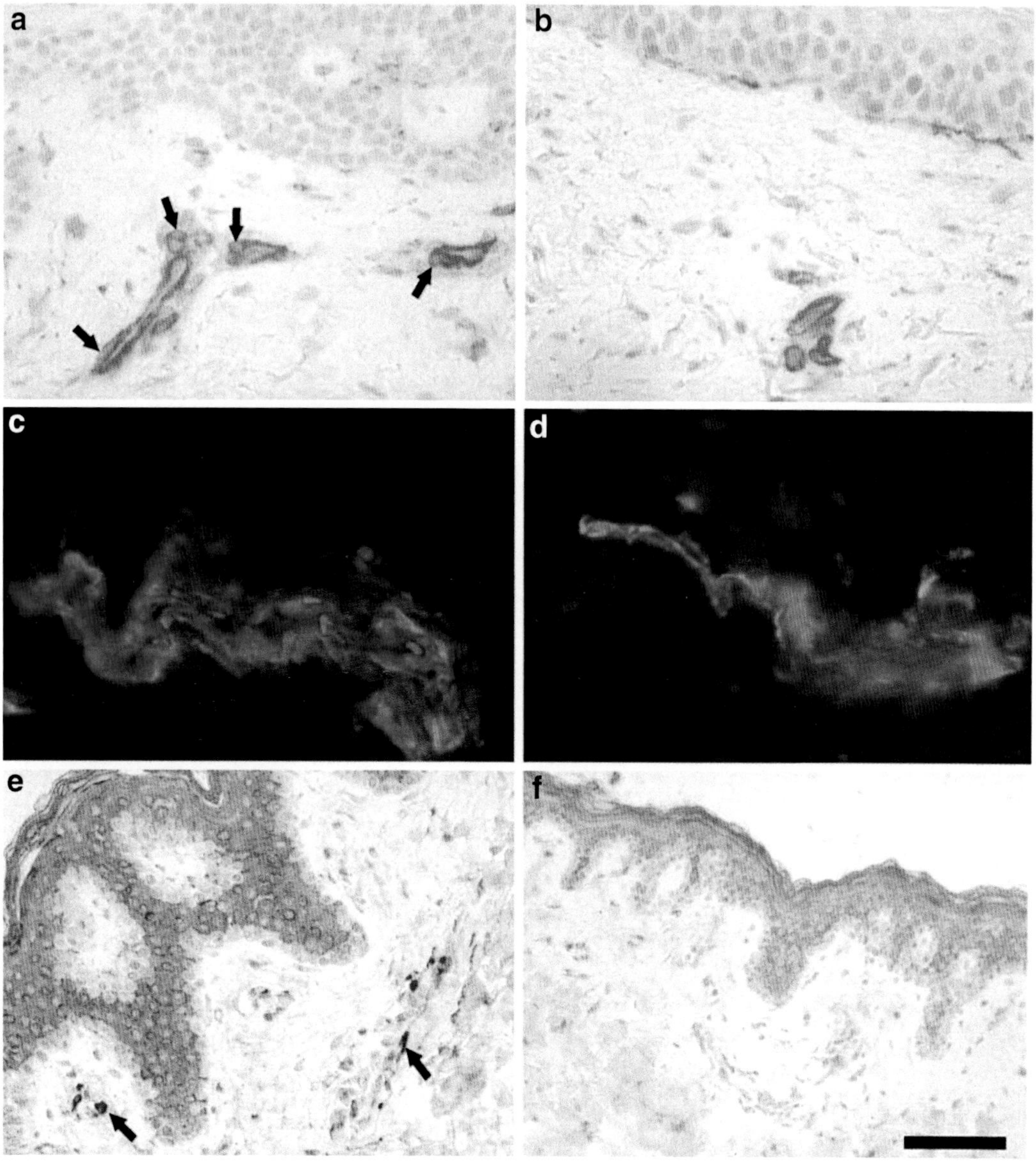

Fig. 1 Age dependency of microvascular density, pericyte-to-endothelial cell ratio (PC/EC), and microvascular TGF-β1 expression. Left column (**a**, **c**, **e**), younger; right column (**b**, **d**, **f**), older skin biopsies. (**a**) Nuclei of microvascular pericytes (*arrows*) are identifiable between the two layers of the collagen IV-positive microvascular basal lamina (*red*) in a collagen IV/hemalaun stained paraffin section of a biopsy of a 21-month-old girl (7.0 capillaries per HPF, PC/EC ratio 0.345). (**b**) Biopsy from the décolleté of a 30-year-old woman with low capillary and pericyte densities (3.1 capillaries per HPF, PC/EC ratio 0.081). (**c**) Fluorescence microphotograph of pericytic surface 3G5 mAB-binding sites (*red*), endothelial cell von Willebrand factor (*green*), and DNA fluorochrome (*blue*). The figure shows a venular capillary of the upper dermis of a 5-year-old boy with almost complete covering of endothelial cells by pericytes (10.75 capillaries per HPF, PC/EC ratio 0.250). (**d**) By contrast, a capillary of the upper dermal plexus of a thoracic biopsy of a 31-year-old woman demonstrates sparse PC density (4.25 capillaries per HPF, PC/EC ratio 0.075). (**e**) High number of microvascular cells express cytoplasmatic TGF-ß1 (*arrows*) in a PC-rich biopsy of a 7-year-old boy (7.1 capillaries per HPF, PC/EC ratio 0.191). (**f**) By contrast, a biopsy from the back of a 20-year-old woman with low microvascular and PC densities is lacking microvascular TGF-ß1 (3.5 capillaries per HPF, PC/EC ratio 0.121). The epidermis serves for intrinsic positive control. Scale bar: A, B = 50 μm, C, D = 15 μm, E = 100 μm, F = 200 μm (Published in Helmbold et al. [1]. Reprinted with permission of J Invest Dermatol)

Results and Discussion

Two periods of vascular aging – childhood and adulthood. Densities of capillaries and venules in the upper dermal plexus showed dramatic decrease during childhood and slow decrease during adulthood. Results showed a mean of 4.9 ± 2.8 capillaries per HPF and 2.4 ± 1.4 venules per HPF. The density of capillaries was highly negatively dependent on chronological age ($r = -0.572$, $p < 0.001$) (Figs. 1a, b and 2). In young children (0–4.99 years), capillary density was 9.7 ± 2.9 per HPF decreasing with adolescence to 4.4 ± 1.5 (15–19.99 years). Thereafter, there was further slow decrease to 2.3 ± 1.4 (range 0.7–5.8) in the age group 70+ years. By contrast, the density of venules showed no significant change during life. At higher ages, the densities of capillaries and venules were comparable.

Pericyte loss during childhood and adult chronological life. Mean PC/EC ratios were 0.125 ± 0.054 and 0.132 ± 0.067 in the capillaries and venules, respectively. There was a negative correlation between chronological age and PC/EC ratio of the capillaries ($r = -0.560$, $p < 0.001$) or venules ($r = -0.594$, $p < 0.001$). Similar to capillary density, the most dramatic changes occurred during adolescence (Fig. 3). In the youngest group (0–4.99 years), PC/EC was twice that in the age group 15–19.99 years, Thereafter, no significant correlation of PC/EC ratio and chronological age was detectable. Studies of the area-based densities of PC and EC showed that the values for PC were highly correlated to the PC/EC ratio, while there was no correlation between total EC counts and PC/EC ratio. It can be concluded that only life-time changes of absolute PC densities (but not changes of EC densities) are responsible for age-dependent decrease in PC/EC ratio. Fluorescence microscopy analysis of PC and EC distribution by anti-pericyte, anti-endothelial antibodies, and DNA fluorochrome (details see above) brought similar results to those shown in the paraffin imbedded material [1].

Photoaging. Body regions that reflect *typical* actinic exposure (photoaging) showed a negative correlation to each of the key microvascular parameters (capillary density: Spearman $r = -0.203$, $p = 0.039$; capillary PC/EC ratio $r = -0.242$, $p = 0.042$; venular PC/EC ratio $r = -0.255$, $p = 0.010$). The effect of photoaging was more clearly demonstrable by a newly introduced technique, the histological scoring of dermal basophilic degeneration (DBD, see ▶ Chap. 2, "Basophilic (Actinic) Degeneration of the Dermis: An Easy Histological Scoring Approach in Dermal Photoaging"). The influence of DBD on key microvascular parameters was studied in 84 biopsies of normal skin of subjects 15 years or older. In connection with chronological aging, additional actinic aging could be demonstrated: the capillary density and the PC/EC ratios of the capillaries or venules showed clear diminution with the degree

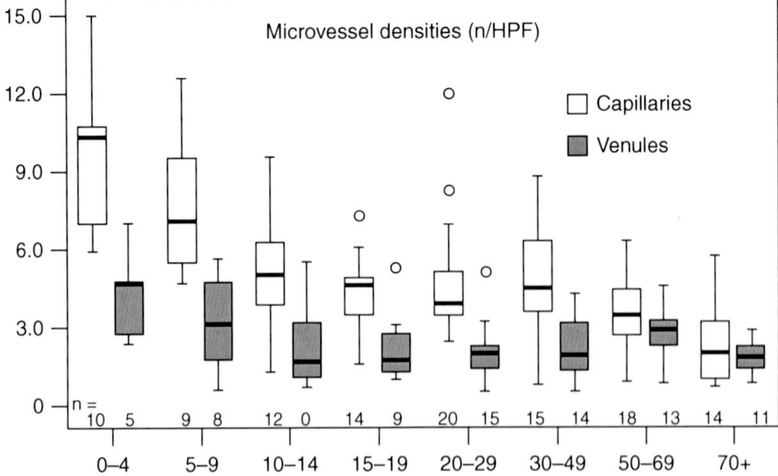

Fig. 2 Age dependency of the densities of capillaries and venules in the upper dermal plexus age groups: "0–4" means 0–4.99 years, etc (Published in Helmbold et al. [1]. Reprinted with permission of J Invest Dermatol)

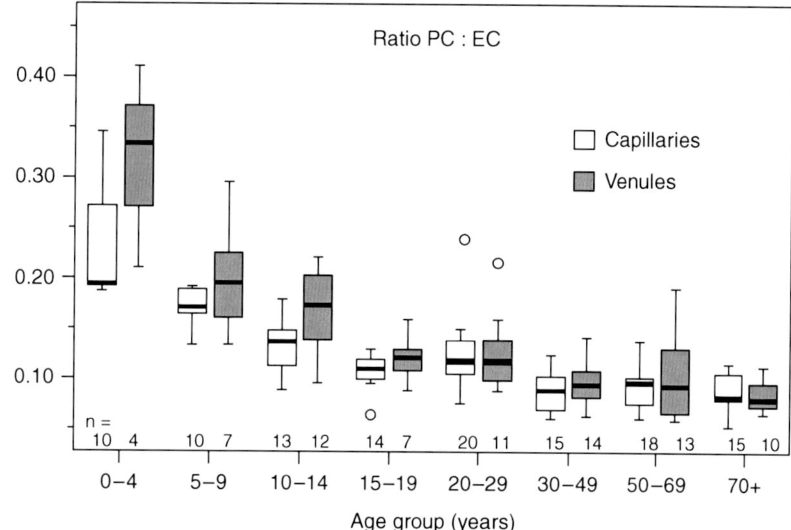

Fig. 3 Age dependency of the pericyte-to-endothelial cell ratios (PC/EC) of the capillaries and venules of the upper dermal plexus age groups: "0–4" means 0–4.99 years, etc (Published in Helmbold et al. [1]. Reprinted with permission of J Invest Dermatol)

of DBD – a significant photoeffect that is "added" individually to the chronological aging (Fig. 4). *Logistic regression* demonstrated that PC/EC ratio of the capillaries and venules was predicted by DBD, and, in contrast to younger ages, the chronological age had only weak independent influence in any subjects 15 years or older [1].

Study of TGF-β, PDGFR, and VEGF expressions showed that there was a correlation between microvascular TGF-β1 expression and the PC/EC ratios of capillaries or venules (Spearman $r = 0.583$, $p = 0.006$, or $r = 0.857$, $p < 0.001$) (Figs. 1e, f and 5), but there was no correlation between the microvascular expression of TGF-β2 and the anatomical parameters of the microvessels. Constitutive microvascular PDGFR-α and -β as well as VEGF expressions were very low and not correlated with any of the microvascular anatomical parameters.

In summary, two key parameters of microvasular aging were identified: capillary density and the quantitative ratio of pericytes to endothelial cells (PC/EC ratio). During the first 15 years of life, the number of capillaries of the upper dermis and the PC/EC ratio of the capillaries and venules decrease dramatically by nearly one half. This is called juvenile aging, which might be a process of maturation. Obviously, this maturation is finished with the end of longitudinal body growth. Nevertheless, decrease in the

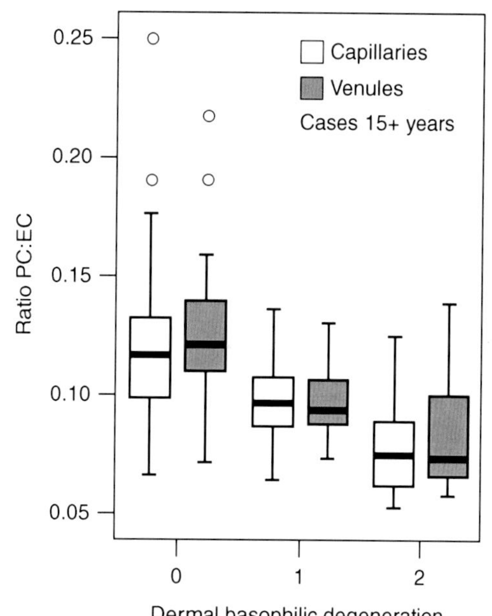

Fig. 4 PC/EC ratios of capillaries and venules of the upper dermal plexus in the context of basophilic degeneration, an indicator of photoaging age groups: "0–4" means 0–4.99 years, etc (Published in Helmbold et al. [1]. Reprinted with permission of J Invest Dermatol)

capacity of wound healing at the same time advocates classification of this process as an early aging process. This would explain the known deceleration of wound healing and angioneogenesis as well as the reduction of local

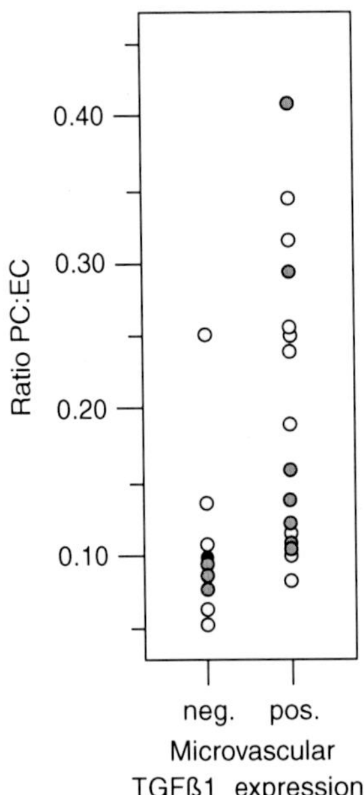

Fig. 5 Microvascular TGF-β1 expression and EC/PC ratios of the capillaries and venules of the upper dermal plexus. White, capillaries; gray, venules. Level 1 and 2 expressions were summarized to "positive" (pos.), and level 0 is represented in the figure as "negative" (neg.) (Published in Helmbold et al. [1]. Reprinted with permission of J Invest Dermatol)

microvascular reactivity due to aging of the skin by reduction of PC-dependent microvascular angioneogenic plasticity and functional loss of physiological microvascular contractility [27–29].

Thereafter, chronological aging alone has a comparatively low influence on both parameters. However, after puberty, the microvascular parameters are modified severely by photoaging, resulting in further decrease of capillary densities and PC/EC ratios. Regarding the capillary densities, this is consistent with previous investigations showing higher influence of photoaging than chronological aging on the upper dermal microvasular plexus during adult life [5, 6, 9]. In summary, two phases of microvascular aging can be postulated in human dermis: a *juvenile phase* finished by the onset of puberty, when an "adult plateau" is reached, and an *adult phase* that highly reflects *photoaging* with interindividual sun-exposure-specific alterations.

Most important, PC loss, but not changes in EC density, is the cause of the changes in the PC/EC ratio in both the juvenile and the photoaging of microvessels. PC expresses several cytokines, particularly TGF-β [30, 31]. The classical members of the TGF-β family belong to a much larger group. In humans, this family consists of almost 30 members, including bone morphogenic proteins, activins, and Mullerian inhibiting substance [32]. These TGF-β family members have effects during development; affect proliferation, differentiation, and cell death; and are important for the development of many tissues. Dermal TGF-β was constitutively active in and around microvessels. A correlation was found between microvascular TGF-β1 expression and the PC/EC ratio. This agrees with previous papers hypothesizing that PCs are the main source of constitutional TGF-β expression within the microvasculature [3, 33].

Conclusion

Thus, it is concluded that TGF-β1 expression reflects the functional state of the microvessels. TGF-β has different effects on microvessels: it inhibits proliferation and migration of endothelial cells, stimulates in vivo angiogenesis in the presence of an inflammatory response, and increases the stability of blood vessels. Furthermore, it has great impact on fibroblasts and connective tissue through chemotaxis of monocytes and fibroblasts, supporting anchorage-independent growth of fibroblasts, production of antiproteolytic activity via modulation of uPA/PAI-1 expression levels, inhibition of the production of proteases, and stimulation of the production of protease inhibitors (data reviewed [33]). Thus, results on microvascular TGF-β expression link the relative and absolute absence of microvascular PC in adult and photoaged skin to proteolytic degradation of dermal connective tissue and reduction of fibroblast function. PC loss might be crucial for dermal connective fiber aging.

In contrast to TGFs, significant expression of PDGFR and VEGF seems to be limited to (neo) angiogenesis or cell proliferation, respectively. There was no evidence for the necessity of these cytokines for physiological microvessel maintenance in normal skin.

Cross-References

▶ Basophilic (Actinic) Degeneration of the Dermis: An Easy Histological Scoring Approach in Dermal Photoaging

References

1. Helmbold P, Lautenschlager C, Marsch W, et al. Detection of a physiological juvenile phase and the central role of pericytes in human dermal microvascular aging. J Invest Dermatol. 2006;126:1419–21.
2. Helmbold P, Wohlrab J, Marsch WC, et al. Human dermal pericytes express 3G5 ganglioside – a new approach for microvessel histology in the skin. J Cutan Pathol. 2001;28:206–10.
3. Helmbold P, Fiedler E, Fischer M, et al. Hyperplasia of dermal microvascular pericytes in scleroderma. J Cutan Pathol. 2004;31:431–40.
4. Helmbold P. Methodische Grundlagen zur Erforschung von Perizyten der Haut. In: Medizinische Fakultät. Halle (Saale): Martin-Luther-Universität Halle, Wittenberg; 2002.
5. Braverman IM. Elastic fiber and microvascular abnormalities in aging skin. Clin Geriatr Med. 1989;5:69–90.
6. Korkushko OV, Sarkisov KG. Age-specific characteristics of microcirculation in middle-and old age. Kardiologiia. 1976;16:19–25.
7. Herrick AL, Moore T, Hollis S, et al. The influence of age on nailfold capillary dimensions in childhood. J Rheumatol. 2000;27:797–800.
8. Leung WC, Harvey I. Is skin ageing in the elderly caused by sun exposure or smoking? Br J Dermatol. 2002;147:1187–91.
9. Chung JH, Yano K, Lee MK, et al. Differential effects of photoaging vs intrinsic aging on the vascularization of human skin. Arch Dermatol. 2002;138:1437–42.
10. Braverman IM. Ultrastructure and organization of the cutaneous microvasculature in normal and pathologic states. J Invest Dermatol. 1989;93:2S–9.
11. Dehouck MP, Vigne P, Torpier G, et al. Endothelin-1 as a mediator of endothelial cell-pericyte interactions in bovine brain capillaries. J Cereb Blood Flow Metab. 1997;17:464–9.
12. Takagi H, King GL, Robinson GS, et al. Adenosine mediates hypoxic induction of vascular endothelial growth factor in retinal pericytes and endothelial cells. Invest Ophthalmol Vis Sci. 1996;37:2165–76.
13. Kim Y, Imdad RY, Stephenson AH, et al. Vascular endothelial growth factor mRNA in pericytes is upregulated by phorbol myristate acetate. Hypertension. 1998;31:511–5.
14. Hirschi KK, D'Amore PA. Pericytes in the microvasculature. Cardiovasc Res. 1996;32:687–98.
15. Lindahl P, Johansson BR, Leveen P, et al. Pericyte loss and microaneurysm formation in PDGF-B-deficient mice. Science. 1997;277:242–5.
16. Hirschi KK, D'Amore PA. Control of angiogenesis by the pericyte: molecular mechanisms and significance. EXS. 1997;79:419–28.
17. de Oliveira F. Pericytes in diabetic retinopathy. Br J Ophthalmol. 1966;50:134–43.
18. Braverman IM, Sibley J, Keh A. Ultrastructural analysis of the endothelial-pericyte relationship in diabetic cutaneous vessels. J Invest Dermatol. 1990;95:147–53.
19. Wallow IH, Bindley CD, Reboussin DM, et al. Systemic hypertension produces pericyte changes in retinal capillaries. Invest Ophthalmol Vis Sci. 1993;34:420–30.
20. Schlingemann RO, Rietveld FJ, Kwaspen F, et al. Differential expression of markers for endothelial cells, pericytes, and basal lamina in the microvasculature of tumors and granulation tissue. Am J Pathol. 1991;138:1335–47.
21. Benjamin LE, Hemo I, Keshet E. A plasticity window for blood vessel remodelling is defined by pericyte coverage of the preformed endothelial network and is regulated by PDGF-B and VEGF. Development. 1998;125:1591–8.
22. Laaff H, Vandscheidt W, Weiss JM, et al. Immunohistochemical investigation of pericytes in chronic venous insufficiency. Vasa. 1991;20:323–8.
23. Lugassy C, Eyden BP, Christensen L, et al. Angiotumoral complex in human malignant melanoma characterised by free laminin: ultrastructural and immunohistochemical observations. J Submicrosc Cytol Pathol. 1997;29:19–28.
24. Tsukamoto H, Mishima Y, Hayashibe K, et al. Alpha-smooth muscle actin expression in tumor and stromal cells of benign and malignant human pigment cell tumors. J Invest Dermatol. 1992;98:116–20.
25. Sundberg C, Ivarsson M, Gerdin B, et al. Pericytes as collagen-producing cells in excessive dermal scarring. Lab Invest. 1996;74:452–66.
26. Braverman IM, Sibley J. Ultrastructural and three-dimensional analysis of the contractile cells of the cutaneous microvasculature. J Invest Dermatol. 1990;95:90–6.
27. Gendron RL. A plasticity for blood vessel remodeling is defined by pericyte coverage of the preformed endothelial network and is regulated by PDGF-B and VEGF. Surv Ophthalmol. 1999;44:184–5.
28. Schönfelder U, Hofer A, Paul M, et al. In situ observation of living pericytes in rat retinal capillaries. Microvasc Res. 1998;56:22–9.
29. Erber R, Thurnher A, Katsen AD, et al. Combined inhibition of VEGF and PDGF signaling enforces tumor vessel regression by interfering with pericyte-mediated endothelial cell survival mechanisms. FASEB J. 2004;18:338–40, Epub 2003 Dec;2004.

30. Sato Y, Rifkin DB. Inhibition of endothelial cell movement by pericytes and smooth muscle cells: activation of a latent transforming growth factor-beta 1-like molecule by plasmin during co-culture. J Cell Biol. 1989;109:309–15.
31. Antonelli-Orlidge A, Saunders KB, Smith SR, et al. An activated form of transforming growth factor beta is produced by cocultures of endothelial cells and pericytes. Proc Natl Acad Sci U S A. 1989;86:4544–8.
32. Massague J, Blain SW, Lo RS. TGFbeta signaling in growth control, cancer, and heritable disorders. Cell. 2000;103:295–309.
33. Papetti M, Herman IM. Mechanisms of normal and tumor-derived angiogenesis. Am J Physiol Cell Physiol. 2002;282:947–70.

Basophilic (Actinic) Degeneration of the Dermis: An Easy Histological Scoring Approach in Dermal Photoaging

2

Peter Helmbold

Contents

Abstract

Chronic ultraviolet (UV) light exposure of skin leads to typical effects: changes in the collagen and elastic tissue matrix are considered the characteristic histological findings in aged skin, followed by visible wrinkling and pigmentary changes. Assessment of the degrees of photoaging by a grading system with low interobserver coefficient of variation seems to be of special interest. Certain methods like "skin surface topography grading" were compared with histological changes like actinic elastosis. Advantages disadvantages of different approaches are listed in this chapter.

Introduction

Chronic ultraviolet (UV) light exposure of skin leads to typical effects: changes in the collagen and elastic tissue matrix are considered the characteristic histological findings in aged skin, followed by visible wrinkling and pigmentary changes. Changes in the epidermis include thinning to atrophy, hyperplasia of melanocytes, and disturbances in the texture of keratinocytes. Assessment of the degrees of photoaging by a grading system with low interobserver coefficient of variation seems to be of special interest. Different clinical methods have been proposed including descriptive grading clinical scales, visual analog scales, and photographic grading scales [1]. Some of these methods like "skin

P. Helmbold (✉)
Department of Dermatology, University of Heidelberg, Heidelberg, Germany
e-mail: peter.helmbold@med.uni-heidelberg.de

M.A. Farage et al. (eds.), *Textbook of Aging Skin*,
DOI 10.1007/978-3-662-47398-6_3

surface topography grading" [2] were compared with histological changes like actinic elastosis. Other studies used histological scoring of dermal aging independent of a noninvasive scoring system. The following approaches were used: quantification of elastic tissue [3], type III procollagen, type III to type I procollagen ratio, quantification of the grenz zone (a wide band of eosinophilic material just beneath the epidermis, devoid of oxytalan fibers) [4], activated fibroblasts with positive procollagen staining [5], acid mucopolysaccharides, improved quality of elastic fibers, and increased density of collagen [6], quantification of changes in the epidermis (thinning of the stratum corneum, granular layer enhancement, and epidermal thickening) [7]. One disadvantage of most of these methods is that actinic and instrinsic aging cannot be distinguished from one another.

Bhawan et al. [8] systematically investigated histological effects of photoaging. The following features proved to be significantly changed in photoaged skin: increase in melanocytes, increase in melanocytic atypia and epidermal melanin, reduced epidermal thickness, more compact stratum corneum, increased granular layer thickness, increased solar elastosis, dermal elastic tissue, melanophages, perivascular inflammation, and perifollicular fibrosis but no change in the number of mast cells or dermal mucin in the photoexposed skin. Of these, actinic elastosis (basophilic degeneration of the dermis) was the single most reliable factor. Basophilic degeneration is very consistent with the clinical sign of wrinkling and with dermal microvasular aging (see ► Chap. 1, "Histology of Microvascular Aging of Human Skin"). Thus, a single-factor scoring system of dermal aging regarding dermal basophilic degeneration (DBD) was developed. It should be mentioned that the knowledge of dermal fiber degeneration is not new and the use of a scoring system is the result of previous work [9,10].

After first experiments with a five-level system, it was found that best interobserver agreement was obtainable with a three-level model (Table 1) together with a histological atlas of the different levels (Fig. 1).

Table 1 Histological scoring of dermal basophilic degeneration (DBD) [11]

No actinic damage (Level 0): No fiber degeneration (Fig. 1a, b).
Moderate actinic damage (Level 1): Fragmentation of fibers of the upper dermis and presence of single basophilic fibers (Fig. 1c, d).
High actinic damage (Level 2): Spotted or band-like basophilic degeneration with conglomerates of basophilic masses in the upper and/or mid-dermis (Fig. 1e, f).

This model was tested in 120 biopsies from normal skin of 87 patients (42 females, 45 males, 27.9 ± 23.7 years [mean ± SD]) from surplus areas (i.e., Burow's triangle) of routinely excised and histologically controlled benign nevus cell nevi of normal skin. Each specimen was characterized by a set of clinical data: age, sex of the patient, and body location of the biopsy with regard to typically solar-exposed skin areas.

The interobserver reliability (agreement among four independent observers) of this technique was 92.2 ± 4.6 % in all biopsies. There was no disagreement of more than one level between the investigators. Correlations were found between DBD and the age of the patient (Spearman $r = 0.662$, $p < 0.001$) as well as DBD and body regions with typical chronic solar exposure (Spearman $r = 0.244$, $p = 0.005$). Sixty-eight biopsies revealed no visible DBD (37 from female, 31 from male patients; age: 19.8 ± 18.4 years), 36 biopsies showed moderate "level 1" DBD (28 females, 10 males, 39.9 ± 19 years), and 16 had a high "level 2" DBD (6 females, 10 males, 64.4 ± 11.9 years). DBD was not observable in patients younger than 15 years.

Conclusion

The advantages of this approach are easy application, use of HE-stained routine sections, fast determination, and sure results with high interobserver agreement. Disadvantages are that this approach cannot "measure" minimal differences and that it reflects only the dermal component of photoaging.

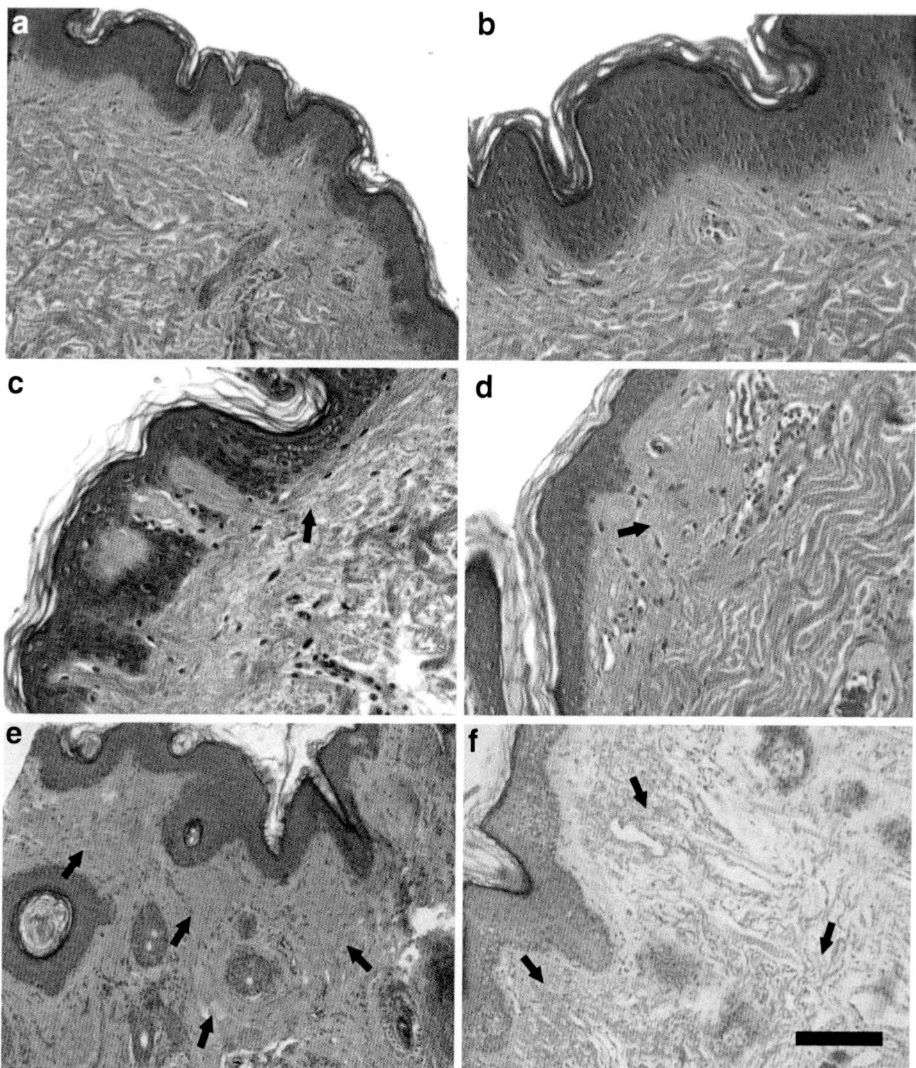

Fig. 1 Scoring of dermal basophilic degeneration (DBD). (**a**, **b**) No fiber degeneration (DBD level = 0). (**c**, **d**) Fragmentation of fibers (*arrows*) of the upper dermis and presence of single basophilic fibers (DBD level = 1). (**e**, **f**) Spotted (**e**) or band-like (**f**) basophilic degeneration (*arrows*) with conglomerates of basophilic masses in the upper and mid-dermis (DBD level = 2). Scale bar: **a**, **c–f** = 200 μm, **b** = 100 μm (Helmbold et al. [11]. Reprinted with permission of J Invest Dermatol)

Thus, the mean application fields are the studies that need reliable classification if there is actinic degeneration (or not). On the other hand, this approach is not suitable for quantification of the effects of an antiaging product or similar studies.

Cross-References

▶ Histology of Microvascular Aging of Human Skin

References

1. Kappes UP. Skin ageing and wrinkles: clinical and photographic scoring. J Cosmet Dermatol. 2004;3:23–5.
2. Battistutta D, Pandeya N, Strutton GM, et al. Skin surface topography grading is a valid measure of skin photoaging. Photodermatol Photoimmunol Photomed. 2006;22:39–45.
3. Chiu AE, Chan JL, Kern DG, et al. Double-blinded, placebo-controlled trial of green tea extracts in the clinical and histologic appearance of photoaging skin. Dermatol Surg. 2005;31:855–60. discussion 860.
4. Seite S, Bredoux C, Compan D, et al. Histological evaluation of a topically applied retinol-vitamin C combination. Skin Pharmacol Physiol. 2005;18:81–7.
5. Rostan E, Bowes LE, Iyer S, et al. A double-blind, side-by-side comparison study of low fluence long pulse dye laser to coolant treatment for wrinkling of the cheeks. J Cosmet Laser Ther. 2001;3:129–36.
6. Ditre CM, Griffin TD, Murphy GF, et al. Effects of alpha-hydroxy acids on photoaged skin: a pilot clinical, histologic, and ultrastructural study. J Am Acad Dermatol. 1996;34:187–95.
7. Newman N, Newman A, Moy LS, et al. Clinical improvement of photoaged skin with 50% glycolic acid. A double-blind vehicle-controlled study. Dermatol Surg. 1996;22:455–60.
8. Bhawan J, Andersen W, Lee J, et al. Photoaging versus intrinsic aging: a morphologic assessment of facial skin. J Cutan Pathol. 1995;22:154–9.
9. Suwabe H, Serizawa A, Kajiwara H, et al. Degenerative processes of elastic fibers in sun-protected and sun-exposed skin: immunoelectron microscopic observation of elastin, fibrillin-1, amyloid P component, lysozyme and alpha1-antitrypsin. Pathol Int. 1999;49:391–402.
10. Lund HZ, Sommerville RL. Basophilic degeneration of the cutis; data substantiating its relation to prolonged solar exposure. Am J Clin Pathol. 1957;27:183–90.
11. Helmbold P, Lautenschlager C, Marsch W, et al. Detection of a physiological juvenile phase and the central role of pericytes in human dermal microvascular aging. J Invest Dermatol. 2006;126:1419–21.

Degenerative Changes in Aging Skin

3

Miranda A. Farage, Kenneth W. Miller, and Howard I. Maibach

Contents

M.A. Farage (✉)
Winton Hill Business Center, The Procter & Gamble Company, Cincinnati, OH, USA
e-mail: farage.m@pg.com

K.W. Miller
Margoshes-Miller Consulting, LLC, Cincinnati, OH, USA
e-mail: 822mbb@gmail.com

H.I. Maibach
Department of Dermatology, University of California, San Francisco, CA, USA
e-mail: maibachh@derm.ucsf.edu

M.A. Farage et al. (eds.), *Textbook of Aging Skin*,
DOI 10.1007/978-3-662-47398-6_4

Abstract

Increased life spans have created a need for greater understanding of the diseases of old age including the integumentary system – the skin. The skin is the largest organ of the human body and performs multiple functions' including homeostatic regulation; prevention of percutaneous loss of fluid, electrolytes, and proteins; temperature maintenance; sensory perception; and immune surveillance. Aging involves both internal aging processes and external stressors to produce consistent changes such as thinning, drying, wrinkling, and uneven pigmentation. Understanding the fundamental physiology of changes in the epidermis, dermis, and hypodermis provides a foundation for progress in understanding the dermatological needs of those whose skin is aging. Physiological changes in aged skin include changes in biochemistry, permeability, vascularization and thermoregulation, response to irritants, immune response, repair capacity and response to injury, and neurosensory perception as well as changes at the genome level. Although aging of the skin, like other systems, is inevitable, research is beginning to define ways to both delay and minimize the troublesome effects of aging on the skin.

Introduction

Medical science, over the last two centuries, has dramatically extended the human life span, more than doubling the average global life expectancy from about 25 (for both sexes) to 68 for men and 73 for women [1]. With that increase, however, has come a pressing need for greater understanding of the diseases of old age. Biological aging consists of a variety of ongoing changes both intrinsic to internal biological processes and produced by external factors acting on body processes. These changes proceed, as the body ages, in every organ system [2], including the integumentary system – the skin.

The skin serves as the bulwark between the body and the environment and is the largest organ of the human body. As a sophisticated and dynamic organ comprising 17 % of the body's weight, the skin primarily acts as the barrier between the internal environment and the world outside. It performs multiple functions beyond simply acting as a barrier [3], including homeostatic regulation; prevention of percutaneous loss of fluid, electrolytes, and proteins; temperature maintenance; sensory perception; and immune surveillance [4].

As such (although incredibly durable), the skin is subjected not only to internal aging processes but also to various external stressors, which in concert lead to distinct structural changes that influence not only the skin's appearance but also its various physiological functions [5–7]. Natural intrinsic aging appears as fine wrinkles, a gradual thinning of the skin with a loss of the fatty tissue that underlies it, and progressive drying of the entire integument [8]. Aging caused by external factors (primarily sunlight) typically produces rough dry skin with coarse wrinkling, spider veins, and irregularities of pigmentation [8].

Skin permeability is deranged in aged skin, as is permeability, angiogenesis, lipid and sweat production, immune function, and vitamin D synthesis; these disturbances in skin function manifest themselves as impaired wound healing, atrophy, vulnerability to external stimuli, and development of several benign and malignant diseases [9].

Distinguishing the precludable aspects of cutaneous aging (primarily hormonal and lifestyle influences) from the inexorable (primarily intrinsic aging) is essential to preventing and treating the ailments of the aging skin. As the population ages, medical care of older skin must shift in focus from cosmetic improvements to reducing morbidity and mortality from the dermatological disorders. This will improve the quality of life for the growing population of elderly adults [10].

Aging involves both intrinsic and extrinsic processes occurring in parallel [11]. Intrinsic aging proceeds at different rates in all organisms at a genetically determined pace. Intrinsic aging has been long believed to be primarily related to a buildup of reactive oxygen species (ROS) as a by-product of cellular metabolism and by ROS-induced damage to critical cellular components like membranes, enzymes, and deoxyribonucleic acid (DNA). Further evidence suggests that intrinsic aging may actually result from an intrinsic activation of signal transduction pathways that trigger an over-activation of normal cellular functions which appear to drive cellular senescence. Cellular senescence, in turn, causes the degenerative diseases associated with aging, as well as age-associated increases in cancer [2]. Skin cells become increasingly senescent as they age [12], and the rate of cell proliferation in the epidermis drops, which contributes to deterioration of skin structure and function [13].

Extrinsic aging is accelerated aging superimposed on the intrinsic aging that occurs as a natural consequences of growing old, i.e., aging that occurs as a result of additional environmental insult to the intrinsically aging skin. Extrinsic aging, then, occurs from generally controllable exposures such as smoking [14–17] or solar radiation [18].

The effects of intrinsic and extrinsic aging combine, as a human ages, to produce consistent changes to the integumentary system. The skin thins, dries, wrinkles, and becomes unevenly pigmented [19]. A loss of subcutaneous fat, as well as underlying bone and cartilage, manifests as sagging skin and fallen nasal tips [20]. Chronic dryness and itching are particularly prevalent; in one study of healthy Japanese over 60 years of age, 95 % suffered dry skin at least part of the year [21]. Irritant contact dermatitis associated with incontinence also rises among older adults [22, 23].

Skin complaints by older adults, particularly women, are largely esthetic – plastic surgery has become the fastest growing medical specialty [19] – but aging of the skin also can produce significant morbidity. In fact, most people over 65 have at least one skin disorder, and many have two or more [24]. Various inflammatory, infectious, and vascular disorders become more common [25], and the prevalence of cutaneous malignancy also rises with age [25, 26].

Distinguishing the precludable aspects of cutaneous aging (primarily hormonal and lifestyle influences) from the inexorable (primarily intrinsic aging) is essential to preventing and treating the ailments of the aging skin. As the population ages, medical care of older skin must shift in focus from cosmetic improvements to reducing morbidity and mortality from the dermatological disorders. This will improve the quality of life for the growing population of elderly adults [10].

Structure and Function of Normal Skin

The skin is composed of three layers: epidermis, dermis, and hypodermis (Fig. 1).

Epidermis

The outer layer of the skin, the epidermis, contains primarily keratinocytes with smaller populations of melanocytes and immune cells (primarily Langerhans cells) [10]. Epidermal thickness, which varies according to anatomic site and individual, averages from 50 to 100 μm [27].

The epidermis is a dynamic system whose structure and metabolism serve two principal functions: to protect the skin from external insult and maintain hydration of internal tissues [28]. Both functions are accomplished primarily by the outermost layer of the epidermis, the

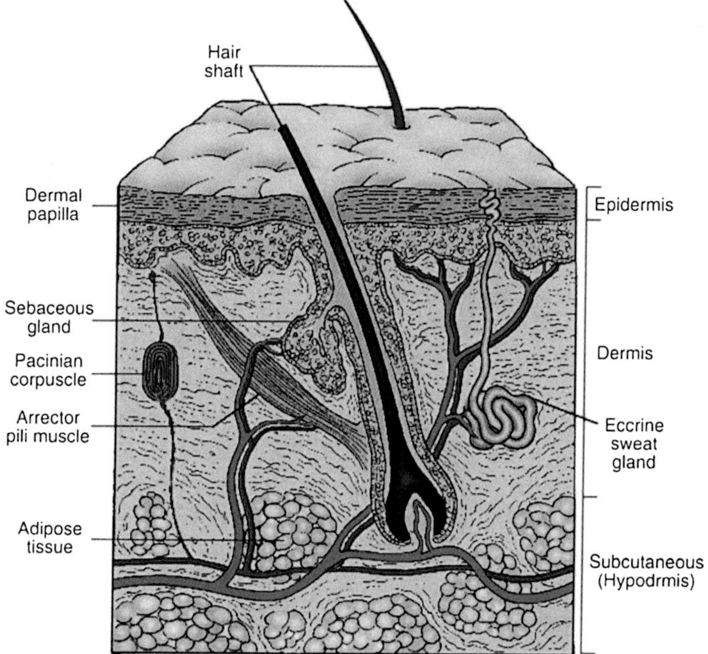

Fig. 1 Normal skin structure showing layers of epidermis, dermis, and hypodermis

stratum corneum [29]. Epidermal keratinocytes originate in a single layer of cells at the basement membrane (the layer between the dermis and the epidermis). Keratinocytes produced at this layer then move upwards; as they ascend, they produce the definitive skin cell protein, keratin, in addition to a variety of lipids.

Keratinocytes also change shape and mature as they move upward toward the skin surface. The stratum corneum (SC), the surface layer of the skin, is composed of the flattened cell bodies of dead keratinocytes, now called corneocytes [30]. This layer of dead keratinocytes averages 15 layers over most of the body but ranges widely from as little as 3 layers in the very thin skin under the eye [31] to more than 50 layers on the palms and soles of the feet [32]. As a dynamic and metabolically interactive tissue [29], the SC comprises about 60 % structural proteins, 20 % water, and 20 % lipids [10, 33].

The corneocytes of the SC are covered by a highly cross-linked and cornified envelope. The extracellular lipid lamellae consist of ceramides, long-chain free fatty acids, and cholesterol. The ceramides strongly adhere to the cornified envelope of the corneocytes, yielding a barrier membrane which, in healthy adults, maintains the water content of the viable portion of the epidermis at about 70 % [34]. The strength of the water barrier also depends on its specific lipid composition [29] and relative proportions of cholesterol, ceramides, and free fatty acids [10, 29]. These intercellular lipids, as well as sebum, natural moisturizing factor (NMF), organic acids, and inorganic ions, impart the water-holding capacity of the SC [30].

Several minor components also contribute to maintaining skin hydration. Hyaluronic acid, a major water-binding component of the dermis, has been recently shown to play a role in the barrier function and hydration of the SC [35]. Glycerol, which acts as an endogenous humectant, has been identified as another component of the SC [36]. In addition, a water-transporting protein named aquaporin-3, expressed from the basal layer up as far as one cell layer below the SC, acts to facilitate the movement of water between the basal layer of the epidermis and the SC in order to maintain a constant level of hydration in the viable epidermis [37].

The water content of the SC (about 20 %) contrasts dramatically with that of the epidermis (about 70 %), a sharp drop observable at the juncture between the stratum granulosum (SG) and the SC [34]. Protein aggregates called tight junction structures, recently identified at the corneo-epidermal junction, prevent water in the epidermis from escaping into the stratum corneum in addition to controlling paracellular permeability [38].

When the barrier function and water-retaining capacity of the SC are compromised [10], pathologic skin dryness can develop, at which point the stratum corneum becomes less flexible and begins to crack or fissure [28]. Skin is considered clinically dry when moisture content of the stratum corneum falls below 10 %. Skin dehydration and cracking may facilitate entry of pathogenic microbes [10].

Dermis

The dermis is a dense and irregular layer of connective tissue, 2–3 mm in thickness, that comprises the most of the skin's thickness (Fig. 1) [39]. Dermal connective tissue contains elastin and collagen; collagen fibers contribute most of the mass of the skin and the bulk of its tensile strength [39]; elastin fibers provide elasticity and resilience [39]. The dermis also contains much of the skin's vasculature, its nerve fibers and sensory receptors, and its primary water-holding components, i.e., hyaluronic acid (responsible for normal turgor of dermis because of its extraordinary water-holding capacity) and supportive glycosaminoglycans [39]. The dermis also serves as the underpinning of the epidermis, binding it to the hypodermis [4].

Hypodermis

The hypodermis is a layer of loose connective tissue below the dermis (Fig. 1), containing the larger blood vessels of the skin, subcutaneous fat (for energy storage and cushioning), and areolar connective tissue. The hypodermis provides cushioning, insulation, and thermoregulation and stabilizes the skin by connecting the dermis to the internal organs (Fig. 1) [40].

Structural Changes in Aged Skin

Changes in the thickness and other characteristics of the epidermis and dermis as skin ages are detailed below (Fig. 2 and Table 1).

Skin Thickness

Skin thickness rises over the first 20 years of life and then (even though the number of cell layers remains stable) [41] begins to thin progressively at a rate that accelerates with age [42]. This phenomenon occurs in all layers of the skin. The epidermis, specifically, decreases in thickness with age [26] when unexposed epidermal skin thins by up to 50 % between the ages of 30 and 80 [43]. Subsidence of epidermal thickness is most pronounced in exposed areas, such as the face, neck, upper part of the chest, and the extensor surface of the hands and forearms [44]. Overall, epidermal thickness decreases at about 6.4 % per decade [42, 45], decreasing faster in women than in men.

The loss of dermal collagen and elastin makes up most of the reduction in total skin thickness in aging adults: for example, in postmenopausal women, a decrease in skin thickness of 1.13 % per year parallels a 2 % decrease per year in collagen content [46]. Dermal thickness decreases at the same rate in both genders [28]. Dermal thickness [42], vascularity, and cellularity also decrease with age [20].

The hypodermis loses much of its fatty cushion as humans age, while the basement membrane, a very small fraction of the total skin thickness, actually increases in thickness with age [47].

Changes in Composition of Aging Skin

Epidermis

As skin ages, epidermal cell numbers [48] and the epidermal turnover rate decrease [40, 49]. With

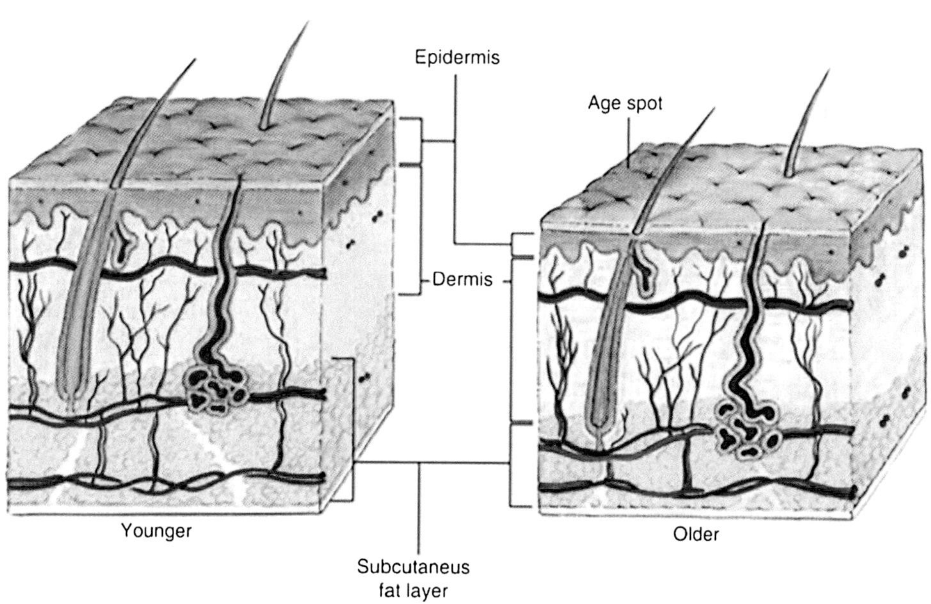

Fig. 2 Differences in skin structure between young and aged skin (With kind permission from Informa Healthcare – Farage et al. [7])

Table 1 Changes in the structure of aged skin

	Observed effect of aging	Reference
	Lower lipid content	[95]
Epidermis	Dermoepidermal junction flattens	[63]
	Number of enzymatically active melanocytes decreases by 8–20 % per decade	[27]
	Number of Langerhans cells decreases	[49]
	Capacity for reepithelization diminishes	[96]
	Number of pores increases	[97]
Dermis	Thickness reduced (atrophy)	[42]
	Vascularity and cellularity decrease	[20]
	Collagen synthesis decreases	[52]
	Pacinian and Meissner's corpuscles degenerate	[52]
	Structure of sweat glands becomes distorted, number of functional sweat glands decreases	[52]
	Elastic fibers degrade	[28]
	Number of blood vessels decreases	[20]
	Number of nerve endings reduced	[13]
Hypodermis	Distribution of subcutaneous fat changes	[52]
	Overall volume decreases	[98]
Appendages	Hair loses normal pigments	[52]
	Hair thins	[52]
	Number of sweat glands decreases	[52]
	Nail plates become abnormal	[52]
	Sebum production reduced	[97]

age, characteristic changes occur in each of the cell types in the epidermis. Cells of the basal layer become less uniform in size, although average cellular size rises [50]. Keratinocytes change shape as the skin ages, becoming shorter and fatter [48]; corneocytes become bigger due to decreased epidermal turnover [41, 51]. Enzymatically active melanocytes decrease at a rate of 8–20 % per decade, resulting in uneven pigmentation in elderly skin [52]. Langerhans cells, like most other epidermal cells, display more uniformity in appearance and function [53]. The number of Langerhans cells in the epidermis also decreases with age, leading to impairment of cutaneous immunity [52]. Langerhans cells that are produced have fewer dendrites and therefore impaired antigen-trapping capability [53]. Although the number of sebaceous glands in the epidermis does not change, sebum production decreases [52]; the evolutionary and biologic significance of this remains unclear.

The water content of aged skin, particularly that of the stratum corneum, is less than that of younger skin [10, 26, 28]. Age-related changes in the amino acid composition [28], in addition, reduce the amount of cutaneous NMF, thereby decreasing the skin's water-binding capacity [10]. The water content of the SC, particularly, decreases progressively with age, eventually dropping below the level necessary for effective desquamation. This abrogation of desquamation causes corneocytes to pile up and adhere to the skin surface, thereby producing the rough, scaly, and flaky skin that accompanies xerosis in aged skin.

The integrity of the SC barrier is dependent on an orderly arrangement of critical lipids [36]. Total lipid content of the aged skin decreases by as much as 65 % [48]. Ceramide levels, particularly ceramide 1 linoleate [54] and ceramide 3 [55], are significantly depleted in older skin. Triglycerides are also reduced, as is the sterol ester fraction of stratum corneum lipids [26]. Although the levels of NMF in the SC are higher in aged skin than in younger (a consequence of the slower rate of epidermal turnover in older individuals [30]), amino acid levels are lower [30]. Corneocytes are fewer but much larger [30], with higher intercorneal cohesiveness [56].

Because permeability does not appear to be significantly increased in the skin of the aged individual, under it has been generally assumed that barrier function does not alter significantly with aging [57]. Some differences in barrier function parameters, however, have been noted: baseline transepidermal water loss (TEWL), a measure of the functional capacity of the stratum corneum to maintain the moisture content of the skin, however, is lower in older patients as compared to younger [26, 58], an observation believed to be due to the reduction of the water content of aged skin (i.e., the elderly have less water to lose) [58]. Recovery of baseline TEWL values after occlusion is also impaired in older skin [26].

It has been demonstrated, in addition, that the permeability barrier of aged skin is also more vulnerable to disruption. In a study which used tape stripping to effect loss of barrier integrity, adults over 80 required only 18 strippings as compared to 31 strippings in young and middle-aged adults. (Tape stripping is a common method of abrogating the SC by removing one layer of skin at a time by applying and then removing a strip of tape.) Recovery of barrier function in the aged subjects also differed dramatically [57]. Only 15 % of those older than 80 had recovered barrier function at 24 h (as assessed by return to baseline TEWL), compared to 50 % of the younger group [57]. Artificially induced water gradients (such as produced by occlusion) were shown to dissipate more slowly in older skin than in younger, again indicating reduced recovery capacity in aged skin [59].

These findings reveal that aging may have a profound impact on barrier integrity even though barrier function appears normal. In the aged skin, a significant disruption of functional capacity is exposed when the epidermal permeability barrier is under stress and barrier function is more easily disturbed and less able to recover. Interestingly, one study found that as skin dries as an inevitable aspect of intrinsic aging, TEWL and the water content of the stratum corneum drop in parallel, while in pathological conditions, TEWL increases even though stratum corneum water content stays low. In stripped skin, both values increase, confirming a derangement of actual barrier function as skin ages [60].

The most widely observed structural change in aged skin is a flattening of the dermoepidermal junction, which occurs as a result of the decreasing numbers and size of dermal papillae [61]. Histological studies reveal that the number of papillae per unit of area decreases dramatically [62], dropping from an average of 40 papillae/mm^2 in young skin to 14 papillae/mm^2 in those aged over 65 [61]. The flattening of the dermoepidermal junction, observed by about the sixth decade [42], creates a thinner epidermis primarily because of retraction of rete pegs [42], decreasing the thickness of the dermoepidermal junction by 35 % [40, 63].

As a consequence of the reduced interdigitation between dermis and epidermis and the flattened dermoepidermal junction, the skin becomes less resistant to shearing forces and more vulnerable to insult [41]. Furthermore, flattening of the dermoepidermal junction results in a smaller contiguous surface between the two layers and reduces communication between the dermis and epidermis; consequently, the supply of nutrients and oxygen to the epidermis diminishes [40, 61]. This flattening also may limit basal cell proliferation and may affect percutaneous absorption [42]. The flattening of the dermoepidermal junction may also contribute to wrinkle formation [41] by increasing the potential for dermoepidermal separation [40, 61].

Dermis

The three major extracellular components of the dermis are collagen, elastin, and hyaluronic acid. All three are depleted in older skin. Collagen content decreases at about 2 % per year [46], primarily because the production of matrix metalloproteinases, which degrade collagen, increases with age [64]. Degradation of dermal collagen by matrix metalloproteinases impairs the structural integrity of the dermis [65]. Mechanical tension or stress on dermal fibroblasts, created by a healthy collagen matrix, is critical for the maintenance of a proper balance between the synthesis of collagen and the synthesis of collagen-degrading enzymes [66]. Fibroblast collapse, due to the accumulation of degraded collagen fibers that prohibit construction of a healthy collagen matrix, causes the ratio of collagen synthesis to collagen degradation to become deranged in a self-perpetuating cycle [65].

Aging is also associated with a decrease in collagen turnover (due to a decrease in fibroblasts and their collagen synthesis) [20]. The relative proportions of collagen types are also disrupted over the life span. The proportion of Type I collagen to Type III collagen in young skin is approximately 6:1, a ratio which drops significantly over the life span as Type I collagen is selectively lost [67], although some increase in collagen Type III synthesis occurs as well [68].

In the aged dermis, collagen fibers become thicker and collagen bundles more disorganized than in younger skin [49]. Collagen cross-links stabilize, reducing elasticity in aged skin. Functional elastin also declines in the dermis with age, as elastin becomes calcified in aged skin and elastin fibers degrade [44]. Elastin turnover also declines [20]. The amount of glycosaminoglycans (GAGs), an important contributor to the structure and water-holding capacity of the dermis, declines with age [40, 61], as does the amount of hyaluronic acid produced by fibroblasts [40, 61] and the amount of interfibrillary ground substance, also a component of a healthy dermal matrix [69].

The loss of structural integrity of the dermis leads to increased rigidity, decreased torsion extensibility [40, 49], and diminished elasticity [28, 39], these properties eroding faster in women than in men [28], with a concomitant increase in vulnerability to shear force injuries [40, 49]. The impact of these changes is dramatic: for example, when skin is mechanically depressed, recovery occurs in minutes in young skin, but takes over 24 h in skin of aged individuals [40, 49]. Perception of pressure and light touch also decrease in aged skin as pacinian and Meissner's corpuscles degenerate. The number of mast cells and fibroblasts in the dermis also decreases [20].

Hypodermis

The overall volume of subcutaneous fat typically diminishes with age, although the overall proportion of subcutaneous fat throughout the body increases until approximately age 70. Fat distribution changes as well; that in the face, hands, and feet decreases, while a relative increase is observed in the thighs, waist, and abdomen. The physiological significance may be to increase thermoregulatory function by further insulating internal organs.

Physiological Changes

Physiological changes in aged skin include changes in (i) biochemistry, (ii) neurosensory perception, (iii) permeability, (iv) vascularization, (v) response to injury, (vi) repair capacity, and (vii) increased incidence of some skin diseases as discussed below (Table 2).

Biochemical Changes

Vitamin D content of aged skin declines: synthesis of this compound slows because the dermis and epidermis lack its immediate biosynthetic precursor (7-dehydrocholesterol), which limits formation of the final product [49].

The surface pH of normal adult skin averages pH 5.5. This cutaneous acidity discourages bacterial colonization; it also contributes to the skin's moisture barrier as amino acids, salts, and other substances in the acid mantle absorb water [62]. The pH of the skin is relatively constant from childhood to approximately age 70 [42], then rises significantly. This rise is especially pronounced in lower limbs, possibly due to impaired circulation [42].

Permeability

The penetration and transit of permeants through the skin involves (i) absorption to the stratum corneum; (ii) diffusion through the stratum corneum, epidermis, and papillary dermis; and (iii) the removal by microcirculation [26]. The

Table 2 Changes in the function of aging skin

Function	Change	Reference
Barrier function	Renewal time of stratum corneum increased by 50 %	[49]
	Baseline TEWL lower in elderly skin	[57]
Sensory and pain perception	Loss in sensitivity, especially after age 50	[41]
	Increased itching	[99]
Thermoregulation	Decreased sweat production	[52]
Response to injury	Lower inflammatory response (erythema and edema)	[41]
	Decreased wound healing	[49]
	Reduced reepithelization	[49]
	Increased vulnerability to mechanical trauma	[49]
Permeability	Decreased percutaneous absorption	[52]
	Decreased sebum production	[49]
	Decreased vascularization	[72]
	Decreased chemical clearance	[49]
Immune function	Decreased number of circulating thymus-derived lymphocytes	[41]
	Decreased risk and intensity of delayed hypersensitivity reactions	[77]
Miscellaneous	Decreased vitamin D production	[52]
	Reduced elasticity	[39]

TEWL transepidermal water loss

first two steps depend on the integrity and hydration of the stratum corneum, which in turn is a function of the level and composition of intracellular lipids [26]. The final step depends on the integrity of the microcirculation [26].

Heightened interest exists in transdermal administration of medications for long-term drug delivery in chronic disease, as this results in fewer side effects and promotes compliance. Consequently, data on percutaneous drug absorption in older adults have gained importance [31]. In general, older adults seem to absorb topical substances more slowly than younger subjects [70]. However, studies on percutaneous absorption in the aged have produced conflicting results. In people over 65, tetrachlorosalicylanilide was absorbed more slowly, but ammonium hydroxide was absorbed more rapidly than in younger adults [41]. Increased permeability of aged skin to fluorescein and testosterone was observed in vitro [40, 49]. Absorption of radiolabeled testosterone was demonstrated to be three times that of younger subjects [31]. However, in a separate in vivo study, no difference between estradiol and testosterone absorption was observed in aged skin, while hydrocortisone and benzoic acid were both absorbed far less readily in aged skin as compared to younger [58].

These conflicting results may reflect compound and body-site differences in the rates of percutaneous absorption [31]. Epidermal penetration of a substance is strongly associated with its hydrophobicity relative to the lipid content of the skin: consequently, hydrophobic compounds penetrate more readily in areas of the body that have high percentage of skin lipids. For example, on the face, where the weight percentage of skin lipids is 12–15 %, hydrophobic compounds (lipophiles) penetrate more readily than hydrophilic ones, whereas on the soles of the feet, where the weight percentage of skin lipids is 1–2 %, hydrophilic compounds penetrate more readily than hydrophobic ones [40, 58].

Using topically applied radiolabeled penetrants, excretion of lipophilic compounds, testosterone, and estradiol was compared to excretion of the more hydrophilic hydrocortisone and benzoic acids. Percutaneous absorption was quantified from urinary excretion profiles of radiolabel. No difference in percutaneous absorption of testosterone and estradiol was noted between younger and older skin, but absorption of both hydrocortisone and benzoic acid were nearly doubled in younger skin [31]. Because aged skin is drier and has a lower lipid content than younger skin, it may be

Table 3 Percutaneous absorption of testosterone, estradiol, hydrocortisone, and benzoic acid in young and elderly people

Compound	Molecular weight[a]	Log K (O/W)[a]	Aqueous solubility	Cumulative % dose excreted in 5 days		
				Young[b]	Older[c]	Elderly[d]
Testosterone	288.4	3.31	Insoluble	13.2 ± 3.0	10.6 ± 5.7	15.2 ± 8.4
				$n = 17$	$n = 8$	$n = 7$
Estradiol	272.4	2.7	Almost insoluble	10.6 ± 4.9	11.5 ± 3.5	9.0 ± 5.6
				$n = 3$	$n = 6$	$n = 6$
Hydrocortisone	362.5	1.93	0.28 g/L	1.87 ± 1.6	0.67 ± 0.58**	0.86 ± 0.5**
				$n = 15$	$n = 8$	$n = 9$
Benzoic acid	122.1	1.87	3.4 g/L	42.6 ± 16.5	27.5 ± 11.6***	23.1 ± 7.0***
				$n = 6$	$n = 8$	$n = 9$

Source: Roskos 1986 [31]
**Significantly different from young control group ($p < 0.01$)
***Significantly different from young control group ($p < 0.05$)
[a]Values taken from the Merck Index; O/W = octanol-water partition
[b]18–35 years
[c]65–75 years
[d]Over 75 years

less amenable to penetration by hydrophilic moieties [31] (Table 3).

Vascularization and Thermoregulation

In older skin, capillaries and small blood vessels regress and become more disorganized [41], blood vessel density diminishes [42], and a 30 % reduction in the number of venular cross sections per unit area of the skin surface occurs in nonexposed areas of the skin [41]. Capillaroscopy measurements using fluorescein angiography and native microscopy suggest a decrease in dermal papillary loops, which house the capillary network [42]. Although the pattern of blood flow through individual capillaries remains unchanged [26], the maximum level of blood flow diminishes as functional capillary plexi are lost.

A significant time delay in autonomic vasoconstriction in the aged (e.g., after postural changes, cold arm challenge, inspiratory gasp, body cooling) [26, 42] is well-documented; this phenomenon is due primarily to declining function of the autonomic nervous system [26].

Eccrine sweating is markedly impaired with age. Spontaneous sweating in response to dry heat was 70 % lower in healthy older subjects compared to young controls, due primarily to decreased output per gland [71]. Vascularity is also lost. Cross sections of photodamaged skin reveal a 35 % reduction in vascularity in the papillary dermis of aged skin [72], as well as reduced blood flow, depleted nutrient exchange, dysfunctional thermoregulation, reduced skin surface temperature, and increased skin pallor [73]. Facial skin temperatures were lower in aged subjects [41], and older people exhibited a wider temperature difference between groin and toes [41].

The elderly are predisposed to both hypothermia and heat stroke, as reduced eccrine sweating rates, lower vasodilation or vasoconstriction of dermal arterioles, and the loss of subcutaneous fat impair thermoregulation [71].

Irritant Response

Inflammatory response to an exogenous agent declines in people over 70 years old [26, 40, 58]. The inflammatory response is slower and less intense, and some clinical signs of skin damage are absent [26, 41] (Fig. 3 **shows the lack of skin response after patch testing with a known irritant in an older person**). Diagnosis of common dermatological problems becomes difficult, and allergic sensitization tests may be

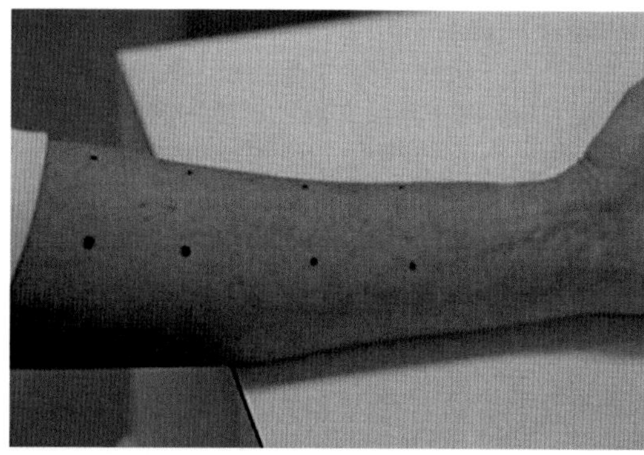

Fig. 3 The inflammatory response is slower and less intense in older people, and some clinical signs of skin damage are visually absent when exposed to a known irritant chemical through patch testing on the forearm

meaningless [41]. Sunburn response also is attenuated and delayed [41]. Fewer inflammatory cells are seen in cantharidin blisters in older subjects [41].

The manifestation of skin irritation is blunted. Patch testing found less erythema, vesicles, pustules, and wheals in aged skin, as well as a decrease in TEWL [40, 58] in response to a range of skin irritants, including toilet soap [41], kerosene [41], dimethyl sulfoxide [DMSO], ethyl nicotinate, chloroform-methanol, and lactic acid [26], chemicals which elicit inflammation by clearly different mechanisms [26]. In some cases, the response is also delayed. Analysis of changes in TEWL after sodium lauryl sulfate (SLS) application to the skin confirmed that in aged skin, the irritation reaction is slower and less frequent in postmenopausal than in premenopausal women [74]. Moreover, although blistering caused by ammonium hydroxide exposure is elicited more rapidly in older people, the time required to attain a full response is much longer than in younger ones [26].

The characteristics of the irritant response may be compound dependent in ways specific to older skin, as chemical irritants induce their effects through different mechanisms. SLS as well as nonanoic acid disrupted keratinocyte metabolism and differentiation, while dithranol induced marked swelling of keratinocytes in the upper epidermis [40, 58]. In a study of croton oil, thymoquinone, and crotonaldehyde on older skin, decreased responsiveness was observed only to croton oil [26, 75].

Immune Response

The immune response of aged skin is generally diminished. Numbers of Langerhans cells in the epidermis decrease by about 50 % between the age of 25 and the age of 70 [49]. The total number of circulating lymphocytes decreases, as does the number of T-cells [40, 49] and B-cells [40, 49], both of which lose functional capacity with age [76].

Delayed hypersensitivity reactions decrease with age: numerous reports have demonstrated a decrease in the capacity for allergic response [40, 49, 77]. For example, healthy older subjects did not develop sensitivity to some known sensitizers and exhibited a lower frequency of positive reactions to standard test antigens compared to young adult controls [40, 49]. The frequency of IgE-mediated, positive prick tests to common allergens declined with age: peak reactivity was observed among people in their twenties, with 52 % of subjects reacting to at least one test allergen; positive response rates dropped steadily with age, declining to 16 % frequency among subjects older than 75 years [26]. Levels of circulating autoantibodies increase with age; this occurs in parallel with a decrease in useful antibodies as the aged individual's existing immunity to specific allergens erodes [40, 49].

Regenerative Capacity and Response to Injury

In healthy skin, about one layer of corneocytes desquamates every day, so that the whole stratum corneum replaces itself about every 2 weeks [30]. In contrast, elderly stratum corneum may take twice as long [78]. Repair of an impaired barrier requires the presence of the three main lipids in appropriate proportions [79] as well as stratum corneum turnover, both of which are suboptimal in older subjects.

Injury repair diminishes with age. Wound healing events begin later and proceed more slowly. For example, a wound area of 40 cm^2, which in 20-year old subjects took 40 days to heal, required almost twice as long – 76 days – in those over 80 [40, 49]. The risk of postoperative wound reopening increased 600 % in people in their mid-80s compared to those in their mid-30s [40, 49]. The tensile strength of healing wounds decreased after the age of 70 [40, 49]. Repair processes like collagen remodeling, cellular proliferation, and wound metabolism are all delayed in the aged [40, 49]. The rate at which fibroblasts initiated migration in vitro following wound initiation was closely related to the age of the cell lines [40, 49, 80].

Barrier function requires twice as long to restore in the aged as compared to younger controls [81]; stratum corneum renewal times were much longer in the aged (about 30 days compared to 20 days in normal skin) [81]. Reepithelialization of the stratum corneum after blistering is also diminished [81], being twice as long for people over 75 than for those aged 25 [40, 49]. The production of messenger ribonucleic acid (mRNA) and interleukin-1 (IL-1) protein is also decreased in the aged, contributing to sluggish barrier recovery [82].

Neurosensory Perception

Itching is reported more frequently by older adults. However, pain perception declines, and pain perception is delayed after age 50 [41]. Consequently, the risk of tissue injury rises, as the most obvious warning signals – pain, erythema, and edema – appear more slowly [41]. This, coupled with longer wound repair times, results in higher morbidity in the aged.

Changes at the Genome Level

Aging brings profound changes in phenotype (the outward appearance) without changing the fundamental genetic sequence encoded by an individual's DNA. It is now known that many of the deleterious changes in skin have their origin in changes to DNA that do not affect the genetic sequence known as epigenetic changes. Epigenetic changes consist of modifications to the DNA packaging and translation into proteins by either covalent modification of histones or methylation of cytosine residues in DNA that changes phenotype, thus acting a kind of arbitrator between the environment and genome. DNA in the aged shows tissue-specific hypermethylation which may be causative in the phenotypic changes associated with aging [83]. MicroRNAs, also recently recognized as a regulator of gene expression, are also believed to play key roles in integumentary processes [84].

The hormonal milieu of the body also has dramatic effects on the skin dependent on the gender of its owner and the sequential hormone changes (i.e., growth hormones, sex-related hormones) to which it is exposed as its owner ages [85].

Falls in hormone levels late in life are associated with skin changes and skin cancer [86].

Aging Skin: Mitigating the Damage

Although aging of the skin, like other systems, is inevitable, research is beginning to define ways to both delay and minimize the troublesome effects of aging on the skin. The impact of various dietary exposures, for example, is the focus of much current research. One study found that sugar consumption (both fructose and glucose) links amino acids in collagen and elastin in the dermis, producing advanced glycation end products (AGES) which produce a cross-linking of collagen fibers that blocks repair. Elevated levels of blood sugar have been shown to accelerate this cross-linking in all body tissues when skin is exposed to ultraviolet light [87]. Analyses have shown that many fruits and vegetables contain antioxidant components like carotenoids, flavonoids, vitamins, and minerals that provide natural antiaging benefits. Antioxidants like phytoestrogens, omega-3 fatty acids, and co-enzyme Q have proven ability to regulate the processes of aging [88].

Excessive exposure to ultraviolet light, known to activate reactive oxygen species that damage DNA and other cellular components resulting in numerous undesirable changes to the skin, should be avoided or protected against (with an awareness that not only ultraviolet (UV)B but UVA rays are now known to cause those changes: sunburn, pigmentation changes, thickening of the skin, and skin cancer) [89]. Interestingly, the body's own mechanisms for ameliorating UV damage are still being uncovered. It was recently shown that 11,14,17-eicosatrienoic acid (ETA) which is significantly increased in photoaged human skin in vivo as well as acutely UV-irradiated human skin in vitro was found to be significantly decreased in intrinsically aged human skin. ETA inhibits matrix metalloproteinase (MMP) expression after UV irradiation, which may be photoprotective [90]. Interestingly, however, sunbathing's role in its most infamous consequence, melanoma, is now being reevaluated, with blame shifting to early genetic processes rather than later environmental exposures, elucidating how urgent the need for greater fundamental understanding of the skin's biology [91].

Pollution (more specifically the airborne particles that comprise it, primarily from auto exhaust) is an increasingly recognized contributor to skin problems. Pollution has been strongly correlated to the degenerative processes of skin aging, particularly pigmentation issues, but also wrinkles [92].

Conclusion

Humans now live to twice their reproductive age, an achievement unique to our species [93]. Although many profound changes occur over a skin's lifetime, the human integument remains relatively functional when protected from excessive environmental insult. The aging skin, nonetheless, with time becomes compromised in many ways [26]. Structural changes lead to undesirable visible characteristics as well as reduced elasticity and resilience. Decreases in neurosensory capacity increase the risk of unrecognized injury, while loss of water and lipids in the skin makes the skin itchy and increasingly uncomfortable. The decrease in the skin's ability to repair itself slows wound repair and reepithelization dramatically and increases the risk of surgical dehiscence.

Understanding the fundamental physiology of the skin provides a foundation for progress in understanding the dermatological needs of those whose skin is aging. Further research will drive better ability to evaluate risk of exposures and provide optimal nutritional foundation for healthy aging skin and medications or ointments that block or even reverse negative epigenetic changes. As the proportion of older adults in the industrialized world increases, the dermatology of aging skin emerges as a focus for research. Furthermore, skin aging becomes increasingly of interest due to a growing awareness that the skin is a window into the overall health of the aging individual, predictive and/or revelatory of internal systemic disease in multiple organ systems [94]. Understanding and learning to care for the problems of aged skin will improve the quality of life in twilight years, as well as facilitate better therapies for dermatological diseases over the life span.

Cross-References

▶ Skin Aging: A Brief Summary of Characteristic Changes

References

1. World Health Organization. World Health Statistics 2014. [News Release] May 15, 2014. http://www.who.int/mediacentre/news/releases/2014/world-health-statistics-2014/en/. Accessed 25 June 2014.
2. Berman AE, Leontieva OV, Natarajan V, McCubrey JA, Demidenko ZN, Nikiforov MA. Recent progress in genetics of aging, senescence and longevity: focusing on cancer-related genes. Oncotarget. 2012;3 (12):1522–32.
3. Monteiro-Riviere NA. Introduction to histological aspects of dermatotoxicology. Microsc Res Tech. 1997;37(3):171.
4. Klassen C, editor. Casarett and Doull's toxicology: the basic science of poisons. New York: McGraw-Hill; 1996. p. 529–46.

5. Farage MA, Miller KW, Elsner P, Maibach HI. Intrinsic and extrinsic factors in skin ageing: a review. Int J Cosmet Sci. 2008;30(2):87–95.
6. Farage MA, Miller KW, Elsner P, Maibach HI. Functional and physiological characteristics of the aging skin. Aging Clin Exp Res. 2008;20(3):195–200.
7. Farage MA, Miller KW, Elsner P, Maibach HI. Structural characteristics of the aging skin: a review. Cutan Ocul Toxicol. 2007;26(4):343–57.
8. Sjerobabski-Masnec I, Situm M. Skin aging. Acta Clin Croat. 2010;49(4):515–8.
9. Gkogkolou P, Böhm M. Advanced glycation end products: key players in skin aging? Dermatoendocrinology. 2012;4(3):259–70.
10. Jackson SM, Williams ML, Feingold KR, Elias PM. Pathobiology of the stratum corneum. West J Med. 1993;158(3):279–85.
11. Ghersetich I, Troiano M, De Giorgi V, Lotti T. Receptors in skin ageing and antiageing agents. Dermatol Clin. 2007;25(4):655–62. xi.
12. Glogau RG. Systemic evaluation of the aging face. In: Bolognia JL, Jorizzo JL, Rapini RP, editors. Dermatology. Edinburgh: Mosby; 2003. p. 2357–60.
13. Puizina-Ivić N. Skin aging. Acta Dermatovenerol Alp Panonica Adriat. 2008;17(2):47–54.
14. Helfrich YR, Yu L, Ofori A, Hamilton TA, Lambert J, King A, et al. Effect of smoking on aging of photoprotected skin: evidence gathered using a new photonumeric scale. Arch Dermatol. 2007;143 (3):397–402.
15. Koh JS, Kang H, Choi SW, Kim HO. Cigarette smoking associated with premature facial wrinkling: image analysis of facial skin replicas. Int J Dermatol. 2002;41(1):21–7.
16. Martires KJ, Fu P, Polster AM, Cooper KD, Baron ED. Factors that affect skin aging: a cohort-based survey on twins. Arch Dermatol. 2009;145(12):1375–9.
17. Doshi DN, Hanneman KK, Cooper KD. Smoking and skin aging in identical twins. Arch Dermatol. 2007;143 (12):1543–6.
18. Gilchrest BA. A review of skin ageing and its medical therapy. Br J Dermatol. 1996;135(6):867–75.
19. Friedman O. Changes associated with the aging face. Facial Plast Surg Clin North Am. 2005;13(3):371–80.
20. Duncan KO, Leffell DJ. Preoperative assessment of the elderly patient. Dermatol Clin. 1997;15 (4):583–93.
21. Hara M, Kikuchi K, Watanabe M, Denda M, Koyama J, Nomura J, et al. Senile xerosis: functional, morphological, and biochemical studies. J Geriatr Dermatol. 1993;1(3):111–20.
22. Farage MA, Miller KW, Berardesca E, Maibach HI. Incontinence in the aged: contact dermatitis and other cutaneous consequences. Contact Dermatitis. 2007;57(4):211–7.
23. Farage MA, Miller KW, Berardesca E, Maibach HI. Psychosocial and societal burden of incontinence in the aged population: a review. Arch Gynecol Obstet. 2008;277(4):285–90.
24. Kligman AM, Koblenzer C. Demographics and psychological implications for the aging population. Dermatol Clin. 1997;15(4):549–53.
25. Farage MA, Miller KW, Berardesca E, Maibach HI. Clinical implications of aging skin: cutaneous disorders in the elderly. Am J Clin Dermatol. 2009;10 (2):73–86.
26. Harvell JD, Maibach HI. Percutaneous absorption and inflammation in aged skin: a review. J Am Acad Dermatol. 1994;31(6):1015–21.
27. Rees JL. The genetics of sun sensitivity in humans. Am J Hum Genet. 2004;75(5):739–51.
28. McCallion R, Li Wan Po A. Dry and photo-aged skin: manifestations and management. J Clin Pharm Ther. 1993;18(1):15–32.
29. Elias PM. Stratum corneum architecture, metabolic activity and interactivity with subjacent cell layers. Exp Dermatol. 1996;5(4):191–201.
30. Tagami H. Functional characteristics of the stratum corneum in photoaged skin in comparison with those found in intrinsic aging. Arch Dermatol Res. 2008;300 Suppl 1:S1–6.
31. Roskos KV, Guy RH, Maibach HI. Percutaneous absorption in the aged. Dermatol Clin. 1986;4 (3):455–65.
32. Ya-Xian Z, Suetake T, Tagami H. Number of cell layers of the stratum corneum in normal skin – relationship to the anatomical location on the body, age, sex and physical parameters. Arch Dermatol Res. 1999;291 (10):555–9.
33. Mathias CG, Maibach HI. Perspectives in occupational dermatology. West J Med. 1982;137(6):486–92.
34. Caspers PJ, Lucassen GW, Puppels GJ. Combined in vivo confocal Raman spectroscopy and confocal microscopy of human skin. Biophys J. 2003;85 (1):572–80.
35. Sakai S, Yasuda R, Sayo T, Ishikawa O, Inoue S. Hyaluronan exists in the normal stratum corneum. J Invest Dermatol. 2000;114(6):1184–7.
36. Verdier-Sévrain S, Bonté F. Skin hydration: a review on its molecular mechanisms. J Cosmet Dermatol. 2007;6(2):75–82.
37. Sougrat R, Morand M, Gondran C, Barré P, Gobin R, Bonté F, et al. Functional expression of AQP3 in human skin epidermis and reconstructed epidermis. J Invest Dermatol. 2002;118(4):678–85.
38. Verdier-Sévrain S. Effect of estrogens on skin aging and the potential role of selective estrogen receptor modulators. Climacteric. 2007;10(4):289–97.
39. Brincat MP, Baron YM, Galea R. Estrogens and the skin. Climacteric. 2005;8(2):110–23.
40. Martini F. Fundamentals of anatomy and physiology. San Francisco: Benjamin-Cummings; 2004.
41. Grove GL. Physiologic changes in older skin. Clin Geriatr Med. 1989;5(1):115–25.
42. Waller JM, Maibach HI. Age and skin structure and function, a quantitative approach (I): blood flow, pH, thickness, and ultrasound echogenicity. Skin Res Technol. 2005;11(4):221–35.

43. Sans M, Moragas A. Mathematical morphologic analysis of the aortic medial structure. Biomechanical implications. Anal Quant Cytol Histol. 1993;15 (2):93–100.
44. Boss GR, Seegmiller JE. Age-related physiological changes and their clinical significance. West J Med. 1981;135(6):434–40.
45. Oriba HA, Bucks DA, Maibach HI. Percutaneous absorption of hydrocortisone and testosterone on the vulva and forearm: effect of the menopause and site. Br J Dermatol. 1996;134(2):229–33.
46. Brincat M, Kabalan S, Studd JW, Moniz CF, de Trafford J, Montgomery J. A study of the decrease of skin collagen content, skin thickness, and bone mass in the postmenopausal woman. Obstet Gynecol. 1987;70 (6):840–5.
47. Vázquez F, Palacios S, Alemañ N, Guerrero F. Changes of the basement membrane and type IV collagen in human skin during aging. Maturitas. 1996;25 (3):209–15.
48. Suter-Widmer J, Elsner P. Age and irritation. In: Agner T, Maibah H, editors. The irritant contact dermatitis syndrome. Boca Raton: CRC Press; 1996. p. 257–65.
49. Fenske NA, Lober CW. Structural and functional changes of normal aging skin. J Am Acad Dermatol. 1986;15(4 Pt 1):571–85.
50. Brégégère F, Soroka Y, Bismuth J, Friguet B, Milner Y. Cellular senescence in human keratinocytes: unchanged proteolytic capacity and increased protein load. Exp Gerontol. 2003;38(6):619–29.
51. Sauermann K, Jaspers S, Koop U, Wenck H. Topically applied vitamin C increases the density of dermal papillae in aged human skin. BMC Dermatol. 2004;4 (1):13.
52. Phillips T, Kanj L. Clinical manifestations of skin aging. In: Squier C, Hill MW, editors. The effect of aging in oral mucosa and skin. Boca Raton: CRC Press; 1994. p. 25–40.
53. Wulf HC, Sandby-Møller J, Kobayasi T, Gniadecki R. Skin aging and natural photoprotection. Micron. 2004;35(3):185–91.
54. Rogers J, Harding C, Mayo A, Banks J, Rawlings A. Stratum corneum lipids: the effect of ageing and the seasons. Arch Dermatol Res. 1996;288 (12):765–70.
55. Zettersten EM, Ghadially R, Feingold KR, Crumrine D, Elias PM. Optimal ratios of topical stratum corneum lipids improve barrier recovery in chronologically aged skin. J Am Acad Dermatol. 1997;37 (3 Pt 1):403–8.
56. Long CC, Marks R. Stratum corneum changes in patients with senile pruritus. J Am Acad Dermatol. 1992;27(4):560–4.
57. Ghadially R, Brown BE, Sequeira-Martin SM, Feingold KR, Elias PM. The aged epidermal permeability barrier. Structural, functional, and lipid biochemical abnormalities in humans and a senescent murine model. J Clin Invest. 1995;95(5):2281–90.
58. Ghadially R. Aging and the epidermal permeability barrier: implications for contact dermatitis. Am J Contact Dermat. 1998;9(3):162–9.
59. Roskos KV, Guy RH. Assessment of skin barrier function using transepidermal water loss: effect of age. Pharm Res. 1989;6(11):949–53.
60. Berardesca E, Maibach HI. Transepidermal water loss and skin surface hydration in the non invasive assessment of stratum corneum function. Derm Beruf Umwelt. 1990;38(2):50–3.
61. Südel KM, Venzke K, Mielke H, Breitenbach U, Mundt C, Jaspers S, et al. Novel aspects of intrinsic and extrinsic aging of human skin: beneficial effects of soy extract. Photochem Photobiol. 2005;81 (3):581–7.
62. Fiers SA. Breaking the cycle: the etiology of incontinence dermatitis and evaluating and using skin care products. Ostomy Wound Manage. 1996;42(3):32–4. 36, 38–40, passim.
63. Neerken S, Lucassen GW, Bisschop MA, Lenderink E, Nuijs TAM. Characterization of age-related effects in human skin: a comparative study that applies confocal laser scanning microscopy and optical coherence tomography. J Biomed Opt. 2004;9(2):274–81.
64. Ashcroft GS, Horan MA, Herrick SE, Tarnuzzer RW, Schultz GS, Ferguson MW. Age-related differences in the temporal and spatial regulation of matrix metalloproteinases (MMPs) in normal skin and acute cutaneous wounds of healthy humans. Cell Tissue Res. 1997;290(3):581–91.
65. Fisher GJ, Varani J, Voorhees JJ. Looking older: fibroblast collapse and therapeutic implications. Arch Dermatol. 2008;144(5):666–72.
66. Varani J, Dame MK, Rittie L, Fligiel SEG, Kang S, Fisher GJ, et al. Decreased collagen production in chronologically aged skin: roles of age-dependent alteration in fibroblast function and defective mechanical stimulation. Am J Pathol. 2006;168(6):1861–8.
67. Oikarinen A. The aging of skin: chronoaging versus photoaging. Photodermatol Photoimmunol Photomed. 1990;7(1):3–4.
68. Savvas M, Bishop J, Laurent G, Watson N, Studd J. Type III collagen content in the skin of postmenopausal women receiving oestradiol and testosterone implants. Br J Obstet Gynaecol. 1993;100(2):154–6.
69. Castelo-Branco C, Figueras F, Martínez de Osaba MJ, Vanrell JA. Facial wrinkling in postmenopausal women. Effects of smoking status and hormone replacement therapy. Maturitas. 1998;29(1):75–86.
70. Kligman AM. The treatment of photoaged human skin by topical tretinoin. Drugs. 1989;38(1):1–8.
71. Ohta H, Makita K, Kawashima T, Kinoshita S, Takenouchi M, Nozawa S. Relationship between dermato-physiological changes and hormonal status in pre-, peri-, and postmenopausal women. Maturitas. 1998;30(1):55–62.
72. Gilchrest BA, Stoff JS, Soter NA. Chronologic aging alters the response to ultraviolet-induced inflammation in human skin. J Invest Dermatol. 1982;79(1):11–5.

73. Baumann L. Skin ageing and its treatment. J Pathol. 2007;211(2):241–51.
74. Elsner P, Wilhelm D, Maibach HI. Sodium lauryl sulfate-induced irritant contact dermatitis in vulvar and forearm skin of premenopausal and postmenopausal women. J Am Acad Dermatol. 1990;23(4 Pt 1):648–52.
75. Coenraads PJ, Bleumink E, Nater JP. Susceptibility to primary irritants: age dependence and relation to contact allergic reactions. Contact Dermatitis. 1975;1 (6):377–81.
76. Szewczuk MR, Campbell RJ. Loss of immune competence with age may be due to auto-anti-idiotypic antibody regulation. Nature. 1980;286(5769):164–6.
77. Robinson MK. Population differences in skin structure and physiology and the susceptibility to irritant and allergic contact dermatitis: implications for skin safety testing and risk assessment. Contact Dermatitis. 1999;41(2):65–79.
78. Baker H, Blair CP. Cell replacement in the human stratum corneum in old age. Br J Dermatol. 1968;80 (6):367–72.
79. Man MQM, Feingold KR, Thornfeldt CR, Elias PM. Optimization of physiological lipid mixtures for barrier repair. J Invest Dermatol. 1996;106 (5):1096–101.
80. Muggleton-Harris AL, Reisert PS, Burghoff RL. In vitro characterization of response to stimulus (wounding) with regard to ageing in human skin fibroblasts. Mech Ageing Dev. 1982;19(1):37–43.
81. Grove GL, Kligman AM. Age-associated changes in human epidermal cell renewal. J Gerontol. 1983;38 (2):137–42.
82. Barland CO, Zettersten E, Brown BS, Ye J, Elias PM, Ghadially R. Imiquimod-induced interleukin-1 alpha stimulation improves barrier homeostasis in aged murine epidermis. J Invest Dermatol. 2004;122 (2):330–6.
83. Grönniger E, Weber B, Heil O, Peters N, Stäb F, Wenck H, et al. Aging and chronic sun exposure cause distinct epigenetic changes in human skin. PLoS Genet. 2010;6(5):e1000971.
84. Ning MS, Andl T. Control by a hair's breadth: the role of microRNAs in the skin. Cell Mol Life Sci. 2013;70 (7):1149–69.
85. Makrantonaki E, Zouboulis CC. Dermatoendocrinology. Skin aging. Hautarzt. 2010;61(6):505–10 [in German].
86. Makrantonaki E, Schönknecht P, Hossini AM, Kaiser E, Katsouli M, Adjaye J. Skin and brain age together: the role of hormones in the ageing process. Exp Gerontol. 2010;45(10):801–13.
87. Danby FW. Nutrition and aging skin: sugar and glycation. Clin Dermatol. 2010;28(4):409–11.
88. Vranesić-Bender D. The role of nutraceuticals in anti-aging medicine. Acta Clin Croat. 2010;49(4):537–44.
89. Situm M, Buljan M, Cavka V, Bulat V, Krolo I, Mihić LL. Skin changes in the elderly people – how strong is the influence of the UV radiation on skin aging? Coll Antropol. 2010;34 Suppl 2:9–13.
90. Kim EJ, Kim M, Jin X, Oh J, Kim JE, Chung JH. Skin aging and photoaging alter fatty acids composition, including 11,14,17-eicosatrienoic acid, in the epidermis of human skin. J Korean Med Sci. 2010;25 (6):980–3.
91. Bataille V. Melanoma. Shall we move away from the sun and focus more on embryogenesis, body weight and longevity? Med Hypotheses. 2013;81(5):846–50.
92. Vierkötter A, Schikowski T, Ranft U, Sugiri D, Matsui M, Krämer U, et al. Airborne particle exposure and extrinsic skin aging. J Invest Dermatol. 2010;130 (12):2719–26.
93. Naftolin F. Prevention during the menopause is critical for good health: skin studies support protracted hormone therapy. Fertil Steril. 2005;84(2):293–4. discussion 295.
94. Makrantonaki E, Bekou V, Zouboulis CC. Genetics and skin aging. Dermatoendocrinology. 2012;4(3):280–4.
95. Saint Léger D, François AM, Lévêque JL, Stoudemayer TJ, Grove GL, Kligman AM. Age-associated changes in stratum corneum lipids and their relation to dryness. Dermatologica. 1988;177 (3):159–64.
96. Holt DR, Kirk SJ, Regan MC, Hurson M, Lindblad WJ, Barbul A. Effect of age on wound healing in healthy human beings. Surgery. 1992;112(2):293–7. discussion 297–8.
97. Rawlings AV. Ethnic skin types: are there differences in skin structure and function? Int J Cosmet Sci. 2006;28 (2):79–93.
98. Puizina-Ivić N, Mirić L, Carija A, Karlica D, Marasović D. Modern approach to topical treatment of aging skin. Coll Antropol. 2010;34(3):1145–53.
99. Buckley C, Rustin MH. Management of irritable skin disorders in the elderly. Br J Hosp Med. 1990;44 (1):24–6. 28, 30–2.

An Overview of the Histology of Aging Skin in Laboratory Models

4

Tapan K. Bhattacharyya

Contents

Abstract

This article is an overview of histomorphological changes documented during various stages of life in many laboratory models utilized in skin aging studies. A bewildering variety in cutaneous aging response has been observed in different strains. The commonly used laboratory models like the rat and the mouse show dissimilar aging changes in skin. There are a few mouse models which seem to resemble the general trend of skin attrition related to advancing age observed in some human studies. Caloric restriction has been observed to modulate skin aging changes in the rat and the mouse. Despite the wide variation in observational studies related to aging changes, some rodent models are useful to aging research and experimental response of aging skin.

Introduction

Human populations worldwide are living longer, and skin from older people becomes more susceptible to diseases and malformations apart from being ravaged by environmental trauma like ultraviolet radiation. The science of clinical dermatology documents numerous diseases of human skin, but scant information has been paid to basic research in the microanatomy of aging skin. This is a subject that invokes biological and evolutionary interest about age-induced involution of the

---

"What lies beneath this aging skin? The untold destruction stealthy creeping, The bones the organs the nerves, the brain, I am breathing, I am functioning, Am I living?"
Julie A. Crippin, 2008

T.K. Bhattacharyya (✉)
Otolaryngology-Head and Neck Surgery, University of Illinois, Chicago, IL, USA
e-mail: tbhatt@uic.edu

M.A. Farage et al. (eds.), *Textbook of Aging Skin*,
DOI 10.1007/978-3-662-47398-6_1

integumentary system. It is logical to introspect about the phenomenon of chronological aging of animal skin from other mammalian species. Despite many descriptive studies published in early literature, there are still many gaps in our knowledge about the patterns of intrinsic aging in various laboratory models. Although animal models may not fully corroborate biochemical data of aging skin and may show inconsistent results, they are still useful tools to interpolate the fundamental etiologies of skin aging and antiaging effects [1].

One reason for the lack of documentation in this area of research is scant availability of animal models of skin aging with clear documentation regarding age or the stages of the life cycle. Animal husbandry for long-term maintenance of aging animals in a disease-free colony is a costly project and is usually beyond the reach of an average laboratory. The aging human skin with increased roughness and wrinkling is sagging, and inelastic, and shows many signs of atrophy, such as epidermal thinning or abnormal collagen and elastic fibers. It is logical to ask if similar or different conditions are observed when a comparative anatomical analysis is extended to different models from the mammalian kingdom. This review explores whether intrinsic aging also affects skin histology in laboratory models in a comparable manner. The data are very limited and were acquired through painstaking investigations by researchers dating back to several decades using classical histological techniques; the reported quantitative data were often uncorroborated by statistical methodology.

The Human Scenario: Skin Aging Histology

Morphological changes of the human integument due to intrinsic aging caused by time-induced physiological changes are understandable, but can be altered due to personal and environmental factors, can vary in different anatomical sites, and are also linked to endocrine factors [2]. Despite these problems, several accounts of intrinsic aging of human skin have been published over the last few decades. Skin atrophy is marked only after the fifth decade of human life and shows a plethora of morphological changes including epidermal thinning, flattening of the dermal-epidermal junction, loss of melanocytes, and immunocompetent Langerhans cells; some physiological functions, such as surface lipid production, and thermoregulation are also affected by the aging process (review in Rittie and Fisher [3]).

There are also dermal changes such as reduced fibroblast population and sebaceous glands. These histopathologic events have been reviewed [4]. Morphometric measurement of collagen fibers from stained human skin biopsies further showed that collagen fiber density started decreasing from around 30–40 years, with thinner and more spaced fibers [5]. Other investigators found no difference in epidermal or dermal thickness in a study of wound healing comparing skin from young and elderly volunteers [6]. The biochemical profile of collagen metabolism of human skin, however, changes with age. A steady decline in synthesis of hydroxyproline in human skin up to the fourth decade has been described [7].

Reports of dermal elastic fiber changes with age including abnormalities and disintegration have been published by some authors. As per the study of Vitellaro-Zuccarello et al. [5], elastic fiber distribution has a different aging pattern in men and women. While the density of elastic fibers in the papillary dermis is not modified as a function of age, in the reticular dermis of both sexes, the fiber density increases in the first decade, followed by a drop only in the female. Biochemically, elastin biosynthesis is stable up to approximately the fourth decade of life [7]. Although reports by different investigators vary in detail due to different kinds of sampling and histological methods employed, a general trend of attrition of the dermal connective tissue fibers is noted as a correlate of the aging process. Histopathologic changes in the epidermis and dermis of human skin in sun-exposed and sun-protected areas have been reviewed by Monteiro-Riviere [8].

Aging in Rodent Models

Some accounts of histological and cellular kinetic changes throughout the life span or representative stages of rodent life span are available. Most of the studies were conducted on the hairless mouse, other strains of mice (CBA, C57131/6NNia, Balb/c), and rats (Wistar rat, Fischer 344). It is difficult to make a meaningful comparison between older studies related to skin aging histopathology, as different authors have reported data on both sexes of various mouse models, which were often based upon limited sample numbers. Some of these important articles lack statistical evaluation. However, some noteworthy findings from early literature on different rodent models are summarized here.

The hairless mouse owes its hairlessness to a homozygous recessive genetic condition, and structural changes of skin accompanying development of hairlessness in this animal were described in the older literature. Age-related modifications in epidermal cell kinetics in this species were described by Iverson and Schjoelberg [9]. Using autoradiography, it was shown that epidermal cell proliferation increased from birth to approximately 20 weeks of age and remained steady. This detailed study could not confirm whether epidermal thickness or cell proliferation rate decreases systematically with increasing age. On the other hand, Haratake et al. [10] presented data showing that the thickness of the epidermis in hairless mice decreases with intrinsic aging. There was also less incorporation of tritiated thymidine in the epidermis in older mice.

The tritiated thymidine technique was used in mice up to 19 months of age, and the data revealed an age-dependent decline in the cell proliferation rate [11]. The data reported from Balb/c mice [12] seemed to indicate epidermal atrophy with age. The epidermis was thinner, with smaller nuclei, in 20-month-old animals compared to 2-month-old animals, although there was no decrease in mitotic activity and DNA labeling index. The loss of epidermal mass was related to a decrease in protein and RNA content of the epidermis. However, similar epidermal changes were not observed in a detailed study in young and old C57B1/6NNia mice [13]. In fact, the epidermis from the ear and footpad showed a statistically significant increase in thickness and augmented cell size. The index of labeling with tritiated thymidine showed no difference between young and old mice. Moreover, in C57BL/6 N mice, the number of epidermal cell layers and the epidermal thickness remained constant from 1 to 22 months of age [14].

Most of the reported studies on mouse skin were mainly concerned with the aging effect on the epidermal cell size or cell kinetics, and scarce attention has been devoted to the morphological changes of the dermal constituents in aging animals. CBA mouse skin was investigated in three age groups (1, 6, and 27 months) from animals procured from NIH colonies [15]. As the rate of skin aging differs in different areas of the body [13], samples were studied from the dorsal, ventral, and pinna skin and the footpad of these young, young adult, and old animals. A negative linear effect of age on epidermal depth with a significant reduction in cell count (cell/mm) and pilosebaceous unit profiles in dorsal skin samples and footpad was observed. The sebaceous glands appeared atrophied with pyknotic nuclei (Figs. 1 and 2). No consistent change in depth of the dermis or area fraction of collagen as determined by histomorphometry was noticed. The dermal elastic fibers in the dorsal skin and footpad showed proliferation in higher age groups in this mouse model. This can be compared with a study in the C57/B16 mice from NIH colonies [16] where decreased dermal cellularity and thickness and decreased epidermal proliferation were reported.

Further investigation of the CBA mice from NIH colonies as described in the previous paragraph [15] was made to compare epidermal morphometry and the index of proliferating cell nuclear antigen (PCNA-I) by immunohistochemistry in respect to the dorsal and pinna skin, ventral skin, and the footpad from other areas of aging experimental animals (Bhattacharyya, unpublished observations). There was an attrition of epidermal thickness in dorsal and ventral skin and the footpad in relation to aging. PCNA-I showed a reduction

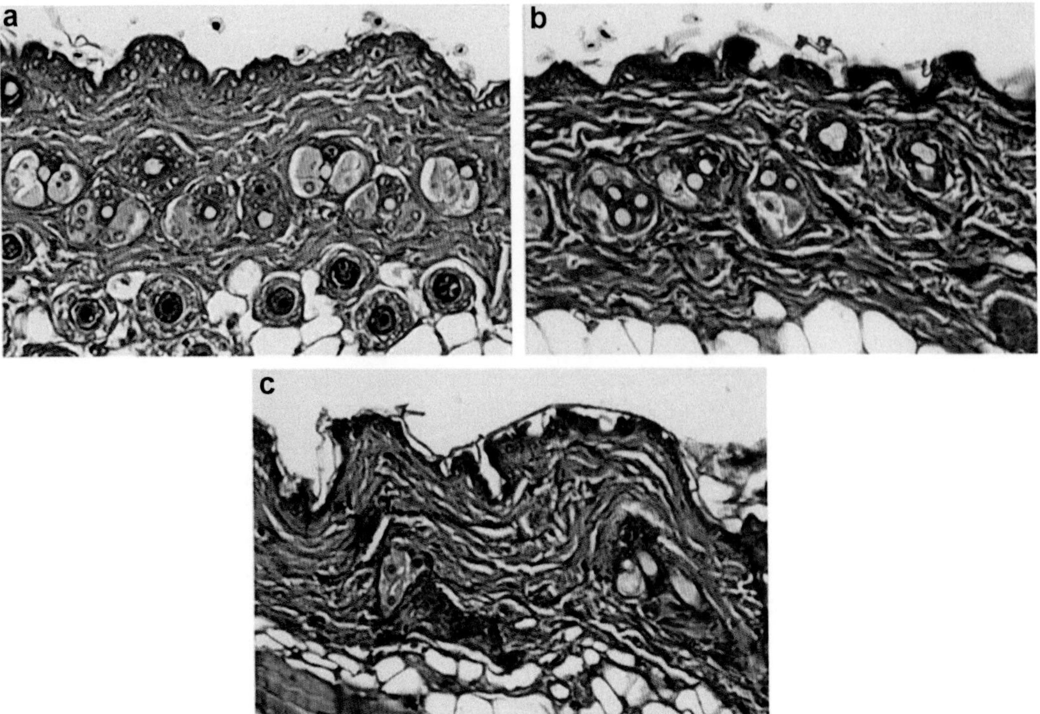

Fig. 1 Histological preparation of the dorsal skin in aging CBA mice in young (**a**), young adult (**b**), and old (**c**) animals, showing increasing atrophy of the epidermis and shrinkage of sebaceous follicles. Dermal elastic fibers can be seen in **c**. Verhoeff-van Giesen stain

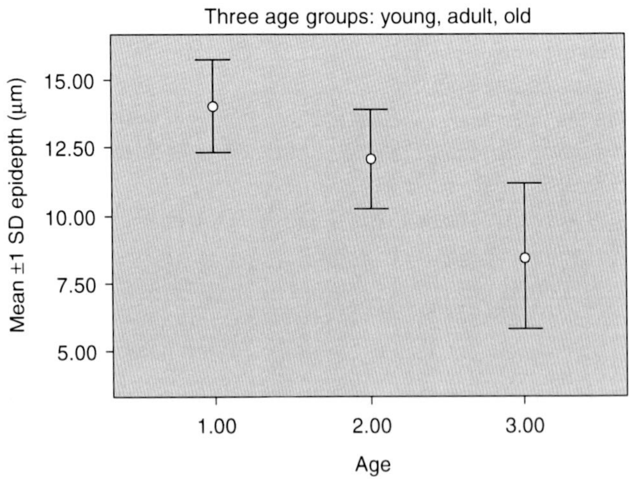

Fig. 2 Error bar chart of epidermal width measurements in three groups of CBA mice

across the ages only in the pinna skin and dorsal surface (Table 1; Figs. 3a–c).

The aging skin in the rat shows nonuniform patterns in different strains when it comes to epidermal and dermal thickness, and the age-associated changes seem to differ from the trend noted in murine species. In an early study of Wistar Institute rats, no significant age-related alteration was noted although the author described many qualitative differences in epidermal layers [17]. In Sprague

Table 1 PCNA-I and epidermal thickness data from aging CBA mice

	PCNA-I	*EPI width* (μm)
DS		
Y	31.9 + 5.0	16.3 + 0.8
AD	32.6 + 5.4	14.1 + 1.0
O	24.1 + 4.3	12.3 + 0.7
	*F 5.46, P 0.01	* F 32.43, P 0.0005
PS		
Y	37.0 + 7.2	15.6 + 1.5
AD	26.8 + 5.3	14.1 + 1.3
O	31.2 + 5.9	13.3 + 3.2
	*F 4.01, P 0.04	
FP		
Y	40.8 + 12.2	88.7 + 11.8
AD	32.6 + 6.5	72.9 + 8.1
O	40.9 + 6.1	55.3 + 8.7
		*F 17.28 P 0.0001
VS		
Y	35.0 + 4.8	14.6 + 0.6
AD	34.8 + 2.7	12.1 + 0.9
O	32.1 + 3.1	9.8 + 0.9
		* F 54.91 P 0.0005

DS dorsal skin, *PS* pinna skin, *FP* footplate, *VS* ventral skin, *Y* young, *AD* adult, *O* old

Dawley rats, the foot epidermis was explored to determine age-related changes in cell kinetics using single-pulse [3H]-thymidine labeling and the percent labeled mitosis technique [18] and led to the conclusion that there is a progressive decline in the rates of cell proliferation associated with age. However, these data were presented from rats only up to the age of 52 weeks. The authors of this chapter referred to five reports published earlier, which showed that rodent epidermal cell proliferation decreased in middle age and then remained constant or increased in senile animals. Skin from aging Wistar rats up to the age of 34 months was studied using histomorphometric analysis by Voros and Robert [19]. Average epidermal and dermal thickness did not show appreciable change with senility in this species. In aging Fischer 344 rats, epidermal thickness remained constant from 3 months of age onward [14]. However, increasing values in epidermal depth and nuclear population were noted in the ventral and dorsal skin and footplate skin samples from young, 1-year-old, and 2-year-old Fischer 344 rats [20, 21]. Earlier, Lapiere [22] commented that instead of becoming atrophic, rat skin increases in size, with more collagen, although the rate of increase is greatly diminished with aging. This is due to reduced collagen biosynthesis and increased degradation of macromolecules, but the balance between synthesis and degradation remains positive in rats.

Aging changes in cells other than epidermal keratinocytes, such as melanocytes or cells of Langerhans, have also been documented in some studies. Ultraviolet radiation has important health consequences on the Langerhans cells of human skin. The numerical density of Langerhans cells in aging inbred mice was studied from epidermal sheets and showed reduction when compared to that in young animals, although cutaneous immunoreactivity was not compromised [23]. Age-related neurodegenerative changes in peripheral nerves are a widespread phenomenon of clinical importance, and rat studies have attested to this inhibitory pattern. Age-associated loss in size of Meissner's corpuscles, with smaller and disorganized axonal processes, was reported in the digital pads of mice aged to the maximum life expectancy [24].

Interpretation of morphological changes of aging skin has many limitations, as discreet biochemical changes underlying such alterations cannot be visualized. In contrast to sparsely available accounts of dermal histochemical or morphological transformations in relation to life history in laboratory models, biochemical studies showing quantitative changes in dermal glycosaminoglycans, hydroxyproline concentration, acid mucopolysaccharides, and skin collagen and elastin changes in aging mice, rats, rabbits, and hamsters have been published. Only a few papers are cited here [25, 26]. Oxidative damage to the lipids and DNA increases with age in Fischer 344 rats, which was studied by measuring antioxidant enzyme activity [27]. In the hairless mouse, however, skin aging was not accelerated due to decreased antioxidant capacity [28]. Such molecular changes of the skin in intrinsically aged laboratory animals can only be revealed by immunohistochemistry as more suitable antibodies become available for research.

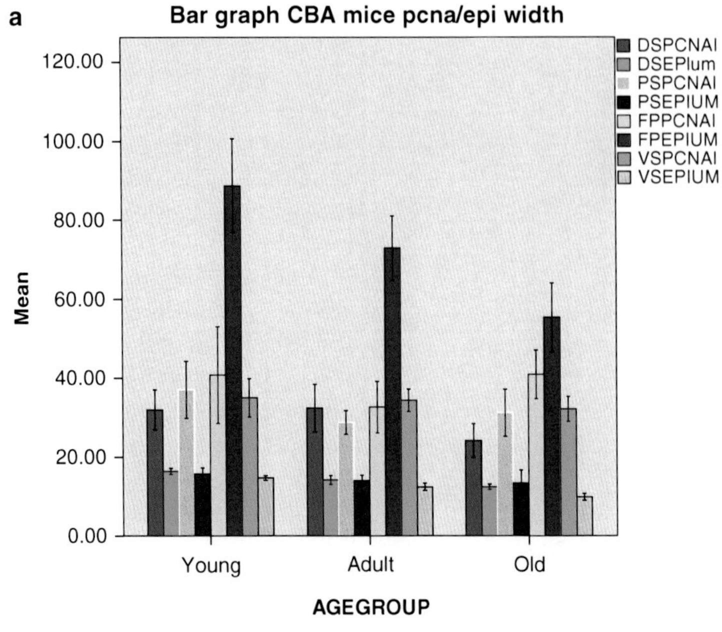

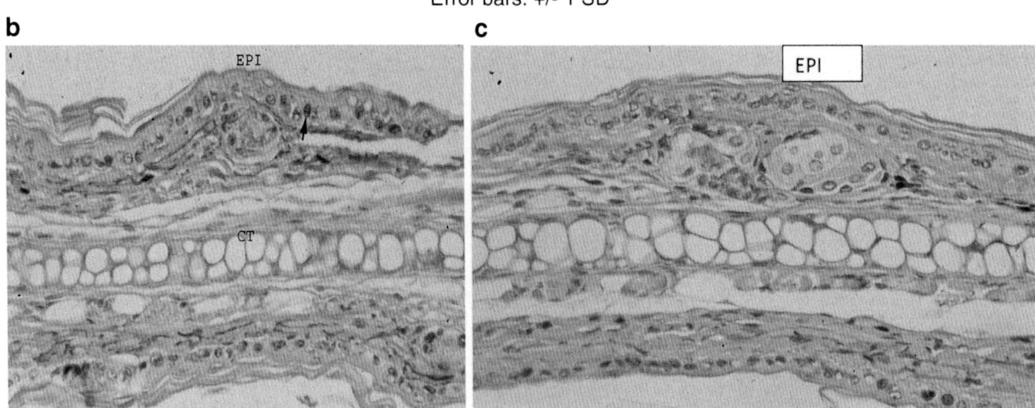

Fig. 3 (**a**) A composite bar diagram showing epidermal width and PCNA-I (PCNA index) in skin samples from dorsal and ventral areas, footpad, and the pinna in three age groups. (**b**). Pinna skin section from a CBA young specimen shows PCNA staining in epidermis (*EPI, arrow*). CT cartilage. (**c**) Pinna skin immunostained for PCNA in an old specimen shows absence of reactive nuclei in a thinner epidermis (EPI)

Morphological Changes with Aging in Other Species

Some sporadic accounts have also been published relating to mammals other than commonly available laboratory rodent models. Age-induced reduction in sebaceous glands was described in sheep by Warren et al. [29]. Epidermal flattening, fewer hair follicles and sebaceous glands, and a decrease in melanocytes were age-related changes in the hairless dog [30]. Veterinary textbooks describe aging changes in skin of domesticated dogs and cats. Senile changes in the skin of old cats and dogs include alopecia, callus formation over pressure points, orthokeratotic hyperkeratosis of the epidermis, and atrophied hair follicles [31]. Due to certain structural similarities with human skin, the pig skin model has been used in many experiments for studying responses to surgical and physiological manipulations [32], but no account is available on aging morphological changes in this species.

Calorie Restriction (CR) and Skin Aging

Calorie restriction (CR) can reverse age-associated alterations in many organs like the heart, the liver, and the brain [33] and has been shown to exert beneficial effects on many skin disorders, although its morphological effect on the aging skin has not been thoroughly explored. Whether CR can modify age-related histomorphological features of the skin in colony-raised rats was evaluated with morphometric procedures in Fischer 344 rats. [20, 21, 34, 35]. Three age groups (young, adult, old) of this strain belonging to ad libitum and CR feeding regimens were obtained from NIH colonies, and skin samples from the dorsum, footpad, and abdominal skin were analyzed with morphometric procedures to evaluate various skin compartments (thickness of stratum corneum, epidermis, PCNA index, dermis, fat layer, percentage fraction of dermal collagen, elastic fibers, fibroblast density, capillary profiles, and staining intensity of dermal glycosaminoglycans). The Fischer 344 rat showed many age-related skin changes, and these were prevented or delayed by CR, presumably due to metabolic alterations imposed by the dietary regimen (Fig. 4).

CR reduces cell proliferation in some tissues, with inhibited pace of DNA replication, and this makes those tissues less susceptible to DNA damage by carcinogens. Epidermal cell proliferation as quantified by immunohistochemistry was also correlated to age-related changes in epidermal thickness in these colony-raised Fischer 344 rats. Just as CR somewhat inhibited the trend of increasing epidermal width in aging rats, the keratinocyte proliferation rate as measured by staining of proliferating cell nuclear antigen (PCNA) was correspondingly lower in aging CR rats. This trend was observed in the epithelium of the dorsal skin as well as the footplate (Figs. 5 and 6) [34]. In C57BL/6 J mice, epidermal cell proliferation was reduced by CR and alternate-day fasting regimens [36]. A study in SENCAR mice also shows that dietary calorie restriction

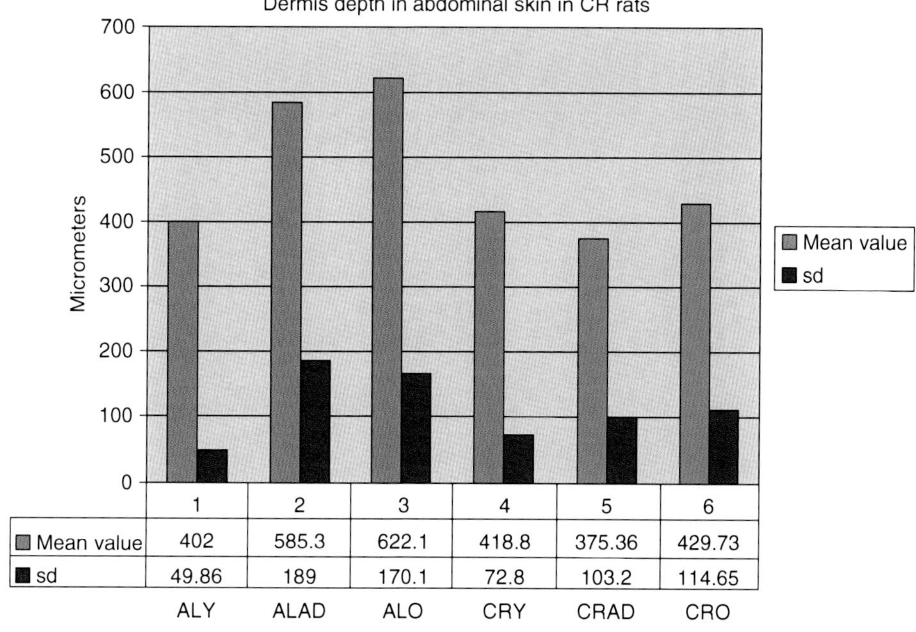

Fig. 4 Bar graph representation of the dermis depth from Fischer 344 rats in CR study. Three age groups of ad libitum (*AL*) and calorie-restricted (*CR*) animals are represented

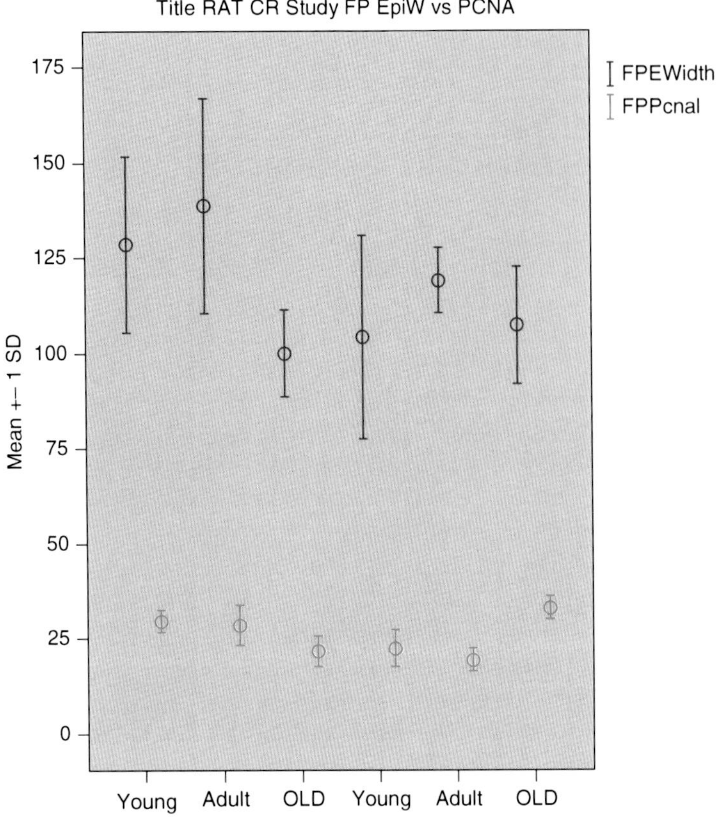

Fig. 5 Representation of epidermal width and PCNA index from footplate (*FP*) in rats from CR study. Three age groups from AL and CR animals are represented

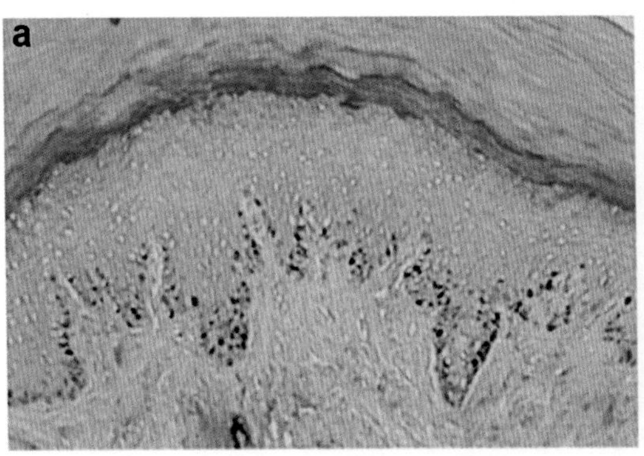

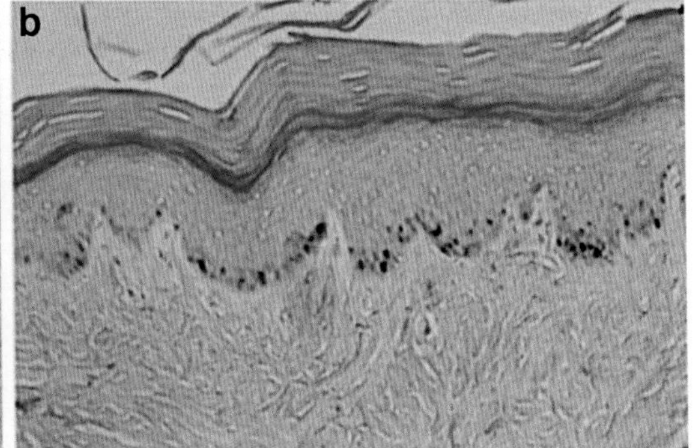

Fig. 6 PCNA staining in footplate epidermis from adult (**a**) and old (**b**) CR rats. (**a**) CR rat, adult group, footplate section. A broad epidermis with a thick cornified layer and brown stained PCNA reactive cells in the basal layer can be observed. (**b**) CR rat, old group. The footplate section shows regression of the epidermis and fewer PCNA positive cells

may inhibit gene expression in skin tissues relevant to cancer risks [37]. CR has been reported to reduce the level of free radicals and prevent accumulation of advanced glycation products and thus may be beneficial to aged skin. On the other hand, loss of subdermal adipose tissue stores, with restricted feeding, may accentuate fine wrinkles in human facial skin. CR can diminish subdermal adipose tissue [21]; therefore, its aesthetic effect on the profile of the aging human face remains to be seen.

Conclusion

Due to the ease of studying skin aging phenomena and age-associated progressive changes in short-lived mammals, published studies were mostly confined to laboratory rodent models. Unfortunately, many earlier descriptions of the histopathologic changes in aging skin in such models did not consider old or senile specimens and therefore lack a proper population sampling. Thus, the story is somewhat incomplete when compared to gerontologic cutaneous changes studied from skin biopsy samples of 90-year-old human patients! It should be noted that rodent life span is also highly variable in different strains. Early literature has recorded that among inbred mice strains used for aging research, a mean life span can vary from a low of 276 days in the AKR/J strain to a maximum of 799 days in the LP/J strain [38]. The lack of availability of suitably aged rodent models is a handicap to such research. This review, however, shows that the mouse model may be more suitable for documenting age-related histological changes that can be compared to human data, despite the caveat that comparing skin from laboratory-grown rodents with a short life span with the human skin assaulted by years of disease and environmental challenge is a rather risky endeavor. Histological deficits in intrinsically aged human skin affect the epidermis, dermal thickness, cellularity, and elastic fiber system. Efforts should be made to search for analogous chronological changes in animal models that can be utilized for studies aimed at rejuvenation of the aged skin. Similarities between human and murine skin have been reported in many studies, making mouse skin a suitable material for studying inflammatory skin diseases. Apart from certain similarities in basic molecular and physiological processes between the mouse and the human [39], the mouse can be maintained under proper husbandry conditions and may be a more suitable animal for studying the process of senescence of the integumentary system. Virtually no data are available on histological changes from intrinsic aging in other animals like the dog, the domestic pig, or the rabbit, although such species are extensively used for biomedical and physiological studies.

Wrinkle formation is a vexing problem of aging human facial skin, and there is little information about skin wrinkles in any animal model at the senile state. Suitable models for studying the histophysiology of wrinkles or their reversal have not been reported, except for one study. Crossbreeding between the Wistar and the wild rat was reported to generate a rat model (the Ishibashi rat) in which skin aging, with wrinkles and furrows, appeared at 12 weeks. Wrinkle formation in this new model was due to a reduction in elastin and collagen contents of the aging skin [40]. This kind of experimental model would prove useful to define the underlying anatomical correlates of skin wrinkle formation, to study its profilometry, and to test the effect of topical anti-wrinkle products for its amelioration [41].

In recent years, stem cells in skin have attracted a lot of scientific introspection due to their potential clinical application in wound healing, burns, and alopecia [42], and these cells can go through self-renewal and terminal differentiation and may regulate tissue aging [43]. It remains to be determined whether stem cells in aging mouse skin can show temporal regression. In vitro studies have shown aged mouse epidermal keratinocytes can function comparably as those cells from young mice [44]. Keratin 15 (K15) promoter activity, which is specific for stem cells, was shown to be active in the hair follicle bulge in murine skin, and the basal epidermal expression of K15 gradually decreased with age [42]. On the other hand, in C57/Bl6 mice from NIH colonies, despite a loss in dermal cellularity and thickness in the dorsal skin associated with skin aging, epidermal stem cells were maintained at normal levels throughout life [16]. Further research will elaborate how stem cells can respond to intrinsic aging in different mouse models and whether they can be pharmacologically stimulated to reverse the process of cutaneous aging.

Acknowledgment The kind support and encouragement provided by Dr. Regan Thomas, MD, Chairman, Department of Otolaryngology – Head and Neck Surgery, UIC, is greatly appreciated. Some of the cited work was partly supported by the Bernstein Grant from the AAFPRS Foundation.

References

1. Hwang K-A, Yi B-R, Choi K-C. Molecular mechanisms and in vivo mouse models of skin aging associated with dermal matrix alterations. Lab Animal Res. 2011;27:1–8.
2. Farage MA, Miller KW, Elsner P. Functional and physiological characteristics of the aging skin. Aging Clin Exp Res. 2008;20:195–200.
3. Rittie L, Fisher GJ. Natural and sun-induced aging of human skin. Cold Spring Harb Perspect Med. 2015;5: a015370. eds. AE Oro,FM Watt.
4. McCullough JL, Kelly KM. Prevention and treatment of skin aging. Ann N Y Acad Sci. 2006;1067:323–31.
5. Vitellaro-Zuccarello L, Cappelletti S, Rossi VDP, et al. Stereological analysis of collagen and elastic fibers in the normal human dermis: variability with age, sex, and body region. Anat Rec. 1994;238:153–62.
6. Thomas DR. Age-related changes in wound healing. Drugs Aging. 2001;18:607–20.
7. Uitto J. The role of elastic and collagen in cutaneous aging: intrinsic aging versus photoexposure. J Drugs Dermatol. 2008;7 Suppl 2:12–6.
8. Monteiro-Riviere NA. Anatomical factors affecting barrier function. In: Zhai H, Wilhelm K-P, Maibach HI, editors. Dermatoxicology. New York: CRC Press; 2008. p. 39–49.
9. Iversen OH, Schjoelberg AR. Age related changes of epidermal cell kinetics in the hairless mouse. Virchows Arch B Cell Pathol Incl Mol Pathol. 1984;46:135–43.
10. Haratake A, Uchida Y, Mimura K, et al. Intrinsically aged epidermis displays diminished UVB-induced alterations in barrier function. J Invest Dermatol. 1997;108:319–23.
11. Cameron IL. Cell proliferation and renewal in aging mice. J Geron Tol. 1972;27:162–72.
12. Argyris TS. The effect of aging on epidermal mass in *Balb/c* female mice. Mech Ageing Dev. 1983;22:347–54.
13. Hill MW. Influence of age on the morphology and transit time of murine stratified squamous epithelia. Arch Oral Biol. 1988;33:221–9.
14. Monteiro-Riviere NA, Banks YB, Birnbaum LS. Laser Doppler measurements of cutaneous blood flow in ageing mice and rats. Toxicol Lett. 1991;57:329–38.
15. Bhattacharyya TK, Thomas JR. Histomorphic changes in aging skin. Observations in the CBA mouse model. Arch Facial Plast Surg. 2004;6:21–5.
16. Giangreco A, Qin M, Pinter JE, et al. Epidermal stem cells are retained in vivo throughout skin aging. Aging Cell. 2008;7:250–9.
17. Andrew W, Andrew W. The anatomy of aging in man and animals. New York: Heinemann Medical Books Ltd/Grune & Statton; 1971.
18. Morris GM, Van den Aardweg GJMJ, Hamlet R, et al. Age-related changes in cell kinetics of rat foot epidermis. Cell Tissue Kinet. 1990;23:113–23.
19. Voros E, Robert AM. Changements histomorphometriques de la peau Rat en fonction de l'age. C R Soc Biol. 1993;187:201–9.
20. Bhattacharyya TK, Merz M, Thomas JR. Modulation of cutaneous aging with calorie restriction in Fischer 344 Rats. Arch Facial Plast Surg. 2005;7:12–6.
21. Thomas JR. Effects of age and diet on rat skin histology. Laryngoscope. 2005;115:405–11.
22. Lapiere CM. The ageing dermis: the main cause for the appearance of "old" skin. Br J Dermaqtol. 1990;122:5–11.
23. Choi KL, Sauder DN. Epidermal Langerhans cell density and contact sensitivity in young and aged BALB/c mice. Mech Ageing Dev. 1987;39:69–79.
24. Nava PB, Mathewson RC. Effect of age on the structure of Meissner corpuscles in murine digital pads. Microsc Res Tech. 1996;34:376–89.
25. Prodi G. Effect of age on acid mucopolysaccharides in rat dermis. J Gerontol. 1964;19:128–31.
26. Murai A, Miyahara T, Shiozawa S. Age-related variations in glycosylation of hydroxylysine in human and rat skin collagens. Biochim Biophys Acta. 1975;404:345–8.
27. Tahara S, Matsuo M, Kaneko T. Age-related changes in oxidative damage to lipids and DNA in rat skin. Mech Ageing Dev. 2001;202:415–26.
28. Lopez-Torres M, Shindo Y, Packer L. Effect of age and molecular markers of oxidative damage in murine epidermis and dermis. J Invest Dermatol. 1994;102: 476–80.
29. Warren GH, James PJ, Neville AM. A morphometric analysis of changes with age in skin surface wax and the sebaceous gland area of Merino sheep. Aust Vet J. 1983;60:238–40.
30. Kimura T, Doi K. Age-related changes in skin color and histologic features of hairless descendents of Mexican hairless dogs. Am J Vet Res. 1994;55:480–6.
31. Scott DW, Miller WH, Griffin CE. Small animal dermatology. New York: W.B. Saunders; 2001. p. 64–5.
32. Alex JC, Bhattacharyya TK, Smyrniotis G, et al. A histologic analysis of three-dimensional vs. two-dimensional tissue expansion in the porcine model. Laryngoscope. 2001;111:36–43.
33. Spindlor SR. Rapid and reversible induction of the longevity, anti- cancer and genomic effects of caloric restriction. Mech Ageing Dev. 2005;126:960–6.
34. Bhattacharyya TK, Jackson P, Thomas JR. Epidermal proliferating cell nuclear antigen in aging rats. Otolaryngol Head Neck Surg. 2008;139:178 (Abs.).
35. Bhattacharyya TK, Jackson P, Patel MK, Thomas JR. Epidermal cell proliferation in calorie-restricted aging rats. Curr Aging Res. 2012;5:96–104.
36. Varady KA, Roohk DJ, McEvoy-Hein BK, et al. Modified alternate- day fasting regimens reduce cell proliferation rates to a similar extent as daily calorie restriction in mice. FASEB J. 2008;22:2090–6.
37. Lu J, Xie L, Sylvester J, et al. Different gene expression of skin tissues between mice with weight controlled by

either calorie restriction or physical exercise. Exp Biol Med (Maywood). 2007;232:473–80.
38. Walford RL. When is mouse "old"? J Immunol. 1976;117:352–3.
39. Demetrius L. Aging in mouse and human systems. Ann N Y Acad Sci. 2006;1067:66–82.
40. Sakuraoka K, Tajima S, Seyama Y, et al. Analysis of connective tissue macromolecular components in Ishibashi rat skin: role of collagen and elastin in cutaneous aging. J Dermatol Sci. 1996;12:232–7.
41. Bhattacharyya TK, Linton J, Thomas JR, et al. Profilometric and morphometric response of murine skin to cosmeceuticals. Arch Fac Plast Surg. 2009;11:332–7.
42. Roh C, Lyle S. Cutaneous stem cells and wound healing. Pediatr Res. 2006;59:100R–3.
43. Rando TA. Stem cells, aging and the quest for immortality. Nature. 2006;441:1080–6.
44. Stern MN, Bickenbach JR. Epidermal stem cells are resistant to cellular aging. Aging Cell. 2007;6:439–52.

Major Changes in Skin Function in the Elderly and Their Contributions to Common Clinical Challenges

5

Jillian Wong Millsop and Anne Lynn S. Chang

Contents

Abstract

The geriatric patient population in dermatology is expected to rise as the elderly population worldwide rapidly increases. By the year 2030, it is estimated that there will be 72.1 million elderly adults. Therefore, it is important to understand the functional skin changes that occur with age and the clinical challenges related to these changes in order to meet the ever-growing geriatric dermatology patient population. This chapter reviews the histological and functional changes that occur with age, including changes in the skin barrier function, immunosenescence, and altered wound healing capacity. Common dermatological challenges that occur because of these functional changes are reviewed.

Introduction

Approximately 13 % of the US population is currently over the age of 65, and the geriatric population is increasing rapidly [1]. The number of older adults will more than double from the year 2000 to 2030, and it is estimated that by year 2030, there will be 72.1 million elderly adults [1]. The study of the geriatric population in dermatology, or dermatogeriatrics, is becoming increasingly popular, as the number of older adult patients cared for in dermatology is expected to rise [2]. Approximately one fourth of the dermatology visits in 2011 at Stanford Hospital and Clinics comprised of the care of elderly patients

J.W. Millsop (✉)
Department of Dermatology, University of California, Davis, Sacramento, CA, USA
e-mail: jmillsop@ucdavis.edu

A.L.S. Chang
Department of Dermatology, Stanford University, School of Medicine, Redwood City, CA, USA
e-mail: alschang@stanford.edu

M.A. Farage et al. (eds.), *Textbook of Aging Skin*,
DOI 10.1007/978-3-662-47398-6_111

Table 1 Overview of histological and physiological changes in the aging skin [4–7, 57]

Epidermal and dermal thinning
Decrease in the number of fibroblasts, melanocytes, and Langerhans cells
Reduction in collagen, elastic fibers, and cutaneous microvasculature
Decreased number of nerve endings
Decline in DNA repair
Decreased hair growth and androgen effects
Decreased nail growth
Reduction in cell turnover
Reduction in the number of sebaceous, sweat, and apocrine glands

Table 2 Overview of skin barrier changes with age

Corneocyte area increases within the stratum corneum
Delayed keratinocyte turnover
Decreased cell replacement
Rete ridges are effaced
Dermal papillae are retracted
Decreased lipid formation
Decreased ceramides
Decreased filaggrin breakdown products
Decreased sebum production and sebaceous gland function
Decreased transepidermal water loss
Loss of NHE1 proton pump antiporter
Decreased expression of aquaporin-3

over the age of 65 [3]. Given the rise of the geriatric patient population in dermatology, it is important to understand the functional skin changes that occur with age and the clinical challenges related to these changes in order to meet the ever-growing geriatric dermatology patient population.

Histologically and physiologically, there are many changes that occur in the aging skin (Table 1). These include thinning of the layers of the skin including the epidermis and dermis [4]. There is also a decrease in the number of fibroblasts, melanocytes, and Langerhans cells and a reduction in collagen, elastic fibers, and cutaneous microvasculature [5–7]. Elderly patients have reduced number of nerve endings and skin appendages, including sebaceous, sweat, and apocrine glands [4].

In this chapter, we will first review the major functional changes of the skin that occur with age. The major functional alterations of the skin include changes in the skin barrier function, immunosenescence, and altered wound healing capacity. Following each description of functional change of the skin, we will then review the major implications of each change on common dermatologic conditions in the elderly.

Changes with Aging in Skin Barrier Function

Over time, the barrier function of our skin becomes compromised (Table 2). The stratum corneum is the outermost epidermal constituent that is integral for barrier protection. The corneocyte area increases within the stratum corneum with age [4]. The epidermis has a slower keratinocyte turnover rate with a decreased rate in cell replacement [8]. This leads to roughness and uneven pigmentation of the skin. The rete ridges become effaced, and there is retraction of the dermal papillae [8]. In addition, there is decreased lipid formation and decreased sebum production, in particular, over the extremities, with age [9]. Sebaceous gland function diminishes due to decreased sex hormones which leads to less endogenous emolliation [5]. These changes individually and taken together lead to increased susceptibility for skin breakdown, trauma, and poor wound repair. Chemicals are able to invade the skin quickly and are removed slowly [10].

On a molecular level, there are also significant cutaneous changes that occur with age. The transepidermal water loss (TEWL) through the epidermis, which is an indicator for skin barrier function, is lower in the elderly compared to adults aged 18–64 [11]. This allows for increased penetration of irritants [7]. In the granular layer, there is a loss of the proton pump antiporter NHE1 (Na^+/H^+ exchanger) which leads to poor acidification of the stratum corneum [5–7, 12–15]. A decrease in NHE1 results in increased stratum corneum pH which subsequently leads to decreased activation of pH-sensitive beta-glucocerebrosidase and therefore poor lipid processing and obstructed maturation of lamellar membranes [14]. Aquaporin-3 is a glycerol and water membrane channel needed for skin hydration by maintaining sufficient glycerol concentration in the stratum corneum. Expression of aquaporin-3, which is linked to filaggrin degradation, is decreased in adults over the age of 60 [16]. Furthermore, filaggrin breakdown products have been reported to decrease with age [17]. The main intercellular component of the stratum corneum, ceramides, which is secreted from lamellar bodies and binds water, also decreases with age [18]. These findings point to the potential for targeted restoration of barrier in older individuals, a subject of ongoing study.

Common Clinical Challenges from Changes in Skin Barrier Function

Xerosis

Xerosis is a major clinical challenge in older adult patients. Its prevalence in the older population ranges between 30 % and 58 % [19], and it affects more than 50 % of adults over the age of 65 [20]. Dry skin typically occurs on the legs as well as the trunk and upper extremities in the elderly [19]. Xerosis is directly related to poor barrier function and decreased water content of the stratum corneum. Xerosis is also related to decreased sweat gland and sebaceous function [4]. The elderly are also more susceptible to xerosis due to a variety of other environmental factors affecting the elderly including overuse of air conditioners and heaters [19]; medical therapies including the use of diuretics, statins, antiandrogen medications, and radiation; and medical conditions including thyroid disease, renal disease, malignancy, neurological disorders causing decreased sweating, and nutritional deficiency lacking essential fatty acids and zinc [4, 19, 21]. Dry skin is susceptible to abrasions and fissures which predispose the patient to infections and contact dermatitis [19].

Pruritus

The most common cause of chronic pruritus is xerosis [19, 22]. Pruritus is reported as a symptom in 1.8 million medical visits annually in the United States in patients over the age of 65 [23]. In addition to xerosis, immunosenescence, which will be covered in the next section, contributes to the eczematous and inflammatory cutaneous disorders in the elderly, which can lead to pruritus [22]. The elderly are at increased risk for pruritus also because of other systemic medical conditions, such as renal or hepatic disease, malignancy, anemia, and neuropathies, and from medications, such as angiotensin-converting enzyme inhibitors, calcium channel blockers, salicylates, and opiates [24]. Furthermore, neurological disorders can contribute to pruritus in the elderly by way of nerve impingement and sensory neuropathy, such as diabetic peripheral neuropathy [25–27]. Pruritus may lead to repetitive scratching which can exacerbate inflammation and lead to the release of histamines, all of which perpetuate an endless itch-scratch cycle.

Management of Xerosis and Xerosis-Related Pruritus

Based on what is known of the structural and functional changes of the aging skin, xerosis can be managed with therapies targeting barrier restoration (Table 3). Ointment-based products including petroleum jelly can serve as an occlusive barrier against microorganisms at sites of small open wounds [28]. Application of alpha-hydroxy acids, such as ammonium lactate lotion, restores the skin pH, decreases skin irritation, accelerates barrier recovery, and promotes keratolysis of hyperkeratotic skin [15]. Alpha-hydroxy acids should not be used on fissured or cracked skin, however. To improve inflammation, topical steroids can be applied. Physiologic lipid mixture vehicles for topical steroids can reduce some of the adverse skin barrier effects of topical steroids [29].

Common daily practices can be instituted to improve the barrier function as well. Patients can decrease the frequency and duration of bathing or showering, limiting water exposure to 5 min a day. Bathing in lukewarm water and avoiding hot

Table 3 Strategies for managing xerosis and xerosis-related pruritus

Apply ointment-based products that have occlusive properties (e.g., petroleum jelly)
Apply alpha-hydroxy acids which can act as humectants (e.g., ammonium lactate lotion)
Limit showering and bathing duration and frequency
Avoid hard detergents and soaps; synthetic detergents ("Syndets") have pH more akin to physiologic skin pH than traditional soaps and may not need to be washed off with water
Avoid skin products with fragrances, antibiotics, propylene glycol, lanolin, and parabens
Moisturize with non-scented creams
Oral antihistamines (cetirizine or other less sedating and less anticholinergic antihistamines)
Phototherapy
Consider patch testing if there is a concern for allergic contact dermatitis

water are ideal. Soap that is used should be nonirritating and moisturizing. Patients can restrict soap to use only over the hair-bearing and soiled areas such as the groin, axillae, and feet. A moisturizing cream should be applied immediately after bathing when the skin is still damp. Patients should avoid any skin products such as soaps and detergents that may cause allergic or irritant contact dermatitis such as fragrances, antibiotics, propylene glycol, lanolin, and parabens [30]. It may be of benefit for patients to undergo patch testing to ensure the patient does not have a contact allergy.

In addition to managing dry skin in the elderly, pruritus can be managed through systemic medications. Oral antihistamines may act centrally to decrease symptoms or prevent histamine release from mast cells by targeting afferent neurons in the peripheral nervous system. Systemic antihistamines increase the risk for sedation, falls, delirium, dry mouth, constipation, and urinary retention, and therefore, caution is advised when prescribing these medications [30]. Nondrowsy fexofenadine may be a good option for elderly patients [31]. Another systemic option for treatment for pruritus is gabapentin. It can be started at 100–300 mg nightly and increased to 1,800 mg in divided doses throughout the day [32].

Phototherapy is also a viable option for management of pruritus in the elderly [33]. It is a good alternative to systemic treatments as it has a low side effect profile. Areas of the body that are at risk for skin cancer can be covered, such as the head, neck, and upper extremities. Ideal patients should be able to stand in a light box and should not be a fall risk.

Immunosenescence

Immunosenescence refers to the changes of the immune system that occur with aging [2]. As a result of the cell-mediated immunological changes that occur with age, there is an increased incidence and severity of infectious disease and malignancy risk in older adult patients [34–37]. There are several mechanisms, including thymus involution, diminished immunocyte function through telomere shortening, and decreased bone marrow mass that lead to changes in immunocytes with aging [38]. There is a relative shift in balance between the T helper 1 (Th1) and Th2 cytokines with age, with older adults having defective Th1 function and enhanced Th2 function [22]. As a result of this shift, older adult patients are more prone to eczematous dermatitis. There is an increase in frequency of cutaneous fungal infections among the elderly which is likely related to these changes [39].

Common Clinical Challenges and Implications of Immunosenescence on Skin in the Geriatric Population

Herpes Zoster and Postherpetic Neuralgia

Herpes zoster is caused by a reactivation of varicella zoster virus (VZV) that may lay dormant in the sensory nerve ganglia for many years, and it presents as a vesicular rash in a unilateral dermatomal distribution. It has a prodrome of pruritus, burning, or pain. Vesicles present for 7–10 days and then typically crust over a period of 2–3 weeks [40]. The risk to the elderly is increased due to a decline of cell-mediated immunity to VZV with age [2]. Approximately 50 % of patients who live to age 85 have had herpes zoster [41]. In addition to immunosenescence, risk for herpes zoster activation is enhanced by immunosuppressive medications, comorbid conditions, infection including HIV, malignancy such as Hodgkin's lymphoma, and organ transplantation [40, 42]. In the United States, the incidence of herpes zoster among adults over the age of 60 is approximately 10 cases per 1,000 individuals per year [43].

Primary prevention for herpes zoster is the administration of the live attenuated herpes zoster vaccine. It is approved for patients ages 50 and over [44]. Herpes zoster is treated with antiviral agents acyclovir, famciclovir, and valacyclovir, which are phosphorylated by viral thymidine kinase to block viral replication [45]. Antiviral therapy should be administered within the first 72 h of onset of vesicle formation [46]. In addition to systemic agents, pain can be treated with topical or oral corticosteroids, nonsteroidal anti-inflammatory drugs (NSAIDs), and gabapentin [45].

Postherpetic neuralgia occurs in 9–34 % of the population [45]. It is defined as persistent neuralgia at least 120 days after the onset of the zoster rash [46]. Though postherpetic neuralgia varies among individuals affected, patients often have an area of sensory loss and scarring surrounded by an area of allodynia and hypersensitivity [47]. A light touch may cause severe discomfort in these patients and can be very debilitating. The severity, incidence, and duration of this condition increases with age, which correlates with declining immunity [48, 49]. Postherpetic neuralgia can lead to poor quality of life, difficulty in carrying out activities of daily living, fatigue, insomnia, and depression [50]. Treatment options for postherpetic neuralgia include antidepressants such as amitriptyline and desipramine, anticonvulsants such as gabapentin and pregabalin, opioids such as tramadol, lidocaine patch, capsaicin patch, intrathecal steroid injection, and nerve block [30, 51].

Dermatophytosis and Cutaneous Candidiasis

Dermatophytosis and cutaneous candidiasis are very common diseases afflicting the geriatric population [39, 52]. A study of nursing home patients in Taiwan found that over half (61.6 %) of the patients had cutaneous fungal infections [39]. Keratinocyte retention, as a result of delayed cell turnover with aging, inhibits desquamation of skin, inhibiting removal of infected skin [53]. In addition to poor barrier function, immunosenescence likely contributes to the increased risk of fungal infections in the elderly. Superficial fungal infections trigger a Th2-dominant response that is similar to the activation of Th2-dominant response in patients with atopic dermatitis [54]. Patients with diabetes are at increased risk for fungal skin disease [55]. Other risk factors include patients receiving chemotherapy, systemic steroids, parenteral nutrition, as well as patients with HIV or who have had organ transplants [56]. Diagnosis is confirmed by potassium hydroxide (KOH) preparation, biopsy, and cultures [57].

Cutaneous candidiasis is regulated by both the cell-mediated and humoral immune systems. With aging, susceptibility to candidiasis is increased as neutrophils have decreased oxidative burst and phagocytotic activity against Candida [38]. Cutaneous candidiasis most commonly presents in the intertriginous areas where the environment is moist. Patients present with erythematous patches with satellite papules. Risk factors for candidiasis include heat, humidity, maceration, diabetes, obesity, chemotherapy, and antibiotic therapy [58]. Candidiasis can be confirmed with culture or direct microscopy for pseudohyphae [57].

A variety of topical and systemic antifungal agents are available for treatment of dermatophytosis and candidiasis. Systemic agents such as fluconazole, itraconazole, and terbinafine are especially helpful [57, 59]. For candidiasis, barrier cream with topical antifungal agent containing allylamine or imidazole can also keep the affected area dry and treat the condition [57].

Altered Wound Healing Capacity

Elderly patients have delayed wound healing as a result of many structural skin changes that occur with age. The skin is susceptible to external trauma as subcutaneous fat progressively deteriorates with age [30]. With atrophy of subcutaneous fat and muscle, there is reduced bony structure support as well. With age, there is an increase in duration for fibroblast replication and a delay in reepithelialization of wounds [60]. Aging fibroblasts have a poor response to transforming growth factor β1 (TGFB1)-mediated activation, which then causes altered proliferation of fibroblasts and defective collagen production [60, 61]. Senescent fibroblasts also have decreased sensitivity to hormones and growth factors [61]. Also with age, there is altered matrix degradation by proteases [60]. Furthermore, poor immune response, decreased vasculature with fragility and a loss of elasticity of blood vessels, and decreased ability of cells to reproduce to regenerate tissue contribute to poor wound healing in the elderly [30]. Altered wound healing capacity in the elderly leads to pressure ulcers. Changes not related to skin alteration such as cognitive and sensory impairment and limited mobility with age also contribute to susceptibility for wounds and poor wound healing.

Pressure ulcers are one of the most common conditions affecting hospitalized elderly and nursing home patients. They are localized injuries to the skin and/or underlying tissue. Typically they occur over a bony structure and occur as a result of pressure, shear forces, and/or friction. Approximately two-thirds of pressure ulcers occur in individuals 70 years of age and over [62]. In acute care hospitals, the incidence of pressure ulcers is 0.4–38.0 %, and in long-term care facilities, the incidence is 2.2–23.9 % [63]. The changes discussed above lead to an increase in pressure ulcers that occur in the elderly population. Prolonged exposure to pressures above the capillary-filling pressure also leads to ulceration [64]. Friction and shear forces perpetuate the effects of pressure. Senescent skin responds to pressure with decreased vasodilation than younger skin [65]. Maceration from incontinent individuals also predisposes the skin to forming a wound by reducing its tensile strength [64]. Obesity, poor nutrition, orthopedic injuries including hip fractures, and neurologic conditions such as cardiovascular infarction increase the risk of pressure ulcers [30]. Patients with comorbidities associated with low oxygen tension of tissues such as congestive heart failure, chronic obstructive pulmonary disease, and myocardial infarction have increased risk for pressure ulcers, as oxygen is needed for wound healing [66]. Pressure ulcers can be very painful, regardless of the depth and stage. It has been estimated that 59 % of patients with pressure ulcers experience pain [67].

There are four stages of ulcers, as created by the National Pressure Ulcer Advisory Panel (NPUAP) (Table 4). In 2007, the NPUAP redefined the stages of pressure ulcers and added two stages describing unstageable pressure ulcers and deep tissue ulcers [68]. Stage I describes nonblanchable erythema. Stage II describes partial thickness. Stage III describes full-thickness skin loss. Stage IV describes full-thickness tissue loss. "Unstageable" describes full-thickness skin or tissue loss but with an unknown depth because it is obscured by slough or eschar on the wound bed. "Suspected deep tissue injury" describes a maroon or purple area of discoloration on intact skin or a blister filled with blood as a result of damage to tissue from shear force or pressure [68].

Many non-pharmacologic measures exist for treatment and prevention of pressure ulcers (Table 5). First, the patient's position should be modified to decrease pressure on the affected site, whether it be over the sacrum, heel, scalp, or other body sites. For a hospitalized patient, the patient can be repositioned and turned every 2 h while recumbent and every 15 min while seated [64]. Patients should limit the time they spend on the bedpan or commode. Heels can be protected with a pillow or wedge device [64]. Foam body support and alternating pressure distribution devices, such as alternating air pressure mattresses, are effective in managing and preventing pressure ulcers [69]. The NPUAP recommends avoiding the often used doughnut seat cushions as they make the focal area of the skin that is in contact with the cushion more susceptible to pressure [68]. Skin barrier protection can be improved with moisturization with barrier creams. For incontinence, barrier

Table 4 National Pressure Ulcer Advisory Panel pressure ulcer staging system – reproduced with permission from the National Pressure Ulcer Advisory Panel

Stage I	**Nonblanchable erythema**	Intact skin with nonblanchable redness of a localized area usually over a bony prominence. Darkly pigmented skin may not have visible blanching; its color may differ from the surrounding area. The area may be painful, firm, soft, warmer, or cooler as compared to adjacent tissue. Category I may be difficult to detect in individuals with dark skin tones. May indicate "at-risk" persons
Stage II	**Partial thickness**	Partial-thickness loss of dermis presenting as a shallow open ulcer with a red-pink wound bed, without slough. May also present as an intact or open/ruptured serum-filled or serosanguineous filled blister. Presents as a shiny or dry shallow ulcer without slough or bruising. This category should not be used to describe skin tears, tape burns, incontinence-associated dermatitis, maceration, or excoriation
Stage III	**Full-thickness skin loss**	Full-thickness tissue loss. Subcutaneous fat may be visible, but bone, tendon, or muscle is *not* exposed. Slough may be present but does not obscure the depth of tissue loss. *May* include undermining and tunneling. The depth of a category/stage III pressure ulcer varies by anatomical location. The bridge of the nose, ear, occiput, and malleolus do not have (adipose) subcutaneous tissue, and category/stage III ulcers can be shallow. In contrast, areas of significant adiposity can develop extremely deep category/stage III pressure ulcers. Bone/tendon is not visible or directly palpable
Stage IV	**Full-thickness tissue loss**	Full-thickness tissue loss with exposed bone, tendon, or muscle. Slough or eschar may be present. Often includes undermining and tunneling. The depth of a category/stage IV pressure ulcer varies by anatomical location. The bridge of the nose, ear, occiput, and malleolus do not have (adipose) subcutaneous tissue, and these ulcers can be shallow. Category/stage IV ulcers can extend into muscle and/or supporting structures (e.g., fascia, tendon, or joint capsule) making osteomyelitis or osteitis likely to occur. Exposed bone/muscle is visible or directly palpable
Unstageable	**Full-thickness skin or tissue loss, depth unknown**	Full-thickness tissue loss in which actual depth of the ulcer is completely obscured by slough (yellow, tan, gray, green, or brown) and/or eschar (tan, brown, or black) in the wound bed. Until enough slough and/or eschar is removed to expose the base of the wound, the true depth cannot be determined; but it will be either a category/stage III or IV. Stable (dry, adherent, intact without erythema, or fluctuance) eschar on the heels serves as "the body's natural (biological) cover" and should not be removed
Suspected deep tissue injury	**Depth unknown**	Purple or maroon localized area of discolored intact skin or blood-filled blister due to damage of underlying soft tissue from pressure and/or shear. The area may be preceded by tissue that is painful, firm, mushy, boggy, warmer, or cooler as compared to adjacent tissue. Deep tissue injury may be difficult to detect in individuals with dark skin tones. Evolution may include a thin blister over a dark wound bed. The wound may further evolve and become covered by thin eschar. Evolution may be rapid exposing additional layers of tissue even with optimal treatment

creams containing zinc oxide, dimethicone, and high-quality silicones can be used [64]. Patients should adhere generally to dry skin care management. The skin barrier can also be protected by preventing bodily fluids such as urine from leading to maceration. Optimization of nutrition and hydration can improve wound healing. This includes incorporating an adequate amount of calories with protein in the patient's diet and supplementing with essential vitamins and minerals.

Table 5 Management of pressure ulcers

Pressure reduction	Turn and reposition patient every 2 h while recumbent and every 15 min while seated Limit time on commode and bedpan Use foam body support and alternating pressure devices Avoid "doughnut" seat or ring cushions
Improving skin barrier protection	Moisturize with barrier cream. For incontinence, barrier creams containing zinc oxide, dimethicone, and high-quality silicones can be used Decrease bath frequency and duration to "non-dirty" areas Protect the skin from contact of bodily fluids, e.g., urine
Optimize nutrition	Adequate hydration Adequate calories with protein Adequate vitamins and minerals
Debridement	Surgical Mechanical (wet to dry dressings, ultrasound laser, high-pressure water irrigation) Enzymatic (collagenase) Biological (maggot and larval therapy)
Dressings	Nonabsorbent, absorbent, debriding, self-adhering Specialized dressings: hydrocolloid, alginate, silver
Manage external factors and comorbidities	Manage diabetes, vascular insufficiency, heart disease, chronic obstructive pulmonary disease Treat underlying infections such as osteomyelitis or cellulitis
Surgery	Grafts Flaps

Ulcer cleaning, debridement, and dressings are important for appropriate wound healing. Surface contamination and dead tissue are necessary to be removed. Typically, debridement involves surgical debridement with a blade, curette, or scissors or mechanical debridement with the use of wet to dry dressings to remove the dead tissue [70]. Other methods for mechanical debridement include high-pressure water irrigation [71], ultrasound [72], and laser [73]. There are also nonconventional methods including enzymatic debridement with enzymes such as collagenase to remove the dead tissue [74] and biological debridement with maggots and larvae [75]. The larvae consume the dead tissue without causing injury to living tissue and maggots release substances to kill bacteria.

For pressure ulcers, a variety of dressings are available for each stage of ulcer including nonabsorbent, absorbent, debriding, and self-adhering [66]. In general, dressings are occlusive and maintain a moist environment for the ulcer to heal appropriately. For dry and clean ulcers, dressings are typically changed weekly or a few times per week. However, for weeping and infected wounds, dressings may need to be changed every few hours or daily. Specialized dressings are used to increase the rate of healing of ulcers. Hydrocolloid dressings have a gel that increases the rate of growth of new cells in the ulcer and maintain a dry environment for the healthy skin [76]. Alginate dressings contain seaweed for which calcium and sodium are key ingredients that increase the rate of wound healing [66]. Silver dressings are effective as the antibacterial property of silver keeps the ulcer clean [77].

For pressure ulcers stages III or IV that are refractory to conservative measures, surgery can be used for treatment. This includes the use of grafts and flaps. Research is currently underway to determine the effectiveness of growth factors and cytokines, hyperbaric oxygen, bioengineered skin, and stem cells [66].

Conclusion

With the growing number of older adults in our population worldwide, it is important to understand the histological and functional changes that occur with age and the clinical challenges specific to the older adult population relating to these changes. Altered skin barrier function, immunosenescence, and poor wound healing capacity are major difficulties encountered in dermatogeriatrics. By understanding the functional changes that occur with senescent skin, management of clinical challenges is made possible. Further research is needed to better understand how to restore the epidermal barrier and maintain and improve skin integrity in the elderly.

References

1. U.S. Administration on aging. Aging statistics. http://www.aoa.acl.gov/Aging_Statistics/index.aspx. Accessed 17 June 2015.
2. Wong JW, Wu JJ, Koo JYM. Diagnosis and management in dermatogeriatrics: a pocketbook for the non-dermatology provider. Newtown: Handbooks in Health Care; 2012.
3. Stanford hospital and clinics, department of dermatology. Patient access database; 2012
4. Norman RA, Menendez R. Diagnosis of aging skin diseases. London: Springer; 2008.
5. Gilchrest BA, Krutmann J. Skin aging. Berlin: Springer; 2006.
6. Zouboulis CC, Makrantonaki E. Clinical aspects and molecular diagnostics of skin aging. Clin Dermatol. 2011;29:3–14.
7. Seyfarth F, Schliemann S, Antonov D, Elsner P. Dry skin, barrier function, and irritant contact dermatitis in the elderly. Clin Dermatol. 2011;29:31–6.
8. Kligman A, Balin A. Aging of human skin. New York: Raven Press; 1989.
9. Young EM, Newcomer VD, Kligman AM. Geriatric dermatology: color atlas and practitioner's guide. Philadelphia: Lea & Febiger; 1992.
10. Fenske NA, Lober CW. Skin changes of aging: pathological implications. Geriatrics. 1990;45:27–35.
11. Kottner J, Lichterfeld A, Blume-Peytavi U. Transepidermal water loss in young and aged healthy humans: a systematic review and meta-analysis. Arch Dermatol Res. 2013;305:315–23.
12. Behne MJ, Meyer JW, Hanson KM, et al. NHE1 regulates the stratum corneum permeability barrier homeostasis. Microenvironment acidification assessed with fluorescence lifetime imaging. J Biol Chem. 2002;277:47399–406.
13. Hachem JP, Behne M, Aronchik I, et al. Extracellular pH controls NHE1 expression in epidermis and keratinocytes: implications for barrier repair. J Invest Dermatol. 2005;125:790–7.
14. Choi EH, Man MQ, Xu P, et al. Stratum corneum acidification is impaired in moderately aged human and murine skin. J Invest Dermatol. 2007;127:2847–56.
15. Jensen JM, Forl M, Winoto-Morbach S, et al. Acid and neutral sphingomyelinase, ceramide synthase, and acid ceramidase activities in cutaneous aging. Exp Dermatol. 2005;14:609–18.
16. Li J, Tang H, Hu X, Chen M, Xie H. Aquaporin-3 gene and protein expression in sun-protected human skin decreases with skin ageing. Australas J Dermatol. 2010;51:106–12.
17. Sandilands A, Sutherland C, Irvine AD, McLean WH. Filaggrin in the frontline: role in skin barrier function and disease. J Cell Sci. 2009;122:1285–94.
18. Boireau-Adamezyk E, Baillet-Guffroy A, Stamatas GN. Age-dependent changes in stratum corneum barrier function. Skin Res Technol. 2014;20:409–15.
19. White-Chu EF, Reddy M. Dry skin in the elderly: complexities of a common problem. Clin Dermatol. 2011;29:37–42.
20. Paul C, Maumus-Robert S, Mazereeuw-Hautier J, Guyen CN, Saudez X, Schmitt AM. Prevalence and risk factors for xerosis in the elderly: a cross-sectional epidemiological study in primary care. Dermatology. 2011;223:260–5.
21. Weismann K, Wadskov S, Mikkelsen HI, Knudsen L, Christensen KC, Storgaard L. Acquired zinc deficiency dermatosis in man. Arch Dermatol. 1978;114:1509–11.
22. Berger TG, Steinhoff M. Pruritus in elderly patients – eruptions of senescence. Semin Cutan Med Surg. 2011;30:113–7.
23. Shive M, Linos E, Berger T, Wehner M, Chren MM. Itch as a patient-reported symptom in ambulatory care visits in the United States. J Am Acad Dermatol. 2013;69:550–6.
24. Chen SC. Pruritus. Dermatol Clin. 2012;30:309–21, ix.
25. Ko MJ, Chiu HC, Jee SH, Hu FC, Tseng CH. Postprandial blood glucose is associated with generalized pruritus in patients with type 2 diabetes. Eur J Dermatol. 2013;23:688–93.
26. Cohen AD, Vander T, Medvendovsky E, et al. Neuropathic scrotal pruritus: anogenital pruritus is a symptom of lumbosacral radiculopathy. J Am Acad Dermatol. 2005;52:61–6.
27. Yamaoka H, Sasaki H, Yamasaki H, et al. Truncal pruritus of unknown origin may be a symptom of diabetic polyneuropathy. Diabetes Care. 2010;33:150–5.
28. Draelos ZD, Rizer RL, Trookman NS. A comparison of postprocedural wound care treatments: do antibiotic-based ointments improve outcomes? J Am Acad Dermatol. 2011;64:S23–9.
29. Lee YB, Park HJ, Kwon MJ, Jeong SK, Cho SH. Beneficial effects of pseudoceramide-containing physiologic lipid mixture as a vehicle for topical steroids. Eur J Dermatol. 2011;21:710–6.
30. Chang AL, Wong JW, Endo JO, Norman RA. Geriatric dermatology review: major changes in skin function in older patients and their contribution to common clinical challenges. J Am Med Dir Assoc. 2013;14:724–30.
31. Yosipovitch G, Greaves MW, Schmelz M. Itch. Lancet. 2003;361:690–4.
32. Yosipovitch G, Bernhard JD. Clinical practice. Chronic pruritus. N Engl J Med. 2013;368:1625–34.
33. Berger TG, Shive M, Harper GM. Pruritus in the older patient: a clinical review. JAMA. 2013;310:2443–50.

34. Pawelec G, Larbi A, Derhovanessian E. Senescence of the human immune system. J Comp Pathol. 2010;142 Suppl 1:S39–44.
35. Weiskopf D, Weinberger B, Grubeck-Loebenstein B. The aging of the immune system. Transpl Int. 2009;22:1041–50.
36. Sandmand M, Bruunsgaard H, Kemp K, Andersen-Ranberg K, Schroll M, Jeune B. High circulating levels of tumor necrosis factor-alpha in centenarians are not associated with increased production in T lymphocytes. Gerontology. 2003;49:155–60.
37. Haynes L, Maue AC. Effects of aging on T cell function. Curr Opin Immunol. 2009;21:414–7.
38. Halter J, Ouslander J, Tinetti M, et al. Hazzard's geriatric medicine and gerontology. New York: McGraw-Hill; 2009.
39. Smith DR, Guo YL, Lee YL, Hsieh FS, Chang SJ, Sheu HM. Prevalence of skin disease among nursing home staff in southern Taiwan. Ind Health. 2002;40:54–8.
40. Oxman MN. Herpes zoster pathogenesis and cell-mediated immunity and immunosenescence. J Am Osteopath Assoc. 2009;109:S13–7.
41. Schmader K. Herpes zoster in older adults. Clin Infect Dis. 2001;32:1481–6.
42. Yenikomshian MA, Guignard AP, Haguinet F, et al. The epidemiology of herpes zoster and its complications in medicare cancer patients. BMC Infect Dis. 2015;15:106.
43. Centers for Disease Control and Prevention. Shingles (Herpes Zoster). 2014. http://www.cdc.gov/shingles/hcp/clinical-overview.html. Accessed 22 June 2015.
44. Centers for disease control and prevention. Update on recommendations for use of herpes zoster vaccine. Morbidity and mortality weekly report. 2014. http://www.cdc.gov/mmwr/preview/mmwrhtml/mm6333a3.htm. Accessed 22 Aug 2014.
45. Gan EY, Tian EA, Tey HL. Management of herpes zoster and post-herpetic neuralgia. Am J Clin Dermatol. 2013;14:77–85.
46. Chen N, Li Q, Zhang Y, Zhou M, Zhou D, He L. Vaccination for preventing postherpetic neuralgia. Cochrane Database Syst Rev. 2011;3, CD007795.
47. Watson CP, Deck JH, Morshead C, Van der Kooy D, Evans RJ. Post-herpetic neuralgia: further post-mortem studies of cases with and without pain. Pain. 1991; 44:105–17.
48. Ragozzino MW, Melton 3rd LJ, Kurland LT, Chu CP, Perry HO. Population-based study of herpes zoster and its sequelae. Medicine. 1982;61:310–6.
49. Dworkin RH, Boon RJ, Griffin DR, Phung D. Postherpetic neuralgia: impact of famciclovir, age, rash severity, and acute pain in herpes zoster patients. J Infect Dis. 1998;178 Suppl 1:S76–80.
50. Gilden DH, Kleinschmidt-DeMasters BK, LaGuardia JJ, Mahalingam R, Cohrs RJ. Neurologic complications of the reactivation of varicella-zoster virus. N Engl J Med. 2000;342:635–45.
51. Johnson RW, McElhaney J. Postherpetic neuralgia in the elderly. Int J Clin Pract. 2009;63:1386–91.
52. Pierard G. Onychomycosis and other superficial fungal infections of the foot in the elderly: a pan-European survey. Dermatology. 2001;202:220–4.
53. O'Quinn DB, Palmer MT, Lee YK, Weaver CT. Emergence of the Th17 pathway and its role in host defense. Adv Immunol. 2008;99:115–63.
54. Al Hasan M, Fitzgerald SM, Saoudian M, Krishnaswamy G. Dermatology for the practicing allergist: Tinea pedis and its complications. Clin Mol Allergy. 2004;2:5.
55. Buxton PK, Milne LJ, Prescott RJ, Proudfoot MC, Stuart FM. The prevalence of dermatophyte infection in well-controlled diabetics and the response to Trichophyton antigen. Br J Dermatol. 1996;134:900–3.
56. Rinaldi MG. Dermatophytosis: epidemiological and microbiological update. J Am Acad Dermatol. 2000;43:S120–4.
57. Jafferany M, Huynh TV, Silverman MA, Zaidi Z. Geriatric dermatoses: a clinical review of skin diseases in an aging population. Int J Dermatol. 2012;51:509–22.
58. Lopez-Martinez R. Candidosis, a new challenge. Clin Dermatol. 2010;28:178–84.
59. Welsh O, Vera-Cabrera L, Welsh E. Onychomycosis. Clin Dermatol. 2010;28:151–9.
60. Fisher GJ, Varani J, Voorhees JJ. Looking older: fibroblast collapse and therapeutic implications. Arch Dermatol. 2008;144:666–72.
61. Simpson RM, Wells A, Thomas D, Stephens P, Steadman R, Phillips A. Aging fibroblasts resist phenotypic maturation because of impaired hyaluronan-dependent CD44/epidermal growth factor receptor signaling. Am J Pathol. 2010;176:1215–28.
62. Decubitus Ulcers. eMedicine. 2005. http://www.emedicine.com. Accessed 25 June 2015.
63. Brandeis GH, Morris JN, Nash DJ, Lipsitz LA. The epidemiology and natural history of pressure ulcers in elderly nursing home residents. JAMA. 1990;264:2905–9.
64. Fleck CA. Pressure ulcers. In: Norman RA, editor. Diagnosis of aging skin diseases. London: Springer; 2008. p. 233–52.
65. Bartus C, Swerlick R. It is better to flush than to break under pressure. J Invest Dermatol. 2010;130:650–1.
66. Bhattacharya S, Mishra RK. Pressure ulcers: current understanding and newer modalities of treatment. Indian J Plast Surg. 2015;48:4–16.
67. Dallam L, Smyth C, Jackson BS, et al. Pressure ulcer pain: assessment and quantification. J Wound Ostomy Continence Nurs. 1995;22:211–5; discussion 7–8.
68. Pressure Ulcer Stages Revised by NPUAP. National Pressure Ulcer Advisory Panel. http://www.npuap.org/resources/educational-and-clinical-resources/npuap-pressure-ulcer-stagescategories/. Accessed 25 June 2015.
69. McInnes E, Jammali-Blasi A, Bell-Syer S, Dumville J, Cullum N. Preventing pressure ulcers – are pressure-redistributing support surfaces effective? A Cochrane

systematic review and meta-analysis. Int J Nurs Stud. 2012;49:345–59.

70. Mosher BA, Cuddigan J, Thomas DR, Boudreau DM. Outcomes of 4 methods of debridement using a decision analysis methodology. Adv Wound Care. 1999;12:81–8.
71. Moore ZE, Cowman S. Wound cleansing for pressure ulcers. Cochrane Database Syst Rev. 2005;3, CD004983.
72. Ramundo J, Gray M. Is ultrasonic mist therapy effective for debriding chronic wounds? J Wound Ostomy Continence Nurs. 2008;35:579–83.
73. Graham JS, Schomacker KT, Glatter RD, Briscoe CM, Braue Jr EH, Squibb KS. Efficacy of laser debridement with autologous split-thickness skin grafting in promoting improved healing of deep cutaneous sulfur mustard burns. Burns. 2002;28:719–30.
74. Ramundo J, Gray M. Enzymatic wound debridement. J Wound Ostomy Continence Nurs. 2008;35:273–80.
75. Sherman RA. Maggot versus conservative debridement therapy for the treatment of pressure ulcers. Wound Repair Regen. 2002;10:208–14.
76. Fletcher J. Understanding wound dressings: hydrocolloids. Nurs Times. 2005;101:51.
77. Jorgensen B, Price P, Andersen KE, et al. The silver-releasing foam dressing, Contreet Foam, promotes faster healing of critically colonised venous leg ulcers: a randomised, controlled trial. Int Wound J. 2005;2:64–73.

Skin Aging: A Brief Summary of Characteristic Changes

6

Cornelia Wiegand, Christina Raschke, and Peter Elsner

Contents

Abstract

Life expectancy in industrialized countries has consistently increased in the last few decades and is predicted to be a continuing process. Like any other organ, the human skin ages and undergoes clearly distinguishable changes due to aging. In aging skin, cell replacement is continuously declining, the barrier function and mechanical protection are compromised, wound healing and immune responses are delayed, thermoregulation is impaired, and sweat and sebum production are decreased. It is evident that environmental factors as well as genetic programs contribute substantially to the processes involved. The long-term exposure of skin to solar UV radiation leads to "photoaging" or "extrinsic" aging and clinically manifests as rough skin textures, wrinkles, laxity, atrophy, pigmentary changes or blotchy dyspigmentation, elastosis, telangiectasia, and precancerous lesions such as actinic keratosis and malignant tumors. In contrast, "intrinsic" aging is genetically determined and characterized by fine wrinkles, a thin and transparent appearance, loss of underlying fat leading to hollowed cheeks and eye sockets, dry and itchy skin, and inability to perspire sufficiently, hair graying, hair loss or hirsutism, and thinning of nail plates. However, both processes may overlap, and the underlying mechanism of both processes is increased oxidative stress, which is probably the single most harmful contributor to skin aging.

C. Wiegand (✉) • C. Raschke
Department of Dermatology, University Hospital Jena, Jena, Germany
e-mail: C.Wiegand@med.uni-jena.de; christina.raschke@med.uni-jena.de

P. Elsner
Department of Dermatology and Dermatological Allergology, Universitätsklinikum Jena, Jena, Germany
e-mail: elsner@derma-jena.de

M.A. Farage et al. (eds.), *Textbook of Aging Skin*,
DOI 10.1007/978-3-662-47398-6_5

Introduction

In the last few decades, life expectancy in many industrialized countries has consistently increased and is predicted to be a continuing process [1]. Today there are more than 227 million people aged ≥80 years [2]. Appropriate care of elderly skin gains increasing medical importance. Since age-dependent effects are so manifest in skin appearance, structure, mechanics, and barrier function, much effort has been placed in research to better understand them. Aging is a consequence of genetic program and cumulative environmental damage, which contribute to a progressive loss of structural integrity and physiological tasks of the skin [3, 4]. The intrinsic aging (physiological-, chronological-, UV-protected aging) of the skin is determined by genetic influences and internal factors such as hormones or metabolic substances [5]. The clinical aspects of intrinsically aged skin are visible on the consistently textile-covered skin areas of elderly persons. Intrinsic aging is mainly controlled by progressive telomere shortening [6]. Telomeres, situated at the ends of eukaryotic chromosomes, are repeated DNA sequences that undergo a base-pair loss during DNA replication. Telomere shortening acts as a mitotic clock, leading to replicative senescence. However, miRNAs may well play a role in cellular aging as recent reports indicate that they can contribute to silencing of proliferation-associated genes [7]. Accumulating experimental evidence further revealed that skin aging may be associated with dysfunctions or loss of certain skin-resident stem/progenitor cells [8]. Extrinsic aging is a similar process that superimposes on the process of intrinsic aging. It is caused by exogenous factors such as ultraviolet (UV) radiation, environmental toxins, and infectious agents that induce DNA alterations and damage the skin [9]. The most important extrinsic factor inducing preterm skin aging is ultraviolet irradiation, which causes photoaging of the skin. UV irradiation accelerates telomere shortening in sun-exposed skin [6]. UV-induced extrinsic aging is visible on chronically UV-exposed skin areas in persons frequently engaged in outdoor activities. Acute and chronic sun exposure induces short-term and long-term effects on the skin, ranging from sunburn (erythema) and suntan up to the development of skin aging and skin cancer. Besides natural sunlight, there is an increasing influence of artificial UV radiation (solarium). The long-wave UVA radiation (320–400 nm) enters the deep dermis, while the more energetic UVB light (290–320 nm) is absorbed mainly in the epidermis, especially in the keratinocytes and melanocytes [10]. The direct interaction of UVB with cellular DNA induces damage of DNA strands [11]. UVA radiation also damages the DNA but less than UVB radiation. UVA damage is induced indirectly, through absorption by other endogenous chromophores that release reactive oxygen species, resulting in lipid peroxidation, activation of transcription factors, and formation of DNA-strand breaks [11, 12].

Age-related physiological changes in elderly skin have clearly distinguishable cutaneous effects (Table 1). In aging skin, cell replacement is continuously declining, the barrier function and mechanical protection are compromised, wound healing and immune responses are delayed, thermoregulation is impaired, and sweat and sebum production are decreased [13]. Clinical experience has shown that elderly people more often suffer from dry skin than young, healthy individuals. This is based on an alteration of the lipid barrier in older people where the content of natural moisturizing factors and lipids in the stratum corneum is reduced leading to decreased lamellar bilayers and poorer water-holding capacity [13]. The drier skin of the aged population is hence reflected by an age-dependent decrease of TEWL [14]. The aging of the skin is also accompanied by an extensive remodeling of extracellular matrix (ECM) in dermal layers, senescence of skin fibroblasts, dramatic upregulation of matrix metalloproteinases (MMPs), and a decrease of collagen production [8].

Clinical Aspects of Aging Skin

The most obvious changes in aged skin include wrinkles, laxity, and pigmentary irregularities (Fig. 1). The formation of a wrinkle in human skin

Table 1 Cutaneous effects of age-related changes in skin physiology [15]

Physiological changes	Cutaneous effects
Decrease in skin lipids and barrier function	Dryness
Decreased cell replacement	Roughness, delayed healing, and uneven pigmentation
Decreased DNA repair	Increased photo-carcinogenesis, malignancies
Fragmentation of collagen and elastic fibers	Wrinkles and lax skin, increased risk of pressure damage, and decubitus ulcers
Reduced support of blood vessels	Purpuric lesions
Decreased sensory perceptions	Increased tendencies to injuries
Impaired thermoregulation	Vulnerability to heat and cold
Reduced hair growth and effects of androgen	Color changes to gray, baldness, and male and female patterns of alopecia, bushier eyebrows, and growth of hair in external auditory meatus in male
Reduced function of apocrine glands	Reduced body odor
Reduced function of sweat glands	Risk of overheating and heat strokes
Reduced function of sebaceous glands	Decreased epidermal lipids
Decreased inflammatory response	Delayed healing and vulnerability to infection
Reduced subcutaneous fat	Increased risk of injury, less natural insulation, increased risk of hypothermia
Flattening of dermal papillae	Increased risk of blister formation and consequent infection
Reduced nail growth	Decreased linear growth, onychogryphosis, longitudinal striations, dull and brittle nails
Decrease in melanocytes	Gray hair, increased susceptibility to solar radiation

has been integrated with marked decreases in skin elasticity. Functional changes in the skin of elderly persons include a decreased growth rate of the epidermis, hair, and nails. The skin of the elderly is characterized by a decreased lipid content with a changed composition of lipids. These changes induce a rough and dry surface of the skin with tendency to irritation and redness and are likely to contribute to the increased susceptibility of aged skin to the disruption of barrier function [16]. Furthermore, formation of dry skin (xerosis) is the most common cause of pruritus in advanced age as integumentary and vascular systems undergo atrophy, leading to suboptimal moisture retention [17]. Decrease of barrier function in the elderly skin alters penetration of contractants and primes the inflammatory response [18]. The secretion of sebaceous and sweat glands is diminished [19]. The immune response is reduced and increases the risk of suffering from age-dependent diseases [20]. Increasing degeneration and disorganization of rarefied capillaries and small vessels in elderly skin induce changes in circulation and thermoregulatory functions with predisposition to hypothermia [21]. The elderly skin is increasingly vulnerable to environmental injury by decelerated wound healing and re-epithelization, resulting in a higher risk of surgical procedures. The susceptibility of the skin to harmful factors is dependent on creating effective repair mechanisms and inflammatory responses [22].

The intrinsically aged skin appears dry and pale and shows an atrophic aspect with fine wrinkles, which are due to the gravitational or conformational forces. Noticeable is a transparent image of the skin with a shining through of underlying vascular structures. Intrinsically aged skin displays a certain degree of laxity and a regular pigmentation and is prone to a variety of benign neoplasms. Clinically and morphologically, the extrinsically aged skin appears in the form of two types of photoaging with either an atrophic or rather a hyperproliferational aspect [10]. The

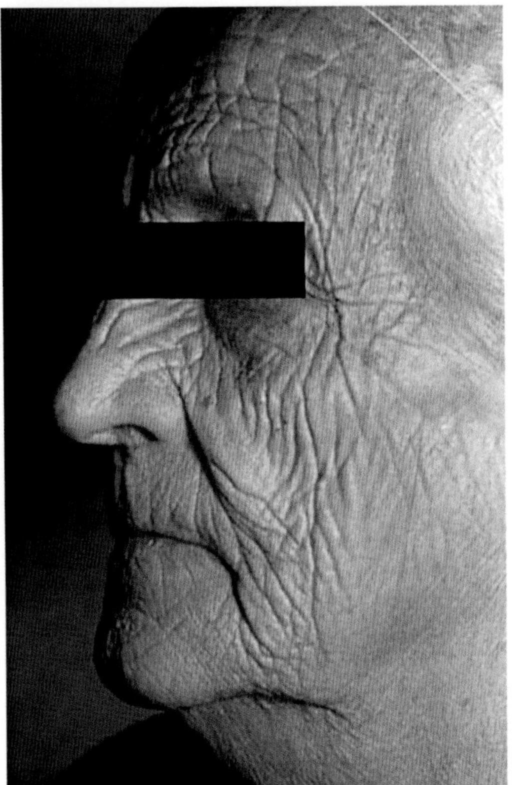

Fig. 1 Obvious signs of aging skin (Courtesy of Department of Dermatology, University Hospital Jena)

atrophic form shows small wrinkles and numerous telangiectasias on skin areas with intensive sun exposure [10]. The hyperproliferational form is thicker with a leather-like image and deeper wrinkles. Favre–Racouchot syndrome is a type of photoaging with the clinical signs of deep furrowing, nodular elastic changes, comedones, and keratinous cysts tending to appear in the periorbital region of the face [23]. Erythrosis interfollicularis colli, a further example for extrinsic skin aging, shows a restricted erythema sparing the hair follicles. Lentigines solaris and seniles located on the forearms and back of the hands are typical signs of photoaging [24]. Melanocytes along the basal membrane vary in reference to size, morphology, and pigmentation inducing the clinical aspect of irregular pigmentation of the so-called photoinduced age spots, hyperpigmentations, and hypomelanosis guttata [25].

Structural Changes of the Aging Skin

Histological analysis is routinely used to diagnose structural changes of skin pathologies. Recent technical progress permits a more precise presentation of the human skin and allows detailed physiological insights into skin changes. Quantitative measurements by bioengineering allow the noninvasive studying of aging skin. Laser Doppler velocimetry analyzes the cutaneous circulation even in vessels of the deeper skin layers [26]. The optical coherence tomography is a pulsed ultrasound technique that enables the fast analysis of the skin thickness [26, 27]. Confocal laser scanning microscopy and multiphoton laser scanning tomography are noninvasive methods for in vivo presentation of the human skin and generate horizontal images parallel to the skin surface [26, 27]. Multiphoton laser scanning tomography allows analysis of skin pathologies by quantifying autofluorescent agents and presenting specific decay rates.

Structurally, the intrinsically aged skin shows a thinning of all layers, the corneocytes are less adherent to one another, and the dermoepidermal junction shows a flattening aspect. Due to the reduced dermoepidermal contact area, the involved layers may dissolve in each other, inducing an increased vulnerability of the skin with the formation of ecchymosis [10]. Progressive decreases in melanocyte and Langerhans cell density occur [20, 28]. The dermis has an atrophic aspect with a loss of cells and extracellular matrix and shows a decline of the vascular network that occupies the dermal papillae [29, 30]. Dermal collagen becomes sparser, and elastin is degraded slowly and accumulates in intrinsically aged skin [26]. In contrast, the extrinsically aged skin shows a completely different histological aspect (Fig. 2). The epidermis becomes acanthotic and dyskeratotic with a high proliferation index of keratinocytes. The epidermis of photoaged skin shows atypia and dysplasia of keratinocytes and melanocytes and a loss of Langerhans cells [31]. The number of hair follicles is reduced more than in intrinsically aged skin, inducing a thinning of the hair [10]. A loss of sebaceous and

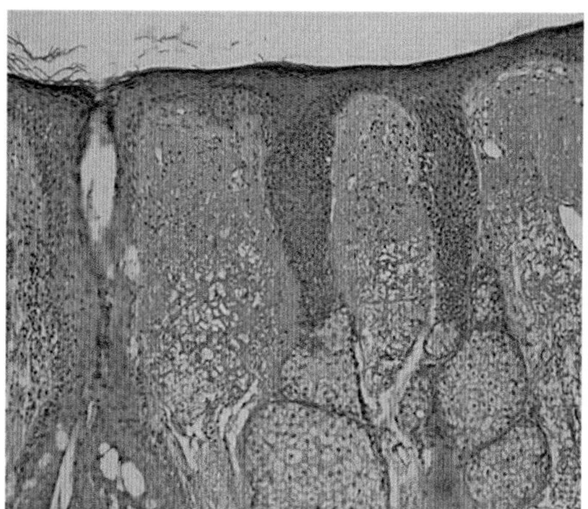

Fig. 2 Histological aspect of photoaged skin. The histological image of photoaged skin includes tight stratum corneum, discrete epidermal atypia, telangiectasias, and solar elastosis (Courtesy of Department of Dermatology, University Hospital Jena)

sweat glands induces increasing dryness of the skin with itching sensations [22]. The histological hallmark of dermal photodamage is the increased synthesis of abnormally structured elastin with its accumulation as elastotic material, termed solar or actinic elastosis. Dermal collagen becomes sparser, degenerated and changed in composition [32]. Other characteristics of extrinsically aged skin are the flattening of the dermis, a histiocyte-lymphocyte perivascular infiltrate, and a loss of rete ridges [31]. Actually the dermal changes in elderly skin may be demonstrated by in vivo autofluorescence and second harmonic generation measurements using multiphoton laser scanning tomography [33].

Biomechanical Changes of Aging Skin

Physical examination readily shows that major changes occur in the mechanical properties of aging skin. For instance, a loss in the elastic recovery of skin in the area of small stress and an increase in the time required for viscoelastic recovery from great stress are found that can be explained by a degenerative change in the elastin network in the dermis [34]. The smooth appearance and fine wrinkles of intrinsically aged skin have been associated with slow fragmentation of the elastic fiber network, whereas extrinsically photoaged skin appears roughened and deeply wrinkled and is histologically characterized by the deposition of disorganized elastic fiber material [35]. In addition, dermal collagen synthesis declines with aging while the stiffness increases leading to a more rigid aged dermis which decreases the ability of the skin to resist shearing forces. Aged skin contains an increased amount of fragmented and disorganized collagen fibrils which results in the reduction of fibroblasts-collagen fibril linkages [36]. Collagen content in extrinsically (photo) aged skin was found to be up to 56 % less than the collagen content in intrinsically aged skin [34]. A decrease in linkages in turn leads to a weakened ECM, a decrease in the amount of mechanical loading experienced by the dermal fibroblasts and a possibly diminished ability of the skin to respond to changes in mechanical load [36]. Mechanical forces greatly influence cellular organization and behavior. Cells respond to applied stress by changes in form and composition; however, without any mechanical stimuli, cells stop to proliferate, discontinue migration, go into cell-cycle arrest, and eventually die [37]. The study of age-associated alterations in cellular mechanotransduction has only recently begun to be appreciated for its potential role in mediating cellular function and dysfunction [36].

Biochemical Changes of Aging Skin

The surface pH of the normal skin averages a slightly acid value of pH 5.5 and increases in the aged skin starting at approximately age 55 [4, 38]. This is initially manifested as a reduced rate of skin barrier repair as the enzymes involved in lipid processing composing the epidermal water barrier require an acid pH [38]. A rise in cutaneous pH value therefore increases susceptibility and suffering of skin damage due to infection, allergy, and irritation [39]. The intrinsic aging is mainly associated with decreasing levels of several hormones. The coincidence of climacteric symptoms and the beginning of intrinsic skin aging suggest that estrogen seems to play a dominant role in this process [40]. Intrinsically aged skin displays a significantly reduced expression of the extracellular matrix protein-1 (ECM-1) in lower and upper epidermal layers inducing potential changes of the normal skin structure and function [41]. Most aging changes, intrinsically and extrinsically caused, are due to molecular damage caused by free radicals [42]. The increase in UV irradiation on the earth due to stratospheric ozone depletion may increase the risk of photooxidative damage induced by the generation of reactive oxygen species (ROS). There are two main sources of ROS: a mitochondrial source that plays the principal role in aging and a non-mitochondrial source, which supposedly has a role in the pathogenesis of age-related diseases [43]. Free radicals are highly reactive due to possession of an unpaired electron. Trans-urocanic acid is a major chromophore for UV radiation in human epidermis that undergoes isomerization to its *cis*-isomer due to UV exposure [44]. Aerobic metabolism generates the superoxide radical, which is metabolized by superoxide dismutase to form hydrogen peroxide and oxygen [45]. Hydrogen peroxide can rapidly generate an extremely reactive hydroxyl radical that damages DNA, proteins, and lipids (Fig. 3). The ultraviolet light-induced reactive oxygen species lead to induction of the transcription factor activator protein-1 (AP-1) [46]. AP-1 induces upregulation of matrix metalloproteinases (MMPs) like collagenase-1 (MMP-1), stromelysin-1 (MMP-3), and gelatinase A (MMP-2), which specifically degrade connective tissue proteins such as collagen and elastin and indirectly inhibit the collagen synthesis in the skin, resulting in the obviously changed photodamaged skin [47–51]. Increasing age reduces the activity of tissue inhibitor of metalloproteinase-1 (TIMP-1), an inhibitor of many members of the MMPs [48]. The balance between collagen synthesis and degradation up to collagen deficiency differs between intrinsic and photoaged skin. The intrinsic aging of the skin seems to be mediated by a reduction in collagen synthesis, while the damage of dermal connective tissue in extrinsically aged skin is more about the induction of matrix metalloproteinases [52]. Skin damage is mediated by imperfect protection mechanisms against reactive oxygen species. The mutations of the DNA may accumulate irreversibly if repair mechanisms such as excision repair or using the enzyme photolyase fail to act [10]. The mutancy of mitochondrial DNA is multiple higher than nuclear DNA, because mitochondria do not contain any repair mechanism [53]. The synthesis of collagen types I and III, mainly structural components of the dermal connective tissue, is diminished in photoaged skin by a downregulation of type I and III procollagen expression [54]. AP-1 has also been shown to negatively regulate type I procollagen gene

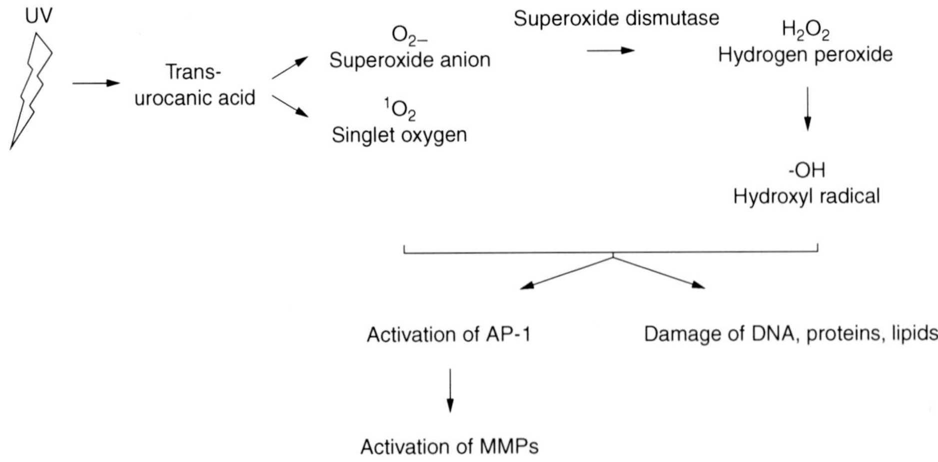

Fig. 3 UVA-induced generation of reactive oxygen species (Figure adapted with permission from Ziemer et al. [10])

expression [55]. There are lot of other environmental damages implicated in the process of extrinsic skin aging like tobacco smoke, infrared light, and ozone. Tobacco smoke is an important inductor of preterm skin aging. Lahmann et al. reported significantly more MMP-1 mRNA in the skin of smokers than nonsmokers, while no difference was seen for the tissue inhibitor of metalloproteinase-1 [56].

Wound Repair in the Aging Skin

Wound healing in healthy old people is delayed, not defective [57]. However, age-related biochemical and biomechanical changes (Table 2) affect wound repair in the elderly impairing healing and underlying chronic wound formation. Aging has been associated with a persistent pro-inflammatory state, while at the same time, there is a decrease in the ability to generate an acute inflammatory response during injury resulting in the lack of synchronization between pro- and anti-inflammatory responses [58]. Clinically, this presents as a higher rate of cutaneous scar formation after wounding with increased patient age, an enhanced risk of postoperative disruption of surgical wounds leading to higher mortality, and a rise in surgical site infections (SSIs) in patients older than 65 years [58]. Studies in animal models demonstrate that proliferation of the cell types responsible for tissue formation such as keratinocytes and fibroblasts is reduced in aging. Furthermore, age-related changes include a decrease in the number of Langerhans cells and melanocytes in the epidermis as well as reduced numbers of macrophages and mast cells in the dermis [57].

Age-Dependent Skin Diseases

The process of skin aging is not only a cosmetic problem but also of medical-dermatological relevance due to a higher incidence of age-dependent skin diseases such as bullous pemphigoid, erysipelas, and herpes zoster (Fig. 4). Many dermatoses of the elderly are presented completely different than in young persons. Herpes zoster is more frequently associated with severe neuralgiform pains, erysipelas appears prevalently in the absence of fever, and atopic syndrome is present in the form of pruriginous eczema. Clinical aspects of the aging skin are pruritus senilis, age-dependent pemphigoid, and atrophic balanitis and vulvitis. Intrinsically aged skin is

Table 2 Changes in wound healing due to aging [57]

Hemostasis	Inflammation	Proliferation	Remodeling
Increased platelet aggregation Increased platelet degranulation	Altered adhesion molecule profile Early increase in neutrophils Delayed monocyte infiltration Increase in mature macrophages Impaired macrophage function: Reduced phagocytic capacity Increased secretion of pro-inflammatory mediators Decreased VEGF production Delayed T cell infiltration	Reduced response to hypoxia: Diminished HIF-1α signaling Decreased SDF-1 expression Delayed angiogenesis Delayed collagen disposition: Reduced fibroblast proliferation Reduced fibroblast migration Reduced responsiveness to TGF-β Delayed re-epithelization: Reduced keratinocyte proliferation Reduced keratinocyte migration	Reduced collagen turnover Increased fibroblast senescence Accelerated maturation Improved scarring

characterized by a higher incidence of benign hyperproliferations of keratinocytes and capillary blood vessels such as seborrheic keratosis and senile hemangiomas [10]. One feature of photoaging is the higher occurrence of benign hyperproliferative skin lesions like lentigines solaris as well as seborrheic keratosis and senile hemangioma (Fig. 5). Lentigines seniles are pigmented maculae in chronically sun-exposed skin, which are due to an increase in the melanin content inside keratinocytes and casual with melanotic hyperplasia [59]. There is strong evidence supporting the direct role of sunlight exposure in the development of skin cancers. The UV-induced free radicals damage the DNA with possible mutations in oncogenes and tumor-suppressor genes or activation of cytoplasmic signal transduction pathways that are related to growth differentiation, senescence, transformation, and tissue degradation [60]. The matrix metalloproteinases have been associated with the process of skin aging and in particular are thought to be critical for tumor invasion and metastasis [61]. An important feature of extrinsically aged skin is the higher incidence of precancerosa such as actinic keratosis or morbus bowen and malignoma-like basal cell carcinoma and squamous cell carcinoma (Fig. 6). Black skin according to Fitzpatrick is less susceptible to sunburn, photoaging, and skin carcinogenesis. A higher melanin content and a different melanosomal dispersion pattern in the epidermis are thought to be responsible for its more resistant

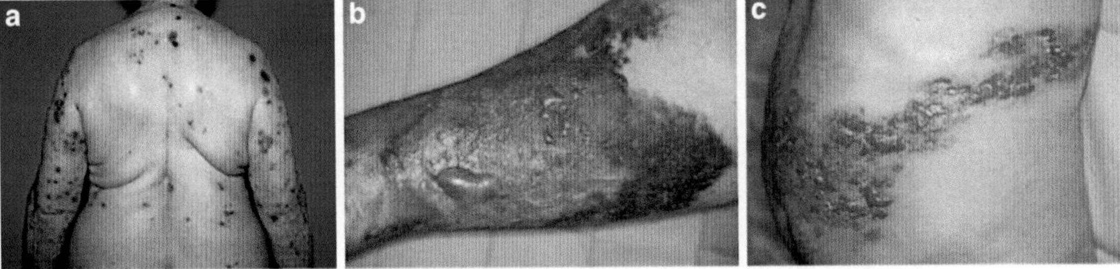

Fig. 4 Typical age-dependent skin diseases. (**a**) Bullous pemphigoid, (**b**) erysipelas, and (**c**) herpes zoster (Courtesy of Department of Dermatology, University Hospital Jena)

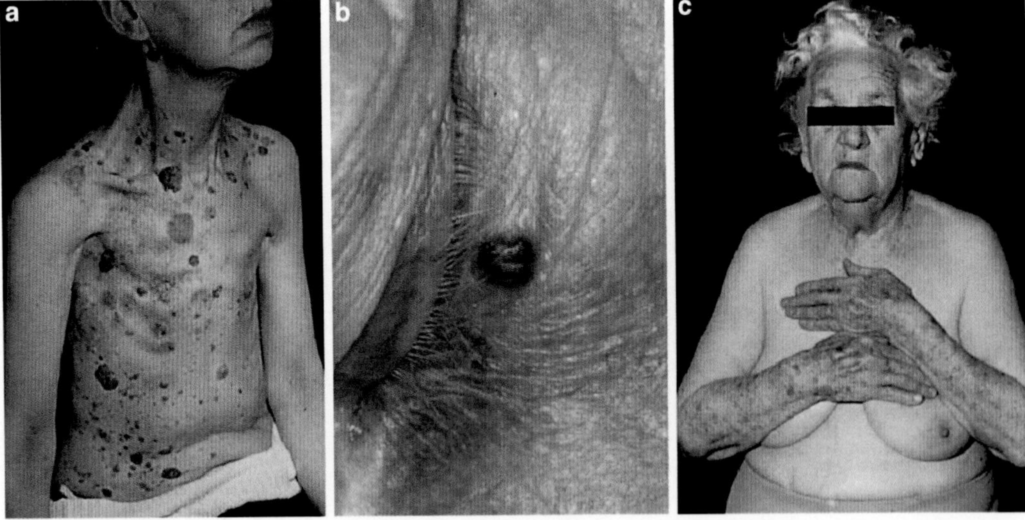

Fig. 5 Age-dependent skin tumors. (**a**) Seborrheic keratosis, (**b**) senile hemangioma, and (**c**) lentigines solares (Courtesy of Department of Dermatology, University Hospital Jena)

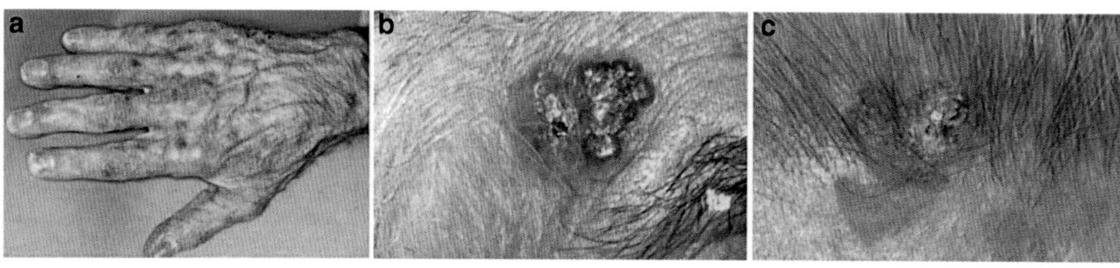

Fig. 6 (Pre)cancerous skin diseases. (**a**) Actinic keratosis, (**b**) basal cell carcinoma, and (**c**) squamous cell carcinoma (Courtesy of Department of Dermatology, University Hospital Jena)

behavior to UV light [62]. Sunscreens with high amounts of sun protection factors protect against solar dermatitis causing a possible decrease in the formation of UV-induced skin malignancies [63].

Conclusion

Human skin, like any other organ, ages and undergoes changes due to aging. It is evident that environmental factors as well as genetic programs contribute substantially to the processes involved. The long-term exposure of skin to solar UV radiation is a severe environmental hazard leading to acute and chronic effects in the human skin caused by the generation of free radicals. This type of skin aging is referred to as "photoaging" or "extrinsic" aging and clinically manifests as rough skin textures, wrinkles, laxity, atrophy, pigmentary changes or blotchy dyspigmentation, elastosis, telangiectasia, and precancerous lesions such as actinic keratosis and malignant tumors. In contrast, "intrinsic" aging is genetically determined. The clinical characteristics of intrinsically aged skin are fine wrinkles, a thin and transparent appearance, loss of underlying fat leading to hollowed cheeks and eye sockets, dry and itchy skin, and inability to perspire sufficiently, hair graying, hair loss or hirsutism, and thinning of nail plates. However, it is very difficult, if not impossible, to separate "intrinsic" aging from a variety of other factors clearly contributing to aging, such as smoking, sun exposure, alcohol consumption, dietary habits, and other environmental and lifestyle factors [43]. In addition, both processes may overlap, and the underlying mechanism of both processes is increased oxidative stress, which is probably the single most harmful contributor to skin aging. The ROS and RNS created induce structural and functional alterations of cutaneous proteins, for example, collagen, elastin, and glycosaminoglycans, and result in DNA damage impairing proper cell function as well as leading to cell senescence.

Cross-References

▶ Degenerative Changes in Aging Skin

References

1. Kligman AM, Koblenzer C. Demographics and psychological implications for the aging population. Dermatol Clin. 1997;15(4):549–53.
2. https://www.census.gov/population/international/data/worldpop/table_population.php. Accessed on 9 June 2015.
3. Farage MA, et al. Structural characteristics of the aging skin: a review. Cutan Ocul Toxicol. 2007;26(4):343–57.
4. Farage MA, et al. Functional and physiological characteristics of the aging skin. Aging Clin Exp Res. 2008;20(3):195–200.
5. Vaillant L, Callens A. Hormone replacement treatment and skin aging. Therapie. 1996;51(1):67–70.
6. Kosmadaki MG, Gilchrest BA. The role of telomeres in skin aging/photoaging. Micron. 2004;35(3):155–9.
7. Ning MS, Andl T. Control by a hair's breadth: the role of microRNAs in the skin. Cell Mol Life Sci. 2013;70(7):1149–69.
8. Mimaeult M, Batra SK. Recent advances on skin-resident stem/progenitor cell functions in skin regeneration, aging and cancers and novel anti-aging and cancer therapies. J Cell Mol Med. 2010;14(1–2):116–34.

9. Menon G, Ghadially R. Morphology of lipid alterations in the epidermis: a review. Microsc Res Tech. 1997;37(3):180–92.
10. Ziemer M, et al. Alterungsprozesse der haut und altersdermatosen. In: Wedding U et al., editors. Medizin des alterns und des alten menschen. 1st ed. Berlin: Verlag Hans Huber; 2007. p. 157–65, Hogrefe AG.
11. Griffiths HR, et al. Molecular and cellular effects of ultraviolet light-induced genotoxicity. Crit Rev Clin Lab Sci. 1998;35(3):189–237.
12. Berneburg M, et al. Photoaging of human skin. Photodermatol Photoimmunol Photomed. 2000;16 (6):239–44.
13. Kottner J, Lichterfeld A, Blume-Peytavi U. Maintaining skin integrity in the aged: a systematic review. Br J Dermatol. 2013;169:528–42.
14. Seyfarth F, Schliemann S, Antonov D, Elsner P. Dry skin, barrier function, and irritant contact dermatitis in the elderly. Clin Dermatol. 2011;29:31–6.
15. Jafferany M, Huynh TV, Silverman MA, Zaidi Z. Geriatric dermatoses: a clinical review of skin diseases in an aging population. Int J Dermatol. 2012;51:509–22.
16. Rogers J, et al. Stratum corneum lipids: the effect of ageing and the seasons. Arch Dermatol Res. 1996;288 (12):765–70.
17. Patel T, Yosipovitch G. The management of chronic pruritus in the elderly. Skin Therap Lett. 2010;15:8.
18. Ghadially R. Aging and the epidermal permeability barrier: implications for contact dermatitis. Am J Contact Dermat. 1998;9(3):162–9.
19. Balin AK, Pratt LA. Physiological consequences of human skin aging. Cutis. 1989;43(5):431–6.
20. Fenske NA, Lober CW. Structural and functional changes of normal aging skin. J Am Acad Dermatol. 1986;15(4 Pt 1):571–85.
21. Horvath SM, Rochelle RD. Hypothermia in the aged. Environ Health Perspect. 1977;20:127–30.
22. Harvell JD, Maibach HI. Percutaneous absorption and inflammation in aged skin: a review. J Am Acad Dermatol. 1994;31(6):1015–21.
23. Patterson WM, et al. Favre-racouchot disease. Int J Dermatol. 2004;43(3):167–9.
24. Schafer T, et al. The epidemiology of nevi and signs of skin aging in the adult general population: results of the kora-survey 2000. J Invest Dermatol. 2006;126 (7):1490–6.
25. Ortonne JP. Pigmentary changes of the ageing skin. Br J Dermatol. 1990;122 Suppl 35:21–8.
26. Waller JM, Maibach HI. Age and skin structure and function, a quantitative approach (I): blood flow, pH, thickness, and ultrasound echogenicity. Skin Res Technol. 2005;11(4):221–35.
27. Neerken S, et al. Characterization of age-related effects in human skin: a comparative study that applies confocal laser scanning microscopy and optical coherence tomography. J Biomed Opt. 2004;9(2):274–81.
28. Fenske NA, Conard CB. Aging skin. Am Fam Physician. 1988;37(2):219–30.
29. Yaar M, Gilchrest BA. Skin aging: postulated mechanisms and consequent changes in structure and function. Clin Geriatr Med. 2001;17(4):617–30. v.
30. Yaar M, et al. Fifty years of skin aging. J Invest Dermatol Symp Proc. 2002;7(1):51–8.
31. Kerscher M, et al. Physiologie der hautalterung. In: Effendy I, Kerscher M, editors. Haut und Alter. 1st ed. Stuttgart: Georg Thieme Verlag KG; 2005. p. 3–10.
32. Schwartz E, et al. Collagen alterations in chronically sun-damaged human skin. Photochem Photobiol. 1993;58(6):841–4.
33. Koehler MJ, et al. In vivo assessment of human skin aging by multiphoton laser scanning tomography. Opt Lett. 2006;31(19):2879–81.
34. Hussain SH, Limthongkul B, Humphreys TR. The biomechanical properties of the skin. Dermatol Surg. 2013;39:193–203.
35. Sherrat MJ. Age-related tissue stiffening: cause and effect. Adv Wound Care. 2013;2(1):11–6.
36. Wu M, Fannin J, Rice KM, Wang B, Blough ER. Effect of aging on cellular mechanotransduction. Ageing Res Rev. 2011;10(1):1–15.
37. Wiegand C, White R. Microdeformation in wound healing. Wound Rep Reg. 2013;21:793–9.
38. Berger TG, Steinhoff M. Pruritus in elderly patients – eruptions of senescence. Semin Cutan Med Surg. 2011;30(2):113–7.
39. Fiers SA. Breaking the cycle: the etiology of incontinence dermatitis and evaluating and using skin care products. Ostomy Wound Manage. 1996;42 (3):32–34, 36, 38–40, passim.
40. Brincat MP, et al. Estrogens and the skin. Climacteric. 2005;8(2):110–23.
41. Sander CS, et al. Expression of extracellular matrix protein 1 (ECM1) in human skin is decreased by age and increased upon ultraviolet exposure. Br J Dermatol. 2006;154(2):218–24.
42. Harman D. Aging: a theory based on free radical and radiation chemistry. J Gerontol. 1956;11(3):298–300.
43. Poljsak B, Dahmane RH, Godic A. Intrinsic skin aging: the role of oxidative stress. Acta Dermatovenerol. 2012;21:33–6.
44. Kaneko K, et al. Cis-urocanic acid initiates gene transcription in primary human keratinocytes. J Immunol. 2008;181(1):217–24.
45. Fridovich I. Superoxide dismutases. An adaptation to a paramagnetic gas. J Biol Chem. 1989;264(14):7761–4.
46. Lo YY, Cruz TF. Involvement of reactive oxygen species in cytokine and growth factor induction of c-fos expression in chondrocytes. J Biol Chem. 1995;270 (20):11727–30.
47. Angel P, et al. Function and regulation of AP-1 subunits in skin physiology and pathology. Oncogene. 2001;20(19):2413–23.
48. Hornebeck W. Down-regulation of tissue inhibitor of matrix metalloprotease-1 (TIMP-1) in aged human skin contributes to matrix degradation and impaired cell

growth and survival. Pathol Biol (Paris). 2003;51 (10):569–73.
49. Varani J, et al. Vitamin A antagonizes decreased cell growth and elevated collagen-degrading matrix metalloproteinases and stimulates collagen accumulation in naturally aged human skin. J Invest Dermatol. 2000;114(3):480–6.
50. Karin M, et al. Ap-1 function and regulation. Curr Opin Cell Biol. 1997;9(2):240–6.
51. Fisher GJ, Voorhees JJ. Molecular mechanisms of photoaging and its prevention by retinoic acid: ultraviolet irradiation induces map kinase signal transduction cascades that induce ap-1-regulated matrix metalloproteinases that degrade human skin in vivo. J Invest Dermatol Symp Proc. 1998;3(1):61–8.
52. Chung JH, et al. Modulation of skin collagen metabolism in aged and photoaged human skin in vivo. J Invest Dermatol. 2001;117(5):1218–24.
53. Richter C. Oxidative damage to mitochondrial DNA and its relationship to ageing. Int J Biochem Cell Biol. 1995;27(7):647–53.
54. Talwar HS, et al. Reduced type I and type III procollagens in photodamaged adult human skin. J Invest Dermatol. 1995;105(2):285–90.
55. Chung KY, et al. An ap-1 binding sequence is essential for regulation of the human alpha2(I) collagen (col1a2) promoter activity by transforming growth factor-beta. J Biol Chem. 1996;271(6):3272–8.
56. Lahmann C, et al. Matrix metalloproteinase-1 and skin ageing in smokers. Lancet. 2001;357(9260):935–6.
57. Sgnoc R, Gruber J. Age-related aspects of cutaneous wound healing: a mini-review. Gerontology. 2013;59:159–64.
58. Bentov I, Reed MJ. Anesthesia, microcirculation and wound repair in aging. Anesthesiology. 2014;120 (3):760–72.
59. Nikkels A, et al. Comparative morphometric study of eruptive puva-induced and chronic sun-induced lentigines of the skin. Anal Quant Cytol Histol. 1991;13(1):23–6.
60. Scharffetter-Kochanek K, et al. UV-induced reactive oxygen species in photocarcinogenesis and photoaging. Biol Chem. 1997;378(11):1247–57.
61. Crawford HC, Matrisian LM. Tumor and stromal expression of matrix metalloproteinases and their role in tumor progression. Invasion Metastasis. 1994;14 (1–6):234–45.
62. Rijken F, et al. Responses of black and white skin to solar-simulating radiation: differences in DNA photodamage, infiltrating neutrophils, proteolytic enzymes induced, keratinocyte activation, and IL-10 expression. J Invest Dermatol. 2004;122 (6):1448–55.
63. Elsner P, et al. Sun protection: possibilities and limitations. J Dtsch Dermatol Ges. 2005;3 Suppl 2: S40–4.

The Stratum Corneum and Aging

7

Anthony V. Rawlings

Contents

Abstract

It is clear that the stratum corneum (SC) maintains its primary protective role throughout life as nobody dies of old skin! However, many skin problems assert themselves in the aged due to changes in the structural and functional biochemistry of dermal and epidermal components. As an example, we now know that dry itchy senile xerotic skin is a problem of faulty epidermal and SC maturation together with reduced desquamation. Decreases in SC lipid levels with aging, especially SC ceramide levels, will affect the lateral and lamellar packing mesophases. In this respect, decreased CER EOS linoleate levels also occur which may affect the presence of the key SC long periodicity phase in aged SC. Decreased SC natural moisturizing factor (NMF) levels occur which are likely to affect SC water holding capacity although some report increases in NMF levels, which may be related to increased corneocyte size and SC thickness. Corneocytes get bigger and flatter and on non-facial body sites, the SC gets thicker all of which should improve transepidermal water loss (TEWL) if it is not compromised by the SC lipid changes. Decreased SC kallikrein 5 activities also occur with aging on non-facial body sites, which probably contributes to the expression of senile xerosis and reduced desquamation. The increased skin surface pH and protease activity lead to reduced SC cohesion with age, but appear not to be affecting superficial

A.V. Rawlings (✉)
AVR Consulting Ltd, Cheshire, UK
e-mail: tonyrawlings@avrconsultingltd.com

M.A. Farage et al. (eds.), *Textbook of Aging Skin*,
DOI 10.1007/978-3-662-47398-6_7

desquamation positively. The increased activities of desquamatory enzymes as well as inflammatory proteases probably contributes to the maintenance of a relatively thin facial SC with elevated TEWL and reduced barrier reserve throughout all ages compared with other body sites. Overall, aged SC functions less well compared with young SC. Measuring TEWL may not reflect these changes but the greater appearance of skin xerosis in the aged indicates that SC biochemistry and that the associated cellular phenotypic response is different. These cellular and biochemical differences are clearly observable when analysing SC tape stripping's

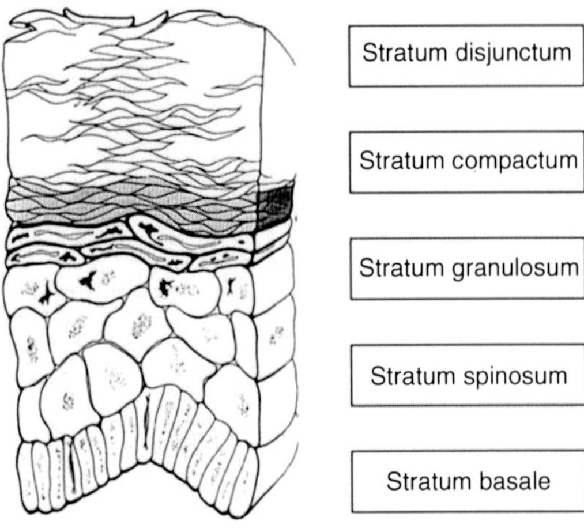

Fig. 1 Schematic of the epidermis and the stratum corneum

Introduction

The father of corneobiology, Albert Kligman [1], wrote in 1979: "No one dies of old skin! No matter how decrepit the integument becomes after a lifetime of assaults, it continues to perform its primary protective role. ... But skin problems abound in the aged!" It is now known that dry itchy senile xerotic skin is a problem of faulty epidermal and stratum corneum (SC) maturation together with desquamation.

The understanding of the changes in the chemistry and function of important stratum corneum (SC) components in aging and dry skin is a result of the tenacity of a plethora of academic and industrial scientists spanning several decades. These include studies on corneocyte size [2–4]; SC lipid levels, especially ceramides [5–9]; lipid ultrastructure and biophysics [10–12]; natural moisturizing factors (NMF) [13, 14]; SC proteases [15, 16]; corneodesmosomal proteins [11, 17, 18]; and finally corneocyte quality [19, 20]. Ultimately, changes in SC cohesion and desquamatory properties were studied by Ronald Marks [21]. Some of these changes, of course, were predicted in 1964 [22].

Key in SC function and maturation, however, is its hydration [23]. It was not until 1994 that the understanding of the perturbation of water gradients in the SC of subjects with xerotic skin was developed [24] and only in 1995 [25] it was shown that water itself was essential for corneodesmosomal degradation and ultimately desquamation. This chapter gives an overview of the latest understanding of the stratum corneum and aging (Fig. 1).

Stratum Corneum Structure

Corneodesmosomes obviously have a big role to play in the cohesion between corneocytes in the stratum compactum and the "apparent" lack of cohesion in the stratum disjunctum (SD) [26]. However, it has been learned in recent years that the interaction between corneocytes in the disjunctum layers is not as "loose" as originally anticipated. Using new high-pressure freezing and freeze-substitution techniques for electron microscopy [27], the SC appeared to be more compact than expected with smaller intercellular spaces and hence tighter intercorneocyte interactions. Equally using novel cryotransmission electron microscopy techniques to image vitreous sections of skin without the use of cryoprotectants [28], a more densely packed stratum corneum was again apparent. The decreased cohesive forces toward the surface layers of the SC, close to the intercorneocyte interaction, must be due to the degradation of corneodesmosomes toward the surface layers, although strong hydrophobic interaction between corneocytes was still observed due to the intercellular and covalently bound lipids. Thus, the basket weave appearance of the SC by histology and the presence of the more widely spaced SD are artifacts from the older methods. However, it is preferable to use the stratum compactum-disjunctum as the term to define their interface, which is probably one of the most biologically active parts of this important barrier tissue.

In addition to the close intercorneocyte interaction, differences in the swellability of corneocytes in the different layers of the SC have also been observed [29, 30]. A lower non-swelling region (LNSR), a swelling region (SR), and an upper non-swelling region (UNSR) have been observed. The differences in the swelling regions of the SC are probably due to a combination of the loss of NMF in the outer layers of the SC, hydrolysis of filaggrin to NMF in the mid layers and lysis of non-peripheral corneodesmosomes, allowing greater intercorneocyte freedom above the stratum compactum, and transglutaminase-mediated maturation and rigidification of corneocytes toward the surface layers of the SC. As will be discussed, many of these events become aberrant in senile dry skin, but these methods need to be more rigorously applied to the study of senile SC.

Stratum Corneum Lipids

All SC lipids are important for barrier function of the skin, but due to their unique structures, properties, and on a weight basis as they constitute approximately 50 % of the SC lipids, ceramides have been the area of most interest in recent years [31]. In fact, 11 classes of ceramides have now been identified. The ceramide head groups are small but can form extensive hydrogen bonds. They differ by head group architecture and fatty acid chain length. Ceramides are classified in general as CER FB, where F indicates the type of fatty acid and B indicates the type of base [32] (Fig. 2 and Table 1). When an ester-linked fatty acid is present, a prefix E is used. Normal fatty acids (saturated or unsaturated), alpha-hydroxy fatty acids, and omega-hydroxy fatty acids are indicated by N, A, and O, respectively, whereas sphingosines, phytosphingosines, and 6-hydroxysphingosine are indicated by S, P, and H. Sphinganine (not previously classified) is proposed to be SP in this nomenclature system. A novel long-chain ceramide containing branched chain fatty acids is also found in vernix caseosa [33]. Typical structures of human ceramides are given in Table 1. Ceramides have also been found attached to the corneocyte envelope. In addition to ceramide A (sphingosine; CEROS) and ceramide B (6-hydroxysphingosine; CEROH), the presence of covalently bound omega-hydroxy fatty acid containing sphinganine and phytosphingosine ceramides has been identified [34]. These covalently bound ceramides should now be named CER OSP and CER OP. However, Hill et al. [35] could only find the presence of CER EOS (72.4 %), CER EOH (19.5 %), and CER OP (8.2 %).

Ceramides are produced as precursors in the epidermis in the form of glucosylceramides, epidermosides, or sphingomyelin (Fig. 3). Epidermosides are glycated precursors of CER EOS, EOH, and EOP together with the ceramides covalently bound to the corneocyte envelope. Sphingomyelin provides a proportion of CER NS and CER AS, whereas the glucosylceramides are precursors to the other classes of ceramides [36]. The chain length distribution of the omega-hydroxy fatty acid portion of CER EOS has recently become a topic of interest. When first identified the omega-hydroxy fatty acid portion of CER EOS was reported to be mainly composed of C30 (63.6 %) to C32 (14.9 %) chain lengths with minor shorter chain length species [37]. However, longer chain variants have been recently identified [38]. Rawlings et al. [39] recently reported that no chain length species were identified below C30 chain length and the bulk was either C32 or C34. Surprisingly more than 27 % of the fatty acids were odd chain length species compared with previous findings of only 16 %. This further heterogeneity in CER EOS composition needs to be understood for its effects on lipid lamellar packing at the molecular level and subsequently on SC function and especially the

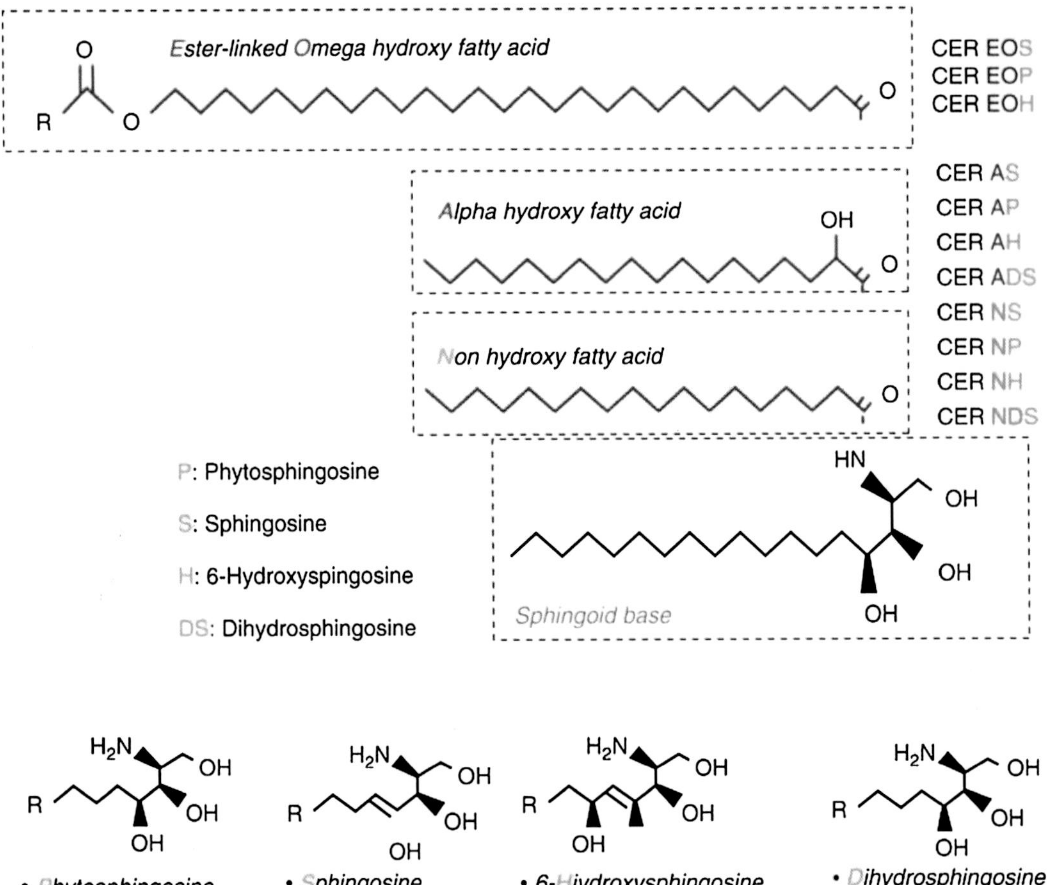

Fig. 2 Nomenclature system of stratum corneum ceramides

impact of aging on these lipid species. Nevertheless, Imokawa et al. [5] first recorded the age-related decline in SC ceramides which will naturally impact on SC functioning. Reductions of all SC lipids with aging were reported slightly later [9] (Fig. 4).

It is the lipid-packing states, however, that influence SC barrier function. Lipids in vivo in the SC appear to exist as a balance between orthorhombic packing (a solid crystalline state) and hexagonal packing (gel). The orthorhombically packed lipids are the most tightly packed conformation and have optimal barrier properties, but a greater proportion of hexagonally packed lipid conformations are known to occur in the outer layers of the SC due to the increased presence of sebum [40]. This is consistent with a weakening of the barrier toward the outer layers of the stratum corneum. It is known that ceramides and cholesterol only form hexagonally packed lipids and it is the long-chain fatty acids that induce the orthorhombic packing states. However, it is possible that an excess of short-chain fatty acids and other lipids derived from sebum contributes to the crystalline to gel transition in the upper stratum corneum layers [41]. Naturally, during aging sebum declines and this transition will be reduced. If sebum influences desquamation in any way, then the age-related reduction in sebum lipids may contribute to the expression of xerotic skin.

A sandwich model for the lamellar lipids consisting of two broad lipid layers with a crystalline structure separated by a narrow central lipid layer with fluid domains has been proposed [42]. It seems that cholesterol and ceramides are important for the formation of the lamellar phase, whereas

Table 1 Eleven classes of human stratum corneum ceramides

	Fatty acid		
Sphingoid	Non-hydroxy fatty acid [N] 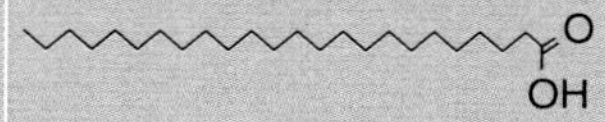	α-Hydroxy fatty acid [A] 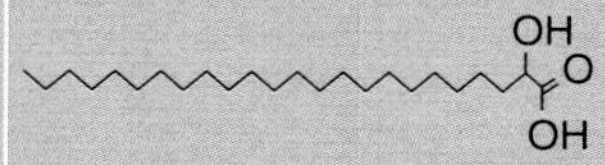	Esterified ω-hydroxy fatty acid [EO] 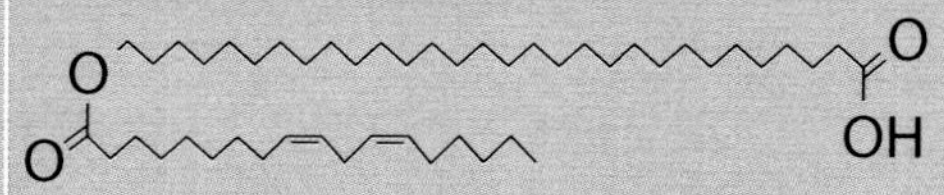
Dihydrosphingosine [DS] 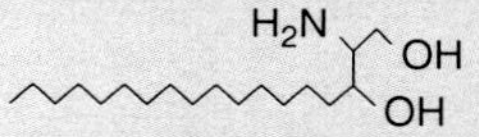	CER [NDS]	CER[ADS]	CER[EODS] (not yet identified in SC)
Sphingosine [S] 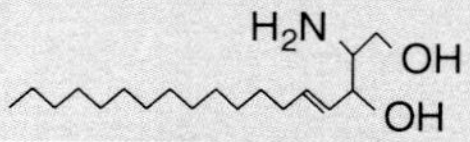	CER[NS]	CER[AS]	CER[EOS]
Phytosphingosine[P] 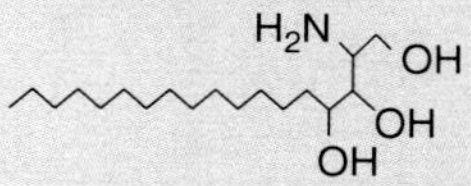	CER[NP]	CER[AP]	CER[EOP]
6-Hydroxy sphingosine [H] 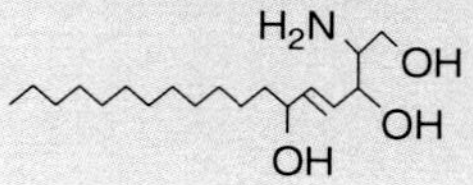	CER[NH]	CER[AH]	CER[EOH]

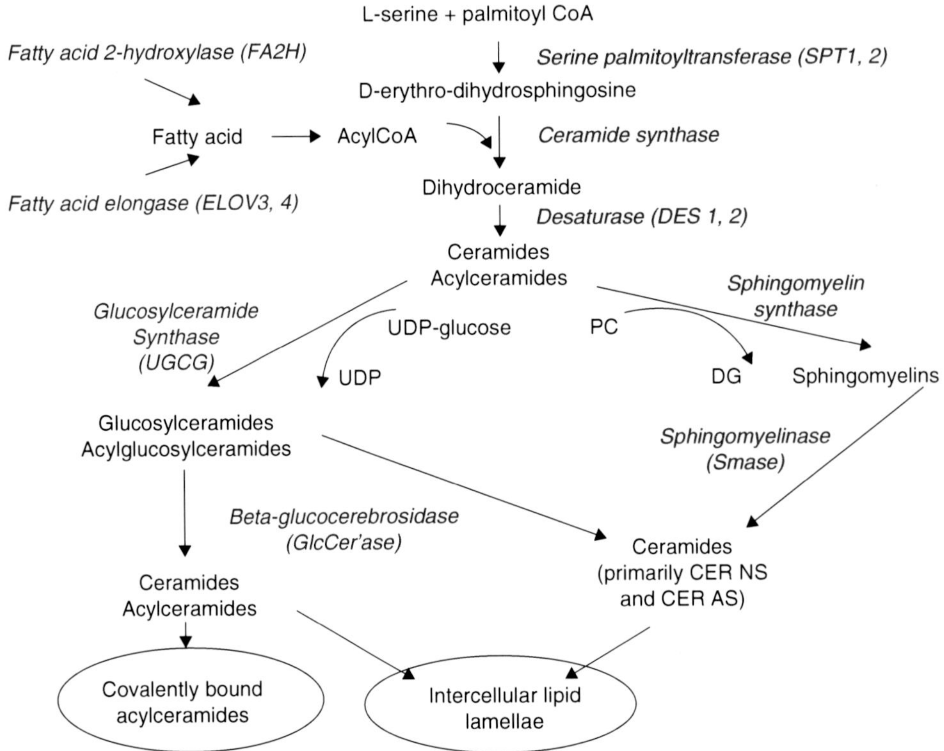

Fig. 3 Summary of main steps in epidermal biosynthesis of ceramides

fatty acids play a greater role in the lateral packing of the lipids. Cholesterol is proposed to be located with the fatty acid tail of CER EOS in the fluid phase. CER EOS, EOH, and EOP play an essential role in the formation of the additional lamellar arrangements. The repeated distances were found to be 13 nm in dimension, composed of two units measuring approximately 5 nm each and one unit measuring approximately 3 nm in thickness. These repeat lamellar patterns were also observed by X-ray diffraction studies and were named the "long periodicity" (LPP) and "short periodicity" (SPP) phases, respectively. In the presence of long-chain fatty acids besides an orthorhombic phase, the lipids also form a liquid phase.

Another important ceramide, ceramide-1 as it used to be called but now known as CER EOS, has a dramatic effect on SC lipid phase behavior. For total lipid mixtures in the absence of CER EOS, mostly hexagonal phases are also observed and equally no LPP phase or liquid phase is formed. Moreover, the importance of ceramide 1 or CER EOS linoleate in facilitating the formation of the LPP has been further elaborated by understanding the influence of the type of fatty acid esterified to the omega-hydroxy fatty acid [43]. As a consequence, greater amounts of the LPP, orthorhombic, and liquid phases are observed mainly with linoleate-containing CER EOS, less with oleate-containing CER EOS, and are totally absent if only stearate-containing CER EOS is present in the lipid mixtures. It seems that the presence of an unsaturated acyl chain is crucial for the formation of these phases and packing states. These studies indicate that for formation of the LPP, a certain fraction of the lipids has to form a liquid phase. If the liquid phase is too high (as with the oleate-containing CER EOS) or too low (as with stearate-containing CER EOS), the levels of the SPP increase at the expense of the LPP. It is important to remember in vivo that the fatty acid composition of CER EOS is highly complex, but it contains a large proportion of linoleic acid. Conti et al. [44] observed decreases

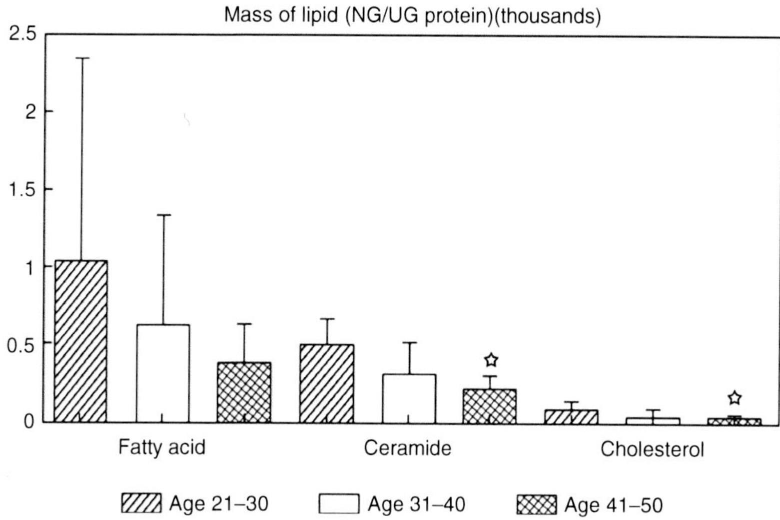

Fig. 4 Age-related reductions in the levels of stratum corneum ceramides, fatty acids, and cholesterol from tape strippings of the human face

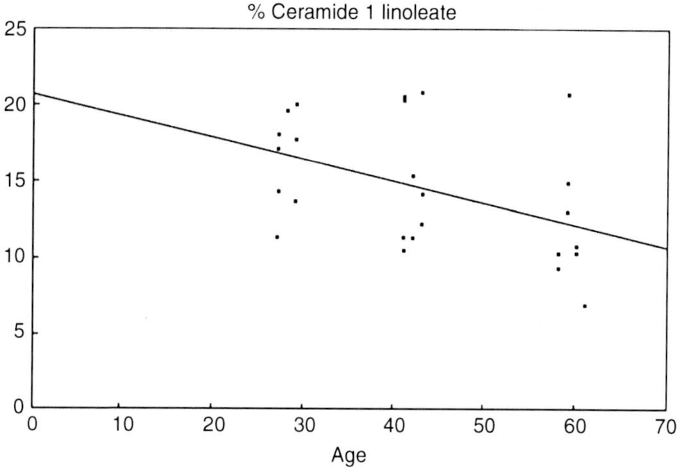

Fig. 5 Age-related reductions in the levels of stratum corneum ceramide-1 (CER EOS) linoleate levels from tape strippings of the human face

in C18:2 and C24 fatty acids with increases in C18:1 and C16:0 in fatty acids of CER EOS in the winter months of the year. Similarly, Rogers et al. [9] demonstrated an age-related decline in the reductions of the linoleate content of SC CER EOS with a trend of increasing oleate levels (Fig. 5). Reductions in the levels of CER EOS linoleate could lead to reductions in both the LPP. It is interesting in this respect that CER EOS directly improves SC flexibility [45] and that it is vital for barrier function [46, 47].

One must not forget the influence of the environment on SC maturation and epidermal differentiation. In the same paper on the aging reductions in CER EOS linoleate levels, Rogers et al. [9] demonstrated that there was a significant reduction in the levels of SC ceramides and fatty acids, together with linoleate-containing CER EOS in subjects in winter compared with summer. Similar differences in scalp lipid levels have been observed between the wet and dry seasons in Thailand [48]. This appears to be related to changes in external humidity. Transepidermal water loss (TEWL) was reduced by approximately 30 % in animals exposed to a dry (<10 % RH) environment due to increased lipid biosynthesis, increased lamellar body extrusion, and a slightly thicker SC layer, whereas, in

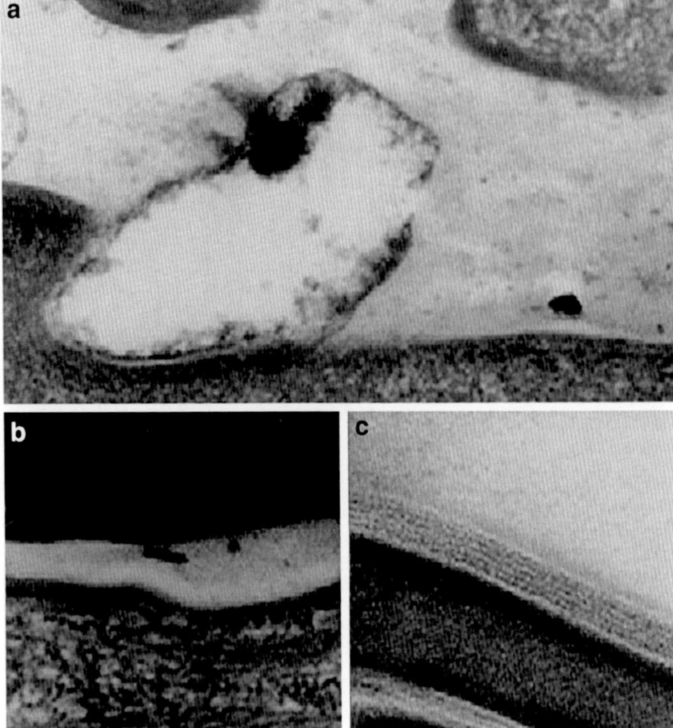

Fig. 6 Organization of stratum corneum lipids in tape strippings of individuals with clinically normal skin. Transmission electron micrographs of tape strippings. Ultrastructural changes in lipid organization toward the surface of the stratum corneum. (**a**) First strip: absence of bilayers and presence of amorphous lipidic material. (**b**) Second strip: disruption of lipid lamellae. (**c**) Third strip: normal lipid lamellae (×200,000)

animals exposed to a high humidity environment (80 % RH), this induction of lipid biosynthesis was reduced [49]. However, abrupt changes in environmental humidity can also influence stratum corneum moisturization [50]. After transferring animals from a humid (80 % RH) to dry (<10 % RH) environment, a sixfold increase in TEWL occurred. Barrier function returned to normal within 7 days due to normal lipid repair processes. These changes did not occur in animals transferred from a normal to dry humidity environment. These changes in barrier function have also been recently reported in a group of Chinese workers who are exposed to very low humidity conditions. However, the changes in barrier function take longer to reach equilibrium than anticipated from the animal studies [51]. These changes are still expected to occur in aged subjects.

Nevertheless, it can be concluded, therefore, that compositional changes in SC lipids could dramatically influence the ordering of lipids in the skin and thereby the condition of the skin. In this respect, using electron microscopy of tape strippings from the outer layers of normal healthy SC, Rawlings et al. [11] first reported complete loss of lamellar ordering (Fig. 6) in 30–40-year-olds which were subsequently confirmed by Warner et al. [52] and more recently by Berry et al. [53]. Focal domains that were depleted or devoid of lipid layers were also reported in aged subjects (>80 years) [19]. Sheu et al. reported that this may not be an aging problem in itself as these changes may be induced by an excess of sebum [54]. However, degradation of CER EOS to its corresponding acyl acid as reported by Wertz and Downing [55] may be the first step in causing a change in the lipid structure for preparing the process of desquamation. Equally, Long et al. [56] reported that the degradation of cholesterol sulfate may be involved in this process. This may be related to the reported distorted orthorhombic phase at the site of cohesive failure [57].

Thus, the relative amounts of SC lipids, sebum, and extent of washing will likely influence the presence of these structures, but they may be more easily visible as one ages. Nevertheless, this phase, that is, no organized lamellar structure, would appear consistently in subjects older than 40 [52].

Desquamation

Over four decades ago, the father of corneobiology [22] suggested that cell cohesion in the SC was dependent upon an "intercellular cement" that was predicted to become less stable near the surface of the skin or to be degraded by enzymes. It was not until 1979 that scientists in Professor Marks group in Cardiff [58, 59] clearly demonstrated reduced intercorneocyte cohesion toward the outer layers of the SC as judged by mechanical cohesography or by using a standardized skin scrub stimulus. While reduced intracorneal cohesion occurs with aging, a trend of reduced desquamation also occurs with increasing age, which seems to be at odds with the reported increased serine protease activity and elevated pH with aging [60]. Nevertheless, changes in desquamation and thereby SC cohesion are likely to be the result of changes in SC lipid organization, corneocyte interdigitation together with corneodesmosome numbers, and their state of degradation.

Corneodesmosomes consist of the cadherin family of transmembrane glycoproteins desmoglein 1 (Dsg 1) and desmocollin 1 (Dsc 1), which bind each other on adjacent corneocytes. Inside the corneocytes, Dsg 1 and Dsc 1 are also linked to keratin microfilaments via corneodesmosomal plaque proteins such as plakoglobin, desmoplakins, and plakophilins. These provide stability and extra-cohesion to the SC "brick wall." Otherwise the only intercorneocyte cohesive force would be that provided by intercellular as well as covalently bound lipids. Another corneodesmosomal protein, corneodesmosin (Cdsn), after secretion within the lamellar bodies with the intercellular lipids and certain proteases (but not all), becomes associated with the desmosomal proteins just before transformation of desmosomes into corneodesmosomes. As all these proteins are cross-linked into the complex by transglutaminase, their controlled disruption must occur by proteolysis to reduce the intermolecular forces between the corneocytes to allow desquamation to proceed. Cdsn is thought to protect Dsg1 and Dsc1 against premature proteolysis. Cdsn undergoes several proteolytic steps. Cleavage of the N terminal glycine loop domain occurs first at the stratum compactum-disjunctum interface (48–46 to 36–30 kDa transition), followed by cleavage of the C terminal glycine loop domain in exfoliated corneocytes (36–30 to 15 kDa transition) [61]. The last step appears to be inhibited by calcium resulting in residual intercorneocyte cohesion. Nevertheless, the presence of oligosaccharides did not protect Cdsn against proteolysis by KLK7 [62, 63]. Duhieu et al. [64] has demonstrated that the extracellular "cores" of epidermal desmosomes contain a highly glycosylated antigen, different from desmosomal cadherins. This protein, recognized by KM48 monoclonal antibody, is likely to be involved in the processes of keratinocyte differentiation, desmosome turnover, and epidermal cohesion. The process of corneodesmosomal degradation in tape strippings of SC from human skin was shown by Rawlings et al. [11] together with the loss of the non-peripheral corneodesmosomes before the peripheral corneodesmosomes were also shown by the same group [17].

Corneodesmolysis, and ultimately desquamation, is facilitated by the action of specific hydrolytic enzymes in the stratum corneum that degrade the corneodesmosomal linkages. Currently, several cysteine and aspartic enzymes are believed to be involved in this process, namely, stratum corneum thiol protease (SCTP, now known as cathepsin L-2), the aspartic proteases cathepsin E and cathepsin D, and the skin aspartic protease [65–70]. But the ones most researched are the kallikreins, and several have now been immunologically identified within the SC (KLK5–KLK8, KLK10–KLK11, and KLK13–KLK14, where KLK5 = stratum corneum tryptic-like enzyme (SCTE) and KLK7 = stratum corneum chymotryptic-like enzyme (SCCE) [71]). Only KLK5, KLK8, and KLK14, however, are capable of degrading Dsg1 [72], but it is known that

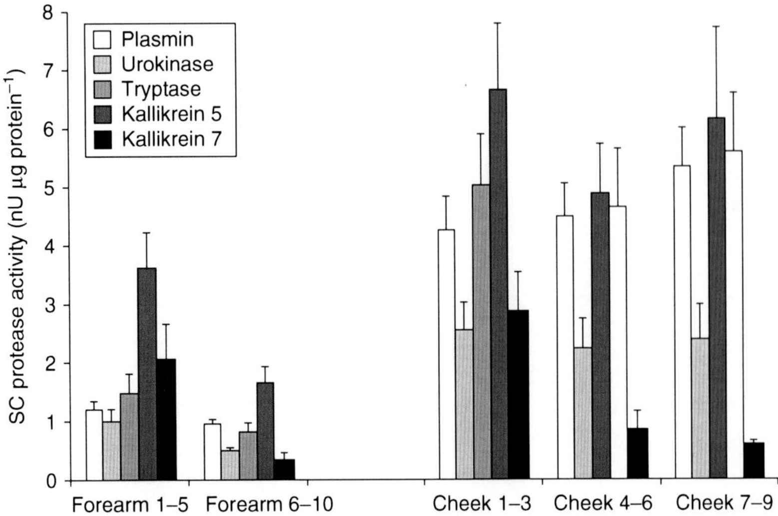

Fig. 7 Protease activity (mean ± SEM) on tape stripping pools of forearm and of cheek in function of depth of stratum corneum

KLK8 also contributes to desquamation [73]. A depth activity profile of these enzymes are reported [66, 74], but Voegeli et al. [75] recently demonstrated a premature activation of and elevated activity levels of KLK5, but not KLK7, on barrier-compromised body sites such as the face but not the forearm (Fig. 7). Elevated activity levels of plasmin, urokinase, and a newly identified SC tryptase-like enzyme were also found. An endoglycosidase, heparanase 1, has been identified within the stratum corneum, which is thought to play a role in the pre-proteolytic processing of the protecting sugar moieties on corneodesmosomal proteins [76].

Some of the desquamatory enzymes are secreted with the lamellar bodies and have been immunolocalized to the intercorneocyte lipid lamellae. Sondell et al. [77] used antibodies that immunoreact precisely with pro-KLK7 to confirm that this enzyme is transported to the stratum corneum extracellular space via lamellar bodies. In later studies, using antibodies to both pro-KLK7 and KLK7, Watkinson et al. [78] demonstrated that the processed enzyme was more associated with the corneodesmosomal plaque. More recently, Igarashi et al. [79] have immunolocalized cathepsin D to the intercellular space, whereas cathepsin E was localized within the corneocytes. Finally, KLK8 has also been reported to be localized to the intercellular spaces of the SC [80]. These enzymes, however, are transported in different lamellar granules to their inhibitor proteins.

Naturally, as some of the desquamatory enzymes are present in the intercellular space, the physical properties of the stratum corneum lipids, together with the water activity in this microenvironment, will influence the activity of these enzymes. In this respect, KLK7 appears to have a greater tolerance to water deprivation than other proteolytic enzymes, and this may be an adaptation to maintain enzyme activity even within the water-depleted stratum corneum intercellular space [81]. Of all the antiproteases found within the SC, it is now thought that only the domains of the lymphoepithelial-Kazal-type 5 inhibitor (LEKTI) of which there are at least 15 inhibitory domains that are spliced from the mature proteins via subtilisin-like enzymes and furin [82] are responsible for attenuating the activity of the kallikreins. Interestingly, the association-disassociation constants between the desquamatory proteins and these inhibitors are influenced by pH [83]. There is a strong association of the inhibitor-enzyme complexes at neutral pH, that is, as the SC is formed, and dissociation of the complexes occurs at low pH, within the outermost surface layers of the SC, where higher activities of the kallikreins are actually observed [75]. As at least pro-KLK7 is processed early in the formation of the SC and that LEKTI is secreted before the enzymes [78], presumably the inhibitors diffuse to the activated enzymes to control the later stages of desquamation. However, KLK5 is also capable of degrading LEKTI and its fragments and may in fact make them pro-inflammatory [84]. Thus, theoretically, at higher skin pHs, there should be reduced desquamation as LEKTI-protease complexes occur. This may account for the apparent reduced cohesion, but not yet relating to increased desquamation.

Like the levels of lipids, the levels of enzymes also change according to the external environment. Declercq et al. [85] have reported an adaptive response in human barrier function, where subjects living in a dry climate such as Arizona (compared with a humid climate in New York) had much stronger barrier function and less dry skin due to increased ceramide levels and desquamatory enzyme levels (KLK5 and KLK7). Reduced kallikrein activity is also reported for aged SC especially for trypsin-like enzyme activity, but not chymotrypsin-like activity (Fig. 8) [15], with KLK8 showing the greatest decline in mass levels [71].

The role of the newly identified skin aspartic protease [86] and caspase 14 [87] in this process is still awaiting clarification and also their relationship to the activities of cathepsins, kallikreins, and intracorneocytic proteases [88]. Nevertheless, it would appear that the reduced levels of trypsin-like enzymes are contributing to senile xerotic skin (photodamaged skin will be considered later).

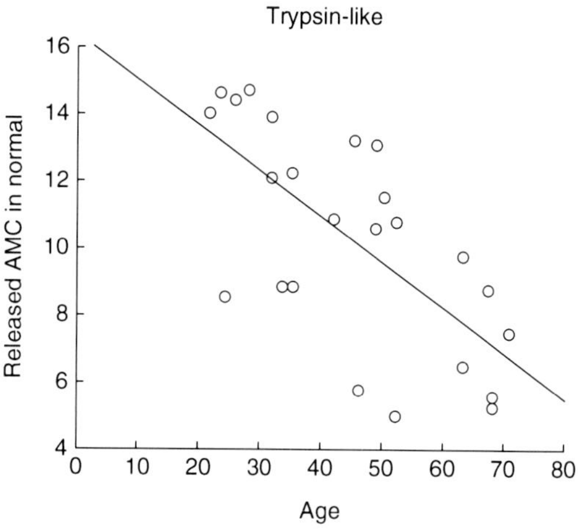

Fig. 8 Age-related reductions in the levels of stratum corneum trypsin-like activity (KLK5-like) from tape strippings of human leg (chymotrypsin-like activity showed no aging changes)

Corneocyte Envelope Maturation

The change in intercorneocyte cohesion from the inner to the outer layers of the SC is also paralleled with changes in corneocyte morphology. In examining changes in corneocytes with increasing depth [89], it was reported that there was an increased folding of the cell surface leading to a more swollen appearance in the deeper depths of the SC. The cells appeared "curled" up, fatter, and less regularly shaped with many microvillous projections. This appeared to be close or within the stratum compactum as "corneocytes were clumped together and desmosomal attachments were seen apparently undisturbed." These results suggested that there was a continuing maturation of these cells during their journey to the surface layers of the SC. Apart from corneodesmolysis and filaggrinolysis (discussed in the next section), changes to the corneocyte envelope can also occur.

The CE is an extremely insoluble cross-linked proteinaceous layered structure. Disulfide, glutamyl-lysine isodipeptide bonds, or glutamyl polyamine cross-linking of glutamine residues of several corneocyte envelope proteins occurs by the action of transglutaminases (TGase) [90]. TGase 1, 3, and 5 isoforms are thought to be involved in this process. Equally, TGase esterifies lipids to involucrin on the CE [91–94]. Serge Michel et al. [19] at CIRD further investigated the morphology and composition of CEs. When viewed by Nomarski microscopy, CEs were shown to have a crumpled surface when isolated from the lower layers of the stratum corneum, named fragile envelopes (CEf), and a smoother, more flattened surface when isolated from the

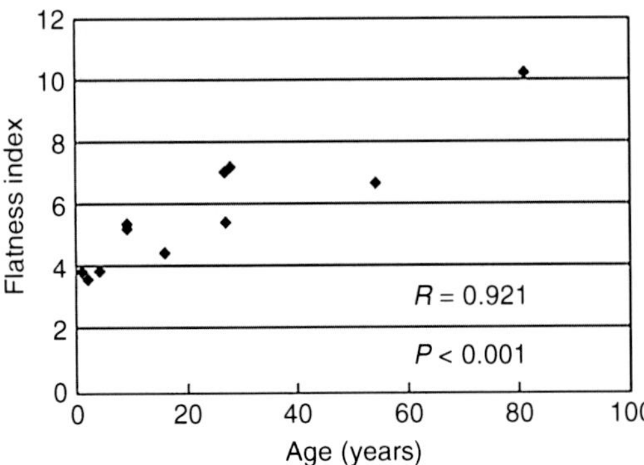

Fig. 9 Positive correlation between corneocyte flatness index and aging

upper stratum corneum rigid envelopes (CEr). This did not appear to be related to any change in the protein composition of the CE, but the authors did speculate on the effect of adding a hydrophobic layer of lipid. Mils et al. [95] reported that about 80 % of corneocytes from volar forearm skin were smooth and rigid, whereas 90 % from foot sole were rough or fragile cells. More recent work by Kashibuchi et al. [96] using atomic force microscopy confirmed these structural changes in corneocytes from the deeper layers of the stratum corneum. However, they reported that there was an age-related reduction in corneocyte thickness and an increase in corneocyte flatness index, that is, corneocytes appear to be getting thinner but longer with age (Fig. 9). This may be to countereffect the known reductions in epidermal lipid synthesis as a balancing mechanism to increase SC tortuosity and maintain "barrier" function, that is, TEWL. Nevertheless, SC function is severely compromised due to the reduced epidermal lamellar granule secretion of lipids and especially desquamatory proteases.

CEs can also be further differentiated by their binding of tetramethylrhodamine isothiocyanate (TRITC), where the rigid envelopes stain to a greater extent [97] or based upon their hydrophobicity (staining with Nile red) and antigenicity (to anti-involucrin) [20]. It is clear from these studies that immature envelopes (CEf) occur in the deeper layers of the stratum corneum (involucrin-positive and weak staining to Nile red or TRITC) and that mature envelopes occur in the surface layers of healthy skin (apparent involucrin staining lessened and increased staining with Nile red or TRITC). The classification of fragile and rigid envelopes has subsequently been found to be a pertinent classification system as, mechanically, they have fragile and rigid characteristics under compressional force. The detection of cumulative TGase-induced cross-links in the CE is an evidence for the role of these enzymes in the maturation of these cells [97] and its activation appears to coincide with filaggrinolysis, that is, above the stratum compactum.

It is also essential to consider the importance of corneocyte size in controlling skin barrier function, which seems to be underestimated. As shown by Marks, the smaller the corneocyte, the greater the TEWL [98]. In addition, recovery of barrier function after scarring is also very much dependent on changes in corneocyte size and maturation and appears to be less so for lipid changes but more characterization is needed [99]. As will be seen later, retention of immature fragile envelopes occurs in barrier-compromised conditions such as dry skin.

Stratum Corneum Natural Moisturizing Factors

Generation of natural moisturizing factors (NMF) is summarized in Fig. 10, which also highlights the importance of peptidylarginine deiminases involved in the processing of filaggrin and thereby allows its hydrolysis to NMF [100]. Under most circumstances, filaggrin is degraded to amino acids in the SC. Nevertheless, Harding and Rawlings [101] recently reported that there was a minor perturbation in filaggrin processing leading to the persistence of a high-molecular-weight filaggrin in the superficial SC. It appears that in some individuals, an imbalance in the activity of peptidyl deiminase (PAD) to general filaggrinase activity may lead to the formation of a form of filaggrin in which complete deimination (through PAD activity) by effectively depleting trypsin-sensitive protease sites (through arginine to

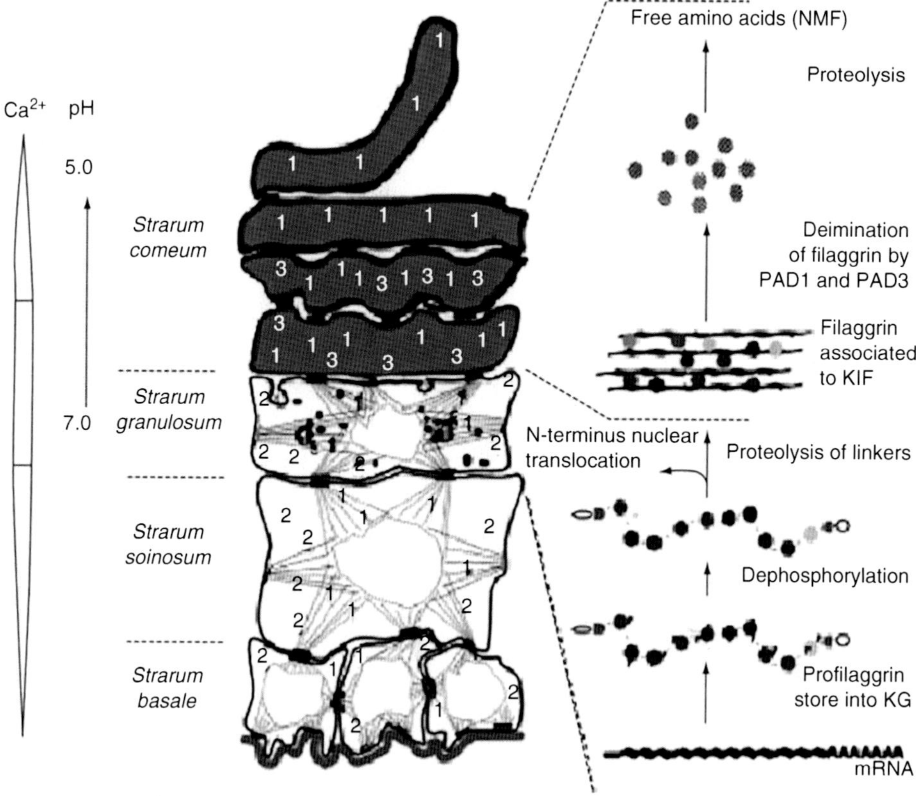

Fig. 10 Schematic representation of profilaggrin catabolism and filaggrin hydrolysis to natural moisturizing factors and activation of peptidylarginine deiminase

citrulline conversion on the filaggrin protein) renders the protein refractive to filaggrinase activity. It has previously been shown that it is the general filaggrinase activity rather than PAD activity that is sensitive to changes in external RH. Changes in filaggrin and NMF levels are expected from changes in the relative humidity the skin is exposed to. Similarly, findings were reported for the water-holding capacity and free amino acid (FAA) content of the SC. Katagiri et al. [102] demonstrated that exposure of mice to a humid environment, and subsequent transfer to a dry one, reduced skin conductance and amino acid levels even after 7 days following transfer; after transfer from a normal environment, however, decreased amino acid levels recovered within 3 days.

It is thought that NMF allows the outermost layers of the SC to retain moisture against the desiccating action of the environment. Traditionally, it was believed that this water plasticized the SC. However, it might be more complicated than this. The general mechanisms by which these NMF components influence SC functionality have been studied extensively [103]. The specific ionic interaction between keratin and NMF, accompanied by a decreased mobility of water, leads to a reduction of intermolecular forces between the keratin fibers and increased elastic behavior, and recent studies have emphasized that it is the neutral and basic free amino acids, in particular, which are important for the plasticization properties of the SC.

A general decline in NMF occurring with age was reported by Rawlings et al. [104] (Fig. 11) and Horii et al. [13]. The latter also examined the effects of xerosis. However, Jacobsen et al. [14] reported that the levels of Ser, Glu, and Gly were increased in aged subjects, whereas the levels of

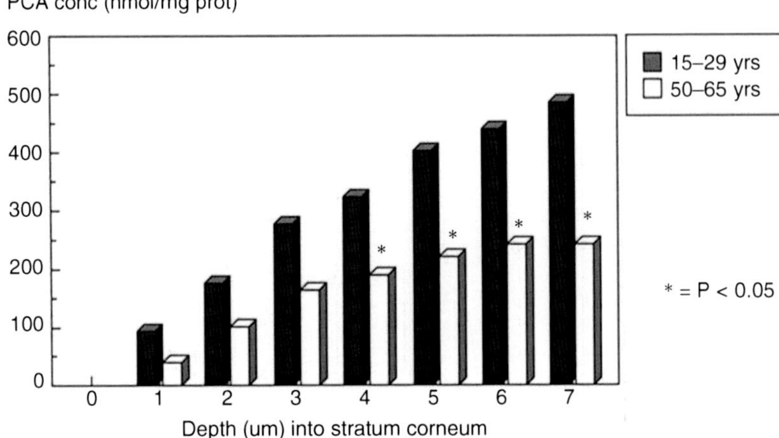

Fig. 11 Depth and age-related reduction in stratum corneum PCA levels

Leu, Phe, Lys, Trp, and Orn were decreased. Gly, Leu, Tyr, Phe, and Lys were elevated in xerotic elderly SC. There were no changes in the total levels of amino acids, but only superficial SC was examined. As shown by the studies of Horii et al. [13] and Rawlings et al. [104], greater differences between young and aged skin are found in the deeper layers of the SC.

However, a recent publication from Takashashi and Tezuka [105] have suggested that the content of FAA in the SC is actually *increased* in both senile xerosis and in "normal" aged skin compared to young. Indeed, these observations are consistent with earlier observations on the age-related increase in the levels of certain FAA primarily found in filaggrin (serine, glutamic acid, glycine) made by Jacobsen [14]. However, in both studies, they were only examining superficial SC, and relatively for the same volume of space there are more cells in old skin compared with young skin.

Hyaluronic acid and glycerol have recently been shown to be present naturally in the SC and are now considered to be part of the skins NMF [106]. Glycerol can also be derived from sebaceous triglyceride breakdown, and again, to emphasize the importance of this molecule, studies by Fluhr et al. [107] have indicated that topically applied glycerol can completely restore the poor quality of SC observed in asebic mice (that are lacking sebaceous secretions) to normal. The importance of glycerol as a natural skin moisturizing molecule has also been shown by Choi et al. [108].

An acid pH within the SC, the "acid mantle," is critical to the correct functioning of this tissue. Studies point to the essential role of free fatty acids generated through phospholipase activity as being vital for SC acidification [109], while Krein and Kermici [110] have recently proposed that urocanic acid (UCA) plays a vital role in the regulation of SC pH. Although this is in dispute, it is likely that all NMF components contribute significantly to the overall maintenance of pH.

Other components of NMF are also not derived from filaggrin, and urea, like lactate, may also be derived in part from sweat. A further understanding of the effects of lactate on SC properties has been recently described. Lactate and potassium were found to be the only components of the NMF analyzed that correlated significantly with the state of hydration, stiffness, and pH in the SC [111].

However, the presence of sugars in the SC primarily represents the activity of the enzyme beta-D-glucocerebrosidase, as it catalyzes the removal of glucose from glucosylceramides to initiate lipid lamellae organization in the deep stratum corneum.

Dry Skin

In dry, flaky skin conditions, corneodesmosomes are not degraded efficiently, and corneocytes accumulate on the skin's surface layer leading to scaling and flaking. Increased levels of

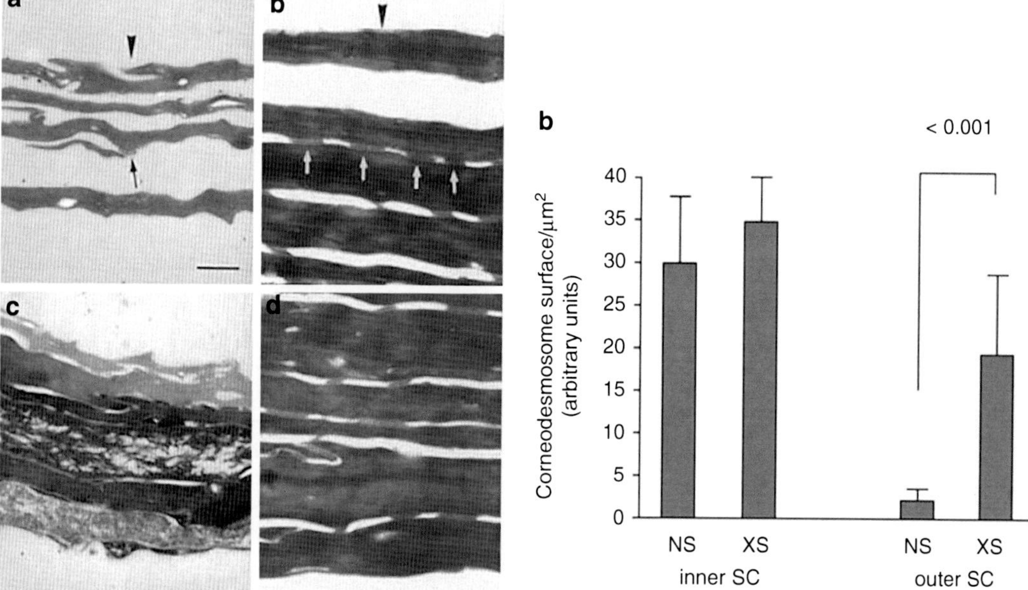

Fig. 12 (**a**) Conventional transmission electron microscopy confirms the persistence of corneodesmosomes in the outer SC of winter xerosis skin. Varnish strippings of normal (*a*, *c*) and winter xerosis (*b*, *d*) skin were analyzed by conventional transmission electron microscopy. Note that, when combined, the micrographs of normal SC correspond to the whole sample. Only part of the total height of xerosis SC, which is much thicker, is shown, however. In the outer SC of normal skin (*a*), corneocytes are loose and corneodesmosomes (*arrows*) are scarcely observed. In the outer SC of xerotic skin (*b*), corneocytes are more cohesive and corneodesmosomes are numerous. In the inner SC of both normal (*c*) and xerotic (*d*) skin, corneodesmosomes are numerous. *Arrowheads* indicate the outer surface of the samples. Scale bar: 0.5 mm. (**b**) Quantification of corneodesmosome density at the surface of corneocytes confirms the reduced degradation of the structures in the outer SC of winter xerosis skin. The corneodesmosome density (area occupied by corneodesmosomes divided by total area of the micrograph) was measured on electron micrographs of the inner SC (two micrographs per individual) and the outer SC (four micrographs per individual) of normal (NS, $n = 2$) and winter xerosis (XS, $n = 3$) skin samples. Histograms representing the mean values show similar densities of corneodesmosomes in the outer SC of xerotic and normal skin. The density of corneodesmosomes in the upper SC of xerotic skin, however, was significantly increased compared with normal skin ($p < 0.001$). Bars, standard deviations

corneodesmosomes in soap-induced dry skin were first reported by Rawlings et al. [11] but have been confirmed more recently by others [18] (Fig. 12a, b). This is consistent with the reported increase in the number of cell layers in the SC, reduced turnover time, and larger corneocytes in senile xerosis [7]. Many corneodesmosomal proteins are now also reported to be increased in the surface layers of xerotic skin [23, 71–73]. Originally, Dsg-1 [11] and Dsc-1 were reported [17]. Interestingly, however, in winter xerosis, the accumulation of the corneodemosomal proteins, Dsg 1 and plakoglobin, correlate with each other [18]. Cdsn protein levels, which were also increased, do not, however, have such an association suggesting that different proteolytic mechanisms occur for the different corneodesmosomal components during desquamation. Simon et al. [18] suggested that, as plakoglobin is a cytoplasmic protein, this would indicate that at least the cytoplasmic domain of Dsg 1 may be cleaved. Perhaps the intracellular portions of Dsg 1 are also degraded within the corneocyte (e.g., by the trypsin-like activity [88] or cathepsin E activity reported within the corneocyte matrix [79]). Conversely, Cdsn and cadherins might be degraded by

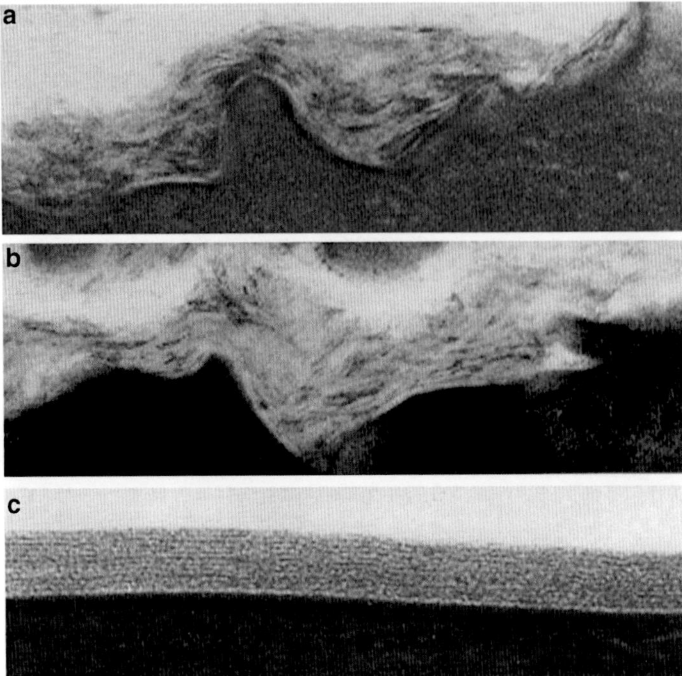

Fig. 13 Organization of stratum corneum lipids in tape stripping of subjects with winter xerosis. Transmission electron micrographs of tape strippings of individuals with severe xerosis. Perturbation in lipid organization toward the surface of the stratum corneum. (**a**) First strip: disorganized lipid lamellae. (**b**) Second strip: disorganized lipid lamellae. (**c**) Third strip: normal lipid lamellae (×200,000)

kallikreins or cathepsin D in the lamellar matrix. This is consistent with the early electron microscope images of Rawlings et al. [11] which show that corneodesmosomes become internally vacuolated, followed by detachment of the protein structures from the corneocyte envelope before their complete degradation.

The lamellar lipid matrix is also perturbed dramatically in dry skin (Fig. 13) [11]. As the main desquamatory enzymes are found within this lipid matrix, the physical properties of the lamellar lipids will, therefore, influence enzyme activity.

Reduced levels of stratum corneum KLK7 (SCCE) were originally reported by Harding et al. [16] in the outer layers of xerotic stratum corneum compared with normal skin (Fig. 14). This has been confirmed recently by others [114] who also found that the equally important stratum corneum KLK5 (SCTE) activities were also reduced.

Conversely, in SLS-induced dry skin, increased activities of these enzymes are reported

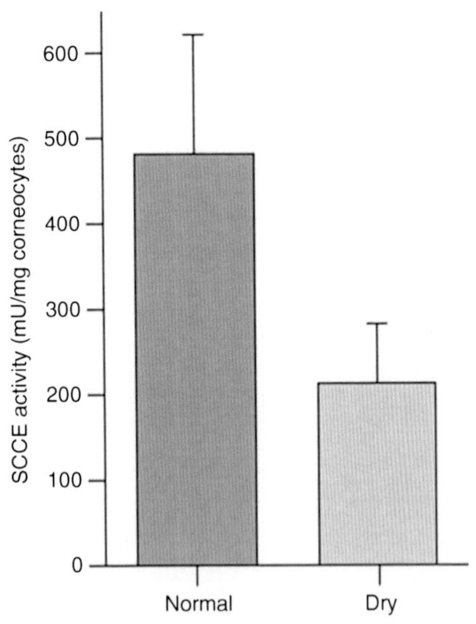

Fig. 14 Reduction in stratum corneum chymotryptic-like enzyme (SCCE) activity in tape strippings of stratum corneum from xerosis

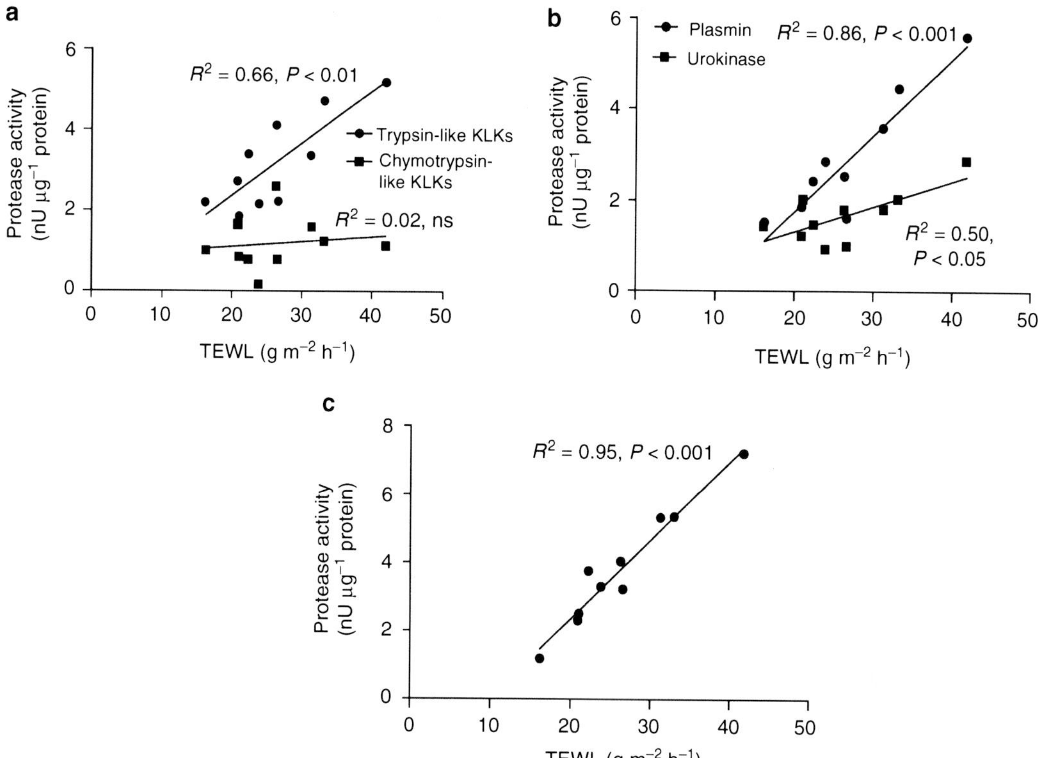

Fig. 15 (**a**) Correlation of kallikrein (KLK) activities and transepidermal water loss (TEWL): SC trypsin-like KLKs, SC chymotrypsin-like KLKs. (**b**) Correlation of inflammatory serine protease activities and TEWL: plasmin and urokinase and (**c**) correlation of SC tryptase-like activity and TEWL

[66, 75]. More recently, the overactivation of the plasminogen cascade has been associated with dry skin. Normally, being observed only in the epidermal basal layers, skin plasmin is widely distributed through the epidermis in dry skin. A urokinase-type plasminogen activator also exists in the stratum corneum [112]. These inflammatory enzymes as well as KLK5 are also increased on barrier-compromised sites such as the face and in fact show a positive correlation with TEWL (Fig. 15) [75]. Clearly, these and other enzymes are potentially involved in the inflammatory and hyperproliferative aspects of dry skin.

It is now well established that, in hyperproliferative disorders such as aged and dry skin (even in dry skin of the aged), an increase in epidermopoiesis is found relative to a younger control group and there is a change in stratum corneum lipid levels and composition. Imokawa et al. [5] first recorded the age-related decline in SC ceramides, in 1992 Rawlings et al. [113] first reported an approximately 50 % decline of ceramides in winter xerosis mainly due to their extraction from the outer layers of the SC, and in 1993 Hara et al. [7] then published the reduced levels of SC ceramides in senile xerosis. Changes in the composition of the ceramide subtypes are reported to occur with a predominance of sphingosine-containing ceramides (at the expense of the phytosphingosine-containing ceramides) observed in the SC of subjects with dry skin [114]. However, Saint-Leger et al. [115] could not find any changes in ceramide levels in dry skin, but found increased fatty acid levels. Likewise, Rawlings et al. [11, 113] demonstrated a positive correlation between xerosis and fatty acids. Conversely, Fulmer and Kramer [8] also showed that

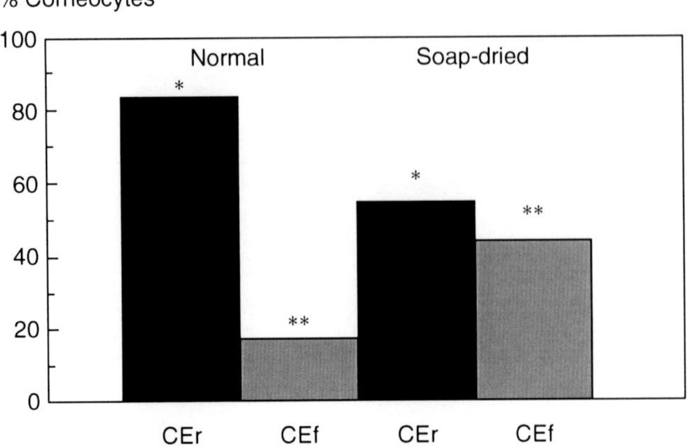

Fig. 16 Changes in the proportion of fragile (CEf) and rigid (CEr) corneocyte envelopes in normal and dry skin

longer chain fatty acid species were lost from the SC samples in their SLS-induced xerosis model versus short-chain fatty acids. Others also observed a shortening and lengthening of the acyl sphingoid bases sphingosine and 6-hydroxysphingosine, respectively, and reduced phytosphingosine-containing ceramides [116]. Imokawa et al. [5] did not find reduced ceramide levels in xerotic skin (but only total SC levels, rather than superficial levels, were measured).

These changes in lipid composition will, of course, influence the lamellar packing of the lipids and a reduction of CER EOS and EOH with increased concentrations of sphingosine-containing ceramides (CER NS and CER AS) and crystalline cholesterol in association with a loss of the LPP in dry skin [117]. However, although the lipid ultrastructure is clearly aberrant in the outer layers of dry skin [11], more work is needed to ascribe a particular lipid phase in senile dry skin.

The proportions of the different corneocyte envelope phenotypes also change in subjects with dry skin [97]. Soap washing leads to a dramatic increase in the levels of the fragile envelope phenotype at the expense of the rigid phenotype (Fig. 16). It is known that stratum corneum transglutaminase activities increase toward the surface of the stratum corneum, particularly the detergent-soluble and particulate fractions. Although the same trend of the relative increase in TGase between the inner and outer corneum is true of dry skin, TGase activities are dramatically lowered in dry skin compared with healthy skin, particularly the detergent-soluble fraction, which contains mainly TGase 1 [118].

Reduced NMF levels are also implicated in dry skin conditions [13]. However, Jacobsen et al. [14] reported relative increases in Gly, Leu, Tyr, Phe, and Lys in xerotic elderly SC. Finally, Ginger et al. [119] reported that the allelic polymorphism recognized in the profilaggrin gene may be linked to a predisposition to dry skin. The profilaggrin gene codes for a 10, 11, or 12 filaggrin repeat, and therefore an individual can be 10:10, 10:11, 11:11, 10:12, 11:11, or 12:12. Using a PCR-based approach, individual profilaggrin allelotypes were determined, and an inverse association between the 12 repeat allele and the frequency of self-perceived dry skin was identified ($n = 89, p = 0.0237$). This novel observation could not be explained by a simple reduction in NMF production and provides further circumstantial evidence for profilaggrin itself (rather than filaggrin or NMF) playing a critical role in epidermal differentiation.

Engelke et al. [120] also reported age-independent decrease of keratins K1 and K10 with an associated increase in the basal keratins K5 and K14. There was also premature expression of involucrin.

In 1987, Leveque et al. [121] reported the "biophysical characterization of dry facial skin" and pointed out that dry skin was related to a slight increase in epidermopoiesis, leading in turn to a less-stretchable stratum corneum, a physical property linked to both stratum corneum water content

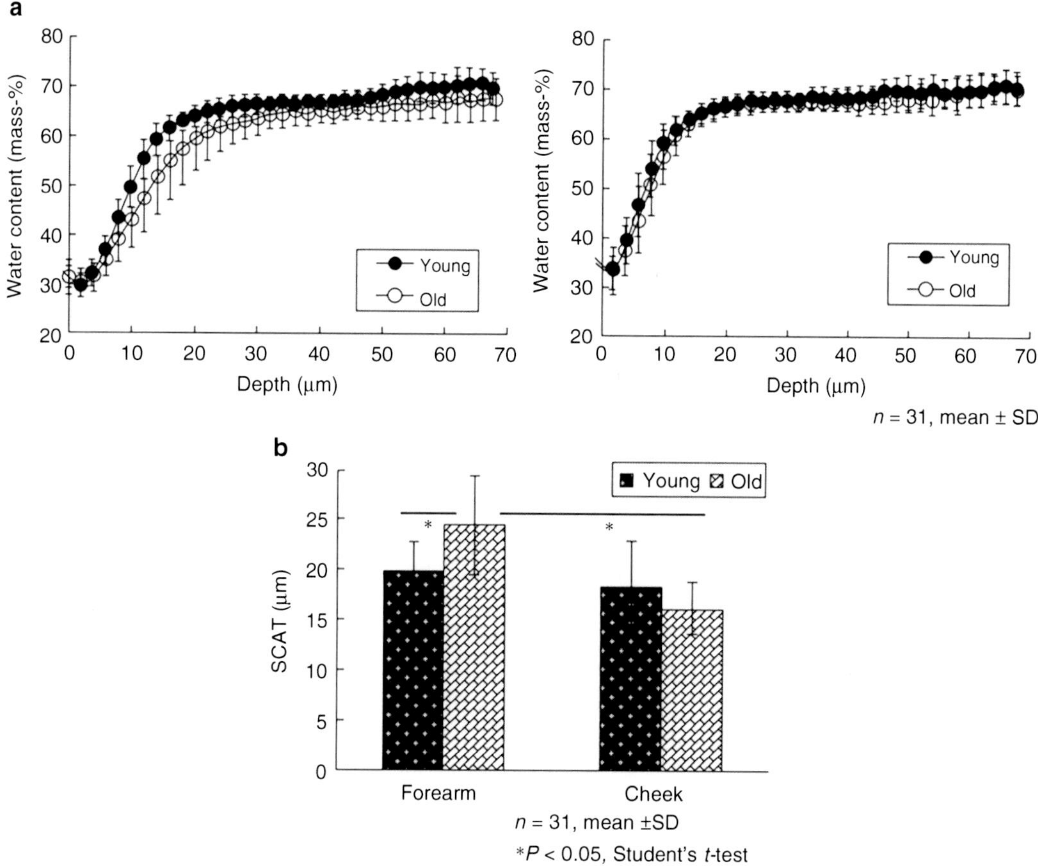

Fig. 17 (**a**) Age-dependent variations in the depth profiles of water content in the stratum corneum of the forearm (*a*) and cheek (*b*) skin. (**b**) Age-dependent changes in the stratum corneum apparent thickness (SCAT) in the forearm and cheek skin

and thickness, but it was less well correlated with impaired barrier function. Nevertheless, the differences in the SC at different body sites should also be considered. For example, Bhwan et al. [122] reported the histopathologic differences in the photoaging process in facial versus arm skin of Caucasians between the ages of 30 and 50 years. The facial skin has a greater number of granular cell layers and a higher degree of keratinocyte atypia. Equally, at the histological level, there was a greater compact SC appearance versus basket weave on the face compared to the forearm skin, which would be consistent with the reduced amount of protein that can be removed from the face by tape stripping [75] and the reduced SC thickness. Although, a reduced SCTE/KLK5 trypsin-like enzyme activity has been reported in the SC derived from calf tissue [15], due to the effects of UV on the face increased proteases may be found. This may be due to the intrinsically inferior barrier function [123] on the face where increased protease activity correlates with TEWL (except KLK7/SCCE chymotrypsin-like enzyme activity) or the direct effects of UV increasing the expression of KLK5/7, while decreasing the expression of LEKTI. Thus, the face may retain a thinner SC throughout life with the appropriate levels of desquamatory proteases, whereas senile xerosis might only occur on the body SC due to reduced proteases. This would be consistent with the work of Egawa et al. [124] showing an aged-related increase in SC thickness, as measured using in vivo confocal Raman microspectroscopy on the forearm but not on the face (Fig. 17a, b).

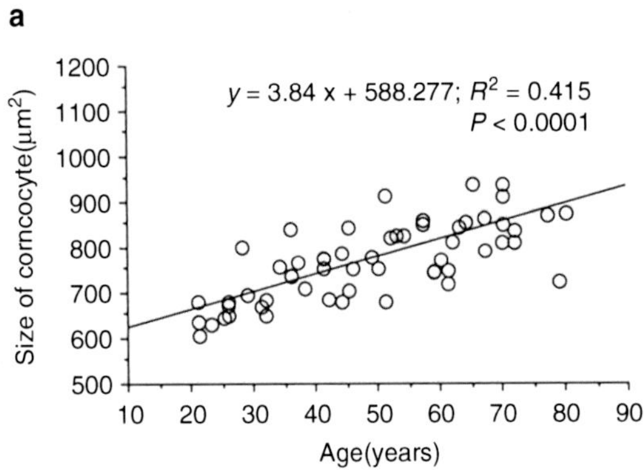

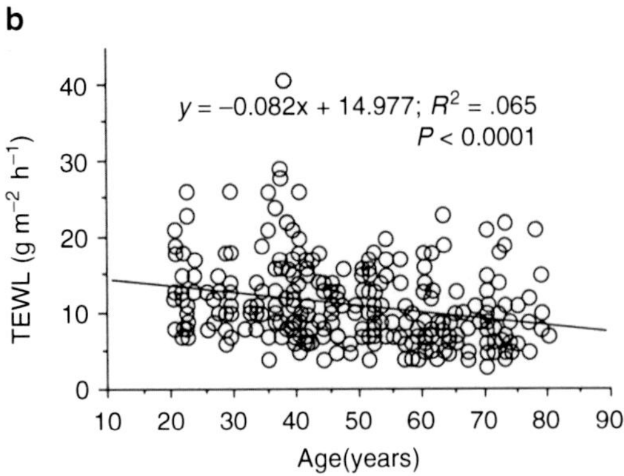

Fig. 18 (**a**) Positive correlation between corneocyte size and aging on the cheek. (**b**) Slight negative correlation with TEWL and aging on the cheek (even TEWL on older subjects, however, is significantly elevated compared to other body sites)

Nevertheless, increased proteases on the face and especially inflammatory proteases may contribute to somatosensory problems. Minimally, however, this would mean that facial skin always has a reduced barrier reserve, as coined by Cork et al. [125], throughout life, that is, the SC is always thinner and the corneocytes are always smaller on the face compared to other body sites, and although there are age-related changes in facial corneocyte size (Fig. 18a), TEWL hardly changes on the face with age unlike other body sites (Fig. 18b). Nevertheless, dry body skin is the highest unmet cosmetic body skincare need across the world [126].

Conclusion

The knowledge of SC biology especially in relation to aging has increased tremendously over the last few decades. Decreases in lipid levels especially ceramides are consistently reported even on the face. In this respect decreased CER EOS linoleate levels occur. Decreased NMF levels occur, although some report increases, which may be related to increased corneocyte size and SC thickness. Corneocytes get bigger and flatter and on non-facial body sites the SC gets thicker. Decreased KLK5/SCTE also occurs with aging on non-facial body sites, which probably contributes to the expression of senile xerosis and reduced desquamation. The increased skin surface pH and protease activity lead to reduced SC cohesion with age, but appear not to be affecting superficial desquamation positively. The increased activities of desquamatory enzymes as well as inflammatory proteases probably contribute to the maintenance of a relatively thin facial SC with elevated TEWL and reduced barrier reserve throughout all ages compared with other body sites.

Cross-References

- ► Corneocyte Size and Cell Renewal: Effects of Aging and Sex Hormones
- ► Physiological Variations During Aging
- ► Stratum Corneum Cell Layers

References

1. Kligman AM. Perspectives and problems in cutaneous gerontology. J Invest Dermatol. 1979;73:39–46.
2. Plewig G, Marples RR. Regional differences of cell sizes in the human stratum corneum. I. J Invest Dermatol. 1970;54(1):13–8.
3. Grove GL. Exfoliative cytological procedures as a nonintrusive method for dermatogerontological studies. J Invest Dermatol. 1979;73(1):67–9.
4. Marks R, Dawber RP. Skin surface biopsy: an improved technique for the examination of the horny layer. Br J Dermatol. 1971;84(2):117–23.
5. Imokawa G, Abe A, Jin Y, et al. Decreased level of ceramides in stratum corneum of atopic dermatitis: an

etiologic factor in atopic dry skin? J Invest Dermatol. 1991;96(4):523–6.
6. Denda M, Hori J, Koyama J. Stratum corneum sphingolipids and free amino acids in experimentally induced scaly skin. Arch Dermatol Res. 1992;284 (6):363–7.
7. Hara M, Kikuchi K, Watanabe M, et al. Senile xerosis: functional, morphological and biochemical studies. J Geriatr Dermatol. 1993;1:111–20.
8. Fulmer AW, Kramer GJ. Stratum corneum lipid abnormalities in surfactant induced dry scaly skin. J Invest Dermatol. 1986;86(5):598–602.
9. Rogers J, Harding CR, Mayo A, et al. Stratum corneum lipids: the effect of ageing and the seasons. Arch Dermatol Res. 1996;288:765–70.
10. Ghadially R, Brown BE, Sequeira-Martin SM, et al. The aged epidermal permeability barrier. Structural, functional, and lipid biochemical abnormalities in humans and a senescent murine model. J Clin Invest. 1995;95(5):2281–90.
11. Rawlings AV, Watkinson A, Rogers J, et al. Abnormalities in stratum corneum structure lipid composition and desmosome degradation in soap-induced winter xerosis. J Soc Cosmet Chem. 1994;45:203–20.
12. Bouwstra JA, Gooris GS, van der Spek JA, et al. Structural investigations of human stratum corneum by small-angle X-ray scattering. J Invest Dermatol. 1991;97(6):1005–12.
13. Horii I, Nakayama Y, Obata M, et al. Stratum corneum hydration and amino acid content in xerotic skin. Br J Dermatol. 1989;121(5):587–92.
14. Jacobson TM, Yüksel JC, Geesin JC, et al. Effects of aging and xerosis on the amino acid composition of human skin. J Invest Dermatol. 1990;95(3):296–300.
15. Koyama J, Nakanishi J, Masuda Y, et al. The mechanism of desquamation in the stratum corneum and its relevance to skin care. Proceedings of the 19th IFSCC Congress, Sydney, 1996.
16. Harding CR, Watkinson A, Rawlings AV. Dry skin, moisturization and corneodesmolysis. Int J Cosmet Sci. 2000;22:21–52.
17. Long S, Banks J, Watkinson A, et al. Desmocollins: a key marker for desmosome processing in stratum corneum. J Invest Dermatol. 1996;106:872.
18. Simon M, Bernard D, Minondo AM, et al. Persistence of both peripheral and non-peripheral corneodesmosomes in the upper stratum corneum of winter xerosis skin versus only peripheral in normal skin. J Invest Dermatol. 2001;116:23–30.
19. Michel S, Schmidt R, Shroot B, et al. Morphological and biochemical characterization of the cornified envelopes from human epidermal keratinocytes of different origin. J Invest Dermatol. 1988;91(1):11–5.
20. Hirao T, Denda M, Takahashi M. Identification of immature cornfield envelopes in the barrier-impaired epidermis by characterization of their hydrophobicity and antigenicities of the components. Exp Dermatol. 2001;10:35–44.
21. Marks R, Black D, Hamami I, et al. A simplified method for measurement of desquamation using dansyl chloride fluorescence. Br J Dermatol. 1984;111(3):265–70.
22. Kligman AM. The biology of the stratum corneum. In: Montagna W, Lobitz WC, editors. The epidermis. New York: Academic; 1964. p. 387–433.
23. Blank IH. Factors which influence the water content of the stratum corneum. J Invest Dermatol. 1952;18:433–40.
24. Warner RR, Lilly NA. Correlation of water content with ultrastructure in the stratum corneum. In: Elsner P, Berardesca E, Maibach HI, editors. Bioengineering of the skin: water and the stratum corneum. Boca Raton: CRC Press; 1994. p. 3–12.
25. Rawlings AV, Watkinson A, Hope J, et al. The effect of glycerol and humidity on desmosome degradation in stratum corneum. Arch Dermatol Res. 1995;287:457–64.
26. Bowser PA, White RJ. Isolation, barrier properties and lipid analysis of stratum compactum, a discrete region of the stratum corneum. Br J Dermatol. 1985;112(1):1–14.
27. Pfeiffer S, Vielhaber G, Vietzke JP, et al. High-pressure freezing provides new information on human epidermis: simultaneous protein antigen and lamellar lipid structure preservation. Study on human epidermis by cryoimmobilization. J Invest Dermatol. 2000;114(5):1030–8.
28. Norlen L. Skin barrier structure and function: the single gel phase model. J Invest Dermatol. 2001;117:830–6.
29. Bouwstra JA, de Graaff A, Gooris GS, et al. Water distribution and related morphology in human stratum corneum at different hydration levels. J Invest Dermatol. 2003;120(5):750–8.
30. Richter T, Peuckert C, Sattler M, et al. Dead but highly dynamic – the stratum corneum is divided into three hydration zones. Skin Pharmacol Physiol. 2004;17(5):246–57.
31. Downing DT, Stewart ME. Epidermal composition. In: Loden M, Maibach HI, editors. Dry skin and moisturizers chemistry and function. Boca Raton: CRC Press; 2000. p. 13–26.
32. Motta SM, Monti M, Sesana S, et al. Ceramide composition of psoriatic scale. Biochim Biophys Acta. 1993;1182:147–51.
33. Oku H, Mimura K, Tokitsu Y, et al. Biased distribution of the branched-chain fatty acids in ceramides of vernix caseosa. Lipids. 2000;35(4):373–81.
34. Chopart M, Castiel-Higounenc I, Arbey E, et al. A new type of covalently bound ceramide in human epithelium. Basel: Stratum Corneum III; 2001.
35. Hill J, Paslin D, Wertz PW. A new covalently bound ceramide from human stratum corneum-ω-hydroxyacylphytosphingosine. Int J Cosmet Sci. 2006;28(3):225–30.
36. Hamanaka S, Hara M, Nishio H, et al. Human epidermal glucosylceramides are major precursors of

stratum corneum ceramides. J Invest Dermatol. 2002;119:416–23.
37. Wertz PW, Miethke MC, Long SA, et al. The composition of the ceramides from human stratum corneum and from comedones. J Invest Dermatol. 1985;84(5):410–2.
38. Farwanah H, Pierstorff B, Schmelzer CEH, et al. Separation and mass spectrometric characterization of covalently bound ceramides using LC/APCI-MS and Nano-ESI-MS/MS. J Chromatogr. 2007;852:562–70.
39. Rawlings AV, Hinder H, Puch P, et al. Composition of human stratum corneum ceramide EOS omega-hydroxy fatty acids. IFSCC Congress, 2008.
40. Pilgram GSK, Engelsma-van Pelt AM, Bouwstra JA, et al. Electron diffraction provides new information on human stratum corneum lipid organisation studied in relation to depth and temperature. J Invest Dermatol. 1999;113:403–9.
41. Brancaleon L, Bamberg MP, Sakamaki T, et al. Attenuated total reflection-Fourier transform infrared spectroscopy as a possible method to investigate biophysical parameters of stratum corneum in vivo. J Invest Dermatol. 2001;116:380–6.
42. Bouwstra J, Pilgram G, Gooris G, et al. New aspects of the skin barrier organization. Skin Pharm Appl Skin Physiol. 2001;14:52–62.
43. Bouwstra J, Gooris GS, Dubbelaar FER, et al. Phase behaviour of stratum corneum lipid mixtures based on human ceramides: the role of natural and synthetic ceramide 1. J Invest Dermatol. 2002;118:606–17.
44. Conti A, Rogers J, Verdejo P, et al. Seasonal changes in stratum corneum ceramide one fatty acid levels and the influence of topical fatty acids. Int J Cosmet Sci. 1996;18:1–12.
45. Rawlings AV, Critchley P, Ackerman C, et al. The functional role of ceramide one in the stratum corneum. 17th IFSCC, Yokohama, Japan, 1992.
46. Oldroyd J, Critchley P, Tiddy GJT, et al. A specialized role for ceramide one in the stratum corneum water barrier. J Invest Dermatol. 1994;102:525.
47. de Jager M, Groenink W, van der Spek J, et al. Preparation and characterization of a stratum corneum substitute for in vitro percutaneous penetration studies. Biochim Biophys Acta. 2006;1758(5):636–44.
48. Meldrum H, et al. The characteristic decrease in scalp stratum corneum lipids in dandruff is reversed by use of a ZnPTO containing shampoo. IFSCC Mag. 2003;6(1):3–6.
49. Denda M, Sato J, Masuda Y, et al. Exposure to a dry environment enhances epidermal permeability barrier function. J Invest Dermatol. 1998;111:858–63.
50. Sato J, Denda M, Chang S, et al. Abrupt decreases in environmental humidity induce abnormalities in permeability barrier homeostasis. J Invest Dermatol. 2002;119:900–4.
51. Chou TC, Lin KH, Wang SM, et al. Transepidermal water loss and skin capacitance alterations among workers in an ultra-low humidity environment. Arch Dermatol Res. 2005;296:489–95.
52. Warner RR, Boissy YL. Effect of moisturizing products on the structure of lipids in the outer stratum corneum of humans. In: Loden M, Maibach HI, editors. Dry skin and moisturisers. Boca Raton: CRC Press; 2000. p. 349–72.
53. Berry N, Charmeil C, Gouion C, et al. A clinical, biometrological and ultrastructural study of xerotic skin. Int J Cosmet Sci. 1999;21:241–9.
54. Sheu HM, Chao SC, Wong TW, et al. Human skin surface lipid film: an ultrastructural study and interaction with corneocytes and intercellular lipid lamellae of the stratum corneum. Br J Dermatol. 1999;140(3):385–91.
55. Wertz PW, Downing DT. Hydroxyacid derivatives in human epidermis. Lipids. 1988;23(5):415–8.
56. Long SA, Wertz PW, Strauss JS, et al. Human stratum corneum polar lipids and desquamation. Arch Dermatol Res. 1985;277(4):284–7.
57. Chen YL, Wiedmann TS. Human stratum corneum lipids have a distorted orthorhombic packing at the surface of cohesive failure. J Invest Dermatol. 1996;107(1):15–9.
58. King CS, Barton SP, et al. The change in properties of the stratum corneum as a function of depth. Br J Dermatol. 1979;100(2):165–72.
59. Marks R, Lawson A, Nicholls S. Age-related changes in stratum corneum structure and function. In: Marks R, editor. The stratum corneum. Cardiff: Stratum Corneum Group; 1986. p. 10–5.
60. Choi EH, Man MQ, Xu P, et al. Stratum corneum acidification is impaired in moderately aged human and murine skin. J Invest Dermatol. 2007;127:2847–56.
61. Serre G, Mils V, Haftek M, et al. Identification of late differentiation antigens of human cornified epithelia, expressed in re-organized desmosomes and bound to cross-linked envelope. J Invest Dermatol. 1991;97:1061–72.
62. Simon M, Jonca N, Guerrin M, et al. Refined characterization of corneodesmosin proteolysis during terminal differentiation of human epidermis and its relationship to desquamation. J Biol Chem. 2001;276:20292–9.
63. Caubet C, et al. Degradation of corneodesmosome proteins by two serine proteases of the kallikrein family. J Invest Dermatol. 2004;122:1235–44.
64. Duhieu S, Laperdrix C, Hashimoto T, et al. Desmosome-binding antibody KM48 recognises an extracellular antigen different from desmosomal cadherins Dsg 1-3 and Dsc 1-3. Eur J Dermatol. 2006;15(2):80–4.
65. Lundstörm A, Egelud T. Cell shedding from human plantar skin in vitro: evidence that two different types of protein structures are degraded by a chymotrypsin-like enzyme. Arch Dermatol Res. 1990;282:234–7.
66. Suzuki Y, Nomura J, Koyama J, et al. The role of proteases in stratum corneum: involvement in stratum

corneum desquamation. Arch Dermatol Res. 1994;286:249–53.
67. Horikoshi T, Igarashi S, Uchiwa H, et al. Role of endogenous cathepsin D-like and chymotrypsin-like proteolysis in human epidermal desquamation. Br J Dermatol. 1999;141:453–9.
68. Horikoshi T, Arany I, Rajaraman S, et al. Isoforms of cathepsin D human epidermal differentiation. Biochimie. 1998;80:605–12.
69. Watkinson A. Stratum corneum thiol protease (SCTP): a novel cysteine protease of late epidermal differentiation. Arch Dermatol Res. 1999;291:260–8.
70. Bernard D, et al. Analysis of proteins with caseinolytic activity in a human SC extract revealed a yet unidentified cysteine protease and identified the so called "SC thiol protease" as Cathepsin L2. J Invest Dermatol. 2003;120:592–600.
71. Komatsu N, Saijoh K, Sidiropoulos M, et al. Quantification of human tissue kallikreins in the stratum corneum: dependence on age and gender. J Invest Dermatol. 2005;125:1182–9.
72. Borgoño CA, Michael IP, Komatsu N, et al. A potential role for multiple tissue kallikrein serine proteases in epidermal desquamation. J Biol Chem. 2007;282 (6):640–52.
73. Kishibe M, Bando Y, Terayama R, et al. Kallikrein 8 is involved in skin desquamation in cooperation with other kallikreins. J Biol Chem. 2007;282 (8):5834–41.
74. Suzuki Y, Nomura J, Hori J, et al. Detection and characterization of endogenous protease associated with desquamation of stratum corneum. Arch Dermatol Res. 1994;285:372–7.
75. Voegeli R, Rawlings AV, Doppler S, et al. Profiling of serine protease activities in human stratum corneum and detection of a stratum corneum tryptase-like enzyme. Int J Cosmet Sci. 2007;29:191–200.
76. Bernard D, Mehul B, Delattre C, et al. Purification and characterization of the endoglycosidase heparanase 1 from human plantar stratum corneum: a key enzyme in epidermal physiology. J Invest Dermatol. 2001;117:1266–73.
77. Sondell B, Thornell LE, Stigbrand T, et al. Immunolocalization of SCCE in human skin. Histo Cyto. 1994;42:459–65.
78. Watkinson A, Smith C, Coan P, et al. The role of Pro-SCCE and SCCE in desquamation. 21st IFSCC Congress, Berlin; 2000. p. 16–25.
79. Igarashi S, Takizawa T, Yasuda Y, et al. Cathepsin D, and not cathepsin E, degrades desmosomes during epidermal desquamation. Br J Dermatol. 2004;151:355–61.
80. Ishida-Yamamoto I, et al. Epidermal lamellar granules transport different cargoes as distinct aggregates. J Invest Dermatol. 2004;122:1145–53.
81. Watkinson A, Harding C, Moore A, et al. Water modulation of stratum corneum chymotryptic enzyme activity and desquamation. Arch Dermatol Res. 2001;293:470–6.
82. Komatsu N, Takata M, Otsuki N, et al. Elevated stratum corneum hydrolytic activity in Netherton syndrome suggests an inhibitory regulation of desquamation by SPINK5-derived peptides. J Invest Dermatol. 2002;118:436–43.
83. Deraison C, Bonnart C, Lopez F, et al. LEKTI fragments specifically inhibit KLK5, KLK7, and KLK14 and control desquamation through a pH-dependent interaction. Mol Biol Cell. 2007;18(9):3607–19.
84. Yamasaki K, Di Nardo A, Bardan A, et al. Increased serine protease activity and cathelicidin promotes skin inflammation in rosacea. Nat Med. 2007;13 (8):975–80.
85. Declercq L, Muizzuddin N, Hellemans L, et al. Adaptation response in human skin barrier to a hot and dry environment. J Invest Dermatol. 2002;119:716.
86. Bernard D, Méhul B, Thomas-Collignon A, et al. Identification and characterization of a novel retroviral-like aspartic protease specifically expressed in human epidermis. J Invest Dermatol. 2005;125 (2):278–87.
87. Fischer H, Stichenwirth M, Dockal M, et al. Stratum corneum-derived caspase-14 is catalytically active. FEBS Lett. 2004;577(3):446–50.
88. Watkinson A, Smith C, Rawlings AV. The identification and localization of tryptic and chymotryptic-like enzymes in human stratum corneum. J Invest Dermatol. 1994;102:637.
89. King CS, Nicholls S, Barton S, et al. Is the stratum corneum of uninvolved psoriatic skin abnormal? Acta Dermatol Venereol Suppl (Stockh). 1979;59 (85):95–100.
90. Watkinson A, Harding CR, Rawlings AV. The cornified envelope: its role on stratum corneum structure and maturation. In: Leyden JJ, Rawlings AV, editors. Skin moisturization. New York: Marcel Dekker; 2002. p. 95–117.
91. Candi E, et al. Transglutaminase cross linking properties of the small proline rich 1 family of cornified envelope proteins. J Biol Chem. 1999;274:7226–37.
92. Kim IG, Gorman JJ, et al. The deduced sequence of the novel protransglutaminase-E (TGase 3) of human and Mouse. J Biol Chem. 1993;268:12682–90.
93. Nemes Z, Marekov LN, Steinert PM. Involucrin cross linking by transglutaminase 1. J Biol Chem. 1999;274:11013–21.
94. Cabral A, Voskamp P, Cleton-Jansen M, et al. Structural organisation and regulation of the small proline rich family of cornified envelope precursors suggest a role in adaptive barrier function. J Biol Chem. 2001;26:19231–7.
95. Mils A, Vincent C, Croute F, et al. The expression of desmosomal and corneodesmosomal antigens shows specific variations during the terminal differentiation of epidermis and hair follicle epithelia. J Histochem Cytochem. 1992;40:1329–37.
96. Kashibuchi N, Hirai Y, O'Goshi K, et al. Three-dimensional analyses of individual corneocytes with

atomic force microscope: morphological changes related to age, location and to the pathologic skin conditions. Skin Res Technol. 2002;8:203–11.
97. Harding CR, Long S, Richardson J, et al. The cornified cell envelope: an important marker of stratum corneum maturation in healthy and dry skin. Int J Cosmet Sci. 2003;25:1–11.
98. Marks R, Nicolls S, King CS. Studies on isolated corneocytes. Int J Cosmet Sci. 1981;3:251–8.
99. Kunii T, Hirao H, Kikuchi K, et al. Stratum corneum lipid profile and maturation pattern of corneocytes in the outermost layer of fresh scars: the presence of immature corneocytes plays a much more important role in the barrier dysfunction than do changes in intercellular lipids. Br J Dermatol. 2003;149 (4):749–56.
100. Mechin MC, Enji M, Nachat R, et al. The peptidylarginine deiminases expressed in human epidermis differ in their substrate specificities and subcellular locations. CMLS DO1 2005;1–12.
101. Harding CR, Rawlings AV. Dry skin and moisturizers. In: Loden M, Maibach H, editors. Dry skin and moisturizers. Boca Raton: CRC Press; 2006. p. 187–209. Chapter 18.
102. Katagiri C, Sato J, Nomura J, et al. Changes in environmental humidity affect the water-holding property of the stratum corneum and its free amino acid content, and the expression of filaggrin in the epidermis of hairless mice. J Dermatol Sci. 2003;31(1):29–35.
103. Jokura Y, et al. Molecular analysis of elastic properties of the stratum corneum by solid-state C-13-nuclear magnetic resonance spectroscopy. J Invest Dermatol. 1995;104:806.
104. Rawlings AV, Scott IR, Harding CR, et al. Stratum corneum moisturization at the molecular level. J Invest Dermatol. 1994;103:731–40.
105. Takahashi M, Tezuka T. The content of free amino acids in the stratum corneum is increased in senile xerosis. Arch Dermatol Res. 2004;295(10):448–52.
106. Sakai S, et al. Hyaluronan exists in the normal stratum corneum. J Invest Dermatol. 2000;114:1184.
107. Fluhr JW, et al. Glycerol regulates stratum corneum hydration in sebaceous gland deficient (Asebia) mice. J Invest Dermatol. 2003;120:728.
108. Choi EH, Man MQ, Wang F, et al. Is endogenous glycerol a determinant of stratum corneum hydration in humans. J Invest Dermatol. 2005;125:288–93.
109. Fluhr JW, et al. Generation of free fatty acids from phospholipids regulates stratum corneum acidification and integrity. J Invest Dermatol. 2001;117:44.
110. Krein PM, Kermici M. Evidence for the existence of a self-regulated enzymatic process within the human stratum corneum- an unexpected role for urocanic acid. J Invest Dermatol. 2000;115:414.
111. Nakagawa N, et al. Relationship between NMF (potassium and lactate) content and the physical properties of the stratum corneum in healthy subjects. J Invest Dermatol. 2004;122:755.
112. Katsura Y, Yoshida Y, Kawai E, et al. Urokinase-type plasminogen activator is activated in stratum corneum after barrier disruption. J Dermatol Sci. 2003;32:55–7.
113. Rawlings AV, Hope J, Rogers J, et al. Mechanisms of desquamation: new insights into dry flaky skin conditions. Proceedings of the 17th IFSCC; 1992, vol. 2, p. 865–880.
114. Van Overloop L, Declercq L, Maes D. Visual scaling of human skin correlates to decreased ceramide levels and decreased stratum corneum protease activity. J Invest Dermatol. 2001;117:811.
115. Saint-Leger D, Francois AM, Leveque JL, et al. Stratum corneum lipids in skin xerosis. Dermatologica. 1989;178:151–5.
116. Chopart M, Castiel-Higounenc C, Arbey E, et al. Quantitative analysis of ceramides in stratum corneum of normal and dry skin. Stratum Corneum III; 2001.
117. Schreiner V, Gooris GS, Pfeiffer S, et al. Barrier characteristics of different human skin types investigated with x-ray diffraction, lipid analysis and electron microscopy imaging. J Invest Dermatol. 2000;114:654–60.
118. Harding CR, Richardson J, Ginger R, et al. Role of transglutaminase in the continued cross linking of cornified envelope protein during stratum corneum maturation. 22nd IFSCC Congress; 2002. p. 139.
119. Ginger RS, Blachford S, Rowland J, et al. Filaggrin repeat number polymorphism is associated with a dry skin phenotype. Arch Dermatol Res. 2005;297 (6):235–41.
120. Engelke M, Jensen JM, Ekanayake-Mudiyanselage S, et al. Effects of xerosis and ageing on epidermal proliferation and differentiation. Br J Dermatol. 1997;137(2):219–25.
121. Leveque JL, Grove G, de Rigal J, et al. Biophysical characterization of dry facial skin. J Soc Cosmet Chem. 1987;82:171–7.
122. Bhawan J, Oh CH, Lew R, et al. Histopathologic differences in the photoaging process in facial versus arm skin. Am J Dermatopathol. 1992;14(3):224–30.
123. Egawa M, Tagami H. Comparison of the depth profiles of water and water-binding substances in the stratum corneum determined in vivo by Raman spectroscopy between the cheek and volar forearm skin: effects of age, seasonal changes and artificial forced hydration. Br J Dermatol. 2008;158(2):251–60.
124. Voegeli R, Rawlings AV, Doppler S, et al. Increased basal transepidermal water loss leads to elevation of some but not all stratum corneum serine proteases. Int J Cosmet Sci. 2008;30(6):435–42.
125. Cork MJ, Robinson DA, Vasilopoulos Y, et al. New perspectives on epidermal barrier dysfunction in atopic dermatitis: gene-environment interactions. J Allergy Clin Immunol. 2006;118(1):3–21. quiz 22-23.
126. Matts PJ, Gray J, Rawlings AV. The "Dry Skin Cycle" – a new model of dry skin and mechanisms for intervention, International Congress and Symposium Series. London: The Royal Society of Medicine Press Ltd; 2005. p. 1–38.

The Extracellular Matrix Protein 1 (ECM1) in Molecular-Based Skin Biology

8

Noritaka Oyama and Joseph Merregaert

Contents

N. Oyama (✉)
Dermatology and Dermato-Allergology, Matsuda General Hospital, Ohno, Fukui, Japan

Department of Dermatology, Fukui University, Fukui, Japan
e-mail: norider@wine.plala.or.jp

J. Merregaert
Laboratory of Molecular Biotechnology, Department of Biomedical Sciences, University of Antwerp, Antwerp, Belgium
e-mail: joseph.merregaert@ua.ac.be

M.A. Farage et al. (eds.), *Textbook of Aging Skin*,
DOI 10.1007/978-3-662-47398-6_8

Abstract

Extracellular matrix protein 1 (ECM1) is an 85-kDa secreted glycoprotein that plays a pivotal role in the structural and homeostatic biology of the skin, particularly in the proliferation and differentiation of epidermal keratinocytes, reconstitution of basement membrane, angiogenesis, malignant transformation, and aging. The multifocal interaction of ECM1 with various extracellular matrix and structural molecules is substantiated by loss-of-function mutations in the *ECM1* gene in an autosomal recessive genodermatosis lipoid proteinosis and circulating IgG autoantibodies to this molecule in a humoral autoimmune condition lichen sclerosus, both of which are now recognized as an immunogenetic disease counterpart sharing comparable skin pathology. A series of underlying insights for the in vivo ECM1 biology, as a binding core and/or a scaffolding protein, arose not only for wide-ranged differentiation properties of the epidermal keratinocytes, acquisition of immune tolerance and allergic responses via particular T cell subsets such as CD4+ CD25+ regulatory T cells and Th2 cells, and various cancers but also from intrinsic and extrinsic aging of the skin.

Introduction

Historical Background: Characterization and Structural Diversity of the *ECM1* Gene and Its Transcripts

The extracellular matrix protein 1 (ECM1) was first identified in 1994 as a novel 85-kDa glycosylated protein secreted in the conditioned medium of the murine osteogenic stromal cell line MN7 [1]. It was discovered amidst various connective tissue proteins including collagens, osteonectin, osteopontin, cathepsins, and bone sialoprotein and was therefore named ECM1, although its potential relevance to extracellular matrix physiology was not immediately apparent. The mouse *Ecm1* gene has been further characterized by cloning and sequencing of its cDNA, analysis of the expression pattern, and genomic localization [2]. The 5-kb-long *Ecm1* gene maps to chromosome 3 and encodes for two distinct splice variants: a complete cDNA clone *Ecm1a*, with an open reading frame of 1,677 bp that encodes for a protein of 559 amino acids (aa) (11-exon gene), and a shorter alternatively spliced *Ecm1b* (lacking exon 8) mRNA of 1.5 kb, coding for a protein of 434 aa [2, 3]. Thereafter, the human *ECM1* gene was isolated in 1997 and mapped to chromosome 1q21.2 [4, 5]. The comparison in the plane structure between mouse and human *ECM1* genes reveals that the human gene contains one exon less than the mouse gene, that is, the sequence homologous to the sixth and shortest mouse exon [4]. The 5′-upstream regulatory sequences of the mouse *Ecm1* gene contain putative binding sites for some major transcription factors, such as GATA, Sp1, AP-1, and ETS family members [3]. These binding motifs are highly conserved with the equivalent portion of the human *ECM1* gene. Of these, the potential binding sites for AP-1 and Sp1 are perfectly conserved, while those for ETS differ in only one nucleotide between both species, with the human sequence conforming even better to the consensus sequence for this transcription factor family. In contrast, the potential GATA-binding sites are not conserved between human and murine *ECM1* genes and are therefore considered functionless in the former [3]. The human *ECM1* gene encodes for four splice variants: the full-length transcript ECM1a (1.8 kb, 540 aa), which is widely expressed in the vast majority of organs, such as the liver, small intestines, lung, ovary, prostate, testis, skeletal muscle, pancreas, kidney, placenta, heart, basal keratinocytes, dermal blood vessels, sebaceous lobules, and adnexal epithelia including the outer root sheath of hair follicles and sweat gland epithelium [3, 4, 6–8]; ECM1b (1.4 kb, 415 aa), which lacks exon 7, has an extremely restricted expression in tonsils and the spinous and granular layers of the epidermis [9]; ECM1c (1.85 kb, 559 aa), which has an extra exon 5a within intron 5, is expressed in the epidermal basal layer [8, 9]; and ECM1d, the fourth splice variant, with an out-of-frame insertion of

71 nucleotides at the 5′ end of exon 2, results in a truncated protein of 57 aa for which the biological relevance is still unclear [10].

The Protein Structure of ECM1

The ECM1 protein has abundant cysteine residues (4.8 %) with a specific distribution according to the CC-(X_{7-10})-C pattern of six cysteine doublets [2]. This characteristic cysteine arrangement, which is also found in serum albumin and sea urchin Endo16 protein, may determine the formation of double-loop structures, specifying putative, important biological protein-protein interactions. ECM1 comprises five different regions: a 19-aa signal sequence for extracellular secretion, an NH_2-terminal cysteine-free domain that is rich in prolines and glutamines, two tandem repeats, and a COOH-terminal region [2, 4] (Fig. 1a). ECM1a contains three double-loop domains, one present in each of the two central tandem repeats and the other in the COOH-terminal domain. It has been hypothesized that the tandem repeat structure allows the ECM1 protein to function as a biotransporter or to be involved in binding of/with various regulatory factor(s) [2]. The three cysteine-rich domains (within two tandem repeats and COOH-terminus) are the most conserved among species; the human pattern is 75 % identical to that of the mouse, whereas the overall identity between the two species reaches 69.4 %. This indicates that the unique arrangement of cysteine residues is critical in maintaining the in vivo structural stability of ECM1. More recently, a rudimentary three-dimensional model was predicted using the third human serum albumin domain as template [11] and divided ECM1a into four distinct domains: an NH_2-terminal domain forming probably α-helical structures (αD1, aa20–aa176), followed by three domains, whose amino acid sequences were highly comparable with the third domain of human serum albumin [*S*erum *A*lbumin *S*ubdomain *L*ike 2 (SASDL2), aa177–aa283; SASDL3, aa284–aa431; and SASDL4, aa432–aa540] [11] (Fig. 1b). More specifically, the last three domains contain a number of typical C-CC-C motifs, which enable to form disulfide bonds, sharing putative double loops. It is possible that these motifs also give rise to "fingerlike" structures, which provide the fatty acid-binding clefts in serum albumin [12]. This characteristic configuration of ECM1a is well conserved between species [2, 4] and also between the splice variants ECM1a–ECM1c, emphasizing the importance of the overall structure and its putative significance in protein-protein interaction of ECM1.

Furthermore, a striking observation for the biological importance of the SASDL subdomains in protein interaction is supported by loss-of-function mutations in the *ECM1* gene as the cause of a rare autosomal recessive genodermatosis lipoid proteinosis (LiP), also known as hyalinosis cutis et mucosae or Urbach-Wiethe disease (OMIM 247100) [13, 14] (see section "Lessons from Lipoid Proteinosis and Lichen Sclerosus in Skin Aging"). Most of the pathogenic mutations in LiP are nonsense or out-of-frame changes and occur frequently within exon 6 and the alternatively spliced exon 7 of *ECM1* [15, 16], coding for SASDL2 and a part of the SASDL3 (Fig. 1c). ECM1 has three putative N-glycosylation sites: Asn354, Asn444, and Asn530 which exist within exon 7 and COOH-terminal domain. Of these three, the two sites Asn354 and Asn444 are N-glycosylated as identified by mass spectrometry analysis. In addition, N-linked glycan at Asn354 negatively regulated secretion of ECM1 in contrast to two LiP patient-derived mutants (Q276X and W359X). Combining the evidence that the three N-glycosylation sites of ECM1 are mostly removed by the upstream mutations in LiP patients (Fig. 1c), therefore, the defect of N-glycosylation is not involved in the aberration of secretion of LiP-derived ECM1 mutants. Although ECM1 has a putative C-mannosylation site at Trp359, this site is not mannosylated by mass spectrometry. On the other hand, ECM1 is O-glycosylated at Ser525 and/or Thr254. The role of O-glycosylation on ECM1 function and its relation to the LiP pathogenesis is not known [17]. The posttranscriptional modification of ECM1 and its interaction with other binding partners (see section "Binding Partners of ECM1") now warrant to be further elucidated.

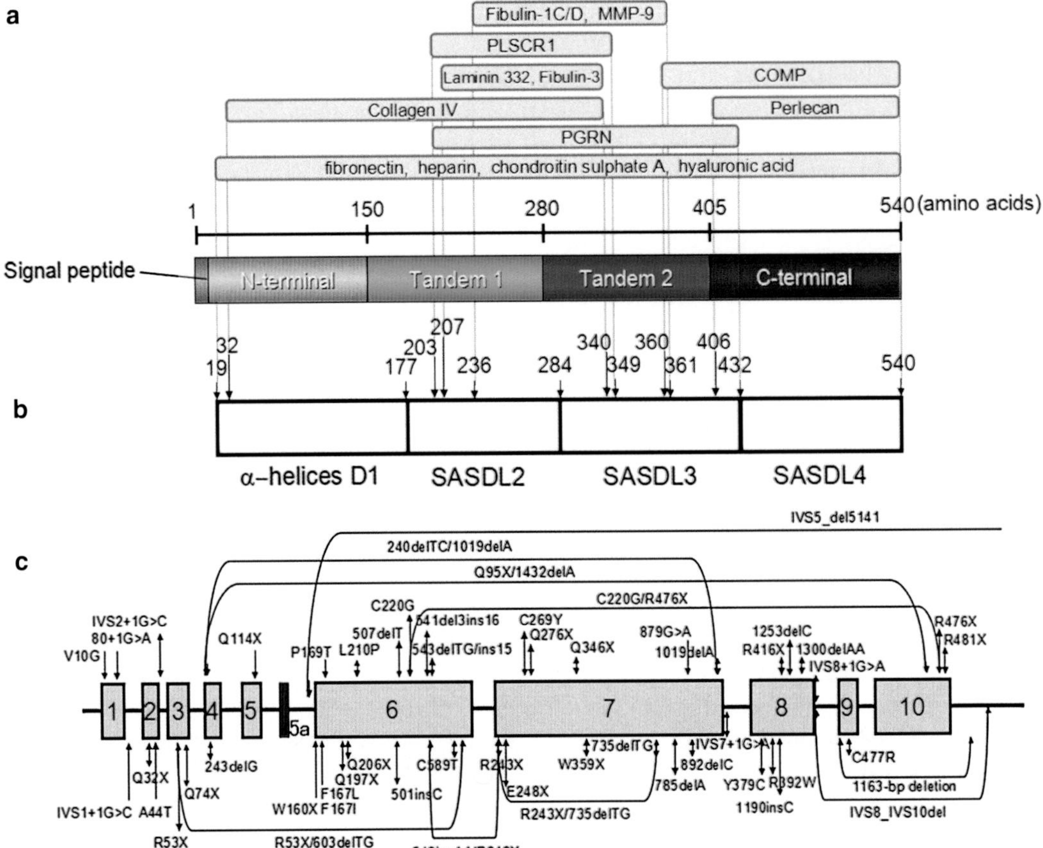

Fig. 1 Gene and domain organization of the human ECM1 and its binding partners. (**a**) Site-specific binding of ECM1a protein to different structural and ECM1 molecules in the skin. A series of in vitro and in vivo binding studies revealed the biological interaction of ECM1 with the following proteins and polysaccharides at different binding sites; perlecan (aa406–aa540 of ECM1a) [8], fibulin-1C/fibulin-1D and MMP-9 (aa236–aa361) [20, 24], type IV collagen (aa32–aa340) [24], laminin 332 and fibulin-3 (aa207–aa340) [11, 24], PLSCR1 (aa203–aa349) [39], PGRN (aa203–aa432) [41, Kong and Liu, unpublished results], and COMP (aa360–aa540) [33]. The binding of the full-length ECM1a with fibronectin, heparin, chondroitin sulfate A, and hyaluronic acid has also been demonstrated [24], but their exact binding sites within ECM1a remained uncharacterized. ECM1a is capable of enhancing the binding of type IV collagen and laminin 332 [24]. (**b**) A predicted secondary structure and its corresponding domains of ECM1a protein. The full-length ECM1a contains a 19-amino acid residue signal peptide and the following four distinct domains: an N-terminal cysteine-free domain, two tandem repeat domains, and a COOH-terminal domain. The latter three domains contain the characteristic cysteine arrangement CC-(X7–10)-C patterns [2, 4], typically observed in the albumin protein family members. This pattern generates double-loop structures that are involved in the protein-protein interactions. The first domain exists of α-helices (αD1), and the remaining three domains are comparable topologically with the subdomain of the third serum albumin domain, named SASDL2, SASDL3, and SASDL4 [11]. The amino acid numbers corresponding with a mature ECM1a precursor protein were indicated. The SASDL2+ region was used to screen a foreskin cDNA library by Yeast two hybridization (Y2H), instrumental in the identification of fibulin-3, laminin 332, and PLSCR1 as putative ECM1-binding partners [11, 24]. (**c**) Schematic representation of human ECM1 gene structure and most updated mutations in LiP patients. *ECM1* gene consists of 10 exons (*boxes*) and alternative introns (*horizontal lines*). All the pathogenic ECM1 mutations thus far reported were depicted [96–105]. The homozygous mutations were indicated as *double arrows*. Note that more than a half of all nonsense and frameshift mutations are located within exon 6 and alternatively spliced exon 7 (Adapted from Oyama and Merregaert [96])

Binding Partners of ECM1

Perlecan

Perlecan is a major heparan sulfate proteoglycan that is involved in the binding and cross-linking with the basement membrane and interstitial dermal components, such as laminins, fibronectin, type IV collagen, fibulin-2, and heparin [18, 19]. The COOH-terminus of ECM1 has been shown to bind specifically with epidermal growth factor-like modules flanking the LG2 subdomain of perlecan domain V [8] (Fig. 1a). These multifocal interactions may play a role in the extracellular matrix assembly around the dermal-epidermal junction and adnexal epithelia in the dermis, as imaged immunohistologically by co-expression of perlecan and ECM1 [8].

MMP-9

Matrix metalloproteinase (MMP)-9 is a proteolytic enzyme, which has a catalytic activity against several extracellular matrix components. The tandem repeat domains of ECM1 can bind with MMP-9 in vitro (Fig. 1a), resulting in a negative regulatory effect on the enzymatic activity, as assessed by a gelatin-based ELISA [20]. In MMP-9 knockout mice, lack of the enzymatic activity reduces the neuronal degeneration evoked by either brain trauma or ischemia, and therefore, MMP-9 is considered an intrinsic factor for the development of epilepsy and neuropsychiatric symptoms, as being similar extracutaneous manifestations in LiP patients [15, 21].

Fibulin-1C,Fibulin-1D and Fibulin-3

Domain III of fibulin-1C/fibulin-1D is capable of binding with the second tandem repeat of ECM1 [22] (Fig. 1a), while fibulin-3 interacts with ECM1 through its SASDL2 domain with a low affinity [11]. Fibulin-1 and fibulin-3 are extracellular matrix protein family members, participating in embryonic development, wound repair, and carcinogenesis. Fibulin-1 is ubiquitously expressed in the basement membrane components of many organs, including the skin. Based on the immunohistochemical data demonstrating the colocalization of fibulin-3 and ECM1, the in vivo binding of both proteins is currently considered to be restricted to the boundary between basal and suprabasal layers in the epidermis [11]. Recently, an angiogenic action of fibulin-3 has been suggested by inhibition of endothelial cell proliferation, invasion, and angiogenic sprouting, as well as the p38 MAPK activation in vascular endothelial growth factor (VEGF)-stimulated endothelial cells [23].

Fibronectin, Laminin 332, and Type IV Collagen

ECM1 can bind to fibronectin, type IV collagen, and laminin 332 (formerly designated as laminin 5) [11, 24]. The SASDL2 domain and the NH_2-terminal portion of ECM1a interact with laminin β3 chain and collagen IV, respectively [11] (Fig. 1a, b). Laminin 332 is a large heterotrimeric glycoprotein consisting of three distinct chains (α3, β3, and γ2) and is a major hemidesmosomal component of the skin basement membrane, bridging between the lamina lucida and lamina densa. It functions as a ligand for α3β1 and α6β4 integrins to regulate adhesion, migration, and morphogenesis of basal keratinocytes. Laminin 332 is broadly expressed in the skin and most other epithelia and plays tissue- and cell-specific roles in the regulation of tumors derived from different tissues [25]. The downregulation of laminin 332 may contribute to the structural failure in forming anchoring filaments and hemidesmosomes, resulting in disturbance of the structural stability in the epithelial-stromal junction, possibly allowing a local invasion of tumor cells into the adjacent tissues. Mutations of laminin 332 (*LAMA3*, *B3*, *or C2*) gene have been known to cause junctional epidermolysis bullosa (OMIM 226650), a lethal and/or incurable blistering genodermatosis [26]. In contrast, circulating autoantibodies against laminin 332 also cause an immuno-bullous disease, mucous membrane pemphigoid, that primarily affects mucous

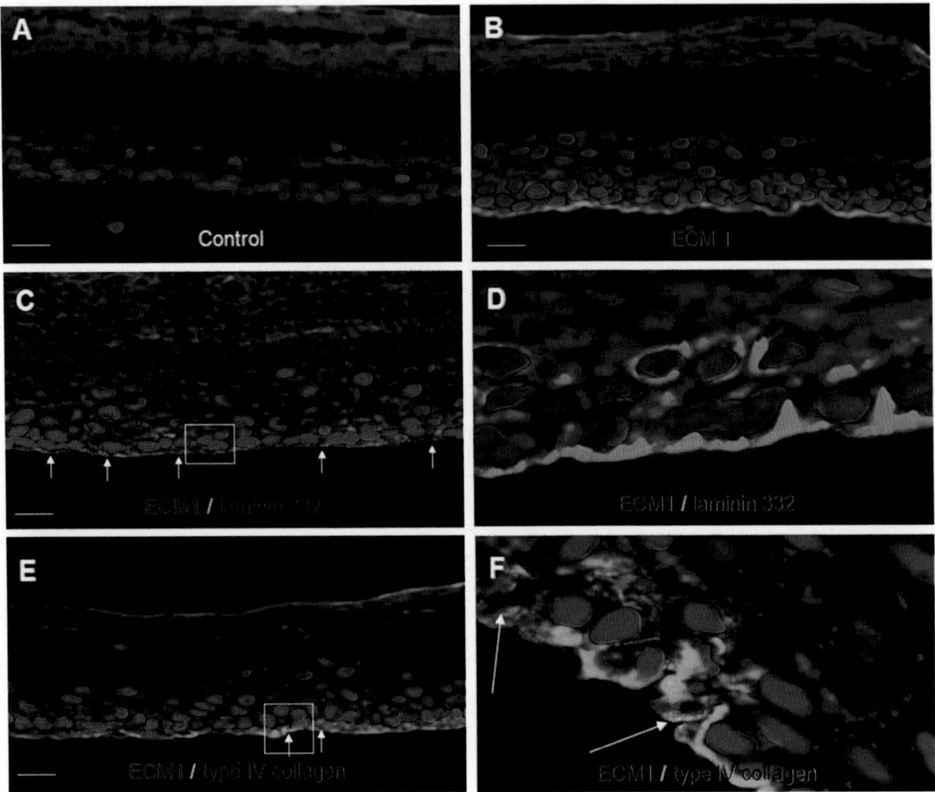

Fig. 2 Colocalization of ECM1 with laminin 332 and collagen type IV in the basal layer of the epidermis. Two-week-old air-exposed organotypic keratinocyte monocultures (**a**), or cocultures (**b–d**), were stained for antibodies against ECM1 (OAP 12516) [24]. Note the colocalization signals (*orange*, *arrows*) of ECM1 (*green*) and laminin 332 (*red*) or type IV collagen (*red*) in the basal cell layer. Scale bar, 50 μm (From Sercu et al. [24])

membranes leading to a scarring phenotype [27]. These findings indicate that laminin 332 plays a vital role in the epidermal-dermal assembly [28]. In situ studies also support the possible in vivo interrelationship between collagen IV and laminin 332 [24]. ECM1 co-localized with collagen IV and laminin 332, as well as perlecan, suggests that ECM1 is exclusively involved in part of two independent suprastructure networks, containing either laminin 332 or collagen IV, at the basal lamina (Fig. 2). Interestingly, in vitro binding experiments have revealed that laminin 332 interacts with collagen IV and that ECM1a is able to enhance this interaction, revealing its involvement in the dermal-epidermal junction [24]. Recently, the recruitment of type IV collagen into the laminin 111-bound extracellular matrices has shown to be mediated through a nidogen bridge, albeit a lesser contribution arising from a direct interaction with laminin 111 [29]. Since collagen IV is linked to laminin 332 through ECM1, which binds to the former two proteins and facilitates their interaction, it is possible that ECM1 functions as a bridging core that stabilizes collagen IV and laminin 332, thereby structurally connecting them to each other in the skin basement membrane presumably via a complex formation between these three molecules.

Cartilage Oligomeric Matrix Protein (COMP)

COMP is a 524-kDa pentameric, disulfide-bonded glycoprotein that represents a prominent non-collagenous component of cartilage extracellular matrix. It is expressed in the tendon, bone (osteoblasts only), and synovium [30, 31].

Mutations in the human *COMP* gene cause the development of pseudoachondroplasia and multiple epiphyseal dysplasia, autosomal dominant forms of short-limb dwarfism characterized by short stature, normal facies, epiphyseal abnormalities, and early onset osteoarthritis [32], thus implicating the pivotal roles of COMP in osteochondrogenesis and matrix mineralization. COMP can bind with a part of the second tandem repeat and COOH-terminus of ECM1 [33] (Fig. 1a).

Phospholipid Scramblase 1 (PLSCR1)

Scramblase is a protein responsible for the translocation of phospholipids between the two monolayers of a lipid bilayer of a cell membrane [34]. In humans, phospholipid scramblases (PLSCRs) constitute a family of five homologous proteins named as hPLSCR1–5. PLSCR1 is an endofacial plasma membrane protein believed to carry out the calcium-dependent nonspecific and bidirectional movement ("scrambling") of phospholipids across the plasma membrane, contributing to cell proliferation/differentiation and apoptosis via direct interaction with epidermal growth factor (EGF), platelet-derived growth factor (PDGF), fibroblast growth factor (FGF7), vascular endothelial growth factor (VEGF), and caspase [35–38]. PLSCR1 can bind with two tandem repeats of ECM1 (Fig. 1a), consisting of SASDL2 and three domains that are frequently affected by the pathogenic mutations in LiP patients (Fig. 1c) [39].

Progranulin Chondrogenic Growth Factor (PGRN)

PGRN is a chondrocyte inductive growth factor and plays a critical role in chondrogenesis during development [40, 41]. ECM1 and PGRN were isolated as binding partners of COMP in a functional genetic screen [33, 41]. Furthermore, ECM1 bound to PGRN in a dose-dependent manner as demonstrated through a solid-phase binding assay and identified the specific domain of ECM1 required for binding to PGRN as aa203–aa432 (Fig. 1a).

Carbohydrates

ECM1-carbohydrate interactions were established through in vitro binding experiments with hyaluronic acid (HA), chondroitin sulfate (CSA), and heparin (Fig. 1a). It is based on the dose-dependent binding of ECM1a to these immobilized extracellular components and the competitive inhibition of this specific binding with unbound equivalents [24].

Biological Functions of ECM1

The biological function of ECM1 has yet to be fully elucidated, but indications for its involvement in important biophysiological processes, including chondrogenesis, skin differentiation and aging, angiogenesis, T cell-dependent allergic reaction, ureteric bud patterning and branching, and various malignancies, have now emerged the following multipotent actions.

Role of ECM1 in Chondrogenesis

The first indication of a putative role of ECM1 in chondrogenesis was provided by Deckers and coworkers [42]. Exogenously added human recombinant ECM1a protein inhibited both alkaline phosphatase activity and mineralization in a dose-dependent manner of mouse embryonic metatarsals in vitro [42]. Therefore, it was proposed that ECM1 is a negative regulator for chondrogenesis. These observations have recently been confirmed by comprehensive in vitro, ex vivo, and in vivo evidences demonstrating that ECM1 acts as a downstream molecule of the PTHrP/AP2 pathway and negatively regulates chondrogenesis through direct interaction and interplay with the cartilage oligomeric matrix protein (COMP) [33, 43] and the progranulin chondrogenic growth factor (PGRN) (see section "Progranulin Chondrogenic Growth Factor

(PGRN)"; Drs. Kong and Liu, personal communication). In conclusion, ECM1, PGRN, and COMP constitute to an interaction network and act in concert in regulating chondrogenesis.

Role of ECM1 in the Dermal-Epidermal Communication

Extracellular matrix molecules, like ECM1, play an important role in fundamental skin biology, such as keratinocyte adhesion and signaling, epidermal differentiation and/or maturation, vascular formation, and in the dermis via extracellular matrix formation.

ECM1a/ECM1c expression has been recently found not only in the epidermal basal layer but also in the network-like suprastructures of the skin basement membrane, containing laminin 332 and collagen type IV [24] (Fig. 2). The structure has an important function in tightly linking the epidermis to the underlying dermis and providing a biological interface to abrupt migration and loss of polarity of the keratinocytes and dermal component cells, such as fibroblasts and endothelial cells, vice versa. Once the basement membrane is assembled, stratification of the epidermis proceeds, with the proliferating cells attached to the basement membrane and the daughter cells migrating into the upper layers. These biological actions in the dermal-epidermal junction have been emphasized by the binding ability of ECM1 with structural and extracellular matrix molecules of the basement membrane zone. ECM1 is capable of binding with laminin 332 and collagen IV, and importantly it also accelerates the direct binding between laminin 332 and collagen IV themselves [24]. Considering the binding activity with a variety of molecules (see section "Binding Partners of ECM1"), ECM1 was suggested to act as a "biological glue" to maintain the structural and biological integrity of the skin basement membrane [16].

On this basis, ECM1 can be a multifunctional binding core and/or a scaffolding protein by its promiscuous interaction with a variety of extracellular and structural proteins, thereby contributing to the maintenance of skin integrity and homeostasis [24]. Hence, the disruption of the ECM1 function may cause the failure of multi-communication among the surrounding skin structural and interstitial molecules, resulting in the torsion of lamina lucida/densa [44] and lamellar or punctuated structures below the basement membrane, accompanied by excess deposition of collagen IV and laminin 332, perlecan, and MMP-9 catalysis-associated extracellular matrixes around the thickening blood vessel walls [44, 45] and disorganization of type VII collagen [44], a major constituent of anchoring fibril for the skin basement membrane, as seen in LiP and LS skin pathology (Fig. 4).

Role of ECM1 in Keratinocyte Differentiation

Preliminary implication opens the functional importance of ECM1 in epidermal differentiation, because the human *ECM1* gene maps to a region on chromosome 1q21.2 centromeric to the gene cluster termed epidermal differentiation complex (EDC) [4, 5]. As assessed by the early (keratin 10) and late markers (involucrin) of epidermal differentiation [9], the full-length *ECM1a* transcript is expressed in cultures of normal human keratinocytes irrespective of their differentiation states, whereas the expression of the alternatively spliced *ECM1b* transcript is restricted exclusively to keratinocyte cultures undergoing late phase of differentiation. This observation is in line with the result from in situ hybridization of isoform-specific *ECM1* mRNA; *ECM1*a mRNA is expressed throughout the epidermis, with the intense expression in the basal and suprabasal layers but much lower expression in the spinous and granular cell layers, while *ECM1*b mRNA is present from suprabasal to granular cell layers [9]. However, in vitro experiments using ECM1a-/ECM1c-deficient (pathogenic mutations outside exon 7) and ECM1b-deficient (pathogenic mutations within exon 7) cultured keratinocytes from LiP patients showed no significant differences in the expression of early and late epidermal differentiation markers, compared with normal human keratinocytes [46]. Moreover, mice overexpressing ECM1a at the basal (keratin 14 promoter-driven) and suprabasal layers (involucrin promoter-driven) have revealed no morphological and histological changes in the skin, comparable with those of wild-type mice. These data indicate that the in vivo ECM1 function can be dispensable or otherwise at least compensable for early and terminal differentiation of keratinocytes in a steady-state condition.

Phorbol ester 12-*O*-tetradecanoylphorbol-13-acetate (TPA), which can efficiently induce terminal differentiation of keratinocytes in vitro, is a potent inducer of *ECM1b* mRNA [9]. TPA also activates the protein kinase C (PKC) signaling pathway that accelerates cell density-induced differentiation of keratinocytes. Of note, the PKC pathway leads, via activation of MAP kinase cascade, to the gene activation of transcription factors AP-1 and/or the ETS family members, whose functional binding motifs are present in the mouse *ECM1* promoter region [3]. Since the activation of these transcription factors by stimulation of the PKC pathway, either by increased cell density or TPA, is most probably responsible not only for the increased expression of *ECM1a* but also that of *ECM1b* in the TPA-stimulated keratinocyte cultures, the PKC pathway might result in the induction or activation of a differentiation-dependent splicing isoform of the *ECM1* gene.

Instead of the ECM1 isoform-dependent differentiation processes in the skin, differences in the expression pattern between ECM1a and ECM1b may affect more structural functions. The ECM1a protein contains a typical CC-(X_{7-10})-C arrangement, which might be responsible for the generation of "double-loop" domains characteristic for the ligand binding [2]. Full-length ECM1a has three serum albumin subdomains, while ECM1b contains only two of the three subdomains [11]. The splicing out of one serum albumin subdomain in ECM1b may explore different binding region(s), which are capable of binding with extracellular matrix molecules other than ECM1a, finally contributing to the structural integrity and proper differentiation (i.e., polarized stratification, keratohyalinization, etc.) of the suprabasal layers of the epidermis. Furthermore, the induction and upregulation of *ECM1b* RNA expression are dependent on the terminal differentiation capacity of the keratinocytes [9]. ECM1b may thus participate in the overall differentiation process in vivo.

Role of ECM1 in Angiogenesis and Vascular Formation

Addition of recombinant human ECM1a/ECM1b has shown to stimulate the proliferation of cultured endothelial cells and promotes the formation of blood vessels in the chorioallantoic membrane of chicken embryos [47]. Since ECM1 is capable of binding with domain V of perlecan (endorepellin) [8] (Fig. 1a and section "Binding Partners of ECM1"), an angiogenesis inhibitor, it is possible that the binding of ECM1 with endorepellin inhibits the anti-angiogenic function of this protein. Another cascade for the angiogenic activity is that ECM1 inhibits the interaction with perlecan, tumstatin, and transforming growth factor (TGF)-β via the inhibition of the proteolytic function of matrix metalloproteinase 9 (MMP-9), leading to a decrease in the local release of these molecules into the skin interstitial matrix [20] and acceleration of tumor growth.

The skin pathology of patients with LiP and LS, both of which genetically and immunologically target ECM1, respectively, shows lack of normal capillary loop network in the upper dermis and abrupt enlargement of the dermal blood vessels [48]. The enlarged vessels are also surrounded by abundant lamellar deposits of type IV collagen-positive material, suggesting that ECM1 contributes to the maintenance of the structural tonus and permeability, via local collagen IV metabolism, in the dermal microvasculature (Figs. 3 and 4).

Role of ECM1 in T Cell-Dependent Allergic Response

DNA microarray assays have disclosed the expression of *ECM1* gene in mouse hematopoietic cells, particularly in T cells [49, 50], although the transcription levels considerably differ in

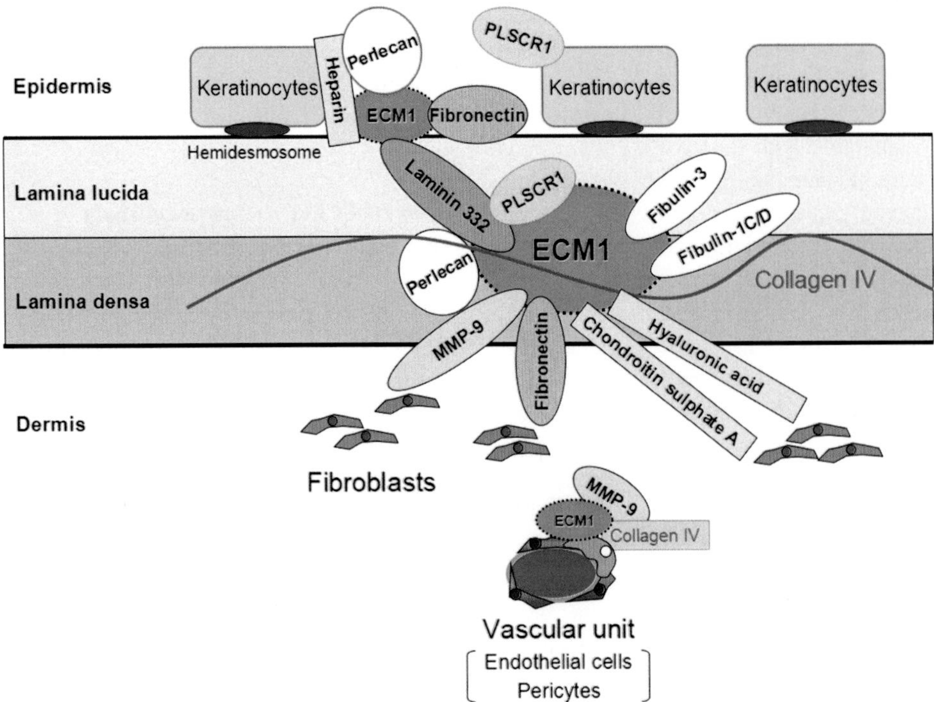

Fig. 3 Summary of the different binding partners of ECM1 in the dermal-epidermal junction. ECM1 binds to a variety of structural and extracellular matrix molecules, forming the stratified epidermis, hemidesmosome, and dermal components in the skin. Most of these molecules are secreted by keratinocytes and fibroblasts, as well as endothelial cells. Laminin 332, fibulin-1, and type IV collagen specifically localize in the basement membrane and dermal blood vessel walls. Major interstitial dermal proteins and polysaccharides contain fibronectin, chondroitin sulfate A, and hyaluronic acid, all of which can bind to ECM1 with different affinities [24]. MMP-9, a proteolytic enzyme for type IV collagen, is capable of binding to ECM1 directly [20], although this specific binding downregulates the enzymatic activity. ECM1 can act as a "biological glue" in the whole basic framework and physical flexibility and stability in the human skin. The remaining proteins that are thought to be currently uninvolved in the ECM1 interactions (i.e., bullous pemphigoid antigens I and II, integrins, etc.) have been omitted

differentiation- and cell lineage-dependent manner; it was much higher in CD4+ helper T cells and CD4+ CD25+ T cells (Tregs) but relatively lower in CD8+ cytotoxic T cells and CD3-negative naïve T cells. Among CD4+ helper T cells, the ECM1 expression was almost restricted to the Th2 cells [51], implicating the possible association between ECM1 and allergic reaction. This was supported by the finding that chimeric BALB/c mice transplanted with *ECM1*-deficient bone marrow cells showed a decrease of inflammatory response in experimentally induced airway allergy, a histology showing fewer infiltration of eosinophils, lymphocytes, and macrophages in the bronchoalveolar lavage [51]. Compared with wild-type mice, the activated CD4+ Th2 cells of *ECM1* chimeric mice, but not other T cell populations including Th1, Th9, Th17, CD8+ T cells, and inducible regulatory T cells (Tregs), were specifically retained in the peripheral lymphoid organs and did not migrate into the inflammatory sites. Functional assays for several T cell lineages from *ECM1* knockout mice exhibited no substantial differences in the proliferation activity, cytokine/chemokine profiles, and polarization of their differentiation, suggesting the direct action of ECM1 in Th2 cell trafficking from lymph nodes into the circulation [51].

In Th2 cells, ECM1 mRNA and protein expression were detectable at 3 days after antigen-dependent engagement of T cell receptor.

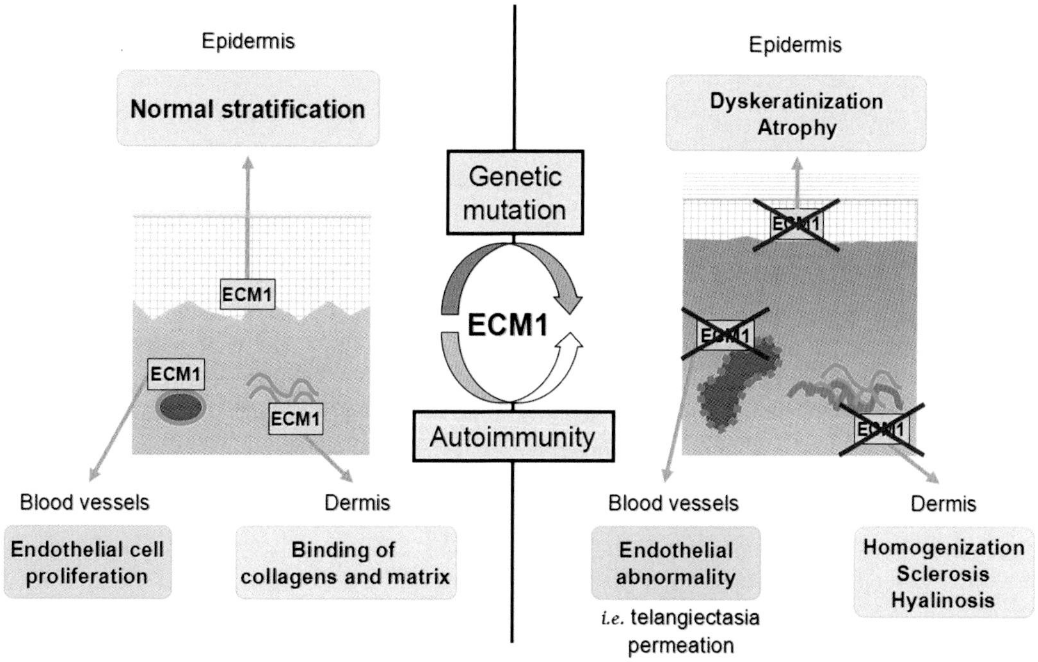

Fig. 4 Localization of ECM1 protein in the human skin and presumable histological changes relevant to in vivo ECM1 damage. ECM1 is ubiquitously expressed in most of the skin components, including the whole living layers of the epidermis (ECM1a/ECM1c in the basal layer and ECM1b in the suprabasal layers), and blood vessel walls and interstitial collagens in the dermis, thus contributing to the overall skin homeostasis. Impairment of ECM1 function, which is caused by genetic ablation (LiP) or autoimmunity (LS), may collapse the multiple assembly with the surrounding skin structural and interstitial molecules, resulting in the clinicopathology characteristics for LiP and LS: hyperkeratosis and atrophy of the epidermis, disruption and duplication of the basement membrane, excess deposition of type IV collagen, perlecan, laminins, and extracellular matrixes around the thickening blood vessel walls with telangiectasia and hyaline changes in the dermis [44, 48, 85, 87]

Subsequently, ECM1 can bind with IL-2 receptor subunit (CD122), but neither with CD25 nor CD132, to inhibit the phosphorylation and activation of the downstream signaling molecules, such as STAT5, KLF2, and S1P1 [51], resulting in the downregulation of Th2 cell trafficking to the local inflammatory sites. On the other hand, both freshly isolated and activated CD4+ CD25+ Tregs have been confirmed to express higher levels of ECM1 transcript [49]. CD4+ CD25+ Tregs are well known to regulate innate and adaptive immune responses, an effective tumor immunity to autologous tumor cells, and a potent anti-inflammatory capacity in autoimmune and chronic inflammatory diseases, such as autoimmune encephalitis, diabetes, thyroiditis, IBDs, and contact skin hypersensitivity [52–56]. Naturally occurring Tregs, the other Treg phenotype, which comprise up to 5 % of the peripheral CD4+ T cell pool, have also shown to express ECM1 [52]. More critically, the ECM1 transcription was significantly increased in naïve T cells by transient transduction of forkhead box P3 (FOXP3), a transcription factor that acts as a master control molecule for the development and function of CD4+ CD25+ Tregs in the thymus and periphery [57].

Role of ECM1 in Carcinogenesis and Tumor Progression

Various types of malignant cell lineages in human express at least any of the three ECM1 variants, ECM1a–ECM1c. In vitro and histochemical studies have revealed the overexpression of ECM1 transcripts and/or protein in osteosarcoma Saos-2 cells [4], squamous carcinoma A431 cells, fibrosarcoma HT1080 cells [8], HaCaT keratinocytes

[39], chondrogenic ATDC5 cells [43], cholangiocarcinoma cells [58], hepatocellular carcinoma cells [59], bone-metastasized lung adenocarcinoma SPCA-1BM cells [60], estrogen receptor-positive breast cancer MCF-7 cells, estrogen receptor-negative bone-metastasized breast cancer MDA-MB-231/MDA-MB-435 cells, Hs578T cells, LCC15 cells [47, 61, 62], embryonic kidney 293 cells [63], and pancreatic cancer SW1990 cells and Capan-2 cells [64]. Altogether, these evidences suggest that ECM1 has an essential role in the vast majority of cell sources, as well as the development and maintenance of malignant potential.

ECM1 expression is a marker for tumorigenesis and is correlated with invasiveness and metastatic potential in various cancers [65–67]. The functional role of ECM1 is still unclear. However, recently two studies by Lee and coworkers contributed significantly to elucidate the role of ECM1 in oncogenic cell signaling in breast cancer. First, they demonstrated that ECM1 regulates breast cell proliferation through its physical interaction with the epidermal growth factor receptor (EGFR) followed by the activation of the Extracellular signal-regulated kinase (ERK) signaling at the transcriptional level leading to EGFR and HER3 protein stabilization. Moreover, ECM1-induced galectin-3 cleavage through the upregulation of MMP-9 not only improved mucin-1 expression but also increased EGFR and human epidermal growth factor 3 protein stability as a secondary signaling [68]. In a follow-up study [69], Lee and coworkers revealed that ECM1 regulates tumor metastasis through the stabilization of beta-catenin. The association between beta-catenin and the mucin-1 cytoplasmic tail was increased by ECM1, enabling mucin to block the degradation of beta-catenin and the nuclear accumulation of beta-catenin [70]. Furthermore, forced expression of beta-catenin altered the gene expression that potentiated epithelial to mesenchymal transition (EMT) and cancer stem cell (CSC) maintenance. Thus, ECM1 may influence the EMT and thus the metastatic potential of breast tumor cells. This is in accordance with reported correlations of ECM1 expression with metastasis in laryngeal carcinoma [71, 72] and cholangiocarcinoma [58]. In addition, ECM1-induced EGF signaling affects also cancer cell metabolism, e.g., the Warburg effect, an oncogenic switch that allows cancer cells to take up more glucose than normal cells and favors anaerobic glycolysis. Indeed, EGF-mediated activation of the EGFR/ERK pathway is linked to the phosphorylation of pyruvate kinase M2 (PKM2) at Ser 37 and induces the expression of HIF-1α, GLUT1, and LDHA. These findings provide evidence that ECM1 plays an important role in promoting the Warburg effect [73].

As far as hepatocellular carcinoma (HCC) is concerned, the underlying HCC development remains poorly understood. Recently, an integrated analysis of DNA methylation and hydroxymethylation identified ECM1 as a candidate tumor suppressor gene, which was confirmed via siRNA experiments to have potentiated anticancer function [74].

Upon the recent wide-genome screening, however, *ECM1* gene loci have yet to be formally associated with any types of primary internal cancers [75], and LiP patients (an ECM1-deficient human model) have no predilection for skin and internal malignancies. The less association between ECM1 and genetic susceptibility for tumor development has yet to be fully characterized [15].

Lessons from Lipoid Proteinosis and Lichen Sclerosus in Skin Aging

Skin aging is an inevitable progressive deterioration of various physiological functions, which are principally divided into intrinsic (chronological) and extrinsic (photo) aging, although the latter is mostly superimposed on the intrinsic mode. The intrinsic aging is slowly progressive occurring in the entire body skin, a morphological feature showing fine shallow wrinkles, lack of elasticity and tensile strength, and hypochromic surface. The skin pathology shows thinner (atrophic) epidermis with degeneration of the underlying connective tissues. These changes are substantiated by reduced expression of extracellular matrix molecules, such as interstitial collagens, elastin, fibulins, and glycosaminoglycans, further accelerated by enhanced release of matrix-degrading metalloproteases and the resultant decrease of extracellular matrices and elastin, fibrillin-1 [76–79]. In contrast, the skin photoaging shows coarse deep wrinkles with yellow-brownish surface, abrupt keratinization and pigmentation, and telangiectasia. Pathologically, it shows irregularly thickened (acanthotic) and atrophic epidermis with loss of keratinocyte polarity and dysregulation of melanocyte density and, more significantly, dermal elastolysis caused by repeated degeneration and production of collagen/elastic fibers and excess deposition of glycosaminoglycans [76, 80–82]. Thus, the skin aging pathology is closely associated with an imbalance of the biological network of extracellular matrix molecules and collagens, being similar to those in LiP patients. From the clinical perspective, warty keratotic and atrophic appearance of the LiP lesional skin is more unlikely to be a direct consequence of deficient ECM1 function but may also result from chronic exposure with extrinsic factors, such as mechanical stress, temperature, dry, or UV [83, 84].

Lipoid Proteinosis as a Human Disease Model for Skin Aging

The skin is the best approachable organ for investigating both intrinsic (i.e., chronogenic) and extrinsic (i.e., photoinduced) aging. Particularly, certain human diseases regarding premature skin aging may simply provide insight for better understanding of intrinsic and extrinsic aging properties. One plausible disease candidate is LiP, an ECM1 knockout human model [13] (see section "The Protein Structure of ECM1"). Clinicopathologically, the disease may represent the prematurely aged condition in various organs; for example, it is characterized with a hoarse cry or voice in early childhood and later develops persisted infiltration and thickening of the skin and mucosa (clinically atrophy and scarring) during the first decade of life (Fig. 5). Hyaline materials can also deposit abruptly on the conjunctivae, cornea, and other ocular components, being similar to the clinical sign of senile cataracts. Other extracutaneous symptoms may include epilepsy and neuropsychiatric abnormalities, sometimes in association with calcification in the central nervous system. Otherwise, disease mortality is less remarkable throughout life. Among a variety of these clinical features, the hallmarks for the skin aging condition include waxy and yellowish papulo-nodules, varicelliform (pox-like) or acneiform scar formation, and profound wrinkling, with generalized atrophoderma [14, 15] (Fig. 5). Hyperkeratosis and pigmentation may appear in area exposed to mechanical friction, such as extremity joints, buttocks, and axillae. Moreover, the patients' skin is easily traumatized, a condition resembling common skin aging in human. Scalp involvement may cause loss of hair, although alopecia and baldness are not of clinical significance. By adolescence, some of these changes become much more obvious, particularly in the sun-exposed skin [83, 84]. Considering these skin manifestations, in vivo ECM1 dysfunction may contribute to the protective action in skin aging and maintenance of the skin homeostasis (Fig. 4).

Lichen Sclerosus as an Autoimmune Counterpart of Lipoid Proteinosis

The unique molecular-based pathology in LiP led to open another window for humoral autoimmunity to this molecule in lichen sclerosus (LS), a disease characterized by circulating IgG autoantibodies directed against the ECM1 protein [6]. LS is an acquired chronic inflammatory disorder that affects the skin and mucous membranes, with highly occurrence in anogenital area [85, 86]. Extragenital LS alone may occur in approximately 15 % of all cases investigated [87, 88]. A constant observation including most recent cross-sectional studies suggests that the disease prevalence ranges from 0.1 % to 0.3 %, with a male to female ratio of 1:10. Clinical features include erosions, pale patches, papulo-plaques, and porcelain-like atrophic scarring with intractable

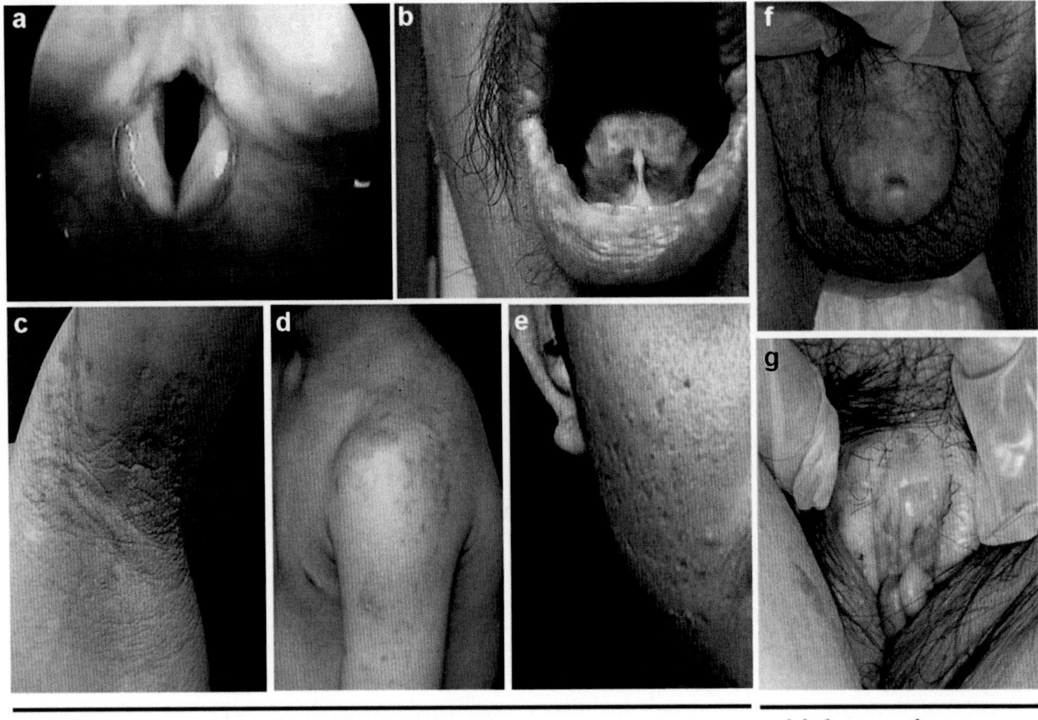

Fig. 5 **Clinical features of lipoid proteinosis and lichen sclerosus**. Patients with lipoid proteinosis show thickening and hardening of vocal cords (**a**), lips and tongue (**b**), and axillae (**c**), caused by persistent infiltration; trauma-induced skin scarring on the trunk and extremity joints (**d**) or punctuated acneiform scarring on the face (**e**). In contrast, male and female patients with lichen sclerosus show atrophic, pale-whitish polygonal lesions in the penile (**f**) and vulval skin (**g**), respectively (**a**: From Hamada et al. [13] with permission; **b** and **e**: From Hamada et al. [106] with permission)

itching and soreness (Fig. 5). There is also an increased risk of squamous cell malignancy in long-standing lesions [87, 89].

More than 70 % of female patients with lichen sclerosus had IgGs reactive with the COOH-terminal part of ECM1a (aa340–aa540), and interestingly, the same patients' sera frequently contained IgGs against the NH_2-terminal part (aa32–aa203) [90]. This heterogeneous IgG reactivity to spared antigenic epitope(s) may efficiently affect the in vivo ECM1 action by targeting all the three functional isoforms, ECM1a, ECM1b, and ECM1c. In contrast, most *ECM1* gene mutations in LiP patients have been detected within exon 7, a region spliced out in ECM1b, while their nonsense or out-of-frame mutations have been found within exons 6 and 7, causing deletion of part of exon 7 and its downstream region [15] (Fig. 1c). One may therefore speculate that anti-ECM1 IgGs in LS interfere with the functional binding of ECM1 at least with collagen IV, COMP, and perlecan, whereas LiP mutations mainly collapse the binding of ECM1 with laminin 332, MMP-9, fibulin-1C/fibulin-1D, fibulin-3, COMP, PLSCR1, PGRN, and perlecan [8, 11, 20, 24, 33, 39] (Fig. 1c). The reaction chain may cause further damages in the interaction between ECM1 and other extracellular matrix components. For example, the micro skin components can be affected by a decrease of ECM1 function/expression or even dominantly an increase of alternative functionless ECM1 (i.e., truncated form). This causes subsequent instability of extracellular matrix and basement membrane assembly in conjunction with decreased

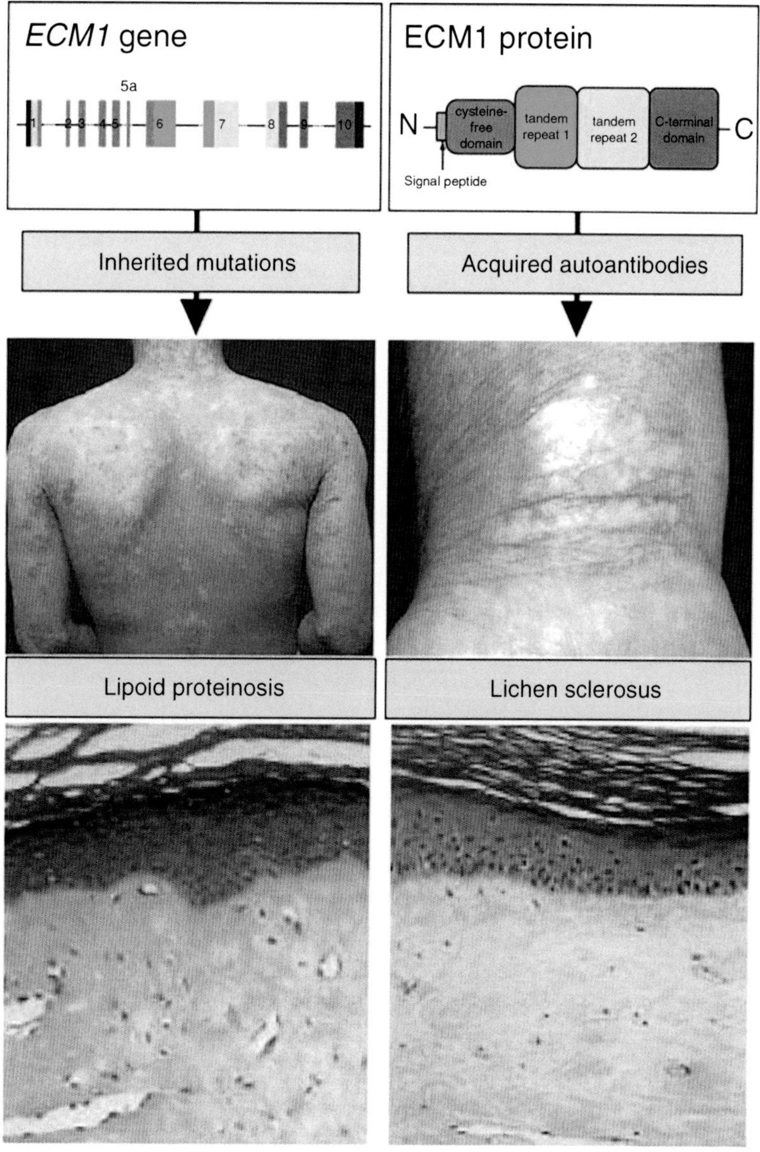

Fig. 6 Lipoid proteinosis and lichen sclerosus are immunogenetic counterparts targeting ECM1. Genetic mutation of ECM1 gene causes lipoid proteinosis (*left column*), whereas the development of humoral autoimmunity to ECM1 causes lichen sclerosus (*right column*). Both diseases have similar skin pathology, including hyperkeratosis, epidermal atrophy, dilated blood vessels, less lymph vascularity, and hyaline (glassy) changes in the upper dermis (From Chan [16]. Reprinted with permission)

enzymatic activity of MMP-9 – via an aberrant increase of collagen IV and laminins, which are both ECM1-binding partners, and disorganization of collagens I, III, IV, and V [86, 91] in the dermal vessels and interstitial – ultimately resulting in the similar clinicopathology in both diseases. To date, there have been no convincing evidence for other functionally compensative molecule(s) equivalent to ECM1, and therefore, ECM1 action is indispensable for maintaining the structural and biological integrity in the skin components. In this context, LS and LiP are immunogenetic counterparts in terms of targeting ECM1 (Fig. 6).

Presumable ECM1 Dysfunction in Premature Aging Disorders

LiP skin never shows any delayed wound healing and mortality with specific organ failures, growth retardation (i.e., lower statue), shortened life span, or increased incidence of malignancies. This clinical setting considerably differs from other representative disorders mimicking prematurely aged condition, such as Werner syndrome, Rothmund-Thomson syndrome, and Alport syndrome. The former two syndromes are rare autosomal recessive "progeroid" disorders caused by loss of the *WRN* [92] and *RECQL4* genes [93], respectively. These are RecQ-like enzymatic nuclear protein family members, which possess helicase and exonuclease activities in repair and replication of DNA double-strand break and telomere maintenance. The absence of both proteins directly leads to genetic instability and cancer predisposition that display many symptoms of premature aging, such as hoarse voice, atrophy (poikiloderma-like), photosensitivity in the skin, baldness or sparse hair, delayed wound healing, cataracts, as well as growth disturbance, part of which resembles the major clinical manifestations of LiP. Both syndromes are currently considered the most proper human models for premature skin aging. Contrary to LiP, most patients with Werner syndrome develop normally until the third decade of life and thereafter gradually establish the mimicry of age-related phenotypes such as atherosclerosis, occasional neoplasia, diabetes mellitus, and osteoporosis by the fifth decade.

Another aged condition, Alport syndrome, is an X-linked inheritance albeit much lesser with the autosomal dominant or recessive form, characterized by nephritis progressing to end-stage kidney failure, a high-tone sensorineural deafness, and retinopathy/corneal dystrophy, by adolescence age [94]. The causative gene is the one coding for the collagen IV family members, a structural axis in the basement membrane of the kidney glomerulus, certain ocular components, as well as epidermal-dermal junction and blood vessels in the skin. The clinical symptoms normally show mild skin scarring with occasional pigmentation. Despite the potential impact of collagen IV-ECM1 network in the skin structural components [24], Alport syndrome does not fulfill the overt skin changes seen in LiP. From the clinicopathological overview between these comparative aging disorders, therefore, ECM1 is not seemingly responsible for the dynamics of cell cycle and DNA metabolism but is explicitly associated with tissue remodeling and integrity via protein-protein interaction as a binding core molecule (see section "Binding Partners of ECM1"). This notion is also true regarding the interrelationship between ECM1 and laminin 332, a causative basement membrane structural molecule for an autosomal recessive genodermatosis junctional epidermolysis bullosa [26] and an autoimmune mucocutaneous blister and scarring condition "mucous membrane pemphigoid," otherwise termed as "anti-epiligrin cicatricial pemphigoid" [27]. Both diseases genetically and immunologically target laminin 332 but do not clearly represent any of premature and photoinduced aging phenotypes. It remains an attractive question how much the functional disturbance of ECM1-binding partners, like collagen IV or laminin 332, can indeed affect the in vivo biological action of ECM1, and vice versa. The molecular-based orchestration in common skin aging properties mediated by ECM1 needs to be updated.

In this context, it is important to note that ECM1 expression is exclusively downregulated in the intrinsically aged skin protected from chronic UV exposure [7], whereas the decreased ECM1 expression in chronologically aged skin may have profound effects on dermal and epidermal homeostasis, leading to the clinical features of skin atrophy, including thinning of the epidermis, rough interstitial connective tissue, and loss of periappendages in the dermis. However, the photoaging pathway(s) mediated by ECM1 remains unclear. The promoter region of the mouse *ECM1* gene contains a functional binding site for the transcription factor AP-1 (composed of the Jun and Fos protein families) well known for its role in skin aging [3]. However, the c-Fos protein expression in young and aged skin is mostly unchanged, while c-Jun is increased in aged skin [95]. ECM1 is capable of binding with MMP-9 to downregulate its bioactivity [20]. Once ECM1 function/expression is reduced, feedback activation of MMP-9 expression and/or function will occur, leading to an enhanced breakdown of interstitial and basement membrane components (e.g., collagen type IV and laminin 332), polysaccharides, HA, and hence to signs of skin aging.

Patients with LiP, an ECM1 knockout human model, from sunny regions have more severe skin phenotypes (i.e., more scarring, pigmentation, and photoaged appearance), compared to those from nonexposed areas [16, 84]. These findings suggest that lack of ECM1 may predispose to increased or accelerated signs of the skin photoaging. Recently, a higher expression of ECM1 was found in the whole epidermal layers, induced by chronically UV exposure [7]. UV irradiation stimulates the production of matrix metalloproteinases, like MMP-1, MMP-3, and MMP-9, and the event subsequently recruits inflammatory cell infiltrates and decreases the number of irregularly dilated blood vessels. Furthermore, MMP-3 degrades important extracellular matrix proteins like collagen IV, laminin 332, fibronectin, and proteoglycans (i.e., perlecan), which are all binding partners of ECM1. ECM1 might thus act as an intrinsic sunscreen via comprehensive regulation with multiple binding partners in skin aging properties.

References

1. Mathieu E, Meheus L, Raymackers J, et al. Characterization of the osteogenic stromal cell line MN7: identification of secreted MN7 proteins using two-dimensional polyacrylamide gel electrophoresis, western blotting, and microsequencing. J Bone Miner Res. 1994;9:903–13.
2. Bhalerao J, Tylzanowski P, Filie JD, et al. Molecular cloning, characterization, and genetic mapping of the cDNA coding for a novel secretory protein of mouse. Demonstration of alternative splicing in skin and cartilage. J Biol Chem. 1995;270:16385–94.
3. Smits P, Bhalerao J, Merregaert J. Molecular cloning and characterization of the mouse Ecm1 gene and its 5′ regulatory sequences. Gene. 1999;226:253–61.
4. Smits P, Ni J, Feng P, et al. The human extracellular matrix gene 1 (ECM1): genomic structure, cDNA cloning, expression pattern, and chromosomal localization. Genomics. 1997;45:487–95.
5. Johnson MR, Wilkin DJ, Vos HL, et al. Characterization of the human extracellular matrix protein 1 gene on chromosome 1q21. Matrix Biol. 1997;16:289–92.
6. Oyama N, Chan I, Neill SM, et al. Autoantibodies to extracellular matrix protein 1 in lichen sclerosus. Lancet. 2003;362:118–23.
7. Sander CS, Sercu S, Ziemer M, et al. Expression of extracellular matrix protein 1 (ECM1) in human skin is decreased by age and increased upon ultraviolet exposure. Br J Dermatol. 2006;154:218–24.
8. Mongiat M, Fu J, Oldershaw R, et al. Perlecan protein core interacts with extracellular matrix protein 1 (ECM1), a glycoprotein involved in bone formation and angiogenesis. J Biol Chem. 2003;278:17491–9.
9. Smits P, Poumay Y, Karperien M, et al. Differentiation-dependent alternative splicing and expression of the extracellular matrix protein 1 gene in human keratinocytes. J Invest Dermatol. 2000;114:718–24.
10. Horev L, Potikha T, Ayalon S, et al. A novel splice-site mutation in ECM-1 gene in a consanguineous family with lipoid proteinosis. Exp Dermatol. 2005;14:891–7.
11. Sercu S, Lambeir AM, Steenackers E, et al. ECM1 interacts with fibulin-3 and the beta 3 chain of laminin 332 through its serum albumin subdomain-like 2 domain. Matrix Biol. 2009;28:160–9.
12. Kragh-Hansen U. Structure and ligand binding properties of human serum albumin. Dan Med Bull. 1990;37:57–84.
13. Hamada T, McLean WH, Ramsay M, et al. Lipoid proteinosis maps to 1q21 and is caused by mutations in the extracellular matrix protein 1 gene (ECM1). Hum Mol Genet. 2002;11:833–40.
14. Urbach EWC. Lipoidosis cutis et mucosae. Virchows Arch Pathol Anat. 1929;273:285–319.
15. Chan I, Liu L, Hamada T, et al. The molecular basis of lipoid proteinosis: mutations in extracellular matrix protein 1. Exp Dermatol. 2007;16:881–90.
16. Chan I. The role of extracellular matrix protein 1 in human skin. Clin Exp Dermatol. 2004;29:52–6.
17. Uematsu S, Goto Y, Suzuki T, et al. N-Glycosylation of extracellular matrix protein 1 (ECM1) regulates its secretion, which is unrelated to lipoid proteinosis. FEBS Open Bio. 2014;4:879–85.
18. Ettner N, Göhring W, Sasaki T, et al. The N-terminal globular domain of the laminin alpha1 chain binds to alpha1beta1 and alpha2beta1 integrins and to the heparan sulfate-containing domains of perlecan. FEBS Lett. 1998;430:217–21.
19. Hopf M, Göhring W, Kohfeldt E, et al. Recombinant domain IV of perlecan binds to nidogens, laminin-nidogen complex, fibronectin, fibulin-2 and heparin. Eur J Biochem. 1999;259:917–25.
20. Fujimoto N, Terlizzi J, Aho S, et al. Extracellular matrix protein 1 inhibits the activity of matrix metalloproteinase 9 through high-affinity protein/protein interactions. Exp Dermatol. 2006;15:300–7.
21. Meletti S, Cantalupo G, Santoro F, et al. Temporal lobe epilepsy and emotion recognition without amygdala: a case study of Urbach-Wiethe disease and review of the literature. Epileptic Disord. 2014;16:518–27.
22. Fujimoto N, Terlizzi J, Brittingham R, et al. Extracellular matrix protein 1 interacts with the domain III of fibulin-1C and 1D variants through its central tandem repeat 2. Biochem Biophys Res Commun. 2005;333:1327–33.

23. Albig AR, Neil JR, Schiemann WP. Fibulins 3 and 5 antagonize tumor angiogenesis in vivo. Cancer Res. 2006;66:2621–9.
24. Sercu S, Zhang M, Oyama N, et al. Interaction of extracellular matrix protein 1 with extracellular matrix components: ECM1 is a basement membrane protein of the skin. J Invest Dermatol. 2008;128:1397–409. Corrigendum J Invest Dermatol. 2009;129:1836–7.
25. Sercu S, Zhang L, Merregaert J. The extracellular matrix protein 1: its molecular interaction and implication in tumor progression. Cancer Invest. 2008;26:375–84.
26. Pulkkinen L, Uitto J. Mutation analysis and molecular genetics of epidermolysis bullosa. Matrix Biol. 1999;18:29–42.
27. Bekou V, Thoma-Uszynski S, Wendler O, et al. Detection of laminin 5-specific auto-antibodies in mucous membrane and bullous pemphigoid sera by ELISA. J Invest Dermatol. 2005;124:732–40.
28. McMillan JR, Akiyama M, Shimizu H. Epidermal basement membrane zone components: ultrastructural distribution and molecular interactions. J Dermatol Sci. 2003;31:169–77.
29. McKee KK, Harrison D, Capizzi S, Yurchenco PD. Role of laminin terminal globular domains in basement membrane assembly. J Biol Chem. 2007;282:21437–47.
30. Di Cesare PE, Fang C, Leslie MP, et al. Expression of cartilage oligomeric matrix protein (COMP) by embryonic and adult osteoblasts. J Orthop Res. 2000;18:713–20.
31. Hedbom E, Antonsson P, Hjerpe A, et al. Cartilage matrix proteins. An acidic oligomeric protein (COMP) detected only in cartilage. J Biol Chem. 1992;267:6132–6.
32. Briggs MD, Hoffman SM, King LM, et al. Pseudoachondroplasia and multiple epiphyseal dysplasia due to mutations in the cartilage oligomeric matrix protein gene. Nature. 1995;10:330–6.
33. Kong L, Tian Q, Guo F, et al. Interaction between cartilage oligomeric matrix protein and extracellular matrix protein 1 mediates endochondral bone growth. Matrix Biol. 2010;29:276–86.
34. Sahu SK, Gummadi SN, Manoj N, Aradhyam GK. Phospholipid scramblases: an overview. Arch Biochem Biophys. 2007;462:103–14.
35. Göhring W, Sasaki T, Heldin CH, Timpl R. Mapping of the binding of platelet-derived growth factor to distinct domains of the basement membrane proteins BM-40 and perlecan and distinction from the BM-40 collagen-binding epitope. Eur J Biochem. 1998;255:60–6.
36. Mongiat M, Taylor K, Otto J, et al. The protein core of the proteoglycan perlecan binds specifically to fibroblast growth factor-7. J Biol Chem. 2000;275:7095–100.
37. Jiang X, Couchman JR. Perlecan and tumor angiogenesis. J Histochem Cytochem. 2003;51:1393–410.
38. Raymond MA, Désormeaux A, Laplante P, et al. Apoptosis of endothelial cells triggers a caspase-dependent anti-apoptotic paracrine loop active on VSMC. FASEB J. 2004;18:705–7.
39. Merregaert J, Van Langen J, Hansen U, et al. Phospholipid scramblase 1 is secreted by a lipid raft-dependent pathway and interacts with the extracellular matrix protein 1 in the dermal epidermal junction zone of human skin. J Biol Chem. 2010;285:37823–37.
40. Feng JQ, Guo FJ, Jiang BC, et al. Granulin epithelin precursor: a bone morphogenic protein 2-inducible growth factor that activates Erk1/2 signaling and JunB transcription factor in chondrogenesis. FASEB J. 2010;24:1879–92.
41. Xu K, Zhang Y, Ilalov K, et al. Cartilage oligomeric matrix protein associates with granulin-epithelin precursor (GEP) and potentiates GEP-stimulated chondrocyte proliferation. J Biol Chem. 2007;282:11347–55.
42. Deckers M, Smits P, Karperien M, et al. Recombinant human extracellular matrix protein 1 inhibits alkaline phosphatase activity and mineralization of mouse embryonic metatarsals in vitro. Bone. 2001;28:14–20.
43. Hoogendam J, Farih-Sips H, van Beek E, et al. Novel late response genes of PTHrP in chondrocytes. Horm Res. 2007;67:159–70.
44. Mirancea N, Hausser I, Beck R, et al. Vascular anomalies in lipoid proteinosis (hyalinosis cutis et mucosae): basement membrane components and ultrastructure. J Dermatol Sci. 2006;42:231–9.
45. Mirancea N, Hausser I, Metze D, et al. Junctional basement membrane anomalies of skin and mucosa in lipoid proteinosis (hyalinosis cutis et mucosae). J Dermatol Sci. 2007;45:175–85.
46. Sercu S, Poumay Y, Herphelin F, et al. Functional redundancy of extracellular matrix protein 1 in epidermal differentiation. Br J Dermatol. 2007;157:771–5.
47. Han Z, Ni J, Smits P, et al. Extracellular matrix protein 1 (ECM1) has angiogenic properties and is expressed by breast tumor cells. FASEB J. 2001;15:988–94.
48. Kowalewski C, Kozłowska A, Górska M, et al. Alterations of basement membrane zone and cutaneous microvasculature in morphea and extragenital lichen sclerosus. Am J Dermatopathol. 2005;27:489–96.
49. Liu Z, Kim JH, Falo Jr LD, You Z. Tumor regulatory T cells potently abrogate antitumor immunity. J Immunol. 2009;182:6160–7.
50. Sugimoto N, Oida T, Hirota K, et al. Foxp3-dependent and -independent molecules specific for CD25 + CD4+ natural regulatory T cells revealed by DNA microarray analysis. Int Immunol. 2006;18:1197–209.
51. Li Z, Zhang Y, Liu Z, et al. ECM1 controls T(H)2 cell egress from lymph nodes through re-expression of S1P(1). Nat Immunol. 2011;12:178–85.

52. Vocanson M, Hennino A, Cluzel-Tailhardat M, et al. CD8+ T cells are effector cells of contact dermatitis to common skin allergens in mice. J Invest Dermatol. 2006;126:815–20.
53. Shapira E, Brodsky B, Proscura E, et al. Amelioration of experimental autoimmune encephalitis by novel peptides: involvement of T regulatory cells. J Autoimmun. 2010;35:98–106.
54. Zhang Y, Bandala-Sanchez E, Harrison LC. Revisiting regulatory T cells in type 1 diabetes. Curr Opin Endocrinol Diabetes Obes. 2012;19:271–8.
55. Marazuela M, García-López MA, Figueroa-Vega N, et al. Regulatory T cells in human autoimmune thyroid disease. J Clin Endocrinol Metab. 2006;91:3639–46.
56. Maul J, Loddenkemper C, Mundt P, et al. Peripheral and intestinal regulatory CD4+ CD25 (high) T cells in inflammatory bowel disease. Gastroenterology. 2005;128:1868–78.
57. Fontenot JD, Gavin MA, Rudensky AY. Foxp3 programs the development and function of CD4 + CD25 + regulatory T cells. Nat Immunol. 2003;4:330–6.
58. Xiong GP, Zhang JX, Gu SP, et al. Overexpression of ECM1 contributes to migration and invasion in cholangiocarcinoma cell. Neoplasma. 2012;59:409–15.
59. Chen H, Jia WD, Li JS, et al. Extracellular matrix protein 1, a novel prognostic factor, is associated with metastatic potential of hepatocellular carcinoma. Med Oncol. 2011;28 Suppl 1:S318–25.
60. Yang S, Dong Q, Yao M, et al. Establishment of an experimental human lung adenocarcinoma cell line SPC-A-1BM with high bone metastases potency by (99m)Tc-MDP bone scintigraphy. Nucl Med Biol. 2009;36:313–21.
61. López-Marure R, Contreras PG, Dillon JS. Effects of dehydroepiandrosterone on proliferation, migration, and death of breast cancer cells. Eur J Pharmacol. 2011;660:268–74.
62. Kenny PA, Enver T, Ashworth A. Receptor and secreted targets of Wnt-1/beta-catenin signalling in mouse mammary epithelial cells. BMC Cancer. 2005;5:3.
63. Breloy I, Pacharra S, Ottis P, et al. O-linked *N,N*-′-diacetyllactosamine (LacdiNAc)-modified glycans in extracellular matrix glycoproteins are specifically phosphorylated at subterminal *N*-acetylglucosamine. J Biol Chem. 2012;287:18275–86.
64. Funahashi H, Okada Y, Sawai H, et al. The role of glial cell line-derived neurotrophic factor (GDNF) and integrins for invasion and metastasis in human pancreatic cancer cells. J Surg Oncol. 2005;91:77–83.
65. Wang L, Yu J, Ni J, et al. Extracellular matrix protein 1 (ECM1) is over-expressed in malignant epithelial tumors. Cancer Lett. 2003;200:57–67.
66. Lal G, Hashimi S, Smith BJ, et al. Extracellular matrix 1 (ECM1) expression is a novel prognostic marker for poor long-term survival in breast cancer: a Hospital-based Cohort Study in Iowa. Ann Surg Oncol. 2009;16:2280–7.
67. Wu QW, She HQ, Liang J, et al. Expression and clinical significance of extracellular matrix protein 1 and vascular endothelial growth factor-C in lymphatic metastasis of human breast cancer. BMC Cancer. 2012;12:47.
68. Lee KM, Nam K, Oh S, et al. Extracellular matrix protein 1 regulates cell proliferation and trastuzumab resistance through activation of epidermal growth factor signaling. Breast Cancer Res. 2014;16:479.
69. Lee KM, Nam K, Oh S, et al. ECM1 regulates tumor metastasis and CSC-like property through stabilization of β-catenin. Oncogene. 2015. doi:10.1038/onc.2015.54.
70. Huang L, Chen D, Liu D, et al. MUC1 oncoprotein blocks glycogen synthase kinase 3beta-mediated phosphorylation and degradation of beta-catenin. Cancer Res. 2005;65:10413–22.
71. Gu M, Guan J, Zhao L, et al. Correlation of ECM1 expression level with the pathogenesis and metastasis of laryngeal carcinoma. Int J Clin Exp Pathol. 2013;6:1132–7.
72. Meng XY, Liu J, Lv F, et al. Study on the correlation between extracellular matrix protein-1 and the growth, metastasis and angiogenesis of laryngeal carcinoma. Asian Pac J Cancer Prev. 2015;16:2313–6.
73. Lee KM, Nam K, Oh S, et al. ECM1 promotes the Warburg effect through EGF-mediated activation of PKM2. Cell Signal. 2015;27:228–35.
74. Gao F, Xia Y, Wang J, et al. Integrated analyses of DNA methylation and hydroxymethylation reveal tumor suppressive roles of ECM1, ATF5, and EOMES in human hepatocellular carcinoma. Genome Biol. 2014;15:533–46.
75. Fisher SA, Tremelling M, Anderson CA, et al. Genetic determinants of ulcerative colitis include the ECM1 locus and five loci implicated in Crohn's disease. Nat Genet. 2008;40:710–2.
76. Wlaschek M, Tantcheva-Poor I, Naderi L, et al. Solar UV irradiation and dermal photoaging. J Photochem Photobiol. 2001;63:41–51.
77. Varani J, Warner RL, Gharaee-Kermani M, et al. Vitamin A antagonizes decreased cell growth and elevated collagen-degrading matrix metalloproteinases and stimulates collagen accumulation in naturally aged human skin. J Invest Dermatol. 2000;114:480–6.
78. Lock-Andersen J, Therkildsen P, de Fine OF, et al. Epidermal thickness, skin pigmentation and constitutive photosensitivity. Photodermatol Photoimmunol Photomed. 1997;13:153–8.
79. Chung JH, Seo JY, Choi HR, et al. Modulation of skin collagen metabolism in aged and photoaged human skin in vivo. J Invest Dermatol. 2001;117:1218–24.
80. Kligman LH, Kligman AM. The nature of photoaging: its prevention and repair. Photodermatology. 1986;3:215–27.
81. de Rigal J, Escoffier C, Querleux B, et al. Assessment of aging of the human skin by in vivo ultrasonic imaging. J Invest Dermatol. 1989;93:621–5.

82. Bernstein EF, Chen YQ, Kopp JB, et al. Long-term sun exposure alters the collagen of the papillary dermis. Comparison of sunprotected and photoaged skin by northern analysis, immunohistochemical staining, and confocal laser scanning microscopy. J Am Acad Dermatol. 1996;34:209–18.
83. Chan I, El-Zurghany A, Zendah B, Benghazil M, et al. Molecular basis of lipoid proteinosis in a Libyan family. Clin Exp Dermatol. 2003;28:545–8.
84. Van Hougenhouck-Tulleken W, Chan I, Hamada T, et al. Clinical and molecular characterization of lipoid proteinosis in Namaqualand, South Africa. Br J Dermatol. 2004;151:413–23.
85. Powell JJ, Wojnarowska F. Lichen sclerosus. Lancet. 1999;353:1777–83.
86. Godoy CA, Teodoro WR, Velosa AP, et al. Unusual remodeling of the hyalinization band in vulval lichen sclerosus by type V collagen and ECM 1 protein. Clinics (Sao Paulo). 2015;70:356–62.
87. Meffert JJ, Davis BM, Grimwood RE. Lichen sclerosus. J Am Acad Dermatol. 1995;32:393–416.
88. Kyriakis KP, Emmanuelides S, Terzoudi S, et al. Gender and age prevalence distributions of morphea en plaque and anogenital lichen sclerosus. J Eur Acad Dermatol Venereol. 2007;21:825–6.
89. Neill SM, Lewis FM, Tatnall FM, Cox NH, British Association of Dermatologists. British Association of Dermatologists' guidelines for the management of lichen sclerosus 2010. Br J Dermatol. 2010;163:672–82.
90. Oyama N, Chan I, Neill SM, et al. Development of antigen-specific ELISA for circulating autoantibodies to extracellular matrix protein 1 in lichen sclerosus. J Clin Invest. 2004;113:1550–9.
91. Kowalewski C, Kozłowska A, Chan I, et al. Three-dimensional imaging reveals major changes in skin microvasculature in lipoid proteinosis and lichen sclerosus. J Dermatol Sci. 2005;38:215–24.
92. Yu CE, Oshima J, Fu YH, et al. Positional cloning of the Werner's syndrome gene. Science. 1996;12:258–62.
93. Kitao S, Shimamoto A, Goto M, et al. Mutations in RECQL4 cause a subset of cases of Rothmund-Thomson syndrome. Nat Genet. 1999;22:82–4.
94. Barker DF, Hostikka SL, Zhou J, et al. Identification of mutations in the COL4A5 collagen gene in Alport syndrome. Science. 1990;248:1224–7.
95. Lener T, Moll PR, Rinnerthaler M, et al. Expression profiling of aging in the human skin. Exp Gerontol. 2006;4:387–97.
96. Oyama N, Merregaert J. The extracellular matrix protein 1 (ECM1) in skin biology: an update for the pleiotropic action. Open Dermatol J. 2013;7:29–41.
97. Chelvan HT, Narasimhan M, Shankaran Subramanian A, et al. Lipoid proteinosis presenting with an unusual nonsense Q32X mutation in exon 2 of the extracellular matrix protein 1 gene. Australas J Dermatol. 2012;53:e79–82.
98. Gao D, Lian P, Wang R, et al. Identification of a novel splicing mutation of ECM1 in a rare lipoid proteinosis family. J Dermatol. 2013;40:675–7.
99. Abbas O, Farooq M, El Khoury J, et al. A novel splice-site ECM1 gene mutation in a Lebanese girl with lipoid proteinosis. Int J Dermatol. 2013;52:824–6.
100. Almeida TF, Soares DC, Quaio CR, et al. Lipoid proteinosis: rare case confirmed by ECM1 mutation detection. Int J Pediatr Otorhinolaryngol. 2014;78:2314–5.
101. Zhang R, Liu Y, Xue Y, et al. Treatment of lipoid proteinosis due to the p.C220G mutation in ECM1, a major allele in Chinese patients. J Transl Med. 2014;12:85.
102. Mondejar R, Garcia-Moreno JM, Rubio R, et al. Clinical and molecular study of the extracellular matrix protein 1 gene in a Spanish family with lipoid proteinosis. J Clin Neurol. 2014;10:64–8.
103. Nasir M, Rahman SB, Sieber CM, et al. Identification of recurrent c.742G > T nonsense mutation in ECM1 in Pakistani families suffering from lipoid proteinosis. Mol Biol Rep. 2014;41:2085–92.
104. Youssefian L, Vahidnezhad H, Daneshpazhooh M, et al. Lipoid proteinosis: phenotypic heterogeneity in Iranian families with c.507delT mutation in ECM1. Exp Dermatol. 2015;24:220–2.
105. Lee MY, Wang HJ, Han Y, et al. Lipoid proteinosis resulting from a large homozygous deletion affecting part of the ECM1 gene and adjacent long non-coding RNA. Acta Derm Venereol. 2015;95:608–10.
106. Hamada T, Wessagowit V, South AP, Ashton GH, Chan I, Oyama N, et al. Extracellular matrix protein 1 gene (ECM1) mutations in lipoid proteinosis and genotype-phenotype correlation. J Invest Dermatol. 2003;120(3):347.

Pathomechanisms of Endogenously Aged Skin

9

Evgenia Makrantonaki and Christos C. Zouboulis

Contents

Abstract

In an ever-aging society a better understanding of the underlying mechanisms accompanying aging skin has become essential. Skin aging can be classified into light-induced aging (photoaging, exogenous aging) and endogenous aging. The latter occurs in nonexposed areas, which are not in direct contact with environmental factors such as ultraviolet (UV) and infrared (IR) irradiation, and is mainly attributed to genetic factors and alterations of the endocrine environment. In this chapter, new insights on the latest findings regarding the pathogenesis of endogenously aged skin are summarized, to what extent intrinsic factors may influence the progress of skin aging and what are the consequences on the morphology and physiology of skin.

Introduction

There has been an unprecedented rapid expansion of the population of elderly people both in the developed and developing world [1]. Since 1840, life expectancy has increased at a rate of about 3 months/year [2], whereas the total worldwide aged population is expected to rise from 605 million in 2000 to 1.2 billion in 2025 and to nearly 2 billion in 2050 [3]. These demographic shifts mandate a better understanding of the aging process and better management strategies for age-associated diseases.

E. Makrantonaki
Departments of Dermatology, Venereology, Allergology and Immunology, Dessau Medical Center, Dessau, Germany

Geriatrics Research Group, Charité Universitätsmedizin Berlin, Berlin, Germany

Department of Dermatology and Allergology, University Medical Center Ulm, Ulm, Germany
e-mail: evgenia.makrantonaki@uni-ulm.de

C.C. Zouboulis (✉)
Departments of Dermatology, Venereology, Allergology and Immunology, Dessau Medical Center, Dessau, Germany
e-mail: christos.zouboulis@klinikum-dessau.de

M.A. Farage et al. (eds.), *Textbook of Aging Skin*,
DOI 10.1007/978-3-662-47398-6_9

Like all other organs, skin suffers progressive morphological and physiological decrement with increasing age and provides the first obvious evidence of the aging process. Skin aging can be classified into light-induced aging (photoaging, exogenous aging) and endogenous aging. The latter occurs in nonexposed areas, which are not in direct contact with environmental factors such as ultraviolet (UV) and infrared (IR) irradiation (e.g., the inner side of the upper arm) [4], and is mainly attributed to genetic factors and alterations of the endocrine environment. In contrast to photoaging, endogenously aged skin reflects degradation processes of the entire organism.

Pathomechanisms of Endogenously Aged Skin

With advancing age the most pronounced changes in endogenously aged skin occur within the epidermis and affect mostly the basal cell layer. As a result, sun-protected aged skin appears thin, finely wrinkled, and dry (reviewed in Table 1) [4]. Although the fundamental mechanisms are still poorly understood, a growing body of evidence points toward the involvement of multiple pathways in the generation of aged skin. Several theories have been proposed including the theory of cellular senescence [5], decrease in cellular DNA repair capacity and loss of telomeres [6–9], point mutations of extranuclear mitochondrial DNA (mtDNA) [10], oxidative stress [11], increased frequency of chromosomal abnormalities [12, 13], and gene mutations. In addition, hormones have also been shown to play a distinct role.

Cellular Senescence

The theory of cellular senescence describes the observed loss of the cell's proliferative potential after a limited number of cell divisions [5]. According to this theory, cells possess a "biological clock," which signals the end of their replicative life span, and as a consequence, they cannot be stimulated to enter the S1 phase by physiological mitogens, arresting at the G1 phase. This process can be partly explained by the selective repression of growth regulatory genes.

Studies on keratinocytes [14], fibroblasts [15], and melanocytes [16] have revealed that they all

Table 1 Morphological and functional changes in intrinsically aged skin [81]

Thinning of epidermis by 10–50 %	Increased vulnerability, fragility
Atrophy of the stratum spinosum	Increased vulnerability, fragility
Increased heterogeneity in size of basal cells	Increased vulnerability, fragility
Decreased mitotic activity, increased duration of cell cycle and migration time	Decreased desquamation, delayed wound healing
Slow replacement of lipids	Disturbed barrier function
Flattening of the dermoepidermal junction	Decrease in surface contact area, increased risk of separation by shearing forces
Decrease and heterogeneity of melanocytes	Graying of hair, guttate amelanosis, lentigines
Decrease of Langerhans cells	Diminished cutaneous immune function
Reduction of dermis thickness, decrease of fibroblasts	Reduced strength and resiliency
Atrophy of the extracellular matrix	Reduced strength and resiliency
Reduction and disintegration of collagen and elastic fibers, deposition of exogenous substances (e.g., amyloid P)	Sensitization to deformational forces, fine wrinkle formation
Reduction of cutaneous microvasculature	Reduction of cutaneous vascular responsiveness, disturbed thermoregulation and supply with nutrients
Decrease of skin appendages and their function (e.g., sebaceous glands, sweat glands, apocrine glands)	Decreased lipid and sweat production, disturbed re-epithelization of deep cutaneous wounds
Thinning of subcutaneous fat	Reduced insulation and energy production
Reduction of nerve endings	Disturbed sensory function

show an age-associated decrease in cumulative population doublings. Fibroblasts, for instance, taken from a normal human tissue go through only about 25–50 population doublings when cultured in a standard mitogenic medium. Toward the end of this time, proliferation slows down and finally stops, and the cells enter a state from which they never recover. The reduction in proliferative capacity of skin-derived cells in culture from old donors and patients with premature aging syndromes and the accumulation in vivo of senescent cells with altered patterns of gene expression also support the theory of cellular senescence.

The Free Radical Theory

Oxygen radicals or reactive oxygen species (ROS) are increasingly considered as the major contributors to aging, and the protective mechanism against oxidative stress is observed as an indispensable function [17]. It has been shown that oxygen radical levels rise and antioxidant activity declines with advancing age [18].

Skin possesses many defensive mechanisms in order to reduce the production of ROS from internal sources. For example, the activity of enzymes that indirectly produce oxygen metabolites can be altered (xanthine oxidase modulation). There is a repair system consisting of enzymes and small molecules, antioxidant enzymes such as catalase and peroxidase, and low-molecular-weight antioxidants such as tocopherols, ascorbic acid, NADH, and carnosine, which can donate an electron and then scavenge ROS.

Excess ROS production leads to accumulation of cellular damage [19, 20], which includes oxidation of DNA resulting in mutations and oxidation of membrane lipids leading to reduced transport efficiency and altered transmembrane signaling, processes whose consequence is the aging phenotype. A disturbed stress response is also known to be associated with a defect in proteolytic systems such as lysosomal activity and ubiquitine-proteosome pathway in somatic cells [21]. As a consequence, altered proteins cannot be eliminated, and this results in accumulation of misfolded and damaged proteins in the cells. Moreover, cumulative evidence suggests that ROS play a crucial role by participating in multiple MAP kinase pathways, which induce AP-1 and in turn the signal cascade, already mentioned above (Fig. 1).

The free radical theory has also been supported by the fact that strategies that reduce metabolism and the production of ROS, such as dietary caloric restriction (DCR), can extend the life span of experimental animals. Studies conducted in animal models demonstrated that DCR can retard the aging process by influencing stress response and altering the expression of metabolic and biosynthetic genes [22]. Cancer prevention due to alterations of hormone metabolism, hormone-related cellular signaling, oxidation status, DNA repair, and apoptosis has been also associated with DCR [23, 24]. In skin tissues of mice with DCR weight control, a palette of genes showed a differential expression when compared to mice receiving normal diet [24]. DCR could show profound inhibitory impact on the expression of genes relevant to cancer risks (e.g., neuroblastoma ras oncogene, neuroblastoma myc-related oncogene 1, Rab40c, myeloblastosis oncogene-like 2, lung carcinoma myc-related oncogene 1, myeloblastosis oncogene, RAB5B, RAP2B, RAB34).

The Telomere Hypothesis

The telomere hypothesis of cellular aging [25] proposes that loss of telomeres due to incomplete DNA replication and absence of telomerase provides a mitotic clock that signals cycle exit, limiting the replicative capacity of the somatic cell [9]. Human telomeres consist of repeats of the sequence TTAGGG/CCCTAA at chromosome end, which are not replicated in the same manner as the rest of the genome but instead are synthesized by the enzyme telomerase [9, 26, 27]. By mechanisms that remain unclear, telomerase also promotes the formation of protein cap structures that protect the chromosome ends. Telomerase is active in germline cells and in humans, and telomeres in these cells are maintained at about

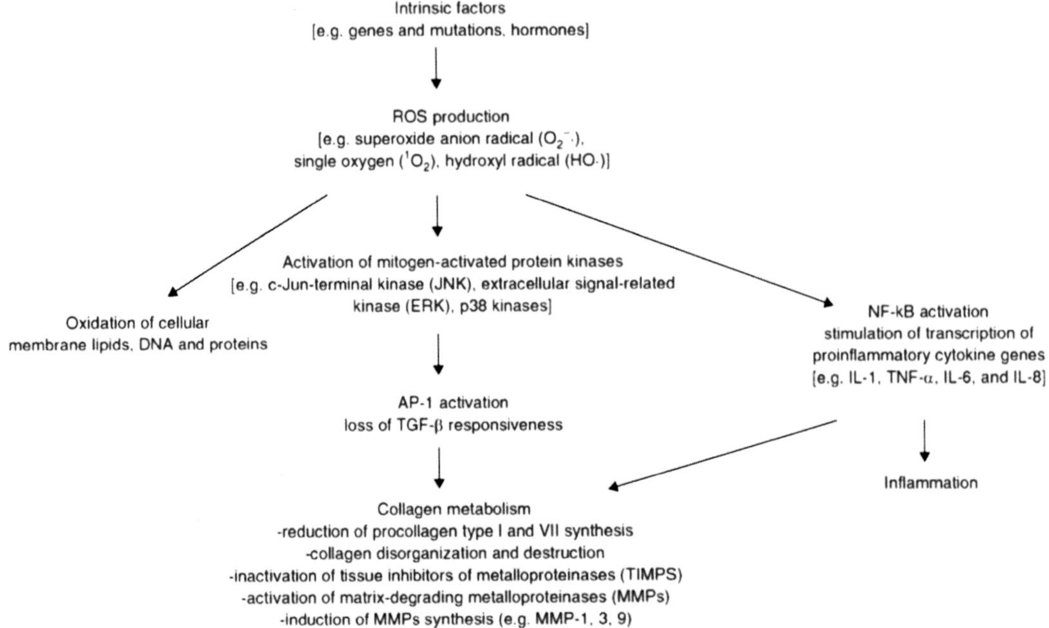

Fig. 1 A schematic overview of major biochemical changes and signaling pathways involved in the generation of endogenously aged skin. In aged skin, mitogen-activated protein (*MAP*) kinase signal transduction pathways play an important role in regulating a variety of cellular functions. Downstream effectors of the MAP kinases include several transcription factors including the c-Jun and c-Fos, which heterodimerize in order to form the activator protein 1 (AP-1) complex. AP-1 is a key regulator of skin aging, as it induces the expression of the MMP family and has been shown to inhibit type I procollagen gene expression through interference with TGF-β signaling pathway. It has been postulated that MAP kinases may be activated by excess production of reactive oxygen species (ROS), which occurs with advanced age and may be superimposed by extrinsic factors (e.g., UV/IR irradiation). Excess ROS production also leads to accumulation of cellular damage, which includes oxidation of DNA resulting in mutations, oxidation of proteins leading to reduced function, and oxidation of membrane lipids resulting in reduced transport efficiency and altered transmembrane signaling. *NF-κB* nuclear factor-kappa B, *TGF-β* transforming growth factor-β, *IL-1* interleukin-1, *IL-6* interleukin-6, *IL-8* interleukin-8

15 kilobase pairs (kbp). In contrast, telomerase is not expressed in most human somatic cells like skin cells [7, 28]. As a result, their telomeres become 50–100 nucleotides shorter with every cell division, and their protective protein caps progressively deteriorate. Eventually, after many cell generations, DNA damage occurs at chromosome ends. The damage activates a p53-dependent cell-cycle arrest that resembles the arrest caused by other types of DNA damage.

The lack of telomerase in most somatic cells has been proposed to help protect humans from the potentially damaging effects of runaway cell proliferation, as occurs in cancer. Telomere loss is thought to control entry into senescence [7, 29, 30].

Genes and Mutations

The mechanisms which seem to be associated with aging are complex [31]. Recent studies on models such as the yeast *Saccharomyces cerevisiae* [32], the nematode *Caenorhabditis elegans* [33], the fly *Drosophila melanogaster* [34–36], the mouse *Mus musculus* [37], and humans [38] show that single gene mutations can contribute to the initiation of aging and induce premature aging syndromes. However, there are no special genes that can cause aging-associated damages. The manifestation of aging is mostly due to the failure of maintenance and repair mechanisms [39, 40].

Studies on human keratinocytes have demonstrated altered expression of growth-regulating molecules with age; there is an increase of the baseline expression of the differentiation-associated genes like SPR2 and interleukin 1 receptor antagonist [41] and EGF binding and receptor phosphorylation is reduced and thought to be the result of age-related changes in a critical downstream signaling element [42].

In senescent fibroblasts, genes like the c-fos proto-oncogene [43], the helix-loop-helix Id-1 and Id-2 genes [44], and components of the E2F transcription factor [45] have been shown to be downregulated, and negative growth regulators are overexpressed including the p21 and p16 inhibitors of cyclin-dependent protein kinases [46]. Other changes seen in senescent skin fibroblasts include increased expression of IL-1 and of the EGF-like cytokine heregulin that modulates the growth and differentiation [47]. Moreover, elastin gene expression is markedly reduced after the age of 40–50, as determined by mRNA steady-state levels [48].

Furthermore, recent studies indicate that endogenous and exogenous aging may share some fundamental pathways, and may have some common mediators. Photoaging is thought to be the superposition of UV irradiation from the sun on intrinsic aging [49].

Some of the similarities are changes in the MAP kinase signaling pathways, like decreases in ERK-dependent MAP kinase activity and increases in stress-activated JNK and p38 kinase [50], which result in reduced cell proliferation, differentiation, and cell survival [51], and enhanced growth arrest, apoptosis, and stress-related responses [51, 52]. As a consequence of the stress-activated MAP kinase pathways, the expression of c-jun and c-Jun N terminal kinase, an upstream activator of c-jun, is elevated in aged compared with young skin [50]. As c-jun is a constituent of the transcription factor AP-1, AP-1 is also elevated and subsequently the AP-1 regulated connective tissue-degrading enzymes MMP-1 (interstitial collagenase), MMP-3 (stromelysin 1), and MMP-9 (gelatinase B). In parallel, there is an observed reduction in the expression of tissue inhibitors of metalloproteinases [53, 54]. Another common feature is the increased insoluble degraded collagen and the reduction of types I and III procollagen synthesis, which may result from the impaired TGFβ signaling pathway [53, 55].

In recent studies, researchers have been focusing on gene mutations accompanying known progeroid syndromes, e.g., Hutchinson-Gilford progeria, Werner's syndrome (WS), Rothmund-Thomson syndrome, Cockayne syndrome, Ataxia teleangiectasia, and Down syndrome. The most common skin disorders of these syndromes, which are characterized by an acceleration of the aging phenotype, are alopecia, skin atrophy and sclerosis, teleangiectasia, poikiloderma, thinning and graying of hair, and several malignancies. Most of these syndromes are inherited in an autosomal recessive way and mostly display defects in DNA replication, recombination, repair, and transcription. Expression gene patterns of skin cells derived from Werner patients [56] and old and young donors showed that 91 % of the analyzed genes had similar expression changes in WS and in normal aging implying transcription alterations common to WS and normal aging represent general events in the aging process.

Ly et al. measured mRNA levels in fibroblasts isolated from young, middle-aged, and elderly patients with progeria and found chromosomal pathologies that lead to misregulation of key structural, signaling, and metabolic genes associated with the aging phenotype [13].

Further studies conducted to investigate changes in gene expression during skin aging have been performed on naturally aged human foreskin obtained from children and elderly males. Some of the mechanisms proposed to be involved in the induction of aging comprise disturbed lipid metabolism, altered insulin and STAT3 signaling, upregulation of apoptotic genes partly due to the deregulation of FOXO1, dowregulation of members of the jun and fos family, differential expression of cytoskeletal proteins (e.g., keratin 2A, 6A, and 16A), extracellular matrix components (e.g., PI3, S100A2, A7, A9, SPRR2B), and proteins involved in cell-cycle control (e.g., CDKs, GOS2) [57].

In own experiments the mechanisms of gender-independent human endogenous skin aging has been examined. Whole genome gene profiling was employed in sun-protected skin obtained from European Caucasian young and elderly females and males, respectively using the Illumina array platform. Only 1.7 % and 1.3 % among all genes examined showed to be regulated with age in women and men, respectively. In total, 39 genes were common in the target lists of significant regulated genes in males and females and these genes could be used as useful biomarkers of endogenous human skin aging. Interestingly, Wnt signaling pathway showed to be significantly downregulated in aged skin with decreased gene and protein expression for males and females, accordingly highlighting for the first time the role of this signaling pathway in the aging process [58].

The analysis of complex methylation patterns in skin samples from young and elderly donors also shows significant differences. A significant increase in the DNA hypermethylation was found in the samples of elderly donors [59]. Additionally, new findings have illustrated the important role of accumulating defective proteins in the skin cells and the associated progressive dysregulated function of proteosome and lysosome with aging [60].

In several studies it has been also pointed out that a dysregulation of adult stem cells in the skin may contribute to aging. A possible cause for this could be a disturbed expression of chromatin regulators such as sirtuins [61], long noncoding RNAs or dysfunctional NF-κB signaling pathways [62].

The Mitochondrial DNA Theory

Genetic damage and instability outside the nuclear genome has been also suggested to contribute to aging [63]. The mtDNA synthesis takes place near the inner mitochondrial membrane, which is the site of formation of ROS, and the fact that mtDNA lacks excision and recombination repair has made many investigators believe that cumulative damage of the mtDNA may play a key role in the pathogenesis of the aging phenotype [10, 11].

Examination of human fibroblast mtDNA in aged individuals revealed point mutations at specific positions in the control region for replication. Notably, a T414G transversion was found in a significantly higher proportion of persons older than 65 years when compared with younger persons [11].

Hormone Decline and Skin Aging

One of the further factors that may play a predominant role in the initiation of skin aging is the physiological hormone decline occurring with age. Over time important circulating hormones decline due to a reduced secretion of the pituitary, adrenal glands and the gonads or due to an intercurrent disease. Among them, growth factors (i.e., growth hormone [GH] and insulin-like growth factor-I [IGF-I]) and sex steroids (e.g., androgens and estrogens) show significant changes in their blood levels.

In animal models, such as in organisms as diverse as the nematode *C. elegans*, the fly *D. melanogaster*, and the mouse *M. musculus*, the importance of hormonal signals on the aging phenotype has already been documented. Suppression of hormones such as insulin-like peptides, growth hormone (GH), and sterols [64] or their receptors can increase life span and delay age-dependent functional decline. Conboy et al. [65] showed that the age-related decline of progenitor cell activity of mice could be reversed by exposure to young serum and that the cells could retain much of their intrinsic proliferative potential even when old, underlining the great importance of the systemic environment. In an in vitro model of human hormonal aging, human skin cells cultured under hormone-substituted conditions showed altered lipid synthesis and metabolism and affected expression of genes being involved in biological processes, such as DNA repair and stability, mitochondrial function, oxidative stress, cell cycle and apoptosis, ubiquitin-induced proteolysis, and transcriptional regulation indicating that these processes may be hormone dependent [66]. These studies illustrate the importance of the hormone environment for deterioration of the human organism and the aging process.

The growth hormone (GH)/insulin-like growth factor-I (IGF-I) axis is considered to be one of the most important signaling pathways involved in aging. Serum levels of IGF-I have been reported to increase from birth to puberty, followed by a slow decline through adulthood. This reduction has been correlated with the progressive decline of GH with advancing age [67].

IGF-I signaling in vitro and in a murine aging model in vivo has been shown to be suppressed in response to accumulation of superoxide anions (O2°-) in mitochondria, either by chemical inhibition of complex I or by genetic silencing of O2°–dismutating mitochondrial Sod2. Consequently, the O2°–dependent suppression of IGF-I signaling may result in decreased proliferation of murine dermal fibroblasts, affects translation initiation factors, and suppresses the expression of α1(I), α1(III), and α2(I) collagen. These results underline the important role of oxidative stress in the regulation of hormonal processes with age [68].

Decreased IGF-I levels have been also associated with a reduced increase in thickness of the epidermis and deficient protective response to UVB irradiation implying that reduced expression of IGF-I in geriatric skin could be an important component in the development of aging-related nonmelanoma skin cancer [69].

Patients with isolated GH deficiency (IGHD), multiple pituitary hormone deficiency (MPHD) including GH, as well as primary IGF-I deficiency (GH resistance, Laron syndrome) present signs of early skin aging such as dry, thin, and wrinkled skin. Other resulting characteristics of GH/IGF-I deficiency are obesity, hyperglycemia, reduced body lean mass, osteopenia, lowered venous access, hypercholesterolemia, cardiovascular diseases, and, subsequently, premature mortality [70–72]. Treatment of normal elderly males with GH resulted in amelioration and reverse of the aging signs and symptoms [73]. However, recent reports of an association of GH substitution and increased risk of prostate, lung, colon, breast cancer, as well as a possible decrease of insulin insensitivity all make further investigations necessary regarding safety and efficacy of GH substitution in the aging population [74].

On the other hand, menopause, which is characterized by a rapid decline of sex steroids, has been associated with a worsening of skin structure and functions, which can be at least partially repaired by hormone replacement therapy or local estrogen treatment [75]. Improvement of epidermal skin moisture, elasticity and skin thickness [76], enhanced production of surface lipids [77], reduction of wrinkle depth, restoration of collagen fibers [78], and increase of the collagen III/I ratio [79] have all been reported under hormone replacement therapy.

In vitro tests that studied the effects of GH, IGF-I androgens, and estrogens at age-specific levels on human skin cells have been documented. IGF-I was shown to play an important role in the regulation of the lipid synthesis in human sebocytes, while 17β-estradiol showed no significant effects on the biological activity of the cells. Dermal fibroblasts showed to be more susceptible to 17β-estradiol treatment, while IGF-I could significantly stimulate fibroblast proliferation. Furthermore, an interplay between the 17β-estradiol and IGF-I signaling pathways was documented in both cell types [80]. These results indicate the importance of IGF-I in the reduction of skin surface lipids and thickness with advanced age.

Conclusion

In summary, several factors may contribute to endogenous skin aging underlining the complexity of this phenomenon. Among these are excess production of reactive oxygen species and impaired scavenge mechanisms, increased frequency of chromosomal abnormalities, telomere loss, and point mutations of extranuclear mitochondrial DNA due to reduced DNA repair capacity. In addition, several genes and their mutations have been correlated with the aging phenotype. Hormones and their physiological decline with time also play a distinct role as shown in several in vitro and in vivo studies.

In addition to internal factors, several environmental factors contribute to this process and sometimes accelerate the onset of aging. Skin functions deteriorate and this results in the development of a palette of diseases, which may jeopardize life quality. Awareness of the pathophysiology of skin aging as well as of preventive measures to avoid skin damage is the first step for successful, healthy aging.

Cross-References

▶ Pathomechanisms of Photoaged Skin

References

1. Diczfalusy E. The third age, the Third World and the third millennium. Contraception. 1996;53(1):1–7.
2. Oeppen J, Vaupel JW. Demography. Broken limits to life expectancy. Science. 2002;296(5570):1029–31.
3. Aleksandrova S, Velkova A. Population ageing in the Balkan countries. Folia Med (Plovdiv). 2003;45 (4):5–10.
4. Makrantonaki E, Zouboulis CC, William J. Cunliffe scientific awards. Characteristics and pathomechanisms of endogenously aged skin. Dermatology. 2007;214(4):352–60.
5. Hayflick L. The limited in vitro lifetime of human diploid cell strains. Exp Cell Res. 1965;37:614–36.
6. Kosmadaki MG, Gilchrest BA. The role of telomeres in skin aging/photoaging. Micron. 2004;35(3):155–9.
7. Bodnar AG, Ouellette M, Frolkis M, et al. Extension of life-span by introduction of telomerase into normal human cells. Science. 1998;279(5349):349–52.
8. Smith JR, Pereira-Smith OM. Replicative senescence: implications for in vivo aging and tumor suppression. Science. 1996;273(5271):63–7.
9. Allsopp RC, Vaziri H, Patterson C, et al. Telomere length predicts replicative capacity of human fibroblasts. Proc Natl Acad Sci U S A. 1992;89 (21):10114–8.
10. Michikawa Y, Mazzucchelli F, Bresolin N, et al. Aging-dependent large accumulation of point mutations in the human mtDNA control region for replication. Science. 1999;286(5440):774–9.
11. Miquel J. An update on the oxygen stress-mitochondrial mutation theory of aging: genetic and evolutionary implications. Exp Gerontol. 1998;33 (1–2):113–26.
12. Benn PA. Specific chromosome aberrations in senescent fibroblast cell lines derived from human embryos. Am J Hum Genet. 1976;28(5):465–73.
13. Ly DH, Lockhart DJ, Lerner RA, et al. Mitotic misregulation and human aging. Science. 2000;287 (5462):2486–92.
14. Gilchrest BA. In vitro assessment of keratinocyte aging. J Invest Dermatol. 1983;81(1 Suppl):184s–9.
15. Cristofalo VJ, Pignolo RJ. Replicative senescence of human fibroblast-like cells in culture. Physiol Rev. 1993;73(3):617–38.
16. Gilchrest BA, Vrabel MA, Flynn E, et al. Selective cultivation of human melanocytes from newborn and adult epidermis. J Invest Dermatol. 1984;83(5):370–6.
17. Barja G. Free radicals and aging. Trends Neurosci. 2004;27(10):595–600.
18. Kohen R. Skin antioxidants: their role in aging and in oxidative stress – new approaches for their evaluation. Biomed Pharmacother. 1999;53(4):181–92.
19. Sohal RS, Weindruch R. Oxidative stress, caloric restriction, and aging. Science. 1996;273 (5271):59–63.
20. Hensley K, Floyd RA. Reactive oxygen species and protein oxidation in aging: a look back, a look ahead. Arch Biochem Biophys. 2002;397(2):377–83.
21. Cuervo AM, Dice JF. How do intracellular proteolytic systems change with age? Front Biosci. 1998;3: d25–43.
22. Lee CK, Klopp RG, Weindruch R, et al. Gene expression profile of aging and its retardation by caloric restriction. Science. 1999;285(5432):1390–3.
23. Kritchevsky D. Caloric restriction and experimental carcinogenesis. Hybrid Hybridomics. 2002;21 (2):147–51.
24. Lu J, Xie L, Sylvester J, et al. Different gene expression of skin tissues between mice with weight controlled by either calorie restriction or physical exercise. Exp Biol Med (Maywood). 2007;232(4):473–80.
25. Harley CB. Telomere loss: mitotic clock or genetic time bomb? Mutat Res. 1991;256(2–6):271–82.
26. Wu KJ, Grandori C, Amacker M, et al. Direct activation of TERT transcription by c-MYC. Nat Genet. 1999;21(2):220–4.
27. Feng J, Funk WD, Wang SS, et al. The RNA component of human telomerase. Science. 1995;269 (5228):1236–41.
28. Kim NW, Piatyszek MA, Prowse KR, et al. Specific association of human telomerase activity with immortal cells and cancer. Science. 1994;266(5193):2011–5.
29. Harley CB, Futcher AB, Greider CW. Telomeres shorten during ageing of human fibroblasts. Nature. 1990;345(6274):458–60.
30. Hastie ND, Dempster M, Dunlop MG, et al. Telomere reduction in human colorectal carcinoma and with ageing. Nature. 1990;346(6287):866–8.
31. Guarente L, Kenyon C. Genetic pathways that regulate ageing in model organisms. Nature. 2000;408 (6809):255–62.
32. Jazwinski SM. The RAS, genes: a homeostatic device in Saccharomyces cerevisiae longevity. Neurobiol Aging. 1999;20(5):471–8.

33. Johnson TE, Henderson S, Murakami S, et al. Longevity genes in the nematode Caenorhabditis elegans also mediate increased resistance to stress and prevent disease. J Inherit Metab Dis. 2002;25 (3):197–206.
34. Rogina B, Reenan RA, Nilsen SP, et al. Extended life-span conferred by cotransporter gene mutations in Drosophila. Science. 2000;290(5499):2137–40.
35. Tatar M, Kopelman A, Epstein D, et al. A mutant Drosophila insulin receptor homolog that extends life-span and impairs neuroendocrine function. Science. 2001;292(5514):107–10.
36. Arking R, Buck S, Hwangbo DS, et al. Metabolic alterations and shifts in energy allocations are corequisites for the expression of extended longevity genes in Drosophila. Ann N Y Acad Sci. 2002;959:251–62 (Discussion 463–255).
37. Kuro-o M, Matsumura Y, Aizawa H, et al. Mutation of the mouse klotho gene leads to a syndrome resembling ageing. Nature. 1997;390(6655):45–51.
38. Yu CE, Oshima J, Fu YH, et al. Positional cloning of the Werner's syndrome gene. Science. 1996;272 (5259):258–62.
39. Rattan SI. Aging, anti-aging, and hormesis. Mech Ageing Dev. 2004;125(4):285–9.
40. Partridge L, Gems D. A lethal side-effect. Nature. 2002;418(6901):921.
41. Gilchrest BA, Garmyn M, Yaar M. Aging and photoaging affect gene expression in cultured human keratinocytes. Arch Dermatol. 1994;130(1):82–6.
42. Yaar M, Eller MS, Bhawan J, et al. In vivo and in vitro SPRR1 gene expression in normal and malignant keratinocytes. Exp Cell Res. 1995;217(2):217–26.
43. Seshadri T, Campisi J. Repression of c-fos transcription and an altered genetic program in senescent human fibroblasts. Science. 1990;247(4939):205–9.
44. Hara E, Yamaguchi T, Nojima H, et al. Id-related genes encoding helix-loop-helix proteins are required for G1 progression and are repressed in senescent human fibroblasts. J Biol Chem. 1994;269(3):2139–45.
45. Simard M, Manthos H, Giaid A, et al. Ontogeny of growth hormone receptors in human tissues: an immunohistochemical study. J Clin Endocrinol Metab. 1996;81(8):3097–102.
46. Noda A, Ning Y, Venable SF, et al. Cloning of senescent cell-derived inhibitors of DNA synthesis using an expression screen. Exp Cell Res. 1994;211 (1):90–8.
47. Jenkins G. Molecular mechanisms of skin ageing. Mech Ageing Dev. 2002;123(7):801–10.
48. Uitto J. Biochemistry of the elastic fibers in normal connective tissues and its alterations in diseases. J Invest Dermatol. 1979;72(1):1–10.
49. Fisher GJ, Kang S, Varani J, et al. Mechanisms of photoaging and chronological skin aging. Arch Dermatol. 2002;138(11):1462–70.
50. Chung JH, Kang S, Varani J, et al. Decreased extracellular-signal-regulated kinase and increased stress-activated MAP kinase activities in aged human skin in vivo. J Invest Dermatol. 2000;115(2):177–82.
51. Xia Z, Dickens M, Raingeaud J, et al. Opposing effects of ERK and JNK-p38 MAP kinases on apoptosis. Science. 1995;270(5240):1326–31.
52. Verheij M, Bose R, Lin XH, et al. Requirement for ceramide-initiated SAPK/JNK signalling in stress-induced apoptosis. Nature. 1996;380(6569):75–9.
53. Zeng G, McCue HM, Mastrangelo L, et al. Endogenous TGF-beta activity is modified during cellular aging: effects on metalloproteinase and TIMP-1 expression. Exp Cell Res. 1996;228(2):271–6.
54. Wick M, Burger C, Brusselbach S, et al. A novel member of human tissue inhibitor of metalloproteinases (TIMP) gene family is regulated during G1 progression, mitogenic stimulation, differentiation, and senescence. J Biol Chem. 1994;269(29):18953–60.
55. Mori Y, Hatamochi A, Arakawa M, et al. Reduced expression of mRNA for transforming growth factor beta (TGF beta) and TGF beta receptors I and II and decreased TGF beta binding to the receptors in in vitro-aged fibroblasts. Arch Dermatol Res. 1998;290 (3):158–62.
56. Kyng KJ, May A, Kolvraa S, et al. Gene expression profiling in Werner syndrome closely resembles that of normal aging. Proc Natl Acad Sci U S A. 2003;100 (21):12259–64.
57. Lener T, Moll PR, Rinnerthaler M, et al. Expression profiling of aging in the human skin. Exp Gerontol. 2006;41(4):387–97.
58. Makrantonaki E, Brink TC, Zampeli V, Elewa RM, Mlody B, Hossini AM, Hermes B, Krause U, Knolle J, Abdallah M, Adjaye J, Zouboulis CC. Identification of biomarkers of human skin ageing in both genders. Wnt signalling – a label of skin ageing? PLoS One. 2012;7(11):e50393.
59. Gronniger E, Weber B, Heil O, Peters N, Stab F, Wenck H, Korn B, Winnefeld M, Lyko F. Aging and chronic sun exposure cause distinct epigenetic changes in human skin. PLoS Genet. 2010;6(5), e1000971.
60. Chondrogianni N, Voutetakis K, Kapetanou M, Delitsikou V, Papaevgeniou N, Sakellari M, Lefaki M, Filippopoulou K, Gonos ES. Proteasome activation: an innovative promising approach for delaying aging and retarding age-related diseases. Ageing Res Rev. 2015;23(Pt A):37–55.
61. Mohrin M, Chen D. Sirtuins, tissue maintenance, and tumorigenesis. Genes Cancer. 2013;4(3–4):76–81.
62. Gilchrest BA, Campisi J, Chang HY, Fisher GJ, Kulesz-Martin MF. Montagna symposium 2014-skin aging: molecular mechanisms and tissue consequences. J Invest Dermatol. 2015;135(4):950–3.
63. Wallace DC. Mitochondrial defects in neurodegenerative disease. Ment Retard Dev Disabil Res Rev. 2001;7 (3):158–66.
64. Tatar M, Bartke A, Antebi A. The endocrine regulation of aging by insulin-like signals. Science. 2003;299 (5611):1346–51.

65. Conboy IM, Conboy MJ, Wagers AJ, et al. Rejuvenation of aged progenitor cells by exposure to a young systemic environment. Nature. 2005;433(7027):760–4.
66. Makrantonaki E, Adjaye J, Herwig R, et al. Age-specific hormonal decline is accompanied by transcriptional changes in human sebocytes in vitro. Aging Cell. 2006;5(4):331–44.
67. Nesbit M, Nesbit HK, Bennett J, et al. Basic fibroblast growth factor induces a transformed phenotype in normal human melanocytes. Oncogene. 1999;18(47):6469–76.
68. Singh K, Maity P, Krug L, Meyer P, Treiber N, Lucas T, Basu A, Kochanek S, Wlaschek M, Geiger H, Scharffetter-Kochanek K. Superoxide anion radicals induce IGF-1 resistance through concomitant activation of PTP1B and PTEN. EMBO Mol Med. 2015;7 (1):59–77.
69. Lewis DA, Travers JB, Somani AK, Spandau DF. The IGF-1/IGF-1R signaling axis in the skin: a new role for the dermis in aging-associated skin cancer. Oncogene. 2010;29(10):1475–85.
70. Laron Z. Effects of growth hormone and insulin-like growth factor 1 deficiency on ageing and longevity. Novartis Found Symp. 2002;242:125–37 (Discussion 137–142).
71. Carroll PV, Christ ER, Bengtsson BA, et al. Growth hormone deficiency in adulthood and the effects of growth hormone replacement: a review. Growth Hormone Research Society Scientific Committee. J Clin Endocrinol Metab. 1998;83(2):382–95.
72. Tomlinson JW, Holden N, Hills RK, et al. Association between premature mortality and hypopituitarism. West Midlands Prospective Hypopituitary Study Group. Lancet. 2001;357(9254):425–31.
73. Rudman D, Feller AG, Nagraj HS, et al. Effects of human growth hormone in men over 60 years old. N Engl J Med. 1990;323(1):1–6.
74. Riedl M, Kotzmann H, Luger A. Growth hormone in the elderly man. Wien Med Wochenschr. 2001;151 (18–20):426–9.
75. Brincat MP. Hormone replacement therapy and the skin. Maturitas. 2000;35(2):107–17.
76. Fuchs KO, Solis O, Tapawan R, et al. The effects of an estrogen and glycolic acid cream on the facial skin of postmenopausal women: a randomised histologic study. Cutis. 2003;71(6):481–8.
77. Sator PG, Schmidt JB, Sator MO, et al. The influence of hormone replacement therapy on skin ageing: a pilot study. Maturitas. 2001;39(1):43–55.
78. Schmidt JB, Binder M, Demschik G, et al. Treatment of skin aging with topical estrogens. Int J Dermatol. 1996;35(9):669–74.
79. Affinito P, Palomba S, Sorrentino C, et al. Effects of postmenopausal hypoestrogenism on skin collagen. Maturitas. 1999;33(3):239–47.
80. Makrantonaki E, Vogel K, et al. Interplay of IGF-I and 17beta-estradiol at age-specific levels in human sebocytes and fibroblasts in vitro. Exp Gerontol. 2008;43(10):939–46.
81. Makrantonaki E, Zouboulis CC. Skin alterations and diseases in advanced age. Drug Discov Today Dis Mec. 2008;5(2):e153–62.

10 Pathomechanisms of Photoaged Skin

Jean Krutmann

Contents

Abstract

Solar UV radiation is the most important in premature skin aging (photoaging). From resent research, it is now clear that both UVB (290–320 nm) and UVA (320–400 nm) radiations contribute to photoaging. UV-induced alterations at the level of the dermis are best studied and appear to be largely responsible for the phenotype of photoaged skin. It is also generally agreed that UVB acts preferentially on the epidermis where it not only damages DNA in keratinocytes and melanocytes but also causes the production of soluble factors including proteolytic enzymes, which in a second step affect the dermis; in contrast, UVA radiation penetrates far more deeply and exerts direct effects on both the epidermal and the dermal compartments. UVA radiation may be at least as important as UVB radiation in the pathogenesis of photoaging.

Introduction

Among all environmental factors, solar UV radiation is the most important in premature skin aging, a process accordingly termed photoaging. Over recent years, substantial progress has been made in elucidating the underlying molecular mechanisms. From these studies, it is now clear that both UVB (290–320 nm) and UVA (320–400 nm) radiations contribute to photoaging. UV-induced alterations at the level of the dermis

J. Krutmann (✉)
Environmental Health Research Institute (IUF), Heinrich-Heine-University, Duesseldorf, Germany
e-mail: krutmann@uni-duesseldorf.de

M.A. Farage et al. (eds.), *Textbook of Aging Skin*,
DOI 10.1007/978-3-662-47398-6_10

are best studied and appear to be largely responsible for the phenotype of photoaged skin. It is also generally agreed that UVB acts preferentially on the epidermis where it not only damages DNA in keratinocytes and melanocytes but also causes the production of soluble factors including proteolytic enzymes, which in a second step affect the dermis; in contrast, UVA radiation penetrates far more deeply on average and hence exerts direct effects on both the epidermal and the dermal compartments (Fig. 1). UVA is also 10–100 times more abundant in sunlight than UVB, depending on the season and time of the day. Therefore, it has been proposed that, although UVA photons are individually far less biologically active than UVB photons, UVA radiation may be at least as important as UVB radiation in the pathogenesis of photoaging [1].

The exact mechanisms by which UV radiation causes premature skin aging are not yet clear, but a number of molecular pathways explaining one or more of the key features of photoaged skin have been described. Some of these models are based on irradiation protocols, which use single or few UV exposures, whereas others take into account the fact that photoaging results from chronic UV damage and, as a consequence, employ chronic repetitive irradiation protocols. Still others rely on largely theoretical constructs rather than experimental observations.

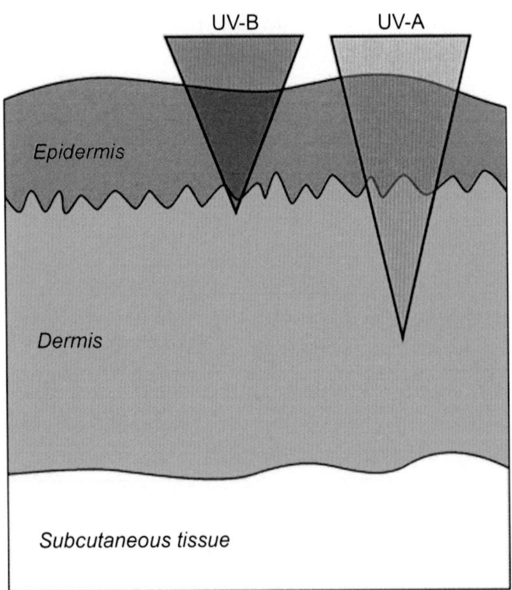

Fig. 1 Wavelength-dependent penetration of UV radiation into human skin

Mechanisms of Photoaging

All organ systems are affected by aging processes, many in organ-specific ways; however, aging uniformly has the effect of reducing maximal function and reserve capacity, as well as the ability to compensate for injury and a hostile environment. Ultimately, such losses are incompatible with life.

Of interest, most, if not all, age-accelerating environmental factors damage DNA either directly or indirectly, often through oxidation. Furthermore, the rate of aging in various species correlates [2] inversely with the rate and fidelity of DNA repair [3], and most progeroid syndromes for which the genetic lesion has been identified have impaired DNA replication and/or DNA damage responses. In combination with the fact that cumulative DNA damage accompanies chronological aging [4], these observations suggest that both the indisputable heritable and the environmental components of aging result in large part from changing DNA status during the individual's lifetime.

The next section develops this intellectual framework and relates it to the phenomenon of skin aging, and particularly photoaging, by focusing on mtDNA [1, 5]. The subsequent sections provide detailed information now available with regard to specific aging targets and signaling pathways responsible for photoaging-associated morphological and functional changes in the skin. These include UV-induced alterations of connective tissue components, vascularization patterns, inflammatory cells, and protein oxidation. Finally, a unifying concept is presented that reconciles with the most recent findings in an attempt to provide a novel and comprehensive model to explain photoaging and provide a framework for future investigations.

Mitochondrial DNA Mutations and Photoaging

Mitochondria are organelles whose main function is to generate energy for the cell. This is achieved by a multistep process called oxidative phosphorylation or electron transport chain. Located at the inner mitochondrial membrane are five multiprotein complexes that generate an electrochemical proton gradient used in the last step of the process to turn ADP and organophosphate into ATP. This process is not completely error-free and ultimately leads to the generation of reactive oxygen species (ROS), making the mitochondrion the site of the highest ROS turnover in the cell. In close proximity to this site lies the mitochondrion's own genomic material, the mtDNA. Human mtDNA is a 16,559-bp long circular double-stranded molecule of which four to ten copies exist per cell. Since mitochondria do not exhibit any repair mechanism to remove bulky DNA lesions, although they do exhibit a base excision repair mechanism and repair mechanisms against oxidative damage, the mutation frequency of mtDNA is approximately 50-fold higher than that of nuclear DNA.

Mutations of mtDNA have been found to play a causative role in degenerative diseases such as Alzheimer's disease, chronic progressive external ophthalmoplegia, and Kearns-Sayre syndrome (KSS) [6]. In addition to degenerative diseases, mutations of mtDNA may play a causative role in the normal aging process with an accumulation of mtDNA mutations accompanied by a decline of mitochondrial functions [7]. Recent evidence indicates that mtDNA mutations are also involved in the process of photoaging [1].

Photoaged skin is characterized by increased mutations of the mitochondrial genome [8–10]. Intraindividual comparison studies have revealed that the so-called common deletion, a 4,977-bp deletion of mtDNA, is increased up to tenfold in photoaged skin as compared with sun-protected skin of the same individuals. The amount of the common deletion in human skin does not correlate with chronological aging [11], and it has therefore been proposed that mtDNA mutations such as the common deletion represent molecular markers for photoaging. In support of this concept, it has been shown that repetitive, sublethal exposure to UVA radiation at doses that may be acquired during a regular summer holiday induces mutations of mtDNA in cultured primary human dermal fibroblasts in a singlet oxygen-dependent fashion [3]. Even more importantly, in vivo studies have revealed that repetitive exposure three times daily of previously unirradiated buttock skin for a total of 2 weeks to physiological doses of UVA radiation leads to an approximately 40 % increase in the levels of the common deletion in the dermal, but not the epidermal, compartment of irradiated skin [12]. Furthermore, it has been shown that, once induced, these mutations persist for at least 16 months in UV-exposed skin. Interestingly, in a number of individuals, the levels of the common deletion in irradiated skin continued to increase with a magnitude up to 32-fold.

It has been postulated for the normal aging process as well as for photoaging that the induction of ROS generates mtDNA mutations, in turn leading to a defective respiratory chain and, in a vicious cycle, inducing even more ROS and subsequently allowing mtDNA mutagenesis independent of the inducing agent [13]. It is the characteristic of vicious cycles that they evolve at ever-increasing speeds. Thus, the increase of the common deletion up to levels of 32-fold, independent of UV exposure, may represent the first in vivo evidence for the presence of such a vicious cycle in general and in human skin in particular.

The mechanisms by which generation of mtDNA mutations by UVA exposure translates into the morphological alterations observed in photoaging human skin are currently being unraveled. In general, a cause-effect relationship between premature aging and mtDNA mutagenesis is strongly suggested by studies employing homozygous knock-in mice that express a proofreading-deficient version of PolgA, the nucleus-encoded subunit of mtDNA polymerase [14]. As expected, these mice develop an mtDNA mutator phenotype with increased amounts of deleted mtDNA. This increase in somatic mtDNA mutations has been found to be associated with a reduced life span and premature onset of aging-related phenotypes such as weight loss, reduced subcutaneous fat, alopecia, kyphosis, osteoporosis, anemia, reduced fertility, and heart enlargement.

In addition, recent studies have demonstrated that UVA radiation-induced mtDNA mutagenesis is of functional relevance in primary human dermal fibroblasts and apparently has molecular consequences suggestive of a causative role for mtDNA mutations in photoaging of human skin as well [15]. Accordingly, induction of the common deletion in human skin fibroblasts is paralleled by a measurable decrease of oxygen consumption, mitochondrial membrane potential, and ATP content, as well as an increase of MMP-1, while tissue-specific inhibitors of MMPs (TIMPs) remain unaltered, an imbalance that is known to be involved in photoaging of human skin (see below). These observations suggest a link not only between mutations of mtDNA and cellular energy metabolism but also between mtDNA mutagenesis, energy metabolism, and a fibroblast gene expression profile that would functionally correlate with increased matrix degradation and thus premature skin aging. In order to provide further evidence for a role of the energy metabolism in mtDNA mutagenesis and the development of this "photoaging phenotype," the effect of creatine was studied in these cells. This applied the hypothesis that generation of phosphocreatine, and consequently ATP, is facilitated if creatine is abundant in cells. This would allow easier binding of existing energy-rich phosphates to the energy precursor creatine. Indeed, experimental supplementation of normal human fibroblasts with creatine normalizes mitochondrial mutagenesis as well as the functional parameters, oxygen consumption, and MMP-1, while an inhibitor of creatine uptake abrogates this effect [15] (Fig. 2).

A second line of evidence for cause-effect relationship between a disturbance of mtDNA integrity and skin aging is provided by a very recent study, in which a phenocopy of cells bearing large-scale deletions of mtDNA was generated by gradually depleting the mtDNA from unirradiated human skin fibroblasts [16].

Gradual depletion of mtDNA caused a gene expression profile, which was a reminiscent of that observed in photoaged skin. Accordingly, in these cells an increased expression of MMP-1 without a concomitant change in tissue inhibitor metalloproteinase-1 as well as a decreased expression of collagen type 1 alpha-1, that is, a gene involved in collagen de novo synthesis, was observed. This altered gene expression resulted from intracellular, mitochondria-derived oxidative stress. These results support the concept that disruption of mt integrity, for example, by UV-induced mtDNA mutagenesis, is of pathogenetic relevance for photoaging of human skin.

Finally, a third line of evidence for a pathogenetic role of mtDNA mutations in photoaging is provided by human in vitro studies employing skin fibroblasts from Kearns-Sayre syndrome (KSS) patients, which constitutionally carry large amounts of the UV-inducible common deletion. Accordingly, human dermal skin equivalent models, which were engineered using KSS skin fibroblasts, developed multiple features of photoaged skin including MMP-1 upregulation and increased collagen breakdown even in the absence of any UV exposure ([17] and Krutmann et al., unpublished observation).

Connective Tissue Alterations in Photoaging: The Role of Matrix Metalloproteinases and Collagen Synthesis

Photoaged skin is characterized by alterations to the dermal connective tissue. The extracellular matrix in the dermis mainly consists of type I and type III collagen, elastin, proteoglycans, and fibronectin. In particular, collagen fibrils are important for the strength and resilience of skin, and alterations in their number and structure are thought to be responsible for wrinkle formation.

In photoaged skin, collagen fibrils are disorganized and abnormal elastin-containing material accumulates [18]. Biochemical studies have revealed that in photoaged skin levels of types I

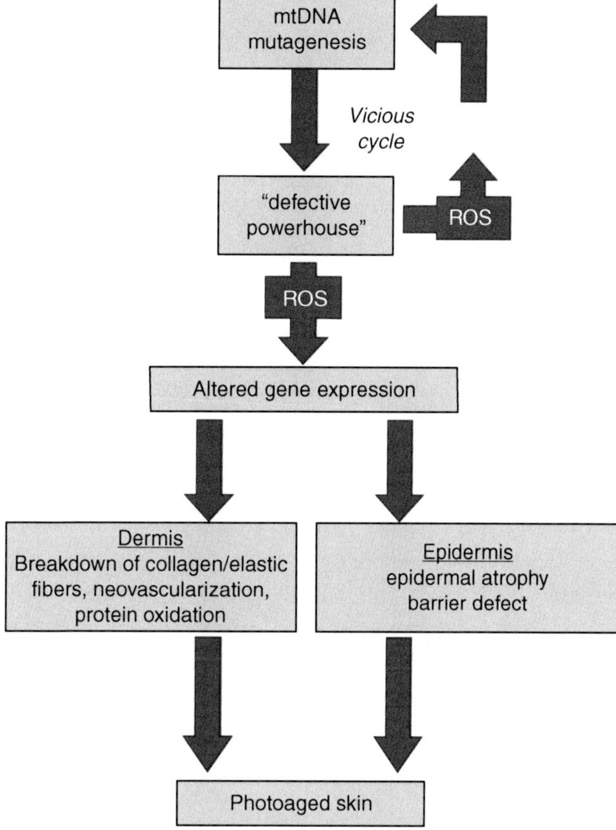

Fig. 2 The defective powerhouse model of (photo)aging of the skin

and III collagen, precursors and cross-links are reduced, whereas elastin levels are increased [19, 20]. How does UV radiation cause these alterations? In principle it is reasonable to assume that UV radiation leads to an enhanced and accelerated degradation and/or a decreased synthesis of collagen fibers, and current knowledge indicates that both mechanisms may be involved.

A large number of studies unambiguously demonstrate that the induction of matrix metalloproteinases (MMPs) plays a major role in the pathogenesis of photoaging. As indicated by their name, these zinc-dependent endopeptidases show proteolytic activity in their ability to degrade matrix proteins such as collagen and elastin. Each MMP degrades different dermal matrix proteins; for example, MMP-1 cleaves collagen types I, II, and III, whereas MMP-9, which is also called gelatinase, degrades collagen types IV and V and gelatin. Under basal conditions, MMPs are part of a coordinated network and are precisely regulated by their endogenous inhibitors, i.e., TIMPs, which specifically inactivate certain MMPs. An imbalance between activation of MMPs and their respective TIMPs could lead to excessive proteolysis.

It is now very well established that UV radiation induces MMPs without affecting the expression or activity of TIMPs [21, 22]. These MMPs can be induced by both UVB and UVA radiations, but the underlying photobiological and molecular mechanisms differ depending on the type of irradiation. In a very simplified scheme, UVA radiation would mostly act indirectly through the generation of ROS, in particular, singlet oxygen, which can subsequently exert a multitude of effects such as lipid peroxidation, activation of transcription factors, and generation of DNA strand breaks [22]. While UVB radiation-induced MMP induction has been shown to involve the generation of ROS as well [23], the main mechanism of action of UVB is by direct interaction with

DNA via the induction of DNA damage. Recent studies have indeed provided evidence that enhanced repair of UVB-induced cyclobutane pyrimidine dimers in the DNA of epidermal keratinocytes through topical application of liposomally encapsulated DNA repair enzymes on UVB-irradiated human skin prevents UVB radiation-induced epidermal MMP expression [24].

The activity of MMPs is tightly regulated by transcriptional regulation, and elegant in vivo studies by Fisher et al. have demonstrated that exposure of human skin to UVB radiation leads to the activation of the respective transcription factors [25]. Accordingly, UV exposure of human skin not only leads to the induction of MMPs within hours after irradiation, but already within minutes, transcription factors AP-1 and NF-κB, which are known stimulatory factors of MMP genes, are induced. These effects can be observed at low UVB dose levels, because transcription factor activation and MMP-1 induction can be achieved by exposing human skin to one tenth of the dose necessary for skin reddening (0.1 minimal erythema dose). Subsequent work by the same group clarified the major components of the molecular pathway by which UVB exposure leads to the degradation of matrix proteins in human skin. Low-dose UVB irradiation induces a signaling cascade, which involves upregulation of epidermal growth factor receptors (EGFR), the GTP-binding regulatory protein p21Ras, extracellular signal-regulated kinase (ERK), c-jun aminoterminal kinase (JNK), and p38. Elevated c-jun together with constitutively expressed c-fos increases activation of AP-1. Identification of this UVB-induced signaling pathway not only unravels the complexity of the molecular basis, which underlies UVB radiation-induced gene expression in human skin, but also provides a rationale for the efficacy of tretinoin (all-*trans*-retinoic acid) in the treatment of photoaged skin. Accordingly, topical pretreatment with tretinoin inhibits the induction and activity of MMPs in UVB-irradiated skin through prevention of AP-1 activation.

In addition to destruction of existing collagen through activation of MMPs, failure to replace damaged collagen is thought to contribute to photoaging as well. Accordingly, in chronically photodamaged skin, collagen synthesis is downregulated as compared to sun-protected skin [26]. The mechanism by which UV radiation interferes with collagen synthesis is not yet known, but a recent study has provided evidence that fibroblasts in severely (photo)damaged skin have less interaction with intact collagen and are thus exposed to less mechanical tension, and it has been proposed that this situation might lead to decreased collagen synthesis [27].

UV-Induced Modulation of Vascularization

There is increasing evidence that cutaneous blood vessels may play a role in the pathogenesis of photoaging. Photoaged skin shows vascular damage; intrinsically aged skin does not. In mildly photodamaged skin, there is venular wall thickening, while in severely damaged skin, the vessel walls are thinned and the supporting perivascular veil cells are reduced in number [28]. The number of vascular cross sections is reduced [29] and there are local dilations, corresponding to clinical telangiectases. Overall, there is a marked change in the horizontal vascularization pattern with dilated and distorted vessels. Studies in humans and in the hairless skh-1 mouse model for skin aging have demonstrated that acute and chronic UVB irradiation greatly increases skin vascularization [30, 31].

The formation of blood vessels from preexisting vessels is tightly controlled by a number of angiogenic factors and factors that inhibit angiogenesis. These growth factors include basic fibroblast growth factor, interleukin-8, tumor growth factor-beta, platelet-derived growth factor, and vascular endothelial growth factor (VEGF). VEGF appears to be involved in chronic UVB damage because UVB radiation-induced dermal angiogenesis in skh-1 mice is associated with increased VEGF expression in the hyperplastic epidermis of these animals [31]. Even more importantly, targeted overexpression of the angiogenesis inhibitor thrombospondin-1 not only prevents UVB radiation-induced skin vascularization and endothelial cell proliferation but also significantly reduces dermal photodamage and wrinkle formation. These studies suggest that UVB radiation-induced angiogenesis plays a direct biological role in photoaging.

Photoaging as a Chronic Inflammatory Process

In contrast to intrinsically aged skin, which shows an overall reduction in cell numbers, photoaged skin is characterized by an increase in the number of dermal fibroblasts, which appear hyperplastic, and also by increased numbers of mast cells, histiocytes, and mononuclear cells. The presence of such a dermal infiltrate indicates the possibility that a chronic inflammatory process takes place in photoaged skin, and in order to describe this situation, the terms heliodermatitis and dermatoheliosis have been coined [32]. More recent studies have shown that increased numbers of CD4 + T cells are present in the dermis, whereas intraepidermally, infiltrates of indeterminate cells and a concomitant reduction in the number of epidermal Langerhans cells have been described [33]. It is currently not known whether the presence of inflammatory cells represents an epiphenomenon or whether these cells play a causative role in the pathogenesis of photoaging, e.g., through the production of soluble mediators, which could affect the production and/or degradation of extracellular matrix proteins.

Protein Oxidation and Photoaging

The aging process is accompanied by enhanced oxidative damage. All cellular components including proteins are affected by oxidation [34]. Protein carbonyls may be formed either by oxidative cleavage of proteins or by direct oxidation of lysine, arginine, proline, and threonine residues. In addition, carbonyl groups may be introduced into proteins by reaction with aldehydes produced during lipid peroxidation or with reactive carbonyl derivatives generated as a consequence of the reaction with reducing sugars or their oxidation products with lysine residues of proteins.

Within the cell, the proteasome is responsible for the degradation of oxidized proteins. During the aging process, this function of the proteasome is diminished and oxidized proteins accumulate. In addition, lipofuscin, a highly cross-linked and modified protein aggregate, is formed. This aggregate accumulates within cells and is able to inhibit the proteasome. These alterations mainly occur within the cytoplasm, and lipofuscin does not accumulate in the nucleus.

In biopsies from individuals with histologically confirmed solar elastosis, an accumulation of oxidatively modified proteins was found specifically within the upper dermis [35]. Protein oxidation in photoaged skin is most likely due to UV irradiation because repetitive exposure of human buttock skin over 10 days to increasing UV doses and in vitro irradiation of cultured dermal fibroblasts with UVB or UVA have been shown to cause protein oxidation. The functional relevance of increased protein oxidation in UV-irradiated dermal fibroblasts, in particular with regard to the pathogenesis of photoaging, is currently not known. Very recent studies, however, indicate that increased protein oxidation, which may result from a single exposure of cultured human fibroblasts to UVA radiation, inhibits proteasomal functions and thereby affects intracellular signaling pathways, which are involved in MMP-1 expression (Krutmann J et al., unpublished observation).

Conclusion and Toward a Unifying Concept

From the above observations, it is evident that major progress has been made recently in identifying molecular mechanisms involved in photoaging. In this regard, the skin has proven to serve as an excellent model organ to understand basic mechanisms relevant for extrinsic aging.

Despite all these progresses, however, a general, unifying concept linking the different mechanisms and molecular targets described in the previous paragraphs is still lacking. In other words, the critical question to answer is: How do mtDNA mutagenesis, neovascularization, protein oxidation, downregulation of collagen synthesis, and increased expression of matrix metalloproteinases together cause photoaging of human skin? Which of these mechanisms are of primary importance and responsible for inducing others? Are some or all of the abovementioned characteristics of photoaged skin merely epiphenomena and, if so, to what extent are they causally related to premature skin aging?

The current state of knowledge does not allow to answer these questions in a definitive manner. Nevertheless, a hypothesis is proposed, which tries to reconcile with most of the research discussed above in one model, for which the term "the defective powerhouse model of skin aging" has been coined [16, 36].

Specifically, the persistence of UV radiation-induced mtDNA mutations and the resulting vicious cycle with further increases in mtDNA mutations lead to a situation resembling a "defective powerhouse" where inadequate energy production leads to chronic oxidative stress. In the dermis, functional consequences of direct DNA damage and aberrant ROS production in human dermal fibroblasts could be (1) an altered gene expression pattern, which would affect neovascularization and collagen metabolism and possibly also the generation of an inflammatory infiltrate, (2) the oxidation of intracellular proteins and inhibition of the proteasome, and (3) possibly also changes in the epidermal compartment such as epidermal atrophy, skin barrier, and dysfunction.

As a consequence, measures to prevent, delay, or even reverse photoaging should target the dermal rather than the epidermal compartment of human skin.

Acknowledgments Part of the work described in this chapter has been supported by the DFG, SFB 728.

Cross-References

▸ Pathomechanisms of Endogenously Aged Skin

References

1. Berneburg M, Plettenberg H, Krutmann J. Photoaging of human skin. Photodermatol Photoimmunol Photomed. 2000;16:239–44.
2. Brash D, Rudolph J, Simon J, Lin A, McKenna G, Baden H, Halperin A, Pontenm JA. Role for sunlight in skin cancer: UV-induced p53 mutations in squamous cell carcinoma. Proc Natl Acad Sci U S A. 1998;88:10124–8.
3. Hart RW, Setlow RB. Correlation between deoxyribonucleic acid excision-repair and life-span in a number of mammalian species. Proc Natl Acad Sci U S A. 1974;71:2169–73.
4. Vijg J. Somatic mutations and aging: a re-evaluation. Mutat Res. 2000;447:117–35.
5. Berneburg M, Grether-Beck S, Kurten V, Ruzicka T, Briviba K, Sies H, Krutmann J. Singlet oxygen mediates the UVA-induced generation of the photoaging-associated mitochondrial common deletion. J Biol Chem. 1999;274:15345–9.
6. DiMauro S, Schon EA. Mitochondrial respiratory-chain diseases. N Engl J Med. 2003;348:2656–68.
7. Wallace DC. Mitochondrial genetics: a paradigm for aging and degenerative diseases? Science. 1992;256:628–32.
8. Berneburg M, Gattermann N, Stege H, Grewe M, Vogelsang K, Ruzicka T, Krutmann J. Chronically ultraviolet-exposed human skin shows a higher mutation frequency of mitochondrial DNA as compared to unexposed skin and the hematopoietic system. Photochem Photobiol. 1997;66:271–5.
9. Birch-Machin MA, Tindall M, Turner R, Haldane F, Rees JL. Mitochondrial DNA deletions in human skin reflect photo- rather than chronologic aging. J Invest Dermatol. 1998;110:149–52.
10. Yang JH, Lee HC, Wei YH. Photoageing-associated mitochondrial DNA length mutations in human skin. Arch Dermatol Res. 1995;287:641–8.
11. Koch H, Wittern KP, Bergemann J. In human keratinocytes the common deletion reflects donor variabilities rather than chronologic aging and can be induced by ultraviolet A irradiation. J Invest Dermatol. 2001;117:892–7.
12. Berneburg M, Plettenberg H, Medve-Konig K, Pfahlberg A, Gers-Barlag H, Gefeller O, Krutmann J. Induction of the photoaging-associated mitochondrial common deletion in vivo in normal human skin. J Invest Dermatol. 2004;12:1277–83.
13. Jacobs HT. The mitochondrial theory of aging: dead or alive? Aging Cell. 2003;2:11–7.
14. Trifunovic A, Wredenberg A, Falkenberg M, Spelbrink JN, Rovio AT, Bruder E, Bohlooly YM, Gidlof S, Oldfors A, Wibom R, Tornell J, Jacobs HT, Larsson NG. Premature ageing in mice expressing defective mitochondrial DNA polymerase. Nature. 2004;429:417–23.
15. Berneburg M, Gremmel T, Kurten V, Schroeder P, Hertel I, Mikecz AV, Wild S, Chen M, Declercq L,

Matsui M, Ruzicka T, Krutmann J. Creatine supplementation normalizes mutagenesis of mitochondrial DNA as well as functional consequences. J Invest Dermatol. 2005;125:213–20.
16. Schroeder P, Gremmel T, Berneburg M, Krutmann J. Partial depletion of mitochondrial DNA from human skin fibroblasts induces a gene expression profile reminiscent of photoaged skin. J Invest Dermatol. 2008;128:2297–303.
17. Majora M, Wittkampf T, Schuermann B, Schneider M, Franke S, Grether-Beck S, Wilichowski E, Bernerd F, Schroeder P, Krutmann J. Functional consequences of mitochondrial DNA deletions in human skin fibroblasts: increased contractile strength in collagen lattices is due to oxidative stress-induced lysyl oxidase activity. Am J Pathol. 2009 Sep;175(3):1019–29. doi:10.2353/ajpath.2009.080832.
18. Smith JG, Davidson EA, Sams WM, Clark RD. Alterations in human dermal connective tissue with age and chronic sun damage. J Invest Dermatol. 1962;39:347–50.
19. Braverman M, Fonferko E. Studies in cutaneous aging: I. The elastic fibre network. J Invest Dermatol. 1982;78:434–43.
20. Talwar HS, Griffioth CEM, Fisher GJ, Hamilton TA, Voorhees JJ. Reduced type I and type III procollagens in photodamaged adult human skin. J Invest Dermatol. 1995;105:285–90.
21. Fisher GJ, Talwar HS, Lin J, et al. Retinoic acid inhibits induction of c-jun protein by ultraviolet radiation that occurs subsequent to activation of mitogen-activated protein kinase pathways in human skin in vivo. J Clin Invest. 1998;101:1432–40.
22. Scharffetter-Kochanek K, Brenneisen P, Wenk J, et al. Photoaging of the skin: from phenotype to mechanisms. Exp Gerontol. 2000;35:307–16.
23. Wenk J, Brenneisen P, Meewes C, Wlaschek M, Peters T, Blaudschun R, Ma W, Kuhr L, Schneider L, Scharffetter-Kochanek K. UV-induced oxidative stress and photoaging. Curr Probl Dermatol. 2001;29:83–94.
24. Dong KK, Damaghi N, Picart SD, Markova NG, Obayashi K, Okano Y, Masaki H, Grether-Beck S, Krutmann J, Smiles KA, Yarosh DB. UV-induced DNA damage initiates release of MMP-1 in human skin. Exp Dermatol. 2008;17:1037–44.
25. Fisher GJ, Wang ZQ, Datta SC, Varani J, Kang S, Voorhees JJ. Pathophysiology of premature skin aging induced by ultraviolet light. N Engl J Med. 1997;337:1419–28.
26. Fisher G, Datta S, Wang Z, Li X, Quan T, Chung J, Kang S, Voorhees J. c-Jun dependent inhibition of cutaneous procollagen transcription following ultraviolet irradiation is reversed by all-trans retinoid acid. J Clin Invest. 2000;106:661–8.
27. Varani J, Schuger L, Dame MK, Leonhard C, Fligiel SEG, Kang S, Fisher GJ, Vorhees JJ. Reduced fibroblast interaction with intact collagen as a mechanism for depressed collagen synthesis in photodamaged skin. J Invest Dermatol. 2004;122:1471–9.
28. Braverman M, Fonfrko E. Studies in cutaneous aging: II. The microvasculature. J Invest Dermatol. 1982;73:59–66.
29. Kligman AM. Perspectives and problems in cutaneous gerontology. J Invest Dermatol. 1979;73:39–46.
30. Bielenberg DR, Bucana CD, Sanchez R, Donawho CK, Kripke ML, Fidler IJ. Molecular regulation of UVB-induced angiogenesis. J Invest Dermatol. 1998;111:864–72.
31. Yano K, Ouira H, Detmar M. Targeted over expression of the angiogenesis inhibitor thrombospondin-1 in the epidermis of transgenic mice prevents ultraviolet-B-induced angiogenesis and cutaneous photodamage. J Invest Dermatol. 2002;118:800–5.
32. Lavker RM, Kligman A. Chronic heliodermatitis: a morphologic evaluation of chronic actinic dermal damage with emphasis on the role of mast cells. J Invest Dermatol. 1988;90:325–30.
33. DeLeo VA, Dawes L, Jackson R. Density of Langerhans cells (LC) in normal versus chronic actinically damaged skin (CADS) of humans. J Invest Dermatol. 1981;76:330–4.
34. Levine RL, Stadtman ER. Oxidative modification of protein during ageing. Exp Gerontol. 2001;36:1495–502.
35. Sander CS, Chang H, Salzmann S, Muller CS, Ekanayake-Mudiyanselage S, Elsner P, Thiele JJ. Photoaging is associated with protein oxidation in human skin in vivo. J Invest Dermatol. 2002;118:618–25.
36. Schroeder P, Krutmann J. Role of mitochondria in photoageing of human skin: the defective powerhouse model. J Investig Dermatol Symp Proc. 2009;14:44.

Proteoglycans in Skin Aging

11

François-Xavier Maquart, Stéphane Brézillon, and Yanusz Wegrowski

Contents

F.-X. Maquart (✉)
Laboratoire de Biochimie, CNRS UMR 7369, Faculté de Médecine, Université de Reims-Champagne-Ardenne, Reims, France

Centre National de la Recherche Scientifique, CNRS UMR 7369, Reims, France

Centre Hospitalier et Universitaire (CHU) de Reims, Reims, France
e-mail: fmaquart@chu-reims.fr

S. Brézillon • Y. Wegrowski
Laboratoire de Biochimie, CNRS UMR 7369, Faculté de Médecine, Université de Reims-Champagne-Ardenne, Reims, France

Centre National de la Recherche Scientifique, CNRS UMR 7369, Reims, France
e-mail: stephane.brezillon@univ-reims.fr; yanusz.wegrowski@univ-reims.fr

M.A. Farage et al. (eds.), *Textbook of Aging Skin*,
DOI 10.1007/978-3-662-47398-6_11

Abstract

Proteoglycans are ubiquitous macromolecules of extracellular matrix, cell surface, and some intracellular granules. They are composed of a glycoprotein core to which one or several glycosaminoglycan chains are attached by covalent linkage. More than 40 different genes encode proteoglycans. Most of them are expressed in skin cells. However, only some of the protein products have been confirmed to reside in skin.

Skin proteoglycans contribute to tissue hydration, resistance and resilience, molecular filtration. They also control cell behavior and cell–cell or cell–matrix interactions. Additionally, by their polyanionic properties, proteoglycans constitute the biological reservoir of many cytokines and growth factors. Such a diversity of functions supposes that any changes of their expression or structure during aging may perturb the tissue homeostasis significantly

In this chapter, we'll review the different types of proteoglycans present in the skin and their main biological functions, with special interest to the alterations of these molecules during aging. The review will show that proteoglycans may play a major role in skin homeostasis and in its functional and architectural properties. Large areas remain, however, unknown at this time and many consequences on skin physiology have still to be investigated. Design of new experimental models, especially in vivo, will permit to better study the implication of proteoglycan alterations in the defects linked to skin aging.

Introduction: Skin Proteoglycans and Skin Aging

Proteoglycans are ubiquitous macromolecules of extracellular matrices, cell surfaces, and some intracellular granules [1]. They are composed of a glycoprotein core to which one or several sulfated glycosaminoglycan chains are attached by covalent linkage. Four different classes of sulfated glycosaminoglycans (GAGs) exist in vertebrates: chondroitin sulfate (CS), dermatan sulfate (DS), keratan sulfate (KS), and heparan sulfate/heparin (HS). Hyaluronic acid is not esterified with sulfate and not linked to a protein core. Glycosaminoglycan properties, structure, and functions are discussed in another chapter.

One protein core may bear one or several types of glycosaminoglycans of the same or different classes. For example, syndecan-1 may contain heparan sulfate only or heparan sulfate and chondroitin sulfate glycosaminoglycan chains. Depending on cell context, the same proteoglycan may be substituted with different GAG chains. For example, serglycin of mast cells is substituted with heparin but serglicyn of macrophages is substituted with chondroitin sulfate.

A third feature of these macromolecules is the possibility of absence of the glycosaminoglycan chain in the same proteoglycan, depending on the organ. Lumican in cornea is a keratan sulfate proteoglycan whereas in skin it is a glycoprotein without any glycosaminoglycan chain. Finally, the presence of GAG may be time dependent in so-called "part-time" proteoglycans. Often, it is done by synthesis of splicing variants lacking the GAG attachment sequence, like in the versican V3 variant.

The GAG chains of galactosaminoglycans (CS/DS) and HS are attached to a serine residue of the core protein via a short common tetrasaccharide, by a beta 1–4 bond in the case of CS/DS and by alpha 1–4 bond in the case of HS. This region is composed of a tetrasaccharide GlcA(β1-3)Gal(β1-3)Gal(β1-4)Xylβ1-*O*-Ser, where GlcA is glucuronic acid, Gal is galactose, and Xyl is xylose. Keratan sulfate chains of aggrecan (KS type II) are also attached to a serine residue via *O*-glycosidic linkage, but the composition of this linkage is similar to those of the *O*-substituted oligosaccharides of glycoproteins. Keratan sulfate chains of lumican or keratocan in cornea (KS I) possess a mannose-rich region attached by *N*-glycosidic linkage to an asparagine, similarly to the *N*-substituted oligosaccharides of glycoproteins. Although the presence of keratan sulfate in skin has been reported [2], no detailed structure of the linkage region of those molecules is known.

Several glyco and sulfotansferases are involved in the assembly of the GAGs on the protein core. The xylosyl-transferases are the enzymes which start the GAG synthesis. Although there is no consensus sequence for a given exported protein to be substituted with GAG chain, the xylosyl-transferases recognize Ser-Gly sequences in the vicinity of acidic amino acids [3]. It seems that the presence of hydrophobic clusters and the general conformation of the protein also contribute to the activity of *N*-acetyl-glucosamine transferase I and *N*-acetyl-galactosamine transferase I, two enzymes which initiate the synthesis of HS or CS/DS, respectively.

Iozzo and Schaefer enumerate 43 genes encoding real (full-time) proteoglycans [1]. The mRNAs of most of them are expressed in skin cells (Table 1) [4]. However, only some of the protein products have been confirmed to reside in skin. The extracellular proteoglycans are regrouped in different groups or classes. First and most abundant class of extracellular matrix proteoglycans of the dermis belongs to the Small Leucine-Rich Proteoglycan (SLRP) family [1]. Although there is no comparative quantification of different proteoglycans of human dermis, decorin seems to be the most abundant representative in skin, associated with collagen fibers. The same localisation concerns lumican which, in skin, carries no GAG chain. Biglycan is present mostly in skin pericellular matrix [5]. Fibromodulin was also reported to be present in epidermis [6].

The second group contains large, aggregating proteoglycans able to bind hyaluronic acid, usually called hyalectans (or lecticans). These proteoglycans are able to form very high molecular mass complexes, composed of numerous proteoglycan molecules settled down on a hyaluronan molecule [1]. From this group, only versican was documented in human dermis and epidermis [7]. Basement membrane of the dermoepidermal junction contains a major heparan sulfate proteoglycan, perlecan but also agrin and collagens type XV and type XVIII. (see below). Some other collagens (type IX, XII, XIII, and XIV) also contain a covalently linked GAG chain. Apart from type IX collagen, they are all expressed in collagen-rich dermis [8]. Testicans form another family of extracellular proteoglycans. Four testican genes have been cloned, but only testican-1 and testican-2 mRNA are expressed in skin, by keratinocytes (Table 1). Among miscellaneous proteoglycans, the mRNA of adlican was reported to be expressed in fibroblasts of very old subjects, but nothing is known about the protein. Another proteoglycan, CSF-1 is expressed by resident skin cells of the immune system, e.g., Langerhans cells [9].

Cell membrane proteoglycans, which are characterized by a very rapid turnover, include two main families of heparan sulfate macromolecules. The family of syndecans (four genes cloned) comprises integral type I membrane proteins, with a transmembrane domain and a short cytoplasmic tail (Table 1). Syndecan-1 is expressed in epidermis including hair follicles [10]. The family of glypicans (six genes cloned) is glycosylphosphatidylinositol-anchored molecules with a glycanic chain attached at the vicinity of plasma membrane [11]. Only the expression of neural glypican-2 was not detected in the skin (Table 1).

Syndecans and glypicans are easily shedded by the action of metalloproteinases and phospholipases, respectively, and are often found in pericellular space. CD-44 and one of its splicing epidermal variants, epican, is an integral plasma membrane proteoglycan which binds hyaluronic acid [12]. Keratinocytes also express the mRNAs of two brain proteoglycans, neuroglycan-C, and phosphacan (Table 1). One of the splicing variants of phosphacan possesses protein tyrosine phosphatase activity. Some proteoglycans characteristics of endothelial cells are also expressed by keratinocytes. The proangiogenic Transforming Growth Factor-beta (TGF-β) coreceptor, endoglin, is expressed in epidermis [13], as well as the thrombin receptor, thrombomodulin [14]. Another TGF-β co-receptor, betaglycan, also known as TGF-beta receptor type III, is also expressed in epidermis at the mRNA level, but the presence of the protein is not documented. Characteristic for embryonic development, the Melanoma-associated Antigen/NG2 is an integral

Table 1 The proteoglycans mRNA expressed by keratinocytes (K) or skin fibroblasts (F) screened by cDNA array obtained from GEO profiles of NCBI [4]

	Gene	NCBI Ref. Seq	mRNA expression	GAG chain
(A) Extracellular Proteoglycans				
S.L.R.P. class				
Decorin	DCN	NM_001920[a]	K/F	DS/CS
Biglycan	BGN	NM_001711	K/F	DS/CS
Asporin	ASPN	NM_017680	K/F	CS
Extracellular matrix protein 2	ECM2	NM_001393	K	
Fibromodulin	FMOD	NM_002023	K	KS
Lumican	LUM	NM_002345	F	KS
Pro/Arg-rich end LRR protein	PRELP	NM_002725[a]	K	CS
Keratocan	KERA	NM_007035	K/F	KS
Osteomodulin	OMD	NM_005014	K	CS
Epiphycan	EPYC	NM_004950	K/F	CS
Osteoglycin	OGN	NM_033014[a]	F	CS
Chondroadherin	CHAD	NM_001267	K	CS
Nyctalopin	NYX	NM_022567	K/F	
Hyalectans				
Versican	VCAN	NM_004385[a]	F	CS/(DS)
Aggrecan	ACAN	NM_013227[a]	K	CS + KS
Neurocan	NCAN	NM_004386	K	CS
Brevican	BCAN	NM_021948[a]	K/F	CS
Basement membrane PGs				
Perlecan (Heparan sulfate proteoglycan 2)	HSPG2	NM_005529	K/F	HS/(CS)
Agrin	AGRN	NM_198576	K/F	HS
Bamacan[b] (Structural maintenance of chromosomes 3)	SMC3	NM_005445	K/F	CS
Leprecan (PRP, Prolyl-3-hydroxylase)[b]	LEPRE1	NM_022356[a]	K/F	CS
Collagens				
Type IX	COL9A2	NM_001852	K	CS
Type XII	COL12A1	NM_004370	F	CS
Type XIV	COL14A1	NM_021110	F	CS
Type XVIII[b]	COL18A1	NM_030582[a]	K/F	HS
Testicans				
Testican 1	SPOCK1	NM_004598	K/F	CS
Testican 2	SPOCK2	NM_014767[a]	K	CS
Miscellaneous				
Adlican	MXRA5	NM_015419	K/F	?
Colony Stimulating Factor-1 (CSF-1, M-CSF)	CSF-1	NM_000757[a]	K/F	CS
(B) Cell Membrane Proteoglycans				
Syndecans				
Syndecan-1	SDC1[a]	NM_001006946	K/F	HS/(CS)
Syndecan-2	SDC2	NM_002998	F	HS
Syndecan-3	SDC3	NM_014654	K/F	HS
Syndecan-4	SDC4	NM_002999	K/F	HS
Glypicans				
Glypican-1	GPC1	NM_002081	K/F	HS
Glypican-3	GPC3	NM_004484	K	HS

(continued)

Table 1 (continued)

	Gene	NCBI Ref. Seq	mRNA expression	GAG chain
Glypican-4	GPC4	NM_001448	K	HS
Glypican-5	GPC5	NM_004466	K	HS
Glypican-6	GPC6	NM_005708	F	HS
Hyalectans				
CD44 (Lymphocyte homing receptor)	CD44	NM_000610[a]	K	CS/HS
Neural PGs				
Neuroglycan C Chondroitin sulfate proteoglycan 5	CSPG5	NM_006574	K	CS
Phosphacan	PTPRZ1	NM_002851	K	CS
Endothelial PGs				
Endoglin (CD105)	ENG,	NM_000118[a]	K/F	CS
Endothelial cell-specific molecule 1 (Endocan)	ESM1	NM_007036[a]	K	DS
Thrombomodulin (CD 141)	THBD	NM_000361	K	HS
Miscellaneous				
NG2, (Melanoma-associated Antigen, MAA) Chondroitin sulfate proteoglycan 4	CSPG4	NM_001897	K/F	CS
Betaglycan	TGFBR3	NM_003243	K	CS
(C) Granules Proteoglycan				
Serglycin	SRGN	NM_002727	K	Heparin/ CS

[a]Different splicing variants or mRNAs
[b]Basement membrane associated proteoglycans

membrane, chondroitin sulfate containing, high molecular mass proteoglycan, overexpressed in aggressive melanoma lesions [15]. NG2 was proposed to be a marker of melanoma invasion in the lymphatic glands. This proteoglycan is also characteristic for stem cell population of hair follicles root sheet and for pericytes [16]. Skin is a niche of mast cells, which contain heparin in their secretory granules. Heparin is linked to the proteoglycan serglycin core protein. This last is also expressed by macrophages and Langerhans cells but, in this case, it is substituted with chondroitin sulfate chains.

The knowledge about the roles of proteoglycans in physiologic and pathologic conditions started when the first demonstration of a dermatan sulfate-protein complex in skin was established [17]. The cloning era, followed by the creation of knockout mice, permitted to this knowledge to expand rapidly. Numerous excellent reviews, either general or devoted to particular class/families of proteoglycans give up-to-date state of the art in this area (cited in [1]). In general, skin proteoglycans retain all the properties and functions of particular glycosaminoglycans, contributing to tissue hydration, resistance and resilience, molecular filtration, cell behavior, and cell–cell or cell–matrix interaction. Additionally, by their polyanionic properties, they contribute to cation exchange and to the retention of all positively charged proteins. As a consequence, they constitute the biological reservoir of many cytokines and growth factors. Recent development of microscale analysis techniques permitted to discover the subtle modulations of glycosaminoglycan structure (i.e., the degree and the positions of sulfatations) in different subtissular compartments. For example, the stem cell niches contain extracellular matrix with poorly sulfated proteoglycans. These subtle modifications of macromolecules results in the different organization of matrix microenvironment, but also in the differences of cell behavior [18]. Such a diversity of functions supposes that any changes of their expression or structure during aging may perturb the tissue homeostasis in important manner.

The clinically relevant morphological changes of the skin during aging can be summarized by the term "senile atrophy." The main changes are a diminished thickness of epidermis with a reduced mitosis rate of epidermal basal cells and a decreased number of fibroblasts and capillaries in the dermis.

The mesenchymal changes in the dermis have been morphologically described by the term "senile elastosis" or "elastoid collagen degeneration," corresponding to a progressive collagen denaturation with aging. Analysis of the glycosaminoglycan content of the senile skin showed a minimal increase of the total content of hexosamines and uronic acids with a significant increase of DS and KS, a decrease of hyaluronic acid, and, also partly, a decrease of chondroitin-4-sulfate and chondroitin-6-sulfate. The neosynthesis of sulfated glycosaminoglycans is only slightly increased in aged skin, whereas the activities of the enzymes specific for the glycosaminoglycan catabolism (beta-glucuronidase, beta-*N*-acetyl-glucosaminidase) are significantly decreased [19].

Proteoglycans of the Dermis Extracellular Matrix

Small Leucine-Rich Proteoglycans

Small Leucine-Rich Proteoglycans (SLRPs) are a family of proteoglycans present in a large number of tissues. They are characterized by their relatively low molecular mass and by the presence of similar structural motifs, the leucine-rich repeats (LRR) [20]. They are presently classified into five distinct classes [1, 21], according to their structural features and chromosomal organization (Table 2).

Table 2 Classification of human SLRPs [1, 20]

SLRP class	Name
I	Biglycan
	Decorin
	Asporin
	ECM2
II	Fibromodulin
	Lumican
	PRELP
	Keratocan
	Chondroadherin
III	Epiphycan
	Opticin
	Osteoglycin
IV	Chondroadherin
	Nyctalopsin
	Tsukushi
V	Podocan
	Podocan-like protein 1

Dermis contains several SLRPs, particularly decorin and biglycan [5], lumican [22], and keratocan [23]. SLRPs play important roles in the regulation of cell activity and in the organization and functional properties of skin connective tissue [24]. Several lines of mice deficient in SLRPs have been generated, particularly for the most prominent and widely expressed SLRPs: decorin, biglycan, fibromodulin, and lumican. All these SLRP deficiencies result in the formation of abnormal collagen fibrils and induce a wide array of diseases in the deficient mice (for review, see [25]). The implication of SLRPs modifications in the alterations of skin function which may occur in skin aging has been suggested by several studies devoted to decorin and, more recently, to lumican.

Decorin

Decorin was the most studied among the SLRP family. It is composed of a 40 kDa protein core, bearing a unique DS/CS chain. It is the most abundant SLRP in adult human dermis, where it is observed in association with collagen fibers. It is synthesized and secreted by dermal fibroblasts and might represent 30–40 % of total proteoglycans of the skin [26].

Previous data from Bernstein et al. [27] reported that decorin was greatly decreased within photoaged skin, as appreciated by immunohistochemical staining and confocal laser scanning microscopy. In addition, Northern blot analysis showed that decorin steady state mRNA levels measured in fibroblasts derived from photoaged skin was decreased by 46 % in cultures derived from photodamaged sites. Since collagen degradation was strongly increased in such areas, and collagen amounts strongly decreased, it is possible, however, that the amount of decorin necessary to bind available collagen fibers may decrease in photoaged skin as collagen degradation takes place.

The decorin alterations in skin chronological aging seem very different from that observed in photoaging. As soon as 1997, Passi et al. [28] studied the modifications of proteoglycans secreted into their growth medium by young and senescent fibroblasts. In this study, senescence was induced in human skin fibroblasts by serial passages in culture, and their proteoglycan synthesis was studied by incorporation of radiolabeled precursors. These authors observed that, whereas the biosynthesis of total proteoglycan fraction was not altered with replicative senescence, the relative proportions of the different proteoglycan populations secreted into the growth medium changed. Particularly, the relative content of small CS/DS-proteoglycans that consisted mainly of decorin, as shown by immunological identification, was increased by 50 % in senescent (28–31 passages) versus young (4–5 passages) fibroblasts. Interestingly, these authors suggested that the increased secretion of decorin into the growth medium by the late passage fibroblasts might contribute to their decline of proliferative capacity, a characteristic common to every aging cell.

In a study of human skin samples from fetal skin, mature skin, and senescent skin, Carrino et al. [29] showed an increase in the proportion of decorin with a concomitant decrease of the large chondroitin-sulfate proteoglycan, versican, in senescent skin. In addition, these authors reported that decorin from postnatal skin is smaller in size than the decorin of mature skin, probably due to shorter glycosaminoglycan chains. More importantly, these authors reported the presence in aged skin of a shortened (Mr about 45 kDa) form of decorin, with a core protein of about 27 kDa only. Analysis of this molecule, named "decorunt" by these authors, indicated that it was a catabolic fragment of decorin, representing the amino terminal 43 % of the mature decorin molecule [30]. Decorunt contains the first four leucine-rich repeats and three amino acids of the fifth leucine-rich repeat. Since decorunt lacks almost half of the collagen-binding domain of decorin, it was expected to have impaired capacity to stabilize collagen fibers. Moreover, since the sixth leucine-rich repeat, the most important for the interaction between decorin and the Epidermal Growth Factor receptor, is lacking, decorunt should be unable to bind to this receptor, which may induce a defect of cell stimulation in aged skin. In addition, the absence of the Transforming Growth Factor-β binding site in decorunt might impair the sequestering of this growth factor in the extracellular matrix.

In an immunohistochemical study of rat dermis, Ito et al. [31], reported that decorin was only faintly visible in young (22 days old) rats, whereas it was abundant on the collagenous network of the dermis of old (24–30 month old) rats. Since decorin was shown to have a growth inhibitory effect, these authors suggested that decorin excess might be one of the cell growth inhibitory factors implicated in skin senescence.

Analysis of rat skin performed by Nomura et al. [32] confirmed that the amount of decorin in rat skin increased with rat's age (postpartus 0.5 days until 90 days of age). Interestingly, these authors noted that the molecular size of decorin decreased during aging, from about 111 kDa in 18.5 days embryo to about 70 kDa at postpartus 90 days. This decrease of size was not due to a decreased size of the core protein but to a decreased length of the glycosaminoglycan chain. The mean length of the chain was 78.58 ± 13.94 nm in the skin of the 18.5 days embryos vs. 54.05 ± 4.79 nm in the 90 days postpartus rat skin. Reducing the length of the decorin glycosaminoglycans was supposed to reduce the distance between the collagen fibers [33].

In a clinical study performed on full thickness punch biopsies obtained from five young (25 – 35 years) and five older (61 – 68 years) volunteers, Lockner et al. [34] reported that decorin mRNA in skin biopsies from older volunteers was approximately twice that in younger volunteers. In contrast, type I and type III collagens mRNAs were decreased. These authors suggested that the resulting decreased collagen to decorin ratio in older skin might be responsible for decreased collagen bundle diameters in aged human skin, which might affect their tensile strength [35, 36]. Intrinsic skin aging-dependent glycosaminoglycan and proteoglycan changes and their possible difference between male and female were investigated by Oh et al. [37]. Immunohistochemical stains of several glycosaminoglycans and proteoglycans were performed in sun-protected buttock skin of young and old, male and female (total $n = 32$) human skin. Decorin stain was decreased in aged skin in both genders. In another study by Li et al. [38], age-related alterations of decorin glycosaminoglycans in human skin were described. Analysis of decorin extracted from young (21–30 years) and aged (>80 years) sun-protected human buttock skin revealed that decorin molecular size in aged skin was significantly smaller than in young skin. The average size of decorin protein did not differ, indicating that size of glycosaminoglycan chains is reduced in aged, compared to young skin. This age-dependent alteration of decorin glycosaminoglycan may contribute to skin fragility of elderly people.

Recently, the effect of age on the integrity of skin was evaluated by an analysis of dermal extracellular and epidermal-dermal junction modifications using matrix-assisted laser desorption/ionization mass spectrometric imaging (MALDI-MSI), in vivo reflectance confocal microscopy (in vivo RCM), echography, and histology [39]. The authors showed that selected proteins (collagen I, collagen IV, collagen VII, collagen XVII, nidogen I) were found to be less abundant in aged group explants versus young group except for decorin.

Solar-stimulated UV irradiation of human skin in vivo stimulated substantial decorin degradation, with kinetics similar to infiltration of polymorphonuclear cells. In addition, neutrophil elastase degraded decorin and this degradation rendered collagen fibrils more susceptible to MMP-1 cleavage [40].

Biglycan

Biglycan and decorin are the predominant proteoglycans expressed in bone and skin, respectively. However, Corsi et al. [41] reported that biglycan deficiency leads to structural abnormality in collagen fibrils in bone, dermis, tendon, and to a "subclinical" cutaneous phenotype with thinning of the dermis but without overt skin fragility. While the immunohistochemical localization of the proteoglycans decorin, biglycan, and versican in human postburn hypertrophic and mature scars was described by Scott et al. [42], no age-related effect on the expression of biglycan mRNA in dermis has been detected.

Lumican

Lumican was first identified as a major proteoglycan of the cornea [43]. It is present in this tissue under the form of a keratan-sulfate (KS)-containing proteoglycan, with a 38 kDa core protein. In adult human skin, however, it is present under the form of a glycoprotein, devoid of glycosaminoglycan chain [44].

As decorin, lumican seems to play an important role in the preservation of skin functional properties. For instance, lumican-null mice showed abnormal collagen fibril assembly, with large and abnormally shaped collagen fibrils and an extremely loose and fragile skin [45].

Vuillermoz et al. [46] studied the expression of SLRPs by early passage cultured fibroblasts, obtained from 36 normal donors of 1 month to 83 years old. By Northern blot analysis, these authors showed a significant negative correlation of lumican mRNA expression with donor's age. By contrast, no correlation with age was found for either decorin or biglycan mRNAs. Immunohistochemistry associated with image analysis quantitation showed that lumican core protein was preferentially located in the superficial, papillary layer of the dermis and that it was strongly decreased (−81 % and −85 % respectively, $p < 0.01$) in aged skin (donors over 50) compared to young (0–15 years old) and adult (16–50 years old) skin.

The strong decrease of lumican expression in aged skin, associated to the increase of decorin, induced important modification of the lumican to decorin ratio. Due to the particular importance of these two SLRPs in dermal organization and properties, the authors suggested that these alterations might be involved in the functional defects which characterize aged skin. Yeh et al. [47] showed that skin of adult Lum (−/−) mice (3 months and older) was much thinner (40 % less) than that of age-matched wild-type. This phenomenon was aggravated in older mice. These authors demonstrated the basic thinner skin phenotypes in Lum (−/−) mice at different time points and the changes in arrangement of collagen fibers by transmission electron microscopy.

Fibromodulin

Fibromodulin, another SLRP belonging to class II, is expressed in human epidermal keratinocytes in culture and in human epidermis in vivo [6]. It has been extensively studied with regards to its role in regulating skin scars [48–51]. Fibromodulin was shown to mediate scarless fetal skin wound repair through, in part, TGF-β modulation [50]. In adult fibromodulin-null mouse model, it was demonstrated that fibromodulin presence is critical for proper temporospatial coordination of wound healing events and normal TGF-β bioactivity [51].

Versican and Other Proteoglycans of the Dermis Extracellular Matrix

Although skin fibroblasts express mRNAs for different proteoglycans (Table 1), only type XII and XIV collagens and versican were studied in the dermis. Collagens are the subject of another chapter in this book and we will only focus on versican here.

Versican, or chondroitin sulfate-glycoprotein 2 (CS-PG2), or PG-M, has a tridomain structure. The amino terminal end, designated as G1, binds to hyaluronan. The carboxy terminal domain, G3, possesses a lectin domain adjacent to two epidermal growth factor domains, and a complement regulatory domain. The central domain (G2) is encoded by two exons that specify CS attachment regions. RNA splicing of these two exons results in four different forms of versican, called V_0 to V_3 (molecular mass 370, 262, 180, and 72 kDa, respectively) with different numbers of GAG attachment domains [52–54]. The distribution of the $V_0 - V_3$ forms in adult varies with tissues and organs. Versican is a widespread ECM component of rodent and human skin and has also been characterized in the kidney in the lamina propria of blood vessels [55].

Versican expression was reported to decrease in aging skin [27, 29]. However, in photoaged skin, an accumulation of versican in elastotic material was reported [56]. After acute UV irradiation, there was a rapid up-regulation of versican mRNA, which persisted up to 72 h after exposure. The accumulation of versican was accompanied by the formation of a truncated molecule which lacked the hyaluronan-binding region of this proteoglycan [57]. In chronic sun exposure, this accumulation of versican led to the decrease of its synthesis, accelerating the loss of the molecule. As versican plays an important role in cell–hyaluronan interaction, the loss of this proteoglycan may substantially contribute to the loss of skin elasticity and resilience, especially in photoaged skin. During photoaging, estradiol was shown to protect dermal hyaluronan/versican matrix by release of epidermal growth factor (EGF) from keratinocytes [58]. Estrogen increases the amount of dermal hyaluronic acid and versican V2 via paracrine release of EGF, which may be implicated in the proliferative and anti-inflammatory effects of estrogen during photoaging.

Versican stain was shown to be increased in human male aged skin, but not in female [37]. These authors suggest that age- and gender-related changes in glycosaminoglycans and proteoglycans in intrinsically aged buttock skin may play important roles in intrinsic skin aging process.

Cell Surface Proteoglycans in Skin Aging

Cell surface proteoglycans may be divided into two main families: the syndecans and the glypicans. The main structural difference between both families is that syndecans have a transmembrane core protein, whereas, for glypicans, the core protein is linked to the cell surface by a glycosylphosphatidylinositol (GPI) anchor. Both families belong to the HS proteoglycans group even if syndecans may carry CS glycosaminoglycan chains in addition to HS.

Since both syndecan and glypican are heparan sulfate proteoglycans, these molecules may bind and modulate the activity of several matrix components, growth factors, proteinases and their activators/inhibitors, cell-cell and cell-matrix adhesion molecules [59]. Such ability likely plays an important role in the regulation of skin cell functions, especially in the aging process. Further investigations have, however, to be performed to better precise the exact place of these molecules in skin physiology.

Syndecans

In vertebrates, the syndecan family is composed of four members: syndecan −1, −2, −3, and −4 (for recent review, see [60]). Each core protein is composed of an extracellular domain bearing three to five chains of HS and sometimes CS, a single-span transmembrane domain and a short cytoplasmic domain. The molecular mass of the four syndecan core proteins are respectively 33 kDa, 23 kDa, 43 kDa, and 22 kDa for syndecans −1, −2, −3, and −4.

The extracellular domains of syndecans are able to interact with a number of extracellular proteins such as fibronectin and growth factors, mainly Fibroblast Growth Factors (FGFs), Vascular Endothelial Growth Factor (VEGF), Transforming Growth Factor-beta (TGF-β), and Platelet-Derived Growth Factor (PDGF). These interactions essentially occur through the heparan-sulfate chains of syndecans. On the other hand, the intracellular domain is able to bind to other syndecan molecules, which permits their multimerization, and to a number of intracellular molecules, involved either in cytoskeleton formation or in signal transduction. Many data indicate that syndecans are involved in complex signaling and cytoplasmic interactions, and are present in membrane microdomains specialized in signal transduction [61].

Syndecan-1 is the most abundant syndecan on epithelial keratinocytes. It is strongly expressed in the suprabasal, differentiating epidermal cells whereas it is expressed at low levels in the basal layer [62, 63]. Its expression is, however, markedly up-regulated in all cell layers of the epidermis during wound healing [64]. Recent data demonstrated that over-expression of syndecan-1 in transgenic mouse epidermis induces epidermal proliferation, as evidenced by increased number of suprabasal cell layers, elevated proliferating cell nuclear antigen (PCNA) expression in both basal and suprabasal cell layers. The expression of terminal differentiation markers, keratin 10, and involucrin was not disrupted in the epidermis of transgenic animals, showing that epidermal differentiation was not altered [65]. On the other hand, the loss of syndecan-1 in syndecan-1-null mice was shown to induce a decreased migration rate, linked to an increased adhesion of syndecan-1 defective keratinocytes [66]. Taken together, these results suggest that syndecan-1 is an important modulator of epidermal cell proliferation, migration, and adhesion and may control the behavior of epithelial cells. It may be suggested that the decreased proliferation potential of keratinocytes in aging epidermis might be linked to a defect in syndecan-1 expression.

Syndecan-4 is another important component of skin. In normal skin, it is detectable in the epidermis but not in the dermis. It is, however, strongly expressed by fibroblasts and endothelial cells in wounded skin [67]. Mice lacking syndecan-4 are characterized by delayed wound repair and impaired angiogenesis [68], which demonstrate that this proteoglycan is essential for skin repair. This finding may be important for understanding the physiopathology of skin aging.

Preliminary data from our laboratory indicated that syndecan-1 expression is decreased during aging. RT-PCR analysis of syndecan-1 mRNA indicated that keratinocytes express syndecans-1, −2, and −4. Syndecan-1 expression was decreased in keratinocytes from donors over 50 years old [69]. That decrease was confirmed by immunocytochemical analysis of syndecan-1 in the epidermis of donors over 50 compared to donors between 16 and 50 years old [70]. Similar decrease was observed by Oh et al. in patients over 70 [37]. Such a decrease in syndecan-1 might alter signalization processes in aged skin.

Glypicans

Glypicans were identified about 15 years ago as phosphatidyl-inositol-anchored membrane heparan sulfate proteoglycans [71]. In mammals, the glypican family is presently composed of 6 members, glypican-1 to glypican-6, with a core protein of 60–70 kDa [11]. The insertion sites for the heparan sulfate chains seem to be restricted to the last 50 amino acids in the C-terminus, placing the chains close to the cell membrane.

Glypicans are predominantly expressed during development [72]. Their main function is to regulate the signaling of Wnts, Hedgehogs, Fibroblast Growth Factors, and Bone Morphogenetic Proteins. Depending on the context, they may have either a stimulatory or inhibitory activity on signaling [11]. Part of glypicans may be shedded from the cell membrane into the extracellular matrix. This shedding is dependent of an extracellular lipase, Notum [73].

Very few data are available about the presence of glypicans in skin and their function. Preliminary data from our laboratory, however, indicated that human keratinocytes may express glypicans -1, -3, -4, -5, and -6 mRNAs [69].

Previous data from Litwack et al. [72] detected glypican-1 mRNA and protein expression in rat skin. Significant glypican-1 protein staining was detected in all layers of epidermis, except *stratum corneum*, and slight expression was found in the dermis. However, no variation of glypican expression during skin aging was reported, up to now.

Betaglycan

Betaglycan, also called TGF-β type III receptor is a membrane-anchored proteoglycan with a high affinity for TGF-β. It is ubiquitously expressed and serves as coreceptor for TGF-β isoforms. The extracellular domain of betaglycan contains two sites for heparan sulfate and chondroitin sulfate chains. The intracellular domain lacks intrinsic enzymatic activity but is able to regulate TGFβ signaling [74, 75]. No studies of betaglycan expression during skin aging were, however, reported.

CD-44

CD-44 is a transmembrane receptor which binds hyaluronic acid and plays an important role in its cellular uptake. Its extracellular domain may carry chondroitin sulfate, heparan sulfate or both types of glycosaminoglycan chains [76]. A decreased expression of CD-44 expression was reported in intrinsic aging, which may contribute to reduced or abnormal function of hyaluronic acid in the aged skin [77].

Proteoglycans of the Dermoepidermal Junction

Components of the dermoepidermal junction include collagen IV, collagen VII, laminin, entactin/nidogen, fibronectin, as well as subepidermal dermal markers (collagen I and fibrillin 1), and proteoglycans (mainly HS proteoglycans). Collagen type IV, HS proteoglycans, laminin, entactin/nidogen, and fibronectin are produced, at least in part, by the epidermal cells of the skin [78].

Heparan-Sulfate Proteoglycans (HS-PGs)

HS-PGs are common constituents of cell surfaces and of the ECM, including the basement membrane [79, 80]. The HS-PGs found in the ECM are perlecan, agrin, and collagen XVIII. HS-PGs are implicated in regulating the integrity of basement membranes, morphogenesis, angiogenesis, tumor metastasis, and tissue repair. These activities are attributed to the ability of HS-PGs to bind mitogenic and angiogenic growth factors [81], and to modulate their biological activities

Severe structural changes, including deterioration of the mechanical properties of the dermis, occur during skin aging. Skin HS-PGs, which regulate cell proliferation and proteolysis as well as matrix adhesion and assembly, decrease during aging and thus, may be implicated in the functional alterations linked to the aging process. They may represent important targets in dermocosmetology for fighting skin aging. For instance, Pineau et al. [82] demonstrated the potential interest of a new C-xylopyranoside derivative (C-beta-D-xylopyranoside-2-hydroxy-propane, simplified as C-Xyloside) to improve HS-PG production in human skin. In an organotypic model of corticosteroid atrophied human skin, characterized by a decrease of PGs expression, treatment with C-Xyloside improved expression of HS-PGs. Improvement of the dermoepidermal junction in human reconstructed skin treated by C-Xyloside was also reported [83].

Basement membranes contain several proteoglycans, and those bearing heparan-sulfate chains such as perlecan and agrin, usually predominate.

Perlecan

Perlecan is a large proteoglycan, with a core protein of 396 kDa, divided into five domains. It is predominantly substituted with HS chains, but on some occasions it may be substituted with CS, DS, hybrid HS/CS, or CS/DS. It may be also secreted as a glycosaminoglycan-free glycoprotein [84, 85].

Perlecan is present in virtually all basement membranes [86, 87]. It interacts with basement membrane components such as laminin-1 and collagen IV, but also with cell adhesion molecules such as β1-integrin [88]. Inactivation of the perlecan gene in mice results in embryonic lethality and prenatal death. Similarly, the functional null-mutation in the perlecan gene is characterized by perinatal death in humans [89]. Perlecan was shown to regulate both the survival and terminal steps of differentiation of keratinocytes: Sher et al. [90] demonstrated that perlecan regulates these processes via controlling the bioavailability of perlecan-binding soluble factors (particularly Keratinocyte Growth Factor or FGF-7), involved in epidermal morphogenesis. Consequently, it may be suggested that perlecan is important for the preservation of skin epithelium. Pineau et al. [82] reported a decreased expression of perlecan during skin aging. Such decrease was later confirmed by Oh et al. [37] in female aged skin. Pain et al. recently reported that perlecan expression was decreased by 81 % in aged skin compared to young skin [91]. This decrease might be involved in the alterations of basement membrane observed in aged skin.

Agrin

Agrin is a ubiquitously expressed proteoglycan, with a 200 kDa core protein [92]. It contains not only HS chains but also CS chains. The synaptic basal lamina, a component of ECM in the synaptic cleft at the neuromuscular junction, is rich in agrin. However, many other structures, which have basal laminae, including skin, also contain agrin. To our knowledge, however, no data on agrin expression in skin aging have been published.

Collagen XVIII

Type XVIII collagen is an ubiquitous basement membrane zone component, occurring prominently at vascular and epithelial basement membranes, including dermoepidermal junction. Whereas it contains collagen domains, it is also a member of the proteoglycan family since it carries heparan-sulfate chains [93].

Endostatin, a proteolytic fragment of type XVIII collagen, has been shown to inhibit angiogenesis, tumor growth, and endothelial cell proliferation and migration. Overexpression of endostatin in the skin [94] induced a widening of the epidermal basement membrane zone, as observed by electron microscopy. Immunoelectron microscopy of the type XVIII collagen in mouse skin showed a polarized orientation of this molecule in the basement membrane, with the C-terminal endostatin region localized in the lamina densa. In transgenic mice overexpressing endostatin, type XVIII collagen was dispersed in the skin, suggesting that the transgene-derived endostatin, might displace the full length collagen XVIII. This may impair the anchoring of the lamina densa to the dermis and thereby lead to loosening of the basement membrane zone, resembling the previously observed situation in collagen XVIII-null mice. It was reported that disorganization of the basement membrane zone was one of the features of aged skin [95].

Chondroitin-Sulfate Proteoglycans (CS-PGs)

Although less abundant than HS-PG, several CS-PG have been described in the basement membrane.

Versican

General characteristics of versican were presented in § 2.2 of the present chapter. Whereas mainly present in the dermis, traces of versican have been found in some basement membranes. No data are available, however, about alterations of versican in the dermoepidermal junction of aging skin.

Leprecan

Leprecan has been described as a CS-PG with a 100-kDa core protein [96]. Immunostaining with polyclonal antibodies showed the localization of its protein core in the basement membrane of the vasculature. Rat-homolog of Gros1, a human growth suppressor gene, was identified to be the leucine-proline-enriched basement membrane-associated proteoglycan leprecan [97]. Leprecan was predicted to be a protein hydroxylase that might be involved in the generation of substrates for protein glycosylation [98]. It was suggested that regulated expression of leprecan coupled with its reported prolyl hydroxylase activity might play a role during basement membrane assembly in the kidney [99]. To our knowledge, however, no data about alterations of leprecan expression during skin aging have been published.

Bamacan

Bamacan is a CS-PG that abounds in basement membranes. Bamacan can occur in certain cell types either as a secreted proteoglycan involved in basement membrane assembly or as an intracellular protein contributing to the structure of chromosome 3 (SMC3) [100]. The entire bamacan core protein is characterized by a Mr of 138 kDa. A stabilizing role for bamacan in the basement membrane has been proposed [101]. To our knowledge, however, no data on bamacan expression during skin aging have been published.

Type XV Collagen

Type XV collagen is a proteoglycan which carries chondroitin sulfate chains, associated in some tissues with heparan-sulfate chains [102]. It is present in the basement membrane zone of all the tissues examined [103]. A specific domain of its C-terminal region, called restin, possesses antiangiogenic properties similar to endostatin [104]. It seems to contribute to the stability of the basement membrane zone. However, no data has been reported up to now about possible alterations of type XV collagen during aging.

Conclusion

It is clear from the data reported in this chapter that proteoglycans may play a major role in skin homeostasis and in the functional and architectural properties of this tissue. Whereas many data are available concerning some particular proteoglycans of the dermal or epidermal compartments, for instance decorin in the dermis or syndecans in the epidermis, large areas remain unknown at the present time. It is particularly the case of the alterations of proteoglycan expression, distribution, or structure, which may occur during the aging process and, more importantly, on their potential consequences on skin physiology. Since these alterations may affect not only the glycosaminoglycan chains but also the core protein of the proteoglycans itself, it will be important to design new experimental models, especially in vivo, which will permit to better study their consequences on skin physiology and their implication in the defects linked to skin aging.

References

1. Iozzo RV, Schaefer L. Proteoglycan form and function: a comprehensive nomenclature of proteoglycans. Matrix Biol. 2015;42:11–55.
2. Zhou J, Haggerty JG, Milstone LM. Growth and differentiation regulate CD44 expression on human keratinocytes. In Vitro. 1999;35:228–35.
3. Esko JD, Zhang L. Influence of core protein sequence on glycosaminoglycan assembly. Curr Opin Struct Biol. 1996;6:663–70.
4. http://www.ncbi.nlm.nih.gov/sites/entrez
5. Bianco P, Fisher LW, Young MF, et al. Expression and localization of the two small proteoglycans, biglycan and decorin in developing human skeletal and non skeletal tissues. J Histochem Cytochem. 1990;38:1549–63.
6. Vélez-Delvalle C, Marsch-Moreno M, Castro-Muñozledo F, et al. Fibromodulin gene is expressed in human epidermal keratinocytes in culture and in human epidermis *in vivo*. Biochem Biophys Res Commun. 2008;371:420–4.
7. Zimmermann DR, Dours-Zimmermann MT, Schubert M, et al. Versican is expressed in the proliferating zone in the epidermis and in association with the elastic network of the dermis. J Cell Biol. 1994;124:817–25.
8. Garrone R, Lethias C, Le Guellec D. Distribution of minor collagens during skin development. Microsc Res Tech. 1997;38:407–12.
9. Ginhoux F, Tacke F, Angeli V, et al. Langerhans cells arise from monocytes *in vivo*. Nat Immunol. 2006;7:265–73.
10. Ojeh N, Hiilesvuo K, Wärri A, et al. Ectopic expression of syndecan-1 in basal epidermis affects keratinocyte proliferation and wound re-epithelialization. J Invest Dermatol. 2008;128:26–34.
11. Filmus J, Capurro M, Rast J. Glypicans. Genome Biol. 2008;9:224.1–6.
12. Kugelman LC, Ganguly S, Haggerty JG, et al. The core protein of epican, a heparan sulfate proteoglycan on keratinocytes, is an alternative form of CD44. J Invest Dermatol. 1992;99:886–91.
13. Quintanilla M, Ramirez JR, Pérez-Gómez E, et al. Expression of the TGF-beta coreceptor endoglin in epidermal keratinocytes and its dual role in multistage mouse skin carcinogenesis. Oncogene. 2003;22:5976–85.
14. Artuc M, Hermes B, Algermissen B, et al. Expression of prothrombin, thrombin and its receptors in human scars. Exp Dermatol. 2006;15:523–9.
15. Campoli MR, Chang CC, Kageshita T, et al. Human high molecular weight-melanoma-associated antigen (HMW-MAA). Crit Rev Immunol. 2004;24:267–96.
16. Kadoya K, Fukushi J, Matsumoto Y, et al. NG2 proteoglycan expression in mouse skin: altered postnatal skin development in the NG2 null mouse. J Histochem Cytochem. 2008;56:295–303.
17. Fujii N, Nagai YJ. Isolation and characterization of a proteodermatan sulfate from calf skin. J Biochem. 1981;90:1249–58.
18. Gattazzo F, Urciuolo A, Bonaldo P. Extracellular matrix: a dynamic microenvironment for stem cell niche. Biochim Biophys Acta. 2014;1840:2506–19.
19. Lindner J, Schönrock P, Nüssgen A, et al. Age-related changes in cell content (DNA) and glycosaminoglycan-degrading enzymes. Z Gerontol. 1986;19:190–205.
20. Iozzo RV. The family of the small leucin-rich proteoglycans: key regulators of matrix assembly and cellular growth. Crit Rev Biochem Mol Biol. 1997;32:141–74.
21. Schaefer L, Iozzo RV. Biological functions of the small leucin-rich proteoglycans: from genetics to signal transduction. J Biol Chem. 2008;283:21305–9.
22. Ying S, Shiraishi A, Kao CW, et al. Characterization and expression of the mouse lumican gene. J Biol Chem. 1997;272:30306–13.
23. Corpuz L, Funderburgh JL, Funderburgh ML, et al. Molecular cloning and distribution of keratocan. Bovine corneal keratan sulfate proteoglycan 37A. J Biol Chem. 1996;271:839–47.
24. Neame PJ, Kay CJ. Small leucine-rich proteoglycans. In: Iozzo RV, editor. Proteoglycans: structure, biology and molecular interactions. New-York, Basel: Marcel Dekker; 2000. p. 201–35.
25. Ameye L, Young MF. Mice deficient in small leucine-rich proteoglycans: novel *in vivo* models for osteoporosis, osteoarthritis, Ehlers-Danlos syndrome, muscular dystrophy and corneal diseases. Glycobiology. 2002;12:107R–16.
26. Longas MO, Fleischmajer R. Immuno-electron microscopy of proteodermatan sulfate in human mid-dermis. Connect Tissue Res. 1985;13:117–25.
27. Bernstein FF, Fisher LW, Richard KL, et al. Differential expression of the versican and decorin genes in photo-aged and sun-protected skin. Lab Invest. 1995;72:662–9.
28. Passi A, Albertini R, Campagnari F, De Luca G. Modifications of proteoglycans secreted into the growth medium by young and senescent human skin fibroblasts. FEBS Lett. 1997;402:286–90.
29. Carrino DH, Sorrell JM, Caplan AI. Age-related changes in the proteoglycans of human skin. Arch Biochem Biophys. 2000;373:91–101.
30. Carrino DA, Onnerfjord P, Sandy JD, et al. Age-related changes in the proteoglycans of human skin. Specific cleavage of decorin to yield a major catabolic fragment in adult skin. J Biol Chem. 2003;278:17566–72.
31. Ito Y, Takeuchi J, Yamamoto K, et al. Age differences in immunohistochemical localizations of large proteoglycan, PG-M/versican, and small proteoglycan, decorin, in the dermis of rats. Exp Anim. 2001;50:159–66.
32. Nomura Y, Abe Y, Ishii Y, et al. Structural changes in the glycosaminoglycan chain of rat skin decorin with growth. J Dermatol. 2003;30:655–64.

33. Nomura Y. Structural change in decorin with skin aging. Connect Tissue Res. 2006;47:249–55.
34. Lockner K, Gaemlich A, Südel KM, et al. Expression of decorin and collagens-I and -III in different layers of human skin *in vivo*: a laser capture microdissection study. Biogerontology. 2007;8:269–82.
35. Kokenyesi R, Woessner Jr JF. Relationship between dilatation of the rat uterine cervix and small dermatan sulfate proteoglycan. Biol Reprod. 1990;42:87–97.
36. Vogel KG, Trotter JA. The effect of proteoglycans on the morphology of collagen fibrils formed *in vitro*. Coll Rel Res. 1987;7:105–14.
37. Oh JH, Kim YK, Jung JY, et al. Changes in glycosaminoglycans and related proteoglycans in intrinsically aged human skin in vivo. Exp Dermatol. 2011;20:545–6.
38. Li Y, Liu Y, Xia W, et al. Age-dependent alterations of decorin glycosaminoglycans in human skin. Sci Rep. 2013;3:2422.
39. Mondon P, Hillion M, Peschard O, et al. Evaluation of dermal extracellular matrix and epidermal-dermal junction modifications using matrix-assisted laser desorption/ionization mass spectrometric imaging, in vivo reflectance confocal microscopy, echography, and histology: effect of age and peptide applications. J Cosmet Dermatol. 2015;14(2):152–60.
40. Li Y, Xia W, Liu Y, et al. Solar ultraviolet irradiation induces decorin degradation in human skin likely via neutrophil elastase. PLoS One. 2013;8(8), e72563.
41. Corsi A, Xu T, Chen XD, et al. Phenotypic effects of biglycan deficiency are linked to collagen fibril abnormalities, are synergized by decorin deficiency, and mimic Ehlers-Danlos-like changes in bone and other connective tissues. J Bone Miner Res. 2002;17(7):1180–9.
42. Scott PG, Dodd CM, Tredget EE, et al. Immunohistochemical localization of the proteoglycans decorin, biglycan and versican and transforming growth factor-beta in human post-burn hypertrophic and mature scars. Histopathology. 1995;26(5):423–31.
43. Funderburgh JL, Conrad GW. Isoform of corneal keratan sulfate proteoglycan. J Biol Chem. 1990;265:8297–303.
44. Grover J, Chen XN, Korenberg JR, Roughley PJ. The human lumican gene. Organization, chromosomal location, and expression in articular cartilage. J Biol Chem. 1995;270:21942–9.
45. Chakravarti S, Magnuson T, Lass JH. Lumican regulates collagen fibril assembly: skin fragility and corneal opacity in the absence of lumican. J Cell Biol. 1998;141:1277–86.
46. Vuillermoz B, Wegrowski Y, Contet-Audonneau JL, et al. Influence of aging on glycosaminoglycans and small leucine-rich proteoglycans production by skin fibroblasts. Mol Cell Biochem. 2005;277:63–72.
47. Yeh JT, Yeh LK, Jung SM, et al. Impaired skin wound healing in lumican-null mice. Br J Dermatol. 2010;163(6):1174–80.
48. Honardoust D, Varkey M, Marcoux Y, et al. Reduced decorin, fibromodulin, and transforming growth factor-β3 in deep dermis leads to hypertrophic scarring. J Burn Care Res. 2012;33(2):218–27.
49. Varkey M, Ding J, Tredget EE. Differential collagen-glycosaminoglycan matrix remodeling by superficial and deep dermal fibroblasts: potential therapeutic targets for hypertrophic scar. Biomaterials. 2011;32(30):7581–91.
50. Zheng Z, Lee KS, Zhang X, et al. Fibromodulin-deficiency alters temporospatial expression patterns of transforming growth factor-β ligands and receptors during adult mouse skin wound healing. PLoS One. 2014;9(6), e90817.
51. Stoff A, Rivera AA, Mathis JM, et al. Effect of adenoviral mediated overexpression of fibromodulin on human dermal fibroblasts and scar formation in full-thickness incisional wounds. J Mol Med (Berl). 2007;85(5):481–96.
52. Dours-Zimmermann MT, Zimmermann DR. A novel glycosaminoglycan attachment domain identified in two alternative splice variants of human versican. J Biol Chem. 1994;269:32992–8.
53. Lemire JM, Braun KR, Maurel P, et al. versican/PG-M isoforms in vascular smooth muscle cells. Arterioscler Thromb Vasc Biol. 1999;19:1630–9.
54. Zhao X, Russell P. Versican splice variants in human trabecular meshwork and ciliary muscle. Mol Vis. 2005;12:603–8.
55. Erickson AC, Couchman JR. Basement membrane and interstitial proteoglycans produced by MDCK cells correspond to those expressed in the kidney cortex. Matrix Biol. 2001;19:769–78.
56. Knott A, Reuschlein K, Lucius R, et al. Deregulation of versican and elastin binding protein in solar elastosis. Biogerontology. 2009;10:181–90.
57. Hasegawa K, Yoneda M, Kuwabara H, et al. Versican, a major hyaluronan-binding component in the dermis loses its hyaluronan-binding ability in solar elastosis. J Invest Dermatol. 2007;127:1657–63.
58. Röck K, Meusch M, Fuchs N, et al. Estradiol protects dermal hyaluronan/versican matrix during photoaging by release of epidermal growth factor from keratinocytes. J Biol Chem. 2012;287(24):20056–69.
59. Jackson RL, Busch SJ, Cardin AD. Glycosaminoglycans: molecular properties, protein interactions and role in physiological processes. Physiol Rev. 1991;71:481–539.
60. Choi Y, Chung H, Jung H, et al. Syndecans as cell surface receptors: unique structure with functional diversity. Matrix Biol. 2011;30:93–9.
61. Multhaupt HA, Yoneda A, Whiteford JR, et al. Syndecan signaling: when, where and why? J Physiol Pharmacol Suppl. 2009;4:31–8.
62. Sanderson RD, Hinkes MT, Bernfield M. Syndecan-1, a cell-surface proteoglycan, changes in size and abundance when keratinocytes stratify. J Invest Dermatol. 1992;99:390–6.

63. Inki P, Larava H, Haapasalmi K, et al. Expression of syndecan-1 is induced by differentiation and suppressed by malignant transformation of human keratinocytes. Eur J Cell Biol. 1994;63:43–51.
64. Elenius K, Vainio S, Laato M. Induced expression of syndecan in healing wounds. J Cell Biol. 1991;114:585–95.
65. Ojeh N, Hiilesvno K, Warri A. Ectopic expression of syndecan-1 in basal epidermis affects keratinocytes proliferation and wound re-epithelialization. J Invest Dermatol. 2008;128:26–34.
66. Stepp MA, Liu Y, Pal-Gosh S, et al. Reduced migration, altered matrix and enhanced TGF-β1 signaling are signatures of mouse keratinocytes lacking Sdc-1. J Cell Sci. 2007;120:2851–63.
67. Gallo R, Kim C, Kokenyesi R, et al. Syndecans -1 and -4 are induced during wound repair of neonatal but not fetal skin. J Invest Dermatol. 1996;107:676–83.
68. Echtermeyer F, Streit M, Wilcox-Adelman S, et al. Delayed wound repair and impaired angiogenesis in mice lacking syndecan -4. J Clin Invest. 2001;107:R9–14.
69. Wegrowski Y, Danoux L, Contet-Audonneau JL, et al. Decreased syndecan-1 expression by human keratinocytes during skin aging. J Invest Dermatol. 2005;125:A5 (abstract).
70. Pauly G, Contet-Audonneau JL, Moussou P, et al. Small proteoglycans in the skin: new targets in the fight against skin aging. IFSCC Mag. 2008;11:21–9.
71. David G, Lories V, Decock V, et al. Molecular cloning of a phosphatidyl-inositol-anchored membrane heparan sulfate proteoglycan from human lung fibroblast. J Cell Biol. 1990;111:149–60.
72. Litwack ED, Ivins JK, Kumbesar A. Expression of the heparan sulfate proteoglycan glypican-1 in the developing rodent. Dev Dyn. 1998;211:72–87.
73. Traister A, Shi W, Filmus J. Mammalian Notum induces the release of glypicans and other GPI-anchored proteins from the cell surface. Biochem J. 2008;410:503–11.
74. Boyd FJ, Cheifetz S, Andres J, et al. Transforming Growth Factor-beta receptors and binding proteoglycans. J Cell Sci Suppl. 1990;13:131–8.
75. Lopez-Casillas F, Payne HM, Andres JL, et al. Betaglycan can act as dual modulator of TGF-beta access to signalling receptors: mapping of ligand binding and GAG attachment sites. J Cell Biol. 1994;124:557–68.
76. Brown TA, Bouchard T, St John T, et al. Human keratinocytes express a new CD44 core protein (CD44E) as a heparan sulfate intrisic membrane proteoglycans with additional exons. J Cell Biol. 1991;113:207–21.
77. Tzellos TG, Sinopidis X, Kyrgidis A, et al. Differential hyaluronan homeostasis and expression of proteoglycans in juvenile and adult human skin. J Dermatol Sci. 2011;61:60–81.
78. Tamiolakis D, Papadopoulos N, Anastasiadis P, et al. Expression of laminin, type IV collagen and fibronectin molecules is related to embryonal skin and epidermal appendage morphogenesis. Clin Exp Obstet Gynecol. 2001;28:179–82.
79. David G. Integral membrane heparan sulfate proteoglycans. FASEB J. 1993;7:1023–30.
80. Erickson AC, Couchman JR. Still more complexity in mammalian basement membranes. J Histochem Cytochem. 2000;48:1291–306.
81. Iozzo RV. Heparan sulfate proteoglycans: intricate molecules with intriguing functions. J Clin Invest. 2001;108:165–77.
82. Pineau N, Bernerd F, Cavezza A, et al. A new C-xylopyranoside derivative induces skin expression of glycosaminoglycans and heparan sulfate proteoglycans. Eur J Dermatol. 2008;18:36–40.
83. Sok J, Pineau N, Dalko-Csiba M, et al. Improvement of the dermal epidermal junction in human reconstructed skin by a new c-xylopyranoside derivative. Eur J Dermatol. 2008;18:297–302.
84. Isemura M, Sato N, Yamaguchi Y, et al. Isolation and characterization of fibronectin-binding proteoglycan carrying both heparan sulfate and dermatan sulfate chains from human placenta. J Biol Chem. 1987;262:8926–33.
85. Iozzo RV, Hassell JR. Identification of the precursor protein for the heparan sulfate proteoglycan of human colon carcinoma cells and its post-translational modifications. Arch Biochem Biophys. 1989;269:239–49.
86. Iozzo RV, Cohen IR, Grässel S, Murdoch AD. The biology of perlecan: the multifaceted heparan sulfate proteoglycan of basement membranes and pericellular matrices. Biochem J. 1994;302:625–39.
87. Murdoch AD, Liu B, Schwarting R, et al. Widespread expression of perlecan proteoglycan in basement membranes and extracellular matrices of human tissues as detected by a novel monoclonal antibody against domain III and by *in situ* hybridization. J Histochem Cytochem. 1994;42:239–49.
88. Brown JC, Sasaki T, Göhring W, et al. The C-terminal domain V of perlecan promotes beta-1 integrin-mediated cell adhesion, binds heparin, nidogen and fibulin-2 and can be modified by glycosaminoglycans. Eur J Biochem. 1997;250:39–46.
89. Arikawa-Hirasawa E, Yamada Y. Roles of perlecan in development and disease: studies in knockout mice and human disorders. Seikagaku. 2001;73:1257–61.
90. Sher I, Zisman-Rozen S, Eliahu L, et al. Targeting perlecan in human keratinocytes reveals novel roles for perlecan in epidermal formation. J Biol Chem. 2006;281:5178–87.
91. Pain S, Dos Santos M, Gaydou A, et al. Restoration of both epithelial and endothelial perlecan/dystroglycan expressions by polygonum bistorta induces skin rejuvenation. IFSCC Mag. 2014;17:31–6.
92. Cole GJ, Halfter W. Agrin: an extracellular matrix heparan sulfate proteoglycan involved in cell

interactions and synaptogenesis. Perspect Dev Neurobiol. 1996;3:359–3711.
93. Hafter W, Dong S, Schurer B, et al. Collagen XVIII is a basement membrane heparan sulfate proteoglycan. J Biol Chem. 1998;372:25404–12.
94. Elamaa H, Sormunen R, Rehn M, et al. Endostatin overexpression specifically in the lens and skin leads to cataract and ultrastructural alterations in basement membranes. Am J Pathol. 2005;166:221–9.
95. Le Varlet B, Chaudagne C, Saunois A, et al. Age-related functional and structural changes in human dermo-epidermal junction components. J Invest Dermatol Symp Proc. 1998;3:172–9.
96. Wassenhove-McCarthy DJ, McCarthy KJ. Molecular characterization of a novel basement membrane-associated proteoglycan, leprecan. J Biol Chem. 1999;274:25004–17.
97. Kaul SC, Sugihara T, Yoshida A, et al. Gros1, a potential growth suppressor on chromosome 1: its identity to basement membrane-associated proteoglycan, leprecan. Oncogene. 2000;19:3576–83.
98. Aravind L, Koonin EV (2001) The DNA-repair protein AlkB, EGL-9, and leprecan define new families of 2-oxoglutarate- and iron-dependent dioxygenases. Genome Biol 2:RESEARCH0007.1-0007.8.
99. Lauer M, Scruggs B, Chen S, et al. Leprecan distribution in the developing and adult kidney. Kidney Int. 2007;72:82–91.
100. Ghiselli G, Siracusa LD, Iozzo RV. Complete cDNA cloning, genomic organization, chromosomal assignment, functional characterization of the promoter, and expression of the murine Bamacan gene. J Biol Chem. 1999;274:17384–93.
101. Wu RR, Couchman JR. cDNA cloning of the basement membrane chondroitin sulfate proteoglycan core protein, bamacan: a five domain structure including coiled-coil motifs. J Cell Biol. 1997;136:433–44.
102. Amenta PS, Scivoletti NA, Newman N, et al. Proteoglycan-collagen XV in human tissues is seen linking banded fibers subjacent to the basement membrane. J Histochem Cytochem. 2005;53:165–76.
103. Myers JC, Dion AS, Abraham V, et al. Type XV collagen exhibits a widespread distribution in human tissues but a distinct localization in basement membrane zones. Cell Tiss Res. 1996;286:493–505.
104. Ramchandran R, Dhanabal M, Volk R, et al. Antiangiogenic activity of restin, NC10 domain of human collagen XV: comparison to endostatin. Biochem Biophys Res Commun. 1999;225:735–9.

Possible Involvement of Basement Membrane Damage by Matrix Metalloproteinases, Serine Proteinases, and Heparanase in Skin Aging Process

12

Satoshi Amano

Contents

Abstract

This paper briefly reviews the characteristics of photoaged skin, and the mechanisms involved in skin photoaging and repair. Sun-exposed skin shows superficial changes, such as wrinkles, sagging, telangiectasis and pigmentary changes, pathological changes such as neoplasia, and also many internal changes in the structure and function of epidermis, basement membrane, and dermis. These changes (so-called photoaging) are predominantly due to the ultraviolet (UV) component of sunlight.

Enzymes such as matrix metalloproteinases (MMPs), urinary plasminogen activator (uPA)/plasmin, and heparanase are increased in epidermis of UV-irradiated skin. These enzymes degrade epidermal basement membrane (BM) components, dermal collagen fibers, and elastic fibers. The BM, which is located at the dermal-epidermal junction, controls dermal-epidermal signaling and is essential for maintaining a healthy epidermis and dermis. Repeated BM damage occurs in sun-exposed skin compared to unexposed skin, leading to epidermal and dermal deterioration and accelerated skin aging. UV-induced skin damage is cumulative and leads to premature aging of skin. However, appropriate daily skin treatment may ameliorate photoaging by inhibiting processes causing damage and enhancing repair processes.

S. Amano (✉)
Shiseido Research Center, Yokohama, Japan
e-mail: satoshi.amano@to.shiseido.co.jp

M.A. Farage et al. (eds.), *Textbook of Aging Skin*,
DOI 10.1007/978-3-662-47398-6_12

Introduction

Skin aging can be classified into two types, intrinsic aging and photoaging [1]. Intrinsic aging is the basic biological process common to all living things and is characterized as an age-dependent deterioration of skin functions and structures, such as epidermal atrophy and epidermal-dermal junctional flattening [2]. Photoaging is well known to be a consequence of chronic exposure of the skin to sunlight. Sun-exposed skin, such as face or neck skin, clearly appears to be "prematurely aged" in comparison with the relatively sun-protected skin of the trunk or thigh and is characterized by various clinical features, including wrinkles, sagging, roughness, sallowness, pigmentary changes, telangiectasis, and neoplasia. The histological features of sun-exposed skin include cellular atypia, loss of polarity, flattening of the dermal epidermal junctions (DEJ), a decrease in collagen, and dermal elastosis [2, 3].

The basement membrane (BM) at the DEJ has many functions, of which the most obvious is to tightly link the epidermis to the dermis [4]. It also determines the polarity of the epidermis and provides a barrier against epidermal migration. Once the BM has been assembled, the epidermal cells recognize the surface adjacent to the BM as the basal surface. Stratification of the epidermis proceeds with the proliferating cells remaining attached to the BM and the daughter cells migrating into the upper layers [5–7]. It is thought that the BM influences epidermal differentiation and maintains the proliferative state of the basal layer. Under normal circumstances, the BM prevents direct contact of epidermal cells with the dermis.

Another important function of the BM derives from the positioning of the structure between the epidermal cells and the dermal cells. The epidermis and the dermis do not function independently [8]. Instead, normal skin homeostasis requires the constant passage of signals back and forth between the two cell types. In general, these signals are small molecules, synthesized in one compartment, that diffuse to the other compartment. In other words, these signals must cross the BM. Components of the BM can selectively facilitate or prevent the passage of these signals. In some cases, the signaling molecules are stored by the BM and only released if the BM is damaged or destroyed. Thus, epidermal-dermal communication through the BM is extremely important.

The BM may be divided into three layers on the basis of morphological studies: the lamina lucida, the lamina densa, and the lamina fibroreticularis [9], as shown in Fig. 1. Lamina densa is a sheet-like structure which is mainly composed of type IV collagen. Lamina lucida is a region between the lamina densa and epithelia, forming electron-dense plaques, hemidesmosomes, which mainly consist of $\alpha6\beta4$ integrin and the bullous pemphigoid antigen 2 (180 kDa). The BM contains unique structures that maintain the attachment of the epidermis. The components of the attachment complex provide links to the intracellular intermediate filament network of basal keratinocytes and to the extracellular matrix of the papillary dermis. One of the key components of the anchoring complex is laminin 5 (332). Past work has shown that laminin 332 is essential to epidermal attachment, as mutations in the genes encoding the laminin 332 chains underlie the severe blistering phenotype of Herlitz' junctional epidermolysis bullosa. Laminin 332 is processed extracellularly to a mature form at the $\alpha3$ and $\gamma2$ chains by BMP-1 and other enzymes [10–12]. It is clear that laminin 332 constitutes the anchoring filaments and binds the transmembrane hemidesmosomal integrin $\alpha6\beta4$, which is known to be the receptor of laminin 332. With regard to binding of laminin 332 with other components of the BM or of the papillary dermis, it has recently been elucidated that (1) laminin 332 directly binds type VII collagen, which forms the anchoring fibrils that insert into the papillary dermis, and (2) laminin 332 forms a covalent complex with laminin 311 or 321, and this laminin 332-311/321 complex interacts with type IV collagen in the BM through nidogen.

The matrix metalloproteinases (MMPs) are zinc-dependent endopeptidases, and they are involved in remodeling of the extracellular matrix and also play important roles in morphogenesis, angiogenesis, arthritis, skin ulcer, tumor invasion, and metastasis [13]. Five families of MMPs have

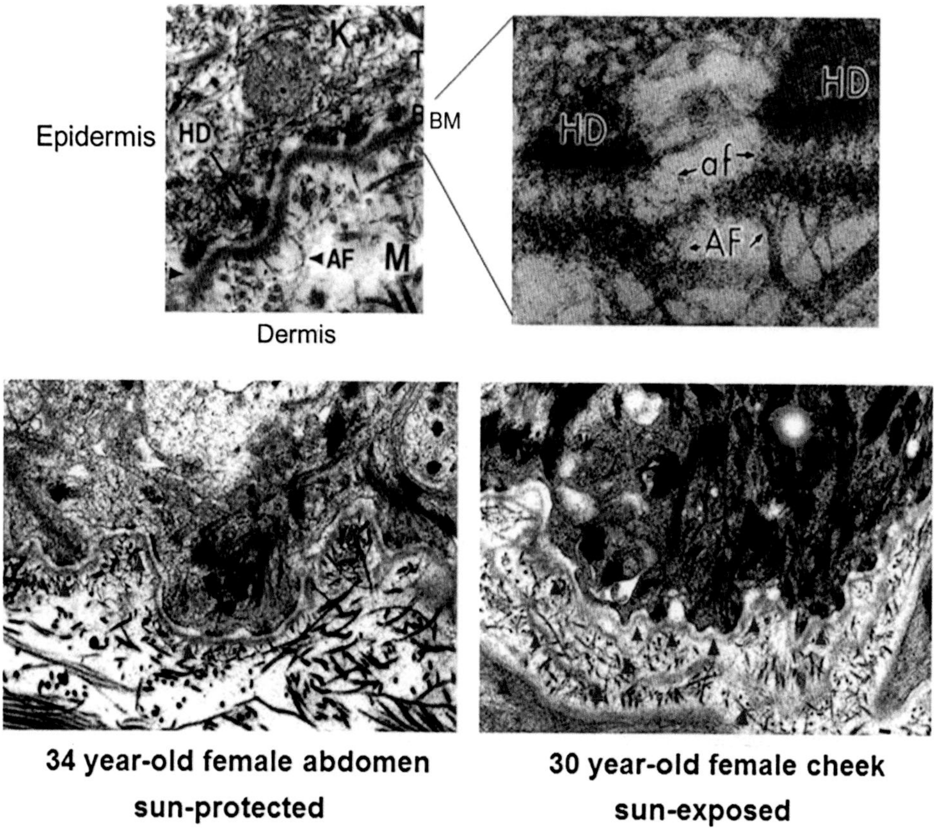

Fig. 1 Basement membrane structure at DEJ and damaged BM structures. In the *top row*, the DEJ is visualized at stepwise magnification in transmission electron microscope scale. Hemidesmosome (*HD*), anchoring filament (*af*), lamina densa, and anchoring fibrils (*Af*) are observed and form the special anchoring complex for the attachment of epidermis to dermis. The *lower* pictures are transmission electron microscopic images of the DEJ of human skin. Disruption and reduplication of the lamina densa can be seen at the DEJ in sun-exposed cheek skin of a 30-year-old female, while neither duplication nor disruption can be observed in sun-protected abdomen skin of a 34-year-old female

been recognized, i.e., collagenases, gelatinases, stromelysins, matrilysins, and membrane-type MMPs. These enzymes are composed of several domains, including propeptide, catalytic, and hemopexin (except for matrilysin) domains. They are involved in the degradation of collagens, proteoglycans, and various glycoproteins [13]. Among them, gelatinase A (MMP-2 or 72 kDa type IV collagenase) and gelatinase B (MMP-9 or 92 kDa type IV collagenase) digest type IV and VII collagens, while stromelysins (MMP-3, MMP-10) degrade laminins of the BM [14]. MMPs are secreted as inactive zymogens (proMMPs), and activation of proMMPs (to active MMPs) is a prerequisite for function. Stimulation or repression of proMMP synthesis is mostly regulated at the transcriptional level by growth factors or cytokines [14]. Furthermore, post-transcriptional regulation of MMP activity is controlled by tissue inhibitors of metalloproteinases (TIMPs), of which TIMP-1, TIMP-2, TIMP-3, and TIMP-4 have been characterized [15]. MMP-2 binds specifically to TIMP-2, whereas MMP-9 binds to TIMP-1 [16]. MMP-2 is constitutively expressed in many cells, including dermal fibroblasts, and has a ubiquitous tissue distribution. ProMMP-2 is activated at the cell surface by a membrane-type MMP known as MT1-MMP.

Plasminogen activators (PAs)/plasmin represent one of the most potent and widely expressed systems for extracellular proteolysis [17]. PAs can be produced by many cell types, including human epidermal keratinocytes [18], and they convert the widely distributed zymogen, plasminogen, to plasmin, which degrades most extracellular proteins either directly or by activating other proteases [18, 19]. Tissue-type PA (tPA) and urokinase-type PA (uPA) are the products of distinct but related genes with different patterns of expression and regulation. Physiologically, tPA is predominantly responsible for fibrinolysis, while uPA appears to be involved in pericellular proteolysis by binding to cell surfaces through a specific, high-affinity, glycosylphosphatidylinositol-anchored plasma membrane receptor [20]. Binding increases the catalytic efficiency and targets generation of plasmin to the immediate pericellular space. In skin, urokinase-type plasminogen activator activity was found to be present in the stratum corneum, as well as the basal layer after barrier disruption [21, 22]. The plasminogen/plasmin system in epidermis is thought to be the major protease activity involved in the delay of barrier recovery [22].

Heparanase is an endo-β-D-glucuronidase and is capable of cleaving heparan sulfate (HS) fragments of quite appreciable size (5–7 kDa) [23]. In normal tissue, heparanase is expressed in placenta, keratinocytes, and platelets but not in connective tissue cells [24]. In normal skin, heparanase is expressed in stratum corneum and hair inner root sheath, and may be involved in differentiation, desquamation, and hair growth [25]. HS proteoglycans are essential for biological processes mediated by HS-binding growth factors [26]. Perlecan, with its large multivalent protein core, is a structural constituent of BM and is a key regulator of these growth factor signaling pathways [27]. HS chains of perlecan at the BM act as a reservoir of heparin-binding growth factors, such as fibroblast growth factors (FGFs) [28], granulocyte-macrophage colony-stimulating factor (GM-CSF) [29], and vascular endothelial growth factor-A (VEGF-A) [30], and serve to prevent uncontrolled diffusion of these factors from the epidermis to the dermis and vice versa [31]. KGF, SCF, and HGF are produced by dermal fibroblasts and act on epidermal keratinocytes and melanocytes.

The first skin-equivalent model was developed in 1981 by Bell et al. [32], who plated human keratinocytes on top of contracted collagen gel containing dermal fibroblasts. It is useful for grafting on wounds [32] or burned skin [32], to explore the dynamics of the BM [33, 34], and for studies of epidermal differentiation, dermal-epidermal interaction, tumor cell invasion, and so on.

Skins of our faces, hands, and arms are usually exposed to air and sun directly. UVB penetrates papillary dermis, and UVA does much deeper, and the UV light induces several kinds of skin damages some of which are shown in the paper. The daily skin damages are accumulated day by day, and then premature aging of skin is facilitated by UV exposure. Therefore, the phoaging process should be controlled by inhibiting the damage process and enhancing the repair of the damages. In this paper the possible involvements of the structural and functional BM damages with enzymes in the process of cutaneous photoaging are discussed.

Ultrastructural Alteration of Epidermal BM in Sun-Exposed Skins

At the DEJ of sun-exposed skin, duplication of lamina densa was reported in both aged adults [2] and mice, and these changes may result in a more fragile epidermal-dermal interface and weaker resistance of the epidermis to shearing forces in aged skin. We observed that, even in cheek (sun-exposed) skin of a 30-year-old female, severe disruption and reduplication of lamina densa were frequently observed beneath keratinocytes and anchoring fibrils were also associated with detached lamina densa, mainly on the dermis side (Fig. 1). On the other hand, in young, sun-protected skin, such as abdominal skin of a 34-year-old female, scarcely any alteration of the epidermal BM structure was apparent at the DEJ

(Fig. 1b). In old sun-exposed skin from cheek of a 60-year-old female, the layer number of reduplicated lamina densa was increased, and laminae densae branched in various directions. In contrast, skin from upper thigh of an 83-year-old female showed very little disruption or reduplication at the DEJ. However, following injury that penetrates or disrupts the BM, the epidermal cells lose contact with the BM and come in contact with naked dermis. Under these conditions, the epidermal cells modify their behavior to cover and close the wound. Such behavior changes include the upregulation of proteolytic enzymes and other changes that accompany conversion to a migratory phenotype [35, 36].

Involvement of Matrix Metalloproteinases in Damage to Epidermal BM in Sun-Exposed Skin

MMPs are considered to be involved in photoaging, since MMPs-1, 2, 3, and 9 were found to be increased by ultraviolet irradiation in experiments using human fibroblasts and human skin [37, 38]. In particular, Fisher et al. demonstrated an increase of MMPs in human skin following exposure even to an extremely low level of UVB [38], and suggested that MMPs are UV-induced aging factors. In fact, gelatinase activities have been detected in the epidermis of forehead skin by in situ gelatin-zymography [39]. For further study, the skin-equivalent was selected as a model for BM damage, which partially mimics the photoaging process because of missing BM structure at the DEJ and the presence of large amounts of MMPs, including gelatinases (MMP-2 and MMP-9), in the culture medium as shown in Fig. 2 [33, 40]. A MMP inhibitor, CGS27023A, enhances the assembly of BM at the DEJ in the skin-equivalent (Fig. 3) [33, 40], suggesting that MMPs play an important role in the degradation of BM components and induce BM structural damage, such as detachment of BM from basal keratinocytes and disruption of lamina densa, which are observed in sun-exposed skin (Fig. 1).

Involvement of Plasminogen Activator/Plasmin in Damage to Epidermal BM, Degradation of Laminin 332, and Reduced Activities of Laminin 332 in Keratinocyte Adhesion and Type VII Collagen Binding

UVB exposure increases the synthesis of urokinase-type plasminogen activator (uPA) [19, 41], as well as matrix metalloproteinases [38, 42]. Both uPA activity and uPA are present in the conditioned medium of skin-equivalents, and the addition of plasminogen enhances the degradation of BM components and impairs the assembly of BM structure at the DEJ even in the presence of MMP inhibitors (Fig. 4) [43]. Aprotinin, a plasmin inhibitor, restores the assembly of BM structure at the DEJ damaged by the addition of plasminogen (Fig. 4).

Since lamina densa structure is detached at the anchoring filament from basal keratinocytes in sun-exposed skin (Fig. 1), laminin 332, a major component of anchoring filament, is a candidate target of plasmin. As expected, plasmin degrades the $\alpha3$ and $\beta3$ chains of laminin 332, although $\gamma2$ is unaffected (Fig. 5). Plasmin cleaves both the amino and carboxy terminals of $\alpha3$ chain, and these cleavages reduce the keratinocyte adhesion activity of laminin 332 (Fig. 6). Similarly, the removal of an amino terminal fragment (domain VI) of the $\beta3$ chain by plasmin (Fig. 5) results in a reduction of its affinity for type VII collagen (Fig. 6). Therefore, degradation of laminin 332 by plasmin may induce BM damage such as the detachment of lamina densa from basal keratinocytes.

Enhanced BM Assembly in the Presence of Laminin 332 and in Response to Increased Synthesis of BM Components in a Skin-Equivalent Model

Damaged BM must be repaired, since BM at the DEJ plays important roles in maintaining a healthy epidermis and dermis. In order to find

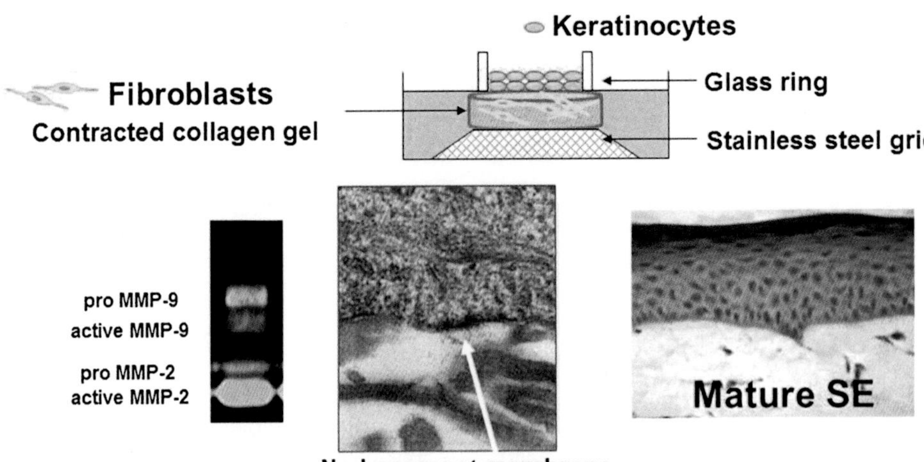

Fig. 2 Skin-equivalent model. Human skin-equivalent models are prepared by using human fibroblasts and keratinocytes. On the *top* of contracted collagen gel containing fibroblasts, keratinocytes are plated, and next day, the keratinocyte layer is exposed to air. Multilayered epidermis with cornified layer, like normal human skin, is formed within a week on the *top*. However, no lamina densa structure is observed at the DEJ. The activities of MMP-2 and MMP-9 are detected in conditioned medium by gelatin-zymography

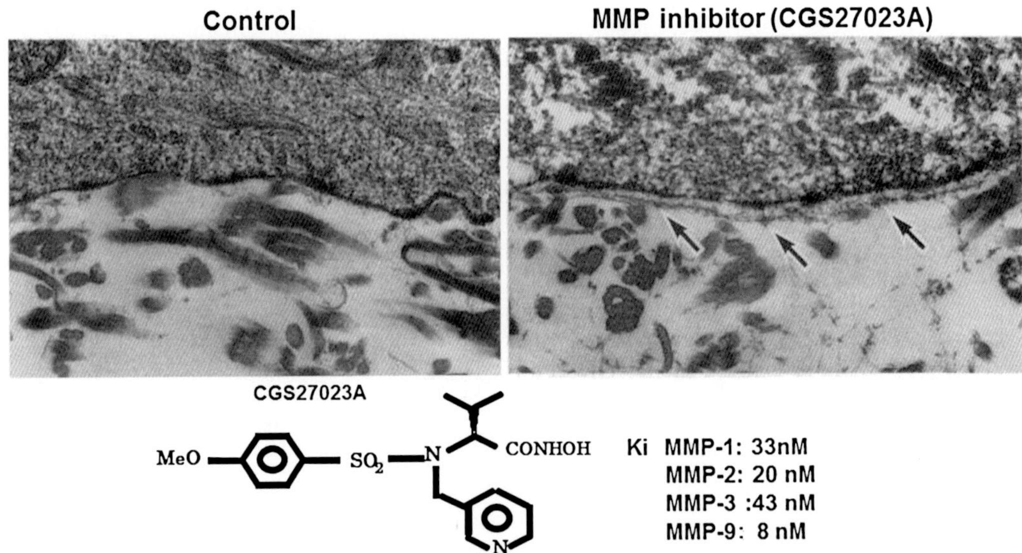

Fig. 3 Protective effects of MMP inhibitors against BM damage at the DEJ. Skin-equivalents were cultured from day 7 through day 14 with or without a synthetic MMP inhibitor, CGS27023A. Each sample was processed for electron microscopy at day 14. Lamina densa (*arrows*) was observed along the DEJ in the presence of CGS27023A

substances which stimulate the repair of damaged BM, we selected for screening purposes a skin-equivalent model, which is suitable for investigating the assembly of BM through cooperation between keratinocytes and fibroblasts. Purified laminin 332, a glycoprotein (MW: 410 kDa) composed of 165 kDa (α3), 140 kDa (β3), and 105 kDa (γ2) chains, enhances the formation of

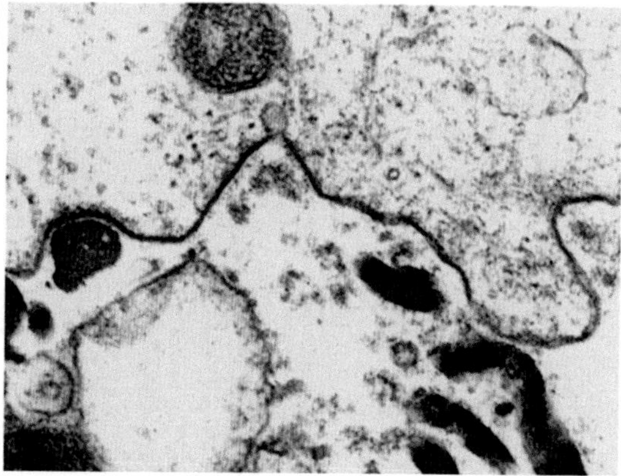

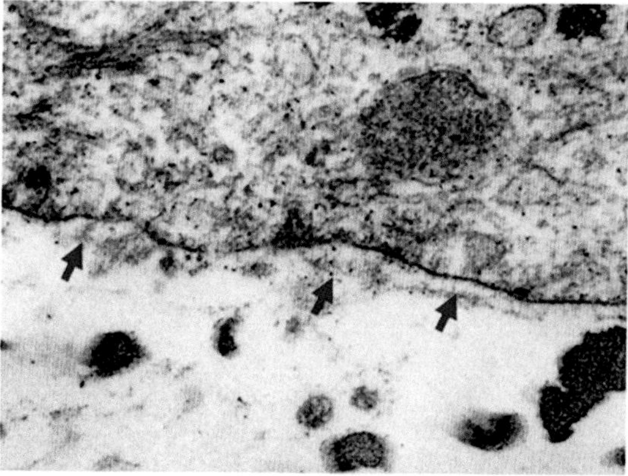

Fig. 4 Ultrastructural analyses of BM structures at the DEJ of SE. At 14 days after plating keratinocytes, SEs were processed for the analysis of BM structures at the DEJ by electron microscopy. CGS27023A (10 μM) enhances the formation of linear and continuous lamina densa-like structure (indicated by *arrows*) at the DEJ just beneath basal keratinocytes. The addition of plasminogen (0.06 μM) impaired the assembly of BM structure at the DEJ. Aprotinin (1.5 μM), a serine proteinase inhibitor, restored the linear and continuous lamina densa-like structures (indicated by *arrows*) at the DEJ

hemidesmosome-like structures and BM at the DEJ in the skin-equivalent [34].

Keratinocytes synthesize BM components, except nidogen [44]. Fibroblasts also produce BM components, other than laminin 332. We recently found that increasing the production of BM components such as laminin 332, collagen IV, and collagen VII in keratinocytes and/or fibroblasts with/without inhibitors of gelatinases and/or serine proteinases is also effective to enhance the repair or assembly of BM at the DEJ.

Involvement of the Degradation of Heparan Sulfate (HS) Chains at BM with Heparanase in the Functional Damage of BM During Photoaging Process

Heparanase is found to increase in inflammatory conditions, such as in UVB-irradiated skin, and is activated in human keratinocytes by UVB exposure and then heparan sulfate (HS) of perlecan is

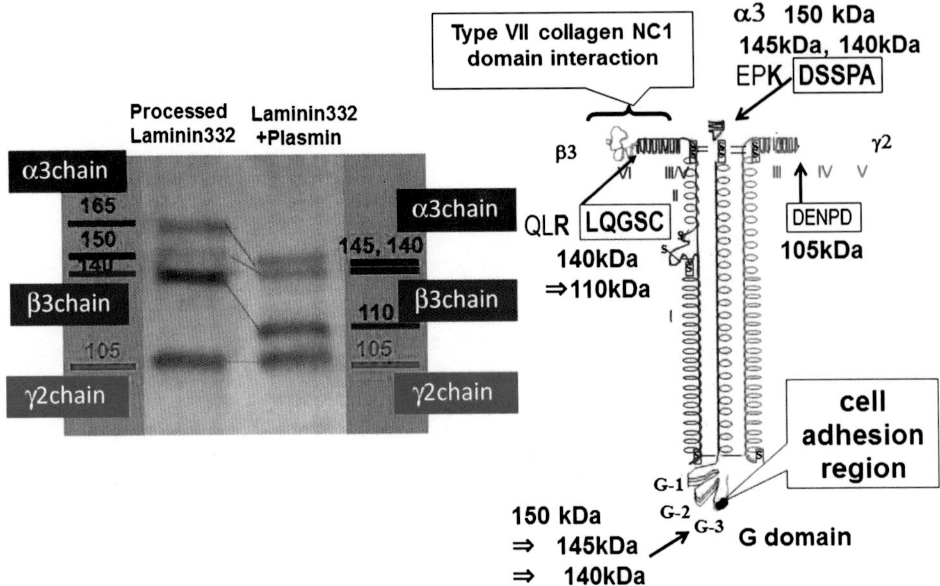

Fig. 5 Degradation of laminin 332 by plasmin and analyses of its cleavage sites of laminin 332. The processed form of laminin 332 was purified from conditioned medium of human keratinocytes and incubated with plasmin for 24 h at 37 °C. SDS-PAGE on 5 % acrylamide gel under reducing conditions and western blotting using polyclonal anti-laminin 332 antibodies were carried out. *Lane 1*, processed form of laminin 332; *lane 2*, plasmin-treated laminin 332. From the N-terminal amino acid sequences of the separated 145, 140, 110, and 105 kDa bands, cleavage sites in α3, β3, and γ2 are indicated by arrows on schematic domain structures of laminin 332. Predicted cleavage sites of α3 chain are shown in G-3. Since the N-terminal sequence of α3 chain is DSSPA, which is the same as that of the 150 kDa fragment of the α3 chain, plasmin cleaved a 5 or 10 kDa fragment from the LG3 domain of the 150 kDa α3 chain, in which the putative cell adhesion region, LRD, is present

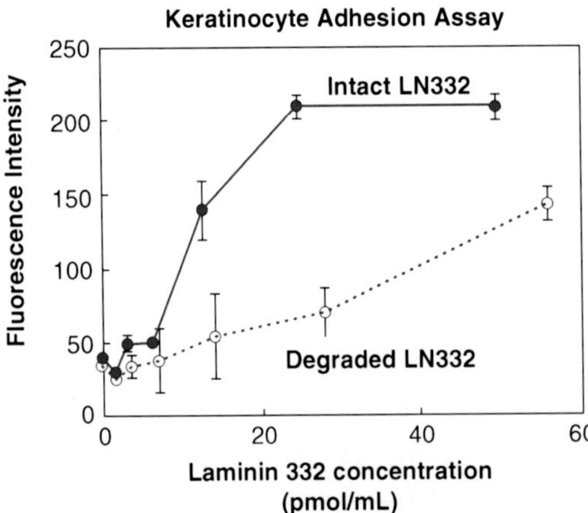

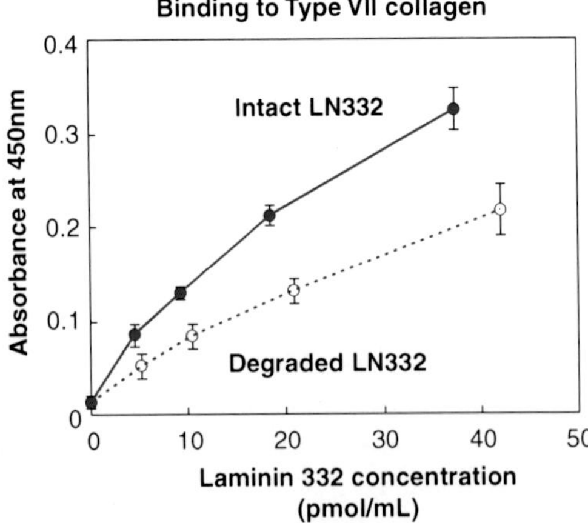

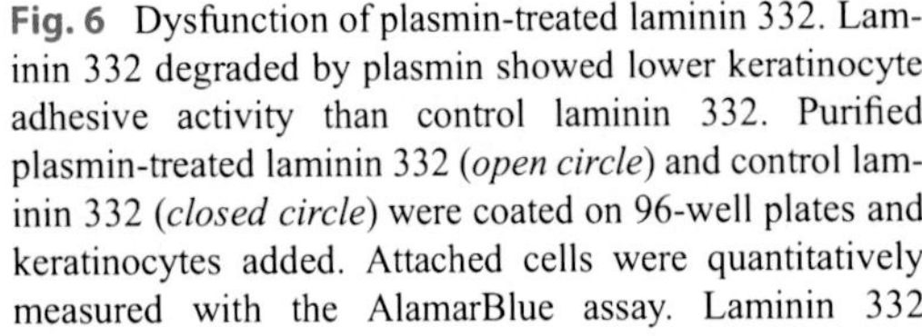

Fig. 6 Dysfunction of plasmin-treated laminin 332. Laminin 332 degraded by plasmin showed lower keratinocyte adhesive activity than control laminin 332. Purified plasmin-treated laminin 332 (*open circle*) and control laminin 332 (*closed circle*) were coated on 96-well plates and keratinocytes added. Attached cells were quantitatively measured with the AlamarBlue assay. Laminin 332 degraded by plasmin (*open circle*) showed reduced binding to type VII collagen as compared with control laminin 332 (*closed circle*). Purified type VII collagen was coated on 96-well plates and purified plasmin-treated laminin 332 (*open circle*) or control laminin 332 (*closed circle*) was added. After washing, bound laminin 332 was detected using polyclonal anti-laminin 332 antibodies

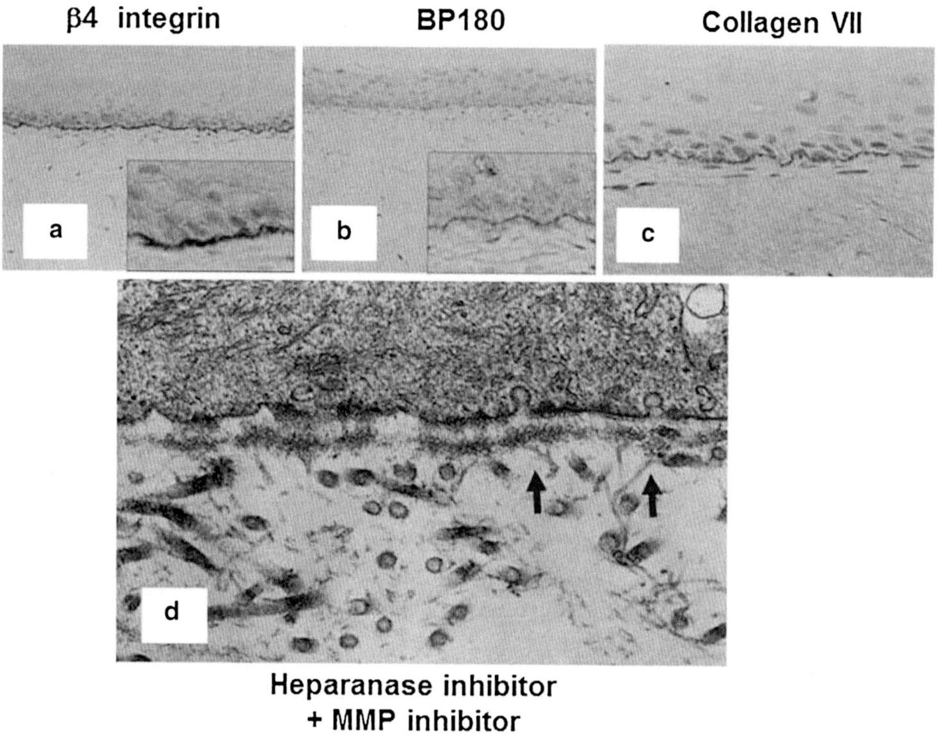

Fig. 7 Role of heparan sulfate chains in assembly of BM structure. β4 Integrin (**a**) and BP180 (**b**) were polarized to the basal surface, while deposition of collagen VII (**c**) was polarized to the basal side and increased by combined treatment with MMP inhibitor and heparanase inhibitor. The inhibitors facilitated assembly of anchoring complex, especially hemidesmosomes and anchoring fibrils (*arrows*), as observed by transmission electron microscopy (**d**)

markedly degraded at the DEJ in UVB-irradiated human skin [45]. Degradation of HS leads to a remarkable reduction in the binding activity of VEGF, FGF-2, and FGF-7 to the BM at the DEJ [46]. The degradation of HS at the DEJ impairs the function of the BM in photoaged skin, altering transfer of several growth factors between epidermis and dermis [45, 46]. Degradation of heparan sulfate was observed not only in acute UVB-irradiated skin but also in daily sun-exposed skin [46]. Since heparan sulfate was degraded in sun-exposed skin but not in sun-protected skin [46], daily UVB exposure activates heparanase, leads to degradation of HS in the BM, and increases growth factor interaction between epidermis and dermis. These changes would facilitate photoaging.

To repair BM damage in sun-exposed skin, it is necessary to control heparanase in addition to MMPs such as gelatinases [33] and/or uPA/plasmin [43]. In the SE model, BP180 and β4 integrin were polarized to the basal side, while deposition of collagen VII was polarized to the basal side and increased by combined treatment with MMP inhibitor and heparanase inhibitor (Fig. 7a–7c), which enhanced the formation of anchoring fibrils and hemidesmosomes as observed by transmission electron microscopy (Fig. 7d) [47]. These inhibitors may protect perlecan, thereby stabilizing BM structure at the DEJ, since perlecan is reported to serve as a connector between laminin- and collagen IV-containing networks at the DEJ [48].

Conclusion

The disruption and reduplication of BM at the DEJ in sun-exposed skins may be associated with increases of BM-damaging enzymes, such as heparanase, plasmin, and MMPs, which

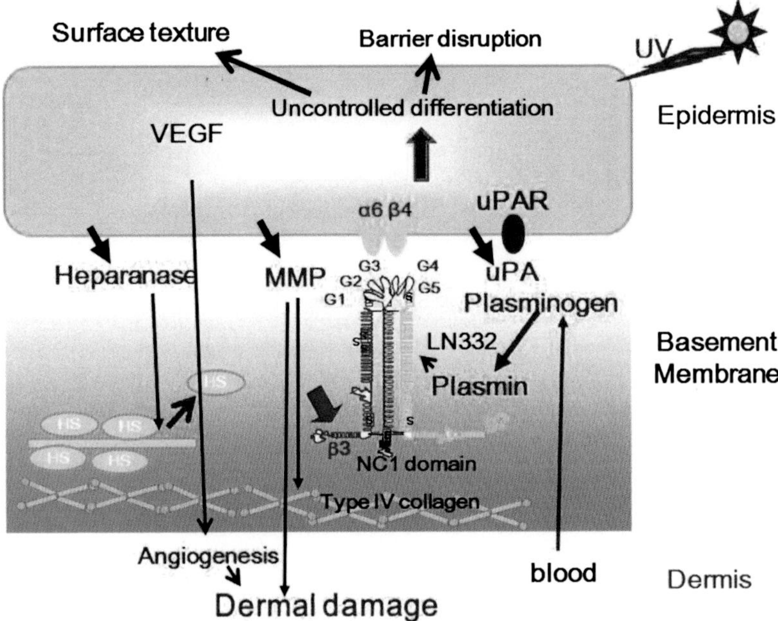

Fig. 8 Schematic illustration of skin-damaging mechanisms associated with photoaging due to repeated UV exposure. The disruption and reduplication of BM at the DEJ in sun-exposed skin may be induced by increased levels of BM-damaging enzymes, such as plasmin, MMPs, and heparanase, through the degradation of BM components: laminin 332, type IV and VII collagens, and perlecan. The impairment of BM structure may be associated with functional changes of epidermal cells and dermal cells and consequently facilitates aging processes by damaging dermal extracellular matrices and inducing keratinocyte abnormality

degrade BM components (HS chains of perlecan, laminin 332, type IV and VII collagens). The impairment of BM structure may be associated with functional changes of epidermal cells and dermal cells and consequently may facilitate photoaging processes by damaging dermal extracellular matrices and inducing keratinocyte abnormality, as summarized in Fig. 8. Laminin 332 is able to enhance BM assembly [34]. Some cosmetic ingredients also promote BM repair by increasing synthesis of BM components such as laminin 332 and type IV and VII collagens in the epidermis and/or the dermis and inhibiting the activities of MMPs and/or heparanase. Therefore, the BM represents a good target for skin-care cosmetics; components that enhance BM repair may improve epidermal-dermal communication and skin homeostasis, thereby strengthening defenses against "skin aging."

References

1. Tagami H. Functional characteristics of the stratum corneum in photoaged skin in comparison with those found in intrinsic aging. Arch Dermatol Res. 2008;300 Suppl 1:S1–6.
2. Lavker RM. Structural alterations in exposed and unexposed aged skin. J Invest Dermatol. 1979;73(1):59–66.
3. Kligman AM, et al. Topical tretinoin for photoaged skin. J Am Acad Dermatol. 1986;15(4 Pt 2):836–59.
4. Ryan MC, et al. The functions of laminins: lessons from in vivo studies. Matrix Biol. 1996;15(6):369–81.
5. Bohnert A, et al. Epithelial-mesenchymal interactions control basement membrane production and differentiation in cultured and transplanted mouse keratinocytes. Cell Tissue Res. 1986;244(2):413–29.
6. Watt FM. Selective migration of terminally differentiating cells from the basal layer of cultured human epidermis. J Cell Biol. 1984;98(1):16–21.
7. Barrandon Y, Green H. Three clonal types of keratinocyte with different capacities for multiplication. Proc Natl Acad Sci U S A. 1987;84(8):2302–6.

8. Hirai Y, et al. Epimorphin: a mesenchymal protein essential for epithelial morphogenesis. Cell. 1992;69(3):471–81.
9. Inoue S. Ultrastructure of basement membranes. Int Rev Cytol. 1989;117:57–98.
10. Amano S, et al. Bone morphogenetic protein 1 is an extracellular processing enzyme of the laminin 5 gamma 2 chain. J Biol Chem. 2000;275(30):22728–35.
11. Goldfinger LE, Stack MS, Jones JC. Processing of laminin-5 and its functional consequences: role of plasmin and tissue-type plasminogen activator. J Cell Biol. 1998;141(1):255–65.
12. Koshikawa N, et al. Membrane-type matrix metalloproteinase-1 (MT1-MMP) is a processing enzyme for human laminin gamma 2 chain. J Biol Chem. 2005;280(1):88–93.
13. Birkedal-Hansen H. Proteolytic remodeling of extracellular matrix. Curr Opin Cell Biol. 1995;7(5):728–35.
14. Reynolds JJ. Collagenases and tissue inhibitors of metalloproteinases: a functional balance in tissue degradation. Oral Dis. 1996;2(1):70–6.
15. Fassina G, et al. Tissue inhibitors of metalloproteases: regulation and biological activities. Clin Exp Metastasis. 2000;18(2):111–20.
16. Goldberg GI, et al. Human 72-kilodalton type IV collagenase forms a complex with a tissue inhibitor of metalloproteases designated TIMP-2. Proc Natl Acad Sci U S A. 1989;86(21):8207–11.
17. Saksela O. Plasminogen activation and regulation of pericellular proteolysis. Biochim Biophys Acta. 1985;823(1):35–65.
18. Morioka S, Jensen PJ, Lazarus GS. Human epidermal plasminogen activator. Characterization, localization, and modulation. Exp Cell Res. 1985;161(2):364–72.
19. Marschall C, et al. UVB increases urokinase-type plasminogen activator receptor (uPAR) expression. J Invest Dermatol. 1999;113(1):69–76.
20. Plow EF, et al. The plasminogen system and cell surfaces: evidence for plasminogen and urokinase receptors on the same cell type. J Cell Biol. 1986;103(6 Pt 1):2411–20.
21. Katsuta Y, et al. Urokinase-type plasminogen activator is activated in stratum corneum after barrier disruption. J Dermatol Sci. 2003;32(1):55–7.
22. Denda M, et al. *Trans*-4-(Aminomethyl)cyclohexane carboxylic acid (T-AMCHA), an anti-fibrinolytic agent, accelerates barrier recovery and prevents the epidermal hyperplasia induced by epidermal injury in hairless mice and humans. J Invest Dermatol. 1997;109(1):84–90.
23. Nakajima M, et al. Metastatic melanoma cell heparanase. Characterization of heparan sulfate degradation fragments produced by B16 melanoma endoglucuronidase. J Biol Chem. 1984;259(4):2283–90.
24. Parish CR, Freeman C, Hulett MD. Heparanase: a key enzyme involved in cell invasion. Biochim Biophys Acta. 2001;1471(3):M99–108.
25. Bernard D, et al. Purification and characterization of the endoglycosidase heparanase 1 from human plantar stratum corneum: a key enzyme in epidermal physiology? J Invest Dermatol. 2001;117(5):1266–73.
26. Friedl A, et al. Differential binding of fibroblast growth factor-2 and -7 to basement membrane heparan sulfate: comparison of normal and abnormal human tissues. Am J Pathol. 1997;150(4):1443–55.
27. Fuki II, Iozzo RV, Williams KJ. Perlecan heparan sulfate proteoglycan. A novel receptor that mediates a distinct pathway for ligand catabolism. J Biol Chem. 2000;275(40):31554.
28. Patel VN, et al. Heparanase cleavage of perlecan heparan sulfate modulates FGF10 activity during ex vivo submandibular gland branching morphogenesis. Development. 2007;134(23):4177–86.
29. Sebollela A, et al. Heparin-binding sites in granulocyte-macrophage colony-stimulating factor. Localization and regulation by histidine ionization. J Biol Chem. 2005;280(36):31949–56.
30. Perrimon N, Bernfield M. Specificities of heparan sulphate proteoglycans in developmental processes. Nature. 2000;404(6779):725–8.
31. Vlodavsky I, et al. Involvement of heparan sulfate and related molecules in sequestration and growth promoting activity of fibroblast growth factor. Cancer Metastasis Rev. 1996;15(2):177–86.
32. Bell E, et al. Living tissue formed in vitro and accepted as skin-equivalent tissue of full thickness. Science. 1981;211(4486):1052–4.
33. Amano S, et al. Importance of balance between extracellular matrix synthesis and degradation in basement membrane formation. Exp Cell Res. 2001;271(2):249–62.
34. Tsunenaga M, et al. Laminin 5 can promote assembly of the lamina densa in the skin equivalent model. Matrix Biol. 1998;17(8–9):603–13.
35. Sarret Y, et al. Constitutive synthesis of a 92-kDa keratinocyte-derived type IV collagenase is enhanced by type I collagen and decreased by type IV collagen matrices. J Invest Dermatol. 1992;99(6):836–41.
36. Sudbeck BD, et al. Collagen-stimulated induction of keratinocyte collagenase is mediated via tyrosine kinase and protein kinase C activities. J Biol Chem. 1994;269(47):30022–9.
37. Koivukangas V, et al. UV irradiation induces the expression of gelatinases in human skin in vivo. Acta Derm Venereol. 1994;74(4):279–82.
38. Fisher GJ, et al. Molecular basis of sun-induced premature skin ageing and retinoid antagonism. Nature. 1996;379(6563):335–9.
39. Inomata S, et al. Possible involvement of gelatinases in basement membrane damage and wrinkle formation in chronically ultraviolet B-exposed hairless mouse. J Invest Dermatol. 2003;120(1):128–34.
40. Amano S, et al. Protective effect of matrix metalloproteinase inhibitors against epidermal basement membrane damage: skin equivalents partially

mimic photoageing process. Br J Dermatol. 2005;153 Suppl 2:37–46.
41. Miralles F, et al. UV irradiation induces the murine urokinase-type plasminogen activator gene via the c-Jun N-terminal kinase signaling pathway: requirement of an AP1 enhancer element. Mol Cell Biol. 1998;18(8):4537–47.
42. Scharffetter K, et al. UVA irradiation induces collagenase in human dermal fibroblasts in vitro and in vivo. Arch Dermatol Res. 1991;283(8):506–11.
43. Ogura Y, et al. Plasmin induces degradation and dysfunction of laminin 332 (laminin 5) and impaired assembly of basement membrane at the dermal-epidermal junction. Br J Dermatol. 2008;159(1):49–60.
44. Fleischmajer R, et al. Skin fibroblasts are the only source of nidogen during early basal lamina formation in vitro. J Invest Dermatol. 1995;105(4):597–601.
45. Iriyama S, et al. Influence of heparan sulfate chains in proteoglycan at the dermal-epidermal junction on epidermal homeostasis. Exp Dermatol 2011;20(10): 810–4.
46. Iriyama S, et al. Activation of heparanase by ultraviolet B irradiation leads to functional loss of basement membrane at the dermal-epidermal junction in human skin. Arch Dermatol Res. 2011;303(4): 53–61.
47. Iriyama S, et al. Key role of heparan sulfate chains in assembly of anchoring complex at the dermal-epidermal junction. Exp Dermatol. 2011;20(11): 953–5.
48. Behrens DT, et al. The epidermal basement membrane is a composite of separate laminin- or collagen IV-containing networks connected by aggregated perlecan, but not by nidogens. J Biol Chem. 2012;287(22):18700–9.

Buffering Capacity Considerations in the Elderly

13

Jacquelyn Levin and Howard I. Maibach

Contents

Abstract

It is known that elderly skin has an increased pH and decreased buffering capacity. These two changes in the physiochemical nature of elderly skin arguably contribute to the fragility of elderly skin by influencing barrier homeostasis, skin integrity/cohesion, susceptibility to infection, and skin sensitivity to topical acids and alkalis. This chapter briefly reviews the basic science of pH, the buffering capacity, and the changes seen in the epidermis of aging skin before presenting a more in-depth review of experimentation investigating the source and characteristics of human skin buffering capacity. These studies are reviewed in an attempt to illuminate the source of the diminished buffering capacity of aged skin.

Experimentation reviewed here suggests that AAs are primarily responsible for the neutralization capacity of the skin. The exact sources of the amino acids as well as the types of AA that are primarily responsible for the neutralization capacity remain still rather speculative. From what is known to date, filaggrin breakdown products may play an important role in skin buffering capacity, and the decrease in filaggrin as we age may explain, at least in part, why the skin buffering capacity decreases with age. Additional components of the epidermis such as sebum and CO_2 seem not to significantly participate as buffering agents of the epidermis, yet they still may play a role

J. Levin (✉)
West Dermatology, Rancho Santa Margarita, CA, USA
e-mail: jlevin@hotmail.com

H.I. Maibach
Department of Dermatology, University of California, San Francisco, CA, USA
e-mail: maibachh@derm.ucsf.edu

M.A. Farage et al. (eds.), *Textbook of Aging Skin*,
DOI 10.1007/978-3-662-47398-6_14

in the protection of skin from the harm of acids and bases.

Introduction

The acidic character of skin was first mentioned by Heuss [1] and later by Schade and Marchionini [2] who introduced the term "acid mantle" for skin's acidic outer surface pH. It has been recognized as playing a crucial role in permeability barrier homeostasis, skin integrity/cohesion, and immune function [3–5]. Given this, it is important for skin to be able to resist acidic/alkaline aggression to some extent (i.e., have buffering capacity) [6]. The pH of skin increases and the ability to buffer the change in skin pH decreases with age [7]. This increase in pH and decreased buffering capacity in elderly skin result in impaired barrier homeostasis and skin integrity/cohesion, increased likelihood for skin infection, and increased sensitivity/irritation to topically applied products [8].

The chapter briefly reviews the basic science of pH and buffering capacity and the deleterious effects of increased pH in the skin of the elderly. In addition, recent experimentation investigating the characteristics of human skin buffering capacity is reviewed. The decrease in buffering capacity in elderly skin will be discussed, firstly by discerning which components of the stratum corneum are most likely responsible for the buffering capacity in skin of all ages and secondly by reviewing the physiologic changes of the stratum corneum that may contribute to the decrease in the buffering capacity detected clinically in elderly skin.

Defining and Measuring the pH and Buffering Capacity of Skin

When dilute aqueous acid or alkaline solutions come into contact with skin, the change in pH is generally temporary, and the original skin pH (a measure of the hydronium ion concentration) is rapidly restored, indicating that skin has significant buffering capacity.

A buffer is a chemical system that can limit changes in pH when an acid or a base is added. Buffer solutions consist of a weak acid and its conjugate base. The system has its optimum buffering capacity when about 50 % of buffer is dissociated or in other words at a pH approximately equal to its pKa [6, 9]. The pKa is the negative of the common logarithm of the acid dissociation constant (Ka) and is a measure for the strength of the acid. The buffer capacity is further dependent on the concentration of the system.

An acid/alkali aggression test is one way to measure the acid/alkali resistance (i.e., buffering capacity) of skin. Alkali/Acidic resistance tests were commonly used in the 1960s to detect workers that may likely develop occupational diseases in certain chemical work environments [6]. A mild variation of the alkali/acidic resistance tests, also called acid/alkali neutralization test, assesses how quickly the skin is able to buffer applied acids/bases without the occurrence of skin corrosion. Repetitive applications of acid or base demonstrate that the skin buffering capacity is limited and may be overcome, as illustrated by the long time required for neutralization [10–13].

Effect of Increase in pH on Elderly Skin Function and Defenses

In a multicenter study on measurement of the natural pH of the skin surface, the values of skin surface pH were 4.9 (arithmetic mean) with a 95 % confidence interval between 4.1 and 5.8 [9]. Ideal acidity for the stratum corneum is a pH of approximately 5.4 [14]. It is well known that an increased skin pH is detected in the elderly skin starting anywhere from age 50 to 80 years [14–18]. Most likely this decreased acidity is due to less efficient mechanisms for skin acidification and more specifically decreased NA + /H + antiporter (NHE1) expression. The NHE1 is one of three highly studied mechanisms for maintaining skin acidity and is assumed to be the predominate mechanism for maintaining skin acidity [18].

Elevation of the skin pH in the elderly alters multiple functions. Those discussed here include impairment of permeability barrier homeostasis, decreased skin integrity/cohesion, and increased susceptibility for microbial infection.

Impaired Permeability Barrier Homeostasis

An acidic pH is critical for permeability barrier homeostasis, in part because of two key lipid-processing enzymes, B-glucocerebrosidase and acid sphingomyelinase which generate a family of ceramides from glucosylceramide and sphingomyelin precursors and exhibit low pH optima [5]. An increased skin pH results in defective lipid processing and delayed maturation of lamellar membranes [18]. These lipids form multi-lamellar sheets amidst the intracellular spaces of the stratum corneum critical to the stratum corneum's mechanical and cohesive properties, enabling it to function as an effective water barrier [18]. This delayed barrier function allows easier penetration of topically applied products and delays barrier recovery after injury or insult to the skin [5, 18].

Decreased Skin Integrity and Cohesion

An acidic pH also clearly promotes stratum corneum integrity and cohesion. In a neutral pH environment, there is an enhanced tendency for the stratum corneum to be removed by tape stripping (integrity) as well as increased amount of protein removed per stripping (cohesion) [18, 19]. The impaired stratum corneum integrity/cohesion is due to pH dependent activation of serine proteases which exhibit neutral pH optima [20]. Serine proteases become activated in the increased pH of elderly skin and lead to the premature degradation of corneodesmosomes and hence increased desquamation [5, 18, 21].

Increased Susceptibility for Skin Infections

The acidic pH of the stratum corneum restricts colonization by pathogenic flora and encourages persistence of normal microbial flora. Pertinently elderly skin, intertriginous areas, and chronically inflamed skin display an increased skin pH [2] and hence reduce resistance to pathogens [14].

In summary, elderly skin commonly has abnormalities in stratum corneum integrity/cohesion, permeability barrier homeostasis, and immune function due to increased skin pH. These abnormalities are attributable to the pH-mediated increase in serine protease-mediated degradation of corneodesmosomes, defect in lipid processing, and decrease in antibacterial activity, respectively.

Discerning Which Components of the Stratum Corneum Contribute to the Skin Buffering Capacity

Both an increased skin surface pH and reduced buffering capacity have been documented for skin of the elderly. The reduced buffering capacity contributes to the increased sensitivity of skin to contact irritants and cleansing procedures [8]. The next section focuses on the aggression tests aimed at discerning which components of the epidermis are responsible for skin buffering capacity.

Free Fatty Acids/Sebum

Early experimentation hypothesized that the sebum contributes to the buffering capacity of skin in two ways: first, it protects the epidermis against the influence of alkali by slowing down the exposure and penetration of acids or alkalis applied to the skin [22–24] and second, the fatty acids in sebum may act as buffer system [25, 26].

Later Lincke et al. [27] refuted the second hypothesis by demonstrating that the sebum had no relevant acid and a negligible alkali buffering capacity around pH 9. Further challenging the hypothesis, a quicker neutralization was observed on delipidized skin than untreated skin [22, 25].

Vermeer concluded similarly when comparing the neutralization on soles and forearm with and without sebum removal, respectively [26]. However, when comparing these different skin regions, differences in sebum content may have also contributed to the observed effect.

Vermeer [24] and Neuhaus [28] believed that the increased rate of neutralization after sebum removal may have been due to increased amounts of carbon dioxide (CO_2) diffusion. This theory, discussed later in detail, is generally not accepted and also not clearly substantiated. After lipid removal, skin starts to increase acid production which may account for the faster neutralization. The same investigators also found that the increase in neutralization after lipid removal is temporary and limited to the first few minutes, which is probably related to the activity of sebaceous glands to produce relevant amounts of sebum.

Due to the negligible buffering capacity of sebum and to standardized experimentation (limit inter- and intraindividual variability), today most neutralization experiments are performed after cleansing the skin with solvents which remove most of the sebum including fatty acids.

Epidermal Water-Soluble Constituents

Vermeer et al. [26] first demonstrated the importance of water-soluble constituents to the skin's buffering ability. Water-soaked skin, where the water-soluble constituents were extracted, demonstrated a significantly reduced neutralization capacity indicating that water-soluble substance constituent(s) of the skin are major contributors to the buffering capacity [12, 26, 29].

The significance of water-soluble constituents of the epidermis to the buffering capacity of skin further supports the theory of minimal contribution from the sebum of skin due to its lipid-soluble nature [26].

Sweat

Eccrine sweat initially accelerates the neutralization of alkalis [10–13, 26, 30, 31]. Spier and Pasher [32] suggest that the main buffering agents of sweat are lactic acid and amino acids. The lactic acid-lactate system in sweat has a highly efficient buffering capacity between pH 4 and pH 5 [23]. However, it has not been completely demonstrated that lactic acid is the main buffering agent in sweat or at the surface of the skin. Conversely, the contribution of amino acids (AAs) to the buffering capacity of sweat and of the horny layer surface has been investigated thoroughly [26, 31].

By comparing sweating and non-sweating persons, Vermeer [26] found that AA plays a significant role in neutralization during the first 5 min, while lactic acid does not. This confirms that AAs are key elements contributing to the buffering capacity of skin.

CO_2

Little is known about the role of CO_2/HCO_3- participating in skin buffering capacity. Burckhardt's studies were the first to suggest that the CO_2 diffusing from the epidermal layer may be responsible for neutralizing alkali in contact with skin [10–13]. He demonstrated that when a 5 min alkali neutralization experiment is repeated subsequently several times on the same skin area, the neutralization times became longer and finally reach an approximately constant time. He suggested that the shorter neutralization times at the beginning were due to acids present on the skin surface rapidly neutralizing the alkali. He further suggested that after successive alkali exposure, the endogenous acids were no longer present on the skin surface resulting in longer neutralization times and diffusing carbon dioxide would take over the role of neutralizing the alkali. At this time, Burckhardt's hypothesis of the role of carbon dioxide as a buffering agent was accepted by others despite the rather weak experimental evidence [27, 33–35].

The decreased neutralization time after lipid removal of the skin surface with the help of soaps or neutral detergents was believed by Burckhardt and others to be the consequence of greater diffusion of CO_2 although this has never been quantified [23, 34, 35]. It was also postulated that a more hydrated stratum corneum retains a greater amount of CO_2 by limiting its diffusion. Therefore, a moderate hydration level was regarded better for effective alkali neutralization; however, this has also never been analyzed in further detail [35].

Knowing that several authors considered CO_2 a relevant contributor in alkali neutralization without having quantitative data to sustain their hypothesis, Vermeer et al. [5] demonstrated that CO_2 is unlikely of great importance for alkali neutralization on skin. His experiment was focused on the first minutes of the neutralization process in contrast to the previous experiments mentioned [28, 33–35], which paid attention to the later neutralization process. For example, Piper [33] analyzed the neutralization process for up to 1 h and concluded that, for the first half hour, alkalis are neutralized on the skin by the skin's own amphoteric substances (such as amino acids) but that in the second half hour, diffusing carbon dioxide takes over. Piper's conclusions are not necessarily contradictory to the results obtained by Vermeer above and may actually be in agreement. According to Piper, "the longer the contact between skin and alkali, the greater the importance of CO_2." This statement is supported by the recent discoveries of relatively low level of carbon dioxide production in the epidermis and the limited activity of the Kreb's Cycle, suggesting that a minimal amount of CO_2 would be available for neutralization [36]. It seems likely that CO_2 does not significantly contribute in the alkali neutralization process. Further studies should further help to clarify the relevance of CO_2 in skin buffering capacity.

The above studies fail to provide quantitative support for their conclusions concerning CO_2 as relevant buffering agent. More likely, the constant neutralization time after successive alkali exposure may be related to the destruction of the "skin barrier" and unlimited penetration of the applied alkali as suggested by others [26, 28].

Free Amino Acids

Free amino acids in the water-soluble portion of the epidermis seem to play a significant role in the neutralization of alkalis within the first 5 min of experimentation [26, 33, 37].

Piper [33] found a good buffering capacity of skin between pH 4 and pH 8 with an optimum at 6.5 well corresponding to the pKa of AA. This observation further indicates that lactic acid may be less relevant in the buffering capacity of skin.

Despite the general agreement about the role of amino acids in the neutralization of alkalis, which amino acids are the key buffering agents remains an open question. The AA composition of the upper stratum corneum was reported by Spier and Pascher [31]. Spier and Pascher reported that the free AA account for 40 % of the water-soluble substances extracted from the stratum corneum removed by tape stripping [32, 38]. Of the amino acids present, the composition was as follows: 20–32 % serine; 9–16 % citrulline; 6–10 % aspartic acid, glycine, threonine, and alanine; and 0.5–2 % glutamic acid.

The water-soluble, free AA on the skin surface may originate from five possible sources:

1. Eccrine sweat

   Sweat contains 0.05 % amino acids which remain on the surface of the skin after evaporation. The specific AA found in sweat was not investigated.
2. Degradation of skin proteins

   Degradation of skin proteins including proteins constituting the desmosomes may be a source for AA such as serine, glycine, and alanine.
3. Hair follicles

   Citrulline is recognized as a constituent of protein synthesized in the inner root sheath and medulla cells of the hair follicle. Specific proteases release citrulline. Citrulline is also found in the membrane of the corneocytes [36].
4. Keratin

   The contribution of keratin to the buffering capacity of skin remains questionable. Keratin is an amphoteric protein with the ability to neutralize acids and alkalis in vitro [8–11, 14, 36, 39] and hence may participate in skin buffering capacity. Scales scraped from normal skin have been shown to bind small amounts of alkali in vitro [32, 40]; however, Vermeer and coworkers showed that water-soluble constituents of the epidermis participate more in skin buffering capacity than the insoluble constituents of the skin such as keratin.

   While insoluble keratin filaments on the skin may have limited buffering capacity [22, 41], keratin hydrolysates and free amino acids might contribute to the water-soluble portion of the epidermis. Yet, the AA composition of keratin [42, 43] does not correspond with the AA composition found in the water-soluble portion of the stratum corneum [27], which implies that keratin is not a major contributor to the pool of free AA.

Despite little evidence of keratin's role in the buffering capacity, a modifying action of keratin is assumed [23]. Without an intact keratin layer, neither a physiological surface pH nor normal neutralization capacity can be maintained [44]. Further research remains to be conducted to determine keratin's role in the buffering capacity of the epidermis.

5. Keratohyalin granule histidine-rich protein: filaggrin

   Urocanic acid and pyrrolidone carboxylic acid in mammalian stratum corneum have been shown to be derived principally or totally from the histidine-rich protein, filaggrin, of the keratohyalin granules. The time course of appearance of free amino acids and breakdown of filaggrin are similar, as are the analyses of the free amino acids and the histidine-rich filaggrin. Quantitative studies show that between 70 % and 100 % of the total stratum corneum-free amino acids are derived from filaggrin [40, 45].

   These results strongly suggest that the free amino acids and/or their metabolites of the stratum corneum might be the final products of a degradation of filaggrin. Further research needs to be completed in order to identify which of these AAs contribute to the buffering capacity of the skin.

Specific Physiologic and Structural Changes in the Stratum Corneum of Elderly Skin: Impact on the Buffering Capacity of Elderly Skin

Lipid Content/Sebum Production

The brick and mortar model is often used to describe the stratum corneum's protein-rich corneocytes embedded in a matrix of ceramides, cholesterol, and fatty acids and smaller amounts of cholesterol sulfates, glucosylceramides, and phospholipids. As stated earlier, these lipids form multi-lamellar sheets amidst the intracellular spaces of the stratum corneum critical to the stratum corneum's mechanical and cohesive properties, enabling it to function as an effective water barrier [18, 45]. Many authors agree that the overall lipid content of human skin decreases with age [46–49], although the proportion of different lipid classes seems to remain fairly constant [7, 49].

Sebaceous gland function is decreased in association with concomitant decrease in endogenous androgen production [50]. This is the likely cause of decreased surface lipid levels in the elderly. In males, sebum levels remain essentially unchanged until the age of 80 years. In women, there is a gradual decrease in sebaceous secretion from menopause through the seventh decade, after which no appreciable change occurs [51].

As discussed in the previous section the lipid layer is presumed to slow down the exposure of any topical insult. Therefore with decreased amount of lipid, any topical insult will more easily overwhelm the buffering system of the stratum corneum.

Water

In young skin, most of the water is bound to proteins and appropriately termed bound water [39]. Bound water is important for the structure and mechanical properties of many proteins and their mutual interactions. Water molecules that are not bound to proteins bind to each other and are called tetrahedron or bulk water [39]. In aged skin, water is mostly found in the tetrahedron form, bound to itself rather than to other molecules [52]. The lack of interaction between water and surrounding molecules in aged skin leads to variation in the water-soluble portion of the stratum corneum and likely contributes to decreased buffering capacity found in elderly skin.

In addition, this chemical change in the water explains why although aged stratum corneum has higher total water content than younger skin, it is often dry and weathered [7].

Proteins

Proteomic profiling has identified at least 30 proteins involved in skin aging. In addition many miRNAs specific to these proteins were shown to be downregulated in aging skin.[53] In particular, filaggrin which assumes an important role in skin hydration, pH, barrier function, and likely buffering capacity (via its breakdown products) has been shown to be decreased 2.7-fold in aged skin [53].

It also has been found that the majority of proteins in young skin are in helical conformation. This is in contrast to aged skin which can show markedly altered protein conformation such as increased protein folding resulting in less exposure to aliphatic residues to water [39, 52]. Increased protein folding and decreased interaction of proteins with water affect the concentration of AA in the stratum corneum which as discussed previously likely plays an important role in the buffering capacity of skin.

In addition the AA composition of proteins and free amino acids in aged skin also differ significantly from that of young skin. There is an increase in the overall hydrophobicity of amino acid in the elderly [41]. As free amino acids are believed to play a key role in stratum corneum buffering capacity, this shift in composition, combined with evidence of altered protein tertiary protein structure, provides insight into the diminished buffering capacity in aged individuals.

It should also be noted that the increase in pH of aged skin will also change the fraction of AA in the stratum corneum that is associated or disassociated. Free AAs work best as a buffer at pH that is equal to their pKa (i.e., the pH at which 50 % of the AA is associated and 50 % disassociated). Because of the increased baseline pH found in elderly skin, the percentage of associated to disassociated AA changes, hence changing the effectiveness of the buffer.

Eccrine Sweat Glands

With aging, the number of active eccrine sweat glands is reduced, and sweat output per gland is diminished in both rate and amount. Morphologically, the secretory cells flatten and become atrophic. A progressive accumulation of lipofuscin is found in the cytoplasm of the glandular epithelium [50, 54].

Therefore, any contribution of eccrine sweat to the buffering capacity would be decreased in aged skin due to the decreased output of sweat overall.

Recent Experimentation Regarding Human Skin Buffering Capacity

A majority of the research presented prior to this section is half a century old. In this section we present more recent investigations in regard to human skin buffering capacity.

In 2008, Ayer and Maibach [55] assessed the possibility of using an in vitro model for evaluating skin buffering capacity. In this study a model base, NaOH, is topically applied to cadaver skin in three different concentrations (0.1 N, 0.05 N, and 0.025 N). pH readings were taken at baseline and again immediately after base application and then at 5, 10, 15, 20, and 25 min after application. After the last reading, the solution was removed, and pH readings were taken immediately and after 5, 10, 15, 20, and 25 min. This procedure was repeated three times using the same skin samples. Unexposed cadaver skin and cadaver skin with deionized water were used as a control.

Ayer and Maibach found a significant difference in the buffering capacity of the cadaver skin with successive applications (P <0.0001). The different NaOH solutions all demonstrated buffer capacity for the two initial successive applications and then showed a significantly diminished buffering ability with the third remaining subsequent application of base. The controls showed no significant variation in pH throughout the experimentation. These results imply a decrease of skin buffering capacity with successive applications of NaOH. Interestingly, the decrease in buffering capacity after successive applications did not differ between the concentrations of the base solution used [55].

After the removal of the alkali, the cadaver skin slowly returned toward baseline skin pH. The ability to restore pH in this experiment did not decrease with successive applications or differ between the three NaOH strengths. Therefore, it is a possibility that the buffering capacity of the skin was overwhelmed in the first portion of the experiment when successive applications of base were applied, and only when the base was removed for a significant period of time, the mechanisms to restore skin pH were able to take effect [55].

Ayer and Maibach [55] offer a good introductory in vitro model adequate for future experimentation and investigation into skin buffering capacity. In 2009, Zhai et al. [56] used the same in vitro model as introduced by Ayer and Maibach [55], to measure the skin buffering capacity against hydrochloric acid (a model acid) and sodium hydroxide (a model base) at concentrations of 0.025, 0.05, and 0.1 N. This experimental design not only serves to verify the reproducibility of the in vitro model proposed by Ayer and Maibach in 2008 [55] but also provides a comparison of human skin buffering capacity upon exposure to acids and bases. pH values of all solutions used were also reported in this experimentation. This is helpful for future experimentation where buffering capacity of chemically different acids and bases can be compared and may discern if the chemical composition of the acid or base in addition to the pH of the solution affects skin buffering capacity.

The results of this experiment showed changes in pH after applications of base or acid that correlated with the increasing concentration of acid or base in the applied solution (i.e., the highest concentration of acid or base caused the largest change in pH). This is not in accord with the previously mentioned Ayer and Maibach study [55], which observed no evidence of a difference between the three strengths of NaOH and suggested that lower concentrations should be examined. Also in contrast to the experiment by Ayer and Maibach, both controls, a phosphate buffer solution (pH = 7.46) and water (pH = 7.41), significantly elevated skin pH ($P < 0.05$) following the washing procedure. This increase in pH may be explained by their alkaline characteristic when compared with untreated acidic skin. Other studies have also shown that the use of plain tap water increases skin pH up to 6 h after application before returning to its "natural" value [57, 58]. The reason for the difference between the two experiments remains unclear.

When comparing pH patterns of acids and bases after solution removal, Zhai et al. [56] reported a significant difference. The authors found that the skin pH normalized relatively faster with acid application when compared with base application and for all cadaver skin exposed to base, the change in the pH values was significantly more ($P < 0.05$) at all time points post-washing compared to the acid-exposed skin. This may imply different inherent buffering mechanisms [56] and perhaps different skin tolerability between bases and acids.

In 2012, Zheng et al. [59] investigated the buffering capacity in three skin layers: the stratum corneum, viable epidermis, and dermis. Zheng et al. used the same in vitro technique on cadaver skin as used in the experiment by Zhai et al. [56] and Ayer and Maibach [55] to evaluate the buffering capacity of different skin layers. Viable epidermis was exposed by removing the SC using 40 continuous tape strippings. The dermis was exposed by heat separating the epidermis in the water bath for 30 s at 60° C [58].

Sodium hydroxide (NaOH) and hydrochloric acid (HCl) solutions at 0.025, 0.05, and 0.1 N were applied to the skin layers (3.18 mL/cm^2). After 30 min, the skin was washed with 1 mL deionized water. TEWL and pH measurements were conducted at baseline (before contact with acid or base) and 0, 10, and 30 min postexposure and continued at 0, 10, and 30 min post-washing [59].

The dermis demonstrated lower pH values at 0 and 10 min post-NaOH exposures in comparison with the intact stratum corneum ($P < 0.001$ at each concentration); different NaOH concentrations presented a similar trend. This observation indicates that within a short time span post-base exposure, the dermis demonstrates the strongest buffering capacity among all three layers [59]. At 30 min post-base dosing, intact skin demonstrated the strongest buffering capacity, while the dermis was ranked the weakest ($P < 0.01$ compared with the other two layers). At 30 min post-washing, the intact skin's pH values declined faster than the other layers ($P < 0.01$ at 0.1 N). However, at that time, the layers did not present a significant difference in the pH values compared with the blank control's pH reading ($P > 0.05$) [59].

The ability of HCl to modify skin pH was comparable with NaOH ability. For HCl, similar to NaOH, the dermis demonstrated the strongest buffering capacity, while at 30 min, intact skin presented the greatest buffering ability [59].

These results from Zheng et al. [59] revealed that skin buffering capacities of different skin layers differ substantially from each other. Future experimentation may help expose specific reasoning and/or mechanisms involved as well as help establish clinical relevance.

Taking a look at these three experiments discussed above, using similar in vitro models to investigate skin buffering capacity, the results demonstrate that cadaver skin retains it buffering capacity and mechanisms involved in restoring skin pH. Cadaver skin before experimentation is stored frozen at −25° C. Freezing the skin at such temperature could compromise the buffering capacity when compared to in vivo living skin [40]. This might be the limitation of cadaver skin (especially the frozen skin), but it needs to be further investigated to discern how great the difference could be.

The authors feel that the reproducibility of the model also needs to be investigated further as each of the three experiments had slightly conflicting results. The first experiment by Ayer and Maibach [55] found no significant difference in pH values between the three concentrations of base, while Zhai et al. [56] found significant differences. Also, while Zhai et al. [59] found significant difference in the amount of pH change after exposure to acid versus base, Zheng et al. [59] found similar modifications in the skin pH. In addition, there were also differences among the controls of each experiment. Whether these differences are from a lack of reproducibility or due to the slight differences in the methodology or statistical analysis remains unclear.

Conclusion

Elderly skin has an increased pH and decreased buffering capacity. These two changes in the physiochemical nature of elderly skin arguably contribute to the fragility of elderly skin by influencing barrier homeostasis, skin integrity/cohesion, susceptibility to infection, and skin sensitivity to topical acids and alkalis.

Skin's exquisite buffering capacity has been widely studied in vitro and in vivo, yet further research is required to better understand the exact mechanisms responsible for the buffering capacity of skin.

Experimentation reviewed here suggests that AAs are primarily responsible for the neutralization capacity of skin. The exact sources of the amino acids as well as the types of AA that are primarily responsible for the neutralization capacity remain still rather speculative; however, it is thought that the AAs may be derived from the keratohyalin granule histidine-rich protein, filaggrin.

In addition, it seems that a sweat component increases the neutralization capacity of the epidermis. Whether the buffering component of sweat is additional, AA or lactic acid remains unknown.

While additional components of the epidermis such as sebum, keratin, and CO_2 seem not to significantly participate as buffering agents of the epidermis, they still may play a role in the protection of skin from the harm of acids and bases. Sebum may slow down the initial penetration of applied substances. Keratin is important for the hydration of the skin and may contribute to the free AA pool responsible for buffering of applied acids/alkalis. Finally, CO_2 may play a role in the buffering capacity of certain compounds under certain circumstances such as after prolonged or repetitive exposure to an alkali.

After thorough review of studies investigating the buffering capacity of skin and studies investigating the endogenous mechanisms for restoring and maintaining skin pH, it is interesting that the two topics have been investigated separately without looking for a commonality. It would not be surprising if the mechanisms responsible for maintaining skin pH influence the processes responsible for maintaining skin buffering capacity. The above rationale may shed light on clinical correlation of increased pH and decreased buffering capacity that is seen in certain skin disease [42] and in elderly skin [7]. This theory is supported by the discovery that 70–100 % of AAs of the stratum corneum are derived from the degradation of histidine-rich protein in keratohyalin granules which is also one of the essential pathways involved in maintaining skin pH [3, 40, 45]. This theory is further supported by the fact that decreasing skin pH in the elderly via acidic topical products has lead to an increased buffering capacity and reduced skin sensitivity [43]. While more research needs to be conducted on the benefit of topical acidic therapy for aged individuals, this application seems reasonable as many authors have demonstrated the use of acidic topic products or washes on patients with increased pH to help restore integrity/cohesion [21] and barrier recovery [21].

The rich experimental literature, even if old at times, leads the way to utilizing several contemporary methods to further refine insights into skin buffering capacity and aging. From more recent experimentation, we have learned that skin pH and its buffering capacity can be easily measured utilizing an in vitro model, and this model may partially replicate the response of in vivo skin buffering capacity. While this model has limitations and cannot completely replace in vivo studies, the in vitro model may be beneficial for pharmacologic and toxicologic studies, as well as for defining mechanisms.

Taken together, we interpret this rich experimental literature, as leading the way to utilization of contemporary methods to further refine our insight into skin buffering capacity. This capacity, when fully understood, may lead not only to the potential for decreasing threat of exogenous acids and bases to aged skin but also for establishing experimental bases for optimal pH in many cosmetic, pharmacologic, metabolic, and toxicologic situations.

References

1. Heuss E. Die Reaktion des Scheisses beim gesunden Menschen. Monatsh Prakt Dermatol. 1892;14:343.
2. Schade H, Marchionini A. Zur physikalischen Chemie der Hautoberflache. Arch Dermatol Syphil. 1928;154:690.
3. Kim M, Patel R, Shinn A. Evaluation of gender difference in skin type and pH. J Dermatol Sci. 2006;41:153–6.
4. Greener B, Hughes A, Bannister N, Douglas J. Proteases and pH in chronic wounds. J Wound Care. 2005;14(2):59–61.
5. Hachem J, Crumrine D, Fluhr J, Brown B, Feingold K, Elias P. pH directly regulates epidermal permeability barrier homeostasis, and stratum corneum integrity/cohesion. J Invest Dermatol. 2003;121:345–53.
6. Agache P. Measurement of skin surface acidity. In: Agache P, Humbert P, Maibach H, editors. Measuring skin. Berlin: Springer; 2004. p. 84–6.
7. Waller JM, Maibach HI. Age and skin structure and function, a quantitative approach (II): protein, glycosaminoglycan, water, and lipid content and structure. Skin Res Technol. 2006;12(3):145–54.
8. Raab W. Skin cleansing in health and disease. Wien Med Wschr. 1990;141(108):4–10.
9. Segger D, Abmus U, Brock M, Erasmy J, Finkel P, Fitzner A, Heuss H, Kortemeier U, Munke S, Rheinlander T, et al. Multicenter study on measurement of the natural PH of the skin surface, IFSCC Magazine. 2007;10(2):107–10.
10. Burckhardt W. Beitrage zur Ekzemfrage. II. Die rolle des alkali in Pathogenese des ekzems speziell des Gewerbeekzems. Arch f Dermat U Syph. 1935;173:155–67.
11. Burckhardt W. Beitrage zur Ekzemfrage. III. Die rolle des alkalischadigung der haut bei der experimentellen Sensibilisierung gengen Nickel. Arch f Dermat U Syph. 1935;173:262–6.
12. Burckhardt W. Neure untersuchungen uber die Alkaliempfindlicjkeit der haut. Dermatologica. 1947;94:73–96.
13. Burckhardt W, Baumle W. Die Beziehungen der saurempfindlichkeit zur Alkaliempfindlicjkeit der haut. Dermatologica. 1951;102:294–300.
14. Fore-Pfliger J. The epidermal skin barrier: implications for the wound care practitioner, part I. Adv Skin Wound Care. 2004;17(8):417–25.
15. Zlotogorski A. Distribution of skin surface pH on forehead and cheek of adults. Arch Dermatol Res. 1987;279:398–401.
16. Thune P, Neilsen T, Hnastad IK, et al. The water barrier function of skin in relation to water content of the stratum corneum, pH and skin lipids. Acta Derm Venerol. 1988;68:277–83.
17. Laufer A, Dikstein S. Objective measurement and self-assessment of skin care treatments. Cosmet Toiletires. 1996;111:91–8.
18. Choi EH, Man MQ, Xu P, Xin S, Liu Z, Crumrine DA, Jiang YJ, Fluhr JW, Feingold KR, Elias PM, Mauro TM. Stratum corneum acidification is impaired in moderately aged human and murine skin. J Invest Dermatol. 2007;127(12):2847–56.
19. Fluhr JW, Kao J, Jain M, Ahn SK, Feingold KR, Elias PM. Generation of free fatty acids from phospholipids regulates stratum corneum acidification and integrity. J Invest Dermatol. 2001;117:44–51.
20. Ekholm E, Egelrud T. Expression of stratum corneum chymotryptic enzyme in relation to other markers of epidermal differentiation in a skin explant model. Exp Dermatol. 2000;9:65–70.

21. Leveque JL, Corcuff P, de Rigal J, Agache P. In vivo studies of the evolution of physical properties of the human skin with age. Int J Dermatol. 1984;23(5):322–9.
22. Dunner M. Der Einfluss des Hauttalges auf die Alkaliabwehr der Haut. Dermatologica. 1950;101:17–28.
23. Fishberg E, Bierman W. Acid base balance in sweat. J Biol Chem. 1932;97:433–41.
24. Vermeer D. The effect of sebum on the neutralization of alkali. Dederl Tijdschr V Geneesk. 1950;94:1530–1.
25. McKenna B. The composition of the surface skin fat (Sebum) from the human forearm. J Invest Dermatol. 1950;15:33–7.
26. Vermeer D, Jong J, Lenestra J. The significance of amino acids for the neutralization by the skin. Dermatologica. 1951;103:1–18.
27. Lincke H. Beitrage zur Chemie und Biologie des Hautoberflachenfetts. Arch f Dermat U Syph. 1949;188:453–81.
28. Neuhaus H. Fettehalt und Alkalineutralisationskahigkeit der haut unter Awendung alkalifrier waschmittel. Arch f Dermat U Syph. 1950;190:57–66.
29. Schmidt P. Uber die Beeinflussung der Wasserstoffionenkonzentration der Hautoberflache durch Sauren. Betrachtungen uber die Funktionen des "Sauremantels". Arch f Dermat U Syph. 1941;182:102–26.
30. Vermeer D. Method for determining neutralization of alkali by skin. Quoted in Yearbook: Dermat & Syph. 1951;415.
31. Wohnlich H. Zur Kohlehydratsynthase der Haut. Arch f Derm Syph. 1948;187:53–60.
32. Spier H, Pascher G. Quantitative Untersuchungen uber die freien aminosauren der hautoberflache – Zur frage Ihrer Genese. Klinische Wochenchrift. 1953;31(41–42):997–1000.
33. Piper H. Das Neutralisationsvermogen der haut gegenuber Laugen und seine Beziehung zur Kohlensauteabgabe. Arch f Dermat U Syph. 1943;183:591–647.
34. Szakall A. Uber die physiologie der obersten Hautschichten und ihre Bedeutung fur die Alkaliresistenz. Arbeitsphysiol. 1941;11:436–52.
35. Szakall A. Die Veranderungen der obersten Hautschichten durch den Dauergebrauch einiger Handwaschmittel. Arbeitsphysiol. 1943;13:49–56.
36. Peterson LL, Wuepper KD. Epidermal and hair follicle transglutaminases and crosslinking in skin. Mol Cell Biochem. 1984;58(1–2):99–111.
37. Steinhardt J, Zaiser E. Combination of wool protein with cations and hydroxyl ions. J Biol Chem. 1950;183:789–802.
38. Green M, Behrendt H. Patterns of skin pH from birth to adolescence with a synopsis on skin growth. Springfield: Charles C Thomas; 1971. p. 93–100.
39. Gniadecka M, Nielsen OF, Christensen DH, Wulf HC. Structure of water, proteins, and lipids in intact human skin hair nail. J Invest Dermatol. 1998;110:393–8.
40. Horii I, Kawasaki K, Koyama J, Nakayama Y, Nakajima K, Okazaki K, Seiji M. Histidine-rich protein as a possible origin of free amino acids of stratum corneum. Curr Probl Dermatol. 1983;11:301–15.
41. Jacobson T, Yuksel Y, Geesin JC, Gordon JS, Lane AT, Gracy RW. Effects of aging and xerosis on the amino acid composition of human skin. J Invest Dermatol. 1990;95:296–300.
42. Kurabayahi H, Tamura K, Machida I, Kubota K. Inhibiting bacteria and skin pH in hemiplegia: effects of washing hands with acidic mineral water. Am J Phys Med Rehabil. 2002;81:40–6.
43. Meigel W, Sepehrmanesh M. Untersuchung der pflegenden wirkung und der vertraglichkeit einer crème/loti bei alteren patienten mit trockenem hautzustand. Dtsch Derm. 1994;42:1235–41.
44. Steinhert P, Freedberg I. Molecular and cellular biology of keratins. In: Goldsmith L, editor. Physiology and molecular biology of the skin. 2nd ed. New York: Oxford University Press; 1991. p. 113–14732.
45. Scott IR, Harding CR, Barrett JG. Histidine-rich protein of the keratohyalin granules. Source of the free amino acids, urocanic acid and pyrrolidone carboxylic acid in the stratum corneum. Biochim Biophys Acta. 1982;719(1):110–7.
46. Rogers J, Harding C, Mayo A, Banks J, Rawlings A. Stratum corneum lipids: the effects of ageing and the seasons. Arch Dermatol Res. 1996;288:765–70.
47. Roskos KV. The effect of skin aging on the percutaneous penetration of chemicals through human skin. Dissertation, UCSF, CA. 1989.
48. Saint Leger D, Francois AM, Leveque JL, Stoudemayer TJ, Grove GL, Kligman AM. Age-associated changes in the stratum corneum lipids and their relation to dryness. Dermatologica. 1988;177:159–64.
49. Ghadially R, Brown BE, Sequeria-Martin SM, Feingold KR, Elias PM. The aged epidermal permeability barrier. J Clin Invest. 1995;95:2281–90.
50. Pollack SV. The aging skin. J Fla Med Assoc. 1985;72(4):245–8.
51. Pochi PE, Strauss JS, Downing DT. Age-related changes in sebaceous gland activity. J Invest Dermatol. 1979;73:108–11.
52. Gniadecka M, Nielsen OF, Wessel S, Heidenheim M, Christensen DH, Wulf HC. Water and protein structure in photoaged and chronically skin. J Invest Dermatol. 1998;11:1129–33.
53. Rinnerthaler M, Duschl J, Steinbacher P, Salzmann M, Bischof J, Schuller M, Wimmer H, Peer T, Bauer JW, Richter K. Age Related changes in the composition of the cornified envelope in human skin. Exp Dermatol. 2013;22:329–35.
54. Selmanowitz VJ, et al. Aging of the skin and its appendages. In: Finch C, Hayflick L, editors. Handbook of the biology of aging. New York: van Nostrand Reinhol; 1977. p. 496–509.
55. Ayer J, Maibach HI. Human skin buffering capacity against a reference base sodium hydroxide: in vitro model. Cutan Ocul Toxicol. 2008;27(4):271–81.

56. Zhai H, Chan HP, Farahmand S, Maibach HI. Measuring human skin buffering capacity: an in vitro model. Skin Res Technol. 2009;15(4):470–5.
57. Jacobi O. Uber die Reaktiosfagigkeit und das Neutralisationsvermogen der lebenden menschlichen Haut. Dermat Wchnschr. 1942;115:733–41.
58. Lustig B, Perutz A. Ube rein einfaches Verfahren zur Bestimmung der Wasserstoffionenkonzentration der normalen menschlichen Hautoberflache. Arch f Dermat U Syph. 1930;162:129–34.
59. Zheng Y, Sotoodian B, Lai W, Maibach HI. Buffering capacity of human skin layers: in vitro. Skin Res Technol. 2012;18(1):114–9.

Considerations for Thermal Injury: The Elderly as a Sensitive Population

14

Donald L. Bjerke

Contents

Abstract

As the "baby boom population" in North America ages, one of the populations at greatest risk of thermal injury continues to expand. According to the US Census Bureau in 2000, the population of US citizens who are 75 years and older was 16,548,000 (6.0 %). In 2010 this figure was projected to be 19,101,000 (6.4 %), and by 2050 it is expected to exceed 54, 094,000 (13.4 %) (Lionelli et al., Burns 31:958–963, 2005). In the United States and Canada, 1.25 million people suffer burn injuries annually (Burn Foundation. Burn incidence and treatment in the United States 1999 Fact Sheet. Philadelphia). Populations identified at increased risk of burns include infants and young children, older adults, and people with any type of disability (Redlick et al., Burn Care Rehabil 23:351–356, 2002; Baptiste and Feck, Am J Public Health 70:727–729, 1980; Petro et al., Geriatrics 44(3):25–48, 1989; Stassen et al., Am Surg. 2001;67:704–708). Many of the burns reported are from scalds. Scald injuries are painful, require prolonged treatment, and may result in lifelong scarring and even death. Most burn injuries happen in the home with tap water scalds occurring in the bathroom or kitchen (Redlick et al., Burn Care Rehabil 23:351–356, 2002; American Burn Association (2000) Scalds: a burning issue. A campaign kit for burn awareness week; Bull and Lawrence, Fire Mater 3(2):100–105, 1979). Burns can also be caused by therapies

D.L. Bjerke (✉)
The Procter & Gamble Company, Central Product Safety, Cincinnati, OH, USA
e-mail: bjerke.dl@pg.com

M.A. Farage et al. (eds.), *Textbook of Aging Skin*,
DOI 10.1007/978-3-662-47398-6_16

in medical treatment facilities (Barillo et al., J Burn Care Rehabil 21:269–273, 2000) or from therapeutic use of heat in the home. This premise is supported by a jointly issued public health advisory in 1995 by the United States Food and Drug Administration and the Consumer Products Safety Commission on electric heating pads. This advisory reported approximately 1,600 heating pad burns treated in the emergency room annually and that approximately 45 % of those patients were over 65 years of age (Burlington DB, Brown A (1995) FDA/CPSC public health advisory: hazards associated with the use of electric heating pads. pp 1–3.

Introduction

As the "baby boom population" in North America ages, one of the populations at greatest risk of thermal injury continues to expand. According to the US Census Bureau in 2000, the population of US citizens 75 years and older was 16,548,000 (6.0 %). In 2010 this figure was projected to be 19,101,000 (6.4 %), and by 2050 it is expected to exceed 54, 094,000 (13.4 %) [1]. In the United States and Canada, 1.25 million people suffer burn injuries annually [2]. Populations identified at increased risk of burns include infants and young children, older adults, and people with any type of disability [3–6]. Many of the burns reported are from scalds. Scald injuries are painful, require prolonged treatment, and may result in lifelong scarring and even death. Most burn injuries happen in the home with tap water scalds occurring in the bathroom or kitchen [3, 7, 8]. Burns can also be caused by therapies in medical treatment facilities [9] or from therapeutic use of heat in the home. This premise is supported by a jointly issued public health advisory in 1995 by the United States Food and Drug Administration and the Consumer Products Safety Commission on electric heating pads. This advisory reported approximately 1,600 heating pad burns treated in the emergency room annually and that approximately 45 % of those patients were over 65 years of age [10, 11].

The American Burn Association classifies the severity of a burn based on the total body surface area affected and the depth of the injury (Table 1).

Not only are the elderly at greater risk of thermal injury, the outcome of that injury can be devastating. Elderly subjects have a higher mortality than younger subjects who have a similar surface area burn. For example, if half the body surface is burned in a young adult, the mortality is about 50 %, whereas a burn of only one-fifth of the body surface in the elderly results in a similar mortality [1, 8]. This increased risk in the elderly is due to many factors as a result of both physical and physiologic differences seen in this population. Diminished senses, impaired mental acuity, slower reaction time, reduced mobility, and bedridden states may lead to the decreased ability of the elderly to identify the severity of the situation as well as their capacity to escape from harm. Physiologic factors include thinner skin, reduced microcirculation, increased susceptibility to infections in the elderly, and higher incidence of premorbid conditions such as chronic disease, alcoholism, medications, senility, and neurological or psychiatric disorders [3, 4]. This, in turn, may lead to an increased total body surface area burn, deeper burns, and more devastating consequences from thermal injury. The present chapter

Table 1 Classification of burn injuries

Major burn injuries are second-degree burns over a body surface area (BSA) greater than 25 % in adults or 20 % in children; all third-degree burns over a BSA of 10 % or greater; all burns involving hands, face, eyes, ears, feet, and perineum; all inhalation injuries; electrical burns; complicated burn injuries involving fractures or other major trauma; and burns on all high-risk patients (i.e., those who are elderly or who have debilitating diseases)
Moderate, uncomplicated burn injuries are second-degree burns over a BSA of 15–25 % in adults or 10–20 % in children, third-degree burns over a BSA of 2–10 %, and burns not involving eyes, ears, face hands, feet, or perineum
Minor burn injuries are second-degree burns over a BSA of 15 % or less in adults or 10 % or less in children, third-degree burns over a BSA of less than 2 %, and burns not involving eyes, ears, face, hands, feet, or perineum. Minor burns exclude electrical injuries, inhalation injuries, and burns on all high-risk patients

discusses the conditions by which thermal injury occurs and the physiologic factors associated with an increased risk in the elderly population.

Background Information on Thermal Injury

The first significant research in the area of thermal injury was conducted by Henriques and Moritz at the Harvard Medical School [12–16] in the 1940s. Prior to this work, remarkably little information existed concerning the mechanism by which hyperthermia leads to irreversible cellular injury; the reciprocal relationships of time and temperature in the production of either cutaneous or systemic injury; the relationship between environmental heat, surface temperature, and the slope of the transcutaneous thermal gradient; the pathogenesis of cutaneous burns; or the physiological mechanisms by which external heat may be responsible for acute disability and death. This research provided information on parameters controlling the flow of heat into the skin and the importance of heat capacity and thermal conductivity and developed an approximate first-order Fourier's law equation to describe the transient heat flow. In vivo factors that affect skin temperature include site variations in the respective thickness of epidermis, dermis, fat, and muscle; variation of existing temperature gradients within the skin with respect to time and/or position of site; average rate of blood flow through the various skin layers and variations of the rate of flow with respect to position of site and temperatures within the site; and the appearance of edema fluid in variable quantities. These factors result in site-specific alterations in the density, heat capacity, thickness, and thermal conductivity of the various layers of skin so affected. Using a pig model (skin similar to humans), Henriques and Moritz brought and held constant the skin at various temperatures until the threshold of irreversible injury occurred. From this, they derived the time–temperature relationship in the layer of basal epidermal cells, which are thought to be the most important cell layer for the production of epidermal injury by heat. Cell death (necrosis) is a result of irreversible thermal denaturation of the protein present within the cell [15, 17]. Because second- and third-degree burns involve cell death at the basal epidermal layer, the distance from the surface of the skin to this basal epidermal layer becomes important for the rate of heat transfer. In other words, a thinner epidermis results in more efficient heat transfer from the surface of the skin to the basal epidermal layer, thus increasing the risk of thermal injury. The in vitro work in pigs was extended to in vivo thermal injury in both pigs and humans. Circulating water at various temperatures was brought in contact with skin on the ventral forearms or anterior thoracic region of presumed young healthy military men. Of particular note is that the time–temperature relationship is not linear, and the rate at which burning occurs is almost doubled for each degree rise in temperature between 44 °C and 51 °C. Discomfort in the form of a stinging sensation occurred between 47.5 °C and 48.5 °C and was variable between subjects with respect to intensity. For example, severe burns were sustained without discomfort at 47 °C, while in other cases, intense discomfort was noted before irreversible injury at temperatures in excess of 48 °C. The lowest temperature resulting in cutaneous burning was 44 °C, and the time required to cause irreversible damage to epidermal cells at this temperature was approximately 6 h. Alternatively, a surface temperature of 70 °C resulted in transepidermal necrosis in less than 1 s. The relationship between temperature and duration of exposure to the extent of skin damage was landmark and has served as a guide for all subsequent work.

Wu extended the work of Moritz and Henriques by adding the heat transfer reaction for a source of high energy [17]. His treatment, assuming contact between two semi-infinite bodies of finite thermal inertia at different temperatures, showed that sources of low inertia (e.g., wood, insulation, some plastics) caused a slower rise in skin temperature than a source of high thermal inertia (e.g., steel and aluminum) at the same temperature. This is explained by high thermal inertia materials that can make more energy available at the surface in a given time than those of lesser thermal inertia.

American Society for Testing and Materials (ASTM) published a document entitled *Standard Guide for Heated System Surface Conditions that Produce Contact Burn Injuries* in October 2003 [18]. Included in this guide is a summary of the Moritz and Henriques 1947 research. The review notes that the earlier work neglected the flow of blood to carry heat away and the physiological changes in skin properties as the damaged zone traverses the outer skin layers. Factors that increase the complexity of predicting burns include: (a) site variations with respect to the thickness of different skin layers; (b) variations of initial conditions within the skin with respect to time, position, and physical condition of the subject; (c) the unknown average rate of blood flow through the skin layers and variations within the layers with respect to location and ambient temperatures (warm ambient causes increased flow near surface and cold ambient results in less flow near surface); and (d) the appearance of watery fluids in variable quantities upon exposure that result in alterations of skin density, heat capacity, thickness, and thermal conductivity. The guide is meant to serve as an estimation of the exposure to which an average individual might be subjected and does not assume to be inclusive of unusual conditions of exposure, physical health variations, or nonstandard ambient condition. The guide applies to contact with heated surfaces only. Importantly, Fig. 1 demonstrates the relationship between skin temperature and time as it relates to thermal injury. The following equations were developed and are reported in the document:

$$T_A = 15.0005 + 0.51907 \times Ln(\text{time} \times 1{,}000) + 352.97/(Ln(\text{time} \times 1{,}000))$$

$$T_B = 39.468 - 0.41352 \times Ln(\text{time} \times 1{,}000) + 190.06/(Ln(\text{time} \times 1{,}000))$$

where

T_A = critical contact temperature for complete transepidermal necrosis, °C
T_B = critical contact temperature for reversible epidermal injury, °C
time = elapsed contact time, s
Ln = natural logarithm

Exposures below the lower curve should not produce permanent injury in normal humans. Exposure between the curves is described as second-degree burns and has intermediate levels

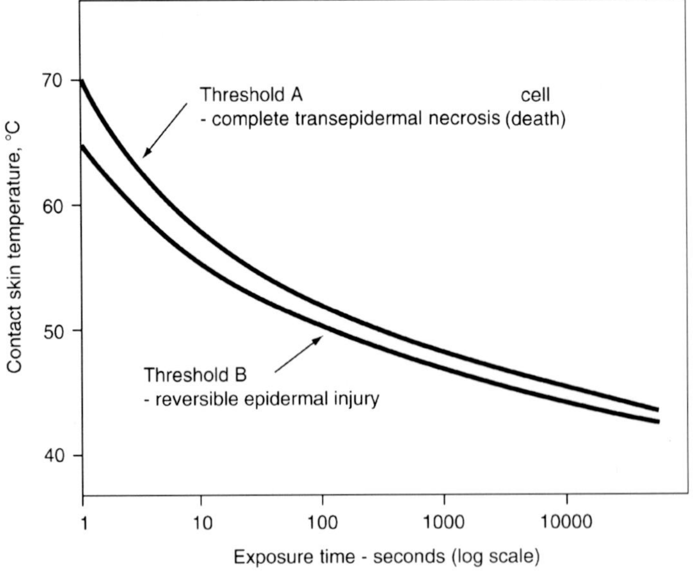

Fig. 1 Temperature-time relationship for burns (From ASTM C 1055-03 [18]. Published October 2003. Copyright ASTM International. Reprinted with permission from ASTM)

of cell damage. Exposures at levels above the top line are defined as third-degree burns that cause deep, permanent cell damage and scarring.

Reported Burn Injuries in the Elderly

Barillo investigated burn injuries in medical treatment facilities [10]. The medical records of 4,510 consecutive admissions to one burn center were reviewed, and a cohort of 54 patients was burned as a result of medical therapy. A number of burns in the home resulted from therapeutic applications of heat, including six patients burned by heating pads, one patient burned by a heat lamp, and four patients burned by contact with hot water bottles or soaks. The average hospital stay for burns resulting from medical therapy (22.9 days) was excessive in comparison to the average total burn size of 3.0 % total body surface area (TBSA). In addition to medical therapies, there were two patients, including one fatality, that were scalded while being bathed in nursing homes. The total body surface area burned by the scalding water was 20.3 % with third-degree burns on 3 % of the body. Contributing factors to thermal injury were advanced age, chronic illness, limited mobility, and altered skin sensation.

More recently, Ghods and colleagues published the results of a survey of 36 burn clinics in Germany with regard to hot air sauna burns [19]. In total, 14 patients were treated in the German burn units between 1999 and 2005 and an additional 2 patients in the author's clinic. Of note, the average age of the individuals was 67 years, and the time spent in the sauna was between 45 and 60 min. In all cases, unconsciousness occurred and was assumed to be a result of orthostatic dysregulation. Deep second- and third-degree burns of the highest-exposed body parts were found in all cases (an average of 14 % TBSA). In two cases, the involved lower extremities had to be amputated; in four cases, primary amputations of toes or fingers were necessary, and four patients died because of multiple system organ failure. Normally, exposure to temperatures up to 120 °C in dry, hot air does not cause damage to the skin because of the low thermal capacity of the air. In the cases presented by the Ghods report, a hypothesis was developed to support a theory for "apex burns." Unconsciousness leads to a declension of the perfusion of the skin with degraded cardiac achievement and low blood pressure. This effect, in turn, results in insufficient cooling of the skin. These two reports clearly demonstrate that conditions that normally do not cause harm in a young healthy population can result in significant thermal injury to older individuals, especially when there are other concomitant factors involved.

Because of the medical significance of burns in the elderly, one encouraging trend is the shift from burn treatment to burn prevention. Behavioral changes include testing water temperature before taking a bath or shower, avoidance of wearing loose sleeves while cooking, having carbon monoxide detectors that are tested regularly, and having smoke detectors that are tested regularly [3]. Additional work by Redlick and colleagues has targeted different mass media channels to promote campaigns targeted at the prevention of burns in the elderly. This groundbreaking work by the Ross Tilley Burn Centre in Toronto along with the Sunnybrook and Women's College Health Sciences Centre and the Toronto Western Hospital has led to an effective burn prevention campaign for older adults [20]. Incorporated into the prevention campaign were previous success stories for lowering hot water heater settings [21] and preventing cigarette burns and contact burns with household radiator heaters [22]. While the campaign was effective at improving burn prevention knowledge, whether this results in a change in burn prevention behavior remains unclear.

Risk Factors for Thermal Injury

It is well accepted that elderly individuals are at greater risk of thermal injury. Physiological factors that contribute to an increased risk include the thinning of the skin, a compromised ability to dilate the vasculature of the skin, and a reduced thermal sensitivity with advancing age. The significance of these changes is that older adults have thinner skin than their younger counterparts, so contact with a hot surface or liquid can cause deeper burns with even brief exposure. To maintain a safe skin temperature upon thermal challenge, the body mobilizes the blood circulation to the periphery to "wick away" the heat by acting as a convective heat exchanger [23]. With aging comes a reduction in the ability to mobilize the circulation to the periphery. In addition, the compromised ability to feel heat may be decreased with aging due to certain medical conditions or medications so the elderly may not realize the thermal insult (e.g., scalding bath or kitchen water) is too hot until injury has occurred. Physical conditions may also contribute to the increased risk of thermal injury. Some older adults have conditions that make them more prone to falls in the bathtub or shower or while carrying hot liquids [8]. The physical factors related to thermal injury are outside the scope of the present chapter. The sections that follow will describe in more detail the literature regarding thinning of skin, compromised microcirculation, and reduced thermal sensitivity that accompany aging.

Thinning Skin

The skin undergoes several structural and functional changes with advancing age. With regard to thermal injury, the significance of the thinning of the skin is that heat applied to the surface can more easily be conducted to the basal layer of the epidermis and beyond because it has less distance to penetrate. Thus, the depth of the thermal injury can be greater in the elderly than in younger individuals exposed to the same temperature. While the thinning of the skin with age has been characterized, there remains an opportunity to examine the effects of changes in skin composition that occur with increasing age in relation to thermal capacity, density, and thermal conductance. In addition, elderly skin is also more prone to blistering from mechanical sheer force, and while controversial, this effect may be exacerbated by thermal challenges.

The process of aging skin is often divided into two components: intrinsic aging which is genetically determined and extrinsic aging which is associated with cumulative damage by UV exposure. Extrinsic aging associated with excess exposure to ultraviolet light is characterized by loss of elasticity, increased roughness and dryness, irregular pigmentation, and deep wrinkling. The epidermis may thin in response to atrophy and may be accompanied with changes in the proportion and/or functionality of the dermal extracellular components [24]. Although there are differences in intrinsic and extrinsic skin aging, it is becoming evident that there are many consistent changes at the molecular level. Changes seen with intrinsic aging such as decreased cellular lifespan, reduced response to growth factors, disruption of matrix synthesis, and elevation of proteolytic activity are all evident in photodamaged skin. The changes are simply more pronounced [24].

Montagna and Carlisle describe aging skin with the undersurface of the epidermis becoming flattened, with little apparent change to the epidermis except for minor alterations in the organization of its cells [25]. The dermis undergoes greater changes with aging as it diminishes in bulk, many of its collagenous elastic fibers are gradually dissolved by enzymes, and the layer of fat becomes thinner. There appears to be a steady decline in the number of fibroblasts and mast cells with advancing age. The upper dermis contains collagenous fiber bundles that are somewhat haphazardly arranged.

Cerimele describes the accompanying physiological changes that occur in aging skin [26]. These include impairment of barrier function, decreased turnover of epidermal cells, reduced keratinocytes and fibroblasts, and a reduced vascular network particularly around hair bulbs and glands. These changes result in fibrosis and atrophy and decreases in hair and nail growth, vitamin D synthesis, and the density of Langerhans cells. Reductions in the immune response and decreased functioning of Meissner's and Pacinian corpuscles are noted. Histological alterations of the microvasculature, including thickening of the basement membrane in the exposed areas of alterations in the veil cells in protected zones, combined with the general reduction in vasculature, are probably responsible for the gradual atrophy of the cutaneous appendages that occurs with time. All of these normal changes with aging impact on the risk of thermal injury [26]. There is also a reduction in the number and biosynthetic capacity of fibroblasts and progressive disappearance of elastic tissue in the papillary dermis. Skin collagen content decreases with age and the fine collagen fibers associated with infancy become increasingly dense and tightly packed and far more randomly oriented [24].

Martin conducted a comprehensive cadaver study of body composition with 13 un-embalmed cadavers aged 59–86 years (six males and seven females) [27]. Measurements were made at 12 sites bilaterally and one central site (abdomen). Skin thickness was measured to a precision of 0.05 mm. Skin thickness varied by subject and site with males having thicker skin than females at all individual sites and overall (1.19 mm compared to 0.96 mm). The mean of all 25 sites ranged from 0.81 to 1.43 mm in males and from 0.73 to 1.10 mm in females. The thinnest site was the bicep (0.76 mm in men and 0.49 mm in women). The thickest skin site was at the subscapular site (2.07 mm in men and 1.76 mm in women). The other body sites measured were triceps, forearm, chest, waist, supraspinal, abdominal, front thigh, medial thigh, rear thigh, patellar, and medial calf. Of note, this study determined the entire skin thickness and concluded that skin likely thins with age.

Moragas and colleagues studied abdominal skin samples from 96 autopsy cases ranging in age from 3.5 months to 86 years [28]. Abdominal skin was chosen as shielded from photoaging and thus, the changes are attributed to intrinsic aging only. Samples, 35 mm by 15 mm, were fixed in 10 % buffered formalin, subsampled and embedded in paraffin wax. Sections 4-μm thick were stained with hematoxylin and eosin. Four characteristics were evaluated in each case. Three were denoted by linear roughness indices: progressive flattening of the epidermal undersurface related to the rete peg profile, effect of shrinkage on the basal layer, and waviness of the interface between the granular and corneum layers due to shrinkage. The fourth variable corresponded to epidermal thickness in micrometers, measured in zones between the rete pegs. When looking at the extreme age groups (0–20 years and 80–100 years), elderly subjects had a 36 % reduction in the roughness index as related to the rete peg profile as compared with younger subjects. In the elderly the epidermis was 49.5 % thinner than in younger individuals. The decreases in shrinkage indices (basal layer and waviness of the interface between the granular and corneum layers) were 6 % and 22 %, respectively. The average epidermal thickness for age groups 0–20, 41–60, and 81–90 were 22.6, 17.9, and 11.4 μm respectively. The reduction in epidermal thickness was not influenced significantly by gender [28].

The progressive decrease in mechanical resistance explains why elderly people complain that they are prone to shear-type skin injuries or show increased blistering [26]. The epidermis makes a major contribution to these changes. The two most striking epidermal features associated with aging are dermoepidermal junction flattening, with effacement of the so-called rete ridges, and epidermal thinning [24, 28]. Epidermal tissue repair also declines with age, whether measured in terms of wound closure time or blister roof regeneration. The flattening of the dermoepidermal junction in the elderly may result in greater separation of the layers and blistering in response to shear force as compared to younger individuals. The effect of heat on pressure ulcers was investigated by Kokate and colleagues [29] in a swine model (considered to have skin similar to humans). Higher skin temperature causes an increase in tissue metabolism and oxygen consumption (about 10 % for a 1 °C rise). The heightened need for nutrients and oxygen cannot be fulfilled because of tissue compression resulting in ischemia and tissue damage. Kokate applied 100 mmHg of pressure and temperatures of 25, 35, 40, and 45 °C for 5 h in the swine model. This model produced both pressure ulcers and injuries consistent with burns. At 35 °C there was deep tissue damage (i.e., pressure damage), while 40 °C resulted in both dermal and deep tissue damage, and 45 °C caused full-thickness cutaneous and deep tissue injuries. In contrast, 25 °C resulted in the absence of damage and was considered protective of pressure ulcers. Thus, the interplay of pressure and temperature should be considered in elderly individuals who develop injuries consistent with pressure ulcers and/or thermal injury, especially in areas of bony prominences.

Decreased Ability for Peripheral Vasodilatation

With advancing age, structural and functional changes take place in the peripheral blood vessels that result in a reduced ability to mobilize blood to the cutaneous vessels when challenged with a heat stimulus. Without the optimal convective heat exchange capacity, the skin temperature can rise more rapidly and thus shorten the time to a skin burn relative to younger individuals. This section will describe the structural and functional changes to the peripheral vasculature with age and the impact on maintaining skin temperature. In addition, studies using pharmacological actives affecting vascular tone to better understand the mechanism by which aging affects peripheral vasodilation in response to thermal stimuli will be presented. These studies will demonstrate that resting blood flow and vascular conductance decrease with age due to increased sympathetic nerve activity, but during exertional heat stress, the diminished blood flow is independent of sympathetic vasoconstriction. With advancing age, there is a decreased nitric oxide-mediated vasodilation and a decreased response to histamine. Thus, the reduced ability to increase blood flow to the peripheral dermal vasculature is multifactorial with effects on structure and function.

Histological changes in cutaneous microvessels with age were investigated by Braverman and by Gunin [30, 31]. The veil cells around normal, diabetic, and aged vessels were reconstructed in three dimensions by a computer graphics system from 120 to 140 serial ultrathin sections. While there did not appear to be any differences in the metabolic capability of the veil cells in the different groups, there were structural differences. The normal vessel was surrounded by a single layer of veil cells which had a wrinkled and pleated surface. The veil cells around aged vessels appeared to have the same length as young veil cells but were underdeveloped in their lateral extensions so that they did not cover the vessel circumferentially as well as the normal veil cells did. In addition, there is an age-related decrease in the number of dermal blood vessels [30, 31, 32].

Moritz and Henriques [13] were two of the first to investigate the importance of blood flow with regard to the protection of the epidermis from reversible injury. Using a pig model, and applying a constant flow of water at 49 °C and 51 °C for durations subthreshold to injury, increasing the pressure from 0 to 80 mmHg (thought to compress the most distal blood vessels) did not result in irreversible transepidermal injury. Thus, the thinness of the epidermis was considered more important than the protective effect of removing heat via the blood circulation. These early conclusions later came under scrutiny. The ASTM review notes that the increased pressure in the Moritz and Henriques study was not sufficient to collapse the blood vessels [18].

The impact of vasodilatation on protecting the surface skin temperature was subsequently demonstrated by Lipkin and Hardy [33] on the human forearm. These authors evaluated thermal inertia, which is a product of thermal conductivity, density, and thermal capacity. They noted that as heating of intact skin progressed, the influence of the increased blood flow became more pronounced, finally causing a decrease in skin temperature in spite of continued irradiation. This phenomenon did not occur when blood flow was occluded as skin temperature continued to increase. Therefore, the values of thermal conductivity, density, and thermal capacity for living skin are not constant and will depend upon blood flow, thickness of the stratum corneum, and possibly upon the state of hydration.

To investigate the effects of age on the response of skin blood flow in the forearm to direct heat [34], 3 groups with 20 male subjects each – young (20–39 years), middle-aged (40–59 years), and older (60–79 years) – had their blood flow measured by laser Doppler flowmeter. The forearm was in a water bath at 30 °C that was elevated to 35 °C and then 40 °C. The older group demonstrated a significantly lower volume in response to 35 °C and 40 °C, and there was a significant reduction in blood flow for both middle-aged and older men at 40 °C. Thus, aging decreases the response of cutaneous blood flow in the forearm to the direct effects of heat. The reduced blood flow suggests that this is mediated by a reduced flow response of individual microvessels in middle-aged and older men. The reduced blood volume data suggests that, in addition, vessel recruitment is depressed in older individuals.

To understand the underlying physiological changes to the peripheral vasculature that occur with aging, several authors have used pharmacologic tools to investigate the sympathetic and parasympathetic nervous system. Dinenno [35] examined hemodynamic changes related to aging. Resting-limb blood flow and vascular conductance are reduced with age in adult humans, and these changes are related to elevations in sympathetic vasoconstrictor nerve activity and reduction in limb oxygen demands. Sixteen young males (28 ± 1 years; mean ± SEM) and 15 older males (63 ± 1 years) were compared for femoral artery blood flow (Doppler ultrasound), vascular conductance, femoral artery resistance, and muscle sympathetic activity. Whole-limb blood flow represents the sum of flow to skeletal muscle, skin, subcutaneous tissue, and bone. The flow to the subcutaneous tissue and bone is thought to be negligible at rest. Data on young adult humans in which relative measurements of whole-forearm blood flow were performed before and after skin flow was abolished with epinephrine iontophoresis suggest that skin blood flow represents 30–35 % of the total flow under these conditions [36]. Femoral artery blood flow was 26 % lower in the older men, despite similar levels of cardiac output. Femoral artery vascular conductance (femoral blood flow/mean arterial pressure) was 32 % lower and femoral vascular resistance (mean arterial pressure/femoral blood flow) was 45 % higher in older men. Muscle sympathetic nerve activity was 74 % higher in the older men and correlated with femoral artery blood flow, vascular conductance, and vascular resistance. Thus, basal whole-leg arterial blood flow and vascular conductance are reduced with age in healthy adult men under resting conditions; these changes are associated with elevations in sympathetic vasoconstrictor nerve activity; and the lower whole-limb blood flow is related to a lower oxygen demand that is independent of tissue mass. The authors raise other possibilities for the findings, including a reduced bioavailability of nitric oxide with age or elevations in locally released (e.g., endothelin) or systemically circulating (e.g., vasopressin) levels of vasoconstrictor agents that may have played a role. While the reduction in whole-limb blood flow of older adults at rest is thought primarily to involve differences in skeletal muscle blood flow, it raises the question as to how well skin blood flow can respond in terms of a thermal challenge. Evidence is accumulating that older adults are limited in their capacity to augment blood flow and vascular conductance in response to acute increases in functional demand imposed by large-muscle dynamic exercise, energy intake, and ambient heat stress [37].

Kenney tested the hypothesis that an attenuated increase in cutaneous vascular conductance in elderly in response to local or reflex-mediated heat stress is due to an augmented or sustained noradrenergic vasoconstriction [38]. Forearm skin perfusion was measured by laser Doppler flowmetry in 15 young (22 + 1 year) and 15 older (66 + 1 years) men who exercised at 50 % peak oxygen uptake in a 36-°C environment. Blood flow was monitored in two sites, one of which it was pretreated with bretylium tosylate (BT) to block the local release of norepinephrine and thus vasoconstriction. Forearm vascular conductance was 40–50 % lower in the older adults. Decreased active vasodilator sensitivity to increasing core temperature, coupled with structural limitations to vasodilation, appears to limit the cutaneous vascular response to exertional heat stress in older subjects. At rest in a thermoneutral environment, human cutaneous vascular conductance is under the tonic influence of noradrenergic vasoconstrictor activity. During dynamic exercise in a warm environment, during which cutaneous vascular conductance can increase more than tenfold, vasoconstriction is withdrawn and the active vasodilator system is activated. For a given mean arterial pressure, under any given set of exercise and environmental conditions, the balance between vasoconstriction and vasodilation activity determines cutaneous vascular conductance. The conclusions of the study were that the diminished cutaneous vascular response in the skin of older subjects during exertional heat stress occurred independent of noradrenergic vasoconstriction. The mechanistic alterations that could explain this diminished vascular response were: (a) a relatively greater vasoconstrictor activity, (b) decreased vasodilator activity, or (c) end-organ response differences, which could be independent of efferent neural activity. The study of Kenney eliminates the first possibility and suggests that a combination of the latter two may be involved [38].

Minson extended the work on the effects of aging on the cutaneous microvasculature by investigating the role of nitric oxide (NO) and the axon reflexes in the skin blood flow response to local heating with advanced age [39]. Two microdialysis fibers were placed in the forearm skin of ten young (22 ± 2 years) and ten older (77 ± 5 years) men and women. Skin blood flow was measured by laser Doppler flowmeter. Both sites were heated to 42 °C for ~60 min while 10 mM N^G-nitro-$_L$-arginine methyl ester ($_L$-NAME) was infused throughout the protocol to inhibit NO synthase (NOS) in one site and 10 mM $_L$-NAME was infused after 40 min of local heating in the second site. Local heating before $_L$-NAME infusion resulted in a significantly reduced initial peak and plateau maximum vasodilation in elderly subjects. This finding suggests that healthy aging impacts the nerves that mediate the axon reflex or vascular responsiveness to the neurotransmitters released from these nerves. When NOS was inhibited after 40 min of heating, vasodilation declined to the same value in the young and older subjects. The initial peak response was significantly lower in the older subjects in both microdialysis sites. These data suggest that age-related changes in both axon reflex-mediated and NO-mediated vasodilation contribute to attenuated cutaneous vasodilator responses in the elderly. This work is supported by Bruning et al. [40] who noted that the production of NO during local heating and cutaneous vasodilation is attenuated even in middle-aged skin [40]. A diminished ability to rapidly increase skin blood flow in response to directly applied heat may make the elderly more susceptible to local tissue damage.

Research by Tur has demonstrated age-related differences in skin blood flow in response to histamine administration [41]. In this study, the cutaneous microvascular response of older individuals (64–74 years) as compared to younger individuals (25–35 years) was slower to peak blood flow and took longer to decay. There were also regional differences such that peak blood flow was greater in the back of the young as compared to the forearm, while both sites were similar in the older cohort.

While heat challenge should produce a vasodilatory response, Khan and others investigated the effect of aging on the vasculature during a cooling challenge and concluded that elderly subjects have diminished sympathetic vasoconstrictor responses [42–44]. This may be a significant factor contributing to thermoregulatory impairment in the elderly, thereby rendering them more susceptible to the harmful effects of cold weather. Using laser Doppler flowmetry sympathetic vascular responses in fingertip skin was evaluated. Indirect body heating was employed to minimize variability. The change in fingertip blood flow produced by inspiratory gasp and contralateral arm cold challenge was determined. The normal response is a rapid vasoconstriction with a subsequent decrease in fingertip blood flow which returns to its pre-stimulus value. The study evaluated 28 elderly (mean age 68 years with SD of 4 years) and 20 younger subjects (mean age 26 years with SD of 5 years). Experiments were conducted in a room set at 25 °C (55 % relative humidity), and the subject's right arm was placed up to the elbow in a water bath maintained at 43 °C. The increase in blood flow is directed mainly through arteriovenous anastomoses, but capillary blood flow also increases, owing to raised local tissue temperature as a consequence of high shunt flow. The inspiratory gasp consisted of a sudden deep breath with the right arm in 43 °C water throughout followed by a transfer of the right arm into a cold water bath at 15 °C. A second experiment took place where subject bodies were placed in a temperature-controlled chamber in a 25 °C room. The chamber was heated to 40 °C to induce central dilation. The chamber was subsequently cooled to 12 °C, which took approximately 10 min and was maintained for another 20 min. The time for blood flow to fall to 75 %, 50 %, and 25 % from steady-state flow was determined. Vasoconstrictor responses were significantly reduced in the elderly group in response to inspiratory gasp and cold challenge, although individual responses varied from normal to absent. The authors concluded that there is a 65 % probability that an otherwise normal elderly person will have a vasoconstrictor response considered abnormal for healthy young subjects. Whole-body cooling yielded similar results in that some elderly subjects demonstrated rapid vasoconstriction, whereas others responded with poor vasoconstrictor ability. Time to minimum blood flow after vasoconstriction was longer in the elderly, but only the time to 25 % blood flow was statistically significant. While specific details on the location and nature of the effect are not clear, diminished vasoconstrictor responses most likely also result from general changes in sympathetic nervous function with age, since fingertip vasoconstriction produced by inspiratory gasp and cold challenge is dependent upon sympathetic nervous activity. There was wide variability among elderly subjects in their response. The authors did not comment on the changes in blood flow with regard to heat challenge. The significance of the findings is that since thermal equilibrium is protected by reflex adjustments of cutaneous blood flow in the extremities, diminished vasoconstrictor response would promote significant heat loss in the elderly during cold exposure. The reduced vasoconstrictor response most probably occurs in the thermoregulatory shunts because a major proportion of the laser Doppler finger blood flow signal arise from flow through arteriovenous anastomoses.

Effects of Aging on Thermoregulation

While increased morbidity and mortality in the elderly population during heat waves have been well documented in several medical reports, relatively few scientific studies have focused on the physiological basis of the aging process in thermoregulation and those that have produced conflicting results. This section examines research on the effects of age on thermal regulation during exertion or exposure to increased ambient temperatures.

Changes in the basic physiological mechanisms of thermoregulation may contribute to a decreased ability to avoid hyperthermia in the elderly. These changes may involve the ability to sweat and the vasomotor response to heat and could result from structural changes in the skin as well as less effective neural regulation of blood flow and sweating. Weiss in 1992 examined the capillary blood flow velocity in the feet of ten young (ages 28–43) and 12 elderly (ages 72–84) men at skin temperatures of 32 °C and 44 °C [45]. The mean peak capillary blood flow in the elderly (102 mV measured by laser Doppler flowmetry) was lower than in the young population (163 mV). Considering that the magnitude, but not the pattern of skin perfusion, varied between the groups, the authors concluded that aging is associated with the loss of capillary plexus functional units, and therefore, skin perfusion is lower in aged people [45].

Martin measured the maximal forearm skin vasodilatory capacity across a group of 74 subjects ranging in age from 5 to 85 years [46]. Maximal forearm skin vascular conductance was the end point of choice and represents the maximum forearm skin blood flow divided by the mean arterial blood pressure. The results demonstrated a progressive decrease in maximum forearm skin vascular conductance with age from young adulthood through old age. The authors note substantial histological and scanning electron micrographic evidence in the underside of the epidermis including the collapse, disorganization, and even total disappearance of vessels comprising the microcirculation. Others report a decrease in the number of superficial capillary loops in the skin as it ages.

Table 2 Effect of heat exposure (40 °C and 40 % relative humidity) on select hemodynamic parameters from Sagawa et al. [48] study

Age group	Control	Onset of sweating	At 95 min
Forearm blood flow (ml/100 ml/min)			
Elderly	1.3 ± 0.2	6.0 ± 1.7	4.6 ± 0.7
Young	2.6 ± 0.4*	7.2 ± 0.9	8.7 ± 1.4*
Forearm vascular conductance (ml/100 ml/min/Torr X 100)			
Elderly	1.3 ± 0.2	7.2 ± 2.4	5.2 ± 0.7
Young	3.0 ± 0.5*	9.3 ± 1.0*	12.2 ± 1.9*

*Significant difference between age groups ($p < 0.05$)

Such changes are consistent with the attenuated maximal skin blood flow response in older adults. However, a reduced blood flow to existing vessels cannot be ruled out as well [47].

To evaluate the effect of age on thermoregulation, Sagawa exposed six older (61–73 years of age) and ten younger (21–39 years of age) Japanese men to 40 °C and 40 % relative humidity (while sitting) for up to 130 min and examined sweat responses, esophageal and skin temperatures, non-evaporative heat exchange, heart rate, cardiac output, blood pressure, forearm blood flow, and metabolic heat production [48]. There was no significant difference in sweat rate or in onset of sweating between the groups (Table 2). Changes in skin temperature, non-evaporative heat exchange, metabolic heat production, heart rate, and cardiac output were the same during heat exposure in both groups. However, forearm blood flow before and after exposure to heat was significantly lower in the elderly group. These data suggest that the greater health risk posed to resting, yet healthy, aged men by hot environments is not a consequence of inadequate sweating but could be associated with retardation of the cutaneous vasodilatation reflex, which can prevent effective transfer of the body heat to its shell, thus resulting in greater heat storage. The impairment of vasomotor function in aged persons is not related to inadequate cardiac response but is perhaps associated with insufficient vasoconstriction of the blood supply to the viscera, resulting in less blood being shunted to the skin. This suggestion is probable because, in old age, the responsiveness of the circulatory system to adrenergic nerve control is known to decrease [49]. Therefore, in elderly individuals, a decreased response to beta stimulation could explain the impaired vasodilatory responses, and a lowered response to alpha stimulation could be the underlying mechanism for diminished vasoconstriction in the viscera.

The effects of age and acclimation on responses to passive heat were studied by Armstrong and Kenney [50]. Six older men (61 ± 1 year) were compared to six young (26 ± 2 years) men in an environmental chamber during a systematic increase in dry-bulb temperature from 28 to 46 °C followed by 30 min in a constant 46 °C environment. If older and younger subjects are matched for VO_2 max, anthropometry (height, weight, and surface area-to-mass ratio), and body composition (skinfold thickness and adiposity), no temperature differences are seen during a passive thermal stress of this magnitude. The authors note that previous studies concluded that older subjects respond to passive heat stress with greater elevations in core temperature than young subjects of the same gender, although this is not a universal finding. Much of the discrepancy can be attributed to subject selection criteria, i.e., such factors as body surface area-to-mass ratio, adiposity, and especially VO_2 max.

The control of heat-induced cutaneous vasodilatation in relation to age was determined in subjects 55–68 years of age as compared to subjects 19–30 years of age [51]. Subjects performed 75-min cycle exercises in a hot environment (37 °C, 60 % relative humidity). Core body temperature and skin temperature rose to the same level in both groups, and there were no differences in the rate of sweating. However, older subjects responded with lower arm blood flow by about 40 % as compared to the younger counterparts.

These results suggest an altered control of skin vasodilatation during exercise in the heat in older individuals. Havenith extended this work by examining the relative influence of age (ranging from 20 to 73 years of age) on cardiovascular and thermoregulatory responses to low intensity cycle exercise (60 W for 1 h) in a warm humid environment (35 °C, 80 % relative humidity) [52]. The results suggest that age is an important contributory factor in cardiovascular effector responses to a humid heat stress test, in particular, for heart rate and skin blood flow (forearm blood flow and forearm vascular resistance), both lower with advancing age. Again, there were no age-related effects on sweating rate. In the warm humid climate chosen for the experiment, in which both dry and evaporative heat loss are minimal, the effect of a reduced skin blood flow on core temperature is likewise minimal. During exercise in warm environments, as core temperature rises, skin blood flow increases to facilitate the convective transfer of heat from core to skin. Both the slope of the skin blood flow–core temperature relationship and the steady-state skin blood flow achieved are attenuated in older subjects. It has been hypothesized that this decreased cutaneous vasodilatory response with aging is due to structural changes in the cutaneous vasculature [27].

Rooke examined the maximum blood flow in elderly men and noted that blood flow does not increase as much when participants were subjected to total body heating and exercise as compared to younger adults [53]. Local heating of the forearm of seven young men (average age 31 years) and seven elderly men (average age 71 years) showed differences between the two age groups. Skin temperature was raised from 32–35 to 42 °C for 60 min. At baseline, skin blood flow in the two age groups (26–37 years and 66–82 years of age) was comparable. During the last 10 min of heating, blood flows as measured by venous plethysmography were much lower in the elderly than in the young subjects (11.1 ± 2.7 vs. 19.9 ± 5.2 ml • min^{-1} • 100 ml^{-1}, respectively). Thus, aging results in a reduction of the maximal conductance of the cutaneous vasculature. The authors suggest that the major limitation of skin blood flow in the elderly is intrinsic to the structure and function of the skin and not due to autonomic dysfunction. Changes in the number, size, and tortuosity of blood vessels in aged skin could be the cause of limited skin blood flow in the elderly. With age, the dermal thickness decreases by 20 % and becomes relatively avascular. The implications are that the elderly appear to be less effective at maintaining normal body temperature than young adults. This applies to both cold exposure and heat exposure, as suggested by a disproportionately high occurrence of hypothermia and heat stroke in the elderly.

Decreased Ability to Feel Heat

Insensate skin and chronic illness such as diabetes mellitus are common risk factors in patients burned by therapeutic heat application [10]. The scald potential from hydrotherapy in patients with diabetic or other neuropathy is well documented [54, 55]. A second group at risk is patients requiring cutaneous, fasciocutaneous, or myocutaneous flap procedures for surgical reconstruction. Transposed flap tissue may be insensate and may also have compromised circulation, which interferes with heat dispersal [56]. Burns have been accidentally produced in anesthetized, unconscious, or immobilized patients by the use of hydrotherapy, heating blankets, hot water bottles, or other warming devices both within the hospital and in the field by emergency medical services. Similarly, the elderly have been identified as a population at greater risk of thermal injury secondary to decreased sensory perception and having a higher threshold for pain [26, 57–61]. This demonstrates the importance of the ability to sense noxious thermal stimuli so as to remove one's self from the burn hazard before extensive damage occurs.

Pacinian and Meissner's corpuscles, which are responsible for pressure and superficial tactile perception, respectively, undergo progressive disorganization and histological degeneration, possibly accompanied by functional loss, with advancing age. Free nerve endings do not seem to be substantially modified. While Buettner [62] reports on the effects of radiant and direct contact heat being similar with a pain threshold at 44.8 °C, this work was done with a small group ($N = 5$) presumably in the general population. Lautenbacher and Strian [63] studied the thresholds for heat pain in 64 healthy persons from 17 to 63 years of age (32 women and 32 men). The stimuli were applied to the thenar and the dorsum pedis with a contact thermode. The thresholds increased significantly with age for the foot, but not the hand. The length of the afferent pathways seems to influence the degree of age-related changes both in heat-pain perception and in thermal sensitivity, resulting in a distal–proximal pattern of age-dependent decline (Table 3).

While the pain threshold for the hand did not show statistical significance with regard to age, there was a positive trend for an elevation in pain threshold with advancing age. Estimated threshold elevations (based on quadratic regression curves) between 15 and 65 years of age are 0.6 °C on the hand and 2.2 °C on the foot. The threshold for determining warmth and coolness on the foot (but not hand) increased significantly with advancing age. The authors note that it is unlikely that the findings of reduced heat pain and thermal sensitivity on the foot are produced only by age changes of the skin: the free nerve endings of the nociceptive and thermoceptive afferents are mainly located near the epidermal–dermal junction. The flattening of the junction and the thinning of the epidermis and dermis with increasing age may indeed result in more frequent damage to the free nerve endings but also in a decrease in the thermal resistance, which would tend to appear as heightened sensitivity.

Chakour investigated the effects of age on pain perception mediated by Aδ-fibers and C-fibers [64]. During pre- and post-nerve block periods, older adults (over 65 years of age) exhibited a significant elevation in thermal pain threshold relative to younger adults (20–40 years of age) in response to a noxious CO_2 laser thermal stimulus. However, when Aδ-fiber function was impaired and only C-fiber information was available, both groups responded similarly. These findings support the notion of a differential age-related change in Aδ-fiber-mediated epicritic pain (phasic pain, sharp and pricking in nature) perception versus C-fiber-mediated protopathic pain (tonic pain, dull, burning, or aching in nature) with older adults having an increased thermal pain threshold (i.e., decreased pain sensitivity) as compared to younger adults. The magnitude of loss in sensitivity to mechanical stimuli is greater than to thermal stimulation, and several authors have suggested that myelinated fiber function may be more prone to the effects of advancing age.

Kenshalo investigated absolute thresholds for six modes of cutaneous stimulation applied to two sites in 27 young (ages 19–31) and elderly (ages 55–84) humans at the thenar eminence (hand) and the plantar foot [65]. The modes were tactile, vibration at 40 and 250 Hz, temperature increases or decreases, and noxious heat (via conductive heat application). For heat-pain threshold, the temperature applied was 40 °C and increased at a rate of 0.3 °C per second until the participant pushed a spring loaded button signifying the detection of heat pain. In this study, no statistically significant differences were found between the hands or feet of the young (mean 44.60 °C and 46.46 °C) and elderly (mean 44.95 °C and 46.69 °C), respectively, in their sensitivity to heat-pain stimulation. In both populations, the hands were more sensitive to a noxious heat stimulus than the

Table 3 Thresholds for detecting cool, warm, and heat pain when the stimulus is applied to the hand or foot of subjects 17–63 years of age, as reported by Lautenbacher and Strin [63]

Modality	Site	Age 17–29 years	Age 30–44 years	Age 45–63 years
Cool	Hand	0.8 ± 0.3 °C	1.0 ± 0.4 °C	0.9 ± 0.4 °C
	Foot	1.4 ± 1.0 °C	1.7 ± 1.0 °C	2.2 ± 1.6 °C
Warm	Hand	1.3 ± 0.7 °C	1.9 ± 1.0 °C	1.6 ± 0.9 °C
	Foot	4.5 ± 1.9 °C	6.1 ± 2.8 °C	6.2 ± 3.2 °C
Pain	Hand	45.6 ± 2.5 °C	45.2 ± 2.5 °C	45.7 ± 1.8 °C
	Foot	44.9 ± 1.5 °C	44.8 ± 1.7 °C	45.7 ± 1.2 °C

Table 4 Thresholds for detecting cool, warm, and heat pain when the stimulus is applied to the chin or lip of subjects 20–89 years of age, as reported by Heft et al. [66]

Modality	Site	Age 30 years[a]	Age 80 years[a]	Change/year (°C)
Cool	Chin	31.5 °C	30.8 °C	0.01
	Lip	32.4 °C	31.9 °C	0.01
Warm	Chin	33.8 °C	36.1 °C	0.05
	Lip	33.8 °C	34.3 °C	0.01
Pain	Chin	43.9 °C	47.1 °C	0.06
	Lip	43.2 °C	45.6 °C	0.05

[a]Predicted by linear regression

feet. A larger study was conducted by Heft that evaluated 179 healthy adults aged 20–89 years who rated threshold and suprathreshold warm, cool, and painful stimuli applied to the upper lip and chin of the face [66]. The results agree with those of Kenshalo in that while there were slight elevations in detection thresholds for cool, warm, and painful stimuli in older subjects, under suprathreshold conditions, there were no statistically significant age differences for the painful stimuli (Table 4). The observed threshold changes and the less consistent changes in suprathreshold performance for the non-noxious stimuli may be related to changes in peripheral nerve function, changes in skin composition, or changes in central nervous system function. Peripheral changes of note would include changes in the underlying innervation of the tissue or changes in the thermal conductivity of the supporting tissues, or both. Free nerve endings, which are associated with the thermal and pain sensations, remain intact into old age [67]. The authors conclude that there is a slight diminution in threshold and suprathreshold thermal performance with increasing age, and they speculate that these changes are best explained at this time by alterations in the skin thermal conductivity. Using linear regression of the data, Heft summarized the thresholds for warming, cooling, and pain conditions at the lip and chin sites in 179 subjects [66].

Burn Prevention

One example of burn prevention is that associated with water heaters in the home. Feldman reported on unsafe bath water temperatures in the Seattle area where 80 % of homes tested had bathtub water temperatures of 54 °C or greater, exposing the occupants to the risk of full-thickness scalds within 30 s exposure [68]. Such burns can be prevented by limiting household water temperatures to less than 52 °C. This work led to educational campaigns and legislation to lower water heater temperatures to 49–54 °C [69, 70]. This work which reduced hot water heater set points from 60 to 65 °C down to 49 °C was effective in reducing the frequency, morbidity, and mortality of tap water burn injuries. The average bath temperature of a group of 20 subjects after lowering the water heater set point was 40.5 °C; with a range from 36 to 42.5 °C. Average shower temperatures (seven subjects) were slightly lower than for baths, 40 °C (range 38.5–41.0 °C) [71]. These and other easy interventions in the home can reduce the risk of injury to elderly individuals.

Conclusions

Thermal injuries in the general population are not uncommon. One particular population at increased risk, the elderly, continues to expand. This increased risk can be explained by several physical and physiological changes that occur with aging. These changes include thinning of the skin, reduced ability to vasodilate the peripheral vasculature in a protective response to a heat stimulus (to remove the heat from the area and maintain a safe skin temperature), and a reduced sensitivity to noxious heat stimuli with advancing age. While the landmark work of Henriques and Moritz has provided data that demonstrates the temporal relationship between skin temperature and thermal injury, additional work is needed to understand this relationship in elderly individuals. Whether advancing age shifts the time–skin–temperature curve relative to a younger population is not known. Regardless, more and more evidence demonstrates that the elderly are less able to defend against a thermal challenge relative to their younger counterparts. Because thermal injury in an elderly population can have more significant consequences with respect to morbidity and mortality, the prevention of these injuries has utmost significance. Burn prevention campaigns thus become very important and effective tools in communicating that older adults are at greater risk of thermal injury, and simple changes in behavior in the home environment can prevent these injuries from occurring [3, 8, 20, 62].

Acknowledgments The author expresses his appreciation and gratitude to Dr. Karen Blackburn, Dr. Rob Rapaport, and Dr. Jim McCarthy for their valuable scientific comments and suggestions.

References

1. Lionelli GT, Pickus EJ, Beckum OK, DeCoursey RL, Korentager RA. A three decade analysis of factors affecting burn mortality in the elderly. Burns. 2005;31:958–63.
2. Burn Foundation. Burn incidence and treatment in the United States 1999 fact sheet. Philadelphia.
3. Redlick F, Cooke A, Gomez M, Banfield J, Cartotto RC, Fish JS. A survey of risk factors for burns in the elderly and prevention strategies. J Burn Care Rehabil. 2002;23:351–6.
4. Kluger N, Laipio J, Virolainen S, Ranki A, Koljonen V. A fatal case of hot air sauna burn in an elderly patient initially misdiagnosed as bullous pemphigoid. Acta Derm Venereol. 2011;91:732–3.
5. Baptiste MS, Feck G. Preventing tap water burns. Am J Public Health. 1980;70:727–9.
6. Petro JA, Belger D, Salzberg CA, Salisbury RE. Burn accidents and the elderly: what is happening and how to prevent it. Geriatrics. 1989;44(3):25–48.
7. Stassen NA, Lukan JK, Mizuguchi NN, Spain DA, Carillo EH, Polk HC. Thermal injury in the elderly: when is comfort care the right choice? Am Surg. 2001;67:704–8.
8. American Burn Association. Scalds: a burning issue. A campaign kit for burn awareness week 2000.
9. Bull JP, Lawrence JC. Thermal conditions to produce skin burns. Fire Mater. 1979;3(2):100–5.
10. Barillo DJ, Coffey EC, Shirani KZ, Goodwin CW. Burns caused by medical therapy. J Burn Care Rehabil. 2000;21:269–73.
11. Burlington, DB, Brown A. FDA/CPSC public health advisory: hazards associated with the use of electric heating pads. 1995. p. 1–3. http://www.fda.gov/MedicalDevices/Safety/AlertsandNotices/PublicHealthNotifications/ucm242866.htm.
12. Henriques FC, Moritz AR. Studies of thermal injury. I: the conduction of heat to and through skin and the temperatures attained therein. A theoretical and experimental investigation. Am J Pathol. 1947;23:531–49.
13. Moritz AR, Henriques FC. Studies of thermal injury. II: the relative importance of time and surface temperature in the causation of cutaneous burns. Am J Pathol. 1947;23:695–720.
14. Moritz AR, Henriques FC, Dutra FR, Weisiger JR. Studies of thermal injury. IV: an exploration of casualty-producing attributes of conflagrations; local and systemic effects of generalized cutaneous exposure to excessive circumambient (air) and circumradiant heat of varying duration and intensity. Arch Pathol. 1947;43:466–88.
15. Henriques FC. Studies in thermal injury. V: the predictability and the significance of thermally induced rate processes leading to irreversible epidermal injury. Arch Pathol. 1947;43:489–502.
16. Henriques FC. Studies of thermal injury VII. Automatic recording calorie applicator and skin tissue and skin surface thermocouples. Rev Sci Instrum. 1947;18:673–680.
17. Wu Y-C. Material properties criteria for thermal safety. J Mater. 1972;1(4):573–9.
18. ASTM Designation: C 1055-03: standard guide for heated system surface conditions that produce contact burn injuries. Published Oct 2003. p. 1–8.
19. Ghods M, Corterier C, Zindel K, Kiene M, Rudolf K, Steen M. Case report. Hot air sauna burns. Burns. 2008;34:122–4.
20. Tan J, Banez C, Cheung Y, Gomez M, Nguyen H, Banfield J, Medeiros L, Lee R, Cartotto R, Fish JS. Effectiveness of a burn prevention campaign for older adults. J Burn Care Rehabil. 2004;25:445–51.
21. Katcher ML. Prevention of tap water scald burns: evaluation of a multi-media injury control program. Am J Public Health. 1987;77:1195–7.
22. Harper RD, Dickson WA. Reducing the burn risk to elderly persons living in residential care. Burns. 1995;21:205–8.
23. Diller KR. Analysis of burns caused by long-term exposure to a heating pad. J Burn Care Rehabil. 1991;12:214–7.
24. Jenkins G. Molecular mechanisms of skin ageing. Mech Ageing Dev. 2002;123:801–10.
25. Montagna W, Carlisle K. Structural changes in ageing skin. Br J Dermatol. 1990;122 Suppl 35:61–70.

26. Cerimele D, Celleno L, Serri F. Physiological changes in ageing skin. Br J Dermatol. 1990;122 Suppl 35:13–20.
27. Martin AD. Skin thickness: caliper measurement and typical values. Boca Raton: CRC Press; 1995. p. 293–6.
28. Moragas A, Castells C, Sans M. Mathematical morphologic analysis of aging-related epidermal changes. Anal Quant Cytol Histol. 1993;15:75–82.
29. Kokate JY, Leland KJ, Held AM, Hansen GL, Kveen GL, Johnson BA, Wilke MS, Sparrow EM, Iaizzo PA. Temperature-modulated pressure ulcers: a porcine model. Arch Phys Med Rehabil. 1995;76:666–73.
30. Braverman IM, Sibley J, Keh-Yen A. A study of the veil cells around normal, diabetic, and aged cutaneous microvessels. J Invest Dermatol. 1986;86:57–62.
31. Gunin AG, Petrov VV, Golubtzova NN, Vasilieva OV, Kornilova NK. Age-related changes in angiogenesis in human dermis. Exp Gerontol. 2014. doi:10.1016/j.exger.2014.04.010.
32. El Nahid MS, El Ashmaui A. The skin microcirculatory changes in the normal and hypertensive elderly. Eur Geriatr Med. 2015;6:7–10.
33. Lipkin M, Hardy JD. Measurement of some thermal properties of human tissues. J Appl Physiol. 1954;7:212–7.
34. Richardson D. Effects of age on cutaneous circulatory response to direct heat on the forearm. J Gerontol. 1989;44:M189–94.
35. Dinenno FA, Jones PP, Seals DR, Tanaka H. Limb blood flow and vascular conductance are reduced with age in healthy humans. Relation to elevations in sympathetic nerve activity and declines in oxygen demand. Circulation. 1999;100:164–70.
36. Detry JMR, Brengelmann GL, Rowell LB, Wyss C. Skin and muscle components of forearm blood flow in directly heated resting man. J Appl Physiol. 1972;32:506–11.
37. Kirby BS, Crecelius AR, Voyles WF, Dinenno FA. Impaired skeletal muscle blood flow control with advancing age in humans: Attenuated ATP release and local vasodilation during erythrocyte deoxygenation. Circ Res. 2012;111(2):220–30.
38. Kenney WL, Morgan AL, Farquahar WB, Brooks EM, Pierzga JM, Derr JA. Decreased active vasodilator sensitivity in aged skin. Am J Physiol. 1997;272: H1609–14.
39. Minson CT, Holowatz LA, Wong BJ, Kenney WL, Wilkins BW. Decreased nitric oxide- and axon reflex-mediated cutaneous vasodilation with age during local heating. J Appl Physiol. 2002;93:1644–9.
40. Bruning RS, Santhanam L, Stanhewicz AE, Smith CJ, Berkowitz DE, Kenney WL, Holowatz LA. Endothelial nitric oxide synthase mediates cutaneous vasodilation during local heating and is attenuated in middle-aged human skin. J Appl Physiol. 2012;112:2019–26.
41. Tur E. Age-related regional variations of human skin blood flow response to histamine. Acta Derm Venereol (Stockh). 1995;75:451–4.
42. Khan F, Spence VA, Belch JJF. Cutaneous vascular responses and thermoregulation in relation to age. Clin Sci. 1992;82:521–8.
43. Holowatz LA, Thompson-Torgerson C, Kenney WL. Aging and the control of human skin blood flow. Front Biosci. 2010;15:718–39.
44. Millet C, Roustit M, Blaise S, Cracowski J-L. Aging is associated with a diminished axon reflex response to local heating on the gaiter skin area. Microvasc Res. 2012;84:356–61.
45. Weiss M, Milman B, Rosen B, Eisenstein Z, Zimlichman R. Analysis of the diminished skin perfusion in elderly people by laser Doppler flowmetry. Age Ageing. 1992;21:237–41.
46. Martin HL, Loomis JL, Kenney WL. Maximal skin vascular conductance in subjects aged 5–85 yr. J Appl Physiol. 1995;79(1):297–301.
47. Holowatz LA, Kenney WL. Peripheral mechanisms of thermoregulatory control of skin blood flow in aged humans. J Appl Physiol. 2010;109:1538–44.
48. Sagawa S, Shiraki K, Yousef MK, Miki K. Sweating and cardiovascular responses of aged men to heat exposure. J Gerontol. 1988;43:M1–8.
49. Roberts J, Steinberg GM. Effects of aging on adrenergic receptors: introduction. Fed Proc. 1986;45:40–1.
50. Armstrong CG, Kenney WL. Effects of age and acclimation on responses to passive heat exposure. J Appl Physiol. 1993;75(5):2162–7.
51. Kenney WL. Control of heat-induced cutaneous vasodilatation in relation to age. Eur J Appl Physiol. 1988;57:120–5.
52. Havenith G, Inoue Y, Luttikholt V, Kenney WL. Age predicts cardiovascular, but not thermoregulatory, responses to humid heat stress. Eur J Appl Physiol. 1995;70:88–96.
53. Rooke GA, Savage MV, Brengelmann GL. Maximal skin blood flow is decreased in elderly men. J Appl Physiol. 1994;77(1):11–4.
54. Katcher ML, Shapiro MM. Lower extremity burns related to sensory loss in diabetes mellitus. J Fam Pract. 1987;24(2):149–51.
55. Balakrishnan C, Rak TP, Meininger MS. Burns of the neuropathic foot following use of therapeutic footbaths. Burns. 1995;21:622–3.
56. Cavadas PC, Bonanad E. Unusual complication in a gracilis myocutaneous free flap. Plast Recontstr Surg. 1996;97:683.
57. Guergova S, Dufour A. Thermal sensitivity in the elderly: a review. Aging Res Rev. 2011;10: 80–92.
58. Van Someren EJW. Chapter 22: Age-related changes in thermoreception and thermoregulation. In: Masoro EJ, Austad SN, editors. Handbook of the biology of aging. 7th ed. New York: Elsevier; 2011. p. 463–78.

59. Heft MW, Robinson ME. Age differences in orofacial sensory thresholds. J Dent Res. 2010;89:1102–5.
60. Heft MW, Robinson ME. Age differences in suprathreshold sensory function. Age. 2014;36:1–8.
61. Tochihara Y, Kumamoto T, Lee J-Y, Hashiguchi N. Age-related differences in cutaneous warm sensation thresholds of human males in thermoneutral and cool environments. J Therm Biol. 2011;36:105–11.
62. Buettner K. Effects of extreme heat and cold on human skin. II. Surface temperature, pain and heat conductivity in experiments with radiant heat. J Appl Physiol. 1951;3:703–13.
63. Lautenbacher S, Strin F. Similarities in age differences in heat pain perception and thermal sensitivity. Funct Neurol. 1991;6:129–35.
64. Chakour MC, Gibson SJ, Bradbeer M, Helme RD. The effect of age on Aδ- and C-fibre thermal pain perception. Pain. 1996;64:143–52.
65. Kenshalo DR. Somesthetic sensitivity in young and elderly humans. J Gerontol. 1986;41:732–42.
66. Heft MW, Cooper BY, O'Brien KK, Hemp E, O'Brien R. Aging effects on the perception of noxious and non-noxious thermal stimuli applied to the face. Aging Clin Exp Res. 1996;8:35–41.
67. Montagna W, Carlisle K. Structural changes in aging human skin. J Invest Dermatol. 1979;73:15–20.
68. Feldman KW, Schaller RT, Feldman JA, McMillon M. Tap water scald burns in children. Pediatrics. 1978;62(1):1–7.
69. Liao C-C, Rossignol AM. Landmarks in burn prevention. Burns. 2000;26:422–34.
70. Erdman TC, Feldman KW, Rivara FP, Heimbach DM, Wall HA. Tap water burn prevention: the effect of legislation. Pediatrics. 1991;88:572–7.
71. Lawrence JC, Bull JP. Thermal conditions which cause skin burns. Inst Mech Eng Eng Med. 1976;5:61–3.

Aging of Epidermal Stem Cells

15

Alexandra Charruyer and Ruby Ghadially

Contents

Abstract

This review discusses the changes in stem and progenitor populations that occur with aging and, more specifically, changes of the epidermis that occur with aging. The consensus of opinion is that changes responsible for aging of tissues occur not only in the stem cell pool itself but also in the transit-amplifying cell compartment and in the stem cell environment. In order to study aging of epidermal stem cells, it is essential to isolate epidermal stem cells at the single cell level to better define them at a molecular level. It will also be important to study the intrinsic and extrinsic changes that occur in the environment/niche of the epidermal stem cell with aging.

Introduction

Advances in biology indicate that stem cells have a crucial role in both organ maturation and in aging. Studies have demonstrated molecular and biochemical changes in tissue-resident progenitor cells and their microenvironments during chronological aging of tissues such as the heart [1], brain [2], and hematopoietic system [3]. In this chapter knowledge in the field of aging and stem cells derived from tissues other than the epidermis is reviewed and the challenges of studying aging stem cells discussed. Subsequently, epidermal stem cells are reviewed and changes in progenitor populations of the epidermis that occur with age

A. Charruyer • R. Ghadially (✉)
Department of Dermatology and Eli and Edythe Broad, Center of Regeneration Medicine and Stem Cell Research, University of California, Veterans Affairs Medical Center, San Francisco, CA, USA
e-mail: acharruyer@gmail.com; ghadiallyr@derm.ucsf.edu; Ruby.Ghadially@ucsf.edu

M.A. Farage et al. (eds.), *Textbook of Aging Skin*,
DOI 10.1007/978-3-662-47398-6_19

discussed. Finally, the body of knowledge specifically related to the aging of epidermal stem cells and the implications of stem cell aging for carcinogenesis are examined.

Aging and Stem Cells

Changes in Stem Cell Frequency with Aging

Information about the impact of aging on stem cells has been obtained from the hematopoietic system, and it remains an ideal system for this type of study as stem and progenitor cells are most well-defined in the hematopoietic system. The loss of immune function and the increased incidence of myeloid leukemia associated with aging were thought to be due to a decrease in hematopoietic stem cell frequency. Research has now contradicted this assumption. Several studies indicate that murine hematopoietic stem cell numbers increase substantially with age [4, 5]. Limiting dilution assays have shown that hematopoietic stem cells from aged mice were more efficient at myeloid reconstitution than hematopoietic stem cells from young mice. Aged hematopoietic stem cells were found to be five times as numerous, but one-quarter as efficient at engrafting, as young hematopoietic stem cells, suggesting a small increase in reconstitution ability [5]. In another study, the relative number of the most primitive stem cells was found to be two- to threefold higher in aged versus young mice, but there was a decrease in the proliferative activity of aged hematopoietic stem cells [4]. In keeping with these findings, the number of adult murine hematopoietic $CD41^{+}$ stem cells increased with age, potentially in order to compensate for the impaired function of stem cells with aging [6]. Thus the majority of studies show an increase in primitive precursors and a decrease in proliferative ability in hematopoietic stem cells with age.

In skeletal muscle, estimates of stem cell (satellite cell) number have produced varying results. Electron microscopy (DNA content and cell count) demonstrated an increase in satellite cell number in aging rats [7]. Using CD34 expression and flow cytometry, there was no difference in satellite cell frequency in aged versus young murine muscles [8]. Additionally, microscopically there was a decrease in $Pax7^{+}$ skeletal stem cells during aging [9–11]. Interestingly, in the same study, despite the decrease in satellite stem cells, muscle regeneration was as effective in aged as in young muscle, indicating that performance of satellite stem cells may not be affected by aging [10, 11]. Different experimental approaches and techniques were used in these studies, including the use of injury [8], and thus a consensus has yet to be reached regarding the effect of aging on skeletal stem cell frequency and proliferative ability.

Intrinsic Cellular Modifications in Stem Cells with Aging

\While changes in stem cell frequency play a role in aging, there is also evidence for intrinsic cellular modifications in stem cells with aging. It is challenging to distinguish intrinsic cellular aging from the effects of the cellular milieu when stem cells are studied in their natural environment, and the isolation of pure stem cell populations is needed (for review, see [12]). Epidermal stem cells, isolated from young and old mice based on their Hoechst dye exclusion, were analyzed for gene expression profile by cDNA arrays. There was similar expression of 422 genes assayed in young and old epidermal stem cells [13]. Expression profiles of highly purified long-term repopulating hematopoietic stem cells showed that aging was associated with a downregulation of genes mediating lymphoid function and upregulation of genes involved in myeloid fate, indicating that the loss of immune function and the increase in leukemia in the elderly are due to intrinsic alterations in hematopoietic stem cells [14]. These latter studies provide evidence that the intrinsic properties of stem cells change with age.

A decrease in Notch signaling has been implicated in the aging of stem cells [15]. Notch can be modified by cytoplasmic proteins such as Numb. Numb interacts with a cytoplasmic domain of Notch and inhibits it [16] and controls asymmetric division of neural progenitor cells [17]. Restoration of Notch activity rejuvenated the regenerative ability of aged muscle stem cells. Aged satellite cells exposed to young serum exhibited restoration of Notch signaling, skeletal muscle stem cell proliferation, and regenerative capacity [15].

Further studies of intrinsic changes with aging showed a cell-autonomous increase in p38 activity resulting in defective self-renewal of aged muscle stem cells. These changes could not be reversed by exposure to a young environment, indicating that intrinsic changes are as important as changes in the stem cell niche [18]. Restoration of p38 activity using pharmacologic inhibition or knockdown restored the maintenance, regeneration, and self-renewal of aged satellite cells after transplantation. Increased p38 activity with aging results in a loss of asymmetric localization of p38 during stem cell divisions and was associated with more committed progenitors and less self-renewal. Inhibition of p38 restored asymmetric divisions in aged muscle stem cells in vitro, as evidenced by increased numbers of $Pax7^+$ quiescent stem cells [18]. In another work, p38 inhibition restored aged muscle stem cell proliferation in vitro and regenerative ability in vivo [19]. Altogether this body of work indicates that muscle stem cells can be rejuvenated not only by rejuvenating the stem niche but also by modulating the intrinsic changes of aging.

Changes in the Stem Cell Niche with Aging

Stem cell homeostasis is not only maintained by intrinsic factors but also extrinsic factors, such as the local environment of the stem cell niche, the surrounding tissue, the systemic milieu of the organism, and the external environment (for review, see [12, 20]). Age-related modifications of extrinsic factors may include alterations in the composition of the extracellular matrix, alterations in membrane proteins and lipids, and alterations in factors that constitute the systemic milieu.

Modifications in the stem cell niche during the aging process have been addressed in *Drosophila*. The *Drosophila* germline stem cells together with the somatic cells present in the niche is one of the most well-defined stem cell niches [21]. In somatic niche cells from older *Drosophila* testes, there is a decrease in expression of a cell adhesion molecule (DE-cadherin) and a self-renewal ligand (unpaired). This was correlated with an overall decrease in stem cell numbers inside the niche [22]. Furthermore, restoring self-renewal (unpaired) resulted in an increase of the number of germline stem cells in older males compared with age-matched controls. Thus modifications of the somatic cells that constitute the niche in aged testes can affect the frequency of stem cells inside the niche. Furthermore, murine spermatogonial stem cells could be serially transplanted in young mice recipients without showing any decline in stem cell number or colony-forming ability for more than 3 years, indicating that a young environment can influence stem cell self-renewal capacity and that failure of niche integrity plays a key role in the reproductive deficit in aged mice [23].

The effect of environment on skeletal muscle satellite cells has been studied [24]. No significant differences were found in mass or maximum force between old muscles grafted into young hosts and young muscle grafted into those same young hosts. Conversely, young muscles grafted into old recipients did not regenerate better than old muscles grafted into the same old hosts, indicating an important role for the environment in muscle regeneration after transplantation. Conditioned medium from differentiated myotubes of young mice exhibited a strong mitogenic action on aged satellite cells in vitro, whereas no mitogenic action was observed from conditioned media of myotubes from aged mice, either on young or on aged satellite cells [25] (for review, see [26]). More recently, systemic influences on aged satellite cells were investigated using parabiotic pairings in which regenerating tissues in aged animals were exposed either to their own serum or that of young mice (isochronic or heterochronic parabioses, respectively) [15]. In this study, exposing injured muscles from old mice to heterochronic parabioses greatly improved muscle regeneration, and myotubule formation was similar to that observed in young mice. The authors concluded that a young systemic environment could improve the impaired regenerative ability of aged skeletal stem cells.

These studies demonstrate the important influence of both the local and systemic environment within which stem cells reside.

Symmetric and Asymmetric Stem Cell Division and Aging

Stem cells in the niche undergo two types of division, symmetric self-renewal divisions leading to two identical daughter cells and asymmetric divisions leading to one daughter cell identical to the original stem cell and another non-stem daughter cell that leaves the niche and undergoes differentiation [21, 27]. It is predicted that aged stem cells would have preserved or increased self-renewal potential (symmetrical divisions) and decreased asymmetrical divisions, and in order to maintain a constant rate of cellular production, the aged will have more proliferation in the transit-amplifying cells [28, 29]. Studies agree with this prediction; in different stem cell compartments including the hematopoietic system and the intestinal crypt, there is an increase in transit-amplifying cells with age [30, 31] (for review, see [28]).

Alterations in Molecular Pathways with Aging

Gatekeepers of genome integrity increase with age, presumably in order to prevent cancer, and have been shown to negatively regulate stem cell function with age [32]. Cellular proliferation and survival are negatively regulated by genes such as $p16^{Ink4a}$, $p19^{Arf}$, and p53 (for review, see [33]). Increasing $p16^{Ink4a}$ and $p19^{Arf}$, by loss of proto-oncogene Hmga2, decreases neural stem cell frequency and self-renewal ability [34]. The cyclin-dependent kinase inhibitor $p16^{Ink4a}$ shows increased expression with aging and has been associated with decreased stem cell number and impaired proliferation in several tissues. In the hematopoietic system, Janzen et al. reported that $p16^{Ink4a}$ was increased in aged hematopoietic stem cells and in the absence of $p16^{Ink4a}$, the repopulation defect was improved and the size of the stem cell pool increased [35]. In the murine brain, the age-associated decline in multipotent progenitor frequency and proliferation ability also correlated with an increase in $p16^{Ink4a}$ [36]. In $p16^{Ink4a}$-deficient mice, the decline in neurogenesis, progenitor number, and self-renewal was less severe than in control mice, indicating the role of $p16^{Ink4a}$ in brain stem cells impairment with age [36].

Non-biased analysis of RNA sequencing of aged versus young keratin 15-positive epidermal stem cells showed that the expression of a core stem cell signature was maintained [37]. However, two pathways, Jak-Stat and Notch, were significantly altered with aging [37]. Inhibition of Jak-Stat with pyridine-6 resulted in reversing aged stem cell clonogenic activity defect, as evidenced by more abundant and faster-growing colonies.

RNA sequencing of hair follicle stem cells in telogen and anagen phases revealed that aged anagen hair follicle stem cells were more similar to young telogen hair follicle stem cells than young anagen hair follicle stem cells, in terms of gene expression [38]. In aged hair follicle stem cells, genes involved in extracellular matrix remodeling, cell proliferation, and survival were downregulated. Nuclear factor of activated T-cell c1 (NFATc1) targets was enriched in the age-related signature, and inhibition of NFATc1resulted in improved hair regeneration [38]. Deficient downregulation of NFATc1 during HFSC activation delays entry into hair cycle and underscores the importance of enhanced BMP/NFATc1 signaling in the age-related changes in hair follicle stem cells [38].

Challenges of Studying Aging and Stem Cells

Issues surrounding the study of aging include the study of aging versus development, the study of animals of an appropriate age, the heterogeneity of aged animals, and the lack of a pure population of stem cells from most tissues. Many studies are confounded by the use of neonatal versus adult or neonatal versus aged tissue. Such studies may not reflect changes of aging, but rather changes occurring during development from birth to adulthood. It is important to keep these studies distinct, and the focus here is on aging of epidermal stem cells from the adult to aged individual.

In aging studies, the age of the aged animals to be studied is of great importance, and guidelines for such studies are limited. The definition of aging varies depending on the physiological system under question. For example, many age-related changes in the immune system are evident by the 70 % survival point and even earlier, while kidney changes start later. The most common age used to model old age is somewhere around thc 50 % survival point, although it may vary from the 70 % survival point to the 30 % survival point. It has been stated that "without epidemic disease or exaggerated or lopsided tumor incidence, the 50 % survival point can be considered as an indicator of the onset of the senescent period" [39]. It is important to note that results from extremely aged animals are not reliable because they may be the consequence of advanced disease rather than aging. The best approach, although often difficult in practice, is to study multiple time points during the senescent period [40].

Aging is also difficult to study because of the heterogeneity that is associated with the aging process. Indeed, the variance in vital characteristics in the elderly is substantially higher compared with other groups of the population [41]. One universal characteristic of aging is the accumulation of molecular damage, which induces alterations in gene expression, genomic instability, mutations, tissue disorganization, and organ dysfunction. Because of the low probability that two molecules will be damaged in the same way and with the same intensity, substantial molecular heterogeneity results, and this leads to clinical heterogeneity in the elderly population [42].

While hematopoietic stem cells can be isolated at a single cell level [43], epidermal stem cell markers that allow isolation of epidermal stem cells at a single cell level have yet to be found. Studying populations of stem cells that are of unknown purity poses a challenge. Furthermore, the lack of a good understanding of the stem cell hierarchy in the epidermis complicates studies further.

In summary, studies of aging and in particular aged epidermal stem cells are profoundly affected by the choice of age for the young cohort, the choice of age for the aged cohort, the heterogeneity of the aged cohort, and the lack of a pure epidermal stem cell population for study.

Characterization of Epidermal Stem Cells

Phenotypic analysis of hematopoietic stem cells has provided the ability to separate long-term repopulating cells from the less primitive cells detected in colony-forming assays [44]. These types of studies have allowed a hierarchy of hematopoietic stem cell differentiation to be determined. Different methods to isolate epidermal stem cells have been proposed, although a hierarchy of progenitors has not been determined in the epidermis.

Stem cells of the epidermis are responsible for maintaining and generating the adult epidermis and its appendages, including hair follicles and sebaceous glands. Different stem cell niches have been described: (i) the follicular stem cell that resides in the hair follicle bulge [45, 46] (for review, see [47]), (ii) the interfollicular stem cell [48] (for review, see [49]), and (iii) the melanocyte stem cell localized in the hair follicle [50].

In the early 1990s, the search began for a molecular signature for the epidermal stem cell, and Jones and Watt showed that high levels of beta1 integrins could be used to characterize highly proliferative keratinocytes in vitro [51]. This pioneer work was followed by dozens of studies aimed at isolating a pure population of epidermal stem cells. The most prevalent methods for isolating putative epidermal stem cells are listed in Table 1, including (i) side population (SP) cells that efflux Hoechst 33342 fluorescent dye [52, 53], (ii) integrin α6 bright/CD71 dim human keratinocytes [54, 55],

Table 1 Putative stem cell markers in epidermis (Adapted from Ghadially R, Journal of Investigative Dermatology, 20l12)

Marker (function)	Stem cel properties
α6 Integrin^{hi} (adhesion)	α6 Integrin^{hi} human keratinocytes were label retaining, quiescent, exhibited high nuclear to cytoplasmic ratio, high colony formation capacity, and had the greatest tissue regeneration capacity [59, 65]
β1 Integrin (adhesion)	Human keratinocytes that adhere rapidly to type IV collagen, a β1 integrin ligand, exhibited high proliferative potential in vitro [51]
BrdU/LRC (incorporated into DNA)	Murine label-retaining cells exhibited high colony-forming efficiency in vitro and the highest integrin levels [66]
CD200^{+} (autoimmunity)	Located in murine follicular bulge. High colony-forming efficiency and in G0/G1 [67]
Side population (SP) (efflux Hoechst 33342)	Using a modified Hoechst 33342 technique, more than 90 % of putative murine stem cells were in G0/G1, and these cells formed larger, more expandable colonies in vitro [68]. Human SP cells were enriched in quiescent cells, were not label-retaining cells, had low expression of surface antigens traditionally thought to mark stem cells [55], expressed the drug transporter ABCG2 [53], exhibited high short- and long-term proliferative potential, and formed a pluristratified epidermis [69]. Murine SP cells expressed keratin 14, β1 integrin, and p63 [70]. Both murine and human SP cells were a subset of α6 integrin + cells
ABCG2^{+} (ATP-binding cassette protein)	Human side population cells expressed the drug transporter ABCG2 [53].
Keratin 19 (structural protein)	Co-localized with label-retaining cells in mice [71]
CD34^{+} (cell-cell adhesion factor)	Marked murine bulge keratinocytes (not human). Predominantly in G0/G1 and expressed high a6 integrin [67]. Refractory to differentiation in culture [72]. Co-localized with label-retaining cells and keratin 15^{+} cells [73]
CD90^{+} (glycophosphatidylinositol-anchored cell surface protein)	Human CD90^{+} cells formed larger clusters than CD90^{-} cells, when injected in NODSCID mice [74]
Lgr5 (leucine-rich G protein-coupled receptor)	Lgr5^{+} murine keratinocytes were actively proliferating and multipotent, able to give rise to new hair follicles for the long term [75]
Lgr6 (leucine-rich G protein-coupled receptor)	Adult Lgr6^{+} murine keratinocytes were capable of long-term wound repair including the formation of new hair follicles [76]
MTS24 (glycoprotein)	MTS24^{+} murine cells expressed a6 integrin and keratin 14 and exhibited a twofold increase in colony formation and colony size over MTS24- cells [77]
Lgr1 (leucine-rich G protein-coupled receptor)	In murine epidermis Lgr1^{+} cells gave rise to all adult epidermal lineages in skin reconstitution assays [78]. In human epidermis, Lgr1 regulated stem cell quiescence [79]
Delta1 (Notch ligand)	Delta1 was expressed in the basal layer of human epidermis with highest expression where stem cells reside [80]. Deletion of Delta1 resulted in a delayed first anagen [81]

(*continued*)

Table 1 (continued)

Marker (function)	Stem cel properties
p63 (p53 homologue)	Holoclones formed using human keratinocytes (in vitro clones that show less than 5 % terminal colonies) showed high expression of p63 [82]
EGFR^{lo} (epidermal growth factor receptor)	Human EGFR^{lo} cells generated pluristratified epidermis in a skin reconstruction model [83]
(MHC) Class I-HLA$^{low/negative}$ (self-nonself discrimination)	There was low/negative expression of MHC Class I-HLA in a subpopulation of basal human keratinocytes [84]. Embryonic stem cells lack MHC Class I antigens
Connexin43 (Cx43^{dim}) (gap junction protein)	10 % of human basal keratinocytes were Cx43^{dim} by flow cytometry. Cx43^{dim} human limbal epithelial cells are small cells, low in granularity, contain high percentage of LRCs, and are p63^{+}, ABCG2^{+}, and integrin β1^{+} [85]. Murine label-retaining cells did not express Cx43 [85]
Desmoglein3 (Dsg3^{dim}) (intercellular junction protein)	High β1 integrin-expressing human keratinocytes were Dsg3^{dim}. Dsg3^{dim} keratinocytes had greater long-term proliferative capacity in vitro than Dsg3^{bright} keratinocytes and showed comparable clonogenicity to α6^{hi}CD71^{lo} cells [86, 87]
CD71^{lo} (transferrin receptor)	Human α6 integrin^{hi} CD71^{hi} keratinocytes have the greatest tissue regeneration capacity [54]
CD146 MCAM (probable adhesion molecule)	Along with multiple other markers, CD146^{lo}, selected for human hair follicle cells with high colony-forming efficiency [88]
CD133 (prominin)	CD133^{+} cells were enriched for long-term repopulating epidermal stem cells, were self-renewing, were multipotent, and were a subset of integrin a6 + CD34^{+} bulge cells [56]
ALDH CD44 (aldehyde dehydrogenase (ALDH^{+}) is a cytosolic enzyme involved in biotransformation of alcohols and aldehydes) (CD44^{+} is a hyaluronic acid receptor)	The ALDH + CD44^{+} population was enriched 12.6-fold for long-term repopulating epidermal stem cells [58]. CD44^{+} ALDH^{+} keratinocytes had self-renewal ability, were holoclone-forming cells in vitro, were multipotent, and 58 ± 7 % were label-retaining cells [58]

(iii) collagen adhesion [51], and (iv) a quantitative epidermal regeneration assay [48, 56–59]. Other methods/markers such as label-retaining cells [60], p63 [61], keratin 19 [62], keratin 15 [63], and elevated levels of β catenin [64] have also been reported as putative stem cell markers. Our laboratory recently added CD133 as a marker of murine epidermal stem cells [56] and ALDH CD44 as a marker of human epidermal stem cells [58].

The study of epidermal stem cells from different sources such as aged versus young or diseased versus healthy would be greatly enhanced by the availability of pure populations of epidermal stem cells. To date techniques have been developed for enriching populations of keratinocytes for early progenitors, but not at the single cell level. Given the difficulty in finding specific stem cell markers, investigation is needed to determine combinations of markers that can enrich for epidermal stem cells at a single cell level. Markers found in stem cells from other tissues, embryonic stem cell markers, or even cancer stem cell markers found in tumorigenic tissues may provide useful strategies for the isolation of normal epidermal stem cells at a single cell level.

Aging and the Keratinocyte Proliferative Compartment

Abundant historical studies in both human and animal models demonstrate that aging of the epidermis is accompanied by decreased proliferation, both basally and in response to proliferative stimuli [89–96]. These studies have led to the concept that epidermal stem cells, which are responsible for the maintenance of the epidermis, are involved in the aging process.

The effect of aging on the keratinocyte proliferative compartment (stem cells and transit-amplifying cells) has been studied in vivo. After skin injury, the regeneration of tissue requires stem cell mobilization [46, 97], which has made wound healing a valuable model for the study of the impact of aging on epidermal stem cells. A battlefield surgeon performed an early study of wound healing and age during World War I [98]. Using a cicatrization index, the biological age of an injured soldier could be determined by measuring the rate of closure of war wounds. Soldiers in their 30s healed more slowly than those in their 20s. Standardized superficial skin wounds were created in young adults (18–25 years) and aged adults (65–75 years) and healing was monitored. By day 28, the younger group had completely restored their original skin markings, while the older cohort took double the time (56 days) [92].

A nonradioactive method, using Dansyl chloride that binds only to nonviable corneocytes, was used to measure stratum corneum transit time. Transit time was increased in aged persons, and there was no difference in the number of horny layers, indicating that the increase in stratum corneum transit time in the aged was a reflection of decreased epidermal proliferation [93]. These studies of stem cells and transit-amplifying cells provide some information on how the proliferative compartment of epidermis changes with aging in vivo, but not specifically on how the stem cell changes.

The effect of aging on keratinocyte proliferation has also been studied using in vitro models of aging. Rheinwald and Green compared the proliferative behavior of seven human newborn-derived keratinocyte cultures with 3-, 12-, and 34-year-old-derived cultures [99]. Newborn-derived cultures were able to undergo 25–51 cell generations versus 20–27 for older person-derived cultures and could be maintained through 3–6 passages versus 2–3 passages. In addition, plating efficiency (colony-forming ability) was up to 15.7 % for the newborn versus 0.7 % for the older person-derived cultures. Another study using newborn human keratinocytes compared with adult human keratinocytes reported that while attachment rate is independent of donor age, plating efficiency was strongly dependent on donor age. Plating efficiency was 2–10 % in newborn cultures and below 0.01 % in adult cultures [91, 100]. It should be noted that the above in vitro studies may reflect development, aging, or a combination of development and aging as they employed newborn human keratinocytes.

Aging and Epidermal Stem Cells

The above in vivo and in vitro observations of aging and proliferation were made on the entire keratinocyte population and not on different proliferative subpopulations. To address the differences in behavior of proliferative keratinocyte subpopulations (stem cells versus transit-amplifying cells), the growth potential of individual proliferative clones from different donors (two neonatal, one 64-year-old, and one 78-year-old) was studied [101]. After plating individual cells, resultant clones were passaged into a second dish. The original clone was classified by the appearance of cells in the secondary dish into holoclones (cells that form large rapidly growing colonies), paraclones (cells that form uniformly small, terminal colonies), and meroclones (cells that form both types of colonies). With age, the number of holoclones (stem cells) decreased and the number of paraclones increased when compared with newborns. The authors concluded that the culture lifetime of a keratinocyte population declines with the age of the donor, as demonstrated by the change in the proportion of the three clone types.

Multiple subsequent studies have now also addressed the influence of aging on epidermal stem cell numbers. Such studies have produced varying results. There were twice as many stem cells in neonatal mouse epidermis (1–2 days) as in adult (8–14 weeks) (8.4 % versus 3.8 %, respectively), using small size and Hoechst fluorescence to define a stem cell [68]. In a study of four human foreskins (from 1-, 4-, 35-, and 61-year-old donors), there was a decrease in the number of putative epidermal stem cells in adult versus neonatal human epidermis, as defined by α6 integrin^{hi} CD71^{lo} expression [102]. Such comparisons of adult and neonatal samples may reveal changes of development and/or aging. While neonatal murine epidermis had three times as many Hoechst dye-excluding cells as adult epidermis, the number of cells that could exclude Hoechst dye was unchanged in aged adult versus young adult murine epidermis [13]. Furthermore, human and mouse keratinocytes that exclude Hoechst dye showed little variability in protein expression profiles in aged versus neonatal epidermis, suggesting that as epidermal stem cells age, they do not substantially change their cellular characteristics [103]. In two studies, using FACS analysis and immunostaining, the same number of integrin a6^{+}/CD34^{+} cells were found in aged murine (22–24 months) and young (2–4 months) keratinocytes [38, 104]. Using keratin 15 reporter mice, there was a significant increase in keratin 15-positive hair follicle stem cells in aged (18 months) versus young (3 months) mice [37]. However aged GFP^{+} stem cells had a diminished CFE ability compared to young GFP^{+} stem cells indicating a decline in stem cell function with aging in vitro [37]. Finally, the epidermal stem cells from young adults and aged adults had similar characteristics in culture, similar gene expression, and did not show extensive loss of telomeres with age. In the same study, epidermal stem cells isolated from 22-month-old transgenic mice that expressed GFP were injected into mouse blastocysts. Six months later, various tissues of the resultant mice contained GFP positive cells, demonstrating that the developmental potency of murine epidermal stem cells is not altered with aging. It was concluded from this study that epidermal stem cells are resistant to cellular aging [13].

The differing findings presented above could result from the study of keratinocytes of varying ages, their human or murine derivation, the possibility that different putative epidermal stem cell markers are not isolating the same population of progenitor cells, or the possibility that different methods have different efficacy in isolating epidermal stem cells. Furthermore, a change in the number of cells expressing stem cell markers in aged versus young tissues may reflect a change in stem cell phenotype rather than a change in stem cell number.

While the previous in vitro studies produced a panoply of results, it has been difficult to study skin aging in vivo due to the lack of relevant models. A recent study attempted to address this issue by studying the effect of aging on keratin 15-positive progenitors from young (2–6 months) and aged (22–26 months) mice [104]. Using whole-mount immunostaining, they observed a similar number of keratin 15-positive bulge stem cells in follicles of both young and aged mice, suggesting that epidermal stem cell frequency is not affected by aging. Surprisingly, there was only a modest, and not statistically significant, decrease in proliferation as measured by Ki67. This is different from previous in vitro studies and suggests that in vivo assays may produce different results in the study of skin aging and epidermal stem cells.

In order to examine in vivo, whether the decreased proliferative ability of aged epidermis could be explained by either quantitative and/or qualitative alterations in the stem and/or transit-amplifying cell proliferative compartments, a quantitative in vivo transplantation assay was used similar to the hematopoietic assays that have been informative about changes in hematopoietic progenitors with aging [5, 105, 106].

In vivo transplantation assays of aged and young adult keratinocytes showed that while no significant difference in epidermal stem cell frequency could be detected, transit-amplifying cell frequency was greater in the aged [31]. With aging there was both an increased growth fraction (proportion of actively cycling cells) and longer cell cycle duration, resulting in prolonged existence of the short-term repopulating cells in vivo. Finally, there was decreased cellular output from both individual epidermal stem cells and transit-amplifying cells with aging (Fig. 1). This suggests that increased cell cycle duration contributes to the decreased cellular output from epidermal progenitors, while the larger growth fraction may be a compensatory mechanism [31].

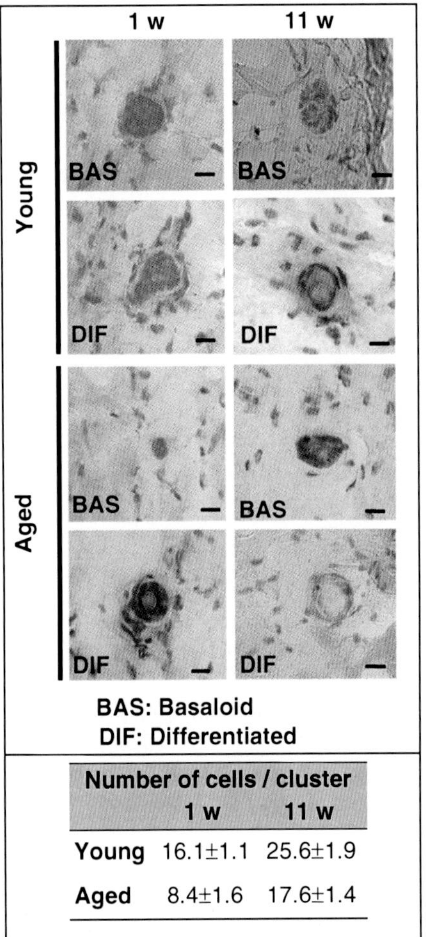

Number of cells / cluster	1 w	11 w
Young	16.1±1.1	25.6±1.9
Aged	8.4±1.6	17.6±1.4

Fig. 1 Epidermal repopulating units from aged repopulating progenitors are smaller and produce less cells than those from young progenitors at 1 and 11 weeks (bar = 10 μm)

Aging, Carcinogenesis, and Stem Cells

Given the role of stem cells in self-renewal, proliferation, and homeostasis, along with the increase in incidence of cancer with aging, it is assumed that stem cells are involved in carcinogenesis. Recently mechanistic links have been made between aging and carcinogenesis.

Because they have the longest life of any cells in the epidermis, it is believed that stem cells are at increased risk of accumulating DNA replication errors and mutations [107]. In addition, it has been shown that senescent cells are more resistant to apoptosis [108] and have impaired DNA repair mechanisms [109]. The resulting genetic instability leads to an increase in carcinogenesis (for review, see [110]).

Stem cells have developed specific mechanisms to protect their genome from accumulating damages. Genome integrity in stem cells involves different mechanisms depending on the tissue. Hematopoietic stem cells have been shown to protect their stem cell DNA by maintaining quiescence [111]. However, while stem cell quiescence minimizes DNA replication-induced mutation, it results in a reduced ability to use the highly accurate homologous recombination repair mechanism, since going through S phase is required for homologous recombination. Intestinal stem cells are highly proliferative cells and have developed other protective mechanisms to avoid the accumulation of DNA damage. Intestinal stem cells in the basal crypt show neutral drifts in clonality that result in selection against mutations in the stem cell compartment [112, 113]. Since intestinal stem cells are going through the cell cycle, they are able to use homologous recombination to repair DNA damage.

Little is known about the mechanism used by epidermal stem cells to maintain their genomic integrity. Like for hematopoietic stem cells, quiescence could be a mechanism of choice for epidermal stem cells to avoid exhaustion and DNA mutation accumulation. Several studies using label retention and cell cycle analysis have demonstrated that bulge epidermal stem cells are more quiescent than transit-amplifying progeny, suggesting quiescence as a protective mechanism used by epidermal stem cells for genome integrity [114–116].

The role of genome integrity in tissue aging and stem cell-induced carcinogenesis remains poorly understood. It is possible that the protective mechanisms used by stem cells to avoid mutations and cancer contribute to the decline in stem cell function with aging. On the other hand, aging can impair the ability of stem cell to proliferate or differentiate, resulting in defects in genome-protective mechanisms and cancer [107].

Conclusion

This review discusses the changes in stem and progenitor populations that occur with aging and, more specifically, changes of the epidermis that occur with aging. The consensus of opinion is that changes responsible for aging of tissues occur not only in the stem cell pool itself but also in the transit-amplifying cell compartment and in the stem cell environment. In order to study aging of epidermal stem cells, it is essential to isolate epidermal stem cells at the single cell level to better define them at a molecular level. It will also be important to study the intrinsic and extrinsic changes that occur in the environment/niche of the epidermal stem cell with aging.

References

1. Anversa P, Kajstura J, Leri A, Bolli R. Life and death of cardiac stem cells: a paradigm shift in cardiac biology. Circulation. 2006;113:1451–63.
2. Galvan V, Jin K. Neurogenesis in the aging brain. Clin Interv Aging. 2007;2:605–10.
3. Rossi DJ, Bryder D, Weissman IL. Hematopoietic stem cell aging: mechanism and consequence. Exp Gerontol. 2007;42:385–90.
4. de Haan G, Van Zant G. Dynamic changes in mouse hematopoietic stem cell numbers during aging. Blood. 1999;93:3294–301.
5. Morrison SJ, Wandycz AM, Akashi K, Globerson A, Weissman IL. The aging of hematopoietic stem cells. Nat Med. 1996;2:1011–6.
6. Gekas C, Graf T. CD41 expression marks myeloid-biased adult hematopoietic stem cells and increases with age. Blood. 2013;121:4463–72.
7. Gibson MC, Schultz E. Age-related differences in absolute numbers of skeletal muscle satellite cells. Muscle Nerve. 1983;6:574–80.
8. Conboy IM, Conboy MJ, Smythe GM, Rando TA. Notch-mediated restoration of regenerative potential to aged muscle. Science. 2003;302:1575–7.
9. Brack AS, Bildsoe H, Hughes SM. Evidence that satellite cell decrement contributes to preferential decline in nuclear number from large fibres during murine age-related muscle atrophy. J Cell Sci. 2005;118:4813–21.
10. Collins CA, Zammit PS, Ruiz AP, Morgan JE, Partridge TA. A population of myogenic stem cells that survives skeletal muscle aging. Stem Cells (Dayton, Ohio). 2007;25:885–94.
11. Shefer G, Van de Mark DP, Richardson JB, Yablonka-Reuveni Z. Satellite-cell pool size does matter: defining the myogenic potency of aging skeletal muscle. Dev Biol. 2006;294:50–66.
12. Rando TA. Stem cells, ageing and the quest for immortality. Nature. 2006;441:1080–6.
13. Stern MM, Bickenbach JR. Epidermal stem cells are resistant to cellular aging. Aging Cell. 2007;6:439–52.
14. Rossi DJ. Cell intrinsic alterations underlie hematopoietic stem cell aging. Proc Natl Acad Sci. 2005;102:9194–9.
15. Conboy IM, et al. Rejuvenation of aged progenitor cells by exposure to a young systemic environment. Nature. 2005;433:760–4.
16. Guo M, Jan LY, Jan YN. Control of daughter cell fates during asymmetric division: interaction of Numb and Notch. Neuron. 1996;17:27–41.
17. Zhong W, Feder JN, Jiang MM, Jan LY, Jan YN. Asymmetric localization of a mammalian numb homolog during mouse cortical neurogenesis. Neuron. 1996;17:43–53.
18. Bernet JD, et al. p38 MAPK signaling underlies a cell-autonomous loss of stem cell self-renewal in skeletal muscle of aged mice. Nat Med. 2014;20:265–71.
19. Cosgrove BD, et al. Rejuvenation of the muscle stem cell population restores strength to injured aged muscles. Nat Med. 2014;20:255–64.
20. Wallenfang MR. Aging within the stem cell niche. Dev Cell. 2007;13:603–4.
21. Xie T, Spradling AC. A niche maintaining germ line stem cells in the *Drosophila* ovary. Science. 2000;290:328–30.
22. Boyle M, Wong C, Rocha M, Jones DL. Decline in self-renewal factors contributes to aging of the stem cell niche in the *Drosophila* testis. Cell Stem Cell. 2007;1:470–8.
23. Ryu B-Y, Orwig KE, Oatley JM, Avarbock MR, Brinster RL. Effects of aging and niche microenvironment on spermatogonial stem cell self-renewal. Stem Cells (Dayton, Ohio). 2006;24:1505–11.
24. Carlson BM, Faulkner JA. Muscle transplantation between young and old rats: age of host determines recovery. Am J Physiol. 1989;256:C1262–6.
25. Mezzogiorno A, Coletta M, Zani BM, Cossu G, Molinaro M. Paracrine stimulation of senescent satellite cell proliferation by factors released by muscle or myotubes from young mice. Mech Ageing Dev. 1993;70:35–44.
26. Gopinath SD, Rando TA. Stem cell review series: aging of the skeletal muscle stem cell niche. Aging Cell. 2008;7:590–8.
27. Potten CS, Loeffler M. Stem cells: attributes, cycles, spirals, pitfalls and uncertainties. Lessons for and from the crypt. Development. 1990;110:1001–20.
28. Lynch MD. Selective pressure for a decreased rate of asymmetrical divisions within stem cell niches may contribute to age-related alterations in stem cell function. Rejuvenation Res. 2004;7:111–25.
29. Meineke FA, Potten CS, Loeffler M. Cell migration and organization in the intestinal crypt using a lattice-free model. Cell Prolif. 2001;34:253–66.

30. Holt PR, Yeh KY, Kotler DP. Altered controls of proliferation in proximal small intestine of the senescent rat. Proc Natl Acad Sci U S A. 1988;85:2771–5.
31. Charruyer A, et al. Transit-amplifying cell frequency and cell cycle kinetics are altered in aged epidermis. J Invest Dermatol. 2009;129:2574–83.
32. He S, Nakada D, Morrison SJ. Mechanisms of stem cell self-renewal. Annu Rev Cell Dev Biol. 2009;25:377–406.
33. Signer RAJ, Morrison SJ. Mechanisms that regulate stem cell aging and life span. Cell Stem Cell. 2013;12:152–65.
34. Nishino J, Kim I, Chada K, Morrison SJ. Hmga2 promotes neural stem cell self-renewal in young but not old mice by reducing p16Ink4a and p19Arf Expression. Cell. 2008;135:227–39.
35. Janzen V, et al. Stem-cell ageing modified by the cyclin-dependent kinase inhibitor p16INK4a. Nature. 2006;443:421–6.
36. Molofsky AV, et al. Increasing p16INK4a expression decreases forebrain progenitors and neurogenesis during ageing. Nature. 2006;443:448–52.
37. Doles J, Storer M, Cozzuto L, Roma G, Keyes WM. Age-associated inflammation inhibits epidermal stem cell function. Genes Dev. 2012;26:2144–53.
38. Keyes BE, et al. Nfatc1 orchestrates aging in hair follicle stem cells. Proc Natl Acad Sci U S A. 2013;110:E4950–9.
39. Walford RL. Letter: when is a mouse 'old'? J Immunol Baltim. 1976;117:352.
40. Miller RA, Nadon NL. Principles of animal use for gerontological research. J Gerontol A Biol Sci Med Sci. 2000;55:B117–23.
41. Hocking T. The physiology of human aging. 2005. at www.ocf.berkeley.edu/~tdhock/science/HumanAging.pdf
42. Rattan SIS. Increased molecular damage and heterogeneity as the basis of aging. Biol Chem. 2008;389:267–72.
43. Uchida N, Fleming WH, Alpern EJ, Weissman IL. Heterogeneity of hematopoietic stem cells. Curr Opin Immunol. 1993;5:177–84.
44. Morrison SJ, Weissman IL. The long-term repopulating subset of hematopoietic stem cells is deterministic and isolatable by phenotype. Immunity. 1994;1:661–73.
45. Oshima H, Rochat A, Kedzia C, Kobayashi K, Barrandon Y. Morphogenesis and renewal of hair follicles from adult multipotent stem cells. Cell. 2001;104:233–45.
46. Taylor G, Lehrer MS, Jensen PJ, Sun TT, Lavker RM. Involvement of follicular stem cells in forming not only the follicle but also the epidermis. Cell. 2000;102:451–61.
47. Ghadially R. In search of the elusive epidermal stem cell. Ernst Schering Res Found Workshop. 2005;54:45–62.
48. Schneider TE, et al. Measuring stem cell frequency in epidermis: a quantitative in vivo functional assay for long-term repopulating cells. Proc Natl Acad Sci U S A. 2003;100:11412–7.
49. Kaur P. Interfollicular epidermal stem cells: identification, challenges, potential. J Invest Dermatol. 2006;126:1450–8.
50. Nishimura EK, et al. Dominant role of the niche in melanocyte stem-cell fate determination. Nature. 2002;416:854–60.
51. Jones PH, Watt FM. Separation of human epidermal stem cells from transit amplifying cells on the basis of differences in integrin function and expression. Cell. 1993;73:713–24.
52. Terunuma A, Jackson KL, Kapoor V, Telford WG, Vogel JC. Side population keratinocytes resembling bone marrow side population stem cells are distinct from label-retaining keratinocyte stem cells. J Invest Dermatol. 2003;121:1095–103.
53. Triel C, Vestergaard ME, Bolund L, Jensen TG, Jensen UB. Side population cells in human and mouse epidermis lack stem cell characteristics. Exp Cell Res. 2004;295:79–90.
54. Li A, Simmons PJ, Kaur P. Identification and isolation of candidate human keratinocyte stem cells based on cell surface phenotype. Proc Natl Acad Sci U S A. 1998;95:3902–7.
55. Terunuma A, et al. Stem cell activity of human side population and alpha6 integrin-bright keratinocytes defined by a quantitative in vivo assay. Stem Cells (Dayton, Ohio). 2007;25:664–9.
56. Charruyer A, et al. CD133 is a marker for long-term repopulating murine epidermal stem cells. J Invest Dermatol. 2012. doi:10.1038/jid.2012.196.
57. Strachan LR, Scalapino KJ, Lawrence HJ, Ghadially R. Rapid adhesion to collagen isolates murine keratinocytes with limited long-term repopulating ability in vivo despite high clonogenicity in vitro. Stem Cells (Dayton, Ohio). 2008;26:235–43.
58. Szabo AZ, et al. The $CD44^{+}$ $ALDH^{+}$ population of human keratinocytes is enriched for epidermal stem cells with long-term repopulating ability. Stem Cells (Dayton, Ohio). 2013;31:786–99.
59. Li A, Pouliot N, Redvers R, Kaur P. Extensive tissue-regenerative capacity of neonatal human keratinocyte stem cells and their progeny. J Clin Invest. 2004;113:390–400.
60. Bickenbach JR. Identification and behavior of label-retaining cells in oral mucosa and skin. J Dent Res. 1981;60 Spec No C:1611–20.
61. Yang A, et al. p63 is essential for regenerative proliferation in limb, craniofacial and epithelial development. Nature. 1999;398:714–8.
62. Stasiak PC, Purkis PE, Leigh IM, Lane EB. Keratin 19: predicted amino acid sequence and broad tissue distribution suggest it evolved from keratinocyte keratins. J Invest Dermatol. 1989;92:707–16.
63. Lyle S, et al. The C8/144B monoclonal antibody recognizes cytokeratin 15 and defines the location of human hair follicle stem cells. J Cell Sci. 1998;111(Pt 21):3179–88.

64. Zhu AJ, Watt FM. Beta-catenin signalling modulates proliferative potential of human epidermal keratinocytes independently of intercellular adhesion. Dev Camb Engl 1999;126:2285–98.
65. Kaur P, Li A. Adhesive properties of human basal epidermal cells: an analysis of keratinocyte stem cells, transit amplifying cells, and postmitotic differentiating cells. J Invest Dermatol. 2000;114:413–20.
66. Braun KM, Watt FM. Epidermal label-retaining cells: background and recent applications. J Investig Dermatol Symp Proc. 2004;9:196–201.
67. Inoue K, et al. Differential expression of stem-cell-associated markers in human hair follicle epithelial cells. Lab Investig J Tech Methods Pathol. 2009;89:844–56.
68. Dunnwald M, Chinnathambi S, Alexandrunas D, Bickenbach JR. Mouse epidermal stem cells proceed through the cell cycle. J Cell Physiol. 2003;195:194–201.
69. Larderet G, et al. Human side population keratinocytes exhibit long-term proliferative potential and a specific gene expression profile and can form a pluristratified epidermis. Stem Cells Dayt Ohio. 2006;24:965–74.
70. Zhou J-X, et al. Enrichment and characterization of mouse putative epidermal stem cells. Cell Biol Int. 2004;28:523–9.
71. Michel M, et al. Keratin 19 as a biochemical marker of skin stem cells in vivo and in vitro: keratin 19 expressing cells are differentially localized in function of anatomic sites, and their number varies with donor age and culture stage. J Cell Sci. 1996;109(Pt 5):1017–28.
72. Sasahara Y, et al. Human keratinocytes derived from the bulge region of hair follicles are refractory to differentiation. Int J Oncol. 2009;34:1191–9.
73. Trempus CS, et al. CD34 expression by hair follicle stem cells is required for skin tumor development in mice. Cancer Res. 2007;67:4173–81.
74. Nakamura Y, et al. Expression of CD90 on keratinocyte stem/progenitor cells. Br J Dermatol. 2006;154:1062–70.
75. Jaks V, et al. Lgr5 marks cycling, yet long-lived, hair follicle stem cells. Nat Genet. 2008;40:1291–9.
76. Snippert HJ, et al. Lgr6 marks stem cells in the hair follicle that generate all cell lineages of the skin. Science. 2010;327:1385–9.
77. Nijhof JGW, et al. The cell-surface marker MTS24 identifies a novel population of follicular keratinocytes with characteristics of progenitor cells. Dev Camb Engl. 2006;133:3027–37.
78. Jensen KB, et al. Lrig1 expression defines a distinct multipotent stem cell population in mammalian epidermis. Cell Stem Cell. 2009;4:427–39.
79. Jensen KB, Watt FM. Single-cell expression profiling of human epidermal stem and transit-amplifying cells: Lrig1 is a regulator of stem cell quiescence. Proc Natl Acad Sci. 2006;103:11958–63.
80. Lowell S, Jones P, Le Roux I, Dunne J, Watt FM. Stimulation of human epidermal differentiation by delta-notch signalling at the boundaries of stem-cell clusters. Curr Biol CB. 2000;10:491–500.
81. Estrach S, Cordes R, Hozumi K, Gossler A, Watt FM. Role of the Notch ligand Delta1 in embryonic and adult mouse epidermis. J Invest Dermatol. 2008;128:825–32.
82. Pellegrini G, et al. p63 identifies keratinocyte stem cells. Proc Natl Acad Sci U S A. 2001;98:3156–61.
83. Fortunel NO, et al. Long-term expansion of human functional epidermal precursor cells: promotion of extensive amplification by low TGF-beta1 concentrations. J Cell Sci. 2003;116:4043–52.
84. Matic M. A subpopulation of human basal keratinocytes has a low/negative MHC class I expression. Hum Immunol. 2005;66:962–8.
85. Chen Z, Evans WH, Pflugfelder SC, Li D-Q. Gap junction protein connexin 43 serves as a negative marker for a stem cell-containing population of human limbal epithelial cells. Stem Cells Dayt Ohio. 2006;24:1265–73.
86. Wan H, et al. Desmosomal proteins, including desmoglein 3, serve as novel negative markers for epidermal stem cell-containing population of keratinocytes. J Cell Sci. 2003;116:4239–48.
87. Wan H, et al. Stem/progenitor cell-like properties of desmoglein 3dim cells in primary and immortalized keratinocyte lines. Stem Cells Dayt Ohio. 2007;25:1286–97.
88. Ohyama M, et al. Characterization and isolation of stem cell-enriched human hair follicle bulge cells. J Clin Invest. 2006;116:249–260.
89. Cerimele D, Celleno L, Serri F. Physiological changes in ageing skin. Br J Dermatol. 1990;122 Suppl 35:13–20.
90. Gerstein AD, Phillips TJ, Rogers GS, Gilchrest BA. Wound healing and aging. Dermatol Clin. 1993;11:749–57.
91. Gilchrest BA. In vitro assessment of keratinocyte aging. J Invest Dermatol. 1983;81:184s–9.
92. Grove GL. Age-related differences in healing of superficial skin wounds in humans. Arch Dermatol Res. 1982;272:381–5.
93. Grove GL, Kligman AM. Age-associated changes in human epidermal cell renewal. J Gerontol. 1983;38:137–42.
94. Haratake A, Uchida Y, Mimura K, Elias PM, Holleran WM. Intrinsically aged epidermis displays diminished UVB-induced alterations in barrier function associated with decreased proliferation. J Invest Dermatol. 1997;108:319–23.
95. Leyden JJ, McGinley KJ, Grove GL, Kligman AM. Age-related differences in the rate of desquamation of skin surface cells [proceedings]. Adv Exp Med Biol. 1978;97:297–8.
96. Roberts D, Marks R. The determination of regional and age variations in the rate of desquamation: a comparison of four techniques. J Invest Dermatol. 1980;74:13–6.
97. Ito M, et al. Stem cells in the hair follicle bulge contribute to wound repair but not to homeostasis of the epidermis. Nat Med. 2005;11:1351–4.

98. Nouy P. Biological Time. 1937.
99. Rheinwald JG, Green H. Epidermal growth factor and the multiplication of cultured human epidermal keratinocytes. Nature publishing group. 1977;265:421–4.
100. Rheinwald JG, Green H. Serial cultivation of strains of human epidermal keratinocytes: the formation of keratinizing colonies from single cells. Cell. 1975;6:331–43.
101. Barrandon Y, Green H. Three clonal types of keratinocyte with different capacities for multiplication. Proc Natl Acad Sci U S A. 1987;84:2302–6.
102. Youn SW, et al. Cellular senescence induced loss of stem cell proportion in the skin in vitro. J Dermatol Sci. 2004;35:113–23.
103. Liang L, et al. As epidermal stem cells age they do not substantially change their characteristics. J Investig Dermatol Symp Proc. 2004;9:229–37.
104. Giangreco A, Qin M, Pintar JE, Watt FM. Epidermal stem cells are retained in vivo throughout skin aging. Aging Cell. 2008;7:250–9.
105. Harrison DE, Astle CM, Stone M. Numbers and functions of transplantable primitive immunohematopoietic stem cells. Effects of age. J Immunol Baltim. 1989;142:3833–40.
106. Sudo K, Ema H, Morita Y, Nakauchi H. Age-associated characteristics of murine hematopoietic stem cells. J Exp Med. 2000;192:1273–80.
107. Falandry C, Bonnefoy M, Freyer G, Gilson E. Biology of cancer and aging: a complex association with cellular senescence. J Clin Oncol. 2014;32:2604–10.
108. Gniadecki R, Hansen M, Wulf HC. Resistance of senescent keratinocytes to UV-induced apoptosis. Cell Mol Biol. 2000;46:121–7.
109. Matta JL, et al. DNA repair and nonmelanoma skin cancer in Puerto Rican populations. J Am Acad Dermatol. 2003;49:433–9.
110. Wulf HC, Sandby-Møller J, Kobayasi T, Gniadecki R. Skin aging and natural photoprotection. Micron. 2004;35:185–91.
111. Trumpp A, Essers M, Wilson A. Awakening dormant haematopoietic stem cells. Nat Rev Immunol. 2010;10:201–9.
112. Schepers AG, et al. Lineage tracing reveals $Lgr5^+$ stem cell activity in mouse intestinal adenomas. Science. 2012;337:730–5.
113. Snippert HJ, Schepers AG, van Es JH, Simons BD, Clevers H. Biased competition between Lgr5 intestinal stem cells driven by oncogenic mutation induces clonal expansion. EMBO Rep. 2014;15:62–9.
114. Blanpain C, Lowry WE, Geoghegan A, Polak L, Fuchs E. Self-renewal, multipotency, and the existence of two cell populations within an epithelial stem cell niche. Cell. 2004;118:635–48.
115. Morris RJ, et al. Capturing and profiling adult hair follicle stem cells. Nat Biotechnol. 2004;22:411–7.
116. Tumbar T. Defining the epithelial stem cell niche in skin. Science. 2004;303:359–63.

Adipose-Derived Stem Cells and Their Secretory Factors for Skin Aging and Hair Loss

16

Byung-Soon Park and Won-Serk Kim

Contents

B.-S. Park (✉)
Cellpark Dermatology Clinic, Seoul, South Korea
e-mail: skinmd@naver.com

W.-S. Kim
Department of Dermatology, Kangbuk Samsung Hospital, Sungkyunkwan University College of Medicine, Seoul, South Korea
e-mail: susini@naver.com

M. A. Farage et al. (eds.), *Textbook of Aging Skin*,
DOI 10.1007/978-3-662-47398-6_20

Abstract

Human mesenchymal stem cells, by virtue of its capability to self-renew and differentiate into a variety of cell types, represent the first pluripotent stem cells to be used in clinical settings related to damage or degeneration. Therefore, there is an urgent need to understand how mesenchymal stem cells and their secretory factors contribute to regenerative medicine. Recent studies on the role of stem cells for skin and hair regeneration by many researchers including the authors have been remarkable. These scientific data enabled us to achieve the cost-effective treatment of skin aging using the legally acceptable cell therapeutic agents and their secretory factors. Objective data on the improvement of diverse aspects of skin aging including wound healing, wrinkle, and melasma due to photoaging have been available. Another progress has been made using the protein extract of the mesenchymal stem cells from the adipose tissue to promote hair growth in vitro, ex vivo, and in vivo by modulating the follicular cell cycles and hair cycle and protecting the follicular cells from androgens and reactive oxygen species. These approaches might mark the first practical application of stem cells among various trials in the field of skin and hair regeneration.

Introduction

The term "stem cell" has attracted increasing attention of the scientific community as well as of the general public. Overcoming confusion and difficulty to understand and interpret information about stem cells, much effort has been made in the field of skin and hair regeneration. They are vital to humans for numerous reasons. Groups of stem cells in some adult tissues give rise to replacement cells for the tissues that are destroyed through injury, disease, or aging [1]. Knowledge relating to how healthy cells replace diseased or otherwise damaged cells would allow development of medical therapies focusing on creation of compatible cell lines to replace aged or diseased cells in the body. The concept of regenerative medicine using the body's own stem cells and growth factors to repair tissue may be realizable as science and clinical experience converge to develop alternative therapeutic strategies to treat the damaged or diseased tissue. Stem cell-based therapies are also being tried in tissue engineering: the aim of tissue engineering is to repair and regenerate damaged organs or tissues using a combination of cells, biomaterials, and cytokines [1–4].

This chapter addresses the human subcutaneous adipose tissue as a promising source of adult mesenchymal stem cells. Adipose-derived stem cells (ADSCs) may offer a solution for the problem of limited availability of human cells that are capable of self-renewal and differentiation. ADSCs can be easily obtained from liposuction of human adipose tissue, cultured in a large scale, and display multi-lineage developmental plasticity. In addition, ADSCs secrete various cytokines and growth factors, which control and manage the damaged neighboring cells, and this has been identified as essential functions of ADSCs [5–7]. As reviewed elsewhere in this book, aging and photoaging are complex processes involving the wound-healing cascade and/or repetitive oxidative stress. Conventional antiaging skin treatments such as light-based or radiofrequency devices and/or peelings have been less than satisfactory because their primary mechanism is mainly inducing new collagen synthesis via activation of dermal fibroblasts. On the basis of previous studies that demonstrated wound healing, antioxidant, anti-wrinkle, and antimelanogenic effects of ADSCs and their secretory factors, they may be good candidates for the treatment of aging [5–9]. Another progress has been made in the field of hair growth using the ADSC protein extract [10, 11]. It was revealed that the protein extract promotes hair growth by modulating the follicular cell cycles and hair cycle and protecting the follicular cells from androgens and reactive oxygen species (ROS) [12, 13]. This chapter compiles the authors' recent research and clinical developments on skin and hair regeneration using ADSCs and their secretory factors.

Stem Cells and ADSCs

Stem cells are a population of immature tissue precursor cells capable of self-renewal and provision of multi-lineage differentiable cells for tissues. Although embryonic stem cell has multipotency, there are many limitations such as difficulties in control of differentiation and issues relating to ethics. As a result, use of adult stem cells with fewer implicating issues is becoming an area of increased interest in stem cell medicine. Given the vast potential of treatments utilizing stem cells, validation and evaluation regarding safety and efficacy will result in greater benefits.

ADSCs and Regeneration

Due to the lack of a specific and universal molecular marker for adult stem cells, functional assays for multiple differentiations must be used to identify stem cells in a tissue. Mesenchymal stem cells (MSCs) were first characterized in bone marrow, but many studies have reported the existence of MSCs in the connective tissue of several organs [14, 15]. The role of these cells is not entirely clear, but they are generally believed to constitute a reserve for tissue maintenance and repair. It was recently demonstrated that the most abundant and accessible source of adult stem cells is adipose tissue. The yield of MSCs from adipose tissue is approximately 40-fold greater than that from bone marrow [16–18].

The following are the highly consistent, although not identical, expression profiles of cell-surface proteins on ADSCs [2, 19]: adhesion molecules, receptor molecules, surface enzymes, extracellular matrix (ECM) proteins, and glycoproteins. However, hematopoietic cell markers such as CD14, CD31, and CD45 are not expressed. Interestingly, the immunophenotype of ADSCs resembles that reported for other adult stem cells prepared from human bone marrow (bone marrow stromal cell [BMSC]) and skeletal muscle [2]. Differentiation of ADSCs is not restricted to the adipocyte lineage, but they can be differentiated into chondrocyte, osteocyte, cardiomyocyte, neuron, etc. [20, 21]. In addition, activity comparison with BMSC revealed a similar regenerative capacity. Therefore, this abundant and accessible cell population has potential clinical utility for regenerating damaged or aged tissue and tissue engineering.

As with many rapidly developing fields, diverse names have been proposed to describe the plastic-adherent cell population isolated from collagenase digests of adipose tissue: adipose-derived stem/stromal cells, adipose-derived adult stem cells, adipose-derived adult stromal cells, adipose stromal cells (ASCs), adipose mesenchymal stem cells (AdMSCs), lipoblast, pericyte, preadipocyte, processed lipoaspirate (PLA) cells, and stromal vascular fraction (SVF) cells. To address the confusion due to diverse nomenclature, the International Fat Applied Technology Society reached a consensus to adopt the term "adipose-derived stem cells" to identify the isolated, plastic-adherent, multipotent cell population. Questioning the validity of the term "stem cell" led to the use of the acronym to mean "adipose-derived stromal cells" [22].

Although studies are limited, the quality and quantity of the ADSCs varies according to interperson differences, the harvest site, harvesting method, and culture conditions. Age and sex are the most obvious of the interperson differences. Stem cell recovery varies between subcutaneous white adipose tissue depots [23, 24]. Yield and growth characteristics of ADSC (Fig. 1) are also affected by the type of surgical procedure used for adipose tissue harvesting. Resection and tumescent liposuction seem to be preferable above ultrasound-assisted liposuction [25].

Mechanism of Action for Regeneration

Stem cell therapy is a safe, practical, and effective source for repair of damaged tissue [26, 27]. Despite rapid translation to the bedside, the

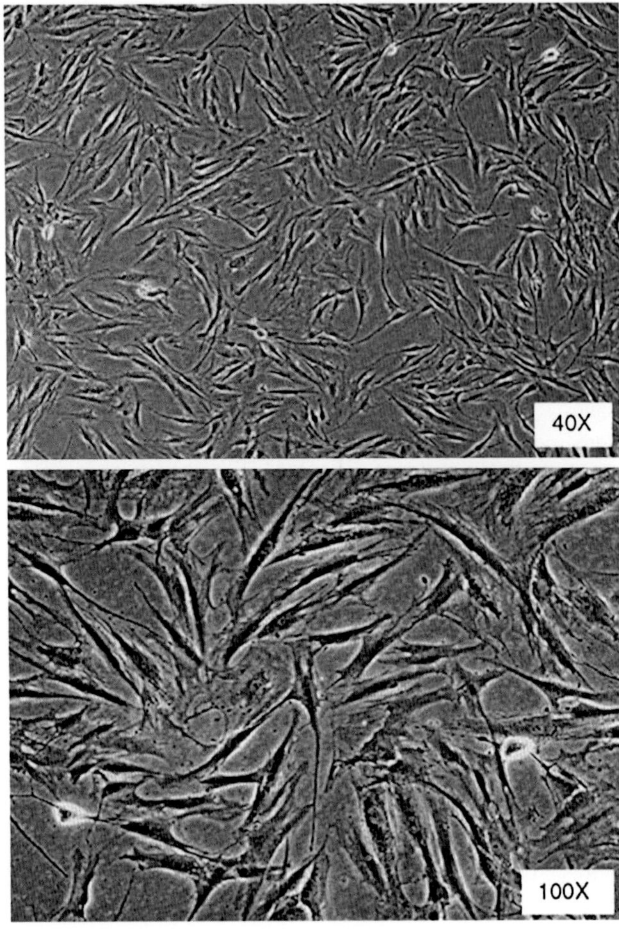

Fig. 1 ADSCs display adherent and fibroblastic morphology. They show abundant endoplasmic reticulum and large nucleus relative to the cytoplasmic volume (Reprinted with permission from Elsevier, Kim et al. [6])

mechanism of action for regeneration is not well characterized. It was initially hypothesized that immature stem cells migrate to the injured area, differentiate into the phenotype of injured tissue, repopulate the diseased organ with healthy cells, and subsequently repair the tissue (building-block function). However, this theory has some drawbacks because the levels of engraftment and survival of engrafted cells are too low to be therapeutically relevant [28]. In addition, acute stem cell-mediated improvement within days or even hours makes it difficult to fully explain the mechanisms by which regeneration occurs [29, 30]. Instead, much of the functional improvement and attenuation of injury afforded by stem cells can be repeated by treatment with cell-free conditioned media derived from ADSCs (ADSC-CM) [31]. Thus, it can be deduced that ADSCs may exert their beneficial effects via complex paracrine actions (manager function) in addition to building-block function.

Proteomic Analysis of ADSCs and Their Secretomes

Proteomics, large-scale studies of proteins, can be used to analyze the intracellular and secretory proteins of ADSCs. For example, Roche et al. conducted a 2-DE gel analysis of BMSCs and ADSCs and confirmed the similarity [32]. Zvonic et al. also analyzed the ADSC-CM by 2-DE gel electrophoresis, detected approximately 300 features from ADSC-CM, and found that secretomes are up-/downregulated by induction of adipogenesis [33]. Although the intracellular and secretory proteins of ADSCs have been analyzed through 2-DE-coupled mass spectrometry or non-gel-based mass spectrometry, the active proteins of ADSCs responsible for the tissue regeneration are not fully identified. This may be due to the fact that studies using proteomics has limitations as this approach is capable of analyzing highly abundant proteins only. Therefore, new mass spectrometry-based proteomic analysis techniques for stem cell proteins in correlation with other state-of-the-art analytical tools and functional study by neutralizing the candidate proteins are needed to clearly characterize the active proteins of regeneration.

Diverse Pharmacologic Actions

Wound-Healing Effect of ADSCs

Several studies of the pathophysiology of photoaging have detected similarities with certain aspects of acute and/or chronic wounds. Histologically, photoaged skin shows marked alterations in ECM composition. Skin wound repair by adult stem cells was originally demonstrated using BMSC. Wu et al. showed that BMSC injection around the wound significantly enhanced wound healing in normal and diabetic mice compared with that of allogeneic neonatal dermal fibroblasts [34]. Sasaki et al. demonstrated that BMSCs can differentiate into multiple skin cell types including keratinocytes, pericytes, and endothelial cells, which contribute to wound repair [35]. Notably, analyses of proteins in conditioned medium of BMSC (BMSC-CM) indicated that BMSCs secret distinctively different cytokines and chemokines compared to dermal fibroblasts [36]. ADSCs have surface markers and gene profiling similar to BMSCs, and their soluble factors are not significantly different [6, 14]. Given their convenient isolation compared with BMSCs and extensive proliferative capacities ex vivo, ADSCs hold great promise for use in wound repair and regeneration. However, there is little evidence demonstrating the wound-healing effects of ADSCs. It was also demonstrated that ADSCs accelerate wound healing, especially with regard to fibroblast activation [6]. They promote proliferation of dermal fibroblasts, not only by direct cell-to-cell contact but also by paracrine activation through secretory factors. This fibroblast-stimulating effect of ADSCs was superior to that of the fibroblasts. Furthermore, ADSC-CM enhanced secretion of type I collagen from dermal fibroblasts and stimulated fibroblast migration in in vitro wound-healing models. ADSCs secreted a variety of growth factors such as basic fibroblast growth factor (bFGF), KGF, TGF-b, hepatocyte growth factor (HGF), and VEGF into the conditioned medium, which might mediate the wound-healing effect of ADSCs. In addition to the in vitro evidence, the wound-healing effect of ADSCs was also verified in an animal study, which showed that topical administration of ADSCs significantly reduced the wound size (34 % reduction) and accelerated the re-epithelialization at the wound edge (Fig. 2). Similar to ADSC treatment,

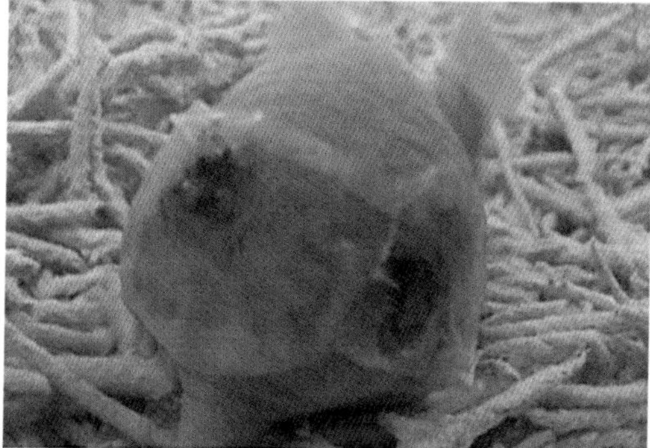

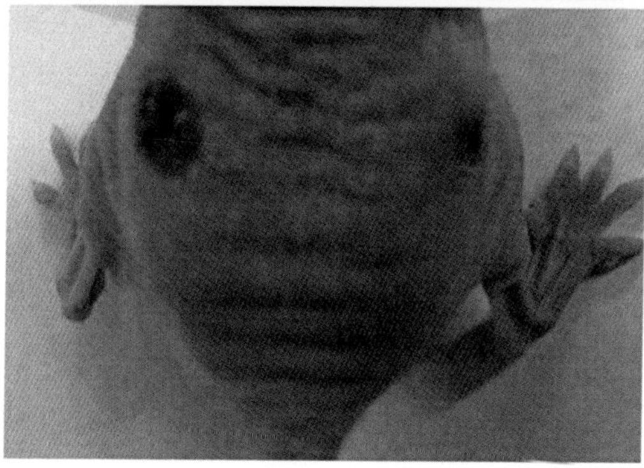

Fig. 2 Wound-healing effect of ADSCs in nude mice. Artificial wounds were made using a 6-mm punch biopsy and ADSCs were topically applied. The wound size was reduced significantly in the ADSC-treated side (*right* side of the back) 7 days after surgery (Reprinted with permission from Elsevier, Kim et al. [6])

ADSC-CM treatment also accelerated wound healing in laser-induced burn mouse models (authors' unpublished data). In this experiment, burn wounds were made by laser surgery in the epidermis, and they were significantly reduced by single and multiple administration of ADSC-CM. As ADSCs are physiologically located beneath dermal fibroblasts, they may interact with dermal fibroblasts. However, ADSCs and secretomes of ADSCs may reach the epidermis in wounded area and may affect the recovery of this layer. As such, ADSC-CM was treated in cultured primary human keratinocytes and shown to increase the proliferation and migration of keratinocytes [37]. This result suggests that secretomes of ADSCs also accelerate the healing of epidermal layer.

Antioxidant and Antimelanogenic Effects of ADSCs

ROS produced in the catalytic reactions by many environmental stimuli may be involved in the pathogenesis of a number of skin disorders including photoaging, photosensitivity diseases, and some types of cutaneous malignancy. Antioxidants, as a popular term in drug and cosmetics, take the form of enzymes, hormones, vitamins, and minerals. In biological systems, the normal processes of oxidation produce highly reactive free radicals, which may continue to damage even the body's own cells. Antioxidants scavenge free radicals before they get a chance to harm the body. As of now, there are few reports on the antioxidant action of stem cells. However, some evidences support the protective role of secretomes of ADSCs against the skin damage induced by reactive oxygen species. For example, IGF reportedly protects fibroblasts and intestinal epithelial cells from free radicals [38, 39]. HGF protects the retinal pigment epithelium against oxidative stress induced by glutathione depletion [40]. Pigment epithelium-derived factor (PEDF) is an anti-angiogenic/neurotropic factor and has been shown to have antioxidant effects [41]. Interleukin-6 (IL-6) reduces the epithelial cell death induced by hydrogen peroxide [42]. In addition, subtypes of superoxide dismutase (SOD) are expressed and secreted from ADSCs [43]. Therefore, antioxidant function of ADSC was investigated in dermal fibroblasts after inducing chemical oxidative stress by the tert-butyl hydroperoxide (tbOOH). Morphological change and cell survival assay revealed that incubation with ADSC-CM aided dermal fibroblasts to resist free radicals induced by tbOOH. In addition, activities of superoxide dismutase (SOD) and glutathione peroxidase (GPx) were enhanced in the dermal fibroblasts treated with ADSC-CM. In a cell cycle analysis, ADSC-CM treatment reversed the apoptotic cell death induced by ROS, which was demonstrated by a significant decrease of sub-G1 phase of dermal fibroblasts [8].

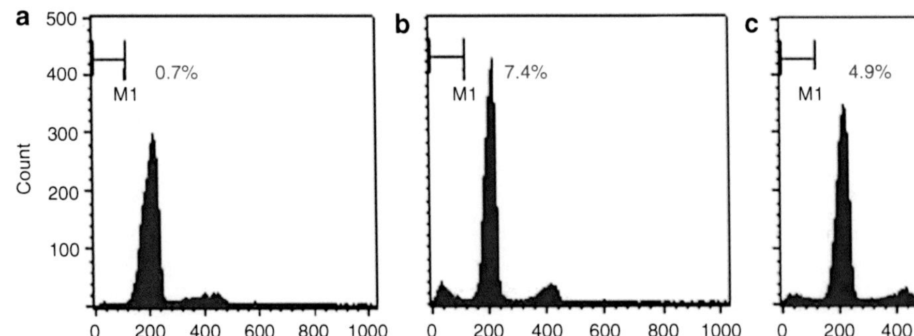

Fig. 3 Antioxidant effect of ADSCs in UVB-irradiated fibroblasts as shown by cell cycle analysis of DNA contents. Untreated fibroblasts showed little or no sub-G1 phases (**a**). However, UVB irradiation significantly increased sub-G1 (apoptotic) cells (**b**), which were reversed by ADSC-CM pretreatment (**c**) (Reprinted with permission from Elsevier, Kim et al. [5])

Photoaging is believed to be responsible for up to almost 80 % of the skin changes commonly attributed to the aging process. The study further investigated the antioxidant and protective effects of ADSCs in the photodamage of the primarily cultured dermal fibroblasts (Fig. 3). In this experiment, ADSC-CM pretreatment significantly reduced the apoptosis of dermal fibroblasts from UVB-induced damage, which was demonstrated by a significant decrease of sub-G1 phase of dermal fibroblasts after ADSC-CM pretreatment. In addition, ADSC-CM treatment increased the production of collagen and reduced the expression of matrix metalloproteinase-1 in the dermal fibroblasts. These results indicated that ADSCs can play a key role in protecting dermal fibroblast from UVB-induced oxidative stress [5].

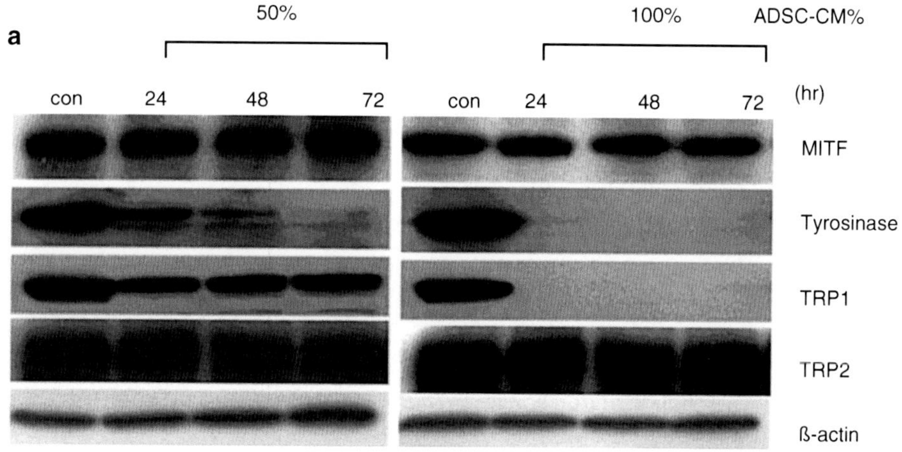

Fig. 4 (**a**) Antimelanogenic effect of ADSC-CM. Expression of MITF and TRP2 remained unchanged, but expressions of tyrosinase and TRP1 were downregulated by ADSC-CM treatment in B16 melanoma cells. (**b**) The inhibitory effect of ADSC on melanin synthesis is schematically represented (Reproduced with permission from Pharmaceutical Society of Japan, Kim et al. [9])

As antioxidants inhibit the chemical reactions leading to melanin formation, change the type of melanin formed, and interfere with the distribution of pigment and melanosome transfer, they are good candidates for skin whitening resources. As ADSC-CM is a free radical scavenger and has potent antioxidant activity, antimelanogenic effect of ADSC was investigated. ADSC-CM treatment inhibited the synthesis of melanin and the activity of tyrosinase in melanoma B16 cells. In addition, expressions of tyrosinase and tyrosinase-relating protein 1 were downregulated by ADSC-CM treatment, which indicated the mechanism of action for antimelanogenic effect of ADSCs and their soluble factors (Fig. 4) [9].

Animal Studies for Skin Aging

To study the effects on in vivo skin, ADSCs (1×10^6 cells) and ADSC-CM were intradermally injected on the back of a micropig, twice in a 14-day interval ($n = 3$). One month after the second injection, skin samples were obtained at the treatment and the control sites of adjacent normal skin. Although the increase in the dermal thickness was not significant, increased collagen expression was noted by Western blot in the ADSC- and ADSC-CM-treated skin samples (Fig. 5) [7].

In another experiment, photodamage was induced by an 8-week UVB irradiation in hairless mice. The irradiation dose was one MED (minimal erythema dose; 60 mJ/cm^2) in the first 2 weeks, two MED in the third week, three MED in the fourth week, and four MED in the fifth through eighth weeks. After wrinkle induction, varying numbers of ADSCs (A group: control; B group: 1×10^3 cells; C group: 1×10^4 cells; and D group: 1×10^5 cells) were subcutaneously injected into the mice ($n = 8$ for each group). In a replica analysis, parameters involving skin roughness were improved with mid-level and higher dose groups of ADSCs (C and D group) (Fig. 6). Dermal thickness was increased in the ADSC-injected groups (16 % and 28 % in C and D groups, respectively) and ECM contents in the dermis were also increased by Masson's trichrome staining results of collagen (blue) in the ADSC-treated groups (Fig. 7). As cell transplantation between species mediates immune rejection, the survival of ADSC from humans was investigated after injection of ADSCs labeled with PKH26

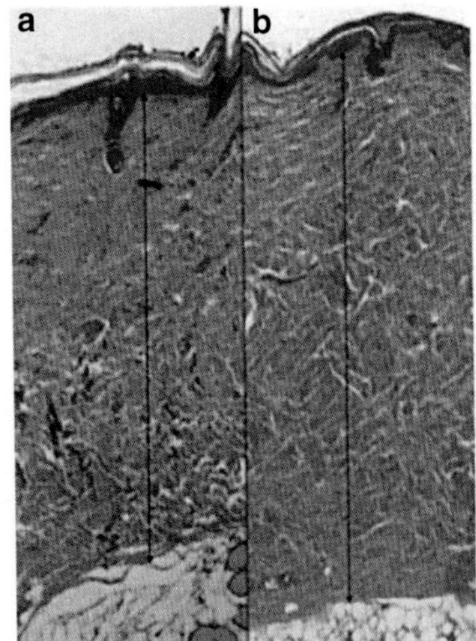

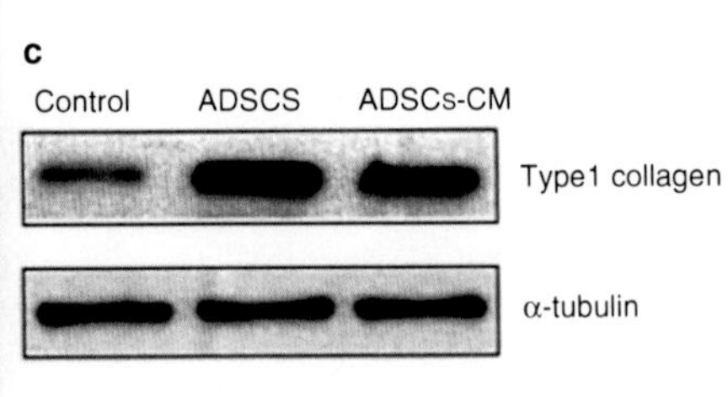

Fig. 5 Micropig experiment shows the change of dermal thickness without (**a**) and with (**b**) intradermal injections of ADSCs. Increased collagen expression was noted by Western blot in the ADSCs- and ADSC-CM-treated skin (**c**) (Reproduced with permission from Wiley-Blackwell, Park et al. [7])

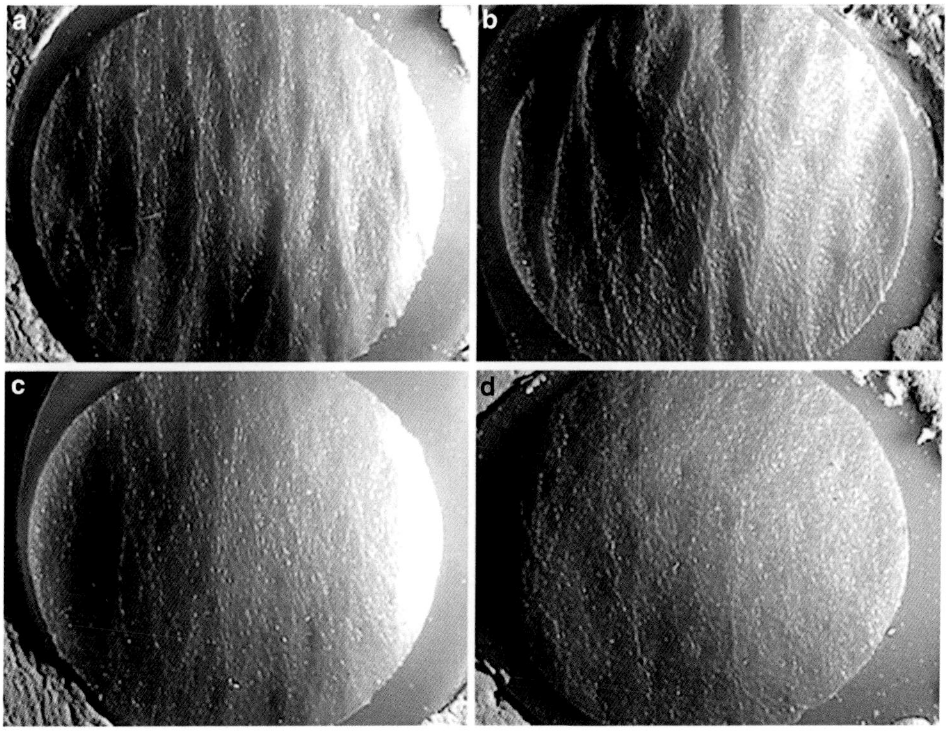

Fig. 6 Anti-wrinkle effects of ADSCs. Photodamage was induced by 8-week UVB irradiation in hairless mice, and ADSCs were intradermally and subcutaneously injected three times. Wrinkles were evaluated by replica analysis. (**a**) Control; (**b**) 1×10^3 cells; (**c**) 1×10^4 cells; (**d**) 1×10^5 cells (Reprinted with permission from Elsevier, Kim et al. [5])

(red color, Fig. 8 inset). As shown in Fig. 8, survival of the ADSCs was clearly demonstrated [5].

Clinical Application for Skin Aging

ADSCs and the ADSC Protein Extract for Skin Aging

As a pilot study, intradermal injections of purified autologous SVF cells (1×10^6 cells), which contain approximately 20–30 % ADSCs, were tried with photoaged skin of one patient [7] after informed consent. The female patient had two successive injections at 2-week intervals. Two months after the second injection, the patient showed improvements in general skin texture and wrinkling as evidenced by medical photographs of periorbital wrinkles. Measurements of dermal thickness by a 20 MHz high-frequency ultrasonographs (Dermascan-C, Cortex, Hadsund, Denmark) also indicated increased thickness (2.054 vs. 2.317 mm) (Fig. 9).

In a large-scale pilot study, the effects of the ADSC protein extract applied transdermally in the treatment of the various signs of skin aging were evaluated: (1) wrinkles, (2) acquired pigmentary lesions, and (3) dilated pores [44]. Korean patients visiting for the treatment of skin aging were recruited during September 2006–August 2007. The population ($n = 235$) aged 28–71 years (mean 41 years) had skin phototypes III and IV with mild to moderate photodamage. The advanced ADSC protein extract (AAPE®; Prostemics Inc., Seoul, Korea) was applied 3–12 times at 2-week intervals. The changes were evaluated objectively by photographic documentation and Robo Skin Analyzer CS100/VA100 (Inforward Inc., Tokyo, Japan) and subjectively by patient questionnaire. The evaluation score was based upon the following scales: 0 = poor/worsened; 1 = no change/no change; 2 = fair/

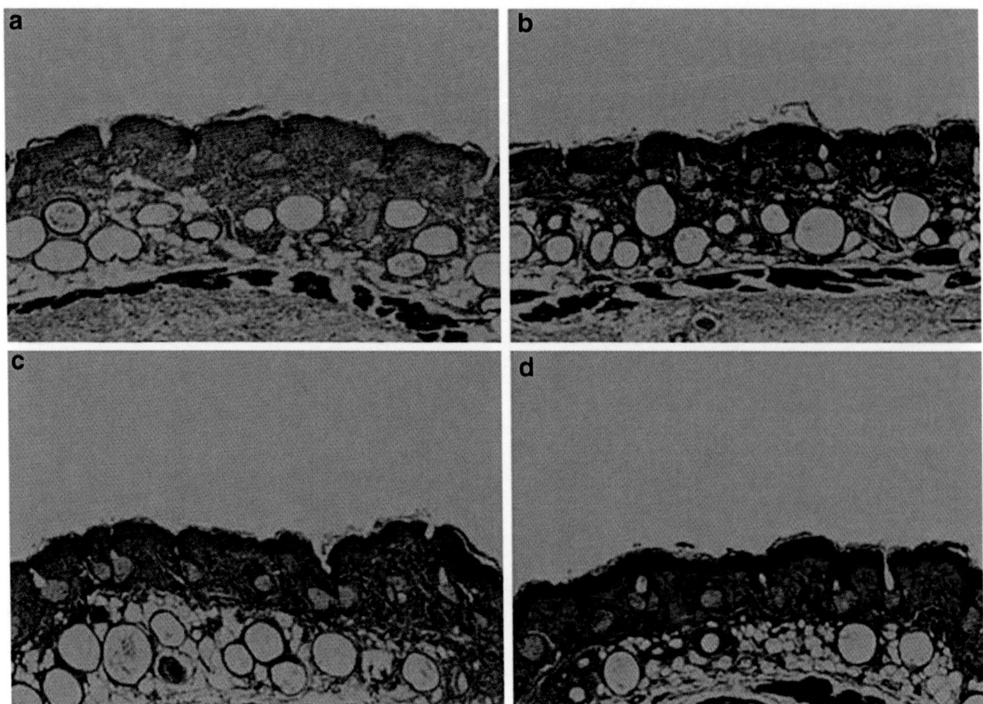

Fig. 7 Massson's trichrome staining shows that collagen contents (*blue*) are significantly increased in the mid-level (**c**) and higher dose (**d**) groups of ADSCs compared with control (**a**) and lower dose group (**b**) in photodamaged hairless mice experiment. (Reprined with permission from Elsevier, Kim et al. [5])

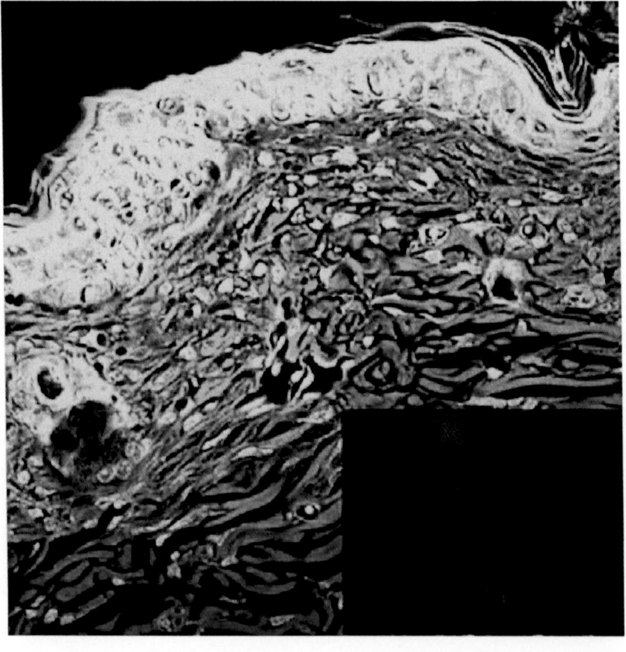

Fig. 8 Survival of ADSCs labeled with PKH26 *(insert)* injected in the skin of hairless mice. Two weeks after injection, mouse skin block was cryosectioned and counterstained with green-fluorescent nucleic acid stain. ADSCs are stained *red* (Reprinted with permission from Elsevier, Kim et al. [5])

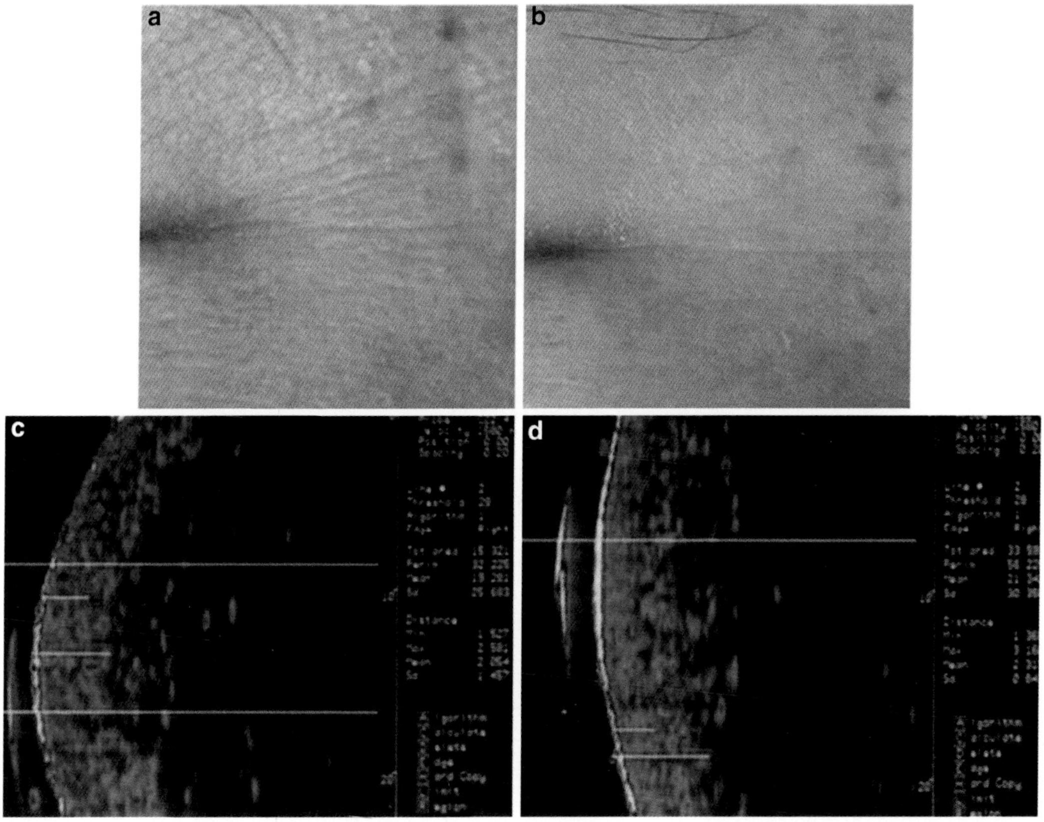

Fig. 9 Clinical study using intradermal injections of purified autologous SVF cells. Medical photographs of periorbital wrinkles were taken before (**a**) and after (**b**) treatment, and dermal thickness was measured by ultrasonographs before (**c**) and after (**d**) treatment. Improved general skin texture and increase thickness (2.054 vs. 2.317 mm) were evident 2 months after two injections (**b**, **d**) (Reprinted with permission from Wiley-Blackwell, Park et al. [7])

mild improvement; 3 = good/moderate improvement; and 4 = excellent/marked improvement. As compared to 47.4 % showing good to excellent improvement in wrinkle, 63 % of the patients were judged to have good to excellent improvement in acquired pigmentary lesions and dilated pores (Fig. 10).

Objective measurement of the periorbital wrinkles was performed with skin surface topography using PRIMOS (Phase Rapid In vivo Measurement of Skin) 3D in vivo optical skin measuring device. Twenty-three healthy females (range, 39–47; ages, mean 43 ± 5 years) applied AAPE® twice daily for 8 weeks. The evaluation was performed before and 4 and 8 weeks after treatment (data not published). There was statistically significant improvement ($p < 0.05$) in the crow's feet (Fig. 11).

Melasma is a multifactorial disorder caused by sun exposure, hormonal imbalance, and genetic predisposition. In many countries including Asia, melasma ranks among the top ten most common skin conditions. Ethnic differences between Asian and other skin types may influence the efficacy and tolerability of melasma treatments. Recent clinicopathologic studies on melasma show that lesional skin showed more prominent solar elastosis when compared to the normal skin [45]. Moreover, it has been suggested that interactions between the cutaneous vasculature and melanocytes might have an influence on the development of pigmentation [46]. The coexistence of telangiectasia and/or solar elastosis with melasma points out that photodamage is closely linked to the pathogenesis of melasma. The actions of ADSCs

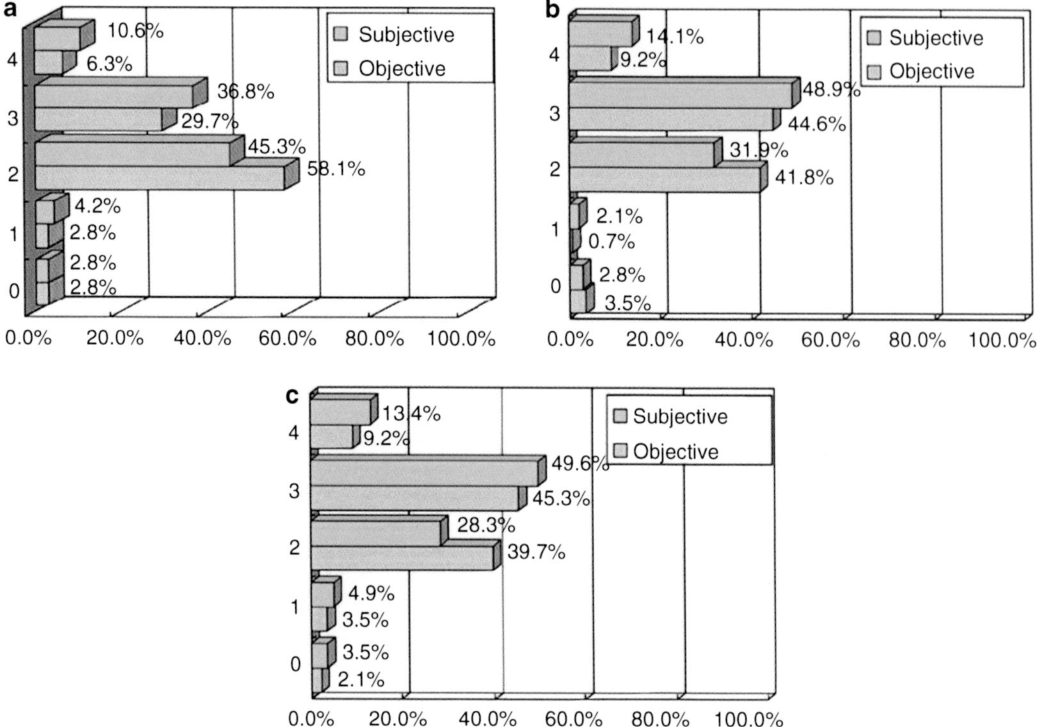

Fig. 10 Objective and subjective evaluation of the ADSC protein extract in a large-scale ($n = 235$) pilot study in terms of: (**a**) wrinkles, (**b**) acquired pigmentary lesions, and (**c**) dilated pores. The evaluation score is based upon the following scales: 0 poor/worsened; 1 no change/no change; 2 fair/mild improvement; 3 good/moderate improvement; and 4 excellent/marked improvement. As compared to 47.4 % showing good to excellent improvement in wrinkle (**a**), 63 % of the patients were judged to have good to excellent improvement in acquired pigmentary lesions (**b**) and dilated pores (**c**)

in wound healing, antioxidation, antimelanogenic effects and the reversal of photodamage in vitro, and in animal models prompted the clinicians to bring these biologic actions to bedside. The representative cases with marked response in melasma were shown in Fig. 12. These clinical results for the past 10 years suggest that the ADSCs and the protein extract are promising rational strategies for melasma and photodamage.

Combination with Other Procedures and Active Transdermal Delivery

Various light source and radiofrequency devices have been used for the treatment of skin aging by selectively heating up the collagen in the dermis to stimulate collagen remodeling. In general, both ablative and nonablative techniques lead to new collagen formation. As ADSCs and their secretory factors promote the wound healing by activating dermal fibroblasts, it can be speculated that when combined, ADSCs and the protein extract might augment the clinical effects beyond the intrinsic fibroblast-stimulatory effect of the various devices.

Based upon the previous documentation of wound-healing and antimelanogenic effects of ADSCs, the efficacy of the ADSC protein extract in reducing healing time and PIH or erythema was investigated after fractional CO_2 laser treatment (MiXto SX®, Lasering, Italy) in a pilot study as prospective, randomized, placebo-controlled, double-blinded, and split-face setting [47]. CO_2 fractional treatments have emerged as one of the new technologies in skin rejuvenation. However, comparatively increased incidence of PIH is problematic especially in dark-skinned patients. In this study, Korean patients of Fitzpatrick skin types III

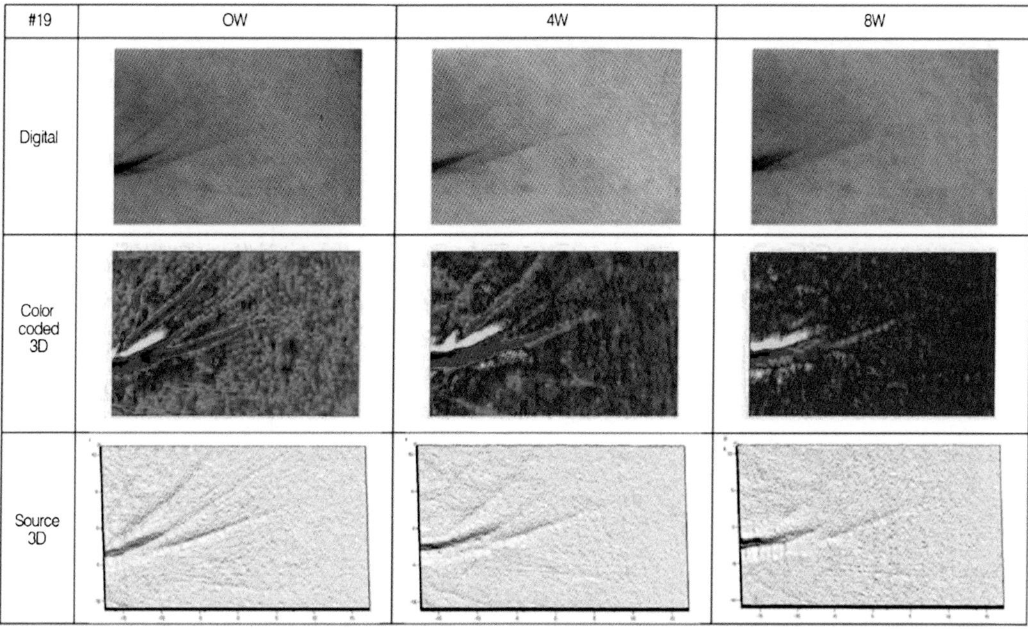

Fig. 11 Images of crow's feet before and after applying AAPE® cream 4 weeks and 8 weeks later (*upper*, fluorescence image; *middle*, color coded 3D image; *lower*, source 3D image)

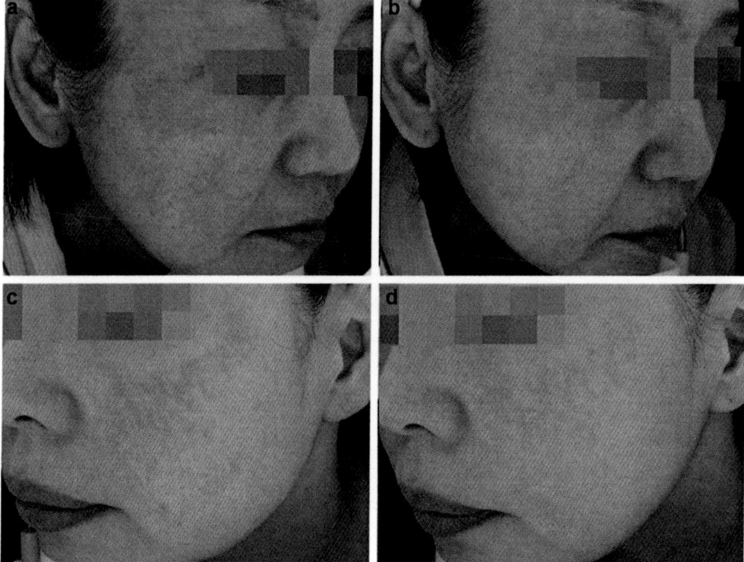

Fig. 12 The representative cases with marked response in whitening of melasma before (**a**, **c**) and after (**b**, **d**) treatment with the ADSC protein extract

and IV (mean age 45.7 years) with facial wrinkles were treated with full-face fractional CO_2 laser (parameter: 8 W, index level 8). All subjects were randomly allocated to split-face application of either the ADSC protein extract or emollient only. Serial photographs were taken at each visit during the treatment and 3-month follow-up period. Marked difference in the duration of erythema and healing was observed (Fig. 13). The quality of wound healing was noted to be improved. This therapy was well tolerated by majority of patients with minimal adverse effects.

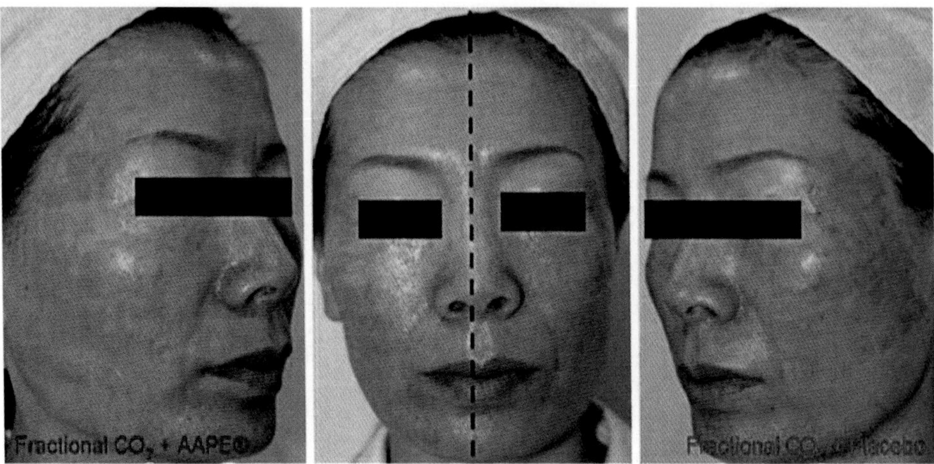

Fig. 13 A split-face comparison shows that the application of the ADSC protein extract results in less intense erythema and microcrusting 2 days after fractional CO_2 laser resurfacing

It was concluded that the ADSC protein extract can be safely and effectively used to prevent PIH and to accelerate wound healing after fractional CO_2 laser treatment in dark skin.

As the secretory factors of ADSCs generally contain ingredients of large molecular weights, various new "active" enhancement technologies designed to transiently circumvent the barrier function of the stratum corneum would be required for transdermal delivery: e.g., iontophoresis, sonophoresis, electroporation, or microneedle arrays or skinstamp.

Basic Mechanism of Hair Regeneration

It was revealed that treatment of the conditioned media of ADSCs (ADSC-CM) enhanced the proliferation of cultured human dermal papilla cells (DPCs) in vitro up to 130 % by activation of both Erk and Akt signaling pathways, which is crucial in enhancing the survival and proliferation of DPCs [12]. In addition, ADSC-CM increased cyclin D1 and CDK2, key cell cycle-related molecules [12]. These results reflect the beneficial efficacy on hair growth because the size and the number of dermal papilla correlate with the hair growth cycle [48]. DPCs are regarded as a key element for regenerating hair cycle [49]. It was revealed that ADSC-CM enhances the elongation of hair shafts by 40 % in ex vivo human hair organ cultures. The length of the cultured human hair follicles in an ADSC-CM-treated group significantly increased, as much as that seen in the follicles treated with 1 mM of minoxidil [12]. In in vivo study, the phase transition from telogen to anagen was found with the topical application of ADSC-CM on C3H/HeN nude mice. It was also revealed that ADSC-CM therapy can protect stressed follicular DPCs against ROS and DHT (Fig. 14) [13]. DHT directly inhibits the proliferation of androgen-sensitive DPCs, and this inhibition can be rescued by ADSC-CM [50]. The proposed mechanism of hair growth with the ADSC-CM treatment is summarized in Table 1.

Furthermore, the efficacy of ADSC-CM in hair growth promotion is potentiated through hypoxic preconditioning. When ADSCs are cultured under hypoxic conditions in vitro, their proliferative and self-renewal capacities are markedly increased [51]. ADSCs in hypoxic conditions produce increased amount of growth factors such as VEGF, PDGF, and insulin-like growth factor-binding protein (IGFBP) [52] which are related to hair growth. It was confirmed that ADSC-CM produced in hypoxic conditions induced the anagen phase of mouse more rapidly than that produced in normoxic conditions [52]. Based on those results of studies, AAPE® is produced under hypoxic conditions by providing 2 % O_2.

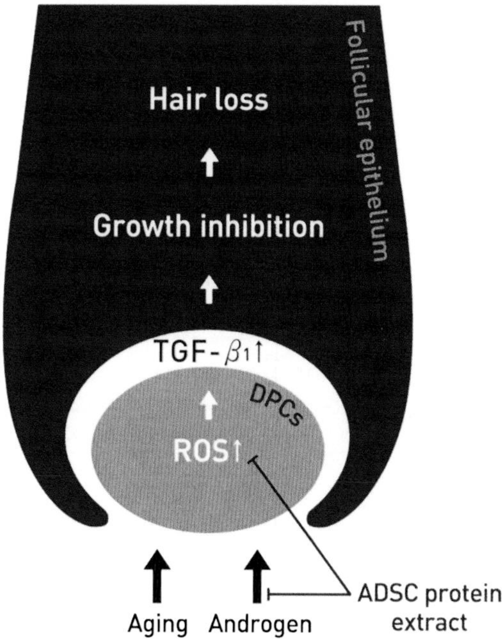

Fig. 14 Currently suggested potential mechanism of action in hair growth by ADSC-CM or the ADSC protein extract. *ADSC* adipose-derived stem cell, *DPCs* dermal papilla cells, *ROS* reactive oxygen species, *TGF* transforming growth factor

Table 1 The proposed mechanism of hair regeneration in the treatment with the ADSC protein extract

Increase the proliferation of hair follicular cells (DPCs, hair follicular epithelium) through modulation of cell cycle
Stimulate the phase transition from telogen to anagen
Protect DPCs from cytotoxic injury by androgen and ROS

Clinical Application for Hair Regeneration

The ADSC Protein Extract for Female Pattern Hair Loss

An observational pilot study was performed to evaluate the efficacy of the ADSC protein extract for the treatment of female pattern hair loss (FPHL) comparing with the baseline status without control [10]. Twenty-seven patients (aged 22–69 years, mean 42 ± 13 years) with FPHL received applications of AAPE® (now termed as NGAL™) for 12 weeks (Fig. 15). Hair density increased from 105.4 to 122.7 counts/cm^2 (P <0.001). Mean hair thickness increased from 57.5 to 64.0 μm (P <0.001). None of the patients reported severe adverse reactions.

The microneedling is widely used to enhance the absorption of topical therapeutics. There has been no report that the use of the microneedle itself ameliorates hair loss [53]. Nine patients among 27 were followed up to 6 months, and one up to 1 year. The clinical improvement was maintained, and they did not complain aggravation of hair loss.

The ADSC Protein Extract for Male Pattern Hair Loss

Another pilot study was performed to evaluate the efficacy of ADSC protein extract for the treatment of male pattern hair loss (MPHL) [11]. This pilot study compared the efficacy with the baseline status without the control group. Twenty-five patients (aged 28–60 years, mean 49 ± 9 years) with MPHL received weekly applications of AAPE® (now termed as NGAL™) without any other treatments such as oral and topical agents. As in the study for FPHL, a microneedle or a mesotherapy gun was used to deliver AAPE® to the scalp. After 12 weeks of therapy, hair density increased from 97.7 to 108.1 counts/cm^2 (P <0.001). Mean hair thickness increased from 65.4 to 71.8 μm (P <0.001). None of the patients reported severe adverse reactions.

These results reveal that the application of the ADSC protein extract could be also effective for MPHL (Fig. 16). The current gold standard treatment for MPHL consists of finasteride medication and topical minoxidil alone or in combination. It remains to be further elucidated whether the ADSC protein extract could completely substitute for the current medical treatment or could be an excellent synergistic tool for patients who feel that the current therapeutic regimen is not fully satisfactory.

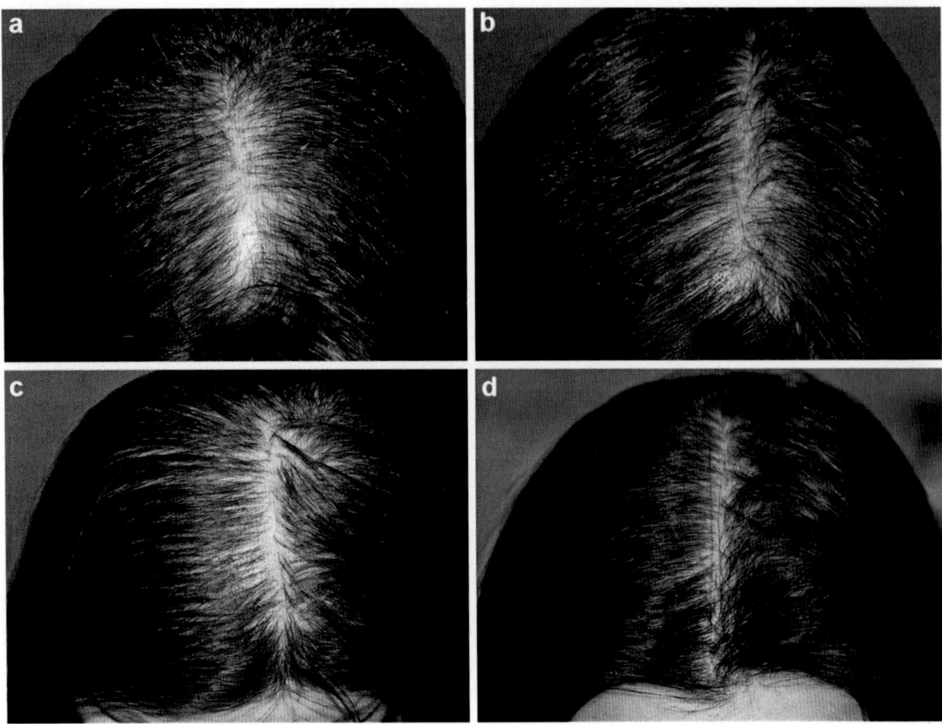

Fig. 15 The representative cases with marked response in hair growth before (**a**, **c**) and after (**b**, **d**) treatment of FPHL with the ADSC protein extract

Split-Scalp Comparison Study Using the ADSC Protein Extract in Patients with MPHL

Split-scalp study was designed to objectively evaluate the effect of the ADSC protein extract on hair loss [11]. Six male healthy patients (aged 20–52 years, mean 36 ± 12 years) with MPHL (Hamilton-Norwood classification type II–IV) were recruited. The scalp was split into the right and left sides: each reference point was shaved to create a circle of 1.0 cm in diameter and then tattooed. AAPE® (now termed as NGAL™) and the vehicle placebo were applied to one half of the scalp weekly, respectively. They had not used any products or taken any drugs that might have affected hair growth for more than 6 months prior to the study.

Close-contact photographic images were taken using a phototrichogram (Folliscope®: LeadM, Seoul, Korea) at a magnification of ×30 at first and 12 weeks after treatment: after 12 weeks, the previously tattooed reference area was shaved again for the follow-up phototrichogram to evaluate the efficacy of the treatment. This phototrichogram comparison study allowed the observer to trace the changes follicle by follicle as each follicle was designated by serial numbers (Fig. 17). This study was more accurate than the previously described studies in which the density and the hair thickness were measured. After 12 weeks of therapy, the total hair count was significantly higher on the AAPE®-treated side of the reference circle than on the vehicle-treated side ($p = 0.002$, paired t-test). The incidence of adverse effects such as pruritus and local irritation was negligible.

Conclusion

The current topics of increasing interest in the dermatological field are anatomical-functional damage to the skin and every possible means to counteract the injurious effects. In the beginning,

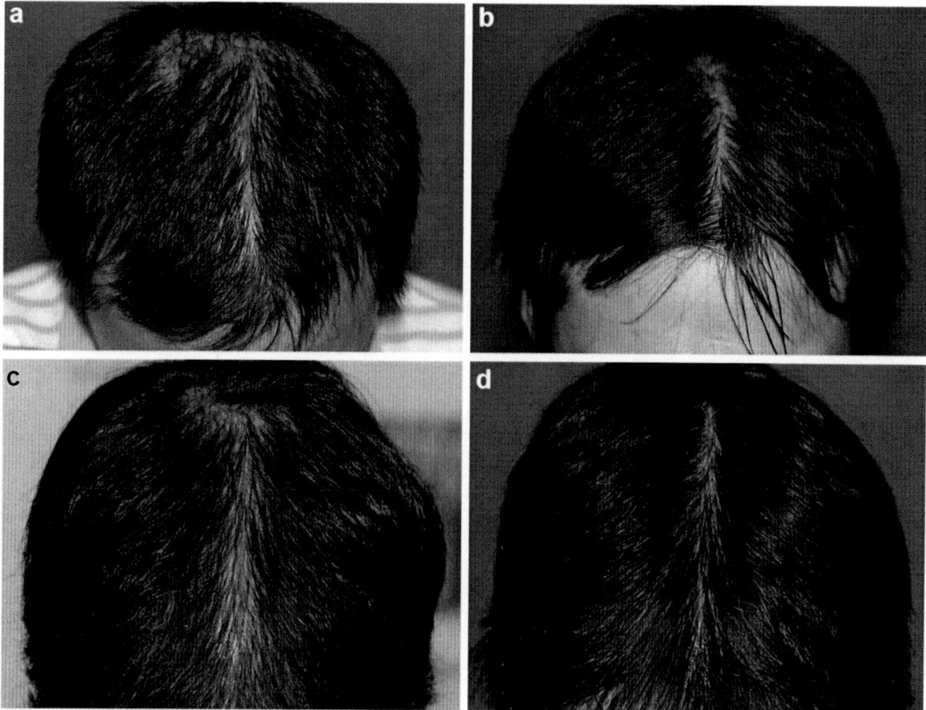

Fig. 16 The representative cases with marked response in hair growth before (**a**, **c**) and after (**b**, **d**) treatment of MPHL with the ADSC protein extract

ADSCs were shown to increase the survival rate in fat transplantation [54]. This chapter explains that ADSCs and their secretory factors have diverse pharmacologic effects for skin aging and hair regeneration. There were some safety concerns on the clinical application of cultured ADSCs and their secretory factors for human skin: the threat of passing on viruses, passing on diseases from other animal source nutrients to cultured stem cells in the laboratory. However, in 2010, Korean Ministry of Food and Drug Safety issued a safety guideline on manufacturing conditioned media from human cells and tissues. The safety guideline includes donor eligibility determination, sanitation and maintenance of cell culture facilities, manufacture of human origin cell/tissue culture media, safety evaluation of human origin cell/tissue culture media, and analytical procedure of human origin cell/tissue culture media [55].

In addition, ADSCs have to overcome the obstacles in that they are difficult both to handle and to commercialize in an industrial point of view: how to store the ADSCs, the containers to store them, how to transport them to the point, and the shelf life in various environments. Therefore, new methods and materials to overcome these limitations are needed. Secretomes of ADSCs have some advantages over cell-based therapies and might have greater potential in skin regeneration, because they can be manufactured in a large scale with long-term stability and they are relatively devoid of safety issues. As such, the study demonstrated that photodamage can be reversed by utilizing the ADSCs/their secretory factors alone [5, 7, 44] or in combination with other devices minimizing unwanted effects [47]. Identification of active proteins will be the next goal, and drug development using these proteins will suggest better strategies for skin aging in the future.

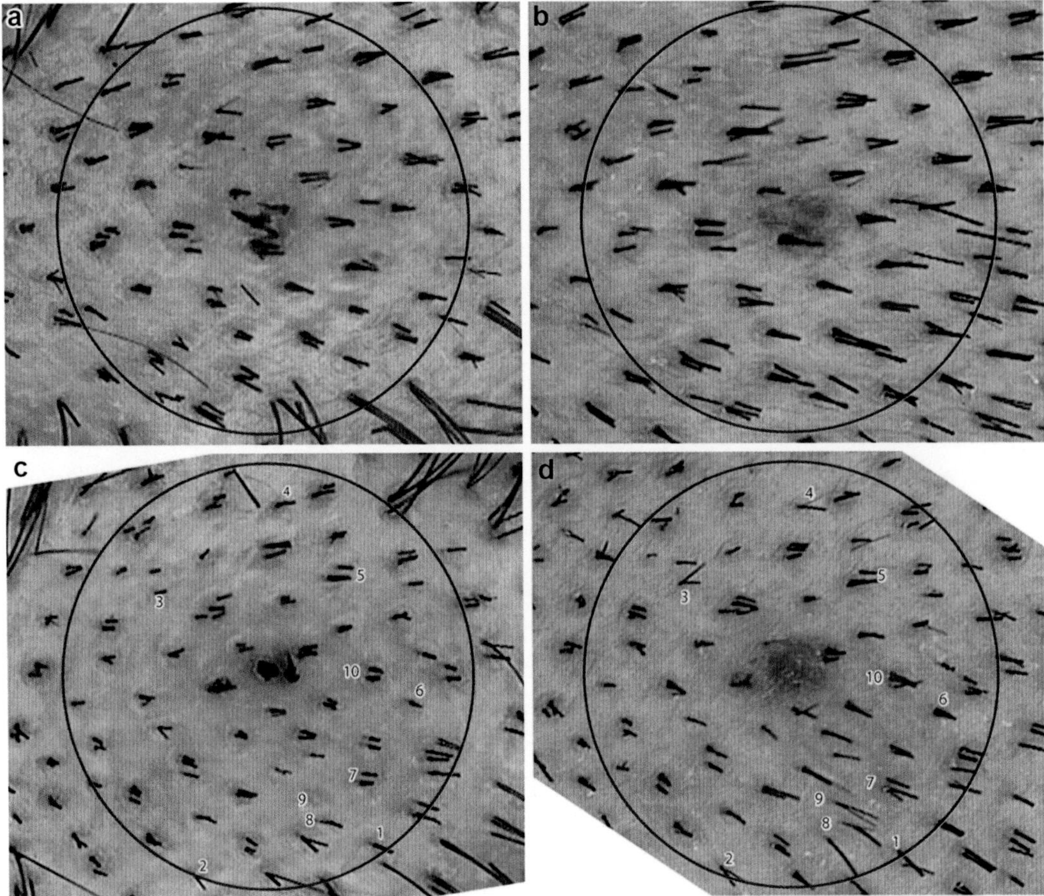

Fig. 17 Phototrichogram analysis of a patient with male pattern hair loss who received split-scalp treatment. Total hair count was measured in the circle of 1 cm diameter. The total hair count remained almost unchanged on the vehicle-treated side before (**a**) and after 12 week-treatment (**b**). By contrast, the total hair count on the AAPE®-treated side increased by 12 after 12 weeks of treatment (**d**) compared with that before treatment (**c**). Split-scalp comparison allowed the observer to trace the changes follicle by follicle as each follicle was designated by serial numbers. *Red* figures indicate the follicle numbers that showed increase in hair counts

References

1. Barry FP, et al. Mesenchymal stem cells: clinical applications and biological characterization. Int J Biochem Cell Biol. 2004;36:568–84.
2. Gimble J, et al. Adipose-derived adult stem cells: isolation, characterization, and differentiation potential. Cytotherapy. 2003;5:362–9.
3. Kinnaird T, et al. Marrow-derived stromal cells express genes encoding a broad spectrum of arteriogenic cytokines and promote in vitro and in vivo arteriogenesis through paracrine mechanisms. Circ Res. 2004;94:678–85.
4. Zuk PA, et al. Human adipose tissue is a source of multipotent stem cells. Mol Biol Cell. 2002;13:4279–95.
5. Kim WS, et al. Antiwrinkle effect of adipose derived stell cell: activation of dermal fibroblast by secretory factors. J Dermatol Sci. 2009;53:96–102.
6. Kim WS, et al. Wound healing effect of adipose-derived stem cells: a critical role of secretory factors on human dermal fibroblasts. J Dermatol Sci. 2007;48:15–24.
7. Park BS, et al. Adipose-derived stem cells and their secretory factors as a promising therapy for skin aging. Dermatol Surg. 2008;34:1323–6.
8. Kim WS, et al. Evidence supporting antioxidant action of adipose-derived stem cells: protection of human dermal fibroblasts from oxidative stress. J Dermatol Sci. 2008;49:133–42.
9. Kim WS, et al. Whitening effect of adipose-derived stem cells: a critical role of TGF-beta 1. Biol Pharm Bull. 2008;31:606–10.

10. Shin H, et al. Clinical use of conditioned media of adipose tissue-derived stem cells in female pattern hair loss: a retrospective case series study. Int J Dermatol. 2015;54(6):730–5.
11. Shin H, et al. Up-to-date clinical trials of hair regeneration using conditioned media of adipose-derived stem cells in male and female pattern hair loss. Curr Stem Cell Res Ther. (accepted for publication).
12. Won CH, et al. Hair growth promoting effects of adipose tissue-derived stem cells. J Dermatol Sci. 2010;57(2):134–7.
13. Won CH, et al. The basic mechanism of hair growth stimulation by mesenchymal stem cells and their secretory factors for the treatment of hair loss. Curr Stem Cell Res Ther. (accepted for publication).
14. Izadpanah R, et al. Biologic properties of mesenchymal stem cells derived from bone marrow and adipose tissue. J Cell Biochem. 2006;99:1285–97.
15. Porada CD, et al. Adult mesenchymal stem cells: a pluripotent population with multiple applications. Curr Stem Cell Res Ther. 2006;1:365–9.
16. Boquest AC, et al. Epigenetic programming of mesenchymal stem cells from human adipose tissue. Stem Cell Rev. 2006;2:319–29.
17. Huang T, et al. Neuron-like differentiation of adipose derived stem cells from infant piglets in vitro. J Spinal Cord Med. 2007;30:35–40.
18. Kern S, et al. Comparative analysis of mesenchymal stem cells from bone marrow, umbilical cord blood, or adipose tissue. Stem Cells. 2006;24:1294–301.
19. Katz AJ, et al. Cell surface and transcriptional characterization of human adipose-derived adherent stromal (hADAS) cells. Stem Cells. 2005;23:412–23.
20. Anghileri E, et al. Neuronal differentiation potential of human adipose-derived mesenchymal stem cells. Stem Cells Dev. 2008;17:909–16.
21. Bunnell BA, et al. Differentiation of adipose stem cells. Methods Mol Biol. 2008;456:155–71.
22. Gimble JM, et al. Adipose-derived stem cells for regenerative medicine. Circ Res. 2007;100:1249–60.
23. Schipper BM, et al. Regional anatomic and age effects on cell function of human adipose-derived stem cells. Ann Plast Surg. 2008;60:538–44.
24. Jurgens WJ, et al. Effect of tissue-harvesting site on yield of stem cells derived from adipose tissue: implications for cell-based therapies. Cell Tissue Res. 2008;332:415–26.
25. Oedayrajsingh-Varma MJ, et al. Adipose tissue-derived mesenchymal stem cell yield and growth characteristics are affected by the tissue-harvesting procedure. Cytotherapy. 2006;8:166–77.
26. Schachinger V, et al. Intracoronary bone marrow-derived progenitor cells in acute myocardial infarction. N Engl J Med. 2006;355:1210–21.
27. Schachinger V, et al. Improved clinical outcome after intracoronary administration of bone-marrow-derived progenitor cells in acute myocardial infarction: final 1-year results of the REPAIR-AMI trial. Eur Heart J. 2006;27:2775–83.
28. Uemura R, et al. Bone marrow stem cells prevent left ventricular remodeling of ischemic heart through paracrine signaling. Circ Res. 2006;98:1414–21.
29. Wang M, et al. Pretreatment with adult progenitor cells improves recovery and decreases native myocardial proinflammatory signaling after ischemia. Shock. 2006;25:454–9.
30. Crisostomo PR, et al. In the adult mesenchymal stem cell population, source gender is a biologically relevant aspect of protective power. Surgery. 2007;142:215–21.
31. Patel KM, et al. Mesenchymal stem cells attenuate hypoxic pulmonary vasoconstriction by a paracrine mechanism. J Surg Res. 2007;143:281–5.
32. Roche S, et al. Comparative proteomic analysis of human mesenchymal and embryonic stem cells: towards the definition of a mesenchymal stem cell proteomic signature. Proteomics. 2009;9:223–32.
33. Zvonic S, et al. Secretome of primary cultures of human adipose-derived stem cells. Mol Cell Proteomics. 2007;6:18–28.
34. Wu Y, et al. Mesenchymal stem cells enhance wound healing through differentiation and angiogenesis. Stem Cells. 2007;25:2648–59.
35. Sasaki M, et al. Mesenchymal stem cells are recruited into wounded skin and contribute to wound repair by transdifferentiation into multiple skin cell type. J Immunol. 2008;180:2581–7.
36. Chen L, et al. Paracrine factors of mesenchymal stem cells recruit macrophages and endothelial lineage cells and enhance wound healing. PLoS One. 2008;3:e1886.
37. Moon KM, et al. The effect of secretory factors of adipose-derived stem cells on human keratinocytes. Int J Mol Sci. 2012;13(1):1239–57. doi:10.3390/ijms13011239. Epub 2012 Jan 23.
38. Baregamian N, et al. IGF-1 protects intestinal epithelial cells from oxidative stress induced apoptosis. Surg Res. 2006;136:31–7.
39. Rahman ZA, et al. Antioxidant effects of glutathione and IGF in a hyperglycaemic cell culture model of fibroblasts: some actions of advanced glycaemic end products (AGE) and nicotine. Endocr Metab Immune Disord Drug Targets. 2006;6:279–86.
40. Shibuki H, et al. Expression and neuroprotective effect of hepatocyte growth factor in retinal ischemia-reperfusion injury. Invest Ophthalmol Vis Sci. 2002;43:528–36.
41. Tsao YP, et al. Pigment epithelium derived factor inhibits oxidative stress-induced cell death by activation of extracellular signal-regulated kinases in cultured retinal pigment epithelial cells. Life Sci. 2006;79:545–50.
42. Kida H, et al. Protective effect of IL-6 on alveolar epithelial cell death induced by hydrogen peroxide. Am J Physiol. 2005;288:342–9.
43. Liochev SI, et al. How does superoxide dismutase protect against tumor necrosis factor: a hypothesis informed by effect of superoxide on "free" iron. Free Radic Biol Med. 1997;23:668–71.

44. Kang SH, et al. Improvement of melasma and scars with the secretory factors from ADSCs. Korean J Dermatol. 2007;45 Suppl 2:136.
45. Kang WH, et al. Melasma: histopathological characteristics in 56 Korean patients. Br J Dermatol. 2002;146:228–37.
46. Kim EH, et al. The vascular characteristics of melasma. J Dermatol Sci. 2007;46:111–6.
47. Park BS, et al. Rejuvenation of aging skin using fractional CO_2 laser resurfacing followed by topical application of ADSC protein extract. Korean J Dermatol. 2008;46 Suppl 1:266–7.
48. Elliott K, et al. Differences in hair follicle dermal papilla volume are due to extracellular matrix volume and cell number: implications for the control of hair follicle size and androgen responses. J Invest Dermatol. 1999;113(6):873–7.
49. Yoon SY, et al. A role of placental growth factor in hair growth. J Dermatol Sci. 2014;74(2):125–34.
50. Shin H, et al. Induction of transforming growth factor-beta 1 by androgen is mediated by reactive oxygen species in hair follicle dermal papilla cells. BMB Rep. 2013;46(9):460–4.
51. Kim JH, et al. The pivotal role of reactive oxygen species generation in the hypoxia-induced stimulation of adipose-derived stem cells. Stem Cells Dev. 2011;20(10):1753–61.
52. Park BS, et al. Hair growth stimulated by conditioned medium of adipose-derived stem cells is enhanced by hypoxia: evidence of increased growth factor secretion. Biomed Res. 2010;31(1):27–34.
53. Lee YB, et al. Effects of topical application of growth factors followed by microneedle therapy in women with female pattern hair loss: a pilot study. J Dermatol. 2013;40(1):81–3.
54. Matsumoto D, et al. Cell-assisted lipotransfer: supportive use of human adipose-derived cells for soft tissue augmentation with lipoinjection. Tissue Eng. 2006;12:3375–82.
55. Park BS. Stem cell cosmetics: development, safety regulation, mechanism and practical application. J Korean Med Soc Cosmetics. 2014;3(2):66–72.

Peroxisome Proliferator-Activated Receptors: Role in Skin Health and Appearance of Photoaged Skin

17

Stacy S. Hawkins, William Shingleton, Jean Adamus, and Helen Meldrum

Contents

Abstract

The outermost layers of the epidermis are critical for providing a barrier against environmental factors. An intact epidermal barrier is critical for preventing moisture loss and maintaining the health. Peroxisome proliferator-activated receptors (PPARs) are ligand-activated transcription factors that belong to the nuclear hormone receptor superfamily. There is evidence that similar to other nuclear receptors, PPARs perform a significant role in skin homeostasis. The emphasis of this chapter will be the role of PPARs in the maintenance and improvement of human epidermal skin conditions.

Introduction

The outermost layers of the epidermis are critical for providing a barrier against environmental factors, such as damage due to chronic UV irradiation and pollutants. An intact epidermal barrier is critical for preventing moisture loss and maintaining the health, function, and attractive appearance of the skin throughout the aging process [1–3]. Peroxisome proliferator-activated receptors (PPARs) are ligand-activated transcription factors that belong to the nuclear hormone receptor superfamily. Other nuclear hormone receptors include steroid hormones, thyroid hormones, and vitamin D hormones, and there is evidence that similar to other nuclear receptors, PPARs perform a significant role in skin homeostasis [4]. Like other

S.S. Hawkins (✉) • J. Adamus • H. Meldrum
Unilever Research and Development, Trumbull, CT, USA
e-mail: stacy.hawkins@unilever.com; jean.adamus@unilever.com; helen.meldrum@uniliver.com

W. Shingleton
General Electric Company, Cardiff, UK
e-mail: bill.shingleton@ge.com

M.A. Farage et al. (eds.), *Textbook of Aging Skin*,
DOI 10.1007/978-3-662-47398-6_21

nuclear receptor superfamily members, PPARs contain both a ligand-binding domain and a DNA-binding domain. On ligand activation, PPARs form a heterodimer with retinoic X receptors (RXRs); the resulting complex then binds to PPAR-response elements (PPREs), leading to either an increase or a decrease in the expression of target genes [4, 5]. Although PPAR target genes have been identified across many clinical applications (e.g., cell proliferation, differentiation, inflammation and angiogenesis, atherosclerosis, lipid and glucose metabolism [4]), the emphasis of this chapter will be the role of PPARs in the maintenance and improvement of human epidermal skin conditions.

PPARs: Role in Epidermal Structure and Function

PPAR-mediated effects on skin homeostasis as well as disease treatment are now well accepted, and it has been shown that activators of PPARs are important regulators of epidermal differentiation. Since the potential roles of PPARs were first identified by Issemann and Green in 1990 [6], three isotypes have been identified in the human epidermis to date: PPARα, PPARβ/δ, and PPARγ [7–9]. Over the past 15 years, PPARs have been studied for many clinical applications in dermatology, such as epidermal permeability barrier development and homeostasis [10, 11], stimulation of epidermal keratinocyte differentiation [5, 12–15], and keratinocyte response to inflammation [16, 17], and for treatment of epidermal disorders characterized by inflammation, keratinocyte hyperproliferation, and abnormal differentiation such as psoriasis [9, 18, 19]. Several pharmaceutical PPAR ligands have been developed; however, the endogenous ligands are naturally occurring fatty acids.

PPAR lipids have also been shown to increase expression of epidermal differentiation proteins in vitro (e.g., transglutaminase [Tgase], involucrin, profilaggrin) and promote cornified cell envelope (CE) maturation in normal human keratinocytes [5]. PPARα agonists have been shown to increase the synthesis of epidermal lipids critical to maintaining a healthy permeability barrier in a living skin equivalent model [20]. Knockout and mutant mouse models have been used to determine the importance of PPARα in epidermal maturation and homeostasis. Analysis has shown that although the barrier function was normal, the stratum granulosum was thinner, with focal parakeratosis, suggesting impaired keratinocyte differentiation, as reflected by a moderate decrease in differentiation markers [21]. A recent study has demonstrated a role for PPAR agonists in improvement in skin barrier in a newborn mouse model, through increased lipid synthesis and acidification [22].

In the skin, induction of PPARγ results in skin inflammatory diseases such as atopic and allergic contact dermatitis or psoriasis. Topical PPARγ agonists troglitazone and ciglitazone increased differentiation markers and promoted epidermal barrier recovery in hairless mice [14], possibly through ERK1/2 and p38 signaling [23]. PPARβ/δ is the most abundant of the three isotypes found in the skin, yet functionally less defined due to its lack of specific ligands [8, 24]. In keratinocytes, it has been shown to be involved in differentiation, lipid accumulation, directional sensing, polarization, and migration [15, 16]. PPARβ/δ may also play a role in the epidermal barrier formation, as evidenced in the LSE model [20] and also in primary keratinocytes [25].

In barrier-compromised skin such as the axillary area, PPAR ligands have been shown to improve epidermal skin condition, as measured by increased involucrin and filaggrin by immunohistochemistry compared to vehicle control, following a repeat patch test [26]. More recently, PPAR lipids have been shown to significantly improve the photoaged appearance after long-term product application [27, 28].

PPARs: Role in Inflammation and Skin Aging

Inflammation is a contributing factor in many aging processes in the human body, from intrinsic aging to the pathogenesis of age-related diseases such as atherosclerosis, Alzheimer's disease, and arthritis. There is a wealth of information in the literature documenting the anti-inflammatory role of PPARs in a variety of animal models, cell types, human tissues, and diseases [29–34]. Therefore, this section of the review focuses on the skin-specific influences of PPARs on inflammation.

In the field of dermatology, inflammation or irritation is associated with many diseases, and activation of PPARs has been shown to have beneficial effects on a number of skin conditions [17, 33, 35–37]. Marketed pharmaceuticals for the treatment of inflammatory skin disorders include agonists to PPARα and PPARγ. The mode of action of these drugs is, in part, through reduction of inflammation. Concomitant with this appears to be a normalization of epidermal turnover [38].

The expression of PPARα and PPARγ in psoriatic skin is unchanged or even reduced; however, PPARβ/δ is upregulated [18]. In mouse skin, PPARβ/δ is upregulated in direct response to the pro-inflammatory cytokine interferon-γ (IFN-γ) [16]. Recently, it has been demonstrated that PPARβ/δ mediates tumor necrosis factor (TNF)-induced survival of activated T cells within psoriatic lesions [39]. This suggests that PPARβ/δ may actually contribute to the pathogenesis of psoriasis. However, in a mouse model of wound healing, TNFα via PPARβ/δ promotes both epidermal differentiation and moderation of inflammation [16]. This mechanism involves ceramide as a second messenger in the TNF signaling cascade leading to upregulation of PPARβ/δ. So the role of PPARβ/δ as a mediator of inflammation and epidermal homeostasis appears to be highly dependent on the environment that the keratinocyte is in (e.g., wounded or inflamed), as well as on the species of animal model or the disease state.

It is interesting to note that ceramide can play a role in the upregulation of PPARβ/δ [16]. It could be speculated that the increased synthesis and secretion of ceramides during epidermal differentiation could concomitantly increase the expression of PPARβ/δ. This may explain why PPARβ/δ is the most abundant PPAR found in normal skin [8, 18].

PPARα agonists such as clofibric acid and WY-14643 appear able to reduce inflammation by preventing inflammatory cell infiltrate. In mouse models of irritant and allergen contact dermatitis, these agonists reduced the amount of pro-inflammatory cytokines, TNFα and interleukin-1 (IL-1) [17]. These cytokines are key drivers of the inflammatory cascades that lead to the migration of inflammatory cells into affected tissues. In this model, the authors comment on the fact that the PPARα agonists were of similar potency as the corticosteroid clobetasol, an indication of the potential for PPAR therapies in treating inflammatory skin disease.

The levels of inflammatory mediators – such as IL-1β, TNFα, IL-6, cyclooxygenase-2 (COX-2), and inducible nitric oxide synthase (iNOS) – increase with age, and aged animals have an increased sensitivity to inflammatory stimuli [34]. A key signaling pathway for both synthesis and activity of pro-inflammatory mediators is the nuclear factor-κB (NK-κB) pathway. Under normal conditions the NF-κB pathway is activated transiently, to enable an appropriate response to the stimulating challenge, such as injury or infection. As resolution of the insult proceeds, the pathway's activity decreases. However, in aged animals there is evidence for constitutive activation of NF-κB, which may contribute to the acceleration of the aging process [40]. Activation of PPARα has been shown to repress NF-κB signaling and reduce production of IL-6 and IL-12 [41]. A recent article has proposed that the inhibitor of NF-κB kinase-alpha (IKKα) is a master regulator of epidermal differentiation [42]. The role of IKKα within the NF-κB signaling pathway is to phosphorylate inhibitors of NF-κB (IκBs), allowing translocation of NF-κB to the nucleus. Exactly how IKKα is involved in keratinocyte differentiation is not completely clear, but these data suggest that keratinocyte hyperproliferation may be driven, in part, by inflammatory pathways. This appears to demonstrate that epidermal homeostasis is very closely linked to the inflammatory status of the skin and that PPARs could be intricately involved in regulation of both.

Exposure to UV light accelerates skin aging, and UV exposure induces skin inflammation, which is a major player in skin aging. While UVB will only penetrate to the epidermis, UVA can penetrate the skin to the dermis, where it will initiate a cascade of events that leads to the degradation of the dermal extracellular matrix. These changes take the form of increased collagen degradation, increased catabolic activity of dermal fibroblasts, and effects on the vasculature that promote the infiltration of inflammatory cells. This infiltrate adds to the catabolic environment within the dermis. Cytokines and chemokines are key to this process, as they orchestrate the response to the UV insult. As discussed above, many of the pro-inflammatory mediators act via the NF-κB intracellular signaling pathway. As such, PPARs are likely to be involved in mediating the inflammatory reaction to UV exposure.

There is evidence that pretreatment of the skin with the PPARα agonist WY-14643 protects against UVB-induced erythema [43]. UVB can only penetrate as far as the epidermis; however, the ultimate effect of UVB irradiation in this model is an increase in erythema, which suggests keratinocyte-induced effects could be driving dermal vasculature changes that lead to the increased blood flow – in other words, an epidermal-induced dermal effect. Potential mediators for this epidermal-driven process could be IL-8 and IL-6. IL-8 is a CXC chemokine known to be expressed by keratinocytes [44], and its function is to draw inflammatory cells out of the vasculature to the seat of an infection or injury. IL-6 is a prominent early-phase cytokine, released in response to insult, which triggers many inflammatory cascades. Expressions of IL-6 and IL-8 were both reduced by WY-14643 in UVB-irradiated keratinocyte cultures [43].

In addition to being induced in response to UV irradiation, IL-6 is known to be upregulated with age [45–47], raising the possibility that IL-6 may play a role in skin aging. IL-6 is a member of a family of cytokines known as the gp130-binding cytokines. They are grouped together as their receptor complexes share a common receptor subunit: gp130. The primary signaling pathway utilized by this family is the Janus kinase/signal transducer and activator of transcription (JAK/STAT) pathway. It is known that members of the IL-6 family, which includes oncostatin M also present in the skin [48, 49], can synergize with IL-1 or TNF to induce matrix-degrading enzymes [50]. Data from this and similar studies [51–53] suggest that low, physiologically relevant levels of the cytokines are enough to induce catabolic events that could contribute to the molecular causes of aged skin. The synergies between these cytokines occur at convergence points within their intracellular signaling pathways. There is evidence in the literature that activation of PPARs can repress the activity of the JAK/STAT pathway [54] and the AP-1 pathway [16]. This evidence, and the fact that PPARs may be able to regulate IL-6 expression in UV-induced inflammation and induce repressive pressures on NF-κB signaling, suggests that intervention or prophylactic treatment with PPAR therapies may be able to ameliorate some of the inflammation-driven causes of premature skin aging.

Many of the natural ligands for PPARs are lipids; therefore, it is not surprising that some members of the bioactive lipid mediator families, prostaglandins, leukotrienes, and thromboxanes, have been identified as PPAR ligands. One such mediator is leukotriene B_4 (LTB_4). The identification of LTB_4 as a PPARα ligand came about during investigations to explore whether induction of PPARα activity would increase the catabolism of LTB_4 [55]. The pro-inflammatory actions of LTB_4 are controlled via its catabolism by peroxisomal enzymes; thus, increasing peroxisomes via PPARs was investigated. This was indeed the case; the authors demonstrated that PPARα knockout mice took longer to resolve LTB_4-induced inflammation.

Prostaglandin E_2 (PGE_2) is a pro-inflammatory mediator that is also derived from the membrane-bound lipid arachidonic acid. Cyclooxygenase enzymes (COX-1 and COX-2) are responsible for the initial cleavage of arachidonic acid, which, via intermediates, leads to the synthesis of PGE_2 and other bioactive lipid mediators. PGE_2 is required for UVB-induced inflammation and is the main prostaglandin produced by keratinocytes [56]. While there is no evidence to date that PGE_2 can bind directly to PPARs, there is evidence in the literature that activation of PPARγ can suppress the transcriptional activation of COX-2 and subsequent synthesis of PGE_2 [57]. The PPARγ ligands tested in this study were ciglitazone, troglitazone, and 15-deoxy-$\Delta^{12,14}$-prostaglandin J_2 (15d-PGJ_2). 15d-PGJ_2 is another member of the prostaglandin family; however, binding of 15d-PGJ_2 to its target receptors tends to elicit anti-inflammatory events. 15d-PGJ_2 is a natural ligand for PPARγ, and its effects on the synthesis of prostaglandins by suppressing the synthesis of COX-2 are PPARγ dependent. 15d-PGJ_2 can also mediate anti-inflammatory activity independent of PPARγ [54]. As discussed above, PPARs can act upon the JAK/STAT pathway to reduce inflammation. It appears that 15d-PGJ_2 can reduce the activity of this pathway [58, 59].

CLA: A Naturally Occurring Lipid with PPAR Activity

Dietary literature suggests that conjugated linoleic acid (CLA) provides a number of physiologic health benefits to the immune system from supplements, which may involve regulation of prostaglandin, cytokine, and PPAR pathways. (For reviews, see [59–61] and references therein.) CLA may be extracted from sunflower or safflower oil and is naturally present in a number of foods, including dairy products (milk, cheese, butter, yogurt) and meats (beef, lamb). CLA is a collective term for positional and geometric (cis/trans) isomers of linoleic acid (C18:2), in which two double bonds are conjugated (e.g., separated by one carbon-carbon single bond). Principal isomers produced from the conjugation of linoleic acid are *cis*-9, *trans*-11 CLA and *trans*-10, *cis*-12 CLA (Fig. 1).

CLA has been shown to be a natural ligand for all three of the PPAR receptors [60, 62, 63]. While most studies on CLA have been directed at understanding the dietary benefits of CLA supplementation, the potential to use CLA as topically applied cosmetic ingredient to improve the appearance of photoaged skin is being investigated.

Previous research has demonstrated that CLA delivers a variety of antiaging benefits to the skin, including a reduction in the appearance of overall photodamage, mottled hyperpigmentation, lines and wrinkles, and coarse wrinkles [28].

Clinical Studies with CLA: Evidence of Antiaging Benefit from Topical Application

Photodamaged Split-Application Facial Studies

Healthy female subjects (ages 40–70 years), with Fitzpatrick skin types I–III and a moderate degree of expert-assessed photodamage, were enrolled in institutional review board-approved, randomized, split-face application studies. A total of 64 subjects were enrolled to complete two facial photodamage studies. Subjects provided informed consent to participate in each study. Subjects were excluded if they had previous reactions to α-hydroxyl acids, retinoids, fragrances, or soaps. Test products were a cream containing 3 % CLA and its vehicle. Subjects applied each test product (approximately 0.35 g for each side at each application) to each side of their face twice daily for 12–16 weeks. Subjects were instructed to use their current cleansing regimen throughout the study and agreed to discontinue the use of their normal moisturizers and other antiaging products (e.g., masks, eye creams, or gels) throughout the study. Expert visual assessment of photodamage attributes in the periorbital region (rated on a 0–9 scale, where 0 = none, 1–3 = mild, 4–6 = moderate, and 7–9 = severe) was performed at baseline and at monthly time points by an expert clinical evaluator. Fine lines in the crow's feet area (periorbital), fine lines under the eye, and overall photodamage were assessed on each side of the face. Analysis of between-treatment differences observed by expert visual assessment was calculated using the Wilcoxon signed-rank test. Digital photos were obtained at baseline and Weeks 12 and 16 for each side of the face (approximately 45° views) to record improvement in the appearance of photodamage using the VISIA-CR® photography system (Canfield Scientific, Inc., Fairfield, NJ, USA). Color calibration cards

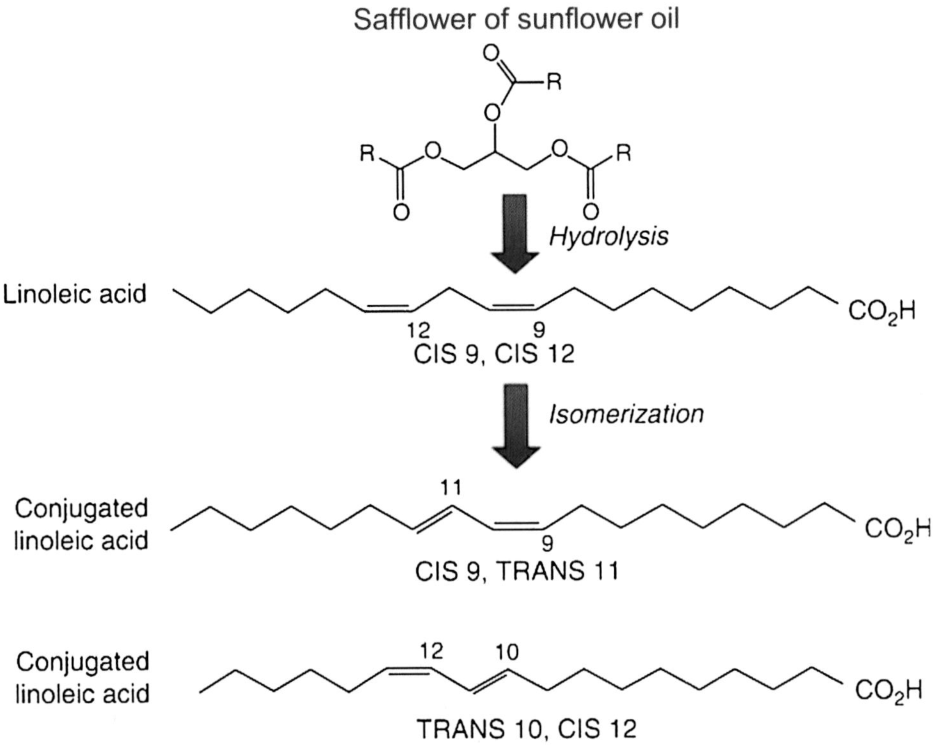

Safflower of sunflower oil

Hydrolysis

Linoleic acid CO_2H

12 9

CIS 9, CIS 12

Isomerization

Conjugated linoleic acid CO_2H

11 9

CIS 9, TRANS 11

Conjugated linoleic acid CO_2H

12 10

TRANS 10, CIS 12

Fig. 1 Conjugated linoleic acid (*CLA*). CLA is a collective term for positional and geometric (cis/trans) isomers of linoleic acid (C18:2), in which two double bonds are conjugated (e.g., separated by one carbon-carbon single bond). Principal isomers produced from the conjugation of linoleic acid are *cis*-9, *trans*-11 CLA and *trans*-10, *cis*-12 CLA

were used to ensure and monitor quality of the images throughout the studies.

Twenty-five subjects completed the first facial study, which was a 16-week double-blind product application study. The CLA cream significantly improved the appearance of photodamage attributes from baseline conditions (Figs. 2, 3, and 4) as assessed by an expert clinical evaluator. Fine lines in the crow's feet and under-eye areas significantly improved from baseline conditions at Weeks 12 and 16 ($p < 0.05$). By Week 12, the CLA cream provided significant improvement in expert visual assessment of photodamage attributes compared to its vehicle cream (Figs. 2, 3, and 4), which continued at Week 16. Sample photos of individual subjects (baseline compared to Week 16) are shown in Figs. 5 and 6. Clinical improvement of fine lines and wrinkles in the periorbital region was observed, as well as improvement in overall appearance.

Thirty-nine subjects completed the second facial study, which was a 12-week double-blind product application study. Expert visual evaluation of photodamage was performed at baseline and after 12 weeks of product application. Objective measurements with 3D facial scans were obtained using the Cyberware™ 3030/HIREZ facial scanner (Cyberware, Inc., Monterey, CA, USA) at baseline and at Weeks 2, 4, 6, 8, and 12. Virtual 3D images were obtained via facial scanning, across a 15-cm vertical line, 90° section, sampled at a rate of 0.2°. The resulting scans captured images approximately from ear to ear on each subject's face. The vertical scan data captured images approximately from subjects' chins upward to mid-forehead, depending on the

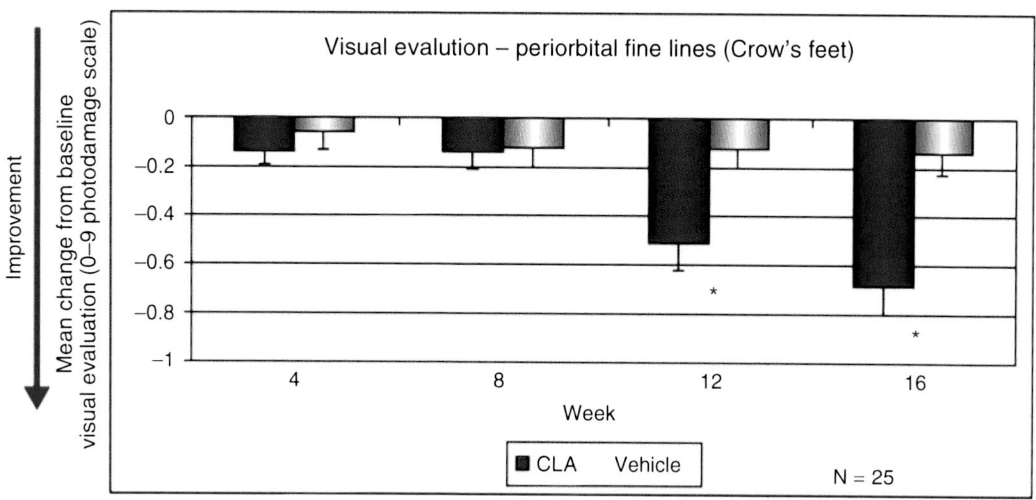

Fig. 2 Clinical evaluation of periorbital fine lines. Compared to its vehicle, CLA cream significantly improved the appearance of periorbital fine lines ($P < 0.05$)

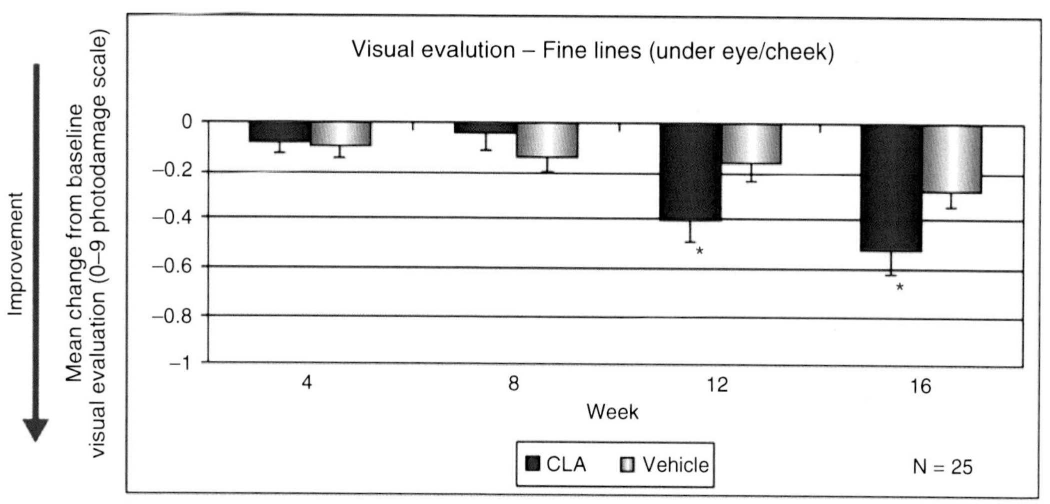

Fig. 3 Clinical evaluation of fine lines under the eye. Compared to its vehicle, CLA cream significantly improved the appearance of fine lines under the eye and on the upper cheek ($P < 0.05$)

size of the individual's face. The nasolabial fold lines, characterized by length and depth parameters, were quantified using Echo-TK/Cyscan™ software.

At Week 12, fine lines in the crow's feet area, under the eye, and overall photodamage significantly improved from baseline condition with the CLA cream (Fig. 7). In addition, the CLA-treated side was significantly more improved than its vehicle-treated control side, and the vehicle-treated side was not significantly improved for any visual assessment at Week 12.

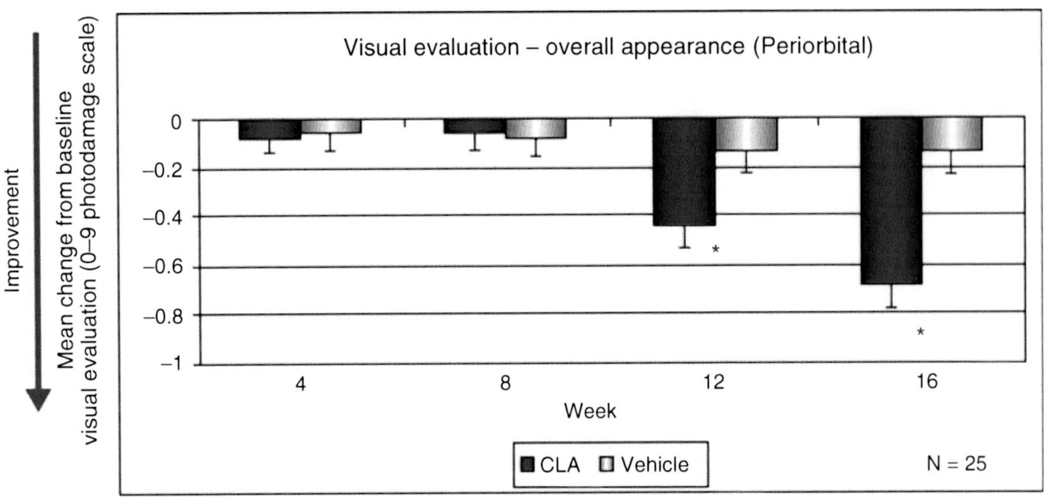

Fig. 4 Clinical evaluation of overall appearance. Compared to its vehicle, CLA cream significantly improved overall appearance ($P < 0.05$)

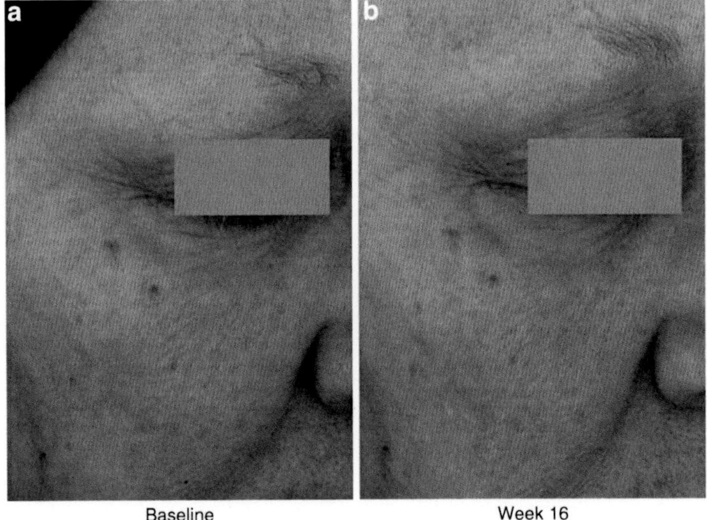

Fig. 5 Courtesy at (**a**) baseline and (**b**) Week 16 for individual subject. CLA cream significantly improved the appearance of photodamage attributes such as fine lines, wrinkles, and overall appearance. Application of the CLA cream has reduced the length and depth of this subject's crow's feet. The fine lines in this subject's under-eye area have also decreased in depth and become less apparent

A subset of the panel ($N = 12$) was measured using objective 3D facial scanning measurements, via measurement of nasolabial fold lines (length in mm). The CLA-treated side showed significant improvement from baseline condition at Weeks 8 and 12; the vehicle-treated side showed no significant improvement at any week (Fig. 8).

Biopsy Study on Photodamaged Forearms

Healthy female subjects (ages 40–65 years), with Fitzpatrick skin types I–III and mild to moderately photodamaged volar forearms, provided informed consent to participate in a 21-day repeat (9×24 h) patch test, followed by a

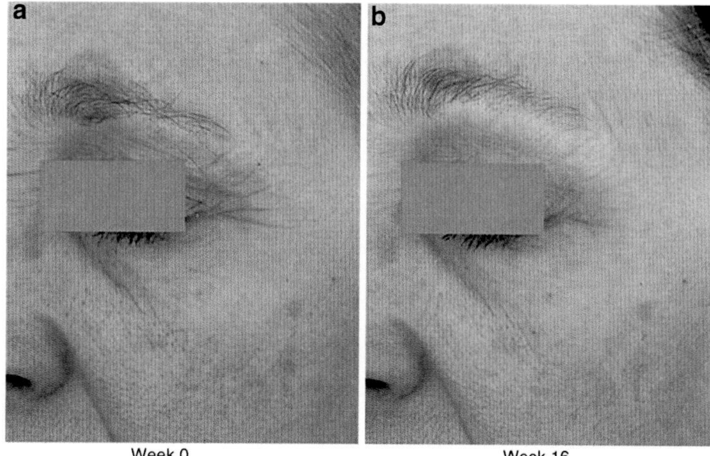

Fig. 6 Courtesy at (**a**) baseline and (**b**) Week 16 for individual subject. CLA cream significantly improved the appearance of photodamage attributes such as fine lines, wrinkles, and overall appearance. The depth of this subject's fine lines in the crow's feet area has greatly decreased with the use of the CLA cream. An improvement in photodamage is also seen in the subject's overall appearance, particularly in the lower cheek area

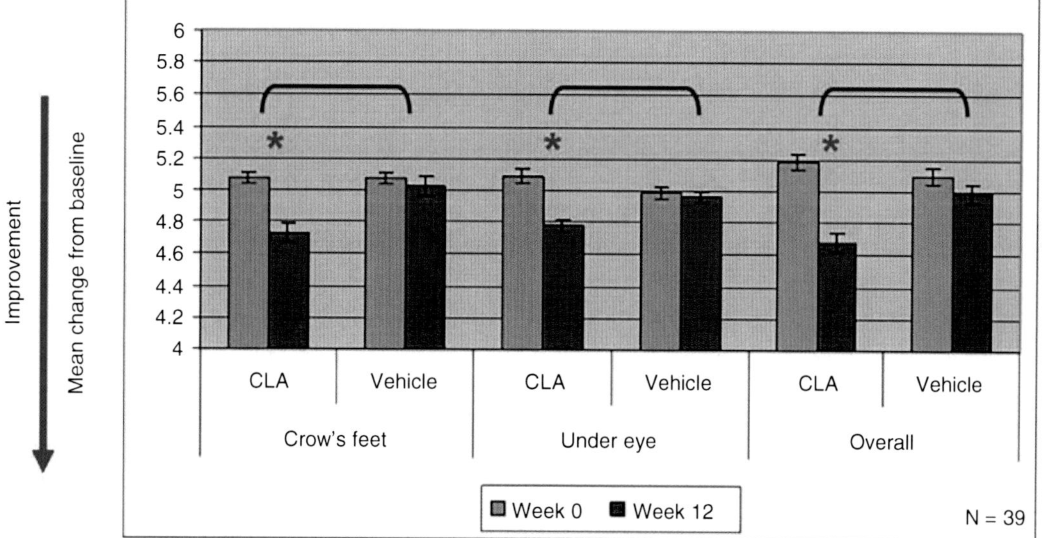

Fig. 7 Clinical evaluation of CLA cream compared to its vehicle at Week 12, by expert assessment of photodamage. Significant improvement was observed with CLA for all attributes, compared to baseline skin condition. Significant improvement favoring CLA over its vehicle was observed for all attributes

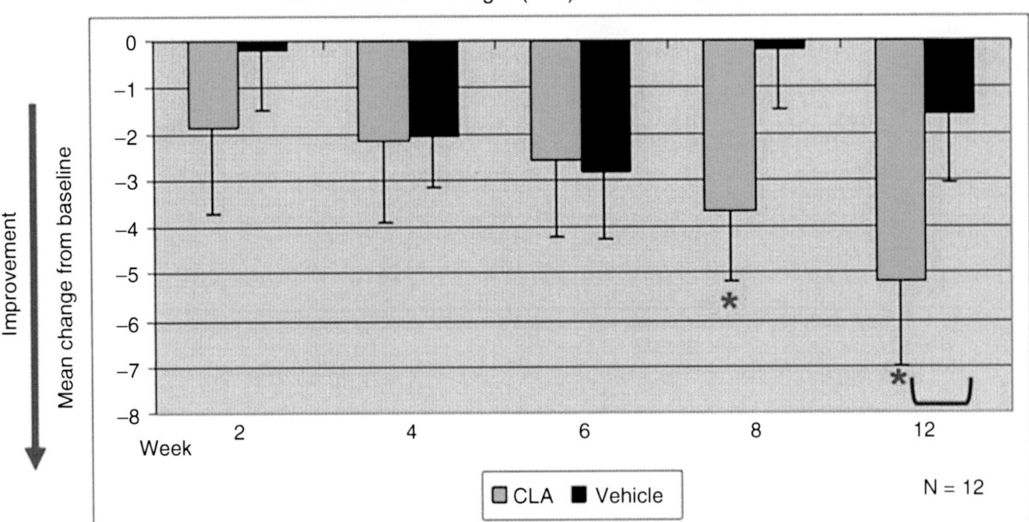

Fig. 8 Objective 3D assessment of CLA compared to its vehicle, using Cyberware facial scanning

dermatologist-collected punch biopsy test. Twelve total subjects were enrolled and completed all phases of the study. The test methodology and evaluation results with CLA were previously described by Shingleton et al. [64].

Test products included CLA formulated into a simple vehicle, the vehicle, and 0.05 % retinoic acid as a positive control. Test products were applied to the skin under occlusive patch for 24 h, with 24-h recovery gaps over the course of 21 days. On the last day of the study, the consulting dermatologist took full-thickness punch biopsies from each site.

Biopsies were formalin-fixed, processed for paraffin wax embedding, and sectioned. Sections were stained for H&E and orcein. Further sections were subjected to immunohistochemical analysis for filaggrin expression. The degree of filaggrin staining was assessed by a trained expert evaluator. The CLA and retinoic acid responses were normalized to degree of staining with the vehicle control and reported as mean increased percentage of responses. Erythema was assessed by the consulting dermatologist on a 0–4 scale (where 0 = none and 4 = severe).

The analysis of biopsies from subjects treated with CLA showed increased keratinocyte proliferation and epidermal thickness (9 out of 12). A significant increase in the expression of filaggrin following CLA cream application was also observed, suggesting a concomitant increase in epidermal differentiation. Detailed histological evaluation of the dermis showed evidence of stimulation of extracellular matrix turnover. In addition, increased removal of elastotic material and a modest increase in damaged collagen degradation were observed in all subjects treated with the CLA cream. After removal of the final patch, there was no significant difference in edema observed between the vehicle and the CLA cream. However, as expected, the retinoic acid control showed significantly increased erythema/edema grades compared to the measured response of the vehicle.

Conclusion

Clinically, CLA – a cosmetic PPAR lipid – has recently been shown to improve the appearance of photodamage [28], such as reduced fine lines and wrinkles, overall appearance, and the appearance of coarse rhytides in the nasolabial fold area, in vehicle-controlled photodamaged facial studies as described above. CLA cream increased epidermal proliferation, leading to an increase in the thickness of the epidermis in a photodamaged forearm test, with no significant edema, whereas application of retinoic acid (0.05 %) induced significant irritation/edema. The increase in keratinocyte proliferation was accompanied by an increase in differentiation, as judged by the significant increase in filaggrin expression and a thickening of the stratum granulosum, which is likely to result in improved epidermal quality. The magnitude of the effects described above is significant and similar to the effects described when PPARs are activated in models of epidermal development and disease. There is an apparent increase in epidermal proliferation [10, 11] and a concomitant increase in differentiation [12, 13].

Evidence of dermal effects following CLA treatment in the photodamaged forearm model is well demonstrated; dermal fibroblasts have been shown to respond to activators of PPARα in vitro [65]; however, there is no evidence to suggest that topically applied PPAR agonists can activate fibroblasts directly. It is possible that by inducing beneficial effects on epidermal homeostasis, CLA also triggers an epidermal-induced dermal response that may lead to the observed dermal changes.

The role of the PPARs in skin homeostasis is now widely accepted, as is their benefit in treating hyperproliferative and inflammatory skin disorders. Keratinocytes can respond to the environment they are in via signaling pathways that utilize PPARs; this includes both cell cycle control and inflammatory pathways. Akin to their role in systemic lipid control, PPARs in the skin could be regarded as the keratinocyte sensors leading to homeostatic control of inflammation as well as differentiation. As such, they have high potential as targets for cosmetic and therapeutic intervention strategies. The significant improvement in photodamaged attributes with no irritation has been summarized here for CLA, a natural ligand for PPAR, in vehicle-controlled, double-blind clinical trials.

Acknowledgment The authors would like to thank Susan Krein, Vickie Foy, Priya Vaidyanathan, and Robert Marriott for their contributions to this research.

References

1. Elias PM. Epidermal lipids, barrier function, and desquamation. J Invest Dermatol. 1983;80:44–9.
2. Harding C. The stratum corneum: structure and function in health and disease. Dermatol Ther. 2004;17:6–15.
3. Rawlings AV. Moisturization and skin barrier function. Dermatol Ther. 2004;17:43–8.
4. Friedmann PS, Cooper HL, Healy E. Peroxisome proliferator-activated receptors and their relevance to dermatology. Acta Derm Venereol. 2005;85:194–202.
5. Komuves LG, Hanley K, Lefebvre AM, Man MQ, Ng DC, Bikle DD, Williams ML, Elias PM, Auwerx J, Feingold KR. Stimulation of PPAR alpha promotes epidermal keratinocyte differentiation in vivo. J Invest Dermatol. 2000;115:353–60.
6. Issemann I, Green S. Activation of a member of the steroid hormone receptor superfamily by peroxisome proliferators. Nature. 1990;347:645–50.
7. Michalik L, Wahil W. Peroxisome proliferator-activated receptors (PPARs) in skin health, repair and disease. Biochim Biophys Acta. 2007;1771:991–8.
8. Westergaard M, Henningsen J, et al. Modulation of keratinocyte gene expression and differentiation by PPAR-selective ligands and tetradecylthioacetic acid. J Invest Dermatol. 2001;116:702–12.
9. Rivier M, Safonova I, Lebrun P, Griffiths CEM, Ailhaud G, Michel S. Differential expression of peroxisome proliferator-activated receptor subtypes during the differentiation of human keratinocytes. J Invest Dermatol. 1998;111:1116–21.
10. Hanley K, Jiang Y, Crumrine D, Bass NM, Appel R, Elias PM, Williams ML, Feingold KR. Activators of the nuclear hormone receptors PPAR alpha and FXR accelerate the development of the fetal epidermal permeability barrier. J Clin Invest. 1997;100:705–12.
11. Hanley K, Komuves LG, Bass NM, He SS, Jiang Y, Crumrine D, Appel R, Friedman M, Bettencourt J, Min K, Elias PM, Williams ML, Feingold KR. Fetal epidermal differentiation and barrier development in vivo is accelerated by nuclear hormone receptor activators. J Invest Dermatol. 1999;113:788–95.
12. Komuves LG, Hanley K, Jiang Y, Elias PM, Williams ML, Feingold KR. Ligands and activators of nuclear hormone receptors regulate epidermal differentiation during fetal rat skin development. J Invest Dermatol. 1998;111:429–33.
13. Hanley K, Komuves LG, Ng DC, Schoonjans K, He SS, Lau P, Bikle DD, Williams ML, Elias PM, Auwerx J, Feingold KR. Farnesol stimulates differentiation in epidermal keratinocytes via PPAR alpha. J Biol Chem. 2000;275:11484–91.

14. Mao-Qiang M, Fowler AJ, Schmuth M, Lau P, Chang S, Brown BE, Moser AH, Michalik L, Desvergne B, Wahli W, Li M, Metzger D, Chambon PH, Elias PM, Feingold KR. Peroxisome proliferator-activated receptor (PPAR)-gamma activation stimulates keratinocyte differentiation. J Invest Dermatol. 2004;123:305–12.
15. Schmuth M, Haqq CM, Cairns WJ, Holder JC, Dorsam S, Chang S, Lau P, Fowler AJ, Chuang G, Moser AH, Brown BE, Mao-Qiang M, Uchida Y, Schoonjans K, Auwerx J, Chambon P, Willson TM, Elias PM, Feingold KR. Peroxisome proliferator-activated receptor (PPAR)-beta/delta stimulates differentiation and lipid accumulation in keratinocytes. J Invest Dermatol. 2004;122:971–83.
16. Tan NS, Michalik L, Noy N, Yasmin R, Pacot C, Heim M, Fluhmann B, Desvergne B, Wahli W. Critical roles of PPAR beta/delta in keratinocyte response to inflammation. Genes Dev. 2001;15:3263–77.
17. Sheu MY, Fowler AJ, Kao J, Schmuth M, Schoonjans K, Auwerx J, Fluhr JW, Man MQ, Elias PM, Feingold KR. Topical peroxisome proliferator activated receptor-alpha activators reduce inflammation in irritant and allergic contact dermatitis models. J Invest Dermatol. 2002;118:94–101.
18. Westergaard M, Henningsen J, Johansen C, Rasmussen S, Svendsen ML, Jensen UB, Schroder HD, Staels B, Iversen L, Bolund L, Kragballe K, Kristiansen K. Expression and localization of peroxisome proliferator-activated receptors and nuclear factor kappaB in normal and lesional psoriatic skin. J Invest Dermatol. 2003;121:1104–17.
19. Mossner R, Kaiser R, Matern P, Kruger U, Westphal GA, Brockmoller J, Ziegler A, Neumann C, Konig IR, Reich K. Variations in the genes encoding the peroxisome proliferator-activated receptors alpha and gamma in psoriasis. Arch Dermatol Res. 2004;296:1–5.
20. Rivier M, Castiel I, Safonova I, Ailhaud G, Michel S. Peroxisome proliferator-activated receptor-alpha enhances lipid metabolism in a skin equivalent model. J Invest Dermatol. 2000;114:681–7.
21. Komuves LG, Hanley K, Man MQ, Elias PM, Williams ML, Feingold KR. Keratinocyte differentiation in hyperproliferative epidermis: topical application of PPARalpha activators restored tissue homeostasis. J Invest Dermatol. 2000;115:361–7.
22. Fluhr JW, Man MQ, Hachem JP, Crumrine D, Mauro TM, Elias PM, Feingold KR. Topical peroxisome proliferator activated receptor activators accelerate postnatal stratum corneum acidification. J Invest Dermatol. 2009;129:365–74.
23. Kobayashi H, Aiba S, Yoshino Y, Tagami H. Acute cutaneous barrier disruption activates epidermal p44/42 and p38 mitogen-activated protein kinases in human and hairless guinea pig skin. Exp Dermatol. 2003;12:734–46.
24. Sertznig P, Seifert M, Tilgen W, Reichrath J. Peroxisome proliferator-activated receptors (PPARs) and the human skin: importance of PPARs in skin physiology and dermatologic diseases. Am J Clin Dermatol. 2008;9:15–31.
25. Degenhardt T, Saramaki A, Malinen M, Rieck M, Vaisanen S, Huotari A, Herzig KH, Muller R, Carlberg C. Three members of the human pyruvate dehydrogenase kinase gene family are direct targets of the peroxisome proliferator-activated receptor beta/delta. J Mol Biol. 2007;372:341–55.
26. Watkinson A, Lee RS, Moore AE, Pudney PDA, Paterson SE, Rawlings AV. Reduced barrier efficiency in axillary stratum corneum. Int J Cosmet Sci. 2002;24:1–11.
27. Mayes AE, Kealahar P, Watson LP, et al. Anti-Aging and skin condition benefits from PPAR alpha activating molecules. Proceedings of the 22nd IFSCC Congress. 2002.
28. Hawkins SS, Feinberg C, Foy V, Usui T, Wada T, Kent J, Green M, Weinkauf R, Marriott R. Clinical and consumer-assessed improvement to photoaged skin with Conjugated Linoleic Acid (CLA): a novel cosmetic PPAR for anti-aging benefits. Proceedings of the 24th IFSCC Congress, Osaka. 2006.
29. Szeles L, Torocsik D, Nagy L. PPAR-gamma in immunity and inflammation: cell types and diseases. Biochim Biophys Acta-Mol Cell Biol Lipids. 2007;1771:1014.
30. Lathion C, Michalik L, Wahli W. Physiological ligands of PPARs in inflammation and lipid homeostasis. Futur Lipidol. 2006;1:191–201.
31. Wahli W. Peroxisome proliferator-activated receptors (PPARs): from metabolic control to epidermal wound healing. Swiss Med Wkly. 2002;132:83–91.
32. Michalik L, Wahli W. Involvement of PPAR nuclear receptors in tissue injury and wound repair. J Clin Invest. 2006;116:598–606.
33. Kersten S, Desvergne B, Wahli W. Roles of PPARs in health and disease. Nature. 2000;405:421–4.
34. Chung JH, Seo AY, Chung SW, Kim MK, Leeuwenburgh C, Yu BP, Chung HY. Molecular mechanism of PPAR in the regulation of age-related inflammation. Ageing Res Rev. 2008;7:126–36.
35. Boyd AS. Thiazolidinediones in dermatology. Int J Dermatol. 2007;46:557.
36. Dahten A, Koch C, Ernst D, Schnoller C, Hartmann S, Worm M. Systemic PPAR gamma ligation inhibits allergic immune response in the skin. J Invest Dermatol. 2008;128:2211.
37. Michalik L, Wahli W. Peroxisome proliferator-activated receptors (PPARs) in skin health, repair and disease. Biochim Biophys Acta-Mol Cell Biol Lipids. 2007;1771:991.
38. Demerjian M, Man MQ, Choi EH, Brown BE, Crumrine D, Chang S, Mauro T, Elias PM, Feingold KR. Topical treatment with thiazolidinediones, activators of peroxisome proliferator-activated receptor-gamma, normalizes epidermal homeostasis in a murine hyperproliferative disease model. Exp Dermatol. 2006;15:154.

39. Al YN, Romanowska M, Krauss S, Schweiger S, Foerster J. PPAR delta is a type 1 IFN target gene and inhibits apoptosis in T cells. J Invest Dermatol. 2008;128:1940.
40. Spencer NF, Poynter ME, Im SY, Daynes RA. Constitutive activation of NF-kappa B in an animal model of aging. Int Immunol. 1997;9:1581–8.
41. Poynter ME, Daynes RA. Peroxisome proliferator-activated receptor alpha Activation modulates cellular redox status, represses nuclear factor-kappa B signaling, and reduces inflammatory cytokine production in aging. J Biol Chem. 1998;273:32833–41.
42. Liu B, Zhu F, Xia X, Park E, Hu Y. A tale of terminal differentiation: IKKalpha, the master keratinocyte regulator. [In process citation]. Cell Cycle (Georgetown, Tex 8). 2009;8(4):527–31.
43. Kippenberger S, Loitsch SM, Grundmann-Kollmann-M, Simon S, Dang TA, Hardt-Weinelt K, Kaufmann R, Bernd A. Activators of peroxisome proliferator-activated receptors protect human skin from ultraviolet-B-light-induced inflammation. J Invest Dermatol. 2001;117:1430–6.
44. Coquette A, Berna N, Vandenbosch A, Rosdy M, De Wever B, Poumay Y. Analysis of interleukin-1 alpha (IL-1 alpha) and interleukin-8 (IL-8) expression and release in vitro reconstructed human epidermis for the prediction of in vivo skin irritation and/or sensitization. Toxicol In Vitro. 2003;17:311–21.
45. Daynes RA, Araneo BA, Ershler WB, Maloney C, Li GZ, Ryu SY. Altered regulation of interleukin-6 production with normal aging. J Immunol. 1993;150: A285.
46. Ershler WB. Interleukin-6 – A cytokine for gerontologists. J Am Geriatr Soc. 1993;41:176–81.
47. Ershler WB, Keller ET. Age-associated increased interleukin-6 gene expression, late-life diseases, and frailty. Ann Rev Med. 2000;51:245–70.
48. Boniface K, Diveu C, Morel F, Pedretti N, Froger J, Ravon E, Garcia M, Venereau E, Preisser L, Guignouard E, Guillet G, Dagregorio G, Pene J, Moles JP, Yssel H, Chevalier S, Bernard FX, Gascan H, Lecron JC. Oncostatin M secreted by skin infiltrating T lymphocytes is a potent keratinocyte activator involved in skin inflammation. J Immunol. 2007;178:4615.
49. Yu M, Kissling S, Freyschmidt PP, Hoffmann R, Shapiro J, McElwee KJ. Interleukin-6 cytokine family member oncostatin M is a hair-follicle-expressed factor with hair growth inhibitory properties. Exp Dermatol. 2008;17:12.
50. Rowan AD, Koshy PJT, Shingleton WD, Degnan BA, Heath JK, Vernallis AB, Spaull JR, Life PF, Hudson K, Cawston TE. Synergistic effects of glycoprotein 130 binding cytokines in combination with interleukin-1 on cartilage collagen breakdown. Arthritis Rheum. 2001;44:1620–32.
51. Cawston TE, Curry VA, Summers CA, Clark IM, Riley GP, Life PF, Spaull JR, Goldring MB, Koshy PJT, Rowan AD, Shingleton WD. The role of oncostatin M in animal and human connective tissue collagen turnover and its localization within the rheumatoid joint. Arthritis Rheum. 1998;41:1760–71.
52. Shingleton WD, Ellis AJ, Rowan AD, Cawston TE. Retinoic acid combines with interleukin-1 to promote the degradation of collagen from bovine nasal cartilage: matrix metalloproteinases-1 and -13 are involved in cartilage collagen breakdown. J Cell Biochem. 2000;79:519–31.
53. Shingleton WD, Jones D, Xu X, Cawston TE, Rowan AD. Retinoic acid and oncostatin M combine to promote cartilage degradation via matrix metalloproteinase-13 expression in bovine but not human chondrocytes. Rheumatology. 2006;45:958.
54. Park EJ, Park SY, Joe EH, Jou I. 15d-PGJ2 and rosiglitazone suppress janus kinase-STAT inflammatory signaling through induction of suppressor of cytokine signaling 1 (SOCS1) and SOCS3 in glia. J Biol Chem. 2003;278:14747–52.
55. Devchand PR, Keller H, Peters JM, Vazquez M, Gonzalez FJ, Wahli W. The PPAR[alpha]-leukotriene B4 pathway to inflammation control. Nature. 1996;384:39–43.
56. Kabashima K, Nagamachi M, Honda T, Nishigori C, Miyachi Y, Tokura Y, Narumiya S. Prostaglandin E2 is required for ultraviolet B-induced skin inflammation via EP2 and EP4 receptors. Lab Invest. 2007;87:49–55.
57. Subbaramaiah K, Lin DT, Hart JC, Dannenberg AJ. Peroxisome proliferator-activated receptor gamma ligands suppress the transcriptional activation of cyclooxygenase-2: evidence for involvement of activator protein-1 and creb-binding protein/p300. J Biol Chem. 2001;276:12440–8.
58. Chen CW, Chang YH, Tsi CJ, Lin WW. Inhibition of IFN-{gamma}-mediated inducible nitric oxide synthase induction by the peroxisome proliferator-activated receptor {gamma} agonist, 15-deoxy-{delta}12,14-prostaglandin J2, involves inhibition of the upstream janus kinase/STAT1 signaling pathway. J Immunol. 2003;171:979–88.
59. Badinga L, Greene ES. Physiological properties of conjugated linoleic acid and implications for human health. Nutr in Clin Pract. 2006;21:367–73.
60. Hwang D. Fatty acids and immune responses: a new perspective in searching for clues to mechanism. Ann Rev Nutr. 2000;20(1):431–56.
61. Belury MA. Dietary conjugated linoleic acid in health: physiological effects and mechanisms of action. Ann Rev Nutr. 2002;22(1):505–31.
62. Moya-Camarena SY, Heuvel J, Blanchard SG, Leesnitzer LA, Belury MA. Conjugated linoleic acid is a potent naturally occurring ligand and activator of PPAR{alpha}. J Lipid Res. 1999;40(8):1426–33.
63. Bassaganya-Riera J, Hontecillas R, Beitz DC. Colonic anti-inflammatory mechanisms of conjugated linoleic acid. Clin Nutr. 2002;21(6):451–9.

64. Shingleton WD, Donovan M, Rogers JS, Feinberg C, Marriott R, Green MR. Conjugated Linoleic Acid (CLA), a cosmetic "PPAR" lipid, promotes epidermal differentiation and dermal matrix turnover without irritation; consistent with its in-vivo skin aging benefits. Proceedings of the 24th IFSCC Congress, Osaka. 2006.
65. Kim SH, Nam GW, Lee HK, Moon SJ, Chang IS. The effects of Musk T on peroxisome proliferator-activated receptor [PPAR]-alpha activation, epidermal skin homeostasis and dermal hyaluronic acid synthesis. Arch Dermatol Res. 2006;298:273–82.

Hyaluronan and the Process of Aging in Skin

18

Diana Alyce Rivers and Robert Stern

Contents

D.A. Rivers • R. Stern (✉)
The Department of Basic Biomedical Sciences, Touro College of Osteopathic Medicine, New York, NY, USA
e-mail: drivers@student.touro.edu; robert.stern@touro.edu

M.A. Farage et al. (eds.), *Textbook of Aging Skin*,
DOI 10.1007/978-3-662-47398-6_22

Abstract

Hyaluronan is a major component of the extracellular matrix of skin and important in the metabolism of both epidermis and dermis. Hyaluronan is responsible for hydration, nutrient exchange, and protects against free radical damage via a multitude of signaling pathways. It is also involved in basic biological processes such as cell renewal, differentiation, and motility. An overview is provided here that provides recent information, bringing up-to-date advances in hyaluronan and matrix biology with a particular emphasis on the process of aging in human skin. The differences between hyaluronan applied exogenously and that occurring naturally in the body are articulated. A brief history is also provided of various commercial hyaluronan-containing skin-care products, including topical applications, as injectable skin fillers, and in nanoparticle delivery systems.

Introduction

The glycosaminoglycan HA (hyaluronic acid, hyaluronan) is the major component of the ECM (extracellular matrix) of skin and plays an important role in the metabolism in both epidermis and dermis. Hyaluronan is responsible for hydration, nutrient exchange, and protects against free radical damage via a multitude of signaling pathways. Hyaluronan and its associated volume of water is a key to skin moisture [1, 2]. Loss of such moisture is one of the hallmarks of aging skin. It is reasonable to assume that loss of HA is the basis of such a decrease in hydration, leading to wrinkling, skin atrophy, and all the other hallmarks of the appearance associated with aging. It is also involved in basic biological processes such as cell renewal, differentiation, and motility. An overview is provided here that provides recent information, bringing up-to-date advances in matrix biology relevant for skin care, with a particular emphasis on skin moisture and the effect of aging in human skin.

Hyaluronan

Glycosaminoglycans (GAGs) are unbranched polysaccharides of the ECM that constitute important workings of connective tissue [3–5]. They are very complex structures with a variety of postsynthetic modifications. Hyaluronan is also one of these straight chain sugar GAG polymers, but in contrast has an exceedingly simple structure, composed entirely of repeating disaccharides of alternating glucuronic acid and *N*-acetylglucosamine connected by β-linkages. HA is involved in multiple aspects of skin biology and despite its simple structure is involved in skin hydration, nutrient exchange, tissue homeostasis, repair processes, protection against free radical damage, cell differentiation, and cell motility [6–8].

Hyaluronan can be up to 10^7 Da in size. At the body's pH, it is one of the most highly charged molecules in biology, which provides HA with some of its unique qualities. A massive cloud of water surrounds the molecule in an attempt to neutralize that charge, 1,000–10,000 times the original volume. It is this particular quality which provides the hydrating functions of HA, with the simultaneous ability to expand tissues and to open spaces for cell movement. The volume of water associated with HA is tightly held, and is not in equilibrium with the remaining water of the body, comprising its own compartment.

Unlike other GAGs, HA is not sulfated, is not covalently attached to proteins, nor is it synthesized in the Golgi but on the cytoplasmic surface of outer cell membranes. Hyaluronan is an extraordinarily large polymer. As an example, the average molecular weight of HA in human synovial fluid is three to four million Da (Daltons), and that purified from the Wharton's jelly of the human umbilical cord is over three million Da. High molecular size HA is considered a sign of normal healthy tissues, while fragmented HA is a reflection of tissues under stress [9, 10].

It would be of intrinsic interest to establish not only the levels of HA in young versus aged skin but also the molecular size of HA in young skin compared to senescent skin, a study that has not yet been carried out. Such studies and other aspects of HA metabolism may provide clues for reversing some of the processes that lead to skin aging, loss of moisture, and wrinkling. It is clear that the "dried" appearance of aging skin is intimately associated with changes in apparent levels and types of HA deposition, dependent on changes in controls of its underlying metabolism.

Because HA is surrounded by water molecules, the charges repel each other, thereby causing the "slippery" viscosity and the ability to hold shape. This is why this molecule is found in abundance in the vitreous humor of the eye, where it provides resilience, in synovial joints functioning as a shock absorber, in Wharton's jelly of the umbilical cord wherein it prevents obstruction of flow through the vessels, and in loose connective tissues.

Hyaluronan in Skin

The 70 kg individual has approximately 15 g of HA, 50 % of which is skin associated. A third of total HA turns over daily. There are numerous reports of decreased amounts of HA in aging skin. These observations are based on histochemical stains, such as Alcian blue, and affinity histochemistry with the HA-binding peptide. However, actual biochemical extraction techniques using progressively potent extraction solutions reveal that the HA content remains constant with age. The difference is that the HA becomes increasingly tissue associated, becoming more and more resistant to extraction [11]. The apparent results from histochemical investigations are perhaps best explained by increasing competition between tissue proteins for HA binding sites and the HA-binding peptide as a function of age. The HA encased within tissue proteins may be restricted from functioning as a hydrating molecule. This proviso also indicates that the HA-staining procedure, as normally performed with an HA-binding peptide, is far not a quantitative procedure.

Distribution of Hyaluronan in Skin

Hyaluronan in skin occurs in both dermis and epidermis, with dermis containing the greater proportion. Epidermal HA is more loosely associated and is more easily extracted from tissue. Formalin, an aqueous fixative, easily removes most of the HA from epidermis. It is less able to extract HA from dermis. Alcoholic formalin enhances histolocalization of epidermal HA and indicates considerable levels are contained therein [12].

Skin HA has a very rapid turnover, with a half-life of 1–2 days in the epidermis. The turnover rate in the dermis is similar, with catabolism occurring in liver and lymph nodes, following lymphatic drainage [13].

The turnover mechanism in the epidermis is not clear and may be a combination of free radical fragmentation stimulated by UV light, and enzymatic degradation (*vide infra*).

Hyaluronan in the Epidermis

Until recently, it was assumed that only mesenchymal cells were capable of synthesizing HA. With newer techniques, evidence for HA being made in the epidermis became apparent. Techniques for separating dermis and epidermis facilitated detection of HA in each compartment. Hyaluronan is most prominent in the upper spinous and granular, where much of it is extracellular. In the basal layer, HA is predominantly intracellular and is not easily eluted out during aqueous fixation. Basal keratinocyte HA is involved in mitotic events, presumably, while extracellular HA in the upper layers of the epidermis is involved in barrier disassociation and sloughing of cells.

Tissue cultures of keratinocytes have facilitated studies of epithelial HA metabolism. These cultured cells synthesize large quantities of HA. When Ca^{++} concentration of the culture medium is increased from 0.05 to 1.20 mM, basal-like cells begin to differentiate, HA synthesis levels drop, and hyaluronidase activity is induced [14, 15]. This increase in calcium that appears to simulate in culture the natural in situ differentiation of basal keratinocytes parallels the increasing calcium gradient observed in the epidermis. There may be intracellular stores of calcium that are released as keratinocytes mature. Alternatively, the calcium stores may be concentrated by lamellar bodies from the intercellular fluids released during terminal differentiation. The lamellar bodies are thought to be modified lysosomes containing hydrolytic enzymes, and a potential source of the hyaluronidase activity.

The lamellar bodies fuse with the plasma membranes of the terminally differentiating keratinocytes, increasing the plasma membrane surface area. Lamellar bodies are also associated with proton pumps that enhance acidity. A proton pump, specifically Na^{+}-H^{+} exchanger1 (NHE1), is part of a complex involved in the internalization and degradation of HA of the ECM [16]. This same pump also creates localized areas of acidity on the cell surface within lipid rafts where CD44, the predominant HA receptor, is localized [17].

The lamellar bodies also acidify, and their polar lipids become partially converted to neutral lipids, thereby participating in skin barrier function. Diffusion of aqueous material through the epidermis is blocked by these lipids synthesized by keratinocytes in the stratum granulosum, the boundary corresponding to the level at which HA staining ends. This constitutes part of the barrier function of skin. The HA-rich area inferior to this layer may obtain water from the moisture-rich dermis. And the water contained therein cannot penetrate beyond the lipid-rich stratum granulosum. The HA-bound water in both the dermis and in the vital area of the epidermis is critical for skin hydration. And the stratum granulosum is essential for maintenance of that hydration, not only for the skin but also for the body in general. Profound dehydration is a serious clinical problem, for example, in severely burned patients, with extensive losses of stratum granulosum.

Hyaluronan of the epidermal ECM forms two different structures: a pericellular coat close to the plasma membrane, forming an intimate pericellular matrix, and HA chains that coalesce into large cables. Such cables, induced by inflammatory agents, bind leukocytes, whereas the pericellular HA does not. Thus, under inflammatory conditions, epidermal keratinocytes are able to form HA cables that can bind leukocytes [18].

Hyaluronan in the Dermis

The HA content of the dermis is far greater than that of the epidermis and accounts for most of the 50 % of total body HA present in skin. The papillary dermis has a more prominent level of HA than does the reticular dermis. The HA of the dermis is in direct continuity with both the lymphatic and vascular systems, which epidermal HA apparently does not.

Exogenous HA is cleared from the dermis and rapidly degraded [13]. The dermal fibroblast provides the synthetic machinery for dermal HA and should be the target for any pharmacological attempts to enhance skin hydration. The fibroblasts of the body, the most banal of cells from a histological perspective, is probably the most diverse of all vertebrate cells with the broadest repertoire of biochemical reactions and potential pathways for differentiation. Much of this diversity is site specific. What makes the papillary dermal fibroblast different from other fibroblasts is not known. However these cells have an HA synthetic capacity similar to that of the fibroblasts that line joint synovium, or the hyalocytes of the eye, responsible for the HA-rich synovial fluid, and the vitreous of the ocular chambers, respectively.

A clue to the vigorous HA synthetic capacity of dermal fibroblasts comes from an unexpected direction. Adiponectin, a cytokine produced by adipose tissue, stimulates HA synthesis in dermal fibroblasts [19]. Sebaceous glands of the skin produce adiponectin as well, and dermal fibroblasts are demonstrated to have specific adiponectin receptors, producing HA by upregulation of their HA synthase 2 (HAS2). The female breast is a modified sebaceous gland, with associated lipid tissue. The body's fat tissue is an endocrine gland that is largely overlooked. The sebaceous glands of the skin may hold a key to the problem of loss of skin moisture, in light of the observation that adiponectin levels decrease markedly with age.

Hyaluronan in the Basal Lamina

Hyaluronan deposition occurs prominently in the basement membrane zone of skin. However, with aging, that HA content decreases. In fact, with time, the entire basal lamina becomes attenuated. Hyaluronan is a component of all basement membranes, but its role in that barrier between dermis and epidermis is entirely unknown. Ultrastructural and immunohistochemical studies have not contributed to our understanding of HA in basement membrane, nor is the relationship between HA and other components of that structure known, such as type IV collagen, laminins, and fibronectin. Stoichiometric measurements make no sense, given that HA is a polymer that varies so widely in size. Decreased levels of HA and decreased thickness of the basal lamina occur in diabetic skin, contributing to "thick skin" syndrome [20].

Addition of exogenous HA to an organotypic keratinocyte-fibroblast coculture model enhances epidermal proliferation resulting in a thicker epidermis. Hyaluronan addition also improves basement membrane assembly as evidenced by an increased expression of laminin-332 and collagen type IV at the epidermal-dermal junction. Furthermore, development of the epidermal lipid barrier structure is enhanced [21]. Presumably, loss of HA would have an opposite effect.

The HA content of skin basal lamina may be greater than in other tissues. Evidence for this is indirect [22]. Goodpastuer's syndrome is a disease that involves rapidly progressive kidney failure as well as hemorrhagic lung disease. It is an autoimmune disorder with autoantibodies directed again a portion of one of the basement membrane-specific collagens. Basal laminas throughout the body share this structure, including those in kidney, lung, and skin, but curiously, skin is rarely involved. High molecular weight HA, a potent immunosuppressive polymer, may be functioning as an immune shield for skin in Goodpasture's syndrome, and be the basis for the anomaly. This also suggests that the HA content of the basal lamina of skin is higher than that in other tissues.

Hyaluronan and Fragment Size

Despite its simple repeating structure, HA has a wide range and occasionally contradictory functions, even though it is without branch points and without sulfation or other secondary modifications. The multiple functions are in part attributed to variations in chain length. In general, high molecular weight HA (up to 2.4×10^4 kDa) occurs in normal healthy tissues, while fragmented HA is highly inflammatory, angiogenic, and immune stimulatory, a reflection of tissues under stress. The large HA polymers are, in marked contrast, anti-inflammatory, antiangiogenic, and immunosuppressive [23, 24]. Smaller fragments have the opposite effect. In fact, various sizes of HA fragments have evolved to become major immune regulators [9]. Such variations in size constitute a rich informational system [25].

A major conundrum remains regarding the hydration properties of HA. The number of water molecules in the hydration shell of HA of different molecular sizes and in the presence of various counterions has not been determined. It is certain to be a nonlinear relationship. Intuitively, it is predicted that large HMW chains of HA are more effective hydrating molecules, that they carry larger numbers of water molecules per disaccharide unit. But this must be demonstrated experimentally. An approach to this question has been described, though no clear relationship was demonstrated [26]. A caveat in such studies and a major experimental problem is that the results are highly dependent upon the methods used to isolate and prepare the HA [27].

Hyaluronan Receptors

CD44

The most predominent receptor for HA is CD44, a transmembrane glycoprotein that occurs in a wide variety of isoforms, products of a single gene with variant exon expression, all inserted into a single extracellular position near the membrane insertion site. CD44 is coded for by 10 constant exons plus from 0 to 10 variant exons. The standard form, CD44s, comprising exons 1–5 and 16–20 contains no variant exons and is distributed exclusively on the cell surface, while variant exon-bearing isoforms can have additional intracellular localization (unpublished observations). CD44 is able to bind a variety of other ligands including fibronectin, collagen, osteopontin, matrix metalloproteinases (MMPs), and heparin-binding growth factors. CD44 is distributed widely, being found on virtually all cells. It participates in cell adhesion, migration, lymphocyte activation and homing, and cancer metastasis. The appearance of HA in dermis and epidermis parallels the histolocalization of CD44. CD44E, a variant containing v8-10, is expressed on epithelial cells.

It is apparent that CD44 is one of the most complex and most intriguing proteins in all of vertebrate biology. It is involved in a myriad of critical functions and underscores the enormous number of biological reactions in which HA participates.

The nature of the CD44 variant exons in skin at each location has not been determined. It would be important to establish whether modulation occurs in CD44 variant exon expression with changes in the state of skin hydration and as a function of age, particularly in wrinkled and UV-exposed skin.

RHAMM

Another receptor for HA is the receptor for HA-mediated motility (RHAMM). This receptor is involved in cell locomotion, focal adhesion turnover, and contact inhibition. RHAMM preceded HA in evolution and is far more ancient. Like CD44, it also is expressed in a number of variant isoforms and occurs as a cell surface receptor as well as having multiple intracellular isoforms. The interactions between HA and RHAMM regulate locomotion of cells by a complex network of signal transduction events and interaction with the cytoskeleton of cells. It is also an important regulator of cell growth.

In a murine system, blocking expression of the RHAMM protein, either by gene deletion or by a blocking reagent, selectively induces the generation of fat cells to replace those lost in the aging process. This has promise as a technique to improve the appearance of aging skin, and a potential source of the adiponectin, as discussed below.

LYVE and HARE

Two other receptors have come into prominence recently, reflecting the ever-increasing role HA is documented to play in biology: lymphatic vessel endothelial hyaluronan receptor (LYVE-1) and hyaluronic acid receptor for endocytosis (HARE), also known as Stabilin-2. HARE mediates systemic clearance of HA, CSs (chondroitin sulfates), and heparin from both the lymphatic and vascular circulation.

Hyaluronan Metabolism

Extrinsic aging in the human skin is associated with alterations in the expression of HA and its metabolizing enzymes [28]. A review of HA metabolism is therefore indicated to fully understand changes in HA with aging.

The Hyaluronan Synthases

Three isoforms of a single enzyme synthesize HA. These are dual-headed transferases that utilize as substrates alternately UDP-glucuronic acid and UDP-*N*-acetylglucosamine. These are membrane proteins, located on the inner surface of the plasma membrane. They extrude their product through the plasma membrane into the extracellular space as the HA is being synthesized. This permits unconstrained polymer growth, without destruction of the cell. There are three synthase genes in the mammalian genome, coding for HAS1, 2, and 3. They are located on three separate chromosomes and are differentially regulated, with each producing a different-size polymer, though they have a high degree of sequence homology [29, 30]. These isoenzymes contain seven membrane-associated regions and a central cytoplasmic domain possessing several consensus sequences that are substrates for phosphorylation by protein kinase C. The HAS1 and 2 genes are upregulated in skin by TGF-β in both dermis and epidermis, but there are major differences in the kinetics of the TGF-β response between HAS1 and 2 and between the two compartments, suggesting that the two genes are regulated independently.

The Hyaluronidases

Hyaluronan is very metabolically active, with a half-life of 3–5 min in the circulation, less than 1 day in skin, and in an apparently an inert a tissue such as cartilage, the HA turns over with a half-life of 1–3 weeks. This catabolic activity is primarily the result of hyaluronidases, endoglycolytic enzymes with a specificity, except for the leech enzyme, for the β1–4 glycosidic bonds. The human genome project has also promoted explication at the genetic level, and a virtual explosion of information has ensued [31].

The mammalian hyaluronidases are endo-β-hexosaminidases and function as hydrolases, in contrast to prokaryotic hyaluronidases that cleave the glycosidic bond using an eliminase mechanism of action. They lack substrate specificity, able to digest chondroitin sulfates (CS), albeit at a slower rate.

Six hyaluronidase-like sequences are present in the human genome, while most other mammals have seven such sequences. All are transcriptionally active with unique tissue distributions. In the human, three genes (*HYAL1*, *HYAL2*, and *HYAL3*) are found tightly clustered on chromosome 3p21.3. Another three genes, *HYAL4*, *PHYAL1* (a pseudogene), and PH20, or sperm adhesion molecule1 (*SPAM1*) are clustered similarly on chromosome 7q31.3.

The enzymes HYAL1 and 2 constitute the major hyaluronidases in somatic tissues. HYAL1, an acid-active lysosomal enzyme, was the first somatic hyaluronidase to be isolated and characterized. Why an acid-active hyaluronidase should occur in plasma is not clear. HYAL1 is able to utilize HA of any size as a substrate and generates predominantly tetrasaccharides. HYAL2 is also acid active, anchored to plasma membranes by a GPI (glycosylphosphatidylinositol)-link. HYAL2 cleaves high molecular weight HA to a limit product of approximately 20 kDa, or about 50 disaccharide units.

Not all tissues that contain HYAL1 activity synthesize that enzyme. Active endocytosis of the protein from the circulation occurs [32]. Monocytes contain no mRNA for HYAL1, yet have very high levels of enzyme activity (unpublished observations). Megakaryocytes and platelets contain no HYAL1 [33], perhaps because they lack the receptors for endocytosis of circulating HYAL1.

A Newly Devised Catabolic Pathway for HA

The hyaluronidase, HYAL2, initiates the degradation of high-molecular size HA into smaller fragments which are then endocytosed and degraded in early lysosomes by HYAL1. These initial cleavages provide substrates for two acid-active exoglycosidases present in lysosomes, β-glucuronidase and *N*-acetylglucosaminidase. The fragments so generated exit the lysosome and become cytoplasmic, where they can participate in other metabolic pathways [34].

The Hyaluronasome

It is possible to invoke the existence of a new and novel organelle, the hyaluronasome. Parallels between glycogen and HA metabolism are the basis of such a formulation. Both are monotonous, unadorned carbohydrate polymers of repeating sugars. A glycogen organelle can be visualized in liver, where it is prominent following a period of starvation, or prolonged intravenous feeding, when the organelles have been emptied of their glycogen substrate.

> Readily visualized by the electron microscope, glycogen granules appear as bead-like structures localized to specific subcellular locales. Each glycogen granule is a functional unit, not only containing carbohydrate, but also enzymes and other proteins needed for its metabolism. These proteins are not static, but rather associate and dissociate, depending on the carbohydrate balance of the tissue. Regulation takes place not only by allosteric regulation of enzymes, but also due to other factors, such as sub-cellular location, granule size, and association with various related proteins. [35]

Such observations may be applicable to HA and the proteins related to its metabolism and regulation in an organelle termed "the hyaluronasome." Indeed, such a complex was described in fibroblasts several decades ago for the synthetic apparatus [36, 37]. This may be a component of an even larger complex that contains not only the synthetic but also the degradative enzymes, associated regulatory proteins and peptides, as well as receptors and other binding proteins. A quasicomplex has been described for the apparatus that brings HA chains into the cells for degradation, containing HA, the CD44 receptor, HYAL2, and a Na^+-H^+ exchanger (NHE1) for creating acidic foci on plasma membrane indentations termed lipid rafts [16]. This putative cell organelle could be a functional unit that provides response mechanisms dependent on the metabolic state of the cell. A search should be taken for such an organelle in the robust HA synthesizing fibroblasts of the papillary dermis.

Suggestive evidence for the existence of the hyaluronasome comes from several sources. Treating cultured cells with very low concentrations of hyaluronidase has the anomalous effect of increasing levels of HA synthesis [38–40]. Even treatment of isolated membrane preparations with low levels of hyaluronidase has a similar effect [38], suggestive of a feedback mechanism that instructs the cell on how much HA has been made. Constant clipping of the polymer as it is being extruded from the cell provides the misinformation that little HA has been deposited into the extracellular space. The plasma membrane-bound receptor CD44 is an ideal candidate for providing such a feedback mechanism.

Treating cells with higher levels of hyaluronidase modulates the expression profile of the variant exons of CD44, thus providing exquisite control mechanisms for the metabolic control of HA deposition [41]. An organelle in which all components are tethered together would provide the structural organization for such reactions to occur with maximum efficiency.

Hyaluronan Protects Against UV Damage

Aging is accelerated in areas exposed to the UV (ultra-violet) radiation of sunlight, a process known as photoaging. There is a combination of short wavelength (UVB) injury to the epidermis and long wavelength (UVA) injury to the dermis.

UVB represents only 0.5 % of the sunlight that reaches the Earth's surface but accounts for much of the acute and chronic sun-related damage to skin. UVB-irradiation accelerates skin aging, in part by disruption of the turnover of its ECM. Among the changes that have been documented are enhanced expression of the MMPs (matrix metalloproteinases), the attendant cleavage of collagen, and reduced levels of HA. The collagen fragments themselves are a component of the mechanism for the suppression of HA deposition; a direct effect on HAS2 expression has been documented [42, 43]. Chronic UVB irradiation causes loss of HA from mouse dermis, because of downregulation of HA synthase expression. Exogenous HA minimizes the effects of UV irradiation when added to cultures of human keratinocytes, protecting against the suppression of CD44 and TLR-2 expression [44].

Hyaluronan Protects Against Damage from Free Radical and Reactive Oxygen Species

There is in vivo evidence for a causal relationship between mitochondrial oxidative damage, cellular senescence, and the aging phenotypes in skin [10]. Reactive oxygen species (ROS) are generated during the metabolic reactions in which oxygen participates. These ROS moieties facilitate the catabolism of HMW HA within dermis and epidermis by mechanisms that are not well understood [45]. The proportion of HA degradation between enzymatic catalysis and ROS scission is also unknown. There are low levels of HYAL1 and 2 in skin, as established in an expression library. Effectiveness of ROS is enhanced by iron and copper ions, as well as by ions of other transition metals, especially in the presence of ascorbic acid. Part of this is offset by the ability of Vitamin C to enhance the activity of hyaluronidase inhibitors [46, 47]. There is apparently an entire system of checks and balances for maintaining levels of HA deposition in skin that is unknown. Many commercial skin serums contain high levels of Vitamin C. Their effectiveness may be due to the ability to tilt the balance toward enhanced HA deposition, an effect achieved entirely by accident.

The ROS free radicals are highly unstable, reactive, and toxic. It is hardly conceivable that they participate as intermediates or as regulatory agents in biological reactions. Yet their high levels in skin and their generation with the constant skin bombardment by UV irradiation suggests their involvement in such reactions occurs through evolutionary forces. Controlled oxidative-reductive degradation of HA chains by the combined effect of oxygen, transition metal cations, and ascorbate is entirely plausible. Reduction of oxidized transitional metal ions occurs in the presence of ascorbate, a reaction that may occur at a greater level in skin than in any other tissue.

It would be of intrinsic interest to examine levels of HA in the skin of severely ascorbate-deficient or anemic patients. Human beings are among the few vertebrates in whom the enzymatic pathway for ascorbate synthesis has been inactivated. Our hairlessness may be the basis of this mutation as a survival mechanism. In humans, the entire pathway is extant, except for the final enzymatic step. Could this inactivation have correlated with loss of body hair in the course of human evolution?

Another concept is that products of enzymatic cleavage of HMW HA generate products that have structures that are, excepting for chain length, identical to the original substrate. The products of free radical cleavage contain oxidized carboxyl and hydroperoxide functional groups [48]. These are reactive moieties that interact with other tissue molecules. This may be the basis of the sequentially more insoluble HA content of skin, the HA that becomes increasingly resistant to extraction as a function of age [11]. This also suggests that the proportion of HA degraded by oxidative reactions generates a greater portion of permanent structural tissue HA than that degraded enzymatically. Further documentation of this sequestering of HA phenomenon as a function of age has been documented. The apparent HA staining of skin decreases with age can be explained [49]. Binding sites on the HA substrate for the biotinylated HA-binding peptide, the basis of the staining reaction, become progressively less available with age.

Extrinsic aging in human skin is associated with alterations in the metabolizing enzymes of HA. There is considerable increase in HA of lower molecular mass with aging, and with UV exposed skin, compared to photoprotected skin of the buttocks. This increase is associated with decreased HAS1 expression and increased expression of HYAL1, 2, and 3. The receptors CD44 and RHAMM are also significantly downregulated [28].

Inspection of the images of HA staining in formalin-fixed skin compared to alcoholic-acid formalin-fixed skin demonstrates that epidermis contains HA that is easily eluted, barely surviving the aqueous formalin fixation. The dermal HA remains more tissue associated, the greater portion remaining present following aqueous fixation. From this, it follows that dermal HA, the more tissue associated, may be the result of a greater proportion being modified by free radicals.

Another proviso is that free radicals and particularly ROS cleave HA, and the fragments generated are more susceptible to subsequent hyaluronidase cleavage than are the parent polymers [50].

Oxidative degradation of polysaccharides might result in nonspecific and/or specific scission of carbohydrate chains. This process could be an alternative and/or supplementary way for glycoside hydrolase-mediated hydrolysis to depolymerize polysaccharides. Indeed, ROS/RNS can degrade polysaccharides and lead to the subsequent enzymatic cleavage of glycosidic bonds. Cellular levels of ROS/RNS can effectively break down polysaccharides, and the data suggest that oxidative cleavage of carbohydrate chains is biologically relevant. It appears that ROS/RNS can also modify the monosaccharide composition of polysaccharides and potentially generate polymer fragments having properties substantially different from those of the original macromolecule. The impact of such changes is unclear but may have major consequences for the aging process, particularly in skin.

Stem Cells of Skin and Hyaluronan

Hyaluronan has a general effect of suppressing differentiation [51]. The concentration of HA is most prominent in tissues undergoing rapid growth and has been identified in the stem cell niche. Hyaluronan provides an environment for maintaining the undifferentiated stem cell state, as well as expansion of the stem cell population. Cells must exit from this HA-rich environment in order to undergo differentiation. The reservoir of stem cells for skin occurs in the bulge regions of hair follicles. They exit the bulge and migrate to areas where skin cell expansion and growth must occur [52]. One of the unsolved mysteries in dermatology is the source of skin stem cells in patients with alopecia areata. They appear to be spared in this disorder.

Retinoids

The synthesis of HA in vitro can be stimulated by several growth factors, including retinoids, dibutyryl cyclic adenosine monophosphate, and peroxisome proliferator-activated receptor-α agonists. The effect of retinyl retinoate, a novel retinol derivative on HA expression, was examined in primary human keratinocyte cultures and in hairless mouse epidermal skin. Histochemistry indicated that topical retinyl retinoate increased HA staining in the murine skin. Moreover, topical retinyl retinoate increased CD44 expression. Using reverse transcription polymerase chain reaction, the expression level of the *HAS2* gene in primary human keratinocytes and in hairless mouse epidermal skin was assessed. It was found that retinyl retinoate upregulates mouse and human *HAS2* mRNAs. Application of retinyl retinoate induced increasing transepidermal water loss less than retinol, retinoic acid, and retinaldehyde. Taken together, retinyl retinoate is more effective on HA production and less of an irritant than other retinoids. But the proper form of Vitamin A for human oral consumption and for maximal effect has still not been established.

Synergistic effects of hyaluronate fragments occur in retinaldehyde-induced skin hyperplasia, which appears to be a CD44-dependent phenomenon [53].

Corticosteroids and Skin Atrophy

Systemic corticosteroids induce skin dehydration and atrophy, as do topical applications. The parallel decrease with HA concentrations indicates a cause and effect relationship, as confirmed in a skin organ culture system [54]. Topical application of glucocorticoids causes a rapid reduction of dermal HA, a phenomenon caused by suppressed HA synthase activity, without an effect on hyaluronidase [55]. Glucocorticoids induce a nearly total inhibition of HAS2 mRNA in dermal fibroblasts, the predominant HA synthase therein [56].

Estrogen Effects

The influence of estrogen on aging has been examined in many organ systems, but there is surprisingly little information on the effect of estrogen on skin HA [57]. As the population ages, interest in skin moisture in postmenopausal women grows proportionately, as does the effect of estrogen on preventing skin aging.

This estrogen effect is best exemplified by the aging and drying of skin after menopause, when ovarian estrogen synthesis ceases. Women with full figures have increased levels of estrogens in their fat stores. These act as estrogen slow-release capsules long after ovaries stop estrogen production. This accounts in part for the moisture and more youthful appearing skin of such women.

Another example of the natural estrogen effect on skin is the sex skin of baboons. The increased redness and fullness of the female sex skin is largely HA and its associated solvent water [58]. From this, it is possible to extrapolate that the fullness of the perineal skin of the sexually aroused female primate is also based on HA. The fullness of the perilabial and perineal skin may also serve the secondary purpose of holding on to the male member more firmly. Direct experimental evidence also comes from observations that HA synthetic levels are induced by estrogens in mouse skin [59].

Vitamin C

Vitamin C (ascorbic acid) is added to many skin preparations that promise moisturizing effects, occurring occasionally at very high concentrations. The mechanisms of action behind such assurances are varied. Vitamin C has pronounced HA-stimulating effects in fibroblasts. The deposition of HA is stimulated when Vitamin C is added to cultured fibroblasts. The most profound changes occur in the compartmentalization of HA. The preponderance of the enhanced HA becomes cell-layer instead of being secreted into the medium [60, 61]. The chemical reactions catalyzed by ascorbic acid that bind HA to cell or matrix components are undefined. Derivatives of Vitamin C and their analogues can function as hyaluronidase inhibitors, in particular L-ascorbic acid-6-hexadecanoate [47]. Some of the ability of Vitamin C to enhance HA deposition may be attributed to its inhibition of hyaluronidase activity. But its oxidizing activity, in the presence of divalent cations, particularly iron and copper, complicates the role of Vitamin C in HA metabolism.

Alpha-Hydroxy Acids

Lactate is part of the anaerobic cycle of glucose metabolism. When lactic acid is added to cultures of human dermal fibroblasts, HA production increases in proportion to the lactate added [1]. Lactic acid is an AHA (α-hydroxy acid). A variety of topical prescription and nonprescription agents containing AHAs are used to enhance the appearance of skin. Such an antiaging effect may be by increasing HA levels in skin. This increases water volume, providing the plumping effect that fills out fine lines and wrinkles [62].

Many AHAs are organic acids derived from a variety of sources including a number of fruits: lactic acid from sour milk, glycolic acid from sugarcane, malic acid from apples, tartaric acid from grape wine, citric acid from citrus fruits, and mandelic acids from apricots, peaches, and almonds. There is a tradition common to many cultures in which fruit compresses are applied to the face in order to improve the appearance of skin. It is suspected that the AHAs contained in these fruit compresses stimulate production of HA and that the volume increase is the mechanism for this cosmetic effect. Of all the AHAs, mandelic acid is the most potent stimulator of HA production when added to cultures of human dermal fibroblasts (B. Neudecker and R. Stern, unpublished experiments).

Hyaluronan-Containing Commercial Skin Products

A great number of HA-containing products have been and continue to be on the market. These reagents have variable amounts of HA and in various widely differing formulations. However, they are all marketed as aids in restoring a youthful appearance. Early in the history of HA in cosmetics, the HA was added because of the "feel good" viscous sensation that it provided when women rubbed it between their fingers. However, within a short time, it became advertised as a natural hydrating reagent.

Topical Applications of Hyaluronan

In 1981, a salon in Paris introduced the very first skin care product to contain HA. Later, that same year, a series of beauty salons in Los Angeles launched another such product. All the HA used in these products, supplied by E. Balazs and J. Denlinger, was an animal product derived from rooster combs.

In 1985, a Japanese cosmetic firm began the production of HA based on bacterial fermentation using *Streptococcus zooepidemicus*. The animal-derived HA provides a much higher molecular weight material, compared to the bacterial. The latter also has the disadvantage that it is extremely difficult to remove the last traces of endotoxin, a bacterial product that is highly inflammatory.

Cross-Linked Hyaluronan and Injectable Fillers

The success of the HA-contaning skin care products led to the development of HA that could be injected under the skin to eliminate or decrease wrinkles. There had been a period prior to this in which collagen was injected under the skin. But these materials were discontinued because of the occasional inflammatory and immune reactions. The need for a substitute became obvious.

Many injectable cosmetic and dermal preparations contain HA in various concentrations and cross-linked using a number of reactions. In order to enhance the stability of the HA, various cross-linking procedures were developed. Some of this technology was an outgrowth of the development of cross-linked HA injectables for the treatment of arthritis. The body's own HA acts like a lubricant and a shock absorber in the synovial fluid of the joint and is needed in order for the joint to work properly. It becomes fragmented during the course of inflammation and age-related degeneration and trauma. The cross-linked injectable forms of rooster-comb HA provide relief from pain, an effect that can last several months.

In its natural state, HA exhibits poor biomechanical properties as a dermal filler. As a soluble polymer, it is cleared rapidly when injected into normal skin. To provide the ability to fill wrinkles in skin, several chemical modifications have been employed. The two most common functional groups that can be modified are the carboxylic acid and the hydroxyl alcohol moieties. Many methods for cross-linking HA are available using these two reactive groups. Biomaterials have been produced through modification of the carboxyl acid group by esterification and through the use of cross-linkers such as dialdehydes and disulfides. The most commonly employed cross-linkers for dermal fillers are divinyl sulfone and diglycidyl ethers, and bis-epoxides. This family of products is the first HA-derived materials to be approved by the FDA for skin injection.

Additional injectable, long-lasting, resorbable HA-modified fillers have recently become available, though the nature or number of the cross-links are not disclosed [63]. The manufacturers claim it is a novel version of the usual HA filers comprised of a homogenized gel that is not a gel-particle suspension. It uses a high concentration of cross-links and manages to retain a gelatinous texture. Interestingly, it has been effective in the treatment of focal steroid atrophy [64].

Another product is an effective treatment modality for moisturizing skin [65–67]. Topical application enhances the moisture of underlying epidermis and extends down into the upper layers of the dermis. A free radical polymerization process is used to cross-link high molecular weight HA polymers into a coil-coil system generating spheres of infinite size. These dry sponge-like spheres, applied to the skin, take on large volumes of water that remain associated with the skin. The nonhydrated spheres are 20–50 um in diameter and grow typically to 400 × 800 um spheres when hydrated, the hydrated sphere being less than 1 % HA, and the rest, i.e., the sponges, take on 100 times their weight in water. The fully hydrated sponges constitute an HA gel system that retains moisture in intimate contact with the skin surface.

There is an intrinsic need to ensure that all such materials do not contain short HA chains that could stimulate an inflammatory response. An additional caution is the generation of short HA fragments that could be cleaved from those cross-linked polymers by endogenous tissue hyaluronidases that could also be highly inflammatory.

Hyaluronan Delivery Through Nanoparticles

A new potential for the application of HA to skin has been initiated with studies on transdermal delivery of nanoparticles. Successful treatment of photodamaged skin was accomplished using nanoscale retinoic acid particles in a novel transdermal delivery system [68]. Whether HA-coated nanoparticles can be used in a similar system to enhance skin moisture and overall appearance of aging and photodamaged skin awaits further studies [69].

In cultured fibroblasts, exogenously added HA is incorporated into fine HA filaments of the pericellular fibroblast matrix. This indicates that soluble HA facilitates assembly of a supramolecular pericellular structure [70]. It would be important to determine whether any topically applied HA to skin in vivo has this effect, whether it is size dependent, and whether any such materials can permeate human skin. Whether cross-linked HA has this property has not been established, nor whether injected stabilized HA or HA delivered through nanoparticles can perform such functions.

Systemic Administration of Hyaluronan

An interesting era of HA biology has begun, with the documentation that systemic administration of HA can have system-wide effects. Intraperitoneal injection of HMW HA stimulates wound healing in diabetic mice [71]. It would be essential that the turnover of such HA be measured in an experimental animal system, accompanied by observations on chain length. Whether the systemic administration of HA can enhance skin hydration to any degree would be the next step.

Oral Administration of Hyaluronan

The literature on the effects of orally administered HA is vast, contradictory, and very confusing. Chain lengths of the polymer used in such studies are often not provided. As documented, this may be the source of much confusion. Controlled, prospective clinical trials are necessary with a need to demonstrate strict dose-dependent effects. It has not been established whether HA survives oral administration, and whether absorption through the small intestine takes place. And whether skin moisture can be modified by oral HA is the critical question.

Conclusion

Skin contains 50 % of body HA. It is a major component of the ECM of skin, appearing in epidermis, dermis, as well as in the basal lamina that lies between. Hyaluronan is also observed intracellularly, where its functions remain unknown. This GAG plays an important role in metabolism, cell turnover, differentiation, cell movement, tissue repair, hydration, nutrient exchange, and protection against free radical damage. Its rapid turnover suggests that it may also be important as a conduit for the removal of toxic materials. It plays key roles in signal transduction pathways, an area of the literature that is so voluminous that it could not be summarized in the present communication. Native HA as well as modified cross-linked HA has been employed to help skin maintain and even regain elasticity, turgor, as well as moisture. The literature on HA is growing rapidly. Dermatology benefits disproportionately as new breakthroughs occur.

References

1. Stern R, Maibach HI. Hyaluronan in skin: aspects of aging and its pharmacologic modulation. Clin Dermatol. 2008;26:106–22.
2. Stern R. Hyaluronan: key to skin moisturization. In: Loden M, Maibach HI, editors. Dry skin and moisturizers: chemistry and function. 2nd ed. Boca Raton: CRC Press; 2005. p. 245–78.
3. Laurent TC, Fraser JR. Hyaluronan. FASEB J. 1992;6:2397–404.
4. Laurent TC, Laurent UB, Fraser JR. Serum hyaluronan as a disease marker. Ann Med. 1996;28:241–53.
5. Laurent TC, Laurent UB, Fraser JR. The structure and function of hyaluronan: an overview. Immunol Cell Biol. 1996;74:1–7.
6. Toole BP. Hyaluronan in morphogenesis. Semin Cell Dev Biol. 2001;12:79–87.
7. Lee JY, Spicer AP. Hyaluronan: a multifunctional, megaDalton stealth molecule. Curr Opin Cell Biol. 2000;12:581–6.
8. Aya K, Stern R. Hyaluronan in wound healing: rediscovering a major player. Wound Repair Regen. 2014;22:579–93.
9. Jiang D, Liang J, Noble PW. Hyaluronan as an immune regulator in human diseases. Physiol Rev. 2011;91:221–64.
10. Jiang D, Liang J, Noble PW. Hyaluronan in tissue injury and repair. Annu Rev Cell Dev Biol. 2007;23:435–61.
11. Meyer LJ, Stern R. Age-dependent changes of hyaluronan in human skin. J Invest Dermatol. 1994;102:385–9.
12. Lin W, Shuster S, Maibach HI, Stern R. Patterns of hyaluronan staining are modified by fixation techniques. J Histochem Cytochem. 1997;45:1157–63.
13. Reed RK, Lilja K, Laurent TC. Hyaluronan in the rat with special reference to the skin. Acta Physiol Scand. 1988;134:405–11.
14. Lamberg SI, Yuspa SH, Hascall VC. Synthesis of hyaluronic acid is decreased and synthesis of proteoglycans is increased when cultured mouse epidermal cells differentiate. J Invest Dermatol. 1986;86:659–67.
15. Tammi R, Säämänen AM, Maibach HI, Tammi M. Degradation of newly synthesized high molecular mass hyaluronan in the epidermal and dermal compartments of human skin in organ culture. J Invest Dermatol. 1991;97:126–30.
16. Bourguignon LY, Singleton PA, Diedrich F, Stern R, Gilad E. CD44 interaction with $Na^{+}-H^{+}$ exchanger (NHE1) creates acidic microenvironments leading to hyaluronidase-2 and cathepsin B activation and breast tumor cell invasion. J Biol Chem. 2004;279:26991–7007.
17. Oliferenko S, Paiha K, Harder T, Gerke V, Schwärzler C, Schwarz H, Beug H, Günthert U, Huber LA. Analysis of CD44-containing lipid rafts: recruitment of annexin II and stabilization by the actin cytoskeleton. J Cell Biol. 1999;146:843–54.
18. Jokela TA, Lindgren A, Rilla K, Maytin E, Hascall VC, Tammi RH, Tammi MI. Induction of hyaluronan cables and monocyte adherence in epidermal keratinocytes. Connect Tissue Res. 2008;49:115–9.
19. Akazawa Y, Sayo T, Sugiyama Y, Sato T, Akimoto N, Ito A, Inoue S. Adiponectin resides in mouse skin and upregulates hyaluronan synthesis in dermal fibroblasts. Connect Tissue Res. 2011;52:322–8.
20. Bertheim U, Engström-Laurent A, Hofer PA, Hallgren P, Asplund J, Hellström S. Loss of hyaluronan in the basement membrane zone of the skin correlates to the degree of stiff hands in diabetic patients. Acta Derm Venereol. 2002;82:329–34.
21. Gu H, Huang L, Wong YP, Burd A. HA modulation of epidermal morphogenesis in an organotypic keratinocyte-fibroblast co-culture model. Exp Dermatol. 2010;19:336–9.
22. Stern A, Stern R. Absence of skin rash in Goodpasture's syndrome: the hyaluronan effect. Med Hypotheses. 2014;83:769–71.
23. McBride WH, Bard JB. Hyaluronidase-sensitive halos around adherent cells. Their role in blocking lymphocyte-mediated cytolysis. J Exp Med. 1979;149:507–15.
24. Delmage JM, Powars DR, Jaynes PK, Allerton SE. The selective suppression of immunogenicity by hyaluronic acid. Ann Clin Lab Sci. 1986;16:303–10.
25. Stern R, Asari AA, Sugahara KN. Hyaluronan fragments: an information-rich system. Eur J Cell Biol. 2006;85:699–715.
26. Prusova A, Smejkolova D, Chytil M, Velebny V, Kucerik J. An alternative DSC (differential scanning colorimetry) approach to study the hydration of hyaluronan. Carbohydr Polym. 2010;52:498–503.
27. Hargitai I, Hargittai M. Molecular structure of hyaluronan: an introduction. Struct Chem. 2008;19:697–717.
28. Tzellos TG, Klagas I, Vahtsevanos K, Triaridis S, Printza A, Kyrgidis A, Karakiulakis G, Zouboulis CC, Papakonstantinou E. Extrinsic ageing in the human skin is associated with alterations in the expression of hyaluronic acid and its metabolizing enzymes. Exp Dermatol. 2009;18:1028–35.
29. Itano N, Sawai T, Yoshida M, Lenas P, Yamada Y, Imagawa M, Shinomura T, Hamaguchi M, Yoshida Y,

Ohnuki Y, Miyauchi S, Spicer AP, McDonald JA, Kimata K. Three isoforms of mammalian hyaluronan synthases have distinct enzymatic properties. J Biol Chem. 1999;274:25085–92.
30. Weigel PH, Hascall VC, Tammi M. Hyaluronan synthases. J Biol Chem. 1997;272:13997–4000.
31. Stern R, Jedrzejas MJ. Hyaluronidases: their genomics, structures, and mechanisms of action. Chem Rev. 2006;106:818–39.
32. Gasingirwa MC, Thirion J, Mertens-Strijthagen J, Wattiaux-De Coninck S, Flamion B, Wattiaux R, Jadot M. Endocytosis of hyaluronidase-1 by the liver. Biochem J. 2010;430:305–13.
33. de la Motte C, Nigro J, Vasanji A, Rho H, Kessler S, Bandyopadhyay S, Danese S, Fiocchi C, Stern R. Platelet-derived hyaluronidase 2 cleaves hyaluronan into fragments that trigger monocyte-mediated production of proinflammatory cytokines. Am J Pathol. 2009;174:2254–64.
34. Stern R. Devising a pathway for hyaluronan catabolism. Are we there yet? Glycobiology. 2003;13:105–15.
35. Shearer J, Graham TE. New perspectives on the storage and organization of muscle glycogen. Can J Appl Physiol. 2002;27:179–203.
36. Mian N. Analysis of cell-growth-phase-related variations in hyaluronate synthase activity of isolated plasma-membrane fractions of cultured human skin fibroblasts. Biochem J. 1986;237:333–42.
37. Mian N. Characterization of a high-Mr plasma-membrane-bound protein and assessment of its role as a constituent of hyaluronate synthase complex. Biochem J. 1986;237:343–57.
38. Philipson LH, Schwartz NB. Subcellular localization of hyaluronate synthetase in oligodendroglioma cells. J Biol Chem. 1984;259:5017–23.
39. Philipson LH, Westley J, Schwartz NB. Effect of hyaluronidase treatment of intact cells on hyaluronate synthetase activity. Biochemistry. 1985;24:7899–906.
40. Larnier C, Kerneur C, Robert L, Moczar M. Effect of testicular hyaluronidase on hyaluronate synthesis by human skin fibroblasts in culture. Biochim Biophys Acta. 1989;1014:145–52.
41. Stern R, Shuster S, Wiley TS, Formby B. Hyaluronidase can modulate expression of CD44. Exp Cell Res. 2001;266:167–76.
42. Dai G, Freudenberger T, Zipper P, Melchior A, Grether-Beck S, Rabausch B, de Groot J, Twarock S, Hanenberg H, Homey B, Krutmann J, Reifenberger J, Fischer JW. Chronic ultraviolet B irradiation causes loss of hyaluronic acid from mouse dermis because of down-regulation of hyaluronic acid synthases. Am J Pathol. 2007;171:1451–61.
43. Röck K, Fischer K, Fischer JW. Hyaluronan used for intradermal injections is incorporated into the pericellular matrix and promotes proliferation in human skin fibroblasts in vitro. Dermatology. 2010;221:19–28.
44. Hašová M, Crhák T, Safránková B, Dvořáková J, Muthný T, Velebný V, Kubala L. Hyaluronan minimizes effects of UV irradiation on human keratinocytes. Arch Dermatol Res. 2011;303:277–84.
45. Agren UM, Tammi RH, Tammi MI. Reactive oxygen species contribute to epidermal hyaluronan catabolism in human skin organ culture. Free Radic Biol Med. 1997;23:996–1001.
46. Mio K, Stern R. Inhibitors of the hyaluronidases. Matrix Biol. 2002;21:31–7.
47. Botzki A, Rigden DJ, Braun S, Nukui M, Salmen S, Hoechstetter J, Bernhardt G, Dove S, Jedrzejas MJ, Buschauer A. L-Ascorbic acid 6-hexadecanoate, a potent hyaluronidase inhibitor. X-ray structure and molecular modeling of enzyme-inhibitor complexes. J Biol Chem. 2004;279:45990–7.
48. Volpi N, Schiller J, Stern R, Soltes L. Role, metabolism, chemical modifications and applications of hyaluronan. Curr Med Chem. 2009;16:1718–45.
49. Oh JH, Kim YK, Jung JY, Shin JE, Chung JH. Changes in glycosamino-glycans and related proteoglycans in intrinsically aged human skin in vivo. Exp Dermatol. 2011;20:454–6.
50. Duan J, Kasper DL. Oxidative depolymerization of polysaccharides by reactive oxygen/nitrogen species. Glycobiology. 2011;21:401–9.
51. Passi A, Sadeghi P, Kawamura H, Anand S, Sato N, White LE, Hascall VC, Maytin EV. Hyaluronan suppresses epidermal differentiation in organotypic cultures of rat keratinocytes. Exp Cell Res. 2004;296:123–34.
52. Underhill CB. Hyaluronan is inversely correlated with the expression of CD44 in the dermal condensation of the embryonic hair follicle. J Invest Dermatol. 1993;101:820–6.
53. Barnes L, Tran C, Sorg O, Hotz R, Grand D, Carraux P, Didierjean L, Stamenkovic I, Saurat JH, Kaya G. Synergistic effect of hyaluronate fragments in retinaldehyde-induced skin hyperplasia which is a CD44-dependent phenomenon. PLoS One. 2010;5:e14372.
54. Agren UM, Tammi M, Tammi R. Hydrocortisone regulation of hyaluronan metabolism in human skin organ culture. J Cell Physiol. 1997;164:240–8.
55. Gebhardt C, Averbeck M, Diedenhofen N, Willenberg A, Anderegg U, Sleeman JP, Simon JC. Dermal hyaluronan is rapidly reduced by topical treatment with glucocorticoids. J Invest Dermatol. 2010;130:141–9.
56. Averbeck M, Gebhardt C, Anderegg U, Simon JC. Suppression of hyaluronan synthase 2 expression reflects the atrophogenic potential of glucocorticoids. Exp Dermatol. 2010;19:757–9.
57. Shah MG, Maibach HI. Estrogen and skin. An overview. Am J Clin Dermatol. 2001;2:143–50.
58. Bentley JP, Brenner RM, Linstedt AD, West NB, Carlisle KS, Rokosova BC, MacDonald N. Increased hyaluronate and collagen biosynthesis and fibroblast estrogen receptors in macaque sex skin. J Invest Dermatol. 1986;87:668–73.
59. Uzuka M, Nakajima K, Ohta S, Mori Y. Induction of hyaluronic acid synthetase by estrogen in the mouse skin. Biochim Biophys Acta. 1981;673:387–93.

60. Huey G, Moiin A, Stern R. Levels of [3H]glucosamine incorporation into hyaluronic acid by fibroblasts is modulated by culture conditions. Matrix. 1990;10:75–83.
61. Kao J, Huey G, Kao R, Stern R. Ascorbic acid stimulates production of glycosaminoglycans in cultured fibroblasts. Exp Mol Pathol. 1990;53:1–10.
62. Ditre CM, Griffin TD, Murphy GF, Sueki H, Telegan B, Johnson WC, Yu RJ, Van Scott EJ. Effects of alpha-hydroxy acids on photoaged skin: a pilot clinical, histologic, and ultrastructural study. J Am Acad Dermatol. 1996;34:187–95.
63. Fischer TC. A European evaluation of cosmetic treatment of facial voume loss with Juvéderm^{TM} Voluma^{TM} in patients previously treated with Restylane SUB-Q^{TM}. J Cosmet Dermatol. 2010;9:291–6.
64. Elliott L, Rashid RM, Colome M. Hyaluronic acid filler for steroid atrophy. J Cosmet Dermatol. 2010;9:253–5.
65. Balazs EA. Hyaluronan-based composition and cosmetic formulations containing same. US Patent #4,303,676. 1981.
66. Phillips GO, du Plessis TA, Al-Assaf S, Williams PA. US Patent #6,610,810. 2003.
67. Phillips GO, du Plessis TA, Al-Assaf S, Williams PA. US Patent #6,841,644. 2005.
68. Yamaguchi Y, Nagasawa T, Nakamura N, Takenaga M, Mizoguchi M, Kawai S, Mizushima Y, Igarashi R. Successful treatment of photo-damaged skin of nano-scale atRA particles using a novel transdermal delivery. J Control Release. 2005;104:29–40.
69. Gupta S, Bansal R, Gupta S, Jindal N, Jindal A. Nanocarriers and nanoparticles for skin care and dermatological treatments. Indian Dermatol Online J. 2013;4:267–72.
70. Röck K, Grandoch M, Majora M, Krutmann J, Fischer JW. Collagen fragments inhibit hyaluronan synthesis in skin fibroblasts in response to UVB: new insights into mechanisms of matrix remodeling. J Biol Chem. 2011;286:18268–76.
71. Galeano M, Polito F, Bitto A, Irrera N, Campo GM, Avenoso A, Calò M, Cascio PL, Minutoli L, Barone M, Squadrito F, Altavilla D. Systemic administration of high-molecular weight hyaluronan stimulates wound healing in genetically diabetic mice. Biochim Biophys Acta. 2011;1812:752759.

Changes in Nail in the Aged

19

Nelly Rubeiz, Ossama Abbas, and Abdul Ghani Kibbi

Contents

N. Rubeiz • O. Abbas • A.G. Kibbi (✉)
Department of Dermatology, American University of Beirut Medical Center, Beirut, Lebanon
e-mail: ngrubeiz@aub.edu.lb; ossamaabbas2003@yahoo.com; agkibbi@aub.edu.lb

M.A. Farage et al. (eds.), *Textbook of Aging Skin*,
DOI 10.1007/978-3-662-47398-6_23

Abstract

Nail abnormalities commonly affect the elderly population. These may represent either normal age-related nail changes or nail dystrophies that tend to be more common in the older population due to several factors. These factors, which include impaired circulation, faulty biomechanics, infections, neoplasms, and dermatological or systemic diseases, may affect the matrix, nail bed, hyponychium, or nail folds with secondary nail plate changes. These nail alterations may be symptomatic and may impair daily activities or may be associated with significant cosmetic problems leading to a negative psychological impact. Knowledge of these age-related nail changes and dystrophies as well as their underlying causes is important in order to effectively reach an accurate diagnosis and thus provide better care for the nail concerns of this large and growing elderly population.

Introduction

Nail complaints are very common among the elderly. These may represent either normal age-related nail alterations or nail dystrophies that tend to be more common in the elderly secondary to several factors including impaired circulation, faulty biomechanics, infections, neoplasms, and dermatological or systemic diseases [1, 2]. Alone or in combination, these factors may affect the matrix, nail bed, hyponychium, or nail folds leading to secondary abnormalities in the nail plate. These nail alterations may be symptomatic and may impair daily activities or may be associated with significant cosmetic problems leading to a negative psychological impact. Knowledge of these age-related nail changes and dystrophies as well as their underlying causes is important in order to effectively reach an accurate diagnosis and thus provide better care for the nail concerns of this large and growing elderly population.

Normal Senile Nail Changes

The age-associated nail changes include characteristic changes in morphology, growth, chemical composition, and histology of the nail unit [1, 2]. The mechanisms underlying these changes are not clear, but may be due to a dysfunctional circulation at the distal extremities or to the ultraviolet radiation effects.

Age-Related Morphological Nail Changes

These include changes in color, contour, surface, and thickness of the nail plate [1, 2]. Among the most common nail color changes observed in elderly people is a yellow to gray discoloration with dull, pale, or opaque appearance. The normally smooth texture of the nail plate tends to become increasingly friable with advancing age leading to splitting, fissuring, and longitudinal superficial or deep striations [1, 2]. In general, nail plates are thicker in men than women, where the normal average thickness of fingernails and toenails is 0.6 and 1.65 mm in men and 0.5 and 1.38 mm in women, respectively. With advancing age, the nail plate thickness may become thicker, thinner, or remain the same [1, 2]. "Neapolitan nails" is a peculiar discoloration observed in up to 20 % of people above 70 years and manifests as three horizontal bands of white (proximal), pink (middle), and opaque (distally) discoloration in addition to an absent lunula [1]. One study found that this peculiar nail alteration is significantly associated with osteoporosis and thin skin and suggested an abnormality in collagen leading to these changes in the nail bed, bone, and skin [3].

Although usually seen in liver cirrhosis and chronic congestive heart failure, Terry's nails, a type of apparent leukonychia characterized by a distal transverse pink band and proximal white band, is occasionally seen as a part of the normal aging process [4]. Senile nail contour changes include an increase in the transverse convexity and a decrease in the longitudinal curvature [1, 2].

Age-Related Nail Growth Rate Changes

The normal average growth rate of fingernails and toenails is 3.0 and 1.0 mm/month, respectively. In elderly people, there is a decrease in this rate of growth by approximately 0.5 %/year after the age of 25 years [1, 2].

Age-Related Changes in the Chemical Composition of the Nail Plate

The nail plate is made up of tightly layered cornified cells that are generated by the nail matrix epithelium and consists mainly of intermediate filamentous proteins or keratins (80–90 % of which are of hard keratins) [5]. The keratins are embedded in a matrix composed of nonkeratin proteins (high-sulfur and high-glycine/tyrosine proteins). Other nail plate constituents include water (7 and 18 %), lipids (0.1–5 %), and trace elements (mainly iron, zinc, calcium, and magnesium) [1, 2, 5–7]. Normally, the nail plate calcium (Ca) content is low (0.2 % by weight), while the sulfur content is high (10 % by weight) [4]. It is believed that the relatively higher-sulfur content to Ca content contributes to nail plate hardness, especially that the former is a reflection of the cysteine disulfide bonds which stabilize fibrous proteins [6]. Even though the Ca content of the nail does not seem to contribute to the hardness of the nail plate, a recent study revealed that both fingernail and toenail Ca concentration decrease with advancing age while magnesium (Mg) concentration tend to increase [6]. Interestingly, this study also showed that measurement of the Ca and Mg contents of the nail plate may be used as an osteoporosis predictor. The iron content usually decreases in senile nails [1, 2]. Another constituent of nail plates are membrane-forming integral lipids such as cholesterol and cholesterol sulfate, which are also present in keratinized skin areas and hair. There is an age-related significant decrease in fingernail cholesterol sulfate levels which has been reported in women and may explain the higher incidence of brittle nails in the elderly category [8].

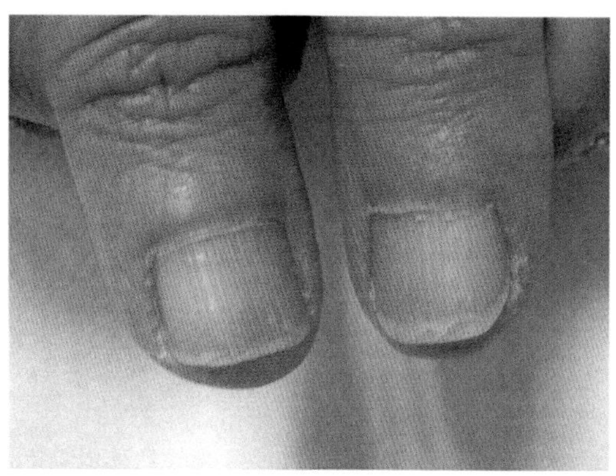

Fig. 1 Brittle nails

Age-Related Changes in Nail Histology

Compared to young individuals, the dermis of the nail bed usually exhibits elastic tissue degeneration and thickening of the blood vessels. In addition, the keratinocytes of the nail plate are commonly enlarged and show increased remnants of keratinocyte nuclei, which are also known as pertinax bodies [1, 2, 9]. To the best of the authors' knowledge, there are no reports describing the changes that may occur in the nail matrix as a result of aging.

Age-Related Nail Dystrophies

Several nail disorders affect the population at large and may appear with advancing age and include, without order of frequency or age-related prevalence, brittle nails, infections (especially onychomycosis), onychauxis, onychocryptosis, onychoclavus, onychogryphosis, onychophosis, splinter hemorrhages, subungual hematoma, and malignancies of the nail apparatus [1, 2, 7–12].

Brittle Nails

Brittle nail disorder is characterized by increased nail plate fragility and is considered to be a polymorphic abnormality affecting about 20 % of the population with higher incidence in women and the elderly [7]. Clinically, brittle nails manifest with onychoschizia and onychorrhexis (Fig. 1), the severity of either may be variable [7]. Onychoschizia, which results from impairment of intercellular adhesion of nail plate corneocytes, usually presents as a lamellar splitting of the distal portion and free edge of the nail plate and a transverse splitting secondary to breakage of the lateral edges. Underlying causes are usually exogenous and include trauma, repetitive cycles of wetting and drying, the action of fungal proteolytic products, and the use of chemicals or cosmetics such as nail enamel solvents, cuticle removers, and nail hardeners, among others.

Onychorrhexis, which results from abnormalities in epithelial growth and keratinization secondary to nail matrix involvement, usually manifests as longitudinal thickening, splitting, or ridging of the nail plate and/or multiple splits leading to triangular fragments at the free edge. Abnormalities of vascularization and oxygenation (such as arteriosclerosis or anemia), dermatological (inflammatory diseases and disorders of cornification), and systemic diseases (endocrine, metabolic, etc.) are among the various factors that may underlie the abnormalities of growth and keratinization responsible for onychorrhexis.

Recently, a composite scoring system assessing the severity of nail brittleness based on the degree of ridging, nail thickness, lamellar, longitudinal, and transverse splitting has been proposed [7].

Management of brittle nails may not be easy or simple [7]. The initial therapeutic approach is to determine the predominance of either onychoschizia or onychorrhexis. Underlying factors should then be identified and if possible, be corrected. After that, general and specific measures may be followed. Nail hydration by 15 min daily soaks of the nail and by the application of emollients rich in phospholipids may be useful. Strengthening the nail plate may be accomplished by the application of nail hardeners containing formaldehyde; however, these should be utilized cautiously because they may lead to brittleness, onycholysis, and subungual hyperkeratosis.

Although enamel application may mechanically protect the nail and fill the fractures; its removal however, may lead to substantial dehydration. Several studies have shown that daily oral intake of biotin (2.5 mg/day) for 1.5–15 months may be beneficial; however, these studies are small and not double-blind placebo controlled [7, 10, 11].

Infections

Infections by different pathogens may affect the nail plate either primarily or through extension from involved adjacent structures such as the nail folds [1, 2, 10–12].

Onychomycosis, a fungal infection of the fingernails and/or toenails, is the most common infection and represents up to half of all nail diseases [12]. It affects 10–20 % of adults, especially the elderly. Multiple factors are associated with an increased risk of onychomycosis including old age, male gender, underlying medical diseases (diabetes, peripheral arterial disease, and immunodeficiency), smoking, and predisposing genetic factors [12]. More than 90 % of onychomycosis cases are caused by dermatophytes, among which *Trichophyton rubrum* and *T. mentagrophytes* are the most common. Other less commonly encountered causative organisms include yeasts such as *Candid*a and nondermatophyte molds such as *Scopulariopsis brevicaulis* and *Scytalidium hyalinum* [12]. Five clinical subtypes of onychomycosis are recognized [12]. Distal and lateral subungual onychomycosis (DLSO), the most common subtype usually caused by *T. rubrum*, manifests as subungual hyperkeratosis, onycholysis, nail thickening, and discoloration secondary to fungal invasion which starts at the hyponychium and spreads proximally along the nail bed (Fig. 2). Superficial onychomycosis usually presents as white (caused by *T. mentagrophytes*) or black (caused by dematiaceous fungi) patchy nail discoloration due to fungal invasion of the dorsal surface of the nail plate. Proximal subungual onychomycosis (PSO) commonly affects immunocompromised individuals and presents clinically as a white spot under the lunula that progresses distally. It results from fungal invasion (usually *T. rubrum*), from the proximal nail fold to the nail plate. Endonyx onychomycosis (EO) is an uncommon form caused by *T. soudanense*; it resembles DLSO; however, the nail thickness is within normal and there is no hyperkeratosis or onycholysis. Total dystrophic onychomycosis (TDO) is an advanced form, characterized by progressive nail plate destruction leaving an exposed abnormally thickened nail bed.

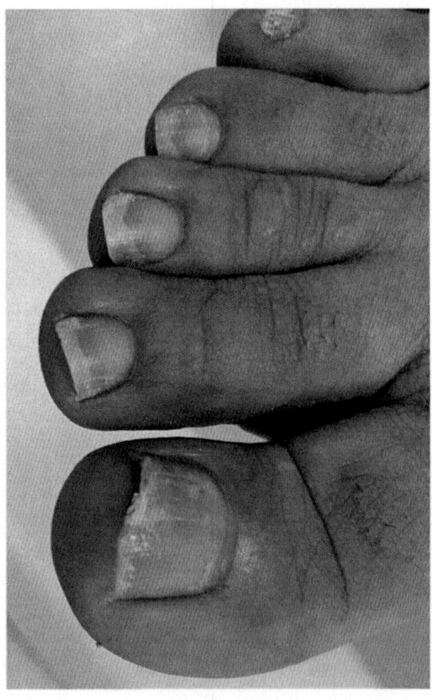

Fig. 2 Distal and lateral subungual onychomycosis

TDO may be observed in immunodeficient patients such as those with chronic mucocutaneous candidiasis and is fairly acute or may be progressive representing an end stage of other forms of onychomycosis.

Effective treatment of onychomycosis entails making an accurate diagnosis and identifying the causative pathogen [12, 13]. Several diagnostic methods including KOH-based microscopy, fungal cultures, and histopathology with PAS may be used alone or in combination, the latter being the most sensitive [12, 13]. The treatment options include oral and/or topical antifungal agents, mechanical or chemical treatments, or a combination of these. The choice of the therapy should be individualized based on several factors such as the causative agent, the potential for drug interactions and side effects, the number of nails involved, the severity of onychomycosis, and the cost. Currently, terbinafine appears to be the most effective oral agent for treating dermatophyte onychomycosis, especially in elderly patients due to its fungicidal action, safety, and low potential for drug interaction [13]. The azoles (ketoconazole, fluconazole, itraconazole) can also be used but are generally considered to be less effective than terbinafine as they are fungistatic rather than fungicidal [13].

Paronychia, seen occasionally in elderly patients, is an acute or chronic infection of the nail folds which may lead to secondary changes in the nail plate [1, 2]. Acute paronychia, usually caused by *Staphylococcus aureus*, most commonly presents as tender erythematous swelling of only one nail and is typically trauma induced. Management includes abscess drainage, warm saline soaks, and the use of topical or systemic antibiotics. Chronic paronychia is commonly caused by *Candida* species or Gram-negative bacteria and presents clinically as red and swollen nail folds with loss of cuticle and multiple secondary transverse ridges in the nail plate (Fig. 3). Keeping the nail fold dry coupled with topical antifungal or antiseptic agents is the treatment of choice.

Elderly patients, similar to infants and immunosuppressed hosts, are prone to uncommon presentations of *Sarcoptes scabiei* infestation in which all skin surfaces such as the scalp and face, as well as nails, may be affected. The mite may inhabit and persist in subungual hyperkeratotic debris, leading to prolonged infestations and/or epidemics among elderly patients and those caring for them in nursing homes. Cutting the nails as much as possible and brushing their tips with a scabicide is an adjunct modality to the antiscabetic treatment [1, 2].

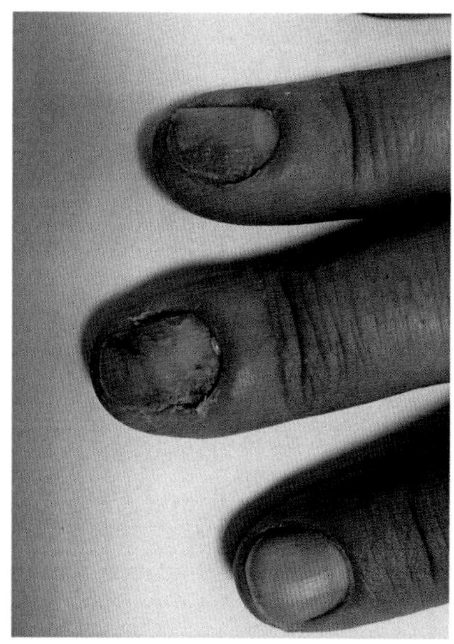

Fig. 3 Chronic paronychia with secondary nail changes

Onychauxis

Onychauxis is a localized hypertrophy of the nail plate which presents clinically as discoloration, hyperkeratosis, loss of nail plate translucency, and often subungual hyperkeratosis [1, 2]. The underlying cause/s may be related to the aging process or to faulty biomechanics that tend to be more common in the geriatric population. Overlapping and underlapping toes, digiti flexi (contracted toes secondary to buckling of toes induced by shortening of the controlling muscles), or foot-to-shoe incompatibility are examples of these faulty mechanics. Onychauxis may be associated with pain and, with time, may be complicated by distal onycholysis, increased risk for onychomycosis, subungual hemorrhage, and/or subungual ulceration.

Partial or total debridement of the thickened nail plate should be done periodically. Other treatment options include the use of electric drills, 40 % or higher urea paste, or nail avulsion. In complicated cases or those with recurrences, chemical or surgical matricectomy may be done to achieve permanent ablation of the affected plate.

Onychoclavus

Onychoclavus, also known as subungual corn, is a hyperkeratotic process most commonly located under the distal nail margins [1, 2]. It results from chronic minor trauma and persistent localized pressure by bony abnormalities such as digiti flexi, rotated fifth toes, foot-to-shoe incompatibility, or hallux valgus (the great toe rotates toward the second toe). It usually presents as a tender dark area under the nail plate (most commonly the great toenail) and may be confused with benign and malignant subungual melanocytic lesions and subungual exostosis [1, 2].

The treatment of this condition is surgical removal of the hyperkeratotic tissue and the correction of the underlying bony abnormality.

Onychogryphosis

Onychogryphosis, also known as ram's horn nail, is a term used to describe thickening and enlargement of the nail plate (Fig. 4), most commonly the great toenails [1, 2]. The affected nail plate is usually brownish to opaque in color, grows faster on one side than the other, may have many grooves and transverse striations, and is commonly associated with nail bed hypertrophy. This nail dystrophy is common among the elderly population and, if untreated, may lead to a walking disability. In patients with diabetes mellitus or peripheral vascular disease, onychogryphosis may be complicated by subungual gangrene due to pressure effects [1]. Infrequent nail cutting, trauma, foot-to-shoe incompatibility, and bony abnormalities such as hallux valgus are responsible for its pathogenesis. Onychogryphosis should be distinguished from hemionychogryphosis, which is characterized by the lateral growth of the nail plate from the onset as a complication of persistent congenital malalignment of the great toenails.

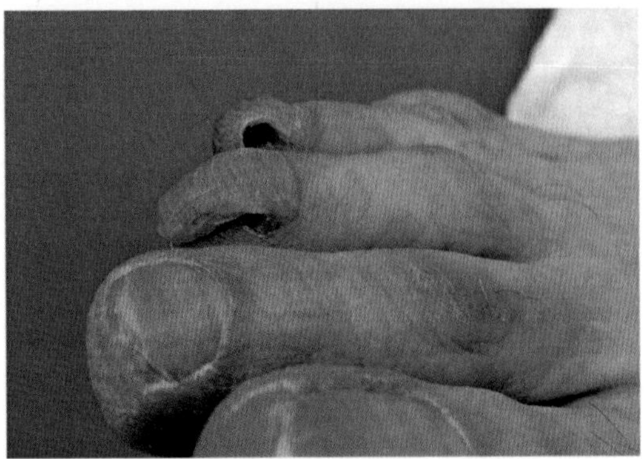

Fig. 4 Onychogryphosis

Beyond cosmetic considerations, treatment of onychogryphosis in the elderly may be mandatory in order to prevent disability and its complications [1, 2]. Conservative management with the use of an electric drill or burr to file the involved nail plate is the initial step followed by removal of subungual hyperkeratosis and subsequent periodic nail plate trimming. Other more radical approaches such as nail avulsion, with or without matricectomy, may be valuable in selected patients.

Onychophosis

Onychophosis is a localized or diffuse hyperkeratosis under the nail plate (subungual), on the lateral or proximal nail folds, or in the space between the nail plate and nail folds [1, 2]. The first and the fifth toes are the digits of predilection. Multiple nail and adjacent soft tissue abnormalities including onychocryptosis, nail fold hypertrophy, and onychomycosis may be the underlying causes of onychophosis. Other external causes such as repeated minor trauma and foot-to-shoe incompatibility may be contributing.

Several treatment modalities may be used to treat onychophosis and include keratolytic agents (urea 20 % or salicylic acid 6–20 %), nail packing, and, if needed, surgical excision. Recurrences may be prevented by wearing appropriate comfortable shoes to minimize pressure effects of the nail plate on surrounding nail folds.

Onychocryptosis (Ingrown Toenail)

Although more commonly observed in young adults, onychocryptosis may occasionally be encountered in the elderly causing significant pain, difficulty walking, and disability [1, 2, 14]. It occurs when the lateral nail plate penetrates the adjacent nail fold (Fig. 5) as a result of nail plate over-curvature, subcutaneous ingrowing toenail, and/or lateral nail fold hypertrophy. Clinically, patients commonly present with tenderness and inflammation of the lateral nail fold, which at times, may be associated with granulation tissue formation and secondary infection. The most common underlying causative factor/s include improper nail cutting, ill-fitting or high-heeled shoes, hyperhidrosis, long toes, prominent nail folds, and bony abnormalities such as hallux valgus.

The management of ingrown toenail consists of treating the acute signs and symptoms and correcting the underlying predisposing factors [1, 2]. There is an evidence that the best chance for complete cure is to excise the lateral nail plate, to curette the granulation tissue, and to perform lateral matricectomy [1, 2, 14]. This procedure may be complicated by postoperative nail bed infection or by regrowth of a nail spicule secondary to incomplete matricectomy. In addition, this procedure, not uncommonly, may lead to recurrences and poor cosmetic results. Recently, surgical decompression of the ingrown toenail without matricectomy has been proven to be very effective. In this approach, a large volume of soft tissue around the nail plate is removed, and the inflammation is relieved [14]. The advantage of this maneuver is complete preservation of the nail anatomy and function with excellent therapeutic and cosmetic results.

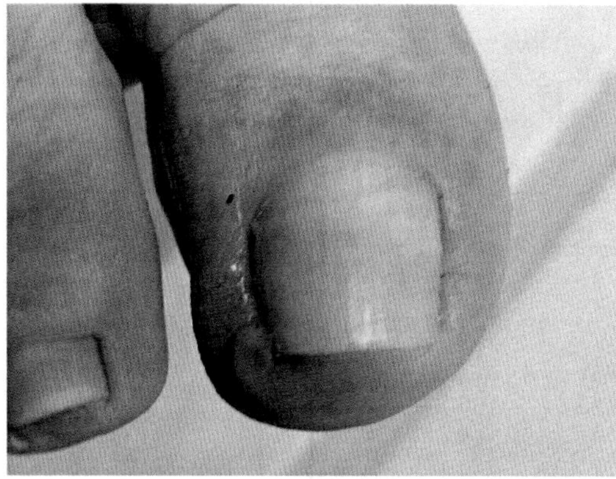

Fig. 5 Ingrown toenail

Splinter Hemorrhages

Splinter hemorrhages are linear discolorations under the nail plate that progress over a period of few days from an initial red color to a dark brown or black color [1, 2]. The location of the splinter hemorrhages may give leads to the underlying pathogenesis. Splinter hemorrhages located in the middle or distal third of the nail plate are usually associated with trauma, while those located proximally are commonly associated with systemic diseases such as infective endocarditis, cholesterol emboli, or connective tissue disorders. Proximal-type splinter hemorrhages especially those associated with systemic diseases are generally more common among young adults, whereas several studies have shown that trauma-associated distal splinter hemorrhages are observed frequently in the elderly population.

Trauma-induced splinter hemorrhages commonly resolve on their own, while the proximal-type splinter hemorrhages require treatment of the underlying systemic disorder.

Subungual Hematomas

Subungual hematomas are common among the elderly and are most frequently induced by trauma, which may or may not be remembered [1, 2]. The event may result in nail bed laceration and bleeding under the nail plate. Amyloidosis, diabetes mellitus, or anticoagulant therapy may also be less common causes of subungual hematomas.

Early on, it presents as a tender red subungual discoloration that tends to move forward and becomes bluish and less painful with time (Fig. 6). The forward and distal movement of this discoloration under the nail plate is a clinical clue that serves to distinguish this lesion from melanocytic proliferations including melanoma. Occasionally, distal onycholysis with subsequent spontaneous nail plate avulsion may occur.

Reassurance and observation of the nail is the main management strategy. However, in acute painful cases, pressure may be relieved by drilling a hole through the nail plate. Chronic cases are best left to heal spontaneously after ruling out melanoma.

Bowen's Disease of the Nail Apparatus

Bowen's disease of the nail unit, also known as in situ epidermoid carcinoma, is a nonaggressive malignancy most commonly originating in the epithelium of the nail folds or grooves [15]. The incidence is highest in patients aged between 50 and 69 years and usually affects the fingers, particularly the thumb [15]. Classical presentations include subungual or periungual ulcerated hyperkeratotic or papillomatous proliferations with associated onycholysis. Rarely, this condition may present as LM or erythronychia. Ulceration or bleeding is usually indicative of invasion which may be deep and reach the underlying contiguous bone in less than 20 % of patients. Distant metastatic rate is usually low.

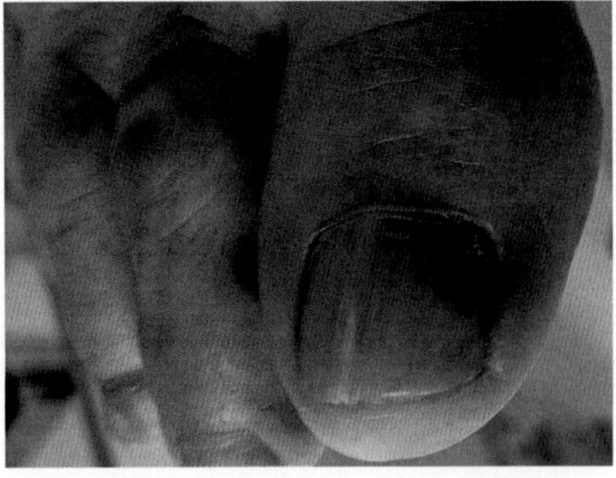

Fig. 6 Subungual hematoma

The etiology remains unclear; trauma, X-ray exposure, arsenic, chronic paronychia, and human papilloma virus (HPV) infection have all been implicated. The latter has been implicated because HPV 16, 34, and 35 have been detected in many cases of in situ and invasive Bowen's disease of the nail apparatus, and this raised speculation about a role for genital-digital transmission of the virus.

Mohs' micrographic surgery is the treatment of choice for this condition [15]. Other less effective modalities have been used and include regular excision, electrosurgery, liquid nitrogen, imiquimod, photodynamic therapy, intra-arterial infusion with methotrexate, and radiation therapy. Amputation of the distal phalanx should be done in case of bone involvement. Regular follow-up is essential in view of the potentially polydactylous nature of this disease.

Nail Apparatus Melanoma

Nail apparatus melanoma (NAM) usually occurs in Japanese and African Americans, with a relative incidence of 23 % and 25 %, respectively [16]. It is rarely observed in the white population. It most commonly occurs in the elderly with a mean age at diagnosis of 60–70 years [16]. The most frequent histogenetic type is acral lentiginous melanoma. The classical presentation is a solitary longitudinal melanonychia (LM) of the thumb, index finger, or big toe. In addition, Hutchinson's sign (brown or black pigment extension from the matrix and nail bed onto the surrounding tissues) may be present and accounts for the radial growth phase of this melanoma. Rarely, a homogeneous or irregular black spot in the matrix or nail bed may be the only sign of a subungual melanoma. Although NAM appears to have a worse prognosis than its cutaneous counterpart, this may be related to the delay in diagnosis of the former.

A strong index of suspicion is required when confronted with an isolated LM, especially in an elderly patient [16]. If a biopsy is obtained and the diagnosis is confirmed, treatment of NAM is then tailored based on the stage of the melanoma. Total excision of the entire nail apparatus or Mohs' surgery is the treatment of choice for in situ melanoma, while invasive melanomas should be managed with distal phalanx amputation. Adjuvant chemotherapy may also be needed in advanced cases.

Other Nail Conditions

Several other conditions should be kept in mind when evaluating nail changes in an elderly patient. These include nail changes associated with cutaneous inflammatory disorders (such as psoriasis or lichen planus) [17], nail cosmetics [18, 19], systemic disorders commonly observed in the elderly (such as renal disease) [20], or medications as the elderly patients are usually on multidrug therapy (such as anticoagulants, anticonvulsants, or beta-blockers) [21].

Conclusion

Elderly patients may complain of nail changes and dystrophies that may be of cosmetic concern, cause pain, affect daily activities, or be malignant. Awareness of these conditions is essential to reach the correct diagnosis and provide appropriate management.

References

1. Cohen PR, Scher RK. Geriatric nail disorders: diagnosis and treatment. J Am Acad Dermatol. 1992;26 (4):521–31.
2. Singh G, et al. Nail changes and disorders among the elderly. Indian J Dermatol Venereol Leprol. 2005;71 (6):386–92.
3. Horan MA, et al. The white nails of old age (Neapolitan nails). J Am Geriatr Soc. 1982;30(12):734–7.
4. Saraya T, et al. Terry's nails as a part of aging. Intern Med. 2008;47(6):567–8.
5. Lynch MH, et al. Acidic and basic hair/nail ('hard') keratins: their colocalization in the upper cortical and cuticle cells of the human hair follicle and their relationship to 'soft' keratins. J Cell Biol. 1986;103:2593–606.
6. Ohgitani S, et al. Nail calcium and magnesium content in relation to age and bone mineral density. J Bone Miner Metab. 2005;23(4):318–22.
7. van de Kerkhof PC, et al. Brittle nail syndrome: a pathogenesis-based approach with a proposed grading system. J Am Acad Dermatol. 2005;53(4):644–51.
8. Brosche T, et al. Age-associated changes in integral cholesterol and cholesterol sulfate concentrations in human scalp hair and finger nail clippings. Aging (Milano). 2001;13(2):131–8.
9. Lewis BL, Montgomery H. The senile nail. J Invest Dermatol. 1955;24(1):11–8.
10. Colombo VE, et al. Treatment of brittle fingernails and onychoschizia with biotin: scanning electron microscopy. J Am Acad Dermatol. 1990;23:1127–32.
11. Hochman LG, et al. Brittle nails: response to daily biotin supplementation. Cutis. 1993;51:303–5.
12. Gupta AK, Ricci MJ. Diagnosing onychomycosis. Dermatol Clin. 2006;24(3):365–9.
13. Gupta AK, Tu LQ. Therapies for onychomycosis: a review. Dermatol Clin. 2006;24(3):375–9.
14. Noel B. Surgical treatment of ingrown toenail without matricectomy. Dermatol Surg. 2008;34(1):79–83.
15. Baran R, Richert B. Common nail tumors. Dermatol Clin. 2006;24(3):297–311.
16. Andre' J, Lateur N. Pigmented nail disorders. Dermatol Clin. 2006;24(3):329–39.
17. Holzberg M. Common nail disorders. Dermatol Clin. 2006;24(3):349–54.
18. Dahdah MJ, Scher RK. Nail diseases related to nail cosmetics. Dermatol Clin. 2006;24(2):233–9.
19. Rich P. Nail cosmetics. Dermatol Clin. 2006;24 (3):393–9.
20. Tosti A, et al. The nail in systemic diseases. Dermatol Clin. 2006;24(3):341–7.
21. Piraccini BM, et al. Drug-induced nail diseases. Dermatol Clin. 2006;24(3):387–91.

Changes in the Composition of the Cornified Envelope During Skin Aging: A Calcium Centric Point of View

20

Maria Karolin Streubel, Mark Rinnerthaler, Johannes Bischof, and Klaus Richter

Contents

M.K. Streubel • M. Rinnerthaler • J. Bischof • K. Richter (✉)
Department of Cell Biology, Division of Genetics, University of Salzburg, Salzburg, Austria
e-mail: klaus.richter@sbg.ac.at

M. A. Farage et al. (eds.), *Textbook of Aging Skin*,
DOI 10.1007/978-3-662-47398-6_112

Abstract

Aging is a complex process that involves a variety of very different factors. Although oxidative stress plays a major role in skin aging, there are many more factors contributing to aging in the skin. In the epidermis, the cornified envelope an extremely complex protein–lipid network provides the barrier function of our skin. It has therefore a crucial function in protecting our body against many hazardous influences from the environment. During aging, the composition of the cornified envelope changes dramatically due to altered expression patterns of genes coding for major components of the cornified envelope. Accordingly, the barrier function of the skin is reduced, leading to an increased susceptibility to mechanical insults. An increased epidermal water loss is prevented by increasing the thickness of the *stratum corneum*. Many of these genes are calcium regulated. In young epidermis, there exists a calcium gradient showing a peak in the *stratum granulosum*. This calcium gradient collapses during aging providing an explanation for the altered gene expression patterns. The reason for the collapse of the calcium gradient is however not known presently and needs further investigation. A rebuilding of the cornified envelope is not specific for aging but can also be observed in. Epidermolysis bullosa, psoriasis, atopic dermatitis, lamellar ichthyosis, ichthyosis vulgaris, bathing suit ichthyosis, Netherton syndrome and loricrin keratoderma

Introduction

In the year 1990, Medvedev collected more than 300 aging theories in his publication *An Attempt at a Rational Classification of Theories of Ageing*. These are in part overlapping and sometimes even contradictory [1]. But not all aging theories apply to each cell type; some of these theories are organ or even cell type specific. However, many of these common aging theories also apply to the skin [2]. One of the most prominent theories is the "free radical theory of aging" published by Denham Harman in 1956 [3]. This theory states that reactive oxygen species (ROS) accumulate with increasing age and damage proteins, leading to protein carbonyls, protein oxidations, lipofuscin, and advanced glycation end products [4–7]. ROS also damage DNA where among many ROS-dependent DNA alterations, 8-oxo-2'deoxyguanosine is the most prominent one [4, 8] and lipids (lipid peroxidation yielding the major degradation products acrolein, malondialdehyde, and 4-hydroxynonenal) [4]. For a long time, mitochondria were believed to be the main source of ROS, but recent studies implicate that other even more important ROS sources can be found in the cell: NADPH oxidases, xanthine oxidoreductases (XOR), several peroxisomal oxidases, enzymes of the cytochrome P450 family, cyclooxygenases, lipoxygenases, and free iron [4]. All these ROS sources are not skin specific and can be found in all organs and all cell types. Like no other organ, the human skin is exposed to very harsh conditions from the environment. Among these are exogenous sources like UV irradiation, oxygen, smoke, and other forms of pollution but also endogenous sources like superoxide and protein aggregates that affect the state of the skin on a daily basis. The skin is, in contrast to any other organ, a target for UV irradiation (UVA, 320–400 nm; UVB, 290–320 nm; UVC, 200–290 nm) which is the main contributor to ROS production in the skin. The process of "photoaging" is mainly driven by UVA. The energy of UVA is absorbed by cellular chromophores and leads to the production of superoxide, hydroxyl radical, singlet oxygen, or hydrogen peroxide [9]. UVB also participates in the process of photoaging. But due to its rapid absorption by many organic compounds, UVB-induced ROS production only exerts its effect on the epidermis, damaging keratinocytes as well as melanocytes [4].

Especially in the dermis, "photoaging" is a main contributor to the aging process. The dermal collagen fibers are ultimately destroyed by processes that are induced by UV irradiation. UVB has a shorter wavelength than UVA (290–320 nm) preventing it from penetrating deeper than the epidermis. UVA, having a longer wavelength (320–400 nm), is able to damage deeper skin layers [10]. Photoaged skin shows a strongly wrinkled appearance, because collagens I and III [11], but also collagen VII [12] and the long collagen fibrils, elastic fibers, glycoproteins, and glycosaminoglycans that are normally interwoven in the extracellular matrix (ECM), are degraded [13]. This degradation is caused by elastases which are secreted by neutrophils that migrate to the dermis after UV exposure [14] as well as by the activation of matrix metalloproteases (MMPs), which are produced by epidermal keratinocytes leading to a degradation of the extracellular matrix in the dermis [15, 16]. Reactive oxygen species, which can also be produced as a result of UV irradiation, increase during the aging process [17] and are able to activate MMPs as well [4]. In old aged skin, it was shown that these MMPs are regularly upregulated, whereas their inhibitors TIMP1 and TIMP3 are downregulated compared to young skin [18, 19].

This chapter will not focus on the dermis but on the epidermis though, in particular on the cornified envelope (CE). Besides ROS and UV irradiation, the small ion calcium plays a major role in the aging process. For this reason, the age-induced collapse of the calcium gradient in the epidermis is the focus of this chapter.

Composition of the Skin with a Main Focus on the Epidermis

The human skin consists of different strata that form three main layers: the hypodermis, also called the subcutaneous tissue, is the innermost skin layer, the dermis is the middle layer, and the epidermis is the outermost layer, forming our barrier to the environment [20, 21]. The dermis is a mesenchymal compartment that derives from the mesoderm; the epidermis is an epithelial component and is a derivative of the ectoderm [22] and the hypodermis, which also has mesodermal origin. The dermis mainly consists of dermal fibroblasts producing an extensive ECM comprising of collagens, elastins, and glycosaminoglycans. A special kind of ECM which is connecting the dermis and epidermis is the basement membrane. The epidermis consists primarily of keratinocytes (more than 95 %), melanocytes, Langerhans cells, and Merkel cells. The keratinocytes originate from epidermal stem cells which are localized in the bottom layer of the epidermis. They are attached to the basal lamina via hemidesmosomes, connecting it to the dermis. The whole epidermis is 100–150 μm thick and can be divided into four sublayers: the *stratum basale* (SB), *stratum spinosum* (SS), *stratum granulosum* (SG), and *stratum corneum* (SC) [20, 21]. Palms and soles have a particularly thick skin, a fact that can be attributed to an additional fifth layer, the *stratum lucidum*.

The epidermal stem cells from the basal layer are constantly dividing asymmetrically, thereby regenerating themselves and generating transit-amplifying (TA) cells. These TA cells are dividing vividly and start their differentiation process. This process leads to the formation of the CE [23], with its ultimate form found in the *stratum corneum*. In this epidermal layer, the keratinocytes are dead; they are called "corneocytes" and are finally shed off. The CE has the most important role as a (1) barrier against pathogens, as a (2) protection against mechanical and chemical stress [21], as a (3) metabolizing layer for molecules coming from the environment, as a (4) UV protectant, and as an (5) important organ for the hydrological balance by controlling the water flow in and out (transepidermal water loss) [24]. After originating from the epidermal stem cells in the basal layer, the transit-amplifying cells lose the ability to adhere and then migrate to the *stratum spinosum* and are connected to each other via desmosomes [23, 25]. A first indication of the start of the differentiation process of keratinocytes is an increase in intracellular keratins [26]. Then the keratinocytes in the *stratum spinosum* start to bud off lipid-enriched lamellar bodies from the Golgi apparatus that are surrounded by a trilaminar membrane. Further on, the cells increase the number of lamellar bodies and flatten their shape during the migration from the *stratum spinosum* to the *stratum granulosum*. In this layer, cytosolic keratohyalin granules are also formed in increasing numbers. This type of granules is filled with histidine- and cysteine-rich proteins that act as a glue for keratin filaments [27]. Lamellar bodies on the other hand are involved in the cornification because they are filled with polar lipids such as glucosylceramides, sphingomyelin, phospholipids, and cholesterol. These molecules serve as precursors of barrier lipids building up the CE-specific lipid enclosure and catabolic enzymes such as β-glucocerebrosidase, sphingomyelinase, and secretory phospholipase A2 [28]. The outermost layer of the epidermis is the *stratum corneum* consisting of terminally differentiated, flattened, and dead keratinocytes that are called corneocytes. The whole differentiation process of keratinocytes from epidermal stem cells to corneocytes can be considered as a kind of apoptotic process and is called cornification. On their journey to the surface, the keratinocytes are constantly changing their shape until they are completely flat. These dead corneocytes are finally shed off the skin as scales, a process that is known as desquamation [27, 29].

The Formation of the CE from Initiation to Desquamation

The cornification is a process that is forming a mega-sized cross-linked protein structure containing also lipids that are replacing the plasma membrane and are completely filling the intracellular space. The cornification of keratinocytes proceeds step-by-step in a very defined, "programmed" way.

The process of "cornification" starts in the keratinocytes that are forming the *stratum spinosum*. An essential step in this process is a rise in intracellular calcium levels that is accompanied by a rise of the expression of mainly three proteins: involucrin [30], periplakin [31], and envoplakin [32]. The enzyme transglutaminase 1 (TG1), adjacent to the inner plasma membrane, is connecting periplakin and envoplakin with involucrin via Nϵ-(γ-glutamyl) lysine-isopeptide bonds [33, 34]. The involucrin–periplakin–envoplakin protein complex forms a protein monolayer at the cytoplasmic side of the lipid bilayer [35]. This protein monolayer is a scaffold for the attachment of further CE-specific proteins that are essential for the process of cornification [36]. Also, other membrane-associated proteins like the desmosomal keratins, K1 and K10, begin to replace the preexisting K5 and K14 intermediate filament bundles (KIFs). At a later stage in the cornification process, junctional proteins and filaments (like desmosomes) are degraded, whereas the K1/K10 KIFs are connected to plakins, loricrin, involucrin, and SPRRs and thereby aggregated into tight bundles [37].

The next step in the cornification process is leading to the formation of lamellar bodies formed by the Golgi apparatus in the *stratum spino*sum and later on in the *stratum granulosum* [38, 39]. These circular granules are characterized by an encircling lipid layer and are filled with a multiplicity of different lipids like glucosylceramides and sphingomyelins [40]. Lamellar bodies also contain lipid-processing enzymes (like glucocerebrosidase, secretory phospholipase A2, acidic sphingomyelinase, and steroid sulfatase) [41, 42], antimicrobial peptides (beta-defensin 2, cathelicidin) [43, 44], proteases and protease inhibitors (e.g., serine proteases SCTE/KLK5/hK5 and SCCE/KLK7/hK7) [45], and the protein corneodesmosin [40, 46]. Corneodesmosin is an adhesive protein which is involved in the corneocyte cohesion and is strictly calcium dependent [47]. After an influx of calcium into keratinocytes, the lamellar bodies fuse with the plasma membrane [48]. This leads to a changed composition of the cellular membrane. The phospholipid bilayer is replaced with ω-OH-ceramides. In a following step, these lipids are cross-linked by TG1 with the involucrin–periplakin–envoplakin protein scaffold, but these membrane-associated ceramides are also cross-linked to other proteins by esterification [27, 37]. One of these proteins that are cross-linked to the involucrin–periplakin–envoplakin scaffold is loricrin. Loricrin is the main component of a fully developed CE (nearly 80 % of its protein mass) and is mainly expressed in the *stratum granulosum* [37]. Attributed to its high insolubility, loricrin is packaged in secluded loricrin granules immediately after its synthesis [49]. The enzymes transglutaminases 1 and 3 are responsible for cross-linking the very insoluble loricrin with itself and members of the small proline-rich repeat (SPRR) protein family, which are characterized by a very high solubility. This way, they act as a bridge to increase the solubility of loricrin. This multigene family consists in humans of ten members and one pseudogene that are clustered in four subgroups: SPRR1 (two members), SPRR2 (six members and a pseudogene), SPRR3, and SPRR4 (each with one member) [50]. TG3 is cross-linking loricrin and SPRRs to a loricrin–SPRR protein complex. In the following, this loricrin–SPRR complex is getting cross-linked to the protein scaffold at the cell membrane by TG1 [51–53].

In the next step, various other CE proteins like trichohyalin, cystatin, and elafin are cross-linked to the multiprotein complex. One of the main components of the CE is the calcium-regulated filaggrin.

Filaggrin is synthesized as a precursor (profilaggrin) and is processed by several cleavage events [54]. Filaggrin is responsible for the bundling of keratins into macrofibrils which leads to the flattened shape of corneocytes and is the most important moisture factor of the skin [21]. Other cross-linked CE proteins are members of the S100 protein family, and some of them are known to serve as a substrate for transglutaminases [52, 55].

In the last step of the cornification, late cornified envelope (LCE) proteins are attached to the protein–lipid complex [56]. Some of these LCEs are expressed in a specific manner [57]. The terminally differentiated keratinocytes are filled with this mega-protein–lipid complex;

they have lost their nuclei, mitochondria, and all other organelles and are finally shedding off as dead corneocytes [58]. The formation of the cornified envelope is summarized schematically in Fig. 1.

The Composition of the CE in Dependence of Age

In the dermis, the aging process manifests itself by a reduction and fragmentation of the extracellular matrix, while in the epidermis the turnover rate of keratinocytes is significantly reduced, and the whole protein composition of the CE changes dramatically. The CE represents the first line of defense against the environment and is therefore especially important in the context of skin aging and, in particular, in the aging process of the epidermis [59].

The expression pattern of the CE-specific genes changes during aging. This statement is not only true for extrinsically aged skin, e.g., UV irradiated, but also for more protected "merely" intrinsically aged skin. Intrinsic aging describes a decrease of the renewal rate of epidermal cells and the aging process without any external influence. In young skin, epithelial cells usually scale off every 28 days, but with increased age this process takes longer. Elderly skin needs 40–60 days from stem cell mitosis to desquamation [60]. The term "extrinsic aging" is used to describe the aging process in dependence of exogenous factors, mostly UV light exposure, but also air pollutants, infrared, and ozone exposure [61].

The first step in cornification, the building of the envoplakin–periplakin–involucrin scaffold, is unaffected by the age of the individual because the expression pattern of envoplakin, periplakin, and involucrin is not changed in old skin compared to young skin [59, 62]. The expression of the enzyme responsible for their cross-linking, transglutaminase 1, is slightly increased, whereas the expression of the loricrin and SPRRs cross-linking enzyme, transglutaminase 3, is nearly unaffected. Loricrin, the major component of the CE, is drastically downregulated in old skin. The loricrin level in the strata of old skin is insignificant compared to young skin. The loss of loricrin might be compensated for increased levels of several SPRRs. All SPRRs with the exception of SPRR2G show increased expression levels. This in part dramatic increase of SPRRs could in fact have another reason than compensation for the loss of loricrin. Like no other organ, the skin has to endure high ROS levels. During the aging process, the ROS level in the epidermis is pushed to even higher levels. But recent research is clearly demonstrating that the CE itself exerts anti-oxidative capabilities and this task is predominantly achieved by the SPRR2 subfamily. Besides proline this protein family is extremely enriched in the amino acid cysteine that has anti-oxidative capabilities [63]. Therefore, it is quite possible that the enormous increase in SPRR levels during aging (more than 100-fold) has its main function in reducing the age-associated ROS burden of the epidermis. Therefore, an increase in SPRRs is not specific for aging but can be observed, for example, after tissue injury, burn injury, or even after heart infarction [64]. Filaggrin which is responsible for the flattening of corneocytes by bundling keratins [21] is also downregulated during aging [65]. This in particular effects hydration and leads to a decreased and reduced water-binding capacity of the skin [66], because filaggrin is degraded to hygroscopic amino acids in the course of the maturation process [67, 68]. On the contrary, many S100 proteins, of which some are known substrates of transglutaminases [52, 55], are upregulated during the aging process.

Other components of the CE like the late cornified envelope proteins (LCEs), which are attached to the protein scaffold at a later stage of the cornification process and which are targets of transglutaminases too [56], are also differentially regulated. LCEs can be divided into three subfamilies [57]. Subfamily one and two are downregulated during aging, whereas subfamily three is upregulated. Members of the subfamily two of the LCEs are expressed in a calcium-dependent manner and are upregulated in cell culture experiments after addition of calcium to the media, whereas the expression of the two other LCE groups is completely unaffected after

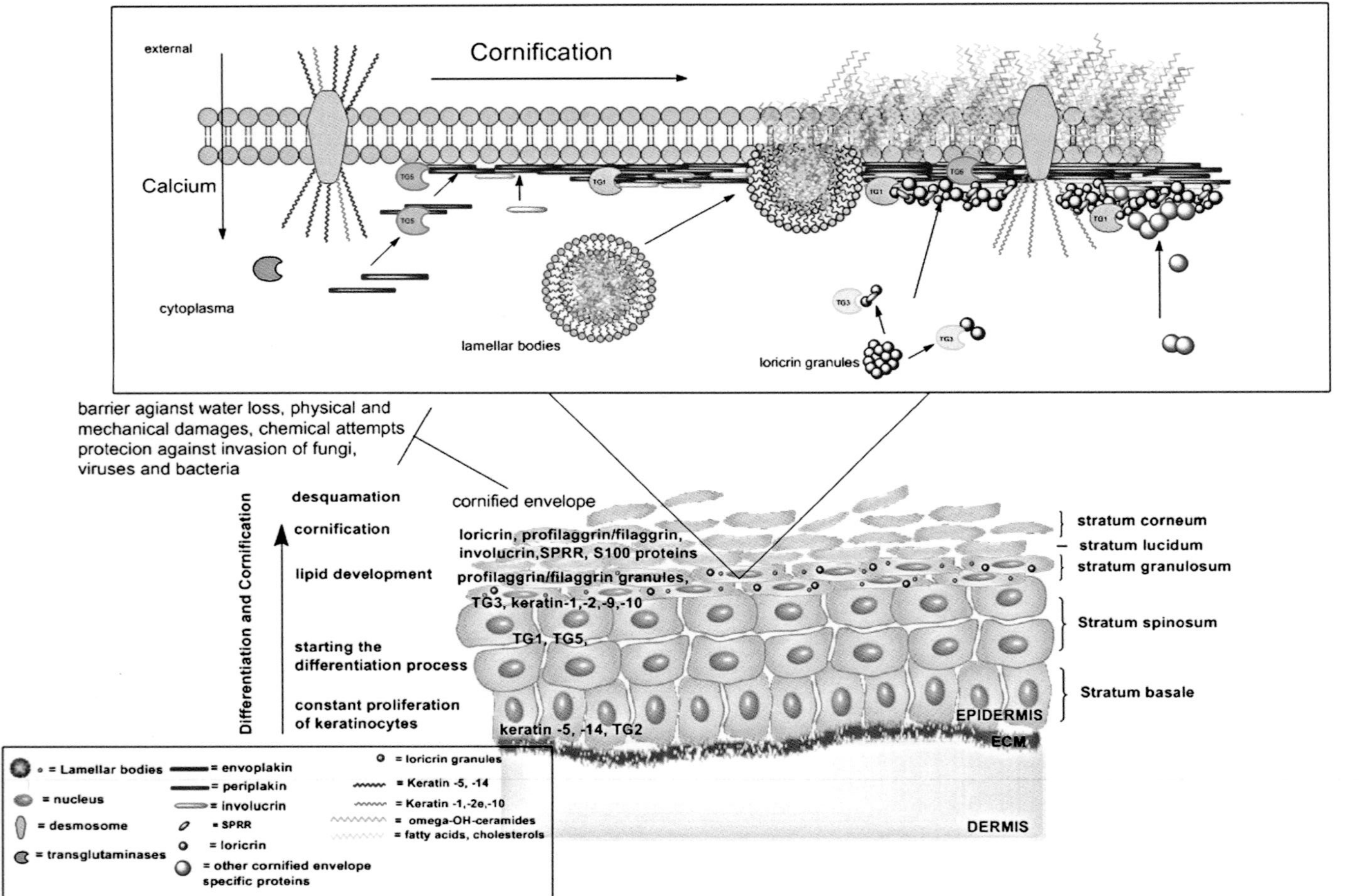

Fig. 1 **Maturation of the cornified envelope on the transition from the stratum spinosum to the stratum corneum**. Involucrin, periplakin, and envoplakin are cross-linked and attached to the plasma membrane. Lamellar bodies are pinched off from the ER and replace the phospholipids in the plasma membrane with ceramides. The apolar loricrin, the main component of the CE, is cross-linked with SPRRs and cross-linked to the growing CE. In a final step, LCEs are attached to the CE. The CE is in close contact to the keratins K1, K2e, and K10. On the way to the periphery, the keratinocytes flatten, lose all organelles including nuclei, and form dead corneocytes

calcium addition [57]. This changed composition of the CE was shown on RNA level, while on the protein level it was confirmed histologically with immunofluorescence [59]. The change of transcription levels during the aging process is summarized in Fig. 2. Due to the complete rebuilding of the CE in the aging process, it has to be expected that main barrier functions are also dramatically affected. But surprisingly transepidermal water loss and the *stratum corneum* hydration level are not significantly changed during aging [69]. This potential controversy can be explained by the fact that the thickness of the *stratum corneum* is constantly increasing over the course of a lifetime to compensate for the gradual rebuilding of the CE. The SC thickness in the dorsal forearm increases from 14.5 μm (age, 20 years) to 20 μm (age, 70 years). Other features of the changed CE cannot be compensated for by increasing the thickness of the *stratum corneum*. Aged epidermis is much more sensitive against tape stripping or treatment with acetone. In addition, the recovery time of the barrier after these insults is drastically extended [70].

The change in the composition is not the only difference in the CE during the aging process. Especially for photoaged skin, it was demonstrated that CE-specific proteins are heavily carbonylated by aldehydes (acrolein, crotonaldehyde, and 4-hydroxy-2-nonenal) originating from lipid peroxidation [71]. This is additionally compromising the function of the CE. By measuring the surface conductance of the skin, a direct indication for the water-holding capacity of the SC, it was demonstrated that protein carbonyls reduce the water-holding capacity of the epidermis substantially [72].

Skin Diseases Affecting the Cornified Envelope

A change in the composition of the CE is not only a hallmark of the aging process of the epidermis but can also be observed in several skin diseases.

In case of recessive dystrophic epidermolysis bullosa, caused by a recessive mutation in the collagen gene (*COL7A1*), such phenotypes as primary lesions, dystrophy of nails, palmoplantar keratoderma, congenital absence of skin, and characteristic nevi can be observed. Many phenotypes of epidermolysis bullosa actually resemble that of aged skin. This includes loss of sweat glands and sebaceous glands, atrophies, and pigmentation abnormalities. Another hallmark of epidermolysis bullosa is a compromised barrier function of the skin identical to aged skin. The reason is a changed CE composition that perfectly mimics the one taking place in aged skin: levels of loricrin and filaggrin are reduced, whereas levels of SPRRs and LCE1B dramatically increase. In addition, a rise of S100A12, S100A7 (psoriasin), S100A7A, S100A8, and S100A9 has been observed [73].

There are several skin diseases that are associated with barrier function defects and resemble this aspect of aging. Some of these diseases will be discussed in the following sections. This list, because of the high number of ichthyosis and palmoplantar keratosis, is not at all complete but shall demonstrate that skin aging and some skin diseases share the same features: a defect in barrier function and changed composition of the CE. As will be discussed later on in this chapter, another shared feature of skin diseases and skin aging is a breakdown of the epidermal calcium gradient.

Besides an impaired skin barrier, both psoriasis and atopic dermatitis share common phenotypes: a hyperproliferation of keratinocytes, a defect in keratinocyte differentiation, an increased transepidermal water loss, and a migration of immunocompetent cells into the dermis and epidermis associated with high expression levels of many cytokines and chemokines. Psoriasis is generally considered as a TH1 and TH17 disease [74], whereas atopic dermatitis is a TH2-polarized disease [75]. In case of psoriasis, high expression levels of LCEs are observed. In addition, it was demonstrated that deletions of LCE3B and LCE3C can lead to psoriasis and increase the risk for psoriatic arthritis and chronic hand eczema with allergic contact dermatitis [76]. Many components of the CE play a crucial role in the development of skin diseases and are

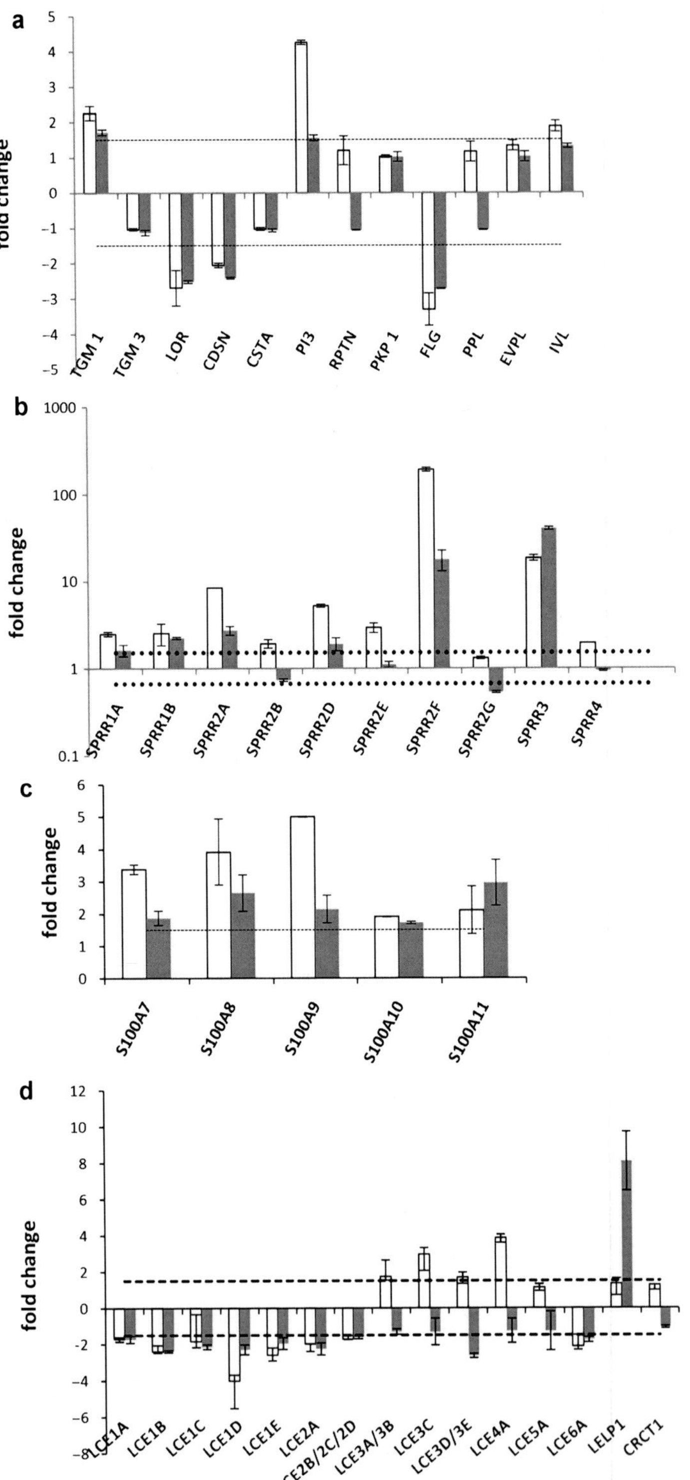

Fig. 2 **Age-dependent change in the composition of the CE**. A comparison between young and old foreskin samples is represented by *white bars*, whereas the *gray bars* stand for a middle-age-old comparison. In (**b**) all members of the *small proline-rich repeat* family can be found, in (**c**) CE-specific S100 proteins can be found, and in (**d**) the *late*

summarized in Table 1. In case of atopic dermatitis, a strong correlation with a loss of filaggrin was found. This also has an impact on the expression of loricrin and many other CE-specific genes. Besides atopic dermatitis, a loss of filaggrin can also lead to food allergy, asthma, and allergic rhinitis [77]. The large group of ichthyosis also shares common features with aging: a defective skin barrier and cornification disorders. For example, in lamellar ichthyosis, a severe congenital skin disorder, the proliferation rate of basal keratinocytes is drastically increased. In extreme cases, the skin of the affected resembles fish scales. A common feature is a thickened epidermis as well as a faster growth of nails and hairs. A genetic basis for this disease can be found in the reduced transglutaminase 1 activity. As a result, the cross-linking of all CE components is impaired, and it can be speculated that the defective barrier function shall be in part compensated for by an increased epidermal thickness [78]. Another congenital ichthyosis with a mutation in the transglutaminase 1 gene is the bathing suit ichthyosis. This form of ichthyosis also leads to scales that are found in the trunk region but are neither present in the face nor at the limbs [79]. In the case of ichthyosis vulgaris, a loss-of-function mutation in the filaggrin gene is involved. Filaggrin fulfills many important functions in the skin. It is synthesized as a proprotein and is cut into up to 12 filaggrin proteins during the maturation of the CE. Besides its cross-linking with the CE, it is also involved in the aggregation of keratin filaments and has an extracellular function as the skin's "natural moisturizing factor." As a result of this skin disease, several phenotypes can be observed: an impaired skin barrier, a reduced skin hydration, scaling of the skin, a palmar and plantar hyperlinearity, and, as expected, a dramatic decrease in the number of keratohyalin granules in which filaggrin is "normally" packed in healthy individuals. To compensate for the loss of loricrin, an epidermal hyperplasia and hyperkeratosis can be observed [80]. Of all these ichthyoses, the harlequin ichthyosis has the most drastic phenotype. The *stratum corneum* is extremely thickened in this autosomal recessive congenital skin disease as is the case with all ichthyosis. The scales in this disease are becoming enormously big and look like white plates separated by red fissures. Besides an impaired movement, the thickened epidermis/*stratum corneum* can lead to necrosis and even auto-amputation of toes. Milder phenotypes have an increased prevalence for sepsis due to the heavily effected skin barrier and an increased transepidermal water loss. The gene affected in this disease is an ATP-binding cassette subfamily, a member 12 with the name ABCA12. The main function of this protein in the *stratum corneum* is the transport of glucosylceramides out of the cells. A direct result is a decreased number of lamellar granules [81]. In the case of the Netherton syndrome, an increased desquamation and hair shaft abnormalities can be observed. In healthy skin, the corneocytes are tightly connected via corneodesmosomes. A protein localized to the corneodesmosomes is corneodesmosin. A key event in the desquamation process is a cleavage of corneodesmosin by the kallikrein-related peptidases KLK5 and KLK7, resulting in the detachment of the corneocytes. Opposing this reaction is the task of the serine protease inhibitor LEKTI, encoded by SPINK5. A mutation in the SPINK5 gene leads to Netherton syndrome and to an increased loss of corneocytes. Further consequences of this mutation are a decreased barrier function of the skin, an increased susceptibility to

Fig. 2 (continued) cornified envelope proteins are shown. In (**a**) several, especially, early markers of the CE are shown. A crossing of the *dotted line* represents a significant change during skin aging. Positive values indicate an increased transcription during aging and negative numbers a transcriptional downregulation. This figure clearly illustrates that the SPRR family and the LCE3 subfamily and the S100 proteins increase their transcription dramatically during aging. A decrease can be observed for loricrin, filaggrin, and the LCE1 and LCE2 subfamily (Adapted from Rinnerthaler et al. [59])

Table 1 **Correlation between CE components and skin diseases**. In this table, the most important CE components, their function, and expression in the epidermis are summarized. This table shall demonstrate that deletions and mutations of these genes have a direct impact on the "wellness" of the skin leading to several diseases

Gene	Process	Function	Expression	Skin-related diseases
Filaggrin	Structural protein in the skin responsible for the cross-linking of keratin filaments, synthesized as precursor profilaggrin, localized in keratohyalin granules	Calcium ion binding, protein binding, structural molecule activity	*Stratum granulosum, stratum corneum*	Ichthyosis vulgaris, atopic dermatitis type 2, dermatitis, eczema herpeticum, lichen planus, x-linked ichthyosis, keratosis, leukoplakia, epidermolysis bullosa
Loricrin	Main component of the cornified envelope	Protein binding (bridging), structural constituent of cytoskeleton, structural molecule activity	*Stratum corneum*	Vohwinkel syndrome, progressive symmetric erythrokeratoderma, keratoderma, epidermolytic hyperkeratosis, psoriasis, endotheliitis, keratosis, epidermolysis bullosa
Involucrin	Cross-linking protein, attached to proteins like loricrin, envoplakin, and periplakin	Protein binding (bridging), structural molecule activity	*Stratum spinosum, stratum granulosum, stratum corneum*	Senile nevus of the skin, clear cell acanthoma, psoriasis, keratosis, leukoplakia, acanthoma
Transglutaminase 1	Responsible for the cross-linking of different CE-specific proteins	Metal ion binding, protein binding, protein-glutamine gamma-glutamyltransferase activity	*Stratum spinosum, stratum granulosum*	Lamellar ichthyosis, nonbullous congenital ichthyosiform erythroderma, autosomal recessive congenital ichthyosis, bathing suit ichthyosis, hypotrichosis
Keratin 1 **An important member of the keratins in connection with skin diseases**	Keratin 1 and keratin 10 belong to the same keratin family; this family consists of mostly basic and neutral proteins; they are arranged in keratin chains	Carbohydrate binding, protein binding, receptor activity, structural molecule activity	*Stratum spinosum, stratum granulosum*	Bullous congenital ichthyosiform erythroderma, epidermolytic ichthyosis, epidermolytic acanthoma, Bowen syndrome, palmoplantar keratosis, epidermolysis bullosa simplex
Keratin 10 **An important member of the keratins in connection with skin diseases**	Keratin 1 and keratin 10 belong to the same keratin family; this family consists of mostly basic and neutral proteins; they are arranged in keratin chains	Structural constituent of the epidermis	*Stratum granulosum, stratum spinosum*	Ichthyosis variegata, epidermolytic hyperkeratosis, palmoplantar keratosis, epidermolysis bullosa, basal cell carcinoma, lichen planus, keratosis, leukoplakia

Transglutaminase 3	Responsible for cross-linking the CE-specific proteins, SPRRs, and loricrin	Calcium ion binding, catalytic activity, protein-glutamine gamma-glutamyltransferase activity, transferase activity, transferring acyl groups	*Stratum granulosum, stratum corneum*	Dermatitis herpetiformis, atopic dermatitis, psoriasis
Desmoplakin	Desmoplakin is responsible for binding intermediate filaments to intact desmosomes	Cell adhesion molecule binding, cell adhesive protein binding involved in bundle of His cell-Purkinje myocyte communication, poly(A) RNA binding, protein binding (bridging), protein kinase C binding, scaffold protein binding, structural constituent of cytoskeleton, structural molecule activity	*Stratum basale, stratum spinosum, stratum granulosum, stratum corneum*	Keratosis palmoplantaris striata, keratoderma
Corneodesmosin	Corneodesmosin is sequentially proteolyzed during cornification and is incorporated in desmosomes	Protein homodimerization activity	*Stratum basale, stratum spinosum, stratum granulosum, stratum corneum*	Hypotrichosis, peeling skin syndrome, psoriasis, atopic dermatitis
ATP-binding cassette transporter 12 (ABCA12)	Important for the lipid development of corneocytes	ATP binding, ATPase activity, coupled to transmembrane movement of substances, apolipoprotein A-I receptor binding, cholesterol transporter activity, lipid transporter activity, lipid-transporting ATPase activity, phospholipid transporter activity, protein binding, receptor binding	*Stratum corneum*	Harlequin syndrome, autosomal recessive ichthyosis
Serine peptidase inhibitor, Kazal type 5 (SPINK5)	A protease inhibitor which is able to inhibit proteins that are responsible for the cleavage of desmosomal proteins in the epidermis and is regulating desquamation	Serine-type endopeptidase inhibitor activity	*Stratum corneum*	Netherton syndrome, ichthyosis linearis circumflexa, atopic dermatitis, psoriasis, dermatitis
S100A7 The most important member of the S100 family in connection with skin diseases	S100 Protein family is important for the differentiation process of keratinocytes but is also immune modulating and cell cycle regulating	RAGE receptor binding, calcium ion binding, protein binding, zinc ion binding	*Stratum corneum*	Atopic dermatitis, psoriasis, genodermatosis

(*continued*)

Table 1 (continued)

Gene	Process	Function	Expression	Skin-related diseases
Envoplakin	Cross-linked to the envoplakin–periplakin–involucrin scaffold	Intermediate filament binding, protein binding (bridging), structural molecule activity	*Stratum spinosum*, *stratum granulosum*, *stratum corneum*	Pemphigus foliaceus, bullous pemphigoid, keratosis, epidermolysis bullosa
Desmoglein 1 **The most important member of the desmogleins in connection with skin diseases**	Desmogleins have the role of connecting keratinocytes with each other	Calcium ion binding, gamma-catenin binding, toxic substance binding	*Stratum basale*, *stratum spinosum*, *stratum granulosum*, *stratum corneum*	Palmoplantar keratosis, dermatitis, Netherton syndrome
Small proline-rich protein 1B (SPRR1B) **The most important member of the SPRR family in connection with skin diseases**	SPRRs are connecting loricrin with each other, and they are attached to the mega-protein scaffold	Protein binding (bridging), structural molecule activity,	*Stratum corneum*	Epidermolysis bullosa, atopic dermatitis
Late cornified envelope 3C (LCE3C) **The most important member of the LCE family in connection with skin diseases**	LCEs are attached to the mega-protein scaffold	Protein binding	*Stratum corneum*	Dermatitis, psoriasis

infections, and a prevalence to atopic dermatitis [82, 83]. Closely related is inflammatory (type B) subtype of the generalized peeling skin syndrome. In this disease, LEKTI is not affected, but the mutation lies directly in the corneodesmosin (CDSN) gene. An inevitable consequence is a decreased desquamation of corneocytes with clinical symptoms comparable to atopic diseases [83, 84]. The last disease with an altered composition of the cornified envelope that will be discussed in this chapter is loricrin keratoderma (Vohwinkel syndrome with ichthyosis). A frameshift mutation in the C-terminal region of the main CE component loricrin is the basic cause of this disease. Some of the numerous associated phenotypes are increased transepidermal water loss due to reduced permeability barrier function, specific knuckle pads due to hypertrophy of the *stratum corneum*, and constricting rings that surround the finger and toes. A benefit from this disease is an increased epidermal barrier recovery [85].

The Epidermal Calcium Gradient and Its Breakdown During the Aging Process

This part will focus on the importance and involvement of calcium in the development of several skin diseases and the change in the composition of the CE during the aging process. Calcium plays a very important role during the cornification process and the expression of CE-specific proteins. In addition, the activity of many enzymes involved in the cornification process is strictly calcium dependent. Calcium is predominantly responsible for driving keratinocytes into differentiation [86]. The dependence of the CE on calcium is summarized in Table 2. The keratinocytes in the epidermis are stuck in a dilemma. On the one hand, calcium is needed to initiate the differentiation/cornification process which proceeds without any further cell division. On the other hand, the epidermis has to maintain a high regenerative capacity. Addition of 1.44 mM calcium chloride leads to an arrest of the cell cycle, induces the expression of CE-specific proteins, and induces the stratification into an up to six-cell-thick layer [87]. Loricrin is only transcribed with 0.35 mM calcium and filaggrin above 0.15 mM calcium in vitro [54]. In the end, the keratinocytes have degraded all organelles including the nuclei, have formed a CE, and are cross-linked by corneodesmosomes. The transition from healthy keratinocytes to dead corneocytes is a prerequisite for the formation of an intact epidermal barrier. The dead corneocytes constantly desquamate. Every 60 days, 80 billion corneocytes are lost and have to be rebuilt [62]. To maintain the proliferative capacity of keratinocytes, a calcium concentration of 0.1 mM is needed. This calcium concentration does not initiate cornification but keeps the cells in a monolayer and a proliferative state [87].

Therefore, the epidermis is in need for different calcium concentrations. Low calcium concentrations are necessary in the *stratum basale* to keep the epidermal stem cells in a proliferative state, and higher calcium concentrations are needed in the *stratum granulosum* to initiate the transition to fully differentiated corneocytes. These different concentrations of calcium are achieved by the establishment of an epidermal calcium gradient: the calcium concentration in the *stratum basale* is very low and constantly increases in direction of the outer periphery. In the *stratum granulosum*, the highest calcium concentration can be detected which declines abruptly in the *stratum corneum* [59, 95, 96]. It is estimated that the calcium concentrations in the stratum corneum drop below a level of 3 μM, whereas in the *stratum granulosum* the calcium concentrations surpass 20 μM [97]. During the aging process, it has been shown that the epidermal calcium gradient collapses, a fact that is directly linked to the age-dependent changes in the composition of the cornified envelope. It has to be noted that the overall calcium concentration in the skin is not changed during aging. It was shown by flame atomic absorption spectroscopy (FAAS) that a calcium concentration of ~117 μg calcium per gram epidermis in middle-aged individuals is not significantly different from ~109 μg calcium per gram epidermis in old individuals (see Fig. 3) [59]. But while the amount of calcium in aged individuals is not changed, the calcium

Table 2 The calcium-dependent activation and expression of CE components

CE-specific gene	Activation	Expression
Involucrin	Is getting cross-linked to the protein scaffold under calcium-dependent manner [34, 88]	Calcium responsiveness of involucrin based on the transcription factor AP-1 and on the protein kinase C isoform delta [89]
Periplakin	Recruitment and attachment to the phospholipid bilayer requires the presence of calcium [33]	
Envoplakin	Recruitment and phospholipid bilayer require the presence of calcium [33]	
Kazrin	The adaptor protein Kazrin is cross-linking between desmoplakin and periplakin at desmosomes and under high calcium (1.8 mM Ca^{2+}) conditions	The expression is twofold increased after 24 h [90]
Loricrin		Synthesized above a calcium concentration of 0.1 mM [49]
SPRRs	Are getting cross-linked with loricrin via TGMs under calcium-dependent regulation [91]	
Transglutaminases	TGMs are calcium-dependent enzymes and need intracellular calcium to get activated [50, 92]	
Filaggrin		At least 0.15 mM calcium is needed for an efficient transcription [93]
S100 proteins	Calcium-regulated EF-hand proteins [50, 55]	
Late cornified envelope proteins	LCE group 2 responds to the addition of external calcium [57]	
E-cadherin	Calcium-dependent cadherin–cadherin interaction [94]	

distribution is dramatically affected. Using cryosections of middle-aged individuals that were stained with the long-wavelength indicator Calcium Green^{TM}-1 AM, it was confirmed that the highest calcium concentration can be found in the *stratum granulosum* (a clear green band wiggling through the epidermis). In old individuals, the peak of calcium in the *stratum granulosum* is lost, and the calcium is equally distributed across the whole epidermis (see Fig. 3) [59, 98]. Because of the complete dependence of the CE components on the presence of high calcium concentrations, the rebuilding of the CE during the aging process is strongly affected by the collapsing epidermal calcium gradient. The failure in the buildup of the calcium gradient is not specific for aging but can also be seen in several other skin diseases: Darier disease, Hailey–Hailey disease, psoriasis, and atopic dermatitis. In the case of Hailey–Hailey disease, the P-type cation transport ATPase ATP2C1, responsible for the transport of calcium into the Golgi apparatus, is affected with the resulting clinical phenotype of reduced keratinocyte adhesion and vesiculation of the epidermis. The basis of Darier disease is a mutation in the P-type Ca^{2+} ATPase ATP2A2/SERCA2, leading to an inefficient transport of calcium from the cytosol to the ER. A loss of cell–cell adhesions, abnormal keratinization patterns, an impaired CE composition, and itchy, malodorous keratotic papules are the results [62]. The clinical manifestations of psoriasis and atopic dermatitis were already discussed previously in this chapter. The reason for the collapse of the ion gradient during the aging process will be difficult to find and track, because until now very little is known about the generation of this gradient. It was shown that an impairment of the epidermal permeability barrier has a direct impact on the calcium gradient. This could indicate a

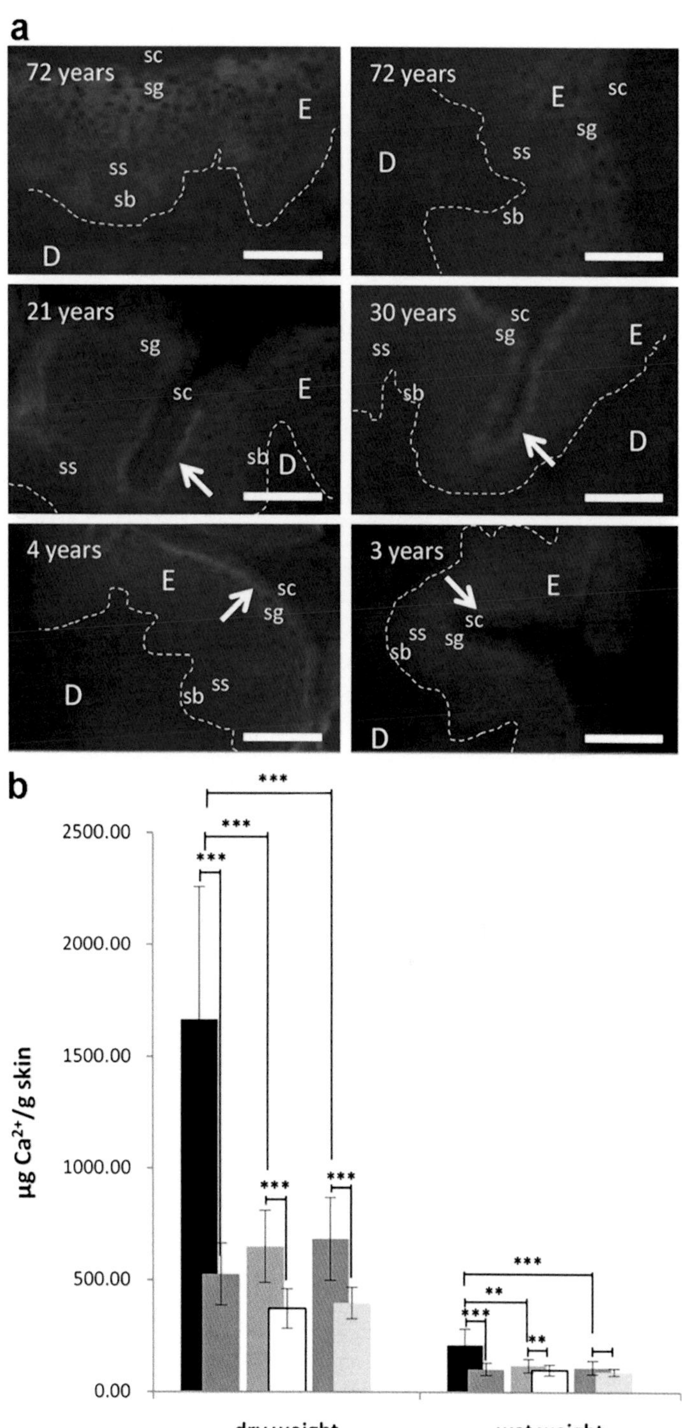

Fig. 3 **The breakdown of the epidermal calcium gradient during aging**. (**a**) In the case of 3- and 4-year-old boys and a 21- and 30-year-old individual, a clear epidermal calcium gradient with a peak in the *stratum granulosum* (indicated by *white arrows*) can be observed. This gradient is completely diminishing in two individuals, 72 years of age. *E* epidermis, *D* dermis, *sc stratum corneum*, *sg stratum granulosum*, *ss stratum spinosum*, and *sb stratum basale*. FAAS measurements of calcium concentrations are shown: young epidermis (*black bars*), young dermis (*gray bars*), middle-aged epidermis (*blue bars*), middle-aged dermis (*white bars*), old epidermis (*green bars*) and old dermis (*yellow bars*) (****P*-value <0.01, ** *P*-value <0.05, * *P*-value <0.1). No significant difference between the calcium concentration of old and young epidermis can be observed. Therefore, it is clear that only the calcium distribution is affected (Adapted from Rinnerthaler et al. [59])

vicious cycle, because an altered calcium gradient would directly affect the CE composition and would lead to further disturbances of the calcium gradient. By a combination of two-photon microscopy, fluorescence-lifetime imaging microscopy and phasor analysis, it was also demonstrated that the epidermal calcium gradient is mainly build up by intracellular calcium stores in the ER and Golgi apparatus and not by extracellular free calcium [97]. This indicates that calcium is released from the intracellular calcium stores or that the calcium import into the cells and/or into the ER and Golgi apparatus is not properly working in aged skin. A first and crucial step in the filling of the intracellular calcium stores is the calcium-sensing receptor CaSR. This receptor is a class C G-protein-coupled receptor which is localized in the plasma membrane of keratinocytes. Binding of extracellular calcium to this receptor initiates a conformational change and then acts as a guanine exchange factor for the Gq protein. Gqα then separates from Gqβγ and activates the phospholipase C, gamma1. This enzyme hydrolyzes phosphatidylinositol 4,5-bisphosphate (PIP_2) to diacylglycerol (DAG) and inositol 1,4,5-trisphosphate (IP_3). DAG activates protein kinase C that shuttles from the cytosol to the plasma membrane. The activation of this kinase stimulates the expression, phosphorylation, and activation of c-FOS and c-JUN that are both forming AP-1 transcription factors (TFs). These TFs drive keratinocyte differentiation because genes like involucrin contain AP-1 binding sites in their promoters. Additionally, IP3 is a second messenger that binds to IP3 receptors (IP3R) found in the membrane of the Golgi and the ER. After binding of the second messenger, IP3R acts as a Ca^{2+} channel transporting calcium into the cytosol. An increase in extracellular calcium is therefore always accompanied by an increase in cytosolic calcium. An emptying of the ER calcium stores activates the stromal interaction molecules 1 and 2 (STIM1 and STIM2). Both are able to sense the calcium concentration via calcium-binding EF hands. A drop of calcium in the ER initiates a translocation of Stim1/Stim2 to the plasma membrane activating the calcium channel ORAI1 and the ion channel "transient receptor potential channel 1" (TRPC1) that are responsible for the import of calcium into the keratinocytes. The cytosolic calcium levels can be reduced by membrane-localized P-type sarco-/endoplasmic reticulum Ca^{2+}-ATPases. These are ATP2A1, ATP2A2, and ATP2A3 that refill the ER stores. A rise in cytosolic calcium also contributes to keratinocyte differentiation by binding to calmodulin. This enzyme further on dephosphorylates and activates the four members of the transcription factor family NFAT. The dephosphorylated transcription factors shuttle to the nucleus where they interact with the AP-1 transcription factors driving the expression of CE proteins such as involucrin, filaggrin, and loricrin [62, 99]. All these genes involved in the calcium metabolism are not differentially expressed during aging as deduced from several studies [73, 100, 101]. Although many data concerning calcium metabolism are available, the disappearance of the calcium gradient remains still mysterious and definitely needs further investigation.

Conclusion

As the aged dermis is associated with specific phenotypes such as degradation of the ECM, also the epidermis shows specific "age markers." One of these signs of aging is a complete rebuilt of the cornified envelope. The hallmarks of this rebuilt are a reduced amount of loricrin and filaggrin. To compensate for this loss of proteins, an increased amount of basically all members of the small proline-rich repeat family can be observed. Therefore, the aged epidermis is much more susceptible to tape stripping or treatment with acetone. A rebuilt of the cornified envelope is not only observed in aged skin but is also a phenotype of such skin diseases as epidermolysis bullosa, psoriasis, atopic dermatitis, several ichthyosis, and loricrin keratoderma. Another sign of aged epidermis is a complete breakdown of the epidermal calcium gradient that could also be the key player in the rebuilding of the CE. The reason for this breakdown remains still mysterious and is in need of further investigation.

References

1. Medvedev ZA. An attempt at a rational classification of theories of aging. Biol Rev. 1990;65:375–98.
2. Farage MA, Miller KW, Elsner P, Maibach HI. Characteristics of the aging skin. Adv Wound Care. 2013;2:5–10.
3. Harman D. Aging – a theory based on free-radical and radiation-chemistry. J Gerontol. 1956;11:298–300.
4. Rinnerthaler M, Bischof J, Streubel MK, Trost A, Richter K. Oxidative stress in aging human skin. Biomolecules. 2015;5:545–89.
5. Dalle-Donne I, Rossi R, Giustarini D, Milzani A, Colombo R. Protein carbonyl groups as biomarkers of oxidative stress. Clin Chim Acta. 2003;329:23–38.
6. Gray DA, Woulfe J. Lipofuscin and aging: a matter of toxic waste. Sci Aging Knowledge Environ. 2005;2005:Re 1.
7. Ahmed N. Advanced glycation endproducts–role in pathology of diabetic complications. Diabetes Res Clin Pract. 2005;67:3–21.
8. Kasai H, Chung MH, Jones DS, Inoue H, Ishikawa H, Kamiya H, Ohtsuka E, Nishimura S. 8-hydroxyguanine, a DNA adduct formed by oxygen radicals: its implication on oxygen radical-involved mutagenesis/carcinogenesis. J Toxicol Sci. 1991;16 Suppl 1:95–105.
9. Prasad A, Pospisil P. Ultraweak photon emission induced by visible light and ultraviolet a radiation via photoactivated skin chromophores: in vivo charge coupled device imaging. J Biomed Opt. 2012;17:085004.
10. Gilchrest BA. Skin aging and photoaging: an overview. J Am Acad Dermatol. 1989;21:610–3.
11. Talwar HS, Griffiths CE, Fisher GJ, Hamilton TA, Voorhees JJ. Reduced type i and type iii procollagens in photodamaged adult human skin. J Invest Dermatol. 1995;105:285–90.
12. Craven NM, Watson RE, Jones CJ, Shuttleworth CA, Kielty CM, Griffiths CE. Clinical features of photodamaged human skin are associated with a reduction in collagen vii. Br J Dermatol. 1997;137:344–50.
13. Naylor EC, Watson RE, Sherratt MJ. Molecular aspects of skin ageing. Maturitas. 2011;69:249–56.
14. Labat-Robert J, Fourtanier A, Boyer-Lafargue B, Robert L. Age dependent increase of elastase type protease activity in mouse skin. Effect of uv-irradiation. J Photochem Photobiol B. 2000;57:113–8.
15. Birkedal-Hansen H, Moore WG, Bodden MK, Windsor LJ, Birkedal-Hansen B, DeCarlo A, Engler JA. Matrix metalloproteinases: a review. Crit Rev Oral Biol Med. 1993;4:197–250.
16. Quan T, Qin Z, Xia W, Shao Y, Voorhees JJ, Fisher GJ. Matrix-degrading metalloproteinases in photoaging. J Investig Dermatol Symp Proc. 2009;14:20–4.
17. Sohal RS, Weindruch R. Oxidative stress, caloric restriction, and aging. Science. 1996;273:59–63.
18. Millis AJ, Hoyle M, McCue HM, Martini H. Differential expression of metalloproteinase and tissue inhibitor of metalloproteinase genes in aged human fibroblasts. Exp Cell Res. 1992;201:373–9.
19. Jenkins G. Molecular mechanisms of skin ageing. Mech Ageing Dev. 2002;123:801–10.
20. Menon GK. New insights into skin structure: scratching the surface. Adv Drug Deliv Rev. 2002;54 Suppl 1:S3–17.
21. Proksch E, Brandner JM, Jensen JM. The skin: an indispensable barrier. Exp Dermatol. 2008;17:1063–72.
22. Gilbert SF. Developmental biology, vol. 8. Sunderland: Sinauer Associates; 2006. p. xviii. 817 p.
23. Segre JA. Epidermal barrier formation and recovery in skin disorders. J Clin Invest. 2006;116:1150–8.
24. Madison KC. Barrier function of the skin: "La raison d'etre" of the epidermis. J Invest Dermatol. 2003;121:231–41.
25. Denecker G, Ovaere P, Vandenabeele P, Declercq W. Caspase-14 reveals its secrets. J Cell Biol. 2008;180:451–8.
26. Leak B, Wei JT, Gabel M, Peabody JO, Menon M, Demers R, Tewari A. Relevant patient and tumor considerations for early prostate cancer treatment. Semin Urol Oncol. 2002;20:39–44.
27. Candi E, Schmidt R, Melino G. The cornified envelope: a model of cell death in the skin. Nat Rev Mol Cell Biol. 2005;6:328–40.
28. Bouwstra JA, Ponec M. The skin barrier in healthy and diseased state. Biochim Biophys Acta. 2006;2080–2095:1758.
29. Lippens S, Denecker G, Ovaere P, Vandenabeele P, Declercq W. Death penalty for keratinocytes: apoptosis versus cornification. Cell Death Differ. 2005;12 Suppl 2:1497–508.
30. Watt FM, Green H. Involucrin synthesis is correlated with cell size in human epidermal cultures. J Cell Biol. 1981;90:738–42.
31. Ruhrberg C, Hajibagheri MA, Parry DA, Watt FM. Periplakin, a novel component of cornified envelopes and desmosomes that belongs to the plakin family and forms complexes with envoplakin. J Cell Biol. 1997;139:1835–49.
32. Ruhrberg C, Hajibagheri MA, Simon M, Dooley TP, Watt FM. Envoplakin, a novel precursor of the cornified envelope that has homology to desmoplakin. J Cell Biol. 1996;134:715–29.
33. Kalinin AE, Idler WW, Marekov LN, McPhie P, Bowers B, Steinert PM, Steven AC. Co-assembly of envoplakin and periplakin into oligomers and ca(2+)-dependent vesicle binding: implications for cornified cell envelope formation in stratified squamous epithelia. J Biol Chem. 2004;279:22773–80.
34. Marekov LN, Steinert PM. Ceramides are bound to structural proteins of the human foreskin epidermal cornified cell envelope. J Biol Chem. 1998;273:17763–70.
35. DiColandrea T, Karashima T, Maatta A, Watt FM. Subcellular distribution of envoplakin and periplakin: insights into their role as precursors of

the epidermal cornified envelope. J Cell Biol. 2000;151:573–86.
36. Sevilla LM, Nachat R, Groot KR, Klement JF, Uitto J, Djian P, Maatta A, Watt FM. Mice deficient in involucrin, envoplakin, and periplakin have a defective epidermal barrier. J Cell Biol. 2007;179:1599–612.
37. Kalinin A, Marekov LN, Steinert PM. Assembly of the epidermal cornified cell envelope. J Cell Sci. 2001;114:3069–70.
38. Chapman SJ, Walsh A. Membrane-coating granules are acidic organelles which possess proton pumps. J Invest Dermatol. 1989;93:466–70.
39. Grayson S, Johnson-Winegar AG, Wintroub BU, Isseroff RR, Epstein Jr EH, Elias PM. Lamellar body-enriched fractions from neonatal mice: preparative techniques and partial characterization. J Invest Dermatol. 1985;85:289–94.
40. Raymond AA, Gonzalez de Peredo A, Stella A, Ishida-Yamamoto A, Bouyssie D, Serre G, Monsarrat B, Simon M. Lamellar bodies of human epidermis: proteomics characterization by high throughput mass spectrometry and possible involvement of clip-170 in their trafficking/secretion. Mol Cell Proteomics. 2008;7:2151–75.
41. Madison KC, Sando GN, Howard EJ, True CA, Gilbert D, Swartzendruber DC, Wertz PW. Lamellar granule biogenesis: a role for ceramide glucosyltransferase, lysosomal enzyme transport, and the golgi. J Investig Dermatol Symp Proc. 1998;3:80–6.
42. Mauro T, Grayson S, Gao WN, Man MQ, Kriehuber E, Behne M, Feingold KR, Elias PM. Barrier recovery is impeded at neutral ph, independent of ionic effects: implications for extracellular lipid processing. Arch Dermatol Res. 1998;290:215–22.
43. Oren A, Ganz T, Liu L, Meerloo T. In human epidermis, beta-defensin 2 is packaged in lamellar bodies. Exp Mol Pathol. 2003;74:180–2.
44. Braff MH, Di Nardo A, Gallo RL. Keratinocytes store the antimicrobial peptide cathelicidin in lamellar bodies. J Invest Dermatol. 2005;124:394–400.
45. Galliano MF, Toulza E, Gallinaro H, Jonca N, Ishida-Yamamoto A, Serre G, Guerrin M. A novel protease inhibitor of the alpha2-macroglobulin family expressed in the human epidermis. J Biol Chem. 2006;281:5780–9.
46. Serre G, Mils V, Haftek M, Vincent C, Croute F, Reano A, Ouhayoun JP, Bettinger S, Soleilhavoup JP. Identification of late differentiation antigens of human cornified epithelia, expressed in re-organized desmosomes and bound to cross-linked envelope. J Invest Dermatol. 1991;97:1061–72.
47. Jonca N, Guerrin M, Hadjiolova K, Caubet C, Gallinaro H, Simon M, Serre G. Corneodesmosin, a component of epidermal corneocyte desmosomes, displays homophilic adhesive properties. J Biol Chem. 2002;277:5024–9.
48. Denda M, Fuziwara S, Inoue K. Influx of calcium and chloride ions into epidermal keratinocytes regulates exocytosis of epidermal lamellar bodies and skin permeability barrier homeostasis. J Invest Dermatol. 2003;121:362–7.
49. Ishida-Yamamoto A, Eady RA, Watt FM, Roop DR, Hohl D, Iizuka H. Immunoelectron microscopic analysis of cornified cell envelope formation in normal and psoriatic epidermis. J Histochem Cytochem. 1996;44:167–75.
50. Eckert RL, Sturniolo MT, Broome AM, Ruse M, Rorke EA. Transglutaminase function in epidermis. J Invest Dermatol. 2005;124:481–92.
51. Steinert PM, Marekov LN. Initiation of assembly of the cell envelope barrier structure of stratified squamous epithelia. Mol Biol Cell. 1999;10:4247–61.
52. Wolf M, Muller KH, Skourski Y, Eckert D, Georgi P, Krause M, Dunsch L. Magnetic moments of the endohedral cluster fullerenes ho3n@c80 and tb3n@c80: the role of ligand fields. Angew Chem Int Ed Engl. 2005;44:3306–9.
53. Ahvazi B, Boeshans KM, Idler W, Baxa U, Steinert PM. Roles of calcium ions in the activation and activity of the transglutaminase 3 enzyme. J Biol Chem. 2003;278:23834–41.
54. Hohl D, Lichti U, Breitkreutz D, Steinert PM, Roop DR. Transcription of the human loricrin gene in vitro is induced by calcium and cell density and suppressed by retinoic acid. J Invest Dermatol. 1991;96:414–8.
55. Robinson NA, Lapic S, Welter JF, Eckert RL. S100a11, s100a10, annexin i, desmosomal proteins, small proline-rich proteins, plasminogen activator inhibitor-2, and involucrin are components of the cornified envelope of cultured human epidermal keratinocytes. J Biol Chem. 1997;272:12035–46.
56. Marshall D, Hardman MJ, Nield KM, Byrne C. Differentially expressed late constituents of the epidermal cornified envelope. Proc Natl Acad Sci U S A. 2001;98:13031–6.
57. Jackson B, Tilli CM, Hardman MJ, Avilion AA, MacLeod MC, Ashcroft GS, Byrne C. Late cornified envelope family in differentiating epithelia–response to calcium and ultraviolet irradiation. J Invest Dermatol. 2005;124:1062–70.
58. Eckhart L, Declercq W, Ban J, Rendl M, Lengauer B, Mayer C, Lippens S, Vandenabeele P, Tschachler E. Terminal differentiation of human keratinocytes and stratum corneum formation is associated with caspase-14 activation. J Invest Dermatol. 2000;115:1148–51.
59. Rinnerthaler M, Duschl J, Steinbacher P, Salzmann M, Bischof J, Schuller M, Wimmer H, Peer T, Bauer JW, Richter K. Age-related changes in the composition of the cornified envelope in human skin. Exp Dermatol. 2013;22:329–35.
60. Grove GL, Kligman AM. Age-associated changes in human epidermal-cell renewal. J Gerontol. 1983;38:137–42.

61. Kohl E, Steinbauer J, Landthaler M, Szeimies RM. Skin ageing. J Eur Acad Dermatol. 2011;25:873–84.
62. Rinnerthaler M, Streubel MK, Bischof J, Richter K. Skin aging, gene expression and calcium. Exp Gerontol. 2015;68:59–65.
63. Vermeij WP, Alia A, Backendorf C. Ros quenching potential of the epidermal cornified cell envelope. J Invest Dermatol. 2011;131:1435–41.
64. Vermeij WP, Backendorf C. Skin cornification proteins provide global link between ros detoxification and cell migration during wound healing. PLoS One. 2010;5(8):e11957.
65. Takahashi M, Tezuka T. The content of free amino acids in the stratum corneum is increased in senile xerosis. Arch Dermatol Res. 2004;295:448–52.
66. Tagami H. Functional characteristics of the stratum corneum in photoaged skin in comparison with those found in intrinsic aging. Arch Dermatol Res. 2008;300 Suppl 1:S1–6.
67. Scott IR, Harding CR. Filaggrin breakdown to water binding compounds during development of the rat stratum corneum is controlled by the water activity of the environment. Dev Biol. 1986;115:84–92.
68. Sandilands A, Sutherland C, Irvine AD, McLean WH. Filaggrin in the frontline: role in skin barrier function and disease. J Cell Sci. 2009;122:1285–94.
69. Luebberding S, Krueger N, Kerscher M. Age-related changes in skin barrier function quantitative evaluation of 150 female subjects. Int J Cosmetic Sci. 2013;35:183–90.
70. Ghadially R, Brown BE, Sequeira-Martin SM, Feingold KR, Elias PM. The aged epidermal permeability barrier. Structural, functional, and lipid biochemical abnormalities in humans and a senescent murine model. J Clin Invest. 1995;95:2281–90.
71. Hirao T, Takahashi M. Carbonylation of cornified envelopes in the stratum corneum. FEBS Lett. 2005;579:6870–4.
72. Iwai I, Hirao T. Protein carbonyls damage the water-holding capacity of the stratum corneum. Skin Pharmacol Physiol. 2008;21:269–73.
73. Breitenbach JS, Rinnerthaler M, Trost A, Weber M, Klausegger A, Gruber C, Bruckner D, Reitsamer HA, Bauer JW, Breitenbach M. Transcriptome and ultrastructural changes in dystrophic epidermolysis bullosa resemble skin aging. Aging. 2015;7:389–411.
74. de Cid R, Riveira-Munoz E, Zeeuwen PLJM, Robarge J, Liao W, Dannhauser EN, Giardina E, Stuart PE, Nair R, Helms C, et al. Deletion of the late cornified envelope lce3b and lce3c genes as a susceptibility factor for psoriasis. Nat Genet. 2009;41:211–5.
75. Guttman-Yassky E, Suarez-Farinas M, Chiricozzi A, Nograles KE, Shemer A, Fuentes-Duculan J, Cardinale I, Lin P, Bergman R, Bowcock AM, et al. Broad defects in epidermal cornification in atopic dermatitis identified through genomic analysis. J Allergy Clin Immun. 2009;124:1235–44.
76. Molin S, Vollmer S, Weiss EH, Weisenseel P, Ruzicka T, Prinz JC. Deletion of the late cornified envelope genes lce3b and lce3c may promote chronic hand eczema with allergic contact dermatitis. J Investig Allergol Clin Immunol. 2011;21:472–9.
77. McAleer MA, Irvine AD. The multifunctional role of filaggrin in allergic skin disease. J Allergy Clin Immunol. 2013;131:280–91.
78. Huber M, Rettler I, Bernasconi K, Frenk E, Lavrijsen SPM, Ponec M, Bon A, Lautenschlager S, Schorderet DF, Hohl D. Mutations of keratinocyte transglutaminase in lamellar ichthyosis. Science. 1995;267:525–8.
79. Benmously-Mlika R, Zaouak A, Mrad R, Laaroussi N, Abdelhak S, Hovnanian A, Mokhtar I. Bathing suit ichthyosis caused by a tgm1 mutation in a tunisian child. Int J Dermatol. 2014;53:1478–80.
80. Thyssen JP, Godoy-Gijon E, Elias PM. Ichthyosis vulgaris: the filaggrin mutation disease. Br J Dermatol. 2013;168:1155–66.
81. Scott CA, Rajpopat S, Di WL. Harlequin ichthyosis: Abca12 mutations underlie defective lipid transport, reduced protease regulation and skin-barrier dysfunction. Cell Tissue Res. 2013;351:281–8.
82. Sun JD, Linden KG. Netherton syndrome: a case report and review of the literature. Int J Dermatol. 2006;45:693–7.
83. De Benedetto A, Kubo A, Beck LA. Skin barrier disruption: a requirement for allergen sensitization? J Invest Dermatol. 2012;132:949–63.
84. Telem DF, Israeli S, Sarig O, Sprecher E. Inflammatory peeling skin syndrome caused a novel mutation in cdsn. Arch Dermatol Res. 2012;304:251–5.
85. Schmuth M, Fluhr JW, Crumrine DC, Uchida Y, Hachem JP, Behne M, Moskowitz DG, Christiano AM, Feingold KR, Elias PM. Structural and functional consequences of loricrin mutations in human loricrin keratoderma (vohwinkel syndrome with ichthyosis). J Invest Dermatol. 2004;122:909–22.
86. Bikle DD, Ng D, Tu CL, Oda Y, Xie Z. Calcium- and vitamin d-regulated keratinocyte differentiation. Mol Cell Endocrinol. 2001;177:161–71.
87. Hennings H, Holbrook KA. Calcium regulation of cell-cell contact and differentiation of epidermal-cells in culture – an ultrastructural-study. Exp Cell Res. 1983;143:127–42.
88. LaCelle PT, Lambert A, Ekambaram MC, Robinson NA, Eckert RL. In vitro cross-linking of recombinant human involucrin. Skin Pharmacol Appl Skin Physiol. 1998;11:214–26.
89. Deucher A, Efimova T, Eckert RL. Calcium-dependent involucrin expression is inversely regulated by protein kinase c (pkc)alpha and pkcdelta. J Biol Chem. 2002;277:17032–40.
90. Sevilla LM, Nachat R, Groot KR, Watt FM. Kazrin regulates keratinocyte cytoskeletal networks, intercellular junctions and differentiation. J Cell Sci. 2008;121:3561–9.
91. Hitomi K. Transglutaminases in skin epidermis. Eur J Dermatol. 2005;15:313–9.

92. Ahvazi B, Boeshans KM, Idler W, Baxa U, Steinert PM. Roles of calcium ions in the activation and activity of the transglutaminase 3 enzyme. J Biol Chem. 2003;278:23834–41.
93. Hohl D, Lichti U, Breitkreutz D, Steinert PM, Roop DR. Transcription of the human loricrin gene in vitro is induced by calcium and cell density and suppressed by retinoic acid. J Invest Dermatol. 1991;96:414–8.
94. Kim SA, Tai CY, Mok LP, Mosser EA, Schuman EM. Calcium-dependent dynamics of cadherin interactions at cell-cell junctions. Proc Natl Acad Sci U S A. 2011;108:9857–62.
95. Mauro T, Bench G, Sidderas-Haddad E, Feingold K, Elias P, Cullander C. Acute barrier perturbation abolishes the ca2+ and k+ gradients in murine epidermis: quantitative measurement using pixe. J Invest Dermatol. 1998;111:1198–201.
96. Menon GK, Elias PM, Lee SH, Feingold KR. Localization of calcium in murine epidermis following disruption and repair of the permeability barrier. Cell Tissue Res. 1992;270:503–12.
97. Celli A, Sanchez S, Behne M, Hazlett T, Gratton E, Mauro T. The epidermal ca2+ gradient: measurement using the phasor representation of fluorescent lifetime imaging. Biophys J. 2010;98:911–21.
98. Denda M, Tomitaka A, Akamatsu H, Matsunaga K. Altered distribution of calcium in facial epidermis of aged adults. J Invest Dermatol. 2003;121:1557–8.
99. Tu CL, Bikle DD. Role of the calcium-sensing receptor in calcium regulation of epidermal differentiation and function. Best Pract Res Clin Endocrinol Metab. 2013;27:415–27.
100. Lener T, Moll PR, Rinnerthaler M, Bauer J, Aberger F, Richter K. Expression profiling of aging in the human skin. Exp Gerontol. 2006;41:387–97.
101. Makrantonaki E, Brink TC, Zampeli V, Elewa RM, Mlody B, Hossini AM, Hermes B, Krause U, Knolle J, Abdallah M, et al. Identification of biomarkers of human skin ageing in both genders. Wnt signalling – a label of skin ageing? PLoS One. 2012;7.

arNOX: A New Source of Aging

21

Dorothy M. Morré and D. James Morré

Contents

D.M. Morré (✉) • D.J. Morré
MorNuCo, Inc, West Lafayette, IN, USA
e-mail: dorothy.morre@gmail.com;
dj_morre@yahoo.com

M. A. Farage et al. (eds.), *Textbook of Aging Skin*,
DOI 10.1007/978-3-662-47398-6_114

Abstract

An aging-related ENOX protein arNOX (ENOX3) of the cell surface and endosomes shed into body fluids increases in activity linearly with age beginning at about 30 years to a maximum at about age 65. Subjects surviving beyond age 65 frequently have reduced arNOX activity. As is characteristic of other ENOX proteins, arNOX proteins reduce molecular oxygen to water and carry out protein disulfide exchange. A property unique to arNOX proteins is the ability to transfer electrons to oxygen to form superoxide during part of the functional cycle. By generating reactive oxygen species at the cell surface and in body fluids (saliva, serum, perspiration, urine), arNOX provides a mechanism to propagate reactive oxygen species at the cell surface to surrounding cells as occurs in skin aging and to circulating serum lipoproteins of importance to atherogenesis. Five family members identified in yeast and humans have been cloned. The arNOX proteins are synthesized as membrane-anchored proteins with their catalytic N-terminus directed toward the cell's exterior. A ca. 30-kDa fragment is shed and enters the blood and other body fluids or is internalized into endosomes. With cells and tissue, the source of electrons and cells would be plasma membrane electron transport. With body fluids, the ultimate source of electrons for the reduction of ferricytochrome c appears to be protein thiols and tyrosines. arNOX proteins share many properties with other ENOX proteins including the oscillatory pattern of activity (26-min period), resistance to N-terminal sequencing and chemical degradation, and a propensity of the purified proteins to aggregate. arNOX proteins are widely distributed among aged systems including late passage cultured cells.

Introduction

Ubiquitous aging-specific cell surface activities that directly generate reactive oxygen species at the point of the age-limiting lesion have long been missing from our information. arNOX proteins, a small subset of cell surface NADH oxidases of the eukaryotic cell surface (ECTO-NOX or ENOX proteins), meet these criteria. Known as arNOX or age-related NOX proteins, they represent a very distinct subset of the ENOX protein family [1]. In this chapter, the ENOX proteins are introduced and described. An accompanying chapter (D. J. Morré and D. M. Morré) is devoted to aging intervention strategies based on modulation of arNOX proteins and their properties.

ECTO-NOX or ENOX (because of their cell surface location) proteins comprise a family of dicopper NAD(P)H oxidases of plants, animals, yeasts, and bacteria that exhibit both oxidative and protein disulfide isomerase (PDI)-like activities (Fig. 1). The two biochemical activities, hydroquinone [NAD(P)H] oxidation and protein disulfide-thiol interchange, alternate, a property unprecedented in the biochemical literature. The constitutive ENOX (CNOX or ENOX1) is ubiquitous, growth related, refractory to drugs and contributes to timing mechanism of the biological clock. A tumor-associated tNOX or ENOX2 is growth related, cancer specific, and cancer drug inhibited. The physiological substrate for the oxidative activity appears to be hydroquinones of the plasma membrane such as reduced coenzymeQ_{10},$^{-}$ .The aging-related NOX (arNOX) ENOX3 or age-related NOX (arNOX) is unique in that it generates superoxide and has roles in both skin aging and cardiovascular disease.

Gorman et al. [2] reported that UV irradiation of HL-60 cells stimulated superoxide production. Diphenyliodonium, a putative-specific inhibitor of NAD(P)H oxidases [3], blocked the production of superoxide to suggest that the UV target was a

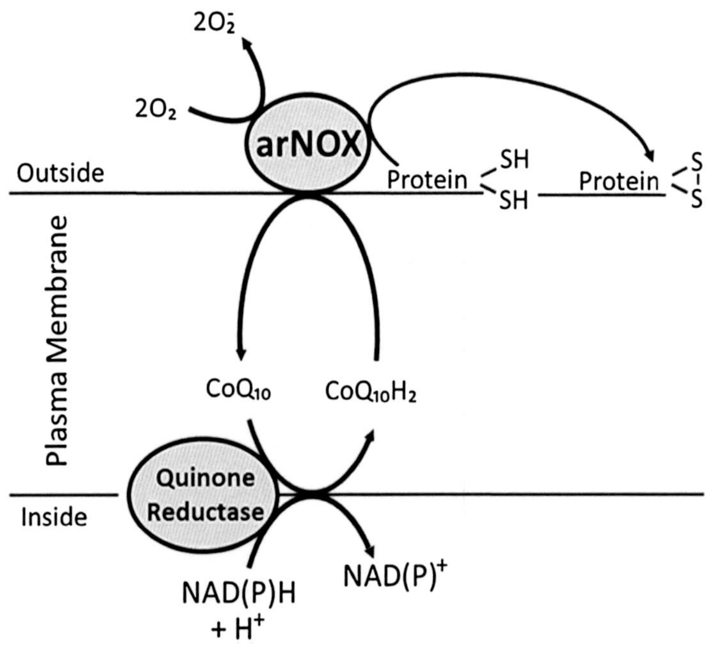

Fig. 1 Generation of superoxide at the cell surface catalyzed by plasma membrane-located arNOX proteins. Illustrated are the spatial relationships between hydroquinones and the external arNOX protein to donate electrons from cytosolic NAD(P)H to molecular oxygen to form superoxide. The arNOX protein also utilizes protein thiols as a source of electrons to generate superoxide as depicted on the *right*

NAD(P)H oxidase. A cell surface location was suggested by reports that plasma membranes generated hydrogen peroxide upon oxidation of NADH [4]. These findings were subsequently confirmed [5] in experiments where superoxide dismutase (SOD)-sensitive reduction of external ferricytochrome c, an impermeant acceptor, was used as described by Butler et al. [6] as an assay for superoxide generation followed by subsequent dismutation to form hydrogen peroxide. Using the SOD-sensitive reduction of ferricytochrome c as the assay, the cell surface NADH oxidase activity was found in sera, saliva, buffy coats, and epidermis of patients beginning at age 30 to a maximum at about age 85. A number of features identified the aging-related superoxide-generating oxidase (arNOX) as an ECTO-NOX. The activity was resistant to protease digestion, including proteinase K, and the activity was resistant to heating to temperatures of up to 80 °C [7]. The superoxide-generating activity was not steady state but exhibited a pattern of oscillations as is a characteristic of ECTO-NOX proteins in general [1]. The period length of the arNOX was about 26 min rather than 24 min [5, 7] as observed for the constitutive ENOX1 protein also present in surface membranes and shed into sera.

Measurement of Superoxide Formation by arNOX

A standard assay for arNOX activity is based on determination using a method described by Butler et al. [6] as an assay for superoxide generation and subsequent dismutations to form hydrogen peroxide to be certain that the rate of ferricytochrome c reduction is superoxide dependent and returns to baseline as a result. Specific assay conditions are given by Morré and Morré [1]. arNOX also may be assayed based on the property of the generated superoxide to reduce tetrazolium salts such as XTT (Na 3′-[(phenylamino)-carbonyl]-3,4-tetrazolium]-bis-(4-methoxy-6-nitro)benzenesulfonic acid) which leads to colored formazan formation [8]. This activity is lacking in other ENOX proteins. arNOX is present in all body fluids (blood, urine, saliva, and perspiration).

Perspiration may be conveniently collected using the Osteopatch™ Sweat Collection Device [9]. This device consists of an absorbent patch which is placed next to the skin to collect the perspiration. When eluted with assay buffer, sufficient arNOX activity to assay is provided. With perspiration, comparisons of different isoforms from specific skin regions topically treated or untreated skin from the same individual may be compared. A response of arNOX in the perspiration may be used to monitor efficacy, dosing, etc. in response to a specific antiaging strategy or to identify responsive and unresponsive individuals or individuals most likely to benefit. Although less specific than super oxidase formation, oxidation of NADH and hydroquinones as well as protein disulfide-thiol exchange also may be assayed as enzymatic activities exhibited by arNOX proteins.

arNOX proteins differ from the constitutive ENOX1 proteins in many ways. arNOX proteins are induced as part of the aging process (Fig. 2). They appear in plasma membranes of red blood cells, at the cell surface of skin explants and cells of the buffy coat fraction of blood and purified lymphocytes, and in serum, saliva, perspiration, and urine age where the activities have been assayed as individuals age. They first appear at about age 30 and increase to a near maximum at about age 55 for women (Fig. 3). Those surviving beyond age 55 usually have reduced arNOX activities compared to age 55. The arNOX activity of males increases to age 55 and beyond to a maximum around age 65–70. As with females, males surviving beyond age 70 may exhibit reduced arNOX activities compared to 65–70-year-olds.

The ECTO-NOX proteins as one consequence of their role as a terminal oxidases in a plasma membrane electron transport (PMET) chain have been postulated to link the accumulation of lesions in mitochondrial DNA to cell surface accumulations of reactive oxygen species during aging [10, 11], Fig. 4. As cells accumulate with functionally deficient mitochondria, their metabolism becomes increasingly anaerobic. As a result, NADH from the glycolytic production of ATP accumulates. An elevated PMET activity is able to maintain the NAD^+/NADH homeostasis

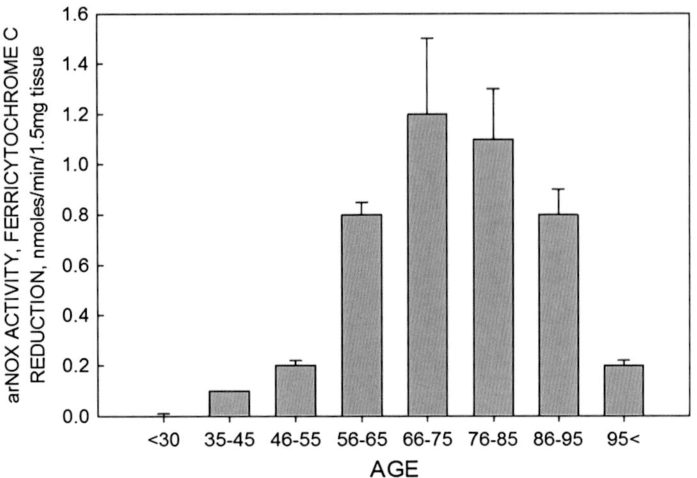

Fig. 2 Serum arNOX correlates with age to a maximum between 66 and 75 years. Individuals reaching age 85 and beyond have reduced levels of serum arNOX

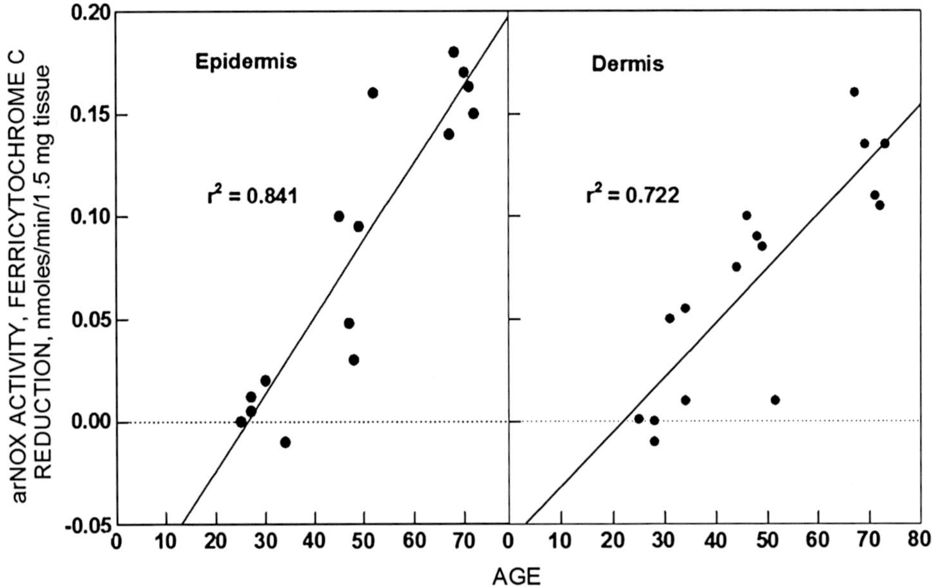

Fig. 3 arNOX activity of epidermal and dermal explants of skin and subject's age are correlated. arNOX activity increases with age beginning about age 30. The subjects were 16 females. Values of activities susceptible to inhibition by SOD did not become measureable until after age 30

essential for survival by regenerating NAD^+. Hyperactivity of the plasma membrane arNOX at the cell surface not only restores NAD^+ but also generates superoxide [5]. The generated superoxide could serve to propagate the aging cascade to adjacent cells as well as to oxidize circulating lipoproteins [12], through action-at-a-distance oxidize collagen and other proteins of the skin matrix [13].

An important identifying characteristic of the ECTO-NOX family of cell surface proteins that also exhibited the arNOX proteins is protease resistance including resistance to digestion by proteinase K along with resistance to heating to temperatures between 70 ° C and 80 ° C [7]. The source of electrons for cell surface arNOX is hydroquinones formed from reduction of NADH. For the circulating arNOX proteins,

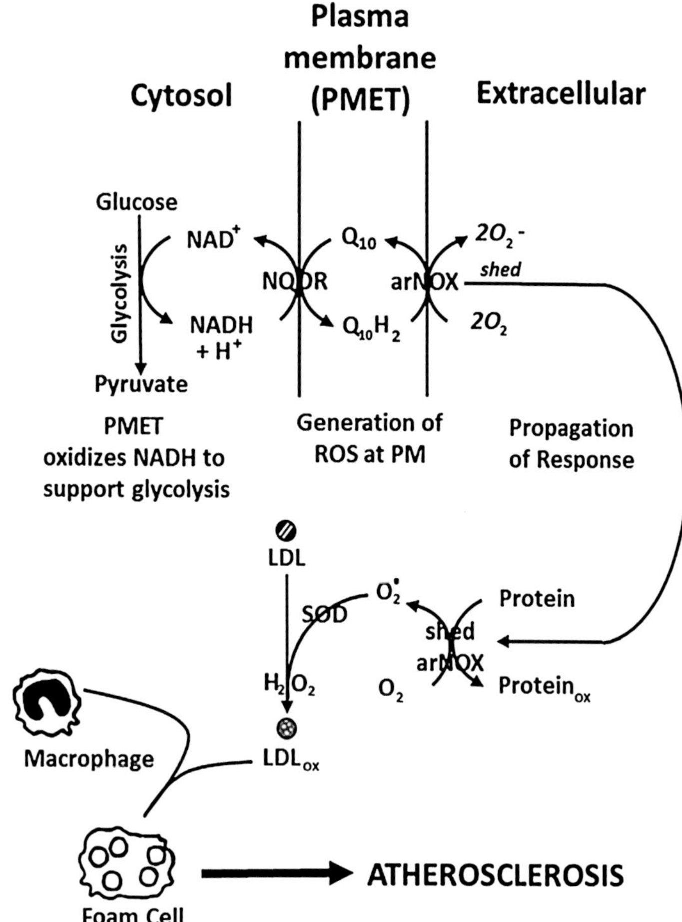

Fig. 4 Hypothesis to explain the mechanism whereby anaerobiosis resulting from mitochondrial lesions, the resultant stimulation of glycolysis, and the enhancement of the plasma membrane oxidoreductase (*PMOR*) system result in the formation of reactive oxygen species (*ROS*) at the cell surface that can be propagated and affect both adjacent cells and circulating blood components. *LDL* low-density lipoprotein

protein thiols were recognized early as a potential source of electrons [7].

Not only do shed arNOX proteins generate superoxide by arNOX proteins but they also oxidize proteins directly. Oxidation of tyrosine residues [14, 15] to form tyrosyl radicals [16] results in formation of intermolecular O,O[1]-dityrosine bonds [17]. The latter increase with aging [18, 19] most likely in response to the aging-related increase in arNOX activities.

arNOX Cloning

arNOX proteins have been cloned [20]. The age-related NADH oxidases of cells and body fluids were difficult to clone in order to determine their genetic origins. This was complicated by human arNOX being not a single protein. Rather it was a complex of at least five related proteins with diverse N-terminal sequences. Additionally, the soluble form was derived from a membrane-associated precursor having 9 transmembrane regions (Fig. 5). As is characteristic of ENOX proteins generally, the shed proteins with arNOX activity formed aggregates when concentrated and were blocked to N-terminal sequencing [20].

While the arNOX (ENOX3) protein family has a relatively divergent, hydrophilic N-terminal domain, its hydrophobic C-terminal domain which contains nine potential membrane-spanning domains, which adopt a type 1 topology, is well conserved. The identification of the immunoreactive yeast arNOX (ENOX3) permitted the cloning of the corresponding cDNAs [21].

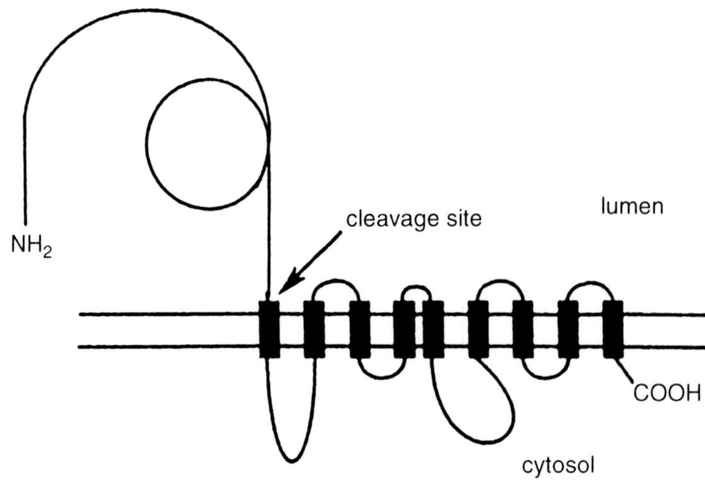

Fig. 5 Representation of the membrane association of the TM9 superfamily members. An N-terminal fragment is cleaved and released into external milieu surrounding cells

Found was a family of proteins designated "TMSF" (transmembrane superfamily) by the Nomenclature Committee. The lead member of the TM9SF family is the *Saccharomyces cerevisiae* EMP70 gene product, a 70-kDa protein that is processed into a 24-kDa (p24a) protein located in the endosomes [22]. Five subtypes of human TM9SF proteins were subsequently distinguished, i.e., TM95F-1 [23], TM95F 1b [24], TM95F2 [25], TM95F-3, and D8744 in D87444, which exhibit 30–40 % amino identity to each other and with the yeast p24a precursor [26].

Based on homology with the yeast arNOX proteins, the five circulating human arNOX were unequivocally identified as isoforms of exfoliated N-termini of the five members of the TM9 family of transmembrane proteins (GenBank NM-006405, NM0001014841, NM-01474742) [20]. The identification was based on cloned TM9SF2 and TM9SF4, two of the family members, and their expression in bacteria. The three additional superfamily members were identified based on the inhibition of their enzymatic activities by specific peptide antisera (Table 1).

The human homolog of the *S. cerevisiae* EMP70 gene product, a precursor protein whose 24-kDa cleavage product (p24) conserved throughout evolution, was found in yeast endosome-enriched membrane fractions [22] and detected in all tissues examined [25]. A ca. 30-kDa fragment normally internalized into endosomes [25] also is shed and enters the blood and other body fluids. The soluble fragments generate superoxide and carry out all of the oxidative functions associated with the cell surface form.

Characterization of Recombinant arNOX Proteins

Recombinant TM9 superfamily human arNOX proteins, TM9SF2 and TM9SF4, were generated from cDNAs corresponding to the exfoliated form of the proteins, both the ca. 30-kDa and 15-kDa N-termini, and were expressed in bacteria [20]. All five of the truncated forms exhibited activities characteristic of endogenous circulating arNOX.

Peptide antibodies were developed for the soluble forms of each of the five isoforms (Table 1). The antibodies identified the 5 isoforms in human skin, sera, and saliva as having sequences appropriate to TM9 superfamily members. RT-PCR probes were generated for each of the isoforms to demonstrate their expression in both human skin explants and human lymphocytes to confirm the genetic origins of the five known arNOX isoforms of human sera, plasma, saliva, and other body fluids as that of the TM9 superfamily of proteins.

The two transcript variants, 1a and 1b of family member 1, are very similar with the exception that the member 1a contains C-terminal residues absent from transcription variant 1b. The different

Table 1 Peptide antibodies were generated in rabbits to the N-terminal sequences of the exfoliated proteins

TM9SF1a & 1b	(aa 72–87)	I	R	H	K	S	K	S	L	G	E	V	L	D	G	D	R			
TM9SF2	(aa 89–104)	G	K	R	P	S	E	N	L	G	Q	V	L	F	G	E	R			
TM9SF3	(aa 70–88)	K	K	S	I	S	H	Y	H	E	T	L	G	E	A	L	Q	G	V	E
TM9SF4	(aa 69–84)	I	T	Y	K	A	E	N	L	G	E	V	L	R	G	D	R			

A cysteine residue was added to the N-terminus of each peptide to facilitate coupling to the carrier protein KLH

```
  1  MATAMDWLPWSLLLFSLMCETSAFYVPGVAPINFHQNDPVEIKAVKLTSSRTQLPYEYYS
 61  LPFCQPSKITYKAENLGEVLRGDRIVNTPFQVLMNSEKKCEVLCSQSNKPVTLTVEQSRL
121  VAERITEDYYVHLIADNLPVATRLELYSNRDSDDKKKEKDVQFEHGYRLGFTDVNKIYLH
181  NHLSFILYYHREDMEEDQEHTYRVVRFEVIPQSIRLEDLKADEKSSCTLPEGTNSSPQEI
241  DPTKENQLVFTYSVHWEE
```

Adenine nucleotide binding site (GXVXXG)
Putative copper sites (YVH, HGY)
Putative protein disulfide interchange site (CXXXC)
Conserved CQ/CE

Fig. 6 Functional motifs of the ca. 30-kDa arNOX form TM9SF4

family members are encoded by different genes and are therefore not splice variants from a single gene as is presumed for the different transcript variants of ENOX2 [27].

Each of the shed forms of arNOX contains functional motifs required of an ENOX protein (Fig. 6). Despite this similarity, sequence identity among the shed N-terminal fragments of different family members was minimal.

The activities of arNOX proteins are resistant to a specific inhibitor of ENOX1, simalikalactone D, and inhibitors of ENOX2, phenoxodiol and capsaicin. The arNOX activity patterns were not phased by addition of melatonin or as is characteristic of ENOX1. However, the period length was increased from 26 min to about 30 min by assay in D_2O in place of water, a general property typical of ENOX proteins.

arNOX as a Biomarker of Aging

While DNA, lipid, and protein oxidation products provide an extensive array of biomarkers for oxidative stress, most appear to be secondary to the actual sources of oxidative damage particularly in aging and provide limited opportunities for intervention. In contrast arNOX is reliably correlated with aging and provides guidance to development of skin care products to slow or prevent skin aging and as oral supplements to reduce protein oxidation leading to coronary artery disease. As such the arNOX biomarkers exhibit a high degree of predictive validity and utility to determine which individuals are most likely to respond to a particular therapeutic or preventive intervention. Additionally the biomarker reflects both long- and short-term exposure to a particular intervention and has the potential to give guidance to clinical trials involving age-related disorders.

Conclusion

Activity of age-related ENOX proteins (arNOX or ENOX3) of the cell surface and endosomes increases linearly with age beginning at about 30 years to a maximum at about age 65. Both males and females surviving beyond age 65 frequently have reduced arNOX activity. arNOX proteins reduce molecular oxygen to water as is characteristic of ENOX proteins in general. In addition the ENOX3 proteins transfer electrons to oxygen to form superoxide. A ca. 30-kDa fragment is shed and enters the blood and other body fluids. By generating reactive oxygen species both at the cell surface and by means of the shed fragment in body fluids (saliva, serum, perspiration, urine), arNOX provides a mechanism to propagate reactive oxygen species generated at the cell surface to surrounding cells as occurs in skin aging and to circulating serum lipoproteins of importance to atherogenesis.

Superoxide formed by arNOX is measured by the ability of superoxide to reduce ferricytochrome c. The superoxide generated is not only active in the reduction of ferricytochrome c but also in the reduction of tetrazolium salts such as XTT (Na 3′-[(phenylamino)-carbonyl]-3,4-tetrazolium]-bis(4-methoxy-6-nitro)benzenesulfonic acid leading to formation of colored formazans. Other NOX proteins lack this activity.

The arNOX protein family, identified in yeast and humans, consists of at least five family members of the transmembrane superfamily (TM9SF), 1a, 1b, 2, 3, and 4. The arNOX proteins are synthesized as membrane-anchored proteins with their catalytic N-terminus directed toward the cell's exterior. With cells and tissues, the source of electrons is plasma membrane electron transport (PMET). With sera, the ultimate source of electrons for the reduction of ferricytochrome c appears to be protein thiols and tyrosines. The arNOX proteins are very stable to heat, proteolysis, and chemical degradation. arNOX proteins are widely distributed among eukaryotic organisms, and in several well-studied examples, activities correlate with the longevity of the organism.

Cross-References

► arNOX: New Mechanisms of Skin Aging and Lipoprotein Oxidation

References

1. Morré DJ, Morré DM. ECTO-NOX proteins, growth, cancer, aging. New York: Springer; 2013. 507 pp.
2. Gorman A, McGowan A, Cutler TG. Role of peroxide and superoxide anion during tumor cell apoptosis. FEBS Lett. 1997;404:27–33.
3. Morré DJ. Preferential inhibition of the plasma membrane NADH oxidase (NOX) activity by diphenyleneiodonium chloride with NADPH as donor. Antioxid Redox Signal. 2002;4:207–12.
4. Ramasarma T, Swaroop A, MacKellar W, Crane FL. Generation of hydrogen peroxide on oxidation of NADH by hepatic plasma membranes. J Bioenerg Biomembr. 1981;13:241–53.
5. Morré DJ, Pogue R, Morré DM. A multifunctional ubiquinol oxidase of the external cell surface and sera. Biofactors. 1999;9:179–87.
6. Butler J, Koppenol WH, Margoliash E. Kinetics and mechanism of the reduction of ferricytochrome c by the superoxide anion. J Biol Chem. 1982;257:10747–50.
7. Morré DM, Guo F, Morré DJ. An aging-related cell surface NADH oxidase (arNOX) generates superoxide and is inhibited by coenzyme Q. Mol Cell Biochem. 2003;264:101–9.
8. Sutherland MW, Learmonth BA. The tetrazolium dyes MTS and XTT provide new quantitative assays for superoxide and superoxide dismutase. Free Radic Res. 1997;27:283–9.
9. Palacios C, Wigertz K, Martin B, Weaver CM. Sweat mineral loss from whole body, patch and arm bag in white and black girls. Nutr Res. 2003;23:401–11.
10. Morré DM, Lenaz G, Morré DJ. Surface oxidase and oxidative stress propagation in aging. J Exp Biol. 2000;203:1513–21.
11. De Grey ADNJ. The mitochondrial free radical theory of aging. Austin: R. G. Landes; 1999. p. 104–10.
12. Morré DJ, Kern D, Meadows C, Knaggs H, Morré DM. Age-related surface oxidases shed into body fluids as targets to prevent skin aging and reduce cardiovascular risk. World J Cardiovasc Dis. 2014;4:119–29.
13. Meadows C, Morré DJ, Morré DM, Draelos ZD, Kern DG. Age-related NADH oxidase (arNOX) catalyzed oxidative damage to skin proteins. Arch Dermatol Res. 2014;306:645–52.
14. Morré DM, Meadows C, Hostetler B, Weston N, Kern D, Draelos Z, Morré DJ. Age-related ENOX protein (arNOX) activity correlated with oxidative skin damage in the elderly. Biofactors. 2009;34:237–44.
15. Morré DM, Meadows C, Morré DJ. arNOX: generator of reactive oxygen species in the skin and sera of aging individuals subject to external modulation. Rejuvenation Res. 2010;13:162–4.
16. van der Vlies D, Wirtz KWA, Pap EHW. Detection of protein oxidation in rat-1 fibroblasts by fluorescently labeled tyramine. Biochemistry. 2001;40:7783–8.
17. Aeschbach R, Amadoò R, Neukom H. Formation of dityrosine cross-links in proteins by oxidation of tyrosine residues. Biochim Biophys Acta. 1976;439:292–301.
18. Leeuwenburgh C, Wagner P, Holloszy JO, Sohal RS, Heinecke JW. Caloric restriction attenuates dityrosine cross-linking of cardiac and skeletal muscle proteins in aging mice. Arch Biochem Biophys. 1997;346:74–80.
19. Well-Knecht MC, Huggins TG, Dyer DG, Thorpe SR, Baynes JW. Oxidized amino acids in lens protein with age. Measurement of 0-tyrosine and dityrosine in the aging human lens. J Biol Chem. 1993;268:12348–52.
20. Tang X, Parisi D, Spicer B, Morré DM, Morré DJ. Molecular cloning and characterization of human age-related NAD oxidase (arNOX) proteins as members of the TM-9 superfamily of transmembrane proteins. Adv Biol Chem. 2013;3:187–97.
21. Dick S, Phung C, Morré DM, Morré DJ. Molecular cloning and characterization of an ECTO-NOX3 (ENOX3) of *Saccharomyces cerevisiae*. Adv Biol Chem. 2013;3:59–69.
22. Singer-Krüger B, Frank R, Crausaz F, Riezman H. Partial purification and characterization of early and late endosomes from yeast. Identification of four novel proteins. J Biol Chem. 1993;268:14376–86.
23. Chluba-de Tapia J, de Tapia M, Jäggin V, Eberle AN. Cloning of a human multispanning membrane protein cDNA: evidence for a new protein family. Gene. 1997;197:195–204.

24. He P, Peng Z, Luo Y, Wang L, Yu P, Deng W, An Y, Shi T, Ma D. High-throughput functional screening for autophagy-related genes and identification of TM9SF1 as an autophagosome-inducing gene. Autophagy. 2009;5:52–60.
25. Schimmöller F, Diaz E, Mühlbauer B, Pfeffer SR. Characterization of a 76 kDa endosomal, multispanning membrane protein that is highly conserved throughout evolution. Gene. 1998;216:311–8.
26. Sugasawa T, Lenzen G, Simon S, Hidaka J, Cahen A, Guillaume J-L, Camoin L, Strosberg AD, Nahmias C. The iodocyanopindolol and SM-11044 binding protein belongs to the TM9SF multispanning membrane protein superfamily. Gene. 2001;273:227–37.
27. Tang X, Tian Z, Chueh P-J, Chen S, Morré DM, Morré DJ. Alternative splicing as the basis for specific localization of tNOX, a unique hydroquinone (NADH) oxidase, to the cancer cell surface. Biochemistry. 2007;46:12337–46.

arNOX: New Mechanisms of Skin Aging and Lipoprotein Oxidation

22

D. James Morré and Dorothy M. Morré

Contents

Abstract

The discovery of a family of cell surface age-related ECTO-NOX proteins, designated as arNOX or ENOX3 capable of generating superoxide which can then dismutase to form hydrogen peroxide as well as the directly oxidized tyrosines and protein thiols, has led to new mechanisms of skin aging applicable, as well, to lipoprotein oxidation and atherogenesis. The arNOX proteins are shed from the cell surface where they enter body fluids and permeate interstitial spaces as a major contributor to skin aging. As introduced in an accompanying chapter, arNOX proteins increase with age beginning about age 30 to a maximum by about age 60. Their activity is reversibly blocked by coenzyme Q and by a variety of herbal infusions including savory, estragon, basil, marjoram, rosemary, and sage as well as their phenolic constituents such as gallic acid. As staples of the French diet, these herbal sources of safe and effective arNOX inhibitors offer a possible explanation for the French paradox of reduced atherogenic risk despite a cholesterol-rich diet high in butter and cheese. Formation of malondialdehyde-like products involved in serum lipoprotein oxidation correlates with arNOX levels.

D.J. Morré (✉) • D.M. Morré
MorNuCo, Inc, West Lafayette, IN, USA
e-mail: dj_morre@yahoo.com;
dorothy.morre@gmail.com

M. A. Farage et al. (eds.), *Textbook of Aging Skin*,
DOI 10.1007/978-3-662-47398-6_115

Introduction

A major contributor to age-related skin deterioration is the accumulation of oxidative damage [1–5]. The sources of this oxidative damage and the manner whereby oxidative damage is directed to specific targets have been inadequately resolved. Aging leads to the accumulation of mitochondrial DNA lesions. However, mitochondria appear not to be a major generator of oxidative damage contributing to skin aging [6–9]. With the discovery of the arNOX proteins, the possibility was raised that reactive oxygen species (ROS) may actually be produced at the cell surface or by shed arNOX proteins of the external milieu [10]. Superoxide anions are generated by single electron reduction of external oxygen using NAD(P)H as the internal electron donor. The superoxide can then dismute (spontaneously or with catalysis by superoxide dismutases) to form hydrogen peroxide.

Role of arNOX in Skin Aging

A major cause of skin aging is the oxidation of proteins of the supporting matrices so important to skin health ([11, 12]; Table 1). Supporting evidence was provided from studies with female subjects where independent graders reviewed photographs of close-ups of the subjects' faces taken at a baseline visit and estimated the age of each subject. The appearance of the skin was scored according to overall skin health, fine wrinkling, deep wrinkling, skin color, skin laxity, pore size, and evenness. The estimates of age by a panel of graders were averaged for comparison to the subject's actual age. arNOX levels were determined from collections of serum, saliva, and perspiration from the same subjects. As summarized in Fig. 1, subjects with high arNOX activity had skin characteristics that made them appear on average 7 years older than their chronological age, whereas subjects with low arNOX activity at the same age had on average 7 years younger-appearing skin than their actual age.

Additional evidence that links arNOX activity levels to oxidative changes during skin aging includes readings of advanced glycation end product (AGE) determined using a Diagnotics (San Diego, CA) fluorescence AGE Reader ([13, 14]; Fig. 2). Fluorescent substances in the tissue are excited by a light source to fluoresce at a wavelength different from the incident light. The major sources of fluorescence are from AGEs linked to protein, mostly collagen that normally accumulates with aging. The latter was determined directly using arNOX purified from human urine in a 96-well plate assay by means of a commercially available protein carbonyl ELISA kit [15].

Also by means of a 96-well plate assay, arNOX-catalyzed oxidation of skin proteins based on oxidation of the amino acid tyrosine was demonstrated with Type I collagen, elastin, and bovine serum albumin ([16]; Table 1). Tyrosines, once oxidized, normally would form dimers to cross-link the proteins. However, in the assay which contained fluorescent tyramine, fluorescent dimers were formed with the oxidized tyrosines as a measure of tyrosine oxidation [17]. That conjugation of the fluorescent tyramine with tyrosyl radical was blocked by arNOX-specific inhibitors and by a mixture of arNOX-directed peptide antibodies provides evidence that tyrosine oxidation was arNOX catalyzed. An arNOX source concentrated from human urine with a specific activity comparable to that of aged skin was employed in the assay. Conjugated tyramine fluorescence increased with time for both collagen and elastin and was proportional to protein amount [16].

To demonstrate in situ arNOX-catalyzed oxidation of skin proteins, cultured primary keratinocytes and fibroblasts as well as frozen sections of human punch biopsies were investigated. Both epidermal keratinocytes and fibroblasts, when reacted overnight with fluorescent tyramine to detect tyrosyl radical formation, exhibited strong fluorescence, whereas fluorescence was blocked by a mixture of arNOX inhibitors [16]. A similar mixture of inhibitors was the basis for Nu Skin's ageLOC technology designed to achieve healthier skin by controlling reactive oxygen species at their source, i.e., superoxide produced by arNOX in body fluids and interstitial

Table 1 In vitro oxidation of proteins by arNOX based on formation of fluorescent dimers by reaction of fluorescent tyramine with the oxidized protein

Target protein	arNOX	SOD	ageLOC Ingredients[c]	Anti-arNOX Antibodies[d]	Relative Fluorescence
None	–	–	–	–	150 ± 28
	+	+	–	–	50 ± 56
BSA	–	–	–	–	320 ± 34
	+	–	–	–	31– ± 43
Collagen[a]	–	–	–	–	664 ± 42
	+	–	–	–	2,208 ± 483
	+	+	–	–	1,321 ± 531
	+	–	+	–	330 ± 203
	+	–	–	+	413 ± 30
Elastin[b]	–	–	–	–	30 ± 24
	+	–	–	–	2,425 ± 591
	+	+	–	–	1,413 ± 1,138
	+	–	+	–	727 ± 378
	+	–	–	+	725 ± 90

[a]Source of collagen was Calbiochem Cat. No. 234138 (collagen type I – human skin)

[b]Source of elastin was Sigma-Aldrich Cat. No. E749202MG, Lot 028 K1161 (elastin from human skin)

[c]To 2.5 mL of assay volume were added 60 μL of an aqueous mixture of 4 mg/mL *Schisandra (Schisandra chinensis)* extract, 9 % schizandrins (Draco, San Jose, CA) plus 1 mg/mL salicin (Sigma, St. Louis, MO), and 20 μL of IBR Dormin (Israeli Biotechnology Research, Ramat Gan, Israel)

[d]In equal mixture of peptide antibodies raised in rabbits to each of the five arNOX isoforms

spaces [18]. Neonatal keratinocytes exhibited low arNOX activities when assayed in parallel and were proportionally less reactive. Results with keratinocytes and fibroblasts were similar [16].

Using frozen sections of skin biopsy material, a group of 16 subjects, 8 females and 8 males, were evaluated for fluorescent tyramine conjugation and arNOX activity and for arNOX activity of saliva and serum as well as for epidermal AGE readings from the same subjects (Table 2). The subjects were in two age groups: young, age 24 ± 3 (20–30-year-olds), and older, age 55 ± 3 (51–59-year-olds). The biopsy specimens were snap frozen, and histological sections of the frozen tissue were examined for fluorescent tyramine conjugation and for arNOX activity by direct biochemical assay. For all subjects, arNOX activity of sera and saliva were closely correlated (r^2 = 0.84). The AGE Index values of the younger subjects (24-year-olds) were 1.4 ± 0.4. That of the older subjects was proportional to tissue arNOX levels (r^2 = 0.64). In half of the young group, arNOX activity could not be detected. arNOX activities of females and males of both age groups were not significantly different.

Fluorescent tyramine formation blocked by arNOX inhibitors was markedly different comparing aged and neonatal keratinocytes with the aged keratinocytes being much more reactive.

In these experiments, inhibition by SOD in the fluorescence assay was complicated by inactivation of SOD in the presence of tyramine where tyrosines of SOD are oxidized by arNOX and dimerized with the tyramine to inactivate the SOD. SODs contain a tyrosine in the active site [19]. Derivatization (e.g., nitration) of active site tyrosines of SOD, in general, leads to enzyme inactivation [20, 21].

Role of arNOX in Oxidation of Serum Lipoproteins

Age and oxidative stress are major risk factors for heart disease [22]. Among these, the oxidation of low-density lipoproteins (LDLs) is most often linked as being causal to atherogenesis ([23]; Fig. 3).

arNOX, both at the cell surface and as a circulating shed form, affords the possibility to

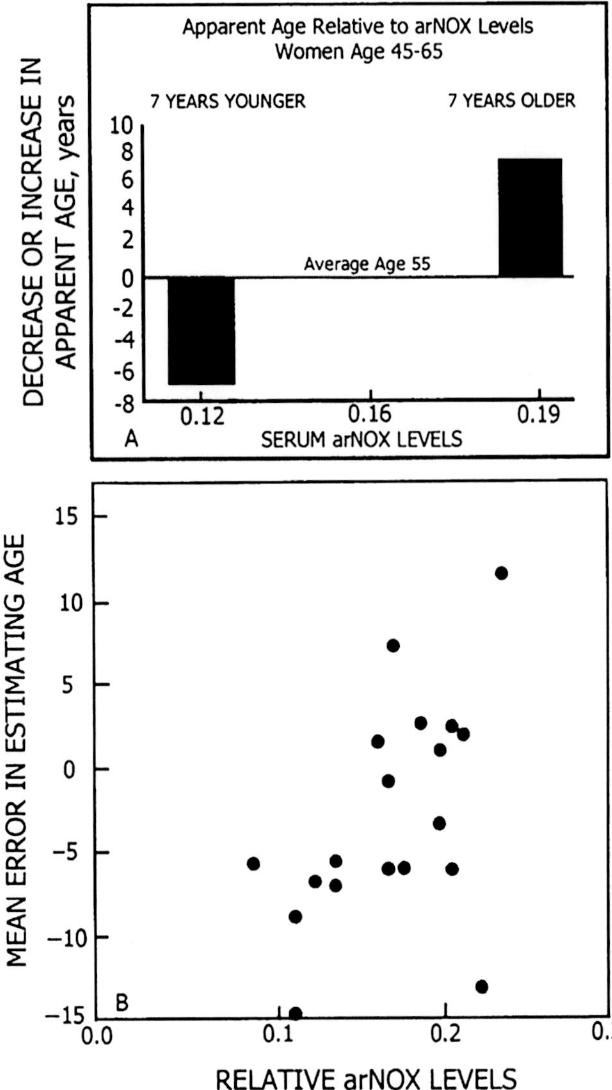

Fig. 1 Serum arNOX activity is correlated with mean error in estimating age. Sera were collected from 25 female subjects and compared to ages estimated from photographs taken at the same time

generate superoxide and reactive oxygen species not only in skin [24] but also in direct contact with circulating lipoproteins as an electron source ([25, 26]; Table 3; Figs. 4 and 5). Through specific oxidation of LDLs, arNOX proteins emerge as major contributors to cardiovascular disease. If LDL oxidation could be prevented or reduced, so might atherogenesis be reduced or prevented. The main destructive action of arNOX is primarily to directly oxidize proteins. While superoxide generation and conversion to H_2O_2 may be less important, the amounts of H_2O_2 generated are sufficient to contribute to lipid oxidation.

The hypothesis is that reactive oxygen species may provide a causal link in the formation of oxidized circulating lipoproteins such as oxidized LDLs and their subsequent clearance by macrophages and delivery to the arterial wall. A link between arNOX and LDL oxidation is provided by evidence that arNOX in the blood is structured as an integral component of the LDL particle. For both sera and plasma, 30–40 % of the arNOX is present in association with lipoprotein particles. During ultracentrifugation, the LDL-associated arNOX floats up through saline or distilled water. It cannot be washed off and

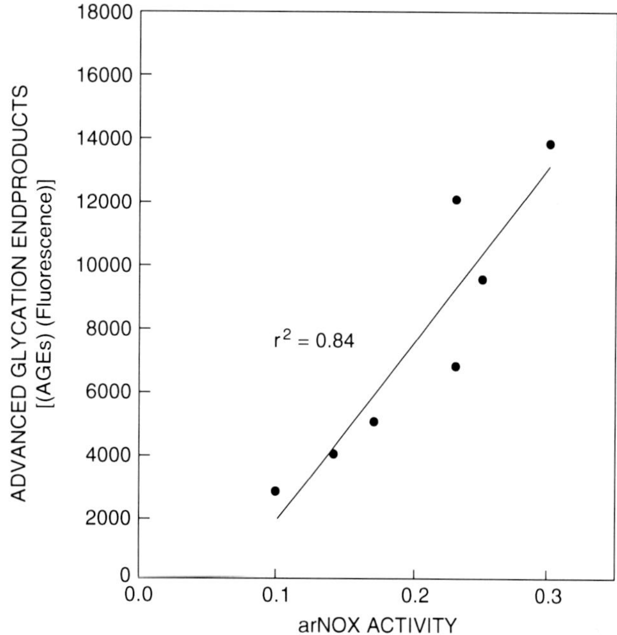

Fig. 2 Advanced glycation oxidation end products rise as arNOX activity of sera increases with increasing age

Table 2 arNOX activity of frozen sections of skin punch biopsies from 16 subjects, 4 males and 4 females in each of two age categories, young and older compared to AGE Index and arNOX activities of saliva and sera of the same subjects

Chronological			*arNOX* activity[b]		
Age (years)	N	Age Index[a]	Saliva	Serum	Tissue
24 ± 3 (20–30)	8	1.4 ± 0.4	0.003 ± 0.013	0.003 ± 0.009	0.004 ± 0.014
55 ± 3 (51–59)	8	2.2 ± 0.8	0.122 ± 0.079[c]	0.124 ± 0.085[c]	0.118 ± 0.030[c]

[a]Arbitrary units (see text)
[b]Units of specific activity are nmol/min/three frozen sections for tissue and nmol/min/200 uL for saliva and sera
[c]Statistically significant ($p < 0.001$)

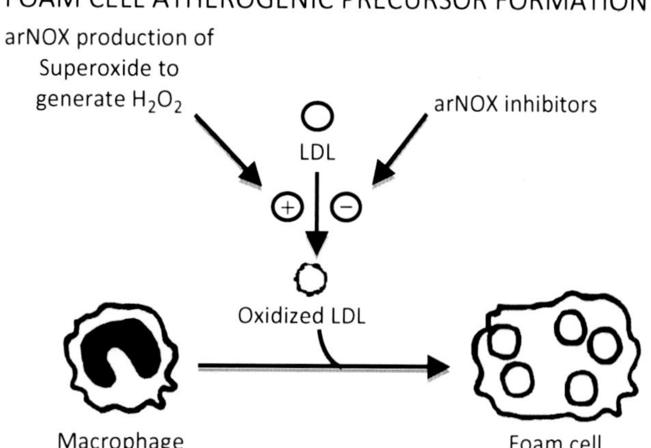

Fig. 3 Foam cell formation by macrophages scavenging oxidized low-density lipoproteins (LDL). Foam cells deliver the oxidized LDLs to the arterial wall resulting in the formation of atherosclerotic plaques

Table 3 arNOX-catalyzed tyrosine oxidation and cross-linking, overnight incubation

	Recombinant arNOX (TM9SF2)		
Substrate	–	+	Fold
Bovine serum albumin	14 ± 1	22 ± 3	1.6
Collagen	70 ± 13	308 ± 56	4.4
apoB	45 ± 11	71 ± 27	1.6

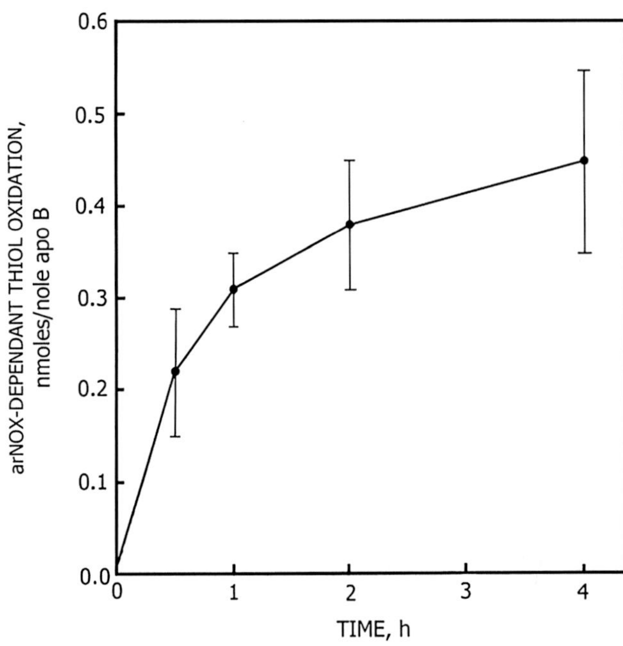

Fig. 4 arNOX-dependent oxidation of thiols in purified human ApB fully reduced with dithiothreitol (DTT), determined by reaction with 5,5′-dithiobis-2-nitrobenzoic acid (DTNB) (Ellman's reagent)

remains associated with serum lipoproteins following an overnight flotation centrifugation (Table 4).

The association of serum arNOX with circulating lipoproteins is supported by the observation that the dominant arNOX isoform of human sera has a 27 amino acid sequence with 40 % similarity to the putative LDL receptor binding surface. Apparently, the arNOX of sera targets the apoB of LDL particles as an electron source for superoxide formation in a relatively stable complex with the apoB target. This much of the oxidative damage is not necessarily due to ROS generation but through direct oxidation of protein thiols and tyrosines.

The pathway of apoB oxidation and subsequent pathology (Fig. 5) involves formation of malondialdehyde-like products (Fig. 6) as obligatory steps [27]. The oxidation of human serum lipoproteins has been correlated with arNOX levels in cell free co-incubation systems [28]. arNOX may contribute as well to the negative correlation between cancer and atherosclerosis [29]. While correlations do not prove cause and effect, the inverse correlation of arNOX with sea urchin life span and decreased levels of arNOX with age in long-lived species [30] is consistent with the idea that reduction of arNOX activity may help reduce the consequences of natural aging.

arNOX Inhibitors

Programs to identify genes associated with the aging process provide targets for antiaging interventions. These interventions may aspire to modulate gene expression at the level of messenger

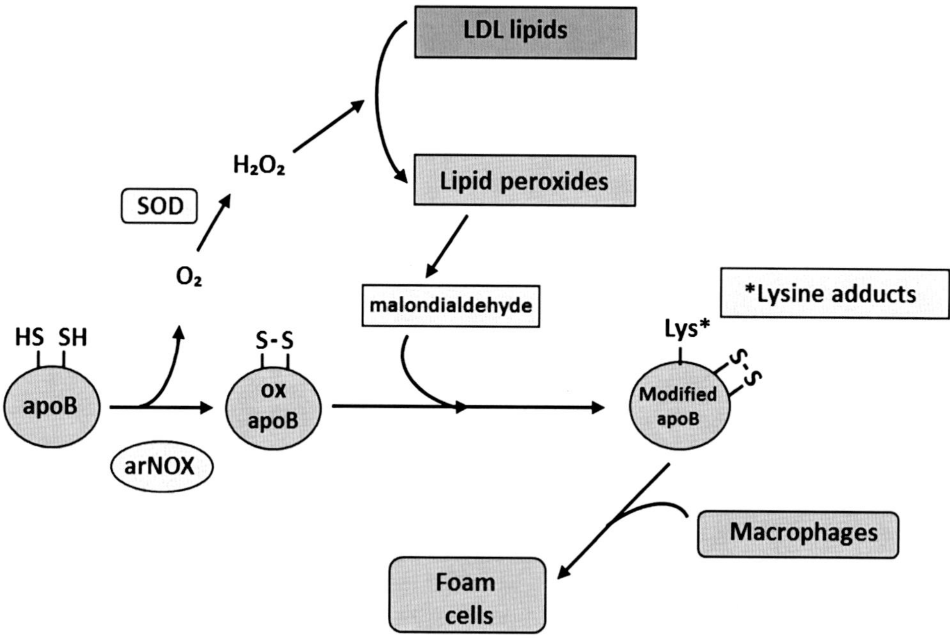

Fig. 5 Summary of the (*apoB* and *lipid*) cascade catalyzed by LDL-bound arNOX leading to LDL (apoB and lipid) oxidation, macrophage recognition, and foam cell formation

Table 4 Lipoprotein-associated arNOX-mediated oxidation of apoprotein B of serum lipoproteins determined from rate of ferricytochrome c reduction with lipoprotein particles isolated by flotation centrifugation of sera and plasma of human subjects comparing low and elevated amounts of LDL

	arNOX activity (nmol/min/mL)		*Lipoprotein bound, % of total activity*	
	Elevated LDL	Low LDL	Elevated LDL	Low LDL
Serum	1.0	0.6	32	20
Plasma	1.2	1.0	43	27

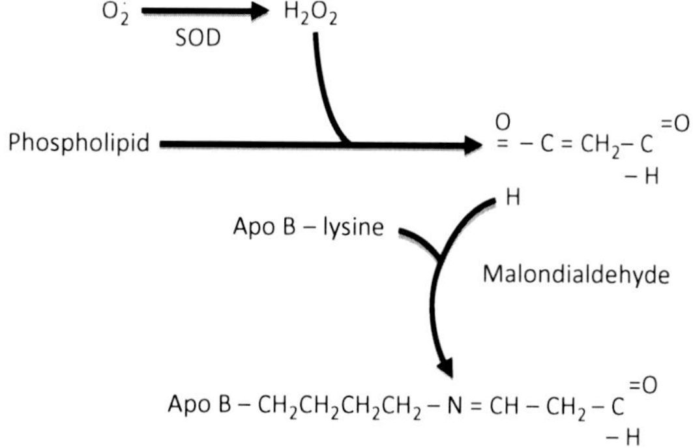

Fig. 6 Formation of lysine-malondialdehyde adducts

RNA or to modulate the protein products of the genes. arNOX genes provide examples of aging genes amenable to such modulation. Additionally, as circulating arNOX activity serves as an age-related indicator of the aging process, arNOX provides both an antiaging target and as a means to access efficacy of arNOX-targeted antiaging interventions.

arNOX generates superoxide and reactive oxygen both in body fluids and at the cell surface to increase significantly the ratio of reactive oxygen species to antioxidant defense molecules. As a result, age-related changes due to lipid and/or protein oxidation may be ablated by agents that reduce arNOX activity and at the same time reduce undesirable cardiovascular changes and prevent oxidation of supporting matrices of importance to skin health [31].

Coenzyme Q

Among the more extensively studied inhibitor of both cell-bound and shed arNOX is oxidized coenzyme Q_{10} (CoQ_{10}) [25, 31]. Administration of CoQ_{10} affords an opportunity to lower arNOX levels pharmacologically in a manner amenable to repeated sampling at short time intervals for real time kinetic analyses. In human intervention trials, measurements of arNOX activity of saliva, as a filtrate of the blood, were initiated as a noninvasive method to monitor arNOX responses that mirror those of the circulation [15].

CoQ_{10} inhibition of arNOX is mediated through the prenyl side chain and is chain length specific [31]. Inhibition occurs with only the N-decaprenyl side chain and without a contribution from the benzoquinone head group (Table 2). The shorter squalene side chain does not inhibit. Oxidation of NADH or protein thiols by arNOX also is inhibited by CoQ_{10}. In contrast, CoQ_{10} is without effect on these activities catalyzed by the constitutive ENOX1 or by the cancer-associated ENOX2.

Over the range of 10–100 μM, CoQ8, CoQ9, and CoQ10 inhibited arNOX, whereas CoQ4 and CoQ6 were without effect [25, 31]. Maximum inhibition was achieved between 100 and 150 μg/ml in the assay [31]. CoQ inhibition of arNOX was reversible and not based on reduction of CoQ. Reduced CoQ_{10} is not produced by arNOX nor does superoxide derived from added KO_2 reduce coenzyme CoQ_{10} at physiological concentrations and pH. On the other hand, superoxide resulting from KO_2 addition to isolated lipoprotein particles does result in formation of malondialdehyde-like lipid oxidation products [28].

Reduction of arNOX activities of sera and saliva in response to CoQ_{10} was correlated as was the activity in sera and perspiration. arNOX activities of sera, saliva, and perspiration increased with age and were reduced to a level comparable to that for subjects age 30 or younger in all subjects receiving CoQ_{10} [15].

A reduction in arNOX activity by oral administration of CoQ_{10} was observed in both male and female subjects, ages 52–72 y (Fig. 7). With a single dose of 30 mg CoQ_{10} (Q gel, Tishcon, NY, USA), the response in saliva was rapid with a half time of < 30 min. The response was reversible and arNOX activity returned to baseline between 8 and 10 h after a single 30 mg dose of CoQ_{10}.

Inhibition of arNOX activity measured after 2 h at the time of maximal response was proportional to dose of CoQ_{10} over the range 0–120 mg. With 120 mg CoQ_{10}, response was more pronounced, was maximal between 2 and 6 h, and returned to baseline at 11 h. Inhibition of salivary arNOX activity was about 70 % at 120 mg. The time of recovery varied from 6 h for 15 mg CoQ_{10} to 11 h for 120 mg CoQ_{10} and was proportional to dose. In these subjects, the arNOX activities of sera and salvia correlate (Fig. 8).

A sustained release containing 50 % CoQ_{10} was prepared and tested with the goal of maintaining arNOX levels at those of a 30-year-old over longer intervals. Single capsules of 240 mg taken twice daily morning and evening reduced arNOX levels to about 30 % of initial and maintained CoQ amounts at that level for 24 h. With eight subjects given the sustained release CoQ_{10} twice daily for 4 days, both serum and salivary arNOX were over 70 % inhibited.

Inhibition of arNOX activity may contribute to skin health benefits attributed by others to CoQ_{10}

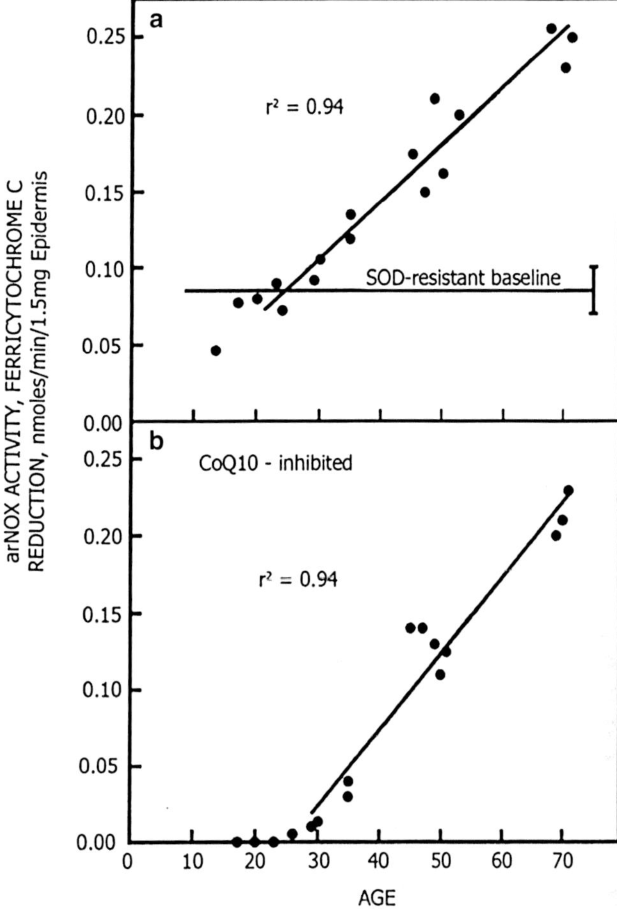

Fig. 7 Superoxide production by epidermal explants of both male and female subjects (**a**) and (**b**) as CoQ_{10}-inhibited activity as a function of chronological age. The CoQ_{10}-inhibited component of the activity was first observed about age 30

[14, 32]. Subjects with aged skin in a randomized, double-blinded, placebo-controlled trial used a skin care preparation containing 1 % CoQ_{10} or its reduced form twice daily for 5 months [32]. Significant reduction of wrinkle grade and an improvement of skin condition were observed. Hoppe et al. [33] showed that topical application of CoQ_{10} for 3 months reduced the depth and area of wrinkles around the eyes in humans. Similar findings were reported by Terada et al. [14] following daily oral supplementation of 60 mg CoQ_{10} for 3 months.

Botanical Sources of arNOX Inhibitors

Unexpected sources of potent arNOX inhibition were herbal infusions of savory, estragon (tarragon), basil, marjoram, rosemary, and sage [12]. Inhibition of arNOX activity varied from 50 to 90 % along with a corresponding inhibition of arNOX-catalyzed lipid oxidation (Table 5). Savory and estragon (tarragon) were effective at concentrations as low as 75 ng/mL. Also effective were tyrosol (Table 5) and phenolic constituents found in botanical ingredients including gallic acid at a final concentration of 0.14 μM (10 ng/mL) and (±)-catechin at 100 μM (300 ng/mL). An arNOX inhibitor cocktail consisting of a blend of botanical ingredients had been investigated previously as a topical application (Table 6).

The inhibition of arNOX by dietary constituents referred to as "Herbes de Provence" (Table 5) provides a possible explanation for the French paradox. The paradox comes about from the reduced atherogenic risk from the French diet or lifestyle despite a cholesterol-rich diet high in cheese and butter. Previous studies attributed the

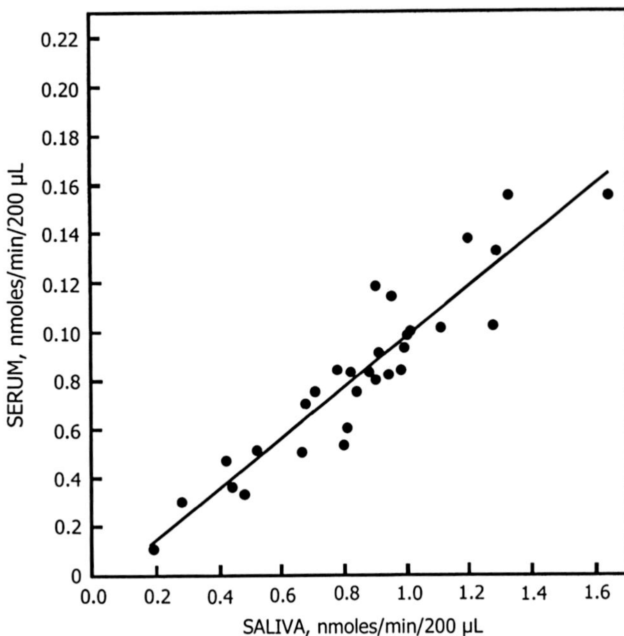

Fig. 8 arNOX activities of sera and saliva correlate

Table 5 arNOX activity inhibition by gallic acid (±)-catechin and by herbal polyphenol sources prepared as hot water infusions at a concentration of 125 mg/mL boiling hot water

Substance or herbal		*Inhibition % arNOX-catalyzed*	
Infusion		arNOX activity	Lipid oxidation
Gallic acid	6 mM	83	84
(±)-Catechin	100 mM	70	80
Savory	Infusion	89	100
Marjoram leaves	Infusion	50	77
Rosemary leaves	Infusion	59	95
Basil	Infusion	82	93
Sage	Infusion	54	70
Estragon (*Tarragon*)	Infusion	82	93

Table 6 Specific inhibitors of arNOX activity

	EC_{50}	
Inhibitor	TM9SF2	TM9SF4
AgeLOC[a]	1:30	1:20
CoQ	30 nM	50 nM
Tyrosol	3 µM	1 µM
Gallic acid	2 µM	2 µM

[a][60 µL of an aqueous mixture of 4 mg/mL *Schisandra chinensis* extract, 9 % schizandrins (Draco, San Jose, CA) plus 1 mg/mL salicin (Sigma, St. Louis, MO), and 20 µL of IBR Dormin (Israeli Biotechnology Research, Ramat Gan, Israel) = AgeLOC (Nu Skin Enterprises, Provo, UT)] added to 2.5 µL of assay volume

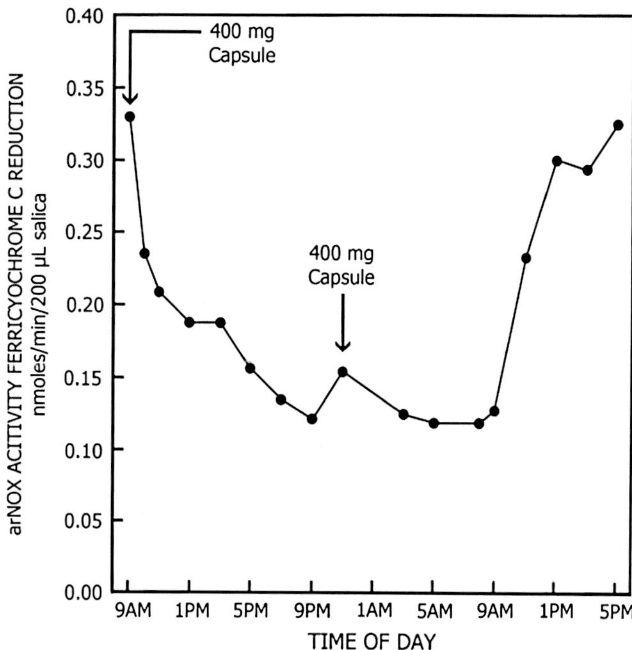

Fig. 9 Inhibition of arNOX-catalyzed superoxide formation of saliva by oral administration of a sustained released preparation of finely ground savory leaves (200 mg savory per 400 mg capsule). Two capsules/day, one in the morning and one in the evening, reduced the salivary arNOX levels to that of a 30-year-old

reduction in risk to consumption of red wine as a natural source of the polyphenol resveratrol [34]. However, the herbs listed in Table 5, which are staples of the French diet, offer a more compelling explanation.

By incorporating the herbal preparations as sustained release formulations, 24 h protection has been attained with just two 400 mg capsules/day (morning and before bedtime) (Fig. 9) and would maintain arNOX levels in an aging population to nearly that of a 30-year-old. It is this aspect that makes possible a therapeutic utility of the arNOX technology of importance to reducing aging-related arterial damage from oxidized circulating lipoproteins as well an overall slowing of age-related skin changes in individuals as they age beyond 30 years.

Besides having destructive properties, hydrogen peroxide may exert beneficial effects by acting as a second messenger molecule to activate specific signal transduction pathways involving phosphatases, protein kinases, and transcription factors [35]. This is especially true of the family of superoxide-generating NADPH oxidases of the inner plasma membrane surface, a well characterized group of at least seven proteins (Nox1 to Nox5, Duox1, and Duox2) named Nox or phox Nox for phagocytic oxidase [36]. Phox Nox proteins are distinct from arNOX proteins and are better positioned strategically for roles in signal transduction. Their spatial orientation is as a complex which facilities a two-step electron flow beginning with electron transfer from NADPH to FAD followed by transfer from FAD to a distal heme group. Finally, electrons move from the distal heme to molecular oxygen with the generation of superoxide anion. The most extensively studied member of the complex is Nox2, expressed in mammalian phagocytes and responsible for superoxide production during engulfment of invading microbes [37, 38]. Usually inactive in resting cells, activation occurs as a result of translocation to the cytosolic plasma membrane surface of a ternary regulatory complex formed by $p47^{phox}$, $p67^{phox}$, and $p40^{phox}$ subunits, as well as of the small GTPase Rac [39]. In concert with other members of the phox Nox family, Nox2 has been implicated in a variety of other biological functions in addition to host defense such as signal transduction, development, angiogenesis, blood pressure regulation, and certain biosynthetic processes [40].

Conclusions

The arNOX proteins, members of the ECTO-NOX (ENOX) family of cell surface proteins, are stable to heat, proteolysis, and chemical degradation and are released into the outer layers of the skin where they convert tyrosines of proteins such as collagen and elastin to tyrosyl radicals which then form cross-links through dityrosyl linkages as a major contributor to alter skin texture and appearance, wrinkle formation, and other degenerative conditions related to skin aging. In the blood, arNOX is bound to low-density lipoprotein (LDL) particles where a particular arNOX family member TM9SF2, with sequence homology to the LDL receptor, contributes to LDL oxidation. LDL oxidation is a prerequisite for internalization by macrophages to form foam cells, the obligate progenitors of atherosclerotic plaques. arNOX proteins actually bind to the ApoB100 proteins of LDLs as a source of electrons for transfer to oxygen to form superoxide. The hydrogen peroxide resulting from the dismutation of the superoxide results in oxidation of the lipid core with formation of malondialdehyde-like adducts. Protein thiols of the LDL coat proteins are oxidized as well to supply electrons to the oxidase.

Cross-References

▶ arNOX: A New Source of Aging

References

1. Hensley K, Maidt ML, Yu Z, Sang H, Markesbery WR, Floyd RA. Electrochemical analysis of protein nitrotyrosine and dityrosine in the Alzheimer brain indicates region-specific accumulation. J Neurosci. 1998;18:8126–32.
2. Smith CD, Carney JM, Starke-Reed PO, Oliver CN, Stadtman FR, Floyd RA, Markesbery WR. Excess brain protein oxidation and enzyme dysfunction in normal aging and in Alzheimer disease. Proc Natl Acad Sci U S A. 1991;88:10540–3.
3. Smith CD, Carney JM, Tatsumo T, Stadtman FR, Floyd RA, Markesbery WR. Protein oxidation in aging brain. Ann N Y Acad Sci. 1992;663:110–9.
4. Stadtman ER, Starke-Reed PE, Oliver CN, Carney JM, Floyd RA. Protein modification in aging. EXS. 1992;62:64–72.
5. Leeuwenburgh C, Hansen P, Shaish A, Holloszy JO, Heinecke JW. Markers of protein oxidation by hydroxyl radical and reactive nitrogen species in tissues of aging rats. Am J Physiol. 1998;274:453–61.
6. Nohl H, Kozlov V, Staniek K, Gille L. The multiple functions of coenzyme Q. Bioorg Chem. 2001;29:1–13.
7. Nohl H, Gille L, Staniek K. Intracellular generation of reactive oxygen species by mitochondria. Biochem Pharmacol. 2005;69:719–23.
8. St. Pierre J, Buckingham J, Roebuck SJ, Brand MD. Topology of superoxide production from different sites in the mitochondrial electron transport chain. J Biol Chem. 2002;277:44784–90.
9. Linnane AW, Kios M, Vitetta L. Healthy aging: regulation of the metabolome by cellular redox modulation and prooxidant signaling systems: the essential roles of superoxide anion and hydrogen peroxide. Biogerentology. 2007;8:445–67.
10. Morré DM, Lenaz G, Morré DJ. Surface oxidase and oxidative stress propagation in aging. J Exp Biol. 2000;203:1513–21.
11. Rehmus WE, Kern D, Janjua R, Morré DM, Morré DJ, Knaggs H. Appearance of skin ageing in healthy women. Correlation with arNOX levels: a potential new mechanism in ageing? Clin Dermatol Retin Other Treat. 2008;24:52–6.
12. Morré DJ, Morré DM, Shelton TB. Aging-related nicotinamide adenine dinucleotide oxidase response to dietary supplementation: the French paradox revisited. Rejuvenation Res. 2010;13:159–61.
13. Reznik AZ, Packer L. Oxidative damage to proteins: spectrophotometric method for carbonyl assay. Methods Enzymol. 1994;223:357–63.
14. Terada T, Takada K, Yamanishi H, Ashida Y. Inhibitory effects of coenzyme Q_{10} on skin aging. In: Abstracts, 5th conference of the International Coenzyme Q_{10} Association. Kobe; 2007. p. 156.
15. Morré DM, Morré DJ, Rehmus W, Kern D. Supplementation with CoQ_{10} lowers age-related (ar) NOX levels in healthy subjects. Biofactors. 2008;32:221–30.
16. Meadows C, Morré DJ, Morré DM, Draelos ZD, Kern DG. Age-related NADH oxidase (arNOX) catalyzed oxidative damage to skin proteins. Arch Dermatol Res. 2014;306:645–52.
17. van der Vlies D, Wirtz KWA, Pap EHW. Detection of protein oxidation in rat-1 fibroblasts by fluorescently labeled tyramine. Biochemistry. 2001;40:7783–8.
18. Kern DG, Draelos ZD, Meadows C, Morré DM, Morré DJ. Controlling reactive oxygen species in skin at their source to reduce skin aging. Rejuvenation Res. 2010;13:165–7.
19. Sorkin DL, Duong DK, Miller AF. Mutation of tyrosine 34 to phenylalanine eliminates the active site pK or reduced iron-containing superoxide dismutase. Biochemistry. 1997;36:368202–8.

20. MacMillan-Crow LA, Crow JP, Thompson JA. Peroxynitrite-mediated inactivation of manganese superoxide dismutase involves nitration and oxidation of critical tyrosine residues. Biochemistry. 1998;37:1613–22.
21. Xu S, Ying J, Jiang B, Guo W, Adachi T, Sharov V, Lazar H, Menzoian J, Knyushko TV, Bigelow D, Schöneich C, Cohen RA. Detection of sequence-specific tyrosine nitration of manganese SOD and SERCA in cardiovascular disease and aging. Am J Physiol Heart Circ Physiol. 2006;290:H2220–7.
22. Schmuck A, Fuller CJ, Devaraj S, Jialal I. Effect of aging on susceptibility of low density lipoproteins to oxidation. Clin Chem. 1995;41:1628–32.
23. Steinberg D. Low density lipoprotein oxidation and its pathobiological significance. J Biol Chem. 1997;272:20963–6.
24. Kern D, Draelos ZD, Morré DM, Morré DJ. Age-related oxidase (arNOX) activity of epidermal punch biopsies correlate with subject age and arNOX activities of serum and saliva. In: Abstracts, Society Investigative Dermatology. Kobe; 2008.
25. Morré DJ, Morré DM. Aging related cell surface ECTO-NOX protein, arNOX, a preventive target to reduce atherogenic risk in the elderly. Rejuvenation Res. 2006;9:231–6.
26. Morré DJ, Kern D, Meadows C, Knaggs H, Morré DM. Age-related surface oxidases shed into body fluids as targets to prevent skin aging and reduce cardiovascular risk. World J Cardiovasc Dis. 2014;4:119–29.
27. Gillotte KL, Hörkkö S, Witztum JL, Steinberg D. Oxidized phospholipids, linked to apolipoprotein B of oxidized LDL, are ligands for macrophage scavenger receptors. J Lipid Res. 2000;41:824–33.
28. Morré DM, Morré DJ. Coenzyme Q and lipid oxidation in aging and cardiovascular disease. In: Abstracts, 41st annual south eastern regional lipid conference. Cashiers;2006. 1–3 Nov 2006, p. 68.
29. Ades LMC, Morré DM, Morré DJ. Age related NADH oxidase (arNOX). Potential link between cancer and reduced cardiovascular risk. J Life Med. 2013;1:38–40.
30. Talbert E, Bodnar A, Morré DM, Morré DJ. Age-related NADH oxidase (arNOX) activity is significantly reduced in coelomic fluid of long-lived sea urchins. Int Aquat Res. 2013;5(2):1–7.
31. Morré DM, Guo F, Morré DJ. An aging-related cell surface NADH oxidase (arNOX) generates superoxide and is inhibited by coenzyme Q. Mol Cell Biochem. 2003;264:101–9.
32. Ichihashi M, Ooe M, Inui M, Omura K, Fugi K. Efficacy evaluation of coenzyme Q_{10} in aged human skin in vivo. In: Abstracts, 5th conference of the International Coenzyme Q_{10} Association. Kobe;2007. p. 88.
33. Hoppe U, Bergemann J, Dienbeck W, Ennen J, Gohla S, Harris L, Jacob J, Kielholz J, Mei W, Pollet D, Schachtschabel G, Sauermann G, Schreiner V, Staband F, Steckel F. Coenzyme Q_{10}, a cutaneous antioxidant and energizer. Biofactors. 1999;9:371–8.
34. Teissedre PL, Waterhouse AL. Inhibition of oxidation of human low density lipoproteins by phenolic substances in different essential ils varieties. J Agric Food Chem. 2000;48:3801–5.
35. Forman JJ, Maiorino M, Ursini F. Signaling functions of reactive oxygen species. Biochemistry. 2010; 49:835–42.
36. Del Principe D, Lista P, Malorni W, Giammarioli AM. Fibroblast autophagy in fibrotic disorders. J Pathol. 2013;229:208–20.
37. Cheng G, Cao Z, Xu X, van Meir EG, Lambeth JD. Homologs of gp92phox: cloning and tissue expression of NOX3, Nox4, and NOX5. Gene. 2001;269:131–40.
38. Sumimoto H. Structure, regulation and evolution of NOX-family NADPH oxidases that produce reactive oxygen species. FEBS. 2008;1175:3249–77.
39. Clark RA, Volpp BD, Leidal KG, Nauseef WM. Translocation of cytosolic components of neutrophil NADPH oxidase. Trans Assoc Am Physicians. 1989;102:224–30.
40. Nauseef WM. Biological roles for the NOX family NADPH oxidases. J Biol Chem. 2008;283:16961–5.

Age-Related Changes in Skin Mechanical Properties

23

Nils Krueger and Stefanie Luebberding

Contents

Abstract

Skin aging is accompanied by a variety of epidermal, dermal, and subcutaneous alterations including changes in pigmentation, volume, skin barrier function and mechanical properties. Although most of these signs of skin aging are somehow linked, the changes in mechanical properties are of special interest as they directly contribute to the development of wrinkles. While skin laxity is often seen first and most prominent at cheeks and neck, the loss of firmness is more general and becomes evident even in sun-protected areas. Although these signs of aging become visible lately, much later than wrinkles, the changes in skin elasticity begin early in life and progress continuously. To treat them most effectively, it is mandatory to understand the underlying dermal processes and how the skin mechanical properties change with aging. In addition, it is important to understand that skin ages differently in men and women due to the gender-related differences in the morphological distinction of dermal tissue. It is further of importance to understand the mechanical properties of the skin as a multiparametric function, influenced by a myriad of factors. It is inevitable to not only recognize all parameters as a whole but also to be able to relate to the measurement technique used to assess skin elasticity.

New data shows that the mechanical properties of the skin progressively decline with

N. Krueger (✉) • S. Luebberding
Rosenpark Research, Darmstadt, Germany
e-mail: nils.krueger@rosenparkresearch.de;
stefanie.luebberding@rosenparkresearch.de

M.A. Farage et al. (eds.), *Textbook of Aging Skin*,
DOI 10.1007/978-3-662-47398-6_116

aging. This aging process affects the elastic ability of the skin to recover after stretching differently than the firmness of the skin. Furthermore, the mechanical properties not only vary significantly between the sexes, they also alter differently in men and women over lifetime. This knowledge can be helpful for a better understanding of the clinical genesis of facial wrinkles and age-related skin laxity as well as for the development and evaluation of effective treatment options for skin aging.

Introduction

Skin aging is a complex biological process associated with increasing functional deficits in the heterogeneous dermal tissue due to structural and molecular alterations [1]. The most visible and obvious morphological sign of skin aging is the development of rhytides or wrinkles [2, 3]. While the fact that wrinkle severity increases with aging is generally known and commonly accepted [4, 5], recent studies [6, 7] have shown that the clinical genesis and onset of facial wrinkles differ between the sexes. The development of facial wrinkles significantly affects men earlier and with greater severity. There is an approximately 15 year earlier onset of visible rhytides compared with women. Furthermore, wrinkle severity linearly increases over lifetime in men whereas women's wrinkles sharply increase with perimenopause [6]. Differences between men and women have further been found regarding the morphology of dermal connective tissue. Histological analyses show a higher volume of elastic fibers in young women but at the same time a stronger decrease with aging. Collagen density and fiber volume in male dermis is, with the exception of male skin between 20 and 40 years of age, lower in comparison to age-matched women [8]. In contrast, Shuster et al. [9] found men to have more collagen, yet others were not able to detect any significant differences between men and women [10].

Although the development of wrinkles might be the most notable sign of skin aging, it is accompanied by a variety of epidermal, dermal, and subcutaneous alterations. These include changes in pigmentation, volume, skin barrier function, and mechanical properties. Although most of these signs of skin aging are somehow linked, the changes in mechanical properties are of special interest as they directly contribute to the development of wrinkles. Therefore, the treatment of skin laxity has become one of the main targets for antiaging procedures including the use of radiofrequency or focused ultrasound devices. To choose the right procedures and to use them most effectively, it is mandatory to understand the underlying dermal processes and how the skin mechanical properties change with aging. In addition, as the number of men requesting skin rejuvenating procedures increase year by year, it is important to understand that skin ages differently in men and women due to the gender-related differences in the morphological distinction of dermal tissue.

It is further of importance to understand the mechanical properties of the skin as a multiparametric function, influenced by a myriad of factors. Therefore, it is inevitable to not only recognize all parameters as a whole but also to be able to relate to the measurement technique used to assess skin elasticity.

Skin Elasticity

The protection against mechanical influences is an important function of the human skin. To serve this function, the skin must exhibit both flexibility and relative resistance to deformation, thus permitting movement and allowing temporary compression and distention of a part [11]. The tensile functional properties of the skin are due to structural and qualitative components of the epidermis, dermis, and subcutis [12, 13]. However, in terms of mechanical properties the human skin can be understood as a five-layer structure. The very top layer is formed by the compact membrane of the stratum corneum. The proximal part of the epidermis with its underlying desmosomes and the dermoepidermal junction represents the second layer. Papillary dermis, which is built of loose connective tissue, is the third layer, whereas the strong connective tissue of the reticular dermis represents the fourth layer. The subcutaneous adipose tissue is the deepest layer [14]. These layers together, consisting of fibers, colloidal substance, motile liquids, and a stiff epidermal layer, determine the mechanical properties of the skin [15]. Because of this complex composition of elastic solids and viscous liquids, the mechanical properties of the skin are neither elastic nor viscous, but rather viscoelastic [16].

Although biophysical measuring methods have been used to assess skin elasticity for more than 30 years it is not yet possible to assign elasticity parameters to one single structural element of the skin. Evidence is given that the elastic fibers permit the skin to return spontaneously to its initial shape after deformation [17, 18]. Thereby, not only the absolute amount of elastic fibers is relevant, but also their orientation. Usually, elastic fibers are vertically oriented to a net and link the dermoepidermal junction with the horizontally oriented collagen fibers. If this architectural structure is impaired due to an excessive and uncontrolled elastin proliferation, the elastic recovery of the skin is partly or totally lost [19]. Collagen fibers do not have any elastic properties but rather are essential for mechanical stability and its resistance to deformation [11]. In unstretched skin, collagen fibers are organized as disordered bundles. As the skin is stretched the bundles unfold, until the collagen fibers reach their maximum length. Therefore, a lack of collagen fibers or a degenerated collagen architecture, due to skin aging or skin disease, results in a high distensibility, slackness, and a higher sensitivity regarding mechanical tension [14, 20]. Besides elastin and collagen fibers, the hydration level of epidermis and dermis also influences skin elasticity. It is known that a moistening of the epidermis with water results in an increase of distensibility and skin fatigue but at the same time skin elasticity decreases. Also, a lack of hydration correlates in clinical evaluation with a loss of elasticity [14]. At the other end, the subcutis, the deepest layer of the skin, is of importance, too, as it serves as a cushioning layer for mechanical shear forces and plastic deformation, but also has an impact on the overlying skin layers.

Quantitative Assessment of Skin Elasticity

The noninvasive assessment of the mechanical properties of the human skin in vivo can be performed by distinct methods mainly characterized by the evaluation of the nature and orientation of skin deformation after an imposed force [11]. Thereby, the available techniques can be grouped into different classes, namely, tensile with electric dynamometers [21], torsion method [22], as well as impact testing (balistometrique technique) [23]. The elevation testing by suction chamber method is currently the most frequently used tool to assess skin mechanics [11, 14].

Tensile Testing

Tensile testing is based on recording skin extension following the imposition of a parallel force to skin's surface [11]. Therefore, tensile testing with electric dynamometers is the oldest commercialized device for investigating mechanical properties of the skin [21]. In this procedure, based on uniaxial tension, a small disk sticks on the skin and is set into forward and backward motion by the electric dynamometers. The stretching of the skin is recorded on the x-axis as superimposed ellipses (Fig. 1). The steepness of the slope of the ellipse gives information about the mechanical properties of the skin such as stiffness and elasticity [24, 25].

Torsion Technique

The measuring probe of the torsion method consists of a central disk and a peripheral ring which are both glued firmly onto the skin with double-sided adhesive tape. Due to a constant torque of the disk, the skin is deformed depending on the mechanical properties of the skin (Fig. 2) [22, 24]. The analysis of the resulting rotation angle (in degrees) of the disk versus time (seconds) gives information about the standard deformation parameters including skin elasticity, firmness, or skin fatigue [26]. The assessment

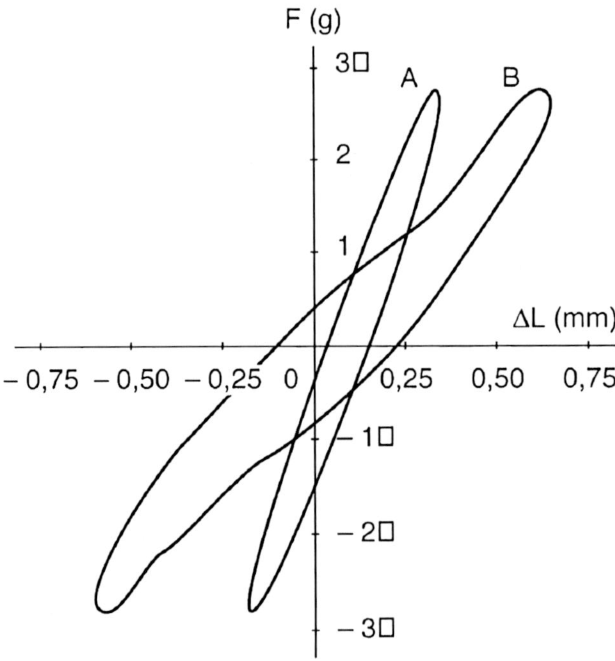

Fig. 1 Typical curve of tensile testing with electric dynamometers

Fig. 2 Schematic overview of skin deformation due to torsion method

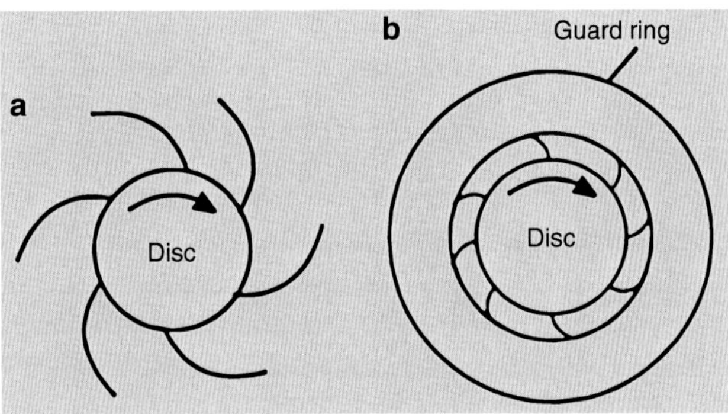

can be adapted by variation of number, duration, intensity, and rhythm of the twisting as well as by the distance between the disc and the ring. To examine the mechanical properties of the epidermis, a distance of 1 mm is used whereas greater distances are used to include underlying skin layers [24].

Impact Technique

The impact testing of the human skin, also called ballistometrique technique, was designed to approach specific tensile functions of the skin involving the deeper skin layers [11]. The balistometrique technique records the successive rebounds of a small hammer being dropped on the skin's surface with defined energy [23, 27]. The more the kinetic energy is transformed into rebound, the more elastic is the surface [24]. Because of the viscoelastic properties of the human skin, parts of the rebounding energy are getting lost with every restitution phase so that height and duration of the hammer lower with every rebound. The induced rebounds are transduced into electrical signals which can be quantified and evaluated in terms of their amplitude and frequency [11]. The main parameter of the balistometrique technique is the so called rebound-coefficient which is calculated from the ratio between the heights of the first and second rebound. The rebound-coefficient depends mainly on skin elasticity and viscosity [11, 24].

Elevation Testing

Elevation testing using suction chamber devices is commonly used to determine noninvasively the mechanical properties of the skin [28–30]. The underlying principle of the suction chamber method is to assess skin extension caused by a negative pressure [14, 31–33]. Based on the measurement of the extension in comparison to the height and the duration of the vacuum, several skin elasticity parameters can be calculated such as skin distensibility, elasticity, or firmness [14].

Besides the Dermaflex® (Cortex Technology, Denmark), the Cutometer® (Courage & Khazaka, Germany) is the most used measuring device to assess skin elasticity in vivo. It measures the vertical deformation of the skin when it is pulled by a controlled vacuum into the probe (Fig. 3). The depth of the penetration is assessed by a contactless, optical measuring method containing an infrared light source, a receiver, and two facing prisms which project the light from sender to receiver. The intensity of the projected light depends on the penetration depth of the skin into the probe [34].

The Cutometer® has a measuring probe which is connected over a hose to the vacuum pump and the measuring system. The opening of the suction probe has a standard diameter of 2 mm; alternatively, probes with a larger diameter up to 8 mm are available. While the 2 mm probe is primarily suitable to assess the elasticity of the epidermis, 4–6 mm can be used to evaluate upper skin layers up to the papillary dermis, and the 8 mm opening can be used to assess all skin layers [34]. The negative pressure can be adjusted between 20 and 500 mbar and the pressure buildup can be generated abruptly or gradually. Suction and relaxing time can vary between 0.1 and 60 s with a maximum repetition up to 99 times.

The suction chamber method represents the deformation of the skin in terms of the time and offers different measurement modes due to pressure variations. In scientific practice, a preset constant negative pressure of 200–500 mbar is commonly used. Therefore, frequent practices are measurements with 3–10 cycles and suction and relaxing time of 2–5 s [16]. Elongation and retraction of the skin is presented on an external monitor already during the measurement.

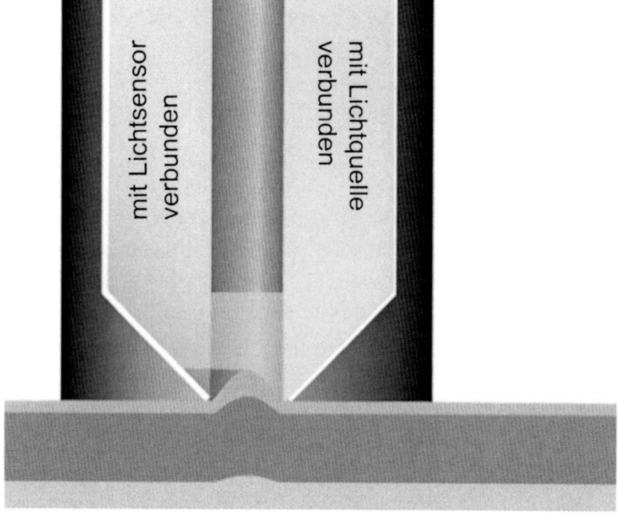

Fig. 3 Schematic representation of the suction chamber method

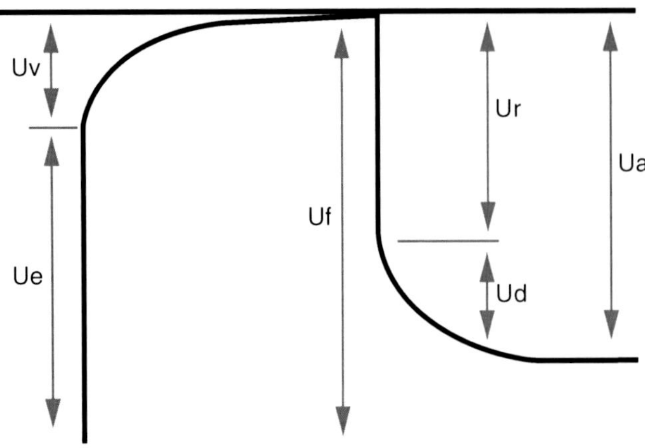

Fig. 4 Skin deformation assessed by suction chamber method

Table 1 Most suitable parameters to evaluate skin aging

Ratio of elastic recovery to distensibility	Ur/Uf
Gross elasticity	Ua/Uf
Net elasticity	Ur/Ue
Maximum recovery	Ua
Immediate recovery	Ur
Skin distensibility of the last curve	Uf5
Skin distensibility	Uf
Immediate distensibility	Ue

A typical measuring curve consists of four phases (Fig. 4). The first phase is characterized by a sharp increase which explains the elastic extension of the skin. The second phase, representing the viscoelastic proportion of extension, is shown by flattening of the curve. Upon pressure discontinuation, the curve sharply declines. This third phase represents the elastic proportion of recovery, which is followed by a flattening of the curve which represents the viscoelastic proportion of recovery.

The evaluation of the stress–strain and strain–time curves obtained with the Cutometer® allows the calculation of several tensile variables representing skin's elasticity, distensibility, or recovery after deformation [11, 35] (Table 1). Parameters that are particularly suitable to assess age-related changes of the skin include the ratio of elastic recovery to distensibility (Ur /Uf) as well as the gross elasticity (Ua/Uf) and net elasticity (Ur/Ue) for evaluation of aging effects on the mechanical properties of skin [36].

Mechanical Properties in Human Skin

While the progress of skin wrinkling is visible to the unaided eye, age-related changes in skin mechanical properties often become visible first at a higher degree of severity as skin laxity and loss of firmness. While skin laxity is often seen first and most prominent at cheeks and neck (see Fig. 5), the loss of firmness is more general and becomes evident even in sun-protected areas. Both findings are common aesthetic complains of people usually starting in their 40s and 50s. Although these signs of aging become visible lately, much later than wrinkles, the changes in skin elasticity begin early in life and progress continuously.

As studies have shown that the clinical genesis and onset of facial wrinkles as well as the morphology of the extracellular matrix differ between the sexes [6, 8, 9], it raises the question of whether the elastic properties of skin differ between men and women, too, and how these characteristics are influenced by skin aging. These questions were answered just recently by Luebberding et al. as her studies, in accordance with previous findings [28, 30, 37], confirm the significant impact of aging on mechanical properties in human skin [38]. All assessed parameters decrease progressively with increasing age. Over lifetime, the skin's distensibility decreases by up to 50 %, while the elasticity, the skin's ability to recover after stretching, decreases by up to 75 %.

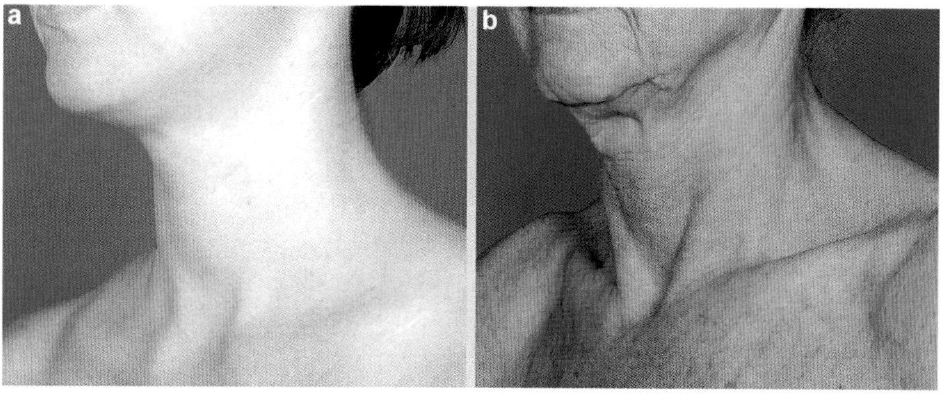

Fig. 5 Neck of a 19-year-old woman (**a**) with no signs of skin laxity and a 66-year-old woman (**b**) with extensive skin laxity

Although it remains elusive to assign skin mechanical parameters to single structural elements of the skin, evidence is given that the elastic fibers permit the skin to return spontaneously to its initial shape after stretching [17, 18], whereas the collagen fiber network is essential for the skin's mechanical stability and tensile strength [11]. It is well known that both the elastic and collagen fibers degenerate and diminish with aging, resulting in increased skin laxity and rhytides [18, 39, 40]. However, study results show that the aging process likely has a stronger influence on the elastic ability of the skin to recover after stretching as opposed to its effect on the firmness of the skin. It seems likely that these results might be due to the different amounts of collagen and elastin in the dermal connective tissue. While collagen makes up 70–80 % of the dry weight of the skin, elastin accounts for only 2–4 % [1]. It seems possible that this quantitative difference in extracellular fiber components led to a relatively faster degeneration of elastic fibers resulting in decreased elasticity. This knowledge is especially relevant for the aesthetic medicine as many antiaging procedures including radiofrequency or focused ultrasound devices target the collagen fibers in the skin to decrease skin laxity. However, how these procedures affect the much more important elastin fibers is virtually unknown.

Considering the known differences in skin physiology in men and women, it seems useful to take a more detailed look at the age-related changes in mechanical properties. The comparison of men and women shows that in fact gender-related differences exist.

While the alterations in female skin occur sharply, the mechanical properties of male skin steadily decline throughout life. In women, the distensibility strongly decreases between the ages of 20–30 years, whereas the elasticity decreases between the ages of 40–50 years. It can be assumed that the abrupt decrease of skin elasticity in women's 40s might be the result of hormonal changes resulting from perimenopause. Hillebrand et al. [41], among others [42], found that alterations in female steroid hormones due to menopausal transition years might highly impact the acceleration of skin wrinkles, compared to a relatively low hormonal status prior to menopause. As the development of wrinkles is strongly linked to skin elasticity [32], this hypothesis may be applicable to the changes in mechanical properties as well. However, further research, including the assessment of hormonal status, is needed for a better understanding of how menopause affects the mechanical properties of female skin.

In addition to the gender-specific decline of mechanical properties over lifetime, differences are also found in skin elasticity and distensibility itself [38]. Study results show that female skin is less distensible but has a higher elasticity (ability to recover after stretching) when compared to male skin. These differences are significant until the age of 40 and equilibrate with increasing age. A probable cause for these results is the gender-related difference in sex hormones. Histological analyses [8] have shown that both the collagen and elastin content in extracellular matrix does not differ significantly between boys and girls until the age of 10. Only with puberty and its hormonal changes, the connective tissue changes gender-specifically resulting in significantly higher collagen content in men and a higher content of elastic fibers in women. These differences remain until the age of 30–40 before they become equal again. Regarding the onset with puberty and the equalization with perimenopause, a connection with women's childbearing capability seems obvious. One plausible explanation may be the need of the abdominal skin to be extensively stretchable during pregnancy and able to recover after birth. However, this may describe the higher elasticity of female skin, but does not explain the higher distensibility in men.

Conclusion

Recently published studies clearly show a progressive decline of the mechanical properties of the skin with aging. The elastic ability of the skin to recover after stretching is more strongly affected by the aging process than the firmness of the skin. Furthermore, the mechanical properties change differently in men and women over lifetime, and female's skin is less distensible but has a higher ability to recover after stretching when compared to male skin. Perimenopause may cause an accelerated decrease in skin elasticity in women.

This knowledge can be helpful for a better understanding of the clinical genesis of facial wrinkles and age-related skin laxity as well as for the development and evaluation of effective treatment options for skin aging.

References

1. Tzaphlidou M. The role of collagen and elastin in aged skin: an image processing approach. Micron. 2004; 35(3):173–7.
2. Callaghan TM, Wilhelm K-P. A review of ageing and an examination of clinical methods in the assessment of ageing skin. Part I: cellular and molecular perspectives of skin ageing. Int J Cosmet Sci. 2008;30(5):313–22.
3. Farage MA, Miller KW, Elsner P, Maibach HI. Intrinsic and extrinsic factors in skin ageing: a review. Int J Cosmet Sci. 2008;30(2):87–95.
4. Friedman O. Changes associated with the aging face. Facial Plast Surg Clin North Am. 2005;13(3):371–80.
5. Kligman AM, Zheng P, Lavker RM. The anatomy and pathogenesis of wrinkles. Br J Dermatol. 1985; 113(1):37–42.
6. Luebberding S, Krueger N, Kerscher M. Life-time development of facial wrinkles of men and women: using three-dimensional fringe projection method and validated assessment scales. Dermatol Surg. 2014;40(1):22–32.
7. Akiba S, Shinkura R, Miyamoto K, Hillebrand G, Yamaguchi N, Ichihashi M. Influence of chronic UV exposure and lifestyle on facial skin photo-aging – results from a pilot study. J Epidemiol Jpn Epidemiol Assoc. 1999;9(6 Suppl):S136–42.
8. Vitellaro-Zuccarello L, Cappelletti S, Dal Pozzo Rossi V, Sari-Gorla M. Stereological analysis of collagen and elastic fibers in the normal human dermis: variability with age, sex, and body region. Anat Rec. 1994;238(2):153–62.
9. Shuster S, Black MM, McVitie E. The influence of age and sex on skin thickness, skin collagen and density. Br J Dermatol. 1975;93(6):639–43.
10. Quaglino DJ, Bergamini G, Boraldi F, Pasquali Ronchetti I. Ultrastructural and morphometrical evaluations on normal human dermal connective tissue – the influence of age, sex and body region. Br J Dermatol. 1996;134(6):1013–22.
11. Rodrigues L. EEMCO guidance to the in vivo assessment of tensile functional properties of the skin. Skin Pharmacol Physiol. 2001;14(1):52–67.
12. Wlaschek M, Tantcheva-Poór I, Naderi L, Ma W, Schneider LA, Razi-Wolf Z, et al. Solar UV irradiation and dermal photoaging. J Photochem Photobiol B. 2001;63(1–3):41–51.
13. Schneider LA, Wlaschek M, Scharffetter-Kochanek K. Skin aging. Clinical aspects and pathogenesis. J Dtsch Dermatol Ges. 2003;1(3):223–32; quiz 233–4.
14. Gniadecka M, Serup J. Suction chamber method for measuring skin mechanical properties: the Dermaflex®. In: Serup J, Jemec G, Grove G, editors. Non-invasive methods and skin. Boca Raton/New York/London: Taylor & Francis; 2006. p. 571–7.
15. Oomens CW, van Campen DH, Grootenboer HJ. A mixture approach to the mechanics of skin. J Biomech. 1987;20(9):877–85.
16. Barel A. Suction chamber method for measurement of skin mechanics. The new digital version of the Cutometer. In: Serup J, Jemec GB, Grove GL, editors. Non-invasive methods and the skin. 2nd ed. Boca Raton/London/New York: Taylor & Francis; 2006. p. 583–91.

17. Oxlund H. Changes in connective tissues during corticotrophin and corticosteroid treatment. Biomechanical and biochemical studies on muscle tendon, skin and aorta in experimental animals. Dan Med Bull. 1984; 31(3):187–206.
18. Oxlund H, Manschot J, Viidik A. The role of elastin in the mechanical properties of skin. J Biomech. 1988; 21(3):213–8.
19. Vieira ACT, Vieira WT, Michalany N, Enokihara M, Freymüller E, Cestari SCP. Elastoderma of the neck in a teenage boy. J Am Acad Dermatol. 2005;53(2 Suppl 1):S147–9.
20. Kolácná L, Bakesová J, Varga F, Kostáková E, Plánka L, Necas A, et al. Biochemical and biophysical aspects of collagen nanostructure in the extracellular matrix. Physiol Res Acad Sci Bohemoslov. 2007; 56 Suppl 1:S51–60.
21. Wan Abas WA, Barbenel JC. Uniaxial tension test of human skin in vivo. J Biomed Eng. 1982;4(1):65–71.
22. Agache P. Twistometry measurement of skin elasticity. In: Serup J, Jemec GBE, editors. Handbook of noninvasive methods and the skin. 1st ed. Boca Raton: CRC-Press; 1995. p. 319–28.
23. Hargens C. Ballistometry. In: Serup J, Jemec GBE, editors. Handbook of non-invasive methods and the skin. 1st ed. Boca Raton: Informa Healthcare; 1995. p. 359–66.
24. Agache P, Varchon D. Mechanical behaviour assessment. In: Agache P, Humbert P, editors. Measuring the skin: non-invasive investigations, physiology, normal constants. 1st ed. Berlin: Springer; 2004. p. 446–67.
25. Cooper EP, Missel PJ, Hannon DP, Albright GB. Mechanical properties of dry, normal, and glycerol-treated skin as measured by the gas-bearing electrodynamometer. J Soc Cosmet Chem. 1985;36:335–48.
26. Bazin R, Fanchon C. Equivalence of face and volar forearm for the testing of moisturizing and firming effect of cosmetics in hydration and biomechanical studies. Int J Cosmet Sci. 2006;28(6):453–60.
27. Adhoute H, Berbis E, Privat Y. Ballistometric properties of aged skin. In: Leveque J-L, editor. Aging skin: properties and functional changes. Illustrated ed. Abingdon (UK): Informa Healthcare; 1993. p. 39 48.
28. Ahn S, Kim S, Lee H, Moon S, Chang I. Correlation between a Cutometer and quantitative evaluation using Moire topography in age-related skin elasticity. Skin Res Technol. 2007;13(3):280–4.
29. Cua AB, Wilhelm KP, Maibach HI. Elastic properties of human skin: relation to age, sex, and anatomical region. Arch Dermatol Res. 1990;282(5):283–8.
30. Ryu HS, Joo YH, Kim SO, Park KC, Youn SW. Influence of age and regional differences on skin elasticity as measured by the Cutometer. Skin Res Technol. 2008;14(3):354–8.
31. Grahame R. A method for measuring human skin elasticity in vivo with observations of the effects of age, sex and pregnancy. Clin Sci. 1970;39(2):223–9.
32. Choi JW, Kwon SH, Huh CH, Park KC, Youn SW. The influences of skin visco-elasticity, hydration level and aging on the formation of wrinkles: a comprehensive and objective approach. Skin Res Technol. 2013;19(1).
33. Mine S, Fortunel NO, Pageon H, Asselineau D. Aging alters functionally human dermal papillary fibroblasts but not reticular fibroblasts: a new view of skin morphogenesis and aging. PLoS One. 2008; 3(12):e4066.
34. O'goshi K-I. Suction chamber method for measurements of mechanics: the Cutometer. In: Serup J, Jemec G, Grove G, editors. Non-invasive methods and skin. Boca Raton/New York/London: Taylor & Francis; 2006. p. 579–82.
35. Agache PG, Monneur C, Leveque JL, De Rigal J. Mechanical properties and Young's modulus of human skin in vivo. Arch Dermatol Res. 1980; 269(3):221–32.
36. Krueger N, Luebberding S, Oltmer M, Streker M, Kerscher M. Age-related changes in skin mechanical properties: a quantitative evaluation of 120 female subjects. Skin Res Technol. 2011;17(2):141–8.
37. Boyer G, Laquièze L, Le Bot A, Laquièze S, Zahouani H. Dynamic indentation on human skin in vivo: ageing effects. Skin Res Technol. 2009;15(1):55–67.
38. Luebberding S, Krueger N, Kerscher M. Mechanical properties of human skin in vivo: a comparative evaluation in 300 men and women. Skin Res Technol. 2014;20(2):127–35.
39. Braverman IM, Fonferko E. Studies in cutaneous aging: I. The elastic fiber network. J Invest Dermatol. 1982;78(5):434–43.
40. Frances C, Branchet MC, Boisnic S, Lesty CL, Robert L. Elastic fibers in normal human skin. Variations with age: a morphometric analysis. Arch Gerontol Geriatr. 1990;10(1):57–67.
41. Hillebrand GG, Liang Z, Yan X, Yoshii T. New wrinkles on wrinkling: an 8-year longitudinal study on the progression of expression lines into persistent wrinkles. Br J Dermatol. 2010;162(6):1233–41.
42. Phillips TJ, Symons J, Menon S. Does hormone therapy improve age-related skin changes in postmenopausal women? A randomized, double-blind, double-dummy, placebo-controlled multicenter study assessing the effects of norethindrone acetate and ethinyl estradiol in the improvement of mild to moderate age-related skin changes in postmenopausal women. J Am Acad Dermatol. 2008;59(3):397–404.e3.

Age-Induced Hair Graying and Oxidative Stress

24

Miri Seiberg

Contents

M. Seiberg (✉)
Seiberg Consulting, LLC, Princeton, NJ, USA
e-mail: mnseiberg@gmail.com

M.A. Farage et al. (eds.), *Textbook of Aging Skin*,
DOI 10.1007/978-3-662-47398-6_117

Abstract

Age-induced hair graying (canities), or the age-induced loss of melanin synthesis and deposition within the hair shafts, is a noticeable and undesired sign of the aging process. Numerous mechanisms contribute to age-induced hair graying, affecting both follicular and stem cell melanocytes and acting at different follicular locations. Many of these processes are induced, directly or indirectly, by oxidative insults and damage. Melanin-producing bulbar melanocytes express high levels of BCL-2 to survive reactive oxygen species (ROS) attacks, which are induced by the melanogenic process itself and by ultraviolet A (UVA) irradiation. With aging, the expression of BCL-2, and possibly of TRP-2, is reduced, and the endogenous, enzymatic antioxidant defense system declines, resulting in greater oxidative stress. In particular, catalase expression and activity are markedly reduced with aging, leading to millimolar accumulation of hydrogen peroxide within the hair follicle and contributing to bulbar melanocyte failure and death. Additionally, exposure of melanocyte stem cells to cumulative oxidative damage, combined with reduced BCL-2 protective levels, results in apoptosis and therefore decreases the number of melanocytes that could repopulate the newly formed anagen follicles. Altogether, oxidative stress may contribute to age-induced hair graying via multiple pathways. Better understanding of the different processes, sources, and types of oxidative stress within the follicular environment, and the different susceptibilities of melanocytes to oxidative stress at the different follicular locations, might yield clues to possible interventions for prevention or reversal of hair graying.

Introduction

While mammalian hair provides protection, temperature control, camouflage, and sexual identity, human hair is kept or removed for cosmetic and social reasons only. Unlike mammalian hair color, the pigmentation of the human hair shaft has no significant biological role, and hair color preferences are socially associated with fashion, youth, health, or maturity. Hair graying (canities) is viewed in many cultures as an undesired consequence of the aging process, as it defies the anticipation of many to look younger than their age. Spelled "gray" by the Americans and "grey" by the British, it is considered a change in hair color that is associated with an older look and feel. The universally believed but inaccurate "Rule of 50" (50 % of 50-year-olds have about 50 % gray hairs) [1] clearly highlights the concern of our society in regard to hair graying.

Numerous strategies have been developed to reduce the visibility, hide, cover, prevent, or reverse hair graying, with hair coloring as the most used approach. Archeological artifacts from as early as about 1500 BC demonstrate the use of plants, minerals, and insects for hair dyeing, and nowadays hair coloring is very popular, with the use of various hair dyes and chemical processes. Additionally, procedures and products for hair coloring "from the inside" are being developed, comprising pigments that are encapsulated in delivery vehicles like liposomes. Currently there is no scientific evidence that any herbal remedy, nutritional supplement, product, or diet could reverse, stop, or slow human hair graying. However, natural products such as amla (Indian gooseberry), coconut oil, curry leaves, amaranth, amino acids, and nutrients are used in certain cultures and societies with claimed efficiency. A known example is He Shou Wu (also named Fo-ti, or "black-haired Mr. He" in Chinese), a water-soluble extract of *Polygonum multiflorum*. In *in vitro* experimental systems like cultured B16 melanoma cells, He Shou Wu induced microphthalmia (MITF) gene expression, tyrosinase activity, and melanin content [2]. *In vivo* He Shou Wu induced anagen and increased hair follicle size and number in telogen C57BL6/N mice [3]. However, its usefulness in affecting human hair graying is yet to be evaluated.

Hair graying could be induced by numerous mechanisms, ranging from the loss or failure of melanocyte stem cells, malfunction of melanocyte stem cell migration, melanocyte death, and failure in melanin synthesis. Better understanding of the biological processes that could induce such destructive processes might provide clues to the initiation of the graying process and might potentially identify targets for the development of technologies that could slow or prevent hair graying. This chapter describes the possible role of oxidative stress in age-induced hair graying. Oxidative stress is induced independently at different follicular locations by melanogenic intermediates, by depletion of the BCL-2 pathway, and by reduced catalase activity, affecting both melanocyte stem cells and bulbar melanocytes (reviewed, e.g., in [4]). This chapter does not wish to review all literature, but rather to connect key observations and seemingly unrelated studies and to provide a possible mechanistic explanation to the early events associated with age-induced hair graying [4].

Hair Pigmentation Is Coupled to the Hair Cycle

The processes of melanin synthesis (melanogenesis) and melanosome transfer are very similar in melanocytes of the epidermis and of the hair follicle. However, while epidermal pigmentation is constant, hair pigmentation is not continuous and is coupled to the hair cycle. The hair cycle [5] constitutes of three major phases of growth (anagen), regression (catagen), and resting (telogen), with melanogenesis taking place only in anagen. Melanocytes of the hair follicle proliferate during early anagen, mature and produce pigment in mid-late anagen, and undergo apoptotic processes during early catagen. The late catagen and the telogen hair follicles are completely devoid of active, melanogenic melanocytes (reviewed, e.g., in [6]). Melanin synthesis, therefore, takes place only during anagen and stops very early in the transition from anagen to catagen, making the club roots of the shed hairs nonpigmented, or "white." Melanogenic activity, such as the expression of tyrosinase and tyrosinase-related protein-1 (TRP-1), or L-3,4-dihydroxyphenylalanine (DOPA)-oxidase activity, is detected in the hair bulb melanocytes from anagen III, but only within a melanin-producing subpopulation of the follicular melanocytes. Tyrosinase, TRP-1, and DOPA-oxidase activity are not detected during the late catagen and telogen phases, and premelanosome protein (pMEL)-17 staining is used to document the inactive melanocytes during these phases [7, 8].

Melanocyte stem cells (reviewed in, e.g., [9–11]) adhere to epithelial hair follicle stem cells within the hair follicle bulge area, or the stem cell niche, at the lower permanent portion of the hair follicle. These stem cells serve as a reservoir of melanocyte for hair pigmentation. At the initiation of a new hair cycle, epithelial and melanocyte stem cells are activated to proliferate, differentiate, and migrate in a coordinated manner to produce a new hair follicle with a pigmented hair shaft. The coordination between the two types of stem cells is crucial to the production of a newly pigmented hair shaft, and impairment in this coordination could affect melanocyte stem cell proliferation and differentiation and could contribute to hair graying (e.g., [12–14]).

Hair follicle melanocytes also differ from epidermal melanocytes in their numbers within their microenvironments. The epidermal melanin unit consists of 1 melanocyte and 36 keratinocytes (reviewed in, e.g., [15, 16]), while only as few as 100 melanocytes could exist in a human scalp hair follicle (reviewed in [17]). Thus it is possible to speculate that follicular melanocyte fatigue and destruction would precede that of epidermal melanocytes, resulting in gray hair but pigmented skin.

Melanogenesis Produces Reactive Oxygen Intermediates and Oxidative Stress

Melanogenesis, or melanin synthesis, is a chemical reaction of oxidative nature [18, 19]. Studies suggest that melanin could be active as either a free radical scavenger or as an oxidant (e.g., [20–24]). In particular, pheomelanin is known to amplify ultraviolet (UV)-induced ROS formation *in vitro*, and mouse skins with melanocortin-1 receptor (MC1R) mutation, which contain pheomelanin only, accumulate significantly more oxidative damage than albino mouse skins [25]. Melanin synthesis intermediates and their induced ROS are involved in several pathological situations, including inflammation, melanoma, and aging (e.g., [26–28]). It is suggested that when the balance between the pro- and antioxidant activities of melanin is impaired, melanocytes become more susceptible to oxidative stress, resulting not only in higher level of "general" oxidative damage but also in specific melanocyte pathologies, malfunction, and death (see examples in [24, 25, 28–30]).

Age-Induced Hair Graying

The aging and graying processes of the human hair (see Fig. 1) are heavily documented (see, e.g., [4, 17, 31–33]). The average time for Caucasian hair to start graying is about 35–40 years, which is roughly about ten hair cycles [34]. Each new hair cycle is linked to the complete renewal and recreation of the hair follicle pigmentary unit. Yet after about the first ten hair cycles, each new hair cycle displays a certain loss of active pigment production, causing an increasing number of hair shafts to display reduced pigment content (gray hairs) or no pigment deposition (white hairs) (reviewed in [31]). Individual hair shafts do not "turn gray" or change their color, but they shed with their original pigmented status. Only the newly grown hair shafts of the new hair cycle are formed as under- or unpigmented. The visual of gray or white hair color (see Fig. 1) is created because of changes in

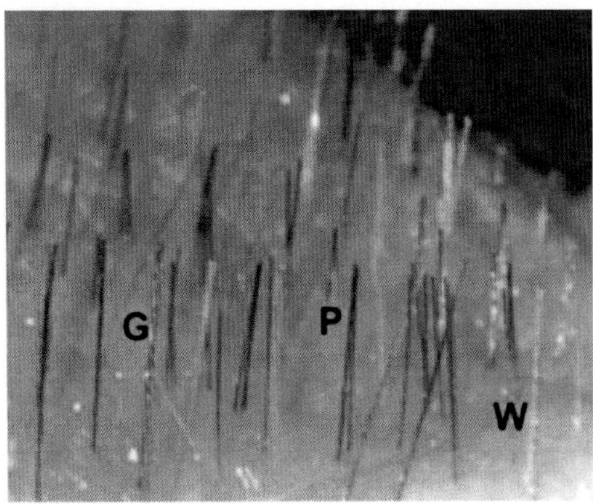

Fig. 1 Macroscopic view of graying scalp with white (*W*), gray (*G*), and pigmented (*P*) hairs (Reprinted with permission of Springer. Tobin [87])

light reflection from these under- or unpigmented hair shafts [35].

One reason for the age-induced decrease in hair shaft melanin production is the decline in bulbar melanocyte numbers with age. It was shown that gray hair bulbs contain lower melanocyte numbers as compared to pigmented hair bulbs from same individuals and that white hair bulbs contain no active melanocytes [33] (see Fig. 2). The gray hair bulbs with their fewer melanocytes still have low but detectable level of DOPA-oxidase activity, documenting their melanogenic potential. The melanocytes residing in the outer root sheath (ORS) of the hair follicle are melanogenic-inactive even in pigmented follicles. Yet their numbers follow the same aging-decline pattern as that of melanin-producing bulbar melanocytes [36]. One remarkable difference in this age-loss pattern is that the ORS amelanotic melanocytes are detected even within the ORS of white hairs, which have no detectable bulbar melanocytes [37]. A schematic representation of the different melanocyte populations of a young, pigmented hair follicle and an aged, "white" hair follicle is shown in Fig. 3. The age-induced progressive loss of follicular melanocytes could result from numerous impaired processes, some of which are described in the following sections.

The Possible Contribution of BCL-2 Depletion to Age-Induced Hair Graying

The B-cell lymphoma 2 gene (BCL-2) was first identified in a chromosomal translocation of follicular lymphoma and was later recognized as a member of the large BCL-2 protein family that regulates apoptosis (programmed cell death). The BCL-2 oncogene interferes with the programmed cell death process, therefore augmenting and prolonging cell survival (reviewed, e.g., in [38]). Mice that are BCL-2 deficient (*bcl-2*$^{-/-}$) were created experimentally for studies of B-cell lymphoma and were unexpectedly found to also exhibit hair graying by the second hair cycle [39, 40]. Unrelated studies of experimental deletion of the phosphate and tensin homologue deleted on chromosome 10 (PTEN) gene resulted in mice with larger melanocytes with increased BCL-2 expression, which were protected from experimentally induced hair graying [41]. These independent studies suggested a role for BCL-2 in the graying phenotype.

BCL-2 expression correlates with the mouse hair cycle [42]. BCL-2 is continuously expressed in the (non-cycling) dermal papilla, while immunohistochemistry staining of the epithelium shows positive staining only during the growth phase. In the *bcl-2*$^{-/-}$ mice, depilation-induced hair cycle led to hair graying, where there were no visible melanin granules, and only very few DOPA-positive melanocytes could be identified. These observations further point to the importance of BCL-2 in melanocyte maintenance and activity [43]. BCL-2 is expressed in normal, long-lived human cells, including melanocytes [44]. ORS melanocytes express BCL-2, suggesting some level of apoptosis resistance [45], which is in agreement with their expression throughout the hair cycle [45]. Bulbar melanocytes, which are likely to undergo apoptosis, differ from apoptosis-resistant melanocytes, which express BCL-2 and are likely to survive. Some BCL-2-expressing melanocytes are detectable during late catagen [45], pointing to a correlation

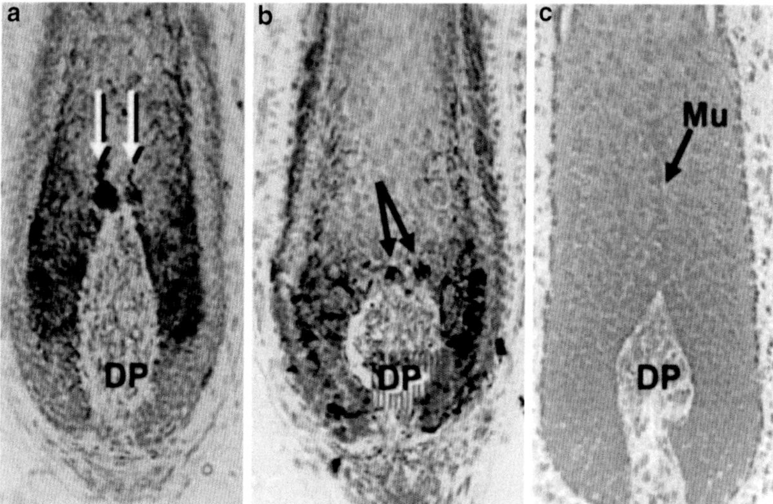

Fig. 2 The progression of melanocyte loss (*left* to *right*, *dark* to *gray* to *white*). Immunohistochemistry staining of human scalp hair bulbs showing gp100-positive melanocytes from three adjacent anagen hair follicles. Note that pigment dilution is greatest in central regions of the hair shaft, reflecting an apparent heightened sensitivity of melanocytes in this region (*DP* follicular dermal papilla, *Mu* Medulla) (Reprinted with permission of Springer-Verlag. Tobin [87])

of melanocyte survival in an apoptotic environment and BCL-2 expression.

It was hypothesized earlier that the hair graying of the *bcl-2*$^{-/-}$ mouse might be related to the effect of BCL-2 on oxidative pathways [39]. BCL-2 had no effect on the generation of ROS, but oxidative damage to affected tissues was reduced upon expressing BCL-2 [46, 47]. Indeed, BCL-2 is localized to areas in the mitochondria, endoplasmic reticulum, and nuclear membranes that generate ROS [48], and an ROS-rescue activity of BCL-2 was demonstrated in numerous, unrelated biological systems. Interestingly, while BCL-2 could fight ROS-induced damage, the stability of the BCL-2 protein itself is impaired by ROS. Superoxide anions induce both the downregulation and the degradation of BCL-2 [49], and exposure of neuronal cell lines to hydrogen peroxide decreases BCL-2 levels by 40 % [50].

The age-induced progressive loss of follicular melanocytes could result from follicular melanocyte apoptosis and/or from defects or depletion of melanocyte stem cells. Both these processes could be initiated and accelerated by ROS damage or by reduced BCL-2 levels (which would lead to increased oxidative stress). Studies of the process of melanocyte stem cell aging are ongoing and progress is continuously reported (reviewed, e.g., in [51]). A defective maintenance process of melanocyte stem cells, which is markedly accelerated with BCL-2 deficiency, was identified during hair graying. This process is accompanied by selective apoptosis of melanocyte stem cells, with no effect on differentiated melanocytes, in both experimental systems and in aging human hair follicles [52].

Altogether, these independent and unrelated studies point to a role of BCL-2 in hair graying. One could assume, therefore, that increasing hair follicle BCL-2 levels could slow, delay, or prevent hair graying. However, such therapeutic approach might be unsafe, as high levels of BCL-2 are associated with possible oncogenic processes (reviewed, e.g., in [53]). It might be more advantageous to study the downstream events of the BCL-2 pathway. Better understanding of the enhanced antioxidant capacity of BCL-2-expressing cells might be a safer approach for the identification of hair graying therapeutic targets.

TRP-2 Might Be Involved in Age-Induced Hair Graying

Tyrosinase-related protein-2 (TRP-2, more commonly named dopachrome tautomerase or DCT) is involved in eumelanin, but not in pheomelanin

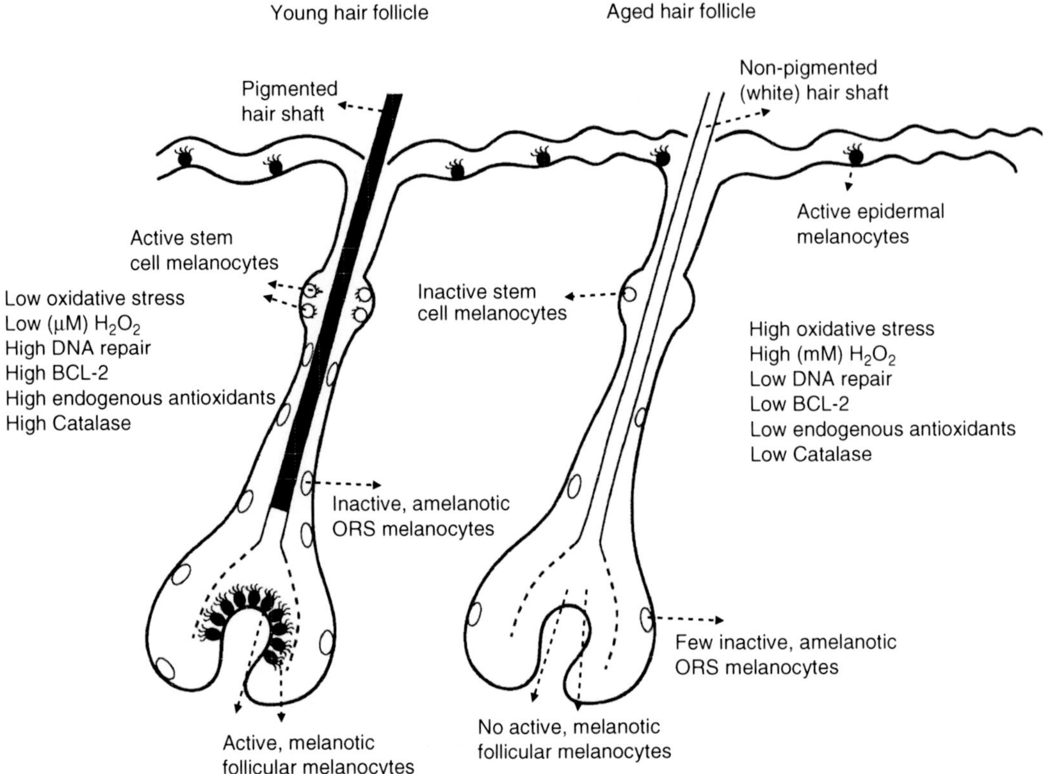

Fig. 3 A schematic representation of young (*left*) and aged (*right*) hair follicles. The young hair follicle (*left*) has active melanocyte stem cells at the bulge area, active follicular melanocytes around the dermal papilla, amelanotic melanocytes at the outer root sheath, and a pigmented hair shaft. The young hair follicle is under a low oxidative stress and has a low (μM) concentration of H_2O_2. BCL-2 expression; the endogenous antioxidant (SOD, catalase, etc.) levels and the level of DNA repair activity are high. The aged hair follicle (*right*) has inactive or no melanocyte stem cells at the bulge area, no active follicular melanocytes around the dermal papilla, very few amelanotic melanocytes at the outer root sheath, and a nonpigmented (white) hair shaft. The aged hair follicle is under a high oxidative stress and has a high (mM) concentration of H_2O_2. BCL-2 expression; the endogenous antioxidant (SOD, catalase, etc.) levels and the level of DNA repair activity are low (Diagram courtesy of Itzuv-Itzuv)

synthesis. TRP-2 is not detected in bulbar melanocytes from lethal yellow mice, which produce mainly pheomelanin, and its experimental deletion results in mice with diluted coat color and reduced hair melanin content [54–59]. TRP-2 is not expressed in cultured hair bulb melanocytes, as compared with cultured epidermal melanocytes, which could potentially explain the premature loss of pigment production in graying hair [60]. Using cultured human, brown and black follicular (anagen) melanocytes from different ethnic origins, it was experimentally difficult to detect or amplify TRP-2, regardless of hair color or origin [60], while pMEL-17, MITF, tyrosinase, and TRP-1 were all detected in these active bulbar melanocytes. Additionally, TRP-2 levels may differ between hair follicles of different anatomical sites. In some *in vitro* experimental systems, TRP-2 expression is detected in bulbar melanocytes from eyelashes, but not in hair bulb melanocytes of the scalp of same individuals [60–62]. Interestingly correlated, individuals with gray and white scalp hairs have reduced or no graying at their eyelashes, as compared to their scalps. These findings suggest that possible differences between hair follicles of these anatomical locations and their graying potential could be related to their TRP-2 expression levels.

TRP-2 is also involved in response to cytotoxic insults [63] and in particular to oxidative stress [64]. TRP-2 overexpression in melanoma cells reduced ROS-induced damage, increased glutathione levels, and reduced sensitivity to oxidative stress, while TRP-2 silencing reversed these protective effects [64]. A more specific role for TRP-2 was identified in epidermal keratinocytes, in protecting from reactive quinone metabolites (dopamine and hydroquinone) [65]. In experimentally deficient TRP-2 mice, chronical exposure to UVA led to elevated ROS levels and to decreased amounts of epidermal eumelanin, as compared to wild type [66]. The possible depletion of TRP-2 from pigmented bulbar scalp melanocytes but not from eyelash melanocytes [60, 62] might represent, therefore, another antioxidant pathway that could possibly affect the degree of sensitivity to hair graying. US patent 8,445,004 associates the absence of TRP-2 with premature disappearance of melanocytes and suggests the restoration of melanocyte metabolism and survival and the arresting or limiting or preventing of the development of canities with compounds that mimic TRP-2 activities. Nonscientific media publications suggest that a large cosmetic company is involved in the development of a gray-prevention pill, which would contain a fruit extract with TRP-2-like activity. Once available at the scientific level, it would be interesting to learn more details about these studies and to assess the potential of TRP-2 as a therapeutic target for hair graying.

The Oxidative Imbalance of Aging Hair Follicles

Oxidative damage is generated by numerous endogenous and environmental processes that create ROS. UV exposure, inflammation, or emotional stress are only few of the biological processes that create reactive intermediates, which destroy or damage biomolecules and induce mutations. Accumulated ROS-induced damage is considered a common mechanism for cellular aging, as described in the "free radical theory of aging" [67] (reviewed in [68]), a theory that correlates cumulative oxidative damage with the degree of aging. To reduce oxidative stress, all cells are armed with a protective antioxidant enzymatic machinery, which includes catalase, glutathione peroxidase, and superoxide dismutase (SOD) (reviewed, e.g., in [69]). Additionally, cells may utilize exogenously supplied antioxidants such as vitamins C and E or CoQ10 to reduce ROS damage (reviewed, e.g., in [70]). The imbalance between ROS production and the ability of the cells to neutralize the reactive intermediates is defined as oxidative stress. Oxidative stress is increased upon aging, as the antioxidant response of the cells slows, mutations accumulate, and cell damage and death increase.

Age-induced oxidative stress is higher in the skin, since UV exposure is a major source of ROS. In melanocytes, in addition to chronological aging and UV exposure, ROS are also generated during melanogenesis. Studies document a high ROS susceptibility in melanogenic-active melanocytes, which is increased with the accumulation of mutations with aging and with graying. The "free radical theory of graying" [71] suggests that the process of melanin synthesis in the anagen follicle generates high oxidative stress, which renders the hair bulb melanocytes a higher susceptibility to free radical-induced aging. Indeed, melanocyte death by oxidative stress is increased in graying follicles, and the "common" mitochondrial DNA deletion, which is a marker of oxidative stress, is detected in graying hair follicles at higher levels than in matched pigmented follicles [71]. Additionally, oxidative stress induces vacuolization, and bulbar melanocytes from gray hairs contain more vacuoles than their pigmented equivalents [72].

A number of studies provide additional connections between oxidative stress and hair graying. Cigarette smoking results in oxidative insult, and an earlier onset of hair graying was demonstrated in smokers [73–75]. A gene expression profile study of nonpigmented and matched, pigmented hair follicles describes a compromised antioxidant activity in the gray hair follicles, with marked reduction in catalase and hydroxyl radical scavenging activities [76]. A double-blind, placebo-controlled human study suggests that a

Pueraria lobata extract, which has antioxidant properties, could prevent new gray hair development [77].

Antioxidative Enzyme Depletion and Hydrogen Peroxide Accumulation in Aging Melanocytes

In cultured normal human melanocytes, catalase expression and activity correlate with the total content of melanin and with *ex vivo* skin color [78]. Comparing race-, age-, and anatomically matched cultures of follicular and cutaneous melanocytes of different age donors, it was suggested that follicular melanocytes age to a higher degree than epidermal melanocytes, by having enhanced oxidative imbalance [79]. Exploring the innate antioxidant defense system decay with aging, it was shown that the expression and activity of catalase are reduced to higher levels in older follicular melanocytes vs. their matched epidermal melanocytes. Interestingly, SOD expression levels did not change with age as significantly in the matched melanocyte cultures. The somewhat reduced SOD activities, combined with the markedly reduced catalase activity, led to higher accumulation of hydrogen peroxide in follicular melanocytes versus in epidermal melanocytes, which would correlate with their enhanced aging process.

Hair graying could be paralleled to vitiligo, a disease of depigmented skin lesions. In vitiligo lesions, catalase expression and activity are reduced, resulting in the accumulation of hydrogen peroxide to millimolar concentrations and in an increase in the oxidative imbalance [80, 81]. Catalase is known to be inactivated by hydrogen peroxide, leading to a cycle of increased oxidative stress and destruction. The vitiligo lesions contain inactive melanocytes, which could be activated *in vitro* to produce melanin upon the experimental elimination of hydrogen peroxide [82, 83]. Similarly, the depigmented lesions of vitiligo patients could be induced to produce pigment and to re-pigment the skin upon the therapeutic elimination of hydrogen peroxide [83]. A UVB-activated pseudocatalase, a bis-manganese III-EDTA-(HCO_3-)2 complex, was shown to induce repigmentation in some, but not all human vitiligo studies [80, 83–85], with variable results per body location. For example, in one children study [84], more than 75 % repigmentation was observed on the face and neck, a little less on the trunk and the extremities, and almost none on the hands and feet. One of these studies [85] also documented the repigmenting of eyelashes of vitiligo patients.

Reduced catalase activity and hydrogen peroxide accumulation to millimolar levels were also documented in a hair graying study, which demonstrated the decline of the innate antioxidant system of the gray hair bulbar melanocytes [86]. Additionally, the oxidative damage induced by the hydrogen peroxide and by the low catalase levels was slow to be repaired, because of low levels of the enzymes methionine sulfoxide reductase (MSR) A and B in the graying follicles. Reduced levels of MSR A and B impair methionine sulfoxide repair, including that of the Met 374 residue in the active site of tyrosinase, which would directly affect pigment production [86]. The reduced BCL-2 levels in graying follicles and the antioxidant activity of BCL-2 were described earlier in this chapter. Interestingly, both BCL-2 and MSR levels are reduced in gray hair follicles, and these enzymes are known to be inactivated by hydrogen peroxide. It is important to note that the decline in catalase and MSR expression and the loss of repair activity were documented not only in the gray hair melanocytes but also throughout the entire gray hair follicles. The schematic representation of a young and an aged hair follicles in Fig. 3 also describes their oxidative microenvironment and the expression and activity of some of the molecular players in the age-induced graying process that were described in this chapter.

The vitiligo-pseudocatalase repigmenting activity and the findings of catalase depletion in gray hair follicles encouraged the development of catalase-based "anti-graying" products. The dietary consumption of catalase-rich foods was suggested for reducing hair graying, and catalase-based nutritional supplements and topical products (containing either catalase or plant extracts that claim to increase catalase activity) were created. As with all other gray hair remedies, the safety and efficacy of these products are yet to be evaluated, and more studies are needed to verify or challenge this anti-graying concept.

Summary and Future Considerations

Numerous unrelated studies point to a strong correlation between oxidative stress and age-induced hair graying (reviewed, e.g., in [4]). Mechanistically, oxidative damage results in the accumulation of mutations and in the decline of the cellular antioxidative protection system (see Fig. 3). As suggested in the "free radical theory of aging" [67, 68], this is the major reason for cellular aging. The additional oxidative stress induced by melanogenesis contributes to the enhanced aging of hair follicles, which contributes to hair graying [71].

Upon aging, melanocyte stem cells reduce BCL-2 expression, accumulate oxidative damage, and lose functionality. The elimination of defective melanocyte stem cells via apoptosis could possibly serve as a protective mechanism to avoid the creation of cancerous processes. However, as the number of functional melanocytes stem cell is reduced with time, the repopulation of newly formed hair follicles is reduced, and therefore more hair shafts are created with reduced or no pigment deposition.

The enzymatic antioxidant defense system of aged follicular melanocytes is significantly impaired, and their BCL-2 levels are reduced. A marked reduction in catalase levels results in hydrogen peroxide accumulation, leading to hair bulb melanocyte death. Interestingly, outer root sheath melanocytes are less affected, possibly because of the lack of melanogenic intermediates, or because of higher BCL-2 levels, and they remain viable longer than the bulbar melanocytes. Nonpigmented (white) hair follicles, therefore, contain no functional melanocyte stem cells and no active bulbar melanocytes, but they still contain live, amelanotic melanocytes at the outer root sheath. These amelanotic melanocytes could possibly be induced to produce melanin, providing a possible avenue for future repigmenting of gray hairs.

The role of oxidative stress in hair graying is likely to be only one part of the whole story. More studies are needed to better understand the graying process and to enable innovative solutions. The understanding of the loss of the enzymatic antioxidant machinery and the specific depletion of catalase could provide gray-preventing strategies. Better understanding of molecular differences at the different follicular locations and their role in the selective susceptibility of melanocytes to ROS could provide indication for relevant pathways and therapeutic targets. The antioxidative pathway downstream of BCL-2 should be better understood, and a possible link between BCL-2 depletion and the specific reduction in catalase should be investigated. The possible role of TRP-2 in hair graying and the relation to its specific antioxidant activities should be further explored. All these anti-graying approaches should be carefully evaluated for their safety and potential undesired effects, with extreme caution for strategies involving the retaining of old melanocyte stem cells. It is desired to affect only a defined melanocyte subpopulation, or to modify only a specific follicular oxidative microenvironment, for the development of new and safe anti-graying products.

References

1. Panhard S, Lozano I, Loussouarn G. Greying of the human hair: a worldwide survey, revisiting the '50' rule of thumb. Br J Dermatol. 2012;167(4):865–73.
2. Jiang Z, Xu J, Long M, Tu Z, Yang G, He G. 2, 3, 5, 4′-tetrahydroxystilbene-2-*O*-beta-D-glucoside (THSG) induces melanogenesis in B16 cells by MAP kinase activation and tyrosinase upregulation. Life Sci. 2009;85(9-10):345–50.
3. Park HJ, Zhang N, Park DK. Topical application of Polygonum multiflorum extract induces hair growth of resting hair follicles through upregulating Shh and β-catenin expression in C57BL/6 mice. J Ethnopharmacol. 2011;135(2):369–75.
4. Seiberg M. Age-induced hair greying – the multiple effects of oxidative stress. Int J Cosmet Sci. 2013; 35(6):532–8.
5. Wolbach SB. The hair cycle of the mouse and its importance in the study of sequences of experimental

carcinogenesis. Ann N Y Acad Sci. 1951; 53(3):517–36.
6. Tobin DJ, Hagen E, Botchkarev VA, Paus R. Do hair bulb melanocytes undergo apoptosis during hair follicle regression (catagen)? J Dermatol. 1998; 111(6):941–7.
7. Slominski A, Paus R, Costantino R. Differential expression and activity of melanogenesis-related proteins during induced hair growth in mice. J Invest Dermatol. 1991;96(2):172–9.
8. Commo S, Bernard BA. Melanocyte subpopulation turnover during the human hair cycle: an immunohistochemical study. Pigment Cell Res. 2000; 13(4):253–9.
9. Nishimura EK. Melanocyte stem cells: a melanocyte reservoir in hair follicles for hair and skin pigmentation. Pigment Cell Melanoma Res. 2011;24(3):401–10.
10. Gola M, Czajkowski R, Bajek A, Dura A, Drewa T. Melanocyte stem cells: biology and current aspects. Med Sci Monit. 2012;18(10):RA155–9.
11. Goldstein J, Horsley V. Home sweet home: skin stem cell niches. Cell Mol Life Sci. 2012;69(15):2573–82.
12. Tanimura S, Tadokoro Y, Inomata K, Binh NT, Nishie W, Yamazaki S, Nakauchi H, Tanaka Y, McMillan JR, Sawamura D, Yancey K, Shimizu H, Nishimura EK. Hair follicle stem cells provide a functional niche for melanocyte stem cells. Cell Stem Cell. 2011; 8(2):177–87.
13. Chang CY, Pasolli HA, Giannopoulou EG, Guasch G, Gronostajski RM, Elemento O, Fuchs E. NFIB is a governor of epithelial-melanocyte stem cell behaviour in a shared niche. Nature. 2013;495(7439):98–102.
14. Rabbani P, Takeo M, Chou W, Myung P, Bosenberg M, Chin L, Taketo MM, Ito M. Coordinated activation of Wnt in epithelial and melanocyte stem cells initiates pigmented hair regeneration. Cell. 2011; 145(6):941–55.
15. Seiberg M. Keratinocyte-melanocyte interactions during melanosome transfer. Pigment Cell Res. 2001; 14(4):236–42.
16. Nordlund JJ. The melanocyte and the epidermal melanin unit: an expanded concept. Dermatol Clin. 2007; 25(3):271–81.
17. Tobin DJ. Aging of the hair follicle pigmentation system. Int J Trichology. 2009;1(2):83–93.
18. Pawelek JM, Lerner AB. 5,6-Dihydroxyindole is a melanin precursor showing potent cytotoxicity. Nature. 1978;276(5688):626–8.
19. Riley PA. Mechanistic aspects of the control of tyrosinase activity. Pigment Cell Res. 1993;6(4 Pt 1):182–5.
20. Korytowski W, Hintz P, Sealy RC, Kalyanaraman B. Mechanism of dismutation of superoxide produced during autoxidation of melanin pigments. Biochem Biophys Res Commun. 1985;131(2):659–65.
21. Korytowski W, Kalyanaraman B, Menon IA, Sarna T, Sealy RC. Reaction of superoxide anions with melanins: electron spin resonance and spin trapping studies. Biochim Biophys Acta. 1986;882(2):145–53.
22. Krol ES, Liebler DC. Photoprotective actions of natural and synthetic melanins. Chem Res Toxicol. 1998; 11(12):1434–40.
23. Bustamante J, Bredeston L, Malanga G, Mordoh J. Role of melanin as a scavenger of active oxygen species. Pigment Cell Res. 1993;6(5):348–53.
24. Denat L, Kadekaro AL, Marrot L, Leachman SA, Abdel-Malek ZA. Melanocytes as instigators and victims of oxidative stress. J Invest Dermatol. 2014; 134(6):1512–8.
25. Mitra D, Luo X, Morgan A, Wang J, Hoang MP, Lo J, Guerrero CR, Lennerz JK, Mihm MC, Wargo JA, Robinson KC, Devi SP, Vanover JC, D'Orazio JA, McMahon M, Bosenberg MW, Haigis KM, Haber DA, Wang Y, Fisher DE. An ultraviolet-radiation-independent pathway to melanoma carcinogenesis in the red hair/fair skin background. Nature. 2012; 491(7424):449–53.
26. Hegedus ZL. The probable involvement of soluble and deposited melanins, their intermediates and the reactive oxygen side-products in human diseases and aging. Toxicology. 2000;145(2-3):85–101.
27. Sarangarajan R, Apte SP. The polymerization of melanin: a poorly understood phenomenon with egregious biological implications. Melanoma Res. 2006; 16(1):3–10.
28. Ranadive NS, Menon IA. S Role of reactive oxygen species and free radicals from melanins in photoinduced cutaneous inflammations. Pathol Immunopathol Res. 1986;5(2):118–39.
29. Meyskens Jr FL, Farmer P, Fruehauf JP. Redox regulation in human melanocytes and melanoma. Pigment Cell Res. 2001;14(3):148–54.
30. Kvam E, Tyrrell RM. The role of melanin in the induction of oxidative DNA base damage by ultraviolet a irradiation of DNA or melanoma cells. J Invest Dermatol. 1999;113(2):209–13.
31. Tobin DJ, Paus R. Graying: gerontobiology of the hair follicle pigmentary unit. Exp Gerontol. 2001; 36(1):29–54.
32. Van Neste D, Tobin DJ. Hair cycle and hair pigmentation: dynamic interactions and changes associated with aging. Micron. 2004;35(3):193–200.
33. Tobin DJ. Human hair pigmentation – biological aspects. Int J Cosmet Sci. 2008;30(4):233–57.
34. Keogh EV, Walsh RJ. Rate of graying of human hair. Nature. 1965;207:877–88.
35. McMullen R, Jachowicz J. Optical properties of hair – detailed examination of specular reflection patterns in various hair types. J Cosmet Sci. 2004;55(1):29–47.
36. Commo S, Gaillard O, Bernard BA. Human hair greying is linked to a specific depletion of hair follicle melanocytes affecting both the bulb and the outer root sheath. Br J Dermatol. 2004;150(3):435–43.
37. Takada K, Sugiyama K, Yamamoto I, Oba K, Takeuchi T. Presence of amelanotic melanocytes within the outer root sheath in senile white hair. J Invest Dermatol. 1992;99(5):629–33.

38. Korsmeyer SJ. Bcl-2: an antidote to programmed cell death. Cancer Surv. 1992;15:105–18.
39. Veis DJ, Sorenson CM, Shutter JR, Korsmeyer SJ. Bcl-2-deficient mice demonstrate fulminant lymphoid apoptosis, polycystic kidneys, and hypopigmented hair. Cell. 1993;75(2):229–40.
40. Nakayama K, Nakayama K, Negishi I, Kuida K, Sawa H, Loh DY. Targeted disruption of Bcl-2 alpha beta in mice: occurrence of gray hair, polycystic kidney disease, and lymphocytopenia. Proc Natl Acad Sci U S A. 1994;91(9):3700–4.
41. Inoue-Narita T, Hamada K, Sasaki T, Hatakeyama S, Fujita S, Kawahara K, Sasaki M, Kishimoto H, Eguchi S, Kojima I, Beermann F, Kimura T, Osawa M, Itami S, Mak TW, Nakano T, Manabe M, Suzuki A. Pten deficiency in melanocytes results in resistance to hair graying and susceptibility to carcinogen-induced melanomagenesis. Cancer Res. 2008;68(14):5760–8.
42. Stenn KS, Lawrence L, Veis D, Korsmeyer S, Seiberg M. Expression of the bcl-2 protooncogene in the cycling adult mouse hair follicle. J Invest Dermatol. 1994;103(1):107–11.
43. Yamamura K, Kamada S, Ito S, Nakagawa K, Ichihashi M, Tsujimoto Y. Accelerated disappearance of melanocytes in bcl-2-deficient mice. Cancer Res. 1996;56(15):3546–50.
44. Klein-Parker HA, Warshawski L, Tron VA. Melanocytes in human skin express bcl-2 protein. J Cutan Pathol. 1994;21(4):297–301.
45. Sharov A, Tobin DJ, Sharova TY, Atoyan R, Botchkarev VA. Changes in different melanocyte populations during hair follicle involution (catagen). J Invest Dermatol. 2005;125(6):1259–67.
46. Korsmeyer SJ, Shutter JR, Veis DJ, Merry DE, Oltvai ZN. Bcl-2/Bax: a rheostat that regulates an anti-oxidant pathway and cell death. Semin Cancer Biol. 1993; 4(6):327–32.
47. Haddad JJ. On the antioxidant mechanisms of Bcl-2: a retrospective of NF-kappaB signaling and oxidative stress. Biochem Biophys Res Commun. 2004; 322(2):355–63.
48. Korsmeyer SJ, Yin XM, Oltvai ZN, Veis-Novack DJ, Linette GP. Reactive oxygen species and the regulation of cell death by the Bcl-2 gene family. Biochim Biophys Acta. 1995;1271(1):63–6.
49. Azad N, Iyer A, Vallyathan V, Wang L, Castranova V, Stehlik C, Rojanasakul Y. Role of oxidative/nitrosative stress-mediated Bcl-2 regulation in apoptosis and malignant transformation. Ann N Y Acad Sci. 2010;1203:1–6.
50. Pugazhenthi S, Nesterova A, Jambal P, Audesirk G, Kern M, Cabell L, Eves E, Rosner MR, Boxer LM, Reusch JE. Oxidative stress-mediated down-regulation of bcl-2 promoter in hippocampal neurons. J Neurochem. 2003;84(5):982–96.
51. Sarin KY, Artandi SE. Aging, graying and loss of melanocyte stem cells. Stem Cell Rev. 2007; 3(3):212–7.
52. Nishimura EK, Granter SR, Fisher DE. Mechanisms of hair graying: incomplete melanocyte stem cell maintenance in the niche. Science. 2005;307(5710):720–4.
53. McDonnell TJ, Marin MC, Hsu B, Brisbay SM, McConnell K, Tu SM, Campbell ML, Rodriguez-Villanueva J. The bcl-2 oncogene: apoptosis and neoplasia. Radiat Res. 1993;136(3):307–12.
54. Furumura M, Sakai C, Potterf B, Vieira WD, Barsh GS, Hearing VJ. Characterization of genes modulated during pheomelanogenesis using differential display. Proc Natl Acad Sci U S A. 1998;95(13):7374–8.
55. Kobayashi T, Vieira WD, Potterf B, Sakai C, Imokawa G, Hearing VJ. Modulation of melanogenic protein expression during the switch from eu- to pheomelanogenesis. J Cell Sci. 1995;108:2301–9.
56. Jackson IJ, Chambers DM, Tsukamoto K, Copeland NG, Gilbert DJ, Jenkins NA, Hearing V. A second tyrosinase-related protein, TRP-2, maps to and is mutated at the mouse slaty locus. EMBO J. 1992; 11(2):527–35.
57. Kroumpouzos G, Urabe K, Kobayashi T, Sakai C, Hearing VJ. Functional analysis of the slaty gene product (TRP2) as dopachrome tautomerase and the effect of a point mutation on its catalytic function. Biochem Biophys Res Commun. 1994;202(2):1060–8.
58. Lamoreux MLM, Wakamatsu K, Ito S. Interaction of major coat color gene functions in mice as studied by chemical analysis of eumelanin and pheomelanin. Pigment Cell Res. 2001;14(1):23–31.
59. Guyonneau L, Murisier F, Rossier A, Moulin A, Beermann F. Melanocytes and pigmentation are affected in dopachrome tautomerase knockout mice. Mol Cell Biol. 2004;24(8):3396–403.
60. Commo S, Gaillard O, Thibaut S, Bernard BA. Absence of TRP-2 in melanogenic melanocytes of human hair. Pigment Cell Res. 2004;17(5):488–97.
61. Kauser S, Westgate G, Green M, Tobin DJ. Age-associated down-regulation of catalase in human scalp hair follicle melanocytes. Pigment Cell Res. 2007;20:432.
62. Thibaut S, De Becker E, Caisey L, Baras D, Karatas S, Jammayrac O, Pisella PJ, Bernard BA. Human eyelash characterization. Br J Dermatol. 2010;162(2):304–10.
63. Balzer M, Lintschinger B, Groschner K. Evidence for a role of Trp proteins in the oxidative stress-induced membrane conductances of porcine aortic endothelial cells. Cardiovasc Res. 1999;42(2):543–9.
64. Michard Q, Commo S, Belaidi JP, Alleaume AM, Michelet JF, Daronnat E, Eilstein J, Duche D, Marrot L, Bernard BA. TRP-2 specifically decreases WM35 cell sensitivity to oxidative stress. Free Radic Biol Med. 2008;44(6):1023–31.
65. Michard Q, Commo S, Rocchetti J, El Houari F, Alleaume AM, Wakamatsu K, Ito S, Bernard BA. TRP-2 expression protects HEK cells from dopamine- and hydroquinone-induced toxicity. Free Radic Biol Med. 2008;45(7):1002–10.
66. Jiang S, Liu XM, Dai X, Zhou Q, Lei TC, Beermann F, Wakamatsu K, Xu SZ. Regulation of DHICA-mediated

antioxidation by dopachrome tautomerase: implication for skin photoprotection against UVA radiation. Free Radic Biol Med. 2010;48(9):1144–510.
67. Harman D. Aging: a theory based on free radical and radiation chemistry. J Gerontol. 1956;11:298–300.
68. Gutteridge JM, Halliwell B. Free radicals and antioxidants in the year 2000: a historical look to the future. Ann NY Acad Sci. 2000;899:136–47.
69. Pugliese PT. The skin's antioxidant systems. Dermatol Nurs. 1998;10(6):401–16.
70. Gašperlin M, Gosenca M. Main approaches for delivering antioxidant vitamins through the skin to prevent skin ageing. Expert Opin Drug Deliv. 2011;8(7):905–19.
71. Arck PC, Overall R, Spatz K, Liezman C, Handjiski B, Klapp BF, Birch-Machin MA, Peters EM. Towards a "free radical theory of graying": melanocyte apoptosis in the aging human hair follicle is an indicator of oxidative stress induced tissue damage. FASEB J. 2006;20(9):1567–9.
72. Sato S, Kukita A, Jimbow K. Electron microscopic studies of dendritic cells in the human gray and white matrix during anagen. Pigment Cell. 1973;1:20–6.
73. Mosley JG, Gibbs AC. Premature grey hair and hair loss among smokers: a new opportunity for health education? BMJ. 1996;313(7072):1616.
74. Zayed AA, Shahait AD, Ayoub MN, Yousef AM. Smokers' hair: does smoking cause premature hair graying? Indian Dermatol Online J. 2013;4(2):90–2.
75. Sabharwal R, Gupta A, Moon N, Mahendra A, Sargaiyan V, Gupta A, Subudhi SK, Gupta S. Association between use of tobacco and age on graying of hair. Niger J Surg. 2014;20(2):83–6.
76. Shi Y, Luo L-F, Liu X-M, Zhou Q, Xu S-Z, et al. Premature graying as a consequence of compromised antioxidant activity in hair bulb melanocytes and their precursors. PLoS One. 2014;9(4):e93589. doi: 10.1371/journal.pone.0093589.
77. Jo SJ, Shin H, Paik SH, Na SJ, Jin Y, Seok WS, Kim SN, Kwon OS. Efficacy and safety of pueraria lobata extract in gray hair prevention: a randomized, double-blind, placebo-controlled study. Ann Dermatol. 2013;25(2):218–22.
78. Maresca V, Flori E, Briganti S, Mastrofrancesco A, Fabbri C, Mileo AM, Paggi MG, Picardo M. Correlation between melanogenic and catalase activity in in vitro human melanocytes: a synergic strategy against oxidative stress. Pigment Cell Melanoma Res. 2007;21 (2):200–5.
79. Kauser S, Westgate GE, Green MR, Tobin DJ. Human hair follicle and epidermal melanocytes exhibit striking differences in their aging profile which involves catalase. J Invest Dermatol. 2011;131:979–82.
80. Schallreuter KU, Moore J, Wood JM, Beazley WD, Gaze DC, Tobin DJ, Marshall HS, Panske A, Panzig E, Hibberts NA. In vivo and in vitro evidence for hydrogen peroxide (H_2O_2) accumulation in the epidermis of patients with vitiligo and its successful removal by a UVB-activated pseudocatalase. J Investig Dermatol Symp Proc. 1999;4(1):91–6.
81. Schallreuter KU, Rübsam K, Gibbons NC, Maitland DJ, Chavan B, Zothner C, Rokos H, Wood JM. Methionine sulfoxide reductases A and B are deactivated by hydrogen peroxide (H_2O_2) in the epidermis of patients with vitiligo. J Invest Dermatol. 2008;128(4):808–15.
82. Tobin DJ, Swanson NN, Pittelkow MR, Peters EM, Schallreuter KU. Melanocytes are not absent in lesional skin of long duration vitiligo. J Pathol. 2000;191(4):407–16.
83. Schallreuter KU, Moore J, Behrens-Williams S, Panske A, Harari M. Rapid initiation of repigmentation in vitiligo with dead sea climatotherapy in combination with pseudocatalase (PC-KUS). Int J Dermatol. 2002;41(8):482–7.
84. Schallreuter KU, Krüger C, Würfel BA, Panske A, Wood JM. From basic research to the bedside: efficacy of topical treatment with pseudocatalase PC-KUS in 71 children with vitiligo. Int J Dermatol. 2008; 47(7):743–53.
85. Schallreuter KU, Salem MA, Holtz S, Panske A. Basic evidence for epidermal H_2O_2/ONOO – mediated oxidation/nitration in segmental vitiligo is supported by repigmentation of skin and eyelashes after reduction of epidermal H_2O_2 with topical NB-UVB-activated pseudocatalase PC-KUS. FASEB J. 2013; 27(8):3113–22.
86. Wood JM, Decker H, Hartmann H, Chavan B, Rokos H, Spencer JD, Hasse S, Thornton MJ, Shalbaf M, Paus R, Schallreuter KU. Senile hair graying: H_2O_2-mediated oxidative stress affects human hair color by blunting methionine sulfoxide repair. FASEB J. 2009;23(7):2065–75.
87. Tobin DJ. Biology of hair follicle pigmentation. In: Blume-Peytavi U, Tosti A, Whiting DA, Trueb R, editors. Hair growth and disorders. Heidelberg: Springer; 2008. p. 51–74.

Appearance and Internal Aging 25

Hidekazu Yamada

Contents

Abstract

Though it may be implicit, appearance has been suggested to serve as an important indicator of aging. Since around 1992, there has been progress in research on evidenced-based physical examination – a clinical analysis method for assessing the results of physical diagnosis by statistics. The twenty-first century is referred to as the "era of images"; the use of image analysis has advanced, and statistical analysis methods are currently used to understand physical findings. The present paper examines the effects of appearance on aging and disease risks by classifying appearance into three distinct components: figure (physique), facial features, and skin.

Importance of Appearance

Stafford [1] has suggested that the arrival of the era of images has had an important influence on the field of social sciences from the late twentieth to the early twenty-first century. With the advancement of science and technology, there has been an increase in the importance of images and other visual data, including photos, movies, as well as data obtained from television and the Internet. The maximum number of pixels that can represent an image continues to increase, and marked progress in television technology is also noted: from analog, to digital, super high vision (HV), 4 K, and finally to 8 K. Furthermore,

H. Yamada
Department of Dermatology of Kinki University, Faculty of Medicine Nara Hospital, Kinki University Antiaging Center, Higashiosaka, Osaka Prefecture, Japan
e-mail: yamadahi@med.kindai.ac.jp

M.A. Farage et al. (eds.), *Textbook of Aging Skin*,
DOI 10.1007/978-3-662-47398-6_118

there has also been progress in holographic technology, with aim of 3D-compatible audio-visual products by 2020. In this context, people are becoming increasingly more concerned of their own figure, appearance, and skin.

It is of interest to examine the reasons that may underlie why people are so concerned of their appearance. Some adults, including the elderly, are dissatisfied with their appearances and report feeling unhappy every time they look into the mirror, which may suggest age-related dissatisfaction, a type of cognitive dissonance defined in the psychology field [2]. There are many people who wish to continue to be beautiful as long as they live, and this point of view is of importance in the study of appearance. Catherine Hakim suggested that appearance is an individual's fourth most important capital [3]. We examined antiaging from the viewpoint of appearances in relation to health.

This field of research was established in response to recent progress in holistic studies. The skin is referred to as a mirror that reflects the condition of the internal organs, mind, and environment. It has been also been established that the skin synthesizes vitamin D and regulates body temperature, while being affected by ultraviolet light, ambient temperature, and humidity, to maintain internal conditions. Therefore, appearance is not only important from a cosmetic perspective but may also serve as a barometer of health.

A basic epidemiological study involving twins attracted wide attention by suggesting an association between appearance and longevity, or telomere length [4]. Caloric restriction delays disease onset and mortality in rhesus monkeys and reduces the incidence of diabetes, cancer, cardiovascular disease, and brain atrophy [5]. The appearance of the monkeys in the caloric restriction group, including facial features (wrinkles around the eyes, nasolabial fold lines, quality of hair, and presence of a "piercing" look), figure (whole body skeleton), and skin (hair loss and skin erosion), was superior. An American study involving identical twins [6, 7] suggested appearances differed depending on lifestyle, and that factors contributing to aging included the duration of time subjects were exposed to ultraviolet light, obesity (subjects under 40 years with a lower body weight appeared to be younger), smoking, and symptoms of depression.

Science of Appearance (Appearance as Physical Findings)

Perception of appearance by humans is thought to be both innate, such as a genetic basis, and based on extrinsic factors due to an association with an acquired social construct (Fig. 1). To better clarify the current understanding of appearance, the present study classified appearance into three components: skin, facial features, and figure or physique. Since 1992, there has been progress in the medical field of a type of clinical analysis conducted based on the sensitivity, specificity, sensitivities prior to and following diagnosis, and likelihood ratio (LR), known as evidence-based physical examination. The JAMA and other journals have introduced many papers on evidence-based physical examination, with

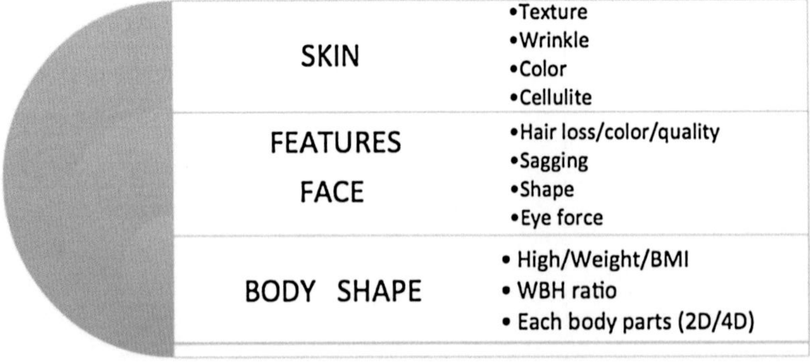

SKIN
•Texture
•Wrinkle
•Color
•Cellulite
FEATURES
FACE
•Hair loss/color/quality
•Sagging
•Shape
•Eye force
BODY SHAPE
• High/Weight/BMI
• WBH ratio
• Each body parts (2D/4D)

Fig. 1 To better clarify appearance, appearance would be clarified into three parts: skin, facial features, and figure or physique

approximately 50 reports, as well as "*Evidenced-based Physical Diagnosis* [8]," a collection of papers, having been published. In addition, an entire chapter in the *Medical Knowledge Self-Assessment Program 1* [4], which was developed and implemented by the American College of Physicians (ACP), was devoted to this subject.

In the dermatology field, it has long been suggested that some dermatological symptoms are associated with cancer, hepatic diseases, and other disorders, and improvements in the quantification of such symptoms (referred to as dermadrome), due to progress in physical analysis, are expected to advance their treatment. Specifically, physical analysis assesses the likelihood ratio (LR) [9, 10], the ratio of the probabilities of people with and without a disorder showing positive examination results and relative risk, the level of association between a factor and occurrence of a disorder. In other words, physical analysis emphasizes the comparison between the exposed and unexposed groups. Furthermore, physical analysis may also utilize objects, and instantaneous diagnosis based on pattern recognition, referred to as snap diagnosis, is also effective.

Table 1 Figure/body shape

Figure/body shape
Height
Women; breast cancer [11]
Cancer
Low height; CVD [12]
Weight
Weight loss > 10 % nutritional disorder [13]
Waist/hip/ratio*men > 1.0 women > 0.85 [14]
Waist/height [15]
Waist; COPD [16] breast cancer [17, 18] DM [19, 20]
BMI; body mass index
BMI > 30 kg/m2 obesity [21]
Ca [17], CVD [22, 23], DMtype 2 [24]
Muscle
Sarcopenia nutritional disorder [25]
Fatty tissue distribution [26–28]
Buffalo hump/moon face [29]
Breast size
Gynecomastia; estrogen/testosterone [30]
Density and breast cancer [31]
Posture and walking
Parkinson disease dementia [32]
Parts
Finger; 2D/4D finger testosterone exposure in pregnancy [33]
Penis [34]

Figure/Body Shape

A person's figure or physique can be categorized by height, weight, circumferences of chest and buttocks, abdominal circumference, sitting height, length of leg, subcutaneous fat, body fat, muscle mass, visceral fat, and contour of the body (Table 1). Previous studies have suggested associations between some of these items and disorders, shown in Table 1. It has been reported that there is a correlation between the height of females and the occurrence of cancer [11] and a negative correlation between the height of subjects and risk of gastric cancer [35]. There have also been studies reporting association between a short height and the following items: hypertension, high LDL-cholesterol levels, and diabetes and other CAD risk factors [12]. Other studies have suggested an association between short height, which is a genetically determined trait, and an increase in coronary artery disease (CAD) risk, as well as with lipid profile, a CAD risk factor. Furthermore, measurement of height is the simplest method to identify osteoporosis, and changes in height are a useful index of longevity, although another study has suggested a correlation between high bone density and increased breast cancer risk. There also exists a diagnostic method in Oriental medicine referred to as "visual examination," which emphasizes the observation of the body in a holistic manner, based on the idea that a person's posture and movement act as biomarkers of health. At the beginning of the twentieth century, Kretschmer's theory of temperament attracted much attention and a classification method based on the physique of people became popular. Simpler 3D analyses are expected to further advance the science of appearance.

Knowledge of the status of metabolic syndrome is thought to be essential for longevity [36]. The relationship between BMI (utilizing both weight and height) and longevity is a common obesity-related subject. Several large-scale studies have suggested that BMI should be maintained between 22 and 25, and there have been an increasing number of studies on the BMI of Asian people in recent years [21, 22]. Furthermore, higher fat distribution in the trunk influences longevity, and BMI, abdominal circumference, and waist/hip ratio are useful for assessing this mortality risk [14].

Because BMI has been associated with some genes (TOMM40-APOE-APOC1, SREBF2, NTRK2, BDNF, MC4R, FTO, SH2B18, and COL4A3BP-HMGCR) [37], distribution of adipose tissue, circumference of the waist, and WHR (waist-to-hip ratio) may be genetically associated with these factors as surrogate markers [38].

An additional study suggested that the circumference of the waist is associated with the risk of COPD [16].

There is a correlation between BMI and mortality, represented by a J-shaped graph. Although there has been an increase in BMI in Japanese males since 1970, BMI of Japanese females remained low, and young Japanese females in particular have been shown to be excessively thin.

According to international criteria, Caucasian, Hispanic, and black people with BMIs of 25–29.9 and 30 or more are regarded as overweight and obese, respectively, whereas Asian people with BMIs of 23–24.9 and 25 or more are regarded as overweight and obese, respectively.

One study was conducted to examine the effectiveness of calorie restriction in monkeys on longevity [5], and the results suggested that obesity prevention measures are important. According to a recent study on changes in blood glucose level of patients with a BMI of 35 or higher immediately following gastrectomy [39], the characteristics of sugar metabolism should be considered not only to prevent obesity but also in consideration of the patient's physique. On the other hand, being underweight may also have adverse effects on longevity. Weight loss (a decrease in muscle mass) in the elderly may cause sarcopenia; as the fast-twitch muscle is replaced by slow-twitch muscle, the proportion of adipose tissue increases and that of the muscle fibers decrease, reducing the ability to exercise and reduces metabolism (an important role of the muscle fibers), which may cause the onset of diabetes. Therefore, it should be noted that assessment of patient appearance is important from the standpoint of health and longevity.

The issue of changes in the physique due to sexual maturation is an important subject in the field of esthetics. According to the results of a study, the size of breasts is associated with the risk of breast cancer [40], suggesting that cancer risks may be associated with sites of fat deposits, although racial differences should be taken into consideration. With advancing globalization, an increasing number of females are becoming interested in liposuction [41]. However, when it comes to obese individuals, metabolic balance is unable to be changed by liposuction, although it may aid in weight loss. Reduction of visceral fat by exercising differs from metabolic activation. When visiting outpatient and other departments for consultation, this point should be taken into consideration because of its impact on the selection of a partner for a relationship, as well as the general impact on society.

Because there is little difference between the length of fertility and longevity in nonhuman simian primates, elderly primates are known to continue breeding. However, humans usually live a long period of time after menopause, so it is necessary to take into consideration factors other than biological ones for discussion of subjects related to appearance. An observational study conducted by Wacoal Corporation [42] examined the changes in the figures of Japanese females born in the 1950s, reporting a significant increase in abdominal circumferences compared to other regions of the body. In particular, the increase in abdominal circumference was very high following menopause. Because an increase in abdominal circumference is associated with future incidence of lifestyle-related diseases, the importance of maintaining a healthy physique has been emphasized [43]. The ratio of subcutaneous to visceral fat presumably varies depending on the disorder, such as diabetes or cancer, warranting further research, focusing on locations of fat deposits.

Research on metabolic syndrome in Japan emphasizes abdominal circumference. However, the validity of its measurement may be suspect due to differences between males and females, measurement methods, and inaccuracy of measurement due to movement of patients, such as breathing.

Furthermore, attention should be paid to the relative amounts of subcutaneous and visceral fat; even if the BMI of two people are the same, their sex, height, weight, and subcutaneous and visceral fat often vary. Whereas visceral fat is insulin,resistant, subcutaneous fat is usually not. In addition, because physiques vary (females in particular) depending on the country (or race), it is necessary to conduct further research in this field while taking into account genetic, cultural, and dietary differences. For example, whereas males usually have a barrel-shaped body with fat in the abdominal area, females are usually pear-shaped with fat at the hips and thighs. Visceral fat has high metabolic activity, releasing fee fatty acids, and is thought to be associated with hyperlipidemia, atheromatous degeneration, and insulin resistance. On the other hand, the metabolic activity of subcutaneous fat in the buttocks and thighs is considered to be low, except during pregnancy or the postpartum period. Chronic inflammation in adipose cells is thought to be the underlying cause of abdominal obesity and a set of metabolic disorders referred to as metabolic syndrome. Therefore, it is useful to take into account the appearance of people as well as any changes.

Regarding metabolic syndrome, males and females whose waist circumferences (generally measured between the lower edge of the ribs and iliac spine, although definitions may vary) are longer than 102 and 88 cm, respectively, are at risk of health problems. However, previous studies have suggested that there are racial differences: 35 in. (90 cm) or longer for Asian males and 31 in. (80 cm) or longer for Asian females [44].

It is difficult to differentiate between people who exercise and those who do not simply by BMI due to variation in muscle mass, and thus mortality risk based on BMI [45] is inappropriately assessed. On the other hand, there is a significant correlation between waist circumference and mortality risk, independent of BMI. Incidence of health problems is significantly higher in males with a WHR (waist-hip ratio) of 1.0 or higher and females with a WHR of 0.85 or higher. The WHR is also correlated with blood-pressure, cholesterol levels, incidence of diabetes and stroke, and total mortality.

Furthermore, symptoms of aging are reflected in posture and present as locomotive syndrome and frailty. It is significant to examine the relationship between the figure of a person and disorders as a subject of research on appearances.

Features of the Face

Results of a previous study shown in Table 2 are biological signs that can be identified from an individual's appearance. Age of a subject was estimated based on photographs and 3D [65] of the face. The study examined whether or not the

Table 2 Features (face)

Sagging
Osteoporosis [46]
Ligament [47]
Nasolabial fold [48]
Position of the eyebrows [49]
Blepharoptosis [50]
Lipoatrophy [51, 52]
Hair
AGA men [53] women [54, 55]
Eyelashes [15]
Eyebrows [56]
Gray hair [57]
Hair quality [58]
Unwanted Hair [59]
Shape
Moon face [29]
Lip [60]
Nail change; finger clubbing /hepatopulmonary syndrome [61]
Dental part
Teeth [62]
Eye
Eye movements [63, 64]

life expectancy was poor of subjects who appeared to be old and attracted much attention. A study conducted in 2009 [4] examined the associations among telomere length, age estimated based on appearance (photos of the face), and longevity. It has been suggested that surface symptoms are associated with the risk of cardiovascular disorders [66, 67]. Previous studies suggested that the earlobe crease referred to as Frank's sign is associated with brain infarction and that alopecia of the head (including the top of the head), wrinkles in the earlobes, and xanthomatosis in the eyelids were significant findings in physical analysis. A study on the contribution of various factors on apparent age (features of the face as well as skin appearance) suggested [48] that appearances are related to the length of nasolabial fold lines, hemoglobin variation/level of heterogeneity, depth, position of eyebrows, distribution and level of hemoglobin, distribution of melanin, and level of skin roughness (in this order). Eyelid ptosis, or the eyelid drooping over the eyeball, is associated with a lack of strength. In addition to aging as the most important risk factor, a previous study suggested other factors: [49] being male, genetic mutation, light skin color, a high BMI score, and continuation of a smoking habit.

Although a study conducted by NIH research group suggested that there were no significant differences in aging-associated appearance due to calorie intake, the effects of calorie control on aging were later supported following the publication of a study by Colman et al. Although this type of study is unable to be conducted using humans as subjects, results of similar studies involving primates may be valid and useful. Regarding the effects of calorie restriction on longevity, it has been reported that decreases in insulin and IGF-1 influence the AKT pathway, blood sugar levels influence the AMPK-mTOR pathway, and NAD influences Sirt-1; essentially, changes in metabolic balance affect these signaling pathways [68].

Previous studies, including an observational study involving twins conducted by Gyiron et al. [6], suggested that differences in appearance are associated with smoking, air pollution, ultraviolet light, obesity, exercise habit, sleep, and depression.

Hairstyles of people vary depending on age and also influence appearance. The results of an interesting study suggested that the site and degree of androgenetic alopecia (AGA) in males younger than 40 years are associated with risk of aggressive prostate cancer [69].

The olfactory nerve, which is involved in one's ability to smell and the ability to gaze at something, is thought to reflect brain function, and examination of these nervous systems may help identify aging of the brain and frailty at early stages. Furthermore, there are associations between facial expressions, eye movements [63], behaviors (temperament [64]), and the brain functions of patients with Alzheimer's disease and dementia.

Skin

In the present study, wrinkles were classified into rough skin; fine, normal, and deep wrinkles; and skin flaps (Table 3). Skin flaps, or sagging skin, are not limited to the face, and infants and elderly people may have skin flaps in the trunk, abdominal area, and arms and legs. Skin flaps are associated with hypertrophied epidermal cells, adipose tissue, decreased muscle mass, and bone thinning due to osteoporosis. Recent studies have suggested that wrinkles in the earlobes, xanthomatosis in the eyelids, and alopecia in the head (including the top of the head) are associated with cardiovascular diseases [67]. An individual is suspected to have xanthoma tuberosum due to hypercholesteremia [80] if an increase in the thickness of the Achilles' tendon is observed, and in some cases, the new concept of dermatoporosis [81] may be applied to thickened Achilles' tendons, taking into account subcutaneous bleeding. It has been pointed out that the frequent occurrence of purpura may be associated with the nerves that control blood vessels or neural reflex.

Hormonal changes may often be determined based on appearance [82], according to the viewpoint of clinical physical analysis. Cushing's

Table 3 Skin

Color
Color homogeneity and age [70]
Pallor and anemia [10]
Redness and ovulation [71]
Jaundice and liver function [9]
Wrinkles
Nasolabial wrinkles and age
Earlobe crease [72] and CVD [67]
Forehead [50] cheek [73]
Telangiectasia
Numbers and liver abnormality [74]
Texture
Texture and aging [75–78]
Thin and cushing [79]

syndrome [83] presents with the following changes in appearance: moon-shaped face, central obesity, "buffalo hump," thin skin, vasodilatation (ruddy face), male pattern alopecia, ecchymosis, striae cutis, acne (dermatological findings), muscle weakness in the arms and legs (thin extremities), and edema. Hypothyroidism presents as dry skin and cold sensation (LH = 4.7), whereas hyperthyroidism presents with moist skin and warm sensation (LR = 6.8).

Recent studies have suggested an association between the number of moles and the risk of breast cancer (HR = 1.35 when the number is 15 or larger) [84, 85], suggesting the effect of hormones. These factors are also thought to be related to longevity.

Photoaging is closely associated with the skin [86] and has a significant influence on people's appearance. The rate of occurrence of photoaging-related symptoms, wrinkles in particular, is high among Caucasians [87] and is also significantly correlated with dullness of the skin and vasodilation. The degree of photoaging one is subject to varies depending on tone of skin, race, residential area (exposure to ultraviolet light), and culture. Furthermore, photoaging significantly contributes to the formation of wrinkles, and a previous study suggested an association between wrinkles due to photoaging and an individual's genetic background [88]. Further research is required to better clarify this association.

In photoaging, it is thought that while UV-A primarily influences the dermis, UV-B affects the epidermis. However, recent studies on solar keratosis have suggested that both UV-A and UV-B influence keratinocytes and fibroblasts, the primary cause of cancer is inflammation, and collagen metabolism and degeneration, in addition to DNA degeneration, are primarily caused by inflammation [89]. In addition to the importance of the prevention of exposure to ultraviolet light, an issue regarding vitamin-D deficiency has arisen in the elderly population. Vitamin-D deficiency has been shown to be not only associated with diabetes, obesity, and osteoporosis but also with depression, and one study suggested that beta-endorphin is produced by ultraviolet light [90]. The development of methods for coping with both the risks and need of ultraviolet light exposure is essential for the promotion of health and longevity. Since 2010, the American Academy of Dermatology has been recommending the intake of vitamin D [91] in addition to the avoidance of exposure to ultraviolet light.

Conclusion

The present paper has classified appearance into distinct components (skin, facial features, and figure) and discussed their association with longevity, including the status of relevant studies. The paper has also discussed subjects associated with exercise, eating, neurological function and sleep, and treatment, as well as basic subjects thought to be important in the antiaging medical field.

References

1. Barbara MS. Visual analogy. Cambridge, MA: MIT Press; 1999.
2. Etcoff N. Survival of the prettiest: the science of beauty. New York: Anchor; 1999 (Reprint).
3. Hakim C. Erotic capital. New York: Basic Books; 2011.
4. Christensen K, Thinggaard M, McGue M, et al. Perceived age as clinically useful biomarker of ageing: cohort study. BMJ. 2009;339:b5262.

5. Colman RJ, Anderson RM, Johnson SC, et al. Caloric restriction delays disease onset and mortality in rhesus monkeys. Science. 2009;325:201–4.
6. Guyuron B, Rowe DJ, Weinfeld AB, Eshraghi Y, Fathi A, Iamphongsai S. Factors contributing to the facial aging of identical twins. Plast Reconstr Surg. 2009;123:1321–31.
7. Martires K, Fu P, Polster A, Cooper K, Baron E. Factors that affect skin aging: a cohort-based survey on twins. Arch Dermatol. 2009;145:1375–9.
8. Mcgee S. Evidenced-based physical diagnosis. 3rd ed. Philadelphia: Saunders; 2014.
9. Udell JA, Wang CS, Tinmouth J, et al. Does this patient with liver disease have cirrhosis? JAMA. 2012;307:832–42.
10. Nardone DA, Roth KM, Mazur DJ, McAfee JH. Usefulness of physical examination in detecting the presence or absence of anemia. Arch Intern Med. 1990;150:201–4.
11. Green J, Cairns BJ, Casabonne D, et al. Height and cancer incidence in the Million Women Study: prospective cohort, and meta-analysis of prospective studies of height and total cancer risk. Lancet Oncol. 2011;12:785–94.
12. Nelson CP, Hamby SE, Saleheen D, et al. Genetically determined height and coronary artery disease. N Engl J Med. 2015;372:1608–18.
13. McGrice M, Don PK. Interventions to improve long-term weight loss in patients following bariatric surgery: challenges and solutions. Diabetes Metab Syndr Obes. 2015;8:263–74.
14. Pischon T, Boeing H, Hoffmann K, et al. General and abdominal adiposity and risk of death in Europe. N Engl J Med. 2008;359:2105–20.
15. Kodama S, Horikawa C, Fujihara K, et al. Comparisons of the strength of associations with future type 2 diabetes risk among anthropometric obesity indicators, including waist-to-height ratio: a meta-analysis. Am J Epidemiol. 2012;176:959–69.
16. Behrens G, Matthews CE, Moore SC, Hollenbeck AR, Leitzmann MF. Body size and physical activity in relation to incidence of chronic obstructive pulmonary disease. CMAJ. 2014;186:E457–69.
17. Bhaskaran K, Douglas I, Forbes H, dos-Santos-Silva I, Leon DA, Smeeth L. Body-mass index and risk of 22 specific cancers: a population-based cohort study of 5 · 24 million UK adults. Lancet. 2014;384:755–65.
18. Gaudet MM, Carter BD, Patel AV, Teras LR, Jacobs EJ, Gapstur SM. Waist circumference, body mass index, and postmenopausal breast cancer incidence in the Cancer Prevention Study-II Nutrition Cohort. Cancer Causes Control. 2014;25:737–45.
19. Schulze MB, Thorand B, Fritsche A, et al. Body adiposity index, body fat content and incidence of type 2 diabetes. Diabetologia. 2012;55:1660–7.
20. Carnethon MR, De Chavez PJ, Biggs ML, et al. Association of weight status with mortality in adults with incident diabetes. JAMA. 2012;308:581–90.
21. Zheng W, McLerran DF, Rolland B, et al. Association between body-mass index and risk of death in more than 1 million Asians. N Engl J Med. 2011;364:719–29.
22. Ni Mhurchu C, Rodgers A, Pan WH, Gu DF, Woodward M, Collaboration APCS. Body mass index and cardiovascular disease in the Asia-Pacific Region: an overview of 33 cohorts involving 310 000 participants. Int J Epidemiol. 2004;33:751–8.
23. Chen Y, Copeland WK, Vedanthan R, et al. Association between body mass index and cardiovascular disease mortality in east Asians and south Asians: pooled analysis of prospective data from the Asia Cohort Consortium. BMJ. 2013;347:f5446.
24. Boffetta P, McLerran D, Chen Y, et al. Body mass index and diabetes in Asia: a cross-sectional pooled analysis of 900,000 individuals in the Asia cohort consortium. PLoS One. 2011;6, e19930.
25. Fry CS, Rasmussen BB. Skeletal muscle protein balance and metabolism in the elderly. Curr Aging Sci. 2011;4:260–8.
26. Shungin D, Winkler TW, Croteau-Chonka DC, et al. New genetic loci link adipose and insulin biology to body fat distribution. Nature. 2015;518:187–96.
27. Chandra A, Neeland IJ, Berry JD, et al. The relationship of body mass and fat distribution with incident hypertension: observations from the dallas heart study. J Am Coll Cardiol. 2014;64:997–1002.
28. Myint PK, Kwok CS, Luben RN, Wareham NJ, Khaw KT. Body fat percentage, body mass index and waist-to-hip ratio as predictors of mortality and cardiovascular disease. Heart. 2014.
29. Jabbour SA. Cutaneous manifestations of endocrine disorders: a guide for dermatologists. Am J Clin Dermatol. 2003;4:315–31.
30. Cuhaci N, Polat SB, Evranos B, Ersoy R, Cakir B. Gynecomastia: clinical evaluation and management. Indian J Endocrinol Metab. 2014;18:150–8.
31. Wang AT, Vachon CM, Brandt KR, Ghosh K. Breast density and breast cancer risk: a practical review. Mayo Clin Proc. 2014;89:548–57.
32. Abdo WF, Borm GF, Munneke M, Verbeek MM, Esselink RA, Bloem BR. Ten steps to identify atypical parkinsonism. J Neurol Neurosurg Psychiatry. 2006;77:1367–9.
33. Manning J, Scutt D, Wilson J, Lewis-Jones D. The ratio of 2nd to 4th digit length: a predictor of sperm numbers and concentrations of testosterone, luteinizing hormone and oestrogen. Hum Reprod. 1998;13:3000–4.
34. Veale D, Miles S, Bramley S, Muir G, Hodsoll J. Am I normal? A systematic review and construction of nomograms for flaccid and erect penis length and circumference in up to 15,521 men. BJU Int. 2015;115:978–86.
35. Thrift AP, Risch HA, Onstad L, et al. Risk of esophageal adenocarcinoma decreases with height, based on consortium analysis and confirmed by mendelian randomization. Clin Gastroenterol Hepatol. 2014;12:1667–76.e1.

36. Haslam DW, James WP. Obesity. Lancet. 2005;366:1197–209.
37. Guo Y, Lanktree MB, Taylor KC, et al. Gene-centric meta-analyses of 108 912 individuals confirm known body mass index loci and reveal three novel signals. Hum Mol Genet. 2013;22:184–201.
38. Yoneyama S, Guo Y, Lanktree MB, et al. Gene-centric meta-analyses for central adiposity traits in up to 57 412 individuals of European descent confirm known loci and reveal several novel associations. Hum Mol Genet. 2014;23:2498–510.
39. Schauer PR, Kashyap SR, Wolski K, et al. Bariatric surgery versus intensive medical therapy in obese patients with diabetes. N Engl J Med. 2012;366:1567–76.
40. Williams PT. Breast cancer mortality vs. exercise and breast size in runners and walkers. PLoS One. 2013;8, e80616.
41. Friedmann DP. A review of the aesthetic treatment of abdominal subcutaneous adipose tissue: background, implications, and therapeutic options. Dermatol Surg. 2015;41:18–34.
42. Aging of the Body (Changes in the Figure due to Aging). 2010. Available from: http://wwww.wacoal.jp/bodyageing/.
43. Ford ES, Maynard LM, Li C. Trends in mean waist circumference and abdominal obesity among US adults, 1999–2012. JAMA. 2014;312:1151–3.
44. Pan WH, Yeh WT, Weng LC. Epidemiology of metabolic syndrome in Asia. Asia Pac J Clin Nutr. 2008; 17 Suppl 1:37–42.
45. Flegal KM, Kit BK, Orpana H, Graubard BI. Association of all-cause mortality with overweight and obesity using standard body mass index categories: a systematic review and meta-analysis. JAMA. 2013;309:71–82.
46. Shaw RB, Katzel EB, Koltz PF, et al. Aging of the facial skeleton: aesthetic implications and rejuvenation strategies. Plast Reconstr Surg. 2010;127(1):374–83.
47. Gierloff M, Stöhring C, Buder T, Gassling V, Açil Y, Wiltfang J. Aging changes of the midfacial fat compartments: a computed tomographic study. Plast Reconstr Surg. 2012;129:263–73.
48. Coma M, Valls R, Mas JM, et al. Methods for diagnosing perceived age on the basis of an ensemble of phenotypic features. Clin Cosmet Investig Dermatol. 2014;7:133–7.
49. Jacobs LC, Liu F, Bleyen I, et al. Intrinsic and extrinsic risk factors for sagging eyelids. JAMA Dermatol. 2014;150:836–43.
50. Ezure T, Amano S. The severity of wrinkling at the forehead is related to the degree of ptosis of the upper eyelid. Skin Res Technol. 2010;16:202–9.
51. Coleman SR, Grover R. The anatomy of the aging face: volume loss and changes in 3-dimensional topography. Aesthet Surg J. 2006;26:S4–9.
52. Coleman S, Saboeiro A, Sengelmann R. A comparison of lipoatrophy and aging: volume deficits in the face. Aesthet Plast Surg. 2009;33:14–21.
53. Smith MR, Halabi S, Ryan CJ, et al. Randomized controlled trial of early zoledronic acid in men with castration-sensitive prostate cancer and bone metastases: results of CALGB 90202 (alliance). J Clin Oncol. 2014;32:1143–50.
54. Sinclair R. Hair shedding in women: how much is too much? Br J Dermatol. 2015; doi: 10.1111/bjd.13873.
55. Fagien S, Maas C, Murphy DK, Thomas JA, Beddingfield FC, Group JLS. Juvederm ultra for lip enhancement: an open-label, multicenter study. Aesthet Surg J. 2013;33:414–20.
56. Choi HI, Choi GI, Kim EK, et al. Hair greying is associated with active hair growth. Br J Dermatol. 2011;165:1183–9.
57. Nishimura EK, Suzuki M, Igras V, et al. Key roles for transforming growth factor beta in melanocyte stem cell maintenance. Cell Stem Cell. 2010;6:130–40.
58. Kmieć ML, Pajor A, Broniarczyk-Dyła G. Evaluation of biophysical skin parameters and assessment of hair growth in patients with acne treated with isotretinoin. Postepy Dermatol Alergol. 2013;30:343–9.
59. Fenske N, Lober C. Structural and functional changes of normal aging skin. J Am Acad Dermatol. 1986;15:571–85.
60. Fink B, Prager M. The effect of incobotulinumtoxin a and dermal filler treatment on perception of age, health, and attractiveness of female faces. J Clin Aesthet Dermatol. 2014;7:36–40.
61. Rodriguez-Roisin R, Roca J. Hepatopulmonary syndrome: the paradigm of liver-induced hypoxaemia. Baillieres Clin Gastroenterol. 1997;11:387–406.
62. Gunn DA, Dick JL, van Heemst D, et al. Lifestyle and youthful looks. Br J Dermatol. 2015;172:1338–45.
63. Anderson TJ, MacAskill MR. Eye movements in patients with neurodegenerative disorders. Nat Rev Neurol. 2013;9:74–85.
64. Choi JE, Vaswani PA, Shadmehr R. Vigor of movements and the cost of time in decision making. J Neurosci. 2014;34:1212–23.
65. Chen W, Qian W, Wu G, et al. Three-dimensional human facial morphologies as robust aging markers. Cell Res. 2015;25:574–87.
66. Christoffersen M, Frikke-Schmidt R, Schnohr P, Jensen GB, Nordestgaard BG, Tybjærg-Hansen A. Xanthelasmata, arcus corneae, and ischaemic vascular disease and death in general population: prospective cohort study. BMJ. 2011;343:d5497.
67. Christoffersen M, Frikke-Schmidt R, Schnohr P, Jensen GB, Nordestgaard BG, Tybjærg-Hansen A. Visible age-related signs and risk of ischemic heart disease in the general population: a prospective cohort study. Circulation. 2014;129:990–8.
68. de Cabo R, Carmona-Gutierrez D, Bernier M, Hall MN, Madeo F. The search for antiaging interventions: from elixirs to fasting regimens. Cell. 2014; 157:1515–26.
69. Zhou CK, Pfeiffer RM, Cleary SD, et al. Relationship between male pattern baldness and the risk of aggressive prostate cancer: an analysis of the prostate, lung, colorectal, and ovarian cancer screening trial. J Clin Oncol. 2014; 33(5). doi: 10.1200/JCO.2014.55.4279

70. Fink B, Matts PJ, D'Emiliano D, Bunse L, Weege B, Röder S. Colour homogeneity and visual perception of age, health and attractiveness of male facial skin. J Eur Acad Dermatol Venereol. 2012;26:1486–92.
71. Burriss RP, Troscianko J, Lovell PG, et al. Changes in women's facial skin color over the ovulatory cycle are not detectable by the human visual system. PLoS One. 2015;10, e0130093.
72. Frank ST. Aural sign of coronary-artery disease. N Engl J Med. 1973;289:327–8.
73. Ezure T, Hosoi J, Amano S, Tsuchiya T. Sagging of the cheek is related to skin elasticity, fat mass and mimetic muscle function. Skin Res Technol. 2009;15:299–305.
74. Li CP, Lee FY, Hwang SJ, et al. Spider angiomas in patients with liver cirrhosis: role of alcoholism and impaired liver function. Scand J Gastroenterol. 1999;34:520–3.
75. Ozdemir R, Kilinç H, Unlü RE, Uysal AC, Sensöz O, Baran CN. Anatomicohistologic study of the retaining ligaments of the face and use in face lift: retaining ligament correction and SMAS plication. Plast Reconstr Surg. 2002;110:1134–47 (discussion 1148–9).
76. Callaghan T, Wilhelm K. A review of ageing and an examination of clinical methods in the assessment of ageing skin. Part 2: clinical perspectives and clinical methods in the evaluation of ageing skin. Int J Cosmet Sci. 2008;30:323–32.
77. Callaghan T, Wilhelm K. A review of ageing and an examination of clinical methods in the assessment of ageing skin. Part I: cellular and molecular perspectives of skin ageing. Int J Cosmet Sci. 2008;30:313–22.
78. McGrath JA, Robinson MK, Binder RL. Skin differences based on age and chronicity of ultraviolet exposure: results from a gene expression profiling study. Br J Dermatol. 2012;166 Suppl 2:9–15.
79. Valassi E, Santos A, Yaneva M, et al. The European Registry on Cushing's syndrome: 2-year experience. Baseline demographic and clinical characteristics. Eur J Endocrinol. 2011;165:383–92.
80. Tsouli SG, Xydis V, Argyropoulou MI, Tselepis AD, Elisaf M, Kiortsis DN. Regression of Achilles tendon thickness after statin treatment in patients with familial hypercholesterolemia: an ultrasonographic study. Atherosclerosis. 2009;205:151–5.
81. Kaya G, Saurat J. Dermatoporosis: a chronic cutaneous insufficiency/fragility syndrome. Clinicopathological features, mechanisms, prevention and potential treatments. Dermatology. 2007;215:284–94.
82. Phillips TJ, Symons J, Menon S, Group HS. Does hormone therapy improve age-related skin changes in postmenopausal women? A randomized, double-blind, double-dummy, placebo-controlled multicenter study assessing the effects of norethindrone acetate and ethinyl estradiol in the improvement of mild to moderate age-related skin changes in postmenopausal women. J Am Acad Dermatol. 2008;59:397–404.e3.
83. Elamin MB, Murad MH, Mullan R, et al. Accuracy of diagnostic tests for Cushing's syndrome: a systematic review and meta-analyses. J Clin Endocrinol Metab. 2008;93:1553–62.
84. Kvaskoff M, Bijon A, Mesrine S, et al. Association between melanocytic nevi and risk of breast diseases: the French E3N prospective cohort. PLoS Med. 2014;11, e1001660.
85. Zhang M, Zhang X, Qureshi AA, Eliassen AH, Hankinson SE, Han J. Association between cutaneous nevi and breast cancer in the Nurses' Health Study: a prospective cohort study. PLoS Med. 2014; 11, e1001659.
86. Baillie L, Askew D, Douglas N, Soyer HP. Strategies for assessing the degree of photodamage to skin: a systematic review of the literature. Br J Dermatol. 2011;165:735–42.
87. Maddin S, Lauharanta J, Agache P, Burrows L, Zultak M, Bulger L. Isotretinoin improves the appearance of photodamaged skin: results of a 36-week, multicenter, double-blind, placebo-controlled trial. J Am Acad Dermatol. 2000;42:56–63.
88. Le Clerc S, Taing L, Ezzedine K, et al. A genome-wide association study in Caucasian women points out a putative role of the STXBP5L gene in facial photoaging. J Invest Dermatol. 2013;133:929–35.
89. Hu B, Castillo E, Harewood L, et al. Multifocal epithelial tumors and field cancerization from loss of mesenchymal CSL signaling. Cell. 2012;149:1207–20.
90. Fell GL, Robinson KC, Mao J, Woolf CJ, Fisher DE. Skin β-endorphin mediates addiction to UV light. Cell. 2014;157:1527–34.
91. American Academy of Dermatology Statement on sun exposure, vitamin D levels and mortality. 2014. Available from: http://www.aad.org/stories-and-news/news-releases/american-academy-of-dermatology-statement-on-sun-exposure-vitamin-d-levels-and-mortality.)

Age-Related Morphometric Changes of Inner Structures of the Skin Assessed by In Vivo Reflectance Confocal Microscopy

26

Katsuhiko Tsuchida and Hidekazu Yamada

Contents

Abstract

The study of skin aging has greatly advanced. The inner structure of the skin can now be studied using various methods. This chapter describes observations on the inner structure of the skin and its age-related changes using in vivo reflectance confocal microscopy (RCM). RCM is a noninvasive method and offers real-time observation.

The human skin is made up of the epidermis and dermis. Each layer has characteristic inner structures. These inner structures and their age-related changes have been observed using RCM. The epidermis is divided into four layers, which differ in thickness and cell shape. The cells of the epidermis are densely arranged. The epidermis and dermis are separated by a basement membrane and form a concave–convex structure known as the dermal papilla. The dermis consists of cellular and stromal components, which form fibrotic tissue.

The inner structures of the epidermis change with age. The depth from the skin surface to the lower end of the dermal papillae and the thickness of the basal layer become thinner with age, and the granular layer becomes thicker with age. The structure of the dermal papillae is evaluated by calculating its parameters. Decrease in number, increase in cross-sectional area, and decrease in the height of the dermal papillae have all been observed with aging. Finally, with age, fibrous structures in

K. Tsuchida
Research and Development Department, Naris Cosmetics Co. Ltd., Osaka, Japan
e-mail: k_tsuchida@naris.co.jp

H. Yamada (✉)
Department of Dermatology of Kinki University, Faculty of Medicine Nara Hospital, Kinki University Antiaging Center, Higashiosaka, Osaka Prefecture, Japan
e-mail: yamadahi@med.kindai.ac.jp

M.A. Farage et al. (eds.), *Textbook of Aging Skin*,
DOI 10.1007/978-3-662-47398-6_119

the dermis change from a cobweb-like pattern to being oriented in the same direction. Elucidating these inner structural changes caused by aging may further the understanding of skin aging.

Introduction

The human skin is consists of three layers: the epidermis, dermis, and subcutaneous tissue [1]. On average, the epidermis is approximately 0.2 mm in thickness, and 95 % of the cells in it are keratinocytes. Epidermal keratinocytes are at different stages of maturation and are densely arranged into layers at four different levels: the horny cell layer (10–20 layers), the granular cell layer (2–3 layers), the suprabasal cell layer (5–10 layers), and the basal cell layer (1 layer). The epidermis and dermis are separated by a basement membrane and form a concave–convex structure. This structure is known as the dermal papilla, and it is believed to play an important role in the skin physiology. The dermis is approximately 15–40 times thicker than the epidermis. The dermis is divided into three layers: the papillary layer, subpapillary layer, and reticular layer. However, its boundary is not clear compared with the epidermis. In addition, the dermis is divided into cellular components, such as fibroblast, and stromal components that form a fibrous structure. The main component of this fibrous structure is the collagen fibril. Thus far, these inner structures of the skin have been observed using skin biopsy [2–6]. However, skin biopsy is invasive and an ex vivo method that requires the tissue to be removed from the skin. Noninvasive methods that do not require the excision of the tissue for evaluating the inner structure of the skin are required. Recently, there have been advances in observational technology for examining the inner structure of the skin. These methods are noninvasive and include ultrasound imaging, magnetic resonance imaging (MRI), and optical coherence tomography (OCT). Ultrasound visualizes structural changes in the acoustic organization of the skin and is used to measure skin thickness and skinfold thickness. MRI visualizes proton density, relaxation time of protons, and blood flow and is used to observe tomographic images as well as the status of tissues. OCT utilizes the coherence of light and offers tomographic images of tissues. However, because of the inadequacy of spatial resolution, it is difficult to apply these methods for the direct measurements of the inner structure of the skin.

3Previous studies have observed the inner structure of the skin using in vivo reflectance confocal microscopy (RCM) [7–10]. RCM is a noninvasive technique used for imaging living skin. Recent reports have suggested that the inner structures of the skin, such as cell size in the granular and the suprabasal layers, thickness of the epidermis and the basal layer, dermal papillae, and collagen bundles, change with age [11–14]. In addition, recent reports have suggested that the structure of the dermal papillae varies depending on the site [15], and it correlates with skin elasticity and the I-value, which represents intensity of light [16].

Skin aging is classified into intrinsic aging and photoaging, each exhibiting characteristic changes [17]. In intrinsic aging, decrease of the skin thickness [18] and lower proliferative rate of the epidermis have been reported. Conversely, in photoaging, increase of the skin thickness [18], increase in the size of corneocytes and wrinkle grade [20, 21], and higher proliferative rate of the epidermis have been reported [19]. These age-related changes may correlate with age-related changes of the inner structure of the skin. Therefore, an observation of the inner structure of the skin may be important in the understanding of skin physiology and aging.

This chapter describes observations on the inner structure and age-related changes of human skin using RCM. Focused around the authors' recent research related to the structure of the dermal papillae, the findings of studies on the inner structure of the skin are presented here.

RCM Apparatus

Confocal microscopy can be used in vivo and is available in fluorescence or reflectance mode. Previously, the fluorescence mode, utilizing a fluorescent probe, has been used to observe the morphology of tissues and depth distribution of substances such as organelles [22, 23]. However, recently, the reflectance mode, known as RCM, utilizing reflected light has been more widely used. RCM allows for the noninvasive observation of living tissue and can be applied to obtain information on the inner structure of the skin. This chapter will focus on RCM.

In contrast to conventional microscopy, in confocal microscopy, only a portion of the focus is brightly imaged, and it is operated by detecting single back-scattered photons from illuminated living tissue [24]. Because light other than that of the focal position is cut by a pinhole, information from only the focal position reaches the detector. Resolution occurs in the depth direction (the Z direction); thus, high contrast and resolution are obtained compared with conventional microscopy. Confocal microscopy can therefore be used to observe horizontal cross-sectional images, every few μm from the tissue surface to the depth direction, by moving a vertically objective lens in real time. However, because RCM utilizes reflected light, signals from deep within the tissues decrease due to scattering and absorption of light. With RCM, imaging is limited to a depth of 200–300 μm.

An expansive image can be obtained by scanning the sample in the horizontal plane (XY plane) keeping a fixed light or scanning light in the horizontal plane keeping the sample. Three-dimensional (3D) images are obtained by reconstructing images in the depth direction on a computer. Most of the light sources used in confocal microscopy are lasers. Lasers can be regarded as a point light source and have high luminance and stable output. The authors' study utilized RCM apparatus with an 830 nm laser, Vivascope 1500/3000 (Lucid Inc., Henrietta, NY).

The contrast of confocal images of the skin is provided by the refractive index differences of intracellular substances, extracellular matrix components, and other microstructures from the background. In the skin, refractive index differences correspond to melanin in the epidermis, collagen and elastin fibers in the dermis, and erythrocytes in the dermal capillaries [25]. Melanin in particular provides strong contrast [26]. It has been reported that various inner structures and cells can be observed using RCM (Table 1).

Table 1 Inner structures and cells observed using RCM

Structures and cells	References
Crista cutis and sulcus cutis	[27]
Thickness of horny cell layer	[13]
Granular cell	[11, 14, 27]
Suprabasal cell	[14, 27]
Thickness of basal cell layer	[11]
Melanin cap	[27]
Melanocyte	[28]
Dermal papilla	[11–14]
Collagen bundle	[13]
Blood vessel and blood cell	[10, 11, 27]
Pore	[29]

Observations using RCM are shown in plane images in the depth direction from the skin surface. Figure 1 shows RCM observations of dermal papillae. In the skin surface, a fissured appearance of the horny cell layer and pores is observed (Fig. 1a). With deepening of the image, a bright spot begins to appear representing the upper end of the dermal papillae (Fig. 1b). Subsequently, the dermal papillae are observed as bright circles (Fig. 1c). The dermal papillae are clearly observed with RCM because the melanin that exists in the basal layer along the dermal papillae offers strong contrast. Pores are observed from the skin surface to the depth direction and can be distinguished from the dermal papillary bright circles.

Imaging of Inner Structures Using RCM

Inner Structure

RCM enables observation from the skin surface to the dermis. The skin surface is not uniformly smooth and is engraved by a number of fine grooves called sulcus cutis. Small ridges surrounded by the sulcus cutis are called the crista cutis. On average, the thickness of the epidermis is approximately 0.2 mm and 95 % of the cells are epidermal keratinocytes. Keratinocytes divide at the lowest layer of the epidermis and migrate to the upper layer as they mature. Keratinocytes at

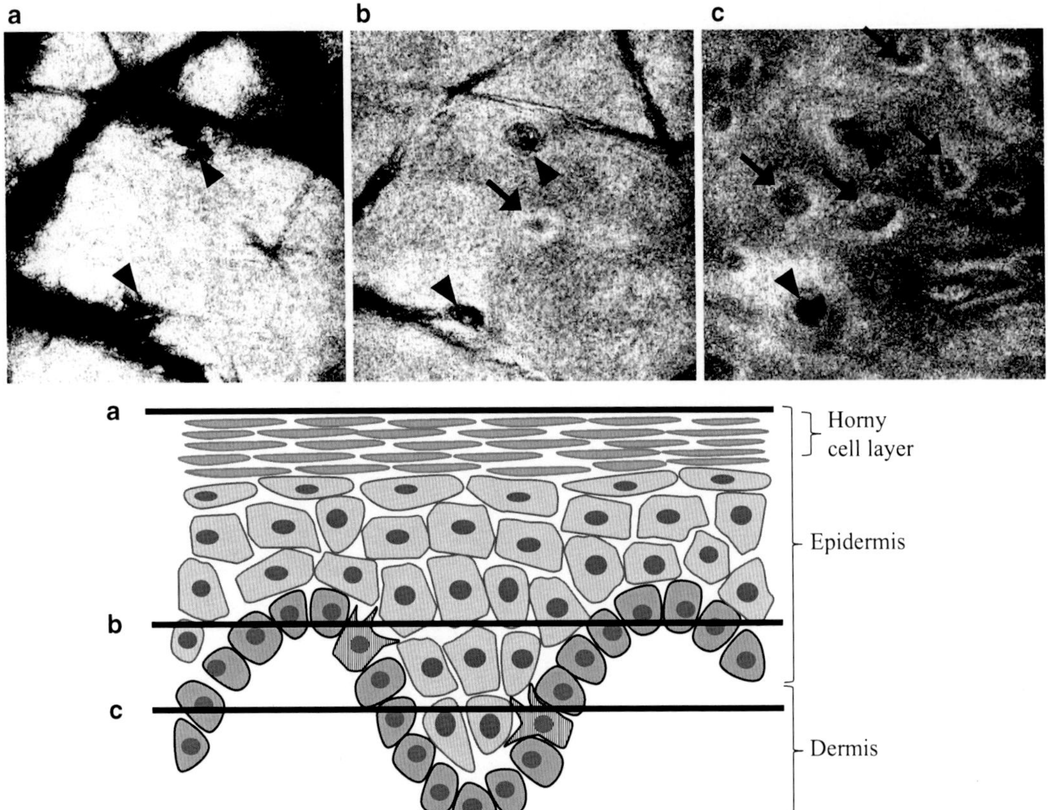

Fig. 1 In vivo RCM images. RCM images from the cheek skin of a 29-year-old man. (**a**) The fissured appearance of the horny layer and the pore (*black arrowhead*) are observed in the skin surface (Z-axis, 0 μm). (**b**) The superior ends of the dermal papillae (*black arrows*) are starting to be seen (Z-axis, 25 μm). (**c**) The cross-sectional surface of the dermal papillae (*black arrows*) is seen (Z-axis, 55 μm). Pore is seen in all images. Image size is 500 × 500 μm

different stages of maturity are arranged in layers and are classified from the depth to the upper layer as follows: the basal cell layer, suprabasal cell layer, granular cell layer, and horny cell layer. Keratinocyte layers and cell sizes can be observed using RCM. The basal cell layer has a thickness of 10–20 μm [11] and the cell forms are cubic and columnar. The diameter of the cells in the suprabasal cell layer is 20–30 μm [14]. In the suprabasal cell layer, lower cells are polygonal and upper cells are flattened. The size of the cells in the granular layer is 800–1000 μm^2 [11], and the cells are flat. The horny cell layer has a thickness of 20–30 μm [13], and the flat cells in the horny layer are stratified.

The epidermis and dermis are in close contact by the basement membrane structure. The boundary of the epidermis and dermis forms a concave–convex structure. The structure by which the dermis is projected toward the epidermis is referred to as the dermal papillary structure. RCM has shown that the thickness between the upper end and the lower end of the dermal papilla is 20–50 μm [13].

The dermis is located below the epidermis across the basement membrane. It is divided into cellular components, such as fibroblast, and stromal components which form fibrotic tissue. The stromal component is composed mostly of collagen fibers and also includes elastic fibers and

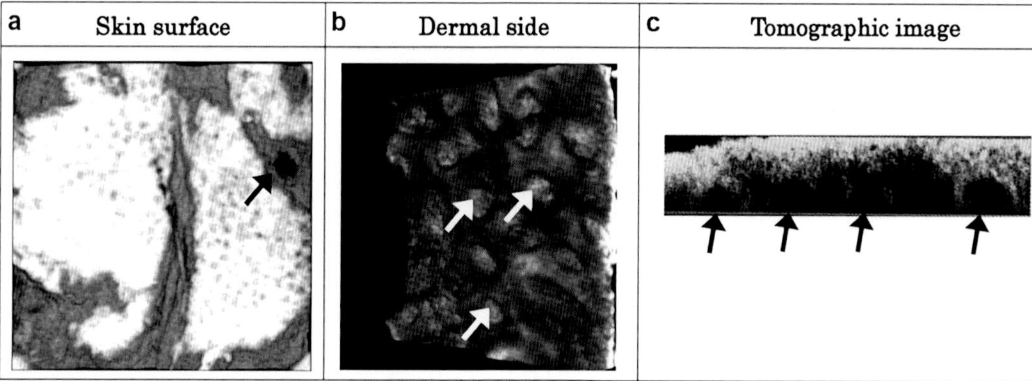

Fig. 2 X-Y horizontal 3D images and X-Z tomographic reconstructed images using RCM. RCM images of the cheek skin were observed. 3D images were obtained by the reconstruction of 100 sheets (500 × 500 μm, X-Y image) from the upper skin surface. (**a**) Sulcus cutis, crista cutis, and pore (*black arrow*) in the skin surface and (**b**) concavity and convexity of the dermal papillae (*white arrow*) on the dermal side are seen. (**c**) A tomographic image (500 × 99 μm, X-Z image) in the vertical direction, and projection of the dermal papillae into the epidermis (*black arrow*) was confirmed

reticular fibers. These are referred to as the extracellular matrix. The dry weight of collagen fibers accounts for 70 % of the dermis. Collagen fibers are very tough and are important as a support organization to keep the mechanical strength of the skin. Collagen fibers are formed to gather into a thin basic unit called a fibril, and the gathered fibers of the fibrils are thick and tough. In the upper dermis (the papillary layer and subpapillary layer), sparse, thin collagen fibers have been observed using RCM at a depth of 90–140 μm from the skin surface [13]. On the other hand, in the lower dermis (the reticular layer), well-developed thick collagen fibers, referred to as collagen fiber bundles or collagen bundles, have been closely observed.

3D Reconstruction Using RCM Image Sequences

RCM image sequences can be used for 3D reconstruction, and dermal papillary structures can be visualized. The 3D imaging can be obtained using Fiji-ImageJ software (NIH, Bethesda, MD) [30], which is an open-source program.

Figure 2 shows a 3D image obtained from RCM image sequences, taken every 1 μm from the surface of the horny cell layer down to 99 μm. The 3D image was rotated, and snapshots at the skin surface (a) and dermal side (b) were taken. The sulcus cutis, crista cutis, and pores in the skin surface (a) and the concavity–convexity structure of the dermal papillae on the dermal side (b) are seen. Tomographic images in the vertical direction show that the dermal papillae project into the epidermis (c).

Parameterization of the Inner Structure

For the evaluation of the dermal papillary structure, the parameters of various structures can be determined using RCM (Fig. 3). Evaluation methods used in the authors' recent study are described below.

Parameters related to the dermal papillary structure include the number of dermal papillae (/mm^2), the cross-sectional area (μm^2) representing broadness of the dermal papillae, and the depth to the upper end of the dermal papillae (μm). In these evaluations, pores were distinguished from the dermal papillae and were excluded. In addition, parameters in the sun-exposed skin sites (cheek and nasolabial fold) were employed for correlation analysis.

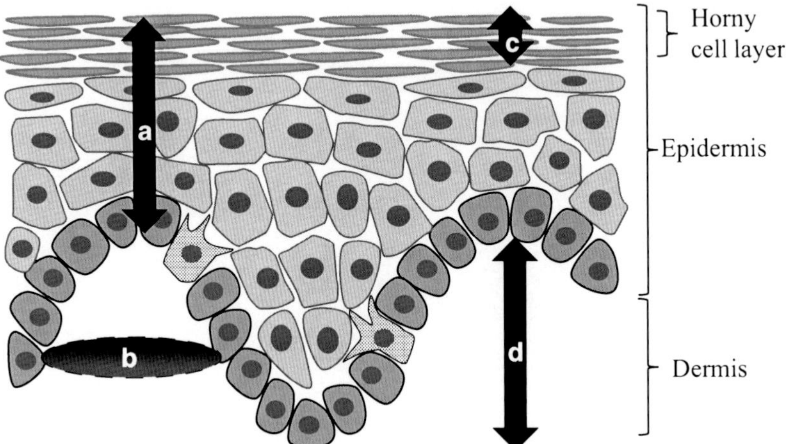

Fig. 3 Parameters of dermal papilla structures. The concave–convex structure in the illustration shows dermal papilla structure. (**a**) The depth to the upper end of the dermal papilla. (**b**) The cross-sectional area of the dermal papilla. (**c**) The thickness of the horny cell layer. (**d**) The height of the dermal papilla. The number of dermal papillae is counted from the cross section of the dermal papillae

Horizontal RCM images, 20–30 μm in depth from the upper end of the dermal papilla, were used for the calculation of these parameters. The number of dermal papillae (/mm^2) was evaluated by counting the dermal papillae in the RCM image. The cross-sectional area (μm^2) of the dermal papillae was calculated using ImageJ software (NIH, Bethesda, MD). The depth to the upper end of dermal papillae (μm) was determined by calculating the depth of the upper end of the dermal papillae from the skin surface.

Parameters of other inner structures have been determined using RCM, including the thickness of the horny cell layer, the thickness from the skin surface to the lower end of the dermal papillae, the thickness of the basal layer, and the height of the dermal papillae [11–13, 15].

Age-Related Changes of the Inner Structure

Structure of the Epidermis

The inner structures of the epidermis can be observed using RCM, including the depth from the skin surface to the lower end of the dermal papillae, thickness of the basal layer, cell size in the granular layer, and thickness of the horny cell layer. These inner structures have been compared between younger and older skin. The depth from the skin surface to the lower end of dermal papillae, including sun-exposed and -protected skin sites, is thinner in older skin than that in younger skin [13]. The thickness of the basal layer, which is a sun-protected skin site, is also thinner in older skin than that in younger skin [11]. However, the thickness of the granular layer, which is a sun-protected site, is thicker in older skin than that in younger skin [11]. The thickness of the horny cell layer does not change with age [11, 13].

Considering decreased skin thickness of sun-protected sites and increased skin thickness of sun-exposed sites with age [18], the pattern of structural change in the epidermis may differ between sun-exposed and sun-protected sites.

Dermal Papillary Structure

The dermal papillary structure has been observed using RCM. Studies have suggested that there are age-related changes in the dermal papillae both in sun-exposed and sun-protected skin sites [11–14]. Using RCM, the authors investigated the

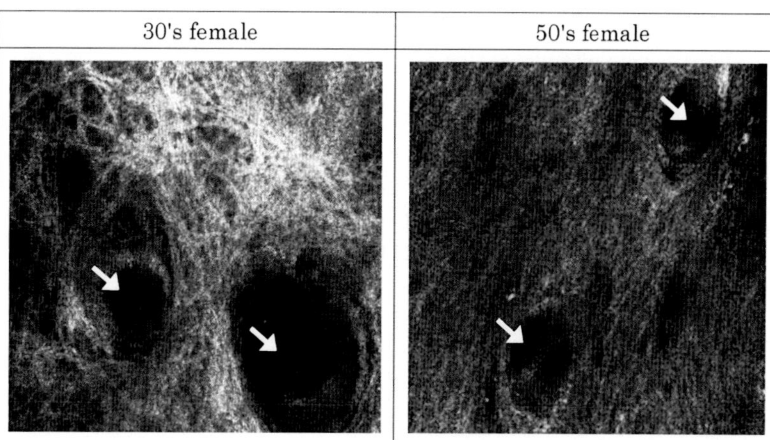

Fig. 4 Age-related changes in fibrous structures observed using RCM. The fibrous structures of cheek skin are shown below. In females in their 30's, they appear as a cobweb-like pattern. In females in their 50's, they are arranged in the same direction. The white arrows indicate pores. Image size is 500 × 500 μm

correlation between age and parameters of the dermal papillary structure. The results are described below.

In facial skin (cheek and nasolabial fold), age had a significantly negative correlation with the number of dermal papillae and a significantly positive correlation with the cross-sectional area of the dermal papillae. There was no correlation between the depth to the upper end of the dermal papillae and age. The number of dermal papillae decreased with age, and the density of the concave–convex structures of the dermal papillae became sparse. The cross-sectional area of dermal papillae increased with age and sharp dermal papillae become broader. These changes suggest flattening of the dermal papillae with age. In addition, it has been reported that dermal papillae decrease in height with age [12, 13], that the depth to the upper end of the dermal papillae increases with age [11], and that vitamin C increases the number of dermal papillae [31].

Age-related changes in dermal papillary structure were shown in the cheek skin of females in their 20s and 60s, using 3D reconstruction of RCM images. On the dermal side, females in their 20s had abundant hole shapes with bright circular patterns indicating dermal papillae. However, females in their 60s had few hole shapes with bright circular patterns. In both groups, pores were observed to pass through from the side of the horny cell layer to the dermal side and were distinguished from the dermal papillary structure. These results using 3D reconstruction of noninvasive RCM images are similar to previous reports in which observations were made by invasive methods [32].

Fibrous Structure of the Dermis

The stromal components of the dermis are fibrotic tissue. Fibrotic tissue is mostly composed of collagen fibers. The collagen fibers form three-dimensional fibrous structures with substrates containing glycosaminoglycan and elastin. These fibrous structures are visible with RCM [13]. Figure 4 shows the fibrous structures in the cheek skin of participants in their 30s compared with those of participants in their 50s. The fibrous structures were arranged in a cobweb-like pattern in participants in their 30s. However, the fibrous structures were arranged in the same direction in participants in their 50s. In addition, anisotropy and clearness of the fibrous structures were shown to change with age [16]. Changes in the level of degraded collagen [33], type I procollagen protein expression [34], and the shape of collagen fibers [35] by photoaging may be related to the changes of fibrous structures in the dermis.

Conclusion

With the development of new observational methods, age-related changes in the inner structure of the skin can now be noninvasively observed. RCM is a suitable method for the noninvasive observation of the inner structure of the epidermis and dermis. Using RCM, the study of the inner structure of the skin has greatly advanced. In particular, the structure of the dermal papillae, which are believed to be involved in the skin physiology, has been observed using RCM. The structure of the dermal papillae changes with age, and it has been suggested that the dermal papillae flatten with age. In addition, the inner structure of the epidermis and fibrous structure of the dermis change with age. Understanding age-related changes of the inner structure of the skin will help to elucidate skin aging and skin physiology.

References

1. Shimizu H. Shimizu's textbook of dermatology. 1st ed. Hokkaido: Hokkaido University Press; 2007. p. 1–26.
2. Freeman RG, Cockerell EG, Armstrong J, et al. Sunlight as a factor influencing the thickness of epidermis. J Invest Dermatol. 1962;39:295–8.
3. Fligiel SE, Varani J, Datta SC, et al. Collagen degradation in aged/photodamaged skin in vivo and after exposure to matrix metalloproteinase-1 in vitro. J Invest Dermatol. 2003;120:842–8.
4. Mine S, Fortunel NO, Pageon H, et al. Aging alters functionally human dermal papillary fibroblasts but not reticular fibroblasts: a new view of skin morphogenesis and aging. PLoS One. 2008; 3. doi: 10.1371/journal.pone.0004066
5. Holbrook KA, Odland GF. Regional differences in the thickness (cell layers) of the human horny cell layer: an ultra structural analysis. J Invest Dermatol. 1974;62:415–22.
6. Contet-Andonneau JL, Jeanmaire C, Pauly G. A histological study of human wrinkle structures: a comparison between sun-exposed areas of the face, with or without wrinkles and sun-protected areas. Br J Dermatol. 1999;140:1038–47.
7. Rajadhyaksha M, González S, Zavislan JM, et al. In vivo confocal scanning laser microscopy of human skin II: advances in instrumentation and comparison with histology. J Invest Dermatol. 1999;113:293–303.
8. Corcuff P, Bertrand C, Leveque JL, et al. Morphometry of human epidermis in vivo by real-time confocal microscopy. Arch Dermatol Res. 1993;285:475–81.
9. Bertrand C, Corcuff P. In vivo spatio-temporal visualization of the human skin by real-time confocal microscopy. Scanning. 1994;16:150–4.
10. González S, González E, White WM, et al. Allergic contact dermatitis: correlation of in vivo confocal imaging to routine histology. J Am Acad Dermatol. 1999;40:708–13.
11. Sauermann K, Clemann S, Jaspers S, et al. Age related changes of human skin investigated with histometric measurements by confocal laser scanning microscopy in vivo. Skin Res Technol. 2002;8:52–6.
12. Mizukoshi K, Yonekura K, Futagawa M, et al. Changes in dermal papilla structures due to aging in the facial cheek region. Skin Res Technol. 2014;0:1–8.
13. Neerken S, Lucassen GW, Bisschop MA, et al. Characterization of age-related effects in human skin: a comparative study that applies confocal laser scanning microscopy and optical coherence tomography. J Biomed Opt. 2004;9:274–81.
14. Kawasaki K, Yamanishi K, Yamada H. Age-related morphometric changes of inner structures of the skin assessed by in vivo reflectance confocal microscopy. Int J Dermatol. 2015;54:295–301.
15. Sakamaki T. In vivo confocal microscopy of normal human skin. Jpn J Dermatol. 2002;112:1501–5.
16. Mizukoshi K, Yonekura K, Goto H, et al. A simple method for assessment of age-related changes in physical properties of facial dermal papilla and fibrous structures. In: 22th IFSCC conference, Rio de Janeiro. 2013, p. 335–46.
17. Farage MA, Miller KW, Elsner P, et al. Intrinsic and extrinsic factors in skin ageing: a review. Int J Cosmet Sci. 2008;30:87–95.
18. Takema Y, Yorimoto Y, Kawai M, et al. Age-related changes in the elastic properties and thickness of human facial skin. Br J Dermatol. 1994;131:641–8.
19. Lavker RM. Cutaneous aging: chronologic versus photaging. In: Gilchrest BA, editor. Photodamage. Cambridge: Blackwell Science; 1995. p. 123–35.
20. Takema Y, Yorimoto Y, Kawai M. The relationship between age-related changes in the physical properties and development of wrinkles in human facial skin. J Soc Cosmet Chem. 1995;46:163–73.
21. Kumagai H, Watanabe H, Kozu T. Physiological and morphological changes in facial skin with aging (I). J Soc Cosmet Chem. 1989;23:9–21.
22. Fink-Puches R, Hofmann-Wellenhof R, Smolle J, et al. Confocal laser scanning microscopy: a new optical microscopic technique for applications in pathology and dermatology. J Cutan Pathol. 1995; 22:252–9.
23. Selim MM, Kelly KM, Nelson JS, et al. Confocal microscopy study of nerves and blood vessels in untreated and treated port wine stains: preliminary observations. Dermatol Surg. 2004;30:892–7.
24. Webb RH. Confocal optical microscopy. Rep Prog Phys. 1996;59:427–71.
25. Dunn AK, Smithpeter C, Welch AJ, et al. Sources of contrast in confocal reflectance imaging. Appl Opt. 1996;35:3441–6.
26. Rajadhyaksha M, Grossman M, Esterowitz D, et al. In vivo confocal scanning laser microscopy of human skin: melanin provides strong contrast. J Invest Dermatol. 1995;104:946–52.
27. Huzaira M, Rius F, Rajadhyaksha M, et al. Topographic variations in normal skin, as viewed by

in vivo reflectance confocal microscopy. J Invest Dermatol. 2001;116:846–52.
28. Yamashita T, Kuwahara T, González S, et al. Non-invasive visualization of melanin and melanocytes by reflectance-mode confocal microscopy. J Invest Dermatol. 2005;124:235–40.
29. Mizukoshi K, Takahashi K. Analysis of the skin surface and inner structure around pores on the face. Skin Res Technol. 2014;20:23–9.
30. Reichelt M, Joubert L, Perrino J, et al. 3D reconstruction of VZV infected cell nuclei and PML nuclear cages by serial section array scanning electron microscopy and electron tomography. PLoS Pathog. 2012;8. doi: 10.1371/journal.ppat.1002740
31. Sauermann K, Jaspers S, Koop U, et al. Topically applied vitamin C increases the density of dermal papillae in aged human skin. BMC Dermatol. 2004;4:13.
32. Hull MT, Warfel KA. Age-related changes in cutaneous basal lamina: scanning electron microscopic study. J Invest Dermatol. 1983;81:378–80.
33. Fisher GJ, Kang S, Varani J, et al. Mechanisms of photoaging and chronological skin aging. Arch Dermatol. 2002;138:1462–70.
34. Varani J, Spearman D, Perone P, et al. Inhibition of type I procollagen synthesis by damaged collagen in photoaged skin and by collagenase-degraded collagen in vitro. Am J Pathol. 2001;158:931–42.
35. Nishimori Y, Edwards C, Pearse A, et al. Degenerative alterations of dermal collagen fiber bundles in photodamaged human skin and UV-irradiated hairless mouse skin: possible effect on decreasing skin mechanical properties and appearance of wrinkles. J Invest Dermatol. 2001;117: 1458–63.

Facial Skin Rheology

27

Gérald E. Piérard, Sébastien L. Piérard, and Trinh Hermanns-Lê

Contents

G.E. Piérard (✉)
Laboratory of Skin Bioengineering and Imaging, Department of Dermatopathology, University Hospital of Liège, Liège, Belgium
e-mail: gerald.pierard@ulg.ac.be

S.L. Piérard
Telecommunication and Imaging Laboratory, INTELSIG, Montefiore Institute, University of Liège, Liège, Belgium
e-mail: pierard@montefiore.ulg.ac.be

T. Hermanns-Lê
Laboratory of Skin Bioengineering and Imaging, Department of Dermatopathology, University Hospital of Liège, Liège, Belgium

Electron Microscopy Unit, Department of Dermatopathology, Unilab Lg, University Hospital of Liège, Liège, Belgium
e-mail: trinh.hermanns@chu.ulg.ac.be

M.A. Farage et al. (eds.), *Textbook of Aging Skin*,
DOI 10.1007/978-3-662-47398-6_27

Abstract

Facial aging expressions include wrinkling, mottled pigmentation, change in lip height, and deepening of nasolabial folds. There is a need for objective assessments of these aging signs. The relationship between the dermal microstructure and the mechanical properties of the facial skin is of utmost importance. It governs the viscoelastic properties of the tissue. They are conveniently assessed by the in vivo suction method as well as the torque method and the measurement of the ultrasound speed propagation. The influences of age, gender, and skin thickness are important to be considered.

Introduction

The appearance of facial aging encompasses distinct clinical features, including wrinkling, mottled pigmentation, change in lip height, and pronounced nasolabial fold [1]. Their crude clinical assessment and any grading system remain highly subjective [2–6] and are awaiting for objective validations. It remains that a higher perceived age is commonly associated with smoking, low socioeconomic class, low body mass index, prominent sunlight exposures, and peculiar genetic influences [7].

There is a global need for improving the objective assessment of physical attributes to the facial skin during aging [8]. The precise determination of the structure physical properties and functions of the facial skin and its constituent parts still remains an open question [9]. By contrast, much more attention has been paid to molecular biology characterization of skin components. In part, this situation reflects the comparatively late development of bioengineering applied to dermometrology and the intrinsic difficulty of obtaining relevant in vivo reproducible physical data from the skin. In addition, some ambient environmental conditions profoundly influence the physical attributes of the skin. As a result, the variations in physical parameters owing to body region, age, gender, and ethnicity greatly outweigh the variability of the corresponding molecular composition of the cutaneous structures.

The term properties of the skin implies assessments similarly to any other physical material. This aspect gives relatively little relevant information about clinical or biological characteristics of in vivo conditions. The qualification of property is more applicable to in vitro testing. By contrast, clinicians and cosmetologists are primarily concerned about a more restricted range of relevant functions rather than overall properties of the skin. It is true that functions are largely dependent on properties, but the conceptual and practical differences are important to consider. Testing a function must be performed in vivo under a fairly narrow range of ambient conditions. However, it does not follow that in vitro testing has no importance for clinicians. By contrast, some data are only obtained by using the in vitro approach, although this requires caution in interpretation.

Skin Structure and Mechanical Functions

The skin is a complex five-layered composite structure (stratum corneum, stratum spinosum or Malpighi layer, papillary dermis, reticular dermis, including hair follicles and sebaceous glands, hypodermis) whose functions depend on some mutual interdependence of the constituent tissues. On the overall, the biomechanical properties and functions of the skin are mainly governed by the dermal and hypodermal connective tissues, with a possible minimal contribution from the stratum corneum [10, 11]. In addition, the skin structures differ largely according to the body site [10, 12]. Thus, regional variations exert profound influences on the biomechanical characteristics. Moreover, a series of chronic and cumulative environmental threats including ultraviolet light and near-infrared radiations [13] exert dissimilar influences over distinct body regions and according to age, phototype, and behavior with regard to sun exposure. The balance between these factors determines and distinguishes the intrinsic and extrinsic aging processes on the skin [14]. In these respects, the facial skin is particularly susceptible to the diverse aspects of weathering and photoaging [15]. Thus, facial skin aging is not similar to that occurring on most other body sites. Such regional anatomical variation was seldom acknowledged in the past [16].

The skin biomechanical properties and functions are time dependent. In addition, they are anisotropic as they differ according to the direction in which a force (load) is applied. Both these characteristics of the skin add complications to determine descriptors of its biomechanical properties and functions. A further major problem in this field is the lack of standardization among investigators. Different research groups have used a variety of devices, measuring units, as well as different conditions of measurement. In addition, they have employed differing test modes for obtaining what was expected to be similar information. It is clear that progress in the field of biomechanical skin bioengineering is only reached when some attempt at uniformity is made. Controlled and standardized practices are welcome.

Facial Skin Aging and Its Physical Attributes

The facial skin is bound to deeper structures, while keeping some mobility. Such condition allows both movements and temporary compression and distension of a part. Flexibility and elasticity are important attributes of the skin, while firmness is another essential component. Such skin properties are relevant to the visual and tactile features of the facial skin [17–19].

Facial skin aging takes place gradually over about four decades. In its early stages, little clinical evidence is present at the exception of the mosaic faint (subclinical) melanoderma [20]. The incipient clinical signs of facial aging are later recognized by individuals with the emergence of discrete furrows and wrinkles, together with a loss of firmness [21, 22]. Additional various cutaneous signs and lesions develop with aging, and some of them result from more severe photoaging. In addition, changes in the deep cutaneous tissues distinct from sun-induced damages are responsible for deepening of facial creases and sagging [22–24].

As a rule, in vivo biomechanical testing of the facial skin proves to be tricky to interpret because of the multiple and complex relationships between the various components of the skin and the ill-defined intrinsic properties of each tissue. In addition, there is commonly an unknown influence of previous mechanical preconditioning at the test sites [10]. Both the biomechanical functions and the surface contours of the skin reflect the structural organization of the tissues [22]. As a result, the combination of rheological and profilometric assessments provided some relevant and noninvasive characterization of the overall aging process of the facial skin [10, 25, 26]. However, the diversity of bioengineering methods of evaluation combined with a wide variation in experimental designs has brought a number of uncertaintics and discrepancies in the literature.

Chief Fibrillar Structures Governing the Skin Mechanical Properties

On a mechanical viewpoint, the dermis has often been compared to rubber, and a series of mechanical tests were adaptations from those used in the rubber industry. In fact, the dermis does not exhibit similar properties and functions.

The bulk of the cutaneous extracellular matrix (ECM) of the connective tissue consists of a network of collagen fibers, the organization of which determines the mechanical characteristics of the tissue and its resistance to deformation [10]. The elastic fibers present in smaller amounts serve to recoil the stretched collagen bundles to their relaxed position. This complex network of fibers is permeated by highly hydrated proteoglycans, glycoproteoglycans, and glycoproteins embedding the connective tissue cells. Fibroblasts and dermal dendrocytes are responsible for maintaining or remodeling the quantitative and structural steady state of both the ECM fibers and the amorphous matrix as well. There are considerable differences in the relative proportions and organization of each of these components in different skin regions, as well as variations during aging and diseases [10].

With respect to the major biomechanical functions of the ECM and to structural features similar to all body regions, the skin connective tissue is conveniently divided into three major superposed layers. The adventitial dermis corresponds to a superficial zone of loose connective tissue adjacent to the epidermis and encasing its follicular structures as well. It corresponds to the papillary and the periadnexal dermis. The rest of the dermis is identified as the reticular dermis because of the netlike appearance of its fiber bundles. Still a third deeper layer corresponds to the connective septae partitioning lobules of adipocytes in the hypodermis. The differences and limits between the three layers are not always sharply identified. It is rather the relative concentration and arrangement of fibers rather than any absolute differences in composition that enable these regions to be distinguished.

In mechanical terms, it is expected that the physical functions of the adventitial dermis somewhat resemble those of the hypodermal septae because they are conditioned by thin collagen fibers arranged in a rather similar loose open meshwork running perpendicular to the surface of the skin. The reticular dermis is more rigid because the collagen fiber bundles are coarser, tightly connected each other, and most often closely packed in planes parallel to the skin surface.

It must be emphasized that this descriptive view of the connective tissue varies tremendously according to the body site. In its structural organization, the dermis of the face, scalp, back, forearm, palms, and soles differs greatly. It should be stressed that the rheological functions of the facial skin are markedly influenced by the presence of a high density of terminal hairs (beard) in men and by abundant and large sebaceous glands. These structures likely put under tension the surrounding fiber networks of the dermis. In addition, facial muscles impose some anisotropic tensions to the skin which are in turn responsible for some wrinkles such as facial frown lines and glabellar rhytids [22, 27, 28]. Moreover, age is important to consider as the skin presents marked differences during fetal life, childhood, perimenopausal period, and senescence [12, 25, 27]. Nonionizing radiations from the environment [13] superimpose their effects on those of the natural chronological aging [14, 29].

Physiological Interferences with Skin Mechanical Properties

The skin withstands various forces originating from the body, and it reacts to those imposed by the environment. These features govern the global skin mechanobiology. The perception of the normal, loose, or stiff skin depends on the ability of the connective tissue to resist and transmit the various forces. When assessing the in vivo skin biomechanical functions, intrinsic tension forces are hardly measurable, and they should ideally be minimized in order to prevent any interference with the testing procedure [10]. This is tentatively achieved by muscle relaxation and a comfortable controlled posture of the concerned body region. These controlled conditions do not abrogate the relaxed skin tension lines and Langer's lines [30–32]. The facial skin is quite unique as far as the skin biomechanical functions are concerned [25, 33–35].

The skin is anisotropic with regard to the variability of mechanical functions according to the direction of the forces applied [30, 36]. There is some complexity associated with sorting out some straightforward relevant information from many vivo testings. In fact, measuring the overall mechanical characteristics of the skin provides a rough estimate of the resultant of multiple features acting on the various parts of the skin. The distinction between the specific dermal and epidermal properties is usually not accessible to accurate and distinctive measurement. One of the major challenges resides in the interpretation of the combination of histological, instrumental, and biological variations that are found [10, 30].

In any circumstance, when a force is applied to the dermis, fibers are first reoriented in parallel to the force. At completion, some elongation is obtained for elastic fibers, while collagen fibers remain almost inextensible. In the physiological range of tensions, the structural organization of collagen bundles, their orientations, the anchorage of bundles together, as well as their relation to elastic fibers and proteoglycans should be considered as predominant in determining the natural tension lines in the skin [31].

When the skin is elongated, the fibers become aligned and slip over one another. With increasing forces, the extensibility of the collagen fibers themselves is being tested. With sustained forces, there is a gradual change in the bonding of the collagen fibers or some other form of molecular realignment. During persistent compression, the interfiber matrix is squeezed out of the site. There are both an alignment of the fiber bundles along the lines of stress and a decrease in their convolution [31]. Most of this first phase is due to straightening of the usually convoluted fibers and not to their lateral contraction.

Basic Skin Viscoelasticity

Basically, the skin exhibits viscoelastic functions and properties. However, the literature occasionally appears quite confusing with regard to the expression and interpretation of mechanical testing of the skin. This situation is due to the absence of a well-recognized nomenclature, of a uniform system of units, and of standardized techniques. However, basic terms and units used in physics should be applied to biology, and these prove to be useful in clinical practice [10].

A series of experimental devices were developed in research laboratories in order to measure the biomechanical functions of the skin perpendicular or parallel to the skin surface. Mechanical functions of the facial skin are conveniently assessed in a noninvasive way using a series of methods. The skin is possibly pulled upward, pressed, twisted, extended parallel to its surface in one or several directions, and submitted to vibrations and to many other types of mechanical stimuli. Forces applied to the skin vary in direction, intensity, and time of application. These different approaches provide different information about the functions of the various connective tissue frameworks.

In practice, the experimental approaches to determining the biomechanical reactions of the skin are divided into six types, namely, the tensile and torsional types as well as those based on elevation, indentation, suction, and vibration. In general, a relevant information is gained with testing the facial skin at low stress. When a force is applied to the skin using a conventional testing device, the tension created is calculated in newtons (N) or in millibars (mbar). In in vitro testing, stress corresponds to the ratio between the force (load) and the cross-sectional area of the skin in a plane at right angles to the direction of the force. It is expressed in N/m^2. Strain is the ratio between elongation and the original length of the tissue submitted to the force. It is dimensionless, since measured as mm per mm.

Most usually the crude information received from an in vivo experiment is the relationship of force (or stress) to deformation (assimilated to strain) over time. However, the maximum deformation for a given force is not gained immediately as some elongation still takes place under stable traction after periods of time. In addition, the deformation is not completely reversed within a short period of time in the absence of compressive force [37–39]. Such features explain the complexity of stress relaxation curves.

The facial skin corresponds to a viscoelastic material characterized by a nonlinear stress-strain properties with hysteresis [10, 40]. This means that the stress-strain curve obtained during loading is not identical to the curve obtained during unloading [37–39]. Furthermore, the deformation of the skin as a function of time shows an immediate incomplete elastic deformation and a creeping viscoelastic deformation followed by an immediate elastic recovery and a creeping recovery with a residual deformation. In any instance, the accuracy, repeatability, and reproducibility of the data rely on strictly controlled and validated experimental conditions. The selection of the most relevant biological viscoelastic parameters benefits from controlled modalities of assessments.

Attempts were made to derive constants from the experimental data. The Hooke constant is obtained in the portion of the curve where a fixed ratio is obtained between load and extension. Young's modulus refers to the value of the stress-strain ratio at a given time during the skin elongation phase.

When the skin is stressed by a load, rapid extension takes place at first but then gives way to a skin condition allowing much less extension. The overall response is nonlinear, although there is a linear portion of the slope. Where extension is directly proportional of the load applied and the tested skin will return to its original length, when the load is removed the relationship is said to be "elastic" or "Hookean." The second phase is typical of an "elastic" material, but the initial one indicates that the skin becomes "stiff." The complex shape of the curve is such that it is difficult to describe it mathematically.

A residual deformation is commonly present at the issue of a stress cycle, and it interferes with subsequent testing at the same site during the next hours. These changes in biomechanical characteristics are referred to as "creep," "viscous extension," or "viscous slip." Hence, the concept of "preconditioning procedure" is achieved by applying a series of preliminary stresses to the tissue before measuring its biomechanical functions. When a series of stress cycles are consecutively applied and removed, slightly different curves are obtained on each occasion. Because of the above considerations, the results of biomechanical testing are clearly time dependent. Indeed, the results obtained depend to some extent on the rate at which the stress is applied, the duration for which it is applied, and the previous stress history of the site.

When performing in vivo biomechanical testing of the skin, relevant information is expected in line with other biological parameters. The measurements should provide data consonant with the usual functions of the skin. In fact, in normal and pathological conditions, the relevant biomechanical functions of the skin represent only a small part of its overall mechanical capacity. Results unrelated to biological functions of the skin should be disregarded. Such approach covers several questions to be answered successively when mechanical testing of the skin is to be performed in vivo:

- What is the relevant range of mechanical function in the condition being studied?
- What is the nature of information expected?
- What is the most relevant parameter to be measured?
- What region of the skin is being tested?
- What section of the skin is being tested?
- How do the tissues respond to the forces exerted?
- What is the interpretation to be given in a four-dimensional concept of skin volume and time?

In the past, many methods were used to assess the mechanical functions of the skin. They measured different parameters, and the data were hardly comparable because they differed considerably by many qualitative and quantitative aspects. Indeed, the crude data must be interpreted with respect to the method used and the type of test performed. Detailed information about the testing conditions is mandatory. It includes any eventual preconditioning, orientation, time of application and magnitude of the force exerted, the deformations gained for several load extents, the body site, and the geometry of the device.

Facial Skin Viscoelasticity Assessed by the Suction Method

One of the most popular methods for measuring skin biomechanics in vivo relies to the so-called suction method [10, 25, 27, 37–39, 41]. On the facial skin, the upper part of the cheeks and the forehead are the sites commonly chosen for the assessments. The Cutometer® SEM 580 (Courage + Khazaka Electronic, Cologne, Germany) is a convenient device equipped with a handheld probe to be applied to the skin at constant pressure. The probe has a central suction aperture of 2–6 mm in diameter. The diameter of the probe and the intensity and duration of the suction are critical parameters influencing the results. The accuracy of measurements reaches 0.01 mm in vertical skin extension under stress.

Two main operating modalities are possible. One is the flu age test using the time/strain mode (Fig. 1). In this mode, for a given aperture of the probe, the choice of vacuum (from 50–500 mbar), the total duration of suction (stress on) and

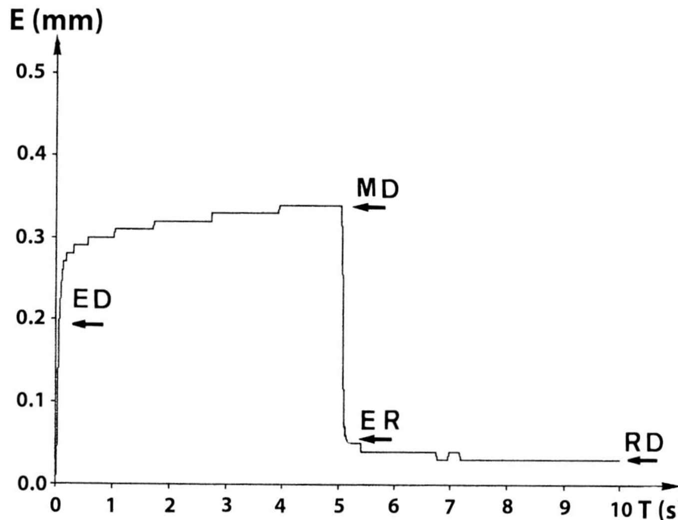

Fig. 1 Fluage test showing the relationship between the skin extension (*E*) and time (*T*). The *curve* shows the effect of a suction applied for 5 s followed by a release of the suction for 5 s. The immediate elastic distension (ED = Ue) is followed by a delayed viscoelastic phase Uv to reach the maximum distension (MD = Uf). The immediate elastic recovery (ER: Uf – Ur) is followed by a delayed viscoelastic phase ending with a residual distension (*RD*) following the Ua recovery

relaxation time (stress off), and the number of measurement cycles are selected. The quantitative parameters describe the elastic deformation and elastic recovery of the skin, the viscoelastic creep after both the initial deformation and the initial recovery, and the residual deformation. U_e is defined as the immediate elastic distention (ED) corresponding to the steep linear part of the curve computed at a very short interval after application of the suction, usually around 0.1 s. U_v refers to the delayed viscoelastic part of the skin deformation (creep). U_f corresponds to the maximum deformation (MD) combining the elastic distention U_e and the following viscoelastic deformation U_v. U_f is computed after various time intervals ranging from 1 to 10 s. This value of maximum deformation depends on the probe aperture and the applied suction. U_r is defined as the immediate elastic recovery (ER) of the skin after removal of the suction. It is measured in the steep linear part of the recovery, mostly 0.1 s after stopping the suction. U_a is equal to the total recovery deformation of the skin at the end point of the recovery phase. RD is the residual deformation of the skin persisting after completion of the stress-off measuring time.

All these determinations of parameters are computed by the device according to a predetermined timing of measurement. The investigator makes the choice and there is no standardized procedure as yet. As a result, caution should be taken before comparing data from different studies.

From the computed biomechanical parameters, different elastic and viscoelastic ratios have been proposed in order to characterize the mechanical functions of the skin:

- U_a/U_f is defined as the overall (biologic) elasticity. It is expressed in %, and it corresponds to the ratio of the total deformation recovery to the total deformation.
- U_r/U_e is defined as the basic elasticity ratio; it corresponds to the ratio of the immediate recovery to the immediate deformation without the contribution of the viscoelastic part.
- U_r/U_f is defined as the relative elastic recovery; it is equal to the ratio of immediate recovery to the total deformation.
- U_v/U_e is defined as the viscoelastic ratio; it is equal to the ratio of the viscoelastic deformation to elastic deformation.

Under repetitive measuring cycles, the deformation versus time curves obtained for the second, third, and subsequent deformation cycles are similar to the first, but they progressively shift upwards as a consequence of the residual deformation. The differential distension (DD, μm) is calculated as the difference between MDs reached at the last and the first cycles. As an example, three

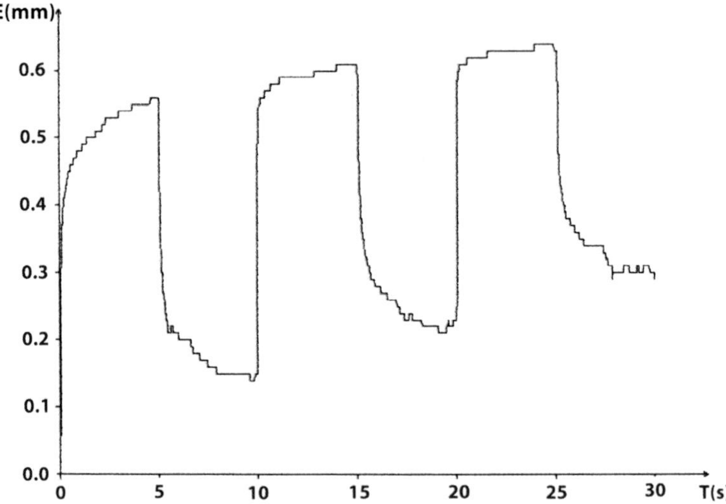

Fig. 2 Repetitive fluage tests showing the effect of preconditioning the skin with a progressive increase in the skin deformation

to five load (traction) cycles of 2–5-s tractions under negative pressure of 400 mbar are separated by identical relaxation periods (Fig. 2).

The second modality test corresponds to the hysteresis procedure using the stress/strain mode [38]. As an example, one cycle of progressively increasing suction at a linear rate of 25 mbar/s for 10–20 s is followed by a release of the depression at the same rate (Fig. 3). In this procedure, nonlinear curves are obtained. The suction curve on loading is not superposed by the relaxation curve. During the relaxation period, the values of strain do not return to zero and the curve intercepts the strain axis. Hysteresis (HY) represents the area delimited by the traction and relaxation curves given by the stress/strain method. It is measured using image analysis of the graphs yielded by the time/strain method.

Facial Skin Viscoelasticity Assessed by the Torque Method

The torque method at low stress provides information that appears quite similar to that described for the suction method. However, the skin layers subjected to the stress are difficult to identify. It was claimed that the contribution of the stratum corneum to the overall mechanical functions of the skin was increased using the torque method.

Ultrasound Speed Propagation and Air-Blown Technique

Subtle variations in tensile functions of the facial skin are conveniently studied by measuring the speed of propagation of ultrasound shear waves. The Reviscometer® RVM 600 (Courage + Khazaka Electronic) is available for that purpose. The resonance running time measurement (RRTM) is inversely correlated with the skin stiffness. Both the dermal mechanical functions and the stratum corneum suppleness/stiffness influence the data [31, 42]. It is assumed that the velocity of ultrasound propagation is affected by the orientation of the resting tension lines or Langer's lines [31].

The air-blown technique is another ingenious procedure for measuring the skin biomechanical functions under low stress [43].

Physiological Changes in Biomechanical Functions

There is general agreement that age, gender, skin thickness, and location on the body are the four main parameters that influence the rheological functions of the skin. They have to be taken into account before interpreting any given physiopathological process.

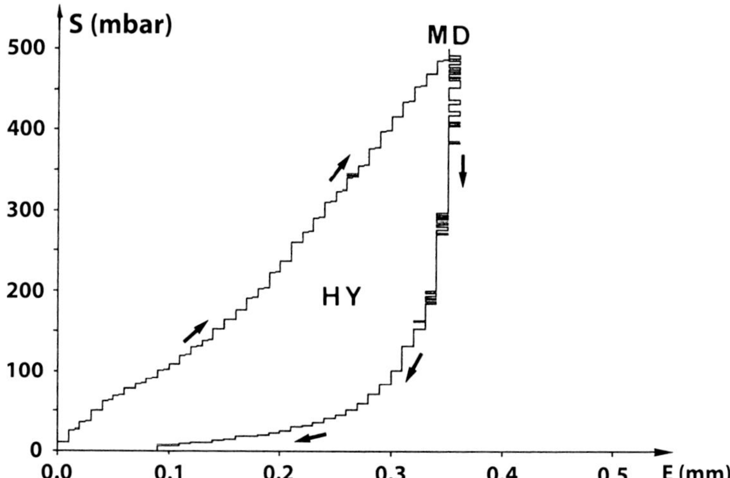

Fig. 3 Hysteresis procedure showing the evolution of the stress (*S*) – skin extension (*E*) under progressive but regular suction until the maximum distension (*MD*) is gained followed by a progressive relaxation phase. Hysteresis (*HY*) represents the area between the suction curve and the relaxation curve

Age Influence

Cutaneous aging encompasses distinct features. Chronologic or intrinsic aging depends on genetic factors, lapse of time, and the sum of various effects of diseases and desmotropic drugs (i.e., corticosteroids, phenitoin), as well as physiologic variations and environmental influences with the exception of sun exposure [14]. Photoaging deals with all these features to which chronic exposure to UV light and near-infrared radiations is superimposed [13, 14]. Some authors regard aging of the facial skin as a single and direct result of actinic insult, but this opinion is probably an oversimplification. In fact, dermatoheliosis is only one aspect of variable importance among subjects of similar age and phototype. On the face, it is superimposed to both the overall intrinsic aging process mainly responsible for tissue atrophy and to unrelated opposite hypertrophic changes consisting of compact solar elastosis. In addition, focal hyperplasia develops in the subcutaneous connective tissue where striated muscles are anchored. Such tissue remodeling resulting from distinct origins is responsible for the progressive deepening of the natural expression lines.

It is clinically obvious that the biomechanical functions of the skin are quite different in children and the elderly [10, 24, 29, 33]. They appear to be correlated with the skin surface patterns and wrinkling [43]. However, measuring them by different test modalities provides controversial findings regarding the nature of the changes and the moment when they take place. From the available information, it is probable that the resistance of the dermis to forces exerted parallel to the skin surface increases with age at least until 60 years. Conversely, the vertical resistances at the dermo-epidermal junction, as well as within the dermis and the hypodermis, progressively weaken.

All age-related changes in the skin obviously influence the biomechanical functions [44]. Moreover, mechanical stimuli applied to the skin throughout life affect the structure of the cutaneous tissues, which in turn modifies the biomechanical functions. Such multiple interrelationships between the various structures of the facial skin, as well as the innumerable factors influencing aging, and the complexity of the biomechanical properties likely preclude any clear-cut understanding of the problem.

Most of the studies on rheological functions of the aging skin were focused on the forearms. Little is known about corresponding changes on the facial skin. It has been shown that the skin elevation following suction depends on the force exerted, the body site, and the area of contact between the probe and the skin. It is particularly difficult to assess the influence of subcutaneous tethering. However, it is likely that the tests using a small hollow probe and producing small elevations of the skin are little influenced by subcutaneous attachments. In these instances, skin extensibility increases while elasticity decreases with aging of the facial skin [10]. However, the bulk of elevation experiments reveals wide variations in the skin deformability in aged individuals. Changes in the elastic rebound of the skin (BE and HY) are more constant, indicating a progressive decrease in these parameters over time.

Gender Influence

The influence of gender on the mechanical functions of the skin is subject of contradictory reports in the literature. Some consider that skin extensibility is higher, or that the modulus of elasticity is lower, in women than in men, but the reverse opinion has been expressed as well. The difference is in part due to different test modalities.

Skin Thickness Influence

The thickness of the dermis is a function of age and gender. It influences the biomechanical functions of the skin [10, 45]. This contention holds true when considering the extracellular matrix of the connective tissue. However, facial skin thickness appears considerably influenced by the density and size of the sebaceous glands. Such a double-component structure exhibits peculiar biomechanical functions. The importance of the facial skin thickness is further complicated by the variable extent in solar elastosis.

Credentiating Antiaging Treatments

During the past decades, the dermocosmetic science applied to the facial skin was considerably influenced by the clinical presentation of aging. Specific cosmetics, cosmeceuticals, and drugs are designed for corrective purposes [46, 47]. A few studies were conducted to assess the rheological changes following the regular use of specific topical treatments [35, 48, 49]. The effects were correlated with the histological nature of wrinkles and improvement of the skin relief.

Other minimally invasive methods are available for improving the appearance of aging face [46]. Among them, the filling procedures, the peelings, the botulinum toxin, the photorejuvenation, and still other nonablative resurfacing procedures are popular. No information is available regarding the induced changes in biomechanical functions of the skin. The same lack of information applies to the effects of skin lifting, lipoaugmentation, and other invasive surgical procedures.

Active cosmetic products, called cosmeceuticals in some countries and quasi-drugs in others, have been rapidly expanding and becoming increasingly sophisticated. The potential value of these formulations for skin health is undisputable. Yet both the consumer and the dermocosmetologist are challenged when evaluating their benefits. Many dermatologic prescriptions fall short of patient expectations, opening the way for the use of cosmeceuticals to enhance the outcome. However, the physician has some guarantee that some pharmaceuticals are at least moderately effective.

When dealing with the facial skin, testing the effects of products on the rheological functions of the skin is difficult to predict when using the suction method on the model of the forearm skin. Only indirect and partial information is obtained.

Conclusion

The evaluation of the biomechanical functions of the skin is useful in dermocosmetic science. A series of different methods using dedicated devices provide different information, although those useful in practice are limited in number. The lack of standardization often precludes the comparison of results obtained by different groups of workers.

In terms of bioengineering, the skin withstands and transmits mechanical forces through specific deformations. Creep and stress relaxation effects are well recognized. This fact implies that the time rate of application of forces onto the skin influences the data when assessing the load transmitting capabilities of the tissue. The comparison between different rheological methods applicable to the face indicates that the progressive increase and release of suction in the stress/strain mode yield the greatest relative variations with age. Hence, this methodology appears well suited to study facial skin aging and the efficacy of products aiming at its correction.

Tests performed in vivo are likely to have the most value for clinical purposes but have special problems of their own:

- The dermis in vivo is under a variable degree of resting tension. Langer's lines are an expression of the state of resting tension in the skin and indicate the orientation of maximum tension.
- There are intimate connections between the dermis, the epidermis, and its pilosebaceous adnexa, as well as between the dermis and the hypodermis. It is virtually impossible to isolate the dermis from its intimately associated neighboring structures when tests are performed in vivo. Inevitably, the tests performed are, in part, testing the epidermal, adnexal, and hypodermal functions as well. It is, however, quite evident that in most cases the results reflect mainly the properties and functions of the dermal collagen fiber bundles. The scope of these tests must be borne in mind when interpreting their results.
- Clearly, the results of biomechanical testing depend on the dimensions of the site being investigated. It is relatively easy to define the length and breadth of the area tested, but the skin thickness decreases with age and is commonly greater in men than women. It is susceptible to a number of endocrine and environmental influences. In addition, the mechanical functions of the dermis are time dependent.

References

1. Nkengne A, et al. Influence of facial skin attributes on the perceived age of Caucasian women. J Eur Acad Dermatol Venereol. 2008;22:982–91.
2. Gunn DA, et al. Perceived age as a biomarker of ageing: a clinical methodology. Biogerontology. 2008;9:357–64.
3. D'Souza R, et al. Enhancing facial aesthetics with muscle retraining exercises-a review. J Clin Diagn Res. 2014;8:ZE09–11.
4. Freund AM, Isaacowitz DM. Aging and social perception: so far, more similarities than differences. Psychol Aging. 2014;29:451–3.
5. Weiss D. What will remain when we are gone? Finitude and generation identity in the second half of life. Psychol Aging. 2014;29:554–62.
6. Zebrowitz LA, et al. Older and younger adults' accuracy in discerning health and competence in older and younger faces. Psychol Aging. 2014;29:454–68.
7. Rexbye H, et al. Influence of environmental factors on facial ageing. Age Ageing. 2006;35:110–5.
8. Witten TM. Introduction to the theory of aging networks. Interdiscip Top Gerontol. 2015;40:1–17.
9. Kawasaki K, et al. Age-related morphometric changes of inner structures of the skin assessed by in vivo reflectance confocal microscopy. Int J Dermatol. 2014;53:e561–6.
10. Piérard GE. EEMCO guidance to the in vivo assessment of tensile functional properties of the skin. Part 1: relevance to the structures and ageing of the skin and subcutaneous tissues. Skin Pharmacol Appl Skin Physiol. 1999;12:352–62.
11. Hendriks FM, et al. The relative contributions of different skin layers to the mechanical behavior of human skin in vivo using suction experiments. Med Eng Phys. 2006;28:259–66.
12. Ryu HS, et al. Influence of age and regional differences on skin elasticity as measured by the Cutometer. Skin Res Technol. 2008;14:354–8.
13. Schroeder P, et al. The role of near infrared radiation in photoaging of the skin. Exp Gerontol. 2008;43:629–32.
14. Farage MA, et al. Intrinsic and extrinsic factors in skin ageing: a review. Int J Cosmet Sci. 2008;30:87–95.
15. Devillers C, et al. Environmental dew point and skin and lip weathering. J Eur Acad Dermatol Venereol. 2010;24:513–7.
16. Piérard-Franchimont C, et al. Immunohistochemical patterns in the interfollicular Caucasian scalps: influences of age, gender, and alopecia. Biomed Res Int. 2013;2013:769489.
17. Ambroisine L, et al. Relationships between visual and tactile features and biophysical parameters in human facial skin. Skin Res Technol. 2007;13:176–83.
18. Wan D, et al. The clinical importance of the fat compartments in midfacial aging. Plast Reconstr Surg Glob Open. 2013;1:e92.
19. Wan D, et al. The differing adipocyte morphologies of deep versus superficial midfacial fat compartments: a cadaveric study. Plast Reconstr Surg. 2014;133:615e–22.
20. Hermanns-Lê T, et al. Scrutinizing skinfield melanin patterns in young Caucasian women. Expert Opin Med Diagn. 2013;7:455–62.
21. Akazaki S, et al. Age-related changes in skin wrinkles assessed by a novel three-dimensional morphometric analysis. Br J Dermatol. 2002;147:689–95.
22. Piérard GE, et al. From skin microrelief to wrinkles. An area ripe for investigation. J Cosmet Dermatol. 2003;2:21–8.
23. Fukuda Y, et al. A new method to evaluate lower eyelid sag using three-dimensional image analysis. Int J Cosmet Sci. 2005;27:283–90.

24. Saito N, et al. Development of a new evaluation method for cheek sagging using a Moire 3D analysis system. Skin Res Technol. 2008;14:287–92.
25. Piérard GE, et al. Ageing and rheological properties of facial skin in women. Gerontology. 1998;44:159–61.
26. Weiss RA, et al. Clinical trial of a novel non-thermal LED array for reversal of photoaging: clinical, histologic, and surface profilometric results. Lasers Surg Med. 2005;36:85–91.
27. Piérard-Franchimont C, et al. Climacteric skin ageing of the face – a prospective longitudinal comparative trial on the effect of oral hormone replacement therapy. Maturitas. 1999;32:87–93.
28. Staloff IA, et al. An in vivo study of the mechanical properties of facial skin and influence of aging using digital image speckle correlation. Skin Res Technol. 2008;14:127–34.
29. Piérard GE, et al. Biomechanical assessment of photodamage. Derivation of a cutaneous extrinsic ageing score. Skin Res Technol. 1995;1:17–20.
30. Piérard GE, Lapière CM. Microanatomy of the dermis in relation to relaxed skin tension lines and Langer's lines. Am J Dermatopathol. 1987;9:219–24.
31. Hermanns-Lê T, et al. Age- and body mass index-related changes in cutaneous shear wave velocity. Exp Gerontol. 2001;36:363–72.
32. Jacquet E, et al. A new experimental method for measuring skin's natural tension. Skin Res Technol. 2008;14:1–7.
33. Takema Y, et al. Age-related changes in the elastic properties and thickness of human facial skin. Br J Dermatol. 1994;131:641–8.
34. Hermanns-Lê T, et al. Skin tensile properties revisited during ageing. Where now, where next? J Cosmet Dermatol. 2004;3:35–40.
35. Piérard-Franchimont C, et al. Tensile properties and contours of aging facial skin. A controlled double-blind comparative study of the effects of retinol, melibiose-lactose and their association. Skin Res Technol. 1998;4:237–43.
36. Khatyr F, et al. Model of the viscoelastic behaviour of skin in vivo and study of anisotropy. Skin Res Technol. 2004;10:96–103.
37. Piérard GE, et al. In vivo evaluation of the skin tensile strength by the suction method: pilot study coping with hysteresis and creep extension. ISRN Dermatol. 2013;2013:841217.
38. Piérard GE, et al. Asymmetric facial skin viscoelasticity during climacteric aging. Clin Cosmet Investig Dermatol. 2014;7:111–8.
39. Piérard GE, et al. Skin viscoelasticity during hormone replacement therapy for climacteric ageing. Int J Cosmet Sci. 2014;36:88–92.
40. Delalleau A, et al. A nonlinear elastic behavior to identify the mechanical parameters of human skin in vivo. Skin Res Technol. 2008;14:152–64.
41. Khatyr F, et al. Measurement of the mechanical properties of the skin using the suction test. Skin Res Technol. 2006;12:24–31.
42. Xhauflaire-Uhoda E, et al. Kinetics of moisturizing and firming effects of cosmetic formulations. Int J Cosmet Sci. 2008;30:131–8.
43. Ahn S, et al. Correlation between a Cutometer and quantitative evaluation using Moire topography in age-related skin elasticity. Skin Res Technol. 2007;13:280–4.
44. Fujimura T, et al. Development of a novel method to measure the elastic properties of skin including subcutaneous tissue: new age-related parameters and scope of application. Skin Res Technol. 2008;14:504–11.
45. Smalls LK, et al. Effect of dermal thickness, tissue composition, and body site on skin biomechanical properties. Skin Res Technol. 2006;12:43–9.
46. Bogle MA. Minimally invasive techniques for improving the appearance of the aging face. Expert Rev Dermatol. 2007;2:427–35.
47. Lee DH, et al. Improvement in skin wrinkles using a preparation containing human growth factors and hyaluronic acid serum. J Cosmet Laser Ther. 2015;17:20–3.
48. Piérard GE, et al. Comparative effect of short-term topical tretinoin and glycolic acid on mechanical properties of photodamaged facial skin in HRT-treated menopausal women. Maturitas. 1996;23:273–7.
49. Uhoda I, et al. Split face study on the cutaneous tensile effect of 2-dimethylaminoethanol (deanol) gel. Skin Res Technol. 2002;8:164–7.

Pathology of Aging Skin

28

Qunshan Jia and J. Frank Nash

Contents

Abstract

Human skin is a dynamic complex organ functioning as both a physical and biochemical barrier to protect the human body from water loss and environmental insults while providing multiple life-sustaining physiological functions. Skin undergoes a chronological aging process accompanied by physical changes, clinical manifestations, and psychological consequences. At the level of epidermis, defects in stratum corneum integrity and subsequent barrier dysfunction following external insults are observed in aged humans. An increase in pH in the stratum corneum of aging skin may decrease the concentration of lipids leading to defects in stratum corneum homeostasis and epidermal barrier function. At the level of upper dermis, fragmentation and reduction in collagen and elastin as well as a collapse in fibroblast morphology underline the majority of the undesired dermal clinical manifestations including the loss of dermal mechanical tension resulting in skin laxity and fine wrinkles. Both intracellular factors including attack by reactive oxygen species, DNA telomere shortening, and damage to DNA repair enzymes and intercellular microenvironmental factors including breakdown of the extracellular matrix and microinflammation are considered important in the process of skin aging.

Q. Jia (✉) • J.F. Nash
The Procter & Gamble Company, Central Product Safety, Cincinnati, OH, USA
e-mail: jia.q.3@pg.com; nash.jf@pg.com

M.A. Farage et al. (eds.), *Textbook of Aging Skin*,
DOI 10.1007/978-3-662-47398-6_28

Introduction

Human skin is the largest and arguably the most complex organ, functioning as a physical and biochemical barrier to protect the human body from water loss as well as environmental insults including pathogens, chemicals, physical agents, and solar ultraviolet radiation (UVR) throughout life. More than that, the skin provides crucial physiological functions including immune defense, thermoregulation, sensory reception, endocrine, as well as metabolism.

Aging is the chronological process accompanied by a progressive loss of physiological function in multiple organs. Skin undergoes an aging process accompanied by physical changes, clinical manifestations, and significant physiological consequences. According to recent statistics, around 25 % of Americans are expected to be 65 years or older by the year 2030 [1]. Therefore, it is important to understand the process of chronological skin aging and its accompanying physiological consequences to anticipate health-related needs in the twenty-first century.

Skin Development and Anatomic Structure

To better understand the pathology and physiology of the aging skin, it is crucial to understand the development, anatomic structure, and physiological function of normal skin.

Structure and Function of Skin

The skin is structurally divided into epidermis and dermis separated by basement membrane. Epidermis is the major protective outer layer with keratinocytes as the major cell population. The epidermis is a stratified epithelium derived from a single layer of ectoderm after gastrulation. Wingless Int (Wnt)/Bone Morphogenetic Proteins (BMP) signaling enables the ectoderm cells to adopt an epidermal fate instead of neurogenesis by inhibiting fibroblast growth factor (FGF) signaling pathways. Over time, the embryonic epidermis will differentiate into epidermal cells under the influences of BMP, Notch signaling, the hair placode, and eventually the hair follicle induced by Wnt signaling and its downstream signaling including SHH, GLI1, PTC. The sebaceous glands are appendages of hair follicles, the origin of which remains unknown [2].

The stratified epidermis is around 100–150 μm thick, which can be further divided into four distinct layers (bottom to top): stratum basale, stratum spinosum, stratum granulosum, and stratum corneum, as illustrated in Fig. 1. The stratum basale consists of epidermal stem cells, a single layer of columnar cells attached to the basal lamina via hemidesmosomes and expressing keratin (K) 14 and K5. Once the cell leaves the basal layer toward the skin surface, it starts to express K1 and K10 in the stratum spinosum. The stratum spinosum, which contains lipid-enriched lamellar bodies, becomes progressively larger due to keratin synthesis and lipogenesis and finally reaches a stage called stratum granulosum with unique lamellar bodies and is ready to differentiate into corneocytes. Finally, intracellular organelles in the corneocyte undergo self-destruction and the lipid packaged in lamellar granules (LG) is released into the intercellular space. The LGs are small organelles full of stacks of lipid lamellae consisting of phospholipids, cholesterol, glucosylceramides, and several enzymes important for the lipid processing including acid hydrolases, ß-glucocerebrosidase, phospholipid A2, and lysosomal acid lipase [3]. Once released from the LGs, the short stacks of lipid membranes will reorganize and transform into an edge-to-edge fusion catalyzed by enzymes released at the same time. In the end, the stratum corneum will form the outermost seal in human skin with 18–21 cell layers 20–40 μm thick consisting mainly of dead corneocytes and the secreted lipids [3].

The brick and mortar structure is a classic model for the organization of the stratum corneum. The most important functions of the stratum corneum is prevention of water loss and percutaneous absorption of xenobiotics [4]. During the final stages of keratinocyte differentiation,

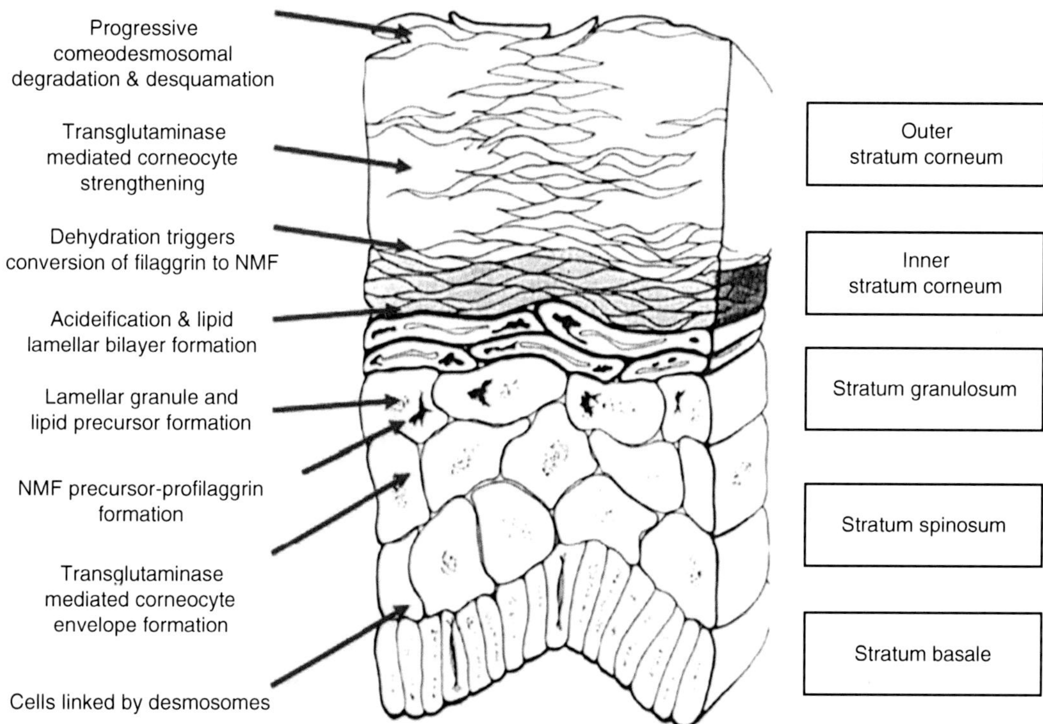

Fig. 1 The structure of the epidermis. The epidermis is made up of the stratum corneum (SC), stratum granulosum, stratum spinosum, and stratum basale from outside to inside. The stratum basale consists of epidermal stem cells, a single layer of columnar cells attached to the basal lamina via hemidesmosomes. The stratum spinosum is rich with lipid-enriched lamellar bodies that become progressively larger due to the keratin synthesis and lipogenesis. The stratum granulosum has unique lamellar bodies and is ready to differentiate into corneocytes. Finally, corneocyte intracellular organelles undergo self-destruction and the lipid packaged in lamellar granules (LG) is released to the intercellular space. The SC forms the outermost seal consisting of dead corneocytes and the secreted lipids. Filaggrin is a key protein required for the formation of the stratum corneum (SC) barrier

the intracellular keratins and filaggrin will interact with each other to form a condensed protein complex, transforming the epidermal cell into a flattened corneocyte. The "bricks" are the multiple layers of protein-enriched dead corneocytes tightly packed and surrounded by a very dense cross-linked protein structure called the cornified envelope. This protein envelope is cross-linked with the surrounding lipid envelope, the "mortar" which is made up of hydrophobic lipid lamellae in the intercellular regions and gives the skin physical protection against water and other molecules [5].

Multiple genes have been identified which play important roles in skin barrier function. For example, aberrant expression of filaggrin will result in multiple barrier defects from atopic dermatitis to flaky skin [6]. Involucrin, loricrin, and trihohyalin are major protein components on the surface of the corneocyte cross-linked by transglutaminases to form a protein envelope. Excessive loss of water and neonatal death has been observed in transglutaminase-deficient mice, illustrating the importance of the stratum corneum's barrier function during development [7]. The specific cell-cell junction between stratum corneum and stratum granulosum, named desmosomes, is also critical, the loss of which disrupts the stratum cell adhesion resulting in barrier function defects [8].

The lipid composition of the stratum corneum is critical for barrier function. Studies have shown that the stratum corneum consists of mainly equimolar ratios of ceramides, cholesterol, and free fatty acids. Ceramides are crucial in the formation of the lipid envelope and a deficiency is associated with atopic dermatitis [9]. Cholesterol is synthesized by the epidermis and is important for intermixing different lipids. The cholesterol efflux is regulated by a membrane transporter named ATP-binding cassette subgroup 1 member transporter or ABCA12. Failure of different enzymes involved in cholesterol synthesis results in significant epidermal barrier defects [6]. Finally, essential fatty acid deficiency will also result in a red, rough skin with significant transepidermal water loss [10, 11] and disruption of gene coding for fatty acid transport protein 4 (FatP4) has been found to result in neonatal death due to disturbed skin permeability [12].

The nucleated lower layers of the epidermis are important for mediating barrier function. The entire loss of the epidermis will lead to life-threatening water loss and rampant microbiological infection, compared to the relatively mild consequences associated with stratum corneum damage [6]. Multiple cell-cell tight junction proteins such as claudins, zonula occludens protein-1, and multi-PDZ protein-1 have been found in the stratum granulosum and the upper stratum spinosum. The importance of these tight junctions is illustrated by extreme water loss in mice with claudin-1 and E-cadherin deficiency.

Adherens and desmosomes are a group of junction proteins essential for stabilizing the cell-cell adhesion in the living layer of the epidermis. Reducing desmoglein-3 and E-caldherin will result in a barrier defect leading to either leaky tight junctions or a lethal dehydration [6]. The intercellular gap junctions are important channels for cell-cell communication. Disturbing such gap junctions, found in connexin 43 loss of function mouse studies, results in barrier defects [6]. Keratins are the major component of intrakeratinocyte filament web which interacts with the junction proteins, desmosomes, and hemidesmosomes. Homozygous K10 knockout mice will develop an extremely delicate epidermis while heterozygous K10 mice will show impaired barrier function repair and skin hydration defects, demonstrating the importance of this differentiation-related protein's effect on epidermal barrier function [6].

Epidermis Homeostasis and Turnover

In healthy skin, the epidermis replenishes itself and maintains a status of homeostasis in response to physical and chemical challenges. In humans, the turnover rate for the epidermis is approximately 4 weeks. During this process, cells in the stratum basale divide and move upward while undergoing differentiation during this progression. Both symmetric and asymmetric models have been used to describe this process. In the symmetric model, the stratum basale daughter cells with lower levels of integrin after mitosis will detach and begin the journey to becoming part of the stratum corneum. Daughter cells with higher levels of integrin will keep their proliferating potential and stay attached to the basement membrane. In the asymmetric model, the mitotic epidermal cells divide disproportionately so that the attached daughter cells receive more integrin and growth factors to keep them attached to the basement membrane and proliferating while the detached suprabasal daughter cells receive less or dissimilar signals such as Notch, leading to differentiation and commitment to stratum corneum replacement [2].

Proliferation and growth of cells in the stratum basale must be tightly controlled to ensure the normal function of the stratum corneum. Studies have found that the extracellular matrix (ECM) and growth factors residing in the basement membrane play a crucial role in controlling cell proliferation in the stratum basale. Two types of junctions are responsible for the cell-ECM connection. The hemidesmosomes containing $\alpha6\beta4$ integrin and the focal adhesions containing $\alpha3\beta1$ integrin control growth and migration through a physical interaction with kinases such as Ras/MAPK signaling. The E-caldherin in cell-cell junctions also contributes to basal cell proliferation and migration through its association with regulatory proteins such as Rho-GTPase. Although the exact mechanisms are unclear, it is accepted that the adherens junction can serve as a signaling center and sense the epidermal cell density and thus provide a feedback loop through specific signaling kinase pathways to control cell activity and proliferation [2].

The epidermal barrier function is also maintained by multiple signaling pathways as indicated by studies of acute skin disruption. For example, proinflammatory cytokines including interleukin-1, interleukin-6, as well as tumor necrosis factors (TNF) have been observed following acute barrier damage. As well, knocking down these genes will delay barrier formation after acute disruption [6]. Recently, a calcium gradient was identified in the epidermis with the highest calcium concentration in stratum granulosum and the lowest concentration in stratum corneum. Calcium is crucial for lamellar body exocytosis and epidermal protein synthesis at the later stage of keratinocyte differentiation and migration in response to barrier permeability damage. In addition, calcium plays important roles for transglutaminase I activity and cell-cell adhesion during epidermal differentiation. The relationship between the calcium level and the transmembrane water loss has been observed in Darier's and Hailey-Hailey diseases caused by the defects of a gene encoding a calcium transporter [6]. Another signaling pathway important in maintaining the barrier is 3′5′-cyclic adenosine monophosphate (cAMP), a secondary messenger in multiple systems. Biochemistry studies have revealed a reverse relationship between the cAMP level and the barrier recovery after acute epidermal damage. Vascular endothelial growth factor (VEGF) generated by the epidermis is also required for the integrity of the barrier function with homozygous VEGF knockout mice showing impaired permeability barrier homeostasis after acute repeated tape striping. Finally, a new mechanism has been suggested for maintaining epidermal homeostasis in which both the lipid matrix and corneocytes are involved. In general, the disruption of stratum corneum will inevitably increase cytokines and calcium concentrations within the epidermis, which in turn will promote lipid synthesis and secretion into the intercellular matrix to facilitate barrier recovery. At the same time, epidermal cornification will be enhanced by serine protease and caspase-14 signaling turned on by protease-activated receptor type 2 (PAR2) in response to acute barrier defects [13].

The fibroblasts located in the dermis can also influence the homeostasis of epidermis. Studies using in vitro reconstructed skin study papillary fibroblasts from aged donors (>75 years old) lose the potential to promote epidermal morphogenesis more than the same cell type taken from young donors [14]. In in vivo studies with nude mice, papillary fibroblasts from young human donors were more potent than corresponding older donors in developing a correctly stratified and differentiated epidermis and formation of normal rete-ridge structure [14]. Dermal fibroblast cells are also required to form cutaneous basement membrane structure in the presence of keratinocyte by producing lamin, type IV, VII collagens and/or by influencing keratinocytes in the formation of basement membrane [15]. Recent data show that keratinocyte proliferation is controlled by the dermal fibroblasts through IL-1 beta signal-mediated AP-1-dependent mitogenic factor which can be inhibited by sIL-1ra under the control of PPAR β/δ [16].

In addition to the keratinocytes, several other cellular populations are found in the epidermis including Langerhans cells, Merkel cells, and melanocytes. Langerhans cells are dendritic cells residing in the epidermis involved in antigen presentation and immunoserveillance [17]. Melanocytes are cells derived from neural crest responsible for skin pigment and hair color through melanin production. They are usually found in the basal layer of epidermis and in hair follicle. Merkel cells are also derived from the neural crest cells and are associated with the sensory nerve endings.

Dermis

The dermis, located below the epidermis basement membrane, is rich with blood supply providing nutrients and circulatory support to the epidermis. In humans, the boundary between the epidermis and dermis undulates due to epidermal protrusions into the dermis resulting in "rete pegs." The cellular populations account for 10 % of the dermal content including the fibrocyte, monocyte, histiocyte, Langerhans cells, lymphocytes, and eosinophils, along with the vascular- and lymphatic-associated cells while the remaining 90 % is mainly connective tissue matrix made up of Type I collagen, elastic fibers, and blood vessels. The collagen in the dermis provides mechanical protection to the body as well as the shape and form by holding all structures together. The blood plexus provides oxygen and nutrients to the living part of the epidermis and removes waste products of metabolism from the epidermis. Body temperature regulation through control of blood flow and sweating as well as the sensations of touch, pain, heat, and cold through the neural fiber embedded in the dermis are all functions that reside in the tissue layer [18].

Skin Physiology

Immune Function

While the skin acts as the principal barrier to protect the body from the water loss, it also serves as a nonspecific defense against infectious organisms. Phagocytic cells such as neutrophils, macrophages, and natural killer cells (NK) present in the skin play a significant role in defense against pathogens. Meanwhile the complement system and cytokines turned on by components of pathogens, e.g., LPS, also contribute to the innate immune response of the skin. Both the innate and adaptive immune responses are equally critical to the host defense against foreign invaders. The skin possesses important peripheral components such as Langerhans cells (LC) and extravasated lymphocytes from circulation for adaptive immune responses. The dendritic LC will process and present an antigen to the resident T lymphocytes which will initiate a cell-mediated acquired immune response [19–22]. Generally, the skin will initiate a rapid cytokine-driven cutaneous inflammation in response to keratinocyte injury followed by a specific adapted immune response to foreign antigens with high specification and immune memory. Recent studies have shown the epidermal keratinocyte cell-cell junctions will promote the immune response after the skin is injured. It has been found that β-catenins in cell-cell junctions function not only as adhesion molecules but also as transcription regulators. Through unknown mechanisms, p120 catenin and α-catenin can affect the transcriptional activity of NF-κB to induce cytokines. It is hypothesized that keratinocyte injury will trigger the catenin/NF-κB signaling cascade, inducing cytokines, chemokines which will recruit immune cells to initiate the innate immune response first and adapted immune response later. Once the epidermis is repaired and the cell-cell junction returns to normal, the inflammation will diminish. This is supported by the findings that chronic inflammation will develop after α-catenin and p120 are mutated [2, 21].

Skin Metabolism

In addition to its physical barrier, the skin also functions as an important extrahepatic organ to metabolically activate or detoxify xenobiotics by virtue of enzymatic activities in epidermis and dermis. Most of the metabolizing enzymes are located in the epidermis [23]. For example, cytochrome P-450 is present in the skin and responsible for the oxidative metabolism of steroid hormones including androgens, estrogens, progesterone, and glucocorticoids, as well as fatty acids. As the major Phase-I enzyme, P-450 plays a critical role in metabolic detoxification or, in some cases, activation. The presence of Phase-II conjugating enzymes such as glucoronyltransferase, sulfotransferase, and glutathione-S-transferase enables the skin to further detoxify and eliminate the metabolites generated from Phase-1 reactions. The major enzymes found in the skin and involved in metabolism are presented in Table 1 [24].

Skin Sensory and Thermoregulation

Advances in immunochemical staining have revealed the presence of neuronal fibers in the epidermis. More than 90 % of these are small-diameter, unmyelinated C-fiber and/or thinly myelinated A-d fibers located in the border between of the basement membrane and

Table 1 Classes of enzymes detected in skin (Adapted from Smith et al. [24])

Phase I enzymes activation/functionalization mechanisms	Function
Microsomal mixed function oxidase	Hydroxylation
Cytochrome P450 with NADPH dehydrogenase	Alcohol oxidation
	Epoxidation
	N-, O- and S-dealkylation oxidative deamination
	N- and S-oxidation
	Dehalogenation
	Reduction of azo and nitro compounds
	Ring cleavage of heterocyclic ring systems
Alcohol dehydrogenases	Interconversion of alcohols and aldehydes
Aldeyde dehydrogenases	Conversion of aldehydes to acids
Flavin-containing monooxygenases	Oxidation of secondary and tertiary amines
	Oxidation of imines and arylamines
Esterases	Ester hydrolysis to yield acid and alcohol
Amidases	Amide hydrolysis
Phase II enzymes and conjugation reactions	
UDP-glucuronosyltransferase	Glucuronidation
Sulphotransferase	Sulphation
Methyltransferase	Methylation
Acetyltransferase	Acetylation
Glutathione S-transferase	Glutathione conjugation at epoxides and halides
Miscellaneous reactions condensation	Amino acid conjugation

epidermis. The major functions of cutaneous neuronal fibers are sensory and integration of incoming signals for pain, itch, and other stimuli. The epidermal nervous system possesses important efferent paracrine and trophic functions that effect cutaneous cells, immune cells, and other axons.

Thermal regulation of the human body is controlled by receptors located in the skin called transient receptor potential (TRP) superfamily which are cation-selective ion channels consisting of six transmembrane subunits. TRPs are activated within a specific temperature range in response to the environmental temperature changes. With the cooperation of central nervous system, healthy individuals will get rid of excess heat by sweating and vasodilation when it is too hot and minimize heat loss through vasoconstriction, and increase heat generation by shivering when it is too cold. The sweat glands dispersed within the skin help control body temperature sweat evaporation. Up to 2 L of sweat can be evaporated in an hour mainly by the eccrine glands. This control for body temperature through sweat production is important for thermal maintenance [25].

Structural and Physiological Changes in Aged Skin

Chronological aging is an inevitable biological process leading to structural and functional changes during the life span of all organisms. This programmed route is inherently determined by genetics and is significantly affected by multiple environmental factors. Dryness, wrinkles, irregular pigmentation are the primary visual event seen in the aging skin of human beings accompanied by histological changes ranging from impaired stratum corneum replenishment to a flattening of the dermal–epidermal junction, a marked loss in elasticity, and atrophy of the dermal connective tissue due to a reduction and disorganization of its major extracellular matrix

Table 2 Characteristic of intrinsic aging (Adapted from Farage et al. [29])

Characteristic	Intrinsic aging
Overall	
Metabolic processes	Slow down
Clinical appearance	Smooth unblemished, loss of elasticity, fine wrinkles
Skin color	Pigment diminishes to pallor
Skin surface marking	Maintains youthful geometric patterns
Onset	Typically 50s–60s (woman earlier than men)
Severity	Only slightly associated to degree of pigmentation
Epidermis	
Thickness	Thins with aging (not consistent)
Proliferative rate	Lower than normal
Keratinocytes	Modest cellular irregularity
Dermo-epidermal junction	Modest reduplication of lamina dense
Dermis	
Elastin	Elastogenesis followed by elastolysis
Elastin matrix	Gradual decline in production of dermal matrix, only modest increase in the number and thickness of elastic fibres in the reticular dermis

components [26–28]. The characteristic histological changes and its impact on barrier function during aging will be reviewed (Table 2).

Anatomic Changes in Aging Skin

Epidermis

The overall histology change in epidermal thickness is neither obvious nor consistent with the conclusion that this structure is "thinner" in aged skin [30]. There is general agreement, however, that the intersection of the epidermis and dermis is flattened in aged skin with a correspondingly diminished connecting surface area leading to increased fragility and reduced nutrient transfer between the dermal and epidermal layers. A 30–50 % decrease in epidermal turnover rate has also been observed in the third to eighth decades of life. Such an impaired epidermal turnover rate might account for some of the pathological findings in aged people [18, 26, 27].

Another significant change in the epidermis of aging skin is in the amount of glycosaminoglycans (GAGs), the primary constituents of skin which hold water up to 1,000 times their weight. Hyaluronic acids (HAs) are a major type of GAGs and are produced by fibroblasts in the dermis and keratinocytes in the epidermis. In the epidermis, HAs are localized in the epidermal intercellular spaces at the middle spinous layer. The total amount of HAs is reduced significantly in the epidermis which may contribute to the reduced water binding and some of the visible changes of the aged skin, including wrinkling, altered elasticity, reduced turgidity, and diminished capacity to support the microvasculature of the skin. However, older and younger subjects have a comparable amount of HAs in dermis [18, 27].

Dermis

In contrast to the epidermis, a consistent lost of 20 % dermal thickness has been observed in aged skin, characterized by reduced cellular components and vascular networks [26]. For example, in aging skin a reduction of collagen due to decreased synthesis by fibroblasts has been observed. As the primary structural component and the most abundant protein found in dermis, collagen is responsible for conferring strength and support to the structure of human skin. In aged skin, the collagen organization is characterized by disarrayed thickened fibrils in rope-like bundles in comparison to the more structured pattern observed in younger skin. The ratio of collagen types also changes with age due to the loss of collagen I in aged skin. Overall, the collagen content per unit area of skin surface is known to decline approximately 1 % per year. The loss of collagen in intrinsically aged skin will lead to an epidermal and dermal atrophy characterized by flattening of the rete ridges and subsequent wrinkle formation (Table 2).

The accumulation of broken elastic fibers has been observed as well. Elastin is a connective tissue protein that allows many tissues in the body to resume their shape after stretching or contracting. An accumulation of amorphous elastin material has been associated with aging and attributed to the increased level of matrix metalloproteinases which are thought to play a role in elastin degradation. The aging dermis has a reduced vascular network in comparison to young skin which will result in reduced blood flow, impaired nutrient exchange, inhibited thermoregulation, and decreased skin surface temperature. Melanocytes, which can synthesize melanin to protect the skin from UV light, are also reduced in older subjects by 8–20 % per decade. For this reason, sun protection remains critically important for elderly patients [18, 26–28].

Changes in Skin Barrier Function

Basal transepidermal water loss (TEWL) has been measured in humans and mice to assess the impact of aging on skin barrier function. The results have revealed no significant change in TEWL in aged subjects (>80 years) compared to the young adult (<30 years) with similar results in mice [31]. Further analysis found no difference in the quantity of laminar bundles in granular cells or the composition of fatty acids in stratum corneum. There was, however, a reduction in total lipid level by 30 % [31, 32].

In spite of the seemingly normal TEWL in older subjects under basal conditions, both barrier function and stratum corneum integrity defects are observed in aged epidermis when stressed. For example, the number of tape strips required to perturb measures of barrier function is about 18 for aged compared to 30 for younger human subjects [31]. Similarly, time for acetone-induced barrier perturbation is less than 10 min in older subjects compared to 30–60 min in younger humans. In addition, the barrier function recovery rate is delayed significantly in older human subjects and hairless mice models compared to their younger cohorts after acute tape stripping. These studies suggest that differences in skin function of older people may only emerge following barrier disruption.

pH and Barrier Function in the Aged Skin

The pH of the stratum corneum is essential for epidermal barrier homeostasis. Stratum corneum acidification has been reported to be impaired in moderately aged human subjects with surface pH in unperturbed skin increasing from 5 to around 5.5. In this regard, a higher pH may result in a reduced level of stratum corneum lipids, which might be the biochemical basis for such defects in older humans [31–33]. Following acute epidermal disruption, an acidic environment is needed for lipid processing enzymes such as ß-glucocerebrosidase and spingomyelinase to function after lamellar bodies (LB) secretion. This association has been confirmed in studies showing delayed barrier recovery at neutral pH and a defective dynamic barrier in neonate stratum corneum having a surface pH around 7.0 [34–36]. Inhibition of the Na^+/K^+ antiporter, NHE1, and sPLA2 will significantly delay postnatal acidification of the skin. These studies suggest that acidic pH is mainly established by endogenous phospholipase and NHE1 through hydrolyzing membrane phospholipids and generating acidifying free fatty acids [36, 37].

Both morphological and biochemical studies have shown that epidermal lipid synthesis was similar in moderately aged (**50–80 years**) and young individuals based on comparable levels of LB in epidermis and mRNA for key enzymes responsible for lipid synthesis. However, defective epidermis lipid processing was observed in the analysis of moderate-aged subjects in contrast to the total lipid synthesis and secretion defects observed within the epidermis in advanced age, i. e., >70 years old [38]. A delayed formation of mature lamellar membrane after 6 h of disruption was found at the SG-SC boundary in the epidermis of moderately aged subjects accompanied by diminished BGC activity revealed by in situ zymography assay. In addition to the lipid processing defects in the epidermis, an increased pH has been proposed to activate a different family of enzymes, namely, the serine proteases, which will degrade the cell–cell junction protein corneodemosomes (CD) disrupting the epidermal integrity in moderately aged subjects. Histological studies in the epidermis of moderately aged subjects revealed a significant correlation between a decrease of CD and the impaired SC integrity. The colocation of NHE1 with the BGC and serine proteases at the SC–GC junction and the decrease of NHE1 activity within the moderately aged epidermis suggested that NHE1 might be responsible for the aging-related pH increase and barrier defects in moderately aged epidermis. NHE1 is the only sodium-proton exchanger class of non-energy-dependent transporters expressed in keratinocytes and in epidermis, which has been shown to affect the intracellular pH. Studies indicated that NHE1 is located at the SG–SC boundary, deletion of which will reduce SG–SC acidification and impair SC barrier function recovery after tape stripping. In addition, an altered SC lipid processing and defects of lamellar membrane maturation has been observed in NHE −/− epidermis [37, 39]. Taken together, these data suggest that the age-related NHE1 downregulation may, in part, account for the pH abnormality found in aged epidermis.

Peroxisome Proliferator Activated Receptors (PPARs)

The downregulation of PPARs with age might also contribute to a defective barrier in aging skin. PPARs are a group of nuclear receptors that heterodimerize with retinoid X receptor (RXR) and are activated by fatty acids, prostaglandins, eicosanoids, as well as other lipid metabolites. Based on in situ hybridization studies, PPARα and γ are expressed in epidermis. Topical application of PPARα activators accelerates SC acidification, which, in turn, significantly improves SC barrier function and epidermal integrity by enhancing LB secretion and lipid processing [40]. It has been reported that serine phospholipase A2 (sPLA2) was activated by PPARα activator, and simultaneous treatment of with PPARα and sPLA2 inhibitors will reverse PPAR-α-induced SC acidification suggesting PPAR/sPLA2 might be important signaling pathways for SC pH regulation [40].

The Estrogens and Barrier Function in Aged Skin

It has been recognized that the continuation of serum estrogen level is important for the maintenance of skin function in females. Age-related loss of estrogen will affect skin collagen content, dermal thickness, and elasticity as well as water content and might result in an impaired skin barrier. Although a recent study showed estrogen will promote epidermal mitotic activities, the exact mechanism(s) by which estrogen influences skin barrier function is unclear [41–44].

Immune Function Change in Aged Skin

The increased prevalence of skin infections in older subjects is suggestive that aging is associated with reduced immune function [22]. Physical barrier function defect, increased pH, skin dehydration, elevated GC level, and accumulated oxidative stress products all contribute to suboptimal function of the skin immune system in older humans. At a cellular level, no significant differences in Langerhans cell abundance or localization between young and aged skin were noticed. However, the panhematopoietic cell antigen CD45 positive cells were found to be reduced and there was a significant loss of T cells and atypical dendritic epidermal T cells (DETCs) in murine aging skin suggesting an impaired immune response [45].

Sensory Function and Thermal Regulation in Aged Skin

As mentioned, skin sensory innervation systems consist of free nerve endings located in the dermis and epidermis which play an important role in skin homeostasis. The function of these sensory nerves is associated with immune function, inflammation, wound healing, thermoregulation, and hair growth. Protein gene product 9.5 (PGP 9.5) immunostaining studies have shown an age-associated decrease in skin sensory innervation networks. In chronological aging, a decrease in skin innervation is associated with the loss of neuronal networks around the sweat glands, and a decrease in perception of thermal stimuli and tactile sensation. However, painful sensation is relatively conserved [46].

Both the adrenergic vasoconstrictor system and an active vasodilator system work in concert to achieve the skin thermoregulation by adjusting skin blood flow. Skin blood flow will increase as the core body temperature increases and sweating and cutaneous active vasodilation (AVD) will occur to increase the evaporation once a threshold is reached. Reflex vasoconstriction (VC) of cutaneous blood vessels in response to cooling will effectively minimize heat loss. It has been found that there is a reduction in the ability to raise skin blood flow during heat stress in older subjects. Evidence from heat stress studies have shown that the attenuated cutaneous reflex vasodilation is mainly due to the attenuated NO-mediated pathways in older (71 ± 6 year) compared to the young (23 ± 2 year) subjects [47, 48]. On the other side, the ability to reduce skin blood flow in response to cooling is also compromised in advanced age which poses a potential health risk for older subjects. Recent studies have shown that the non-noradrenergic-mediated VC mechanisms are mainly responsible for the age-related defects in reflex cutaneous VC [49, 50].

Possible Intracellular Molecular Mechanisms and Chronological Skin Aging

Telomere shortening

It is well recognized that cellular proliferation is accompanied by a progressive shortening of the telomere structure at the end of chromosomes. Telomeres are the tandem repetitive DNA sequences at ends of mammal chromosomes which generally consist of several thousand base pairs with the 3′ strand overhanging by 75–300 bases, i.e., $(TTAGGG)_n$. The major function of the telomeric repeats is to protect the chromosome by shortening during cell proliferation. It has been found that telomere length decreases with every cell division, which in all likelihood is inversely related to the individual's physiological age [51, 52]. At the same time, the single-stranded telomere overhang can also form a loop structure by telomeric repeat binding factor 2 (TRF2) to provide further protection of DNA integrity. Loop disruption will result in digestion of the overhanging sequence and various DNA damage responses including cellular apoptosis and senescence. This may occur naturally after critical telomere shortening or DNA damage. Dominant negative TRF2 transfection will disrupt the telomere loop structure and promote cell senescence. As the telomere reaches a threshold length after proliferation, the cells may become old and lose normal physiological function. It has been reported that the telomere length plays an important role in controlling the age-associated transcript profile and cellular capacities during aging [51, 53–55].

The length of telomeres is dynamic and maintained by ribonucleoprotein enzyme telomerase which can lengthen the terminal regions of telomeric DNA by addition of tandemly repeated telomeric sequences. The teleomeric balance between lengthening and shortening is influenced by genetic, developmental, and physiological factors [56, 57]. In an epidemiology study, a continuous loss of the telomere DNA during the aging process was observed in individuals ranging from 0 to 90 years old in peripheral hematopoietic cells suggesting a negative correlation between chronological aging and telomere length [58].

The relationship between telomere shortening and skin aging has also been observed in several studies. For example, analysis of DNA samples from sun-protected epidermis obtained from 52 subjects ranging from 0 to 101 years old in Japan showed a rate of 36 bp reduction per year in epidermis with the estimated telomere lengths in the epidermis around 13.3 kb at birth. In another study, the length of the telomeric TTAGGG repeat sequences in skin sample from 21 human subjects between 0 and 92 years of age showed a statistical reduction of telomere length by a rate of 19.8 bp/year [52]. In another study, telomere length was measured in the skin of nine elderly patients (age range 73–95 years) and found to be an average of 7.8– kb (7,792 ± 596 bp). An inverse relationship between the age and telomere length was also detected in skin specimens with an average of reduction about 79 bp [52]. The yearly telomere reduction rate in the epidermis ranges from 19 to 75 bp a year. It did not match with the high turnover rate of the epidermis which is roughly every 4 weeks. So, in skin, the lengthening of telomeres may exist. It has to be mentioned here that the epidermis telomere length measured in above studies never fell below the critical size as 5.6– kb identified in previous studies even in advanced age subjects. However, since the current technology cannot measure the exact telomere length in single cells and for a single chromosome, it cannot be excluded that the telomere either in a subpopulation of the cells or a subgroup of the chromosome is shorter than the critical size. So, how the telomere shortening affects cell senescence in skin remains to be established [52, 55, 59].

Although the normal epidermis contained no or only slight telomerase activity determined by the TRAP assay, epidermal cells reserve the potential to increase telomerase activity in response to stressors such as UV light to maintain chromosome stability. For example, only one of seven specimens from sun-protected epidermis in adults showed detectable human telomerase RNA, whereas the epidermal basal cells in all samples obtained from sun-exposed areas showed moderate human telomerase RNA signals. Thus, sun-exposed skin contains higher levels of telomerase activity than sun-protected skin which suggests telomerase is expressed by epidermal cells and can function as a protective mechanism in response to environmental stresses. Although age-related decrease in telomerase activities has been observed in previous studies, it would be very interesting to confirm this relationship in epidermis with more robust experimental data in the future. Generally, basal cells in normal epidermis have been reported to possess telomerase activity [55, 59].

Although more data are needed to clarify how the telomere/telomerase activity affects the skin barrier function during the progress of aging, all current data suggest a correlation between the normal skin function and the skin telomere integrity/telomerase activity.

Reduced DNA Repair

DNA repair capacity is impaired in primary dermal fibroblasts of older subjects. Cells possess DNA repair mechanisms to remove damaged segments mainly through nucleotide excision repair (NER) or base excision repair (BER) pathways during the G1 and G2 phase; otherwise the cell will undergo apoptosis to protect the organism from potential cancerous transformation. In a UV-induced model, the cell repair capacity in the primary dermal fibroblast cell was compared between young and old subjects. The results showed that initially, UV exposure will induce similar levels of DNA damage in both groups and this will remain at 20 % after 6 h in "young" group. In contrast, the residue level remains high, around 60–80 %, in the aged subjects suggesting there is a significant difference in terms of the DNA repair capacity in fibroblast taken from the young and old subjects. At the same time, FACS assay revealed a significant decrease in S phase population in aged dermal fibroblast cells, suggesting that the cellular replicative potential is impaired in aged dermal fibroblast cells as well. However, it is surprising to find no changes in cellular antioxidant system in aged fibroblast compared to the young ones [60]. In a similar study, a lower DNA repair capacity for strand breaks has also been observed in aged dermal fibroblasts in response to acute oxidative stress [60, 61]. Overall the lower repair capacity might account for accumulated DNA damage found in skin of older subjects and this might result in the chromosome instability, cellular growth arrest, apoptosis, as well as the chronic dermal inflammation induced by the oxidative stress.

Oxidative Stress

It has been very well accepted that oxidative stress is one of the most important driving factors in the aging process [62]. Both endogenously and exogenously generated free radicals will produce oxidative damage to cellular components including DNA during the lifetime, which in turn will accumulate and disturb normal cellular function. To maintain normal cell function, cells are also equipped with antioxidant defenses including nonenzymatic antioxidants such as glutathione and several enzymes such as superoxide dismutase (SOD), catalase (CAT), and glutathione peroxidases (GPx) to scavenge the Reactive Oxygen Species (ROS).

The concentration of carbonyl groups and advanced glycation end products (AGEs) serves as a good measure of ROS-mediated protein oxidation. Recent studies have shown that oxidized proteins may lose their structure and aggregate to form protein complexes. Since the antioxidant capacity of tissues decreases during aging, the accumulation of oxidative damage to cells resulting from aerobic metabolism is the molecular basis for the free radical theory of aging process. This has been supported by experimental data showing an accumulation of oxidative damage such as 8-oxo-2′-deoxyguanosine (8-oxodG) residues from DNA, AGEs from proteins, and hydroperoxides and thiobarbituric acid-reacting substances (TBARS) from lipids in the tissues of aged animals [63–68].

Since skin is continuously exposed to oxidative stress from environmental factors and endogenous aerobic metabolism, the damage likely accumulates. It has been found that, in aged rat skin, the oxidized lipid phosphatidylcholine hydroperoxide (PCOOH) increases as does from TBARS the free 7-hydro-peroxycholesterol (ChOOH) content and oxidized DNA. Although the skin possesses efficient antioxidant activities, the increased ROS products in aged skin suggest chronic accumulation effects during the lifetime [69–71].

The Extracellular Microenvironmental Factors and Chronological Skin Aging

Other than intrinsic cellular processes, a wealth of evidence indicates that dermal extracellular microenvironment including fragmented collagen and microinflammation play an important role in skin aging through a variety of cellular processes including signal transduction, gene expression, and tissue homeostasis.

Breakdown in Collagen and Elastin

Collagen is the major fibrous protein found in dermis providing tissue tensile strength [72]. There are different types of collagen with Type I and III being the most abundant structural proteins in skin comprising > 90 % of the skin's dry weight [73, 74] while Type IV collagen is rich in dermal–epidermal junction (DEJ) [75]. The stratum basale and the dermis are fixed to DEJ via anchoring fibrils which are composed mainly of Type VII collagen [76]. The microfibril extensions of the elastic fiber system termed oxytalan fibers also pass through the DEJ vertically and help secure the dermis to DEJ [72]. Thus a breakdown of these anchoring fibrils will result in the flattening of dermoepidermal junction and the formation of wrinkles due to the loss of bonding and stability between the epidermal and dermal layers [26]. A reduction of more than 50 % in the number of interdigitations per unit area of the skin between 30 and 90 years old has been reported [77].

In the dermis of younger subjects, collagen fibrils are intact, lengthy, abundant, tightly packed, well organized, and appear relatively thin in upper dermis and thicker in reticular dermis [77]. In the aging process, superficial collagen in the dermis undergoes fragmentation and finally lyses with the thinnest fibers being affected first. Throughout life, a considerable amount of collagen is degraded and fragmented. Disorganized collagen fibrils and the appearance of amorphous open space are the prominent, histological characteristic of aged human skin [77]. Quantitative analysis reveals that the amount of fragmented collagen is 4.3-fold greater in aged (>80 years old) compared with young (21–30 years old) human dermis [78]. Therefore, the gradual lysis of connective fibers results in a gradual thinning of the uppermost dermis. Histologically, in some people over the age of 75–80 years, the remaining collagen fibers appear thick but gradually lose their typical dense aspect, becoming loose and "teased" in appearance [77]. At the same time, the synthesis of new collagen is reduced. Dermal fibroblasts are the primary cells responsible for collagen production with each fibroblast synthesizing approximately 3.5 million molecules of collagen/day [79]. The number of fibroblasts from 80+-year-old individuals is reduced by 35 % based on morphometric analysis [80]. The enzymes prolyl hydroxylase and lysyl hydroxylase, both involved in the formation of collagen, decrease with age and might contribute to reduction of the total amount of collagen produced throughout the body too [72]. In the end, Type I collagen synthesis was reported to decrease by 68 % in old compared to young skin [81].

Elastic fibers are the second most important structural elements in the skin which allow it to stretch and recoil repeatedly [82]. The alternating hydrophobic lysine domain in tropoelastin generates hydrophobic interactions between turns in three-dimensional structure during protein assembly and gives the elastic fiber most of its elasticity [83]. Elastic fibers are primarily composed of elastin and microfibrils with an "elastic" core fiber formed by cross-linking of a monomeric secreted tropoelastin on a microfibril scaffold. The amorphous elastin polymer is the primary component (~90 %) and microfibrils are composed primarily by fibrillins [84]. In the reticular dermis, large-diameter elastic fibers lie parallel to the skin surface. These fibers are connected to smaller-diameter elaunin fibers in the papillary dermis which eventually transform into oxytalan fibers and connect with the dermal–epidermal junction (DEJ) through microfibril extensions [85].

The elastic fibers appear thin and long at the level of the superficial (papillary) dermis, being oriented in several directions and mostly parallel to the skin surface in young dermis. After the age of 55 years, the superficial dermis becomes more and more dense and is thinning gradually with elastic fibers appearing more and more fragmented and even visibly reduced quantitatively. Elastin fragmentation becomes more and more obvious during the process of aging and with vast majority of elastic fibers being fragmented and few fibers maintaining elongated appearance after >70 years [77]. The appearance of fine wrinkles in intrinsically aged skin is associated with a gradual fragmentation of the elastic fiber network [85].

Collapse in Extracellular Collagen Matrix: Loss of Structural Integrity

The characteristically histological feature of chronological aged human skin is fragmentation of collagen fibrils and elastic fibers [77, 78]. Clinically, these impairments manifest as fine wrinkles, loss of tissue compliance and resilience, and delayed wound healing [74]. Both collagen and elastin fibers are produced by fibroblasts and persist with minimal turnover throughout adulthood making them vulnerable to attack over time [86]. Both protein glycation and increased matrix metalloproteinase (MMP) activity contribute to the accumulation of protein fragments in aged skin. Nonenzymatic glycation occurs when a sugar molecule covalently binds with a protein. Endogenously high serum glucose concentrations lead to increased glycation while tighter glycemic control can reduce glycated collagen by 25 % in 4 months [87]. There is a gradual accumulation of glycated protein over time that depends on glucose concentration [88, 89]. In general, glycated collagen is first observed at the age of 20 and accumulates with a yearly rate of approximately 3.7 % reaching to 130–150 % of that observed at 20 when at the age of 80 [90, 91]. Exogenous glycosylation of proteins occurs when the reactive carbonyl group of sugar reacts with the amine free function of an amino acid (lysine, arginine) of a protein in foods, which can be absorbed into systemic circulation significantly [87]. Once formed, glycated proteins are highly stable and almost impossible to eradicate from the body [87]. Glycated collagen or elastin can undergo further oxidation, polymerization, and oxidative breakdown to form advanced glycoxidation end products (AGEs). Data also show that AGEs can stimulate fibroblast cell apoptosis [86]. Thus, the accumulation of AGEs not only modifies the mechanical properties of human skin through loss of elasticity and strength tensile and increased stiffening by cross-linking collagen but also impairs the function of fibroblast cell in the dermis [87, 92, 93]. It has been reported that AGEs can also significantly inhibit the hyaluronic acid (HA) synthesis in fibroblasts which in turn will contribute to the loss of skin hydration in aged skin [93].

Elevated collagenase (MMP-1) is largely responsible for initiation of collagen fragmentation and the phenotype of aged human skin [94, 95]. In human skin, MMP-1 concentration increases as does the number of cross-linked collagen fibers which are resistant to complete proteolytic cleavage. Consequently, age-dependent cross-linked collagen fragments accumulate [90, 91]. Transgenic mice expressing active hMMP-1 in the epidermis recapitulate some of the prominent features of aged human skin, including fragmentation/disorganization of collagen fibrils, reduced fibroblast attachment, and contracted fibroblast morphology [96]. It is reported that dermal fibroblasts express increased levels of collagen-degrading MMP-1 in aged (>80 years old) compared with young (21–30 years old) human skin [94]. As well, transcription factor AP-1, a key regulator of MMP-1 expression, is elevated in fibroblasts in aged human skin in vivo [95]. MMP-1 mRNA, MMP-1 protein level, and collagenase activity were all significantly elevated in aged compared with young human dermis. Increased MMP-1 expression in aged human skin was predominantly localized to fibroblasts in the upper dermis [94]. Expression of this linkage establishes a self-perpetuating cycle of damage whereby collagen fragmentation elevates MMP-1 expression, which in turn results in more collagen fragmentation.

The loss of normal fibroblast function followed by the collapse of ECM is believed to underline the age-dependent phenotypic alterations. At the cellular level during aging, the collapsed collagen fibril microenvironment deleteriously alters fibroblast morphology and function as collagen binding sites are lost and mechanical resistance to traction forces is reduced. [73, 95]. It is reported that fibroblast contact with collagen fibrils is reduced 80 % in aged human dermis, and cross-sectional fibroblast surface area is reduced 75 % [81]. As a consequence, fibroblasts have collapsed with little cytoplasm, and less direct association with collagen fibrils and reduced spreading. The concept that cell spreading/mechanical force, along with ECM tissue microenvironment, is critical for dermal fibroblast function is indirectly supported by the effects dermal fillers have in aged human skin. Injection of dermal filler (i.e., cross-linked hyaluronic acid) into the skin of individuals over 80+ years of age stimulates fibroblast collagen production and proliferation, expands vasculature, and increases epidermal thickness which is associated with local increase of mechanical forces and enhancement of the structural integrity as indicated by fibroblast spreading and new collagen deposition [73, 97]. Thus, fibroblasts in aged human skin retain their capacity for functional activation, which can be restored by enhancing structural and mechanical support of the ECM [73, 95].

In the upper dermis of young subjects, dermal fibroblasts firmly attach to the intact ECM substrate through matrix adhesion contact/intergin receptors on the cell surface, while their cytoplasmic tails firmly interact with intracellular actin cytoskeleton. The connectivity of structural elements is all the way from ECM to the nucleus through Plakins and Nesprins. This physical link between the ECM and the cytoskeleton across the cell surface allows propagating mechanical forces in both directions: (1) matrix adhesion contacts transmit forces derived from the ECM substrate to the interior, and (2) cytoskeleton generated forces to the exterior of the cells. Due to these dynamic interactions, fibroblasts can use their adhesion contacts as sensors to probe the mechanical properties of their extracellular environment. The sensing mechanism depends on actomyosin contractility, which is largely controlled by the RhoA/ROCK pathway [98]. There is increasing evidence that mechanical stimulation can be converted directly into multiple chemical signaling including calcium-dependent signaling, ROS/nuclear factor kappa-B pathway, Ras/mitogen-activated protein kinase pathway, and small GTPase/Rho signaling [98].

Current data suggest that reduced cellular spreading/mechanical force induces c-Jun, which in turn elevates MMP-1 expression in aged human skin [95]. The mechanisms by which cell spreading/mechanical force induces c-Jun/AP-1 are not well understood. But it is known that AP-1 activity is regulated by a wide range of stimuli including ROS [99]. Recent studies have found fibroblasts, which have reduced spreading/mechanical force due to fragmentation of surrounding collagen fibrils, display increased levels of ROS suggesting AP-1 elevation is mediated by ROS in the aging process [94]. However, failure of short-term

MitoQ10 (antioxidant) treatment to fully normalize MMP-1 expression indicates that although oxidative stress is a contributing factor, it is not the sole determinant of MMP-1 overexpression by fibroblasts in fragmented collagen lattices [94]. This conclusion suggests that the benefit of antioxidant therapy alone may have limited potential, and better understanding of mechanosensing mechanisms is needed to develop more effective therapies. Given that AP-1 functions as a major driving force for multiple MMPs and potent negative regulator of type I procollagen expression, it is conceivable that AP-1 activity induced by a fragmented collagen microenvironment significantly contributes to elevated MMPs and loss of type I collagen expression [100].

In summary, the quality of the extracellular matrix environment instead of intrinsic intracellular factors is a more important determinant of fibroblast function and cellular aging in vivo based on the facts that (1) increased MMP-1 levels are seen in dermal fibroblasts in aged skin in vivo but the difference was not found in in vitro cultured fibroblasts from young or aged individuals [94]; (2) fibroblasts cultured in partially fragmented collagen lattices have increased MMP-1 and cellular oxidant levels, independent of the age of fibroblast donor; [94] and (3) fibroblast collagen production is stimulated in vivo by injection of dermal filler (cross-linked hyaluronic acid) in individuals over 80+ years [97].

It has also been observed that mechanical stress can regulate ECM genes through the secretion and activation of TGF-β, a prominent growth factor required for myofibroblast differentiation and ECM production [101]. Mechanical stress can lead to the paracrine release and activation of TGF-β within ECM and fibroblasts [102, 103]. In return, TGF-β will induce procollagen α1(I) via classical signaling pathways [103]. The association of integrins with growth factor receptors at matrix adhesion contacts on the fibroblast surface allows cells to integrate mechanical with growth factor derived signals, resulting in anchorage-dependent growth and anoikis [98]. In a recent study, Type I procollagen mRNA in upper dermis was found to be reduced by >75 % in upper dermis in aged compared to young skin which is correlated with a reduction of Type I procollagen mRNA and protein in the same location. As expected, TGFß1 mRNA and protein level in upper dermis fibroblasts were reduced by 70 % and the TGFß1gene expression in the same region was reduced by 87 %. CTGF (connective tissue growth factor) is expressed in upper dermis fibroblast and regulates procollagen expression depending on TGF signaling pathway but not through direct activation of TGF pathway. CTGF mRNA in upper dermis region and in fibroblast localized in this region was reduced by 50 %. Downregulation of TGFβ/Smad/CTGF axis likely mediates the reduced type I procollagen due to the collapse of ECM structure in aged skin. In contrast to the in vivo data, the expression of TGFβ, CTFG, and procollagen in cultured dermal fibroblast from old donors and young donors remains to be seen, suggesting tissue ECM microenvironment instead of intracellular intrinsic factors plays a critical role in fibroblast function and age-dependent decline of TGFbeta/SMAD/CTGF/procollagen originates from altered structural and mechanical properties [104].

In summary, the collapse of the extracellular collagen matrix leads to a functional decline in fibroblasts and results in an increase in MMP-1 and decrease in TGFβ signaling which further breaks down collagen and reduces collagen deposition finally exacerbating the loss in elasticity and mechanical tension. This spiraling decline in ECM is reflected in the most predominant signs of skin aging.

The Microinflammatory Model and Chronological Skin Aging

More and more evidences support a critical role of chronic low-grade asymptomatic inflammation in skin aging. In one genomic study, immune and inflammatory responses were the dominant themes with most of the genes upregulated in old (60–67) versus young (18–20 years old) accompanied by the upregulated extracellular matrix genes [105]. It was noticed that intercellular adhesion molecule-1 (ICAM-1) in the dermis endothelium was always induced by the factors that promote skin aging. This adhesion molecule enables circulating monocytes and granulocytes to roll over, adhere, and diapedese through the endothelial wall of blood vessels. Once in the dermis, both macrophages and monocytes can secrete collagenase and ROS to damage the extracellular ECM and nearby fibroblasts or kerotinocytes which will further trigger a cascade of arachidonic acid and prostaglandin release to activate resident mast cells to produce TNF alpha and histamine. In return, these will further induce ICAM-1 and maintain the inflammatory responses. In the end, the imbalance in the degradation and synthesis of elastin and collagen fibers results in skin aging [72, 106].

Among the multiple factors, the aforementioned glycated collagen and elastin play important roles in the microinflammation model of skin aging. Glycated protein has been shown to induce ICAM and trigger the cycle of a self-sustaining inflammatory response [106] [107]. AGEs by themselves can promote a proinflammatory response through their interaction with specific receptors (RAGE). The binding of AGEs to RAGE will activate many proinflammatory genes through multiple signaling pathways including mitogen-activated protein kinases (MAPKs), extracellular signal-regulated kinases (ERK) 1 and 2, phosphatidyl-inositol 3 kinase, p21Ras, stress-activated protein kinase/c-Jun-N-terminal kinase, and the janus kinases resulting in the activation of the transcription factor nuclear factor kappa-B (NFκB). AGE-activated NFκB is characterized by a sustained and self-perpetuating action by increasing further expression of RAGE, which itself further stimulates NFκB, forming a vicious cycle of self-renewing and perpetuating proinflammatory signals. RAGE activation is found associated with the induction of oxidative stress by activating nicotinamide adenine dinucleotide phosphate (NADPH)-oxidase (NOX), decreasing activity of superoxide dismutase (SOD), catalase, and by reducing cellular antioxidant defenses, like GSH and ascorbic acid indirectly [90].

To date, elastin fragments (EFs) or elastin degradation products (EDPs) are the best-characterized matrikines which can elicit diverse biological functions including chemotaxis, gene transcription, and cell cycle regulation [108]. Although the mature elastic fibers do not display chemotactic properties, all EDPs with the hydrophobic motifs GXXPG or XGXPG possess chemotactic properties. In the progress of inflammation, elastases from macrophages and neutrophils can break intact elastic fibers into EDPs which in turn can attract multiple cells including macrophage, neutrophils, and lymphocytes (consequences of elastosis) into the reaction site. Exposure of human skin fibroblasts to VGVAPG (EDP) has been shown to induce MMP1 and MMP3 [109] expression. Thus a self-maintained inflammatory reaction in a vicious positive feedback can be created.

Finally, intrinsically aged skin has structural changes in the vasculature which might also contribute to the low level of uncontrolled chronic inflammation observed in a skin of aged people. In human skin samples obtained from 33- to 80-year-old individuals, fluorescence microscopy analyses revealed that the total area covered by CD31+ vessels (marker of blood vessel) was apparently reduced in the dermis of aged buttock skin and NG2+ (marker of pericyte) CD31+ vessels in the buttock skin gradually decreased by 66 % in 75–89 years group compared with 30–44 years group. The significant loss of pericyte-covered vessels in aged skin might contribute to impaired vessel function with an increase of leakiness resulting in inflammation [110]. The vascular permeability will also be impaired as the endothelial cells were observed to undergo granular degeneration, became swollen, and tended to detach in aged skin with the smallest vessels being affected mostly. Consequently, the larger quantities of extravasated fluid observed in aged skin might also contribute to the skin inflammation [77].

Summary and Conclusion

The primary function of the skin is to serve as a barrier. To this end, the structure of the epidermis is highly regulated in coordinated, dynamic balance between proliferation, differentiation, and

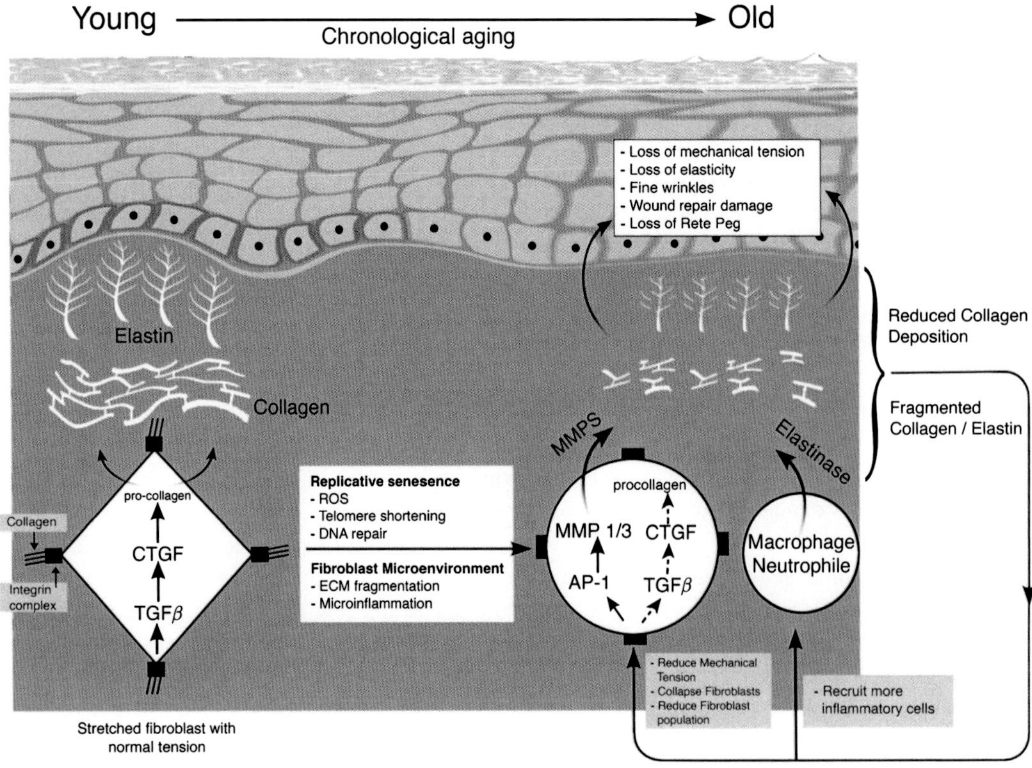

Fig. 2 Both extracellular and intracellular events are involved in chronological skin aging

desquamation. An acidic pH is required to maintain the barrier function by providing an optimal environment for the function of enzymes involved in lipid production/processing. In addition to its barrier function, the skin also has a role in immunosurveillance, metabolism, and sensory reception/transmission.

Figure 2 presents an oversimplified depiction of events associated with the intrinsic aging process in skin. This chronological skin aging is an intrinsic ongoing progress which will lead to the loss of normal skin mechanical tension/elasticity gradually accompanied by an increase of fine wrinkles, impaired barrier function, and many other unfavorable physiological changes, which could be accelerated by environmental factors such as UV light. It has been very well documented that cellular replicative senescence induced by ROS damage, DNA telomere shortening, and cellular DNA damage plays important roles in skin chronological aging. However, recent studies have shown undesirable dermal extracellular microenvironment including fragmented collagens, and microinflammation is a prominent feature in aged skin and is directly linked to the morphology and impaired barrier function. In summary, the chronological fragmentation of dermal ECM will initiate the collapse of fibroblasts which, in turn, will induce the increase of MMP-1 production and decrease of procollagen synthesis through AP-1/MMP-1 and TGFbeta/CTGF/procollagen signaling pathways. In addition, the glycated collagen and elastin fragments can induce a low-grade asymptomatic inflammation in skin aging by recruiting macrophages and neutrophils which will further degrade the dermis ECM through secreted elastinases. All these signaling pathways are woven together to maintain a vicious self-perpetual positive feedback loop accelerating skin aging.

References

1. Waite LJ. The demographic faces of the elderly. Popul Dev Rev. 2004;30:3–16.
2. Fuchs E. Scratching the surface of skin development. Nature. 2007;445:834–42. doi:10.1038/nature05659.
3. Madison KC. Barrier function of the skin: "la raison d'être" of the epidermis. J Invest Dermatol. 2003; 121:231–41. doi:10.1046/j.1523-1747.2003.12359.x.
4. Elias PM. The skin barrier as an innate immune element. Semin Immunopathol. 2007;29:3–14.
5. Menon GK. New insights into skin structure: scratching the surface. Adv Drug Deliv Rev. 2002;54 Suppl 1:S3–17.
6. Proksch E, Brandner JM, Jensen J-M. The skin: an indispensable barrier. Exp Dermatol. 2008; 17:1063–72.
7. Matsuki M, Yamashita F, Ishida-Yamamoto A, Yamada K, Kinoshita C, Fushiki S, et al. Defective stratum corneum and early neonatal death in mice lacking the gene for transglutaminase 1 (keratinocyte transglutaminase). Proc Natl Acad Sci U S A. 1998;95:1044–9.
8. Descargues P, Deraison C, Bonnart C, Kreft M, Kishibe M, Ishida-Yamamoto A, et al. Spink5-deficient mice mimic Netherton syndrome through degradation of desmoglein 1 by epidermal protease hyperactivity. Nat Genet. 2005;37:56–65. doi:10.1038/ng1493.
9. Macheleidt O, Kaiser HW, Sandhoff K. Deficiency of epidermal protein-bound omega-hydroxyceramides in atopic dermatitis. J Invest Dermatol. 2002; 119:166–73. doi:10.1046/j.1523-1747.2002.01833.x.
10. Jackson SM, Wood LC, Lauer S, Taylor JM, Cooper AD, Elias PM, et al. Effect of cutaneous permeability barrier disruption on HMG-CoA reductase, LDL receptor, and apolipoprotein E mRNA levels in the epidermis of hairless mice. J Lipid Res. 1992;33:1307–14.
11. Proksch E, Feingold KR, Elias PM. Epidermal HMG CoA reductase activity in essential fatty acid deficiency: barrier requirements rather than eicosanoid generation regulate cholesterol synthesis. J Invest Dermatol. 1992;99:216–20.
12. Herrmann T, van der Hoeven F, Grone H-J, Stewart AF, Langbein L, Kaiser I, et al. Mice with targeted disruption of the fatty acid transport protein 4 (Fatp 4, Slc27a4) gene show features of lethal restrictive dermopathy. J Cell Biol. 2003;161:1105–15. doi:10.1083/jcb.200207080.
13. Demerjian M, Hachem J-P, Tschachler E, Denecker G, Declercq W, Vandenabeele P, et al. Acute modulations in permeability barrier function regulate epidermal cornification: role of caspase-14 and the protease-activated receptor type 2. Am J Pathol. 2008;172:86–97. doi:10.2353/ajpath.2008.070161.
14. Mine S, Fortunel NO, Pageon H, Asselineau D. Aging alters functionally human dermal papillary fibroblasts but not reticular fibroblasts: a new view of skin morphogenesis and aging. PLoS One. 2008;3:e4066. doi:10.1371/journal.pone.0004066.
15. Lee D-Y, Cho K-H. The effects of epidermal keratinocytes and dermal fibroblasts on the formation of cutaneous basement membrane in three-dimensional culture systems. Arch Dermatol Res. 2005;296:296–302. doi:10.1007/s00403-004-0529-5.
16. Chong HC, Tan MJ, Philippe V, Tan SH, Tan CK, Ku CW, et al. Regulation of epithelial-mesenchymal IL-1 signaling by PPARbeta/delta is essential for skin homeostasis and wound healing. J Cell Biol. 2009;184:817–31. doi:10.1083/jcb.200809028.
17. Haschek WM, Rousseaux CG, Wallig MA. Fundamentals of toxicologic pathology. London: Academic; 2009.
18. Fore J. A review of skin and the effects of aging on skin structure and function. Ostomy Wound Manage. 2006;52:24–35; quiz 36–37.
19. Bos JD. The skin as an organ of immunity. Clin Exp Immunol. 1997;107 Suppl 1:3–5.
20. Strid J, Strobel S. Skin barrier dysfunction and systemic sensitization to allergens through the skin. Curr Drug Targets Inflamm Allergy. 2005;4:531–41.
21. Sugita K, Kabashima K, Atarashi K, Shimauchi T, Kobayashi M, Tokura Y. Innate immunity mediated by epidermal keratinocytes promotes acquired immunity involving Langerhans cells and T cells in the skin. Clin Exp Immunol. 2007;147:176–83. doi:10.1111/j.1365-2249.2006.03258.x.
22. Debenedictis C, Joubeh S, Zhang G, Barria M, Ghohestani RF. Immune functions of the skin. Clin Dermatol. 2001;19:573–85.
23. Hikima T, Tojo K, Maibach HI. Skin metabolism in transdermal therapeutic systems. Skin Pharmacol Physiol. 2005;18:153–9. doi:10.1159/000085860.
24. Smith Pease CK, Basketter DA, Patlewicz GY. Contact allergy: the role of skin chemistry and metabolism. Clin Exp Dermatol. 2003;28:177–83.
25. Schepers RJ, Ringkamp M. Thermoreceptors and thermosensitive afferents. Neurosci Biobehav Rev. 2009;33:205–12. doi:10.1016/j.neubiorev.2008.07.009.
26. Baumann L. Skin ageing and its treatment. J Pathol. 2007;211:241–51. doi:10.1002/path.2098.
27. Calleja-Agius J, Muscat-Baron Y, Brincat MP. Skin ageing. Menopause Int. 2007;13:60–4. doi:10.1258/175404507780796325.
28. Kappes UP. Skin ageing and wrinkles: clinical and photographic scoring. J Cosmet Dermatol. 2004;3:23–5. doi:10.1111/j.1473-2130.2004.00092.x.
29. Farage MA, Miller KW, Elsner P, Maibach HI. Intrinsic and extrinsic factors in skin ageing: a review. Int J Cosmet Sci. 2008;30:87–95. doi:10.1111/j.1468-2494.2007.00415.x.
30. Whitton JT, Everall JD. The thickness of the epidermis. Br J Dermatol. 1973;89:467–76.
31. Elias PM, Ghadially R. The aged epidermal permeability barrier: basis for functional abnormalities. Clin Geriatr Med. 2002;18:103–20. vii.

32. Ghadially R. Aging and the epidermal permeability barrier: implications for contact dermatitis. Am J Contact Dermat Off J Am Contact Dermat Soc. 1998;9:162–9.
33. Ghadially R, Brown BE, Sequeira-Martin SM, Feingold KR, Elias PM. The aged epidermal permeability barrier. Structural, functional, and lipid biochemical abnormalities in humans and a senescent murine model. J Clin Invest. 1995;95:2281–90. doi:10.1172/JCI117919.
34. Behne MJ, Barry NP, Hanson KM, Aronchik I, Clegg RW, Gratton E, et al. Neonatal development of the stratum corneum pH gradient: localization and mechanisms leading to emergence of optimal barrier function. J Invest Dermatol. 2003;120:998–1006.
35. Fluhr JW, Mao-Qiang M, Brown BE, Hachem J-P, Moskowitz DG, Demerjian M, et al. Functional consequences of a neutral pH in neonatal rat stratum corneum. J Invest Dermatol. 2004;123:140–51. doi:10.1111/j.0022-202X.2004.22726.x.
36. Fluhr JW, Behne MJ, Brown BE, Moskowitz DG, Selden C, Mao-Qiang M, et al. Stratum corneum acidification in neonatal skin: secretory phospholipase A2 and the sodium/hydrogen antiporter-1 acidify neonatal rat stratum corneum. J Invest Dermatol. 2004;122:320–9. doi:10.1046/j.0022-202X.2003.00204.x.
37. Behne MJ, Meyer JW, Hanson KM, Barry NP, Murata S, Crumrine D, et al. NHE1 regulates the stratum corneum permeability barrier homeostasis. Microenvironment acidification assessed with fluorescence lifetime imaging. J Biol Chem. 2002;277:47399–406. doi:10.1074/jbc.M204759200.
38. Choi E-H, Man M-Q, Xu P, Xin S, Liu Z, Crumrine DA, et al. Stratum corneum acidification is impaired in moderately aged human and murine skin. J Invest Dermatol. 2007;127:2847–56. doi:10.1038/sj.jid.5700913.
39. Hachem J-P, Behne M, Aronchik I, Demerjian M, Feingold KR, Elias PM, et al. Extracellular pH Controls NHE1 expression in epidermis and keratinocytes: implications for barrier repair. J Invest Dermatol. 2005;125:790–7. doi:10.1111/j.0022-202X.2005.23836.x.
40. Fluhr JW, Man M-Q, Hachem J-P, Crumrine D, Mauro TM, Elias PM, et al. Topical peroxisome proliferator activated receptor activators accelerate postnatal stratum corneum acidification. J Invest Dermatol. 2009;129:365–74. doi:10.1038/jid.2008.218.
41. Stevenson S, Sharpe DT, Thornton MJ. Effects of oestrogen agonists on human dermal fibroblasts in an in vitro wounding assay. Exp Dermatol. 2009;18:988–90. doi:10.1111/j.1600-0625.2009.00864.x.
42. Verdier-Sévrain S, Bonté F, Gilchrest B. Biology of estrogens in skin: implications for skin aging. Exp Dermatol. 2006;15:83–94. doi:10.1111/j.1600-0625.2005.00377.x.
43. Brincat MP, Baron YM, Galea R. Estrogens and the skin. Climacteric J Int Menopause Soc. 2005; 8:110–23. doi:10.1080/13697130500118100.
44. Thornton MJ. The biological actions of estrogens on skin. Exp Dermatol. 2002;11:487–502.
45. McCullough JL, Kelly KM. Prevention and treatment of skin aging. Ann N Y Acad Sci. 2006;1067:323–31. doi:10.1196/annals.1354.044.
46. Besné I, Descombes C, Breton L. Effect of age and anatomical site on density of sensory innervation in human epidermis. Arch Dermatol. 2002; 138:1445–50.
47. Holowatz LA, Thompson CS, Minson CT, Kenney WL. Mechanisms of acetylcholine-mediated vasodilatation in young and aged human skin. J Physiol. 2005;563:965–73. doi:10.1113/jphysiol.2004.080952.
48. Holowatz LA, Houghton BL, Wong BJ, Wilkins BW, Harding AW, Kenney WL, et al. Nitric oxide and attenuated reflex cutaneous vasodilation in aged skin. Am J Physiol Heart Circ Physiol. 2003;284: H1662–7. doi:10.1152/ajpheart.00871.2002.
49. Thompson CS, Kenney WL. Altered neurotransmitter control of reflex vasoconstriction in aged human skin. J Physiol. 2004;558:697–704. doi:10.1113/jphysiol.2004.065714.
50. Scremin G, Kenney WL. Aging and the skin blood flow response to the unloading of baroreceptors during heat and cold stress. J Appl Physiol Bethesda Md 1985. 2004;96:1019–25. doi:10.1152/japplphysiol.00928.2003.
51. Kosmadaki MG, Gilchrest BA. The role of telomeres in skin aging/photoaging. Micron Oxf Engl 1993. 2004;35:155–9. doi:10.1016/j.micron.2003.11.002.
52. Lindsey J, McGill NI, Lindsey LA, Green DK, Cooke HJ. In vivo loss of telomeric repeats with age in humans. Mutat Res. 1991;256:45–8.
53. Boukamp P. Skin aging: a role for telomerase and telomere dynamics? Curr Mol Med. 2005;5:171–7.
54. Shariftabrizi A, Eller MS. Telomere homolog oligonucleotides and the skin: current status and future perspectives. Exp Dermatol. 2007;16:627–33. doi:10.1111/j.1600-0625.2007.00580.x.
55. Sugimoto M, Yamashita R, Ueda M. Telomere length of the skin in association with chronological aging and photoaging. J Dermatol Sci. 2006;43:43–7. doi:10.1016/j.jdermsci.2006.02.004.
56. Smogorzewska A, de Lange T. Different telomere damage signaling pathways in human and mouse cells. EMBO J. 2002;21:4338–48.
57. Blackburn EH. Switching and signaling at the telomere. Cell. 2001;106:661–73.
58. Rufer N, Brümmendorf TH, Kolvraa S, Bischoff C, Christensen K, Wadsworth L, et al. Telomere fluorescence measurements in granulocytes and T lymphocyte subsets point to a high turnover of hematopoietic stem cells and memory T cells in early childhood. J Exp Med. 1999;190:157–67.

59. Nakamura K-I, Izumiyama-Shimomura N, Sawabe M, Arai T, Aoyagi Y, Fujiwara M, et al. Comparative analysis of telomere lengths and erosion with age in human epidermis and lingual epithelium. J Invest Dermatol. 2002;119:1014–9. doi:10.1046/j.1523-1747.2002.19523.x.
60. Hazane F, Sauvaigo S, Douki T, Favier A, Beani J-C. Age-dependent DNA repair and cell cycle distribution of human skin fibroblasts in response to UVA irradiation. J Photochem Photobiol B. 2006;82:214–23. doi:10.1016/j.jphotobiol.2005.10.004.
61. Sauvaigo S, Bonnet-Duquennoy M, Odin F, Hazane-Puch F, Lachmann N, Bonté F, et al. DNA repair capacities of cutaneous fibroblasts: effect of sun exposure, age and smoking on response to an acute oxidative stress. Br J Dermatol. 2007;157:26–32. doi:10.1111/j.1365-2133.2007.07890.x.
62. Callaghan TM, Wilhelm K-P. A review of ageing and an examination of clinical methods in the assessment of ageing skin. Part I: cellular and molecular perspectives of skin ageing. Int J Cosmet Sci. 2008;30:313–22. doi:10.1111/j.1468-2494.2008.00454.x.
63. Trouba KJ, Hamadeh HK, Amin RP, Germolec DR. Oxidative stress and its role in skin disease. Antioxid Redox Signal. 2002;4:665–73. doi:10.1089/15230860260220175.
64. Sander CS, Chang H, Hamm F, Elsner P, Thiele JJ. Role of oxidative stress and the antioxidant network in cutaneous carcinogenesis. Int J Dermatol. 2004;43:326–35. doi:10.1111/j.1365-4632.2004.02222.x.
65. Bickers DR, Athar M. Oxidative stress in the pathogenesis of skin disease. J Invest Dermatol. 2006;126:2565–75. doi:10.1038/sj.jid.5700340.
66. Kohen R. Skin antioxidants: their role in aging and in oxidative stress – new approaches for their evaluation. Biomed Pharmacother. 1999;53:181–92. doi:10.1016/S0753-3322(99)80087-0.
67. Kaneko T, Tahara S, Taguchi T, Kondo H. Accumulation of oxidative DNA damage, 8-oxo-2-′-deoxyguanosine, and change of repair systems during in vitro cellular aging of cultured human skin fibroblasts. Mutat Res. 2001;487:19–30.
68. Meyer F, Fiala E, Westendorf J. Induction of 8-oxo-dGTPase activity in human lymphoid cells and normal fibroblasts by oxidative stress. Toxicology. 2000;146:83–92.
69. Sivonová M, Tatarková Z, Duracková Z, Dobrota D, Lehotský J, Matáková T, et al. Relationship between antioxidant potential and oxidative damage to lipids, proteins and DNA in aged rats. Physiol Res Acad Sci Bohemoslov. 2007;56:757–64.
70. Tahara S, Matsuo M, Kaneko T. Age-related changes in oxidative damage to lipids and DNA in rat skin. Mech Ageing Dev. 2001;122:415–26.
71. Lasch J, Schönfelder U, Walke M, Zellmer S, Beckert D. Oxidative damage of human skin lipids. Dependence of lipid peroxidation on sterol concentration. Biochim Biophys Acta. 1997;1349:171–81.
72. Calleja-Agius J, Brincat M, Borg M. Skin connective tissue and ageing. Best Pract Res Clin Obstet Gynaecol. 2013;27:727–40. doi:10.1016/j.bpobgyn.2013.06.004.
73. Fisher GJ, Varani J, Voorhees JJ. Looking older: fibroblast collapse and therapeutic implications. Arch Dermatol. 2008;144:666–72. doi:10.1001/archderm.144.5.666.
74. Naylor EC, Watson REB, Sherratt MJ. Molecular aspects of skin ageing. Maturitas. 2011;69:249–56. doi:10.1016/j.maturitas.2011.04.011.
75. Fleischmajer R, Utani A, MacDonald ED, Perlish JS, Pan TC, Chu ML, et al. Initiation of skin basement membrane formation at the epidermo-dermal interface involves assembly of laminins through binding to cell membrane receptors. J Cell Sci. 1998;111 (Pt 14):1929–40.
76. Christiano AM, Anhalt G, Gibbons S, Bauer EA, Uitto J. Premature termination codons in the type VII collagen gene (COL7A1) underlie severe, mutilating recessive dystrophic epidermolysis bullosa. Genomics. 1994;21:160–8. doi:10.1006/geno.1994.1238.
77. Bonta M, Daina L, Muţiu G. The process of ageing reflected by histological changes in the skin. Romanian J Morphol Embryol Rev Roum Morphol Embryol. 2013;54:797–804.
78. Fisher GJ, Kang S, Varani J, Bata-Csorgo Z, Wan Y, Datta S, et al. Mechanisms of photoaging and chronological skin aging. Arch Dermatol. 2002;138: 1462–70.
79. McAnulty RJ. Fibroblasts and myofibroblasts: their source, function and role in disease. Int J Biochem Cell Biol. 2007;39:666–71. doi:10.1016/j.biocel.2006.11.005.
80. Varani J, Warner RL, Gharaee-Kermani M, Phan SH, Kang S, Chung JH, et al. Vitamin A antagonizes decreased cell growth and elevated collagen-degrading matrix metalloproteinases and stimulates collagen accumulation in naturally aged human skin. J Invest Dermatol. 2000;114:480–6. doi:10.1046/j.1523-1747.2000.00902.x.
81. Varani J, Dame MK, Rittie L, Fligiel SEG, Kang S, Fisher GJ, et al. Decreased collagen production in chronologically aged skin: roles of age-dependent alteration in fibroblast function and defective mechanical stimulation. Am J Pathol. 2006;168:1861–8. doi:10.2353/ajpath.2006.051302.
82. Boraldi F, Annovi G, Tiozzo R, Sommer P, Quaglino D. Comparison of ex vivo and in vitro human fibroblast ageing models. Mech Ageing Dev. 2010;131:625–35. doi:10.1016/j.mad.2010.08.008.
83. Baldock C, Oberhauser AF, Ma L, Lammie D, Siegler V, Mithieux SM, et al. Shape of tropoelastin, the highly extensible protein that controls human tissue elasticity. Proc Natl Acad Sci U S A. 2011;108:4322–7. doi:10.1073/pnas.1014280108.

84. Vrhovski B, Weiss AS. Biochemistry of tropoelastin. Eur J Biochem FEBS. 1998;258:1–18.
85. Sherratt MJ. Age-related tissue stiffening: cause and effect. Adv Wound Care. 2013;2:11–7. doi:10.1089/wound.2011.0328.
86. Pageon H. Reaction of glycation and human skin: the effects on the skin and its components, reconstructed skin as a model. Pathol Biol (Paris). 2010;58:226–31. doi:10.1016/j.patbio.2009.09.009.
87. Draelos ZD. Aging skin: the role of diet: facts and controversies. Clin Dermatol. 2013;31:701–6. doi:10.1016/j.clindermatol.2013.05.005.
88. Park H-Y, Kim J-H, Jung M, Chung CH, Hasham R, Park CS, et al. A long-standing hyperglycaemic condition impairs skin barrier by accelerating skin ageing process. Exp Dermatol. 2011;20:969–74. doi:10.1111/j.1600-0625.2011.01364.x.
89. Dunn JA, Patrick JS, Thorpe SR, Baynes JW. Oxidation of glycated proteins: age-dependent accumulation of N epsilon-(carboxymethyl)lysine in lens proteins. Biochemistry (Mosc). 1989; 28:9464–8.
90. Gkogkolou P, Böhm M. Advanced glycation end products: key players in skin aging? Dermatoendocrinol. 2012;4:259–70. doi:10.4161/derm.22028.
91. Corstjens H, Dicanio D, Muizzuddin N, Neven A, Sparacio R, Declercq L, et al. Glycation associated skin autofluorescence and skin elasticity are related to chronological age and body mass index of healthy subjects. Exp Gerontol. 2008;43:663–7. doi:10.1016/j.exger.2008.01.012.
92. Crisan M, Taulescu M, Crisan D, Cosgarea R, Parvu A, Cãtoi C, et al. Expression of advanced glycation end-products on sun-exposed and non-exposed cutaneous sites during the ageing process in humans. PLoS One. 2013;8:e75003. doi:10.1371/journal.pone.0075003.
93. Okano Y, Masaki H, Sakurai H. Dysfunction of dermal fibroblasts induced by advanced glycation end-products (AGEs) and the contribution of a nonspecific interaction with cell membrane and AGEs. J Dermatol Sci. 2002;29:171–80.
94. Fisher GJ, Quan T, Purohit T, Shao Y, Cho MK, He T, et al. Collagen fragmentation promotes oxidative stress and elevates matrix metalloproteinase-1 in fibroblasts in aged human skin. Am J Pathol. 2009;174:101–14. doi:10.2353/ajpath.2009.080599.
95. Qin Z, Voorhees JJ, Fisher GJ, Quan T. Age-associated reduction of cellular spreading/mechanical force up-regulates matrix metalloproteinase-1 expression and collagen fibril fragmentation via c-Jun/AP-1 in human dermal fibroblasts. Aging Cell. 2014; 13:1028–37. doi:10.1111/acel.12265.
96. Xia W, Hammerberg C, Li Y, He T, Quan T, Voorhees JJ, et al. Expression of catalytically active matrix metalloproteinase-1 in dermal fibroblasts induces collagen fragmentation and functional alterations that resemble aged human skin. Aging Cell. 2013; 12:661–71. doi:10.1111/acel.12089.
97. Quan T, Wang F, Shao Y, Rittié L, Xia W, Orringer JS, et al. Enhancing structural support of the dermal microenvironment activates fibroblasts, endothelial cells, and keratinocytes in aged human skin in vivo. J Invest Dermatol. 2013;133:658–67. doi:10.1038/jid.2012.364.
98. Chiquet M, Gelman L, Lutz R, Maier S. From mechanotransduction to extracellular matrix gene expression in fibroblasts. Biochim Biophys Acta. 2009;1793:911–20. doi:10.1016/j.bbamcr.2009.01.012.
99. Shaulian E, Karin M. AP-1 as a regulator of cell life and death. Nat Cell Biol. 2002;4:E131–6. doi:10.1038/ncb0502-e131.
100. Quan T, Little E, Quan H, Qin Z, Voorhees JJ, Fisher GJ. Elevated matrix metalloproteinases and collagen fragmentation in photodamaged human skin: impact of altered extracellular matrix microenvironment on dermal fibroblast function. J Invest Dermatol. 2013;133:1362–6. doi:10.1038/jid.2012.509.
101. Desmoulière A, Chaponnier C, Gabbiani G. Tissue repair, contraction, and the myofibroblast. Wound Repair Regen Off Publ Wound Heal Soc Eur Tissue Repair Soc. 2005;13:7–12. doi:10.1111/j.1067-1927.2005.130102.x.
102. Wipff P-J, Rifkin DB, Meister J-J, Hinz B. Myofibroblast contraction activates latent TGF-beta1 from the extracellular matrix. J Cell Biol. 2007;179:1311–23. doi:10.1083/jcb.200704042.
103. Lindahl GE, Chambers RC, Papakrivopoulou J, Dawson SJ, Jacobsen MC, Bishop JE, et al. Activation of fibroblast procollagen alpha 1(I) transcription by mechanical strain is transforming growth factor-beta-dependent and involves increased binding of CCAAT-binding factor (CBF/NF-Y) at the proximal promoter. J Biol Chem. 2002;277:6153–61. doi:10.1074/jbc.M108966200.
104. Quan T, Shao Y, He T, Voorhees JJ, Fisher GJ. Reduced expression of connective tissue growth factor (CTGF/CCN2) mediates collagen loss in chronologically aged human skin. J Invest Dermatol. 2010;130:415–24. doi:10.1038/jid.2009.224.
105. Bennett MF, Robinson MK, Baron ED, Cooper KD. Skin immune systems and inflammation: protector of the skin or promoter of aging? J Investig Dermatol Symp Proc Soc Investig Dermatol Inc Eur Soc Dermatol Res. 2008;13:15–9. doi:10.1038/jidsymp.2008.3.
106. Giacomoni PU, Rein G. A mechanistic model for the aging of human skin. Micron Oxf Engl 1993. 2004;35:179–84. doi:10.1016/j.micron.2003.11.004.
107. Schmidt AM, Hori O, Chen JX, Li JF, Crandall J, Zhang J, et al. Advanced glycation endproducts interacting with their endothelial receptor induce expression of vascular cell adhesion molecule-1 (VCAM-1) in cultured human endothelial cells and in mice. A potential mechanism for the accelerated vasculopathy of diabetes. J Clin Invest. 1995; 96:1395–403. doi:10.1172/JCI118175.

108. Duca L, Floquet N, Alix AJP, Haye B, Debelle L. Elastin as a matrikine. Crit Rev Oncol Hematol. 2004; 49:235–44. doi:10.1016/j.critrevonc.2003.09.007.
109. Brassart B, Fuchs P, Huet E, Alix AJ, Wallach J, Tamburro AM, et al. Conformational dependence of collagenase (matrix metalloproteinase-1) up-regulation by elastin peptides in cultured fibroblasts. J Biol Chem. 2001;276:5222–7. doi:10.1074/jbc.M003642200.
110. Kajiya K, Kim YK, Kinemura Y, Kishimoto J, Chung JH. Structural alterations of the cutaneous vasculature in aged and in photoaged human skin in vivo. J Dermatol Sci. 2011;61:206–8. doi:10.1016/j.jdermsci.2010.12.005.

Biology of Stratum Corneum: Tape Stripping and Protein Quantification

29

Hanjiang Zhu, Ali Alikhan, and Howard I. Maibach

Contents

Abstract

Stratum corneum (SC) adhesive tape stripping has been utilized in the measurement of stratum corneum mass, barrier function, drug reservoir, and percutaneous penetration of topical substances. The process involves a methodical, relatively noninvasive layer-by-layer removal of the SC. SC removal may rely on the interaction between the adhesive stripping force and the cohesive intercellular force. This chapter goes through the process methodologies.

Introduction

Stratum corneum (SC) adhesive tape stripping has been utilized in the measurement of stratum corneum mass, barrier function, drug reservoir, and percutaneous penetration of topical substances. The process involves a methodical, relatively noninvasive layer-by-layer removal of the SC, which comprises the outermost epidermal cell layers. Complete SC removal may require over 70 tape strips [1, 2]. The quantity of SC harvested diminishes with each sequential strip, possibly due to increased SC cohesiveness in deeper layers. Thus, the mass of any single strip depends on the mass removed by the prior strip [3]. SC removal may rely on the interaction between the adhesive stripping force and the cohesive intercellular force [3].

H. Zhu
Department of Dermatology, UC San Francisco, San Francisco, CA, USA
e-mail: sunnie.zhu@foxmail.com

A. Alikhan (✉)
Department of Dermatology, University of Cincinnati, Cincinnati, OH, USA
e-mail: alialikhan1@yahoo.com

H.I. Maibach
Department of Dermatology, University of California, San Francisco, CA, USA
e-mail: maibachh@derm.ucsf.edu

M.A. Farage et al. (eds.), *Textbook of Aging Skin*,
DOI 10.1007/978-3-662-47398-6_40

Tape Stripping Studies

Tape stripping was first devised in the 1940s and examined by Pinkus in 1951. Pinkus demonstrated a remarkable burst of mitotic epidermal activity poststripping, concluding that the lost horny layer is replaced by basal mitotic division [4]. The degree of hyperplasia correlates with the level and duration of barrier disruption [5]. Nevertheless, mitotic rate may remain five times greater than baseline 6 days after stripping [6]. Keratinocyte hyperproliferation may be a response to water barrier disruption or cytokine release secondary to epidermal injury [5, 6]. Adhesive stripping increases: epidermal lipid synthesis, lamellar body production/secretion in the stratum granulosum, epidermal DNA synthesis, epidermal cytokine production, dermal inflammation, and presence of TNF and IL-1α in skin [6]. Conversely, occlusion of stripped human skin via adhesive application suppresses mitotic activity; adhesive occlusion may provide artificial restoration of the lost barrier [6]. Similar experiments in mice do not support these findings [6].

The SC is essential to life, protecting the human body from desiccation and external penetration of deleterious agents. The SC is composed of nucleated, keratin-rich corneocytes embedded in an extracellular multilamellar lipid matrix organized into membrane-like bilayers; intercorneocyte communication occurs through desmosomes [7]. Many other SC models exist but none of them fully integrate all aspects of the skin barrier function. The SC is thin, less than 20 μm thick, and composed of about 10–15 tightly stacked layers, depending on the location [8]. Ceramides, cholesterol, and free fatty acids comprise the lipid matrix of the SC, providing invaluable roles in the barrier structure and function [7]. Their synthesis is required for barrier homeostasis; as with DNA, a burst of lipid synthesis (due to synthesis of their rate-limiting enzymes) occurs, following barrier perturbation [9]. Lipid levels decrease in aged human skin, possibly due to SC pH increases and subsequent lipid processing impairment; this is described further, below [7].

The SC provides the rate determining step for the passage of most molecules across skin [10]. Therefore, topical agent concentration within the SC is directly related to that in the epidermis and dermis, the typical target sites. Additionally, corneocytes and intercellular lipids are responsible for preventing insensible water loss [11]. The transepidermal water loss can be measured with an evaporimeter and frequently used to assess skin barrier integrity [11]. Anatomically, regional SC variations in percutaneous drug absorption, lipid composition, TEWL measurements, mean thickness, and number of cell layers have been described. Despite its structural heterogeneity, each layer of SC equally contributes in preventing water loss [11]. In doing so, the SC behaves as a membrane compatible with Fick's laws of passive diffusion [11].

TEWL increase as a function of tape strip number depends on the factors including: anatomical site, pressure, pressure duration, and tape removal rate [12]. Loffler et al. demonstrated that TEWL increased fastest on the forehead, followed by the back, and finally, the forearm [12]. These findings may be explained by the differences in SC thickness, differences in spontaneous desquamation (SC cohesion), and pressure resistance because of inherent viscoelasticity and type of tissue underlying the skin [12]. Rapid removal (vs. slow), shorter pressure duration (2 vs. 10 s), and higher pressure (330 g cm^{-2} vs. 165 cm^{-2}) all produced earlier TEWL increases [12].

A similar study by Breternitz et al. revealed the highest rise of TEWL on the cheek, compared to the back, upper arm, and forearm [13]. Interestingly, the cheek also demonstrated the greatest increase in SC hydration after stripping [13]. Breternitz et al. further established greater, earlier TEWL increase with higher pressure (7 N stamp vs. 2 N) and longer application (10 vs. 2 s) [13]. Moreover, using the thumb, stretching the skin, and utilizing a roller or stamp all result in varying quantities of harvested SC [13]. The use of thumb removed most of SC and produced the highest TEWL, even when compared with usage of a roller or skin stretching [13]. Occlusion of the test site prior to the stripping procedure resulted in higher TEWL values [13]. Occlusion results in water retention and degradation of the intercellular proteins [13]. In conclusion, reliable, reproducible results depend on standardization of the aforementioned variables.

Kalia et al. found that initial tape strips removed thicker layers of the SC, relating this to decreased number of desmosomes closer to the skin surface [10]. Kalia et al. demonstrated decreased impedance with increasing depth achieved, theorizing that removal of the upper corneocyte layers and lipid matrix diminishes structural opposition to ion flow, facilitating ion transport [10]. Yagi et al. determined the change of SC lipid structural order along with a sequence of tape stripping, and found less structurally ordered lipids in the outermost SC layers, whereas tighter structure of inner SC layers [14]. Depth profiling of SC lipid composition showed a sharp decline of free fatty acid from skin surface to tape stripping number 4 [15, 16]. In addition, TEWL increased disproportionally with later tape strips; removing only the upper SC layers was insufficient to significantly enhance the water loss [10]. Removal of 6–8 μm of SC (deeper layers) typically resulted in significant TEWL increases [10]. Removal of the outermost layers affected impedance more than TEWL, with a 40 % decrease in impedance after removal of only 4 μm of SC. Nonetheless, a correlation between TEWL increase and impedance decrease was observed. Upon completion of the tape stripping experiment, full return to the basal values of impedance occurred after 3 days, while TEWL recovery time was 5–6 days [10]. External layers, more crucial in impedance, are formed prior to deep compact layers [10].

The aforementioned findings suggest a gradation in water-regulating ability within the SC, with the deepest layers most responsible for controlling water flux [10]. However, via simple mathematical deduction, these results, in fact, support a Fickian model [10]. Though structurally heterogeneous and complex, the SC behaves as a homogenous barrier to water in vivo [10]. The water transport route may be homogeneous throughout SC, with each layer contributing equally to the barrier [10]. The best fit curve plotting experimental values of TEWL as a function of tape stripping frequency closely resembled a theoretical curve based on Fick's first law of diffusion [17]. The first half of the theoretical curve fit the actual curve; in the second half, experimental data show slightly higher TEWL values than Fick's theoretical values [17]. The authors of the study offer plausible explanations for this discrepancy [17].

In contrast to most studies, Schwindt et al. demonstrated that quantity of harvested SC was constant with each strip in a given anatomical site and volunteer [11]. Schwindt et al. found a linear relationship (in all anatomical sites) between 1/TEWL and the total mass of removed SC, further establishing that the SC acts as a Fickian membrane for steady state water diffusion [11]. It also appears that intercellular lipids, not corneocytes, are the determining factor for SC water diffusion [11]. This linear relationship was also described by another group, plotting 1/TEWL as a function of SC thickness (13 subjects examined) [18]. Table 1 summarizes the results from three studies quantifying SC thickness.

Tape construction influences outcome [13]. Three brands of adhesive tapes, utilized in vivo, displayed statistically equivalent mean water diffusion coefficients, SC permeability, and SC mass/thickness removal [3]. After 40 strips, however, a proprietary adhesive stripped the most, while a rayon adhesive stripped the least [3]. TEWL increased significantly as deeper SC layers were reached with proprietary and polyethylene adhesives but not with rayon tape [3]. Tape properties, subject properties, or a combination may account for variation in barrier disruptive properties. Variation may also be accounted for by unique adhesive systems; adhesives of different tape brands may bind similarly to cellular SC but differently to extracellular components of the SC barrier. These extracellular components (e.g., free fatty acids, ceramides, and lipids) are essential to barrier function. Furthermore, apparently 5–7 μm of SC removal resulted in significant TEWL elevations, a depth unobtainable by the rayon tape (Table 2) [3]. This implies that structural elements of the water barrier may not be

Table 1 Calculations of SC thickness in vivo in man

Authors	No. of subjects	Anatomical site	No. of strips	Mean total SC thickness (μm)
Kalia et al. [10]	3	Forearm	22–28	12.7 ± 3.3
Schwindt et al. [11]	6	Lower back	Up to 35	11.2
		Abdomen	Up to 35	7.7
		Thigh	Up to 35	13.1
		Forearm (ventral)	Up to 35	12.3 ± 3.5
Pirot et al. [18]	13	Forearm (ventral)	15	12.6 ± 5.3

Thickness appears to be a function of anatomical site

Table 2 Relationship between protein removal and TEWL from Bashir et al. [3]

Tape type	Location (forearm)	No. of strips	Mean thickness removed (μg)	TEWL (g m^{-1} h^{-1})
Proprietary	Dorsal	40	8.10	30.33
	Ventral	40	5.83	30.80
Polyethylene	Dorsal	40	7.25	31.98
	Ventral	40	4.96	30.83
Rayon	Dorsal	40	4.99	13.4
	Ventral	40	2.99	11.95

There are significant differences in TEWL and mean thickness removed depending on tape construction. The dorsal forearm, in all cases, had greater SC thickness removed than the ventral forearm

homogeneously distributed. In some subjects, neither the proprietary adhesive nor the polyethylene adhesive disrupted the water barrier; these individuals experienced no barrier disruption at any of six tested sites, suggesting variation of water barrier disruption to be a function of the individual.

Demonstrating that removal of the same amount of SC from different individuals does not result in similar increases in TEWL, Kalia et al. asked whether this variation was secondary to interindividual differences in intact membrane thickness [19]. Kalia et al. demonstrated that once interindividual differences in the thickness of the intact SC are corrected for (by normalizing the SC thickness removed with respect to calculated total SC thickness), the same degree of barrier disruption induces the same increase in TEWL in each individual [19]. Stated differently, removal of the same percentage of SC in two individuals results in equivalent barrier disruption. TEWL rises considerably only after about 75 % of the SC has been removed, presenting a very consistent barrier to water loss in the healthy human population [19].

As number of tape stripping does not linearly correlate with amount of SC removal [10], tape stripping numbers cannot be directly applied in dermatopharmacokinetic studies of topical formulations; normalized SC depth determined by TEWL measurements allowed the determination of SC concentration-depth profiles and the estimation of total chemical concentration in SC [20–22]. The mathematical fit of SC concentration-depth profile derives SC-vehicle partition coefficient (K) of chemical solute and its "diffusion kinetic" (D/L^2), which are useful parameters to characterize the extent and rate of chemical absorption across SC [20].

Tape Stripping and Aging

Aged skin demonstrates increased susceptibility to the xerosis, exogenous, and environmental insults, and diminished ability to recover from these insults, indicating a suboptimal epidermal barrier. It is believed that no definitive studies have compared aged versus normal SC thickness; nonetheless, some authors believe aged SC to be thicker, with decreased lipid content and deficient water-binding capacity [8]. TEWL is decreased in the aged, as is topical absorption [8]. The aging barrier was elegantly examined by Ghadially et al.; results are summarized below.

Aged humans (>80 years) have prolonged barrier recovery rates after tape stripping or acetone application compared to control subjects (20–30 years) [23]. Twenty-four hours after acetone treatment, 50 % recovery occurred in control subjects compared to 15 % in aged subjects [23]. Photoaging, in combination with this chronologic aging, may further delay recovery [9]. Furthermore, delays in SC lipid reappearance after barrier disruption have been described in aged murine epidermis [23].

Additionally, tape stripping studies have revealed decreased cohesiveness in aged skin [9]. In fact, barrier perturbation (TEWL $\geq$20 g m^{-2} h^{-1}) occurred after 18 $\pm$ 2 strippings in aged skin versus 31 $\pm$ 5 strippings in control skin [23]. Fortunately, topical lipid formulations, containing predominantly cholesterol, may accelerate barrier recovery in aged human skin [24].

The above findings may be explained by reduced delivery of secreted lipids to the epidermal surface in the elderly. There is a global diminution ($\approx$30 %) of ceramide, cholesterol, and free fatty acid contents in the aged murine skin [23]. This reduction could be due to the decreased production and/or increased destruction; cytokines (e.g., IL-1α) and growth factors may play a role [9]. Additionally, decreased secretion of lamellar body contents (at stratum granulosum-stratum corneum interface) with fewer extracellular lamellar bilayers (at stratum corneum interstices) contributes to a more porous extracellular SC matrix [23].

Ghadially et al. further examined the effect of lipids on SC barrier function [25]. As described previously, SC of aged mice displays decreased lipid content and extracellular bilayers. This may result in impaired barrier recovery after a tape stripping insult (18.7 vs. 60.8 % recovery by 24 h in aged vs. young mice). Upon further examination, Ghadially et al. determined that cholesterol synthesis is decreased significantly under basal conditions. Furthermore, sterologenesis fails to reach absolute levels obtained in young epidermis following tape stripping perturbation. A 40 % decrease in activity of HMG-CoA reductase, the rate-limiting enzyme in sterologenesis, was observed under basal conditions in aged mice. Despite a greater than 100 % increase in HMG-CoA reductase activity after barrier perturbation in aged mice, absolute levels did not attain those reached in treated, young epidermis.

Ghadially et al. also supplemented aged murine SC with an equimolar mixture of SC physiological lipids (cholesterol, ceramide, linoleic acid, palmitic acid) or cholesterol alone [25]. Either mixture applied once enhanced the recovery after barrier disruption. Additionally, after four applications of either mixture, electron microscopy demonstrated repletion of extracellular spaces with normal lamellar bilayer structures.

Further work examining the role of aging on the SC remains to be done. Tape stripping and TEWL studies of aged skin are currently underway.

Protein Quantification

After harvesting of SC onto adhesives is complete, protein can be measured via several methods. For decades, weighing (gravimetry) was the preferred method, despite its inherent inconvenience (weighing before and after stripping under constant hydration conditions). Additionally, results were subjected to inflation secondary to absorption of exogenous (topically applied) or endogenous (sebum, sweat, and interstitial fluid) substances within the SC. Initial strips were most affected by this absorption.

One decade ago, a novel colorimetric method was developed and validated by Dreher et al. [26]. This colorimetric method relies on a protein assay similar to one developed by Lowry et al. over half a century ago. Lowry's method involved measurement of protein with a folin phenol reagent after alkaline copper treatment [27]. It was demonstrated to be simple, sensitive, specific, and easily adaptable to small scale analyses, making it suitable for measurement of miniscule absolute protein amounts [27]. Dreher's method relies on spectrophotometry and colorimetry, based on the calibration of stained SC proteins to the corneocyte mass [28]. Drawbacks include time-consuming preparation of tape strips with necessary destruction of the original strips.

The Bradford dye reaction, which relies on Coomassie Brilliant Blue G-250 dye, is similar to Dreher's method. The dye binds protein, resulting in ionic and hydrophobic reactions, with a spectral shift from reddish-brown to blue. Maximal absorption for the bound form of the dye is 595 nm, the optimal wavelength for colorimetric measurement once the reaction has occurred. Despite disadvantages (e.g., serial dilutions), it is a fast and generally reliable method for protein quantification.

Dreher's colorimetric method has been successfully adapted to 96-well microplates, effectively shortening analysis time [29]. Note that limited areas of adhesive tape are not predictive of SC removal on the entire tape [29]. Alternatively stated, SC distribution on tape is not homogeneous [29].

A pivotal study examined direct spectroscopic SC protein quantification via absorption in the visible range (595 and 600 nm), with and without staining of corneocyte aggregates, and the UV range (278 nm) [30]. Correlation coefficients R^2 were 0.71 and 0.74, respectively. The results demonstrated weak SC protein absorption with immense light scattering [30]. The Coomassie brilliant blue protein coloring did not increase light absorption by SC proteins, and thus could not decrease the interference secondary to light scattering [30]. The absorption techniques utilized in this study cannot accurately predict corneocyte aggregate quantity.

Latter studies utilizing wavelengths of 430 nm have established optical spectroscopy in the visible range as a sensitive and reproducible method of protein quantification [2]. Absorbance in this range depends exclusively on quantity of corneocyte aggregates and adequately reflects SC mass [2]. Corneocyte aggregates, adhering to tape strips, decrease transmission of visible light by scattering, reflection, and diffraction. The resulting pseudo-absorption has been successfully correlated with mass of removed SC particles [2]. Absorbance measurement allows facile determination of absolute mass from corneocyte aggregates harvested via tape stripping. Topically applied substances do not interfere with the spectroscopic measurements as they do with gravimetric measurements, explaining mass differences in the most superficial strips (when compared with gravimetry) [31].

Practically comparing spectrally measured quantity (absorbance) with corneocyte aggregate weight requires correction for: topical applications in upper SC layers, interstitial fluid in deeper SC layers, the "stack effect" which decreases absorbance, and the tape stripping procedure itself (e.g., nonhomogeneous removal of tape or incomplete tape contact with skin) [2]. Once these factors are corrected for (primarily by excluding analysis of the most superficial and deep strips), $R^2 = 0.93$, demonstrating proportionality between quantification methods [2].

A multicenter study involving 24 subjects found a correlation coefficient of $R^2 = 0.94$ when comparing UV/VIS spectroscopy (430 nm) with conventional weight determination [31]. Superficial (first five) and deep (19–23) strips were excluded on the basis of weight enhancement; application on an oil–water emulsion (part of the study) inflated superficial strip weight and intrinsic interstitial fluid increased deep strip weight [31]. Nonhomogeneous strips and those subjected to handling errors were excluded [31]. Only 66 % of total strips were utilized to determine the correlation coefficient [31]. Weigmann et al. explain that pseudo-absorption/weight correlation can be extrapolated to the deepest layers of the SC [31].

A recent study demonstrated strong correlation ($R^2 = 0.92$ and $R^2 = 0.95$) between pseudo-absorption at 430 nm and both protein absorption at 278 nm and absorption of Trypan blue-stained proteins at 652 nm [28]. However, protein absorption at 278 nm was characterized by a weak band, implying application limited to tape strips with high amounts of corneocytes [28]. Mass determination based on the UV absorption is further limited by the potential superpositioning of strong absorption bands from exogenous substances and/or tape components in the same spectral range. Unlike the previous study, correlation was

Table 3 Studies using infrared densitometry method to quantify protein content on tape strips

Authors	Body site	Ethnicity	Age	Regression equation[a]	R^2
Voegeli et al. [32]	Forearm	Caucasian	38.8 ± 8.6	y = 0.62x + 2.70	0.85
Hahn et al. [33]	Volar forearm	Caucasian	24–50	y = 0.61x + 2.07	0.63
	Volar forearm/abdominal skin	Caucasian	24–50	y = 0.45x + 4.8	0.57
Raj et al. [35]	Forearm	Caucasian	44.6 ± 3.1	y = 0.72x + 0.12	0.91
		Black African	38.2 ± 2.3	y = 0.68x + 1.19	0.77
	Cheek	Caucasian	44.6 ± 3.1	y = 0.63x + 0.70	0.69
		Black African	38.2 ± 2.3	y = 0.87x − 2.40	0.86

[a]y is tape stripping absorption (%) at 850 nm; x is protein content (μg/cm^2) measured by colorimetric method

described using all the tape strips (superficial and deep), regardless of adherent exogenous or endogenous components [28].

Lademann et al. tested an inexpensive, easily reproducible optical device ("corneocyte density analyzer"), based on a slide projector, which also measures corneocyte pseudo-absorption at 430 nm [1]. When compared with standard UV-visible spectrometric measurements, a correlation factor of $R^2 = 0.95$ was demonstrated [1]. The device may simplify calculation of removed SC, without messy chemistry or an expensive spectrometer; it includes a mechanical autofeed system, well suited for the handling of tape strips [1].

More recently, an infrared densitometry method was designed for quantifying protein on tape stripping samples. Overall linear regression between absorption at 850 nm and protein content determined by colorimetric method were established for in vivo and in vitro studies [32–35]. Table 3 presents regression equations and correlation coefficients obtained from various anatomical sites of human subjects with different ethnicities in vivo. Protein content measured by this infrared method was also correlated with SC weight removed by tape stripping with $R^2 = 0.65$ [36]. In vitro tape stripping study on human surgical skin showed freezing and storage of skin may change the cohesiveness of SC [33]. This fast and nondestructive method was used to quantify SC removed by sequence of tape stripping, and thus characterize the penetration of topically applied chemicals [37].

Colorimetric Bioassay of Keratolytic Efficacy

The desquamating effects of three keratolytics are presented in table format (Table 4) using the data obtained from colorimetric protein assays described by Dreher et al. (mentioned above) [20]. The process begins with cutaneous application of the agent; the agent is placed on a patch and taped onto the subject's skin for a predetermined number of hours. After this period, placement and removal of tape strips (number varies by study) onto the site of topical treatment are performed. The assay involves immersion and shaking of SC adhering tapes in sodium hydroxide solution resulting in extraction of the soluble SC protein fraction. The solution, now containing SC protein, is neutralized with hydrogen chloride, as the assay is ineffective under strongly alkaline conditions. The protein assay is performed using the Bio-Rad Detergent Compatible Protein Assay Kit and following the prescribed microassay procedure. This assay is similar to the Lowry assay and is based on the reaction of protein with an alkaline copper tartrate solution and Folin reagent. Finally, absorbance at 750 nm is measured using a Hitachi U-2001 UV–vis spectrophotometer. This method allows for quantification of microgram amounts of SC, diminishing confounding factors, namely, vehicle and water uptake by the SC.

The protein measured using the assay described can be compared among groups, with statistical analysis allowing determination of

Table 4 Studies using colorimetric protein assay to measure keratolytic potential

Authors	Drug	Result
Bashir et al. [38]	Aqueous solution 2 % Salicylic Acid – 3 formulations	Statistically significant mass of SC removed after 6 h and 20 tape strips in all three experimental groups (salicylic acid pH 3.3, salicylic acid pH 3.3 w/menthol, and salicylic acid pH 6.95) compared to vehicle, untreated, and untreated but occluded groups.
Waller et al. [40]	Aqueous solutions of 0.05 % all-trans RA, 2 % BPO, and 2 % SA	Statistically significant mass of SC removed after 6 h and 25 tape strips in all three experimental groups compare to vehicle, untreated, and occluded groups. The first 10 tape strips from SA group removed more protein than the other groups; at 10–15 strips, treatments were comparable; at 16–25 strips, protein removed from BPO sites was greatest.

All agents tested demonstrated significant efficacy in SC removal. SA had superior superficial removal, while BP had superior deep removal

strong and weak keratolytics. SC removal via tape stripping in treatment and control groups is attributable to keratolytic mechanisms, which loosen SC cohesion. The disintegrated SC is subsequently collected by the adhesive.

In the first keratolytic bioassay using this technique, salicylic acid was examined [38]. Keratolytic efficacy of salicylic acid was determined as a function of pH. The test preparations were: aqueous vehicle control of pH 7.4, 2 % SA aqueous solution of pH 3.3, 2 % SA aqueous solution of pH 3.3 with menthol, and 2 % SA aqueous solution of pH 6.95 [38]. A statistically significant mass of SC was removed after 6 h and 20 tape strips in all three experimental groups compared to vehicle, untreated, and untreated but occluded groups [38]. However, after 10 strips, the SA pH 3.3 solution with menthol and the SA pH 6.95 solution removed significantly more SC than any other group, including the SA pH 3.3 solution [38]. These data suggest that a neutral preparation of SA results in a pronounced keratolytic effect. Moreover, the neutral preparation was associated with the least skin irritation among treatment groups [38]. This finding differs from that of a previous study, which demonstrated superior SA skin penetration in an acidic solution compared to neutral solution [39].

In the second bioassay using the aforementioned technique, salicylic acid, benzoyl peroxide (BPO), and retinoic acid were examined [40]. The test preparations were: 0.05 % all-trans retinoic acid, 2 % salicylic acid at pH 6.95, 2 % BPO, vehicle, untreated skin, and occluded but untreated skin [40]. After 3 h of treatment, only BPO treatment removed significantly more SC on 25 strips than untreated skin, while the other treatments did not achieve statistical significance [40]. At 3 h, SA had greater SC amounts removed in the first 10 (superficial) strips, while deeper strips (11–25) demonstrated BPO to have the greatest SC removal [40].

Statistically significant masses of SC were removed after 6 h and 25 tape strips in all three experimental groups when compared to vehicle, untreated, and occluded groups [40]. At 6 h, the first 10 tape strips from the SA group removed more protein than the other groups; at 10–15 strips, all treatments were comparable; at 16–25 strips, BPO removed the most protein [40].

These in vivo human results indicate that all treatments tested are effective keratolytics, which may account for their effectiveness against acne vulgaris. Furthermore, it appears that salicylic acid may be a more suitable treatment for mild, superficial acne while BPO may be optimal for deeper, inflammatory acne. BPO's ability to loosen SC at deeper levels complements its antimicrobial/anti-inflammatory properties, resulting in an effective anti-inflammatory agent for papulo-pustular acne. Additionally, BPO appears to be effective even with short-term administration. RA had inferior SC disruption at 3 h but significant disruption at 6 h, indicating time-dependent keratolytic effects, consistent with its complex nuclear receptor interactions and alteration of gene transcription.

Conclusion

Taken together, the SC is beginning to reveal some of its secrets. Much remains to be done.

Cross-References

- ▶ Corneocyte Size and Cell Renewal: Effects of Aging and Sex Hormones
- ▶ Stratum Corneum Cell Layers
- ▶ The Stratum Corneum and Aging

References

1. Lademann J, Ilgevicius A, Zurbau O, Liess HD, Schanzer S, Weigmann HJ, Antoniou C, Pelchrzim RV, Sterry W. Penetration studies of topically applied substances: optical determination of the amount of stratum corneum removed by tape stripping. J Biomed Opt. 2006;11(5):054026.
2. Weigmann H, Lademann J, Meffert H, Schaefer H, Sterry W. Determination of the horny layer profile by tape stripping in combination with optical spectroscopy in the visible range as a prerequisite to quantify percutaneous absorption. Skin Pharmacol Appl Skin Physiol. 1999;12(1–2):34–45.
3. Bashir SJ, Chew AL, Anigbogu A, Dreher F, Maibach HI. Physical and physiological effects of stratum corneum tape stripping. Skin Res Technol. 2001;7(1):40–8.
4. Pinkus H. Examination of the epidermis by the strip method of removing horny layers. I. Observations on thickness of the horny layer, and on mitotic activity after stripping. J Invest Dermatol. 1951;16(6):383–6.
5. Denda M, Wood LC, Emami S, Calhoun C, Brown BE, Elias PM, Feingold KR. The epidermal hyperplasia associated with repeated barrier disruption by acetone treatment or tape stripping cannot be attributed to increased water loss. Arch Dermatol Res. 1996;288(5–6):230–8.
6. Fisher LB, Maibach HI. Physical occlusion controlling epidermal mitosis. J Invest Dermatol. 1972;59(1):106–8.
7. Jungersted JM, Hellgren LI, Jemec GB, Agner T. Lipids and skin barrier function – a clinical perspective. Contact Dermatitis. 2008;58(5):255–62.
8. Tagami H. Functional characteristics of the stratum corneum in photoaged skin in comparison with those found in intrinsic aging. Arch Dermatol Res. 2008;300 Suppl 1:1–6.
9. Elias PM, Ghadially R. The aged epidermal permeability barrier: basis for functional abnormalities. Clin Geriatr Med. 2002;18(1):103–20, vii.
10. Kalia YN, Pirot F, Guy RH. Homogeneous transport in a heterogeneous membrane: water diffusion across human stratum corneum in vivo. Biophys J. 1996;71(5):2692–700.
11. Schwindt DA, Wilhelm KP, Maibach HI. Water diffusion characteristics of human stratum corneum at different anatomical sites in vivo. J Invest Dermatol. 1998;111(3):385–9.
12. Loffler H, Dreher F, Maibach HI. Stratum corneum adhesive tape stripping: influence of anatomical site, application pressure, duration and removal. Br J Dermatol. 2004;151(4):746–52.
13. Breternitz M, Flach M, Prassler J, Elsner P, Fluhr JW. Acute barrier disruption by adhesive tapes is influenced by pressure, time and anatomical location: integrity and cohesion assessed by sequential tape stripping. A randomized, controlled study. Br J Dermatol. 2007;156(2):231–40.
14. Yagi ER, Sakamoto K, Nakagawa K. Depth dependence of stratum corneum lipid ordering: a slow-tumbling simulation for electron paramagnetic resonance. J Invest Dermatol. 2007;127(4):895–9.
15. Bonte F, Saunois A, Pinguet P, Meybeck A. Existence of a lipid gradient in the upper stratum corneum and its possible biological significance. Arch Dermatol Res. 1997;289(2):78–82.
16. Weerheim A, Ponec M. Determination of stratum corneum lipid profile by tape stripping in combination with high-performance thin-layer chromatography. Arch Dermatol Res. 2001;293(4):191–9.
17. van der Valk PG, Maibach HI. A functional study of the skin barrier to evaporative water loss by means of repeated cellophane-tape stripping. Clin Exp Dermatol. 1990;15(3):180–2.
18. Pirot F, Berardesca E, Kalia YN, Singh M, Maibach HI, Guy RH. Stratum corneum thickness and apparent water diffusivity: facile and noninvasive quantitation in vivo. Pharm Res. 1998;15(3):492–4.
19. Kalia YN, Alberti I, Sekkat N, Curdy C, Naik A, Guy RH. Normalization of stratum corneum barrier function and transepidermal water loss in vivo. Pharm Res. 2000;17(9):1148–50.
20. Herkenne C, Naik A, Kalia YN, Hadgraft J, Guy RH. Dermatopharmacokinetic prediction of topical drug bioavailability in vivo. J Invest Dermatol. 2007;127(4):887–94.
21. Herkenne C, Naik A, Kalia YN, Hadgraft J, Guy RH. Effect of propylene glycol on ibuprofen absorption into human skin in vivo. J Pharm Sci. 2008;97(1):185–97.
22. Alberti I, Kalia YN, Naik A, Bonny JD, Guy RH. In vivo assessment of enhanced topical delivery of terbinafine to human stratum corneum. J Control Release. 2001;71(3):319–27.
23. Ghadially R, Brown BE, Sequeira-Martin SM, Feingold KR, Elias PM. The aged epidermal permeability barrier. Structural, functional, and lipid biochemical abnormalities in humans and a senescent murine model. J Clin Invest. 1995;95(5):2281–90.

24. Zettersten EM, et al. Optimal ratios of topical stratum corneum lipids improve barrier recovery in chronologically aged skin. J Am Acad Dermatol. 1997;37(3 Pt 1):403–8.
25. Ghadially R, Brown BE, Hanley K, Reed JT, Feingold KR, Elias PM. Decreased epidermal lipid synthesis accounts for altered barrier function in aged mice. J Invest Dermatol. 1996;106(5):1064–9.
26. Dreher F, Arens A, Hostynek JJ, Mudumba S, Ademola J, Maibach HI. Colorimetric method for quantifying human Stratum corneum removed by adhesive-tape stripping. Acta Derm Venereol. 1998;78(3):186–9.
27. Lowry OH, Rosebrough NJ, Farr AL, Randall RJ. Protein measurement with the Folin phenol reagent. J Biol Chem. 1951;193(1):265–75.
28. Lindemann U, Weigmann HJ, Schaefer H, Sterry W, Lademann J. Evaluation of the pseudo-absorption method to quantify human stratum corneum removed by tape stripping using protein absorption. Skin Pharmacol Appl Skin Physiol. 2003;16 (4):228–36.
29. Dreher F, Modjtahedi BS, Modjtahedi SP, Maibach HI. Quantification of stratum corneum removal by adhesive tape stripping by total protein assay in 96-well microplates. Skin Res Technol. 2005;11(2):97–101.
30. Marttin E, Neelissen-Subnel MT, De Haan FH, Bodde HE. A critical comparison of methods to quantify stratum corneum removed by tape stripping. Skin Pharmacol. 1996;9(1):69–77.
31. Weigmann HJ. UV/VIS absorbance allows rapid, accurate, and reproducible mass determination of corneocytes removed by tape stripping. Skin Pharmacol Appl Skin Physiol. 2003;16(4):217–27.
32. Voegeli R, Heiland J, Doppler S, Rawlings AV, Schreier T. Efficient and simple quantification of stratum corneum proteins on tape strippings by infrared densitometry. Skin Res Technol. 2007;13(3):242–51.
33. Hahn T, Hansen S, Neumann D, Kostka KH, Lehr CM, Muys L, Schaefer UF. Infrared densitometry: a fast and non-destructive method for exact stratum corneum depth calculation for in vitro tape-stripping. Skin Pharmacol Physiol. 2010;23(4):183–92.
34. Klang V, Schwarz JC, Hartl A, Valenta C. Facilitating in vitro tape stripping: application of infrared densitometry for quantification of porcine stratum corneum proteins. Skin Pharmacol Physiol. 2011;24(5):256–68.
35. Raj N, Voegeli R, Rawlings AV, Gibbons S, Munday MR, Summers B, Lane ME. Variation in stratum corneum protein content as a function of anatomical site and ethnic group. Int J Cosmet Sci. 2015. doi:10.1111/ics.12274.
36. Mohammed D, Yang Q, Guy RH, Matts PJ, Hadgraft J, Lane ME. Comparison of gravimetric and spectroscopic approaches to quantify stratum corneum removed by tape-stripping. Eur J Pharm Biopharm. 2012;82(1):171–4.
37. Cadavona, JJP, Zhu H, Hui X, Jung, EC, and Maibach HI, Depth-dependent stratum corneum permeability in human skin in vitro. J Appl Toxicol. 2016. doi:10.1002/jat.3289.
38. Bashir SJ, Dreher F, Chew AL, Zhai H, Levin C, Stern R, Maibach HI. Cutaneous bioassay of salicylic acid as a keratolytic. Int J Pharm. 2005;292(1–2):187–94.
39. Leveque N, Makki S, Hadgraft J, Humbert P. Comparison of Franz cells and microdialysis for assessing salicylic acid penetration through human skin. Int J Pharm. 2004;269(2):323–8.
40. Waller JM, Dreher F, Behnam S, Ford C, Lee C, Tiet T, Weinstein GD, Maibach HI. "Keratolytic" properties of benzoyl peroxide and retinoic acid resemble salicylic acid in man. Skin Pharmacol Physiol. 2006;19(5):283–9.

Corneocyte Size and Cell Renewal: Effects of Aging and Sex Hormones

30

Razvigor Darlenski, Enzo Berardesca, and Joachim W. Fluhr

Contents

R. Darlenski (✉)
Department of Dermatology and Venereology, Tokuda Hospital Sofia, Sofia, Bulgaria
e-mail: darlenski@gmail.com

E. Berardesca
San Gallicano Dermatological Institute, Rome, Italy
e-mail: berardesca@berardesca.it

J.W. Fluhr
Department of Dermatology, Charité University Clinic, Berlin, Germany
e-mail: Joachim.Fluhr@charite.de

M.A. Farage et al. (eds.), *Textbook of Aging Skin*,
DOI 10.1007/978-3-662-47398-6_36

Abstract

Epidermal barrier function resides almost entirely in the outermost skin layer – stratum corneum (SC). Aging process results in certain structural and functional changes in SC morphology. The epidermis shows a linear decrease in thickness with age. The reduction in epidermal population size suggests that there may be also a decrease in the rate on production of epidermal cells and the apparent lengthening of the SC renewal time. The lengthening of the turnover implies a reduction in the desquamation rate, but this is not as large as thought. The reason for this might be the increase of corneocyte size during aging. There is a correlation and an inverse relationship between SC turnover and dimensions of corneocytes.

Sex hormones exhibit certain effects on SC structure and functions. A decreased sebum content of the forehead in menopausal women and higher SC hydration of the forehead in late menopausal women were observed. SC sphingolipid content and synthesis were decreased with the decrease of the effect of sex hormones with age. Aged epidermal permeability barrier shows decreased cohesion as well as delayed barrier repair with age under stress conditions. Significantly smaller corneocytes in premenopausal women vs. postmenopausal women or men were witnessed and are likely to be attributed to the different levels of female sex hormones.

These effects were decreased when hormone replacement therapy was introduced in post-menopausal women.

Introduction: Epidermal Organization and Cell Turnover

The stratum corneum (SC) responsible for the epidermal barrier function is viewed currently as a layer of protein-enriched corneocytes embedded in a lipid-enriched, intercellular matrix [1], the so-called "bricks and mortar" model. The "bricks" are corneocytes surrounded by a cornified cell envelope made up of proteins, mainly loricrin, filaggrin, and involucrin, and covalently bound to the hydroxyceramide molecules of a lipid envelope. The "bricks" are embedded in a "mortar" of lipid bilayers [2–4]. The so-called mortar contains a variety of intercellular lipids including ceramides, free sterols and sterol esters, cholesterol sulfate, and free fatty acids. The SC continually renews itself with a steady state between the proliferation and differentiating process of keratinocytes and desquamation of corneocytes.

Two important forces are responsible for the adherence of corneocytes and build the functional barrier of the skin: the corneodesmosomes as a morphomechanical force and the intercellular lipids as a functional force. Entering the process of differentiation, keratinosomes containing lamellar structured lipid bilayers are reaching from the center of the cytosol in the stratum spinosum to the apical cell pole and are extruded at the border between the stratum granulosum and SC. In the intercellular space, lipids form bi- and multilamellar structures adhering to the corneocytes [1, 3]. Apart from an intact barrier function, the water content of the epidermis depends on so-called natural moisturizing factors (NMF). These are amino acids, lactic acid, pyrrolidone carboxylic acid, and urea which are released after the breakdown of filaggrin in the midportion of the stratum corneum corneocytes, exhibiting an osmotic force and thus binding water.

The effect of age on the thickness of skin strata is one of the more controversial topics among dermatological researchers. Comparing measures of skin layer thickness between individuals (and between studies) is especially challenging because of significant variation in measurements between individuals and between sites within each individual. Light and electron microscopic studies have provided important evidence for morphological changes in skin strata with age, even though there is a general agreement that skin thickness (in terms of epidermis, dermis, and also SC) decreases with age (Fig. 1).

Changes in SC with Age

There have been few attempts to measure the rate of corneocyte loss and desquamation in relation to the aging process. Corneocyte size and renewal (or turnover) depend not only on the rate of input into the system (epidermopoiesis) but also on the rate at which cells are lost (desquamation). The epidermis shows a linear decrease in thickness with age, both in absolute terms and in cell number [5, 6]. The reduction in epidermal population size suggests that there may be also a decrease in the rate on production of epidermal cells, and the apparent lengthening of the SC renewal time [7] seems to confirm it [8]. In addition, there is some evidence that the rate of reepithelialization of wounds decreases with age. Using tritiated thymidine and an autoradiographic labeling method, Kligman [9] reported a reduced value for an elderly cohort compared to a younger group; in a study comparing the effects of aging between sun-exposed and nonexposed sites, this has not been detected [10]. In a more sensitive but complicated assay using the fluorescence activated cell sorting (FACS) fluorescent assay, an age-related decrease in the DNA synthesis and so in a longer cell cycle through the SC was demonstrated [11]. SC cell turnover and replacement time have been evaluated using the dansyl chloride staining technique. Dansyl chloride is a fluorescent dye which penetrates the full thickness of the SC and, when applied topically to the skin in vivo, becomes florescent under Wood's light [12]. The time the fluorescence takes to disappear corresponds to the turnover cycle of the SC. These

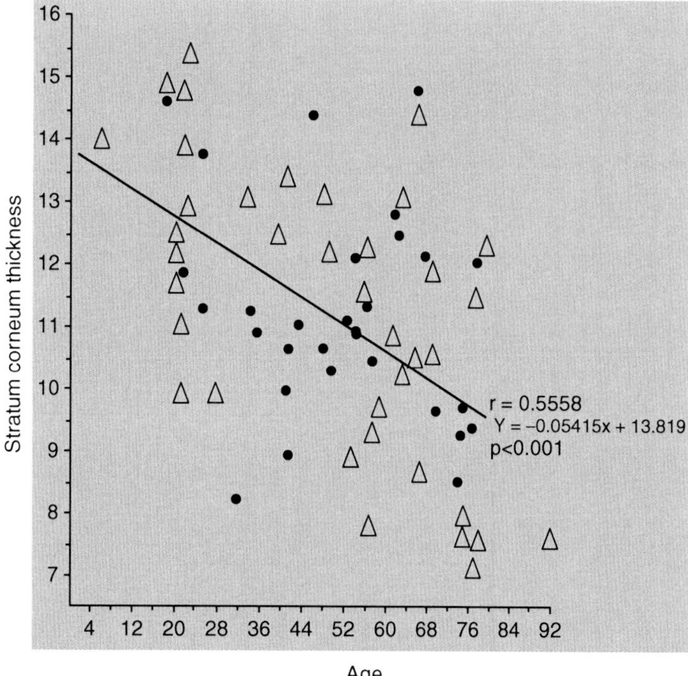

Fig. 1 Correlation between thickness of the stratum corneum and age [14]

studies have shown a progressive increase in the turnover time of the SC associated with increasing age [13]. The lengthening of the turnover implies a reduction in the desquamation rate, but this is not as large as thought. The reason for this is the increase of corneocyte size during aging. Thus, there are fewer corneocytes in an old individual's SC compared to a young one per volume unit (Fig. 2). Studies measuring the release of corneocytes from the skin showed also that there is a decrease of corneocyte loss at least measured under these experimental conditions [14].

The evolution of corneocyte size during the aging process has been studied by several authors; there is a consensus that the size progressively increases with age, even though there are body site variations and seasonal variations (changes due to hormonal status will be discussed later in this document). The more investigated sites are the arm and the forearm, and data shows a progressive increase of corneocyte size from birth to age (Fig. 3) [15–18].

Some differences have been reported between sun-exposed and non-sun-exposed areas (Fig. 4) [19] where in general UV irradiation increases epidermal turnover leading to smaller corneocytes compared to a similar photoprotected site. Indeed, seasonal variations in corneocyte size have been reported with smaller corneocytes in summer as a consequence of prolonged solar irradiation [4, 20]. In a study on professional cyclists, it was found that the size of corneocytes from the area of the arm protected by the shirt was "normal," while in the adjacent exposed area, the area of the cells was significantly smaller [21].

In conclusion there is a correlation and an inverse relationship between SC turnover and dimensions of corneocytes (Fig. 5).

Influence of Sex Hormones

The influences of sex hormones on morphologic and functional parameters of the epidermis are of increasing interest. The effects of hormones and aging on SC structure, function, and composition are not yet known in detail. Although age-dependent factors have been studied, few data are available concerning changes in perimenopausal women [22] with a significantly decreased sebum content of the forehead in menopausal women and higher SC hydration of the

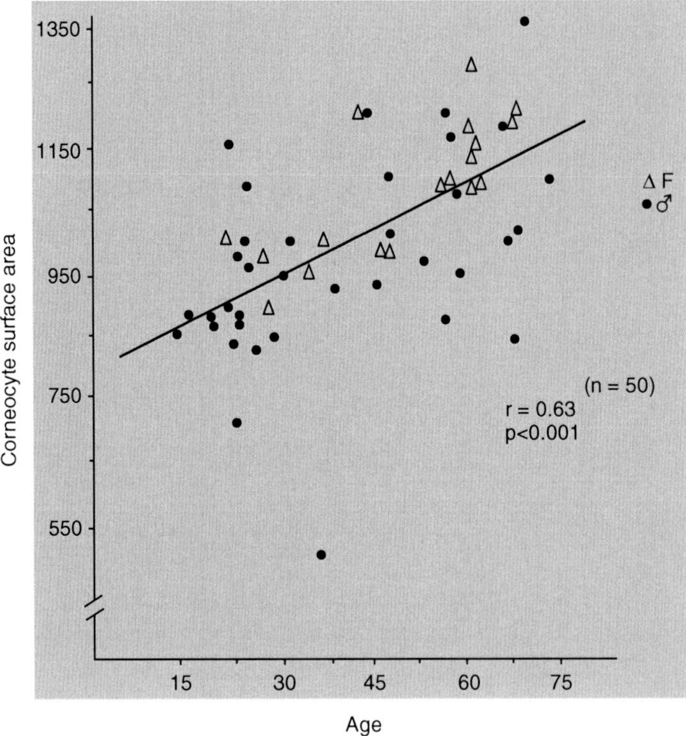

Fig. 2 Corneocyte surface area and age. There is a significantly positive correlation [18]

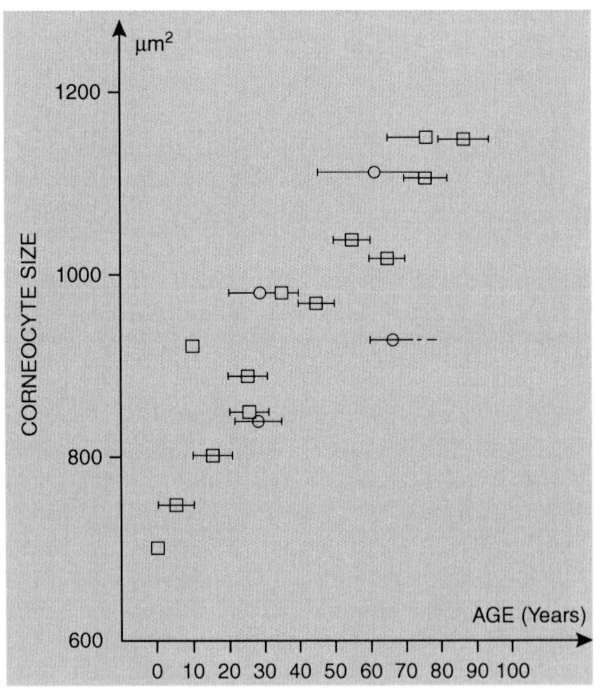

Fig. 3 Evolution of the corneocyte size versus age on the forearm. Data of different groups from references [11] (*solid squares*), [12] (*solid circles*), [13] (*open circles*), and [14] (*open squares*)

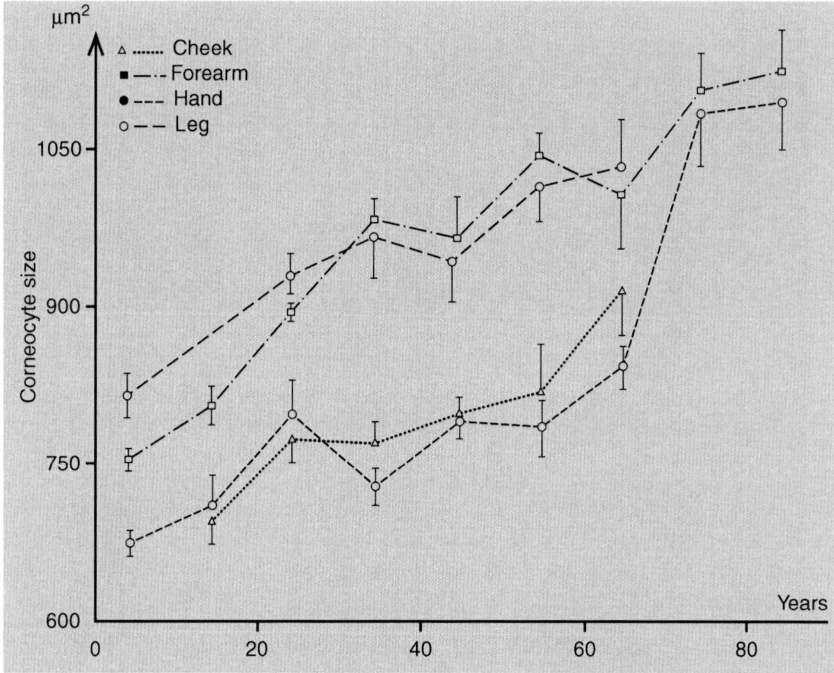

Fig. 4 Comparative evolution of corneocyte size at different body sites (From Ref. [15])

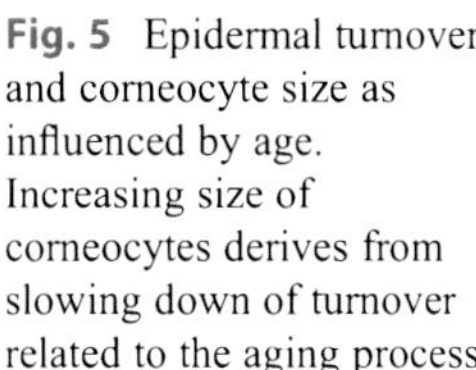
Fig. 5 Epidermal turnover and corneocyte size as influenced by age. Increasing size of corneocytes derives from slowing down of turnover related to the aging process

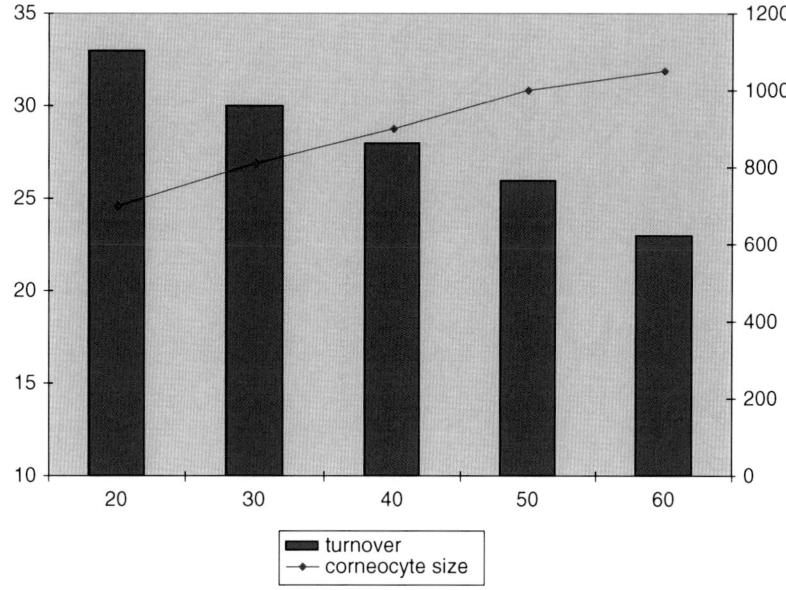

forehead in late menopausal women. Influences of female hormones on the composition of SC sphingolipids have been described, as well as the negative impact of age on the biosynthesis of sphingolipids [23]. With age, a decline occurs in hormone levels, especially in sex hormones like estrogen, testosterone, dehydroepiandrosterone, and growth hormones [24, 25]. Hormone replacement therapy leads to an increase in collagen content [26]. Under basal conditions, the

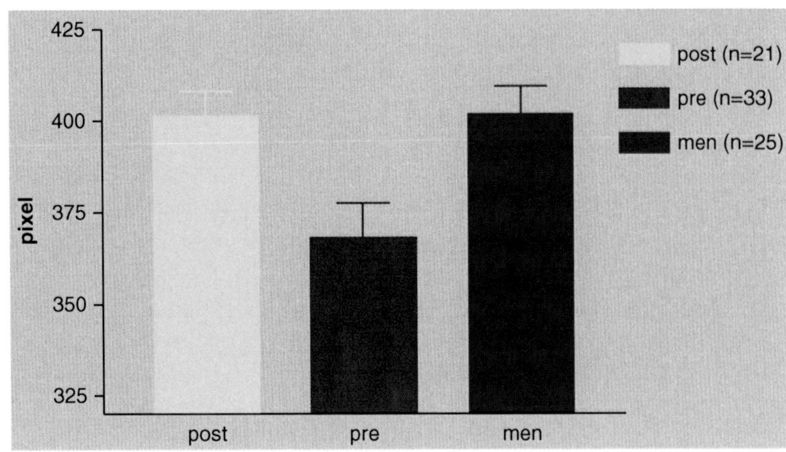

Fig. 6 Corneocyte size pre- and postmenopause as compared to men of the same age. Menopause induces an increase in corneocyte size comparable to men of the same age (Pixel as surface unit of the corneocyte size; mean ± SD) [29]

physiologic functions of SC seem to remain unchanged with age. Under stressed conditions, however, aged skin is more susceptible to barrier disruption than younger skin, i.e., an aged epidermal permeability barrier shows decreased cohesion as well as delayed barrier repair with age under stress conditions [27, 28].

Corneocyte size in pre- and postmenopausal women of the same age group (40–50 years age range) was investigated and compared to men of the same age range using a videomicroscopic technique [29]: despite the close age range, the significantly smaller corneocytes in premenopausal women vs. postmenopausal women or men are likely to be attributed to the different levels of female sex hormones (Fig. 6). The detected differences support the hypothesis that sexual hormones have an impact on corneocyte surface area. Female sex hormone levels of premenopausal women are supposed to be higher than those of nonhormonal substituted postmenopausal women or men, and thus the smaller corneocyte surface area could be explained by the influence of female sex hormones. The barrier function and the SC hydration parameters are not involved in this mechanism as no correlation between these parameters and corneocyte surface area was detectable. In this study, no other major differences in barrier function or SC water-holding properties have been detected (at least for the close chronological age range of the investigated groups), even though there are some reports in the literature on the positive impact of hormone replacement therapy on cutaneous mechanical properties and water-holding capacity [30, 31]. Further investigation is necessary to study the physiology of perimenopausal skin especially under stress conditions. The role of hormonal replacement therapy (HRT) has been documented in a study [32] where menopausal women had been treated for at least 5 or 10 years; the biophysical measurements were significantly higher for the parameters evaluating hydration and sebum secretion, which generally decrease after the menopause, associated with higher values for the yellow intensity parameter and the skin relief parameters on the forehead. The skin relief parameters on the forehead were significantly higher in menopausal women since at least 5 years taking HRT. This study could show an effect of HRT on skin color assessed by colorimetry and on skin relief with an increase of the roughness parameters on the forehead. A further investigation assessed the effect of HRT on the skin, using high-frequency diagnostic ultrasound combined with computerized image analysis [33]. The study was a cross-sectional observational study carried out on 84 women (comprising 34 HRT users, 25 postmenopausal controls, and 25 premenopausal controls). The time period of HRT varied from 6 months to 6 years. The skin was thicker in the HRT group than in the postmenopausal control group [33]. An additional study evaluating the severity of facial wrinkling by an eight-point photographic scale in Korean women assessed the HRT impact among 85 postmenopausal women, comprising 15 taking HRT. HRT was associated with a lower risk for facial wrinkling in the postmenopausal group [34]. These results support the subjective impression and the clinical evaluation concerning the impact of HRT on the development and the severity of some properties associated with skin aging after menopause.

Conclusions

The aging process, associated with hormonal changes in women during menopause, has a significant impact on the physiology of the skin and the SC. In particular, corneocytes are larger due to the slowing of metabolic processes and to the slower keratinocyte turnover. This can cause changes in the physical properties of the upper layers causing some "cosmetic" effects such as decreased brightness and reduction of transcutaneous penetration. Cell renewal is slower, even though desquamation rate seems to be constant. Hydration of the SC seems not to change significantly during early aging, despite contradictory reports: probably, this is related to an uneven distribution of the water profile on skin surface which can be investigated today by new imaging techniques [35].

Cross-References

▸ Stratum Corneum Cell Layers
▸ The Stratum Corneum and Aging

References

1. Landmann L. The epidermal permeability barrier. Anat Embryol (Berl). 1988;178(1):1–13.
2. Steven AC, Steinert PM. Protein composition of cornified cell envelopes of epidermal keratinocytes. J Cell Sci. 1994;107(Pt 2):693–700.
3. Swartzendruber DC, et al. Evidence that the corneocyte has a chemically bound lipid envelope. J Invest Dermatol. 1987;88(6):709–13.
4. Wertz PW, Downing DT. Covalently bound omega-hydroxyacylsphingosine in the stratum corneum. Biochim Biophys Acta. 1987;917(1):108–11.
5. Haftek M. 'Memory' of the stratum corneum: exploration of the epidermis' past. Br J Dermatol. 2014;171 Suppl 3:6–9.
6. Fluhr JW, et al. Development and organization of human stratum corneum after birth: electron microscopy isotropy score and immunocytochemical corneocyte labelling as epidermal maturation's markers in infancy. Br J Dermatol. 2014;171(5):978–86.
7. Chu M, Kollias N. Documentation of normal stratum corneum scaling in an average population: features of differences among age, ethnicity and body site. Br J Dermatol. 2011;164(3):497–507.
8. Furukawa F, et al. Effects of adenosine 5′-monophosphate on epidermal turnover. Arch Dermatol Res. 2008;300(9):485–93.
9. Kligman AM. Perspectives and problems in cutaneous gerontology. J Invest Dermatol. 1979;73(1):39–46.
10. Marks R. The effects of photoageing and intrinsic ageing on epidermal structure and function. G Ital Chir Dermatol Oncol. 1987;2:252–63.
11. Marks R. The epidermal engine: a commentary on epidermopoiesis, desquamation and their interrelationships. Int J Cosmet Sci. 1986;8(3):135–44.
12. Jansen LH, Hojyo-Tomoko MT, Kligman AM. Improved fluorescence staining technique for estimating turnover of the human stratum corneum. Br J Dermatol. 1974;90(1):9–12.
13. Roberts D, Marks R. The determination of regional and age variations in the rate of desquamation: a comparison of four techniques. J Invest Dermatol. 1980;74(1):13–6.
14. Marks R. Measurement of biological ageing in human epidermis. Br J Dermatol. 1981;104(6):627–33.
15. Grove G, et al. Use of nonintrusive tests to monitor age associated changes in human skin. J Soc Cosmet Chem. 1981;32:15–26.
16. Leveque JL, et al. In vivo studies of the evolution of physical properties of the human skin with age. Int J Dermatol. 1984;23(5):322–9.
17. Marks R, Nicholls S, King CS. Studies on isolated corneocytes. Int J Cosmet Sci. 1981;3(6):251–9.
18. Plewig G. Regional differences of cell sizes in the human stratum corneum. II. Effects of sex and age. J Invest Dermatol. 1970;54(1):19–23.
19. Corcuff P, Leveque JL. Corneocyte changes after acute UV irradiation and chronic solar exposure. Photodermatol. 1988;5(3):110–5.
20. Hermann S, Scheuber E, Plewig G. Exfoliative cytology: effects of seasons. In: Marks R, Plewig G, editors. Stratum corneum. Berlin: Springer; 1983. p. 181–5.
21. Leveque J, et al. Influence of chronic sun exposure on some biophysical parameters of the human skin; an in vivo study. J Cutan Aging Cosmet Dermatol. 1988;1:123–7.
22. Ohta H, et al. Relationship between dermato-physiological changes and hormonal status in pre-, peri-, and postmenopausal women. Maturitas. 1998;30(1):55–62.

23. Denda M, et al. Age- and sex-dependent change in stratum corneum sphingolipids. Arch Dermatol Res. 1993;285(7):415–7.
24. Roshan S, Nader S, Orlander P. Review: ageing and hormones. Eur J Clin Invest. 1999;29(3):210–3.
25. Tazuke S, Khaw KT, Barrett-Connor E. Exogenous estrogen and endogenous sex hormones. Medicine (Baltimore). 1992;71(1):44–51.
26. Sauerbronn AV, et al. The effects of systemic hormonal replacement therapy on the skin of postmenopausal women. Int J Gynaecol Obstet. 2000;68(1):35–41.
27. Ghadially R, et al. The aged epidermal permeability barrier. Structural, functional, and lipid biochemical abnormalities in humans and a senescent murine model. J Clin Invest. 1995;95(5):2281–90.
28. Reed JT, Ghadially R, Elias PM. Skin type, but neither race nor gender, influence epidermal permeability barrier function. Arch Dermatol. 1995;131(10):1134–8.
29. Fluhr JW, et al. Differences in corneocyte surface area in pre- and post-menopausal women. Assessment with the noninvasive videomicroscopic imaging of corneocytes method (VIC) under basal conditions. Skin Pharmacol Appl Skin Physiol. 2001;14 Suppl 1:10–6.
30. Pierard GE, et al. Effect of hormone replacement therapy for menopause on the mechanical properties of skin. J Am Geriatr Soc. 1995;43(6):662–5.
31. Pierard-Franchimont C, et al. Skin water-holding capacity and transdermal estrogen therapy for menopause: a pilot study. Maturitas. 1995;22(2):151–4.
32. Guinot C, et al. Effect of hormonal replacement therapy on skin biophysical properties of menopausal women. Skin Res Technol. 2005;11(3):201–4.
33. Chen L, et al. The use of high-frequency diagnostic ultrasound to investigate the effect of hormone replacement therapy on skin thickness. Skin Res Technol. 2001;7(2):95–7.
34. Youn CS, et al. Effect of pregnancy and menopause on facial wrinkling in women. Acta Derm Venereol. 2003;83(6):419–24.
35. Batisse D, Giron F, Leveque JL. Capacitance imaging of the skin surface. Skin Res Technol. 2006;12(2):99–104.

Stratum Corneum Cell Layers

31

Hachiro Tagami

Contents

H. Tagami (✉)
Department of Dermatology, Tohoku University School of Medicine, Sendai, Japan
e-mail: hachitagami@ybb.ne.jp

M.A. Farage et al. (eds.), *Textbook of Aging Skin*,
DOI 10.1007/978-3-662-47398-6_37

Abstract

Although the stratum corneum (SC) exhibits disordered features when observed with conventional histologic sections, its cryostat section clearly shows the uniquely compact structure consisting of orderly overlapped layers of flattened corneocytes, supporting its important role in the skin barrier as well as in its water-binding capacity to keep the smooth and soft normal skin surface. Moreover, the SC is not uniform all over the body, showing big differences in its number of densely overlapped layers of corneocytes, reflecting the respective role unique for each body location. Thus, the SC of the thick palmoplantar skin shows nearly 50 cell layers of corneocytes in contrast to that of the genital skin or facial skin covered by thin SC consisting of less than 10 cell layers of flattened corneocytes. In such a way they exert their respective unique functional characteristics at each body location. By contrast, the hydration state of the SC seems to be influenced not only by the number of SC cell layers but also by other factors such as sweat and sebum secretion in addition to the turnover speed of the SC.

Introduction

Despite its most important role in the skin as a barrier membrane, the structural intactness of the stratum corneum (SC) has rather been neglected in histological examination because of its disordered features when prepared in ordinary histological specimens. Although the SC is only an extremely thin membrane covering the skin surface, it plays the most important and vital role of the skin in maintaining life, a skin barrier preventing loss of water from the underlying fully hydrated living tissue even in an extremely dry atmosphere. Hence, it is natural that the SC can also protect the body from invasion by various injurious exogenous chemicals and microorganisms from the environment [1].

Moreover, it keeps skin surface smooth and soft by binding water even under very dry conditions. These characteristics definitely require the structural intactness of the SC in vivo on the skin surface. The SC produced under pathological conditions such as various lesional skins is not only deficient in the barrier function but also presents a dry, scaly clinical appearance.

Functional studies of the SC have demonstrated that even normal healthy skin shows a great difference in its water-holding capacity as well as in the barrier function depending on the anatomical locations [2]. For example, the face is often affected by steroid-induced dermatitis after inadvertent prolonged usage of potent topical steroids. In fact, the barrier function of the facial skin is much less capable than that of abdominal skin [3, 4]. However, it is hard to demonstrate these differences in an ordinary histological specimen except for that of the palmoplantar skin, which shows closely packed layers of corneocytes even in the ordinary histological preparations because of the strong adhesiveness of the corneodesmosomes between the corneocytes to construct a tough and thick SC structure.

The Uniqueness of the Palmoplantar Stratum Corneum

The palmoplantar SC is remarkably thick to be able to resist even a strong external force. However, it exhibits unbelievably poor barrier function as compared with the SC of other locations [5]. Recently developed Raman spectroscopy has revealed that, except for the narrow, deepermost portion close to the viable epidermis, most of its thick outer and mid portions show a lower hydration state in contrast to the thin SC found in other bodily locations [6].

Electron microscopic study demonstrated that, in contrast to the SC of other bodily portions, the plantar SC is accompanied by unique intercellular spaces occupied by corneodesmosomes rather than by the intercellular lipids that play an important role in providing the SC with its barrier function [7]. The palmoplantar skin is covered by a uniquely thick SC distinct from that of other locations to execute its specific function, to withstand the strong external physical forces, even that which is required to sustain heavy body weight with their small surface areas. The mechanical role is more important than the biological role of barrier function here. Its barrier function should rather be poor enough to allow sufficient water from the deeply located viable epidermis to the skin surface to make the latter soft and flexible.

Differences in Barrier Function of the SC at Various Anatomical Locations

Although the SC covering most parts of the skin surface is extremely thin, in general less than 15 μm thick, they are far more efficient in its barrier function as well as in water-holding capacity than the palmoplantar SC [2, 5, 8]. In contrast to the latter, the SC covering most parts of the body is highly rich in its unique intercellular lipids crucial for the barrier function [1]. However, they are easily extracted during the preparatory process required for the production of ordinary histological specimens.

The data obtained measuring percutaneous permeation of chemicals demonstrated a parallel variation with those data recorded in vivo measuring transepidermal water loss (TEWL). Such data strongly supports that TEWL can be employed as a parameter of skin barrier function [4]. TEWL takes place between the water-saturated living epidermis and the dry environmental atmosphere through the SC under nonsweating condition, namely at the ambient condition of 20 °C and 40–50 % relative humidity. It can be used as an endogenous standard for the SC barrier function. Various types of scaly skin lesions such as those found in atopic dermatitis and psoriasis covered by pathological SC always reveal higher TEWL due to impaired barrier function [8].

However, even on the normal skin, in vivo measurement of TEWL clearly demonstrates great variations among various body regions, reflecting the differences in thickness as well as the degree of the structural integrity due to maturity of the SC. The facial SC shows the feature of immaturity in their composing corneocytes [9]. Usually, freshly produced immature corneocytes existing in the deepest SC portion are covered by a cornified envelope composed of protein components such as involucrin, loricrin, and small proline-rich proteins. However, as they become maturated with upward movement, they acquire hydrophobicity, because of covalent attachment of omega-hydroxyceramides of the intercellular lipids to the extracelluar surface of CE. In fact, the SC covering normal facial skin shows rather rapid turnover similar to that noted in mildly irritated hyperproliferative epidermis. Scattered immature corneocytes can be detected even in the superficial SC cell layer of normal facial skin, but not on the normal skin covering the trunk and the limbs, where slow turnover of the SC takes place. These findings suggest that the corneocytes of the facial skin tend to desquamate even in the immature state to maintain its thin SC cell layer as compared to those of the volar forearm.

Reflecting such immaturity of the corneocytes composing the facial SC, the TEWL value measured on the facial skin is more than 10 g/m^2/h, being much higher than those of the forearm and upper arm whose TEWL is around 5 g/m^2/h similar to those measured on the trunk and the lower extremity [5, 8]. Likewise, TEWL measured on the scalp [10] or on the axilla [11] is around 7 g/m^2/h, while that on the female vulva reaches 25 g/m^2/h, because the SC of the genital skin is the thinnest on the body [12]. Such a high level of TEWL corresponds to that of the acutely inflamed, eczematous facial lesions of atopic dermatitis [8].

The nape (12 g/m^2/h) and elbow (11 g/m^2/h) reveal unexpectedly high TEWL values, even though they are regarded to constitute a part of the trunk and the extremities. Both are the body locations characterized by frequent bending and stretching movement. In contrast, the skin of the knee covering another highly movable joint does not show any such high TEWL values. Likewise, the antecubital fossa or the popliteal fossa, the flexor surfaces of the joint regions, does not show any specifically higher TEWL than other sites of the extremities, although they constitute one of the predilection sites for atopic dermatitis like the neck [8].

In contrast, despite the relatively high TEWL observed in the facial skin, its SC lipid content is not lower than that of the SC of other anatomical locations. Thus, it is presumed that their poor barrier function reflects their extremely thin SC structure [13, 14], as well as the unique rapid turnover speed that does not allow the sufficient maturation process for the corneocytes [9].

Differences in the Hydration State of the Stratum Corneum Composing the Skin Surface

Because the lower portion of the SC can receive an ample supply of water from the underlying hydrated living epidermal tissue, it is the water content in the superficial portion of the SC, only several microns in depth, which keeps the skin smooth and soft. To evaluate such a skin surface hydration state, the high-frequency impedance measurement of the skin [15] is used conventionally. Between the two components of high-frequency impedance, i.e., conductance and capacitance, conductance is more suitable for the measurement of the hydrated state of the skin surface [15]. Thus, it is also fitted for the measurements of the efficacy of various moisturizers and skin care cosmetics. The pattern of the increase in high-frequency conductance with the depth of the SC also corresponds to the water distribution in the SC directly estimated by recently developed in vivo Raman spectroscopy [6]. There exists an exponential increase in water concentration from the skin surface to the fully hydrated viable epidermis [6]. Such a water gradient in the SC can also be observed with conductance measurements after serial stripping of the SC, but is difficult to demonstrate with capacitance measurements [15, 16]. In contrast, while capacitance measurements are less sensitive to evaluate the hydrated skin surface, they are more sensitive for the evaluation of dry skin conditions as noted in various skin diseases.

Among various anatomical locations of the adult Japanese, the measurements of the skin surface hydration state demonstrated that high-frequency conductance values were highest on the anterior neck, amounting to 225 micro-Siemens (μS) on average, being followed by the nape of the neck, with 123 μS as compared to 108 μS measured on the cheek [9]. While the seborrheic areas such as the cheek in adults definitely showed high skin surface lipid levels (117 AU) when measured with a Sebumeter (Courage & Khazaka, Cologne, Germany), the lipid levels were much lower on the frontal neck (44 AU) or the nape (21 AU). Such moderate sebum excretion alone does not seem to account for the remarkably high hydration state of the neck skin.

Other flexural areas of the extremities such as the antecubital fossa with 91 μS and popliteal fossa with 85 μS were also relatively well hydrated. In fact, they rarely develop dry skin even in winter. Their hydration levels were significantly higher than those of the volar forearm with 47 μS or the calf with 33 μS ($P < 0.001$).

In contrast, the extensor surfaces of the joint regions such the elbow (28 μS) and the knee (25 μS) were demonstrated to be poorly hydrated sites even compared with the volar forearm. In fact, they easily develop dry skin in children and the elderly in dry and cold winter.

Materials and Methods for Visualizing the SC Cell Layer in Normal Skin Specimens

For the demonstration of the cellular layer nature of the SC of other skin areas, Chistophers and Kligman [17] utilized frozen sections expanded in alkaline solutions, which allow such counting of the SC cell layer. However, in the past available data were based only on the findings in a small number of skin specimens that were obtained from a limited area of the body such as the trunk and the proximal extremities [18, 19].

Ya-Xian et al. [20] have also tried to use biopsy specimens of normal skin from various parts of the body including the face, scalp, genitals, and acral regions of the extremities, the locations where biopsy is not easy to perform in normal individuals. Hence, an uninvolved area of the surgical margin of excised skin tumors was used at various locations of the body of 301 Japanese patients, who had complaints of either benign or malignant tumors; the complaints led to an analysis of the relation of the SC cell layer to age, sex, and anatomical locations. In addition to these study samples, a small portion of normal skin specimens was included, which was obtained from certain areas such as the abdomen and anterior aspect of the thigh that frequently served as a donor site for a skin graft.

As the nature of the sampling method depended totally on the chance of surgery, sufficient numbers of samples could not be collected for all the locations of the body to analyze the SC. However, the counting of the cell layers in the SC in a large number of samples was successfully completed; skin specimens were obtained from a total of 158 males and 143 females, ranging from 1 to 97 years of age with the mean age of 42 ± 26 years.

Preoperative procedures of the skin consisted of applying povidone-iodine with gauze, which was subsequently wiped off with gauze soaked in 0.02 % chlorhexidine gluconate solution. The skin samples were frozen quickly and 6-μm-thick cryostat sections were prepared by cutting them in a plane perpendicular to the skin surface. The method to determine the number of cell layers in the SC is based on that reported by Christophers and Kligman [17] in principle and modified from that described by Blair [18]. In short, a cryostat section was at first stained with 1 % aqueous solution of safranin for 1 min and then flooded with 2 % potassium hydroxide (KOH) aqueous solution. The safranin produces clear reddened intensification of the intercellular portions of the SC even in the presence of the KOH solution. The number of swollen corneocyte layers over the epidermis was counted at several spots avoiding the sites of sweat pores and follicular ostium, to obtain the mean value [20].

The obtained data was statistically analyzed with Sheffe's F procedure for comparisons of the SC cell layers at various locations, Mann–Whitney test for comparisons of functional data of the SC, and Fisher's r to z transformations to check the correlation between age and the number of corneocyte layers.

Anatomical Differences in SC Cell Layer

The typical features of histological specimens consisted of a compact feature of the SC, which helped in easy counting of the number of flattened cell layers in the SC (Fig. 1). The number of cell layers was smallest in the genital (both for the penis and the scrotum of the male genitalia and the vulva of the female genitalia) skin (6 ± 2; $n = 9$), whereas it was between 10 and 20 in most locations of the trunk and the extremities.

The obtained data are summarized for various anatomical locations of the body. In general, the SC of the face, neck, and scalp skin tended to be smaller than that of the trunk. Although they look similar, the SC of the extremities showed higher number of cell layers than the trunk ($P < 0.01$).

The facial skin showed statistically significant smaller numbers of cell layers (9 ± 2; $n = 84$) than those of the extremities (15 ± 4; $n = 55$) ($P < 0.05$). From the smallest number found in the genital skin (6 ± 2; $n = 9$), they could be put in order by placing the face (9 ± 2; $n = 84$) next and then from the neck (10 ± 2; $n = 5$), scalp (12 ± 2; $n = 12$), trunk (13 ± 4; $n = 94$), and extremities (15 ± 4; $n = 55$) to the acral regions, namely the palms and the soles (47 ± 24; $n = 42$). Among them, the heel showed the largest numbers (86 ± 36; $n = 5$) (Table 1).

The SC cell layers of the face, neck, and scalp skin tended to be smaller than that of the trunk. The facial skin showed statistically significant smaller numbers of cell layers (9 ± 2; $n = 82$) than those of the extremities (15 ± 4; $n = 55$) ($P < 0.05$).

Even among the facial skin, there were some differences depending upon the location. The eyelid (8 ± 2; $n = 8$), nasolabial fold (7; $n = 2$), and the ear lobe (7 ± 2; $n = 8$) showed lower numbers. In contrast, the forehead (9 ± 1; $n = 8$), nose (10; $n = 2$), cheek (10 ± 3; $n = 43$), preauricular region (10 ± 3; $n = 30$, and the lip (10; $n = 2$) exhibited somewhat higher numbers.

The skin of the trunk showed similar SC cell layer numbers ranging from 12 ± 4 ($n = 20$) on the buttock to 14 ± 4 on the abdomen ($n = 44$). On the other hand, the extremities revealed some differences between those of the extensor upper arm (13 ± 4; $n = 13$), flexor upper arm (14; $n = 2$), flexor forearm (16 ± 4; $n = 4$), and extensor thigh (16 ± 4; $n = 31$), and the flexor surface of the leg (18 ± 5; $n = 5$).

In contrast, it was remarkably thick in the distal portion of the extremities, such as the dorsa of the hands (25 ± 11; $n = 10$) and those of the feet (30 ± 6; $n = 7$) and particularly the palms

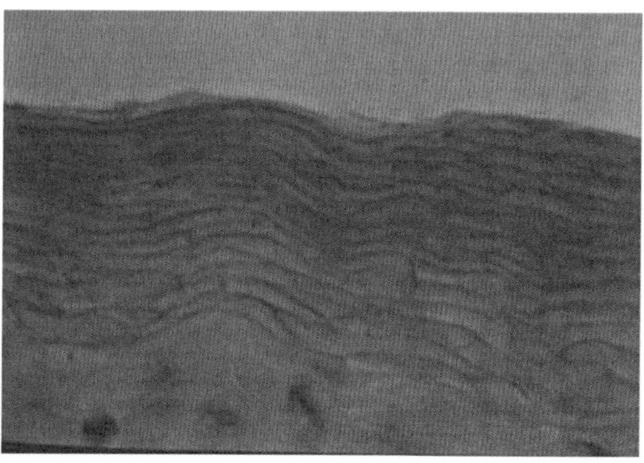

Fig. 1 Stratum corneum of the back (×400)

Table 1 Comparison of the number of cell layers of the SC at various anatomical locations

Location	Number of cell layers (mean ± SD)
Face	9 ± 2 (n = 84)
Forehead	9 ± 1 (n = 8)
Eyelid	8 ± 2 (n = 16)
Cheek	10 ± 3 (n = 43)
Nose	10 (n = 2)
Nasolabial fold	7 (n = 2)
Lip	10 (n = 2)
Ear	7 ± 2 (n = 8)
Periauricular region	10 ± 3 (n = 3)
Scalp	12 ± 2 (n = 12)
Neck	10 ± 2 (n = 5)
Trunk	13 ± 4 (n = 94)
Shoulder	13 ± 2 (n = 3)
Chest	13 ± 4 (n = 9)
Back	13 ± 3 (n = 18)
Abdomen	14 ± 4 (n = 44)
Buttock	12 ± 4 (n = 20)
Genital	6 ± 2 (n = 9)
Extremities	15 ± 4 (n = 55)
Extensor surface, upper arm	13 ± 4 (n = 13)
Flexor surface, upper arm	14 (n = 2)
Flexor surface, forearm	16 ± 4 (n = 4)
Thigh	16 ± 4 (n = 31)
Flexor surface, leg	18 ± 5 (n = 5)
Acral region	47 ± 24 (n = 42)
Dorsum of the hand	25 ± 11 (n = 10)
Dorsum of the foot	30 ± 6 (n = 7)
Palm	50 ± 10 (n = 8)
Sole	55 ± 14 (n = 12)
Heel	86 ± 36 (n = 5)

(n = 50 ± 10; n = 8) and the soles (55 ± 14; n = 12). As mentioned above, the heel showed the largest numbers (86 ± 36; n = 5).

Differences in SC Cell Layer Due to Age, Sex, and Race

In regard to age, their numbers could be compared at four different skin regions, i.e., the cheek, back, abdomen, and the anterior surface of the thigh, where sufficient numbers of samples were available for such analysis. The results showed a significant increase in the SC cell layers with increasing age only in the cheek skin of the males with the correlation coefficient of 0.67 ($P < 0.05$). Such a tendency was not found in the females. There is no clear-cut explanation for these findings. In the skin of the back, the SC cell layers showed an increased with age both in male and female individuals ($r = 0.63$; $P < 0.05$). However, the increase was much more prominent in males than in females (Fig. 2).

By contrast when the skin from elderly individuals with senile xerosis was studied mainly on the extensor surface of the legs in winter, there was a significant increase in the SC cell layers in those with senile xerosis versus the young healthy individuals [21].

A comparative study was conducted between different sexes at the sites where such comparison was possible. Surprisingly, there was no significant difference in the number of corneocyte layers due to sex.

Although there was a great individual difference in the number of cell layers in the SC even from the same location, in general, the skin of the trunk and that of the extremities of the Japanese are covered by the SC with relatively similar numbers of cell layers ranging from 10 to 20. These numbers generally agree well with those reported previously using a small number of samples from other countries [17–19], ruling out the influence of racial difference.

Comparison of the Number of SC Cell Layer with Functional Properties of the SC In Vivo

Finally, when a comparison of these histological data of the SC with its functional data, the values of in vivo measured TEWL, was made, the latter seemed to correlate with the number of the SC cell layer except for the palmoplantar SC. The obtained TEWL values were close to each other in representative areas of the trunk and the extremities, where the numbers of cell layers of the SC were also close to each other. By contrast, they were remarkably high on the face as compared

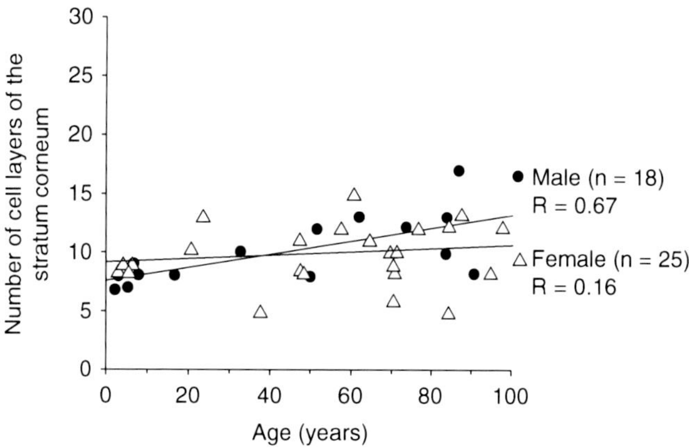

Fig. 2 The number of corneocyte layers in the stratum corneum of the check versus age (cited from [20])

with the trunk and limbs, being double to triple on the cheek and the eyelid.

In contrast, using high-frequency conductance, the parameter of the water content in the outer SC did not show any correlation with the number of the SC cell layers. There is a water concentration gradient from the skin surface exposed to the dry atmosphere to the lowermost layer of the SC facing the hydrated epidermal tissue [6]. Thus, when the SC is serially removed with adhesive cellophane tape stripping, there occurs a gradual increase in high-frequency conductance [15].

Although their SC cell layers were almost comparable in number, the hydration values were statistically higher on the back than on other portions of the trunk and limb ($P < 0.05$) [20]. Hence, it is likely that the water content of the outer SC is influenced not only by the thickness of the SC but also by other factors such as sweat and sebum secretion, as well as by the physicochemical properties of the SC themselves [22]. It is well known that even a simple application of effective moisturizing agents produces a prominent increase in water content of the SC without any change in the number of SC cell layers.

In fact, on the facial skin covered with thin SC layers, the site rich in skin surface lipids such as the nose tends to show significantly higher conductance levels than other regions [23]. Moreover, the areas covered with larger mature corneocytes such as the eyelid skin reveal higher conductance than those sites covered by smaller immature corneocytes such as the cheek, nasolabial fold, and forehead [24]. The size of the corneocytes conversely correlates with the turnover speed of the SC [25].

Clinical Implications

From the obtained data, it is clear that the genital skin and certain parts of the facial skin such as the eyelid, ear, and nasolabial portion showed small numbers of SC cell layers. These findings seem to explain well that these skin regions are sensitive to topical applications of irritants or lipid solvents. These areas are also the sites often affected by contact dermatitis [26]. The frequently experienced but poorly understood intolerance of the face or neck skin to various topical formulations [27, 28] can also be in part understood from their relatively thin corneocyte layers. Such skin areas with thin SC are also the predilection sites for atopic dermatitis, contact dermatitis, and seborrheic dermatitis, because they are not only rich in skin appendages but also are more permeable to various environmental substances including irritants, haptens, aeroallergens, and microorganisms.

Moreover, these findings also correspond well to the experimental observations that the barrier function of the scrotal skin, face, and neck is much less effective than that of abdominal skin [3], although no obvious histological differences can be found in ordinary histology specimens. The face is also the site where the development of steroid-induced dermatitis is often observed clinically, because even uninvolved skin allows penetration of ample amounts of potent steroids as compared to that of the trunk and extremities.

Conclusion

To count the number of cell layers in the SC of normal skin taken from different anatomical locations of the body, normal skin samples were collected from 301 individuals with various ages. Frozen sections of 6 μm thickness that were stained with 1 % safranin aqueous solution and observed under microscope after application of 2 % KOH solution showed that there were great variations in the SC cell layers (mean ± SD) according to the location and among different individuals. The smallest number was found in the genital skin (6 ± 2), being followed in order by the face (9 ± 2), neck (10 ± 2), scalp (12 ± 2), trunk (13 ± 4), extremities (15 ± 4), and the acral regions (47 ± 24). Among them, the heel showed the largest numbers (86 ± 36). No definite correlation of the number of corneocyte layers was found with sex of the individuals, whereas there was a slight increase in the number with age in the skin of the cheek and back, particularly in males. Comparison of these data with those of functional assessment of the SC showed that TEWL, a parameter of SC barrier function, reflects the number of corneocyte cell layers. In contrast, high-frequency conductance, a parameter for the hydration state of the outer SC, does not seem to be influenced only by it.

As compared with other methods that have been utilized to measure the thickness and numbers of cell layers in the SC, the technique used in the present study is simple and not time consuming, that enables the study of a large number of skin samples. It does not require any wide laboratory space or special facilities except for an ordinary microscope and cryostat.

Cross-References

- ▶ Corneocyte Size and Cell Renewal: Effects of Aging and Sex Hormones
- ▶ The Stratum Corneum and Aging

References

1. Elias PM, Feingold KR, editors. Skin barrier. New York: Taylor & Francis; 2006.
2. Tagami H. Location-related differences in structure and function of the stratum corneum with special emphasis on those of the facial skin. Int J Cosmet Sci. 2008;30:413–34.
3. Feldman RJ, Maibach HI. Regional variation in percutaneous penetration of ^{14}C cortisol in man. J Invest Dermatol. 1967;48:181–3.
4. Rougier A, Lotte C, Maibach HI. In vivo percutaneous penetration of some organic compounds related to anatomic site in humans: predictive assessment by the stripping method. J Pharm Sci. 1987;76:451–4.
5. Wilhelm KP, Cua AB, Maibach HI. Skin aging. Effect on transepidermal water loss, stratum corneum hydration, skin surface pH, and casual sebum content. Arch Dermatol. 1991;127:1806–9.
6. Egawa M, Hirao T, Takahashi M. In vivo estimation of stratum corneum thickness from water concentration profiles obtained with Raman spectroscopy. Acta Dermatol Venereol. 2007;87:4–8.
7. Egelrud T, Lundström A. Intercellular lamellar lipids in plantar stratum corneum. Acta Dermatol Venereol. 1991;71:369–72.
8. O'goshi K, Okada M, Iguchi M, Tagami H. The predilection sites for chronic atopic dermatitis do not show any special functional uniqueness of the stratum corneum. Exog Dermatol. 2002;1:195–202.
9. Hirao T, Denda M, Takahashi M. Identification of immature cornified envelopes in the barrier-impaired epidermis by characterization of their hydrophobicity and antigenicities of the components. Exp Dermatol. 2001;10:35–44.
10. O'goshi K, Iguchi M, Tagami H. Functional analysis of the stratum corneum of scalp skin: studies in patients with alopecia areata and androgenetic alopecia. Arch Dermatol Res. 2000;292:605–11.
11. Watkinson A, Lee RS, Moore AE, Pudney PDA, Patterson SE, Rawlings AV. Reduced barrier efficiency in axillary stratum conreum. Int J Cosmet Sci. 2002;24:151–61.
12. Warren R, Bauer A, Greif C, Wigger-Alberti W, Jones MB, Roddy MT, Seymour JL, Hansmann MA, Elsner P. Transepidermal water loss dynamics of human vulvar and thigh skin. Skin Pharmacol Physiol. 2005;18:139–43.
13. Lampe MA, Burlingame AL, Whitney J, Williams ML, Brown BE, Roitman E, Elias PM. Human stratum corneum lipids: characterization and regional variations. J Lipid Res. 1983;24:120–30.
14. Yoshikawa N, Imokawa G, Akimoto K, Jin K, Higaki Y, Kawashima M. Regional analysis of ceramides within the stratum corneum in relation to seasonal changes. Dermatology. 1994;188:207–14.
15. Tagami H, Ohi M, Iwatsuki K, Kanamaru Y, Yamada M, Ichijo B. Evaluation of the skin surface

hydration in vivo by electrical measurement. J Invest Dermatol. 1980;75:500–7.

16. Hashimoto-Kumasaka K, Takahashi K, Tagami H. Electrical measurement of the water content of the stratum corneum in vivo and in vitro under various conditions. Comparison between skin surface hygrometer and corneometer in evaluation of the skin surface hydration state. Acta Dermatol Venereol (Stockh). 1993;73:335–9.
17. Christophers E, Kligman AM. Visualization of the cell layers of the stratum corneum. J Invest Dermatol. 1964;42:407–9.
18. Blair C. Morphology and thickness of the human stratum corneum. Br J Dermatol. 1968;80:430–43.
19. Holbrook KA, Odland GF. Regional differences in the thickness (cell layers) of the human stratum corneum: an ultrastructural analysis. J Invest Dermatol. 1974;62:415–22.
20. Ya-Xian Z, Suetake T, Tagami H. Number of cell layers of the stratum corneum in normal skin – relationship to the anatomical location on the body, age, sex and physical parameters. Arch Dermatol Res. 1999;291:555–9.
21. Hara M, Kikuchi K, Watanabe M, Denda M, Koyama J, Nomura J, Horii I, Tagami H. Senile xerosis: functional, morphological, and biochemical studies. J Geriatr Dermatol. 1993;1:111–20.
22. Egawa M, Tagami H. Comparison of the depth profiles of water and water-binding substances in the stratum corneum determined in vivo by Raman spectroscopy between the cheek and volar forearm skin: effects of age, seasonal changes and artificial forced hydration. Br J Dermatol. 2008;158:251–60.
23. Kobayashi H, Tagami H. Distinct locational differences observable in biophysical functions of the facial skin: with special emphasis on the poor functional properties of the stratum corneum of the perioral region. Int J Cosmet Sci. 2004;26:91–101.
24. Pratchyapruit W, Kikuchi K, Gritiyarangasan P, Aiba S, Tagami H. Functional analyses of the eyelid skin constituting the most soft and smooth area on the face: contribution of its remarkably large superficial corneocytes to effective water-holding capacity of the stratum corneum. Skin Res Technol. 2007;13:169–75.
25. Hölzle E, Plewig GJ. Effects of dermatitis, stripping, and steroids on the morphology of corneocytes. A new bioassay. J Invest Dermatol. 1977;68:350–6.
26. Ockenfels HM, Seemann U, Goos M. Contact allergy in patients with periorbital eczema: an analysis of allergens. Dermatology. 1997;195:119–24.
27. Shriner DL, Maibach HI. Regional variation of nonimmunologic contact urticaria. Functional map of the human face. Skin Pharmacol. 1996;9:312–21.
28. Berardesca E, Fluhr JW, Maibach HI. Sensitive skin syndrome. New York: Taylor & Francis; 2006.

Aging and Melanocytes Stimulating Cytokine Expressed by Keratinocyte and Fibroblast

32

Mutsumi Okazaki

Contents

Abstract

In the skin pigmentation, the actinic damage plays a major role, but the effect of chronologic cellular aging is also critical. Melanocytes, keratinocytes, and fibroblasts, whose paracrine effects on melanocytes play an important role in the epidermal pigmentation. The relationship of aging a cytokine secretion will be discussed in this chapter.

Introduction

In the skin pigmentation, the actinic damage plays a major role [1], but the effect of chronologic cellular aging is also an important factor. The chief cellular components of the skin other than melanocytes are keratinocytes and fibroblasts, whose paracrine effects on melanocytes (rather than melanocyte itself) play an important role in the epidermal pigmentation [2–11]. Human keratinocytes express several melanogenic cytokines, such as endothelin-1 (ET-1) [2–4], granulocyte macrophage colony-stimulating factor (GM-CSF) [5], stem cell factor (SCF), and basic fibroblast growth factor (bFGF) [7–9]. Human fibroblasts, on the other hand, secrete several melanogenic cytokines such as bFGF, HGF, and SCF [6, 10, 11]. Further, interleukin-1α (IL-1α), a pro-inflammatory cytokine, stimulates the production of ET-1 by keratinocytes and of HGF by

M. Okazaki (✉)
Department of Plastic and Reconstructive Surgery, Graduate School of Science, Tokyo Medical and Dental University, Bunkyo-ku, Tokyo, Japan
e-mail: okazaki-m@umin.ac.jp

M.A. Farage et al. (eds.), *Textbook of Aging Skin*,
DOI 10.1007/978-3-662-47398-6_38

fibroblasts [3, 12–14]. It has been reported that the overexpression of these melanogenic cytokines is responsible for the age-related pigmentary cutaneous disorders [15–17]. The age-associated change was studied in cytokine secretion by keratinocytes and fibroblasts based upon this paracrine cytokine network within the skin for epidermal pigmentation mechanisms.

Correlation Between Age and Secretion of Melanogenic Cytokine

Studies were planned to elucidate whether the aging of keratinocytes and fibroblasts was related to the potential to secrete several melanogenic cytokines. In the first experiment, the keratinocytes and fibroblasts derived from the skin of different chronological ages were cultured, and the secretions of melanogenic cytokines were evaluated by enzyme-linked immunosorbent assay (ELISA). The series of study were carried out with the informed consent of the person whose skin samples were used.

Fibroblast

Normal skin specimens were taken from Japanese patients (disused skin during plastic surgery, i.e., after the dog-ear correction). Informed consent was obtained from all patients. Fibroblasts were cultured from 19 specimens (age = 26.7 ± 15.6, from 7 to 65 years old, 8 males, 11 females). The methods of isolation and culture of fibroblasts were reported previously [18]. Fibroblasts were grown in the fibroblast growth medium (FGM), which consists of Dulbecco's Modified Eagle's Medium (DMEM), 0.6 mg/mL glutamine, and 10 % fetal calf serum (FCS). The third cultures of fibroblasts were used for the experiments. Fibroblasts were seeded in a 60 mm culture dish at a density of 5×10^5 cells/5 mL and cultured in FGM. After human fibroblasts had been cultured for 96 h at 37 °C under a 5 % CO_2 atmosphere, the medium was collected to quantify HGF, SCF, and bFGF, respectively, by ELISA.

Keratinocyte

Normal skin specimens were obtained from Japanese patients, and keratinocytes were cultured from 16 specimens (age = 28.0 ± 17.1, from 7 to 64 years, six males, ten females). The methods of isolation and culture of keratinocytes were reported previously [18]. Keratinocytes were grown in the serum-free keratinocyte growth medium (KGM; Kyokuto Seiyaku, Tokyo) which consists of MCDB153 with high concentrations of amino acids, transferrin (final concentration 10 μg/mL), insulin (5 μg/mL), hydrocortisone (0.5 μg/mL), phosphorylethanolamine (14.1 μg/mL), and bovine pituitary extract (40 μg/mL). The final concentration of Ca^{2+} in the medium was 0.03 mM. The second cultures of keratinocytes were used for the experiment. Keratinocytes were seeded in a 60 mm culture dish at a density of 1.5×10^5 cells/5 mL and cultured in KGM supplemented with 0.5 % FCS. After human keratinocytes had been cultured at 37 °C under a 5 % CO_2 atmosphere for 72 h, the keratinocyte-conditioned medium was collected to quantify IL-1α, ET-1, and GM-CSF, respectively, by ELISA.

The comparison of the cytokine concentration between male and female was carried out using unpaired *t*-test. And the scatter diagrams showing the relationship between age and cytokine concentration were drawn, and simple linear regression equations were calculated, and simple linear regression test was used to determine whether there was any correlation between age and concentration of cytokine. A value of $P < 0.05$ was considered statistically significant.

1. Cytokine secretion by fibroblasts

   No gender differences in the donor age and cytokine concentration were found between male and female. There was no correlation between age and cytokine concentration (*R* coefficient of determination; HGF $R = 0.0054$, $P = 0.98$; SCF, $R = 0.19$, $P = 0.44$; bFGF $R = 0.0064$, $P = 0.98$) (Fig. 1a–c).

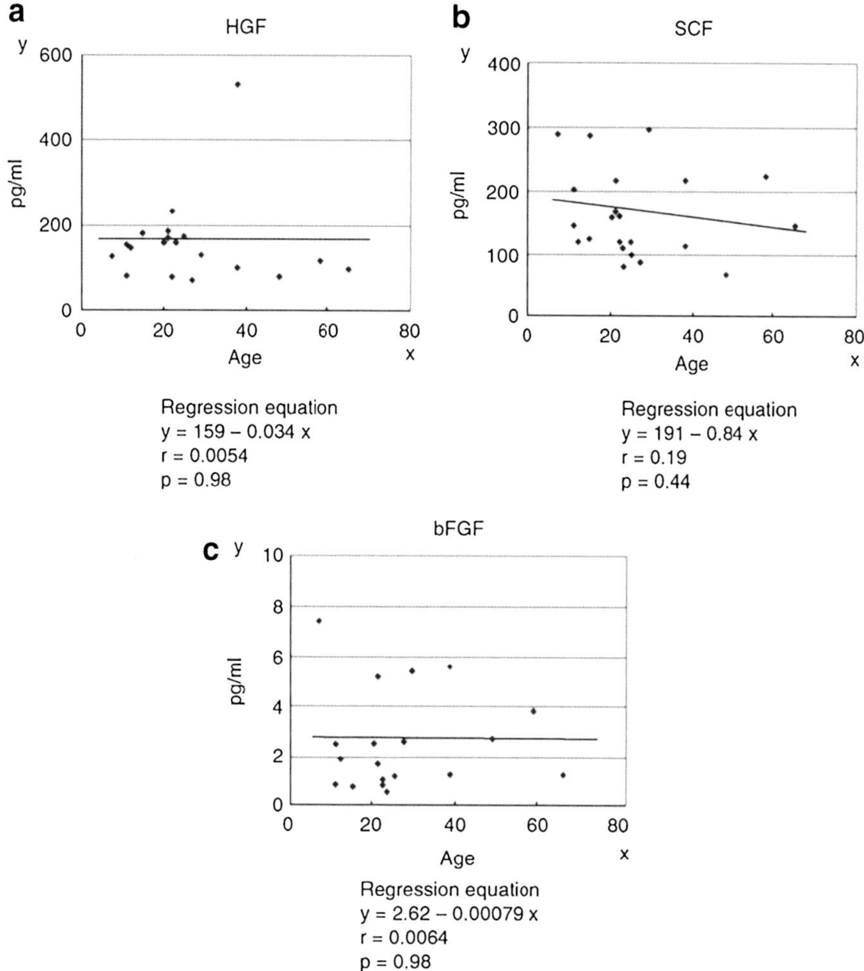

Fig. 1 Scatter diagram showing the relationship between donor age and value of cytokine concentration in fibroblasts. The *lines* represent the linear regression equation ($n = 19$; R, coefficient of determination). (**a**) HGF $y = 159–0.034x$, $R = 0.0054$, $P = 0.98$; (**b**) SCF $y = 191–0.84x$, $R = 0.19$, $P = 0.44$; (**c**) bFGF $y = 2.62 - 0.00079x$, $R = 0.0064$, $P = 0.98$

2. Cytokine secretion of keratinocytes

No gender differences in the donor age and cytokine concentration were found between male and female. There was a significant correlation between age and IL-1α concentration ($R = 0.71$, $P = 0.002$). There was a relatively weak correlation between age and ET-1 concentration, but the correlation was not significant ($R = 0.41$, $P = 0.051$). No correlation existed between age and GM-CSF concentration ($R = 0.32$, $P = 0.23$) (Fig. 2a–c).

In the second experiment, the secretions of IL-1α and ET-1 by keratinocytes were compared between the second and fifth cultures. In this study, the fifth cultures of keratinocytes derived from nine donors who were less than 30 years old were used. Cell cultures and ELISA assay were performed in the same way as the first experiments. A comparison of the cytokine concentrations between the second and fifth culture keratinocytes was carried out using paired t-test. A value of $P < 0.05$ was considered statistically significant.

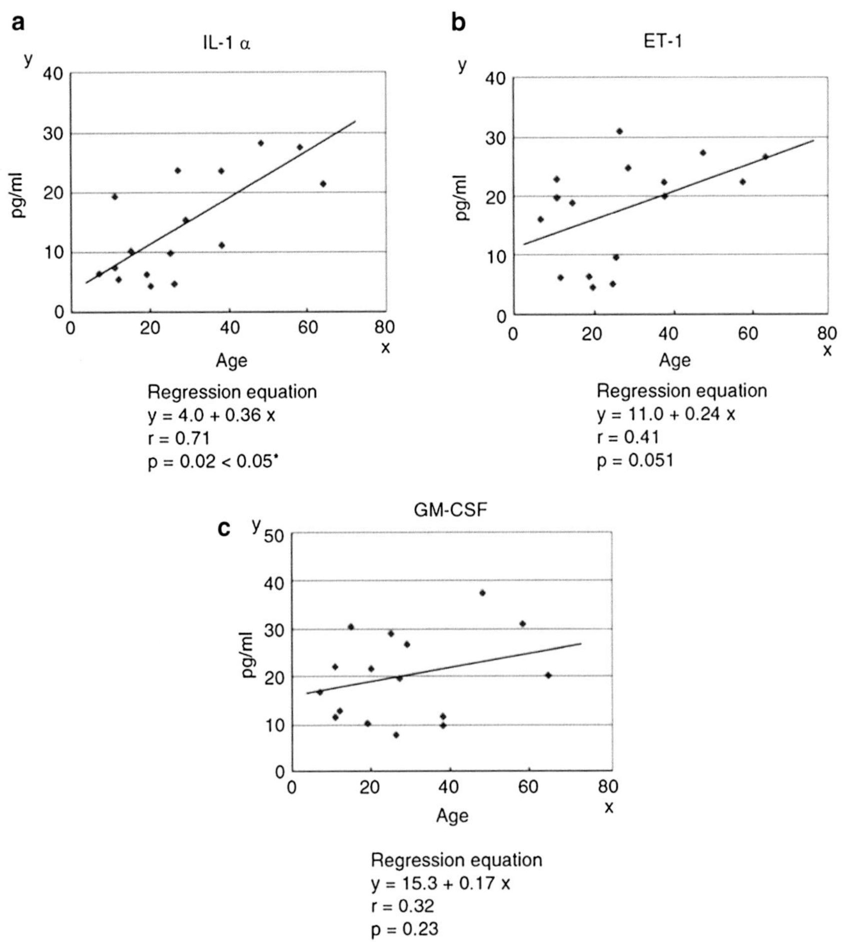

Fig. 2 Scatter diagram showing the relationship between donor age and value of cytokine concentration in keratinocytes. The *lines* represent the linear regression equation ($n = 16$; R, coefficient of determination). (**a**) IL-1α y $= 4.0 + 0.36x$, $R = 0.71$, $P = 0.002$*; (**b**) ET-1 $y = 11.0 + 0.24x$, $R = 0.41$, $P = 0.051$; (**c**) GM-CSF $y = 15.3 + 0.17x$, $R = 0.32$, $P = 0.23$

The concentration of IL-1α was significantly increased in the fifth cultures compared with the second cultures ($P < 0.005$), but the levels of ET-1 did not differ significantly ($P = 0.52$) (Fig. 3a, b).

Conclusion

The results suggest that increasing secretion (occurring as the cell ages) of IL-1α by keratinocytes may play a role in the age-associated skin change. Because IL-1α stimulated the ET-1 production by keratinocytes [3], and ET-1 induced an increase in tyrosinase activity and stimulated melanocyte proliferation [2–4], the increasing secretion of IL-1α by keratinocytes may be responsible for the accentuated cutaneous pigmentation associated with aging. In the study, however, the correlation between age and ET-1 secretion by keratinocytes was not significant, although there was a weak correlation ($R = 0.41$, $P = 0.051$). One of the possible reasons for this is small sample size, and another is that the autocrine stimulation by IL-1α might not be as efficient on the aged keratinocytes under the specific culture condition. This is supported by the second experiment; the levels of ET-1 secretion

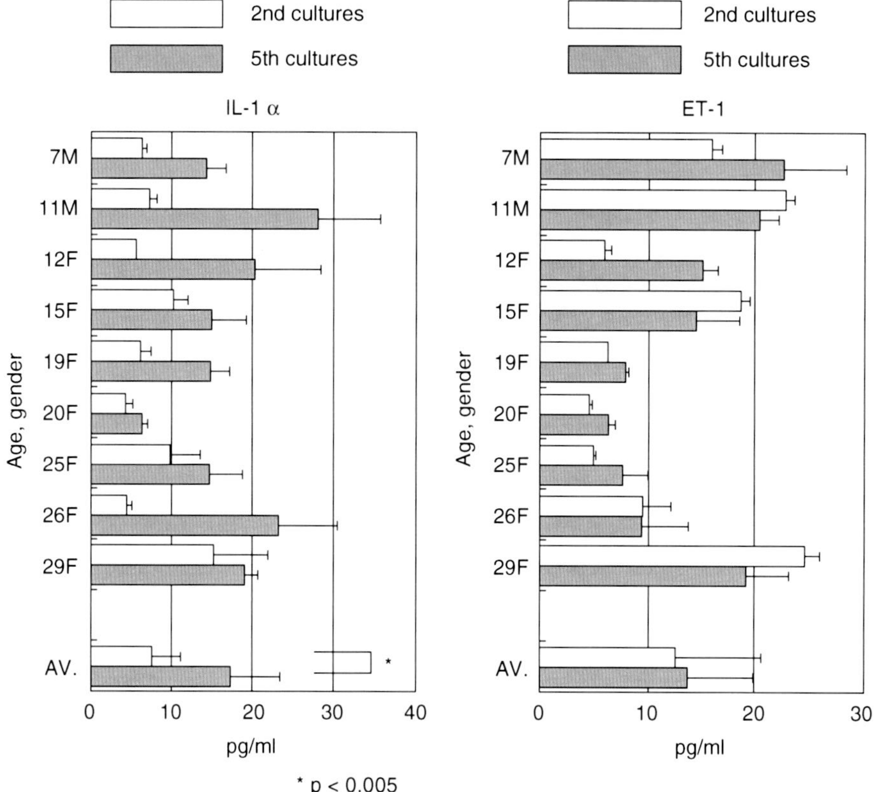

Fig. 3 Comparison of IL-1α and ET-1 secretion by keratinocytes between the second and fifth cultures. Each ELISA values (values are means ± SD derived from three wells of each specimens) of nine donors and average values (*AV*) are shown. **P* <0.005 to second cultures. (**a**) IL-1α; (**b**) ET-1

did not differ significantly, although IL-1α secretion was significantly increased in old (the fifth) cultures compared with young (the second) cultures.

In the culture methods used, keratinocytes derived from aged skin (approximately older than 30 years of age) can no longer proliferate vigorously after three to four serial subcultures. In a preliminary study, the keratinocytes derived from a 1-year-old child could be cultivated serially for about seven to eight passages under these culture conditions when they are subcultured every 7 days. At the seventh or eighth cultures, most of the cultures were composed of enlarged and flattened cells, and such cultures were considered senescent, and subculturing was not continued. These findings were consistent with those reported by Boyce and Ham [19], and the chronologic cellular age of the fifth culture can be estimated 30–40 years older than that of the second culture. It was reported that after irradiation with ultraviolet B (UVB), ET-1 production by keratinocytes increased accompanied by significant secretion of IL-1α [3]. The study suggests that melanocytes in the aged skin are stimulated persistently by keratinocytes via IL-1α-ET-1 cascade, as if the skin were irradiated with UVB. Thus, epidermal pigmentation might be persistently accentuated in the aged skin.

The study also suggests that there was no correlation between secretions of melanogenic cytokine by fibroblasts and cellular age. It was reported that human dermal fibroblasts from aged donors (over 80 years) produced more HGF than fibroblasts from young and middle-aged donors, and the production of HGF by human embryonic lung fibroblasts increased sharply after about 70 % completion of their

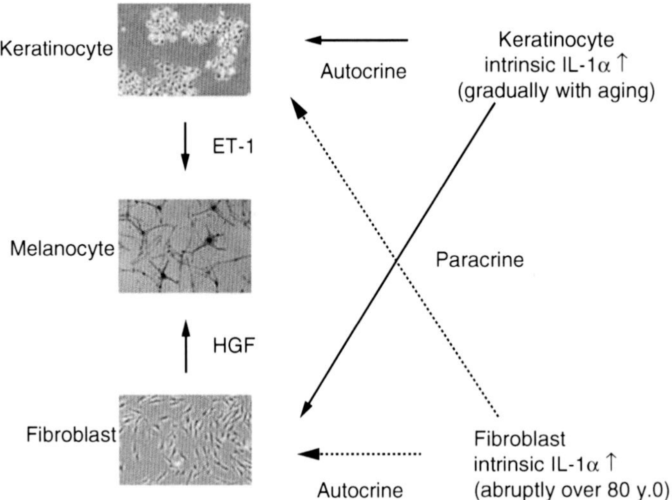

Fig. 4 Schematic showing the hypothesis of the accentuated pigmentation in the aged skin. The secretion of IL-1α by keratinocytes gradually increases with age, which stimulates ET-1 production by keratinocytes autocrinely and HGF production by dermal fibroblasts paracrinely, and these cytokines stimulate melanocyte proliferation and induce an increase of tyrosinase activity in melanocytes. On the other hand, the production of IL-1α by fibroblast would increase abruptly from the age about 70–80, which stimulates HGF production by dermal fibroblasts autocrinely and ET-1 production by keratinocytes paracrinely

lifespan in culture, which is mainly due to autocrine stimulation by IL-1α [20]. IL-1α was reported to stimulate the expression of HGF in the fibroblasts [12–14]. In this study, however, there was no correlation between age and HGF secretion, probably because the age of donor ranged from 7 to 65 years old.

One hypothesis concerning age-associated cutaneous pigmentation can be proposed (Fig. 4); the secretion of IL-1α by keratinocytes gradually increases with age, which stimulates ET-1 production by keratinocytes autocrinely and HGF production by dermal fibroblasts paracrinely, and these cytokines stimulate melanocyte proliferation and induce an increase of tyrosinase activity in melanocytes. On the other hand, the production of IL-1α by fibroblast would increase abruptly from the age of about 70 to 80 years, which stimulates HGF production by dermal fibroblasts autocrinely and ET-1 production by keratinocytes paracrinely.

One of the limitations of the study is that skin specimens were obtained from various sites of the body; site-specific differences of cytokine secretion could not be assessed because of small number of specimen involved. It is an essential variable whether the specimen was obtained from sun-exposed or sun-protected sites. To exclude the influence of acute sunlight exposure to the skin on the cytokine secretion, the isolated skin cells were used in culture (not use freshly isolated cells). Conversely, it was inevitable that biological age of the cultured cells used in the study is larger than the age of donors (as was mentioned above, it is estimated that the 7-day culture of keratinocyte corresponds to about 10–12 years of age). Another limitation of the study is that only Japanese specimens were used. There are some reports describing the differences of pigmentation, or response to ultraviolet radiation, in the skin of different ethnic groups [21, 22]. It is probable that the general tendency for age-related change in the melanogenic cytokine secretion is common in all ethnic groups, but there may be some ethnic difference.

Because cytokine expression was evaluated with ELISA (protein level) in the study, the expression of membrane-bound SCF (m-SCF) of keratinocyte was not assessed; in epidermal keratinocyte, SCF is expressed as a membrane-bound form, not in a secretory or soluble cytokine form such as ET-1 [23]. Even in stimulated conditions such as following UVB exposure, only the expression of m-SCF is accentuated in epidermal keratinocytes [23]. In the evaluation of the expression of m-SCF, mRNA might reveal a different mechanism of accentuated cutaneous pigmentation.

It was reported that accentuated epidermal pigmentation in lentigo senilis and seborrheic keratosis is attributed to a larger amount of secretion of ET-1 by keratinocytes [15, 17]. The study suggests the probability that formations of such lesions in the older person are associated with an increasing production of IL-1α by epidermal keratinocyte. Furthermore, because IL-1α is a primary mediator that responds to inflammation and injury [24], the transcription of genes involved in skin inflammation may be persistently induced in the aged skin. Thus, it is probable that the aged skin is always exposed to the conditions like inflammation, and the increased potential to secrete IL-1α in aged keratinocytes is associated with various skin aging in addition to the epidermal pigmentation.

References

1. Leyden JJ. Clinical features of aging skin. Br J Dermatol. 1990;122(35):1–3.
2. Yada Y, Higuchi K, Imokawa G. Effect of endothelins on signal transduction and proliferation in human melanocytes. J Biol Chem. 1991;266:18352–7.
3. Imokawa G, Yada Y, Miyagishi M. Endothelins secreted from human keratinocytes are intrinsic mitogens for human melanocytes. J Biol Chem. 1992;267:24675–80.
4. Imokawa G, Miyagishi M, Yada Y. Endothelin-1 as a new melanogen: coordinated expression of its gene and the tyrosinase gene in UVB-exposed human epidermis. J Invest Dermatol. 1995;105:32–7.
5. Imokawa G, Yada Y, Kimura N, et al. Granulocyte/macrophage colony-stimulating factor is an intrinsic keratinocyte-derived growth factor for human melanocytes in UVA-induced melanosis. Biochem J. 1996;313:625–31.
6. Grabbe J, Welker P, Dippel E, et al. Stem cell factor, a novel cutaneous growth factor for mast cells and melanocytes. Arch Dermatol Res. 1994;161:78–84.
7. Halaban R, Langdon R, Birchall N, et al. Basic fibroblast growth factor from human keratinocytes is a natural mitogen for melanocytes. J Cell Biol. 1988;107:1611–9.
8. Puri N, van der Weel MB, de Wit FS, et al. Basic fibroblast growth factor promotes melanin synthesis by melanocytes. Arch Dermatol Res. 1996;288:633–5.
9. Scott G, Stoler M, Sarkar S, et al. Localization of basic fibroblast growth factor mRNA in melanocytic lesion by in situ hybridization. J Invest Dermatol. 1991;96:318–22.
10. Matsumoto K, Tajima H, Nakamura T. Hepatocyte growth factor is a potent stimulator of human melanocyte DNA synthesis and growth. Biochem Biophys Res Commun. 1991;176:45–51.
11. Imokawa G, Yada Y, Morisaki N, et al. Characterization of keratinocyte- and fibroblast-derived mitogens for human melanocytes – their roles in stimulated cutaneous pigmentation. Melanogenesis and malignant melanoma. In: Hori Y, Hearing VJ, Nakayama J, editors. Biochemistry, cell biology, molecular biology, pathophysiology, diagnosis and treatment. Amsterdam: Elsevier; 1996. p. 35–48.
12. Matsumoto K, Okazaki H, Nakamura T. Up-regulation of Hepatocyte growth factor gene expression by interleukin-1 in human skin fibroblasts. Biochem Biophys Res Commun. 1992;188:235–43.
13. Maas-Szabowski N, Fusenig N. Interleukin-1-induced growth factor expression in postmitotic and resting fibroblasts. J Invest Dermatol. 1996;107:849–55.
14. Mildner M, Mlitz V, Gruber F, et al. Hepatocyte growth factor establishes autocrine and paracrine feedback loops for the protection of skin cells after UV irradiation. J Invest Dermatol. 2007;127:2637–44.
15. Kadono S, Manaka I, Kawashima M, et al. The role of the epidermal endothelin cascade in the hyperpigmentation mechanism of lentigo senilis. J Invest Dermatol. 2001;116:571–7.
16. Hattori H, Kawashima M, Ichikawa Y, et al. The epidermal stem cell factor is over-expressed in lentigo senilis: Implication for the mechanism of hyperpigmentation. J Invest Dermatol. 2004;122:1256–65.
17. Teraki E, Tajima S, Manaka I, et al. Role of endothelin-1 in hyperpigmentation in seborrheic keratosis. Br J Dermatol. 1996;135:918–23.
18. Okazaki M, Yoshimura K, Uchida G, et al. Correlation between age and the secretions of melanocyte-stimulating cytokines in cultured keratinocytes and fibroblasts. Br J Dermatol. 2005;153(s3):23–9.
19. Boyce ST, Ham RG. Calcium-regulated differentiation of normal human epidermal keratinocytes in chemically defined clonal culture and serum-free serial culture. J Invest Dermatol. 1983;81.
20. Miyazaki M, Gohda E, Kaji K, et al. Increased Hepatocyte growth factor production by aging human fibroblasts mainly due to autocrine stimulation by interleukin-1. Biochem Biophys Res Commun. 1998;246:255–60.
21. Tadokoro T, Yamaguchi Y, Batzer J, et al. Mechanisms of skin tanning in different racial/ethnic groups in response to ultraviolet radiation. J Invest Dermatol. 2005;124:1326–32.

22. Wagner JK, Parra EJ, Norton HL. Skin responses to ultraviolet radiation: effects of constitutive pigmentation, sex, and ancestry. Pigment Cell Res. 2002;15:385–90.
23. Hachiya A, Kobayashi A, Ohuchi A, et al. The paracrine role of stem cell factor/c-kit signaling in the activation of human melanocytes in ultraviolet B-induced pigmentation. J Invest Dermatol. 2001;116:578–86.
24. Murphy JE, Robert C, Kupper TS. Interleukin-1 and Cutaneous inflammation: a crucial link between innate and acquired immunity. J Invest Dermatol. 2000;114:602–8.

Cyanoacrylate Skin Surface Strippings 33

Claudine Piérard-Franchimont and Gérald E. Piérard

Contents

C. Piérard-Franchimont
Laboratory of Skin Bioengineering and Imaging, Department of Dermatopathology, University Hospital of Liège, Liège, Belgium

Department of Dermatology, Regional Hospital of Huy, Huy, Belgium
e-mail: claudine.franchimont@ulg.ac.be

G.E. Piérard (✉)
Laboratory of Skin Bioengineering and Imaging, Department of Dermatopathology, University Hospital of Liège, Liège, Belgium
e-mail: Gerald.pierard@ulg.ac.be

M.A. Farage et al. (eds.), *Textbook of Aging Skin*,
DOI 10.1007/978-3-662-47398-6_39

Abstract

The cyanoacrylate skin surface stripping (CSSS) is a minimally invasive method for harvesting the superficial part of the horny layer. Under regular conditions, CSSSs are painless and do not induce adverse events. CSSSs are scrutinized under controlled and appropriate methods of analytical morphology. These procedures apply to a series of clinical conditions including xerosis grading, comedometry, corneodynamics, corneomelametry, corneosurfametry, and corneoxenometry. With each of the designed analytical methods, CSSSs provide specific salient information. In particular, CSSSs appear valuable and complementary in assessing any changes in the human skin structure. A set of quantitative analytical methods applicable to the minimally invasive and low-cost CSSS procedures allow for a sound assessment of the horny layer in dermatology and dermocosmetic science.

Introduction

The human stratum corneum (SC) is a superficial continuous membrane composed of tightly stacked corneocytes parted by multilamellar lipid sheets. In its most widely recognized positioning, the SC exerts a major barrier function protecting from ultraviolet (UV) light, the biocene or microbiome environment, a diversity of oxidants, and a set of other toxic xenobiotics. In addition, it prevents from loss of water and electrolytes from the body. Despite its own restricted metabolic activity, the SC corresponds to a highly specialized structure showing continuous renewal keeping ideally a steady state in its structure and thickness. However, it is heterogeneous in its molecular composition and structure. In addition, it acts as a unique sophisticated biosensor transmitting signals to the underlying epidermis. Such mechanism responds to a series of external stresses.

At most locations on the body surface, the SC is typically composed of about 12–16 layers of flattened corneocytes. The loose superficial portion of the SC is referred to as the stratum disjunctum, and the deep cohesive part is named stratum compactum. The whole structure participates in a progressive maturation process during its maturation to the skin surface. This process ends with the physiological imperceptible desquamation.

The superficial corneocytes are about 1 μm thick and have a mean area of approximately 1,000 μm^2. However, the surface area varies with age, anatomical location, and conditions. These parameters influence the epidermal renewal by means of chemical signals and UV light irradiations. In particular, the average corneocyte size apparently increases with aging. This is generally assumed to be related to an increased cell transit time inside the SC. Each corneocyte contains a water-insoluble protein complex corresponding to a highly organized keratin microfibrillar matrix. The intracellular structure is encapsulated in a protein- and lipid-enriched shell. The cornified cell envelope exhibits some differences in maturation among corneocytes. Basically, two distinct types of cornified corneocyte envelopes are distinguished. They correspond to "fragile" or "immature" and "rigid" or "mature" membranes, respectively [1, 2].

Discrete alterations in the corneocyte organization commonly lead to the presence of parakeratosis. Various other aspects are possibly additional clues to the disturbance of the SC physiology. In some skin conditions, the SC homeostasis is altered. In particular, the SC is the repository of many biological events that occurred beneath in previous days. The SC structure is further altered by diverse and repeated external threats. Clearly, the genetic background, nutritional status, some physical agents, as well as drugs, cosmetics, toiletries, and other chemical xenobiotics represent a variety of major modulators of the SC organization. Knowledge about the fine SC structure is crucial in many aspects of the dermocosmetic science, particularly when dealing with age-related xerosis and effects of surfactants, emollients, and squamolytic agents [3, 4].

Critical Factors for CSSS Collection

Cyanoacrylate skin surface stripping (CSSS) formerly called skin surface biopsy and follicular biopsy is a time-honored method [5] that was developed for diagnostic purposes in various fields in dermatology and cosmetology [4, 6, 7]. It represents a regular way for collecting the stratum disjunctum.

The CSSS method consists of depositing a drop of cyanoacrylate liquid adhesive onto a supple transparent sheet of terephthalate polyethylene, 175 μm thick, cut to the approximate size of a conventional coverslip (1.5 × 6 cm). The material (3S-biokit, CK Technology, Visé, Belgium) is pressed firmly on the target site [7]. It is possible to get a perfect modeling of curved areas on the body. In addition, the adhesion of the SC to the ethylene sheet is such that it prevents its detachment during the laboratory procedure. After approximately 15–30 s, a sheet of SC of uniform thickness is gently lifted and conveniently harvested (Fig. 1). Because the adhesion mechanism of cyanoacrylate relies on a chemical polymerization, the thickness of the removed SC is determined by the depth of penetration of the adhesive before it hardens. The cleavage level is exclusively located inside the SC. Oozing and eroded lesions are not adequately studied using CSSS. The sampling procedure is minimally invasive and is often painless and bloodless. Anesthesia and antiseptic procedures are unnecessary.

The next laboratory procedures are simple and not time-consuming. The CSSS cost is minimal.

CSSSs are conveniently harvested from any part of the body, with, however, two main provisos. On the one hand, CSSS sampling from a hairy area is painful because of pulling out of hairs. In addition, such CSSS quality is frequently inadequate owing to the erratic contact of the sampling material with the SC. It is therefore advisable to shave these areas before harvesting for CSSS. On the other hand, intercorneocyte cohesion on the palms and soles is normally stronger than the cyanoacrylate bond, thus impairing the collection of an undisrupted sheet of corneocytes. However, any CSSS sampling from these sites is possible in certain physiopathological conditions associated with a compromised texture and cohesion of the SC.

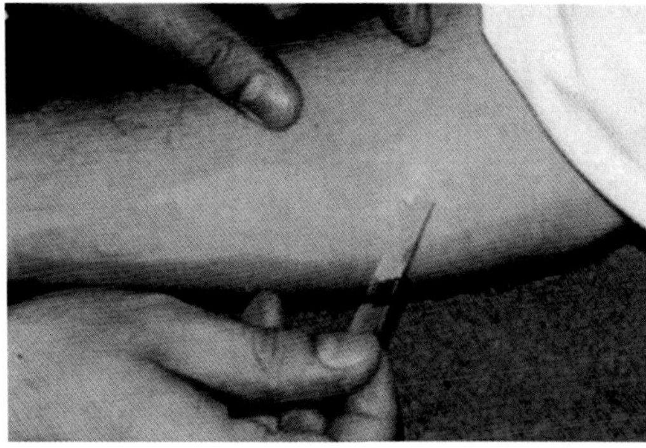

Fig. 1 CSSS sampling

Global Aspect of Normal Skin on CSSS

CSSS is conveniently observed under the microscope and by scanning electron microscopy as well. CSSS of healthy skin reveals a regular network of high-peaked crests corresponding to the skin surface hollow furrows forming the so-called first- and second-order lines. Their pattern of distribution is typical for specific parts of the body and is subject to changes with age [6]. The primary lines of the skin surface correspond to shallow depressions in the latticework papillary relief at the dermoepidermal junction [3]. In young individuals, regular crisscross orientations of the primary and secondary lines delimit regularly shaped polyhedral plateaus (Fig. 2a). Aging remodels this innate network which progressively loses its configuration. The primary lines become in their great majority oriented along the skin tension lines (Fig. 2b). The process ends with the disappearance of the shallow patterned creases [8]. It is therefore possible to indirectly assess the texture of the superficial dermis on CSSS. Accordingly, dermatoporosis in dermal aging and corticosteroid-induced atrophy, as well as sclerosis, striae distensae, scars, and many other changes in the connective tissue, are readily visible in a noninvasive way using CSSS. Such morphological assessment of the skin microrelief is conveniently quantified using computerized image analysis and any regular profilometric method [3].

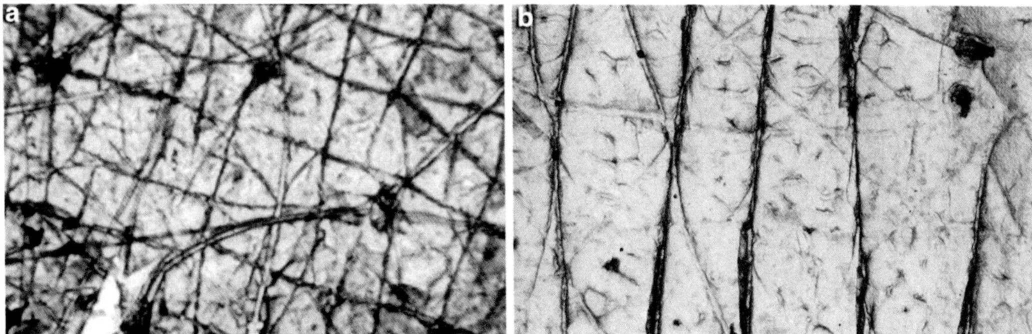

Fig. 2 CSSS age-related global aspect. (**a**) Regular crisscross pattern of primary and secondary order lines of the skin surface. (**b**) Reshaping of the order lines during aging

Vellus hairs are commonly captured in CSSS. In addition, CSSS collects follicular casts corresponding to the horny material present at the opening of the pilosebaceous follicles near the skin surface [8]. It is therefore possible to assess the density of the follicles per unit of surface area and to observe the presence of follicular hyperkeratosis (kerosis) comedones, *trichostasis spinulosa*, as well as intrafollicular bacteria and mites [3, 5, 8–10].

Cytological characteristics of corneocytes are hardly visible on CSSS unless cytological/histochemical dyes are used [5, 7]. A number of staining procedures are suitable for that purpose. The most convenient and simple stain conveniently handled in a regular office setting is a mixture of toluidine blue and basic fuchsin in 30 % ethanol. Normal skin shows a regular cohesive pattern of adjacent anucleated corneocytes. Their boundaries are clearly identified as a thin polyhedral rim (Fig. 3a). Their aspect is also identified by scanning electron microscopy (Fig. 3b). Parakeratotic cells are usually rare and dispersed singly on normal skin. They are recognized by the presence of a nucleus central to the polyhedral corneocyte.

Resident saprophytic microorganisms present at the skin surface are forming the regular biocene, also called biocenosis or microbiome. Most of them are encased within the cyanoacrylate bond during sampling, and they are not reached by the staining procedure. As a result, only a portion of the surface microflora is observed on CSSS [5]. By contrast, microorganisms present inside follicular casts are collected distinctly from the skin surface biocene by scraping out these horny spiky structures appending to the CSSS. Viability of the intrafollicular bacteria is assessed using flow cytometry [11] or any other relevant method exploring the follicular microbiome [12].

Analytical Morphology of CSSS

Various skin conditions and treatments alter the SC presentation. Analytical morphology applied to CSSS provides diverse quantitative, semiquantitative, or binary information. Image analysis, optical profilometry, reflectance colorimetry, and light transmission assessments are among the most salient procedures applicable to CSSS. Four main types of assessments are targeted, including (a) the appraisal of the SC structure, (b) the assessment of the SC dynamics, (c) the evaluation of the skin surface microbiome, and (d) the use of CSSS as a substrate in a series of ex vivo bioassays.

Analytical morphology of CSSS deals with quantitative methods providing statistically assessable data. Meaningful evaluation relies on careful sampling procedures. The challenge of analytical assessments of CSSS both in

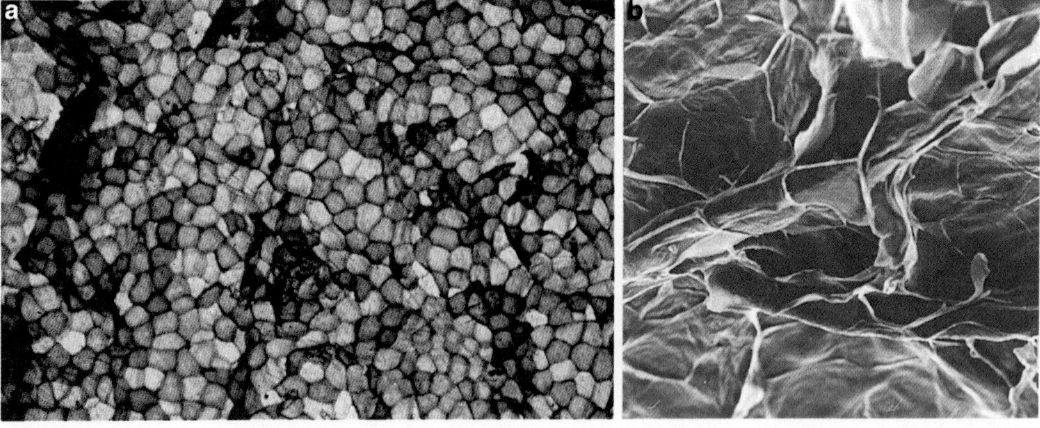

Fig. 3 CSSS: regular corneocyte paving. (**a**) Optical microscopy of the stratum corneum. (**b**) Scanning electron microscopy showing the cohesive pattern of corneocytes

dermatology and cosmetology is to quantify some selected aspects of the structure and functions of the SC. The procedures are respectively named corneomelametry, corneodynamics, corneofungimetry, comedometry, corneosurfametry, and corneoxenometry.

CSSS in Inflammatory Conditions

CSSSs are used as nearly noninvasive methods, and they prove to be useful for diagnostic purpose in a number of skin conditions. Obviously the diagnostic indications for CSSS only apply to disorders characterized by changes taking place in the SC. A number of common dermatoses are conveniently diagnosed using CSSS [3, 4, 6, 7, 13].

Straightforward diagnoses can be established in various superficial infectious and parasitic skin diseases. Some morphological examinations, possibly combined with fungal cultures, can be carried out to identify these dermatoses (Fig. 4a–c). By essence, infectious agents that are made visible on CSSS are not those adhering on top of the skin surface (see above) but rather those invading the SC. Fungi, including yeasts and dermatophytes, exhibit typical aspects forming clusters or a network of globular or filamentous structures (Fig. 4a–c).

In the group of parasitic disorders, scabies occasionally sets a difficult problem at the time of sampling. In fact, the accurate diagnosis is only established when the mite, its eggs, or its dejecta are present in the sample. Duplicate CSSS should therefore be sampled from a typical scabies burrow. The first one removes the roof of the burrow, and the second one allows to collect the parasite. Any sample taken outside such lesion, for instance, from unspecific prurigo, will be unhelpful because the observation will only suggest the presence of a spongiotic dermatitis [6, 7, 14]. Demodex mites are conveniently recognized [6, 14] and highlighted in the follicular casts using the Fite stain.

Noninfectious erythemato-squamous disorders conveniently assessed using CSSS include spongiotic (Fig. 5a) and parakeratotic dermatoses

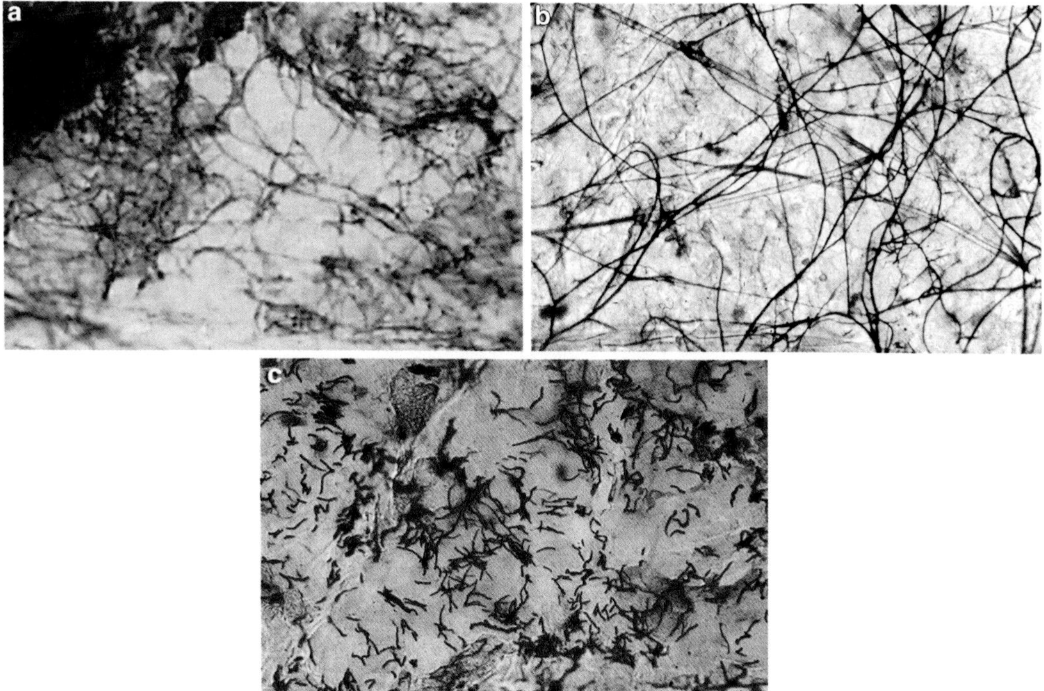

Fig. 4 CSSS of a dermatomycoses. (**a**) Fungal hyphae are clearly identified at the PAS stain. (**b**) Fungal hyphae at the Gomori-Grocott stain. (**c**) *Malassezia* spp. in pityriasis versicolor

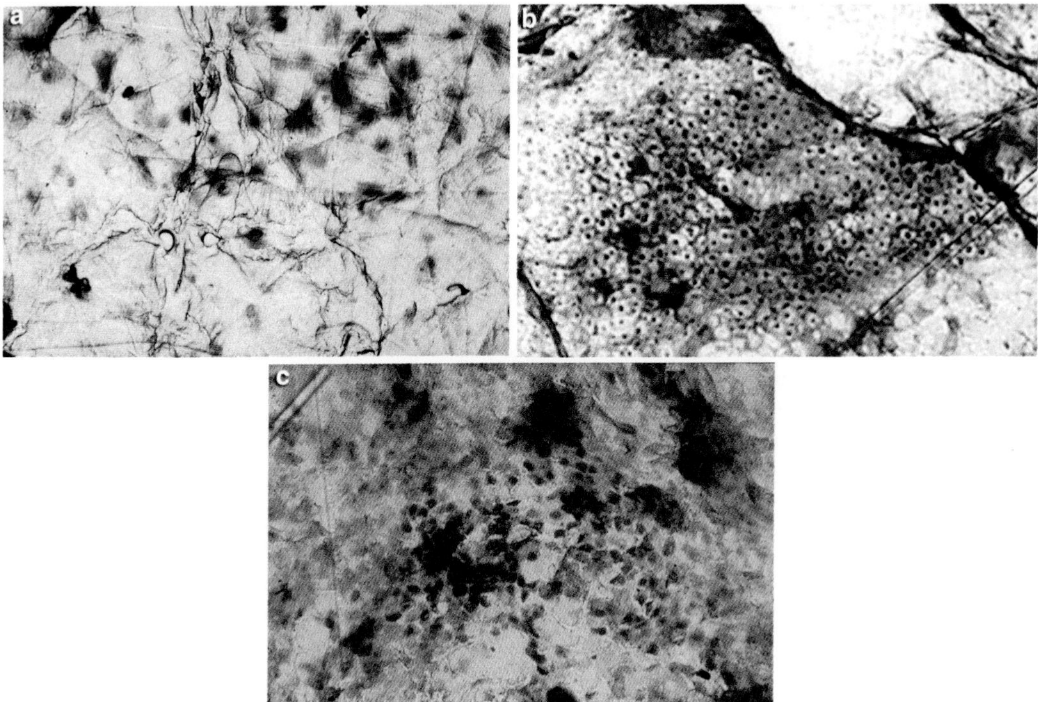

Fig. 5 CSSS in inflammatory dermatosis. (a) Serum deposits in the stratum corneum. (b) Sheet of parakeratotic cells. (c) Dispersed parakeratotic cells

(Fig. 5b) and xeroses [3, 6, 7, 14]. Spongiotic dermatoses represent superficial inflammatory reactions responsible for spongiosis, microvesiculation, and serosity leakage inside the SC. Contact dermatitis, atopic dermatitis, and pityriasis rosea are examples that belong to the spongiotic group. Parakeratotic dermatoses encompass id reactions, chronic eczema, and stable psoriasis. The parakeratotic cells are clustered in sheets or in thicker bulks (Fig. 5b, c). Seborrheic dermatitis also comes within this parakeratotic category particularly in cases when *Malassezia* yeasts are rare. In active psoriasis, clusters of neutrophils are found on top of parakeratotic foci [14].

CSSS in Cutaneous Neoplasms

Some epithelial neoplasms display typical aspects on CSSS. Seborrheic keratoses show spotty lenticular foci of soft hyperkeratosis (Fig. 6a, b). Widening shallow furrows with hyperkeratosis are often present [6]. Samples of actinic keratosis often exhibit uneven thickness with foci of interfollicular parakeratosis and xerosis. The perifollicular rim is by contrast featureless. Basal cell carcinomas and squamous cell carcinomas commonly exhibit unspecific features or at best suggest some clues on CSSS. Actinic porokeratosis is revealed by a rim of cornoid lamellation and loss of the normal microrelief inside the lesion [6]. Verrucous surfaces overlying melanocytic nevi and dermatofibromas are less pathognomonic, but sharp circumscription with normal surrounding skin and uniform changes in the texture of the SC are commonly present in such benign neoplasms.

In melanocytic neoplasms, melanin is found inside corneocytes and eventually in atypical melanocytes. Melanin restricted only inside corneocytes is a characteristic of benign neoplasms such as lentigines and melanocytic nevi (Fig. 7a). By contrast, the presence of atypical

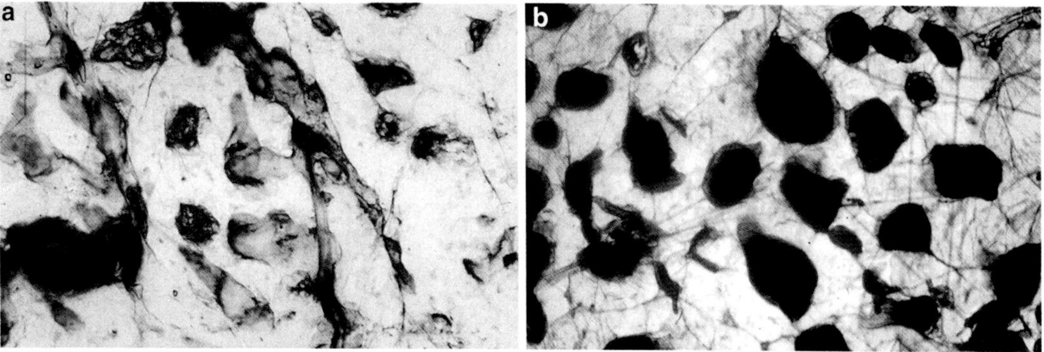

Fig. 6 CSSS from a seborrheic keratosis. (**a**) Hyperkeratotic foci. (**b**) Hyperkeratotic melanized foci

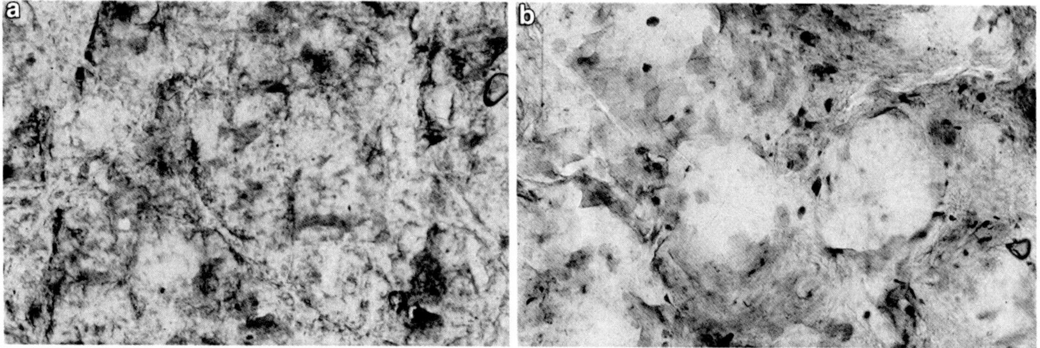

Fig. 7 CSSS of pigmented tumors. (**a**) Melanized corneocytes in a benign melanocytic nevus. (**b**) Melanocytes in the stratum corneum of a malignant melanoma

melanocytes inside the SC strongly suggests a malignant melanoma (Fig. 7b) but also, in rare instances, a benign melanoacanthoma [6, 13–15]. Thus, CSSS proves to be sensitive and specific for distinguishing most malignant melanomas from benign melanocytic tumors such as common melanocytic nevi, dysplastic nevi, or pigmented seborrheic keratoses [13]. For investigative purposes, karyometry of neoplastic melanocytes is possibly performed on CSSS [15].

CSSS Assessment of Disease Severity and Therapeutic Activity

Disease severity and therapeutic improvement are possibly assessed noninvasively on CSSS exhibiting specific features in the SC. For instance, xeroses correspond to various forms of predominantly orthokeratotic hyperkeratosis [3]. Such condition encompasses what is commonly referred by the laity as reactive (sensitive) skin or dry skin, but this appearance also corresponds to a more severe stage in a diversity of ichthyoses [3, 4, 6, 7, 14].

Several grades of orthokeratotic hyperkeratosis are distinguished on CSSS [3, 6, 14]. Type 0 is the absence of hyperkeratosis, except for some discrete focal accumulation of corneocytes in the primary order lines of the skin. Type 1a corresponds to a continuous linear hyperkeratosis of the primary lines. Type 1b is characterized by hyperkeratosis predominant at the site of adnexal openings either at hair follicles or at acrosyringia. Type 2 shows focal hyperkeratosis of the skin surface plateaus covering less than 30 % of the surface of the sampling. Type 3 resembles type 2, but with an extension of the xerotic area over 30 % of the CSSS. Type 4 is defined by a homogeneous and diffuse hyperkeratosis with persistence of the trace of primary order lines. Type 5a resembles type 4, but with loss of recognizable primary lines. Type 5b corresponds to the most heterogeneous and diffuse hyperkeratosis with loss or marked remodeling of the primary line network.

Corneomelametry

Normal corneocytes of phototype V and VI individuals contain melanin. In addition, lighter phenotypes exhibit focal clusters of melanin-loaded corneocytes at the site of clinically pigmented lesions. The dusty load can be specifically revealed using argentaffin-staining procedures. The relative darkness of these CSSS can be assessed using corneomelametry [4, 7, 16, 17]. This method consists of measuring the reduction of light transmission through the CSSS using a photomicroscope equipped with an internal photodensitometer device. On a cytological viewpoint, it is important to distinguish melanin-laden anucleated corneocytes from neoplastic dendritic melanocytes after their migration into the SC covering a malignant melanoma.

Corneodynamics

Corneodynamics was initially the combination of CSSS with the dansyl chloride (DC) test as an attempt at assessing the SC turnover [4]. The overall time for fluorescence extinction depends on both the transit rate of corneocytes through the SC and the thickness of that layer. Such a clinical test proved to be difficult to interpret on clinical grounds due to the uneven fade-out of fluorescence at the skin surface. An improved method [18] was introduced by the examination of CSSS harvested from a DC test area (Fig. 8). It was further refined by replacing DC with the browning dihydroxyacetone (DHA) agent [19].

Corneodynamics is assessed using CSSS from DC and DHA test sites at a predetermined time of a trial. Accordingly, at about day 10, CSSSs are examined under a fluorescent light microscope because both DC and DHA are fluorescent. Image analysis applied to such pictures allows quantification of the nonfluorescent versus fluorescent areas of the SC. This ratio is an indicator of the rate of SC turnover. However, both the DC and DHA tests are dramatically influenced by cleansing agents and skincare products [20]. The extraction of the dyes from the SC by these products is tentatively used to predict irritancy potential [20].

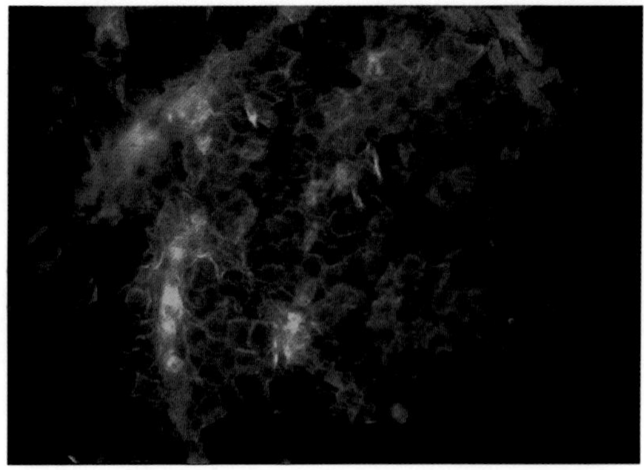

Fig. 8 Fluorescent CSSS from a dansyl chloride test

An inverse relationship has been suggested between the size of corneocytes and the speed of epidermal turnover. This aspect is possibly studied on skin strippings, particularly CSSS during corneodynamics.

Corneofungimetry

In superficial dermatomycoses, fungal cells are readily visible on CSSS. In experimental settings, some assessments of disease severity and therapeutic activity on dermatomycoses are conveniently performed using computerized image analysis of CSSS.

In an in vitro procedure, microscopy fungi are conveniently cultured using corneocytes [21] and particularly CSSS as growth substrates [22, 23]. Quantifications of the restricted fungal growth after application of antifungals in experimental dermatomycosis are conveniently performed using corneofungimetry [22, 24–26]. The oral or topical antifungals are administered to healthy volunteers for a given period of time (usually a couple of days). CSSSs are sampled afterward. A controlled amount of fungal cells collected from a primary culture is deposited onto the CSSS supposedly impregnated with the test antifungal. After a given time (usually 7–10 days) of culture in a clean environment, the CSSS are stained for revealing fungi. Computerized image analysis is used to fine-tune the quantification of the mycelium growing on CSSS. The comparison with control untreated CSSS allows to derive the percentage of inhibition of the fungal growth.

Corneofungimetry has several advantages over conventional in vitro evaluation of antifungals: (a) the treatment is applied in vivo in conditions normally encountered by patients, (b) the initial fungal load is controlled, (c) the growth medium is only composed of keratinocytes without any artificial compounds, and (d) any influence of keratinocytes including natural antimicrobial peptides is respected.

Comedometry

Comedometry allows the computerized quantification of the number and size of follicular casts present on CSSS. This method finds application on the face and the back in the assessment of comedogenesis-related disorders and in their treatments [10, 11, 27]. The method reflects the balance between comedo formation and lysis. Acne is the major indication for this method.

In vivo comedometry on human skin appears more relevant than animal models of comedogenesis. The sensitivity of the method is such that microcomedolysis is possibly objectivated by computerized image analysis after a few weeks of treatment. Comedometry predicts comedogenic risks linked to some xenobiotics and conversely to quantify any comedolytic activity of cosmetic compounds [4].

Corneosurfametry and Corneoxenometry

The interaction between the SC and various chemical xenobiotics is conveniently assessed on CSSS. Corneosurfametry (CSM) refers to the effects of surfactants and wash solutions [3, 28–30]; CSSSs are harvested from healthy volunteers. A solution of the test product is sprayed on the CSSS which is placed in covered plastic trays. After a given period of incubation at controlled temperature, the samples are thoroughly rinsed in tap water, dried, and stained for 3 min in a toluidine blue-basic fuchsin solution. The samples are then copiously rinsed with water and dried prior to color determination using reflectance colorimetry. Indeed, surfactants remove lipids and denaturate corneocyte proteins, thus revealing sites available for staining deposition. A combined dotted and rimmed pattern is visible at the microscopic examination (Fig. 9a–c).

Using quantitative reflectance colorimetry, mean luminancy (L*) and Chroma C* are calculated from measurements made at three sites on each sample placed on a white reference plate. Mild surfactants with little effect on corneocytes give high L* values and low Chroma C* values. L* decreases and Chroma C* increases with the irritancy potential of the product. The differences between L* and Chroma C* values of each sample give colorimetric indices of mildness (CIM). The CSM index (CSMI) of the test product corresponds to the color difference between water-treated control samples and those exposed to the test product. It is conveniently calculated according to the following formula:

$$\mathrm{CSMI} = \left[(\Delta L*)^2 + (\Delta C*)^2\right]^{0,5}.$$

Microwave CSM is a more rapid procedure [31]. CSSSs are immersed in a flask containing the test surfactant solution. Samples are then placed in a microwave oven with a 500 ml water load. Microwave CSM is typically run at 750 W for 30 s. The next steps are identical to the standard CSM procedure.

Responsive CSM is a variant of the method where skin has been pretreated before CSSS sampling [32]. The method is based on repeat subclinical injuries by surfactants monitored in a controlled forearm immersion test. At completion of the in vivo procedure, CSSSs are harvested for a regular or microwave CSM bioassay using the same surfactant as in the preliminary in vivo procedure. Preconditioning the skin by this way

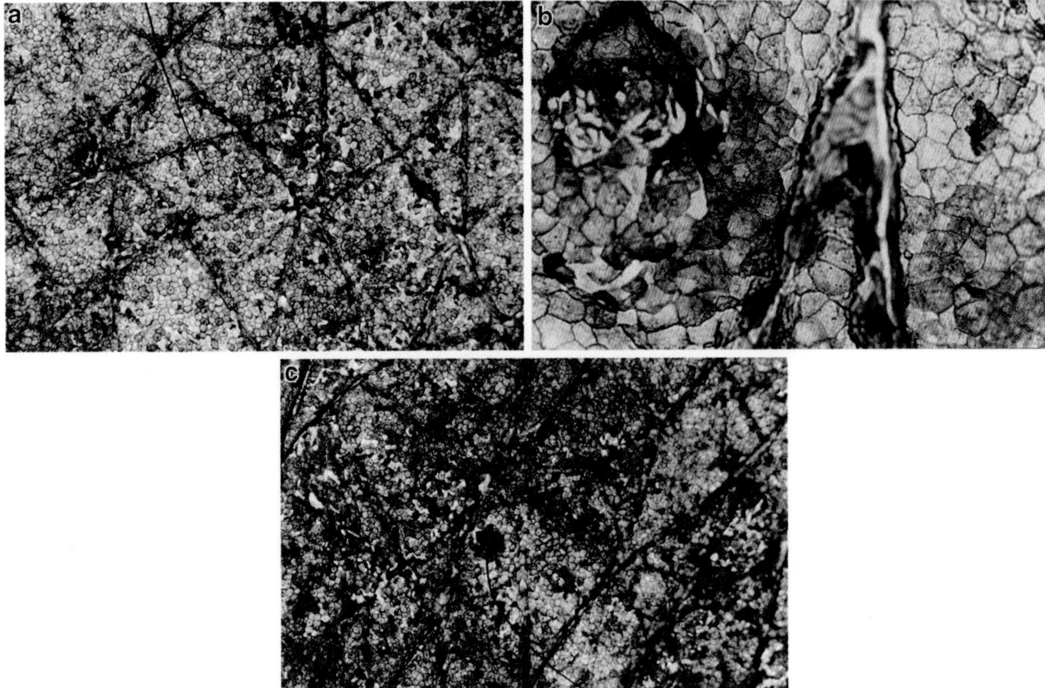

Fig. 9 CSSS bioassay: corneocyte alterations following contact with surfactants. (**a**) Medium grade alteration with focal increase in stratum corneum stainings. (**b**) Higher magnification showing the heterogeneity in the corneocyte alterations. (**c**) Higher response of the horny layer to a surfactant

increases CSM sensitivity to discriminate among mild surfactants [32].

Shielded CSM is used for testing skin protective products (SPP) [33]. SPP claiming for being barrier creams should be shields against noxious agents. In shielded CSM, the CSSSs are first covered by the test SPP before performing regular CSM using a reference surfactant. Comparative screenings of SPP are conveniently performed using shielded CSM without exposing volunteers to hazards linked to in vivo testing.

Animal CSM is performed [34] in a way similar to human CSM. The method is available for safety testing of cleansing products specifically designed for some animal species. In addition, interspecies differences in surfactant reactivity of the skin to surfactants are conveniently assessed [34].

The corneoxenometry (CXM) bioassay is used for testing any chemical xenobiotic other than surfactants [33, 35, 36]. The basic procedure is similar to CSM and its variants. One main indication is found in any case of putative skin irritation while avoiding the in vivo hazards. Another indication concerns the comparative assessment of penetration enhancers commonly used in topical formulations [35].

Conclusions

The SC holds a large account of information about skin biology and the internal milieu itself. Beside conventional biopsies and cytology of exudates, imprints, and scrapings, CSSSs provide useful information in the field of dermatopathology and cosmetology. This simple, rapid, cheap, and minimally invasive method allows the clinician to avoid conventional biopsy within limits of well-defined indications. Less than 3 min is necessary between CSSS sampling and examination. There are evident features and subtle characteristics discernible in the structure of the SC that enable a diagnosis to be made in a variety of skin diseases. It is important to stress that no single criterion should usually be relied upon for a definitive diagnosis, but rather a constellation of clues should be sought. Quantifications are made possible on CSSS using computer-assisted image analysis and other analytical examinations.

Meaningful analytical morphologic aspects are open to CSSS samplings. A series of derived methods have been designed for investigative purposes. When performed under controlled procedures, the information appears reproducible and sensitive. In many instances, the procedures help to bypass animal testing and to avoid a number of hazards bound to in vivo human trials.

References

1. Hirao T, et al. Identification of immature cornified envelopes in the barrier-impaired epidermis by characterization of their hydrophobicity and antigenicities of the components. Exp Dermatol. 2001;10:35–44.
2. Harding CR, et al. The cornified cell envelope: an important marker of stratum corneum maturation in healthy and dry skin. Int J Cosmet Sci. 2003;25:157–67.
3. Piérard GE. EEMCO guidance for the assessment of dry skin (xerosis) and ichthyosis: evaluation by stratum corneum strippings. Skin Res Technol. 1996;2:3–11.
4. Piérard GE, et al. From observational to analytical morphology of the stratum corneum: progress avoiding hazardous animal and human testings. Clin Cosmet Investig Dermatol. 2015;8:113–25.
5. Marks R, Dawber RP. Skin surface biopsy: an improved technique for the examination of the horny layer. Br J Dermatol. 1971;84:117–23.
6. Piérard-Franchimont C, Piérard GE. Assessment of aging and actinic damages by cyanoacrylate skin surface strippings. Am J Dermatopathol. 1987; 9:500–9.
7. Piérard GE, et al. Cyanoacrylate skin surface stripping and the 3S-Biokit advent in tropical dermatology: a look from Liege. Sci World J. 2014;2014:462634.
8. Uhoda E, et al. The conundrum of skin pores in dermocosmetology. Dermatology. 2005;210:3–7.
9. Pagnoni A, et al. Determination of density of follicles on various regions of the face by cyanoacrylate biopsy: correlation with sebum output. Br J Dermatol. 1994;131:862–5.
10. Letawe C, et al. Digital image analysis of the effect of topically applied linoleic acid on acne microcomedones. Clin Exp Dermatol. 1998;23:56–8.
11. Piérard-Franchimont C, et al. Lymecycline and minocycline in inflammatory acne: a randomized, double-blind intent-to-treat study on clinical and in vivo antibacterial efficacy. Skin Pharmacol Appl Skin Physiol. 2002;15:112–9.
12. Grice EA. The skin microbiome: potential for novel diagnostic and therapeutic approaches to cutaneous disease. Semin Cutan Med Surg. 2014;33:98–103.
13. Piérard GE, et al. Cyanoacrylate skin surface stripping: an improved approach for distinguishing dysplastic nevi from malignant melanomas. J Cutan Pathol. 1989;16:180–2.
14. Piérard-Franchimont C, Piérard GE. Skin surface stripping in diagnosing and monitoring inflammatory, xerotic, and neoplastic diseases. Pediatr Dermatol. 1985;2:180–4.
15. Piérard GE, et al. Karyometry of malignant melanoma cells present in skin strippings. Skin Res Technol. 1995;1:177–9.
16. Thirion L, et al. Whitening effect of a dermocosmetic formulation: a randomized double-blind controlled study on melasma. Int J Cosmet Sci. 2006;28:263–7.
17. Piérard-Franchimont C, et al. Analytic quantification of the bleaching effect of a 4-hydroxyanisole-tretinoin combination on actinic lentigines. J Drugs Dermatol. 2008;7:873–8.
18. Piérard GE. Microscopic evaluation of the dansyl chloride test. Dermatology. 1992;185:37–40.
19. Piérard GE, Piérard-Franchimont C. Dihydroxyacetone test as a substitute for the dansyl chloride test. Dermatology. 1993;186:133–7.
20. Paye M, et al. Dansyl chloride labelling of stratum corneum: its rapid extraction from skin can predict skin irritation due to surfactants and cleansing products. Contact Dermatitis. 1994;30:91–6.
21. Faergemann J. A new model for growth and filament production of Pityrosporum ovale (orbiculare) on human stratum corneum in vitro. J Invest Dermatol. 1989;92:117–9.
22. Rurangirwa A, et al. Culture of fungi on cyanoacrylate skin surface strippings – a quantitative bioassay for evaluating antifungal drugs. Clin Exp Dermatol. 1989;14:425–8.
23. Aljabre SH, et al. Germination of Trichophyton mentagrophytes on human stratum corneum in vitro. J Med Vet Mycol. 1992;30:145–52.
24. Piérard GE, et al. Comparative study of the activity and lingering effect of topical antifungals. Skin Pharmacol. 1993;6:208–14.
25. Arrese JE, et al. Euclidean and fractal computer-assisted corneofungimetry: a comparison of 2%

ketoconazole and 1% terbinafine topical formulations. Dermatology. 2002;204:222–7.
26. Piérard-Franchimont C, et al. Activity of the triazole antifungal r126638 as assessed by corneofungimetry. Skin Pharmacol Physiol. 2006;19:50–6.
27. Uhoda E, et al. Comedolysis by a lipohydroxyacid formulation in acne-prone subjects. Eur J Dermatol. 2003;13:65–8.
28. Piérard GE, et al. Surfactant-induced dermatitis: comparison of corneosurfametry with predictive testing on human and reconstructed skin. J Am Acad Dermatol. 1995;33:462–9.
29. Henry F, et al. Regional differences in stratum corneum reactivity to surfactants. Quantitative assessment using the corneosurfametry bioassay. Contact Dermatitis. 1997;37:271–5.
30. Xhauflaire-Uhoda E, et al. Skin capacitance imaging and corneosurfametry. A comparative assessment of the impact of surfactants on stratum corneum. Contact Dermatitis. 2006;54:249–53.
31. Goffin V, Piérard GE. Microwave corneosurfametry and the short-duration dansyl chloride extraction test for rating concentrated irritant surfactants. Dermatology. 2001;202:46–8.
32. Uhoda E, et al. Responsive corneosurfametry following in vivo skin preconditioning. Contact Dermatitis. 2003;49:292–6.
33. Xhauflaire-Uhoda E, et al. Skin protection creams in medical settings: successful or evil? J Occup Med Toxicol. 2008;3:15.
34. Goffin V, et al. Comparative surfactant reactivity of canine and human stratum corneum: a plea for the use of the corneosurfametry bioassay. Altern Lab Anim. 1999;27:103–9.
35. Goffin V, et al. Penetration enhancers assessed by corneoxenometry. Skin Pharmacol Appl Skin Physiol. 2000;13:280–4.
36. Xhauflaire-Uhoda E, et al. Effects of various concentrations of glycolic acid at the corneoxenometry and collaxenometry bioassays. J Cosmet Dermatol. 2008;7:194–8.

Vaginal Secretions with Age

34

Paul R. Summers

Contents

P.R. Summers (✉)
University of Utah School of Medicine, Salt Lake City, UT, USA
e-mail: paul.summers@hsc.utah.edu

M.A. Farage et al. (eds.), *Textbook of Aging Skin*,
DOI 10.1007/978-3-662-47398-6_24

Abstract

Vaginal secretions are influenced by the dynamics of female hormones as well as local pathology. As an intended defense against infection, secretions contain innate "natural antibiotic" chemicals that at least regulate normal vaginal flora. Anaerobic metabolism of glucose into lactate by the genital tract epithelium as well as anaerobic or facultative microbes maintains a mildly acidic pH that is important for normal skin metabolism. Characteristic changes in the exfoliated epithelial content of vaginal secretions can indicate local inflammatory skin disorders such as mucus membrane graft vs host disease, lichen planus, lichen simplex, or lichen sclerosus.

The Source of Vaginal Secretions

In the developing fetus, the vaginal epithelium is transformed from columnar to squamous prior to term birth. With the exclusion of the vaginal epithelium, most mucosal surfaces in the human body that demonstrate this type of squamous metaplasia during fetal development retain specific secretory glands. In spite of an absence of secretory subdermal glands, it is significant that the vaginal epithelial cells retain a remarkable secretory ability.

Vaginal mucosa contains a microscopic intercellular network of secretory pathways. Intercellular channels are found between the

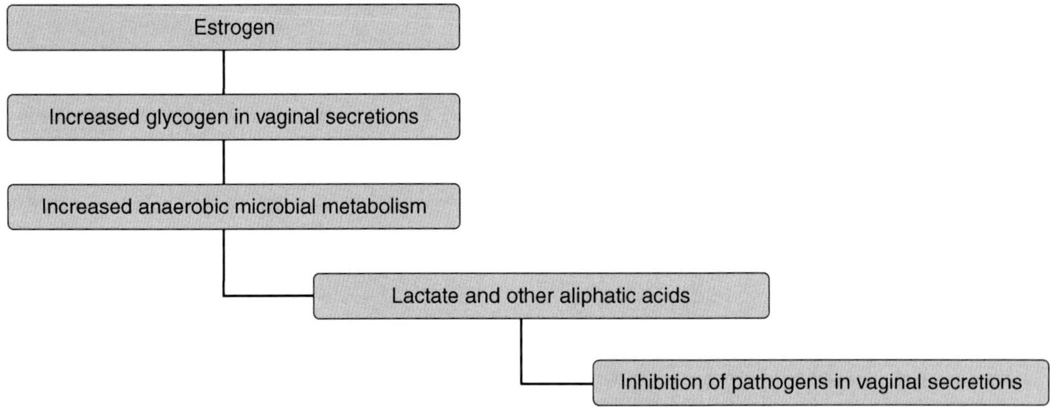

Fig. 1 Theory of microbial inhibition proposed in the early twentieth century

tight junctions in the intermediate cell layer of the mucosa. These areas of dilation start as clefts in the parabasal cell layer of the epithelium, and appear as pores that can be seen at the mucosal surface using scanning electron microscopy [1]. The entire vaginal surface is, then, a secretory structure. The mucosal secretions of the female lower genital tract fulfill several important roles in the process of reproduction, ranging from lubrication, to microbial inhibition, to sperm facilitation.

In a manner similar to mucosa at other body sites, it is presumed that vaginal secretions trap potentially pathogenic bacteria. The constant daily drainage of approximately 2 cm^3 of secretions during the reproductive years may, in this case, contribute somewhat to the removal of these adverse microbes [2]. More important, the confluent coating of secretions may restrict pathogens from contacting the mucosal surface, to prevent the essential first step in the establishment of infection. This mucosal barrier is lost with the postmenopausal decline in estrogen.

The most widely recognized constituent of vaginal mucosal secretions is the lactobacillus. More recent nonculture-based data have shown a number of acid-producing bacteria that may be present with or instead of lactobacillus [3, 4]. Normal vaginal secretions favor the growth of the various lactobacillus and other acid-producing bacteria strains that are considered normal flora. A mildly acidic pH and the presence of glycogen are two key factors for these strains. Metabolically restricted to anaerobic glycolysis, the lactobacillus strains release significant amounts of lactic acid into the vaginal mucosal secretions. Tradition attributes a protective role for the lactobacillus against potential pathogens, although clinical experience suggests this presumed defensive action of the lactobacillus is strikingly inadequate. In spite of the essentially ubiquitous presence of acid-producing bacteria in normal vaginal secretions, the vaginal mucosa remains susceptible to a wide range of pathogenic microbes.

During the antiseptic era of the early twentieth century, it was presumed that the lactate content of vaginal secretions contributed a significant antiseptic action to prevent infection (Fig. 1). Although this simplistic view of vaginal antisepsis still remains popular, modern research has disclosed other constituents of vaginal secretions that present a more plausible explanation for antimicrobial action in the vaginal secretions.

Human epithelial cells are highly active in the production of a wide range of metabolic products. In this regard, the vaginal mucosa is no exception. Many of these chemical products are released into the vaginal secretions, in some cases presumably to carry out a protective role. More than 40 different organic substances have been identified in normal vaginal secretions. Lactate is the primary acid that contributes to the low vaginal pH, but other normal constituents range from 15 typical aliphatic acids (such as acetic, myriatic, linoleic) to alcohols, glycols, and various aromatic compounds [5]. There is an important role for various elements of the innate and humoral immune systems, such as defensins and small amounts of IgA and IgG, in the vaginal fluid (refer to the chapter on immunology of the female lower genital tract). Unfortunately, vaginal pathogens are often able to evade the potential immune and mechanical barriers presented by the coating of mucosal secretions. For example, the polymicrobial pathogens of *bacterial vaginosis* produce hydrolytic enzymes that lyse the protein base of vaginal mucosal secretions so that pathogenic bacteria can reach the mucosa [6].

Hormone Influence upon the Vaginal Mucosal Secretions

Hormone production regulates the quantity and character of vaginal mucosal secretions. Under the influence of estrogen, the glycogen-rich intermediate cell layer of the mucosa is the area of greatest metabolic and secretory activity. Basal and superficial cell regions are less metabolically important. Under the influence of cyclic hormone changes, constituents of vaginal secretions change significantly during the menstrual cycle [7]. Lactic acid and urea content is greatest between 48 h prior to 24 h after the luteinizing hormone (LH) surge. Mid-cycle changes probably reflect increased mucosal metabolic activity at that time [8]. After menopause, the metabolically active intermediate cell layer of the mucosa is lost, with a simultaneous decline in secretory products [9]. Furthermore, vaginal subdermal blood flow is decreased after menopause, resulting in less mucosal transudate [10].

pH and Vaginal Secretions

Tradition has assigned an acid pH around 4.5 to be the main regulatory parameter for the vagina (see Chart). Lactic acid is the major source of hydrogen ions in vaginal secretions during the reproductive years [5]. Although the common literature tends to attribute vaginal lactic acid production solely to the lactobacillus, the vaginal mucosa also releases lactate as an end result of glycolysis. A significant amount of lactic acid is a by-product of normal anaerobic vaginal mucosal metabolism [9]. Lactobacilli are not the only source of vaginal lactate, and actually may not be the primary source.

Lactate from *Lactobacillus* Versus Mucosal Glycolysis

Early studies demonstrated the dual sources of vaginal lactate, and even suggested mucosal glycolysis as the primary source. There is no direct correlation between the pH of vaginal mucosal secretions and the presence of lactobacilli, nor is there a correlation between the amount of glycogen substrate for growth of lactobacilli and the actual amount of lactobacillus [11, 12]. In the absence of a significant vaginal colonization with lactobacillus, the pH may still be in the normal acid pH range. For example, a newborn has significant lactate in the initially sterile vaginal secretions, with a pH of around 5, prior to any colonization with lactobacillus [13]. With declining maternal estrogen influence, the vaginal pH of the infant rises to the neutral range as the metabolic activity of the vaginal mucosa declines by 6 weeks of life. The vagina does not become colonized with lactobacillus until puberty. The neutral vaginal pH after menopause is associated with a significant lack of lactate as a result of diminished glycolysis in the intermediate cell layer of the mucosa, as well as a lack of lactobacillus. In view of this early research, it is surprising that the idea that the lactobacillus is the single source of lactate prevails in the current common understanding.

Recent research also suggests that lactate from gylcolysis in the vaginal mucosa may have the chief regulatory role for vaginal pH. For example, pH in the vaginal fornices has been shown to be lower than the pH in the mid vagina, in spite of a relatively uniform distribution of lactobacillus [14]. Lactate from lactobacillus would not explain the observation that mucosal secretion during sexual stimulation appears to contain the same concentration of lactate that is found in the nonstimulated state [5]. It is also unlikely that transient alterations in lactobacillus metabolism

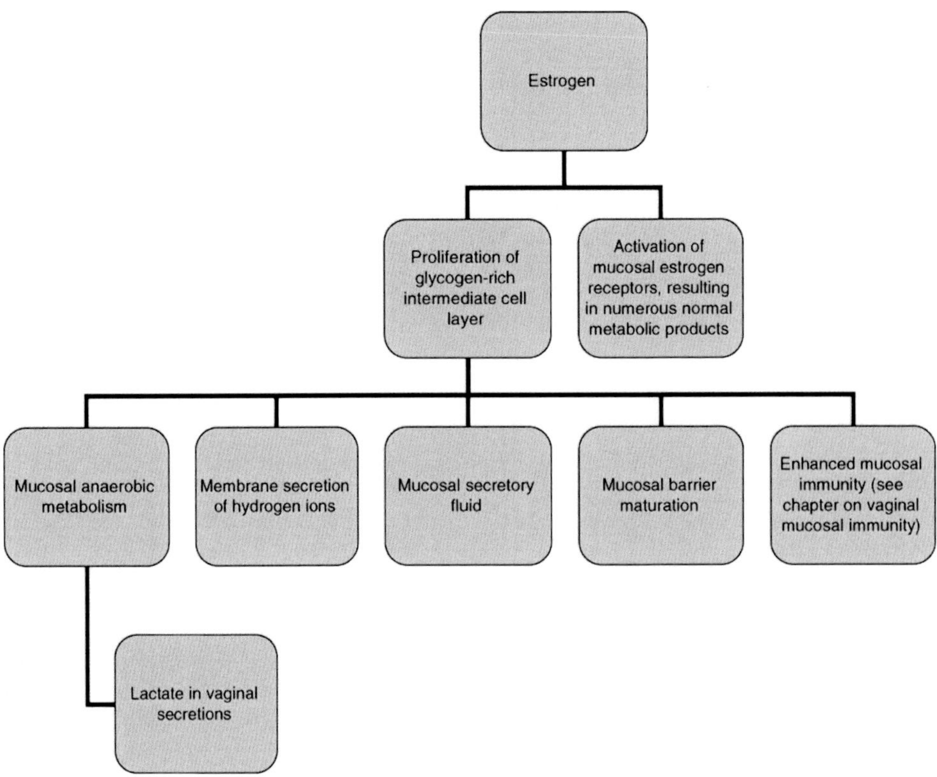

Fig. 2 Vaginal pH and other mucosal effects of estrogen

or growth, with resulting release of excess lactate, could explain the brief decline in pH at the time of ovulation [9].

Estrogen directly and indirectly regulates vaginal mucosal metabolism, mucosal secretions, and pH (Fig. 2). Microbial sources of lactate are dependent upon estrogen-induced glycogen as an energy source. Similarly, vaginal mucosal anaerobic metabolism is estrogen dependent. Possibly, a separate mechanism for vaginal mucosal pH regulation has been identified. Under the influence of estrogen, superficial vaginal mucosal cells may secrete hydrogen ions into the vaginal lumen in a manner similar to gastric chief cells [15]. A direct link with intraepithelial lactate production was not reviewed in this study, but anaerobic metabolism of glycogen remains the prime source of intracellular hydrogen ions. Decreased mucosal metabolism after menopause alters content as well as quantity of normal mucosal secretions.

Either vaginal glycogen increases under the influence of estrogen [16], or it is subjected to increased metabolism to lactate [17]. In either case, estrogen contributes to increased lactate. The vaginal pH fluctuates with the menstrual cycle, with its lowest average value around the time of ovulation. Presumably, this would be evidence of maximal anaerobic skin metabolism and lactate release. Sperm survive best in an anaerobic environment. It is reasonable to speculate that this enhanced anaerobic environment at the time of ovulation may contribute to sperm survival [7].

Vaginal pH With Age

The vaginal pH is not just important for microbe control, but a mildly acid pH is also ideal for normal vaginal skin metabolism, including the production of various proteins that are important for vaginal immune defenses. The rise in vaginal pH after menopause results in a loss of natural skin defenses, with an increased rate of urinary tract infection [18]. Topical application of estrogen to the menopausal vagina restores a normal pH and lowers the risk for bladder infection [19]. It is clear that skin barrier function is compromised by the typically neutral menopausal vaginal pH. This rise in pH increases the susceptibility to contact dermatitis [20]. A menopausal rise in skin pH results in defective enzyme function and vulvar skin ceramide deficiency [21]. Stratum corneum acidity is known to be essential for a normal inflammatory response and for optimal skin barrier function [22]. This concept most likely also applies to vaginal mucosa. Application of neutral pH buffers to skin in general results in decreased stratum corneum integrity and cohesion [23]. It is only reasonable to conclude that this concern also applies to the neutral vaginal pH in the menopausal state. It is of interest to note that the vaginal pH is mildly alkaline during menses. It is possible that this transient neutral or alkaline vaginal pH during menses also contributes to a risk for contact dermatitis from menstrual sanitary pads, with special concern if the bleeding episode is prolonged.

Cellular Content of Vaginal Secretions

Exfoliated cells from the lower female genital tract are captured in the vaginal secretions. The character of these exfoliated cells reflects estrogen status, as well as vulvovaginal dermatopathology in some cases. Estrogen promotes maturation of genital tract epithelial cells. Parabasal cells, immature cells in the vaginal fluid that lack the action of estrogen, are prominent prior to puberty and after menopause. These cells are round or oval with a relatively large nucleus. Such immature cells reflecting no maturation beyond the parabasal layer of the epithelium are seen in a high power view in Fig. 3. In contrast, Fig. 4 shows well estrogenized flat mature epithelial cells found in the vaginal fluid during the reproductive years.

Inflammation that promotes epithelial cell proliferation [24] may be evident in the vaginal secretions. Severe inflammation from disorders such as mucus membrane graft vs host disease or lichen planus can cause such rapid turnover of the vaginal epithelium that exfoliated cells show no estrogen effect. With these disorders in the genital tract, immature parabasal epithelial cells and white blood cells are the dominant findings in the vaginal fluid as seen in Fig. 3.

The common papular vulvovaginal disorders of lichen simplex and lichen planus are characterized by flaking of the surface, hence the characterization in the name, "lichen." Such flakes of desquamated epithelium can be found in vaginal secretions as also seen in Fig. 4. Flakes of epithelium found in the vaginal secretions range from thin to thick and few to numerous, based upon the degree of lichenification of the associated

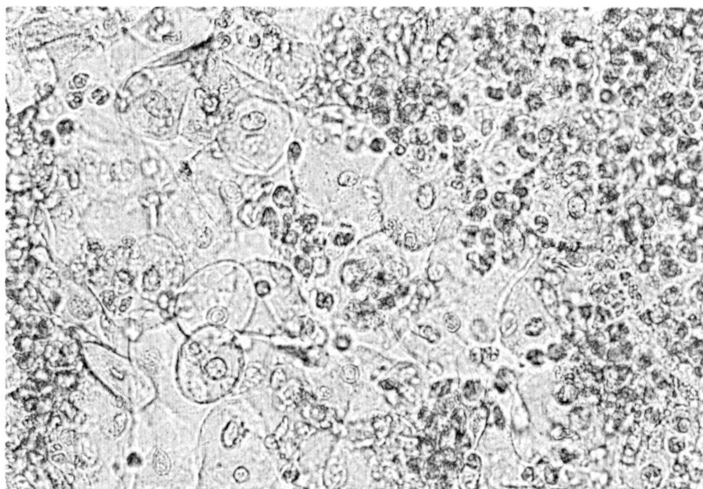

Fig. 3 High power view of immature paarabasal squamous cells and numerous white blood cells

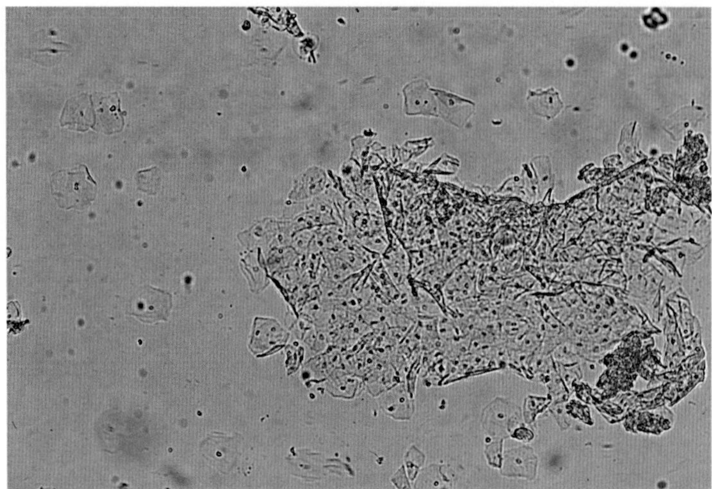

Fig. 4 Mature squamous epithelial cells and a skin flake

vulvovaginal skin disorder. Vulvovaginal skin barrier function is naturally further compromised by either lack of maturation of the epithelium or by lichenification, as reflected by the cellular content of the vaginal secretions.

Conclusion

Vaginal mucosal metabolism is uniquely estrogen dependent (Table 1). During the reproductive years, estrogen stimulates the maturation of a metabolically active intermediate cell layer within the vaginal epithelium. This glycogen-rich cell layer is the source for much of the complex content of the mucosal secretions. Constituents of the mucosal secretions, as well as support for normal microbial flora, remain almost totally estrogen dependent. The characteristically low vaginal pH is directly linked to anaerobic vaginal mucosal metabolism, as well as to the traditionally recognized lactobacilli and other acid-producing vaginal microflora. A low estrogen level prior to puberty and after menopause results in inactive vaginal mucosa with little production of secretions. Vaginal pH rises with the metabolic decline in mucosal and microbial glycogen-dependent anaerobic glycolysis. The resulting neutral pH after menopause most likely results in further loss of vulvovaginal skin barrier function.

Table 1 Menopausal effects

Decreased glycogen to support lactobacillus and other microbes
Decreased glycogen to support mucosal metabolism in the intermediate cell layer
Significant loss of the metabolically active intermediate cell layer
Decline in protective mucosal secretion
Decline in hydrogen ions and other secretory products in the vaginal fluid

References

1. Burgos MH. Roig de vargas-Linares CE. Cell junctions in the human vaginal epithelium. Am J Obstet Gynecol. 1970;108(4):565–7.
2. Wagner G, Levin RJ. Vaginal fluid. In: Hafez ESE, Evans TN, editors. The human vagina. New York: North-Holland; 1978. p. 123.
3. Zhou X, Bent SJ, Schneider MG, et al. Characterization of vaginal microbial communities in adult healthy women using cultivation-independent methods. Microbiology. 2004;150:2565–73.
4. Zhou X, Brown CJ, Abdo Z, et al. Differences in the composition of vaginal microbial communities found in healthy Caucasian and black women. ISME J. 2007;1:121–33.
5. Huggins GR, Preti G. Volatile constituents of human vaginal secretions. Am J Obstet Gynecol. 1976; 126(1):129–36.
6. Cauci S, Hitti J, Noonan C, Agnew K, Quadrifoglio F, Hillier SL, Eschenbach DA. Vaginal hydrolytic enzymes, immunoglobulin against Gardnerella vaginalis toxin, and early risk of preterm birth among

women in preterm labor with bacterial vaginosis or intermediate flora. Am J Obstet Gynecol. 2002; 187:877–81.

7. Preti G, Huggins GR. Cyclical changes in volatile acidic metabolites of human vaginal secretions and their relation to ovulation. J Chem Ecol. 1975; 1:361–76.
8. Preti G, Hugins GR. Organic constituents of vaginal secretions. In: Hafez ESE, Evans TN, editors. The human vagina. New York: North-Holland; 1978. p. 162–3.
9. Gross M. Biochemical changes in the reproductive cycle. Fertil Steril. 1961;12(3):245–62.
10. Society of Obstetricians and Gynecologists of Canada. The detection and management of vaginal atrophy. Int J Gynecol Obstet. 2004;88:222–8.
11. Weinstein L, Howard JH. The effect of estrogenic hormone on the H-ion concentration and the bacterial content of the human vagina with special reference to the Doederline bacillus. Am J Obstet Gynecol. 1939; 37:698–703.
12. Weinstein L, Bogin M, Howard JH, Finkelstone BB. A survey of the vaginal flora at various ages with special reference to the Doederline bacillus. Am J Obstet Gynecol. 1936;32:211–8.
13. Raskoff AE, Feo LG, Goldstein L. The biologic characteristics of the normal vagina. Am J Obstet Gynecol. 1943;47:467–94.
14. Tsai CC, Semmens JP, Semmens EC, Lam CF, Lee FS. Vaginal physiology in postmenopausal women: pH value, transvaginal electropotential difference, and estimated blood flow. South Med J. 1987;80:987–90.
15. Gorodeski GI, Hopfer U, Liu CC, Margles E. Estrogen acidifies vaginal pH by up-regulation of proton secretion via the apical membrane of vaginal-ectocervical epithelial cells. Endocrinology. 2005;146 (2):816–24.
16. Bo WJ. The effect of progesterone and progesterone-estrogen on the glycogen deposition in the vagina of the squirrel monkey. Am J Obstet Gynecol. 1970; 107:524–30.
17. Ayre WB. The glycogen-estrogen relationship in the vaginal tract. J Clin Endocrinol Metab. 1951; 11:103–10.
18. Weisberg E, Aytin R, Darling G, et al. Endometrial and vaginal effects of dose-related estradiol delivered by vaginal ring or vaginal tablet. Climacteric. 2005; 8:83–92.
19. Kunin CM, Evans C, Barhholomew D, Bates G. The antimicrobial defense mechanism of the female urethra: a reassessment. J Urol. 2002;168:413–9.
20. Berg RW, Milligan MC, Sarbaugh FC. Association of skin wetness and pH with diaper dermatitis. Pediatr Dermatol. 1994;11:18–20.
21. Fluhr JW, Kao J, Jain M, et al. Generation of free fatty acids from phospholipids regulates stratum corneum acidification and integrity. J Invest Dermatol. 2001; 117:44–51.
22. Mauro TM. SC pH: measurement, origins, and functions. In: Elias PM, Feingold KR, editors. Skin barrier. New York: Taylor & Francis; 2006. p. 225.
23. Hachem JP, Crumrine D, Fluhr J, Brown BE, Feingold KR, Elias PM. pH directly regulates epidermal permeability barrier homeostasis and stratum corneum integrity/cohesion. J Invest Dermatol. 2003;121:345–53.
24. Falabella AF, Falanga V. Wound Healing. In: Freinkel RK, Woodley DT, editors. The biology of the skin. New York: Parthenon Publishing; 2001. p. 281–97.

Unique Skin Immunology of the Lower Female Genital Tract with Age

35

Paul R. Summers

Contents

Abstract

Although generally overlooked in clinical medicine, the complex and important immune system of the lower female genital tract plays a significant role in fertility, defense against infection, and the relatively common dermatologic disorders of this area. Unique immune characteristics help to facilitate sperm survival. Infectious genital tract pathogens typically have mechanisms to avoid the natural immune defenses. Vulvovaginal skin disorders reflect aberrant immune responses. An understanding of basic lower genital tract immunology provides a helpful foundation for clinical medical care.

Introduction

It has been long recognized that the genital tract must be able to defend against significant microbial exposures. In this area of medicine, old theories that may have even acquired some attributes of folklore must be revised to include new knowledge. Through the last century, popular ideas regarding mechanisms of microbial defenses in the genital tract have reflected the medical thinking of each era. In the time of antisepsis of the early twentieth century, lactic acid from the lactobacillus was proposed as the chief regulatory vaginal antiseptic. Subsequently, the possibility of antiseptic action from hydrogen peroxide-producing lactobacilli was considered, although little

P.R. Summers (✉)
University of Utah School of Medicine, Salt Lake City, UT, USA
e-mail: paul.summers@hsc.utah.edu

M.A. Farage et al. (eds.), *Textbook of Aging Skin*,
DOI 10.1007/978-3-662-47398-6_25

hydrogen peroxide would be expected to be produced in the naturally anaerobic environment of the vaginal lumen. With the influence of the more recent antibiotic era, research interest has focused upon bacteriocins, unique but relatively weak lactobacillus-derived antibiotics. Theories of microbial defense have evolved further in the current, more enlightened era of immunology. Rapid advances in the area of immunology have now disclosed complex immune defenses in the genital epithelium that do have a significant antimicrobial impact, moderated by estrogen and progesterone.

Immunology of reproduction has also evolved into an area of extensive knowledge. Significant immune involvement is evident in the normal physiology of all areas of the female reproductive system. From the immune standpoint, the lower genital tract has the following competing roles: (1) to facilitate the various aspects of reproduction and (2) to simultaneously prevent the access of locally resident microbes to the upper genital tract and to the peritoneal cavity. To match the needs of a primary function in reproduction, the immune responsiveness of the lower female genital tract is blunted. Ovulation, fertilization, pregnancy, labor, and delivery of the infant are all mediated by immune mechanisms that may not be optimal for microbial defense. A blunted humoral immune response may be compensated by an active innate or cell-mediated response. For example, sperm may be highly immunogenic. If sperm are detected by the humoral immune system, the development of antisperm antibodies can reduce fertility [1]. It is important for the vaginal immune system to identify potential pathogens, but not to target sperm or the fetus, or to disrupt the immune mechanisms of fertility.

Microbial and immune events in the female urethra mirror the status of the vaginal vestibule [2]. The immune function and microbial flora of the vaginal vestibule and urethra change in a parallel fashion in response to the effects of aging and hormone cycles. Hormone changes alter the morphology and mucosal defenses. Menopausal decline in innate immune defenses in the vaginal mucosa allows colonization with potential uropathogens and increases the risk for bladder infection.

Recent decades have shown growing research interest in immunology of the male and female genital tracts, in part due to the HIV epidemic. This is a previously somewhat neglected but highly significant aspect of human immunology. Unfortunately, current educational efforts still direct little attention to the extensive knowledge base that has developed in the area of urogenital immunology. This clinically important topic is totally omitted in most major textbooks of obstetrics and gynecology. Fortunately, educational efforts have now reached the point where textbooks that focus on immunology of the genital tract are now in publication [3].

Humoral Immunity

The humoral immune system associated with vaginal mucosa is unique. Mucosal surfaces outside the genital tract develop in conjunction with lymphoid tissue that predominantly produces IgA. At other body sites, IgA may have a significant role in mucosal defense against microbes. With the absence of associated lymphoid tissue, vaginal mucosa releases only limited quantities of any category of immunoglobulin at all stages of life. IgG is present in vaginal secretions. The relatively small amount of IgG is serum derived as well as locally produced in the vaginal and cervical mucosa [4]. With the relative absence of a local source of IgA, more IgG than IgA is detected in vaginal secretions [5]. The converse is true for mucosal surfaces elsewhere in the body.

Cervical secretions have a higher concentration of IgA than vaginal secretions [6]. This finding is consistent with the presumed protective role of cervical mucus to prevent ascent of microbes into the endometrial cavity. The concentration of IgA in vaginal secretions declines by 90 % after hysterectomy, so the upper genital tract may be assumed to be the primary source of the small quantity of IgA that is present in the vaginal lumen [7]. It is reasonable to assume a similar decline in lower genital tract immunoglobulins after the menopause, with the minimal production of cervical mucus and vaginal secretions at that time in life. Cervical secretion of IgG and IgA into the vaginal pool varies during the menstrual cycle with the highest levels prior to ovulation during the proliferative phase, but with an 80 % decline at the time of ovulation [8]. The limited amount of immunoglobulin in vaginal secretions may lower the risk for the development of antisperm antibodies. It is reasonable to speculate that sperm survival may be enhanced in some fashion by the further decline in immunoglobulins around the time of ovulation.

Disruption of vaginal immunoglobulin homeostasis can be harmful. Electrical loop excision of the cervical transformation zone (LEEP) may allow an unregulated humoral immune response at that site. Serum antisperm antibodies have been identified in women who are sexually active while the cervical LEEP site is healing [9].

Innate Immunity

The innate immune system has major importance in preventing invasion of potentially pathogenic microbes normally found in the lower genital tract and on the perirectal skin. During the reproductive years, an active innate immune response compensates somewhat for the blunted humoral and cell-mediated immune response in the lower female genital tract (Table 1). Sexually transmitted diseases develop when sexually acquired pathogens have the ability to evade these standing defenses [10]. Human beta defensins (HBD) 1, 2, 3, and 5, secretory leukocyte protease inhibitor (SLPI), elafin, and mannose-binding lectin (MBL) have been demonstrated in vaginal secretions [10]. The highest concentration of SLPI is in the cervical mucus plug, although it is expressed in secretions throughout the female genital tract. SLPI blocks the action of various destructive enzymes that may be released by pathogens. Elafin is an important protein that inhibits inflammation-related tissue damage by blocking elastase, which may be released by activated neutrophils. Elafin also has antimicrobial activity. Leukocytes and vaginal epithelial cells are the main sources of defensins [11]. Defensins are antibiotic substances that are active against various bacteria and yeast. Surfactant proteins in vaginal mucosal secretions (SP-A, SP-D) protect against viral infections, including HIV-1 and herpes simplex virus (HSV) [12]. Human neutrophil peptides (HNP 1–3) also suppress HSV in vaginal secretions [13]. These secretory products of the innate immune system are considered to be estrogen dependent, since many are the result of local mucosal metabolism, and the secretory fluid that contains these substances requires estrogen stimulation. Menopause results in a decline in the mucosal-dependent elements of the innate immune system.

Table 1 Important characteristics of the cervical transformation zone during the reproductive years

High concentration of elements of cell-mediated immunity to interact with viruses and to prevent ascent of bacteria into the upper genital tract and peritoneum
Macrophages are involved in cervical ripening prior to labor
Macrophages and granulocytes are involved in cervical dilation during labor

Minor congenital defects in the innate immune system, such as polymorphisms which result in deficiency of mannose-binding lectin (MBL), increase the risk of symptomatic infection [14]. MBL provides a target for complement activation by binding to the cell surface of pathogenic microbes. MBL is produced mainly in the liver and most likely arrives in the vaginal secretions as a transudate from the bloodstream. MBL is a significant factor in vaginal mucosal defense against pathogens, although the MBL level in vaginal secretions is much lower than the level normally found in the systemic circulation. It is not clear whether MBL is produced by vaginal mucosal cells.

During the reproductive years, toll-like receptors (TLRs) 1, 2, 3, 5, and 6 are expressed in vaginal mucosal cells. TLR 1, 2, and 5 mainly target bacteria. TLR 3 is directed against virus, and TLR 6 controls fungi [10]. The expression of TLRs is estrogen dependent. This may explain the prepubertal and possibly postmenopausal increased mucosal susceptibility to pathogens such as streptococcus or *Neisseria gonorrhea*.

Cell-Mediated Immunity

Langerhans cells are abundant in vaginal and cervical mucosa [15]. In the lower female genital tract, T cells and Langerhans cells are most prevalent in the normal cervical transformation zone, so the cervical transformation zone is assumed to be the major site for cell-mediated immune reactions in this area of the human body [16]. The likely immune consequences of excision of this important area by extensive LEEP or cervical cone biopsy have not been determined (Table 1). If the human skin is considered to be a major immune organ, then the cervix should be considered to have special immune function in that organ. Chronic cervicitis, often detected on cervical biopsy in asymptomatic women, is actually a misnomer, as the normal cervical transformation zone is a site of significant immune activity in normal health. Pathogenic microbes can activate cervical inflammation, but the presence of numerous immune cells is actually physiologic. The increased vulnerability of the relatively fragile transitional epithelium in the transformation zone may require better standing defenses to prevent ascending infection.

During the reproductive years, and to a greater extent during pregnancy, estrogen downregulates antigen-presenting cells. This results in a shift toward a Th2 immune response [17–19]. Although this has not been studied with specific reference to the female lower genital tract, a Th2 response downregulates the defensins and other secretory products of the innate immune system [20]. This relative immune compromise is presumed to be important for normal fertility and pregnancy. However, there are consequences, such as an increased risk for allergic contact dermatitis, as well as increased susceptibility to yeast, viruses, and other pathogens. Sexually transmitted diseases typically have mechanisms to avoid cell-mediated immunity [21].

The abundant macrophages and granulocytes in the cervical transformation zone are regulated by hormone changes of pregnancy. Reflecting the immune suppression of pregnancy, the number of macrophages in the cervical transformation zone declines in early pregnancy and then increases in preparation for labor. Macrophages are involved in cervical ripening just prior to the onset of labor, and macrophages and granulocytes have a significant role in cervical dilation [22].

Immune Changes with Age

Innate immune defenses of the vaginal mucosa are compromised with aging. Estrogen influences the expression of TLRs in vaginal mucosa [23, 24] (Tables 2 and 3). This loss of TLR expression increases the risk for colonization with pathogens. The postmenopausal lack of epithelial cell maturation results in loss of vaginal surface-barrier function. Pathogens can invade the more readily traumatized fragile epithelium. Estrogen deficiency leads to a decline in mucosal secretions that contain the antimicrobial constituents of the innate immune system. The neutral vaginal pH after the menopause reflects loss of the acid defense as well as a significant decline in vaginal mucosal metabolic ability.

Cell-mediated immunity is estrogen and age dependent. Langerhans cells are most prevalent in vulvar skin during the reproductive years [25]. Estrogen receptors on dendritic cells moderate the maturation of functional dendritic cells from precursor cells [26]. There is a decline in Langerhans cell function with aging, as well as a decreased Langerhans cell count by approximately 50 % [27, 28]. A decreased response to cytokines is also characteristic of aging [19]. The immunologically active cervical transformation zone is gradually eliminated by the aging process of squamous metaplasia.

Table 2 Characteristics of the lower female genital tract under the influence of estrogen

Innate immunity	TLR 1, 2, 3, 5, 6; HBD 1, 2, 3, 5; SLPI MBL SP-A SP-D; etc.
Humoral immunity	Very low IgA; very low IgG (IgG > IgA)
Cell-mediated immunity	Depressed Th1 tendency for enhanced Th2

TLR toll-like receptor, *HBD* human beta defensin, *SLPI* secretory leukocyte protease inhibitor, *MBL* mannose-binding lectin, *SP* surfactant proteins

Table 3 Characteristics of the lower female genital tract in the absence of estrogen

Innate immunity	Decreased expression of TLRs decrease in all secretory products
Humoral immunity	Further decline in IgA with decreased cervical secretions
Cell-mediated immunity	Decline in Langerhans cell count, decline in cytokine responsiveness, and estrogen-associated suppression of Th1 response is eliminated

TLR toll-like receptor, *HBD* human beta defensin, *SLPI* secretory leukocyte protease inhibitor, *MBL* mannose-binding lectin, *SP* surfactant proteins

Antigen-presenting cells are still present in the vaginal mucosa after menopause [29]. Postmenopausal estrogen replacement can reactivate deficient vaginal mucosal cell-mediated immune function. Asthma is a good example of the estrogen effect upon cell-mediated immunity. Asthma is influenced by the estrogen-related shift of cell-mediated immunity from a Th1 to a Th2 environment. Asthma is more prevalent in males than females prior to puberty but higher in females with the rise in estrogen after puberty [30]. Asthma may become less severe after menopause following the decline in Th1 suppression [31]. Hormone replacement therapy after menopause may make asthma worse [32]. Similarly, topical postmenopausal estrogen replacement may restore a Th2 environment that favors vaginal colonization with yeast. An increased susceptibility to microbial colonization and pathogen invasion with decline in hormones after menopause is well documented [33].

Current hormone replacement regimens are directed toward the lowest dose and shortest reasonable course for prevention of osteoporosis and menopausal hot flashes. Concerns about breast cancer and deep venous thrombosis restrict hormone administration after menopause. Thus, the postmenopausal dose of oral or topical hormones that would be required to more fully restore female immune function is not known and is not a current therapeutic goal. Various studies have demonstrated a potential benefit from postmenopausal hormone replacement for various autoimmune conditions [34] and even some malignancies [35]. Hormone replacement does restore a degree of immune function [36]. Unfortunately, generalization is difficult since each estrogenic product has its own unique pattern of estrogen receptor activation or inhibition throughout the body, depending upon the unique chemical structure or each estrogen.

Conclusion

Lower female genital tract immune defenses are complex and are not yet completely understood. Clearly, the immune system plays a major role in regulating vaginal microflora, but unfortunately, many pathogens have mechanisms to evade the immune defenses. Estrogen promotes the innate system, but suppresses the cell-mediated response in the lower genital tract. Humoral immunity appears to play only a small role in this portion of the female body. Immune function during the reproductive years reflects a balance between the need to protect against infection and the requirements of reproduction.

References

1. Hjort H. Do antisperm antibodies reduce fecundity? A mini review in historical perspective. Am J Reprod Immunol. 1998;40:215–22.
2. Kunin CM, Evans C, Bartholomew D, Bates G. The antimicrobial defense mechanism of the female urethra: a reassessment. J Urol. 2002;168:413–9.
3. Weissenbacher ER, Wirth M, Mylonas I, Ledger W, Witkin SS. Immunology of the female genital tract. Heidelberg: Springer; 2015.
4. Brandtzaeg P. Mucosal immunity in the female genital tract. J Reprod Immunol. 1997;36(1):23–50.
5. Quesnel A, Cu-Uvin S, Murphy D, Ashley RL, Flanigan T, Neutra MR. Comparative analysis of methods for collection and measurement of immunoglobulins in cervical and vaginal secretions of women. J Immunol Methods. 1997;202:153–61.
6. Crowley-Nowick PA, Bell MC, Brockwell R, Edwards RP, Chen S, Partridge EE, Mestecky J. Rectal immunization for induction of specific antibody in the genital tract of women. J Clin Immunol. 1997;17:370–9.
7. Jalanti R, Isliker H. Immunoglobulin in human cervicovaginal secretions. Int Arch Allergy Appl Immunol. 1977;53:402–8.

8. Nardelli-Haefliger D, Wirthner D, Schiller JT, Lowy DR, Hildesheim A, Ponci F, De Grandi P. Specific antibody levels at the cervix during the menstrual cycle of women vaccinated with human papillomavirus 16 virus-like particles. J Natl Cancer Inst. 2003;95 (15):1128–37.
9. Nicholson SC, Robindson TN, Sargent IC, Hallan NF. Does large loop excision of the transformation zone of the cervix predispose to the development of antisperm antibodies in women? Fertil Steril. 1996;65 (4):871–3.
10. Horne AW, Stock SJ, King AE. Innate immunity and disorders of the female reproductive tract. Reproduction. 2008;135:739–49.
11. Klotman ME, Chang TL. Defensins in innate antiviral immunity. Nat Rev Immunol. 2006;6:447–56.
12. Meschi J, Crouch EC, Skolnik P, Yahya K, Holmskov U, Leth-Larsen R, Tornoe I, Tecle T, White MR, Hartshorn KL. Surfactant protein D bonds to human immunodeficiency virus (HIV) envelope protein GP120 and inhibits HIV replication. J Gen Virol. 2005;86:3097–107.
13. John M, Keller MJ, Fam EH, Cheshenko K, Kasowitz A. Cervicovaginal secretions contribute to innate resistance to herpes simplex virus infection. J Infect Dis. 2005;192:1731–40.
14. Babula O, Lazdane G, Kroica J, Ledger WJ, Witkin SS. Relation between recurrent vulvovaginal candidiasis, vaginal concentrations of mannose-binding lectin, and a mannose-binding lectin gene polymorphism in Latvian women. Clin Infect Dis. 2003;37:733–7.
15. Bjercke S, Scott H, Braathen LR, Thorsby E. HLA-DR-expressing Langerhans-like cells in vaginal and cervical epithelium. Acta Obstet Gynecol Scand. 1983;62:585–9.
16. Pudney J, Quayle AJ, Anderson DL. Immunological microenvironments in the human vagina and cervix: mediators of cellular immunity are concentrated in the cervical transformation zone. Biol Reprod. 2005;73:1253–63.
17. Wira CR, Rossoll RM, Kaushic C. Antigen-presenting cells in the female reproductive tract: influence of estradiol on antigen presentation by vaginal cells. Endocrinology. 2000;141(8):2877–85.
18. Wira CR, Rossoll RM. Antigen-presenting cells in the human reproductive tract: influence of sex hormones on antigen presentation in the vagina. Immunology. 1995;84:505–8.
19. Faas M, Bouman A, Moes H, Heineman MJ, Leij L, Schuiling G. The immune response during the luteal phase of the ovarian cycle: a Th2-type response. Fertil Steril. 2000;74:1008–13.
20. Thivolet J, Nicolas JF. Skin aging and immune competence. Br J Immunol. 1990;122:77–81.
21. Chang JH, Ryang YS, Morio T, Lee SK, Chang EJ. *Trichomonas vaginalis* inhibits proinflammatory cytokine production in macrophages by suppressing NF-kappaB activation. Mol Cells. 2004;18:177–85.
22. Sakamoto Y, Moran P, Bulmor JN, Searle RF, Robson SC. Macrophages and not granulocytes are involved in cervical ripening. J Reprod Immunol. 2005;66:161–73.
23. Pioli PA, Amiel E, Schaefer TM, Connolly JE, Wira CR, Guyre PM. Differential expression of toll-like receptors 2 and 4 in tissues of the human female reproductive tract. Infect Immun. 2004;72:5799–806.
24. Sonnex C. Influence of ovarian hormones on urogenital infection. Sex Transm Infect. 1998;74:11–9.
25. Harper WF, McNicol EM. A histological study of normal vulval skin from infancy to old age. Br J Dermatol. 1977;96:249–53.
26. Paharkova-Vatchkova V, Maldonado R, Kovats S. Estrogen preferentially promotes the differentiation of $CD11c^{+}$ $CD11b^{intermediate}$ dendritic cells from bone marrow precursors. J Immunol. 2004;172:1426–36.
27. Nomura I, Goleva E, Howell MD, et al. Cytokine milieu of atopic dermatitis, as compared to psoriasis, skin prevents induction of innate immune response genes. J Immunol. 2003;171:3262–9.
28. Gilchrest B, Murphy G, Soter N. Effect of chronological aging and ultraviolet irradiation on Langerhans cells in human epidermis. J Invest Dermatol. 1982;79:85–8.
29. Fahey JV, Prabhala RH, Guyre PM, Wira CR. Antigen-presenting cells in the human female reproductive tract: analysis of antigen presentation in pre- and postmenopausal women. Am J Reprod Immunol. 1999;42:49–57.
30. Yawn BP, Wollan P, Kurland MJ, Scanlon P. A longitudinal study of asthma prevalence in a community population of school age children. J Pediatr. 2002;140 (5):576–81.
31. Balzano G, Fuschillo S, Melillo G, Bonini S. Asthma and sex hormones. Allergy. 2001;56(1):13–20.
32. Kos-Kudla B, Ostrowska Z, Marek B, et al. Effects of hormone replacement therapy on endocrine and spirometric parameters in asthmatic postmenopausal women. Gynecol Endocrinol. 2001;15(4):304–11.
33. Olsen NJ, Kovacs WJ. Gonadal steroids and immunity. Endocr Rev. 1996;17:369–84.
34. Cutolo M, Capellino S, Sulli A, Serioli B, Secchi ME, Villagio B, Straub RH. Estrogens and autoimmune diseases. Ann N Y Acad Sci. 2006;1089:538–47.
35. Gameiro CM, Romao F, Castelo-Branco C. Menopause and aging: changes in the immune system – a review. Maturitas. 2010;67:316–20.
36. Kamada M, Irahar M, Maegawa M, Ohmoto Y, Takeji T, Yasui T, Toshihiro A. Postmenopausal changes in serum cytokine levels and hormone replacement therapy. Am J Obstet Gynecol. 2001;184:309–14.

Aging Genital Skin and Hormone Replacement Therapy Benefits

36

William J. Ledger

Contents

W.J. Ledger (✉)
Department of Obstetrics and Gynecology, The New York-Presbyterian Hospital, Weill Medical College of Cornell University, New York, NY, USA
e-mail: wjledger@med.cornell.edu

M.A. Farage et al. (eds.), *Textbook of Aging Skin*,
DOI 10.1007/978-3-662-47398-6_26

Abstract

Menopause is heralded by dramatic changes: the cessation of menses, a loss of fertility, and a precipitous drop in the level of estrogen. These alterations in body functions create new concerns for a woman, including bone thinning and cardiovascular and cerebrovascular maladies, as well as continued surveillance for breast, ovarian, uterine, and cervical cancers. Add to this quality-of-life issues, including lower genital tract epithelial atrophy, one result of low estrogen. These problems often get short shrift from the physicians caring for these women.

Introduction

The most precise word that can be used to describe menopause is change. The most dramatic alteration in body function for older women is the cessation of menses, the usual monthly flow of bloody vaginal fluid. This obviously easily perceived and recognized phenomenon announces a new era for aging women; a new life passage with a loss of fertility and a growing awareness with new symptoms of the inexorable process of aging.

Currently in American medicine, preventive health care of menopausal women has too narrowly focused upon bone thinning, cardiovascular and cerebrovascular health, as well as surveillance for breast, ovarian, uterine, and cervical cancer. These ignore the quality-of-life issues associated with a relative lack of endogenous estrogen. There are also major concerns about hormone replacement therapy (HRT) because of studies showing a lack of protection against cardiovascular and cerebrovascular disease as well as an associated increased risk of breast cancer [1]. There has been a rush to the therapeutic bandwagon of nonhormonal agents for these women, including alendronate and raloxifene to prevent bone loss and the statins for cardiovascular protection.

Estrogen

The lack of the female hormone estrogen means the loss of hormonal activity that maintains the health of lower genital tract tissue. This loss results in the many changes that confront postmenopausal women. This absence is not an abrupt shift; the curtain does not suddenly fall one evening as the human drama of reproductive life ends, with the new playbill, postmenopausal existence beginning the next day. Instead, perimenopause, the transition period's new name, describes the very gradual changes in the years or decades before the cessation of menses. This is a slow and inexorable process in which minute bodily alterations occur over months and years that are perceived by the woman involved. Although early on, menstruation continues unabated, there is a drastic falloff in reproductive success. Assisted reproductive physicians note a stunning drop after the age of 42 in the ability of women to become pregnant and those few who succeed have a high number of spontaneous first-trimester pregnancy losses [2]. Subsequently, these perimenopausal women notice changes in their menstrual cycle, which can vary from too frequent and heavier periods to less frequent and lighter periods. Along with these menstrual changes, these women become aware of "hot flashes," i.e., vasomotor instability, trouble sleeping, decreased libido, and a dry and less lubricated vagina that makes intercourse uncomfortable.

Vaginal Changes

This diminishment in estrogen levels dramatically changes the vagina. There is a major decrease in the amount of vaginal secretion and a loss in both the elasticity and capacity of the vagina. These changes become very apparent to women. The annual or biannual visit to the gynecologist becomes an unwelcome chore, for it is increasingly uncomfortable, even when a pediatric speculum is used. Socially, intercourse can change from a pleasurable sensation to a painful event with a subsequent drop in libido, a loss accentuated by a drop in testosterone production. Parallel to these unpleasant alterations, the vaginal pH becomes more alkaline.

Upon microscopic examination of the vaginal secretion in a saline preparation, menopausal women have smaller, more rounded immature vaginal squamous cells and a markedly diminished number of acid-producing bacteria, such as the *Lactobacilli* (Fig. 1). These microscopic changes in the bacterial flora can be confirmed by culture. One report shows a marked diminishment in the number of probiotic *Lactobacilli*, with *Lactobacilli* the dominant vaginal species in only 13 % of the menopausal subjects [3]. Anaerobes become the dominant species. The numbers of these organisms were previously held in check by the dominance of the *Lactobacilli* and other organisms that produce lactic acid. There are clinical consequences of these changes in the vaginal

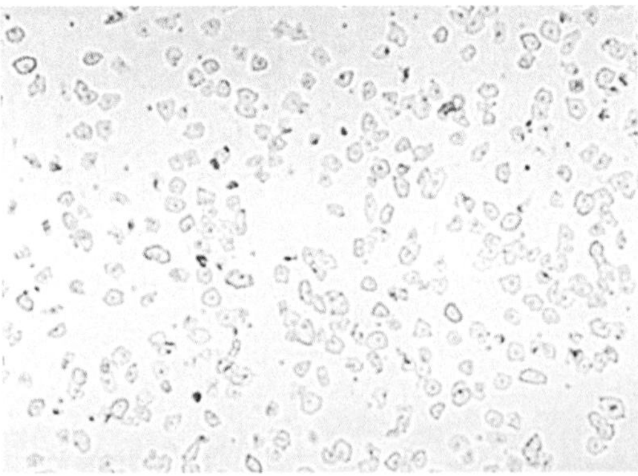

Fig. 1 Microscopic examination of vaginal secretions of an asymptomatic postmenopausal woman

bacterial flora that can result in lifestyle alterations for these women.

Perimenopausal and particularly postmenopausal women are colonized by *Escherichiae coli* at an increased incidence, and this is inversely related to the presence of *Lactobacilli* [4]. These vaginal bacterial changes make women much more susceptible to lower urinary tract infection due to *E. coli* [5]. The protective effect of organisms producing lactic acid which keep the numbers of these gram-negative aerobes in check has been lost and the relatively short female urethra becomes an easy transit site for these urinary tract pathogens. The perimenopausal woman is also much more prone to suffer from a grossly purulent and persistent vaginitis, named desquamative inflammatory vaginitis (DIV) [6]. The hallmarks of this troublesome syndrome, seen most commonly in women over the age of 40, are an alkaline pH, a negative whiff test when a drop of vaginal secretion is placed in a 10 % potassium hydroxide mixture, the absence of *Lactobacilli*, an increase in other bacterial forms, many immature vaginal squamous cells, and most significantly an outpouring of inflammatory white cells. These vaginal changes make older women more susceptible to urinary tract and vaginal infections.

Vulvar Changes

There are visually apparent alterations in the vulva of postmenopausal women. The tremendous reduction in the levels of estrogen results in a loss of tissue elasticity and an obvious thinning of the vulvar tissue (Fig. 2). This thinning, apparent to the naked eye, is accompanied by other significant subcutaneous changes. These become more noticeable when the V-600 Syris imaging system is used, which allows the observer to view the tissue two cell layers beneath the surface [7].

Using this system of cross-polarized light visualization, there is decreased vascularity, more dryness, and more subdermal inflammation. On the surface, the vulvar skin becomes retracted with the tissue demarcations between the labia majora and labia minora blunted. These changes are particularly apparent using the magnification of the colposcope. This thinner tissue area is much more fragile and more prone to splitting and cracking, at times leaving the distressed patient with a painful, slow-healing vulvar cut. Some women of this age group who are susceptible will develop a chronic inflammatory skin disease, lichen sclerosis, which predominantly affects the skin and mucous membranes of the vulvar and rectal area. This thinned vulvar skin also loses much of its natural surface defense mechanisms and is more likely to become and stay inflamed.

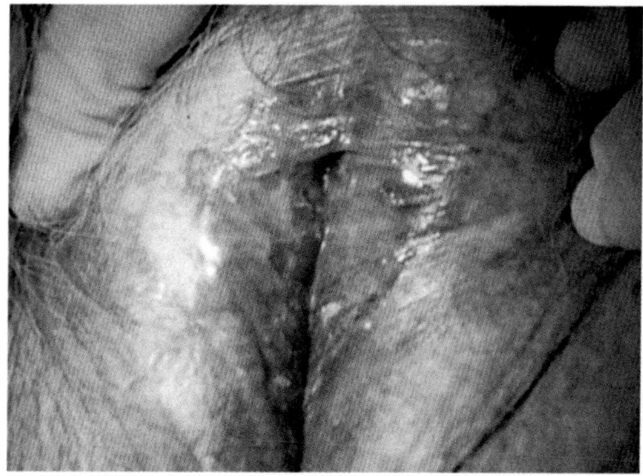

Fig. 2 Superficial tissue changes of postmenopausal woman not on hormone replacement therapy

Postmenopausal women, not taking estrogen, have higher induced levels of the proinflammatory cytokine interleukin-1, interleukin-6, and tumor necrosis factor α when compared to women in their reproductive years [8]. The body's response to this new inflammation is a repair process with new tissue formation. This new tissue regeneration at an inflammatory site is accompanied by vulvar and perineal itching. This initiates a vicious cycle. The itching leads to scratching, often when the patient is asleep and unaware of her response. The scratching increases the tissue inflammation, and the cycle begins anew. This is a constant source of symptomatology leading to patient frustration.

The thinning of the keratin layer of the labia majora and labia minora also diminishes the protection normally afforded against bacterial and fungal adhesion to this tissue site. The epithelial cells of reproductive-age women also produce

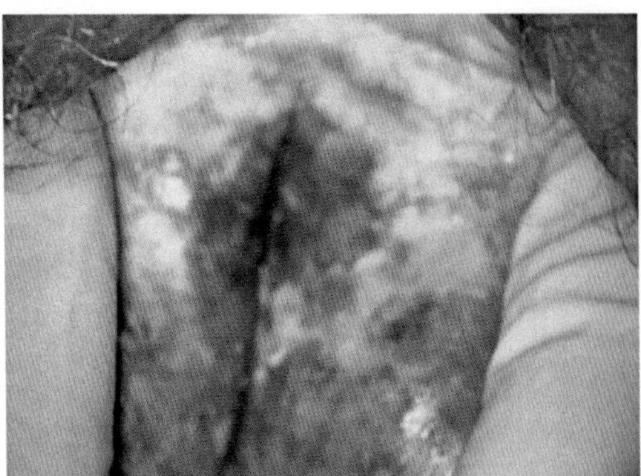

Fig. 3 *Candida albicans* infection of vulva of postmenopausal woman

many substances, such as peptides [9], that can kill potential bacterial or fungal pathogens. Lessened production of these substances in menopausal women increases the chances of infection. The resulting skin infections add to the inflammation. The suspicion of a Candida infection of the vulva can be confirmed by a scraping of the coated white area of the vulva with a portion sent for culture. Another portion added to a drop of 10 % potassium hydroxide solution and examined under the microscope reveals the presence of pseudohyphae.

Vulvar fungal infections occur commonly in this aging population (Fig. 3) and if not eradicated by treatment contribute to the cycle of inflammation, itching, scratching, and more inflammation. Bacterial infection of the vulva can be a life-threatening problem in postmenopausal women, particularly in diabetics in whom synergistic bacterial vulvar infections can occur, with tissue death requiring operative intervention for survival [10]. These women have pain, but suspicion of possible necrotizing fasciitis can be confirmed when pinprick stimulation of this tissue evokes no response. Operative intervention needs to be done as soon as possible.

Outside Influences: Male

The television advertisements of the American pharmaceutical industry are dominated by concerns about both male urinary function and sexual prowess. The theme of male erectile dysfunction captures the attention of the male drug consumer. The models in the ads blend the knowing smiles of the older but still physically rugged and vigorous male with the "come hither" looks of their very attractive female partners. For the viewer, the obvious result will be the nirvana of continued sexual satisfaction.

For the postmenopausal sexual partner of these newly invigorated older males, there can be a tremendous downside for vaginal and vulvar skin health. The resulting increase in heterosexual activity can cause vaginal and/or vulvar lacerations because of the dryness and decreased elasticity of the lower genital tract skin and mucous membranes. This genital tract pain sets in place a cascade of continuing problems. Pain will reduce vaginal secretion and the memory of prior discomfort can result in heightened pelvic floor muscle contraction when insertion is attempted, making a prior unpleasant sexual experience even more uncomfortable. Reflex attempts to modify this response by using commercially available, over-the-counter lubricants can have unintended results. These products contain propylene glycol, a chemical preservative to which some women with inflamed mucous membranes can develop sensitivities. This contact dermatitis increases even more the local inflammation and pain. To avoid this possibility, these couples should be advised to use mineral oil or olive oil as a precoital lubricant. They are unquestionably messy, but do not dry out over time with firm residual kernels of commercial products that can be an additional source of irritation, and they contain no chemicals that could cause a local tissue reaction.

Outside Influences: Hormone Replacement Therapy (HRT)

Since the changes in the health of the vagina and vulva in perimenopausal and menopausal women are related to a lessened production of estrogen, estrogen supplementation would be an aid for these women. This is true. Estrogen therapy is most helpful as a preventive measure. It is usually beneficial if given before the aging vaginal and vulvar tissue changes of thinning, loss of turgor and elasticity have become grossly apparent. It either prevents or markedly slows these genital skin and mucous membrane alterations. In the vagina of women receiving estrogen supplementation, the pH is more acidic than it was before the treatment, and the dominant bacterial flora contains bacteria that produce lactic acid. If the progressive tissue changes of thinning, inflammation, or lacerations occur, estrogen is much less effective. It can accelerate the healing of these cuts and decrease inflammation, but it does not return the tissue to a premenopausal state. These are not formulae for the "fountain of youth," but they do halt further deterioration.

Other pharmaceutical agents, topical adrenocortical steroids, are much better in combating local tissue inflammation and are frequently prescribed as an additional therapy in women with inflammatory vulvar changes. Despite these shortcomings, the lifestyle of women taking supplemental estrogen is usually much improved. They experience less discomfort with intercourse and have fewer lower urinary tract infections. All of these are positive observations. The reader should reflexively wonder why there has not been a deluge of television advertisements for the improvement in female well-being and pleasure with estrogen replacement therapy to parallel the onslaught of ads trumpeting male well-being. This would give equal time to the current focus upon male sexual satisfaction. Instead, there is an absence of these ads and market evidence of a decrease in the current use of hormone replacement therapy (HRT) in American women. Why?

This phenomenon of the current less frequent use of HRT in the United States has been largely driven by the publicity surrounding the results of Women's Health Initiative (WHI) studies. These studies, sponsored by the National Institutes of Health (NIH), have highlighted the potential dangers for women taking systemic HRT. There is a small but increased risk of developing breast cancer in women taking HRT for 5 years or more [1]. This had been previously reported in earlier studies [11]. Other unexpected adverse outcomes were noted in asymptomatic menopausal women taking HRT. They had a greater chance of having either a heart attack or a stroke as compared to the population of women taking a placebo [1]. This was a surprise, for prior studies of HRT had shown beneficial effects, with a lowering of blood lipids [12]. This had been the basis for the medical dogma of the 1980s that HRT had cardiovascular and cerebrovascular benefits for all postmenopausal women. These WHI studies raised doubts about that hypothesis and led to a precipitous drop in the numbers of American women using HRT.

There were some major problems in the WHI postmenopausal women study design that have been too often overlooked. The focus of the WHI study was upon asympotomatic menopausal women. This in itself was appropriate, for if symptomatic women had been studied, there would have been an inordinate loss of women recruited for the study who were given the placebo. Their symptoms would have continued, and they would have been more likely to drop out of the study. Using asymptomatic women avoided this, but to recruit this population, one-third of the women had been menopausal for over 5 years and another third had been menopausal for over 10 years. This fact should raise some concerns about the interpretation of the study. This is not the usual target group for HRT. The focus should be upon women who become symptomatic with perimenopause, with symptoms becoming more pronounced as they become menopausal.

For the skin, the greatest benefits from estrogen treatment result from the prevention or slowing of the skin-aging process and not from the treatment of established aging skin changes. This goal of HRT therapy – prevention, not treatment – was not reached in two-thirds of the WHI study population. An interesting aside is that the minority one-third of these WHI study patients who received HRT within the first 5 years of menopause did not have the increased cardiovascular and cerebrovascular risks noted in the other two-thirds.

There are dangers of the use of systemic HRT for women, particularly an increased risk of breast cancer [13] but these have been overemphasized to include local estrogren products while downplaying the benefits. Many women with vaginal or vulvar symptoms due to skin aging will benefit from a wide variety of local estrogen products, including creams, vaginal tablets, or a vaginal ring, none of which to date have been associated with any of the systemic risks that have been attributed to systemic HRT.

The concerns about HRTs have been widely publicized. All too often, many women will avoid these potentially beneficial local medications for they have been led to believe that the risks associated with systemic HRT apply to all estrogen products. This is unfortunate, because for many women, these agents improve their sense of worth for they help to modify at least some of the pitfalls of aging. Most of the older women using estrogen look and feel better. They are a selected population, for they were symptomatic prior to the use of these hormones. For them, the hormones improve their daily lives and the quality of their social interactions. These benefits for women should be cited as they have been for men. Males, taking drugs for erectile dysfunction, have an increased risk of heart attacks and blindness, both serious medical problems. These have not been the primary focus in discussion as have been the concerns about the risks for HRT for women.

There are medical problems with the lack of estrogen. Lack of estrogen and a resulting higher vaginal pH lowers the numbers of *Lactobacilli* present as well as other good bacteria that produce lactic acid. Nonculture studies of the vaginal flora of normal healthy women have cast doubt on the potential significance of hydrogen peroxide-producing *Lactobacilli,* for its most commonly identified species, *Lactobacillus iners*, does not produce hydrogen peroxide [14]. In addition, a study from Johns Hopkins indicates that cervical vaginal fluid and semen block the microbicidal activity of hydrogen peroxide [15]. In addition, healthy women without *Lactobacilli* present in the vagina have other organisms present that produce lactic acid. This is the protective factor maintaining vaginal health.

The incidence of lower urinary tract infection is much higher in these postmenopausal women, not on HRT [16]. This is not a straightforward cause-and-effect guide to therapy. There is an interplay of factors. Topical vaginal estrogen treatment results in an increase in the numbers of good bacteria, *Lactobacilli,* and others that produce lactic acid. These will subsequently reduce the numbers of gram-negative aerobes with the potential to ascend and cause lower urinary tract infections. All of these effects are good and should reduce the incidence of infection [5]. However, this local estrogen improves vaginal health and lubrication function, making intercourse a more frequent event. Intercourse is a separate factor that can increase the incidence of urinary tract infection [17]. It does in younger women and the same factors apply in older women, with a more youthful vagina related to local estrogen therapy.

Vulvar discomfort is a common symptom in this population. It can present in many forms. The lack of estrogen results in thinning of the vulvar skin and a loss of tissue elasticity. There is decreased vascularity and this dryer epithelium is more prone to tears and is less likely to resist inflammation. This tissue inflammation is manifested by local discomfort and itching.

Vulvar itching: a common and hated symptom. The itching is constant and it occurs in an area where reflexive scratching is not acceptable social behavior. The symptoms parallel the itching that occurs after a torso sunburn when a superficial layer of skin peels and increased new epithelial tissue is formed. New tissue formation is part and parcel of the body's response to vulvar inflammation. Unfortunately, too often this symptom of vulvar itching is interpreted as a Candida infection and subsequent antifungal treatment does not provide relief. Local estrogen will increase the health and thickness of the vulvar epithelium while a local steroid will diminish the inflammation. This estrogen deprived vulvar region is more susceptible to local infection, occasionally bacterial or viral but more commonly Candida in origin. The diagnosis requires a physical examination, scraping the surface of the lesion to obtain a specimen for microscopic study, plus appropriate culture studies. In addition to itching, these women can have pain, the result of fissures, often large, related to the loss of elasticity of the vulvar tissues. These fissures usually require more than local estrogen for a cure. That is an important first step, but local steroids to lessen inflammation are also usually required.

Multiple vaginal problems are seen that are related to estrogen lack. At the entrance of the vagina, the uretheral orifice often assumes a distinctive worrisome look, with a prominent outpouching of the bright red columnar epithelium of the uretheral canal. Usually, this startling altered appearance is not accompanied by symptomatology, but occasionally, patients have some associated voiding discomfort or point tenderness to touch. In symptomatic patients, local or systemic, estrogen therapy usually returns this uretheral site to a more normal appearance as supporting structures are enhanced and relieve the symptomatology. If this is not effective, surgical excision of the protruding tissue can be considered and it does provide tissue for microscopic examination. Uretheral cancers are very rare, but if present, are not visually distinguishable from uretheral caruncles.

Treatment of a postmenopausal woman with vaginal symptoms can be very helpful for these patients. With limited levels of estrogen available to these patients before treatment, there are a multiplicity of changes in the vagina. Some are visible. Vaginal color becomes much paler, vaginal rugae are much less prominent, the cervix becomes less prominent and is flush with the vagina. These women find uncomfortable any pelvic examination, even with the smallest speculum, and they avoid intercourse. Other, nonvisible changes are also prominent. The vaginal pH is more alkaline and *Lactobacilli* are reduced in numbers, often absent, replaced by other organisms, particularly gram-negative aerobes, which have the potential to become pathogens for the urinary tract. Vaginal and vulvar pallor is related to the decrease in blood flow to the lower genital region. This can be increased by an elevation in the amount of estrogen delivered to that tissue.

Fortunately, there are a variety of therapeutic approaches. Each has its advantages and disadvantages, and the treatment choice should be tailored to the specific needs of the individual patient.

Systemic estrogen therapy by either the oral route or a skin patch can be very effective. There can be problems. If the patient still has her uterus, periodic or continuous progestational therapy needs to be instituted to present endometrial hyperplasia from unopposed estrogen, but these progestational agents are sometimes poorly tolerated and bleeding often results, usually not a welcome symptom in these postmenopausal women. In addition, there is a justified concern that HRT increases the risk of breast cancer.

The other alternative is local estrogen, in which the low levels of absorbed estrogens do not lead to endometrial hyperstimulation. For the woman whose problem is a dry vagina, the periodic use of a vaginal estrogen cream is often very helpful. There are drawbacks. Many women detest the messiness of the cream and some women develop a contact dermatitis to the chemical preservative, propylene glycol, an ingredient of this cream. They have severe vaginal burning and if this occurs, it should end that therapeutic approach. There are vaginal estradiol tablets that can be given periodically and are helpful. If few vaginal secretions are present, these vaginal tablets dissolve incompletely, which is unacceptable. There are plastic vaginal rings available that release low levels of estrogen continuously. They need replacing every three months and while insertions are usually easy, removal may require a visit to the doctor.

For women in whom estrogen is anathema, because of a history of estrogen-dependent breast cancer, there are helpful alternatives. There are jellies that will provide an acidic vaginal pH. Alternatively, there are moisturizing agents that are helpful. Finally, in younger women with breast cancer who are estrogen-depressed, intercourse can be eased with the use of local lubricants such as olive oil. They have the advantage over commercial products for they contain no chemical preservatives.

Conclusion

There is a gender gap here. For women, downplay benefits and stress the risks; for men, emphasize pleasure and gloss over the risks. This is a curious commentary upon the current American scene.

Cross-References

► Biological Effects of Estrogen on Skin
► Perimenopausal Aging and Oral Hormone Replacement Therapy

References

1. Rossouw TE, Anderson GL, Prentice RL, et al. Risks and benefits of estrogen plus progestin in healthy post-menopausal women: principal results from the Women's Health Initiative randomize controlled trial. JAMA. 2002;288:321–33.
2. American Society for Reproductive Medicine. Age and fertility: a guide for patients (patient information series). Birmingham: American Society for Reproductive Medicine; 2003.
3. Hillier SL, Lau RJ. Vaginal microflora in post-menopausal women who have not received estrogen replacement therapy. Clin Infect Dis. 1997;25 Suppl 2: S123–6.
4. Pabich WL, Fihn SD, Stamm WE, et al. Prevalence and determinants of vaginal flora alternations in post-menopausal women. J Infect Dis. 2003;188:1054–8.
5. Raz R, Stamm WE. A controlled trial of intravaginal estriol in post-menopausal women with recurrent urinary tract infection. N Engl J Med. 1993;329:753–6.
6. Sobel JD. Desquamative inflammatory vaginitis: a new subgroup of purulent vaginitis responsive to topical 2% clindamycin therapy. Am J Obstet Gynecol. 1994;171:1215–20.
7. Farage M, Singh M, Ledger WJ. Investigation of the sensitivity of a cross-polarized light visualization system to detect subclinical erythema and dryness in women with vulvovagintis. Am J Obstet Gynecol. 2009;201:1e1–6.
8. Pfeilschifter J, Kodtiz R, Pfohl M, et al. Changes in proinflammatory cytokine activity after menopause. Endocr Rev. 2002;23:90–119.
9. Hancock REW. Lationic peptides: effectors in innate immunity and novel antimocrobials. Lancet Infect Dis. 2001;1:156–64.
10. Addison WA, Livengood III CH, Hill GB, et al. Necrotizing fasciitis of vulvar origin in diabetes patients. Obstet Gynecol. 1984;63:473–9.
11. Hulley S, Grady B, Bush T, et al. Randomized trial of estrogen plus progestin for secondary prevention of coronary heart disease in post-menopausal women. JAMA. 1998;280:605–13.
12. Rossouw JE, Prentice RL, Manson JE, et al. Postmenopausal hormone therapy and risk of cardiovascular disease by age and years since menopause. JAMA. 2007;297:1465–77.
13. Chlebowski RT, Kuller LH, Prentice RL, et al. Breast cancer after use of estrogen plus progestin in post-menopausal women. N Engl J Med. 2009;360:573–82.
14. Zhou X, Bent SJ, Schneider MG, et al. Characterization of vaginal microbial communities in adult healthy women using cultivation-independent methods. Micro. 2004;150:2565–73.
15. O'Hanlon DE, Lanier BR, Moench TR, et al. Cervicovaginal fluid and semen block the microbicidal activity of hydrogen peroxide produced by vaginal Lactobacilli. BMC Infect Dis. 2010;10:120.
16. Stamm WE, Raz R. Factors contributing to susceptibility of post-menopausal women to recurrent urinary tract infections. Clin Infect Dis. 1999;28:723–5.
17. Hooton TM, Schoks D, Hughes HP, et al. A prospective study of risk factors for symptomatic uninary tract infections in young women. N Engl J Med. 1996;335:468–74.

Platinum and Palladium Nanoparticles Regulate the Redox Balance and Protect Against Age-Related Skin Changes in Mice

37

Shuichi Shibuya, Kenji Watanabe, Koutaro Yokote, and Takahiko Shimizu

Contents

S. Shibuya • K. Watanabe • T. Shimizu (✉)
Department of Advanced Aging Medicine, Chiba University Graduate School of Medicine, Chiba, Japan
e-mail: shimizut@chiba-u.jp

K. Yokote
Department of Clinical Cell Biology and Medicine, Chiba University Graduate School of Medicine, Chiba, Japan

Abstract

Skin aging is defined by two skin phenotypes: photoaging-induced hypertrophy and intrinsic aging-associated atrophy. Accumulating evidence suggests that impaired reactive oxygen species metabolism induces oxidative damage and causes age-related changes in the skin. To prevent the morphological changes from oxidative injuries, cells possess multiple antioxidative components, such as superoxide dismutase (SOD), catalase, and glutathione peroxidase. Noble metal nanoparticles, such as platinum (Pt) and palladium (Pd) nanoparticles, are considered to function as antioxidants due to their strong catalytic activity. Pt nanoparticles show apparent SOD and catalase activity, while Pd nanoparticles exhibit weak activity. Interestingly, Pd nanoparticles prevent the oxidative deterioration of Pt nanoparticles, which helps to extend the SOD/catalase activity. A transdermal treatment with a mixture of Pt and Pd nanoparticles, called PAPLAL, completely reversed skin thinning associated with the normalization of lipid peroxidation in $Sod1^{-/-}$ mice, which exhibited aging-like skin atrophy accompanied by the imbalance of extracellular matrix homeostasis. Furthermore, PAPLAL normalized the expression of extracellular matrix-related genes in the skin of $Sod1^{-/-}$ mice. Other materials, such as vitamin C derivative, collagen peptides, and resveratrol, also attenuate age-related skin pathologies via the

M.A. Farage et al. (eds.), *Textbook of Aging Skin*,
DOI 10.1007/978-3-662-47398-6_120

normalization of reactive oxygen species metabolism in the skin. These findings suggest that redox regulation in the skin is a beneficial strategy for the treatment of aging-related skin diseases caused by oxidative damage.

Introduction

The skin is the largest and outermost organ of the body, and it functions as a protective barrier against external damage. The skin is constantly exposed to external stress and the progression of aging. Skin aging manifests as two main symptoms: photoaging induced by environmental stress, such as sunlight, which leads to skin hypertrophy and intrinsic aging induced by chronologic or intrinsic factors, which leads to skin atrophy [1]. The amount of skin collagen components decrease in an age-dependent manner in both males and females, resulting in age-related skin thinning in older individuals [2, 3]. Evidence suggests that oxidatively modified proteins, DNA and lipids in the skin and other organs are progressively accumulated during aging [4]. To prevent structural changes caused by oxidative damage, cells possess multiple antioxidative components, such as vitamins C (VC) and E as well as glutathione, and enzymes such as superoxide dismutase (SOD), catalase, and glutathione peroxidase. SODs play a central role in superoxide ($O_2^{\cdot -}$) metabolism in vivo due to their ability to catalyze the dismutation of cellular $O_2^{\cdot -}$ to O_2 and hydrogen peroxide (H_2O_2). In mammals, there are three SOD isoforms: CuZn-SOD (SOD1), which exists in the cytoplasm; Mn-SOD (SOD2), which exists in the mitochondrial matrix; and extracellular SOD (SOD3), which is localized in the extracellular fluids such as lymph, synovial fluids, and plasma [5, 6]. *Sod1*-deficient (*Sod1*$^{-/-}$) mice exhibit increased intracellular $O_2^{\cdot -}$ levels and various aging-associated organ phenotypes [7]. The aged *Sod1*$^{-/-}$ mice showed a higher degree of kyphosis and decreased bone mass compared with those of age-matched *Sod1*$^{+/+}$ mice [7]. We also reported that a mouse model for Alzheimer's disease lacking *Sod1* showed exacerbation of memory loss and behavioral abnormalities associated with accelerated plaque formation and amyloid accumulation [8, 9]. Additionally, age-related macular degeneration [10], fatty deposits in the liver [11, 12], dry eye [13, 14], infertility in females [15], and rotator cuff degeneration [16] spontaneously occur in *Sod1*$^{-/-}$ mice. Notably, *Sod1* insufficiency resulted in both epidermal and dermal atrophies, which are associated with the downregulation of the extracellular matrix-related genes, including type I collagen (*Col1a1*) and hyaluronan synthase 2 (*Has2*) [17–19]. Therefore, *Sod1*$^{-/-}$ mice represent a suitable model for studying skin aging in elderly people.

Noble metal nanoparticles, including platinum (Pt), palladium (Pd), and gold (Au) nanoparticles, have strong catalytic activities, such as hydrogenation, hydration, and oxidation, due to their large surface area and the high proportion of metal atoms located on their surface [20–22]. Because of the catalytic activity of such noble metal nanoparticles, they are considered to function as antioxidants and are potentially useful in material science and clinical therapy. In this review, we describe the strong antioxidant activities of Pt and Pd nanoparticles and how they protect against age-related skin changes in mice, which may have implications in delaying skin aging in humans.

Platinum Nanoparticles Show Strong SOD and Catalase Activities

A number of studies have reported that Pt nanoparticles exhibit a strong ability to scavenge reactive oxygen species (ROS) [23–25]. We biochemically assessed the SOD and catalase activities of Pt nanoparticles (Fig. 1a). Platinum nanoparticles possess strong SOD activity (2,142.3 ± 423.1 U) and also exhibit robust catalase activity (68.7 ± 15.5 U) (Fig. 1b, c). We then assessed the antioxidant effects of Pt nanoparticles on *Sod1*$^{-/-}$ fibroblasts, which enhance intracellular $O_2^{\cdot -}$ generation in the cytoplasm [26, 27]. Platinum nanoparticles effectively decreased $O_2^{\cdot -}$ generation by 23.3 % in the mutant fibroblasts [19], suggesting beneficial

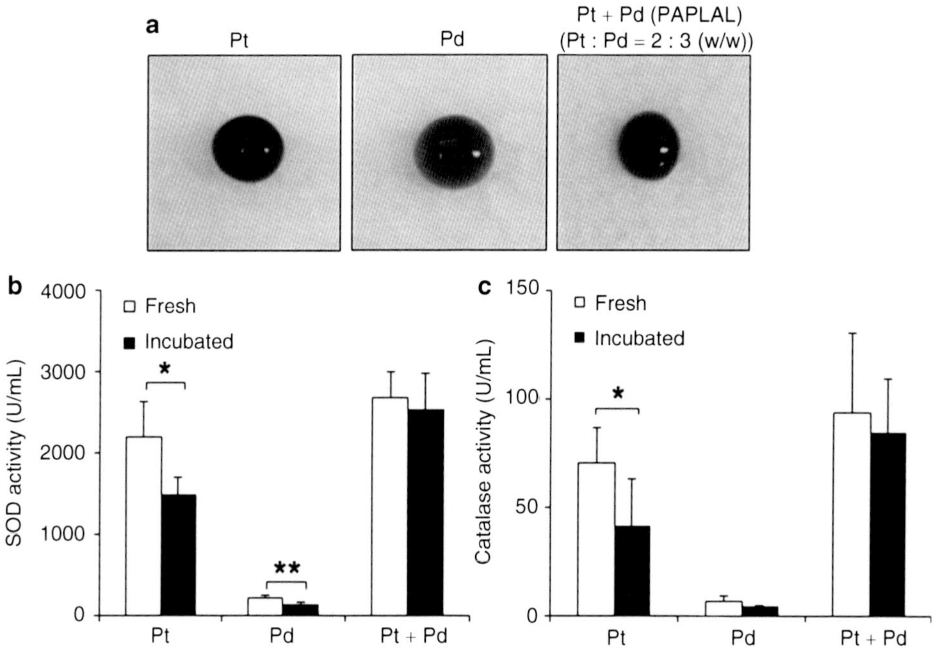

Fig. 1 (**a**) A solution of Pt nanoparticles (1.03 mM Pt), Pd nanoparticles (2.82 mM Pd), and a Pt and Pd nanoparticle mixture called PAPLAL (1.03 mM Pt and 2.82 mM Pd). The SOD (**b**) and catalase (**c**) activities of Pt nanoparticles, Pd nanoparticles, and PAPLAL. An open column represents a fresh preparation, while a solid column represents an air incubation for 24 h, indicating oxidized preparation. Data are presented as the mean ± SD: $^{*}p < 0.05$

effects for oxidative damage-induced organ changes *in vivo*. In a lifespan analysis of *Caenorhabditis elegans*, Kim et al. reported that Pt nanoparticles extended the lifespan of wild-type N2 and short-lived *mev-1* nematodes, in which intracellular ROS accumulated due to respiratory impairment [28]. Takamiya et al. also reported that Pt nanoparticles attenuate brain disorders induced by the transient middle cerebral artery occlusion by reducing the intracellular $O_2^{\cdot -}$ generation in mice [29].

Notably, when Pt nanoparticles were exposed to air for 24 h, the SOD and catalase activities were significantly decreased (Fig. 1b, c). Okamoto et al. reported that Pt nanoparticles were oxidized to PtO by oxygen in the air, which resulted in a time-dependent increase in their ability to degrade vitamin C (VC) [30]. Because Larese Filon et al. reported that oxidation induces nanoparticle aggregation [31], oxidation-induced aggregation of Pt nanoparticles might reduce the antioxidant activity because of a reduction in the superficial area.

Palladium Nanoparticles Prevent the Oxidative Deterioration of Pt Nanoparticles

Palladium has been mainly used in industry due to its strong catalytic activity. Many studies have demonstrated that the Pd complex has diverse biological activities such as antitumor, antimicrobial, anti-inflammatory, and antiviral activities [32, 33]. Li et al. reported that the Pd-mediated deprotection reaction activated a protein within living cells due to biocompatible and efficient catalysts of Pd that cleave the propargyl carbamate group of a protected lysine analog to generate a free lysine [34]. There are few reports describing the antioxidant activity of Pd nanoparticles, which is something we have investigated (Fig. 1a). Compared to the Pt nanoparticles, the Pd nanoparticles displayed weak SOD activity (77.8 ± 11.7 U) (Fig. 1b). Notably, the Pd nanoparticles also displayed low catalase activity (6.7 ± 2.7 U) (Fig. 1c).

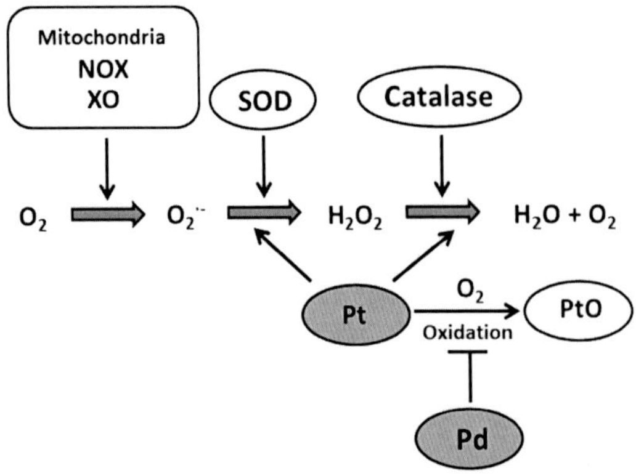

Fig. 2 A schematic diagram of the antioxidative effects of the Pt and Pd nanoparticles. H_2O_2 hydrogen peroxide, NOX nicotinamide adenine dinucleotide phosphate oxidase, $O_2^{\cdot -}$ superoxide, PtO oxidized platinum, SOD superoxide dismutase, XO xanthine oxidase

Treatment with Pd nanoparticles failed to reduce intracellular $O_2^{\cdot -}$ generation in *Sod1*$^{-/-}$ fibroblasts [19], further demonstrating the low antioxidant activity of Pd. These results suggest that Pd nanoparticles cannot catalyze $O_2^{\cdot -}$ directly.

Okamoto et al. also reported that Pd had a lower oxidation and reduction potential than Pt, and that Pd reduced Pt^{2+} to Pt in solution [30]. In contrast with Pt alone, a mixture of Pt and Pd nanoparticles exposed to air retained its SOD and catalase activities, indicating that the oxidative deterioration of the Pt nanoparticles was inhibited (Fig. 1b, c). Importantly, the mixture of Pd and Pt nanoparticles with a molar ratio of 3 or 4 to 1 continued to exhibit SOD and catalase activities after oxidation [19], indicating that Pd nanoparticles prevent the oxidative deterioration of Pt nanoparticles (Fig. 2). Indeed, Pt nanoparticles, but not Pt/Pd mixtures, that had been oxidized in air failed to suppress intracellular $O_2^{\cdot -}$ generation in *Sod1*$^{-/-}$ mice [19]. Recently, Elhusseiny and Hassan reported that a complex of Pt and Pd nanoparticles demonstrated highly potent antimicrobial and antitumor activities [35]. Because long-term storage accelerates the oxidative deterioration of Pt nanoparticles and other antioxidants under normal conditions, the addition of Pd nanoparticles to such antioxidants might efficiently maintain their bioactivity under oxidative conditions.

Sod1 Loss Exhibits Age-Related Skin Pathologies in Mice

Over the course of 10 years, we have investigated pathophysiological phenotypes in *Sod1*$^{-/-}$ mice. *Sod1*$^{-/-}$ mice showed age-related changes in various organs, including the skin [17–19, 26, 27]. In the skin, *Sod1*$^{-/-}$ loss showed a typical aging-like skin atrophy (Fig. 3a). When we prepared histological sections of the skin on the backs of mice, significant atrophic changes were observed in the epidermis and dermis of *Sod1*$^{-/-}$ mice (Fig. 3b, c). Furthermore, the mRNA level of *Col1a1* in *Sod1*$^{-/-}$ was significantly reduced, while that of matrix metalloproteinase 2 (*Mmp2*) was significantly increased, compared with those of *Sod1*$^{+/+}$ mice (Fig. 3d). This indicated that collagen biosynthesis was impaired in the *Sod1*$^{-/-}$ mice. Moreover, the mRNA expression of *Has2* was significantly downregulated in the skin of the *Sod1*$^{-/-}$ mice. In contrast, the mRNA expression level of *Decorin* and *Ki67* did not differ between the *Sod1*$^{+/+}$ and *Sod1*$^{-/-}$ mice (Fig. 3d). These results suggested that *Sod1* deficiency causes skin thinning due to deregulation of the extracellular matrix, including collagen and hyaluronic acid. The *Sod1*$^{-/-}$ skin also exhibited significantly higher expression levels of inflammatory cytokines, including *Tnf-α* and *Il-6* (Fig. 3d). These results suggest a pathological link between inflammation and skin thinning in *Sod1*$^{-/-}$ skin. TNF-α regulates type I collagen expression via the c-Jun N-terminal kinase and nuclear factor kappa-light-chain-enhancer of activated B cells (NF-κB) pathways in skin fibroblasts [36]. Additionally, Galera et al. reported that NF-κB directly suppresses *COL1A1* gene transcription in the human dermal fibroblasts [37] and accumulates in the nuclei of aged human fibroblasts in association with the downregulation of the *COL1A1* gene [38]. An IκB kinase-β inhibitor has also been shown to suppress interleukin-1β-induced collagen

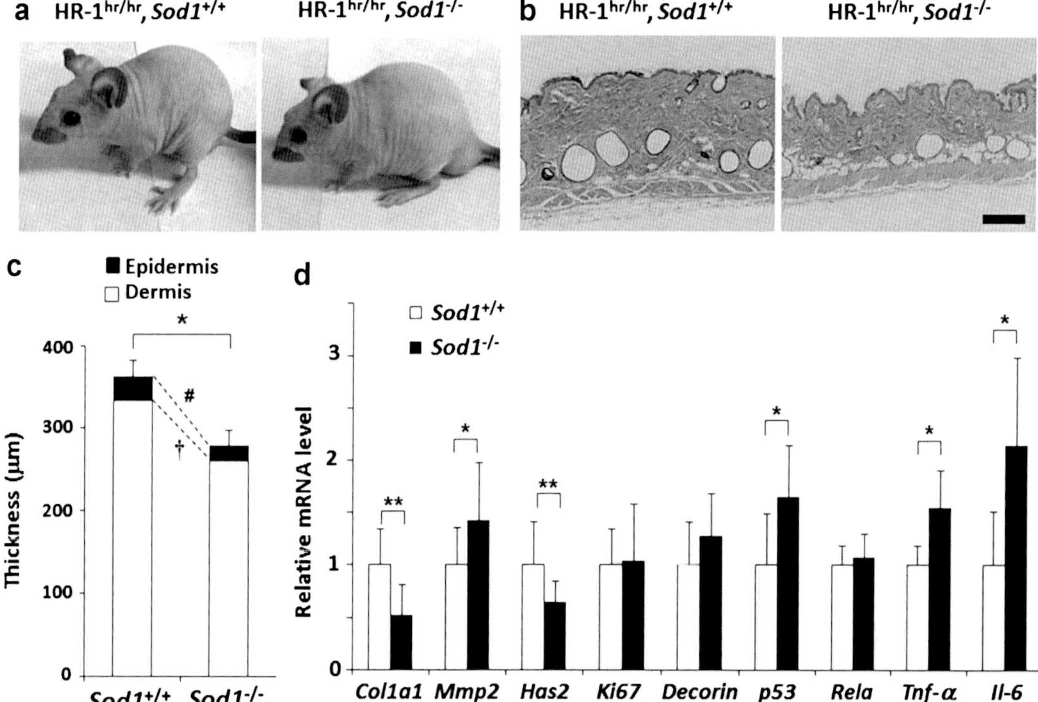

Fig. 3 (**a**) A hairless, *Sod1*$^{+/+}$ mouse (HR-1$^{hr/hr}$, *Sod1*$^{+/+}$, *left*) and a hairless, *Sod1*$^{-/-}$ mouse (HR-1$^{hr/hr}$, *Sod1*$^{-/-}$, *right*). (**b**) Hematoxylin and eosin staining of the skin on the backs of HR-1$^{hr/hr}$, *Sod1*$^{+/+}$ (*left*) and HR-1$^{hr/hr}$, *Sod1*$^{-/-}$ mice (*right*). The scale bar represents 200 μm. (**c**) The thickness of the epidermal (*black*) and dermal layers (*white*) of the skin on the backs of HR-1$^{hr/hr}$, *Sod1*$^{+/+}$ and HR-1$^{hr/hr}$, *Sod1*$^{-/-}$ mice. Data are presented as the mean ± SD: $^*p < 0.05$ in the total skin layer, $^{\#}p < 0.05$ in the epidermis, and $^{\dagger}p < 0.05$ in the dermis. (**d**) The relative mRNA expression levels of *Col1a1*, *Mmp2*, *Has2*, *Ki67*, *Decorin*, *p53*, *Rela*, *Tnf-α*, and *Il-6*. Each mRNA expression level was determined using quantitative RT-PCR. Data are presented as the mean ± SD: $^*p < 0.05$, $^{**}p < 0.01$

degradation by inhibiting the activation of NF-κB and upregulation of matrix metalloproteinases [39]. Taken together, the inflammatory response controls the collagen homeostasis via transcriptional mechanisms in fibroblasts. Furthermore, the expression of the tumor suppressor *p53* gene, which is known to be associated with DNA damage [40] and skin aging [41], was significantly upregulated in the *Sod1*$^{-/-}$ mice (Fig. 3d). When the *Sod1*$^{-/-}$ dermal fibroblasts were cultured under 20% O_2 conditions, they showed significantly increased intracellular $O_2^{\cdot -}$ generation with decreased viability and increased apoptotic cell death [26]. Collectively, a redox imbalance in the skin caused by SOD1 depletion leads to skin inflammation and an impaired repair process.

A Mixture of Pt and Pd Nanoparticles, Called PAPLAL, Improves Skin Atrophy in the *Sod1*-Deficient Mice

Interestingly, PAPLAL, which is a mixture of Pt and Pd nanoparticles, has been used to treat patients with burns, frostbite, hives, lung inflammation, gastric ulcers, and rheumatoid arthritis in Japan over the past 60 years. Additionally, PAPLAL has been shown to have various beneficial effects on chronic disease [42] and was approved as a treatment for acute gastric inflammation and chronic gastric catarrh in Japan under the Pharmaceutical Affairs Law and patented as an antioxidant with the Japan Patent Office (Patent No. 341195, 2003). *In vitro* studies have

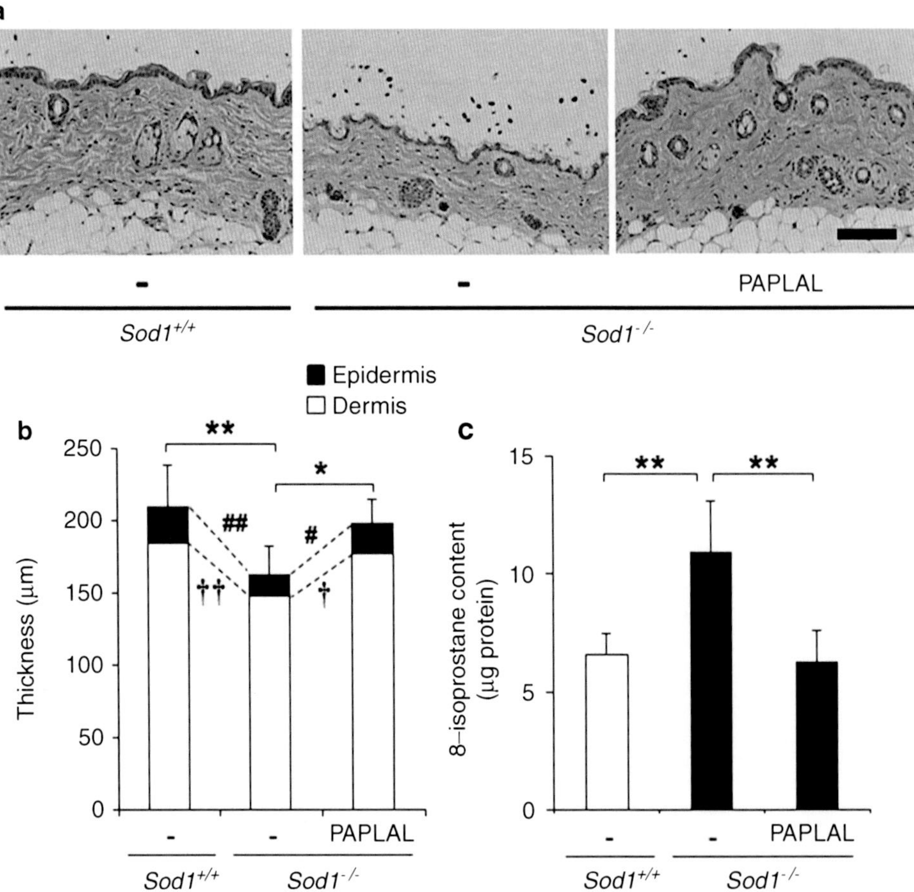

Fig. 4 (**a**) Hematoxylin and eosin staining of the skin on the backs of HR-1$^{hr/hr}$, *Sod1*$^{+/+}$ and HR-1$^{hr/hr}$, *Sod1*$^{-/-}$ mice treated with PAPLAL. The scale bar represents 100 μm. (**b**) The thickness of the epidermal and dermal layers of the skin on the backs of HR-1$^{hr/hr}$, *Sod1*$^{+/+}$ and HR-1$^{hr/hr}$, *Sod1*$^{-/-}$ mice treated with PAPLAL. Data are presented as the mean ± SD: $*p < 0.05$ in the total skin layer, $**p < 0.01$ in the total skin layer, $^{\#}p < 0.05$ in the epidermis, $^{\#\#}p < 0.01$ in the epidermis, $^{\dagger}p < 0.05$ in the dermis, and $^{\dagger\dagger}p < 0.01$ in the dermis. (**c**) 8-Isoprostane content of the skin on the backs of HR-1$^{hr/hr}$, *Sod1*$^{+/+}$ and HR-1$^{hr/hr}$, *Sod1*$^{-/-}$ mice treated with PAPLAL. Data are presented as the mean ± SD: $**p < 0.01$

reported that PAPLAL exhibits antioxidant activity against $O_2^{\cdot-}$ anions and hydroxyl radicals [19, 43, 44].

In an *in vitro* experiment, PAPLAL was transdermally administered to the skin on the backs of 4-month-old *Sod1*$^{-/-}$ and wild-type mice daily for 4 weeks. The skin on the backs of the *Sod1*$^{-/-}$ mice that were treated with PAPLAL was significantly thicker than that of the *Sod1*$^{-/-}$ mice treated with the control (Fig. 4a, b). To examine the degree of oxidative damage in the skin of the *Sod1*$^{-/-}$ mice, we measured the concentration of 8-isoprostane as a representative of lipid peroxidation products. The 8-isoprostane content, which was an oxidative stress marker, of the *Sod1*$^{-/-}$ skin was 65.4 % higher than that of the *Sod1*$^{+/+}$ mice, which indicated the accumulation of lipid peroxidation products (Fig. 4c). Meanwhile, treatment with PAPLAL significantly decreased the 8-isoprostane content of the *Sod1*$^{-/-}$ mice skin compared with that of the *Sod1*$^{-/-}$ mice skin treated with the control (Fig. 4c). Notably, PAPLAL does not produce adverse effects during its clinical use as a treatment for chronic diseases in human [42]. Indeed, no significant differences in skin thickness were observed among the *Sod1*$^{+/+}$ mice treated with or without PAPLAL [19]. Additionally, no abnormalities, such as cell infiltration or PAPLAL deposition, were detected in the skin of the *Sod1*$^{+/+}$ mice [19], suggesting that PAPLAL does not have any adverse effects on the skin, at least in the short term. Nojiri et al. reported that the administration of VC significantly attenuated bone loss and fragility in *Sod1*$^{-/-}$ mice [45]. Likewise, the transdermal administration of VC derivatives was demonstrated to normalize the skin thinning in *Sod1*$^{-/-}$ mice [17, 26, 27]. Furthermore, Iuchi et al. reported that oral *N*-acetylcysteine treatment mitigates hemolytic anemia in *Sod1*$^{-/-}$ mice by suppressing ROS generation in red blood cells [46]. These results suggest that antioxidants, including PAPLAL, can improve *Sod1* loss-induced organ pathologies.

To investigate the mechanism by which PAPLAL treatment counters skin atrophy in *Sod1*$^{-/-}$ mice, we analyzed the expression patterns of extracellular matrix-related genes in the skin. Treatment with PAPLAL significantly normalized the mRNA levels of *Col1a1*, *Mmp2*, and *Has2* (data not shown), suggesting that PAPLAL treatment increases skin thickness by increasing the concentration of extracellular components, such as collagen and hyaluronic acid. This treatment also significantly downregulated the mRNA expression levels of *Tnf-α* and *Il-6* in the skin of the *Sod1*$^{-/-}$ mice (data not shown). Onizawa et al. reported that the intranasal administration of Pt nanoparticles reduced NF-κB activity and inhibited pulmonary inflammation in mice exposed to cigarette smoke [47]. Rehman et al. also reported that Pt nanoparticles have anti-inflammatory effects on the lipopolysaccharide-induced inflammatory response by downregulating the expression of *IL-1β*, *TNF-α* and *IL-6* in macrophages [48]. Collectively, these findings suggest that PAPLAL and Pt nanoparticles suppress the inflammatory response, resulting in improvements in the anabolic and catabolic regulation of collagen homeostasis. Furthermore, PAPLAL treatment significantly normalized the mRNA expression level of *p53* in *Sod1*$^{-/-}$ mice (data not shown), suggesting that PAPLAL delays skin aging by inhibiting *p53* upregulation in *Sod1*$^{-/-}$ mice.

Nanoparticle Absorption in the Skin

The skin acts as the first barrier to xenobiotics. Permeation of noble metal nanoparticles into the skin is associated with size, shape, charge, and surface properties [31]. Watkinson et al. reported that nanoparticles about 1 nm in diameter can efficiently permeate the intact skin [49]. However, many reports demonstrated that even larger nanoparticles (more than 100 nm in diameter) can cross the skin barrier, albeit with lower efficiency than smaller nanoparticles [50, 51]. In a recent study involving electron microscopy, Okamoto et al. reported that the Pt and Pd nanoparticles in PAPLAL were 1.93 ± 0.34 nm and 3.59 ± 0.56 nm, respectively, in diameter [30]. The grain size of these particles was the same as that of hemoglobin molecules (5.2 nm) [52]. The grain size of Pt and Pd nanoparticles in PAPLAL is smaller than that of metal nanoparticles used in other studies (Au: 5–198 nm, Ag: 9.8–70 nm) [31], suggesting Pt and Pd could more efficiently enter the skin. A previous study has revealed that cells treated with Pt nanoparticles exhibited increased cellular Pt concentrations compared with control cells [25]. In an inductively coupled plasma mass spectrometry-based study of *Caenorhabditis elegans*, Sakaue et al. reported that treatment with Pt nanoparticles increased the internalization of Pt in nematodes [53]. Taken together with our data, PAPLAL and/or Pt nanoparticles might be able to enter skin cells transdermally.

Interestingly, Larese Filon et al. reported that metal nanoparticles were incorporated more in damaged skin than in intact skin [31]. Furthermore, quantum dots can permeate the skin when the skin was damaged by H_2O_2 or UVB [31]. In an *in vitro* study, Arora et al. also reported that UVB exposure enhanced the cellular internalization of Ag nanoparticles in human keratinocytes [54]. These results suggest that a damaged skin barrier allows the penetration and permeation of nanoparticles. However, it is unclear how UVB radiation promotes the uptake of nanoparticles in damaged skin and cells. It is possible that exposure to external stimuli such as UVB and ROS might induce pore formation in the cell membranes [54]. We previously investigated the ability of PAPLAL to promote wound healing in aged murine skin (17 months of age). Although the areas of the wounds treated with or without PAPLAL did not differ at 2 days after wounding, the wounds treated with PAPLAL were significantly smaller than those treated with the control at 4 and 6 days after wounding [19]. These results suggest that aged skin with accumulated damage, such as ROS and UVB injuries, increases permeation of nanoparticles into the skin, resulting in more protective effects against age-related skin changes. A further analysis is necessary to clarify the underlying mechanism regulating the entry of Pt and Pd nanoparticles into the skin.

Protective Effects of Various Agents Against Aging-Like Skin Atrophy

Because VC exhibits low stability and liposolubility, it does not easily absorb into the skin. L-Ascorbyl 2-phosphate 6-palmitate trisodium salt (APPS), a VC derivative, is more stable than VC and exhibits permeability through cell membranes because of its conjugated long hydrophobic chain (Fig. 5). When APPS was transdermally administered to the skin of *Sod1*$^{-/-}$ mice daily, the thinning of the skin was completely reversed likely due to an increase in collagen and elastin contents [17, 26, 27]. In an in vitro study, pretreatment with APPS effectively suppressed $O_2^{\cdot -}$ generation and increased the number of *Sod1*$^{-/-}$ fibroblasts. Meanwhile, L-ascorbyl 2-phosphate trisodium salt failed to attenuate the skin pathologies of the *Sod1*$^{-/-}$ mice, suggesting that the permeability of VC derivatives is an essential factor for transdermal treatment [26]. These reports suggest that VC derivatives, including APPS, are likely to be more efficient in terms of their pharmacological activities, due to their higher stability and permeability. Recently, Massip et al. implied that VC supplementation delayed premature aging caused by mutations in WRN, a RecQ-like DNA helicase in mice [55]. These data suggest that VC therapy can be applied to treat age-related and premature aging disorders. We reported that a co-treatment with APPS and collagen peptides significantly increased the epidermal and dermal skin thickness in the *Sod1*$^{-/-}$ mice compared to a treatment with APPS alone [18]. This report suggests that the use of combination therapy, such as that involving antioxidants and an active substance, provides a novel strategy for treating age-related tissue damage.

Melinjo (Indonesian name; *Gnetum gnemon* Linn) is an arboreal dioecious plant that is widely cultivated in Southeast Asia. Its fruits and seeds are used as food products in Indonesia. Melinjo seeds contain various stilbenoids including

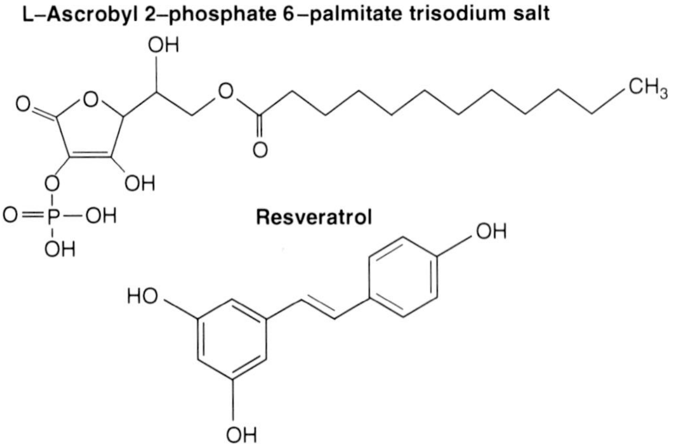

Fig. 5 The structures of L-ascorbyl 2-phosphate 6-palmitate trisodium salt and resveratrol

trans-resveratrol (3,5,4′-trihydroxy-trans-stilbene, RSV) (Fig. 5), its glucoside, resveratrol dimer (gnetin C), and resveratrol dimer glucoside (gnetin L, gnemonoside A, gnemonoside C, and gnemonoside D) [56]. Trans-resveratrol has been identified as a *Sirt1* activator that can protect various organs against aging [57, 58]. *Sirt1* is a key modulator of cellular pathways involved in inherited dermatologic diseases and skin cancers [59], suggesting that *Sirt1* activation is a molecular target for dermatological therapy. The skin on the backs of $Sod1^{-/-}$ mice that had been provided with a melinjo seed extract (MSE) and RSV diet was significantly thicker with higher collagen contents compared with that of $Sod1^{-/-}$ mice provided with the control diet [60]. Consistent with a histological analysis, MSE and RSV treatment significantly normalized mRNA levels of *Col1a1* in $Sod1^{-/-}$ skin. Interestingly, we revealed that MSE and RSV treatment also significantly upregulated *Sirt1* expression, suggesting the molecular link between *Sirt1* expression and skin thinning in $Sod1^{-/-}$ mice. Administration of MSE and RSV to $Sod1^{-/-}$ mice also reduced the 8-isoprostane content in plasma and the intracellular ROS level in bone marrow cells. These data indicated that MSE and RSV defused oxidative damage in $Sod1^{-/-}$ mice. The melinjo seed extract is useful as a nutrient source of RSV and as a safe antioxidant for delaying skin aging in humans.

Conclusion

PAPLAL, which is composed of Pd and Pt nanoparticles, exhibits potent SOD and catalase activities and attenuates age-related skin changes *in vivo*. This mixture has been found to have few adverse effects on skin morphology in transdermally treated mice. Consistent with these results, no previous study has found that PAPLAL induces adverse effects, despite its use in Japan for over 60 years to treat patients with chronic conditions. Therefore, PAPLAL is considered to be a safe and valuable antioxidant for delaying skin aging in humans.

References

1. Glogau RG. Physiologic and structural changes associated with aging skin. Dermatol Clin. 1997;15:555–9.
2. Shuster S, Black MM, McVitie E. The influence of age and sex on skin thickness, skin collagen and density. Br J Dermatol. 1975;93:639–43.
3. Naylor EC, Watson RE, Sherratt MJ. Molecular aspects of skin ageing. Maturitas. 2011;69:249–56. doi:10.1016/j.maturitas.2011.04.011.
4. Finkel T, Holbrook NJ. Oxidants, oxidative stress and the biology of ageing. Nature. 2000;408:239–47.
5. Miao L, St Clair DK. Regulation of superoxide dismutase genes: implications in disease. Free Radic Biol Med. 2009;47:344–56.
6. Fattman CL, Schaefer LM, Oury TD. Extracellular superoxide dismutase in biology and medicine. Free Radic Biol Med. 2003;35:236–56.
7. Watanabe K, et al. Superoxide dismutase 1 loss disturbs intracellular redox signaling, resulting in global age-related pathological changes. Biomed Res Int. 2014;2014:140165. doi:10.1155/2014/140165.
8. Murakami K, et al. SOD1 (copper/zinc superoxide dismutase) deficiency drives amyloid beta protein oligomerization and memory loss in mouse model of Alzheimer disease. J Biol Chem. 2011;286:44557–68.
9. Murakami K, et al. Cytoplasmic superoxide radical: a possible contributing factor to intracellular Abeta oligomerization in Alzheimer disease. Commun Integr Biol. 2013;5:255–8. doi:10.4161/cib.19548.
10. Imamura Y, et al. Drusen, choroidal neovascularization, and retinal pigment epithelium dysfunction in SOD1-deficient mice: a model of age-related macular degeneration. Proc Natl Acad Sci U S A. 2006;103:11282–7. doi:10.1073/pnas.0602131103.
11. Uchiyama S, Shimizu T, Shirasawa T. CuZn-SOD deficiency causes ApoB degradation and induces hepatic lipid accumulation by impaired lipoprotein secretion in mice. J Biol Chem. 2006;281:31713–9. doi:10.1074/jbc.M603422200.
12. Kondo Y, et al. Senescence marker protein-30/superoxide dismutase 1 double knockout mice exhibit increased oxidative stress and hepatic steatosis. FEBS Open Bio. 2014;4:522–32. doi:10.1016/j.fob.2014.05.003.
13. Kojima T, et al. Age-related dysfunction of the lacrimal gland and oxidative stress: evidence from the Cu, Zn-superoxide dismutase-1 (Sod1) knockout mice. Am J Pathol. 2012;180:1879–96.
14. Ibrahim OM, et al. Oxidative stress induced age dependent meibomian gland dysfunction in cu, zn-superoxide dismutase-1 (sod1) knockout mice. PLoS One. 2014;9:e99328. doi:10.1371/journal.pone.0099328.
15. Noda Y, Ota K, Shirasawa T, Shimizu T. Copper/zinc superoxide dismutase insufficiency impairs progesterone secretion and fertility in female mice. Biol Reprod. 2012;86:1–8.

16. Morikawa D, et al. Contribution of oxidative stress to the degeneration of rotator cuff entheses. J Shoulder Elbow Surg. 2014;23:628–35. doi:10.1016/j.jse.2014.01.041.
17. Murakami K, et al. Skin atrophy in cytoplasmic SOD-deficient mice and its complete recovery using a vitamin C derivative. Biochem Biophys Res Commun. 2009;382:457–61.
18. Shibuya S, et al. Collagen peptide and vitamin C additively attenuate age-related skin atrophy in *Sod1*-deficient mice. Biosci Biotechnol Biochem. 2014;78:1212–20.
19. Shibuya S, et al. Palladium and platinum nanoparticles attenuate aging-like skin atrophy via antioxidant activity in mice. PLoS One. 2014;9:e109288. doi:10.1371/journal.pone.0109288.
20. Lewis L, Lewis N. Platinum-catalyzed hydrosilylation-colloid formation as the essential step. J Am Chem Soc. 1986;108:7228–31.
21. Toshima N, Yonezawa T. Bimetallic nanoparticles-novel materials for chemical and physical applications. New J Chem. 1998;22:1179–201.
22. Roucoux A, Schulz J, Patin H. Reduced transition metal colloids: a novel family of reusable catalysts? Chem Rev. 2002;102:3757–78.
23. Yoshihisa Y, et al. Protective effects of platinum nanoparticles against UV-light-induced epidermal inflammation. Exp Dermatol. 2010;19:1000–6.
24. Kajita M, et al. Platinum nanoparticle is a useful scavenger of superoxide anion and hydrogen peroxide. Free Radic Res. 2007;41:615–26.
25. Yoshihisa Y, et al. SOD/catalase mimetic platinum nanoparticles inhibit heat-induced apoptosis in human lymphoma U937 and HH cells. Free Radic Res. 2011;45:326–35.
26. Shibuya S, Kinoshita K, Shimizu T. Protective effects of vitamin C derivatives on skin atrophy caused by *Sod1* deficiency. In: Preedy BS, editor. Handbook of diet, nutrition and the skin. Wageningen: Academic; 2011. p. 351–64.
27. Shibuya S, Nojiri H, Morikawa D, Koyama H, Shimizu T. Protective effects of vitamin C on age-related bone and skin phenotypes caused by intracellular reactive oxygen species. In: Preedy BS, editor. Oxidative stress and dietary antioxidants. New York: Academic; 2014. p. 137–44.
28. Kim J, et al. Effects of a potent antioxidant, platinum nanoparticle, on the lifespan of *Caenorhabditis elegans*. Mech Ageing Dev. 2008;129:322–31.
29. Takamiya M, et al. Neurological and pathological improvements of cerebral infarction in mice with platinum nanoparticles. J Neurosci Res. 2011;89:1125–33. doi:10.1002/jnr.22622.
30. Okamoto H, Horii K, Fujisawa A, Yamamoto Y. Oxidative deterioration of platinum nanoparticle and its prevention by palladium. Exp Dermatol. 2012;21:5–7.
31. Larese Filon F, Mauro M, Adami G, Bovenzi M, Crosera M. Nanoparticles skin absorption: new aspects for a safety profile evaluation. Regul Toxicol Pharmacol. 2015;72:310–22. doi:10.1016/j.yrtph.2015.05.005.
32. Bharti N, Shailendra SS, Naqvi F, Azam A. New palladium(II) complexes of 5-nitrothiophene-2-carboxaldehyde thiosemicarbazones. synthesis, spectral studies and in vitro anti-amoebic activity. Bioorg Med Chem. 2003;11:2923–9.
33. Brudzinska I, Mikata Y, Obata M, Ohtsuki C, Yano S. Synthesis, structural characterization, and antitumor activity of palladium(II) complexes containing a sugar unit. Bioorg Med Chem Lett. 2004;14:2533–6. doi:10.1016/j.bmcl.2004.02.095.
34. Li J, et al. Palladium-triggered deprotection chemistry for protein activation in living cells. Nat Chem. 2014;6:352–61. doi:10.1038/nchem.1887.
35. Elhusseiny AF, Hassan HH. Antimicrobial and antitumor activity of platinum and palladium complexes of novel spherical aramides nanoparticles containing flexibilizing linkages: structure–property relationship. Spectrochim Acta A Mol Biomol Spectrosc. 2013;103:232–45. doi:10.1016/j.saa.2012.10.063.
36. Verrecchia F, Mauviel A. TGF-beta and TNF-alpha: antagonistic cytokines controlling type I collagen gene expression. Cell Signal. 2004;16:873–80. doi:10.1016/j.cellsig.2004.02.007.
37. Beauchef G, et al. The p65 subunit of NF-kappaB inhibits COL1A1 gene transcription in human dermal and scleroderma fibroblasts through its recruitment on promoter by protein interaction with transcriptional activators (c-Krox, Sp1, and Sp3). J Biol Chem. 2012;287:3462–78. doi:10.1074/jbc.M111.286443.
38. Bigot N, et al. NF-kappaB accumulation associated with COL1A1 transactivators defects during chronological aging represses type I collagen expression through a -112/-61-bp region of the COL1A1 promoter in human skin fibroblasts. J Invest Dermatol. 2012;132:2360–7. doi:10.1038/jid.2012.164.
39. Kondo Y, Fukuda K, Adachi T, Nishida T. Inhibition by a selective IkappaB kinase-2 inhibitor of interleukin-1-induced collagen degradation by corneal fibroblasts in three-dimensional culture. Invest Ophthalmol Vis Sci. 2008;49:4850–7. doi:10.1167/iovs.08-1897.
40. Lopez-Otin C, Blasco MA, Partridge L, Serrano M, Kroemer G. The hallmarks of aging. Cell. 2013;153:1194–217. doi:10.1016/j.cell.2013.05.039.
41. Tyner SD, et al. *p53* mutant mice that display early ageing-associated phenotypes. Nature. 2002;415:45–53.
42. Ishizuka S. Creation of PAPLAL. Japan: Juseikai; 1956, In Japanese.
43. Tajima K, Watabe R, Kanaori K. Antioxidant activity of PAPLAL a colloidal mixture of Pt and Pd metal to superoxide anion radical as studied by quantitative spin

trapping ESR measurements. Clin Phamacol Ther. 2005;15:635–42.

44. Tajima K, et al. Chemical reactivity of Pd-, and Pt-colloid involved in PAPLAL to solvated oxygen and hydroxyl radical. Clin Phamacol Ther. 2009;19:397–404.
45. Nojiri H, et al. Cytoplasmic superoxide causes bone fragility owing to low-turnover osteoporosis and impaired collagen cross-linking. J Bone Miner Res. 2011;26:2682–94.
46. Iuchi Y, et al. Elevated oxidative stress in erythrocytes due to a SOD1 deficiency causes anaemia and triggers autoantibody production. Biochem J. 2007;402:219–27. doi:10.1042/BJ20061386.
47. Onizawa S, Aoshiba K, Kajita M, Miyamoto Y, Nagai A. Platinum nanoparticle antioxidants inhibit pulmonary inflammation in mice exposed to cigarette smoke. Pulm Pharmacol Ther. 2009;22:340–9. doi:10.1016/j.pupt.2008.12.015.
48. Rehman MU, Yoshihisa Y, Miyamoto Y, Shimizu T. The anti-inflammatory effects of platinum nanoparticles on the lipopolysaccharide-induced inflammatory response in RAW 264.7 macrophages. Inflamm Res. 2012;61:1177–85. doi:10.1007/s00011-012-0512-0.
49. Watkinson AC, Bunge AL, Hadgraft J, Lane ME. Nanoparticles do not penetrate human skin – a theoretical perspective. Pharm Res. 2013;30:1943–6. doi:10.1007/s11095-013-1073-9.
50. Sonavane G, et al. In vitro permeation of gold nanoparticles through rat skin and rat intestine: effect of particle size. Colloids Surf B Biointerfaces. 2008;65:1–10. doi:10.1016/j.colsurfb.2008.02.013.
51. Labouta HI, Schneider M. Interaction of inorganic nanoparticles with the skin barrier: current status and critical review. Nanomedicine. 2013;9:39–54. doi:10.1016/j.nano.2012.04.004.
52. Gu H, Yu A, Chen H. Direct electron transfer and characterization of hemoglobin immobilized on a Au colloid–cysteamine-modified gold electrode. J Electroanal Chem. 2001;516:119–26.
53. Sakaue Y, Kim J, Miyamoto Y. Effects of TAT-conjugated platinum nanoparticles on lifespan of mitochondrial electron transport complex I-deficient Caenorhabditis elegans, nuo-1. Int J Nanomedicine. 2010;5:687–95.
54. Arora S, et al. Silver nanoparticles protect human keratinocytes against UVB radiation-induced DNA damage and apoptosis: potential for prevention of skin carcinogenesis. Nanomedicine. 2015;11:1265–75. doi:10.1016/j.nano.2015.02.024.
55. Massip L, et al. Vitamin C restores healthy aging in a mouse model for Werner syndrome. FASEB J. 2010;24:158–72.
56. Kato E, Tokunaga Y, Sakan F. Stilbenoids isolated from the seeds of Melinjo (*Gnetum gnemon* L.) and their biological activity. J Agric Food Chem. 2009;57:2544–9. doi:10.1021/jf803077p.
57. Baur JA, Sinclair DA. Therapeutic potential of resveratrol: the *in vivo* evidence. Nat Rev Drug Discov. 2006;5:493–506. doi:10.1038/nrd2060.
58. Hubbard BP, Sinclair DA. Small molecule SIRT1 activators for the treatment of aging and age-related diseases. Trends Pharmacol Sci. 2014;35:146–54. doi:10.1016/j.tips.2013.12.004.
59. Serravallo M, Jagdeo J, Glick SA, Siegel DM, Brody NI. Sirtuins in dermatology: applications for future research and therapeutics. Arch Dermatol Res. 2013;305:269–82. doi:10.1007/s00403-013-1320-2.
60. Watanabe K, Shibuya S, Ozawa Y, Izuo N, Shimizu T. Resveratrol derivative-rich melinjo seed extract attenuates skin atrophy in *Sod1*-deficient mice. Oxid Med Cell Longev. 2015;2015:391075. doi:10.1155/2015/391075.

Skin Aging: An Immunohistochemical Evaluation

38

Moetaz El-Domyati and Walid Medhat

Contents

Abstract

Aging of the skin is a multifactorial phenomenon, in which ongoing intrinsic changes combine the cumulative effects of chronic exposure to the elements, primarily ultraviolet radiation, in a synergistic fashion, causing decreased skin thickness and elasticity with subsequent wrinkle formation. Understanding the mechanisms by which the skin ages has been increasing significantly, along with considerable progress on the way to prevent and reverse the visible signs of aging. However, there are still several mysterious factors concerning the aging process and why we all appear to age differently. The skin is mostly important because of its social impact and as it is visible, making it an appropriate model for studying the aging phenomenon. As the skin ages, multiple histological changes occur throughout the epidermis, dermis, and subcutaneous tissue which manifest via distinct skin alterations in appearance. There is general agreement that cutaneous aging is a complex biological process, which affects various layers of the skin; however, the major changes are seen in the dermis. This chapter discusses the main histological and immunohistochemical changes observed in aging skin.

M. El-Domyati (✉) • W. Medhat
Department of Dermatology, Al-Minya University, Al-Minya, Egypt
e-mail: moetazeldomyati@yahoo.com; moetazeldomyati@gmail.com; d_waleed@yahoo.com

M.A. Farage et al. (eds.), *Textbook of Aging Skin*, DOI 10.1007/978-3-662-47398-6_121

Introduction

Aside from being the largest organ of human body, the skin is also the only organ continually exposed to the surrounding world, interacting with the environment and reflecting general health condition and age changes. Such changes are largely determined by skin color, texture, firmness, and smoothness. The quality of skin features is greatly affected by aging; as skin ages, it tends to become uneven in color, roughened, lax, and wrinkled [1].

The skin is a dynamic and ever-changing organ which accounts for 12–16 % of body weight with a surface area of ~2 m^2. It contains many specialized cells and structures divided into three key regions: epidermis, dermis, and subcutaneous tissue. The epidermis, a cell-rich layer, mainly a keratinized stratified squamous epithelium, is the most superficial layer of the skin and is approximately 100 μm thick. Basement membrane separates the epidermis from the dermis. Ultrastructurally, it is composed of two main layers, the upper (lamina lucida) which is attached directly to the plasma membrane of the basal keratinocytes and the lower layer (lamina densa), which interacts with the mesenchymal matrix of the upper dermis. The junction is characterized by downward folds of the epidermis called epidermal ridges or rete which interdigitate with upward projections of the dermis called dermal papillae. This structure of the dermo-epidermal junction (DEJ) contributes to minimizing the risk of dermo-epidermal separation by shearing forces [2, 3].

The dermis is formed of connective tissue to which the epidermis is attached; it is typically subdivided into two zones, a papillary and a reticular dermis, and primarily contains supporting matrix or ground substance in which polysaccharides and protein coexist. The dermis supports the vascular network to supply the epidermis with nutrients and plays an important function in thermoregulation. Fibroblasts (master cells) are the key cells of the dermis which are responsible for the synthesis of collagen, elastin, and other extracellular matrix (ECM) proteins that promote elasticity as well as the structural support of the skin [3, 4].

Collagen fibers, the main protein of ECM, are responsible for the tensile properties of the dermis and allow skin to serve as a protective organ against external trauma. Collagen has been classified into 29 (from I to XXIX) families, according to the order in which they were discovered. Dermal collagen comprises different types of collagen family: types I, III, IV, V, VI, VII, XVII, and XXIX collagen. The most abundant protein in skin connective tissue is type I collagen (80–85 %), while type III (10–15 %) is the second major fibrillar collagen found in the skin. Type IV collagen is a basement membrane collagen present within the dermo-epidermal junction (lamina densa) as well as in the vascular basement membranes. Type V collagen is present on the surface of large collagen fibers; it regulates the lateral growth of these fibers, thus contributing to connective tissue stability. Type VI collagen is a relatively minor collagen in human dermis where it assembles into thin microfibrils independent of the large collagen fibers. Type VII collagen is located at the dermo-epidermal junction and is considered as a constituent of the basement membrane zone (BMZ). The main role of type VII collagen fibers, the main component of anchoring fibrils, is anchoring the epidermis to the dermis [5–7].

Elastic fibers form an interconnecting network that provides elasticity and resilience to the normal skin. The third component is the glycosaminoglycan (GAG)/proteoglycan macromolecules which comprise only a small percentage of the dry weight of the skin. Although it is a minor component, it plays an important role in providing hydration to the skin [7–9].

Aging is a process perhaps best defined as decreased maximal function and reserve capacity in all body organs, resulting in an increased likelihood of disease and death. Like all other tissues, skin unavoidably ages, a process that affects the function and appearance of the skin. There are two clinically and biologically distinct aging processes affecting the skin. The first is intrinsic aging, "the biological clock," which affects the skin by slow, irreversible tissue degeneration [10]. The second is extrinsic aging, "photoaging," which was first described in 1986 as the effect of chronic exposure to the elements, primarily ultra violet (UV) radiation on the skin [11–13]. Intrinsically aged skin is smooth and shows wrinkles due to gravitational or conformational forces. In contrast, photoaged skin often shows deep wrinkles and has a leathery yellow appearance. This coarse leathery quality of the skin and deep furrowing and deep wrinkle formation is predominantly due to the process of dermal elastosis. Damaging effects of UV radiation on the dermis are also greatly responsible for increased skin fragility, blister formation, decreased wound healing, and vascular changes, including telangiectasia. Both intrinsic and photoinduced aging processes have quantitative and qualitative effects on collagen and elastic fibers in the skin [10].

Photoaging describes those clinical histological and physiological changes that occur in the habitually sun-exposed skin of older individuals and represents a superimposition of chronic cumulative photodamage on the innate or intrinsic aging process. Chronological aging, or intrinsic aging, affects the skin in a manner similar to other organs and can best be defined as a loss of maximal functional capacity in tissues and organs throughout the body. This intrinsic aging has only a minor impact on the appearance of skin, while it has important functional implications. Most of the unwanted changes in skin appearance that occur with age are due to the process of photoaging. It has been estimated that photoaging accounts for more than 90 % of the skin's age-associated cosmetic problems, which in turn dramatically impact an individual's self-esteem [14, 15].

Skin Aging and Wrinkles

One of the telltale signs of aging is increased wrinkling of the face, which are configurational changes in skin surface in the form of creases and furrows. There are secondary factors causing these wrinkles of the face, including constant pull of gravity, frequent and constant positional pressure on the skin of the face (e.g., during sleep), and repeated facial movements caused by contractions of mimetic muscles of facial expression. Dermatologists can distinguish between two types of facial wrinkles: static and dynamic. Static wrinkles are always visible even when all facial muscles are resting, while dynamic wrinkles are visible only on muscle movements. Static wrinkles showed some histological and immunohistochemical differences in the wrinkle site when compared to adjacent photoaged skin; which may help in understanding the pathophysiology of facial wrinkling as well as its ideal way of management [16].

Qualitative evaluation of dermal elastic fibers revealed haphazard distributions, in which the transverse plexus was seen clumped as densely stained elastotic material losing its fibrillar nature in the upper dermis, and this material was separated from the epidermis by a thin unstained zone. In the wrinkle site, the elastotic material under the wrinkle bottom appeared less than those on each side of the wrinkle-forming real pads. This result was confirmed by quantitative evaluation of elastin, which revealed a statistically significant lower level at the bottom of the wrinkle when compared to nearby photoaged skin. Moreover, tropoelastin showed a statistically significant lower level at the bottom of the wrinkle in relation to nearby photoaged skin. As regards collagen fibers, they were distributed as randomly and loosely grouped fibers with clearly visible interfibrillary spaces throughout the whole dermis but tend to be more condensed just beneath the epidermis, in which a densely stained band was seen with no fibrillar structure. With the advance of age, there is loss of collagen fibers so that only sparse amounts of collagen were seen in these areas [16].

Quantitative evaluation of collagen I and III in the upper dermis demonstrated no statistically significant difference in their amounts in wrinkle site when compared to surrounding photoaged skin. On the other hand, collagen VII showed statistically significant lower level at the bottom of the wrinkle in relation to nearby photoaged skin [16].

Skin Thickness

Skin thickness rises over the first 20 years of life; even though the number of cell layers remains stable [17], adult skin thins progressively at a rate that accelerates with age. This phenomenon occurs in all layers of the skin. The epidermis decreases in thickness with age [18]. The unexposed epidermis thins by up to 50 % between the ages of 30 and 80, but changes in epidermal thickness are most pronounced in exposed areas, such as the face, neck, upper part of the chest, and the extensor surface of the hands and forearms [19]. Overall, epidermal thickness decreases at about 6.4 % per decade, decreasing faster in women than in men. Dermal thickness, vascularity, and cellularity also decrease with age. In sun-protected skin, the loss of dermal collagen and elastic fibers makes up most of the reduction in total skin thickness in elderly adults: for example, in postmenopausal women, a decrease in skin thickness of 1.13 % per year parallels a 2 % decrease per year in collagen content. Dermal thickness decreases at the same rate in both genders [19, 20].

Aging of the Epidermis

As skin ages, epidermal cell numbers and the epidermal turnover rate decrease. Characteristic changes occur in each of the cell types in the epidermis. Cells of the basal layer become less uniform in size, although average cellular size rises. Keratinocytes change shape as skin ages, becoming shorter and thicker [10]; corneocytes become bigger due to decreased epidermal turnover [21]. Enzymatically active melanocytes decrease at a rate of 8–20 % per decade, resulting in uneven pigmentation in elderly skin. Langerhans cells, like other epidermal cells, display more heterogeneous appearance and function. The number of Langerhans cells in the epidermis also decreases with age, leading to impairment of cutaneous immunity [22].

The most prominent and consistent histological change is the flattening of the dermo-epidermal junction, leading to a substantially smaller surface between the dermis and epidermis and probably less communication and nutrient transfer [23]. Histological studies reveal that the number of papillae per unit of area decreases dramatically, from an average of 40 papillae/mm^2 in young skin down to 14 papillae/mm^2 in those aged over 65 [24]. The flattening of the dermo-epidermal junction, observed by about the sixth decade, creates thinner epidermis primarily because of retraction of rete pegs, decreasing the thickness of the dermo-epidermal junction by 35 % [25].

Dermo-epidermal separation has been demonstrated to occur more readily in old skin under experimental conditions. A change in epidermal thickness is probably observed with advancing age, but variability in thickness and in individual keratinocyte size increases [23]. With increasing age, average thickness and degree of compaction of the stratum corneum appear perpetual, although individual corneocytes become larger. Examination of skin surface pattern shows slight age-related loss of regularity. There is also an age-associated decrease in the barrier function of intact stratum corneum as measured by percutaneous absorption of some substances [26].

An age-associated decrease in epidermal renewal rate of approximately 30–50 % between the third and eighth decades has been shown by a study of desquamation rates for corneocytes at selected body sites, with a corresponding 100 % prolongation in stratum corneum replacement rate. In addition, there is an increased involucrin level and decreased integrin 1, type VII collagen and fibrillin 1 expression [27].

Intrinsic skin aging is characterized mainly by functional alterations rather than by gross morphological changes in the skin. Chronologically aged skin appears pale and dry with fine wrinkles with a definite degree of laxity and is prone to a variety of benign neoplasms [28].

In intrinsically aged skin, there are various histological changes throughout the epidermal layers; the DEJ becomes flattened because of the decrease in the number of dermal papillae [29]. It is thought that such a loss of DEJ surface area may contribute to the increased fragility of the skin associated with age and may also lead to reduced nutrient transfer between the dermis and epidermis. A gradual decline in the number of Langerhans cells and melanocytes also occurs together with irregularities in pigment distribution [30]. With accelerating age skin loses its structural and morphological characteristics, and as a consequence all skin functions are deteriorated (Table 1).

A prominent feature of photodamaged skin is a pronounced thickening of stratum corneum. Epidermal changes include variability in thickness accompanied by disorganized maturation and some cytological atypia. Another prominent feature of photodamaged skin is so-called "Sunburn" cells. These cells show pyknotic nuclei and a necrotic, eosinophilic cytoplasm. These cells are now referred to as apoptotic cells. It was found that epidermal inclusion cyst may also be a sign of chronic UV damage. Follicular epithelial retention hyperkeratosis and comedone formation are other well-recognized features of chronic photodamage [31] (Table 2).

Exposure to UV light is a major environmental cause of DNA damage and skin neoplasia, to which skin responds by activation of the checkpoint protein p53 which is involved in the mechanisms protecting cells from malignant transformation [31]. The p53 protein is responsible for the decision whether the cells should cease replication and continue to repair their DNA or undergo programmed cell death (apoptosis) [32, 33].

Apoptosis is an important cellular process that may play a key role in photoaging, maintaining proliferative homeostasis within the skin, as well as regulating the associations between cells [34]. High doses of UV radiation to the epidermis cause mutations in the p53 gene, a tumor-suppressor gene which is located on the short arm of chromosome 17 and consequently leads to loss of p53 function to trigger programmed cell death [32]. Thus, elevated expression of p53 mutations may be considered as a marker for both photodamaged skin and an increased risk of developing cutaneous carcinoma, and this can be assessed through mutation analysis [33, 35–38].

P53 expression in sun-exposed skin is higher in older ages when compared to younger ones which may reflect a cumulative accumulation over the years; also, p53 expression in exposed skin is higher when compared to nonexposed skin [33, 36]. This could be partially interpreted by the

Table 1 Morphological and functional changes in intrinsically aged skin

Morphological appearance	Functional changes
Epidermal thinning by 10–50 %	Increased weakness, fragility
Decreased stratum spinosum	Increased weakness, fragility
Heterogeneity in size of basal cells	Increased weakness, fragility
Decreased mitotic activity, increased duration of cell cycle and migration time	Reduced desquamation, delayed wound healing
Slow replacement of lipids	Disturbed barrier function
Flattening of the dermo-epidermal junction	Reduced surface area, with risk of separation by shearing forces
Reduced number and heterogeneity of melanocytes	Graying of hair, guttate amelanosis, lentigines
Reduced number of Langerhans cells	Diminished immune function
Reduced dermis thickness and fibroblasts	Decreased strength and resiliency
Decreased extracellular matrix	Decreased strength and resiliency
Reduction and disintegration of collagen and elastic fibers	Sensitization to deformational forces, fine-wrinkle formation
Reduction of cutaneous microvasculature	Disturbed thermoregulation and supply with nutrients
Decrease of skin appendages and their function (e.g., sebaceous glands, sweat glands, apocrine glands)	Reduced lipid and sweat production, disturbed reepithelization of deep cutaneous wounds
Reduction of nerve endings	Disturbed sensory function
Thinning of subcutaneous fat	Decreased insulation and energy production

Table 2 Histological and clinical manifestations of photoaging

Histological features	Clinical signs
Thickening of stratum corneum and micro-fissures	Dry, flaky rough skin
DNA damage to basal cells (keratinocytes dysplasia and neoplasia)	Actinic keratosis, BCC and SCC
Hyperplasia and dysplasia of melanocytes	Lentigens
Epidermal inclusion cysts	Milia
Follicular epithelial hyperplasia	Solar comedones
Reduced collagen with thickened, disorganized elastic fibers	Wrinkles
Dilated tortuous dermal blood vessels	Telangiectasia and sallowness
Hypertrophy of sebaceous gland	Sebaceous hyperplasia

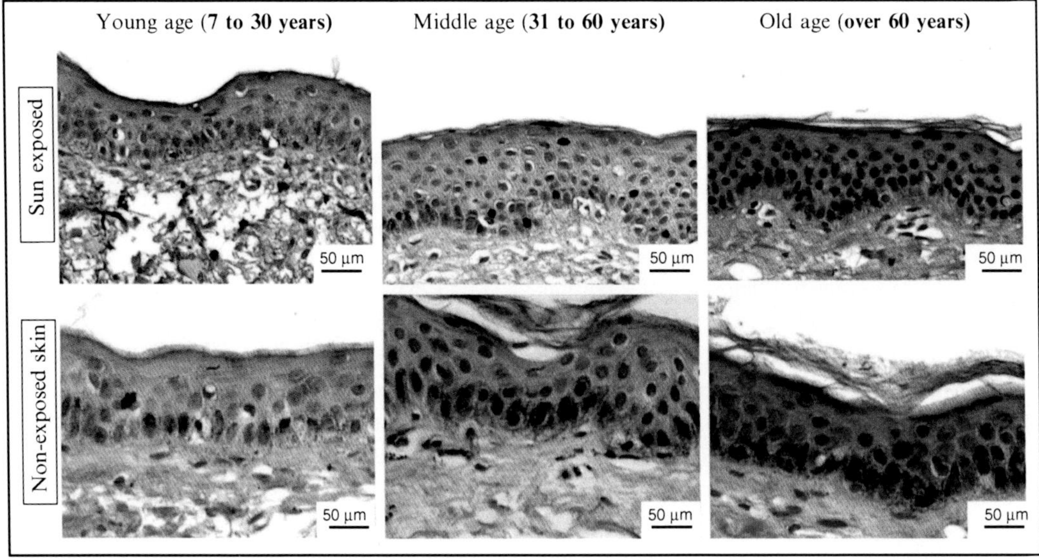

Fig. 1 Expression of p53 protein showing increased level in sun-exposed versus sun-protected skin. Meanwhile, the level of p53 in sun-exposed skin is higher in old-age group when compared to young- and middle-age groups **(Immunoperoxidase (IP), X 300 "sun-exposed" and X 400 "nonexposed skin")**

possibility of accumulation of wild-type p53 in photoaged skin which is related to altered keratinocyte differentiation [39] (Fig. 1).

A decrease of p53 expression has been reported after ablative and non-ablative facial resurfacing suggesting the beneficial effect of these modalities [36–38, 40]. Such decrease in p53 expression may play a role in mediating the effects of such treatment modalities on the epidermis, as well as prevention of actinic neoplasia by adjusting any disturbance in the proliferation/apoptosis balance observed in photoaged skin [36–38].

In extrinsic aging, the outermost portion of the epidermis, the stratum corneum, and the epidermal keratinocytes become disorganized and less effective as a protective barrier to the external environment with hyperkeratosis and comedone formation [41]. Stratum corneum transit time was reported to be 20 days in young adults and 30 or more days in older adults [29]. Such a cell cycle lengthening in older adults coincides with a prolonged stratum corneum desquamation rate, slower wound healing, and often cellular atypia and dysplasia [42].

There is controversy regarding the effect of aging, whether intrinsic or extrinsic, on epidermal thickness. Some studies have suggested that intrinsic aging tends to cause a slight overall thinning of the viable epidermis [43, 44]; meanwhile,

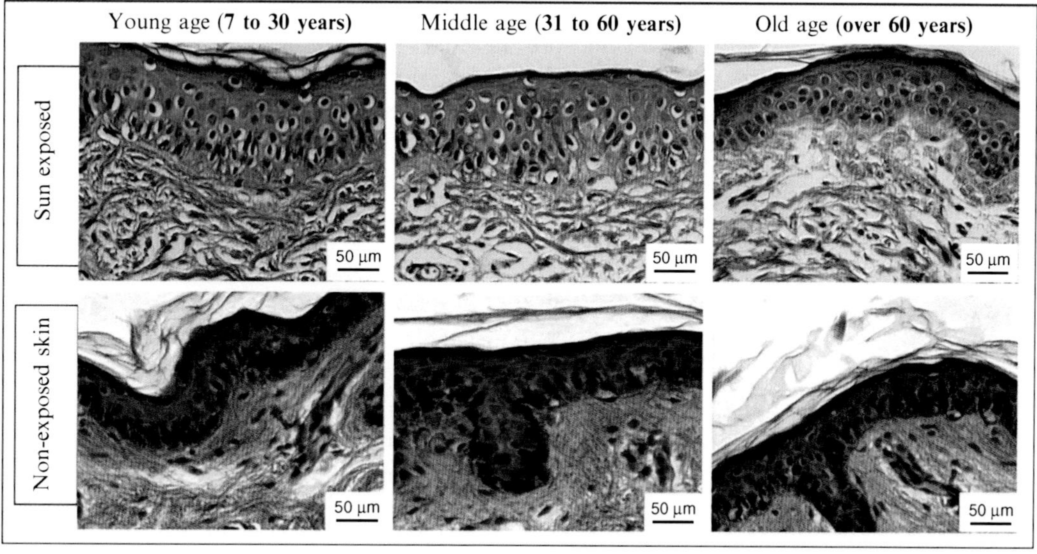

Fig. 2 Epidermal thickness showing no differences in both sun-exposed and protected areas in different age groups, while the epidermis of sun-exposed skin is significantly thicker than that of the nonexposed skin **(H&E, X 300)**

others have found that extrinsic aging tends to cause irregular thickening of the epidermis [45]. In a study comparing the effects of intrinsic and extrinsic aging, a histopathological examination of 83 biopsies from sun-exposed and protected skin in healthy volunteers aged 6–84 years revealed epidermal thickness to be constant across the decades in both sun-exposed and protected skin, with the thickness found to be greater in sun-exposed skin [10] (Fig. 2); additionally, Whitton and Everall found that there is remarkable uniformity of the epidermal thickness with increasing age [46].

Aging of the Dermis

The major extracellular components of the dermis are collagen and elastin which are depleted in chronologically aged skin. Collagen content decreases at about 2 % per year, primarily because the production of matrix metalloproteinases, which degrade collagen, increases with age. Degradation of dermal collagen by matrix metalloproteinases impairs the structural integrity of the dermis. Fibroblast collapse, due to the accumulation of degraded collagen fibers that prohibit construction of a healthy collagen matrix, causes the ratio of collagen synthesis to collagen degradation to become deranged in a self-perpetuating cycle [1, 47].

The main structural and most abundant extracellular matrix component of the skin is collagen (80–85 %) [48]. In adult skin, the most abundant type of collagen is type I collagen, followed by type III collagen. Type I collagen constitutes 80–85 % of the collagen in the skin and is the main structural protein in the body. The second most abundant type of collagen in adult skin is type III collagen that constitutes 10–15 % of the collagen in the skin. Type III collagen is also known as fetal collagen, owing to its abundance in fetal tissues [49].

Elastic fibers are critical to the ability of skin and other organs to stretch and recoil. In contrast to the large bulk of collagen in the dermis, elastic fibers compose only 1–2 % of the dry weight of sun-protected skin [13]. Mature elastic fibers are composed of amorphous elastin that stretches and recoils and a more fibrillar protein, appropriately named fibrillin. Elastic fibers are analogous to a bungee cord, in which elastin represents the stretchy inner core and the fibrillins the more rigid outer string wrapping [48]. In sun-protected skin, elastic fibers in the papillary dermis appear as thin structures that run perpendicular to the dermo-epidermal junction and that connect the basal lamina to the dermal elastic tissue. These fibers are composed of microfibrils and are termed oxytalan fibers. They subsequently branch to form a horizontal network in the upper reticular dermis where they contain small amounts of elastin (so-called elaunin fibers). Still deeper in the dermis are the fully mature elastic fibers, composed of structural glycoproteins arranged around a core of elastin [10, 50].

Elastin is the final, fibrillar polymeric substance resulting from the complicated process of fibrillogenesis which refers to this insoluble fibrillar material. The soluble precursor of elastin fibers is tropoelastin [51]. Elastin is synthesized as a precursor, tropoelastin, with a characteristic composition. Elastin contains unique amino acid derivatives, desmosine and isodesmosine, its isoform. These amino acids are unique to elastic fibers of mammalian proteins and thus can be used to measure the amount of cross-linked elastic fibers present in skin [52]. With age, in sun-protected skin, the newly formed fibers are rather loosely assembled [53], together with a loss of fibers in the superficial dermis and a degradation of deeply located mature fibers; ultrastructurally, fragmentation of the fibers may result in the formation of lacunae and cystic spaces [54].

Loss of dermal thickness approaches 20 % in elderly individuals, although in sun-protected sites, significant thinning occurs only after the eighth decade [55]. The dermis displays loss of extracellular matrix, loss of fibroblasts and vascular network, and in particular loss of the capillary loops that occupy the dermal papillae [56]. It also has a somewhat "washed-out" appearance with sparsity of fibroblasts. Subepidermal microvessels are scanty and small and adventitial cells are sparse. The most prominent changes are noted in the elastic and collagen fibers in different age groups. In intrinsic aging, there is a decrease in the elastic and collagen fibers particularly in the eighth and ninth decades [10].

On the other hand, the histological landmark of photoaged skin is dermal elastosis, which largely consists of gradual accumulation of thickened, tangled and ultimately granular amorphous elastic structures [10].

Extrinsic aging results in histological changes that are distinct from those caused by intrinsic aging [10]. Intrinsically aged skin is characterized by loss of elastic tissue and a reduction in cellularity, while photodamaged skin is characterized by elastosis, the overgrowth of abnormal elastic fibers, and increased populations of mast cells, histiocytes, and fibroblasts [57]. This elastotic material is postulated to result from direct UV-mediated damage to the dermal fibroblasts which then produce abnormal elastin, or it may result from chronic low-grade enzymatic digestion of extracellular matrix by proteases elicited by inflammatory mediators [58].

On histological analysis, the process starts with an increase of slightly thickened elastic fibers in the papillary dermis; with time, thickened, curled, and fragmented fibers accumulate in the papillary and reticular dermis in the form of basophilic material that may assume a homogeneous appearance. Capillaries, embedded in this material, become telangiectatic. On electron microscopic analysis, the thickened microfibrils have an irregular, fuzzy outline and are more electron dense; finally, the material becomes granular and disrupted, and electron-lucent areas appear [53]. The accumulation of elastotic material is accompanied by quantitative changes in collagen biosynthesis which are reflected by steady decline in collagen content approximately 1 % per year [9, 59].

Chronologically aged elastic fibers become shorter, thicker, and disorganized with loss of fiber integrity; however, the fibrillar nature of individual elastic fibers is preserved. Reduction of the oxytalan fibers has been observed during chronological aging. The elaunin plexus is gradually thinned out with age, and the oxytalan fibers become gradually shortened [10, 60]. However, from the sixth decade on, the amount of oxytalan fibers was noted to decrease, and this change progressed gradually until the ninth decade when only scanty oxytalan fibers could be seen [10] (Tables 1 and 2) (Fig. 3).

Aging is also associated with a decrease in collagen turnover (due to a decrease in fibroblasts

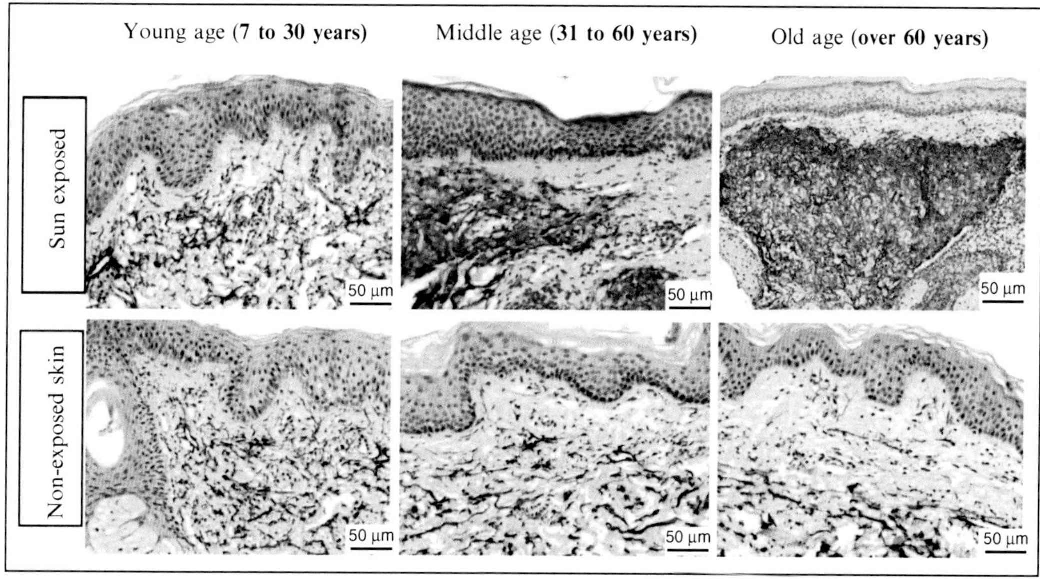

Fig. 3 Total elastin showing increased level in sun-exposed versus sun-protected areas. Meanwhile, total elastin in sun-exposed skin is higher in older-age groups when compared to younger age **(IP, X 200)**

and their collagen synthesis). The relative proportions of collagen types are also disrupted over the lifespan. The proportion of type I collagen to type III collagen in young skin is approximately 6:1, a ratio which drops significantly over the lifespan as type I collagen is selectively lost, although some increase in collagen type III synthesis occurs as well [10, 61]. In the aged dermis, collagen fibers become thicker and collagen bundles more disorganized than in younger skin [62].

Evaluation of tropoelastin in sun-exposed skin of different age groups showed statistically significantly higher expression in young age (7–30 years), when compared to middle (31–60 years) and old ages (over 60 years). In addition, the level of tropoelastin in nonexposed skin was significantly higher in young-age, group if compared to middle- and old-age groups. The tropoelastin level was always significantly higher in the sun-exposed skin when compared to nonexposed skin (Fig. 4).

Meanwhile, there was a statistically significant increase in quantitatively normal tropoelastin level after radiofrequency (RF), electro-optical synergy (ELOS), neodymium:yttrium-aluminum garnet (Nd: YAG) 1320 nm and Erbium: YAG 2940 nm mini-peel treatments [6, 7, 14, 63].

Collagen bundles are formed by the secretion of newly synthesized procollagen into the dermal extracellular space, where it undergoes enzymatic processing, arranging itself into a triple-helix configuration. Regularly arranged fibrillar structures are formed by the association of the triple-helix complexes with other ECM proteins, such as leucine-rich small proteoglycans [64, 65]. When tissues are stained with picrosirius red and viewed under polarized microscope, large collagen fibers stain red while the thinner ones, which represents the newly synthesized fibers, are stained yellow to orange [63, 66, 67].

Newly synthesized collagen showed statistically significantly higher level in sun-exposed skin of young age, if compared to middle-age and old-age skin. Additionally, the level of newly formed collagen in nonexposed skin is significantly higher in young age when compared to middle- and old-age groups. The level of newly synthesized collagen was always higher in nonexposed skin when compared to sun-exposed skin (Fig. 5). Meanwhile, volunteers treated with RF; Nd: YAG 1320 nm and Erbium: YAG 2940 nm mini-peel; and ELOS showed statistically significantly higher level of newly synthesized

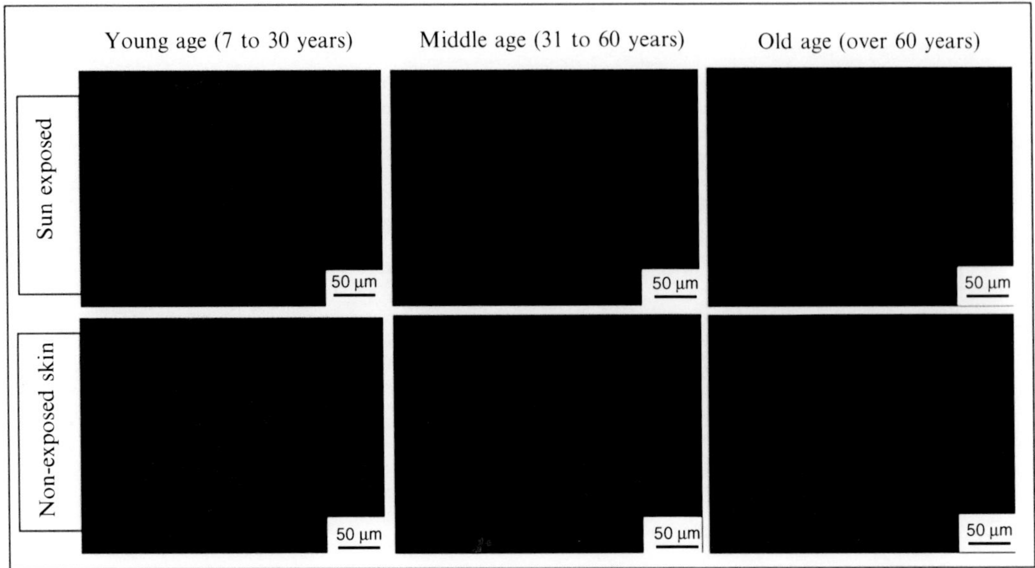

Fig. 4 Tropoelastin showing higher level in young-age sun-exposed skin than middle and old ages. The expression of tropoelastin is higher in sun-exposed than nonexposed skin in all ages **(Immunofluorescence (IF), X 200)**

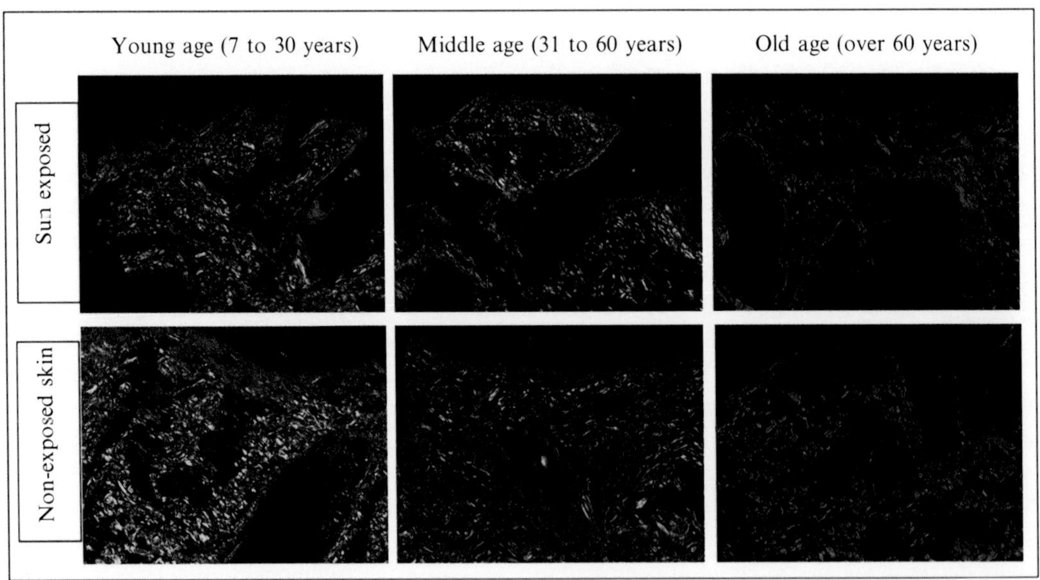

Fig. 5 Newly formed collagen showing higher level in young age than middle and old ages. Expression of newly synthesized collagen is higher in nonexposed than sun-exposed skin in all age groups **(Picrosirius red, polarized light, X 200)**

collagen content after treatment when compared to sun-exposed skin of middle and old ages, while no statistically significant difference was observed when compared to young age [6, 14, 63].

In intrinsic aging, there is a reduction in the number of fibroblasts, mast cells, and blood vessels. The production of types I and III procollagen is decreased which inhibits the synthesis of

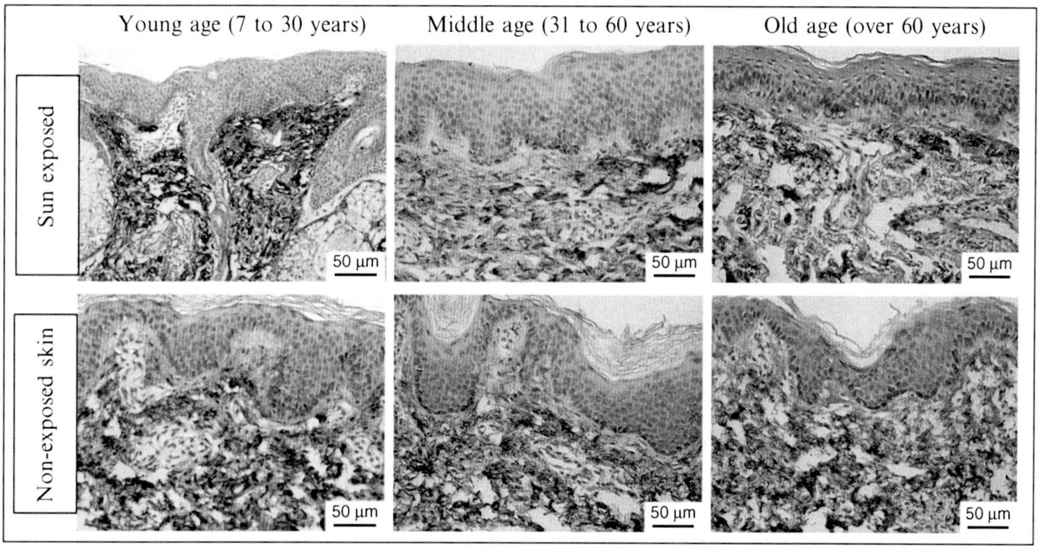

Fig. 6 Collagen type I showing higher level in young-age sun-exposed skin than middle and old ages. Expression of collagen I showing no significant difference in content in nonexposed skin in all ages **(IP, X 200)**

collagen and induces its degradation; this results in alteration in collagen orientation as well as organization [68]. The collagen fibers become thinner with atrophy of collagen bundles [9]. However, in extrinsic aging, the deposited elastin replaces the degenerated collagen leading to collective decrease in dermal collagen content [10] (Figs. 6 and 7). Changes in collagen type VII at the DEJ with increased age have been recorded: there is reduced production with increased degradation [45, 56] (Fig. 8). Quantitatively, the amount of collagen is decreased so that in the eighth and ninth decades only sparse amounts of collagen can be seen. The zone of densely stained collagen just beneath the epidermis could still be identified in the sun-exposed skin even in old age. However, from the fifth to ninth decades, the amounts of collagen are always significantly lower in sun-exposed skin than in nonexposed skin [10]. Previous studies showed that collagen type VII was reduced in sun-exposed skin which is reflected by significant reduction in the anchoring fibrils [68, 69].

In both types of skin aging, the ground substance and matrix metalloproteinases are also affected. Whereas total GAGs synthesis is decreased in aged skin, the metalloproteinases as collagenase and gelatinase are elevated [41, 70]. Skin aging is associated with decreased number of eccrine glands and terminal hairs; however, the sebaceous glands become hyperplastic. Pacinian and Meissner's corpuscles, the cutaneous end organs responsible for pressure perception, light, and touch, progressively decrease. There is also a loss of sensory nerve endings in the epidermis and dermis. This makes older people less able to detect changes in environmental stimuli and thus more prone to injury [22, 71, 72].

It has been shown that expression of type VII collagen is regulated by several cytokines which includes transforming growth factor-β (TGF-β) and various pro-inflammatory cytokines, such as tumor necrosis factor-α (TNF- α) and interleukin-1 (IL-1) [73].

Transforming growth factor-beta with its known isoforms TGF-β 1, TGF-β 2, and TGF-β 3 is a multifunctional cytokine that acts as inhibitor of cell proliferation and facilitates cellular differentiation in a wide variety of cells; it also plays an important role in tissue remodeling and repair. TGF-β acts by inhibiting the action of growth stimulators (e.g., TGF-α) and promoting the expression of ECM components [74, 75]. Collagen is one of the main structures of ECM responsible for the skin's strength. Dermal fibroblasts produce collagen under control of two

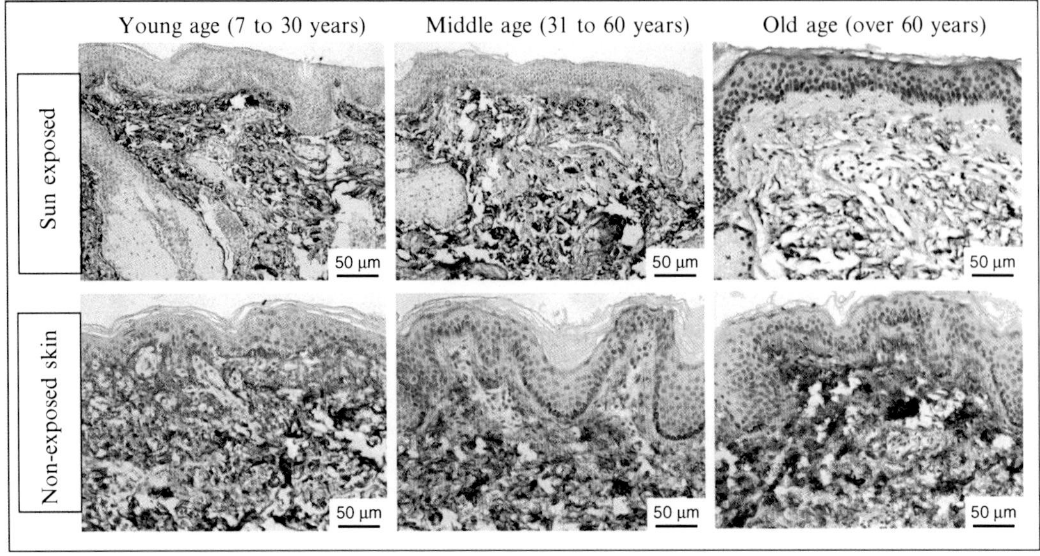

Fig. 7 Collagen type III showing higher level in sun-exposed skin of young age when compared to middle and old ages. Expression of collagen III showing no significant differences in content in nonexposed skin in all ages **(IP, X 200)**

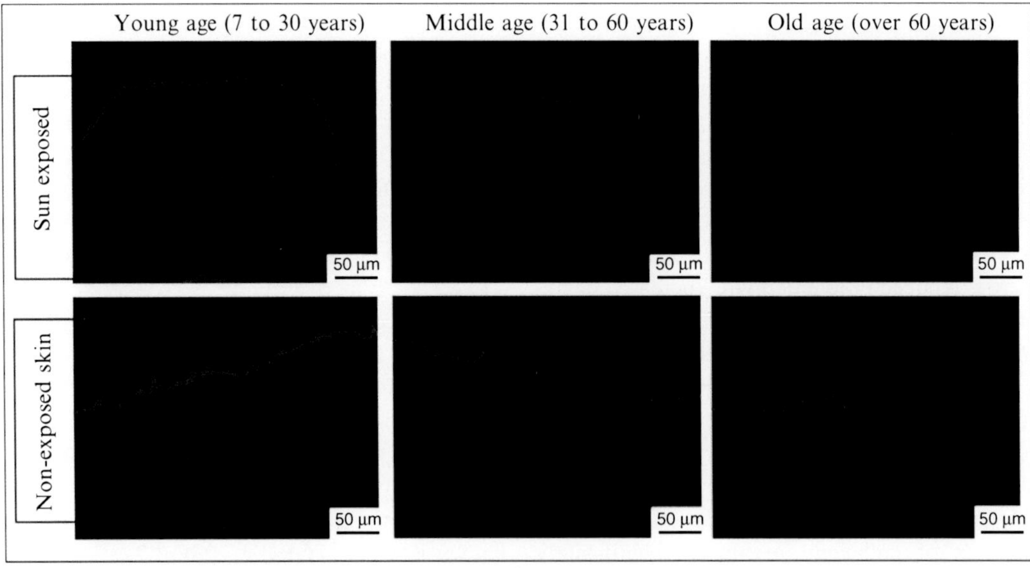

Fig. 8 Collagen type VII at DEJ showing higher levels in young-age group when compared to middle- and old-age groups. The expression of collagen type VII is higher in sun-protected than sun-exposed skin in all age groups **(IF, X 200)**

important proteins: TGF-β which promotes collagen formation, and activator protein-1 (AP-1) is a transcription factor that inhibits collagen production and enhances its breakdown via upregulating enzymes like matrix metalloproteinases (MMPs) [12, 56, 76].

Analysis of TGF-β in subjects with different age groups showed statistically significantly higher level in sun-exposed skin in young age (7–30 years) when compared to middle (31–60 years) and old age (over 60 years). In addition, the level of TGF-β in nonexposed skin was significantly higher in young age if compared to middle- and old-age groups. The levels of TGF-β were higher in nonexposed skin when compared to sun-exposed skin in all groups [76].

The expression of TGF-β at the end of Nd: YAG 1320 nm and Erbium: YAG nm mini-peel only showed statistically significantly higher levels when compared to middle and old ages (31–60 and over 60 years, respectively); meanwhile, no statistically significant differences were observed when compared to young age (7–30 years). The expression of TGF-β, 3 months posttreatment, showed statistically significantly higher levels in response to RF and ELOS treatments when compared to middle-age (31–60 years) and old-age (over 60 years) groups, while Nd: YAG 1320 nm and Erbium: YAG mini-peel showed statistically significantly lower levels. The levels of TGF-β after treatments in all groups were statistically significantly lower than young age (7–30 years), except for ELOS group which did not show any difference of statistical significance [76].

A reduction of the cutaneous microvasculature has been observed in the skin of older individuals, leading to reduced nutritional support of aged skin [77, 78]. Moreover, there are obliterated vessels which have been associated with disturbances of the normal architecture of the vascular plexus in the dermis [79, 80]. Previous studies of the cutaneous vasculature in intrinsically aged and photoaged skin have almost exclusively focused on end-stage dermal changes, whereas a detailed study of the sequence of vascular alterations occurring over decades has been lacking. In particular, the sequential vascular changes occurring during distinct stages of photoaging have remained unclear [56, 79, 80].

The volume of subcutaneous fat diminishes with age, which means its role in thermoregulation by limiting conductive heat loss is impaired. The distribution of subcutaneous fat also changes with age. For example, it decreases in parts of the face and hands and increases in the thigh and abdomen. Muscle wasting and increased bone fragility are also noticed to be a major consequence of aging process [71, 81].

In conclusion, skin aging is a complex biological phenomenon affecting different constituents of the skin; however, aging processes, whether intrinsic or extrinsic, have a definite qualitative and quantitative effect on both dermal collagen and elastin.

References

1. Fisher GJ, Varani J, Voorhees JJ. Looking older: fibroblast collapse and therapeutic implications. Arch Dermatol. 2008;144:666–72.
2. Farage MA, Miller KW, Berardesca E, Maibach HI. Clinical implications of aging skin: cutaneous disorders in the elderly. Am J Clin Dermatol. 2009;10:73–86.
3. Callaghan TM, Wilhelm KP. A review of ageing and an examination of clinical methods in the assessment of ageing skin. Part I: cellular and molecular perspectives of skin ageing. Int J Cosmet Sci. 2008;30:313–22.
4. Mukherjee S, Date A, Patravale V, Korting HC, Roeder A, Weindl G. Retinoids in the treatment of skin aging: an overview of clinical efficacy and safety. Clin Interv Aging. 2006;1:327–48.
5. Chung HJ, Uitto J. Type VII collagen: the anchoring fibril protein at fault in dystrophic epidermolysis bullosa. Dermatol Clin. 2010;28:93–105.
6. El-Domyati M, El-Ammawi TS, Medhat W, Moawad O, Mahoney MG, Uitto J. Multiple minimally invasive Erbium:YAG laser mini-peels for skin rejuvenation: an objective assessment. J Cosmet Dermatol. 2012;11:122–30.
7. El-Domyati M, El-Ammawi TS, Medhat W, Moawad O, Brennan D, Mahoney MG, et al. Radiofrequency facial rejuvenation: evidence-based effect. J Am Acad Dermatol. 2011;64:524–35.
8. El-Domyati M, Attia S, Saleh F, Ahmad H, Uitto J. Trichloroacetic acid peeling versus dermabrasion: a histometric, immunohistochemical, and ultrastructural comparison. Dermatol Surg. 2004;30:179–88.
9. Uitto J. The role of elastin and collagen in cutaneous aging: intrinsic aging versus photoexposure. J Drugs Dermatol. 2008;7:s12–6.
10. El-Domyati M, Attia S, Saleh F, Brown D, Birk DE, Gasparro F, et al. Intrinsic aging vs. photoaging: a comparative histopathological, immunohistochemical, and ultrastructural study of skin. Exp Dermatol. 2002;11:398–405.
11. Kligman LH, Kligman AM. The nature of photoaging: its prevention and repair. Photodermatol. 1986;3:215–27.
12. Helfrich YR, Sachs DL, Voorhees JJ. Overview of skin aging and photoaging. Dermatol Nurs. 2008;20:177–83.
13. Uitto J, Fazio MJ, Olsen DR. Molecular mechanisms of cutaneous aging. Age-associated connective tissue alterations in the dermis. J Am Acad Dermatol. 1989;21:614–22.
14. El-Domyati M, El-Ammawi TS, Medhat W, Moawad O, Mahoney MG, Uitto J. Electro-optical

synergy technique: a new and effective nonablative approach to skin aging. J Clin Aesthet Dermatol. 2010;3:22–30.
15. El-Domyati M, Medhat W. Minimally invasive facial rejuvenation: current concepts and future expectations. Expert Rev Dermatol. 2013;8:565–80.
16. El-Domyati M, Medhat W, Abdel-Wahab HM, Moftah NH, Nasif GA, Hosam W. Forehead wrinkles: a histological and immunohistochemical evaluation. J Cosmet Dermatol. 2014;13:188–94.
17. Grove GL. Physiologic changes in older skin. Clin Geriatr Med. 1989;5:115–25.
18. Harvell JD, Maibach HI. Percutaneous absorption and inflammation in aged skin: a review. J Am Acad Dermatol. 1994;31:1015–21.
19. Wehrli NE, Bural G, Houseni M, Alkhawaldeh K, Alavi A, Torigian DA. Determination of age-related changes in structure and function of skin, adipose tissue, and skeletal muscle with computed tomography, magnetic resonance imaging, and positron emission tomography. Semin Nucl Med. 2007;37:195–205.
20. Waller JM, Maibach HI. Age and skin structure and function, a quantitative approach (II): protein, glycosaminoglycan, water, and lipid content and structure. Skin Res Technol. 2006;12:145–54.
21. Bregegere F, Soroka Y, Bismuth J, Friguet B, Milner Y. Cellular senescence in human keratinocytes: unchanged proteolytic capacity and increased protein load. Exp Gerontol. 2003;38:619–29.
22. Wulf HC, Sandby-Moller J, Kobayasi T, Gniadecki R. Skin aging and natural photoprotection. Micron. 2004;35:185–91.
23. Montagna W, Carlisle K. Structural changes in aging human skin. J Invest Dermatol. 1979;73:47–53.
24. Sudel KM, Venzke K, Mielke H, Breitenbach U, Mundt C, Jaspers S, et al. Novel aspects of intrinsic and extrinsic aging of human skin: beneficial effects of soy extract. Photochem Photobiol. 2005;81:581–7.
25. Neerken S, Lucassen GW, Bisschop MA, Lenderink E, Nuijs TA. Characterization of age-related effects in human skin: a comparative study that applies confocal laser scanning microscopy and optical coherence tomography. J Biomed Opt. 2004;9:274–81.
26. Holtkotter O, Schlotmann K, Hofheinz H, Olbrisch RR, Petersohn D. Unveiling the molecular basis of intrinsic skin aging. Int J Cosmet Sci. 2005;27:263–9.
27. Bosset S, Barré P, Chalon A, Kurfurst R, Bonté F, André P, et al. Skin ageing: clinical and histopathologic study of permanent and reducible wrinkles. Eur J Dermatol. 2002;12:247–52.
28. Makrantonaki E, Zouboulis CC. William J. Cunliffe Scientific Awards. Characteristics and pathomechanisms of endogenously aged skin. Dermatology. 2007;214:352–60.
29. Fusco FJ. The aging face and skin: common signs and treatment. Clin Plast Surg. 2001;28:1–12.
30. Calleja-Agius J, Muscat-Baron Y, Brincat MP. Skin ageing. Menopause Int. 2007;13:60–4.
31. Berardesca E, Bertona M, Altabas K, Altabas V, Emanuele E. Reduced ultraviolet-induced DNA damage and apoptosis in human skin with topical application of a photolyase-containing DNA repair enzyme cream: clues to skin cancer prevention. Mol Med Rep. 2012;5:570–4.
32. Van der Pols JC, Xu C, Boyle GM, Parsons PG, Whiteman DC, Green AC. Expression of p53 tumor suppressor protein in sun-exposed skin and associations with sunscreen use and time spent outdoors: a community-based study. Am J Epidemiol. 2006;163:982–8.
33. El-Domyati M, Attia S, Saleh F, Galaria N, Ahmad H, Gasparro F, et al. Expression of p53 in normal sun-exposed and protected skin (type IV-V) in different decades of age. Acta Derm Venereol. 2003;83:98–104.
34. Pustisek N, Situm M. UV-radiation, apoptosis and skin. Coll Antropol. 2011;35 Suppl 2:339–41.
35. de Gruijl FR. p53 mutations as a marker of skin cancer risk: comparison of UVA and UVB effects. Exp Dermatol. 2002;11 Suppl 1:37–9.
36. El-Domyati M, Attia S, Saleh F, Ahmad H, Gasparro F, Uitto J. Effect of topical tretinoin, chemical peeling and dermabrasion on p53 expression in facial skin. Eur J Dermatol. 2003;13:433–8.
37. El-Domyati M, Attia S, Esmat A, Ahmad H, Abdel-Wahab H, Badr B. Effect of laser resurfacing on p53 expression in photoaged facial skin. Dermatol Surg. 2007;33:668–75.
38. El-Domyati M, El-Ammawi TS, Medhat W, Moawad O, Mahoney MG, Uitto J. Expression of p53 protein after non-ablative rejuvenation: the other side of the coin. Dermatol Surg. 2013;39:934–43.
39. Fung CY, Fisher DE. p53: from molecular mechanisms to prognosis in cancer. J Clin Oncol. 1995;13:808–911.
40. Orringer JS, Johnson TM, Kang S, Karimipour DJ, Hammerberg C, Hamilton T, et al. Effect of carbon dioxide laser resurfacing on epidermal p53 immunostaining in photodamaged skin. Arch Dermatol. 2004;140:1073–7.
41. Bosset S, Bonnet-Duquennoy M, Barré P, Chalon A, Kurfurst R, Bonté F, et al. Photoageing shows histological features of chronic skin inflammation without clinical and molecular abnormalities. Br J Dermatol. 2003;149:826–35.
42. Baumann L. Skin ageing and its treatment. J Pathol. 2007;211:241–51.
43. Lavker RM. Structural alterations in exposed and unexposed aged skin. J Invest Dermatol. 1979;73:59–66.
44. Branchet MC, Boisnic S, Frances C, Robert AM. Skin thickness changes in normal aging skin. Gerontology. 1990;36:28–35.
45. Gilchrest B. Skin aging 2003: recent advances and current concepts. Cutis. 2003;72:5–10.
46. Whitton JT, Everall JD. The thickness of the epidermis. Br J Dermatol. 1973;89:467–76.
47. Ashcroft GS, Horan MA, Herrick SE, Tarnuzzer RW, Schultz GS, Ferguson MW. Age-related differences in

the temporal and spatial regulation of matrix metalloproteinases (MMPs) in normal skin and acute cutaneous wounds of healthy humans. Cell Tissue Res. 1997;290:581–91.

48. Bernstein EF, Andersen D, Zelickson BD. Laser resurfacing for dermal photoaging. Clin Plast Surg. 2000;27:221–40.
49. El-Domyati M, Abd-El-Raheem T, Abdel-Wahab H, Medhat W, El-Fakahany H, Hosam W, et al. Fractional versus ablative erbium:yttrium-aluminum-garnet laser resurfacing for facial rejuvenation: an objective evaluation. J Am Acad Dermatol. 2013;68:103–12.
50. Cotta-Pereira G, Guerra Rodrigo F, Bittencourt-Sampaio S. Oxytalan, elaunin, and elastic fibers in the human skin. J Invest Dermatol. 1976;66:143–8.
51. Mahoney MG, Brennan D, Starcher B, Faryniarz J, Ramirez J, Parr L, et al. Extracellular matrix in cutaneous ageing: the effects of 0.1 % copper-zinc malonate-containing cream on elastin biosynthesis. Exp Dermatol. 2009;18:205–11.
52. Uitto J. Molecular pathology of collagen in cutaneous diseases. Adv Dermatol. 1991;6:265–86.
53. Braverman IM, Fonferko E. Studies in cutaneous aging: I. The elastic fiber network. J Invest Dermatol. 1982;78:434–43.
54. Tsuji T, Hamada T. Age-related changes in human dermal elastic fibres. Br J Dermatol. 1981;105:57–63.
55. de Rigal J, Escoffier C, Querleux B, Faivre B, Agache P, Leveque JL. Assessment of aging of the human skin by in vivo ultrasonic imaging. J Invest Dermatol. 1989;93:621–5.
56. Yaar M, Gilchrest BA. Photoageing: mechanism, prevention and therapy. Br J Dermatol. 2007;157:874–87.
57. Sadick NS. Overview of ultrasound-assisted liposuction, and body contouring with cellulite reduction. Semin Cutan Med Surg. 2009;28:250–6.
58. Lavker RM, Kligman AM. Chronic heliodermatitis: a morphologic evaluation of chronic actinic dermal damage with emphasis on the role of mast cells. J Invest Dermatol. 1988;90:325–30.
59. Sadick NS, Weiss R. Intense pulsed-light photorejuvenation. Semin Cutan Med Surg. 2002;21:280–7.
60. Nishimori Y, Edwards C, Pearse A, Matsumoto K, Kawai M, Marks R. Degenerative alterations of dermal collagen fiber bundles in photodamaged human skin and UV-irradiated hairless mouse skin: possible effect on decreasing skin mechanical properties and appearance of wrinkles. J Invest Dermatol. 2001;117:1458–63.
61. Oikarinen A. The aging of skin: chronoaging versus photoaging. Photodermatol Photoimmunol Photomed. 1990;7:3–4.
62. Sauermann K, Jaspers S, Koop U, Wenck H. Topically applied vitamin C increases the density of dermal papillae in aged human skin. BMC Dermatol. 2004;4:13.
63. El-Domyati M, El-Ammawi TS, Medhat W, Moawad O, Mahoney MG, Uitto J. Effects of the Nd: YAG 1320-nm laser on skin rejuvenation: clinical and histological correlations. J Cosmet Laser Ther. 2011;13:98–106.
64. Bernstein EF, Uitto J. The effect of photodamage on dermal extracellular matrix. Clin Dermatol. 1996;14:143–51.
65. Makrantonaki E, Zouboulis CC. The skin as a mirror of the aging process in the human organism – state of the art and results of the aging research in the German National Genome Research Network 2 (NGFN-2). Exp Gerontol. 2007;42:879–86.
66. Whittaker P, Kloner RA, Boughner DR, Pickering JG. Quantitative assessment of myocardial collagen with picrosirius red staining and circularly polarized light. Basic Res Cardiol. 1994;89:397–410.
67. Rich L, Whittaker P. Collagen and picrosirius red staining: a polarized light assessment of fibrillar hue and spatial distribution. Braz J Morphol Sci. 2005;22:97–104.
68. Varani J, Dame MK, Rittie L, Fligiel SE, Kang S, Fisher GJ, et al. Decreased collagen production in chronologically aged skin: roles of age-dependent alteration in fibroblast function and defective mechanical stimulation. Am J Pathol. 2006;168: 1861–8.
69. Amano S, Ogura Y, Akutsu N, Nishiyama T. Quantitative analysis of the synthesis and secretion of type VII collagen in cultured human dermal fibroblasts with a sensitive sandwich enzyme-linked immunoassay. Exp Dermatol. 2007;16:151–5.
70. Vuillermoz B, Wegrowski Y, Contet-Audonneau JL, Danoux L, Pauly G, Maquart FX. Influence of aging on glycosaminoglycans and small leucine-rich proteoglycans production by skin fibroblasts. Mol Cell Biochem. 2005;277:63–72.
71. Fore J. A review of skin and the effects of aging on skin structure and function. Ostomy Wound Manage. 2006;52:24–35.
72. Flynn C, McCormack BA. Simulating the wrinkling and aging of skin with a multi-layer finite element model. J Biomech. 2009;43:442–8.
73. Villone D, Fritsch A, Koch M, Bruckner-Tuderman L, Hansen U, Bruckner P. Supramolecular interactions in the dermo-epidermal junction zone: anchoring fibril-collagen VII tightly binds to banded collagen fibrils. J Biol Chem. 2008;283:206–13.
74. Roberts WE, Sporh M. Transforming growth factor beta. Adv Cancer Res. 1988;51:107–45.
75. Martinez-Ferrer M, Afshar-Sherif AR, Uwamariya C, de Crombrugghe B, Bhowmick NA. Dermal transforming growth factor-beta responsiveness mediates wound contraction and epithelial closure. Am J Pathol. 2010;176:98–107.
76. El-Domyati M, El-Ammawi TS, Medhat W, Moawad O, Mahoney MG, Uitto J. Expression of transforming growth factor-beta after different non-invasive facial rejuvenation modalities. Int J Dermatol. 2015;54:396–404.
77. Kligman AM. Perspectives and problems in cutaneous gerontology. J Invest Dermatol. 1979;73:39–46.

78. Yaar M, Eller MS, Gilchrest BA. Fifty years of skin aging. J Investig Dermatol Symp Proc. 2002;7:51–8.
79. Chung JH, Yano K, Lee MK, Youn CS, Seo JY, Kim KH, et al. Differential effects of photoaging vs intrinsic aging on the vascularization of human skin. Arch Dermatol. 2002;138:1437–42.
80. Quatresooz P, Piérard GE. Immunohistochemical clues at aging of the skin microvascular unit. J Cutan Pathol. 2009;36:39–43.
81. Ezure T, Hosoi J, Amano S, Tsuchiya T. Sagging of the cheek is related to skin elasticity, fat mass and mimetic muscle function. Skin Res Technol. 2009;15:299–305.

Advanced Age Pruritus

39

Afton Metkowski, Rodrigo Valdes-Rodriguez, and Gil Yosipovitch

Contents

Abstract

Chronic itch is a common and debilitating symptom in the elderly. Skin xerosis, immunosenescence, and neuropathic changes are common causes of itch in the elderly. Cutaneous diseases, systemic conditions, and psychogenic disorders can also increase and augment an elderly patient's itch. Determining the cause of itch can be difficult, and, in some cases, elderly pruritus is idiopathic. Treatments should address the changes in the skin that are specific to aging, in addition to treating underlying cutaneous, systemic, or psychogenic itch-inducing conditions. Treatment can include topical medications, systemic medications, and psychological treatments. Appropriate treatment can be determined by understanding the pathophysiology of itch in the elderly.

Introduction

Pruritus, or itch, was first defined by a German Dermatologist Samuel Hafenreffer as "the unpleasant sensation that provokes the desire to scratch" [1]. Chronic itch is defined as itch that lasts for more than 6 weeks [2]. The reported prevalence of chronic itch in the elderly population ranges between 7 % and 37 % in different countries [3]. In a recent study on the prevalence and characteristics of itch in a geriatric Hispanic population, a prevalence of 25 % was reported [3].

A. Metkowski • R. Valdes-Rodriguez • G. Yosipovitch (✉)
Department of Dermatology and Itch Center, Temple University School of Medicine, Philadelphia, PA, USA
e-mail: afton.metkowski@temple.edu; rodrigo@temple.edu; Gil.Yosipovitch@tuhs.temple.edu

M.A. Farage et al. (eds.), *Textbook of Aging Skin*,
DOI 10.1007/978-3-662-47398-6_158

The mean itch intensity reported was 6 ± 2.1, which is considered moderate to severe [3]. Chronic itch is a common problem in the elderly and has negative impact on a patient's quality of life [3, 4]. Itch can result from the aging process, as well as cutaneous, systemic, and psychogenic causes. The correct assessment of chronic itch in an elderly patient is important and, in some cases, requires laboratory and imaging studies to make a correct diagnosis. Treatment is also an important consideration because of the polypharmacy present in the vast majority of cases [5].

Pathophysiology of Chronic Itch

A better understanding of the underlying itch mechanisms has been achieved in recent years. The main peripheral fibers that carry the itch sensation from the skin are the C fibers. These small, unmyelinated, itch-specific nerves can be histamine dependent or histamine independent [6]. Various other processes occur in skin when C fibers are stimulated, including neurogenic inflammation with microvascular changes and immune changes that can further impact a patient's pruritus [7]. The C fibers form synapses with second-order projections in the dorsal horn. The itch signal ascends in the contralateral spinothalamic tract with projections to the thalamus. From the thalamus, itch is transmitted to several regions of the brain that are involved in sensation, evaluative processes, emotion, reward, and memory [6]. Similar to the itch fibers in the skin, central itch also has histamine-dependent and histamine-independent pathways which have unique but occasionally overlapping networks in the brain [8]. Patients experiencing chronic itch may have a component of peripheral or central hypersensitization, including alloknesis and hyperknesis, that contributes to the perception of itch [6, 8]. Because of the various different interactions on a cellular, tissue, and organ level that are required to generate the sensation of itch, the pathophysiology of itch is complex and requires more research.

Aging Changes that Predispose to Itch

The aging process can contribute to the presence of chronic pruritus through three different mechanisms: skin xerosis (dry skin), neuropathic (neural changes), and immunologic changes.

Skin xerosis, or dry skin, is the most common underlying agent responsible for causing pruritus in the elderly [3]. Xerosis commonly presents as cracked, dry skin that may be scaling, fissured, and pruritus in some cases [9–11]. Although xerosis is typically not associated with a rash, the scratching of itchy skin may cause secondary lesions [10]. It is thought that xerosis develops in the elderly because of a combination of (i) defective desquamation, (ii) changed function of proteases, (iii) changes in surface lipids, (iv) changes in pH, and (v) decreased estrogen [4, 9, 10].

There are several components that appear to be integral to the process of desquamation [10]. In order to shed the keratinocytes from the stratum corneum (SC), corneodesmosomes are required to break apart [10]. In elderly patients with xerosis, the corneodesmosomes do not break apart as they do in normal skin [10]. It has been proposed that defective desquamation in xerosis may be attributed to ineffective proteolysis of the corneodesmosomes [12]. A study by Rawlings et al. showed that while some proteases play a role in desquamation by degrading cadherins and corneodesmosomes, there are other proteases that may work against the shedding of skin cells; additional studies could help clarify the role of proteases in desquamation [13].

As a person ages, the water content of the SC decreases. A lack of hydration in elderly skin interferes with desquamation, leading to an increased flaking, roughness, and xerosis [9]. Hydration also serves in maintaining the flexibility of keratinocytes so that the SC does not become brittle [13]. However, it is important to note that skin hydration, while linked to xerosis, has not been shown to directly impact pruritus [9].

Lipids in the SC can also contribute to desquamation [10, 14] While there seems to be consensus that total lipid content is decreased in aged skin, there are conflicting reports on how the lipid components impact xerosis in the elderly population [14, 15].

Squalene, a molecule that is a marker for sebaceous activity, was found to be decreased in xerotic skin. Elderly patients are known to have a decreased sebaceous gland activity, as well as a high prevalence of xerosis. This commonality suggests that the decreased sebaceous gland activity may help to explain the high incidence of xerosis in the aging population [10, 14].

As we age, our skin pH tends to be more alkaline. Skin alkalization can affect the enzymatic activity within the upper layers of the epidermis, leading to dry skin and chronic itch. Decreased pH can cause dry skin by affecting the production of natural moisturizing factor, the activity of ceramide-forming enzymes, and lamellar secretion. Furthermore, chronic itch has been related to changes in pH because it increases the activity of serine proteases leading to activation of protease-activated receptor 2 (PAR2). For those reasons, it is important to consider treatments that can reduce the pH in xerotic and itchy elderly skin [16].

Decreased levels of estrogen in postmenopausal woman have been related to skin changes that predisposed to dryness and possible itch. These skin changes can be divided in epidermal and dermal. Epidermal changes include thinning of the epidermis, decreased hydration, increased TEWL, and change in lipid composition. Dermal changes include decreased glycosaminoglycans and loss of collagen [17]. While it is thought that some of these changes may be related to itch pathology, further investigations may help determine exactly how decreased estrogen plays a role in chronic itch [18].

Immunologic. As we age, the immune system undergoes a process of senescence [19]. Interestingly, a relation between immunosenescence and nonspecific itchy rashes that evolved into bullous pemphigoid (BP) has been made [20]. BP is an autoimmune disorder that most commonly affects the elderly. It is caused by IgG and occasionally IgE and IgA autoantibodies that target the basal membrane. Patients typically present with pruritic tense bullae and/or pruritic urticarial plaques [20]. The state of immunosenescence can lead to a process of autoreactivity of the immune system. As a consequence, Th2 cells can have increased levels of IL-4 and IL-5 [21]. Furthermore, similar interleukins IL-4, IL-5, and IL-13 have been found in patients with BP [22]. These findings lead to the hypothesis that the state of autoreactivity and nonspecific itchy rashes is a preclinical stage of bullous pemphigoid. It is important to be aware of this possible relation when evaluating a nonspecific itchy rash in elderly patients.

Furthermore in aging skin, the number of Langerhans cells found in the epidermis is not only decreased, but the Langerhans cells themselves have fewer dendrites. This could interfere with antibody trapping. T-cell dysregulation also occurs with age and such changes may lead to an increase in autoimmune events secondary to a loss of self-tolerance [20, 90].

Neuropathic itch (NI) in the elderly occurs when neurons responsible for detecting, transmitting, or processing itch are damaged [7, 23]. Thus, chronic neuropathic itch can be caused by lesions in the peripheral nervous system or the central nervous system [7]. Of note, another manifestation of age-related neuropathy involves a delay of pain, erythema, and edema after scratching, making pruritic elderly patients more susceptible to severe self-induced skin injury.

Brachioradial pruritus is a neuropathic itch that usually affects the dorsolateral arm, either unilaterally or bilaterally, but can also involve the shoulder, neck, back, chest, and upper arm [24]. In addition to an itching sensation, patients may also experience burning, tingling, or stinging sensations over the affected areas. The cause of the neuropathic itch in brachioradial pruritus is mainly attributed to cervical spinal stenosis and compression in C5–C8 [25]. Another potential exacerbating factor may be sun exposure [24]. Both theories involve potential confounding factors relating to age, and further research needs to be done to clarify the etiology [8, 24].

Notalgia paresthetica is another form of neuropathic itch which mainly affects those in middle to older age. In a retrospective study conducted by Huesmann et al. examining the characteristics of patients with NP, it was found that 73.8 % of patients were above 40 years old at the onset of their disease [26]. Patients with NP typically complain of unilateral itch between their shoulder blades [26]. Huesmann et al. found that half of the pruritic dermatomes were located within T1–T5, with T2, T4, and T5 being the most commonly affected. Skin changes are common, although not always present, and can appear as a circumscribed hyperpigmented macule or patch and may be accompanied by a yellow- or brown-colored pigmented lesion secondary to scratching, known as macular amyloidosis [8, 26]. Like with BR, the etiology of NP is not fully understood. Some theories revolve around spinal nerve damage or spinal abnormalities as a possible cause, suggesting that a compression of the dorsal rami is to blame for the neuropathic pruritus [8, 26]. A second proposed etiology is that NP is caused by damage to the peripheral nerves [26].

Shingles is a reactivation of the varicella zoster virus in older age that causes chicken pox during childhood. It presents with a vesicular, unilateral skin rash that may be preceded by a tingling or burning sensation for several days before rash onset [27]. Typically self-limited, the rash remains present for up to 2 weeks [27]. A common complication of shingles is postherpetic neuralgia (PHN). Oaklander reviewed data from postherpetic patients at several different sites and found that many patients experience chronic itch after their Shingles episode [28]. This pruritus has been called postherpetic itch, and it is believed that it has a similar pathophysiology to PHN, with damage occurring to the neurons involved with itch sensation [7].

Post stroke itch is a common problem within the geriatric population [29]. Massey presented a study of nine patients who developed pruritus mainly on the affected side 3–6 weeks after experiencing a stroke [30]. The patients' strokes involved either the internal capsule or the middle cerebral artery; five of the lesions included deep structures of the brain, such as the thalamus and subcortical areas [30]. When damage occurs specifically in the lateral medulla, it is called Wallenberg syndrome and patients present with a constellation of itching, painful thermoalgic hypoesthesia and contralateral trigeminal hypoesthesia, cerebellar dysfunction, nausea, and vomiting [8].

Diabetes mellitus (DM) is a common cause of pruritus in the elderly, and while it is a systemic disease, it can also be classified as a type of neuropathic itch [31, 32]. One proposed mechanism of diabetic pruritus is small fiber polyneuropathy [7]. A study by Yamaoka H. et al. suggested that truncal pruritus of unknown origin is seen more often in diabetic patients than healthy controls and may be associated with diabetic polyneuropathy [32].

Scalp itch is a common problem among the geriatric population, specifically in those who suffer from DM [3]. The cause of scalp itch in elderly diabetic patients is believed to be related to small fiber neuropathy [33]. Scalp itch may be the first presenting symptom in a diabetic elderly patient, and DM should be considered as a potential diagnosis [3].

Trigeminal trophic syndrome is a rare neuropathic itch linked to the trigeminal nerve skin distribution. Causes can be central or peripheral. It is important to consider this diagnosis in elderly patients who present with chronic itch in an area innervated by the trigeminal nerve [7].

Cutaneous Causes

Multiple cutaneous conditions have been related to chronic itch in the elderly. It is important to note that these conditions can increase the itch intensity [3]. Therefore, it is important to address any underlying skin rash that cause itch in this population.

Seborrheic dermatitis (SD) has a very high prevalence in the elderly population. SD results from an abnormal inflammatory process that affects lipid-rich skin areas including but not limited to the eyebrows, around the nose and ears, scalp, axillae, parts of the chest and back, and the groin. The dermatitis presents as erythemic patches or red-brown papules with a greasy yellow scale. The disease has also been observed to occur more frequently in patients who have neurological disorders, like CNS diseases or Parkinson's disease, both of which can affect the elderly [27].

Contact dermatitis (CD) is an inflammatory reaction of the skin secondary to direct interaction with a specific substance. CD can be a cause of chronic itch in the elderly [3]. There are two types of contact dermatitis: irritant and allergic [34]. Irritant contact dermatitis (ICD) is more common than allergic contact dermatitis (ACD). The pathogenesis varies between ICD and ACD. ICD is the result of a nonspecific inflammatory reaction and does not require prior sensitization or genetic predisposition to allergy, compared to ACD, which is an immune reaction to a specific substance mediated by memory T cells [34]. Clinically, it is difficult to differentiate ACD from ICD. Lesions may range from acute signs, like erythema and a papular or vesicular rash, to subacute signs, like scaling and serous exudate, to chronic lesions, which display characteristic hyperkeratosis, fissures, and lichenification [34]. Diagnosis is made because of the distribution of the symptoms, patient's history, and patch test [34]. It has been proposed that age-related skin changes, like alterations in epidermal lipids, impaired barrier function, and increased time necessary for epidermal barrier recovery, contribute to the formation of contact dermatitis [34, 35]. As mentioned previously, the common elderly malady, xerosis, can facilitate irritant and allergen exposure [34]. The immune system of elderly demonstrates a decrease in Langerhans cells and pro-inflammatory cytokines, which may diminish an inflammatory response. Because of the slower onset for reactivity and decreased intensity of reaction during patch testing, results must be interpreted carefully in the elderly population [34]. Additional predisposing factors common to the elderly population include stasis dermatitis, extremity ulcers, implanted devices, denture or hearing aid material, incontinence, and ostomies [34].

Lichen simplex chronicus (LSC) presents clinically with lichenification that develops as a consequence of continuous scratching. LSC is a common cause of chronic itch in the elderly [3]. Common areas of involvement include the genital area, particularly scrotal itch in men and vulvar itch in women, scalp, neck, arms, ankles, and shins [27]. Although the pathogenesis is not clear, the origin of LSC has been suspected to involve either a neuropathic origin or dry skin. Of note, LSC has been associated with depression [36, 37]. Therefore, it is important to correctly diagnose patients presenting with LSC and evaluate them for depression.

Nummular eczema is more prevalent in older people [27]. Patients have a varied presentation ranging from erythemic patches with vesicles to dry scaly patches, but lesions are typically coin shaped and 1–5 cm in diameter [27]. The lesions present with significant itching. Their etiology is unknown. However, a previous study on nummular eczema and skin innervation showed that the skin within nummular eczema lesions exhibits a decrease in epidermal nerve fibers when compared to uninvolved skin, suggesting either nerve damage or the role of other inflammatory markers as a possible explanation for the pruritus [38].

Stasis dermatitis and varicose veins are common problems among geriatric population resulting from a deficient venous drainage from the lower extremities [39]. It can cause chronic pruritus and should be considered as a possible cause of chronic itch in the lower extremities of elderly patients [3].

Psoriasis is a common skin condition in the elderly [40, 41]. Clinically, psoriasis presents as erythematous plaques covered with a silvery scale typically located on the extensor surfaces of elbows and knees, as well as on the back and scalp [42]. Koebnerization, or development of psoriatic lesions at sites of trauma, can be found around eyeglasses or hearing aids in elderly patients [42]. The etiology of psoriasis is thought to be related to a dysregulated immune system and activation of cytokines [42]. The disease can be associated with comorbidities, including psoriatic arthritis, cardiovascular disease, malignancy, and metabolic syndrome [41]. Itch is the most common symptom in elderly psoriatic patients [43]. The exact pathophysiology of itch on psoriasis is not well understood. However, multiple cytokines and neuropeptides have been associated with psoriasis itch such as nerve growth factor, substance P, neurokinin A, and cytokines like TNF-alpha, interleukin-2, interleukin-23, and interleukin-17 [44, 45]. As mentioned earlier, the elderly are commonly exposed to polypharmacy, and some medications may incite psoriasis [41]. A few of these iatrogenic agents associated with exacerbations include ACE inhibitors, Β-blockers, antimalarials, lithium, and a sudden cessation of glucocorticoids [42].

Transient acantholytic dermatosis or the Grover disease (GD) most commonly affects elderly Caucasian men. It is characterized by very pruritic papules and papulovesicles affecting the trunk and proximal limbs. Exposure to sunlight, hot temperatures, sweat, malignancies, and reaction to cutaneous infection have all been related to GD. Although tumor necrosis factor alpha (TNF-α) and other inflammatory mediators have been related to itch in these patients, the exact cause remains unclear [46].

Scabies usually presents as a pruritic papular or vesicular dermatitis affecting the intertriginous areas, hands and wrists, feet, and elbows [47]. It is caused by a mite, S*arcoptes scabiei*, and outbreaks are known to occur in long-term elderly care facilities [47]. A retrospective study by Wilson et al. examined an outbreak in a nursing home and found that the time of diagnosis from onset of symptoms averaged 38 days [47]. While many of the patients had a papulosquamous rash, the majority did not complain of itching, which may have delayed diagnosis [47]. Patients had a more generalized distribution of scabies lesions [47]. Age-related immune changes, dementia, and being bedridden with contractures may have contributed to the decreased itch complaints [47]. Additionally, Wilson et al. note that in elderly skin, the epidermal tissue flattens and has less undulations. They suggest that this trait may allow the mite to cover more skin distance quicker and may help explain why the scabies lesions are more widespread and generalized in the elderly [47].

Skin cancers: basal cell carcinoma is the most common skin cancer followed by squamous cell carcinoma. In a large prospective study, it was found that itch and pain may accompany these skin cancers. The authors discovered that itch is more associated with superficial lesions, like basal cell carcinoma, whereas pain is associated with deeper lesions that are seen more commonly with squamous cell carcinoma. There was also a correlation between inflammation and intensity of itch or pain, with moderate to marked inflammation being associated with more pain and itch. They also found that neutrophil and eosinophil presence coincided with greater itch and pain [48].

Cutaneous T-cell lymphoma (CTCL) is a T-cell neoplasm that grows within the skin and occurs most commonly in patients over 50 years of age. Intense pruritus is often present in CTCL patients [49]. Two of the most common types of CTCL are mycosis fungoides, which presents with various lesions from patches to plaques to tumors with pronounced and advanced infiltration, and Sezary syndrome, which can present as generalized pruritic erythroderma and occurs when the peripheral blood and lymph nodes also contain the abnormal T cells. Sezary syndrome is known to be more aggressive [50]. Recent research suggests that one possible explanation of chronic itch in these patients is the presence of interleukin (IL)-31 [50].

Systemic Causes

Chronic itch in systemic conditions can present with or without primary rash. Diabetes mellitus, cholestatic pruritus, chronic kidney disease, HIV, thyroid dysfunction, malignancy, and medications are common systemic conditions that have been related to chronic itch in the elderly.

Chronic kidney disease pruritus occurs in a significant percentage of patients with advanced renal disease, including those on dialysis. Up to 90 % of patients receiving dialysis can experience pruritus. Because dialysis is being used commonly in elderly patients to prolong their life and chronic kidney disease has been increasing in incidence and prevalence and the trend is expected to continue, we can expect an increase in number of chronic itch patients [51, 52].

Patients present with either a localized or generalized pruritus, most commonly on the back. These symptoms may occur daily or be more spread out and are often worse at nighttime [52].

Patients with CKD-associated pruritus also have a decreased quality of their sleep that leads to negative effects on the patient's quality of life [52]. It has been hypothesized that the pathophysiology may involve neuropathic damage, as well as changes in the immune system. A study by Papiou et al. compared fMRIs of end-stage renal disease patients to healthy patients [53]. The authors' findings are suggestive of a possible central neuropathy component to the pathophysiology of CKD-associated pruritus, with activation seen in certain areas of the brain (S1, SPL, precuneus, insula, and ACC) in chronic kidney disease patients [53].

The authors also acknowledged an increase in gray matter density in parts of the limbic system (nucleus accumbens, hippocampus, amygdala) and brain stem [53]. They suggest that the alterations in nucleus accumbens function may have some role in the sleep disturbances experienced by patients with end-stage renal disease pruritus [53]. Uremic pruritus has also been associated with an elevation in several immune molecules, including high-sensitivity C-reactive protein, interleukin-2, and interleukin-6 [54]. In a cross-sectional study, Ko et al. demonstrated a correlation between uremic pruritus and increased interleukin-31, a cytokine that has been associated with itch in various other pruritic skin conditions like atopic dermatitis and allergic contact dermatitis [54]. Further studies must be done to explore the immune system and its possible role in the pathophysiology of CKD-associated pruritus [54]. Additional possible contributors to the pruritus experienced by CKD patients include imbalances in the opioidergic system (specifically an increased activity of u-opioid receptors), changes in calcium-phosphate balances, anemia, hyperparathyroidism, and increased histamine [52].

Cholestatic pruritus. Itch is a common and debilitating symptom among patients with hepatobiliary diseases and negatively impacts their quality of life. Reports suggest that the prevalence of itch in this disease ranges from 15 % to 69 %, depending on the underlying pathology. Recently, the underlying pathophysiology of cholestatic pruritus has been attributed to autotaxin and lysophosphatidic acid [55, 56].

HIV. Chronic itch is a common symptom and will affect most HIV patients at some time during the course of their disease. HIV is becoming of increasing importance in the geriatric population because HIV patients are living longer and new cases of HIV have been diagnosed in the 65-and-older population. In this population, chronic itch usually presents with an underlying skin condition such as xerosis, superficial fungal infections, or seborrheic dermatitis. Although the exact mechanism of itch in this population is not known, it is important to better understand the pathophysiology of itch in order to provide appropriate medications to patients. Because many are taking multiple medications, thoughtful prescribing is necessary to avoid drug interactions and side effects [57, 58].

Thyroid dysfunction (TD) has been related to chronic itch. A study by Arantas et al. found that pruritus occurs more in patients with thyroid dysfunction compared to healthy subjects. The exact prevalence of chronic itch in elderly population with thyroid dysfunction, as well as the incidence of chronic itch in hypo- and hyperthyroid elderly patients, specifically, has not been reported and could be examined with further research [59]. Furthermore, it would be of interest to better understand the role of thyroid hormones on itch in the elderly population [56].

Malignancy. With increasing age comes an increased risk of developing cancer [60]. Although rare, a recent study that examined patients recently diagnosed with malignancy suggested that 5.9 % of them had generalized pruritus. The Special Interest Group (SIG) of the International Forum on the Study of Itch (IFSI) has defined paraneoplastic itch (PI) as "the sensation of itch as a systemic (not local) reaction to the presence of a tumor or a hematological malignancy neither induced by the local presence of cancer cells nor by tumor therapy." The SIG also notes that the itch usually subsides when the tumor disappears and can reappear if the tumor relapses and that the itch may be a single symptom or associated with a variety of clinical signs and symptoms [61]. The pruritus may present with specific or nonspecific skin eruptions [62]. Various malignancies can present with paraneoplastic itch. Fett et al. demonstrated that chronic pruritus without primary dermatologic rash is a risk factor for undiagnosed hematologic and bile duct malignancies, but not other solid tumor malignancies [63]. Several other cancers, like polycythemia vera and lymphoma, can have itch as an associated symptom [61]. Various associations with differing pathways have been suggested, but the pathogenesis of PI is still generally unknown.

Medications. The elderly are often subjected to polypharmacy due to the high frequency of chronic diseases in their age group [5]. Many medications have been found to cause itch. Some drugs that may be implicated include MU opioids, antihypertensives such as angiotensin-converting enzyme inhibitors, antidiabetics, hypolipemics, antibiotics, chemotherapeutics, psychotropic drugs, antiepileptics, and cytostatics [64]. The newer targeted anticancer biologics such as EGFR inhibitors (cetuximab, erlotinib, panitumumab), a RAF kinase inhibitor (vemurafenib), and a monoclonal antibody (ipilimumab) have been demonstrated to have a high incidence of patients developing pruritus as a side effect [65]. Another interesting connection between drugs and pruritus can be seen in a study by Joly et al., which suggested that calcium channel blockers may be associated with chronic eczematous eruptions in the elderly [66].

Because these are commonly used medications and the elderly are exposed to polypharmacy, medication-induced pruritus should be considered as part of a differential for chronic itch in the elderly.

Psychogenic

Psychogenic itch has been related to multiple underlying psychological/psychiatric abnormalities. Although the prevalence of psychogenic pruritus in elderly population is not known, both an increase in life expectancy in patients with mental disorders and a high prevalence of mental disorders among elderly population may play a role in the number of aging patients with psychogenic pruritus. Clinically, patients present with an excessive impulse to scratch, gouge, or pick at normal skin. Moreover, patients with severe dementia may pick at their skin, exacerbating the itch-scratch cycle. Itch in some dermatological conditions like nummular eczema, psoriasis, and lichen simplex chronicus can be exacerbated by anxiety or stress. It is important to consider a psychiatric consultation in elderly population with normal skin and after excluding systemic causes [23].

Workup

When an elderly patient presents with itch, it is important to elicit a detailed medical history with a thorough review of systems and medication list as well as conduct a proper physical examination. In some cases, skin biopsy, laboratory studies, and imaging are required to achieve a diagnosis [6]. Figure 1 shows a proposed workup for elderly.

When obtaining the history of present illness, it is important to consider certain itch characteristics that may aid in making the correct diagnosis, such as duration of itch (acute vs. chronic), intensity of itch (visual analogue scale [VAS]), localized (hands or scalp) vs. generalized itch, timing of itch intensity (what part of day the itch is at its worst – morning vs. day vs. night), alleviating factors, and aggravating factors. In particular, it is important to assess the intensity of itch (VAS, NRS, or VRS) on a scale from 0 (least intense) to 10 (most intense) in every visit as an important tool to monitor the response to treatment [67]. When an elderly patient has new onset pruritus (within the past 6 months), it is important to consider paraneoplastic itch.

Obtaining a detailed past medical history and social history during the patient interview is important when attempting to determine the cause of chronic itch. The presence of some systemic conditions, such as diabetes mellitus, significant kidney and liver insufficiency, HIV, or history of neck or spinal trauma, can predispose an elderly patient to chronic itch. When taking a social history, eliciting a patient's use of alcohol, drug abuse, and sexual habits can suggest a specific disease as a possible origin of chronic itch.

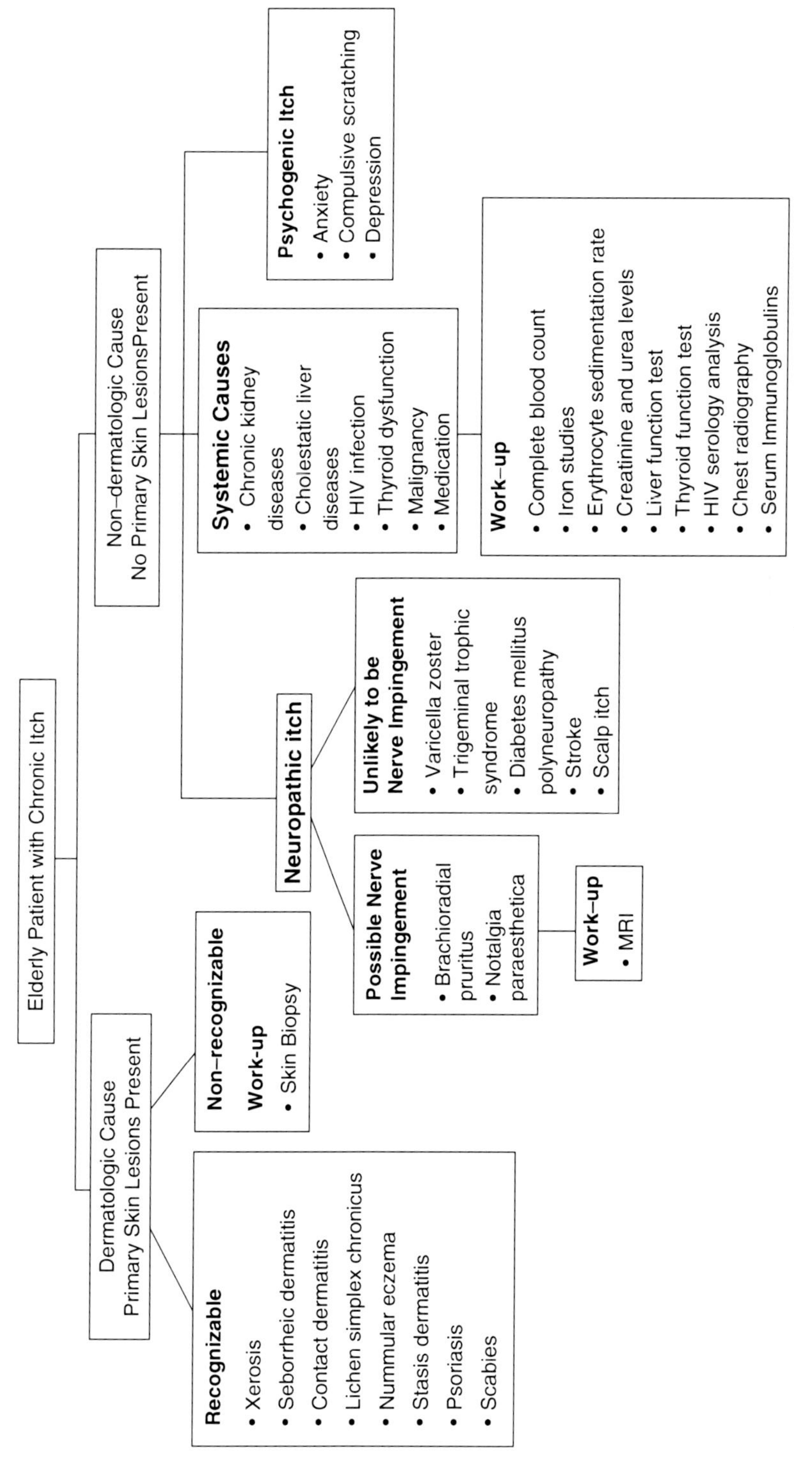

Fig. 1 Proposed workup for elderly patients with chronic itch. MRI magnetic resonance imaging, HIV human immunodeficiency virus

Another aspect of the social history involves screening the patient for clues that would suggest scabies as a causative agent by asking about living arrangements (e.g., nursing homes), and whether other family members, friends, or caretakers are also experiencing itch. Many of the chronic itchy conditions described above cause sleep abnormalities that should always be addressed during the workup of chronic itch and should be questioned about their sleep hygiene.

During the physical examination, it is important to determine if the cause is dermatologic or non-cutaneous. Part of determining the diagnosis may involve distinguishing whether the patient's rash is primary or secondary. Primary lesions result from the same pathology that is causing the itch, whereas secondary lesions are caused by repetitive scratching from the itch itself, and the secondary lesion is unrelated to the original itch pathophysiology.

When considering systemic malignancy as a cause of chronic itch, it is important to evaluate lymph nodes as part of the physical exam [6].

When a patient does not present with a characteristic, identifiable rash or lesion, a biopsy may help determine the diagnosis. Immunohistochemistry and immunofluorescence can be useful in the diagnosis of some skin conditions [20].

It is important to consider laboratory studies to assess for systemic causes of itch including a full blood count, iron studies, blood urea and creatinine, liver function tests, thyroid function tests, erythrocyte sedimentation rate, and serum immunoglobulins [56]. When suspecting a paraneoplastic itch, special tests for screening can be considered [63].

Imaging studies should be considered on a case-dependent basis. When evaluating itch localized to a specific dermatome, from suspected spinal degeneration, magnetic resonance imaging should be considered. A chest x-ray should be ordered when paraneoplastic itch is on the differential.

When aging, cutaneous, and systemic causes have been ruled out, psychological/psychiatric evaluation can be implemented as part of the assessment.

Treatment

As demonstrated above, there are many different causes of itch in the elderly. If an underlying cause is apparent, the first step in treating the itch is to treat the underlying disease [6, 56]. With the polypharmacy, physical impairments, and comorbidities that come with age, an elderly patient requires a treatment for itch that is individualized to accommodate his/her overall health and daily activities [56]. Fortunately, there are many different treatments available ranging from topical medications to systemic medications to psychological therapies.

Topical Therapy

There are many topical treatments that can be used when an elderly patient has chronic itch.

Table 1 presents a summary of topical treatments.

Topical moisturizers/emollients are commonly used for xerosis and mild, localized itch [6]. Moisturizers/emollients have multiple benefits when used continuously, such as reducing itch, being topical steroid-sparing agents, and preventing water loss [6].

Topically applied humectants (urea and glycerin) have the ability to retain water and replenish some of the lipids around keratinocytes on the stratum corneum. The use of topical humectants has been shown to be beneficial in multiple pruritic conditions, including xerosis [68, 69].

Multiple studies have demonstrated the beneficial effect of oatmeal on xerosis and itch control. These anti-inflammatory and antipruritic effects are thought to be related to a decrease in multiple anti-inflammatory mediators, such as TNF-alpha, nuclear factor kappa B (NF-kappa B), IL-8, and histamine [69].

Topical salicylic acid has some keratolytic and emollient effects, which serve to counteract scratch-induced thickening of the skin. Its antipruritic effect may be related to local desensitization of itch fibers. In previous studies, it has been shown to decrease itch in patients with LSC [70].

Table 1 Topical treatment

Medication	Mechanism of action	Therapeutic indications
Emollients/moisturizers	Prevent water loss, promotes epidermal repair	Xerosis, mild localized itch, adjuvant to other treatments for more intense itch
Humectants (Urea and glycerin)	Replenish lipids in SC Promotes water retention	Xerosis, various pruritic conditions
Oatmeal	Decreases inflammatory mediators	Xerosis, various pruritic conditions
Salicylic acid	Keratolytic and emollient agent Local desensitization of itch fibers	LSC, psoriasis
Menthol	Acts on TRPM8, TRPA1, TRPV3	Various pruritic conditions
Wet pajama	Moisturizing, breaks itch-scratch cycle	Various pruritic conditions
Capsaicin	TRPV1 agonist	CKD itch, BRP, stasis dermatitis
Corticosteroids	Anti-inflammatory agents	Inflammatory skin diseases
Pimecrolimus, tacrolimus	Calcineurin inhibitors, changes in T-cell regulation, decreased release of inflammatory cytokines, over-activation of TRPV1	Inflammatory skin diseases
Pramoxine	Local anesthetic, stabilizes the neuronal membrane	CKD itch
Lidocaine and prilocaine	Local anesthetic	NP, pretreatment for capsaicin
Strontium	Depolarization of C fibers	Xerosis, neuropathic itch, LSC
Topical ketamine with amitriptyline and lidocaine	Local inhibition of sensitized A and C fibers	Neuropathic itch (BRP, NP, postherpetic itch)

LSC lichen simplex chronicus, *SC* stratum corneum, *TRPM8* transient receptor potential melastatin 8, *TRPV1 and TRPV3* transient receptor potential vanilloid 1 and 3, *TRPA1* transient receptor potential cation channel, subfamily A, *CKD* chronic kidney disease, *H1 H2* histamine receptor 1 and 2, *BRP* brachioradial pruritus, *NP* notalgia paresthetica, *TCA* tricyclic antidepressant

Topical menthol has been used for itch control. It is believed that the itch reduction is mediated by its cooling effect. The cooling effect is related to a low concentration of topical menthol (1–5 %) and is thought to be mediated by transient receptor channels, particularly TRPM8, TRPA1, and TRPV3 [6, 71].

In some cases, the treatment with topical medications can be further enhanced with the use of occlusive bandaging [56]. Not only does the bandaging allow for better delivery of the topical medication, but it also is a physical barrier against scratching, which may prevent further exacerbation of the itch-scratch cycle [56]. Bandages can also be dampened or medicated to sooth itchy skin which can help to keep the skin hydrated [56]. An example of this type of treatment approach is using the "wet pajama" treatment: An emollient with or without a low-potency topical glucocorticoid is applied to itchy skin. Cotton pajamas are dipped into water and wrung out so that they are damp. The patient then puts them on over the topical treatments, places another dry set of pajama over top, and wears them during the night [6]. Treatment with the wet pajamas with topical steroids should be limited to 1 week of use at a time due to fears of increased absorption of glucocorticoids and folliculitis [6].

Topical capsaicin has been used for itch in multiple conditions. Capsaicin is thought to work by binding to the TRPV1 ion channel on the C fibers and depleting pruritogenic neuropeptides such as substance P from the nerve fibers [72]. Intense burning and erythema are common during the beginning of treatment. The use of topical anesthetics (EMLA) before the application of capsaicin can help improve those undesirable symptoms [69]. Capsaicin has been used on uremic itch, brachioradial pruritus, and stasis dermatitis (lipodermatosclerosis) [72].

Topical steroids have been used for itch relief for more than 50 years. The mechanism of action is thought to be related to an anti-inflammatory effect. One of the most common side effects of topical corticosteroids is skin thinning. Because the skin of the elderly subjects is thinner and fragile, it is important to avoid exacerbating the thinning with chronic steroid use [56]. Furthermore, as the elderly have accumulated sun damage to their skin over the course of their lifetime, it is highly recommended that patients avoid long-term topical steroid use.

Topical calcineurin inhibitors (TCI) include tacrolimus and pimecrolimus [6]. There are several mechanisms of action that have been proposed for the control of itch, including changes in the regulation of T cells, decreased release of inflammatory cytokines, and over-activation of TRPV1 in cutaneous nerve fibers. Because TCIs do not have skin thinning as a side effect, they can theoretically be used as a substitute for steroids [56].

Several topical anesthetics have been used for the control of itch. Pramoxine (1 % or 2 % cream) is thought to exert its antipruritic effect by stabilizing the neuronal membrane and has been used in patients with CKD. The combination of lidocaine and prilocaine (EMLA®) has been used for notalgia paresthetica and pretreatment for capsaicin [6, 73, 74].

Topical strontium (4 %) helps relieve itch, but the exact antipruritic effect of strontium is not well understood. It is thought to act through depolarization of C-type nerve fibers. Previous studies demonstrated that a topical gel containing 4 % strontium had an antipruritic effect on histamine-induced itch [75]. Furthermore, a recent double-blind, vehicle-controlled trial showed that topical strontium is effective in reducing non-histaminergic itch induced by cowhage itch in humans [76]. We have used this topical for itch secondary to xerosis, NI, and LSC.

The combination of topical amitriptyline and ketamine has been used for localized pruritus of neuropathic origin. The antipruritic effect of amitriptyline is thought to be related to its antihistaminic and anticholinergic properties. The exact antipruritic effect of ketamine is not well understood. However, this topical combination is thought to act through local inhibition of sensitized A and C fibers. Conditions for which amitriptyline and ketamine have been showed to have an effect are BRP, NP, and postherpetic itch [77]. The addition of lidocaine to this formulation has been used in clinical practice with beneficial results.

Systemic Treatments

Elderly patients pose a particular challenge due to age-related pharmacokinetic and pharmacodynamic issues, comorbid conditions, and polypharmacy, as well as frailty and cognitive decline. Whenever prescribing systemic medications, it is important to be aware of the patient's other medications to prevent drug-to-drug interactions and adverse effects. Table 2 presents a summary of the systemic treatments.

Antihistamines are often prescribed first line for chronic itch. Unfortunately, first-generation antihistamines (hydroxyzine and diphenhydramine) and second-generation antihistamines (cetirizine, fexofenadine, loratadine) have a limited effect in chronic itchy diseases other than urticaria. Second generation has been used for chronic urticaria. Because the soporific effect of first-generation antihistamines, they have been used for nocturnal itch. Drowsiness, confusion, dry mouth, and urinary retention are some of their side effects [6, 56].

Analogues of gamma-aminobutyric acid (GABA) include the medications gabapentin and pregabalin, have antinociceptive effects, and are also helpful for treating chronic itch. Dosing of gabapentin can range from low doses of 300 mg at nighttime to a maximum of 3000 mg in divided doses. Pregabalin doses range from 25 mg up to 150 mg twice daily to be helpful in treating neuropathic itch. These medications can also be used in patients with chronic kidney disease-related pruritus [6].

Systemic immunosuppressants can be used in elderly patients suffering from chronic itch.

Table 2 Systemic treatments

Medication	Mechanism of action	Therapeutic indication	Side effects
Antihistamines			
First generation	H1 receptor antagonists	Nocturnal itch, paraneoplastic itch	Sedation, dry mouth
Second generation		Chronic urticaria	Headache, dry mouth, urinary retention
Antidepressants			
Mirtazapine	NaSSA	CTCL, nocturnal itch, inflammatory skin disease	Dry mouth, weight gain, drowsiness
Paroxetine, fluvoxamine, sertraline	SSRI	Solid carcinomas, cholestatic itch, atopic dermatitis, systemic lymphoma	Insomnia, dry mouth, sexual dysfunction
Amitriptyline Doxepin	TCA, H1 receptor antagonist, anticholinergic	Neuropathic itch, psychogenic itch	Urinary retention, constipation, dizziness, dry mouth, cardiac abnormalities, blurred vision
Immunomodulatory agents			
MTX, AZA, glucocorticoids, mycophenolate mofetil	Immune suppressants	Various chronic itch	
Thalidomide	Central and peripheral nerve depressant, decreases TNF-α secretion	CKD itch Prurigo nodularis	Somnolence, dizziness, paresthesia
Opioid receptor agonists and antagonists			
Naltrexone	Mu-opioid antagonist	Cholestasis, atopic dermatitis	Nausea, loss of appetite, diarrhea, hepatotoxicity, reversal of analgesia
Butorphanol	Mu-opioid antagonist, kappa-opioid agonist	Intractable pruritus	Drowsiness, dizziness, nausea, Nightmares
Nalfurafine	Kappa-opioid agonist	CKD itch	Headache, insomnia
Antiepileptics			
Gabapentin Pregabalin	GABA agonist	CKD itch, neuropathic itch	Drowsiness, weight gain, leg swelling
Substance P antagonists			
Aprepitant	NKR1 antagonist	CTCL, paraneoplastic itch, drug-induced itch, BRP	Weakness, dizziness
Phototherapy			
UV phototherapy	Immunomodulatory	Various cutaneous disease, CKD itch	Increased risk of skin cancer
Behavioral therapy			
Habit reversal training Relaxation Cognitive behavioral therapy	Breaks itch-scratch cycle	Various chronic itch	

H1 and H2 histamine receptor 1 and 2, *SNRI* selective norepinephrine reuptake inhibitor, *SSRI* selective serotonin reuptake inhibitors, *TCA* tricyclic antidepressants, *GABA* gamma-aminobutyric acid, *NaSSA* noradrenergic and specific serotonergic antidepressant, *CKD* chronic kidney disease, *MTX* methotrexate, *AZA* azathioprine, *TNF* tumor necrosis factors, *NK1* neurokinin 1 receptor, *CTCL* cutaneous T-cell lymphoma, *UV* ultraviolet

Usually, the decision to use immunosuppressants is based on the cause and pathophysiology of a patient's itch. A myriad of different immunomodulators has been used for different cutaneous and systemic itchy conditions, including cyclosporine, methotrexate, azathioprine, glucocorticoids, and mycophenolate mofetil [69].

Thalidomide also has immunosuppressive and anti-inflammatory activity. Its anti-itch effect is thought to be the result of a decrease in TNF-α secretion, as well as possible action as a central and peripheral nerve depressant. Thalidomide has been used to treat prurigo nodularis and uremic pruritus [75, 78].

Mirtazapine is a noradrenergic and specific serotonergic antidepressant (NaSSA). In doses of 7.5–15 mg daily, it has been used to alleviate nocturnal itch of various types. Itch improvement has been reported in case series and case reports in patients with inflammatory skin disease [6]. Furthermore, the use of mirtazapine in combination with either gabapentin or pregabalin has been reported to improve itch in a case series of patients with cutaneous T-cell lymphoma [6, 79].

The selective serotonin reuptake inhibitors (SSRIs) include fluvoxamine and paroxetine. These medications may work as antipruritic by increasing 5-HT (serotonin). Elevated 5-HT may have a suppressive effect on T cells and may reduce some of the inflammatory markers related to itch [80]. A prospective study showed SSRIs to have an antipruritic effect in patients with atopic dermatitis, systemic lymphoma, or solid carcinomas [81]. Sertraline has been used to control itch in patients with chronic liver disease in a randomized, double-blind, placebo-controlled trial [82]. Some of the side effects of SSRIs may include insomnia, dry mouth, and sexual dysfunction.

Tricyclic antidepressants, which were discussed earlier in topical medications, can also be used systemically to suppress itch. The antipruritic effect of amitriptyline and doxepin may be related to their antagonist effects on H1 and H2 receptors and anticholinergic properties [6]. Side effects for these medications include urinary retention, constipation, dizziness, dry mouth, cardiac conduction abnormalities, and blurred vision. These medications may be used to treat nocturnal itch and psychogenic itch [4].

Aprepitant is an oral selective neurokinin-1 receptor antagonist (NKR1 antagonist). It works by blocking the effects of substance P. Substance P is an important mediator of itch that exerts its effects by binding to the receptor neurokinin-1. Aprepitant has been shown to have some antipruritic effect in various case series and case reports for patients with drug-induced pruritus, paraneoplastic pruritus, CTCL, and brachioradial pruritus [83, 84]. Other NK-1 antagonists have been tested recently in clinical trials such as serolipitant.

Naltrexone, a mu-opioid receptor antagonist, may be used systemically to combat chronic pruritus. At a low dose (up to 25 mg a day), naltrexone has been shown to reduce itch associated with cholestasis and atopic dermatitis in randomized controlled trials. In elderly patients, its use is limited due to its side effects of nausea, loss of appetite, diarrhea, hepatotoxicity, and reversal of analgesia [85].

Butorphanol is a kappa-opioid agonist and mu-opioid antagonist that is used to decrease itch. Intranasal butorphanol has shown antipruritic effect in a small case series [86]. Butorphanol is an efficacious treatment for intractable itch. A common dose of butorphanol is 1–4 mg inhaled at bedtime. Some side effects include nightmares, drowsiness, dizziness, nausea, and vomiting [6].

Nalfurafine is a kappa-opioid agonist. It has been shown to reduce itch in patients with uremic pruritus in a randomized placebo-controlled trial. This medication is only approved in Japan for severe pruritus on hemodialysis patients [87].

Phototherapy

Ultraviolet A radiation (UVA), ultraviolet B radiation (UVB), and narrowband ultraviolet B radiation (NBUVB) alone, or the combination, have been used to improve several cutaneous diseases that increase elderly pruritus as well as help alleviate chronic kidney disease-induced itch [6]. It is important to note that in the beginning of phototherapy of both UVB and NBUVB may experience itch because of erythema from photo irradiation. However, this adverse effect subsides after 1–2 weeks of phototherapy with relative few short-term adverse effects [88]. The long-term use of ultraviolet radiation should be used with extreme caution in sun-damaged skin and in patients with history of skin cancers.

Behavioral Treatments

The aforementioned treatments may be augmented by psychological interventions. Developing coping mechanisms such as habit reversal, relaxation (stress reduction), and cognitive behavioral therapy can assist in breaking the itch-scratch cycle. Unfortunately, there is limited data on how alterations in behavior influence itch, and more studies need to be done [6, 89].

Special Considerations

Treating xerosis itch. A combination of moisturizers, steroids, and keratolytics is typically used to treat xerosis. Patients should apply topical moisturizing agents like alpha-hydroxy acid moisturizers after soaking in warm water to aid in corneodesmosome degradation [10]. It is thought that emollients can act as replacements for lost lipid components in the epidermis and help keep water from escaping into the environment [11]. Irritating soaps and very hot water should be avoided when bathing [10, 11]. A keratolytic agent, like ammonium lactate 12 % lotion, can be used to improve dry flaking skin [10]. Steroid ointments like triamcinolone can also be used for 4–5 days to treat the inflammatory component [10].

Treating neuropathic itch. As discussed previously, neuropathic itch can be caused by many etiologies within either the PNS or the CNS [8]. A few steps can be taken to treat neuropathic pruritus in general. These include preventing dry skin, as was discussed earlier in the section on xerosis, and avoiding irritation to the skin [8]. The use of topical compounded medicated cream consisting of amitriptyline (5 %), ketamine (1–5 %), and lidocaine in lipoderm base could be a good option because good tolerability, safety, and less side effects. Gabapentin and pregabalin, as well as low-dose tricyclics such as amitriptyline, may be helpful in treatment neuropathic itch [8]. Special consideration should be related to dose adjustments.

Conclusions

Chronic itch in the aging population has multiple causes including cutaneous, systemic neuropathic, and psychogenic. It is important to better understand the pathophysiology of chronic itch in the elderly in order to provide target treatments and avoid polypharmacy.

References

1. Weisshaar E, Grull V, Konig A, Schweinfurth D, Diepgen TL, Eckart WU. The symptom of itch in medical history: highlights through the centuries. Int J Dermatol. 2009;48(12):1385–94.
2. Stander S, Weisshaar E, Mettang T, Szepietowski JC, Carstens E, Ikoma A, et al. Clinical classification of itch: a position paper of the International Forum for the Study of Itch. Acta Derm Venereol. 2007;87(4):291–4.
3. Valdes-Rodriguez R, Mollanazar NK, Gonzalez-Muro J, Nattkemper L, Torres-Alvarez B, Lopez-Esqueda FJ, et al. Itch prevalence and characteristics in a Hispanic geriatric population: a comprehensive study using a standardized itch questionnaire. Acta Derm Venereol. 2015;95(4):417–21.
4. Valdes-Rodriguez R, Stull C, Yosipovitch G. Chronic pruritus in the elderly: pathophysiology, diagnosis and management. Drugs Aging. 2015;32(3):201–15.
5. Reich A, Stander S, Szepietowski JC. Pruritus in the elderly. Clin Dermatol. 2011;29(1):15–23.
6. Yosipovitch G, Bernhard JD. Clinical practice. Chronic pruritus. N Engl J Med. 2013;368(17):1625–34.
7. Oaklander AL. Neuropathic itch. Semin Cutan Med Surg. 2011;30(2):87–92.
8. Misery L, Brenaut E, Le Garrec R, Abasq C, Genestet S, Marcorelles P, et al. Neuropathic pruritus. Nat Rev Neurol. 2014;10(7):408–16.
9. Yosipovitch G. Dry skin and impairment of barrier function associated with itch – new insights. Int J Cosmet Sci. 2004;26(1):1–7.
10. Norman RA. Xerosis and pruritus in the elderly: recognition and management. Dermatol Ther. 2003; 16(3):254–9.

11. White-Chu EF, Reddy M. Dry skin in the elderly: complexities of a common problem. Clin Dermatol. 2011;29(1):37–42.
12. Simon M, Bernard D, Minondo AM, Camus C, Fiat F, Corcuff P, et al. Persistence of both peripheral and non-peripheral corneodesmosomes in the upper stratum corneum of winter xerosis skin versus only peripheral in normal skin. J Invest Dermatol. 2001;116 (1):23–30.
13. Rawlings AV, Voegeli R. Stratum corneum proteases and dry skin conditions. Cell Tissue Res. 2013; 351(2):217–35.
14. Saint-Leger D, Francois AM, Leveque JL, Stoudemayer TJ, Kligman AM, Grove G. Stratum corneum lipids in skin xerosis. Dermatologica. 1989;178(3):151–5.
15. Ghadially R, Brown BE, Sequeira-Martin SM, Feingold KR, Elias PM. The aged epidermal permeability barrier. Structural, functional, and lipid biochemical abnormalities in humans and a senescent murine model. J Clin Invest. 1995;95(5):2281–90.
16. Ali SM, Yosipovitch G. Skin pH: from basic science to basic skin care. Acta Derm Venereol. 2013; 93(3):261–7.
17. Guinot C, Malvy D, Ambroisine L, Latreille J, Mauger E, Guehenneux S, et al. Effect of hormonal replacement therapy on skin biophysical properties of menopausal women. Skin Res Technol. 2005; 11(3):201–4.
18. Rimoin LP, Kwatra SG, Yosipovitch G. Female-specific pruritus from childhood to postmenopause: clinical features, hormonal factors, and treatment considerations. Dermatol Ther. 2013;26(2):157–67.
19. Sunderkotter C, Kalden H, Luger TA. Aging and the skin immune system. Arch Dermatol. 1997; 133(10):1256–62.
20. Schmidt T, Sitaru C, Amber K, Hertl M. BP180- and BP230-specific IgG autoantibodies in pruritic disorders of the elderly: a preclinical stage of bullous pemphigoid? Br J Dermatol. 2014;171(2):212–9.
21. Malaguarnera L, Ferlito L, Imbesi RM, Gulizia GS, Di Mauro S, Maugeri D, et al. Immunosenescence: a review. Arch Gerontol Geriatr. 2001;32(1):1–14.
22. Rico MJ, Benning C, Weingart ES, Streilein RD, Hall 3rd RP. Characterization of skin cytokines in bullous pemphigoid and pemphigus vulgaris. Br J Dermatol. 1999;140(6):1079–86.
23. Yosipovitch G, Samuel LS. Neuropathic and psychogenic itch. Dermatol Ther. 2008;21(1):32–41.
24. Mirzoyev SA, Davis MDP. Brachioradial pruritus: Mayo Clinic experience over the past decade. Br J Dermatol. 2013;169(5):1007–15.
25. Kwatra SG, Stander S, Bernhard JD, Weisshaar E, Yosipovitch G. Brachioradial pruritus: a trigger for generalization of itch. J Am Acad Dermatol. 2013;68(5):870–3.
26. Huesmann T, Cunha PR, Osada N, Huesmann M, Zanelato TP, Phan NQ, et al. Notalgia paraesthetica: a descriptive two-cohort study of 65 patients from Brazil and Germany. Acta Derm Venereol. 2012; 92(5):535–40.
27. Farage MA, Miller KW, Berardesca E, Maibach HI. Clinical implications of aging skin: cutaneous disorders in the elderly. Am J Clin Dermatol. 2009; 10(2):73–86.
28. Oaklander AL, Bowsher D, Galer B, Haanpaa M, Jensen MP. Herpes zoster itch: preliminary epidemiologic data. J Pain. 2003;4(6):338–43.
29. Krishnamurthi RV, Feigin VL, Forouzanfar MH, Mensah GA, Connor M, Bennett DA, et al. Global and regional burden of first-ever ischaemic and haemorrhagic stroke during 1990–2010: findings from the Global Burden of Disease Study 2010. Lancet Glob Health. 2013;1(5):e259–81.
30. Massey EW. Unilateral neurogenic pruritus following stroke. Stroke. 1984;15(5):901–3.
31. Tseng H-W, Ger L-P, Liang C-K, Liou H-H, Lam H-C. High prevalence of cutaneous manifestations in the elderly with diabetes mellitus: an institution-based cross-sectional study in Taiwan. J Eur Acad Dermatol Venereol. 2015;29(8):1631–5.
32. Yamaoka H, Sasaki H, Yamasaki H, Ogawa K, Ohta T, Furuta H, et al. Truncal pruritus of unknown origin may be a symptom of diabetic polyneuropathy. Diabetes Care. 2010;33(1):150–5.
33. Bin Saif GA, Ericson ME, Yosipovitch G. The itchy scalp–scratching for an explanation. Exp Dermatol. 2011;20(12):959–68.
34. Prakash AV, Davis MDP. Contact dermatitis in older adults: a review of the literature. Am J Clin Dermatol. 2010;11(6):373–81.
35. Seyfarth F, Schliemann S, Antonov D, Elsner P. Dry skin, barrier function, and irritant contact dermatitis in the elderly. Clin Dermatol. 2011;29(1):31–6.
36. Solak O, Kulac M, Yaman M, Karaca S, Toktas H, Kirpiko O, et al. Lichen simplex chronicus as a symptom of neuropathy. Clin Exp Dermatol. 2009; 34(4):476–80.
37. Konuk N, Koca R, Atik L, Muhtar S, Atasoy N, Bostanci B. Psychopathology, depression and dissociative experiences in patients with lichen simplex chronicus. Gen Hosp Psychiatry. 2007;29(3):232–5.
38. Maddison B, Parsons A, Sangueza O, Sheehan DJ, Yosipovitch G. Retrospective study of intraepidermal nerve fiber distribution in biopsies of patients with nummular eczema. Am J Dermatopathol. 2011; 33(6):621–3.
39. Jafferany M, Huynh TV, Silverman MA, Zaidi Z. Geriatric dermatoses: a clinical review of skin diseases in an aging population. Int J Dermatol. 2012; 51(5):509–22.
40. Duque MI, Yosipovitch G, Chan YH, Smith R, Levy P. Itch, pain, and burning sensation are common symptoms in mild to moderate chronic venous insufficiency with an impact on quality of life. J Am Acad Dermatol. 2005;53(3):504–8.

41. Grozdev IS, Van Voorhees AS, Gottlieb AB, Hsu S, Lebwohl MG, Bebo BFJ, et al. Psoriasis in the elderly: from the Medical Board of the National Psoriasis Foundation. J Am Acad Dermatol. 2011;65(3):537–45.
42. Potts GA, Hurley MY. Psoriasis in the geriatric population. Clin Geriatr Med. 2013;29(2):373–95.
43. Kwon HH, Kwon IH, Youn JI. Clinical study of psoriasis occurring over the age of 60 years: is elderly-onset psoriasis a distinct subtype? Int J Dermatol. 2012; 51(1):53–8.
44. Nedoszytko B, Sokolowska-Wojdylo M, Ruckemann-Dziurdzinska K, Roszkiewicz J, Nowicki RJ. Chemokines and cytokines network in the pathogenesis of the inflammatory skin diseases: atopic dermatitis, psoriasis and skin mastocytosis. Postepy Dermatol Alergol. 2014;31(2):84–91.
45. Chang S-E, Han S-S, Jung H-J, Choi J-H. Neuropeptides and their receptors in psoriatic skin in relation to pruritus. Br J Dermatol. 2007;156(6):1272–7.
46. Quirk CJ, Heenan PJ. Grover's disease: 34 years on. Australas J Dermatol. 2004;45(2):83–8.
47. Wilson MM, Philpott CD, Breer WA. Atypical presentation of scabies among nursing home residents. J Gerontol A Biol Sci Med Sci. 2001;56(7):M424–7.
48. Yosipovitch G, Mills KC, Nattkemper LA, Feneran A, Tey HL, Lowenthal BM, et al. Association of pain and itch with depth of invasion and inflammatory cell constitution in skin cancer: results of a large clinicopathologic study. JAMA Dermatol. 2014;150(11):1160–6.
49. Singer EM, Shin DB, Nattkemper LA, Benoit BM, Klein RS, Didigu CA, et al. IL-31 is produced by the malignant T-cell population in cutaneous T-Cell lymphoma and correlates with CTCL pruritus. J Invest Dermatol. 2013;133(12):2783–5.
50. Cedeno-Laurent F, Singer EM, Wysocka M, Benoit BM, Vittorio CC, Kim EJ, et al. Improved pruritus correlates with lower levels of IL-31 in CTCL patients under different therapeutic modalities. Clin Immunol. 2015;158(1):1–7.
51. Sorensen SS. Rates of renal transplantations in the elderly-data from Europe and the US. Transplant Rev. 2015. [Epub ahead of print] doi:10.1016/j.trre.2015.04.005
52. Patel TS, Freedman BI, Yosipovitch G. An update on pruritus associated with CKD. Am J Kidney Dis. 2007;50(1):11–20.
53. Papoiu ADP, Emerson NM, Patel TS, Kraft RA, Valdes-Rodriguez R, Nattkemper LA, et al. Voxel-based morphometry and arterial spin labeling fMRI reveal neuropathic and neuroplastic features of brain processing of itch in end-stage renal disease. J Neurophysiol. 2014;112(7):1729–38.
54. Ko M-J, Peng Y-S, Chen H-Y, Hsu S-P, Pai M-F, Yang J-Y, et al. Interleukin-31 is associated with uremic pruritus in patients receiving hemodialysis. J Am Acad Dermatol. 2014;71(6):1151–9.e1.
55. Kremer AE, van Dijk R, Leckie P, Schaap FG, Kuiper EMM, Mettang T, et al. Serum autotaxin is increased in pruritus of cholestasis, but not of other origin, and responds to therapeutic interventions. Hepatology. 2012;56(4):1391–400.
56. Lonsdale-Eccles A, Carmichael AJ. Treatment of pruritus associated with systemic disorders in the elderly: a review of the role of new therapies. Drugs Aging. 2003;20(3):197–208.
57. Kaushik SB, Cerci FB, Miracle J, Pokharel A, Chen SC, Chan YH, et al. Chronic pruritus in HIV-positive patients in the southeastern United States: its prevalence and effect on quality of life. J Am Acad Dermatol. 2014;70(4):659–64.
58. Nasi M, Pinti M, De Biasi S, Gibellini L, Ferraro D, Mussini C, et al. Aging with HIV infection: a journey to the center of inflammAIDS, immunosenescence and neuroHIV. Immunol Lett. 2014;162(1 Pt B):329–33.
59. Artantas S, Gul U, Kilic A, Guler S. Skin findings in thyroid diseases. Eur J Intern Med. 2009;20(2):158–61.
60. Berger NA, Savvides P, Koroukian SM, Kahana EF, Deimling GT, Rose JH, et al. Cancer in the elderly. Trans Am Clin Climatol Assoc. 2006;117:146–7.
61. Weisshaar E, Weiss M, Mettang T, Yosipovitch G, Zylicz Z. Paraneoplastic itch: an expert position statement from the Special Interest Group (SIG) of the International Forum on the Study of Itch (IFSI). Acta Derm Venereol. 2015;95(3):261–5.
62. Yosipovitch G. Chronic pruritus: a paraneoplastic sign. Dermatol Ther. 2010;23(6):590–6.
63. Fett N, Haynes K, Propert KJ, Margolis DJ. Five-year malignancy incidence in patients with chronic pruritus: a population-based cohort study aimed at limiting unnecessary screening practices. J Am Acad Dermatol. 2014;70(4):651–8.
64. Reich A, Stander S, Szepietowski JC. Drug-induced pruritus: a review. Acta Derm Venereol. 2009; 89(3):236–44.
65. Fischer A, Rosen AC, Ensslin CJ, Wu S, Lacouture ME. Pruritus to anticancer agents targeting the EGFR, BRAF, and CTLA-4. Dermatol Ther. 2013; 26(2):135–48.
66. Joly P, Benoit-Corven C, Baricault S, Lambert A, Hellot MF, Josset V, et al. Chronic eczematous eruptions of the elderly are associated with chronic exposure to calcium channel blockers: results from a case–control study. J Invest Dermatol. 2007; 127(12):2766–71.
67. Phan NQ, Blome C, Fritz F, Gerss J, Reich A, Ebata T, et al. Assessment of pruritus intensity: prospective study on validity and reliability of the visual analogue scale, numerical rating scale and verbal rating scale in 471 patients with chronic pruritus. Acta Derm Venereol. 2012;92(5):502–7.
68. Pan M, Heinecke G, Bernardo S, Tsui C, Levitt J. Urea: a comprehensive review of the clinical literature. Dermatol Online J. 2013;19(11):20392.
69. Mollanazar NK, Smith PK, Yosipovitch G. Mediators of chronic pruritus in atopic dermatitis: getting the itch out? Clin Rev Allergy Immunol. 2015. [Epub ahead of print] doi: 10.1007/s12016-015-8488-5

70. Yosipovitch G, Sugeng MW, Chan YH, Goon A, Ngim S, Goh CL. The effect of topically applied aspirin on localized circumscribed neurodermatitis. J Am Acad Dermatol. 2001;45(6):910–3.
71. Leslie TA, Greaves MW, Yosipovitch G. Current topical and systemic therapies for itch. Handb Exp Pharmacol. 2015;226:337–56.
72. Gooding SMD, Canter PH, Coelho HF, Boddy K, Ernst E. Systematic review of topical capsaicin in the treatment of pruritus. Int J Dermatol. 2010;49(8):858–65.
73. Layton AM, Cotterill JA. Notalgia paraesthetica–report of three cases and their treatment. Clin Exp Dermatol. 1991;16(3):197–8.
74. Yosipovitch G, Maibach HI, Rowbotham MC. Effect of EMLA pre-treatment on capsaicin-induced burning and hyperalgesia. Acta Derm Venereol. 1999; 79(2):118–21.
75. Zhai H, Hannon W, Hahn GS, Harper RA, Pelosi A, Maibach HI. Strontium nitrate decreased histamine-induced itch magnitude and duration in man. Dermatology. 2000;200(3):244–6.
76. Papoiu ADP, Valdes-Rodriguez R, Nattkemper LA, Chan Y-H, Hahn GS, Yosipovitch G. A novel topical formulation containing strontium chloride significantly reduces the intensity and duration of cowhage-induced itch. Acta Derm Venereol. 2013;93(5):520–6.
77. Gupta MA, Guptat AK. The use of antidepressant drugs in dermatology. J Eur Acad Dermatol Venereol. 2001;15(6):512–8.
78. Wu JJ, Huang DB, Pang KR, Hsu S, Tyring SK. Thalidomide: dermatological indications, mechanisms of action and side-effects. Br J Dermatol. 2005;153(2):254–73.
79. Hundley JL, Yosipovitch G. Mirtazapine for reducing nocturnal itch in patients with chronic pruritus: a pilot study. J Am Acad Dermatol. 2004;50(6):889–91.
80. Kim K. Neuroimmunological mechanism of pruritus in atopic dermatitis focused on the role of serotonin. Biomol Ther. 2012;20(6):506–12.
81. Stander S, Bockenholt B, Schurmeyer-Horst F, Weishaupt C, Heuft G, Luger TA, et al. Treatment of chronic pruritus with the selective serotonin re-uptake inhibitors paroxetine and fluvoxamine: results of an open-labelled, two-arm proof-of-concept study. Acta Derm Venereol. 2009;89(1):45–51.
82. Mayo MJ, Handem I, Saldana S, Jacobe H, Getachew Y, Rush AJ. Sertraline as a first-line treatment for cholestatic pruritus. Hepatology. 2007;45(3):666–74.
83. Stander S, Luger TA. NK-1 antagonists and itch. Handb Exp Pharmacol. 2015;226:237–55.
84. Borja-Consigliere HA, Lopez-Pestana A, Vidal-Mancenido MJ, Tuneu-Valls A. Aprepitant in the treatment of refractory pruritus secondary to cutaneous T-cell lymphoma. Actas Dermosifiliogr. 2014;105(7):716–8.
85. Phan NQ, Bernhard JD, Luger TA, Stander S. Antipruritic treatment with systemic mu-opioid receptor antagonists: a review. J Am Acad Dermatol. 2010;63(4):680–8.
86. Dawn AG, Yosipovitch G. Butorphanol for treatment of intractable pruritus. J Am Acad Dermatol. 2006; 54(3):527–31.
87. Inui S. Nalfurafine hydrochloride to treat pruritus: a review. Clin Cosmet Investig Dermatol. 2015;8:249–55.
88. Anderson TF, Waldinger TP, Voorhees JJ. UV-B phototherapy. An overview. Arch Dermatol. 1984; 120(11):1502–7.
89. Lavda AC, Webb TL, Thompson AR. A meta-analysis of the effectiveness of psychological interventions for adults with skin conditions. Br J Dermatol. 2012; 167(5):970–9.
90. Wulf HC, Sandby-Møller J, Kobayasi T, Gniadecki R. Skin aging and natural photoprotection. Micron. 2004;35(3):185–91.

Physiological Variations During Aging

40

Gérald E. Piérard, Claudine Piérard-Franchimont, Philippe Delvenne, and Jean-Luc Nizet

Contents

G.E. Piérard (✉)
Laboratory of Skin Bioengineering and Imaging, Department of Dermatopathology, University Hospital of Liège, Liège, Belgium
e-mail: Gerald.pierard@ulg.ac.be

C. Piérard-Franchimont
Laboratory of Skin Bioengineering and Imaging, Department of Dermatopathology, University Hospital of Liège, Liège, Belgium

Department of Dermatology, Regional Hospital of Huy, Huy, Belgium
e-mail: claudine.franchimont@ulg.ac.be

P. Delvenne
Department of Dermatopathology, University Hospital of Liège, Liège, Belgium
e-mail: p.delvenne@ulg.ac.be

J.-L. Nizet
Department of Plastic Surgery, University Hospital of Liège, Liège, Belgium
e-mail: jlnizet@chu.ulg.ac.be

M.A. Farage et al. (eds.), *Textbook of Aging Skin*,
DOI 10.1007/978-3-662-47398-6_6

Abstract
In any individual, physical growth and senescence are characterized by cumulative progression of interlocking biological events. There is evidence that aging progresses differently among individuals of similar age. In addition, each and every organ of the human body develops and progressively fails at its own rate, which is referred to as its biological age. Clinically relevant skin aging mechanisms include chronological influence, environmental aging and photoaging, phototype and ethnicity-related aging (genetic type), endocrine aging, catabolic aging, and gravitational aging. All individuals perceive a global appearance of skin aging. By contrast, prevention and correction of skin aging typically benefit from targeting some of the specific underlying biologic processes.

Introduction

In affluent societies of the developed world, an extraordinary shift in the age distribution of the populations has taken place over the past decades. Indeed, older people progressively represent a rising segment of the overall demographic profile. Such an evolution where nobody escapes from aging is correlated with the progressive individual decrease in youthful appearance, which in turn has important social implications. As a result, any newer medical, cosmeceutical, and cosmetic antiaging modality is avidly watched by aging individuals. In addition, some middle-aged and younger subjects already show a craze for cosmetic dermatology beginning with the early incipient signs of wear and tear. Hopefully, real breakthroughs in dermocosmetic procedures including novel treatments fulfill some of the expectations and promises. In addition, technological advances at the forefront for the management of skin aging are supported by an increased understanding of the relationships between skin biology, skin physiology, and the ultimate clinical appearance.

Physical growth and senescence are both characterized by cumulative progression of interlocking biological events. They in part proceed at some time in life, seemingly evolving in tandem. Globally, aging is a physiological process corresponding to a progressive impairment in the homeostatic and adaptive homeodynamic capacities of the body systems, ultimately increasing the susceptibility and vulnerability to some environmental threats and internal changes. While aging is associated with a slower rate in cutaneous wound healing, it is paradoxically associated with an improvement in the quality of scarring.

The global aging process is quite complex. It becomes severe in cases where the impaired skin has lost most of its protective biological and mechanical functions. In these circumstances, skin atrophy becomes considerably disabling when the aspect of the so-called transparent skin, atrophoderma, or "dermatoporosis" is reached [1]. The corresponding clinical manifestations encompass a series of markers of fragility including senile purpura, stellate pseudoscars, and skin thinning. Skin fragility leads to frequent lacerations following minor traumas. A variable combination of delayed wound healing, nonhealing atrophic ulcers, subcutaneous bleeding, and dissecting hematomas is at the origin of large necrotic areas.

From Global to Molecular Aging and Back Again

All living organisms are engaged in a combination of multifaceted aging processes showing interspecies variations. Two complementary classifications of life histories are of major importance in the biologic definition of aging. The first classification distinguishes species that, on the one hand, show a clear distinction between germ cells and somatic tissues from those, on the other hand, that do not. The second classification distinguishes the semelparous species reproducing only once in their lifetime from the iteroparous species that reproduce repeatedly. It is mistaken to regard the post-reproductive end of life of semelparous species, which usually occurs in a highly determinate fashion, as being comparable with the more protracted process of senescence in iteroparous species.

There is evidence that aging progresses differently among individuals of similar age. In addition,

Table 1 Core age markers of each of the body system (After Braverman [2])

Aging type	Decline in	Average onset age
Electropause	Electrical activity of brain waves	45
Biopause	Neurotransmitters	Dopamine 30, acetylcholine 40, GABA 50, serotonin 60
Pineal pause	Melatonin	20
Pituitary pause	Hormone feedback loops	30
Sensory pause	Touch, hearing, vision, taste, and smell sensitivity	40
Psychopause	Personality health and mood	30
Thyropause	Calcitonin and thyroid hormone levels	50
Parathyropause	Parathyroid hormone	50
Thymopause	Glandular size and immune system	40
Cardiopause/ vasculopause	Ejection fraction and blood flow	50
Pulmonopause	Lung elasticity and function with increase in blood pressure	50
Adrenopause	DHEA	55
Nephropause	Erythropoietin level and creatinine clearance	40
Somatopause	Growth hormone	30
Gastropause	Nutrient absorption	40
Pancropause	Blood sugar level	40
Insulopause	Glucose tolerance	40
Andropause	Testosterone in men	45
Menopause	Estrogen, progesterone, and testosterone in women	40
Osteopause	Bone density	30
Dermopause	Collagen, vitamin D synthesis	35
Onchopause	Nail growth	40
Uropause	Bladder control	45
Genopause	DNA	40

each and every organ of the human body develops and progressively fails at its own rate, which is referred to as its biological age [2]. Senescence is heterogeneous at other levels including tissues, cells, and subcellular structures [3]. Intracellular and extracellular molecular compounds are involved differently by aging. However, within each organ system, aging manifests as a progressive almost linear reduction in maximal function and reserve capacity. Although some aspects of aging appear as a predetermined programmed process, many of the age-associated physiological decrements result in part from environmental insults and/or from endogenous failures.

The global but heterogeneous aging process occurs throughout the entire body from the time of about 30–45 years of age (Table 1). To further make the situation more complex, some regional variability is present in skin aging over the body. It is indeed quite evident that at any time in adult life, distinct body sites show different manifestations or stages of aging. In addition, scrutinizing skin aging at the tissue level (epidermis, dermis, hypodermis, hair follicle) and further at the cellular level (keratinocyte, melanocyte, fibroblast, dermal dendrocyte, endothelial cells, etc.) shows a patchwork of aging severity.

Cellular Senescence in Perspective

Several basic cellular mechanisms are involved in the aging process, namely, the telomere shortening, the oxidative stress, the mitochondrial dysfunction, and a series of genetic mechanisms [4].

Granted that death is the ultimate failure of the organisms, the aging process itself is considered to bring about the termination of the replicative ability of cells when the individual becomes progressively older. The age of any tissue appears to be reflected in the behavior of their cultured cells [5]. Replicative senescence of human cells is thus related to and perhaps caused by the exhaustion of their proliferative potential. At each cell division, cells lose some of their telomere repeats corresponding to specific DNA sequences at the end of linear DNA [6]. According to the telomere hypothesis, somatic cells lack a sustained activity of telomerase to maintain the telomere repeats allowing replication. The telomere shortening is attributed to the accumulation of DNA single-strand breaks induced by oxidative stress. Since telomere length predicts the replicative capacity of cells, it is thought to provide one of the best biomarkers for cellular aging [7].

Aging is associated to free radical damages by a variety of reactive oxygen species (ROS) including superoxide and hydroxyl radicals, as well as other activated forms of oxygen such as hydrogen peroxide and singlet oxygen [8]. In the intracellular machinery, mitochondriae are the primary sites of ROS production. Oxidative injury is minimized by superoxide dismutase, catalase, glutathione peroxidase, glutathione transferases, thiol-specific antioxidant enzymes, and other compounds including melatonin [4]. In addition, ROS play a role in normal signaling processes. Their generation is essential to maintain homeostasis and cellular responsiveness [9].

The so-called stress-induced premature senescence (SIPS) occurs following a series of sublethal stresses including those induced by hydrogen peroxide and a variety of other ROS [10]. Of note, cells engaged in replicative senescence share common features with cells involved in SIPS [10]. Thus, SIPS could be a mechanism of the in vivo accumulation of senescent-like cells in the skin [11].

Mitochondriae are both producers and targets of oxidative stress thus forming the basis for the mitochondrial theory of aging. With advanced age, the activity of the mitochondrial respiratory system declines, eventually leading to apoptosis [12–14]. It is acknowledged that alterations in the mechanisms of apoptosis result from genetically programmed features and oxidative stress as well [15, 16].

Cellular senescence and cancer are closely related by several biologic aspects including p53 mutation [17, 18], telomere shortening [6, 19], vitamin A depletion [20], and defects in intercellular communications [21]. The age-related mottled faint (subclinical) melanoderma might be a predictive sign for a skin carcinoma-prone condition [22, 23].

Clinically Relevant Skin Aging Mechanisms

In the past, human aging was perceived as one single chronologic process of physiologic decline with age. However, this process exhibits multiple facets altering differently the organs and their tissues and cells. This is particularly obvious in the skin. For years, the understanding of aging skin has benefited from the distinction between the intrinsic chronological aging and photoaging [24, 25]. According to this concept, the changes observed in the aging skin appearance reflect two main processes (Table 2). First, the intrinsic changes in the aging skin are caused by the passage of time modulated by hereditary factors, along with modifications occurring inherently in the structure, physiology, and mechanobiology. Second, photodamage is a result of the cumulative exposure of the skin to ultraviolet (UV) light [25] and near-infrared (NIR) radiations [26]. Clinically, these two distinct types of aging manifest differently, with intrinsic aging being responsible for dry-looking, pale, and smooth to finely wrinkled skin. By contrast, photoaging gives rise to coarse, roughened, and deeply wrinkled skin accompanied by pigmentary changes such as solar lentigines and mottled melanosis [22]. Differences between such duality in aging types can be seen in given individuals when comparing an area of skin commonly exposed to the sun, for example, the face, the neck, and the dorsal hands, with an area commonly masked from the sun, for example, buttock skin.

Table 2 Comparison of intrinsic aging and photoaging

Feature	Intrinsic aging	Photoaging
Clinical appearance	Smooth texture, unblemished surface	Nodular, leathery surface Sallow complexion yellowish mottled pigmentation
	Fine wrinkles	Coarse wrinkles
	Some deepening of skin surface markings	Severe loss of elasticity
	Some loss of elasticity, redundant skin	
Epidermis	Thin and viable	Marked acanthosis, cellular atypia, skin field carcinogenesis, most skin cancers
Elastic tissue	Increased, but almost normal	Tremendous increase, altered as elastotic amorphous mass
Collagen	Thick, disoriented bundles	Marked decrease of bundles and fibers
Glycosaminoglycans	Slightly decreased	Markedly increased
Reticular dermis	Thinner	Thickened, elastosis
	Fibroblasts decreased, inactive	Fibroblasts increased, hyperactive
	Mast cells decreased, no inflammation	Mast cells markedly increased, mixed inflammatory infiltrate
Papillary dermis	No grenz zone	Solar elastosis with grenz zone
Microvasculature	Moderate loss	Great loss, abnormal and telangiectatic
Subcutaneous fat	Focal shrinkage	Unaffected
	Focal hypertrophy	
Hair	Hair thinning	Discoloration
	Graying hair	
	Hypertrichosis	

This concept based on a duality in skin aging has been challenged because it appears as an oversimplification in clinical practice [27]. In addition, recent evidence indicates that chronologically aged and UV-irradiated skin share important molecular features [8, 9, 28, 29]. Oxidative stress is thought to play a central role in initiating and driving the signaling events that lead to cellular response following UV and IR exposures. These features suggest that nonionizing radiations accelerate many key aspects of the chronological aging process in human skin [26].

In order to better cope with the diversity of clinical presentations of skin in the elderly, another classification of skin aging in seven distinct types was offered (Table 3). The most important categories included the endocrine and overall metabolic status, the past and present lifestyle, and several environmental threats, including cumulative UV and IR exposures, as well as repeated mechanical prompting by muscles and gravitational forces [27]. In this framework, the past history of the subject is emphasized. Accordingly, the global aging is considered to represent the cumulative or synergistic effects of specific features, each of them being independent from the others. Such a concept allows to individualize or integrate typical processes including among others perimenopausal aging and smoking effects.

Table 3 Cutaneous aging types (After Piérard [26])

Aging type	Determinant factor
Genetic	Genetic (premature aging syndromes, phototype-related, ethnic background)
Chronologic	Time
Actinic	Ultraviolet and infrared irradiations
Behavioral	Tobacco, alcoholic abuse, drug addiction, facial expressions
Endocrinological	Pregnancy, physiological and hormonal influences (ovaries, testes, thyroid)
Catabolic	Chronic intercurrent debilitating disease (infections, cancers), nutritional deficiencies
Gravitational	Earth gravity

Increased awareness of the distinct age-associated physiological changes in the skin allows for more effective and specific preventive measures, skin care regimens, and dermatological treatment strategies in the elderly. As a consequence, the immutability of diverse factors in skin aging was challenged [3, 30]. However, factors of skin aging share some common mechanisms [31]. For instance, molecular mechanisms imply hyaluronate-CD44 pathways in the control and maintenance of epithelial growth, and the viscoelastic properties of the ECM offer new opportunities for preventive interventions [1].

Environmental Aging and Photoaging

Environment produces obvious alterations in the texture and quality of the skin, the major extrinsic insults being chronic exposures to UV and IR [26]. The action spectrum of photodamages is not fully characterized. The cumulative effects from repeated exposures to suberythemal doses of UVB, UVA, and IRA in human skin are involved in these processes [26, 32, 33].

In photoaging, the role of UVB in elastin promoter activation is established. In addition, UVA significantly contributes to long-term actinic damage, and the spectral dependence for cumulative damages does not parallel the erythemal spectrum for acute UV injury in human beings. The earliest detectable response of the skin cell to UV irradiation is the activation of multiple cell surface receptors to cytokines and growth factors including epidermal growth factor receptor (EGF-R). TNF-α receptor, platelet activating factor (PAF) receptor, insulin receptor, interleukin (IL)-1 receptor, and platelet-derived growth factor (PDGF) receptor [28].

Nonionizing radiations initiate a number of cellular responses, including ROS production within both dermal and epidermal cells. The so-called SIPS (stress-induced parameter senescence) phenomenon is engaged [10]. More specifically, cultures of keratinocytes derived from donors of different ages and from paired sun-exposed and sun-protected sites of older donors demonstrate that both chronological aging and photoaging affect quite distinctly some gene expressions. For instance, chronological aging strikingly increases the baseline expressions of the differentiation-associated gene SPR2 (small proline-rich protein) and of the IL-1 receptor antagonist gene. By contrast, it has relatively little effect on the UV inducibility of several other genes including the protooncogenes c-myc and c-fos, the GADD 153, a gene inducible by growth arrest and DNA damage, and the IL-1α and 1L-β genes. Photoaging appears different because it increases the UV inducibility of c-fos while decreasing the baseline expression of the differentiation-associated genes IL-1ra and SPR2 [34, 35]. The physiological consequences of photodamages occur at variable pace on the different skin structures. For instance, both skin loosening and solar elastosis exhibit clinical manifestations independently from the severity in the mottled faint melanoderma [22].

IR radiations are nonionizing, electromagnetic radiations accounting for more than half of the solar energy reaching human skin. The IR wavelengths range between 760 nm and 1 mm and are further divided into IRA, IRB, and IRC. While IRB and IRC do not penetrate deeply into the skin, more than 65 % of IRA reaches the dermis. Human skin is increasingly exposed to IRA radiation. The most relevant sources are (a) natural solar radiation consisting of over 30 % IRA, (b) artificial IRA sources used for therapeutic or wellness purposes, and (c) artificial UVA sources supplemented with IRA. As part of natural sunlight, IRA significantly contributes to extrinsic photoaging.

Photoaging affects both the epidermis and dermis. The epidermis becomes more atrophic than on sun-protected areas often with disordered keratinocyte maturation. This probably represents an early step in actinic field carcinogenesis [23]. Key histological features of photoaged skin are most apparent in the dermis where the ECM is altered in its composition [36]. The collagen network is responsible for most skin strength and resiliency and is intimately involved in the expression of photoaging. The major fibrillar collagen component of the dermal ECM belongs to the type I and III collagens. In photoaged human skin, precursors of both proteins are markedly reduced in the papillary dermis, and their reduction correlates with the clinical severity of photoaging [37]. This reduction results from a combination of decreased procollagen biosynthesis contrasting with an increased enzymatic breakdown by matrix metalloproteinases (MMPs) [38]. Furthermore, collagen breakdown products negatively influence the procollagen biosynthesis by fibroblasts [39]. Fibrillar collagens are closely associated with decorin, a small chondroitin sulfate proteoglycan. Its distribution closely mirrors that of type I collagen in the dermis, regardless of level of extrinsic aging [40]. Decorin makes connections between the fibrillar collagens and the microfibril-forming type VI collagen with further interaction with type IV collagen in the basement membrane at the dermoepidermal junction. Therefore, type VI collagen is likely to play an important physiological role in the organization of the dermal ECM. It is abundant in the papillary dermis, and it seems little affected by photoaging [41]. Type VII collagen is the major constituent of anchoring fibrils below the basement membrane providing cohesiveness between the epidermis and dermis. In photoaged skin, the number of anchoring fibrils along the basement membrane is reduced, thus increasing the potential for fragility and blistering in photoaged skin [42]. It was reported to be involved in the mechanism of wrinkle formation.

The elastic fiber network is responsible for recoil and elasticity to the skin. The process of elastic fiber formation is under tight developmental control, involving tropoelastin deposition on a preformed framework made of fibrillin-rich microfibrils. Mature elastic fibers are encased in fibrillin and form a continuous network throughout the dermis. The elastic fiber network comprises thick elastin-rich fibers within the reticular dermis, finer fibers with reduced elastin content in the lower papillary dermis, and a meshwork of discrete fibrillin-rich microfibrillar bundles, with only discrete elastin, in the upper papillary dermis merging with the dermoepidermal junction. Fibrillin is both a product of fibroblasts and keratinocytes. The elastic fiber network is considerably disrupted and clumped in chronically photoaged skin. First, photoaged skin contains abundant amounts of dystrophic elastotic material in the reticular dermis [43], which is immunopositive for tropoelastin, fibrillin, lysozyme, and immunoglobulins [44] Versican, a large chondroitin sulfate proteoglycan, appears to be regulated along with dystrophic elastin resulting in a relative increase in photoaging. The fibrillin-rich microfibrils are markedly altered since the early stages of photoaging [45].

All structural changes found in the dermis particularly affect the biomechanical properties of the skin. A cutaneous extrinsic aging score was derived from the difference between comparative photoexposed and photoprotected areas [46].

Phototype and Ethnicity-Related Aging

The most obvious ethnic skin difference relates to skin color which is dominated by the presence of melanin [47, 48] affording relative photoprotection. The rate of skin aging commonly varies between different racial groups, although none of the groups escapes the photoaging process. Generally, Caucasians present an earlier onset and a deeper skin wrinkling and sagging than other skin phototypes. In general, increased pigmentary problems develop in skin of color, although East Asians living in Europe and North America exhibit less pigment spots with age. Induction of a melanotic response to sun exposure is thought to occur through signaling by the protease-activated receptor (PAR)-2 which together with its activating protease is increased in the epidermis of subjects with skin of color [49]. Changes in skin biophysical properties with age demonstrate that subjects of dark complexion keep younger skin properties compared with the more lightly pigmented individuals.

Endocrine Aging

Skin is recognized as a hormone-dependent organ [50–52]. Irrespective of age, most of the skin components are under the physiological control of endocrine and neuroendocrine factors (Table 4). The whole endocrine system is affected

Table 4 Neuroendocrine receptors active in the skin

1. Adrenergic receptors
2. Androgen and estrogen receptors
3. Calcitonin gene-related peptide receptor (CGRP-R)
4. Cholinergic receptors
5. Corticotropin-releasing hormone and urocortin receptors (CRH-R)
6. Glucocorticoid and mineralocorticoid receptors
7. Glutamate receptors
8. Growth hormone receptor (GH-R)
9. Histamine receptors
10. Melanocortin receptors (MC-R)
11. Miscellaneous neuropeptide receptors
12. Miscellaneous receptors
13. Neurokinin receptors (NK-R)
14. Neurotrophin receptors (NT-R)
15. Opioid receptors
16. Parathormone (PTH) and PTH-related protein (PTHrP) receptors
17. PRL and LH/CG receptors (LH/CG-R)
18. Serotonin receptors
19. Thyroid hormone receptors
20. Vasoactive intestinal peptide receptor (VIP-R)
21. Vitamin D receptor (VDR)

by the global aging process. Like any other system in the body, aging of the hormonal functions basically results in deteriorations expressed by deficiencies which in turn influence the aging machinery operative in the skin. Quite distinct are the skin manifestations of some endocrinopathies which mimic or interfere with skin aging [50–52]. They are mostly related to the declined activity of the pituitary gland, adrenal glands, ovaries, and testes.

Some hormones and neurotransmitters are synthesized by nerves, as well as by epithelial and dermal cells in the skin (Table 5). A number of environmental and intrinsic factors regulate the level of the cutaneous neuroendocrine system activity. Solar radiation, temperature, environmental moisture, as well as diverse chemical and biological xenobiotics represent important environmental factors. Some internal mechanisms affecting the neuroendocrine system of the skin are possibly generated in reaction to some environmental signals or result from local biological rhythms or from local or general disease processes [51].

Table 5 Hormones and neurotransmitters produced by the skin

1. Hypothalamic and pituitary hormones
2. Neuropeptides and neurotrophins
3. Neurotransmitters/neurohormones
4. Other steroid hormones
5. Parathormone-related protein
6. Sex steroid hormones
7. Thyroid hormones

The paradigm of deleterious hormonal effects is represented by the induction of skin atrophy by corticosteroids. Cushing syndrome and iatrogenic effects of topical and systemic corticotherapy are equally involved. Corticosteroids are known to regulate the expression of genes encoding collagens I, III, IV, V, decorin; elastin; MMPs 1, 2, and 3; tenascin; and tissue inhibitors of MMPs 1 and 2 [53]. However, the precise molecular mechanisms of skin atrophy induced by corticosteroids remain unsettled. The corticosteroid-induced atrophy can be one of the most severe forms of skin aging corresponding to dermatoporosis [1].

The most important endocrine compound produced by the skin is vitamin D, which is a regulator of the calcium metabolism and exhibits other systemic effects as well. For example, epidemiological evidence suggests that sunlight deprivation with associated reduction in the circulating level of vitamin D_3 apparently results in increased incidence of carcinomas of the breast, colon, and prostate [54]. Vitamin D_3 and its analogues also modulate the biology of keratinocytes and melanocytes of the skin in vivo [55].

Growth hormone (GH) is secreted by the pituitary gland under the control of several hypothalamic and peripheral modulators that exert either positive or negative influences [42]. The final balance among the modulating factors determines the pulsatile and circadian secretion of GH. Moreover, physiological changes occurring during aging affect the GH secretion. The peripheral effects of GH are mainly exerted by insulin-like growth factor (IGF)-1, produced by the liver upon GH stimulation. The circulating IGF-1 is bioavailable and functionally active depending upon its binding with the IGF-binding proteins (IGF-Bps).

Skin is a target of the GH-IGF system that exerts a significant influence on the dermal and epidermal physiology [56]. GH, IGF-1, IGF-2, and IGF-Bps are present in the skin and are involved in its physiologic homeostasis, including the dermoepidermal cross-talking. Thus, systemic paracrine and/or autocrine cutaneous activity of the GH-IGF system contributes to skin homeostasis [56, 57]. The global GH system is abated during aging. GH supplementation induces skin changes, a part of which may correspond to some corrective effects on aging skin [58, 59].

The progressive decline in DHEA serum concentration with age and conversely its supplementation has not demonstrated prominent effects on the skin except on sebum production.

Sex hormones manifest a variety of biological and immunological effects in the skin [60]. In responsive women, estrogen, alone or together with progesterone, has been reported to prevent or reverse skin atrophy, dryness, and wrinkles associated with chronological aging or photoaging. In responsive women, estrogen and progesterone stimulate proliferation of keratinocytes, while estrogen suppresses apoptosis and thus prevents epidermal atrophy. Estrogen also enhances collagen synthesis, and estrogen and progesterone suppress collagenolysis by reducing MMP activity in fibroblasts, thereby maintaining skin thickness. Estrogen maintains skin moisture by increasing hyaluronic acid levels in the dermis. Progesterone increases sebum excretion.

Both the perimenopause and the andropause decade negatively affect the skin [60–62]. Hormone replacement therapy (HRT) during perimenopause helps limit these changes [63–65]. However, there is a limitation because it seems to exist good and poor responders [66]. Smoking habit possibly interferes with the treatment result [67].

Catabolic Aging

The elderly is often accompanied by a substandard diet deficiency in many of the nutrients thought to be essential for maintaining health. Protein-containing foods such as meat and fish tend to be too expensive or troublesome to prepare. Dietary faddism, confusional states, and forgetfulness are also responsible for an inadequate diet. These conditions predispose to skin changes that often amplify the alterations induced by age-related deficiencies.

Any insufficient intake of fresh fruit and/or vegetables leads to vitamin C deficiency and ultimately to scurvy. It is responsible for a defect in coagulation and purpura, particularly in a typical punctate perifollicular pattern on the legs. In the elderly, iron deficiency is common and potentially leads to anemia, generalized pruritus, and diffuse hair loss.

Essential fatty acid and vitamin A deficiencies due to dietary faddism or deprivation in the elderly are responsible for xerosis [68]. Many of the elderly are also deficient in zinc, and this may impair wound healing. Zinc supplementation, however, does not improve healing.

Chronic hemodialysis is another model of catabolic aging affecting the mechanical properties of the skin [69, 70].

Gravitational Aging

Skin of any part of the body is subjected to intrinsic and extrinsic mechanical forces. Among them, earth gravitation influences skin folding and sagging during aging. Any force generated by the skin or applied to it transduces information to cells that may in turn respond to it [71, 72]. The effects of mechanobiology are particularly evident in fibroblasts, dermal dendrocytes, keratinocytes, and melanocytes [73–75]. Gravitational forces involve mechanotransduction in the skin [76] and affect cell tensegrity and the cell mechanosensitive ion channels. As a result, the structure of the dermal extracellular matrix is affected.

Diversity of Wrinkles

There is evidence that wrinkles are not related to the genuine microrelief [77, 78]. In addition, the microanatomical support of wrinkles is varied

[77–80]. It depends on subtle changes in the structure of the superficial dermis, as well as elastotic deposits in the upper reticular dermis, loosening of the hypodermal connective tissue strands, or, conversely, on focal hypertrophic binding of the dermis to the underlying facial muscles [78, 80]. The wrinkle severity rating [81] is influenced by the nature of the altered connective tissue. Similarly, the skin mechanical properties are under such influences [82, 83].

Photoaged facial skin does not always present clinically with characteristic wrinkling. In some individuals, usually of light phototype, smooth unwrinkled skin and telangiectasia predominate. These people appear to be more at risk of developing basal cell carcinomas on sun-exposed facial skin [84, 85]. There is an apparent inverse relationship between the degree of facial wrinkling and the occurrence of facial basal cell carcinomas [85]. Mechanistically, little is known regarding how these two clinical outcomes occur in response to the same sun exposure stimulus.

Smoking effects on skin aging are probably mediated by the increased production of collagenase, and elastase is an additional cause of wrinkling [86–88]. Degradation of elastic fibers by ROS and repeated mechanical promptings by some muscle contractions play a putative role in the formation of the so-called smoker's wrinkles.

Conclusions

Aging is apparent at all levels of the physiology and anatomy of the body. Organs, tissues, cells, and molecules have their own aging processes which differ in their clinical relevance. Since the introduction of in vivo reflectance confocal microscopy, this method is open to improve the perception of aging in the superficial layers of the skin [89–92]. All individuals perceive a global appearance of skin aging. By contrast, prevention and correction of skin aging typically benefit from targeting some of the specific underlying biologic processes as structural changes. So-called rejuvenation of skin modulated by stem cells [93, 94] could possibly interfere with the present concepts about aging in a near future.

Cross-References

► The Stratum Corneum and Aging

References

1. Piérard-Franchimont C, et al. Dermatoporosis, a vintage for atrophoderma and transparent skin. Rev Med Liege. 2014;69:210–3.
2. Braverman ER. Ageprint for anti-ageing medicine. J Eur Anti-ageing Med. 2005;1:7–8.
3. Piérard GE. Ageing across the life span: time to think again. J Cosmet Dermatol. 2004;3:50–3.
4. Slominski AT, et al. Local melatoninergic system as the protector of skin integrity. Int J Mol Sci. 2014;15:17705–32.
5. Campisi J. From cells to organisms: can we learn about aging from cells in culture? Exp Gerontol. 2001;36:607–18.
6. Kim Sh SH, et al. Telomeres, aging and cancer: in search of a happy ending. Oncogene. 2002;21:503–11.
7. Orren DK. Werner syndrome: molecular insights into the relationships between defective DNA metabolism, genomic instability, cancer and aging. Front Biosci. 2006;11:2657–71.
8. Rattan SI. Theories of biological aging: genes, proteins, and free radicals. Free Radic Res. 2006;40:1230–8.
9. Martindale JL, Holbrook NJ. Cellular response to oxidative stress: signaling for suicide and survival. J Cell Physiol. 2002;192:1–15.
10. Toussaint O, et al. Cellular and molecular mechanisms of stress-induced premature senescence (SIPS) of human diploid fibroblasts and melanocytes. Exp Gerontol. 2000;35:927–45.
11. Hadshiew IM, et al. Skin aging and photoaging: the role of DNA damage and repair. Am J Contact Dermat. 2000;11:19–25.
12. Lesnefsky EJ, Hoppel CL. Oxidative phosphorylation and aging. Ageing Res Rev. 2006;5:402–33.
13. Linford NJ, et al. Oxidative damage and aging: spotlight on mitochondria. Cancer Res. 2006;66:2497–9.
14. Paquet P, Piérard GE. Toxic epidermal necrolysis: revisiting the tentative link between early apoptosis and late necrosis (review). Int J Mol Med. 2007;19:3–10.
15. Orrenius S, et al. Mitochondrial oxidative stress: implications for cell death. Annu Rev Pharmacol Toxicol. 2007;47:143–83.
16. Warner HR. Is cell death and replacement a factor in aging? Mech Ageing Dev. 2007;128:13–6.
17. Itahana K, et al. Regulation of cellular senescence by p53. Eur J Biochem. 2001;268:2784–91.
18. Campisi J. Between Scylla and Charybdis: p53 links tumor suppression and aging. Mech Aging Dev. 2002;123:567–73.

19. Campisi J, et al. Cellular senescence, cancer and aging: the telomere connection. Exp Gerontol. 2001; 36:1619–37.
20. Saurat JH. Skin, sun, and vitamin A: from aging to cancer. J Dermatol. 2001;28:595–8.
21. Krtolica A, et al. Senescent fibroblasts promote epithelial cell growth and tumorigenesis: a link between cancer and aging. Proc Natl Acad Sci U S A. 2001;98:12072–7.
22. Petit L, et al. Regional variability in mottled subclinical melanoderma in the elderly. Exp Gerontol. 2003;38:327–31.
23. Quatresooz P, et al. Crossroads between actinic keratosis and squamous cell carcinoma, and novel pharmacological issues. Eur J Dermatol. 2008;18:6–10.
24. Farage MA, et al. Intrinsic and extrinsic factors in skin ageing: a review. Int J Cosmet Sci. 2008;30:87–95.
25. Sanches Silveira JE, Myaki Pedroso DM. UV light and skin aging. Rev Environ Health. 2014;29:243–54.
26. Schroeder P, et al. The role of near infrared radiation in photoaging of the skin. Exp Gerontol. 2008;43:629–32.
27. Piérard GE. The quandary of climacteric skin ageing. Dermatology. 1996;193:273–4.
28. Matsumura Y, Ananthaswamy HN. Short-term and long-term cellular and molecular events following UV irradiation of skin: implications for molecular medicine. Expert Rev Mol Med. 2002;4:1–22.
29. Sander CS, et al. Photoaging is associated with protein oxidation in human skin in vivo. J Invest Dermatol. 2002;118:618–25.
30. de Grey AD, et al. Time to talk SENS: critiquing the immutability of human aging. Ann N Y Acad Sci. 2002;959:452–62. discussion 463–55.
31. Giacomoni PU, Rein G. Factors of skin ageing share common mechanisms. Biogerontology. 2001;2:219–29.
32. Pierard GE. Ageing in the sun parlour. Int J Cosmet Sci. 1998;20:251–9.
33. Piérard SL, et al. Greenhouse gas-related climate changes and some expected skin alterations. Austin J Dermatol. 2014;1:3.
34. Bender K, et al. UV-induced signal transduction. J Photochem Photobiol B. 1997;37:1–17.
35. Yaar M, Gilchrest BA. Aging versus photoaging: postulated mechanisms and effectors. J Investig Dermatol Symp Proc. 1998;3:47–51.
36. Ma W, et al. Chronological ageing and photoageing of the fibroblasts and the dermal connective tissue. Clin Exp Dermatol. 2001;26:592–9.
37. Talwar HS, et al. Reduced type I and type III procollagens in photodamaged adult human skin. J Invest Dermatol. 1995;105:285–90.
38. Varani J, et al. Inhibition of type I procollagen production in photodamage: correlation between presence of high molecular weight collagen fragments and reduced procollagen synthesis. J Invest Dermatol. 2002;119:122–9.
39. Varani J, et al. Inhibition of type I procollagen synthesis by damaged collagen in photoaged skin and by collagenase-degraded collagen in vitro. Am J Pathol. 2001;158:931–42.
40. Bernstein EF, et al. Differential expression of the versican and decorin genes in photoaged and sun-protected skin. Comparison by immunohistochemical and northern analyses. Lab Invest. 1995;72:662–9.
41. Watson RE, et al. Distribution and expression of type VI collagen in photoaged skin. Br J Dermatol. 2001;144:751–9.
42. Watson RE, Griffiths CE. Pathogenic aspects of cutaneous photoaging. J Cosmet Dermatol. 2005;4:230–6.
43. Sellheyer K. Pathogenesis of solar elastosis: synthesis or degradation? J Cutan Pathol. 2003;30:123–7.
44. Piérard-Franchimont C, et al. Androgenic alopecia and stress-induced premature senescence by cumulative ultraviolet light exposure. Exog Dermatol. 2002;1:203–6.
45. Watson RE, et al. Fibrillin-rich microfibrils are reduced in photoaged skin. Distribution at the dermal-epidermal junction. J Invest Dermatol. 1999;112:782–7.
46. Piérard GE, et al. Biomechanical assessment of photodamage. Derivation of a cutaneous extrinsic ageing score. Skin Res Technol. 1995;1:17–20.
47. Wesley NO, Maibach HI. Racial (ethnic) differences in skin properties: the objective data. Am J Clin Dermatol. 2003;4:843–60.
48. Rawlings AV. Ethnic skin types: are there differences in skin structure and function? Int J Cosmet Sci. 2006;28:79–93.
49. Seiberg M, et al. The protease-activated receptor 2 regulates pigmentation via keratinocyte-melanocyte interactions. Exp Cell Res. 2000;254:25–32.
50. Kanda N, Watanabe S. Regulatory roles of sex hormones in cutaneous biology and immunology. J Dermatol Sci. 2005;38:1–7.
51. Slominski A. Neuroendocrine system of the skin. Dermatology. 2005;211:199–208.
52. Szepetiuk G, et al. Biometrology of physical properties of skin in thyroid dysfunction. J Eur Acad Dermatol Venereol. 2008;22:1173–7.
53. Schoepe S, et al. Glucocorticoid therapy-induced skin atrophy. Exp Dermatol. 2006;15:406–20.
54. Giovannucci E, et al. Prospective study of predictors of vitamin D status and cancer incidence and mortality in men. J Natl Cancer Inst. 2006;98:451–9.
55. Piérard-Franchimont C, et al. Smoothing the mosaic subclinical melanoderma by calcipotriol. J Eur Acad Dermatol Venereol. 2007;21:657–61.
56. Edmondson SR, et al. Epidermal homeostasis: the role of the growth hormone and insulin-like growth factor systems. Endocr Rev. 2003;24:737–64.
57. Hyde C, et al. Insulin-like growth factors (IGF) and IGF-binding proteins bound to vitronectin enhance keratinocyte protein synthesis and migration. J Invest Dermatol. 2004;122:1198–206.
58. Rudman D, et al. Effects of human growth hormone in men over 60 years old. N Engl J Med. 1990;323:1–6.
59. Piérard-Franchimont C, et al. Mechanical properties of skin in recombinant human growth factor abusers among adult bodybuilders. Dermatology. 1996;192:389–92.

60. Piérard GE, et al. Effect of hormone replacement therapy for menopause on the mechanical properties of skin. J Am Geriatr Soc. 1995;43:662–5.
61. Paquet F, et al. Sensitive skin at menopause; dew point and electrometric properties of the stratum corneum. Maturitas. 1998;28:221–7.
62. Raine-Fenning NJ, et al. Skin aging and menopause: implications for treatment. Am J Clin Dermatol. 2003;4:371–8.
63. Quatresooz P, Piérard GE. Downgrading skin climacteric aging by hormone replacement therapy. Expert Rev Dermatol. 2007;2:373–6.
64. Sator PG, et al. A prospective, randomized, double-blind, placebo-controlled study on the influence of a hormone replacement therapy on skin aging in postmenopausal women. Climacteric. 2007;10:320–34.
65. Verdier-Sevrain S. Effect of estrogens on skin aging and the potential role of selective estrogen receptor modulators. Climacteric. 2007;10:289–97.
66. Piérard GE, et al. Comparative effect of hormone replacement therapy on bone mass density and skin tensile properties. Maturitas. 2001;40:221–7.
67. Castelo-Branco C, et al. Facial wrinkling in postmenopausal women. Effects of smoking status and hormone replacement therapy. Maturitas. 1998;29:75–86.
68. Uhoda E, et al. Ultraviolet light-enhanced visualization of cutaneous signs of carotene and vitamin A dietary deficiency. Acta Clin Belg. 2004;59:97–101.
69. Deleixhe-Mauhin F, et al. Influence of chronic haemodialysis on the mechanical properties of skin. Clin Exp Dermatol. 1994;19:130–3.
70. Uhoda I, et al. Effect of haemodialysis on acoustic shear wave propagation in the skin. Dermatology. 2004;209:95–100.
71. Wang N, et al. Mechanotransduction across the cell surface and through the cytoskeleton. Science. 1993;260:1124–7.
72. Silver FH, et al. Mechanobiology of force transduction in dermal tissue. Skin Res Technol. 2003;9:3–23.
73. Ingber DE. Tensegrity: the architectural basis of cellular mechanotransduction. Annu Rev Physiol. 1997;59:575–99.
74. Hermanns-Lê T, et al. Factor XIII a-positive dermal dendrocytes and shear wave propagation in human skin. Eur J Clin Invest. 2002;32:847–51.
75. Quatresooz P, et al. Mechanobiology and force transduction in scars developed in darker skin types. Skin Res Technol. 2006;12:279–82.
76. Nizet JL, et al. Influence of body posture and gravitational forces on shear wave propagation in the skin. Dermatology. 2001;202:177–80.
77. Piérard GE, et al. From skin microrelief to wrinkles. An area ripe for investigation. J Cosmet Dermatol. 2003;2:21–8.
78. Quatresooz P, et al. The riddle of genuine skin microrelief and wrinkles. Int J Cosmet Sci. 2006;28:389–95.
79. Bosset S, et al. Skin ageing: clinical and histopathologic study of permanent and reducible wrinkles. Eur J Dermatol. 2002;12:247–52.
80. Piérard GE, Lapière CM. The microanatomical basis of facial frown lines. Arch Dermatol. 1989;125:1090–2.
81. Day DJ, et al. The wrinkle severity rating scale: a validation study. Am J Clin Dermatol. 2004;5:49–52.
82. Hermanns-Lê T, et al. Age- and body mass index-related changes in cutaneous shear wave velocity. Exp Gerontol. 2001;36:363–72.
83. Hermanns-Lê T, et al. Skin tensile properties revisited during ageing. Where now, where next? J Cosmet Dermatol. 2004;3:35–40.
84. Kricker A, et al. Sun exposure and non-melanocytic skin cancer. Cancer Causes Control. 1994;5:367–92.
85. Brooke RC, et al. Discordance between facial wrinkling and the presence of basal cell carcinoma. Arch Dermatol. 2001;137:751–4.
86. Ernster VL, et al. Facial wrinkling in men and women, by smoking status. Am J Public Health. 1995;85:78–82.
87. Koh JS, et al. Cigarette smoking associated with premature facial wrinkling: image analysis of facial skin replicas. Int J Dermatol. 2002;41:21–7.
88. Raitio A, et al. Levels of matrix metalloproteinase-2, -9 and -8 in the skin, serum and saliva of smokers and non-smokers. Arch Dermatol Res. 2005;297:242–8.
89. Kawasaki K et al. Age-related morphometric changes of inner structures of the skin assessed by in vivo reflectance confocal microscopy. Int J Dermatol. 2014.
90. Longo C, et al. Skin aging: in vivo microscopic assessment of epidermal and dermal changes by means of confocal microscopy. J Am Acad Dermatol. 2013;68:e73–82.
91. Piérard GE. In vivo confocal microscopy: a new paradigm in dermatology. Dermatology. 1993;186:4–5.
92. Corcuff P, et al. In vivo confocal microscopy of human skin: a new design for cosmetology and dermatology. Scanning. 1996;18:351–5.
93. Lee HJ, et al. Efficacy of microneedling plus human stem cell conditioned medium for skin rejuvenation: a randomized, controlled, blinded split-face study. Ann Dermatol. 2014;26:584–91.
94. Tan KK, et al. Characterization of fetal keratinocytes, showing enhanced stem cell-like properties: a potential source of cells for skin reconstruction. Stem Cell Rep. 2014;3:324–38.

Neurotrophins and Skin Aging

41

Mohamed A. Adly, Hanan Assaf, and Mahmoud R. Hussein

Contents

M.A. Adly (✉)
Department of Zoology, Faculty of Science, Sohag University, Sohag, Egypt
e-mail: m.adly@yahoo.com

H. Assaf
Department of Dermatology, Saudi German Hospital, Jeddah, Saudi Arabia
e-mail: assaf_hanan@yahoo.com

M.R. Hussein
Department of Pathology, Assir Central Hospital, and Assuit University, Assuit, Egypt
e-mail: mrcpath17@gmail.com

M.A. Farage et al. (eds.), *Textbook of Aging Skin*,
DOI 10.1007/978-3-662-47398-6_15

Abstract

Cutaneous aging is a complex biological phenomenon that consists of two superimposed components: intrinsic (true aging) and extrinsic (photoaging) aging. Intrinsic aging is largely genetically determined and represents an inevitable change attributable to the passage of time alone. The intrinsic rate of skin aging in any individual is influenced by personal and environmental factors (primarily to UV). Detailed mechanisms for each of intrinsic and extrinsic factors will be discussed in this chapter.

Introduction

Cutaneous aging is a complex biological phenomenon that consists of two superimposed components: intrinsic (true aging) and extrinsic (photoaging) aging. Intrinsic aging is largely genetically determined and represents an inevitable change attributable to the passage of time alone. It resembles aging that is seen in most internal organs and its underlying mechanisms probably involve decreased proliferative capacity, leading to cellular senescence and altered biosynthetic activity of skin-derived cells. Intrinsic aging is manifested primarily by physiologic alterations with subtle but undoubtedly important consequences for both healthy and diseased skin. The morphologic changes of intrinsic aging include smoothing and thinning of the skin with exaggeration of the expression lines. The intrinsic rate of skin aging in any individual is dramatically influenced by personal and environmental factors, particularly the amount of exposure to ultraviolet light (UV), that is, intrinsic and extrinsic aging are superimposed processes. Extrinsic aging is caused by environmental exposure, primarily to UV. It is observed in the sun-exposed areas (photoaging) and is manifested by the presence of skin wrinkles, pigmented lesions, patchy hypopigmentations, and actinic keratoses. It involves changes in the cellular biosynthetic activity and usually leads to gross disorganization of the dermal matrix. Photodamage, which considerably accelerates the visible aging of skin, also greatly increases the risk of cutaneous neoplasia.

The molecular mechanisms underlying skin aging are poorly understood. They seem to be a multifaceted process influenced by various factors affecting different body sites at variable degrees. This chapter discusses the possible roles of some molecules involved in cutaneous aging, namely neurotrophins (NTs).

Overview of Neurotrophins

Neurotrophins (NTs) are a family of structurally and functionally related polypeptides, which show about 50 % amino acid sequence homology. NTs belong to a family of growth factors, which control the development, maintenance, and apoptotic death of neurons. They also have multiple regulatory functions outside the peripheral and central nervous systems [1–3]. The NTs family consists of four structurally and functionally related proteins known as nerve growth factor (NGF), brain-derived neurotrophic factor (BDNF), neurotrophin-3 (NT-3), and neurotrophin-4 (NT-4). It is well known that all four members of the NTs family are synthesized as precursors which are cleaved by intracellular proteases to release the C-terminal mature proteins [4]. Mature NT proteins are approximately 13 kDa in size and share about 50 % of amino acid sequence homology. They exert their biological effects as dimers interacting with specific receptors. High-affinity receptors for NTs belong to the tyrosine kinase family. Tyrosine kinase receptor A (TrkA) is the high-affinity receptor for NGF, tyrosine kinase receptor B (TrkB) is the high-affinity receptor for BDNF and NT-4, and tyrosine kinase receptor C (TrkC) is the high-affinity receptor for NT-3 [5]. However, NT-3 may also bind to TrkA and TrkB receptors but with low affinity. All four NTs interact with the low-affinity p75 kDa NT receptor (p75NTR), which is a member of the tumor necrosis factor family of receptors containing the cytoplasmic "death" domain, involved in mediating a number of responses independently or in association with Trk receptors [4, 6].

By interacting with Trk receptors and/or p75NTR, NTs induce a variety of biological responses in neurons as well as in nonneuronal cells. They control proliferation, differentiation, and survival, whereby these interactions occur. The signals promoting survival or differentiation are generated by NT interaction with Trk receptors and require receptor dimerization, autophosphorylation, and the subsequent involvement of a number of adaptor molecules coupling Trk receptors to the distinct intracellular signal transduction pathways [5]. NTs modulate synaptic transmission via Trk-associated regulation of intracellular Ca^{2+} and promote survival via phosphorylation and inactivation of several proapoptotic substrates including Bad. They promote differentiation via activation of the Ras/Raf/ERK kinase/mitogen-activated protein kinase cascade [5].

p75NTR performs distinct functions depending on whether it is coexpressed with Trk receptors and/or selected other growth factor receptors (sortilin, Nogo receptor complex), or whether it is expressed alone. The coexpression of p75NTR with Trk receptors increases high-affinity NT binding, enhances Trk ability to discriminate a preferred ligand from the other NTs, and promotes survival effects of the NTs [4, 6]. When p75NTR is coexpressed with sortilin (a non-G-protein-coupled neurotensin receptor), NT precursor proteins (pro-NTs) interacting with p75NTR-sortilin complex induce apoptotic death [7]. In case of coexpression of p75NTR with the Nogo receptor complex, Nogo induces growth inhibition [4]. When p75NTR is expressed alone on the cell surface, mature NT peptides or selected non-NT ligands (beta-amyloid or a fragment of the prion protein) are capable of inducing apoptosis or promote survival depending on the intracellular adaptor molecules present in target cells [4, 8]. Apoptotic signaling via p75NTR requires the presence of intracellular adaptor molecules (NT receptor-interacting factors 1 and 2, NT receptor-interacting MAGE homolog, and NT-associated death executor) that link p75NTR signaling with the JNK-p53-Bax proapoptotic pathway. However, signaling through p75NTR expressed alone – besides inducing apoptosis – may also promote cell survival. Intracellular adaptor molecules interacting with the C-terminus of p75NTR (TNF receptor-associated factor 6, Fas-associated phosphatase-1, and receptor-interacting protein-2) link p75NTR with the NF-κβ pathway and can thus promote survival. However, mechanisms involved in controlling the expression and preferential engagement of adaptor molecules in distinct cell types remain to be clarified.

NT Family Members Are Expressed in the Mammalian Skin

NTs were originally discovered in the nervous system where they were found to be involved in the differentiation and survival of the neurons. However, they were found to be expressed in a variety of tissues outside the nervous system where they have nonneuronal targets in the skin [3, 9–11], kidney, tooth, muscle, and heart [12].

In mice, NTs are expressed very early during embryonic development (E9.5–E10.5) in both the skin epithelium and the cutaneous mesenchyme [13]. The onset of NT expression in embryonic skin coincides with the time point of appearance of K5 and K14 in the epidermis (E9.5), whereas maximal NT synthesis coincides with the beginning of vibrissa development in facial skin (E12.5), and with the initiation of tylotrich hair follicle (HF) induction in dorsal murine skin (E14.5) [13]. This raises the hypothesis that NTs fulfill multiple nonneurotrophic functions during skin development.

In murine postnatal skin, NTs and their receptors are differentially distributed in distinct cell populations. NGF and NT-3 are expressed by basal epidermal keratinocytes in mice and humans [12, 14–21] (Fig. 1). They are also produced by fibroblasts in vitro, and NGF stimulates fibroblast migration [14, 15]. In situ, BDNF and NT-3 are expressed in cutaneous nerve fibers and myocytes of the arrector pili and panniculus carnosus muscles of mice [16, 17]. In adult human skin, NGF and NT-3 are also expressed by fibroblasts, arrector pili muscle, sebaceous and sweat glands, and hair follicles [15, 16] (Figs. 2 and 3). NT receptors (TrkA, TrkC, and p75NTR) have been detected on human epidermal keratinocytes [12, 14–19]. In murine skin, only TrkA and TrkB isoforms are seen in epidermal keratinocytes, whereas TrkC and p75NTR are expressed in cutaneous nerves and in the HF [16, 17].

NTs and Epidermal Homeostasis

Work over the past 10 years has indicated that NTs possess a range of functions outside the nervous system [12, 18, 19] and can be considered as growth factors in epithelial tissue homeostasis. It was demonstrated that normal human keratinocytes synthesize and secrete biologically active NGF [14, 20, 21]. In human skin, NGF is released in increasing amounts by proliferating keratinocytes, whereas secretion ends in more differentiated cells [22, 23]. Both exogenous and endogenous NGFs are capable of inducing keratinocyte proliferation [12, 14–19]. On the other hand, in the presence of their normal mesenchymal environment, exogenous NGF can indeed either stimulate or inhibit murine epidermal and HF keratinocyte proliferation in situ, depending on whether the keratinocytes are in a state of relative quiescence or are already maximally proliferating [24]. The proliferative effects of autocrine NGF on human keratinocytes are also confirmed by the use of the natural alkaloid K252a, an inhibitor of TrkA phosphorylation. Indeed, K252 blocks keratinocyte proliferation, in the absence of exogenous NGF [18]. Moreover, human keratinocytes transfected with NGF

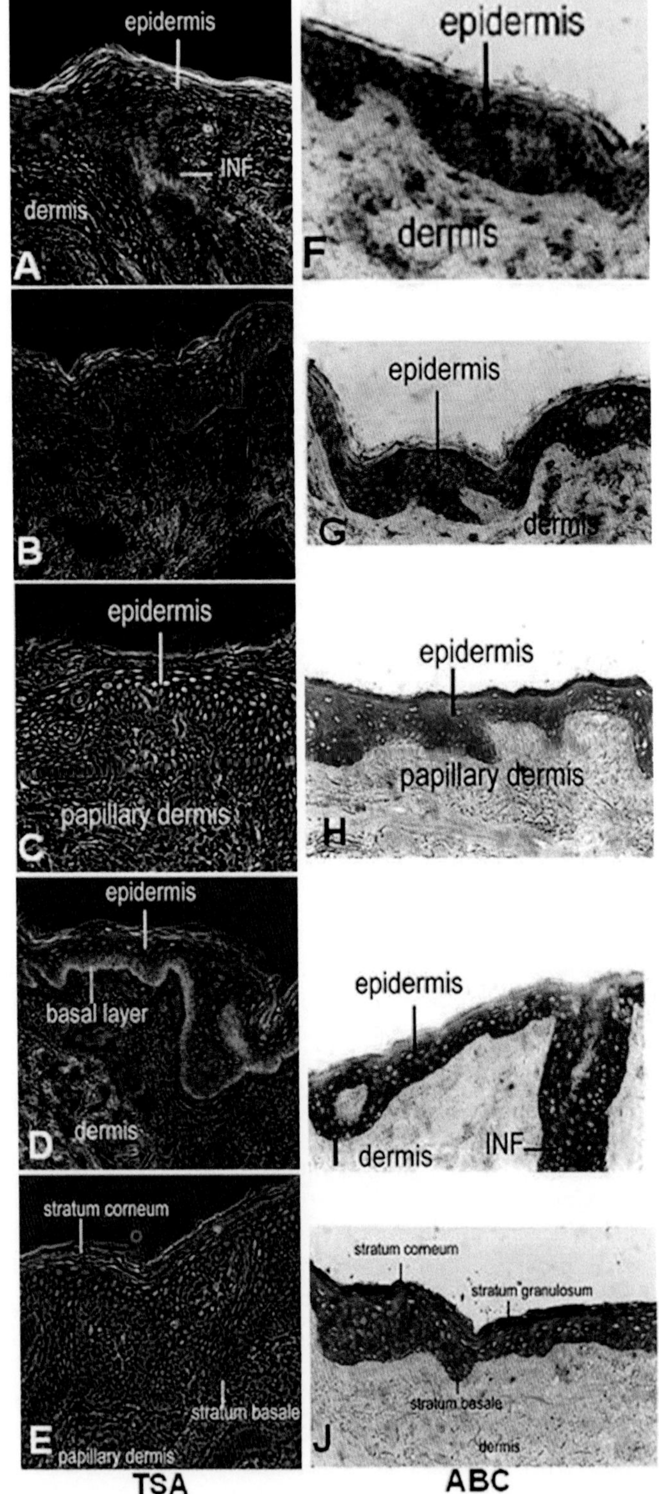

Fig. 1 Expression of NTs and their receptors in normal human skin shown in *red* color with tyramide signal amplification (TSA) and avidin-biotin complex (ABC) immunostaining techniques. (**a**) Nerve growth factor (NGF) (200×), (**b**) NT3 (200×), (**c**) Tyrosine kinase A (TrkA) (200×), (**d**) TrkC (200×), (**e**): p75NTR (200×), (**f**, **g**, **h**, **i** and **j**) refer to as the expressions of NGF, NT-3, TrK A, TrK C, and p75NTR, respectively, confirmed with ABC immunostaining. (INF) Infundibulum (Adapted from Adly et al. [17, 21] © 2005, 2006, Wiley-Blackwell and Reprinted with permission from Adly et al. [32] © 2009, Elsevier)

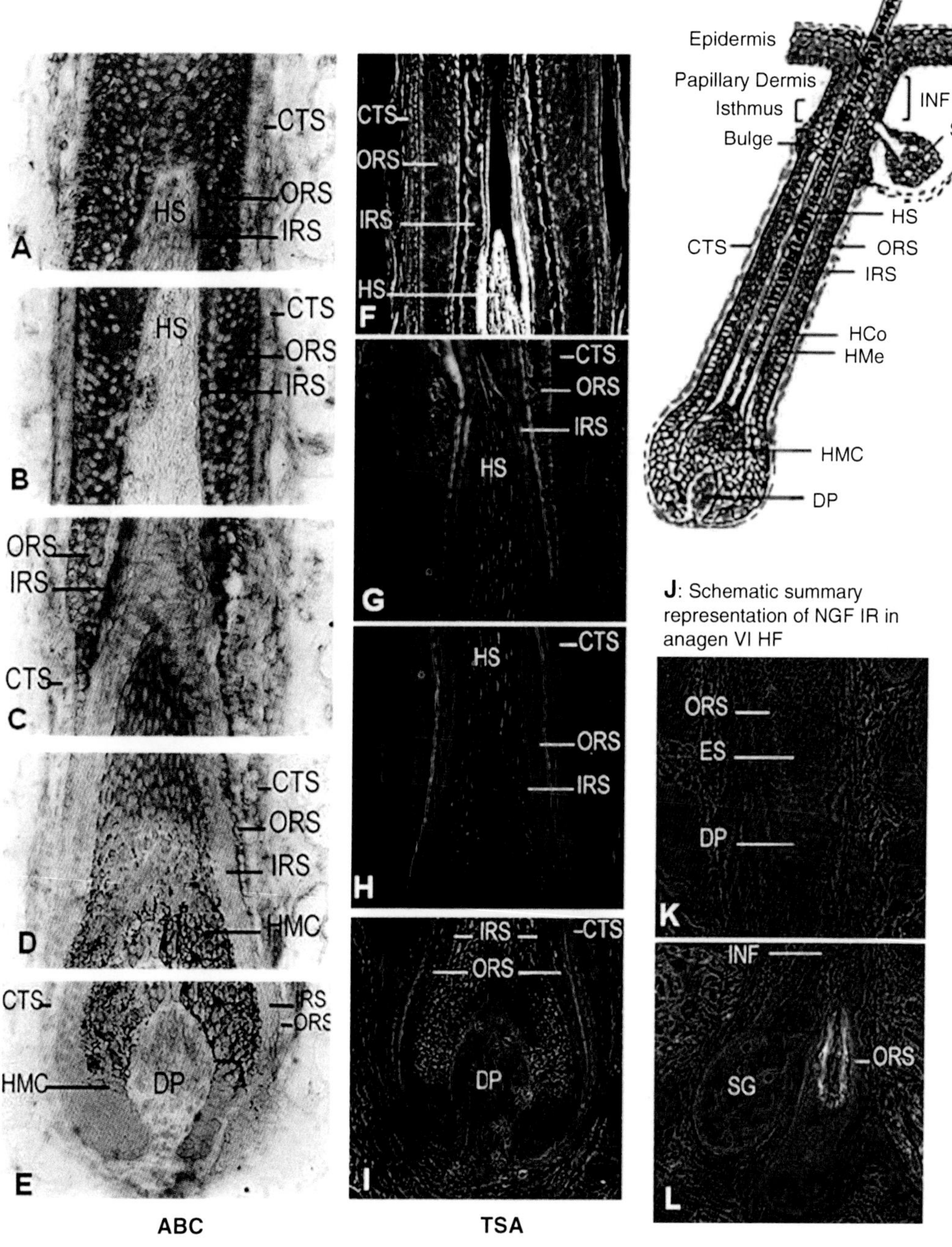

Fig. 2 Immunoreactivity of nerve growth factor (NGF) protein in adult human scalp anagen VI HF (hair follicle), shown in *red* color with avidin-biotin complex (ABC) and tyramide signal amplification (TSA) techniques. (**a**, **b**, **f**, and **g**) show IR in the distal region of HF. (**c**, **d**, and **h**) show immunoreactivity (IR) in the mid region of hair follicle (HF). (**e** and **i**) show IR in the proximal bulb region of HF. (**j**) is a schematic summary representation of IR in the whole HF shown in *red* color. (**k**) shows IR in catagen HF. (**l**) shows IR in telogen HF. *CTS* connective tissue sheath, *DP* dermal papilla, *HCo* hair cortex, *HMe* hair medulla, *HMC* hair matrix cells, *HS* hair shaft, *INF* infundibulum, *IRS* inner root sheath, *ORS* outer root sheath (Reprinted with permission from Adly et al. [21] © 2006, Wiley-Blackwell)

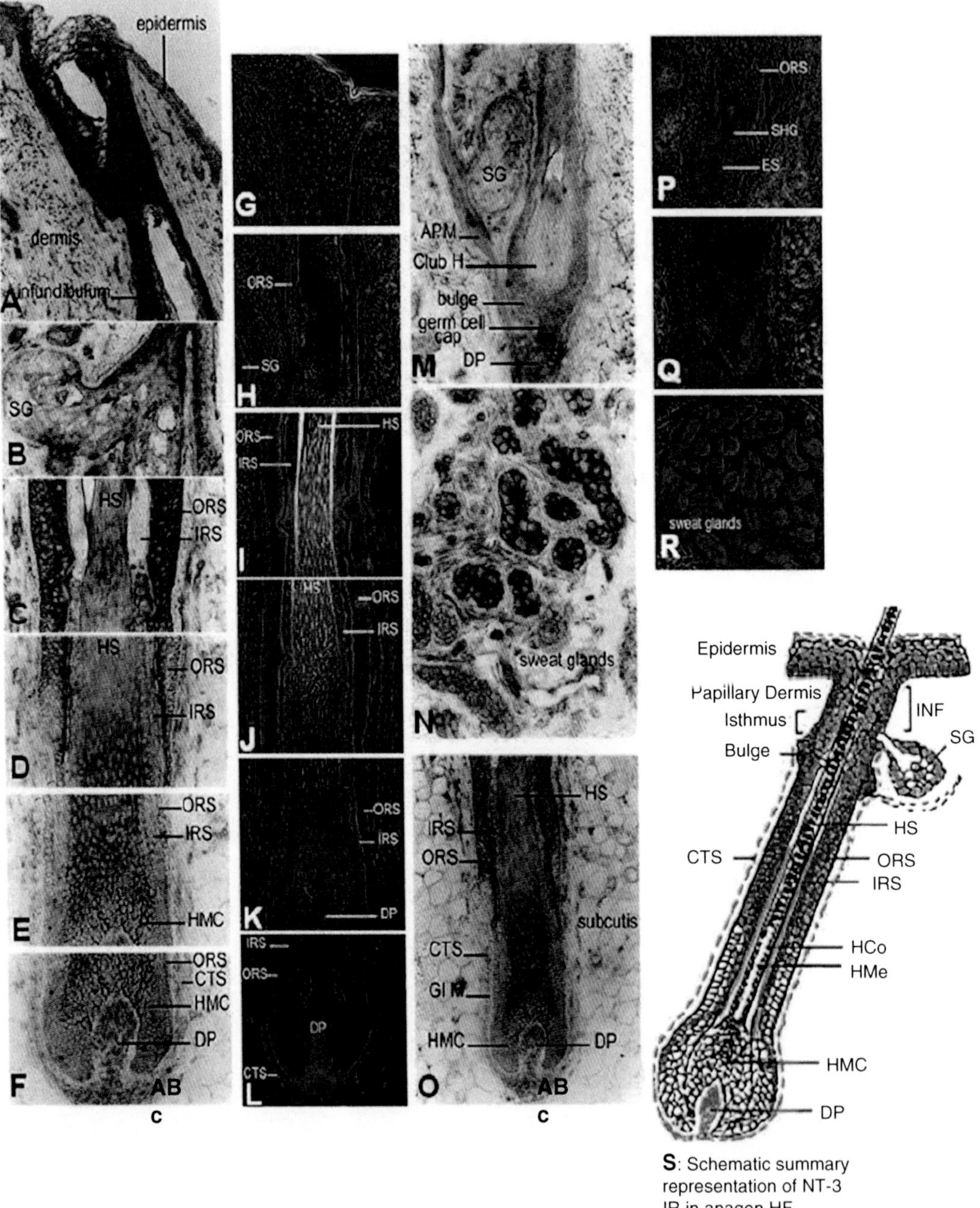

Fig. 3 Immunoreactivity of NT-3 in human scalp skin and HF, shown in *red* color with avidin-biotin complex (ABC) and tyramide signal amplification (TSA) techniques. (**a** and **g**) show the epidermis. (**b**–**f**) (*panel 1*) and (**h**–**l**) (*panel 2*) show IR in anagen VI HF. (**c** and **j**) show IR in the sebaceous gland (SG). (**n** and **r**) show IR in the sweat gland. (**o**) shows IR in the early anagen, some fibroblasts in the dermis, and adipocytes in subcutis. (**m**) and (**p**) show IR in telogen HF. (**q**) shows IR in catagen HF. (**s**) is a schematic summary representation of IR in anagen VI HF shown in *red* color. *APM* arrector pili muscle (Reprinted with permission from Adly et al. [15] © 2005, Wiley-Blackwell)

proliferate to a significantly greater extent than mock-transfected cells [25].

Keratinocytes express and release NTs, other than NGF [16, 17, 26], and BDNF, NT-3, and NT-4 stimulate murine epidermal keratinocyte proliferation in situ [16, 17]. NGF is secreted at highest levels as compared to the other NTs, whereas NT-3 and NGF upregulate each other's secretion in human keratinocytes. NGF expression is downregulated by UVB irradiation [23, 25], whereas NT-3 release is augmented by UVA.

At the skin level, TrkA and TrkC mediate NGF- and NT-3-induced keratinocyte proliferation, respectively. Indeed, keratinocytes overexpressing TrkA proliferate significantly better than controls [27], and increasing concentrations of anti-NT-3 antibody inhibit keratinocyte proliferation [26]. In mouse skin, epidermal keratinocytes express TrkA and TrkB, and all NTs are capable of stimulating their proliferation in ex vivo-cultured skin explants [16, 17, 24]. In human skin, epidermal keratinocytes express TrkA, TrkB, and TrkC proteins in different intensities [21], and NTs can stimulate keratinocyte proliferation and epidermal homeostasis.

Apoptosis plays a fundamental role in epidermal homeostasis by counterbalancing cell proliferation, and apoptotic cells are consistently present in normal human epidermis [28–30]. In vitro, NGF, but not the other NTs, can rescue human epidermal keratinocytes from spontaneous and UVB-induced apoptosis via TrkA [25, 28, 29]. Although UVB downregulates NGF and TrkA in human keratinocytes, NGF-overexpressing keratinocytes are protected from UVB-induced apoptosis [25].

NGF protects keratinocytes from cell death via the Bcl-2 family of apoptosis inhibitors. Indeed, K252a fails to induce apoptosis in keratinocytes overexpressing Bcl-2, and UVB causes a decrease in Bcl-2 and Bcl-xL expression in mock-transfected keratinocytes but not in NGF-overexpressing cells. NGF prevents the cleavage of the enzyme poly (ADP-ribose) polymerase, a substrate for caspases, which is induced in human keratinocytes by UVB [25]. These observations are consistent with a model whereby autocrine NGF protects human keratinocytes from apoptosis through its high-affinity receptor TrkA by maintaining constant levels of Bcl-2 and Bcl-xL, which in turn block caspase activation [25].

The above-mentioned observations clearly show that NTs mediate proliferative and survival signals in epidermal keratinocytes through their high-affinity Trk receptors. Still, the role of the low-affinity p75NTR in NGF signaling in keratinocytes remains to be clarified. Although TrkA is evenly distributed in the basal keratinocyte layer (Fig. 1c), p75NTR is expressed in basal keratinocytes with an irregular pattern (Fig.1e). As human keratinocytes lack functional TrkB [25], BDNF and NT-4 obviously signal through p75NTR in these cells. Indeed, BDNF and NT-4 induce apoptosis in cultured human keratinocytes. This is in agreement with the observation of a similar function of p75NTR in the catagen phase of the hair cycle [31] and the strong expression of p75NTR protein in the anagen-catagen transition and early catagen stages of the human hair follicle cycle [32]. Therefore, a balance between the low- and the high-affinity NT receptors exists in keratinocytes. However, the exact stimuli and conditions whereby NGF and other NTs signal life or death in keratinocytes are yet to be defined. In addition, it should also be determined whether NTs and their receptors could play a role in the development of nonmelanoma skin cancers by stimulating proliferation and inhibiting apoptosis, in a manner similar to what has been shown for prostate [33] and breast neoplasia [34].

NTs and Melanocytes

During skin development, neural crest-derived melanoblasts migrate into the skin and differentiate into melanocytes, which populate the basal layer of the epidermis and the HFs. Together with other paracrine signaling molecules (fibroblast growth factor [FGF], bone morphogenetic proteins, noelin-1, stem cell factor, hepatocyte growth factor, endothelins), NTs play an important role in the control of melanoblast migration, viability, and differentiation [14, 29]. Normal human melanocytes also express p75NTR [32], and its expression level is upregulated by a variety of stimuli including UV irradiation [35]. Keratinocyte-derived NGF, whose expression is also upregulated by UV irradiation [20, 36], may influence epidermal melanocytes in a paracrine manner. In vitro, NGF is chemotactic for melanocytes and stimulates melanocyte dendrite formation [14]. Although under optimal basal culture conditions there is no effect of NGF on melanocyte cell yields or melanogenesis, both NGF and NT-3, the latter expressed by dermal fibroblasts [15], increase melanocyte survival when the cells are maintained in medium depleted of growth factors [15, 37].

Interestingly, phorbol 12-tetra decanoate 13 acetate, a strong activator of protein kinase C, upregulates the expression of p75NTR and induces the expression of TrkA in melanocytes [15]. Although the exact mechanism that regulates phorbol 12-tetra decanoate 13 acetate-induced p75NTR and TrkA upregulation is not known, phorbol 12-tetra decanoate 13 acetate is recognized to have a striking effect also on melanocyte dendricity. It is possible that this differentiated morphology of melanocytes is part of an integrated complex of differentiated functions that includes induction of receptors to NGF. In contrast with TrkA expression that requires induction, melanocytes constitutively express TrkC, albeit the expression is likely to be low as it was detected by the sensitive reverse transcriptase-PCR methodology [15]. Also, in contrast with TrkA expression, TrkC expression is decreased after phorbol 12-tetra decanoate 13 acetate, suggesting that although melanocytes can bind both NGF and NT-3, different signals that preferentially induce a specific high-affinity receptor determine which NT would exert its effect. Thus, the effects of NGF and NT-3 on melanocytes may be influenced by outside signals through modulations of their high-affinity receptor expression.

Indeed, using UV-irradiated cultured melanocytes and human melanoma cells, NGF supplementation enhances cell survival, markedly reduces apoptotic cell death, and increases the level of the antiapoptotic Bcl-2 protein, which is expressed strongly by melanocytes in vivo even in the absence of UV irradiation [23, 37]. The data suggest that NGF, which is constitutively produced by neighboring epidermal keratinocytes, may preserve the population of cutaneous melanocytes that would otherwise be depleted by sun exposure. In contrast, NT-3, which is strongly expressed by nonproliferating fibroblasts [15], like those in the dermal compartment of nondamaged human skin, could help in melanocyte maintenance during steady state conditions.

NTs Expression in Human Skin Decreases with Aging

Recent studies have revealed that the expression of NTs and Trk receptors within the human skin decreases with aging. NGF is a member of a family of structurally and functionally related polypeptides known as the neurotrophins (NTs) [38]. Since its discovery, NGF is known to guide and sustain neuronal development and differentiation within peripheral neural networks. NGF can regulate tissue morphogenesis, remodeling, proliferation, and apoptosis [3]. The common neuroectodermal origin of the cutaneous epithelium and the nervous system makes it reasonable to hypothesize that the same growth factors, which govern the development, and maintenance, of neurons are also involved in skin morphogenesis [3]. The NGF is established locally in the skin by glia cells, epithelial cells, fibroblasts, and Merkel cells. The skin is a rich source of NGF, and the epidermis is recognized as a site of NGF expression. Shortly thereafter, it became clear that epidermal keratinocytes are not only important NGF sources but also are NT targets expressing NT receptors. In murine skin organ cultures, NGF is produced by keratinocytes. Also, NGF stimulates the proliferation and inhibits the apoptosis in cultured human epidermal keratinocytes. Interestingly, NGF is critical for proper innervation of this peripheral sensory organ. Thus, defects in NTs singling are associated with severe sensory skin disorders that inhibit wound healing [3].

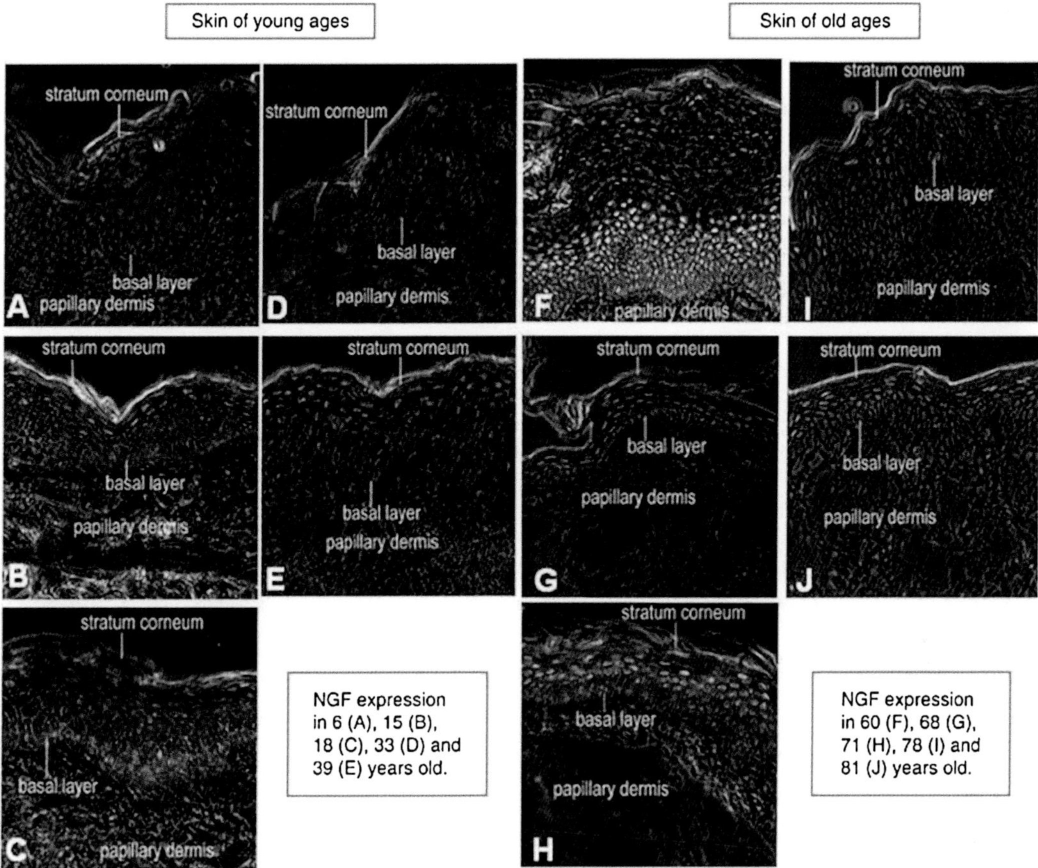

Fig. 4 Nerve growth factor protein expression in human skin derived from different aged donors shown in *red* color with tyramide signal amplification (TSA) technique. (**a**–**e**) Young age group (5–39 years). (**a**) 6Y, (**b**) 15Y, (**c**) 18Y, (**d**) 33Y, and (**e**) 39Y. (**f** and **g**) Old age group (60–81 years). (**f**) 60Y, (**g**) 68Y, (**h**) 71Y, (**i**) 78Y, and (**j**) 81Y. Magnification: 200× (Reprinted with permission from Adly et al. [3])) © 2006, Elsevier)

Downregulation of NGF Protein Expression with Aging

The expression pattern of NGF was examined previously in different age groups. NGF protein expression exhibited striking age-associated changes within the human epidermis [3]. In sun-protected skin specimens derived from young individuals (<40 years), NGF expression was very strong and was prominent in the most epidermal layers, particularly in the stratum basale, stratum spinosum, and stratum granulosum (Fig. 4). In contrast, in the skin derived from old donors (>60 years), no or only a weak NGF expression was detected (Fig. 4). Semiquantitative analysis of NGF immunostaining revealed that NGF protein expression values were significantly higher in young ages than in old ages (Tables 1 and 2). NGF immunoreactivity was strongest in the ages 6, 15, and 18 years and decreased gradually in the ages 33 and 39 years (Fig. 4). In the young ages, the expression was detected in all layers of the epidermis except for the stratum corneum (Fig. 4a–c), whereas in the middle ages (33 and 39 years) the expression was confined to the Malpighian layer and stratum spinosum (Fig. 4d, e).

In the old ages (>60 years), NGF expression was dramatically reduced and the expression was detected mainly in the stratum basale (Fig. 4f–j). Among old ages (60–81 years), the expression was strongest in the age of 60 years (Fig. 4f), whereas it

Table 1 Nerve growth factor protein expression in human skin of different ages. The staining results were examined by the authors and were scored as (−) for absent, (+) for weak, (++) for medium, and (+++) for intense nerve growth factor (NGF) protein expression

Age (years)	Stratum basale	Stratum spinosum	Stratum granulosum	Stratum corneum
6	+++	+++	+++	−
8	+++	+++	+++	−
11	+++	+++	+++	−
13	+++	+++	+++	−
15	+++	+++	+++	−
18	+++	+++	+++	−
32	+++	++	++	−
33	+++	++	++	−
34	+++	++	++	−
36	+++	++	++	−
37	+++	++	++	−
39	+++	++	++	−
60	++	+	−	−
64	+	+	−	−
68	+	−	−	−
71	+	−	−	−
74	+	−	−	−
76	+	−	−	−
78	+	−	−	−
81	+	−	−	−

Table 2 Expression values of nerve growth factor in human skin of different ages. The immunoreactivity score (IR score) was evaluated by multiplying the percentage of positive cells (PP%) and the staining intensity (SI). First, the PP% was scored as 0 for <5 %, 1 for 5–25 %, 2 for 25–50 %, 3 for 50–75 %, and 4 for >75 %. Second, the SI was scored as 1 for weak, 2 for medium, and 3 for intense staining, following other groups. Values between brackets represent the standard errors of mean

Age groups (years)	Basal layer			Spinous layer			Granular layer		
	SI	PP	IRS	SI	PP	IRS	SI	PP	IRS
6–18	2.8 {0.2}	3.8 {0.2}	11.0 {1.0}	2.8 {0.1}	3.8 {0.2}	11.0 {1.0}	2.8 {0.2}	3.7 {0.2}	10.5 {1.0}
19–50	2.8 {0.1}	3.7 {0.3}	6.8 {1.1}	1.8 {0.1}	3.1 {0.1}	5.7 {0.3}	1.7 {0.3}	2.6 {0.4}	5.1 {0.8}
51–81	1.0 {0.0}	1.8 {0.1}	1.8 {0.1}	1.1 {0.1}	1.4 {0.4}	1.4 {0.4}	0.75 {0.1}	0.70 {0.1}	0.9 {0.1}

was greatly diminished in older ages (Fig. 4g–i) until it became completely negative in the age of 81 years (Fig. 4j). Although NGF expression was seen in the stratum granulosum of the skin derived from certain old ages (68- and 78-year-old donors), its immunoreactivity was weak (Fig. 4g, i). The level of NGF protein in the sweat glands does not apparently differ with aging (Fig. 5).

The age-related decrease of NGF protein expression in the human epidermis is parallel with its level in the nervous system. There was a gradual reduction of NGF levels with aging in the brain and thymus of rats and a low amount of NGF protein in the plasma of old subjects. Also, the administration of NGF in rats can reduce age-related atrophy of the neurons. Similarly in human, administration of

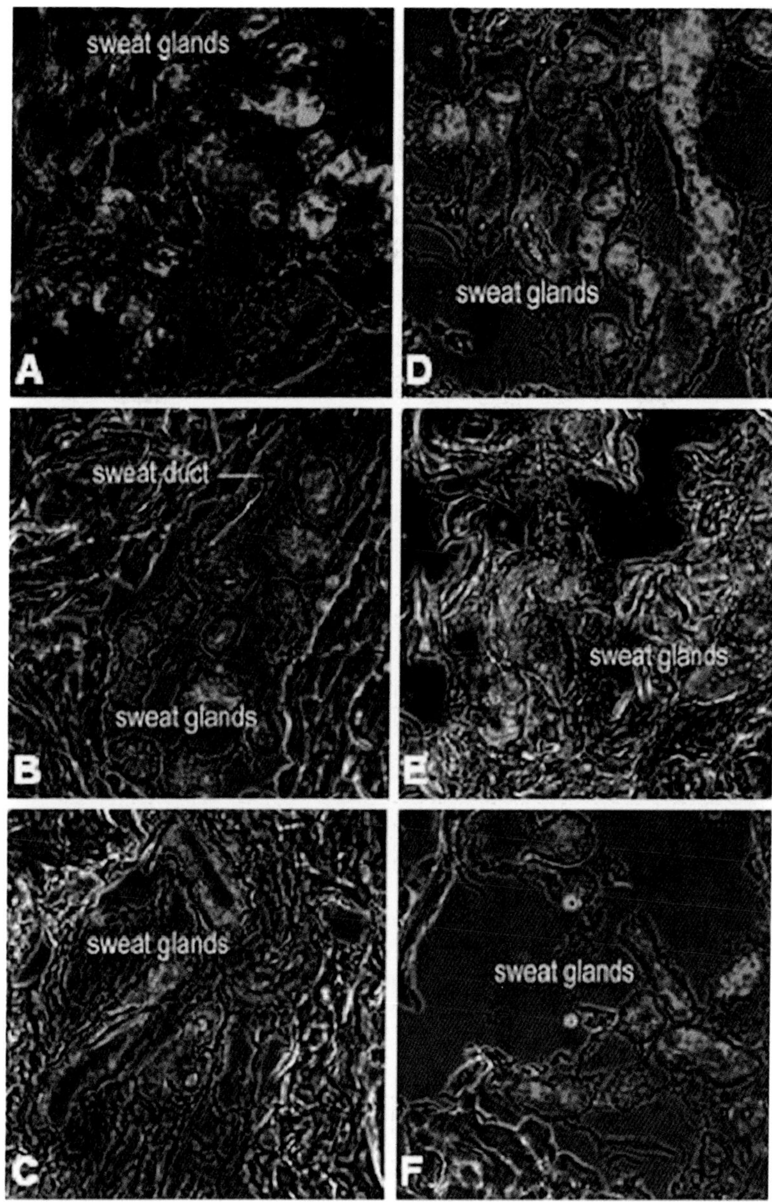

Fig. 5 Nerve growth factor protein expression in sweat glands derived from different aged donors. The reactivity appeared as *red* color (tyramide signal amplification [TSA] technique). Nerve growth factor (NGF) expression in the following ages in years (Y). (**a**) 6Y, (**b**) 33Y, (**c**) 39Y, (**d**) 71Y, (**e**) 78Y, and (**f**) 81Y (Reprinted with permission from Adly et al. [3] © 2006, Elsevier)

NGF can delay retinal degeneration in patients with retinitis pigmentosa [39, 40].

The strong expression of NGF protein in the skin of young individuals may be due to an increased receptor-mediated internalization of NGF proteins released by nerve endings [41, 42] or altered expression of certain cytokines, such as tumor necrosis factor alpha (TNF-α), that influence the synthesis of NGF. In transgenic mice, the basal level of brain NGF can be influenced negatively or positively by local expression of TNF-α [19, 43]. The decrease of NGF protein expression in aged skin may reflect impairment of these mechanisms or a reduction in the number of high-affinity NGF-binding sites. Indeed, as women age, they become hypoestrogenic; therefore, a hypothesis to be tested is that NGF changes with aging might by related to hormonal change and not as much with aging. To test this hypothesis, NGF protein expression in skin of male subjects need to be examined in this type of studies.

Downregulation of NT-3 Protein Expression with Aging

Similarly, NT-3 protein expression in human skin underwent age-associated decrease [32]. In young ages, NT-3 expression was very strong and immunoreactivity was detected in almost all layers of the epidermis, including the stratum corneum in the ages below 20 years. Alternatively, in old ages, the NT-3 expression was very weak or completely absent.

Conclusion

The neurotrophins are a family of polypeptide growth factors. These proteins are critical not only for the development but also for the maintenance of the vertebrate nervous system. Recently, several leads indicate that these factors could have a broader role than their name might suggest, in particular, the putative role of NGF and its receptor TrkA and NT-3 in cutaneous homeostasis and in skin aging. To date knowledge about the expression pattern of neurotrophins in skin remains rudimentary. This chapter discussed the expression of neurotrophins and their receptors in different cutaneous structures based on the data obtained from the studies of the human scalp skin. The clinical and therapeutic ramifications of these studies are open for further investigations.

References

1. Botchkareva NV, Botchkarev VA, Welker P, Airaksinen M, Roth W, Suvanto P, Muller-Rover S, Hadshiew IM, Peters C, Paus R. New roles for glial cell line-derived neurotrophic factor and neurturin: involvement in hair cycle control. Am J Pathol. 2000;156(3):1041–53.
2. Botchkarev VA, Botchkareva NV, Peters EM, Paus R. Epithelial growth control by neurotrophins: leads and lessons from the hair follicle. Prog Brain Res. 2004;146:493–513.
3. Adly MA, Assaf H, Hussein MR. Age-associated decrease of the nerve growth factor protein expression in the human skin: preliminary findings. J Dermatol Sci. 2006;42(3):268–71.
4. Teng KK, Hempstead BL. Neurotrophins and their receptors: signaling trios in complex biological systems. Cell Mol Life Sci. 2004;61(1):35–48.
5. Segal RA. Selectivity in neurotrophin signaling: theme and variations. Annu Rev Neurosci. 2003;26:299–330.
6. Dechant G, Barde YA. The neurotrophin receptor p75 (NTR): novel functions and implications for diseases of the nervous system. Nat Neurosci. 2002;5 (11):1131–6.
7. Nykjaer A, Willnow TE, Petersen CM. p75NTR – live or let die. Curr Opin Neurobiol. 2005;15(1):49–57.
8. Yaar M, Zhai S, Fine RE, Eisenhauer PB, Arble BL, Stewart KB, Gilchrest BA. Amyloid beta binds trimers as well as monomers of the 75-kDa neurotrophin receptor and activates receptor signaling. J Biol Chem. 2002;277(10):7720–5.
9. Peters EM, Hansen MG, Overall RW, Nakamura M, Pertile P, Klapp BF, Arck PC, Paus R. Control of human hair growth by neurotrophins: brain-derived neurotrophic factor inhibits hair shaft elongation, induces catagen, and stimulates follicular transforming growth factor beta2 expression. J Invest Dermatol. 2005;124(4):675–85.
10. Peters EM, Hendrix S, Golz G, Klapp BF, Arck PC, Paus R. Nerve growth factor and its precursor differentially regulate hair cycle progression in mice. J Histochem Cytochem. 2006;54(3):275–88.
11. Botchkareva NV, Botchkarev VA, Albers KM, Metz M, Paus R. Distinct roles for nerve growth factor and brain-derived neurotrophic factor in controlling the rate of hair follicle morphogenesis. J Invest Dermatol. 2000;114(2):314–20.
12. Sariola H. The neurotrophic factors in non-neuronal tissues. Cell Mol Life Sci. 2001;58(8):1061–6.
13. Ernfors P, Lee KF, Jaenisch R. Target derived and putative local actions of neurotrophins in the peripheral nervous system. Prog Brain Res. 1994;103:43–54.
14. Yaar M, Grossman K, Eller M, Gilchrest BA. Evidence for nerve growth factor-mediated paracrine effects in human epidermis. J Cell Biol. 1991;115(3):821–8.
15. Yaar M, Eller MS, DiBenedetto P, Reenstra WR, Zhai S, McQuaid T, Archambault M, Gilchrest BA. The trk family of receptors mediates nerve growth factor and neurotrophin-3 effects in melanocytes. J Clin Invest. 1994;94(4):1550–62.
16. Botchkarev VA, Metz M, Botchkareva NV, Welker P, Lommatzsch M, Renz H, Paus R. Brain-derived neurotrophic factor, neurotrophin-3, and neurotrophin-4 act as "epitheliotrophins" in murine skin. Lab Invest. 1999;79(5):557–72.

17. Adly MA, Assaf HA, Nada EA, Soliman M, Hussein M. Human scalp skin and hair follicles express neurotrophin-3 and its high-affinity receptor tyrosine kinase C, and show hair cycle-dependent alterations in expression. Br J Dermatol. 2005;153 (3):514–20.
18. Bonini S, Rasi G, Bracci-Laudiero ML, Procoli A, Aloe L. Nerve growth factor: neurotrophin or cytokine? Int Arch Allergy Immunol. 2003;131(2):80–4.
19. Aloe L. Nerve growth factor, human skin ulcers and vascularization. Our experience. Prog Brain Res. 2004;146:515–22.
20. Marco E, Di Marchisio PC, Bondanza S, Franzi AT, Cancedda R, De Luca M. Growth-regulated synthesis and secretion of biologically active nerve growth factor by human keratinocytes. J Biol Chem. 1991;266 (32):21718–22.
21. Adly MA, Assaf HA, Nada EA, Soliman M, Hussein M. Expression of nerve growth factor and its high-affinity receptor, tyrosine kinase A proteins, in the human scalp skin. J Cutan Pathol. 2006;33(8):559–68.
22. Pincelli C, Sevignani C, Manfredini R, Grande A, Fantini F, Bracci-Laudiero L, Aloe L, Ferrari S, Cossarizza A, Giannetti A. Expression and function of nerve growth factor and nerve growth factor receptor on cultured keratinocytes. J Invest Dermatol. 1994;103 (1):13–8.
23. Stefanato CM, Yaar M, Bhawan J, Phillips TJ, Kosmadaki MG, Botchkarev V, Gilchrest BA. Modulations of nerve growth factor and Bcl-2 in ultraviolet-irradiated human epidermis. J Cutan Pathol. 2003;30(6):351–7.
24. Paus R, Luftl M, Czarnetzki BM. Nerve growth factor modulates keratinocyte proliferation in murine skin organ culture. Br J Dermatol. 1994;130(2):174–80.
25. Marconi A, Vaschieri C, Zanoli S, Giannetti A, Pincelli C. Nerve growth factor protects human keratinocytes from ultraviolet-B-induced apoptosis. J Invest Dermatol. 1999;113(6):920–7.
26. Marconi A, Terracina M, Fila C, Franchi J, Bonte F, Romagnoli G, Maurelli R, Failla CM, Dumas M, Pincelli C. Expression and function of neurotrophins and their receptors in cultured human keratinocytes. J Invest Dermatol. 2003;121(6):1515–21.
27. Pincelli C. Nerve growth factor and keratinocytes: a role in psoriasis. Eur J Dermatol. 2000;10(2):85–90.
28. Pincelli C, Haake AR, Benassi L, Grassilli E, Magnoni C, Ottani D, Polakowska R, Franceschi C, Giannetti A. Autocrine nerve growth factor protects human keratinocytes from apoptosis through its high affinity receptor (TRK): a role for BCL-2. J Invest Dermatol. 1997;109(6):757–64.
29. Pincelli C, Yaar M. Nerve growth factor: its significance in cutaneous biology. J Investig Dermatol Symp Proc. 1997;2(1):31–6.
30. Wehrli P, Viard I, Bullani R, Tschopp J, French LE. Death receptors in cutaneous biology and disease. J Invest Dermatol. 2000;115(2):141–8.
31. Botchkarev VA, Botchkareva NV, Albers KM, Chen LH, Welker P, Paus R. A role for p75 neurotrophin receptor in the control of apoptosis-driven hair follicle regression. FASEB J. 2000;14(13):1931–42.
32. Adly MA, Assaf HA, Hussein MR. Expression pattern of p75 neurotrophin receptor protein in the human scalp skin and hair follice: hair cycle-dependent expression. J Am Acad Dermatol. 2009;60(1):99–109.
33. Krygier S, Djakiew D. The neurotrophin receptor p75NTR is a tumor suppressor in human prostate cancer. Anticancer Res. 2001;21(6A):3749–55.
34. Nakagawara A. Trk receptor tyrosine kinases: a bridge between cancer and neural development. Cancer Lett. 2001;169(2):107–14.
35. Peacocke M, Yaar M, Mansur CP, Chao MV, Gilchrest BA. Induction of nerve growth factor receptors on cultured human melanocytes. Proc Natl Acad Sci U S A. 1988;85(14):5282–6.
36. Marco E, Di Mathor M, Bondanza S, Cutuli N, Marchisio PC, Cancedda R, De Luca M. Nerve growth factor binds to normal human keratinocytes through high and low affinity receptors and stimulates their growth by a novel autocrine loop. J Biol Chem. 1993;268 (30):22838–46.
37. Zhai S, Yaar M, Doyle SM, Gilchrest BA. Nerve growth factor rescues pigment cells from ultraviolet-induced apoptosis by upregulating BCL-2 levels. Exp Cell Res. 1996;224(2):335–43.
38. Alleva E, Petruzzi S, Cirulli F, Aloe L. NGF regulatory role in stress and coping of rodents and humans. Pharmacol Biochem Behav. 1996;54 (1):65–72.
39. Alberch J, Perez-Navarro E, Arenas E, Marsal J. Involvement of nerve growth factor and its receptor in the regulation of the cholinergic function in aged rats. J Neurochem. 1991;57(5):1483–7.
40. Garcia-Suarez O, Germana A, Hannestad J, Perez-Perez M, Esteban I, Naves FJ, Vega JA. Changes in the expression of the nerve growth factor receptors TrkA and p75LNGR in the rat thymus with ageing and increased nerve growth factor plasma levels. Cell Tissue Res. 2000;301 (2):225–34.
41. Backman C, Rose GM, Hoffer BJ, Henry MA, Bartus RT, Friden P, Granholm AC. Systemic administration of a nerve growth factor conjugate reverses age-related cognitive dysfunction and prevents cholinergic neuron atrophy. J Neurosci. 1996;16 (17):5437–42.
42. Amendola T, Aloe L. Developmental expression of nerve growth factor in the eye of rats affected by inherited retinopathy: correlative aspects with retinal structural degeneration. Arch Ital Biol. 2002;140 (2):81–90.
43. Aloe L. Rita Levi-Montalcini: the discovery of nerve growth factor and modern neurobiology. Trends Cell Biol. 2004;14(7):395–9.

Cluster of Differentiation 1d (CD1d) and Skin Aging

42

Mohamed A. Adly, Hanan Assaf, and Mahmoud R. Hussein

Contents

M.A. Adly (✉)
Department of Zoology, Faculty of Science, Sohag University, Sohag, Egypt
e-mail: m.adly@yahoo.com

H. Assaf
Department of Dermatology, Saudi German Hospital, Jeddah, Saudi Arabia
e-mail: assaf_hanan@yahoo.com

M.R. Hussein
Department of Pathology, Assir Central Hospital, and Assuit University, Assuit, Egypt
e-mail: mrcpath17@gmail.com

M.A. Farage et al. (eds.), *Textbook of Aging Skin*,
DOI 10.1007/978-3-662-47398-6_18

Abstract

CD1d is a member of CD1 family of transmembrane glycoproteins which represent a third lineage of antigen-presenting molecules. CD1 molecules have evolved to bind lipids and glycolipids. The gene for CD1d is located on chromosome 1 in humans. This chapter will go into detail about the different CDI family function, expression and regulations.

Introduction

CD1d is a member of CD1 family of transmembrane glycoproteins which represent a third lineage of antigen-presenting molecules. These molecules are distantly related to the classical major histocompatibility complex (MHC) molecules in the immune system [1–4]. However, unlike the first and second lineages of antigen-presenting molecules (the classical MHC class I and class II molecules) that bind peptide antigens, CD1 molecules have evolved to bind lipids and glycolipids [5–7]. CD1 family molecules are closely related to MHC class Ia and Ib proteins by sequence homology, domain organization ($\alpha 1$, $\alpha 2$, $\alpha 3$, and $\beta 2m$), and association with $\beta 2$ microglobulin rather than to class II molecules [2, 6]. In contrast to MHC class I molecule which is polymorphic, CD1 molecules are not polymorphic [1–3] and are encoded by linked genes outside the MHC complex; the gene for CD1d is located on chromosome 1 in humans

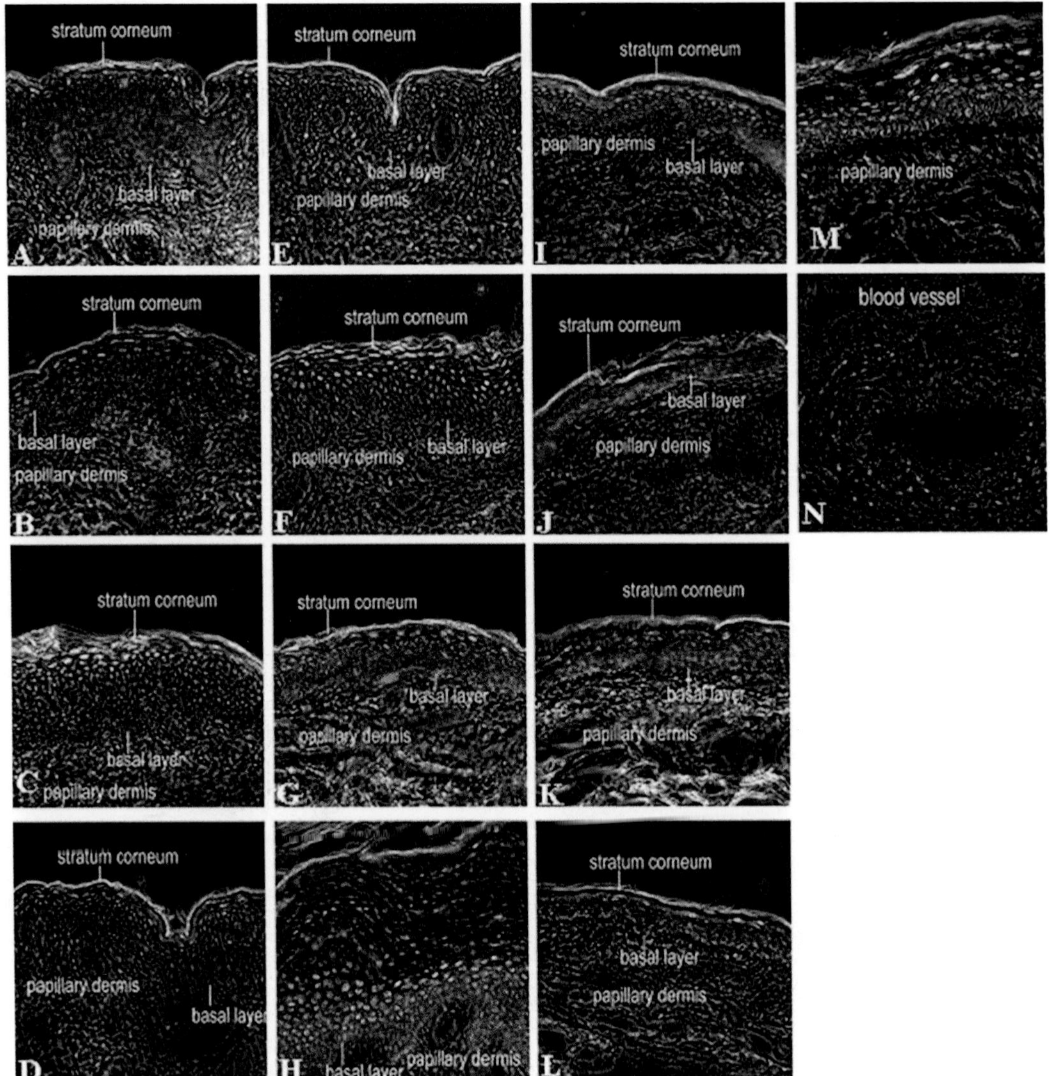

Fig. 1 Immunoreactivity of CD1d protein in human skin of 6 (**a**), 15 (**b**), 18 (**c**), 33 (**d**), 39 (**e**), 53 (**f**), 57 (**g**), 60 (**h**), 68 (**i**), 71 (**j**), 78 (**k**), and 81 (**l**) years old individuals, shown in *red* color with TSA technique. *M* negative control; *N* positive control shows CD1d expression in a blood vessel. At the age of 6 years, CD1d immunoreactivity was not only strong, but also seen in all layers of the epidermis except the stratum corneum (**a**). In the ages between 10 and 30 years old, CD1d immunoreactivity decreased and was detected in the Malpighian layer, stratum spinosum, and a few layers of stratum granulosum (**b**–**c**). In the ages between 30 and 40 years old, CD1d had moderate expression that was mainly seen in the stratum basale (**d**–**e**). In the ages between 40 and 60 years, CD1d protein expression was moderate immunoreactivity, and localized to the basal and granular layers (**f**). In the skin derived from 57-year-old donors, the immunoreactivity was, however, stronger, and the expression was apparent both in the basal and granular layers (**g**). In the old ages, the expression of CD1d was confined to the stratum basale (**h**). Sometimes, CD1d protein expression was seen in the stratum spinosum and some cells of the stratum granulosum, in addition to the basal layer (**i**–**l**) (Reprinted with permission from Adly et al. [23, 25] © 2005, 2006, Wiley-Blackwell)

[1–4]. The CD1 family is divided into two groups by sequence homology: group I which consists of CD1a, -b and -c isotypes and groupII which includes CD1d [8]. Only the group II CD1d isotypes are preserved in human, mouse, rat, rabbit, and monkey [4, 9]. Sequence similarity is substantially higher for the same isotype from different species than for different isotypes within

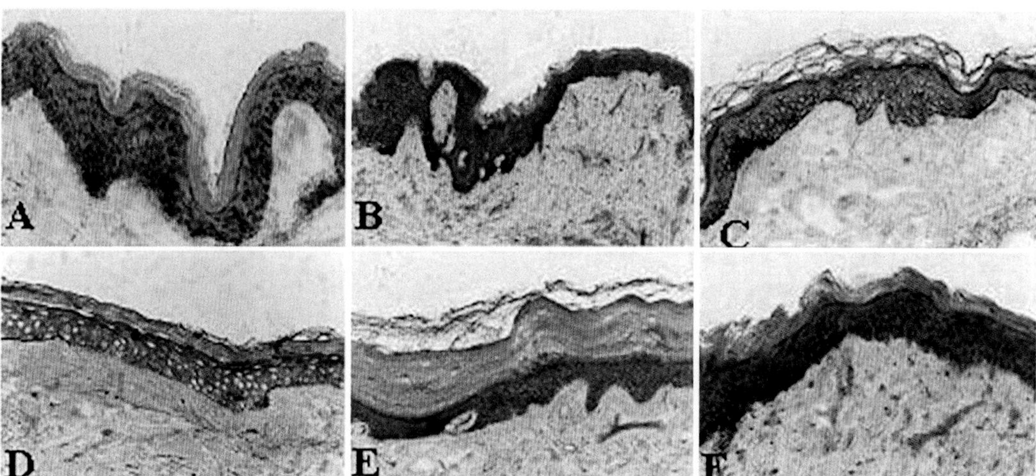

Fig. 2 Immunoreactivity of CD1d protein in human skin of 6 (**a**), 18 (**b**), 33 (**c**), 53 (**d**), 60 (**e**), and 71 (**f**) years old individuals, shown in *red* color with ABC technique. At the age of 6 years, CD1d immunoreactivity was not only strong but also seen in all layers of the epidermis except the stratum corneum (**a**). In the ages between 10 and 30 years old, CD1d immunoreactivity decreased and was detected in the Malpighian layer, stratum spinosum, and a few layers of stratum granulosum (**b**). In the ages between 30 and 40 years old, CD1d had moderate expression that was mainly seen in the stratum basale (**c**). In the ages between 40 and 60 years, CD1d protein expression was moderate immunoreactivity and localized to the basal and granular layers (**d**) (Reprinted with permission from Adly et al. [23, 25] © 2005, 2006, Wiley-Blackwell)

the same species [1–3, 10], suggesting that each group of CD1 molecules could have a different function [4].

CD1d binds glycol- and phospholipid antigens and is essential for the development and activation of a subset of T cells known as natural killer T (NK-T) cells which are characterized by the expression of receptors used by NK cells [1–3, 6, 11] and invariant Vα-Jα TCRs, such as Vα24-JαQ TCR in humans and Vα14Jα281 TCR in mice [12]. NK-T cells recognize self or nonself glycolipids presented by CD1d molecule and respond by secretion of cytokines, most notably IFN-γ and IL-4 [1–3, 6, 13]. The synthetic glycolipid molecule α-galactosylceramide (α-GalCer) was shown to stimulate human and mouse NK-T cells in a CD1d-restricted manner [14–16]. CD1d plays, therefore, via the production of cytokines secreted by NK-T cells, a critical role in performing a number of immunoregulatory functions within the human and mammalian body including protection against autoimmune diseases, microbial infection, and cancer. In mice, it was shown that CD1d regulates UV-induced carcinogenesis by inhibiting apoptosis to prevent elimination of potentially malignant keratinocytes and fibroblasts [17, 18].

CD1d Expression in the Human Skin

Recently, CD1d expression and NK-T cells were demonstrated in the epidermis of acute and chronic psoriatic plaques [19–22]. Not only did CD1d show expression in psoriatic skin, but also in normal sun-protected and scalp skin [22–25]. Moreover, it was found that CD1d is expressed on human scalp hair follicle keratinocytes and that its expression undergoes hair cycle-associated changes, suggesting a role in hair follicle cycle regulation.

CD1d Expression in Human Skin Undergoes Age-Associated Changes

The expression pattern of CD1d in different age groups was examined recently and variable profiles found [25]. CD1d had a strong expression in the skin of young (between 6 and 18 years

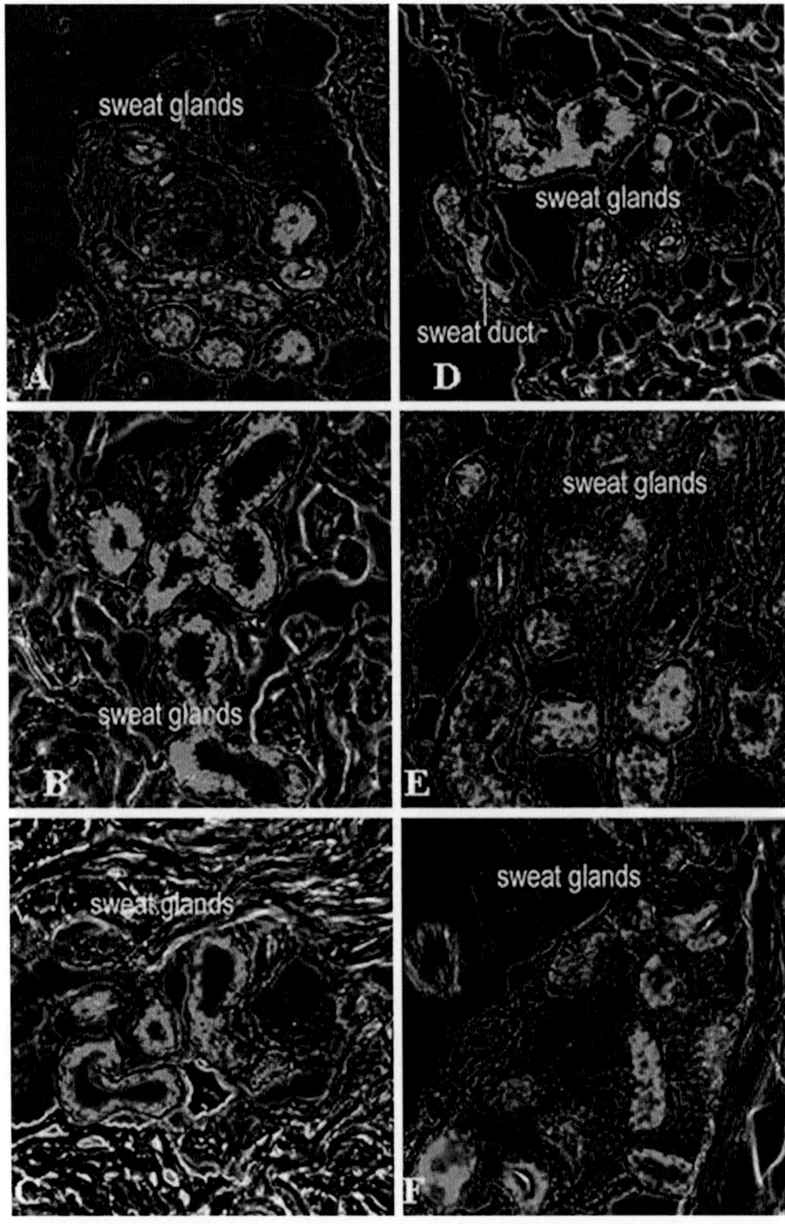

Fig. 3 Immunoreactivity of CD1d protein in sweat glands of human skin derived from 6 (**a**), 33 (**b**), 39 (**c**), 64 (**d**), 71 (**e**), and 78 (**f**) years old individuals, shown in *red* color with TSA technique. CD1d protein expression was strong in sweat glands of all ages (Reprinted with permission from Adly et al. [23, 25] © 2005, 2006, Wiley-Blackwell)

old), but it declined in the skin of mid (between 30 and 40 years old) and old (50–81) age groups. In the epidermis, CD1d was expressed in all layers except in the stratum corneum (Figs. 1, 2, 3, 4, and 5). However, its expression had different intensities, with strong immunoreactivity in the stratum basale and stratum spinosum but weak immunoreactivity in the stratum granulare, particularly in old individuals (Table 1).

The findings of age-related decrease of CD1d protein expression in the human epidermis agree with other groups [26, 27]. Decreased density and function of epidermal dendritic cell populations were found in aged C57BL/6 J mice. However, the capacity of the dendritic cells to transport antigen from the skin to the draining lymph nodes was found in vivo to be comparable to that of young mice. The strong expression of CD1d protein in the skin of children and young

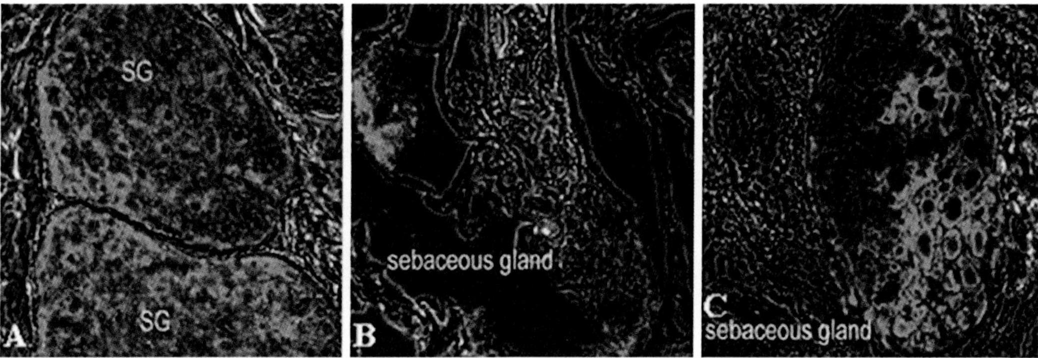

Fig. 4 Immunoreactivity of CD1d protein in sebaceous glands of human skin derived from 15 (**a**), 39 (**b**), and 71 (**c**) years old individuals, shown in *red* color with TSA technique. In sebaceous glands, CD1d protein expression was strong in all ages. Interestingly, CD1d protein was comparable to that in the epidermis, i.e., it was strong in children, moderate in young adults, and weak with aging (Reprinted with permission from Adly et al. [23, 25] © 2005, 2006, Wiley-Blackwell)

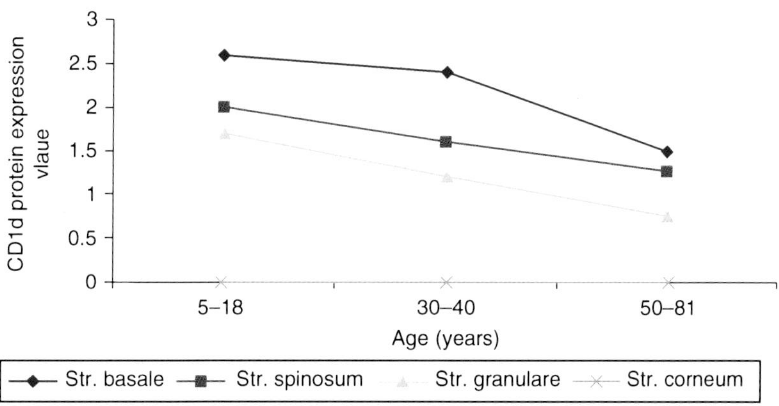

Fig. 5 Immunoreactivity of CD1d protein in different ages (Reprinted with permission from Adly et al. [23, 25] © 2005, 2006, Wiley-Blackwell)

Table 1 CD1d protein expression in the normal human skin: all the specimens were batch-stained in the same run

Age groups (years)	Stratum basale	Stratum spinposum	Stratum granulare	Stratum corneum	Dermis
6–18	2.6 ± 0.3	2.0 ± 0.5	1.7 ± 0.3	0.0	2.6 ± 0.3
30–40	2.4 ± 0.2	1.6 ± 0.3	1.2 ± 0.2	0.0	2.6 ± 0.3
50–81	1.5 ± 0.3	1.25 ± 0.2	0.75 ± 0.2	0.0	2.7 ± 0.3

The immunostaining experiments were repeated at least three times. The staining results were examined by the authors and were scored as (–) for absent, (1) for weak, (2) for moderate, and (3) for intense staining, following other groups

individuals may be due to increased recruitment, tissue accessibility, and local proliferatioin of CD1d + cells (Table 1). Molecular signaling of three distinct pathways of apoptosis, namely the death receptor pathway, the mitochondrial pathway, and the endoplasmic reticulum stress pathway may be involved in CD1d + cells apoptosis [28–31].

Conclusion

CD1d plays, therefore, via the production of cytokines secreted by NK-T cells, a critical role in performing a number of immunoregulatory functions within the human and mammalian body including protection against autoimmune diseases, microbial infection, and cancer. In mice, it was shown that CD1d regulates UV-induced carcinogenesis by inhibiting apoptosis to prevent elimination of potentially malignant keratinocytes and fibroblasts.

References

1. Porcelli SA. The CD1 family: a third lineage of antigen-presenting molecules. Adv Immunol. 1995;59:1–98.
2. Porcelli SA, Segelke BW, Sugita M, Wilson IA, Brenner MB. The CD1 family of lipid antigen-presenting molecules. Immunol Today. 1998;19(8):362–8.
3. Porcelli SA, Modlin RL. The CD1 system: antigen-presenting molecules for T cell recognition of lipids and glycolipids. Annu Rev Immunol. 1999;17:297–329.
4. Zeng Z, Castano AR, Segelke BW, Stura EA, Peterson PA, Wilson IA. Crystal structure of mouse CD1: an MHC-like fold with a large hydrophobic binding groove. Science. 1997;277 (5324):339–45.
5. Hong S, Scherer DC, Singh N, Mendiratta SK, Serizawa I, Koezuka Y, Van Kaer L. Lipid antigen presentation in the immune system: lessons learned from CD1d knockout mice. Immunol Rev. 1999;169:31–44.
6. Exley M, Garcia J, Balk SP, Porcelli S. Requirements for CD1d recognition by human invariant Valpha24 + CD4-CD8- T cells. J Exp Med. 1997;186(1):109–20.
7. Sidobre S, Kronenberg M. CD1 tetramers: a powerful tool for the analysis of glycolipid-reactive T cells. J Immunol Methods. 2002;268(1):107–21.
8. Calabi F, Jarvis JM, Martin L, Milstein C. Two classes of CD1 genes. Eur J Immunol. 1989;19 (2):285–92.
9. Kashiwase K, Kikuchi A, Ando Y, Nicol A, Porcelli SA, Tokunaga K, Omine M, Satake M, Juji T, Nieda M, Koezuka Y. The CD1d natural killer T-cell antigen presentation pathway is highly conserved between humans and rhesus macaques. Immunogenetics. 2003;54(11):776–81.
10. McMichael AJ. Lymphocytes. 1. Function. Genetic restrictions in the immune response. J Clin Pathol Suppl (R Coll Pathol). 1979;13:30–8.
11. Brossay L, Chioda M, Burdin N, Koezuka Y, Casorati G, Dellabona P, Kronenberg M. CD1d-mediated recognition of an alpha-galactosylceramide by natural killer T cells is highly conserved through mammalian evolution. J Exp Med. 1998;188 (8):1521–8.
12. Dellabona P, Padovan E, Casorati G, Brockhaus M, Lanzavecchia A. An invariant V alpha 24-J alpha Q/V beta 11 T cell receptor is expressed in all individuals by clonally expanded CD4-8- T cells. J Exp Med. 1994;180(3):1171–6.
13. Fujii S, Shimizu K, Steinman RM, Dhodapkar MV. Detection and activation of human Valpha24 + natural killer T cells using alpha-galactosyl ceramide-pulsed dendritic cells. J Immunol Methods. 2003;272 (1-2):147–59.
14. Spada FM, Koezuka Y, Porcelli SA. CD1d-restricted recognition of synthetic glycolipid antigens by human natural killer T cells. J Exp Med. 1998;188 (8):1529–34.
15. Kawano T, Cui J, Koezuka Y, Toura I, Kaneko Y, Motoki K, Ueno H, Nakagawa R, Sato H, Kondo E, Koseki H, Taniguchi M. CD1d-restricted and TCR-mediated activation of valpha14 NKT cells by glycosylceramides. Science. 1997;278(5343):1626–9.
16. Nieda M, Nicol A, Koezuka Y, Kikuchi A, Takahashi T, Nakamura H, Furukawa H, Yabe T, Ishikawa Y, Tadokoro K, Juji T. Activation of human Valpha24NKT cells by alpha-glycosylceramide in a CD1d-restricted and Valpha24TCR-mediated manner. Hum Immunol. 1999;60(1):10–9.
17. Matsumura Y, Moodycliffe AM, Nghiem DX, Ullrich SE, Ananthaswamy HN. Resistance of CD1d−/− mice to ultraviolet-induced skin cancer is associated with increased apoptosis. Am J Pathol. 2004;165(3):879–87.
18. Matsumura Y, Moodycliffe AM, Nghiem DX, Ullrich SE, Ananthaswamy HN. Inverse relationship between increased apoptosis and decreased skin cancer in UV-irradiated CD1d−/− mice. Photochem Photobiol. 2005;81(1):46–51.
19. Nickoloff BJ, Wrone-Smith T, Bonish B, Porcelli SA. Response of murine and normal human skin to injection of allogeneic blood-derived psoriatic immunocytes: detection of T cells expressing receptors typically present on natural killer cells, including CD94, CD158, and CD161. Arch Dermatol. 1999;135(5):546–52.
20. Nickoloff BJ, Wrone-Smith T. Injection of pre-psoriatic skin with CD4 + T cells induces psoriasis. Am J Pathol. 1999;155(1):145–58.
21. Nickoloff BJ, Bonish B, Huang BB, Porcelli SA. Characterization of a T cell line bearing natural killer receptors and capable of creating psoriasis in a SCID mouse model system. J Dermatol Sci. 2000;24 (3):212–25.
22. Bonish B, Jullien D, Dutronc Y, Huang BB, Modlin R, Spada FM, Porcelli SA, Nickoloff BJ. Overexpression of CD1d by keratinocytes in psoriasis and CD1d-dependent IFN-gamma production by NK-T cells. J Immunol. 2000;165(7):4076–85.
23. Adly MA, Assaf HA, Hussein M. Expression of CD1d in human scalp skin and hair follicles: hair cycle related alterations. J Clin Pathol. 2005;58 (12):1278–82.
24. Adly MA, Assaf HA, Nada EA, Soliman M, Hussein M. Human scalp skin and hair follicles express neurotrophin-

3 and its high-affinity receptor tyrosine kinase C, and show hair cycle-dependent alterations in expression. Br J Dermatol. 2005;153(3):514–20.
25. Adly MA, Assaf HA, Hussein MR, Neuber K. Age-associated decrease of CD1d protein production in normal human skin. Br J Dermatol. 2006;155 (1):186–91.
26. Sunderkotter C, Kalden H, Luger TA. Aging and the skin immune system. Arch Dermatol. 1997;133 (10):1256–62.
27. Gilchrest BA, Murphy GF, Soter NA. Effect of chronologic aging and ultraviolet irradiation on Langerhans cells in human epidermis. J Invest Dermatol. 1982;79 (2):85–8.
28. Fainboim L, Salamone Mdel C. CD1: a family of glycolypid-presenting molecules or also immunoregulatory proteins? J Biol Regul Homeost Agents. 2002;16 (2):125–35.
29. Fenske NA, Lober CW. Structural and functional changes of normal aging skin. J Am Acad Dermatol. 1986;15(4 Pt 1):571–85.
30. Fenske NA, Conard CB. Aging skin. Am Fam Physician. 1988;37(2):219–30.
31. Sprecher E, Becker Y, Kraal G, Hall E, Harrison D, Shultz LD. Effect of aging on epidermal dendritic cell populations in C57BL/6J mice. J Invest Dermatol. 1990;94(2):247–53.

The Genetics of Skin Aging

43

David A. Gunn

Contents

D.A. Gunn (✉)
Unilever R&D, Colworth Science Park, Sharnbrook, Bedfordshire, UK
e-mail: david.gunn@unilever.com

M.A. Farage et al. (eds.), *Textbook of Aging Skin*,
DOI 10.1007/978-3-662-47398-6_171

Abstract

The sequencing of the human genome in 2001 was a revolutionary milestone in human genetics and heralded the arrival of the genome-wide association study (GWAS). The GWAS approach identifies which DNA sequence variants across the human genome associate with a particular aging phenotype. Such DNA sequence variants can have marked or subtle effects on the regulation and function of nearby genes and, as a result, affect how cells and tissues age. Indeed, twin studies indicate that approximately half of the variation in the appearance of skin aging features can be attributable to such DNA variants. The GWAS approach has now been applied to the variation in skin pigmentation, skin cancer prevalence, and the presence of skin aging features (e.g., pigmented age spots, skin sag), predominately in northern European populations. The identity of the genes tagged by the DNA variants that associated with these phenotypes is presented in this chapter. As DNA sequence variants do not change over time, the GWAS approach is more likely to identify causal biological mechanisms of aging rather than mechanisms that result from (i.e., consequence of) the aging process. In effect, the GWAS findings have identified proteins and biological pathways that can be targeted to negate the skin aging process. Further advances in genetic technologies (e.g., lower sequencing costs), larger GWASs (to identify rare gene variant effects), and complementary epigenetic studies will further advance the identification of causal mechanisms of skin aging and, as a result, be instrumental in the advancement of new antiaging technologies.

Introduction

One of the most notable characteristics of skin aging is how different the appearance of skin can be between individuals of the same age. While some individuals can display severe wrinkling and hyperpigmentation, others can display little wrinkling but severe skin sagging and skin hypopigmentation [1]. Such variation is reflective of the range of environmental and genetic factors that can influence the way skin ages. Over the past several years, there have been a multitude of genome-wide association studies (GWASs) that have attempted to identify the DNA sequence variants that underlie the genetic variation in aging phenotypes/traits within populations. These findings are having a significant impact on understanding the etiology of age-related diseases, and the GWAS approach is starting to reverberate into the skin aging field, a trend likely to accelerate in the coming years.

The draft sequencing of the human genome in 2001 was a milestone in genetic research [2]. It was the forerunner to and facilitated GWAS – epidemiological investigations into whether variations in the sequence of DNA nucleotide codes in and around genes (herein termed gene variants) associate with the presence of a particular phenotype. Initially, there was much optimism on the value of being able to screen human populations for gene variants that linked to disease presence. Indeed, over the last few years, a plethora of findings linking gene variants with numerous diseases have been published; for example, over 60 gene variants have now been found to link to the presence of diabetes [3]. Although the GWAS approach for skin aging is at an early phase, there have been many recent GWASs published on skin pigmentation and cancer which have uncovered a multitude of genes linked to the underlying biology of these traits. Hence, GWAS is an important tool in understanding the complex biology underlying many human traits.

Here, the current findings for GWAS of skin aging phenotypes are reviewed, and the implications for such findings for understanding the underlying biology of skin aging and for therapeutic solutions are discussed.

Heritability of Skin Aging Phenotypes

To determine whether genetic variation underlies a substantial proportion of phenotype variation within a population, heritability studies can be performed. These heritability estimates involve the use of monozygotic (identical) and dizygotic (nonidentical) twins. As only environmental factors can influence differences between monozygotic twins, if a phenotype displays considerable variability within dizygotic but not monozygotic twins, then genetic variation must be responsible for the variance of that phenotype. In contrast, if the phenotype variability is similar in the dizygotic and monozygotic twins, then environmental factors will be the main cause of the variation. The use of twin studies has been applied widely in estimating the heritability of diseases and human longevity [4].

The first twin study of skin pigmentation found a high heritability estimate for the variation in skin color at a sun-protected site and lower estimates in sun-exposed sites [5]. This finding was as expected because genetic factors tend to have a stronger influence (penetrance) on phenotypes where environmental influences are weak. The first twin study of a skin aging phenotype was carried out by Shekar et al., who estimated that 62 % of the variation in deterioration in the pattern of the stratum corneum on the back of the hand was due to genetic factors [6]. In a study of Danish female twins, genetic factors were estimated to influence 55 %, 41 %, and 61 % of the variation in facial wrinkling, pigmented spots, and perceived facial age, respectively [7]. For sag, the degree to which the skin around the eyebrow sagged across the eye was estimated at 61 % [8], again giving a considerable estimate to the influence of genetic factors. It is perhaps surprising that a relative high genetic estimate was found for these skin aging features given the strong influence of environmental factors on these body sites (particular sun exposure) and the relative homogenous nature of the populations studied (i.e., restricted to those from each country's ancestral population). Hence, taken together, the twin studies performed to date suggest a sizeable genetic component to the variation in skin aging features and support the use of GWAS for studying skin aging.

GWAS and Skin Aging

There have been very few candidate gene studies investigating common gene variants which have found variants that reproducibly associate with a skin aging phenotype, although they have been used with success for identifying the phenotype associations for *MC1R* variants [9] and in identifying rare gene variants that cause skin diseases within families. For example, mutations in the *CDKN2a* gene have been found to be responsible for a number of familial melanoma cases [10]. The advent of GWAS, though, has enabled the genetics of skin aging to be studied much more intensively. Indeed, a large number of GWASs of skin pigmentation and cancer have been published in the last 10 years.

Skin Color and Skin Tanning

The first genome-wide association study that was published on skin color focused on skin reflectometry using L*a*b* skin scores [11] in a population with Indian ancestry but living in the UK. Associations were found between skin color and variants in the genes *SLC24A5*, *TYR*, and *SLC45A2* [12]. Differences in skin color (also via skin reflectometry) between indigenous Americans and Europeans were also found to be associated with *SLC24A5* and *SLC45A2* variants along with associations for *OPRM1* and *EGFR* [13]; these latter two findings have yet to be replicated. The gene variant in *SLC24A5* (rs1426654) had the largest effect on skin color in both the Indian population and the indigenous Americans and Europeans. In addition, one allele of this SNP is fixed in populations with European ancestry and pale white skin, and the other allele fixed in populations from sub-Saharan Africa with black skin. Therefore, this gene variant can be arguably viewed (at least to date) as the common variant with the strongest effect on skin color in humans.

In Caucasians, Han et al. [14] found variants in five genomic loci that associated with hair color and then tested the association of these variants with skin color and tanning ability. Those that associated ($P < 0.05$) with skin color were in or near the genes *HERC2/OCA2*, *IRF4*, *MC1R*, and *SLC45A2*. In the same study, these genes were also found to associate with tanning ability along with gene variants in *SLC24A4* [14]. Two further GWASs on skin tanning response/skin sensitivity to the sun in Europeans [15, 16] confirmed the associations for *ASIP*, *HERC2/OCA2*, *IRF4*, *MC1R*, *SLC24A4*, *SLC45A2*, and *TYR*. The most recent and largest study of skin color to date [17] confirmed the association between five gene loci (*ASIP*, *HERC2/OCA2*, *IRF4*, *MC1R*, *SLC45A2*) with skin color and gave supporting evidence for three others (*BNC2*, *SLC24A4*, *TYR*) in those with northern European ancestry.

A GWAS on skin color variation in black-skinned/sub-Saharan ancestral populations has yet to be performed but should give insights into gene variant influences on the wider range of skin pigmentation levels, similar to the detection of *SLC24A5*. Differences between individuals in their tanning response and base skin color have also yet to be established. Although the two overlap, it is possible that the response to UV radiation and then the subsequent reduction of melanin production to basal levels requires protein interactions not required for normal basal levels of melanin. Hence, GWASs on in vivo measurement of skin color changes post-UV exposure of skin (rather than self-report) would be a good way to dissect any differences between these two phenotypes.

Other genes have been found to associate with skin pigmentation diseases through candidate gene approaches. For example, gene variants in *KITLG* have been found to be responsible for hypo- and hyperpigmentation disorders [18]. However, although this study pinpointed this gene's importance for correct skin color development into adulthood, it is unclear whether this gene is also important for variation in normal skin color or age-related decline in even pigmentation. Indeed, Sulem et al. found no association for variants in this gene with sensitivity of skin to the sun [19]. Hence, all pigmentation genes might not all necessarily influence the changes to skin pigmentation with age.

Pigmented Spots

The term "pigmented spots" covers a wide range of skin aging phenotypes. Whereas freckles and nevi/moles develop during childhood, solar lentigines and seborrheic keratosis develop as a result of skin aging. In addition, solar lentigines are strongly associated with sun exposure, whereas seborrheic keratoses can be commonly found on sun-protected body sites. Such underlying biological differences for these three types of pigmented spots might be reflected by differences in the gene variants that influence their prevalence.

In the only two GWASs on freckles to date, Sulem et al. [19] found associations between freckles and gene variants in/near *IRF4*, *MC1R*, and *TYR*, and in a follow-up study, they found evidence for association between *ASIP* and freckles [20]. Despite the different life-stage prevalence of senile lentigines and freckles, the gene variants associated with freckles were also found to associate with facial pigmented spots in an elderly population [21]. The similarity in findings likely points to the importance of eumelanin in preventing damage occurring in skin from sun exposure whether in childhood (for freckles) or during adult life (for solar lentigines). However, the association between these gene variants and pigmented spots was independent of basal skin color, reflecting findings for these gene variants with actinic keratosis and skin cancer [22, 23]. It is unclear, though, whether this skin color independence indicates these gene variants influence a melanin-independent pathway or are linked to tanning response rather than basal melanin production or that there is residual confounding (i.e., that the measures of skin color did not capture the full variation of skin color present in the population). Larger GWAS is required, along with more accurate measures of skin color, tanning responses, and measurements of spot subtypes (e.g., no GWAS has yet been performed on melasma spots) to determine whether mechanisms other than those related to melanin production or eumelanin/pheomelanin ratio are causing the development of pigmented spots with age. In support of the involvement in other biological mechanisms, pigmented spots in an elderly population have been associated with health independently of sun exposure [24] suggesting intrinsic biological mechanisms are also associated with their development.

Melanoma

As melanoma can have severe health consequences, it is of little surprise that of all the skin aging phenotypes, GWAS has been strongly focused on this disease. There is evidence that variants in or near *ATM*, *ARNT*, *ASIP*, *CASP8*, *CDKN2A/MATP*, *FTO*, *HERC2/OCA2*, *MC1R*, *MX2*, *NID1*, *PLA2G6*, *SLC45A2*, *TERT*, *TYR*, and *TYRP1* associate with melanoma prevalence (e.g., [25–28]). A recent large GWAS of melanoma [29] also identified variants in *AGR3*, *CCND1*, *CDKAL1*, *CYP1B1*, *OBFC1*, *RAD23B*, and *PARP1*, but failed to replicate *NID1* and *TRYP1* associations. The identity of these genes highlights the predominant pathways that are involved in melanoma development. For example, a number of these genes are involved in melanin production (*ASIP*, *HERC2*, *MC1R*, *SLC45A1*, *TYR*, and *TYRP1*), DNA damage (*ATM*, *MC1R*, *TERT1*, *OBFC1*, *PARP1*, and *RAD23B*), and cell senescence and apoptosis (*ATM*, *CASP8*, *CCND1*, *CDKN2A*, and *TERT1*). In support of this, Ingenuity (http://www.ingenuity.com) analysis of all the genes tagged by DNA sequence variants detected pigmentation/melanin, DNA, and cell-cycle-linked pathways (Fig. 1). These findings indicate that a lack of UV

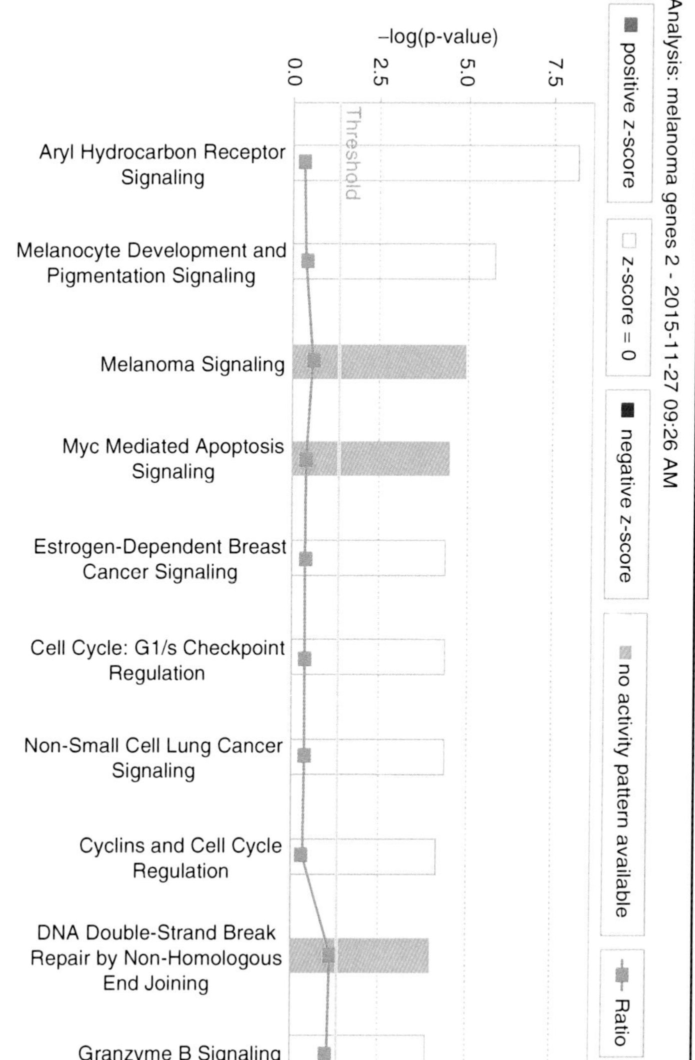

Fig. 1 Ingenuity canonical analysis of the genes tagged by DNA sequence variants through melanoma GWASs highlights the pigmentation/melanin, DNA repair, apoptosis, and cell-cycle/senescence pathways as key mechanisms preventing melanocytes turning into melanoma. The top ten canonical pathways are given. The analysis identified the pathways from the Qiagen Ingenuity Pathways Analysis library of canonical pathways (IPA®,QIAGEN Redwood City, www.qiagen.com/ingenuity) that were most significant to the data set. The significance of the association between the data set and the canonical pathway was measured in two ways: (1) A ratio of the number of molecules from the data set that map to the pathway divided by the total number of molecules that map to the canonical pathway is displayed. (2) Fisher's exact test was used to calculate a P value determining the probability that the association between the genes in the data set and the canonical pathway is explained by chance alone

protection from melanin leads to the accumulation of DNA damage in cells, which can lead to melanocytes becoming cancerous unless prevented through apoptosis or cell senescence. Hence, reducing sun exposure and DNA damage and promoting cellular senescence or apoptosis become logically melanoma prevention strategies. However, cellular senescence is possibly also a driver of skin aging [30], indicating apoptosis is likely a better outcome for the future health of the skin.

Nevi are generally benign conditions that occur mainly during childhood and adolescence. However, it has been known for many years that the number of nevi is associated with an increased risk of melanoma. Recent GWAS has started to uncover the reason for these overlaps. For example, gene variants in *PLA2G6* [31] and *SLC45A2* [31, 32] are associated with nevus numbers and also melanoma. Hence, GWAS is helping identify the biological reasons why there are common occurrences between particular skin phenotypes.

Rare gene variants that are not tested in GWAS can also cause melanoma. For example, familial forms of melanoma are due to rare gene variants/mutations in the *CDN2KA* [10] and *MITF* [33] genes, with the latter gene yet to be detected in a GWAS. Thus, genes tagged by rare gene variants can be just as important for understanding the etiology of skin aging. Further GWASs can help identify rare gene variant associations with melanoma, but would require very large numbers of cases and controls (>100,000). Such large-scale studies will only be possible through global collaborations between genetic epidemiology groups and large-scale recruitment of subjects for new or current epidemiology studies.

Basal Cell Carcinoma (BCC) and Squamous Cell Carcinoma (SCC)

Although under less scrutiny than melanoma, GWAS of BCC has been performed with particular focus in the Icelandic population. Gene variants found to associate with basal cell carcinoma are *CASP8*, *CDKN2a*, *GATA3*, *IRF4*, *KLF14*, *KRT5*, *MC1R*, *MYCN*, *PADI6-RCC2*, *RGS22*, *RHOU*, *SLC45A2*, *TERT-CLPTM1L*, *TGM3*, *TP53*, *UBAC2*, and *ZFHX4* (e.g., [34–36]). *UBAC2* is the only gene of the group whose association was not replicated in the largest GWAS to date [35] highlighting the robustness of the GWAS approach. A pathway analysis approach using BCC GWAS data [37], at that time, identified (along with pigmentation and BCC risk pathway terms) the pathways heparan sulfate biosynthesis, mCalpain, Rho cell motility signaling, and nitric oxide. Pathway analysis can highlight where numerous gene variants effect the same pathway which, even if each variant has only a weak effect, can add up to a strong accumulative effect on the biological function of the pathway. It also highlights other proteins in the pathway that could be influencing the development of the trait whether tagged by gene variants or not (e.g., Fig. 1). For BCC, the influence of pathways independent of sun exposure is clearly evident and points to routes other than sun avoidance/protection for intervention.

Squamous cell carcinoma has come under less scrutiny than BCC, and a large-scale GWAS on cutaneous SCC has yet to be performed. However, some evidence exists for association of gene variants in/near *IRF4* [36], *KRT5* [38], *SLC45A2* [38], and *UBAC2* [36] with SCC.

For the GWASs of the three types of skin cancer, there are some differences between the results. For example, *TERT-CLPTM1L* is associated with melanoma and BCC [34, 38] but not SCC [38]. In addition, whereas *CDKN2a* is associated with both BCC and melanoma, *TB53* is only associated with BCC. This perhaps indicates that the *TB53*-induced senescence pathway is not an important cell-cycle checkpoint in melanocytes. Although yet to be performed, statistical comparisons between the different pathways tagged by GWAS results for melanoma and BCC might give insight into how keratinocytes and melanocytes age differently due the specific nature of each cell type.

Due to recent advances in DNA sequencing, it is also now possible to sequence the genome of cells from skin to a sufficient depth of coverage to determine how genetic mutations might be accumulating with age. A landmark study on eyelid skin [39] identified many DNA mutations within the skin cell populations (2–6 mutations per Mb of DNA per cell – which approximates to 100–300 per cell per year), many of which had the hallmarks of UV-induced DNA damage. Mutations in *NOTCH1-3*, *FAT1*, *RBM10*, and *TP53* were particularly enriched in the sun-exposed skin, and mutations in *NOTCH1*, *TP53*, and *FGFR3* were associated with the greatest clonal expansion of cells. This study highlights how the accumulation of mutations within the DNA of skin cells drives cell expansion when the mutations occur in particular genes and increases the chances of the cells becoming cancerous. Indeed, the genes enriched for mutations were similar to those detected in SCC samples. Although these genes were also mutated in BCC samples, the *PTCH1* gene was less mutated and is the most common mutated gene in BCC samples [40]. As BCC is three times more prevalent than SCC, it would have been expected that elderly skin would also accumulate mutations in *PTCH1*. It is feasible, though, that *PTCH1* represents part of the last control/defense mechanism for preventing BCC (similar to *CDKN2a* in melanocytes) and hence that mutated forms are unlikely in BCC-free skin.

These sequencing studies of genetic mutations help identify genes involved in aging which might not be normally detected by GWAS, possibly because there is evolutionary selection against inherited variants within some genes due to their critical role in development, for example; in support of this, *PTCH* and *NOTCH* are well-known developmental genes. How the accumulation of mutations in cells affects other skin functions beyond cell proliferation (e.g., melanin production) remains to be determined but will be critical for understanding other skin aging phenotypes.

Skin Sag

To date, the only GWAS of skin sagging was performed in the Rotterdam study, which focused on sagging of upper eyelid skin [21]. This study found a variant in *DLGAP1* and near the gene *TGIF1* (linked to cell senescence and elastin repair) to associate with eyelid sag. This variant was the only one found to be significantly associated with eyelid sag despite the relatively large numbers of subjects used (>5,000), suggesting that the heritability (60 %) of this trait is due to many common variants with weak influences or rarer variants not yet tested. Hence, much larger studies will be required to identify other gene variants that associate with skin sag in the future.

Stretch marks are a phenotype that could have some commonality with skin sag, as both are related to the elastic properties of skin. In a GWAS of stretch marks, associations were found for variants in the genes *ELN*, *SRPX*, *HMCN1*, and *TMEM18*, and nominal associations were found for variants in/near *PNPLA1*, *FN1*, and *NPIPL2* [41]. The link with the elastin (*ELN*) and fibronectin (*FN1*) genes is particularly relevant findings, as these genes are known to be important in the normal functioning of elastin fibers. Candidate gene studies using the variants tagged to stretch marks can now be performed to determine whether these gene variants could also be playing a role in skin sag. However, an overlap between these two phenotypes cannot be assumed as the accumulation of elastin fiber damage with age could be quite a different phenomenon to the inability of elastin fibers to recoil after maximal loads.

Skin sag is a phenotype that can be measured in many ways, from human judgment to technical twisting or punching of skin followed by measurement of the skin recall. The difficulty with trying to compare the different ways of measuring sag is that it is unclear to what degree subcutaneous tissues influence each measure and how this varies between body sites. For example, modern face lift techniques target the connective tissue underneath the skin, indicating its importance in producing facial sag in the first place [42]. However, as there has only been one GWAS of skin sagging to date, it is not yet possible to determine whether different genes influence skin sagging in different parts of the face and body.

Skin Wrinkling

There are currently no published GWASs on skin wrinkling despite many publications focused on the epidemiology of wrinkles (e.g., [43]). There have been, though, two GWASs published on global measures of skin aging which included wrinkling as a major component. The first to be published was by Le et al. [44] who found variants in/near the genes STXBP5L and FBXO40 associated with photoaging and both are known to be expressed in skin. In a study of a composite skin age score [45], variants in/near KCND2 (a potassium channel gene important for nerve signaling), DIAPH2 (linked to ovary development), and EDEM1 (involved in endoplasmic reticulum degradation of glycoproteins) were found to significantly associate. There was no concordance in the findings between these two studies, and due to the composite nature of each skin aging measure, it is difficult to determine to what extent these findings could be related to skin wrinkling. In addition, relative to the recent GWAS on skin color and melanoma, the subject sizes of these studies were low ($n \leq 500$) making it difficult to determine how reproducible these findings were.

The principle of using a global/composite measure of skin aging rather than individual phenotypes could help detect gene variants which might have a weak effect on any one skin aging feature but due to a ubiquitous biological function (e.g., DNA repair) are important for skin aging per se and effect many skin aging phenotypes. Indeed, *MC1R* could be viewed as such a gene as it has been associated with skin color, nevi, freckles, pigmented spots, melanoma, and BCC. Whether this is related to the fact *MC1R* is involved in DNA repair as well as melanin production [46] is yet to be proven beyond doubt, but highlights the possibility that gene variants that affect multiple skin aging phenotypes could be found through pursing global skin aging measures. Weakness to using such global measures of skin aging is discussed below.

Application of GWAS Findings

Gene Variant Mechanism of Action

DNA sequence variants can influence gene function through many different routes. Severe changes to the amino acid structure of a protein can result from variants which produce frameshift mutations in the DNA sequence of a gene. For example, familial melanoma cases have been linked to a severely truncated *CDKN2a* protein (p16INK4a) due to a 19 bp deletion in exon 2 of the gene [47]. In effect, this mutation prevents p16INK4a from functioning, thereby preventing damaged melanocytes from becoming senescent and increasing the risk of them turning cancerous. Changes to one amino acid in the sequence of a protein can also influence its function. A change to the amino acid sequence in the NCKX5 protein (produced from the *SLC24A5* gene), for example, has been shown to impair its ion exchange function and reduce melanin production in melanocytes [12].

Other variant influences can be more subtle, particularly where they are not located within the exons of a gene. These sequence variants tend to influence the way a gene's transcription levels are regulated via the binding of transcription factors to DNA and can be located many Kbs away from the gene they influence; this makes it difficult to assign the variant effects to one particular gene. Gene variants identified from GWAS that were initially difficult to attribute with certainty to one gene were those in/near the *ASIP* locus, *CDKN2a/MTAP* locus, and *HERC2/OCA2* locus. Gene variants in the introns of *IRF4* and *HERC3* influence transcription of *IRF4* and *OCA2*, respectively, by interacting with transcription factors that form a chromatin loop between their introns and the promoter regions of the latter genes [48, 49]. The different alleles of these gene variants affect the ability of the transcription factors to form this chromatin loop and thereby influence the transcription of the nearby genes from their promoter regions. Some gene variants attributed to the effects of *CDKN2a* are actually located in the *MTAP* [50] gene, which has yet to be ruled out to be at least partly responsible for some of the melanoma variation. For the *ASIP* pigmentation gene, there are other genes that could be influencing the association of the SNPs at 20q11.22 with skin color. For example, the expression of the nearby genes *EIF2S2* and *GSS* was found to be correlated with melanin levels [17] suggesting that the gene variants in this region could be influencing more than one gene. Hence, the follow-up investigative work to GWAS findings is key for further understanding of gene regulation and its control of skin aging.

Pros and Cons of GWAS Approach for Skin Aging

There are substantial benefits to utilizing a GWAS approach for investigating skin aging. Perhaps the main advantage of genetic research over transcriptomic and proteomic research, for example, is the issue of cause versus consequence. It is difficult to distinguish between mRNA and protein changes that drive the aging process (cause) and those that result from the aging process (consequence). As gene variants are not modified over the life span, then their association with a phenotype cannot be as a result of the occurrence of that phenotype. This means that genetic evidence enriches for genes involved in causing variation in the way skin ages and can help identify protein targets for antiaging (see next section for discussion).

Another advantage to the GWAS approach is when large numbers of genes are found to associate with a skin aging phenotype through larger and larger GWASs. The identification of multiple genes involved in a phenotype of interest helps pinpoint enrichment of particular cellular pathways in the etiology of the phenotype. For example, although the *aryl hydrocarbon receptor* (*AhR*) gene has not been identified in melanoma GWAS, the AhR signaling pathway is highlighted from the pathway analysis of melanoma GWAS results (Fig. 1) indicating it could be an important factor in melanoma susceptibility. Indeed, AhR has been shown to modulate melanogenesis [51] and, therefore, could be an important aspect of melanocyte aging. Hence, GWAS helps identify the key biological pathways that influence natural variation in skin aging, helping target potential biological mechanisms in the body for therapeutic purposes.

Although GWASs are valuable in helping identify potential antiaging targets, there are also a number of weaknesses. For example, if particular gene variants are not found to associate with a phenotype, this does not mean it is not important in the development of that phenotype. There might be, for example, no gene variants in the population under study that effect the gene function strongly enough for their effects to be detected. For example, a gene could be involved in skin pigmentation, but if also critical in a particular development process, then there could have been an evolutionary selection against any variants in the gene locus that affect its function (as per the *NOTCH* and *PCTH* gene example discussed above). In addition, the gene variants available for study will vary by population. For example, *SLC24A5* would not have been found by carrying out a GWAS in either European or African ancestral populations separately, as the functional alleles in this gene are fixed in both populations due to selection pressures on the gene variants in each of these ancestral populations.

Another weakness is that the genetic variation underpinning the prevalence of common diseases and phenotypes is being found to be more complex than many first envisaged. In particular, the variation in disease prevalence within a population that gene variants can explain was lower than anticipated. The multitude of environmental factors that influence a phenotype are likely one of the reasons that gene variants have small effect sizes – i.e., a gene variant might only have an effect given a specific set of environmental circumstances. To detect gene variant effects on skin aging then due to the range of environmental factors (particularly sun exposure) that influence it [52] GWASs might need to accommodate within any statistical analyses the main environmental influences on the skin phenotype under study. In addition, global aging phenotypes (composites of many individual phenotypes [53]) might have a lower probability of finding gene variants due to the fact any one gene variant might only influence one individual skin aging phenotype rather than them all. Studies of gene variants that influence human longevity, for example, have yielded little progress compared to individual diseases [54]. Hence, GWAS of global phenotypes should be accompanied by GWAS of the component phenotypes to help identify variants with global effects alongside those with effects only on specific component aging features.

Skin Antiaging Technology

GWAS findings can be valuable in determining a potential antiaging protein target. For example, a variant in the gene *HMGCR* associates with cholesterol levels, but its effect on cholesterol levels is small [55]. However, the protein made from this gene (HMGCoA) is the target of statins, one of the most profitable and widely used drugs in health care, which have strong effects on lowering cholesterol levels. Hence, the tagging of genes by GWAS helps identify the proteins that can be targeted by antiaging technologies irrespective of the effect size of the DNA sequence variant. In support of this, a recent review of current drug targets relative to GWAS findings for disease phenotypes indicated that the success rate of drug development could be doubled if genetic evidence is included in the screening of potential targets [56].

GWAS can also help indicate what could be the knock-on consequences of targeting a particular protein on other phenotypes. For example, variants in *IRF4* have strong effects on pigmented spots and melanoma risk suggesting that this gene/protein target could be a potential target for reducing the prevalence of pigmented spots and, as a result, also reduce melanoma risk. Whether *IRF4* is a good/practical target or not, being able to verify which other traits a gene variant is associated with might help determine likely side effects (beneficial or detrimental) for any particular technology intervention. Indeed, an atlas of genetic correlations between phenotypes is being developed [57] and could prove invaluable in the future for assessing a protein target for any widespread tissue effects.

To invent and generate new technologies for skin aging, it is first best to decide whether the technology will be for preventing the development of a particular phenotype or treating it once developed. For treatment of skin cancers, for example, it might be best to target proteins that are heavily expressed within the cancer cells compared to surrounding cells, even if that protein did not cause the development of the cancer in the first place. In this situation, proteomic and transcriptomic studies or sequencing studies of the cancer cells would be particularly useful for identifying such targets, whereas GWAS is less so. For example, boosting melanin production through TYR function (which associates with melanoma in GWAS) would help reduce UV damage in healthy cells but likely have little effect on the treatment of melanoma cells. However, it is still possible some genes tagged by GWAS could also be involved in the progression of the cancer and, therefore, might also make good targets for treatment. Hence, GWAS findings are more appropriate for preventative technologies, although they should not automatically be ruled out for treatment (of disease) purposes as well.

One common myth of genetic findings is that because it is (at least currently [58]) unrealistic to change the sequence of DNA within cells, then there is nothing that can be done to change one's susceptibility to particular phenotypes. Although it is true that the gene variants themselves cannot be changed, the function and activity of the gene it influences can be targeted. A good example (as well as the *Hmg-CoA* example above) is the way pigmentation genes and sun exposure interact. If an individual carries a particular set of gene variants that makes them susceptible to sun damage, for example, then keeping out the sun will help mitigate the effect of their gene variants on skin aging and reduce the prevalence of such features. In effect, the individual has adapted their environment to their genetic profile and changed the way their gene variants influence their skin. This is a far removed scenario than that believing that genetics fixes one's fate.

One of the biggest hurdles for preventative approaches to skin antiaging is the behavior changes that are normally required for the preventative approaches. For example, the best way to avoid skin sun damage is to avoid the sun and to use sun protection factor creams. Although this approach has been proven to reduce skin aging (e.g., wrinkles [59]) and indeed the message has been adopted by many, there is still a large segment of European populations who prefer the short-term appearance benefits of a tan [60] and possibly the effects of endorphins [61] to the longer-term detrimental effects on skin aging. Hence, preventative approaches can suffer from the realities of modern behaviors irrespective of the long-term benefits such approaches can bring. However, these barriers also offer opportunities for health care and the cosmetics industry – to determine how tanning could be induced without the need of skin exposure to harmful UV radiation. There is also the controversial area of the benefits of vitamin D production in skin. However, this debate is population dependent with some populations clearly suffering too much exposure (e.g., Australians of northern European ancestry) and others too little (e.g., women consistently wearing clothing [62] over skin when outside). Hence, advice should be tailored dependent on the person's sun exposure through the seasons.

There has been much interest into whether the identification of associations between genetic variants and skin phenotypes enables a genetic personalization approach for the skin-care industry.

However, there are currently a number of hurdles in realizing such an approach. For many common age-related traits, gene variants have been found to only explain a small fraction of the natural variation within populations (e.g., see [63] for a review of this in relation to obesity), indicating the actual prognostic value of genetic personalization for common aging traits is low. In addition, the advice given alongside any genetic testing would have to add value over and above current recommendations – as it is not yet even clear how many gene variants exert their effects on various skin aging phenotypes, it is difficult to see how current advice could be changed until greater understanding is gained. There are also many traits where the genetic predisposition to a trait is already evident to the individual (e.g., skin color) limiting the extra value of genetic prognostic tests, although predisposition to aging traits in young to middle-aged populations could be relevant. Future findings might help overcome some of these hurdles (e.g., epigenetics [64]), and investment in research to determine which gene variants associate with a particular trait and how they exert their influence (i.e., understanding the etiology of a phenotype) is likely the best current approaches to the genetics of skin aging.

Epigenetics

The epigenetics field is primarily the study of chemical modifications (e.g., methylation and acetylation) to DNA and histones which can be inherited across cell divisions. These modifications are, generally, much more stable in tissues over time compared to mRNA and protein levels. In addition, epigenetic modifications can be influenced by environmental and genetic factors. Taken together, epigenetic modifications are a good measure of historical environmental and genetic influences on cells which subsequently influence how gene transcription is regulated. Recently, new technologies have facilitated studies of epigenetic changes that occur due to human aging within different tissues, including skin [65, 66]. Such technologies offer a new way to investigate the modification of gene regulation with age and will likely highlight new routes for antiaging technologies.

Correlations between DNA methylation levels in different human tissues with age have identified many gene loci that are differentially methylated, some of which are consistently differentially methylated across many tissues including skin [67]. These findings have enabled the concept of an epigenetic clock [68] – methylation changes with age that predict the degree to which a particular tissue has aged. However, whether such changes relate to the susceptibility of skin to develop a particular aging phenotype remains to be tested. Also, although a direct comparison between epigenetic and genetic prediction models (for predicting the risk a particular disease or phenotype develops by a certain age) has yet to be performed, epigenetic measures can be predicted to have better prognostic value as they are influenced by the environmental as well as genetic factors – in effect acting as a measure of the influence of both on cellular function. Indeed, DNA methylation differences in skin between sun-exposed and protected body sites as well as between young and old were found at particular gene loci [66], suggesting that they could act as a marker of the amount of damage that has occurred to skin. In addition, it is now becoming clear that many gene variants influence the methylation levels of gene loci (e.g., [69]) indicating that one of the routes gene variants influence gene regulation is through their effects on the epigenetic control of gene transcription. Hence, although at an early stage, epigenetic research will help determine some of the routes through which gene variants are able to influence cellular function and how such effects impact skin aging.

Conclusions

The GWAS approach to skin aging has only just begun, and already we are seeing the identification of many genes that associate with skin pigmentation and cancer. However, the number of studies is still relatively small compared to those carried out for most age-related diseases, and their use outside of northern European populations has been limited. For example, only two skin pigmentation GWASs [13, 70] have been carried out in those without northern European ancestry. Hence, expansion of GWAS is likely to give new findings and insights into the etiologies of many skin aging phenotypes across global populations.

It is striking that a number of GWAS investigations into many aspects of skin appearance are yet to be published (e.g., skin wrinkling) suggesting that the next 5–10 years could be a "golden" period for genetic research into skin aging. Indeed, future GWASs will likely encompass large numbers of subjects (e.g., >10,000), use whole genome sequencing to investigate rarer variants, be carried out in different ancestral populations, and integrate with epigenetic and transcriptomic approaches to understand gene regulation and the dynamic temporal interactions between genes. Genetic studies are proving to be invaluable in understanding why there is such a large variation in the appearance of skin within populations and will offer new biological insights that will help seed skin antiaging technologies for the future.

References

1. Griffiths CEM. The clinical identification and quantification of photodamage. Br J Dermatol. 1992;127:37–42.
2. Lander ES, et al. Initial sequencing and analysis of the human genome. Nature. 2001;409:860–921.
3. Morris AP, et al. Large-scale association analysis provides insights into the genetic architecture and pathophysiology of type 2 diabetes. Nat Genet. 2012;44:981–90.
4. vB Hjelmborg J, et al. Genetic influence on human lifespan and longevity. Hum Genet. 2006; 119:312–21.
5. Clark P, et al. A twin study of skin reflectance. Ann Hum Biol. 1981;8:529–41.
6. Shekar SN, et al. Genetic and environmental influences on skin pattern deterioration. J Invest Dermatol. 2005;125:1119–29.
7. Gunn DA, et al. Why some women look young for their age. PLoS One. 2009;4, e8021.
8. Jacobs LC, et al. Intrinsic and extrinsic risk factors for sagging eyelids. JAMA Dermatol. 2014;150 (8):836–43.
9. Elfakir A, et al. Functional MC1R-gene variants are associated with increased risk for severe photoaging of facial skin. J Invest Dermatol. 2010;130(4):1107–15.
10. van der Rhee JI, et al. Clinical and histologic characteristics of malignant melanoma in families with a germline mutation in CDKN2A. J Am Acad Dermatol. 2011;65:281–8.
11. Alaluf S, et al. The impact of epidermal melanin on objective measurements of human skin colour. Pigment Cell Res. 2002;15:119–26.
12. Ginger RS, et al. SLC24A5 encodes a trans-Golgi network protein with potassium-dependent sodium-calcium exchange activity that regulates human epidermal melanogenesis. J Biol Chem. 2008;283:5486–95.
13. Quillen EE, et al. OPRM1 and EGFR contribute to skin pigmentation differences between Indigenous Americans and Europeans. Hum Genet. 2012;131:1073–80.
14. Han J, et al. A genome-wide association study identifies novel alleles associated with hair color and skin pigmentation. PLoS Genet. 2008;4, e1000074.
15. Nan H, et al. Genome-wide association study of tanning phenotype in a population of European ancestry. J Invest Dermatol. 2009;129:2250–7.
16. Sulem P, et al. Two newly identified genetic determinants of pigmentation in Europeans. Nat Genet. 2008;40:835–7.
17. Liu F, et al. Genetics of skin color variation in Europeans: genome-wide association studies with functional follow-up. Hum Genet. 2015;134 (8):823–35.
18. Picardo M, et al. The genetic determination of skin pigmentation: KITLG and the KITLG/c-Kit pathway as key players in the onset of human familial pigmentary diseases. J Invest Dermatol. 2011;131:1182–5.
19. Sulem P, et al. Genetic determinants of hair, eye and skin pigmentation in Europeans. Nat Genet. 2007;39:1443–52. doi:10.1038/ng.2007.13.
20. Sulem P, et al. Two newly identified genetic determinants of pigmentation in Europeans. Nat Genet. 2008;40:835–7. doi:10.1038/ng.160.
21. Jacobs LC, et al. A Genome-wide association study identifies the skin color genes IRF4, MC1R, ASIP, and BNC2 influencing facial pigmented spots. J Invest Dermatol. 2015;135(7):1735–42.
22. Kosiniak-Kamysz A, et al. Potential association of single nucleotide polymorphisms in pigmentation genes with the development of basal cell carcinoma. J Dermatol. 2012;39(8):693–8.
23. Jacobs LC, et al. IRF4, MC1R and TYR genes are risk factors for actinic keratosis independent of skin color. Hum Mol Genet. 2015;24(11):3296–303.
24. van Drielen K, et al. Markers of health and disease and pigmented spots in a middle-aged population. Br J Dermatol. 2015;173(6):1550–2.
25. Barrett JH, et al. Genome-wide association study identifies three new melanoma susceptibility loci. Nat Genet. 2011;43:1108–13.
26. Gudbjartsson DF, et al. ASIP and TYR pigmentation variants associate with cutaneous melanoma and basal cell carcinoma. Nat Genet. 2008;40:886–91.

27. Law MH, et al. Meta-analysis combining new and existing data sets confirms that the TERT-CLPTM1L locus influences melanoma risk. J Invest Dermatol. 2012;132:485–7.
28. Iles MM, et al. A variant in FTO shows association with melanoma risk not due to BMI. Nat Genet. 2013;45:428–32. 432e1.
29. Law MH, et al. Genome-wide meta-analysis identifies five new susceptibility loci for cutaneous malignant melanoma. Nat Genet. 2015;47(9):987–95.
30. Waaijer ME, et al. P16INK4a Positive cells in human skin are indicative of local elastic fiber morphology, facial wrinkling, and perceived age. J Gerontol A Biol Sci Med Sci. 2015; doi: 10.1093/gerona/glv114.
31. Falchi M, et al. Genome-wide association study identifies variants at 9p21 and 22q13 associated with development of cutaneous nevi. Nat Genet. 2009;41:915–9.
32. Newton-Bishop JA, et al. Melanocytic nevi, nevus genes, and melanoma risk in a large case–control study in the United Kingdom. Cancer Epidemiol Biomarkers Prev. 2010;19:2043–54.
33. Yokoyama S, et al. A novel recurrent mutation in MITF predisposes to familial and sporadic melanoma. Nature. 2011;480:99–103.
34. Yang X, et al. Association between TERT-CLPTM1L rs401681[C] allele and NMSC cancer risk: a meta-analysis including 45,184 subjects. Arch Dermatol Res. 2012;305:49-52.
35. Stacey SN, et al. New basal cell carcinoma susceptibility loci. Nat Commun. 2015;6:6825.
36. Nan H, et al. Genome-wide association study identifies novel alleles associated with risk of cutaneous basal cell carcinoma and squamous cell carcinoma. Hum Mol Genet. 2011;20:3718–24.
37. Zhang M, et al. Pathway analysis for genome-wide association study of basal cell carcinoma of the skin. PLoS One. 2011;6, e22760.
38. Stacey SN, et al. New common variants affecting susceptibility to basal cell carcinoma. Nat Genet. 2009;41:909–14.
39. Martincorena I, et al. Tumor evolution. High burden and pervasive positive selection of somatic mutations in normal human skin. Science. 2015;348 (6237):880–6.
40. Jayaraman SS, et al. Mutational landscape of basal cell carcinomas by whole-exome sequencing. J Invest Dermatol. 2014;134(1):213–20.
41. Tung JY, et al. Genome-wide association analysis implicates elastic microfibrils in the development of nonsyndromic striae distensae. J Invest Dermatol. 2013;133:2628–31.
42. Ozdemir R, et al. Anatomicohistologic study of the retaining ligaments of the face and use in face lift: retaining ligament correction and SMAS plication. Plast Reconstr Surg. 2002;110:1134–47.
43. Cosgrove MC, et al. Dietary nutrient intakes and skin-aging appearance among middle-aged American women. Am J Clin Nutr. 2007;86:1225–31.
44. Le CS, et al. A genome-wide association study in Caucasian women points out a putative role of the STXBP5L gene in facial photoaging. J Invest Dermatol. 2013;133(4):929–35.
45. Chang AL, et al. Identification of genes promoting skin youthfulness by genome-wide association study. J Invest Dermatol. 2014;134(3):651–7.
46. Hauser JE, et al. Melanin content and MC1R function independently affect UVR-induced DNA damage in cultured human melanocytes. Pigment Cell Res. 2006;19(4):303–14.
47. Gruis NA, et al. Homozygotes for CDKN2 (p16) germline mutation in Dutch familial melanoma kindreds. Nat Genet. 1995;10(3):351–3.
48. Visser M, et al. HERC2 rs12913832 modulates human pigmentation by attenuating chromatin-loop formation between a long-range enhancer and the OCA2 promoter. Genome Res. 2012;22(3):446–55.
49. Visser M, et al. Allele-specific transcriptional regulation of IRF4 in melanocytes is mediated by chromatin looping of the intronic rs12203592 enhancer to the IRF4 promoter. Hum Mol Genet. 2015;24(9):2649–61.
50. Amos CI, et al. Genome-wide association study identifies novel loci predisposing to cutaneous melanoma. Hum Mol Genet. 2011;20:5012–23.
51. Luecke S, et al. The aryl hydrocarbon receptor (AHR), a novel regulator of human melanogenesis. Pigment Cell Melanoma Res. 2010;23(6):828–33.
52. Gunn DA, et al. Lifestyle and youthful looks. Br J Dermatol. 2015;172(5):1338–45.
53. Guinot C, et al. Relative contribution of intrinsic vs extrinsic factors to skin aging as determined by a validated skin age score. Arch Dermatol. 2002;138:1454–60.
54. Deelen J, et al. Genome-wide association study identifies a single major locus contributing to survival into old age; the APOE locus revisited. Aging Cell. 2011;10:686–98.
55. Aulchenko YS, et al. Loci influencing lipid levels and coronary heart disease risk in 16 European population cohorts. Nat Genet. 2009;41:47–55.
56. Nelson MR, et al. The support of human genetic evidence for approved drug indications. Nat Genet. 2015;47(8):856–60.
57. Bulik-Sullivan B, et al. An atlas of genetic correlations across human diseases and traits. Nat Genet. 2015;10.
58. LaFountaine JS, et al. Delivery and therapeutic applications of gene editing technologies ZFNs, TALENs, and CRISPR/Cas9. Int J Pharm. 2015;494(1):180–94.
59. Hughes MC, et al. Sunscreen and prevention of skin aging: a randomized trial. Ann Intern Med. 2013;158:781–90.
60. Chung VQ, et al. Hot or not–evaluating the effect of artificial tanning on the public's perception of attractiveness. Dermatol Surg. 2010;36:1651–5.
61. Fell GL, et al. Skin beta-endorphin mediates addiction to UV light. Cell %19. 2014; 157(7):1527–34.
62. Buyukuslu N, et al. Clothing preference affects vitamin D status of young women. Nutr Res. 2014;34(8):688–93.

63. Loos RJ. Genetic determinants of common obesity and their value in prediction. Best Pract Res Clin Endocrinol Metab. 2012;26:211–26.
64. Zbiec-Piekarska R, et al. Development of a forensically useful age prediction method based on DNA methylation analysis. Forensic Sci Int Genet. 2015;17:173–9.
65. Raddatz G, et al. Aging is associated with highly defined epigenetic changes in the human epidermis. Epigenetics Chromatin. 2013;6:36.
66. Gronniger E, et al. Aging and chronic sun exposure cause distinct epigenetic changes in human skin. PLoS Genet. 2010;6, e1000971.
67. Horvath S. DNA methylation age of human tissues and cell types. Genome Biol. 2013;14:R115.
68. Marioni RE, et al. The epigenetic clock is correlated with physical and cognitive fitness in the Lothian Birth Cohort 1936. Int J Epidemiol. 2015;44(4):1388–96.
69. Kato N, et al. Trans-ancestry genome-wide association study identifies 12 genetic loci influencing blood pressure and implicates a role for DNA methylation. Nat Genet. 2015;47(11):1282–93.
70. Stokowski RP, et al. A genomewide association study of skin pigmentation in a South Asian population. Am J Hum Genet. 2007;81:1119–32.

Skin Aging and Health

44

David A. Gunn and Kaare Christensen

Contents

D.A. Gunn (✉)
Unilever Research and Development, Colworth Science Park, Sharnbrook, Bedfordshire, UK
e-mail: david.gunn@unilever.com

K. Christensen
The Danish Twin Registry and The Danish Aging Research Center, Department of Public Health, University of Southern Denmark, Odense C, Denmark
e-mail: KChristensen@health.sdu.dk

M.A. Farage et al. (eds.), *Textbook of Aging Skin*,
DOI 10.1007/978-3-662-47398-6_172

Abstract

Skin aging research usually aims to uncover the causes of skin cancer and to improve the appearance of skin for cosmetic purposes. Skin aging could also offer a route to study systemic aging and health, for which the skin has a number of advantages such as its accessibility for measurement. However, this would partly depend on whether the biological mechanisms driving variation in human health also drive skin aging variation. Here, evidence is found that indeed some skin aging features associate with specific aspects of health (e.g., skin wrinkling and pulmonary disease), and perceived age, a measure of facial aging, consistently associates with survival and markers of systemic aging. Furthermore, as potential drivers of these links, lifestyle factors such as smoking, pollution, and diet associate with both advanced skin aging and disease. Hence, the study of skin and facial aging does offer a way to study systemic aging mechanisms, such as the effects of glucose, cortisol, IGF-1, estrogen, and cell senescence which associate with skin and facial aging features. However, pigmented spots associate with better metabolic health, obesity associates with reduced facial wrinkling, and sun exposure boosts vitamin D levels (essential for bone health) but drives advanced skin aging. Hence, while some variation in skin and facial aging mirrors systemic aging, other variations link inversely (i.e., advanced skin aging, better health). The causal mechanisms responsible for these links now need elucidating to enable the study of their mechanism of action in the skin and further the understanding of systemic aging and human health.

Introduction

It's written on your face – one of the clearest manifestations of the aging process is the change in facial appearance that occurs over the decades of life. There are many features of appearance that become visible over time such as skin wrinkling, pigmented age spots, and sagging skin. The majority of these changes have little known consequence for health and function and have, therefore, received little attention in medical research outside cutaneous oncology and plastic surgery. This is despite the fact that the physical and functional properties of skin are relatively easy to measure and, thus, offer a practical way to study human aging. The main focus historically for skin aging research has been the link between skin cancer and features of skin aging, for example, the association between the presence of photodamage and melanoma. These studies have investigated whether such features can help classify the likelihood individuals will develop skin cancer and glean insights into skin cancer etiology. The other area of research commonly reported in the literature and attributable to the cosmetic industry is the formation and reduction of skin wrinkling or uneven pigmentation. There has been little work, though, focusing on why individuals of the same age can have large differences in the appearance of skin aging features and whether this variation reflects variance in systemic aging and, therefore, predicts the occurrence of various diseases.

Recently, progress has been made in not only identifying links between appearance and health but also in identifying molecular factors that associate with both. Such findings are highlighting the potential for using skin to investigate the aging process per se – i.e., systemic aging. However, the findings relate to many different features of appearance (e.g., skin versus facial appearance, wrinkling versus pigmented spots) as well as parameters of health (e.g., bone mineral density, BMD, versus chronic obstructive pulmonary disease, COPD) making it difficult to compare between the findings. Here, we review which features of skin and facial aging associate with which parameters of health, the biological mechanisms that could be underpinning the links, and if lifestyle could be partly driving the associations.

Biological Age

Biological age can be defined as a measure of how well somebody is aging relative to others of the same age and should reflect the physiological function and capacity of tissues as well as the degree to which molecular and tissue damage has occurred. Biological age received much attention in the 1970s and 1980s but with little impact into mainstream research in the following years [1]. This was mainly because the field was fragmented (no one goal or outcome was widely studied); for example, gerontology research focused on how to identify those who maintain their health with age (healthy agers), whereas most medical disciplines focused on a measure of risk for a specific disease event. In addition, no marker of biological age was proven to be more predictive of mortality or disease than risk factors already known (e.g., chronological age, smoking, body mass index [BMI], etc.). Hence, the study of biological age gained little momentum in the 1990s.

Over the last 10 years, the study of biological age has gained momentum. For example, the Framingham cardiovascular disease (CVD) risk score has been proven to predict those that are most likely to have a CVD risk event in 10 years of follow-up [2]. This score enabled the concept of "heart age" [3] and has become a valid and popular marker for the biological age of cardiovascular tissue. Momentum is also gaining in the study of molecular markers of aging such as telomere length leading to companies selling an "aging predictor" based on measures of telomere length [4]. Many companies claim to be able to measure biological age, despite only limited studies comparing the various methodologies for their prognostic value for either specific disease outcomes or survival. Hence, further progress in this field will require comparisons between methods to help determine the true clinical value of any particular biological age method beyond knowing a person's age, BMI, and smoking habits, which are easy to determine.

The use of appearance as a way to measure biological age has gained much attention in the last decade. The focus on appearance has wide-ranging advantages to aging research, particularly where human aging is the focus. One advantage of using the skin as a measure of biological age is that it is readily visible and accessible (e.g., for measuring its structure or histology through biopsies) making it the most practical human tissue choice for study. Another advantage is that the skin can be studied in vitro at the level of the cell (monocultures), for interactions between cell types (cocultures), using 3D models of the skin (tissue equivalents) and using ex vivo skin (e.g., cosmetic surgical discards). Hence, the practical and mostly noninvasive nature of human skin research offers great potential in being able to study mechanisms of human aging from in vitro to in vivo. If evidence can be gained into what aspects of skin aging mirror systemic aging, it offers a route for the use of skin aging research outside its dominant use in the study of skin cancer and in cosmetic research.

Perceived Age as a Measure of Biological Age

How old a person looks in a photograph (their perceived age) has had the most attention for its value as a measure of biological age. Humans can estimate age in others to help determine, for example, the fitness/fecundity of potential mates or rivals. Although the type of human assessor used for age perception studies has varied greatly (reviewed in [5]), it has been found that if large numbers of assessors are used, then resulting age estimations for subjects are generally similar irrespective of assessor variables such as age or sex [5, 6]. A much larger influence on age perception is the type of photographic image used to generate the perceived age estimates: photographs of individuals fully clothed from the waist up, photographs of the whole head, and frontal facial photographs (i.e., minus neck and scalp [7]) have all been commonly used. The manipulation of images to reduce or increase the presence of a feature has enabled studies into which aging features have a causal influence on age perception. For example, skin color homogeneity has been demonstrated to have a causal relationship with perceived age through image manipulations [8]. Thus, the use of perceived age has a number of advantages: features driving the perception of age can be identified through image modifications, large numbers of age assessors ensures a reproducible estimate of age, and different types of images can be used dependent on which facial features the investigators want to study (e.g., whether hair cues are included in images or not).

Perceived age best reflects facial aging if images of subjects are tailored to the "naked" face. This can be achieved by cropping photographs of subjects around the scalp hairline and neck (to remove hair and clothing cues) and by ensuring the subjects wear no makeup. As a result, the only cues in the photographs that can be used for the judgment of age relate to the anatomy of the face (bar grooming/shaping of the facial hair such as the eyebrows, mustache) and the appearance of the skin. Indeed, perceived age generated in this manner has been shown to be a measure of skin wrinkling [9], pigmented spots (in Chinese women) [10], lip size, and aspects of facial sag (e.g., the degree of presence of the nasolabial fold) [9] demonstrating it is a measure of anatomical changes that have occurred to various facial tissues with age. All these findings were independent of/controlled for chronological age indicating that perceived facial age is a measure of the biological age of the face.

Perceived Age and Health

If a feature of skin aging is a marker of systemic aging, it should associate with markers of aging in various body tissues in cross-sectional studies or predict an age-related disease outcome and/or survival in longitudinal studies [11]. Perceived age was first investigated as a marker of systemic aging by Bulpitt et al. in 1983. They found a significant association between cholesterol levels and perceived age [12], although this failed to replicate in a Dutch population [13]. In the first prospective study of perceived age (of Danish twins in passport-type images) and survival, individuals over 70 years of age who looked old for their age had a significant increased risk of dying within 7 years of the photograph being taken compared to younger looking individuals [6, 14]. In addition, perceived age was shown to be associated with cognitive and physical function as well as telomere length in leukocytes [6]. In a follow-up study, the link with survival was shown to be due to facial rather than hair and clothing cues in the passport-type images, and perceived age was still found linked to survival for those still alive 7 years after the photograph was taken for a further 5 years of survival follow-up [15]. Hence, it is unlikely that the link between perceived age and survival was just because those who looked old for their age had an illness at the time their image was taken. This Danish twin study was the first to provide strong evidence of a link between perceived age and survival and has since been replicated in an independent study [16].

Support for the link between perceived age and health has also been found in middle-aged and young populations. Using facial images for the generation of perceived age in middle-aged to elderly subjects, it was found that men from long-lived families (the offspring of siblings greater than 90 years of age [17]) looked younger than aged-matched controls, whereas perceived age in middle-aged women was a marker of CVD risk through its association with systolic blood pressure. Although there are no other studies of appearance in long-lived families, a relationship between perceived age and CVD was also found by Kido et al., specifically carotid atherosclerosis in Japanese subjects [18]. In a longitudinal study of aging, the change in blood biomarkers of aging between the subject ages of 26 and 38 years of age correlated strongly with subject perceived ages at 38 [19]. Hence together, these studies underline that there are links between facial appearance and systemic aging at all ages. However, as each study focused on either a different age group, ethnicity, or marker of disease, then replication of each finding is warranted.

Mechanisms Linking Perceived Age to Health

High levels of glucose can lead to advanced aging in tissues due to its link to insulin sensitivity, the formation of advanced glycated endpoints (AGE), and increased fat mass. High glucose levels have been associated with a higher perceived age [20]. The route through which perceived age is linked to glucose levels could be via the accumulation of AGE in the skin. AGE has been shown to be higher in the skin of those with high CVD risk, in diabetics, in those with kidney disease and impaired cognition, and in sun-exposed compared to protected skin (e.g., [21] and [22]). The accumulation of AGE in the skin is also predictive of their accumulation in blood vessels and with vessel stiffness [23], highlighting a potential direct route through which an aging mechanistic process is impacting skin aging and CVD risk. Hence, skin AGEs are a good marker of AGE in blood vessels, particularly in diabetics, and is one route through which skin aging reflects aging mechanisms occurring elsewhere in the body.

A higher perceived age, greater skin wrinkling, and pigmented spots are all linked to lower IGF-1 levels in blood (e.g., [24–26]). In addition, injection of IGF-1 into the skin of subjects older than 65 years of age improved the response of their skin to ultraviolet (UV) radiation exposure, as reflected by reduced numbers of proliferating keratinocytes with DNA damage [27]. The IGF-1 receptor influences a number of downstream pathways, from cell proliferation through to apoptosis. As well as being present in blood, IGF-1 is also expressed in skin fibroblasts, whereas the receptor is mainly expressed in keratinocytes [28]. As IGF-1 promotes cell proliferation and differentiation, it is likely to be a key growth factor for normal epidermal turnover, and lower levels with age could well reduce epidermal thickness by slowing keratinocyte growth and differentiation. How such effects lead to specific phenotypes such as skin wrinkling or pigmented spots though is less clear, but the role of IGF-1 in skin's response to UV exposure warrants further investigation.

High IGF-1 levels are linked to shorter life span in rodent models of aging, and caloric restriction (which increases rodent life span) reduces IGF-1 levels in blood. One might predict, therefore, that high levels of IGF-1 reflect reduced skin aging but poorer health in humans (i.e., an inverse association, Fig. 1). However, cross-sectional studies indicate that high IGF-1 levels associate with longer rather than shorter telomeres in white blood cells [29], low and high levels of IGF-1 are linked to poorer health [30], and caloric restriction in humans does not lower IGF-1 levels [31]. Due to the dramatic drop in IGF-1 blood levels with age, it is unclear to what degree cross-sectional IGF-1 levels reflect levels in early adulthood or more their reduction with age. In addition, IGF-1 binding proteins determine how much IGF-1 levels are available to tissues and also have variable associations with health [32], questioning to what degree IGF-1 levels per se reflect the availability of this hormone to cells. Measures of IGF-1 and its binding proteins during early adulthood in the skin as well as blood and their subsequent reduction with age are required to further understand this complex link between IGF-1, skin aging, and health.

Links between estrogen blood measures and perceived age were first observed by Wildt and Sir-Petermann [33] who found a strong negative correlation between estradiol serum concentration and lower perceived age in women attending an outpatient clinic. Although there hasn't been any replication of this finding, Smith et al. [34] did find estrogen levels were associated with perceived facial femininity, attractiveness, and health, and this association was ameliorated in women wearing makeup. In addition, estrogen levels in blood are associated with reduced skin wrinkling, and women on hormone replacement therapy (HRT) have thicker skin (e.g., [35]). HRT has also been shown to provide both protective and detrimental effects for CVD risk which seems to depend on the age of the women taking the HRT [36]. A clearer benefit of estrogens is their link to bone health; for example, HRT use associates with reduced bone fractures and gene variants in the estrogen receptor associate with bone mineral density (BMD) [37]. Hence, higher estrogen levels likely reduce

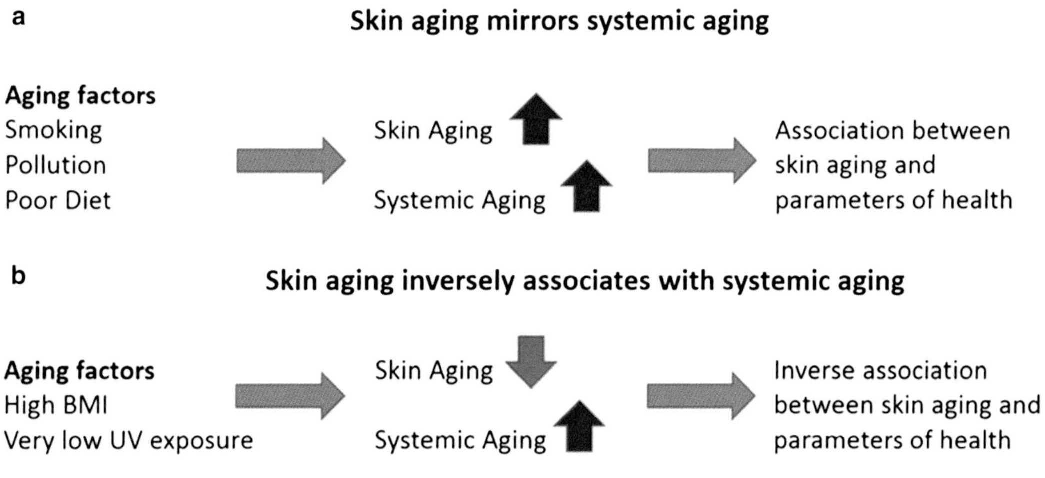

a
Skin aging mirrors systemic aging

Aging factors
Smoking
Pollution
Poor Diet
Skin Aging
Systemic Aging
Association between skin aging and parameters of health

b
Skin aging inversely associates with systemic aging

Aging factors
High BMI
Very low UV exposure
Skin Aging
Systemic Aging
Inverse association between skin aging and parameters of health

Fig. 1 Schematic to illustrate skin aging mirroring systemic aging (**a**) as opposed to having an inverse relationship with (**b**). Note that a high BMI is not proven to reduce skin aging at a molecular level, but more associates with less facial wrinkling likely through a "filler effect"

the rate of skin aging and BMD loss in women. The factors that influence the variance in estrogen level bioavailability are largely unknown, and thus, the identification of these factors should help determine how changes to estrogen levels with age influence skin aging and bone health.

High cortisol levels in morning blood samples, an indicator of psychological stress, associate with a higher perceived age [38]. Psychological stress is associated with poor health and with elevated cortisol levels in the blood [39]. Chronic treatment of the skin with synthetic analogs of cortisol (e.g., dexamethasone) thins the skin, and patients with Cushing's syndrome (caused by prolonged exposure to cortisol) show signs of advanced skin aging, including thinner skin [40]. In addition, cortisol can be made in the skin via 11β-hydroxysteroid dehydrogenase type 1 (11β-HSD1), which increases with age, and is elevated in sun-exposed compared to protected skin, and its inhibition gives improved wound healing in mice [41]. Hence, as the skin thins with age, this in part could be due to elevated cortisol levels in the skin and could reflect similar effects in other tissues. Better profiling of cortisol levels in the skin with age and its association with specific skin aging phenotypes is needed, however, to better determine whether cortisol is directly affecting particular skin aging phenotypes or more a proxy of correlated factors.

Skin Aging Phenotypes and Health

Skin Wrinkling

A wide range of changes occur to skin with age, with the most prominent being skin wrinkling. Skin wrinkling is strongly linked to sun exposure and is predominantly found in sun-exposed body sites. In addition, obesity is associated with reduced skin wrinkling and with poorer health. Hence, those with a high BMI and lower vitamin D levels would be expected to have fewer skin wrinkles but poorer health – an inverse association (Fig. 1). Indeed, the links between perceived age and glucose [20], cortisol [26], long-lived families [13], and CVD risk [13] were all independent of facial wrinkling. However, wrinkling has been associated with lung function tests and COPD, although there is conflicting data on how much this is confined to smokers [42] or not [43]. The lungs have a similar functional role to the skin in terms of an epithelial barrier to extrinsic factors (e.g., pollution, see below) and underlying extracellular matrix support. In support of this commonality, genetic variants in extracellular matrix genes have been found to underlie the link between wrinkling and lung function [43], although this finding has yet to be replicated. Hence, facial wrinkling could well signpost susceptibility to advanced lung aging, although any prognostic value in the clinic needs further investigation.

Subcutaneous fat can act similarly to a cosmetic filler, pushing skin outward and reducing the appearance of wrinkles. This is the most likely reason that BMI associates reduced wrinkling [44]. Hence, those with a high BMI would be expected to have less wrinkles but a higher risk of metabolic-related diseases, such as diabetes. However, there is also evidence that a high fat mass could be having a detrimental effect on skin aging. For example, once the influence of wrinkling on perceived age is removed, a high BMI is associated with a higher perceived age [44]. Furthermore, whereas in all age groups a high BMI (in the form of obesity) is linked to less wrinkling and poorer health, in elderly populations a low BMI is also linked to reduced survival [45]. Hence, the exact link between skin wrinkling and health, particularly metabolic health, is likely driven through fat mass levels and is dependent on the age group under study.

The wrinkling of skin in other parts of the body can be quite different to that on the face. In particular, wrinkling on sun-protected parts with little influence from contouring by underlying musculature tends to be finer in nature and more related to the loss of epidermal curvature than large-scale dermal changes. Reduced changes to the pattern/wrinkling of the skin at this site with age have been linked to health [46] and to individuals from long-lived families [47]. Hence, upper inner arm skin wrinkling is a good biomarker of familial longevity and possibly health per se. As a potential mechanism for these links, it was also found that there were less senescent (p16INK4a positive) melanocytes in upper inner arm skin in long-lived families, and they associated with perceived age and facial wrinkling independently of age, smoking, and sun exposure [48]. Thus, the number of senescent melanocytes in upper inner arm skin was indicative of facial aging and familial longevity. Senescent cells are known to damage surrounding cells and tissue structures [49], suggesting that once formed they advance the aging process. Hence, if there are genetic or environmental factors that drive cellular senescence formation in individuals, then cellular senescence could be a route explaining (at least in part) links between skin aging and health. Further work investigating whether cellular senescence in other parts of the body (e.g., p16INK4a positive cells found in kidney) is associated with melanocyte senescence in sun-protected skin would help confirm whether these cells drive links between skin aging and health due to a correlation between senescent cell numbers across tissues.

Pigmented Age Spots

Pigmented skin spots can be categorized into senile lentigines, seborrheic keratosis, melasma, and ephelides/freckles. Seborrheic keratoses increase with age in sun-protected as well as sun-exposed sites, whereas senile lentigines more strongly associate with sun-exposed sites with age, melasmas associate with sun-exposed sites and pregnancy, and freckles associate with childhood and skin type [50]. Diabetics, those with hypertension and a higher BMI, have been shown to have reduced numbers of pigmented spots on the face in Dutch Europeans [24]. Although senile lentigines tend to be more prevalent on the face of elderly subjects, it is uncertain which type of pigmented spot drove the link with these metabolic syndrome risk factors. As this is the first common feature of skin aging that associates with better metabolic health, replication of these findings in other populations is warranted.

Face Shape Changes

Along with the skin, there is increasing evidence that changes with age to subcutaneous facial tissues have large influences on appearance. Evidence from the plastic surgery field indicates that changes to facial fat pads, the subcutaneous musculoaponeurotic system (SMAS), and the bone all influence facial appearance. For example, changes in the position of the malar cheek fat pad with age have been shown to be associated with an increase in the appearance of the nasal-labial fold [51]. In addition, modern cosmetic procedures commonly involve augmentation of the SMAS, particularly for face lifts [52], indicating the importance of subcutaneous tissues in facial sagging. As subcutaneous tissues of the face are less affected by extrinsic factors, then it would be expected that these changes are linked to aspects of health. Data linking face shape changes to health are lacking though, although previous reported links between perceived age and health (as above) could be due to such changes [47]. Hence, measures of changes to face shape with age and their relationship with perceived age and health now need evaluating.

Lifestyle Effects on Health and Appearance

Environmental influences on skin aging phenotypes are consistently estimated at around 40–60 % of the variance in various skin aging phenotypes (e.g., [9] and see Chap. 43, "The Genetics of Skin Aging") and at around 75 % of the variance in human life span [53]. Along with stochastic influences and measurement errors, environmental influences include lifestyle which can have effects on both health and appearance and can partly explain the links between the two.

Sun Exposure

The evidence that sun exposure causes skin aging is compelling. Skin wrinkling and pigmented spots are found predominantly on sun-exposed skin sites, and those who are commonly in the sun have greater skin wrinkling than those that avoid it [54]. In a longitudinal study of sun-protection factor use, an increase in wrinkles was observed for those who did not consistently apply such products compared to those who did [55]. In addition, a whole host of cellular and tissue damage has been found to result from UV radiation exposure. For example, DNA is particularly susceptible to UV-induced damage such as pyrimidine dimers. Other damage includes the cross-linking of collagen fibers in the dermis and increases in cellular oxidative damage (e.g., [56]). While sun exposure drives skin aging, its links to health (aside from its direct link to melanoma) have mainly focused on the beneficial production of vitamin D through skin UV exposure. Vitamin D is important for the normal turnover of the bone, and vitamin D deficiency is responsible for the bone disease rickets. Links to other diseases, though, remain controversial with many citing links between low vitamin D levels with bowel and prostate cancers (e.g., [57]) and others finding no benefit for high vitamin D levels with CVD [58]. Overall, as vitamin D has some health benefits, then it might be expected that those with high levels of skin sun damage could be healthier through greater vitamin D production – i.e., an inverse association (Fig. 1). However, only small doses of UV exposure (e.g., less than 15 min under a summer midday sun) are needed to give adequate doses of vitamin D [59], although this depends on skin type, geographical location, and the time of day and year. Hence, those with large amounts of skin sun damage are unlikely to be much healthier than those with low to moderate sun damage, but further studies of the exact doses of UV that individuals receive, through wrist-worn monitors, for example, should help determine the UV exposure levels (per skin type) that associate with health benefits. In addition, the role of UVa to UVb doses will be required to accurately access the true effects of UV exposures [56].

Smoking and Pollution

Smokers are more likely to look older for their age [60] and have more skin wrinkles (e.g., [44]). In addition, smoking causes lung cancer, cardiovascular disease, and reduced survival. It is therefore clear that smoking is detrimental to both skin and health. As well as the systemic effects of smoking, there are also likely to be localized and extrinsic effects on the skin, particularly around the mouth. Smoking can affect skin by impairing blood supply [61] and lowering the availability of important food nutrients [62]. Indeed, as skin microvasculature degrades with age, it would be important to understand whether this degradation is associated with similar changes to microvasculature in the rest of the body and the degree to which smoking drives such changes. In support of this, those with a higher risk of CVD had an impaired microvasculature blood flow in the skin [63], and such links in smokers would indicate that the microvasculature could be the key mechanism linking smoking effects on both CVD risk and skin aging.

Pollution effects on human health are of particular concern in urban areas. The lungs and skin are the main routes through which pollution can enter the body, and there is now mounting evidence that pollution levels link with COPD, skin sensitivities (e.g., rashes, eczema), as well as skin aging phenotypes (reviewed in [64]). In addition, pollution is associated with aging in other tissues such as the brain (reviewed in [65]), indicating skin aging in response to pollution might reflect wider pollution effects in the body. Identifying the pollutants underlying the aging in tissues needs further elucidation as fine particulate matter (PM 2.5), coarse matter (PM 10), as well as gases (e.g., NO_2) all associate with aging phenotypes (e.g., [66]), and their presence can be highly correlated to each other. Once identified, however, then their mechanism of action on skin aging could give wider understanding on how pollution drives aging in other tissues.

Oral Care

The number of teeth and the condition of the surrounding gums and bones are known to be important for the appearance of the outside of the face. For example, lip size, the appearance of facial skin, and looking younger have all been linked to the support given from within the mouth (e.g., [67]). Furthermore, better oral care in Chinese and Caucasians associates with a younger perceived age in subjects with their mouths closed [44, 68]. These findings highlight the importance of the teeth and gums in supporting the skin above and influencing facial appearance. Oral care has also been strongly linked with cardiovascular disease, possible through the reduction of harmful bacteria in the mouth that could have systemic health implications [69]. Poor oral care is also linked, though, to poor nutritional intake and smoking making it a marker of other lifestyle factors. Hence, further research is required to disentangle to what degree oral care helps prevent the decline in facial appearance around the mouth with age or is more a marker of other healthy lifestyles such as nutritional intake.

Diet

Links between diet and skin aging phenotypes have highlighted the importance of fruit and vegetable intake for reducing the rate of skin aging. For example, in a cross-sectional study, vegetables, olive oil, and legumes were found to associate with reduced skin wrinkling [70]. Vitamin C intake, which is considered a proxy of fruit and vegetable intake, has also been linked to reduced skin wrinkling and skin dryness [71]. Vitamin C, though, is required for collagen production in the skin and, as well as a proxy of fruit and vegetable intake, could also be having direct skin benefits. In support of this, dietary supplements rich in vitamin C have been shown to reduce the signs of skin aging (e.g., [72]), and vitamins C and E have been demonstrated to increase UV-induced minimal erythema dose (MED) [73]. Such UV beneficial effects have also been found for other plant compounds such as carotenoids which also link with health benefits in the elderly [74]. Hence, antioxidant benefits for UV-induced oxidative stress could also be indicative of similar antioxidant benefits of nutrients across tissues. However, while it is clear that low levels of antioxidants are linked to advanced skin aging and poorer health, taking high levels of the same nutrients does not necessarily drive any extra benefits (e.g., [75]).

A high cholesterol and saturated fat dietary intake have been linked to increased risk of CVD [2, 76]. In addition, a higher fat and saturated fat intake is linked to greater skin wrinkling [70, 71]. In contrast, linoleic acid consumption (found in vegetable oils), which cannot be synthesized by the body, associates with reduced skin dryness and thinning [71] as well as reduced risk of coronary heart disease (CHD) [77]. Hence, the evidence to date points to a diet rich in fruit and vegetables and vegetable oils rather than animal fats as an optimal diet for reduced skin aging and good health. However, future research should also consider whether other associated socioeconomic, lifestyle, and nutrient factors are confounding the epidemiological results.

Sleep

It is known that severe lack of sleep affects facial appearance and skin barrier function (e.g., [78]). In addition, sleep disorders are associated with many types of diseases (e.g., CVD [79]). Outside the effects of sleep disorders and acute sleep deprivation, there is evidence that sleeping problems affect health and survival [80]. Circadian rhythms help determine the sleep-wake cycle and this rhythm is disrupted with age, including in the skin [81]. However, it is difficult to determine what comes first – the disruption of circadian gene regulation (e.g., through cellular damage) or disruption to sleep that then affects circadian gene regulation. Hence, longitudinal investigations into whether changes to circadian gene regulation precede changes to sleep or vice versa are required to understand the underlying etiology of the link between sleep, skin aging, and health.

Alcohol

There is currently no evidence that variation of alcohol consumption within recommended intake levels affects skin aging (e.g., [82]). However, low to moderate alcohol consumption are linked to better systemic aging [83], whereas high levels associate with disease prevalence. In addition, alcoholics are known to present with a wide range of skin conditions (e.g., rosacea). Hence, it would be logical to conclude low to moderate amounts of alcohol are likely best for skin and systemic aging. Low to moderate amounts of alcohol, though, are still associated with an increased risk of some cancers and with no beneficial effects (relative to abstinence) in low-income countries [84]. As the current reported studies for alcohol intake and skin aging phenotypes had relatively low power to detect associations, then larger studies are required to prove whether low to moderate alcohol consumption can give small beneficial or detrimental effects to skin aging and how this might reflect similar effects in other bodily tissues.

Conclusions

For research into skin aging to have a wider interest outside oncology and the cosmetics industry, it will be important for the recent findings linking facial appearance and skin aging phenotypes to health to be replicated across different age groups and ethnicities, as most studies used different appearance and health measures to investigate these links. The easy accessibility of skin tissue, the many practical noninvasive ways to measure skin aging phenotypes, and the range of in vitro models of skin aging offer one of the most feasible ways to investigate human mechanisms of aging. Furthermore, testing to what degree quick and easy assessments of skin and facial aging phenotypes could highlight potential health issues in the clinic would confirm the utility of using skin and/or facial aging as part of a general health assessment. However, the causal mechanisms responsible for the links between skin aging and health are still unclear. Hence, the identification of these mechanisms will enable their study using skin as an aging model, leading to insights into their mechanism of action within tissues, which should help explain some of the variation in parameters of health within human populations.

References

1. Bulpitt CJ. Assessing biological age – practicality – discussion. Gerontology. 1995;41:315–21.
2. D'Agostino Sr RB, et al. General cardiovascular risk profile for use in primary care: the Framingham Heart Study. Circulation. 2008;117:743–53.
3. Soureti A, et al. Evaluation of a cardiovascular disease risk assessment tool for the promotion of healthier lifestyles. Eur J Cardiovasc Prev Rehabil. 2010;17(5):519–23.
4. Wolinsky H. Testing time for telomeres. Telomere length can tell us something about disease susceptibility and ageing, but are commercial tests ready for prime time? EMBO Rep. 2011;12(9):897–900.
5. Gunn DA, et al. Perceived age as a biomarker of ageing: a clinical methodology. Biogerontology. 2008;9:357–64.
6. Christensen K, et al. Perceived age as clinically useful biomarker of ageing: cohort study. BMJ. 2009;339: b5262.
7. Warren R, et al. Age, sunlight, and facial skin – a histologic and quantitative study. J Am Acad Dermatol. 1991;25:751–60.
8. Matts PJ, et al. Color homogeneity and visual perception of age, health, and attractiveness of female facial skin. J Am Acad Dermatol. 2007;57:977–84.
9. Gunn DA, et al. Why some women look young for their age. PLoS One. 2009;4:e8021.
10. Mayes A, et al. Ageing appearance in China: biophysical profile of facial skin and its relationship to perceived age. J Eur Acad Dermatol Venereol. 2009;24(3):341-8.
11. Levine ME. Modeling the rate of senescence: can estimated biological age predict mortality more accurately than chronological age? J Gerontol A Biol Sci Med Sci. 2013;68(6):667–74.
12. Bulpitt CJ, et al. Why do some people look older than they should? Postgrad Med J. 2001;77:578–81.
13. Gunn DA, et al. Facial appearance reflects human familial longevity and cardiovascular disease risk in healthy individuals. J Gerontol A Biol Sci Med Sci. 2013;68:145–52.
14. Christensen K, et al. "Looking old for your age": genetics and mortality. Epidemiology. 2004;15:251–2.
15. Gunn DA, et al. Mortality is written on the face. J Gerontol A Biol Sci Med Sci. 2015;glv090. doi:10.1093/gerona/glv090
16. Dykiert D, et al. Predicting mortality from human faces. Psychosom Med. 2012;74:560–6.
17. Westendorp RG, et al. Nonagenarian siblings and their offspring display lower risk of mortality and morbidity than sporadic nonagenarians: the Leiden Longevity Study. J Am Geriatr Soc. 2009;57:1634–7.
18. Kido M, et al. Perceived age of facial features is a significant diagnosis criterion for age-related carotid atherosclerosis in Japanese subjects: J-SHIPP study. Geriatr Gerontol Int. 2012;12:733–40.

19. Belsky DW, et al. Quantification of biological aging in young adults. Proc Natl Acad Sci U S A. 2015;112: E4104–10.
20. Noordam R, et al. High serum glucose levels are associated with a higher perceived age. Age (Dordr). 2013;35(1):189-95.
21. Rajaobelina K, et al. Autofluorescence of skin advanced glycation end products: marker of metabolic memory in elderly population. J Gerontol A Biol Sci Med Sci. 2015;70(7):841–6.
22. Crisan M, et al. Expression of advanced glycation end-products on sun-exposed and non-exposed cutaneous sites during the ageing process in humans. PLoS One. 2013;8(10):e75003.
23. Semba RD, et al. Serum carboxymethyl-lysine, an advanced glycation end product, is associated with increased aortic pulse wave velocity in adults. Am J Hypertens. 2009;22(1):74–9.
24. van Drielen K, et al. Markers of health and disease and pigmented spots in a middle-aged population. Br J Dermatol. 2015;173:1550–2.
25. Noordam R, et al. Serum insulin-like growth factor 1 and facial ageing: high levels associate with reduced skin wrinkling in a cross-sectional study. Br J Dermatol. 2013;168:533–8.
26. van Drielen K, et al. Disentangling the effects of circulating IGF-1, glucose, and cortisol on features of perceived age. Age (Dordr). 2015;37(3):9771.
27. Lewis DA, et al. The IGF-1/IGF-1R signaling axis in the skin: a new role for the dermis in aging-associated skin cancer. Oncogene. 2010;29(10):1475–85.
28. Rudman SM, et al. The role of IGF-I in human skin and its appendages: morphogen as well as mitogen? J Invest Dermatol. 1997;109(6):770–7.
29. Barbieri M, et al. Higher circulating levels of IGF-1 are associated with longer leukocyte telomere length in healthy subjects. Mech Ageing Dev. 2009;130:771–6.
30. van Bunderen CC, et al. Serum IGF1, metabolic syndrome, and incident cardiovascular disease in older people: a population-based study. Eur J Endocrinol. 2013;168(3):393–401.
31. Fontana L et al. Effects of 2-year calorie restriction on circulating levels of IGF-1, IGF-binding proteins and cortisol in nonobese men and women: a randomized clinical trial. Aging Cell. 2016;15(1):22-7.
32. Maggio M, et al. Insulin-like growth factor-1 bioactivity plays a prosurvival role in older participants. J Gerontol A Biol Sci Med Sci. 2013;68(11):1342–50.
33. Wildt L, et al. Oestrogen and age estimations of perimenopausal women. Lancet. 1999;354:224.
34. Law-Smith MJ, et al. Facial appearance is a cue to oestrogen levels in women. Proc R Soc B Biol Sci. 2006;273:135–40.
35. Callens A, et al. Does hormonal skin aging exist? A study of the influence of different hormone therapy regimens on the skin of postmenopausal women using non-invasive measurement techniques. Dermatology. 1996;193:289–94.
36. Vitale C, et al. Gender differences in the cardiovascular effects of sex hormones. Fundam Clin Pharmacol. 2010;24:675–85.
37. Rivadeneira F, et al. Twenty bone-mineral-density loci identified by large-scale meta-analysis of genome-wide association studies. Nat Genet. 2009;41(11):1199–206.
38. Noordam R, et al. Cortisol serum levels in familial longevity and perceived age: the Leiden Longevity Study. Psychoneuroendocrinology. 2012;37:1669–75.
39. Phillips KM, et al. Stress management intervention reduces serum cortisol and increases relaxation during treatment for nonmetastatic breast cancer. Psychosom Med. 2008;70:1044–9.
40. Newell-Price J, et al. Cushing's syndrome. Lancet. 2006;367(9522):1605–17.
41. Tiganescu A, et al. 11beta-Hydroxysteroid dehydrogenase blockade prevents age-induced skin structure and function defects. J Clin Invest. 2013;123(7):3051–60.
42. Patel BD, et al. Smoking related COPD and facial wrinkling: is there a common susceptibility? Thorax. 2006;61(7):568–71.
43. Vierkotter A, et al. MMP-1 and -3 promoter variants are indicative of a common susceptibility for skin and lung aging: results from a cohort of elderly women (SALIA). J Invest Dermatol. 2015;135(5):1268–74.
44. Gunn DA, et al. Lifestyle and youthful looks. Br J Dermatol. 2015;172(5):1338–45.
45. Wierup I, et al. Low anthropometric measures and mortality – results from the Malmo Diet and Cancer Study. Ann Med. 2015;47(4):325–31.
46. Purba MB, et al. Can skin wrinkling in a site that has received limited sun exposure be used as a marker of health status and biological age? Age Ageing. 2001;30:227–34.
47. Gunn DA, et al. Facial appearance reflects human familial longevity and cardiovascular disease risk in healthy individuals. J Gerontol A Biol Sci Med Sci. 2013;68:145–52.
48. Waaijer ME, et al. P16INK4a positive cells in human skin are indicative of local elastic fiber morphology, facial wrinkling, and perceived age. J Gerontol A Biol Sci Med Sci. 2015;glv114. doi:10.1093/gerona/glv114
49. Campisi J. Senescent cells, tumor suppression, and organismal aging: good citizens, bad neighbors. Cell. 2005;120:513–22.
50. Bastiaens M, et al. Solar lentigines are strongly related to sun exposure in contrast to ephelides. Pigment Cell Res. 2004;17:225–9.
51. Yousif NJ, et al. The nasolabial fold – an anatomic and histologic reappraisal. Plast Reconstr Surg. 1994;93:60–9.
52. Castello MF, et al. Modified superficial musculoaponeurotic system face-lift: a review of 327 consecutive procedures and a patient satisfaction assessment. Aesthetic Plast Surg. 2011;35:147–55.
53. vB Hjelmborg J, et al. Genetic influence on human lifespan and longevity. Hum Genet. 2006;119:312–21.

54. Griffiths CEM. The clinical-identification and quantification of photodamage. Br J Dermatol. 1992;127:37–42.
55. Hughes MC, et al. Sunscreen and prevention of skin aging: a randomized trial. Ann Intern Med. 2013;158:781–90.
56. Premi S, et al. Photochemistry. Chemiexcitation of melanin derivatives induces DNA photoproducts long after UV exposure. Science. 2015;347(6224):842–7.
57. Lee JE, et al. Circulating levels of vitamin D and colon and rectal cancer: the Physicians' Health Study and a meta-analysis of prospective studies. Cancer Prev Res (Phila). 2011;4(5):735–43.
58. Brondum-Jacobsen P, et al. No evidence that genetically reduced 25-hydroxyvitamin D is associated with increased risk of ischaemic heart disease or myocardial infarction: a Mendelian randomization study. Int J Epidemiol. 2015;44(2):651–61.
59. Terushkin V, et al. Estimated equivalency of vitamin D production from natural sun exposure versus oral vitamin D supplementation across seasons at two US latitudes. J Am Acad Dermatol. 2010;62:929.
60. Rexbye H, et al. Influence of environmental factors on facial ageing. Age Ageing. 2006;35:110–5.
61. Avery MR, et al. Age and cigarette smoking are independently associated with the cutaneous vascular response to local warming. Microcirculation. 2009;16:725–34.
62. Stryker WS, et al. The relation of diet, cigarette smoking, and alcohol consumption to plasma beta-carotene and alpha tocopherol levels. Am J Epidemiol. 1988;127:283–96.
63. IJzerman RG, et al. Individuals at increased coronary heart disease risk are characterized by an impaired microvascular function in skin. Eur J Clin Invest. 2003;33:536–42.
64. Krutmann J, et al. Pollution and skin: from epidemiological and mechanistic studies to clinical implications. J Dermatol Sci. 2014;76(3):163–8.
65. Weuve J. Invited commentary: how exposure to air pollution may shape dementia risk, and what epidemiology can say about it. Am J Epidemiol. 2014;180(4):367–71.
66. Shah AS, et al. Short term exposure to air pollution and stroke: systematic review and meta-analysis. BMJ. 2015;350:h1295.
67. Ismail SF, et al. Three-dimensional assessment of the effects of extraction and nonextraction orthodontic treatment on the face. Am J Orthod Dentofacial Orthop. 2002;121:244–56.
68. Mayes AE, et al. Environmental and lifestyle factors associated with perceived facial age in Chinese Women. PLoS One. 2010;5:e15270.
69. Hyvarinen K, et al. A common periodontal pathogen has an adverse association with both acute and stable coronary artery disease. Atherosclerosis. 2012;223(2):478–84.
70. Purba MB, et al. Skin wrinkling: can food make a difference? J Am Coll Nutr. 2001;20:71–80.
71. Cosgrove MC, et al. Dietary nutrient intakes and skin-aging appearance among middle-aged American women. Am J Clin Nutr. 2007;86:1225–31.
72. Jenkins G, et al. Wrinkle reduction in post-menopausal women consuming a novel oral supplement: a double-blind placebo-controlled randomized study. Int J Cosmet Sci. 2014;36(1):22–31.
73. Eberlein-Konig B, et al. Protective effect against sunburn of combined systemic ascorbic acid (vitamin C) and d-alpha-tocopherol (vitamin E). J Am Acad Dermatol. 1998;38(1):45–8.
74. Klipstein-Grobusch K, et al. Dietary antioxidants and risk of myocardial infarction in the elderly: the Rotterdam Study. Am J Clin Nutr. 1999;69(2):261–6.
75. Ye Y, et al. Effect of antioxidant vitamin supplementation on cardiovascular outcomes: a meta-analysis of randomized controlled trials. PLoS One. 2013;8(2):e56803.
76. Hooper L, et al. Reduction in saturated fat intake for cardiovascular disease. Cochrane Database Syst Rev. 2015;6:CD011737.
77. de Goede J, et al. N-6 and N-3 fatty acid cholesteryl esters in relation to fatal CHD in a Dutch adult population: a nested case–control study and meta-analysis. PLoS One. 2013;8(5):e59408.
78. Altemus M, et al. Stress-induced changes in skin barrier function in healthy women. J Invest Dermatol. 2001;117:309–17.
79. Wang X, et al. Obstructive sleep apnea and risk of cardiovascular disease and all-cause mortality: a meta-analysis of prospective cohort studies. Int J Cardiol. 2013;169(3):207–14.
80. Li Y, et al. Association between insomnia symptoms and mortality: a prospective study of U.S. men. Circulation. 2014;129(7):737–46.
81. Sporl F, et al. Kruppel-like factor 9 is a circadian transcription factor in human epidermis that controls proliferation of keratinocytes. Proc Natl Acad Sci U S A. 2012;109(27):10903–8.
82. Nagata C, et al. Association of dietary fat, vegetables and antioxidant micronutrients with skin ageing in Japanese women. Br J Nutr. 2010;103:1493–8.
83. Khaw KT, et al. Combined impact of health behaviours and mortality in men and women: the EPIC-Norfolk prospective population study. PLoS Med. 2008;5:e12.
84. Smyth A, et al. Alcohol consumption and cardiovascular disease, cancer, injury, admission to hospital, and mortality: a prospective cohort study. Lancet. 2015;386:1945–54.

Influence of Exogenous Factors on Skin Aging

45

Avani Ahuja, Neha Singh, Prashant Gupta, Shivangi Mishra, and Vibha Rani

Contents

A. Ahuja • N. Singh • P. Gupta • S. Mishra • V. Rani (✉)
Department of Biotechnology, Jaypee Institute of Information Technology, Noida, UP, India
e-mail: a10avani@gmail.com; a3neha@gmail.com; prashantg050795@gmail.com; shivangi.m27@gmail.com; vibha.rani@jiit.ac.in

M.A. Farage et al. (eds.), *Textbook of Aging Skin*,
DOI 10.1007/978-3-662-47398-6_173

Abstract

Being the most superficial organ, skin is constantly exposed to various insults in the surrounding majorly including ultraviolet rays (UVR), air pollutants, heavy metals, and cigarette smoke. Additionally, chemical ingredients in most of the cosmetic and dermatological products applied on the skin for its maintenance and protection negatively impact by contributing in the process of degeneration of skin cells. These exogenous factors further enhance the release of reactive oxygen species (ROS) triggering the activation of matrix metalloproteinases (MMPs) and inflammatory responses, hence damaging the extracellular matrix (ECM) components by stimulating skin aging through intrinsic factors. Certain UVR-sensitive genes also get activated by ROS, resulting in DNA damage and with compromised repair pathway, the cell undergoes the process of apoptosis. The alterations a cell undergoes after being exposed to environmental toxins contribute in its morphological and physiological deterioration resulting in dark spots, wrinkles, decreased elasticity, and dryness: characterizing aged skin. The present chapter discusses some of the major environmental pollutants and chemicals which influence the process of accelerated skin aging.

List of Abbreviations

ECM	Extracellular matrix
HRT	Hormone replacement therapy
IR	Infra –red radiation
MMP	Matrix metalloproteinases
MMP-1	Matrix metalloproteinase-1
MWF	Metal working fluids
NO	Nitrogen oxide
PAH	Poly-aromatic hydrocarbons
PM	Particulate matter
RNS	Reactive nitrogen species
RNS	Reactive nitrogen species
ROS	Reactive oxygen species
ROS	Reactive oxygen species
TCDD	2,3 7, 8-tetrachlorodibenzo-p-dioxin
UV	Ultraviolet radiation
UVR	Ultraviolet radiation
VOC	Volatile organic compounds

Introduction

Skin is the largest and most superficial protection of an organism from environmental toxicants. Consisting of mesenchymal cells and pigmentation factor melanin by melanocytes, it has three layers, i.e., epidermis, dermis, and hypodermis. Skin cells are at constant exposure to a wide range of intrinsic and extrinsic factors which leads to their multisystem degeneration hence enhancing aging effects. Intrinsic factors basically are the genetically programmed changes; however, the wear and tear effects on the skin as a result of exposure to gerontogens such as ultraviolet radiation (UVR), polyhydrocarbons, and cigarette smoke are the extrinsic factors [1].

Skin aging has been a major dermatologic concern in the society since ages and various theories have been provided to study the causes and their consequences.

Wear and Tear Theory (1882)

The theory by biologist Dr. August Weissman suggests that accumulation of damages to a cell, tissue, and organ over time eventually leads to its degeneration and death. Beginning at the molecular level, as the DNA sustains repeated damage from toxins and radiations it loses its repairing capacity and consequently the damages accumulate progressively, causing visible wrinkles and dark spots.

The Cross-Linking Glycosylation Theory (1941)

Dr. Johan Bjorksten observed that with age, protein and other molecular structures begin to cross-link by forming covalent bonds to create larger polymeric molecules having reduced elasticity and mobility. Thus, the protein gets damaged leading to its inefficiency. Additionally, exposure to extrinsic factors generates excess ROS (reactive oxygen species) which interact with glucose, proteins, and DNA and elevate cross-linking of collagen resulting in dry, leathery, and yellow skin along with the appearance of wrinkles and decreased skin elasticity.

The Neuroendocrine Theory (1954)

The theory is a continuation of wear and tear theory first addressed by Dr. Vladimir Dilman. According to this theory, with age hypothalamus loses its ability to precisely regulate the release of hormones while the hormone receptors become less sensitive. The secretion of key hormones declines and their efficacy is reduced by an increase in cortisol, one of the few hormones that increases with age, resulting in enhanced catabolism, breaking down of muscle tissue, as well as degradation of collagen.

The Free Radical Theory (1950s)

One of the deep-rooted and most well-known theories of aging, by Dr. Denham Harmon, focuses on the association of free radicals with skin degeneration. Excess ROS attack the structure of our cell membranes, creating waste products, including pigments known as lipofuscins, which accumulate to give an appearance of "age spots." Lipofuscins interfere with the cells' ability to repair and reproduce themselves, disturb DNA and RNA synthesis, inhibit protein synthesis, degrade collagen and elastin, and destroy cellular enzymes. This kind of damage begins at birth but its effects are not detrimental in juvenile phase due to the body's natural repair mechanisms. With age, the accumulated effects of free radicals slow down the cell function therefore reducing the body's self-repair capabilities eventually leading to wrinkles, sagging skin, and "age spots."

The Telomere Theory of Aging (1972)

The findings of Alexei Olovnikov and John Watson suggest that aging is divided into two categories:

Intrinsic Aging (chronological aging)
Intrinsic aging is a natural process with numerous interlinked pathways involved. Production of collagen and elastin fibers, responsible for providing mechanical strength, support, and elasticity to skin, slows down and hence skin loses its flexibility. Hence, it becomes thinner and the dermal-epidermal junction compresses and begins to collapse, eventually resulting in decreased skin cell turnover causing cell death. The visual signs of intrinsic aging are dry/flaky skin, fine lines, wrinkles, and sagging/lax skin.

Extrinsic Aging (premature or photoaging)
Extrinsic aging is caused by environmental factors such as air pollutants including cigarette smoke and vehicle exhaust but the most common cause is exposure to UVR. Continual sun exposure not only hinders the skin's ability to repair but continues to break down and debilitate the synthesis of collagen in addition to the degradation of elastin fibers. The perceivable results of photoaging are hyperpigmentation, leathery appearance, dry skin, and deep wrinkles.

Extrinsic skin aging process is characterized by striking morphological and physiological changes enhancing premature aging of the skin. Prominent manifestations of the extrinsic skin aging process are coarse wrinkles, solar elastosis, and pigment irregularities. The rate of extrinsic skin aging varies strikingly among individuals and ethnic populations (Fig. 1) [2].

Sun Exposure and Skin Aging

Sun exposure is the most damaging environmental factor responsible for wrinkles, dark spots, and rough skin. Epidemiological and clinical studies have identified excessive sun exposure as a primary causal factor in various skin diseases including premature aging, inflammatory conditions, melanoma,

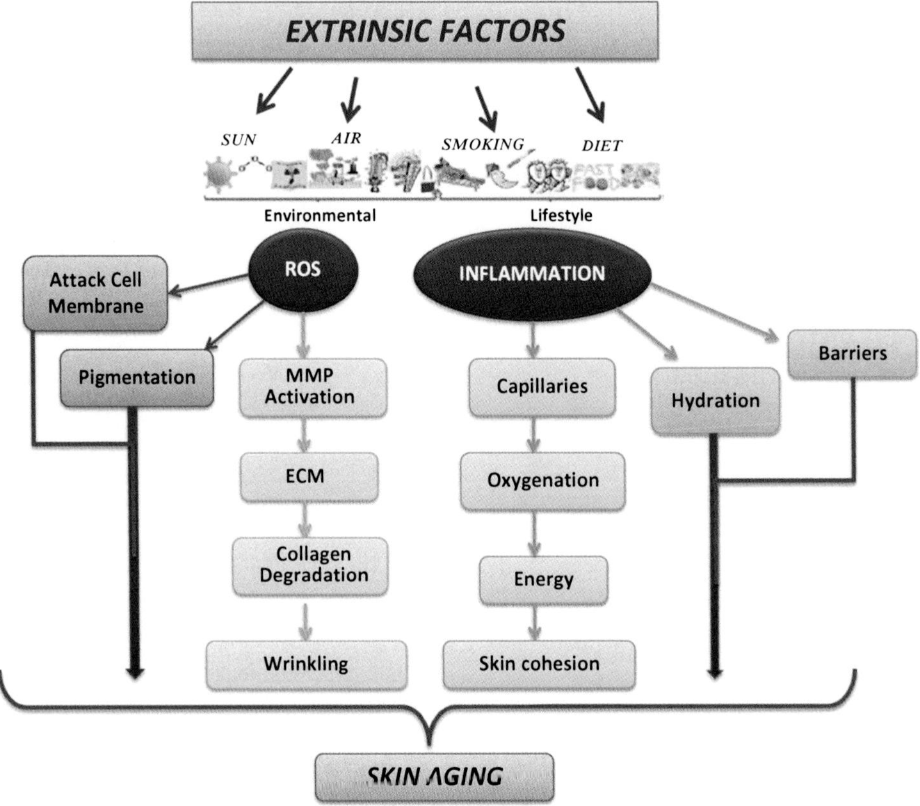

Fig. 1 Numerous extrinsic factors, linked to environment and lifestyle that undergo different mechanisms and affect the appearance of skin aging

and nonmelanoma skin cancers [3]. Chronic sun exposure damages the dermal connective tissue and alters normal skin metabolism, in addition to a reduction in immunity while stimulating oxidative stress and inflammation. Radiations from sun especially UVR induce collagen breakdown while enhancing synthesis of malformed elastin and make the morphological alterations more evident causing spots, wrinkles, and dehydrated skin. The destruction of collagen is a major contributor to the loss of skin flexibility and structure that occurs with advancing age. This process of premature aging as a result of a series of deleterious biochemical reactions occurring within the skin with the exposure to excess UV radiation is referred to as ***Photoaging***. UVR majorly targets the surface epidermal layers which results in the depletion of antioxidants such as alpha-tocopherol (vitamin E) and ascorbic acid (vitamin C), decreasing the overall antioxidant capacity within the skin. Secondarily to the depletion of vital antioxidant molecules in the epidermis, intrinsic antioxidant defence systems such as the activity of antioxidant enzymes superoxide dismutase, catalase, and glutathione-*S*-transferase trim down.

The solar spectrum has shown to affect skin according to the wavelength of various radiations, wherein short-wavelength radiations in the UV range with higher energy are potentially more damaging (Fig. 2) [4].

UVC

Ultraviolet C (200–280 nm) radiation is efficiently absorbed by cellular and mitochondrial DNA; however, it does not reach the surface of the earth and gets absorbed by stratospheric ozone layer. UVC radiation emitted from artificial light sources

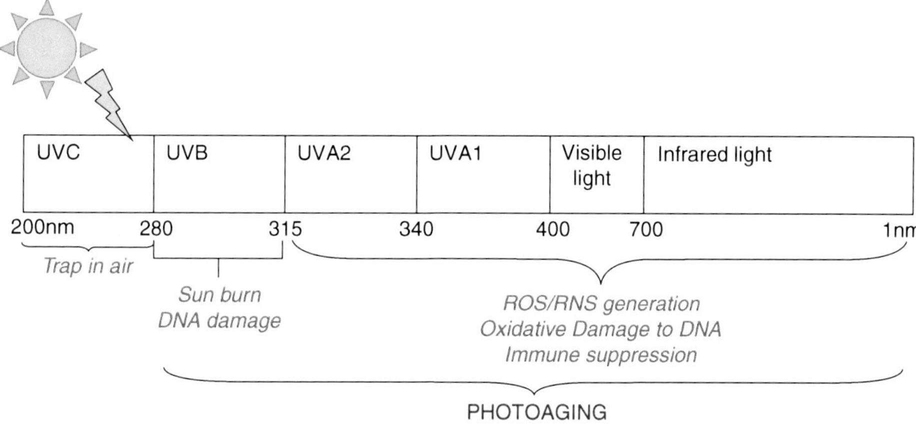

Fig. 2 The solar radiation spectrum and its effects on skin. All solar wavelengths contribute altogether to skin ageing and wrinkling

can cause DNA damage in cells to the level of spinous layers, but it does not penetrate the basal layer. Hence it is the least harmful for skin cells.

UVB (Midwave)

UVB rays (280–315 nm) are partially filtered by the ozone layer. It compromises only about 5 % of the total UVR and is highly damaging to DNA and epidermal keratinocytes. UVB being biologically active penetrates the superficial layers of skin down to the basal layer of the epidermis, where it generates reactive oxygen species and reactive nitrogen species (ROS and RNS respectively), causing inflammation, sunburn, skin aging, and in some cases nonmelanoma skin cancer. The high-energy photons of UVB can also be absorbed directly by DNA bases that cause mutagenic lesions that cannot be repaired inducing the cell to undergo apoptosis and hence misbalancing the turnover of topmost skin layer. This contributes to the dead skin cells in the superficial layer making it appear aged.

UVA (Long Wave)

Less energetic than UVB, but constituting about (90–95 %) of total UVR, UVA radiation (315–400 nm) can penetrate deeper into the epidermis and dermis of the skin than UVB (Fig. 3). It activates melanin pigmentation in the topmost layer of the skin and creates tanning appearance for shorter time duration. However, with its penetration potential, it can damage the connective tissues and blood vessels along with other major skin components including extracellular matrix (ECM). As a result the skin gradually loses its elasticity and starts to wrinkle leading to premature aging. UVA damages the DNA in keratinocytes in the basal layer of the epidermis compromising the repair mechanism and hence the cell undergoes apoptosis and eventually dies. In severe cases of mutation and cell cycle continuation, keratinocytes become a major site for the onset of most of the skin cancer.

Visible Light

Of even lesser energy, visible light (400–700 nm) accounts for approximately 50 % of the total solar spectrum. It penetrates deeply into biological tissues and about 20 % reaches the hypodermis. However, visible light is considered to be beneficial to the living system and thus seems inoffensive.

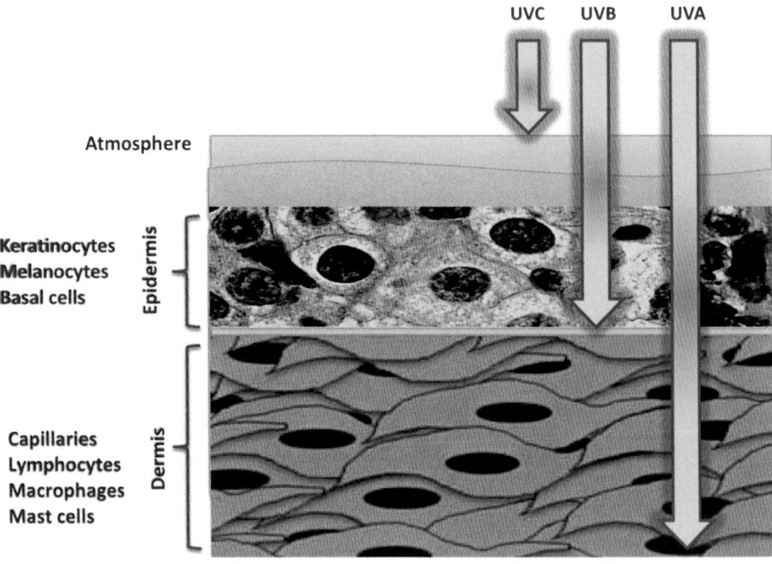

Fig. 3 The penetration potential of UVA and UVB in skin

Infrared Radiation

IR with the lowest energy contributes around 45 % to the solar spectrum reaching human skin. IR comprises IRA (700–1400 nm), IRB (1400–3000 nm), and IRC (3000 nm–1 mm), where only IRA deeply penetrates the skin. It represents about 30 % of IR radiation, of which 65 % reaches the dermis and 10 % the hypodermis wherein the radiation increases the production of matrix metalloproteinases, particularly MMP-1, a collagenase in dermal fibroblasts, which is critical to skin's vitality and juvenile appearance. MMP-1 digests several types of collagen (I, II, III, VII, and X) and thus a balance is necessary for the maintenance of skin morphology as well as for its remodeling after injury [4]. Abnormally high level of MMP-1 is evident during IR exposure, causing excessive collagen destruction, which leads to weakening of the skin matrix, formation of wrinkles, and thinning of the dermis – all hallmarks of skin aging. Other proaging effects of IRA include activation of inflammatory reactions, excessive cell division and hence accelerated accumulation of senescent cells, and excessive growth of blood vessels leading to persistent skin redness.

Effect of Air Pollutants on Skin Aging

Air pollutants found in the form of gases and finely divided solid and liquid aerosols are divided into two categories, i.e., primary and secondary [5]. Primary air pollutants are emitted directly into the atmosphere, however secondary air pollutants are formed as a result of reactions between primary pollutants and other elements in the atmosphere, such as ozone (Fig. 4).

Benzoapyrene

Benzo[a]pyrene, $C_{20}H_{12}$, is a polycyclic aromatic compound, having mutagenic and highly carcinogenic metabolites and its exposure leads to skin cancer and inflammatory skin diseases due to oxidative stress. Hence, its potential role in skin aging has also been hypothesized. Residual wood burning is the major source of benzo[a] pyrene, while it is also found in coal tar, automobile exhaust fumes (especially from diesel engines), and in smoke resulting from the combustion of organic material (including cigarette smoke).

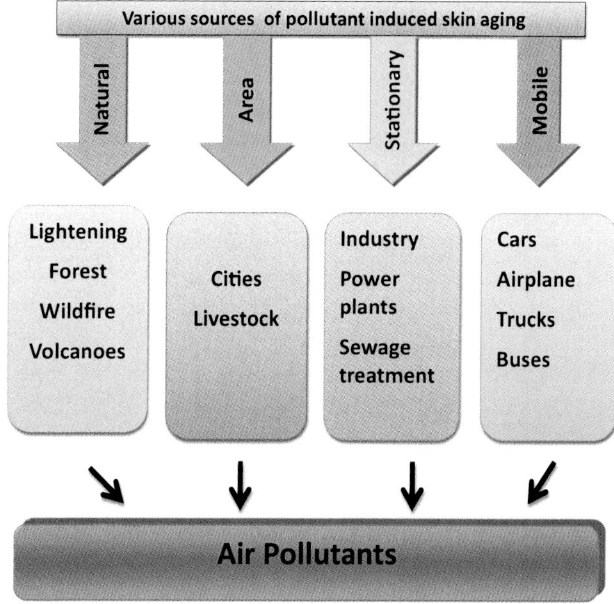

Fig. 4 Different sources of air pollution affecting skin aging

Polyaromatic Hydrocarbons (PAHs)

Poly-aromatic hydrocarbons, PAHs, are converted into quinines, redox-cycling chemicals that produce ROS by activating the xenobiotic metabolism, key compounds in particulate matter (PM). Long-term-exposed skin to PM-bound PAHs, which is either through hair follicle or transepidermal absorption, may cause oxidative stress further contributing to skin aging. Ambient particles such as soot may be able to reach melanocytes and directly affect the function of cutaneous cells by releasing surface-bound PAHs. Activated PAHs produce epoxides and diols that bind to DNA and initiate cutaneous carcinogenesis [6].

2, 3, 7, 8-TetraChloroDibenzo-p-Dioxin (TCDD)

2, 3, 7, 8-tetrachlorodibenzo-p-dioxin a polychlorinated dibenzo-p-dioxin ($C_{12}H_4C_{14}O$) is a colorless solid with no distinguishable odor at room temperature. The most potent member of the group of polyhalogenated aromatic hydrocarbons, it is formed as a side product of organic synthesis and burning of organic materials. Being a persistent environmental contaminant it is usually present in a complex mixture of dioxin-like compounds and acts as a carcinogen. The greatest production of TCDD occurs from waste incineration, metal production, and combustion of fossil fuel and wood. It activated the aryl hydrocarbon receptor (AHR) which is known to cause tumors of the skin [7].

Chloracnegens (Halogenated Aromatic Hydrocarbons)

Chloracnegens (halogenated aromatic hydrocarbons) are fat-soluble compounds which cause Chloracne, a systemic toxic disease characterized by acneiform skin lesions such as comedones and cysts mainly on the face (outer sides of the eye and behind the ears) and neck. The chloracnegens ligands, for example, polychlorobiphenyls, polychlorodibenzofurans, dioxins, and azoxybenzenes, bind to cell nucleus and DNA where they alter translation of genes [8]. These alterations are causal factors of induced skin aging with the appearance of age spots on skin.

Volatile Organic Compounds (VOCs)

Volatile organic compounds are organic chemicals with a high vapor pressure at ordinary room temperature which results from a low boiling point causing a large number of molecules to evaporate or sublimate from the liquid or solid form of the compound and enter the surrounding. Originating from the use of organic solvents in paints, varnishes (e.g., aliphatic hydrocarbons, ethyl acetate, glycol ethers, methylene chloride, and acetone), vehicle refinishing products in repairing car paint, environmental tobacco smoke, stored fuels, exhaust from cars (e.g., benzene), and emissions from industrial facilities (e.g., tetrachloroethene) with the presence of sunlight and NOx, these compounds cause the formation of photochemical oxidant products such as O_3 at ground level which is also referred as summer photochemical smog. Study on cultured keratinocytes has showed that exposure to VOCs increases cytokines, which could then favor the development of inflammatory and allergic reaction as atopic dermatitis or eczema by the induction of vascular hyperpermeability, which is an initiator of skin inflammation [9].

Nitrogen Oxides (NO)

Nitric oxide is a colorless gas, with a distinct sharp, biting odor, produced along with NO_2 with the combustion of fuels. Initially almost 90 % of NOX combustion product is in the form of NO which is further oxidized to nitrogen dioxide (NO_2) in the presence of air.

Nitrogen oxides are emitted mainly from mobile and stationary combustion sources and react with O_3 or radicals in the atmosphere, forming NO_2. Amongst NOx, NO_2 is known to cause oxidative damage resulting in the generation of free radicals that may oxidize amino acids in tissue proteins and initiate lipid peroxidation of polyunsaturated fatty acids. Human skin contains photolabile nitric oxide derivates like nitrite and S-nitroso thiols, which after UVA irradiation decompose and lead to the formation of vasoactive NO [10].

Atmospheric Sulfur Dioxide (SO_2)

Sulfur dioxide is a colorless gas with a pungent, suffocating odor. Atmospheric sulfur dioxide can be formed from both anthropogenic (fuel combustion from power generation and industrial processes) and natural sources (volcanic activity, forest fires). Sulfur contents in fossil fuels range between 0.1 % and 4 % in oil, oil by-products, and coal, while up to 40 % in natural gas. Marine phytoplankton produce dimethyl sulfide (DMS) which is then oxidized to SO_2 in the atmosphere. Additionally, the decay process in soil and vegetation releasing H_2S or volcanic eruptions also adds up to the SO_2 level. Around 90 % of all natural sulfur emissions come in the form of DMS. Sulfur dioxide being corrosive to organic components leads to impairment of the hydrolipidic film which makes the skin irritated and sensitive and can even cause burns.

Carbon Monoxide (CO)

CO is an air pollutant which is a product of incomplete combustion from mobile sources. Carbon monoxide acts on cell metabolism through hypoxic and nonhypoxic modes of action, resulting from its ability to bind to heme and alter its function and metabolism. It slows down the skin's metabolism and causes a dull complexion, premature aging, and dryness of the skin [11].

Particulate Matter (PM)

Particulate matter is the general term used for a mixture of solid particles and liquid droplets in the air. It includes aerosols, smoke, fumes, dust, ash, and pollen. Factories, power plants, refuse incinerators, automobile, construction activities, fires, and natural windblown dust are some of the main sources of PM.

Major components of PM include metals, organic compounds, material of biological origin, ions, reactive gases, and the particle carbon core. Particles in the nanosize range, especially those from traffic sources, are considered among the most harmful components of ambient PM, since their physical properties make them highly reactive toward biological surfaces and structures and induce oxidative stress in human skin. The generation of oxidative stress by PM contributes to extrinsic skin aging [12].

Research says than an increase in soot, an increase in particles from traffic, and higher PM_{10} background concentrations were associated with more pigment spots on the face and more pronounced nasolabial folds.

Occupational Exposure to Heavy Metals

Heavy metals constitute a very heterogeneous group of elements widely varied in their chemical properties and biological functions. They are found naturally in the earth, and become concentrated as a consequence of mining and industrial wastes, vehicle emissions, lead-acid batteries, fertilizers, paints, and treated woods and further potentially harms the living system via air inhalation, diet, and manual handling. Motor vehicle emissions are a major source of airborne contaminants including arsenic, cadmium, cobalt, nickel, and lead. Water sources (groundwater, lakes, streams, and rivers) can be polluted by heavy metals through leaching from industrial and consumer waste and acid rain can exacerbate this process by releasing heavy metals trapped in soils. Plants are exposed to heavy metals through the uptake of water, animals eat these plants, and ingestion of plant- and animal-based foods is the largest source of heavy metals in humans. Absorption through skin contact with soil is another potential source of heavy metal contamination. Heavy metals can accumulate in organisms as they are hard to metabolize [13]. Some of the heavy metals that are stated environment pollutant and affect human health are

Lead

Lead is a naturally occurring toxic metal found in the Earth's crust. Its widespread use has resulted in extensive environmental contamination, human exposure, and significant public health problems in many parts of the world. Some of the major sources of lead are contaminated soil, which is found near busy streets as lead was an ingredient in gasoline until the late 1970s, houses painted with lead-based paint, water through old lead pipes or faucets, food stored in bowls glazed or painted with lead or imported from countries that use lead to seal canned food, some toys, jewellery, hobby, and sports objects such as stained glass, ink, paint, and plaster. Dermal exposure plays a role for exposure to organic lead among workers, but is not considered a significant pathway for the general population. Organic lead, for example, tetramethyl lead, is more likely to be absorbed through the skin than inorganic lead and hence people who work with lead are most susceptible to dermal exposure which not just enhances the process of premature aging but in chronic exposure cases can cause skin cancer.

Arsenic

Arsenic poisoning is a medical condition caused by elevated levels of arsenic in the body. The dominant basis of arsenic poisoning is from groundwater that naturally contains high concentrations of arsenic. Long-term exposure to arsenic in drinking water is mainly related to increased risks of skin cancers in addition to skin lesions such as hyperkeratosis and pigmentation changes contributing to premature skin aging.

Apart from heavy metals, chlorine exposure affects skin by stripping it off its top protective layer, making it dry or itchy, a common phenomenon that also occurs after exiting a traditional swimming pool. The outermost layer of our skin contains a dense network of protein and keratins that help keep it hydrated and prevent water evaporation. These cells absorb water and help skin achieve its "springy" natural shape. Chlorine reacts with skin cells and leaves behind a layer on the top; while exiting the swimming pool, skin is still sufficiently covered in chlorine and is usually left dry, sticky, or flaky. Chlorine is a harsh pool chemical and repeated exposure can cause signs of premature aging. Moreover, shower with hot water after exiting the pool causes the pores to open and chlorine seeps further into the layers of skin causing it to be stripped off natural oils, leading to dryness, cracking, and wrinkles.

Metal Working Fluids (MWFs)

People working with heavy metals remain exposed for longer duration and hence are more prone to skin aging. One of the most common examples is metal working fluids (MWFs), which are industrial coolants and lubricants used to reduce friction and heat generated due to the machining, grinding lubrication, and fabrication operations of metal products. These fluids have additives that are corrosion inhibitors, emulsifiers, antifoaming agents, preservatives, and biocides. MWFs can be irritating to the skin. Skin problems include mechanical trauma to the skin, infections, oil acne, folliculitis, and irritant and allergic dermatitis. Small cuts to the skin from metal shavings (swarf) are a common injury, which can lead to serious infection as a result of contact with MWFs contaminated with microbial organisms. Direct contact to oils can result in folliculitis (inflammation of the hair follicles), which results in blocked skin follicles causing red irritation around hair follicles and small black plugged pores to large pustules. This problem can be found on the neck, hands, arms, and thighs. Exposure to MWFs can also worsen acne and even cause irritant dermatitis, the most common type of skin problem due to exposure to MWFs [14].

Soluble and synthetic metal working fluids are strong alkaline solutions (pH of approximately 9) containing numerous additives and solvents. These solutions remove protective oils in the skin and damage proteins in its outer layer resulting in damage to the natural skin barrier, which causes a decrease in the water content of the skin leading to a dry, thickened, fissured, and inflamed skin and shows the sign of premature aging.

Infrequently, very small fluid-filled blisters can also develop on the hands and fingers. Small cuts in the skin from metal pieces allow more penetration of irritant fluids and contribute to irritant dermatitis. The type and concentration of fluid used, duration of exposure during the work period, and the presence of preexisting skin disease (eczema or severe dry skin) all contribute to the development of dermatitis. Longer exposure to MWFs then thus can ultimately lead to premature skin aging.

Cosmetic Ingredients in Skin Aging

Most of the skin care products and cosmetics contain ingredients that are not only harmful to the structure and morphology of the skin, but also their adverse effects can be seen at later stages of life. Many of these ingredients are known carcinogens and are used by the cosmetic industries, although in a very less amount, simply because of being less expensive as compared to the organic compounds extracted from plants or microbes. These toxic ingredients in beauty products negatively affect the production of collagen, hence disturb the balance of collagenase and collagen making the skin sag and less elastic. Some of the toxic chemicals in cosmetics and dermatological products have been discussed further (Fig. 5).

Sodium Lauryl Sulfate (SLS) and Ammonium Lauryl Sulfate (ALS)

Often described as being "derived from coconut" to disguise their toxic nature, these chemicals are commonly used in shampoos, toothpaste, foaming facial and body cleansers, and bubble bath. SLS and ALS, easily absorbed into the body, can cause severe skin irritation and their building up in the brain, heart, lungs, and liver can lead to the expression of cytokines and proto-oncogenes in photoaged and intrinsically aged human keratinocytes [15].

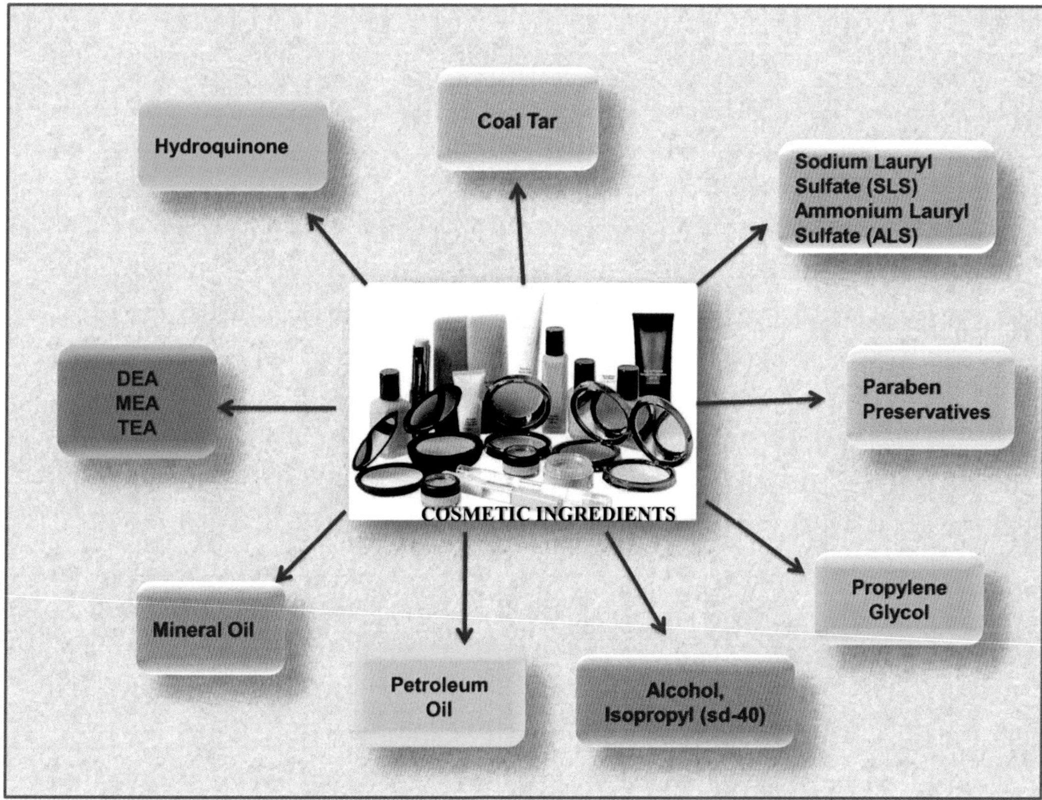

Fig. 5 Harmful constituents of cosmetics causing skin aging

Paraben Preservatives

These are widely used in cosmetic products to prolong their shelf life. They are known to be highly toxic causal factors for rashes and allergic reactions. A subgroup, methylparabens, has been shown to chemically react with UVB rays when applied to the skin, thereby intensifying the effects of UVB skin damage, resulting in premature skin aging [16].

Alcohol, Isopropyl (sd-40)

It is made from propylene, a petroleum derivative, and is found in many skin and hair products, fragrance, antibacterial hand washes, as well as shellac and antifreeze. A very drying and irritating solvent and dehydrator, it strips our skin's moisture and natural immune barrier, making the skin more vulnerable to bacteria, molds, and viruses. It acts as a "carrier" accelerating the penetration of other harmful chemicals into the skin, promoting brown spots and premature aging of skin [17].

Petroleum Oil

Found in an overwhelming number of products like baby oil, mascara, moisturizers, etc. it seals off the skin creating a barrier which feels slick, but doesn't allow the skin to breath, which is essential for the proper functioning of this organ, so it slows down skin's function and normal cell development, resulting in premature aging and many other health and skin disorders such as contact dermatitis [18].

Mineral Oil

Mineral oil is a petroleum derivative that coats the skin like saran wrap, which prevents the skin from breathing, absorbing, and excreting. It also slows the skin's natural cell development, causing to age prematurely.

DEA (Diethanolamine), TEA (Triethanolamine), and MEA (Monoethanolamine)

These substances are harsh solvents and detergents that are used in cosmetics and face and body creams as an emollient. Owing to the allergic reactions caused by the use of these ingredients, the long-term use of DEA-based products can further be linked to an increase in the incidence of liver and kidney cancer [19].

Hydroquinone

Commonly used in skin lighteners. It is linked to cancer and organ-system toxicity. In addition to its use in skin lighteners, hydroquinone is a possible impurity of tocopheryl acetate (synthetic Vitamin E) which is very common in facial and skin cleansers, facial moisturizers, and hair conditioners. Hydroquinone works by decreasing the production and increasing the degradation of melanin pigments in the skin. This increases the skin's exposure to UVA and UVB rays, increasing the risk of premature aging and skin cancer [20].

Coal Tar

Coal tar is a known carcinogen derived from burning coal. It is a complex mixture of hundreds of compounds, many of which are polycyclic aromatic hydrocarbons (PAHs). Coal tar is used in food, textiles, cosmetics, and personal care products. Experimental studies have found that the exposure to coal tar produces skin tumors and neurological damage.

Some of the studies also show that not only the use of these toxic ingredients which are found in cosmetics causing skin aging but also the amount and duration of skin and cosmetic contact is of concern, as a good portion of makeup is actually absorbed by the skin throughout the day, from the dermal layers into the blood, in the same way nicotine skin patches deliver nicotine into the blood. Using cosmetics regularly can hence cause the absorbed chemicals to accumulate in epidermal (skin) tissue, fatty tissue, and throughout the body as the blood carries and deposits them in various cells and organs, accelerating the aging process and encouraging the onset of disease as these chemicals produce their toxic effects. In this regard natural products can be of great significance having antioxidative properties and less toxicity [21].

Effect of Extreme Temperatures on Skin Aging

Whether it's cold, dry, hot, or humid, climatic conditions affect the skin, causing various skin problems from acne breakouts to itchy dry patches. Extremes in weather can exacerbate some existing skin conditions or even trigger the onset of new ones. Colder climates can be harsh as low temperatures cause low humidity, which dries out skin. Bitterly cold wind can also strip its moisture leading to rough, red, tightened, cracked, or peeling skin because of dryness. Furthermore, dry weather is found to be responsible for skin conditions, such as eczema. However, warmer climate with increased heat and humidity leads to sweating, resulting in breakouts, especially for oily skin types. Salicylic acid can help to dry up some of the oil, but it can also make our skin more sensitive to sunlight. Additionally heat also results in heat rash, which happens when sweat ducts get closed off, trapping the moisture under the skin and leading to a rash made up of blisters or bumps [22].

Smoking and Skin Aging

Cigarette smoking is strongly associated with elastosis in both sexes, and telangiectasia (red spots on skin) in men. Smoking causes skin damage primarily by decreasing capillary blood flow to the skin, which, in turn, creates oxygen and nutrient deprivation in cutaneous tissues. It has been shown that those who smoke have fewer collagen and elastin fibers in the dermis, which causes skin to become slack, hardened, and less elastic. It alters extracellular matrix turnover in the skin, leading to an imbalance between biosynthesis and degradation of dermal connective tissue proteins [23]. This reduced mechanical tension in fibroblasts results in increased intracellular levels of oxidants which in turn stimulate further expression of MMP-1. While smoking downregulates synthesis of type I and type III collagens, a major factor for accelerated skin aging, it also elevates tropoelastin and increases collagen degradation. It increases keratinocyte dysplasia and skin roughness. A clear dose–response relationship between wrinkling and smoking has been identified, with smoking being a greater contributor to facial wrinkling than even sun exposure. It was demonstrated to be an independent risk factor for premature wrinkling even when age, sun exposure, and pigmentation were controlled. Although hormone replacement therapy (HRT) was demonstrated to reverse wrinkling, the skin of long-time smokers did not respond [24]. Wrinkle scores were three times greater in smokers than in nonsmokers, with a significant increase in the risk of wrinkles after 10 pack-years. Pack-years are calculated by multiplying the number of packs of cigarettes smoked per day to the number of years the person has smoked. Smoking also increases free radical formation and is an important risk factor in cutaneous squamous cell carcinoma.

Research shows that the skin-aging effects of smoking may be due to increased production of an enzyme that breaks down collagen in the skin and causes it to sag (Fig. 6). Over time, as collagen is reduced squinting in response to the irritating nature of the smoke and the puckering of the mouth when drawing on a cigarette causes wrinkling around the eyes (known as Crow's feet) and mouth. Smokers in their 40s often have as many facial wrinkles as nonsmokers in their 60s. Skin damage caused by smoking may not be immediately visible to the naked eye but is still happening

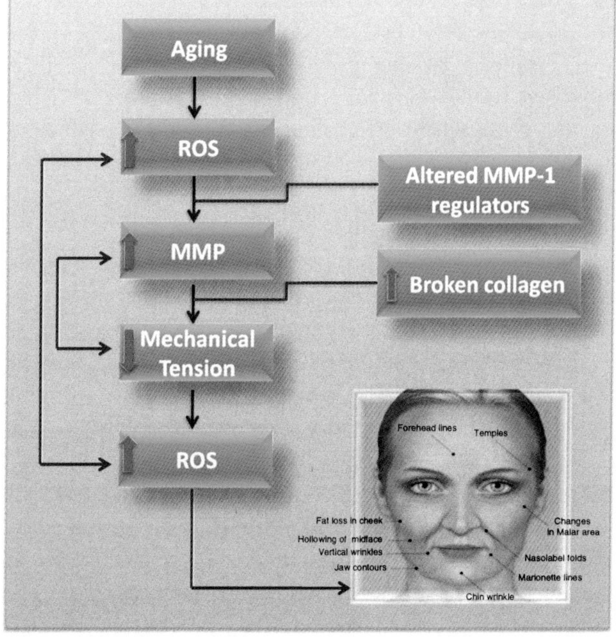

Fig. 6 Mechanism of smoking-induced precocious aging along with aging effects on the face

and can start to be detected in one's 20s or 30s. The most common manifestation of smoking, and perhaps the most socially distressing, is precocious aging. A "smoker's face" characteristically has prominent wrinkles, a gauntness of facial features with prominence of the underlying bony contours, an atrophic, gray appearance of the skin, and a plethoric complexion. This risk is higher in women as compared to men [25]. The appearance of wrinkles is exaggerated by direct contact of cigarette smoke, which reduces moisture levels in the stratum corneum and induces a mild inflammatory reaction. Skin exposed to cigarette smoke is thin and fragile, tending to sag. While cigarette smoking is an independent risk factor for the increase of elastic fibers in the reticular dermis of nonexposed causing skin wrinkling, there is a synergistic effect with sun exposure on skin aging. This increase results from degradation of elastic material in an additive manner, as in solar elastosis [26].

Nicotine with a half-life of about 2 h can enter the human body by smoke inhalation, ingestion, intranasal spray, transdermal patch, topical cream, or enema [27] although occurring naturally in small quantities in certain foods such as tomato, potato, and eggplant. It can be absorbed through the oral cavity, lung, bladder, gastrointestinal tract, and skin. Seventy to eighty percent of nicotine absorbed from the gastrointestinal tract is converted to its principal metabolite, cotinine, via first-pass hepatic metabolism. It is absorbed through skin and mucous membranes in a dose-dependent manner [28].

There are many dermatological hazards of tobacco use that can affect the skin both directly on the epidermis and indirectly via the bloodstream. Tobacco smoke is comprised of a solid particulate phase, including the alkaloid, nicotine, and a volatile gas phase. There are many mutagens and carcinogens in tobacco smoke, notably polycyclic aromatic hydrocarbons, nitrosamines, and heterocyclic amines. The main toxic constituents of the solid phase include nicotine, phenol, catechol, quinoline, aniline, toluidine, nickel, *N*-nitrosodimethylamine, benzopyrenes, benzanthracene, and 2-naphthylamine. The main toxic constituents of the gas phase include carbon dioxide, carbon monoxide, hydrogen cyanide, nitrogen oxides, acetone, formaldehyde, acrolein, ammonium, pyridine, 3-vinylpyridine, *N*-nitrosodimethylamine, and *N*-nitrosopyrrolidine. Studies of gene expression in the skin revealed that tobacco constituents upregulate 14 different genes involved in xenobiotic metabolism, oxidative stress, and stress response [29]. Smoking may exhaust cellular defense and repair functions, resulting in an accumulation of damage due to mutations and malfunctioning proteins. Hence, it induces the intrinsic factors also to contribute in the accelerated aging of skin.

Heavy smokers can typically be identified by characteristic cutaneous and mucosal manifestations. Classic findings include a yellow discoloration of light-colored mustaches and fingernails that are stained by tobacco by-products [30]. With smoking cessation, a demarcation appears between the distal pigmented nail and growth of the normal nail. This is termed a Harlequin nail, or quitter's nail. The duration of smoking cessation may be deduced by the length of normal nail growth. Chronic heating from holding lit cigarettes may also discolor the fingertips due to postinflammatory hyperpigmentation.

Conclusion

With advancement in technologies, concern about health and appearance is growing. However, lifestyle is somewhere negatively affecting society. Environmental pollution adds up to that, with the exposure to various toxic substances in the surrounding, including UVR and heavy metals. Skin being the window of human health, showing the most obvious signs of aging, has triggered the research into this field. Attempts are still going on to find the exact mechanism behind the role of exogenous factors in premature skin aging. As reactive oxygen species holds the central position in enhancing the aging process, antioxidant therapies and treatments need to be elucidated to overcome the accelerated aging process of skin.

References

1. Dayan N, et al. Market evolution of topical anti-aging treatments. In: Skin aging handbook: an integrated approach to biochemistry and product development. 1st ed., Norwich, NY: William Andrew 2008, pp. 4–14.
2. Dayan N, et al. Market evolution of topical anti-aging treatments. In: Skin aging handbook: an integrated approach to biochemistry and product development. 1st ed., Norwich, NY: William Andrew 2008, pp. 16–31.
3. Trojahn C, et al. The skin barrier function: differences between intrinsic and extrinsic aging. G Ital Dermatol Venereol. 2015;150:687–92.
4. Anna B, et al. Mechanism of UV-related carcinogenesis and its contribution to nevi/melanoma. Expert Rev Dermatol. 2007;2:451–69.
5. Burke KE, et al. Synergistic damage by UVA radiation and pollutants. Toxicol Ind Health. 2009;25:219–24.
6. Penning TM, et al. Dihydrodiol dehydrogenase and poly- cyclic aromatic hydrocarbon activation: generation of reactive and redoxactiveo-quinones. Chem Res Toxicol. 1999;12:1–18.
7. Lin S, et al. Hippocampal metabolomics reveals 2, 3, 7, 8-tetrachlorodibenzo-p-dioxin toxicity associated with ageing in Sprague–Dawley rats. Talanta. 2011;85:1007–12.
8. Drakaki E, et al. Air pollution and the skin. Front Environ Sci. 2014;2:11–6.
9. Baudouin C, et al. Environmental pollutants and skin cancer. Cell Biol Toxicol. 2002;18:341–8.
10. Katsitadze A, et al. Nitric oxide dependent skin aging mechanism in postmenopausal women. Georgian Med News. 2012;209:66–71.
11. Vierkötter A, et al. Airborne particle exposure and extrinsic skin aging. J Invest Dermatol. 2010;130:2719–26.
12. Vierkötter A, et al. Environmental influences on skin aging and ethnic-specific manifestations. Dermatoendocrinol. 2012;4:227–31.
13. Katsouyanni K, et al. Ambient air pollution and health. Br Med Bull. 2003;68:143–56.
14. Duruibe O, et al. Heavy metal pollution and human bio toxic effects. Int J Phys Sci. 2007;2:112–8.
15. Suh DH, et al. Effects of 12-O-tetradecanoyl-phorbol-13-acetate and sodium lauryl sulphate on the production and expression of cytokines and proto-oncogenes in photo aged and intrinsically aged human keratinocytes. J Invest Dermatol. 2001;117:1225–33.
16. Ishiwatari S, et al. Effects of methyl paraben on skin keratinocytes. J Appl Toxicol. 2007;27:1–9.
17. Sgarbossa A, et al. Dolichol: a solar filter with UV-absorbing properties which can be photo enhanced. Biogerontology. 2003;4:379–85.
18. Dika E, et al. Causal relationship between exposure to chemicals and malignant melanoma? A review and study proposal. Rev Environ Health. 2010;25:255–9.
19. Knaak JB, et al. Toxicology of mono-, di-, and triethanolamine. Rev Environ Contam Toxicol. 1997;149:1–86.
20. Hung CF, et al. The risk of hydroquinone and sunscreen over-absorption via photo damaged skin is not greater in senescent skin as compared to young skin: nude mouse as an animal model. Int J Pharm. 2014;25:135–45.
21. Tanuja Y, et al. Anticedants and natural prevention of environmental toxicants induced accelerated aging of skin. Environ Toxicol Pharmacol. 2015;39:384–91.
22. Kenney WL, et al. Heat waves, aging, and human cardiovascular health. Med Sci Sports Exerc. 2014;46:1891–9.
23. Endo K, et al. Establishment of the MethyLight assay for assessing aging, cigarette smoking, and alcohol consumption. Biomed Res Int. 2015;2015:45–51.
24. Morita A, et al. Molecular basis of tobacco smoke-induced premature skin aging. J Investig Dermatol Symp Proc. 2009;14:53–5.
25. Farage MA, et al. Intrinsic and extrinsic factors in skin ageing: a review. Int J Cosmet Sci. 2008;30:87–95.
26. Ribera M, et al. Effect of smoking on skin elastic fibres: morphometric and immunohistochemical analysis. Br J Dermatol. 2007;156:85–91.
27. Ishibashi MH, et al. Age-related changes in nicotine response of cholinergic and non-cholinergic later dorsal tegmental neurons: implications for the heightened adolescent susceptibility to nicotine addiction. Neuropharmacology. 2014;85:263–83.
28. Benowitz NL, et al. Nicotine chemistry, metabolism, kinetics and biomarkers. Hand Exp Pharmacol. 2009;192:29–60.
29. Craighead, T. et al.: Chemistry and toxicology of cigarette smoke and biomarkers of exposure and harm. In : A report of the surgeon general centres for disease control and prevention. US, 2010; pp. 784–93.
30. Daniell HW. Smoker's wrinkles. A study in the epidemiology of "crow's feet". Ann Intern Med. 1971;75:873–80.

Impact of Dietary Supplements on Skin Aging

46

Utkrishta L. Raj, Garima Sharma, Shweta Dang, Sanjay Gupta, and Reema Gabrani

Contents

U.L. Raj • G. Sharma • S. Dang • S. Gupta • R. Gabrani (✉)
Department of Biotechnology, Jaypee Institute of Information Technology, Noida, UP, India
e-mail: utkrish11@gmail.com; garimash.sharma777@gmail.com; shweta.dang@jiit.ac.in; reema.gabrani@jiit.ac.in; rmgabrani@gmail.com

M.A. Farage et al. (eds.), *Textbook of Aging Skin*,
DOI 10.1007/978-3-662-47398-6_174

Abstract

Skin, known to be the largest organ, consists of epidermis and dermis. Any physiological change associated with age is ultimately reflected by a person's skin. Two major factors responsible for premature aging are intrinsic, i. e., involvement of genes, and extrinsic that covers exposure of skin to ultraviolet (UV) radiation. UV rays induce the oxidative stress and consequently cause the loss of cellular regulation. Dietary nutriments may help the body to fight against signs of early aging as antioxidants and by regulating keratinocytes proliferation and differentiation. Main ingredients of these dietary supplements include several vitamins, minerals, phytochemicals, omega-3 fatty acids, amino acids, and probiotics. Vitamin A, C, D, and E assist in maintaining skin veracity. Zinc, copper, and selenium are the main minerals which are involved in sustenance of healthy skin. Phytochemicals consisting of flavonoids, terpenoids, and alkaloids with antibacterial, antifungal, and antioxidative property may benefit the texture and physiological parameters of skin delaying its aging. Amino acids like arginine, proline, ornithine, and glutamine alone as well as in combination support the healthy being of skin. The probiotic bacteria like *Lactobacillus johnsonii* and *Lactobacillus plantarum* commonly found in intestine aid in delaying aging by hydrating the skin as well as by showing protective effect on UV-exposed area. Though many clinical studies favor the role of dietary substances in prevention of early skin aging there is a need to cover the wider population and understand the various contributory factors.

Introduction

Skin, the largest organ of the body, plays an important role in maintaining homeostasis between external environment and internal tissues thus providing protection against microorganisms, ultraviolet radiation, toxic agents, or mechanical insults. It plays a vital role in maintaining neurosensory, circulatory, and immunological functions at the body surface. Skin consists of two major layers: epidermis and dermis [1]. Epidermis, the outer layer, is a stratified squamous epithelium and consists of mainly basal and differentiated keratinocytes which gradually lead to the formation of stratum corneum, the outermost layer of dead cells. Epidermis also consists of melanocytes for the production of melanin, langerhans cells as antigen presenting cells, and merkel cells interacting with nerve endings. Basically, dermis acts as a supportive connective tissue between the epidermis and the underlying subcutis. It is a fibrous and elastic tissue that gives skin its flexibility and strength consisting of sweat glands, hair roots, blood, and lymph vessels. Dermis is made up of fibroblast which produces extracellular matrix protein like collagen mainly of type I and type III. Extracellular matrix comprises of hyaluronic acid and dermatan sulfate as heteropolysaccharides along with collagen fiber network. Hyaluronic acid consists of alternating units of *N*-acetylglucosamine and glucuronic acid, and maintains elasticity, viscosity, and skin moisture by retaining water. Subcutis is the layer of loose connective tissue and fat beneath the dermis [2, 3].

In order to maintain a healthy skin the structural and functional integrity of the skin should be maintained throughout the epidermis, dermis, and hypodermis. Various factors for skin stability include skin thickness, lipid content, proper barrier function, and hydration level. The functional integrity is associated with maintenance of acidic pH, vitamin D level, neurosensory function, percutaneous absorption, adequate vascularization, immune surveillance, temperature regulation, and capacity for injury repair [1].

Aging is a biological process which leads to progressive decline in the organism's fitness and cellular function. In terms of skin, aging is characterized by formation of lines and wrinkles, increased pigmentation, loss of elasticity and firmness, and dull skin due to both intrinsic and extrinsic factors [4]. Intrinsic aging is due to genetic factors and corporal changes that occur/appear during the normal aging process like production of reactive oxygen species (ROS) and estrogen deficiency whereas extrinsic aging focuses on aging process accelerated by environmental influences like physiological stress and exposure to excessive ultraviolet light (UV). Other factors like smoking, air pollution are critical chronic stresses that impact skin aging and along with exposure to UV light can cause premature elderly look. Airborne particles, exposure to traffic has been associated with significant increase in pigmentation, spots, and facial wrinkles [3, 5]. Telomere is the DNA at the end of chromosome which shortens with every cell division leading to senescence and premature cellular aging [2]. Telomerase shortening has also emerged as another factor influencing skin aging and linked to chronic psychological stress. The poor quality of sleep has showed increased sign of aging including fine lines, uneven pigmentation, and reduced elasticity.

Aged skin undergoes progressive structural and functional degeneration making it prone to various diseases like eczema, contact and allergic dermatitis, seborrheic dermatitis, autoimmune diseases with cutaneous manifestations, and various forms of neoplasms, such as basal and squamous cell carcinoma and malignant melanoma [1]. Progerin, a mutant of lamin A, is one of the known physiological biomarkers of aging process which begins at age 30. It interacts with cellular environment ensuing alteration in chromatin remodeling, transcription factors, DNA repair, antioxidant proteins and impact cell proliferation, arrest cell apoptosis, and may lead to dysfunction

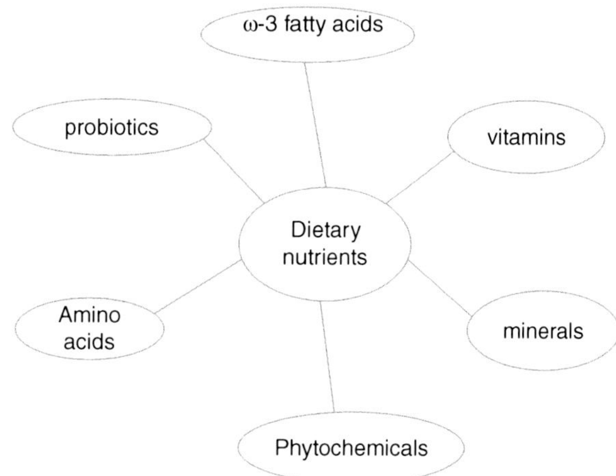

Fig. 1 Dietary components used in supplementary food products

of tissue and organs. There are also other biomarkers of skin aging such as lipofuscin and lactic acid, which are results of dysfunctional cell processes [6].

Dietary Role in Skin Aging

Diet taken by an individual can also play an important role in maintaining the health of a skin by controlling age-related diseases. Normal diet consumed by an individual includes vegetables, fruits, dairy products, fish, meat which fulfills the essential requirement of vitamins, minerals, micro–macro nutrients. Surveys conducted have shown that the normal diet consumed by the population does not completely fulfill the nutrient requirement and therefore has led to the development of alternate approach. Food supplemented with necessary nutrients like functional food is available in the market which can be consumed on the daily basis. Apart from nutritional value, functional food also consists of health-promoting components [7].

Dietary supplements as defined by World Health Organisation (WHO) consists of vitamins, minerals, herbs, and plant components (Fig. 1) which can be formulated into tablets, pills, capsules, or liquid and can be added to the normal diet but cannot be a substitute to food. Micronutrients like vitamin A, E, C, and B, iron, copper, phosphorous, manganese are the active ingredients of dietary supplements. Apart from these omega-3 fatty acids (eicosapentaenoic acid and docosahexaenoic acid), flavonoids (phytoestrogen), free radical quenching compounds like coenzyme Q10, other substances like carotenoids, lycopene, lutein, and zeaxanthin are imperative nutrient supplements as they possess antioxidant properties [8, 9]. Herbs and spices like oregano, cinnamon, cloves, garlic, ginger and lipoic acids from fruits and vegetables play vital role in maintaining the normal glucose level as its higher concentration may lead to reduced elasticity and increased stiffness in skin [8, 10]. Research has proven that the western diet can be a potential cause of acne due to the high glycemic load diet [8]. Amino acids like arginine, proline, and glutamate help to regulate the collagen production and damage caused due to UV exposure. Lipids are another major component of epidermal region consisting mainly of ceramide (vital lipid constituent), cholesterol, and fatty acids where ceramide toxic level due to high exposure to UV radiations leads to apoptosis and the subtoxic levels decrease apoptosis [11].

Nutrient Components and Skin Aging

Vitamins

Vitamins are the group of organic components which are required in minute quantities and cannot be synthesized by human beings except niacin and vitamin D and thus need to be taken

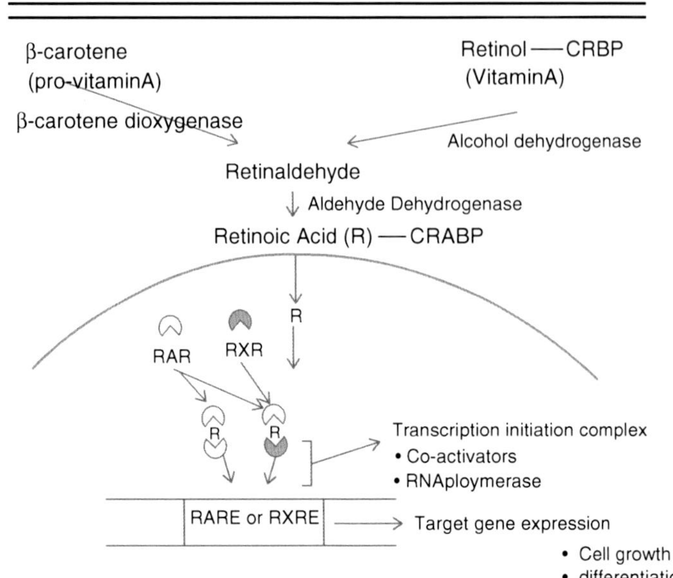

Fig. 2 Vitamin A signalling pathway. *RAR* retinoic acid receptor, *RXR* retinoid X receptor, *RARE* retinoic acid response element, *RXRE* retinoid X response element, *MMPs* matrix metalloproteinases, *CRABP* cellular retinoic acid binding protein, *CRBP* cellular retinol binding protein

externally. Vitamins are required for proper functioning and maintenance of healthy being and the body needs are fulfilled by consuming varied and balanced diet. The diseases originating due to deficiency of vitamins are well known and have led to the development of a huge vitamin industry. Vitamins A, C, D, and E have been implicated to play a vital role in maintaining the skin integrity.

Vitamin A, the unsaturated group of organic compounds, consists of two major derivatives: retinoid (from animals) and carotenoids (from plants); both are involved in maintaining various processes in humans like regulation of cell proliferation, apoptosis, and differentiation in cells including skin cells. Carotenoids are the natural antioxidants and help maintain the skin integrity mainly through scavenging ROS whereas retinoids bind to nuclear hormone receptor and regulate the transcription of target genes. Retinoids are 20-carbon molecules with cyclohexane ring, a side chain, and an alcohol group. Nuclear hormone receptors, retinoic acid receptors (RAR), and retinoid X receptors (RXR) form homo (RXR/RXR) or hetero (RAR/RXR) dimers after being activated by retinoids. These dimers further bind to retinoic acid response elements or retinoid X response elements (consensus DNA regions) in the promoter region of target gene, facilitating the assembly of transcription complex and ensue transcription of genes (Fig. 2). Retinoid receptors are mostly expressed in both epidermal keratinocytes and dermal fibroblasts, thus affecting their proliferation and differentiation. Retinoids also help in repairing the damage of skin caused due to UV radiation due to increased protein and extracellular matrix content and nuclear lamina stabilization. Tretinoin is a retinoid approved by Food and Drug Administration (FDA) for topical application for the treatment of wrinkles and preventing serious effects of UV rays. Deficiency of retinoid may lead to conditions like xerosis and follicular hyperkeratosis and delayed healing [12, 13]. Retinoic acid is used as a gold standard for the treatment of photoaging.

Vitamin C also known as ascorbic acid plays an important role to preserve skin integrity. This water-soluble vitamin acts as powerful antioxidant and mainly prevents the production of ROS induced by UV light exposure. There are two types of UV lights namely UVA (in range 320–400 nm) and UVB (in range 290–320 nm). UVA can penetrate deep into the skin and therefore is mainly responsible for the production of ROS and can modify DNA. UVB has limited

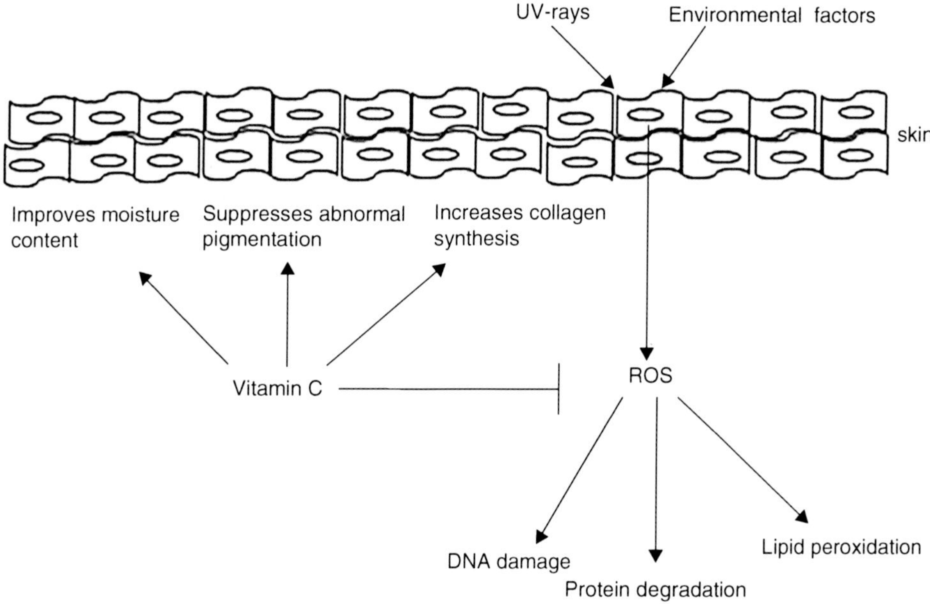

Fig. 3 Vitamin C and its role against UV and environmental factor induced skin damage

penetration and can act only on epidermal cells thus damaging keratinocytes and melanocytes. Excessive UV irradiation exposure may lead to degradation of collagen and elastin content resulting in wrinkles, coarse texture and pigmentation. Vitamin C mainly helps in the stimulation of collagen synthesis by acting as a cofactor during the hydroxylation of the amino acids proline and lysine. It also helps in wound healing, improving moisture content thus skin hydration (Fig. 3) [14, 15].

Vitamin D, synthesised by skin or taken in diet, is important for preventing the problems related to skin aging [16]. The active form of vitamin D, 1,25-dihydroxyvitamin D_3 (1,25$(OH)_2$D), is not directly synthesized in the body but follows a series of enzymatic reactions which involves the photochemical cutaneous synthesis of vitamin D_3. Vitamin D_3 (cholecalciferol) is synthesized from 7-dehydrocholesterol in the skin due to the action of UV light. The active form of vitamin D is generated by its first conversion into 25-hydroxyvitamin D_3 (25OHD) by the enzyme 25-hydroxylase in the liver and then to the 1,25 $(OH)_2$D or calcitriol by enzyme 1-α-hydroxylase present in the kidney. Subsequently this active form is carried into circulation by binding to the vitamin D-binding protein (DBP). 1,25 $(OH)_2$ D binds to Vitamin D receptors (VDR) besides retinoid X receptor (RXR) which regulates calcium and phosphate homeostasis, immune system, cell proliferation and induce differentiation (Fig. 4). Vitamin D has also shown to upregulate the level of cathelicidin antimicrobial peptide to protect against bacterial infection, modulate angiogenesis, and promote wound healing. Aging may affect the overall production of vitamin D owed to decrease in VDR, reduced renal production of 1, 25 $(OH)_2$ D, and Vitamin D syntheses in skin [16, 17]. It has been shown to protect the keratinocytes against the hazardous effect of UV rays, suppress apoptosis, and prevent the DNA damage and facilitate repair [18]. Moreover, vitamin D has been implicated to protect the skin against aging by inhibiting UV-B-mediated cleavage of Poly (ADP-Ribose)-Polymerase, a key DNA repair enzyme, and inducing the synthesis of methallothionein, an antioxidant [19]. Depletion of vitamin D can also be a marker of oxidative stress induced by UV rays and environmental factors.

The lipophilic vitamin E which consists of tocopherols and tocotrienols protects the body

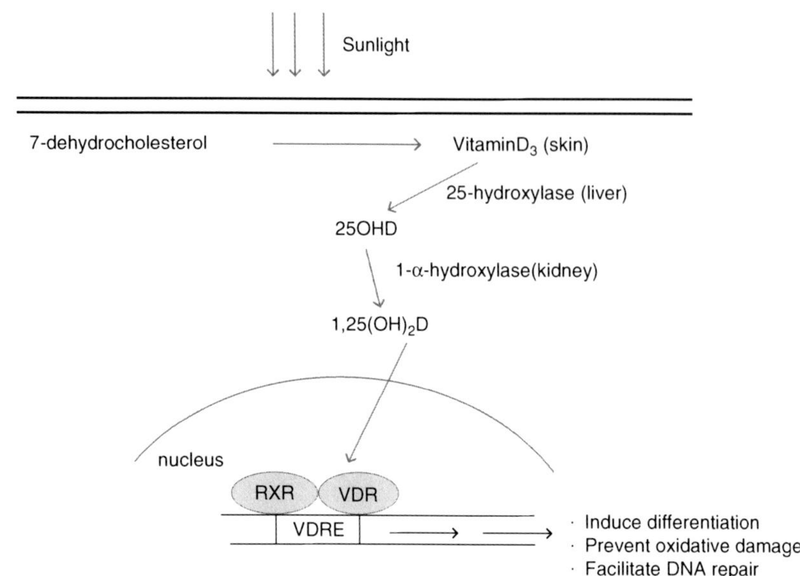

Fig. 4 Vitamin D signalling pathway. *VDR* vitamin D receptor, *25OHD* 25-hydroxyvitamin D_3, *1,25 (OH)$_2$D* 1,25-hydroxyvitamin D_3

against oxidative stress caused by various environmental factors and UV exposure [7]. Vitamin E deficiency may lead to keratosis, premature skin aging, and delayed wound healing. Vitamin E has been identified as crucial antioxidant which reinforces collagen synthesis, reduces MMPs concentration, and also plays an important role in apoptosis and modulating immune response [20]. The isomer of vitamin E tocotrienol was able to effectively prevent damage to human skin fibroblasts due to oxidative stress by upregulating collagen [21]. The supplementary drink consisting of soy isoflavons, lycopene, vitamin C, vitamin E with fish oil capsule exhibited wrinkle reduction in postmenopausal women through increase in deposition of collagen fibers in the dermal region [22].

Minerals

These are the group of substances occurring naturally like zinc, copper, selenium which play an important role in maintaining skin health. Zinc is one of the important cofactors for various metalloenzymes that protect skin by absorbing UV radiation [23]. Copper is crucial in maintaining body functions like building strong tissue, controlling blood volume, and producing energy in cells. It is important for maintaining skin elasticity and pigmentation as it acts as a stimulant for collagen maturation and melanin synthesis. Selenium is a trace mineral which protects keratinocytes and melanocytes from oxidative stress, induced by UVB radiation, by stimulating the activity of antioxidant enzyme like glutathione peroxidase and thioredoxin reductase [24]. Their deficiency may lead to problems like epidermolysis bullosa in case of zinc, steely hair syndrome for copper, and recessive dystrophic epidermolysis bullosa for selenium [25]. These minerals can be obtained from various sources like whole-grain cereals, seafood, garlic, and eggs, oysters, lean meat, and poultry.

Amino Acids

Amino acid is the building block of protein and plays a major role in protein metabolism. Many studies indicate the role of various amino acids like arginine, proline, ornithine, glutamine, or a mixture of amino acids in improving the quality of skin [26]. Proline and its precursors like glutamate and pyrroline-5-carboxylate stimulate type1 procollagen expression and collagen biosynthesis, respectively, in fibroblast cells [27]. Arginine [28], ornithine [29], and amino acid mixture [30] aid in wound healing and collagen deposition. L-arginine, a precursor for synthesis of urea, polyamines, proline, glutamate, creatine, and agmatine, was shown to have antiaging effect in a pilot study conducted in 2010 on 21 subjects of age-group 41–75 suffering from various health issues [31]. A study demonstrated that the mixture of amino acids such as branched-chain amino acid (BCAA) in combination with arginine and glutamine, BCAA + glutamine and BCAA + proline resulted in increased fraction of collagen whereas these components when given in isolation did not improve the synthesis rate of skin tropocollagen [26].

Reflex cutaneous vasoconstriction, an easy response to whole body cold exposure, generally attenuated in older adults due to absence of noradrenaline, a synthetic neurotransmitter, can be overcome by the supplementation of tyrosine or tetrahyrdrobioprotein (BH4) [32]. L-arginine and ascorbate supplementation have also shown improved attenuated reflex cutaneous vasodilation in aged human skin [33, 34]. In yet another study the dimethylaminoethanol (DMAE), a vitamin B choline and precursor of acetylcholine, in combination with amino acid increased the dermal and epidermal thickness, and upregulated collagen type I, II, and matrix metalloproteinase MMP-1 expression in D-galactose-induced aging skin in rats [35].

Phytochemicals

Phytochemicals are grouped under different categories: flavonoids, terpenoids, alkaloids which display certain properties including antioxidant, antibacterial, antifungal, and antiaging. The phytochemicals may protect skin as anitioxidants, scavenge free radicals, and prevent transdermal water loss, therefore protecting skin from wrinkles and leading to a glowing and healthy skin [36]. Dietary source of these phytochemicals can be from onions consisting of flavonols; cocoa consisting of catechin; grape seeds consisting of proanthocyanidins; tea, apples, and red wine consisting of flavonols and catechins; citrus fruits consisting of flavanones; berries and cherries consisting of anthocyanidins; and soy consisting of isoflavons [37]. Isoflavonoids like equol produce their antiaging effect by increasing the collagen and elastin synthesis and decrease in metalloproteinase gene expression [38].

Ellagic acid and 4-*O*-xyloside of ellagic acid, a phytochemical from *Platycarya strobilacea,* reduce expression of matrix metalloproteinase-1 (MMP-1), enhance type 1 collagen synthesis, and possess free-radical scavenging property and elastase inhibitory activity [39]. Resveratrol are polyphenols found in grapes, peanuts, pistachios, blueberries, cranberries and have been shown to prevent oxidative stress in human primary keratinocytes by increasing AMP-activated protein kinases and Forkhead box O3. This pathway regulates the senescence and proliferation ability of the cells [40].

Curcumin also acts as a strong antioxidant by inhibiting the ROS formation and lipid peroxidation and is one of the best known antiaging supplements [41]. Catechins contained in the green tea are also powerful antioxidants and have shown to protect fibroblasts against oxidative stress-induced death probably by downregulating MAP kinase pathway and inducing caspase 3, required for apoptosis [42]. Lycopene, a carotenoid from *Lycopersicon esculentum* (tomatoes), is another powerful antioxidant [43]. Some other naturally occurring compounds associated with inhibiting the early signs of aging are listed in Table 1.

Quercetin, a flavonoid found in fruits and green tea, possesses antioxidant properties that promote survival of primary human fibroblasts. It improves the proteasomal degradation activity and promotes the efficient removal of normal and degraded proteins [55]. Dietary intake of soy isoflavone aglycone has been shown to significantly improve the fine wrinkles [56] in a study conducted on middle-aged women ($n = 26$) without any adverse symptoms. Galangin flavonoid obtained from *Alpinia officinarum* and *Helichrysum aureonitens* was found to work against UVB-induced oxidative harm to human keratinocytes [57].

Probiotics

Probiotics have found usage in maintaining the beneficial microbiota of intestine. It has been

Table 1 List of various naturally occurring compounds from different plant sources associated with the inhibition of skin aging

Compound	Source	Function	References
Lutein	Fruits and green leafy vegetables	Antioxidant, inhibition of MMPs	[44]
Polypodium leucotomos	Tropical Fern plant	Inhibit proliferation and expression of MMPs	[45]
Nordihydroguaiaretic acid	*Larrea tridentata*	Prevents UV induced skin damage by inhibiting UV-B induced c-fos and AP-1 trans activation	[46]
Xanthohumol	*Humulus lupulus*	Inhibits MMPs and elastase activities, increased expression of type I, III and V collagen, fibrillin-2	[47]
Epigallactocatechin-3-gallate	Green white and black tea and in some amount in apples	Strong antioxidant protects skin from UV damage by reducing lipid peroxidation	[48]
Safranal and Crocin	*Crocus sativus*	Antioxidant, anti-inflammatory, wound healing activities	[49]
Ginsensoside Rb1	*Panax quinquefolius*	Increases antioxidant production and collagen synthesis, inhibits MMPs expression	[50]
Genistein	Soybeans	Decreases transforming growth factor β1, tissue trans glutaminase 2 and vascular endothelial growth factor (VEGF)	[51]
Carnosic acid	Rosemarry (*Rosmarinus offinalis L.*)	Enhances nerve growth factor, decrease in MMP-1 mRNA levels	[52]
Aloesin	Aloe plant	Inhibit *Clostridium histolyticum* collagenase reversibly and non-competitively. Both aloe gel and aloin are also effective inhibitors of stimulated granulocyte MMPs	[53]
Curcuma longa	Turmeric	Inhibit expression and activity of MMP-9, ERK activation and AP-1 DNA binding activity in UV-induced skin inflammation	[54]

postulated that probiotics can modulate local and systemic immune system and can also help to preserve skin homeostasis. The probiotic *Lactobacillus johnsonii* showed protective effect on UV-induced damage to skin in a clinical trial on 54 subjects. The possible mechanism could be the absorption of dietary nutrients that uphold the skin homeostasis, synthesize the structural and functional components of the skin, boost the immune system, and help fight the inflammatory response [58]. In yet another clinical study (110 middle-aged women) *Lactobacillus plantarum* HY7714 strain was found useful in increasing skin hydration, reduction in transdermal water loss and wrinkle depth, and improved skin elasticity by 13.17 % after 4 weeks and by 21.73 % after 12 weeks. *L. plantarum* HY7714 was also shown to inhibit the phosphorylation of Jun N-terminal kinase, type of mitogen-activated protein (MAP) kinase pathway and thus expression of c-Jun [59, 60]. Transcription factor c-Jun along with Fos forms AP-1 which is the major stimulatory factor for transcription of MMP, involved in the degradation of collagen, contributing to skin aging.

Clinical Trials for Dietary Supplements Related to Skin Aging

The link between dietary intake and its impact on skin aging has been assessed through various observational and experimental studies and it has been shown that there is a positive correlation between various supplements and skin aging [61].

Cosgrove et al. studied the effect of vitamin C and linoleic acid intake on skin-aging appearance among middle-aged American women (n = 4025). Independent of age, race, sunlight exposure, and body mass index, vitamin C was associated with reduced chance of wrinkled appearance and dryness. Linoleic acid was also associated with lower possibility of senile dryness and skin atrophy [62]. Dietary supplements containing combination of probiotic *Lactobacillus johnsonii* and specific doses of carotenoids were shown to prevent UV-induced skin damage (n = 139). The combination reduced dermal inflammatory cells as determined by histology and immunohistochemistry. The study indicates the long-term favorable effect of supplement intake on skin photoaging [63].

Green tea known to have significant antioxidative and anti-inflammatory effect was studied for its effect on photoaging skin in women (n = 40). The intake of green tea and application of green tea cream did not elicit any difference in clinical grading; however, histological grading of skin biopsies showed improved elasticity in the skin indicating that long-term consumption might be beneficial [64]. The effect of Skin Health Experimental Product supplement food of mixture containing ascorbic acid, ω-3 fatty acids, mixed carotenoids, zinc rice chelate, luetin, pyridoxine, pantothenate, niacin, and coenzyme Q10, was studied on skin health of 76 subjects (61 women and 15 men). The skin hydration, antioxidant levels, texture was assessed experimentally and showed considerable decrease in fine lines, improved skin texture, and carotenoid levels in selected areas indicating the positive effect on skin health [65].

The result of oral intake of a novel formulation (Imedeen Prime Renewal™) that consists of soy extract, fish protein polysaccharides, extracts from white tea, grape seed and tomato, vitamins C and E, as well as zinc and chamomile extract, was analyzed on postmenopausal women skin health. Imedeen Prime Renewal™ elicited significant improvement in overall appearance with decreased wrinkles and improvement in firmness of the skin [66].

Oral dietary supplements including antioxidants, minerals, and glycosaminoglycans were analyzed for efficacy on cutaneous aging on women aged 35–60 years (n = 60). The surface evaluation of skin showed 21.2 % improvement in fine wrinkles and depth of skin roughness in the treatment group, whereas the placebo group indicated the benefit in 1.7 %. This difference was found to be statistically significant ($P < 0.001$). No change in skin color was observed in the treatment group [67].

Collagen synthesis in the skin has been linked to the reduction in wrinkles on the skin. Thus the effect of Red ginseng root containing various ginsenosides having antioxidant and immunostimulatory properties exhibited reduction in facial wrinkles and it was linked to increased type I procollagen synthesis, reduction in matrix metalloproteinase (MMP)-9 gene expression, and increase in length of fibrillin-1 fibers. On the other hand the extract did not have any impact on facial elasticity, pigmentation, and thickness of epidermis [68].

The effect of squalene was also studied on type I procollagen synthesis in 40 female subjects aged more than 50. The decrease in facial wrinkles was linked to increased type I procollagen mRNA levels and reduction in matrix metalloproteinase 1 expression. UV-induced apoptosis in keratinocytic and thymine dimer formation was also found to be reduced. However the side effect in terms of loose stool was observed [69].

Overall studies indicate toward the positive link between dietary supplements and its effect on skin aging in terms of wrinkles, texture, and thickness of epidermal layer. Certain limitations need to be considered. Most of the clinical studies conducted are of short duration and also have low participant burden. These studies have been restricted to only females thus reducing the application to wider populations. The reports related to the side effects are very limited thus making it difficult to monitor the toxicity.

Overall the beneficial effects of taking the supplements supersede the side effects. However, most of the studies have been supported by the commercial players involved in manufacture and marketing of the nutraceuticals. There is an urgent need to conduct independent studies covering the wider population of both the sexes to draw conclusions.

Mechanism of Action of Antiaging Dietary Supplements

The process of aging involves the loss of regulation of various genes associated with different cellular mechanisms that help maintain the healthy human being. These may include the genes related to antioxidant status, cellular detoxification, inflammatory pathways, and the accumulation of damaging by-product [70]. Nuclear factor erythroid 2-related factor 2 is a transcriptional factor which is involved in the induction and expression of antioxidant response element regulated genes like gluthathione and glutathione S-transferase 1. Glutathione occurs in two forms namely the reduced sulfhydryl (GSH) and oxidized disulfide gluthathione (GSSG). Glutathione S-transferase 1, a detoxification enzyme, is involved in the detoxification of stressors and can irreversibly bind to GSH [71]. Vitagenes, another category of genes including heme oxygenase 1, a rate-limiting enzyme, is also impaired during aging. Apart from these genes involved in the regulation are glutamate-cystein ligase, a rate-limiting enzyme of GSH synthesis, Glutathione reductase, a central enzyme in cellular antioxidant system which maintains GSH/GSSG ratio, glutathione peroxidase that catalytically removes hydrogen peroxide, and also transcriptional factor NF-κB [70].

The mice exposed to either acute or chronic UVB irradiation were given dietary grape seed proanthocyanidins (0.2–0.5 %, w/w) which sustained antioxidant defense system by maintaining the levels of glutathione peroxidase, catalase, and glutathione. Thus, they prevented photo-oxidative damage by downregulating UVB-induced hydrogen peroxide, lipid peroxidation in mouse skin [72]. The oral administration of green tea in the drinking water of mice has also been shown to inhibit UVB radiation-induced depletion of antioxidant defense enzymes, such as catalase, glutathione peroxidase, superoxide dismutase, and glutathione [73]. The green tea also reduced the levels of biomarkers of cellular proliferation including proliferating cell nuclear antigen and cyclin D1.

Green tea polyphenols, resveratrol, grape seed proanthocyanidins, and silymarin are polyphenols which have shown to reduce UVB-induced cyclooxygenase-2 expression and a subsequent increase in the production of prostaglandin metabolites in the skin which are the characteristic response of keratinocytes to acute or chronic exposure to UVB radiation [37, 74]. Silymarin has also been shown to inhibit the expression of ornithine decarboxylase, an enzyme required for polyamine biosynthesis, which has a role in tumor promotion in UVB-exposed skin [37].

Conclusion

Skin maintains homeostasis between external environment and internal tissues and provides a defense system to whole body from microorganisms, ultraviolet radiation, any toxic agents, or mechanical insults. It consists of two major layers: epidermis and dermis. Epidermis is the outer layer consisting mainly of keratinocytes and dermis is made up of fibroblast which produces extracellular matrix protein like collagen including type I and type III and its functional integrity must be maintained to live a healthy life. Term aging is a biological process which affects the quality of skin and is reflected by the signs like dullness, wrinkled skin, patches, dryness, increased pigmentation, loss of elasticity and firmness. Aging gets accelerated by genetic and molecular changes, UV exposure, and physiological stress. Dietary supplements have long been implicated in improving skin health. Numerous studies indicate several micronutrients, minerals, phytochemicals, and amino acids, alone and in combination, help in delaying skin aging. Vitamins A, C, D, and E have been shown to prevent the UV damage to skin and increase the levels of collagen. Vitamin A includes carotenoids and retinoids; carotenoids are the natural antioxidant and help maintain the skin integrity mainly through scavenging ROS whereas retinoids regulate the cellular proliferation, differentiation and repair. Vitamin C is essential for collagen synthesis, scavenges free radicals, and preserves firmness of skin. Vitamin D controls skin homeostasis and prevents genomic instability, DNA damage, and UV-B-mediated apoptosis. Studies based on the clinical trials have shown that the use of dietary supplements maintain the cell integrity by regulating the cellular mechanism encompassing antioxidants, cellular detoxification, inflammation, and the accumulation of damaging by-products to control skin aging. There has been ample evidence that diet taken by an individual can play an important role in maintaining the health of a skin by controlling age-related diseases. Combinatorial studies incorporating various vitamins, phytochemicals as nutraceuticals have shown great potential in mitigating aging-associated changes by targeting oxidative damage, modulating immune system, improving collagen, and promoting differentiation of keratinocytes. The various constraints encountered in designing and conducting of the nutritional studies include human rights, patient compliance, time, and cost. Moreover one size doesn't fit all and the individual metabolic differences could result in a very varied response and may require personalized nutrition. Further studies are required to cover the wider population and understand the biochemical and molecular changes elicited by the combinatorial nutraceuticals.

References

1. Farage MA, et al. Characteristics of the aging skin. Adv Wound Care Prog. 2012;2(1):5–10. doi:10.1089/wound.2011.0356.
2. Ivi NP. Skin aging. Acta Dermatovenerol Alp Panonica Adriat. 2008;17(2):47–53.
3. Rinnerthaler M, et al. Oxidative stress in aging human skin. Biomolecules Prog. 2015;5:545–89. doi:10.3390/biom5020545.
4. Dunn JH, et al. Psychological stress and skin aging: a review of possible mechanisms and potential therapies. Dermatol Online J. 2013;19(6):1.
5. Thornton MJ. Estrogen and aging skin. Dermato-Endocrinology. 2013;5(2):264–70.
6. Skoczyńska A, et al. New look at the role of progerin in skin aging. Przeglad Menopauzalny. 2015;14(1):53–8. doi:10.5114/pm.2015.49532.
7. Szyszkowska B, et al. The influence of selected ingredients of dietary supplements on skin condition. Postep Dermatol Alergol. 2014;31(3):174–81. doi:10.5114/pdia.2014.40919.
8. Katta R, Desai SP. The role of dietary intervention in skin disease. J Clin Aesth Dermatol. 2014;7(7):46–51.
9. Danby FW. Nutrition and aging skin: sugar and glycation. Clin Dermatol. 2010;28(4):409–11.
10. Spravchikov N, et al. Glucose effects on skin keratinocytes. Diabetics. 2001;50:1627–35.
11. Park K. Role of micronutrients in skin health and function. Biomol Ther. 2015;23(3):207–17.
12. Mukherjee S, et al. Retinoids in the treatment of skin aging: an overview of clinical efficacy and safety. Clin Interv Aging. 2006;1(4):327–48.
13. Lee DD, et al. Retinoid-responsive transcriptional changes in epidermal keratinocytes. J Cell Physiol. 2009;220(2):427–39. doi:10.1002/jcp.21784.
14. Godic A, et al. The role of antioxidants in skin cancer prevention and treatment. Oxidative Med Cell Longev. 2014;2014:6. doi:10.1155/2014/860479.
15. Pandel R, et al. Skin photo aging and the role of antioxidants in its prevention. Int Sch Res Not Dermatol. 2013;2013:11. Article ID 930164. doi:10.1155/2013/930164.
16. Gallagher JC. Vitamin D and aging. Endocrinol Metab Clin North Am. 2013;42(2):319–32. doi:10.1016/j.ecl.2013.02.004.
17. Gombart AF, et al. Human cathelicidin antimicrobial peptide (CAMP) geneis a direct target of the vitamin D receptor and is strongly up-regulated in myeloid cells by 1, 25-dihydroxyvitamin D3. Fed Am Soc Exp Biol. 2005;19:1067–77. doi:10.1096/fj.04-3284com.
18. Trémezaygues L, et al. 1,25-dihydroxyvitamin D3 protects human keratinocytes against UV-B-induced damage. Dermato-Endocrinologyi. 2009;1(4):239–45.
19. Reichrath J. The role of vitamin D in skin aging. Dermato-Endocrinology. 2012;4(3):241–4.
20. Ricciarelli R, et al. Age-dependent increase of collagenase expression can be reduced by alpha-tocopherol via protein kinase C inhibition. Free Radic Biol Med. 1999;27(7–8):729–37. doi:10.1016/S0891-5849(99)00007-6.
21. Makpol F, et al. Modulation of collagen synthesis and its gene expression in human skin fibroblasts by tocotrienol-rich fraction. Arch Med Sci. 2011;7(5):889–95. doi:10.5114/aoms.2011.25567.
22. Jenkins G, et al. Wrinkle reduction in post-menopausal women consuming a novel oral supplement: a double-blind placebo-controlled randomized study. Int J Cosmet Sci. 2014;36:22–31. doi:10.1111/ics.12087.
23. Mitchnick MA, et al. Microfine zinc oxide (Z-cote) as a photostable UVA/UVB sunblock agent. J Am Acad Dermatol. 1999;40(1):85–90.
24. Rafferty TS, et al. Differential expression of selenoproteins by human skin cells and protection by selenium from UVB-radiation-induced cell death. Biochemical J. 1998;332:231–6.
25. Pickart L, et al. The human tripeptide GHK-Cu in prevention of oxidative stress and degenerative

conditions of aging: implications for cognitive health. Oxid Med Cell Longev. 2012;2012:8. Article ID 324832, 8 p. doi:10.1155/2012/324832.

26. Murakami H, et al. Importance of amino acid composition to improve skin collagen protein synthesis rates in UV-irradiated mice. Amino Acids. 2012;42:2481–9. doi:10.1007/s00726-011-1059-z.
27. Curi R, et al. Molecular mechanisms of glutamine action. J Cell Physiol. 2005;204:392–401.
28. Shi HP, et al. Supplemental L-arginine enhances wound healing in diabetic rats. Wound Repair Regen. 2003;11(3):198–203.
29. Shi HP, et al. Effect of supplemental ornithine on wound healing. J Surg Res. 2002;106(2):299–302.
30. Badiu DL, et al. Amino acids from mytilus galloprovincialis (L.) and rapana venosa molluscs accelerate skin wounds healing via enhancement of dermal and epidermal neoformation. Protein J. 2010;29:81–92. doi:10.1007/s10930-009-9225-9.
31. Gad MZ. Anti-aging effects of L-arginine. J Adv Res. 2010;1:169–77. doi:10.1016/j.jare.2010.05.001.
32. Lang JA. Localized tyrosine or tetrahydrobiopterin supplementation corrects the age-related decline in cutaneous vasoconstriction. J Physiol. 2010;588 (8):1361–8. doi:10.1113/jphysiol.2009.185694.
33. Holowatz LA, et al. L-arginine supplementation or arginase inhibition augments reflex cutaneous vasodilatation in aged human skin. J Physiol. 2006;574 (2):573–81. doi:10.1152/ajpheart.00648.2006.
34. Holowatz LA, Thompson CS, Kenney WL. Acute ascorbate supplementation alone or combined with arginase inhibition augments reflex cutaneous vasodilation in aged human skin. Am J Physiol Heart Circ Physiol. 2006;291:H2965–70.
35. Liu S, et al. Effects of dimethylaminoethanol and compound amino acid on D-galactose induced skin aging model of rat. Sci World J. 2014;2014;7. Article ID 507351. doi:10.1155/2014/507351.
36. Mukherjee PK, et al. Bioactive compounds from natural resources against skin aging. Phytomedicine. 2011;19:64–73. doi:10.1016/j.phymed.2011.10.003.
37. Nichols JA, Katiyar SK. Skin photoprotection by natural polyphenols: anti-inflammatory, anti-oxidant and DNA repair mechanisms. Arch Dermatol Res. 2010;302(2):71. doi:10.1007/s00403-009-1001-3.
38. Gopaul R, et al. Biochemical investigation and gene analysis of equol: a plant and soy derived isoflavonoid with antiaging and antioxidant properties with potential human skin applications. Biofactors. 2012;38 (1):44–52. doi:10.1002/biof.191.
39. Kim JH, et al. Anti-wrinkle activity of *Platycarya strobilacea* extract and its application as a cosmeceutical ingredient. J Cosmet Sci. 2010;61:211–23.
40. Ido Y, et al. Resveratrol prevents oxidative stress-induced senescence and proliferative dysfunction by activating the AMPK-FOXO3 cascade in cultured primary human Kerstinocytes. PLoS One. 2015;10 (2):1–18. doi:10.1371/journal.pone.011534.
41. Bala K, et al. Neuroprotective and anti-aging effects of curcumin in aged rat brain regions. Biogerontology. 2006;7:81–9. doi:10.1007/s10522-006-6495-x.
42. Tanigawa T, et al. (+)-Catechin protects dermal fibroblasts against oxidative stress-induced apoptosis. BMC Complement Altern Med. 2014;14:133. doi:10.1186/1472-6882-14-133.
43. Anunciato TP, et al. Carotenoids and polyphenols in nutricosmetics, nutraceuticals, and cosmeceuticals. J Cosmet Dermatol. 2012;11(1):51–4.
44. Philips N, et al. Regulation of the extracellular matrix remodeling by lutein in dermal Wbroblasts, melanoma cells, and ultraviolet radiation exposed fibroblasts. Arch Dermatol Res. 2007;299:373–9. doi:10.1007/s00403-007-0779-0.
45. Philips N, et al. Beneficial regulation of matrixmetalloproteinases and their inhibitors, Wbrillar collagens and transforming growth factor by *Polypodium leucotomos*, directly or in dermal Wbroblasts, ultraviolet radiated Wbroblasts, and melanoma cells. Arch Dermatol Res. 2009;301:487–95. doi:10.1007/s00403-009-0950-x.
46. Philips N, et al. Beneficial regulation of matrix metalloproteinases for skin health. Enzyme Res. 2011;2011;4. Article ID 427285. doi:10.4061/2011/427285.
47. Philips N, et al. Direct inhibition of elastase and matrixmetalloproteinases and stimulation of biosynthesis of fibrillar collagens, elastin, and fibrillins by xanthohumol. J Cosmet Sci. 2010;61 (2):125–32.
48. Huang CC, et al. Protective effects of (_)-epicatechin-3-gallate on UVA-induced damage in HaCaT keratinocytes. Arch Dermatol Res. 2005;269:473–81.
49. Assimopoulou AN. Radical scavenging activity of *Crocus sativus* L. extract and its bioactive constituents. Phytother Res. 2005;19:997–1000. doi:10.1002/ptr.1749.
50. Kimura Y, Sumiyoshi M, Sakanaka M. Effects of ginsenoside Rb1 on skin changes. J Biomed Biotechnol. 2012;2012:11. Article ID 946242. doi:10.1155/2012/946242.
51. Polito F, et al. Genistein aglycone, a soy-derived isoflavone, improves skin changes induced by ovariectomy in rats. Br J Pharmacol. 2012;165:994–1005. doi:10.1111/j.1476-5381.2011.01619.x.
52. Elmhdwi MF, Attitalla IH. Antioxidant and free radical scavenging activity of essential oil extracted from *Rosmarinus officinalis*. J Biol Sci Opin. 2015;3 (5):223–9. doi:10.7897/2321-6328.03549.
53. Jones K, et al. Modulation of melanogenesis by aloesin: a competitive inhibitor of tyrosinase. Pigment Cell Res. 2002;15(5):335–40. doi:10.1034/j.1600-0749.2002.02014.x.
54. Mamgain RK. Acne vulgaris and its treatment by indigenous drugs SK-34 (Purim) and SK-235 (Clarina). Antiseptic. 2000;97(3):76–8.

55. Chondrogianni N, et al. Anti-aging and rejuvenating effects of quercetin. Exp Gerontol. 2010;45:763–71. doi:10.1016/j.exger.2010.07.001. Epub 7 July 2010.
56. Izumi T, et al. Oral intake of Soy Isoflavone Aglycone improves the aged skin of adult women. J Nutr Sci Vitaminol. 2007;53:57–62.
57. Hewage SRKM, et al. Galangin (3, 5, 7-trihydroxyflavone) shields human keratinocytes from ultraviolet B-induced oxidative stress. Biomol Ther. 2015;23(2):165–73.
58. Guéniche A, et al. Probiotics for photoprotection. Dermato-Endocrinology. 2009;1(5):275–9.
59. Lee DE, et al. Clinical evidence of effects 1 of *Lactobacillus plantarum* HY7714 on skin aging: a randomized, double blind, placebo-controlled study. J Microbiol Biotechnol. 2015;25(12):2160–8. doi:10.4014/jmb.1509.09021.
60. Kim HM, et al. Oral administration of *Lactobacillus plantarum* HY7714 protects hairless mouse against ultraviolet B-induced photo aging. J Microbiol Biotechnol. 2014;24(11):1583–91. doi:10.4014/jmb.1406.06038.
61. Pezdirc K, et al. Can dietary intake influence perception of and measured appearance? A systematic review. Nutr Res. 2015;35(3):175–97. doi:10.1016/j.nutres.2014.12.002.
62. Cosgrove MC, et al. Dietary nutrient intakes and skin-aging appearance among middle aged American women. Am J Clin Nutr. 2007;86(4):1225–31.
63. Bouilly-Gauthier D, et al. Clinical evidence of benefits of a diatery supplement containing probiotics and carotenoids on ultraviolet- induced skin damage. Br J Dermatol. 2010;163(3):536–43. doi:10.1111/j.1365-2133.2010.09888.x.
64. Chiu AE, et al. Double-blinded, placebo-controlled trial of green tea extracts in the clinical and histologic appearance of photo aging skin. Dermatol Surg. 2005;31:855–60.
65. Dayan SH, et al. A phase 2, double-blind, randomized, placebo-controlled trial of a novel nutritional supplement product to promote healthy skin. J Drugs Dermatol. 2011;10(10):1106–14.
66. Skovgaard GR, et al. Effect of a novel dietary supplement on skin aging in post-menopausal women. Eur J Clin Nutr. 2006;60(10):1201–6.
67. Udompataikul M, et al. An oral nutraceuticals containing antioxidant, minerals and glycosaminoglycans improves skin roughness and fine wrinkles. Int J Cosmet Sci. 2009;31(6):427–35.
68. Cho S, et al. Red ginseng root extract mixed with Torilus fructus and Corni fructus improves wrinkles and increase type I procollagen synthesis in human skin: a randomized, double-blind, placebo-controlled study. J Med Food. 2009;12(6):1252–9. doi:10.1089/jmf.2008.1390.
69. Cho S, et al. High dose squalene ingestion increases type I procollagen and decreases ultraviolet induced DNA damage in human skin in vivo but is associated with transient adverse effects. Clin Exp Dermatol. 2009;34(4):500–8. doi:10.1111/j.1365-2230.2008.03133.x.
70. Mastaloudis A, Wood SM. Age-related changes in cellular protection, purification, and inflammation-related gene expression: role of dietary phytonutrient. Ann N Y Acad Sci. 2012;1259:112–20. doi:10.1111/j.1749-6632.2012.06610.x.
71. McElwee JJ, et al. Evolutionary conservation of regulated longevity assurance mechanisms. Genome Biol. 2007;8(7):R132. doi:10.1186/gb-2007-8-7-r132.
72. Sharma SD, et al. Dietary grape seed proanthocyanidins inhibit UVB-induced oxidative stress and activation of mitogen-activated protein kinases and nuclear factor-KB signaling in in vivo SKH-1 hairless mice. Mol Cancer Ther. 2007;6(3):995–1005.
73. Vayalil PK, et al. Treatment of green tea polyphenols in hydrophilic cream prevents UVB-induced oxidation of lipids and proteins, depletion of antioxidant enzymes and phosphorylation of MAPK proteins in SKH-1 hairless mouse skin. Carcinogenesis. 2003;24(5):927–36. doi:10.1093/carcin/bgg025.
74. Meeran SM, et al. Inhibition of UVB-induced skin tumor development by drinking green tea polyphenols is mediated through DNA repair and subsequent inhibition of inflammation. J Investig Dermatol. 2009;129(5):1258–70. doi:10.1038/jid.2008.354.

Part II

Molecular Biology and Metabolism

Alterations of Energy Metabolism in Cutaneous Aging

47

Thomas Blatt, Horst Wenck, and Klaus-Peter Wittern

Contents

T. Blatt (✉) • H. Wenck • K.-P. Wittern
The Beiersdorf Research Center, Hamburg, Germany
e-mail: thomas.blatt@beiersdorf.com; horst.wenck@beiersdorf.com; klaus-peter.wittern@beiersdorf.com

M.A. Farage et al. (eds.), *Textbook of Aging Skin*,
DOI 10.1007/978-3-662-47398-6_29

Abstract

Energy metabolism plays an important role in cutaneous aging. Cellular energy levels deciline during intrinsic and extrinsic aging and consequently the capacity of the skin to encounter environmental stress declines with aging. More detail on this relationship is presented in this chapter.

Introduction

Aging is understood as the result of a complex interaction of biological processes that are caused by both environmental processes (extrinsic aging) and genetic processes (intrinsic aging). Research into the biology of aging has provided detailed insight into the molecular mechanisms of age-related changes in organs, tissues, and cells. Most information relating to intrinsic aging processes comes from tissues other than the skin. This is in part due to the fact that clinically manifest diseases such as type 2 diabetes or neurodegenerative disease are often correlated with aging of cells. In part it is also due to the fact that substantial amounts of primary cells and organelles for biochemical analyses can be more easily isolated from other organs such as the muscle, brain, or liver, as compared with skin. Nevertheless, intrinsic aging is based on general biological processes that apply more or less to all proliferating cells and terminally differentiated cells as well.

Therefore, general intrinsic aging processes seen in a liver cell, muscle cell, or neuron can be expected also to apply more or less to skin cells. In fact, most of the aging processes identified and studied with other cells could also be confirmed with keratinocytes or dermal fibroblasts, even though some downstream details may be different. Extrinsic aging processes have been intensively studied in the skin though. This applies especially to a process called photoaging, which is induced by the skin's most dominant stressor – UV light. In contrast to skin, UV light is an irrelevant stressor to other tissues. Researchers have developed a battery of slightly invasive or non-invasive biophysical measurement procedures to study UV-induced stress and aging-related damage in situ even in small skin samples. Furthermore, many in vitro methods are available to study photoaging based on cultured cells or three-dimensional cultured skin models. Besides UV light, there are many other extrinsic stressors, encompassing, for example, environmental chemicals, nutritional conditions, or even hormonal imbalances which may induce extrinsic aging of the skin and other organs as well.

This overview will focus on aspects of energy metabolism in cutaneous aging. These aspects are especially important since human skin tissue, being exposed to a plethora of endogenous and environmental stress factors, is highly dependent on energy supply in order to combat cellular deregulation and/or to repair damage. As detailed below, cellular energy levels decline during intrinsic and extrinsic aging as well, and consequently the capacity of the skin to counteract environmental stress declines with aging. Decreased compensation of environmental stress and insufficient repair, in turn, accelerate skin aging, which consequently leads to further decline of cellular energy levels in the skin. Breaking this feedback loop by sustaining cellular energy levels in the skin is thought to decelerate, stop, or even reverse intrinsic and extrinsic skin aging, with compounded interest over time.

Phenomenology of Energetic Factors Associated with Skin Aging

The energy demand of skin cells is supplied by two major primary sources – mitochondrial oxidative phosphorylation and glycolysis. In addition to these major primary sources, skin cells may also utilize a major secondary energy store for situations of acute high energy demand – the creatine/phosphocreatine system. As detailed below, all three major energy sources are affected by intrinsic and extrinsic skin aging and offer potential entry points for intervention strategies to decelerate the aging process.

Aging Effects on Mitochondrial Function

The mitochondria, as small oxidative power plants in the cells, play a pivotal role in energy supply. Beyond energy production, mitochondria can perform other pivotal cellular functions such as regulation of programmed cellular death (apoptosis). These organelles contain their own genetic material, mitochondrial DNA (mtDNA), which is maternally inherited. Although much smaller than the nuclear genome, mtDNA is equally important, as it has been shown to play a crucial role in aging, as discussed in detail in the section "Genetic Damage to Mitochondria" of this overview. This central organelle of energy metabolism and control of cell death is supposed to be a target for aging and a promoter of aging as well [1].

Within living cells, mitochondria are observed as small sausage-shaped organelles, longer snake-like tubules, branched reticula, extended filaments, and networks or clusters that are connected via intermitochondrial junctions. Mitochondrial morphology is regulated in many cultured eukaryotic cells by fusion and fission, and a tightly controlled balance between fission and fusion events is supposed to ensure normal mitochondrial ultrastructure as well as mitochondrial and cellular functions. Mitochondria of old endothelial cells show a significant and equal decrease of both fusion and fission activity [2], indicating that these processes are sensitive to aging and are likely to contribute to the accumulation of damaged mitochondria during aging [3]. Aging of cells is also associated with aberrations of mitochondrial morphology and ultrastructure. Typical changes of mitochondrial ultrastructure during aging, as can be seen by electron microscopy in cultured fibroblasts, are loss of branched mitochondria in old cells, enlargement of mitochondria, matrix vacuolization, shortened cristae, and loss of dense granules [4]. Furthermore, cystic blebs are evident in mitochondria of some cells with an apparent increase in old cells. These blebs appear to be due to the weakening of the inner membrane, allowing dilatation of the outer membrane which otherwise appears intact. Similar ultrastructural changes of mitochondria as seen in aged cells are also seen in cultivated skin fibroblasts of patients with point mutations in mitochondrial DNA (mtDNA) affecting the energy metabolism of the organelles. The changes encompass partially swollen mitochondria with unusual and sparse cristae, heterogeneity of cristae in size and shapes or their absence, as well as almost complete absence of branched mitochondria [5]. Furthermore, similar changes in mitochondrial ultrastructure as seen in aged fibroblasts are also seen in photoaged keratinocytes chronically exposed to low doses of UV-B irradiation [6]. Thus, ultrastructural changes of mitochondria in intrinsically aged cells are similar to those seen in mitochondria from skin cells damaged by intrinsic genetic defects or damaged by exogenous stressors leading to photoaging. Since morphological features typical of mitochondria from aged cells can also be induced in mitochondria from otherwise normal cultured primary skin fibroblasts by inhibition of energy metabolism with drugs targeting the respiratory chain [7], changes of the mitochondrial ultrastructure can be hypothesized to be a cause and consequence of altered mitochondrial energy metabolism as well.

The central function of the mitochondrial network in the cell is the production of adenosintriphosphate (ATP) by transfer of electrons from digested food to carrier molecules such as nicotinamide adenine dinucleotide (NAD^+) and flavin adenine dinucleotide (FAD^+), thus generating NADH and FADH, and subsequent delivery of the electrons to the respiratory oxidative phosphorylation generates mitochondrial ATP by means of five multiple subunit enzyme complexes (I through V) plus the adenine nucleotide translocator (ANT), all localized within the mitochondrial inner membrane. Complexes I–IV constitute the electron transport chain. Reduced NADH is oxidized by Complex I (NADH dehydrogenase), and succinate is oxidized by Complex II (succinate dehydrogenase); the electrons are transferred to ubiquinone (coenzyme Q_{10}) to yield ubiquinol. The electrons from ubiquinol are transferred to Complex III (ubiquinol/cytochrome c oxidoreductase), then to cytochrome c, then to Complex IV (cytochrome c oxidase), and finally to oxygen. The energy released is used to pump protons out of the mitochondrial inner membrane through Complexes I, III, and IV, and the resulting electrochemical gradient is exploited by Complex V (ATP synthase) to condense adenosindiphosphate (ADP) and inorganic phosphate to form ATP. Both ATP and ADP are exchanged across the mitochondrial inner membrane by ANT. The five protein complexes of the electron transport chain work as an integrated system, with mitochondrial DNA (mtDNA) encoding 13 of the proteins and nuclear DNA encoding approximately 60. The formation of these complexes is a complicated procedure based on the coordinated transport and assembly of components from two different genomes and compartments [8].

As an organism ages, either by extrinsic or intrinsic aging, there is a significant decline in mitochondrial function and cellular energy balance [9, 10]. This applies especially to mitochondrial membrane potential which is key to mitochondrial function [11]. Assessment methods to monitor the mitochondrial respiration rate and membrane potential, even on a single intact cell level, are discussed in the section "Energetic Effects of Creatine" of this overview. The decrease of mitochondrial function during aging has been described as a general feature in many in vitro systems. These descriptions encompass the loss of mitochondrial membrane potential of old and postmitotic human umbilical vein endothelial cells [2] or lower respiration rates of spleen lymphocytes isolated from old mice as compared with lymphocytes from young mice [12], just to mention a few. In fact, the general decline of mitochondrial respiratory functions with age has also been described in human studies, for example, in hepatocytes investigated in a study enrolling subjects of 31–76 years old, where a significant negative correlation between age and respiratory control and ADP/O ratios was observed [13]. The decline in skeletal muscle mitochondrial respiratory chain function has also been investigated in isolated intact skeletal muscle mitochondria in a study enrolling subjects aged 16–92 years. State 3 (activated) mitochondrial respiration rates showed a significant negative correlation between respiration rate and age. A similar trend was seen for respiratory enzyme activities assayed in muscle homogenate [14]. These findings demonstrate a substantial fall in mitochondrial function in aging muscle and liver cells and suggest that a fall in mitochondrial oxidative capacity and membrane potential in aging cells may be an important general contributor to the aging process.

Loss of mitochondrial membrane potential has also been reported in human dermal fibroblasts aged in vitro by serial passage [15]. Furthermore, a marked aging-related decline in efficiency of oxidative phosphorylation was observed in human skin fibroblasts isolated from a large group of subjects ranging in age between 20 weeks fetal and 103 years [16]. In the latter study, the analysis of endogenous respiration rate revealed a significant decrease in the age range from 40 to 90 years and a tendency to uncoupling in the samples from subjects above 60 years. These findings clearly pointed to a dramatic mitochondrial dysfunction, which would lead to a decrease in ATP synthesis rate in skin fibroblasts with increasing age. The impact of intrinsic aging on the mitochondrial oxidative capacity and mitochondrial membrane potential of skin cells is furthermore supported by a number of indirect studies discussed in this review, addressing the effects of aging on the generation of reactive oxygen species (ROS) in skin cells from young and old donors or the effect of energy enhancers. Besides intrinsic aging effects on the mitochondrial capacity of skin cells, a substantial decline of the mitochondrial membrane potential can be observed following UV irradiation of keratinocytes in vitro, which is the dominant stressor leading to photoaging of cells [17, 18]. A decline of mitochondrial membrane potential after UV irradiation has also been reported in situ using suction blisters taken from irradiated and nonirradiated skin areas of healthy old volunteers with an average age of 65.2 years [17].

Aging Effects on Anaerobic Energy Pathways

The loss of mitochondrial function represents an inherent part in modern theories trying to explain the cutaneous aging process. The number of damaged mitochondria increases with aging, and as a consequence an impaired mitochondrial ATP synthesis can be observed. To assure survival of a cell, any decrease in mitochondrial energy production due to impaired mitochondrial function has to lead to compensatory actions in cellular metabolism which result in higher energy production via non-mitochondrial pathways such as glycolysis. This goes along with reports from several in vitro studies demonstrating a higher glucose uptake and lactate production at advanced cellular age in fibroblasts [10, 19].

As a special feature of the skin, atmospheric oxygen may be directly taken up by the human epidermis, and in theory, the flux of oxygen from the environment should be sufficient to fully cover its oxygen demand [20]. A rather surprising hypothesis, stimulated by a study from Ronquist et al. [21], is that human epidermis works to a substantial extent in an anaerobic manner. In cell culture, keratinocytes contain more lactate than do most other cell types. Their lactate production in vitro is vigorous and independent of oxygen and most of it is released to the medium. During autoincubation of the epidermis under starved conditions, energy charge values are low and comparable with those reported for smooth muscle. Moreover, the overwhelming majority of the keratinocytic mitochondria have an appearance markedly deviating from those in other cells, such as Langerhans cells, melanocytes, and fibroblasts, and, above all, are characterized by an enormous reduction of the inner membrane. Ronquist concludes from these findings that epidermal energy metabolism is predominantly anaerobic in spite of the formal presence of mitochondria and sufficient oxygen.

According to not yet published data generated in at the authors' institution, significant age-dependent differences in mitochondrial function can be observed in keratinocytes isolated from skin biopsies of young and old donors. The data suggest that energy metabolism shifts to a predominantly non-mitochondrial pathway and is therefore functionally anaerobic with advancing age. Primary keratinocytes derived from old donors show a higher glucose uptake compared to the cells obtained from a young donor panel, and the increased lactate production in keratinocytes from the old age group clearly indicates a suboptimal utilization of glucose and a shift in metabolism toward an increased glycolysis. The data generated so far show no differences in mitochondrial content and structure during aging in skin keratinocytes, indicating that the number of mitochondria does not change but rather their function. This decline of mitochondrial function may explain the observed age-associated glycolytic activity as some kind of compensatory counterregulation. Simulation of mitochondrial dysfunction by inhibition of ATP synthase in keratinocytes from young donors leads to a comparable rise in glucose uptake and lactate production as seen in the basic, unstressed state of keratinocytes from the old age group.

In fact, the energy metabolism of keratinocytes is a subject of controversy, and it is unclear why keratinocytes express a metabolic status that is, as compared with fibroblasts or endothelial cells, partially shifted to an anaerobic status. It was found that keratinocytes respire as much oxygen as fibroblasts, even though maximal activities of the respiratory chain complexes are two- to five-fold lower, whereas expression levels of respiratory chain proteins are similar. Congruent with this, superoxide anion levels are much higher in keratinocytes, and keratinocytes display higher lipid peroxidation levels and a lower reduced glutathione/oxidized glutathione ratio, indicating enhanced oxidative stress [22]. Thus, it seems that keratinocytes actively use the mitochondrial respiratory chain not only for adenosine 5' triphosphate synthesis but also for the accumulation of superoxide anions, even at the expense of mitochondrial functional capacity. The reason for this behavior of keratinocytes is not clear, but it may indicate that superoxide-driven processes might be a prerequisite for keratinocyte differentiation, even though the lack of energy supply via oxidative phosphorylation has to be compensated via glycolysis then.

Aging Effects on Extramitochondrial Energy Stores

Precise coupling of spatially separated intracellular ATP-producing and ATP-consuming processes is fundamental to the bioenergetics of living organisms, ensuring a fail-safe operation of the energetic system over a broad range of cellular functional activities, thereby securing the cellular economy and energetic homeostasis under stress [23]. Beside the mitochondrial energy supply and glycolysis as primary sources for energy, cells also have a secondary energy storage system named the creatine/phosphocreatine (Cr/PCr) pathway. This is also established in the human skin and is responsible for an extremely fast energy supply in situations of high temporal energy demand when ATP is used up faster than can be produced from primary sources [17, 24, 25] or when energy supply from primary sources is temporarily interrupted, such as in situations of short-term hypoxia or anoxia [26].

The free energy of ATP, which itself cannot be stored efficiently, is stored and transported in the form of PCr from subcellular sites of energy production, e.g., mitochondria, to places of high energy requirements, where creatine kinase (CK) activity can rapidly replenish cellular ATP in situ [27–29]. Predominant isoforms of CK consist of cytosolic mm-CK (muscle type), mainly found in muscle cells, as well as cytosolic bb-CK (brain type) and ubiquitous mitochondrial mt-CK, with the last two mainly located in the brain but also present in the skin [30, 31]. Creatine kinases catalyze the following reversible reaction:

$$\mathrm{Mg} - \mathrm{ATP} + \mathrm{Cr} \leftrightarrow \mathrm{PCr} + \mathrm{Mg} - \mathrm{ADP} + \mathrm{H}^{+}.$$

The mt-CKs form octamers assembled from four dimers each, but only the octameric form can interact with both inner and outer mitochondrial membranes through the adenine nucleotide translocator (ANT) and the voltage-dependent anion channel (VDAC). The mt-CK activity couples the oxidative phosphorylation to mitochondrial PCr production by catalyzing the conversion of Cr to PCr at expenses of the intramitochondrially produced ATP. The PCr is exported to the cytosol, whereas the produced ADP is pumped back to the mitochondrial matrix via ANT. Cells attain their physiological levels of creatine, either by biosynthesis from the amino acids arginine, glycine, and methionine in the kidney, liver, and pancreas of vertebrates including humans and/or alternatively by ingestion of meat and fish. Creatine is transported via the blood circulation and is taken up into cells by the Na- and Cl-dependent creatine transporter (CRT) protein [32, 33]. Once inside a cell, creatine can be stored at high concentrations (e.g., 40 mM for muscle cells).

In skin, oxidative damage of cellular and extracellular components activates intrinsic repair mechanisms, which necessarily require ATP for full functionality. The PCr/CK system together with the recently discovered epidermal creatine transporter (CRT) [30] provides human skin with an important tool to cope efficiently with such conditions of high energy demand. In fact, both creatine kinase subtypes, bb-CK and mt-CK, and CRT are expressed in human skin [17], showing high levels in the epidermis but less in the dermis, with the highest enzyme activity found in keratinocytes, which are generally shifted to a more anaerobic state of metabolism, as discussed in the section "Aging Effects on Anaerobic Energy Pathways".

Results from experiments using skeletal muscle and heart muscle clearly show that both PCr amount [34–36] and CK activity decrease with age [35, 37]. Also in the skin, a reduction in the cellular concentration of creatine can be determined from the age of about 30 [38], paralleled by a slightly reduced CK activity in skin cells from older donors [17]. This decline in skin CK activity may be caused by the generation of ROS during cutaneous aging. This is supported by the fact that CK, specifically mt-CK, is a primary target for ROS, especially peroxynitrite [39]. Moreover, cutaneous cells may show signs of a declining creatine level, probably caused by a stress and age-related decline of dermal vascularization [40].

Mechanisms of Skin Aging Related to Energy Metabolism

Mitochondrial Impairment by Its Own Oxidation By-Products

Free reactive oxygen species (ROS) are generated in the skin by several different processes [41], with exogenous stress following UV irradiation being the most dominant generator of ROS in UV-exposed skin. Other important contributions include proteins within the plasma membrane, such as the growing family of NADPH oxidases. Furthermore, the generation of H_2O_2 as a by-product of fatty acid degradation in peroxisomes has to be taken into account as an endogenous source of ROS. The same holds for the generation of ROS by oxidative burst of phagocytes during inflammatory reactions, as well as the activity of various cytosolic enzymes such as cyclooxygenases. Although all these sources contribute to the overall oxidative burden of a cell, the vast majority of cellular ROS (estimated at approximately 90 %) which is generated in cells independently of UV stress can be traced back to the mitochondria as by-products of impaired mitochondrial respiration [42], and oxidants generated by mitochondria are supposed to be the major source of the oxidative lesions that accumulate with age [43]. The continuous threat of oxidant damage to the cell, tissue, and organism as a whole is underscored by the existence of an impressive array of cellular defenses that have evolved to battle these reactive oxidants [44]. The cell is equipped with a variety of defense mechanisms to remove ROS. Superoxide dismutases convert superoxide into hydrogen peroxide, which in turn can be transformed into water by catalase or glutathione peroxidase. The cell also contains nonenzymatic scavengers such as ascorbate, pyruvate, flavonoids, carotenoids, and glutathione which may inactivate potentially damaging ROS. However, these defenses are not perfect and, consequently, cellular macromolecules become oxidatively damaged.

Relevant to mitochondrial function is the efficiency of electron movement through the electron transport chain and its coupling to oxidative phosphorylation to produce ATP. The coupling efficiency can be measured experimentally by determining ADP/O ratio and by determining whether the mitochondria are in State 3 or State 4, whereby State 3 represents a condition where the rate of oxidative phosphorylation is not limited by ADP concentration, and State 4 represents a condition where the level of ADP limits oxidative phosphorylation. State 4 is associated with a reduced respiratory chain, leading to an "electron jam" and increased formation of ROS by-products. When the rate of electron flow is slow, electrons tend to accumulate in the respiratory chain, and electrons escaping from the somewhat "leaky" electron transport chain (ETC) can reduce oxygen to form the highly reactive free-radical superoxide anion ($O_2\bullet^-$), which, in turn, can be further reduced to hydroxyl radical (OH•) and hydrogen peroxide (H_2O_2). Furthermore, the superoxide anion can initiate the oxidation of sulfite or nitric oxide, resulting in ROS such as sulfur pentoxy anion or peroxynitrite. Overall, mitochondrial ROS generation is high during resting respiration, but when electrons flow quickly through the respiratory chain reducing O_2 to water, the rate of ROS production is usually lower. It has been estimated that about 10^{12} O_2 molecules are processed by each cell daily and that the leakage of partially reduced oxygen molecules is about 2 %, yielding about 2×10^{10} $O_2\bullet^-$ and H_2O_2 molecules per cell per day [45]. In addition to the toxic electron transport chain reactions of the inner mitochondrial membrane, the mitochondrial outer membrane enzyme monoamine oxidase catalyzes the oxidative deamination of biogenic amines and is a quantitatively large source of H_2O_2 that contributes to a further increase in the steady-state concentrations of reactive species within both the mitochondrial matrix and cytosol [46].

High ROS concentrations, resulting from either increased production or decreased detoxification, can cause oxidative damage to various cellular components, ultimately leading to cell death [47]. Beyond damage to mitochondria, which will be discussed in detail below, age-related features often associated with excess ROS are the accumulation of oxidized intracellular proteins with age [48], the decrease of fluidity of cellular membranes with age [49], or even malfunctioning of the connective tissue remodeling process due to increased activity of extracellular matrix-degrading metalloproteinases [50], just to mention a few. Toxic reactions exerted by ROS, and imbalances in the production and removal of ROS, significantly contribute to the aging process and are the basis of the "The Free Radical Theory of Aging" [51], postulating that the production of intracellular reactive oxygen species is the major determinant of life span [42].

The hypothesis that rate of intracellular ROS production is associated with the rate of aging was tested by Sohal [52], comparing the rate of H_2O_2 generation by mitochondria in houseflies. The rate of mitochondrial H_2O_2 release was found to be associated with remaining life expectancy or the physiological age of flies. At the same chronological age, mitochondria from flies with a shorter remaining life expectancy had a markedly higher rate of H_2O_2 generation than those with a longer life expectancy. In another experimental model of aging – the senescence-accelerated mouse (SAM) – animals exhibit a shortened life span (about 18 months) as compared with normal mice, as well as early manifestation of various signs of senescence including changes in physical activity, skin, and spinal curvature. In the SAM the respiratory control ratio and the ATP/O – an index of ATP synthesis – decrease more rapidly as compared with the unaffected wild-type mice. Furthermore, uncoupled respiration in liver mitochondria is markedly decreased with aging in SAM [53]. Cultured dermal fibroblasts from SAM produce more ROS within the mitochondria than do cells from wild-type control mice, coinciding with an increase in the mass of the mitochondria, degenerative mitochondrial morphology with longer culture periods, and lower membrane potential as compared with the controls [54]. Another study supporting the hypothesis that rate of intracellular ROS production is associated with the rate of aging used genetically modified mice with impaired mtDNA repair function. Secondary to the impaired mtDNA repair function, all such mice exhibit a significant reduction in respiratory chain activity and ATP generation in postmitotic tissue such as the heart, as well as a significantly shortened life span and the appearance of a number of age-related phenotypes, including hair loss, kyphosis, and reduced fertility [55]. These findings suggest that damaged mitochondria, which produce an excess of ROS, can accelerate the aging process in a kind of feedback loop.

In fact, the mitochondria seem to be highly susceptible to harm exerted by ROS, including those produced by themselves, and increasing levels of oxidative damage in various compartments of the mitochondrion can be observed during cellular aging. Damages to mitochondrial DNA (mtDNA) – which contributes a substantial part of the proteins of the respiratory chain – isolated from rat liver or various human brain regions are at least tenfold higher than those of nuclear DNA. These higher levels of oxidative damage and mutation in mtDNA have been ascribed to the location of the DNA near the inner mitochondrial membrane sites where oxidants are formed. The extent of damage and mutation of mtDNA may be further aggravated by lack of protective histones and lack of DNA repair activity in mitochondria. Oxidative lesions in mtDNA accumulate as a function of age, which has been well described for the human diaphragm muscle [56], human brain [57]), and rat liver [58].

As in the case of oxidative damage to DNA, an age-associated increase in oxidative damage to mitochondrial protein is also observed [59]. The accumulation of oxidized dysfunctional protein with reactive carbonyl groups can lead to inter- and intramolecular cross-links with protein amino groups and may cause loss of biochemical and physiological function in mitochondria. Thus, the age-related accumulation of protein oxidation products in mitochondria may also lead to loss of energy production and increased production of oxidants.

Increased oxidants may also contribute to alterations in mitochondrial membrane fluidity and phospholipid composition that occur during aging. These in turn can affect the ability of mitochondria to transport substrates and to generate sufficient proton motive force to meet cellular energy demands. With regard to lipids, part of the increased sensitivity of mitochondria to oxidants appears to be due to peculiarities in membrane lipid composition [60] which is characterized by the presence of cardiolipin. Cardiolipin serves as an insulator and stabilizes the activity of protein complexes important to the electron transport chain, and it also "glues" them together. Because cardiolipin plays a pivotal role in facilitating the activities of key mitochondrial inner membrane enzymes, it would be expected that changes that increase its susceptibility to oxidative damage would be deleterious to normal mitochondrial function [43]. Cardiolipin is solely synthesized in the mitochondria and is typically present in the membranes of mitochondria, mostly in the inner membrane, which consists roughly 20 % of its lipids. Cardiolipin acquires an increasing percentage of polyunsaturated fatty acids with the increasing age of an organism (substitution 18:2 to 22:4 and 22:5), which renders it even more susceptible to oxidative damage. In fact, mitochondrial cardiolipin content has been reported to decrease with age in a number of tissues, including the heart, the liver, nonsynaptic brain mitochondria, and epithelial cells [61–64], presumably due to oxidative damage. The decrease of cardiolipin with age is associated with a decrease in State 3/State 4 ratio. This loss of cardiolipin by increased susceptibility to oxidation could play a critically important role in the age-related decrements in mitochondrial function.

In addition to the established role of the mitochondria in energy metabolism, regulation of cell death has emerged as a second major function of these organelles. This seems also to be intimately linked to their generation of ROS [65]. Mitochondrial regulation of apoptosis occurs by mechanisms, which have been conserved through evolution, involving the release of cytochrome c into the cytoplasm which may be initiated by the oxidation of cardiolipin. Oxidation of cardiolipin, which occurs at higher rates in aged cells, reduces cytochrome c binding to mitochondrial inner membranes and increases the level of soluble cytochrome c in the intermembrane space. Subsequent release of the hemoprotein into the cytoplasm, which starts the apoptotic machinery via activation of caspases, occurs by pore formation mediated by proapoptotic Bcl-2 family proteins or opening of mitochondrial permeability transition pores (MPTP). Various factors enhance the likelihood of MPTP opening, among them are dissipation of the difference in voltage between the inside and outside of mitochondrial membranes (known as permeability transition), or the presence of free radicals, both typical features of mitochondria in aged cells.

ROS are also known as signaling molecules under subtoxic conditions which may activate cytoplasmic signal transduction pathways that are related to growth, differentiation, senescence, transformation, and tissue degradation [66–68]. Hydrogen peroxide, for example, has been shown in different cultured cell lines to induce either apoptosis at high concentrations or features of senescence at subtoxic concentrations [69], with cellular senescence being defined as the loss of proliferative capacity of primary cell lines, characterized by cell cycle arrest, reduced DNA synthesis, increased cell size, granularity, and size heterogeneity [70, 71]. Senescent cells enter a terminally nondividing state in which they can stay for long periods before dying. Thus, in the case of stress-induced premature senescence, ROS are considered important intermediates contributing to the phenotype. The data of Zwerschke et al. [10] suggest the occurrence of significant metabolic imbalances in human fibroblasts rendered senescent by exposition to ROS. There is a drastic deregulation of the carbohydrate metabolism in senescent cells, characterized by an imbalance of glycolytic enzyme activities and the failure to maintain ATP levels. This leads to an upregulation of adenylate kinase activity and the levels of AMP, which acts as a growth-suppressive signal that induces premature senescence. The activities of several glycolytic enzymes are strongly upregulated. Moreover, the function of the malate-aspartate shuttle is reduced in senescent cells, preventing the transport of hydrogen into the mitochondria, where it could be used for ATP production. Instead, senescent cells activate LDH and take up pyruvate to get rid of hydrogen. Thus, ATP-consuming steps of glycolysis are enhanced, whereas the ATP-producing steps are inhibited, and this leads to a severe reduction of the intracellular concentration of both ATP and GTP. Senescent keratinocytes and fibroblasts were also described by Campisi [72] to accumulate with age in human skin, likely due to the impact of increased endogenous oxidative stress in aged skin.

Genetic Damage to Mitochondria

The mitochondrial genome is very small and economically packed, and the expression of the whole genome is essential for the maintenance of mitochondrial bioenergetic function. Thus, even small genetic alterations may have tremendous effects on mitochondrial function. In the past decade, more than 100 mtDNA mutations have been found in patients with mitochondrial disease, and some of them also occur in aging human tissues [73]. Thus, it may be hypothesized that accumulation of mitochondrial DNA deletions may be an important factor in intrinsic aging.

At higher age, several independently acquired types of mtDNA mutations, accumulating clonally in certain cells, can even be found in different tissues of the same subject [74]. The incidence and abundance of mutant mtDNAs are increased with age and much more than for nuclear DNA mutations [75, 76]. Studies of sequence heterogeneity of mitochondrial DNA from rat and mouse tissues derived from young adult and senescent animals have revealed that about 1 % of the native mtDNA population in adult liver and about 5 % in senescent liver are having deleted/inserted segments [77]. In humans it was found that normal heart muscle and brain from adult human individuals contain low, though substantial, levels of a specific mitochondrial DNA deletion, previously found only in patients affected with certain types of neuromuscular disease. This deletion was not observed in fetal heart or brain [78]. In a further human study focusing on the prevalence of mtDNA deletions in tumorous and surrounding healthy tissue, mtDNA mutations were found to be abundant in margin tissue specimens from older patients, and their number correlated with the patient age. Significantly fewer deletions were detected in the tumors than the margins, and the tumors often had no deletions [79], implying a potential selection for full-length mtDNA or perhaps a protective role for mtDNA deletions in the process of tumorigenesis.

Concerning photoaging, also photoaged skin is characterized at the molecular level by increased amounts of large-scale deletions of the mitochondrial genome such as the 4977 bp common deletion encompassing the deletion of four genes for subunits of complex I, one gene for complex IV, two genes for complex V, and several genes for mitochondrial tRNAs [80, 81]. The common deletion can be generated in dermal fibroblasts through repetitive ultraviolet UV-A irradiation [82]. For example, in a human study, previously unirradiated skin of 52 normal human individuals was repetitively exposed to physiological doses of UV-A light, and repetitive UV exposure led to an approximately 40 % increase in the levels of the common deletion in skin tissue. Nine individuals were examined up to 16 months after cessation of UV exposure, and some showed accumulation up to 32-fold [83]. In another human study focusing on extrinsic photoaging, several types of mtDNA length mutations including the common 4977 bp deletion were investigated in normal human skin tissues. It was found that the incidences of these deletions and tandem duplications of mtDNA in sun-exposed skin were all significantly higher than those in nonexposed skin [84]. Moreover, these mutations started to appear in the third decade of life, and the age at which the mutations could be detected in sun-exposed skin was substantially younger than in nonexposed skin. In another human study focusing on mtDNA aberrations in skin tissue, the frequency of a so-called T414G mutation within the control region of mtDNA has been demonstrated to accumulate in both chronologically and photoaged skin using cultured dermal fibroblasts from donors of different age [85]. Thus, there is a strong correlation of extrinsic and intrinsic cellular aging with the accumulation of aberrations of mtDNA, and increasing evidence suggests that, due to a negative feedback loop, damaged mtDNA is a cause and consequence of aging as well.

The causative role of mtDNA mutations and resulting mitochondrial dysfunction for intrinsic and extrinsic aging has been demonstrated in several experimental models and human studies. Premature aging has, for example, been reported in knock-in mice expressing a defective mitochondrial DNA polymerase. These knock-in mice develop an mtDNA mutator phenotype with a threefold to fivefold increase in the levels of point mutations, as well as increased amounts of deleted mtDNA, associated with reduced life span and premature onset of age-related phenotypes such as weight loss, reduced subcutaneous fat, alopecia (hair loss), kyphosis (curvature of the spine), osteoporosis, anemia, reduced fertility, and heart enlargement [55]. The results thus provide a causative link between mtDNA mutations and aging phenotypes in mammals. It is plausible that the accumulation of mtDNA mutations leads to decreased gene expression, resulting in a decline in oxidative phosphorylation, and inefficient electron transport, which consequently increases the generation of ROS [86]. A direct link between the amount of mtDNA aberrations and oxidative stress has been demonstrated using a series of the cybrids harboring varying proportions of mtDNA with the common 4977 bp deletion. The population doubling time was longer for the cybrids containing higher proportions of 4977 bp-deleted mtDNA. In addition, the respiratory function was decreased with the increase of the portion of aberrant mtDNA in the cybrids. The results also showed that the specific contents of typical cellular oxidation products stemming from ROS in cybrids harboring >65 % of the aberrant mtDNA were significantly increased as compared with those of the cybrids containing undetectable mutant mtDNA [80, 87]. In a study on human fibroblasts, gradual large-scale deletion of the mtDNA from unirradiated human skin fibroblasts was found to induce a gene expression profile reminiscent of photoaged skin. The modified cells exhibited an altered gene expression profile resulting from intracellular, mitochondria-derived oxidative stress, dominated by high expression of matrix metalloproteinase-1 (MMP-1) which is known to be expressed in response to oxidative stress [95].

Vice versa, the increase in ROS production is a likely promotor for additional mtDNA damage and accumulation of mtDNA mutations. The causative role of oxidative stress for the increased frequency of mitochondrial DNA aberrations has been demonstrated in a variety of experimental models and in human studies. For example, oxidative damage elicited by the imbalance of free-radical scavenging enzymes and its association with large-scale mtDNA deletions in aging human skin has been suggested using skin tissue derived from donors of different age. In subjects above the age of 60 years, elevated oxidative stress was caused by an imbalance between the production and removal of ROS and free radicals and was paralleled by an increase of the proportion of mtDNA with the 4977 bp deletion [88]. The causative role of singlet oxygen in mediating UV-A-induced generation of the photoaging-associated mitochondrial common deletion has been demonstrated in a pivotal study by Berneburg et al. [89]. Normal human fibroblasts were repetitively exposed to sublethal doses of UV-A radiation and assayed for the common deletion. There was a time- and dose-dependent generation of the common deletion, attributable to the generation of singlet oxygen, since the common deletion was diminished when irradiating in the presence of singlet oxygen quenchers but increased when enhancing singlet oxygen half-life by deuterium oxide. The induction of the common deletion by UV-A irradiation was mimicked by treatment of unirradiated cells with singlet oxygen produced by the thermodecomposition of an endoperoxide. These studies provide direct evidence for the involvement of reactive oxygen species in the generation of aging-associated mtDNA lesions in human cells.

Side Effects of Anaerobic Energy Pathways

High glycolytic fluxes and glucose accumulation may be a last resort when oxidative energy capacity of mitochondria declines during aging, but they are also sources of endogenous damage by themselves. In fact, both aging and diabetes are characterized by the formation of so-called advanced glycation end products (AGEs), though due to different reasons. Most glycolytic intermediates favor the formation of AGEs via reactive carbonyl groups that are able to modify protein amino groups in the cytosol based on the Maillard reaction. This reaction is termed glycation or nonenzymatic glycosylation. AGEs constitute a heterogeneous group of structures, whereby N'--(carboxymethyl)lysine (CML) adducts are the most prevalent AGEs present in vivo. Methylglyoxal, glyoxal, and other autooxidated derivatives of sugars induce AGEs that negatively affect essential features of skin cells and extracellular matrix proteins. It has been reported that AGE formation results in a loss of contractile capacity and cytoskeleton integrity in human skin fibroblasts, which possibly affects tissue cohesion and leads to visible effects of skin aging. Vimentin was identified as a major target in skin glycation besides other long-lived proteins such as fibronectin, laminin, collagen, and elastin [90]. Strikingly, the accumulation of modified vimentin can be found in skin fibroblasts of elderly donors in vivo, bringing AGE modifications in skin into strong relationship with loss of organ contractile functions associated with aging. It is also reported that the intracellular concentration of the glycating agents – such as highly reactive methylglyoxal, which is formed from dihydroxyacetone and glyceraldehyde-3-phosphates, and rapidly glycates proteins – damages mitochondria [91], and AGEs may even induce apoptosis by the enhancement of the expression of proapoptotic genes and stimulation of apoptosis through cytoplasmic and mitochondrial pathways [92]. Furthermore, intracellular AGEs induce oxidative stress, activate NF-κB and heme oxygenase, produce lipid peroxidation products, and cross-link proteins [93].

Monitoring Methods for Energetic Processes in Skin Cells

Monitoring of Mitochondrial and Glycolytic Activity in the Skin

There is no direct method available to measure mitochondrial or glycolytic activity in the skin in situ. In any case, dermal cells have to be isolated from skin biopsies or suction blisters, or cultured dermal cell lines have to be employed.

The assessment of the mitochondrial membrane potential is then possible through the availability of redistribution potentiometric radioactive compounds such as tetraphenylphosphonium bromide or redistribution potentiometric dyes such as rhodamine 123 (R123) or tetramethylrhodamine methyl ester (TMRM). These substances are lipophilic cations accumulated by mitochondria in proportion to the membrane potential ($\Delta\Psi$). Whereas the use of tetraphenylphosphonium bromide requires isolation of the mitochondria for uptale analysis [94], the dyes may be used also with living intact cells. Upon accumulation in the cytoplasm, R123 and TMRM exhibit a red shift in both their absorption and fluorescence emission spectra. The fluorescence intensity is quenched when the dyes are accumulated by mitochondria. These properties can be used to monitor membrane potentials even in single cells or in isolated mitochondria [95]. Rhodamine 123 and TMRM have also been used to monitor the mitochondrial membrane potential of intact human skin fibroblasts [96, 97], down to the single organelle level [98]. Another way to monitor the mitochondrial membrane potential is the use of redox indicators such as safranine or the tetrazolium dye 5,5',6,6'-tetrachloro-1,1',3,3'-tetraethyl-benzimidazol-carbocyanine iodide (JC-1). The latter is taken up by cells and exists as a monomer in the cytosol (green). The negative charge established by the intact mitochondrial membrane potential allows the lipophilic dye to enter the mitochondrial matrix where it accumulates. When the critical concentration is exceeded as the mitochondrial membrane becomes more polarized, J-aggregates form, which become fluorescent red and can be monitored photometrically. JC-1 has also been used to monitor the mitochondrial membrane potential on the level of single intact cells, for example, by flow cytometry [99].

Another method to determine the energy flux in mitochondria is the estimation of the amount of ATP in relation to the amount of oxygen consumed, also called the P/O ratio. If mitochondria or permeabilized cells are incubated in an oxygraph apparatus (oxygen electrode) in an isotonic medium containing substrate and phosphate, then the addition of ADP causes a sudden burst of oxygen uptake as the ADP is converted into ATP. The actively respiring state is referred to as State 3 respiration, while the slower rate after all the ADP has been phosphorylated to form ATP is referred to as State 4. The ratio [State 3 rate]/[State 4 rate] is called the respiratory control index and indicates the tightness of the coupling between respiration and phosphorylation. It is possible to calculate P/O ratio by measuring the decrease in oxygen concentration during the rapid burst of State 3 respiration after adding a known amount of ADP [16]. In parallel, the degree of glycolytic activity in a given cell suspension can be assessed by comparing the glucose uptake of cells with the amount of lactate produced.

Monitoring of Reactive Oxygen Species

Although many enzymatic and chemical methods have been developed for evaluating ROS, in cell homogenates and in cell suspensions down to the single cell level, evaluation methods for ROS generation in situ are quite limited. Intracellular ROS production in single cells, for example, can be measured by a fluorometric assay based on deacetylation and oxidation of nonfluorescent dichlorodihydrofluoresceindiacetate (DCHF-DA), which penetrates the plasma membrane followed by enzymatic cleavage of the acetate groups and which specifically reacts with peroxides to the fluorescent dichlorofluorescein (DCF). Dihydrocalcein (H_2-calcein) is another probe for intracellular ROS detection. In contrast to dichlorodihydrofluorescein, its fluorescent oxidation product calcein is thought not to leak out of cells. Other methods to monitor ROS in cells rely on luminescence enhancers such as luminol-, coelenterazine-, or lucigenin-enhanced chemiluminescence, which have been used extensively as indicators of $O_2\bullet^-$ generation in intact cells and homogenates. Luminescence in this case is based on the activation of the probes by $O_2\bullet^-$ and subsequent release of photons which can be measured in a luminometer.

In situ, oxidative modification of dermal biomolecules induces ultraweak photon emission (UPE) as a by-product. Such light signals, which can be recorded in a noninvasive way, are supposed to contain valuable information regarding the extent of chemical damage and the nature of the oxidative modifications and might be employed as a sensitive tool to monitor the efficacy of cosmetic or dermatological antioxidative intervention regimens. Data generated indicate that UPE is induced by oxidative damage especially in deeper (living) skin layers, where antioxidants must be active in order to interfere with accelerated skin aging [100, 101].

Energetic Entry Points for Intervention

There are several entry points for cosmetic intervention with intrinsic and extrinsic skin aging. Many of them refer to the topical application of antioxidants aimed at neutralizing free ROS, which are the central noxious effector molecules in both intrinsic and extrinsic aging processes. Typically used antioxidants, such as vitamin C, vitamin E, vitamin A, and carotenes, have only indirect effects on energy metabolism, as they may reduce the ROS exposition of skin cells. These typical antioxidants will not be discussed in detail in this chapter because they are discussed extensively elsewhere in this book.

There are, however, two compounds that may be topically used in cosmetic applications and dermatology, which interfere directly with the energy metabolism of skin cells – creatine and coenzyme Q_{10}. Both compounds are in the very scope of this chapter and deserve in-depth discussion.

Energetic Effects of Creatine

Creatine (Cr), a body-inherent amino acid derivative, is known to play a pivotal role in organ energy supply, because it acts like an energy store which can fastly provide energy in situations of high energy demand. After cellular uptake, creatine is phosphorylated to phosphocreatine (PCr) by the creatine kinase (CK) reaction using ATP. At subcellular sites with high energy requirements, e.g., at the myofibrillar apparatus during muscle contraction, CK catalyzes the transphosphorylation of PCr to ADP to regenerate ATP, thus preventing a depletion of ATP levels. PCr is thus available as a secondary energy source, serving not only as an energy buffer but also as an energy transport vehicle. In humans, the major part of the total creatine content is located in skeletal muscle, of which approximately a third is in its free form. The remainder is present in the phosphorylated form. It is supposed, for example, that the energy required for a 100-m sprint is entirely delivered from the creatine/phosphocreatine battery. Numerous scientific studies indicate that nutritional creatine supplementation favorably affects long-endurance exercise [Vandenberghe et al. (102)] and exerts protective effects in many clinical disorders, presumably caused by its energetic capacity.

Creatine is normally metabolized to creatinine which is cleared via renal excretion, and daily turnover of creatine to creatinine for a 70-kg male has been estimated to be around 2 g. Cells attain their physiological levels of creatine, either by biosynthesis from the amino acids arginine, glycine, and methionine in the kidney, liver, and pancreas of vertebrates including humans and/or alternatively by ingestion of meat and fish. Creatine is transported via the blood circulation and is taken up into cells by a Na- and Cl-dependent CRT protein [32, 33, 103]. Once inside a cell, creatine can be stored at high concentrations (e.g., 40 mM for muscle cells). Creatine can be synthesized in human cells, but from the age of about 30, a reduction in the cellular concentration in the skin can be determined [38].

Highly interesting with regard to aging processes is that mitochondrial creatine kinase activity prevents reactive oxygen species generation due to a kind of "antioxidant" role of mitochondrial kinase-dependent ADP recycling activity. Of course, creatine is not a radical scavenger in itself. The activation of the mitochondrial creatine kinase (mt-CK) by creatine and ATP or ADP rather induces a State 3-like respiration in mitochondria, which represents a condition where the rate of oxidative phosphorylation is not limited by ADP concentration [104]. Thus, supplementation of cells with creatine may reduce the electron "jam" in the respiratory chain by providing a sink for free ATP-coupled energy by building up phosphocreatine (PCr) stores and consequently increasing the pool of available ADP for phosphorylation.

Supplementation of skin cells with creatine has been described to reduce the amount of cellular damage induced by UV-A irradiation or chemical oxidants per se [17]. This protective effect is most likely due to the general energy-recharging effect of creatine and may have further implications in modulating processes which are involved in premature skin aging and skin damage. In contrast to the protective effect of creatine supplementation, the inhibition of cytosolic and mitochondrial creatine kinase by siRNA in HaCaT and HeLaS3 cells, as performed at the authors' institution, affects cell viability and mitochondrial morphology negatively [105].

Besides its role on energy metabolism, it has recently been demonstrated that the activation of mt-CK by creatine inhibits the mitochondrial permeability transition (MPT), a process that is involved in apoptosis [106]. The postulated protective mechanism of mt-CK activity against MPT pore opening lies on the one hand on functional coupling between the mt-CK reaction and oxidative phosphorylation. It is known that MPT can be directly induced by mitochondrial ROS, and it is conceivable that the protective role of mt-CK activity against MPT may occur through the reduction of ROS generation by keeping ADP phosphorylation. On the other hand, octamer-dimer transitions of mt-CK as well as different creatine kinase substrates have a profound influence on controlling mitochondrial permeability transition (MPT). Kinetic analyses suggested a functional interaction between the mt-CK, outer membrane pore protein, and inner membrane adenylate translocator (ANT). Permeability transition-pore-like functions are not observed unless the creatine kinase octamer is dissociated, which is facilitated in the absence of creatine [107–109].

As a zwitterion, creatine is also able to penetrate skin remarkably well and is able to replenish energy stores of epidermal cells. Several research data clearly demonstrate that only when enough creatine is available, skin cells function perfectly, all repair and protection systems work faultlessly, and the metabolism runs at full performance. For example, supplementation of keratinocytes in vitro with creatine has marked protective effects against oxidative stress, and, in clinical trials conducted at the authors' institution, exogenous supplementation of the skin with creatine in a topical formulation had marked protective against UV-induced damage [17]. In these studies, healthy old volunteers with an average age of 65.2 years were topically treated with a stabilized creatine formulation twice a day for 4 weeks on their upper arm. Afterwards, epidermal cells were isolated via suction blister to examine the mitochondrial membrane potential in response to UV irradiation. Epidermal cells from placebo-treated skin sites showed a substantial and statistically significant decline in their mitochondrial membrane potential compared with nonirradiated control cells. In contrast, cells from the creatine/creatinine-treated skin sites showed a statistically significant maintenance of their mitochondrial membrane potential even after irradiation compared with the irradiated placebo control cells. Thus, topically applied creatine significantly protects human epidermal cells from a UV-induced decline in mitochondrial energy metabolism.

Moreover, experimental results indicate that creatine promotes protection and repair of mitochondrial DNA to ensure the maintenance of healthy cells. As discussed in the section "Genetic Damage to Mitochondria" of this overview, mitochondrial mutations are thought to be mediated by ROS and persist in human skin as long-term biomarkers of UV exposure. In a pivotal study by Berneburg et al. [110], UV-induced mitochondrial mutagenesis of skin cells, as assessed by the frequency of the common deletion, as well as functional consequences on mitochondrial energy metabolism, could be normalized by increasing intracellular creatine levels.

All these data clearly indicate that human skin cells energetically recharged with creatine both in vitro and in vivo are better protected against a variety of cellular stress conditions by reversing deficiencies in cutaneous energy supply [25]. So far there are no reports of harmful side effects of topical Cr loading of human skin.

Energetic Effects of Coenzyme Q_{10}

Coenzyme Q_{10} (CoQ_{10}, ubiquinone) is a lipophilic vitamin-like substance which is present in most eukaryotic cells, primarily in the mitochondria [111]. The CoQ_{10} found in humans is a benzoquinone with a polyisoprene chain containing ten isoprene units. It is a component of the electron transport chain, where CoQ_{10} has a unique function since it transfers electrons from the primary substrates to the oxidase system at the same time that it transfers protons to the outside of the mitochondrial membrane, resulting in the proton gradient across the mitochondrial membrane which is employed by Complex IV to generate ATP. It is known that Complex I (NADH-ubiquinone reductase) and Complex II (succinate-ubiquinone reductase) are found to be the predominant generators of ROS during prolonged respiration under uncoupled conditions, whereas complex III (ubiquinol/cytochrome c reductase) plays a less dominant role for mitochondrial ROS production. Complex II, in particular, appears to contribute most to the basal production of ROS in cells [112]. It is obvious that the reduction of CoQ_{10} in a cell impairs the respiratory chain in mitochondria, resulting in electron "jam" and excess production of ROS.

By the reduction of the quinone to quinol, a carrier of protons and electrons is produced. Thus, in addition to its "antioxidative" role in the respiratory chain, the reduced form of CoQ_{10}, ubichinol-10, is itself a real lipid-soluble radical scavenger molecule. It could be demonstrated in this context that ubiquinone reduced to ubiquinol through the electron transport chain strongly inhibits lipid peroxidation in isolated mitochondria [113, 114]. Thus, reduced CoQ_{10} interferes also as an antioxidant with some of the basic age-associated processes in mitochondria such as destruction on cardiolipin. Ubiquinol-10 is about as effective in preventing peroxidative damage to lipids as vitamin E, which is considered the best lipid-soluble antioxidant in humans. In contrast to vitamin E, ubiquinol-10 is not recycled by ascorbate. However, it is known that ubiquinol-10 can be recycled by electron transport carriers present in various biomembranes and possibly by some enzymes [115]. In addition to direct antioxidant radical scavenging, the quinol can rescue tocopheryl radicals produced by reaction with lipid or oxygen radicals by direct reduction back to tocopherol (vitamin E). Without CoQ_{10} in a membrane, regeneration of tocopherol is very slow. The regeneration of tocopherol can also be observed in low-density lipoprotein where a small amount of CoQ_{10} protects a larger amount of tocopherol [111].

In normal healthy individuals, CoQ_{10} is synthesized in all cells from tyrosine (or phenylalanine) and mevalonate, and supplementation with CoQ_{10} does not increase tissue levels above normal. However, CoQ_{10} contents in cells decline during aging, which has been shown, for example, in muscle cells [116]. Previously it has been shown that levels of CoQ_{10} are also lowered in skin cells from aging donors [117], suggesting that a decrease in mitochondrial CoQ_{10} content is an integral aspect of skin aging. In some tissue, such as aged skin, supplemental CoQ_{10} can restore normal levels. In fact, it was demonstrated that CoQ_{10} penetrates into the viable layers of the epidermis and reduces the basal level of oxidation measured by weak photon emission. Furthermore, a reduction in wrinkle depth following CoQ_{10} application was shown in clinical studies [117]. It is further known that UV irradiation depletes CoQ_{10} as well as other antioxidants in the skin and causes oxidative damage [118]. In studies using nude mice, supplementation with CoQ10 was found to reduce the acute oxidative stress response following UV irradiation, as characterized by reduced induction of manganese superoxide dismutase and glutathione peroxidase following irradiation in the presence of topical CoQ10 supplementation [119]. In studies by the authors, supplemental CoQ_{10} was also shown to be effective against UV-A-mediated oxidative stress in human keratinocytes in terms of thiol depletion, modulation of specific phosphotyrosine kinases, and prevention of oxidative mtDNA damage [117]. CoQ_{10} was also able to significantly suppress the expression of collagenase in human dermal fibroblasts following UV-A irradiation. In another study, conducted in the author's institution, healthy volunteers were topically treated with a CoQ_{10}-containing cream formulation twice a day in a 7-day period. Afterward, epidermal primary keratinocytes were isolated via suction blister, irradiated and examined for mitochondrial membrane potential. CoQ_{10} application clearly resulted in a significant amelioration (+44 %) of mitochondrial membrane potential after irradiation compared to the untreated control. These results indicate that CoQ_{10} has the efficacy to prevent many of the detrimental effects of photoaging and has general "energizing" effects in skin [117, 120].

Conclusion

Cutaneous aging is characterized by a decline in energy metabolism of skin cells partially caused by detrimental changes in mitochondrial respiration. The processes involved seem to be predominantly mediated by free-radical actions known to be generated either by exogenous noxes, such as UV light, or by endogenous processes such as impaired mitochondrial respiration associated with electron "jam" and generation of ROS by leakage of electrons from the respiratory chain. It is widely accepted that alterations in mitochondrial respiration can be regarded as both a reason as well as an important consequence for aging. Any lack of mitochondrial function impairs cellular ATP synthesis, reducing the "fuel supply" for repair mechanisms. It does further induce the formation of ROS as by-products of an impaired mitochondrial respiration. The accumulation of ROS may, in turn, damage neighboring mitochondrial complexes, membranes, and mtDNA and further accelerate the aging process in a kind of feedback loop. Once the damage of macromolecules has reached the level of mtDNA, leading to mutations, the energetic age of a mitochondrion, and thus of a cell, is carved in stone.

Basically, any loss of mitochondrial energetic capacity is attempted to be compensated by energy generation from other sources. This is either the exploitation of intracellular energy stores for high energy demands in a short term or the switch to anaerobic pathways for energy supply, such as glycolysis, as a last resort in a long term. In this context glycolysis, used by a cell as last resort, is associated with the generation of reactive glycolytic intermediates which favor the formation of advanced glycation end products (AGEs) via reactive carbonyl groups. These AGEs may harm a cell by processes ranging from the generation of unfunctional cytoskeletal proteins up to the induction of apoptosis. Thus, it is important to keep tissues from anaerobiosis by keeping mitochondrial energy generation upright. Furthermore, it is important to supply a cell with

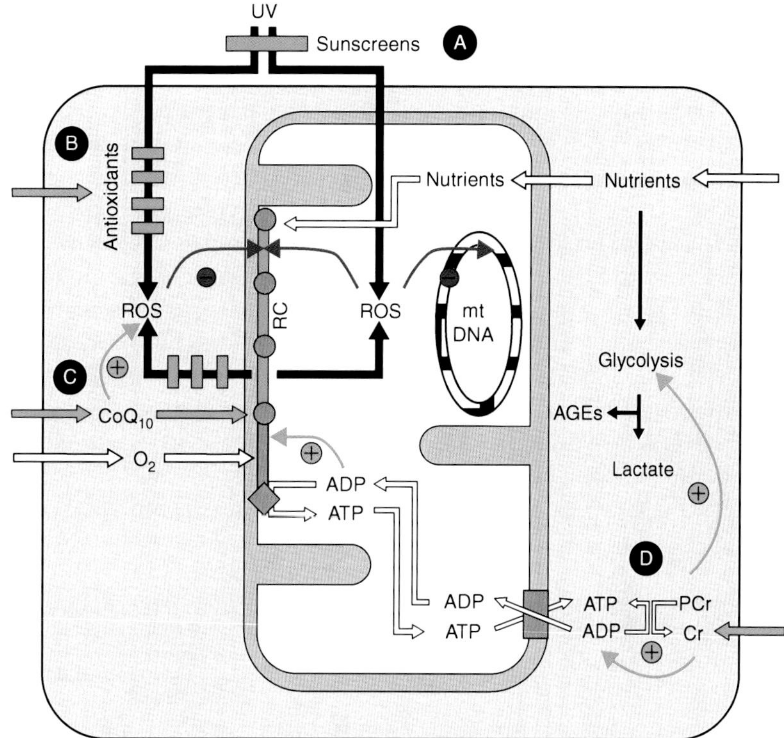

Fig. 1 Pathways leading to aging of skin cells. Processes (A)-(D) are described in detail in the "Conclusion" of this overview. *Blue arrows* marked with a (+) sign represent beneficial processes for the cell with antiaging efficacy. *Red arrows* marked with a (−) sign represent detrimental processes for a cell, which are associated with accelerated aging (*ROS* reactive oxygen species, *AGE* advanced glycation end product, *RC* respiratory chain, *CoQ_{10}* Coenzyme Q_{10}, *mtDNA* mitochondrial DNA, *Cr* creatine, *PCr* phosphocreatine)

substantial energy stores to be filled with energy in phases of baseline activity, which can be used in situation of high energy demand without the need to switch to glycolysis.

There are several entry points to affect skin aging from an energetic perspective. Besides sunscreens to protect the skin from the most important ROS-generating insult, UV light (Fig. 1a), the first and most obvious entry point is to keep the antioxidant system of a cell working. This will result in protection against ROS from whatever sources and thus targets the key effector molecules of skin aging (Fig. 1b). Antioxidants are beyond the scope of this overview. However, it should be mentioned that one antioxidant which has been proven to be especially potent in pathological dermatological situations characterized by excessive deregulation of ROS generation, such as polymorphous light eruption (PLE), is α-glucosylrutin [121–123], a potent plant-derived antioxidant with excellent bioavailability in the skin.

The next energetically relevant entry point with regard to skin aging is to keep the respiratory chain in skin cells working, in order to avoid electron "jam" and subsequent generation of ROS. This can be done by supplementation with coenzyme Q_{10}, which is a key component of the respiratory chain. CoQ_{10} declines with age but can be effectively replenished in skin by topical formulations (Fig. 1c). In addition to its central role as a structural component of the respiratory chain, CoQ_{10} is also a potent radical scavenger which protects important membrane proteins of the respiratory chain, such as cardiolipin, from oxidative damage.

In addition to this, supplementation of the skin with creatine is an important entry point for intervention with aging processes. Creatine levels and activities of creatine kinases in skin decline with age, reducing the available energy store for short-term demand. Skin cells that are energetically recharged with sufficient creatine are better protected against a variety of cellular stressors, age-dependent deficiencies in cellular functions, or oxidative and free-radical-induced cell damage. This is also due to a kind of "antioxidant" activity of the creatine/phosphocreatine system, which results from its capacity to form a sink for ATP, keeping the amount of available ADP for phosphorylation by the mitochondrial respiratory chain high (Fig. 1d). This, in turn, keeps the mitochondrion in a kind of unrestricted State 3 respiration.

At first sight, it might be tempting to speculate that supplementation of skin with additional oxygen might also enforce the capacity of the respiratory chain to generate energy. This, however, could not yet be proven in experimental systems or clinical trials, and it might be due to the fact that skin can directly take up atmospheric oxygen in sufficient amounts and thus is generally not in a situation of hypoxia as other organs might be [20]. Nevertheless, beneficial effects of short-term oxygen pulses on the activity of skin cells have been observed, but these are supposed to be related to some yet unknown signal transduction effects of oxygen rather than on enhanced energy metabolism (publication in preparation). The energetic pathways leading to skin aging, as well as the possible intervention strategies, as discussed in this overview, are summarized in Fig. 1.

In conclusion, biological science has advanced the ability to directly target skin aging. The declining energy metabolism has turned out as a high-priority field of antiaging interventions such as creatine and CoQ_{10} (Figs. 2 and 3).

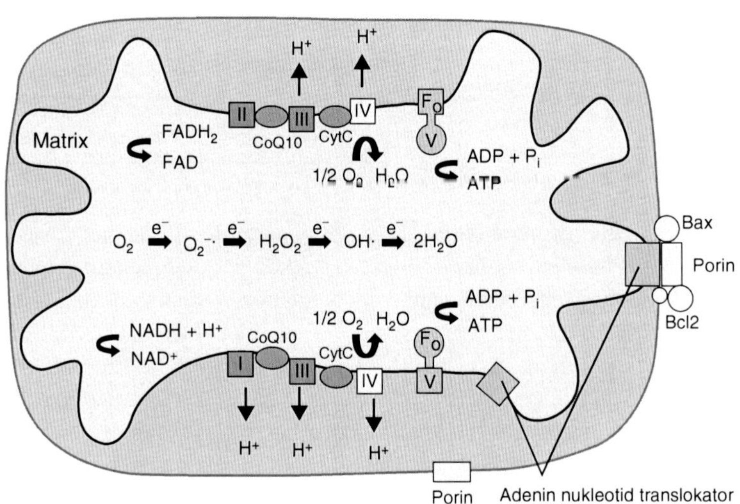

Fig. 2 Mitochdonrial enzyme topography

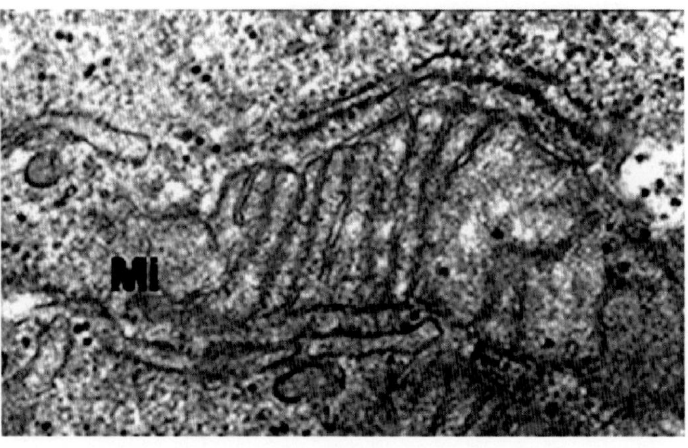

Fig. 3 Electron microscopy of a mitochondrium

References

1. Birch-Machin MA. The role of mitochondria in ageing and carcinogenesis. Clin Exp Dermatol. 2006;31:548–52.
2. Jendrach M, Pohl S, Voth M, et al. Morpho-dynamic changes of mitochondria during ageing of human endothelial cells. Mech Ageing Dev. 2005;126:813–21.
3. Hansford RG. Bioenergetics in aging. Biochim Biophys Acta. 1983;726:41–80.
4. Goldstein S, Moerman EJ, Porter K. High-voltage electron microscopy of human diploid fibroblasts during ageing in vitro. Morphometric analysis of mitochondria. Exp Cell Res. 1984;154:101–11.
5. Brantova O, Tesarova M, Hansikova H, et al. Ultrastructural changes of mitochondria in the cultivated skin fibroblasts of patients with point mutations in mitochondrial DNA. Ultrastruct Pathol. 2006;30:239–45.
6. Feldman D, Bryce GF, Shapiro SS. Mitochondrial inclusions in keratinocytes of hairless mouse skin exposed to UVB radiation. J Cutan Pathol. 1990;17:96–100.
7. Guillery O, Malka F, Frachon P, et al. Modulation of mitochondrial morphology by bioenergetics defects in primary human fibroblasts. Neuromuscul Disord. 2008;18:319–30.
8. Lazarou M, McKenzie M, Ohtake A, Thorburn DR, Ryan MT. Analysis of the assembly profiles for mitochondrial- and nuclear-DNA-encoded subunits into complex I. Mol Cell Biol. 2007;27:4228–37.
9. Papa S. Mitochondrial oxidative phosphorylation changes in the life span. Molecular aspects and physiopathological implications. Biochim Biophys Acta. 1996;1276:87–105.
10. Zwerschke W, Mazurek S, Stockl P, et al. Metabolic analysis of senescent human fibroblasts reveals a role for AMP in cellular senescence. Biochem J. 2003;376:403–11.
11. Sugrue MM, Tatton WG. Mitochondrial membrane potential in aging cells. Biol Signals Recept. 2001;10:176–88.
12. Rottenberg H, Wu S. Mitochondrial dysfunction in lymphocytes from old mice: enhanced activation of the permeability transition. Biochem Biophys Res Commun. 1997;240:68–74.
13. Yen TC, Chen YS, King KL, Yeh SH, Wei YH. Liver mitochondrial respiratory functions decline with age. Biochem Biophys Res Commun. 1989;165:944–1003.
14. Trounce I, Byrne E, Marzuki S. Decline in skeletal muscle mitochondrial respiratory chain function: possible factor in ageing. Lancet. 1989;1:637–9.
15. Mammone T, Gan D, Foyouzi-Youssefi R. Apoptotic cell death increases with senescence in normal human dermal fibroblast cultures. Cell Biol Int. 2006;30:903–9.
16. Greco M, Villani G, Mazzucchelli F, et al. Marked aging-related decline in efficiency of oxidative phosphorylation in human skin fibroblasts. FASEB J. 2003;17:1706–8.
17. Lenz H, Schmidt M, Welge V, et al. The creatine kinase system in human skin: protective effects of creatine against oxidative and UV damage in vitro and in vivo. J Invest Dermatol. 2005;124:443–52.
18. Paz ML, Gonzalez Maglio DH, Weill FS, Bustamante J, Leoni J. Mitochondrial dysfunction and cellular stress progression after ultraviolet B irradiation in human keratinocytes. Photodermatol Photoimmunol Photomed. 2008;24:115–22.
19. Jongkind JF, Verkerk A, Poot M. Glucose flux through the hexose monophosphate shunt and NADP(H) levels during in vitro ageing of human skin fibroblasts. Gerontology. 1987;33:281–6.
20. Stucker M, Struk A, Altmeyer P, et al. The cutaneous uptake of atmospheric oxygen contributes significantly to the oxygen supply of human dermis and epidermis. J Physiol. 2002;538:985–94.
21. Ronquist G, Andersson A, Bendsoe N, Falck B. Human epidermal energy metabolism is functionally anaerobic. Exp Dermatol. 2003;12:572–9.
22. Hornig-Do HT, von Kleist-Retzow JC, Lanz K, et al. Human epidermal keratinocytes accumulate superoxide due to low activity of Mn-SOD, leading to mitochondrial functional impairment. J Invest Dermatol. 2007;127:1084–93.
23. Dzeja PP, Terzic A. Phosphotransfer networks and cellular energetics. J Exp Biol. 2003;206:2039–47.
24. Bessman SP, Carpenter CL. The creatine-creatine phosphate energy shuttle. Annu Rev Biochem. 1985;54:831–62.
25. Blatt T, Lenz H, Koop U, et al. Stimulation of skin's energy metabolism provides multiple benefits for mature human skin. Biofactors. 2005;25:179–85.
26. Wilken B, Ramirez JM, Probst I, Richter DW, Hanefeld F. Creatine protects the central respiratory network of mammals under anoxic conditions. Pediatr Res. 1998;43:8–14.
27. Bessman SP. The creatine phosphate energy shuttle–the molecular asymmetry of a "pool". Anal Biochem. 1987;161:519–23.
28. Wallimann T, Wyss M, Brdiczka D, Nicolay K, Eppenberger HM. Intracellular compartmentation, structure and function of creatine kinase isoenzymes in tissues with high and fluctuating energy demands: the 'phosphocreatine circuit' for cellular energy homeostasis. Biochem J. 1992;281(Pt 1):21–40.
29. Wyss M, Smeitink J, Wevers RA, Wallimann T. Mitochondrial creatine kinase: a key enzyme of aerobic energy metabolism. Biochim Biophys Acta. 1992;1102:119–66.
30. Schlattner U, Mockli N, Speer O, Werner S, Wallimann T. Creatine kinase and creatine transporter in normal, wounded, and diseased skin. J Invest Dermatol. 2002;118:416–23.
31. Zemtsov A. Skin phosphocreatine. Skin Res Technol. 2007;13:115–8.

32. Snow RJ, Murphy RM. Creatine and the creatine transporter: a review. Mol Cell Biochem. 2001;224:169–81.
33. Speer O, Neukomm LJ, Murphy RM, et al. Creatine transporters: a reappraisal. Mol Cell Biochem. 2004;256–257:407–24.
34. McCully KK, Forciea MA, Hack LM, et al. Muscle metabolism in older subjects using 31P magnetic resonance spectroscopy. Can J Physiol Pharmacol. 1991;69:576–80.
35. Steinhagen-Thiessen E, Hilz H. The age-dependent decrease in creatine kinase and aldolase activities in human striated muscle is not caused by an accumulation of faulty proteins. Mech Ageing Dev. 1976;5:447–57.
36. Verzar F, Ermini M. Decrease of creatine-phosphate restitution of muscle in old age and the influence of glucose. Gerontologia. 1970;16:223–30.
37. Bogatskaia LN, Shegera VA. Creatine kinase activity and isoenzymic spectrum of myocardium creatine kinase in rats of different age. Ukr Biokhim Zh. 1981;53:71–4.
38. Ponticos M, Lu QL, Morgan JE, et al. Dual regulation of the AMP-activated protein kinase provides a novel mechanism for the control of creatine kinase in skeletal muscle. EMBO J. 1998;17:1688–99.
39. Stachowiak O, Schlattner U, Dolder M, Wallimann T. Oligomeric state and membrane binding behaviour of creatine kinase isoenzymes: implications for cellular function and mitochondrial structure. Mol Cell Biochem. 1998;184:141–51.
40. Chung JH, Eun HC. Angiogenesis in skin aging and photoaging. J Dermatol. 2007;34:593–600.
41. Ames BN, Shigenaga MK, Hagen TM. Oxidants, antioxidants, and the degenerative diseases of aging. Proc Natl Acad Sci U S A. 1993;90:7915–22.
42. Balaban RS, Nemoto S, Finkel T. Mitochondria, oxidants, and aging. Cell. 2005;120:483–95.
43. Shigenaga MK, Hagen TM, Ames BN. Oxidative damage and mitochondrial decay in aging. Proc Natl Acad Sci U S A. 1994;91:10771–8.
44. Wei YH, Lu CY, Wei CY, Ma YS, Lee HC. Oxidative stress in human aging and mitochondrial disease-consequences of defective mitochondrial respiration and impaired antioxidant enzyme system. Chin J Physiol. 2001;44:1–11.
45. Chance B, Sies H, Boveris A. Hydroperoxide metabolism in mammalian organs. Physiol Rev. 1979;59:527–605.
46. Cadenas E, Davies KJ. Mitochondrial free radical generation, oxidative stress, and aging. Free Radic Biol Med. 2000;29:222–30.
47. Droge W. Free radicals in the physiological control of cell function. Physiol Rev. 2002;82:47–95.
48. Stadtman ER. Protein oxidation and aging. Science. 1992;257:1220–4.
49. Huber LA, Xu QB, Jurgens G, et al. Correlation of lymphocyte lipid composition membrane microviscosity and mitogen response in the aged. Eur J Immunol. 1991;21:2761–5.
50. Nelson KK, Melendez JA. Mitochondrial redox control of matrix metalloproteinases. Free Radic Biol Med. 2004;37:768–84.
51. Harman D. Aging: a theory based on free radical and radiation chemistry. J Gerontol. 1956;11:298–300.
52. Sohal RS. Hydrogen peroxide production by mitochondria may be a biomarker of aging. Mech Ageing Dev. 1991;60:189–98.
53. Mori A, Utsumi K, Liu J, Hosokawa M. Oxidative damage in the senescence-accelerated mouse. Ann N Y Acad Sci. 1998;854:239–50.
54. Chiba Y, Yamashita Y, Ueno M, et al. Cultured murine dermal fibroblast-like cells from senescence-accelerated mice as in vitro models for higher oxidative stress due to mitochondrial alterations. J Gerontol A Biol Sci Med Sci. 2005;60:1087–98.
55. Trifunovic A, Wredenberg A, Falkenberg M, et al. Premature ageing in mice expressing defective mitochondrial DNA polymerase. Nature. 2004;429:417–23.
56. Hayakawa M, Torii K, Sugiyama S, Tanaka M, Ozawa T. Age-associated accumulation of 8-hydroxydeoxyguanosine in mitochondrial DNA of human diaphragm. Biochem Biophys Res Commun. 1991;179:1023–9.
57. Mecocci P, MacGarvey U, Kaufman AE, et al. Oxidative damage to mitochondrial DNA shows marked age-dependent increases in human brain. Ann Neurol. 1993;34:609–16.
58. Ames BN, Shigenaga MK, Gold LS. DNA lesions, inducible DNA repair, and cell division: three key factors in mutagenesis and carcinogenesis. Environ Health Perspect. 1993;5 Suppl 101:35–44.
59. Sohal RS, Dubey A. Mitochondrial oxidative damage, hydrogen peroxide release, and aging. Free Radic Biol Med. 1994;16:621–6.
60. Laganiere S, Yu BP. Modulation of membrane phospholipid fatty acid composition by age and food restriction. Gerontology. 1993;39:7–18.
61. Dumas M, Maftah A, Bonte F, et al. Flow cytometric analysis of human epidermal cell ageing using two fluorescent mitochondrial probes. C R Acad Sci III. 1995;318:191–7.
62. Paradies G, Ruggiero FM. Age-related changes in the activity of the pyruvate carrier and in the lipid composition in rat-heart mitochondria. Biochim Biophys Acta. 1990;1016:207–12.
63. Paradies G, Ruggiero FM. Effect of aging on the activity of the phosphate carrier and on the lipid composition in rat liver mitochondria. Arch Biochem Biophys. 1991;284:332–7.
64. Ruggiero FM, Cafagna F, Petruzzella V, Gadaleta MN, Quagliariello E. Lipid composition in synaptic and nonsynaptic mitochondria from rat brains and effect of aging. J Neurochem. 1992;59:487–91.
65. Orrenius S, Gogvadze V, Zhivotovsky B. Mitochondrial oxidative stress: implications for cell death. Annu Rev Pharmacol Toxicol. 2007;47:143–83.

66. Ha MK, Chung KY, Bang D, Park YK, Lee KH. Proteomic analysis of the proteins expressed by hydrogen peroxide treated cultured human dermal microvascular endothelial cells. Proteomics. 2005;5:1507–19.
67. Scharffetter-Kochanek K, Wlaschek M, Brenneisen P, et al. UV-induced reactive oxygen species in photocarcinogenesis and photoaging. Biol Chem. 1997;378:1247–57.
68. Suzuki YJ, Forman HJ, Sevanian A. Oxidants as stimulators of signal transduction. Free Radic Biol Med. 1997;22:269–85.
69. Davies KJ. The broad spectrum of responses to oxidants in proliferating cells: a new paradigm for oxidative stress. IUBMB Life. 1999;48:41–7.
70. Bladier C, Wolvetang EJ, Hutchinson P, de Haan JB, Kola I. Response of a primary human fibroblast cell line to H_2O_2: senescence-like growth arrest or apoptosis? Cell Growth Differ. 1997;8:589–98.
71. Chen Q, Ames BN. Senescence-like growth arrest induced by hydrogen peroxide in human diploid fibroblast F65 cells. Proc Natl Acad Sci U S A. 1994;91:4130–4.
72. Campisi J. The role of cellular senescence in skin aging. J Investig Dermatol Symp Proc. 1998;3:1–5.
73. Wallace DC. Mitochondrial genetics: a paradigm for aging and degenerative diseases? Science. 1992;256:628–32.
74. Pang CY, Lee HC, Yang JH, Wei YH. Human skin mitochondrial DNA deletions associated with light exposure. Arch Biochem Biophys. 1994;312:534–8.
75. Linnane AW, Marzuki S, Ozawa T, Tanaka M. Mitochondrial DNA mutations as an important contributor to ageing and degenerative diseases. Lancet. 1989;1:642–5.
76. Richter C. Oxidative damage to mitochondrial DNA and its relationship to ageing. Int J Biochem Cell Biol. 1995;27:647–53.
77. Piko L, Hougham AJ, Bulpitt KJ. Studies of sequence heterogeneity of mitochondrial DNA from rat and mouse tissues: evidence for an increased frequency of deletions/additions with aging. Mech Ageing Dev. 1988;43:279–93.
78. Cortopassi GA, Arnheim N. Detection of a specific mitochondrial DNA deletion in tissues of older humans. Nucleic Acids Res. 1990;18:6927–33.
79. Eshaghian A, Vleugels RA, Canter JA, et al. Mitochondrial DNA deletions serve as biomarkers of aging in the skin, but are typically absent in nonmelanoma skin cancers. J Invest Dermatol. 2006;126:336–44.
80. Porteous WK, James AM, Sheard PW, et al. Bioenergetic consequences of accumulating the common 4977-bp mitochondrial DNA deletion. Eur J Biochem. 1998;257:192–201.
81. Shoffner JM, Lott MT, Voljavec AS, et al. Spontaneous Kearns-Sayre/chronic external ophthalmoplegia plus syndrome associated with a mitochondrial DNA deletion: a slip-replication model and metabolic therapy. Proc Natl Acad Sci U S A. 1989;86:7952–6.
82. Schroeder P, Gremmel T, Berneburg M, Krutmann J. Partial depletion of mitochondrial DNA from human skin fibroblasts induces a gene expression profile reminiscent of photoaged skin. J Invest Dermatol. 2008;128:2297–303.
83. Berneburg M, Plettenberg H, Medve-Konig K, et al. Induction of the photoaging-associated mitochondrial common deletion in vivo in normal human skin. J Invest Dermatol. 2004;122:1277–83.
84. Yang JH, Lee HC, Wei YH. Photoageing-associated mitochondrial DNA length mutations in human skin. Arch Dermatol Res. 1995;287:641–8.
85. Birket MJ, Passos JF, von Zglinicki T, Birch-Machin MA. The relationship between the aging- and photo-dependent T414G mitochondrial DNA mutation with cellular senescence and reactive oxygen species production in cultured skin fibroblasts. J Invest Dermatol. 2009;129(6):1361–6.
86. Bandy B, Davison AJ. Mitochondrial mutations may increase oxidative stress: implications for carcinogenesis and aging? Free Radic Biol Med. 1990;8:523–39.
87. Wei YH, Lee CF, Lee HC, et al. Increases of mitochondrial mass and mitochondrial genome in association with enhanced oxidative stress in human cells harboring 4,977 BP-deleted mitochondrial DNA. Ann N Y Acad Sci. 2001;928:97–112.
88. Lu CY, Lee HC, Fahn HJ, Wei YH. Oxidative damage elicited by imbalance of free radical scavenging enzymes is associated with large-scale mtDNA deletions in aging human skin. Mutat Res. 1999;423:11–21.
89. Berneburg M, Grether-Beck S, Kurten V, et al. Singlet oxygen mediates the UVA-induced generation of the photoaging-associated mitochondrial common deletion. J Biol Chem. 1999;274:15345–9.
90. Kueper T, Grune T, Prahl S, et al. Vimentin is the specific target in skin glycation. Structural prerequisites, functional consequences, and role in skin aging. J Biol Chem. 2007;282:23427–36.
91. Hipkiss AR. Does chronic glycolysis accelerate aging? Could this explain how dietary restriction works? Ann N Y Acad Sci. 2006;1067:361–8.
92. Alikhani Z, Alikhani M, Boyd CM, et al. Advanced glycation end products enhance expression of pro-apoptotic genes and stimulate fibroblast apoptosis through cytoplasmic and mitochondrial pathways. J Biol Chem. 2005;280:12087–95.
93. Kasper M, Funk RH. Age-related changes in cells and tissues due to advanced glycation end products (AGEs). Arch Gerontol Geriatr. 2001;32:233–43.
94. Rugolo M, Lenaz G. Monitoring of the mitochondrial and plasma membrane potentials in human fibroblasts by tetraphenylphosphonium ion distribution. J Bioenerg Biomembr. 1987;19:705–18.

95. Scaduto Jr RC, Grotyohann LW. Measurement of mitochondrial membrane potential using fluorescent rhodamine derivatives. Biophys J. 1999;76:469–77.
96. Koopman WJ, Visch HJ, Smeitink JA, Willems PH. Simultaneous quantitative measurement and automated analysis of mitochondrial morphology, mass, potential, and motility in living human skin fibroblasts. Cytometry A. 2006;69:1–12.
97. Plasek J, Vojtiskova A, Houstek J. Flow-cytometric monitoring of mitochondrial depolarisation: from fluorescence intensities to millivolts. J Photochem Photobiol B. 2005;78:99–108.
98. Distelmaier F, Koopman WJ, Testa ER, et al. Life cell quantification of mitochondrial membrane potential at the single organelle level. Cytometry A. 2008;73:129–38.
99. Cossarizza A, Baccarani-Contri M, Kalashnikova G, Franceschi C. A new method for the cytofluorimetric analysis of mitochondrial membrane potential using the J-aggregate forming lipophilic cation 5,5′6,6-′-tetrachloro-1,1′3,3-′-tetraethylbenzimidazolcarbocyanine iodide (JC-1). Biochem Biophys Res Commun. 1993;197:40–5.
100. Hagens R, Khabiri F, Schreiner V, et al. Non-invasive monitoring of oxidative skin stress by ultraweak photon emission measurement. II: biological validation on ultraviolet A-stressed skin. Skin Res Technol. 2008;14:112–20.
101. Khabiri F, Hagens R, Smuda C, et al. Non-invasive monitoring of oxidative skin stress by ultraweak photon emission (UPE)-measurement. I: mechanisms of UPE of biological materials. Skin Res Technol. 2008;14:103–11.
102. Vandenberghe K, Goris M, Van Hecke P, et al. Long-term creatine intake is beneficial to muscle performance during resistance training. J Appl Physiol. 1997;83:2055–63.
103. Daly MM, Seifter S. Uptake of creatine by cultured cells. Arch Biochem Biophys. 1980;203:317–24.
104. Meyer LE, Machado LB, Santiago AP, et al. Mitochondrial creatine kinase activity prevents reactive oxygen species generation: antioxidant role of mitochondrial kinase-dependent ADP re-cycling activity. J Biol Chem. 2006;281:37361–71.
105. Lenz H, Schmidt M, Welge V, et al. Inhibition of cytosolic and mitochondrial creatine kinase by siRNA in HaCaT- and HeLaS3-cells affects cell viability and mitochondrial morphology. Mol Cell Biochem. 2007;306:153–62.
106. O'Gorman E, Beutner G, Dolder M, et al. The role of creatine kinase in inhibition of mitochondrial permeability transition. FEBS Lett. 1997;414:253–7.
107. Brdiczka D, Beutner G, Ruck A, Dolder M, Wallimann T. The molecular structure of mitochondrial contact sites. Their role in regulation of energy metabolism and permeability transition. Biofactors. 1998;8:235–42.
108. Dolder M, Walzel B, Speer O, Schlattner U, Wallimann T. Inhibition of the mitochondrial permeability transition by creatine kinase substrates. Requirement for microcompartmentation. J Biol Chem. 2003;278:17760–6.
109. Dolder M, Wendt S, Wallimann T. Mitochondrial creatine kinase in contact sites: interaction with porin and adenine nucleotide translocase, role in permeability transition and sensitivity to oxidative damage. Biol Signals Recept. 2001;10:93–111.
110. Berneburg M, Gremmel T, Kurten V, et al. Creatine supplementation normalizes mutagenesis of mitochondrial DNA as well as functional consequences. J Invest Dermatol. 2005;125:213–20.
111. Crane FL. Biochemical functions of coenzyme Q_{10}. J Am Coll Nutr. 2001;20:591–8.
112. McLennan HR, Degli EM. The contribution of mitochondrial respiratory complexes to the production of reactive oxygen species. J Bioenerg Biomembr. 2000;32:153–62.
113. Lopez-Lluch G, Barroso MP, Martin SF, et al. Role of plasma membrane coenzyme Q on the regulation of apoptosis. Biofactors. 1999;9:171–7.
114. Mellors A, Tappel AL. The inhibition of mitochondrial peroxidation by ubiquinone and ubiquinol. J Biol Chem. 1966;241:4353–6.
115. Frei B, Kim MC, Ames BN. Ubiquinol-10 is an effective lipid-soluble antioxidant at physiological concentrations. Proc Natl Acad Sci U S A. 1990;87:4879–83.
116. Lass A, Kwong L, Sohal RS. Mitochondrial coenzyme Q content and aging. Biofactors. 1999;9:199–205.
117. Hoppe U, Bergemann J, Diembeck W, et al. Coenzyme Q_{10}, a cutaneous antioxidant and energizer. Biofactors. 1999;9:371–8.
118. Podda M, Traber MG, Weber C, Yan LJ, Packer L. UV-irradiation depletes antioxidants and causes oxidative damage in a model of human skin. Free Radic Biol Med. 1998;24:55–65.
119. Kim DW, Hwang IK, Yoo KY, et al. Coenzyme Q_{10} effects on manganese superoxide dismutase and glutathione peroxidase in the hairless mouse skin induced by ultraviolet B irradiation. Biofactors. 2007;30:139–47.
120. Stab F, Wolber R, Blatt T, Keyhani R, Sauermann G. Topically applied antioxidants in skin protection. Methods Enzymol. 2000;319:465–78.
121. Hadshiew IM, Treder-Conrad C, v Bulow R, et al. Polymorphous light eruption (PLE) and a new potent antioxidant and UVA-protective formulation as prophylaxis. Photodermatol Photoimmunol Photomed. 2004;20:200–4.
122. Rippke F, Wendt G, Bohnsack K, et al. Results of photoprovocation and field studies on the efficacy of a novel topically applied antioxidant in polymorphous light eruption. J Dermatolog Treat. 2001;12:3–8.
123. Wolber R, Stab F, Max H, et al. Alpha-glucosylrutin, a highly effective flavonoid for protection against oxidative stress. J Dtsch Dermatol Ges. 2004;2:580–7.

Cellular Energy Metabolism and Oxidative Stress

48

Shujiang (Suzie) Cheng, Regina Hourigan, Zeenat Nabi, and Laurence Du-Thumm

Contents

S.S. Cheng • R. Hourigan (✉) • Z. Nabi • L. Du-Thumm
Colgate-Palmolive Company, Piscataway, NJ, USA
e-mail: suzie_cheng@colpal.com; regina_hourigan@colpal.com; zeenat_nabi@colpal.com; laurence_du-thumm@colpal.com

M.A. Farage et al. (eds.), *Textbook of Aging Skin*,
DOI 10.1007/978-3-662-47398-6_30

Abstract
The skin's energy metabolism systems lead to a decline in function and hence contribute to skin aging. This chapter discusses how the skin uses energy to maintain its appearance followed by a background on energy production in cells. Defects in energy production are part of the mitochondrial theory of aging. Recent advances in understanding how UV radiation contribute to skin aging will be discussed in this chapter, as well as antiaging therapies that improve or maintain metabolic functions of the skin are given.

Introduction

The objective of this chapter is to provide an overview of how changes to the skin's energy metabolism systems lead to a decline in function and hence contribute to skin aging. This chapter first discusses how the skin uses energy to maintain its appearance followed by a background on energy production in cells. Defects in energy production are part of the mitochondrial theory of aging, which will be introduced next. Skin-specific examples that support this theory of aging will be given as well as evidence that questions this theory. The examples are divided into chronological skin aging and extrinsic skin aging. Recent advances in understanding how environmental stresses, such as UV radiation, especially in the regions of ultraviolet-A (UVA), visible and near infrared (NIR), contribute to skin aging will be discussed. Lastly, examples of antiaging therapies that improve or maintain metabolic functions of the skin are given.

This chapter intends to also provide areas for discussion or debate, as there is a cyclic nature to the role of mitochondria in aging. It is not clear if aging causes mitochondrial defects or if mitochondrial defects cause aging. Similarly, while oxidative stress can cause mitochondrial defects, mitochondrial defects can also generate oxidative stress. It is in fact this cyclic nature which may progressively lead to more damage.

Energy Metabolism and the Role of Mitochondria in the Skin

As the largest organ of the body that covers all body surfaces, skin exerts a protective function against external insults. In order to maintain protection, it is constantly sacrificing while also regenerating itself. As such, the skin is composed of layers of proliferating cells which require high energy supply. For example, suprabasal layers of the epidermis and cells within the root of the hair follicle have high metabolic activity associated with the synthesis of keratin and the cornified envelopes. The energy to support such biosynthetic activities in skin, cells, or essentially all other types of cells is called adenosine triphosphate (ATP). It is required for proliferation as a result of mitogenic stimuli, collagen synthesis, and DNA repair. It supports functions that maintain skin turnover and the extracellular matrix. As skin ages, a decline or dysfunction in ATP production impacts the skin's functions and ultimately its appearance.

Mitochondria, the primary locations of ATP production, also have an impact on the skin through keratinocyte differentiation. In cell cultures, mitochondria-mediated cell death can trigger keratinocyte differentiation. Characteristics of differentiation (flattened morphology, stratification, and keratin 10 expression) are detected after a reactive oxygen species (ROS)-induced release of cytochrome *c* and apoptosis-inducing factor (AIF) [1].

Background on Mitochondria Structure and Function

This section briefly describes the mitochondrial mechanisms for energy production and provides a brief background for the later discussions. Mitochondria utilize the nutrients ingested, including carbohydrates, fats, and proteins, along with oxygen to generate ATP, which is used as chemical energy for most eukaryotic cells. They also control cell functions related to cell death, differentiation, and cell signaling. Mitochondria have their own DNA called mitochondrial DNA (mtDNA), while most other DNA of the cell reside in the nucleus.

The mitochondria are composed of several compartments, enclosed by an inner and outer membrane. The outer membrane contains a protein called porin, which forms aqueous channels allowing for transportation of molecules 10 kDa or less through the membrane. The more complex inner membrane is folded to create a large internal space, where the electron transport chain (ETC) is taking place to produce ATP. The components of ETC include five enzymatic complexes, called complexes I, II, III, IV, and V. These complexes use molecules derived from fuel sources to produce oxygen. The starting molecules are electron donators, reduced nicotinamide adenine dinucleotide (NADH), and reduced flavin adenine dinucleotide ($FADH_2$). The NADH enters at complex I and $FADH_2$ enters at complex II. Both complex I and II provide substrate for complex III, which through electron transfer produces substrate for complex IV. The output of complex IV is oxygen, which combines with the electrons and protons to form water. Electron transfer through complexes I–IV is managed by the complexes and electron carriers, such as coenzyme Q10 (CoQ10) and cytochrome *c*. The flow of electrons and ATP production are continuous within tissues containing mitochondria [2].

The exchange of electrons from a high-energy state to a lower-energy state generates an electrochemical proton gradient. This gradient provides the energy to drive the phosphorylation of adenosine diphosphate (ADP) to ATP. This process, in which ADP is converted to ATP using inorganic phosphate with the assistance of ATP synthase, is called oxidative phosphorylation (OxPHOS). It occurs in complex V. The ATP is then available for use as chemical energy for the cell [2].

ROS and Mitochondria

Through the mitochondrial respiratory chain, majority of electrons travel successfully to successive enzymatic complexes, but some electrons can leak from the ETC. These electrons readily react with the available oxygen to form the ROS. In fact, the locations for the highest ROS production in cells are mitochondria. It is thought that about 1–3 % of the O_2 reduced in the mitochondria may form superoxide [2]. The mitochondria contain antioxidant defenses to control the level of ROS. Superoxide anion, the primary ROS produced by mitochondria, is converted to hydrogen peroxide and water catalyzed by the antioxidant enzyme superoxide dismutase. The hydrogen peroxide is converted to water and molecular oxygen by catalase, glutathione peroxidase, or thioredoxin peroxidase from the mitochondrial antioxidant systems [3]. Although at times detrimental, ROS is also used for cell signaling [2], for example, for apoptosis of the cell [4]. Damage to the mitochondria increases ROS, which triggers the release of cytochrome *c* and apoptosis-inducing factor (AIF). Their release initiates the caspase-dependent and caspase-independent cell death pathways to remove the damaged cell [4].

ROS poses various damages to mitochondria, including protein carbonylation, lipid peroxidation, and mtDNA damage. The damaged mitochondria decline in function, which in turn generate more ROS. This is known as the "vicious cycle" where ROS are both a cause and a consequence of mtDNA mutations. The "vicious cycle" creates an amplifying feedback loop which sustains the damaging effects, even with a small amount of initial insult. The "vicious cycle" is believed to create ongoing elevated levels of stress, such as those found with aging [5, 6]. The ROS and its resulting "vicious cycle" are the foundations of the mitochondrial theory of aging.

Mitochondrial Theory of Aging

The free radical theory of aging (FRTA) was formed by Harman, in 1950s [7]. The FRTA proposes that the underlying source of aging is the accumulation of oxidative damage caused by free radicals in macromolecules and tissues. Later in 1970s, Harman proposed that the mitochondria's production of the ROS may be central to the FRTA [8]. This is called the mitochondrial theory of aging. A fundamental part of this theory is that mtDNA is at particular risk of ROS damage. This is proposed because of the proximity of mtDNA to the ROS-producing mitochondrial matrix.

The mitochondrial theory of aging is supported by evidence of age-related ROS accumulation and mitochondrial changes. There is an increase in ROS produced from the ETC with aging [9, 10]. Protein complexes I, II, and III are considered to be the sites of excessive ROS [11–14]. As tissues age, there is lower flux through the ETC and reduced ATP production [15]. The lower flux causes more free electrons to escape and form ROS [16, 17].

The increased ROS with age can directly damage the crucial structures of the mitochondria itself, such as proteins, lipids, and mtDNA [18–20]. ROS damages mtDNA by creating strand breaks within the mtDNA. Studies of the respiration-dependent mitochondrial processes conclude that mtDNA damage is related to a decline in respiratory processes. These processes include mitochondrial protein synthesis, oxygen consumption, and ATP generation. For example, as the amount of mtDNA damage increases, the mitochondria membrane potential lowers and cannot be maintained. Maintaining membrane potential is critical to the electrochemical proton gradient and OxPHOS. In parallel, cytochrome *c* is released into the cytoplasm, which activates caspases leading to premature apoptosis [21]. The compromised respiratory processes elevate ROS levels further, creating the above-mentioned "vicious cycle." As a result, accumulated oxidative DNA damage contributes to the aging process, which serves as evidence of the mitochondrial theory of aging.

However, it has been debated whether the accumulation of such oxidative damage is a cause or a consequence of aging. In 2007, Muller et al. reviewed the topic of whether oxidative stress determines life span. They conclude that the case for oxidative stress as a life span determinant may be tentatively made for *Drosophila melanogaster*, but is not certain in humans or mice [22]. Speakman et al. reported that a small European cave salamander (*Proteus anguinus*) possesses exceptionally long life span, but at the same time its protective ability against oxidative stress is not profound at all [23]. Kujoth et al. have proposed accumulation of mtDNA mutations, which promote that apoptosis may be a mechanism driving mammalian aging [24]. Recent work by Doonan et al. found that there is no impact on basal life span with increased levels of superoxide dismutase (through gene manipulation of *Caenorhabditis elegans*) [25]. While basal life span was not changed, improving organisms' ability to cope with elevated oxidative stress can lengthen life span. Supplying *C. elegans* with antioxidant mimetics extended their life span and normalized prematurely aged organisms' life spans, during exposure to oxidative stress [26]. The mitochondrial ROS production is not the only contributing factor of aging and might be more prominent in some particular model organisms than others. Coping with such cellular stress is critical to survival and longevity. It should be noted that other factors related to coping with stresses, such as inflammation or repair mechanisms, are also critical determinants of longevity. In the skin, stressful environments can clearly cause oxidative damage that leads to extrinsic aging, and there is likely a place for the mitochondrial theory of aging. Mitochondrial ROS production might be a cause of symptoms such as loss of skin elasticity [27].

Skin Energy Metabolism and Chronological Aging

Like every other organ, skin is aged through biological aging in a chronological fashion. Since skin is in direct contact with the external environment, external stress, such as ultraviolet radiation (UVR), also contributes significantly to the aging of skin. There are mainly three resources supplying energy to skin: mitochondrial oxidative phosphorylation, glycolysis, and the creatine/phosphocreatine system, which all undergo influence from chronological and extrinsic aging. This section discusses the chronological aging of skin, related to energy metabolism, and will be followed by a separate discussion on extrinsic skin aging and energy metabolism.

One approach to studying chronological aging is harvesting the skin cells from variously aged human donors and comparing their functions. When skin cells are collected in this manner, differences in the metabolic functions of age groups have been observed. According to Greco et al., in 2003, human dermal fibroblasts from 51 donors aged 1–103 years showed a clear reduction in mitochondrial processes with age. These included mitochondrial protein synthesis, respiration rate, and coupling of respiration to ATP production. In individuals above 40 years' age, there was a significant decline in the mitochondrial protein synthesis. There was also a significant decrease in endogenous native respiration rate within the age range of 40–90 years. Human skin fibroblasts also had a significant age-dependent decrease in the efficiency of respiration and phosphorylation. The ratio of skin cell's rate of respiration in the presence of ADP to that in the absence of ADP (RCR) is a measure of the OxPHOS's control of respiration efficiency. This ratio significantly decreased with the age of the donor [28]. In the skin cells, particularly from donors over the age of 40, metabolic functions decline as a function of age.

The loss of function of fibroblast cells may have been due to multiple causes experienced over their life span. Another study looked at the targeted influence of older mtDNA on cell functions. In this study, mitochondria from fibroblasts of 21 individuals between the ages of 20 weeks and 103 years were inserted into human mtDNA-less cells. An age-dependent decrease in growth rate and a decline in respiratory rate were detected in the cells receiving the older mitochondria [29]. Therefore, although the number of mitochondria in skin cells does not change as they age [30], chronologically aged mitochondria can cause characteristics of aging, such as reduced cell growth and respiratory functions.

The amount of available energy metabolites in the skin may be thought to be related to the age of the skin, that is, younger skin contains more energetic materials – yet that is not the case observed in vivo. There are no differences in the skin's basal levels of energy metabolites with age [31]. Using ^{31}P nuclear magnetic resonance spectroscopy, young and old skin (ventral aspect of the wrist) from panelists did not show differences in baseline levels of phosphocreatine, inorganic phosphate, adenosine triphosphate, phosphomono, and phosphodiesters. However, what is significantly different is how the age groups respond to stress. After single exposure to a low, suberythema level of UVA irradiation, there were significant differences in the response and recovery of energy metabolism. The older skin showed slower response and recovery than younger skin [31]. This is an indication of the importance of evaluating skin aging characteristics in basal as well as stressed conditions. This is an important consideration when evaluating therapies related to energy metabolism. An antiaging material may not influence the basal characteristics of the skin but may be influential in reducing stresses or upregulating repair, thereby preventing extrinsic aging.

The mitochondria and its functions play both causative and effective roles in cell dysfunctions and senescence (cells stop proliferation). Senescent human cell cultures are a model for chronological aging [32]. The loss of mitochondrial functions, as passage number increases, can cause premature senescence in skin cells. It induces a senescent phenotype likely with the increase in ROS. This has been demonstrated by a reduction in the level of OxPHOS in fibroblasts causing a reduction in cell proliferation and premature senescence in human fibroblasts [33].

On one hand, the mitochondria dysfunction can lead to senescence, but on the other changes that occur with senescence can effect mitochondrial respiration. With increasing passage number, senescent fibroblasts show a loss of membrane potential along with notably higher ROS levels [34] and a decline in ATP production [35]. This may be due to inefficient removal of mitochondrial damage in the cells as proteasomes activity declines.

Proteasome inhibition is emerging as a common factor, based on in vitro and in vivo experiments, in aging and age-related diseases. Proteasomes are part of the protein removal system for most eukaryotic cells. At the molecular level, aging in one way is reflected in the accumulation of altered proteins, such as oxidized proteins. This could potentially lead to protein damage. Proteasomes contain proteases, which degrade damaged or unnecessary proteins from the cell. Proteasome activity declines with age in the human epidermis [36]. Keratinocytes that undergo replicative senescence are known to have a reduction in proteasome levels [37]. While oxidative damage has been known to cause proteasome dysfunction during aging, Torres and Perez later showed that proteasome inhibition is a mediator of oxidative stress and ROS production by affecting mitochondrial function. They proposed that a progressive decrease in proteasome function during aging can promote mitochondrial damage and ROS accumulation [38]. For fibroblasts collected from human donors of different age groups, significant decline of proteasome activity has been observed from young-aged groups (23–29 years old) to middle-aged groups (60 $\pm$ 8 years old). In human fibroblast cells, there is functional interplay between the mitochondrial and proteasomal systems, as the pharmacological inhibition can cause the drop in mitochondrial function, and vice versa. [39]

Skin Energy Metabolism and Extrinsic Aging

The change in skin appearance from external insults is called extrinsic aging. These insults can include UVR, pollution, and smoking. The major cause of extrinsic aging is UVR, referred to as photoaging, which accounts for up to 80 % of the environmental factors to aging [40]. UVA (320–400 nm) and UVB (290–320 nm) are the two major wavelengths that the skin is exposed to, while UVC gets absorbed in the ozone layer. The sunlight emits 10–100 times more UVA than UVB; therefore, UVA accounts for the majority of the skin damage as it also penetrates deeper into skin dermis. Although far less abundant, UVB radiation is considered highly damaging to skin DNA [41]. Photoaged skin has many well-accepted characteristics, such as loss of elasticity, reduced hydration, greater barrier damage, to mention a few. The UVR induces theses changes by interacting with and damaging skin structures, that is, the proteins, DNA, and lipids of the skin. mtDNA can also be damaged by UVR. Greater accumulations of mtDNA damage are found in sun-exposed skin compared to protected skin [42–49]. The most prominent mtDNA damage/mutation is called common deletion (CD). It is thought that mtDNA CD caused by UVR are mediated by ROS, particularly superoxide.

The 4,977-base pair (bp) mitochondrial CD and 3,895-bp mitochondrial CD are among the recognized mtDNA deletions related to skin photoaging [44, 47, 48, 52]. The 4,977-bp deletion is called the common deletion because it is the most prevalent marker of mtDNA damage in humans and is found in several types of tissues. Its increase is associated with age in several tissues [50]. The 3,895-bp deletion, which is less reported, may also play a role in skin photoaging [48].

The 4,977-bp deletion occurs in both in vitro and in vivo skin studies and relates to UVR exposure. The common deletion was found in human skin fibroblasts treated with a repeated, sublethal dose of UVA [43]. It is generated by singlet oxygen induced by UVA [51]. Studies with keratinocytes are less numerous, but have also indicated a link between UVR and mitochondrial damage. A single dose of UVB exposure to keratinocytes induced two mtDNA deletions: the 4,977-bp and a novel 5,128-bp deletion [52]. In vivo, the common deletion can be induced in the dermal tissue of living skin after repeated exposure to UVA radiation. UVA induced a 40 % increase in CD in the dermis, but not in the epidermis of the irradiated skin [44].

There are differing findings on the presence of the 4,977-bp deletion in chronologically aged skin. There is evidence for an age-related increase in the 4,977-bp type of deletion in skin mtDNA. The 4,977-bp deletion was not found in skin samples from donors under the age of 60 years. The frequency of this deletion in skin did increase with age for individuals who were 60–90 years old [44]. Keratinocytes-induced 4,977-bp deletion has, in other cases, not corresponded to the chronological age of the donors (30–78 years). Koch et al. noted slower cell proliferating body sites, that is, blood, brain, and skeletal tissues, and showed correlation between chronological age and increasing mtDNA deletion [47].

The 3,895-bp deletion corresponds to broad-spectrum UV exposure in both in vitro and in vivo studies. HaCaT cells (engineered keratinocytes as experimental models) exposed to repeated UVA/UVB doses were found to have the mtDNA 3,895-bp deletion [48]. Among skin samples from 42 skin donors, the 3,895-bp deletion was found at a higher amount in "usually" sun-exposed body sites (face, ears, neck, and scalp) compared with "occasionally" exposed sites (shoulders, back, and chest). The deletion was not detected in the body sites that were "rarely" exposed to sunlight. The 3,895-bp deletion induction was in both the epidermis and the dermis of the exposed sites. In the usually exposed sites, the level was almost equal in the epidermis and the dermis. Therefore, mitochondrial damage may serve as a biomarker for cumulative sun exposure [48].

In summary, UV-induced ROS can cause mtDNA damage, which serves as a marker of skin damage. Moreover, a 23-fold increase in mtDNA copy number has also been observed in sun-exposed skin versus less exposed skin. Indicating copy number could also be served as a potential biomarker for UV exposure [51]. These genetic changes also lead to a decline in mitochondrial function, especially in energy supply. The UVA-induced common deletion in human dermal fibroblasts corresponds to decreases in oxygen consumption, mitochondrial membrane potential, and ATP content [53]. This leads to compromised mitochondrial respiration.

Once compromised in this manner, the mitochondrial respiration causes an increase in ROS produced by the ETC. The intracellular mitochondrial oxidative stress generated under these conditions upregulates matrix metalloproteinase-1 (MMP-1) [53]. MMP-1 is an accepted indicator of aged and damaged skin. MMP-1 is the major enzyme that is counted responsible for collagen degradation in photoaged skin [54], the skin of tobacco smokers [55], and chronologically aged (sun-protected) skin [56]. Skin fibroblast studies have shown that in the absence of UVA, a deletion of 4,977-bp causes an increase of MMP-1. UVA-induced common deletion also corresponds to an increase in the expression of MMP-1 without an increase of the tissue-specific MMP inhibitors [53]. The cascade of UV stress, ROS generation, mtDNA damage, and elevated ROS from compromised respiration leads to collagen degradation, a direct factor in the appearance of aged skin.

While this cascade has a linear sequence of events, there is also a feedback loop (the "vicious cycle" mentioned earlier) created by the ROS. The ROS that cause mitochondrial respiratory dysfunction lead to more ROS being produced by the cell. There has been recent evidence of the "vicious cycle" in the skin as measured by sustained mtDNA damage. The common deletion was found in in vivo experimental treatment to remain in UV-exposed skin for up to 16 months. In some cases, the deletion continued to increase after UV exposure has ceased [44]. This increase after exposure and sustained level of mtDNA deletion may be due to the ongoing cycle of ROS generation and mtDNA mutations. This "vicious cycle" may be a source of chronic oxidative stress within the skin. The chronic stress may be a factor in premature aging as the ROS may then interact with skin proteins, initiate inflammation, and promote extracellular matrix degradation (Fig. 1).

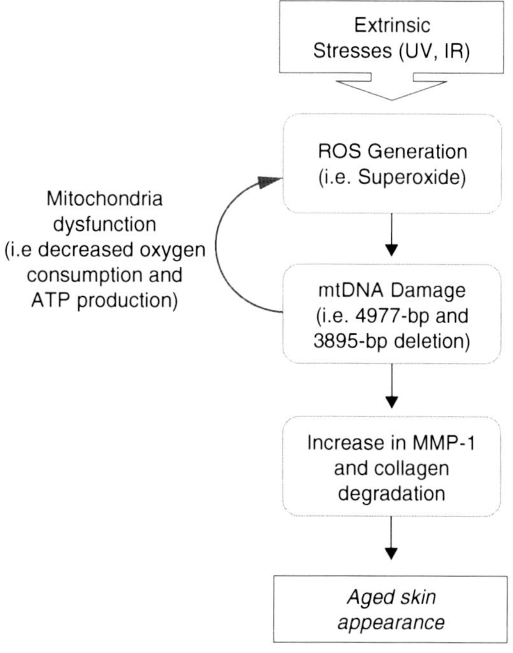

Fig. 1 The potential vicious cycle of mitochondrial damage and skin aging

While ultraviolet radiation has been well studied for its impact on skin photoaging, recent studies are now showing an emerging role for infrared radiation (IR) in photoaging. IR accounts for more than half of the solar energy that reaches the human skin [57]. It is divided into IRA (Infrared Radiation A), IRB (Infrared Radiation B), and IRC (Infrared Radiation C). IRB and IRC do not penetrate deeply into the skin, while more than 65 % of IRA reaches the dermis [57]. Near IRA (760–1,440 nm) can induce MMP-1 expression in ex vivo fibroblast cells [58]. Similar to UVA, IRA radiation induces collagen breakdown [41]. The production of ROS from IRA stress originates from the mitochondrial ETC. Cultured fibroblasts treated with antioxidants are protected from the IRA radiation and do not upregulate MMP-1 expression [58]. In vivo studies also show that skin responds to IRA radiation with upregulation of MMP-1 in the dermis [59]. In conclusion, on the molecular level, photoaging includes the alterations of inflammatory cells and protein oxidation caused by UV, as well as the IRA-induced retrograde signaling cascades [41].

Select Topical Antiaging Approaches

This section highlights select antiaging approaches targeting at cellular metabolism. As mentioned above, one protective approach is with antioxidants. DNA, lipids, and proteins are known to be protected by the application of antioxidants on the skin. Antioxidants can regulate the transfer of electrons or quench the free radicals escaping from the ETC. This can mitigate the effects of photoaging through the prevention of oxidative damage and the related damage to mitochondrial functions. Some examples of antioxidants are glutathione, CoQ10, and *N*-acetyl cysteine (NAC).

At low concentrations of the antioxidant glutathione, UVB-induced mtDNA deletions have been prevented [52], giving further evidence that mtDNA damage by UVR is mediated by ROS. At higher levels of glutathione, when it acts as a reductive antioxidant (electron donor) and hence a deleterious agent, the protective effect ceases and the mtDNA deletions return [52].

CoQ10 is a known antioxidant found in the mitochondria and serves to carry electrons in the ETC. Its level in the skin declines with age and UV stress [60]. A series of in vitro and in vivo experiments by Hoppe et al. have shown the benefits of CoQ10 in prevention of skin aging. Topical application of CoQ10 reduced wrinkle depth and level of oxidation in vivo. CoQ10 is also effective in protecting the DNA of keratinocytes from UVA-induced oxidative stress and reducing the expression of collagenase in dermal fibroblasts following UVA irradiation [61].

N-Acetyl cysteine (NAC) is an antioxidant which increases the intracellular concentration of glutathione (GSH) [62]. Lipoic acid and NAC supplementation of Alzheimer's patient's fibroblasts protected the mitochondria from oxidative stress in vitro [63]. Although not performed with skin cells, NAC oral supplementation of mice increases the mitochondrial respiration of senescent liver cells. The liver cells' ETC complexes had higher activity, while levels of protein carbonyls, a marker of protein oxidation, were reduced [64].

The second group of topical actives include cell regulators such as retinols, peptides, and botanicals [65]. These molecules directly stimulate the collagen metabolism and thus provide the skin with antiaging benefits. Retinol, also known as vitamin A, promotes collagen synthesis in photoaged skin. In one clinical study, 53 individuals in their 80s were treated with 1 % retinol topically for 1 week. It was found that a number of proteases involved in the breakdown of collagen, including collagenase, matrix metalloproteinase, were all downregulated, resulting in increased fibroblast growth and collagen synthesis [66]. This is one of the many studies that prove the efficacy of retinol, the retinol derivative, and the retinoid family in treatment of aging.

Another therapy for the improvement of skin's energy metabolism is to provide the skin with energy supplementation. One approach is with the amino acid creatine. Creatine is the precursor to phosphocreatine. Phosphocreatine is synthesized in the mitochondria by creatine kinases. Phosphocreatine can donate a phosphate group to ADP to produce ATP. This provides an additional reserve of ATP that can be used by cells for metabolic activity. Creatine does not offer direct UV protection, rather its protective effect is from increasing cell energy reserves. Lenz et al. observed the photoprotective effect of creatine on human skin cells in vitro and in vivo [67]. Supplementation of normal human fibroblasts with creatine during repeated UVA exposure showed a mitigation of mtDNA mutations as well as the normalization in oxygen consumption and MMP-1 production [53]. Creatine also prevents the common deletion, and inhibitors of creatine block these effects [53]. These data show that while UVA reduces mitochondrial function, supplementation with creatine can mitigate these effects. The researchers suggest that the prevention of UVA-induced common deletion may be from creatine's ability to normalize the cell's energy status. This prevents an upregulation of a deleterious respiratory chain, which generates more ROS [53].

Supplementation with energy precursors also allows for more efficient repair. Maes et al. have shown, in a skin model, that DNA repair from UV stress exposure is enhanced with creatine [68]. In human clinicals, with a formulation containing creatine, acetyl-L-carnitine, and NADH, reduced the appearance of aging [69]. The researchers believed that the enhanced repair was due to the increased availability of ATP that the creatine provided. Under the stress of UV, the cells can synthesize the needed repair enzymes using this additional ATP [68, 69].

Combinations of the above therapies are also effective. In vivo, a combination of CoQ10 and a stabilized form of creatine in a topical emulsion improved signs of skin aging, including density of the dermal papillae [70]. Protecting cellular energy metabolism of skin can improve protection from UV stress, provide energy for repair systems during stress, and cause positive changes to the skin morphology.

Conclusion

Aging is a complex topic involving all of the functions of the skin, and its underlying mechanism is difficult to attribute to any single biological source. Multiple studies give evidence that mitochondrial damage is either the cause or a marker of age-related dysfunctions in the skin. The damage, and related decline in mitochondrial functions, can create aged skin appearance. The contribution of mitochondrial damage to skin aging may be amplified by the presence of a vicious cycle. Mitigation and prevention of this mitochondrial damage alleviates the signs of skin aging. While by no means the only factor in skin aging, alterations to the skin's energy metabolism systems lead to a decline in function and hence contribute to skin aging.

Cross-References

▶ Alterations of Energy Metabolism in Cutaneous Aging

References

1. Tamiji S, et al. Induction of apoptosis-like mitochondrial impairment triggers antioxidant and Bcl-2-dependent keratinocyte differentiation. J Invest Dermatol. 2005;125:647–58.
2. Halliwell B, Gutteridge JMC. Free radicals in biology and medicine. 4th ed. New York: Oxford University Press; 2007.
3. Marchi S, et al. Mitochondria-Ros crosstalk in the control of cell death and aging. J Signal Transduct. 2012;2012:329635.
4. Danial NN, Korsmeyer SJ. Cell death: critical control points. Cell. 2004;116:205–19.
5. Linnane A, et al. Mitochondrial DNA mutations as an important contributor to ageing and degenerative diseases. Lancet. 1989;1:642–5.
6. Bandy B, Davison AJ. Mitochondrial mutations may increase oxidative stress: implications for carcinogenesis and aging? Free Radic Biol Med. 1990;8:523–39.
7. Harman D. Aging: a theory based on free radical and radiation chemistry. J Gerontol. 1956;11(3):298–300.
8. Harman D. The biologic clock: the mitochondria? J Am Geriatr Soc. 1972;20(4):145–7.
9. Barja G. Mitochondrial free radical production and aging in mammals and birds. Ann N Y Acad Sci. 1998;854:224–38.
10. Moghaddas S, Hoppel C, Lesnefsky EJ. Aging defect at the QO site of complex III augments oxyradical production in rat heart interfibrillar mitochondria. Arch Biochem Biophys. 2003;414:59–66.
11. Chen Q, et al. Production of reactive oxygen species by mitochondria central role of complex III. J Biol Chem. 2003;278(38):36027–31.
12. Turrens JF. Superoxide production by the mitochondrial respiratory chain. Biosci Rep. 1997;17(1):3–8.
13. Turrens JF. Mitochondrial formation of reactive oxygen species. J Physiol. 2003;552(2):335–44.
14. Barja G. Mitochondrial oxygen radical generation and leak: sites of production in states 4 and 3, organ specificity, and relation to aging and longevity. J Bioenerg Biomembr. 1999;31(4):347–66.
15. Harper ME, et al. Age-related increase in mitochondrial proton leak and decrease in ATP turnover reactions in mouse hepatocytes. Am J Physiol Endocrinol Metab. 1998;275:197–206.
16. Qian T, Nieminen AL, Herman B, Lemasters JJ. Mitochondrial permeability transition in

pH-dependent reperfusion injury to rat hepatocytes. Am J Physiol. 1997;273:C1783–92.
17. Chen Q, Lesnefsky EJ. Depletion of cardiolipin and cytochrome *c* during ischemia increases hydrogen peroxide production from the electron transport chain. Free Radic Biol Med. 2006;40:976–82.
18. Chen JJ, Yu BP. Alterations in mitochondrial membrane fluidity by lipid peroxidation products. Free Radic Biol Med. 1994;17:411–8.
19. Sohal RS, Dubey A. Mitochondrial oxidative damage, hydrogen peroxide release, and aging. Free Radic Biol Med. 1994;16:621–6.
20. Agarwal S, Sohal RS. DNA oxidative damage and life expectancy in houseflies. Proc Natl Acad Sci U S A. 1994;91:12332–5.
21. Mandavilli BS, Santos JH, Van Houten B. Mitochondrial DNA repair and aging. Mutat Res. 2002;509:127–51.
22. Muller F, et al. Trends in oxidative aging theories. Free Radic Biol Med. 2007;43(4):477–503.
23. Speakman JR, et al. The free-radical damage theory: accumulating evidence against a simple link of oxidative stress to ageing and lifespan. Bioessays. 2011;33 (4):255–9.
24. Kujoth GC, et al. Mitochondrial DNA mutations, oxidative stress, and apoptosis in mammalian aging. Science. 2005;309:481–4.
25. Doonan R, et al. Against the oxidative damage theory of aging: superoxide dismutases protect against oxidative stress but have little or no effect on life span in *Caenorhabditis elegans*. Genes Dev. 2008;-22:3236–41.
26. Melov S, et al. Extension of life-span with superoxide dismutase/catalase mimetics. Science. 2000;289 (5484):1567–9.
27. Brand MD, et al. The role of mitochondrial function and cellular bioenergetics in ageing and disease. Br J Dermatol. 2013;169:1–8.
28. Greco M, et al. Marked aging-related decline in efficiency of oxidative phosphorylation in human skin fibroblasts. FASEB J. 2003;17:1706–8.
29. Laderman KA, et al. Aging-dependent functional alterations of mitochondrial DNA (mtDNA) from human fibroblasts transferred into mtDNA-less cells. J Biol Chem. 1996;271:15891–7.
30. Quinlan CL, et al. The role of mitochondrial function and cellular bioenergetics in aging and disease. Br J Dermatol. 2013;169(02):1–8.
31. Declercq L, et al. Age-dependent response of energy metabolism of human skin to UVA exposure: an *in vivo* study by 31P nuclear magnetic resonance spectroscopy. Skin Res Technol. 2002;8:125–32.
32. Cristofalo VJ, et al. Use of the fibroblast model in the study of cellular senescence. In: Barnett Y, Barnett C, editors. Aging methods and protocols. Totowa: Humana Press; 2000. p. 26.
33. Stockl P, et al. Sustained inhibition of oxidative phosphorylation impairs cell proliferation and induces premature senescence in human fibroblasts. Exp Gerontol. 2006;41:674–82.
34. Mammone T, Gan D, Foyouzi-Youss R. Apoptotic cell death increases with senescence in normal human dermal fibroblast cultures. Cell Biol Int. 2006;30:903–9.
35. Zwerschke W, et al. Metabolic analysis of senescent human fibroblasts reveals a role for AMP in cellular senescence. Biochem J. 2003;376(Pt 2):403–11.
36. Bulteau AL, Petropoulos I, Friguet B. Age-related alterations of proteasome structure and function in aging epidermis. Exp Gerontol. 2000;35:767–77.
37. Petropoulos I, et al. Increase of oxidatively modified protein is associated with a decrease of proteasome activity and content in aging epidermal cells. J Gerontol Biol Sci Med Sci. 2000;55:B220–7.
38. Torres CA, Perez VI. Proteasome modulates mitochondrial function during cellular senescence. Free Radic Biol Med. 2008;44:403–14.
39. Jansen-Durr P, et al. Functional interplay between mitochondrial and proteasome activity in skin aging. J Invest Dermatol. 2011;131:594–603.
40. Poljsak B. General overview of skin: extrinsic (external) and intrinsic (free radical mediated internal) factors. In Skin aging, free radicals and antioxidants. Nova Science Publishers; pp. 39–66.
41. Krutmann J. Skin aging. In Nutrition for healthy skin. Springer-Verlag Berlin Heidelberg; 2011 pp. 15–24.
42. Yang JH, Lee HC, Lin J, Wei YH. A specific 4977-bp deletion of mitochondrial DNA in human ageing skin. Arch Dermatol Res. 1994;286:386–90.
43. Berneburg M, et al. Singlet oxygen mediates the UVA-induced generation of the photoaging-associated mitochondrial common deletion. J Biol Chem. 1999;274(22):15345–9.
44. Berneburg M, et al. Induction of the photoaging-associated mitochondrial common deletion *in vivo* in normal human skin. J Invest Dermatol. 2004;122 (5):1277–83.
45. Birch-Machin MA, et al. Mitochondrial DNA deletions in human skin reflect photo-rather than chronologic aging. J Invest Dermatol. 1998;111 (4):709–10.
46. Ray A, et al. The spectrum of mitochondrial DNA deletions is a ubiquitous marker of ultraviolet radiation exposure in human skin. J Invest Dermatol. 2000;115:674–9.
47. Koch H, Wittern K-P, Bergemann J. In human keratinocytes the common deletion reflects donor variabilities rather than chronologic aging and can be induced by ultraviolet a irradiation. J Invest Dermatol. 2001;117:892–7.
48. Krishnan K, Harbottle A, Birch-Machin MA. The use of a 3895 bp mitochondrial DNA deletion as a marker for sunlight exposure in human skin. J Invest Dermatol. 2004;123:1020–4.
49. Eshaghian A, et al. Mitochondrial DNA deletions serve as biomarkers of aging in the skin, but are typically

absent in nonmelanoma skin cancers. J Invest Dermatol. 2006;126:336–44.
50. Ji F, et al. Novel mitochondrial deletions in human epithelial cells irradiated with an FS20 ultraviolet light source in vitro. J Photochem Photobiol. 2006;184(3):340–6.
51. Cortopassi GA, et al. A pattern of accumulation of a somatic deletion of mitochondrial DNA in aging human tissues. Proc Natl Acad Sci U S A. 1992;89:7370–4.
52. Gebhard D et al. Mitochondrial DNA copy number – but not a mitochondrial tandem CC to TT transition – is increased in sun-exposed skin. Exper Dermatol. 2014;23(3):209–11.
53. Berneburg M, et al. Creatine supplementation normalizes mutagenesis of mitochondrial DNA as well as functional consequences. J Invest Dermatol. 2005;125:213–20.
54. Brennan M, et al. Matrix metalloproteinase-1 is the major collagenolytic enzyme responsible for collagen damage in UV-irradiated human skin. Photochem Photobiol. 2003;78(1):43–8.
55. Lahmann C, et al. Matrix metalloproteinase-1 and skin ageing in smokers. Lancet. 2001;357(9260):935–6.
56. Varani J, et al. Vitamin A antagonizes decreased cell growth and elevated collagen-degrading matrix metalloproteinases and stimulates collagen accumulation in naturally aged human skin. J Invest Dermatol. 2000;114:480–6.
57. Schroeder P, Haendeler J, Krutmann J. The role of near infrared radiation in photoaging of the skin. Exp Gerontol. 2008;43:629–32.
58. Schroeder P, et al. Cellular response to infrared radiation involves retrograde mitochondrial signaling. Free Radic Biol Med. 2007;43(1):128–35.
59. Schroeder P, et al. Infrared radiation-induced matrix metalloproteinase in human skin: implications for protection. J Invest Dermatol. 2008;128:2491–7.
60. Podda M, et al. UV radiation depletes antioxidants and causes oxidative damage in a model of human skin. Free Radic Biol Med. 1998;24:55–65.
61. Hoppe U, et al. Coenzyme Q10, a cutaneous antioxidant and energizer. Biofactors. 1999;9(2–4):371–8.
62. Zafarullah M, et al. Molecular mechanisms of *N*-acetylcysteine actions. Cell Mol Life Sci. 2003;60 (1):6–20.
63. Moreira P, et al. Lipoic acid and *N*-acetyl cysteine decrease mitochondrial-related oxidative stress in Alzheimer disease patient fibroblasts. J Alzheimer's Dis. 2007;12(2):195–206.
64. Miquel J, et al. *N*-Acetylcysteine protects against age-related decline of oxidative phosphorylation in liver mitochondria. Eur J Pharmacol. 1995;292:333–5.
65. Ganceviciene R, et al. Skin anti-aging strategies. Dermatoenocrinol. 2012;4(3):308–19.
66. Mukherjee S, et al. Retinoids in the treatment of skin aging: an overview of clinical efficacy and safety. Clin Interv Aging. 2006;1(4):327–48.
67. Lenz H, et al. The creatine kinase system in human skin: protective effects of creatine against oxidative and UV damage in vitro and in vivo. J Invest Dermatol. 2005;124:443–52.
68. Maes D, et al. Improving cellular function through modulation of energy metabolism. IFSCC Mag. 2002;2:121–6.
69. Declerq L, et al. Cosmetic benefits from modulation of cellular energy metabolism. In: Wille JJ, editor. Energy skin delivery systems: transdermals, dermatologicals, and cosmetic actives. 1st ed. Ames: Wiley-Blackwell; 2006. p. 117–24.
70. Blatt T, et al. Stimulation of skin's energy metabolism provides multiple benefits for mature skin. The Fourth Conference of the International Coenzyme Q10 Association. BioFactors Special Issue. 2005;25 (1–4):179–85.

DNA Damage and Repair in Skin Aging 49

Daniel B. Yarosh

Contents

D.B. Yarosh (✉)
The Estee Lauder Companies, Inc., Melville, NY, USA
e-mail: dyarosh@danyarosh.com

M.A. Farage et al. (eds.), *Textbook of Aging Skin*,
DOI 10.1007/978-3-662-47398-6_31

Abstract

Skin aging reflects the accumulation of damage to DNA from both internal and environmental sources. While solar UV induces the most frequent modifications of DNA, air pollution and tobacco smoke have also been demonstrated to induce the cascade of repair responses triggered by DNA damage. Cells use complexes of proteins to remove or reverse DNA damage, but if the lesions are not repaired, a sequence of proteins is activated that invokes wound-healing reactions or cell death. If these reactions are not sufficient to control the DNA damage, the skin risks immunosuppression, destruction of the collagen support structure, and even cancer. Genetic mutations in DNA repair genes can cause hereditary cancer diseases, while simple polymorphisms in some DNA repair genes in apparently healthy people may also predispose them to cancer. Methods to defend against DNA damage include melanin, sunscreens, antioxidants, and administration of DNA repair enzymes.

Introduction

DNA has many roles in skin cell function, including directing metabolism, storing the information of heredity, and sensing cell danger. Damage to DNA is correlated with, and probably a major cause of, aging in general and skin aging in specific [1]. Our natural repair system offers significant protection, and new compounds offer the promise of augmenting DNA repair.

This chapter will focus to a large extent on UV damage to DNA because solar UV is by far the greatest danger to DNA. Sun exposure is a major public health concern and has been directly linked to most of the more than 3.5 million new skin cancers that arise in the USA each year [2]. Over the past 20 years, the incidence rates of nonmelanoma skin cancer and melanoma have consistently increased [3]. DNA damage caused by solar UV has been directly linked to these skin cancers, as the cancers contain in their inactivated tumor suppressor gene mutations that are characteristic of UV [4]. Other important contributors to DNA damage that cause skin aging are tobacco smoking and air pollution.

Sources of DNA Damage

DNA damage comes from two sources: the intrinsic metabolism of the cell and environmental insult.

Intrinsic Metabolism. During aerobic energy generation, about 2 % of all the oxygen burned ends up as reactive oxygen species (ROS). DNA is damaged by ROS most frequently by the oxidation of the guanine base to form 8-oxoguanine (8oxoG), which is often misread by the DNA replication machinery causing a mutation. This is particularly serious for mitochondria, whose DNA is closest to the source of the short-lived ROS. Stress, caused by, e.g., long working hours, is associated with increased levels of 8oxoGua in urine [5]. In addition, disruption of the circadian rhythm by our modern lifestyles and normal aging can also increase the accumulation of DNA damage by disrupting DNA repair [6].

Environmental insult. By far the most serious damage to skin DNA is from the sun, because DNA readily absorbs photons in the UV region producing modified DNA bases. These modified bases cause a characteristic type of DNA mutation produced by no other carcinogen, and these signature mutations are frequently found in key cancer genes in squamous and basal cell carcinomas. This is the smoking gun that connects sun exposure to this sign of premature aging. Solar UV may indirectly damage DNA by creating reactive oxygen species that then react with DNA. Additional environmental sources of DNA damage to skin come from pollutants carried in the air, particularly in urban areas.

Sun Damage to DNA

Wavelengths of Sunlight that Damage DNA

DNA readily absorbs photons in the UV portion of the solar spectrum. Although the shorter UVC wavelengths (200–280 nm) do not actually reach the earth's surface due to their absorption by the ozone layer, the longer-wavelength UVB (280–320 nm) is still relatively efficient in causing direct damage to the DNA bases and penetrates largely only into the epidermis [7]. The even longer-wavelength UVA (320–400 nm) penetrates into the dermis; however, since these photons carry less energy, they are relatively less efficient in producing direct damage to DNA than UVB and create proportionately more reactive oxygen species in the skin cells that indirectly damage DNA [8]. Recent evidence suggests that very high fluences of visible light can produce indirect DNA damage through the formation of reactive oxygen species [9].

Photoproducts

Solar UV directly causes an instantaneous photochemical reaction in DNA that links together adjacent pyrimidine bases (cytosine or thymine) [10]. This *cyclobutane pyrimidine dimer* (CPD) is the most common form of DNA damage and is formed by all UV wavelengths, including UVA, UVB, and UVC [11]. After a sunburn dose, on the order of 100,000 CPDs are formed in the DNA of every sun-exposed cell. In a much less common reaction, solar UV can directly link together these bases by a single twisted bond, resulting in a *6-4-photoproduct* (<6-4 > PP) [11].

Solar UV can also cause DNA damage by an indirect method, through the formation of reactive oxygen species that attack DNA, particularly the guanine base. This oxidation reaction most often results in 8-oxo-guanosine (8oGua), but even after UVA exposure, CPDs are much more common than 8oGua [12]. Oxidation of DNA can also result in single-stranded breaks, but under physiological conditions, these are very difficult to detect. When single-stranded breaks are found after UV irradiation, they are almost all caused by DNA repair enzymes cutting the DNA in an intermediate step in repair.

Recently, a new pathway has been described wherein fragments of melanin are excited by UV-induced reactive oxygen and nitrogen species and then transfer the energy to DNA to form CPDs even in the dark [13].

Air Pollution Damage to DNA

Pollutants carried in the air are becoming a serious source of DNA damage in urban environments. Carcinogens in tobacco smoke attach an alkyl group to DNA. The most prevalent are at the 7-position of guanine (N^7-alklylGua) and to the phosphates of the DNA backbone, but a much less common form of damage, alkylation of the 6-position of guanine (O^6-alkylGua) is the most mutagenic and hence the most dangerous. Polyaromatic hydrocarbons coating the surface of air pollutants, particularly 2.5 μm particulates (PM2.5), are becoming a significant source of 8oGua [14]. Ground-level ozone is also capable of damaging the DNA of keratinocytes [15].

Mechanisms of DNA Repair

DNA is the rare biomolecule that is not discarded when it is damaged, but rather is repaired. Human cells have developed two fundamental repair strategies to restore DNA to its native sequence and conformation.

Nucleotide Excision Repair

More than 20 different proteins participate in this multistep process, and many of these proteins also participate in RNA transcription and/or DNA synthesis. In a typical day, a cell may have to repair 10,000 damaged bases and after sun exposure each cell of the skin may have to remove 100,000 lesions! This process consumes cellular stores of nicotinamide adenine dinucleotide (NAD), which are used to tag sites of single-stranded breaks and other damages. The depletion of NAD can endanger cell energy reserves, so niacin and niacinamide, members of the vitamin B family and precursors of NAD, are necessary to replenish the NAD reservoir.

Major damage to DNA, such as CPDs or <6-4 > PPs, interferes with its coding ability and must be repaired in order for the nucleotide sequence to function. Each of these is removed in a patch of about 30 DNA nucleotides by a process termed *nucleotide excision repair* (NER) [16]. A dozen or more proteins may cooperate to complete NER. One subset of these proteins recognizes CPDs throughout the genome because they distort the regular turns of the DNA helix, and they initiate *global genomic repair* (GGR). However, an additional set of proteins are especially responsive to RNA transcription forks which are stalled at sites of CPDs in the coding sequence, and they are able to more quickly mobilize the NER machinery to these regions of DNA vital to cell function to initiate *transcription-coupled repair* (TCR).

Once these recognition proteins bind to the site of DNA damage, they recruit additional enzymes that unwind the DNA, make a single-stranded break on either side of the CPD, and release the 30-nucleotide piece of DNA. The single-strand gap is then filled in by DNA polymerases using the opposite strand of the DNA as a template. Each cell has several varieties of DNA polymerases and most of them copy DNA very accurately. However, a few types are much more error prone and when they are called into service, they introduce mutations by incorporating incorrect bases into the patch [17].

NER of CPDs is not a very efficient process. After UV exposure that produces a sunburn in human skin, it takes about 15 h to remove 50 % of the CPD and 5 h to remove 50 % of the <6-4 > PPs [18]. This is due to the fact that <6-4 > PPs are less frequent, and they so greatly distort DNA that they are easier for the NER proteins to locate and excise.

Base Excision Repair

Damage to single bases such as 8oGua distorts DNA much less and is repaired by a second pathway termed *base excision repair* (BER) [16]. Here a DNA repair enzyme termed an *oxoguanine glycosylase-1* (OGG1) specifically recognizes 8oGua and releases it from the DNA backbone, leaving a vacant (abasic) site. A second enzyme recognizes this baseless site and makes a single-stranded break. A few bases on either side of the break are removed, and the short patch is again resynthesized using the opposite strand as a template. This is a speedy process, and half of the 8oGua introduced by solar UV are repaired in about 2 h [19].

In human cells, CPDs are not repaired by BER because there is no glycosylase to recognize them. However, the bacteriophage enzyme *T4 endonuclease V* recognizes CPDs and clips one side of the CPD from the DNA, initiating BER. Amazingly, when delivered into human cells, this enzyme functions quite well to initiate repair of CPDs by BER [20].

Photoreactivation

An additional pathway of DNA repair is used by plants, fish, reptiles, and amphibians, but it is not present in humans or other mammals. This repair is accomplished by the enzyme *photolyase* by directly reversing CPD. It captures long-wavelength UV and visible light and uses the energy to split the bonds that bind together the pyrimidine bases in a CPD [21]. This restores the DNA to normal without producing a single-stranded break or removing any DNA. Once again, while human cells have no photolyase enzymes, when these enzymes are introduced into human cells, they function quite well in repairing CPDs [22].

Diseases of DNA Repair

Much has been learned by studying rare genetic diseases with defects in DNA repair and other diseases in which skin cancer rates are elevated. This has not only clarified the function of many of the DNA repair proteins but has also revealed that many DNA repair proteins have multiple functions in the cell.

Xeroderma Pigmentosum, Trichothiodystrophy, Cockayne Syndrome

Xeroderma pigmentosum (XP) is characterized by mild to extreme photosensitivity, often with areas of hypo- and hyperpigmentation, an increased risk of skin cancer, and a shortened life expectancy [23]. There are seven complementation groups of XP (A-G), corresponding to defects in one of the seven genes that code for proteins involved in NER, and a variant group with a defect in repair synthesis. Stringent photoprotection from an early age can greatly reduce actinic damage, but does not prevent neurological defects that are a hallmark of some of the complementation groups. This may be because some of these genes are also involved in non-DNA repair gene transcription.

Trichothiodystrophy (TTD) patients have a defect in the same gene as XP-D patients, but at different locations within the gene, so they manifest photosensitivity, stunted growth, and brittle hair, but not an increase in skin cancer [23]. This highlights that subtle differences in a DNA repair protein can produce drastic differences in human development and morphology. Patients with Cockayne Syndrome (CS) have mutations in one of the two genes that code for proteins controlling TCR, and they also have growth and developmental abnormalities, but surprisingly little increased risk of skin cancer [23].

Solid Organ Transplant Patients

Organ transplant patients have an elevated rate of skin cancer on sun-exposed skin during the period in which they are on immunosuppressive therapy [24]. There is no doubt that suppression of the immune system plays a significant role in allowing nascent skin cancers to grow out. However, there is increasing evidence that these drugs also impair DNA repair in the skin [25]. The two most widely used drugs, CsA and tacrolimus, target the phosphatase calcineurin. Calcineurin dephosphorylation of the nuclear transcription factor NFAT allows NFAT to localize in the nucleus, where it is a key activator of transcription of several immunoregulatory genes. Immobilization of calcineurin sequesters NFAT in the cytoplasm and shuts down transcription of these genes. Other transcription factors, such as TFHII, are vital to the preferential repair of DNA by targeting the repair machinery to sites of stalled transcription complexes. NFAT may also participate in recovery from transcription blocks. Switching immunosuppressors to those that do not target calcineurin reduces rates of skin cancer [26].

DNA Repair Gene Polymorphisms

The genes implicated in DNA repair deficiency genetic diseases code for proteins that participate not only in DNA repair but in other routine developmental programs and cell functions. The general population carries many forms of these genes with other, less serious, mutations and these forms are called *genetic polymorphisms*. While some of these polymorphisms are innocuous, some gene forms increase the risk of cancer, including skin cancer [27]. A growing body of evidence suggests that polymorphisms in base excision repair genes contribute to diseases of aging [28].

One such DNA repair gene polymorphism is in the OGG1 gene coding for the glycosylase that releases 8oGua from DNA. The OGG1 polymorphism S326C has been associated with an increased risk of several types of cancer [29]. However, three separate in vitro biochemical studies of the activity of the protein produced by the variant gene failed to identify any deficit in activity or reduced DNA repair of oxidatively damaged DNA [30–32]. The S326C variant polymorphism in the OGG1 gene is linked to increased risk of cancers such as prostate cancer, but the protein produced by the variant gene does not have any obvious biochemical defects. The variant polymorphic genotype, however, is the most sensitive to cell killing by cytotoxic agents, and the heterozygous genotype was most resistant [33]. The delivery of exogenous OGG1 enzyme to cells increased repair of 8-oxoguanine in the homozygous variants [19]. Thus, subtle changes in DNA repair genes may alter their activity in cells and increase susceptibility to endogenous and exogenous damage.

Prevention of DNA Damage

Melanin

The first line of defense against DNA damage is the pigment deposited by melanocytes at the surface of the skin. Melanocytes are pigment-producing cells that are found in the basal layer of the epidermis and disperse melanosomes, containing melanin, among the surrounding keratinocytes. These melanosomes encapsulate two main classes of pigment found in the human skin: eumelanin, which is brown or black, and pheomelanin, which is reddish brown. The relative amounts of these two pigments, and the size and density of the melanosomes, largely determine the differences in skin color among humans.

The constitutive pigment that is associated with racial groups is deposited by melanocytes above the nuclei of keratinocytes, thereby shielding them from UV. Skin color has an enormous effect on the risk of skin cancer because this constitutive melanin absorbs and reflects a broad spectrum of UVR. Thus, UV exposure to dark skin produces less DNA damage than in light skin. The induced pigmentation in tanned skin, however, is significantly dispersed as pigment granules, rather than capping nuclei. The result is that tanned skin is much less protective against DNA damage than the equivalent in constitutive color.

As noted previously, new research suggests that fragments of melanin, particularly red pheomelanin, can actually produce DNA damage itself by catalyzing the formation of cyclobutane pyrimidine dimers even in the absence of light [13]. This may well counterbalance the protective effects of melanin, especially in lightly or red pigmented people.

Sunscreens

Sunscreens are an additional defense against DNA damage by reflecting or absorbing UV at the skin surface. The absorbed energy is released from the sunscreen molecules mostly as fluorescence or heat. Sunscreens are either inorganic physical sunscreens that largely reflect light or chemical sunscreens that mostly absorb light. Some sunscreens are less photostable than others and lose their absorption capacity during UV exposure. Some of the energy absorbed by sunscreen molecules can cause the release ROS, and this is true of both physical and chemical sunscreens. Recent advances in sunscreen development have been designed to reduce or eliminate these possibilities. To date, there is no evidence that ROS released by sunscreens in skin cause significant levels of DNA damage. Of far greater concern is that sunscreens are usually not used properly or in the right amounts, and despite their application, significant DNA damage still results [34].

The most frequently used physical UV filters are the inorganic micropigments, zinc oxide or titanium dioxide, in the range of 10–100 nm in diameter. These micropigments are capable of reflecting a broad spectrum of UV rays in the UVA and UVB region. Major disadvantages of micropigments are that they also reflect visible light, creating the so-called "ghost" effect on skin, and they are difficult to formulate, often resulting in disagreeable preparations in which the micropigments have a strong tendency to agglomerate, which greatly decrease their efficacy.

Chemical UV filters have the capacity to absorb short-wavelength UV photons and to transform them into heat by emitting long-wavelength photons (infrared radiation) which are much less likely to damage DNA. Most chemical filters absorb in a relatively small wavelength range. In general, chemical filters may be divided into molecules which absorb primarily in the UVB region (290–310 nm) and those which primarily absorb in the UVA region (320–400 nm). Only a few efficiently absorb both UVB and UVA photons. Although these are relatively easier to formulate into cosmetically elegant textures, combinations of chemical filters are required in order to meet regulatory standards for sun protection.

Antioxidants

A third protection against the formation of DNA damage is antioxidants. Antioxidants absorb ROS and thereby prevent oxidative DNA damage, primarily 8oGua. The natural skin antioxidant system is composed of lipophilic antioxidants such as vitamin E and CoQ_{10} and hydrophilic antioxidants such as vitamin C and glutathione and the enzymes catalase and superoxide dismutase. An exciting new finding is that the powerful antioxidant ergothioneine and its receptor (OCNT-1) are found in the suprabasal layer of the epidermis, as well as in dermis. This implicates ergothioneine as a new natural component of the human skin antioxidant system.

Antioxidants cooperate to regenerate each other after reacting with ROS. For example, oxidation of vitamin C leads to its fast degradation, but vitamin E can generate oxidized vitamin C. In the same way, vitamin C can regenerate ergothioneine. Complete antioxidant protection requires many types of antioxidants, since ROS can be in the form of singlet oxygen, superoxides, or peroxides, as well as others. They can also be sequestered in the water or lipid compartment of cells. Therefore, the examination of the antioxidant protection system of skin requires consideration of all the antioxidants as a network.

Cellular Effects of DNA Damage

A complex system regulates the cell's progression through division to insure that only undamaged ones replicate, in order to avoid genetic instability and cancer [35, 36]. As cells approach commitment to DNA synthesis (S phase), proteins encoded by checkpoint genes delay entry if DNA damage is present. DNA protein kinases, such as ATM (ataxia-telangiectasia mutated) and ATR (ataxia-telangiectasia mutated and Rad3 related), then initiate signaling cascades resulting in DNA damage responses that include activation of the p53 protein. This tumor suppressor plays a central role in whether a cell repairs the damage [16] or is diverted into programmed cell death (apoptosis), cell cycle arrest, or senescence [35]. New insights reveal that the AKT/mTOR pathway opposes the p53-controlled pathways, inhibiting apoptosis and increasing proliferation even in the face of DNA damage [37].

Mitochondrial DNA is damaged largely as a result of oxidative damage secondary to the production of excess ROS by UV or normal metabolism. Sufficient levels of this damage cause release of mitochondrial factors, such as cytochrome C, which binds to the apoptotic protease-activating factor 1 (Apaf-1), resulting in the formation of the apoptosome. This critical event leads to the activation of caspase-9 and the initiation of the mitochondrial apoptotic pathway through caspase-3 activation [38]. Apoptosis is a critical event preventing damaged cells from progressing to malignancy.

One new photoprotection strategy is to selectively target DNA-damaged cells for apoptosis while leaving normal cells unaffected. Oral administration of caffeine or green tea (which often contains high levels of caffeine) in amounts equivalent to three to five cups of coffee per day to UVB-exposed mice increased levels of p53, slowed cell cycling, and increased apoptotic sunburn cells in the epidermis [39]. Human studies confirm that coffee has a modest protective effect against melanoma [40] and basal cell carcinoma [41].

Signal Transduction

These dramatic events that follow DNA damage indicate that DNA is an important sensor of environmental insult and is able to trigger a variety of cell responses. The molecular mechanisms for this sensor-effector mechanism are being unraveled.

The UV-induced cyclobutane pyrimidine dimers and pyrimidine [4–6] pyrimidone photoproducts cause distortions in the DNA helix and halt RNA polymerase II (RNA-PII) transcription of DNA. Protein kinases that activate their downstream targets via phosphorylation play an important role in signal transduction. A group of protein kinases that interact with DNA (ATR, Chk2, DNA-PK) are implicated in the molecular cascade that detects and responds to several forms of DNA damage caused by genotoxic stress [42]. ATR (ATM-Rad3-related kinase) is a primary DNA sensor and essential for UV-induced phosphorylation of several G1/S checkpoint proteins. ATR was also shown to bind UVB-damaged DNA, with a resulting increase in its kinase activity, with many proteins as its target [43].

One such target is the RNA-PII itself, where phosphorylation represses further transcription initiation. This stalled RNA polymerase II leads to recruitment of the nucleotide excision repair complex. Another target of ATR is p53. Following phosphorylation, the half-life of the p53 protein is increased drastically, leading to a quick accumulation of p53 in stressed cells. Next, a conformational change forces p53 to take on an active role as a transcriptional regulator in these stressed cells. p53 is able to transactivate a plethora of genes with an active role in cell cycle arrest, global genomic DNA repair, apoptosis, and cytokine release.

Systemic Effects of DNA Damage

Cytokines

DNA in skin acts like a sensor for UV damage on behalf of both exposed and unexposed cells in distal parts. DNA damage triggers the production and release of cytokines that act on the cell itself, as well as other cells with such cytokine receptors, to activate characteristic UV responses, such as wound healing and immunosuppression [44]. Keratinocytes are the main source of these cytokines. Other epidermal cells, like Langerhans cells (LHC), and melanocytes, together with infiltrating leukocytes, are also active contributors to changed cytokine profile after UV exposure. Keratinocytes are able to secrete a wide variety of pro-inflammatory cytokines upon UV exposure, including interleukins IL-1α, IL-1β, IL-3, IL-6, and IL-8, granulocyte colony stimulating factor (G-CSF), granulocyte macrophage–CSF (GM-CSF), interferon gamma (INF-γ), platelet-derived growth factor (PDGF), transforming growth factor alpha (TGF-α), TGF-β, and tumor necrosis factor-α (TNFα) [45–47].

Cytokines such as IL-1 and TNFα then induce a cascade of other cytokines that can activate collagen-degrading enzymes, suppress the immune system, dilate blood vessels, and attract inflammatory T cells [48]. In this way, cells with DNA photodamage, even if they are destined to die, have profound effects on cells in the skin and elsewhere that may not have been UV exposed.

IL-12 plays a curious role in photoprotection. It is an immunostimulatory cytokine that is released by keratinocytes at late times after UV in order to counteract the suppressive effects of IL-10 [49]. Recently, it has also been reported to stimulate the repair of CPDs in the DNA of keratinocytes in a manner yet to be understood [50].

Immunosuppression

UV-induced immunosuppression is an essential event for skin cancer formation [51]. It is important to note that this is not generalized immunosuppression, but a reduced ability to respond to antigens presented just after exposure. There may be a genetic susceptibility to UV-induced suppression, because skin cancer patients are more easily UV suppressed than cancer-free controls [52]. At lower UV doses, the primary target is the Langerhans cells, which flee the epidermis, and those with DNA damage have impaired antigen-presenting ability [53]. Higher doses produce systemic immunosuppression, mediated by the generation of suppressor T cells, in which non-exposed skin becomes hampered in responding to antigens [51]. In several experimental models, including humans, reducing DNA damage decreases the degree of immunosuppression [54].

Wound Healing and Photoaging

UV-induced DNA damage also triggers a wound-healing response in skin, as it tries to eliminate damaged cells and stimulate cell division to replace them. UVR directly to fibroblasts, as well as signals from damaged keratinocytes, causes the release of metalloproteinase (MMP-1) which selectively degrades large collagen cables [55]. Soluble factors released by keratinocytes, including IL-1, IL-6, and TNFα, are principle actors in this paracrine effect [56]. DNA damage is directly related to the release of soluble mediators since enhanced repair of keratinocyte DNA reduced the release of the mediators and lowered the release of MMP-1 by unirradiated fibroblasts [57].

As part of this response, MMP-2 and MMP-9, which are responsible for digesting small collagen fragments, are downregulated by UVR. This results in the accumulation of collagen fragments, which severs the anchorage of fibroblasts, inhibits their ability to produce new collagen, and degrades the dermal elastic fiber network [58]. This is followed by hyperproliferation among keratinocytes, and together these responses are designed to fill in sites of skin wounds.

Repeated rounds of this type of imperfect wound healing produce many of the microscopic hallmarks of photoaged skin, including a corresponding decrease in the biophysical properties of the skin [59], reflected in a loss of both skin strength and elasticity, flattening of the rete ridges, and the appearance of wrinkles and skin folds. Additionally, there are degradative vascular changes in the dermis resulting in telangiectasia and decreases in the capillary network and in skin blood flow [60]. These small changes accumulate after repeated rounds of DNA damage to form what is readily recognized as aged skin.

These connections, from DNA damage to stalled transcription complexes, resulting in kinase cascades activating metalloproteinases which degrade skin collagen, explain why photoaging is a product of unrepaired DNA lesions. It is likely that other sources of DNA damage, such as tobacco smoke and air pollution, induce similar cascades resulting in premature skin aging.

Mutations and Skin Cancer

Mutations

Most of the solar UV-induced DNA damage distorts the double helix. In attempting to replicate past CPD lesions, the cell often makes the same mistake of misincorporating two consecutive bases, resulting in mutations characteristic of UV damage [4]. In many cases, these mutations have no effect on the cell, but if they occur at critical locations in tumor suppressor genes, they abrogate apoptosis and initiate the process of carcinogenesis. These UV "signature" mutations are often found in mutated p53 genes, a key tumor suppressor gene, in human squamous cell carcinoma and basal cell carcinoma [4]. This is the key link between UV exposure and skin cancer and directly implicates CPDs in carcinogenesis. These p53 signature mutations are also frequently found in precancerous actinic keratosis, suggesting that these mutations are an early step in the process of forming squamous cell carcinomas and that later steps, such as additional gene mutations and immunosuppression, determine if a cell goes on to malignancy.

The situation is less clear in melanoma. There appears to be many different tumor suppressor genes that can be mutated in melanoma, and the frequency of signature mutations is not as common as in squamous cell carcinoma [61].

Mitochondria generate energy for the cell, and they contain DNA that encodes many of the crucial proteins in the energy production machinery. This DNA is also subject to mutations, and mitochondria develop a peculiar type of mutation called the *common deletion*, in which a particular 477 base pair section of the DNA is deleted. The frequency of the common deletion in the mitochondria of human skin cells does not correlate with chronological age, but rather with sun exposure and photoaging [62]. This implies that solar UV is responsible for the formation of the common deletion, and its contribution to the signs of photoaging is an active area of research.

Prevention of Skin Cancer with DNA Repair Enzymes

The inevitable consequence of the accumulation of DNA damage over a lifetime is an increased incidence of mutations and an elevated risk of skin cancer. The primary strategy for reducing this risk is the attenuation of the UV dose striking the skin, by sun avoidance, pigmentation, and sunscreens. Antioxidants have become a part of the defense by scavenging ROS before they can oxidize DNA. The next step in intervention is the enhanced repair of DNA damage before it can fix as a mutation and increase the probability of malignant transformation.

Over the past 40 years, the field of DNA repair has identified many enzymes that recognize and initiate removal of DNA damage, either by nucleotide excision repair, base excision repair, or direct reversal. The use of some of these enzyme activities for photoprotection became practical with the development of liposomes specifically engineered for delivery into skin [63].

The small protein T4 endonuclease V from bacteriophage recognizes the major form of DNA damage produced by UVB, which is the cyclobutane pyrimidine dimer (CPD). Liposomal delivery of T4 endonuclease V to UV-exposed human skin increased repair from 10 % of CPD to 18 % over 6 h but dramatically reduced or eliminated the release of cytokines such as IL-10 and TNFα [64]. In a randomized clinical study of the effects of the daily use of this liposomal T4 endonuclease V in XP patients, the rate of premalignant actinic keratosis and basal cell carcinoma was reduced by 68 % and 30 %, respectively, compared to the placebo control [65].

Associations with Aging Signs

Sun exposure is the greatest and best understood contributor to skin aging. However, two other external sources of DNA damage are responsible for accelerated skin aging. Cigarette smokers look old for their age, and they have elevated levels of MMP-1 in their skin [66]. More recently, the degree of air pollution has been positively correlated with signs of skin aging, such as wrinkles and pigment spots [67]. Air pollution particles coated with polyaromatic hydrocarbons are particularly dangerous because they can also compromise the barrier function of skin [68] allowing deeper penetration of DNA-damaging compounds.

Conclusion

During a lifetime, skin is exposed to chemical challenges generated by its own metabolism as well as the environment, particularly solar UV. There are a variety of defenses, such as skin color, sunscreens, and antioxidants, to counteract these. Inevitably, however, cells sustain damage.

DNA serves the cell not only as the master controlled of cell function, and the storehouse of heredity information, but also as a sensor of damage and consequently a sentinel for danger to the cell and the organism. It is able to convert the distortion caused by altered nucleic acid bases into signals that arrest and redirect its own cell machinery. It also converts that distortion into notification of adjoining cells, whether damaged or not, that significant lesions have occurred. The purpose of these signals is to evoke repair and healing responses.

DNA is a unique macromolecule in carrying with it the toolkit for its own repair. DNA repair is focused at the site of actively transcribed DNA by a complex of enzymes, some of which are specifically adapted to recognize modified DNA and some borrowed from the transcription machinery itself. The repair may have the task of repairing hundreds of thousands of lesions daily, and while it is an efficient process, it is not perfect. The resulting mutations in the DNA sequence are the necessary components for the development of skin cancer.

Skin aging, therefore, can be viewed as the accumulation of imperfections from repeated rounds of DNA damage and repair, as well as rounds of wounding and healing. Skin cancer is just one manifestation of these cycles. Viewed in this way, it is likely that properly conceived efforts to alleviate skin aging will also have the benefit of reducing rates of skin cancer. Since over long periods of time, people are more motivated by improving their physical appearance than lowering their perceived risk of disease, the most successful anticancer efforts will arrive as treatments for skin aging.

Cross-References

▸ Fibulin-5 Deposition in Human Skin: Decrease with Aging and UVB Exposure and Increase in Solar Elastosis

References

1. Freitas A, de Magalhaes J. A review and appraisal of the DNA damage theory of ageing. Mutat Res. 2011;728:12–22.
2. Rogers H, et al. Incidence estimate of nonmelanoma skin cancer in the United States, 2006. Arch Dermatol. 2010;146:283–7.
3. Jou P, Tomecki K. Sunscreens in the United States: current status and future outlook. Adv Exp Med Biol. 2014;810:464–84.
4. Brash D. Sunlight and the onset of skin cancer. Trends Genet. 1997;13:410–4.
5. Irie M, et al. Occupational and lifestyle factors and urinary 8-hydroxydeoxyguanosine. Cancer Sci. 2005;96:600–6.
6. Kettner NM, Katchy CA, Fu L. Circadian gene variants in cancer. Ann Med. 2014;46:208–20.
7. Yarr M, et al. Photoageing: mechanism, prevention and therapy. Br J Dermatol. 2007;157:874–87.
8. Cadet J, et al. Ultraviolet radiation -mediated damage to cellular DNA. Mutat Res. 2005;571:3–7.
9. Mahmoud BH, et al. Effects of visible light on the skin. Photochem Photobiol. 2008;84:450–62.
10. Schreier W, et al. Thymine dimerization in DNA is an ultrafast photoreaction. Science. 2007;315:625–9.
11. Yoon J-H, et al. The DNA damage spectrum produced by simulated sunlight. J Mol Biol. 2000;299:681–93.
12. Courdavault S, et al. Larger yield of cyclobutane dimers than 8-oxo-7, 8-dihydroguanine in the DNA of UVA-irradiated human skin cells. Mutat Res. 2004;556:135–42.
13. Premis S, et al. Chemiexcitation of melanin derivatives induces DNA photoproducts long after UV exposure. Science. 2015;347:842–7.
14. Huang HB, et al. Traffic-related air pollution and DNA damage: a longitudinal study. PLoS One. 2012;7:e37412.
15. McCarthy JT, et al. Effects of ozone in normal human epidermal keratinocytes. Exp Dermatol. 2013;22:360–1.
16. Sancar A, et al. Molecular mechanisms of mammalian DNA repair and the DNA damage checkpoints. Ann Rev Biochem. 2004;73:39–85.
17. Christmann M, et al. Mechanisms of human DNA repair: an update. Toxicology. 2003;193:3–34.
18. Bykov VJ, et al. *In situ* repair of cyclobutane pyrimidine dimers and 6-4 photoproducts in human skin exposed to solar simulating radiation. J Invest Dermatol. 1999;112:326–31.
19. Yarosh D, et al. After sun reversal of DNA damage: enhancing skin repair. Mutat Res. 2005;571:57–64.
20. Tanaka K, et al. Restoration of ultraviolet-induced unscheduled DNA synthesis of xeroderma pigmentosum cells by the concomitant treatment with bacteriophage T4 endonuclease V and HVJ (Sendai virus). Proc Natl Acad Sci U S A. 1975;72:4071–5.
21. Carell T, et al. The mechanism of action of DNA photolyases. Curr Opin Chem Biol. 2001;5:491–8.
22. Stege H, et al. Enzyme plus light therapy to repair DNA damage in ultraviolet-B-irradiated human skin. Proc Natl Acad Sci U S A. 2000;97:1790–5.
23. Cleaver J. Cancer in xeroderma pigmentosum and related disorders of DNA repair. Nat Rev. 2005;5:564–73.
24. Randle H. The historical link between solid-organ transplantation, immunosuppression, and skin cancer. Dermatol Surg. 2004;30:595–7.
25. Yarosh D, et al. Calcineurin inhibitors decrease DNA repair and apoptosis in human keratinocytes following ultraviolet B irradiation. J Invest Dermatol. 2005;125:1020–5.
26. Wheless L, et al. Skin cancer in organ transplant recipients: more than the immune system. J Am Acad Dermatol. 2014;71:359–65.
27. Au W, Navasumrit P, et al. Use of biomarkers to characterize functions of polymorphic DNA repair genotypes. Int J Hyg Environ Health. 2004;207:301–4.
28. Wilson D, et al. Variation in base excision repair capacity. Mutat Res. 2011;711:100–12.
29. Goode E, Ulrich C, Potter J. Polymorphisms in DNA repair genes and associations with cancer risk. Cancer Epidemiol Biomarkers Prev. 2002;11:1513–30.
30. Kohno T, et al. Genetic polymorphisms and alternative splicing of the hOOG1 gene, that is involved in the repair of 8-hydroxyguanine in damaged DNA. Oncogene. 1988;16:3219–25.
31. Dherin C, et al. Excision of oxidatively damaged DNA bases by the human α-hOGG1 protein and the polymorphic α-hOGG1(Ser326Cys) protein which is frequently found in human populations. Nucleic Acids Res. 1999;27:4001–7.
32. Janssen K, et al. DNA repair activity of 8-oxoguanine DNA glycosylase I (OGG1) in human lymphocytes is

not dependent on genetic polymorphism Ser^{326}/Cys^{326}. Mutat Res. 2001;486:207–16.
33. Yarosh D, et al. DNA repair gene polymorphisms affect cytotoxicity in the National Cancer Institute Human Tumour Cell Line Screening Panel. Biomarkers. 2005;10:188–202.
34. Mahroos AI, et al. Effect of sunscreen application on UV-induced thymine dimers. Arch Dermatol. 2002;138:1480–5.
35. Funk JO. Cell cycle checkpoint genes and cancer. Encyclopedia of Life Sciences. John Wiley & Sons Ltd 2005. pp. 1–5.
36. Harper JW, et al. The DNA damage response: ten years after. Mol Cell. 2007;28:739–45.
37. Strozyk E, Kulms D. The role of AKT/mTOR pathway in stress response to UV-irradiation: implication in skin carcinogenesis by regulation of apoptosis, autophagy and senescence. Int J Mol Sci. 2013;14:15260–85.
38. Guzman E, et al. Mad dogs, Englishmen and apoptosis: the role of cell death in UV-induced skin cancer. Apoptosis. 2003;8:315–25.
39. Lu Y-P, et al. Effect of caffeine on the ATR/Chk1 pathway in the epidermis of UVB-irradiated mice. Cancer Res. 2008;68:2523–9.
40. Loftfield E, et al. Coffee drinking and cutaneous melanoma risk in the NIH-AARP diet and health study. J Natl Cancer Inst. 2015;107:dju421.
41. Ferrucci L, et al. Tea, coffee, and caffeine and early-onset basal cell carcinoma in case–control study. Eur J Cancer Prev. 2014;23:296–302.
42. Zhou BB, et al. The DNA damage response: putting checkpoints in perspective. Nature. 2000;408:433–9.
43. Unsal-Kacmaz K, et al. Preferential binding of ATR protein to UV-damaged DNA. Proc Natl Acad Sci U S A. 2002;99:6673–8.
44. Kondo S. The roles of keratinocyte-derived cytokines in the epidermis and their possible responses to UVA-irradiation. J Investig Dermatol Symp Proc. 1999;4:177–83.
45. Ansel J, et al. Cytokine modulation of keratinocyte cytokines. J Invest Dermatol. 1990;94:101S–7.
46. Luger TA, et al. Evidence for an epidermal cytokine network. J Invest Dermatol. 1990;95:100S–4.
47. Enk A, et al. Early molecular events in the induction phase of contact sensitivity. Proc Natl Acad Sci U S A. 1992;89:1398–402.
48. Heck DE, et al. Solar ultraviolet radiation as a trigger of cell signal transduction. Toxicol Appl Pharmacol. 2004;195:288–97.
49. Barr R, et al. Suppressed alloantigen presentation, increased TNF-α, IL-1, IL-1RA, IL-10, and modulation of TNF-R in UV-irradiated human skin. J Invest Dermatol. 1999;112:692–8.
50. Schwarz A, et al. Interleukin-12 suppresses ultraviolet radiation-induced apoptosis by inducing DNA repair. Nat Cell Biol. 2002;4:26–31.
51. Kripke M. Immunologic unresponsiveness induced by ultraviolet radiation. Immunol Rev. 1984;80:87–102.
52. Streilein J. Immunogenetic factors in skin cancer. N Engl J Med. 1991;325:884–7.
53. Vink A, et al. The inhibition of antigen-presenting activity of dendritic cells resulting from UV irradiation of murine skin is restored by *in vitro* photorepair of cyclobutane pyrimidine dimers. Proc Natl Acad Sci U S A. 1997;94:5255–60.
54. Kuchel J, et al. Cyclobutane pyrimidine dimer formation is a molecular trigger for solar-simulated ultraviolet radiation-induced suppression of memory immunity in humans. Photochem Photobiol Sci. 2005;4:577–82.
55. Brennan M, et al. Matrix metalloproteinase-1 is the major collagenolytic enzyme responsible for collagen damage in UV-irradiated human skin. Photochem Photobiol. 2003;78:43–8.
56. Wlaschek M, et al. UVA-induced autocrine stimulation of fibroblast-derived collagenase/MMP-1 by interrelated loops of interleukin-1 and interleukin-6. Photochem Photobiol. 1994;59:550–6.
57. Dong K, et al. UV-Induced DNA damage initiates release of MMP-1 in human skin. Exp Dermatol. 2008;17:1037–44.
58. Fisher GJ, et al. Looking older. Fibroblast collapse and therapeutic implications. Arch Dermatol. 2008;144:666–72.
59. Leveque J-C, et al. Aging skin: properties and functional changes. Aulnoy-sous Bois, France: Informa Health Care; 1993.
60. Ryan T. The ageing of the blood supply and the lym phatic drainage of the skin. Micron. 2004;35:161–71.
61. High W, et al. Genetic mutations involved in melanoma: a summary of our current understanding. Adv Dermatol. 2007;23:61–79.
62. Berneburg M, et al. Induction of the photoaging-associated mitochondrial common deletion *in vivo* in normal human skin. J Invest Dermatol. 2004;122:1277–83.
63. Yarosh D, et al. Localization of liposomes containing a DNA repair enzyme in murine skin. J Invest Dermatol. 1994;103:461–8.
64. Wolf P, et al. Topical treatment with liposomes containing T4 endonuclease V protects human skin *in vivo* from ultraviolet-induced upregulation of interleukin-10 and tumor necrosis factor-α. J Invest Dermatol. 2000;114:149–56.
65. Yarosh D, et al. Effect of topically applied T4 endonuclease V in liposomes on skin cancer in xeroderma pigmentosum: a randomized study. Lancet. 2001;357:926–9.
66. Lahmann C, et al. Matrix metalloproteinase-1 and skin ageing in smokers. Lancet. 2001;357:935–6.
67. Vierkotter A, et al. Airborne particle exposure and extrinsic skin aging. J Invest Dermatol. 2010;130:2719–26.
68. Pan TL, et al. The impact of urban particulate pollution on skin barrier function and the subsequent drug absorption. J Dermatol Sci. 2015;78:51–60.

Fibulin-5 Deposition in Human Skin: Decrease with Aging and UVB Exposure and Increase in Solar Elastosis

50

Satoshi Amano

Contents

S. Amano
Shiseido Research Center, Yokohama, Japan
e-mail: satoshi.amano@to.shiseido.co.jp

M.A. Farage et al. (eds.), *Textbook of Aging Skin*,
DOI 10.1007/978-3-662-47398-6_32

Abstract

The aim of this study was to explore the changes of fibulin-5 and elastic fibers during the skin aging process and to clarify the role of fibulin-5 in the formation of elastic fibers. We analyzed fibulin-5 expression in both normal and actinically damaged skins compared with expression of elastin, fibulin-2, and fibrillin-1. Fibulin-5 decreased in an age-dependent manner in the reticular dermis, and the reduction was enhanced by UVB irradiation. Moreover, acute UVB irradiation markedly reduced fibulin-5. However, fibulin-5 was also found to accumulate in solar elastosis, together with other elastic fiber components, such as elastin, fibulin-2, and fibrillin-1. On the other hand, an increase of fibulin-5 synthesis by dermal fibroblasts was effective for elastic fiber regeneration. Fibulin-5 could facilitate the elastic fiber assembly in in vitro condition These results indicated that fibulin-5 is an early marker of skin aging and that the early loss of fibulin-5 in the dermis may prefigure the age-dependent reduction of other elastic fiber components and furthermore that fibulin-5 may be effective on the repair of elastic fiber.

Introduction

Skin aging is classified into two types: intrinsic aging and photoaging. Intrinsic aging is a basic biological process common to all living things and can be characterized as age-dependent deterioration of skin functions and structures, such as epidermal atrophy and epidermal-dermal junction flattening [1]. Histologically, intrinsically aged skin has an atrophied extracellular matrix with a reduced amount of elastin [2]. On the other hand, photoaging is well known to be a consequence of chronic exposure to sunlight. Sun-exposed skin, such as the skin on the face or neck, is apparently prematurely aged compared with the relatively sun-protected skin of the trunk and is characterized by various clinical features, including wrinkles, sagging, roughness, sallowness, pigmentary changes, telangiectasia, and neoplasia [3, 4], and histological features of sun-exposed skin including cellular atypia, loss of polarity, epidermal-dermal junction flattening, a decrease in collagen, and dermal elastosis, with abnormal deposition of elastotic material in the dermis [1, 5]. Damage to skin collagen and elastin (extracellular matrix) is the hallmark of long-term exposure to solar ultraviolet irradiation and is believed to be responsible for the wrinkled appearance of sun-exposed skin [5].

The fibulin gene family comprises five distinct genes that encode more than eight protein products via alternative splicing [6]. Fibulins are widely expressed secreted proteins found in the blood and in the basement membranes and stroma of most tissues, where they self-associate [7, 8] and/or interact with a variety of extracellular matrix components, including fibronectin, laminin, nidogen, aggrecan, versican, endostatin, fibrillin, and elastin [6, 9–11]. Fibulins are thought to be involved in the assembly and stabilization of extracellular matrix structures and have also been implicated in regulating organogenesis, vasculogenesis, fibrogenesis, and tumorigenesis [12–14].

Fibulin-5 (known as EVEC [15] or DANCE [16]), a 448-amino acid glycoprotein, is one of the components of microfibrils and contains an integrin-binding RGD motif, six calcium-binding epidermal growth factor-like repeats, a Pro-rich insert in the first calcium-binding epidermal growth factor-like repeat, and a globular C-terminal domain [15, 16]. Functionally, fibulin-5 binds $\alpha v\beta 3$, $\alpha v\beta 5$, and $\alpha 9\beta 1$ integrins [10] and mediates endothelial cell adhesion via its RGD motif [16]. Inactivation of the fibulin-5 gene in mice produces profound elastinopathy in the skin, lung, and vasculature [10, 11]. In humans, mutations in fibulin-5 have been found to cause cutis laxa [17].

Elastic fibers are composed of an amorphous elastin core surrounded by a peripheral mantle of microfibrils. Soluble tropoelastin monomers are polymerized and cross-linked to form insoluble elastin and which process is essential for the assembly of elastic fibers [18]. However, self-association of tropoelastin monomers alone is not sufficient to form elastic fibers indicating the need for other processes or substances. Microfibrils are 10–12 nm filaments in the extracellular matrices and composed of many proteins such as fibrillin-1 and fibrillin-2 [19–21], microfibril-associated glycoproteins (MAGPs) [22, 23], and latent transforming growth factor β-binding proteins (LTBPs) [24, 25]. Microfibrils are considered to provide a scaffold for the polymerization of elastin and play an essential role in elastogenesis.

In this study, the changes of fibulin-5 and elastic fibers in both normal and actinically damaged skins during the skin aging process were examined, and the role of fibulin-5 in the formation of elastic fibers was clarified.

Localization of Fibulin-5 in the Dermis of Young Human Sun-Protected Skin

In the reticular dermis of young sun-protected skin from the upper arm of a 17-year-old female, fibulin-5 was co-localized with other elastic fiber components, such as elastin, fibrillin-1, and fibulin-2 (Fig. 1a–d). In contrast with fibrillin-1, fibrillin-2 was not detected in the skin from children and adults (data not shown). In the papillary dermis, fibulin-5 showed candelabra-like structures perpendicular to the epidermis, resembling those of other elastic fiber components (Fig. 1a–d). In areas just beneath the epidermis, fibulin-5 does not go up to the dermal-epidermal junction like fibrillin-1 which was observed there as fiber structures which may be inserted into the epidermal

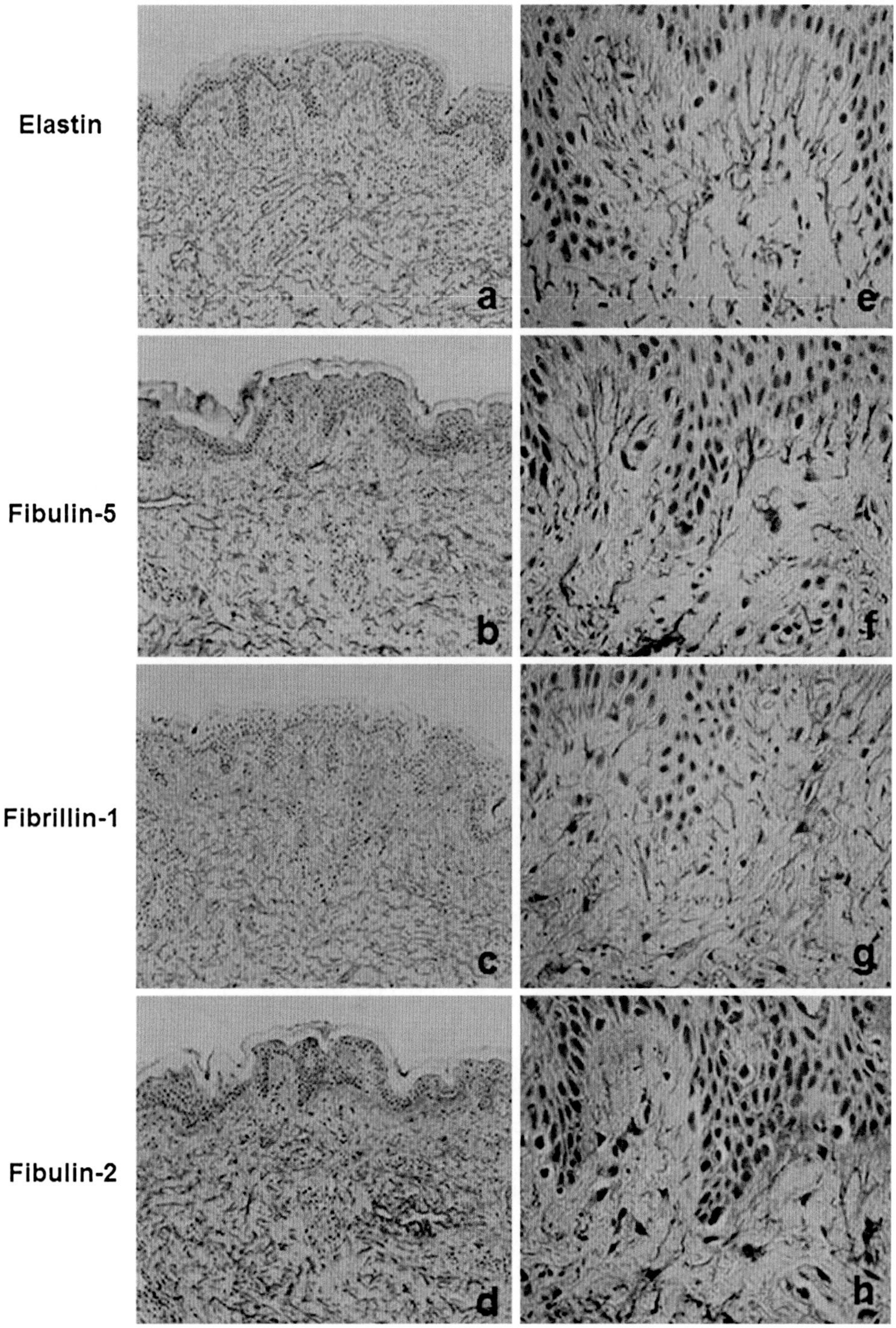

Fig. 1 Localization of elastin, fibulin-5, fibrillin-1, and fibulin-2 in the dermis of young human sun-protected skin. The localization of elastin (**a**), fibulin-5 (**b**), fibrillin-1 (**c**), or fibulin-2 (**d**) in sun-protected skin from the upper arm of a 17-year-old female was examined by means of immunohistochemistry using specific antibodies, as described in materials and methods

basement membrane [26, 27] (Fig. 1b, c). The fiber structure of fibulin-2 was not as sharp in the papillary dermis (Fig. 1a) as those of elastin, fibrillin-1, or fibulin-5 (Fig. 1a–c), although it was clearer in the reticular dermis (Fig. 1d).

Age-Dependent Changes of Fibulin-5 Distribution in the Dermis of Sun-Protected or Sun-Exposed Skin

In the dermis of sun-protected thigh skin from 5-, 13-, and 16-year-old subjects, fibulin-5 showed candelabra-like structures in the papillary dermis and was associated with elastic fibers composed of other elastic fiber components, such as elastin, fibrillin-1, and fibulin-2 (Fig. 2a–l) in the reticular dermis. However, the staining intensity of fibulin-5 (Fig. 2n) was reduced as compared with that of other elastic fiber components (Fig. 2m, o, p) in the reticular dermis of the skin from a 34-year-old subject. Fibulin-5 (Fig. 2r) was almost absent in the reticular dermis of the skin from a 75-year-old women. Similarly, fibulin-5 associated with elastic fibers was reduced in the reticular dermis of sun-protected upper arm skin from a 36-year-old subject as compared with those from 11-, 17-, and 24-year-old subjects (data not shown). Moreover, fibulin-5 associated with elastic fibers was markedly reduced as compared with fibrillin-1 and fibulin-2 in the reticular dermis of the abdomen skin from 34- and 75-year-old subjects (data not shown). On the other hand, in the papillary dermis, fibulin-5 maintained its staining intensity, although the number of stained fibers seemed to be reduced with age (Fig. 2n, r), whereas elastin was age-dependently reduced much more markedly in the papillary dermis than in reticular dermis (Fig. 2m, q).

In sun-exposed skin, fibulin-5 was mostly lost in the dermis of the cheek skin even from 20- and 45-year-old subjects (Fig. 3b, f), and this change occurred much earlier than that in sun-protected skin (Fig. 2). Elastic fiber structures in the dermis of 45-year-old skin (Fig. 3e, g, h) appeared to be thicker than those of 20-year-old skin (Fig. 3a, c, d) and were intermediate in pattern between the 20-year-old skin and the elastic fibers observed in the dermis of a 76-year-old subject (Fig. 3i, k, j), suggesting that the 45-year-old skin may be progressing to solar elastosis. However, while increased deposition of fibulin-5 was observed in solar elastosis (Fig. 3j), as was observed for other elastic fiber components, fibulin-5 decreased with age in sun-exposed skin before solar elastosis appeared (Fig. 3b, f).

Fibulin-5-deficient mice were reported to develop marked elastinopathy owing to the disorganization of elastic fibers, resulting in loose skin, vascular abnormalities, and emphysematous lung [10, 11]. Since fibulin-5 has an integrin-binding N-terminal domain, fibulin-5 is thought to stabilize the attachment of cells to elastic fibers and to contribute to the organization of elastic fibers [10]. Recently, fibulin-5 is reported to be a key protein for the induction of elastic fiber formation, and the full intact form of fibulin-5 diminishes with age [28]. Therefore, the loss of fibulin-5 may decrease the stability of elastic fibers by disturbing the interactions between dermal cells and elastic fibers or among elastic fiber components and may contribute to the atrophy of elastic fibers during aging.

The hallmark of actinic damage of the skin is changes associated with deposition of elastotic materials in the dermis [1]. Previous immunohistochemical studies reported an increased deposition of elastin, versican, hyaluronic acid, fibrillin, and fibulin-2 in areas of solar elastosis [29–31]. In this study, we found that fibulin-5 deposition was also increased in solar elastosis. The mechanism of the increase in the expression of these elastic fiber components, leading to abnormal deposition in the dermis of actinically damaged skin, remains unknown. However, since all elastic fiber components, including fibulin-5, are increased in solar elastosis, the mechanism may activate the elastic fiber developmental program. Since fibulin-5 was observed to be extremely reduced in the aging dermis, it is possible that the control of gene expression, protein synthesis, or deposition of fibulin-5 may be different from those of other elastic fiber components. Further studies are needed to clarify the role of fibulin-5 in normal aging and in the pathogenesis of solar elastosis.

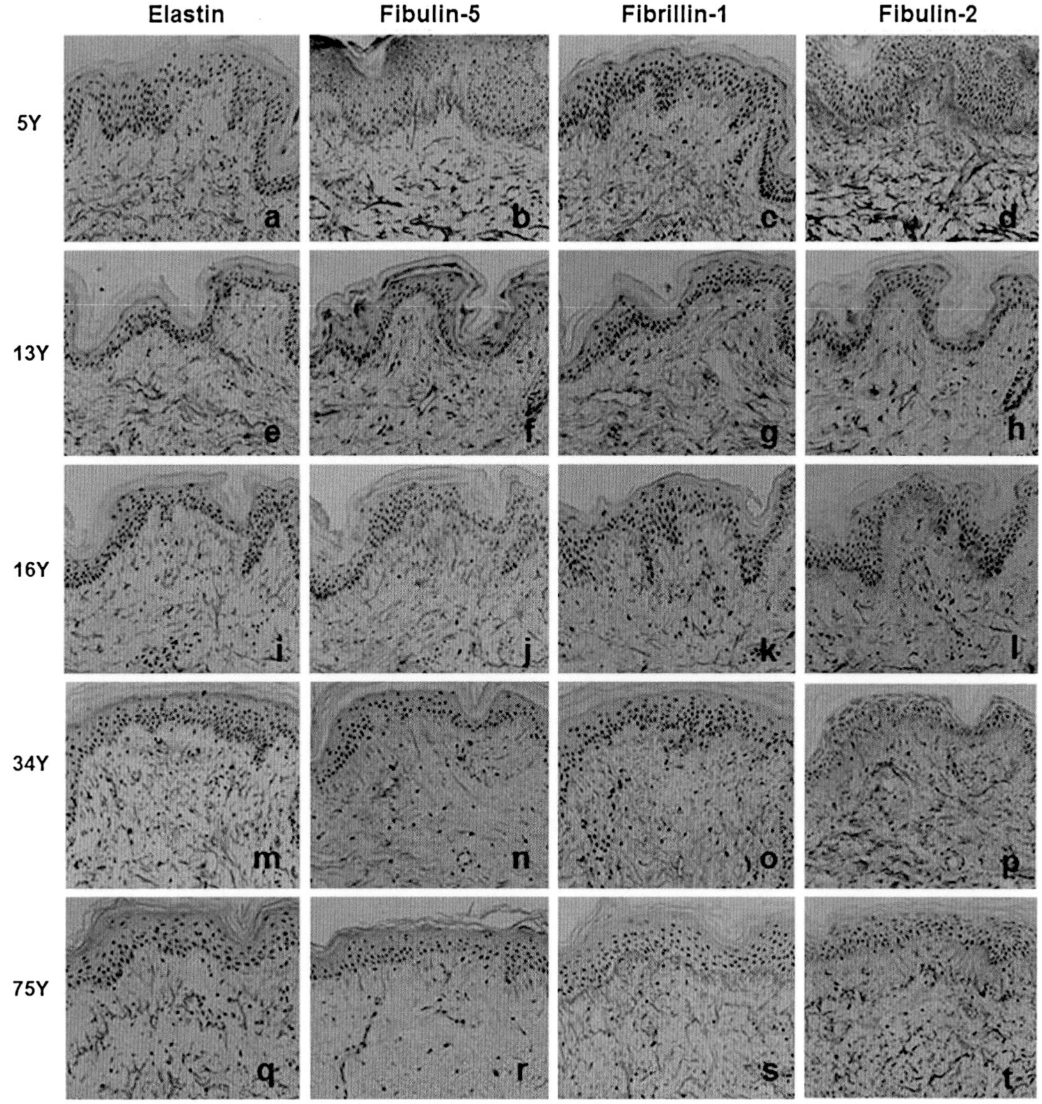

Fig. 2 Age-dependent changes of expression of elastin, fibulin-5, fibrillin-1, and fibulin-2 in the dermis of sun-protected skins. The localization of elastin (**a e**, **i**, **m**, and **q**), fibulin-5 (**b**, **f**, **j**, **n**, and **r**), fibrillin-1 (**c**, **g**, **k**, **o**, and **s**), or fibulin-2 (**d**, **h**, **l**, **p**, and **t**) in the dermis of sun-protected thigh skin was examined by means of immunohistochemistry using specific antibodies, as described in materials and methods. Age-dependent changes of the elastic fiber components were examined in the dermis of skins from subjects in the age range from 5 to 75 years old. It should be noted that fibulin-5 decreased especially markedly in the reticular dermis with aging (Image reproduced, with permission, from Br. J. Dermatol. 2005, 153(3):607–612)

Reduction of Fibulin-5 in the Dermis After UVB Irradiation

Since fibulin-5 in the dermis was reduced in sun-exposed skin earlier than that in sun-protected skin, we explored the effect of UVB irradiation on the fibulin-5 distribution in the buttock skin from two male volunteers. A single UVB irradiation at 2 MED decreased fibulin-5 (Fig. 4i, j), fibulin-2 (Fig. 4k, l), and elastin (Fig. 4g, h) levels in the dermis markedly, moderately, and weakly, respectively, as compared with those in non-treated skin (Fig. 4a–f).

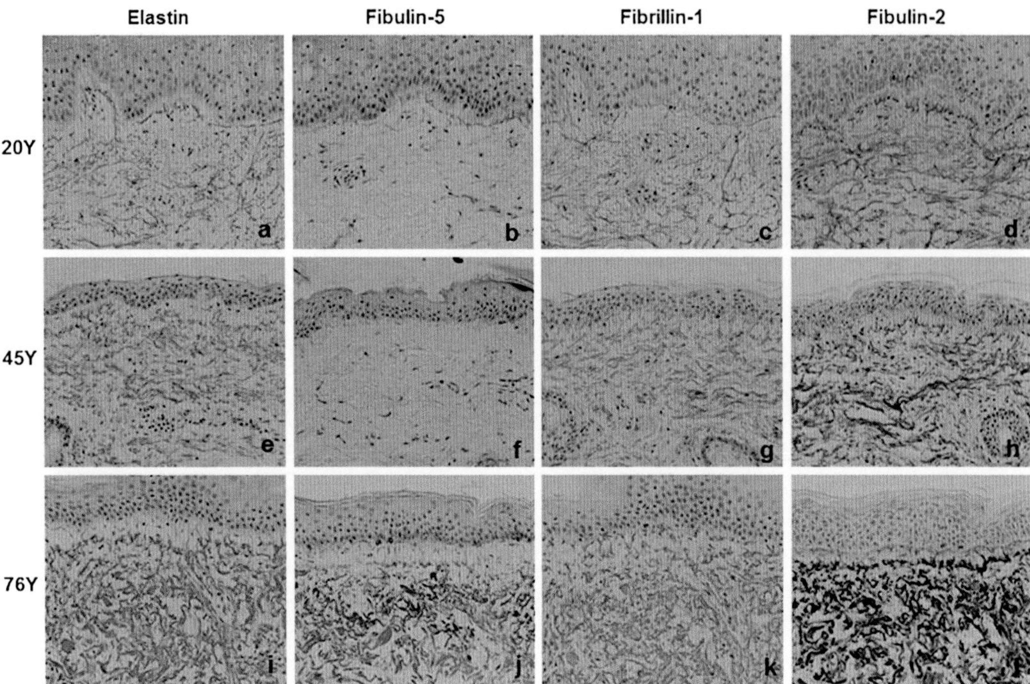

Fig. 3 Age-dependent changes of expression of elastin, fibulin-5, fibrillin-1, and fibulin-2 in the dermis of sun-exposed skin. The localization of elastin (**a**, **e**, and **i**), fibulin-5 (**b**, **f**, and **j**), fibrillin-1 (**c**, **g**, and **k**), or fibulin-2 (**d**, **h**, and **l**) in the dermis of sun-exposed cheek skins was examined by means of immunohistochemistry using specific antibodies, as described in materials and methods. Age-dependent changes of the elastic fiber components were examined in the dermis of skins from subjects in the age range from 20 to 76 years old. It should be noted that the reduction of fibulin-5 in the reticular dermis occurred earlier in sun-exposed skin than in sun-protected skin. Increased deposition of fibulin-5, as well as the other elastic fiber components, was observed in solar elastosis (Image reproduced, with permission, from Br. J. Dermatol. 2005, 153(3):607–612)

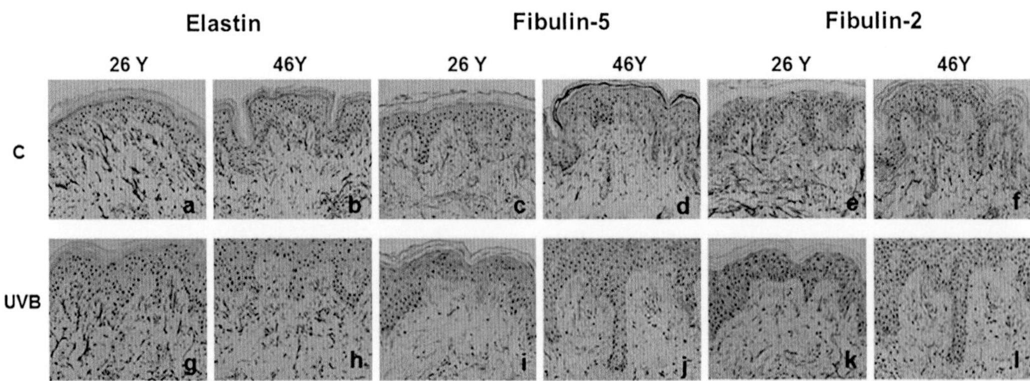

Fig. 4 Reduction of fibulin-5 in the dermis after UVB irradiation. The localization of elastin (**a**, **b**, **g**, and **h**), fibulin-5 (**c**, **d**, **i**, and **j**), or fibulin-2 (**e**, **f**, **k**, and **i**) in the dermis of buttock skin was compared between non-treated sites (**a**–**f**) and UVB-irradiated sites (**g**–**l**) by means of immunohistochemistry using specific antibodies, as described in materials and methods. It should be noted that fibulin-5 was markedly reduced in the dermis by UVB irradiation (Image reproduced, with permission, from Br. J. Dermatol. 2005, 153(3):607–612)

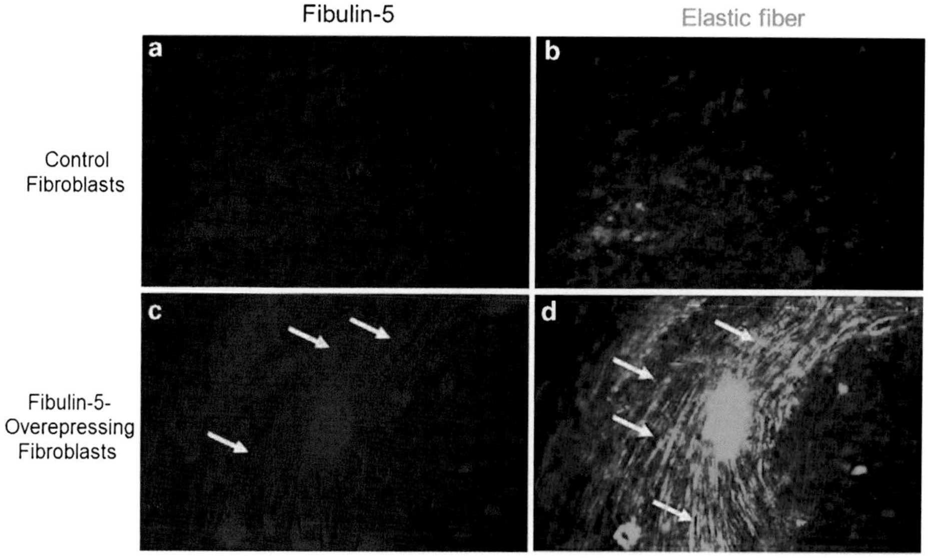

Fibulin-5 | Elastic fiber
Control Fibroblasts
Fibulin-5-Overepressing Fibroblasts
a b c d

Fig. 5 Overexpressed fibulin-5 enhanced elastic fiber assembly. Human foreskin fibroblasts were transfected with a retroviral vector containing the CMV promoter and human fibulin-5 cDNA (pRevCMV2-FBLN-5) or CMV promoter (pRevCMV2) only as control. The selected transduced cells were cultured on slide chambers. At 2 weeks after reaching confluency, the cells were fixed with acetone. Fibulin-5 deposited around the cells was stained red with anti-fibulin-5 antibody (**a**, **c**). Deposited elastin was stained green with anti-elastin antibody (**b**, **d**). It should be noted that overexpression of fibulin-5 enhanced the elastic fiber assembly (**c**, **d**)

Fibulin-5 deposition decreased much earlier in sun-exposed skins than in sun-protected skins. Furthermore, UVB irradiation induced the degradation of fibulin-5 deposited in the dermis. Matrix-degrading metalloproteinase messenger RNAs, proteins, and activities are known to be induced in the human skin in vivo within hours of exposure to UVB irradiation and may degrade collagen and elastin in the skin [32]. Fibulin-2 was reported to be degraded by matrix metalloproteinases (stromelysin, matrilysin), circulating proteases (thrombin, plasmin, kallikrein), leukocyte elastase, and mast cell chymase [33]. Smaller degradation products of fibulin-2 were also detected in actinic elastosis, presumably reflecting increased proteinase activity in photodamaged skin [31].

Acceleration of the Assembly of Elastic Fibers by Increased Fibulin-5 in Human Fibroblasts

To examine the effect of fibulin-5 on the assembly of elastic fibers, a retroviral vector containing the cytomegalovirus (CMV) promoter and human fibulin-5 cDNA (pRevCMV-FBLN-5) or tropoelastin cDNA (pRevCMV-ELN) [34] was constructed. Human foreskin fibroblasts were transduced with either pRevCMV-ELN, pRevCMV-FBLN-5, or both vectors. The transduced cells were selected in media containing the appropriate antibiotics. The gene expression of tropoelastin and fibulin-5 was confirmed to be upregulated by quantitative PCR [34]. The overexpression of tropoelastin by pRevCMV-ELN did not affect the gene expression of fibulin-5 [34]. Each cell line was then cultured in DMEM/10 % FBS in slide chambers. Two weeks after reaching confluency, the culture was immunostained using anti-elastin mouse monoclonal antibody and antihuman fibulin-5 rabbit polyclonal antibodies with the appropriate secondary antibody. The tropoelastin-overexpressing cells did not deposit elastic fibers (Fig. 5b) as seen in culture with the cells transduced with the control vectors pRevCMV and pRevCMV2 (data not shown). On the other hand, fibulin-5-overexpressing cells showed an increase in elastic fiber assembly (Fig. 5d). Cells overexpressing both tropoelastin and fibulin-5 had similar levels of elastic fiber as cells overexpressing only fibulin-5, suggesting that fibulin-5 is a critical component in the control of elastic fibers by dermal fibroblasts, which is consistent with the finding by Drs. Hirai and Nakamura [28].

Conclusion

In this study, we demonstrated that the fibulin-5 content in the reticular dermis decreases with age and decreases earlier than other elastic fiber components, such as elastin, fibrillin-1, and fibulin-2. The reduction of fibulin-5 was enhanced by UVB exposure and occurred in sun-exposed skin much earlier than in sun-protected skin. Therefore, UVB is likely to be one of the major factors causing impairment of elastic fibers during aging, and the early loss of fibulin-5 may signal the later changes of elastic fibers during aging, especially photoaging. Therefore, fibulin-5 is proposed to be a good marker of skin aging, especially photoaging. Interestingly, fibulin-5 deposition is enhanced in solar elastosis, suggesting that solar elastosis involves the global activation of genes for elastic fiber components.

Moreover, we found that fibulin-5-overexpressing cells enhanced the assembly of elastic fibers in cultured normal human dermal fibroblasts, suggesting that fibulin-5 was an important microfibril constituent for the assembly of elastic fibers. Thus, fibulin-5 may be a potential target to prevent or delay the deterioration of elastic fibers during the skin aging process in human.

Cross-References

► DNA Damage and Repair in Skin Aging

References

1. Lavker RM. Structural alterations in exposed and unexposed aged skin. J Invest Dermatol. 1979;73(1):59–66.
2. Braverman IM, Fonferko E. Studies in cutaneous aging: I. The elastic fiber network. J Invest Dermatol. 1982;78(5):434–43.
3. Gilchrest BA. Skin aging and photoaging: an overview. J Am Acad Dermatol. 1989;21(3 Pt 2):610–3.
4. Griffiths CE. The clinical identification and quantification of photodamage. Br J Dermatol. 1992;127 Suppl 41:37–42.
5. Kligman AM, et al. Topical tretinoin for photoaged skin. J Am Acad Dermatol. 1986;15(4 Pt 2):836–59.
6. Timpl R, et al. Fibulins: a versatile family of extracellular matrix proteins. Nat Rev Mol Cell Biol. 2003;4(6):479–89.
7. Balbona K, et al. Fibulin binds to itself and to the carboxyl-terminal heparin-binding region of fibronectin. J Biol Chem. 1992;267(28):20120–5.
8. Pan TC, et al. Structure and expression of fibulin-2, a novel extracellular matrix protein with multiple EGF-like repeats and consensus motifs for calcium binding. J Cell Biol. 1993;123(5):1269–77.
9. Aspberg A, et al. Fibulin-1 is a ligand for the C-type lectin domains of aggrecan and versican. J Biol Chem. 1999;274(29):20444–9.
10. Nakamura T, et al. Fibulin-5/DANCE is essential for elastogenesis in vivo. Nature. 2002;415(6868):171–5.
11. Yanagisawa H, et al. Fibulin-5 is an elastin-binding protein essential for elastic fibre development in vivo. Nature. 2002;415(6868):168–71.
12. Zhang HY, et al. Fibulin-1 and fibulin-2 expression during organogenesis in the developing mouse embryo. Dev Dyn. 1996;205(3):348–64.
13. Tran H, et al. The interaction of fibulin-1 with fibrinogen. A potential role in hemostasis and thrombosis. J Biol Chem. 1995;270(33):19458–64.
14. Roark EF, et al. The association of human fibulin-1 with elastic fibers: an immunohistological, ultrastructural, and RNA study. J Histochem Cytochem. 1995;43(4):401–11.
15. Kowal RC, et al. EVEC, a novel epidermal growth factor-like repeat-containing protein upregulated in embryonic and diseased adult vasculature. Circ Res. 1999;84(10):1166–76.
16. Nakamura T, et al. DANCE, a novel secreted RGD protein expressed in developing, atherosclerotic, and balloon-injured arteries. J Biol Chem. 1999;274(32):22476–83.
17. Loeys B, et al. Homozygosity for a missense mutation in fibulin-5 (FBLN5) results in a severe form of cutis laxa. Hum Mol Genet. 2002;11(18):2113–8.
18. Urry DW. Entropic elastic processes in protein mechanisms. II. Simple (passive) and coupled (active) development of elastic forces. J Protein Chem. 1988;7(2):81–114.
19. Sakai LY, Keene DR, Engvall E. Fibrillin, a new 350-kD glycoprotein, is a component of extracellular microfibrils. J Cell Biol. 1986;103(6 Pt 1):2499–509.
20. Zhang H, Hu W, Ramirez F. Developmental expression of fibrillin genes suggests heterogeneity of extracellular microfibrils. J Cell Biol. 1995;129(4):1165–76.
21. Zhang H, et al. Structure and expression of fibrillin-2, a novel microfibrillar component preferentially located in elastic matrices. J Cell Biol. 1994;124(5):855–63.

22. Gibson MA, et al. The major antigen of elastin-associated microfibrils is a 31-kDa glycoprotein. J Biol Chem. 1986;261(24):11429–36.
23. Gibson MA, et al. Further characterization of proteins associated with elastic fiber microfibrils including the molecular cloning of MAGP-2 (MP25). J Biol Chem. 1996;271(2):1096–103.
24. Gibson MA, et al. Bovine latent transforming growth factor beta 1-binding protein 2: molecular cloning, identification of tissue isoforms, and immunolocalization to elastin-associated microfibrils. Mol Cell Biol. 1995;15(12):6932–42.
25. Taipale J, et al. Human mast cell chymase and leukocyte elastase release latent transforming growth factor-beta 1 from the extracellular matrix of cultured human epithelial and endothelial cells. J Biol Chem. 1995;270(9):4689–96.
26. McGrath JA, et al. Immunoelectron microscopy of skin basement membrane zone antigens: a pre-embedding method using 1-nm immunogold with silver enhancement. Acta Derm Venereol. 1994;74(3):197–200.
27. Haynes SL, Shuttleworth CA, Kielty CM. Keratinocytes express fibrillin and assemble microfibrils: implications for dermal matrix organization. Br J Dermatol. 1997;137(1):17–23.
28. Hirai M, et al. Fibulin-5/DANCE has an elastogenic organizer activity that is abrogated by proteolytic cleavage in vivo. J Cell Biol. 2007;176(7):1061–71.
29. Bernstein EF, et al. Differential expression of the versican and decorin genes in photoaged and sun-protected skin. Comparison by immunohistochemical and northern analyses. Lab Invest. 1995;72(6):662–9.
30. Bernstein EF, et al. Chronic sun exposure alters both the content and distribution of dermal glycosaminoglycans. Br J Dermatol. 1996;135(2):255–62.
31. Hunzelmann N, et al. Increased deposition of fibulin-2 in solar elastosis and its colocalization with elastic fibres. Br J Dermatol. 2001;145(2):217–22.
32. Fisher GJ, et al. Molecular basis of sun-induced premature skin ageing and retinoid antagonism. Nature. 1996;379(6563):335–9.
33. Sasaki T, et al. Different susceptibilities of fibulin-1 and fibulin-2 to cleavage by matrix metalloproteinases and other tissue proteases. Eur J Biochem. 1996;240(2):427–34.
34. Katsuta Y, et al. Fibulin-5 accelerates elastic fibre assembly in human skin fibroblasts. Exp Dermatol. 2008;17(10):837–42.

Cutaneous Oxidative Stress and Aging 51

Thomas G. Polefka and Thomas A. Meyer

Contents

Abstract

The earliest known microfossil records suggest that microorganisms existed on the earth approximately 3.8 billion years ago. With the aid of sunlight, these photosynthetic organisms began to generate molecular oxygen (O_2) and fundamentally changed the earth's atmosphere and direction of evolution. Paradoxically, an atmosphere of ~20 % oxygen offers aerobic organisms both benefits and challenges. As the outermost boundary, the skin is continuously exposed to various environmental stresses ranging from O_2 itself to solar radiation, air pollution, and lifestyle excesses, all of which can produce oxidative stress. This chapter summarizes almost 60 years of research and provides a "60,000 ft" perspective on cutaneous oxidative stress. Topics reviewed include: What are free radicals and reactive oxidizing species (ROS)? Where do they come from and how are they formed? What is their chemistry and molecular targets? What are their roles in health and disease in general and the skin in particular? How does the skin protect itself from these reactive species? And finally, what roles do ROS and oxidative stress play in the aging process?

Introduction

Fossil records suggest that life first arose on the earth approximately 3.8 billion years ago [1]. By 2.5 billion years, photosynthetic organisms were

T.G. Polefka (✉)
Life Science Solutions, LLC, Somerset, NJ, USA
e-mail: tpolefka@lifescisolutions.com

T.A. Meyer
Bayer Healthcare, Memphis, TN, USA
e-mail: thomas.meyer3@bayer.com

M.A. Farage et al. (eds.), *Textbook of Aging Skin*,
DOI 10.1007/978-3-662-47398-6_123

already using the energy inherent in sunlight to split water into hydrogen and oxygen [2]. The hydrogen, along with available atmospheric CO_2 and N_2, was used to drive metabolism and build complex living communities, while oxygen was discarded to the atmosphere, changing earth's biosphere forever. Ultimately, enough O_2 accumulated to generate a somewhat protective stratospheric ozone layer and, equally important, allowing the evolution of new life forms [2, 3].

Life in an oxygenated environment offers benefits and consequences [4–6]. The key benefit is that oxidative metabolism allows aerobic organisms an opportunity to generate 38 moles of ATP from each mole of glucose metabolized, whereas those organisms using anaerobic metabolism (i.e., fermentation) produce only 2 moles of ATP per mole glucose [7]. However, one consequence of aerobic life is that O_2 can be toxic. As organisms evolved in the primordial aerobic environment, so did their ability to neutralize and protect themselves from the deleterious effects of reactive oxygen/nitrogen species [8]. The objective of this chapter is to provide a "60,000 ft" perspective on cutaneous oxidative stress as it relates to health, disease, and aging.

What Are Free Radicals and Reactive Oxygen Species (ROS)?

A free radical is any species capable of independent existence that contains one or more unpaired electrons occupying an atomic or molecular orbital [9]. For example, molecular oxygen (O_2) is a free radical since it has two unpaired electrons and two molecular orbitals of equal energy [10]. Because electrons normally like to be paired, radicals carrying extra electrons have two choices to achieve chemical stability: (1) donate an unpaired electron to another molecule (i.e., oxidation reaction) or (2) accept an electron from another molecule (i.e., reduction reaction). Of particular relevance to the skin is the oxidation of key biomolecules such as DNA [11], proteins [12], and lipids [13].

Related to free radicals is a group of reactive oxygen-, nitrogen-, and sulfur-centered non-radical oxygen species [8]. To avoid confusion, the acronym ROS will be used in this chapter to describe all the reactive oxidizing species, not just the oxygen-centered ones. By definition, oxidation is a reaction where a compound either adds oxygen or accepts an electron from another molecule. Conversely, reduction is the reaction where a compound loses oxygen or gains electrons [14]. A simple oxidation-reduction reaction (redox reaction) is shown in Fig. 1. Life as we know it is based on redox reactions [2]. Figure 2 shows the ROS resulting from the incomplete reduction of oxygen.

Biologically Relevant ROS

Table 1 lists some of the more biologically relevant ROS and provides some facts about each [15, 17]. Although half-life is not a direct measure of reactivity, it is a useful predictor. For example, hydroxyl radical (•OH) and singlet oxygen ($^1O_2$) are characterized by the shortest half-lives and are the most reactive [15]. In contrast to this, hydrogen peroxide (H_2O_2) is much weaker and more

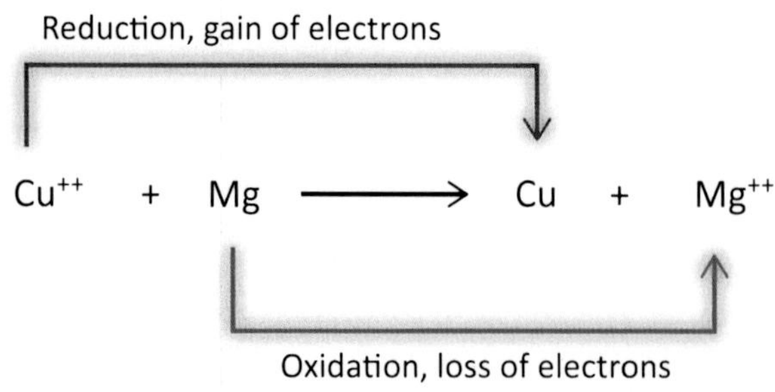

Fig. 1 Schematic diagram of simple oxidation-reduction (redox) reaction. Oxidation is the loss of electrons (shown in *blue*), whereas reduction is the gain of electrons (shown in *red*). In the reaction shown, Cu^{++} is reduced to Cu, while Mg is oxidized to Mg^{++}

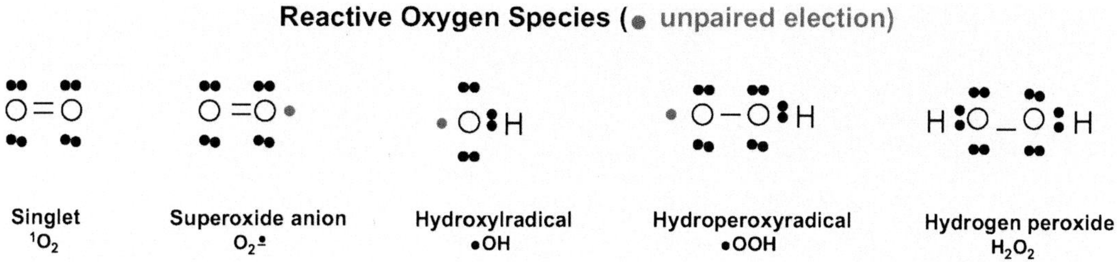

Reactive Oxygen Species (• unpaired election)

Singlet $^1O_2$ | Superoxide anion $O_2^{\bullet -}$ | Hydroxylradical •OH | Hydroperoxyradical •OOH | Hydrogen peroxide H_2O_2

Fig. 2 **Oxygen-based reactive oxygen species** (Modified and used with the permission from rbowen@colostate.edu)

Table 1 Key reactive oxidizing species relevant to the skin

ROS	Symbol	Sources	Half-life (seconds)
Triplet oxygen	$^3O_2$	Molecular oxygen	Long
Singlet oxygen	$^1O_2$	UV radiation	10^{-6}
Hydrogen peroxide	HOOH	Metabolism	Long
Superoxide anion	$\bullet O_2^-$	Metabolism UV radiation	Long
Hydroxyl radical	•OH	Metal catalysis	10^{-9}
Alkyl radical	R•	2nd chemical reaction	10^{-6}
Alkyl peroxyl radical	ROO•	2nd chemical reaction	1–10
Hypochlorite	OCl^-	Metabolism (myeloperoxidase) Anthropogenic	Short
Thiyl radical	RS•	Metabolism	10^{-6}
Nitric oxide	NO•	Metabolism (iNOS) Anthropogenic	1–10
Peroxynitrite	$ONOO^-$	Anthropogenic	1
Ozone	O_3	Anthropogenic	Short

Sources: Refs. [15, 16]

selective in its reactions [18], oxidizing molecules with redox potentials lower than itself (E° ~320 mV) [19].

Biological Sources of Reactive Oxidizing Species (ROS)

All living organisms are susceptible to endogenous and exogenous ROS [8]. In most cases, the production of these reactive molecules is tightly controlled. Approximately 98 % of the oxygen metabolized by the cells is handled by a single enzyme located in the mitochondria, namely, cytochrome oxidase [14]. Uniquely, this enzyme is capable of carrying out the chemically difficult task of simultaneously transferring four electrons to completely reduce oxygen to water [14]. However, leakage from the electron transport chain, various cellular oxidases, and various environmental factors can give rise to ROS (Fig. 3). Table 2 presents an overview of the sources and functions of some key cellular ROS. However, organisms, in general, and the skin, in particular, have little control over the ROS generated as a consequence of exposure to ionizing radiation (e.g., x-rays, γ-radiation) [33], non-ionizing radiation (e.g., solar radiation) [34], air pollutants (ozone, VOCs) [35], and photoreactive xenobiotic agents (e.g., tetracycline, chlorpromazine, retinoids, etc.) [36].

Figure 4 shows the key biochemical pathways leading to and away from various ROS [37]. One of the most striking features of Fig. 4 is the number of pathways that converge on the superoxide anion ($\bullet O_2^-$). In most cells, it represents the

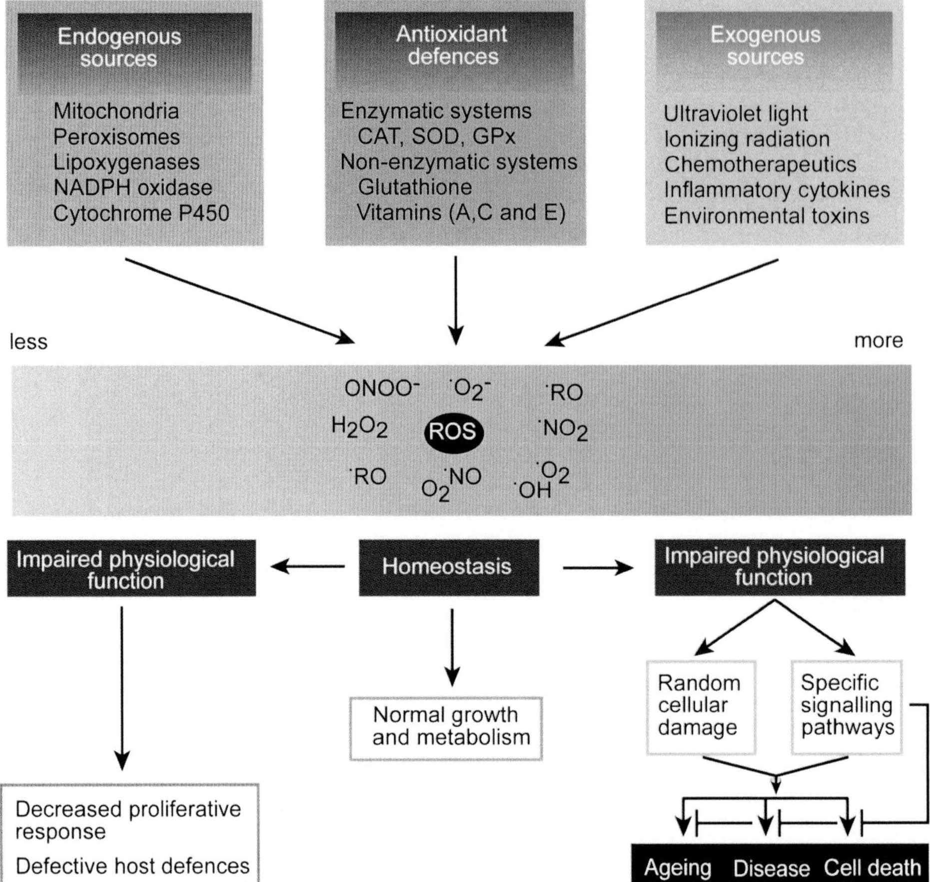

Fig. 3 Sources and cellular response to reactive oxidizing species (*ROS*). ROS are a consequence of normal cellular metabolism and the impact of exogenous environmental factors. The total amount of ROS generated is finely regulated by the cell's antioxidant defense system, composed of low molecular weight nonenzymatic antioxidants and highly efficient antioxidant enzymes. Dysregulation of the antioxidant defense system is associated with alterations in cell growth and proliferation, morbidity, aging, and cell death (apoptosis) (Reprinted from Finkel and Holbrook [20] with the permission from the Nature Publishing Group)

dominant ROS [23]. Although there are several ways to generate $\bullet O_2^-$, leakage from the mitochondrial respiratory chain (representing ~1–2 % of the O_2) appears to be the dominant source [20, 38]. As will be discussed later, superoxide anion is at the heart of several theories of aging. Another explanation for the central role of superoxide anion is that at low concentrations, it functions beneficially as a signaling molecule, modulator of various biochemical pathways, and protein modifier and in antimicrobial defense [39, 40]. For example, all nucleated cells use the xanthine oxidase pathway and the $\bullet O_2^-$ generated to degrade purine nucleotides to uric acid for excretion [41]. Other cells have specialized organelles, peroxisomes, where $\bullet O_2^-$-generating enzymes (D-amino acid oxidase, uric oxidase, etc.) help to detoxify xenobiotic compounds [42]. Finally, other cells, particularly those involved in host defense, use NADPH oxidase (highlighted in blue) to generate $\bullet O_2^-$ for the specific purpose of killing or neutralizing bacteria and viruses [17] and enhancing wound healing [43].

Of particular relevance to the skin is the pathway directly above the superoxide anion (Fig. 4, highlighted in red). Accordingly, endogenous and exogenous photosensitizer molecules absorb photons of solar radiation (320–1400 nm) and

Table 2 Source and function of reactive oxygen/nitrogen species

Primary ROS/RNS	Sources	Function/comment
$^1O_2$	UVR photodynamic processes	UVR-induced toxicant
O_3	Air pollution	Powerful oxidizing toxicant
$\bullet O_2^-$	Mitochondria ETC and other enzymes Peroxisome; xanthine oxidase, monooxygenase (e.g., cytochrome P450)	2nd messenger; regulates cell growth and proliferation Activates oxidative stress response, gene transcription, inflammation, many other pathways
•OH	$H_2O_2 + M^{n+}$ Ionizing radiation Hydroperoxide decomposition	Putative antimicrobial, antiviral, and antitumor [21] Because of reactivity, generally viewed as indiscriminant toxicant
H_2O_2	Mitochondria and cytosol superoxide dismutase of $\bullet O_2^-$ Nonenzymatic dismutation of $\bullet O_2^-$ Oxidases: xanthine, glucose, NADPH [22], oxalate, peroxisome oxidase, monooxygenase (cytochrome P450), etc.	2nd messenger; cell growth, proliferation, cell senescence, and death Activates oxidative stress response, gene transcription, inflammation, various pathways Involved in melanogenesis
•NO	Nitric oxide synthetase	2nd messenger; cell growth, proliferation, cell senescence, and death Vascular tone and neurotransmitter regulator
ONOO-	Reaction between $\bullet O_2^- + \bullet NO$ Air pollution	Putative antimicrobial, antiviral, and antitumor [21] Putative 2nd messenger via protein tyrosine nitration
HOCl	Myeloperoxidase	Antimicrobial, antiviral activity

Sources: Refs. [23–32]

generate via a photodynamic reaction singlet oxygen, $^1O_2$ [24, 44]. Examples of endogenous photosensitizers include melanin, porphyrins, riboflavin, and tryptophan derivatives [24, 45, 46]. Some of the better-known exogenous photosensitizers include drugs, tetracycline, psoralen, azathioprine, and retinoic acid [47]. Singlet oxygen ($^1O_2$) is an electronically excited form of molecular oxygen (Table 1) that reacts indiscriminately with almost any molecule, including water [25]. Once formed, $^1O_2$ reacts rapidly in one of two main ways: (1) by donating an electron to molecular oxygen, which in turn gives rise to $\bullet O_2^-$, or (2) by abstracting a hydrogen atom from a nearby unsaturated fatty acid giving rise to a lipid radical (R•) and alkyl peroxide (ROO•) [11].

Aside from directly interacting with key biomolecules such as proteins, lipids, nucleic acids, and low molecular weight antioxidants, $\bullet O_2^-$ is readily dismutated to H_2O_2 by the enzyme superoxide dismutase [48]. Since H_2O_2 is much less reactive than superoxide anion (Table 1), it frequently functions as an intracellular 2nd messenger (Table 2; cf. section on "Redox Signaling Overview") [18]. However, should concentrations of this ROS – or any other ROS – exceed some cell-defined threshold, redox balance will shift from a normally reduced state to a prooxidant state, frequently referred to as oxidative stress. Originally coined by Sies [49], oxidative stress reflects a disturbance in the balance between cellular oxidants and antioxidants, favoring the former. Not surprisingly, should a state of oxidative stress persist for an extended period, not only will key biomolecules be damaged, but also the cell may initiate apoptosis or programmed cell death [26].

As previously mentioned, H_2O_2 is one of the least potent ROS [19]. However, when produced in the presence of transition metals such as Fe^{++} or Cu^+, H_2O_2 accepts an electron from these metal ions generating the highly reactive hydroxyl radical (•OH) (cf. Fig. 4). This chemical reaction is known as the Fenton reaction ($Fe^{++} + H_2O_2 \rightarrow Fe^{+++} + OH^- + \bullet OH$) [8]. As can be seen in Table 1, the

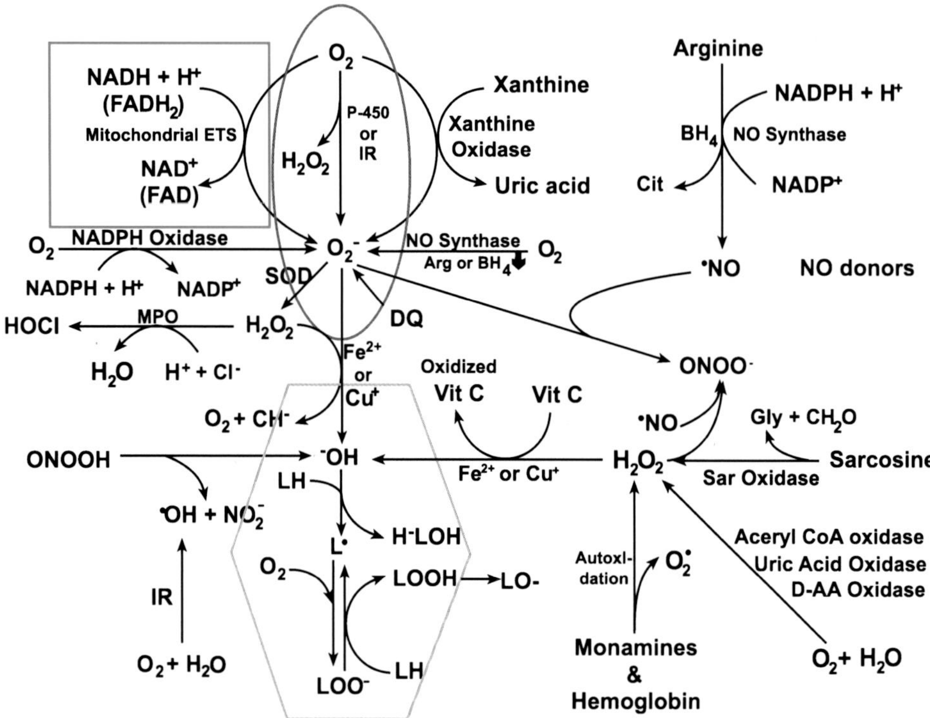

Fig. 4 Biochemistry of reactive oxidizing species in mammalian cells. Production of oxygen and nitrogen free radicals and other reactive oxidizing species in mammalian cells. *AA* amino acid, *Arg* L-arginine, BH_4 (6R)-5,6,7,8-tetrahydro-L-biopterin, CH_2O formaldehyde, *Cit* L-citrulline, *DQ* diquat, *ETS* electron transport system, *FAD* flavin adenine dinucleotide (oxidized), $FADH_2$ flavin adenine dinucleotide (reduced), *Gly* glycine, H_2O_2 hydrogen peroxide, *HOCl* hypochlorous acid, *H•LOH* hydroxyl lipid radical, *IR* ionizing radiation, *L•* lipid radical, *LH* lipid (unsaturated fatty acid), *LO•* lipid alkoxyl radical, *LOO•* lipid peroxyl radical, *LOOH* lipid hydroperoxides, *MPO* myeloperoxidase, NAD^+ nicotinamide adenine dinucleotide (oxidized), *NADH* nicotinamide adenine dinucleotide (reduced), $NADP^+$ nicotinamide adenine dinucleotide phosphate (oxidized), *NADPH* nicotinamide adenine dinucleotide phosphate (reduced), *•NO* nitric oxide, $•O_2$ superoxide anion radical, *•OH* hydroxyl radical, $ONOO^-$ peroxynitrite, *P450* cytochrome P450, *PDG* phosphate-dependent glutaminase, *Sar* sarcosinate, *SOD* superoxide dismutase, *Vit C* vitamin C (ascorbic acid), *Vit E* vitamin E (α-tocopherol) (Reprinted from Fang et al. [37] with the permission from Elsevier)

•OH is so reactive that its half-life is measured in nanoseconds. UV-induced liberation of free iron has been shown to contribute to accelerated skin aging [50–52]. To prevent this reaction, cellular iron is tightly complexed to specific enzymes and/or transport/storage proteins such as ferritin or hemosiderin [53]. Nevertheless, once formed, •OH has several options depending on its environment: (1) abstract a hydrogen, (2) donate an electron and act as a reducing agent, (3) accept an electron and act as an oxidizing agent, or (4) react with a biomolecule to generate another radical, usually of lower reactivity [54]. Because of its reactivity, all biomolecules are potential targets for •OH.

Molecular Targets and Reactions Mediated by ROS

The skin, like most organs of the body, must contend with the ROS generated *intrinsically* through normal biological processes. However, unlike other organs, the skin is also exposed to various *extrinsic* environmental insults/stresses such as solar radiation [34], cigarette smoking [55], and volatile and nonvolatile chemical pollutants (e.g., ozone, diesel exhaust, etc.) [35] that induce the formation of ROS above and beyond intrinsic levels. When the level of these reactive species exceeds the neutralization capacity of the endogenous antioxidant defense system (to be discussed subsequently), oxidative stress results with potentially deleterious effects [56]. Described below are some of interactions between ROS and their molecular targets. For more details, the reader is referred to several review articles [9, 57–59].

ROS-Mediated DNA Effects

Not surprisingly, nuclear and mitochondrial DNA represent key molecular targets for ROS. In general, two types of oxidative lesions are seen, oxidation of nucleotides and single-strand breaks [11, 60]. One of the most characterized oxidatively induced DNA lesions is the conversion of guanosine to 8-oxo-7,8-dihydro-2-deoxyguanosine (8-oxodGuo) [61]. This reaction is mediated by the highly reactive $^1O_2$ or •OH. As noted in Table 2, $^1O_2$ is produced via a photodynamic reaction involving UVA, visible, or IR radiation and a wavelength-specific photosensitizer. In contrast to this, hydroxyl radicals are generally formed by reactions involving the relatively abundant H_2O_2 and a transition metal such as Fe^{++} (Fig. 4) [11]. Although the formation of 8-oxodG is not overtly lethal because these lesions are rapidly repaired, the modified base is highly mutagenic [60, 62]. If not repaired by base excision repair enzymes, the 8-oxodG lesion could cause the misincorporation of adenine into the replicating chain, producing a C:G to A:T transversion mutation [63]. Two other pyrimidine lesions arise from the interaction of •OH with the methyl group of thymine and the hydroxymethyl group of uracil [60]. Finally, the *N*-glycosidic bonds that form the DNA backbone are susceptible to attack and cleavage by •OH, producing single-strand breaks [60]. The consequences of nuclear DNA damage are largely determined by the location of the DNA lesions and the efficiency of DNA repair mechanisms [61, 64]. For example, mutations in noncoding sections of DNA may have little effect on cell function. However, damage to any of the known proto-oncogenes (e.g., *C-KIT, EGFR, MITF*, various ras oncogenes, etc.), tumor suppressor genes (e.g., *p53, p16, PTEN, PTCH*, etc.), or replication control genes (e.g., *mTERT*) may lead to carcinogenesis [62, 65–67].

Another type of DNA lesion, cyclobutane pyrimidine dimers (CPDs), is associated with the direct absorption of UVB radiation (280–320 nm) by pyrimidine bases [11]. This reaction is independent of oxygen (and ROS) and is associated with several skin cancers, especially basal cell and squamous cell carcinoma [68]. Recently, however, Premi et al. [69] described a novel UVA-mediated oxidative pathway leading to the generation of CPDs. According to this "chemiexcitation" process (Fig. 5), UVA exposure induces the enzymatic generation of NO• and $•O_2^-$. These ROS react to form another moderately reactive ROS, peroxynitrite ($ONOO^-$), which in turn initiates the degradation of cytosolic melanin into small molecular weight derivatives, capable of diffusing into the nucleus. Here, melanin precursors and/or melanin breakdown products are excited to short-lived, triplet-state intermediates (e.g., dioxetane) by excess $ONOO^-$ and almost immediately degrade, yielding triplet-state carbonyls which transfer their energy to pyrimidines, generating CPDs hours after UVR exposure (Fig. 4) [69]. Although historically viewed as a protective molecule, melanin appears to also have a "dark side" [46, 70].

Keratinocyte and fibroblast mitochondria are not only a major source of ROS [71] but also a target for light-induced ROS formation [24, 72]. Recently, Krutmann and associates not only provided evidence that infrared radiation (IR) is responsible for generating ROS but also presented evidence showing that topical antioxidants can mitigate the resulting oxidative stress and retrograde signaling [73] (▶ Chapter 53, "Infrared A-Induced Skin Aging"). Paradoxically, mitochondrial DNA (mtDNA) is particularly susceptible to oxidative stress, largely because mtDNA lack histones and the mitochondrial enzymatic repair mechanisms appear less efficient than that found in the nucleus [74, 75]. Birch-Machin and colleagues [76] report that the mtDNA mutation rate is tenfold greater than nuclear DNA. Exposure to UVR is associated with several different mtDNA lesions including 4799-bp common deletion and 3895-bp deletion, base oxidation, point mutations, and strand breaks [72, 76, 77]. Despite having many mitochondria

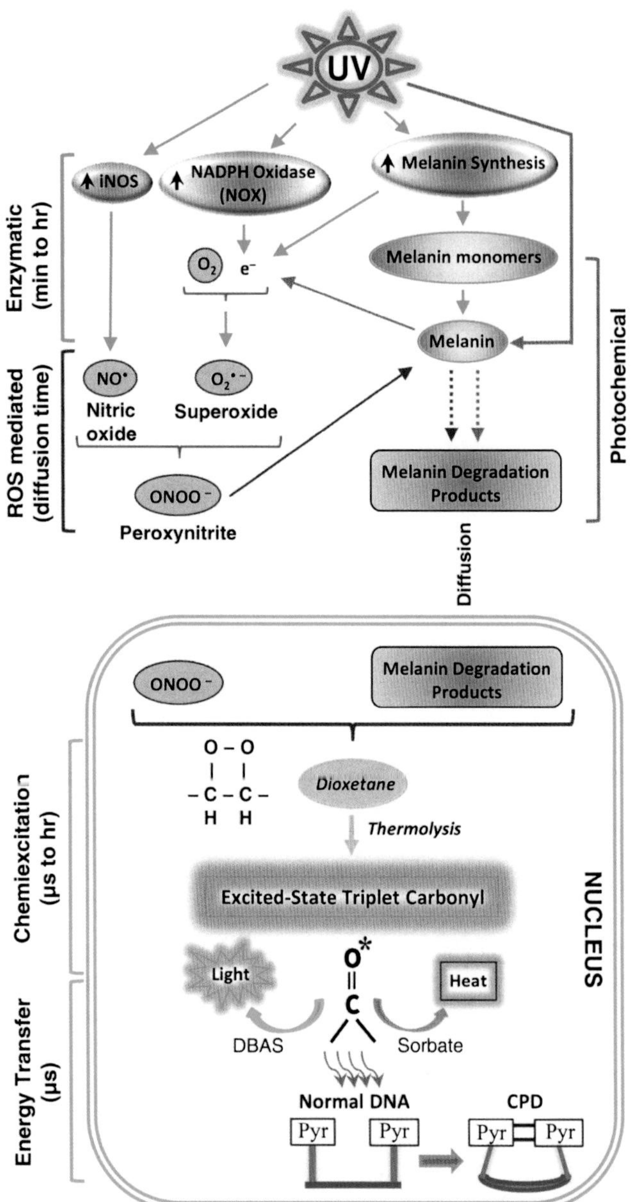

Fig. 5 Formation of cyclobutane pyrimidine dimers by chemiexcitation. UVA exposure induces the enzymatic generation of NO• and $\bullet O_2^-$. These ROS react to form a moderately reactive oxidizing specie, peroxynitrite ($ONOO^-$), which in turn initiates the degradation of cytosolic melanin into small molecular weight derivatives, capable of diffusing into the nucleus. Here, the melanin derivatives are excited to the triplet state by excess $ONOO^-$ and almost immediately thermolyze, yielding triplet-state carbonyls that transfer their energy to pyrimidines and generate CPDs long after UVR exposure (Reprinted from Premi et al. [69] with permission from The American Association for the Advancement of Science)

(heteroplasmy), chronic cellular oxidative stress leads to not only premature aging but also lipomas, pigmentation disorders, and alopecia [74, 78].

ROS-Mediated Lipid Damage

The highly unsaturated skin lipids – a mixture of sebaceous and epidermal lipids – represent an obvious oxidation target [79]. These lipids include palmitoleic acid (C16:1), oleic acid (C18:1), linoleic acid (C18:2), linolenic acid (C18:3), arachidonic acid (C20:4), sebaleic acid (C18:2), squalene, and cholesterol [79]. Peroxidation of lipids can occur via two routes, nonenzymatic – typically ROS-mediated – and enzymatic [80].

Nonenzymatic, ROS-mediated lipid peroxidation consists of three stages; initiation, propagation, and termination [81]. The reaction is initiated by any chemical species with sufficient reactivity to abstract a hydrogen atom from the methylene group adjacent to a fatty acid double bond [82]. Although this reaction can be initiated by molecular oxygen (re: O_2 is also a radical) given sufficient time and/or elevated temperature, in most biological systems, it involves a more reactive oxidizer (Fig. 4). As noted above, the ROS abstracts a hydrogen atom leaving behind a fatty acid (FA) alkyl radical (cf. Table 1, R•) with one unpaired electron. This R• can react with molecular oxygen to generate a lipid peroxyl radical (ROO•) – a slightly less reactive species (Table 1) – or it can abstract a hydrogen atom from another FA, generating another R• and propagating the chain reaction [82]. This reaction continues until the lipid radicals deplete available substrate or are neutralized by antioxidant [80].

The enzymatic generation of lipid peroxides is mediated by the lipoxygenases (LOX), cyclooxygenases (COX), and cytochrome P450 [83]. The end products are a class of bioactive lipid mediators known as eicosanoids [84]. In general, three fatty acids, derived largely from the plasma membrane, serve as substrates for these enzymes, arachidonic acid (C20:4), γ-linolenic acid (C20:4), and eicosapentaenoic acid (C20:5) [83]. Depending on the substrate and enzyme, a wide variety of bioactive lipid mediators are produced (reviewed in [84]). In general, the eicosanoids (prostaglandins and leukotrienes) are short-lived and regulate the local immune response, pain, and inflammation [85]. Recently, Li et al. [86] reported an age-related increase in PGE_2 (prostaglandin E_2), COX2, and PTGES1 (prostaglandin E synthase) in sun-protected skin, especially in the dermis. These results provide a rational explanation for degradation of the dermal matrix, since elevated levels of PGE_2 are known to suppress collagen synthesis and enhance the expression of matrix metalloproteases [86].

Although it is not surprising to observe elevated levels of eicosanoids and other pro-inflammatory mediators (e.g., cytokines, stress hormones, etc.) in individuals with inflammatory dermatoses (e.g., atopic dermatitis and psoriasis), it is surprising to see these inflammatory mediators elevated in healthy, but aged, skin [86]. To rationalize age-related inflammation, Franceschi et al. [87] coined the term *inflamm-aging*. Accordingly, *inflamm-aging* describes a shift toward a chronic pro-inflammatory state, characterized by the dysregulation of the immune system, leading to immunosenescence [88]. The development of this state is largely determined by genetics, age, and exposure to external stresses [89]. Since oxidative stress is known to trigger inflammation, it is a likely contributor to aging (discussed later). However, it is unclear at this time whether the age-related inflammation is a consequence of aging or a cause of aging [89].

Although there is good evidence to support the involvement of ROS and oxidative stress in several skin diseases [57, 90], the specific role of lipid hydroperoxides in skin morbidity is not well established [91]. Acute exposure of mice to ozone failed to show significant effects on transepidermal water loss [92]. This may be related to the self-renewing nature of the stratum corneum (i.e., desquamation), which limits damage. Nevertheless, there is substantial evidence that indicates that FA radicals (R•) decompose to reactive aldehydes (e.g., 4-hydroxynonenal (4-HNE), malondialdehyde (MDA), acrolein, etc.) which in turn react with proteins and dramatically affect their function (cf. next section) [93]. Squalene, a major component of sebum, is highly susceptible to the oxidizing effects of UVR [94] and ozone [95]. Valacchi suggests that ozone-generated peroxides function as 2nd messengers, activating various biochemical pathways without inducing overt damage [55, 96]. Nevertheless, lipid peroxides and their degradation product continue to serve as useful biomarkers of oxidative stress [97].

ROS-Mediated Protein Damage

ROS-mediated protein oxidation has been studied extensively [42, 81, 98–100] and reviewed recently [101]. Cellular oxidative stress can modify proteins by several different ROS-mediated reactions including the oxidization of sensitive amino acid residues, protein-adduct formation, covalent protein-protein cross-links, and peptide bond cleavage [100, 102]. While some of these oxidation reactions are reversible, others are irreversible and may contribute to cellular damage disease, and aging [91, 103].

The reversible oxidation of amino acid thiols (e.g., cysteine, methionine, selenocysteine) by the relatively abundant H_2O_2 may represent one of the most common protein modifications [104]. Because of its ability to undergo reversible oxidation/reduction (redox), cysteine uniquely serves as a molecular switch, regulating enzyme activity, gene expression, and numerous biochemical pathways [105]. The molecular consequences of protein thiol oxidation include alterations in protein folding, catalytic activity, and interaction with other key biomolecules [105]. The importance of protein thiols to cell function is supported by a recent genomic analysis, which estimates that the human proteome contains 20,000–40,000 redox-sensitive peptidyl-cysteine residues [105].

In contrast to the thiol-containing amino acids, modification of the aromatic amino acids (i.e., histidine, tryptophan, and phenylalanine) requires the action of a more potent ROS, such as •OH, generated via metal-catalyzed reactions or ionizing radiation [54, 100]. These reactions can lead to peptide bond cleavage or protein-protein cross-links. The consequences of these reactions include misfolding, decreased solubility, lost function and activity, aggregation, fragmentation, and increased/decreased susceptibility to proteolysis. Although mildly cross-linked proteins are readily degraded by the proteasome [106], extensively cross-linked or aggregated proteins appear to be poor substrates for degradation by proteases or proteasomes [107–109]. These cross-linked/aggregated proteins not only promote the generation of additional ROS [110] but also impose a significant bioenergetic cost on the cell in terms of disposal, repairing, and/or replacing.

Excessive accumulation of damaged proteins is associated with many age-related pathologies [12, 59, 91, 100, 101, 108]. In a recent study, Meadows et al. [111] observed not only a correlation between the amount of cross-linked proteins in the epidermis and dermis with age but also a correlation between the activity of age-related NADH oxidase (arNOX) – a superoxide generator – and cross-linked protein (cf. chapter entitled ▶ 22, "arNOX: New Mechanisms of Skin Aging and Lipoprotein Oxidation" and ▶ 21, "arNOX: A New Source of Aging").

Several amino acid residues (e.g., arginine, lysine, proline, and histidine) are susceptible to ROS-mediated carbonylation [91]. As noted earlier, lipid peroxidation frequently generates reactive aldehydes such as MDA and 4-HNE that readily react via a Michael addition reaction with side-chain amine groups, generating protein adducts (Fig. 6) [12]. Measurement of protein carbonyls is frequently used as a biomarker of cutaneous oxidative stress [97]. For example, Thiele et al. [113] showed that exposing stratum corneum to ozone, hypochlorite, or solar-simulated UV radiation generated protein carbonyls in a dose-dependent fashion.

Photoaged skin, a consequence of excessive exposure to sunlight (discussed later), exhibits significantly higher levels of protein carbonyls than sun-protected skin [114, 115]. Fisher and colleagues confirmed this finding, showing that aged skin is significantly more oxidized than young skin [116]. Most recently, Larroque-Cardoso and coworkers [117] showed that repeated exposure of mice to UVA induced not only the formation of ROS, but also 4-NHE, which was shown to react with elastin, reducing its digestion by leukocyte elastase. Since the accumulation of elastotic material is a hallmark of photoaged skin (discussed later), this study provides another mechanism connecting oxidative stress to accelerated skin aging.

Advanced glycation end products (AGEs) represent a specific type of reaction (Maillard reaction; reviewed in [118]) between an aldehyde and the amine group of proteins (Fig. 6). This reaction generates a heterogeneous group of compounds that polymerize into yellow-brown, autofluorescent aggregates, known as lipofuscin [119, 120]. These pigment granules are responsible for yellow hue seen in aging skin. Formation of this pigment not only correlates with intrinsic aging [121] but appears to be accelerated by extrinsic factors that induce oxidative stress such as the various conditions associated with metabolic syndrome [122] and lifestyle excesses (e.g.,

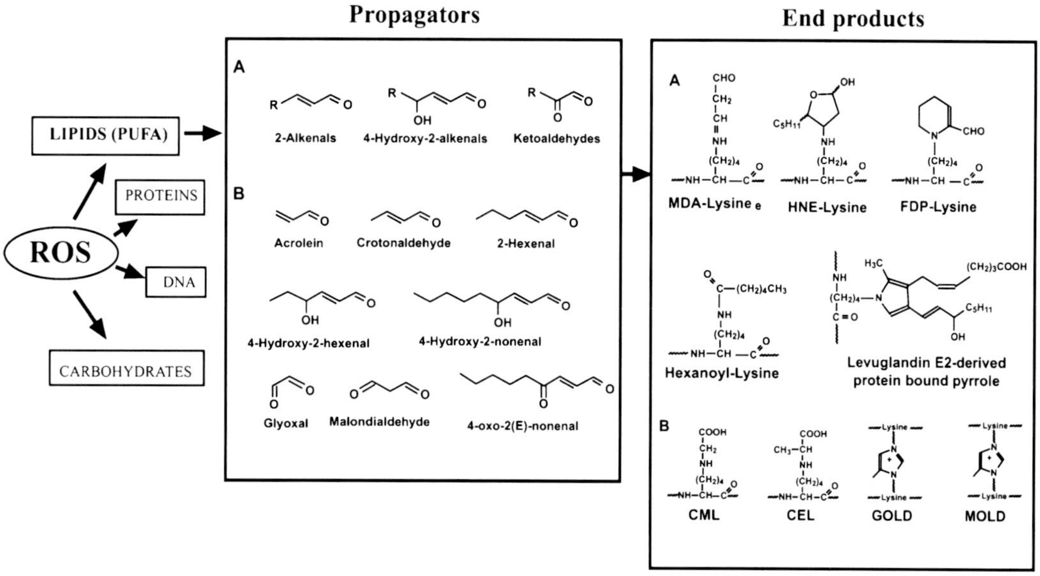

Fig. 6 Formation of advanced glycation end products (*AGEs*). ROS generated by any of the mechanisms shown in Fig. 4 attack key biomolecules and generate various substrate-specific reactive aldehydes. These aldehydes subsequently react with the abundant protein lysine and arginine residues via Maillard reaction to form various types of AGEs (Reprinted from Hulbert et al. [112] with permission from The American Physiology Society)

sun exposure, cigarette smoking, alcohol consumption) [119, 123–125]. Once formed, AGEs can interact with a specific pattern recognition receptor known as RAGE (receptor for advanced glycation end products) found on many cells, including keratinocytes, fibroblasts, dendritic cells, and mononuclear cells [110, 126, 127]. Once RAGE is activated, cells initiate a multitude of cell-specific responses (cf. Table 3 in [119]). One of the most studied RAGE-mediated responses is inflammation [132]. Deletion of this receptor in mice has been shown to impair inflammation and to protect against the development of skin tumors [132]. The various cell-specific RAGE-mediated signaling pathways are reviewed in Kierdorf and Fritz [133]. Cutaneous AGE formation is associated with hyperpigmentation (cf. ► Chaps. 77, "Hyperpigmentation in Aging Skin," and ► 79, "The New Face of Pigmentation and Aging"), increased skin laxity, and visible wrinkling [134–136]. However, it should be noted that the increase in skin autofluorescence reflects not only environmental stresses on the skin but also systemic diseases such as diabetes and renal failure. In fact, skin autofluorescence represents a potentially useful biomarker for diabetes [137].

The last ROS-mediated protein modification is the hydrolysis of the peptide bond and fragmentation of the protein. This reaction requires a highly energetic ROS, typically singlet oxygen ($^1O_2$) or •OH [81, 100]. Mechanistically, •OH mediates the abstraction of the α-hydrogen atom from any one of the amino acid residues in a protein, creating a carbon-centered radical that subsequently reacts with molecular oxygen, resulting in peptide bond cleavage [100]. Although in vivo evidence supporting protein fragmentation is generally lacking – largely because damaged proteins are rapidly degraded by proteases and proteasomes [106] – in vitro studies clearly show that •OH depolymerizes collagen [116, 138].

Cutaneous Antioxidant Defense System

Although all aerobic organisms require oxygen to sustain life, an overabundance can lead to the deleterious reactions discussed in the previous

Table 3 Nonenzymatic antioxidants in human skin

Antioxidant	Concentration Epidermis/stratum corneum	Dermis
Ascorbic acid[a]	3798	723
Uric acid[a]	1071	182
Glutathione (total)[a]	484	84
Tocopherol (total)[a]	34.2	18.0
Ubiquinol (total)[a]	7.7	3.2
Retinoids[b]	~2.0	–
β-Carotene[b]	13.7	–
Protein thiols	Keratins [128], cell envelope [129]	Cytoplasmic proteins
Metal-binding proteins (ferritin, metallothioneins, etc.)	NA	NA

[a]nmol/g tissue [130]
[b]μg/mg protein [131]

section. Moreover, unlike many organs, the skin is exposed to oxygen from both the atmosphere and the capillary bed. In a recent study, Meinke and associates [139] showed that greater quantities of ROS are generated in vivo than ex vivo skin by UVR. This result suggests that most of the oxygen in the skin is derived from the circulatory system. Nevertheless, the skin has evolved a sophisticated and extensive antioxidant defense system, focused on two goals: (1) prevent the formation of ROS and (2) neutralize those ROS that are formed.

One approach to prevent the formation of ROS is to expend metabolic energy to generate and maintain a "reduced" cellular environment. In general, three redox couples maintain cellular redox state: nicotinamide adenine dinucleotide phosphate ($NADPH/NADP^+$), glutathione (GSH/GSSG), and thioredoxin (TRX_{red}/TRX_{ox}) [140]. These reducing agents readily donate electrons to neutralize ROS. Another preventive approach, and arguably a critical one, is the synthesis of highly efficient peptide chelators such as ferritin, transferrin, lactoferrin, and metallothioneins [54]. These proteins bind transition metal ions such as Fe^{++} and Cu^+, making them unavailable to participate in the Fenton reaction and the generation of highly reactive •OH (Fig. 4) [53].

Despite the limited approaches to prevent radical formation, most cells, and the skin in particular, have evolved an elaborate endogenous antioxidant defense system (reviewed in [57, 141, 142]). By definition, an antioxidant is any substance that significantly delays or prevents the oxidation of an oxidizable substrate despite being present in concentrations lower than the substrate [9]. Most antioxidants are characterized by having one or more hydroxy or thiol groups, frequently associated with an aromatic structure [143].

In most organisms, redox balance and control of ROS are achieved through two distinct systems: nonenzymatic antioxidants and enzymatic antioxidant reactions (Fig. 7) [37]. The nonenzymatic antioxidant system is subdivided into two classes, defined largely by their solubility properties. The water-soluble antioxidants, such as ascorbic acid, glutathione, cysteine, dihydrolipoic acid, and uric acid, are responsible for eliminating ROS from the aqueous compartments, whereas the lipid-soluble antioxidants such as the tocopherols (α, β, γ, δ), ubiquinol (CoQ_{10}), retinoids and the various carotenoids obtained from the diet function largely in the lipid compartment. Table 3 lists the key cutaneous antioxidants and their relative distribution between the epidermis/stratum corneum and dermis [130, 131]. Despite its low water content, the stratum corneum exhibits a surprisingly high level of water-soluble antioxidants such as ascorbate, urate, and glutathione. These antioxidants represent functional remnants from the metabolically active basal keratinocytes. They provide the stratum corneum an antioxidant regenerating system (Fig. 8).

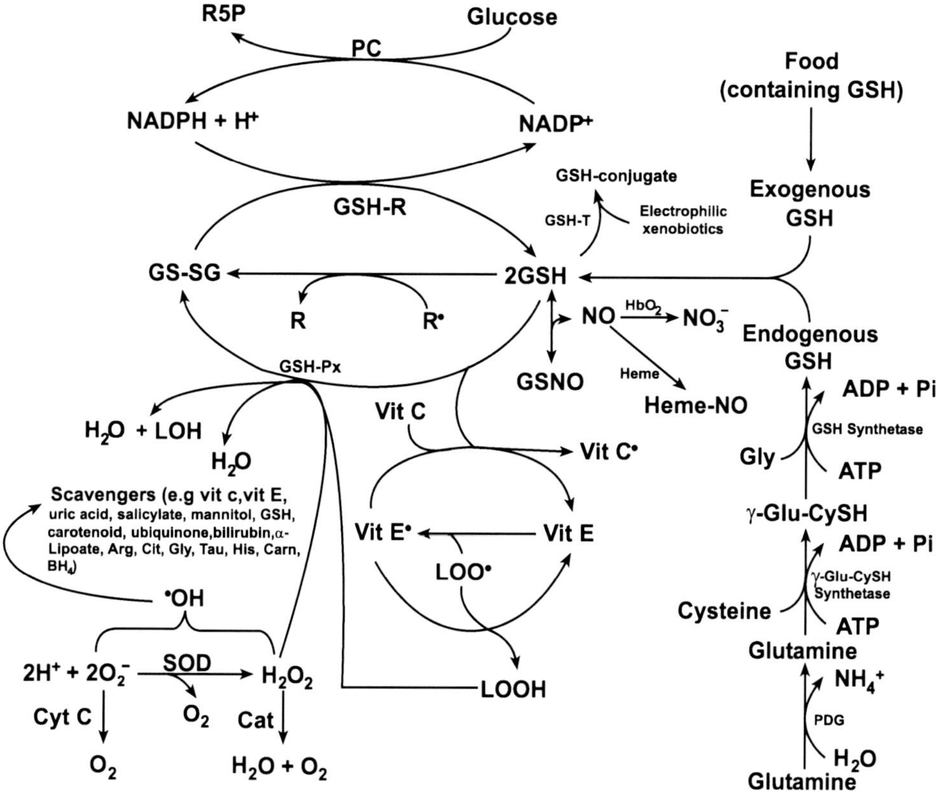

Fig. 7 Removal of reactive oxidizing species from mammalian cells. *ADP* adenosine diphosphate, *Arg* arginine, *BH_4* (6R)-5,6,7,8-tetrahydro-L-biopterin, *Carn* carnosine, *Cat* catalase, *Cit* citrulline, *Cyt C* cytochrome C, *ETS* electron transport system, *Glu* L-glutamate, *Gly* glycine, *γ-Glu-cySH* γ-glutamylcysteine, *GS-SH* oxidized glutathione (glutathione disulfide), *GSH* glutathione (reduced form), *GSH-Px* glutathione peroxidase, *GSH-R* glutathione reductase, *GSH-T* glutathione S-transferase, *GSNO* nitrosylated glutathione, *HbO_2* oxyhemoglobin, *Heme-NO* heme-nitric oxide, *His* histidine, *LOH* lipid alcohol, *LOO•* lipid peroxyl radical, *LOOH* lipid hydroperoxides, *•NO* nitric oxide, *NO_3^-* nitrate, *$•O_2$* superoxide anion radical, *•NOO* peroxynitrite, *PC* pentose cycle, *R•* radicals, *R* non-radicals, *R5P* ribulose-5-phosphate, *SOD* superoxide dismutase, *Tau* taurine, *Vit C* vitamin C (ascorbic acid), *Vit C•* vitamin C radical, *vit E* vitamin E (α-tocopherol), *Vit E•* vitamin E radical (Reprinted from Fang et al. [37] with the permission from Elsevier)

Although present at lower levels and confined largely to the epidermis (Table 3), the carotenoids (β-carotene, lycopene, and lutein) represent key contributors to the skin's antioxidant defense system [145, 146]. Studies from the Lademann lab have established the carotenoids as the skin's primary scavengers of solar radiation-induced singlet oxygen [147, 148]. Topical application of carotenoids has been shown to mitigate the solar radiation-induced oxidative stress [149–152]. Carotenoids are particularly important since they provide protection at wavelengths beyond the functioning of current sunscreens, namely, visible and IR [153]. It is also worth noting that phytonutrients (green tea polyphenols/flavonoids, grape seed proanthocyanidins, milk thistle silymarin, Polypodium leucotomos, etc.) derived from the diet play a key role in mitigating oxidative stress in the skin [154–158, also Cf. Impact of dietary supplements on skin aging].

Since many stratum corneum structural proteins (e.g., keratins and cornified envelope proteins) contain thiols, they too may function as effective ROS "sinks" [128]. Vermeij et al. [129, 159] recently demonstrated that the cornified envelope in general, and the cysteine-enriched

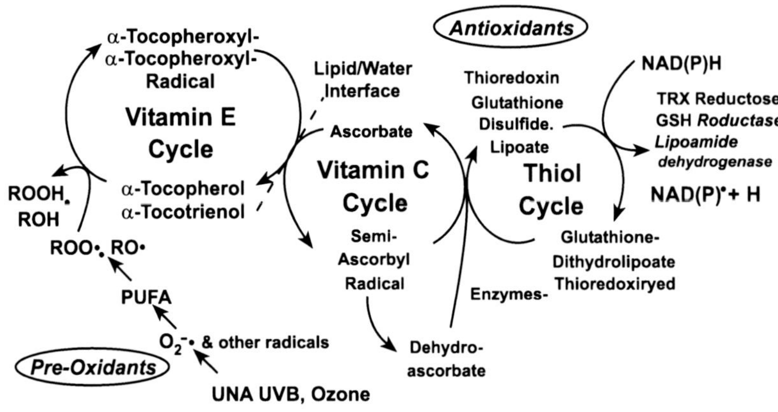

Fig. 8 **Antioxidant network**. Cutaneous antioxidant network showing the relationship between vitamin E cycle, vitamin C cycle, and thiol cycle (Reprinted from Packer et al. [144] with permission from The American Society for Nutritional Sciences)

Table 4 Human skin enzymatic antioxidant defense system

Antioxidant	Enzyme activity (units/g tissue) Epidermis	Dermis
Superoxide dismutase [130] $2H^+ + 2{\bullet}O_2^- \rightarrow H_2O_2 + O_2$	816	361
Catalase [130] $2H_2O_2 \rightarrow 2H_2O + O_2$	2912	355
Glutathione peroxidase [130] (1) $ROOH + 2GSH \rightarrow RHO + GSSG + 2H_2O$ (2) ${\bullet}O_2^- + NADPH + H^+ + GSH \rightarrow GSSH + NADP^+ + H_2O_2$	0.71	0.44
Glutathione reductase [130] $G\text{-}SS\text{-}G + NADPH + H^+ \rightarrow 2GSH + NADP^+$	0.63	0.20
Thioredoxin reductase [160] $R\text{-}SS\text{-}R + NADPH + H^+ \rightarrow 2RSH + NADP^+$	Detected	Detected
Methionine sulfoxide reductase [161–163] Peptidyl-Met-SO-CH_3 + thioredoxin + H_2O → Peptidyl-Met-S-CH_3 + thioredoxin disulfide	Detected	Detected
Heme oxygenase-1 [164–166] Heme + O_2 + NADPH → biliverdin + Fe^{++} + CO + NADP + H_2O	Detected	Detected
Peroxiredoxins Prx (red) + H_2O_2 → Prx (oxid) + $2H_2O$	Detected	Detected

small-proline rich proteins in particular, represent a first-line antioxidant defense against environmentally-induced oxidative stress.

The second component of the cellular antioxidant defense system is based on enzymes. Some researchers believe that the antioxidant enzymes represent the most efficient mechanism since they are specific, function catalytically, and are not generally consumed in the reaction [14]. Table 4 lists some of the key antioxidant enzymes, their distribution, and the reactions that define the cutaneous enzymatic antioxidant defense system [130, 161, 167–169]. Superoxide dismutase and catalase represent two of the most active enzymes, reflecting the importance of regulating cellular levels of ${\bullet}O_2^-$ and H_2O_2 (cf. Fig. 3) [170]. Glutathione peroxidase is a membrane-bound enzyme that plays a key role in limiting the chain reaction in lipid peroxidation [80]. Of equal importance is the role glutathione reductase plays in regenerating reduced glutathione (GSSH → 2GSH) and providing reducing equivalents [80].

Since two key antioxidants are also vitamins (vitamins E and C) and their availability may be limited by diet and/or disease, nature has evolved an ingenious system to ensure the regeneration of these antioxidants. The *antioxidant network* was a concept (Fig. 8) advanced by Packer and associates [171]. Vitamin E (tocopherol) functions as the major chain-breaking antioxidant within the lipid compartment (cf. Table 3). To overcome dietary limitation, vitamin E can be catalytically regenerated by ascorbic acid (vitamin C). Not only is ascorbic acid present in greater amounts (cf. Table 3), but it is also a much more effective reducing agent [19]. Finally, to ensure adequate quantities of reduced ascorbate, the cell uses metabolic energy to generate thiols, such as glutathione (GSH), dihydrolipoate (DHL), and thioredoxin (THX), to catalytically reduce the semi-ascorbyl radical to ascorbate [144]. Overall, this process conserves the limited amounts of tocopherol and ascorbic acid located in the various skin compartments.

Redox Signaling Overview

The medical community's views on the involvement of ROS in health and disease have evolved over the past decade [172, 173]. Originally, these highly reactive molecules were viewed as something that must be avoided and/or eliminated at all costs. However, more recent thinking suggests that ROS play an indispensible role in cellular signaling, homeostasis, and inducing an adaptive response [174]. Not surprisingly, the paradoxical effects of ROS depend on several factors including the nature of the ROS, concentration, location, persistence, and the effectiveness of the antioxidant defenses. Although a thorough review of redox signaling is beyond the scope of this chapter, several regulatory mechanisms will be highlighted. However, for a more thorough review on cellular redox signaling, the reader is referred to several excellent reviews [26, 40, 172, 173, 175–179].

Cellular redox state reflects the balance between the rate of ROS formation and rate of removal by the antioxidant defense system [42]. Under normal conditions, each cell is characterized by a cell-specific redox state [26, 180]. Redox homeostasis is maintained within a narrow range by the cell's antioxidant systems and the following redox couples: GSH/GSSG, $NADPH/NADP^+$, thioredoxin (reduced)/thioredoxin (oxidized), and peroxiredoxin (reduced)/peroxiredoxin (oxidized) [181, 182]. Because of its abundance and relatively low redox value ($E^\circ \sim -200$ to -260 mV), the 2GSH/GSSG couple represents one of the most versatile redox buffers [180, 182].

Five distinct redox mechanisms have been proposed to regulate cell function: transcriptional regulation, direct oxidative modification, regulation of redox-sensitive interacting proteins, regulation of redox-sensitive modifying enzymes, and regulation of protein turnover [18, 179]. Table 5 describes these redox mechanisms and provides several relevant biochemical examples.

Of particular importance to the skin is Keap1-Nrf2. Keap1-Nrf2 (Kelch-like ECH-associated protein 1-nuclear factor erythroid 2-related factor 2) is a redox-sensitive transcription factor that regulates the expression of antioxidant genes [183–186]. Under normal cellular redox conditions (Fig. 9), Keap1 is complexed to Nrf2, marking the Keap1-Nrf2 complex for continuous proteasomal degradation. However, upon exposure to ROS (e.g., H_2O_2, •NO, lipid peroxides, etc.) or electrophiles (e.g., acetaminophen, aromatic hydrocarbons, paraquat, pentachlorophenol, heavy metals, etc.), one or more Keap1 cysteines are modified, releasing Nrf2 from the complex and allowing it to translocate to the nucleus [187]. Once in the nucleus, the activated Nrf2 protein binds to an antioxidant response element (ARE) and promotes the transcription of genes encoding for antioxidant enzymes (Table 4), enzymes responsible for generating reducing equivalents and/or synthesis of low molecular weight antioxidants (Table 3), and various cytoprotective proteins that detoxify electrophiles or scavenge redox-active metals (Table 3) (e.g., cytochrome P450, proteasome components) [183, 185, 188]. Although constitutively expressed, recent research suggests the Keap1-Nrf2 can be enhanced by topical application of

Table 5 Redox-mediated mechanisms that regulate protein function

Type of regulation	Mechanism of regulation	Examples
Transcription	Transcription factors containing a redox-sensitive Cys/Met in DNA-binding domain	NFκB, AP-1, HIF-1α, p53, FOXO
Direct oxidative modification	Activity of enzyme is posttranslationally modified by the oxidation of one or more amino acids (Cys, Met, Tyr), via nitration/nitrosylation (•NO) or carbonylation	MAPK, JNK, PKC, ANT, Hsp, BCL2, PTEN
Redox-sensitive accessory proteins	Transcription factor stabilized by association with redox-sensitive accessory protein	Keap1-Nrf2, ASK1-TRX, JNK, p53-JNK,
Redox-sensitive modifying enzyme	Protein is posttranslationally modified (phosphorylated/ dephosphorylated) by another enzyme that is redox-sensitive (phosphatase and kinase)	Phosphotyrosine kinase, protein tyrosine phosphatases
Protein turnover	Redox-mediated protein modification (e.g., phosphorylation, ubiquitination, glutathionylation, etc.) promotes the proteasome-mediated degradation of protein	IκB, Bcl-2, p53

Source: Ref. [179]

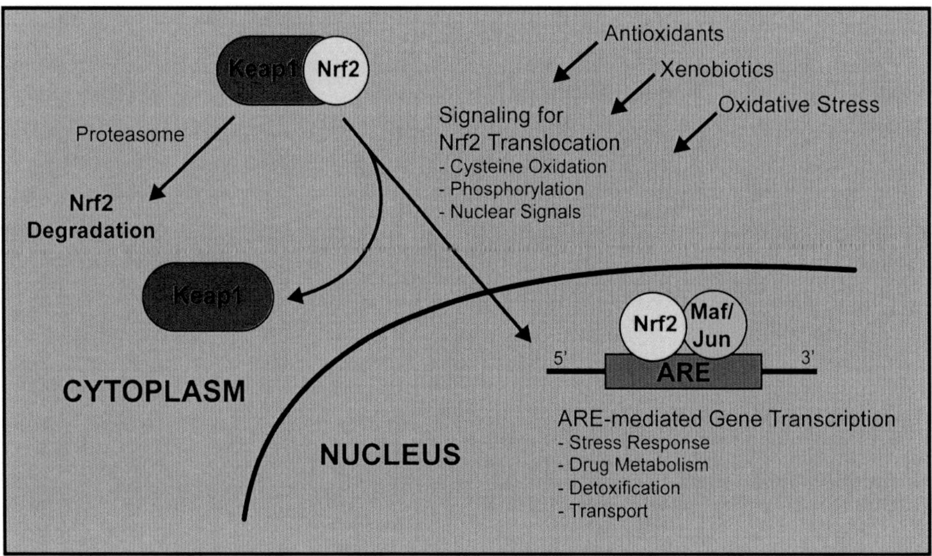

Fig. 9 Redox regulation of the Keap1-Nrf2. Under normal cell conditions (normoxia), Nrf2 is associated with Keap1. However, continuous ubiquitination of Keap1 marks the Keap1-Nrf2 complex for proteasomal degradation. Upon exposure to electrophilic compounds and/or conditions of oxidative stress, several key Keap1 cysteine residues are modified [187], resulting in the dissociation of Keap1-Nrf2 complex. The uncomplexed Nrf2 migrates to the nucleus where it binds to the antioxidant response element (*ARE*) and stimulates gene expression (Reprinted from Aleksunes and Manautou [186] with permission from Sage Publication)

phytochemicals (licochalcone A, sulforaphane, and soybean tar). For more information on Keap1-Nrf2, the interested reader is directed to several reviews [17, 183, 185, 188–190].

In summary, it is clear that nature employs physiologically low levels of ROS as intracellular 2nd messengers to regulate a myriad of cell processes (Table 5). Indeed, even critical processes such as epidermal differentiation and follicle development are regulated by H_2O_2 [191, 192]. However, as will be discussed in the next section, this form of communication comes with some risks.

Introduction to the Free Radical Theory of Aging

Aging is defined as a progressive loss of physiological integrity, leading to impaired function and an increased vulnerability to death [193]. Many theories have been proposed to explain the aging process [194]. Not surprisingly, most have been abandoned in light of recent findings, while several others continue to drive research in this area.

Denham Harman first advanced the *Free Radical Theory of Aging* in the 1950s [195]. According to this theory, intrinsic aging results from the accumulation of oxidative damage, largely as a result of normal cellular processes. Despite its many attractive features – it provides a biochemical mechanism for cell damage and implies a rational approach for intervention via antioxidant supplementation – it suffers from some serious limitations (reviewed in [196]). Many years later, Harman [197] proposed and Miquel and colleagues [198] refined the *mitochondrial free radical theory of aging*, which proposed that the mitochondria were the major source for cellular ROS (cf. ▶ Chap. 48, "Cellular Energy Metabolism and Oxidative Stress"). Earlier research by Cadenas and Davies [38] provided evidence that the electron transport chain was less than 100 % efficient and a key source of $\bullet O_2^-$. Unless neutralized by the antioxidant defenses, this and other ROS were responsible for oxidatively damaging mtDNA. Consequently, as mtDNA damage accumulates, the mitochondrial function deteriorates, creating a vicious cycle (cf. ▶ Chaps. 47, "Alterations of Energy Metabolism in Cutaneous Aging" and ▶ 48, "Cellular Energy Metabolism and Oxidative Stress"). Ultimately, mitochondrial dysfunction leads to reduced cellular ATP, changes in cell metabolism and redox status, [199] and potentially to apoptosis [76].

Over the years, the *mitochondrial free radical theory of aging* has gained much support, based largely on the following: (1) a strong correlation between chronological age and the amount of ROS generated and oxidative damage produced, (2) mitochondrial function declines with age, (3) inhibitor studies and gene manipulation studies appear to enhance ROS removal, and (4) several age-dependent diseases are associated with oxidative stress [200]. However, despite numerous studies supporting the free radical theories of aging, a growing body of evidence suggests that these theories are inconsistent with many observable facts [201]. For example, Gladyshev [202] notes that anaerobically grown yeast generate little ROS, but yet exhibit signs of aging. Additionally, the various versions of the *Free Radical Theories of Aging* do not explain the life-extending benefits of caloric/dietary restriction, exercise, and nutrient sensing (i.e., TOR, target of rapamycin), which tend to increase the formation of ROS [200, 202–206]. Most importantly, these theories fail to reconcile what is referred to as the "antioxidant paradox" [207]. The antioxidant paradox is based on the finding from numerous intervention studies that show dietary supplementation with antioxidants and/or genetic manipulations that enhance the expression of antioxidant enzymes fail in most cases – with some notable exceptions such as some cancers, diabetes, neurodegenerative diseases, inflammatory bowel disease, and skin aging – to provide measurable improvement in aging outcome [208]. Finally, and most significantly, numerous studies with *Caenorhabditis elegans*, yeast, and fruit flies show that a transient prooxidant state (e.g., H_2O_2) produced beneficial effects, including life extension [204, 209–212].

To rationalize the beneficial effects of oxidative stress, several hypotheses have been advanced. Tapia's *Mitohormesis* concept suggests that low levels of ROS exert a beneficial, pro-survival effect, by stimulating an adaptive response [209]. According to this theory, "what doesn't kill you; makes you stronger." Equally valid is the concept that ROS regulate the actions of longevity/senescence genes such as *p66shc*, *SIRT*, *FOXO*, and *Klotho* [213, 214]. According to Jones' *Redox Hypothesis* [182], oxidative stress is a consequence of the disruption of specific thiol redox circuits – largely, by the more prevalent non-radical oxidants – which normally function in cell signaling and physiological regulation. In a related concept, Sohal and Orr [181] proposed the *Redox Stress Hypothesis* which suggests that aging reflects a process whereby cellular redox status shifts from a reducing environment to one that is decidedly oxidizing, leading to dysfunctional redox signaling [181]. This hypothesis is supported by observations made across many different species and tissues that old cells are characterized by higher amounts of oxidized protein thiols and mixed disulfides compared to young cells [181, 182].

Clearly, organismal aging is a complex process, impacted by various endogenous and exogenous factors [193]. As highlighted above, the results to date in animal models appear conflicting; low levels of oxidative stress appear to promote beneficial outcomes, whereas high levels are consistent with disease and accelerated aging [182].

Oxidative Stress and Skin Aging

Like any other organ the skin ages intrinsically with the passage of time [215]. As noted in the previous section, intrinsic aging is complex and not fully understood. However, unlike any other organ, the skin is exposed to various environmental conditions that induce oxidative stress such as solar radiation [215], air pollution [35], tobacco smoke [216], and endogenous or exogenous photosensitizing compounds [45]. Skin that is protected from sun exposure (e.g., buttock, underarm, etc.) typically ages under the influence of intrinsic or chronological aging mechanisms such as those described above. Intrinsically/chronologically aged skin is characterized by modest loss of function and changes in visual appearance (e.g., elasticity, uniform coloration, texture, etc.) (cf. ► Chaps. 3, "Degenerative Changes in Aging Skin," ► 5, "Major Changes in Skin Function in the Elderly and Their Contributions to Common Clinical Challenges," ► 28, "Pathology of Aging Skin," ► 9, "Pathomechanisms of Endogenously Aged Skin," ► 6, "Skin Aging: A Brief Summary of Characteristic Changes," and ► 62, "Aging and Intrinsic Aging: Pathogenesis and Manifestations"). However, if one superimposes the effects of habitual exposure to environmental stresses (e.g., solar radiation and air pollution) and/or lifestyle excesses (e.g., tobacco usage) onto endogenous intrinsic aging process, the skin ages prematurely.

Photoaging, a term coined by Kligman in 1969, describes clinical, histological, and functional changes in skin that is chronically exposed to sunlight (e.g., face, chest, hands, forearms) [217, 218]. Unlike intrinsically/chronologically aged skin, photoaged skin is characterized by deep wrinkles, irregular pigmentation, significant loss of skin elasticity/resilience, and overall poor quality (cf. ► Chaps. 3, "Degenerative Changes in Aging Skin," ► 28, "Pathology of Aging Skin", ► 10, "Pathomechanisms of Photoaged Skin," and ► 6, "Skin Aging: A Brief Summary of Characteristic Changes"). The molecular mechanism by which solar radiation causes photoaging is complex and more fully discussed by Krutmann (► Chap. 10, "Pathomechanisms of Photoaged Skin") and Bernerd and Marionnet (New Insights in Photoageing Process Revealed by in vitro Reconstructed Skin Models). Recent research suggests that all wavelengths of sunlight, UVB (280–320 nm), UVA (320–400 nm), visible (400–770 nm), and infrared radiation (IR, 700–1400 nm) contribute to photoaging (Fig. 10) [17, 44]. UVB induces direct damage to DNA, whereas UVA, visible, and infrared radiation appear to induce the formation of ROS via photodynamic reactions [44, 219, 220]. Most recently, Wolf and associates [221] created a transgenic mouse that expressed a redox-sensitive green fluorescent protein. Exposing these mice to physiological relevant levels of UVA produced a clear fluorescent signal, indicating generation of ROS and cutaneous oxidative stress [221]. Moreover, studies in humans show that daily use of broad-spectrum sunscreens for 4.5 years significantly reduces the visible signs of aging by 24 % [222]. In another human study, topical application of a sunscreen containing a cocktail of antioxidants mitigated the induction of metalloproteinase-1 by infrared A radiation [73]. Taken together, these studies and others (cf. ► Chaps. 10, "Pathomechanisms of Photoaged Skin," ► 53, "Infrared A-Induced

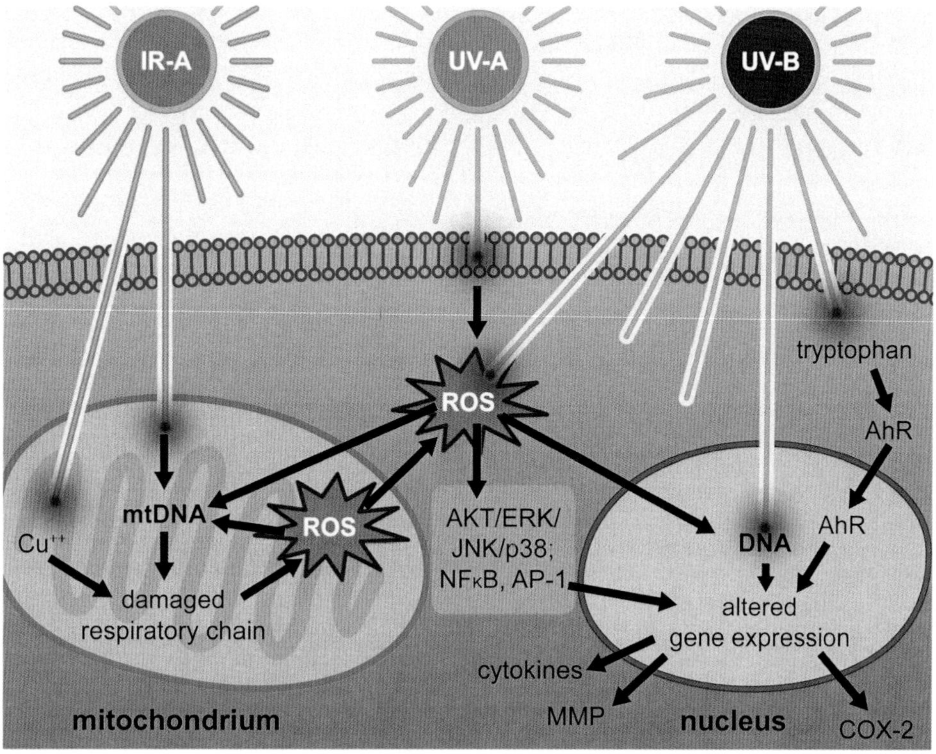

Fig. 10 **Photoinduced reactive oxygen oxidizing and their targets**. UVB radiation directly damages DNA. UVA is absorbed by an endogenous chromophore and photodynamically generates ROS. Similar to UVA, IRA radiation is absorbed by a mitochondrial respiratory chain chromophore and photodynamically produces ROS. Regardless of their source, the ROS attack nuclear and mtDNA, activate signaling pathways, alter gene expression, and promote inflammation and further destruction of key biomolecules (Reprinted from Wolfle et al. [17] with permission from Karger AG)

Skin Aging," ► 55, "Skin Photodamage Prevention: State of the Art and New Prospects," and ► 102, "New Insights in Photoaging Process Revealed by In Vitro Reconstructed Skin Models.") Support a role of oxidative stress in the premature aging of the skin.

In addition to chronic exposure to solar radiation, tobacco smoking is also strongly associated with premature aging (cf. ► Chap. 57, "Tobacco Smoke and Skin Aging"). Moreover, recent studies from the Krutmann laboratory indicate that the exposure to air pollutants such as airborne particulate matter is highly associated with premature skin aging [35, 223–225]. Another emerging pollutant, ozone, has also been implicated with cutaneous oxidative stress [35, 226, 227] and may be associated with premature skin aging (cf. chapter entitled ► 52, "Cutaneous Responses to Tropospheric Ozone exposure"). Taken together, there appears to be little doubt that ROS and oxidative stress accelerate skin aging [58, 228].

Concluding Remarks

Life in an aerobic environment offers benefits and consequences. The benefits include more efficient energy generation and intracellular communication, which may be counterbalanced by oxidative stress, loss of function, disease, cancer, and aging. Nevertheless, nature has provided aerobic organisms with a sophisticated antioxidant defense system, which under normal circumstances is highly effective in maintaining the skin's redox balance. Clearly we cannot live without ROS and the vital functions they perform. Paradoxically however, a lifetime exposure to these reactive species may contribute to morbidity and, ultimately, to our demise. It is for this reason that ROS and oxidative stress will continue to drive biomedical and aging research [211].

References

1. Des Marais DJ. When did photosynthesis emerge on earth? Science. 2000;289(5485):1703–5.
2. Falkowski PG, Godfrey LV. Electrons, life and the evolution of Earth's oxygen cycle. Philos Trans R Soc Lond B Biol Sci. 2008;363(1504):2705–16.
3. Graham JB, Aguilar NM, Dudley R, Gans C. Implications of the late Palaeozoic oxygen pulse for physiology and evolution. Nature. 1995;375 (6527):117–20.
4. Wright CJ, Dennery PA. Manipulation of gene expression by oxygen: a primer from bedside to bench. Pediatr Res. 2009;66(1):3–10.
5. Maltepe E, Saugstad OD. Oxygen in health and disease: regulation of oxygen homeostasis – clinical implications. Pediatr Res. 2009;65(3):261–8.
6. Auten RL, Davis JM. Oxygen toxicity and reactive species: the devil is in the details. Pediatr Res. 2009;66(2):121–7.
7. Voet D, Voet JG. Biochemistry. 4th ed. New York: Wiley; 2010.
8. Halliwell B. Reactive species and antioxidants. Redox biology is a fundamental theme of aerobic life. Plant Physiol. 2006;141(2):312.
9. Halliwell B, Gutteridge J. Free radicals in biology and medicine. 4th ed. Oxford/New York: Oxford University Press; 2007.
10. Kalyanaraman B. Teaching the basics of redox biology to medical and graduate students: oxidants, antioxidants and disease mechanisms. Redox Biol. 2013;1(1):244–57.
11. Cadet J, Douki T, Ravanat J-L. Oxidatively generated damage to cellular DNA by UVB and UVA radiation. Photochem Photobiol. 2015;91(1):140–55.
12. Davies MJ. The oxidative environment and protein damage. Biochim Biophys Acta. 2005;1703(2):93–109.
13. Peres PS, Terra VA, Guarnier FA, Cecchini R, Cecchini AL. Photoaging and chronological aging profile: understanding oxidation of the skin. J Photochem Photobiol B Biol. 2011;103(2):93–7.
14. McCord JM. The evolution of free radicals and oxidative stress. Am J Med. 2000;108(8):652–9.
15. Sies H. Strategies of antioxidant defense. Euro J Biochem. 1993;215(2):213–9.
16. Stoyanovsky DA, Maeda A, Atkins JL, Kagan VE. Assessments of thiyl radicals in biosystems: difficulties and new applications. Anal Chem. 2011;83 (17):6432–8.
17. Wölfle U, Seelinger G, Bauer G, Meinke MC, Lademann J, Schempp CM. Reactive molecule species and antioxidative mechanisms in normal skin and skin aging. Skin Pharmacol Physiol. 2014;27 (6):316–32.
18. Marinho HS, Real C, Cyrne L, Soares H, Antunes F. Hydrogen peroxide sensing, signaling and regulation of transcription factors. Redox Biol. 2014;2:535–62.
19. Buettner GR. The pecking order of free radicals and antioxidants: lipid peroxidation, alpha-tocopherol, and ascorbate. Arch Biochem Biophys. 1993;300 (2):535–43.
20. Finkel T, Holbrook NJ. Oxidants, oxidative stress and the biology of ageing. Nature. 2000;408(6809):239–47.
21. Petibois C, Gionnet K, Goncalves M, Perromat A, Moenner M, Deleris G. Analytical performances of FT-IR spectrometry and imaging for concentration measurements within biological fluids, cells, and tissues. Analyst. 2006;131(5):640.
22. Leung TH, Zhang LF, Wang J, Ning S, Knox SJ, Kim SK. Topical hypochlorite ameliorates NF-κB–mediated skin diseases in mice. J Clin Invest. 2013;123(12):5361–70.
23. Radi R. Peroxynitrite, a stealthy biological oxidant. J Biol Chem. 2013;288(37):26464–72.
24. Wondrak GT, Jacobson MK, Jacobson EL. Endogenous UVA-photosensitizers: mediators of skin photodamage and novel targets for skin photoprotection. Photochem Photobiol Sci. 2006;5 (2):215–37.
25. Ogilby PR. Singlet oxygen: there is still something new under the sun, and it is better than ever. Photochem Photobiol Sci. 2010;9(12):1543–60.
26. Circu ML, Aw TY. Reactive oxygen species, cellular redox systems, and apoptosis. Free Radic Biol Med. 2010;48(6):749–62.
27. del Río LA. Peroxisomes as a cellular source of reactive nitrogen species signal molecules. Arch Biochem Biophys. 2011;506(1):1–11.
28. Sena L, Chandel N. Physiological roles of mitochondrial reactive species. Mol Cell. 2012;48(2):158–67.
29. Giorgio M, Trinei M, Migliaccio E, Pelicci PG. Hydrogen peroxide: a metabolic by-product or a common mediator of ageing signals? Nat Rev Mol Cell Biol. 2007;8(9):722–8.
30. Hill BG, Dranka BP, Bailey SM, Lancaster Jr JR, Darley-Usmar VM. What part of NO don't you understand? Some answers to the cardinal questions in nitric oxide biology. J Biol Chem. 2010;285 (26):19699–704.
31. Freinbichler W, Colivicchi MA, Stefanini C, Bianchi L, Ballini C, Misini B, et al. Highly reactive species: detection, formation, and possible functions. Cell Mol Life Sci. 2011;68(12):2067–79.
32. Nathan C, Cunningham-Bussel A. Beyond oxidative stress: an immunologist's guide to reactive species. Nat Rev Immunol. 2013;13(5):349–61.

33. Ryan JL. Ionizing radiation: the good, the bad, and the ugly. J Invest Dermatol. 2012;132:985–93.
34. Polefka TG, Meyer TA, Agin PP, Bianchini RJ. Effects of solar radiation on the skin. J Cosmet Dermatol. 2012;11(2):134–43.
35. Krutmann J, Liu W, Li L, Pan X, Crawford M, Sore G, et al. Pollution and skin: from epidemiological and mechanistic studies to clinical implications. J Dermatol Sci. 2014;76(3):163–8.
36. Kovacic P, Somanathan R. Dermal toxicity and environmental contamination: electron transfer, reactive species, oxidative stress, cell signaling, and protection by antioxidants. Rev Environ Contam Toxicol. 2010;203:119–38.
37. Fang YZ, Yang S, Wu G. Free radicals, antioxidants, and nutrition. Nutrition. 2002;18(10):872–9.
38. Cadenas E, Davies KJ. Mitochondrial free radical generation, oxidative stress, and aging. Free Radic Biol Med. 2000;29(3–4):222–30.
39. Alfadda AA, Sallam RM. Reactive oxygen species in health and disease. J Biomed Biotechnol. 2012;2012:936486.
40. Ray PD, Huang B-W, Tsuji Y. Reactive oxygen species (ROS) homeostasis and redox regulation in cellular signaling. Cell Signal. 2012;24(5):981–90.
41. Droge W. Free radicals in the physiological control of cell function. Physiol Rev. 2002;82(1):47–95.
42. Valko M, Leibfritz D, Moncol J, Cronin MT, Mazur M, Telser J. Free radicals and antioxidants in normal physiological functions and human disease. Int J Biochem Cell Biol. 2007;39(1):44–84.
43. Fitzmaurice SD, Sivamani RK, Isseroff RR. Antioxidant therapies for wound healing: a clinical guide to currently commercially available products. Skin Pharmacol Physiol. 2011;24(3):113–26.
44. Grether-Beck S, Marini A, Jaenicke T, Krutmann J. Photoprotection of human skin beyond ultraviolet radiation. Photodermatol Photoimmunol Photomed. 2014;30(2–3):167–74.
45. Park SL, Justiniano R, Williams JD, Cabello CM, Qiao S, Wondrak GT. The tryptophan-derived endogenous aryl hydrocarbon receptor ligand 6-formylindolo[3,2-b]carbazole is a nanomolar UVA photosensitizer in epidermal keratinocytes. J Invest Dermatol. 2015;135:1649–58.
46. Chiarelli-Neto O, Ferreira AS, Martins WK, Pavani C, Severino D, Faiao-Flores F, et al. Melanin photosensitization and the effect of visible light on epithelial cells. PLoS One. 2014;9(11):e113266.
47. Dawe RS, Ibbotson SH. Drug-induced photosensitivity. Dermatol Clin. 2014;32(3):363–8.
48. Buettner GR. Superoxide dismutase in redox biology: the roles of superoxide and hydrogen peroxide. Anticancer Agents Med Chem. 2011;11(4):341–6.
49. Sies H. Oxidative stress: from basic research to clinical application. Am J Med. 1991;91(3c):31–8.
50. Bissett DL, Chatterjee R, Hannon DP. Chronic ultraviolet radiation-induced increase in skin iron and the photoprotective effect of topically applied iron chelators. Photochem Photobiol. 1991;54(2):215–23.
51. Bissett DL, McBride JF. Iron content of human epidermis from sun-exposed and non-exposed body sites. J Soc Cosmet Chem. 1992;43:215–7.
52. Bissett DL, McBride JF. Synergistic topical photoprotection by a combination of the iron chelator 2-furildioxime and sunscreen. J Am Acad Dermatol. 1996;35(4):546–9.
53. Aroun A, Zhong JL, Tyrrell RM, Pourzand C. Iron, oxidative stress and the example of solar ultraviolet A radiation. Photochem Photobiol Sci. 2012;11(1):118–34.
54. Jomova K, Baros S, Valko M. Redox active metal-induced oxidative stress in biological systems. Transit Met Chem. 2012;37(2):127–34.
55. Valacchi G, Sticozzi C, Pecorelli A, Cervellati F, Cervellati C, Maioli E. Cutaneous responses to environmental stressors. Ann NY Acad Sci. 2012;1271(1):75–81.
56. Poljsak B, Dahmane R. Free radicals and extrinsic skin aging. Dermatol Res Pract. 2012;4. doi:10.1155/2012/135206.
57. Bickers DR, Athar M. Oxidative stress in the pathogenesis of skin disease. J Invest Dermatol. 2006;126(12):2565–75.
58. Starr JM, Starr RJ. Skin aging and oxidative stress, Chapter 2. In: Preedy VR, editor. Aging: Oxidative Stress and Dietary Antioxidants. Oxford, UK, and Waltham, MA, USA, Academic Press; 2014. p. 15–22.
59. Kammeyer A, Luiten RM. Oxidation events and skin aging. Ageing Res Rev. 2015;21:16–29.
60. Kryston TB, Georgiev AB, Pissis P, Georgakilas AG. Role of oxidative stress and DNA damage in human carcinogenesis. Mutat Res. 2011;711(1–2):193–201.
61. Jena NR. DNA damage by reactive species: mechanisms, mutation and repair. J Biosci. 2012;37(3):503–17.
62. Pfeifer GP, Besaratinia A. UV wavelength-dependent DNA damage and human non-melanoma and melanoma skin cancer. Photochem Photobiol Sci. 2012;11(1):90–7.
63. van Loon B, Markkanen E, Hübscher U. Oxygen as a friend and enemy: how to combat the mutational potential of 8-oxo-guanine. DNA Repair. 2010;9(6):604–16.
64. Rastogi RP, Richa, Kumar A, Tyagi MB, Sinha RP. Molecular mechanisms of ultraviolet radiation-induced DNA damage and repair. J Nucleic Acids. 2010;32. doi:10.4061/2010/592980.
65. Brash DE. UV signature mutations. Photochem Photobiol. 2015;91(1):15–26.
66. Boukamp P. Non-melanoma skin cancer: what drives tumor development and progression? Carcinogenesis. 2005;26(10):1657–67.
67. Chial H. Proto-oncogenes to oncogenes to cancer. Nat Educ. 2008;1(1):33.

68. Marrot L, Meunier JR. Skin DNA photodamage and its biological consequences. J Am Acad Dermatol. 2008;58(5):S139–48.
69. Premi S, Wallisch S, Mano CM, Weiner AB, Bacchiocchi A, Wakamatsu K, et al. Chemiexcitation of melanin derivatives induces DNA photoproducts long after UV exposure. Science. 2015;347(6224):842–7.
70. Taylor J-S. The dark side of sunlight and melanoma. Science. 2015;347(6224):824.
71. Murphy MP. How mitochondria produce reactive species. Biochem J. 2009;417(Pt 1):1–13.
72. Birch-Machin MA, Swalwell H. How mitochondria record the effects of UV exposure and oxidative stress using human skin as a model tissue. Mutagenesis. 2010;25(2):101–7.
73. Grether-Beck S, Marini A, Jaenicke T, Krutmann J. Effective photoprotection of human skin against infrared A radiation by topically applied antioxidants: results from a vehicle controlled, randomized study. Photochem Photobiol. 2015;91(1):248–50.
74. Wallace DC. Mitochondrial DNA, mutations in disease and aging. Environ Mol Mutagen. 2010;51(5):440–50.
75. Gredilla R, Bohr VA, Stevnsner T. Mitochondrial DNA repair and association with aging – an update. Exp Gerontol. 2010;45(7–8):478–88.
76. Birch-Machin MA, Russell EV, Latimer JA. Mitochondrial DNA damage as a biomarker for ultraviolet radiation exposure and oxidative stress. Br J Dermatol. 2013;169(Suppl S2):9–14.
77. Gebhard D, Mahler B, Matt K, Burger K, Bergemann J. Mitochondrial DNA copy number – but not a mitochondrial tandem CC to TT transition – is increased in sun-exposed skin. Exp Dermatol. 2014;23(3):209–11.
78. Birch-Machin MA. Mitochondria and skin disease. Clin Exp Dermatol. 2000;25(2):141–6.
79. Niki E. Lipid oxidation in the skin. Free Rad Res. 2015;49(7):827-834.
80. Niki E, Yoshida Y, Saito Y, Noguchi N. Lipid peroxidation: mechanisms, inhibition, and biological effects. Biochem Biophys Res Commun. 2005;338(1):668–76.
81. Valko M, Morris H, Cronin MT. Metals, toxicity and oxidative stress. Curr Med Chem. 2005;12(10):1161–208.
82. Halliwell B, Chirico S. Lipid peroxidation: its mechanism, measurement, and significance. Am J Clin Nutr. 1993;57(Suppl):715S–25.
83. Kendall AC, Pilkington SM, Massey KA, Sassano G, Rhodes LE, Nicolaou A. Distribution of bioactive lipid mediators in human skin. J Invest Dermatol. 2015;135:1510–20.
84. Nicolaou A. Eicosanoids in skin inflammation. Prostaglandins Leukot Essent Fatty Acids. 2013;88(1):131–8.
85. Kendall AC, Nicolaou A. Bioactive lipid mediators in skin inflammation and immunity. Prog Lipid Res. 2013;52(1):141–64.
86. Li Y, Lei D, Swindell WR, Xia W, Weng S, Fu J, et al. Age-associated increase in skin fibroblast-derived prostaglandin E2 contributes to reduced collagen levels in elderly human skin. J Invest Dermatol. 2015;135:2181–2188.
87. Franceschi C, Bonafe M, Valensin S, Olivieri F, De Luca M, Ottaviani E, et al. Inflamm-aging: an evolutionary perspective on immunosenescence. Ann NY Acad Sci. 2000;908(1):244–54.
88. Cevenini E, Monti D, Franceschi C. Inflamm-ageing. Curr Opin Clin Nutr Metab Care. 2013;16(1):14–20.
89. Cannizzo ES, Clement CC, Sahu R, Follo C, Santambrogio L. Oxidative stress, inflamm-aging and immunosenescence. J Proteomics. 2011;74(11):2313–23.
90. Xu F, Yan S, Wu M, Li F, Xu X, Song W, et al. Ambient ozone pollution as a risk factor for skin disorders. Br J Dermatol. 2011;165(1):224–5.
91. Avery SV. Molecular targets of oxidative stress. Biochem J. 2011;434(2):201–10.
92. Thiele JJ, Dreher F, Maibach HI, Packer L. Impact of ultraviolet radiation and ozone on the transepidermal water loss as a function of skin temperature in hairless mice. Skin Pharmacol Appl Skin Physiol. 2003;16(5):283–90.
93. Fritz KS, Petersen DR. An overview of the chemistry and biology of reactive aldehydes. Free Radic Biol Med. 2013;59:85–91.
94. Mudiyanselage SE, Hamburger M, Elsner P, Thiele JJ. Ultraviolet A induces generation of squalene monohydroperoxide isomers in human sebum and skin surface lipids in vitro and in vivo. J Invest Dermatol. 2003;120(6):915–22.
95. Wisthaler A, Weschler CJ. Reactions of ozone with human skin lipids: sources of carbonyls, dicarbonyls, and hydroxycarbonyls in indoor air. Proc Natl Acad Sci U S A. 2010;107(15):6568–75.
96. De Luca C, Valacchi G. Surface lipids as multifunctional mediators of skin responses to environmental stimuli. Mediators Inflamm. 2010; doi:10.1155/2010/321494, 11 pg.
97. Dalle-Donne I, Rossi R, Colombo R, Giustarini D, Milzani A. Biomarkers of oxidative damage in human disease. Clin Chem. 2006;52(4):601–23.
98. Stadtman ER. Protein oxidation and aging. Science. 1992;257(5074):1220–4.
99. Stadtman ER. Metal ion-catalyzed oxidation of proteins: biochemical mechanism and biological consequences. Free Radic Biol Med. 1990;9(4):315–25.
100. Stadtman ER, Berlett BS. Reactive oxygen-mediated protein oxidation in aging and disease. Chem Res Toxicol. 1997;10(5):485–94.
101. Cecarini V, Gee J, Fioretti E, Amici M, Angeletti M, Eleuteri AM, et al. Protein oxidation and cellular homeostasis: emphasis on metabolism. Biochim Biophys Acta. 2007;1773(2):93–104.
102. Jung T, Höhn A, Grune T. The proteasome and the degradation of oxidized proteins: part II – protein

oxidation and proteasomal degradation. Redox Biol. 2014;2:99–104.
103. Moller IM, Rogowska-Wrzesinska A, Rao RS. Protein carbonylation and metal-catalyzed protein oxidation in a cellular perspective. J Proteomics. 2011;74(11):2228–42.
104. Rudyk O, Eaton P. Biochemical methods for monitoring protein thiol redox states in biological systems. Redox Biol. 2014;2:803–13.
105. Go YM, Jones DP. The redox proteome. J Biol Chem. 2013;288(37):26512–20.
106. Manton C, Chandra J. Oxidative stress and the proteasome: mechanisms and therapeutic relevance. In: Dou QP, editor. Resistance to proteasome inhibitors in cancer. Switzerland Springer International Publishing; 2014. p. 249–74.
107. Grune T, Reinheckel T, Davies KJ. Degradation of oxidized proteins in mammalian cells. FASEB J. 1997;11(7):526–34.
108. Dunlop RA, Brunk UT, Rodgers KJ. Oxidized proteins: mechanisms of removal and consequences of accumulation. IUBMB Life. 2009;61(5):522–7.
109. Jung T, Grune T. The proteasome and the degradation of oxidized proteins: part I – structure of proteasomes. Redox Biol. 2013;1(1):178–82.
110. Ott C, Jacobs K, Haucke E, Navarrete Santos A, Grune T, Simm A. Role of advanced glycation end products in cellular signaling. Redox Biol. 2014;2:411–29.
111. Meadows C, Morré DJ, Morré DM, Draelos ZD, Kern D. Age-related NADH oxidase (arNOX)-catalyzed oxidative damage to skin proteins. Arch Dermal Res. 2014;306(7645–852):1–8.
112. Hulbert AJ, Pamplona R, Buffenstein R, Buttemer WA. Life and death: metabolic rate, membrane composition, and life span of animals. Physiol Rev. 2007;87(4):1175–213.
113. Thiele JJ, Traber MG, Re R, Espuno N, Yan LJ, Cross CE, et al. Macromolecular carbonyls in human stratum corneum: a biomarker for environmental oxidant exposure? FEBS Lett. 1998;422(3):403–6.
114. Sander CS, Chang H, Salzmann S, Muller CSL, Ekanayake-Mudiyanselage S, Elsner P, et al. Photoaging is associated with protein oxidation in human skin in vivo. J Invest Dermatol. 2002;118(4):618–25.
115. Hirao T, Takahashi M. Carbonylation of cornified envelopes in the stratum corneum. FEBS Lett. 2005;579(30):6870–4.
116. Fisher GJ, Quan T, Purohit T, Shao Y, Cho MK, He T, et al. Collagen fragmentation promotes oxidative stress and elevates matrix metalloproteinase-1 in fibroblasts in aged human skin. Am J Pathol. 2009;174(1):101–14.
117. Larroque-Cardoso P, Camare C, Nadal-Wollbold F, Grazide M-H, Pucelle M, Garoby-Salom S, et al. Elastin modification by 4-hydroxynonenal in hairless mice exposed to UV-A. Role in photoaging and actinic elastosis. J Invest Dermatol. 2015;135:1873–81.
118. Thorpe SR, Baynes JW. Maillard reaction products in tissue proteins: new products and new perspectives. Amino Acids. 2003;25(3–4):275–81.
119. Gkogkolou P, Böhm M. Advanced glycation end products: key players in skin aging? Derm Endocrinol. 2012;4(3):1–12.
120. Singh R, Barden A, Mori T, Beilin L. Advanced glycation end-products: a review. Diabetologia. 2001;44(2):129–46.
121. Jeanmaire C, Danoux L, Pauly G. Glycation during human dermal intrinsic and actinic ageing: an *in vivo* and *in vitro* model study. Br J Dermatol. 2001;145(1):10–8.
122. Hopps E, Noto D, Caimi G, Averna MR. A novel component of the metabolic syndrome: the oxidative stress. Nutr Metab Cardiovasc Dis. 2010;20(1):72–7.
123. Crisan M, Taulescu M, Crisan D, Cosgarea R, Parvu A, Cătoi C, et al. Expression of advanced glycation end-products on sun-exposed and non-exposed cutaneous sites during the ageing process in humans. PLoS One. 2013;8(10):e75003.
124. Nomoto K, Yagi M, Arita S, Ogura M, Yonei Y. Skin accumulation of advanced glycation end products and lifestyle behaviors in Japanese. J Anti-Aging Med. 2012;9(6):165–73.
125. Ichihashi M, Yagi M, Nomoto K, Yonei Y. Glycation stress and photo-aging in skin. J Anti-aging Med. 2011;8(3):23–9.
126. Sorci G, Riuzzi F, Giambanco I, Donato R. RAGE in tissue homeostasis, repair and regeneration. Biochim Biophys Acta. 2013;1833(1):101–9.
127. Xie J, Méndez JD, Méndez-Valenzuela V, Aguilar-Hernández MM. Cellular signalling of the receptor for advanced glycation end products (RAGE). Cell Signal. 2013;25(11):2185–97.
128. Thiele JJ, Schroeter C, Hsieh SN, Podda M, Packer L. The antioxidant network of the stratum corneum. Curr Probl Dermatol. 2001;29:26–42.
129. Vermeij WP, Alia A, Backendorf C. ROS quenching potential of the epidermal cornified cell envelope. J Invest Dermatol. 2011;131:1435–41.
130. Shindo Y, Witt E, Han D, Epstein W, Packer L. Enzymic and non-enzymic antioxidants in epidermis and dermis of human skin. J Invest Dermatol. 1994;102(1):122–4.
131. Vahlquist A, Lee JB, Michaelsson G, Rollman O. Vitamin A in human skin: II concentrations of carotene, retinol and dehydroretinol in various components of normal skin. J Invest Dermatol. 1982;79(2):94–7.
132. Leibold JS, Riehl A, Hettinger J, Durben M, Hess J, Angel P. Keratinocyte-specific deletion of the receptor RAGE modulates the kinetics of skin inflammation in vivo. J Invest Dermatol. 2013;133(10):2400–6.
133. Kierdorf K, Fritz G. RAGE regulation and signaling in inflammation and beyond. J Leukoc Biol. 2013;94(1):55–68.

134. Naylor EC, Watson REB, Sherratt MJ. Molecular aspects of skin ageing. Maturitas. 2011;69(3):249–56.
135. Corstjens H, Dicanio D, Muizzuddin N, Neven A, Sparacio R, Declercq L, et al. Glycation associated skin autofluorescence and skin elasticity are related to chronological age and body mass index of healthy subjects. Exp Gerontol. 2008;43(7):663–7.
136. Hori M, Yagi M, Nomoto K, Shimode A, Ogura M, Yonei Y. Inhibition of advanced glycation end product formation by herbal teas and its relation to anti-skin aging. Anti-Aging Med. 2012;9:135–48.
137. Antonios V. Drivers of redox status & protein glycation. PhD thesis. Glasgow: University of Glasgow; 2014. http://encore.lib.gla.ac.uk/iii/encore/record/C__Rb3083853?lang=eng
138. Uchida K, Kato Y, Kawakishi S. Metal-catalyzed oxidative degradation of collagen. J Agric Food Chem. 1992;40(1):9–12.
139. Meinke MC, Müller R, Bechtel A, Haag SF, Darvin ME, Lohan SB, et al. Evaluation of carotenoids and reactive species in human skin after UV irradiation: a critical comparison between *in vivo* and *ex vivo* investigations. Exp Dermatol. 2015;24(3):194–7.
140. Filomeni G, Rotilio G, Ciriolo MR. Disulfide relays and phosphorylative cascades: partners in redox-mediated signaling pathways. Cell Death Differ. 2005;12(12):1555–63.
141. Thiele J, Dreher F, Packer L. Antioxidant defense system in skin. In: Elsner P, Maibach H, editors. Cosmeceuticals-drugs vs cosmetics. New York: Marcel Dekker; 2000. p. 145–88.
142. Pinnell S. Cutaneous photodamage, oxidative stress, and topical antioxidant protection. J Am Acad Dermatol. 2003;48(1):1–19.
143. Tiwari A. Imbalance in antioxidant defence and human diseases: multiple approach of natural antioxidants therapy. Curr Sci. 2001;81(9):1179–87.
144. Packer L, Weber SU, Rimbach G. Molecular aspects of alpha-tocotrienol antioxidant action and cell signalling. J Nutr. 2001;131(2):369s–73.
145. Darvin ME, Fluhr JW, Caspers P, van der Pool A, Richter H, Patzelt A, et al. *In vivo* distribution of carotenoids in different anatomical locations of human skin: comparative assessment with two different Raman spectroscopy methods. Exp Dermatol. 2009;18(12):1060–3.
146. Lademann J, Meinke MC, Sterry W, Darvin ME. Carotenoids in human skin. Exp Dermatol. 2011;20(5):377–82.
147. Darvin ME, Haag SF, Lademann J, Zastrow L, Sterry W, Meinke MC. Formation of free radicals in human skin during irradiation with infrared light. J Invest Dermatol. 2009;130(2):629–31.
148. Darvin M, Haag S, Meinke M, Zastrow L, Sterry W, Lademann J. Radical production by infrared A irradiation in human tissue. Skin Pharmacol Physiol. 2010;23(1):40–6.
149. Darvin ME, Fluhr JW, Meinke MC, Zastrow L, Sterry W, Lademann J. Topical beta-carotene protects against infra-red-light–induced free radicals. Exp Dermatol. 2011;20(2):125–9.
150. Darvin M, Zastrow L, Sterry W, Lademann J. Effect of supplemented and topically applied antioxidant substances on human tissue. Skin Pharmacol Physiol. 2006;19(5):238–47.
151. Meinke MC, Friedrich A, Tscherch K, Haag SF, Darvin ME, Vollert H, et al. Influence of dietary carotenoids on radical scavenging capacity of the skin and skin lipids. Eur J Pharm Biopharm. 2013;84(2):365–73.
152. Lademann J, Schanzer S, Meinke M, Sterry W, Darvin ME. Interaction between carotenoids and free radicals in human skin. Skin Pharmacol Physiol. 2011;24(5):238–44.
153. Lademann J, Darvin M, Weigmann H-J, Schanzer S, Zastrow L, Douchet O, et al. Sunscreens – UV or light protection. IFSCC Mag. 2014;4:23–8.
154. Svobodova A, Psotova J, Walterova D. Natural phenolics in the prevention of UV-induced skin damage. A review. Biomed Pap Med Fac Univ Palacky Olomouc Czech Repub. 2003;147(2):137–45.
155. Katiyar SK. Proanthocyanidins from grape seeds inhibit UV radiation-induced immune suppression in mice: detection and analysis of molecular and cellular targets. Photochem Photobiol. 2015;91(1):156–62.
156. Nichols J, Katiyar S. Skin photoprotection by natural polyphenols: anti-inflammatory, antioxidant and DNA repair mechanisms. Arch Dermatol Res. 2010;302(2):71–83.
157. Katiyar S, Elmets C. Green tea and skin cancer: photoimmunology, angiogenesis and DNA repair. J Nutr Biochem. 2007;18(5):287–96.
158. Yusuf N, Irby C, Katiyar S, Elmets C. Photoprotective effects of green tea polyphenols. Photodermatol Photoimmunol Photomed. 2007;23:48–56.
159. Vermeij WP, Backendorf C, Bridger JM. Skin cornification proteins provide global link between ROS detoxification and cell migration during wound healing. PLoS One. 2010;5(8):996–9.
160. Schallreuter KU, Wood JM. The role of thioredoxin reductase in the reduction of free radicals at the surface of the epidermis. Biochem Biophys Res Commun. 1986;136(2):630–7.
161. Schallreuter KU, Rubsam K, Gibbons NC, Maitland DJ, Chavan B, Zothner C, et al. Methionine sulfoxide reductases A and B are deactivated by hydrogen peroxide (H_2O_2) in the epidermis of patients with vitiligo. J Invest Dermatol. 2008;128(4):808–15.
162. Schallreuter KU. Functioning methionine-S-sulfoxide reductases A and B are present in human skin. J Invest Dermatol. 2006;126(5):947–9.
163. Ogawa F, Sander CS, Hansel A, Oehrl W, Kasperczyk H, Elsner P, et al. The repair enzyme peptide methionine-S-sulfoxide reductase is expressed in human epidermis and upregulated by UVA radiation. J Invest Dermatol. 2006;126(5):1128–34.

164. Tyrrell RM. Solar ultraviolet A radiation: an oxidizing skin carcinogen that activates heme oxygenase-1. Antioxid Redox Signal. 2004;6(5):835–40.
165. Tyrrell RM. Modulation of gene expression by the oxidative stress generated in human skin cells by UVA radiation and the restoration of redox homeostasis. Photochem Photobiol Sci. 2012;11(1):135–47.
166. Gozzelino R, Jeney V, Soares MP. Mechanisms of cell protection by heme oxygenase-1. Annu Rev Pharmacol Toxicol. 2010;50:323–54.
167. Schallreuter KU, Wood JM. Thioredoxin reductase – its role in epidermal redox status. J Photochem Photobiol B. 2001;64(2–3):179–84.
168. Ogawa F, Sander CS, Hansel A, Oehrl W, Kasperczyk H, Elsner P, et al. The repair enzyme peptide methionine-S-sulfoxide reductase is expressed in human epidermis and upregulated by UVA Radiation. J Invest Dermatol. 2006;126(5):1128–34.
169. Rhie G, Shin MH, Seo JY, Choi WW, Cho KH, Kim KH, et al. Aging-and photoaging-dependent changes of enzymic and nonenzymic antioxidants in the epidermis and dermis of human skin *in vivo*. J Invest Dermatol. 2001;117(5):1212–7.
170. Lee J, Koo N, Min DB. Reactive oxygen species, aging, and antioxidative nutraceuticals. Compr Rev Food Sci Food Saf. 2004;3(1):21–33.
171. Constantinescu A, Han D, Packer L. Vitamin E recycling in human erythrocyte membranes. J Biol Chem. 1993;268(15):10906–13.
172. Holmstrom KM, Finkel T. Cellular mechanisms and physiological consequences of redox-dependent signalling. Nat Rev Mol Cell Biol. 2014;15(6):411–21.
173. Schieber M, Chandel Navdeep S. ROS function in redox signaling and oxidative stress. Curr Biol. 2014;24(10):R453–62.
174. Yan L-J. Positive oxidative stress in aging and aging-related disease tolerance. Redox Biol. 2014;2:165–9.
175. Collins Y, Chouchani ET, James AM, Menger KE, Cochemé HM, Murphy MP. Mitochondrial redox signalling at a glance. J Cell Sci. 2012;125(4):801–6.
176. Schulz E, Wenzel P, Munzel T, Daiber A. Mitochondrial redox signaling: interaction of mitochondrial reactive species with other sources of oxidative stress. Antioxid Redox Signal. 2014;20(2):308–24.
177. Wagener FA, Carels CE, Lundvig DM. Targeting the redox balance in inflammatory skin conditions. Int J Mol Sci. 2013;14(5):9126–67.
178. Bito T, Nishigori C. Impact of reactive species on keratinocyte signaling pathways. J Dermatol Sci. 2012;68(1):3–8.
179. Trachootham D, Lu W, Ogasawara MA, Nilsa RD, Huang P. Redox regulation of cell survival. Antioxid Redox Signal. 2008;10(8):1343–74.
180. Schafer FQ, Buettner GR. Redox environment of the cell as viewed through the redox state of the glutathione disulfide/glutathione couple. Free Radic Biol Med. 2001;30(11):1191–212.
181. Sohal RS, Orr WC. The redox stress hypothesis of aging. Free Radic Biol Med. 2012;52(3):539–55.
182. Jones DP. Radical-free biology of oxidative stress. Am J Physiol Cell Physiol. 2008;295(4):C849–68.
183. Beyer TA, auf dem Keller U, Braun S, Schafer M, Werner S. Roles and mechanisms of action of the Nrf2 transcription factor in skin morphogenesis, wound repair and skin cancer. Cell Death Differ. 2007;14(7):1250–4.
184. Bhatia M, Karlenius TC, Trapani GD, Tonissen KF. The interaction between redox and hypoxic signalling pathways in the dynamic oxygen environment of cancer cells. In: Tonissen K, editor. Carcinogenesis: Intechopen. 2013. http://www.intechopen.com/books/carcinogenesis/the-interaction-between-redox-and-hypoxic-signalling-pathways-in-the-dynamic-oxygen-environment-of-c. p. 125–52.
185. Osburn WO, Kensler TW. Nrf2 signaling: an adaptive response pathway for protection against environmental toxic insults. Mutat Res. 2008;659(1–2):31–9.
186. Aleksunes LM, Manautou JE. Emerging role of Nrf2 in protecting against hepatic and gastrointestinal disease. Toxicol Pathol. 2007;35(4):459–73.
187. Holland R, Fishbein JC. Chemistry of the cysteine sensors in Kelch-like ECH-associated protein 1. Antioxid Redox Signal. 2010;13(11):1749–61.
188. Kaspar JW, Niture SK, Jaiswal AK. Nrf2:INrf2 (Keap1) signaling in oxidative stress. Free Radic Biol Med. 2009;47(9):1304–9.
189. Kansanen E, Kuosmanen SM, Leinonen H, Levonen A-L. The Keap1-Nrf2 pathway: mechanisms of activation and dysregulation in cancer. Redox Biol. 2013;1(1):45–9.
190. Li Y, Paonessa JD, Zhang Y. Mechanism of chemical activation of Nrf2. PLoS One. 2012;7(4):e35122.
191. Hamanaka RB, Chandel NS. Mitochondrial metabolism as a regulator of keratinocyte differentiation. Cell Logist. 2013;3(1):e25456.
192. Hamanaka RB, Glasauer A, Hoover P, Yang S, Blatt H, Mullen AR, et al. Mitochondrial reactive species promote epidermal differentiation and hair follicle development. Sci Signal. 2013;6(261):ra8.
193. López-Otín C, Blasco MA, Partridge L, Serrano M, Kroemer G. The hallmarks of aging. Cell. 2013;153(6):1194–217.
194. Medvedev ZA. An attempt at a rational classification of theories of ageing. Biol Rev. 1990;65(3):375–98.
195. Harman D. Aging: a theory based on free radical and radiation chemistry. J Gerontol. 1956;11(3):298–300.
196. Brieger K, Schiavone S, Miller FJ, Krause K-H. Reactive oxygen species: from health to disease. Swiss Med Wkly. 2012;142:w13659.
197. Harman D. Free radical theory of aging: dietary implications. Am J Clin Nutr. 1972;25(8):839–43.
198. Miquel J, Economos AC, Fleming J, Johnson JE. Mitochondrial role in cell aging. Exp Gerontol. 1980;15(6):575–91.
199. Massudi H, Grant R, Braidy N, Guest J, Farnsworth B, Guillemin GJ. Age-associated changes

in oxidative stress and NAD^+ metabolism in human tissue. PLoS One. 2012;7(7):e42357.
200. Hekimi S, Lapointe J, Wen Y. Taking a "good" look at free radicals in the aging process. Trends Cell Biol. 2011;21(10):569–76.
201. Salmon AB, Richardson A, Pérez VI. Update on the oxidative stress theory of aging: does oxidative stress play a role in aging or healthy aging? Free Radic Biol Med. 2010;48(5):642.
202. Gladyshev VN. The free radical theory of aging is dead. Long live the damage theory! Antioxid Redox Signal. 2013;20(4):727–31.
203. Bratic A, Larsson N-G. The role of mitochondria in aging. J Clin Invest. 2013;123(3):951–7.
204. Ristow M, Schmeisser S. Extending life span by increasing oxidative stress. Free Radic Biol Med. 2011;51(2):327–36.
205. Newgard CB, Sharpless NE. Coming of age: molecular drivers of aging and therapeutic opportunities. J Clin Invest. 2013;123(3):946–50.
206. Sanz A, Stefanatos RK. The mitochondrial free radical theory of aging: a critical view. Curr Aging Sci. 2008;1(1):10–21.
207. Halliwell B. The antioxidant paradox: less paradoxical now? Br J Clin Pharmacol. 2013;75(3):637–44.
208. Halliwell B. Free radicals and antioxidants: updating a personal view. Nutr Rev. 2012;70(5):257–65.
209. Tapia PC. Sublethal mitochondrial stress with an attendant stoichiometric augmentation of reactive species may precipitate many of the beneficial alterations in cellular physiology produced by caloric restriction, intermittent fasting, exercise and dietary phytonutrients: "Mitohormesis" for health and vitality. Med Hypotheses. 2006;66(4):832–43.
210. Ristow M, Zarse K. How increased oxidative stress promotes longevity and metabolic health: the concept of mitochondrial hormesis (mitohormesis). Exp Gerontol. 2010;45(6):410–8.
211. Liochev SI. Reactive oxygen species and the free radical theory of aging. Free Radic Biol Med. 2013;60:1–4.
212. Ristow M. Unraveling the truth about antioxidants: mitohormesis explains ROS-induced health benefits. Nat Med. 2014;20(7):709–11.
213. Afanas'ev I. Reactive oxygen species and age-related genes p66shc, sirtuin, FOX03 and klotho in senescence. Oxid Med Cell Longev. 2010;3(2):77–85.
214. Prather AA, Epel ES, Arenander J, Broestl L, Garay BI, Wang D, et al. Longevity factor klotho and chronic psychological stress. Translat Psychiatry. 2015;5:e585.
215. Rittié L, Fisher GJ. Natural and sun-induced aging of human skin. Cold Spring Harb Perspect Med. 2015;5(1):a015370. doi:10.1101/cshperspect.a015370.
216. Morita A. Tobacco smoke and skin aging. In: Farage M, Miller K, Maibach H, editors. Textbook of aging skin. Berlin/Heidelberg: Springer; 2010. p. 447–50.
217. Kligman AM. Early destructive effect of sunlight on human skin. JAMA. 1969;210(13):2377–80.
218. Kligman L, Kligman A. Photoaging. Manifestations, prevention, and treatment. Dermatol Clin. 1986;4(3):517.
219. Wondrak GT. Let the sun shine in: mechanisms and potential for therapeutics in skin photodamage. Curr Opin Investig Drugs. 2007;8(5):390–400.
220. Mahmoud BH, Hexsel CL, Hamzavi IH, Lim HW. Effects of visible light on the skin. Photochem Photobiol. 2008;84(2):450–62.
221. Wolf AM, Nishimaki K, Kamimura N, Ohta S. Real-time monitoring of oxidative stress in live mouse skin. J Invest Dermatol. 2014;134:1701–9.
222. Iannacone MR, Hughes MCB, Green AC. Effects of sunscreen on skin cancer and photoaging. Photodermatol Photoimmunol Photomed. 2014;30(2–3):55–61.
223. Vierkoetter A, Li M, Ma C, Deng B, Matsui M, Krutmann J, et al. Indoor air pollution from cooking with coal or firewood accelerates skin aging in northern Chinese women. J Invest Dermatol. 2014;132(S51):Abs # 296.
224. Vierkötter A, Krutmann J. Environmental influences on skin aging and ethnic-specific manifestations. Derm Endocrinol. 2012;4(3):227–31.
225. Vierkötter A, Schikowski T, Ranft U, Sugiri D, Matsui M, Krämer U, et al. Airborne particle exposure and extrinsic skin aging. J Invest Dermatol. 2010;130(12):2719–26.
226. He QC, Tavakkol A, Wietecha K, Begum-Gafur R, Ansari SA, Polefka T. Effects of environmentally realistic levels of ozone on stratum corneum function. Int J Cosmet Sci. 2006;28(5):349–57.
227. Drakaki E, Dessinioti C, Antoniou CV. Air pollution and the skin. Front Environ Sci. 2014;2:1–6.
228. Allerhand M, Ting Ooi E, Starr RJ, Alcorn M, Penke L, Drost E, et al. Skin ageing and oxidative stress in a narrow-age cohort of older adults. Eur Geriatr Med. 2011;2(3):140–4.

Part III

Endogenous and Exogenous Factors

Cutaneous Responses to Tropospheric Ozone Exposure

52

Giuseppe Valacchi

Contents

G. Valacchi (✉)
Department of Life Sciences and Biotechnology, University of Ferrara, Ferrara (FE), Italy

Department of Food and Nutrition, Kyung Hee University, Seoul, South Korea
e-mail: vlcgpp@unife.it

M.A. Farage et al. (eds.), *Textbook of Aging Skin*,
DOI 10.1007/978-3-662-47398-6_41

Abstract

Living organisms are continuously exposed to environmental pollutants. Because the skin is an interface between the body and the environment, it is chronically exposed to several forms of stress (UV, O_3). Ozone (O_3) represents one of the major oxidants in photochemical smog, levels being highest in heavily polluted areas where exposure to UV is also high. Correlation between O_3 exposure and the development of skin pathologies as well as its effects will be discussed in detail.

Introduction

Living organisms are continuously exposed to environmental pollutants. Depending on their state, pollutants can be taken up by ingestion, inhalation, or contact with the skin. Because the skin is an interface between the body and the environment, it is chronically exposed to several forms of stress such as ultraviolet (UV) radiation and other environmental oxidants such as cigarette smoke and ozone (O_3). UVB and, to a lesser degree, UVA induce various skin pathological conditions, including erythema, edema, hyperplasia, "sunburn cell" formation, photoaging, and photocarcinogenesis. There is abundant information that reactive oxygen species (ROS) such as hydroxyl radicals are involved in UV-induced skin damage, both by direct effects of UV and by subsequent phagocyte infiltration and activation. Oxidative environmental pollutants, such as cigarette smoke, O_3, and oxides of nitrogen that have been studied in the respiratory tract [1], also represent a potential oxidant stress to the skin. In order of importance, the skin is the second most frequent route by which chemicals can enter into the body. The skin is the major target of liquid and gaseous pollutants, and the pollutant that reacts most specifically with the cutaneous tissues, besides UV radiation, hydrocarbon, and organic compounds, is O_3. Ozone represents one of the major oxidants in photochemical smog, levels being highest in heavily polluted areas where exposure to UV is also high. In the last decade, many studies have shown the toxic effect of O_3 on the skin [2–4].

Ozone: A Double-Edge Molecule

The word ozone derives from the Greek word δεω, which means "to give off a smell." It is an unstable gas of a soft sky-blue color, with a pungent, acrid smell already perceptible at a concentration of 0.01 ppb. The molecule is composed of three oxygen atoms (O_3) and has a molecular weight of 48 g mol^{-1}. It has a cyclical structure assessed by the spectrum absorption in the infrared region, with a distance of 1.26 Å among oxygen atoms. O_3 does not have a stable structure but exists in several mesomeric states in dynamic equilibrium. In the liquid and solid states, O_3 is highly explosive, and among oxidant agents, it is the third strongest (O_3, $E° = +2.076$ V) after fluorine (+3.0353 V) and persulfate (+2.866 V).

O_3 is naturally present in the atmosphere surrounding the Earth. In the upper part of the atmosphere, the stratosphere, 20–30 km from the Earth's surface, the O_3 layer can reach the concentration of 10 ppm. The O_3 occurring in the stratosphere, where the majority of atmospheric ozone is found, forms a "filtering layer" that acts as a barrier to the dangerous radiations from the sun.

In contrast, O_3 present within the lower troposphere (10 miles from the ground level) is hazardous and dangerous to the terrestrial health. It is a ubiquitous pollutant of the urban environment, and it is not emitted directly by any man-made source in significant quantities.

With increasing populations, more automobiles, and more industry, there's more ozone in the lower atmosphere. Since 1900 the amount of ozone near the Earth's surface has more than doubled. Tropospheric ozone is formed by the interaction of sunlight, particularly ultraviolet light, with hydrocarbons and nitrogen oxides, which are emitted by automobiles, gasoline vapors, fossil fuel power plants, refineries, and certain other industries.

The photochemistry involved in the generation of O_3 usually comprises several reactions such as photoactivation, photodecomposition, and free radical chain reaction [5]. The most common molecules that lead to O_3 formation at the ground level are nitric oxides (NO_x). NO_2 can be photolyzed by solar UV resulting in NO and the atomic oxygen that can react with molecular oxygen, leading to the formation of O_3. Ozone can also be destroyed by nitric oxide. NO can react with O_3 to form NO_2 and O_2. Under these steady-state conditions, the concentration of O_3 cannot increase until most of NO has been converted to NO_2 by additional reactions occurring within the complex. This accumulation occurs as the rate of NO_2 photolysis is much faster than that of O_3.

Other species in photochemical smog also undergo photodecomposition to yield free radicals that may participate either directly or indirectly in the conversion of NO to NO_2. Hydroxyl and hydroperoxyl radicals are the examples of compounds that can react with nitrogen radicals with the destruction of O_3 by NO.

The average tropospheric amount of ozone ought to be far less than 40 ppb, which is much lower than that present in the stratosphere. Yet in large metropolises such as Mexico City, and also in European cities such as Rome, Milan, and Paris, O_3 can reach toxic concentrations (0.8 ppm) especially during the summer. Anthropogenic emissions, mainly of NO_x and also methane (CH_4), carbon monoxide (CO), and sulfuric compounds, have caused a progressive increase of O_3 concentration up to 1,000 ppb or more [6].

In urban areas in the Northern Hemisphere, high ozone levels usually occur during the warm, sunny summer months (from May through September). Typically, ozone levels reach their peak in mid to late afternoon, after the sun has had time to react fully with the exhaust fumes from the morning rush hours. A hot, sunny, still day is the perfect environment for ozone pollution production. In early evening, the sunlight's intensity decreases and the photochemical production process that forms ground-level ozone begins to subside.

The majority of US citizens live in areas that are impacted by tropospheric ozone pollution. They are familiar with "smog alerts," local government pleas to reduce vehicle traffic, and news reports about cities that have failed to meet EPA standards for ozone pollution levels. At the street level, O_3 has become the main toxicant not only for the respiratory tract but also for other tissues such as the skin.

Ozone in Life: History and Future

Reports of hazardous effects induced by smog reach as far back as the thirteenth century when, during the reign of Richard III (1377–1399), human diseases were attributed to severe air pollution. Trends in tropospheric O_3 are poorly documented. The O_3 level in the northern hemisphere increased significantly during the periods of industrialization. In the late nineteenth century, O_3 was measured near Paris (Montsouris) to follow a seasonal cycle and to be in the range of 10–20 ppb. Such values are considerably lower than present-day $O_3$with background concentration values of 40–50 ppb observed over the continents in the Northern Hemisphere. The presence of O_3 in air was well recognized in Los Angeles during the early 1940s, based on its damaging effects on rubber products (http://www.who.int/en/). In the 1950s, London and other major cities in the UK suffered a series of smog episodes that caused the death of 4,000 people in a week [7]. During pollution episodes, O_3 mixing ratios higher than 80 ppb can be observed locally in the industrialized regions of North America, Europe, and Asia. It is likely that, on an average, the O_3 abundance has increased by a factor of 2 or more since the preindustrial era (http://www.who.int/en/), and it is, therefore, conceivable that oxidizing power of the atmosphere has changed during the same period. It has been estimated by Zeng and Pyle that the level of tropospheric O_3 will be increased fivefold at the end of this century because of the increase of cars and industrial fumes, leading to dangerous consequences to the terrestrial life [8].

The average environmental O_3 levels that vary considerably for many reasons need to be known, in order to understand the effects of a daily 8-h O_3 exposure (April–October). The US Clean Air Act has set an O_3 level of 0.075 ppm (160 $\mu g/m^3$) as an 8-h mean concentration to protect the health of workers (US Environmental Protection Agency, 2008). Evaluation of recent studies [9, 10] allows establishing an average environmental O_3 concentration of 90 $\pm$ 10 ppb. However, O_3 concentration in urban air can exceed 800 ppb in high-pollution conditions [11], reducing not only pulmonary functions and enhancing the risk of cardiovascular death but also affecting skin physiology. For these reasons recently (October 2015), EPA strengthened the National Ambient Air Quality Standards (NAAQS) for ground-level ozone to 70 parts per billion (ppb), based on extensive scientific evidence about ozone's effects on public health and welfare. The updated standards will improve public health protection, particularly for at-risk groups including children, older adults, and people of all ages who are active outdoors.

Ozone as an Oxidant

It is generally understood that, although O_3 is not a radical species per se, the toxic effects of O_3 are mediated through free radical reactions and they are achieved either directly by the oxidation of biomolecules to give classical radical species (hydroxyl radical) or by driving the radical-dependent production of cytotoxic, nonradical species (aldehydes) [12].

Furthermore, the formation of the oxidation products by O_3, characteristic of damage from free radicals, has been shown to be prevented by the addition of the antioxidant vitamins E and C, though the mechanism is not fully understood. The target specificity of O_3 toward certain compounds together with its physicochemical properties of fairly low aqueous solubility and diffusivity must be taken into account when a target tissue like the skin is exposed to O_3.

As it was hypothesized [13], O_3 does not penetrate the cells but oxidizes available antioxidants and reacts instantaneously with surfactant's polyunsaturated fatty acids (PUFAs) present at the air-cellular interface to form reactive oxygen species (ROS), such as hydrogen peroxide and a mixture of heterogeneous lipid oxidation products (LOPs) including lipoperoxyl radicals, hydroperoxides, malondialdehyde, isoprostanes, the ozonide radical, O_3^- [14], and alkenals, particularly 4-hydroxy-2,3-trans-nonenal (HNE) [15]. As cholesterol is a component of the upper layer of the skin and because its double bond is readily attacked by O_3, it can give rise to biologically active oxysterols [16]. For instance, a major ozonation product of cholesterol, 3β-hydroxy-5-oxo-5,6-secocholestan-6-al, induces apoptosis in H9c2 cardiomyoblasts, implying a role for O_3 in myocardial injury. Furthermore, 3β-hydroxy-5-oxo-5,6-secocholestan-6-al has been also implicated in pulmonary toxicity, Alzheimer's disease, and atherosclerosis.

Ozone Targets

Because of its chemo-physical properties, it is easy to understand that several are the target tissues of ozone. Besides lung tissues, of which the ozone toxicity has been clearly demonstrated [5, 10, 12], other tissues such as the cornea and skin are continuously exposed to this pollutant. Indeed, it has recently been shown that O_3 exposure can also affect healthy ocular surface [17]. In vivo experiments revealed that O_3 is able to compromise the corneal epithelial integrity, decreases the number of mucin-secreting cells, and promotes the production of inflammatory cytokines, without altering tear volume [17]. Moreover, in conjunctival epithelial cells after O_3 exposure, the nuclear translocation of NF-κB, as well as increased κB-dependent transcriptional activity, NF-κB inhibitor α (IκBα) proteolysis, and expression of phosphorylated IκBα (p-IκBα), has been observed. In addition, O_3 induced the expression of inflammatory cytokines, Toll-like receptors, and C-C chemokine receptors, but decreased the expression of mucins. Furthermore, inhibition of NF-κB with pyrrolidine dithiocarbamate before exposure of cultured human conjunctival epithelial cells to ozone prevented changes in IκBα and p-IκBα levels in association with a decrease in the levels of inflammatory cytokines [17]. Therefore, these results suggest that O_3 exposure interferes with ocular surface integrity and induces inflammation involving NF-κB-mediated processes at the level (and/or upstream) of IκBα.

The Stratum Corneum as the First Cutaneous Target of Environmental Stressors

Within the skin, the SC has been identified as the main target of oxidative damage. As the outer skin barrier, the SC has important functions, limiting transepidermal water loss and posing a mechanical barrier to penetration by exogenous chemicals and pathogens. It comprises a unique two-compartment system consisting of protein-enriched corneocytes (structural, nonnucleated cells) embedded in a lipid-enriched intercellular matrix, forming stacks of bilayers that are rich in ceramides, cholesterol, and free fatty acids. The effects of O_3 on cutaneous tissues have been evaluated using a murine model and in a few studies using even human subjects [18, 19]. While no effect of O_3 on endogenous antioxidants was observed in full-thickness skin (dermis, epidermis, and SC), it could be demonstrated that a single high dose of O_3 (10 ppm for 2 h) significantly depleted topically applied vitamin E. When the skin was separated into upper epidermis, lower epidermis, papillary dermis, and dermis, O_3 induced a significant depletion of tocopherols and ascorbate followed by an increase in the lipid peroxidation measured as malondialdehyde (MDA) content. O_3 is known to react readily with biomolecules and does not penetrate through the cells; therefore, it was hypothesized that O_3 mainly reacts within the SC [20].

This hypothesis was supported by further experiments, where hairless mice were exposed to varying levels of O_3 for 2 h. Depletion of SC lipophilic (tocopherols) as well as hydrophilic (ascorbate, urate, GSH) antioxidants was detected upon O_3 exposure, and it was accompanied by a rise in lipid peroxidation as an indicator of increased oxidative stress. Furthermore, a recent study has shown the increase of 4-hydroxylnonenal (4-HNE) content in murine SC using both Western blot and immunohistochemical analysis. Finally, the increase of protein oxidation was also shown in in vivo studies [20, 21].

It is well known that oxygen radicals and other activated oxygen species generated as by-products of cellular metabolism or from environmental sources like O_3 cause modification of the amino acids of proteins and therefore modify their functions. Besides the modification of amino acid side chains, oxidation reactions can also alter the protein cross-linking with peptides. Protein carbonyls may be formed by oxidative cleavage of proteins or by direct oxidation of lysine, arginine, proline, and threonine residues. In addition, carbonyl groups may be introduced into proteins by reaction with aldehydes (4-HNE) produced during lipid peroxidation generated as a consequence of O_3 reactivity with the cutaneous tissues. This explains the use of carbonyl formation as a marker of oxidative stress. Protein oxidation has been also associated with skin aging and other skin pathologies.

Thiele et al. were able to detect protein carbonyl formation in the upper layer of the SC and in whole skin homogenates exposed to environmental insults. The main protein oxidized was keratin 10 and it showed an increasing level of oxidation from the lower SC to the upper level. This protein oxidation gradient was inversely correlated with the gradient of the antioxidant vitamin E. There are studies that have shown that protein oxidation can be quenched by antioxidants such as tocopherol and thiols. Of note is the fact that the keratin in SC contained dramatically more carbonyl groups than the keratin present in keratinocytes, indicating that the baseline levels of keratin oxidation are considerably higher in the SC as compared to the epidermal layers.

Furthermore, the oxygen partial pressure, a rate-limiting factor for the formation of reactive oxygen intermediates in the skin, decreases gradually from the outer to the inner SC layers.

All these effects may have important implications in the desquamation process of the SC because of the role that the proteins in corneodesmosomes play in cell cohesion. It should also be taken into account that while protein degradation increases proteolytic susceptibility up to a protein-specific degree, further damage actually causes a decrease in proteolytic susceptibility and leads to cross-linking and aggregation [20, 21].

Another major component of skin surface lipids is squalene [22]. Squalene takes part in reactions with indoor oxidants such as O_3 and NO_3 and can protect the skin against oxidation; in fact it is shown to account for about 40 % of O_3 removal by the human skin and hair [23]. However, as supported by recent studies, the reaction of squalene with O_3 also results in generation of harmful secondary products [24]. Among these, volatile aldehydic and ketonic products are known to have adverse health effects as asthma triggers and sensitizers [25]. Although the most part of these oxidation products is volatile and may be respiratory irritants, a large fraction of the less volatile products remain on the surface of the skin and may be skin irritants [26–29].

Cell membranes and their lipids are relevant potential targets of environmental stressors such as O_3. Using a spin-trapping technique, the formation of radicals in the stratum corneum (SC) upon exposure to O_3 was detected.

The spin adduct could arise from an alkoxyl radical formed during lipid peroxidation. Furthermore, lipid radicals (L·) are generated in epidermal homogenates that have been exposed to environmental stressors. The organic free radical L · reacts with O_2, forming peroxyl radical LOO · and hydrolipoperoxides (LOOH). Transition metals, and in particular iron, play a key role in the reactions of LOOH and in the subsequent generation of alkoxyl radicals (RO · can amplify the lipid peroxidation process).

Moreover, the toxicity is certainly augmented by the presence of NO_2, CO, SO_2, and particles (PM10). On this basis, it appears clear how the O_3-generated ROS and LOPs at the tissue level, after being only partly quenched by the antioxidants, will act as cell signals able to activate transcription factors, such as nuclear factor-kappa B (NF-κB), NO synthase, and some protein kinases, thus enhancing the synthesis and release of proinflammatory cytokines (TNFα, IL-1, IL-8, IFNγ, and TGFβ) and the possible formation of nitrating species. With a possible increasing inflow into the cutaneous tissues of neutrophils and activated macrophages, a vicious circle will start, perpetuating the production of an excess of ROS including also hypochlorous acid [30], LOPs, isoprostanes, tachykinins, cytokines, and proteases, which will self-maintain the inflammation after O_3 exposure.

Skin Antioxidant Defenses

To protect itself against oxidative stress, the skin is equipped with an elaborate system of antioxidant substances and enzymes that includes a network of redox-active antioxidants. Antioxidant enzymes such as glutathione reductases and peroxidases, superoxide dismutases, and catalase interact with the low-molecular-weight antioxidant substances such as vitamin E isoforms, vitamin C, glutathione (GSH), and ubiquinol [31]. The presence of tocopherol, ascorbate, urate, and glutathione has been demonstrated in the SC [31]. Interestingly, the distribution of antioxidants in the SC is not uniform but follows a gradient with higher concentrations in deeper layers and decreasing concentrations toward the skin surface. This may be explained by the fact that SC layers move up in time as a part of the physiological turnover and are replaced by newly differentiated keratinocytes. Therefore, the superficial layer has been exposed longer to chronic oxidative stress than a deeper layer.

Compared with the SC, the surface lipids contain high levels of tocopherol due to the secretion of vitamin E by sebaceous glands [32]. Eventually, the uppermost layer of the SC desquamates and the remaining antioxidants and reaction products will be eliminated from the body.

In general, the outermost part of the skin, the epidermis, contains higher concentrations of antioxidants than the dermis. In the lipophilic phase, tocopherol is the most prominent antioxidant, while vitamin C and GSH have the highest abundance in the cytosol.

Ozone-Induced Cutaneous Cellular Responses

Inflammatory Responses

Ozone, like many other environmental challenges, is able to activate redox-sensitive transcriptional factors such as nuclear factor-kappa B (NF-κB). This transcriptional factor acts as an activator for a multitude of proinflammatory genes (IL-8, TNFα, and TGFβ) and adhesion molecules (ICAM and VCAM). It has been assessed that O_3 is able to activate NF-κB using both in vitro and in vivo systems. Thiele et al., using an immortalized human keratinocytes (HaCaT cells), were able to show that O_3 induced the activation of NF-κB by electrophoretic mobility shift assay (EMSA). O_3 induced a dose-dependent activation of the transcription factor. This effect was likely to be mediated by ROS because it was inhibited by the incubation of the cells with lipid soluble antioxidants (tocopherol).

Finally, using a murine model, an increase of proinflammatory marker cyclooxygenase-2 (COX-2) was detected confirming the role that O_3 can play in skin inflammation [18].

Induction of Heat Shock Protein

As mentioned above, O_3 exposure was shown to induce antioxidant depletion as well as lipid and protein oxidation in the SC. Recent studies have investigated the effects of O_3 in the deeper functional layers of the skin. To evaluate the effect on cutaneous tissues of O_3 exposure, hairless mice were exposed for 6 days to 0.8 ppm of O_3 for 6 h/day, and the skin responses were analyzed using the whole skin homogenates. Under these experimental conditions, an increase in the protein level of heat shock protein (HSP)32, also known as hemoxygenase-1 (HO-1), confirms that HSPs are sensitive markers of O_3-induced stress in cutaneous tissues.

The author's group was the first to document the upregulation of HSPs 27, 32, and 70 in homogenized murine skin upon O_3 exposure. HSP27 showed the earliest (2 h) and highest (20-fold) response to O_3 compared with the delayed induction (12 h) of HSP70 and HO-1. Increased expression of HSP27 has been demonstrated following heating of both keratinocyte cell lines and organ-cultured human skin. HSP27 is expressed predominantly in the suprabasal epidermis in the human skin, whereas HSP70 predominates in the dermis compared with the epidermis. These differences in location between HSP27 and HSP70 might explain the different time course of induction of these stress proteins upon O_3 exposure. Interestingly, O_3 induction of HO-1 showed a delayed time course compared with that for HSP27 and HSP70, in line with a previous study, which showed a peak of HO-1 induction at 18–24 h in rat lungs after O_3 treatment [18]. It is therefore possible that bioactive compounds generated by the products of O_3exposure may be responsible for the induction of HO-1 as was also shown after UV radiation.

As HSPs are involved in cell proliferation, apoptosis, and inflammatory response, O_3-mediated HSP induction can affect normal skin physiology. Thus, HSPs might provide an adaptive cellular response to O_3; enhancing the expression of HSPs might turn out to be a new way to deal with the immediate and long-term consequences of O_3 exposure. A prerequisite for the utilization of this concept is the development of nontoxic HSP inducers and their evaluation for clinical efficacy and safety.

Ozone and MMPs

Among the multiple systems altered in the skin by environmental pollutants, MMPs are among the major targets. Indeed, O_3 exposure is able to affect their synthesis and/or activity with logical consequences on tissue remodeling and wound healing. Within the MMP family, MMP-2 and MMP-9 are the only members able to degrade type IV collagen of the basal membranes [33]. MMP-2 is involved in pathological processes such as photoaging and precancerous/cancerous skin lesions after UV exposure; moreover, MMP-2 is capable of cleaving other substrates, in addition to type IV collagen, including other MMPs, and therefore can (indirectly) control extracellular matrix degradation and remodeling.

MMP-9, like MMP-2, plays a role in human skin aging and tumor development as well as in other cutaneous lesions such as psoriasis and dermatitis [34]. In a recent study, it was demonstrated that the environmental pollutant O_3 was able to affect specific types of MMP activity in whole skin homogenates from hairless mice. Specifically, the exposure to 0.25 ppm of O_3 for 4 days (6 h/day) clearly induced MMP-2 activity in cutaneous tissues. In this case, the generation of ROS can be the cause of such activation, as it has been shown that MMPs can be activated by reactive oxygen species. It has been also demonstrated that O_3 is able to induce NO production via the activation of iNOS in cutaneous tissues. NO, while playing regulatory roles in the skin at physiological levels, when produced in excess, may combine with superoxide to form peroxynitrite (derived from other sources) that can activate MMPs especially MMP-9. Thus, the increase of oxidative stress after O_3 exposure, plus the interaction between oxygen and nitrogen active molecules, might be the main mechanism that leads to the enhanced MMP activities in skin tissues. It has been shown in a number of cases that photoaging and precancerous/cancerous lesions can result from an imbalance between MMPs and their endogenous inhibitors, the tissue inhibitors of metalloproteinases (TIMPs) [34].

In fact the activities of MMPs are regulated by TIMPs, which can be produced by a multitude of cell types present in the cutaneous tissue. While MMP activity resulted to be altered by the O_3, neither TIMP-1 nor TIMP-2 level expression was affected. The lack of changes in TIMP-1 and TIMP-2 levels, combined with the increased activity of MMPs, suggests that O_3 can cause a net increase in matrix degradation.

Furthermore, there are other MMPs involved in skin diseases; for example, MMP-12, the human macrophage metalloelastase, accumulates in skin granuloma and in other inflammatory skin diseases such as dermatitis herpetiformis and pityriasis lichenoides. Moreover, MMP-7 or matrilysin is very efficient in elastin degradation, and increased elastolytic activity by both MMP-12 and MMP-7 has been reported upon oxidative stress exposure in hairless mice skin. Enhanced MMP-7 expression has also been detected in benign sweat gland tumors and aggressive basal and squamous cell carcinomas.

Skin Age-Related Responses to O_3 Exposure: MMPs

It is well known that oxidative stress occurring after oxidant stressor such as O_3 or UV radiation is implicated in the pathogenesis of skin-related diseases and that the levels of antioxidant defenses decrease with aging. Consistently, it has been reported that aged mice are more susceptible to oxidative stress than young mice [35], and previous reports have suggested that oxidant pollutant exposure and age interact and potentiate each other [21].

Therefore, it can be concluded that among the multiple consequences of oxidative stress, an increase in the MMP/TIMP ratio also occurs. The question of whether a cause-effect relationship exists between oxidative stress and MMP release or they are two independent responses is not still clear and needs further studies to be better demonstrated. However, by integrating the results from recent works, the redox-associated signal transduction pathways that lead to MMP induction can be easily reconstructed. Indeed, oxidative stress, through both receptor and non-receptor protein tyrosine kinases (PTK), activates several signaling proteins, such as ERK and PKB, which, in turn, mediate the transcriptional regulation of MMPs, via Ap-1, Ets, and NF-κB [36]. In closing, it is now documented that the interaction between aging and oxidative pollutant exposure can impair resistance of cutaneous tissues to environmental oxidative stress in elderly subjects.

Skin Age-Related Responses to O_3 Exposure: Wound Healing

Wound healing is a critical process in the skin and has been known to be affected by oxidative stress and also to decline with increasing age. Although the exact sequence of wound healing is not completely understood, cutaneous wound healing begins with wounding-induced signaling factor-based transformation of stationary keratinocytes into cells capable of both replication and migration. Upon transformation, these cells express a host of molecules that promote the invasion of the injured epithelial matrix and re-epithelialization of the wound surface. Delayed wound healing in the elderly has been well described [37]. Among the elderly, the SC transit time was delayed 10 days compared to young adults. More recently, Hellemans and coworkers published that older skin, subjected to UVA-induced deactivation of catalase, requires a longer time to replenish the antioxidant capacity than in younger skin; furthermore, it was shown that aged skin strongly differs from young skin in the ability to cope with oxidative environmental insults [21, 31–38].

In the recent literature, it has been shown that hydrogen peroxide (H_2O_2) (molecules involved in the induction of oxidative stress) induced vascular endothelial growth factor (VEGF) expression in human keratinocytes and therefore can be able to stimulate wound healing [39].

As mentioned above, O_3 exposure is also associated with activation of transcription factor NF-κB, which is important to regulate inflammatory responses and eventually entire wound healing. O_3 exposure increased levels of tumor growth factor (TGFβ) that is a critical factor in tissue remodeling [40]. The roles of the multiple, coordinated processes involved in the injured skin repair, as well as the signals that initiate and terminate skin responses, remain ill-defined. Furthermore, the age-related differences in the response of the skin wound healing to particular environmental insults are poorly documented. Given the documented role of oxidants in wound healing [39], the potential effects of O_3 on cutaneous wound healing in combination with aging represent a poorly understood area. It has been suggested that O_3 as an oxidant might also stimulate wound healing, but aging with O_3 would be detrimental due to increased oxidative stress and have biological as well as practical implications.

In a recent study, the detrimental effects of O_3 on cutaneous wound healing in the aged animals were demonstrated. In fact when young hairless mice (8 weeks old) and aged mice (18 months old) with full-thickness excisional wounds were exposed to 0.5 ppm O_3 for 6 h/day, the rate of wound closure was significantly delayed in the aged group. It was also shown that O_3 exposure induces protein and lipid oxidation assessed as changes in protein oxidation (carbonyls) and lipid peroxidation (4-hydroxynonenal, HNE adducts) in the old mice compared to the young mice during the later stage of cutaneous wound healing. The extent of wound closure in young and old animals with full-thickness excisional wounds exposed to a relevant concentration of O_3 was monitored until day 9 (complete wound closure) [21]. These data suggest that O_3 exposure has different effects depending on the age of the mice. In fact, it significantly delayed wound closure in old mice, while in young mice, it had no significant effect, although an accelerated trend during the first few days of the exposure was detected. This might be attributed to the antibacterial properties of O_3, as it has been shown that application of hydropressive ozonization provides fast cleansing of wound surface from pyonecrotic masses, promotes elimination of infection, and thus substantially reduces the period of treatment of the patients. Recently, clinical treatments using hyperbaric oxygen therapy demonstrated that increased oxygen tension at the wound site increases the formation of granulation tissue and enhanced accelerated wound closure and ameliorated impairs dermal wound healing; therefore, accelerated trend of wound closure shown in young population may be due to decreased bacterial infection and/or increased oxygen tension by O_3exposure in wound area [41].

One of the possible driving processes of the effect of O_3 on wound healing can be, also in this case, the modulation of the transcription factor NF-κB. Although NF-κB is an immune regulator in inflammatory stage, it may be critical to modulate later stage of healing process in injury. Consistent with this one, a recent study reported that human airway epithelium inflammatory response to inhaled O_3 has been shown to be in part controlled by free radical-mediated NF-κB activation. Further, very recently, it has been reported that overexpression of superoxide dismutase not only prevents O_3-related changes in bronchoalveolar lavage fluid protein, macrophage content, and 4-hydroxyalkenals but also O_3-dependent activation of NF-κB [42]. These researchers have also reported that O_3-induced lung injury is mediated by NF-κB. These results clearly link O_3 exposure to NF-κB activation and suggest that intracellular oxidants such as superoxide and related free radicals are important components of these responses. Interestingly, the dose-effect relationship between level of oxidative stress and NF-κB exhibits a biphasic profile: while moderate levels of oxidative stress activate NF-κB through an IkB kinase-independent mechanism, extremely high levels of oxidative stress have been shown to inhibit NF-κB activation by blocking IkBα phosphorylation. Furthermore, the levels of oxidative stress were increased in aged rats and the content of activated forms, p50 and p65 subunits, of NF-κB increased with age. One potential explanation for the differential effect of O_3 in the older animals is that the level of oxidative stress generated by O_3 exposure combined with aging causes levels of oxidative stress that inhibits IkBα phosphorylation, thereby resulting in a decline in NF-κB activation. The existence of a higher basal level of oxidative stress in old mice is proved by the higher levels of protein carbonyls and 4-HNE. These data fit with studies that have shown that old rats had higher lipid peroxides and superoxide dismutase activity tended to decrease. This finding is consistent with what is mentioned previously that O_3 exposure induced skin antioxidant depletion. In addition, Gilhar and coworkers have reported that the human epidermis showed reduced proliferation and increased keratinocyte apoptosis with aging [43]. This could be interpreted as an additional evidence of increased load of oxidative stress burdens in the keratinocytes of old mice, as apoptosis has been linked to elevated levels of cellular oxidants. The evidences and considerations reported above are controversial because the levels of cutaneous oxidative stress in response to O_3 treatment should be higher in aged skin and these levels may be further increased by O_3 exposure so as to raise levels of skin oxidative stress in old mice to levels above those that maximally evoke NF-κB activation. This study suggests that although O_3 exposure increased NF-κB activation in the young and old mice, it may differently modulate wound healing process by aging. Furthermore, NF-κB also has important roles in later tissue remodeling stage as well as in initial inflammatory stage during cutaneous wound healing.

This interpretation is also bolstered by the data on TGFβ, a crucial modulator of tissue remodeling, and is linked to both NF-κB status and levels of oxidative stress during the entire wound healing process. The reduced TGFβ levels in both air- and O_3-exposed old mice, as well as the lower induction of TGFβ by O_3 exposure in the old animals, suggest that the noted delays in wound closure might be related to defects in oxidative stress-dependent NF-κB status as well as levels of oxidative stress and TGFβ signaling in aged mice during later stage of wound healing.

In summary, given the role of oxidative stress in wound healing, an interaction between O_3 and aging is of great interest to be explored in cutaneous wound healing process. The ability of O_3 to alter wound healing indicates that environmental effects of pollutants need to be taken into account when damaged skin repair is explored in human subjects.

Ozone Potentiates UV-Induced Oxidative Stress in the Skin

Although exposure of cutaneous tissues to either UV or O_3 alone is known to deplete vitamin E and induce lipid peroxidation, it is of interest to evaluate the possible additive effects of sequential or simultaneous exposure of the skin to these important environmental oxidant stresses. It should be taken into consideration that the skin is continuously exposed to several environmental pollutants each day and UV and O_3 are among the most toxic and noxious of them.

While UV radiation penetrates into the epidermis (UVB) or into the dermis (UVA), and is known to induce the release of tissue-degrading enzymes even at suberythemal levels, O_3 oxidizes biological systems only at the surface. Therefore, since O_3 and UV cooperatively damage SC components, it can be speculated that they exert an additive effect in the deeper layers of the epidermis. Products of O_3-induced lipid oxidation penetrate the outer skin barrier and cause effects to constituents of the deeper epidermis. This can lead to the activation of NF-κB. On the other hand, NF-κB activation has also been implicated in the expression of collagenases by solar-simulated UV radiation and in cutaneous responses to wounding. UV radiation has been shown to compromise the skin barrier. O_3 may enhance this phenomenon by perturbing SC lipid constituents in the SC, which are known to be critical determinants of the barrier function. Thus, O_3 may cause a disturbance of the barrier function, increase the transepidermal water loss, and provoke epidermal repair responses, as can be also seen after barrier perturbation. Since O_3 enhances UV-induced oxidation in the SC, it cannot be excluded that potentially O_3 also enhances other UV effects such as photoaging [44].

In conclusion, the "additive" data demonstrate that O_3 and UV radiation, two common sources of environmental oxidant stressors, exhibit additive effects in terms of oxidative damage to the skin barrier.

Health Implication

Being lipids, the first target of O_3, the consequent induction of lipid peroxidation in the upper layers of the skin can affect the physiology of cutaneous tissues. In fact, oxidation of the lipids present in the SC will change the skin barrier integrity, and this has been shown to be a leading factor for several skin pathologies such as psoriasis, atopic dermatitis, and irritant dermatitis. The increase of peroxidation markers such as 4-HNE, MDA, and TBARS in the upper layers of the skin after O_3 exposure is a consequence of the PUFA peroxidation like arachidonic acid and linolenate, and this could consequently affect also the lower layers of the skin trigging all a cascade of noxious biological processes. The toxicity of O_3 is the result from the effects of a cascade of products that are produced in the reactions of O_3 with target molecules that lie close to the air-tissue interface. Ozone is too reactive to penetrate far into the tissue, only a small fraction of environmentally relevant doses of O_3 is believed to pass through a bilayer membrane, and none pass through the cell. Therefore, the products that derive from the oxidation of the SC, which have longer lifetime and lower reactivity, will transmit the effect of O_3 beyond the air-tissue interface. Peroxidation products such as 4-HNE and alkenals are relatively stable and can damage or alter cells and tissues at more distant sites not directly exposed to O_3.

Clinical Evidences of Ozone Toxicity

Recent evidences have highlighted that the exposure to ambient ozone (O_3) may be associated with various skin conditions [4].

Based on the previous indicated mechanisms of ozone impact on the skin, i.e., oxidative stress and inflammation, it can be assumed that exposure to this ambient pollutant can cause susceptibility to viral or bacterial infections at level of the epithelial barriers. In fact, a recent epidemiological study based on a case-crossover analysis of the emergency department visits in 5 Canadian hospitals during the decade 1992–2002 revealed a clear positive association between cellulitis and pharyngitis episodes and ambient ozone exposure [45]. These results reinforce the knowledge about the detrimental effects of ozone in terms of the ability to facilitate bacterial invasion in the skin and mucous membranes [45].

Similarly, a significant association between emergency-room visits for skin conditions and

O_3 exposure emerged in a study conducted during a period of circa 700 days in the Department of Dermatology of a Shanghai hospital [4]. Using a time series analysis, the authors demonstrated that an increase of 10 μg m^{-3} in the 7-day average O_3 corresponds to an enhanced risk of several skin conditions including urticaria, eczema, contact dermatitis, rash /other nonspecific eruption, infected skin disease, and other skin diseases, whereas other pollutants, such as particulate matter with aerodynamic diameter of 10 lm or less (PM10), sulfur dioxide (SO2), and nitrogen dioxide (NO2), were not significantly associated with ER visits for skin conditions [4]. We should take into consideration that the study by Xu et al. did not analyze the effect of particles with a diameter below 2.5 μm, possibly toxic also to cutaneous tissues [46].

Therapeutic Approaches

Because the SC is the main target of O_3 reactivity, therapeutic strategies should involve the more accessible skin layers via a topical antioxidant application. In a murine model, topical application of vitamin E reduced the peroxidation induced by O_3 exposure, demonstrating that topical application could be a way to counteract ozone-induced skin toxicity.

This indicates a key role for vitamin E both as an indicator and in the prevention of skin oxidative damage. In addition to physical or chemical measures for protection against environmental stressors consistent with the "free radical theory of aging," the use of low-molecular-weight antioxidants for preventing premature skin aging and skin disease seems appropriate. Vitamin E and other antioxidants can only be supplied to the skin to some extent via a diet rich in fruits and vegetables. Moreover, vitamin E supplementation and/or its topical administration will substantially enhance skin vitamin E concentrations. Since oxidant skin alteration occurs mainly in the SC and outer epidermal layers, this is relevant for a preventive and/or therapeutic approach.

Conclusion

The results summarized in this chapter support the concept first advanced by Pryor et al. [12] that O_3 exposures to noncellular constituents of surface epithelial cells are capable of generating potentially toxic peroxidation products. Extrapolation of this concept to cutaneous tissues would suggest that O_3 reacts directly with SC lipids that contribute to cutaneous tissue protective barrier, generating products that are able to penetrate the SC and target keratinocytes. It is concluded that O_3 not only affects antioxidant levels and oxidation markers in the SC but also induces cellular responses in the deeper layers of the skin (Fig. 1a, b).

It is recognized that exposure of the skin to environmental stressors causes injury to the skin due to oxidants and free radicals, which leads to "oxidative stress," also defined as imbalance between oxidants and antioxidants.

Low-molecular-weight antioxidants are present in high concentrations especially in the epidermis. Oxidative stress can overwhelm the skin antioxidants and increase the formation of oxidized cell components. Topical exposure to tropospheric O_3 induces skin oxidative stress. Oxidative damage to the SC may result in a barrier perturbation and in the production of lipid oxidation products that can act as "second messengers" in the deeper layers of the skin, which, in turn, elicits repair responses and/or the induction of defense enzymes such as HSPs. Oxidative injury to the outermost layers of the skin may initiate localized inflammatory responses, resulting in the recruitment of phagocytes and their cell-specific, tightly regulated NAD(P)H-oxidase systems for generating oxidants, thus amplifying oxidative stress and inducing activation of MMPs.

Cross-References

- ▶ Climate Change and Its Dermatologic Impact on Aging Skin
- ▶ Skin Photodamage Prevention: State of the Art and New Prospects

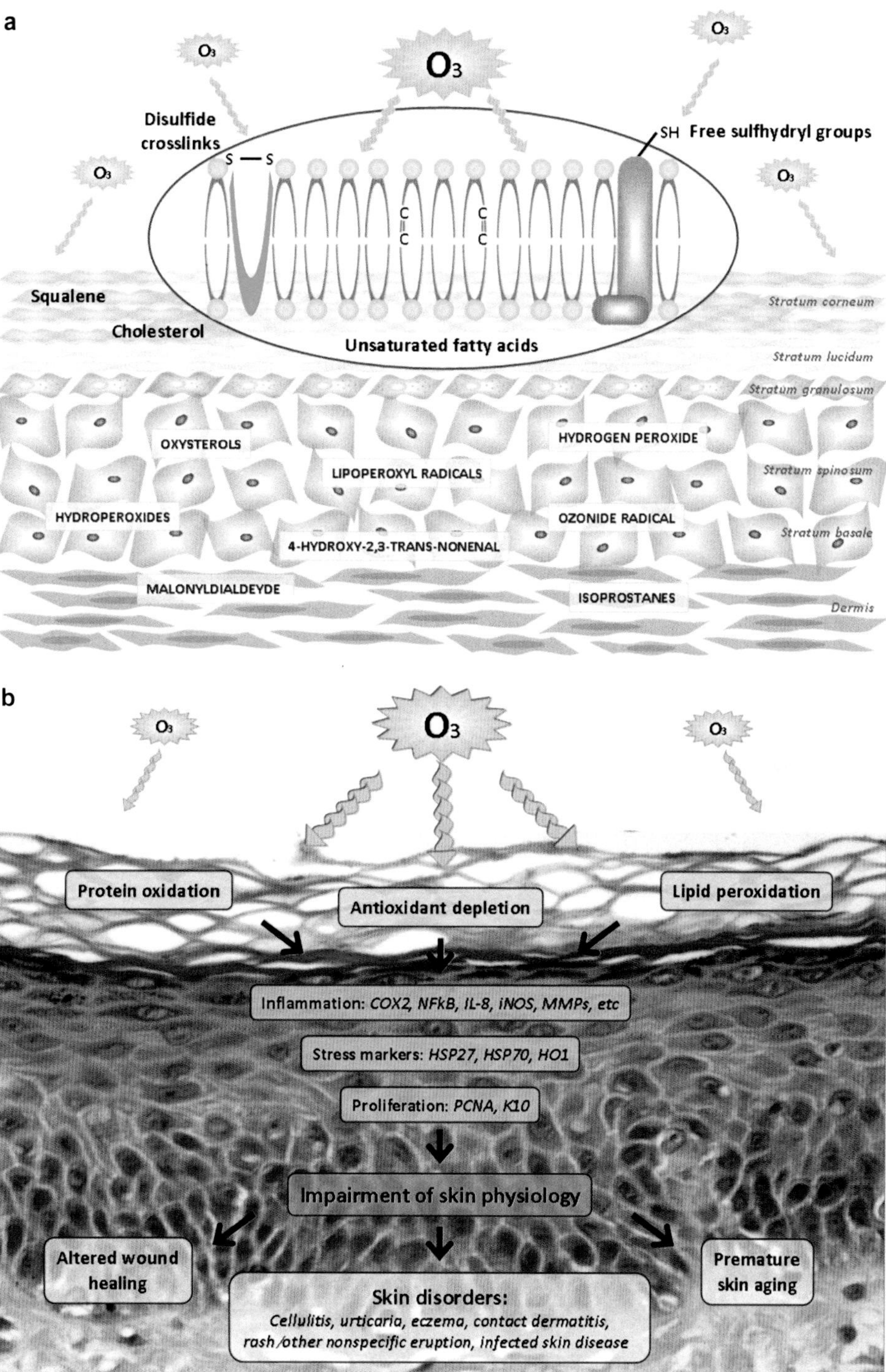

Fig. 1 (**a**) Scheme summarizing the main effects of ozone exposure on cutaneous lipids (stratum corneum), with the consequent generation of bioactive compounds, such as aldehydes and H_2O_2, that are the "carrier" of the oxidative effects to the deeper layers of the skin. (**b**) Some pathways triggered by the harmful effects of ozone exposure on the stratum corneum components (lipids and cell membranes), leading to the alterations of normal skin physiology and to the development of the skin disorders

References

1. Kelly FJ, et al. Air pollution and the elderly: oxidant/antioxidant issues worth consideration. Eur Respir J Suppl. 2003;40:70s–5.
2. Valacchi G, et al. Induction of stress proteins and MMP-9 by 0.8 ppm of ozone in murine skin. Biochem Biophys Res Commun. 2003;305(3):741–6.
3. Valacchi G, et al. The dual action of ozone on the skin. Br J Dermatol. 2005;153(6):1096–100.
4. Xu F, et al. Ambient ozone pollution as a risk factor for skin disorders. Br J Dermatol. 2011;165(1):224–5.
5. Mudway IS, et al. Ozone and the lung: a sensitive issue. Mol Aspects Med. 2000;21(1–2):1–48.
6. Zimmermann PH. Tracing the sources of tropospheric ozone, Proceedings of the International Ozone Symposium, 21 and 22 October 1999. Basel (IOA – EA3G Ed), 1999, p. 157–160.
7. Weber SU, et al. Ozone: an emerging oxidative stressor to skin. Curr Probl Dermatol. 2001;29:52–61.
8. Dentener F, et al. The global atmospheric environment for the next generation. Environ Sci Technol. 2006;11:3586–94.
9. Mortimer KM, et al. The effect of ozone on inner-city children with asthma: identification of susceptible subgroups. Am J Respir Crit Care Med. 2000;162(5):1838–45.
10. Tager IB, et al. Chronic exposure to ambient ozone and lung function in young adults. Epidemiology. 2005;16(6):751–9.
11. Mustafa MG. Biochemical basis of ozone toxicity. Free Radic Biol Med. 1990;9(3):245–65.
12. Pryor WA. Mechanisms of radical formation from reactions of ozone with target molecules in the lung. Free Radic Biol Med. 1994;17(5):451–65.
13. Pryor WA, et al. The cascade mechanism to explain ozone toxicity: the role of lipid ozonation products. Free Radic Biol Med. 1995;19(6):935–41.
14. Ballinger CA, et al. Antioxidant-mediated augmentation of ozone-induced membrane oxidation. Free Radic Biol Med. 2005;38(4):515–26.
15. Esterbauer H, et al. Chemistry and biochemistry of 4-hydroxynonenal, malonaldehyde and related aldehydes. Free Radic Biol Med. 1991;11(1):81–128.
16. Sathishkumar K, et al. A major ozonation product of cholesterol, 3beta-hydroxy-5-oxo-5,6-secocholestan-6-al, induces apoptosis in H9c2 cardiomyoblasts. FEBS Lett. 2005;597(28):6444–50.
17. Lee H, et al. Effects of ozone exposure on the ocular surface. Free Radic Biol Med. 2013;63:78–89.
18. Valacchi G, et al. In vivo ozone exposure induces antioxidant/stress-related responses in murine lung and skin. Free Radic Biol Med. 2004;36(5):673–81.
19. He QC, et al. Effects of environmentally realistic levels of ozone on stratum corneum function. Int J Cosmet Sci. 2006;28(5):349–57.
20. Thiele JJ, et al. The antioxidant network of the stratum corneum. Curr Probl Dermatol. 2001;29:26–42.
21. Lim Y, et al. Modulation of cutaneous wound healing by ozone: differences between young and aged mice. Toxicol Lett. 2006;160(2):127–34.
22. Nicolaides N. Skin lipids: their biochemical uniqueness. Science. 1974;186:19–26.
23. Wisthaler A, et al. Reactions of ozone with human skin lipids: sources of carbonyls, dicarbonyls, and hydroxycarbonyls in indoor air. Proc Natl Acad Sci U S A. 2010;107(15):6568–75.
24. Fooshee DR, et al. Atmospheric oxidation of squalene: molecular study using COBRA modeling and high-resolution mass spectrometry. Environ Sci Technol. 2015;49(22):13304–13.
25. Anderson SE, et al. Evaluation of the contact and respiratory sensitization potential of volatile organic compounds generated by simulated indoor air chemistry. Toxicol Sci. 2007;97(2):355–63.
26. Pham DM, et al. Oxidization of squalene, a human skin lipid: a new and reliable marker of environmental pollution studies. Int J Cosmet Sci. 2015;37(4):357–65.
27. Thiele JJ, et al. Ozone-exposure depletes vitamin E and induces lipid peroxidation in murine stratum corneum. J Invest Dermatol. 1997;108:753–7.
28. Thiele JJ, et al. Tropospheric ozone: an emerging environmental stress to skin. Biol Chem. 1997;378:1299–305.
29. Podda M, et al. Influence of environmental polluting ozone on the skin. Hautarzt. 2004;55:1120–4.
30. Spickett CM, et al. The reactions of hypochlorous acid, the reactive oxygen species produced by myeloperoxidase, with lipids. Acta Biochim Pol. 2000;47(4):889–99.
31. Packer L, et al. Antioxidants and the response of skin to oxidative stress: vitamin E as a key indicator. Skin Pharmacol Appl Skin Physiol. 2002;15(5):282–90.
32. Thiele JJ, et al. Sebaceous gland secretion is a major physiologic route of vitamin E delivery to skin. J Invest Dermatol. 1999;113(6):1006–10.
33. Brenneisen P, et al. Ultraviolet-B irradiation and matrix metalloproteinases: from induction via signaling to initial events. Ann N Y Acad Sci. 2002;973:31–43.
34. Hofmann UB, et al. Matrix metalloproteinases in human melanoma. J Invest Dermatol. 2000;115(3):337–44.
35. Stadtman ER. Role of oxidant species in aging. Curr Med Chem. 2004;11(9):1105–12.
36. Galis ZS. Matrix metalloproteinases in vascular remodeling and atherogenesis: the good, the bad, and the ugly. Circ Res. 2002;90(3):251–62.
37. Crooks A. How does ageing affect the wound healing process? J Wound Care. 2005;14(5):222–3.
38. Fortino V, et al. Cutaneous MMPs are differently modulated by environmental stressors in old and young mice. Toxicol Lett. 2007;173(2):73–9.
39. Sen CK, et al. Oxidant-induced vascular endothelial growth factor expression in human keratinocytes and

cutaneous wound healing. J Biol Chem. 2002;277 (36):33284–90.
40. Valacchi G. Studies on the biological effects of ozone: 11. Release of factors from human endothelial cells. Mediators Inflamm. 2000;9(6):271–6.
41. Gajendrareddy PK, et al. Hyperbaric oxygen therapy ameliorates stress-impaired dermal wound healing. Brain Behav Immun. 2005;19(3):217–22.
42. Fakhrzadeh L. Ozone-induced production of nitric oxide and TNF-alpha and tissue injury are dependent on NF-kappaB p50. Am J Physiol Lung Cell Mol Physiol. 2004;287(2):L279–85.
43. Gilhar A, et al. Ageing of human epidermis: the role of apoptosis, fas and telomerase. Br J Dermatol. 2004;150 (1):56–63.
44. Valacchi G, et al. Ozone potentiates vitamin E depletion by ultraviolet radiation in the murine stratum corneum. FEBS Lett. 2000;466(1):165–8.
45. Valacchi G, et al. Ambient ozone and bacterium streptococcus: a link between cellulitis and pharyngitis. Int J Occup Med Environ Health. 2015;28(4):771–4.
46. Magnani ND, et al. Skin damage mechanisms related to airborne particulate matter exposure. Toxicol Sci. 2016;149(1):227–36.

Infrared A-Induced Skin Aging

53

Peter Schroeder and Jean Krutmann

Contents

Abstract

Extrinsic skin aging can be attributed to infrared radiation, especially infrared. This chapter will summarize the current knowledge about the epidemiological evidence, molecular principles, and prevention/protection, as it concerns skin aging induced by infrared A.

Introduction

Extrinsic skin aging has, for many years, been mainly attributed to ultraviolet (UV) radiation. Recently, it has become evident that other parts of the solar electromagnetic spectrum contribute as well. Among these, infrared radiation, especially infrared A, has received increasing attention. This chapter will summarize the current knowledge about the epidemiological evidence, molecular principles, and prevention/protection, as it concerns skin aging induced by infrared radiation.

P. Schroeder (✉) • J. Krutmann
Environmental Health Research Institute (IUF), Heinrich-Heine-University, Duesseldorf, Germany
e-mail: peet@gmx.de; krutmann@uni-duesseldorf.de

M.A. Farage et al. (eds.), *Textbook of Aging Skin*,
DOI 10.1007/978-3-662-47398-6_42

Infrared Radiation

Physical Basics and Natural and Artificial Sources

Solar radiation is filtered by the earth's atmosphere; the part reaching the earth surface includes the wavelengths from 290 to 4,000 nm and is divided into three bands: ultraviolet radiation (UV, 290–400 nm), visible light (400–760 nm), and infrared radiation (IR, 760–4,000 nm). Infrared radiation is further subdivided into IRA (λ = 760–1,440 nm), IRB (λ = 1,440–3,000 nm), and IRC (λ = 3,000 nm–1 mm).

While the photon energy of IR is lower than that of UV, the total amount of solar energy reaching human skin contains approximately 54 % IR, while UV only accounts for 7 % [1]. Most of the IR radiation lies within the IRA band (~30 % of total solar energy), which deeply penetrates the human skin, while IRB and IRC only affect the upper skin layers (Fig. 1). In comparison, IRA penetrates better than UV into the skin, with approximately 50 % reaching the dermis [1–3].

The main source of IR radiation is the sun; the actual solar dose reaching the skin is influenced by several factors: ozone layer, position of the sun, latitude, altitude, cloud cover, and ground reflections. Based on these parameters, it should be noted that the overall composition of sunlight, e.g., in terms of the UV/IRA ratio, is changing throughout the day. In addition to natural sunlight, artificial IR sources are constantly gaining importance; they are used for therapeutic as well as for lifestyle purposes. While therapeutic use of IRA provides beneficial effects, for example, in wound healing, lifestyle-motivated applications of IRA, e.g., for "wellness" irradiations or for means of skin rejuvenation, appear to be quite paradoxical [4].

Infrared Radiation and Skin Aging

The role of IR radiation in premature skin aging was described over 20 years ago by L. Kligman

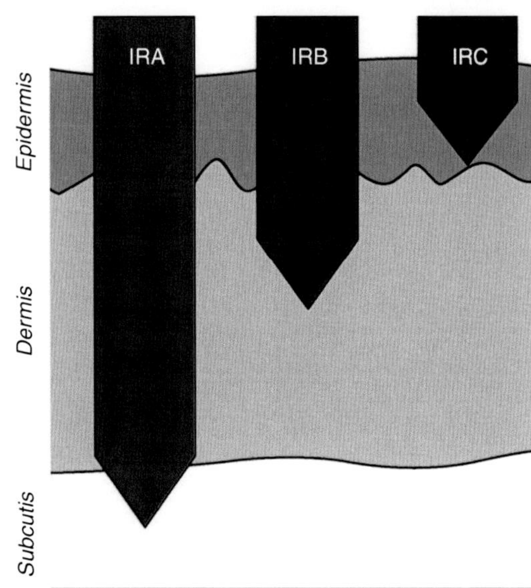

Fig. 1 Skin penetration of infrared radiation. Different wavelengths of natural and artificial radiations have different penetration capabilities. IRA penetrates well into the skin, approximately 50 % of IRA is absorbed in the dermis. IRB reaches the dermis as well, while IRC is nearly completely absorbed in the epidermis

[5]. She was the first to report that infrared radiation enhances UV-induced skin damage in guinea pigs. This prompted her to investigate the effect of IR alone; as a consequence, she could demonstrate that IR leads to elastosis, with "IR inducing the production of many fine, feathery fibers" and "a large increase in ground substance, a finding also seen in actinically damaged human skin." From these observations, she has concluded that IR radiation contributes to skin aging. It took, however, almost 20 years until the underlying molecular mechanisms could be identified.

Molecular Mechanisms

Schieke et al. reported in 2002 that low, physiologically relevant doses of IRA lead to a disturbance of the dermal extracellular matrix. IRA irradiation results in an induction of matrix metalloproteinase-1 (MMP-1) in vitro in human dermal fibroblasts, while expression of the respective tissue inhibitor TIMP-1 was not increased. This finding has, since then, been confirmed in independent studies by different workgroups in vitro and in vivo [6, 7].

Matrix metalloproteinases (MMPs) are zinc-dependent endopeptidases responsible for the degradation of extracellular matrix components such as collagen and elastin. Under physiological conditions, MMPs are part of a coordinate network and are precisely regulated by their endogenous inhibitors, tissue inhibitors of MMPs (TIMPs). The unbalanced activity of MMPs with excessive proteolysis is thought to be a major pathophysiological factor in extrinsic skin aging. The increased expression of MMPs without a respective increase in TIMP expression results in the cleavage of fibrillar collagen and thus impairs the structural integrity of the dermis [8–10].

This impairment can be partially countered by an increased expression of collagen itself. It is therefore important to note that IRA has recently been found to decrease the expression of the dominant human collagen gene Col1a1 in vitro and in vivo [6, 11].

Taken together, IRA disturbs the collagen equilibrium of the skin in two ways: (1) by increasing the amount/activity of MMP-1, which results in an increased collagen degradation, and (2) by decreasing de novo synthesis of collagen.

While the biological endpoints of IRA irradiation resemble those found after UV irradiation, the underlying cellular molecular processes are completely different. This is particularly evident if UVA and IRA are being compared: the primal event in both cases is an increased amount of reactive oxygen species (ROS), which on a first glare seems to indicate a similarity rather than a difference. More detailed analysis – however – revealed huge differences between UVA and IRA. UVA induces an increased production of ROS by NADPH-oxidases, which are located in the cytoplasmic membrane [12], and in addition repetitive UVA irradiation results in damage to the mitochondrial DNA (mtDNA) [13]. IRA, on the other hand, acts via a disturbance of the mitochondrial electron transport chain (mtETC). This multiprotein facility, driven by reduction equivalents (NADH/H + and FADH2), is responsible for energy conservation by transferring electrons to oxygen while building up an electrochemical proton gradient across the inner mitochondrial membrane, which in turn fuels the production of ATP from ADP and Pi. As this process is not error-free, relatively small amounts of ROS are always generated. Upon IRA irradiation this amount is significantly increased [4].

ROS are often recognized only as damaging agent, but they are well known to function in terms of cellular signaling. Reactive oxygen species (ROS) can serve to trigger molecular signaling responses and several studies indicate that ROS cause an inactivation of protein-tyrosine phosphatases (PTPs) by oxidizing conserved cysteine residues in the active sites of PTPs and thereby lead to a net increase in kinase phosphorylation/activation [14].

After IRA irradiation, not only the mitochondrial levels but also the cellular ROS levels are increased and a disturbance of the cellular glutathione (GSH) equilibrium is observed [15]. GSH is one of the most important endogenous antioxidants; it can prevent or repair oxidative damage, and as a consequence it is oxidized itself, forming the glutathione dimer (GSSG). In this regard, IRA irradiation leads to a significant shift of the GSH/GSSG equilibrium toward the oxidized form [15].

IRA-induced ROS production is not just a by-product of the irradiation but of functional relevance because boosting the cellular antioxidative defense by increasing the cellular GSH content abrogated the IRA-induced upregulation of MMP-1 [15]. In addition, use of specific antioxidants in cell culture has also been shown to decrease the IRA-induced effects [7].

Mitochondria are known to act as a hub for cellular signaling with disruption of the mtETC being a prominent inducer of such retrograde (i.e., from mitochondria to nucleus) signaling [16]. In contrast to anterograde signaling processes, here the nuclear gene expression is regulated by events originating in the mitochondria. The IRA-induced increase in mitochondrial ROS was recently found to initiate such a retrograde signaling cascade (Fig. 2).

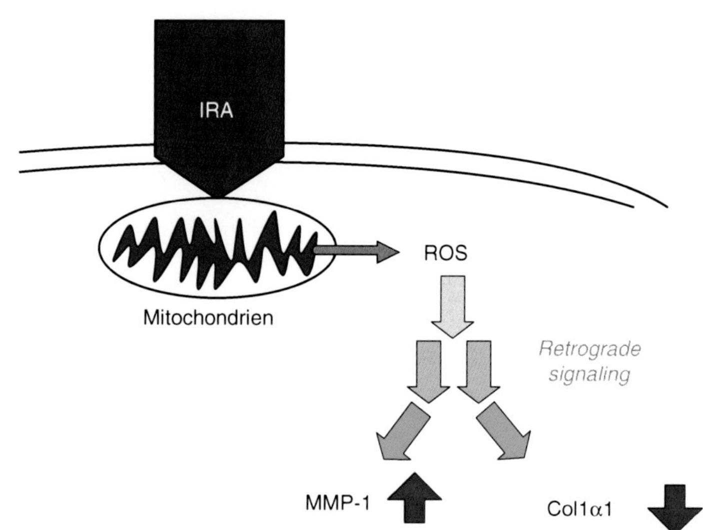

Fig. 2 Infrared A-induced signal transduction. IRA radiation leads to an increased amount of mitochondrial ROS, which in turn leads to initiation of retrograde signaling, finally resulting in an increased expression of MMP-1 mRNA and protein and a decreased expression of Col1α1

Downstream of mitochondrial ROS, the IRA radiation-induced signaling pathway relevant for MMP-1 induction has been found to involve the activation of MAPKinases. Three distinct MAPK pathways have been characterized: the extracellular signal-regulated kinase 1/2 (ERK1/2) pathway (Raf-MEK1/2-ERK1/2), the c-Jun N-terminal kinase pathway (MEKK1/3-MKK4/7-JNK1/2/3), and p38 (MEKK-MKK3/6-p38 a-d) pathway also termed stress-activated protein kinases (SAPKs). The ERK1/2 pathway is primarily induced by mitogens such as growth factors, whereas the SAPK pathways are predominantly induced by inflammatory cytokines as well as environmental stress such as UV, heat, and osmotic shock. Activated MAPKs translocate to the nucleus, where they phosphorylate and activate transcription factors such as c-Jun, c-Fos, ATF-2, and ternary complex factors (TCF) leading to the formation and activation of homo- or heterodimeric forms of the transcription factor AP-1. The promoter region of MMP-1 carries multiple AP-1-binding sites. For IRA, it has been demonstrated that ERK1/2 and p38 are activated in dermal fibroblasts, but that only inhibition of ERK1/2 activation subdues the IRA-induced increase of MMP-1 (reviewed in [17]).

Although up to now the main research focus has been on MMP-1 and Col1a1, it is very likely that the IRA-induced activation of MAPKinases affects the regulation of other genes as well. Indeed, several additional effects of IRA are known: Kim et al. reported that infrared exposure is involved in neoangiogenesis in human skin, because IRA induces an angiogenic switch by altering the balance between the angiogenic inducer VEGF and the angiogenic inhibitor TSP-2 [18]. Interestingly, increased neoangiogenesis is a prominent feature of photoaged human skin [19]. Others found that IRA irradiation led to a decrease in epidermal proliferation, Langerhans cell density, and contact hypersensitivity reaction in mice [20], and a subsequent study by the same group indicates that IRA influences cutaneous wound repair by altering the levels of transforming growth factor (TGF)-b1 and MMP-2 [21]. Yet another study showed an influence of IRA on protein expression of ferritin: an increased ferritin expression was detected after IRA irradiation of keratinocytes and fibroblasts [22]. Ferritin is involved in the cellular antioxidative defense and the induction of this putative defense system in human skin most likely reflects a cellular response to oxidative processes triggered by IRA. Frank et al. showed that IRA interferes with apoptotic pathways, namely, the mitochondrial apoptosis pathway [23], and reported that IRA signals via p53 [24]. The abrogating effect of IRA on apoptosis induced by lethal doses of extrinsic factor has recently been confirmed by another study [25].

Dosimetry of IRA

Human dermal fibroblasts withstand IRA doses up to at least 1,200 J/cm^2 [26], but the gene regulatory effects can already be observed at much lower, physiologically relevant dosage, i. e., 54 [8], 240 [4], or 360 J/cm^2 [15]. Increased levels of cytosolic and mitochondrial ROS were detected even after a treatment with 30 J/cm^2 [15].

IRA Chromophores

While the endogenous chromophores for IR are very likely to be part of the mtETC [27] and remain to be identified, several exogenous chromophores for IR are known. They are used for therapeutic purposes, e.g., in photodynamic therapy, and include palladium-bacteriopheophorbide and indocyanine green [28, 29].

Protection Against IRA

Up to now, photoprotection of human skin has focused against UVB and/or UVA radiation. The studies discussed above indicate, however, that protection against IRA radiation has to be included in order to achieve complete protection.

In this regard, antioxidants appear to be promising. Based on the fact that mtROS are functionally relevant in the IRA-induced effects, antioxidants that target the mitochondria theoretically represent potential IRA protective substances. Indeed, it has been demonstrated in vitro and in vivo that such specific antioxidants protect against detrimental IRA effects, e.g., IRA-induced MMP-1 expression [7].

In contrast, there are currently no chemical or physical UV filters available, which are suited for commercial suncare products and which have been shown to provide IRA protection.

The protective effect of textiles remains to be evaluated in terms of IRA protection. There is, however, data available showing that use of a black cloth at least partially provides IRA protection [18].

Finally, the topic of avoidance has to be discussed. Until now, there is no information source available that would provide a measure on the actual IRA load that would be comparable to the well-established UV index. Establishing a respective IRA index might be a considerable contribution.

Conclusion

As skin aging is a complex process, it is not surprising that ongoing research efforts uncover more and more environmental factors enfolding detrimental effects on the skin. Regarding natural sunlight or artificial sources of its components, there is a major doubt that whether in addition to UV, IRA protection also has to be taken into account.

IRA photoprotection requires specialized strategies with topical application of mitochondrially targeted antioxidants being a promising option.

References

1. Kochevar IE, Taylor CR, Krutmann J. Fundamentals of cutaneous photobiology and photoimmunology. In: Wolff K, Austen KF, Goldsmith LA, Katz SI, Gilchrest BA, Paller AS, Leffel DJ, editors. Fitzpatrick's dermatology in general medicine. New York: McGraw-Hill; 2007.
2. Cobarg CC. Physikalische Grundlagen der wassergefilterten Infrarot-A-Strahlung. In: Vaupel P, Krüger W, editors. Wärmetherapie mit wassergefilterter Infrarot-A-Strahlung. Stuttgart: Hippokrates Verlag; 1995. p. 19–28.
3. Hellige G, Becker G, Hahn G. Temperaturverteilung und Eindringtiefe wassergefilterter Infrarot-A-Strahlung. In: Vaupel P, Becker G, editors. Wärmetherapie mit wassergefilterter Infrarot-A-Strahlung. Stuttgart: Hippokrates Verlag; 1995. p. 63–80.
4. Schroeder P, Haendeler J, Krutmann J. The role of near infrared radiation in photoaging of the skin. Exp Gerontol. 2008;43:629–32.
5. Kligman LH. Intensification of ultraviolet-induced dermal damage by infrared radiation. Arch Dermatol Res. 1982;272:229–38.
6. Kim MS, Kim YK, Cho KH, Chung JH. Regulation of type I procollagen and MMP-1 expression after single or repeated exposure to infrared radiation in human skin. Mech Ageing Dev. 2006;127:875–82.
7. Schroeder P, Lademann J, Darvin ME, Stege H, Marks C, Bruhnke S, Krutmann J. Infrared radiation-induced matrix metalloproteinase in human skin: implications for protection. J Invest Dermatol. 2008;128:2491–7.
8. Brenneisen P, Sies H, Scharffetter-Kochanek K. Ultraviolet-B irradiation and matrix

metalloproteinases: from induction via signaling to initial events. Ann N Y Acad Sci. 2002;973:31–43.
9. Fisher GJ, Kang S, Varani J, Bata-Csorgo Z, Wan Y, Datta S, Voorhees JJ. Mechanisms of photoaging and chronological skin aging. Arch Dermatol. 2002;138:1462–70.
10. Fisher GJ, Wang ZQ, Datta SC, Varani J, Kang S, Voorhees JJ. Pathophysiology of premature skin aging induced by ultraviolet light. N Engl J Med. 1997;337:1419–28.
11. Buechner N, Schroeder P, Kunze K, Maresch T, Calles C, Krutmann J, Haendeler J. Changes of MMP-1 and collagen type alpha1 by UVA, UVB and IRA are differentially regulated by Trx-1. Exp Gerontol. 2008;43(7):633–637.
12. Schauen M, Hornig-Do HT, Schomberg S, Herrmann G, Wiesner RJ. Mitochondrial electron transport chain activity is not involved in ultraviolet A (UVA)-induced cell death. Free Radic Biol Med. 2007;42:499–509.
13. Berneburg M, Plettenberg H, Medve-Konig K, Pfahlberg A, Gers-Barlag H, Gefeller O, Krutmann J. Induction of the photoaging-associated mitochondrial common deletion in vivo in normal human skin. J Invest Dermatol. 2004;122:1277–83.
14. Cross JV, Templeton DJ. Regulation of signal transduction through protein cysteine oxidation. Antioxid Redox Signal. 2006;8:1819–27.
15. Schroeder P, Pohl C, Calles C, Marks C, Wild S, Krutmann J. Cellular response to infrared radiation involves retrograde mitochondrial signaling. Free Radic Biol Med. 2007;43:128–35.
16. Butow RA, Avadhani NG. Mitochondrial signaling: the retrograde response. Mol Cell. 2004;14:1–15.
17. Schieke SM, Schroeder P, Krutmann J. Cutaneous effects of infrared radiation: from clinical observations to molecular response mechanisms. Photodermatol Photoimmunol Photomed. 2003;19:228–34.
18. Kim MS, Kim YK, Cho KH, Chung JH. Infrared exposure induces an angiogenic switch in human skin that is partially mediated by heat. Br J Dermatol. 2006;155:1131–8.
19. Yaar M. Clinical and histological features of intrinsic versus extrinsic skin aging. In: Gilchrest BA, Krutmann J, editors. Skin aging. New York: Springer; 2006. p. 9–21.
20. Danno K, Sugie N. Effects of near-infrared radiation on the epidermal proliferation and cutaneous immune function in mice. Photodermatol Photoimmunol Photomed. 1996;12:233–6.
21. Danno K, Mori N, Toda K, Kobayashi T, Utani A. Near-infrared irradiation stimulates cutaneous wound repair: laboratory experiments on possible mechanisms. Photodermatol Photoimmunol Photomed. 2001;17:261–5.
22. Applegate LA, Scaletta C, Panizzon R, Frenk E, Hohlfeld P, Schwarzkopf S. Induction of the putative protective protein ferritin by infrared radiation: implications in skin repair. Int J Mol Med. 2000;5:247–51.
23. Frank S, Oliver L, Lebreton-De Coster C, Moreau C, Lecabellec MT, Michel L, Vallette FM, Dubertret L, Coulomb B. Infrared radiation affects the mitochondrial pathway of apoptosis in human fibroblasts. J Invest Dermatol. 2004;123:823–31.
24. Frank S, Menezes S, Lebreton-De Coster C, Oster M, Dubertret L, Coulomb B. Infrared radiation induces the p53 signaling pathway: role in infrared prevention of ultraviolet B toxicity. Exp Dermatol. 2006;15:130–7.
25. Jantschitsch C, Majewski S, Maeda A, Schwarz T, Schwarz A. Infrared radiation confers resistance to UV-induced apoptosis via reduction of DNA damage and upregulation of antiapoptotic proteins. J Invest Dermatol. 2009;129(5):1271–9, Epub 27 Nov 2008.
26. Schieke S, Stege H, Kurten V, Grether-Beck S, Sies H, Krutmann J. Infrared-A radiation-induced matrix metalloproteinase 1 expression is mediated through extracellular signal-regulated kinase 1/2 activation in human dermal fibroblasts. J Invest Dermatol. 2002;119:1323–9.
27. Karu T. Primary and secondary mechanisms of action of visible to near-IR radiation on cells. J Photochem Photobiol B. 1999;49:1–17.
28. Koudinova NV, Pinthus JH, Brandis A, Brenner O, Bendel P, Ramon J, Eshhar Z, Scherz A, Salomon Y. Photodynamic therapy with Pd-Bacteriopheophorbide (TOOKAD): successful in vivo treatment of human prostatic small cell carcinoma xenografts. Int J Cancer. 2003;104:782–9.
29. Tseng WW, Saxton RE, Deganutti A, Liu CD. Infrared laser activation of indocyanine green inhibits growth in human pancreatic cancer. Pancreas. 2003;27:e42–5.

Climate Change and Its Dermatologic Impact on Aging Skin

54

Young Hui, Haw-Yueh Thong, and Howard I. Maibach

Contents

Y. Hui (✉)
University of California, San Diego, CA, USA
e-mail: Young_Hui@comcast.net

H.-Y. Thong • H.I. Maibach
Department of Dermatology, University of California, San Francisco, CA, USA
e-mail: hythong@stanfordalumni.org; maibachh@derm.ucsf.edu

M.A. Farage et al. (eds.), *Textbook of Aging Skin*,
DOI 10.1007/978-3-662-47398-6_43

Abstract

According to the Fifth Assessment Report issued by the United Nations Intergovernmental Panel on Climate Change (IPCC) in 2014, the average combined land and ocean surface temperature across the globe rose approximately 0.85 °C over the period of time from 1880 to 2012. The 30-year period from 1983 to 2012 was the warmest in the last thirteen centuries. Current climate models predict that global surface temperatures will rise another 0.3–0.7 °C between 2016 and 2035, culminating in a total increase of 1.5–2 °C by the end of the twenty-first century (IPCC, Climate change 2014: synthesis report. In: Core Writing Team, Pachauri RK, Meyer LA (eds) Contribution of working groups I, II and III to the fifth assessment report of the Intergovernmental Panel on Climate Change. IPCC, Geneva, 151 pp, 2014). There is a scientific consensus that this change is due to anthropogenic causes, namely, the atmospheric accumulation of greenhouse gases: carbon dioxide (CO_2), methane (CH4), chlorofluorocarbons (CFCs), and nitrous oxide (NO). The impact of global warming on the environment will potentially be felt in multiple areas, including sea level rises, the spread of disease vectors, and altered severe weather patterns. These and other effects will challenge public health and medical care, among them the field of dermatology. Doctors and other healthcare professionals need to be aware of the risks. Efforts to meet these challenges remain a work in progress (Andersen, Int J Dermatol 51:656–661, 2012).

Introduction

Strong evidence links anthropogenic carbon emissions to global warming. As a greenhouse gas, carbon dioxide helps trap infrared radiation from the sun. The increasing atmospheric concentration of carbon dioxide comes from human activities such as burning fossil fuels and deforestation. This rising concentration of CO_2 drives the changes in global surface temperatures witnessed in modern times.

Some of the potential consequences of climate change are more severe weather, increased UV exposure, and changing habitats. For dermatology, climate change may lead to increased incidence of skin cancer due to rising temperatures and more UV exposure, more cases of skin infection due to extreme weather events, and altered disease vector patterns due to climate shifts.

The human skin, particularly the outer layer of the epidermis, is a barrier that protects the internal body, but by the same token it is the most exposed part of the body and bears the brunt of any changes in the external environment. The skin's protective ability is not unlimited, and problems arise when exposure to abnormal environmental stresses exceeds the skin's limits. Stress can come from natural factors or anthropic pollutants. Depending on the nature of these pollutants and the skin's integrity, the mode of penetration may vary. Alterations that disturb the skin's barrier function, in either the stratum corneum lipid metabolism or protein components of corneocytes, are implicated in the development of various skin diseases [1].

Factors that affect the skin include ultraviolet radiation (UVR), as well as major air pollutants such as polycyclic aromatic hydrocarbons (PAHs), volatile organic compounds (VOCs), nitrogen oxide (NOx), particulate matter (PM), and cigarette smoke. Air pollutants may interfere with the normal functioning of lipids, DNA, and proteins in the human skin via oxidative damage [2–8], leading to skin cancer, skin aging, and inflammatory or allergic conditions such as atopic dermatitis, psoriasis, and acne [9, 10]. Their effects are amplified when multiple factors work in conjunction, such as UVR interacting with air pollutants or the presence of several air pollutants at once. These combinations are major active components of pro-oxidant smog [5, 9, 11].

Climate Change and Ozone

The rapid pace of climate change has created an urgent need for a greater understanding of how climate and pollution impact human health. The effects of climate change on the skin, the organ that stands between human bodies and the outside environment, are of particular concern due to the sensitivity of cutaneous diseases to local environmental conditions [12]. Despite the importance of this angle, the number of studies that have investigated this link is limited [13]. From the available reports, several effects of climate change on the skin can be observed.

One climate effect that directly impacts the human skin is ultraviolet (UV) radiation. Lack of exposure to UV radiation has been linked to vitamin D deficiency, while excessive exposure is linked to increased incidence of carcinoma, nonmelanoma, malignant melanoma, and other types of skin cancer [14]. Rising temperatures may amplify UV exposure, increasing the effective UV dose by approximately 2 % per degree Celsius [15].

Other climate factors which impact skin cancer rates include aerosols and behavioral changes due to weather. Improvements in air quality, while welcome on their own merits, will as a side effect increase solar radiation and thus UV exposure. On the other hand, changes in cloud cover may decrease UV exposure in high northern latitudes [16]. But the greatest impact could come from behaviors associated with higher temperatures, such as recreational sports and outdoor activities. These may increase UV exposure significantly [17].

Another important factor in UV exposure is the atmospheric ozone layer. The ozone layer is part of the Earth's stratosphere, serving as a shield that protects the surface from UV radiation. During the twentieth century, this layer was damaged by ozone-depleting chemicals spread by pollution. Ozone depletion has been linked to increased surface UV radiation [18]. The Montreal Protocol has helped restore atmospheric ozone by taking steps to eliminate these pollutants [14]. But while international cooperation has yielded results, the ozone layer has yet to recover to pre-1970s levels, and climate change may yet imperil ozone recovery efforts [19]. Full restoration of the ozone layer is not projected to occur until the end of the twenty-first century or later if other factors such as geoengineering come into play [16]. By impairing the ozone layer's ability to absorb UV radiation, ozone depletion leads to an increase in melanoma and nonmelanoma skin cancer [20].

Solar UV and Skin Exposure

Efforts have been made over the years to raise public awareness of the effects of UV radiation. Concerns have focused on depletion of the ozone layer, as well as social trends such as sunbathing and tanning parlors, but climate change may also affect levels of UV exposure. In addition, rising temperatures may increase the carcinogenic effectiveness of UV radiation. As early as the mid-twentieth century, studies on mice showed that elevated temperatures enhanced UV-induced carcinogenesis. Studies of humans suggest similar effects, with each °C rise corresponding to an estimated equivalent impact of +2 % in effective UV dose [15].

Such effects will be intertwined with those of changing social patterns, from growth in outdoor leisure activities to countervailing trends to remain indoors. Humans have always had a large say in the matter of their own health. But even and especially in an age of anthropogenic climate change, human behavior may prove the greatest determinant of outcomes. Behavior associated with climate change, as Diffey proposed for the UK population, may have a larger impact on UV exposure and consequent skin cancer than ozone depletion [21,17]. In other regions, climate change may compel people to limit their outdoor activities, as predicted by Maloney and Forbes in Australia, increasing the number of days unsuitable for labor or strenuous exercise [22].

Air Pollution and the Skin

Increasing air pollution has major effects upon the human skin [23]. Along with ultraviolet radiation (UVR), the skin is exposed to environmental air pollutants such as polycyclic aromatic hydrocarbons (PAHs), volatile organic compounds (VOCs), nitrogen oxide (NOx), particulate matter (PM), ozone (O_3), and other substances such as those found in cigarette smoke. Although the human skin acts as a biological shield against pro-oxidative chemical and physical air pollutants, prolonged or repetitive exposure to high levels of pollutants may have profound negative consequences for dermatological health.

Air pollutants may severely interfere with the normal functions of lipids, DNA, and proteins in the human skin via oxidative damage [2–8]. Skin exposure to air pollutants has been linked to inflammatory or allergic skin conditions such as atopic dermatitis, eczema, psoriasis, and acne, as well as skin aging and most seriously skin cancer [9, 10]. A slight benefit is that some air pollutants (e.g., O_3, nitrogen dioxide, and sulfur dioxide) and the scattering of particulate matter (clouds and soot) in the troposphere reduce exposure to short-wavelength UVR, leading to significant reductions in UV irradiance in polluted urban areas, though this does not balance the other negative effects.

Polycyclic Aromatic Hydrocarbons

Polycyclic aromatic hydrocarbons (PAHs) are widespread organic pollutants [24–26]. The main source of atmospheric PAH benzo[a]pyrene is residual wood burning [27]. Other sources include diesel exhaust and smoke from combusting organic material (e.g., cigarettes). PAHs may bind to the surface of particulate matter (PM) from combustion or PM suspended in urban areas [28]. Via conversion into quinines, redox-cycling chemicals that produce reactive oxygen species [29], PAHs can coat the surface of PM with toxic pollutants.

PAHs have been implicated in the development of skin cancer, as well as inflammatory and allergic disorders. Activated PAHs produced epoxides and diols, which bind to DNA and initiate cutaneous carcinogenesis [30–32, 9]. The carcinogenic action of benzo[a]pyrene is enhanced by interaction with UVA [30, 33]. PAHs are believed to be irritants and allergens, with reactive oxygen species generated from oxygenated PAHs serving as exacerbating factors. PAHs may also contribute to inflammation by activating aryl hydrocarbon receptor-mediated transcription. This inflammation from PAHs may play a role in disorders such as asthma, rhinitis, and dermatitis [34].

PAHs may also play a role in skin pigmentation (tanning) in the absence of UV radiation and skin aging [35]. PAHs can cause tanning in mice by inducing melanocyte proliferation [36]. Skin aging and oxidative stress may result from long-term exposure of skin to PAHs bound to PM, via transepidermal absorption or through hair follicles [37]. Via ambient particles such as soot, PAHs bound to their surface may reach melanocytes or affect cutaneous cells directly [36].

Acneiform eruptions may result from exposure to certain halogenated aromatic hydrocarbons [9]. A potent polyhalogenated aromatic hydrocarbon is 2,3,7,8-tetrachlorodibenzo-p-dioxin (TCDD), which is a product of waste incineration, metal production, wood burning, fossil fuel use, and other types of combustion. Exposure to chloracnegens, halogenated aromatic hydrocarbons, can result in chloracne, a systemic toxic disease characterized by acneiform skin lesions such as comedones and cysts on the face and neck, as well as fatigue, liver dysfunction, neuropathy, and arthritis [38].

Extreme Weather and Climatological Disasters

The frequency of events is rising over time (Lancet Commission on Health and Climate Change). Previous estimates of the toll of climate change may need to be updated, and earlier World Health Organization and IPCC predictions may be inaccurate in the face of new data. Recent years have witnessed many natural disasters, from the Indian Ocean tsunami, to Hurricane Katrina, to heat waves in India and Pakistan. While individually their links to climate change are difficult to confirm, collectively they illustrate the impending challenges society and health professionals face from changing weather patterns.

The spread of natural disasters has changed the literature on skin infections. After Hurricane Katrina in 2005, the Centers for Disease Control and Prevention (CDC) reported on wound infections with methicillin-resistant *Staphylococcus aureus* (MRSA), *Vibrio vulnificus*, and *Vibrio parahaemolyticus* among local residents and tinea corporis, folliculitis, miliaria, and arthropod bites among rescue personnel [39]. Rhoads also reported on cases of *V. vulnificus* causing problems, including septic shock, for victims [40].

The Indian Ocean tsunami of December 2004 provided the literature with new cases of dermatologic conditions associated with massive flooding. Multidrug-resistant diseases, polymicrobial infections, and other unusual pathogens, such as *Burkholderia pseudomallei*, *Cladophialophora bantiana*, and *Mycobacterium* abscesses, were found following exposure to freshwater contaminated by flooding [41–43]. In another report, Hiransuthikul et al. found that 515 (66.3 %) tsunami survivors with traumatic wounds were diagnosed with skin and soft-tissue infections, with the most common isolated being *Aeromonas* species [44]. In May 2016, Indian heat waves saw temperatures rise up to 47 °C, causing 2200 deaths. Subsequent waves of heat caused further fatalities. Such challenges may become more familiar to dermatologists if these weather trends continue.

Global Warming and Infectious Skin Diseases

Environmental changes wrought by global warming may alter disease patterns and dynamics [45, 46]. Along with globalization and demographic shifts, climate change will be one of the largest factors influencing future pathogen outbreaks.

Warming climates will drive diseases previously confined to lowlands and the tropics into higher elevations and northern latitudes [47, 48]. Treating outbreaks of such diseases, potentially resistant to antimicrobials, will be a test for health professionals including dermatologists. Patterns of drought and rainfall will change, causing associated problems. For example, a lack of water for personal hygiene may lead to infectious skin diseases such as scabies and impetigo [49]. Drought may also increase algae blooms, which can lead to symptoms such as rashes, lesions, blisters, vomiting, headaches, and diarrhea in those who come into contact with high levels of microcystins in water due to increased cyanobacteria levels [50].

Various authors have explored the potential effects of climate change upon vector-borne diseases such as malaria, dengue, leishmaniasis, and tick-borne pathogens [51–54]. An example of the relationships between vector-borne diseases and climate variation is the report from Cardenas et al. on the impact of the El Niño Southern Oscillation on incidences of leishmaniasis in Columbia from 1985 to 2002, which show an increase during El Niño and decrease during La Niña phases [55]. However, the existing literature may not present sufficient evidence to support a causal relationship between global warming and increased incidence for all vector-borne diseases; despite the potential impact of climate change, Randolph finds that it has not been proven to be the cause of increases in tick-borne diseases [56]. As is often the case, more research is necessary, and knowledge will have a major impact on the ability to cope with climate change [57].

Adapting to climate change will be an imposing task that demands a new arsenal of tools. Dermatology will need to advance to meet the challenge of treating the largest human organ, in knowledge and practice. The skin, like the gastrointestinal tract, is heavily colonized. Recently, dermatologists have learned to appreciate the complexity of this biota and improve their investigations [58]. Such new molecular identification tools, still in their infancy, should provide fertile insights into the role of microbes in health and disease. The implications as they relate to climate control call for detailed investigation.

Conclusions

According to the Intergovernmental Panel on Climate Change, globally averaged combined land and ocean surface temperature rose approximately 0.85 °C from 1880 to 2012. From 1983 to 2012 the northern hemisphere witnessed the warmest 30-year period since the seventh century CE. From 2016 to 2035, climate models predict another rise of 0.3–0.7 °C, culminating in a rise of 1.5–2 °C by the end of the twenty-first century. The scientific evidence for anthropogenic causes is stronger than ever, via the atmospheric accumulation of greenhouse gases such as carbon dioxide, methane, chlorofluorocarbons (CFCs), and nitrous oxide. Global warming's potential impact on the environment may include sea level rise due to melting ice caps as well as an increase in severe weather [59]. These effects and others may pose challenges for skin disease and healthcare in the future [60]. Awareness of these issues is spreading among medical professionals and dermatologists, with progress building [61–65].

Both humans and the natural world will face serious challenges over the course of the coming century, with climate patterns shifting and millions of species facing potential extinction [66–68]. Science and medicine must step up to the challenge [69]. In order to care for patients and do their part to prepare society for the demands imposed by climate change, dermatologists will need every tool at their disposal.

References

1. Valacchi G, Sticozzi C, Pecorelli A, Cervellati F, Cervellati C, Maioli E. Cutaneous responses to environmental stressors. Ann N Y Acad Sci. 2012;1271(1): 75–81.
2. Adelman R, Saul RL, Ames BN. Oxidative damage to DNA: relation to species metabolic rate and life span. Proc Natl Acad Sci. 1988;85(8):2706–8.

3. Ames BN, Gold LS, Willett WC. The causes and prevention of cancer. Proc Natl Acad Sci. 1995; 92(12):5258–65.
4. Halliwell B, Gutteridge JMC. Protection against oxidants in biological systems: the superoxide theory of oxygen toxicity. In: Free radicals in biology and medicine. Oxford: Clarendon Press; 1989. p. 86.
5. Kampa M, Castanas E. Human health effects of air pollution. Environ Pollut. 2008;151(2):362–7.
6. Menzel DB. The toxicity of air pollution in experimental animals and humans: the role of oxidative stress. Toxicol Lett. 1994;72(1):269–77.
7. Stadtman ER. Protein oxidation and aging. Science. 1992;257(5074):1220–4.
8. Valko M, Rhodes CJ, Moncol J, Izakovic MM, Mazur M. Free radicals, metals and antioxidants in oxidative stress-induced cancer. Chem Biol Interact. 2006; 160(1):1–40.
9. Baudouin C, Charveron M, Tarroux R, Gall Y. Environmental pollutants and skin cancer. Cell Biol Toxicol. 2002;18(5):341–8.
10. Kohen R. Skin antioxidants: their role in aging and in oxidative stress – new approaches for their evaluation. Biomed Pharmacother. 1999;53(4):181–92.
11. Katsouyanni K. Ambient air pollution and health. Br Med Bull. 2003;68(1):143–56.
12. Balato N, Ayala F, Megna M, Balato A, Patruno C. Climate change and skin. Giornale italiano di dermatologia e venereologia: organo ufficiale, Societa italiana di dermatologia e sifilografia. 2013;148(1): 135–46.
13. Balato N, Megna M, Ayala F, Balato A, Napolitano M, Patruno C. Effects of climate changes on skin diseases Expert Rev Anti Infect Ther. 2014;12(2):171–81.
14. Lucas RM, Norval M, Neale RE, Young AR, de Gruijl FR, Takizawa Y, van der Leun JC. The consequences for human health of stratospheric ozone depletion in association with other environmental factors. Photochem Photobiol Sci. 2015;14(1):53–87.
15. van der Leun JC, Piacentini RD, de Gruijl FR. Climate change and human skin cancer. Photochem Photobiol Sci. 2008;7:730–3.
16. Bais AF, McKenzie RL, Bernhard G, Aucamp PJ, Ilyas M, Madronich S, Tourpali K. Ozone depletion and climate change: impacts on UV radiation. Photochem Photobiol Sci. 2015;14(1):19–52.
17. Diffey B. Climate change, ozone depletion and the impact on ultraviolet exposure of human skin. Phys Med Biol. 2004;49:R1.
18. Lemus-Deschamps L, Makin JK. Fifty years of changes in UV Index and implications for skin cancer in Australia. Int J Biometeorol. 2012;56(4):727–35.
19. Makin J. Implications of climate change for skin cancer prevention in Australia. Health Promot J Austr. 2011;22(4):39–41.
20. Fabbrocini G, Triassi M, Mauriello MC, Torre G, Annunziata MC, Vita VD, … Monfrecola G. Epidemiology of skin cancer: role of some environmental factors. Cancers. 2010;,2(4):1980–9.
21. Diffey BL. Solar ultraviolet radiation effects on biological systems. Phys Med Biol. 1991;36(3):299.
22. Maloney SK, Forbes CF. What effect will a few degrees of climate change have on human heat balance? Implications for human activity. Int J Biometeorol. 2011;55:147–60.
23. Drakaki D, Dessinioti C, Antoniou CV. Air pollution and the skin. Front Environ Sci. 2014. doi:10.3389/fenvs.2014.00011.
24. Samanta SK, Singh OV, Jain RK. Polycyclic aromatic hydrocarbons: environmental pollution and bioremediation. TRENDS Biotechnol. 2002;20(6):243–8.
25. Epstein JH, Ormsby A, Adams RM. Occupational skin cancer. In: Adams RM, editor. Occupational skin disease. 3rd ed. WB Saunders; 1999. p. 142–64.
26 English JS, Dawe RS, Ferguson J. Environmental effects and skin disease. Brit Med Bull. 2003;68 (1):129–42.
27. Burke KE, Wei H. Synergistic damage by UVA radiation and pollutants. Toxicol Ind Health. 2009;25(4–5): 219–24.
28. Menichini E. Urban air pollution by polycyclic aromatic hydrocarbons: levels and sources of variability. Sci Total Environ. 1992;116(1):109–35.
29. Penning TM, Burczynski ME, Hung CF, McCoull KD, Palackal NT, Tsuruda LS. Dihydrodiol dehydrogenases and polycyclic aromatic hydrocarbon activation: generation of reactive and redox active o-quinones. Chem Res Toxicol. 1999;12(1):1–8.
30. Kelfkens G, de Gruijl FR, van der Leun JC. Tumorigenesis by short-wave ultraviolet A: papillomas versus squamous cell carcinomas. Carcinogenesis. 1991;12(8):1377–82.
31. Fernandez AO, Banerji AP. Inhibition of benzopyrene induced forestomach tumors by field bean protease inhibitors. Carcinogenesis. 1995;16:1843–6.
32. Hecht SS, McIntee EJ, Cheng G, Shi Y, Villalta PW, Wang M. New aspects of DNA adduct formation by the carcinogens crotonaldehyde and acetaldehyde. In: Biological reactive intermediates VI. Springer US; 2001. p. 63–71.
33. Wei X, Decker JM, Wang S, Hui H, Kappes JC, Wu X, … Shaw GM. Antibody neutralization and escape by HIV-1. Nature. 2003;422(6929):307–12.
34. Tauchi M, Hida A, Negishi T, Katsuoka F, Noda S, Mimura J, Hosoya T, Yanaka A, Aburatani H, Fujii-Kuriyama Y, Motohashi H, Yamamoto M. Constitutive expression of aryl hydrocarbon receptor in keratinocytes causes inflammatory skin lesions. Mol Cell Biol. 2005;25(21):9360–8.
35. Tschachler E, Morizot F. Ethnic differences in skin aging. In: Skin aging. Berlin/Heidelberg: Springer; 2006. p. 23–31.
36. Vierkötter A, Schikowski T, Ranft U, Sugiri D, Matsui M, Krämer U, Krutmann J. Airborne particle exposure and extrinsic skin aging. J Invest Dermatol. 2010;130(12):2719–26.
37. Lademann IJ, Schaefer H, Otberg N, Teichmann A, Blume-Peytavi U, Sterry W. Penetration von

Mikropartikeln in die menschliche Haut. Der Hautarzt. 2004;55(12):1117–9.
38. Tindall JP. Chloracne and chloracnegens. J Am Acad Dermatol. 1985;13(4):539–58.
39. CDC. Infectious disease and dermatologic conditions in evacuees and rescue workers after Hurricane Katrina – multiple states. MMWR Morb Mortal Wkly Rep. 2005;54:961–4.
40. Rhoads J. Post-Hurricane Katrina challenge: *Vibrio vulnificus*. J Am Acad Nurse Pract. 2006;18(7): 318324.
41. Garbino J, Garzoni C. Unusual pathogens and multidrug-resistant bacteria in tsunami survivors. Clin Infect Dis. 2006;42(6):889.
42. Nieminen T, Vaara M. Burkholderia pseudomallei infections in Finnish tourists injured by the December 2004 tsunami in Thailand. Euro Surveill. 2005;10(3): E050303.
43. Petrini B, Farnebo F, Hedblad MA, Appelgren P. Concomitant late soft tissue infections by *Cladophialophora bantiana* and *Mycobacterium* abscesses following tsunami injuries. Med Mycol. 2006;44(2):189–92.
44. Hiransuthikul N, Tantisiriwat W, Lertutsahakul K, Vibhagool A, Boonma P. Skin and soft-tissue infections among tsunami survivors in southern Thailand. Clin Infect Dis. 2005;41(10):e93.
45. Wang X, Towers S, Panchanathan S, Chowell G. A population based study of seasonality of skin and soft tissue infections: implications for the spread of CA-MRSA. PLoS One. 2013;8(4):e60872.
46. Yildirim A, Erdem H, Kilic S, Yetiser S, Pahsa A. Effect of climate on the bacteriology of chronic suppurative otitis media. Ann Otol Rhinol Laryngol. 2005;114(8):652–5.
47. Ogden NH, Maarouf A, Barker IK, Bigras-Poulin M, Lindsay LR, Morshed MG, O'callaghan CJ, Ramay F, Waltner-Toews D, Charron DF. Climate change and the potential for range expansion of the Lyme disease vector Ixodes scapularis in Canada. Int J Parasitol. 2006;36(1):63–70.
48. Pounds JA, Bustamante MR, Coloma LA, Consuegra JA, Fogden MPL, Foster PN, La Marca E, Masters KL, Merino-Viteri A, Puschendorf R, et al. Widespread amphibian extinctions from epidemic disease driven by global warming. Nature. 2006;439(7073):161–7.
49. Thacker S, Music S, Pollard R, Berggren G, Boulos C, Nagy T, Brutus M, Pamphile M, Ferdinand R, Joseph V. Acute water shortage and health problems in Haiti. Lancet. 1980;315(8166):471–3.
50. Walker SR, Lund JC, Schumacher DG, Brakhage PA, McManus BC, Miller JD, Augustine MM, Carney JJ, Holland RS, Hoagland KD, Holz JC. Nebraska experience. In: Cyanobacterial harmful algal blooms: state of the science and research needs. New York: Springer; 2008. p. 139–152.
51. Bormane A, Lucenko I, Duks A, Mavtchoutko V, Ranka R, Salmina K, Baumanis V. Vectors of tick-borne diseases and epidemiological situation in Latvia in 1993–2002. Int J Med Microbiol Suppl. 2004;293:3647.
52. Kołodyński J, Malinowska A. Impacts of climate change on infectious diseases. Wiad Parazytol. 2001;48(1):29–37.
53. Kovats RS, Campbell-Lendrum DH, McMichel AJ, Woodward A, Cox JSH. Early effects of climate change: do they include changes in vector-borne disease? Philos Trans R Soc Lond B Biol Sci. 2001; 356(1411):1057.
54. Sutherst RW. Global change and human vulnerability to vector-borne diseases. Clin Microbiol Rev. 2004;17 (1):136–73.
55. Cárdenas R, Sandoval CM, Rodríguez-Morales AJ, Franco-Paredes C. Impact of climate variability in the occurrence of leishmaniasis in northeastern Colombia. Am J Trop Med Hyg. 2006;75(2):273–7.
56. Randolph SE. Evidence that climate change has caused 'emergence' of tick-borne diseases in Europe? Int J Med Microbiol Suppl. 2004;293:5–15.
57. Jessup CM, Balbus JM, Christian C, Haque E, et al. Climate change, human health, and biomedical research: analysis of the national institutes of health research portfolio. Environ Health Perspect. 2013; 121(4):399–404.
58. Scharschmidt TC, List K, Grice EA, Szabo R, NISC Comparative Sequencing Program, Renaud G, Lee CCR, Wolfsberg TG, Bugge TH, Segre JA. Matriptase-deficient mice exhibit ichthyotic skin with a selective shift in skin microbiota. J Invest Dermatol. 2009;129(10):2435–42.
59. IPCC. Climate change 2014: synthesis report. In: Core Writing Team, Pachauri RK, Meyer LA, editors. Contribution of working groups I, II and III to the fifth assessment report of the Intergovernmental Panel on Climate Change. Geneva: IPCC; 2014. 151 pp.
60. Patz JA, Frumkin H, Galloway T, Vimont DJ, Haines A. Climate change: challenges and opportunities for global health. JAMA. 2014;312(15):1565–80. doi:10.1001/jama.2014.13186.
61. Andersen LK. Global climate change and its dermatological diseases. Int J Dermatol. 2011;50(5):601–3.
62. Epstein PR. Climate change and human health. N Engl J Med. 2005;353(14):1433–6.
63. Grover S. Global warming and its impact on skin disorders. Indian J Dermatol Venereol Leprol. 2009;75(4):337.
64. Llamas-Velasco M, García-Díez A. Climatic change and skin: diagnostic and therapeutic challenges. Actas Dermosifiliogr (English Edition). 2010;101(5): 401–10.
65. Thong HY, Maibach HI. Global warming and its dermatologic implications. Int J Dermatol. 2008;47 (5):522–4.
66. Thomas CD, Cameron A, Green RE, Bakkenes M, Beaumont LJ, Collingham YC, Erasmus BFN, De Siqueira MF, Grainger A, Hannah L, et al. Extinction risk from climate change. Nature. 2004;427(6970): 145–8.

67. Hall L, Hagens W. The oak processionary caterpillar and public health: the Dutch approach. Chem Hazards Poisons Rep. 2014;2014(24):80–3.
68. Bauchner H, Fontanarosa PB. Climate change: a continuing threat to the health of the world's population. JAMA. 2014. doi:10.1001/jama.2014.13094.
69. Roulin, A. Melanin-based colour polymorphism responding to climate change. Glob Chang Biol. 2014;20(11):3344–50.

Skin Photodamage Prevention: State of the Art and New Prospects

55

Denize Ainbinder and Elka Touitou

Contents

Abstract

Human skin aging is caused by a number of factors. UV radiation is responsible for up to 90 % of visible skin aging. However, the effects of the sunlight on skin include not only dryness, loss of elasticity, wrinkles, discoloration, and changes in texture but also increased incidence in various precancerous conditions and skin malignancies. This chapter will go through state-of-the-art skin photodamage preventions.

Introduction

Human skin aging is caused by a number of factors. One of the most important and influential factors is the exposure of the skin to UV radiation, which leads to the damage of the skin's structure and integrity. UV radiation is responsible for up to 90 % of visible skin aging. However, the effects of the sunlight on the skin include not only dryness, loss of elasticity, wrinkles, discoloration, and changes in texture but also increased incidence in various precancerous conditions and skin malignancies.

The prominent dermatologist Prof. Albert Kligman once said, "Wear a sunscreen every day of your life, or live as shady a life as possible." In this chapter the state of the art in skin photodamage prevention by the use of sunscreens

D. Ainbinder (✉) • E. Touitou
Institute of Drug Research, School of Pharmacy, The Hebrew University of Jerusalem, Jerusalem, Israel
e-mail: Denizekib@gmail.com; touitou@mail.huji.ac.il

M.A. Farage et al. (eds.), *Textbook of Aging Skin*,
DOI 10.1007/978-3-662-47398-6_44

and the latest technologies in this field will be reviewed.

The Mechanism of Skin Photodamage

In order to understand the need for preventing skin damage, which is a result of exposure to UV radiation, one must first explore the underlying mechanisms of UV-induced skin damage.

UV radiation is composed of three main wavelength ranges: UVC (100–290 nm) which is largely blocked by the ozone layer and has little impact on skin; UVB (290–320 nm) which penetrates mostly into the dermis and is responsible for both severe acute sunburn damage and keratinocyte mutations; and UVA (320–400 nm), which for years was considered to be irrelevant to skin damage but is now held responsible for most of the skin damage in the dermis causing skin aging and prolonged pigmentation [1] (Fig. 1).

The molecular mechanisms underlying the UV-induced human skin aging process have been extensively investigated in the last two decades. It is now clear that UV irradiation invokes a complex cascade of molecular responses which eventually alter the structure of dermal extracellular matrix causing wrinkle formation, loss of skin elasticity, increased skin fragility, and impaired barrier function of the skin.

Upon exposure to UV, as a primary event, the light interacts with a suitable chromophore, which could be either an exogenous agent or an endogenous compound, including porphyrins, flavins, DNA bases, amino acids, and their derivatives such as urocanic acid. As a result, the chromophore may be damaged directly or may act as a photosensitizer, leading to the generation of reactive oxygen species (ROS) in the presence of oxygen. Increased ROS concentration initiates a number of signal transduction pathways through activation of cell surface receptors, including receptors for epidermal growth factor (EGF), interleukin -1 (IL-1), insulin, keratinocyte growth factor (KGF), and tumor necrosis factor-α (TNF-α). Activated cell surface receptors stimulate intracellular kinases (p38, *c*-Jun) leading to upregulation of the expression and functional activation of the nuclear transcription factor, AP-1 (composed of Jun and Fos proteins). AP-1 activation blocks the effect of transforming growth factor-β (TGF-β) resulting in reduced collagen gene

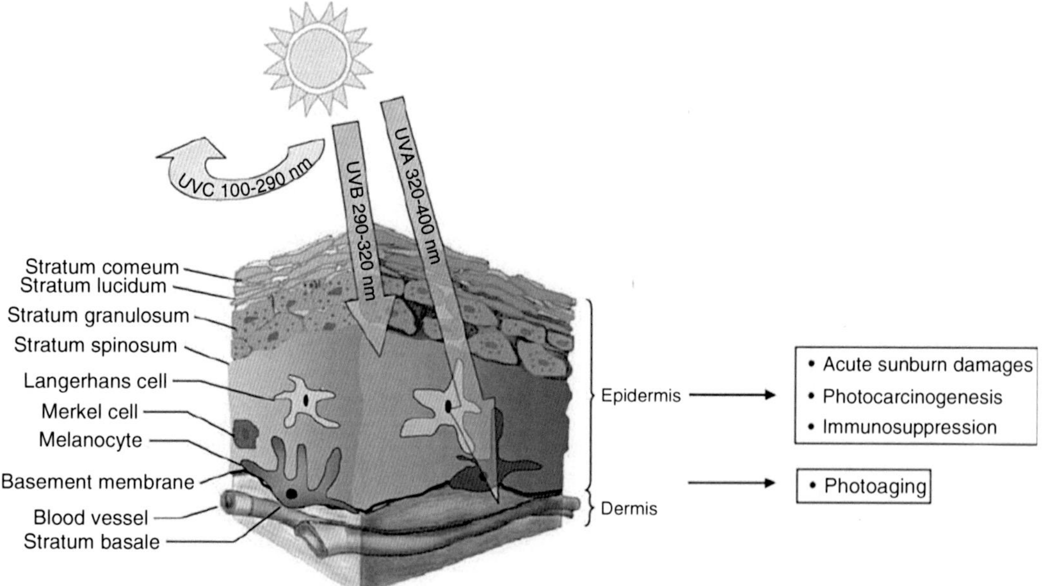

Fig. 1 The effects of UV radiation on the skin

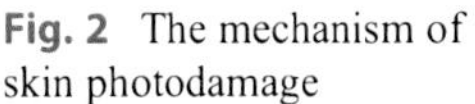

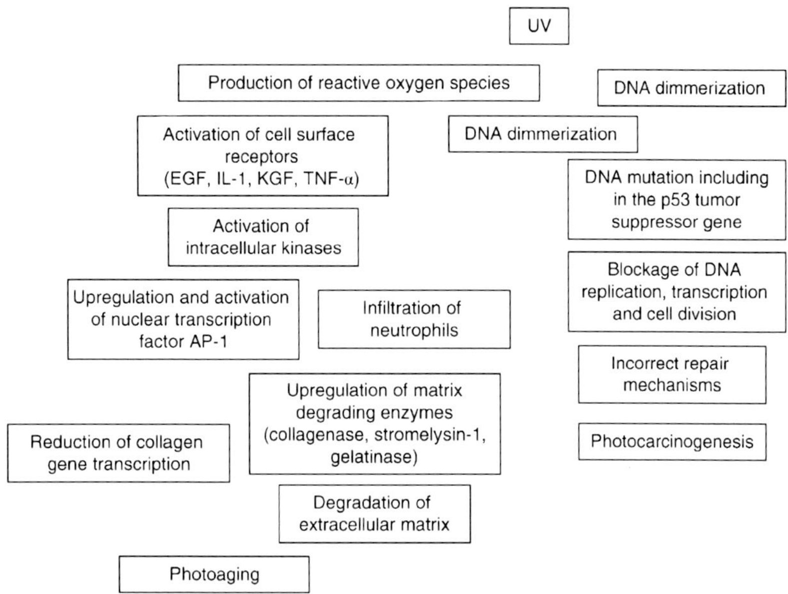

Fig. 2 The mechanism of skin photodamage

transcription. Moreover, activation of AP-1 stimulates transcription of genes for matrix-degrading enzymes such as matrix metalloproteinase 1 (MMP-1 - collagenase), MMP-3 (stromelysin 1), and MMP-9 (92-kd gelatinase). These MMPs together can degrade collagenous and noncollagenous molecules in the extracellular matrix, thereby impairing the structural integrity of the skin. Following repeated exposure to UV irradiation, MMP-mediated collagen damage accumulates and contributes excessively to the phenotype of photoaged human skin [2, 3].

Ultraviolet irradiation also activates the transcription factor NF-Kb which positively regulates gene transcription of 92 k-gelatinase and proinflammatory cytokine genes, including IL-1β, TNF-α, IL-6, and IL-8. UV-induced cytokine gene products act to trigger AP-1 and NF-Kb, thereby amplifying the UV damage. Additionally, stimulation of the expression of the proinflammatory cytokine genes IL-1 and TNF-α is partly responsible for the recruitment of inflammatory cells from the circulation into the skin, notably neutrophils. Infiltration of neutrophils into the UV-damaged skin is accompanied by an increase in MMP-8 (neutrophil collagenase) protein levels, which in turn contribute to dermal degradation in addition to the AP-1 regulated MMPs.

Collagen degradation as a result of exposure to UV irradiation is generally incomplete, leading to the accumulation of partially degraded collagen fragments in the dermis. These large collagen fragments reduce the structural integrity of the skin and negatively regulate new collagen synthesis [3]. The result is formation of sagging skin and wrinkles. Besides the deteriorating effect of UV on skin elasticity, it also decreases the number of Langerhans cells present in the dermis and induces photodermatoses such as lupus erythematosus and polymorphous light eruption (PMLE) [4] (Fig. 2).

UV radiation is also responsible for cellular damage resulting in precancerous and cancer skin conditions. UVA toxicity to the cells depends mainly on indirect mechanisms through generation of ROS, which in turn cause the destruction of DNA and other cellular components. UVB light causes DNA damage by the formation of dimmers between adjacent pyrimidine bases on the same strand, generating the cyclobutyl pyrimidine dimmer (CPD) and pyrimidine (6-4) pyrimidinone photoproducts. This dimerization of pyrimidines leads to the distortion of DNA structure, accounting for about 95 % of all DNA lesions. The result is a blockage of DNA replication, cell division, and DNA transcription needed for messenger RNA synthesis. Moreover, as a consequence of repeated exposure to UV light, the number of DNA distortions increases so that the normal repair mechanisms of the cells are unable to correct them. Thus, continuous exposure to UV irradiation generates DNA mutations in the epidermal cells, which cause the development of skin cancer [5, 6].

Recent studies have shown that one of the targets of UV-induced DNA damage is the p53 tumor suppressor gene. Fifty percent of epidermal tumors exhibit DNA mutations at bipyrimidine sites in the p53 gene. Under normal circumstances, p53 is activated as a transcription factor in response to accumulation of DNA alterations. It can then cause cell cycle arrest or apoptosis of the damaged cell. When p53 gene undergoes mutation, the ability to discharge these cells is lost and a tendency toward the selection of highly damaged cells with p53 gene mutations occurs. Eventually, this increasing mass of mutated cells progresses into cancer [5, 6].

Photodamage Prevention

Sunscreens as the Gold Standard for Photodamage Prevention

Although it is currently impossible to prevent or reverse the genetic processes responsible for intrinsic skin aging and cutaneous cancers, skin changes associated with extrinsic aging and photocarcinogenesis are largely avoidable. Protection from UV rays decreases photoaging and reduces the risks of age-related skin diseases. The "gold standard" for skin protection from UV radiation is topical application of sunscreens.

The history of sunscreens began around 1928, when the first commercial sunscreen became available as a formulation of benzyl salicylate and benzyl cinnamate. Later, in the 1940s, the FDA (Food and Drug Administration) began to regulate sunscreen formulations. From the 1980s until now, the development of sunscreens has focused on finding broader-spectrum sunscreens with higher stability and minimal toxicity [4].

In 1993, a sunscreen active ingredient was defined by the FDA as: "an active ingredient that absorbs at least 85 % of radiation in the UV range at wavelengths from 290 to 320 nm (UVB), but may or may not transmit radiation at wavelengths longer than 320 nm" [7]. Later, due to the acknowledgment of the harmful effects of UVA radiation on the skin, this definition was modified to include sunscreen active ingredients whose absorption maximum is within the UVA range of 320–400 nm [8].

So what should the requirements of an optimal modern sunscreen be?

- It should absorb and/or reflect UV radiation and provide absorption over a wide spectrum of UV. Protection of the skin against both UVA and UVB is crucial in order to prevent sun-induced damage, including erythema and sunburn, photoaging, the possibility of carcinogenesis, and immunosuppression.
- It must be stable on the human skin despite exposure to heat and sunlight. Decomposition of the UV-filter decreases the expected UV-protective capacity. Moreover, photodegradation could result in toxic by-products.
- It must remain on the skin surface without penetrating into and through the skin, exposing the whole body to the active agent.
- It should also be water resistant, colorless, and suited for formulation in cosmetic preparations [9].

Currently, no sunscreen, which encompasses all the above requirements, exists. Therefore, to enable better coverage of both UVA and UVB wavelength range, sunscreen formulations usually combine a number of UV-filters, selecting those with favorable stability and safety properties.

The number of approved sunscreen active ingredients and their concentrations in use differs considerably around the world. In Europe, 27 active sunscreen agents are permitted, while only 16 UV-filters are approved for use by the FDA. This discrepancy could be explained by the fact that sunscreen agents are treated like drugs in the USA but as cosmeceutical products in Europe. The sunscreens can be subdivided according to whether they are organic or inorganic agents, as well as by the range of their UV absorption and by their chemical structure. Table 1 lists all the organic FDA-approved sunscreens and their properties.

Unlike organic sunscreens which absorb UV radiation, inorganic sunscreens mainly reflect/scatter UV, but depending on the particle size may also absorb UV. Titanium dioxide (TiO_2) and zinc oxide (ZnO), the most commonly used inorganic sunscreens, are regarded as photostable, nontoxic, and nonallergenic. They are used at a concentration of up to 25 % to protect the skin in the UVA and UVB region, with maximum absorption at around 400 nm, depending on particle size [4, 9–11]. Until recently, metal oxides have been promoted as safer alternatives to organic sunscreens, based on the belief that they do not penetrate beyond the stratum corneum of the skin thus negating the possibility of systemic absorption. Effective protection by inorganic sunscreens requires thick coating of the systems on the skin. As a consequence of large particle size, topical application of systems containing metal oxides resulted in an opaque whitish layer on the skin. Reduction of the size of metal oxide particles to nanoscale was developed in order to improve their undesirable cosmetic appearance. The advantages and drawbacks of this technology will be discussed later in this chapter.

Innovations in Sunscreen Delivery

In spite of all the benefits, the use of sunscreens is not without drawbacks. One of the major concerns, besides skin reactions, is the possibility of skin penetration and as a result of that toxic systemic effects. This alarm should be considered heavily, especially in view of the fact that sunscreen active ingredients are available in a range of different cosmetic products such as shampoos, conditioners, skin moisturizers, and lipsticks and may be applied over large skin areas repeatedly as in the case of beach-type application, or may be applied on a daily basis to the face and other more restricted areas of skin when using nonbeach products.

It has been suggested that the organic UV sunscreens could be absorbed by the skin because of their lipophilic nature. Their hydrophobic character ensures their ability to resist removal by water and tends to reduce diffusion of the active into the viable epidermis and deeper skin layers. However, as for other lipophilic substances applied topically it should be anticipated that sunscreens will eventually enter the systemic circulation. Watkinson and his group predicted skin absorption of various sunscreens 12 h following application and found that some of the sunscreens might undergo systemic absorption which could be significant if the sunscreen is to be applied over large surface areas for prolonged periods of time [12]. Thus, there is clearly a need for new strategies to ensure sunscreen safety by minimizing its penetration into viable tissues.

Another issue associated with the use of sunscreens is their photostability. Upon exposure to UV radiation some of the organic sunscreens can undergo structural transformation or degradation, while the filter loses its absorption capacity. Other, even worse scenarios could include interactions of the excited molecules with other ingredients of the sunscreen product or skin components leading to the production of undesirable toxic reactive species [9].

Several methods for increasing the efficiency, preventing penetration into the skin, and increasing the photostability of sunscreen agents have been developed and tested over the last few years: encapsulation of sunscreens has been applied to both decrease their possible skin absorption and increase their photostability; sunscreen particle size reduction to nanoscale has been used to increase the appearance of metal oxide sunscreen formulations and improve the efficacy of existing sunscreen actives; new combinations of sunscreens with antioxidants were developed to prevent photoaging and to decrease the incidence of photocarcinogenesis.

Encapsulation of UV Absorbers in Particles

Various methods based on particulate systems have been used to increase the efficiency and stability of the sunscreens and to decrease

Table 1 Currently Food and Drug administration (FDA) approved organic sunscreens and their properties [4, 10, 11]

Chemical group	Sunscreen active	Synonyms and abbreviations	Maximum approved concentration (%)	Absorption (nm)	Comments
Aminobenzoates					
	PABA	4-aminobenzoic acid	15	283–289	Nearly insoluble, highly substantive, photoallergic reactions in 4 % of the population, skin discoloration
	Pamidate O	2-Ethylhexyl 4-dimethylaminobenzoate, octydimethyl PABA	8	290–310	Possible mutagenicity and carcinogenicity
	Meradimate	Methyl-2-aminobenzoate, methyl anthranilate	5	286, 335	
Cinnamates					
	Octinoxate	Octyl methoxycinnamate, ethylhexyl methoxycinnamate, Parsol MCX, OMC	7.5	311	Most commonly used, low skin irritancy potential
	Cinoxate	2-ethoxyethyl p-methoxycinnamate	3	289	
Salicylates					
	Octisalate	2-ethylhexyl salicylate, octyl salicylate	5	307	Weak UVB absorbers, highly substantive, safe and photostable
	Homosalate	Homomethyl salicylate, HMS	15	306	
	Trolamine salicylate	Triethanolamine salicylate	12	260–355	
Benzophenones					
	Oxybenzone	Benzopehnone-3, BENZ-3, Eusolex 4360	6	288, 325	Highest percents of contact dermatitis, low photostability. Presence in blood and urine after topical application (up to 10 %)
	Sulisobenzone	2-Hydroxy-4-methoxybenzophenone-5-sulfonic acid, Benzophenone-4, BENZ-4	10	288, 366	
	Dioxybenzone	Benzophenone-8	3	288, 352	
Dibenzoylmethane					
	Avobenzone	1-(4-tert-butylphenyl)-3 (4-methoxyphenyl) propane-1,3-dione, butyl methoxy dibenzomethane, BMDBM, Parsol 1789, Eusolex 9020	3	360	Broad UV absorption spectrum (up to 380 nm), highly photounstable, combined with other sunscreens for increased photostability
Miscellaneous					
	Octocrylene	2-cyano-3,3-diphenyl acrylic acid, 2-ethyl hexyl ester, Eusolex OCR	10	303	
	Ensulizole	2-phenylbenzimidazole-5-sulfonic acid, PBSA, Eusolex 232, Parsol HS	4	310	

(*continued*)

Table 1 (continued)

Chemical group	Sunscreen active	Synonyms and abbreviations	Maximum approved concentration (%)	Absorption (nm)	Comments
	Ecamsule	Terephthalylidene dicamphor sulfonic acid, TDSA, Mexoryl SX	10	345	Broad UV absorption spectrum (290–390 nm), photostable, low systemic absorption

skin penetration of the existing sunscreen actives.

In 2003, Sol-Gel Technologies Ltd published their new technology for reducing skin absorption, improving safety profile, and increasing the Sun Protection Factor (SPF) of the sunscreen. They have used the sol-gel silica glasses to function as an entrapping matrix. In this system, the sunscreen, which is usually a lipophilic compound, composes the core that is entrapped within a silica shell. The sol-gel sunscreen containing systems are then incorporated into a suitable cosmetic vehicle, enabling high UV protection together with reduced penetration into the skin. The investigators have tested systems containing combinations of OMC, benzophenone-3, butyl methoxy dibenzomethane (BMDBM), and methyl benzylidene camphor to achieve systems with a broad UV absorption spectrum. OMC encapsulated into sol-gel microcapsules showed a close to zero percent leaching profile, while other OMC systems like OMC absorbed to cosmetic grade silica showed a leaching profile of more than 50 %. Skin absorption of free OMC formulation was about three times higher than that of encapsulated OMC system. The sol-gel technology enabled encapsulation of high levels of sunscreen actives resulting in high SPF values. Reduction of the contact between the actives and the human tissue resulted in decreased skin absorption of the sunscreen and thus decreased possibility of toxic effects [13].

Wissing and Müller have proposed a novel sunscreen system based on tocopherol acetate incorporated into solid lipid nanoparticles (SLNs). SLNs have been shown to form a protective and occlusive film on the skin. Previous studies have shown that tocopherol acetate has a UV-blocking efficacy in the UVB region. Moreover, it reduces the skin damage caused by UV radiation and increases both cell proliferation and moisture content of the skin. SLNs with tocopherol acetate were prepared and tested against placebo SLNs, tocopherol acetate emulsion, and placebo emulsion. Investigation of the UV-blocking capacity showed that tocopherol SLNs were at least twice as effective as the reference emulsions. Placebo SLNs showed even greater blocking efficiency than tocopherol acetate emulsions. Thus incorporation of tocopherol acetate into SLNs prevented chemical degradation of the active and increased its UV-blocking capacity [14].

Scalia et al. prepared 4-methylbenzyldiene camphor (4-MBC) solid lipid microparticles in order to prevent systemic absorption of the sunscreen after topical application. Systemic absorption of 4-MBC has raised safety issues based on in vitro and animal studies showing that 4-MBC has estrogenic activity; moreover, permeation of the sunscreen leaves the skin surface unprotected. Microparticles containing various lipids (tristearin, cetyl palmitate, glyceryl behenate) and surfactants (hydrogenated phosphatidylcholine, polysorbate 60) were prepared and tested by the researchers. The results of the study showed that the use of microparticles resulted in a decreased release rate of the sunscreen compared to its dissolution rate. In vivo tape-stripped human skin penetration experiments showed that emulsion containing the 4-MBC microparticles decreased, by 33 %, the amount of the sunscreen penetrating into the stratum corneum when compared with the use of emulsion alone [15].

Another technique for improved efficacy of UV-filters, the SunSpheres, was introduced by adding nonabsorbing material to sunscreens. The nonabsorbing material, developed by Rohm and Haas, is a styrene/acrylates copolymer manufactured by emulsion polymerization. The polymer does not absorb UV light and is designed to scatter the UV light on the skin surface thereby increasing its probability of coming into contact with the sunscreen active. SunSpheres are filled with water, which migrates out of the spheres when the system is applied on the skin, leaving microscopic hollow beads. As UV radiation hits these hollow beads, it is scattered on the skin surface traveling sideways, resulting in the increased probability of the sunscreen reacting with UV radiation. The SunSpheres technology is claimed to increase the SPF of sunscreen by 50–70 %, by thus enabling the use of a decreased amount of active in the formulation without compromising its photoprotective effect [16].

Sunscreen Particle Size Reduction to Nanoscale

In order to overcome the whitening effect associated with topical application of metal oxides for sun protection, micronized powders of both titanium dioxide and zinc oxide were produced with an average particle size of 10–50 nm. Decreasing the particle size into the micronized or ultrafine form has considerably improved cosmetic acceptability by reducing the scattering of visible light and making the new formulations transparent; it is important to take into consideration that it has also shifted the protection toward shorter wavelengths (Fig. 3).

An additional disadvantage of micronized sunscreens was found in their tendency to agglomerate because of the electrostatic effects, and thus losing their dispersive properties and becoming opaque once again. A solution to this problem was found by coating the microparticles with dimethicone or silica to keep them in dispersion [4].

Although until recently metal oxides have been promoted as safe sunscreens, in vitro studies showed that titanium dioxide nanoparticles can induce free radical formation in the presence of UV. Incubation of titanium dioxide solutions with pyrimidine and purine bases, together with DNA and RNA, under artificial mercury light exposure produced damage to DNA and RNA through free radical generation [17].

The possibility of systemic toxicity of metal oxides and their reduced particle size have raised concerns about the safety of their use. In a recent review by Nohynek et al., a comprehensive assessment of metal oxide nanoparticle skin absorption and safety was carried out. Most of the studies evaluating skin absorption of metal oxide nanoparticles have shown no or negligible penetration beyond the stratum corneum layer of the skin. However, several works have shown the presence of nanoparticles in the hair follicles.

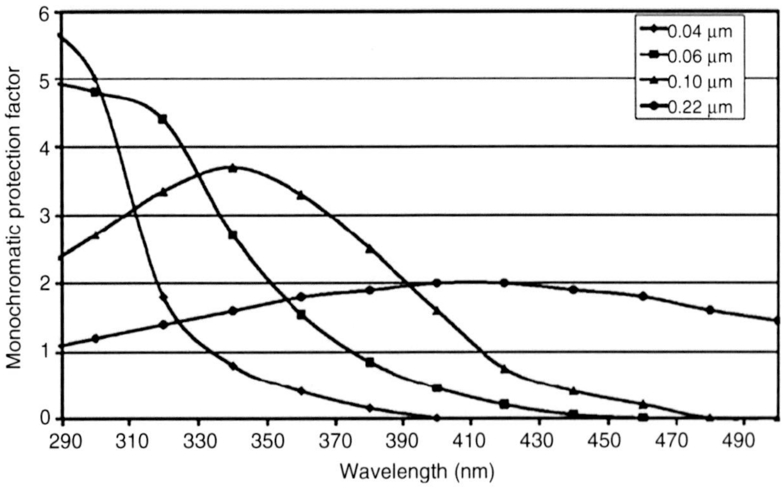

Fig. 3 Influence of primary particle size on absorption spectra of water in oil emulsions containing 4 % titanium dioxide (Forestier [9], with permission)

Based on the current knowledge and on the results of various works, Nohynek and his group concluded that there is no evidence that metal oxide nanoparticles penetrate into or through human skin [18].

While accessing the skin absorption of metal oxide nanoparticles, it is important to bear in mind that skin absorption of actives can be influenced by system composition. Bennat and his colleagues evaluated the skin absorption of microfine titanium dioxide from oily and aqueous dispersions. They found that titanium dioxide penetrated deeper into the skin from an oily dispersion with octyl palmitate than from an aqueous one. Further, the penetration depth of microfine titanium dioxide from an oil-in-water emulsion containing carboxymethylcellulose sodium to stabilize the micropigment was tested by tape-stripping technique. The results showed that after nine strips titanium dioxide was no longer detectable. Since liposomal vesicles have the possibility to stabilize titanium dioxide formulation and prevent agglomeration of the micropigments, micropigments incorporated into liposomes were also investigated. The amount of titanium dioxide in the strips following application of liposomal formulation was higher compared to the emulsion, with penetration depth comparable to that from oily dispersion (up to 15 strips) [19].

Despite these encouraging reports on low skin absorption of metal oxide nanoparticles, concerns regarding the safety of their use in sunscreen products have been raised. Just recently, a number of environmental and consumer-oriented organizations have urged the FDA and other regulatory authorities worldwide to reevaluate thoroughly the safety of sunscreens containing nanoparticles. In 2007, the Scientific Committee on Consumer Products (SCCP) published an opinion on the safety of nanomaterials in cosmetic products [20]. The committee concluded that based on the current knowledge there is no conclusive evidence for skin penetration into viable tissues by 20 nm or larger nanoparticles, which are used in metal oxide sunscreens. However, they emphasize that the current validated methods are unable to detect small quantities of nanoparticles in the skin and there is an urgent need for new methodologies to assess skin absorption. Further, it is important to note that the studies for the evaluation of metal oxide nanoparticle skin absorption were performed on healthy skin and no information is present for skin with impaired barrier function as in the case of atopic or sunburn skin. The 2007 SCCP opinion concludes that there is a need to review the safety of the insoluble nanomaterials (i.e.,; metal oxides) used in sunscreen formulations.

Reduction of particle size to nanoscale is applied not only for inorganic sunscreens. In the endless search for a better UV-filter, a system enabling the combination of both organic and inorganic sunscreen properties was developed [21]. In this system, Methylene-bis-benzotriazolyl tetramethylbutylphenol (MBBT or Tinosorb™), a UV-filter, is presented as microfine organic particles (<200 nm) in aqueous dispersion. The result is a broad-spectrum sunscreen, which absorbs, scatters, and reflects UV, by combining the properties of both organic and inorganic filters. As for micronized titanium dioxide and zinc oxide, the physical properties of these organic particles are also dependent on particle size. At a particle size of 160 nm, 85 % of the UV radiation is absorbed and the other 15 % is scattered forward or backward. As a result of this triple action, these organic UV particles are highly efficient, possess photostability, and have low systemic absorption due to the large molecular size.

Increasing the Photostability of Existent Sunscreens

Octinoxate (OMC) is one of the most popular sunscreens in the world. Upon exposure to UV light it can undergo trans to cis isomerization, resulting in a decreased photoprotective efficiency. Encapsulation of a sunscreen agent in nanoparticles was shown to result in increased photostability. Vettor and his group have evaluated the effect of OMC encapsulation in poly (D,L-lactide) (PLA) nanoparticles on the sunscreen photostability. They also hypothesized that encapsulation of the sunscreen in PLA nanoparticles (which are crystalline and highly hydrophobic) will decrease OMC leakage from the nanoparticles and reduce its contact with the skin limiting photoallergic contact reactions. Photostability studies of nanoencapsulated OMC showed a significant reduction in photoisomerization degree with a 36–70 % stabilizing effect dependent on OMC concentration in the system. The results supported the hypothesis that OMC is protected in nanoparticles and that PLA nanoencapsulation could be used to prevent photoisomerization. An in vitro filter efficacy experiment demonstrated that no SPF could be associated to the nanoparticles whereas the obtained protective effect by OMC was not altered by encapsulation of the sunscreen in nanoparticles [22].

Another popular sunscreen which suffers from the disadvantage of insufficient photostability is avobenzone. Since its discovery, avobenzone has been one of the most used sunscreens because of its ability to filter UV radiation in the UVA I range. However, it was found to be highly unstable and degrading within 1 h following exposure to UV. Yang et al. investigated the possibility to increase the stability and prevent absorption, through the skin, of avobenzone by complexing it with hydroxypropyl-β-cyclodextrin (HPCD). HPCD is a chemically modified cyclodextrin, which enables formation of inclusion complexes with active substances by modifying their physicochemical properties. As a result of its large molecular weight and its hydrophilic nature, cyclodextrin molecules do not readily penetrate into the skin. Complexations of avobenzone with 10 %, 20 %, and 30 % of HPCD were tested for skin absorption and photostability. The results of the experiments showed that at all concentrations tested HPCD caused an increase in skin absorption of avobenzone after 24 h; however, skin absorption of the system containing 30 % HPCD was the lowest. This decrease in skin absorption of avobenzone in spite of the increased HPCD concentration was explained by a shift in the theoretical equilibrium of the complexation reaction toward the complexed form, thereby diminishing the amount of free avobenzone available for skin absorption. The 30 % HPCD-avobenzone system was the most photostable following UVA exposure at various regimens and also enabled better photoprotective efficiency in vivo, evidenced by lower levels of sunburn cell and skin edema induction [23].

New Sunscreens: A Dual Approach

There is accumulated evidence of a causal relationship between UV light-induced intracellular damage and skin malignancies. Therefore, to increase skin protection against photocarcinogenesis, one should also aim to prevent or reverse the intracellular UV damage.

To protect against ROS generated by sunlight the skin uses natural antioxidants which undergo depletion process. Some of them cannot be synthesized in the human body and must be supplied through diet. Thus, it would be advantageous to increase the existing skin reservoir of antioxidants in order to improve its defense against UV-induced damage. Topical application would achieve this purpose with the advantage of targeting the chemicals directly at the skin, and thus decreasing the amount of antioxidants needed for effective protection, as compared to oral supplementation [24]. However, topical delivery of antioxidants to the skin has several obstacles: antioxidants must penetrate into the skin and moreover into the cells in order to reach their site of action [25]; they are highly unstable compounds which make them difficult to formulate; and many of them are deeply colored adding to the complexity of producing an acceptable formulation for cosmetic use.

Previous works have shown that incorporation of free radical scavengers into topical applications may be beneficial in delaying the aging process of the skin by preventing photodamage [26]. Classical antioxidants include vitamin C, vitamin E, and beta-carotene, whose photoprotective effects against UVB and UVA are well characterized.

A dual approach, based on concomitant use of both sunscreen and antioxidant, was investigated for enhanced skin photodamage prevention.

Damiani and his colleagues have designed UV absorbers with a built-in antioxidant function [27]. A new sunscreen based on OMC derivative with an attached nitroxide moiety, OC-NO (4-(1-oxyl-2,2,5,5-tetramethyl-1,5-dihydro-1H-pyrr ol-3-yl) methoxycinnamic acid ethylhexyl ester) was synthesized and studied. For broad UV spectr um coverage, OC-NO was combined with two commonly used UVA filters: BMDBM (butylmethoxy dibenzoylmethane) and DHHB (diethylamino hydr oxybenzoyl hexylbenzoate). The combination OC-NO + BMDBM lost absorbance in the entire UVA spectrum after UVA exposure, due to lack of p hotostability of BMDBM. On the other hand, the combination with DHHB was photostable without significant modifications in the spectral shape or the molecular extinction. Evaluation of nitrosamine antioxidant activity in OC-NO complex showed that at a concentration of 40 Mm OC-NO totally inhibited UVA-induced lipid peroxidation in phosp hatidylcholine multilamellar liposomes. The antioxidant activity of OC-NO was comparable to the effect of other commonly used antioxidants: vitamin E and BHT. A reduction of cellular membrane lipid peroxidation was observed with OC-NO and OC-NO + DHHB complexes. The conclusion of this study was that OC-NO + DHHB is a promising photostable broad-spectrum UV-filter combination which is also able to reduce UV-induced free radical damage.

The development of OC-NO complex presents an interesting approach for skin photoprotection. For efficient photoprotection the sunscreen needs to reside on the skin surface, while the target site of the antioxidant is in the viable epidermis, deeper in the skin. Another dual approach for efficient skin photoprotection was proposed based on a new sunscreen that does not permeate the skin and a carrier that enables enhanced skin and intracellular penetration of free radical scavengers (Fig. 4) [28].

The concept of skin Non-Permeating SUNscreens (NPSUN) was to immobilize UV-absorbing moieties in the structure of a jojoba backbone. Jojoba oil is an ester of polycarbonous fatty acids and alcohols (C18-22), widely used as an ingredient in cosmetic and pharmaceutical formulations. It was chosen as the backbone structure because of its high molecular weight (600–700) and high lipophilicity: the two characteristics which ensure accumulation of the molecule in the outermost upper layers of the skin where the sunscreen is aimed to act. Due to its structure two to four UV-sunscreen actives could be linked to the backbone via ester bonds, and thus enabling the design of UVA, UVB, or UVA-UVB systems (Fig. 5).

Methoxycinnamate (MC) was chosen as a model sunscreen active. NPSUNs containing two or four MC units were synthesized and characterized by ^{1}H-NMR, UV-spectroscopy, FTIR, mass spectroscopy, and elemental analysis. The UV absorption spectrum of the MC-NPSUNs was similar to OMC and the modified sunscreen could be easily formulated in standard cosmeceutical and pharmaceutical topical products. In vitro permeation experiments showed absolutely no permeation of MC-NPSUN across the skin in 24 h (Fig. 6). Moreover, MC-NPSUNs were found to exhibit high substantivity on the skin and thereby decrease the need for repetitive applications.

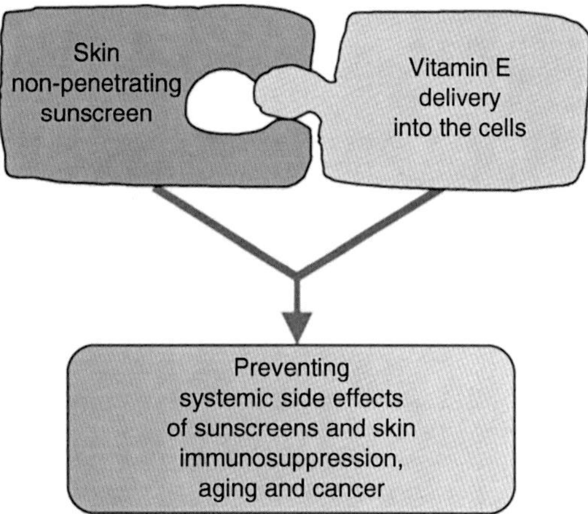

Fig. 4 The dual approach for efficient protection from UV induced skin damage

Results obtained so far point toward a high applicability of NPSUNs given the significant advantage of skin nonpenetrability. The nonpenetrating characteristics of NPSUNs are a major improvement over the currently used sunscreens and can be seen as meeting one of the most important safety requirements of sunscreens.

Another arm of this dual approach is an antioxidant delivered into the deep skin, intracellularly by an efficient carrier. Vitamin E (α-tocopherol) was chosen since it is the major lipid phase antioxidant of the body and has a number of activities. It acts as a free radical scavenger, enables photoprotection due to UV-light absorption with a maximum at 295 nm and suppression of the risk of skin cancer, and inhibits the activity of cyclooxygenase (COX). Vitamin E has a lipophilic nature that makes it attractive for topical application. The effectiveness of topically

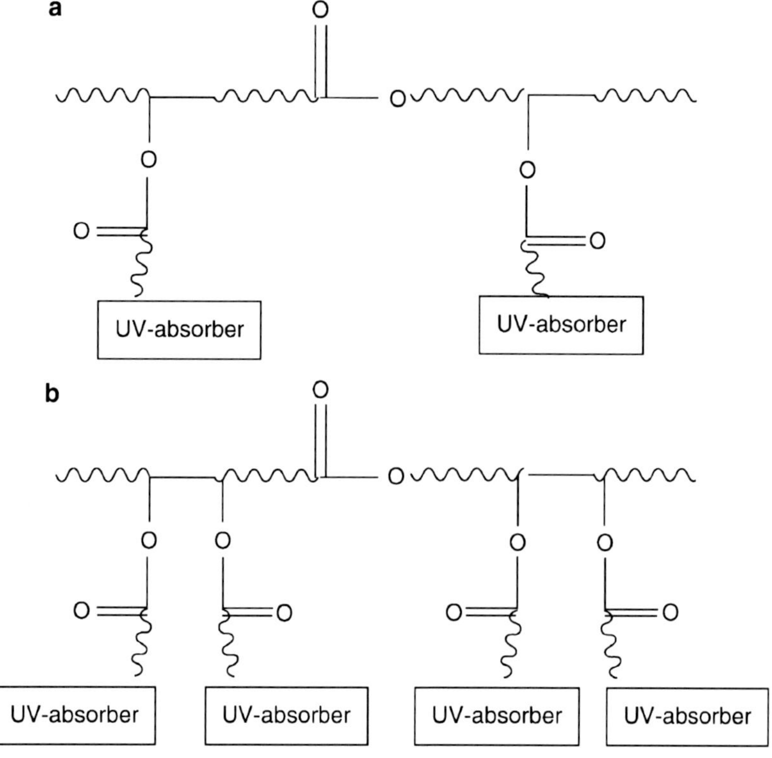

Fig. 5 Structure of NPSUN derivatives with two (**a**) and four (**b**) UV absorbing units (Reprinted with permission from Venditi et al. [27])

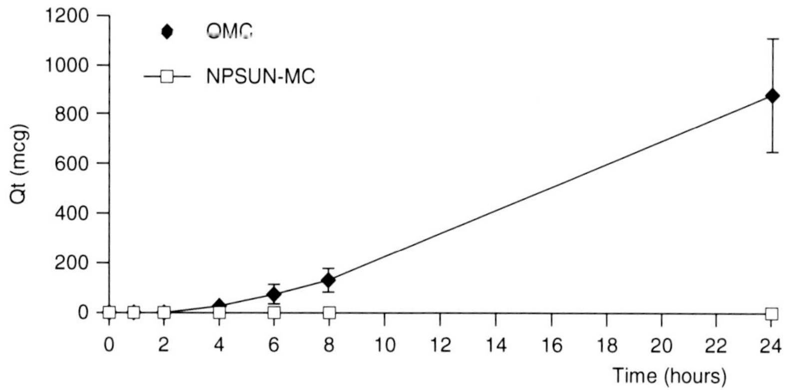

Fig. 6 Permeation profile of OMC and NPSUN-MC across nude mice skin after application of 10 mg of the sunscreens on skin surface (Reprinted with permission from Venditi et al. [27])

applied vitamin E was tested in various studies. It was shown to protect rabbit skin against UV-induced erythema and mice against UV-induced skin lipid peroxidation, photoaging, immunosuppression, and photocarcinogenesis. Studies on the mechanism of photocarcinogenesis prevention by vitamin E have revealed that it inhibits pyrimidine dimmer formation in mouse skin cells. Vitamin E has also shown a protective effect against melanogenesis by inhibition of melanin formation in human melanoma cells.

As with other nonenzymatic antioxidants, vitamin E's primary site of action is within the cells, especially in the cellular membrane. Thus, intracellular uptake of tocopherol is necessary for optimal photoprotection effect and prevention of malignant processes [25]. Tocopherol carrier systems were tested for skin penetration and intracellular delivery. Skin penetration experiments showed that 55 % of the applied α-tocopherol accumulated in full thickness skin after 24 h. Quantification of the intracellular delivery of α-tocopherol has showed an efficient intracellular delivery of the vitamin.

These results demonstrate that the proposed carriers are able to efficiently entrap α-tocopherol and deliver it into the skin as well as through cellular membranes into the cells, pointing toward a high potential of this delivery system to enhance skin photoprotective effects of the antioxidant.

A new skin nonpermeating sunscreen based on OMC combined with jojoba oil backbone was synthesized and a dual approach for increased skin photoprotection which encompasses the use of skin nonpenetrating sunscreens together with intracellularly delivered antioxidants from carriers is proposed. In the proposed approach, prevention of systemic absorption of sunscreens will diminish the possible toxic side effects of these compounds, while powerful delivery of α-tocopherol to the site of its action, in the deep dermal layers and inside the cells, will increase its efficiency in inhibiting UV-induced carcinogenic processes.

Conclusion

A good clinical strategy would be the use of nonpenetrating sunscreens to prevent UV radiation damages upon exposure to sunlight followed by application of α-tocopherol carrier systems after short- or long-term solar radiation in order to prevent the UV-induced cellular damage.

Cross-References

- ▶ Climate Change and Its Dermatologic Impact on Aging Skin
- ▶ Cutaneous Responses to Tropospheric Ozone exposure
- ▶ In Vitro Method to Visualize UV-induced Reactive Oxygen Species in a Skin Equivalent Model

References

1. Farage M, et al. Intrinsic and extrinsic factors in skin ageing: a review. Int J Cosmet Sci. 2008;30:87–95.
2. Pillai S, et al. Ultraviolet radiation and skin aging: roles of reactive oxygen species, inflammation and protease activation, and strategies for prevention of inflammation-induced matrix degradation – a review. Int J Cosmet Sci. 2005;27:17–34.
3. Fisher G, et al. Mechanisms of photoaging and chronological skin aging. Arch Dermatol. 2002;138:1462–70.
4. Palm M, O'Donoghue M. Update on photoprotection. Dermatol Ther. 2007;20:360–76.
5. Marrot L, Meunier JR. Skin DNA photodamage and its biological consequences. J Am Acad Dermatol. 2008;58:s139–48.
6. Matsumura Y, Ananthaswamy H. Toxic effects of ultraviolet radiation on the skin. Toxicol Appl Pharmacol. 2004;195:298–308.
7. Federal Register. Sunscreen drug products over-the-counter human use; tentative final monograph; proposed rule. Fed Regist. 1993;58:28194–320.
8. Federal Register. Sunscreen drug products over-the-counter human use; amendment to the tentative final monograph. Fed Regist. 1996;61:48645.
9. Forestier S. Rationale for sunscreen development. J Am Acad Dermatol. 2008;58:S133–8.
10. Gonzalez S, et al. The latest on skin photoprotection. Clin Dermatol. 2008;26:614–26.
11. Nash JF. Human safety and efficacy of ultraviolet filters and sunscreen products. Dermatol Clin. 2006;24:35–51.
12. Watkinson AC. Prediction of the percutaneous penetration of ultra-violet filters used in sunscreen formulations. Int J Cosmet Sci. 1992;14:265–75.
13. Lapidot N, et al. Advanced sunscreens: UV absorbers encapsulated in sol-gel glass microcapsules. J Sol-Gel Sci Technol. 2003;26:67–72.
14. Wissing SA, Muller RH. A novel sunscreen system based on tocopherol acetate incorporated into solid lipid nanoparticles. Int J Cosmet Sci. 2001;23:233–43.
15. Scalia S, et al. Influence of solid lipid microparticle carriers on skin penetration of the sunscreen agent, 4-methylbenzylidene camphor. J Pharm Pharmacol. 2007;59:1621–7.
16. Jones CV. Use of SunSpheres™ technology to increase the effective SPF and UVA absorbance of personal care products containing UV actives. 2005. www.rohmhaas.com/assets/attachments/business/pcare/formulations/SunSpheres_%20PCIA-Bangkok.pdf
17. Serpone N, et al. Deleterious effects of sunscreen titanium dioxide nanoparticles on DNA: efforts to limit DNA damage by particle surface modification. Proc SPIE. 2001;4258:86–98.
18. Nohynek GJ, et al. Grey Goo on the skin? Nanotechnology, cosmetic and sunscreen safety. Crit Rev Toxicol. 2007;37:251–77.
19. Bennat C, Müller-Goymann CC. Skin penetration and stabilization of formulations containing microfine

titanium dioxide as physical UV filter. Int J Cosmet Sci. 2000;22:271–83.
20. SCCP (Scientific Committee on Consumer Products). Safety of nanomaterials in cosmetic products. SCCP/1147/07; 2007. p. 1–63.
21. Muller S, et al. Microfine organic particles – a new type of "physical" sunscreen actives. Presented at the 63th annual meeting of the American Academy of Dermatology, New Orleans; 2005. doi:10.1016/j.jaad.2004.10.171.
22. Vettor M, et al. Poly(D, L-lactide) nanoencapsulation to reduce photoinactivation of a sunscreen agent. Int J Cosmet Sci. 2008;20:219–27.
23. Yang J, et al. Influence of hydroxypropyl-β-cyclodextrin on transdermal penetration and photostability of avobenzone. Eur J Pharm Biopharm. 2008;69:605–12.
24. Pinnell SR. Cutaneous photodamage, oxidative stress, and topical antioxidant protection. J Am Acad Dermatol. 2003;48:1–19.
25. McVean M, Liebler DC. Prevention of DNA photodamage by vitamin E compounds and sunscreens: roles of ultraviolet absorbance and cellular uptake. Mol Carcinog. 1999;24:169–76.
26. Dreher F, Maibach H. Protective effects of topical antioxidants in humans. In: Thiele J, Elsner P, editors. Oxidants and antioxidants in cutaneous biology, vol. 29. Basel: Karger; 2001. p. 157–64.
27. Venditti E, et al. In vitro photostability and photoprotection studies of a novel 'multi-active' UV-absorber. Free Radic Biol Med. 2008;45:345–54.
28. Touitou E, Godin B. Skin nonpenetrating sunscreens for cosmetic and pharmaceutical formulations. Clin Dermatol. 2008;26:375–9.

Environmental and Genetic Factors in Facial Aging in Twins

56

David J. Rowe and Bahman Guyuron

Contents

Abstract

The causes of facial aging can be divided into two broad categories: intrinsic and extrinsic aging. Intrinsic aging is that which occurs as a response to the deterioration of tissues over time. Intrinsic changes of the face include those to the skin, subcutaneous tissue, dermal appendages, facial musculature, as well as the facial skeleton. The process of extrinsic facial aging is, theoretically, a distinct entity. Typically, extrinsic aging is induced by external factors, such as UV radiation, causing progressive damage at both the molecular and cellular levels. Unlike intrinsic aging, most extrinsic factors exert their effect at the skin level only. The chapter also discuss aging and possible risk factors in twin investigational studies.

Introduction

The etiologic factors contributing to facial senescence have been investigated for decades if not centuries. In essence, the causes of facial aging can be divided into two broad categories: intrinsic and extrinsic [1]. Intrinsic aging is that which occurs as a response to the deterioration of tissues over time [2]. This process is ubiquitous throughout all organs and tissues, although the methods of "deterioration" may vary from system to system. Intrinsic changes of the face include those to the skin, subcutaneous tissue, dermal appendages, facial musculature, as well as the facial skeleton.

D.J. Rowe (✉)
University Hospitals, Case Western Reserve University, Cleveland, OH, USA
e-mail: David.Rowe1@uhhospitals.org

B. Guyuron
Department of Plastic Surgery, University Hospitals of Cleveland, Case Western Reserve University, Cleveland, OH, USA
e-mail: bguyuron@aol.com

M.A. Farage et al. (eds.), *Textbook of Aging Skin*,
DOI 10.1007/978-3-662-47398-6_45

The process of extrinsic facial aging is, theoretically, a distinct entity. Typically, extrinsic aging is induced by external factors, such as UV radiation, causing progressive damage at both the molecular and cellular levels. Unlike intrinsic aging, most extrinsic factors exert their effect at the skin level only.

Discriminating between the levels of involvement of both aging processes, extrinsic and intrinsic, is problematic. As both processes continually occur, the ability for the body to resist change depends on the amount of cumulative damage of each individual process. Furthermore, there may be a dynamic interplay between extrinsic and intrinsic modalities that lead to variable amounts of aging depending on the levels of each and the ability of the body to repair or resist these. For example, a minor intrinsic defect, such as that in a DNA repair mechanism, may cause slightly accelerated aging from an intrinsic standpoint; however, it could cause an uncommonly aberrant response for extrinsic factors.

A preponderance of information exists on the presence and types of extrinsic factors that may influence aging; however, the intrinsic causes are likely as important or more important on skin and facial aging. Multiple genetic disorders exist that corroborate the fact that premature aging can be genetic. Diseases with defects in DNA repair mechanisms, such as xeroderma pigmentosum, Werner syndrome, and Cockayne syndrome, all show accelerated aging [3]. Hutchinson-Gilford progeria syndrome is caused by a defect in lamin A, a protein used in the cell nuclear envelope, leading to abnormal morphology in the cell nucleus. This too leads to an accelerated aging phenotype. Theoretically, variable penetrance, or a less severe genetic aberration, may either increase or decrease the signs of aging, independent of external factors.

Most data regarding the influence of external factors on aging have been conducted as epidemiological collections on specific patient populations. Epidemiological studies have intimated associations between environmental factors and aging; however, the influence of genetic differences cannot be controlled when dealing with a diverse genetic population. One research tool that may be implemented in the study of skin aging is the investigation of twin sets. Examination of monozygotic, as well as dizygotic twins, allows a unique opportunity to control for genetic differences. In the analysis of facial senescence, this gives the investigator the ability to control for most of the causes of intrinsic aging. Despite the relative benefit of genetic control, the statistical study of twins requires a relatively large patient population, as many twin sets have very similar lifestyles.

The rest of the chapter attempts to analyze the findings of the several twin investigations in the current literature and identify possible risk factors for extrinsic aging.

Extrinsic Causes of Aging

Smoking

The association of skin aging with smoking was first scientifically proposed in 1856 when Solly postulated that facial appearance in smokers is markedly different than nonsmokers [4]. Since this time, epidemiological data have shown a possible correlation between smoking and facial aging, although the amount of associated aging due to smoking has been debated. Results have been equivocal, with several investigations showing little to no aging difference due to smoking status [5, 6], while others have seen a significant association [7–12].

Several analyses of twins have corroborated the influence of smoking on facial aging (Fig. 1). Doshi et al. reported a significant difference in facial aging of a singular set of twins [13]. Each of the twins in this report had similar lifestyles, body habitus, and sun exposure; however, one of the twins had a greater than 50-pack-year history of smoking. The differences with regard to superficial and deep rhytides, lentigines, tissue laxity, and pigmentary changes were disparate. Antell and Taczanowski also provided anecdotal evidence on 34 sets of identical twins, showing a possible correlation to smoking differences [14].

Rexbye et al., in an investigation of 1826 Danish twin sets over the age of 70, demonstrated

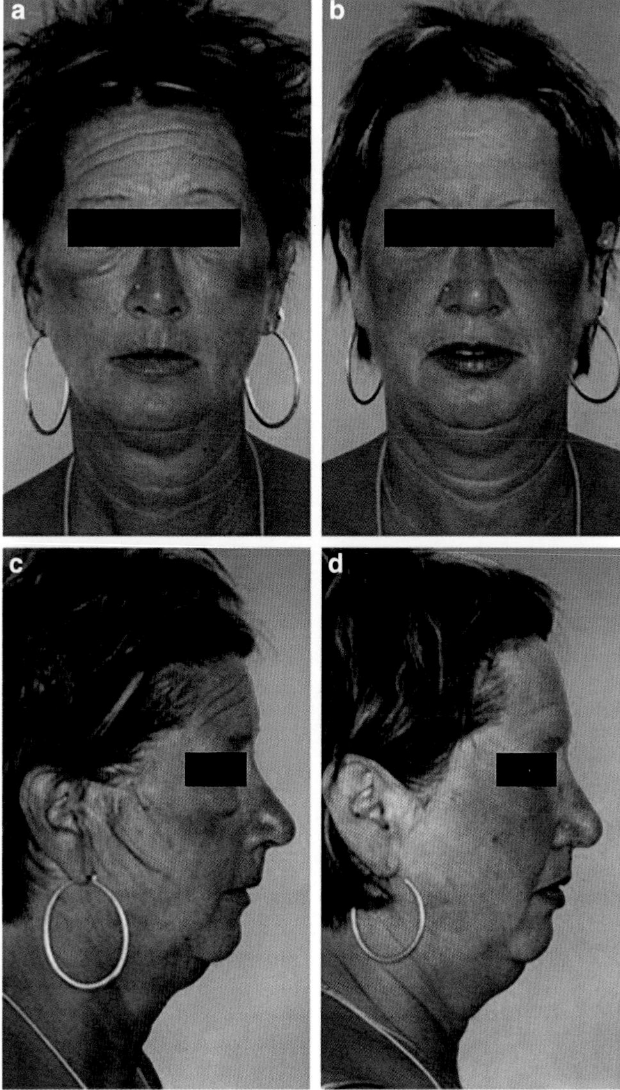

Fig. 1 Twins (natural age 52) with difference in smoking history. Twin (**a**, **c**) had a 20-year greater smoking history than twin (**b**, **d**). Perceived age difference of the twins was 6.25 years

that smoking was a significant determinant of facial aging in men, yet less so in women [15]. Smoking 20 cigarettes per day per year for 20 years increased perceived age by 1 year. For women, this number was increased to 20 cigarettes per day for 40 years (Fig. 2). The authors attribute this discrepancy to the difference of smoking habits between the sexes in the Netherlands. Fewer women were smokers, and those who did smoke actually smoked less than their male counterparts.

Guyuron et al. conducted an investigation of 186 sets of identical twins at an annual international festival for twins [16]. Females from the ages of 18 to 76 were analyzed in this study. A comprehensive questionnaire was filled out, and standardized high-resolution photographs were taken of each twin set. Smoking was found to be significantly correlated with perceived facial age. In analysis of the data, approximately 10 years of smoking difference led to a 2½ years older appearance.

The mechanism for smoking induced damage in the skin is unclear, although many theories exist. One postulate is that the increase of matrix

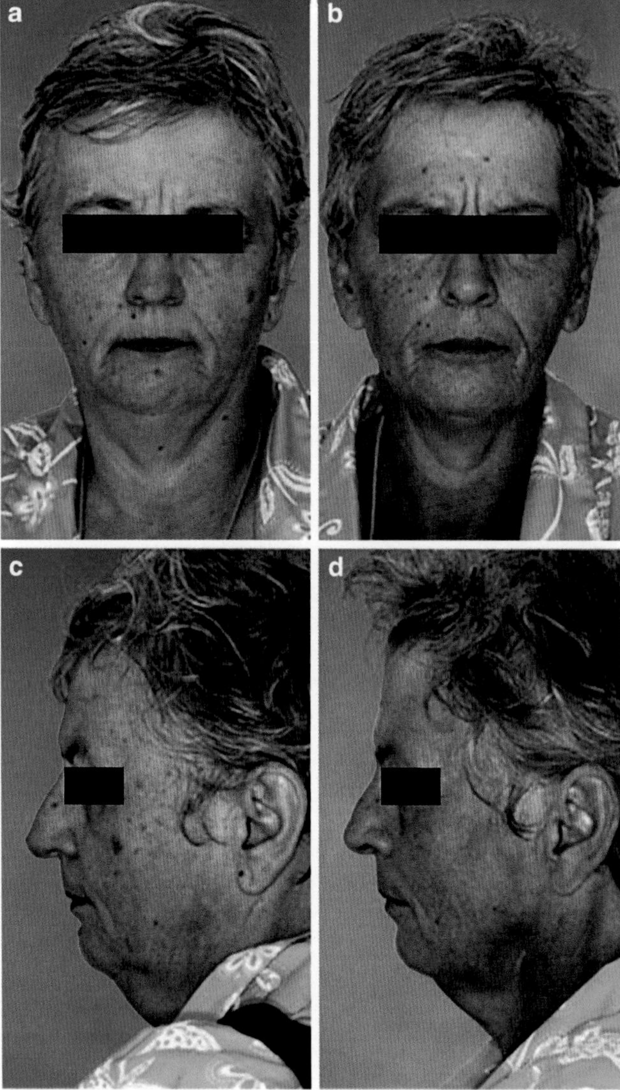

Fig. 2 Twins (natural age 57) with difference in smoking history. Twin (**b**, **d**) had a 40 year greater smoking history than Twin (**a**, **c**). Twin (**a**, **c**) had 2 years of hormone replacement therapy. The perceived age difference was 8.25 years

metalloproteinases (MMPs) in the skin of smokers contributes to skin damage [17]. Matrix metalloproteinases are proteases responsible for degrading dermal collagen and other extracellular matrix material. This effect may be synergistic with the effects of UV radiation, as irradiation also induces MMPs. Other likely changes include the decrease of the skin microvasculature, leading to the increase of reactive oxygen species and thus free radicals [13, 18]. These processes are also known to occur in the face of photodamage; therefore, there may be additive effects of sun and smoking on skin aging.

Sun Exposure

Sun exposure is perhaps the most investigated cause of extrinsic aging. There is incontrovertible evidence that ultraviolet irradiation damages the skin and induces premature aging. The pathophysiology of photodamage is multifactorial, involving the upregulation of matrix metalloproteinases, reversible and irreversible damage to DNA, and creation of reactive oxygen species [18]. Details on these and other mechanisms are beyond the scope of this chapter and are discussed in subsequent chapters.

Controversy does exist, however, on the importance of sun damage on perceived age. Chronological or intrinsic skin aging shares many of the features and possible mechanisms of photoaged skin. In both photoaging and chronological aging of the skin, elevated concentrations of degraded collagen are present. Furthermore, both mechanisms of aging have been theorized to occur as a result of oxidative damage [19]. Although the actual pathways involved in chronological aging may be distinct from those in photoaging, the two may share common central mediators.

Many studies have been performed evaluating the importance of photoaging with respect to skin changes and alteration of perceived age [20]. While there is no question that UV irradiation induces age-related changes in the skin, the amount of change is a topic of considerable debate. When evaluating an elderly (>60 years) population, Leung and Harvey found that sun exposure alone did not have a considerable effect on perceived age [2]. In their multivariate regression analysis, 30 years of sun exposure for 5 h a day only produced 1.5 years of perceived age difference. Guinot et al., in designing a skin age score in a prospective analysis of Caucasian women from 18 to 80 years of age, found that visual signs of chronic photodamage did not contribute significantly to the age score [21]. These investigations do not refute the contribution of ultraviolet irradiation in skin aging but they do underscore the difficulty in attributing visible skin changes to a singular extrinsic or intrinsic cause.

One method to investigate the importance of photoaging, and control for chronological (intrinsic) aging, is the analysis of identical twins. The analysis of twin sets has shown significant perceived differences in aging with respect to sun exposure (Fig. 3). Guyuron et al. investigated hours of sun exposure as well as the participation in outdoor hobbies and the use of sunscreen [16]. The increase in sun exposure as well as the participation in outdoor activities both significantly increased perceived age. The use of sunscreen did significantly decrease perceived age; however, the level of SPF used was not assessed.

Sun exposure was also correlated with increased perceived age in a study of elderly (70+) Danish twins [15]. Here, sun exposure was evaluated on the type of employment the individual performed during the longest period of working. Interestingly, sun exposure was statistically significant in men, however, not in women. The authors attributed this effect to the likely high rate of sun exposure in working men. Only 8.3 % of women in this study were exposed to sun during the working hours of the day.

Diet (BMI)

BMI may have a not-so-indirect effect on perceived age, although this may not necessarily be due to changes at the skin level. For years, plastic surgeons have recognized that facial atrophy and soft tissue descent are harbingers for an increase in perceived facial age. Various surgical and injectable modalities have been introduced that restore facial volume and resuspend tissues to their previous anatomical position.

Several studies have identified an inverse relationship between BMI and facial wrinkling. Guinot et al. prospectively analyzed a cohort of 361 white females in the process of developing a skin age score [21]. They found that body mass index did significantly affect their skin age score in an inverse relationship. Purba et al. evaluated skin wrinkling in elderly (>70) patients from multiple countries [22]. As with the previous study, this investigation found that wrinkling was significantly negatively correlated with BMI.

Analysis of twins' data has further substantiated these findings. In Guyuron et al.'s study, the influence of body mass index was highly dependent on the age of the twin set [16]. In twins that were younger than 40 years of age, a four-point increase in BMI was associated with a perceived older appearance. A four-point increase in BMI in twins older than 40 years of age, however, was associated with a perceived younger appearance (Fig. 4). The latter finding was supported by the Rexbye et al. investigation [15]. Here, an increase of BMI in both elderly men and women was associated with a younger appearance. A decrease

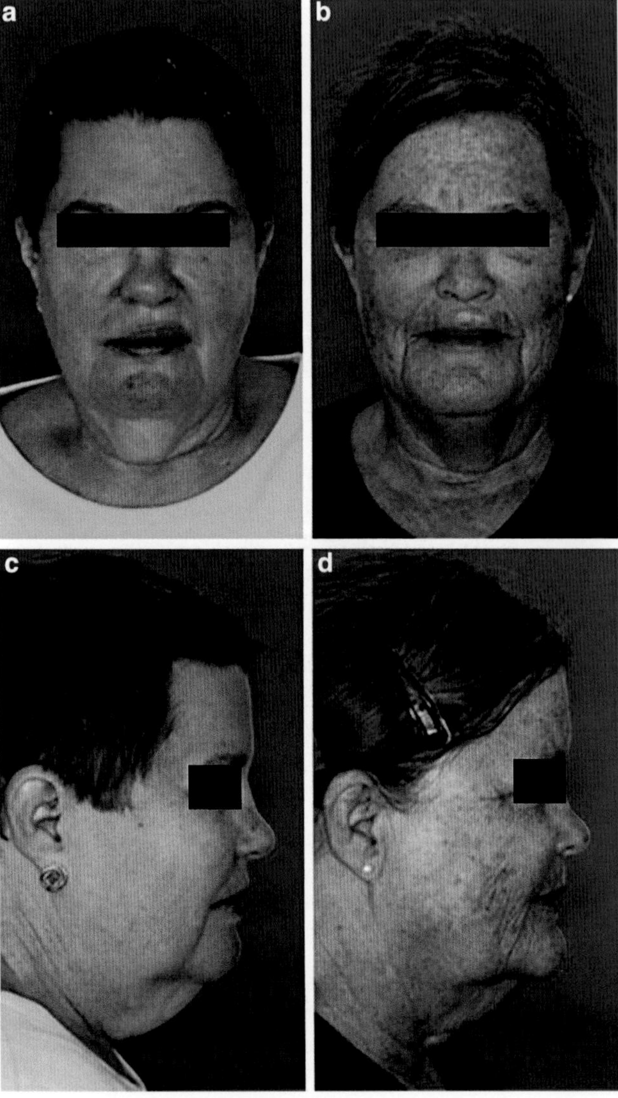

Fig. 3 Twins (natural age 61) with significant difference in sun exposure. Twin (**b**, **d**) had approximately 10 h/week greater sun exposure than twin (**a**, **c**). Twin (**a**, **c**) had a BMI 2.7 points higher than twin (**b**, **d**). The perceived age difference was 11.25 years

of BMI of 2 in males and 7 in females was associated with a 1 year older perceived age.

Hormone Replacement Therapy (HRT)

Estrogens have a profound effect on the skin, as evidenced by the cutaneous alterations in skin characteristics following menopause. Although the mechanisms are poorly understood, a decrease in circulating estrogen is associated with decreased skin elasticity, decreased dermal thickness, as well as increased dryness [23]. Conversely, analyses of estrogen replacement therapy have suggested possible increases in the dermal thickness, concentration of dermal collagen, elasticity, and fewer fine wrinkles [24]. Epidemiological investigations have nonetheless been equivocal in their findings of hormone replacement therapy on perceived aging.

With regard to twins' analysis, hormone replacement therapy has been associated with a younger perceived age [16]. In addition, the effect of HRT on age increased as the age of the twin sets increased and as the difference of years of treatment increased (Fig. 5).

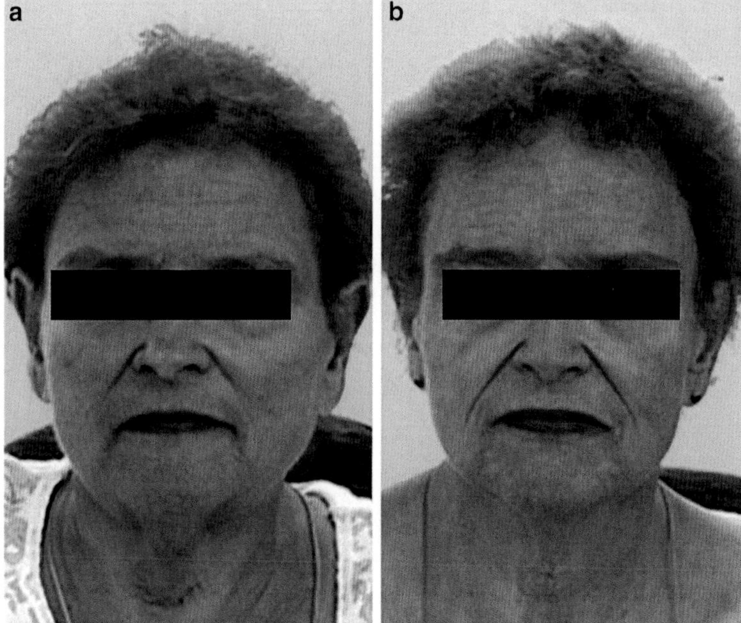

Fig. 4 Twins (natural age 58) with differences in BMI. Twin a, c had a 14.7 point higher BMI than twin b, d. No other differences were discerned from the questionnaire. Perceived age difference was 5.25 years

Adverse Social Factors

External social factors have been found to significantly alter biological aging. Several aspects that have been associated with aging include depression, divorce, socioeconomic status, and alcohol consumption [25, 26]. Additionally, there is usually an interaction or intermingling of these deleterious social factors. Osler et al. investigated the role of marital status, BMI, depression, and smoking in 1,175 sets of identical Danish twins [27]. The twins that were divorced, widowed, or never married had higher depression scores and smoked more than their married counterparts.

It is no surprise that perceived facial aging may also be adversely affected by these same factors. Limited epidemiological data exists on perceived facial aging and skin aging relating to factors such as depression, divorce, and alcohol consumption. However, several of the twin investigations previously discussed in this chapter have evaluated these social facets and will be discussed below.

Depression

In the Guyuron et al. study, depression was indirectly investigated by measuring the utilization of antidepressants. Here, the use of antidepressants, either current or past, led to an increase in perceived age [16]. Rexbye et al. used a depression symptomatology score to analyze depression in their study [15]. They found that an increase in the depression score was significantly associated with an increase in perceived age. Specifically, an increase in depression symptomatology score from 17 to 49 was associated with a perceived age increase of 2.4 years for men and 3.9 years for women.

The length and type of depression, however, have not been investigated with relation to facial aging. In both of these studies, only the presence of depression, either in the past or current, was analyzed.

Alcohol Consumption

A significant amount of data on the effects of alcohol on twins does not exist. Guyuron et al. investigated alcohol avoidance, but did not quantify alcohol consumption [16]. Despite this caveat, the twins who "avoided alcohol" had a younger perceived age. Rexbye et al. did not notice a significant effect of substantial alcohol consumption; however, their number of positive responders was small enough to limit the power of this study [15].

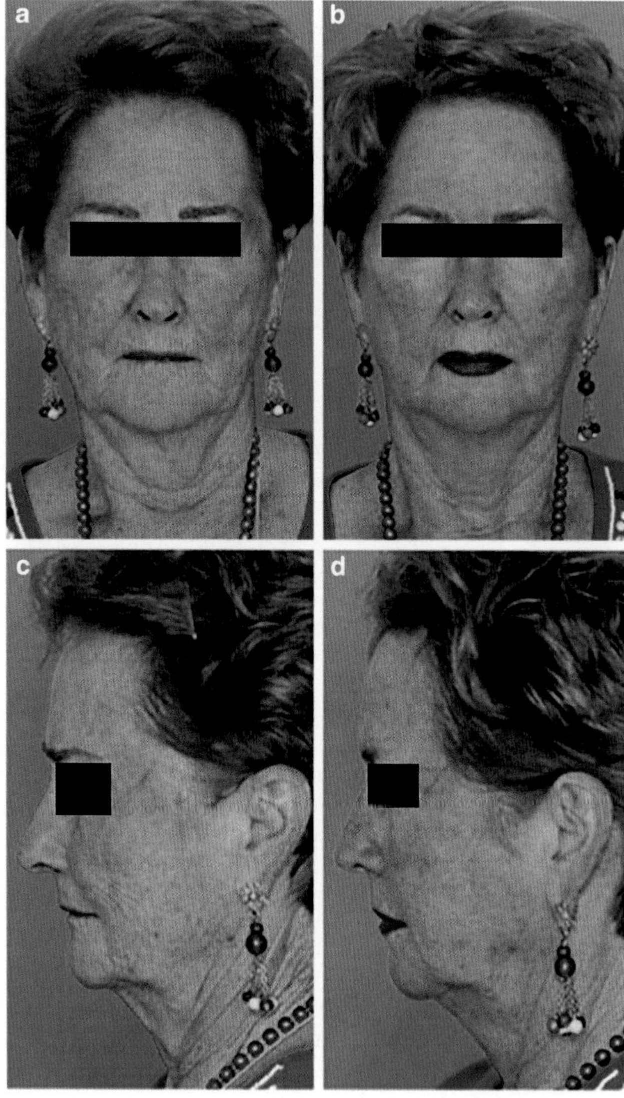

Fig. 5 Twins (natural age 71) with difference in HRT. Twin (**b**, **d**) had 22 more years of HRT than twin (**a**, **c**). Twin (**b**, **d**) had a 1.2 lower BMI. Perceived age difference was 7.25

Marital Status

In the analysis of twins, women who were divorced were perceived to be approximately 1.7 years older than those who were either single or married [16]. Interestingly, widows appeared approximately 2 years younger than their non-widowed counterparts. Although Rexbye et al. also reported a 1.9-year difference in age between married and unmarried women, this was not statistically significant.

Conclusion

The etiological delineation of skin and facial aging is complicated, given the large number of possible contributing factors. Epidemiological data has been helpful; however, it does not allow for control of the intrinsic factors of aging that are inherently different in all individuals. The analysis of twins gives the investigator the ability to control for genetic causes. In the study of skin and perceived facial aging, one is able to investigate purely the environmental causes of skin and facial aging, extrinsic aging.

From the data presented in the several twin investigations in the current literature, there appear to be several factors important to extrinsic skin aging and perceived facial age. Smoking and sun exposure, the two most epidemiologically studied factors, do appear to have a significant role in perceived age. Other factors such as hormone replacement therapy, BMI, depression, and the use of alcohol also have an influence on facial aging. Larger series of twins' analyses are needed to further delineate the importance of each of these facets.

Cross-References

- ▶ Climate Change and Its Dermatologic Impact on Aging Skin
- ▶ Cutaneous Responses to Tropospheric Ozone exposure
- ▶ In Vitro Method to Visualize UV-induced Reactive Oxygen Species in a Skin Equivalent Model
- ▶ Skin Photodamage Prevention: State of the Art and New Prospects
- ▶ Tobacco Smoke and Skin Aging

References

1. Uitto J. Understanding premature skin aging. New Eng J Med. 1997;337:1419–28.
2. Leung W, Harvey I. Is skin ageing in the elderly caused by sun exposure or smoking? Br J Dermatol. 2002;147 (6):1187–91.
3. Pesce K, Rothe M. The premature aging syndromes. Clin Dermatol. 1996;14:161–70.
4. Solly S. Clinical lectures on paralysis. Lancet. 1856;130(2):167–73.
5. O'Hare P, et al. Tobacco smoking contributes little to facial wrinkling. J Eur Acad Dermatol Venereol. 1999;12(2):133–9.
6. Allen H, Johnson B. Diamond S Smokers wrinkles? JAMA. 1973;225:1067–9.
7. Daniell H. A study in the epidemiology of 'crows feet'. Ann Intern Med. 1971;75(6):873–80.
8. Model D. Smoker's face: an underrated clinical sign? BMJ. 1985;291(6511):1760–3.
9. Ernster V, et al. Facial wrinkling in men and women, by smoking status. Am J Public Health. 1995;85:78–82.
10. Keadunce D, et al. Cigarette smoking: risk factor for premature facial wrinkling. Ann Intern Med. 1991;114 (10):840–4.
11. Chung J, et al. Cutaneous photodamage in Koreans: influence of sex, sun exposure, smoking, and skin color. Arch Dermatol. 2001;137(8):1043–51.
12. Helfrich Y, et al. Effect of smoking on aging of photoprotected skin: evidence gathered using a new photonumeric scale. Arch Dermatol. 2007;143 (5):397–402.
13. Doshi D, Hanneman K, Cooper K. Smoking and skin aging in identical twins. Arch Dermatol. 2007;143 (12):1543–6.
14. Antell D, Taczanowski E. How environment and lifestyle choices influence the aging process. Ann Plast Surg. 1999;43:585–8.
15. Rexbye H, et al. Influence of environmental factors on facial ageing. Age Ageing. 2006;35(2):110–5.
16. Guyuron B, et al. Factors contributing to the facial aging of identical twins. Plast Reconstr Surg. 2009;123:1–11.
17. Lahmann C, et al. Matrix Metalloproteinase-1 and skin ageing in smokers. Lancet. 2001;357:935–6.
18. Fisher G, et al. Mechanisms of photoaging and chronological skin aging. Arch Dermatol. 2002;138 (11):1462–70.
19. Sohal R, Weindruch R. Oxidative stress, caloric restriction, and aging. Science. 1996;273:59–63.
20. Fisher G, et al. Pathophysiology of premature skin aging by ultraviolet light. New Engl J Med. 1997;337:1463–5.
21. Guinot C, et al. Relative contribution of intrinsic vs extrinsic factors to skin aging as determined by a validated skin age score. Arch Dermatol. 2002;138 (11):1454–60.
22. Purba M, et al. Can skin wrinkling in a site that has received limited sun exposure be used as a marker of health status and biological age? Age Ageing. 2001;30:227–34.
23. Pierard G, et al. Effect of hormone replacement therapy for menopause on the mechanical properties of the skin. J Am Geriatr Soc. 1995;43(6):662–5.
24. Callens A, et al. Does hormonal skin aging exist? A study of the influence of different hormone therapy regimens on the skin of postmenopausal women using non-invasive measurement techniques. Dermatology. 1996;193(4):289–94.
25. Nilsson P, et al. Adverse social factors predict early ageing in middle-aged men and women: the Ebeltoft Health Study. Denmark Scand J Public Health. 2003;31(4):255–60.
26. Demakakos P, et al. Socioeconomic status and health: the role of subjective social status. Soc Sci Med. 2008;67(2):330–40.
27. Osler M, et al. Marital status and twins' health and behavior: an analysis of middle-aged Danish twins. Psychosom Med. 2008;70(4):482–7.

Tobacco Smoke and Skin Aging

57

Akimichi Morita

Contents

Abstract

Tobacco smoke has deleterious effects on skin, such as the induction of wrinkles, pigmentation, and other signs of skin aging. Epidemiologic studies indicate that tobacco smoking is a strong independent predictor of facial wrinkle formation and other aspects of premature skin aging. Recent in vivo studies in humans and mice provided the first direct evidence that tobacco smoke causes premature skin aging and has begun to elucidate the molecular changes in the skin that occur in response to tobacco smoke. Water-soluble tobacco smoke extract, which predominantly produces oxidative stress when applied to cultured skin fibroblasts, impairs collagen biosynthesis. Matrix metalloproteinases, which degrade collagen, are induced dose dependently by tobacco smoke extract and other constituents that trigger the aryl hydrocarbon receptor (AhR), a ligand-dependent transcription factor that mediates the toxicity of several environmental contaminants, including photoproducts in the body generated by ultraviolet (UV) B radiation. Tobacco smoke contains many non-water-soluble constituents that also activate the AhR pathway. Hexane-soluble tobacco extract activates the AhR pathway to induce the premature skin aging effects of tobacco smoke exposure. Based on the results of several studies, it is now widely accepted that tobacco (cigarette) smoking is an environmental factor that induces premature skin aging

A. Morita (✉)
Department of Geriatric and Environmental Dermatology, Nagoya City University Graduate School of Medical Sciences, Nagoya, Japan
e-mail: amorita@med.nagoya-cu.ac.jp

M.A. Farage et al. (eds.), *Textbook of Aging Skin*,
DOI 10.1007/978-3-662-47398-6_46

Introduction and Epidemiologic Study

As early as 1971, Daniell [1] reported that tobacco smoking has deleterious effects on the skin, and smoker's wrinkles are typical clinical features of patients who smoke. A recent epidemiologic study demonstrated that tobacco smoking is one of several factors that contribute to premature skin aging, which is dependent on age, sex, pigmentation, sun exposure history, alcohol consumption, and other factors [2–5]. In a cross-sectional study, sun exposure, pack years of smoking history, and potential confounding variables were assessed by questionnaire. Facial wrinkles were quantified using the Daniell score. Logistic statistical analysis of the data revealed that age, pack years, and sun exposure independently contributed to facial wrinkle formation [6]. The association between wrinkle formation and tobacco smoking was investigated using silicone rubber replicas combined with computerized image processing, which is an objective measurement of the skin's topography. The skin replicas of 63 enrolled volunteers were assessed to elucidate the association between tobacco smoking and wrinkles [7]. The replica analysis indicated that the depth (*R* **z**) and variance (*R* **v**) of furrows (*R* **v**) were significantly greater in subjects with a smoking history ($\geq$35 pack years) than in nonsmokers ($P < 0.05$). The lines of furrows (*R* **l**) in subjects with a smoking history were significantly lower than those in nonsmokers ($P < 0.05$) [7, 8]. Tobacco smoking, which is considered an important environmental factor, potentially causes "tobacco wrinkles" [1], although chronic exposure of skin to ultraviolet (UV) radiation also results in marked alterations in the structure and composition of the epidermis and dermis, i.e., photoaging [9–11]. Based on previous studies, tobacco smoking per se or smoking combined with UV exposure is a strong predictor of skin aging [12].

Tobacco-Induced Skin Aging

Tobacco smoking likely exerts its deleterious effects on the skin directly on the epidermis through its irritant components and indirectly on the dermis via the blood circulation [3, 13]. The decreased stratum corneum moisture of the face contributes to facial wrinkling because of the direct toxicity of the smoke. Pursing the lips during smoking with contraction of facial muscles and squinting because of the irritation of smoke may cause the formation of wrinkles around the mouth and in the crow's foot area [14]. Changes in macromolecular metabolism in the dermis have been brought into focus as a major factor leading to skin aging [15]. Specifically, the accumulation of elastosis material is accompanied by the degradation of matrix protein, which is mediated by matrix metalloproteinases (MMPs) in skin aging. Molecular alterations in the dermis include a decrease in collagen synthesis, induction of MMPs, and an abnormal accumulation of elastic fibers and proteoglycans [16–18].

Effects of Tobacco Smoke on Skin Models In Vitro

The biosynthesis of new collagen is significantly decreased by tobacco smoke extracts in cultured skin fibroblasts [18]. Studies using Western blot analysis have also demonstrated that the production of both procollagen types I and III, collagen precursors, from the supernatant of cultured fibroblasts treated with tobacco smoke extracts, is significantly decreased [18]. This finding indicates that the final production of collagen secreted into the medium is reduced, regardless of the rate of collagen synthesis in the cell, as tested using 3H-proline incorporation.

Although elastic fibers account for only 2–4 % of the extracellular matrix, they provide elasticity and resilience to normal skin. Tobacco smoke extracts induce a significant increase in tropoelastin mRNA in cultured skin fibroblasts. Accumulation of abnormal elastic material (termed solar elastosis) is the prominent histopathologic alteration in photoaged skin [19, 20]. Boyd et al. [21] reported that tobacco smoking promotes elastosis in subjects with an average of 42 pack years of tobacco smoking. In an in vitro study using cultured skin fibroblasts, tobacco smoke extracts induced an elevation of tropoelastin, which might cause premature skin aging.

Expression of *MMP-1* and *MMP-3* mRNA, extracellular matrix-associated members of the MMP gene family, was induced in cultured skin fibroblasts stimulated with tobacco smoke extracts in a dose-dependent manner [18]. The findings support the concept that MMPs are primary mediators of connective tissue damage in skin exposed to tobacco smoke extracts and of premature skin aging. In addition, expression of *tissue inhibitor of metalloproteinase-1* and *tissue inhibitor of metalloproteinase-3* remained unchanged [18]. By inducing the expression of *MMP-1* and *MMP-3*, but not tissue inhibitor of MMPs, tobacco smoke extracts could alter their ratio in favor of the induction of MMPs, resulting in a more degradative environment with loss of cutaneous collagen [18]. MMPs comprise a family of degradative enzymes that lead to the deterioration of extracellular matrix components, such as native collagen, elastin fibers, and various proteoglycans. MMP-3 and MMP-7 may have a key role in the degradation of elastin and proteoglycans [22], and MMP-7 is increased in fibroblasts exposed to tobacco smoke extract [18].

Effect of Tobacco Smoke in Human and Mouse Models

In a clinical study, significantly higher levels of MMP-1 mRNA were observed in the buttock skin of smokers compared with nonsmokers, based on quantitative real-time polymerase chain reaction [23]. High levels of MMP-1 mRNA result in the degradation of collagen, elastic fibers, and proteoglycans. Therefore, observations in dermal connective tissue treated with tobacco suggest an imbalance between biosynthesis and degradation, with less repair capacity in the face of ongoing degradation, which leads to the loss of collagen and elastic fibers, manifesting clinically as an aging appearance of skin.

Although staining of skin specimens and biochemical analysis of photodamaged skin demonstrate that sun-damaged skin has a high glycosaminoglycan content, the underlying molecular pathogenesis is unclear. Versican, a large chondroitin sulfate (CS) proteoglycan, is present in the dermis in association with elastic fibers, which contain a hyaluronic acid-binding domain. The core protein is postulated to have a role in the molecular interactions and, specifically, to facilitate the binding of these macromolecules to other matrix components or cytokines such as transforming growth factor (TGF) [24]. Decorin, a small CS proteoglycan, co-distributes with collagen fibers and is postulated to function in cell recognition, possible by connecting extracellular matrix components and cell surface glycoproteins [25]. Targeted disruption of decorin synthesis in mice significantly reduces the tensile strength of the skin [26]. Carrino et al. [27] reported a decrease in the proportion of large CS proteoglycans (versican) and a concomitant increase in the proportion of small dermatan sulfate proteoglycans (decorin) as a function of age. Ito et al. [28] also observed that versican is strongly stained in young rats and only faintly in old rats. On the other hand, decorin is faintly stained in young rats and distinctly stained in old rats. Proteoglycans change due to photoaging, especially UVB irradiation [29, 30]. Analysis of newly synthesized proteoglycans revealed a marked increase after UVB radiation in mice [30]. Versican and decorin immunostaining are increased in photoaged tissue samples, accompanied by similar alterations in gene expression [29]. Tobacco smoke extracts decrease versican protein and mRNA levels, whereas they significantly increase decorin levels in cultured skin fibroblasts. These findings are similar to those observed in photoaging.

Molecular Mechanisms of Tobacco-Induced Skin Aging via Reactive Oxygen Species Generation and Cytokines

Based on experimental evidence, a working model for UVA damaged skin was proposed, in which UV irradiation-induced gene expression is mediated via the generation of singlet oxygen through a pathway involving the activation of transcription factor AP-2 [10]. To determine whether reactive oxygen species were involved in the upregulation of MMPs induced by tobacco, we used sodium azide (NaN3), L-ascorbic acid, and vitamin E, which are potent quenchers of singlet oxygen and other reactive oxygen species [18]. NaN3, L-ascorbic acid, and vitamin E blocked the induction of MMPs in fibroblasts exposed to tobacco smoke extract [18]. Among the antioxidant reagents, L-ascorbic acid most obviously diminished the increase in MMP-1 expression in fibroblasts exposed to tobacco smoke extracts [18]. These findings suggest that reactive oxygen species are responsible for the enhanced induction of MMPs by tobacco smoke extract.

TGF-β1 is a multifunctional cytokine that regulates cell proliferation and differentiation, tissue remodeling, and repair [31]. TGF-β1 is a potent growth inhibitor in the epidermis with an important role in maintaining tissue homeostasis. In the dermis, however, TGF-β1 acts as a positive growth factor, inducing the synthesis of extracellular matrix proteins. TGF-β signals through a heteromeric complex of type I/II TGF-β receptors to initiate signal transduction [32, 33]. A recent report demonstrated that UV irradiation downregulates TGF-β type II receptor mRNA and protein and induces Smad7 mRNA and protein in human skin [34]. Tobacco smoke extracts induce the latent form of TGF-β, not the active form, based on enzyme-linked immunosorbent assay of supernatants from cultured skin fibroblasts [35]. The induction of endogenous TGF-β1 from tobacco-exposed cells contributes to the intracellular defense capacity. Fibroblast responses to TGF-β1 are mediated through binding of its active form to the cell surface receptor. Tobacco smoke extracts block cellular responsiveness to TGF-β1 through the induction of the nonfunctional latent form and downregulation of TGF-β1 receptors [35]. Exogenous addition of TGF-β1 might be useful for stimulating collagen production or to protect against the deleterious effects of tobacco smoke.

Molecular Mechanisms of Tobacco-Induced Skin Aging via Aryl Hydrocarbon Receptors

Tobacco smoke contains more than 3800 constituents, including numerous water-insoluble polycyclic aromatic hydrocarbons that trigger aryl hydrocarbon receptor (AhR) signaling pathways. To analyze the molecular mechanisms involved in tobacco smoke-induced skin aging, we exposed primary human fibroblasts and keratinocytes to tobacco smoke extracts. Hexane- and water-soluble tobacco smoke extracts significantly induced MMP-1 mRNA in both human cultured fibroblasts and keratinocytes in a dose-dependent manner. To clarify the involvement of the AhR pathway, we used a stable AhR-knockdown HaCaT cell line. AhR knockdown abolishes the increased transcription of the AhR-dependent genes CYP1A1/CYP1B1 and MMP-1 that is induced by either of the tobacco smoke extracts [36]. Furthermore, the tobacco smoke extracts induced 7-ethoxyresorufin-*O*-deethylase activity, which was almost completely abolished by AhR knockdown. Likewise, treating fibroblasts with AhR pathway inhibitors, i.e., the flavonoids 3-methoxy-4-nitroflavone and α-naphthoflavone, blocked the expression of CYP1B1 and MMP-1 [36]. These findings suggest that the tobacco smoke extracts induce MMP-1 expression in human fibroblasts and keratinocytes via activation of the AhR pathway. Thus, the AhR pathway may be pathogenetically involved in extrinsic skin aging.

It is widely recognized that tobacco smoke causes skin pigmentation. No studies, however, have directly evaluated the mechanisms underlying the effects of smoking on skin pigmentation. When cultured with water-soluble tobacco smoke extract, human epidermal melanocytes grew to a large size and produced more melanins. Melanocyte activation was analyzed by quantifying microphthalmia-associated transcription factor expression by real-time polymerase chain reaction [37]. Microphthalmia-associated transcription factor expression was significantly and dose-dependently increased by exposure to tobacco smoke extract. The Wnt/β-catenin signaling pathway seemed to mediate the tobacco smoke extract-induced melanocyte activation. Immunocytochemical studies revealed that the activated melanocytes actively express AhR around the nuclear membrane. Tobacco smoke extract-induced microphthalmia-associated transcription factor activation is inhibited by RNA silencing of the AhR [37]. This study provided evidence that tobacco smoke enhances pigmentation in vitro and that the increase in pigmentation may be due, at least in part, to β-catenin and AhR-mediated mechanisms inside human melanocytes.

Deleterious Effects of Tobacco Smoke Beyond Skin Aging

Environmental factors contribute to the increased prevalence of autoimmune disease via the activation of T helper type 17 cells (Th17). Tobacco smoke increases the risk and severity of psoriasis, but the underlying mechanisms are unclear. Tobacco smoke contains low levels of AhR agonists. AhR is a ligand-dependent transcription factor that mediates cellular events in response to halogenated aromatic hydrocarbons and non-halogenated polycyclic aromatic hydrocarbons. AhR is expressed in human Th17 and activation of AhR during the generation of Th17 leads to a marked increase in Th17. Differentiation of Th17 from naïve $CD4^+$ T cells requires the presence of interleukin (IL)-6 and TGF-β and is further enhanced by IL-1β and IL-21. In addition, IL-1β and IL-6 induce excessive secretion of IL-17A from central memory T cells (Tcm). There are two distinct populations of memory T cells. The first, called effector memory T cells, is similar to effector cells. Effector memory T cells target tissues and rapidly produce cytokines upon restimulation. The other subset, the Tcm, acts as a reservoir of antigen-specific T cells that can expand upon rechallenge and become effector T cells. Tcm express CD62L, which promotes their ability to interact with antigen-presenting dendritic cells.

IL-1β, IL-1β/IL-6, and TGF-β/IL-21 induce IL-17 expression, as described above, and tobacco smoke extract significantly increases IL-17 expression in the presence of these cytokines. Tobacco smoke extract also induces IL-22 expression in the presence of IL-1β and IL-1β/IL-6, even in the absence of the cytokines. These findings indicate that tobacco smoke extract promotes Th17 differentiation from Tcm, probably via AhR stimulation, and induces Th17 to express IL-17 and IL-22. The same Th17 produces IL-17 and IL-22, but distinct mechanisms regulate the production of these cytokines at the molecular level. Our findings suggest that tobacco smoke induces the expression of Th17 from Tcm. Tcm differentiate into a variety of helper T cells depending on the types of cytokines present [38]. AhR agonists in smoke might drive Tcm to differentiate into Th17, which results in a higher proportion of Th17 among the peripheral blood mononuclear cells of psoriasis patients that are smokers compared with those that are nonsmokers.

Conclusion

Tobacco smoke contains numerous compounds with at least 3800 constituents [39]. The specific constituents in tobacco smoke that cause damage to the connective tissue, however, remain unclear. Our recent studies revealed that reactive oxygen species, cytokines, and the AhR pathway are some of the molecular mechanisms underlying these skin-damaging effects of tobacco smoke. Tobacco-induced skin aging provides a tool for studying the effects of smoking. Detailed knowledge of these effects may provide motivation to stop smoking, especially among those who are more concerned with their appearance than the potential internal damage associated with smoking.

References

1. Daniell HW. Smoker's wrinkles: a study in the epidemiology of "crow's feet". Ann Intern Med. 1971;75:873–80.
2. Ernster VL, Grady D, Miike R, et al. Facial wrinkling in men and women, by smoking status. Am J Public Health. 1995;85:78–82.
3. Frances C. Smoker's wrinkles: epidemiological and pathogenic considerations. Clin Dermatol. 1998;16:565–70.
4. Grady D, Ernster V. Does cigarette smoking make you ugly and old? Am J Epidemiol. 1992;135:839–42.
5. Kadunce DP, Burr R, Gress R, et al. Cigarette smoking: risk factor for premature facial wrinkling. Ann Intern Med. 1991;114:840–4.
6. Yin L, Morita A, Tsuji T. Skin aging induced by ultraviolet exposure and tobacco smoking: evidence from

epidemiological and molecular studies. Photodermatol Photoimmunol Photomed. 2001;17:178–83.
7. Yin L, Morita A, Tsuji T. Skin premature aging induced by tobacco smoking: the objective evidence of skin replica analysis. J Dermatol Sci. 2001;27 Suppl 1:S26–31.
8. Yin L, Morita A, Tsuji T. Tobacco smoking: a role of premature skin aging. Nagoya Med J. 2000;43: 165–71.
9. Fisher GJ, Talwar HS, Lin J, et al. Molecular mechanisms of photoaging in human skin in vivo and their prevention by all-*trans*-retinoic acid. Photochem Photobiol. 1999;69:154–7.
10. Grether-Beck S, Buettner R, Krutmann J. Ultraviolet A radiation-induced expression of human genes: molecular and photobiological mechanisms. Biol Chem. 1997;378:1231–6.
11. Wenk J, Brenneisen P, Meewes C, et al. UV-induced oxidative stress and photoaging. Curr Probl Dermatol. 2001;29:83–94.
12. Leung W-C, Harvey I. Is skin ageing in the elderly caused by sun exposure or smoking? Br J Dermatol. 2002;147:1187–91.
13. Lofroth G. Environmental tobacco smoke: overview of chemical composition and genotoxic components. Mutat Res. 1989;222:73–80.
14. Smith JB, Fenske NA. Cutaneous manifestations and consequences of smoking. J Am Acad Dermatol. 1996;34:717–32.
15. Uitto J, Fazio MJ, Olsen DR. Molecular mechanisms of cutaneous aging: age-associated connective tissue alterations in the dermis. J Am Acad Dermatol. 1989;21:614–22.
16. Fisher GJ, Voorhees JJ. Molecular mechanisms of photoaging and its prevention by retinoic acid: ultraviolet irradiation induces MAP kinase signal transduction cascades that induce Ap-1-regulated matrix metalloproteinases that degrade human skin in vivo. J Investig Dermatol Symp Proc. 1998;3:61–8.
17. Shuster S. Smoking and wrinkling of the skin. Lancet. 2001;358:330.
18. Yin L, Morita A, Tsuji T. Alterations of extracellular matrix induced by tobacco smoke extract. Arch Dermatol Res. 2006;292:188–94.
19. Montagna W, Kirchner S, Carlisle K. Histology of sun-damaged human skin. J Am Acad Dermatol. 1989;21:907–18.
20. Tsuji T. Ultrastructure of deep wrinkles in the elderly. J Cutan Pathol. 1987;14:158–64.
21. Boyd AS, Stasko T, King Jr LE, et al. Cigarette smoking-associated elastotic changes in the skin. J Am Acad Dermatol. 1999;41:23–6.
22. Saarialho-Kere U, Kerkela E, Jeskanen L, et al. Accumulation of matrilysin (MMP-7) and macrophage metalloelastase (MMP-12) in actinic damage. J Invest Dermatol. 1999;113:664–72.
23. Lahmann C, Bergemann J, Harrison G, et al. Matrix metalloprotease-1 and skin ageing in smokers. Lancet. 2001;357:935–6.
24. Fisher LW, Termine JD, Young MF. Deduced protein sequence of bone small proteoglycan I (biglycan) shows homology with proteoglycan II (decorin) and several nonconnective tissue proteins in a variety of species. J Biol Chem. 1989;264:4571–6.
25. Zimmermann DR, Ruoslahti E. Multiple domains of the large fibroblast proteoglycan, versican. EMBO J. 1989;8:2975–81.
26. Danielson KG, Baribault H, Homes DF, et al. Targeted disruption of decorin leads to abnormal collagen fibril morphology and skin fragility. J Cell Biol. 1997;136:729–43.
27. Carrino DA, Sorrell JM, Caplan AI. Age-related changes in the proteoglycans of human skin. Arch Biochem Biophys. 2000;373:91–101.
28. Ito Y, Takeuchi J, Yamamoto K, et al. Age differences in immunohistochemical localizations of large proteoglycan, PG-M/versican, and small proteoglycan, decorin, in the dermis of rats. Exp Anim. 2001;50:159–66.
29. Bernstein EF, Fisher LW, Li K, et al. Differential expression of the versican and decorin genes in photoaged and sun-protected skin: comparison by immunohistochemical and northern analyses. Lab Invest. 1995;72:662–9.
30. Margelin D, Fourtanier A, Thevenin T, et al. Alterations of proteoglycans in ultraviolet-irradiated skin. Photochem Photobiol. 1993;58:211–18.
31. Massague J. TGF-beta signal transduction. Annu Rev Biochem. 1998;67:753–91.
32. Kadin ME, Cavaille-Coll MW, Gertz R, et al. Loss of receptors for transforming growth factor beta in human T-cell malignancies. Proc Natl Acad Sci U S A. 1994;91:6002–6.
33. Piek E, Heldin CH, Ten Dijke P. Specificity, diversity, and regulation in TGF-beta superfamily signaling. FASEB J. 1999;13:2105–24.
34. Quan T, He T, Voorhees JJ, et al. Ultraviolet irradiation blocks cellular responses to transforming growth factor-beta by down-regulating its type-II receptor and inducing Smad. J Biol Chem. 2001;276:26349–56.
35. Yin L, Morita A, Tsuji T. Tobacco smoke extract induces age-related changes due to the modulation of TGF-β. Exp Dermatol. 2003;12:51–6.
36. Ono Y, Torii K, Fritsche E, et al. Role of the aryl hydrocarbon receptor in tobacco smoke extract induced-matrix metalloproteinase-1 expression. Exp Dermatol. 2013;22:349–53.
37. Nakamura M, Ueda Y, Hayashi M, et al. Tobacco smoke-induced skin pigmentation is mediated by the aryl hydrocarbon receptor. Exp Dermatol. 2013;22:556–8.
38. Torii K, Saito C, Furuhashi T, et al. Tobacco smoke is related to Th17 generation with clinical implications for psoriasis patients. Exp Dermatol. 2011;20:371–3.
39. Bartsch H, Malaveille C, Friesen M, et al. Black (air-cured) and blond (flue-cured) tobacco cancer risk IV: molecular dosimetry studies implicate aromatic amines as bladder carcinogens. Eur J Cancer. 1993;29A:1199–207.

Sebum Production

58

Claudine Piérard-Franchimont, Marianne Lesuisse, Justine Courtois, Caroline Ritacco, and Gérald E. Piérard

Contents

C. Piérard-Franchimont
Laboratory of Skin Bioengineering and Imaging, Department of Dermatopathology, University Hospital of Liège, Liège, Belgium

Department of Dermatology, Regional Hospital of Huy, Huy, Belgium
e-mail: claudine.franchimont@ulg.ac.be

M. Lesuisse
Department of Dermatology, Unilab Lg, Regional Hospital Citadelle, Liège, Belgium

Department of Dermatology, Regional Hospital of Huy, Huy, Belgium
e-mail: marianne.lesuisse@chrcitadelle.be

J. Courtois • C. Ritacco • G.E. Piérard (✉)
Laboratory of Skin Bioengineering and Imaging, Department of Dermatopathology, University Hospital of Liège, Liège, Belgium
e-mail: justine.courtois@student.ulg.ac.be; caroline.ritacco@student.ulg.ac.be; Gerald.pierard@ulg.ac.be

M.A. Farage et al. (eds.), *Textbook of Aging Skin*,
DOI 10.1007/978-3-662-47398-6_33

Abstract
Sebum produced by sebaceous glands is progressively altered during its transit in the sebaceous duct. Sebaceous gland dynamics involves four successive features including sebum productive and storage, sebum delivery at the skin surface, and the sebum resorption by the stratum corneum. The excretion rate at the skin surface is indeed different from the secretion rate by the gland. The skin microbiome is globally influenced by sebum that promotes anaerobic and lipophilic microorganisms. The lipid composition of sebum exerts profound influences on epithelial tissues.

Introduction

Sebum is produced exclusively by the sebaceous glands. It serves as a vehicle for odors involved in sexual and social attraction. By a similar mechanism, the newborn child commonly recognizes his/her mother's body odor. The reciprocal recognition between the newborn and the mother likely develops during the first weeks of life when the sebaceous glands are active in the newborn. In addition, it is noteworthy that the individual sebum-driven scents of each human being are commonly detected by dogs on the skin and clothes. Other volatile compounds corresponding to pheromones are produced by mammalian skin in a mixture of apocrine sweat and sebum. In addition, sebum brings vitamin E, the α-melanocyte-stimulating hormone (α-MSH) isotype, and other various compounds to the stratum corneum (SC).

Sebum interferes with the skin microbiome [1]. In particular, it is fungistatic to dermatophyte species. Tinea capitis caused by *Microsporum* or *Trichophyton* spp. typically occurs only before puberty when sebum production is minimal to absent. In addition, sebum exhibits some bacteriostatic properties. By contrast, sebum promotes the growth of specific anaerobic and lipophilic microorganisms and parasites including *Propionibacterium* spp. [2], *Staphylococcus epidermidis*, *Malassezia* spp., and *Demodex* mites [3]. Interestingly enough, some specific follicular bacteria, particularly *Propionibacterium acnes*, release porphyrins that are identifiable by their fluorescence [4, 5]. They are seen clinically using a special camera (Visiopor, CK Electronic, Cologne, Germany) revealing fluorescent follicular ostia (Fig. 1). Other fields of biology are influenced by sebum. The high squalene content in sebum supposedly represents, after resorption, a substrate for cholesterol and vitamin D synthesis by the epidermis.

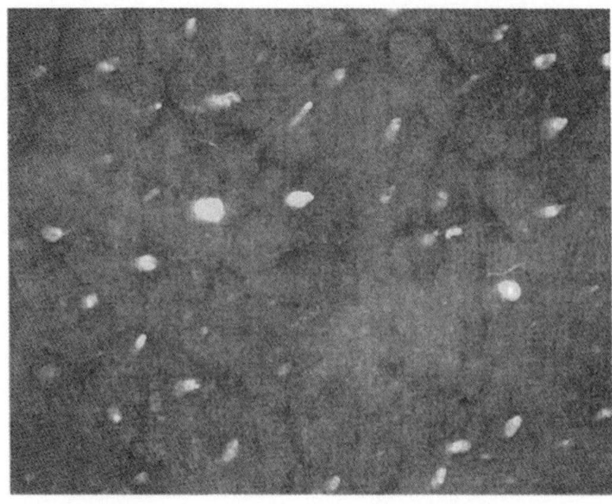

Fig. 1 Fluorescent follicular openings under Visiopor® examination

Plasticity and cohesion between corneocytes are somewhat related to the sebum amount. Sebum protects the skin and the hair shaft from damage induced by mild acid solutions and friction. Indeed, combing and hairdressing generate friction effects on the cuticular cells. Skin and hair surfaces that are primarily hydrophobic and paradoxical become more wettable by a series of sebum components including free fatty acids [6]. In fact, surface wettability is involved in various protective functions of the SC including biocenosis preservation, smoothness, resiliency, and barrier effect to various xenobiotics.

Sebum production shows large interindividual differences. Nonetheless, there are global influences of age and gender. In adults, the critical period in life regarding sebum production begins after menopause and andropause. In older subjects, the sebum flow at the skin surface usually runs dry. In a global perspective aging of the sebaceous glands appears quite complex.

Seborrhea in Cosmetic Perspective

Sebum production shows large interindividual variations as well as intraindividual fluctuations with age. Any excess in sebum output defines seborrhea that leads to unpleasant cosmetic aspects, and possibly fuels specific disorders. Most seborrheic subjects exhibit both greasy hair and oily skin on the forehead and nose. However, some relative differences are possibly found between these locations. After wiping or washing the skin, the sebum coating is often quickly restored. Hence, seborrhea commonly represents a matter of concern to the affected individual.

Observing the skin under ultraviolet light (Visioscan, CK Electronic, Cologne, Germany) discloses specific subclinical or faint mosaic patterns of perifollicular melanosis [7]. Typically, speckled perifollicular melanotic rims (SPMR) are disclosed on the face and scalp of seborrheic individuals (Fig. 2), in particular those with androgenic alopecia [7]. SPMR are evidenced well before the development of distinct patterns of photodamage-related melanosis. In addition, SPMR are absent in children when sebaceous glands are quiescent. It is also absent in nonseborrheic parts of the body, including sun-exposed areas. It has been postulated that SPMR on the seborrheic skin resulted from the melanocyte activation by α-MSH produced by the follicular infundibulum and present in sebum [7].

Greasy hair has lost its natural luster, and it looks dull, darker, and moist. Hair shafts are weighted down with leaking sebum which makes them adherent and flattens all hairstyles in thick masses on the scalp. They are hard to comb. Sebum appears to exert similar effect as a humid environment on hair hold. Sebum is left on the fingers and clothes. When feeling the oily tresses of sticky hairs, their limpness is perceptible, and it is difficult to separate the individual hairs. The possibility to render translucent a piece of paper helps to distinguish sweaty and greasy hair. On heating, an aqueous impregnation disappears rapidly by evaporation, while lipids remain. It should be noted that sustained sweating may be associated with increased seborrhea.

A scaly dermatitis is commonly present on seborrheic scalp. This condition is sometimes associated with pruritus or slight discomfort during the days preceding a shampoo. While these symptoms disappear with a regular shampoo, dandruff become more visible, since scales are no longer stuck to the scalp by sebum, and they are more easily shed on to the clothes and pillow.

Structure of the Sebaceous Gland

Mature sebaceous glands are holocrine lobulated structures distributed all over the skin except on the palms and soles (Fig. 3). Apart from

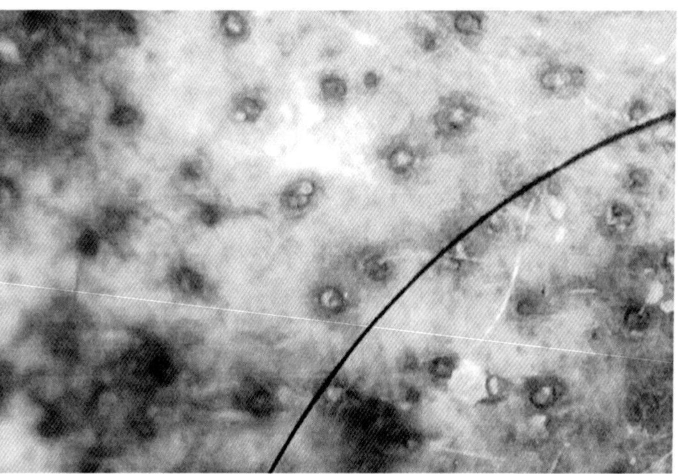

Fig. 2 Speckled perifollicular melanotic rims under Visioscan® examination

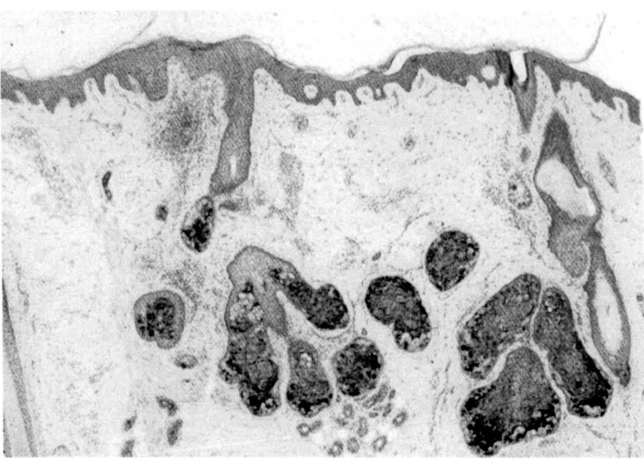

Fig. 3 Sebaceous glands highlighted by an anti-EMA (epithelial membrane antigen) antibody

specialized sites such as the eyelids and prepuce, sebaceous glands open indirectly at the skin surface via the hair follicle [8, 9]. The density of sebaceous glands differs from site to site on the body, being higher on the face and scalp followed by the back, chest, abdomen, arms, and legs. The face contains about 300–1,500 glands/cm^2, the scalp about 300–500 glands/cm^2, and other sites present 100 glands/cm^2 or less.

Three distinct types of pilosebaceous follicles are identified according to the volume of the sebaceous glands and the size of associated hairs. They are termed terminal hair follicle, vellus hair follicle, and sebaceous follicle, respectively. Terminal hair follicles are present on the scalp and beard region in men. The corresponding hair shaft is thick, and the sebaceous gland is of medium to large size reaching about 1 mm^3. Vellus hair is found over the entire body surface except on the palms, soles, and areas with terminal hair follicles. In vellus hair follicle, the hair shaft is short and thin, and the sebaceous gland is tiny when present. The sebaceous follicle is only found in humans. The gland is quite large, whereas the hair shaft is miniature and does not reach the skin surface.

The holocrine process of sebum production begins with the proliferation of basaloid undifferentiated cells located at the periphery of the acini as well as in transglandular partitioning epithelial strands. During sebocyte maturation and lipid synthesis, cells enlarge up to 150-fold in volume, and they express the epithelial membrane antigen (EMA). They move toward the ostia of the glands. Finally, the cell wall ruptures. The lipid content and the cellular remnants form the sebum that is discharged into the sebaceous duct and further to the pilosebaceous infundibulum and finally to a hair follicle opening (skin pore) [8, 9].

The pilosebaceous infundibulum forms a reservoir which commonly contains a sizable amount of sebum. The overall transit time of sebocytes takes about 2–3 weeks within the gland and a further week or so through the follicular reservoir before reaching the SC surface. The SC acts as a sponge trapping part of the sebum and eventually resorbing it [10, 11]. In these respects, the bulk of lipids present at the skin surface depends on so many variables that it does not directly reflect the metabolic events taking place in the glands themselves.

Lipid Composition of the Sebum

Skin surface lipids originate from two distinct sources, namely, the keratinizing epithelium and sebum. The composition of lipids from these two origins greatly differs. Native sebum is composed of triglycerides, wax esters, squalene, and cholesterol esters (Table 1). In mature sebocytes, vacuoles almost filling the cytoplasm contain two components that appear clearly distinct on electron microscopy. One looks opaque, cloudy, and osmium positive, probably enriched in squalene.

Table 1 Average lipid composition of sebum (%)

Component	Native sebum	Skin surface
Triglycerides	57	30–40
Wax esters	25	22–25
Squalene	15	12
Cholesterol esters	3	7
Diglycerides	0	2
Free fatty acids	0	16–25
Ceramides	0	2

The other component appears translucent and osmium-negative reflecting the presence of saturated lipids. Heparan sulfate contributes to the sebaceous gland morphogenesis [12].

Synthesis of the various components of sebum involves two different pathways including (a) squalene synthesis following the classical mevalonate and farnesyl pyrophosphate route and (b) fatty acid [13] and wax ester synthesis. Cholesterol is only present in trace amounts in native sebum because it is part of the structural compounds of the cell rather than to the sebum itself. Indeed, sebocytes do not contain the required enzymatic equipment for synthesizing cholesterol from squalene. Wax esters or squalene is generally a marker of sebum excretion helping to differentiate the sebum contribution from epidermal lipids.

Fatty acids of the triglycerides are varied, corresponding to either saturated or unsaturated compounds that are branched or not. They show straight hydrocarbon chains with even or odd numbers of carbon atoms. Wax esters contain the longest chains, with the C16 and C18 fatty acids being the most abundant.

During its transit up to the skin surface, the sebum composition is altered by oxidative processes and biodegradation partly induced by specific microorganisms [6]. Indeed, triglyceride hydrolysis by bacterial lipases gives rise to free fatty acids and mono- and diglycerides. At the skin surface, epidermal lipids are admixed with the sebum forming a spotty or continuous lipid film. In adults, the relative contribution of epidermal lipids over the SC is minimal in areas rich in sebaceous glands, although it affects the surface lipid composition on the limbs and trunk away from the midline. On the scalp and forehead, for example, epidermal lipids amount to 5–10 $\mu g/cm^2$ of the skin, whereas sebum is present at 100–700 $\mu g/cm^2$ [14].

Quantitative variations in sebum production following drug intake (e.g., retinoids, antibiotics, etc.) are likely associated with subtle changes in its molecular composition which in turn possibly alter the infundibulum cornification and be a key factor for comedogenesis.

Sebum Excretion and Spreading

Sebaceous gland dynamics involves four basic distinct and successive steps represented by sebum production (a secretion rate function), storage (a volume function), skin surface output (a delivery rate function), and SC permeation (an influx rate function). The oily appearance of the skin and hair results from an excess of sebum excretion, spreading and interacting with sweat, SC, and the hair.

On the scalp, sebum often appears as discrete droplets emerging from follicular outlets, and partly as a surface coating. The droplets are unevenly spread on the hair. In seborrheic subjects, the whole hair shaft appears to be fully coated with sebum. On the skin surface, sebum is usually accumulated in the follicular funnels from where it flows out. Sebum permeates the superficial layers of SC, but a homogenous film is only found in seborrheic subjects. Sebum migration occurs between contiguous hairs or in a swatch, due to capillary forces. After degreasing hairs, the initial refatting rate reaches about 2–3.5 mm/min.

Methods for Sebum Excretion Measurement

Subjective methods for evaluating skin and hair greasiness are available based on tactile and visual scales. Their correlation with an overall rating into five classes (very dry, dry, medium, greasy, very greasy) is convenient. These assessments are useful for the appraisal of sebum-controlling products.

Objective measurements of the sebum excretion provide better evidence of greasy skin and hair. Over the years, a wide variety of ingenious methods have been developed for measuring the amount of sebum excreted at the skin surface and present on the hair [6]. Indeed, scalp and hair sebum amounts must be distinguished because they commonly differ. Estimating the amount of scalp sebum needs a miniature sampling method, and the hair must be shaved 24–30 h before measurement. The sebum amount present at the skin surface is conveniently measured in vivo using photometric assessment and lipid-sensitive tapes. A reproducibility of about 10 % and a sensitivity threshold in the 5 μg range of lipid amounts are usually considered to be satisfactory [6].

Sebum production and secretion are not measurable in the gland itself. In contrast, sebum excretion at the skin surface after its transit within the storage and delivery units corresponding to the infundibulum reservoir is routinely measured. Several major methods contributed over the years in the evaluation of certain parameters quantifying the sebum bulk and rheology. It should be kept in mind that components of the excreted sebum are partly trapped as any xenobiotic by the SC. Hence, part of sebum is free inside the infundibulum and at the skin surface, while another part permeates onto the SC before eventually being metabolized and further resorbed.

Photometric Method

The basic principle of the photometric method relies on the fact that opalescent glass, sapphire plate, or lipid-sensitive tapes of a given opacity to light become translucent when their surfaces are coated with lipids. The photometric procedure is time-saving and highly reproducible and does not require specially trained scientific staff.

The Sebumeter® SM810 (CK Electronic) is a device that has reached popularity [6]. Sebum is absorbed into a piece of matted plastic strip 0.1 mm thick placed on a roller which is manually rewound before each measurement. The probe is pressed under constant pressure against the skin surface. Pitfalls arise from skin microrelief and roughness impairing the close contact between the probe and the SC. After the probe has been in contact with the skin surface for 30 s, measured by an internal timer, it is placed back into the main unit of the Sebumeter®. Transparency of the plastic film is measured by a photocell linked to a microprocessor after the emitted light has passed back and forth through the strip. It is acknowledged that the measures are in good agreement with the actual amount of lipids present on the strip. In fact, it is estimated that an average of about 40 % of total skin surface lipids is absorbed with one sampling. The digital readout displayed as μg/cm^2 gives the estimated total amount of lipids on the skin. In order to get valid data, it is necessary to take several samples within a given area in order to avoid the problematic heterogeneity in sebaceous gland activity. However, the calculated amounts are possibly underestimated when seborrhea is intense due to a saturation effect of the plastic strip.

The photometric method yields a single global estimate of the casual bulk of lipids present on a given surface of the skin at one point in time. The test area is large compared to the size of the ostia of sebaceous follicles. Thus, any difference between the activities of individual sebaceous follicles remains impossible to assess through this method. A few overactive sebaceous follicles releasing a large amount of sebum contribute to a disproportionate large effect on measurements.

Sebum-Sensitive Tape Method

The method using standardized hydrophobic lipid-absorbent tapes relies on opaque, open-celled, microporous polymeric films [6, 15, 16]. It is considered as complementary to and as useful as the photometric method [6, 17, 18]. The tape material has to be affixed to the skin by gentle pressure ensuring the elimination of any air bubbles. When the sebum-sensitive tape is placed on a skin area possibly moved by muscles, the investigator should periodically check that the uniform contact between tape and SC is maintained throughout the test.

Two proprietary tapes are currently available. One type is the regular Sebutape® (Cuderm Corp., Dallas, Texas) characterized by the presence of an adhesive coat on one side of the tape designed to adhere tightly to the SC. Such adhesive coat likely impairs the swift penetration of sebum into the tape. The other type of lipid-sensitive tape is designed to be applied for only a very short time to the skin surface without interfacing any adhesive coating. These commercially available tapes are the Instant Sebutape® (Cuderm Corp.) and the Sebufix® (CK Electronic).

Depending on the study design, the skin is prepared or not prior to the timed collection by removing sebum from the skin surface. The collection time should be determined according to the type of tape. With the regular Sebutape®, the adhesive interposed between the lipid-sensitive film and the skin is a limiting factor to the transfer of lipids. This is of importance when the rate of sebum excretion is low and/or when the duration of the test is short. On the other hand, a saturation effect occurs on regular Sebutape® when evaluating intense seborrhea during a test period beyond about 30 min. The amount of sebum collected over uninterrupted period of time is in fact lower than the addition of shorter sebum collections for a similar cumulative period of time. This is associated with confluence of sebum droplets and inaccuracy in identifying each spot as a single sebaceous follicle. These features are the main reasons why sebum samplings longer than about 30 min should be avoided when using regular Sebutape®. When using one of the uncoated sebum-sensitive tapes, a contact time of 30 s or so is appropriate.

During the procedure, each follicular outlet enriched in sebum pours out lipids which fill pores of the tape rendering it focally transparent. The size of the clear spots is proportional to the amount of sebum delivered. The number of spots reflects the number of sebum-rich follicular ostia. These parameters are conveniently evaluated by visual inspection alone. Looking at samples against a black background in reflectance mode results in a black and white pattern that can be assessed using an ordinal scale. The method allows to obtain a rough but reasonable estimate of skin greasiness without requiring sophisticated equipment.

Better quantitative assessments are achieved using computerized image analysis [16–21], which represents the most sensitive and accurate method (Fig. 4) when offering the possibility of recording the number and size of individual spots and calculating the mean and total area of spots (TAS). The free sebum content of follicular reservoir is conveniently assessed using Sebufix® tapes affixed onto a recording video camera working under ultraviolet light illumination (Visioscan VC 98®, CK Electronic). Computer-assisted image analysis provides proper readings [21]. A

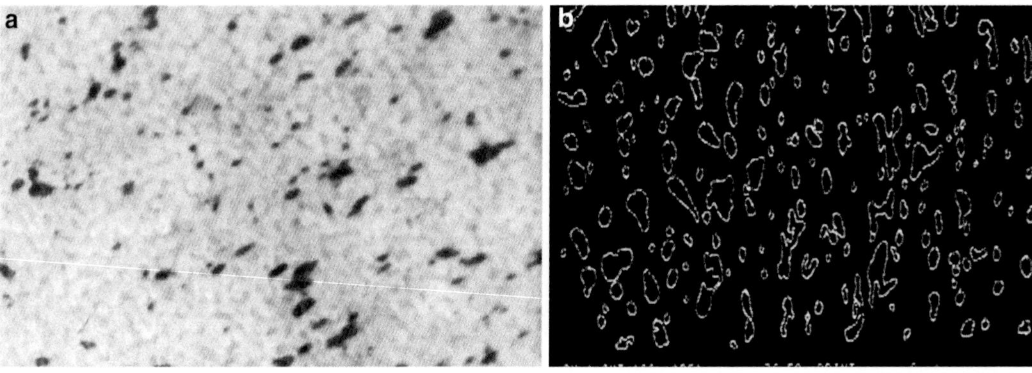

Fig. 4 Aspect of a computerized image from a lipid-sensitive tape. (**a**) The *black dots* represent the sebum output at the follicular orifices. (**b**) Higher magnification of the *dots* allowing measurements of sizes and shapes

built-in microprocessor providing such information is present in the device.

A photometric evaluation obtained by measuring the intensity of light transmitted through the samples is an alternative rapid approach [19] and is roughly equivalent to the TAS value obtained by image analysis. A variant is represented by reflectance colorimetric assessment of the samples placed against a colored background [20]. However, such overall quantitative approaches lose one of the main benefits of the lipid-absorbent tape method, namely, the evaluation of sebum excretion at single individual sebaceous follicles.

A similar quantitative method was designed aiming at collecting data any time during the tape application onto the skin [21]. The basic principle relies on the measurement of the color modifications of the tape that occur when it becomes transparent. It shifts the natural "white" color of the tape to a color closer to that of the skin itself. Reflectance colorimetry is conveniently expressed as DE*ab. The benefit of such an approach is the ability to obtain multiple measurements without removing the tape and therefore to explore a continuous reading of the kinetics of sebum output.

There are some limitations to the proper interpretation of the data. Some are specifically related to the material itself. Sebum spots are subject to changes in their size and transparency depending on storage time and temperature. At 20 °C or so, they should be evaluated at a defined time after removal, preferably within 24 h. When immediate evaluation is not possible, storage in a freezer at −30 °C is advisable.

Combined Methods

When using lipid-sensitive tapes alone, the interpretation of the number and size of lipid droplets with regard to the sebaceous glands is occasionally uncertain. In fact, it is not valid to ascribe a single follicular outlet to each spot, particularly when the latter is large. In order to solve such uncertainty, a two-step method was designed [11]. Before removing the sebum-sensitive tape from the skin, its outlines are delineated on the SC with an ink mark. In a second step, a cyanoacrylate skin surface stripping [22] using a cyanoacrylate-coated polyester film (3S-Biokit, CK Technology, Visé, Belgium) is collected from that site. The CSSS conveniently exhibits follicular casts and microcomedones [6, 8, 22, 23]. The ink marks of the outlines of sebum-sensitive film are harvested on this material. The skin surface stripping and the corresponding lipid-sensitive tape are then exactly superposed using the ink imprint as an adjusting mark. This dual material is examined under the microscope and processed in a computerized image analyzer. This method allows simultaneous assessment of the size of lipid droplets and that of the corresponding follicular ostia and microcomedones [17].

A surrogate method relies on examination using a video camera working under ultraviolet light illumination (Visioscan VC98®, CK Electronic). A frame designed to precisely attach and locate the camera is first affixed onto the test site. The aspect of the skin surface and follicular outlets is recorded. In a second step, a Sebufix® is interposed between the SC and the camera. The picture of lipid droplets is recorded after a 45-s collection. The comparison of both pictures identifies sebum-poor and sebum-rich follicles [21, 23].

Quantitative Parameters of Sebum Excretion

The various sampling procedures of sebum provide information about a series of specific parameters. As a rule, the values obtained for these parameters commonly differ among subjects by a tenfold coefficient, but each value is a representative of a given subject in a precise environment.

Sebum Casual Level

Sebum casual level (CL) is defined as the lipid amount present at equilibrium when the skin surface remains untouched for several hours. It is a global estimate of skin greasiness. For practical reasons, most researchers record CL generally after a 4-h lag time following uncontrolled removal of the sebum film from the skin surface. It is expected but uncertain that such CL measurement reflects a plateau value. CL is not recommended as a single parameter for in-depth studies of the sebaceous system. Therefore, CL is believed to represent a rough estimate of a constant value for each normal adult. In contrast, interindividual variations are large as shown by CL ranging from 100 to 700 μg/cm^2 on the forehead of healthy subjects. Similar wide variations are found on the scalp.

Sebum Excretion Rate

Sebum excretion rate (SER) refers to the amount of sebum excreted on a given skin area during a defined period of time [6]. The duration of the collection period is important because SER progressively decreases over the first hours after degreasing the skin. SER of the first hour sampling from the forehead usually ranges from 0.5 to 2.5 μg/cm^2/min. On the scalp, it varies from 0.1 to 0.8 μg/cm^2/min. TAS values yielded by the lipid-sensitive tape method represent a surrogate of SER evaluations.

SER is expected to be roughly correlated with CL. A linear relationship is commonly yielded between four successive 1-h SER and TAS measurements at least in the medium range of severity of seborrhea. The correlation is lost when the sebum output is either very low or quite high. This finding indicates that these parameters are related to the delivery of the pool of sebum already secreted by the gland and stored in the sebum reservoir corresponding to the distal portion of pilosebaceous duct. Thus, it is clear that an initial 3–4-h collection is a measurement of sebum excretion rather than sebum secretion.

Sebum Replacement Time

Sebum replacement time appears to be a cumbersome parameter difficult to manage. It refers to the expected time duration needed to recover CL after sebum removal from the skin surface. It has been reported to take about 4 h in subjects with sebum excretion in the medium range.

Density in Sebum-Enriched Reservoirs

The number of spots over a lipid-sensitive tape is a rough indicator of the density of follicular reservoirs enriched in sebum. Such a figure is usually lower than the number of sebaceous glands present on that area of the skin. This information can be confirmed by staining CSSS for lipids. The sebum delivery at a given follicular ostium represents a clue for the presence of an actively secreting sebaceous gland. It occasionally represents the site of a follicular reservoir passively filled by the sebum coming from the skin surface. It is clear using the combination of lipid-sensitive tape and CSSS that many follicular ostia neither store sebum nor represent a route for sebum outflow. It is also possible that one single droplet corresponds to a merging of several smaller ones. The size of the follicular outlet at the skin surface is not correlated with the presence or absence of sebum [17].

Instant Sebum Delivery

SER and TAS decrease almost linearly during the initial hours of collection time. Calculating the regression line for the cumulative data at hourly intervals allows to extrapolate a theoretical value for instant sebum delivery (ISD) at T0. This parameter supposedly reflects the spontaneous leakage of free sebum from the follicular reservoirs. ISD is not always correlated with SER. Information similar to ISD is provided by the Sebufix® tape applied to the skin for a few seconds.

Follicular Excretion Rate

The slope of the above-mentioned regression line between cumulative TAS over time has been coined follicular excretion rate (FER). It is a measure of the delivery rate of sebum from the follicular reservoirs. FER is frequently related to the first hour TAS value, although physiological influences and some topical compounds interfere with such a relationship.

Factors Affecting Sebum Excretion

Physicochemical Regulation

SER and FER are influenced by the physicochemical characteristics of sebum. Environmental and skin temperatures and the balance between the sebum molecular components affect the viscosity and rheology of lipids at the skin surface [24]. This could explain in part some chronobiological variations in SER and FER including seasonal fluctuations [25–27] as well as the influence of the ovarian cycle [28, 29] and perhaps other chronobiological rhythms of unknown periodicity. A circadian rhythm has been suggested for sebum output being optimal in the midmorning and minimal during late evening and early morning hours [29].

The width of follicular ostium greatly influences sebum rheology. There is an inverse relationship between the fluid flux and the fourth power of the radius of the tube in which the fluid passes through. Hence, variations in corneocyte accumulation and swelling at the lips of follicular outlets, occurring during the ovarian cycle or after occlusion, probably influence sebum rheology [28, 29].

Skin surface energy phenomena result from molecular interactions. They are involved in sebum and sweat dispersion. Sweating is indeed an important confounding factor in rating sebum excretion. Even in dry-skinned subjects, intensive or continuous sweating increases the CL. The sebum of seborrheic subjects appears as an oily and homogeneous fluid barely emulsified with water at ordinary temperatures. However, in some instances, it can be emulsified with sweat though it generally takes several hours.

The theory of a continuous sebum excretion is opposed to the concept of a discontinuous excretion with a feedback control by the CL. SER appears to decline progressively as CL returns to its initial value. This observation supported the hypothesis of a feedback mechanism controlling sebaceous excretion by the lipid film developed on the skin surface. This concept was further strengthened by the fact that the amounts of sebum collected at constant time intervals seem to increase with the number of degreasing procedures. Sebum excretion stops spontaneously even in highly seborrheic subjects if the area, although isolated, remains uncovered. However, the plateau effect in excretion kinetics is only apparent and due to the sebum spreading over a larger surface or to its permeation into the upper layers of the SC. It is concluded that the initial phase of sebaceous secretion is likely continuous or fluctuating as a result of the combination of chronobiological rhythms. Any feedback mechanism from CL could only affect the sebum excretion thus modifying sebum storage rather than sebum production.

Shampoos dedicated to greasy hair are commonly used as sebum-controlling products for the scalp. Some chitosan-derived molecules hinder sebum coating of the hair shaft. Particles of dry shampoos adhere to the hair, retain lipids, and exert electrostatic forces repulsing the hair shafts. Frequent regular shampoos do not appear to increase the sebum output on the scalp and do not influence the sebum coating of the hair. By contrast, cationic polymers and silicone oils used in some shampoos facilitate sebum spreading. Regreasing studies on the scalp and hair show general differences according to the level of greasiness. Hair sebum amount is typically lower than the accumulation of scalp sebum. Scalp CL recovers completely after 1–4 days following hair washing, at least for greasy hair types [30], and the aspect remains fairly constant in the following days. Scalp SER has been reported to progressively increase until 24 h after shampooing when it reaches its maximum value.

Hormonal Regulation

The human skin, in particular the sebaceous glands, receives, produces, and coordinates hormone activation and inactivation through various molecular signals. The involved physiological mechanisms belong to the endocrine, paracrine, juxtacrine, autocrine, and intracrine hormonal repertoire.

Free testosterone and 3α-dihydrotestosterone (DHT) are considered to exert a major boosting and dose-related effect on sebocyte proliferation and sebum secretion in man [31]. The levels of type 1 isoform of 5α-reductase are significantly higher in sebaceous glands than in other skin structures [31, 32]. Cells of the infundibulum are also reported to be sensitive to the same hormones. In women, the most important androgen is Δ^4-androstenedione, which is produced by adrenal gland and ovaries. It is possibly converted into testosterone, but it has some intrinsic androgenic activity. The 5α-androstane-3β, 17β-diol compound is a potent androgen and is the main metabolite of testosterone in the back and scalp skin. Other androgen precursors of purely adrenal origin such as dehydroepiandrosterone (DHEA) explain sebaceous development in the fetus, in the newborn, and in the prepubertal years [33]. DHEA is converted into androstenedione and testosterone inside the sebocytes. By contrast, conversion of DHEA sulfate to DHEA only occurs with the assistance of monocytes exhibiting steroid sulfatase activity. The amount of circulating androgens is important to consider. However, the local production of sexual steroids provides autonomous control adjusting sexual steroid metabolism according to the body area. Facial and scalp sebocytes are particularly involved in this mechanism.

The glucocorticoid receptor is another nuclear steroid receptor present in sebocytes. Glucocorticoids have been reported to stimulate sebocyte proliferation [31].

The second group of nuclear receptors, namely, the thyroid receptor family, encompasses different soluble receptors in sebocytes. They correspond to the thyroid hormone receptor isotype β1, the estrogen receptor β, the retinoic acid receptor (RAR) isotypes α and γ, retinoid X receptor (RXR) isotypes α, β, and γ, and the peroxisome proliferator-related receptor (PPAR) isotypes α, δ, and γ. PPAR ligands augment the androgen stimulation of sebocyte differentiation [34].

Estrogens exert the opposite effect of androgens but with a much weaker potency. However, any decrease in size and excretion of sebaceous glands is only achieved with high doses of estrogens that are nonphysiological in women and feminizing in men. It is thus unlikely that normal estrogen levels play any role in inhibiting sebaceous gland activity. Following estrogen suppression, administration of testosterone restores sebum secretion. Estrogens at sebum-suppressive doses have been shown to reduce plasma and urine levels of testosterone. They also inhibit gonadotropin-releasing hormone synthesis and 5α-reductase activity.

There is no established relationship between the growth rate of vellus hairs and sebum excretion. By contrast, the intensity of seborrhea and severity of evolving androgenic alopecia are often related. In this condition, GH and IGF-1 might play a role.

Neuropeptide Regulation

A neurovegetative nerve plexus surrounds the sebaceous gland, but acetylcholine and adrenaline do not seem to influence sebum secretion. Sympathectomy has no effect on the level of surface lipids. A localized neurological lesion conversely induces seborrhea in the involved site. Several types of neuropeptide receptors are present in sebocytes. They include the μ-opiate receptor which binds β-endorphin, the vasoactive intestinal polypeptide (VIP) receptor, the neuropeptide Y receptor, and the calcitonin gene-related peptide (CGRP) receptor.

Psychotropic drugs, often dopamine inhibitors, increase sebaceous secretion considerably. The same observation is present in Parkinson's disease [35] perhaps due to high α-MSH serum levels. During treatment with levodopa, seborrhea decreases, although the drug is inactive on sebaceous excretion in normal subjects.

Ethnic, Gender, and Age Effects

Some specific attributes related to sebum excretion have been ascribed to ethnic groups [36]. Such observation awaits for confirmation.

As a consequence of the diversity of hormonal signals, sebum excretion varies according to age, gender, and the perimenopausal period [37–39]. At any given age in men and women, both sebum excretion and secretion rates differ between individuals over a wide range. In addition, there is a huge overlap between data gained in both genders. Hence, it is not the amount of circulating androgens, but rather the receptivity of the target tissues that accounts for interindividual differences in sebum excretion. It is clear that other additional factors are likely to be involved.

SER and FER values remain high in men until the eighth decade. In women the rates remain unchanged until menopause. During the perimenopausal period, seborrhea either increases or steadily decreases with age. Using the lipid-sensitive tapes, it is possible to distinguish distinct patterns according to age and physiopathological conditions [36]. The size of follicular reservoirs and pores shows no tendency to shrink with age.

A series of endocrine imbalances and a few drug treatments aiming or not at direct or indirect hormonal effects affect the activity of sebaceous apparatus. The most potent inhibitor of sebum excretion is the synthetic retinoid 13-*cis*-retinoic acid or isotretinoin, which at oral doses of 0.1–1 mg/kg/day inhibits sebum production by up to 80 % within 6–8 weeks. Isotretinoin reduces cell renewal and lipid formation in the sebaceous gland. Isotretinoin reduces not only SER but also the follicular reservoir, and both remain significantly suppressed for up to 1 year after therapy. Topical products are far less potent although of cosmetic interest [40, 41].

Conclusions

The current knowledge of sebaceous gland physiology and sebum rheology on the glabrous skin, scalp, and hair shaft has made some progress, leading to the introduction of new antiseborrheic agents. This breakthrough was made possible through the development of qualitative and quantitative methods for measuring the amounts of excreted sebum and evaluating its lipid composition.

Seborrhea on the scalp and forehead possibly represents a single phenomenon or be part of a more complex system of multiple disturbances. As an interesting index of neuroendocrine physiology, it plays an increasing role in the understanding of biology, mainly due to the reliability of its measurement.

The sebum flow is altered with aging. In any study in this field, ethnicity, age range, gender, adequate skin profile, and test area on the body must be appropriate for a relevant design. The environmental conditions including seasons, relative humidity, and temperature should be controlled. In addition, skin temperature affects sebum rheology. A number of other physiological parameters modulate sebum excretion, and some of them are responsible for chronobiological variations. Despite clever experimental designs, it should be stressed that panelists, subjective perceptions, clinical gradings, and biometrological measurements are not always matched.

Several objective methods have been devised for measuring the greasiness of skin, most of which involve the collection of sebum once it runs off the sebaceous apparatus. Preconditioning the skin by prior removal of sebum from the skin surface is a common procedure. Part of the sebum present inside the follicular reservoir is potentially ignored by measurements. Uncontrolled depletion of the sebum pool impedes collection of reliable data.

Conceptually, aging of the sebum production in women begins in the perimenopausal period after menopause. It is obvious in men well after entering the andropause period. In both genders, the early changes are often erratic, and they progressively evolve to a reduction of the sebum flow.

References

1. Grice EA. The skin microbiome: potential for novel diagnostic and therapeutic approaches to cutaneous disease. Semin Cutan Med Surg. 2014;33:98–103.
2. Jahns AC, et al. Propionibacterium species and follicular keratinocyte activation in acneic and normal skin. Br J Dermatol. 2015;172:981–987.

3. Porta Guardia CA. Demodex folliculorum: its association with oily skin surface rather than rosacea lesions. Int J Dermatol. 2015;54:e14–7.
4. Szepetiuk G, et al. Recent trends in specular light reflectance beyond clinical fluorescence diagnosis. Eur J Dermatol. 2011;21:157–61.
5. Piérard-Franchimont C, et al. Sun addiction, its death blow and the multitude of sunscreens. Rev Med Liege. 2013;68:321–5.
6. Piérard GE, et al. EEMCO guidance for the in vivo assessment of skin greasiness. The EEMCO Group. Skin Pharmacol Appl Skin Physiol. 2000;13:372–89.
7. Petit L, et al. Subclinical speckled perifollicular melanosis of the scalp. Eur J Dermatol. 2002;12:565–8.
8. Uhoda E, et al. The conundrum of skin pores in dermocosmetology. Dermatology. 2005;210:3–7.
9. Kim SJ, et al. Pore volume is most highly correlated with the visual assessment of skin pores. Skin Res Technol. 2014;20:429–34.
10. Blanc D, et al. An original procedure for quantitation of cutaneous resorption of sebum. Arch Dermatol Res. 1989;281:346–50.
11. Piérard-Franchimont C, et al. Sebum rheology evaluated by two methods in vivo. Split-face study of the effect of a cosmetic formulation. Eur J Dermatol. 1999;9:455–7.
12. Coulson-Thomas VJ, et al. Heparan sulfate regulates hair follicle and sebaceous gland morphogenesis and homeostasis. J Biol Chem. 2014;289:25211–26.
13. Akaza N, et al. Fatty acid compositions of triglycerides and free fatty acids in sebum depend on amount of triglycerides, and do not differ in presence or absence of acne vulgaris. J Dermatol. 2014;41:1069–76.
14. Boncheva M. The physical chemistry of the stratum corneum lipids. Int J Cosmet Sci. 2014;36:505–15.
15. Nordstrom KM, et al. Measurement of sebum output using a lipid absorbent tape. J Invest Dermatol. 1986;87:260–3.
16. Piérard GE. Follicule to follicule heterogeneity of sebum excretion. Dermatologica. 1986;173:61–5.
17. Piérard GE. Rate and topography of follicular sebum excretion. Dermatologica. 1987;175:280–3.
18. Pagnoni A, et al. An improved procedure for quantitative analysis of sebum production using Sebutape. J Soc Cosmet Chem. 1994;45:221–5.
19. Piérard GE, Piérard-Franchimont C. Effect of a topical erythromycin-zinc formulation on sebum delivery. Evaluation by combined photometric-multi-step samplings with Sebutape. Clin Exp Dermatol. 1993;18:410–3.
20. Piérard GE, et al. Kinetics of sebum excretion evaluated by the Sebutape – Chromameter technique. Skin Pharmacol. 1993;6:38–44.
21. Piérard-Franchimont C, Piérard GE. Postmenopausal aging of the sebaceous follicle: a comparison between women receiving hormone replacement therapy or not. Dermatology. 2002;204:17–22.
22. Piérard GE, et al. Cyanoacrylate skin surface stripping and the 3S-Biokit advent in tropical dermatology: a look from Liege. Sci World J. 2014;2014:462634.
23. Piérard GE, et al. Digital image analysis of microcomedones. Dermatology. 1995;190:99–103.
24. El Khyat A, et al. Skin critical surface tension. A way to assess the skin wettability quantitatively. Skin Res Technol. 1996;2:91–6.
25. Piérard-Franchimont C, et al. Seasonal modulation of sebum excretion. Dermatologica. 1990;181:21–2.
26. Youn SW, et al. Regional and seasonal variations in facial sebum secretions: a proposal for the definition of combination skin type. Skin Res Technol. 2005;11: 189–95.
27. Song EJ, et al. A study on seasonal variation of skin parameters in Korean males. Int J Cosmet Sci. 2015;37:92–7.
28. Piérard-Franchimont C, et al. Rhythm of sebum excretion during the menstrual cycle. Dermatologica. 1991;182:211–3.
29. Verschoore M, et al. Circadian variations in the number of actively secreting sebaceous follicles and androgen circadian rhythms. Chronobiol Int. 1993;10:349–59.
30. Black D, et al. An improved method for the measurement of scalp sebum. Curr Probl Dermatol. 1998;26:61–8.
31. Thiboutot D, et al. Activity of the type 1 5 alpha-reductase exhibits regional differences in isolated sebaceous glands and whole skin. J Invest Dermatol. 1995;105:209–14.
32. Zouboulis CC, et al. The human sebocyte culture model provides new insights into development and management of seborrhoea and acne. Dermatology. 1998;196:21–31.
33. Rutkowski K, et al. Dehydroepiandrosterone (DHEA): hypes and hopes. Drugs. 2014;74:1195–207.
34. Rosenfield RL, et al. Mechanisms of androgen induction of sebocyte differentiation. Dermatology. 1998;196:43–6.
35. Martignoni E, et al. Is seborrhea a sign of autonomic impairment in Parkinson's disease? J Neural Transm. 1997;104:1295–304.
36. Nouveau-Richard S, et al. Oily skin: specific features in Chinese women. Skin Res Technol. 2007;13:43–8.
37. Piérard GE, et al. Patterns of follicular sebum excretion rate during lifetime. Arch Dermatol Res. 1987;279 (Suppl):S104–7.
38. Callens A, et al. Does hormonal skin aging exist? A study of the influence of different hormone therapy regimens on the skin of postmenopausal women using non-invasive measurement techniques. Dermatology. 1996;193:289–94.
39. Caisey L, et al. Influence of age and hormone replacement therapy on the functional properties of the lips. Skin Res Technol. 2008;14:220–5.
40. Piérard GE, Cauwenbergh G. Modulation of sebum excretion from the follicular reservoir by a dichlorophenyl-imidazoldioxolan. Int J Cosmet Sci. 1996;18:219–27.
41. Piérard GE, et al. New insight into the topical management of excessive sebum flow at the skin surface. Dermatology. 1998;196:126–9.

Perimenopausal Aging and Oral Hormone Replacement Therapy

59

Trinh Hermanns-Lê, Claudine Piérard-Franchimont, and Gérald E. Piérard

Contents

T. Hermanns-Lê
Laboratory of Skin Bioengineering and Imaging, Department of Dermatopathology, University Hospital of Liège, Liège, Belgium

Electron Microscopy Unit, Department of Dermatopathology, Unilab Lg, University Hospital of Liège, Liège, Belgium
e-mail: trinh.hermanns@chu.ulg.ac.be

C. Piérard-Franchimont
Laboratory of Skin Bioengineering and Imaging, Department of Dermatopathology, University Hospital of Liège, Liège, Belgium

Department of Dermatology, Regional Hospital of Huy, Huy, Belgium
e-mail: claudine.franchimont@ulg.ac.be

G.E. Piérard (✉)
Laboratory of Skin Bioengineering and Imaging, Department of Dermatopathology, University Hospital of Liège, Liège, Belgium
e-mail: Gerald.pierard@ulg.ac.be

M.A. Farage et al. (eds.), *Textbook of Aging Skin*,
DOI 10.1007/978-3-662-47398-6_34

Abstract
Healthy aging in women is a physiological process modulated by special features particularly occurring during the perimenopausal period. The dermal extracellular matrix is involved in this process linked to hypoestrogenemia. In these instances, the skin presentation is occasionally indicative of some distinct internal failures. Measuring the in vivo mechanical functions of skin represents a convenient means for quantifying the perimenopausal skin changes. Such assessments have shown a beneficial effect of hormone replacement therapy on the skin status.

Introduction

Healthy aging in humans is a physiological process characterized by a progressive decrement in homeostatic capacity of the organism, ultimately increasing the vulnerability to a series of environmental threats and to certain disease status. Obviously, the clinical expression of the healthy aging process evolves at different rates among individuals of similar ages. Genders distinctly influence this process. In addition, any given subject shows a variety of aging status among his/her organs and among each of their constituent tissues, cells, and subcellular structures, as well as in the extracellular matrix (ECM) [1]. Some molecular aspects of skin aging are progressively uncovered [2]. Within each organ system, aging usually manifests as progressive and almost linear regression changes in maximal function and reserve capacity.

The global woman appearance is particularly appreciated through her skin aspect, reflecting in part her global health. Menopause represents a specific time initiated by the permanent cessation of menstruations following the failure of ovarian activity. It represents a turning point of importance in women's life. In addition, the menopause effects on skin are intermingled with age-associated physiologic decrements resulting from acute and chronic environmental insults [3–5]. Hence, menopause appears to spot a decline in skin qualities [6, 7]. Any skin tissue is subject to alterations, including the epidermis, dermis, hypodermis, and hair.

A progressive transition phase takes place from regular ovulatory cycles to the menopausal status. A series of peculiar hormonal and clinical alterations reflect the decline in ovarian activity. Perimenopause represents the period of time separating the reproductive period of life from the postmenopausal years. It includes the last years preceding menopause when typical endocrine and biologic changes associated with menopause are occurring, as well as the first year following menopausal amenorrhea. Postmenopause is defined as the time thereafter.

In general, life expectancy of women is substantially longer than that of men, but women commonly experience greater burdens of morbidity and disability. In many social groups, the rapid trend in the proportion of the aging population, combined with the increasing feminization of aging, contributes to the need for a sharp focus on gender issues in this matter. As the proportion of older women grows at rapid rates in the global population, the challenges of learning more about the skin condition of this group is welcome. Menopause exerts a potential etiological role in some age-related diseases and particular physiological conditions. One of the medical priorities concerns research about the physiology and treatment of perimenopause [8–10]. Risk factors of specific diseases and health needs are both likely to change as women enter that period of life. The continuing increase of woman life expectancy has resulted in a marked increase of women living years beyond menopause. Indeed, women nowadays expect to live one third of their lives in a potential deficient hormonal status. Using age 50 as a proxy for menopause, about 25 million women presently undergo menopause each year. By 2030, the world population of postmenopausal women is expected to increase to about 1.2 billion, with 50 million or so new entrants each year [6].

Menopause in the Overall Aging Process

Menopause probably represents a milestone in the women aging process. It corresponds to a universal and global evolution showing many different presentations. Physical growth and senescence are both characterized by cumulative progression of potentially interlocking biologic events. They are not always separated in the timetable of life, and they occasionally proceed in tandem. There is evidence that depletion in estrogens exerts a prominent influence on aging of a series of body systems including bones, the cardiovascular system, and skin [11]. For years, the rationale for hormone replacement therapy (HRT) designed for menopausal women appeared straightforward for many physicians. Such replenishment therapy convincingly showed evidence for alleviating some aspects of skin atrophy and xerosis in peri- and postmenopausal women [6, 11–13].

Conceptually, healthy global aging in humans was initially perceived as one single basic physiological decline progressing with age. Over the past decades, the understanding of aging skin considerably expanded, with emphasis on differentiating intrinsic chronological aging from photoaging resulting from habitual chronic sun exposures [3]. The action spectrum of photodamages is not fully characterized, but it is acknowledged that the cumulative effects from repeated exposures to suberythemal doses of ultraviolet (UV) B and UVA on human skin are responsible for photoaging. The role of UVB in elastin promoter activation in photoaging is clearly established. In addition, UVA radiations contribute largely to long-term actinic damages. The spectral dependency for cumulative damages does not parallel the erythema spectrum for acute UV injury on human skin. Near-infrared (IR) radiations bring additional deleterious effects contributing to skin aging.

Such a concept based on a dual process in skin aging has been challenged because it appeared as an oversimplification in the reality of life. Another more diversified classification of skin aging in seven distinct types was offered [14]. In that model, the most important causative variables include the past and present lifestyle, the endocrine and overall metabolic status, several environmental threats including cumulative UV light and IR radiations, as well as repeated mechanical solicitations originating from muscles and external gravitational forces (Table 1). In such a framework, perimenopausal aging is individualized and emphasized as a major endocrine facet of aging. Healthy global aging is considered to result from the cumulative or synergistic effects of each abovementioned specific cause. Increased awareness of the distinct age-associated physiological changes in the skin including menopause effects allows for promoting more effective preventive measures, skin care regimens, and cutaneous treatment strategies. The immutability of skin aging is challenged by this way.

In such a context, skin aging appears as a notoriously complex process. In particular, the ideal appearance, structural integrity, and functional capacity of the skin require an adequate balance between a series of hormonal influences. Any alteration in this controlled system results in significant changes in skin qualities. Among hormones, estrogens and the other sex steroids exert profound influences on both skin development and composition [6, 7, 11, 13–15]. The relative hypoestrogenemia associated with menopause contributes to and probably exacerbates any other deleterious effect of age. Therefore, a gender perspective is required for a full understanding of skin aging. Both from the physiologic and psychosocial viewpoints, the determinants of global aging are closely related to the skin aspect and to the gender. The two past decades or so has

Table 1 Types of cutaneous aging

Aging type	Determinant factor
Genetic	Genetic (premature aging syndromes, phototype related)
Chronologic	Time
Actinic	Ultraviolet and infrared irradiations
Behavioral	Diet, tobacco, alcoholic abuse, drug addiction, facial expressions
Endocrine	Pregnancy, physiological and hormonal influences (ovaries, testes, thyroid)
Catabolic	Chronic intercurrent debilitating disease (infections, cancers)
Gravitational	Earth gravity

witnessed progresses in understanding the hormonal involvement in the global aging process [1, 7, 14].

Gender-Linked Aging

The effects of estrogens have been extensively studied on several body systems including the skin [6, 11–13]. Since their introduction as therapeutic agents, estrogens were acknowledged to exhibit some antiaging effects on women skin because several critical functions of the skin are hormone dependent. In particular, estrogen receptors and their associated proteins are involved [6, 15].

The regular ovarian cycle results from complex interactions between the hypothalamus, pituitary gland, and ovaries. It is further modulated by higher cortical centers, the thyroid gland, the adrenals, and some peripheral hormonal productions. The ovulatory cycle starts with the recruitment of a series of follicles from which one becomes dominant and is the source of ovulation. From puberty to menopause, about 200,000 follicles give rise to 500 mature ovocytes or so. Hence, atresia appears as a dominant and continuous process in ovarian physiology. This process is a key element leading to menopause [6]. During the regular menstrual cycle, estradiol acts as the dominant estrogen, reaching a peak level at the time of ovulation. Circulating levels of FSH and LH are characterized by a mid-cycle surge. During perimenopause, the function of the ovaries is progressively disturbed and failing.

The transition phase from regular ovulatory cycles to the perimenopause is characterized by variations in the ovarian cycle length and bleeding pattern. Women who experience menopause at a young age usually have a short transition phase. By contrast, menopause of later occurrence is commonly associated with a variety of long and short intermenstrual bleeding episodes, combined with an overall increased mean cycle length. During the transition phase of perimenopause, there is a large variability in sex steroid production including estrogen release. The amount in circulating estradiol varies from cycle to cycle, probably representing varying degrees of follicular maturation and function.

The perimenopausal ovaries require greater amounts of FSH to stimulate estrogen production. The most sensitive clue for declining ovarian function during perimenopause relies on the assessments of serum gonadotropins, particularly FSH. The initial dramatic rise of FSH during perimenopause is followed by a slow decline over the ensuing decades. Of note, LH levels commonly remain unaltered in the face of elevated FSH.

Contrary to an older belief, estradiol levels do not gradually wane in the years preceding menopause, but remain in the normal range until follicular growth and development cease [6]. In contrast to estrogens and progestins, androgen levels remain stable during the transitional period. Androstenedione, testosterone, dehydroepiandrostenedione (DHEA), and DHEA-sulfate (DHEAS) do not show any change in circulating concentrations during the time prior to menopause.

Skin Perimenopausal Aging

Estrogens and other sex steroids exert profound influences on both skin biology and structure. It is acknowledged that adequate hormone levels are required for controlling the skin structural integrity and functional capacity. Sex steroids clearly exert a key role in the skin aging process as evidenced by the decline in skin appearance from the perimenopausal years onward. Histological aspects have demonstrated the presence of estrogen and progesterone receptors in the skin and a relative decline in their expression from the time of perimenopause [15, 16]. In addition, aromatase activity is present in fibroblasts, adipocytes, and sebocytes in postmenopausal women. As a result, androgens are possibly switched in situ to estrogens.

Estrogen receptors are present in epidermal and dermal cells [6]. However, their regional distribution within the skin varies considerably in keeping with the concentrations present within the female genital tract. A high estrogen/androgen receptor ratio is present in the vagina, and a reverse ratio with an increase in androgen receptors and a decrease in both estrogen and progesterone receptors is present in the vulva.

Menopause and the effects of its suited HRT still leave a great many challenges unresolved particularly in the skin. The issues of HRT effects are not yet resolved on a series of physiological functions of the epidermis and dermis. In that field, dissensions and controversies are rife, and glaring discrepancies remain present in the current literature. In a global view, HRT appears to markedly improve perimenopausal changes in many organs including the skin [7, 17, 18]. The bulk of recent studies confirm that both estrogens and estro-progestins effectively suppress the perimenopausal syndrome, the genital atrophy, and they significantly decrease the risk of osteoporotic fractures.

The influence of menopause on skin and its correction by HRT and specific topical treatments are frequently difficult to objectively notice by clinical inspection alone. However, several relevant aspects are conveniently rated in a semiquantitative manner. The visual and tactile perceptions of skin characteristics represent valuable tools in clinical dermocosmetology. However, they lack sensitivity and reproducibility when comparative assessments are performed over prolonged periods of time. In addition, the clinical skin appearance is sometimes misleading compared to the actual changes induced by HRT. By contrast, noninvasive and analytic objective methods of biometrology are more suited for improving the reliability and preciseness of assessments.

Some skin changes of perimenopausal aging are detected early in this age period, at a stage when HRT might be of benefit to control them well before the postmenopausal stage. A series of cutaneous changes observed in the decade following menopause are both age and hormone related [7, 8, 17]. A number of postmenopausal women commonly complain of xerosis, easily bruising, and wrinkled skin. Dermal thickness seemingly decreases with time after menopause. It has been reported that the decline in dermal collagen content occurred at a rapid rate soon after menopause and became more gradual thereafter [6]. Approximately 30 % of skin collagen was reported to be lost in the first 5 years after menopause, with an average decline of about 2 % each postmenopausal year over a period of 20 years [6]. In this context, it is difficult to distinguish the consequences of menopause from age-associated changes related to a decline in growth hormone (GH). Indeed, both estrogen and GH depletions are combined in aging women [1].

The relative estrogen reduction at perimenopause contributes to and exacerbates the negative effects of age. As a consequence, the effects of HRT on skin have deservedly attracted much interest [6, 8, 18], although the issue remains somewhat controversial [8, 19, 20]. Anyway, the bulk of the literature indicates that hypoestrogenemia has a detrimental effect on skin collagen content, which is partially addressed by HRT. The maximum effect at preventing dermal aging appears to occur when HRT is initiated early in the perimenopausal years [6]. By contrast, short-term treatments fail to bring significant improvements of the skin condition [19, 20]. Some controversial data are found in the literature [8].

HRT and the Dermal Extracellular Matrix

The dermis contains a tough ECM supporting various structures embedded in it. Extracellular matrix (ECM) contains highly stable fiber networks, predominantly made of collagen and elastin. Fibrillar collagen represents about 80 % of the dry weight of adult skin. It exhibits high tensile strength and prevents the skin from being torn by overstretching. Elastic fibers compose about 5 % of the dermis and serve to recoil the skin to its initial shape after deformation. Fibroblasts and dermal dendrocytes synthesize and control the ECM components. Optical and electron microscopy reveals that the collagen fibrous network on sun-protected skin areas is thinner and less compact in aged people. The interstitial material interposed between collagen bundles contains hyaluronic acid and other glycosaminoglycans.

Molecular biology, histomorphology, and ultrastructure have deferred comprehension of important structural changes in the collagen network during aging. It commonly becomes considerably distorted by lifelong mechanical stresses. Moreover, the number of dermal cells progressively declines with age, and their shape evokes shrunken fibrocytes, becoming narrower with much cytoplasm, suggesting a decreased metabolic activity [21].

A number of studies about HRT effects on the dermis focused on changes in the tissue thickness, its collagen content, and mechanical functions [18, 22, 23]. HRT administration modalities were clearly different among a variety of trials. Distinct estrogens were used in combination or not with cyclic administration of progesterone derivatives for preventing endometrial hyperplasia. Most often, the information has been discussed collectively without distinguishing the effects of estrogens from those of estrogens and progesterone derivatives in combination [6].

Globally, the dermal collagen content and the dermal thickness appeared to be maintained in HRT receivers compared to age-matched untreated women [6, 7, 17]. In women with a decreased skin collagen content, estrogen replenishment is believed to be initially of corrective, and later of prophylactic value, while in those women with mild reduction of collagen content in the early menopausal years, estrogens are of prophylactic value only [6]. Thus, a depletion in skin collagen is expected to be in part corrected, although not overcorrected. The replenishment in skin collagen content possibly shows some regional variability with a more pronounced effect expected on the abdomen than on the thighs [6]. It remains that at present, no consensus has been reached about the value of HRT on perimenopausal aging of the dermis. Some authors denied any significant effect [19, 20]. Others feel that there exist different levels of skin response with good and poor responders [18, 24]. The latter poor responsive result presumably corresponds to women who have recently entered the menopausal period and have not yet lost estrogen-replaceable collagen [6].

The water content stored in the dermis is bound to hydrophilic glycosaminoglycans. Such a feature helps in protecting the skin against excessive tissue compression and maintains its suppleness. Estrogens increase dermal hygroscopic properties, probably through enhanced synthesis of dermal hyaluronic acid and versican [21].

During aging, the reduced quantitative changes and the decrease in compactness of the collagen bundles in the dermal ECM lead to progressive skin slackness. The resulting aging aspect is characterized by a progressive increase in skin distensibility associated with a reduction in elasticity [18, 25, 26]. Some wrinkles are correlated with these functional changes [5]. The perimenopausal period appears to be responsible for wrinkles particularly on the forearms and face. The benefit of HRT for mitigating some of these changes has been acknowledged in many instances. Fine wrinkling, dermal atrophy, and a progressive deepening of facial creases are then decreased [27]. The increase in skin distensibility commonly occurring in untreated perimenopausal women appears limited by HRT which therefore helps preventing skin slackness. Hence, HRT possibly exerts a beneficial effect on the facial skin by reducing the age-related rheological changes without, however, limiting the number and depth of established wrinkles [7, 27]. The maximal effect at preventing skin aging appears to occur when HRT is started early [17].

HRT and the Dermal Microvasculature

Flushes at menopause appear to be caused by prominent and transient vascular ectasias particularly on the face, neck, chest, palms, and soles. Their prevalence during the early perimenopausal years is in part, explained by the impairment of peripheral vascular control following estrogen deficiency. This phenomenon is corrected by HRT administration. Indeed, estrogens appear to enhance both endothelium-dependent and endothelium-independent vasodilation in the skin of women [28, 29]. A quantitative biometrological study showed higher red color intensity values (parameter a*) in the skin of menopausal women receiving HRT for at least 1 year [8]. The maximum inducible vasodilation in the forearm skin was reported to be reduced in postmenopausal women receiving estrogen replacement and in premenopausal women, compared with untreated postmenopausal women [28]. The beneficial effect of HRT on the skin blood flow was, however, challenged. HRT was reported to reduce the occurrence of chronic leg ulcers and pressure-induced ulcers [30]. Estrogen therapy possibly increases the wound healing rate in the elderly. This finding warrants confirmation before recommending HRT to improve wound healing.

HRT and Skin Epithelia

Stress-induced premature senescence (SIPS) occurs following many different sublethal stresses such as those induced by hydrogen peroxide, other oxygen species, and a variety of chemicals. The estrogen depletion possibly promotes SIPS. Cells engaged in replicative senescence share common features with cells involved in SIPS, including morphology, senescence-associated β-galactosidase activity, cell cycle regulation, gene expression, and telomere shortening. Telomere shortening is then attributed to the accumulation of DNA single-strand breaks induced by oxidative stress. Thus, SIPS could be responsible for in vivo accumulation of senescent-like cells in the skin, and DNA damage plays a key role in skin aging and photoaging.

Xerosis corresponds to an alteration of the stratum corneum (SC) which is known as "dry skin" to the laity. This condition results from an altered desquamation process often associated with a decreased hydration of the upper layers of the SC and with a weakening in the barrier function of the skin. The SC moisture, water-holding capacity, and barrier function appear to be increased following HRT intake [8, 31, 32].

Lip structure and properties are quite distinct from those of the face and other body areas. Lip tissues are subjected to frequent mechanical stresses as well as other physical and chemical annoyances [33]. Age-related changes in lip shape have been reported with resulting alterations in distensibility and contractibility [34]. In addition, marked differences were disclosed in the hydration level of the epithelial surface as the upper lip commonly appeared more hydrated than the lower one. It was claimed without any evidence that hormonal effects were unlikely in age-related changes in lip surface hydration and lip mechanical properties [34].

HRT and Pilosebaceous Follicles

Hair loss, particularly the frontal fibrosing alopecia, is apparently associated with menopause, but it is not corrected by HRT. Tibolone which is an alternative to HRT has been reported to increase the severity of diffuse alopecia and to induce facial hypertrichosis [35]. Sebum excretion on facial skin shows large interindividual differences. In nonsupplemented menopausal women, sebum excretion was reported to be increased during perimenopausal, but later on declined with chronological aging [7, 34, 36]. HRT-treated women show less prominent variations. However, the HRT benefit differs among women, and it remains hardly predictable.

Sebaceous glands are privileged targets for sex steroids, particularly 5α-dihydroxytestosterone. Other hormonal controls and neuropeptides are also operative on sebocytes. As a result, the sebum production is commonly regarded as a marker of some specific hormonal changes. The sebaceous gland apparatus is an androgen target exhibiting the highest androgen receptor density in human skin. During perimenopausal aging, changes are expected in the sebocyte proliferation, intracellular lipid synthesis, sebum transit time in the follicle, storage in the infundibulum reservoir, rheology, and capture at the surface and inside the SC. The modifications in the balance in sex hormones at the menopause are often believed to initiate the observed changes in sebum physiology. The decline in estrogen combined with a minimal decrease in androgens results in a relative increase in the androgen-estrogen balance. This should theoretically not hinder the sebocyte activity. In addition, these hormonal changes affect other segments of the sebaceous follicle, in particular the size of the sebum reservoir. This is indeed evidenced by the progressive enlargement of the follicular openings. Although sex hormones are tentatively offered as the agents responsible for the objective changes, other hormones and nonhormonal aspects of aging cannot be dismissed.

Globally, HRT possibly increases the casual sebum level, but there is a lack of consensus about that aspect. There are indeed quite few objective studies evaluating the amount of sebum released at the skin surface during perimenopause. In addition, in many instances, the number of subjects was too limited and precluded any sound conclusion. Some studies showed that sebum excretion decreased with aging. In particular, sebum excretion in menopausal women appeared lower than in nonmenopausal women [34]. By contrast, it was claimed to increase in menopausal women under HRT [7, 8, 34]. Contrasting data were reported in another controlled study involving large numbers of women [37]. Data showed that the sebum excretion changes in postmenopausal women were more likely related to hormones than to aging [37]. There was a large diversity among individual values of sebum output at the skin surface. In untreated women, a significant decline in sebum excretion rate accompanied by an increase in both the sebum replacement time and the mean pore size was evidenced during the first decade after menopause. The sebum excretion rate and casual level showed a wide range of interindividual differences in early postmenopause. These physiological changes were less prominent in women receiving HRT. It was concluded that postmenopausal aging affected the sebum production, but HRT did not significantly control the complex process of seborrhea. However, HRT appeared to mitigate the progressive enlargement of the openings of the sebum follicular reservoir.

As a consequence of the diversity of hormonal signals to the sebaceous apparatus, sebum excretion varied according to age, gender, pregnancy, and postmenopause. However, at any given age in both genders, the sebum excretion rate differed between individuals over a wide range. In addition, there was a huge overlap between data gained in both genders. Hence, it is not the amount of circulating androgens, but rather the receptivity of the target tissues that accounts for interindividual differences in sebum excretion. It is clear that additional factors are likely to be operative.

The effect of the peri- and postmenopausal age upon the sebaceous gland function has not been thoroughly and adequately studied using recent biometrological methods. It was generally acknowledged that the sebum dynamics varied throughout adult life. In women, it was reported that the sebum production remained almost stable over about three decades and dropped significantly in the age range of 50–59 years. However, those views were challenged.

HRT appears to reduce moderately the effects of postmenopausal aging on the sebum rheology. In addition, the follicular pores are kept narrower compared to the skin of untreated women. Indeed, estrogens unquestionably suppress human sebaceous secretion at high pharmacological dosages. It is debatable, however, whether they have any significant effect at physiological levels and whether they play any sizeable part in normal control of the gland. It should be stressed that contraceptives show a moderate sebosuppressive activity in acne-prone young women suffering from increased seborrhea. It is possible that HRT has no effect when seborrhea is absent or discrete. This does not exclude the possibility of an effect in severe cases. Nevertheless, it should be noted that chronological aging by itself likely mitigates seborrhea.

HRT, Skin and Bones

Menopause has been shown to have a potential role in the etiology of some major age-related diseases including osteoporosis. The one area that has fulfilled the hope of the HRT research has been the changes occurring in the skin and bones. The changes present in the dermis and bone, both in the perimenopause and in HRT recipients, apparently parallel each other [13, 16, 38]. There is also a correlation between some skin biomechanical properties and bone density [24, 38]. It is probably the combination of skin thickness, dermal biomechanical functions [39], and bone mineral density that presents the greater sensitivity and specificity in identifying women vulnerable to osteoporotic fractures after menopause.

Conclusion

Most women associate the middle years of life with a negative experience. In particular, it is generally acknowledged that a series of skin changes occur when women traverse the menopause and the years beyond. A gender perspective is indispensable for a full understanding of sex-hormone-sensitive cells of the skin. Yet until recently, some of these aspects have rather been neglected by biomedical researchers. However, the concept of perimenopausal and postmenopausal aging affecting the skin has progressively emerged in recent years. It was particularly studied at the level of the tensile strength of the dermis affected by atrophy and wrinkling. Perimenopausal xerosis is also recognized and most probably represents the consequence of a defect in the process of desquamation.

The administration of HRT appears both safe and effective, provided adequate patient selection is made, and contraindications and appropriate use of hormones (nature, dosages, regimens, routes of administration) are respected. HRT increases the well-being as well as some somatic features in menopausal women. It remains that at present, the pros and cons of HRT make it a complex issue for the physicians taking care of skin changes. All the foregoing findings indicate that chronological aging, the perimenopausal estrogen deficiency, and HRT exert profound effects on various parts of the skin. In many cases, the deleterious effects of low estrogenemia on the skin are reflected in the internal organs.

It is acknowledged that skin during perimenopausal suffers from some decline in its aspect and physical properties. HRT appears to protect in part the skin from some of the negative changes. HRT acts on the skin at several different sites and thus exhibits a multifactorial effect. The effects can be mediated by a direct hormonal effect on cells enriched in the adequate receptors. These stimulated cells can further produce some paracrine signals to other cells which are thus indirectly influenced by HRT. It is the interplay between the various skin cell types and their signaling pathways that probably control the skin aspect and healthy look. At least the skin represents the one target organ where the HRT benefits are readily visible to the woman and her relatives.

References

1. Piérard GE, et al. Skin ageprint: the causative factors. In: Barel AO, Paye M, Maibach HI, editors. Handbook of cosmetic science and technology. 4th ed. New York: Publ Informa Healthcare; 2014. p. 235–43.
2. Naylor EC, et al. Molecular aspects of skin ageing. Maturitas. 2011;69:249–56.
3. Farage MA, et al. Intrinsic and extrinsic factors in skin ageing: a review. Int J Cosmet Sci. 2008;30:87–95.
4. Mac-Mary S, et al. Assessment of cumulative exposure to UVA through the study of asymmetrical facial skin aging. Clin Interv Aging. 2010;5:277–84.
5. Piérard GE, et al. Asymmetric facial skin viscoelasticity during climacteric aging. Clin Cosmet Investig Dermatol. 2014;7:111–8.
6. Raine-Fenning NJ, et al. Skin aging and menopause: implications for treatment. Am J Clin Dermatol. 2003;4:371–8.
7. Farage MA, et al. Gender differences in skin aging and the changing profile of the sex hormones with age. J Steroids Horm Sci. 2012;3:1000109.
8. Guinot C, et al. Effect of hormonal replacement therapy on skin biophysical properties of menopausal women. Skin Res Technol. 2005;11:201–4.
9. Piérard GE, et al. Revisiting the cutaneous impact of oral hormone replacement therapy. Biomed Res Int. 2013;2013:971760.
10. Windler E et al. Is postmenopausal hormone replacement therapy suitable after a cardio- or cerebrovascular event? Arch Gynecol Obstet. 2015;291:213–7.
11. Verdier-Sevrain S, et al. Biology of estrogens in skin: implications for skin aging. Exp Dermatol. 2006;15:83–94.
12. Dunn LB, et al. Does estrogen prevent skin aging? Results from the First National Health and Nutrition Examination Survey (NHANES I). Arch Dermatol. 1997;133:339–42.

13. Piérard-Franchimont C, et al. Climacteric skin ageing of the face – a prospective longitudinal comparative trial on the effect of oral hormone replacement therapy. Maturitas. 1999;32:87–93.
14. Piérard GE. The quandary of climacteric skin ageing. Dermatology. 1996;193:273–4.
15. Nelson LR, Bulun SE. Estrogen production and action. J Am Acad Dermatol. 2001;45:S116–24.
16. Shah MG, Maibach HI. Estrogen and skin. An overview. Am J Clin Dermatol. 2001;2:143–50.
17. Sauerbronn AV, et al. The effects of systemic hormonal replacement therapy on the skin of postmenopausal women. Int J Gynaecol Obstet. 2000;68: 35–41.
18. Piérard GE, et al. Skin viscoelasticity during hormone replacement therapy for climacteric ageing. Int J Cosmet Sci. 2014;36:88–92.
19. Oikarinen A. Systemic estrogens have no conclusive beneficial effect on human skin connective tissue. Acta Obstet Gynecol Scand. 2000;79:250–4.
20. Phillips TJ, et al. Does hormone therapy improve age-related skin changes in postmenopausal women? A randomized, double-blind, double-dummy, placebo-controlled multicenter study assessing the effects of norethindrone acetate and ethinyl estradiol in the improvement of mild to moderate age-related skin changes in postmenopausal women. J Am Acad Dermatol. 2008;59:397–404.
21. Piérard-Franchimont C, et al. Immunohistochemical patterns in the interfollicular caucasian scalps: influences of age, gender, and alopecia. Biomed Res Int. 2013;2013:769489.
22. Krueger N, et al. Age-related changes in skin mechanical properties: a quantitative evaluation of 120 female subjects. Skin Res Technol. 2011;17:141–8.
23. Firooz A, et al. Variation of biophysical parameters of the skin with age, gender, and body region. Sci World J. 2012;2012:386936.
24. Piérard GE, et al. Comparative effect of hormone replacement therapy on bone mass density and skin tensile properties. Maturitas. 2001;40:221–7.
25. Piérard GE, et al. Effect of hormone replacement therapy for menopause on the mechanical properties of skin. J Am Geriatr Soc. 1995;43:662–5.
26. Hermanns-Lê T, et al. Skin tensile properties revisited during ageing. Where now, where next? J Cosmet Dermatol. 2004;3:35–40.
27. Henry F, et al. Age-related changes in facial skin contours and rheology. J Am Geriatr Soc. 1997;45:220–2.
28. Arora S, et al. Estrogen improves endothelial function. J Vasc Surg. 1998;27:1141–6. discussion 1147.
29. Lim SC, et al. The effect of hormonal replacement therapy on the vascular reactivity and endothelial function of healthy individuals and individuals with type 2 diabetes. J Clin Endocrinol Metab. 1999;84:4159–64.
30. Margolis DJ, et al. Hormone replacement therapy and prevention of pressure ulcers and venous leg ulcers. Lancet. 2002;359:675–7.
31. Piérard-Franchimont C, et al. Skin water-holding capacity and transdermal estrogen therapy for menopause: a pilot study. Maturitas. 1995;22:151–4.
32. Paquet F, et al. Sensitive skin at menopause; dew point and electrometric properties of the stratum corneum. Maturitas. 1998;28:221–7.
33. Devillers C, et al. Environmental dew point and skin and lip weathering. J Eur Acad Dermatol Venereol. 2010;24:513–7.
34. Caisey L, et al. Influence of age and hormone replacement therapy on the functional properties of the lips. Skin Res Technol. 2008;14:220–5.
35. Roux C, et al. Randomized, double-masked, 2-year comparison of tibolone with 17beta-estradiol and norethindrone acetate in preventing postmenopausal bone loss. Osteoporos Int. 2002;13:241–8.
36. Sator PG, et al. The influence of hormone replacement therapy on skin ageing: a pilot study. Maturitas. 2001;39:43–55.
37. Piérard-Franchimont C, Piérard GE. Postmenopausal aging of the sebaceous follicle: a comparison between women receiving hormone replacement therapy or not. Dermatology. 2002;204:17–22.
38. Piérard GE, et al. Relationship between bone mass density and tensile strength of the skin in women. Eur J Clin Invest. 2001;31:731–5.
39. Piérard GE, et al. In vivo evaluation of the skin tensile strength by the suction method: pilot study coping with hysteresis and creep extension. ISRN Dermatol. 2013;2013:841217.

Biological Effects of Estrogen on Skin

60

Christina Phuong and Howard I. Maibach

Contents

Abstract

Skin aging involves progressive degenerative change, such as gradual dryness, thinning, fragility, atrophy, wrinkling, a progressive increase in extensibility, and a reduction in elasticity, becoming more susceptible to injury. The average woman spends about a third of her life after the onset of menopause. Estrogen replacement therapy (ERT) has been regularly prescribed, which reduces symptoms associated with menopause. Much data exists regarding estrogen's role in aging skin and evidence of ERT on ameliorating postmenopausal aging, which have been analyzed with multiple perspectives. Numerous studies reported increases in collagen skin thickness and skin elasticity, thus reducing wrinkling, and increases in skin moisture after ERT. Estrogen also affects wound healing and scarring, but much remains to be elucidated regarding the mechanisms by which estrogen acts. There may be limitations on the benefits of ERT, though, depending on the type of skin damage accumulated. A limited number of studies contradict these benefits of ERT. Due to a lack of standardized methods, not all studies are comparable, and the power of each study differs. Overall, it seems clear that there is a role of the therapeutic use of estrogen on skin. Selective estrogen receptor modulators (SERMS) are a viable option that should be further explored. Increased research should be directed at the clinical pharmacology of estrogen and medical prescription, such as

C. Phuong (✉)
Department of Dermatology, University of California San Francisco, San Francisco, CA, USA
e-mail: cphuong49@gmail.com

H.I. Maibach
Department of Dermatology, University of California, San Francisco, CA, USA
e-mail: maibachh@derm.ucsf.edu

M.A. Farage et al. (eds.), *Textbook of Aging Skin*,
DOI 10.1007/978-3-662-47398-6_35

determining the form of estrogen to administer as well as delivery and application methods.

Introduction

Changes in skin aging and function occur at variable rates and are influenced by environmental, hormonal, and genetic factors unique to each individual. Skin aging involves progressive degenerative changes, such as gradual dryness, thinning, fragility, atrophy, and wrinkling. Over time, the skin experiences a progressive increase in extensibility and a reduction in elasticity, thereby becoming more frail and susceptible to trauma. This in turn leads to an increased risk of skin injury (e.g., lacerations, tears, ulcerations, bruising) and an impairment of wound healing.

Improvements in nutrition, sanitation, quality and provision of health care, and other related factors have led to a dramatic increase in life expectancy for human beings over the past century. The average life expectancy of women in the United States has increased from about 50 years in 1900 [1] to 79.56 years in 2014 [2]. As the developing world catches up, a similar but much more significant trend in average global longevity is projected to occur. The number of women age 60 and over worldwide is expected to increase from about 336 million in 2000 to just over 1 billion by 2050 [3]. Since the average woman in a developed nation spends about one third of her life after the onset of menopause, the benefits and risks of estrogen replacement therapy (ERT) – also known as hormone replacement therapy (HRT) and menopausal hormone therapy (MHT) – have become major areas of focus for research.

ERT has been regularly prescribed by physicians for postmenopausal women since the 1940s to reduce symptoms associated with menopause, such as hot flashes, night sweats, vaginal dryness, and sleep disturbances [4]. In the intervening period, the risks and benefits of ERT have been and continue to be debated. In terms of benefits to ERT, estrogen has been demonstrated to ameliorate menopausal maladies such as vasomotor symptoms, mood changes, atrophy of reproductive organs, and sleep disturbances [5].

Particularly in light of the increasing life expectancy of women throughout the world, health workers need to more fully understand the physiology and treatment of menopause. To this end, this chapter focuses on the biological effects of estrogen on the skin of postmenopausal women with regard to skin thickness, moisture, wrinkling, wound healing, and scarring and briefly discusses future estrogen therapies, such as selective estrogen receptor modulators (SERMS).

Studies have uncovered various mechanisms by which estrogen may affect skin aging and function. Research indicates that topical and systemic ERT leads to a statistically significant improvement in many aging skin problems [6]. ERT increases skin collagen content and preserves thickness, thereby reducing wrinkling. Skin moisture content improves with ERT, as it increases the skin's hyaluronic acid, acid mucopolysaccharides, and sebum levels and possibly maintains stratum corneum barrier function. ERT benefits likely differ depending on the type of damage on skin.

Beyond its impact on aging, topical ERT accelerates and improves cutaneous wound healing in elderly individuals, possibly by regulating the levels of a cytokine and through estrogen receptors. Conversely, a lack of estrogen (i.e., hypoestrogenism) or addition of tamoxifen – the first SERM developed – may improve the quality of scarring, though the relationship between estrogen and scarring is more ambiguous.

ERT intervention in postmenopausal women is still debated, though the detailed knowledge of estrogen's mechanism of action remains unclear. Different experimental parameters, such as skin location, years since menopause, race, and much more, may help explain varying results. In addition, detrimental effects may result from long-term ERT use. Possible increased risks include breast cancer, stroke, and thromboembolic disease. Thus, more in-depth knowledge with more standardized methods and noting changes in experimental parameter is necessary before proper dosing and use can be administered. Overall, there is a clear role for the therapeutic use of estrogen on aging skin. Going forward, factors such as the form of estrogen to use, delivery methods, and timing of use should be determined.

Skin Aging Perspectives

Numerous reports support the notion that physiological changes are not simply a result of senescence but also due to hormonal changes in the body. Copious studies have been performed detailing ERT/HRT's effect on the skin, especially after menopause. As such, multiple reviews in the recent decade have attempted to organize the existing information and analyze the complex influence of hormones, with an emphasis on estrogen, on aging.

In 2005, Hall and Phillips detailed the biochemistry of estrogen, including pathways, mechanisms, and regulation of synthesis. Understanding estrogen's role and interaction with other molecules at the molecular level is a major area of study, which begins by understanding estrogen biosynthesis [7]. Calleja-Agius et al. detail the various structural elements of skin, changes due to aging – notably the effect on collagen – and various treatment options, hormonal and nonhormonal [8].

Pierard et al. note that the transition period between the end of women's reproductive life and beginning of menopause, known as the perimenopausal phase or climacteric phase (WCA), is a unique stage in women's lives [9]. The body undergoes numerous changes; therefore, it may respond differently to HRT during WCA compared to during pre-/postmenopausal stages. Thus, HRT studies should take women's postmenopausal age into consideration while conducting and analyzing studies.

Samaras et al. review the role of various hormones in the aging process, along with the risks and benefits of supplementation [10]. They pose the question: should hormonal decline be considered normal or actively treated? They take the position endorsing hormone supplementation as a part of geriatric care; however, large-scale, in-depth studies are still necessary to define proper treatment regimens. Emmerson and Hardman focus on aging's effect on efficient wound healing and the beneficial role of estrogen [11]. They believe that understanding ER-mediated signaling changes can significantly aid our ability to use estrogen to counteract poor wound healing in the elderly.

Skin aging and estrogen's role are complex processes. These reviews show that much data is known about hormonal influence on aging, and there are many potential benefits of ERT; however, there is still a lot that needs to be understood. Molecular mechanisms involved in aging still remain unclear, and the possible health risks still exist. Thus, ongoing debates regarding the safety and detailed effects of estrogen are still present today.

Thickness and Collagen

Collagen is the primary protein of connective tissue in mammals, comprising about 25–35 % of total body protein content. Collagen has a high tensile strength and is a major component of fascia, cartilage, ligaments, tendons, bone, and skin. At least 30 different collagen genes have been identified and described. These collagen genes combine to form over 20 different types of collagen fibrils, of which, Types I, II, and III are the most common [12]. Human skin contains over 14 types of collagen that are responsible for skin strength. Eighty percent of the collagen is Type I collagen, which is more responsible for the strength of skin, while 15 % is Type III, which is more responsible for the elastic properties of skin.

Collagen becomes progressively sparse, disordered, and atrophied as skin ages – one of the chief reasons for the skin transformations resulting from aging. Copious studies establish that menopause leads to estrogen deficiency, and research over the past 60 years demonstrates that skin thickness, estrogen content, and skin collagen are closely correlated (Table 1).

In 1941, Albirght et al. first noticed that elderly women with osteoporotic fractures – an injury closely correlated with menopause – had visibly thinner skin. Correlation between skin thickness and estrogen content was first noted by

Table 1 Selected studies on skin thickness and ERT

Date	Study	Type of measurement	Hormones used	Duration	Results
1969	Rauramo and Punnomen	Skin biopsy analysis (measured by calipers)	Estradiol succinate 2.0 mg	6 months	Improvement in skin thickness
1987	Brincat et al.	Skin biopsy analysis	Estradiol implant and percutaneous estradiol gel	2–10 years	Increase in skin thickness by 30 %; average linear decline of 1.13 % skin thickness and 2.1 % collagen per year in the first 15–18 postmenopausal years without ERT
1992	Castelo-Branco et al.	Skin biopsy analysis	Conjugated equine estrogens or transdermal 17b- estradiol	12 months	Increase in skin collagen by 1.8–5.1 %
1994	Maheux et al.	Skin thickness (measured by ultrasonography)	Conjugated estrogen 0.625 mg	12 months	Increase in skin thickness by 11.5 %
1995	Varila et al.	Skin biopsy analysis	Topical 17β-estradiol	3 months	Increase in hydroxyproline by 38 %
1996	Callens et al.	Skin thickness (measured by ultrasonography at five skin locations)	17β-estradiol gel or estradiol patches	Mean of 4.8 years	Increase in skin thickness by 7–15 % in all locations
2000	Sauerbronn et al.	Skin biopsy analysis	2.0 mg valerate estradiol, cycled with 1.0 mg cyproterone acetate	6 months	Increase in skin collagen by 6.49 %
2007	Sator et al.	Sebumeter, the Corneometer, and high-frequency ultrasound	2.0 mg 17β-estradiol/ 10 dydrogesterone	7 months	Significant improvements in skin elasticity, skin hydration, and skin thickness
1993	Sawwas and Laurent	Skin biopsy analysis	Subcutaneous estradiol and testosterone	3–14 years	Significantly greater levels of collagen Type III
1997	Haapasaari et al.	Skin biopsy analysis	17β-estradiol and norethisterone acetate; estradiol valerate	12 months	No significant change in skin collagen or thickness
2012	Pingel et al.	Microdialysis-urine, blood, dialyzate samples	Estrogen patch (50 μg/24 h estradiol hemihydrate)	5 days	No significant changes in overall serum PINP. Serum PINP significantly higher at day 5 vs day 2 preexercise. Increased muscle PINP but not peritendinous PINP

Bullough's 1941 study on mice [13]. McConkey et al. posited in 1963 that the "transparent skin" described by Albright was caused by a decrease in dermal collagen Type I [14]. In 1970, Black et al. [15] demonstrated that thickness is in fact proportional to collagen content – as McConkey et al. had suggested – utilizing the 1964 radiographic technique for measuring skin thickness employed by Meema et al. [16].

The above studies established that the estrogen deficiency associated with menopause leads to skin collagen degradation and decreasing skin thickness. Thus, future studies should focus on deciphering the effects of reproductive hormones on skin collagen. In 1969, Rauramo and Punnomen noted that ERT had a favorable effect on human skin [17]. Their study involved 6 months of treatment with 2.0 mg estradiol succinate and showed improvement in skin thickness of biopsies measured using calipers.

A subsequent 1987 study by Brincat et al. corroborated Rauramo and Punnomen's findings, showing a decrease in skin thickness and collagen content after menopause. Their study demonstrated an increase in skin thickness for women receiving an estradiol implant or percutaneous estradiol gel. Using radiographic techniques, Brincat et al. found an average increase in skin thickness by 30 % for those on ERT. Additionally, Brincat et al. found that 30 % of collagen is lost within the first 5 years of menopause and witnessed an average linear decline of 1.13 % in skin thickness and 2.1 % in collagen per year in the first 15–18 postmenopausal years for those not on ERT. The study also noted that skin collagen decline was correlated specifically to the duration of estrogen deficiency (i.e., postmenopausal years) and not chronological age [18].

In a 1992 study, Castelo-Branco et al. similarly found that ERT – both oral and transdermal – increased skin collagen content. Their study used conjugated equine estrogens and transdermal 17-β-estradiol over a 12-month period and showed an increase in skin collagen content of 1.8–5.1 %, varying based on the type of ERT administered. Unlike Brincat et al., Castelo-Branco et al. observed a higher correlation between skin collagen content and chronological age, though they still recognize a statistically significant correlation between skin collagen content and time since the onset of menopause [19]. Subsequent studies by Affinito et al. and others have achieved the same results as Brincat et al. and showed postmenopausal years to be the determining factor [20]. The likely cause of this aberration in the Castelo-Branco et al. study was that many participants were in their initial postmenopausal years, with a short history of estrogen deprivation. This problem with study participants has plagued other studies (e.g., [21, 22]) and has contributed to some of the controversy surrounding the effects of ERT on skin aging.

A 1994 study by Maheux et al. controlled for some of the factors which complicate the measurement of skin aging (e.g., smoking and exposure to solar radiation), thereby focusing more specifically on the effects of conjugated estrogens. Maheux et al. employed a randomized, double-blind, placebo-controlled study of postmenopausal nuns. Their study used conjugated estrogen 0.625 mg over a 12-month period and showed an increase in skin thickness, as measured by ultrasonography, of 11.5 % for the group receiving ERT [23].

Varila et al. studied the effect of topical ERT on collagen content, as measured by skin hydroxyproline, in a 1995 study. Hydroxyproline is a major component of collagen and is found in few proteins other than collagen. The only other mammalian protein that includes hydroxyproline is elastin. For this reason, hydroxyproline content has been used as an indicator to determine collagen or gelatin amount. Via skin biopsy analysis, Varila et al. measured an increase in hydroxyproline of 38 % following administration of topical 17β-estradiol for 3 months. The study also observed increased levels of the carboxyterminal propeptide of human Type I procollagen and of the aminoterminal propeptide of human Type III procollagen, thus showing that estrogen increases collagen synthesis [24].

Subsequent studies by Callens et al. [25], Sauerbronn et al. [26], Sator [27], and others have further substantiated the aforementioned studies' claims. Callens et al. found that ERT increased skin thickness by 7–15 % in postmenopausal women utilizing estradiol gel patches or an estradiol transdermal system. Sauerbronn et al. focused on skin collagen rather than thickness. Following 6 months of treatment with estradiol valerate and cyproterone acetate, their study observed a 6.49 % increase in collagen fibers in the dermis and no significant change in epidermal thickness. Sator noted significant improvements in skin elasticity, skin hydration, and skin thickness after 7 months of treatment. This corroborates a 2005 Sumino et al. study which showed that after menopause, skin elasticity declined 0.55 % per year and that 12 months of ERT increased elasticity by 5.2 % [28].

Oxidative stress is a major component of aging. Progressive radical damage accumulation occurs within the body according to the free radical theory of aging [29]. Reactive oxygen species (ROS), such as superoxide, hydroxyl radical, and hydrogen peroxide, have long-term effects on the body. One detrimental effect includes induction of matrix metalloproteinases (MMPs), which degrade collagen. ERT could potentially increase collagen in part by reducing oxidative stress. Bottai et al. found that 17β-estradiol stimulated procollagen-I synthesis in skin fibroblast and could interfere with oxidative stress-induced collagen decrease [30]. They showed that pretreatment with 17β-estradiol protected dermal fibroblasts and HaCaT against H_2O_2-induced lipoperoxidation.

However, there also exist studies that debate the effectiveness of ERT in increasing collagen content and skin thickness. Utilizing immunohistochemistry and colorimetric methods, Haapasaari et al. detected no increase in skin collagen content following 1 year of systemic estrogen therapy. The investigators hypothesized estrogen affects collagen turnover rather than skin collagen [22]. A more likely explanation, however, is that the low median postmenopausal age of 12 months among the study participants did not provide adequate time to show the effects of low estrogen levels. Recently, Pingel et al. studied the effect of transdermal ERT and exercise on collagen synthesis in postmenopausal women by measuring the levels of procollagen Type I NH2-terminal propeptide (PINP), a marker for Type I collagen synthesis [31]. They found that exercise and ERT together, compared with each alone, significantly increased muscle PINP but not peritendinous PINP; however, this may be due to physiological and methodological limitations in the study design. In disagreement with previous studies though, they found no difference in overall serum PINP levels between the control and ERT period. However, serum PINP was significantly higher at day 5 than at day 2 preexercise only in the ERT period. Because of the short time frame, these results may possibly be explained as observing only the initial phase of ERT before the beneficial effects take place such as on bone mass [32].

While ERT increases skin thickness, there are limits to the potential for ERT to reverse skin aging. Savvas and Laurent conducted research in 1993 which, in accordance with the 1987 Brincat et al. study, suggests that ERT produces no additional increase in skin collagen content after 2 years. Their study focused specifically on collagen Type I and Type III and found increased collagen content in postmenopausal women receiving estradiol and testosterone implants. However, beyond 3 years, they found no increase in the proportion of collagen Type III [33].

Beneficial ERT effects may also be limited to photo-protected skin. In 2010, Neder showed that immunohistochemical expression of MMP-1 enzyme in keratinocytes, endothelial cells, and fibroblasts did not decrease in photo-exposed skin after using topical estradiol 0.05 % for 30 days [34]. MMP-1 levels may actually increase. Yoon et al. showed a large induction of MMP-1 mRNA after estrone cream treatment [35]. This could help explain why induction of Type I procollagen protein was not observed despite detecting increase in Type I procollagen and fibrillin-1 mRNA. It is possible that there are different regulatory mechanisms between photo-protected and photo-exposed skin. Thus, further investigation is necessary to elucidate the mechanism by which ERT affects collagen synthesis.

Lastly, as seen earlier by the wide range of improvement, it is difficult to quantify the real effects of ERTs on skin thickness and collagen content. Some factors, such as individual skin history, are extremely difficult to correct for when studied. For example, Lee et al. highlighted the need to standardize the methods of measuring skin atrophy and thickness so that results are more comparable across studies [36].

Moisture

Studies show that the loss of moisture, which leads to dry skin, is another age-related skin condition. In 1996, Schmidt et al. noted an increase in skin moisture among perimenopausal and postmenopausal women after using topical estradiol 0.01 % and estriol 0.3 % (systemic) for 6 months [37]. Dunn et al. compiled results from a much larger population-based cohort study in 1997 –

the first National Health and Nutrition Examination Survey (NHNES), a Center for Disease Control and Prevention (CDC) program of studies designed to assess the health and nutritional status of adults and children in the United States – and showed that postmenopausal women on ERT were significantly less likely to experience dry skin [38].

Research provides the following possible explanations as to why topical and systemic estrogen therapies preserve skin moisture: increased acid mucopolysaccharides and hyaluronic acid in the dermis, higher sebum levels, increased water-holding capacity of the stratum corneum, and changes in the corneocyte surface area.

First, Grossman et al. observed increased acid mucopolysaccharides and hyaluronic acid in the skin of mice treated with estrogen in the early 1970s. Hyaluronic acid is known to have a high water-holding capacity, which supports an increase in dermal water content [39, 40].

Second, the 1996 study by Callens et al. demonstrated a 35 % increase in sebum levels among women on estrogen [25]. This study suggests that ERT may prevent the decrease in glandular secretions that Pochi et al. noted in postmenopausal women in their 1979 study [41].

Third, the ability of skin to retain water is largely associated with the stratum corneum lipids, which maintain skin barrier function. In 1995, Pierard-Franchimont et al. suggested that estrogen may play a role in stratum corneum barrier function, noting that women on transdermal ERT showed increased water-holding capacity of the stratum corneum [42]. Similarly, Paquet et al. demonstrated in 1998 that estrogen also improves the ability of the stratum corneum to prevent water loss by observing a decrease in the rate of water accumulation in postmenopausal women [43].

Lastly, ERT may lead to changes in the corneocyte surface area, thereby further enhancing the epidermal barrier function.

Wrinkling

Skin wrinkling is the result of lost skin elasticity [44], dermal thickening, and elastic deterioration caused by a variety of degenerative environmental, hormonal, and genetic factors. Histological studies of wrinkles by Contet-Audonneau et al. [45] and Bosset et al. [46] showed alterations of dermal collagen and elastic fibers, as well as a marked decrease in glycosaminoglycans. Numerous studies have shown that ERT can improve fine wrinkles, prevent development of skin wrinkles, and decrease existing wrinkle depth.

Creidi et al. studied the effect of conjugated estrogen cream on postmenopausal women in a double-blind, placebo-controlled study utilizing clinical evaluation by dermatologists. This study found significant improvement in fine wrinkles [47]. Dunn et al. employed the NHNES to control for age, body mass index, and subexposure and found that postmenopausal women on ERT were less likely to develop wrinkles in the first place [26]. Schmidt et al. further demonstrated that existing wrinkle depth can be decreased using topical ERT [37].

In contradiction to these studies, a 2008 study by Phillips et al. found no improvement in age-related skin changes from topical ERT. However, this study was limited in that it utilized low-dose estrogen (i.e., 1 mg norethindrone acetate and 5–10 μg ethinyl estradiol) for only 48 weeks and in women with an average of only five postmenopausal years [22].

Wolff et al. investigated race/ethnicity differences in skin wrinkles and rigidity in the face and neck of the Kronos Early Estrogen Prevention Study (KEEPS) population with women only recently in their menopausal stage [48]. The data, utilizing the Lemperle scale, showed Black women had the fewest wrinkling at all facial locations except the neck. This supports previous studies that reported racial/ethnic difference in skin properties [49]. However, a significant relationship between wrinkles and time since menopause was not observed. A durometer was used to measure skin rigidity [50]. While there were no significant differences in skin rigidity among races/ethnicities or chronological age, skin rigidity was more correlated with time since menopause in the White subpopulation [48]. As a side, only wrinkles at the neck correlated with skin rigidity, indicating possible differences in neck and face skin physiology.

The impact of ERT on wrinkling likely relates partially to its impact on collagen, namely, its capacity to increase the proportion of collagen III in skin. Punnonen et al. noted the elastic fibers in the papillary dermis following local estriol treatment had thickened, increased slightly in number, and become better oriented [51]. Furthermore, the increase in hyaluronic acid noted by Grosman increases water capacity and thus skin turgor, thereby reducing the ability to develop wrinkles and the appearance of any wrinkles present [52]. An interesting side note, however, is that a study by Castelo-Branco et al. found that ERT does not appear to reduce wrinkling in those with a history of over 10 years smoking. Thus, it seems ERT cannot reverse some of the damage done by smoking, such as destruction of the ground substance, decreased blood flow in the skin, and direct toxic effects [52]. In addition, Yoon et al. measured wrinkles using skin replicas and Visiometer SV 600 and skin elasticity using Cutometer MPA 580 after 24 weeks of topical estrone cream treatment [35]. They found no significant differences in facial wrinkles or skin elasticity between treatment and control groups. Differences between estrone and estradiol may have impacted the differing results between this study and prior ones [53]. Further, this study focused on facial skin; thus, photo exposure is another variable to be considered when determining effects of ERT.

Wound Healing

Natural aging significantly impacts wound healing by increasing susceptibility to trauma, bruising, and chronic wounds. The role of estrogen and effect of ERT to wound healing is still unclear, largely because most early studies were performed using animal models that produced conflicting results. Differences in species, duration of treatment, and methodologies employed likely led to the inconsistent findings in animal studies conducted during the 1960s and 1970s [54].

Studies on wound healing have focused primarily on the molecular role of estrogen on the cells and metabolic processes involved in wound repair. Age-related impairment of wound healing has been partially attributed to low levels of transforming growth factor-β1 (TGF-β1), decreased collagen synthesis, and increased presence of proteases (specifically elastase). Furthermore, estrogen's presence on fibroblasts, the main cell type involved in wound healing, indicates it may directly modify their function [54].

Studies by Ashcroft et al. suggest estrogen positively affects wound repair by causing TGF-β1 secretion by fibroblast – not by increasing fibroblast production in a wound – increasing collagen content, and reducing collagenolysis [55–57]. The 1997 Ashcroft et al. study used rats to demonstrate that topical ERT was associated with significantly accelerated acute wound healing as shown by decreased reepithelialization time, decreased wound width, and increased collagen deposition. The 1999 and 2003 Ashcroft et al. studies demonstrated that topical ERT reduces the activity of protease elastase in cutaneous wounds in humans, thereby improving healing as shown by decreased wound sizes, faster increases in collagen levels, increased fibronectin levels, and enhanced strength. Furthermore, the latter study suggested topical ERT might even be useful on a prophylactic basis, though more work needs to be done in this area.

The detailed mechanism by which estrogen modulates skin repair is still unclear. Estrogen signaling occurs via two nuclear hormone receptors, ERα and ERβ, each with its own diverse role in body tissue and differing roles in cutaneous healing. These receptors bind to the estrogen response element (ERE) to initiate gene transcription [58]. Estrogen is likely to affect skin through ERE-dependent and ERE-independent signaling pathways [59].

While ERα is more predominant in most tissue, Campbell et al. showed that epidermal ERβ is crucial to mediating skin wound healing [60]. Skin repair wounds treated with ERβ agonist, DPN, significantly reduced wound area similar to 17β-estradiol treatment. Treating with ERα agonist, PPT, though, had no effect on healing. In fact, without ERβ, ERα may be detrimental to wound healing. Furthermore, estrogen's wound healing effect is specific to epidermal ERβ and interestingly seems to be irrespective of the anti-inflammatory activity of ERα and ERβ.

Emmerson et al. found that wound tissue treated with 17β-estradiol induced strong peri-wound activation of ERE, which reversed the delayed healing of estrogen-deficient mice [61]. Less ERE activation was found at the wound center. It is possible that the strong periphery signal activation detected comes from the basal and suprabasal keratinocytes, neutrophils, monocytes, and other cells that are recruited from the wound margins in response to damage [62, 63].

Novotny et al. investigated different roles of ERα and ERβ in rat skin and suggested that ERα would better treat incisional skin wounds while ERβ would better treat excisional wounds [64]. ERβ was more effective in achieving higher wound tensile strength in all groups, while ERα showed decreased wound tensile strength after 5 days and was only significantly higher than the control group after 10 days. ERα stimulated the transition of fibroblasts to myofibroblast, while ERβ stimulated higher amounts of new collagen. Both led to high number of vessels in granulation tissues. Interestingly, both ERα and ERβ increased the amount of proenzymes of MMP-2 and MMP-9 but not their active forms.

Much data emphasize a beneficial role of ERT in skin repair; however, specific mechanisms of skin wound repair remain unclear. The role of molecules associated with wound healing still need to be elucidated before ERT can be properly used for skin healing.

Scarring

The cellular and subcellular sites and mechanisms involved in the scarring process are poorly understood. Whitby et al. conducted a study comparing the differences between fetal and adult wound healing. Fetal scars tend to be superior in that they are pale and flat, rather than pigmented and everted as in adults. Their study found fetal wounds deficient in the inflammatory cytokine TGF-β1, whereas adult skin typically had a large amount of TGF-β1 [65].

As mentioned in the section on wound healing, postmenopausal women in a hypoestrogenic state tend to be deficient in TGF-β1; thus, they should produce scarrings that are better both macroscopically and microscopically. A study by Shah et al. supports this supposition and suggests that estrogen antagonists may be effective in limiting scarring [66].

Selective Estrogen Receptor Modulators (SERMS)

SERMS act at the level of the estrogen receptors, either mimicking positive estrogen effects or blocking negative estrogen effects, depending on the tissue. This tissue specificity allows for targeted ERT treatments. For example, tamoxifen has an antiestrogenic effect on breast tissue but an estrogenic effect on bone and is used to treat breast cancer and prevent postmenopausal osteoporosis simultaneously. Hu et al. demonstrated that tamoxifen also inhibits collagen wound contraction and mechanism for the inhibition of wound contraction could be the inhibition of fibroblasts or fibroblast proliferation [67]. Surazynski et al. found that in fibroblasts, a SERM currently used for the treatment of postmenopausal osteoporosis known as raloxifene has a stronger positive stimulating effect on collagen synthesis than estradiol [68].

Intensive research is currently underway to develop new SERMs specifically for the purpose of targeting the skin without incurring systemic side effects [69]. Thus, these drugs will likely become an important means of controlling scarring and other effects of skin aging.

Conclusion

New studies continue to support the above conclusions that both topical and systemic ERTs have positive impacts on skin aging as it relates to thickness, moisture, wrinkling, wound healing, and scarring [70–72]. ERT's ability to slow skin aging is largely due to estrogen's ability to repair and prevent a decline in skin collagen, increase skin turgor and water-holding capacity, improve epidermal barrier function, and decrease changes in skin elasticity over time.

Other areas remain to be explored further, such as optimal methods for administering ERT, determining the impact of ERT on men and premenopausal women, understanding the effect of estrogen on melanocyte function, and ascertaining the role of estrogen in skin cancer prevention, if any. ERT also affects skin and skin appendages in ways not discussed in this chapter, such as hair growth during pregnancy and hair loss during menopause [73–75].

Although much research indicates that estrogen has a large impact on skin in postmenopausal women, detailed mechanisms of action are still unclear. Further, estrogen's impact possibly differs depending on the type of damage that accumulated in skin, such as from smoking or sunlight.

When determining if ERT is appropriate, the benefits and risks of ERT must be weighed by patients and health-care workers in light of the potential side effects, particularly from systemic ERT. At this point in time, treatment of skin aging should not be the sole basis for systemic ERT, at least until it is understood what minimum concentration of estrogen can achieve the best local effects without systemic hormonal side effects. Most topical ERTs (e.g., estradiol creams) may not be significantly systemically absorbed [76]. Since topical ERT may present a safe and effective treatment for skin aging, menopausal women not receiving systemic ERT are candidates for this treatment when administered by a dermatologist educated in endocrinology. Finally, SERMs may present another future means of achieving the benefits of estrogen therapy without the systemic risks.

Estrogen's role in skin care has been an ongoing investigation. While a large majority of evidence strongly supports its use, few studies do exist which cautions people. However, limitations of the studies must be considered. Continued research is necessary with standardized methods to more definitively compare studies. It is believed that it is clearly conceivable that there is a role for the therapeutic use of estrogen in aging skin. Many factors still need to be taken into consideration, such as skin condition and race. Further, optimal delivery method and application location need to be investigated. Taken together, current experimental data supports using topical estrogens to ameliorate skin aging. Going forward, increased research should be directed at the clinical pharmacology of estrogen and medical prescription, such as determining the form of estrogen to administer as well as delivery and application methods.

Cross-References

▶ Aging Genital Skin and Hormone Replacement Therapy Benefits

References

1. Our World in Data. Life expectancy. 2015. http://ourworldindata.org/data/population-growth-vital-statistics/life-expectancy/
2. Central Intelligence Agency. The world factbook. 2014. https://www.cia.gov/library/publications/the-world factbook/rankorder/2102rank.html
3. Women, ageing and health: a framework for action. World Health Organization. 2007. http://www.who.int/ageing/publications/Women-ageing-health-lowres.pdf
4. Shah M, Maibach H. Estrogen and skin, an overview. Am J Clin Dermatol. 2001;2(3):143.
5. Palacios S. Current perspectives on the benefits of HRT in menopausal women. Maturitas. 1999;33:S1–3.
6. Stevenson S, Thornton J. Effects of estrogen on skin aging and the potential role of SERMs. Clin Interv Aging. 2007;2(3):283–97.
7. Hall G, Phillips TJ. Estrogen and skin: the effects of estrogen, menopause, and hormone replacement therapy on the skin. J Am Acad Dermatol. 2005;53(4):569–72.
8. Calleja-Agius J, Brincat M, Borg M. Skin connective tissue and ageing. Best Pract Res Clin Obstet Gynaecol. 2013;27(5):727–40.
9. Pierard GE, Humbert P, Berardesca E, et al. Revisiting the cutaneous impact of oral hormone replacement therapy. Biomed Res Int. 2013;2013:971760.
10. Samaras N, Papadopoulou M, Samaras D, et al. Off-label use of hormones as an antiaging strategy: a review. Clin Interv Aging. 2014;9:1175–86.
11. Emmerson E, Hardman MJ. The role of estrogen deficiency in skin ageing and wound healing. Biogerontology. 2012;13(1):3–20.
12. King M. The Medical biochemistry page. IU School of Medicine. http://themedicalbiochemistrypage.org/extracellularmatrix.html. Last modified 11 June 2008.

13. Bullough HF. Cyclical changes in the skin of the mouse during estrous cycle. J Endocrinol. 1943;3:280–7.
14. McConkey B, Fraser GM, Bligh AS, et al. Transparent skin and osteoporosis. Lancet. 1963;I:693–5.
15. Black MM, Bottoms E, Shuster S. Changes in skin collagen and thickness in endocrine disease. Eur J Clin Invest. 1970;1:127.
16. Meema HE, Sheppard RH, Rapoport A. Roentgenographic visualization and measurement of skin thickness and its diagnostic application in acromegaly. Radiology. 1964;82:411.
17. Rauramo L, Punnomen R. Wirkung einer oralen ostrogenotherapie mit ostriolsuccinat auf die Hautt kastrierter Frauen. Z Haut Geschl Kr. 1969;44:463–70.
18. Brincat M, Yuen AW, Studd JW, et al. Response of skin thickness and metacarpal index to estradiol therapy in postmenopausal women. Obstet Gynecol. 1987;70 (4):538–41.
19. Castelo-Branco C, Duran M, Gonzales-Merlo J. Skin collagen and bone changes related to age and hormone replacement therapy. Maturitas. 1992;14:113–19.
20. Affinito P, Palomba S, Sorrentino C, et al. Effects of postmenopausal hypoestrogenism on skin collagen. Maturitas. 1999;33:239–47.
21. Phillips TJ, Symons J, et al. Does hormone therapy improve age-related skin changes in postmenopausal women? A randomized, double-blind, double-dummy, placebo-controlled multicenter study assessing the effects of norethindrone acetate and ethinyl estradiol in the improvement of mild to moderate age-related skin changes in postmenopausal women. J Am Acad Dermatol. 2008;59(3):397–404, e3.
22. Haapasari K, Raudaskoski T, Kallioinen M, et al. Systemic therapy with estrogen or estrogen with progestin has no effect on skin collagen in postmenopausal women. Maturitas. 1997;27:153–62.
23. Maheux R, Naud F, Rioux M, et al. A randomized, double-blind, placebo-controlled study on the effect of conjugated estrogens on skin thickness. Am J Obstet Gynecol. 1994;170:642–9.
24. Varila E, Rantala I, Oikarinen A, et al. The effect of topical estradiol on skin collagen of postmenopausal women. Br J Obstet Gynaecol. 1995;102(12):985–9.
25. Callens A, Valliant L, Lecomte P, et al. Does hormonal skin aging exist? A study of the influence of different hormone therapy regimens on the skin of postmenopausal women using non-invasive measurement techniques. Dermatology. 1996;193:289–94.
26. Sauerbronn AVD, Fonseca AM, Bagnoli VR, et al. The effects of systemic hormone replacement therapy on the skin of the postmenopausal women. Int J Gynecol Obstet. 2000;68:35–41.
27. Sator PG, Sator MO, Schmidt JB, et al. A prospective, randomized, double-blind, placebo-controlled study on the influence of a hormone replacement therapy on skin aging in postmenopausal women. Climacteric. 2007;10:320–34.
28. Sumino H, Ichikawa S, et al. Effects of aging, menopause, and hormone replacement therapy on forearm skin elasticity in women. J Am Geriatr Soc. 2004;52:945–9.
29. Hardman D. Free radical theory of aging. Mutat Res. 1992;275(3):257–66.
30. Bottai G, Mancina R, Muratori M, et al. 17β-estradiol protects human skin fibroblasts and keratinocytes against oxidative damage. J Eur Acad Dermatol Venereol. 2013;27:1236–43.
31. Pingel J, Langberg H, Skovgard D, et al. Effects of transdermal estrogen on collagen turnover at rest and in response to exercise in postmenopausal women. J Appl Physiol. 2012;113(7):1040–7.
32. Garnero P, Tsouderos Y, Marton I, et al. Effects of intranasal 17β-estradiol on bone turnover and serum insulin-like growth factor I in postmenopausal women. J Clin Endocrinol Metab. 1999;84:2390–7.
33. Savvas M, Laurent G. Type III collagen content in the skin of postmenopausal women receiving estradiol and testosterone implants. Br J Obstet Gynaecol. 1993;100:154–6.
34. Neder L. Topical estradiol does not interfere with the expression of the metalloproteinase-1 enzyme in photo exposed skin cells. An Bras Dermatol. 2012;87 (1):70–5.
35. Yoon H, Lee S, Chung JH. Long-term topical oestrogen treatment of sun-exposed facial skin in post-menopausal women does not improve facial wrinkles or skin elasticity, but induced matrix metalloproteinase-1 expression. Acta Derm Venereol. 2014;94(1):4–8.
36. Lee JY, Maibach HI. Corticosteroid skin atrophogenicity: assessment methods. Skin Res Technol. 1998;4:161–6.
37. Schmidt J, Binder M, Demschik G, et al. Treatment of skin aging with topical estrogens. Int J Dermatol. 1996;35:669–74.
38. Dunn L, Damesyn M, Moore A, et al. Does estrogen prevent skin aging? Results from the First National Health and Nutritional Examination Survey. Arch Dermatol. 1997;133:339–42.
39. Grosman N, Hridbey E, Schon J. The effect of estrogenic treatment on the acid mucopolysaccharide pattern in the skin of mice. Acta Pharmacol Toxicol. 1971;30:458–64.
40. Grosman N. Studies on the hyaluronic acid protein complex the molecular size of hyaluronic acid and the exchangeability of chloride in skin of mice before and after estrogen treatment. Acta Pharmacol Toxicol. 1973;33:201–8.
41. Pochi PE, Strauss JS, Downing D. Age related changes in sebaceous gland activity. J Invest Dermatol. 1979;73:108–11.
42. Pierard-Franchimont C, Letawe C, Goffin V, et al. Skin water- holding capacity and transdermal estrogen therapy for menopause: a pilot study. Maturitas. 1995;22:151–4.
43. Paquet F, Pierard-Franchimont C, Fuman I, et al. Sensitive skin at menopause; dew point and electrometric properties of the stratum corneum. Maturitas. 1998;28:221–7.

44. Sumino H, Ichikawa S, Abe M, et al. Effects of aging and postmenopausal hypoestrogenism on skin elasticity and bone mineral density in Japanese women. Endocr J. 2004;51:159–64.
45. Contet-Audonneau JL, Jeanmaire C, Pauly G. A histological study of human wrinkle structures: comparison between sun-exposed areas of the face, with or without wrinkles, and sun-protected areas. Br J Dermatol. 1999;140:1038–47.
46. Bosset S, Barre P, Chalon A, et al. Skin ageing: clinical and histopathologic study of permanent and reducible wrinkles. Eur J Dermatol. 2002;12(3):247–52.
47. Creidi P, Faivre B, Agache P, et al. Effect of a conjugated estrogen (Premarin) cream on ageing facial skin. A comparative study with a placebo cream. Maturitas. 1994;19:211–23.
48. Wolff E, Pal L, Altun T, et al. Skin wrinkles and rigidity in early postmenopausal women vary by race/ethnicity: baseline characteristics of the skin ancillary study of the KEEPS trial. Fertil Steril. 2011;95(2):658–62.
49. Wesley NO, Maibach HI. Racial (ethnic) differences in skin properties. In: Barel AO, Paye M, Maibach HI, editors. Handbook of cosmetic science and technology. 2nd ed. Boca Raton: CRC Press, Taylor and Francis Group; 2006. p. 15–44. Chp 3.
50. Kissin EY, Schiller AM, Gelbard RB, et al. Durometry for the assessment of skin disease in systemic sclerosis. Arthritis Rheum. 2006;55:603–9.
51. Punnonen R, Vaajalahti P, Teisala K. Local estriol treatment improves the structure of elastic fibers in the skin of postmenopausal women. Ann Chir Gynaecol. 1987;202(Suppl):39–41.
52. Castelo-Branco C, Figueras F, Martinez de Osaba M, et al. Facial wrinkling in postmenopausal women. Effects of smoking status and hormone replacement therapy. Maturitas. 1998;29:75–86.
53. Watson CS, Jeng YJ, Kochukov MY. Nongenomic actions of estradiol compared with estrone and estriol in pituitary tumor cell signaling and proliferation. FASEB J. 2008;22:3328–36.
54. Brincat MP, Muscat Baron Y, Galea R. Estrogens and the skin. Climacteric. 2005;8:110–23.
55. Ashcroft GS, Dodsworth J, van Boxtel E, et al. Estrogen accelerates cutaneous wound healing associated with an increase in TGF-b1 levels. Nat Med. 1997;3:1209–15.
56. Ashcroft GS, Greenwell-Wild T, Horan MA, Wahl SM, Ferguson MW. Topical estrogen accelerates cutaneous wound healing in aged humans associated with an altered inflammatory response. Am J Pathol. 1999;155:1137–46.
57. Ashcroft GS, Ashworth JJ. Potential role of estrogens in wound healing. Am J Clin Dermatol. 2003;4(11):737–43.
58. Tremblay GB, Tremblay A, Copeland NG, et al. Cloning, chromosomal localization, and functional analysis of the murine estrogen receptor beta. Mol Endocrinol. 1997;11:353–65.
59. Verdier-Sevrain S, Yaar M, Cantatore J, et al. Estradiol induces proliferation of keratinocytes via a receptor mediated mechanism. FASEB J. 2004;18:1252–4.
60. Campbell L, Emmerson E, Davies F, et al. Estrogen promotes cutaneous wound healing via estrogen receptor β independent of its antiinflammatory activities. J Exp Med. 2010;207(7):1825–33.
61. Emmerson E, Rando G, Meda C, et al. Estrogen receptor-mediated signalling in female mice is locally activated in response to wounding. Mol Cell Endocrinol. 2013;375(1-2):149–56.
62. Matsuzaki K, Inoue H, Kumagai N. Re-epithelialisation and the possible involvement of the transcription factor, basonuclin. Int Wound J. 2004;1(2):135–40.
63. Werner S, Grose R. Regulation of wound healing by growth factors and cytokines. Physiol Rev. 2003;83:835–70.
64. Novotny M, Vasilenko T, Varinska L, et al. ER-α agonist induces conversion of fibroblasts into myofibroblasts while ER-β agonist increases ECM production and wound tensile strength of healing skin wounds in ovariectomised rats. Exp Dermatol. 2011;20:703–8.
65. Whitby DJ, Ferguson MWJ. Immunohistochemical localization of growth factors in fetal wound healing. Dev Biol. 1991;147:207–15.
66. Shah M, Foreman DM, Ferguson MWJ. Control of scarring in adult wounds by neutralizing antibody to transforming growth factor B. Lancet. 1992;339:213–14.
67. Hu D, Hughes MA, Cherry GW. Topical tamoxifen – a potential therapeutic regime in treating excessive dermal scarring? Br J Plast Surg. 1998;51(6):462–9.
68. Surazynski A, Jarzabek K, Haczynski J, Laudanski P, Palka J, Wolczynski S. Differential effects of estradiol and raloxifene on collagen biosynthesis in cultured human skin fibroblasts. Int J Mol Med. 2003;12:803–9.
69. Osborne K, Zhao HH, Fuqua SAW. Selective estrogen receptor modulators: structure, function, and clinical use. J Clin Oncol. 2000;18:3172–86.
70. Hall GK, Phillips TJ. Skin and hormone therapy. Clin Obstet Gynecol. 2004;47(2):437–49.
71. Kanda N, Watanabe S. Regulatory roles of sex hormones in cutaneous biology and immunology. J Dermatol Sci. 2005;38(1):1–7.
72. Schmidt JB. Perspectives of estrogen treatment in skin aging. Exp Dermatol. 2005;14(2):156.
73. Thornton MJ. Estrogen functions in skin and skin appendages. Expert Opin Ther Targets. 2005;9(3):617–29.
74. Lynfield YL. Effect of pregnancy on the human hair cycle. J Invest Dermatol. 1960;35:323–7.
75. Whiting DA. Diagnosis of alopecia. Current concepts. Kalamazoo: A Scope Publication, The Upjohn; 1990.
76. Burger H. Hormone replacement therapy in the post-Women's Health Initiative era. Report of a meeting held in Funchal, Madeira, February 24–25. Climacteric. 2003;6 Suppl 1:11–36.

DNA Biomarkers in Aging Skin

61

Kimberly G. Norman, Alex Eshaghian, and James E. Sligh

Contents

K.G. Norman (✉)
Institute for In Vitro Sciences, Gaithersburg, MD, USA
e-mail: knorman@iivs.org

A. Eshaghian
AE Skin, Encino, CA, USA
e-mail: aeshaghian@salud.unm.edu

J.E. Sligh
Medicine, Dermatology, The University of Arizona, Tucson, AZ, USA
e-mail: jsligh@azcc.arizona.edu

M.A. Farage et al. (eds.), *Textbook of Aging Skin*,
DOI 10.1007/978-3-662-47398-6_47

Abstract

Mitochondrial DNA (mtDNA) mutations are thought to be involved in the photoaging phenotype based upon the observation that chronically UV-exposed skin with clinical signs of photoaging has a high frequency of mtDNA damage, including the 4977 bp deletion, as compared to UV-protected skin. Of the UV light that reaches the skin, short-wavelength UVB (280–320 nm) is mostly absorbed by keratinocytes in the epidermis and induces nuclear DNA and mtDNA damage via the formation of pyrimidine dimers. Longer wavelength UVA (320–400 nm) is able to penetrate the actively dividing basal layer of the epidermis where mtDNA changes may be initiated indirectly through the generation of reactive oxygen species (ROS). Mitochondria are the site of highest cellular ROS levels because of the inherent errors of oxidative phosphorylation, and increased levels of ROS mediated by UVA have been shown to generate signature mtDNA deletions in the human skin and cultured cells. This evidence indicates that mtDNA changes may be involved in the photoaging phenotype and serve as biomarkers of aging in the skin.

Introduction

Aging in the skin is the result of both the intrinsic chronological aging process and extrinsic damage caused by environmental factors. A major role of the skin is that of protection from external environmental factors. Ultraviolet radiation (UVR) is the most significant environmental insult to the skin. UVR comprises the spectrum of electromagnetic radiation between the wavelengths of 200 and 400 nm. UVR is subdivided into three categories, each of which has distinct biological effects: UVA (320–400 nm), UVB (280–320 nm), and UVC (200–280 nm). The stratospheric ozone blocks radiation whose wavelength is below 290 nm, effectively preventing the entire UVC spectrum and part of the UVB spectrum from reaching the human skin. The UVR that does reach the human skin can cause molecular defects including DNA damage, lipid peroxidation, and protein cross-linking, which can lead to premature skin aging or photoaging. Photoaging is a term used to describe the clinical and histological features of chronically UV-exposed skin [1].

Photoaging occurs more frequently in people with fair skin and tends to be located in sun-exposed areas such as the head, neck, hands, and forearms. Sun-exposed areas of the skin exhibit characteristic features of aging in common with sun-protected, chronologically aged skin as well as with other chronologically aged tissues. However, certain features of sun-exposed skin are exclusive to this tissue. Hence, the term photoaging refers to the physiologic and pathological changes that occur specifically in aged tissue that has experienced chronic sun exposure over time. Clinical symptoms of photoaging include dry skin, formation of lentigines and nevi, hyperpigmentation, telangiectasia, leathery appearance, increased wrinkle formation, reduced recoil capacity, increased skin fragility, blister formation, and impaired wound healing ability [1, 2]. UVR also causes histological changes in the skin including hyperkeratosis, thickening of the basement membrane, irregular melanocyte distribution, elastosis, dermal intercellular and perivascular edema, and perivascular infiltration [1]. Further changes include deposition of glycosaminoglycans, fragmented elastic fibers, and interstitial collagen.

Of the UV light that reaches the skin, UVB is mostly absorbed in the epidermis, whereas UVA penetrates through the epidermis and into the dermis. Therefore, UVB affects keratinocytes in the epidermis, and UVA affects keratinocytes in the epidermis and fibroblasts in the dermis. UVB most commonly causes damage in the form of cyclobutane pyrimidine dimers (Fig. 1). The characteristic hallmarks of UVB damage are C to T and CC to TT DNA changes. These occur in semiconservative DNA replication due to the A rule, which states that when DNA polymerase comes across uninterpretable changes, it inserts A residues by default. Thus two A residues are inserted into DNA on strands opposite to cyclobutane-type cytosine-cytosine dimers, leading to two TT residues on the template strand. UVA, on the other hand, primarily causes DNA damage indirectly by the production of short-lived reactive oxygen species (ROS) such as singlet oxygen ($O^{\cdot -}$), $O_2^{\cdot -}$, and H_2O_2 via endogenous photosensitizers. ROS lead to single-stranded DNA breaks, nucleotide changes, and DNA-protein cross-links. Potential sites of ROS-induced DNA damage are shown in Fig. 2, and the formation of 8-hydroxyguanine, the most common altered base due to ROS, is shown in

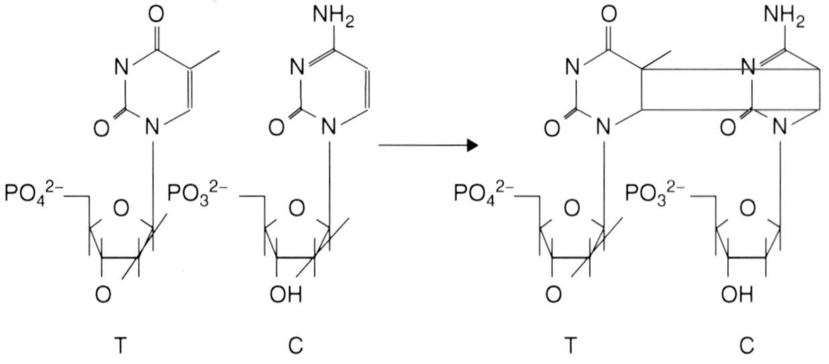

Fig. 1 Cyclobutane-type pyrimidine dimer formation. The formation of cyclobutane-type pyrimidine dimers as a result of UVB is shown between thymidine (T) and cytosine (C) nucleotides

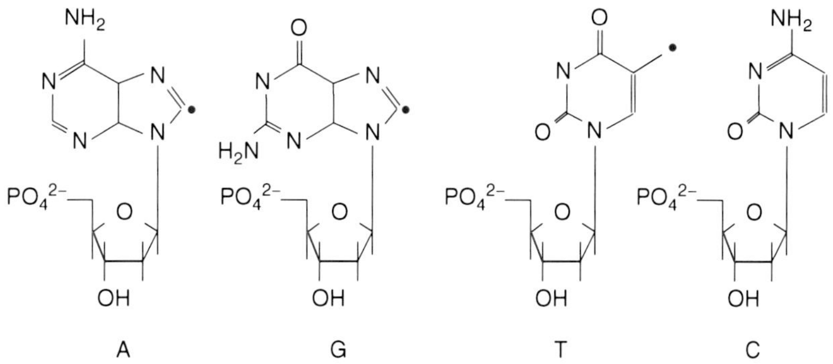

Fig. 2 Potential sites of oxidative DNA damage. The sites of potential DNA damage due to ROS are shown in *red* on the four deoxyribonucleotides. *A* adenosine, *G* guanosine, *T* thymidine, *C* cytosine

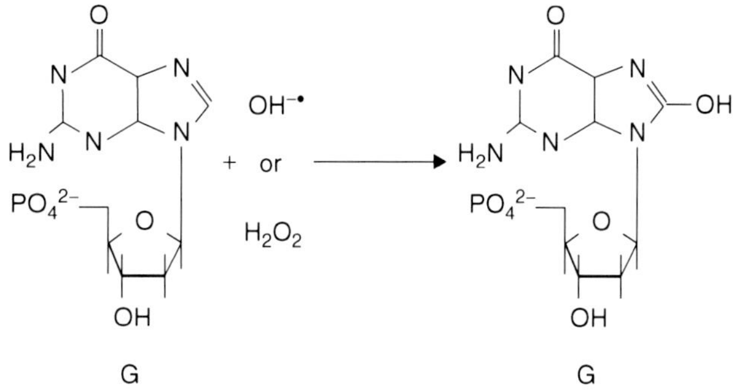

Fig. 3 8-Hydroxyguanine formation. The formation of 8-hydroxyguanine is the most common DNA defect as a result of ROS. 8-Hydroxyguanine can be formed when a hydroxide radical ($OH^{-\bullet}$) or H_2O_2 reacts with guanosine (G)

Fig. 3. 8-Hydroxyguanine lesions are employed as a DNA marker of overall oxidative stress in the cell and UV damage in the skin. Singlet oxygen produced by UVA light has been shown to cause strand breaks in the mitochondrial DNA (mtDNA) which resulted in mtDNA deletions [3]. mtDNA deletions are thought to be involved in the photoaging phenotype and serve as biomarkers of aging in the skin, based upon the observation that chronically UV-exposed skin with clinical signs of photoaging has a high frequency of mtDNA deletions as compared to UV-protected skin [4, 5].

Mitochondrial Implications in Photoaging

Mitochondria have well-recognized roles both in the generation of cellular energy and as mediators of cellular events such as apoptosis. Mitochondria contain their own genome, a maternally inherited, circular, double-stranded DNA of 16,569 bp encoding 22 tRNAs, two rRNAs, and 13 polypeptides, all of which are subunits in the electron transport chain [6–8]. The remainder of the proteins that function in the mitochondrion are encoded in the nucleus and imported into the mitochondrion. Because the mitochondria contain multiple copies of the mtDNA and cells may contain thousands of mitochondria, newly acquired somatic mutations are heteroplasmic, or mixed with wild-type, in nature. However, replicative segregation may allow mutant mtDNA molecules in some cells to become prominent or even to become the exclusive mtDNA in the cell, a condition known as homoplasmy.

The mitochondrion serves as the major site for production of ATP through the process of oxidative phosphorylation (OXPHOS). ROS, natural by-products of this pathway, can damage lipids, proteins, and DNA [9, 10]. mtDNA has a high mutation rate due to its lack of histones, decreased capacity for repair, and close proximity to the site of ROS formation [11]. Imbalances between oxidative stress and free radical scavenging enzymes have been suggested as the underlying causes of most of the mtDNA damage [12, 13]. There is emerging evidence for mtDNA changes in the complex processes of cellular aging and neoplasia [14–16]. The mitochondrial theories of aging hold as their basic principles that OXPHOS produces a main source of cellular energy in the form of ATP and that there is an age-related decline in OXPHOS. The mtDNA may be particularly important in this energetic decline because its mutation rate is thought to be at least 10-fold higher than that of the nuclear genome [17]. A multitude of factors are likely responsible for this increased mutation rate including the lack of protective histones and a less sophisticated system of proofreading than that present in the nucleus [18]. Also, mtDNA is exposed to higher concentrations of oxygen free radicals as a consequence of their liberation from natural events occurring in the electron transport chain. Continued exposure of the mtDNA to oxidative damage results in an accumulation of somatic mtDNA mutations over time. These mutations may further decrease the efficiency of OXPHOS and increase the likelihood of additional oxygen free radical production with further subsequent mtDNA damage. This cycle results in a progressive decline in the energy-generating capacity of the cell. Disease ensues when energy output falls below the minimum energetic threshold for normal tissue function. mtDNA changes have been associated with a variety of inherited and acquired human neurodegenerative disorders, myopathies, and endocrinopathies. Common characteristics of these clinical phenotypes are both delayed-onset and age-related progression [16]. Age-related onset and a history of sun exposure are typical for acquired cases of nonmelanoma skin cancer, which is the most common malignancy of older individuals and is one of the most frequently occurring health problems requiring surgical procedures in the elderly. Although there is substantial data correlating mtDNA changes with aging, in general, and with photoaging in the skin, there is no evidence of mtDNA mutations directly causing these phenotypes.

Mitochondrial DNA Mutations and Photoaging

In contrast to other tissues, the skin is subject to both chronological aging and environmental insult in the form of UVR. The resulting genetic changes may lead to specific phenotypes of aging skin: photodamage and neoplasia. Changes in the mtDNA in the skin are well recognized in association with photoaging [19–21]. The most common mutation found in aging tissues is the 4977 bp "common" deletion [22–28]. In autopsy specimens, the common deletion has been found primarily in sun-exposed areas, and not in sun-protected areas [29]. Imbalances between oxidative stress and free radical scavenging enzymes have been suggested as the underlying causes of most of the mtDNA damage [12, 13]. The common deletion has been shown to be inducible both in vitro and in vivo in the human skin and is thought to occur as a result of mtDNA damage mediated through singlet oxygen [3, 30]. Additionally, the 4977 bp "common" deletion has been proposed to be a biomarker of photoaged skin because the level of heteroplasmy in the sun-exposed skin increases with age, while such levels are not increased in sun-protected skin [29]. In a study by Ray et al., many mtDNA deletions in addition to the common deletion were identified in the epidermis of the skin from older individuals, and these deletions were strongly associated with UVR [4]. A report of 200 bp and 260 bp duplications in the noncoding D-loop adds another class of mtDNA rearrangements that have been observed in aged human skin [31]. Additionally, an mtDNA deletion of 3895 bp was identified as a quantitative marker for sunlight exposure in the human skin [32, 33], and the aging-dependent T414G mutation within the control region of mtDNA was found to accumulate in UVR-damaged skin [34]. It was also discovered that the T414G mutation, which may serve as both a marker for chronological aging and photoaging, was commonly identified within a 3895 bp deleted mtDNA population.

In a study in our lab to examine mtDNA mutations in photoaging, mtDNA from photodamaged skin was screened for the presence of deletions using long-extension PCR. mtDNA deletions were found to be abundant in photoaged skin specimens from older patients, and their number correlated with the patient age, supporting the use of mtDNA mutations as biomarkers of photoaging in the skin [35]. These mtDNA deletions were typically absent in the paired nonmelanoma skin cancers. The observed DNA deletions from the skin were often unreported (19 of 21 deletions) but usually shared structural features with mtDNA deletions reported in other tissues in that they generally contain short direct or indirect repeats at the breakpoints, and a single copy of the repeat is left behind in the deleted molecule. The structural similarities between the mtDNA deletions observed in the skin and those seen in tissues not exposed to UVR [36] imply a potential common factor in their generation or resolution. Some of the identified deletions were detected from the numerous skin samples, including 3715 bp and 6278 bp deletions. Interestingly, the frequency of these newly identified deletions approached that of the well-characterized 4977 bp deletion. We found a consistently higher level of heteroplasmy of the 4977 bp "common" deletion in the dermis as compared to the epidermis in our split samples, consistent with previous studies [29]. Furthermore, the number of novel deletions in photoaged skin not reported in other tissues suggests that the skin may be more vulnerable to such mutations via direct exposure to UVR.

The mechanism of formation of such mtDNA deletions has been proposed to be a slipped mispairing of the repeats during replication [3, 13, 37, 38]. In order for such a mutation to occur, however, both breakpoints must be single stranded simultaneously, which does not normally occur. However, the sequences flanking the repeats or the sequences within the repeats may render the DNA susceptible to structural conformations allowing mispairing [39]. Our findings show that most deletions identified contain such repeats, supporting the slip replication model. The novel 3715 and 6278 bp deletions contain 10 and 11 bp direct repeats, respectively, similar in size to that of the 4977 bp "common" deletion (13 bp). Additionally, the novel 6278 bp deletion contains a homopolymeric track of seven consecutive cytosine residues interrupted by a single adenosine residue within its repeated breakpoint sequence. Such sequences have been proposed to take on structural characteristics allowing for mispairing to occur [40]. These features may explain the reason why the frequencies of detection of the novel 3715 and 6278 bp deletions approached that of the 4977 bp "common" deletion. It has been proposed that ROS, which are normally generated in response to UVR [41], play a role in the generation of the 4977 bp "common" deletion [3]. Thus it is not surprising that so many unreported mtDNA deletions were identified in photoaged skin given its role as a barrier to UVR. As mtDNA deletions accrue in photoaged skin, they may be useful as biomarkers of the combined effects of chronological aging and UV exposure. Additionally, specific mtDNA deletions may complement other deletions, and the potential level of a single mtDNA deletion may plateau with time as it adversely affects the bioenergetic properties of the cell. Measurement of a panel of deletions may be a more useful assay of photodamage than heteroplasmy levels of any single deletion alone. Quantitative analysis of other deletions, in addition to the 4977 bp "common" deletion, may be useful for this purpose.

Concluding Remarks

While the 4977 bp "common" deletion has been proposed to be a biomarker for photoaging, it may reflect only a small portion of total mtDNA damage. The 3715 bp, 6278 bp, and 3895 bp deletions and T414G mutation may prove valuable as additional markers of photoaging in the skin. Furthermore, in our study, the photoaged skin contained an abundance of various deletions beyond the aforementioned mtDNA changes. Thus the use of the 4977 bp "common" deletion as a biomarker for photoaged skin may indeed be the tip of the iceberg.

References

1. Berneburg M, Plettenberg H, Krutmann J. Photoaging of human skin. Photodermatol Photoimmunol Photomed. 2000;16:239–44.
2. Scharffetter-Kochanek K. Photoaging of the connective tissue of skin: its prevention and therapy. Adv Pharmacol. 1997;38:639–55.
3. Berneburg M, Grether-Beck S, Kurten V, Ruzicka T, Briviba K, Sies H, Krutmann J. Singlet oxygen mediates the UVA-induced generation of the photoaging-associated mitochondrial common deletion. J Biol Chem. 1999;274:15345–9.
4. Ray AJ, Turner R, Nikaido O, Rees JL, Birch-Machin MA. The spectrum of mitochondrial DNA deletions is a ubiquitous marker of ultraviolet radiation exposure in human skin. J Invest Dermatol. 2000;115:674–9.
5. Berneburg M, Krutmann J. Mitochondrial DNA deletions in human skin reflect photo- rather than chronologic aging. J Invest Dermatol. 1998;111:709–10.
6. Anderson S, Bankier AT, Barrell BG, de Bruijn MH, Coulson AR, Drouin J, Eperon IC, Nierlich DP, Roe BA, Sanger F, Schreier PH, Smith AJ, Staden R, Young IG. Sequence and organization of the human mitochondrial genome. Nature. 1981;290:457–65.
7. Andrews RM, Kubacka I, Chinnery PF, Lightowlers RN, Turnbull DM, Howell N. Reanalysis and revision of the Cambridge reference sequence for human mitochondrial DNA. Nat Genet. 1999;23:147.
8. Giles RE, Blanc H, Cann HM, Wallace DC. Maternal inheritance of human mitochondrial DNA. Proc Natl Acad Sci U S A. 1980;77:6715–9.
9. Shigenaga MK, Hagen TM, Ames BN. Oxidative damage and mitochondrial decay in aging. Proc Natl Acad Sci U S A. 1994;91:10771–8.
10. Richter C. Oxidative damage to mitochondrial DNA and its relationship to ageing. Int J Biochem Cell Biol. 1995;27:647–53.
11. Wallace DC, Lott MT, Shoffner JM, Brown MD. Diseases resulting from mitochondrial DNA point mutations. J Inherit Metab Dis. 1992;15:472–9.
12. Lu CY, Lee HC, Fahn HJ, Wei YH. Oxidative damage elicited by imbalance of free radical scavenging enzymes is associated with large-scale mtDNA deletions in aging human skin. Mutat Res. 1999;423:11–21.
13. Shoffner JM, Lott MT, Voljavec AS, Soueidan SA, Costigan DA, Wallace DC. Spontaneous Kearns-Sayre/chronic external ophthalmoplegia plus syndrome associated with a mitochondrial DNA deletion: a slip-replication model and metabolic therapy. Proc Natl Acad Sci U S A. 1989;86:7952–6.
14. Copeland WC, Wachsman JT, Johnson FM, Penta JS. Mitochondrial DNA alterations in cancer. Cancer Invest. 2002;20:557–69.
15. Eng C, Kiuru M, Fernandez MJ, Aaltonen LA. A role for mitochondrial enzymes in inherited neoplasia and beyond. Nat Rev Cancer. 2003;3:193–202.
16. Wallace DC. Mitochondrial diseases in man and mouse. Science. 1999;283:1482–8.
17. Kujoth GC, Hiona A, Pugh TD, Someya S, Panzer K, Wohlgemuth SE, Hofer T, Seo AY, Sullivan R, Jobling WA, Morrow JD, Van Remmen H, Sedivy JM, Yamasoba T, Tanokura M, Weindruch R, Leeuwenburgh C, Prolla TA. Mitochondrial DNA mutations, oxidative stress, and apoptosis in mammalian aging. Science. 2005;309:481–4.
18. Croteau DL, Bohr VA. Repair of oxidative damage to nuclear and mitochondrial DNA in mammalian cells. J Biol Chem. 1997;272:25409–12.
19. Pang CY, Lee HC, Yang JH, Wei YH. Human skin mitochondrial DNA deletions associated with light exposure. Arch Biochem Biophys. 1994;312:534–8.
20. Yang JH, Lee HC, Lin KJ, Wei YH. A specific 4977-bp deletion of mitochondrial DNA in human ageing skin. Arch Dermatol Res. 1994;286:386–90.
21. Yang JH, Lee HC, Wei YH. Photoageing-associated mitochondrial DNA length mutations in human skin. Arch Dermatol Res. 1995;287:641–8.
22. Brierley EJ, Johnson MA, Lightowlers RN, James OF, Turnbull DM. Role of mitochondrial DNA mutations in human aging: implications for the central nervous system and muscle. Ann Neurol. 1998;43:217–23.
23. Cortopassi GA, Shibata D, Soong NW, Arnheim N. A pattern of accumulation of a somatic deletion of mitochondrial DNA in aging human tissues. Proc Natl Acad Sci U S A. 1992;89:7370–4.
24. Cortopassi GA, Arnheim N. Detection of a specific mitochondrial DNA deletion in tissues of older humans. Nucleic Acids Res. 1990;18:6927–33.
25. Wallace DC. Mitochondrial genetics: a paradigm for aging and degenerative diseases? Science. 1992;256:628–32.
26. Ikebe S, Tanaka M, Ohno K, Sato W, Hattori K, Kondo T, Mizuno Y, Ozawa T. Increase of deleted mitochondrial DNA in the striatum in Parkinson's disease and senescence. Biochem Biophys Res Commun. 1990;170:1044–8.
27. Nagley P, Wei YH. Ageing and mammalian mitochondrial genetics. Trends Genet. 1998;14:513–7.
28. Sciacco M, Bonilla E, Schon EA, DiMauro S, Moraes CT. Distribution of wild-type and common deletion forms of mtDNA in normal and respiration-deficient muscle fibers from patients with mitochondrial myopathy. Hum Mol Genet. 1994;3:13–9.
29. Birch-Machin MA, Tindall M, Turner R, Haldane F, Rees JL. Mitochondrial DNA deletions in human skin

reflect photo- rather than chronologic aging. J Invest Dermatol. 1998;110:149–52.

30. Berneburg M, Plettenberg H, Medve-Konig K, Pfahlberg A, Gers-Barlag H, Gefeller O, Krutmann J. Induction of the photoaging-associated mitochondrial common deletion in vivo in normal human skin. J Invest Dermatol. 2004;122:1277–83.
31. Durham SE, Krishnan KJ, Betts J, Birch-Machin MA. Mitochondrial DNA damage in non-melanoma skin cancer. Br J Cancer. 2003;88:90–5.
32. Harbottle A, Birch-Machin MA. Real-time PCR analysis of a 3895 bp mitochondrial DNA deletion in nonmelanoma skin cancer and its use as a quantitative marker for sunlight exposure in human skin. Br J Cancer. 2006;94:1887–93.
33. Krishnan KJ, Harbottle A, Birch-Machin MA. The use of a 3895 bp mitochondrial DNA deletion as a marker for sunlight exposure in human skin. J Invest Dermatol. 2004;123:1020–4.
34. Birket MJ, Birch-Machin MA. Ultraviolet radiation exposure accelerates the accumulation of the aging-dependent T414G mitochondrial DNA mutation in human skin. Aging Cell. 2007;6:557–64.
35. Eshaghian A, Vleugels RA, Canter JA, McDonald MA, Stasko T, Sligh JE. Mitochondrial DNA deletions serve as biomarkers of aging in the skin, but are typically absent in nonmelanoma skin cancers. J Invest Dermatol. 2006;126:336–44.
36. Kogelnik AM, Lott MT, Brown MD, Navathe SB, Wallace DC. MITOMAP: a human mitochondrial genome database. Nucleic Acids Res. 1996;24:177–9.
37. Mita S, Rizzuto R, Moraes CT, Shanske S, Arnaudo E, Fabrizi GM, Koga Y, DiMauro S, Schon EA. Recombination via flanking direct repeats is a major cause of large-scale deletions of human mitochondrial DNA. Nucleic Acids Res. 1990;18:561–7.
38. Schon EA, Rizzuto R, Moraes CT, Nakase H, Zeviani M, DiMauro S. A direct repeat is a hotspot for large-scale deletion of human mitochondrial DNA. Science. 1989;244:346–9.
39. Hou JH, Wei YH. The unusual structures of the hot-regions flanking large-scale deletions in human mitochondrial DNA. Biochem J. 1996;318 (Pt 3):1065–70.
40. Fullerton SM, Bernardo Carvalho A, Clark AG. Local rates of recombination are positively correlated with GC content in the human genome. Mol Biol Evol. 2001;18:1139–42.
41. Scharffetter-Kochanek K, Wlaschek M, Brenneisen P, Schauen M, Blaudschun R, Wenk J. UV-induced reactive oxygen species in photocarcinogenesis and photoaging. Biol Chem. 1997;378:1247–57.

Aging and Intrinsic Aging: Pathogenesis and Manifestations

62

Hanan Assaf, Mohamed A. Adly, and Mahmoud R. Hussein

Contents

H. Assaf (✉)
Department of Dermatology, Saudi German Hospital, Jeddah, Saudi Arabia
e-mail: assaf_hanan@yahoo.com

M.A. Adly
Department of Zoology, Faculty of Science, Sohag University, Sohag, Egypt
e-mail: m.adly@yahoo.com

M.R. Hussein
Department of Pathology, Assir Central Hospital, and Assuit University, Assuit, Egypt
e-mail: mrcpath17@gmail.com

M.A. Farage et al. (eds.), *Textbook of Aging Skin*,
DOI 10.1007/978-3-662-47398-6_13

Abstract

As the population ages, dermatological focus must shift from ameliorating the cosmetic consequences of skin aging to decreasing the genuine morbidity associated with problems of the aging skin. Therefore, a better understanding of both the intrinsic and extrinsic influences on the aging of the skin, as well as distinguishing the retractable aspects of cutaneous aging (primarily hormonal and lifestyle influences) from the unretractable cutaneous aging (primarily intrinsic aging), is critical to solve the problem of aging.

Introduction

Cutaneous aging is a complex biological phenomenon consisting of two components: intrinsic aging and extrinsic aging. Intrinsic aging is also termed true aging which is an inevitable change attributable to the passage of time alone and is manifested primarily by physiologic alterations with subtle but undoubtedly important consequences for both healthy and diseased skin and is largely genetically determined [1]. Extrinsic aging is caused by environmental exposure, primarily to UV light, and more commonly termed photoaging. In sun-exposed areas, photoaging involves changes in cellular biosynthetic activity that lead to gross disorganization of the dermal matrix [2]. The intrinsic rate of skin aging in any individual can be dramatically influenced by personal and environmental factors, particularly the amount of exposure to ultraviolet light. Photodamage, which considerably accelerates the visible aging of skin, also greatly increases the risk of cutaneous neoplasms. So, the processes of intrinsic and extrinsic aging are superimposed. As the population ages, dermatological focus must shift from ameliorating the cosmetic consequences of skin aging to decreasing the genuine morbidity associated with problems of the aging skin. Therefore, a better understanding of both the intrinsic and extrinsic influences on the aging of the skin, as well as distinguishing the retractable aspects of cutaneous aging (primarily hormonal and lifestyle influences) from the irretractable cutaneous aging (primarily intrinsic aging), is very important to solve the problem of aging [2].

Pathogenesis of Intrinsic Aging

Logic dictates that one or more molecular events must underlie the aging process. These changes are now beginning to be unraveled and are discussed. As these mechanisms are identified, further insights into the underlying processes of skin aging should emerge and better strategies to prevent the undesirable effects of age on skin appearance should follow. The process of intrinsic skin aging resembles that seen in most internal organs and an explanation is thought to involve decreased proliferative capacity leading to cellular senescence and altered biosynthetic activity of skin derived cells [2].

The molecular mechanisms partly underlying skin aging comprise a multifaceted process influenced by various factors affecting different body sites at variable degrees. A stochastic process that implies random cell damage as a result of mutations during metabolic processes due to the production of free radicals is also implicated [2–4]. As the molecular mechanisms leading to human senescence are complex processes, different research approaches are used to study aging including studies of monogenic segmental progeroid syndromes. Two progeria syndromes, Werner's syndrome (WS) and Hutchinson-Gilford progeria syndrome (HGPS), which are characterized by clinical features mimicking physiological aging at an early age, provide insights into the mechanisms of natural aging. They suggest a model of human aging. Based on recent findings on WS and HGPS, human aging can be triggered by two main mechanisms: telomere shortening and DNA damage. In telomere-dependent aging, telomere shortening and dysfunction may lead to DNA damage responses which induce cellular senescence. In DNA damage-initiated aging, DNA damage accumulates, along with DNA repair deficiencies, resulting in genomic instability and accelerated cellular senescence. In addition, aging due to both mechanisms (DNA damage and telomere shortening) is strongly dependent on p53 status. These two mechanisms can also act cooperatively to increase the overall level of genomic instability, triggering the onset of human aging phenotypes [3, 5].

Data from another trial revealing the molecular changes of intrinsic skin aging were analyzed by applying "serial analysis of gene expression" (SAGE(TM)) to skin biopsies of young and aged donors. The analysis resulted in several hundred differentially expressed genes with varying statistical significance. Of these, several genes were identified that either have never been described in skin aging before (e.g., APP) or have no identified function (e.g., EST sequences). This is the first time that intrinsic skin aging has been analyzed in such a comprehensive manner, offering a new and partially unexpected set of target genes that have to be analyzed in more detail in terms of their contribution to the skin aging process [4, 6]. Moreover, normal human fibroblasts undergoing serial passaging have been extensively used to identify genes linked with aging. Most of the isolated genes relate to growth retardation signals and the failure of homeostasis that accompanies aging and senescence. In contrast, there is still limited knowledge regarding the nature of the genes that influence positively the rate of aging and longevity. Healthy centenarians represent the best example of successful aging and longevity. Studies using samples from these individuals have proved very valuable for identifying a variety of factors that contribute to successful aging [5, 7].

Manifestation of Skin Aging

Various expressions of intrinsic aging include smooth, thinning skin with exaggerated expression lines. Extrinsically aged skin is characterized by photodamage as wrinkles, pigmented lesions, patchy hypopigmentations, and actinic keratoses [2].

The Wrinkle and Its Measurement

There is a new method for the measurement of the size and function of the wrinkle, called "profilometric" method. Facial wrinkles are not a single groove but comprise an anatomical and functional unit (the "wrinkle unit") along with the surrounding skin. This wrinkle unit participates in the functions of a central neuromuscular system of the face responsible for protection, expression, and communication. Thus, the wrinkle unit, the superficial musculoaponeurotic system (superficial fascia of the face), and the underlying muscles controlled by the CNS and psyche are considered to be a "functional psycho-neuro-muscular system of the face for protection, expression, and communication." The three major functions of this system exerted in the central part of the face and around the eyes are: (1) to open and close the orifices (eyes, nose, and mouth), contributing to their functions; (2) to protect the eyes from sun, foreign bodies, etc.; and (3) to contribute to facial expression, reflecting emotions (real, pretended, or theatrical) during social communication. These functions are exercised immediately and easily, without any opposition ("wrinkling ability") because of the presence of the wrinkle unit that gives (a) the site of refolding (the wrinkle is a waiting fold, ready to respond quickly at any moment for any skin mobility need) and (b) the appropriate skin tissue for extension or compression (this reservoir of tissue is measured by the parameter of WTRV). The "wrinkling ability" of a skin area is linked to the wrinkle's functions and can be measured by the parameter of "skin tissue volume compressed around the wrinkle" in cubic millimeter per 30 mm wrinkle during maximum wrinkling. The presence of wrinkles is a sign that the skin's "recovery ability" has declined progressively with age. The skin's "recovery ability" is linked to undesirable cosmetic effects of aging and wrinkling. This new profilometric method can be applied in studies where the effectiveness of antiwrinkle preparations or the cosmetic results of surgery modalities are tested, as well as in studies focused on the functional physiology of the wrinkle unit [6]. Nevertheless, the gradual physiologic decline of aging skin is well documented [7, 8].

Aging of the Epidermis

The most striking and consistent histologic change is flattening of the dermoepidermal junction, a considerably smaller surface between the two compartments and presumably less communication and nutrient transfer [9]. Dermal-epidermal separation has been demonstrated to occur more readily in old skin under experimental conditions. Inter-rete epidermal thickness probably remains constant with advancing age, but variability in epidermal thickness and in individual keratinocyte size increases [9].

Average thickness and degree of compaction of the stratum corneum appears constant with increasing age, although individual corneocytes become larger. The skin surface pattern examination reveals slight age-associated loss of regularity. There is also an age-related decrease in the barrier function of intact stratum corneum as measured by percutaneous absorption of at least some substances. Subsequent work suggests that age effects on percutaneous absorption depend, in part, on drug structure, with hydrophilic substances being less well absorbed through the skin of old subjects, but hydrophobic substances being equally well absorbed [1]. More recent work indicates that there is an age-associated decrease in percutaneous absorption for hydrophilic substances like hydrocortisone and benzoic acid, but no change for hydrophobic substances like testosterone and estradiol [10].

An age-associated decrease in epidermal turnover rate of approximately 30–50 % between the third and eighth decades has been determined by a study of desquamation rates for corneocytes at selected body sites. The thymidine-labeling index of the epidermis in vivo has been reported to decline nearly 50 % with age [1]. There is also a corresponding 100 % prolongation in stratum corneum replacement rate and a decrease in the linear growth rates for hair and nails. A study of epidermal wound healing showed that the repair rate in the skin likewise declines with age, as restoration of normal skin surface markings in deroofed subcorneal blister sites required a median of approximately 3 weeks in subjects aged 18–25 years, but 5 weeks in subjects aged 65–75 years. Healing was essentially complete in all young subjects who were healed by 7 weeks and the last by 8 weeks [11]. Clinical observations suggest that the development of chronic wounds frequently associate with persistent low tissue oxygen supply (hypoxia). The prolonged tissue hypoxia exposes wounds to bacterial infection, a prolonged inflammatory response, and eventually tissue necrosis. The elderly population accounts for a large portion of this morbidity [12]. Consistent with clinical observations, compelling evidence from laboratory studies has shown that age affects wound healing in several aspects: sprouting of aged microvessels was significantly less than the sprouting of young microvessels [13], increased gelatinase and collaginase levels in skin of aged donors and in wound fluid from chronic leg ulcers, and decreased TIMP (tissue inhibitor of matrix metalloproteinase) levels in the skin of aged donors as well as reduced deposition of matrix components and reepithelialization [14–16]. A novel study about wound healing with increasing age done by Yu-Ping Xia et al. (2001) [17] revealed that keratinocytes isolated from elderly donors, in contrast to those from young individuals, had depressed migratory activity when they were exposed to hypoxia [17]. Analysis of underlying biochemical changes demonstrated a differential activation of matrix metalloproteinases by hypoxia in keratinocytes isolated from young and old ages. Matrix metalloproteinases-1 and matrix metalloproteinases-9 and tissue inhibitor of matrix metaloproteinases-1 were strongly upregulated by hypoxia in young cells, whereas no induction was observed in aged cells. Furthermore, transforming growth factor-β1 signaling appears to be involved in keratinocyte differential response to hypoxia, as transforming growth factor-β type 1 receptor was upregulated by hypoxia in young cells, while there was no induction in aged cells. Transforming growth factor-β neutralizing reagents blocked hypoxia-induced matrix metalloproteinase-1, matrix metalloproteinase-9 expression, and hypoxia-induced cell migration as well. These results introduced by Yu-Ping Xia et al. [17] suggest that an age-related decrease in response to hypoxia plays a crucial part in the pathogenesis of related reepithelialization in wounds [17].

A decrease in the number of the enzymatically active melanocytes per unit surface area of the skin, approximately 10–20 % of the remaining cell population each decade, has been repeatedly documented [8]. It is not known whether the cells truly disappear or simply become undetectable by ceasing to produce pigment, but in either case the protective barrier of the body against ultraviolet radiation presumably is reduced. The number of melanocytic nevi (moles) also progressively decreases with age from a peak of 15–40 in the third and fourth decade to an average of four per person after age 50; moles are rarely observed in persons above age 80 [18]. The contribution of extracellular matrix components to intrinsic skin aging has been investigated thoroughly; however, there is little information as to the role of the cytoskeletal proteins in this process. Therefore, the new studies highlight the importance of the cellular compartment in this process and demonstrate that special attention has to be given to RNA as well as protein normalization in aging studies. Oender et al. (2008) demonstrated that the mRNA levels of the genes for K1, K3, K4, K9, K13, K15, K18, K19, and K20 are downregulated in aged skin, K5 and K14 are unchanged, and K2, K16, and K17 are upregulated in aged skin. The mRNA data were confirmed on the protein level. This diverse picture is in contrast to other cytoskeletal proteins including components of the desmosome (JUP), microtubuli (TUBA), and microfilaments (ACTB) – often regarded as house-keeping genes – that were all reduced in aged skin [19].

The incidence of cancers, infectious diseases, and autoimmune disorders increases with advancing age [20]. In addition, aging is accompanied by a number of changes in immune function such as decreased lymphocyte proliferative responses to both mitogens and antigens, reduced delayed type hypersensitivity reactions, and decreased antibody responses to vaccination and infection [19]. Murine models of aging have demonstrated that there is an age-associated dysregulation in cytokine production, as evidenced by consistently decreased production of interleukin-2 (IL-2) and generally increased production of interleukin-4 [21]. These data, coupled with the increased incidence of cancer and the recurrence of latent viral infection in aged humans, have led to the hypothesis that the process of aging per se induces a switch from a predominantly type 1 cytokine (IL-2, INF-γ, IL-12) profile, supporting a dominant cell-mediated immune response, to a predominantly type 2 cytokine (IL-4, IL-5, IL-6, IL-10) profile, promoting a dominant humoral response. A 20–50 % reduction in the number of morphologically identifiable epidermal Langerhans cells occurs between early and late adulthood and may account in part for the age-associated decrease in immune responsiveness observed in the skin [7, 8].

In principle, inhibition of aging should delay cancer. But the question which arises is whether it is possible to slow aging. As recently proposed, the nutrient-sensing TOR (target of rapamycin) pathway is involved in cellular and organismal aging. In rodents, certain conditions that interfere with the TOR pathway slow aging and prevent cancer. Retrospective analysis of clinical data reveals that in animals, from worms to mammals, caloric restrictions, life-extending agents, and numerous mutations that increase longevity all converge on the TOR pathway. And, in humans, cell hypertrophy, hyperfunction, and hyperplasia, typically associated with activation of TOR, contribute to diseases of aging. Theoretical and clinical considerations suggest that rapamycin may be effective against atherosclerosis, hypertension, and hypercoagulation (thus, preventing myocardial infarction and stroke), osteoporosis, cancer, autoimmune diseases and arthritis, obesity, diabetes, macular degeneration, and Alzheimer's and Parkinson's diseases. Finally, the extended life span will reveal new causes for aging (e.g., ROS, "wear and tear", Hayflick limit, stem cell exhaustion) that play a limited role now, in relation to TOR. So, there is a potential clinical use of TOR inhibitors in order to slow aging and delay cancer [22]. Richardson et al. (2004) also emphasized that regulation of growth and proliferation in higher eukaryotic cells results from an integration of nutritional, energy, and mitogenic signals [23]. Biochemical processes underlying cell growth and proliferation are governed by the phosphatidylinositol 3-kinase (PI3K) and TOR signaling pathways. The importance of the interplay between these two pathways is underscored by the discovery that the TOR inhibitor rapamycin is effective against tumors caused by misregulation of the PI3K pathway.

Moreover, one of the recent breakthrough studies in TOR signaling resulted in the identification of the tuberous sclerosis complex gene products, TSC1 and TSC2, as negative regulators for TOR signaling. Furthermore, the discovery that the small GTPase Rheb is a direct downstream target of TSC1-TSC2 and a positive regulator of the TOR function has significantly advanced the understanding of the molecular mechanism of TOR activation. So, the regulation of TOR signaling is very important to control cell growth during normal development and tumorigenesis [24].

Vitamin D production, which is an important endocrine function of human epidermis, is suspected to decline with age. With advancing age, bone mass decreases markedly, especially in postmenopausal women, predisposing to trabecular bone fractures. Osteoporosis, or lack of cortical and trabecular bone, is a prominent factor, but some elderly individuals also have osteomalacia, since the decreased mineralization of bone is classically associated with vitamin D deficiency. Although avoidance of dairy products, the principal dietary source of vitamin D, insufficient sun exposure, and sun screen use undoubtedly contribute to vitamin D deficiency in the elderly [25]. The level of epidermal 7-dehydrocholesterol per unit skin surface area also appears to decrease linearly by approximately 75 % between early and late adulthood suggesting that lack of its

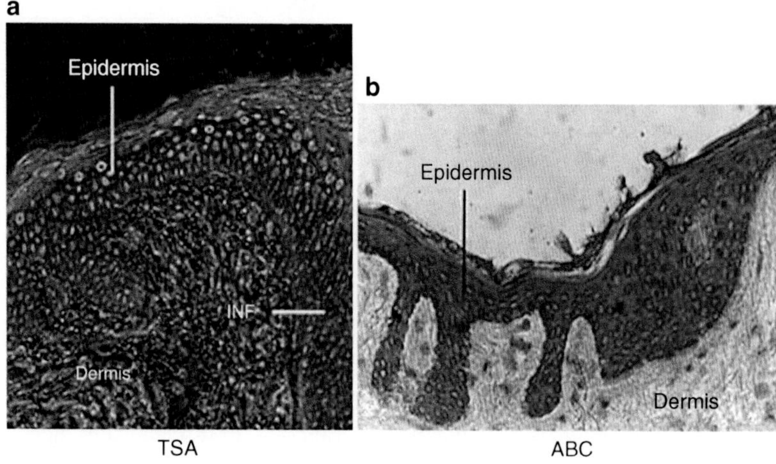

Fig. 1 Expression of Hsp27 protein in normal human skin. A moderate to strong expression is found in most epidermal layers, including the stratum corneum. (**a**) Tyramid signal amplification (TSA) technique (200×), (**b**) avidin-biotin complex (ABC) technique (200×) (Reprinted with permission from Adly et al. [47].) © 2006, Elsevier

immediate biosynthetic precursor may also limit vitamin D production. In one study, old adult volunteers exposed to total body UV irradiation produced far less vitamin D3, over the ensuing week, than did complexion-matched young adult volunteers exposed to the same UV dose [2].

Neoplasia is associated with aging in virtually all organ systems but is especially characteristic for aged skin. Acrochorrdon, cherry angioma, seborrheic keratosis, lentigo, and sebaceous hyperplasia are benign epidermal tumors; one or more of these benign epidermal tumors is present in nearly every adult beyond age 65 years, and most individuals have dozens of lesions [20]. Actinically induced basal cell carcinoma and squamous cell carcinoma are by far the most common human malignancies. These benign and malignant neoplasms almost certainly reflect in part the loss of proliferative homeostasis with age.

Epidermal Proteins and Skin Aging

Recent studies revealed by gel electrophoresis of healthy human skin (sun-protected skin) from donors of different ages that there are age-associated changes in five proteins, which were identified as keratin 10, involucrin, prealbumin, Hsp 27, and Rho B. More recently, it was found by the tool of immunohistochemistry that these epidermal proteins are expressed in the human skin epidermis and that their expression patterns undergo age-associated changes [26]. Examination of cryosections from healthy sun-protected skin derived from individuals ranging from the first decade of life until the ninth decade revealed that keratin 10, involucrin, prealbumin, Hsp 27, and Rho B proteins are present in high density nearly in all layers of young epidermis (Fig. 1). In contrast, the expression of the investigated epidermal proteins is reduced as a function of age. In some skin specimens from very old individuals, the proteins were not detectable [26].

All five proteins are known to be closely related to differentiation and proliferation of keratinocytes. Moreover, prealbumin, Hsp27, and Rho B have been demonstrated to play a crucial role in tumor cell biology. Thus, decreased expression of these proteins could be one reason for the increased prevalence of skin cancer in old individuals. Additionally, these proteins are possible marker proteins for intrinsic aging of the epidermis [26]. Additionally, Hsp27 and other epidermal proteins were found to be expressed in the human skin hair follicles and involved in hair follicle cycle control [26] (Fig. 2).

Aging of the Dermis

Loss of dermal thickness approaches 20 % in elderly individuals, although in sun-protected sites significant thinning occurs only after the

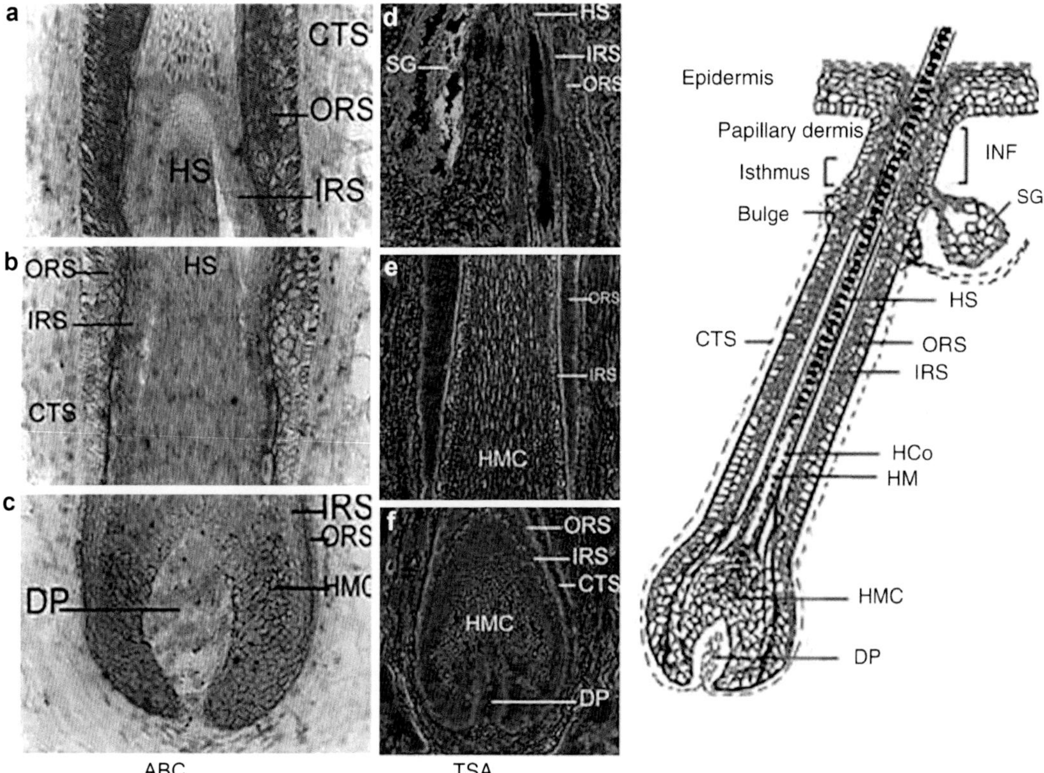

Fig. 2 Expression of Hsp27 protein in normal human scalp skin anagen VI hair follicle, immunostained with (ABC) and (TSA) techniques. (**a** and **d**) show the distal region (200×), (**b** and **e**) show the central region (200×), (**c** and **f**) show the proximal bulb region (200×). (**d**) shows schematic representation of anagen VI hair follicle (Reprinted with permission from Adly et al. [47].) © 2006, Elsevier

eighth decade [27]; the remaining tissue is relatively acellular and avascular [1, 9]. Precise histologic concomitants of wrinkling, if any, are unknown, although the age-related loss of normal elastin fibers may be contributory [9]. Deep expression lines seem to result from contractions of connective tissue septae within the subcutaneous fat. In one study, an approximately 50 % reduction in mast cells and a 30 % reduction in venular cross sections were noted in the papillary dermis of buttock skin from elderly adults compared to that from young adult controls, associated with a corresponding reduction in histamine released and other manifestations of the inflammatory response following UV radiation exposure [7]. The striking age-associated loss of vascular bed, especially of the vertical capillary loops that occupy the dermal papillae in young skin, is felt to underlie many of the physiologic alterations in old skin. Reduction in the vascular network surrounding hair bulbs and eccrine, apocrine, and sebaceous glands may contribute to their gradual atrophy and fibrosis with age [1]. An age-associated decrease in dermal clearance of transepidermally absorbed materials has been reported and is probably due to alterations in both the vascular and extracellular matrix. A previous study showed that wheal resorption after intradermal saline injection required almost twice as long on average in elderly versus young adult subjects [1]. Controversely, the time required for development of a tense blister after topical application of 50 % ammonium hydroxide is nearly twice as long in older subjects, suggesting a decreased transduction rate with age in injured skin. Impaired transfer of cells as well as solutes between the extravascular and intravascular dermal compartments is suggested by several studies to occur by age, but it is difficult to isolate these components in a complex inflammatory reaction. Decreased vascular responsiveness in the skin of older individuals has been documented clinically assessing vasodilation and transudation after application of standardized irritants, histamine, and the mast cell degranulating agent 48/80 [11].

Intensity of erythema following a standardized UV exposure is also decreased with age in normal skin, although factors other than decreased vascular responsiveness may also contribute [7]. A previous study that assessed cutaneous vascular response to the vasodilator methyl nicotinate concluded that there was no difference between young adult and old adult subjects after correction for rate of drug absorption [28]. Compromised thermoregulation, which predisposes the elderly to sometimes fatal heat stroke or hypothermia may be due in part to reduced vascularity of dermal arterioles, and in the latter instance, to loss of subcutaneous fat as well. The skin of healthy older subjects is less sensitive to dinitrochlorobenzene (DNCB) and to standard recall antigens, compared to the skin of young adult controls [29]. This decrease undoubtedly reflects the well-documented decrease in total number of circulating thymus-derived lymphocytes and in their responsiveness to standard mitogens.

The elastic fibers in the skin are less well studied but have been reported to show progressive cross-linkage and calcification with age in adult skin. On average, older skin has thicker elastic fibers than young skin, and elastic fiber alterations extend deeper into the dermis with advancing age [30, 31]. Small cysts and lacuna are common in aging elastic fibers, sometimes progressing to complete fragmentation. Similar changes can be produced experimentally by incubation of dermal slices with elastase or chymotrypsin (but not collagenase) in vitro, suggesting that enzymatic degradation of elastin may be a mechanism of normal dermal aging [30, 31]. The dermal microvasculature in middle-aged or elderly subjects may show mild vascular wall thickening; vascular wall thinning to less than half of the normal young adult measurement associated with absent or reduced perivascular veil cells has been reported in skin of very old subjects and probably contributes to vascular fragility [30, 31]. Significant decrease in thrombomodulin-positive cells and vascularity were evidenced in the aged group. Specific subsets of the dermal dendrocyte populations and the blood microvasculature appear affected by aging. Capsaicin may limit these aging effects [32].

Biochemical changes in collagen, elastin, and dermal ground substance that have been described during fetal and early postnatal development are far greater than those that have been described with advancing age during adulthood. With advancing adult age, rat tail collagen does manifest a slight increase in the force of contraction (isometric tension), when heated above its shrinkage temperature, consistent with increasing cross-linkage of the collagen molecule [33]. Both rat tail tendon and human skin display a progressive decrease in the ratio of soluble to insoluble collagen [34]. The predominant cross-links in skin have been reported to decrease and virtually disappear with age in mature animals, however, using techniques that measure borohydride reducible cross-links, despite evidence of increasing mechanical stability This suggests that some collagen cross-links in vivo may be progressively reduced or oxidized and are, therefore, no longer measurable. Certain nonenzymatic cross-links in connective tissue, such as histidinoalanine and the Millard reaction product, do show a strong positive correlation with adult age and have been suggested to contribute to age-associated changes in the dermis [1]. The proportion of recently synthesized dermal collagen, as determined by neutral salt extraction, is small and does not vary with age in adult [35, 36]. However, there is a significant decrease with age in the percent of total collagen that is released by pepsin digestion, and hence incompletely cross-linked, from approximately 25 % at 30 years to approximately 10 % at 75 years with a proportionate increase in the percent of insoluble collagen from approximately 70–88 %. The amount of ketoamine-linked glycosylation of insoluble dermal collagen also increases with age, possibly related to slower collagen turnover or higher average glucose levels in the tissue [35, 36]. Prolyl- and lysyl-hydroxylase, enzymes necessary for intercellular stabilization of the collagen triple helix and for its intermolecular cross-linking, show an age-associated decline in activity in human skin, although these coenzyme activities in cultured dermal fibroblasts from donors ranging in age from a few months to 94 years do not. This apparent contradiction could be explained by an age-associated decrease in either dermal fibroblast number in vivo or fibroblast responsiveness to a serum-derived enzyme stimulating factor in vitro.

There is some data concerning the possible postmaturational age-associated changes in mucopolysaccharides (glycosaminoglycans and proteoglycans) or other molecules of the ground substance in which collagen and elastic fibers are embedded. There appears to be a slight decrease with age in mucopolysaccharide content relative to dry weight or collagen content of the skin, especially for hyaluronic acid. Although mucopolysaccharides constitute only 0.1–0.3 % of dry weight for whole skin, their decrease may adversely influence skin turgor as proteoglycans bind a high volume of water in the dermis [37, 38].

Mechanical properties of the skin also change with age. Uniaxial and biaxial tension tests performed on excised abdominal skin stripes demonstrate progressive loss of elastic recovery, consistent with gradual destruction of the dermal elastin network, and the time required for excised skin to return to its original thickness after 50 % compression is markedly prolonged [39]. This early work, which has been confirmed and extended by in vivo studies of ventral forearm skin of 133 volunteers in each decade of life, showed linear declines of approximately 25 % in both men and women for elasticity and extensibility. Loss of elasticity began in childhood and continued through the ninth decade, while extensibility was constant through the sixth decade and then declines more rapidly thereafter. Overall, a picture emerges of aging dermis as an increasingly rigid, inelastic, and unresponsive tissue, less capable of undergoing modification in response to stress. IGF-I is a key regulator of human skin aging and declining IGF-I levels with age may play a significant role in the reduction of skin surface lipids and thickness [40].

Nerves and Appendages

By the end of the fifth decade, approximately half the population has at least 50 % grey (white) body hair with an even higher proportion of depigmented scalp hair, and virtually everyone has some degree of greying due to progressive and eventually total loss of melanocytes from the hair bulb. Loss of melanocytes is believed to occur more rapidly in hair than in skin because the cells proliferate and manufacture melanin at maximal rates during the anagen phase of the hair cycle, while epidermal melanocytes are comparatively inactive throughout their lifespan. Scalp hair may gray more rapidly than other body hair because its anagen to telogen ratio is considerably greater than that of other body hair. Advancing age is also accompanied by a modest decrease in number of hair follicles. Remaining hairs may be smaller in diameter and grow more slowly. The process called balding results primarily from the androgen-dependent conversion of the relatively dark thick scalp hairs to lightly pigmented short fine hairs similar to those on the ventral forearm. Bitemporal hair line recession begins during late adolescence in most women and virtually all men. Assessment of baldness is hampered by lack of a precise definition, but by certain criteria advanced bitemporal and occipital hair loss in men increases in prevalence, respectively, from 20 % and 30 % at the end of the third decade to more than 60 % by the seventh decade. Eccrine glands decrease approximately 15 % in average number during childhood in most body sites. Spontaneous sweating in response to dry heat is further reduced by more than 70 % in healthy old subjects as compared to young controls, attributable primarily to a decreased output per gland. Maximal sweat production has not been quantified in the elderly but is almost certainly reduced and probably predisposes to heat stroke in this age group [41]. Similar studies have not been performed for apocrine glands, although the apparently decreased requirement for underarm deodorants in the elderly suggests decreased function. Lipofuscin gradually accumulates with age in the secretory cells of both eccrine and apocrine glands.

Sebaceous gland size and number appear not to change with age [9]. The exponential decrease in sebum production of approximately 23 % per decade beginning in the second decade in both men and women, approximately 60 % over the adult lifespan, is attributed to the concomitant decrease in production of gonadal or adrenal androgen to which sebaceous glands are exquisitely sensitive. The clinical effects of decreased sebum production, if any, are unknown. There is no direct relationship to xerosis or seborrheic dermatitis [42].

Pacinian and Meissner's corpuscles, the cutaneous end organs responsible for pressure perception, light and touch, progressively decrease to approximately one third of their initial average density between the second and ninth decades of life and display greater size variation. There are very few histologically demonstrable aging-related changes in Merkel corpuscles or in free nerve endings. Decreased sensory perception was documented in old skin more than three decades ago by several techniques. Cutaneous pain threshold has been reported to increase up to 20 % with advancing age [43]. The available data do not permit differentiation among an age-associated increase in the prevalence of peripheral neuropathy, a true aging change in healthy subjects, increased rate of heat dispersion in old skin due to age-associated dermal alterations, an increased peripheral nerve threshold to painful stimuli, and an increased central threshold to pain perception [43]. The many psychological and social factors influencing an individual reaction to pain may also be presumed to vary with age. In any case, either decreased awareness of, or reaction to, noxious stimuli would facilitate wounding and irritation of old skin. Sympathetic nervous system activity is altered in aging.

Aging and Skin Diseases

Disorders of the skin are known to be common and bothersome in the elderly, but existing incidence and morbidity figures are suspect [44]. Few dermatologic disorders occur predominantly in the elderly, and none is restricted to this age group. Perhaps the prototypic disease of old skin is bullous pemphigoid, characterized by subepidermal blister formation with fixation of complement and immunoglobulins along the basement membrane. Its predilection for the elderly may partially explained by the age-associated increase in circulating autoantibodies and ease of dermal-epidermal separation, although other autoimmune and blistering dermatoses are not more common in old age. Possibly age-associated changes in the basement membrane itself render it specifically vulnerable to the disease process. More than two thirds of herpes zoster cases occur after the fifth decade, with an age-adjusted annual incidence rate of approximately 0.25 % at 20–50 years versus more than 1 % at age 80 years [45]. Postherpetic neuralgia, uncommon in patients less than 40 years old, occurs frequently in older patients, more than half of those beyond age 60 years. In one large series this altered response to varicella virus has been established; however, no mechanism explaining this altered response to varicella virus has been found. Recurrent herpes simplex infection also involves reactivation of latent virus in regional ganglia and T cell-mediated host defenses but is more common in young adults and indeed rare among immunocompetent elders. The general phenomenon of impaired wound healing in the elderly may account for slower resolution of the acute eruption, but its relevance, if any, to postherpetic neuralgia is unclear [45]. Age-associated muting of the inflammatory response might indeed be expected to reduce the risk of neuralgia, since prophylactic use of anti-inflammatory corticosteriods is often successful.

Xerosis, the dry rough quality of old skin, may be attributable to a subtle disorder of epidermal maturation, although histologic studies reveal little alteration of either the viable epidermis or the stratum corneum with age. Available data fails to support water loss [1], decreased stratum corneum lipids [42], or altered amino acid composition as etiologic factors [42]. The surface irregularity may also be attributed simply to slower transit of corneocytes through the stratum corneum, allowing accumulation of damage in situ. Similarly, there is no explanation for the pruritus that often accompanies xerosis. Unsupported hypotheses include frequent penetration of irritants through an abnormal stratum corneum and an altered sensory threshold due to subtle neuropathy. Many dermatoses more commonly observed in the elderly reflect the higher prevalence of systemic diseases such as diabetes, vascular insufficiency, and various neurologic syndromes in this population. In the case of chronic leg ulcers, for example, healing of previously recalcitrant lesions can sometimes be achieved by use of neonatal epidermal allograft, postulated to elaborate needed growth factors and/or matrix materials that the surrounding senescent host epithelium is incapable of producing. The allegedly increased incidence of other disorders such as tinea pedis or seborrheic dermatitis may reflect reduced local skin care with subsequent exacerbation of previously unapparent problems, rather than an age-associated change in the skin itself. Alternatively, subtle changes in the immune status may be responsible in analogy to the increased prevalence and severity of those disorders in patients with acquired immunodeficiency syndrome [1]. Reduced tolerance to systematically administrated drugs is well documented in the elderly due to the decrements in lean body mass and metabolism and renal excretion of the active ingredients [46]. Comparable data for topically applied medication do not exist, but it is tempting to postulate that retarded dermal clearance of absorbed material reduced dermal mass and cellularity, and possibly altered metabolic capacity may render old skin more susceptible to both beneficial and adverse effects of topical medications, or at least alter the optimal dosage frequency [1]. In the case of corticosteriod preparations, relative vascular unresponsiveness may render blanching of erythema as an unreliable indicator of other effects in old skin.

Conclusion

A better understanding of both the intrinsic and extrinsic influences on the aging of the skin, as well as distinguishing the retractable aspects of cutaneous aging (primarily hormonal and lifestyle influences) from the irretractable cutaneous aging (primarily intrinsic aging), is very important to solve the problem of aging.

Cross-References

▶ Degenerative Changes in Aging Skin

References

1. Balin AK, Pratt LA. Physiological consequences of human skin aging. Cutis. 1989;43(5):431–6.
2. Puizina-Ivic N. Skin aging. Acta Dermatovenerol Alp Panonica Adriat. 2008;17(2):47–54.
3. Ding SL, Shen CY. Model of human aging: recent findings on Werner's and Hutchinson-Gilford progeria syndromes. Clin Interv Aging. 2008;3(3):431–44.
4. Holtkotter O, Schlotmann K, Hofheinz H, Olbrisch RR, Petersohn D. Unveiling the molecular basis of intrinsic skin aging(1). Int J Cosmet Sci. 2005;27(5):263–9.
5. Chondrogianni N, de Simoes D CM, Franceschi C, Gonos ES. Cloning of differentially expressed genes in skin fibroblasts from centenarians. Biogerontology. 2004;5(6):401–9.
6. Hatzis J. The wrinkle and its measurement – a skin surface Profilometric method. Micron. 2004;35(3):201–19.
7. Gilchrest BA, Stoff JS, Soter NA. Chronologic aging alters the response to ultraviolet-induced inflammation in human skin. J Invest Dermatol. 1982;79(1):11–5.
8. Gilchrest BA. Age-associated changes in the skin. J Am Geriatr Soc. 1982;30(2):139–43.
9. Montagna W, Carlisle K. Structural changes in aging human skin. J Invest Dermatol. 1979;73(1):47–53.
10. Roskos KV, Maibach HI, Guy RH. The effect of aging on percutaneous absorption in man. J Pharmacokinet Biopharm. 1989;17(6):617–30.
11. Grove GL. Age-related differences in healing of superficial skin wounds in humans. Arch Dermatol Res. 1982;272(3–4):381–5.
12. Van de Kerkhof PC, Van Bergen B, Spruijt K, Kuiper JP. Age-related changes in wound healing. Clin Exp Dermatol. 1994;19(5):369–74.
13. Arthur WT, Vernon RB, Sage EH, Reed MJ. Growth factors reverse the impaired sprouting of microvessels from aged mice. Microvasc Res. 1998;55(3):260–70.
14. Ashcroft GS, Horan MA, Ferguson MW. Aging is associated with reduced deposition of specific extracellular matrix components, an upregulation of angiogenesis, and an altered inflammatory response in a murine incisional wound healing model. J Invest Dermatol. 1997;108(4):430–7.
15. Ashcroft GS, Herrick SE, Tarnuzzer RW, Horan MA, Schultz GS, Ferguson MW. Human ageing impairs injury-induced in vivo expression of tissue inhibitor

of matrix metalloproteinases (TIMP)-1 and −2 proteins and mRNA. J Pathol. 1997;183(2):169–76.
16. Ashcroft GS, Kielty CM, Horan MA, Ferguson MW. Age-related changes in the temporal and spatial distributions of fibrillin and elastin mRNAs and proteins in acute cutaneous wounds of healthy humans. J Pathol. 1997;183(1):80–9.
17. Xia YP, Zhao Y, Tyrone JW, Chen A, Mustoe TA. Differential activation of migration by hypoxia in keratinocytes isolated from donors of increasing age: implication for chronic wounds in the elderly. J Invest Dermatol. 2001;116(1):50–6.
18. Maize JC, Foster G. Age-related changes in melanocytic naevi. Clin Exp Dermatol. 1979;4(1):49–58.
19. Oender K, Trost A, Lanschuetzer C, Laimer M, Emberger M, Breitenbach M, Richter K, Hintner H, Bauer JW. Cytokeratin-related loss of cellular integrity is not a major driving force of human intrinsic skin aging. Mech Ageing Dev. 2008;129(10):563–71.
20. Blagosklonny MV. Prevention of cancer by inhibiting aging. Cancer Biol Ther. 2008;7(10):1520–4.
21. Albright JW, Mease RC, Lambert C, Albright JF. Trypanosoma musculi: tracking parasites and circulating lymphoid cells in host mice. Exp Parasitol. 1999;91(2):185–95.
22. Blagosklonny MV. Aging: ROS or TOR. Cell Cycle. 2008;7(21):3344–54.
23. Richardson CJ, Schalm SS, Blenis J. PI3-kinase and TOR: PIKTORing cell growth. Semin Cell Dev Biol. 2004;15(2):147–59.
24. Inoki K, Ouyang H, Li Y, Guan KL. Signaling by target of rapamycin proteins in cell growth control. Microbiol Mol Biol Rev. 2005;69(1):79–100.
25. Matsuoka LY, Wortsman J, Hanifan N, Holick MF. Chronic sunscreen use decreases circulating concentrations of 25-hydroxyvitamin D. A preliminary study. Arch Dermatol. 1988;124(12):1802–4.
26. Hussein MR. Analysis of p53, BCL-2 and epidermal growth factor receptor protein expression in the partial and complete hydatidiform moles. Exp Mol Pathol. 2009;87(1):63–9. doi:10.1016/j.yexmp.2009.03.005. Epub 2009 Apr 5
27. de Rigal J, Escoffier C, Querleux B, Faivre B, Agache P, Leveque JL. Assessment of aging of the human skin by in vivo ultrasonic imaging. J Invest Dermatol. 1989;93(5):621–5.
28. Roskos KV, Bircher AJ, Maibach HI, Guy RH. Pharmacodynamic measurements of methyl nicotinate percutaneous absorption: the effect of aging on microcirculation. Br J Dermatol. 1990;122(2):165–71.
29. Wayne SJ, Rhyne RL, Garry PJ, Goodwin JS. Cell-mediated immunity as a predictor of morbidity and mortality in subjects over 60. J Gerontol. 1990;45(2): M45–8.
30. Braverman IM, Fonferko E. Studies in cutaneous aging: II. The microvasculature. J Invest Dermatol. 1982;78(5):444–8.
31. Braverman IM, Fonferko E. Studies in cutaneous aging: I. The elastic fiber network. J Invest Dermatol. 1982;78(5):434–43.
32. Quatresooz P, Pierard GE. Immunohistochemical clues at aging of the skin microvascular unit. J Cutan Pathol. 2009;36(1):39–43.
33. Escoffier C, de Rigal J, Rochefort A, Vasselet R, Leveque JL, Agache PG. Age-related mechanical properties of human skin: an in vivo study. J Invest Dermatol. 1989;93(3):353–7.
34. Miyahara T, Murai A, Tanaka T, Shiozawa S, Kameyama M. Age-related differences in human skin collagen: solubility in solvent, susceptibility to pepsin digestion, and the spectrum of the solubilized polymeric collagen molecules. J Gerontol. 1982;37(6): 651–5.
35. Schnider SL, Kohn RR. Effects of age and diabetes mellitus on the solubility and nonenzymatic glucosylation of human skin collagen. J Clin Invest. 1981;67(6):1630–5.
36. Schnider SL, Kohn RR. Effects of age and diabetes mellitus on the solubility of collagen from human skin, tracheal cartilage and dura mater. Exp Gerontol. 1982;17(3):185–94.
37. Lipson MJ, Silbert JE. Acid mucopolysaccharides of tadpole tail fin and back skin. Biochim Biophys Acta. 1965;101(3):279–84.
38. Kondo K, Seno N, Anno K. Mucopolysaccharides from chicken skin of three age groups. Biochim Biophys Acta. 1971;244(3):513–22.
39. Daly CH, Odland GF. Age-related changes in the mechanical properties of human skin. J Invest Dermatol. 1979;73(1):84–7.
40. Makrantonaki E, Vogel K, Fimmel S, Oeff M, Seltmann H, Zouboulis CC. Interplay of IGF-I and 17beta-estradiol at age-specific levels in human sebocytes and fibroblasts in vitro. Exp Gerontol. 2008;43(10):939–46.
41. Silver AF, Chase HB. An in vivo method for studying the hair cycle. Nature. 1966;210(5040):1051.
42. Downing DT, Stewart ME, Strauss JS. Changes in sebum secretion and the sebaceous gland. Dermatol Clin. 1986;4(3):419–23.
43. Procacci P, Zoppi M, Maresca M. Experimental pain in man. Pain. 1979;6(2):123–40.
44. Beauregard S, Gilchrest BA. A survey of skin problems and skin care regimens in the elderly. Arch Dermatol. 1987;123(12):1638–43.
45. Hope-Simpson RE. The nature of herpes zoster: a long-term study and a new hypothesis. Proc R Soc Med. 1965;58:9–20.
46. Vestal RE. Aging and pharmacology. Cancer. 1997;80 (7):1302–10.
47. Adly MA, Assaf HA, Hussein MR. Expression of the heat shock protein-27 in the adult human scalp skin and hair follicle: hair cycle-dependent changes. J Am Acad Dermatol. 2006;54(5):811–7.

Infrared Radiation: Mechanisms, Implications, and Protection

63

Kasra Soltani Nia and Howard I. Maibach

Contents

K.S. Nia (✉)
Department of Dermatology, University of California, School of Medicine, San Francisco, CA, USA
e-mail: kasra101@gmail.com

H.I. Maibach
Department of Dermatology, University of California, San Francisco, CA, USA
e-mail: maibachh@derm.ucsf.edu

M.A. Farage et al. (eds.), *Textbook of Aging Skin*,
DOI 10.1007/978-3-662-47398-6_175

Abstract

Skin damage, as a result of solar radiation, has long been associated to exposure of UV radiation (UVB and UVA) on human skin. However, this damage can also be attributed to longer wavelengths, specifically infrared radiation (IR). Infrared A radiation (IRA; 760 nm–1440 nm) has been shown to induce skin damage in two significant ways: upregulation of the enzyme matrix metalloproteinase (MMP-1), responsible for the degradation of proteins in the extracellular matrix, and an increase in free radical production, specifically reactive oxygen species (ROS). Protection against IRA is currently centered around the use of antioxidants to neutralize ROS production, leading to the downregulation of MMP-1 mRNA and protein expression. Thus, the sunscreen of the future should provide protection for the entire solar spectrum.

Introduction

Human skin is exposed to solar radiation daily with UV being the main focus of photoaging and inflammation. The consequences of UV irradiation to human fibroblasts as well as the need for effective protection against it has been the main

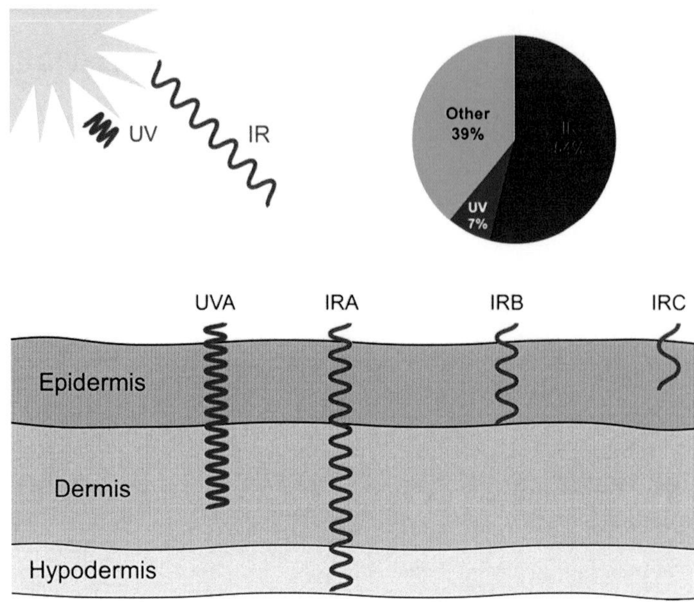

Fig. 1 Ratio of IR in comparison to UV taken from total solar radiation in addition to the categorization of IR as it relates to dermal components. IRA penetrates deeply into the skin reaching the hypodermis, while IRB and IRC only penetrate the epidermis

topic of photoaging in the past. However, recent studies have shown that infrared radiation may also have a profound role in inflammation and photoaging. Infrared radiation has a wavelength of 760 nm–1 mm and is categorized, similar to UV, into infrared A irradiation (IRA; 760–1,440 nm), infrared B irradiation (IRB; 1,440–3,000 nm), and infrared C irradiation (IRC; 3,000 nm–1 mm). Infrared radiation accounts for 54 % of the total energy transferred by the sun, the largest part being IRA, which accounts for 30 % of total solar energy, while UV only contributes 7 % [1]. IRA penetrates deeply into human skin reaching both the deep dermis and hypodermis while IRB and IRC only affect the epidermis. Additionally, IRA penetrates the skin more effectively in comparison to UV, with approximately 50 % reaching the dermis [1–3] (Fig. 1). Solar radiation is influenced by a variety of factors including ozone layer, position of the sun, latitude, altitude, cloud cover, and ground reflections. Therefore, it should be noted that most studies discussed in this chapter use artificial sources of IR at specifically set doses for specific times. This chapter examines the contemporary knowledge through the analysis of recent studies which provide evidence for the underlying mechanisms of IR, implications of IR in regard to photoaging, and protection as it pertains to IR-induced skin aging.

Skin Damage by Infrared Radiation

The direct implications of IRA are best demonstrated by observation of the changes in the transcriptome of primary human skin fibroblasts through Microarray analysis [4]. Approximately 600 genes were found to be activated by IRA, and these genes were clustered into the four categories: extracellular matrix, calcium homeostasis, stress signaling, and apoptosis [4]. Among these genes that were significantly upregulated in primary human skin fibroblasts was that coding for MMPs, specifically MMP-1 [4]. Increased MMP-1 mRNA expression occurred in human skin fibroblasts without the upregulation of its tissue specific inhibitor TIMP-1, indicating the possibility that IRA may cause increased MMP-1 activity, and the degradation of the extracellular matrix leading to the breakdown of collagen fibers, which would ultimately cause the formation of coarse wrinkles and photoaged skin [7].

Matrix metalloproteinase (MMPs) are zinc-dependent calcium-containing endopeptidases mainly responsible for the degradation of proteins in the extracellular matrix, in this case, dermal fibers, collagen, and elastin. MMPs are primarily deployed after dermal wounds in order to break down the damaged extracellular matrix, allowing new extracellular matrix components to assimilate congruously with the intact extracellular matrix. The MMPs are then regulated by specific endogenous tissue inhibitors of MMPs (TIMPS), which encompass four protease inhibitors. The upregulation of MMPs without a parallel increase in TIMP expression results in the degradation of the healthy components in the extracellular matrix essential in maintaining the mechanisms of the dermis [5, 6].

IRA upregulates MMP-1 protein and mRNA expression resulting in the modifications to the extracellular matrix both in vitro on fibroblasts and in vivo on human skin [7, 8]. Using normal buttock skin of 32 healthy human volunteers, a single dose (360 or 720 J/cm^2) of IRA prompted increased MMP-1 mRNA expression and protein release ex vivo [7]. Similarly, fibroblasts exposed to a single dose of IRA (162 J/cm^2) for 1 h and incubated for 24 h in vitro reflected a clear increase in MMP-1 mRNA expression and protein release under low to moderate doses of IRA irradiation [8].

Collagen itself, a component of the extracellular matrix, can be used in order to counteract the degradation of MMPs; however, IRA exposure results in a decrease in the expression of collagen type 1 and in some cases, more specifically, alpha 1 (Col1a1) [8–10]. The reduction in collagen was detected 72 h after IRA exposure through immunostaining [8]. Similar results were also observed after the buttocks of 16 healthy volunteers (aged 24–43 years, ten male and six female) were irradiated with a 1.1–3 minimal erythema dose (MED) of natural sunlight [9]. Likewise, human dermal fibroblasts were isolated from the foreskin of three donors and then irradiated exposed to a single dose of IRA (240 J/cm^2) for 15 min, then immunoblotted with antibodies directed against Col1a1 [10].

IRA has also been found to increase the number of MAST cells, indicating its photoaging ability as this also occurs with UV radiation [11]. Using buttock skin taken from young volunteers and testing for upregulated tryptase expression using immunohistochemical staining of mast cell-specific tryptase and chymase, both UV or IRA resulted in a clear increase in MAST cells [11].

The upregulation of MMP-1 by IRA is also similar to UV in terms of collagen equilibrium, but the rudimentary mechanisms are substantially different [12, 13]. IRA utilizes mitochondrial reactive oxygen species (ROS) as the initiating episode to alter the expression of the MMP-1 gene via activation of the MAP kinases ERK1/2 [13, 14]. This event occurs in the mitochondria due to the components of the mitochondrial respiratory chain which absorb IRA [15]. This instigates a disturbance in mitochondrial electron flow, increasing mitochondrial ROS production. The implications of this event stimulate retrograde signaling mechanisms that are directly related to nuclear gene expression [16] (Fig. 2).

Following IRA irradiation, both cells and mitochondria experience an increase in free radical production in vitro on normal human fibroblasts as well as in vivo on human skin [8, 13, 17]. This was confirmed under low dosages of irradiation (20-160 J/cm^2) in vitro on various fibroblast samples from the cheek, face, breast, and eyelids through incubation of cells with dichlorofluorescein diacetate at 100 uM for 30 min [8]. Additionally, ROS production was detected in vitro on monolayer fibroblast cultures derived from the foreskins of healthy donors aged 3–8 years through reactive oxygen species (ROS)-sensitive fluorescent probes [13]. In vivo, IRA radiation-induced free radical production through electron paramagnetic resonance spectroscopy [17]. IRA has also been found to deplete normal levels of skin antioxidants, such as cellular glutathione (GSH), β-carotene, and lycopene [13, 18]. GSH is an important endogenous antioxidant as a result of its ability to reduce disulfide bonds by serving as an electron donor and oxidizing itself into glutathione dimer (GSSG). Similarly, β-carotene is one of the most important carotenoids due to its ability to act as an antioxidant and be a precursor of Vitamin A. The oxidation of GSH levels were observed in vitro on monolayer fibroblast cultures utilizing the glutathione

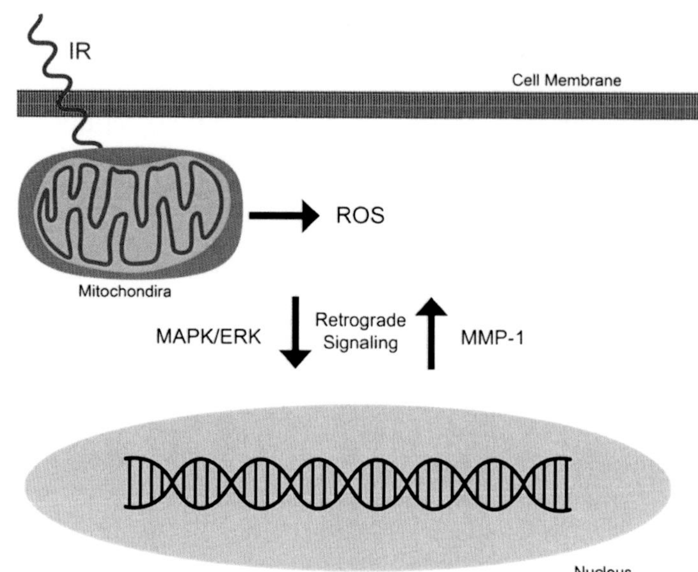

Fig. 2 IRA-induced ROS production altering the expression of the MMP-1 via activation of the MAP kinases ERK1/2, stimulating retrograde signaling mechanisms related to nuclear gene expression

recycling assay [13]. The depletion of β-carotene and lycopene levels were measured in vivo on the flexor forearms of 12 healthy volunteers (three men and nine women) who all had skin type II and were aged 25–35 years through resonance Raman spectroscopy [18]. Collectively, these independent studies provide clear evidence that IRA causes photoaging (Table 1).

Protection Against IRA Skin Damage

IRA-induced skin damage is currently centered around the use of antioxidants to neutralize ROS production which leads to the downregulation of MMP-1 mRNA and protein expression. However, IR range protection requires specific mitochondria-targeted antioxidants in order to provide maximum efficacy. Several protection methods for IR have been tested including the use of topical antioxidants and sunscreen antioxidant mixtures such as vitamin E, grape seed extract, ubiquinone, *N*-acetylcysteine, MitoQ ascorbic acid, as well as physical and chemical filters [7, 13, 18–20].

Currently there are no specific chemical or physical filters available against IRA, but existing physical filters such as titanium dioxide have shown significant IRA reflection [19]. Using pig ear skin analyzed through EPR spectroscopy after being irradiated with a duplicate dose (72 J/cm^2, 120 mW/cm^2) for 10 min, several creams containing different combination mixtures of titanium dioxide, organic UV filters, hydrophilic antioxidants, and lipophilic antioxidants were found to reduce radical formation in the IR range significantly to 65 % [19]. Regardless of its effectiveness, it should be noted that physical filters like titanium dioxide may not be a realistic protection method due to cosmetic issues, specifically a change in skin color after topical application [19].

In regard to antioxidants, the combination of *N*-acetylcysteine and MitoQ ascorbic acid has been shown to provide effective protection against IRA-induced upregulation of MMP-1 in vitro [13]. Another antioxidant mixture consisting of grape seed extract, ubiquinone, vitamin C, and vitamin E was later tested in vivo on the buttock skin of nine volunteers, six of which exhibited significant MMP-1 mRNA expression, and in which, topical application of the antioxidant mixture diminished this IRA response in six out of six individuals [7]. Furthermore, an SPF 30 sunscreen was compared to the same sunscreen supplemented with the antioxidant cocktail used previously on two sites of the buttock skin (with 2 mg/cm^2 of either mixture) on 30 healthy human volunteers (11 males, mean age

Table 1 Skin damage by infrared radiation

Findings	Obtained by	Subjects	Conclusions
Infrared radiation influences skin fibroblast transcriptome [4]	Microarray analysis and real-time PCR	Human dermal fibroblasts isolated from the foreskin of three donors	Approximately 600 genes are affected by IRA, significantly the coding for matrix metalloproteinase 1 (MMP-1)
Increased MMP-1 mRNA expression does not upregulate tissue specific inhibitor TIMP-1 [7]	Biopsies of three volunteers after irradiation with an intensity of 105 mW/cm^2 and single dose of 360–720 J/cm^2 for 57–114 min	Buttock skin of 32 healthy human subjects	IRA may cause MMP-1 activity and the degradation of the extracellular matrix
Increased MMP-1 mRNA expression and MMP-1 protein release in vivo [7]	Irradiation of buttock skin with an intensity of 105 mW/cm^2 and single dose of 360–720 J/cm^2 for 57–114 min	Buttock skin of 23 healthy human subjects	IRA leads to skin aging
Increased MMP-1 mRNA expression and MMP-1 protein release in vitro [8]	Irradiation of different body sites with an intensity of 45 mW/cm^2 exposed to a single dose of 20–160 J/cm^2 for 1 h and incubated for 24 h in vitro	Normal human skin fibroblasts from biopsies of donors aged 40–54 years from different body sites (cheek, face, breast, eyelid)	IRA leads to skin aging
Reduction in type 1 collagen [8]	Immunostaining 72 h after IRA irradiation of different body sites (with an intensity of 45 mW/cm^2 exposed to a single dose of 20–160 J/cm^2 for 1 h)	Normal human skin fibroblasts from biopsies of donors aged 40–54 years from different body sites (cheek, face, breast, eyelid)	Single IRA exposure downregulated the expression of type 1 collagen both at the mRNA and protein level
Reduction in type 1 collagen [9]	Irradiation of buttock skin with a 1.1–3 minimal erythema dose (MED) of natural sunlight	Buttocks of 16 healthy volunteers (aged 24–43 years, ten male and six female)	Single IRA exposure downregulated the expression of type 1 collagen both at the mRNA and protein level
Reduction in collagen type 1 alpha 1 (Col1a1) [10]	Irradiation of foreskin exposed to a single dose of IRA (240 J/cm^2) for 15 min	Three donors	Expression of Col1a1 is regulated by IRA
Increased number of MAST cells and upregulated tryptase expression [11]	Immunohistochemical staining of mast cell-specific tryptase and chymase	Buttock skin taken from young volunteers	Mast cells and tryptase expression may be activated and recruited by IR and
IRA radiation-induced free radical production in vitro on monolayer fibroblast cultures [8]	Incubation of cells with dichlorofluorescein diacetate at 100 uM for 30 min	Normal human skin fibroblasts from biopsies of donors aged 40–54 years from different body sites (cheek, face, breast, eyelid)	From 40 J/cm^2 a significant increase in ROS production is observed
Cellular response to infrared radiation involves retrograde mitochondrial signaling from induced free radical production [13]	Reactive oxygen species (ROS)-sensitive fluorescent probes	Skin fibroblasts from the foreskins of healthy donors aged 3–8 years	Retrograde mitochondrial signaling processes in human dermal fibroblasts contribute to actinic damage of human skin
IRA radiation-induced free radical production in vivo on monolayer fibroblast cultures [17]	Electron paramagnetic resonance spectroscopy	Flexor forearms of 12 healthy volunteers (three males, nine females)	Free radicals are produced by IRA of the skin

(continued)

Table 1 (continued)

Findings	Obtained by	Subjects	Conclusions
		aged between 25 and 35 years	
Change in oxidation levels of glutathione (GSH) to glutathione dimer (GSSG) [13]	Glutathione recycling assay	Skin fibroblasts from the foreskins of healthy donors aged 3–8 years	
Depletion of normal levels of skin antioxidants, such as β-carotene and lycopene, in vivo [18]	Resonance raman spectroscopy	Flexor forearms of 12 healthy volunteers (three males, nine females) aged between 25 and 35 years	

Table 2 Protection against IRA skin damage

Finding	Obtained by	Subjects	Conclusions
Creams containing different combination mixtures of titanium dioxide, organic UV filters, hydrophilic antioxidants, and lipophilic antioxidants provide protection in the IR range [19]	EPR spectroscopy after irradiation with an intensity of 120 mW/cm^2 with a duplicate dose of 72 J/cm^2 for 10 min	Pig ear skin	The physical filter titanium dioxide was best for protection because of its high IR range reflectability
Combination of N-acetylcysteine and MitoQ ascorbic acid provides effective protection against IR range [13]	Biopsies after reactive oxygen species (ROS)-sensitive fluorescent probes	Skin fibroblasts from the foreskins of healthy donors aged 3–8 years	Provided effective protection
Combination of grape seed extract, ubiquinone, vitamin C, and vitamin E provide effective protection against IR range [7]	Biopsies of three volunteers after irradiation with an intensity of 105 mW/cm^2 and single dose of 360–720 J/cm^2 for 57–114 min	Buttock skin of nine volunteers, six of which exhibited significant MMP-1 mRNA expression	Antioxidant mixture is highly protective and reproducible
Topical application of SPF 30 sunscreen or SPF 30 sunscreen supplemented with the antioxidant cocktail containing grape seed extract, ubiquinone, vitamin C, and vitamin E (2 mg/cm^2) [20]	4 mm punch biopsies 24 h after being irradiated with an intensity of 105 mW/cm^2 with an intensity of exposed to 360 J/cm^2 of IRA	30 healthy human volunteers (11 males, mean age 45.0 years; 19 females, mean age 51.2 years)	Sunscreen with antioxidant mixture proved to be most effective.
Topical application of the antioxidant β-carotene (2 mg/cm^2) provided protection [18]	Resonance raman spectroscopy after being exposed to a 30 min dose 190 mW/cm^2 intensive IRA.	Flexor forearm of 12 healthy volunteers (three men and nine women)	β-carotene protects against IR-induced free radicals

45.0 years; 19 females, mean age 51.2 years) receiving 4 mm punch biopsies 24 h after being irradiated (360 J/cm^2, 105 mW/cm^2) with IRA. Although the SPF 30 sunscreen diminished some of the MMP-1 mRNA expression, the SPF 30 antioxidant mixture proved to be the most effective method for diminishing MMP-1 mRNA expression [20]. Additionally, topical application of the antioxidant β-carotene (2 mg/cm^2) provided protection for human flexor forearm skin of 12 healthy volunteers (three men and nine women) through resonance Raman spectroscopy when exposed to a 30 min dose of (190 mW/cm^2) IRA [18] (Table 2).

Conclusion

The process of IRA-induced skin aging is as complex as, if not more than, UV, and as a result it is imperative that new and ongoing research efforts provide more substantiations, explanations, and resolutions in regard to its mechanisms, implications, and obstruction of IRA. Collectively, contemporary evidence exemplifies the main implications of IRA irradiation: (1) MMP-1 protein and mRNA expression is upregulated prompting the degradation of the extracellular matrix and (2) ROS free radical production stimulates retrograde signaling mechanisms that are directly related to nuclear gene expression. Therefore, the sunscreen of the future should provide protection for the entire solar spectrum, including UVB and UVA filters for the UV range, physical filters for the entire range, as well as antioxidants for the IR range.

References

1. Kochevar IE, Taylor CR, Krutmann J. Fundamentals of cutaneous photobiology and photoimmunology. In: Wolff K, Austen KF, Goldsmith LA, Katz SI, Gilchrest BA, Paller AS, Leffel DJ, editors. Fitzpatrick's dermatology in general medicine. New York: McGraw-Hill; 2007. 1.
2. Cobarg CC. Physikalische Grundlagen der wassergefilterten Infrarot- A-Strahlung. In: Vaupel P, Kru¨ger W, editors. Wa¨rmetherapie mit was- sergefilterter Infrarot-A-Strahlung. Stuttgart: Hippokrates Verlag; 1995. p. 19–28.
3. Hellige G, Becker G, Hahn G. Temperaturverteilung und Eindringtiefe wassergefilterter Infrarot-A-Strahlung. In: Vaupel P, Becker G, editors. Wa ¨rmetherapie mit wassergefilterter Infrarot-A-Strahlung. Stuttgart: Hippokrates Verlag; 1995. p. 63–80.
4. Krutmann J, Morita A, Chung JH. Sun exposure: what molecular photo- dermatology tells us about its good and bad sides. J Invest Dermatol. 2012;132:-976–84. 2.
5. Brenneisen P, Sies H, Scharffetter-Kochanek K. Ultraviolet-B irradiation and matrix metalloproteinases: from induction via signaling to intial events. Ann N Y Acad Sci. 2002;973:31–43. 3.
6. Fisher GJ, Kang S, Varani J, Bata-Csorgo Z, Wan Y, Datta S, Voorhees JJ. Mechanisms of photoaging and chronological skin aging. Arch Dermatol. 2002;138:1462–70. 4.
7. Schroeder P, Lademann J, Darvin ME, Stege H, Marks C, Bruhnke S, Krutmann J. Infrared radiation-induced matrix metalloproteinase in human skin: implications for protection. J Invest Dermatol. 2008;128:2491–7. 5.
8. Robert C, Bonnet M, Marques S, Numa M, Doucet O. Low to moderate doses of infrared A irradiation impair extracellular matrix homeostasis of the skin and contribute to skin photodamage. Skin Pharmacol Physiol. 2015;28:196–204. 6.
9. Cho S, Lee MJ, Kim MS, Lee S, Kim YK, Lee DH, Lee CW, Cho KH, Chung JH. Infrared plus visible light and heat from natural sunlight participate in the expression of MMPs and type I procollagen as well as infiltration of inflammatory cell in human skin in vivo. J Dermatol Sci. 2008;50(2):123–33. 7.
10. Buechner N, Schroeder P, Kunze K, Maresch T, Calles C, Krutmann J, Haendeler J. Thioredoxin-1 protects from MMP-1 upregulation and collagen type Ia1 downregulation: implication for photoaging. Exp Gerontol. 2008;43:633–37.
11. Kim MS, Kim YK, Lee DH, Seo JE, Cho KH, Eun HC, Chung JH. Acute exposure of human skin to ultraviolet or infrared radiation or heat stimuli increases mast cell numbers and tryptase expression in human skin in vivo. Br J Dermatol. 2009;160(2):393–402. 9.
12. Krutmann J, Schroeder P. Role of mitochon- dria in photoageing of human skin: the de- fective powerhouse model. J Investig Dermatol Symp Proc. 2009;14:44–9. 10.
13. Schroeder P, Pohl C, Calles C, Marks C, Wild S, Krutmann J. Cellular response to infrared radiation involves retrograde mitochondrial signaling. Free Radic Biol Med. 2007;43:128–35. 11.
14. Schieke S, Stege H, Kurten V, Grether-Beck S, Sies H, Krutmann J. Infrared-A radiation-induced matrix metalloproteinase 1 expression is mediated through extracellular signal-regulated kinase 1/2 activation in human dermal fibroblasts. J Invest Dermatol. 2002;119:1323–9. 12.
15. Karu T. Primary and secondary mechanisms of action of visible to near-IR radiation on cells. J Photochem Photobiol B. 1999;49:1–17. 13.
16. Butow RA, Avadhani NG. Mitochondrial signaling: the retrograde response. Mol Cell. 2004;14:1–15. 14.
17. Darvin ME, Haag S, Meinke M, Zastrow L, Sterry W, Lademann J. Radical production by infrared A irradiation in human tissue. Skin Pharmacol Physiol. 2010;23:40–6. 15.
18. Darvin ME, Fluhr JW, Meinke MC, Zastrow L, Sterry W, Lademann J. Topical beta-carotene protects against infra-red-light-induced free radicals. Exp Dermatol. 2011;20:125–9. 16.

19. Grether-Breck S, Marini A, Jaenicke T, Krutmann J. Effective photoprotection of human skin against infrared A radiation by topically applied antioxidants: results from a vehicle controlled double-blind, randomized study. Photochem Photobiol. 2015;91:248–50. 17.
20. Meinke MC, Syring F, Schanzer S, Hagg SF, Graf R, Loch M, Gersonde I, Groth N, Pflüker F, Lademann J. Radical protection by differently composed creams in UV/VIS and IR spectral ranges. Photochem Photobiol. 2013;89:1079–84. 18.

Textbook of Aging Skin

Miranda A. Farage • Kenneth W. Miller
Howard I. Maibach
Editors

Textbook of Aging Skin

Second Edition

Volume 2

With 574 Figures and 224 Tables

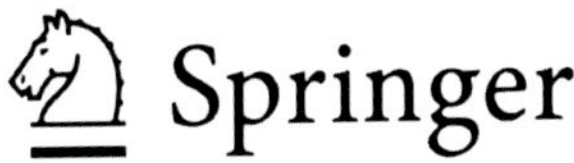

Editors
Miranda A. Farage
Winton Hill Business Center
The Procter and Gamble Company
Cincinnati, OH, USA

Kenneth W. Miller
Margoshes-Miller
Consulting, LLC
Cincinnati, OH, USA

Howard I. Maibach
Department of Dermatology
University of California
San Francisco, CA, USA

ISBN 978-3-662-47397-9 ISBN 978-3-662-47398-6 (eBook)
ISBN 978-3-662-47399-3 (print and electronic bundle)
DOI 10.1007/978-3-662-47398-6

Library of Congress Control Number: 2009938632

Printed on acid-free paper

This Springer imprint is published by Springer Nature
The registered company is Springer-Verlag GmbH Germany
The registered company address is: Heidelberger Platz 3, 14197 Berlin, Germany

Dedication
To a forgotten and sometimes lonely and scary aging journey –
Much more dignity and respect are deserved for all of you. MAF,
KWM, and *HIM*

When things go wrong as they sometimes will,
When the road you're trudging seems all uphill,
When the funds are low and the debts are high,
And you want to smile but you have to sigh,
When care is pressing you down a bit
Rest if you must, but don't you quit.
Success is failure turned inside out,
The silver tint on the clouds of doubt,
And you can never tell how close you are,
It may be near when it seems afar.
So, stick to the fight when you're hardest hit
It's when things go wrong that you mustn't quit.

—*Unknown*

Foreword

We mourn the loss of Professor Albert Kligman – a man whose energy, enthusiasm and intelligence benefited the specialty and many of us. His remarks below are as cogent today – as when written for the first Edition in December 2009.

Editors
MAF, KWM and HIM

The population is aging rapidly. Centenarians are no longer a rarity. The fastest growing segment of the population in the United States is people over 80. In the next 25 years, half of the population in the United States will be aged over 50.

These shifts will have a tremendous impact on the delivery of healthcare to the elderly and will require a new awareness of how cutaneous disorders affect the quality of life, comprising a heavy burden on health and wellbeing.

Physicians and healthcare workers are woefully ignorant of the distress, discomfort, and anxieties of people afflicted by disorders of the skin. There exists a widespread misconception that skin disorders are simply cosmetic nuisances that can be self-treated by a great assortment of anti-aging creams and lotions available at the local drug store. Most of these include high-sounding ingredients such as antioxidants, vitamins, nutrients, botanicals, and ancient folkloristic remedies, the efficacy and safety of which have never been tested. They offer little more than hope in a bottle. The fact is that common skin diseases may not often be lethal but can ruin enjoyment of life. Chronic itchy rashes can be maddening, lowering one's self-esteem, embarrassing, interfering with sleep, and often accompanied by depression, social isolation, and deterioration of appearance; they can also be uncomfortable, and, not least, costly to treat.

The elderly commonly take 15–20 oral supplements daily to fight the ailments of old age. These are generally useless and may be harmful, often interacting adversely with prescription drugs. The elderly often resort to alternative medicines instead of seeing their doctor to obtain FDA-approved drugs, and also often skip their daily doses to save money. Noncompliance is common. Misdiagnosis and mistreatment of the elderly by health-care workers are common. National surveys show that skin diseases increase steadily throughout our life-span. Old people may have as many as 5–10 coexistent cutaneous problems that are worthy of medical attention. Moreover, the clinical manifestations of skin diseases in the aged often have different

appearances than in the young, confounding diagnosis. Importantly, healing of chronic lesions, especially ulcers, is impaired in the elderly. Immunity is weakened, increasing susceptibility to infections. Response to treatment is slower, leading to noncompliance. Adverse drug reactions are common and too commonly not suspected. Management of chronic conditions is difficult and frustrating.

The above litany of problems makes this textbook edited by Farage, Miller, and Maibach a welcome addition to the literature. It is invaluable as a reference resource covering exhaustively an enormous number of clinical conditions. No topic is neglected including cosmetic treatments. The numerous contributions are by highly qualified experts who have a published record of expertise.

This comprehensive volume is also practical and relevant to the everyday world of clinical practice. The information will be useful to physicians, manufacturers of drugs and skincare products, educators, investigators, nursing home personnel, estheticians, and federal regulators.

This first edition is up to date, including much new material that belongs to the shelves of every library, which deals with geriatric problems. Dermatologists especially will be remiss if they do not put this volume within easy reach for consultation as they encounter a swelling clientele of aging patients.

University of Pennsylvania
Philadelphia, PA, USA

Albert M. Kligman M.D., Ph.D.
Professor Emeritus

Preface

The skin is a portal of knowledge on aging. From its softness and smoothness in infancy, through its suppleness in youth, to its wrinkled texture in elders, the skin displays the most visible and accessible manifestations of aging.

Due to falling birth rates and rising life expectancies in industrialized countries, the average age of the population is increasing. People are more preoccupied with looking and "staying" young, and research into the process of aging has expanded.

Although excellent compendia exist on the subject of aging skin, the body of knowledge is burgeoning and we still have more to learn. The purposes of this textbook are: (1) to compile the most current information into one comprehensive reference (it covers a range of topics, from the basics of skin structure and function to the cellular and molecular mechanisms of aging, to the latest bioengineering instruments used to assess age-related changes in the skin); (2) to guide on how to utilize skin as a tool for insights into the remainder of organs; and (3) to encourage the rapidly expanding universe of aging research in a more holistic aspect (heart, lung, brain, etc., as well as laboratories and investigators/foundations/government agencies) to utilize the readily available skin as an entry/surrogate for research on other organs.

Contributors are internationally recognized experts from multiple disciplines germane to this topic. We gratefully acknowledge all contributors for sharing their time and expertise.

We expect this second edition of the textbook to be valuable to researchers and students with an interest in aging skin, and the aging process in general. Because research progress in this area is rapid, we hope to update this compendium periodically as advances in the field dictate.

The editors welcome suggestions for the third edition.

Miranda A. Farage
Kenneth W. Miller
Howard I. Maibach

Acknowledgments

Deep appreciation and grateful thank yous are extended to the many experts who contributed both knowingly and indirectly to this book.

A special thank you to Drs. N. Enane-Anderson, G. Collier, P. Schofield, R. Leboeuf, Mr. Ron Visscher, and Mr. John Cooper, who generously offered their time and expertise to peer-review relevant chapters and for their support of this book. No praise is excessive for their efforts, and they have our heartfelt gratitude.

Many thanks go to the significant efforts of all the contributors of this book and the valuable time they dedicated preparing their chapters. This book represents the fruits of a jointly conceived and executed venture and has benefited from global and diverse partners.

We would also like to single out Ms. Sunali Mull (Springer Editorial-India) for a special recognition. Her great efforts, time, discipline, and dedication helped moved this book forward on a timely and organized manner. In addition, we would like to thank Mr. S. Klemp, Mr. A. Baroi, Ms. R. Amos, Ms. A. Singh, Ms. S. Friedrichsen, and Ms. S. Westendorf (Springer Office) for their help in moving this book forward. We acknowledge the usefulness of the new "SpringerMeteor" system which helped contributors and editors get the first glance of the future of electronic information/submission/editing.

In addition, Dr. D. A. Hutchins, Ms. Z. Schwen, Ms. W. Wippel, Ms. G. Entrup, Dr. T. L. Nusair, and Ms. P. Fifth (Rest in Peace our dear friend; your memories will always be with us) have all assisted with this book.

Above all, our everlasting gratitude, thanks, and love go to our parents who inspired us and to our families and children who supported, helped, and encouraged us all the way with their incredible patience. Your continuous care, unconditional love, and sacrifice made all this possible and easier to achieve.

MAF, *KWM*, and *HIM*

Contents

Volume 1

Volume 2

About the Editors

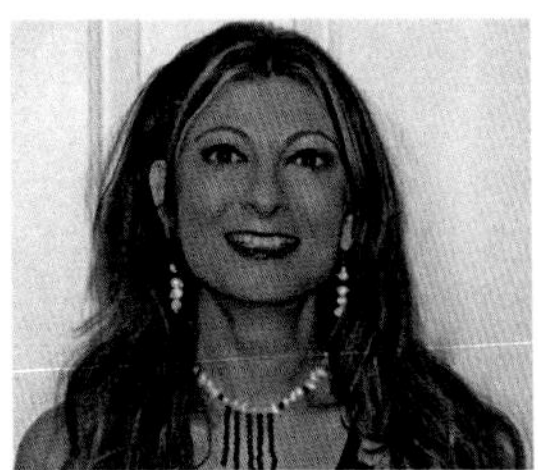

Miranda A. Farage is a Research Fellow in the Global Clinical Sciences Innovation at the Procter & Gamble Company, Cincinnati, Ohio. Dr. Farage leads global research on genital health, dermatological testing and claims, new clinical methods development, sensitive skin, physiology, clinical toxicology, women's health, quality of life, and related fields. Dr. Farage has invented novel state-of-the-art clinical test methods that have resulted in efficient ways of assessing new technologies and products as well as the filing of 15 patent applications. She has published more than 200 manuscripts and chapters in peer-reviewed journals and medical books. She is the Editor-in-Chief of several books such as *The Vulva*; *Textbook of Aging Skin*, first edition; *Topical Application and the Mucosa*; and *Skin, Mucosa and Menopause: Management of Clinical Issues*.

Dr. Farage is a member of many scientific societies including the American Academy of Dermatology, the European College of Society of Vulva Diseases, the National Vulvodynia Association, the American Society for Testing and Materials (ASTM) International, and the Science Advisory Board. Currently, she is serving on the editorial boards of more than a dozen scientific, dermatology, and medical journals. She received a Ph.D. in Medical Sciences and a master degree (MS) in Biology from the University of Illinois, Urbana-Champaign. Before joining Procter & Gamble, she was a faculty member at the Virginia Polytechnic Institute and State University (Virginia Tech).

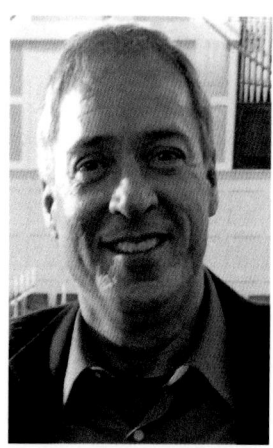

Kenneth W. Miller

- Principal Consultant, Margoshes Miller Consulting LLC, for Product Safety, Toxicology, and Regulatory Strategy (June 2015 to present).
- Associate Director, The Procter & Gamble Company (July 1984–June 2015), with global safety and regulatory experience in medical devices, OTC health care products, and food products.
- Diplomate, American Board of Toxicology (1986–2006).
- Postdoctoral Fellow, University of Medicine and Dentistry of New Jersey (June 1982–July 1984), Nutritional Biochemistry.
- Doctoral degree (Ph.D.): Cornell University, 1982, Toxicology and Food Chemistry.
- Master's degree (M.S.): Cornell University, 1979, Toxicology and Food Chemistry.
- Bachelor's degree (B.S.): Iowa State University, 1977, Biology.
- Dr. Miller has published over 50 manuscripts in the area of toxicology in peer-reviewed journals plus numerous abstracts, book chapters, and presentations at meetings of scientific societies. He is a member of several scientific and professional societies.

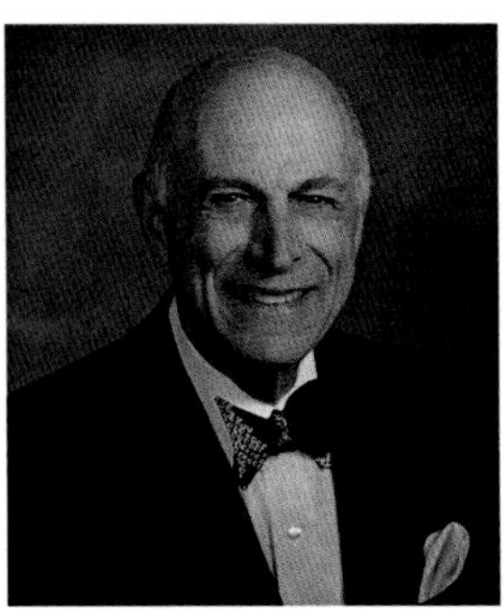

Howard I. Maibach
Present Title: Professor

Education	Degree
Tulane University, New Orleans, LA	A.B.
Tulane University, New Orleans, LA	M.D.
USPHS, Hospital of the University of Pennsylvania	Resident/Fellow

Honorary degrees	Degree	Year
L'Universite de Paris-Sud, France	Ph.D.	1985
Université Claude Bernard Lyon 1, France	Ph.D.	2008
University of Southern Denmark	M.D.	2010

Dr. Howard Maibach joined the University of California Faculty as Assistant Professor and is currently Professor of Dermatology.

Dr. Maibach, an expert in contact and occupational dermatitis, sees patients at the Environmental Dermatoses Clinic, which is part of the Dermatology Clinic at UCSF. His most active fields of research are in dermatopharmacology, dermatotoxicology, and environmental dermatoses. He has been doing human subject research for 45 years.

He has been on the editorial board of more than 30 scientific journals. His bibliography includes more than 2790 publications and 100 books.

He is member of 19 professional societies including the American Academy of Dermatology (AAD), San Francisco Dermatological Society (SFDS), North American Contact Dermatitis Group (NACDG), American Contact Dermatitis Society (ACDS), International Contact Dermatitis Research Group (ICDRG), Society of Toxicology (SOT), European Environmental and Contact Dermatitis Research Group (EECDRG), and the Internal Commission on Occupational Health. He is a consultant to government, academia, and industry worldwide.

Dr. Howard Maibach was honored as the 2013 recipient of The Master Dermatologist Award by The American Academy of Dermatology's 71st Annual Conference held in Miami, Florida. This prestigious award recognizes an Academy member's significant contributions to the field of dermatology and to the American Academy of Dermatology.

In March 2015, The International League of Dermatological Societies (ILDS) awarded Dr. Maibach their 2014 ILDS Certificate of Appreciation in recognition of his outstanding contribution to dermatology, both nationally and internationally, through his work, research, publications, and teaching in the USA and over 60 countries.

Contributors

Rami Abadi Department of Dermatology, American University of Beirut Medical Center, Beirut, Lebanon

Ossama Abbas Department of Dermatology, American University of Beirut Medical Center, Beirut, Lebanon

Jihane Abou Rahal Department of Dermatology, American University of Beirut Medical Center, Beirut, Lebanon

Jean Adamus Unilever Research and Development, Trumbull, CT, USA

Mohamed A. Adly Department of Zoology, Faculty of Science, Sohag University, Sohag, Egypt

Avani Ahuja Department of Biotechnology, Jaypee Institute of Information Technology, Noida, UP, India

Denize Ainbinder Institute of Drug Research, School of Pharmacy, The Hebrew University of Jerusalem, Jerusalem, Israel

A. Deniz Akkaya Department of Dermatology, Koç University Hospital, Istanbul, Turkey

Department of Dermatology, V.K. Foundation, American Hospital of Istanbul, Istanbul, Turkey

Ali Alikhan Department of Dermatology, University of Cincinnati, Cincinnati, OH, USA

Satoshi Amano Shiseido Research Center, Yokohama, Japan

Marco Ardigò Clinical Dermatology, IFO San Gallicano Dermatological Institute, Rome, Italy

Melina C. Armenaka Department of Dermatology and Venereology, University of Athens, A. Sygros Hospital, Athens, Greece

Hanan Assaf Department of Dermatology, Saudi German Hospital, Jeddah, Saudi Arabia

Daniel Asselineau L'Oreal, Research and Innovation, Aulnay-sous-bois, France

Carmela Rita Balistreri Department of Pathobiology and Medical Biotechnologies, University of Palermo, Immunosenescence Unit, Palermo, Italy

Elma Baron Department of Dermatology, Case Western Reserve University, Cleveland, OH, USA

Leslie S. Baumann Baumann Cosmetic and Research Institute, Miami, FL, USA

Enzo Berardesca San Gallicano Dermatological Institute, Rome, Italy

Françoise Bernerd L'Oreal Research and Innovation, Aulnay-sous-bois, France

Christiane Bertin SkinCare R&D, Johnson & Johnson Santé Beauté France, Issy-les-Moulineaux, France

Marianne Berwick Internal Medicine, Division of Epidemiology, University of New Mexico, Albuquerque, NM, USA

Tapan K. Bhattacharyya Otolaryngology-Head and Neck Surgery, University of Illinois, Chicago, IL, USA

Emil Bisaccia Columbia University College of Physicians and Surgeons, New York, NY, USA

Johannes Bischof Department of Cell Biology, Division of Genetics, University of Salzburg, Salzburg, Austria

Donald L. Bissett Beauty Technology Division, The Procter & Gamble Company, Sharon Woods Innovation Center, Cincinnati, OH, USA

Donald L. Bjerke The Procter & Gamble Company, Central Product Safety, Cincinnati, OH, USA

Thomas Blatt The Beiersdorf Research Center, Hamburg, Germany

Miroslav Blumenberg The R.O. Perelman Department of Dermatology, NYU Langone Medical Center, New York, NY, USA

Department of Biochemistry and Molecular Pharmacology, NYU Langone Medical Center, New York, NY, USA

Ulrike Blume-Peytavi Department of Dermatology and Allergy, Clinical Research Center for Hair and Skin Science, Charité-Universitätsmedizin Berlin, Berlin, Germany

Markus Böhm Department of Dermatology, Laboratory for Neuroendocrinology of the Skin and Interdisciplinary Endocrinology, University of Münster, Münster, Germany

Carol Bosko Unilever Research and Development, Trumbull, CT, USA

Mario Bramante Product Safety and Regulatory Affairs, Procter & Gamble Service GmbH, Schwalbach am Taunus, Germany

Douglas E. Brash Departments of Therapeutic Radiology, Genetics, and Dermatology, Yale School of Medicine, New Haven, CT, USA

Stéphane Brézillon Laboratoire de Biochimie, CNRS UMR 7369, Faculté de Médecine, Université de Reims-Champagne-Ardenne, Reims, France

Centre National de la Recherche Scientifique, CNRS UMR 7369, Reims, France

Carla Abdo Brohem R&D Department, Grupo Boticário, São José dos Pinhais, PR, Brazil

Robert L. Bronaugh Office of Cosmetics and Colors, Center for Food Safety and Applied Nutrition, Food and Drug Administration, College Park, MD, USA

John Jay P. Cadavona Department of Dermatology, University of California, San Francisco, CA, USA

Fernanda Camozzato Department of Dermatology, Brazilian Center for Studies in Dermatology, Porto Alegre, RS, Brazil

Giuseppina Candore Department of Pathobiology and Medical Biotechnologies, University of Palermo, Immunosenescence Unit, Palermo, Italy

Calogero Caruso Department of Pathobiology and Medical Biotechnologies, University of Palermo, Immunosenescence Unit, Palermo, Italy

Anne Lynn S. Chang Department of Dermatology, Stanford University School of Medicine, Redwood City, CA, USA

Duane L. Charbonneau The Procter & Gamble Company, Cincinnati, OH, USA

Alexandra Charruyer Department of Dermatology and Eli and Edythe Broad, Center of Regeneration Medicine and Stem Cell Research, University of California, Veterans Affairs Medical Center, San Francisco, CA, USA

Adele Chedraoui Department of Dermatology, Lebanese American University, Beirut, Lebanon

Ying Chen Global R&D, Equity and Claims, Reckitt Benckiser, Montvale, NJ, USA

Shujiang (Suzie) Cheng Colgate-Palmolive Company, Piscataway, NJ, USA

Raymond J. Cho Department of Dermatology, University of California, San Francisco, CA, USA

Yun-Hee Choi Anti-aging Research Institute of BIO-FD&C Co. Ltd., Incheon, Republic of Korea

Departments of Pharmacology and Global Medical Science, Institute of Lifestyle Medicine and Nuclear Receptor Research Consortium, Wonju College of Medicine, Yonsei University, Wonju, Republic of Korea

Kaare Christensen The Danish Twin Registry and The Danish Aging Research Center, Department of Public Health, University of Southern Denmark, Odense C, Denmark

Jin Ho Chung Department of Dermatology, Seoul National University College of Medicine, Seoul, Korea

Maria Grazia Cifone Life, Health and Environmental Sciences, University of L'Aquila, L'Aquila, Italy

Benedetta Cinque Life, Health and Environmental Sciences, University of L'Aquila, L'Aquila, Italy

Daniele Corridoni Division of Gastroenterology and Liver Disease, Department of Medicine, Case Western Reserve University School of Medicine, Cleveland, OH, USA

Giovanni Corsetti Department of Clinical and Experimental Sciences, Division of Human Anatomy and Physiopathology, University of Brescia, Brescia, Italy

Gertrude-Emilia Costin The Institute for In Vitro Sciences, Inc. (IIVS), Gaithersburg, MD, USA

Justine Courtois Laboratory of Skin Bioengineering and Imaging, Department of Dermatopathology, University Hospital of Liège, Liège, Belgium

Jonathan M. Crowther JMC Scientific Consulting Ltd, Surrey, UK

Shweta Dang Department of Biotechnology, Jaypee Institute of Information Technology, Noida, UP, India

Razvigor Darlenski Department of Dermatology and Venereology, Tokuda Hospital Sofia, Sofia, Bulgaria

Nancy C. Dawes The Procter and Gamble Company, Cincinnati, OH, USA

Philippe Delvenne Department of Dermatopathology, University Hospital of Liège, Liège, Belgium

Céline Deneuville L'Oreal, Research and Innovation, Aulnay-sous-bois, France

Luisa Di Marzio Department of Pharmacy, University of Chieti - Pescara "G d'Annunzio", Chieti - Pescara, Italy

Francesco S. Dioguardi Department of Internal Medicine and Community Health, University of Milan, Milan, Italy

Luisa A. DiPietro Center for Wound Healing and Tissue Regeneration, College of Dentistry, University of Illinois at Chicago, Chicago, IL, USA

Department of Biology, DePaul University, Chicago, IL, USA

Alexander S. Donath Cincinnati Facial Plastic Surgery, Cincinnati, OH, USA

Frank Dreher MERZ North America, Inc., San Mateo, CA, USA

Laurence Du-Thumm Colgate-Palmolive Company, Piscataway, NJ, USA

Christine Duval L'Oreal Research and Innovation, Aulnay-sous-bois, France

Kimberly M. Eickhorst Dermatology Associates Of W CT, Danbury, CT, USA

Moetaz El-Domyati Department of Dermatology, Al-Minya University, Al-Minya, Egypt

Akram Elmahdy Department of Dermatology, University of California, San Francisco, CA, USA

Peter Elsner Department of Dermatology and Dermatological Allergology, Universitätsklinikum Jena, Jena, Germany

Alex Eshaghian AE Skin, Encino, CA, USA

Khaled Ezzedine Department of Dermatology, CHU Saint-André, Bordeaux, France

Miranda A. Farage Winton Hill Business Center, The Procter & Gamble Company, Cincinnati, OH, USA

Susan P. Felter The Procter & Gamble Company, Cincinnati, OH, USA

Vincenzo Flati Department of Biotechnological and Applied Clinical Sciences, University of L'Aquila, L'Aquila, Italy

Sara Flores Department of Dermatology, University of Cincinnati, Cincinnati, OH, USA

Joachim W. Fluhr Department of Dermatology, Charité University Clinic, Berlin, Germany

Reema Gabrani Department of Biotechnology, Jaypee Institute of Information Technology, Noida, UP, India

Mary Carmen Gasco-Buisson P&G Brand Creation and Innovation, Procter & Gamble, Cincinnati, OH, USA

Licia Genovese Minerva Research Labs Ltd, London, UK

G. Frank Gerberick Human Safety Department, Procter and Gamble Company, Cincinnati, OH, USA

Ruby Ghadially Department of Dermatology and Eli and Edythe Broad, Center of Regeneration Medicine and Stem Cell Research, University of California, Veterans Affairs Medical Center, San Francisco, CA, USA

Paolo U. Giacomoni Elan Rose Int., Tustin, CA, USA

Sarah Girardeau-Hubert L'Oreal, Research and Innovation, Aulnay-sous-bois, France

Maurizio Giuliani Life, Health and Environmental Sciences, University of L'Aquila, L'Aquila, Italy

Francesca Giusti Department of Dermatology, University of Modena and Reggio Emilia, Modena, Italy

Paraskevi Gkogkolou Department of Dermatology, Laboratory for Neuroendocrinology of the Skin and Interdisciplinary Endocrinology, University of Münster, Münster, Germany

Farzam Gorouhi Department of Dermatology, University of California, Davis, CA, USA

James C. Grotting Department of Plastic Surgery, University of Alabama, Birmingham, AL, USA

Linna Guan Department of Dermatology, Case Western Reserve University, Cleveland, OH, USA

Christiane Guinot Biometrics and Epidemiology Unit, CE.R.I.E.S., Neuilly-sur-Seine, France

David A. Gunn Unilever Research and Development, Colworth Science Park, Sharnbrook, Bedfordshire, UK

Madhulika A. Gupta Department of Psychiatry, Schulich School of Medicine and Dentistry, University of Western Ontario, London, ON, Canada

Prashant Gupta Department of Biotechnology, Jaypee Institute of Information Technology, Noida, UP, India

Sanjay Gupta Department of Biotechnology, Jaypee Institute of Information Technology, Noida, UP, India

Varun Gupta Department of Plastic Surgery, Vanderbilt University, Nashville, TN, USA

Bahman Guyuron Department of Plastic Surgery, University Hospitals of Cleveland, Case Western Reserve University, Cleveland, OH, USA

Elisabeth Hahnel Department of Dermatology and Allergy, Clinical Research Center for Hair and Skin Science, Charité-Universitätsmedizin Berlin, Berlin, Germany

Tomohiro Hakozaki Beauty Technology Division, The Procter & Gamble Company, Mason Business Center, Mason, OH, USA

Stacy S. Hawkins Unilever Research and Development, Trumbull, CT, USA

Valerie Haydont L'Oreal, Research and Innovation, Aulnay-sous-bois, France

Timothy P. Heffernan Departments of Therapeutic Radiology, Genetics, and Dermatology, Yale School of Medicine, New Haven, CT, USA

Peter Helmbold Department of Dermatology, University of Heidelberg, Heidelberg, Germany

Trinh Hermanns-Lê Laboratory of Skin Bioengineering and Imaging, Department of Dermatopathology, University Hospital of Liège, Liège, Belgium

Electron Microscopy Unit, Department of Dermatopathology, Unilab Lg, University Hospital of Liège, Liège, Belgium

Doris Hexsel Department of Dermatology, Brazilian Center for Studies in Dermatology, Porto Alegre, RS, Brazil

Department of Dermatology, Pontificia Universidade Católica do Rio Grande do Sul (PUC-RS), Porto Alegre, RS, Brazil

K. Kye Higdon Department of Plastic Surgery, Vanderbilt University, Nashville, TN, USA

Greg Hillebrand Amway Corporation, Ada, MI, USA

Tetsuji Hirao Faculty of Pharmacy, Chiba Institute of Science, Choshi, Japan

Regina Hourigan Colgate-Palmolive Company, Piscataway, NJ, USA

Christopher R. Hughes Internal Medicine, Division of Epidemiology, University of New Mexico, Albuquerque, NM, USA

Michael F. Hughes U.S. Environmental Protection Agency, Office of Research and Development, National Health and Environmental Effects Research Laboratory, Research Triangle Park, NC, USA

Young Hui University of California, San Diego, CA, USA

Mahmoud R. Hussein Department of Pathology, Assir Central Hospital, and Assuit University, Assuit, Egypt

Qunshan Jia The Procter & Gamble Company, Central Product Safety, Cincinnati, OH, USA

Mary B. Johnson Beauty Technology Division, The Procter & Gamble Company, Sharon Woods Innovation Center, Cincinnati, OH, USA

Nancy Karapasha The Procter & Gamble Company, Cincinnati, OH, USA

Alexandra Katsarou Department of Dermatology and Venereology, University of Athens, A. Sygros Hospital, Athens, Greece

Linda M. Katz Office of Cosmetics and Colors, Center for Food Safety and Applied Nutrition, Food and Drug Administration, College Park, MD, USA

Abdul Ghani Kibbi Department of Dermatology, American University of Beirut Medical Center, Beirut, Lebanon

Christine C. Kim Dermatology Institute and Skin Care Center, Santa Monica, CA, USA

Hyeong-Sik Kim Anti-aging Research Institute of BIO-FD&C Co. Ltd., Incheon, Republic of Korea

Ki Woo Kim Departments of Pharmacology and Global Medical Science, Wonju College of Medicine, Yonsei University, Wonju, Republic of Korea

Institute of Lifestyle Medicine and Nuclear Receptor Research Consortium, Wonju College of Medicine, Yonsei University, Wonju, Republic of Korea

Won-Serk Kim Department of Dermatology, Kangbuk Samsung Hospital, Sungkyunkwan University College of Medicine, Seoul, South Korea

Mayumi Komine Department of Dermatology, Jichi Medical University, Shimotsuke, Tochigi, Japan

Jan Kottner Department of Dermatology and Allergy, Clinical Research Center for Hair and Skin Science, Charité-Universitätsmedizin Berlin, Berlin, Germany

Aleksandar Krbanjevic Department of Dermatology, Indiana University School of Medicine, Indianapolis, IN, USA

Shalini Krishnasamy University of California, Los Angeles, CA, USA

Nils Krueger Rosenpark Research, Darmstadt, Germany

Jean Krutmann Environmental Health Research Institute (IUF), Heinrich-Heine-University, Duesseldorf, Germany

Atul Kulkarni Anti-aging Research Institute of BIO-FD&C Co. Ltd., Incheon, Republic of Korea

School of Mechanical Engineering, Sungkyunkwan University, Suwon, South Korea

Mazen Kurban Department of Dermatology, American University of Beirut Medical Center, Beirut, Lebanon

Department of Biochemistry and Molecular Genetics, American University of Beirut Medical Center, Beirut, Lebanon

Department of Dermatology, Columbia University, New York, NY, USA

Cristina La Torre Life, Health and Environmental Sciences, University of L'Aquila, L'Aquila, Italy

S. Lahtinen Active Nutrition, DuPont Nutrition and Health, Kantvik, Finland

Samuel M. Lam Willow Bend Wellness Center, Lam Facial Plastic Surgery Center and Hair Restoration Institute, Plano, TX, USA

William J. Ledger Department of Obstetrics and Gynecology, The New York-Presbyterian Hospital, Weill Medical College of Cornell University, New York, NY, USA

Jeong Hun Lee Anti-aging Research Institute of BIO-FD&C Co. Ltd., Incheon, Republic of Korea

Marianne Lesuisse Department of Dermatology, Unilab Lg, Regional Hospital Citadelle, Liège, Belgium

Department of Dermatology, Regional Hospital of Huy, Huy, Belgium

Jacquelyn Levin West Dermatology, Rancho Santa Margarita, CA, USA

Davina A. Lewis Department of Anatomic Pathology and Histology, Covance CLS, Indianapolis, IN, USA

Aikaterini I. Liakou Departments of Dermatology, Venereology, Allergology and Immunology, Dessau Medical Center, Dessau, Germany

University of Athens Medical School, Athens, Greece

Andrea Lichterfeld Department of Dermatology and Allergy, Clinical Research Center for Hair and Skin Science, Charité-Universitätsmedizin Berlin, Berlin, Germany

Low Chai Ling The Sloane Clinic, Singapore, Singapore

Chengxu Liu The Procter & Gamble Company, Cincinnati, OH, USA

Jane Y. Liu Department of Dermatology, University of California, School of Medicine, San Francisco, CA, USA

Márcio Lorencini R&D Department, Grupo Boticário, São José dos Pinhais, PR, Brazil

Isabelle Lorthois Centre LOEX de l'Université Laval, Québec, QC, Canada

Stefanie Luebberding Rosenpark Research, Darmstadt, Germany

Judit Lukács Klinik für Hautkrankheiten, Universitätsklinikum Jena, Jena, Germany

John Lyga Avon Global R&D, Suffern, NY, USA

Howard I. Maibach Department of Dermatology, University of California, San Francisco, CA, USA

Robert Maidof Avon Global R&D, Suffern, NY, USA

Evgenia Makrantonaki Departments of Dermatology, Venereology, Allergology and Immunology, Dessau Medical Center, Dessau, Germany

Geriatry Research Group, Charité Universitaetsmedizin Berlin, Berlin, Germany

Department of Dermatology and Allergology, University Medical Center Ulm, Ulm, Germany

Denis Malvy EA 3677 and Centre René-Labusquière, Université Victor Segalen, Bordeaux, France

Department of Internal Medicine and Tropical Diseases, University Hospital Center, Bordeaux, France

Valéria Maria Di Mambro R&D Department, Grupo Boticário, São José dos Pinhais, PR, Brazil

François-Xavier Maquart Laboratoire de Biochimie, CNRS UMR 7369, Faculté de Médecine, Université de Reims-Champagne-Ardenne, Reims, France

Centre National de la Recherche Scientifique, CNRS UMR 7369, Reims, France

Centre Hospitalier et Universitaire (CHU) de Reims, Reims, France

Anna Margolina Research and Development, Skin Biology, Bellevue, WA, USA

Claire Marionnet L'Oreal Research and Innovation, Aulnay-sous-bois, France

Slaheddine Marrakchi Department of Dermatology, Hedi Chaker Hospital, Sfax, Tunisia

Daniel S. Marsman The Procter & Gamble Company, Cincinnati, OH, USA

Jean-Yves Mary INSERM U717, Biostatistics and Clinical Epidemiology, DBIM, Saint-Louis Hospital, University Paris 7, Paris, France

Paul J. Matts Procter & Gamble, Greater London Innovation Centre, Egham, Surrey, UK

Walid Medhat Department of Dermatology, Al-Minya University, Al-Minya, Egypt

Reena Mehra Sleep Medicine Center, The Cleveland Clinic, Cleveland, OH, USA

Esterina Melchiorre Life, Health and Environmental Sciences, University of L'Aquila, L'Aquila, Italy

Helen Meldrum Unilever Research and Development, Trumbull, CT, USA

Joseph Merregaert Laboratory of Molecular Biotechnology, Department of Biomedical Sciences, University of Antwerp, Antwerp, Belgium

Afton Metkowski Department of Dermatology and Itch Center, Temple University School of Medicine, Philadelphia, PA, USA

Thomas A. Meyer Bayer Healthcare, Memphis, TN, USA

Gianfranca Miconi Life, Health and Environmental Sciences, University of L'Aquila, L'Aquila, Italy

Kenneth W. Miller Margoshes-Miller Consulting, LLC, Cincinnati, OH, USA

Jillian Wong Millsop Department of Dermatology, University of California, Davis, Sacramento, CA, USA

Shivangi Mishra Department of Biotechnology, Jaypee Institute of Information Technology, Noida, UP, India

Sang Hyun Moh Anti-aging Research Institute of BIO-FD&C Co. Ltd., Incheon, Republic of Korea

Akimichi Morita Department of Geriatric and Environmental Dermatology, Nagoya City University Graduate School of Medical Sciences, Nagoya, Japan

D. James Morré MorNuCo, Inc, West Lafayette, IN, USA

Dorothy M. Morré MorNuCo, Inc, West Lafayette, IN, USA

Zeenat Nabi Colgate-Palmolive Company, Piscataway, NJ, USA

Kouichi Nakagawa Department of Radiological Life Sciences, Graduate School of Health Sciences, Hirosaki University, Hirosaki, Aomori, Japan

J. Frank Nash The Procter & Gamble Company, Central Product Safety, Cincinnati, OH, USA

Dany Nassar Department of Dermatology, American University of Beirut Medical Center, Beirut, Lebanon

Department of Anatomy, Cell Biology and Physiological Sciences, American University of Beirut Medical Center, Beirut, Lebanon

Véronique Neiveyans L'Oreal, Research and Innovation, Aulnay-sous-bois, France

Isaac M. Neuhaus Department of Dermatology, University of California, San Francisco, CA, USA

Paul Nghiem Departments of Therapeutic Radiology, Genetics, and Dermatology, Yale School of Medicine, New Haven, CT, USA

Kasra Soltani Nia Department of Dermatology, University of California, School of Medicine, San Francisco, CA, USA

Georgios Nikolakis Departments of Dermatology, Venereology, Allergology and Immunology, Dessau Medical Center, Dessau, Germany

John Nip Unilever Research and Development, Trumbull, CT, USA

Jean-Luc Nizet Department of Plastic Surgery, University Hospital of Liège, Liège, Belgium

Alex Nkengne Clarins Laboratories, Pontoise, France

Kimberly G. Norman Institute for In Vitro Sciences, Gaithersburg, MD, USA

John Oblong Beauty Technology Division, The Procter & Gamble Company, Sharon Woods Innovation Center, Cincinnati, OH, USA

Mutsumi Okazaki Department of Plastic and Reconstructive Surgery, Graduate School of Science, Tokyo Medical and Dental University, Bunkyo-ku, Tokyo, Japan

Yasemin Oram Department of Dermatology, V.K. Foundation, American Hospital of Istanbul, Istanbul, Turkey

A. C. Ouwehand Active Nutrition, DuPont Nutrition and Health, Kantvik, Finland

Noritaka Oyama Dermatology and Dermato-Allergology, Matsuda General Hospital, Ohno, Fukui, Japan

Department of Dermatology, Fukui University, Fukui, Japan

Herve Pageon L'Oreal, Research and Innovation, Aulnay-sous-bois, France

Paola Palumbo Life, Health and Environmental Sciences, University of L'Aquila, L'Aquila, Italy

Apostolos Pappas The Johnson & Johnson Skin Research Center, CPPW, a Division of Johnson & Johnson Consumer Companies, Inc, Skillman, NJ, USA

Byung-Soon Park Cellpark Dermatology Clinic, Seoul, South Korea

Evasio Pasini "S. Maugeri Foundation", IRCCS, Cardiology Rehabilitative Division, Medical Centre of Lumezzane, Brescia, Italy

Paula C. Pennacchi Department of Clinical Chemistry and Toxicology, School of Pharmaceutical Sciences, University of Sao Paulo, Sao Paulo, Brazil

Jerrold Scott Petrofsky Department of Physical Therapy, Loma Linda University, Loma Linda, CA, USA

School of Allied Health, Loma Linda University, Loma Linda, CA, USA

Christina Phuong Department of Dermatology, University of California San Francisco, San Francisco, CA, USA

Loren Pickart Research and Development, Skin Biology, Bellevue, WA, USA

Gérald E. Piérard Laboratory of Skin Bioengineering and Imaging, Department of Dermatopathology, University Hospital of Liège, Liège, Belgium

Sébastien L. Piérard Telecommunication and Imaging Laboratory, INTELSIG, Montefiore Institute, University of Liège, Liège, Belgium

Claudine Piérard-Franchimont Laboratory of Skin Bioengineering and Imaging, Department of Dermatopathology, University Hospital of Liège, Liège, Belgium

Department of Dermatology, Regional Hospital of Huy, Huy, Belgium

Raimondo Pinna Plastic and Reconstructive Surgery and Burns Centre, Brotzu Hospital, Cagliari, Italy

Thomas G. Polefka Life Science Solutions, LLC, Somerset, NJ, USA

S. Brian Potterf Unilever Research and Development, Trumbull, CT, USA

Tarl W. Prow Dermatology Research Centre, School of Medicine, The University of Queensland, Princess Alexandra Hospital, Translational Research Institute, Brisbane, QLD, Australia

Prashant Rai L'Oreal China, Shanghai, China

Utkrishta L. Raj Department of Biotechnology, Jaypee Institute of Information Technology, Noida, UP, India

Vibha Rani Department of Biotechnology, Jaypee Institute of Information Technology, Noida, UP, India

Matthew J. Ranzer Center for Wound Healing and Tissue Regeneration, College of Dentistry, University of Illinois at Chicago, Chicago, IL, USA

Department of Biology, DePaul University, Chicago, IL, USA

Anthony P. Raphael Dermatology Research Centre, School of Medicine, The University of Queensland, Princess Alexandra Hospital, Translational Research Institute, Brisbane, QLD, Australia

Wellman Center for Photomedicine, Massachusetts General Hospital, Harvard Medical School, Boston, MA, USA

Christina Raschke Department of Dermatology, University Hospital Jena, Jena, Germany

Suresh I. S. Rattan Laboratory of Cellular Ageing, Department of Molecular Biology and Genetics, Aarhus University, Aarhus C, Denmark

Anthony V. Rawlings AVR Consulting Ltd, Cheshire, UK

Glen Rein Innovative Biophysical Technologies, Ridgway, CO, USA

Klaus Richter Department of Cell Biology, Division of Genetics, University of Salzburg, Salzburg, Austria

Sylvie Ricois L'Oreal, Research and Innovation, Aulnay-sous-bois, France

Mark Rinnerthaler Department of Cell Biology, Division of Genetics, University of Salzburg, Salzburg, Austria

Caroline Ritacco Laboratory of Skin Bioengineering and Imaging, Department of Dermatopathology, University Hospital of Liège, Liège, Belgium

Diana Alyce Rivers The Department of Basic Biomedical Sciences, Touro College of Osteopathic Medicine, New York, NY, USA

Michael K. Robinson Global Biotechnology and Life Sciences Technology Platform, The Procter & Gamble Company, Mason Business Center, Mason, OH, USA

Sheila Rocha Unilever Research and Development, Trumbull, CT, USA

Igor Roganin DAO Clinic, Moscow, Russia

Claudia Romano Department of Clinical and Experimental Sciences, Division of Human Anatomy and Physiopathology, University of Brescia, Brescia, Italy

David J. Rowe University Hospitals, Case Western Reserve University, Cleveland, OH, USA

Nelly Rubeiz Department of Dermatology, American University of Beirut Medical Center, Beirut, Lebanon

Anna Rufo Department of Biotechnological and Applied Clinical Sciences, University of L'Aquila, L'Aquila, Italy

Cindy A. Ryan The Procter and Gamble Company, Cincinnati, OH, USA

Shingo Sakai Basic Research Laboratory, Kanebo Cosmetics Inc., Kanagawa, Japan

Salah Salman Department of Dermatology, American University of Beirut Medical Center, Beirut, Lebanon

Preamjit Saonanon Department of Ophthalmology, King Chulalongkorn Memorial Hospital, The Thai Red Cross Society, Chulalongkorn University, Bangkok, Thailand

Giovanni Scapagnini Department of Health Sciences, University of Molise, Campobasso, Italy

Richard Scarborough University Hospitals Case Medical Center, Cleveland, OH, USA

Dwight Scarborough Clinical Assistant Professor of Medicine, Division of Dermatology, The Ohio State University Wexner Medical Center, Columbus, OH, USA

Megan E. Schrementi Center for Wound Healing and Tissue Regeneration, College of Dentistry, University of Illinois at Chicago, Chicago, IL, USA

Department of Biology, DePaul University, Chicago, IL, USA

Peter Schroeder Environmental Health Research Institute (IUF), Heinrich-Heine-University, Duesseldorf, Germany

Miri Seiberg Seiberg Consulting, LLC, Princeton, NJ, USA

Stefania Seidenari Department of Dermatology, University of Modena and Reggio Emilia, Modena, Italy

Hyo Hyun Seo Anti-aging Research Institute of BIO-FD&C Co. Ltd., Incheon, Republic of Korea

Garima Sharma Department of Biotechnology, Jaypee Institute of Information Technology, Noida, UP, India

Susan N. Sherman SNS Research, Cincinnati, OH, USA

Shuichi Shibuya Department of Advanced Aging Medicine, Chiba University Graduate School of Medicine, Chiba, Japan

Takahiko Shimizu Department of Advanced Aging Medicine, Chiba University Graduate School of Medicine, Chiba, Japan

William Shingleton General Electric Company, Cardiff, UK

Sara Sibilla Minerva Research Labs Ltd, London, UK

Neha Singh Department of Biotechnology, Jaypee Institute of Information Technology, Noida, UP, India

James E. Sligh Medicine, Dermatology, The University of Arizona, Tucson, AZ, USA

Jack Sobel Infectious Diseases, Wayne State University, Detroit, MI, USA

Mi Young Song Anti-aging Research Institute of BIO-FD&C Co. Ltd., Incheon, Republic of Korea

Yuli Song The Procter & Gamble Company, Mason Business Center, Mason, OH, USA

Dan F. Spandau Departments of Dermatology and Biochemistry and Molecular Biology, Indiana University School of Medicine, Indianapolis, IN, USA

Georgios N. Stamatas SkinCare R&D, Johnson & Johnson Santé Beauté France, Issy-les-Moulineaux, France

Robert Stern The Department of Basic Biomedical Sciences, Touro College of Osteopathic Medicine, New York, NY, USA

Maria Karolin Streubel Department of Cell Biology, Division of Genetics, University of Salzburg, Salzburg, Austria

Paul R. Summers University of Utah School of Medicine, Salt Lake City, UT, USA

Cheri L. Swanson The Procter & Gamble Company, Sharon Woods Innovation Center, Cincinnati, OH, USA

Hachiro Tagami Department of Dermatology, Tohoku University School of Medicine, Sendai, Japan

Haw-Yueh Thong Department of Dermatology, University of California, San Francisco, CA, USA

Kirsti Tiihonen Active Nutrition, DuPont Nutrition and Health, Kantvik, Finland

Danielle Tokarz Wellman Center for Photomedicine, Massachusetts General Hospital, Harvard Medical School, Boston, MA, USA

Princess Margaret Cancer Centre, University Health Network, Toronto, ON, Canada

Marjana Tomic-Canic Wound Healing and Regenerative Medicine Research Program, Department of Dermatology and Cutaneous Surgery and Hussman Institute of Human Genomics, University of Miami Miller Medical School, Miami, FL, USA

Salina M. Torres Department of Pathology, Center for HPV Prevention, University of New Mexico, Albuquerque, NM, USA

Elka Touitou Institute of Drug Research, School of Pharmacy, The Hebrew University of Jerusalem, Jerusalem, Israel

Jeffrey B. Travers Departments of Pharmacology and Toxicology and Dermatology, Boonshoft School of Medicine at Wright State University, Dayton, OH, USA

Joel Tsevat Division of General Internal Medicine, Department of Internal Medicine, University of Cincinnati College of Medicine and Cincinnati VA Medical Center, Cincinnati, OH, USA

Katsuhiko Tsuchida Research and Development Department, Naris Cosmetics Co. Ltd., Osaka, Japan

Gabe Tzeghai Wyoming, OH, USA

Efstratios Vakirlis Department of Dermatology and Venereology, Aristotle University of Thessaloniki, Thessaloniki, Greece

Giuseppe Valacchi Department of Life Sciences and Biotechnology, University of Ferrara, Ferrara (FE), Italy

Department of Food and Nutrition, Kyung Hee University, Seoul, South Korea

Rodrigo Valdes-Rodriguez Department of Dermatology and Itch Center, Temple University School of Medicine, Philadelphia, PA, USA

Fabien Valet Biostatistics Department, Institut Curie, Paris, France

Jessica Michelle Vasquez-Soltero Research and Development, Skin Biology, Bellevue, WA, USA

Annika Vogt Clinical Research Center for Hair and Skin Science, Department of Dermatology and Allergy, Charité-Universitätsmedizin Berlin, Berlin, Germany

Shilpa Vora Unilever Research and Development, Bangalore, India

Kenji Watanabe Department of Advanced Aging Medicine, Chiba University Graduate School of Medicine, Chiba, Japan

Yanusz Wegrowski Laboratoire de Biochimie, CNRS UMR 7369, Faculté de Médecine, Université de Reims-Champagne-Ardenne, Reims, France

Centre National de la Recherche Scientifique, CNRS UMR 7369, Reims, France

Horst Wenck The Beiersdorf Research Center, Hamburg, Germany

Katherine M. Whipple Envision Eye and Aesthetics, Fairport, NY, USA

Cornelia Wiegand Department of Dermatology, University Hospital Jena, Jena, Germany

Julian Winocour Department of Plastic Surgery, Vanderbilt University, Nashville, TN, USA

Klaus-Peter Wittern The Beiersdorf Research Center, Hamburg, Germany

Hidekazu Yamada Department of Dermatology of Kinki University, Faculty of Medicine Nara Hospital, Kinki University Antiaging Center, Higashiosaka, Osaka Prefecture, Japan

Paul S. Yamauchi Dermatology Institute and Skin Care Center, Santa Monica, CA, USA

David Geffen School of School of Medicine at UCLA, Los Angeles, CA, USA

Daniel B. Yarosh The Estee Lauder Companies, Inc., Melville, NY, USA

Max Yeslev Department of Plastic Surgery, Vanderbilt University, Nashville, TN, USA

Koutaro Yokote Department of Clinical Cell Biology and Medicine, Chiba University Graduate School of Medicine, Chiba, Japan

Hyun Sun Yoon Department of Dermatology, Seoul National University Boramae Hospital, Seoul, Korea

Gil Yosipovitch Department of Dermatology and Itch Center, Temple University School of Medicine, Philadelphia, PA, USA

Sidra Younis The R.O. Perelman Department of Dermatology, and Department of Biochemistry and Molecular Pharmacology, NYU Langone Medical Center, New York, NY, USA

Department of Biochemistry, Quaid-i-Azam University, Islamabad, Pakistan

Efterpi Zafiriou Department of Dermatology and Venereology, University of Thessaly, Larissa, Greece

Hanjiang Zhu Department of Dermatology, UC San Francisco, San Francisco, CA, USA

Ying Zou Department of Dermatology, UC San Francisco, San Francisco, CA, USA

Christos C. Zouboulis Departments of Dermatology, Venereology, Allergology and Immunology, Dessau Medical Center, Dessau, Germany

Helene Zucchi L'Oreal, Research and Innovation, Aulnay-sous-bois, France

Part IV

Disease State/Conditions with Aging

Nonneoplastic Disorders of the Aging Skin

64

Miranda A. Farage, Kenneth W. Miller, Enzo Berardesca, and Howard I. Maibach

Contents

M.A. Farage (✉)
Winton Hill Business Center, The Procter & Gamble Company, Cincinnati, OH, USA
e-mail: farage.m@pg.com

K.W. Miller
Margoshes-Miller Consulting, LLC, Cincinnati, OH, USA
e-mail: 822mbb@gmail.com

E. Berardesca
San Gallicano Dermatological Institute, Rome, Italy
e-mail: berardesca@berardesca.it

H.I. Maibach
Department of Dermatology, University of California, San Francisco, CA, USA
e-mail: maibachh@derm.ucsf.edu

M.A. Farage et al. (eds.), *Textbook of Aging Skin*,
DOI 10.1007/978-3-662-47398-6_54

Abstract

Diseases and disorders of the skin increase in prevalence in older people. Most people over 65 have at least one skin disorder, and many have two or more conditions which can create substantial morbidity and mortality and deterioration in quality of life in older adults. Primary care providers must monitor the condition of the patient's skin and refer to the dermatologist as needed. It is estimated that cutaneous diseases occur in more than 50 % of otherwise healthy older adults. Common conditions include dry skin (xerosis and pruritus), inflammatory scaling dermatoses (eczema, contact dermatitis, and seborrheic dermatitis), cutaneous expression of autoimmune disorders (bullous pemphigoid, benign mucous membrane pemphigoid, pemphigus vulgaris, paraneoplastic pemphigus, and lichen sclerosis), vascular disorders (pressure ulcer and rosacea), and viral infection (specifically herpes zoster or shingles). Management of skin disease in the elderly must take into account variables pertinent to the older patient and accurate diagnosis is key. Diagnosis of drug reactions is critical before the any underlying cutaneous disorder can be identified. Topical treatment must take into account the fragility of aged skin compromised by structural degeneration and comorbidities. Psychosocial issues must also be considered in treatment decisions to assess whether the patient will be able to comply with the therapy regimen.

Introduction

The skin serves as a barrier between the vulnerable internal tissues and a plentitude of potentially injurious environmental factors [1]. Degenerative processes inherent to aging produce the characteristic thinning, drying, and sagging of elderly skin [2] as well as a progressive deterioration in skin function [3] at a rate influenced by many factors including ethnicity and gender [4]. Most of the visible changes in aged skin [4] however, as well as most pathological changes, are due to a lifetime exposure to external environmental insult [1]. Degenerative processes that occur in aging skin and their clinical significance are shown in Table 1.

It is estimated that 7 % of all physician visits in the elderly involve skin disorders [5] and that treatable (but often untreated) cutaneous diseases occur in more than 50 % of otherwise healthy older adults [5]. Most people over 65 have at least two skin diseases worthy of treatment [6] and 10 % of those over 70 years of age have more than ten concurrent complaints [7]. Although the stigma of "looking old" drives global industry anticipated to surpass $290 billion by 2014 [8], skin aging is far more than just a cosmetic complaint. Disorders of the skin, in particular xerosis and pruritus, account for as many as 80 % of skin complaints in the aged [9], producing significant suffering for those afflicted and causing a substantial loss in quality of life (QoL) in the later years [10]. Effective management of skin disease in old age must take into account the frailness of some patients as well as personal and social issues that affect them [11, 12].

The Problem of Dry Skin

The two most common conditions of dry skin are xerosis and pruritus.

Xerosis

As the skin ages, the epidermis becomes thinner, the water and lipid content of the skin diminish, and sebum production and sweating decline. This results in dryer skin (Fig. 1) [13]. Along with these changes, the process of keratinocyte maturation and adhesion degenerates. These changes, together, result in skin that is dry, rough, and scaly, a condition called xerosis [14]. Xerosis (or asteatosis) is the most common dermatosis in older patients, occurring at equal rates in men and women [9], with incidences as high as 85 % [15]. By age 70, nearly all adults are affected [16]. Because xerosis is aggravated by low humidity [14], its onset is often linked to the

Table 1 The clinical implications of aging skin

Physiological change	Pathological change	Clinical significance
Thinning of epidermis and dermis	Increased vulnerability to mechanical trauma, especially shearing and friction	Increased incidence of skin tears and decubitus ulcers
Flattening of dermal papillae	Increased risk of blister formation	Increased susceptibility of infection
Slowdown in epidermal turnover rate; decreased ratio of proliferative to differentiated keratinocytes	Delayed cellular migration and proliferation	Increased time to re-epithelialization
		Longer healing times after injury or surgery
	Decreased wound contraction	Longer healing times after injury or surgery
Decrease in elastin fibers	Loss of elasticity	Lax skin, wrinkling
Decrease in vascularity and supporting structures in dermis	Blood vessels fragile, easily broken	Skin easily bruised (senile purpura)
	Decreased wound capillary growth	Increased risk of wound dehiscence
Decrease in vascular plexus, blunted capillary loops	Loss of thermoregulatory ability	Hypothermia, heat stroke
Changes in and loss of collagen and elastin fibers	Decreased tensile strength, lower skin layers more susceptible to injury	Increased risk of pressure damage to elderly skin, decubitus ulcers
	Delayed collagen remodeling	Longer healing times after injury or surgery
Impaired immune response	Impaired inflammatory response	Impaired wound healing
	Impaired delayed contact hypersensitivity reaction	Increased risk of severe injury from irritants and contact sensitizers
	Decreased production of cytokines	Diminished immune function
	Decrease in numbers of Langerhans cells	Increased susceptibility to photocarcinogenesis, false-negative results in patch tests for delayed contact hypersensitivity
Impaired neurological responses	Reduced sensation	Increased risk of thermal or other accidental injury
Decreased skin thickness	Loss of cushioning and support	Increased risk of pressure damage, decubitus ulcers
		Increased susceptibility to skin tears, bruising
	Decreased production of vitamin-D precursor	Osteoporosis and bone fractures
Atrophy of sweat glands	Decreased sweating	Impaired thermoregulation; hypothermia
		Dry skin, xerosis
Reduced stratum corneum lipids	Decreased ability to retain water	Dry skin, xerosis
Structural changes in stratum corneum	Altered barrier function	Variable response to topical medications, altered sensitivity to irritants
Reduced water movement from dermis to epidermis	Reduced epidermal hydration	Dry skin, xerosis
Decrease in melanocytes	Loss of ability to tan, more susceptible to solar radiation	Cutaneous neoplasms
	Graying hair	Loss of self-esteem

Table 1 summarizes findings from References [5, 19, 122, 145, 146]

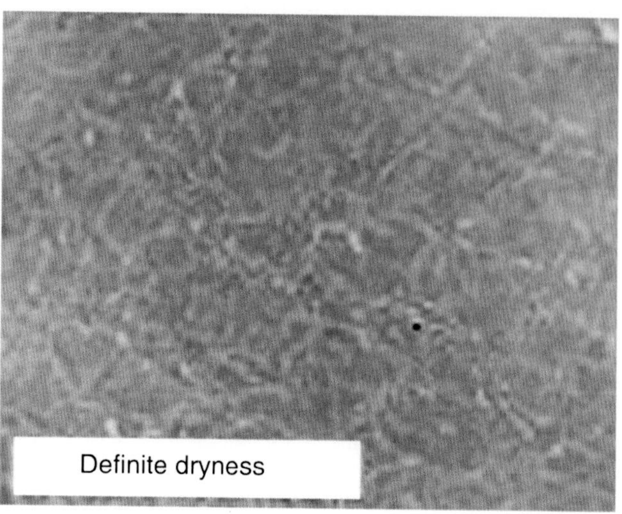

Fig. 1 Xerosis: skin that is dry, rough, and scaly

initiation of home heating [16], leading to the nickname "winter itch" [17]. Surface irritants, such as harsh soaps and other cleansers, can further aggravate the problem [14]. Xerotic skin causes considerable discomfort and distress in the older patient. Moreover, xerosis, and other common disorders that compromise skin integrity, may increase skin permeability to environmental allergens. This factor is now recognized to contribute to recalcitrant skin disorders in the elderly, such as nummular eczema.

The key to managing xerosis in the aging patient is to rehydrate the skin and lock in hydration [18]. A relative humidity level of 60 % is required for atmospheric moisture to supplement stratum corneum hydration [19]; the use of room humidifiers, especially in the winter months, is advisable [16]. Applying humectant moisturizers also can increase epidermal water content [18]. Bathing, which has traditionally been discouraged in those suffering from xerosis, actually rehydrates the stratum corneum [20]. Tepid baths should be indulged in [19], soaking for at least 10 min to enable the stratum corneum to absorb water [15]. Use of soaps should be minimal and limited to gentle, nonirritant preparations [13]. Moisturizers should be applied liberally immediately after bathing. This fills the spaces between the keratinocytes with lipid [18] and encourages corneosome degradation of the corneodesmosome [21]. Petrolatum products also help to prevent transepidermal water loss (TEWL), thus maintaining skin hydration [22, 23]. Lotions containing ammonium lactate have also proven effective in the treatment of xerosis [24], and topical corticosteroids can be prescribed for especially severe cases [14].

Pruritus (Itch)

Pruritus is a common dermatological problem in the aged and increasing [25], with reported prevalence as high as 29 % [26]. It is more common in men than in women [27]. Itching, which can be intense, may be accompanied by sensations of tingling or burning [28]. Severity, due to a nocturnal rise in internal body temperature, often increases at night [29]. Chronic scratching causes the skin to become thickened and hyperpigmented, a process known as lichenification [30]. The lichen simplex chronicus, which often is the result, is a skin condition, common on itchy sites accessible to scratching, marked by the appearance of lichenified scaly plaques [16] or thick raised papules with linear excoriations from scratching [31]. Lichen simplex chronicus is more prevalent in women than in men and generally clears quickly where scratching is avoided [31].

Xerosis is the most common cause of pruritus (in one survey, almost 40 % of all patients have pruritus [9]), associated with a thickened and cracked stratum corneum [32]. Patients with pruritus have clinically drier skin than matched controls; the severity of the itch is directly linked to the degree of xerosis, skin surface conductance, and presence of intracorneal adhesions. This suggests that an abnormality of keratinization may be involved [32]. Recent evidence suggests that senile pruritus may be an immune phenomenon as immune aging causes a loss of tolerance to cutaneous autoantigens [25].

The causes and mechanisms of itching are diverse. One study in 149 elderly patients identified the most common disorders associated with senile pruritus, in order of prevalence, as xerosis, inflammatory eczematous disorders, lichen simplex chronicus, skin infections, psoriasis vulgaris, urticaria, reactions to various drugs, and insect bites [9]. Therefore, elucidation of the cause of an individual patient's suffering, which can drive some patients to consider suicide, can be very challenging [30].

Effective management of pruritus requires a systematic approach to discovering the causative factors [30]. About half of pruritus cases occur without any physical signs, making diagnosis difficult [26]. Nevertheless, the patient's subjective complaints are accompanied by nocturnal scratching: a direct correlation has been established between the severity of itching that the patient reports and measurable nocturnal limb movement [26]. Several types of medications produce pruritus in varying degrees. These include: antibiotics, diuretics, nonsteroidal antiinflammatory drugs (NSAIDs), and calcium channel blockers [26]. Resolution of symptoms may take several weeks after drug withdrawal [33]. Idiopathic pruritus increases in both frequency and severity with increasing age [32]; 69 % of idiopathic pruritus in one study involved patients older than age 60 [26].

Generalized pruritus often coincides with the onset of emotional or psychological stress [26]; stress acts to increase the perception of itch [26]. Older patients may have severe and intractable emotional issues such as financial pressures, chronic health issues, boredom, bereavement, and loneliness [26] which should not be discounted as possible contributors to idiopathic itching [34].

With sudden onset of generalized persistent itching, aggressive pursuit of the etiology should be initiated, with a minimum of complete blood count (CBC), urinalysis, thyroid evaluation, tests of renal function, and a chest X-ray to rule out evidence of other internal disease (Table 2) [35]. The origin of pruritus, in fact, often proves to be multifactorial [36].

Table 2 Pruritus screen for underlying disease

Laboratory analysis	Abnormal finding	Possible etiology of pruritus
Complete blood count (CBC)	Anemia	Lymphoma/leukemia, myelodysplastic syndrome, iron deficiency
	Eosinophilia	Drug reaction, helminthic infestation
	Lymphopenia	Leukemia, AIDS
	Polycythemia	Polycythemia vera
Plasma viscosity	Out of normal range	Myeloma, infection, malignancy
Ferritin	Iron deficiency	Anemia
Electrolytes	Out of normal range	Impaired renal function
Liver function test	Out of normal range	Obstructive jaundice (gallstones, tumor, primary biliary cirrhosis)
Thyroid function	Out of normal range	Hypothyroidism, hyperthyroidism
Autoantibodies	Out of normal range	Thyroid disease, primary biliary cirrhosis
Renal function	Elevated blood creatinine levels	Diabetes mellitus
Chest X-ray	Mass	Carcinoma of the bronchus
	Mediastinal lymph nodes	Lymphoma

Table 2 summarizes findings from References [11, 30]
AIDS acquired immune deficiency syndrome

Treatment depends on the specific source of each patient's symptoms. Treatment for pruritus of xerotic origin has been described above. Topical and systemic corticosteroids and antihistamines, as well as topical cooling agents and anesthetics, have been employed. Physical therapies include phototherapy, acupuncture, thermal stimulation, and transcutaneous electrical nerve stimulations (TENS) [30].

Oral antihistamines are the most commonly prescribed therapy for pruritis [36]; systemic corticosteroids are used in approximately 30 % of cases [36]. Antihistamines may be sedating in the older patient, and corticoids can accentuate atrophy in skin already compromised by sun damage [37]. In addition, topical preparations used to treat pruritus may cause contact sensitivity, which should be suspected if a weeping, vesicular, crusting dermatitis develops [38].

Resolution of the older patient's symptoms can at times prove elusive, as histamine release can induce a repetitive cycle [39]. Senile insomnia makes nighttime scratching more common.

Inflammatory Scaling Dermatoses

Inflammatory dermatoses are common and include a variety of clinical conditions such as eczema, contact dermatitis, and seborrheic dermatitis. Accurate histological diagnosis of the underlying conditions, which can sometimes be difficult, is important for successful clinical management.

Eczema

Atopic eczema is less common in older adults, but nummular (discoid) eczema, gravitational eczema, and asteatotic eczema occur almost exclusively among the aged [1]. Epidermal inflammation with predominant intracellular edema is common to these conditions. Edematous fluid collects in surface vesicles, which may weep (Fig. 2) [40]. Diagnostic difficulties arise when there are secondary manifestations caused by scratching or by infection. However, the three hallmark signs of eczematous inflammation should be recognized: erythema, scaling, and vesicles [41]. Eczematous inflammation is virtually always accompanied by itching [41]. Most eczematous diseases, if left untreated and neither scratched nor irritated, will resolve without complication. Unfortunately, this situation is almost never achieved [41], as virtually all patients will scratch (even during sleep [41]), and attempts at self-treatment with over-the-counter (OTC) topical drugs are very common [42].

The clinical development of eczema has been divided into three phases, although the disease may present at any phase. The acute phase of eczema includes erythematous lesions and pain, heat, and tenderness [43]. The skin may sting, burn, or itch intensely and vesicles and blisters may develop [43]. Epidermal thickening is present in the acute phase of all forms of eczema [40]. Skin biopsies show inflammatory cells and swelling.

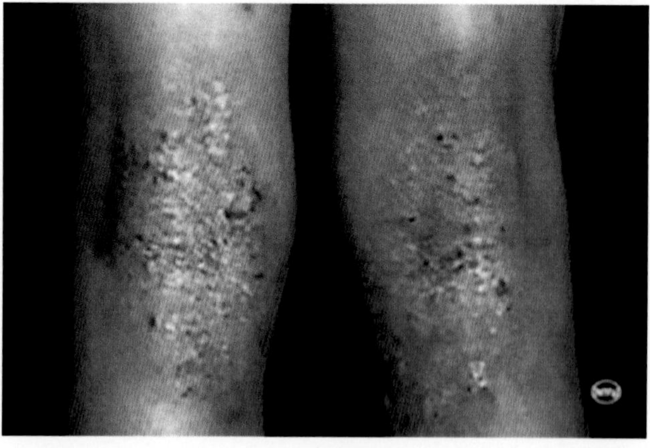

Fig. 2 Eczema (atopic dermatitis) (Reproduced with permission from the American Academy of Dermatology, Copyright© 2008. All rights reserved)

The subacute phase of eczema does not exhibit pronounced swelling but rather reddened, scaly, and fissured skin that appears parched or scalded [41]. The subacute phase tends to be characterized by itching rather than pain [43].

Chronic eczema is defined by the presence of lesions for more than 3 months [41]; itching is pronounced, and scratching often exacerbates existing lesions [43]. In the chronic stage the skin is thickened and lichenified, often with marked excoriation and/or fissuring [41]. Symptoms tend to worsen in the winter months due to low humidity in the home or office [44].

Asteatotic Eczema

Xerotic skin, particularly in men, may exhibit stratum corneum fissuring in a cracked porcelain pattern, particularly on the lower legs. This condition, initially termed "eczema craquelé," is now known as asteatotic eczema [13]. Fissures can be deep enough to disrupt dermal capillaries, causing bleeding [13]. The affliction is often accompanied by intense itching [14] and subsequent scratching can result in secondary lesions [13].

The cause of asteatotic eczema is believed to be a combination of intrinsic, environmental, and lifestyle factors. Skin dries naturally with old age, as keratin synthesis and sebaceous gland activity wanes [2]; low humidity and cold intensify dryness and exacerbate the condition in northern winters [45]. Frequent bathing in hot water with use of degreasing soaps, combined with infrequent use of emollients, can promote the condition [41]. Treatment consists primarily of avoiding soaps and hot baths but indulging in warm baths and applying alpha hydroxy acid preparations after bathing to preserve skin hydration [45]. Short-term use of a steroid ointment, such as triamcinolone (for 4–5 days), is indicated in more serious cases [45].

In most patients, asteatotic eczema is an irksome but not a dangerous condition, although if not adequately treated, it can compromise skin integrity and increase the risk of contact dermatitis or infection [45]. In some cases, however, the disorder may be the external manifestation of a more serious internal problem. Asteatotic eczema may be linked to a deficiency of zinc or essential fatty acids [46, 47], thyroid disease [48], and various forms of cancer [49, 50]. In a recent prospective observational study of 68 patients hospitalized with asteatotic eczema, concurrent cancers were discovered in 47 % of the patients [51]. These concurrent cancers were strongly associated with specific clinical characteristics of the eczema: deep red fissures, widespread lesions (particularly on the trunk), and resistance to topical steroid treatment were significantly associated with internal malignancy [51].

Nummular (Discoid) Eczema

Nummular eczema occurs most often in elderly men, usually on the extremities. The presentation of nummular eczema varies widely, from a sudden onset of florid patches of erythema with vesicles and swelling to slow-growing, dry patches of scale [52]. Lesions are coin-shaped macules, papules, or vesicles that ooze and crust over and are superimposed on scaly or raw inflamed skin [53]. Lesions, which vary greatly in number, are generally between 1 and 5 cm in diameter and may be mistaken for ringworm or psoriasis [52]. Scale is usually thin and sparse [41]. Papules or vesicles eventually coalesce to form nummular plaques that within a few days become dry and scaly, often with central clearing. Plaques eventually turn brown and flatten into macules, which may persist as hyperpigmented areas [54]. Nummular eczema often recurs, with new lesions appearing in the same area as former ones [54]. The lesions are frequently secondarily infected [54].

The pathophysiology of nummular eczema is not well understood. The association with xerotic skin [55], irritant or atopic skin reactions [56, 57], recent loss of skin integrity [54], and interferon or necrosis factor-alpha blocking therapies [58, 59] is beginning to shed light on the possible origins of nummular eczema. Xerotic skin of the elderly may cause, particularly in winter or other adverse environmental conditions, a cracking and fissuring of the skin's surface [55]. Initial dryness and skin damage produce pruritus and subsequent scratching exacerbates damage, with a breach of skin integrity that allows skin permeation of a variety of environmental allergens. The penetration of environmental allergens past the stratum corneum results in the eczematous changes characteristic of nummular eczema, seemingly an expression of delayed hypersensitivity despite advanced age [55].

Significant temperature changes, low humidity, and stress may worsen symptoms [52]. In the acute phase, inflammation and itching can be alleviated by applying cool wet dressings: evaporative cooling produces vasoconstriction and serum production. Dressings should be replaced every 30 min [41]. When lesions are intense or widespread, oral corticosteroids (prednisone) can be added at a dosage of least 30 mg bid (with no tapering) for at least 3 days; up to 3 weeks may be necessary for adequate control [41]. Antihistamine relieves itching and facilitates sleep. Systemic antibiotics are indicated when signs of secondary infection are present [41].

For subacute presentations, high-potency topical corticosteroids, applied two to four times per day, are the first-line therapy [38, 41]. Topical tacrolimus is efficacious without being associated with skin atrophy [33]. Nummular eczema is often chronic, with some cases very recalcitrant to treatment [41].

Gravitational Eczema (Stasis Dermatitis)

Gravitational eczema (also known as stasis dermatitis) is a recurrent swelling with characteristic of skin eruptions of the feet and ankles, particularly in older men [14], associated with disorders of chronic venous insufficiency (CVI) [60]. Risk factors are a familial disposition, prolonged standing or sitting, and concomitant vascular disease [18]. Up to six million people have CVI in the United States, while approximately 500,000 have venous ulcers [60]. The prevalence of CVI is increasing [60].

Initial skin damage in gravitational eczema results from microvascular changes; later pathology is often associated with bacterial vasculitis [61]. Venous insufficiency in these patients produces a cyanotic erythema of the distal extremities, either unilaterally or bilaterally [14]. Impairment of the main veins and venules causes pulmonary hypertension; microthrombi that form in the capillaries cause microinfarctions and micronecrosis [62]; the resulting endothelial damage produces interstitial tissue edema [62], which, in turn, promotes an itchy inflammation with a greater risk of ulceration [37].

The condition may be acute, subacute, chronic, or recurrent [41]. Subacute dermatitis begins with edema of the ankles [63]. Typically, inflammation begins in winter as the skin of the lower extremities becomes dry and scaly [41]. Brown staining of the skin, caused by deposition of hemosiderin by extravasated red blood cells, may spread slowly [62]. Scratching induces eczematous inflammation, often self-treated with medications. Potential contact sensitizers in these treatments can exacerbate and prolong the inflammation [41].

In the acute phase, pruritic plaques appear most commonly in the medial perimalleolar area [14]. They are characterized by poorly demarcated erythema and possible scaling [14]. Weeping and crusting may occur and a vesicular eruption – the id reaction – may appear on the palms, trunk, and extremities [41]. Untreated, the disorder creates hyperpigmented areas with focal purpura, which may ulcerate [64]. These ulcers, often extremely painful, are distinctly marginated erosions that heal with ivory-white plaques called "atrophie blanche" [65].

Gravitational eczema can be persistent, recurring even after apparently successful treatment [1]. Chronic inflammation begins when episodic inflammation further compromises the integrity of affected tissues, typically presenting as a cyanotic red plaque over the medial malleolus [41]. This development is typically followed by a condition called lipodermatosclerosis with a characteristic production of fibrous scar tissue of the reticular dermis made up of collagen bundles [66]. The resulting scleroderma-like hardening of skin is a consequence of intense proteolytic activity that degenerates the extracellular matrix of both dermis and epidermis. The result is ulceration, a refractory condition in which the epidermis is completely destroyed and the matrix structures of the upper dermis partially degraded [66]. At this point, the physiologic mechanisms are no longer able to repair damage [62]. Lipodermatosclerosis typically begins on the medial side of the ankle and then spreads, possibly as far as thighs and trunk [67].

The ulcerated tissues of gravitational eczema occasionally give rise to secondary neoplasms, although prevalence rates are uncertain [68]. Vascular ulcers should be monitored for malignant growth. In an evaluation of 85 cases of histologically confirmed malignancies that occurred as complications of ulcerated legs, 98 % were observed to be squamous cell carcinomas (SCC) and 2 % basal cell carcinomas (BCC). SCC ulcers in the leg appear as a rolled, partially keratinized lesions with eversion raised borders; they have a 30 % metastasis rate [62]. Any ulcer that, with treatment, continues to resist healing should be suspected [62, 69].

Stasis ulceration is responsible for prolonged hospitalization of many older people who are otherwise healthy [70]; effective treatment depends on considering the whole pathophysiological process [63]. Support stockings, which act to minimize edema, have been the mainstay of prevention; they are effective in the short term but do not represent a long-term solution [63]. Once edema develops, it must be treated promptly to prevent rapid deterioration of the skin. Legs should be elevated and compression continued [38]. Topical corticoids of mild to moderate potency are commonly prescribed. Topical medications should be used judiciously to avoid further complication by contact sensitization. (Potential sensitizers may be present in moisturized, medicated dressings, preservatives, and topical antimicrobials and antibiotics [71].) The cutaneous scale prevalent in this disorder can harbor abundant microbial life. It should be treated by soaking followed by a gentle rub with emollient to soften and lift it off [72].

Oral antibiotics are appropriate and effective where ulceration has resulted in infection [38]. Because this disease often is recalcitrant to standard therapies, much research effort is being devoted toward new approaches to promote healing, such as maggot debridement therapy [73], honey (as a natural antiseptic) [74], cellulose and collagen dressings [75], therapeutic ultrasound [76], mesh grafts with vacuum-assisted closure [77], hyperbaric oxygen therapy [78], and the stimulation of cytokine release by dermal dendrocytes [61]. In severe and recalcitrant cases, a surgical approach may be indicated. The prospective, randomized, multicenter trial of 80 chronic leg ulcer patients treated by ambulatory compression therapy, as well as subfascial, endoscopic, perforating vein surgery combined with superficial vein ligation, produced a higher healing rate than in patients treated with compression only (83 % vs 73 %), although the difference was not significant [79]. Seventy-two percent of surgically treated patients remained ulcer-free after 29 months, compared to only 53 % in the compression-treated group; this difference did not reach statistical significance.

Contact Dermatitis

Contact dermatitis, which includes both irritant and allergic reactions, occurs in as much as 11 % of the elderly population (Figs. 3 and 4) [18]. In both types, the appearance of lesions is accompanied by burning and itching, which can be intense [80]. Older patients generally display less inflammation with vesiculation but more scaling than younger subjects, and hyperpigmentation may be an early feature of the eruption [80]. Contact dermatitis tends to be more persistent in the elderly [80].

Older adults are predicted to be less susceptible to allergic contact dermatitis [81], as they are less able to mount a delayed-type hypersensitivity reaction because of reduced numbers of Langerhans cells [82] and T-cells and lower vascular reactivity [81]. Nonetheless, several investigators found an increase in positive patch tests in older patients [42, 83, 84], with higher rates in women than in men [9]. This phenomenon is due to the frequent use of common topical medicaments by older people [84]. For example, up to 81 % of patients being treated for chronic leg ulcers exhibit allergic reactions to topical medications [42].

Patch testing before prescribing topical medications may be beneficial, especially in high-risk patients, such as those being treated for dermatitis or ulceration of the lower extremities [85]. Decades of exposure to potential sensitizers [86] and increased use of medications and topical

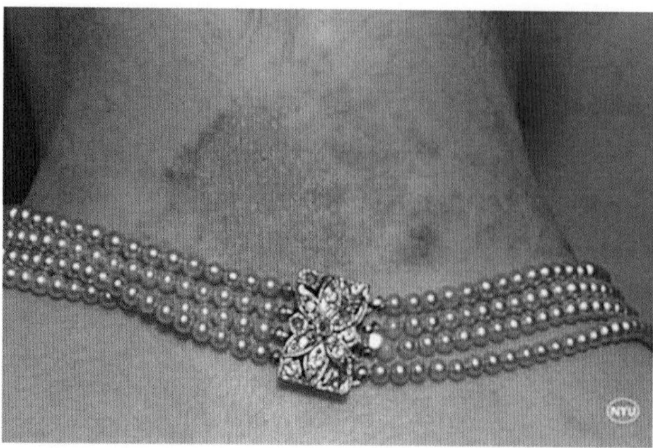

Fig. 3 Contact dermatitis caused by nickel (Reproduced with permission from the American Academy of Dermatology, Copyright© 2008. All rights reserved)

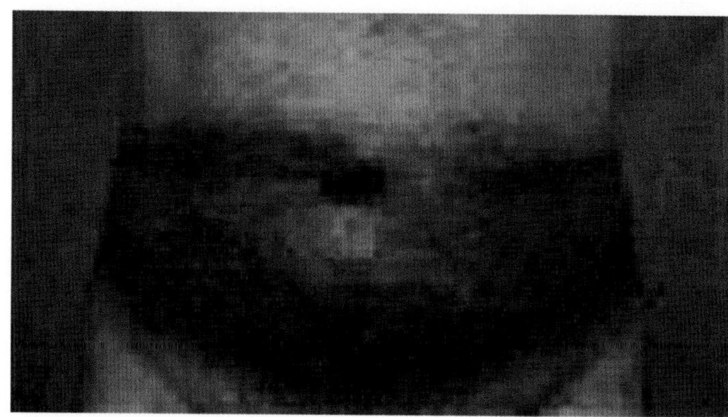

Fig. 4 A severe reaction to rubber (Reproduced with permission from the American Academy of Dermatology, Copyright© 2008. All rights reserved)

products account for the high prevalence of allergic contact sensitivity in the geriatric population [87]. Common allergens include lanolin, paraben esters, dyes, plants, balsams, rubber, nickel, and topical medications [16]. Patch testing of older patients should include components of medicaments and dressings, dental prostheses, and medications for ocular disease [85].

While aged patients are susceptible to allergic contact dermatitis, they may be less likely to develop irritant contact dermatitis [88] because of limited occupational exposure to irritants [1] and because these patients are less able to mount an inflammatory response [5]. Irritant contact dermatitis present as erythema, with edematous plaques and potentially vesicles [16]. It begins at the site of contact but may spread. In the elderly, signs of irritant contact dermatitis may represent thermal injury [5]. Patients should be advised not to use strong soaps and to avoid contact with household cleaners and other products that have the potential to irritate their skin [5].

Management of contact dermatitis requires first identification and removal of the offending agent [88]. Treatment consists of administering topical corticosteroids [89, 90], adding oral antihistamines where needed [88–90].

Seborrheic Dermatitis

Seborrheic dermatitis is a common inflammatory disorder thought to result from chronic infection of the lipid-rich areas of the skin. *Malassezia* yeasts are believed to be the causative organism; these fungi are components of the endogenous skin microflora to which some individuals apparently have an abnormal host response [91]. Its incidence in older patients is reportedly as high as 31 % [18]. Seborrheic dermatitis occurs slightly more often in men than in women. It affects areas of the skin where sebaceous glands are most prominent: the eyebrows, paranasal area, pre- and postauricular regions, presternal and intrascapular areas, scalp (dandruff is a form of this disorder), axillae, and groin [92]. Affected women tend to have more severe symptoms than men [93].

Seborrheic dermatitis is characterized by inflammatory changes (erythema) with greasy red-brown papules [35] covered by scaly yellow flakes and plaques [92]. Chronic dermatitis with pruritus, resembling psoriasis, may develop in seborrheic areas [92]. The disorder disproportionately affects patients with neurological disorders like Parkinson's disease, epilepsy, and diseases or trauma of the central nervous system [94]; the association with neurological disorders is unclear [92]. The dermatitis may intensify during times of increased stress and fatigue [70].

Seborrheic dermatitis does not have serious physiological consequences, but can be distressing. Therapies include antiinflammatory preparations (e.g., steroids or calcineurin inhibitors), keratolytic agents (e.g., pyrithione zinc, sulfur, coal tar, salicylic acid), and antifungal medications (e.g., ketoconazole); keratolytic agents and antifungal medications are often administered in the form of medicated shampoos. Shampoos should be regularly applied by being lathered abundantly, rubbed into scalp, and left on for about 5 min [92]. Ciclopirox olamine, piroctone olamine, and climbazole are also used outside the United States [92].

Cutaneous Expression of Autoimmune Disorders

Older adults have a higher frequency of autoimmune disease, possibly linked to the senescence of the immune system [95]. The prevalence of polypharmacy in the elderly also increases the risk of drug-induced autoimmune cutaneous eruptions [95]. Cutaneous autoimmune eruptions include bullous pemphigoid, benign mucous membrane pemphigoid, pemphigus vulgaris, paraneoplastic pemphigus, and lichen sclerosis.

Bullous Pemphigoid

Bullous pemphigoid occurs in people over 60 and exhibits no ethnic or gender difference in prevalence [96]. It is a life-threatening disorder whose incidence is increasing [97] for reasons yet unknown [98]. Risk factors identified include cognitive impairment, Parkinson's disease, bipolar or unipolar disorder, being bedridden, or chronic use of spironolactone or some phenothiazines. Chronic use of analgesics was associated with a decreased risk [97].

This autoimmune disease produces chronic eruptions of multiple bullae, either on otherwise normal skin or on an urticarial base (Figs. 5 and 6) [99]; polymorphic pruritic lesions may be a prodromal phase [100]. Pruritic lesions may initially present as hives accompanied by intense itching [101]. Blisters result when basal epidermal keratinocytes detach from the dermis at the level of the lamina lucida [102]. Cutaneous blisters are large, tense, and tough enough to resist minor trauma [35]. About a third of people with this condition have oral blisters [38, 64], which are

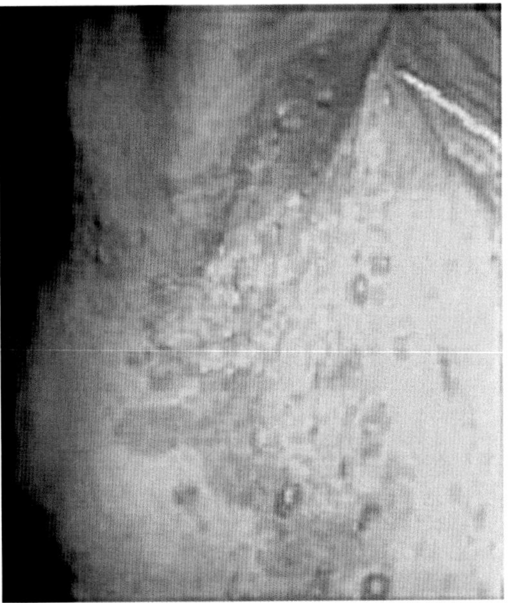

Fig. 5 Bullous pemphigoid on trunk and extremities (Reproduced with permission from the American Academy of Dermatology, Copyright© 2008. All rights reserved)

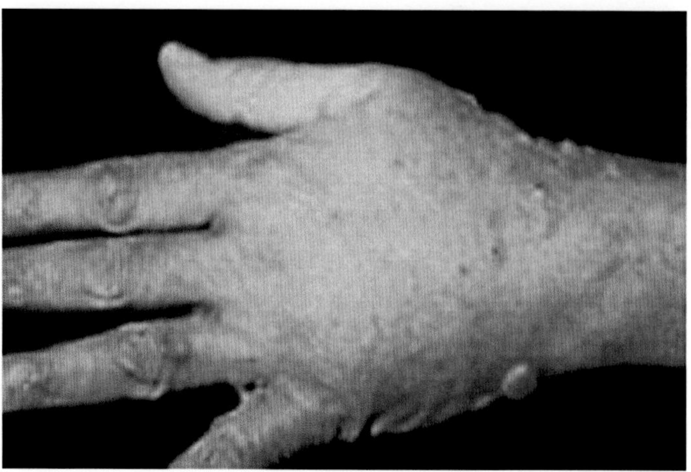

Fig. 6 Bullous pemphigoid on the hand (Reproduced with permission from the American Academy of Dermatology, Copyright© 2008. All rights reserved)

exquisitely painful. The disease may be preceded by a long period of generalized itching or eczema. If large areas of skin are denuded, a significant loss of fluids and vital electrolytes may result [67].

Bullous pemphigoid is associated with circulating and tissue-associated [38, 99] antibodies to hemidesmosomal proteins BP180-BP230 [103], which are present in the basement membrane of stratified squamous epithelia [104]. IgE recognition of the BP autoantigens appears to be an early pathogenetic event [103]. Antibodies may be the result of a deregulation of antibody production caused by immune senescence [25]. The antibodies are produced specifically against a 230 kDa antigen located in the lamina lucida region of the dermoepidermal junction and produce separation of the epidermis from the dermis with a subsequent blister [99]. Bullous pemphigoid is confirmed by histology, immunofluorescence, electron microscopy, and molecular biology techniques [99] and has been associated with both solid organ tumors and the paraneoplastic myelodysplastic syndrome [105]. Potent topical corticosteroids have been employed for first-line therapy, with tetracycline, alone or with nicotinamide, for patients who cannot tolerate corticosteroids or as corticosteroid-sparing therapy following steroid use [99]. In recent research, however, methotrexate produced better results with fewer side effects compared to prednisone [106].

Benign Mucous Membrane Pemphigoid

Benign mucous membrane pemphigoid, an autoimmune disease in which the antibodies produced attack the attachment fibrils of the basement membrane, occurs primarily in the older adults. Blisters and erosions appear primarily in the mouth, on the conjunctivae, and in the nose. In 20–30 % of cases, blisters also occur on the head, neck, and upper trunk. The disease can lead to blindness due to optic keratitis caused by occlusion of the lacrimal ducts. If left untreated, within 3–5 years both eyes may be affected.

Patients diagnosed with mucous membrane pemphigoid should be promptly referred to an ophthalmologist. Mouthwashes containing topical steroids may be employed for oral lesions, and corticoid-containing artificial tears can be used to treat the eyes [107]. However, ocular disease is difficult to treat, and management usually involves systemic therapy with immunomodulators to control inflammation and prevent progression to irreversible blindness; surgical intervention may be indicated in advanced disease. Recent advances in treatment, including methotrexate, mycophenolate mofetil, monoclonal antibodies, and topical tacrolimus therapies, are promising [108].

Pemphigus Vulgaris

Pemphigus vulgaris is the most serious blistering disease in older adults (Fig. 7). Onset typically occurs after the age of 65 [98]. Oral blisters erupt initially, followed by blistering of the trunk, limbs, face, and scalp. Lesions progressively ooze, become crusted, and lichenify (Fig. 7) [38].

The condition is readily identified by the Nikolsky's sign: lateral pressure with the thumb at the edge of the blister will produce an erosion [38]. Histological evaluation reveals intraepidermal blister formation and acantholytic cells within the lesion. Indirect immunofluorescence reveals intercellular deposition of immunoglobulin (Ig) conjugates and complement 3 (C3); on occasion, other immunoglobulins and complement components are present [38]. Serum antibodies, particularly to desmoglein-3, are helpful for diagnosis; serial titers can help monitor progress of disease [109].

Pemphigus vulgaris is a serious chronic disorder with the potential for fatality due to secondary electrolyte imbalance or secondary infection [38]. The risk of death in people with the condition is three times that of age-matched controls [98]. Treatment requires systemic therapy with corticosteroids, which should be started as early as possible [38]. Morbidity and mortality from chronic corticosteroid use, however, are considerable [110]; lower doses of corticosteroid (80–120 mg/day) [38], adjunct use of immunosuppressive drugs, tetracycline with nicotinamide [38], or sublesional corticosteroid injections [111] can be considered as alternative therapies. Recent studies have shown adjuvant therapies, particularly azathioprine, to be useful in reducing steroid dosage [112].

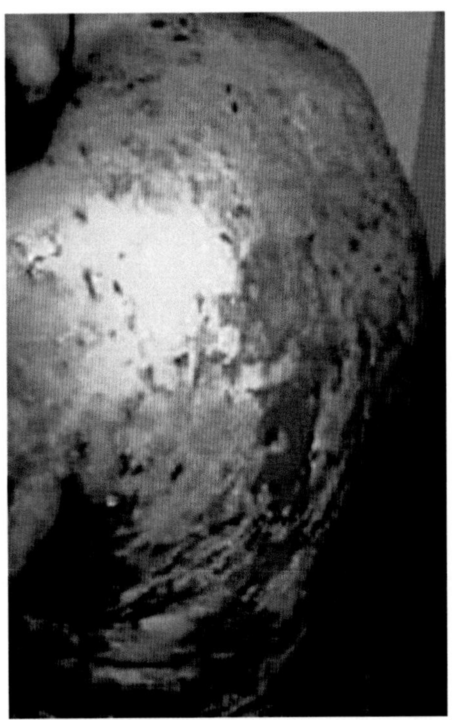

Fig. 7 Pemphigus vulgaris on the back (Reproduced with permission from the American Academy of Dermatology, Copyright© 2008. All rights reserved)

Paraneoplastic Pemphigus

The elderly are especially susceptible to paraneoplastic pemphigus [104]. Paraneoplastic pemphigus occurs in conjunction with several neoplasms, most commonly chronic lymphocytic leukemia [113], but also with Castleman's tumor, non-Hodgkin's lymphoma, thymoma, and follicular dendritic cell sarcoma. The condition is seen primarily in those over 60 and twice as often in men than in women.

Paraneoplastic pemphigus exhibits extensive and painful mucocutaneous erosions that usually arise in the oral mucosa. Histological analysis reveals acantholysis, basal cell vacuolation and clefts, and scattered necrotic keratocytes as unique features of the erosions [113]. Direct immunofluorescence locates intercellular and basement membrane IgG and C3 both within the epidermal spaces and at the epidermal basement membrane. Indirect immunofluorescence demonstrates circulating antibodies specific for stratified squamous or transitional epidermal epithelium [96]. Autoantibodies against epidermal proteins are produced by the associated tumors [113]. Paraneoplastic pemphigus is often complicated by bronchiolitis obliterans, which leads eventually to respiratory failure [113]. Successful treatment depends on early detection and removal of associated tumor as well as intravenous administration of immunoglobulin [113].

Lichen Sclerosis

In older men, cutaneous issues of the genitalia are generally limited to those who are uncircumcised. However, genital lesions are not uncommon among elderly women [114]. Lichen sclerosis (LS) is an apparently autoimmune dermatosis in women, with a predilection for the genital skin. Known formerly as kraurosis vulvae or leukoplakia of the vulva, LS produces well-demarcated, porcelain-white papules and plaques among areas of bruising; lesions occur throughout the genital area with the exception of the genital mucosa [115]. Itching is the principal symptom, which creates the potential for secondary lichenification due to scratching [115].

LS creates rare but potentially debilitating complications. Lichenified scars or adhesions may cause the introitus to narrow or close; this interferes with micturition and intercourse and occasionally requires subtotal or total circumcision [115]. Additionally, LS is associated with an increased incidence of invasive squamous cell carcinoma of the anogenital area [115]. The ultra-potent topical corticosteroid, clobetasol propionate, is a first-line therapy [116]. It produces improvement in as many as 96 % of patients [117]. There is some concern that corticosteroid use may induce oncogenic human papillomavirus (HPV), which is carried by 20 % of LS patients [115].

Vascular Disorders

Several vascular changes occur in aged skin. The capillaries and small vessels regress and become more disorganized [12], blood vessel densities diminish [85], and the number of venular cross sections per 3 mm^2 of skin surface in non-exposed areas is reduced by 30 % [12]. Intravital capillaroscopy measurements in 26 subjects, using fluorescein angiography and native microscopy, suggest a decrease in dermal papillary loops [85]. Because of loss of functional capillary plexi, the maximum amount of blood pumped is reduced, although in individual capillary units the blood-flow pattern remains unchanged [99].

Loss of collagen and elastin fibers in the dermis (associated with an overall derangement of organization) decreases the tensile strength of the skin. This makes aged skin more susceptible to injury (especially the lower layers) [11, 70] and results in a collapse of structural support for the cutaneous vasculature. Where initial skin injury occurs, impaired wound healing significantly increases the risk of complication [35, 99].

Vascular disorders common in the aged include pressure ulcers and rosacea.

Pressure Ulcers

Elderly patients who lose functional mobility become susceptible to pressure ulcers (bedsores), a localized area of tissue necrosis that affects the skin, subcutaneous tissue, muscle, and bone. People aged 70–75 have double the risk of pressure ulcers compared to those aged 55–69 [118]. Up to 14 % of patients in acute care facilities [119], 25 % of patients in skilled-nursing facilities, and 12 % of patients in home care suffer from pressure ulcers [120].

Pressure ulcers occur most often over bony prominences: the sacrum, ischial tuberosities, greater trochanters, heels, and lateral malleoli [64]. The first sign of pressure damage is blanchable erythema (indicating the presence of a mild, perivascular, lymphocytic infiltrate and edema in the papillary dermis). This is followed by nonblanchable erythema, due to red blood cell engorgement of the capillaries and venules and degeneration of pilosebaceous structures and subcutaneous fat. At this stage there is no observable effect in the epidermis [119].

Pressure ulcer dermatitis subsequently manifests as marked redness, with scaling or bullae. Initial ulceration is due to loss of the epidermis and acute inflammation of papillary and reticular dermis. Chronic ulcers display a diffusely fibrotic dermis [119]. Early pressure damage may go unnoticed by caregivers [121], as damage first destroys deeper structures while the surface of the skin exhibits only erythema [119]. High interstitial pressures are created at the bone/muscle interface, causing substantial deep tissue injury with relatively little superficial damage [122]. Multiple factors contribute to the formation of pressure ulcers: prolonged immobilization; pressure upon bony prominences, combined with shear forces; a compromised vasculature; heightened skin moisture in patients with urinary incontinence; poor nutritional status; impaired wound healing; and possible sensory deficits in the patient.

Institutionalized patients are most at risk; the composition of many hospital beds produces twice the pressure required to produce necrosis in a 2-h period [119]. Immobile patients, therefore, must be regularly repositioned, a practice that caregivers find difficult to perform regularly [123]. Nutrition is also important: pressure ulcers were significantly less likely in at-risk patients taking oral nutritional augmentation than in a similar population receiving appropriate routine care without nutritional supplement [124]. Smoking also increases risk [119].

Management of pressure ulcers should focus on prevention, with nutritional supplementation, regular pressure relief, and fastidious perineal hygiene in patients who are incontinent [119]. Seating systems that provide pressure relief and blood-flow stimulation, and/or passive standing capability, reduce the risk of pressure ulcers and enhance the patient's functioning [119].

Rosacea

Rosacea is a chronic inflammatory disorder characterized by acneiform papules, pustules, and dilation of the capillaries. It appears primarily on the cheeks, nose, forehead, and chin (Fig. 8). Its onset is intermittent in middle age, but later becomes persistent. Prevalence is 12 % among people over age 64 [14, 16]. Hyperplasia of the sebaceous glands may be present [14], and in more than 90 % of all patients there is ocular involvement [14].

Histology reveals telangiectasias and a perivascular lymphocytic inflammatory infiltrate with dermal edema [16]. The etiology is not well understood: mites, vascular instability, and vitamin deficiencies have been proposed [16]. The pathology involves, at least in part, atrophy of the papillary dermis that allows easier visualization of dermal capillaries [16]. Triggers include spicy foods, sun exposure, some medications, and facial products that contain known irritants [125].

Recently, the observation that rosacea correlates with gastrointestinal disorders [16] has been strengthened by the association of rosacea with *Helicobacter pylori* (HP) infection [126]. Eradication of *H. pylori* when identified in rosacea patients produced significant improvement in rosacea symptoms in 66 % of treated

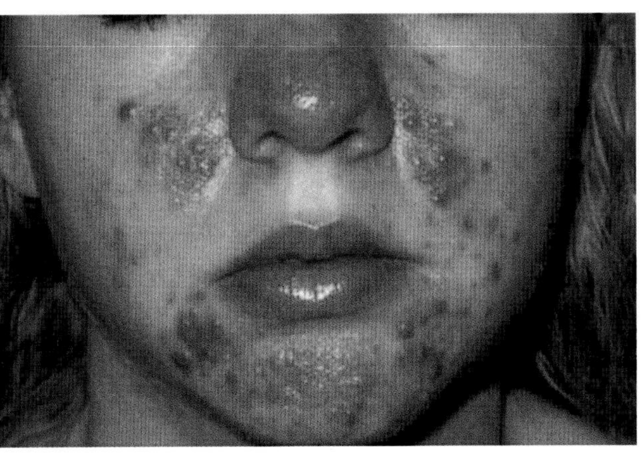

Fig. 8 Rosacea on the face (Reproduced with permission from the American Academy of Dermatology, Copyright© 2008. All rights reserved)

patients and complete resolution in 33 % [127]. Moreover, rosacea also has been associated with an increase in the generation of reactive oxygen species (ROS) in vivo [128] and tentatively proposed to be an antioxidant system defect [129]. *H. pylori* is known to increase the generation of reactive oxygen species in the gastric mucosa; further research is needed to elucidate the role of this microorganism in the progression of rosacea [130].

Often chronic, rosacea deteriorates the skin over time [38] and should be treated to avoid disfigurement (e.g., of the nasal area in men.) [125] Patients should be instructed to avoid triggers [125]. Metronidazole is the topical treatment of choice [38]; antibiotics (topical and oral) may be useful as well. Azelaic acid, topical retinaldehyde, and vitamin C also are efficacious [125]. Speculation regarding a possible antioxidant-deficit etiology for rosacea prompted a recent trial of a macrolide antibiotic, azithromycin, evaluated in 17 patients with papulopustular rosacea against healthy controls. Rosacea patients had higher ROS levels in facial skin biopsies at baseline than healthy controls, which normalized significantly in rosacea patients after 4-week treatment with azithromycin ($p < 0.001$) [131].

Viral Infection: Herpes Zoster

Herpes zoster (shingles) is a reactivation of *Varicella zoster* (the chicken pox virus) [38]. Involvement of the major sensory nerve ganglion accompanies skin eruptions [38] generally characterized by ipsilateral one or two dermatomal distribution [132], although extensive disseminated rash is common in immune-compromised patients and may occur in elderly patients who are immunocompetent [132]. Two-thirds of cases occur in patients older than 50 [70], with highest prevalence in patients 60 years and older [16]. A tingling or itching sensation (sometimes with pain) precedes a unilateral vesicular [11] cutaneous eruption by several days [38]. Vesicles persist for up to 2 weeks and eventually form dry hemorrhagic crusts with possible scarring. Secondary bacterial infections are common [16]. Reactivation sites, in decreasing order of frequency, are the thoracic, cervical, and trigeminal nerves and the lumbosacral segments [67].

Shingles is usually self-limiting [66]. Serious sequelae occur only in immunosuppressed patients (in whom the virus can easily disseminate) or when the optic nerve is involved, which occurs more often in older patients [38]. Vesicles on the side of the nose often occur in association with corneal involvement [11].

Postherpetic neuralgia (acute chronic pain along involved nerves) is a complication in about half the patients over the age of 60 with herpes-zoster reactivation. Risk of this complication increases with age [38]; increased risk is also associated with severe pain during zoster reactivation, pain more than 72 h before the rash appears, severe rash, and female gender [133]. Although the pain gradually abates over time, it is frequently disabling and refractory to typical pain medications. This can significantly affect QoL in the older patient [67]. The severity and duration of postherpetic neuralgia [62, 134], particularly in older patients [135], can be reduced by prompt and aggressive treatment of the acute infection with oral antiviral drugs (such as acyclovir) before virus spreads beyond the initially damaged nerve. Vaccination of the elderly against varicella zoster is effective and can prevent serious complications of varicella zoster virus infection [136], which can be particularly dangerous in the very old [137]; depression, however, common in the elderly, has been shown to lessen efficacy of the vaccine [138]. Treatment with antidepressant medication, however, normalizes vaccine response [138]. Zoster vaccine has been shown to be safe in the elderly population [139] and to offer effective prevention of shingles for at least 5 years [140].

In a randomized, double-blind, placebo-controlled, prospective trial in more than 38,000 senior adults, a new vaccine composed of live, attenuated *Varicella zoster* virus reduced incidence of postherpetic neuralgia by 66.5 % [141]. Morbidity due to herpes zoster was markedly reduced with few side effects (principally mild dermatological reactions at the injection sites). Discussion of the cost-effectiveness of the vaccine in the target populations is ongoing [142].

Management of Cutaneous Disorders in the Elderly

Management of skin disease in the elderly must take into account variables pertinent to the older patient. Accurate diagnosis is key. In the elderly, diagnosis is complicated by the use of multiple medications in this age group: drug eruptions, which can simulate almost any dermatological disease (Table 3), must be distinguished from cutaneous eruptions of other etiologies [33]. Diagnosis of drug reactions is critical before the any underlying cutaneous disorder can be identified. Moreover, prompt withdrawal of the culprit drug may be necessary to avoid complications [143].

Topical treatment must take into account the fragility of aged skin [70]. Aged skin is compromised with structural degeneration and comorbidities [72]. Consequently, second-line therapies may be more advisable at earlier treatment stages [11].

Psychosocial issues must also be considered in treatment decisions. Older patients may suffer from memory loss, impaired vision, hearing, or mobility and sometimes, dementia [11, 12]. They may lack attentive caregivers and adequate housing or nutrition [11]. The patient's ability to comply with therapy should be considered, though often it is not [72]. Physicians need to consider whether compliance with the regimen prescribed is actually feasible for the patient: simple regimens should be advised whenever possible to maximize compliance [72]. Clinicians or care providers should follow-up to ensure that medications were applied as required [33].

Conclusions

Diseases and disorders of the skin increase in prevalence in older people [70]. Most people over 65 have at least one skin disorder, and many have two or more [6] conditions which can create substantial morbidity and mortality and deterioration of QoL in older adults [14, 119, 144]. For optimal care of skin disease in the

Table 3 Cutaneous eruptions and possible drug etiology by classification of lesions

Type of rash or eruption	Possible drug etiology
Exanthems	Beta-lactam antibiotics, sulfonamides, erythromycin, gentamicin, anticonvulsants, gold salts
Eczema, lichenification	Antiarrhythmic agents, anticonvulsive agents, antituberculosis agents, gold, quinidine, methyldopa
Acne-like	Corticosteroids, bromides, iodides
Urticaria and angioedema	Converting enzyme (ACE) inhibitors, NSAIDs, opiates, curare, antibiotics (esp penicillins), blood products
Bullous	Penicillamine, bleomycin, iodides
Fixed drug	Penicillins, phenolphthalein, tetracycline, nalidixic acid, barbiturates, sulfonamides, gold salts
Exfoliation	Gold
Anticoagulant skin necrosis	Warfarin, heparin
Nodular eruption	Sulfathiazole, salicylates, oral contraceptives
Rash on sun-exposed areas	Coal-tar derivates, psoralen, chlorpromazine, tetracycline, doxycycline, NSAIDs, phenothiazines, chlorothiazide, demeclocycline, griseofulvin, oral hypoglycemics, sulfonamides
Erythema multiforme target lesions, SJS, TEN	Allopurinol, barbiturates, dapsone, digitalis, phenobarbital, carbamazepine, phenytoin, gold, hydralazine, salicylates, sulfonamides, penicillin, quinolone, cephalosporins, NSAIDs, tetracycline, trimethoprim-sulfamethoxazole

Table 3 is modified from References [147, 148]

ACE angiotensin-converting enzyme, *NSAIDs* nonsteroidal antiinflammatory drugs, *SJS* Stevens-Johnson syndrome, *TEN* toxic epidermal necrolysis

elderly, primary care providers most monitor the condition of their patient's skin and distinguish lesions that are a normal part of aging from more clinically significant lesions that may require specialized intervention [5], prompting referral to the dermatologist as needed [5]. Treatment decisions should consider the patient's housing, presence or lack of caregivers, nutritional status, clothing, heating, mobility, hearing, and vision [11]. Prompt and thoughtful treatment of any clinically significant cutaneous disorder can substantially improve the aging patient's QoL in their latter years [144].

References

1. Marks R. Skin disease in old age. New York: Taylor & Francis; 1999.
2. Farage MA, Miller KW, Elsner P, et al. Structural characteristics of the aging skin: a review. Cutan Ocul Toxicol. 2007;26:343–57.
3. Farage MA, Miller KW, Elsner P, et al. Functional and physiological characteristics of the aging skin. Aging Clin Exp Res. 2008;20:195–200.
4. Farage MA, Miller KW, Elsner P, et al. Intrinsic and extrinsic factors in skin ageing: a review. Int J Cosmet Sci. 2008;30:87–95.
5. Gilchrest BA. Geriatric skin problems. Hosp Pract (Off Ed). 1986;21:55. 59–65.
6. Kligman AM, Koblenzer C. Demographics and psychological implications for the aging population. Dermatol Clin. 1997;15:549–53.
7. Kligman AM. Psychological aspects of skin disorders in the elderly. Cutis. 1989;43:498–501.
8. Global Industry Analysts Inc. Global anti-aging products market to reach $291.9 billion by 2015, according to new report by Global Industry Analysts. http://www.prweb.com/releases/2009/02/prweb2021254.htm. Accessed 4 Sept 2014.
9. Thaipisuttikul Y. Pruritic skin diseases in the elderly. J Dermatol. 1998;25:153–7.
10. Farage MA, Miller KW, Elsner P, et al. Characteristics of the aging skin. Adv Wound Care (New Rochelle). 2013;2:5–10.
11. Bleiker TO, Graham-Brown RA. Diagnosing skin disease in the elderly. Practitioner. 2000;244:974–81.
12. Laube S, Farrell AM. Bacterial skin infections in the elderly: diagnosis and treatment. Drugs Aging. 2002;19:331–42.
13. Norman RA. Xerosis and pruritus in elderly patients, part 1. Ostomy Wound Manage. 2006;52:12–4.
14. Wolff K, Johnson R, Suurmond R. Fitzpatrick's color atlas & synopsis of clinical dermatology. 5th ed. New York: McGraw-Hill Professional; 2005.
15. Resnick B. Dermatologic problems in the elderly. Lippincotts Prim Care Pract. 1997;1:14–30; quiz 31–2.
16. Kleinsmith DM, Perricone NV. Common skin problems in the elderly. Dermatol Clin. 1986;4:485–99.
17. Peters S. Dermatologic issues in the elderly. Examining common problems. Adv Nurse Pract. 1999;7:63–4.
18. Fitzpatrick JE. Common inflammatory skin diseases of the elderly. Geriatrics. 1989;44:40–6.
19. Haroun MT. Dry skin in the elderly. Geriatr Aging. 2003;6:41–4.
20. Shwayder T. Ichthyosis in a nutshell. Pediatr Rev. 1999;20:5–12.
21. Harding C, Watkinson A, Rawlings A, et al. Dry skin, moisturization and corneodesmoloysis. Int J Cosmet Sci. 2000;22:21–52.
22. Loden M, Maibach H, editors. Dry skin and moisturizers: chemistry and function. Boca Raton: CRC Press; 2006.
23. Leyden JJ, Rawlings AV. Skin moisturization. New York: Marcel Dekker; 2002.
24. Jennings MB, Alfieri D, Ward K, et al. Comparison of salicylic acid and urea versus ammonium lactate for the treatment of foot xerosis. A randomized, double-blind, clinical study. J Am Podiatr Med Assoc. 1998;88:332–6.
25. Schmidt T, Sitaru C, Amber K, et al. BP180- and BP230-specific IgG autoantibodies in pruritic disorders of the elderly: a preclinical stage of bullous pemphigoid? Br J Dermatol. 2014;171:212–9.
26. Fleischer ABJ. Pruritus in the elderly. Adv Dermatol. 1995;10:41–60.
27. Waisman M. A clinical look at the aging skin. Postgrad Med. 1979;66:87–93, 96.
28. Yosipovitch G. Assessment of itch: more to be learned and improvements to be made. J Invest Dermatol. 2003;121:xiv–xv.
29. Perkins P. The management of eczema in adults (continuing education credit). Nurs Stand. 1996;10:49–53; quiz 55–6.
30. Braun M, Lowitt MH. Pruritus. Adv Dermatol. 2001;17:1–27.
31. Rogers C. Lichen simplex chronicus. Dermatol Nurs. 2003;15:271.
32. Long CC, Marks R. Stratum corneum changes in patients with senile pruritus. J Am Acad Dermatol. 1992;27:560–4.
33. Lim SPR, Abdullah A. Managing skin disease in elderly patients. Practitioner. 2004;248:100–4. 106, 108–9.
34. Gupta MA, Gupta AK. Medically unexplained cutaneous sensory symptoms may represent somatoform dissociation: an empirical study. J Psychosom Res. 2006;60:131–6.
35. Shelley WB, Shelley ED. The ten major problems of aging skin. Geriatrics. 1982;37:107–13.
36. Fleischer ABJ. Pruritus in the elderly: management by senior dermatologists. J Am Acad Dermatol. 1993;28:603–9.

37. Webster GF. Common skin disorders in the elderly. Clin Cornerstone. 2001;4:39–44.
38. Tierney L, McPhee S, Papadakis M. Current medical diagnosis and treatment. New York: McGraw Hill; 2000.
39. DeWitt S. Nursing assessment of the skin and dermatologic lesions. Nurs Clin North Am. 1990;25:235–45.
40. Marks R. Skin disease in old age. London: Martin Dunitz; 1987.
41. Habif T. Clinical dermatology: a color guide to diagnosis and treatment. St. Louis: Mosby; 2004.
42. Tavadia S, Bianchi J, Dawe RS, et al. Allergic contact dermatitis in venous leg ulcer patients. Contact Dermatitis. 2003;48:261–5.
43. MacKie R. Clinical dermatology: an illustrated textbook. Oxford: Oxford University Press; 1987.
44. Hall J. Sauer's manual of skin diseases. Philadelphia: Lippincott, Williams and Wilkins; 2000.
45. Norman R, editor. Diagnosis of aging skin diseases. London: Springer; 2008.
46. Weismann K, Wadskov S, Mikkelsen HI, et al. Acquired zinc deficiency dermatosis in man. Arch Dermatol. 1978;114:1509–11.
47. Akimoto K, Yoshikawa N, Higaki Y, et al. Quantitative analysis of stratum corneum lipids in xerosis and asteatotic eczema. J Dermatol. 1993;20:1–6.
48. Warin AP. Eczéma craquelé as the presenting feature of myxoedema. Br J Dermatol. 1973;89:289–91.
49. Guillet MH, Schollhammer M, Sassolas B, et al. Eczema craquelé as a pointer of internal malignancy – a case report. Clin Exp Dermatol. 1996;21:431–3.
50. van Voorst Vader PC, Folkers E, van Rhenen DJ. Craquelé-like eruption in angioimmunoblastic lymphadenopathy. Arch Dermatol. 1979;115:370.
51. Sparsa A, Boulinguez S, Liozon E, et al. Predictive clinical features of eczema craquelé associated with internal malignancy. Dermatology. 2007;215:28–35.
52. Soter NA. Nummular eczematous dermatitis. In: Freedberg IM, Eisen AZ, Wolff K, Austen KF, Goldsmith LA, Katz SI, Fitzpatrick TB, editors. Fitzpatrick's dermatology in general medicine. New York: McGraw-Hill; 1999.
53. du Vivier A. Atlas of clinical dermatology. Kidlington: Churchill Livingston; 2002.
54. Miller J. Nummular dermatitis. http://emedicine.medscape.com/article/1123605-print. Accessed 6 Sept 2014.
55. Aoyama H, Tanaka M, Hara M, et al. Nummular eczema: an addition of senile xerosis and unique cutaneous reactivities to environmental aeroallergens. Dermatology. 1999;199:135–9.
56. Adachi A, Horikawa T, Takashima T, et al. Mercury-induced nummular dermatitis. J Am Acad Dermatol. 2000;43:383–5.
57. Le Coz C. Contact nummular (discoid) eczema from depilating cream. Contact Dermatitis. 2002;46:111–2.
58. Flendrie M, Vissers WHPM, Creemers MCW, et al. Dermatological conditions during TNF-alpha-blocking therapy in patients with rheumatoid arthritis: a prospective study. Arthritis Res Ther. 2005;7:R666–76.
59. Shen Y, Pielop J, Hsu S. Generalized nummular eczema secondary to peginterferon Alfa-2b and ribavirin combination therapy for hepatitis C infection. Arch Dermatol. 2005;141:102–3.
60. White JV, Ryjewski C. Chronic venous insufficiency. Perspect Vasc Surg Endovasc Ther. 2005;17:319–27.
61. Quatresooz P, Henry F, Paquet P, et al. Deciphering the impaired cytokine cascades in chronic leg ulcers (review). Int J Mol Med. 2003;11:411–8.
62. Leu AJ, Leu HJ, Franzeck UK, et al. Microvascular changes in chronic venous insufficiency – a review. Cardiovasc Surg. 1995;3:237–45.
63. Coleridge Smith PD. Deleterious effects of white cells in the course of skin damage in CVI. Int Angiol. 2002;21:26–32.
64. Shai A, Maibach HI. Wound healing and ulcers of the skin: diagnosis and therapy – the practical approach. New York: Springer; 2005.
65. Trent JT, Falabella A, Eaglstein WH, et al. Venous ulcers: pathophysiology and treatment options. Ostomy Wound Manage. 2005;51:38–54; quiz 55–6.
66. Herouy Y, Nockowski P, Schöpf E, et al. Lipodermatosclerosis and the significance of proteolytic remodeling in the pathogenesis of venous ulceration (review). Int J Mol Med. 1999;3:511–5.
67. Buckley C, Rustin MH. Management of irritable skin disorders in the elderly. Br J Hosp Med. 1990;44:24–6. 28, 30–2.
68. Combemale P, Bousquet M, Kanitakis J, et al. Malignant transformation of leg ulcers: a retrospective study of 85 cases. J Eur Acad Dermatol Venereol. 2007;21:935–41.
69. Gilchrest B, Krutmann J, editors. Skin aging. New York: Springer; 2006.
70. Carter DM, Balin AK. Dermatological aspects of aging. Med Clin North Am. 1983;67:531–43.
71. Machet L, Couhé C, Perrinaud A, et al. A high prevalence of sensitization still persists in leg ulcer patients: a retrospective series of 106 patients tested between 2001 and 2002 and a meta-analysis of 1975–2003 data. Br J Dermatol. 2004;150:929–35.
72. Smoker A. Skin care in old age. Nurs Stand. 1999;13:47–53.
73. Chan DCW, Fong DHF, Leung JYY, et al. Maggot debridement therapy in chronic wound care. Hong Kong Med J. 2007;13:382–6.
74. Jull AB, Cullum N, Dumville JC, Westby MJ, Deshpande S, Walker N. Honey as a topical treatment for wounds (a Review). The Cochrane Collaboration. Published by John Wiley & Sons, Ltd. 2015;3:1–132.
75. Coelho S, Amarelo M, Ryan S, et al. Rheumatoid arthritis-associated inflammatory leg ulcers: a new treatment for recalcitrant wounds. Int Wound J. 2004;1:81–4.

76. Taradaj J, Franek A, Brzezinska-Wcislo L, et al. The use of therapeutic ultrasound in venous leg ulcers: a randomized, controlled clinical trial. Phlebology. 2008;23:178–83.
77. Körber A, Franckson T, Grabbe S, et al. Vacuum assisted closure device improves the take of mesh grafts in chronic leg ulcer patients. Dermatology. 2008;216:250–6.
78. Kranke P1, Bennett MH, Martyn-St James M, Schnabel A, Debus SE, Weibel S. Hyperbaric oxygen therapy for chronic wounds. Cochrane Database Syst Rev. 2015;6:CD004123. doi: 10.1002/14651858.CD004123.pub4. Page 1–19.
79. van Gent WB, Hop WC, van Praag MC, et al. Conservative versus surgical treatment of venous leg ulcers: a prospective, randomized, multicenter trial. J Vasc Surg. 2006;44:563–71.
80. Beacham BE. Common dermatoses in the elderly. Am Fam Physician. 1993;47:1445–50.
81. Piaserico S, Larese F, Recchia GP, et al. Allergic contact sensitivity in elderly patients. Aging Clin Exp Res. 2004;16:221–5.
82. Ghadially R, Brown BE, Sequeira-Martin SM, et al. The aged epidermal permeability barrier. Structural, functional, and lipid biochemical abnormalities in humans and a senescent murine model. J Clin Invest. 1995;95:2281–90.
83. Goh CL, Ling R. A retrospective epidemiology study of contact eczema among the elderly attending a tertiary dermatology referral centre in Singapore. Singapore Med J. 1998;39:442–6.
84. Green CM, Holden CR, Gawkrodger DJ. Contact allergy to topical medicaments becomes more common with advancing age: an age-stratified study. Contact Dermatitis. 2007;56:229–31.
85. Nedorost ST, Stevens SR. Diagnosis and treatment of allergic skin disorders in the elderly. Drugs Aging. 2001;18:827–35.
86. Mangelsdorf HC, Fleischer AB, Sherertz EF. Patch testing in an aged population without dermatitis: high prevalence of patch test positivity. Am J Contact Dermat. 1996;7:155–7.
87. Spencer SK, Kierland RR. The aging skin: problems and their causes. Geriatrics. 1970;25:81–9.
88. Chew AL, Maibach HI, editors. Irritant dermatitis. Berlin: Springer; 2005.
89. Levin C, Zhai H, Bashir S, et al. Efficacy of corticosteroids in acute experimental irritant contact dermatitis? Skin Res Technol. 2001;7:214–8.
90. Levin C, Zhai H, Maibach H. Corticosteroids of clinical value in lipid-soluble-chemical-induced irritation in man? Exog Dermatol. 2002;1:97–101.
91. Sandström Falk MH, Tengvall Linder M, Johansson C, et al. The prevalence of Malassezia yeasts in patients with atopic dermatitis, seborrhoeic dermatitis and healthy controls. Acta Derm Venereol. 2005;85:17–23.
92. Schwartz RA, Janusz CA, Janniger CK. Seborrheic dermatitis: an overview. Am Fam Physician. 2006;74:125–30.
93. Schwartz JR, Cardin CW, Dawson TLJ. Dandruff and seborrheic dermatitis. In: Baran R, Maibach HI, editors. Textbook of cosmetic dermatology. London: Martin Dunitz; 2004.
94. Mastrolonardo M, Diaferio A, Logroscino G. Seborrheic dermatitis, increased sebum excretion, and Parkinson's disease: a survey of (im)possible links. Med Hypotheses. 2003;60:907–11.
95. Loo WJ, Burrows NP. Management of autoimmune skin disorders in the elderly. Drugs Aging. 2004;21:767–77.
96. Bickle K, Roark TR, Hsu S. Autoimmune bullous dermatoses: a review. Am Fam Physician. 2002;65:1861–70.
97. Bastuji-Garin S, Joly P, Lemordant P, et al. Risk factors for bullous pemphigoid in the elderly: a prospective case-control study. J Invest Dermatol. 2011;131:637–43.
98. Langan SM, Smeeth L, Hubbard R, et al. Bullous pemphigoid and pemphigus vulgaris – incidence and mortality in the UK: population based cohort study. BMJ. 2008;337:a180.
99. Walsh SRA, Hogg D, Mydlarski PR. Bullous pemphigoid: from bench to bedside. Drugs. 2005;65:905–26.
100. Feliciani C, Caldarola G, Kneisel A, et al. IgG autoantibody reactivity against bullous pemphigoid (BP) 180 and BP230 in elderly patients with pruritic dermatoses. Br J Dermatol. 2009;161:306–12.
101. Brodell LA, Beck LA. Differential diagnosis of chronic urticaria. Ann Allergy Asthma Immunol. 2008;100:181–8; quiz 188–90, 215.
102. Stanley J. Bullous pemphigoid. In: Freedberg IM, Eisen AZ, Wolff K, Austen KF, Goldsmith LA, Katz SI, Fitzpatrick TB, editors. Fitzpatrick's dermatology in general medicine. New York: McGraw-Hill; 1999.
103. Fania L, Caldarola G, Müller R, et al. IgE recognition of bullous pemphigoid (BP)180 and BP230 in BP patients and elderly individuals with pruritic dermatoses. Clin Immunol. 2012;143:236–45.
104. Mutasim DF. Autoimmune bullous dermatoses in the elderly: diagnosis and management. Drugs Aging. 2003;20:663–81.
105. Lee YY, Bee PC, Lee CK, et al. Bullous pemphigoid in an elderly patient with myelodysplastic syndrome and refractory anemia coupled with excess of blast. Ann Dermatol. 2011;23:S390–2.
106. Kjellman P, Eriksson H, Berg P. A retrospective analysis of patients with bullous pemphigoid treated with methotrexate. Arch Dermatol. 2008;144:612–6.
107. Sollecito TP, Parisi E. Mucous membrane pemphigoid. Dent Clin N Am. 2005;49:91–106. viii.
108. Laforest C, Huilgol SC, Casson R, et al. Autoimmune bullous diseases: ocular manifestations and management. Drugs. 2005;65:1767–79.
109. Li Z, Zhang J, Xu H, et al. Correlation of conventional and conformational anti-desmoglein antibodies with

phenotypes and disease activities in patients with pemphigus vulgaris. Acta Derm Venereol. 2014. doi:10.2340/00015555-1961 [Epub ahead of print].

110. da Silva AV, Valones MA, Guimaraes RP, et al. Pemphigus vulgaris: a therapeutic option for disease control. Gen Dent. 2008;56:700–3.
111. Tehranchi-Nia Z, Qureshi TA, Ahmed AR. Pemphigus vulgaris in older adults. J Am Geriatr Soc. 1998;46:92–4.
112. Chams-Davatchi C, Esmaili N, Daneshpazhooh M, et al. Randomized controlled open-label trial of four treatment regimens for pemphigus vulgaris. J Am Acad Dermatol. 2007;57:622–8.
113. Zhu X, Zhang B. Paraneoplastic pemphigus. J Dermatol. 2007;34:503–11.
114. Farage MA, Maibach HI, editors. The vulva: anatomy, physiology, and pathology. New York: Informa Healthcare; 2006.
115. Neill SM, Tatnall FM, Cox NH. Guidelines for the management of lichen sclerosus. Br J Dermatol. 2002;147:640–9.
116. Lorenz B, Kaufman RH, Kutzner SK. Lichen sclerosus. Therapy with clobetasol propionate. J Reprod Med. 1998;43:790–4.
117. Cooper SM, Gao X, Powell JJ, et al. Does treatment of vulvar lichen sclerosus influence its prognosis? Arch Dermatol. 2004;140:702–6.
118. Berlowitz DR, Wilking SVB. Pressure ulcers in the nursing home. In: Reubentein L, Wieland D, editors. Improving care in the nursing home: comprehensive reviews of clinical research. Newbury Park: Sage Publications; 1993.
119. Edlich RF, Winters KL, Woodard CR, et al. Pressure ulcer prevention. J Long Term Eff Med Implants. 2004;14:285–304.
120. National Pressure Ulcer Advisory Panel T. Pressure ulcers prevalence, cost, and risk assessment: consensus development conference statement. Decubitus. 1989;2:24–8.
121. Nola GT, Vistnes LM. Differential response of skin and muscle in the experimental production of pressure sores. Plast Reconstr Surg. 1980;66:728–33.
122. Baranoski S. Skin tears: the enemy of frail skin. Adv Skin Wound Care. 2000;13:123–6.
123. Baeke JL. Hospital-acquired pressure ulcers: an epidemic. Plast Reconstr Surg. 2000;106:945–6.
124. Stratton RJ, Ek A, Engfer M, et al. Enteral nutritional support in prevention and treatment of pressure ulcers: a systematic review and meta-analysis. Ageing Res Rev. 2005;4:422–50.
125. Cohen AF, Tiemstra JD. Diagnosis and treatment of rosacea. J Am Board Fam Pract. 2002;15:214–7.
126. Diaz C, O'Callaghan CJ, Khan A, et al. Rosacea: a cutaneous marker of Helicobacter pylori infection? Results of a pilot study. Acta Derm Venereol. 2003;83:282–6.
127. Boixeda de Miquel D, Vázquez Romero M, Vázquez Sequeiros E, et al. Effect of *Helicobacter pylori* eradication therapy in rosacea patients. Rev Esp Enferm Dig. 2006;98:501–9.
128. Tisma VS, Basta-Juzbasic A, Jaganjac M, et al. Oxidative stress and ferritin expression in the skin of patients with rosacea. J Am Acad Dermatol. 2009;60(2):270–6. doi:10.1016/j.jaad.2008.10.014. Epub 2008 Nov 25.
129. Oztas MO, Balk M, Ogüs E, et al. The role of free oxygen radicals in the aetiopathogenesis of rosacea. Clin Exp Dermatol. 2003;28:188–92.
130. Baz K, Cimen MYB, Kokturk A, et al. Plasma reactive oxygen species activity and antioxidant potential levels in rosacea patients: correlation with seropositivity to *Helicobacter pylori*. Int J Dermatol. 2004;43:494–7.
131. Bakar O, Demirçay Z, Yuksel M, et al. The effect of azithromycin on reactive oxygen species in rosacea. Clin Exp Dermatol. 2007;32:197–200.
132. Yoon KJ, Kim SH, Lee EH, et al. Disseminated herpes zoster in an immunocompetent elderly patient. Korean J Pain. 2013;26:195–8.
133. McKendrick MW, Ogan P, Care CC. A 9 year follow up of post herpetic neuralgia and predisposing factors in elderly patients following herpes zoster. J Infect. 2009;59:416–20.
134. Niv D, Maltsman-Tseikhin A, Lang E. Postherpetic neuralgia: what do we know and where are we heading? Pain Physician. 2004;7:239–47.
135. Johnson R. Herpes zoster – predicting and minimizing the impact of post-herpetic neuralgia. J Antimicrob Chemother. 2001;47(Suppl T1):1–8.
136. van Lier A, van Hoek AJ, Opstelten W, et al. Assessing the potential effects and cost-effectiveness of programmatic herpes zoster vaccination of elderly in the Netherlands. BMC Health Serv Res. 2010;10:237.
137. Studahl M, Petzold M, Cassel T. Disease burden of herpes zoster in Sweden – predominance in the elderly and in women – a register based study. BMC Infect Dis. 2013;13:586.
138. Irwin MR, Levin MJ, Laudenslager ML, et al. Varicella zoster virus-specific immune responses to a herpes zoster vaccine in elderly recipients with major depression and the impact of antidepressant medications. Clin Infect Dis. 2013;56:1085–93.
139. Morrison VA, Oxman MN, Levin MJ, et al. Safety of zoster vaccine in elderly adults following documented herpes zoster. J Infect Dis. 2013;208:559–63.
140. Schmader KE, Oxman MN, Levin MJ, et al. Persistence of the efficacy of zoster vaccine in the shingles prevention study and the short-term persistence substudy. Clin Infect Dis. 2012;55:1320–8.
141. Oxman MN, Levin MJ, Johnson GR, et al. A vaccine to prevent herpes zoster and postherpetic neuralgia in older adults. N Engl J Med. 2005;352:2271–84.
142. Koplan JP, Harpaz R. Shingles vaccine: effective and costly or cost-effective? Ann Intern Med. 2006;145:386–7.

143. Bachot N, Roujeau J. Differential diagnosis of severe cutaneous drug eruptions. Am J Clin Dermatol. 2003;4:561–72.
144. Liao YH, Chen KH, Tseng MP, et al. Pattern of skin diseases in a geriatric patient group in Taiwan: a 7-year survey from the outpatient clinic of a university medical center. Dermatology. 2001;203:308–13.
145. Fletcher K. Skin: geriatric self-learning module. Medsurg Nurs. 2005;14:138–42.
146. Boss GR, Seegmiller JE. Age-related physiological changes and their clinical significance. West J Med. 1981;135:434–40.
147. Kooken A, Tomecki K. Drug eruptions. http://www.clevelandclinicmeded.com/medicalpubs/diseasemanagement/dermatology/drug-eruptions/. Accessed 2 Sept 2014.
148. Kauppinen K, Alanko K, Hannuksela M, et al. Skin reactions to drugs. Boca Raton: CRC Press; 1998.

Neoplastic Skin Lesions in the Elderly Patient

65

Miranda A. Farage, Kenneth W. Miller, Enzo Berardesca, Howard I. Maibach, and Isaac M. Neuhaus

Contents

M.A. Farage (✉)
Winton Hill Business Center, The Procter & Gamble Company, Cincinnati, OH, USA
e-mail: farage.m@pg.com

K.W. Miller
Margoshes-Miller Consulting, LLC, Cincinnati, OH, USA
e-mail: bbbns2@fuse.net

E. Berardesca
San Gallicano Dermatological Institute, Rome, Italy
e-mail: berardesca@berardesca.it

H.I. Maibach • I.M. Neuhaus
Department of Dermatology, University of California, San Francisco, CA, USA
e-mail: maibachh@derm.ucsf.edu; neuhausi@derm.ucsf.edu

M.A. Farage et al. (eds.), *Textbook of Aging Skin*,
DOI 10.1007/978-3-662-47398-6_55

Abstract

As the proportion of the elderly in the United States increases steadily, the costs of treating cutaneous disorders also rise. Proliferative disorders of the skin are particularly common in the aged, and the risk of malignancy increases with age with possible catastrophic consequences. Nonmalignant proliferative disorders (e.g., skin tags, seborrheic keratosis) are not likely to be fatal but can produce significant disfigurement and discomfort. The burden of benign skin neoplasms, when disfiguring, should be recognized, and older patients should be monitored by all their physicians for the development of potentially dangerous neoplastic disease, particularly the recognized precursor of squamous cell carcinoma, actinic keratosis, and the three cutaneous neoplasms that represent half of all skin cancers – basal cell carcinoma, squamous cell carcinoma, and melanoma. Newer therapies, particularly ones that target molecular and/or genetic pathways to carcinogenesis, are also improving patient outcomes.

Introduction

As the proportion of the aged in the US population increases, so does the burden of cutaneous disease [1]. Cutaneous disease in the elderly is the source of significant morbidity and not infrequent mortality, with many patients having multiple skin conditions [2]. Hyperproliferative disorders, common in older

Table 1 Malignant potential in hyperproliferative diseases of the aged skin

Benign	Premalignant	Malignant
Skin tags	Actinic keratosis (AK)	Basal cell carcinoma (BCC)
Senile lentigo (lentigines)	Lentigo maligna	Squamous cell carcinoma (SCC)
Seborrheic keratoses	Leukoplakia	Bowen's disease (SCC in situ)
Cherry hemangiomas (de Morgan's spots)	Atypical nevi	Keratoacanthoma (SCC in situ)
Corns		Malignant melanoma

Table 1 summarizes findings from [37, 40–43, 49, 52]

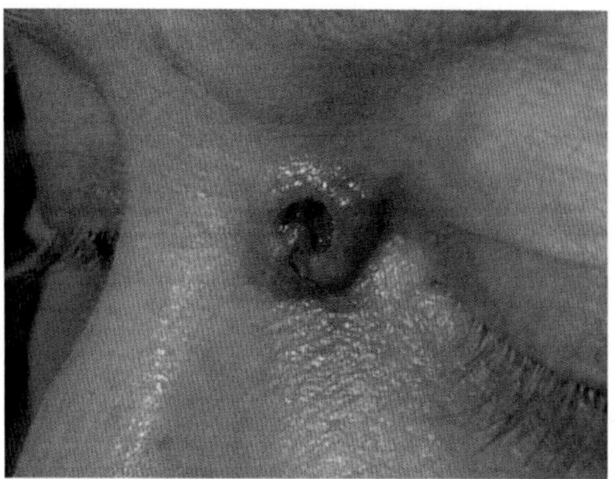

Fig. 1 Picture of basal cell carcinoma (BCC)

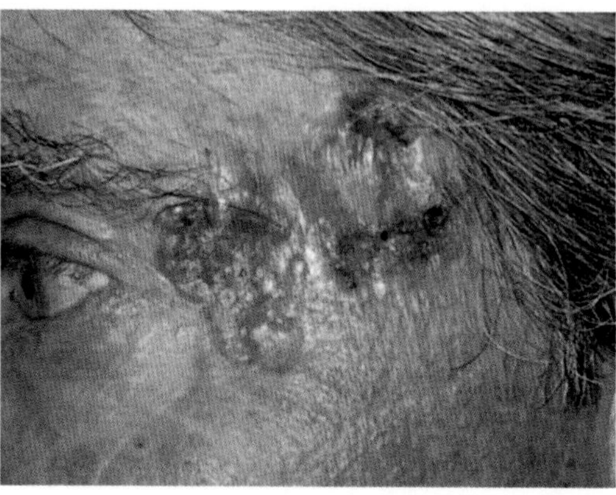

Fig. 2 Picture of basal cell carcinoma (BCC)

adults, are strongly associated with exposure to solar radiation [3]. Although nonmalignant growths are far more common than those that are malignant, skin cancers represent about 6 % of all dermatology visits [4], and the costs of treating patients with cancers are considerable: the total cost of melanoma treatment in the US population is an estimated $249 million annually [5], with per patient lifetime costs reaching more than $28,000. The prevalence of cutaneous malignancies, moreover, increases with age [6] (Table 1).

The most common cutaneous neoplasms are basal cell carcinoma (BCC) (Figs. 1 and 2), squamous cell carcinoma (SCC) (Fig. 3), and malignant melanoma. These three skin cancers account for almost half of all human cancers [7]. Increases in skin cancer rates have paralleled a cultural shift toward recreational ultraviolet (UV) exposure [8]. As a result, skin cancers are appearing at alarming rates in young adults. Because the risk of skin cancer recurrence is directly related to the length of time of past initial diagnosis, dramatic leaps in skin cancer rates in young people may well precede a steep increase of future skin cancers in old age [9].

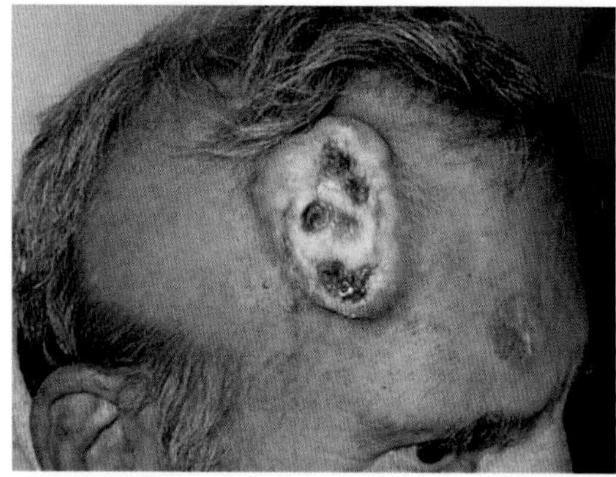

Fig. 3 Squamous cell carcinoma (SCC)

The major factor contributing to skin cancer in humans is lifetime cumulative exposure to cancer-causing agents, including UV radiation, decreased melanocyte protection, diminished DNA repair, and decreased immunosurveillance [10]. The strong correlation observed between age and increasing rates of skin cancers, however, is not well understood [11]. Evidence suggests that age-related susceptibility to skin cancers may be associated with an age-related accumulation of senescent stromal cells that, in turn, create a tumor-promoting environment involving the receptor for insulin-like growth factor-1 (IGF-1R). Keratinocytes for which IGF-1 has been inactivated abnormally proliferate when ultraviolet-B (UVB) damage has occurred. More than 90 % of all skin cancers, however, are believed to have direct origin in exposure to the sun's ultraviolet rays [8].

A major function of the skin is the absorption of UV radiation. Virtually, all ultraviolet-B (UVB) is absorbed by the upper layers of the epidermis, with only 20 % reaching the dermoepidermal junction. Ultraviolet-A (UVA) penetrates deeper, releasing up to 50 % of its energy in dermal stratum papillare [12]. Despite its inability to penetrate beyond the epidermis, UVB is far more mutagenic than UVA [12]. Induction of squamous cell carcinoma has been observed to be 1000 times more efficient with UVB (300 nm) than with UVA (380 nm) [13]. Constitutive levels of melanin in the skin, an inherited contributor to UV risk, play a major role in the capacity of UV insult to affect DNA mutation. Twenty percent of Caucasians, more accurately described as Fitzpatrick skin types I, II, and III, will suffer some form of skin cancer over their lifetimes [14]. People with darker skin, Fitzpatrick types IV and V, benefit from the substantial protection that melanin density offers: a 500-fold level of protection from UV radiation (based on skin cancer rates) between white and black skin [15].

The appearance of a cutaneous malignancy is the culmination of an accumulation of genetic abnormalities, some inherited and some acquired. The types of mutations and the number accumulated will define malignant potential [16]. Genetic abnormalities caused by UV radiation represent a spectrum of damage. The ability of ultraviolet light (UVL) to cause point mutations has been long recognized [17]. More recently, UV-induced deletions [18] and micronuclei [19] have also been observed in irradiated skin cells. In addition, the presence of aneuploidy has been observed in every type of skin cancer; aneuploidy increases as the tumor progresses and robustly correlates with the malignant potential of the lesion [16].

Epidermal cells bear the brunt of environmental insult to the body, and multiple mutations occur in every epidermal cell every day. The vast majority will be quickly repaired and do not lead to malignant transformation. In cases where accumulation of unrepaired genetic abnormalities occurs in a particular cell over time, impaired normal function can result [16]. The accrual of genetic damage in particular genes – those related to cell cycle control, ongoing DNA repair, upregulation of proliferation, or induction of apoptosis – can result in cell transformation with subsequent tumor initiation [16]. Ultimately, transformation is a multistep process requiring distinct damage events, creating the typical latency period between initial insult and appearance of cancerous lesion [12].

UV insult causes damage with a dual action of creating mutation in the DNA and suppressing intrinsic immunity through disruption of tumor surveillance [12]. UVL acts both as tumor initiator and promoter [20]. Mutation in the gene that produces p53 is considered a hallmark of UV-induced genome modification. P53 in healthy cells is involved in tumor suppression, arresting the cell cycle in the G1 phase in order to allow for DNA repair before mitosis ensues [12]. Most UV-induced DNA damage is repaired by p53 [21]. If genetic damage in the cell is extensive, p53 will initiate apoptosis [22]. Mutation in p53 aborts the progression to apoptosis, permitting the mutated cell to continue to divide [12]. Cells carrying p53 mutations are ubiquitous in every type of skin cancer [23]. Another regulator of apoptosis, CD95 (fas) is also inhibited by chronic UV exposure [24].

UV exposure also has been demonstrated to increase the population of tumor-permissive macrophages, depress Langerhans cell numbers, reduce Langerhans cell function, induce cytotoxic T cells to undergo apoptosis, and activate suppressor T cells [20]. A resident malignancy can affect immunosuppression as well. The capacity for DNA repair after UV exposure was observed to be lower in patients with basal cell carcinoma (BCC) than in controls without skin cancer [25].

In addition, in a population of nonmelanoma skin cancer (NMSC) patients, 90 % exhibited a decreased immune response in delayed hypersensitivity skin testing [20]. Organ transplant recipients receiving immunosuppressive therapy have dramatically increased risk for all types of skin cancers [26]. Skin cancer patients therefore can be at higher risk for additional cancers [27].

The efficacy of DNA repair is an additional factor in carcinogenesis. Three levels of cellular DNA repair exist. Base excision repair (BER) removes lesions in DNA bases caused by oxidation; nucleotide excision repair (NER) acts as the main repair mechanism for UV-induced lesions; and mammalian mismatch repair (MMR) is responsible for removal of mismatched bases [28]. The importance of these processes in preventing carcinogenesis is reflected in the 100-fold increase in mutation frequency observed in cells that lack MMR [28] and the 2,000-fold increase in cancers in xeroderma pigmentosum (XP) patients who lack NER [28]. A defect in MMR recently found in tumor cells indicates that MMR is affected by a repair protein hMSH2, which is regulated by p53 [29]. Mutation in p53 produces dysfunctional hMSH2, acting as second step toward transformation [12].

An additional factor that may influence carcinogenesis in the skin is nutritional status. High fat diets [30] and low levels of vitamin C [31], beta carotene [31], cruciferous vegetables [31], vitamin E [32], vitamin D [33], and selenium are associated with elevated skin cancer risk [34]. In a population of elderly men (mean age, 73), men with the highest levels of 25-hydroxy vitamin D (25 [OH] D) levels (>40 ng/mL) had 40 % lower occurrences of having nonmelanoma skin cancer [33]. Concurrent infection with oncogenic human viruses may also play a role. Human papillomavirus (HPV) infection, for example, appears to promote NMSC [35].

Nonmalignant Hyperproliferative Conditions

Skin growths without malignant potential include seborrheic keratoses, cherry hemangiomas, senile lentigines, and skin tags [36]. Almost every adult over 65 has at least one benign neoplastic growth, with seborrheic keratoses being the most common [3].

Seborrheic Keratoses

Seborrheic keratoses (SKs) are tan to black growths, which appear to be stuck on the skin and vary from a few millimeters to over 4 cm in diameter. They occur in all ages, but 88 % of all those affected are over 65 [37]; the incidence in men is higher than in women. Lesions most often appear on the trunk and can occur anywhere on the body, but generally avoid the palms [33], soles, and mucous membranes [38, 39]. People with SKs often have a family history of the condition and can have numerous lesions (50 % have greater than ten lesions [37], and some have hundreds [40]). The sudden appearance of numerous pruritic SKs may be associated with internal malignancy (sign of Leser-Trelat) [37, 41]. SKs can become irritated and sore, but they pose no risk of malignant transformation. Careful cutaneous exam is required to ensure that SKs do not obscure a distinct malignant skin lesion which may be missed. No treatment is medically necessary, but cryotherapy or curettage can be used to remove unwanted lesions [39].

Skin Tags and Angiomas

Skin tags (soft, flesh-colored, pedunculated papules on the neck and upper eyelids) and cherry hemangiomas (bright-red nodules several millimeters in size) are both very common in older adults. Benign growths are treated for cosmetic reasons or if their location makes them susceptible to irritation [39].

Actinic Keratoses

Actinic keratoses (AK) arise from UVB damage to the genetic material in keratinocytes; this damage induces clones of malignant keratinocytes that are confined to the epidermis [37]. Mutation in the

Table 2 Differential diagnosis of actinic keratoses

Description of lesions	Population and prevalence	Growth	Common sites	Size of lesion	Invasive	Metastasis	Danger sign
Flesh or tan colored papules with marked scaling and well-defined borders. Rough texture	Caucasian, especially fair skinned	Usually appears in multiple lesions	Strong correlation with sun exposure: face, hands, forearms, bald scalp	Few millimeters to more than an inch in diameter. Usually less than 1 cm	No	No	Palpable nodularity under scale, infiltration, elevation, rapid growth, tenderness
	Onset typically greater than age 50 in northern latitudes, younger ages in southern	May wax and wane with seasons			But up to 20 % become invasive SCC		
	Prevalence: near 100 % in Caucasian populations of aged individual with lifelong sun exposure						

Source: American Cancer Society 2004
SCC squamous cell carcinoma

p53 gene is the most important pathogenetic event [12]. Left untreated, an occurrence of AK has a minor risk of extending into the dermis, becoming invasive squamous cell carcinoma (SCC) [42]. Patients with AKs often have numerous lesions [43]. Since approximately 1 out of every 1,000 AKs progresses to invasive skin cancer per year [42], patients with many AKs have a more significant risk of eventually having at least one lesion becoming invasive [16, 44]. AKs represent the earliest recognizable manifestation of SCC as a premalignant lesion [45, 46].

AK is very common in elderly Caucasians (Fitzpatrick skin types I–III), with a higher prevalence in men [42]. The incidence of AK increases steadily with age, from approximately 10 % in people in their 20s to more than 80 % in people older than 70 [47]. These growths have a strong association with sun exposure, both in terms of geographic region and the individual's degree of sun exposure [38]. Lesions occur almost exclusively on photodamaged sites: i.e., the neck, face, dorsal surface of the hands, forearms, and the bald scalp [48]. Extensive involvement of the lip can occur and is termed actinic cheilitis [49].

Although AK lesions typically remain inactive for years, approximately 10 % will eventually invade the dermis as SCC [50]. Some patients have numerous keratoses that never transform, while, for unknown reasons, some will have numerous AKs that undergo rapid change simultaneously [48].

AKs are more likely to progress to SCC if mutations exist in the p16 gene (which codes an additional tumor suppression protein) [47]. The presence of AK lesions signifies a high risk for other skin cancers in the future; regular follow-up and the strongest measures of prevention should be encouraged [43]. The use of sunscreen may not only prevent further lesions but also may hasten regression of existing ones [47]. Further details on AK are presented in Table 2.

AKs often multiply within a specific region of the skin, a phenomenon now considered to be field cancerization. Skin that appears clinically normal but surrounding existing AKs is believed to be genetically vulnerable, damaged skin in which lurk clinically invisible precancerous changes, with progression to AK likely [51]. Topical applications are a good choice as the entire susceptible field can be simultaneously treated [52, 53].

Patients with numerous lesions have been treated simultaneously with intermittent topical applications including 5 % fluorouracil cream, diclofenac sodium, and imiquimod. A newer field therapy, ingenol mebutate gel (often combined with photodynamic therapy) causes necrosis and subsequent destruction of residual disease cells through a neutrophil-mediated and antibody-dependent process [54–56] that persists beyond the initial application [57]. The brief length of actual treatment (2 or 3 days) both decreases the burden of the disease and increases compliance. In several multicenter trials, ingenol mebutate demonstrated higher clearance rates of AK as compared to both vehicle and to cryotherapy. Ingenol mebutate was also well tolerated and without any associated adverse events at 12 months post treatment [58]. Of those subjects who experienced complete clearance of AK after ingenol mebutate treatment, 87 % had no recurrence 1 year later [59]. A first-in-class therapy, ingenol mebutate research will likely spur further ingenol products [59].

Photodynamic therapy (PTD) activates photosensitizers with visible light [51] to form reactive and cytotoxic singlet oxygen. The site is photosensitized by topical application of gamma – 5-aminolevulinic acid or its methyl esters; it is then irradiated with visible light, causing phototoxic destruction of superficial layers of skin [60]. Cure rates are as high as 91 % [53, 61–64], similar to that with cryotherapy but with improved cosmetic results [51].

Nonmelanoma Skin Cancers

The incidence of nonmelanoma skin cancers (NMSC) is increasing steadily and now represents more than 33 % of all cancers in the United States [23]. Rigorous and substantial evidence supports the assertion that the vast majority of NMSCs result directly from cumulative unprotected sun exposure, particularly occurring before the age of 18 [65]: they develop primarily in pale, sun-exposed skin [66]; frequency is related to the degree of sun exposure and also directly related to latitude [67]; sun avoidance and the use of sunscreen decrease the frequency of NMSC [68]; these cancers are readily produced experimentally by UV exposure [69]; and their frequency is greatly increased in XP, a condition in which the repair process for UV damage to DNA is compromised [70]. The incidence of NMSCs is approximately 20 times the incidence of melanoma [23].

The most important factor in skin cancer prognosis is early diagnosis [71], including accurate classification of the malignant lesion. It can be clinically difficult to distinguish from proliferative AK and early invasive SCC [51], to distinguish among the different classifications of BCC, and sometimes even to distinguish among the three major classifications themselves, particularly in patients of color [72]. Ideally, histopathologic classification should accurately identify subtypes and therefore predict tumor behavior. Immunohistochemical adjuvants such as marker Melan-A improve traditional histology; the use of Melan-A increased successful differential diagnosis of melanocytic tumors from among actinic keratosis and solar lentigines also evaluated [73]. Optical coherence tomography, positron emission tomography, and computed tomography also can improve diagnostic capabilities. A new technique, computer-assisted nuclear morphometry, was able to predict recurrence and disease-free survival rates in BCC [74].

Biopsies have been relied on for prognostic information, but the advent of less invasive therapies demands noninvasive diagnostics as well [71]. Much research effort, therefore, has focused on technological improvements in traditional diagnosis and prognostic methods. A comparison of common therapies for neoplastic lesions is shown in Table 3.

Dermatoscopic evaluation of the suspicious lesion can improve differential diagnosis [75]. Ultrasound shows promise for determining three-dimensional size and margin characteristics, as well as information about homogeneity and tissue health of inner structures [71]. Ultrasound can also be employed for identification of metastasis in the sentinel node [76].

Table 3 Comparison of common therapies for neoplastic lesions

Treatment	Lesion	Protocol	Efficacy	Advantages	Disadvantages	Reference
Curettage	AK	Standard		Tissue available for histological examination	Sometimes pigment changes, scarring, poor wound healing. Potential for nerve damage	[47]
	nBCC, sBCC	Standard	5 years no recurrence rate 86–97 %	Less expensive, easier technically than Mohs	Higher risk of recurrence	[112]
Cryotherapy	AK	Standard		Preserves dermal nerves, blood vessels, collagen	Possibility of hypopigmentation	[47]
	BCC	Standard	5 years no recurrence as high as 96–83 %	Inexpensive, few side effects, quick recovery	Pain, scarring, dyspigmentation	[112]
Photodynamic therapy	AK	20 % ALA, two treatments, 14–18 h exposure, blue light, 12-month follow-up	78 % cure rate	Very good cosmetic results Useful for treatment of large areas (field cancerization)	Painful	[53]
		20 % ALA, two treatments, 14–18 h exposure, blue light, 3-month follow-up	89 % cure rate	Very good cosmetic results Useful for treatment of large areas (field cancerization) [53]	Painful [53]	[63]
Photodynamic therapy, cont.	AK, cont.	20 % ALA, two treatments, 14–18 h exposure, red light, 2-month follow-up	85 % cure rate	Very good cosmetic results Useful for treatment of large areas (field cancerization)	Painful [53]	[64]
		16 % MAL, 3 h exposure, two treatments, and 3-month follow-up	89–91 % cure rate	Very good cosmetic results Useful for treatment of large areas (field cancerization) [53]	Painful [53]	[62]
	sBCC[a]	20 % ALA, one treatment, 4 h exposure, red light	91 % cure rate	Very good cosmetic results Useful for treatment of large areas (field cancerization) [53]	Painful [53]	[146]
		16 % MAL, red light, two treatments, and 3-month follow-up	92 % cure rate	Very good cosmetic results Useful for treatment of large areas (field cancerization) [53]	Painful [53]	[147]

(continued)

Table 3 (continued)

Treatment	Lesion	Protocol	Efficacy	Advantages	Disadvantages	Reference
5-Fluorouracil topical cream (DNA synthesis inhibitor) [92]	AK	$N = 21$ 0.5 %, once per day, opposite side of face as control for 4 weeks	78 % reduction in lesions	Comparatively short treatment period needed for efficacy	Erythema, dryness, temporarily disfigurement, and pain so high rate of noncompliance [47]	[148]
5-Fluorouracil topical cream (DNA synthesis inhibitor) [92] cont.	AK, cont.	$N = 21$ 5 %, twice per day, opposite side of face as control for 4 weeks	60 % reduction in lesions	Comparatively short treatment period needed for efficacy [148]	Erythema, dryness	[148]
		$N = 177$ 0.5 %, once per day for 4 weeks	78 % reduction in lesions	Comparatively short treatment period needed for efficacy [148]	Erythema, dryness	[149]
Diclofenac sodium (appears to boost immunosurveillance [92])	AK	$N = 120$ 3 %, twice a day, for 3 months	50 % subjects cleared	Higher tolerability than 5-FU	Pruritus, erythema, dryness, relatively long treatment period for efficacy	[150] [47]
		$N = 195$ 3 %, twice a day, for 2 months	33 % subjects cleared	Higher tolerability than 5-FU [47]	Pruritus, erythema, dryness	[151]
		$N = 20$ 3 % once per day for 3 months	9.3 % cleared, 64.7 reduced in size	Higher tolerability than 5-FU [47]	Minimal irritation	[152]
Colchicine (mitosis inhibitor [92])	AK	$N = 20$ 1 % gel twice a day for 10 days, monitored 2 months	70 % cleared	Prolonged effect noted	Little to no irritation reported	[153]
		$N = 16$ 0.5 % cream twice a day for up to three 10-day cycles	87.5 % cleared	Higher tolerability than 5-FU [47]	Little to no irritation reported	[154]
		$N = 16$ 1 % cream twice a day for up to three 10-day cycles	75 % cleared	Higher tolerability than 5-FU [47]	Little to no irritation reported	[154]

Imiquimod (toll-like receptor 7 agonist, boosts immune response)	AK	$N = 52$ 5 % cream three times a week for up to 12 weeks	84 % cleared	Reveals previously undetectable AKs	Mild to severe erythema, erosions, edema vesicles, pruritus	[155]
		$N = 25$ 5 % cream three times a week for 4 weeks, 4-week rest, cycle repeated three times	82 % cleared (figure achieved by end of second cycle)	Prolonged effect noted	Mild to severe erythema, erosions, edema vesicles, pruritus. Efficacy proportional to intensity of site reaction	[156]
Imiquimod (toll-like receptor 7 agonist, boosts immune response), cont.	AK, cont.	N = 22 5 % cream three times a week for 8 weeks, opposite of face as control	33 % reduction in lesions	Reveals previously undetec/AKs [155] Prolonged effect noted [156]	Mild to severe erythema, erosions, edema vesicles, pruritus. Efficacy proportional to intensity of site reaction	[157]
		$N = 436$ 5 % cream twice a week for 16 weeks	45 % cleared at 24 weeks	Reveals previously undetectable AKs [155] Prolonged effect noted [156]	Mild to severe erythema, erosions, edema vesicles, pruritus. Efficacy proportional to intensity of site reaction	[158]
		$N = 286$ 5 % cream three times a week for 16 weeks	57 % cleared at 24 weeks	Reveals previously undetectable AKs [155] Prolonged effect noted [156]	Mild to severe erythema, erosions, edema vesicles, pruritus. Efficacy proportional to intensity of site reaction	[100]
		$N = 492$ 5 % cream three times a week for 16 weeks	48 % cleared at 24 weeks	Reveals previously undetectable AKs [155] Prolonged effect noted [156]	Mild to severe erythema, erosions, edema vesicles, pruritus. Efficacy proportional to intensity of site reaction	[158]
	BCC (80 % superficial, 20 % nodular)	$N = 35$ 5 %, once or twice daily three times a week for 16 weeks	Three times a week: 100 % clearance at 16 weeks. Twice a week, clearance dropped to 60 %	Reveals previously undetectable AKs [155] Prolonged effect noted [156]	Mild to severe erythema, erosions, edema vesicles, pruritus. Efficacy proportional to intensity of site reaction	[159]
Imiquimod (toll-like receptor 7 agonist,	sBCC	$N = 99$ 5 %, once or twice daily for 6 weeks	Twice daily, three times a week: 100 % clearance at 6 weeks	Reveals previously undetectable AKs [155] Prolonged effect noted [156]	Mild to severe erythema, erosions, edema vesicles, pruritus. Efficacy	[160]

(*continued*)

Table 3 (continued)

Treatment	Lesion	Protocol	Efficacy	Advantages	Disadvantages	Reference
boosts immune response), cont.			(once daily, three times a week, clearance dropped to 70 %)		proportional to intensity of site reaction	
		$N = 128$ 5 %, once or twice daily three–five times per week for 12 weeks	Twice daily, five times a week: 100 % clearance at 12 weeks (once daily, three times a week, clearance dropped to 52 %)	Reveals previously undetectable AKs [155] Prolonged effect noted [156]	Mild to severe erythema, erosions, edema vesicles, pruritus. Efficacy proportional to intensity of site reaction	[161]
		$N = 364$ 5 %, five or seven times per week for 6 weeks	Five times weekly, 82 % clearance, seven times weekly, 79 % clearance	Reveals previously undetectable AKs [155] Prolonged effect noted [156]	Mild to severe erythema, erosions, edema vesicles, pruritus. Efficacy proportional to intensity of site reaction	[162]
Imiquimod (toll-like receptor 7 agonist, boosts immune response), cont.	nBCC	$N = 99$ 5 %, once daily for 6 weeks	71 % clearance	Reveals previously undetectable AKs [155] Prolonged effect noted [156]	Mild to severe erythema, erosions, edema vesicles, pruritus. Efficacy proportional to intensity of site reaction	[163]
		$N = 92$ 5 %, once daily for 12 weeks	76 % clearance	Reveals previously undetectable AKs [155] Prolonged effect noted [156]	Mild to severe erythema, erosions, edema vesicles, pruritus. Efficacy proportional to intensity of site reaction	[163]
Ingenol mebutate	AK	$N = 547$ 0.015 %, once daily for 3 days Face and scalp	42 % complete clearance 64 % partial clearance	Short duration of therapy, improved patient adherence	Erythema, flaking or scaling, crusting, swelling, vesiculation or postulation, and erosion or ulceration	[58]
		$N = 458$ 0.05 %, once daily for 2 days Trunk and extremities	34 % complete clearance 49 % partial clearance	Short duration of therapy, improved patient adherence	Erythema, flaking or scaling, crusting, swelling, vesiculation or postulation, and erosion or ulceration	[58]

Mohs micrographic surgery	BCC	Standard	5 years no recurrence rate greater approaches 100 % [112]	Lowest risk of recurrence, good cosmetic result	Bony invasion, risk of loss of function or deformity, ongoing positive margins, surgical procedure	[92]
	SCC	Standard	5 years no recurrence rates, 92 %	Lowest risk of recurrence, good cosmetic result	Bony invasion, risk of loss of function or deformity, ongoing positive margins, surgical procedure	[112]
Radiation therapy	BCCs	Standard	5 years no recurrence rates, 92.6 %	Useful for large tumors or tumors in difficult locations, older patients	Risk of inducing malignancy in younger patients, not cosmetically favorable	[112]
Radiotherapy	SCC	Standard	Tumor control rates, 70–100 %	Useful when surgery refused or impossible	Cartilaginous areas susceptible to necrosis, not advised in immunocompromised patients	[112]
Vismodegib	BCC	$N = 41$ 150 mg daily, 18 months planned, actual ranged 1–15 months (mean 8 months)	90 % reduction of hedgehog target-gene expression 83 % clearance	Significantly reduced the rate of new BCC; and reduced surgically eligible BCC, some to clinical resolution	Most BCCs regrew once the drug was stopped. Loss of taste, muscle cramps, hair loss, weight loss	[99]
	BCC, metastatic	$N = 33$ 150 mg daily, 7.6 months	30 % response rate	Tumor shrinkage	Muscle spasms, alopecia, dysgeusia (taste disturbance), weight loss, fatigue	[98]
	BCC, locally advanced	$N = 63$ 150 mg daily, 7.6 months	43 % objective response rate, 21 % complete response	Tumor shrinkage, prevention and treatment of basal cell carcinomas in patients with the basal cell nevus syndrome	Muscle spasms, alopecia, dysgeusia (taste disturbance), weight loss, fatigue	[98]

AK actinic keratoses, *ALA* aminolevulinic acid, *BCC* basal cell carcinoma, *MAL* methyl aminolevulinate, *nBCC* nodular basal cell carcinoma, *sBCC* superficial basal cell carcinoma 5-FU=5-fluorouracil

[a]Not recommended for nodular or morpheaform BCC due to tendency to increase rate of recurrence

Analysis of genetic markers also promises to increase prognostic ability, particularly with regard to obtaining tumor karyotypes [16]. The frequency of aneuploidy in skin cancer suggests that it has at least some etiologic role in carcinogenesis and therefore can indicate malignant potential [16]. Aneuploidy is generally detected through the use of flow cytometry, and the level of aneuploidy correlates well with staging criteria and therefore prognosis. For example, in melanoma, while aneuploidy was found in only 3 % of melanocytic nevi, it was found in 34 % of level IV melanomas and 100 % of level V [77]. Assessing level of aneuploidy may therefore aid in prognostic consideration.

Basal Cell Carcinoma

Basal cell carcinoma (BCC) (Figs. 1 and 2), which arises from cells in the basal layer of the epidermis, is the most common form of skin cancer [12, 43]. BCCs account for 80 % of all skin cancers [78]. Although clonal expansion of mutant p53s is often expressed in and around BCCs on sun-exposed skin [79], these UV-fingerprint mutations are much more rare in BCC than in SCC [12]. The seminal event in the development of sporadic BCC appears to be mutation in the gene PTCH1, a hedgehog pathway gene mutation with broad control of embryonic proliferation [12]. Other regulatory defects have been observed in association with BCC lesions: mutation in the H-ras gene (also involved in cell division) occurs at increased frequency [80], mutations in c-fos (a proto-oncogene) are reduced [81], and mutations in p16, a tumor suppressor gene, are also observed [82]. Induction of IL-4 and IL-10 by UV irradiation reduces tumor surveillance [83] as well as interstitial collagenase, which facilitates invasion of the tumor into the surrounding tissue [84].

The most typical presentation of BCC is a papule or nodule with a central umbilication, distinguished by a generally pearly or translucent appearance with telangiectasia and a characteristic rolled boarder. Central crusting and bleeding is often seen [85]. Other presentations can also be seen and include an erythematous, scaly, flat patch (superficial BCC variant) or a pale scar-like lesion without distinct borders (morpheaform variant) [10]. Tumors resemble hair follicle structures morphologically, so BCC is believed to be a malignant tumor of the follicular germinative cells (these germinative cells are referred to as trichoblasts) [86].

The clinical presentation of BCC in its various forms makes classification difficult and aggressiveness and recurrence difficult to predict; recurrence sometimes occurs even when excision is performed with clearly free margins [74]. Over 50 % of BCC lesions that occur in people of color are pigmented versus only 6 % of lesions found in Caucasians [72]. Most BCCs are visually distinguishable from squamous cell carcinomas (SCC), but biopsy should nonetheless be performed [87]. Although the BCCs rarely metastasize, they are invasive, with a high rate of recurrence [87].

BCC is strongly associated with sun exposure. Tumors occur most frequently on sun-exposed sites [25], 85 % of the time on the head and neck [51] BCC is far more common in those with fair complexions and significantly more common in those exposed to UVL, including phototherapy [25]. It has been observed to occur at less frequently, however, on certain body sites that nevertheless have strong sun exposure (e.g., the dorsal hand), and its relative frequency on diverse facial sites is not strongly correlated to UVL exposure [25], even when topographical anatomy and other possible cofounders are considered [25].

Some correlation exists between a high frequency of BCC and concave shape, reduced skin tension, and marked skinfolds, which may reflect areas of high matrix metalloproteinases (MMP) expression; MMPs are responsible for tissue breakdown as tumor expansion proceeds, and they are present at increased levels in and around BCCs [84]. Integrins, which regulate MMPs, have been observed to be greatly reduced in BCCs [88].

The frequent occurrence of BCC on nonexposed sites implies a potential for multiple mechanisms in BCC development [86]. Arsenic, x-rays, grenz ray exposure, and mustard gas are known contributors to some specific BCCs [86]. The role of an additional causative agent in

BCC is suggested by the observations that sunscreens with a high skin protection factor reduce the risk of SCC, but prospective studies have found no protective effect on BCC [89]; Li-Fraumeni syndrome, caused by an inherited point mutation in p53, does not raise BCC risk [90]; and truncal BCCs on the trunk appear to be specifically associated with variations in the gene for the enzymes glutathione S-transferase (three forms) and cytochrome P450 [86].

It is considered likely that immunosuppression may play a significant role in the development of BCC, as BCCs occur frequently in immunosuppressed patients (only SCCs have a higher prevalence in this population). In fact, the risk of BCC in organ transplant recipients is considerably higher (reported at anywhere from 6 % to 100 % higher [86]) than in the general population. Basal cell tumors, particularly morpheaform BCC, also have dramatically elevated mast cell indices which do not correlate to levels of sun exposure [91]. The observation that elevation of mast cell indices does correlate with cigarette use supports the hypothesis that BCC development is multifactorial, with some part of its etiology susceptible to influence by lifestyle factors [91]. Further details on BCC are presented in Table 4.

The rate of recurrence of basal cell carcinomas is directly related to tumor size, location, and histologic subtype as well as the presence of residual transformed cells after treatment [92]. The chosen therapy will depend on the patient's age, lesion size and site, and histologic subtype and whether it is a primary lesion or a recurrence [42]. Surgical excision with suturing has a recurrence rate of less than 5 % [43, 93]. The recurrence rate drops to 1 % [43, 93] with Mohs micrographic surgical excision. Mohs surgery evaluates horizontal sections with 100 % margin control. The neoplasm is mapped and additional sections are taken until clear margins are achieved.

Imiquimod appears to be a potentially useful adjuvant in BCC: one study found no recurrence after 34 months when imiquimod was used as adjuvant therapy after Mohs [94], and another observed 94 % of lesions to have histologically cleared at 3 months after curettage [95]. Another study evaluated treatment of BCC with three cycles of curettage against treatment with electrodesiccation followed by 5 % imiquimod cream for 1 month. At 8 weeks, 1/11 (9 %) of imiquimod treated group had residual tumor compared to 4/11 (36 %) of controls [96]. Patients with a previous BCC should be fastidiously examined by a physician yearly for signs of recurrence [43].

Photodynamic therapy (PTD), which activates photosensitizers with visible light [51] to form reactive and cytotoxic singlet oxygen, has shown potential efficacy in early clinical trials [51]. The site is photosensitized by topical application of gamma – 5-aminolevulinic acid or its methyl esters – and then irradiated with visible light, causing phototoxic destruction of superficial layers of skin [60]. Cure rates are similar to that with cryotherapy but with improved cosmetic results [51]; efficacy, however, has been limited to superficial BCC [51].

Only recently approved by the FDA (2012) in the treatment of BCC, vismodegib is indicated for locally advanced as well as metastatic BCC. Vismodegib, developed in response to the realization that BCC is often associated with aberrant signaling in the hedgehog pathway that regulates embryonic development [59], acts as a hedgehog pathway inhibitor, frequently resulting in dramatic clearance of multiple severe lesions in patients with both BCC [97] and Gorlin syndrome, which also causes lesions [98, 99].

Squamous Cell Carcinoma

Squamous cell carcinoma (SCC) is the second most common cutaneous neoplasm. SCC has significant risk of metastasis and accounts for 20 % of deaths from skin cancer [100]. SCC arises from the keratinizing Malpighian cells of the squamous layer [16] of the skin and mucous membranes [52]. P53 mutation is thought to be the primary mutagenic event [12]. Other tumor suppressor genes mutated in SCC include p16 (INK4a) and p14 (ARF).

SCC is associated with chronic, long-term photodamage and is most commonly seen in exposed skin and mucous membranes [87]. Chronic sunburn is more strongly implicated

Table 4 Differential diagnosis of basal cell carcinoma

Type of growth	Description of lesions	Population and prevalence	Growth	Common sites	Size of lesion	Invasive	Metastasis	Danger sign
80 % of all nonmelanoma skin cancers	Small, dome-shaped pimple-like growth, often pearly in color. Usually single lesion	90 % Caucasian, especially fair skinned. Onset greater than 50 years, men higher incidence than women	Relatively slow	Head, neck account for 85 %, 30 % of these on nose. Most subtypes strongly associated with sun exposure	1–2 cm	Yes	Rarely, when metastasis occurs, it appears in lymph nodes, lungs Recurs in 40–50 % within 5 years	Ulcer that won't heal and bleeds when scratched
Nodular	Smooth, flesh colored, translucent nodule with pearly border, telangiectasias, and slight central umbilication. Sometimes accompanied by itch	60 % of BCC Caucasian, especially fair skinned	Slow Usually appears as single nodule Nests push into dermis	Good correlation with sun exposure	Few millimeters to a few centimeters	Yes, even bone, nerves, cartilage	No	Ulcer that won't heal and bleeds when scratched
Superficial	Slightly raised, erythematous, scaling patch, with threadlike periphery and atrophy in center	Caucasian, especially fair skinned	Slow to ulcerate Nests restricted to epidermis	Trunk and other nonexposed sites. Not correlated with sun exposure	As large as greater than 4 cm in diameter	Not readily	No	Ulcer that won't heal and bleeds when scratched
Morpheaform	Indurated yellow to flesh-colored plaque with poorly defined margins. Resembles a scar	Caucasian, especially fair skinned	Infiltrate, tumor nests diffuse, and irregularly spread, often subcutis	Good correlation with sun exposure		Yes	No, but recurrence common	Scat that ulcerates, oozes, or bleeds when scratched

Source: American Cancer Society 2004 [51]

in SCC than sunburns in childhood [101]. Other risk factors include prior trauma, frostbite, psoralen plus ultraviolet (PUVA) therapy, exposure to ionizing radiation or chemical carcinogens, viral oncogenesis, and chronic immunosuppression [43].

SCC often presents as a firm, discrete nodule or plaque which arises on an erythematous elevated base. With time, the tumor can progress and become fungating, exophytic, with overlying crust. SCC in situ more typically presents as an erythematous scaly patch or plaque with clear margins. Both forms of SCC are commonly associated with surrounding actinic damage. Clinicians should keep in mind that, though relatively rare in black patients, SCC is nevertheless the most common skin cancer in that population and more likely to occur in damaged or chronically inflamed skin that in sun-exposed areas [102]. Like all skin cancers, diagnosis is often delayed in more heavily pigmented skin [103].

SCC In Situ

Two forms of SCC may represent developing SCC in situ. Bowen's disease lesions occur on nonexposed sites; they become more aggressive SCCs than those which arise from AK [52]. An association with internal malignancy typically signals arsenic occupational exposure as an etiological agent [104].

Keratoacanthoma

Keratoacanthomas (Fig. 4), whose classification as SCC is more controversial, are single dome-shaped nodules with a central keratin plug that typically arise in a hair follicle in a sun-exposed location [103]. These tumors grow rapidly for about 8 weeks and then remain static for about the same period before spontaneously regressing [42]. Recurrences are common, however, and typically more invasive than the initial tumor [42]. Once thought to be benign and self-limiting, keratoacanthomas both clinically and histopathologically resemble well-differentiated SCC [103] and are now believed to represent SCC in progress [87]. The term *infundibular squamous cell carcinoma* [105] has been proposed to classify keratoacanthomas as a well-differentiated variant of SCC that arises from an alternative follicular-based, etiologic pathway, as distinct from SCCs that more commonly arise from solar keratoses. Further details on SCC are presented in Table 5. Treatment for squamous cell carcinoma (SCC) employs many similar treatment options as for BCC. Surgical excision is the treatment of choice. As with BCC, the use of Mohs surgery for treatment of SCC results in a lower recurrence rate as compared to standard excision (3 % vs. 8 %) [43]. In the rare case of extensive SCC, topical treatments may be considered. Follow-up should be frequent and thorough, beginning at 3 months. Most recurrences (70 %) occur within the first 2 years [43] and should be managed aggressively [87]. Use of high SPF sunblock has been persuasively demonstrated to reduce the risk of squamous cell carcinoma [106].

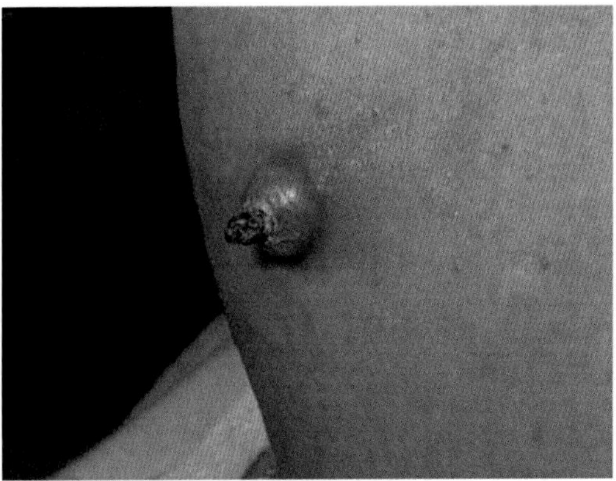

Fig. 4 Keratoacanthoma

Melanomas

Malignant Melanoma

Melanoma has been labeled a "near epidemic" with a strong and direct association with solar radiation [10]. Melanoma accounts for less than 2 % of skin cancer cases, but the vast majority of skin cancer deaths [107]. Older melanoma patients (the majority) present with thicker tumors [108] and in general tend to be more often diagnosed with advanced stages of disease.

Table 5 Differential diagnosis of squamous cell carcinoma

Type of growth	Description of lesions	Population and prevalence	Growth	Common sites	Size of lesion	Invasive	Metastasis	Danger sign
Squamous cell carcinoma (unspecific)	Crusted or scaly patches with red inflamed-based, nonhealing ulcer, or enlarging growth, typically heaped up, cauliflower appearance	Caucasian, especially fair skinned Higher incidence in men than women Average onset, 60 years Prevalence: 250,000 new cases/year, 2500 deaths	Rapid	Primarily	1–5 cm	Yes Lips, nose, ears, more so	Yes to lungs or lymph nodes	
				Head 75 %, back of hands, arms 15 %, t5:5 others 10 % Strong correlation with sun exposure			Lips, ears, vulva, and penis have higher rates of metastasis	
							Skin, 3 %, lip, 11 %	
							SCC in burn scars, radiation scars, ulcers, up to 30 %	
Verrucous	Warty growth	Caucasian, especially fair skinned	Relatively slow	Plantar foot, anogenital region	Less than 1 cm			
				No correlation with sun-exposed sites				
Bowen's disease (SCC in situ)	Round or oval erythematous plaques with well-defined margins and scaling. Loss of polarity gives windblown appearance	Greater than 60 years of age	Grows gradually with continuous peripheral extension, typically present for many years before suspicion of danger arises	Usually lower half of body: more often on nonexposed sites. Some cases related to arsenic exposure	As large as several inches	No, but about 5 % becomes invasive SCC	When invasive, more likely to metastasize than SCC arising in AKs	Occurrence on nonexposed sites carries association with internal malignancy
	55 % occurs as multiple growths							
Keratoacanthoma	Large nodular growth with epidermal lipping around keratin-filled crater. Usually appears as single nodule	Caucasian, onset in 60s or 70s. Higher incidence in men than women	Grows very rapidly for about 6–8 weeks, then stops	Face, back of hands. Strong association with sun exposure	Greater than 1 in. in diameter	Yes	Rarely, but often recurs	

Source: American Cancer Society 2004

AK actinic keratoses, *SCC* squamous cell carcinoma

Consequently, lesions exhibit a higher grade at presentation and worse prognosis [109].

Melanoma is classified according to the TNM system, which evaluates the thickness of the tumor (known as the Breslow depth), the amount of ulceration present, the evidence of presence in the lymph nodes, and the presence of metastatic lesions in other tissues (perineural or perivascular involvement) or organs. Stage III reflects evidence of in-transit or regional nodal metastasis or both; the presence of distant metastasis is defined as Stage IV [110]. Once melanoma has metastasized, 5-year survival is about 10 % [111]. Tumor thickness is the most important prognostic factor [23]. Staging by sentinel lymph node biopsy, which identifies micrometastatic disease, has become common practice over the last few years as a prognostic tool, replacing elective lymph node dissection. Significant survival advantage has yet to be proven in large randomized multicenter trials, and effective adjuvant therapies for patients demonstrated to carry micrometastatic disease are lacking [112]. The tumor site, however, has some prognostic influence, with location on the lower legs, upper arms, and head being associated with better outcomes than location on the chest, back, and shoulders [113]. Women, in addition, have a better long-term prognosis than men [114].

This malignancy arises from melanocytes in basal layer of the epidermis [16]. Although malignant melanomas may arise within two premalignant states, lentigo maligna or an existing mole mostly arises de novo. People who have dysplastic nevi benign moles are at increased risk of developing single or multiple melanomas. The higher the number of these moles someone has, the higher the risk; those who have ten or more have 12 times the risk of developing melanoma compared to the general population [107]. Risk factors for malignant melanoma include a light complexion, family history of melanoma, a history of sunburns as a child, and carriage of a high number of melanocytic or clinically atypical nevi [101].

Lentigo maligna are large brown macules on sun-exposed skin that resemble large, permanent freckles. Lesions enlarge, but very slowly. Lentigo maligna melanoma, typically seen in older patients, arises from lentigo maligna on sun-exposed areas when malignant melanocytes penetrate the dermis [111]; however, most patients of advanced age carrying lentigo maligna lesions will die before any malignant changes occur [10, 52]. Superficial spreading melanoma, the most common form of malignant melanoma, occurs primarily on the torso (men) and legs (women). Nodular melanoma enlarges rapidly in a typically darkened papule, although unpigmented nodules occasionally may arise [111]. Nodular and lentiginous melanoma are both more common in the elderly [108, 115], whereas superficial spreading melanoma is more common in younger patients. Acral-lentiginous melanoma, common in blacks (though rare in other ethnic groups), develops primarily on palmar, plantar, or subungual skin [111]. A melanotic melanoma is a nonpigmented lesion which is frequently misdiagnosed clinically as a BCC. It presents as a pink- or flesh-colored nodule. The prevalence of melanoma at specific anatomic sites depends on age; nearly 80 % of melanoma lesions in those over 80 occur on the head and neck. Despite a lower incidence of metastasis in the geriatric melanoma population, 5-year survival rates in that population are worse [116]. Although the risk of any one lesion becoming malignant is small, premalignant conditions should be watched carefully [87].

The exact role of solar radiation in the pathogenesis of malignant melanoma has been controversial for decades [117] and is still being debated [70, 118]. The majority opinion is that solar exposure is the principal carcinogen in melanoma, supported by the observation that its incidence is much higher in lighter-skinned individuals [119]. A correlation exists between sun exposure and melanoma incidence [119, 120]; this correlation is strengthened by association with gender-specific patterns of exposure (trunk in men, lower extremities in women) [121]. XP patients, who carry a mutation that eradicates repair of UV-induced damage to the DNA, are 1000-fold more likely than the general public to develop melanoma [122]. UV-specific mutations P16/INK4a and ras are frequently observed in melanoma cells [123]. Comparison of melanoma risk between blacks and whites suggests that 96 % of melanoma in men and 92 % of melanoma in women could be contributed to UV exposure [124].

Persuasive arguments against a principal role of sunlight in the development of melanoma also exist, particularly by comparing data that support a role of UV in the etiology of BCC and SCC but are lacking or conflicting with respect to malignant melanoma. For perspective, the following observations support the role of sunlight in the carcinogenesis of BCC and SCC: they occur primarily in pale, sun-exposed skin [66]; they have a strong association with the degree of sun exposure and latitude [67]; they are effectively prevented by sun protection [68, 69]; they are readily UV-induced experimentally [69]; and they are dramatically increased in patients with XP, in which UV-specific DNA repair is compromised [70].

By comparison, these lines of evidence are lacking with regard to melanoma. The variation of risk for melanoma is more ethnic [125–127] than pigmentary [128]; 75 % of lesions occur on nonexposed sites [119], especially on the feet in dark-skinned subjects [126, 127]; and the correlation of melanoma incidence to latitude is small and inconsistent in major geographic areas such as Europe and the United States [129]. Moreover, in numerous studies, melanoma incidence and mortality rates are inversely related to sun exposure levels; moreover, melanoma risk does not correlate strongly with the use of tanning beds [130], nor is melanoma readily induced by UV exposure in the lab [131]. Although melanoma incidence is higher in XP patients, the elevation is far lower than for nonmelanoma skin cancers.

It has also been observed that albino African-Americans rarely have cutaneous malignant melanoma, although BCC and SCC are prevalent in this group [117]. In addition, very little solar elastosis is found around CMM lesions in African-American albinos [117]. Epidemiological data records that the incidence of melanoma decreases in association with occupational limitation of sun exposure as well as higher national gross domestic product (GDP) [117].

Case-controlled studies indicate that intermittent sun exposure with sunburn, particularly in childhood, may be a primary risk factor for melanoma. This would offer some explanation for apparent contradictions in the literature regarding UV exposure as a risk factor [118]. The role of intermittent sun exposure and childhood sunburn is postulated to explain the lack of correlation between overall sun exposure and melanoma; however, a strong association of lesion site with burn site would be expected, yet is not observed [70, 126, 128].

The efficacy of sunblock in preventing malignant melanoma is still unproven. The incidence of melanoma has risen despite widespread use of high sun protection factor (SPF) sunblock since the early 1980s [132]. The comparative rarity of this form of skin cancer has hindered extensive prospective studies [106], and even retrospective data are limited. Consequently, the available data are inconclusive. In many studies, sunscreen had no demonstrable preventative power, and in others sunscreen use actually seemed to increase melanoma risk [106]. One explanation may be that chemical screens are primarily designed to avoid sunburns, blocking UVB while admitting virtually all of UVA radiation. Sunscreen use may thus allow people to spend more time in the sun than they would have otherwise, thereby increasing exposure to potentially mutagenic UVA [132].

More than one molecular mechanism may lead to the formation of malignant melanoma [133]. It has long been recognized that some melanomas arise from precursor nevi, while some arise spontaneously [133]. In addition, it has been observed that those with chronic solar exposure have a lower risk of melanoma compared to those with intermittent exposures [133]. Indeed, the B-raf oncogene (BRAF) mutation, although quite common in lesions on intermittently exposed skin, is quite rare on areas with extensive chronic sun damage, which strongly suggests divergent molecular pathways [134]. In black skin, melanoma typically does not occur in sun-exposed sites, but does appear on less pigmented sites [102].

It has been hypothesized that after UV exposure, the most severely damaged keratinocytes undergo apoptosis, while the remaining cells upregulate DNA-repair capacity [10]. The skin tans and thickens, providing additional protection. Subsequent exposure, if frequent, will perpetuate adaptive protection. Sporadic high-dose exposures, however, may cause substantial damage but not apoptosis, so that mutated melanocytes survive and continue to divide. Certain mutations may enable such melanocytes to cross the basement membrane into the dermis, where they proliferate and give rise to junctional nevi as a prelude to full-scale melanoma [23]. Further details on malignant melanomas are presented in Table 6.

The best treatment for melanoma is early detection, followed by biopsy to determine both the nature and depth of penetration of the lesion [111]. If the melanoma is still confined to the epidermis, surgical excision has a good prognosis [87]. If the melanoma has invaded the dermis and spread, surgical removal may be supplemented with additional therapies [110]. Adjuvant chemo- and radiotherapies have recently been joined by immuno-based therapies like alpha interferon, particularly in cases where metastasis has reached the lymph nodes and has resulted in significant improvement in remission and long-term survival rates [111, 135]. Surgery for melanoma metastases using18-fluorodeoxyglucose positron emission tomography (FDG-PET) and FDG-PET/computed tomography (FDG-PET/CT), both capable of providing highly sensitive tumor demarcation, provides for precise surgical margins [37, 39, 112]. Three 12-month randomized controlled trials of high-dose regimens of interferon alpha demonstrated a significant increase in recurrence-free survival in stage III disease, so adjuvant interferon in intermediate and high-risk CMM patients should be standard care [112]. One cytostatic drug, temozolomide (TMZ), has demonstrated significant improvement in progression-free survival in CMM [112].

Management requires adroit use of the available adjuvant diagnostic and therapeutic options. Chemotherapy, immunostimulants, and vaccines have failed as adjuvants in stage II–III disease. Interferon staves off relapses, but does not influence overall survival [76]. More accurate initial characterization of the tumor can greatly influence ultimate outcome, and emerging techniques show significant potential to improve diagnostic capabilities. Topical adjuvants can increase cure rates and are particularly beneficial when field cancerization has occurred.

Merkel Cell Carcinoma

Merkel cell carcinoma (MCC) arises from Merkel cells in the epidermis. It represents a particularly aggressive form of melanoma. Regional metastasis occurs in up to two-thirds of patients, with distant metastasis in one-third [38]. MCC often is initially misdiagnosed as other small-cell tumors [43] but histological and immunocytochemistry can assist in correct diagnosis [43]. Merkel cell carcinoma recurs in up to 44 % of patients, usually within 4 months. The 3-year survival rate, with appropriate excision and adjuvant chemotherapy, is only 55 % [43].

AKs are commonly treated by application of liquid nitrogen (cryotherapy) as an effective method of eradication [136], with an 8-year cure rate of 98.8 % [42].

Conclusion

Cutaneous lesions are not uncommon in older adults [4]. Increasing numbers of nonmalignant cutaneous lesions in older people, along with the pigmentation changes common to old age [87], can make identification of potential malignancies difficult even for dermatologists. Although very few lesions in an older person will likely become malignant, cutaneous malignancy can carry a significant risk of mortality [137].

Although most skin growths are benign, sun exposure plays a crucial role in the development and progression of several types of cutaneous malignancies. Consequently, patients should consistently be made aware of the dangers of unprotected exposure to solar radiation [65]. Current evidence suggests that sunscreen use dramatically reduces the risk of SCC, but may have less ability to protect against BCC and melanoma. Relying on sunscreen alone to lower the risk of skin cancers may thus be inadvisable [106]: patients should be

Table 6 Differential diagnosis of malignant melanoma

Type of growth	Description of lesions	Population and prevalence	Growth	Common sites	Size of lesion	Invasive	Metastasis	Danger sign
Malignant melanoma (unspecific)	Highly pigmented macule or papule, colors brown black, red, white, gray, pink, or blue	Caucasian, especially fair skinned. Highest incidence greater than 65 years. Incidence equal in men and women, although women better survival rate. Prevalence: 54, 200 cases/year, 7,600 deaths in United States in 2003 [23]				Yes	Yes	Appearance of blue pigment in lesion, increase in size, peripheral halo of pigment, ulceration, hemorrhagic exudation, local satellite nodules
Superficial spreading melanoma	Multicolored pigmented lesion with notched irregular margin, associated with acute sun exposure	Caucasian, especially fair skinned. Over 65 in men, younger in women Prevalence: 70 % of all malignant melanomas	Slowly, up to 24 months before onset of invasive behavior	Sun-exposed sites, trunk significantly more common in men, legs in women		Yes	Yes, but less likely than other forms	Formation of nodule with lesion, ulceration
Lentigo maligna (melanotic freckle)	Large flat variegated plaque of brown black. Usually single lesion Associated with chronic sun exposure	Caucasian, especially fair skinned Prevalence: 5 % of all melanomas	Very slow, decades before becomes invasive	Head and neck account for 92 %, most common site, cheek; strong correlation with sun exposure	May reach more than 3 cm	Yes	Yes	Appearance of black macules or papules within lesion, induration, ulceration, nodule formation

Acral-lentiginous melanoma	Flat tan-brown stain with irregular borders Usually single lesion	Men more than women, highest incidence in blacks, Asians, and Hispanics. Primarily in those older than 65 Prevalence: 10 % of all melanomas	Grows slowly, but since occurs in occult locations often overlooked until in advanced stages	Plantar foot, more rarely genitalia, mucous membranes		Yes	Yes	Variegation in pigment, oozing, and crusting
Nodular	Multicolored nodule with ulceration. Usually single lesion Associated with acute sun exposure		Fast, no radial growth phase		Less than 2 cm in size	Yes	Yes	
Desmoplastic melanoma	Nodule with unpredictable pigment and irregular features. Usually single lesion	Greater than 65 years of age, men more often than women	Extends along peripheral nerves	Head and neck, strong association with sun damage		Yes, often nerves	Yes, but less aggressively than other melanomas	Typically long delay in correct diagnosis due to unusual features
Merkel cell carcinoma	Shiny, indurated, pink, bluish-red or red-brown nodule	Greater than 65 years of age. Primarily Caucasians	Relatively slowly	Head, neck, extremities, buttocks, trunk	Typically 0.5–5 cm, lesions up to 15 cm reported	Yes	Yes, frequently	Often not diagnosed before metastasis occurs
Leukoplakia	Rough white patches with sharp borders	Greater than 65 years		Oral and genital mucosa				Erosion, ulceration, or fissures

Source: 2004 American Cancer Society

instructed to wear hats and sunglasses and to avoid short sleeves or shorts if they anticipate spending an extended period of time in the sun [132]. Clinicians must emphasize the risk of recurrence to all skin cancer patients and communicate that avoidance of further UV exposure is critical [47].

Older patients should be encouraged to bring to a physician's attention any new or changed skin lesions, but family practitioners should also assume responsibility for identifying any potentially malignant skin changes [49]. Physical examinations should include the entire surface of the skin, with special attention to places with chronic sun exposure, particularly overlooked sites like eyelids, folds of nose, earlobes, and lips [87]. The relatively low risk of skin cancer in African-Americans should not reduce importance of thorough examination, as all skin cancers carry higher mortality rates in this population due to delayed detection.

In addition, wider education is needed of all physicians who care for elderly subjects with respect to differences in the incidence and presentation of different cancers in the elderly [108, 115, 138]. Life-threatening cutaneous neoplasms are not infrequently diagnosed in the elderly population [139–141]. Nevus spilus, particularly, should be monitored in the elderly patient for possible transformation to melanoma [142].

Available therapies for skin cancers, particularly the NMSC, are highly effective, yet recurrence is substantial, creating significant morbidity for the patient as well as a significant burden on the health-care system. These effects will only increase as the proportion of older people in the population rises [26]. Clinicians should emphasize to their patients the very real risk of recurrence and stress that regular checkups are critical in order for patients to remain skin cancer-free [47].

Clinical management of skin malignancies has relied primarily on cryotherapy or surgical excision and on avoidance of sun exposure. Although excision results in a 95 % overall cure rate, skin malignancies still kill about 10,000 Americans each year. Sunscreen, although a practical and safe approach to preventing many lesions with malignant potential, is not universally effective; moreover, and because sunscreen use promotes longer UV exposure times, it may actually increase the risk for some skin cancers [143]. For at least some malignancies, carcinogenesis involves additional factors besides sun exposure [25, 86]. Confounding factors in all studies of sunscreen efficacy are that sunscreen application is difficult to both verify and quantify and that latency periods (believed to be as much as four or five decades) are longer than any studies yet completed [143]. The relative contributions to the process of carcinogenesis of sun-induced DNA damage, a compromised immunologic response to nascent changes in the cell, and the individual's personal risk factors continue to be investigated on a molecular level; better understanding of the actual pathologic mechanisms of cancer formation will undoubtedly lead to better therapeutic approaches.

Numerous efficacious topical treatments have been developed over the last decade or so, but none yet exceeds the efficacy of traditional excision. The use of these topical medicaments as adjuvants may increase survival rates. Immunotherapies, vaccines, adoptive immunotherapies, manipulation of cytokines, blockage of signaling pathways, and modulation of T-cell function have been, so far, largely unsuccessful [20]. Monoclonal antibodies as yet have also not lived up to initial expectations, although only a small fraction of possible antigens have been studied. The ongoing identification of critical molecular events in carcinogenesis provides many more potential approaches both for targeted therapies and for preventative treatments [144].

Improvement in therapies remains somewhat elusive, yet many novel approaches to better diagnosis and for predicting malignant potential have been described. A comparison of etiologic and diagnostic parameters for cutaneous malignancies is shown in Table 7. Although of significant benefit in research, it is yet to be seen if these new laboratory tools will become cost effective for physicians [71]. In general, curative therapies are much less frequently provided to elderly skin cancer patients due to overestimation of operative risk in these subjects; evidence demonstrates,

Table 7 Comparison of etiologic and diagnostic parameters in cutaneous malignancy

Lesion	Estimated lifetime risk in fair-skinned individuals	Increased risk in fair-skinned individuals as compared to blacks	Increased risk in OTR patients	Percentage containing p53 mutations	Percent containing aneuploid cells	Percentage on sun-exposed skin
AK	100 % in some geographical areas [38]	Virtually nonexistent in blacks [164]	50 % [165]	80 % [166]	69 % [16]	80 % [47]
BCC	33 % [167, 168]	80-fold [102]	100-fold [86]	56 % [169]	Up to 40 % [16]	80 [170]
SCC	11 % [167, 168] cancer: clinical	65-fold [72]	82-fold [171]	90 % [23, 172]	Up to 80 % [16]	82 % [173]
CMM	1.3 % US [174] 4 % AUSy	50-fold [23]	8-fold [20]	20 % [175]	100 % of stage 5 [16]	Varies by age group, 80 % in those over 80 years of age [176]

AK actinic keratoses, *AUS* Australia, *BCC* basal cell carcinoma, *CMM* cutaneous malignant melanoma, *OTR* organ transplant recipient, *SCC* squamous cell carcinoma, *US* United States

however, that curative therapies in the elderly are both safe and effective [138].

Early diagnosis has enabled success in maintaining mortality rates for melanoma constant even though incidence has soared. Early diagnosis should remain the frontline focus – the diligent and meticulous examination of the older patient's skin – yet few clinicians do this [145]. Moreover, since presentation and course of skin cancer can differ in older subjects, further testing of suspected neoplasms is warranted [115]. Consistent proactive surveillance of aging skin will not only prolong life but also significantly improve the aged patient's quality of life.

Cross-References

▶ Melanoma and Skin Aging

References

1. Liao YH, Chen KH, Tseng MP, et al. Pattern of skin diseases in a geriatric patient group in Taiwan: a 7-year survey from the outpatient clinic of a university medical center. Dermatology. 2001;203:308–13.
2. Kligman AM, Koblenzer C. Demographics and psychological implications for the aging population. Dermatol Clin. 1997;15:549–53.
3. Fenske NA, Lober CW. Structural and functional changes of normal aging skin. J Am Acad Dermatol. 1986;15:571–85.
4. Bergfeld WF. The aging skin. Int J Fertil Womens Med. 1997;42:57–66.
5. Seidler AM, Pennie ML, Veledar E, et al. Economic burden of melanoma in the elderly population: population-based analysis of the Surveillance, Epidemiology, and End Results (SEER) – Medicare data. Arch Dermatol. 2010;146:249–56.
6. Harvell JD, Maibach HI. Percutaneous absorption and inflammation in aged skin: a review. J Am Acad Dermatol. 1994;31:1015–21.
7. Webster GF. Common skin disorders in the elderly. Clin Cornerstone. 2001;4:39–44.
8. Armstrong BK, Kricker A. How much melanoma is caused by sun exposure? Melanoma Res. 1993;3:395–401.
9. Christenson LJ, Borrowman TA, Vachon CM, et al. Incidence of basal cell and squamous cell carcinomas in a population younger than 40 years. JAMA. 2005;294:681–90.
10. Gilchrest B, Krutmann J, editors. Skin aging. New York: Springer; 2006.
11. Lewis DA, Travers JB, Somani A, et al. The IGF-1/IGF-1R signaling axis in the skin: a new role for the dermis in aging-associated skin cancer. Oncogene. 2010;29:1475–85.
12. Rass K, Reichrath J. Damage and DNA repair in malignant melanoma and nonmelanoma skin cancer. In: Reichrath J, editor. Sunlight, vitamin D and skin cancer. Austin: Landes Bioscience; 2008.
13. de Gruijl FR, Van der Leun JC. Estimate of the wavelength dependency of ultraviolet carcinogenesis in humans and its relevance to the risk assessment of a stratospheric ozone depletion. Health Phys. 1994;67:319–25.
14. Fields KA. Skin breakthroughs in the year 2000. Int J Fertil Womens Med. 2000;45:175–81.
15. Rees JL. The genetics of sun sensitivity in humans. Am J Hum Genet. 2004;75:739–51.
16. Carless M, Griffiths L. Cytogenetics of melanoma and nonmelanoma skin cancer. In: Reichrath J, editor. Sunlight, vitamin D and skin cancer. Austin: Landes Bioscience; 2008.
17. Sarasin A. The molecular pathways of ultraviolet-induced carcinogenesis. Mutat Res. 1999;428:5–10.
18. Matsumura Y, Ananthaswamy HN. Toxic effects of ultraviolet radiation on the skin. Toxicol Appl Pharmacol. 2004;195:298–308.
19. Emri G, Wenczl E, Van Erp P, et al. Low doses of UVB or UVA induce chromosomal aberrations in cultured human skin cells. J Invest Dermatol. 2000;115:435–40.
20. Domingo DS, Baron DB. Melanoma and nonmelanoma skin cancers and the immune system. In: Reichrath J, editor. Sunlight, vitamin D and skin cancer. Austin: Landes Bioscience; 2008.
21. Erb P, Ji J, Kump E, Mielgo A, Wernli M. Apoptosis and pathogenesis of melanoma and nonmelanoma skin cancer. In: Reichrath J, editor. Sunlight, vitamin D and skin cancer. Austin: Landes Bioscience; 2008.
22. Donehower LA, Bradley A. The tumor suppressor p53. Biochim Biophys Acta. 1993;1155:181–205.
23. Letier U, Garbe C, et al. Epidemiology of melanoma and nonmelanoma skin cancer – the role of sunlight. In: Reichrath J, editor. Sunlight, vitamin D and skin cancer. Austin: Landes Bioscience; 2008.
24. Filipowicz E, Adegboyega P, Sanchez RL, et al. Expression of CD95 (Fas) in sun-exposed human skin and cutaneous carcinomas. Cancer. 2002;94:814–9.
25. Heckmann M, Zogelmeier F, Konz B. Frequency of facial basal cell carcinoma does not correlate with site-specific UV exposure. Arch Dermatol. 2002;138:1494–7.
26. Auborn KJ. Carcinogenesis: current trends in skin cancer research. In: Zhai H, Wilhelm KP, Miabach H, editors. Marzulli and Maibach's dermatotoxicology. Boca Raton: CRC Press LLC; 2008.

27. Addeo R, Napolitano A, Montella L, et al. Squamous cell carcinoma of the tongue in a female with advanced breast cancer: a case report of an elderly patient presenting with two types of cancer. Oncol Lett. 2014;8:235–7.
28. Heywood LA, Burke JF. Mismatch repair in mammalian cells. Bioessays. 1990;12:473–7.
29. Peltomäki P, Aaltonen LA, Sistonen P, et al. Genetic mapping of a locus predisposing to human colorectal cancer. Science. 1993;260:810–2.
30. Jaax S, Scott LW, Wolf JEJ, et al. General guidelines for a low-fat diet effective in the management and prevention of nonmelanoma skin cancer. Nutr Cancer. 1997;27:150–6.
31. Lamberg L. Diet may affect skin cancer prevention. JAMA. 1998;279:1427–8.
32. Davies TW, Treasure FP, Welch AA, et al. Diet and basal cell skin cancer: results from the EPIC-Norfolk cohort. Br J Dermatol. 2002;146:1017–22.
33. Tang JY, Parimi N, Wu A, et al. Inverse association between serum 25(OH) vitamin D levels and non-melanoma skin cancer in elderly men. Cancer Causes Control. 2010;21:387–91.
34. Clark LC, Combs GFJ, Turnbull BW, et al. Effects of selenium supplementation for cancer prevention in patients with carcinoma of the skin. A randomized controlled trial. Nutritional Prevention of Cancer Study Group. JAMA. 1996;276:1957–63.
35. Biliris KA, Koumantakis E, Dokianakis DN, et al. Human papillomavirus infection of non-melanoma skin cancers in immunocompetent hosts. Cancer Lett. 2000;161:83–8.
36. Bleiker TO, Graham-Brown RA. Diagnosing skin disease in the elderly. Practitioner. 2000;244:974–81.
37. Carter DM, Balin AK. Dermatological aspects of aging. Med Clin N Am. 1983;67:531–43.
38. Kelly R. Dermatoses in geriatric patients. Aust Fam Physician. 1977;6:36. 38-41, 43-4, PASSIM.
39. Kleinsmith DM, Perricone NV. Common skin problems in the elderly. Dermatol Clin. 1986;4: 485–99.
40. Shelley WB, Shelley ED. The ten major problems of aging skin. Geriatrics. 1982;37:107–13.
41. Spencer SK, Kierland RR. The aging skin: problems and their causes. Geriatrics. 1970;25:81–9.
42. Lin AN, Carter DM, Balin AK. Nonmelanoma skin cancers in the elderly. Clin Geriatr Med. 1989;5:161–70.
43. Keller KL, Fenske NA, Glass LF. Cancer of the skin in the older patient. Clin Geriatr Med. 1997;13:339–61.
44. Frost C, Williams G, Green A. High incidence and regression rates of solar keratoses in a queensland community. J Invest Dermatol. 2000;115:273–7.
45. Bickle K, Roark TR, Hsu S. Autoimmune bullous dermatoses: a review. Am Fam Physician. 2002;65:1861–70.
46. Cockerell CJ, Wharton JR. New histopathological classification of actinic keratosis (incipient intraepidermal squamous cell carcinoma). J Drugs Dermatol. 2005;4:462–7.
47. Chia A, Moreno G, Lim A, et al. Actinic keratoses. Aust Fam Physician. 2007;36:539–43.
48. Cole HNJ. Skin tumors in the elderly. Postgrad Med. 1968;43:188–91.
49. Lynch PJ. Tumors of the skin. Premalignment and malignant. Minn Med. 1974;57:780–7.
50. Knox JM, Freeman RG. Diagnosis and treatment of skin tumors in the AGED. Geriatrics. 1967; 22:143–55.
51. Ericson MB, Wennberg A, Larkö O. Review of photodynamic therapy in actinic keratosis and basal cell carcinoma. Ther Clin Risk Manag. 2008;4:1–9.
52. Pollack SV. Skin cancer in the elderly. Clin Geriatr Med. 1987;3:715–28.
53. Tschen EH, Wong DS, Pariser DM, et al. Photodynamic therapy using aminolaevulinic acid for patients with nonhyperkeratotic actinic keratoses of the face and scalp: phase IV multicentre clinical trial with 12-month follow up. Br J Dermatol. 2006;155:1262–9.
54. Ogbourne SM, Suhrbier A, Jones B, et al. Antitumor activity of 3-ingenyl angelate: plasma membrane and mitochondrial disruption and necrotic cell death. Cancer Res. 2004;64:2833–9.
55. Hampson P, Kavanagh D, Smith E, et al. The antitumor agent, ingenol-3-angelate (PEP005), promotes the recruitment of cytotoxic neutrophils by activation of vascular endothelial cells in a PKC-delta dependent manner. Cancer Immunol Immunother. 2008; 57:1241–51.
56. Challacombe JM, Suhrbier A, Parsons PG, et al. Neutrophils are a key component of the antitumor efficacy of topical chemotherapy with ingenol-3-angelate. J Immunol. 2006;177:8123–32.
57. Rosen RH, Gupta AK, Tyring SK. Dual mechanism of action of ingenol mebutate gel for topical treatment of actinic keratoses: rapid lesion necrosis followed by lesion-specific immune response. J Am Acad Dermatol. 2012;66:486–93.
58. Lebwohl M, Swanson N, Anderson LL, et al. Ingenol mebutate gel for actinic keratosis. N Engl J Med. 2012;366:1010–9.
59. Sligh JEJ. New therapeutic options for actinic keratosis and basal cell carcinoma. Sem Cutan Med Surg. 2014;33:S76–80.
60. Braathen LR, Szeimies RM, Basset-Seguin N, Bissonnette R, Foley P, Pariser D, Roelandts R, Wennberg AM, Morton CA, International Society for Photodynamic Therapy in Dermatology. Guidelines on the use of photodynamic therapy for nonmelanoma skin cancer: an international consensus. International Society for Photodynamic Therapy in Dermatology, 2005. J Am Acad Dermatol. 2007; 56(1):125–43.
61. Freeman M, Vinciullo C, Francis D, et al. A comparison of photodynamic therapy using topical methyl aminolevulinate (Metvix) with single cycle

cryotherapy in patients with actinic keratosis: a prospective, randomized study. J Dermatol Treat. 2003; 14:99–106.
62. Pariser DM, Lowe NJ, Stewart DM, et al. Photodynamic therapy with topical methyl aminolevulinate for actinic keratosis: results of a prospective randomized multicenter trial. J Am Acad Dermatol. 2003; 48:227–32.
63. Piacquadio DJ, Chen DM, Farber HF, et al. Photodynamic therapy with aminolevulinic acid topical solution and visible blue light in the treatment of multiple actinic keratoses of the face and scalp: investigator-blinded, phase 3, multicenter trials. Arch Dermatol. 2004;140:41–6.
64. Sandberg C, Stenquist B, Rosdahl I, et al. Important factors for pain during photodynamic therapy for actinic keratosis. Acta Derm Venereol. 2006; 86:404–8.
65. Epstein E. Does intermittent "pulse" topical 5-fluorouracil therapy allow destruction of actinic keratoses without significant inflammation? J Am Acad Dermatol. 1998;38:77–80.
66. Urbach F. Ultraviolet radiation and skin cancer. In: Smith K, editor. Topics in photomedicine. Philadelphia: Plenum Press; 1984.
67. Gordon D, Siverstone H. Worldwide epidemiology of pre-malignant and malignant cutaneous lesions. In: Andrade R, editor. Cancer of the skin. Philadelphia: Saunders; 1976.
68. Hill D. Efficacy of sunscreens in protection against skin cancer. Lancet 1999;354:699–700.
69. Ananthaswamy HN, Ullrich SE, Mascotto RE, et al. Inhibition of solar simulator-induced p53 mutations and protection against skin cancer development in mice by sunscreens. J Invest Dermatol. 1999;112:763–8.
70. Shuster S. Is sun exposure a major cause of melanoma? No. BMJ. 2008;337:a764.
71. Mogensen M, Jemec GBE. Diagnosis of nonmelanoma skin cancer/keratinocyte carcinoma: a review of diagnostic accuracy of nonmelanoma skin cancer diagnostic tests and technologies. Dermatol Surg. 2007;33:1158–74.
72. Gohara MA. Skin cancer in skins of color. J Drugs Dermatol. 2008;7:441–5.
73. Helm K, Findeis-Hosey J. Immunohistochemistry of pigmented actinic keratoses, actinic keratoses, melanomas in situ and solar lentigines with Melan-A. J Cutan Pathol. 2008;35(10):931–4.
74. Cheretis C, Angelidou E, Dietrich F, et al. Prognostic value of computer-assisted morphological and morphometrical analysis for detecting the recurrence tendency of basal cell carcinoma. Med Sci Monit. 2008;14:MT13–9.
75. Peris K, Micantonio T, Piccolo D, et al. Dermoscopic features of actinic keratosis. J Dtsch Dermatol Ges. 2007;5:970–6.
76. Eggermont AM, Voit C. Management of melanoma: a European perspective. Surg Oncol Clin N Am. 2008;17:635–48. x.
77. von Roenn JH, Kheir SM, Wolter JM, et al. Significance of DNA abnormalities in primary malignant melanoma and nevi, a retrospective flow cytometric study. Cancer Res. 1986;46:3192–5.
78. Bikle DD. Vitamin D, receptor, UVR, and skin cancer: a potential protective mechanism. J Invest Dermatol. 2008;128:2357–61.
79. Shea CR, McNutt NS, Volkenandt M, et al. Overexpression of p53 protein in basal cell carcinomas of human skin. Am J Pathol. 1992;141:25–9.
80. Amstad PA, Cerutti PA. Ultraviolet-B-light-induced mutagenesis of C-H-ras codons 11 and 12 in human skin fibroblasts. Int J Cancer. 1995;63:136–9.
81. Urabe A, Nakayama J, Taniguchi S, et al. Expression of the fos oncogene in basal cell carcinoma. J Dermatol Sci. 1994;8:50–3.
82. Eshkoor SA, Ismail P, Rahman SA, et al. p16 gene expression in basal cell carcinoma. Arch Med Res. 2008;39:668–73.
83. Kim J, Modlin RL, Moy RL, et al. IL-10 production in cutaneous basal and squamous cell carcinomas. A mechanism for evading the local T cell immune response. J Immunol. 1995;155:2240–7.
84. Goslen JB, Bauer EA. Basal cell carcinoma and collagenase. J Dermatol Surg Oncol. 1986;12:812–7.
85. Lear JT, Smith AG. Basal cell carcinoma. Postgrad Med J. 1997;73:538–42.
86. Roewert-Huber J, Lange-Asschenfeldt B, Stockfleth E, et al. Epidemiology and aetiology of basal cell carcinoma. Br J Dermatol. 2007;157 Suppl 2:47–51.
87. Tierney L, McPhee S, Papadakis M. Current medical diagnosis and treatment. New York: McGraw Hill; 2000.
88. Stamp GW, Pignatelli M. Distribution of beta 1, alpha 1, alpha 2 and alpha 3 integrin chains in basal cell carcinomas. J Pathol. 1991;163:307–13.
89. Green A, Williams G, Neale R, et al. Daily sunscreen application and betacarotene supplementation in prevention of basal-cell and squamous-cell carcinomas of the skin: a randomised controlled trial. Lancet. 1999;354:723–9.
90. Brash DE, Ziegler A, Jonason AS, et al. Sunlight and sunburn in human skin cancer: p53, apoptosis, and tumor promotion. J Investig Dermatol Symp Proc. 1996;1:136–42.
91. Erbagci Z, Erkiliç S. Can smoking and/or occupational UV exposure have any role in the development of the morpheaform basal cell carcinoma? A critical role for peritumoral mast cells. Int J Dermatol. 2002;41:275–8.
92. Newman MD, Weinberg JM. Topical therapy in the treatment of actinic keratosis and basal cell carcinoma. Cutis. 2007;79:18–28.
93. Frisch M, Hjalgrim H, Olsen JH, et al. Risk for subsequent cancer after diagnosis of basal-cell carcinoma. A population-based, epidemiologic study. Ann Intern Med. 1996;125:815–21.
94. Thissen MRTM, Kuijpers DIM, Krekels GAM. Local immune modulator (imiquimod 5% cream) as

adjuvant treatment after incomplete Mohs micrographic surgery for large, mixed type basal cell carcinoma: a report of 3 cases. J Drugs Dermatol. 2006;5:461–4.
95. Wu JK, Oh C, Strutton G, et al. An open-label, pilot study examining the efficacy of curettage followed by imiquimod 5% cream for the treatment of primary nodular basal cell carcinoma. Australas J Dermatol. 2006;47:46–8.
96. Spencer JM. Pilot study of imiquimod 5% cream as adjunctive therapy to curettage and electrodesiccation for nodular basal cell carcinoma. Dermatol Surg. 2006;32:63–9.
97. Von Hoff DD, LoRusso PM, Rudin CM, et al. Inhibition of the hedgehog pathway in advanced basal-cell carcinoma. N Engl J Med. 2009;361:1164–72.
98. Sekulic A, Migden MR, Oro AE, et al. Efficacy and safety of vismodegib in advanced basal-cell carcinoma. N Engl J Med. 2012;366:2171–9.
99. Tang JY, Mackay-Wiggan JM, Aszterbaum M, et al. Inhibiting the hedgehog pathway in patients with the basal-cell nevus syndrome. N Engl J Med. 2012;366:2180–8.
100. Szeimies R, Gerritsen MP, Gupta G, et al. Imiquimod 5% cream for the treatment of actinic keratosis: results from a phase III, randomized, double-blind, vehicle-controlled, clinical trial with histology. J Am Acad Dermatol. 2004;51:547–55.
101. Kennedy C, Bajdik CD, Willemze R, et al. The influence of painful sunburns and lifetime sun exposure on the risk of actinic keratoses, seborrheic warts, melanocytic nevi, atypical nevi, and skin cancer. J Invest Dermatol. 2003;120:1087–93.
102. Garrett AB. Skin cancer in people of color. In: Snow N, Mikhail GR, editors. Mohs micrographic surgery. Madison: University of Wisconsion Press; 2004.
103. Mueller CS, Reichrath J. Histology of melanoma and nonmelanoma skin cancer. In: Reichrath J, editor. Sunlight, vitamin D and skin cancer. Austin: Landes Bioscience; 2008.
104. Akhdari N, Amal S, Ettalbi S. Bowen disease. CMAJ. 2006;175:739.
105. Kossard S, Tan K, Choy C. Keratoacanthoma and infundibulocystic squamous cell carcinoma. Am J Dermatopathol. 2008;30:127–34.
106. Gallagher RP. Sunscreens in melanoma and skin cancer prevention. CMAJ. 2005;173:244–5.
107. Skin Cancer Foundation. Skin cancer facts: melanoma. http://www.skincancer.org/skin-cancer-information/skin-cancer-facts#melanoma. Accessed 19 Aug 2014.
108. Manganoni AM, Pavoni L, Sereni E, et al. Role of occasional evaluation of the skin in early detection of melanoma in elderly patients. Indian J Dermatol Venereol Leprol. 2012;78:664.
109. Giles GG, Armstrong BK, Burton RC, et al. Has mortality from melanoma stopped rising in Australia? Analysis of trends between 1931 and 1994. BMJ. 1996;312:1121–5.
110. McCartney RA. Malignant melanoma. In: Thackery E, editor. Gale encyclopedia of cancer. Farmington Hills: Thomson Gale Publishing; 2002.
111. Beers MH, Berkow BR. Dermatologic disorders: malignant tumors. In: Beers MH, Berkow R, editors. The Merck manual of diagnosis and therapy. Whitehouse Station: Merck Research Laboratories; 2002.
112. Rass K, Tilgen W. Treatment of melanoma and nonmelanoma skin cancer. In: Reichrath J, editor. Sunlight, vitamin D and skin cancer. Austin: Landes Bioscience; 2008.
113. Gillgren P, Brattström G, Frisell J, et al. Effect of primary site on prognosis in patients with cutaneous malignant melanoma. A study using a new model to analyse anatomical locations. Melanoma Res. 2005;15:125–32.
114. Cochran AJ, Elashoff D, Morton DL, et al. Individualized prognosis for melanoma patients. Hum Pathol. 2000;31:327–31.
115. Newman MD, Mirzabeigi M, Gerami P. Chromosomal copy number changes supporting the classification of lentiginous junctional melanoma of the elderly as a subtype of melanoma. Mod Pathol. 2009;22:1258–62.
116. Macdonald JB, Dueck AC, Gray RJ, et al. Malignant melanoma in the elderly: different regional disease and poorer prognosis. J Cancer. 2011;2:538–43.
117. Moan J, Porojnicu A, Dahlback A. Ultraviolet radiation and malignant melanoma. In: Reicharth J, editor. Sunlight, vitamin D and skin cancer. Austin: Landes Biosciences; 2008.
118. Menzies SW. Is sun exposure a major cause of melanoma? Yes. BMJ. 2008;337:a763.
119. Armstrong BK, Kricker A. The epidemiology of UV induced skin cancer. J Photochem Photobiol B. 2001;63:8–18.
120. Bulliard J, De Weck D, Fisch T, et al. Detailed site distribution of melanoma and sunlight exposure: aetiological patterns from a Swiss series. Ann Oncol. 2007;18:789–94.
121. Tsao H, Sober AJ. Ultraviolet radiation and malignant melanoma. Clin Dermatol. 1998;16:67–73.
122. Kraemer KH, Lee MM, Andrews AD, et al. The role of sunlight and DNA repair in melanoma and nonmelanoma skin cancer. The xeroderma pigmentosum paradigm. Arch Dermatol. 1994;130:1018–21.
123. Hussein MR. Ultraviolet radiation and skin cancer: molecular mechanisms. J Cutan Pathol. 2005;32:191–205.
124. Armstrong BK, Kricker A. Skin cancer. Dermatol Clin. 1995;13:583–94.
125. Cress RD, Holly EA. Incidence of cutaneous melanoma among non-hispanic whites, Hispanics, Asians, and blacks: an analysis of California cancer registry

data, 1988–93. Cancer Causes Control. 1997;8:246–52.
126. Garsaud P, Boisseau-Garsaud AM, Ossondo M, et al. Epidemiology of cutaneous melanoma in the French West Indies (Martinique). Am J Epidemiol. 1998;147:66–8.
127. Rolón PA, Kramárová E, Rolón HI, et al. Plantar melanoma: a case-control study in Paraguay. Cancer Causes Control. 1997;8:850–6.
128. Le Marchand L, Saltzman BS, Hankin JH, et al. Sun exposure, diet, and melanoma in Hawaii Caucasians. Am J Epidemiol. 2006;164:232–45.
129. Crombie IK. Variation of melanoma incidence with latitude in north America and Europe. Br J Cancer. 1979;40:774–81.
130. Gallagher RP, Spinelli JJ, Lee TK. Tanning beds, sunlamps, and risk of cutaneous malignant melanoma. Cancer Epidemiol Biomarkers Prev. 2005;14: 562–6.
131. Setlow RB, Woodhead AD, Grist E. Animal model for ultraviolet radiation-induced melanoma: platyfish-swordtail hybrid. Proc Natl Acad Sci U S A. 1989;86:8922–6.
132. Garland CF, Garland FC, Gorham ED. Rising trends in melanoma. An hypothesis concerning sunscreen effectiveness. Ann Epidemiol. 1993;3:103–10.
133. Rivers JK. Is there more than one road to melanoma? Lancet. 2004;363:728–30.
134. Maldonado JL, Fridlyand J, Patel H, et al. Determinants of BRAF mutations in primary melanomas. J Natl Cancer Inst. 2003;95:1878–90.
135. Kirkwood JM, Strawderman MH, Ernstoff MS, et al. Interferon alfa-2b adjuvant therapy of high-risk resected cutaneous melanoma: the Eastern Cooperative Oncology Group Trial EST 1684. J Clin Oncol. 1996;14:7–17.
136. Callen JP, Bickers DR, Moy RL. Actinic keratoses. J Am Acad Dermatol. 1997;36:650–3.
137. Kurban RS, Kurban AK. Common skin disorders of aging: diagnosis and treatment. Geriatrics. 1993;48:30–1. 35-6, 39-42.
138. Gugić J, Strojan P. Squamous cell carcinoma of the head and neck in the elderly. Rep Pract Oncol Radiother. 2012;18:16–25.
139. Gulati HK, Deshmukh SD, Anand M, et al. Low-grade malignant proliferating pilar tumor simulating a squamous-cell carcinoma in an elderly female: a case report and immunohistochemical study. Int J Trichol. 2011;3:98–101.
140. Jung HJ, Jun JH, Kim HY, et al. Pigmented basal cell carcinoma of the nipple-areola complex in an elderly woman. Ann Dermatol. 2011;23: S201–4.
141. Kanitakis J, Arbona-Vidal M, Faure E. Extensive pigmented vulvar basal-cell carcinoma presenting as pruritus in an elderly woman. Dermatol Online J. 2011;17:8.
142. Corradin MT, Giulioni E, Fiorentino R, et al. In situ malignant melanoma on nevus spilus in an elderly patient. Acta Dermatovenerol Alpina Pannonica Adriat. 2014;23:17–9.
143. Berwick M. Counterpoint: sunscreen use is a safe and effective approach to skin cancer prevention. Cancer Epidemiol Biomarkers Prev. 2007;16:1923–4.
144. Xie J. Molecular biology of basal and squamous cell carcinomas. In: Reichrath J, editor. Sunlight, vitamin D and skin cancer. Austin: Landes Bioscience; 2008.
145. Wartman D, Weinstock M. Are we overemphasizing sun avoidance in protection from melanoma? Cancer Epidemiol Biomarkers Prev. 2008;17:469–70.
146. Wennberg AM, Lindholm LE, Alpsten M, et al. Treatment of superficial basal cell carcinomas using topically applied delta-aminolaevulinic acid and a filtered xenon lamp. Arch Dermatol Res. 1996;288:561–4.
147. Horn M, Wolf P, Wulf HC, et al. Topical methyl aminolaevulinate photodynamic therapy in patients with basal cell carcinoma prone to complications and poor cosmetic outcome with conventional treatment. Br J Dermatol. 2003;149:1242–9.
148. Loven K, Stein L, Furst K, et al. Evaluation of the efficacy and tolerability of 0.5% fluorouracil cream and 5% fluorouracil cream applied to each side of the face in patients with actinic keratosis. Clin Ther. 2002;24:990–1000.
149. Weiss J, Menter A, Hevia O, et al. Effective treatment of actinic keratosis with 0.5% fluorouracil cream for 1, 2, or 4 weeks. Cutis. 2002;70:22–9.
150. Wolf JEJ, Taylor JR, Tschen E, et al. Topical 3.0% diclofenac in 2.5% hyaluronan gel in the treatment of actinic keratoses. Int J Dermatol. 2001;40:709–13.
151. Rivers JK, Arlette J, Shear N, et al. Topical treatment of actinic keratoses with 3.0% diclofenac in 2.5% hyaluronan gel. Br J Dermatol. 2002;146:94–100.
152. Fariba I, Ali A, Hossein SA, et al. Efficacy of 3% diclofenac gel for the treatment of actinic keratoses: a randomized, double-blind, placebo controlled study. Indian J Dermatol Venereol Leprol. 2006;72:346–9.
153. Grimaître M, Etienne A, Fathi M, et al. Topical colchicine therapy for actinic keratoses. Dermatology. 2000;200:346–8.
154. Akar A, Bülent Taştan H, Erbil H, et al. Efficacy and safety assessment of 0.5% and 1% colchicine cream in the treatment of actinic keratoses. J Dermatol Treat. 2001;12:199–203.
155. Stockfleth E, Meyer T, Benninghoff B, et al. A randomized, double-blind, vehicle-controlled study to assess 5% imiquimod cream for the treatment of multiple actinic keratoses. Arch Dermatol. 2002; 138:1498–502.
156. Salasche SJ, Levine N, Morrison L. Cycle therapy of actinic keratoses of the face and scalp with 5% topical imiquimod cream: an open-label trial. J Am Acad Dermatol. 2002;47:571–7.
157. Persaud AN, Shamuelova E, Sherer D, et al. Clinical effect of imiquimod 5% cream in the treatment of actinic keratosis. J Am Acad Dermatol. 2002;47:553–6.

158. Lebwohl M, Dinehart S, Whiting D, et al. Imiquimod 5% cream for the treatment of actinic keratosis: results from two phase III, randomized, double-blind, parallel group, vehicle-controlled trials. J Am Acad Dermatol. 2004;50:714–21.
159. Beutner KR, Geisse JK, Helman D, et al. Therapeutic response of basal cell carcinoma to the immune response modifier imiquimod 5% cream. J Am Acad Dermatol. 1999;41:1002–7.
160. Marks R, Gebauer K, Shumack S, et al. Imiquimod 5% cream in the treatment of superficial basal cell carcinoma: results of a multicenter 6-week dose-response trial. J Am Acad Dermatol. 2001; 44:807–13.
161. Geisse JK, Rich P, Pandya A, et al. Imiquimod 5% cream for the treatment of superficial basal cell carcinoma: a double-blind, randomized, vehicle-controlled study. J Am Acad Dermatol. 2002;47:390–8.
162. Sterry W, Ruzicka T, Herrera E, et al. Imiquimod 5% cream for the treatment of superficial and nodular basal cell carcinoma: randomized studies comparing low-frequency dosing with and without occlusion. Br J Dermatol. 2002;147:1227–36.
163. Shumack S, Robinson J, Kossard S, et al. Efficacy of topical 5% imiquimod cream for the treatment of nodular basal cell carcinoma: comparison of dosing regimens. Arch Dermatol. 2002;138:1165–71.
164. Spencer J. Actinic keratoses. http://www.emedicine.com/derm/topic9.htm. Accessed 18 Jan 2015.
165. Ulrich C, Busch JO, Meyer T, et al. Successful treatment of multiple actinic keratoses in organ transplant patients with topical 5% imiquimod: a report of six cases. Br J Dermatol. 2006;155:451–4.
166. Ortonne J. From actinic keratosis to squamous cell carcinoma. Br J Dermatol. 2002;146 Suppl 61:20–3.
167. Weinstock MA. Epidemiology of nonmelanoma skin cancer: clinical issues, definitions, and classification. J Invest Dermatol. 1994;102:4S–5.
168. Weinstock MA. Epidemiologic investigation of nonmelanoma skin cancer mortality: the Rhode Island Follow-Back Study. J Invest Dermatol. 1994;102: 6S–9.
169. Soehnge H, Ouhtit A, Ananthaswamy ON. Mechanisms of induction of skin cancer by UV radiation. Front Biosci. 1997;2:d538–51.
170. Leman JA, McHenry PM. Basal cell carcinoma: still an enigma. Arch Dermatol. 2001;137:1239–40.
171. Moloney FJ, Comber H, O'Lorcain P, et al. A population-based study of skin cancer incidence and prevalence in renal transplant recipients. Br J Dermatol. 2006;154:498–504.
172. Zhang H, Ping XL, Lee PK, et al. Role of PTCH and p53 genes in early-onset basal cell carcinoma. Am J Pathol. 2001;158:381–5.
173. Scotto J, Fears TR, Fraumeni JF. Incidence of non-melanoma skin cancer in the United States. US Department of Health and Human Services, Bethesda MD: National Institutes of Health. 1983.
174. Rigel DS, Carucci JA. Malignant melanoma: prevention, early detection, and treatment in the 21st century. CA Cancer J Clin. 2000;50:215–36. quiz 237–40.
175. van der Pols JC, Williams GM, Pandeya N, et al. Prolonged prevention of squamous cell carcinoma of the skin by regular sunscreen use. Cancer Epidemiol Biomarkers Prev. 2006;15:2546–8.
176. Hoersch B, Leiter U, Garbe C. Is head and neck melanoma a distinct entity? A clinical registry-based comparative study in 5702 patients with melanoma. Br J Dermatol. 2006;155:771–7.

Cutaneous Effects and Sensitive Skin with Incontinence in the Aged

66

Miranda A. Farage, Kenneth W. Miller, Enzo Berardesca, and Howard I. Maibach

Contents

M.A. Farage (✉)
Winton Hill Business Center, The Procter & Gamble Company, Cincinnati, OH, USA
e-mail: farage.m@pg.com

K.W. Miller
Margoshes-Miller Consulting, LLC, Cincinnati, OH, USA
e-mail: bbbns2@fuse.net

E. Berardesca
San Gallicano Dermatological Institute, Rome, Italy
e-mail: berardesca@berardesca.it

H.I. Maibach
Department of Dermatology, University of California, San Francisco, CA, USA
e-mail: maibachh@derm.ucsf.edu; Howard.Maibach@ucsf.edu

M.A. Farage et al. (eds.), *Textbook of Aging Skin*,
DOI 10.1007/978-3-662-47398-6_64

Abstract

Urinary and fecal incontinence affects a significant portion of the elderly population. While reported prevalence rates vary widely, incontinence tends to increase with age and becomes a relatively common affliction in those over 50. Although urinary and fecal incontinence increases with age, neither are natural sequelae of aging, but disorders which could be treated. Occlusion of the skin, often induced by incontinence pads or other containment devices, has a profound influence on the skin surface. Incontinence in aged skin has the potential to produce chemical irritation, mechanical injury, and increased susceptibility to incontinence dermatitis, dermal infections (both fungal and bacterial), intertrigo, vulvar folliculitis, pruritus ani, and pressure ulcers. Urinary incontinence also represents a psychosocial burden and is associated with a variety of psychiatric disorders. Dermatologists who are knowledgeable about geriatric issues can help to maintain the health and quality of life of their older patients.

Introduction

Urinary and fecal incontinence affects a significant portion of the elderly population. The increase in the incidence of incontinence is not only dependent on age but also on the onset of concomitant aging issues such as infection, polypharmacy, and decreased cognitive function. If incontinence is left untreated, a host of dermatologic complications can occur, including incontinence dermatitis, dermatological infections, intertrigo, vulvar folliculitis, and pruritus ani.

The presence of chronic incontinence can produce a vicious cycle of skin inflammation due to the loss of cutaneous integrity. Minimizing skin damage caused by incontinence is dependent on the successful control of excess hydration, maintenance of proper pH, minimization of interaction between urine and feces, and prevention of secondary infection. Even though incontinence is common in the aged, it is not an inevitable consequence of aging but a disorder that can and should be treated. Appropriate clinical management of incontinence can help seniors continue to lead vital, active lives as well as avoid the cutaneous sequelae of incontinence.

Table 1 Contributing factors in fecal incontinence

Intrinsic factors (concomitant diseases)
Anorectal dysfunction [7]
Arthritis [8]
Cancer [7]
Dementia [9]
Diabetes [7]
Fecal impaction [9]
Gastrointestinal infections [7]
Inflammatory bowel disease [7]
Liver failure [7]
Neuromuscular dysfunction [9]
Neurosensory dysfunction [10]
Stroke [8]
External factors
Obstetrical injury [6]
Patient restraint [8]

With kind permission from Wiley-Blackwell publisher adapted from Farage et al. [11]

Prevalence of Incontinence

As part of the aging process, the bladder becomes more irritable, holds less, and empties less efficiently [1]. These normal changes, when accompanied by concomitant illnesses or medications, obstetrical injury, dementia, or changes in nutrition or hormonal status, can produce incontinence [1, 2].

While reported prevalence rates vary widely, incontinence tends to increase with age and becomes a relatively common affliction in those over 50 [3]. A community-based study of American women over 50 found that 48.4 % experienced urinary incontinence, 15.2 % suffered from fecal incontinence, and 9.4 % experienced both [4, 5]. Studies have reported the prevalence of fecal incontinence in nursing homes to be as high as 50 % [6]. Risk factors include advancing age, female gender, and multiparity [6]; the numerous underlying causes of fecal incontinence are shown in Table 1. Chronic conditions such as hypertension, diabetes, and obesity may also be associated with urinary incontinence [12]. Incontinence is thus an important clinical problem in the elderly today and one that is expected to grow.

Incontinence: Cutaneous Effects

Although urinary and fecal incontinence increases with age, neither are natural sequelae of aging, but disorders which could be treated [9]. After 6 months, transient incontinence is more likely to be established as chronic, with a decreased prognosis for long-term resolution [1]. Incontinence of any type creates a hostile environment for the skin [1].

The skin's ability to provide a barrier between the internal and external environment depends on the integrity of the skin and its histological structure, the presence of intra- and extracellular lipids, and the skin's pH [13]. Genital hygiene is of particular importance to the health and well-being of older women, as perineal dermatitis is frequently encountered in patients with urinary and/or fecal incontinence [10]. Moreover, the risk of pressure ulcers and incontinence dermatitis can be significant when older women suffer impaired mobility and urinary or fecal incontinence [3].

Occlusion of the skin, often induced by incontinence pads or other containment devices, has a profound influence on the skin surface as shown in Table 2. Historically, skin occluded by

Table 2 Dermatological effects of occlusion

Parameter measured	Influence of occlusion
pH	Increases pH [14]
Integrity of stratum corneum	Disrupts lipid organization and metabolism [14]
	Prevents expected increase in epidermal lipid synthesis [15]
	Increases TEWL [15]
	Increases hydration of stratum corneum [16]
Bacterial counts	Increased [17]
Function of stratum corneum	Prevents recovery of elevated TEWL [15]
	Increases permeability, especially to nonpolar lipids [14, 18]
	Inhibits barrier restoration [19]
Carbon dioxide emission rate	Increased [17]
Cellular function	Decreases mitotic activity [20]
	Inhibits DNA synthesis [21]
	Induces intercellular adhesion molecule 1 [22]
	Increases CD3+ epidermal lymphocytes [22]
	Inhibits increase in epidermal cell proliferation [23]
	Reduces epidermal pool of IL-1α [24]
	Increases skin surface temperature [25]
Visible changes	Deepens skin furrows [16]
	Increases inflammation [22]
	Increases frequency of hydration dermatitis [26]

With kind permission from Wiley-Blackwell publisher adapted from Farage et al. [11]
DNA deoxyribonucleic acid, *TEWL* transepidermal water loss

diapering is wetter, with higher pH, bacterial count, and susceptibility to erosion [17]. Barrier permeability, as well as molecular and cellular homeostasis [25], is affected as well. Improved pad design with changes in the absorption core has shown lower pH levels [27].

Aged skin is additionally compromised [28]. Skin becomes drier, with more tendency to crack [29]. It also becomes thinner, more fragile, and less resistant to infection. Loss of elasticity leaves it more susceptible to injury, while its ability to repair itself diminishes. Skin aging also results in less surface sensory perception, increasing the risk of injuries like pressure ulcers [28].

Incontinence in aged skin has the potential to produce chemical irritation, mechanical injury, and increased susceptibility to infection. Chemical irritation can be defined as an imbalance of moisture, salts, enzymes, or other chemicals [10]. The pH of normal health skin ranges from 4.0 to 6.8, with an average of approximately 5.5. With exposure to excess moisture, pH can increase to as much as 7.5; pH with exposure to urine can reach 8.0 [10]. The associated disruption of the acid mantle interferes with the production of lipids and enzymes critical for barrier integrity, as well as keratinization critical to the repair of damage caused by prolonged exposure to urine or feces [10, 30].

The acid mantle of the skin provides significant resistance against dehydration as well as bacterial invasion [31]. Disruption of the acid mantle by incontinence allows for secondary infection [32]. *Staphylococcus*, indigenous to perineal skin, is the most common culprit [10]. Secondary infection by *Candida albicans*, a common resident of the gastrointestinal (GI) tract, is also common [10]. In those with impaired immune function, the overgrowth of cutaneous pathogens, or invasion of fecal bacteria, is more likely to be a complication [3].

Exposure to excess water alone can cause damage in 48 h, with multiple possible effects as displayed in Table 3. Stool and urine contain numerous substances with the potential to further irritate skin: ammonia, which raises pH; urea, which gets converted to ammonia in the presence of bacteria-containing feces [37]; and digestive enzymes that are erosive to skin [10], creating

Table 3 Dermatological effects of water

Parameter measured	Influence of water
Visible changes	Increases erythema [33, 34]
	Increases irritation [25]
Function of stratum corneum	Trend to increased cutaneous blood flow [33, 34]
	Increases TEWL [33, 34]
	Increases permeability to low molecular weight irritants [35]
	Increases frictional coefficient, causing increased susceptibility to trauma [32, 35]
Pathogenesis	Increases risk of pressure ulcers [31]
	Increases risk of loss of skin integrity [31, 35]
	Increases susceptibility to bacterial colonization [32, 35]
pH	Increase in pH [36]

With kind permission from Wiley-Blackwell publisher adapted from Farage et al. [11]
TEWL transepidermal water loss

increased erythema, transepidermal water loss (TEWL), and susceptibility to fungal infection [38]. A 3-week exposure to physiological concentrations of fecal enzymes and bile salts in vivo produced significant barrier disruption and erythema in one human model [38].

Excess moisture on the skin will eventually produce mechanical damage. Twice as much energy is required to produce frictional erosions on dry skin as on skin subjected to 24-h water exposure [39]; therefore, incontinence is a major risk factor in pressure ulcers [40]. Skin hydration following occlusion is significantly higher and slower to dissipate in aged skin [41].

Overhydrated skin is also more vulnerable to tearing, particularly when immobile patients are moved [32, 39]. In addition, overzealous scrubbing during cleansing procedures on fragile elderly skin can strip away the protective horny layer, an event usually limited to epidermis, but which may involve huge areas of skin [10]. Any breach of skin integrity in an elderly individual can become a serious injury due to the potential for infection, loss of fluid and electrolytes, decreased thermoregulatory function, and impaired metabolism and communication [3].

Incontinence Dermatitis

Perineal dermatitis, or incontinence dermatitis, is a broad term describing skin problems in patients with urinary or fecal incontinence. The condition creates much pain and discomfort in elderly sufferers, causing inflammation and tissue damage to the vulva, perineum, perianal region, and buttocks [3]. The prevalence of risk of perineal dermatitis, predictably, increases as mobility declines. Frequency of incontinence, baseline skin condition, overall health, management of excess moisture [42], cognitive impairment, and concurrent medications are also factors, as shown in Fig. 1 [43–49].

Sixty percent of fecal matter is comprised of microorganisms [50]. Urine and feces in contact with the dry, cracked skin characteristic of the elderly are absorbed into the crevices, providing an excellent environment for bacterial growth [35, 40, 51, 52]. When urine and stool mix, bacteria present in the stool convert urea to ammonia [53], which raises the pH of the skin thus destroying the acid mantle and facilitating penetration of irritants. Feces also contain proteolytic and lipolytic digestive enzymes, normally deactivated in the digestive tract [31], which are reactivated in the presence of ammonia, with the potential to erode skin [38, 53].

Perineal dermatitis is thus more likely when stool and urine are simultaneously present [54], as pathogens in stool overwhelm the skin's defenses, leading to breakdown and subsequent colonization [55]. In a study of geriatric psychiatric patients, all patients with both urine and fecal incontinence developed perineal dermatitis within 2 days [54].

Incontinence dermatitis in older people begins with mild erythema of the skin, which may worsen and develop into blistering and erosion [10]. Severe or improperly managed cases can result in full-thickness wounds [56]. Initial inflammation may be harder to detect in darker skin. With urinary incontinence, dermatitis begins between the labial folds; dermatitis associated with fecal incontinence originates in the perianal area and progresses to the posterior aspect of the upper thighs [10]. Unusual patterns may reflect occlusion of the skin by a containment device [10].

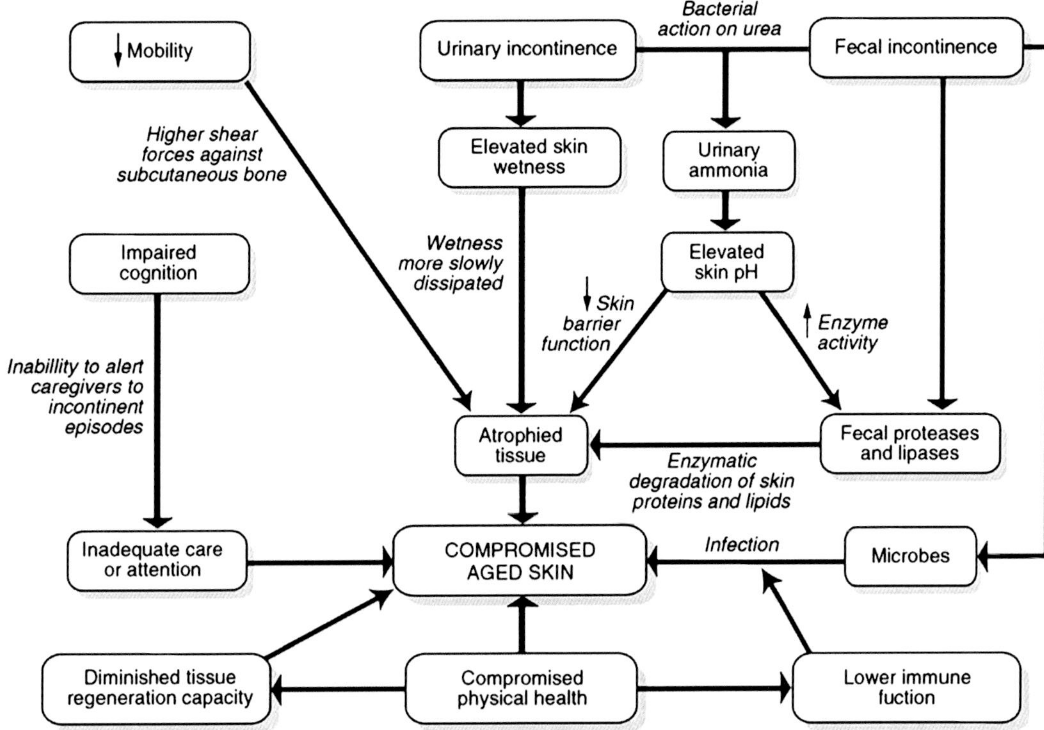

Fig. 1 (Copyright (2006) from Farage and Bramante [3]. Reproduced with kind permission of Routledge/Taylor & Francis Group, LLC) Factors Contributing to the Morbidity of Incontinence Dermatitis in Elderly People

Selection of proper treatment must take into account the fragility of elderly skin [39], as additional tissue injury is an all too common sequelae of cleansing [44]. Treatment for incontinence dermatitis must be carefully considered to avoid further unintentional damage [57, 58]. Although the use of products such as vegetable shortening, shaving cream, or veterinary supplies is common, legal liability makes this practice unsupportable [31].

Dermal Infections

Fungal Infections

Fungal infections of the skin related to incontinence involve primarily one of the two organisms: tinea and *C. albicans*. Tinea is a fungal infection of the vulvar skin folds, more commonly known as ringworm. Though rare, its prevalence rises in older women because of diminished cellular immune response [29, 59]. Characteristic presentation is a ring-shaped eruption with an actively advancing border but healing center. Any pruritic, scaly eruption of the vulva, however, should be scraped for microscopic examination and treated with antifungal therapy, if appropriate. Avoiding overhydration of the skin will generally prevent this condition [3].

Secondary infection with *C. albicans* will result in erythematous, punctuate pustules with a central confluence; satellite lesions may be visible at the border of the infection [60]. Lesions can take on a macular appearance from friction [10]. Yeast may extend into the groin and thigh folds [43], with curd-like plaques on mucous membranes [2]. Even mild inflammation is accompanied by significant burning, requires pain management [43], and can be accompanied by intense pruritus of affected areas [2]. Chronic infection can cause darkened or reddened skin which may be mistaken for a pressure ulcer [10].

The gastrointestinal tract is an important reservoir of *C. albicans*, and fecal incontinence increases the risk of *Candida* colonization [61]. Routine administration of amoxicillin doubled the counts of *C. albicans* observed from both the rectum and skin, with an associated increase in the risk of dermatitis [62]. Treatment for candidiasis consists principally of topical antifungal agents [2]. The use of systemic antibiotics should be discontinued, when possible [2], while affected areas are kept dry and, as much as possible, exposed to air [2]. There is recent evidence that caprylic acid may also be a good treatment option for infections caused by *C. albicans*, *Helicobacter pylori*, and other microorganisms [63].

Bacterial Infections

A primary skin function is the prevention of invasion by external pathogens. Compromised skin may be less effective, allowing the proliferation and invasion of microbials [35]. *Staphylococcus* can readily colonize skin already compromised by incontinence dermatitis [61]. About 20 % of cases of necrotizing fasciitis, a particularly destructive necrosis of the skin and deeper tissues, have been associated with the presence of infected hair follicles [64]. In addition, the use of incontinence therapies such as trans-obturator and vaginal tape has a demonstrated association with both necrotizing fasciitis and cellulitis [65, 66].

Intertrigo and Vulvar Folliculitis

Exposure to excess moisture and excretory products associated with incontinence encourages the development of both intertrigo and vulvar folliculitis in the genital area. Intertrigo, a maceration of the tissue due to heat, moisture, and friction [2], affects areas with opposing skin surfaces such as the labia, perineum, and genitocrural folds [67].

Vulvar folliculitis, a result of bacterial infection in the presence of increased moisture, warmth, and decreased hygiene, is the development of red, tender pus-filled papules surrounding the hair follicles which may be associated with general staphylococcal or streptococcal infection. Both conditions respond to fastidious hygiene and keep the perineal area dry [3].

Pruritus Ani

Anogenital pruritus, characterized by perianal itching, can be the result of minor incontinence but can also result from overzealous cleansing with harsh soaps [2]. It is characterized by intense itching accompanied by erythema and/or excoriation. Chronic scratching may result in perianal inflammation and skin damage, particularly in the presence of impaired mental function [43].

Pressure Ulcers

Pressure, or decubitus, ulcers are an area of localized cutaneous damage typically associated with pressure from bony protuberances on aged skin (Fig. 2) [68, 69]. Overhydration of the skin, typically in the form of incontinence, increases the susceptibility of the skin to this type of injury [32, 40]. Skin needs to be as dry as possible and patients repositioned frequently [28]. The frequency of pad changes for incontinent patients is directly related to the risk of Stage II pressure ulcers [70]. Adequate nutritional status should be maintained [28].

Little research, however, has been performed with regard to an effective skin care regimen for decubitus ulcer prevention. One retrospective

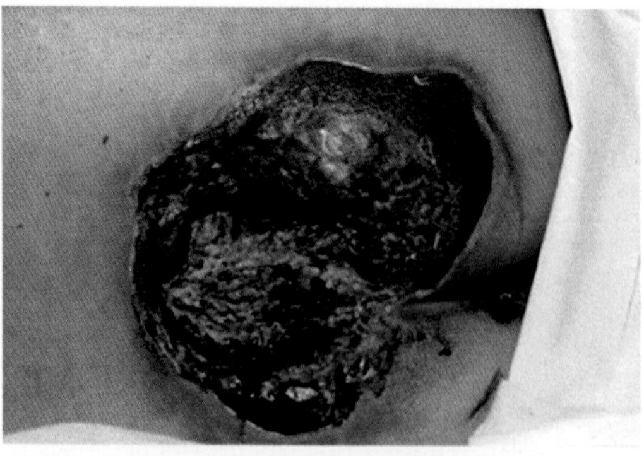

Fig. 2 Pressure Ulcer in the Sacral Area. A Patient Laying in the Bed After Spinal Injury

study demonstrated that the use of a combined skin cleanser/protectant product on residents with incontinence decreased the incidence of nosocomial pressure ulcers in the sacral/buttock area [71]. A 6-month prospective study found that the use of a body wash and skin protectant with incontinence patients reduced the risk of Stage I and II pressure ulcers from 11.3 % to 4.8 % [72].

Management of Incontinence

Few systematic trials document the impact of specific cleansing regimens on the prevention or treatment of incontinence dermatitis. The only published prospective study of preventative care was a preliminary trial of structured intervention in 15 institutionalized patients with dementia [54]. An equal number of developed dermatitis (two in the structured care intervention group and three in the unstructured care group) regardless of whether cleansers, moisturizers, or moisture-barrier preparations were used. Dermatitis developed only in those with urofecal incontinence and followed more than four incontinent episodes in 24 h. None of the patients were capable of informing caregivers of incontinent episodes. The small number of subjects and their poor mental health limit the conclusions that can be drawn from this study.

Thus, patients who are incapable of reporting incontinent episodes should be monitored closely and promptly cleansed. Wet or soiled garments should be changed promptly and skin cleansing should follow every incontinent episode [31]; efforts should be made to prevent further moisture from reaching the skin [44, 73].

Skin cleansing must be performed using cleansers specifically formulated for incontinent patients, which have an acidic pH and a no-rinse formulation [44] in order to avoid frictional forces during cleansing [31]. Where possible, air-drying of the skin is optimal [31]. The pH of cleansing products should be verified before use, as many common products, even when supposedly appropriate for incontinent patients, have pH outside the recommended range [31].

Skin should be kept dry [31] by using superabsorbent incontinence pads [35]. Barrier ointments, which protect the skin from contact with moisture while at the same time preventing friction from diapers and bed linens, should also be used [74]. Case reports have supported their effectiveness [7, 27, 75–77].

Moisturizers can contain medicating ingredients which bind moisture, thus helping to heal damaged skin and prevent drying [31, 44]. Topical antibiotics and antimicrobials should be employed only when an infection is actually present [44]. Antifungal powders and creams can be applied underneath barrier creams or ointments where needed to control incontinence-associated fungal rashes [44].

The chronically incontinent person should be monitored closely for signs of impending loss of skin integrity, with particular attention to skin folds and creases. In women who are obese, skin folds of the lower abdomen must also be exposed and examined, particularly in women who are diabetic or immunocompromised [10].

In elderly women with urinary incontinence, targeted clinical assessment including digital vaginal palpation should be performed in order to detect pelvic floor muscle dysfunction and to optimize therapeutic measures [78]. Incontinence-associated dermatitis (IAD) management is an important challenge for community nurses. It is important to understand the pathophysiology of IAD, the differentiation between IAD and pressure ulcers, and the recommendations thereof for prevention/treatment of IAD [79, 80].

Sensitive Skin with Incontinence

Incontinence in the aged population is quite common, with a prevalence of about 50 % both in community [4] and institutionalized [6] populations. In addition, the majority of women in industrialized countries (50–90 %, depending on the population studied), as well as a rapidly increasing percentage of men in those countries, believe that they have sensitive skin [81]. As the proportion of the elderly continues to increase in industrialized nations, the numbers of individuals who suffer from both incontinence and sensitive skin are likely to increase as well. It is possible that this population may experience more serious dermatological effects related to incontinence than those individuals without sensitive skin.

The physiological changes that occur as skin ages would predict an increased susceptibility to irritants, including urine and feces [82]. Existing studies, however, are ambiguous with regard to the influence of age on skin sensitivity. Clinical assessment of the erythematous response to irritants in older people suggests that susceptibility generally decreases with age [83]. However, objective signs of irritation often show little correlation with the intensity of subjective complaints [83]. A study of sensory perceptions of sensitive skin conducted on 1,039 individuals in Ohio stratified subjects into four age groups (subjects under 30, subjects in their 30s, subjects in their 40s, and those over 50) and evaluated subjective data according to age [83]. Those over 50 were more likely to claim sensitive skin than younger adults and more likely to perceive genital skin (to the exclusion of other body sites) to be more sensitive [83]. Older adults also stated that their skin had become more sensitive over time (46 %) [83]. In a large Italian study including over 100 elderly subjects that performed lactic acid sting tests on every subject, the intensity of the stinging response was inversely proportional to the age of the patient [84].

Urinary incontinence, however, represents a substantial psychosocial burden and is associated with a variety of psychiatric disorders, including depression, anxiety, decreased self-esteem, reduced social and personal interaction, and other psychological disorders [85–89]. It is possible, then, that incontinence may modulate these individual's perceptions of skin sensitivity, particularly in the genital area.

The vulva, formed partially from embryonic endoderm, differs from skin at exposed body sites [90] and displays differences in irritant potential which seem to be dependent on the relative permeability of irritants in vulvar skin: vulvar skin was shown to be significantly more reactive than forearm skin to benzalkonium chloride and maleic acid [91], but less reactive than the forearm to sodium lauryl sulfate [90, 92]. The non-keratinized skin of the vulva, however, exhibits clearly increased permeability [90] related to the absence of keratin, a loosely packed, less structured lipid barrier and a relative thinness as compared to keratinized skin [90]. Buccal tissue, similar in structure, is often employed in a surrogate model for vulvar testing; buccal skin has been demonstrated to be ten times more permeable than keratinized skin [93].

Although the vulvar area may be particularly susceptible to cutaneous irritation [94], little objective published data exists on the relationship between repeated exposure to habitual vulvar irritants and sensitive skin [95]. When tested, the vulvar area was less responsive to both venous blood and the products of menses than the upper arm [90, 92]. The contribution to irritation by topical agents is substantial [96, 97] and often underestimated [98]. In fact, 29 % of patients with chronic vulvar irritation were demonstrated to have contact hypersensitivity, and 94 % of those were determined to have developed secondary sensitization to topical medications [99]. Thus, incontinence may aggravate overlying issues in an aged patient as well, with sequelae which may differ in intensity in those with sensitive skin.

Recent studies have evaluated skin sensitivity in the vulvar area with regard to sensory responses to consumer products meant for the vulvar area. It was hypothesized that patients with erythema related to a previous genital infection may represent a population of sensitive subjects; however, no increase in sensory effects to exposure to feminine hygiene pads was observed [95]. In a similar population, however, in which observed erythema was evaluated against perceived sensory effects, women who perceived themselves as particularly susceptible to facial erythema were significantly more likely to have vulvar erythema, a potential indicator of an underlying biological origin [95].

Interestingly, a separate study evaluated perceptions of sensitive skin in women with urinary incontinence, expecting to observe an increased sensitivity of genital skin [100]. Increased sensitivity specific to the genital area was not observed, but incontinent women were significantly more likely to assess themselves as having overall skin sensitivity than continent subjects ($p = 0.014$; 86.2 % in incontinent subjects versus 68.3 % in controls) [100].

Summary

The economics of incontinence reflect its impact on older adults in the USA: $1.1 billion/year is spent on incontinence-related products and $16.4 billion/year on incontinence-related care [101]. Restoring normalcy to the lives of incontinent seniors and offering proper clinical care will greatly decrease the risk for serious dermatologic, social, and psychological problems in the aging population [1, 89]. Dermatologists who are knowledgeable about geriatric issues can help to maintain the health and quality of life of their older patients. Additional prospective clinical trials are needed to study the long-term efficacy of preventive hygiene measures as well as therapeutic interventions [3].

Cross-References

- ▶ Atopic Dermatitis in the Aged
- ▶ Effects of Aging on skin reactivity
- ▶ Irritant Contact Dermatitis
- ▶ Perceptions of Sensitive Skin with Age
- ▶ Solutions and Products for Managing Female Urinary Incontinence
- ▶ Susceptibility to Irritation in the Elderly

References

1. Millard RJ, Moore KH. Urinary incontinence: the Cinderella subject. Med J Aust. 1996;165:124–5.
2. Geriatric medicine. In: Tierney L, McPhee S, Papadakis M, editors. Geriatric medicine. In Current medical diagnosis and treatment 2000. New York: 39th McGraw Hill; 1999;62.
3. Farage MA, Bramante M. Genital hygiene: culture, practices, and health impact. In: Farage M, Maibach H, editors. The vulva: anatomy, physiology, and pathology. New York: LLC, Routledge/Taylor & Francis Group; 2006.
4. Roberts RO, Jacobsen SJ, Reilly WT, et al. Prevalence of combined fecal and urinary incontinence: a community-based study. J Am Geriatr Soc. 1999;47:837–41.
5. Gorina Y, Schappert S, Bercovitz A, et al. Prevalence of incontinence among older Americans. Vital Health Stat. 2014;3:1–33.
6. Cooper ZR, Rose S. Fecal incontinence: a clinical approach. Mt Sinai J Med. 2000;67:96–105.
7. Haugen V. Perineal skin care for patients with frequent diarrhea or fecal incontinence. Gastroenterol Nurs. 1997;20:87–90.
8. Nelson RL, Furner SE. Risk factors for the development of fecal and urinary incontinence in Wisconsin nursing home residents. Maturitas. 2005;52:26–31.
9. Stevens TK, Soffer EE, Palmer RM. Fecal incontinence in elderly patients: common, treatable, yet often undiagnosed. Cleve Clin J Med. 2003;70:441–8.
10. Gray M. Preventing and managing perineal dermatitis: a shared goal for wound and continence care. J Wound Ostomy Continence Nurs. 2004;31:S2–9. quiz S10–2.
11. Farage MA, Miller KW, Berardesca E, et al. Incontinence in the aged: contact dermatitis and other cutaneous consequences. Contact Dermatitis. 2007;57:211–7.
12. Burti JS, Santos AMB, Pereira RMR, et al. Prevalence and clinical characteristics of urinary incontinence in elderly individuals of a low income. Arch Gerontol Geriatr. 2012;54:e42–6.
13. Chew AL, Maibach HI, editors. Irritant Dermatitis. Berlin/Heidleberg Springer; 2005.
14. Rippke F, Schreiner V, Doering T, et al. Stratum corneum pH in atopic dermatitis: impact on skin barrier function and colonization with staphylococcus aureus. Am J Clin Dermatol. 2004;5:217–23.
15. Grubauer G, Elias PM, Feingold KR. Transepidermal water loss: the signal for recovery of barrier structure and function. J Lipid Res. 1989;30:323–33.
16. Zhai H, Maibach HI. Occlusion vs. skin barrier function. Skin Res Technol. 2002;8:1–6.
17. Aly R, Shirley C, Cunico B, et al. Effect of prolonged occlusion on the microbial flora, pH, carbon dioxide and transepidermal water loss on human skin. J Invest Dermatol. 1978;71:378–81.
18. Zhai H, Maibach H. Effects of occlusion: percutaneous absorption. In: Bronaugh R, Maibach H, editors. Percutaneous absorption, drug-cosmetics-mechanisms-methodology. Boca Raton: Taylor and Francis; 2005.
19. Taljebini M, Warren R, Mao-Oiang M, et al. Cutaneous permeability barrier repair following various types of insults: kinetics and effects of occlusion. Skin Pharmacol. 1996;9:111–9.
20. Fisher LB, Maibach HI, Trancik RJ. Variably occlusive tape systems and the mitotic activity of stripped human epidermis. Effects with and without hydrocortisone. Arch Dermatol. 1978;114:727–9.
21. Proksch E, Feingold KR, Man MQ, et al. Barrier function regulates epidermal DNA synthesis. J Clin Invest. 1991;87:1668–73.

22. Emilson A, Lindberg M, Forslind B, et al. Quantitative and 3-dimensional analysis of Langerhans' cells following occlusion with patch tests using confocal laser scanning microscopy. Acta Derm Venereol. 1993;73:323–9.
23. Proksch E, Brasch J, Sterry W. Integrity of the permeability barrier regulates epidermal Langerhans cell density. Br J Dermatol. 1996;134:630–8.
24. Wood LC, Elias PM, Calhoun C, et al. Barrier disruption stimulates interleukin-1 alpha expression and release from a pre-formed pool in murine epidermis. J Invest Dermatol. 1996;106:397–403.
25. Zhai H, Maibach HI. Skin occlusion and irritant and allergic contact dermatitis: an overview. Contact Dermatitis. 2001;44:201–6.
26. Kligman A. Hydration injury to human skin. In: Van der Valk P, Maibach H, editors. The irritant contact dermatitis syndrome. Boca Raton: CRC Press; 1996.
27. Beguin A, Malaquin-Pavan E, Guihaire C, et al. Improving diaper design to address incontinence associated dermatitis. BMC Geriatr. 2010;10:86.
28. Zulkowski K. Protecting your patient's aging skin. Nursing. 2003;33:84.
29. Waller JM, Maibach HI. Age and skin structure and function, a quantitative approach (I): blood flow, pH, thickness, and ultrasound echogenicity. Skin Res Technol. 2005;11:221–35.
30. Cerruto MA, D'Elia C, Aloisi A, et al. Prevalence, incidence and obstetric factors' impact on female urinary incontinence in Europe: a systematic review. Urol Int. 2013;90:1–9.
31. Fiers SA. Breaking the cycle: the etiology of incontinence dermatitis and evaluating and using skin care products. Ostomy Wound Manage. 1996;42:32–4. 36, 38–40, passim.
32. Zimmerer RE, Lawson KD, Calvert CJ. The effects of wearing diapers on skin. Pediatr Dermatol. 1986;3:95–101.
33. Andersen PH, Maibach HI. Skin irritation in man: a comparative bioengineering study using improved reflectance spectroscopy. Contact Dermatitis. 1995;33:315–22.
34. Nangia A, Andersen PH, Berner B, et al. High dissociation constants (pKa) of basic permeants are associated with in vivo skin irritation in man. Contact Dermatitis. 1996;34:237–42.
35. Berg RW, Buckingham KW, Stewart RL. Etiologic factors in diaper dermatitis: the role of urine. Pediatr Dermatol. 1986;3:102–6.
36. Berg RW. Etiologic factors in diaper dermatitis: a model for development of improved diapers. Pediatrician. 1987;14 Suppl 1:27–33.
37. Berg RW, Milligan MC, Sarbaugh FC. Association of skin wetness and pH with diaper dermatitis. Pediatr Dermatol. 1994;11:18–20.
38. Andersen PH, Bucher AP, Saeed I, et al. Faecal enzymes: in vivo human skin irritation. Contact Dermatitis. 1994;30:152–8.
39. Sivamani R, Wu G, Maibach H, et al. Tribological studies on skin: measurement of the coefficient of friction. In: Serup J, Jemec B, Grove G, editors. Handbook of non-invasive methods and the skin. Boca Raton: Taylor and Francis; 2006.
40. Panel for the prediction and prevention of pressure ulcers in adults. Pressure ulcers in adults: prediction and prevention. US Department of Health and Human Services, Agency for Health Care Policy and Research; 1992.
41. Roskos KV, Guy RH. Assessment of skin barrier function using transepidermal water loss: effect of age. Pharm Res. 1989;6:949–53.
42. Brown DS. Perineal dermatitis: can we measure it? Ostomy Wound Manage. 1993;39:28–30. 31.
43. Fiers S, Thayer D. Management of intractable incontinence. In: Doughty D, editor. Urinary and fecal incontinence: nursing management. St. Louis: Mosby; 2000.
44. Scardillo J, Aronovitch SA. Successfully managing incontinence-related irritant dermatitis across the lifespan. Ostomy Wound Manage. 1999;45:36–40. 42–4.
45. Long MA, Reed LA, Dunning K, et al. Incontinence-associated dermatitis in a long-term acute care facility. J Wound Ostomy Continence Nurs. 2012; 39:318–27.
46. Gray M, Beeckman D, Bliss DZ, et al. Incontinence-associated dermatitis: a comprehensive review and update. J Wound Ostomy Continence Nurs. 2012;39:61–74.
47. Gray M. Context for WOC practice: peristomal recurrence of Crohn's disease, hospital-acquired pressure ulcers, negative pressure wound therapy, and incontinence-associated dermatitis. J Wound Ostomy Continence Nurs. 2012;39:227–9.
48. Kirss F, Lang K, Toompere K, et al. Prevalence and risk factors of urinary incontinence among Estonian postmenopausal women. Springerplus. 2013; 2:524.
49. Bliss DZ, Harms S, Garrard JM, et al. Prevalence of incontinence by race and ethnicity of older people admitted to nursing homes. J Am Med Dir Assoc. 2013;14:451.e1–7.
50. Whitman D. Intra-abdominal infections: pathophysiology and treatment. Frankfurt: Hoechst; 1991.
51. Lutz J. Etiology of adult incontinence dermatitis. Pre-conference workshop: device use and skin care management of incontinence. Multispecialty Nursing Conference on Urinary Continence in Adults. Phoenix. 20 Jan 1984.
52. Rohwer K, Bliss DZ, Savik K. Incontinence-associated dermatitis in community-dwelling individuals with fecal incontinence. J Wound Ostomy Continence Nurs. 2013;40:181–4.
53. Shannon ML, Lehman CA. Protecting the skin of the elderly patient in the intensive care unit. Crit Care Nurs Clin North Am. 1996;8:17–28.

54. Lyder CH, Clemes-Lowrance C, Davis A, et al. Structured skin care regimen to prevent perineal dermatitis in the elderly. J ET Nurs. 1992;19:12–6.
55. Skin bacteria and their role in infection. New York: McGraw-Hill; 1965.
56. Miller J, Hoffman E. The causes and consequences of overactive bladder. J Womens Health (Larchmt). 2006;15:251–60.
57. Sibbald RG, Campbell K, Coutts P, et al. Intact skin – an integrity not to be lost. Ostomy Wound Manage. 2003;49:27–8. 30, 33 passim, contd.
58. Bardsley A. Prevention and management of incontinence-associated dermatitis. Nurs Stand. 2013;27:41–6.
59. Shenefelt PD, Fenske NA. Aging and the skin: recognizing and managing common disorders. Geriatrics. 1990;45:57–9. 63-6.
60. Maibach HI, Kligman AM. The biology of experimental human cutaneous moniliasis (*Candida albicans*). Arch Dermatol. 1962;85:233–57.
61. LeLievre S. Skin care for older people with incontinence. Elder Care. 2000;11:36–8.
62. Krasner D. Alterations in skin integrity related to continence management/incontinence: some problems and solutions. Ostomy Wound Manage. 1990;28:62–3.
63. Omura Y, O'Young B, Jones M, et al. Caprylic acid in the effective treatment of intractable medical problems of frequent urination, incontinence, chronic upper respiratory infection, root canalled tooth infection, ALS, etc., caused by asbestos & mixed infections of *Candida albicans*, *Helicobacter pylor* i & *Cytomegalovirus* with or without other microorganisms & mercury. Acupunct Electrother Res. 2011;36:19–64.
64. Scheinfeld N. Infections in the elderly. Dermatol Online J. 2005;11:8.
65. Caquant F, Collinet P, Deruelle P, et al. Perineal cellulitis following trans-obturator sub-urethral tape Uratape. Eur Urol. 2005;47:108–10.
66. Connolly TP. Necrotizing surgical site infection after tension-free vaginal tape. Obstet Gynecol. 2004;104:1275–6.
67. Nathan L. Vulvovaginal disorders in the elderly woman. Clin Obstet Gynecol. 1996;39:933–45.
68. Edlich RF, Winters KL, Woodard CR, et al. Pressure ulcer prevention. J Long Term Eff Med Implants. 2004;14:285–304.
69. Temkin-Greener H, Cai S, Zheng NT, et al. Nursing home work environment and the risk of pressure ulcers and incontinence. Health Serv Res. 2012;47:1179–200.
70. Fader M, Clarke-O'Neill S, Cook D, et al. Management of night-time urinary incontinence in residential settings for older people: an investigation into the effects of different pad changing regimes on skin health. J Clin Nurs. 2003;12:374–86.
71. Clever K, Smith G, Bowser C, et al. Evaluating the efficacy of a uniquely delivered skin protectant and its effect on the formation of sacral/buttock pressure ulcers. Ostomy Wound Manage. 2002;48:60–7.
72. Thompson P, Langemo D, Anderson J, et al. Skin care protocols for pressure ulcers and incontinence in long-term care: a quasi-experimental study. Adv Skin Wound Care. 2005;18:422–9.
73. Beeckman D, Woodward S, Rajpaul K, et al. Clinical challenges of preventing incontinence-associated dermatitis. Br J Nurs. 2011;20:784–6. 788,790.
74. Bryant R. Acute and chronic wounds: nursing management. St. Louis: Mosby; 1992.
75. Corcoran E, Woodward S. Incontinence-associated dermatitis in the elderly: treatment options. Br J Nurs. 2013;22:450–2. 454–7.
76. Beldon P. Incontinence-associated dermatitis: protecting the older person. Br J Nurs. 2012;21:402. 404–7.
77. Nix D, Haugen V. Prevention and management of incontinence-associated dermatitis. Drugs Aging. 2010;27:491–6.
78. Talasz H, Jansen SC, Kofler M, et al. High prevalence of pelvic floor muscle dysfunction in hospitalized elderly women with urinary incontinence. Int Urogynecol J. 2012;23:1231–7.
79. Beeckman D, Woodward S, Gray M. Incontinence-associated dermatitis: step-by-step prevention and treatment. Br J Community Nurs. 2011;16:382–9.
80. Gray M. Optimal management of incontinence-associated dermatitis in the elderly. Am J Clin Dermatol. 2010;11:201–10.
81. Farage MA, Maibach HI. Sensitive skin: new findings yield new insights. In: Baran R, Maibach HI, editors. Textbook of cosmetic dermatology. New York: Informa Healthcare; 2010.
82. Farage MA, Miller KW, Maibach HI. Degenerative changes in aging skin. In: Farage MA, Miller KW, Maibach HI, editors. Textbook of aging skin. Berlin/Heidleberg: Springer; 2010.
83. Farage MA. Perceptions of sensitive skin with age. In: Farage MA, Miller KM, Maibach HI, editors. Textbook of aging skin. Berlin/Heidleberg: Springer; 2010.
84. Sparavigna A, Di Pietro A, Setaro M. 'Healthy skin': significance and results of an Italian study on healthy population with particular regard to 'sensitive' skin. Int J Cosmet Sci. 2005;27:327–31.
85. Stach-Lempinen B, Hakala A, Laippala P, et al. Severe depression determines quality of life in urinary incontinent women. Neurourol Urodyn. 2003;22:563–8.
86. Perry S, McGrother CW, Turner K. An investigation of the relationship between anxiety and depression and urge incontinence in women: development of a psychological model. Br J Health Psychol. 2006;11:463–82.
87. Jackson S. The patient with an overactive bladder – symptoms and quality-of-life issues. Urology. 1997;50:18–22. discussion 23–4.

88. Specht JKP. 9 myths of incontinence in older adults: both clinicians and the over-65 set need to know more. Am J Nurs. 2005;105:58–68. quiz 69.
89. Farage MA, Miller KW, Berardesca E, et al. Psychosocial and societal burden of incontinence in the aged population: a review. Arch Gynecol Obstet. 2008;277:285–90.
90. Farage MA, Maibach HI. The vulvar epithelium differs from the skin: implications for cutaneous testing to address topical vulvar exposures. Contact Dermatitis. 2004;51:201–9.
91. Britz MB, Maibach HI, Anjo DM. Human percutaneous penetration of hydrocortisone: the vulva. Arch Dermatol Res. 1980;267:313–6.
92. Farage MA, Warren R, Wang-Weigand S. The vulva is relatively insensitive to menses-induced irritation. Cutan Ocul Toxicol. 2005;24:243–6.
93. Squier CA, Hall BK. The permeability of skin and oral mucosa to water and horseradish peroxidase as related to the thickness of the permeability barrier. J Invest Dermatol. 1985;84:176–9.
94. Farage MA, Stadler A, Elsner P, et al. Safety evaluation of modern feminine hygiene pads: two decades of use. Female Patient. 2004;29:23–30.
95. Farage MA, Bowtell P, Katsarou A. The relationship among objectively assessed vulvar erythema, skin sensitivity, genital sensitivity, and self-reported facial skin redness. J Appl Res. 2006;6:272.
96. Lee CH, Maibach HI. The sodium lauryl sulfate model: an overview. Contact Dermatitis. 1995;33:1–7.
97. Basketter DA, Wilhelm KP. Studies on non-immune immediate contact reactions in an unselected population. Contact Dermatitis. 1996;35:237–40.
98. Farage MA. Vulvar susceptibility to contact irritants and allergens: a review. Arch Gynecol Obstet. 2005;272:167–72.
99. Marren P, Wojnarowska F, Powell S. Allergic contact dermatitis and vulvar dermatoses. Br J Dermatol. 1992;126:52–6.
100. Farage MA. Perceptions of sensitive skin: women with urinary incontinence. Arch Gynecol Obstet. 2009;280:49–57.
101. Agency for Health Care Policy and Research (AHCPR). Overview: urinary incontinence in adults, clinical practice guideline update. http://www.ahrq.gov/clinic/uiovervw.htm. Accessed 18 Jan 2015.

Aging Skin as a Diagnostic Tool for Internal Diseases: A Chance for Dermatology

67

Georgios Nikolakis, Evgenia Makrantonaki, and Christos C. Zouboulis

Contents

Abstract

Aged skin is an easily accessible and cost-effective model for the determination of aging of the whole human organism and eventually for the prediction of other age-related comorbidities. Its endogenous variable is called intrinsic aging, while the effect of external factors, such as UV radiation, is termed extrinsic aging. In this overview, key hallmarks, which determine intrinsic aging and extrinsic aging, are mentioned. These include aging of the cellular components of the skin, as well as of the dermal components, i.e., the extracellular matrix. Furthermore, the most common age-related diseases are presented. At last, evidence for the predicting value of aged skin for the development or course of certain pathological conditions is elucidated.

Introduction

Aging is defined as a natural, gradual process of biochemical events, leading to gradual damage accumulation and resulting in disease and death [1]. Such changes are hidden as far as the inner organs are concerned and, therefore, the skin appears as the first and main teller of these gradual alterations [2]. Moreover, the easy and cost-effective accessibility of this organ, as well as the detection or isolation of its main cellular (keratinocytes, fibroblasts, hair follicle and sebaceous cells, mast cells, Langerhans cells, etc.) and

G. Nikolakis • C.C. Zouboulis (✉)
Departments of Dermatology, Venereology, Allergology and Immunology, Dessau Medical Center, Dessau, Germany
e-mail: nikolakisgeorgios@gmail.com; christos.zouboulis@klinikum-dessau.de

E. Makrantonaki
Departments of Dermatology, Venereology, Allergology and Immunology, Dessau Medical Center, Dessau, Germany

Geriatry Research Group, Charité Universitaetsmedizin Berlin, Berlin, Germany

Department of Dermatology and Allergology, University Medical Center Ulm, Ulm, Germany
e-mail: makrant@yahoo.com

M.A. Farage et al. (eds.), *Textbook of Aging Skin*,
DOI 10.1007/978-3-662-47398-6_125

noncellular components (extracellular matrix, collagen, elastin), provides a model for the assessment and determination of the involved molecular mechanisms [3]. For this, it can be considered the "key hole" to observe the aging process of the whole organism.

Skin has long been recognized to protect organisms against deleterious environmental factors and is important for the homeostasis of temperature, electrolyte, and fluid balance of the body [4].

Skin Aging: A Different Pathophysiology Leads to A Different Phenotype

Aged skin is characterized by a phenotype of a disturbed lipid barrier, angiogenesis, production of sweat, gradual deterioration of the epidermal immune response and production of calcitriol, cellular heterogeneity, as well as the tendency toward development of various benign or malignant diseases [5, 6]. These biological processes include endogenous variables such as genetic predisposition, impairment of cellular metabolic pathways, and qualitative and quantitative hormonal alterations, termed intrinsic aging. At the other end of the spectrum, exogenous factors, such as ultraviolet (UV) irradiation, chemicals and toxins, and pollution, lead to extrinsic aging [7]. Based on this knowledge, two experimental models of human skin were developed and utilized in order to express the two main axes of skin aging (patho)physiology: The model for intrinsic aging is the skin deriving from areas which are not sun exposed, such as the inner side of the upper arm and the gluteal region, while for the model for extrinsic aging, it involves constantly UV-exposed skin regions, such as the facial skin. The phenotype of intrinsically aged skin appears macroscopically thin and atrophic and exhibits fine wrinkles, subcutaneous fat loss, prominent dryness, and reduced elasticity [8]. In contrast, extrinsically photoaged skin exhibits deeper wrinkles, thickening of the epidermis, dullness, roughness, and mottled discoloration. Telangiectasias and pigmentary discoloration might also be observed in advanced and severe degrees of photoaging [8–13].

The phenotype of aging shows considerable variations between different ethnical groups. Caucasians have greater skin wrinkle formation and sagging in comparison to other skin phenotypes, while the manifestations have an earlier onset [14]. Furthermore, Caucasians are more prone to skin desquamation, which is dependent of age [15]. Afro-American and Caucasian women are both having a higher prevalence of age-related dryness compared to other ethnicity groups [16]. Chinese women have more severe periorbital wrinkles in comparison to women from Japan, while Thai women were characterized by severe wrinkling of the lower half of their faces [17]. Caucasian females have a higher prevalence of sagging in the subzygomatic area [14]. Wrinkling in each facial area has a later onset in Chinese women in comparison to French women, although age-related pigment spot intensity is the cardinal sign of aging in Chinese women [18]. Lastly, although Asian skin seems to have similar transepidermal water loss and ceramide levels to Caucasian skin, the stratum corneum barrier appears to be more susceptible to mechanical stimuli. Asian skin is more sensitive to exogenous chemicals because of the thinner stratum corneum barrier, higher eccrine gland intensity, and smaller pore areas in comparison to other ethnic groups, indicating the correlation of the latter to the sebaceous gland activity [14]. Since skin aging phenotype varies according to the population, not universal but ethnicity-specific aging characteristics could only be correlated with age-associated diseases. Photographic severity scales and other clinical methods are developed to assess the severity of skin aging features [8, 19].

Intrinsic Aging

Current experimental research led to the development of different theories in order to determine different pathophysiological key aspects of aging. Among them are the theory of cellular senescence, telomere shortening and decreased proliferative capacity, the inflammation theory, mitochondrial DNA single mutations, and the free radical theory [20–25].

Cellular Senescence

Senescence is the term used to describe the decrease of regenerative potential of cells or tissues through an individual's lifetime. The mechanisms involved in these processes involve response to numerous cellular stresses, including production of reactive oxygen species and telomere shortening. Lately, the role of microRNAs has been highlighted as fine tuners of the balance between proliferative capacity and replicative senescence of skin key cellular components, such as keratinocytes and fibroblasts [26].

Human dermal fibroblasts were shown to exhibit enlarged cell bodies after many series of passages in vitro. Furthermore, they were more often stained positive for the myofibroblast marker α-smooth actin, the senescence markers β-galactosidase, and p16, in comparison to early passage fibroblasts. The fibroblasts were in a subsequent step involved in the creation of in vitro reconstructed skin or human skin equivalents (HSE). HSE formation with late passage fibroblasts resulted in an altered phenotype mimicking intrinsic aging in vivo with thinner dermis and reduced matrix formation, and weaker expression of the differentiation marker keratin 10 [27], highlighting the effects of aging in ECM quality, keratinocyte differentiation, and strata formation. However, the changes regarding epidermal proliferation and the basement membrane, which are observed in vivo, were missing [28].

Both matrix degradation and pro-inflammatory responses are involved in skin aging. Recent studies compared the genome of human sebocytes and whole skin and the secretome of normal human fibroblasts isolated from intrinsically aged skin of young, middle-aged, and old donors. Thirty-nine genes and 70 proteins depicted an age-dependent pattern. Twenty-seven of the proteins were isolated exclusively from intrinsically aged skin and are associated with processes such as metabolism and adherence junction interactions. These present a distinct pattern related to intrinsic aging mechanisms, thus differing from the classical senescent-associated secretory phenotype of cellular senescence, mentioned later in "immunological impairment" [29].

High-passage fibroblasts deriving from the papillary and reticular dermis were utilized for the reconstruction of artificial skin in vitro [30]. The HSE which were formed from reticular fibroblasts showed impaired differentiation patterns and areas of impaired epidermal strata formation. More specifically, a more prominent expression of the epidermal differentiation markers loricrin, filaggrin, and small proline-rich protein 2 in the stratum granulosum and corneum of the HSE deriving from papillary fibroblasts in comparison to reticular fibroblast-derived ones was observed. In addition, the presence of papillary fibroblasts resulted in a higher number of Ki67-positive basal keratinocytes. Papillary fibroblast senescence led to a more reticular-like fibroblast phenotype [30].

Another approach to assimilate intrinsic aging is to use normal human fibroblasts and prolong the culture time of HSEs for up to 120 days. The phenotypic changes resembled the ones of in vivo intrinsic aging with a significant decrease of the epidermis thickness and the number of basal keratinocytes expressing the proliferation marker Ki67. Moreover, differentiation markers were also strongly decreased, while as the senescence marker p16INK4a was significantly increased [31].

Immunological Alterations

Aging is usually associated with a gradual deterioration of the immune system and immunological swifts named immunosenescence. In contrast, it is also reported to correlate to a hyper-inflammatory state, termed inflamm-aging [2, 32]. The impairment of the aged immune system makes it susceptible to certain infections, autoimmune diseases, and malignancies. The age-relating processes in this case are not exclusively intrinsic, but extrinsic factors such as UV damage are also being involved [33]. Damaged cells secrete inflammatory mediators, such as prostaglandins and leukotrienes, inducing the release of tumor necrosis factor-α (TNF-α) and histamine from resident mast cells. This leads to the release of P-selectins and the upregulation of adhesion molecules, as well as interleukin-1 dysregulation. Molecules which can promote the intercellular adhesion molecule-1 (ICAM-1) synthesis and the subsequent recruitment of circulating immune cells in the dermis are aging factors. On a subsequent step, these inflammatory cells release proteases and radical oxygen species, which provoke long-term damage in cutaneous cells [33–37]. Surface oxidative damage leads to formation of squalene peroxide, which correlates with extrinsic aging factors, mainly UV damage [33]. Senescent cells are believed to force the surrounding cells in acquiring the so-called senescent-associated secretory phenotype by the secretion of various pro-inflammatory factors [38]. Furthermore, there is increasing evidence that chronic inflammation correlates with normal aging and impairs stem cell dysfunction [39].

Disruption of Epidermal Barrier

With advancing age, the epidermis develops an abnormality of the barrier homeostasis, which is even more prominent in photoaged skin [2, 40]. This is due to an overall reduction of stratum corneum lipids and a disturbance regarding the cholesterol and fatty acid synthesis [41]. Alterations in the cell membrane lipids are observed with human cell aging, such as the decrease in the polyunsaturated fatty acid content of phospholipids and the increase in cholesterol levels. Modulation of peroxisome proliferator-activated receptor gamma (PPARγ) in human dermal fibroblasts partially reduces the effects of stressed induced senescence through 8-methoxypsoralen plus UVA irradiation, such as such cytoplasmic enlargement, the expression of senescence-associated-beta-galactosidase, matrix-metalloproteinase-1, cell cycle proteins, and cell membrane lipid alterations [42]. Not only the "mortar" of the skin barrier but the bricks as well are affected by aging: Genes associated with keratinocyte differentiation, including keratins and cornified envelope components, undergo an age-related downregulation [43]. Sebaceous lipids are also implicated in skin aging. The potential release of sebaceous lipids was highlighted in the recent development of a co-culture model of ex vivo skin with immortalized sebocytes. Although the sebaceous glands of the ex vivo skin were rapidly degenerated, co-culture of the latter with immortalized sebocytes led to a partial prevention of age-related events of the explant epidermis, namely, basal keratinocyte proliferation and apoptosis of epidermal cells [44].

Intrinsic Aging of Other Skin Cell Types

Not only the major components composing the skin but other cell types, such as the ones comprising the skin appendages, undergo age-related changes through intrinsic and/or extrinsic aging. A premium example is the sebaceous gland. Sebaceous gland cells also show a profound decrease of sebaceous lipid release, which is age related, as well as a decrease of the size of sebaceous cells [45–47], after an initial increase, i.e., senile sebaceous gland hyperplasia, in order to compensate the reduction of the single-cell capacity to produce lipids [47]. These particular in vivo observations were confirmed after in vitro treatment of human sebocytes with a hormone mixture of androgens, estrogens, and growth factor levels correlating to the average serum levels of 20-year-old and 60-year-old women. Significant reduction of sebaceous lipogenesis was the result of the treatment with the 60-year-old hormone mixture in comparison to the former, showing remarkable correlation to the phenotypical changes observed in vivo. Differences in gene expression were reported, according to the age correspondence of the mixture used. These differences included the regulation of genes, which were shown to be regulated and were implicated in DNA repair and stability, oxidative stress, mitochondrial processes, ubiquitin-induced proteolysis, cell cycle and apoptosis, and other pathways. The most significantly altered pathway was that of tumor growth factor-β, known for its association with malignancies [48]. Moreover, genes which are associated with the development of neurodegenerative diseases were reported to be expressed in human sebaceous cells, also prone to regulation through hormone treatment. These results are supported from the common embryogenic origin of the skin and the neuronal tissue and suggest interesting perspectives for the skin and rejuvenation research: Taking into account the fact that the skin and the nervous system both derive from the ectoderm, this finding led to the logical assumption that skin may be used as a tool for investigating aging of the nervous system. Additional experiments, in which the whole genome of human skin biopsies from young and elderly males and females was investigated, confirmed this hypothesis. Skin expresses several genes associated with age-associated diseases of the nerve system, and these genes are regulated with increasing age, may be due to the accompanying hormone decline [49].

The hair follicle is also susceptible to intrinsic and extrinsic aging mechanisms. There is a specialized mesenchymal population, called the dermal papilla, the number and senescence of which is correlated with follicular decline [50]. The dermal papilla, located in the hair follicle, is capable to express androgen receptors and plays an important role in hair growth. Dermal papilla cells deriving from patients with androgenetic alopecia were reported to have an increased expression of senescence marker p16INK4a. The fact that the treatment of these cells with androgens led to p16INK4a upregulation suggests a major role of the androgen/androgen receptor complex in the pathogenesis of hair follicle aging. Interestingly, these effects are observed from non-balding frontal and transitional zone of balding scalp follicles but not in beard follicles [51]. Hair graying is known also a hallmark of aging, with a pathophysiology ranging from follicular melanocyte stem cell defects to follicular melanocyte death [52, 53]. Oxidative damage leads to selective apoptosis of melanocyte stem cells, through depletion of the antiapoptotic B-cell lymphoma 2 gene (BCL-2). BCL-2 is known to be expressed in order for melanocytes to evade UVA-induced ROS damage [54]. Aging hair follicle stem cells of the mouse epidermis showed increased amounts of 53BP1-foci, independent of telomere shortening, suggesting increased number of double-stand breaks in these cells [55].

Dermal Aging

The number and composition of skin glycosaminoglycans (GAGs) change, as it was depicted in corneal keratinocytes and skin-derived fibroblasts. Hyaluronan appears to have a prominent role among the different components involved [56, 57]. Hyaluronan is a GAG which has the ability to bind and retain water molecules [58], contributing direly to skin hydration [59]. It was shown to affect the expression of metalloproteinases (MMPs). MMPs are special proteases implicated in physiological and pathological skin processes, prime examples of which are skin morphogenesis, tissue remodeling, wound healing, and tumorigenesis [60]. Different proteases such as trypsin and plasmin regulate the MMP activity in the level of transcription and level of activation of the inactive zymogen forms. Hyaluronan increases expression and activation of MMP-2 and MMP-9 of skin explant cultures [61]. Epidermal hyaluronan disappears from aged skin, while reduction of the size of polymers may also result in an overall reduction of skin moisture [62, 63]. The expression of hyaluronan and its surface receptor drastically decreases after prolonged culture ex vivo in an HSE [31]. miR-23a-3p microRNA, which targets the enzyme hyaluronan synthase-2, was upregulated in the skin of old mice compared to young ones [64]. As far as skin explant cultures are concerned, other ECM components, such as dermatan sulfate, keratan sulfate, and chondroitin sulfate, can upregulate MMP-9 activation, thus being of pathophysiological significance for skin remodeling [65].

The ECM of the skin comprises different complex components such as collagen proteins, glycosaminoglycan-rich proteoglycans, and elastic fibers. The ECM is constantly under structural modification and remodeling, with main components the collagen I and III, which offer skin its tensile strength [2]. Skin elasticity is due to various other ECM molecules with slow turnover rate, mainly elastin and fibrillin-1, which form an elastin core and a microfibrillar scaffold. Fibrillin-1 is one of the potential biomarkers for the objective assessment of aging [66, 67]. The fact that many ECM molecules are not rapidly regenerating makes them excellent potential immunohistochemical targets for quantifying dermal aging.

Glycation

Glycation is the nonenzymatic reaction between sugars and proteins, and lipids and nucleic acids. A long-standing high level of sugar in rats was shown to decrease epidermal lipid synthesis, lamellar body production, and antimicrobial peptide expression [68]. The impact of advanced glycation end products (AGEs) and in aging has been highlighted over the recent years. Their formation is a stepwise process and starts with the Maillard reaction, which ends to the production of a non-stable Schiff base (or an Amadori product after further rearrangements) after reaction of the sugar carbonyl groups with amino groups of protein amino acid residues [69]. Stable products might result also after protein adduct formation or cross-linking of Schiff base or Amadori products. AGEs exert their actions both per se and through interaction with specific receptors (receptor for AGEs – RAGE). This is a pattern recognition receptor, binding also various other molecules such as S100, β-amyloids, and β-sheet fibrils [70, 71]. Binding of AGEs leads to activation of NFκB and transcription of various inflammatory genes [72]. AGEs are accumulated gradually with aging. Increased levels of AGEs are the result of diseases such as diabetes mellitus, the excessive production of ROS, dietary factors, and smoking [71, 73]. AGEs deposition in peripheral tissues is implicated in many diseases, such as diabetes-related macular degeneration, osteoarthritis, and diabetic angiopathy [74–77]. AGEs contribute to the impairment of the arterial wall content, through their accumulation together with gradual elastin reduction [78, 79]. AGEs significantly increased TGF-β1 and metalloproteinase-2 expression in cardiac fibroblasts, which are implicated in aging and ECM remodeling, respectively [80]. Total content of AGEs accumulated in the organism is also defined from their removal rate, in which the glutathione-dependent system of glyoxalase I and II, as well as the fructosyl amine oxidases and the fructosamine kinases [81, 82]. Proteins with a slow turnover rate, like collagen types I and IV, are mainly susceptible to glycation during intrinsic aging [83, 84]. Collagen glycation leads to intermolecular cross-link formation of adjacent collagen fibers, leading to decreased flexibility and stiffness [85]. Moreover, AGE-induced collagen modification makes collagen resistant to MMP proteolysis, thus hindering its degradation and substitution with new and functional fibers [86]. Other ECM protein targets are elastin and fibronectin [83, 84, 87]. AGEs mediate their effects also directly on cells, by reducing the proliferation and inducing the premature senescence apoptosis of dermal fibroblasts [88], decreasing keratinocyte cell viability and migration [89], and the premature cellular senescence of both [90–92]. In a recent study, AGE-associated skin autofluorescence was reported to mirror the vascular function. The authors analyzed the AGE modifications in collagens obtained from residual bypass graft material via hydroxyproline assay and AGE intrinsic fluorescence and correlated their findings with skin autofluorescence measured by an autofluorescence reader. In addition, they measured pulse wave velocity which reflects vessel stiffness and correlated the findings. They found that skin autofluorescence and pulse wave velocity significantly correlate with the content of AGE in graft material so that both methods could be utilized as predictive markers of vessel function in patients suffering from coronary heart disease [93, 94]. Recently, a glycated reconstructed skin equivalent was assembled from glycation-induced extracellular matrix, in order to facilitate the investigation [95].

Furthermore, nonenzymatic glycation substantially affects the collagen's ability to dissipate energy in bony tissue. Glycation-related alterations of bone's organic matrix, mostly collage type I, reduce its capacity to withstand strain forces typically associated with fall (3000–5000 μstrain) [96]. Moreover, there is evidence that it leads to age-related anemia and hematopoietic stem cell exhaustion [97], ocular neovascularization [98], compromised lymph flow [99], etc. Series of experiments are needed to correlate skin AGE accumulation with the previously mentioned comorbidities, in order to provide robust models of global aging in the near future.

Skin Stem Cell Aging

Stem cells are cells able to undergo self-regeneration by multiple cycles of division, while retaining their undifferentiated phenotype [100, 101]. Embryonic stem cells are multipotent cells and are able to give rise to all other cell types, while adult stem cells have more restricted potentials. The latter have also high proliferative capacity and are required for tissue renewal throughout the organism life span [102]. As far as the skin is concerned, epidermal stem cells are located in the stratum basale and differentiate to transient amplifying cells (TA-cells) and differentiating progenitors, forming functional epidermal proliferative units (EPUs), and extending from the basal to the corneal layer [103]. Furthermore, dermal stem cells are also of great importance for skin homeostasis, since they produce the progeny responsible for ECM synthesis and growth factors. Although they are of mesodermal origin, they can give rise to endodermal liver cells and ectodermal nerve cells, suggesting the potential for giving birth to a broader palette of cell type progenitors [102, 104, 105]. Since they comprise the pool of tissue regeneration, stem cells also came in focus of the aging research as a potential target of intrinsic and extrinsic aging factors, which could potentially affect the number and the function of these cells. On the other hand, the potential therapeutic effects of utilization of stem cells, and especially the abundant and easy way to access adipose-derived stem cells, are also being examined [106, 107].

The epidermal turnover rate is 28 days in young individuals, while it varies between 40 and 60 days in the elderly [108]. Epidermal stem cells are considered unique in comparison to other adult stem cells in their ability to resist aging. They show no effects associated with increased ROS levels, perhaps as a result of maintaining high levels of superoxide dismutase [109]. Interestingly, stem cell numbers do not necessarily decline with age [110]. However there are studies suggesting a functional deficit to produce differentiated progeny [111]. Wound healing is a prime example, since keratinocytes isolated from older donors give rise to a lower proportion of holoclones, in comparison to younger ones [112]. Higher levels of the senescence marker p16INK4A in human epidermal cells of senior individuals [113] suggest an impairment of stem cell mobilization with age, as well as the inability to respond to proliferating signals. Furthermore, epidermal stem cells of older individuals express lower levels of the stem cell markers β1-integrin and melanoma chondroitin sulfate proteoglycan (MCSP), which are correlated with the higher self-renewal capacity [114].

Multiple mechanisms are involved in stem cell exhaustion. DNA repair mechanism deficits are considered one of the main causes. Deletion of the DNA repair gene ataxia–telangiectasia and rad3-related (ATR) protein resulted in progeroid phenotypes in adult mice, involving alopecia, kyphosis, osteoporosis, thymic involution, and fibrosis [115]. Experiments with mouse skin have shown that epidermal stem cells are resistant to cellular aging [116, 117], highlighting the role of the microenvironment (stem cell niche) in age-related stem cell exhaustion [102, 110, 118]. Accumulation of 53BP1 foci throughout the highly compacted heterochromatin of aged hair follicle stem cells confirmed that DNA damage is between the primary mechanisms of stem cell exhaustion [55].

Jak-Stat and Notch pathways are involved to age-associated epidermal stem cell alterations [119]. More specifically, cells of the aging epidermis as well as the epidermal stem cell population express high levels of phosphorylated Stat3, which is also involved in tumor progression [119–122], whereas skin was used as a model to provide insights in the way that aging is linked with age-associated pathophysiologic events, including inflammation and tumorigenesis. The Wnt and mTOR pathways are also involved in skin aging. Persistent expression of Wnt1 led to rapid growth of hair follicles, followed by epithelial stem cell senescence, apoptosis, and epidermal stem cell exhaustion [123]. Lastly, the PI3K-Akt pathway is involved in the senescence of embryonic neural crest- or somite-derived multipotent progenitor cells with properties of stem cells of the dermal compartment, termed skin-derived precursors. These cells were shown to contribute to wound healing, maintenance of the dermis, and hair follicle morphogenesis [124]. Separation of these cells from their niche led to accelerated senescence together with a profound decrease of Akt activity. Similar cell phenotypes were obtained after blocking the aforementioned pathway with several inhibitors [125].

The p63 protein in both its isoforms, with (TAp63) and without (ΔNp63) in its transactivation domain, was demonstrated to have multiple functions during skin development and a protective role against premature aging through maintenance of SKPs, as well as a fundamental role in cardiac development. TAp63−/− mice display a phenotype with severe ulcerations, kyphosis, hair loss, and impaired wound healing. Interestingly, siRNA-specific knockdown of Tap63 prevented the formation of beating cardiomyocytes in mice [126–128].

Although mechanisms related to age-related defects in stem cell polarity and asymmetrical damage protein segregation have been described in bacteria and yeast, data from humans are still lacking [129, 130].

Extrinsic Aging

Chronic Photodamage

Chronic photodamage of the skin is the prime factor leading to skin aging, exerting its manifestations through induction of DNA damage and UV-mediated ROS. ROS formation facilitates the expression of the transcription factor c-Jun via mitogen-activated protein kinases, leading to an overexpression of MMP-1, MMP-3, and MMP-9 and inhibition of procollagen-1 [131]. The cutaneous manifestations of this process are pigmentary changes and wrinkling [58]. A main difference in the phenotype of extrinsic from intrinsically aged skin is the thickened epidermis and the hyperplasia of the elastic tissue, termed solar elastosis [6, 12]. The level of sun exposure determines the level of hyperplastic response, with the accumulation of abundant dystrophic elastotic material in the dermis considered to be pathognomonic for this condition [132, 133]. Photoaged skin accumulates more mutations of mitochondrial DNA in comparison to photo-protected skin [134]. The role of the 1000-fold repeats of TTAGGG sequences, termed telomeres, has been implicated in photoaging, since the photo-exposed epidermis exhibits shorter telomere length in the epidermis than in the dermis [135].

UV radiation interferes with the cutaneous immune system action, which has also therapeutic implications in many cases in dermatology. On the other hand, inhibition of action of certain immune cells (Langerhans cells, T cells) might hinder the blocking mechanisms of early cell tumorigenic progression [136].

Smoking

Smoking is a widely accepted factor, which accelerates extrinsic aging [137–139], targeting mainly the elastin network of the skin [140]. Cigarette smokers' wrinkle formation depicts a distinctive pattern with prominent perioral lines and sharply contoured crow's feet, termed the "smoker's face." The physical movement of the lips and face while inhaling the smoke is the natural explanation for their formation. Facial wrinkles radiate typically at right angles from the lips and eyes and a thinning of the facial features are also observed [138, 141].

Glycation

The development of AGEs is also a result of extrinsically aged skin. In young individuals, AGE accumulation is mainly co-localized with solar elastosis, indicating that UV irradiation affects AGE precipitation in vivo [72, 84, 87]. Using photo-exposed and photo-protected skin specimens, a significant increase of lower molecular mass of hyaluronan was observed in photo-exposed skin, with a concomitant downregulation of its receptors CD44 and RHAMM [142].

Age-Associated Skin Diseases

Aging, both intrinsic and extrinsic, comprises a major variable of many cutaneous manifestations.

There is a number of important skin functions, which deteriorate with increasing age, like epidermal regeneration capacity, synthesis of sebum and sweat, dermoepidermal adhesion, wound healing, thermoregulation, and the speed of natural elimination of potentially hazardous chemical factors [143]. In addition, several age-associated diseases such as diabetes, arterial hypertension, and malignancies indicate their subtle manifestation through skin, e.g., through disturbance of wound-healing processes and chronic ulcerations or paraneoplastic syndromes.

Based on these characteristics, we present below some common age-associated skin diseases or diseases whose prevalence and manifestation have specific characteristics when appearing in elderly patients.

Wound Healing

The prevalence of leg ulcers, as a result of an end-stadium venal insufficiency affects a great number of elderly patients, with 4 % of the population suffering from healed or active venous ulcers. Apart from the chronic pain, immobility of the patients, depression, and decreased quality of life characterize the disease [144–146]. Multimedication of the elderly can be also the cause for their development [147]. Leg ulcers and decubital ulcers consist a major financial problem for the health system, since they require a longer inpatient care, until they are sufficiently treated, compared to other age-related skin disorders [148].

Skin Infections

Skin and soft tissue infections are frequent in senior patients, also because of the impaired epidermal skin barrier. *Staphylococcus aureus* and β-hemolytic streptococci are often the causative organisms leading to infections such as impetigo, folliculitis, furunculosis, carbunculosis, and erysipelas. Comorbidities such as lymphedema and deep vein thrombosis play an important role in facilitating skin infections. Excoriations caused from pruritus of the elderly as a result of the barrier impairment or underlined conditions such as renal disease or diabetes mellitus might provide the ground for bacterial superinfections [149]. Zoster manifests itself after reactivation of the *Varicella zoster* virus, usually following a "blow" to the immune system (e.g., infection, operation) on a basis of already existing age-related immune alterations [150].

Immunological Diseases

The increase of certain immunologic skin disorders, correlated to age-related immune system alterations, is a possible explanation for the prevalence of such diseases. A prime example is the T cell-mediated shift from the naïve to the memory phenotype, their reduced proliferation following activation, Langerhans cell number reduction, and the cytokine profile alterations, which make skin cells more susceptible to endotoxins [151, 152]. Bullous pemphigoid is clinically characterized by tense skin blistering and crusts usually on an erythematous skin [153], and pemphigus vulgaris is a chronic blistering disease characterized histologically by intraepidermal bulla formation. Pemphigus vulgaris mostly affects older adults of 40–70 years, while bullous pemphigoid peaks at 80 years [143, 154, 155]. On the other hand, immunological skin senescence might explain why the manifestations of inflammatory skin diseases such as psoriasis or lupus erythematosus of the elderly are mild in comparison to young patients. Erythrodermic psoriasis has a higher prevalence in those patients, while the scalp skin of the elderly patients with plaque psoriasis is more frequently affected. In contrast, younger patients usually present with erythematosquamous plaques on the knees and elbows [143, 156–158].

Pigmentary Disorders

Vitiligo is a disorder of progressive loss of melanocytes from the skin and hair follicle. It was recently shown that melanocytes in vitiligo are accumulating an increased number of p16, which does not correlate to the age of the donor, and several active proteins of the senescence-associated secretory phenotype, implying a pathophysiologic mechanism of premature cellular senescence [159].

Skin Tumors

A high rate of skin cancers (90 %) is attributed to sun exposure [160]. Among them, a common form of noninvasive intraepithelial skin neoplasm, namely, actinic keratosis, is characterized by atypical proliferation of suprabasal keratinocytes and a frequent reason for dermatological consultation. This lesion might evolve to squamous cell carcinoma (SCC) and is currently defined as an in situ SCC [161]. Actinic keratoses occur in UV-exposed skin and develop in older, fair skin individuals [162]. The frequency of actinic keratosis correlates with lighter skin phototypes. Apart from sun exposure, drugs, such as thiazide diuretics, are also contributing to the genesis of the lesions [163].

Basal cell carcinoma (BCC) and SCC appear on a sun-exposed skin, and Fitzpatrick type II and III skin types are more prone to their development [136]. BCC is the most common skin cancer of the Caucasians and comprises a usually only locally invasive cancer, deriving from the basaloid cells, resembling the undifferentiated basal cells of the epidermis and its appendages. Eighty-five percent of all BCCs are localized on the head and neck area [164]. Its prevalence is increasing with age and sun exposure [165]. SCC is the second most common nonmelanoma skin cancer, occurring more often in men in comparison to women. It is characterized by the malignant transformation of suprabasal keratinocytes. It shows a higher metastatic potential than the BCC, and its incidence rises after the age of 40. Factors correlated with UV exposure, such as agricultural work, sunburns, solarium, and PUVA therapy, play an important role in its pathogenesis, as well as factors such as ionizing radiation, chemical carcinogens, immunosuppression/immunosenescence [166], and human papillomavirus infection [143, 167].

Malignant melanoma is a tumor deriving from the epidermal melanocytes. Melanoma is also more prevalent in senior patients, since half of the patients with the disease in Europe, the USA, and Australia are over 65 years old [168–170]. A retrospective study of 610 patients showed that patients over 70 years appear to have thicker melanomas, higher local/transit metastases, and a higher mitotic ratio [171]. For all histological subtypes except of lentigo maligna melanoma, men of more than 50 years of age were most likely to be diagnosed with thick (≥2.0 mm) tumors [172]. In contrast, younger women had fewer thick melanomas in all histological subtypes. In addition, ulceration is more common in the aged population. Interestingly, de novo melanomas are more common in the elderly, whereas it is more probable that a malignant tumor will develop on the basis of a preexisting single nevus in the elderly, also due to the decrease of nevus counts in this population [172]. Older age is considered an independent poor prognostic factor, while it is unclear that conditions, such as impaired host defenses and a change in the disease's pathophysiology, have a confounding role [173].

The Skin as a Tool for Understanding Global Aging

Apart from the skin-associated intrinsic and extrinsic alterations and the skin diseases usually related to the aging process, there is an ongoing interest of the utilization of the skin as a model for age associated pathologic conditions of various systems, such as the nervous and endocrine system. The way that skin can efficiently mirror inner organ alterations or deficiencies coming with age is also highlighted by the prominent skin signs of genetic diseases, which resemble aspects of aging at a very early age.

Hormone Deficiency

Increasing age leads to decrease of insulin growth factor (IGF) and this has a reflection to the skin, since it affects sebaceous differentiation and epidermal thickness [174]. Patients suffering from conditions of multiple hormone deficiency or IGF-1 deficiency present with a phenotype of prematurely aged skin. Important aspects of the growth hormone/IGF-1 deficiency are hyperglycemia, obesity, osteopenia, hypercholesterolemia, decrease of lean mass, cardiovascular diseases, and premature mortality [23, 175–177].

Neurodegenerative Diseases

In addition to the common ectodermal origin of the nervous system and the skin, the use of the second as a model of detection of hormone-associated aging has been recently highlighted.

cDNA microarray analysis of immortalized sebocytes treated with a hormonal mixture of growth factors and sex steroids resembling one of 20- and 60-year-old women resulted in the regulation of 899 genes, which have been related to significant metabolic pathways related to aging [4, 49]. Furthermore, specific genes associated with the pathomechanism of neurodegenerative diseases, such as Parkinson's disease, Huntington disease, Alzheimer's disease, dentatorubral-pallidoluysian atrophy, and amyotrophic lateral sclerosis were also documented to alter their expression. Amyloid precursor protein was expressed and found to play a role in human epidermis [178], while the expression of β-amyloid and tau protein was detected in skin mast cells, bearing another proof of skin reflecting neural degeneration [179]. Moreover, skin melanocytes undergo apoptosis after treatment of β-amyloid, while nerve growth factor attenuates the action of the latter and exerts a protective effect [180]. Induction of pluripotent stem cell-derived neuronal cells from normal human fibroblasts of an 82-year-old patient with Alzheimer's disease led to expression of the p-tau and GSK3B, a physiological kinase of tau, which are involved in Alzheimer's disease pathophysiology. This model could provide a useful skin-derived tool for a better understanding of Alzheimer's disease and for the future development of therapeutic strategies against it [181].

MMP regulation seems to play a very important role for neurodegenerative disorders, such as Alzheimer's disease, Parkinson's disease, and Huntington's disease. MMPs and the tissue inhibitors of MMPs are highlighted in neuronal aging since they remodel the extracellular matrix of the central nervous system [182]. A possible correlation in the dysregulation of these remodeling mechanisms might provide valuable markers of skin ECM degradation or remodeling impairment as tools to assess age-related neural degeneration.

Progeria Syndromes: Disease Models for Aging

Hutchinson–Gilford progeria syndrome (HGPS) is a rare genetic disorder with clinical features of premature aging. Clinical symptoms of this syndrome include scleroderma-like skin changes, bone abnormalities, alopecia, lack of subcutaneous fat, growth retardation, bone abnormalities, and joint stiffness. The average life span of HGPS patients is 13 years, with atherosclerotic heart disease being between the most common cause of death [183, 184]. The disease occurs due to a single-nucleotide mutation, which results in the production of a truncated mRNA transcript encoding a prelamin A protein with an internal deletion of 50 amino acids, known as progerin. Surprisingly, the discovery of progerin in normal cells suggests mechanisms of progeria in normal aging [185, 186]. The way that progerin builds up in normal skin with age and is detected in the papillary dermis, spreading to reticular dermis with age and a few terminally differentiated keratinocytes in the elderly, confirms how skin can accurately function as a model, reflecting human aging [187]. In vivo and in vitro data implicate the premature exhaustion of stem cells as a major reason for the progeria phenotype. Skin was again the means to confirm stem cell impairment, since cells isolated from all known stem cell-rich skin areas of a progeria mouse model (bulge region, sebaceous gland) showed reduced clonogenic capacity in comparison to controls. In addition, progeria skin keratinocytes exhibited lower levels of the stem cell markers α6-integrin and CD34 [188]. HGPS skin fibroblasts exhibit nuclear defects, such as altered gene expression, nuclear blebbing, disorganization of the underlying heterochromatin, stem cell dysfunction, increased DNA damage, cellular senescence, and high p16INK4A levels [189].

Werner syndrome is a premature aging disorder, associated with increased occurrence of inflammatory diseases, cataract, diabetes mellitus type II, and atherosclerosis. Surprisingly, skin manifestations and hair graying precede the inner organ defects. Skin fibroblasts in vitro are characterized by premature cellular senescence correlated to genomic instability resulting in stress kinase activation, such as p38 [190]. Restrictive respiratory disease, hyperuricemia, proteinuria, and primary hypogonadism are also findings of premature aging syndromes [191].

These and several other syndromes associated with premature aging phenotypes (Bloom syndrome, Cockayne syndrome, trichothiodystrophy, ataxia–telangiectasia, Rothmund–Thomson syndrome, and xeroderma pigmentosum) have contributed to important findings regarding aging and cancer [189].

Metabolic Diseases

Diabetes mellitus is a common disease affecting multiple organs of the elderly and skin can be an attractive model of combining the cutaneous manifestations of uncontrolled chronic hyperglycemia with skin defects. Chronic hyperglycemia leads to an increase of AGEs, thus enhancing the aging process [72]. Specifically, the impairment of the skin barrier, namely, decreased epidermal lipid synthesis and antimicrobial peptide expression, was shown to be correlated with hemoglobin A1c levels in a chronic hyperglycemia mouse model [68]. Diabetic mice exhibit a reduced hydration state of the stratum corneum and a decrease of the activity of the sebaceous gland, resembling senile xerosis [192]. Diabetic skin depicts abnormalities of the elastic cutaneous network, resulting in age-associated laxity [193]. Diabetic skin, as well as aged skin, showed reduction of blood flow in rest and in response to sustained heat [194, 195]. Skin autofluorescence as a measure of AGEs in skin is a marker, which was reported to correlate with hyperglycemia, age, adiposity, vascular damage, and the metabolic syndrome [196], suggesting a promising noninvasive method for patients in risk for developing complications [197].

Conclusion

This chapter presents key mechanisms involved in skin aging and confirms the fact that aging skin can reflect accurately age-related comorbidities. Proper correlation of age-related skin and inner organ defects can provide reproducible, easily accessible, and cost-effective predictors of diseases such as cancer, coronary disease, and diabetes. In a future step, it could determine the time points for the initiation of specific treatments for these diseases and lastly provide reproducible follow-up markers to monitor the patient's response.

References

1. Vina J, et al. Theories of ageing. IUBMB Life. 2007;59:249–54.
2. Nikolakis G, et al. Skin mirrors human aging. Horm Mol Biol Clin Investig. 2013;16:13–28.
3. Ganceviciene R, et al. Skin anti-aging strategies. Dermatoendocrinol. 2012;4:308–19.
4. Makrantonaki E, et al. Genetics and skin aging. Dermatoendocrinol. 2012;4:280–4.
5. Kinn PM, et al. Age-dependent variation in cytokines, chemokines, and biologic analytes rinsed from the surface of healthy human skin. Sci Rep. 2015;5:10472.
6. Zouboulis CC, Makrantonaki E. Clinical aspects and molecular diagnostics of skin aging. Clin Dermatol. 2011;29:3–14.
7. Cevenini E, et al. Human models of aging and longevity. Expert Opin Biol Ther. 2008;8:1393–405.
8. Callaghan TM, Wilhelm KP. A review of ageing and an examination of clinical methods in the assessment of ageing skin. Part 2: clinical perspectives and clinical methods in the evaluation of ageing skin. Int J Cosmet Sci. 2008;30:323–32.
9. El-Domyati M, et al. Intrinsic aging vs. photoaging: a comparative histopathological, immunohistochemical, and ultrastructural study of skin. Exp Dermatol. 2002;11:398–405.
10. Kligman LH. Photoaging. Manifestations, prevention, and treatment. Clin Geriatr Med. 1989; 5:235–51.
11. Lock-Andersen J, et al. Epidermal thickness, skin pigmentation and constitutive photosensitivity. Photodermatol Photoimmunol Photomed. 1997; 13:153–8.
12. Makrantonaki E, Zouboulis CC. Molecular mechanisms of skin aging: state of the art. Ann N Y Acad Sci. 2007;1119:40–50.
13. Moragas A, et al. Mathematical morphologic analysis of aging-related epidermal changes. Anal Quant Cytol Histol. 1993;15:75–82.
14. Rawlings AV. Ethnic skin types: are there differences in skin structure and function? Int J Cosmet Sci. 2006;28:79–93.
15. Chu M, Kollias N. Documentation of normal stratum corneum scaling in an average population: features of differences among age, ethnicity and body site. Br J Dermatol. 2011;164:497–507.
16. Diridollou S, et al. Comparative study of the hydration of the stratum corneum between four ethnic groups: influence of age. Int J Dermatol. 2007;46 Suppl 1:11–4.
17. Tsukahara K, et al. Comparison of age-related changes in wrinkling and sagging of the skin in Caucasian females and in Japanese females. J Cosmet Sci. 2004;55:351–71.
18. Nouveau-Richard S, et al. Skin ageing: a comparison between Chinese and European populations. A pilot study. J Dermatol Sci. 2005;40:187–93.

19. Valet F, et al. Assessing the reliability of four severity scales depicting skin ageing features. Br J Dermatol. 2009;161:153–8.
20. Allsopp RC, et al. Telomere length predicts replicative capacity of human fibroblasts. Proc Natl Acad Sci U S A. 1992;89:10114–8.
21. Dimri GP, et al. A biomarker that identifies senescent human cells in culture and in aging skin in vivo. Proc Natl Acad Sci U S A. 1995;92:9363–7.
22. Harman D. The free radical theory of aging. Antioxid Redox Signal. 2003;5:557–61.
23. Makrantonaki E, et al. Skin and brain age together: the role of hormones in the ageing process. Exp Gerontol. 2010;45:801–13.
24. Medvedev ZA. An attempt at a rational classification of theories of ageing. Biol Rev Camb Philos Soc. 1990;65:375–98.
25. Michikawa Y, et al. Aging-dependent large accumulation of point mutations in the human mtDNA control region for replication. Science. 1999;286:774–9.
26. Mancini M, et al. MicroRNAs in human skin ageing. Ageing Res Rev. 2014;17:9–15.
27. Janson D, et al. Effects of serially passaged fibroblasts on dermal and epidermal morphogenesis in human skin equivalents. Biogerontology. 2013;14:131–40.
28. Gilhar A, et al. Ageing of human epidermis: the role of apoptosis, Fas and telomerase. Br J Dermatol. 2004;150:56–63.
29. Waldera Lupa DM, et al. Characterization of skin aging-associated secreted proteins (SAASP) produced by dermal fibroblasts isolated from intrinsically aged human skin. J Invest Dermatol. 2015; 135:1954–68.
30. Janson D, et al. Papillary fibroblasts differentiate into reticular fibroblasts after prolonged in vitro culture. Exp Dermatol. 2013;22:48–53.
31. Dos Santos M, et al. In vitro 3-D model based on extending time of culture for studying chronological epidermis aging. Matrix Biol. 2015;47:85–97.
32. Franceschi C, et al. Human immunosenescence: the prevailing of innate immunity, the failing of clonotypic immunity, and the filling of immunological space. Vaccine. 2000;18:1717–20.
33. Giacomoni PU, et al. Aging of human skin: review of a mechanistic model and first experimental data. IUBMB Life. 2000;49:259–63.
34. Linton PJ, Dorshkind K. Age-related changes in lymphocyte development and function. Nat Immunol. 2004;5:133–9.
35. Plackett TP, et al. Aging and innate immune cells. J Leukoc Biol. 2004;76:291–9.
36. Plowden J, et al. Innate immunity in aging: impact on macrophage function. Aging Cell. 2004;3:161–7.
37. Ye J, et al. Alterations in cytokine regulation in aged epidermis: implications for permeability barrier homeostasis and inflammation. I. IL-1 gene family. Exp Dermatol. 2002;11:209–16.
38. Coppe JP, et al. Senescence-associated secretory phenotypes reveal cell-nonautonomous functions of oncogenic RAS and the p53 tumor suppressor. PLoS Biol. 2008;6:2853–68.
39. Freund A, et al. Inflammatory networks during cellular senescence: causes and consequences. Trends Mol Med. 2010;16:238–46.
40. Elias PM, Ghadially R. The aged epidermal permeability barrier: basis for functional abnormalities. Clin Geriatr Med. 2002;18:103–20. Vii.
41. Tsutsumi M, Denda M. Paradoxical effects of beta-estradiol on epidermal permeability barrier homeostasis. Br J Dermatol. 2007;157:776–9.
42. Briganti S, et al. Modulation of PPARgamma provides new insights in a stress induced premature senescence model. PLoS One. 2014;9:e104045.
43. Robinson MK, et al. Genomic-driven insights into changes in aging skin. J Drugs Dermatol. 2009;8:s8–11.
44. Nikolakis G, et al. Ex vivo human skin and SZ95 sebocytes exhibit a homoeostatic interaction in a novel coculture contact model. Exp Dermatol. 2015;24:497–502.
45. Engelke M, et al. Effects of xerosis and ageing on epidermal proliferation and differentiation. Br J Dermatol. 1997;137:219–25.
46. Pochi PE, et al. Age-related changes in sebaceous gland activity. J Invest Dermatol. 1979;73:108–11.
47. Zouboulis CC, Boschnakow A. Chronological ageing and photoageing of the human sebaceous gland. Clin Exp Dermatol. 2001;26:600–7.
48. Makrantonaki E, et al. Age-specific hormonal decline is accompanied by transcriptional changes in human sebocytes in vitro. Aging Cell. 2006;5:331–44.
49. Makrantonaki E, et al. Identification of biomarkers of human skin ageing in both genders. Wnt signalling – a label of skin ageing? PLoS One. 2012;7:e50393.
50. Chi W, et al. Dermal papilla cell number specifies hair size, shape and cycling and its reduction causes follicular decline. Development. 2013;140:1676–83.
51. Yang YC, et al. Androgen receptor accelerates premature senescence of human dermal papilla cells in association with DNA damage. PLoS One. 2013; 8:e79434.
52. Arck PC, et al. Towards a "free radical theory of graying": melanocyte apoptosis in the aging human hair follicle is an indicator of oxidative stress induced tissue damage. FASEB J. 2006;20:1567–9.
53. Peters EM, et al. Graying of the human hair follicle. J Cosmet Sci. 2011;62:121–5.
54. Seiberg M. Age-induced hair greying – the multiple effects of oxidative stress. Int J Cosmet Sci. 2013;35:532–8.
55. Schuler N, Rube CE. Accumulation of DNA damage-induced chromatin alterations in tissue-specific stem cells: the driving force of aging? PLoS One. 2013;8: e63932.
56. Inoue M, Katakami C. The effect of hyaluronic acid on corneal epithelial cell proliferation. Invest Ophthalmol Vis Sci. 1993;34:2313–5.
57. Toole BP. Hyaluronan in morphogenesis. J Intern Med. 1997;242:35–40.

58. Baumann L. Skin ageing and its treatment. J Pathol. 2007;211:241–51.
59. Papakonstantinou E, et al. Hyaluronic acid: a key molecule in skin aging. Dermatoendocrinol. 2012;4:253–8.
60. Shapiro SD. Matrix metalloproteinase degradation of extracellular matrix: biological consequences. Curr Opin Cell Biol. 1998;10:602–8.
61. Isnard N, et al. Regulation of elastase-type endopeptidase activity, MMP-2 and MMP-9 expression and activation in human dermal fibroblasts by fucose and a fucose-rich polysaccharide. Biomed Pharmacother. 2002;56:258–64.
62. Longas MO, et al. Evidence for structural changes in dermatan sulfate and hyaluronic acid with aging. Carbohydr Res. 1987;159:127–36.
63. Meyer LJ, Stern R. Age-dependent changes of hyaluronan in human skin. J Invest Dermatol. 1994;102:385–9.
64. Rock K, et al. miR-23a-3p causes cellular senescence by targeting hyaluronan synthase 2: possible implication for skin aging. J Invest Dermatol. 2015; 135:369–77.
65. Isnard N, et al. Effect of sulfated GAGs on the expression and activation of MMP-2 and MMP-9 in corneal and dermal explant cultures. Cell Biol Int. 2003;27:779–84.
66. Langton AK, et al. A new wrinkle on old skin: the role of elastic fibres in skin ageing. Int J Cosmet Sci. 2010;32:330–9.
67. Naylor EC, et al. Molecular aspects of skin ageing. Maturitas. 2011;69:249–56.
68. Park HY, et al. A long-standing hyperglycaemic condition impairs skin barrier by accelerating skin ageing process. Exp Dermatol. 2011;20:969–74.
69. Paul RG, Bailey AJ. Glycation of collagen: the basis of its central role in the late complications of ageing and diabetes. Int J Biochem Cell Biol. 1996; 28:1297–310.
70. Bierhaus A, et al. Understanding RAGE, the receptor for advanced glycation end products. J Mol Med (Berl). 2005;83:876–86.
71. Fleming TH, et al. Reactive metabolites and AGE/RAGE-mediated cellular dysfunction affect the aging process: a mini-review. Gerontology. 2011; 57:435–43.
72. Gkogkolou P, Bohm M. Advanced glycation end products: key players in skin aging? Dermatoendocrinol. 2012;4:259–70.
73. Cerami C, et al. Tobacco smoke is a source of toxic reactive glycation products. Proc Natl Acad Sci U S A. 1997;94:13915–20.
74. Glenn JV, et al. Confocal Raman microscopy can quantify advanced glycation end product (AGE) modifications in Bruch's membrane leading to accurate, nondestructive prediction of ocular aging. FASEB J. 2007;21:3542–52.
75. Sell DR, et al. Differential effects of type 2 (non-insulin-dependent) diabetes mellitus on pentosidine formation in skin and glomerular basement membrane. Diabetologia. 1993;36:936–41.
76. Stitt AW. Advanced glycation: an important pathological event in diabetic and age related ocular disease. Br J Ophthalmol. 2001;85:746–53.
77. Vlassara H, et al. Inflammatory mediators are induced by dietary glycotoxins, a major risk factor for diabetic angiopathy. Proc Natl Acad Sci U S A. 2002;99:15596–601.
78. Thijssen DH et al. Arterial structure and function in vascular ageing: "Are you as old as your arteries?". J Physiol. 2015.
79. Wang Y, et al. Effect of glucose on the biomechanical function of arterial elastin. J Mech Behav Biomed Mater. 2015;49:244–54.
80. Fang M, et al. Advanced glycation end-products accelerate the cardiac aging process through the receptor for advanced glycation end-products/transforming growth factor-beta-Smad signaling pathway in cardiac fibroblasts. Geriatr Gerontol Int. 2015;28:12499.
81. Wu X, Monnier VM. Enzymatic deglycation of proteins. Arch Biochem Biophys. 2003;419:16–24.
82. Xue M, et al. Glyoxalase in ageing. Semin Cell Dev Biol. 2011;22:293–301.
83. Dyer DG, et al. Accumulation of Maillard reaction products in skin collagen in diabetes and aging. J Clin Invest. 1993;91:2463–9.
84. Jeanmaire C, et al. Glycation during human dermal intrinsic and actinic ageing: an in vivo and in vitro model study. Br J Dermatol. 2001;145:10–8.
85. Avery NC, Bailey AJ. The effects of the Maillard reaction on the physical properties and cell interactions of collagen. Pathol Biol (Paris). 2006; 54:387–95.
86. Degroot J, et al. Age-related decrease in susceptibility of human articular cartilage to matrix metalloproteinase-mediated degradation: the role of advanced glycation end products. Arthritis Rheum. 2001;44:2562–71.
87. Mizutari K, et al. Photo-enhanced modification of human skin elastin in actinic elastosis by N(epsilon)-(carboxymethyl)lysine, one of the glycoxidation products of the Maillard reaction. J Invest Dermatol. 1997;108:797–802.
88. Alikhani Z, et al. Advanced glycation end products enhance expression of pro-apoptotic genes and stimulate fibroblast apoptosis through cytoplasmic and mitochondrial pathways. J Biol Chem. 2005; 280:12087–95.
89. Zhu P, et al. Impairment of human keratinocyte mobility and proliferation by advanced glycation end products-modified BSA. Arch Dermatol Res. 2011;303:339–50.
90. Berge U, et al. Sugar-induced premature aging and altered differentiation in human epidermal keratinocytes. Ann N Y Acad Sci. 2007;1100:524–9.
91. Ravelojaona V, et al. Expression of senescence-associated beta-galactosidase (SA-beta-Gal) by

human skin fibroblasts, effect of advanced glycation end-products and fucose or rhamnose-rich polysaccharides. Arch Gerontol Geriatr. 2009;48:151–4.
92. Sejersen H, Rattan SI. Dicarbonyl-induced accelerated aging in vitro in human skin fibroblasts. Biogerontology. 2009;10:203–11.
93. Hofmann B, et al. Advanced glycation end product associated skin autofluorescence: a mirror of vascular function? Exp Gerontol. 2013;48:38–44.
94. Yamagishi S, et al. Evaluation of tissue accumulation levels of advanced glycation end products by skin autofluorescence: a novel marker of vascular complications in high-risk patients for cardiovascular disease. Int J Cardiol. 2015;185:263–8.
95. Pennacchi PC, et al. Glycated reconstructed human skin as a platform to study pathogenesis of skin aging. Tissue Eng Part A. 2015;1:1.
96. Poundarik AA, et al. A direct role of collagen glycation in bone fracture. J Mech Behav Biomed Mater. 2015;50:82–92.
97. Sestier B. [Hematopoietic stem cell exhaustion and advanced glycation end-products in the unexplained anemia of the elderly]. Rev Esp Geriatr Gerontol. 2015;50:223–31.
98. Kandarakis SA, et al. Dietary glycotoxins induce RAGE and VEGF up-regulation in the retina of normal rats. Exp Eye Res. 2015;137:1–10.
99. Zolla V, et al. Aging-related anatomical and biochemical changes in lymphatic collectors impair lymph transport, fluid homeostasis, and pathogen clearance. Aging Cell. 2015;14:582–94.
100. Fuchs E, Chen T. A matter of life and death: self-renewal in stem cells. EMBO Rep. 2013;14:39–48.
101. Thomson JA, et al. Embryonic stem cell lines derived from human blastocysts. Science. 1998;282:1145–7.
102. Zouboulis CC, et al. Human skin stem cells and the ageing process. Exp Gerontol. 2008;43:986–97.
103. Potten CS. The epidermal proliferative unit: the possible role of the central basal cell. Cell Tissue Kinet. 1974;7:77–88.
104. Biernaskie JA, et al. Isolation of skin-derived precursors (SKPs) and differentiation and enrichment of their Schwann cell progeny. Nat Protoc. 2006;1:2803–12.
105. Chen FG, et al. Clonal analysis of nestin(−) vimentin (+) multipotent fibroblasts isolated from human dermis. J Cell Sci. 2007;120:2875–83.
106. Kim J-H, et al. Adipose-derived stem cells as a new therapeutic modality for ageing skin. Exp Dermatol. 2011;20:383–7.
107. Yang YI, et al. Ex vivo organ culture of adipose tissue for in situ mobilization of adipose-derived stem cells and defining the stem cell niche. J Cell Physiol. 2010;224:807–16.
108. Grove GL, Kligman AM. Age-associated changes in human epidermal cell renewal. J Gerontol. 1983;38:137–42.
109. Racila D, Bickenbach JR. Are epidermal stem cells unique with respect to aging? Aging (Albany NY). 2009;1:746–50.
110. Conboy IM, et al. Rejuvenation of aged progenitor cells by exposure to a young systemic environment. Nature. 2005;433:760–4.
111. Sharpless NE, Depinho RA. How stem cells age and why this makes us grow old. Nat Rev Mol Cell Biol. 2007;8:703–13.
112. Barrandon Y, Green H. Three clonal types of keratinocyte with different capacities for multiplication. Proc Natl Acad Sci U S A. 1987; 84:2302–6.
113. Ressler S, et al. p16INK4A is a robust in vivo biomarker of cellular aging in human skin. Aging Cell. 2006;5:379–89.
114. Giangreco A, et al. Human skin aging is associated with reduced expression of the stem cell markers beta1 integrin and MCSP. J Invest Dermatol. 2010;130:604–8.
115. Ruzankina Y, et al. Deletion of the developmentally essential gene ATR in adult mice leads to age-related phenotypes and stem cell loss. Cell Stem Cell. 2007;1:113–26.
116. Giangreco A, et al. Epidermal stem cells are retained in vivo throughout skin aging. Aging Cell. 2008;7:250–9.
117. Stern MM, Bickenbach JR. Epidermal stem cells are resistant to cellular aging. Aging Cell. 2007;6:439–52.
118. Asumda FZ. Age-associated changes in the ecological niche: implications for mesenchymal stem cell aging. Stem Cell Res Ther. 2013;4:47.
119. Doles J, et al. Age-associated inflammation inhibits epidermal stem cell function. Genes Dev. 2012;26:2144–53.
120. Bromberg JF, et al. Stat3 as an oncogene. Cell. 1999;98:295–303.
121. Demaria M, et al. STAT3 can serve as a hit in the process of malignant transformation of primary cells. Cell Death Differ. 2012;19:1390–7.
122. Demaria M, Poli V. Pro-malignant properties of STAT3 during chronic inflammation. Oncotarget. 2012;3:359–60.
123. Castilho RM, et al. mTOR mediates Wnt-induced epidermal stem cell exhaustion and aging. Cell Stem Cell. 2009;5:279–89.
124. Biernaskie J, et al. SKPs derive from hair follicle precursors and exhibit properties of adult dermal stem cells. Cell Stem Cell. 2009;5:610–23.
125. Liu S, et al. The PI3K-Akt pathway inhibits senescence and promotes self-renewal of human skin-derived precursors in vitro. Aging Cell. 2011;10:661–74.
126. Beaudry VG, Attardi LD. SKP-ing TAp63: stem cell depletion, senescence, and premature aging. Cell Stem Cell. 2009;5:1–2.
127. Paris M, et al. Regulation of skin aging and heart development by TAp63. Cell Death Differ. 2012;19:186–93.
128. Su X, Flores ER. TAp63: the fountain of youth. Aging (Albany NY). 2009;1:866–9.

129. Bufalino MR, et al. The asymmetric segregation of damaged proteins is stem cell-type dependent. J Cell Biol. 2013;201:523–30.
130. Florian MC, Geiger H. Concise review: polarity in stem cells, disease, and aging. Stem Cells. 2010;28:1623–9.
131. Chung JH, et al. Decreased extracellular-signal-regulated kinase and increased stress-activated MAP kinase activities in aged human skin in vivo. J Invest Dermatol. 2000;115:177–82.
132. Bernstein EF, et al. Enhanced elastin and fibrillin gene expression in chronically photodamaged skin. J Invest Dermatol. 1994;103:182–6.
133. Mitchell RE. Chronic solar dermatosis: a light and electron microscopic study of the dermis. J Invest Dermatol. 1967;48:203–20.
134. Berneburg M, et al. Chronically ultraviolet-exposed human skin shows a higher mutation frequency of mitochondrial DNA as compared to unexposed skin and the hematopoietic system. Photochem Photobiol. 1997;66:271–5.
135. Sugimoto M, et al. Telomere length of the skin in association with chronological aging and photoaging. J Dermatol Sci. 2006;43:43–7.
136. Gilchrest BA. A review of skin ageing and its medical therapy. Br J Dermatol. 1996;135:867–75.
137. Ernster VL, et al. Facial wrinkling in men and women, by smoking status. Am J Public Health. 1995; 85:78–82.
138. Kadunce DP, et al. Cigarette smoking: risk factor for premature facial wrinkling. Ann Intern Med. 1991;114:840–4.
139. Yin L, et al. Skin aging induced by ultraviolet exposure and tobacco smoking: evidence from epidemiological and molecular studies. Photodermatol Photoimmunol Photomed. 2001;17:178–83.
140. Just M, et al. Effect of smoking on skin elastic fibres: morphometric and immunohistochemical analysis. Br J Dermatol. 2007;156:85–91.
141. Model D. Smoker's face: an underrated clinical sign? Br Med J (Clin Res Ed). 1985;291:1760–2.
142. Tzellos TG, et al. Differential hyaluronan homeostasis and expression of proteoglycans in juvenile and adult human skin. J Dermatol Sci. 2011; 61:69–72.
143. Makrantonaki E, et al. Skin diseases in geriatric patients. Epidemiologic data. Hautarzt. 2012;63:938–46.
144. Eklof B, et al. Updated terminology of chronic venous disorders: the VEIN-TERM transatlantic interdisciplinary consensus document. J Vasc Surg. 2009;49:498–501.
145. Nicolaides AN, et al. Management of chronic venous disorders of the lower limbs: guidelines according to scientific evidence. Int Angiol. 2008;27:1–59.
146. Rabe E, et al. Epidemiology of chronic venous disorders in geographically diverse populations: results from the Vein Consult Program. Int Angiol. 2012;31:105–15.
147. Dissemond J. Medications. A rare cause for leg ulcers. Hautarzt. 2011;62:516–23.
148. Theisen S, et al. Pressure ulcers in older hospitalised patients and its impact on length of stay: a retrospective observational study. J Clin Nurs. 2012;21:380–7.
149. Laube S, Farrell AM. Bacterial skin infections in the elderly: diagnosis and treatment. Drugs Aging. 2002;19:331–42.
150. Na CR, et al. Elderly adults and skin disorders: common problems for nondermatologists. South Med J. 2012;105:600–6.
151. Gilchrest BA, et al. Effect of chronologic aging and ultraviolet irradiation on Langerhans cells in human epidermis. J Invest Dermatol. 1982;79:85–8.
152. Sunderkotter C, et al. Aging and the skin immune system. Arch Dermatol. 1997;133:1256–62.
153. Schmidt E, Zillikens D. Diagnosis and clinical severity markers of bullous pemphigoid. F1000 Med Rep 1. 2009.
154. Ingen-Housz-Oro S, et al. Pemphigus in elderly adults: clinical presentation, treatment, and prognosis. J Am Geriatr Soc. 2012;60:1185–7.
155. Langan SM, et al. Bullous pemphigoid and pemphigus vulgaris–incidence and mortality in the UK: population based cohort study. BMJ. 2008;337:a180.
156. Ejaz A, et al. Presentation of early onset psoriasis in comparison with late onset psoriasis: a clinical study from Pakistan. Indian J Dermatol Venereol Leprol. 2009;75:36–40.
157. Ferrandiz C, et al. Psoriasis of early and late onset: a clinical and epidemiologic study from Spain. J Am Acad Dermatol. 2002;46:867–73.
158. Kwon HH, et al. Clinical study of psoriasis occurring over the age of 60 years: is elderly-onset psoriasis a distinct subtype? Int J Dermatol. 2012;51:53–8.
159. Bellei B, et al. Vitiligo: a possible model of degenerative diseases. PLoS One. 2013;8:e59782.
160. Gallagher RP. Sunscreens in melanoma and skin cancer prevention. CMAJ. 2005;173:244–5.
161. Goldberg LH, Mamelak AJ. Review of actinic keratosis. Part I: etiology, epidemiology and clinical presentation. J Drugs Dermatol. 2010;9:1125–32.
162. Schmitt JV, Miot HA. Actinic keratosis: a clinical and epidemiological revision. An Bras Dermatol. 2012;87:425–34.
163. Traianou A, et al. Risk factors for actinic keratosis in eight European centres: a case–control study. Br J Dermatol. 2012;167 Suppl 2:36–42.
164. Baxter JM, et al. Facial basal cell carcinoma. BMJ. 2012;345:e5342.
165. Bath-Hextall F, et al. Trends in incidence of skin basal cell carcinoma. Additional evidence from a UK primary care database study. Int J Cancer. 2007; 121:2105–8.
166. Perrotta RE, et al. Non-melanoma skin cancers in elderly patients. Crit Rev Oncol Hematol. 2011; 80:474–80.
167. Samarasinghe V, Madan V. Nonmelanoma skin cancer. J Cutan Aesthet Surg. 2012;5:3–10.

168. Chamberlain AJ, et al. Nodular type and older age as the most significant associations of thick melanoma in Victoria, Australia. Arch Dermatol. 2002; 138:609–14.
169. Chang AE, et al. The National Cancer Data Base report on cutaneous and noncutaneous melanoma: a summary of 84,836 cases from the past decade. The American College of Surgeons Commission on Cancer and the American Cancer Society. Cancer. 1998;83:1664–78.
170. Lasithiotakis KG, et al. The incidence and mortality of cutaneous melanoma in Southern Germany: trends by anatomic site and pathologic characteristics, 1976 to 2003. Cancer. 2006;107:1331–9.
171. Macdonald JB, et al. Malignant melanoma in the elderly: different regional disease and poorer prognosis. J Cancer. 2011;2:538–43.
172. Swetter SM, et al. Melanoma in the older person. Oncology (Williston Park). 2004;18:1187–96; discussion 1196–1187.
173. Tsai S, et al. Epidemiology and treatment of melanoma in elderly patients. Nat Rev Clin Oncol. 2010;7:148–52.
174. Makrantonaki E, et al. Interplay of IGF-I and 17beta-estradiol at age-specific levels in human sebocytes and fibroblasts in vitro. Exp Gerontol. 2008;43:939–46.
175. Laron Z. Do deficiencies in growth hormone and insulin-like growth factor-1 (IGF-1) shorten or prolong longevity? Mech Ageing Dev. 2005;126:305–7.
176. Tomlinson JW, et al. Association between premature mortality and hypopituitarism. The Lancet. 2001;357:425–31.
177. Zouboulis CC, et al. Sexual hormones in human skin. Horm Metab Res. 2007;39:85–95.
178. Herzog V, et al. Biological roles of APP in the epidermis. Eur J Cell Biol. 2004;83:613–24.
179. Kvetnoi IM, et al. Expression of beta-amyloid and tau-protein in mastocytes in Alzheimer disease. Arkh Patol. 2003;65:36–9.
180. Yaar M, Gilchrest BA. Human melanocytes as a model system for studies of Alzheimer disease. Arch Dermatol. 1997;133:1287–91.
181. Hossini AM, et al. Induced pluripotent stem cell-derived neuronal cells from a sporadic Alzheimer's disease donor as a model for investigating AD-associated gene regulatory networks. BMC Genomics. 2015;16:015–1262.
182. Mukherjee A, Swarnakar S. Implication of matrix metalloproteinases in regulating neuronal disorder. Mol Biol Rep. 2015;42:1–11.
183. Debusk FL. The Hutchinson-Gilford progeria syndrome. Report of 4 cases and review of the literature. J Pediatr. 1972;80:697–724.
184. Merideth MA, et al. Phenotype and course of Hutchinson-Gilford progeria syndrome. N Engl J Med. 2008;358:592–604.
185. Scaffidi P, Misteli T. Lamin A-dependent misregulation of adult stem cells associated with accelerated ageing. Nat Cell Biol. 2008;10:452–9.
186. Wenzel V, et al. Naive adult stem cells from patients with Hutchinson-Gilford progeria syndrome express low levels of progerin in vivo. Biol Open. 2012;1:516–26.
187. Mcclintock D, et al. The mutant form of lamin A that causes Hutchinson-Gilford progeria is a biomarker of cellular aging in human skin. PLoS One. 2007;2:e1269.
188. Rosengardten Y, et al. Stem cell depletion in Hutchinson-Gilford progeria syndrome. Aging Cell. 2011;10:1011–20.
189. Capell BC, et al. From the rarest to the most common: insights from progeroid syndromes into skin cancer and aging. J Invest Dermatol. 2009;129:2340–50.
190. Davis T, et al. The role of cellular senescence in Werner syndrome: toward therapeutic intervention in human premature aging. Ann N Y Acad Sci. 2007;1100:455–69.
191. Winkelspecht K, et al. Metageria–clinical manifestations of a premature aging syndrome. Hautarzt. 1997;48:657–61.
192. Sakai S, et al. Functional properties of the stratum corneum in patients with diabetes mellitus: similarities to senile xerosis. Br J Dermatol. 2005; 153:319–23.
193. Braverman IM. Elastic fiber and microvascular abnormalities in aging skin. Clin Geriatr Med. 1989;5:69–90.
194. Petrofsky J, et al. The influence of aging and diabetes on heat transfer characteristics of the skin to a rapidly applied heat source. Diabetes Technol Ther. 2010;12:1003–10.
195. Petrofsky JS, et al. Skin heat dissipation: the influence of diabetes, skin thickness, and subcutaneous fat thickness. Diabetes Technol Ther. 2008;10:487–93.
196. Monami M, et al. Skin autofluorescence in type 2 diabetes: beyond blood glucose. Diabetes Res Clin Pract. 2008;79:56–60.
197. Lutgers HL, et al. Skin autofluorescence as a noninvasive marker of vascular damage in patients with type 2 diabetes. Diabetes Care. 2006;29:2654–9.

Carcinogenesis: UV Radiation

68

Douglas E. Brash, Timothy P. Heffernan, Paul Nghiem, and Raymond J. Cho

Contents

This chapter is adapted with permission from Ch. 112 of Wolff, E, Goldsmith, L, Katz, S, Gilchrest, B, Paller, A and Leffell, D (eds.), Fitzpatrick's Dermatology in General Medicine, 7th ed., vol. 1, pp 999–1006, Mc-Graw-Hill, 2007.

D.E. Brash • T.P. Heffernan • P. Nghiem
Departments of Therapeutic Radiology, Genetics, and Dermatology, Yale School of Medicine, New Haven, CT, USA
e-mail: douglas.brash@yale.edu; timothy_heffernan@dfci.harvard.edu; pnghiem@u.washington.edu

R.J. Cho (✉)
Department of Dermatology, University of California, San Francisco, CA, USA
e-mail: ChoR@derm.ucsf.edu

M.A. Farage et al. (eds.), *Textbook of Aging Skin*,
DOI 10.1007/978-3-662-47398-6_56

Abstract

The incidence of human skin cancers collectively outnumbers that of all other cancers combined. Ultraviolet radiation (UVR) has long been understood to produce photoproducts in DNA, some of which give rise to specific somatic mutations capable of driving epithelial and melanocytic cancers. Accordingly, the vast numbers of somatic point mutations found in melanoma and basal and squamous cell carcinoma are predominantly base changes associated with UVR. While *TP53* and *NOTCH1* mutation have emerged as hallmarks of squamous cell carcinomas, as have *PTCH* mutations in basal cell carcinoma, large-scale sequencing projects are illuminating dozens of other known tumor suppressors and oncogenes mutated at low frequency in both melanomas and nonmelanoma skin cancer. Thus, cells tolerating DNA damage without triggering apoptosis eventually acquire mutations favoring clonal growth, and these populations in turn accumulate additional, lower frequency mutations enhancing oncogenic cell behavior. The process of UV-driven transformation in skin cancers is markedly accelerated not only by deficiencies in DNA repair, but also by immunodeficiency, suggesting that surveillance mechanisms actively eliminate UV-damaged cells, perhaps through T-cell detection of neoepitopes. Genetic factors modulating risk of UV carcinogenesis include resistance conferred by melanin and susceptibility associated with impaired free-radical clearance. Epidemiological efforts have begun validating systemic chemopreventatives, such as caffeine, which may be deployed, in concert with sun protection and avoidance, to further delay UV carcinogenesis.

Introduction

Skin cancer offers a uniquely integrated portrait of how a carcinogen causes human neoplasia. The basic principles of carcinogen exposure and slow development – discovered when Sir Percivall Pott traced scrotal cancers in adults to childhood employment as a chimney sweep – also apply to sunlight-induced cancers [1, 2]. The process begins with carcinogen exposure, DNA damage, and failure to repair DNA or apoptotically eliminate the damaged cell [3–6]. A mutant gene arises in a single cell, which then expands into a mutant clone [7]. Rare cells of this clone repeat the carcinogenesis cycle to generate mutations in additional genes. Sunlight acts at each of these steps.

Epidemiologic Observations

The lifetime incidence of skin cancer in Australia is ~60 %. In the southern US and Hawaii, nonmelanoma skin cancers exceed all other cancers combined. Basal and squamous cell carcinomas (BCC and SCC), and an SCC precursor, actinic keratosis (AK) are most frequent on sun-exposed skin, in outdoor workers, and at lower latitudes. SCCs increase more quickly with dose and low latitude than BCC, and occur later in life, implying that SCC require more sun-related steps. In contrast, one third of BCC occur on body sites having only intermittent sun exposure, such as the trunk and legs.

Melanoma also depends on sunlight. The relation to latitude is clear. Predilection of melanomas for the back and lower legs may simply reflect their considerable surface area. When expressed as lesions per unit area, melanomas are 10–20-fold more frequent on the face and male ears than on intermittently exposed sites, such as the lower legs in women, shoulders, back, or neck [8]. The slow-growing lentigo maligna melanoma and its precursor, lentigo maligna (Hutchinson's freckle), occur on exposed body sites of light-skinned individuals. Melanomas are rare on the buttocks and soles.

Melanoma appears to have two distinct origins:

1. A chronic sun damage (CSD) etiology affects the head and neck and is associated with chronic elastosis – a classic indicator of chronic sun damage – as well as gene

amplification of the cell cycle genes *CDK4* and *CCND1* [9].

2. A non-CSD route involves intermittent sun exposure of sites such as the trunk. Non-CSD melanomas carry mutations in the *BRAF* or *NRAS* oncogene – upstream regulators of cell cycle genes – and the patients have variant alleles of the melanocortin 1 receptor [10]. Intermittently exposed body sites are the locations of the melanoma increase in recent decades, melanomas in patients under age 50, and the additional melanomas seen near the equator [8]. Recreational sunburn may explain these and the twofold higher melanoma incidence in office workers compared to outdoor workers.

Sunlight is also implicated by the susceptible population: both classes of skin cancer are more frequent in light-skinned individuals with blonde or red hair who burn rather than tan. Compared to black-skinned individuals, nonmelanoma skin cancer risk rises ~10-fold in Asians and ~100-fold in Caucasians, with a further 2–12-fold for blonde or, especially, red hair. The divergence is less for melanoma, about 1:1:15. In black skin, BCC is rare even in patients with the hereditary nevoid basal cell carcinoma syndrome (NBCCS or Gorlin syndrome). Skin tumors in black patients are often scar-related, but these may be associated with sunlight as well. These effects result from less melanin in light skin [11], less shielding by pheomelanin than eumelanin, and greater production of photosensitized reactive oxygen from pheomelanin.

Molecular epidemiology has provided the most direct evidence for UV as the active component of sunlight: UVB signature mutations are present in human BCC, SCC, and AK (see section "UV Signature Mutations"). Mutant cells are associated with elastotic dermis, indicating chronic sun exposure. UVB partially penetrates the ozone layer and stratum corneum, enhancing absorption by DNA [12]. The ozone layer absorbs all but one part per million of UVC (used in germicidal bulbs), which otherwise would be lethal; UVA penetrates well but is poorly absorbed by DNA. Nevertheless, chronic UVA can induce tumors in mice and malignantly transforms predisposed human cells. The cumulative dose of sunlight required to cause BCC or SCC in adults is fairly large, approximately 10,000 and 70,000 h of exposure, respectively. Psoriasis patients who had low PUVA (psoralen + UVA) exposure and received <100 UVB treatments had a risk of SCC or BCC on sun-shielded sites slightly above background, but risk was threefold higher with >300 UVB treatments.

Some melanomas appear to be independent of sunlight: tumors of the mucosa, palms, soles, and nailbeds are equally frequent in whites and blacks and have remained constant, while melanomas of the skin have become epidemic, and are not associated with precursor nevi. Ocular melanomas are more frequent in whites than blacks, but do not depend on latitude and have not increased in the last few decades.

The Skin Cancer Epidemic

The incidence of melanoma and nonmelanoma skin cancers has doubled each decade since the 1930s [8]. AK, lentigo maligna, and lentigo maligna melanoma – typically lesions of the middle-aged and elderly – are now seen in young adults. But because cancer requires several events, it is not guaranteed that this increase in skin cancer is caused by an increase in one of the sun-related events. The best evidence for sun is that increases have been greatest for intermittently sun-exposed sites such as the trunk and limbs, with little change in melanomas of the head and neck. Increased recreational exposure is usually blamed. Another suspect has been ozone depletion; because of a steep absorption curve in the UVB region, small changes in ozone concentration greatly affect UVB penetration. (UVC is fortunately still blocked.) The Antarctic ozone hole caused a 50 % ozone reduction over southern Chile and Argentina in the last two decades, with UVB increasing up to 40-fold. Yet, skin cancers in these areas are increasing at the same rate as elsewhere. The Arctic ozone hole has been offset by screening from air pollutants, yet skin cancers in Scandinavia are rising.

An iatrogenic source of increased skin cancer incidence is PUVA (psoralen + UVA) therapy for psoriasis, which increases the risk of SCC eight-fold; in some patient cohorts, it raises melanoma >14-fold; BCC is not affected. Cancer is now increasing as a result of tanning beds. Individuals whose first sunbed exposure occurred as a young adult, or who had long durations or high frequencies of tanning bed exposure, already have a 70 % higher risk of melanoma [13].

Characteristics of UV-Induced Cancers and Precancers

In the US, ~1,000,000 BCCs are diagnosed annually, as well as 100,000 SCCs and 60,000 melanoma. Survival differs strikingly. Fewer than one in 10,000 BCCs will metastasize and threaten the patient. This number increases to 1 in 40 for SCC, with clinical experience indicating that SCCs on sun-exposed skin are less likely to metastasize than those arising in scars. One in seven invasive melanomas is lethal. Merkel cell carcinoma is a sun-induced cutaneous neuroendocrine cancer that will kill one in three patients diagnosed with it. Its incidence has tripled in the past 15 years to approximately 1,000 per year in the US.

The type of exposure preferentially leading to each malignancy differs. Cumulative lifetime sun exposure is strongly associated with SCC incidence. BCC and AK instead seem to depend on reaching a certain threshold of UV exposure, often attained in youth, such that sensitive individuals develop BCC at a relatively early age and the incidence does not increase with further exposure. Case-control studies link melanoma with intense exposure early in life, with one or two blistering sunburns doubling the melanoma risk. This effect may be an underestimate if, as mentioned above, melanoma has two origins, one depending on chronic sun damage and one on intermittent exposure and sunburn.

Children are particularly sensitive to sunlight: moving from England to Australia before age 20 confers the higher Australian incidence of AK, SCC, BCC, and melanoma, but the risk is much less when adults immigrate. This is not simply due to children spending more time outdoors, as <25 % of lifetime exposure occurs before age 18. One explanation may be that mutant cells created in youth have more years in which to acquire the additional genetic requirements for cancer.

Precursor lesions for SCC (AK) and melanoma (nevi) are also usually related to sun exposure. Accounting for roughly three million physician visits each year in the US, AK are the fourth leading cause for a visit to a dermatologist. They typically manifest as 1–3 mm scaly papules that involve erythema but often are easier felt than seen. They proceed to SCC in ~1 % of cases if left untreated. Actinic chelitis is an analogous precancerous state on the sun-exposed lip. The importance of ongoing sun exposure is made apparent by clinical studies indicating that reducing sun exposure can reduce the number of AK over a span of months. In randomized sunscreen studies, statistically significant decreases in AK were seen in the sunscreen group over brief periods. Common nevi and especially clinically atypical nevi can be precursors of malignant melanoma, with abundant nevi conferring a tenfold risk for cancer. Acquired melanocytic nevi begin to appear at age 1–5 in proportion to sunlight exposure and are most frequent in individuals with freckles and red hair. Acquired nevi carry the *BRAF* mutations seen in non-CSD melanomas, but congential nevi instead harbor *NRAS* mutations.

UV-Induced Genetic Alterations

UV-Induced DNA Damage and Repair

DNA Photoproducts

The first molecular step in sunlight-induced carcinogenesis occurs when UVB photons induce DNA photoproducts. UVB and UVC tend to be absorbed at the 5–6 double bond of pyrimidines (thymine and cytosine), allowing the bond to open [14]. If two adjacent pyrimidines are activated, their open bonds crossreact. Creating two single bonds (5–5 and 6–6) results in a cyclobutane pyrimidine dimer (Fig. 1). The most frequent is TT, but TC and CC cyclobutane dimers are also

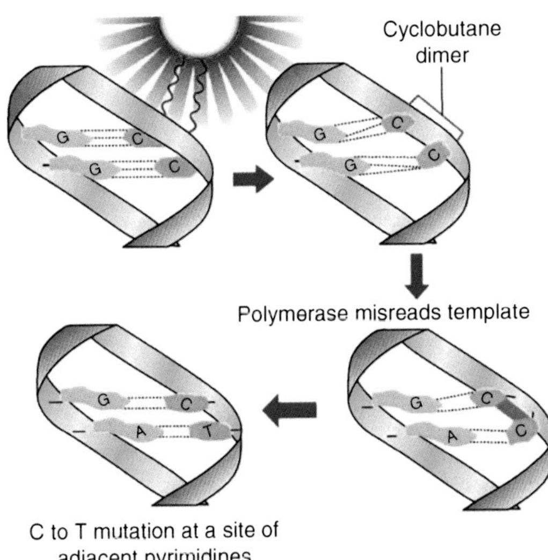

Fig. 1 UV-induced C to T "signature mutation." UV radiation causes adjacent pyrimidines on the same strand to form a cyclobutane dimer. If not repaired, the C in the dimer can be misread by the DNA polymerase or can degrade to uracil; in either case, it erroneously pairs with adenine. The net change is that a cytosine in the sequence is converted to thymine. If both cytosines mutate, the result is CC to TT

made. A single bond between the six position of one pyrimidine and the exocyclic group of the other instead creates a pyrimidine-pyrimidone (6–4) photoproduct. Both photoproducts distort the DNA helix and are recognized by DNA repair enzymes.

UVA is 20-fold more frequent in sunlight but requires 1,000-fold greater doses for its biological effect. UVA induces T-containing cyclobutane dimers and lesser numbers of oxidized purines and pyrimidines and single-strand breaks [15]. UVA generates these lesions indirectly by photosensitization. UVA also efficiently photoisomerizes UVB-induced (6–4) photoproducts to their poorly repaired and highly mutagenic Dewar isomers.

Photosensitized Reactive Oxygen Species

Both UVB and UVA can be absorbed by cytoplasmic ring-containing molecules such as NADH, riboflavin, quinones, tryptophan and tyrosine, and the heme group of catalase. The resulting energetic molecule can interact with DNA to produce a T-containing cyclobutane dimer [15] or can produce reactive oxygen species. In the latter pathway, the chromophore's energy is transferred to oxygen, resulting in singlet oxygen ($^1O_2$; an excited state of oxygen) or, if an electron is transferred, superoxide ($O_2\bullet^-$). In the presence of water, these lead to hydrogen peroxide (H_2O_2) and thence, in the presence of Fe^{+2}, to the hydroxyl radical (•OH). Hydroxyl radicals produce oxidative DNA damage resembling that after gamma radiation. Reactive oxygen species react with lipid membranes and the redox-sensitive catalytic site of phosphatases (see section "Cytoplasmic Signaling," below). Their production of 8-hydroxy-deoxyguanosine in DNA probably accounts for the occasional non-UV-like mutations after UVB. UV also upregulates nitric oxide (NO), a more stable radical species that can participate in similar reactions after diffusing long distances and traversing lipid membranes.

Excision Repair

Nucleotide excision repair (NER) is the key protection mechanism against the lethal and mutagenic effects of UV-induced cyclobutane dimers and (6–4) photoproducts. Two NER pathways have been identified, global genome repair (GGR) and transcription coupled repair (TCR). GGR removes DNA lesions throughout the genome, whereas TCR is specialized for DNA lesions in the transcribed strand of transcriptionally active genes. In humans, excision repair requires the concerted action of six repair factors (XPA, RPA, XPC, TFIIH, XPG, and XPF-ERCC1) composed of nearly 20 polypeptides, some identified and named according to the seven complementation groups of xeroderma pigmentosum (XP). The enzymatic steps of NER include: recognizing damaged DNA, forming dual incisions that bracket the UV lesion, removing the damaged oligomer (24–32 nucleotides in length), gap filling by DNA synthesis, and ligating the repaired strand [16]. Global NER is considered error-free because the complementary undamaged strand is used as a template for repair synthesis. In fact, XPC protein appears commonly inactivated in spontaneous SCCs, although the genetic mechanisms are not clear [17].

This core machinery of GGR is also used by TCR in active genes. Whereas in GGR the XPC protein recognizes distortions in the DNA double helix, the damage recognition signal for TCR is an RNA polymerase II complex stalled at a UV lesion, which attracts the core GGR machinery. RNA pol II sterically hinders the accessibility of NER factors and so is removed from the damage site by the CSA and CSB proteins. CSA and CSB are the genes mutated in Cockayne's syndrome (CS), an autosomal recessive disorder characterized by cutaneous photosensitivity and physical and mental retardation. Induction of these repair factors is genetically regulated (see section "DNA Damage Signalling"). The GGR machinery has also recently been suggested to be specifically excluded from regions of tightly packaged chromatin, contributing to differential mutation rates observed in skin and other cancer genomes [18]. A genome-wide map of DNA repair, based on sequencing 30-mer nucleotide excision products, indicates that cyclobutane dimer repair occurs preferentially at transcribed regions, whereas (6–4) photoproduct repair occurs uniformly throughout the genome [19].

UV Signature Mutations

UV leaves a characteristic signature when it interacts with DNA, and this signature remains in the tumor decades later. It has been used to answer many questions about the origin of cancer. A cyclobutane dimer or (6–4) photoproduct can lead to a mutation in two ways (Fig. 1). When the lesion is copied during DNA replication, the DNA polymerase may read a damaged cytosine as a thymine and insert an adenine opposite it. At the next round of replication, the polymerase correctly inserts thymine across from adenine with the result being a C → T substitution. Although the TT cylobutane pyrimidine dimer is the best known and most frequent photoproduct, the thymines are not mutagenic because the *XPV* gene encodes a specialized polymerase (Pol eta) that adds adenines across from a T-containing cyclobutane dimer. Alternatively, a mutation can arise because cyclobutane dimers accelerate deamination of their cytosines to uracil (or 5-methylcytosine to thymine), leading to a C → T substitution; no polymerase error is involved. In either case, C → T mutations occur only where a cytosine lies next to a thymine or another cytosine, because the major UV photoproducts join adjacent pyrimidines. If two adjacent cytosines mutate, the result is CC → TT. This distinctive pattern of mutation, C → T where the C lies next to another pyrimidine, including CC → TT, is unique to UV radiation and is called the UV signature [20].

UV signature mutations provide a tool for deducing backward from mutations found in tumors to the original carcinogen. Nearly all experimentally created UVB or UVC mutations occur at adjacent pyrimidines, and about two thirds are signature mutations. The remaining third, typically C → A and T → C substitutions or 1–2 base insertions or deletions, are still caused by UV but probably arise by photosensitized production of reactive oxygen. Because this oxidative class is caused by many carcinogens, these mutations cannot identify whether their source was UVB, UVA, tobacco smoke, or intracellular oxidative phosphorylation. A set of tumors carrying the classic UV signature mutations must, however, also have some tumors with these UV-induced oxidative mutations. UVA, in contrast, only weakly induces UVB signature mutations by photosensitization but also generates oxidation-like mutations and T → G changes. The latter are rare with UVB or other carcinogens and have been proposed to represent a UVA fingerprint.

p53

UV signature mutations identified *p53* as critical for preventing SCC and BCC but not melanoma. The P53 protein is a transcription factor that controls genes involved in the cell cycle, apoptosis, and DNA repair; it also acts directly on apoptosis proteins [6]. The *p53* gene is mutated in about half of all human cancers and is termed a tumor suppressor gene because cancer arises from losing its normal function rather than gaining an abnormal function as oncogenes do. Over 90 % of SCC in US patients contain these mutations, as well as three quarters of AK. Although nearly all BCC overexpress P53 protein, only half carry *p53* mutations. Each mutation changes the amino acid, indicating that the mutation was selected for and contributed to tumor development, rather than being simply an indicator of sun exposure. These *p53* mutations are most frequent at nine mutation hotspots in important functional regions of the protein. Compared to internal cancers, some skin cancer hotspots displace several nucleotides to lie at a site of adjacent pyrimidines. Some sites may be hotspots because repair is slower there [21]. Other skin hotspots, like internal cancer hotspots, lie at 5-methylCG sites where body temperature slowly deaminates 5-methylcytosine to thymine; UV accelerates this process.

The *p53* mutations in AK indicate that these dysplasias are clonal rather than toxic reactions; patients with multiple AK's have different mutations in each lesion [22]. The similarity of AK and SCC mutations supports the idea that AKs can progress to SCC. Aggressive skin tumors from patients exposed to both sun and chemicals contain multiple unrelated *p53* mutations, as if multiple tumors arose in an abnormal field and merged. XP tumors contain very frequent CC → TT mutations, perhaps because slow repair allows more time for cytosine deamination. Double-base mutations are also seen in conjunctival SCC, a tumor associated with HIV in sunny areas. Sunscreens reduce the level of UV signature mutations. In contrast, arsenic-induced BCC and SCC have non-UV *p53* mutations; *p53* mutations in BCCs from sun-shielded body sites resemble those seen with oxidative damage.

Sunlight mutates *p53* early. Normal sun-exposed skin carries ~60,000 clones of p53-mutant keratinocytes, 3–3,000 cells in size [23]. By hematoxylin-eosin staining, the cells in these mutant clones appear completely normal. The early appearance of *p53* mutations makes it possible to trace lineages in tumor development. Microdissecting lesions containing AK, carcinoma in situ, and SCC reveal that each stage contains the same *p53* mutation. Although this result shows that each stage arose from the same founder lesion, it does not show that the stages derived from each other. To show a lineage, it is necessary to find additional mutations that appear in succession. In microdissected BCCs, one *p53* mutation is present throughout the tumor, with various second mutations in different regions of the tumor. Once both *p53* alleles are mutated, the cell is prone to aneuploidy, increasing the likelihood of a mutator phenotype.

Hedgehog Pathway

Nearly all sporadic BCC's have inactivating mutations in the *PTCH* tumor suppressor gene, a part of the hedgehog pathway; the remainder have activating mutations in its target, *SMO*. The hedgehog pathway appears to be a "gatekeeper" for basal cell carcinogenesis, needing to be mutated early in BCC: minute BCCs have *PTCH* mutations, as do all histological subtypes; no BCCs have loss on other chromosomes without involvement of *PTCH*; and a congenital lesion that can progress to BCC, the sebaceous nevus, has *PTCH* allelic loss in 40 % of cases [24].

In sporadic BCCs about three quarters of *PTCH* mutations are UV-like (either UV signature mutations or the expected UV-induced oxidative mutations), and a further 15 % are one- or two-base insertions or deletions, often adjacent to a C → T at a dipyrimidine site. BCCs from XP patients contain UV-like *PTCH* and *SMO* mutations, with CC → TT mutations overrepresented. About 20 % of the mutations in sporadic BCCs are not UV-like and resemble germline mutations seen in Gorlin syndrome patients – deletions or insertions larger than 2 bp. This finding may relate to the clinical observation that one third of BCCs occur on parts of the body that are not chronically sun-exposed, as well as the correlation between truncal BCC and defects in the glutathione radical-scavenging system (see section "Genetic Risk Factors for UV Carcinogenesis"). *PTCH* mutations tend to code for stop codons or frameshifts that completely inactivate the protein. In hereditary BCCs, nearly all tumors arose after losing the normal allele. This allelic loss appears related to sunlight, since NBCCS tumors are most frequent on sun-exposed skin and are rare in blacks. UVB rarely causes this type of large genetic rearrangement so, in analogy to the x-ray sensitivity of NBCCS patients,

UVA-photosensitized reactive oxygen may be important.

Psoralen + UVA (PUVA)

Psoralen irradiated with UVA forms adducts at TA, TG, or TT sequences, as well as crosslinks between the two DNA strands at these sites. In human PUVA-induced keratoses, SCCs, and BCCs, about one-quarter of mutations in *p53* or *HRAS* are psoralen-like mutations at the T of TA, TG, or TT; this proportion increases as the PUVA dose increases. The majority of mutations, however, are UV signature mutations. These UV-like mutations could have arisen from the UVA in PUVA, separate UVB treatments for psoriasis, or environmental UVB.

Melanoma Mutations

Despite the correlation between melanoma and sunlight, genes with UV signature mutations are not prevalent. The *CDKN2A* locus is frequently mutated or deleted in familial and sporadic melanoma. Its two distinct tumor suppressor proteins, INK4A (also known as P16) and ARF, inhibit cell cycle progression via RB and P53, respectively. INK4A inhibits CDK4/6's inactivation of the retinoblastoma protein, RB. ARF inhibits MDM2-mediated degradation of P53. Germline mutations in *CDKN2A* are observed in ~25–40 % of familial melanomas. In sporadic melanoma, allelic loss of *CDKN2A* is more common than the rare *INK4A* inactivating mutations or inactivation of *INK4A* by promoter methylation.

The wealth of sequencing studies in melanoma have identified a trove of predominantly UV-induced point mutations, both rare and common, in coding and regulatory regions of established oncogenes in both CSD and non-CSD melanomas [25–29]. Mutations are most common in the RAS-BRAF-MEK-ERK mitogen-activated protein kinase (MAPK) signaling pathway. This signaling cascade is normally activated upon growth factor stimulation, and its sequential phosphorylation regulates cell proliferation and differentiation. Activating mutations in MAPK signaling remove the growth factor requirement. *RAS* mutations are present in 10–20 % of melanomas and have been correlated with UV exposure. The most prevalent RAS pathway mutations in melanomas are in the *BRAF* gene, particularly the *BRAF* V600E point mutation that renders the kinase constitutively active and enhances ERK activation [30]. This mutation is present in nearly ~80 % of acquired melanocytic nevi, suggesting a potential early role of *BRAF* in melanoma development. The V600E mutation is not UV-like and is associated with intermittent sunlight exposure.

UV-Induced Steps in Cancer and Cancer Prevention

Skin tumors arise on a background of sun-damaged skin. To prevent sun damage, the skin reacts to acute and chronic UV exposure by multiple stress responses. Although the most well-studied stress responses appear activated via DNA damage, UVB also generates ligand photoproducts such as (AhR) ligand 6-formylindolo[3,2-b] carbazole, which enhance EGFR-dependent ERK1/2 signaling and the downstream stress response [31].

DNA Damage Signaling

A cell with damaged DNA upregulates normal P53 protein. UV signaling is initiated by cyclobutane dimers and (6–4) photoproducts specifically in the small minority of actively-transcribed genes, with stalled RNA polymerase not only recruiting excision repair proteins but also initiating signaling [5, 6]. In an unknown way, this activates ATR and CHK1 kinases, which phosphorylate P53 at sites that make it resistant to proteasomal degradation mediated by HDM2. P53 then transcriptionally activates a large repertoire of genes, including the repair proteins P48, which is required for GGR and is defective in XP group E, and GADD45. Additionally, P53 functions as a chromatin accessibility factor, modifying the structure of damaged DNA and making it more accessible to repair factors. P53 also transactivates the cell cycle arrest protein P21, although in keratinocytes UV induces P21 even without P53. UV primarily slows down S phase ("S phase delay") and induces a modest G2 arrest, unlike ionizing radiation, which uses P53 to induce G1 arrest. It is often said that cell cycle arrest facilitates DNA repair and survival, but there is little evidence supporting this concept; deleting the P21 cell cycle arrest protein has no effect on repair after UV. These "guardian of the genome" roles of P53 are complemented by a "cellular proofreading" role in which P53 erases aberrant cells by apoptosis rather than repairing them [22]: it transcriptionally activates the death receptor Fas and proapoptotic effectors Bax, Bak, Bid, and PUMA; it directly activates Bax protein at the mitochondrion; and it inactivates E2F1, which otherwise inhibits anti-apoptotic Bcl-2 [7]. This suite of UV responses is lost when P53 is mutated by sunlight. DNA damage also activates the cytoplasmically-sequestered transcription factor NFćB, which then activates proinflammatory cytokines such as IL-10, growth signals, and antiapoptotic signals. Finally, DNA photoproducts trigger UV-induced systemic immunosuppression and suppression of dendritic cell antigen-presenting activity, but not inflammatory edema.

Cytoplasmic Signaling

"The UV response" initially referred to the P53-independent activation of JNK, its target c-JUN, and via the FOS-JUN transcription factor AP-1, induction of genes for collagenase, metallothionein, and c-JUN and c-FOS themselves [32]. The signal begins when reactive oxygen species generated by UVB or UVA photosensitization inactivate phosphatases by converting a highly sensitive cysteine residue in the catalytic site to sulfenic acid [33]. Dephosphorylation of growth factor receptor dimers and death receptor trimers is slowed, leading within minutes to more phosphorylated active receptors. Activated death receptors (involved in apoptosis) such as Fas and TNFα receptor then cluster even without a ligand, recruiting the adapter proteins DAXX and FADD and activating cytoplasmic kinases and scaffold proteins. These activate ASK1 and MEKK 4,7 kinases and their target, JNK [34]. Phosphatase inhibition can activate JNK directly. In parallel, AP-1 also induces genes for the death receptor ligands, FasL and TNFα. These ligands, together with UV upregulation of FAS receptor via P53, create a delayed feedback loop that, as with ionizing radiation, appears to prolong the rapid but transient response triggered by UV's inactivation of phosphatases. Without this prolongation, UV-activated NFćB quickly terminates the JNK response. This loop is important because transient JNK activation leads to cell proliferation, but constitutive JNK activation induces apoptosis. AP-1 also induces immunomodulatory cytokines such as IL-12, which facilitates nucleotide excision repair [35]; the AP-1-induced metalloproteinases degrade dermal extracellular matrix molecules such as collagen and may contribute to photoaging [36]. UV also blocks initiation of protein translation, via kinases that inactivate elongation factor eIF2α.

Cellular Responses

Apoptosis

UV signaling generates sunburn cells – basal and suprabasal keratinocytes with dense, pycnotic nuclei and intensely eosinophilic cytoplasm. This apoptotic morphology is accompanied by pathognomic DNA double-strand breaks and cleaved caspase 3. UV-induced apoptosis requires signals from both DNA damage and the cytoplasm: DNA photoproducts in active genes trigger P53 and its regulator Mdm-2, but apoptosis also requires JNK and is partially blocked by antioxidants. Although TNFα is required, injecting TNFα does not lead to sunburn cells so UV-induced cytoplasmic signaling is not sufficient. In fibroblasts, keratinocytes, or melanocytes with normal P53 and irradiated with physiologic UVB or UVC doses, apoptosis proceeds through the intrinsic mitochondrial pathway rather than the death-receptor/caspase 8 pathway.

Apoptosis then prevents cancer by removing UV-damaged cells, termed "cellular proofreading". Mice accumulate mutations at a rapid rate if they are defective in apoptosis due to a defect in *p53* or Fas ligand, or due to overexpressing the

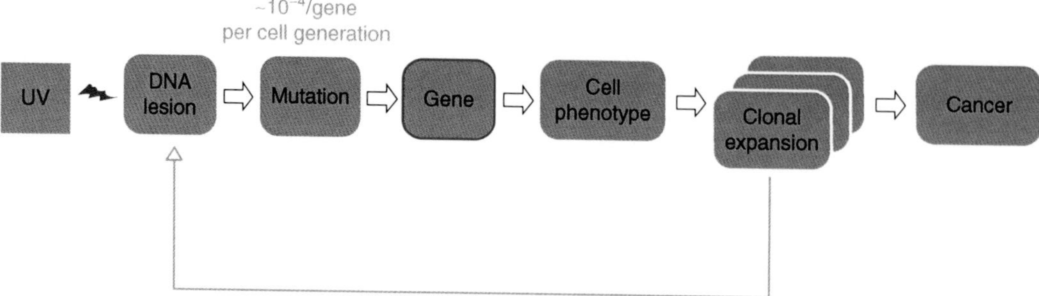

Fig. 2 The carcinogenesis cycle UV makes chemical changes in DNA that create mutations when DNA is copied. Some mutations alter the function of the gene in which they occur and lead to a new cell phenotype. The abnormal cell expands into a clone that becomes the target of further DNA damage

antiapoptotic protein Survivin [7, 37]. In the case of Survivin, this increases SCC. The epidermal hyperplasia that occurs several days after UV may replace cells lost by apoptosis or may remove additional damaged or mutant cells by desquamation. The signal for hyperplasia involves both DNA photoproducts and the EGF receptor.

Stem-Cell Populations

In chronically UVB-exposed human skin, *p53*-mutant clones are found at the two sites of epidermal stem cells: the hair follicle, whose bulge region contributes to follicle development and transiently to wound repair, and the interfollicular epidermis, which maintains epidermal homeostasis and can also generate follicles [38]. SCC are thought to originate in interfollicular epidermis, whereas histological evidence and the expression pattern of PTCH indicate that BCC originate in the follicles [39]. Hedgehog signaling through PTCH is crucial for maintaining skin stem cell populations, and for regulating hair follicle and sebaceous gland development. Chronically UV-irradiated human or mouse skin contains scattered basal cells with unusually high levels of DNA photoproducts. The tumor promoter TPA, which induces skin stem cells to proliferate, causes these cells to disappear and be replaced by clusters of p53-mutant keratinocytes. This behavior resembles that of stem cells that are quiescent and poorly repaired, at least on the parental DNA strand, until triggered to divide. However, meta-analysis indicates that withdrawal of UVB irradiation stabilizes expansion of *p53*-mutant cell populations, suggesting preneoplastic clones arise not from mutant stem cells, but from progenitors whose cell fate is random [40].

Clonal Expansion of Mutant Cells

A single mutant cell must clonally expand to reach a clinical size. Less obviously, clonal expansion facilitates the multiple genetic hit mechanism of cancer. Physiologic UV doses create mutations at a frequency of ~10^{-4}/gene per cell division (Fig. 2). The specific mutations needed to activate an oncogene would be rarer. Spontaneous mutations, which reflect errors by the replication machinery or DNA damage due to body temperature, are also rare, on the order of 10^{-5}. The probability of mutating five genes, such as an oncogene and both alleles of two particular tumor suppressor genes, is then at best 10^{-20}. With 10^6 proliferating keratinocytes per cm^2 in human skin, and ~1 m^2 exposed, fewer than one person in 10^{10} would have a tumor. Accounting for the 60 % lifetime expectation of skin cancer in Australia solely in terms of genetic hits in one cell is impossible. In contrast, clonal expansion increases by 1,000-fold the number of targets for the next mutation.

A stem cell's clonal expansion is normally limited to its stem cell compartment [41]. Sunlight is a key driver of clonal expansion beyond this point. Sequencing studies show that a large range of known oncogenes are activated by UV-damage in phenotypically normal skin, producing focal clonal proliferations that may precede skin cancer [42]. The *p53*-mutant clones in human skin, the first to be thus characterized, are larger in chronically sun-exposed skin. In mice, clones stop growing and regress when UVB treatment ends, indicating that clone expansion is due to a UV-induced physiological event rather than an irreversible mutation. One of these physiological events is UV-induced apoptosis [7]. Once a p53 mutation arises, the cellular proofreading mechanism backfires. Subsequent UV exposures eliminate damaged normal cells but spare apoptosis-resistant mutants. A mutant normally restrained within its stem cell compartment then escapes to colonize the newly-vacated compartment. Repeating this process results in quantized clonal expansion. Apoptosis retards or accelerates skin cancer depending on the stage. It prevents new *p53* mutations, accelerates the expansion of p53-mutant clones and papillomas, and prevents the mutations that convert a papilloma to SCC.

Cell–Cell Communication

Cell–cell interactions prevent abnormal cells from proliferating inappropriately. In human autotransplant experiments, BCC's transferred from their original site regressed – suggesting that an abnormal underlying dermis is required for the tumor to persist. Dermal fibroblasts suppress transformed keratinocytes by secreting TGFβ that induces squamous differentiation. Normal keratinocytes also suppress their transformed neighbors, and UV interferes with these signals. Normal human keratinocytes eliminate adjacent transformed keratinocytes (universally mutated in p53 and Notch receptors [43, 44] and more rarely in *HRAS*) by inducing cell cycle arrest and differentiation. Physiologic doses of UVB cause apoptosis and differentiation in the normal cells, but not in the transformed keratinocytes, allowing the latter to clonally expand [45]. Other intercellular signals are mediated by integrins – membrane receptors for extracellular matrix proteins such as collagen ($\alpha_2\beta_1$ integrin), laminin ($\alpha_3\beta_1$), and fibronectin ($\alpha_5\beta_1$). Keratinocytes bound to such ligands provide a "do not differentiate" signal through MAP kinase pathways, suppressing keratinocyte apoptosis and allowing a stem-cell pool to be maintained. Integrin receptors are often dysregulated in tumors. UVB irradiation downregulates the β_1 integrin subunit; UVA downregulates the gap junction communication protein connexin 43, resembling the action of the tumor promoter TPA.

Melanocyte proliferation is normally regulated by keratinocytes via cell–cell adhesion receptors such as E-cadherin, P-cadherin, and desmogleins; these receptors are lost in vertical growth phase melanomas. UV stimulates keratinocytes to secrete endothelin-1, which then downregulates melanocyte E-cadherin and upregulates their N-cadherin. This E to N-cadherin switch diverts melanocyte interactions away from keratinocytes and toward fibroblasts and melanocytes.

Immune Surveillance

In humans, the primary evidence cited for immune surveillance in preventing UV-induced skin cancer is the 10–20-fold increase in AK and SCC on previously sun-exposed skin in transplant patients receiving chronic immune suppression to prevent organ rejection. In one Australian study, 27 % of deaths in a heart transplant cohort were due to skin cancer. The increase begins months to a few years after immune suppression is initiated, and both the AK and SCC are unusually aggressive. Melanomas are also increased. Several lines of evidence mar the interpretation as immune surveillance: Cyclophosphamide is a well-known mutagen. Cyclosporine promotes tumor growth in vitro and in immune deficient mice where there is no immune system to be suppressed. Azathioprine (Imuran) is a mutagen when followed by UVA irradiation. HIV patients do have a modestly increased incidence of SCC, but these tumors at sun-shielded sites are associated with human papilloma virus. Skin cancers are often said to develop in patients who are immunodeficient due to leukemia or lymphoma. Most published reports lack controls or patient data, but an eight-fold elevation in chronic lymphocytic leukemia seems valid. Most of these patients had received immunosuppressive drugs, or radiation, so the mutagenicity caveat applies. In contrast, Merkel cell carcinoma may be truly sensitive to immune function because its incidence increases 10–20-fold not only in solid-organ transplant recipients but also in HIV patients (~13-fold) and in chronic lymphocytic leukemia.

Animal Models of Skin Cancer

UV Radiation Wavelengths and Carcinogenesis

Showing causality requires manipulating an experimental system, which usually cannot be done in humans. Early experiments generated fibrosarcomas by irradiating mouse ears. SCC are generated by irradiating back skin daily for about 4 months with doses of UVB several-fold above the minimal erythemal dose. The sequence of events resembles that in humans, with p53-mutant clones appearing early, followed by reddish lesions that resemble AKs both visibly and histologically. SCC induced by UVB contain UV signature p53 mutations. p53-mutant clones may be a precursor lesion for SCC because (a) the relationship between UVB dose and induction time for an AK equals that for a p53-mutant clone plus an additional similar event and (b) mutant clones and SCC have the same sensitivity to DNA repair knockouts. Growth of an existing SCC no longer depends on UV.

The action spectrum for carcinogenesis in the hairless mouse closely approximates that for erythema in human skin and edema in murine skin, with the most effective wavelengths at 295–305 nm in the UVB region. Calculations show that this peak is the product of the 260 nm DNA absorption peak and absorption by the skin [12]. Activity decreases sharply at wavelengths above this range. The UVA used in tanning beds can also cause skin tumors in mice; p53 mutations are rare. Some evidence indicates that because of an attenuated antigenotoxic response between the UVA and UVB wavelengths near 315 uM, such "border" wavelengths may actually prove maximally mutagenic [46].

UVB acts as both initiator and promoter for mouse skin papillomas and UVA acts as a promoter. Tumor promoters are agents that increase the frequency of tumors, but only when delivered after the initiator mutagen and only while the promoter is present. Initiation is considered to contribute irreversible genetic events, whereas promotion stimulates reversible growth acceleration. The promotion concept developed from studies of chemically-induced papillomas, especially those now known to be mutated at *Hras* and at low risk for conversion to SCC, which are transiently increased after treating with a chemical such as phorbol ester. Similarly, 90 % of UVB-initiated *p53*-mutant clones regress within 3 weeks after UVB is terminated; T or B cells are not required. AKs also often regress once irradiation stops but SCCs do not, indicating that invasive tumors no longer need a promoter. Because it is now clear that tumorigenesis consists of multiple cycles of mutation and growth, dividing cancer development into initiation and promotion phases has been largely superseded by a focus on the timing of specific genetic and cellular mechanisms.

Studies in mice also revealed that: cyclobutane dimers are responsible for UVB-induced apoptosis, hyperplasia, p53-mutant clones, and SCC [47]; repairing the UVB-induced oxidative lesion 8-OH dG reduces SCC by half; $p53^{-/-}$ mice are highly susceptible to UV-induced AK and SCC, whereas UV induces BCC in $Ptch^{+/-}$ mice; and basaloid budding and BCC can be induced by overexpressing the hedgehog pathway [39]. Physiological status also affects tumor development: exposure to stress (fox urine) reduces the latency of UV-induced SCC from 21 weeks to 8 weeks.

Modeling melanoma has been more challenging. A melanoma-susceptible fish demonstrated the ability of UVA-induced reactive oxygen to induce melanomas. In the opossum *Monodelphis domestica*, UVB + UVA induces melanomas and melanocytic hyperplasia, and UVA can itself induce melanocytic hyperplasia. Generating melanomas in mice requires genetic manipulation. Ocular and dermal melanomas arise without UV when the SV40 virus early region sequences are put under the control of the tyrosinase promoter. When the metallothionein promoter drives hepatocyte growth factor, melanocytes are produced in the epidermis – not their normal location in mice – and a single high dose of sunlamp UV in the neonate, but not adult, generates melanomas months later. When the tyrosinase promoter is used to drive mutant *HRAS* in a mouse deleted for the *ARF* gene, melanomas arise months later but sooner if the mice receive a single high neonatal UV dose. Half the UV-induced tumors carry amplified *CDK6*, reminiscent of chronic sun damage melanomas in humans. It is crucial to realize, however, that both metallothionein and tyrosinase promoters are UV-inducible, so the single UV dose used here is not guaranteed to model the role of UV in causing human melanoma.

Immune Function and Skin Cancer

The mouse model reveals an important immunological component to tumor progression. Murine UV-induced tumors are highly immunogenic, but early in the course of chronic UV radiation, before primary tumors are evident, mice lose their ability to reject UV-induced tumors. UV therefore has a systemic immunosuppressive effect. Natural killer T lymphocytes are the suppressor T cells responsible [48]. However, it has also been shown that immune cells may metabolize and thus potentiate carcinogens, such as 7,12-dimethylbenz[a]anthracene (DMBA) in mice, highlighting more complex relationships with oncogenesis [49].

Genetic Risk Factors for UV Carcinogenesis

Pigmentation and Initial Damage

Melanin has a large role in resistance to skin cancer. The Fitzpatrick skin types are determined not only by baseline pigmentation but also by a person's response to UV (always burns, tans easily, or rarely burns). This simple UV skin response scale can account for up to a 100-fold difference in susceptibility to skin cancers. Similarly, the many molecular etiologies of oculocutaneous albinism, which result in a deficiency of normal melanin, markedly increase the risk of skin cancer. Increased skin cancer among albinos is mostly nonmelanoma skin cancer but melanomas seem elevated as well. Another hereditary risk factor, red or blonde hair, is now understood at a molecular level as commonly caused by polymorphisms in the melanocortin-1 receptor. This receptor is a G-protein coupled receptor that binds melanocyte stimulating hormone (MSH) and lies at a key point in melanogenesis. Certain mutations in this receptor render it insensitive to normal pigmentation signals, resulting in pheomelanin instead of eumelanin. This is an important distinction in terms of skin cancer prevention. Red or yellow pheomelanin is a markedly less effective free radical scavenger; indeed, UV exposed pheomelanin is degraded with a net formation of superoxide [11]. Therefore, pheomelanin can act as a photosensitizer, even inducing apoptosis in nearby cells [50]. Decreased protection and increased damage from pheomelanin in the epidermis may partly underlie the markedly increased risk of skin cancer associated with red-haired individuals. However, cyclobutane dimers may also result from energy transfer to DNA from melanin hours after UVA exposure has ceased [51] highlighting complexities in the protective functions of skin pigmentation.

Reactive oxygen species are largely absorbed by radical scavengers such as glutathione before they cause significant membrane or DNA damage. Specific polymorphisms in the genes for glutathione S-transferase confer a twofold risk for truncal AK, SCC, and BCC [52]. This genetic risk increases to sixfold in patients with high sun exposure and 12-fold in sun-exposed transplant patients.

DNA Repair and Apoptosis

Xeroderma pigmentosum highlights the association between DNA repair capacity and skin cancer. Although defects in any of the XP genes result in some defect in NER, the severity of the XP disorder – number of skin tumors and life expectancy – correlates with DNA repair capacity [16]. The correlation between repair capacity and cancer incidence is also present in the general population. Patients with AK have 30–50 % reduced excision repair in their normal fibroblasts or lymphocytes. These data suggest that relatively subtle variability in DNA repair capacity contributes to an individual's risk of developing skin cancer.

Viral Sensitivity

In the rare inherited sensitivity to HPV infection termed epidermodysplasia verruciformis, roughly one-half of patients will develop SCC. These SCC are typically on sun-exposed body sites and occur decades earlier than in the general population. HPV may be important in UV carcinogenesis in immunosuppressed transplant patients, as it is detected twice as frequently in SCCs from these patients as in immunocompetent controls.

Prevention

The potential of education and sunscreen to control skin cancer remains largely unproven due to the long latency between sun exposure and skin cancer appearance. Adult sunscreen use can reduce AK by twofold. Randomized studies of school children who aggressively applied sunscreen indicate that common nevi can be reduced. A regimen of sun protection longer than the typical 2–4-year study would likely decrease nevi and subsequent melanoma risk more impressively. Encouraging data are emerging from Australia where education campaigns, covered sidewalks, and covered playgrounds at schools have led to a stabilization of the incidence of nonmelanoma skin cancers. Clearly, an effective campaign to reduce skin cancer needs to begin with school-age children. This is due to the combined factors that children under the age of 18 spend a significant portion of their time in outdoor recreation, and sun damage sustained early in life has more time to contribute to UV carcinogenesis.

One could ask "how much sun is too much?" The answer will vary immensely depending on many factors such as pigmentation, whether sun exposure occurs in modest doses or large exposures, the immune status of the individual, and subtle differences in DNA repair capacity. Small studies have suggested that behavioral responses to sun exposure share addiction-like features [53, 54]. Although highly controversial, there may be some benefit to sun exposure. Several studies have suggested twofold better survival following a diagnosis of invasive melanoma among patients with extensive sun exposure as compared to those with less exposure. A potential explanation is greater vitamin D synthesis induced by UV.

Conclusion

Despite the use of suncreens and public awareness of the effects of long-term exposure to UV, the incidence of both melanoma and nonmelanoma skin cancers continues to increase. This has led to investigation of novel chemopreventive agents that interfere with the development of cancer through diverse mechanisms. Perhaps the most important recent advance in this area is the use of imiquimod (Aldara), an activator of the innate immune system through the TLR7 receptor. Imiquimod has recently been approved for treating AKs and superficial BCCs, and reports of imiquimod effects also exist for atypical melanocytic proliferations such as lentigo maligna.

In terms of foods, tea appears to have chemopreventive activity. Orally administered green or black tea reduces UV-induced skin cancers in mice to less than half of control levels. Polyphenols and caffeine appear to be the major chemopreventive components. Epidemiological studies suggest that caffeine intake correlates with decreased risk of both melanoma and nonmelanoma skin cancers [55–57].

Low fat diets have been well studied as an approach to preventing skin cancer. Animal studies have shown that high fat diets shorten the time between UV exposure and tumor formation and markedly increase the number of tumors per animal. In human trials of patients with nonmelanoma skin cancer, restricting calories from fat reduced the appearance of AKs by two thirds and the development of new nonmelanoma skin cancers by one- half.

A recent development in the area of chemoprevention is the ability to augment normal DNA repair pathways. If one could increase DNA repair capacity, the mutations, chromosomal aberrations, and cell death known to be causal for skin tumors should be reduced. The most direct application of this concept is the use of a viral enzyme (T4 endonuclease V) capable of recognizing cyclobutane dimers and accelerating the initial incision step of the nucleotide excision repair pathway. This enzyme has been formulated into a liposomal preparation allowing penetration into the relevant layers of skin. Indeed, studies in XP patients have shown efficacy in decreasing the residual DNA damage, as well as the number of actinic keratoses. There are thus diverse emerging approaches by which chemopreventive therapies may increasingly serve as an adjunct to classical UV protection with sunscreens and avoidance of UV exposure to skin.

Cross-References

- ▶ Melanoma and Skin Aging
- ▶ Sunlight Exposure and Skin Thickness Measurements as a Function of Age: Risk Factors for Melanoma

References

1. Leigh I, Newton-Bishop JA, Kripke ML. Skin cancer, Cancer surveys, vol. 26. Plainview: Cold Spring Harbor Laboratory Press; 1996. p. 361.
2. Brash DE, Pontén J. Skin precancer. In: Pontén J, editor. Precancer: biology, importance, and possible prevention. Cold Spring Harbor: Cold Spring Harbor Press; 1998. p. 69–113.
3. Brash DE. Sunlight and the onset of skin cancer. Trends Genet. 1997;13:410–4.
4. de Gruijl FR, Ananthaswamy HN. Biological effects of ultraviolet radiation, Mutation research, vol. 571. Amsterdam: Elsevier; 2005 (special issue).
5. Hussein MR. Ultraviolet radiation and skin cancer: molecular mechanisms. J Cutan Pathol. 2005; 32(3):191–205.
6. Latonen L, Laiho M. Cellular UV damage responses – functions of tumor suppressor p53. Biochim Biophys Acta. 1755;2005:71–89.
7. Raj D, Brash DE, Grossman D. Keratinocyte apoptosis in epidermal development and disease. J Invest Dermatol. 2006;126:243–57.
8. Green A, MacLennan R, Youl P, Martin N. Site distribution of cutaneous melanoma in Queensland. Int J Cancer. 1993;53:232–6.
9. Curtin JA, Fridlyand J, Kageshita T, Patel HN, Busam KJ, Kutzner H, Cho KH, Aiba S, Brocker EB, LeBoit PE, Pinkel D, Bastian BC. Distinct sets of genetic alterations in melanoma. N Engl J Med. 2005; 353(20):2135–47.
10. Landi MT, Bauer J, Pfeiffer RM, Elder DE, Hulley B, Minghetti P, Calista D, Kanetsky PA, Pinkel D, Bastian BC. MC1R germline variants confer risk for BRAF-mutant melanoma. Science. 2006;313 (5786):521–2.
11. Kollias N, Sayre RM, Zeise L, Chedekel MR. Photoprotection by melanin. J Photochem Photobiol B. 1991;9(2):135–60.
12. Freeman SE, Hacham H, Gange RW, Maytum DJ, Sutherland JC. Wavelength dependence of pyrimidine dimer formation in DNA of human skin irradiated in *situ* with ultraviolet light. Proc Natl Acad Sci U S A. 1989;86:5605–9.
13. Gallagher RP, Spinelli JJ, Lee TK. Tanning beds, sunlamps, and risk of cutaneous malignant melanoma. Cancer Epidemiol Biomarkers Prev. 2005;14(3):562–6.
14. Wang SY. Photochemistry and photobiology of nucleic acids, vol. I. New York: Academic; 1976, 596 pp.
15. Douki T, Reynaud-Angelin A, Cadet J, Sage E. Bipyrimidine photoproducts rather than oxidative lesions are the main type of DNA damage involved in the genotoxic effect of solar UVA radiation. Biochemistry. 2003;42(30):9221–6.
16. Cleaver JE. Cancer in xeroderma pigmentosum and related disorders of DNA repair. Nat Rev Cancer. 2005;5(7):564–73.
17. Cleaver JE, Feeney L, Tang JY, Tuttle P. Xeroderma pigmentosum group C in an isolated region of Guatemala. J Invest Dermatol. 2007;127(2):493–6.
18. Zheng CL, et al. Transcription restores DNA repair to heterochromatin, determining regional mutation rates in cancer genomes. Cell Rep. 2014;9(4):1228–34.
19. Hu J, Adar S, Selby CP, Lieb JD, Sancar A. Genome-wide analysis of human global and transcription-coupled excision repair of UV damage at single-nucleotide resolution. Genes Dev. 2015;29(9):948–60.
20. Brash DE, Rudolph JA, Simon JA, Lin A, McKenna GJ, Baden HP, Halperin AJ, Pontén J. A role for sunlight in skin cancer: UV-induced p53 mutations in squamous cell carcinoma. Proc Natl Acad Sci U S A. 1991;88:10124–8.
21. Tornaletti S, Pfeifer GP. Slow repair of pyrimidine dimers at *p53* mutation hotspots in skin cancer. Science. 1994;263:1436–8.
22. Ziegler A, Jonason AS, Leffell DJ, Simon JA, Sharma HW, Kimmelman J, Remington L, Jacks T, Brash DE. Sunburn and p53 in the onset of skin cancer. Nature. 1994;372:773–6.
23. Jonason AS, Kunala S, Price GJ, Restifo RJ, Spinelli HM, Persing JA, Leffell DJ, Tarone RE, Brash DE. Frequent clones of p53-mutated keratinocytes in normal human skin. Proc Natl Acad Sci U S A. 1996;93:14025–9.
24. Gailani MR, Bale SJ, Leffell DJ, DiGiovanna JJ, Peck GL, Poliak S, Drum MA, Pastakia B, McBride OW, Kase R, Greene M, Mulvihill JJ, Bale AE. Developmental defects in Gorlin syndrome related to a putative tumor suppressor gene on chromosome 9. Cell. 1992;69:111–7.
25. Hodis E, et al. A landscape of driver mutations in melanoma. Cell. 2012;150(2):251–63.
26. Berger MF, et al. Melanoma genome sequencing reveals frequent PREX2 mutations. Nature. 2012; 485(7399):502–6.
27. Krauthammer M, et al. Exome sequencing identifies recurrent somatic RAC1 mutations in melanoma. Nat Genet. 2012;44(9):1006–14.
28. Cancer Genome Atlas Network. Genomic classification of cutaneous melanoma. Cell. 2015;161(7):1681–96.
29. Huang FW, et al. Highly recurrent TERT promoter mutations in human melanoma. Science. 2013; 339(6122):957–9.

30. Davies H, Bignell GR, Cox C, Stephens P, Edkins S, Clegg S, Teague J, Woffendin H, Garnett MJ, Bottomley W, Davis N, Dicks E, Ewing R, Floyd Y, Gray K, Hall S, Hawes R, Hughes J, Kosmidou V, Menzies A, Mould C, Parker A, Stevens C, Watt S, Hooper S, Wilson R, Jayatilake H, Gusterson BA, Cooper C, Shipley J, Hargrave D, Pritchard-Jones K, Maitland N, Chenevix-Trench G, Riggins GJ, Bigner DD, Palmieri G, Cossu A, Flanagan A, Nicholson A, Ho JW, Leung SY, Yuen ST, Weber BL, Seigler HF, Darrow TL, Paterson H, Marais R, Marshall CJ, Wooster R, Stratton MR, Futreal PA. Mutations of the BRAF gene in human cancer. Nature. 2002;417 (6892):949–54.
31. Fritsche E, et al. Lightening up the UV response by identification of the arylhydrocarbon receptor as a cytoplasmatic target for ultraviolet B radiation. Proc Natl Acad Sci U S A. 2007;104(21):8851–6.
32. Bender K, Blattner C, Knebel A, Iordanov M, Herrlich P, Rahmsdorf HJ. UV-induced signal transduction. J Photochem Photobiol B. 1997;37:1–17.
33. Tonks NK. Redox redux: revisiting PTPs and the control of cell signaling. Cell. 2005;121:667–70.
34. Devary Y, Rosette C, DiDonato JA, Karin M. NF-kB activation by ultraviolet light not dependent on a nuclear signal. Science. 1993;261:1442–5.
35. Schwarz A, Stander S, Berneburg M, Bohm M, Kulms D, van Steeg H, Grosse-Heitmeyer K, Krutmann J, Schwarz T. Interleukin-12 suppresses ultraviolet radiation-induced apoptosis by inducing DNA repair. Nat Cell Biol. 2002;4:26–31.
36. Fisher GJ, Datta SC, Talwar HS, Wang ZQ, Varani J, Kang S, Voorhees JJ. Molecular basis of sun-induced premature skin ageing and retinoid antagonism. Nature. 1996;379:335–9.
37. Hill LL, Ouhtit A, Loughlin SM, Kripke ML, Ananthaswamy HN, Owen-Schaub LB. Fas ligand: a sensor for DNA damage critical in skin cancer etiology. Science. 1999;285:898–900.
38. Levy V, Lindon C, Harfe BD, Morgan BA. Distinct stem cell populations regenerate the follicle and interfollicular epidermis. Dev Cell. 2005;9(6):855–61.
39. Oro AE, Higgins KM, Hu Z, Bonifas JM, Epstein EH, Scott MP. Basal cell carcinomas in mice overexpressing sonic hedgehog. Science. 1997;276:817–21.
40. Klein AM, Brash DE, Jones PH, Simons BD. Stochastic fate of p53-mutant epidermal progenitor cells is tilted toward proliferation by UV B during preneoplasia. Proc Natl Acad Sci U S A. 2010; 107(1):270–5.
41. Zhang W, Remenyik E, Zelterman D, Brash DE, Wikonkal NM. Escaping the stem cell compartment: sustained UVB exposure allows p53-mutant keratinocytes to colonize adjacent epidermal proliferating units without incurring additional mutations. Proc Natl Acad Sci U S A. 2001;98:13948–53.
42. Martincorena I, et al. Tumor evolution. High burden and pervasive positive selection of somatic mutations in normal human skin. Science. 2015;348(6237):880–6.
43. Durinck S, et al. Temporal dissection of tumorigenesis in primary cancers. Cancer Discov. 2011;1(2):137–43.
44. Wang NJ, et al. Loss-of-function mutations in Notch receptors in cutaneous and lung squamous cell carcinoma. Proc Natl Acad Sci U S A. 2011;108:17761–6, 201114669.
45. Mudgil AV, Segal N, Andriani F, Wang Y, Fusenig NE, Garlick JA. Ultraviolet-B irradiation induces expansion of intraepithelial tumor cells in a tissue model of early cancer progression. J Invest Dermatol. 2003;121:191–7.
46. Ikehata H, et al. Action spectrum analysis of UVR genotoxicity for skin: the border wavelengths between UVA and UVB can bring serious mutation loads to skin. J Invest Dermatol. 2013;133(7):1850–6.
47. Jans J, Schul W, Sert YG, Rijksen Y, Rebel H, Eker AP, Nakajima S, van Steeg H, de Gruijl FR, Yasui A, Hoeijmakers JH, van der Horst GT. Powerful skin cancer protection by a CPD-photolyase transgene. Curr Biol. 2005;15(2):105–15.
48. Moodycliffe AM, Nghiem D, Clydesdale G, Ullrich SE. Immune suppression and skin cancer development: regulation by NKT cells. Nat Immunol. 2000; 1(6):521–5.
49. Modi BG, et al. Langerhans cells facilitate epithelial DNA damage and squamous cell carcinoma. Science. 2012;335(6064):104–8.
50. Takeuchi S, Zhang W, Wakamatsu K, Ito S, Hearing V, Kraemer KH, Brash DE. Melanin acts as a potent UVB sensitizer to cause an atypical mode of cell death in murine skin. Proc Natl Acad Sci U S A. 2004;101:15076–81.
51. Premi S, et al. Photochemistry. Chemiexcitation of melanin derivatives induces DNA photoproducts long after UV exposure. Science. 2015; 347(6224):842–7.
52. Ramsay HM, Harden PN, Reece S, Smith AG, Jones PW, Strange RC, Fryer AA. Polymorphisms in glutathione S-transferases are associated with altered risk of nonmelanoma skin cancer in renal transplant recipients: a preliminary analysis. J Invest Dermatol. 2001;117:251–5.
53. Harrington CR, et al. Addictive-like behaviours to ultraviolet light among frequent indoor tanners. Clin Exp Dermatol. 2011;36(1):33–8.
54. Kaur M, et al. Induction of withdrawal-like symptoms in a small randomized, controlled trial of opioid blockade in frequent tanners. J Am Acad Dermatol. 2006; 54(4):709–11.
55. Song F, Qureshi AA, Han J. Increased caffeine intake is associated with reduced risk of basal cell carcinoma of the skin. Cancer Res. 2012;72(13):3282–9.
56. Abel EL, et al. Daily coffee consumption and prevalence of nonmelanoma skin cancer in Caucasian women. Eur J Cancer Prev. 2007;16(5):446–52.
57. Loftfield E, et al. Coffee drinking and cutaneous melanoma risk in the NIH-AARP diet and health study. J Natl Cancer Inst. 2015;107(2). doi:10.1093/jnci/dju421.

Melanoma and Skin Aging

69

Salina M. Torres, Christopher R. Hughes, and Marianne Berwick

Contents

S.M. Torres (✉)
Department of Pathology, Center for HPV Prevention, University of New Mexico, Albuquerque, NM, USA
e-mail: storres@salud.unm.edu

C.R. Hughes • M. Berwick
Internal Medicine, Division of Epidemiology, University of New Mexico, Albuquerque, NM, USA
e-mail: mberwick@salud.unm.edu

M.A. Farage et al. (eds.), *Textbook of Aging Skin*,
DOI 10.1007/978-3-662-47398-6_57

Abstract

The interaction between skin aging and melanoma derives from the contributions of chronologic aging and photoaging and the subsequent changes that occur in each scenario in the skin. The resultant changes in skin dynamics and their impact on melanoma development and progression are the focus of this chapter.

Introduction

The interaction between skin aging and melanoma derives from the contributions of chronologic aging and photoaging and the subsequent changes that occur in each scenario in the skin. The resultant changes in skin dynamics and their impact on melanoma development and progression are the focus of this chapter.

During the past 50 years, the world has seen an increase in the incidence and mortality of cutaneous malignant melanoma (CMM). CMM accounts for nearly 85 % of all skin cancer mortality [1]. The American Cancer Society estimates that in 2015, 73,870 Americans will be diagnosed with melanoma, resulting in approximately 9,940 deaths [2]. Several studies have found tumor thickness to be the most important prognostic factor in cutaneous malignant melanoma [3, 4]. Tumor thickness, referred to as Breslow thickness, is the depth of a melanoma lesion measured from the basement membrane of the epidermis to the deepest identified melanoma tumor cell [5]. The 5-year survival rate for patients diagnosed with early melanoma, Breslow thickness of <1.0 mm, is about 93 %; however, in patients with very thick melanoma lesions, Breslow thickness of >4 mm, the survival rate is about 40 % [6, 7]. In addition to thickness, ulceration, mitotic index, and the presence of metastases are also strong prognostic indicators [1, 8, 9]. Risk factors for melanoma development include age, phenotype, genetic and family history, numbers and types of nevi, and immune system status [10]. Melanoma, like other cancers, is a complex disease: Lachiewicz and colleagues describe it as a heterogeneous cancer with different biological mechanisms having different survival patterns [11]. Sex and behavior also contribute to the intricacy of this disease lending itself to complex prognostic challenges.

Aging is a significant risk factor in the development of skin cancer. Older individuals are among the highest risk of developing CMM [12]. The incidence of skin tumors has been found to increase with age; with more than one million new cases each year, basal cell carcinoma, squamous cell carcinoma, and melanoma combined account for almost half of all cancer diagnoses [13]. Worldwide, a threefold surge in melanoma among the elderly has been observed, and almost half of melanoma diagnoses come from this population [14]. Over three decades (1969–1999), mortality rates from melanoma have increased 157 % in men aged 65 and older [15]. The continual increase in the incidence of skin cancer during adulthood strongly relates risk to chronologic age; further, basal cell carcinoma, squamous cell carcinoma, and melanoma are strongly associated with photoaging [16]. The age-adjusted incidence rate of malignant melanoma is increasing faster than any other cancer. Combined with the fact that adult populations of advanced age continue to increase because of greater life expectancy and individuals born in years with high birth rates are growing older, the number of adults diagnosed with melanoma will continue to be a significant public health concern.

Independent of the population structure, it should be noted that some proportion of the increase might be due to better methods of, and attention to, early detection. Other studies suggest incidence rates have increased independently of early detection [17]. However, as the mortality rate among males increases, detection is not the entire answer.

Although younger Americans are experiencing improved survival and stabilizing incidence rates of melanoma, older individuals continue to encounter increasing melanoma incidence and mortality [18]. Older adults tend to develop different subtypes of melanoma, have reduced access to medical specialists, and have comorbidities that affect their ability to undergo treatment for advanced disease [19]. The age–cancer relationship is dependent on increasing opportunities for cancer to develop from old or aging cells because these cells have had more time to acquire tumorigenic mutations [20]. Age-induced reductions in DNA repair capacity may also be responsible for tumorigenesis. In the case of melanoma among older individuals, melanocytes have been exposed for decades to ultraviolet (UV) radiation and other environmental exposures. These exposures allow for the accumulation of mutations that bypass cellular DNA repair mechanisms and increase susceptibility to disease.

Epidemiology of Melanoma in Relation to Chronologic Age

Several epidemiologic studies have been conducted to evaluate the relationship between age and melanoma. A number of these studies are listed in Table 1. Lachiewicz and colleagues utilized the National Cancer Institute Surveillance, Epidemiology, and End Results (SEER) data for analyses of 51,704 non-Hispanic white adults diagnosed with a first invasive CMM between 1992 and 2003 [21]. The objective of their study was to compare the anatomic site of melanoma with prognosis. In their analyses, older age was found to independently predict more aggressive rates of melanoma-related death [22]. Further analyses of age-specific incidence patterns in melanoma cases in non-Hispanic white adults diagnosed between 2000 and 2004 revealed a peak in age-specific incidence rates among patients 70–79 years of age [11]. The incidence

Table 1 Epidemiologic studies evaluating the relationship between age and melanoma

Study population	Age group(s)	Findings	Reference
Florida population of melanoma patients $n = 442$	Separated into ≤65 or >65	Geriatric patients with melanoma had a worse prognosis	Austin et al. [24]
Non-Hispanic white adults diagnosed 1969–1999	20–65+	Fivefold increase in the incidence in men ≥65 years of age	Geller et al. [15]
Adults diagnosed 1988–1999 $n = 23{,}068$	≥65	Older age independently associated with greater risk of death from melanoma	Reyes-Ortiz et al. [25]
Cutaneous head and neck melanoma patients diagnosed 1994–2002 $n = 2{,}218$	66 (mean age)	Increased age had a significantly higher risk of death	Golger et al. [26]
Non-Hispanic white adults diagnosed 2000–2004 $n = 48{,}673$	20–80+	Age-specific incidence rate of melanomas increased with age	Lachiewicz et al. [11]
Non-Hispanic white adults diagnosed 1992–2003 $n = 51{,}704$	20–65+	Older age predicted faster rates of melanoma-related death	Lachiewicz et al. [21]
Spanish Mediterranean consecutive melanoma patients 2000–2015 $n = 1122$	40–65+	Melanoma development in younger population is due to genetic factors, while environmental variables play a major role in older patients	Montero et al. [27]
SEER 2003–2011 sentinel lymph node biopsies $n = 47{,}577$	0–80+	Older patients have higher mortality rates but are less likely to have positive sentinel lymph nodes	Cavanaugh-Hussey et al. [28]

rate in this age group was 5.9 times higher than in patients aged 20–29 years. Age-specific incidence rate curves and age distribution curves were plotted for all cases of melanoma as well as by anatomic site. The curve for age-specific incidence rates of all cases of melanoma showed a rapid increase until age 55–59 at which point it continued to rise at a slower rate before an eventual decline. The age distribution plot for all cases of melanoma displayed early- and late-onset peak frequencies at ages 54 and 74 years, respectively [11]. Trunk melanoma age-specific incidence rates increased until age 55–59, then plateaued, and subsequently declined [11]. Similar to the age distribution plot for all cases of melanoma, the age distribution for trunk melanoma demonstrated an early-onset peak around 44 and 54 years in females and males, respectively. Melanoma on anatomical areas that are continually exposed to UV radiation – the face and ears – exhibited age-specific incidence rates that drastically increased with age and peaked in the distribution plot at age 78 [11]. These two reports of SEER data analyses reveal an association between age and melanoma mortality and incidence. Lachiewicz and colleagues hypothesized that their findings of a multimodal age distribution of melanoma in their population are indicative of a "divergent pathway" model, originally proposed by Whiteman and colleagues [22]. In this model, people with inherently low propensity for melanocyte proliferation develop melanoma after chronic sun exposure to habitually exposed sites like the face and ears (late onset); in contrast, people with a high propensity for melanocyte proliferation develop melanoma on anatomical sites with less intermittent solar damage and/or unstable melanocytes like the trunk (early onset) [22]. The existence of divergent age-specific incidence patterns provides support for the idea that more than one causal pathway exists for melanoma and the existence of distinct melanoma genotypes [11]. This divergent pathway may be partially explained by somatic mutations occurring in two oncogenes – BRAF and NRAS [23]. However, their exact mechanisms remain unknown. Other epidemiological and animal studies have demonstrated that epidermal melanocytes are predominantly initiated and transformed by exposure to sunlight in early life [22]. These findings led Whiteman and colleagues to conclude that melanoma development, like other cancers, is dependent upon host phenotype and environmental conditions [22].

The divergent pathway model of melanoma development is important to consider when evaluating the relationship between age and melanoma. Nevus-prone/early-onset individuals are hypothesized to have melanocytes initiated by sunlight followed by proliferation to a neoplasm without additional sun exposure; these tend to occur on the trunk of the body [22]. In the case of nevus-resistant/late-onset individuals, melanocytes from this phenotype are hypothesized to require heavy doses of ongoing sun exposure to develop melanoma; these tend to occur on sun-exposed anatomical sites among older ages. Understanding the differing etiologies of melanoma and their relationship to sun exposure at various points throughout the life of an individual is a crucial component for the development of appropriate prevention and early detection strategies.

Intense UV exposure among older individuals is thought to be responsible for the fast-increasing incidence of melanoma over other cancers [24]. Austin and colleagues evaluated the role of age as a prognostic factor for malignant melanoma in a population of 442 melanoma patients residing in Florida. They determined that increasing age was a significant predictor for disease-free survival, with a worse prognosis seen in older melanoma patients. The outcome of older patients with malignant melanoma is generally poor, and treatment can include the use of biological agents with elevated toxicities. Often, elderly patients and their families will choose to opt out of aggressive treatments that younger patients might otherwise receive [1]. This might account for some age-associated prognostic indicators being skewed toward older demographics.

A large population-based survey in Germany was conducted to understand the epidemiology of nevi and signs of skin aging. Nevi are of interest as they are the strongest indicators of melanoma risk [19]. The prevalence of signs of skin aging like dermal elastosis, cutis rhomboidalis nuchae, Morbus Favre–Racouchot, lentigines solaris, lentigines seniles, and actinic keratosis increased significantly with age. In contrast, after age 25, the prevalence of nevi (including atypical nevi) declined significantly with age. The decrease in nevi with age is thought to be due to induction of new antigens by sunlight or cell-mediated immunity, each of which elicits an immune response capable of eliminating the nevi [19]. Findings from studies confirm speculations that signs of skin aging are frequent and increase with age in contrast to common and atypical nevi, which decrease with age, all of which are associated with melanoma risk.

The American Joint Committee on Cancer (AJCC) established a large international melanoma database, which was analyzed to determine the effect of patient age as a prognostic factor for melanoma survival [29]. In the study population of 13,581 patients with localized melanoma and a group of 4,750 patients with regional nodal metastasis, following thickness and ulceration, age was the third most important determinant of prognosis. Several factors have been identified to explain differences in prognosis in older patients. Some of which include undertreatment with increasing age because of narrower surgical margins, interference of other medical conditions, difficulty with skin self-examination because of failing eyesight or poor health, differences in reporting signs and symptoms as compared to younger populations, inaccessibility to adequate health care, and lack of a social network to provide support for at-home health-care maintenance among those being treated for melanoma [18].

It has been well established that socioeconomic status (SES) influences cancer survival. Interestingly, melanoma incidence increases in populations with higher SES, but lower SES populations display greater mortality [30]. SES impacts access to health care, insurance status, exposure to carcinogenic agents, and cancer screening practices and attitudes – all of which can have an impact on survival. Generally, SES impacts survival through biological characteristics of the tumor, thickness at diagnosis, host factors, and treatment [25]. Older patients are more likely to experience differences in access to health-care resources [31]. Reyes-Ortiz and colleagues utilized SEER data from 23,680 melanoma patients aged 65 and older diagnosed between 1988 and 1999 [25]. They sought to determine the association between SES and survival in older melanoma patients. Findings from this study revealed that subjects residing in lower-income areas had significantly lower 5-year survival rates than subjects residing in higher-income areas [25]. Further, an interaction effect between SES and ethnicity and melanoma survival was found in this population, which was demonstrated by improved 5-year survival rates in nonwhites and whites but enhanced for nonwhites as income increased. Similar to other reports, this study found older age to be independently associated with greater risk of death from melanoma. The lower survival in older melanoma patients has been attributed to older patients who are screened less, present with later stages of melanoma, have a greater percentage of ulcerated melanomas, and tend to have more melanomas with a high potential for metastases – increasing the probability of recurrence and mortality [18, 25]. In addition, older patient outcome is also affected by the loss of a spouse and social relationships [1].

Research on the costs of skin cancer suggests that annual spending for skin cancer is rapidly increasing and imposing a significant economic burden [32]. That burden may make it more difficult to access health care especially for elderly populations. These studies provide another demonstration of the association between age and melanoma and also illustrate the interaction between other demographic factors commonly associated with aging (i.e., SES) that impact melanoma.

Biological Factors

The relationship between age and cancer is a result of the interaction of several biological and environmental factors: decreased DNA repair capacity, decreased immune function, and in the case of skin cancer, cumulative exposure to UV radiation [33]. Elderly patients have a propensity for thicker lesions, which correlates with a poorer prognosis, especially in cases that are diagnosed at an advanced stage [34]. Increased incidence, long diagnostic delays, and poor prognosis experienced by elderly melanoma patients are of great concern. Sex is also an important biological factor. There is a distinct survival advantage for females diagnosed with invasive melanoma. 10-year survival rates significantly favor female patients independent of demographic, clinical, and stage factors [35]. However, the female survival advantage is temporarily lost from ages 46–59 and reacquired after age 60 [35]. This indicates that hormones may influence melanoma survivorship and the onset of menopause may normalize some of the biological influences between sexes.

DNA repair mechanisms and cell cycle regulation also contribute and are the cell's means of handling UV-induced DNA damage. Cumulative DNA damage over decades, mainly attributed to UV radiation, alongside age-associated decreases in DNA repair capacity is thought to play a central role in progression to melanoma [16]. Moriwaki and colleagues sought to demonstrate in vitro the association between DNA repair capacity and aging by measuring the ability of cells from individuals of different ages to repair new UV-induced DNA damage and establishing a cellular model for age-related changes in the processing of damaged DNA [36]. Their study of primary skin fibroblasts from donors aged 3–96 years and their ability to repair damage in plasmid DNA identified an age-related decline in post-UV DNA repair capability and a corresponding increase in post-UV mutagenesis. Earlier studies by the same research group demonstrated a 0.6 % per annum decline in post-UV DNA repair capacity of circulating T lymphocytes in control populations over four decades from 20 to 60 years of age [37]. Findings from this study indicate that the ability to process new UV-induced DNA damage decreases with age and that this reduction in repair followed by an increase in DNA mutability is evident in cultured cells of the skin and blood [36]. The mirrored increase in DNA mutability has been hypothesized to arise from accumulation of DNA damage over time, a decreased ability to process new DNA damage, or a combination of both [36]. In a similar study, Yamada and colleagues demonstrated an age-associated decline in nucleotide excision repair of UV-induced cyclobutane-type pyrimidine dimmers (CPD) [38]. In their study UV-exposed skin biopsies of younger men removed CPDs within 4 days after irradiation compared to biopsies of older men in which CPDs were removed within 7–14 days following irradiation. Their results suggest that age and its concomitant decline in DNA repair capacity are linked to the high risk of UV-associated skin cancer [38]. Further, long-lasting DNA damage has the potential to influence mutational events required for tumor progression [36].

Aging is an intrinsic component of many initiating events in melanoma: alterations in the melanocyte cell cycle, aberrant signal transduction pathways, and activation/deactivation of melanoma-relevant oncogenes, all of which are associated with tumor formation, are all susceptible to biological alterations in response to aging [13]. The interactions between melanocytes and their microenvironment, which can change with age, may play a critical role in tumor progression as well as a diminished immune surveillance as a consequence of age [13, 16]. Further, the biological response to sun exposure is dependent upon the physiological age of the skin more than the chronological age [39].

Cells have an inherent ability to repair damage to DNA. However, with age, the proficiency of these repair mechanisms/enzymes declines with a concomitant increase in DNA mutability. Malignant transformation can still be avoided if cells with accumulated mutations are directed toward apoptosis via p53 mechanisms or senescence via the retinoblastoma (RB) system [13]. Melanocytes, cells responsible for the synthesis of pigment, which provides protection from UV radiation, decrease in number, life span, and response to growth factors with age [40]. Further, melanocyte mutations in the B-RAF kinase initiate proliferation and the formation of nevi, and this cellular stress activates the RB/p16^{INK4a} pathway resulting in irreversible growth arrest and senescence to prevent further proliferation and acquisition of additional mutations [13]. This mechanism explains why nevi stop growing once they reach a certain size and why they rarely develop into melanomas [20].

In melanocytes, senescence functions in vivo as a potent tumor suppressor mechanism [13]. Senescence can be thought of as a double-edged sword, although senescence of melanocytes affords these cells the capacity to suppress tumorigenesis, their cellular physiology is changed. Senescent melanocytes have been found to have altered melanin chemistry, increasing their susceptibility to DNA damage [13]. Specifically, in vitro investigations of senescent human melanocytes have revealed a reduction in the microphthalmia-associated transcription factor (*MITF*), a transcription factor critically involved in commitment, proliferation, and survival of melanocytes, as well as a downregulation of dopachrome tautomerase, an enzyme involved in the melanin pathway [13]. The consequences of these alterations and resultant susceptibility to DNA damage in senescent melanocytes remain to be elucidated. Although these cells no longer proliferate, they may play a role in melanoma progression.

Immunology of the Skin and Age

Immunosenescence refers to decreased immune competence as a result of advancing age. Immunologic competencies of the skin in general are difficult to assess because of the numerous influences on the immune system that affect individuals to different extents. Evaluating these competencies in the context of age adds another level of complexity. It is generally believed that the immune system in elderly patients functions poorly in comparison to younger populations [41]. Underlying diseases or comorbidities, such as diabetes mellitus, malnourishment, increased scratching, or pruritic desiccated skin, alter immune function; thus, their individual contribution to the skin immune system is difficult to distinguish. The influence of age-associated physiologic changes on the immune system cannot be evaluated separately from intrinsic changes such as decreased DNA repair capacity and/or extrinsic changes like UV exposure [42]. Skin that is chronically sun exposed exhibits immunologic changes that are not encountered in all aging individuals [42]. Thus, it is difficult to assess whether an immunologic parameter associated with melanoma progression is associated with aging, chronic sun exposure, or both.

The effects of decreased immune function on the skin as a consequence of aging are thought to be related to changes in skin-specific immune cells. The number of Langerhans cells, skin-specific antigen-presenting cells, in the epidermis decreases by 20–50 % with age. In addition, the antigen-presentation function of these cells has also been shown to be reduced with age [40, 42]. The functional capacity of T cells is also known to be altered with age. Specifically, a decrease in the proliferative response, cytolytic activity, and repertoire of the T cell antigen receptors has been demonstrated [42]. Keratinocytes, which provide barrier function, mechanical protection, cytokine production, and cell signaling, decrease in proliferation and differentiation with age (reviewed in [40]). In addition, the barrier function in response to injury is compromised with age and cell signaling, and growth factor response is decreased with age in keratinocytes. Alterations in the immune system of the skin in response to aging affect detection and removal of abnormal skin cells, which may favor the emergence of skin cancers [13]. This underscores the adaptive arm of the immune system and the age-associated decrease in immune response that is key to understanding elderly melanoma incidence and survival.

Photoaging

The effect of long-term UV exposure and sun damage superimposed on intrinsically aged skin is referred to as photoaging [40]. Cutaneous malignancies are one of the many clinical hallmarks associated with photoaging. Ultraviolet radiation causes damage indirectly by inducing the formation of free radicals as well as directly causing cellular injury [40]. UV radiation also causes molecular and genetic changes, vascular alterations, and immunosuppression and has effects on pigmentation and the extracellular matrix. Several inherent cellular mechanisms exist to minimize UV-induced damage – among them are DNA repair and apoptosis. However, these mechanisms decline with age, and, after a lifetime of assault, these devices may fail, making melanocytes vulnerable to the deleterious effects of UV exposure leading to photoaging and melanoma [40]. However, evidence is now emerging that suggests UV exposure may positively contribute to elderly patient health – especially in relation to vitamin D synthesis [43]. Traditionally, older patients present with lower serum levels of vitamin D and may benefit from carefully mediated UV exposure although the causality of pathological associations of nonmelanoma diseases remains controversial [43].

Solar elastosis, a sign of photoaging positively associated with age, is the deposit and accumulation of elastotic material in the upper and middle dermis that is thought to absorb sunlight [10]. Since solar elastosis increases with skin age, it has been considered as a surrogate for the cumulative dose of absorbed UV radiation. This protective biological response to long-term sun exposure has been found to be a favorable prognostic indicator in melanoma [3, 44]. The presence or absence of solar elastosis can be used to differentiate between melanomas that developed following higher cumulative absorbed doses of UV from those that develop after a lower dose of UV, respectively [10].

A study of 1,200 patients diagnosed between 1980 and 1990 at a melanoma clinic in North Carolina was conducted to evaluate the relationship between elastosis as a result of long-term cumulative UV exposure and cutaneous melanoma. The presence of solar elastosis was significantly related to patient age, and melanomas with elastosis were found to occur at later stages than melanomas without elastosis [10]. Vollmer speculated that (i) elastosis is simply a surrogate for older age and thus accounts for the reason why melanomas with elastosis occur at older ages, (ii) elastosis may not be involved in the development of melanoma, or (iii) the etiology of melanomas with elastosis differs from those without. In this study, once melanoma developed, elastosis did not appear to affect thickness, mitotic rate, ulceration, or overall survival when compared to tumors in which elastosis was not present. Thus, the importance of elastosis appears to be prior to melanoma development and is associated with age.

In contrast, two population-based studies have measured solar elastosis. In Western Australia, Heenan et al. found a dose–response association between solar elastosis and improved 5-year survival from melanoma [3]. In 2005, Berwick et al. reported a 50 % decrease in risk of dying from melanoma associated with the presence of solar elastosis [44]. The contradictory evidence presented could be the result of study design (hospital based vs. population based), analytic technique (univariate vs. multivariate), or some other important factor that was not measured in the studies. The role of sun exposure in photoaging is complex. Overtime, photoaged skin becomes chronically hyperpigmented and contains melanocyte densities that are almost twice that in comparable body sites [46]. Prolific melanocyte production, in conjunction with chronic aging factors, likely contributes to melanomagenesis, although a precise association is not clear.

Lentigo Maligna Melanoma

Older individuals are disproportionately affected by lentigo maligna (LM) melanoma. Solar lentigines, also referred to as "age spots," are benign pigmented lesions that are commonly present in older Caucasian individuals. The presence of these lesions predisposes these individuals to a higher incidence of a preinvasive form of melanoma associated with chronic sun exposure, known as lentigo maligna [13]. Lentigo maligna (LM) usually presents as large, flat, discolored patches on the face; the in situ component of this lesion can remain dormant for many years before the vertical growth phase nodular component develops [34]. This subtype of melanoma is often evaluated separately in epidemiologic studies because of its specificity for elderly people, slow growth, and link with cumulative sun exposure [47]. A double case–control study was designed to compare risk factors for LM and other melanomas in elderly people; in general, this study revealed that the risk factors for LM were similar to those for other melanomas (sunburns, light skin, and tendency to freckle). Contrary to other melanomas, this epidemiologic study revealed the absence of an association between lentigo maligna and the presence of nevi and/or genetic propensity to develop nevi [47]. These findings agree with those of an earlier study conducted by the same research group, in which their case–control study designed to identify epidemiologic factors associated with skin aging characterized by multiplication of senile lentigos also did not identify a relationship with the number of nevi [48]. A correlation between these studies and the decrease in the number of nevi and an increase in the incidence of lentigo maligna seen in older individuals is evident. Although associated with chronic sun exposure, the risk of lentigo maligna has not been found to increase with the cumulative dose of sun exposure in epidemiologic studies [48].

Another form of melanoma, the most rare, acral lentiginous melanomas (ALM) are not related to ongoing sun exposure; in fact, they usually develop on the skin of the lower limb. In a comprehensive study of 1,413 acral lentiginous melanomas using the SEER data from 1986 to 2005, 78 % of these melanomas were found on the skin of the lower limb with 22 % on the skin of the upper limbs. These melanomas, although rare and unlikely associated with sun exposure, are somewhat more aggressive than other melanomas. In this study the mean age of diagnosis was 62.8 years, and a significant increase in incidence was seen with each year of advancing age [49]. In addition, the proportion of ALMs is greatest in people of color – being more common among blacks [49].

Conclusion

Skin aging and melanoma are uniquely intertwined in a complex continuum of cancer. Advanced chronologic age and skin age have been demonstrated biologically and epidemiologically to be associated with melanoma development and progression. This intricate relationship needs to be taken into consideration in future investigations of melanoma as well as during development of prevention and intervention strategies. The observed increase in melanoma incidence along with the growing population of elderly adults establishes the importance of early detection in elderly populations as well as a further understanding of the etiology of melanomas in this population.

Cross-References

▶ Carcinogenesis: UV Radiation
▶ Neoplastic Skin Lesions in the Elderly Patient

References

1. Hegde UP, Chakraborty N, Mukherji B, Grant Kels JM. Metastatic melanoma in the older patient: immunologic insights and treatment outcomes. Expert Rev Pharmacoecon Outcomes Res. 2011;11(2):185–93. doi:10.1586/erp.11.14.
2. American Cancer Society. Cancer facts and figures 2015. http://www.cancer.org/cancer/skincancer-melanoma/detailedguide/melanoma-skin-cancer-key-statistics (2015)
3. Heenan PJ, English DR, Holman CDJ, Armstrong BK. Survival among patients with clinical stage I cutaneous malignant melanoma diagnosed in Western Australia in 1975–1976 and 1980/1981. Cancer. 1991;68:2079–87.
4. Rosso S, Sera F, Segnan N, Zanetti R. Sun exposure prior to diagnosis is associated with improved survival in melanoma patients: results from a long-term follow-up study of Italian patients. Eur J Cancer. 2008;44:1275–81.
5. Breslow A. Thickness, cross-sectional area, and depth of invasion in the prognosis of cutaneous melanoma. Am Surg. 1970;66:527–31.
6. Finley JW, Rodriguez LM, Letourneau R, Driscoll D, Kraybill W. Pathologic and clinical features influencing outcome of thin cutaneous melanoma: correlation with newly proposed staging system. Am Surg. 2000;66:527–31.
7. Buzaid CM, Ross MI, Balch CM, et al. Critical analysis of the current American Joint Committee on Cancer staging system for cutaneous melanoma and proposal of a new staging system. J Clin Oncol. 1997;15:1039–51.
8. Balch CM. Cutaneous melanoma: prognosis and treatment results worldwide. Semin Surg Oncol. 1992;8:400–14.
9. Gershenwald JE, Thompson W, Mansfield PF, et al. Multi-institutional melanoma lymphatic mapping experience: the prognostic value of sentinel lymph node status in 612 stage I or II melanoma patients. J Clin Oncol. 1999;17:976–83.
10. Volmer RT. Solar elastosis in cutaneous melanoma. Am J Clin Pathol. 2007;128:260–4.
11. Lachiewicz AM, Berwick M, Wiggins CL, Thomas NE. Survival differences between patients with scalp or neck melanoma and those with melanoma of other sites in the Surveillance, Epidemiology, and End Results (SEER) program. Arch Dermatol. 2008;144:515–21.
12. Hegde UP, Grant-Kels JM. Metastatic melanoma in the older patient: special considerations. Clin Dermatol. 2013 ;31(3):311–6. doi:10.1016/j.clinderma-tol.2012.08.011.
13. Desai A, Krathen R, Orengo I, Medrano EE. The age of skin cancers. Sci Aging Knowl Environ. 2006;9:pe13.
14. Sabel MS, Kozminski D, Griffith K, Chang AE, Johnson TM, Wong S. Sentinel lymph node biopsy use among melanoma patients 75 years of age and older. Ann Surg Oncol. 2015;22(7):2112–9. doi:10.1245/s10434-015-4539-7.
15. Geller AC, Miller DR, Annas GD, et al. Melanoma incidence and mortality among US whites, 1969–1999. JAMA. 2002;288:1719–20.
16. Yaar M, Gilchrest BA. Ageing and photoageing of keratinocytes and melanocytes. Clin Exp Dermatol. 2001;26:583–91.
17. Beddingfield FC. The melanoma epidemic: res ipsa loquitur. Oncologist. 2003;8(5):459–65. doi:10.1634/theoncologist.8-5-459.
18. Sweeter SM, Geller AC, Kirkwood JM. Melanoma in the older person. Oncology. 2004;18:1187–96.
19. Schafer T, Merkl J, Klemm E, Wichmann HE, Ring J. KORA study group. The epidemiology of nevi and signs of skin aging in the adult general population: results of the KORA-survey 2000. J Invest Dermatol. 2006;126:1490–6.
20. Sage J. Making young tumors old: a new weapon against cancer? Sci Aging Knowl Environ. 2005;2005(33):pe25.
21. Lachiewicz AM, Berwick M, Wiggins CL, Thomas NE. Epidemiologic support for melanoma heterogeneity using the Surveillance, Epidemiology, and End Results program. J Invest Dermatol. 2008;128:243–5.
22. Whiteman DC, Watt P, Purdie DM, Hughes MC, Hayward NK, Green AC. Melanocytic nevi, solar keratoses, and divergent pathways to cutaneous melanoma. J Natl Cancer Inst. 2003;95:806–12.
23. Whiteman DC. Testing the divergent pathway hypothesis for melanoma: recent findings and future challenges. Expert Rev Anticancer Ther. 2010;10(5):615–8. doi:10.1586/era.10.42.
24. Austin PF, Cruse CW, Lyman G, Schroer K, Glass F, Reintgen DS. Age as a prognostic factor in the malignant melanoma population. Ann Surg Oncol. 1994;1:487–94.
25. Reyes-Ortiz CA, Goodwin JS, Freeman JL, Kou YF. Socioeconomic status and survival in older patients with melanoma. JAGS. 2006;54:1758–64.
26. Golger A, Young DS, Ghazarian D, Neligan PC. Epidemiologic features and prognostic factors of

cutaneous head and neck melanoma. Arch Otolaryngol Head Neck Surg. 2007;133:442–7.
27. Montero I, et al. Age-related characteristics of cutaneous melanoma in a Spanish Mediterranean population. Int J Dermatol. 2015;54(7):778–84.
28. Cavanaugh-Hussey MW, Mu EW, Kang S, Balch CM, Wang T. Older age is associated with a higher incidence of melanoma death but a lower incidence of sentinel lymph node metastasis in the SEER databases (2003–2011). Ann Surg Oncol. 2015;22(7):2120–6. doi:10.1245/s10434-015-4538.
29. Balch CM, Soong SJ, Gershenwald JE, et al. Prognostic factors analysis of 17,600 melanoma patients: validation of the American Joint Committee on Cancer Melanoma Staging System. J Clin Oncol. 2001;19:3622–34.
30. Jiang AJ, Rambhatla PV, Eide MJ. Socioeconomic and lifestyle factors and melanoma: a systematic review. Br J Dermatol. 2015;172(4):885–915. doi:10.1111/bjd.13500.
31. Balch CM. Decreased survival rates of older-aged patients with melanoma: biological differences or undertreatment? Ann Surg Oncol. 2015;22(7):2101–3. doi:10.1245/s10434-015-4540-1.
32. Guy GP, Machlin SR, Ekwueme DU, Yabroff KR. Prevalence and costs of skin cancer treatment in the U.S., 2002–2006 and 2007–2011. Am J Prev Med. 2015;48(2):183–7. doi:10.1016/j.amepre.2014.08.036.
33. Syrigos KN, Tzannou I, Katirtzoglou N, Georgiou E. Skin cancer in the elderly. In Vivo. 2005;19:643–52.
34. Kaplan RP. The aging skin. Comp Ther. 1991;17:59–67.
35. Khosrotehrani K, Dasgupta P, Byrom L, Youlden DR, Baade PD, Green AC. Melanoma survival is superior in females across all tumour stages but is influenced by age. Arch Dermatol Res. 2015. doi:10.1007/s00403-015-1585-8.
36. Moriwaki SI, Ray S, Tarone RE, Kraemer KH, Grossman L. The effect of donor age on the processing of UV-damaged DNA by cultured human cells: reduced DNA repair capacity and increased DNA mutability. Mutat Res. 1996;364:117–23.
37. Wei Q, Matanoski GM, Farmer ER, Hedayati MA, Grossman L. DNA repair and aging in basal cell carcinoma: a molecular epidemiology study. Proc Natl Acad Sci U S A. 1993;90:1614–8.
38. Yamada M, Udono MU, Hori M, Hirose R, Sato S, Mori T, Nikaido O. Aged human skin removes UVB-induced pyrimidine dimmers from the epidermis more slowly than younger adult skin in vivo. Arch Dermatol Res. 2006;297:294–302.
39. Uitto J. The role of elastin and collagen in cutaneous aging: intrinsic aging versus photoexposure. J Drugs Dermatol. 2008;7:12–6.
40. Rabe JH, Mamelak AJ, McElgunn PJS, Morison WL, Sauder DN. Photoaging: mechanisms and repair. J Am Acad Dermatol. 2006;55:1–19.
41. Hegde UP, Chakraborty N, Kerr P, Grant-Kels JM. Melanoma in the elderly patient: relevance of the aging immune system. Clin Dermatol. 2009;27 (6):537–44. doi:10.1016/j.clindermatol.2008.09.012.
42. Sunderkotter C, Kalden H, Luger TA. Aging and the skin immune system. Arch Dermatol. 1997;133:1256–62.
43. Wright F, Weller RB. Risks and benefits of UV radiation in older people: More of a friend than a foe? Maturitas. 2015. doi:10.1016/j.maturitas.2015.05.003.
44. Berwick M, Armstrong BK, Ben-Porat L, Fine J, Kircker A, Barnhill RL. Sun exposure and mortality from melanoma. J Natl Cancer Inst. 2005;97:1–5.
45. Landi et al. MC1R germline variants confer risk for BRAF-mutant melanoma. Science. 28: Supporting Online Material. 2006. http://www.sciencemag.org/cgi/content/full/1127515/DC1
46. Yaar M, Gilchrest BA. Aging and photoaging of keratinocytes and melanocytes (Alterung Und Lichtalterung von Keratinozyten Und Melanozyten). H + G Zeitschrift Fur Hautkrankheiten. 2001;76(10):623–9.
47. Gaudy-Marqueste C, Madjlessi N, Guillot B, Avril MF, Grob JJ. Risk factors in elderly people for lentigo maligna compared with other melanomas. Arch Dermatol. 2009;145:418–23.
48. Monestier S, Gaudy C, Gouvernet J, Richard MA, Grob JJ. Multiple senile lentigos of the face, a skin ageing pattern resulting from a life excess of intermittent sun exposure in dark-skinned Caucasians: a case–control study. Br J Dermatol. 2006;154:438–44.
49. Bradford PT, Goldstein AM, McMaster ML, Tucker MA. Acral lentiginous melanoma incidence and survival patterns in the United States, 1986–2005. Arch Dermatol. 2009;145:427–34.

Aging-Associated Nonmelanoma Skin Cancer: A Role for the Dermis

70

Davina A. Lewis, Aleksandar Krbanjevic, Jeffrey B. Travers, and Dan F. Spandau

Contents

D.A. Lewis
Department of Anatomic Pathology and Histology, Covance CLS, Indianapolis, IN, USA
e-mail: davlewis@iupui.edu

A. Krbanjevic
Department of Dermatology, Indiana University School of Medicine, Indianapolis, IN, USA
e-mail: alexkrba@iu.edu

J.B. Travers
Departments of Pharmacology and Toxicology and Dermatology, Boonshoft School of Medicine at Wright State University, Dayton, OH, USA
e-mail: jeffrey.travers@wright.edu

D.F. Spandau (✉)
Departments of Dermatology and Biochemistry and Molecular Biology, Indiana University School of Medicine, Indianapolis, IN, USA
e-mail: dspanda@iupui.edu

M.A. Farage et al. (eds.), *Textbook of Aging Skin*,
DOI 10.1007/978-3-662-47398-6_58

Abstract

The cocktail of sun's ultraviolet (UVB) rays, and the hands of father time, can significantly increase the risk of skin cancers. However, genetic predisposition, certain skin diseases, and some viral infections can also increase the risk of skin cancers. Nonmelanoma skin cancer (NMSC), including basal cell (BCC) and squamous cell carcinoma (SCC), is thought to be based on a life time exposure to risk factors such as UV radiation combined with little sun protection in that life time. In fact, over 80 % of all skin cancers are found in people over the age of 60. NMSC tends to occur on highly visible areas such as the head, face, and neck. The treatment of these NMSC represents both a significant economic burden to health services and can cause significant morbidity especially as these occur on highly visible areas. Treatment is often invasive surgery which often leads to scaring and affects quality of life. Other treatments are based on chemotherapeutic, immunotherapies that can also affect quality of life. While very effective standard treatments have been developed to treat NMSC, very little is understood about the underlying cellular causes, and as such, alternative methods of treatment have not readily been developed. In this chapter, we explore the mechanisms of UVB-induced effects on skin and exciting new possible methods to treat NMSC.

Introduction

The American Cancer Society estimates that well over two million patients are diagnosed with skin cancer each year, representing over half of all invasive and in situ cancers that occur in the USA each year [1]. The magnitude of these statistics suggests that the treatment of skin cancer in the USA is a problem both for patients and for the healthcare system. Despite the relatively low mortality associated with squamous cell carcinoma, nearly the same numbers of patients die from melanoma and squamous cell carcinoma each year [2]. Conclusive evidence has demonstrated that the main environmental risk factor for developing skin cancer is exposure to the ultraviolet components in sunlight, primarily ultraviolet B wavelengths (UVB) [3–7]. Although skin cancer can occur at any age, there is a strong correlation between the development of skin cancer and advancing age [8]. In fact, the majority of *skin cancers* are found in people over the age of 60; therefore, age is also a risk factor for the development of skin cancer [1, 8]. While the correlation between aged epidermis and skin cancer is obvious, the mechanism responsible for this relationship remains obscure. Recent in vitro evidence, as well as epidemiological data, suggests one possible mechanism may involve alterations in the insulin-like growth factor-1 receptor (IGF-1R) signaling network [9–12]. In the skin, keratinocytes express the IGF-1 R, but they do not synthesize IGF-1 [13, 14]. Dermal fibroblasts support the proliferation of keratinocytes in the epidermis by secreting IGF-1 [13, 14]. Interestingly, as dermal fibroblasts age, their capacity to produce IGF-1 is severely diminished; therefore, aged skin keratinocytes are provided with a reduced supply of IGF-1 [12]. This drop in IGF-1 expression is critically important for nonmelanoma skin carcinogenesis because adequate levels of IGF-1 are required to prevent potential UVB-induced mutations in replicating keratinocytes. In vitro and in vivo studies have shown that IGF-1R activation protects the epidermis from initiating carcinogenic events [9–12]. The chapter will discuss the relationship between aging and cancer, the critical features of nonmelanoma skin cancer (NMSC), and the newly proposed role for the dermis in driving the development of aging-associated NMSC.

Aging and Carcinogenesis

Evidence accumulated thus far definitively links increasing age and the onset of cancer; in fact, the greatest risk factor for developing cancer is age [15]. At least 80 % of *all neoplasia* occur in individuals over the age of 50 [15, 16], and the incidence of cancer rises with increasing age until the age of 90 [16]. In general, cancer is a disease that primarily afflicts geriatric patients. However, the mechanisms behind the link between cancer and aging are only beginning to be understood. Many explanations defining the relationship between aging and carcinogenesis have been postulated, but few have been conclusively proven. A common theory describes the long passage of time required between the creation of initiated cells containing fixed DNA mutations and the phenotypic appearance of tumors containing the descendent clones of the original initiated cells [17]. This theory suggests that the sequential changes seen in the carcinogenic process require many years if not decades to develop, ensuring that apparent diagnosable tumors arise in older patients [17]. Separate studies have shown that the ability of individuals to effectively prevent the occurrence of initiated cells through DNA repair mechanisms declines with age [17–19]. Aging cells have an increased number of somatic mutations, probably through a combination of DNA damage as a result of environmental factors and an enhanced rate of errors occurring during DNA replication [16, 17]. As the capability to repair DNA lesions diminishes, the frequency of newly initiated potentially neoplastic cells increases as well as the probability of identifiable neoplasia. More recently, studies have identified age-dependent changes in stromal tissue which provide a favorable growth environment for initiated cells to thrive [17, 20–22]. As cells in these support tissues age, they frequently begin to lose control of normal gene expression and cellular function [20–22]. Increasingly they express genes characterized by an inflammatory phenotype that can promote the growth of previously initiated cells or enhance the progression of newly initiated tumorigenic cells [20, 21].

Nonmelanoma Skin Cancer: The Epidermis

Cancers of the skin are the most common cancers to afflict Caucasians in the USA [1, 23]. The significant morbidity and exorbitant healthcare costs associated with the management of skin cancer provide substantial evidence of the need for research in this field. The primary environmental factor influencing the development of skin cancer is exposure to ultraviolet wavelengths in sunlight [3–6, 24–26]. Because 80 % of all skin cancers are found in people over the age of 60, age is also a risk factor for the development of skin cancer. Despite this explicit correlation between aged epidermis and NMSC, it remains to be determined why aged skin is more sensitive to UVB-induced carcinogenesis. The historical explanation for the correlation between skin cancer and aging argues that UVB damage inflicted on skin during adolescence initiates mutations in keratinocytes that are selectively enriched over many decades until enough genetic changes have gradually accumulated in these keratinocytes that they become carcinogenic. In fact, this mechanism has been proposed to explain the long latency period observed in other types of cancers where there is also a correlation between the development of cancer and age [27, 28]. However, recent data have suggested a modification of this theory based on the altered function of aged stromal cells (i.e., fibroblasts) affecting epithelial cells [20, 21]. This hypothesis states that the selection of initiated epithelial cells is accelerated in aged tissue due to altered gene expression in senescent fibroblasts supporting epithelial cell growth [22, 29, 30]. In addition, the aged state of cells may play a greater role in the initiation of carcinogenic DNA mutations than was previously thought to occur [31]. These new ideas on the origins of cancer have led to a new paradigm to explain nonmelanoma skin carcinogenesis. In order to explain the rationale for this theory of skin carcinogenesis, the following paragraphs will summarize the current understanding of the effect of ultraviolet B (UVB) irradiation on skin, aging-associated NMSC risk factors, and how cellular senescence influences NMSC carcinogenesis.

Effects of UVB Irradiation on the Skin

Sunlight is composed of a variety of wavelengths of light, which can be divided into infrared, visible, and ultraviolet light, arranged from the longest wavelengths to the shortest. The ultraviolet (UV) spectrum can be further divided into three classifications, UVA (320–400 nm), UVB (280–320 nm), and UVC (200–280 nm) [4]. Wavelengths of light in the UVC range have the potential to cause the most damage to living organisms; however, nearly all UVC wavelengths are absorbed in the atmosphere and never reach the surface of the Earth [4]. UVA radiation is the most abundant ultraviolet light to penetrate the atmosphere, although the data are still inconclusive as to the exact role that UVA radiation plays in human skin cancer [32]. Even though UVB radiation makes up only 0.3 % of the total light that reaches the surface of the earth [5], exposure of human cells to the UVB component in sunlight can directly damage DNA and lead to the development of cancer [6]. In general, UVB radiation only penetrates the epidermal layer of the skin. Therefore, the primary cells at risk of potential UVB-induced damage reside in the epidermis, where keratinocytes are the predominant cell type. UVB irradiation of the epidermis leads to UVB-induced DNA damage in keratinocytes [33, 34]. Exposure to UVB produces distinctive signature mutations in keratinocyte DNA due to the direct absorption of energy. This DNA damage consists predominantly of cytosine (C) to thymidine (T) transitions at dipyrimidine sites, including CC → TT dimerization between adjacent pyrimidines takes place on the same DNA strand. If these mutations are allowed to persist, this DNA damage may be propagated to daughter cells perhaps giving rise to proliferative diseases including basal cell carcinoma (BCC) and squamous cell carcinoma (SCC). The importance of cellular proliferation with DNA damage in carcinogenesis is elegantly illustrated by organisms composed largely of postmitotic cells which do not develop cancers, such as the nematode *C. elegans* and the fruit fly *D. melanogaster* [35–37]. In contrast, tissues from organisms containing replicatively mitotic cells do develop cancers [36, 37]. The dose and duration of UVB received determines how the epidermis responds [32, 38, 39]. Brief exposures to UVB will arrest keratinocyte proliferation to allow for the repair of DNA damage before the keratinocyte reenters the cell cycle. However, if the exposure to UVB is prolonged, a combination of several outcomes can occur: (1) DNA damage is not repaired and keratinocytes undergo apoptosis, (2) keratinocytes become senescent as a tumor evasion mechanism, or (3) damage may be misrepaired or partially repaired and cells continue to proliferate, propagating potentially mutagenic DNA damage. The first two observations, UVB-induced apoptosis and UVB-induced senescence, are part of the normal protective response of human skin to UVB exposure that maintains the integrity of the protective barrier function of the epidermis while ensuring that UVB-damaged keratinocytes are not permitted to replicate with DNA mutations (the appropriate UVB response). The third observation, the failure of UVB-induced senescence leading to replication in keratinocytes containing UVB-damaged DNA, represents flawed protection from UVB damage, and the consequences of failed UVB protection may include the stabilization of initiating DNA mutations that could lead to the malignant transformation of keratinocytes (an inappropriate UVB response). Acquired mutations in key tumor suppressor genes such as p53 and RB are targets of UVB exposure [33, 40, 41]. Keratinocytes harboring p53 mutations fail to undergo UVB-induced senescence [11], become resistant to the fail-safe apoptotic response, and acquire a growth advantage [32, 40–42]. This growth advantage allows for clonal expansion of mutant p53 cells over time contributing to the development of premalignancies and malignancies in skin [32, 40–43]. Importantly, p53 mutation hot spots are common in NMSC at dipyrimidine sites [40, 43]. In addition to causing gene mutations, UVB exposure also induces immunosuppression [44, 45]. Reports show that UVB exposure inhibits the antigen presenting capabilities of epidermal Langerhans cells and stimulates the release of keratinocyte immunosuppressive and pro-inflammatory lipids and cytokines [38, 46–48]. The importance of this UV-induced immunosuppression and inflammation in relation to skin malignancies is logical since development of cancers requires escape from immune system function and inflammatory changes [33, 38, 46, 49]. Along with

UVB-induced mutations, immunesuppression and inflammation, UVB is known to cause a change in epidermal architecture and biochemistry. In skin chronically exposed to the sun, there is an increase in actinic damage along with a disorganization of collagen bundles [50]. UVB-induced alterations in skin biochemistry include deregulation of growth factors and their receptors, for example IGF-1, erbB1, erbB2, activation of mitogenic signaling pathways such as RAS, p38, and JNK MAPKs, and inappropriate activation of transcription factors such as NF-κB [10, 51, 52].

Aging-Related Risk Factors for Developing NMSC

As noted previously, there is a strong correlation between the development of skin cancer and advancing age. Childhood exposure to UV is believed to be one of the most critical risk factors in the development of skin cancers in adults [53]. One explanation for this correlation is that epidermal keratinocytes acquire UV-induced tumorigenic mutations in childhood which accumulate over time in selected populations of cells that manifest as skin cancers later in adult life [8, 31, 36, 54]. This explanation adheres to the multistage theory of carcinogenesis where initiating mutations occurring in target genes require promotional events to expand and form clones of mutated cells, eventually progressing and developing into cancers. People are exposed daily to oxidative stressors which cause DNA damage that has the potential to be fixed as mutations [55–57]. Furthermore, as human beings age, there also appears to be an increase in the production of reactive oxygen species (ROS) that may in turn increase the potential for damage to DNA [56–58]. Along with this, a decline in the function of the p53 protein has been reported in the aging process that could contribute to an increase in the frequency of mutations and tumorigenesis [31]. Furthermore, with aging, the fidelity of DNA repair mechanisms declines and, therefore, may accelerate the accumulation of mutations over time [58–60]. Mutations in cancer cells are so numerous that almost certainly other factors must contribute to their development. Indeed, aging is also associated with a decreased immune function [61, 62]. Investigations have demonstrated that age-related changes in human T-lymphocytes contributed to a decrease in immunity against infections and neoplasms as well as causing an increase in autoimmune diseases [62, 63]. The combination of increased ROS production, decreased immune function, decreased p53 function, and a decreased fidelity in DNA repair mechanisms with advancing age does indeed provide a provocative environment for developing cancers.

Cellular Senescence and NMSC

Cellular senescence is defined as an irreversible arrest in cellular replication in otherwise metabolically active cells. First identified as a phenomenon controlling the longevity of cells cultured in vitro [64], it is now known that replicative senescence in vitro is caused by the erosion of telomeres and an ensuing DNA-damage response [65–67]. Characteristics of senescent cells in vitro include irreversible growth arrest, increased resistance to apoptotic signals, and changes in cell functions such as secretion of growth factors, cytokines, degrading enzymes, an overexpression of proteins and oncogenes, and chromatin reorganization. Factors leading to senescence include finite replicative capacity via telomere shortening, DNA damage, or overexpression of mitogenic signals [35, 64, 68]. Although senescent cells cannot initiate DNA replication in response to physiological mitogens, they remain viable and continue to be metabolically active. There is compelling evidence suggesting that senescent cells accumulate in aged tissues [69–71]. In order to assess the contribution of senescent cells to aging and cancer, several markers have been employed such as senescence-associated β-galactosidase, high levels of HIRA (a heterochromatin protein), and damaged telomeres. In one study examining cultured human fibroblasts and keratinocytes, the senescent phenotype was absent in terminally differentiated keratinocytes, quiescent fibroblasts, presenescent cells, or immortalized cell lines

[69]. In this same report, an age-related increase in senescent dermal fibroblasts and epidermal keratinocytes in human skin was observed [69]. Up to 80 % of the fibroblasts examined in geriatric primate skin have senescent markers such as damaged telomeres and high levels of HIRA [70, 71]. Recent reports have indicated up to 60 % of fibroblasts in geriatric human dermis are senescent [72]. Given this age-associated accumulation of senescent cells, it is reasonable to propose that cellular senescence may contribute to age-related cancers by altering the surrounding tissue into a neoplastic promoting environment. The paradoxical effect of cellular senescence on an organism's well-being has been called antagonistic pleiotropy [36, 73]. On one hand, cellular senescence is a powerful tumor suppressor limiting cell lifespan and removing damaged cells from a proliferative state preventing formation of clonal tumors [22, 43, 74]. On the other hand, the accumulation of senescent cells may contribute to aging and provide a tumor-promoting environment due to their altered properties such as stromal matrix reorganization and/or degradation and secretion of growth factors and inflammatory cytokines [21, 36]. Inflammation is an important factor promoting carcinogenesis. For example, lesions visually described to be solar keratosis were identified as squamous cell carcinoma histologically when inflammation was present [49]. Simply put, the accumulation of senescent cells in aging tissue may serve to maintain tissue architecture but inadvertently due to their altered function, change the surrounding tissue milieu to an environment where damaged and mutated cells can more easily become malignant. Evidence to substantiate this hypothesis comes from investigations in which human senescent fibroblasts were found to stimulate premalignant and malignant cells to proliferate in culture and form tumors in mice due in part to senescence-induced secretion of soluble and insoluble factors [20, 21, 75]. A study using a conditional mouse oncogenic *K-rasV12* model for cancer initiation showed that senescent cells only existed in premalignant and not malignant tumors, suggesting senescence may be an indicator in the diagnosis and prognosis of cancers [76].

Nonmelanoma Skin Cancer: The Dermis

Historically, aging-associated NMSC is believed to be caused by the accumulation of damaged cells over decades. For example, one of the first signs of precancerous NMSC in aged individuals has been the appearance of actinic lesions. These lesions are readily apparent in the epidermis and are treated at the level of the keratinocyte. However, what if arising actinic damage could be prevented, and thereby NMSC, by detecting changes before they have reached the epidermis? The answer to this question may lay underneath the epidermis in the dermis. Considering the essential role the dermis has on epidermal function, it is surprising that it was only a decade ago that attention was drawn to age-related changes in the dermis. Therefore, although the target cell of NMSC resides in the epidermis, it is necessary to reexamine the role the dermis may play in the development of NMSC.

Dermal and Epidermal Synergism

The proper functioning and well-being of the skin is reliant on synergistic interactions between the dermal fibroblasts and epidermal keratinocytes. The integration of all signals received by a keratinocyte will determine the specific path that a cell takes at any given time during differentiation. The dermis contains a variety of cell types including fibroblasts, macrophages, mast cells, dendritic cells, and dermal T-lymphocytes. Composed of extracellular matrix, collagen, and elastin fibers, the stroma and some basement membrane components are synthesized by dermal fibroblasts, which produce soluble factors promoting survival and growth of the tissue. When it is necessary to remodel or repair the tissue, fibroblasts produce a mixture of degrading enzymes, cytokines, and growth factors. The influence of the dermis on the epidermis, and vice versa, is far reaching. In studies where site-matched papillary or reticular dermal fibroblasts were used to construct in vitro skin equivalents, the epidermal morphology, the formation of the basement membrane, and the terminal differentiation status were influenced by the type of fibroblast used [77]. When the dermis was composed of papillary fibroblasts, epidermal keratinocytes were morphologically symmetrical and all levels of terminal differentiation were expressed, whereas skin equivalents constructed using reticular fibroblasts impeded the formation of the basement membrane and terminal differentiation in the epidermis [77]. Furthermore, the number of fibroblasts used to construct the dermal matrix of skin equivalents also appears to be essential in establishing normal epidermal growth [78].

The Dermis, the Immune System, and Inflammation

What about the role of the dermis in skin immunity? The dermis has its own armory of weapons to impede the progress of any invader which has compromised the epidermis. Acting as a sentinel, the epidermis defends against environmental insults and pathogenic invasion. The epidermis is equipped with Langerhans cells and T-cell receptor-expressing dendritic epidermal T-cells (DETC) to cope with incoming insults. A substantial list of dermatologic diseases can cause epidermal immunity to go awry, such as psoriasis, atopic dermatitis [79], which may upset the balance between epidermis and dermis. DETC produce and respond to insulin-like growth factor I (IGF-1). In mice that are deficient for DETC, the epidermal balance is tipped from proliferation to apoptosis and levels of insulin-like growth factor receptor (IGF-1R) are decreased [80]. Addition of either DETC or IGF-1 can correct this imbalance highlighting the influence of the immune system on growth factors in the epidermal–dermal relationship, skin homeostasis, and wound repair [80]. Fibroblasts are the most abundant cells of the dermis and have a key role in the structural integrity, mechanical strength, and landscape of the extracellular matrix (ECM). Fibroblasts secrete both collagen and matrix metalloproteases that regulate ECM turnover. Adding to their resume, fibroblasts have also been shown to trigger and alter the inflammatory response as well as aid in wound healing [81–84]. Additionally, in some tissue, suppression of the immune response may be driven in part by fibroblasts [85]. "Activated" or "cancer associated" fibroblasts are known to produce (tissue specific) pro-inflammatory cytokines, chemokines, and growth factors [81, 86, 87]. Inflammation leads to further activation of fibroblasts and the production of more inflammatory mediators [86]. This persistent vicious cycle has been well established for fibroblasts and results in chronic inflammation. Chronic inflammation can be started and sustained by disease states, cancer, and activated fibroblasts. Chronic inflammation is also well known to be involved in all stages of carcinogenesis. In many cases, inflammation is therapeutically treated at the level of an immune cell or blockade of the offending cytokine [86]. However, the discovery that fibroblasts can indeed initiate, promote, and sustain inflammation should make them attractive new target for anti-inflammatory and anticancer therapeutics.

Dermal Aging, Senescence, and Cancer

In 1956, Harman et al. suggested that free radicals were involved with the deterioration of human biochemistry with age and degenerative diseases [88]. Furthermore, reactive oxygen species (ROS) were shown to cause DNA damage and indeed promote the aging process [89]. Organism aging is therefore thought to be at least in part due to accumulation of this free radical damage over time (aging) indirectly and directly causing DNA damage [90, 91]. Fortunately the skin has powerful antioxidant defense mechanisms preventing or scavenging ROS formed and repairing DNA damage. Currently, aging-associated skin cancer has been hypothesized to be a direct result of DNA damage accumulating over time until a threshold is reached overwhelming the tissue resulting in skin cancers [8, 31, 37, 54, 55]. One powerful mechanism employed in response to stress is a state of arrested growth and altered function called senescence.

Senescence was observed by Hayflick in 1961 [64] as a cell that had reached the end of its proliferative capacity in culture. Even though these cells had lost their proliferative capacity, they remained viable. Some of the characteristic of senescent cells are growth arrest, resistance to apoptotic signals, and altered gene expression [87, 92]. In tissues where homeostasis hinges on precise interactions between epithelial and mesenchymal cells, presence of senescent cells may disrupt the proper function of the tissue and may have far reaching effects [93]. In fact, the targeted deletion of senescent cells in a mouse model for aging ameliorated most of the phenotypes associated with advanced age [94].

As humans age, there are many significant changes that occur in the body, of these the most outwardly visible are the changes to the skin. Loss of tone/elasticity, increased pigmentation, and transparency are all commonly visible in aging [95]. However, what are not visible are the underlying biological, chemical, and molecular changes going on under those outwardly visible changes. Cellular senescence appears to play a role in aging [74]. Brought on by DNA damage, oncogene dysfunction, other forms of stress, chromatin damage, and telomere shortening (accelerated by oxidative damage), senescent cells are also found to accumulate in during normal epidermal aging [69–71]. The degree to which senescent cells help or disrupt the normal functioning of skin is unknown. What effect they have on the surrounding tissue microenvironment, adjacent cells, as well as the role they have in disease processes such as skin cancer is only just beginning to be unearthed. Some of the changes, such as secretion of growth factors, cytokines, and degrading enzymes as well as changes in gene expression, have been seen in senescent cells.

A New Role for the Dermis in Aging-Associated NMSC

As discussed, the central dogma correlating the link between skin cancer and aging is that UVB-induced skin damage during childhood and early adolescence initiates mutations in keratinocytes. Subsequently, these keratinocytes containing mutations acquire a growth advantage and become carcinogenic only after many decades have passed. However, can it be presumed that time is the sole contributor to UVB-induced skin cancers? It is reasonable then to consider that the physiology of aging may also lend a hand to carcinogenic events. Recent data from a variety of labs have led to a modification on the origin of aging-associated skin cancer based on the accumulation of senescent dermal fibroblasts in geriatric skin [12]. This new paradigm further substantiates the importance of the interaction between dermal fibroblasts and epidermal keratinocytes in preventing the initiation of carcinogenic events. These interactions are dependent on IGF-1/IGF-1R signaling which play an important role in aging and the response of skin to UVB irradiation [9–12].

Role of the IGF-1R and IGF-1 in the Skin

The stroma and some basement membrane components are synthesized by stromal fibroblasts which also produce soluble factors that promote survival and growth of the tissue. When it is necessary to remodel or repair the tissue, stromal fibroblasts produce a mixture of degrading enzymes, cytokines, and growth factors. The health and proper functioning of the skin is highly dependent on the synergistic interactions between the dermal fibroblasts and epidermal keratinocyte. One factor regulating the interaction between dermal fibroblasts and epidermal keratinocytes is IGF-1 [13, 14]. In human skin, keratinocytes express the IGF-1R but do not synthesize IGF-1. Dermal fibroblasts support the proliferation of epidermal keratinocytes by secreting IGF-1. The mature IGF-1R consists of four subunits: two identical extracellular alpha and two identical transmembrane beta subunits. The two alpha and alpha-beta subunit structures are maintained by disulphide bridges. IGF-1, IGF-2, and high concentrations of insulin can activate the IGF-1R, resulting in tyrosine kinase activity. Subsequently, binding or phosphorylation of cellular substrates in close proximity via SH2 binding domain leads to downstream signaling. The importance of IGF-1R signaling in skin carcinogenesis is clearly evident from a variety of studies. Transgenic mice overexpressing IGF-1 in the basal layer of skin epidermis exhibited epidermal hyperplasia, hyperkeratosis, and papillomas [96–98]. Conversely, IGF-1R knockout mice demonstrate severe hypoplasia [97]. The IGF-1R has also been shown to be important in normal epidermal differentiation [99]. Therefore, the activation of the IGF-1R can influence all stages of epidermal homeostasis. The control of longevity has also demonstrated a critical role for the insulin/IGF-1 signaling pathway in invertebrate and mammalian animal models [100–102]. Furthermore, reports have identified a key role for the IGF-1R in regulating the response of cells to oxidative stress [103].

The IGF-1R-Dependent UVB Response of Human Keratinocytes

Experiments that assessed the role of various growth factors on the response of keratinocytes to UVB irradiation identified that the activation status of the IGF-1R was a critical component affecting UVB-induced apoptosis in vitro (Fig. 1) [9]. Inhibition of the IGF-1R, via ligand withdrawal, treatment with neutralizing antibodies, or treatment with IGF-1R-specific small molecule inhibitors prior to irradiation increased the sensitivity of keratinocytes to UVB-induced apoptosis [9–12]. Studies identified that the functional activation of the IGF-1R provided protection to human keratinocytes from UVB-induced apoptosis. However, an equally important observation was that although the activation of the IGF-1R prevents cell death, the surviving keratinocytes cannot replicate and become senescent (Fig. 1) [9, 11]. The induction of senescence in response to UVB irradiation is a tumor evasion mechanism that maintains the important barrier function of the epidermis while ensuring keratinocytes cannot proliferate in the presence of irreparable UVB-induced DNA damage. This appropriate response to UVB irradiation prevents the propagation of potentially neoplastic keratinocytes. In contrast, when the IGF-1R is functionally inactive at the time of UVB irradiation, a portion of the keratinocytes will undergo apoptosis; however, keratinocytes that survive do not become senescent, do not repair UVB-damaged DNA, and continue to proliferate with the potential of converting the damaged DNA into initiating carcinogenic mutations [11]. This scenario would be an inappropriate response to UVB-induced DNA damage, leading to carcinogenesis [11, 12].

Aging and NMSC

The important in vitro discovery that epidermal keratinocytes IGF-1R activation status was crucial in response to UVB led to a hypothesis that reduced activation of the IGF-1R may be correlated to an increased susceptibility to skin cancer in vivo. In a retrospective epidemiological study, it was found that type 2 diabetic patients using insulin to treat their disease had a 2.5-fold decreased risk of developing nonmelanoma skin cancer over the control group and type 2 diabetic patients using noninsulin medicines to treat their disease [104]. This study is important because insulin and IGF-1 have very similar molecular structures and high concentrations of insulin will activate the IGF-1R. Intriguingly, the protective effect of insulin use increased with age, implying that insulin was somehow protecting against the age-associated increase in nonmelanoma skin cancer [104]. Since high levels of insulin activate the IGF-1R, these important data suggested the clinical relevance for the involvement of the IGF-1R signaling pathway in NMSC in vivo. Recently, the age-related changes in the IGF-1/IGF-1R signal transduction pathway have been examined in vivo. The production of IGF-1 diminishes as fibroblasts become senescent [72, 105]. Given the critical role of dermal fibroblasts in supplying IGF-1 to epidermal keratinocytes, an age-related decrease in fibroblast IGF-1 may result in keratinocytes in aged epidermis having functionally deficient activation of IGF-1R and thereby respond inappropriately to UVB irradiation. Analysis of IGF-1 in samples of geriatric individuals showed a significant reduction in IGF-1 levels when compared to young adults [72]. Accordingly, keratinocyte-activated IGF-1R levels were high in young adult compared to virtual absence in geriatric individuals [72].

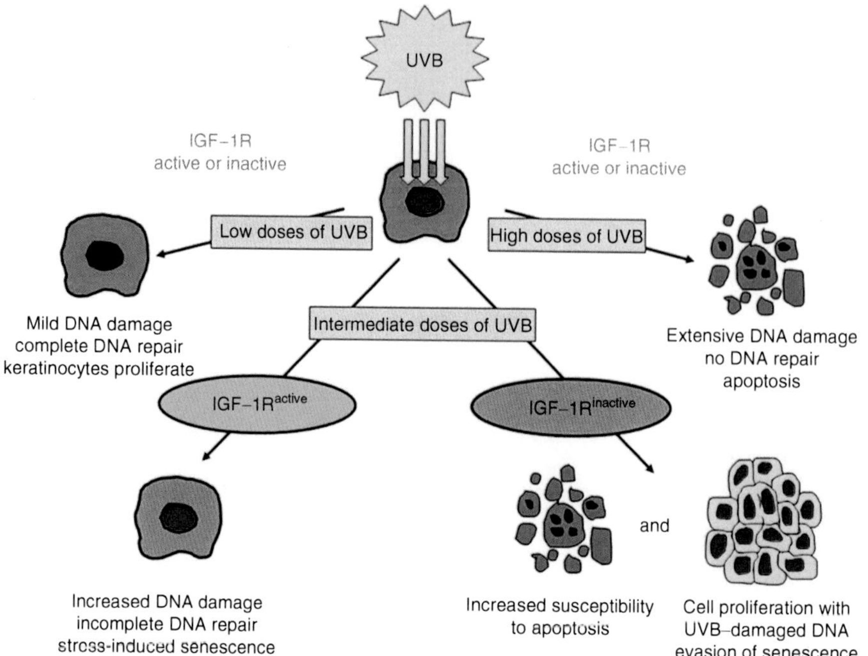

Fig. 1 **Keratinocyte IGF-1R-dependent UVB response.** This cartoon demonstrates the consequences of UVB exposure to normal human keratinocytes in vitro and the role of the IGF-1R. At low doses of UVB irradiation, keratinocytes sustain mild DNA damage which can be completely repaired via normal cellular processes. These keratinocytes continue to proliferate unabatedly. High doses of UVB cause extensive DNA damage that the keratinocyte cannot repair resulting in cell death via apoptosis, or even necrosis if the UVB dose is high enough. Keratinocyte responses to both low and high doses of UVB irradiation are independent of the IGF-1R activation status. However, the keratinocyte response to a wide range of intermediate doses of UVB is completely dependent on the activation status of the IGF-1R. UVB irradiation of keratinocytes with activated IGF-1Rs incurs substantial DNA damage that cannot be completely repaired. Because of the persistence of UVB-induced DNA damage, these keratinocytes become senescent, thus preventing the replication of UVB-damaged DNA. It is important to note that when the IGF-1R is activated, no keratinocytes containing UVB-induced DNA lesions will be replicating. Unfortunately, when the IGF-1R is inactive in keratinocytes, this restriction on cellular replication with DNA damage is not in effect. Keratinocytes with functionally inactive IGF-1Rs that are exposed to UVB irradiation are more likely to undergo apoptosis; however, surviving keratinocytes can continue to proliferate, thus establishing mutations from unrepaired DNA in the daughter cells

It has been reported that the difference between UVB-induced DNA damage repair in young verses aged human skin is the rate at which DNA damaged is cleared [59]. However, the most important point is that *any* DNA damage existing while cell proliferation continues leaves the possibility for the propagation of mutations. In young adult skin where IGF-1 levels are high, the proliferation of keratinocytes containing UVB-damaged DNA will be prevented by a combination of DNA repair, apoptosis, and stress-induced senescence. This response to UVB irradiation which prevents the creation of tumor-initiated keratinocytes is called the appropriate UVB response. The goal of the appropriate UVB response is to ensure the integrity of the epidermis while preventing the proliferation of keratinocytes that contain UVB-induced DNA damage [12]. Because geriatric skin contains reduced levels of IGF-1, the normal UVB response is altered in aged skin [12, 72]. Following UVB exposure, keratinocytes that are proliferating despite the presence of UVB-damaged DNA can be found in geriatric skin (i.e. an inappropriate response) [72]. The role of the IGF-1R in the appropriate UVB response is demonstrated by the restoration of the appropriate UVB response in geriatric skin via treatment with exogenous

IGF-1 prior to UVB irradiation [72]. Therefore, the age-related decrease in IGF-1 expression, IGF-1R inactivation, and proliferation with DNA damage are major components in the development of NMSC seen in geriatric patients (Fig. 2).

It is important to distinguish between the role that IGF-1 plays in the *initiation* of UVB-induced skin cancer [12] and the previously well-documented activity that IGF-1 plays in *promoting* a variety of epithelial tumors [106–109]. In geriatric skin, diminished expression of IGF-1 leads to uncharacteristically decreased activation of the IGF-1R in the epidermis. When keratinocytes are exposed to UVB in the absence of IGF-1R activation, the normal protective response to UVB is altered, so that keratinocytes with DNA damage fail to undergo stress-induced senescence and are capable of replicating chromosomes containing the UVB-damaged DNA. Therefore, the lack of IGF-1R activation at the time of UVB irradiation increases the probability of a cancer-*initiating* event. Previous reports of IGF-1-increasing carcinogenesis were in the context of *promoting* the growth of previously initiated cells, a distinctly different process. [12].

In tissues where homeostasis is dependent on precise interactions between epithelial and mesenchymal cells, the accumulation of senescent cells can disrupt the proper function of the tissue. The skin is one of these tissues where the dermal and epidermal components are interdependent on each other for the proper functioning of the organ. Therefore, cellular senescence affects the UVB response of keratinocytes in the epidermis through two distinct and opposite mechanisms: one mechanism suppresses UVB-induced transformation of keratinocytes and the second mechanism promotes keratinocyte carcinogenesis. On the positive side, keratinocytes use stress-induced senescence as a tumor evasion mechanism. The advantage to cellular senescence versus UVB-induced apoptosis is that senescence maintains the cellularity of the epidermis, thus preserving the barrier function. In other words, widespread UVB-induced keratinocyte apoptosis in the epidermis will severely compromise the epidermal barrier function, while UVB-induced keratinocyte senescence will not. In this manner, the induction of senescence in UVB-irradiated keratinocytes suppresses carcinogenesis. On the negative side, cellular senescence in dermal fibroblasts will promote UVB-induced carcinogenesis in aging skin. IGF-1 expression by dermal fibroblasts is critical for the appropriate response of keratinocytes to UVB irradiation. The silencing of IGF-1 expression by senescent fibroblasts contributes to an increased initiation of transformed keratinocytes by UVB exposure. Furthermore, the altered inflammatory phenotype of senescent fibroblasts may promote the expansion of clones of initiated keratinocytes.

Clinical Implications of Dermal Involvement in NMSC

Given the magnitude of NMSC incidence with its associated morbidity and cost, the prevention of these tumors has significant clinical importance. Still the lack of understanding of its causes, risk factor roles and obscure pathogenesis, renders the prevention of NMSC a challenging goal for basic and clinical science. Past commonly practiced (and still valuable) strategies for the tumor prevention included avoiding excessive UVB exposure [110–112]. In the light of recent translational cutaneous biology research discussed in this review, a novel hypothesis of NMSC photocarcinogenesis has emerged, as well as new potentially preventive and therapeutically promising strategies. Several dermal wounding therapies have recently been tested to restore endogenous levels of IGF-1 and collagen I expression in geriatric dermal fibroblasts that alleviate dysfunctional signaling in geriatric epidermis. Two dermal rejuvenation treatments, dermabrasion and fractionated laser resurfacing, have been shown to reinstate the young adult UVB response in geriatric skin.

Dermabrasion is a cosmetic method of creating a skin ablation using rough sandpaper. The skin wound extends through epidermis deeply into the papillary dermis. It represents a first historical wounding therapy tested, and the known principle behind it is stimulation of the production of new collagen by initiating "wounding skin response" [113]. Until recently, the cellular and molecular

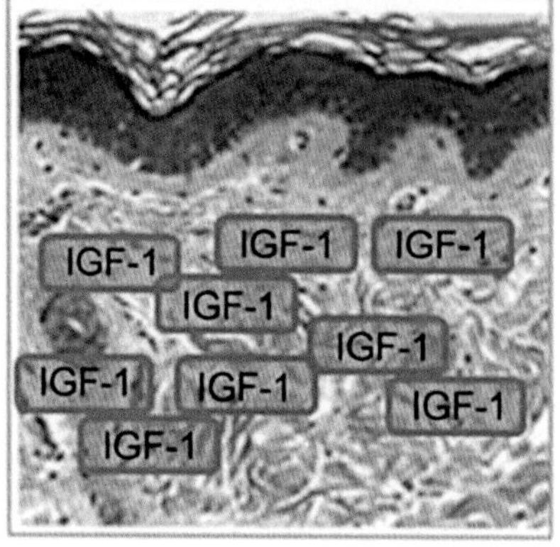

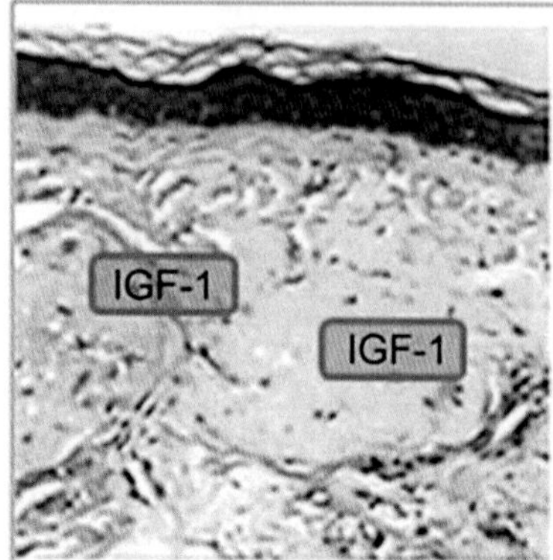

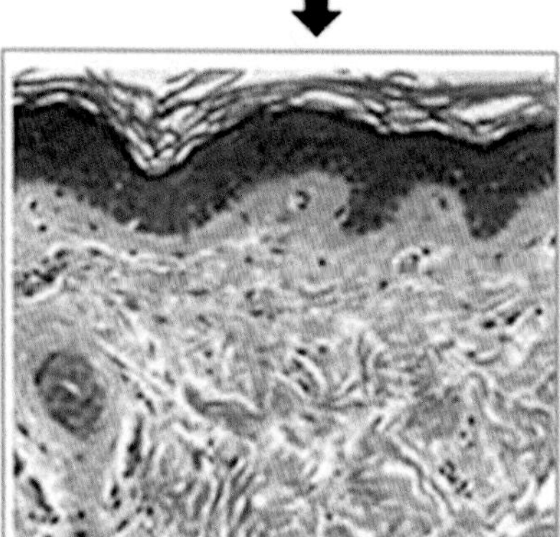

Fig. 2 Skin IGF-1/IGF-1R-dependent UVB response. This illustration compares the response of young skin and old skin to UVB irradiation. The dermis of young adults produces sufficient levels of IGF-1 to activate the IGF-1R on epidermal keratinocytes. The appropriate activation of the IGF-1R on keratinocytes leads to the induction of stress-induced senescence following sufficient UVB exposure. In young skin exposed to UVB, replicating keratinocytes will never contain UVB-damaged DNA; if UVB-irradiated keratinocyte cannot repair all of the UVB-induced DNA damage, they become senescent. UVB-induced senescence is a tumor evasion mechanism to prevent the establishment of initiated neoplastic keratinocytes. In contrast, the expression of IGF-1 is silenced in aged dermis. The consequence of diminished dermal fibroblast IGF-1 expression is a lack of IGF-1R activation in epidermal keratinocytes. Instead of undergoing stress-induced senescence, the aged keratinocytes are able to proliferate in the presence of UVB-damaged DNA. In contrast to young skin, keratinocytes possessing UVB-induced DNA lesions can replicate in geriatric skin. This decrease in IGF-1 expression with advancing age, the subsequent decrease in IGF-1R activity, and the evasion of the normal skin UVB response contribute to the increase in nonmelanoma skin cancer seen in geriatric patients

mechanisms of this skin response have not been fully elucidated. In older healthy (age <65) volunteers, a 3-month-old dermabraded skin was exposed to a standardized dose of UVB irradiation and skin punch out biopsies were analyzed. Wounding using dermabrasion produces a histological skin changes with increase in dermal fibroblast density, accumulation of more elliptical fibroblast replicating nuclei, restoration of collagen fiber dermal layers, reversal of aging-associated atrophy of the papillary dermis, recovery of undulating dermal-epidermal border, and increased numbers of replicative keratinocytes all similar to a young skin. Molecularly, this modality produced increased synthesis of collagen and decrease in markers of DNA-damage response in dermal fibroblasts suggesting loss of senescent fibroblasts and several-fold higher levels of IGF-1 messenger RNA levels. These values in wounded geriatric skin were similar to those found in skin from younger (age <30) volunteers. Noteworthy, when this geriatric dermabraded skin was exposed to UV light, the number of basal layer keratinocytes that co-expressed proliferation (Ki67) markers and UVB-induced DNA damage markers was tenfold lower than in geriatric UVB-irradiated nondermabraded skin. These findings provided the first evidence that dermal rejuvenation in addition to upregulation of IGF-1 mRNA also normalizes abnormal (pro-carcinogenic) UVB response in geriatric skin [72].

Interestingly, dermabrasion as a method to prophylactically treat actinic keratosis and NMSC was introduced into clinical practice over 40 years ago. Numerous reports from clinical settings proved that dermabrasion can reduce the incidence of actinic keratosis and NMSC in up to 95 % of disease-prone individuals for many years after treatment. Nonetheless, the use of dermabrasion has fallen out of favor as a primary method for the prevention of actinic keratosis and NMSC in spite of the fact that novel treatment modalities like topical chemotherapy (imiquimod, 5-fluorouracil) have never achieved the same level of potency as dermabrasion [114–118]. In point of fact, clinical studies that assessed these modalities often use dermabrasion as the gold standard for NMSC prevention.

Though the early research on dermabrasion proved a success in NMSC prevention, the molecular mechanisms that underlie it remained obscure. Initial hypothesis was that dermabrasion was effective due to physical removal of previously initiated carcinogenic keratinocytes. This idea, though sensible, has never been tested. However, if this idea is true, then other ablative methods should be, just as successful in treating NMSC as dermabrasion, but they were not. Recent studies support the identification of a new mechanism by which dermabrasion can prevent actinic keratosis and NMSC [72]. Their focus is on dermal fibroblasts signaling in aged skin and state that accumulation of senescent fibroblasts in aged dermis modifies the susceptibility of keratinocytes to gather and fix UVB-induced mutations. Though dermabrasion has its limitations, it has helped to enlighten pathogenic mechanisms that can be used to develop novel clinical methods of prevention and hopefully treatment of NMSC in elderly population.

Though the results of dermabrasion studies were promising, the use of dermabrasion for widespread areas of skin as a preventive strategy renders it impractical due to the drastic physical and psychological morbidity of the procedure. Thus, the ability of a less-aggressive photorejuvenation treatment to influence the UVB response in geriatric skin was examined. In addition to dermabrasion, the most commonly used and quite successful technique is fractionated laser resurfacing (FLR). FLR uses a laser beam that delivers brief pulses of high-energy light to skin chromophores and water. The light energy in interaction with skin molecules is converted to heat energy; the heat vaporizes skin sections layer by layer causing mini wounds. These mini wounds induce localized "wounding reaction" in skin causing a new skin to repopulate the damaged one. This procedure is manifested with skin tightening rather than with significant superficial skin ablation present in dermabrasion [119]. Though the cosmetic aspect of laser remains the ultimate goal, the cellular and molecular mechanism of its action on skin remains for so many decades unknown. The recent work of several groups clarifies the mechanism of this cosmetic procedure and proposes a novel role of lasers in NMSC prevention. Preclinical work in animal models of NMSC demonstrated that FLR reduces the size and time of first occurrence of skin tumors in animals exposed to FLR treatment and UVB irradiation in comparison with animals exposed to UVB irradiation only. Pathohistological analysis of animal skin exposed to both FLR and UV light demonstrated development of low-grade skin tumors (benign papilloma or dysplastic papilloma). On contrary, control UVB-only irradiated animals developed high-grade invasive squamous cell carcinoma. Moreover, skin exposed to FLR and UVB light demonstrated significantly higher and thicker elastic and collagen content compared with the UV-only treated group where decrease in normal collagen amount and drastic loss of elastic fibers were observed [120]. Noteworthy in human volunteers, similar findings were observed. Following FLR treatment, histological changes manifested in the reduction of senescent fibroblasts that due to normal skin aging accumulate in dermal papillae. Interestingly, this reduction in number of senescent fibroblast was only partially dependent on skin UV exposure, suggesting that an intrinsic aging appears to be as important as extrinsic aging in the studied population. Molecular analysis of geriatric skin treated with FLR shows results similar to dermabrasion; on either sun-protected or sun-exposed skin, FLR treatment significantly increased IGF-1 expression in the geriatric dermis. The level of IGF-1 expression in FLR-treated skin was equivalent to the skin of young adult controls. Moreover, FLR treatment virtually eliminated the inappropriate UVB response shown in matched geriatric control tissue. Importantly, this reduction in the inappropriate UVB response outpaces that previously noticed in dermabraded geriatric skin. Furthermore, FLR treatment appears to reverse the age-dependent decrease in UVB-induced DNA repair response seen in geriatric skin. These observations demonstrate that the benefits of FLR treatment exceeds the previously described therapeutic ability of dermabrasion in restoring the appropriate UVB response in aging skin. FLR thus has an additional benefit of obtaining the desired results without the broad tissue damage observed in dermabrasion [121].

Conclusion

One possible new treatment strategy would be to develop methods to rejuvenate the fibroblasts to allow production of factors such as IGF-1. Though marketed for cosmetic purposes, skin damaging agents ranging from chemical peels, laser resurfacing, heating of the skin, and other "wounding" procedures could have this benefit [122, 123] and should be explored. Indeed, dermal wounding which would result in upregulation of fibroblast genes (e.g., procollagen) should also result in the upregulation of IGF-1. It should be noted that a recent study demonstrated that the topical chemotherapeutic agent 5-fluorouracil results in the induction of dermal procollagen [124]. The ability of this chemotherapeutic agent to both remove precancerous keratinocytes and induce dermal wounding that could protect against future UV exposure could result in an improved effect. Other therapeutic strategies that could possibly share these "dual effects" of both the removal of mutated keratinocytes and the induction of dermal rejuvenation would include photodynamic therapy and topical imiquimod. Future studies should examine the dermal effects of these chemotherapeutic therapies.

Since there appears to be a protective effect of exogenous insulin in skin cancer development [104], systemic treatment with IGF-1 could have a use in protecting high-risk populations. Currently used for short-stature syndromes, IGF-1 has an established side effect profile and should also be studied [125]. Thus, this new paradigm of the role of aging in the development of skin cancer could have significant clinical implications.

References

1. ACS Cancer Facts and Figures 2015.
2. Karia PS, Han J, Schmults CD. Cutaneous squamous cell carcinoma: estimated incidence of disease, nodal metastasis, and deaths from disease in the United States, 2012. J Am Acad Dermatol. 2013;68:957–66.
3. Kripke ML. Carcinogenesis: ultraviolet radiation. In: Fitzpatrick TB, Eisen AZ, Wolff K, Freedberg IM, Austen KF, editors. Dermatology in general medicine. New York: McGraw-Hill; 1993. p. 797–804.

4. Tyrrell RM. The molecular and cellular pathology of solar ultraviolet radiation. Mol Aspects Med. 1994;15:1–77.
5. Clingen PH, Arlett CF, Roza L, Mori T, Nikaido O, Green MHL. Induction of cyclobutane pyrimidine dimers, pyrimidine(6-4) pyrimidone photoproducts, and Dewar valence isomers by natural sunlight in normal human mononuclear cells. Cancer Res. 1995;55:2245–8.
6. Wikonkal NM, Brash DE. Ultraviolet radiation induced signature mutations in photocarcinogenesis. J Investig Dermatol Symp Proc. 1999;4:6–10.
7. Brash DE, Heffernan T, Nghiem P. Carcinogenesis: ultraviolet radiation. In: Wolff K, editor. Fitzpatrick's dermatology in general medicine. 6th ed. New York: McGraw-Hill Professional; 2003.
8. Kraemer KH. Sunlight and skin cancer: another link revealed. Proc Natl Acad Sci U S A. 1997;94:11–4.
9. Kuhn C, Kumar M, Hurwitz SA, Cotton J, Spandau DF. Activation of the insulin-like growth factor-1 receptor promotes the survival of human keratinocytes following ultraviolet B irradiation. Int J Cancer. 1999;80:431–8.
10. Lewis DA, Spandau DF. UVB-induced activation of NF-κB is regulated by the IGF-1R and dependent on p38 MAPK. J Invest Dermatol. 2008;128:1022–9.
11. Lewis DA, Yi Q, Travers JB, Spandau DF. UVB-induced senescence in human keratinocytes requires a functional IGF-1R and p53. Mol Biol Cell. 2008;19:1346–53.
12. Lewis DA, Travers JB, Spandau DF. A new paradigm for the role of aging in the development of skin cancer. J Invest Dermatol. 2008;129:787–91.
13. Barreca A, De Luca M, Del Monte P, Bondanza S, Damonte G, Cariola G, et al. In vitro paracrine regulation of human keratinocyte growth by fibroblast derived insulin-like growth factors. J Cell Physiol. 1992;151:262–8.
14. Tavakkol A, Elder JT, Griffiths CE, Cooper KD, Talwar H, Fisher GJ, et al. Expression of growth hormone receptor, insulin-like growth factor 1 (IGF-1) and IGF-1 receptor mRNA and proteins in human skin. J Invest Dermatol. 1992;99:343–9.
15. Campisi J. Aging and cancer cell biology, 2008. Aging Cell. 2008;7:281–4.
16. Vasto S, Carruba G, Lio D, Colonna-Romano G, Di Bona D, Candore G, Caruso C. Inflammation, ageing and cancer. Mech Ageing Dev. 2009;130:40–5.
17. Anisimov VN. Carcinogenesis and aging 20 years after. Escaping horizon. Mech Ageing Dev. 2009;130:105–21.
18. Moriwaki S, Ray S, Tarone RE, Kraemer KH, Grossman L. The effect of donor age on the processing of UV-damaged DNA by cultured human cells: reduced DNA repair capacity and increased DNA mutability. Mutat Res. 1996;364:117–23.
19. Ouhtit A, Ueda M, Nakazawa M, Dumaz N, Sarasin A, Yamasaki H. Quantitative detection of ultraviolet-specific p53 mutations in normal skin from Japanese patients. Cancer Epidemiol Biomarkers Prev. 1997;6:433–8.
20. Krtolica A, Parrinello S, Lockett S, Desprez P-Y, Campisi J. Senescent fibroblasts promote epithelial cell growth and tumorigenesis: a link between cancer and aging. Proc Natl Acad Sci U S A. 2001;98:12072–7.
21. Parrinello S, Coppe J-P, Krtolica A, Campisi J. Stromal-epithelial interactions in aging and cancer: senescent fibroblasts alter epithelial cell differentiation. J Cell Sci. 2005;118:485–96.
22. Campisi J. Senescent cells, tumor suppression, and organismal aging: good citizens, bad neighbors. Cell. 2005;120:513–22.
23. Jemal A, Tiwari RC, Murray T, et al. Cancer statistics. CA Cancer J Clin. 2004;54:8–29.
24. Fuchs E, Raghavan S. Getting under the skin of epidermal morphogenesis. Nat Rev Genet. 2002;31:199–209.
25. Mullenders LHF, Van Hoffen A, Vreeswijk MP, Gruven HJ, Vrieling H, van Zeeland AA. Ultraviolet-induced photolesions: repair and mutagenesis. Recent Results Cancer Res. 1997;143:89–99.
26. Yuspa SH, Dlugosz AA. Cutaneous carinogenesis: natural and experimental. In: Goldsmith LA, editor. Physiology, biochemistry and molecular biology of the skin. New York: Oxford University Press; 1991. p. 1365–402.
27. Vogelstein B, Kinzler KW. Cancer genes and the pathways they control. Nat Med. 2004; 10:789–99.
28. Sjoblom T, Jones S, Wood LD, Parsons DW, Lin J, Barber TD, Mandelker D, Leary RJ, Ptak J, Stillman N, Szabo S, Buckhaults P, Farrell C, Meeh P, Markowitz SD, Willis J, Dawson D, Willson JKV, Gazdar AF, Hartigan J, Wu L, Liu C, Parmigiani G, Park BH, Bachman KE, Papadopoulos N, Vogelstein B, Kinzler KW, Velculescu VE. The consensus coding sequences of human breast and colorectal cancers. Science. 2006;314:268–74.
29. Campisi J. Suppressing cancer: the importance of being senescent. Science. 2005;309:886–7.
30. Dimri GP. What has senescence got to do with cancer? Cancer Cell. 2005;7:505–12.
31. Feng Z, Hu W, Teresky AK, Hernando E, Cordon-Cardo C, Levine AJ. Declining p53 function in the aging process: a possible mechanism for the increased tumor incidence in older populations. Proc Natl Acad Sci U S A. 2007;104:16633–8.
32. Melnikova VO, Ananthaswamy HN. Cellular and molecular events leading to the development of skin cancer. Mutat Res. 2005;571:91–106.
33. Ichihashi M, Ueda M, Budiyanto A, Bito T, Oka M, Fukunaga M, et al. UV-induced skin damage. Toxicology. 2003;189:21–37.
34. Nishigori C. Cellular aspects of photocarcinogenesis. Photochem Photobiol Sci. 2006;5:208–14.
35. Mathon NF, Lloyd AC. Cell senescence and cancer. Nat Rev Cancer. 2001;1:203–13.

36. Krtolica A, Campisi J. Cancer and aging: a model for the cancer promoting effects of the aging stroma. Int J Biochem Cell Biol. 2002;34:1401–14.
37. Campisi J. Cancer and ageing: rival demons? Nat Rev Cancer. 2003;3:339–49.
38. Matsumura Y, Ananthaswammy HN. Toxic effects of ultraviolet radiation on the skin. Toxicol Appl Pharmacol. 2004;195:298–308.
39. Ramos J, Villa J, Ruiz A, Armstrong R, Matta A. UV dose determines key characteristics of non-melanoma skin cancer. Cancer Epidemiol Biomarkers Prev. 2004;13:2006–11.
40. Brash DE. Roles of the transcription factor p53 keratinocyte carcinomas. Br J Dermatol. 2006; 154:8–10.
41. Benjamin CL, Anathaswamy HN. p53 and the pathogenesis of skin cancer. Toxicol Appl Pharmacol. 2007;224:241–8.
42. Jonason AS, Kunala S, Price GJ, Restifo RJ, Spinelli HM, Persing JA, et al. Frequent clones of p53 -mutated in keratinocytes in normal skin. Proc Natl Acad Sci U S A. 1996;93:14025–9.
43. Rodier F, Campisi J, Bhaumik D. Two faces of p53: aging and tumor suppression. Nucleic Acids Res. 2007;35:7475–84.
44. Halliday GM, Rana S. Wave band and dose dependency of sunlightinduced immunomodulation and cellular changes. Photochem Photobiol. 2008; 84:35–46.
45. Zhang Q, Yao Y, Konger RL, Sinn A, Cai S, Pollok KE, Travers JB. Platelet-activating factor mediates ultraviolet B radiation-mediated inhibition of delayed-type contact hypersensitivity reactions. J Invest Dermatol. 2008;128:1780–7.
46. Aubin F. Mechanisms involved in ultraviolet light-induced immunesuppression. Eur J Dermatol. 2003;13:515–23.
47. Schwartz T. Photoimmunosupression. Photodermatol Photoimmunol Photomed. 2002;18:141–5.
48. Marathe GK, Johnson C, Billings SD, Southall MD, Pei Y, Spandau DF, Murphy RC, Zimmerman GA, McIntyre TM, Travers JB. Ultraviolet B radiation generates platelet-activating factor-like phospholipids underlying cutaneous damage. J Biol Chem. 2005;280:35448–57.
49. Halliday GM. Inflammation, gene mutation and photoimmunosuppression in response to UVR-induced oxidative damage contributes to photocarcinogenesis. Mutat Res. 2005;571:107–20.
50. Chung JH, Hanft VN, Kang S. Aging and photoaging. J Am Acad Dermatol. 2003;49:690–7.
51. Cooper SJ, Bowen GT. Ultraviolet B regulation of transcription factor families: role of the nuclear factor-kappa B (NF-κB) and activator protein-1 (AP-1) in UVB-induced skin carcinogenesis. Curr Cancer Drug Targets. 2007;7:325–34.
52. Madson JG, Hansen LA. Multiple mechanisms of erbB2 action after ultraviolet irradiation of the skin. Mol Carcinog. 2007;46:624–8.
53. Gallagher RP, Hill GB, Bajdik CD, Fincham S, Coldman AJ, McLean DI, Threlfall WJ. Sunlight exposure, pigmentary factors, and risk of nonmelanocytic skin cancer I. Basal cell carcinoma. Arch Dermatol. 1995;131:157–63.
54. MacKie RM. Long-term health risk to the skin of ultraviolet radiation. Prog Biophys Mol Biol. 2006;92:92–6.
55. Bickers DR, Athar M. Oxidative stress in the pathogenesis of skin disease. J Invest Dermatol. 2006;126:2565–75.
56. Chen J-H, Hales N, Ozanne SE. DNA damage, cellular senescence and organismal ageing: causal or correlative. Nucleic Acids Res. 2007;35:7417–28.
57. Bertram C, Hass R. Cellular responses to ROS-induced DNA damage and aging. Biol Chem. 2008;389:211–20.
58. Burhans WC, Weinberger M. DNA replication stress, genome instability and aging. Nucleic Acids Res. 2007;35:7545–56.
59. Yamada M, Udono M, Hori M, Hirose R, Sato S, Mori T, et al. Aged human skin removes UVB-induced pryimidine dimers from the epidermis more slowly than younger adult skin in vivo. Arch Dermatol Res. 2006;297:294–302.
60. Kenyon J, Gerson SL. The role of DNA damage repair in aging of adult stem cells. Nucleic Acids Res. 2007;35:7557–65.
61. Sunderkotter C, Kalden H, Luger TA. Aging and the skin immune system. Arch Dermatol. 1997; 133:1256–62.
62. Gruver AL, Hudson LL, Sempowski GD. Immunosenescence of ageing. J Pathol. 2007;211:144–56.
63. Witkowski JM, Soroczynska-Cybula M, Bryl E, Smolenska Z, Jozwik A. Klotho-a common link in physiological and rheumatoid arthritis related aging of human CD4 lymphocytes. J Immunol. 2007;178:771–7.
64. Hayflick L, Moorhead P. The serial cultivation of human diploid cell strains. Exp Cell Res. 1961;25:385–621.
65. Harley CB, Futcher AB, Greider CW. Telomeres shorten during ageing of human fibroblasts. Nature. 1990;345:458–60.
66. Ben-Porath I, Weinberg RA. The signals and pathways activating cellular senescence. Int J Biochem Cell Biol. 2005;2005(37):961–76.
67. Blackburn EH. Telomeres and telomerase: their mechanisms of action and the effects of altering their function. FEBS Lett. 2005;579:859–62.
68. Herbig U, Jobling WA, Chen BPC, Chen DJ, Sedivy JM. Telomere shortening triggers senescence of human cells through a pathway involving ATM, p53 and p21CIP1 but not p16INK4a. Mol Cell. 2004;14:501–13.
69. Dimiri GP, Lee X, Basile G, Acosta M, Scott G, Roskelley C, et al. A biomarkers that identifies senescent human cells in culture and in aging skin in vivo. Proc Natl Acad Sci U S A. 1995; 92:9363–7.

70. Herbig U, Ferreira M, Carey D, Sedivy JM. Cellular senescence in aging primates. Science. 2006; 311:1257.
71. Jeyapalan JC, Ferreira M, Sedivy JM, Herbig U. Accumulation of senescent cells in mitotic tissue of aging primates. Mech Ageing Dev. 2007;128:36–44.
72. Lewis DA, Travers JB, Machado C, Somani AK, Spandau DF. Reversing the aging stromal phenotype prevents carcinoma initiation. Aging. 2011;3:407–16.
73. Williams GC. Pleiotropy, natural selection, and the evolution of senescence. Evolution. 1957; 11:398–411.
74. Hornsby PJ. Senescence as an anticancer mechanism. J Clin Oncol. 2007;14:1852–7.
75. Dilley T, Bowden G, Chen Q. Novel mechanisms of sublethal oxidant toxicity: induction of premature senescence in human fibroblasts confer tumor promoter activity. Exp Cell Res. 2003;290:38–48.
76. Collado M, Blasco MA, Serrao M. Cellular senescence in cancer and aging. Cell. 2007;130:223–31.
77. Sorrell JM, Baber MA, Caplan AI. Site-matched papillary and reticular human dermal fibroblasts differ in their release of specific growth factors/cytokines and in their interaction with keratinocytes. J Cell Physiol. 2004;200:134–45.
78. El-Ghalbzouri A, Gibbs S, Lamme E, Van Blitterswijk CA, Ponec M. Effect of fibroblasts on epidermal regeneration. Br J Dermatol. 2002; 147:230–43.
79. Kneilling M, Rocken M. Mast cells: novel clinical perspectives from recent insights. Exp Dermatol. 2009;18:488–96.
80. Sharp L, Jameson J, Cauvi G, Havran W. Dendritic epidermal T cells regulate skin homeostasis through local production of insulin-like growth factor 1. Nat Immun. 2004;6:73–9.
81. Coppe JP, Patil CK, Rodier F, Sun Y, Munoz DP, Goldstein J, Nelson PS, Desprez PY, Campisi J. Senescence associated secretory phenotypes reveal cell non-autonomous functions of oncogenic RAS and p53 tumor suppressor. PLoS Biol. 2008;6:2853–68.
82. Nolte SV, Xu Weiguo W, Rennekampff HO, Rodemann HP. Diversity of fibroblasts – a review on implications for skin tissue engineering. Cell Tissues Organs. 2008;187:165–76.
83. Eming Sabine A, Krieg T, Davidson JM. Inflammation in wound repair: molecular and cellular mechanisms. J Invest Dermatol. 2007;127:514–25.
84. Spiekstra SW, Breetveld M, Rustemeyer T, Scheper RJ, Gibbs S. Wound-healing factors secreted by epidermal keratinocytes and dermal fibroblasts in skin substitutes. Wound Repair Regen. 2007; 15:708–17.
85. Haniffa MA, Wang XN, Holtick U, Rae M, Isaacs JD, Dickinson AM, Hilkens CMU, Collin MP. Adult human fibroblasts are potent immunoregulatory cells and functionally equivalent to mesenchymal stem cells. J Immunol. 2007;179:1595–604.
86. Flavell SJ, Hou TZ, Lax AD, Salmon M, Buckley CD. Fibroblasts as novel therapeutic targets in chronic inflammation. Br J Pharmacol. 2008;153: s241–6.
87. Campisi J, Fagagna F. Cellular senescence: when bad things happen to good cells. Mol Cell Biol. 2007;8:729–40.
88. Harman D. Aging: a theory based on free radical and radiation chemistry. J Gerontol. 1956;11:298–300.
89. Sohal RS, Orr WC. Oxidative stress may be a causal factor in senescence. Age. 1998;21:81–2.
90. Hamilton ML, Remmen HV, Drake JA, Yang H, Guo ZM, Kewitt K, Walter CA, Richardson A. Does oxidative damage to DNA increase with age? Proc Natl Acad Sci U S A. 2001;98:10469–74.
91. Lin MT, Flint BM. The oxidative theory of aging. Clin Neurosci Res. 2003;2:305–15.
92. Shelton DN, Chang E, Whittier PS, Choi D, Funk WD. Microarray analysis of replicative senescence. Curr Biol. 1999;9:939–45.
93. Wall IB, Moseley R, Briard DM, Kipling D, Giles P, Laffafian I, et al. Fibroblast dysfunction is a key factor in non-healing of chronic venous leg ulcers. J Invest Dermatol. 2008;128:2526–40.
94. Baker DJ, Wijshake T, Tchkonia T, LeBrasseur NK, Child BG, van de Sluis B, et al. Clearance of p16Ink4a-positive senescent cells delays ageing-associated disorders. Nature. 2011;479:232–6.
95. Farage MA, Miller KW, Elsner P, Maibach HI. Intrinsic and extrinsic factors in aging: a review. Int J Cosmet Sci. 2008;30:87–95.
96. Bol DK, Kigucji K, Gimenez-Conti I, Rupp T, DiGiovanni J. Overexpression of the insulin-like growth factor-1 induces hyperplasia, dermal abnormalities and spontaneous tumor formation in transgenic mice. Oncogene. 1997;14:1725–34.
97. Wilker E, Bol D, Kiguchi K, Rupp T, Beltran L, Di Giovanni J. Enhancement for susceptibility to diverse skin tumor promoters by activation of the insulin-like growth factor-1 receptor in the epidermis of transgenic mice. Mol Carcinog. 1999;25:122–31.
98. DiGiovanni J, Bol DK, Wilker E, Beltran L, Carbajal S, Moats S, et al. Constitutive expression of insulin-like growth factor-1 in epidermal basal cells of transgenic mice leads to spontaneous tumor promotion. Cancer Res. 2000;60:1561–70.
99. Sadagurski M, Yakar S, Weingarten G, Holzenberger M, Rhodes C, Breikreutz D, et al. Insulin-like growth factor receptor signaling regulates skin development and inhibits skin keratinocyte differentiation. Mol Cell Biol. 2006;26:2675–87.
100. Lin K, Hsin H, Libina N, Kenyon C. Regulation of the *Caenorhabditis elegans* longevity protein DAF-16 by insulin/IGF1 and germline signaling. Nat Genet. 2001;28:139–45.
101. Holzenberger M, Dupont J, Ducos B, Leneuve P, Geloen A, Even PC, et al. IGF-1 receptor regulates lifespan and resistance to oxidative stress in mice. Nature. 2003;21:182–7.

102. Kruso H, Yamamoto M, Clark JD, Pastor JV, Nandi A, Gurnani P, et al. Suppression of aging in mice by the hormone Klotho. Science. 2005;309:1829–33.
103. Ikushima M, Rakugi H, Ishidawa K, Maedawa Y, Yamamoto K, Ohta J, et al. Anti-apoptotic and anti-senescent effects of Klotho on vascular endothelial cells. Biochem Biophys Res Commun. 2006; 339:827–32.
104. Chuang T-Y, Lewis DA, Spandau DF. Decreased incidence of nonmelanoma skin cancer in patients with type 2 diabetes mellitus using insulin: a pilot study. Br J Dermatol. 2005;153:552–7.
105. Ferber A, Chang C, Sells C, Ptasznik A, Cristofalo V, Hubbard K, et al. Failure of senescent human fibroblasts to express insulin-like growth factor-1 gene. J Biol Chem. 1993;268:17883–8.
106. Pollak M. Insulin and insulin-like growth factor signaling in neoplasia. Nat Rev Cancer. 2008;8:915–28.
107. Lann D, LeRoith D. The role of endocrine insulin-like growth factor-1 and insulin in breast cancer. J Mammary Gland Biol Neoplasia. 2008;13:371–9.
108. Dziadziuszko R, Camidge DR, Hirsch FR. The insulin-like growth factor in lung cancer. J Thorac Oncol. 2008;3:815–8.
109. Donovan EA, Kummar S. Role of the insulin-like growth factor-1R system in colorectal carcinogenesis. Crit Rev Oncol Hematol. 2008;66:91–8.
110. Thompson SC, Jolley D, Marks R. Reduction of solar keratosis by regular sunscreen use. N Engl J Med. 1993;329:1147–51.
111. Green A, Williams G, Neale R, Hart V, Leslie D, Parsons P, Marks G, Gaffney P, Battistath D, Frost C, Lang C, Russell A. Daily sunscreen application and betacarotene supplementation in prevention of basal-cell and squamous-cell carcinomas of the skin: a randomized controlled trial. Lancet. 1999;354:723–9.
112. Neale R, Williams G, Green A. Application patterns among participants randomized to daily sunscreen use in a skin cancer prevention trial. Arch Dermatol. 2002;138:1319–25.
113. Travers JB, Spandau DF, Lewis DA, Machado C, Kingsley M, Mousdicas N, Somani AK. Fibroblast senescence and squamous cell carcinoma: how wounding therapies could be protective. Dermatol Surg. 2013;39:967–73.
114. Cooley JE, Casey DL, Kauffman CL. Manual resurfacing and trichloracetic acid for the treatment of patients with widespread actinic damage. Dermatol Surg. 1997;23:373–9.
115. Hantash BM, Stewart DB, Cooper AZ, Rehmus WE, Koch RJ, Setter SM. Facial resurfacing for nonmelanoma skin cancer prophylaxis. Arch Dermatol. 2006;142:976–82.
116. Ostertag JU, Quaedvlieg PJF, Neumann MHAM, Kerkels GA. Recurrence rates and long-term follow-up after laser resurfacing as a treatment for widespread actinic dermatoses in the face and on the scalp. Dermatol Surg. 2006;32:261–7.
117. Halachmi S, Lapidoth M. Lasers in skin cancer prophylaxis. Expert Rev Anticancer Ther. 2008; 8:1713–5.
118. Love WE, Bernhard JD, Bordeaux JS. Topical imiquimod or fluorouracil therapy for basal and squamous cell carcinoma. Arch Dermatol. 2009; 145:1431–8.
119. Loesch MM, Somani AK, Kingsley MM, Travers JB, Spandau DF. Skin resurfacing procedures: new and emerging options. Clin Cosmet Investig Dermatol. 2014;28:231–41.
120. Gye J, Ahn SK, Kwon JE, Hong SP. Use of fractional CO_2 laser decreases the risk of skin cancer development during ultraviolet exposure in hairless mice. Dermatol Surg. 2015;41:378–86.
121. Spandau DF, Lewis DA, Somani AK, Travers JB. Fractionated laser resurfacing corrects the inappropriate UVB response in geriatric skin. J Invest Dermatol. 2012;132:1591–6.
122. Meshkinpour A, Ghasri P, Pope K, Lyubovitsky JG, Risteli J, Krasieva TB, Kelly KM. Treatment of hypertrophic scars and keloids with a radiofrequency device: a study of collagen effects. Lasers Surg Med. 2005;37:343–9.
123. DeHoratius DM, Dover JS. Nonablative tissue remodeling and photorejuvenation. Clin Dermatol. 2007;25:474–9.
124. Sachs DL, Kang S, Hammerberg C, Helfrich Y, Karimipour D, Orringer J, Johnson T, Hamilton TA, Fisher G, Voorhees JJ. Topical fluorouracil for actinic keratoses and photoaging: a clinical and molecular analysis. Arch Dermatol. 2009;145:659–66.
125. Collett-Solberg PF, Misra M, Drug and Therapeutics Committee of the Lawson Wilkins Pediatric Endocrine Society. The role of recombinant human insulin-like growth factor-I in treating children with short stature. J Clin Endocrinol Metabol. 2008;93:10–8.

71 Nonsurgical Modalities of Treatment for Primary Cutaneous Cancers

Rami Abadi, Salah Salman, and Ossama Abbas

Contents

Abstract

Skin cancer, including melanoma and nonmelanoma skin cancers (NMSCs), is the most common malignancy affecting humans. The incidence of these cutaneous malignancies increases with age, making the elderly population most prone to the development of these cancers. Although surgery is usually the treatment of choice for cutaneous malignancies, it may not be the most appropriate solution. Not only does surgery cause major disfigurement and functional impairment, but also the patient may be a poor surgical candidate, necessitating use of other modalities of treatment. The choice of the treatment modality to be utilized should be tailored according to specific cancer characteristics (type, size, location) and patient factors (age, comorbidities, use of multiple drugs, including anticoagulants). This is especially true if elderly patients have an increased incidence of other medical comorbidities that may have an adverse effect on surgery. In such circumstances, alternatives to surgery may be the preferred choice. This chapter aims at reviewing the currently available evidence on the various nonsurgical therapeutic modalities for the different types of skin cancer. These include topical, intralesional, and systemic treatments, as well as physical treatment modalities. Furthermore, certain dietary and herbal supplements may also have a role in the prevention of skin cancers.

R. Abadi • S. Salman • O. Abbas (✉)
Department of Dermatology, American University of Beirut Medical Center, Beirut, Lebanon
e-mail: rami_abadi@hotmail.com; salmanderm@gmail.com; ossamaabbas2003@yahoo.com

M.A. Farage et al. (eds.), *Textbook of Aging Skin*,
DOI 10.1007/978-3-662-47398-6_59

Introduction

Skin cancer, which includes melanoma and nonmelanoma skin cancers (NMSCs), is the most common malignancy affecting humans [1–4]. Basal cell carcinoma (BCC) represents the most common cutaneous malignancy (comprising approximately 75 % of NMSCs), followed by squamous cell carcinoma (SCC), which comprises around 20 % of NMSCs [1–4]. The incidence of these cutaneous malignancies increases with age, making the elderly population most prone to the development of these cancers [1–4].

Although surgery, particularly Mohs micrographic surgery, is usually the treatment of choice in the management of cutaneous malignancies in terms of margin control and cure rates, it may not be the most appropriate solution because of its disadvantages [1–4]. The choice of the treatment modality to be utilized should be tailored according to specific cancer characteristics (such as type, size, location) and patient factors (age, comorbidities, use of multiple drugs, including anticoagulants) [1–4]. Not only does surgery cause major disfigurement and functional impairment, but also the patient may be a poor surgical candidate, necessitating use of other modalities of treatment [1–4]. This is especially true in elderly patients who are not only characterized by an increased incidence of cutaneous malignancies but also by an increased incidence of other medical comorbidities that may have an adverse effect on surgery [1–4]. In such circumstances, alternatives to surgery may be the preferred choice.

The chapter aims at reviewing the currently available evidence on the various nonsurgical therapeutic modalities for the different types of skin cancer. These include topical, intralesional, and systemic treatments, as well as physical treatment modalities. Furthermore, certain dietary and herbal supplements may also have a role in the prevention of skin cancers.

Topical Therapies

Several topical agents have been used in the treatment of cutaneous malignancies, including imiquimod, 5-fluorouracil, tazarotene, ingenol mebutate, diclofenac, and cidofovir [1–4]. The use of these agents should be guided by evidence on their effectiveness in the treatment of specific types of skin cancers, patient profile, and the medication's side effects. The use of topical agents has several advantages such as ease of use, convenience (as the medication can be applied at home), and ability to treat larger lesions and critical sites and may usually lead to better cosmetic outcomes. However, several disadvantages should be noted, the most important of which is the initial irritating inflammatory response, which can affect patient's compliance and subsequently the final results. In addition, the expensive cost of some of these agents (such as imiquimod) may limit its use.

Imidazoquinoline Compounds (Imiquimod and Resiquimod)

Several studies have shown that the mechanism of action of imidazoquinoline compounds (imiquimod and resiquimod) as immunomodulators is mediated by the activation of Toll-like receptors 7 and 8 (TLR7, TLR8), which leads to the production of interferon-alpha (IFN-a) and other cytokines, including interleukin (IL)-12 and IL-18 [1, 5]. These then mediate the antitumoral effect through their enhancement of the cell-mediated immunity. Also, the antitumoral effect is mediated through upregulation of the opioid growth factor receptor (OGFr) that, in turn, stimulates the interaction of the OGF–OGFr axis, which is an inhibitory pathway regulating cell proliferation [6].

There is now plenty of evidence on the effectiveness of the imiquimod 5 % cream in the treatment of multiple primary cutaneous malignancies. Currently, it is US Food and Drug Administration (FDA) approved for the treatment of superficial BCCs (especially those that are smaller than 2 cm on the trunk, neck, or extremities) and actinic keratoses (AKs) [1, 2, 5].

Different studies have shown that the rate of clinical and histological clearance of superficial BCCs treated with imiquimod 5 % cream (applied

5 or 7 days/week for 6–12 weeks) is greater than 90 %. Although less evidence based, the use of imiquimod in the treatment of nodular BCCs has also proven to be effective (clearance rate ranged between 70 % and 100 % based on different studies) [1, 2, 5].

As in the case of superficial BCCs, imiquimod is also FDA approved for treating AKs of the head and neck region. This has been supported by several studies that have shown a 50 % complete clearance rate of AKs (compared to 5 % of AKs in patients treated with placebo) that were treated with imiquimod 5 % cream (applied 3 days/week for 12–16 weeks) [1, 2]. Recently, a new standard for AK management has been set with the target being detection and clearance of clinical and subclinical AKs across the entire sun-exposed field. This concept has used imiquimod 3.75 % cream (daily on two 2-week treatment cycles that are separated by a 2-week treatment-free interval) and reduction in lesions from Lmax (maximum lesion count during treatment). This treatment resulted in 92 % median percentage reduction in AK lesions with sustained lesion clearance for at least 1 year and acceptable tolerability profile [7]. Based on these data, imiquimod 3.75 % was suggested as a first-choice treatment for patients with AK.

Although there is currently less evidence supporting the use of topical imiquimod in the treatment of other skin malignancies – including Bowen's disease or squamous cell carcinoma in situ (SCCIS), invasive SCC, or lentigo maligna – anecdotal reports and small studies have shown that imiquimod may be quite effective [1, 2]. This can thus be used in those patients who are poor surgical candidates.

Adverse reactions most commonly encountered with the use of topical imiquimod include erythema, ulceration, edema, and/or scaling, and these are usually limited to the application site. These reactions can be intense, especially with increased application frequency and especially in patients being treated for AK or BCC [1, 2, 5]. Flu-like symptoms such as fever, fatigue, and myalgias are systemic adverse effects that have been reported in approximately 1–2 % of patients.

5-Fluorouracil (5-FU)

The mechanism of action of 5-FU derives from it being a structural analog of thymine. 5-FU acts as an antimetabolite and interferes with DNA synthesis by inhibiting thymidylate synthetase. It acts mainly on rapidly dividing cells such as tumor cells [1–4].

First used in clinical practice in the 1960s, topical 5-FU is now present in different formulations including solutions (1 %, 2 %, and 5 %) and creams (0.5 %, 1 %, 2 %, and 5 %). They are approved by the FDA for the treatment of AKs. The 5 % cream has been approved by the FDA for treating superficial BCCs. Its effectiveness in the treatment of AKs has been shown to be comparable to imiquimod [1, 2]. Anecdotal reports have also shown that 5-FU may be effective in the treatment of SCCIS [1]. The usual application regimen is once or twice daily for up to 4 weeks.

Adverse reactions commonly described with the topical use of 5-FU include local irritation, allergic contact dermatitis, pain, erythema, edema, pruritus, dyspigmentation, and photosensitivity [1–4]. Uncommon reactions such as onychodystrophy and the appearance of telangiectasias may also occur. Rarely, systemic absorption may lead to systemic side effects such as nausea, myelosuppression, diarrhea, cardiac abnormalities, and neurologic toxicity [1–4].

Tazarotene

Tazarotene is a third-generation retinoid that usually exerts its effect on keratinocyte differentiation and proliferation, mainly through its interaction with RAR-β and d receptors [1]. However, the underlying mechanism of its confirmed effect in the treatment of NMSCs in a few small studies is still not well understood [1].

One study showed that the daily use of 0.1 % tazarotene gel for the treatment of BCC resulted in a complete clearance rate of 53 %. The duration of treatment in this study ranged between 5 and 8 months [1]. Similarly, 0.1 % tazarotene gel used daily for up to 6 months in the treatment of SCCIS resulted in a clearance rate of 47 % [1].

Like the other topical retinoids, the most common adverse reaction observed with tazarotene is skin irritation, manifesting in the form of redness, scaling, dryness, and pruritus, in addition to a burning, stinging sensation. This reaction tends to be most severe during the first weeks of therapy, with gradual recession later on [1]. Other less common adverse effects include dyspigmentation and allergic contact dermatitis.

Ingenol Mebutate

Ingenol mebutate is a macrocyclic diterpene ester and a natural extract from the sap of *Euphorbia peplus*. It has a dual mechanism of action: induces rapid cell death that occurs few hours after application and also elicits an inflammatory response within days that eliminates residual tumor cells [8, 9]. Two formulations are available and FDA approved for AKs. A 0.015 % gel for the face and scalp is applied once daily for 3 days and may cover a 5 × 5 cm surface area. A 0.05 % gel is used for the trunk and extremities once daily for 2 days. It offers the advantage of increasing compliance because it is applied for a short period of time. Phase 3 trials on efficacy showed that the proportion of patients who achieved complete clearance (100 %) and partial clearance (>75 %) of AKs on the face or scalp was significantly higher with ingenol mebutate than with vehicle: 42.2 % versus 3.7 % and 63.9 % versus 7.4 %, respectively, ($P < 0.001$) [8, 9]. In the studies of AK on the trunk or extremities, results for the primary end point of complete clearance also demonstrated significantly higher clearance rates with ingenol mebutate versus vehicle: 34.1 % versus 4.7 % ($P < 0.001$). Partial clearance rates (ingenol mebutate versus vehicle, 49.1 % versus 6.9 %; $P < 0.001$) and median lesion count reduction (ingenol mebutate versus vehicle, 75 % versus 0 %) were significantly higher for ingenol mebutate than for vehicle and confirmed the efficacy of ingenol mebutate for the treatment of AK on the trunk or extremities.

Adverse effects include erythema, scaling, crusting, pruritus, infection, blister formation, postulation, erosions, and ulcerations [8, 9]. They are usually transient and healing occurs within 2–4 weeks of application.

Other Topical Agents

Case reports and small studies have also documented the effect of other topical agents such as cidofovir and diclofenac in the treatment of cutaneous malignancies [1].

In one study, cidofovir, which is a purine nucleotide analog of deoxycytidine, resulted in a 75 % clearance rate of BCC when used as a 1 % cream applied daily over a period of 2 months [1]. No significant side effects were observed in the study, and the treatment was well tolerated by patients. The underlying mechanism of action of cidofovir is thought to be an antineoplastic and antiangiogenic effect.

Diclofenac, a nonsteroidal antiinflammatory drug (NSAID), usually exerts its antitumor effect through the inhibition of the cyclooxygenase (COX II). This is believed to inhibit angiogenesis and tumor invasion, leading to a decrease in the rate of epithelial tumor growth. One double-blind, placebo-controlled study showed that twice-daily diclofenac application in the form of a 3 % gel resulted in a 33 % complete clearance of AKs [1]. Local irritation was observed as a side effect, but was much less severe than that observed with either 5-FU or imiquimod [1].

Intralesional Agents

Multiple agents in an intralesional form have proven their efficacy in the management of cutaneous malignancies, including bleomycin, 5-FU, and interferon-a (IFN-a) [1, 10, 11]. Advantages of this form of therapy include the ease of delivery, the ability to use it as an adjuvant treatment to surgery, and good cosmetic results in general. Disadvantages include the currently sparse amount of evidence supporting their use, their high costs, and the usual need for multiple treatment sessions [1, 10].

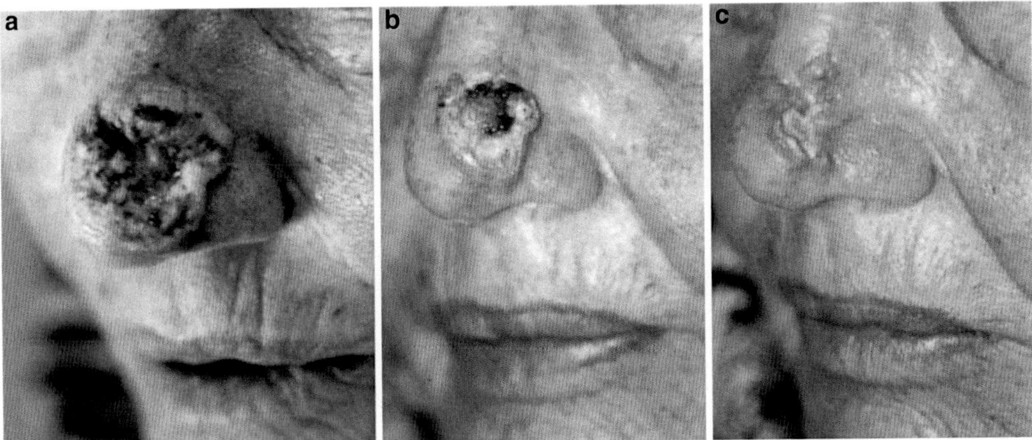

Fig. 1 Elderly woman with keratoacanthoma over the nose treated with intralesional IFN-a: (**a**) before treatment, (**b**) after one injection, and (**c**) after two injections

Bleomycin

Several mechanisms mediate the antitumor effect of bleomycin, a cytotoxic antibiotic produced by *Streptomyces verticillatus*, including its inhibition of DNA ligase preventing repair of DNA, its effect on the G2 and S phases of the cell cycle of fast-dividing cells resulting in SS DNA breakage, and promotion of apoptosis and epidermal necrosis [1, 10].

Individual case reports have described the efficacy of intralesional bleomycin in the treatment of BCCs and keratoacanthomas [1, 10]. Adverse effects that have been described with the intralesional use of bleomycin include local pain, swelling, dyspigmentation, ulceration, superficial scarring, flu-like symptoms, and, rarely, flagellate hyperpigmentation [1, 10].

5-Fluorouracil

There is now evidence that 5-FU as an intralesional preparation can be quite effective in the treatment of BCC, SCC, and keratoacanthomas [1]. In one study, intralesional injection of 0.5 mL of 5-FU/epi gel three times weekly for 2 weeks resulted in 100 % clearance of BCCs. Another study on the treatment of SCCs showed that 1.0 mL weekly injection of 5-FU/epi gel for up to 6 weeks achieved a 96 % clearance rate.

Although excellent cosmetic results may be achieved with its use, intralesional 5-FU may be locally complicated by pain, erosion, ulceration, and dyspigmentation [1].

Interferon-a (IFN-a)

Intralesional interferon-a (IFN-a) can be quite effective in the treatment of keratoacanthomas (Fig. 1), BCCs, and SCCs [1, 2, 11]. This effect of IFN-a is thought to be mediated by the enhancement of cell-mediated immunity against malignant cells through increasing the antigen-presenting cell function, stimulating the activity of natural killer cells, and promoting the development of T-helper (Th)-1 response while at the same time suppressing the production of Th-2 cytokines [1, 11].

One study showed complete clearance of all BCCs and SCCs that were treated with intralesional IFN-a given in a dose of 1×10^6–2×10^6 IU three times weekly for 3 weeks. Adverse reactions most commonly encountered with the use of IFN-a include flu-like symptoms and local injection-site reactions. Laboratory abnormalities may also be observed, such as elevation in hepatic transaminases and decrease in white blood cell count [1, 11]. Given that the relative contraindications for the use of IFN-a include a history of cardiovascular, renal, hepatic, or central nervous system disorders, its use in the elderly population should be undertaken with extra caution, as these patients usually have multiple comorbidities.

Systemic Agents

A problem in treating transplant patients is to provide effective immunosuppression while at the same time not promoting cancer development. Mammalian target of rapamycin (mTOR) inhibitors have both immunosuppressive and tumor-suppressive functions [12].

For the most part, there are insufficient data to draw clear conclusions on the effectiveness of mTOR inhibitors against cancer in humans. However, there are hints that these drugs may be very useful in transplant recipients. Multiple groups have reported on calcineurin inhibitor (CNI) immunosuppressed renal transplant recipients with Kaposi's sarcoma, demonstrating tumor regression after switching from CNIs to sirolimus, which is an mTOR inhibitor [12]. Tumor regression occurred in the face of full immunosuppression with sirolimus, thus not increasing the risk for organ allograft rejection.

Physical Modalities of Treatment

Many treatment modalities fall under this category, including cryotherapy, electrodessication and curettage (ED&C), radiotherapy, photodynamic therapy (PDT), and laser ablation [1, 2]. Most of these have plenty of evidence to support their use, with each of them having its advantages and disadvantages.

Cryotherapy

Cryotherapy has historically been the classical alternative treatment for cutaneous malignancies when surgery is not an option. There is now plenty of evidence to support the use of cryotherapy in the treatment of AK, SCCIS, and BCC (Fig. 2) [1, 2, 13]. It is suitable for the treatment of single or multiple tumors, especially in patients who are old, debilitated, using pacemakers, or maintained on anticoagulation [1, 2, 13]. Excellent cure rates, ranging from 97 % to 99 %, have been achieved upon treatment of these different tumor types with cryotherapy; however, cryotherapy is usually associated with higher recurrence rates (reaching

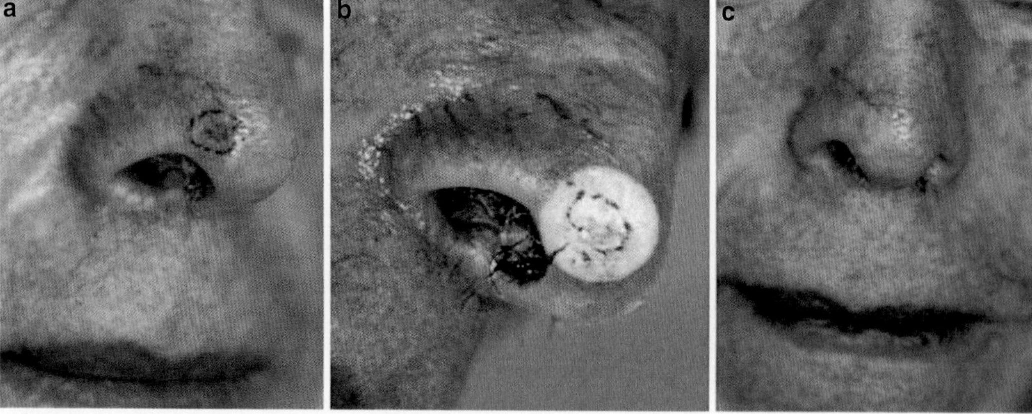

Fig. 2 Elderly man with BCC over the nose treated with cryotherapy: (**a**) before treatment, (**b**) during treatment, and (**c**) after treatment

Common adverse effects observed with PDT include stinging, itching, and burning during treatment, subsequently followed by erythema and edema [1, 2, 15, 16].

Laser Therapy

Ablative lasers such as the carbon dioxide (CO2) or erbium:yttrium–aluminum–garnet (erbium: YAG) vaporize tissue reaching to the level of the papillary dermis. By controlling the depth of injury, we may reduce the risk of scarring and the risk of permanently altered pigmentation [1, 17]. When considering treatment of cutaneous malignancies with laser ablation, the physician should consider the type of malignancy, as well as its location and the skin phototype of the patient. The advantages of using laser ablation in the treatment of primary cutaneous malignancies include the ability to treat large surface areas, the hemostatic nature of the procedure, the prophylactic effects, and the added potential cosmetic result of rejuvenation [1, 17]. Disadvantages include risk of scarring, expensive costs of the procedure, and the inability to treat hyperkeratotic or elevated lesions. Several studies have shown that laser ablation is quite effective in the treatment of AKs (reducing the number of AKs by up to 94 %), superficial and nodular BCCs (up to 97 % clearance), and SCCIS [1, 17]. However, laser ablation should not be used for thick hyperkeratotic lesions. Laser ablation as a full-face resurfacing procedure has also been shown to prevent the appearance of new NMSCs [1, 17].

Pulsed-dye lasers (PDL) and Nd:YAG lasers that target the vasculature have been also used for the treatment of superficial and nodular BCCs [18, 19]. In a study by Jalian et al., 75 % of tumors less than 1 cm in diameter responded to combined treatment with both lasers [18]. In a study by Ortiz et al., the Nd:YAG laser was used for the treatment of BCCs on the trunk and extremities on lesions with a diameter less than 1.5 cm and achieved clearance rates of >90 % proven by histopathology [19].

Chemical Peels

Not only has chemical peeling proven its efficacy in improving photodamaged skin, but a few studies have also shown satisfactory effects in the treatment of AKs (Fig. 3) [1, 20, 21]. Chemical peeling involves the controlled application to the skin of one or more exfoliating agents, resulting in different levels of peeling (superficial, medium depth, deep) depending on the agents used and techniques followed.

Advantages of using chemical peeling in the treatment of AKs include, in addition to the reduction in the number of lesions, the diffuse nature of the treatment and the added skin rejuvenation effect [1, 20]. In fact, one study showed that

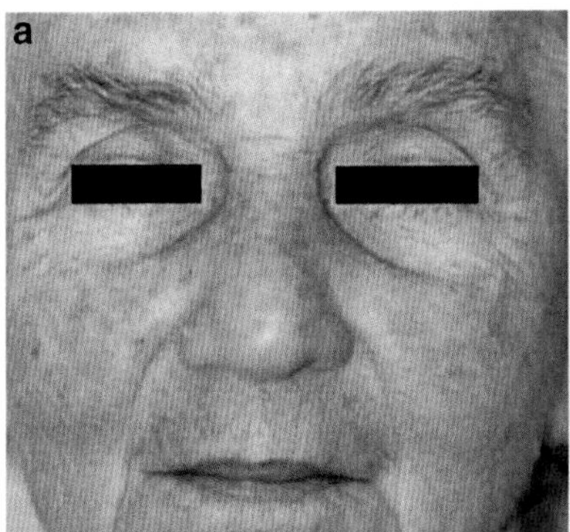
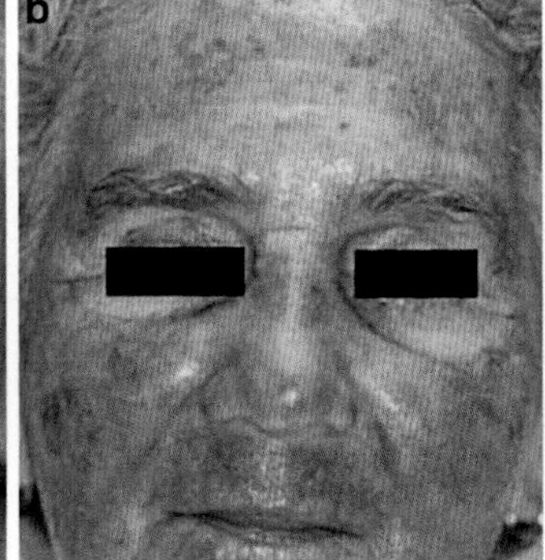
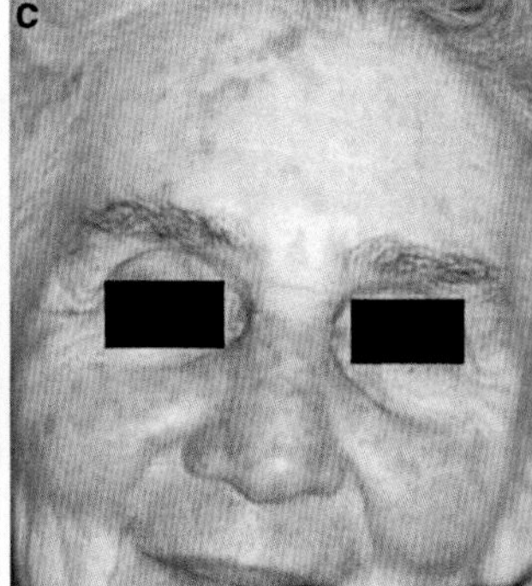

Fig. 3 Elderly woman with extensive AKs over the face treated with chemical peeling: (**a**) before treatment, (**b**) during treatment, and (**c**) after treatment

medium-depth peeling (Jessner's solution followed by 35 % trichloroacetic acid) was as effective as 5 % 5-FU cream applied twice daily for 3 weeks. In another study, Kaminaka et al., used 100 % phenol on 46 patients with AKs and Bowen's disease with 84.8 % clearance response after a 1-year follow-up [22].

Disadvantages of chemical peeling include prolonged healing time and the self-pay nature of the procedure. Adverse effects depend on the depth of injury reached by the chemical peel and include persistent erythema, secondary infection, dyspigmentation, and scarring, as well as cardiac, renal, and hepatic toxicity (associated with deep phenol peels) [1, 20, 21].

Dietary and Herbal Effects

Recently, there has been great interest in the presumed benefits provided by dietary modifications and herbal supplements in the prevention or even treatment of cutaneous malignancies [3]. Extensive work has been done, with only a few studies showing significant benefit. In one study, a low-fat diet was associated with significantly lower incidence of actinic keratosis development compared to a high-fat diet. However, more recent larger RCT studies have shown no association between low-fat diets and prevention of NMSCs [23]. Other studies on animal models have shown that the polyphenols from black and green tea may inhibit UV-induced photocarcinogenesis. In addition, more recent studies suggest a benefit for prevention of NMSCs with resveratrol (found in grapes, red wines, berries, and peanuts) and lycopene (found in red fruits and vegetables) [23].

Conclusion

Elderly people constitute a special, expanding patient population that is more prone to develop cutaneous malignancies. Although surgery is usually considered the first-line management option for the treatment of cutaneous malignancies, elderly patients are, not uncommonly, found to be poor surgical candidates because of multiple causes, including age and associated medical comorbidities, among others. In such cases, alternative modalities of treatment may be of great benefit. The unique properties of the different modalities should be known, as well as the characteristics of the tumor (size, type, and location) and the patient profile, in order to choose the best modality to treat our patients. In the future, more randomized controlled trials are needed in order to reach standard guidelines for the use of these different modalities and also to test new therapies that are continuously emerging.

References

1. Tull S, et al. Nonsurgical treatment modalities for primary cutaneous malignancies. Dermatol Surg. 2008; 34(7):859–72.
2. Neville JA, et al. Management of nonmelanoma skin cancer in 2007. Nat Clin Pract Oncol. 2007; 4(8):462–9.
3. Chakrabarty A, Geisse JK. Medical therapies for non-melanoma skin cancer. Clinics in dermatology. Clin Dermatol. 2004;22(3):183–8.
4. Martinez JC, Otley CC. The management of melanoma and nonmelanoma skin cancer: a review for the primary care physician. Mayo Clin Proc. 2001;76:1253–65.
5. Papadavid E, et al. Imiquimod: an immune response modifier in the treatment of precancerous skin lesions and skin cancer. Expert Opin Pharmacother. 2007; 8(11):1743–55.
6. Zagon IS, et al. Imiquimod upregulates the opioid growth factor receptor to inhibit cell proliferation independent of immune function. Exp Biol Med (Maywood). 2008;233(8):968–79.
7. Stockfleth E. Lmax and imiquimod 3.75%: the new standard in AK management. J Eur Acad Dermatol Venereol. 2015;29:9–14.
8. Fidler B, Goldberg T. Ingenol mebutate gel (picato): a novel agent for the treatment of actinic keratoses. PT. 2014;39(1):40–6.
9. Martin G, Swanson N. Clinical findings using ingenol mebutate gel to treat actinic keratoses. J Am Acad Dermatol. 2013;68:S39–48.
10. Saitta P, et al. Bleomycin in dermatology: a review of intralesional applications. Dermatol Surg. 2008; 34(10):1299–313.
11. Kim KH, et al. Intralesional interferon alpha-2b in the treatment of basal cell carcinoma and squamous cell carcinoma: revisited. Dermatol Surg. 2004;30:116–20.
12. Gaumann A, et al. Immunosuppression and tumor development in organ transplant recipients: the

emerging dualistic role of rapamycin. Transpl Int. 2008;21(3):207–17.

13. Kuflik EG. Cryosurgery for skin cancer: 30-year experience and cure rates. Dermatol Surg. 2004; 30:297–300.
14. Sheridan A, Dawber R. Curettage, electrosurgery, and skin cancer. Australas J Dermatol. 2000;41:19–30.
15. MacCormack MA. Photodynamic therapy in dermatology: an update on applications and outcomes. Sem Cutan Med Surg. 2008;27(1):52–62.
16. Morton CA, et al. Guidelines for topical photodynamic therapy: update. Br J Dermatol. 2008;159(6):1245–66.
17. Iyer S, et al. Full face laser resurfacing: therapy and prophylaxis for actinic keratoses and non-melanoma skin cancer. Lasers Surg Med. 2004;34:114–9.
18. Jalian HR, et al. Combined 585 nm pulsed-dye and 1,064 nm Nd:YAG lasers for the treatment of basal cell carcinoma. Lasers Surg Med. 2014;46(1):1–7.
19. Ortiz AE, et al. 1064 nm long-pulsed Nd:YAG laser treatment of basal cell carcinoma. Lasers Surg Med. 2015;47(2):106–10.
20. Hantash BM, et al. Facial resurfacing for nonmelanoma skin cancer prophylaxis. Arch Dermatol. 2006;142:976–82.
21. Lawrence N, et al. A comparison of the efficacy and safety of Jessner's solution and 35% trichloroacetic acid vs 5% fluorouracil in the treatment of widespread facial actinic keratoses. Arch Dermatol. 1995;131:176–81.
22. Kaminaka C, et al. Phenol peels as a novel therapeutic approach for actinic keratosis and Bowen disease: prospective pilot trial with assessment of clinical, histologic, and immunohistochemical correlations. J Am Acad Dermatol. 2009;60(4):615–25.
23. Bronsnick T, et al. Diet in dermatology: part I. Atopic dermatitis, acne, and nonmelanoma skin cancer. J Am Acad Dermatol. 2014;71(6):1039.e1–2.

Sunlight Exposure and Skin Thickness Measurements as a Function of Age: Risk Factors for Melanoma

72

Akram Elmahdy and Howard I. Maibach

Contents

A. Elmahdy (✉) • H.I. Maibach
Department of Dermatology, University of California, San Francisco, CA, USA
e-mail: Akram.elmahdy@ucsf.edu; maibachh@derm.ucsf.edu

M.A. Farage et al. (eds.), *Textbook of Aging Skin*,
DOI 10.1007/978-3-662-47398-6_60

Abstract

Epidermal thickness is used for studying tissue weight, protein, and/or DNA content since epidermal metabolism occurs at the level of single keratinocytes and varies significantly over anatomic sites but not significantly from person to person. Epidermal thickness is greater in males than in females and can be further evaluated in regard to risk factors for melanoma. The effects of sunlight exposure and aging will be discussed in this chapter.

Introduction

Epidermal thickness is used for studying tissue weight, protein, and/or DNA content since epidermal metabolism occurs at the level of single keratinocytes [1] and varies significantly over anatomic sites but not significantly from person to person [2]. Epidermal thickness is greater in males than in females [2] and can be further evaluated in regard to risk factors for melanoma. In fact, centuries ago, heliotherapy via intense sun exposure was used to treat illness [3].

Aging, which produces dermal damage to elastic and collagen fibers that releases thickened, stiff, tangled, and degraded nonfunctional fibers of skin, is a continuous process that decreases rapid production of keratinocytes and is enhanced by sun exposure [4]. Outward signs of skin aging, as determined by photogoaging [5–7] or simply by sun exposure [8], are seen as a decrease in size of appendages and subcutaneous fat [8]. These changes are a result of local regulatory factors not operating as accurately as they once did in younger skin – examples include loss, thinning, and depigmentation of hair, decreased secretion of sebum, increased dryness, and thinning and atrophy of the epidermis [8].

Sun Exposure

Sun exposure parameters have often demonstrated a positive correlation between the development of melanoma and the recollection of short-term intense UVR exposure, particularly burning, in childhood [7]; yet, Ackerman [3] suggests evidence has not yet convincingly shown that sunlight in excessive exposures is the determinant in the development of most melanomas. Photoaging is triggered by receptor-initiated signaling, mitochondrial damage, protein oxidation, and consequences of telomere-based DNA damage [6]. The aforementioned variations result in differing thickness displayed by photodamaged skin. Epidermal thickness is used as a variable to measure cutaneous melanoma (CM) risk.

UVR is considered a foremost environmental cause for CM risk. The number of sunburns acquired over a lifetime, measured by acute and intense sun exposure, is also an important risk factor for CM [5]. Since sunburn measurements are easily acquired by looking at regions of excessive redness after exposure to the sun and measurement of penetration of UVR, they are commonly used by investigators for CM risk research. However, they still present the limitation of being a retrospective tool, as discussed later in the article. DNA repair shows circadian changes in mice, therefore more risk for sunburns and DNA alterations in early morning. However, there is still limitation regarding public health recommendation due to differences between mice and human circadian clock [30].

Sunburns and Risk for Melanoma

Elevated risk for CM was found to be associated with the history of childhood sunburns, with the highest risk groups as those exposed to sunlight in early life, even if the period of exposure was relatively brief [9–12]. In fact, a significant increase in the risk of adult cutaneous melanoma acquisition corresponded to the number of weeks spent on holiday at the beach, such as Australia or California, as a child [9, 10]. Events occurring during the first few decades of life have a special role in determining melanoma risk for that same adult (Tables 1 and 2). In adults older than 20, there was a significant negative correlation

Table 1 Odds ratio of melanoma by sunburns in childhood and severe sunburns lifelong (Autier and Dore [12])

Factor	Category	Melanoma cases[a]	Controls[a]	Odds ratio (reference category)	(95 % confidence interval)
Sunburns in childhood					
	Never	186	382	1[b]	
	Sometimes	48	26	4.4	(2.5–7.5)
	Often	26		12	(4.6–31.0)
	X^2_1 (trend)			58.7;	
				$P < 0.001$	
	Mild	21	15	3.2	(1.5–1.6)
	Severe	41	16	6.5	(3.4–12.3)
	X^2_1 (trend)			43.8;	
				$P < 0.001$	
Severe	Never	180	328	1[b]	
Sunburns	1	50	53	1.7	(1.1–2.6)
Lifelong	≥2	24	29	1.5	(0.8–2.7)
	X^2_1 (trend)			4.5;	
				$P = 0.04$	

[a]Some strata do not add up to the total because of missing values
[b]Adjusted for sex and category

Table 2 Interaction between sunburns in childhood and severe sunburns lifelong on melanoma risk (Autier and Dore [12])

	Odds ratio (95 % confidence interval)[a]			
	Severe sunburns lifelong			
Sunburns in childhood		Never	Ever	Adjusted odds ratio (95 % CI)[b]
Never	Cases	143	40	
	Controls	316	64	
	OR	1 (reference)	1.4	1 (reference)
	(95 % CI)		(0.9–2.2)	
Ever	Cases	37	35	
	Controls	13	18[c]	
	OR	8	4.9	5.3
	(95 % CI)	(3.9–16.5)	(2.6–9.2)	(3.3 8.6)
Adjusted		1 (reference)	1.2	
			(0.8–1.8)	

[a]Adjusted for sex and age in decades
[b]Adjusted for sunburns in childhood or severe sunburns lifelong in addition to sex and decade
[c]Strata do not add up because of missing values

between age and number of sunburns per sun-year. In subjects younger than 20, there was a significant positive correlation between age and number of sunburns [13]. There is misconception among the public that indoor tanning can reduce risk for CM; on the contrary, tanning beds can have adverse effect on CM outcomes [31].

For this study, damage to the skin does not correspond with age, but, instead, with the amount of UV penetration and sun exposure [3, 6]. Severe or frequent sunburns in childhood conferred a two- to threefold increased risk for melanoma acquisition [6] – the number of sunburns is interpreted as an indicator of sun damage during that age frame, as influenced by sun exposure, habits, and individual sun sensitivity. Tissues that undergo postnatal development are especially vulnerable to environment carcinogen exposure in childhood [10]. Within the melanoma paradigm, there are grounds for inferring that the period of peak melanocytic activity occurs in early life and might therefore be a period of vulnerability to the adverse effects of solar radiation [10]. Biologically, this finding may suggest that melanocytes in children are more sensitive to the sun or that, in the context of the multistage model of carcinogenesis, early exposure to the purported carcinogen (i.e., solar radiation) may increase the changes of completing the remaining stages in subsequent life periods [9]. Contradictory evidence [3] suggests that skin lesions or sunburns are not correlated to melanoma acquisition because these skin lesions occur on sites directly exposed to sunlight and are numerous, and none of these descriptions are true for melanoma.

Sun Protection and Risk for Melanoma

Research on sun protection results in an increased risk for CM in adults who did not have appropriate sun protection as children – sun avoidance during childhood would have a greater impact on decreasing melanoma risk than sun avoidance during adulthood [12]. Sun protection includes recently photoprotective clothing, avoidance of the sun for high risk group, and use of sunscreens with a high sun protection factor (SPF) "+15" [33]. Sunscreens help to protect from sunburn through absorbing, reflecting, and/or scattering UV light [32]. The melanoma risk associated with a given level of sun exposure during adulthood increased with higher sun exposure during childhood, meaning that high sun exposure during childhood constitutes a significant risk factor for melanoma [12]. Adults with current low or moderate sun exposure but high childhood sun exposure may well be at higher risk to develop malignant melanoma than adults with high current sun exposure, but with low childhood sun exposure. Thus, sun protection during childhood has a greater impact on melanoma risk than sun protection during adulthood [12], ultimately reiterating the conclusion of increased CM risk with increased childhood sun exposure and sunburn [9–12].

When considering sun protection, other research [3, 14] suggests no association with overall sunscreen amount used with CM [14] or an increase in CM [3]; yet it is the never or rare use of sunscreen that increases CM risk. Some [14] suggest that the propensity to sunburn, ability to tan, skin type, density of facial freckling, hair color, and eye color over the course of an individual's lifetime are all significantly associated with melanoma acquisition. Yet, the only period for which there was an association with sunscreen use and melanoma was under 5 years of age, where the risk of melanoma was doubled for those who never/rarely used sunscreen versus often/always used sunscreen. Additional research [3] correlates sunscreen use with the development of melanoma since sunscreen might lure individuals into believing that they are allowed to be in the sun longer, increasing the length of exposure to solar radiation and thus risk for developing melanoma. Other research [15] suggests that the concept of a "critical period" for melanoma acquisition is not true – in fact, there is an additive effect that begins at an "early age" with respect to melanoma and sun exposure. In 2010, Green and colleagues studied the effect of regular sunscreen use on the CM risk; they found a 50 % reduction in new primary melanomas and 73 % reduction in invasive melanoma rates among participants of the sunscreen group. Some researchers argue with the fact that sunburn is not the main factor in developing melanoma, and it is better to focus on the individual risk characteristics [34].

Skin Thickness

Research about epidermal thickness differences in children versus adults suggests increased melanoma occurrences in individuals who have had childhood sunburns. Contradictory evidence suggests that either photoaging [6, 14] or solely sunlight exposure [3] is responsible for most aging changes in skin appearance. Photoaging can be associated with mitochondrial damage (the most common deletion in mtDNA, which is tenfold less common than sun-protected areas, is found in photodamaged skin), telomere-based DNA damage, protein oxidation, and receptor-initiated signaling [6]. Long-term stress and old age are also common causes of epidermal chalone mitotic depression in basal cells [16]. Epidermal thickness is important because it is a uniformly accessible measure and can be measured in relation to anatomic site, age, gender, pigmentation, blood content, and smoking [2].

Table 3 Epidermal thickness using backward multiple regression analyses is not significant when measuring stratum corneum and cellular epidermis thickness

	Stratum corneum	Cellular epidermis
Body site	>0.0001	>0.0002
Age	Ns	Ns
Gender	0.048	>0.0001

Ns Nonsignificant

Skin thickness and pigmentation do not significantly increase or decrease in specific anatomic sites of individuals as they age during adulthood [1, 2, 4, 17] (Table 3), where "adulthood" is measured as different periods of the 20–68-year-old age group (1), the 50–72-year-old age group (2), and/or the 23–47-year-old age group (3). These data suggest that, as expected, the stratum corneum and stratum granulosum are significantly thicker in sun-protected than in sun-exposed sites, where the latter sites show a greater variability [17].

Contradictory results [18] (Fig. 1) from research done thirty years prior that take proposed cell shrinkage measurements into account suggest an increase epidermal thickness in the arms and leg sites of adults in the 15–89-year-old age group. Such research [18] suggests it is commonly believed that the epidermis in an older person is thinner than in a younger person. This may be because skin looks thinner and measurements that fail to correct for shrinkage would show an apparent thinning of epidermis with advancing age. This thin appearance occurs because skin becomes less elastic. Additional results [19]

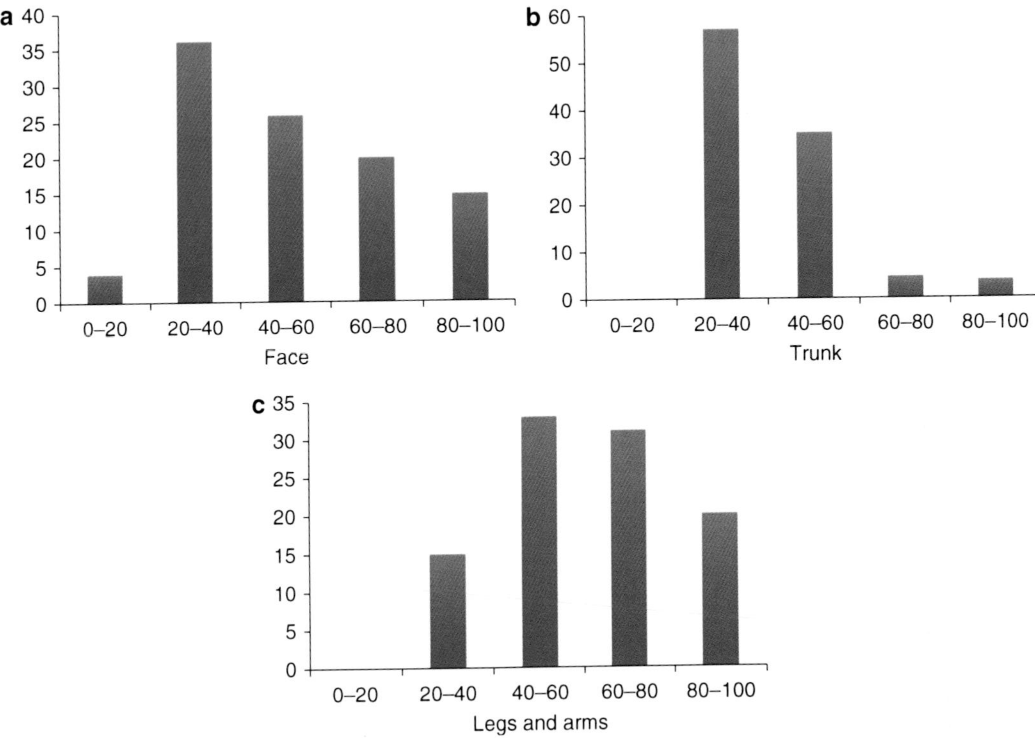

Fig. 1 Distribution of average epidermal thickness on three regions is about half those recorded by negative shrinkage (Whitton 1973). Average epidermal thickness (micrometer) measured against percentage (male and female) per 20 μm increments

suggest no change in epidermal thickness during the young adult phase (age group 18–25), but an increased epidermal thickness during the older age group (adults over 65).

Recent studies focus on noninvasive ways to estimate skin thickness from hyperspectral imaging validated by echography; however, the limitation to the study was that only one physician was used to create the gold standard [35]. Over the last few years, confocal microscopy was successfully applied to detect in vivo skin changes either in chronologically aging skin or photodamaged skin. This study [36] which measured epidermal thickness using confocal microscopy revealed significant decrease in thickness in age group >65 years.

Multiphoton laser tomography (MLT) has also emerged as noninvasive way to investigate dermatologic changes in photodamaged skin including epidermal thickness [37]. However, in a study of differences of epidermal thickness among group of women aged 20 till 70 years old using optical coherence tomography (OCT), it has been noted no remarkable difference in epidermal thickness between UV light exposed areas and other covered areas of skin [38].

Discussion

Skin cancer is a common malignancy [11] and requires great attention to be paid per patient for appropriate care. Many changes in aging skin are produced or aggravated by ionizing or ultraviolet radiation [8]. Photoaging, change accentuated by the sun, accounts for much of these age-related changes in skin appearance [6] and is represented by chronic degenerative changes including freckles (ephelides), solar lentigines, nevi, solar keratoses, and melanoma [4, 28]. Chronic sunlight exposure can induce an impediment of normal maturation of human dermal collagen resulting from a degradation of mature collagen cross-links [4, 6, 8, 20]. These cells' histological photodamage of degradation and remodeling of collagen is related to individual cumulative ultraviolet radiation (UVR) exposure. As a function of age, nonfibrous protein and soluble collagen decrease, while insoluble collagen increases, ultimately increasing total collagen with respect to age [20]. Senescent cells have an increased resistance to apoptosis (natural cell death) and survive for very long periods of time without division, allowing for DNA and protein damage accumulation and, eventually, cumulative cellular damage [4, 8].

Absorption accounts for more than 93 % of why light does not pass through skin [21]. Excessive absorption of sunlight can create sunburns, which, some suggest, play an important role in the development of skin cancer, especially malignant melanoma [13]. In contrast to earlier views of dependence on the stratum corneum's thickness for filtration of harmful UV rays, studies show [22] that the epidermal pigment is largely responsible for such filtration. The filtration and absorption ratios are evaluated in regard to sun exposure. Sunburns occurring during childhood are often cited as posing the greatest risk for cutaneous malignant melanoma [5]. Since melanoma is a common malignancy [11], studies are conducted for further knowledge on the disease.

While skin thickness data are often difficult to interpret [23], it remains a widely used parameter to evaluate the influences of different variables on skin aging, including sunlight exposure, elasticity, and absorption [23, 24]. Whole skin thickness increases in youth [23, 24], remains constant during adulthood, and decreases in the elderly, beginning at age ~70 [24]. Others maintain that photoexposed areas thicken with age, whereas protected areas become thinner, or that skin thickness changes with age are related to location on the extremities or axially as opposed to sun exposure [23]. Regardless, further evaluation of skin thickness, melanoma, and childhood exposure to the sun must be acquired to better understand relations to melanoma occurrences in adulthood.

The only period for which there was an association of melanoma with sunscreen use was under 5 years of age, when risk of melanoma was doubled for those who never/rarely used sunscreen at home versus often/always [14]. Participants with many sunburns during childhood also tend to have more sunburns later in life than those with only few or no sunburns during childhood and ultimately have a higher risk for acquiring adulthood melanoma [15]. When relating epidermal thickness to age with respect to adult melanoma acquisition, conclusions suggest that since epidermal thickness measurements do not change as an individual ages [1, 2, 4, 17], skin thickness cannot currently influence the increased risk of childhood sunburns on adult melanoma.

While aforementioned data suggest a relationship between melanoma and UVR exposure, some research [3] proposes that the notion of melanoma in Caucasians being a consequence of the effects of the dose of cumulative UVR received by the skin is without merit in prepubescent children. The association of melanoma as the result of intermittent UVR exposure over the course of years, specifically in Caucasians, is baseless [3] because the melanoma acquired in these individuals was in places not in the direct path rays of the sun.

Problems with Data

A possible confound when measuring epidermis thickness is shrinking of the skin during fixation, which is required to measure epidermal thickness [1, 25, 26]. To offset shrinkage, acetic acid is often used. The belief that the epidermis of an older individual is thinner than that of a younger individual is due to the inability of some researchers to correct such cell shrinkage [18]. The apparent thinning of the epidermis with advancing age occurs because skin becomes less elastic with age. The method by which sun exposure (and ultimately skin thickness) is measured and the concept of shrinkage leads to strikingly different conclusions regarding the association of sun exposure at specific ages and consequent risks of adulthood melanoma [10].

For several studies, data were acquired by asking patients to recall past circumstances. Recall and retrospective data acquisition [15, 27] can create biased responses by patients and, consequently, altered data. Additionally, interviewers and questioners can cause patients to feel either overly comfortable or awkward, thus further skewing responses. When applicable in certain studies of adolescent or older individuals, patients also kept a diary of daily events [13], which could have allowed individuals to learn from their mistakes, showing that sun behavior changes with age and maturity [5] – again, an extraneous variable that is not consistent throughout the research. It has also been suggested that melanoma patients tend to over-report past sun-exposure habits in an attempt to explain and/or justify why they received the diagnosis of malignant melanoma [27].

The inability to keep participant environment the same could affect data in other ways as well. Some suggest [9] a significant increase in the risk of cutaneous melanoma is also associated with the number of weeks spent on holiday at the beach as an adult and as a child. However, others [10] propose that individuals who spent their youth in places similar to California (where excessive outdoor play is the norm) were at increased risk of melanoma compared with those born and raised elsewhere, even after many decades of cohabitation. Thus, the amount of time spent in the sun as a child appears to be a significant risk factor for melanoma – not increased age or decreased skin thickness.

Vitamin D and Sun Exposure

UV exposure is the most important environmental risk factor for the development of nonmelanoma skin cancer [7]. Clothing is efficient in absorbing all UV-B radiation, thereby preventing any UV-B photons from reaching the skin; additionally, a vitamin D supplement can also be effective in melanoma prevention [7]. Approximately, 90 % of all requisite vitamin D is attained via sunlight; thus, strict sun protection procedures to prevent melanoma may induce the severe health risk of vitamin D deficiency [7]. To help alleviate this challenge, physicians suggest daily administrations of 15 min of sunlight exposure or oral consumption of vitamin D [7]. There is no evidence to support the role of vitamin D in prevention of melanoma, but recent data found inherited variation in vitamin D receptor (VDR) gene is associated with melanoma risk [39]. A healthy balance must be reached and publicly advertised in order to minimize acquisition of malignant melanoma.

Future Implications

Sunburns may play an important role in the development of skin cancer [13] and should be further investigated as a means to prevent melanoma occurrences. Preventing intermittent sunburns during childhood has the strongest correlation with decreased malignant melanoma occurrences later in life [9–12]. Such prevention measures include appropriate sun block usage and control of the amount of time spent in the sun and outdoors, depending on risk factors of the individual, such as sun sensitivity, white skin, fair hair, light eyes, tendency to freckle, family history of melanoma, dysplastic nevi, increased numbers of typical nevi, large congenital nevi, and immunosuppression [11, 28]. Since UVR exposure is the most important environmental risk factor for the development of skin cancer [7], it is important to protect early childhood skin from exposure to excessive sunlight to ultimately protect them from adulthood melanoma acquisition.

Conclusion

In relation to the study of age thickness as a function of time, future studies would be benefited by increased standardization of skin sites tested, methodology, and sample size. Great differences in the study method, population, and anatomic site are likely to account for markedly different results from different researchers, which obscure reasonable conclusions. Since the effect of age on thickness of skin strata is one of the more controversial topics among dermatological scientists [23, 29], further research needs to be done to synchronize data and create a standard method for both acquiring and interpreting such data.

Cross-References

▶ Carcinogenesis: UV Radiation

References

1. Bergstresser PR, Pariser RJ, Taylor JR. Counting and sizing of epidermal cells in normal skin. J Invest Dermatol. 1978;70(5):280–4.
2. Sandy-Moller J, Poulsen T, Wulf HC. Epidermal thickness at different body sites: relationship to age, gender, pigmentation, blood content, skin type, and smoking habits. Acta Dermato-Venereologica. 2003;83(6):410–3.
3. Ackerman B. The Sun and the "epidemic" of melanoma: myth on myth! New York: Ardor Scribendi; 2008.
4. Wulf HC, Sandby-Møller J, Kobayasi T, Gniadecki R. Skin aging and natural photoprotection. Micron. 2004;35(3):185–91.
5. Dennis LK, Vanbeek MJ, Beane Freeman LE, Smith BJ, Dawson DV, Coughlin JA. Sunburns and risk of cutaneous melanoma: does age matter? A comprehensive meta-analysis. Ann Epidemiol. 2008;18(8):614–27.
6. Yaar M, Gilchrest BA. Photoageing: mechanism, prevention and therapy. Br J Dermatol. 2007;157(5):874–87.
7. Reichrath J. The challenge resulting from positive and negative effects of sunlight: how much solar UV exposure is appropriate to balance between risks of vitamin D deficiency and skin cancer? Prog Biophys Mol Biol. 2006;92(1):9–16.
8. Daniels Jr F. Sun exposure and skin aging. N Y State J Med. 1964;64:2066–9.
9. Zanetti R, Franceschi S, Rosso S, Colonna S, Bidoli E. Cutaneous melanoma and sunburns in childhood in a southern European population. Eur J Cancer. 1992;28A(6–7):1172–6.
10. Whiteman DC, Whiteman CA, Green AC. Childhood sun exposure as a risk factor for melanoma: a systematic review of epidemiological studies. Cancer Causes Control. 2001;12(1):69–82.
11. Rager EL, Bridgeford EP, Ollila DW. Cutaneous melanoma: update on prevention, screening, diagnosis, and treatment. Am Fam Physician. 2005;72(2):269–76.
12. Autier P, Dore JF. Influence of sun exposure during childhood and during adulthood on melanoma risk. EPIMEL and EORTC Melanoma Cooperative Group. European, Organization for Research and Treatment of Cancer. Int J Cancer. 1998;77(4):533–7.
13. Thieden E, Philipsen PA, Sandby-Moller J, Wulf HC. Sunburn related to UV radiation exposure, age, sex, occupation, and sun bed use based on time-stamped personal dosimetry and sun behavior diaries. Arch Dermatol. 2005;141(4):482–8.
14. Youl P, Aitken J, Hayward N, Hogg D, Liu L, Lassam N, Martin N, Green A. Melanoma in adolescents: a case–control study of risk factors in Queensland. Australia Int J Cancer. 2002;98(1):92–8.
15. Pfahlberg A, Kolmel KF, Geffeller O. Timing of excessive ultraviolet radiation and melanoma: epidemiology does not support the existence of a critical period of high susceptibility to solar ultraviolet radiation-induced melanoma. Br J Dermatol. 2001;144(3):471–5.
16. Bullough WS. The control of epidermal thickness. Br J Dermatol. 1972;87(3):187–99.
17. Huzaira M, Rius F, Rajadhyaksha M, Anderson RR, Gonzalez S. Topographic variations in normal skin, as viewed by in vivo reflectance confocal microscopy. J Invest Dermatol. 2001;116(6):846–52.
18. Whitton JT, Everall JD. The thickness of the epidermis. Br J Dermatol. 1973;89(5):467–76.
19. Sauermann K, Clemann S, Jaspers S, Gambichler T, Altmeyer P, Hoffmann K, Ennen J. Age related changes of human skin investigated with histometric measurements by confocal laser scanning microscopy in vivo. Skin Res Technol. 2002;8(1):52–6.
20. Smith Jr JG, Davidson EA, Sams Jr WM, Clark RD. Alterations in human dermal connective tissue with age and chronic sun damage. J Invest Dermatol. 1962;39:347–50.
21. Na R, Stender IM, Henriksen M, Wulf HC. Autofluorescence of human skin is age-related after correction for skin pigmentation and redness. J Invest Dermatol. 2001;116(4):536–40.
22. Mitchell RE. The effect of prolonged solar radiation on melanocytes of the human epidermis. J Invest Dermatol. 1963;41:199–212.
23. Waller JM, Maibach HI. Age and skin structure and function, a quantitative approach (I): blood flow, pH, thickness, and ultrasound echogenicity. Skin Res Technol. 2005;11(4):221–35.
24. Serup J, editor. Handbook of non-invasive methods and the skin. Boca Ratton: Taylor & Francis; 2006. p. 512–3.
25. Zinabu GM, Thomas B. The effects of formalin and Lugol's iodine solution on protozoan cell volume. Limnolog Ecol Manage Inland Waters. 2000;30(1):59–63.
26. Ohno N, et al. Application of cryobiopsy to morphological and immunohistochemical analysisÉvessels. Cancer. 2008;113:1068–79.
27. Westerdahl J, Olsson H, Ingvar C. At what age do sunburn episodes play a crucial role for the development of malignant melanoma. Eur J Cancer. 1994;30A(11):1647–54.
28. Elwood JM, Whitehead SM, Davison J, Stewart M, Galt M. Malignant melanoma in England: risks associated with naevi, freckles, social class, hair colour, and sunburn. Int J Epidemiol. 1990;19(4):801–10.
29. Linos E, Swetter SM, Cockburn MG, Colditz GA, Clarke CA. Increasing burden of melanoma in the United States. J Invest Dermatol. 2009;129(7):1604–6.
30. Gaddameedhi S, Selby CP, Kemp MG, et al. The circadian clock controls sunburn apoptosis and erythema in mouse skin. J Invest Dermatol. 2015;135:1119–27.
31. Vogel RI, Ahmed RL, Nelson HH et al. Exposure to indoor tanning without burning and melanoma risk by sunburn history. J Natl Cancer Inst. 2014;106.

32. Mancebo SE, Hu JY, Wang SQ. Sunscreens: a review of health benefits, regulations, and controversies. Dermatol Clin. 2014;32:427–38. x.
33. Poon F, Kang S, Chien AL. Mechanisms and treatments of photoaging. Photodermatol Photoimmunol Photomed. 2015;31:65–74.
34. Berwick M. Counterpoint: sunscreen use is a safe and effective approach to skin cancer prevention. Cancer Epidemiol Biomarkers Prev. 2007;16:1923–4.
35. Vyas S, Meyerle J, Burlina P. Non-invasive estimation of skin thickness from hyperspectral imaging and validation using echography. Comput Biol Med. 2015;57:173–81.
36. Longo C, Casari A, Beretti F, et al. Skin aging: in vivo microscopic assessment of epidermal and dermal changes by means of confocal microscopy. J Am Acad Dermatol. 2013;68:e73–82.
37. Koehler MJ, Vogel T, Elsner P, et al. In vivo measurement of the human epidermal thickness in different localizations by multiphoton laser tomography. Skin Res Technol. 2010;16:259–64.
38. Tsugita T, Nishijima T, Kitahara T, Takema Y. Positional differences and aging changes in Japanese woman epidermal thickness and corneous thickness determined by OCT (optical coherence tomography). Skin Res Technol. 2013;19:242–50.
39. Randerson-Moor JA, Taylor JC, Elliott F, et al. Vitamin D receptor gene polymorphisms, serum 25-hydroxyvitamin D levels, and melanoma: UK case–control comparisons and a meta-analysis of published VDR data. Eur J Cancer. 2009;45 (18):3271–81.

Influence of Race, Gender, Age, and Diabetes on Blood Flow

73

Jerrold Scott Petrofsky

Contents

Abstract

While the circulation is controlled by local (metabolic) and neurogenic control, it is modulated by a number of factors. Estrogen, which varies during the normal menstrual cycle, causes circulation in the skin to peak near ovulation. With birth control pills, this change is abolished as it is with menopause. Other conditions like diabetes not only alter circulation but lead to endothelial dysfunction and numerous secondary diseases like heart disease, kidney failure, and retinopathy. Skin circulation in people with diabetes can be as little as one-third normal. This predisposes skin damage and burns. One of the principal factors leading to diabetes-related endothelial cell dysfunction is cellular inflammation. This can be caused by high-fat diets, obesity, cigarette smoking, and a generally poor diet. Some races are more susceptible to endothelial cell damage. A thrifty gene found in all Asians causes cellular inflammation and reduced endothelial response with even a single high-fat meal. Aging causes a natural senescence of the skin circulation and is partly due to increased free radicals in the body causing endothelial dysfunction. Thus all of these factors are important in understanding the circulation in the skin in man.

J.S. Petrofsky (✉)
Department of Physical Therapy, Loma Linda University, Loma Linda, CA, USA

School of Allied Health, Loma Linda University, Loma Linda, CA, USA
e-mail: jpetrofsky@llu.edu

M.A. Farage et al. (eds.), *Textbook of Aging Skin*,
DOI 10.1007/978-3-662-47398-6_61

Introduction

The vascular endothelial cell is the center of the control of the circulation in the body. In the arteries they release vasodilator and vasoconstrictor substances that moderate blood flow. In the capillaries, the endothelial cell adjusts the permeability to small molecules and proteins and can vary widely in permeability to such substances as histamine. It is also a barrier that allows for the movement of nutrients, waste products, oxygen, and carbon dioxide from the cells through the interstitial space. In the veins, the endothelial cells release venodilators and venoconstrictors to adjust venous return, altering the capacitance of the veins in the body.

All of these functions are altered by race, inflammation, sex hormones in women, aging, and a variety of factors that modulate circulation and can cause senescence of the endothelial cells and lead to endothelial dysfunction and cardiovascular disease. This chapter will examine many of these factors.

Gender and Circulation

The menstrual cycle is divided into the follicular and luteal phases, during which the reproductive hormones estrogen and progesterone fluctuate cyclically [1]. The follicular phase of the cycle can be subdivided into early follicular and late follicular phases. In the early follicular phase, after the onset of bleeding (days 1–7), estrogen and progesterone concentrations in the blood are low; in the late follicular phase (days 8–14), the estrogen concentration in blood increases due to the effect of follicular stimulating hormone (FSH) [1].

The luteal phase that follows ovulation can be subdivided into early and late luteal phases. During the early luteal phase (days 15–21), formation of the corpus luteum promotes a rise in levels of progesterone and estrogen; in the late luteal phase (22–28), both hormones gradually decrease reaching their lowest concentration in blood at day 28 of the menstrual cycle [2].

In premenopausal women, cyclical fluctuations in estrogen and progesterone influence the thermoregulatory system [3, 4]. Core temperature in the body increases by an average of 0.3–0.5 °C during the mid-luteal phase, altering the threshold for sweating and skin blood flow in response to exercise or to whole-body heating [5]. For example, in premenopausal women, local cooling of the hand to 15 °C causes more vasoconstriction during the luteal phase compared to follicular phase [6, 7]. The vascular response in the forearm skin to arterial occlusion also is attenuated during the luteal phase [8]. In addition, resting skin blood flow and skin blood flow during exercise are modulated by the menstrual cycle [5].

The menstrual cycle also affects irritant susceptibility of the skin. Skin exposure to the irritant, sodium lauryl sulfate, produces a higher blood flow response the first day of the menstrual cycle than during the ninth or tenth day [9]. The severity of existing skin diseases changes throughout the menstrual cycle. For example, atopic dermatitis is exacerbated on the first day of the menstrual cycle [10]. Evidence exists that the response of the microvasculature to local stimuli may be caused by a local vascular response to hormones rather than central sympathetic activity. Specific receptors for estrogen have been identified throughout the arterial system [11]. These receptors are believed to modulate the skin blood flow response to local stimuli based on estrogen concentrations in plasma. Many of these changes in blood flow over the menstrual cycle are lost when women are given the birth control pill or in older women who go through menopause [12]. In addition, resting and exercising skin blood flow are altered during the menstrual cycle [13, 14]; these changes are abolished with the birth control pills (Fig. 1).

Clinical evidence strongly suggests that estrogen plays a role in both angiogenesis and in modulating tissue blood flow [15]. Endothelial progenitor cells or EPCs are generally derived from the bone marrow and are mobilized in response to tissue damage and/or cytokines in blood. In adults, EPCs isolated from peripheral blood create foci for neovascularization; this effect varies during the menstrual cycle [16].

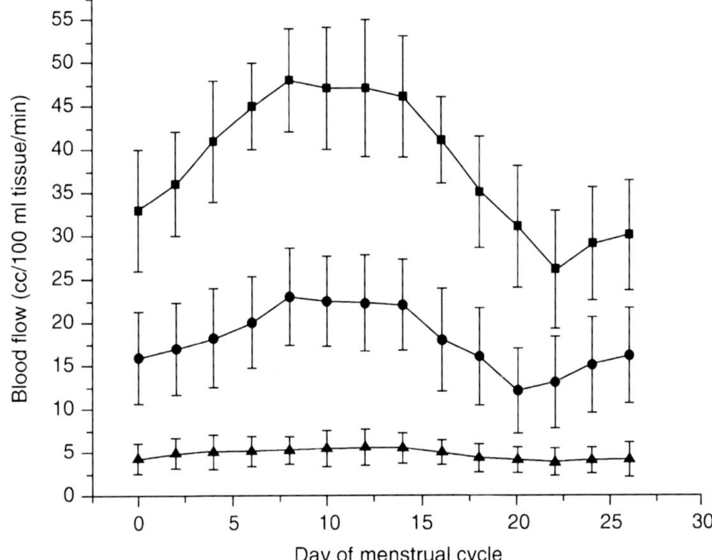

Fig. 1 This figure shows limb blood flow in cc per minute per 100 ml tissue measured every other day of the menstrual cycle at the end of fatiguing isometric contractions at 20 % (*squares*), 40 % (*circles*), and 60 % (*triangles*) of the subject's strength on eight subjects (From Petrofsky et al. [5])

Mature vascular endothelial cells in humans and a variety of species express at least two different estrogen receptors: ER-alpha and ER-beta [17]. Different genes encode ER-alpha and ER-beta. The receptors act as ligand-dependent transcription factors [18, 19]. Human EPCs express ER-alpha but not ER-beta [20]. In humans, the activity of ER-alpha receptors mediates the response of blood vessel walls to estrogen; this response includes accelerated re-endothelialization and elevated release of endothelial nitric oxide [21]. Consequently, the activity of ER-alpha contributes to gender differences in the protection from cardiovascular disease [22].

The signaling pathway by which estrogen affects levels of EPCs is not known [22, 23]. Several studies indicate that the activation of phosphoinositide 3-kinase (PI3K/Akt) pathways may be involved [24, 25]. If PI3K/Akt is activated by estrogen, this would in turn activate nitric oxide synthetase [26, 27].

Estrogen has direct effects on vascular genesis and also angiogenesis mediated by VEGF [27]. Vascular genesis is the formation of new blood vessels in the body and is mediated by stem cells in the bone marrow. Angiogenesis differs in that it involves the extension of existing blood vessels and is under the control of a compound, vascular endothelial growth factor (VEGF), released by endothelial cells. Estrogen has been associated with wound healing in some experimental models. In animal models, male organs such as the penis have been shown to have estrogen receptors [28–30], and estrogen will increase the rate of healing of a wound [31]. Part of the healing process is increased reactivity of VEGF induced by estrogen [32].

Role of Estrogen in Pulmonary Hypertension

Studies on isolated pulmonary arteries show that estrogen upregulates nitric oxide production [33]. Both endogenous and exogenous estrogens decrease pulmonary arterial vasoconstriction under normoxic and hypoxic conditions [33, 34]. This is not surprising, because acute and chronic hypoxic pulmonary hypertension (as well as systemic hypertension) is less common and less pronounced in females than males [33, 35].

However, the response to estrogen may be dose dependent. Studies on the effect of sex hormones on blood flow have produced conflicting results. For example, cutaneous vasodilatation to local warming increased in young users of oral contraceptives [3]. In men, testosterone may inhibit, rather than stimulate, nitric oxide-dependent vasodilatation [36]. When small doses of estrogen (lower than those used in a birth control pill) were administered together with testosterone to a group of subjects, the degree of vasodilation caused by local warming of the skin did not change relative to the response of untreated subjects [37]. Conversely, in young men and women, testosterone reduced the blood flow response to local heat, whereas estrogen increased the blood flow response to local heat if given in physiological concentrations [3]. However, this result was not reproduced when older people were studied [37]. It is well known that aging causes a decrease in the cutaneous vasodilator response [38]. Perhaps aging alters the activity of estrogen receptors in vascular endothelial cells as well, although diminished production or bioavailability of nitric oxide may play a role [38]. One hypothesis is that the diminished response to estrogen and testosterone [36] in older individuals could be the result of defective nitric oxide transduction by estrogen in the aged.

In people with diabetes, the nitric oxide pathway in vascular endothelial cells is defective. Not surprisingly, estrogen has little or no effect on endothelial dysfunction in postmenopausal women with diabetes. Aging and diabetes both affect signaling pathways mediated by ER-alpha and ER-beta receptors on vascular endothelial cells. Hence estrogen exerts its greatest effects on blood flow in younger women.

The Influence of Diabetes on Skin Circulation

Both type 1 diabetes (sometimes called juvenile diabetes) and type 2 diabetes (sometimes called metabolic syndrome) have similar effects on the autonomic nervous system. Type 1 diabetes is an autoimmune disease. Autonomic dysfunction is due to high glucose concentrations in blood plasma [39–41]. Type 2 diabetes causes damage to endothelial cells due to high plasma glucose, oxidative and inflammatory stressors, and insulin resistance [42–45]. In type 2 diabetes, hyperinsulinemia is common early in the disease, because the pancreas must overproduce insulin to compensate for high cellular insulin resistance. The resistance stems not from a defect in the insulin receptor itself but from impaired signal transduction from the receptor in activating phosphatidylinositol 3-kinase. In type 2 diabetes, insulin levels usually rise to such a degree that the pancreas is unable to sustain production and the pancreatic beta-cells finally fail and insulin production decreases or stops completely over a number of years [46, 47].

Activation of phosphatidylinositol 3-kinase is the critical step in cellular activation of the glucose transporter, GLUT-4. The inability of the cell to transport glucose into the cytosol shifts cellular metabolism from carbohydrates to lipids [42]. Chronic lipid metabolism damages the cell due to oxidative by-products which cause chronic cellular inflammation [48].

It was once thought that the best predictor of damage to the autonomic nervous system and blood vessels associated with diabetes was the average body burden of glucose over many months (as assessed by a measure called HbA1c). Recently, it has been shown that spikes in blood glucose concentration over the course of the day (especially postprandial) are more damaging to endothelial cells than the average concentration of glucose in the blood itself [49]. Large spikes in glucose cause immediate damage to the autonomic nervous system forcing a type of shock such that autonomic function is impaired for over 24 h [49].

Because vascular endothelial cells are exquisitely sensitive to high glycemic concentrations, damage to these cells usually occurs before type 1 or type 2 diabetes is clinically diagnosed [42, 50, 51]. Thus, at the time of diagnosis, young children and adults with diabetes already have autonomic damage and impaired blood flow responses to stress [42]. Damage to blood vessels of the skin is twofold. First, in type 2 diabetes, the sympathetic ganglia are damaged [109] although the ability of the blood vessels to constrict is unimpaired. Secondly, in both type 1 and type 2 diabetes, vasodilation is impaired through direct damage to endothelial cells [42, 52]. Clinically, damage to the parasympathetic and sympathetic nervous systems centrally or at the ganglia is quantified by changes in heart rate variability [42, 53]. Normally, vasomotor rhythm in the sympathetic and parasympathetic system causes the heart rate to vary continuously on a breath-by-breath and minute-by-minute basis [42]. Heart rate changes are evident on analysis of the EKG. In diabetes, progressive damage to the sympathetic and parasympathetic ganglia diminishes heart rate variability to such a degree that eventually little variation in heart rate occurs with a change in body position, breathing, or with exercise [45].

The loss of the skin's ability to adequately dilate limits the response to global heat and other physiological stressors such as emotions [46]. For example, the response to vascular occlusion is severely limited in people with diabetes as shown in Fig. 2. Here, as shown in this figure, the response to vascular occlusion of the skin is reduced by as much as two-thirds in people with diabetes compared to age-matched control subjects [54]. The most damage caused by diabetes occurs directly on endothelial cells. Several pathways in endothelial cells are damaged by diabetes. First, nitric oxide is less bioavailable. In type 2 diabetes, some studies indicate that high glycemic levels damage either the enzyme, nitric oxide synthetase, or the TRPV-4 calcium channels [50]. The result is that less nitric oxide is produced by vascular endothelial cells in response to a given vasodilator stimulus. Further, nitrergic neurons might also be damaged by high glycemic levels. This reduced production of nitric oxide by endothelial cells or by neurons alters the balance between vasodilation and vasoconstriction favoring vasoconstriction [55]. Other studies show that diabetes reduces the bioavailability of arginine, thereby altering the ability of the endothelial cells to produce nitric oxide. Some studies point to a third mechanism in which the high free radical concentration in the body associated with both obesity and diabetes bioconverts nitric oxide into peroxynitrite, thereby reducing the bioavailability of nitric oxide as a vasodilator [42, 56]. Probably all three mechanisms are present to various extents in different populations of patients with diabetes. The combined effects of reduced nitric oxide bioavailability are to reduce active vasodilatation in blood vessels. These reactions can be further exacerbated by reduction in l-arginine bioavailability due to destruction of l-arginine or lack of availability due to diet- or age-related

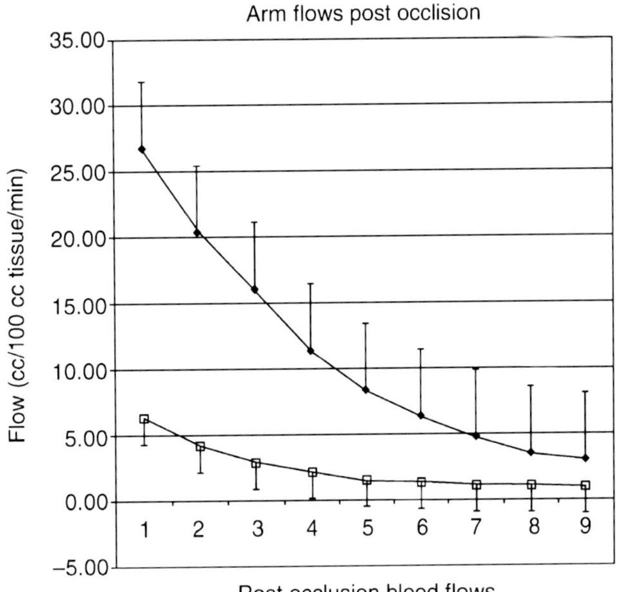

Fig. 2 Illustrated here is the forearm blood flow in age-matched controls (*upper curve*) and subjects with diabetes (*lower curve*) after 4 min of vascular occlusion of the arm [54]

impairment in intestinal absorption [55, 57]. Decreased l-arginine also increases production of the superoxides, damaging the cell even further [58, 59]. Further with tetrahydrobiopterin (BH4) depletion (a nitric oxide synthetase cofactor) as can occur in diabetes and aging, ENOS is also uncoupled and produces superoxides instead of nitric oxide [58, 60].

Nitric oxide release can be elicited by vasodilation due to acetylcholine from the sympathetic nervous system, or endothelial nitric oxide synthetase can be activated by stimuli like local heat to produce a change in local pressure or tissue osmolarity or shear stress in the blood vessel. The response of endothelial cells to all of these stimuli is blunted in diabetes [56]. The impairment in blood flow in response to these stimuli, however, is greater than would be expected by a loss in vasodilation alone. This may be due to additional diabetes-related impairments.

Insulin is a vasodilator. In nondiabetic subjects, insulin reduces inflammation and causes vasodilation as well as enhancing glucose transport. Insulin accomplishes this by activating the phosphatidylinositol 3-kinase/Akt pathway, activating both ENOS and GLUT-4 glucose transport. But insulin also activates a mitogen-activated kinase pathway (MAPK). This pathway causes vasoconstriction of vascular smooth muscle. Normally, vasodilation overwhelms constriction and blood vessels dilate in response to insulin. But in diabetes, the MAPK pathway overwhelms the PI3K pathway, and insulin, which is present in high plasma concentrations in diabetes, becomes a vasoconstrictor stimulus, further reducing blood flow to tissue and causing additional microvascular damage.

Microvascular damage to the kidneys in diabetes causes the release of renin, a renal enzyme which is involved in the regulation of sodium in the blood. Renin converts blood angiotensinogen to angiotensin I. In most tissues in the body, angiotensin-converting enzyme converts angiotensin I to angiotensin II. Angiotensin II is a potent vasoconstrictor and overwhelms endothelial vasodilation and is also proinflammatory. It also impairs insulin signaling.

Morphological changes in the endothelial cell-smooth muscle interfaces are also observed in diabetes [56]. Normally, small cellular attachments (electrotonic connections) exist between endothelial cells and vascular smooth muscle. Thus, in addition to vasodilators and vasoconstrictors affecting the surrounding smooth muscle in blood vessels, there is direct electrical contact. When endothelial cells depolarize or hyperpolarize, the electrotonic connection through these gap junctions helps coordinate electrical activity between endothelial cells and the surrounding vascular smooth muscle. When vasodilator effectors bind to the endothelial membrane, the endothelial cell hyperpolarizes through an increase in potassium permeability. This increase in potassium permeability hyperpolarizes the vascular smooth muscle, making it harder for action potentials to develop and thus aiding in the process of vasodilatation [56, 61–63]. In people with diabetes, these electrotonic connections are destroyed; consequently some of the ability of the endothelial cell to relax vascular smooth muscle is lost [64].

The overall effect of all of these factors is that, due to a predominant vasoconstriction, resting blood flow in the skin is reduced (by almost 66 %) in people with diabetes. Consequently, blood flow responses to global and local heat are reduced; therapeutic modalities such as contrast baths, which normally cause a large increase in blood flow in the skin, are ineffective in people with diabetes [45, 46, 65].

As shown in Fig. 3a, b, whereas control subjects show a much greater increase in skin blood flow to a contrast bath than a constant warm bath, the response is lost in people with diabetes.

The blood flow response to stressors such as electrical stimulation, when used clinically for therapy or wound healing, is also diminished [66, 67]. Because modulation of the skin circulation depends to a greater degree on nitric oxide in older individuals, as people with diabetes age, blood flow responses in the skin worsen disproportionately.

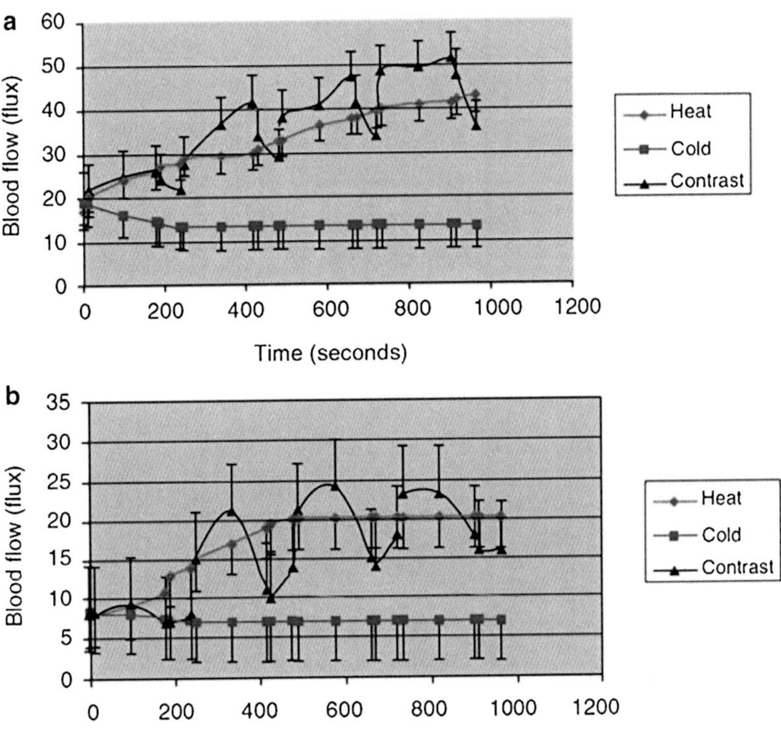

Fig. 3 (**a**) This figure illustrates the blood flow in the skin (flux) measured over the experimental period in control subjects during immersion in contrast baths (*triangles*), continuous passive heating (*diamonds*), and continuous cold immersion (*squares*). All data is the mean +/− the SD [13]. (**b**) This figure illustrates the blood flow in the skin (flux) in subjects with diabetes during immersion in contrast baths (*triangle*), continuous passive heating (*diamond*), and continuous cold immersions (*squares*) [13]

Lifestyle, Race, and Endothelial Function

Recently, several studies have shown that lifestyle factors such as obesity [119, 120] and cigarette smoking [68], as well as race [69], are associated with changes in vascular endothelial cells connected to cardiovascular disease.

Lifestyle

Adipose tissue expresses a variety of cytokines, such as interleukin-6 (IL-6) and tumor necrosis factor-alpha (TNF-alpha) [70], that increase the production of C-reactive protein (CRP) [71]. These cytokine-mediated inflammatory processes are involved in the early stages of atherogenesis [72–74]. Damage occurs to endothelial and other cells in the body [75]. IL-6 and TNF-alpha cause the release of endothelial adhesion molecules and impair insulin action by interfering with the insulin signaling cascade [76]. CRP, elevated in response to inflammatory cytokines, impairs endothelium-dependent vasodilatation by interfering with either endothelial nitric oxide synthetase (ENOS) or endothelial nitric oxide bioavailability [77]. Endothelial damage, especially in capillaries, precedes serious cardiovascular disease [78, 79]. Vascular endothelial damage can be measured by biomarkers such as E-selectin and soluble vascular adhesion molecule (sVCAM-1) [78, 80].

Environmental factors, such as smoking, also damage vascular endothelial cells [81]. Smoking is a major risk factor for atherogenesis and vascular disease. Tobacco smoke contains more than 4,000 chemicals, many of which cause pathological changes in endothelial cells [132]. Oxygen free radicals from tobacco smoking increase cellular oxidation and can limit the bioavailability of nitric oxide [82]. These radicals oxidize nitric oxide to chemicals such as peroxynitrite, a superoxide that can further damage tissue by lipid peroxidation of membranes [81]. Smoking increases sympathetic vasoconstrictor nerve activity and thus contributes to increased vascular tone arteries. Smoking also increases concentration of the protein fibrinogen, resulting in prothrombotic effects [83]. Thus, smoking has multiple effects on the health of vascular endothelial cells [84].

Other environmental agents, such as air and water pollutants, may impair endothelial vascular function. Recent studies show that particulate matter from diesel engines can activate the JNK pathway and damage endothelial function [85]. Cigarette smoke [86] and air pollution in general [87] exert their effects through the ENOS pathway. Further, since both age and diabetes increase oxidation in the body, both increase endothelial dysfunction [88].

Race

The impact of race is complex. Studies of the effect of race on the vasculature have measured reactivity to various challenges such as vascular occlusion [69]. This is done by examining the effect of ischemia on blood flow in vessels in the skin (by using a laser Doppler imaging) or on larger arteries, such as the brachial artery, by ultrasound [69]. Tests of vascular function also employ agonists of sympathetic activity (such as acetylcholine or methylcholine) to activate muscarinic receptors on vascular endothelial cells. This increases intracellular calcium, increases ENOS activity, and releases nitric oxide [89, 90]. Bradykinin also activates ENOS [90].

The impact of race on nitric oxide-dependent vasodilatation was recently reviewed [69]. A decrease in nitric oxide-dependent vasodilatation is evident in many populations. Young, healthy African American subjects exhibit a lower vasodilatory response to methylcholine and albuterol than do Caucasians. Among African Americans, 30 % of deaths in men and 20 % of deaths in women are caused by hypertension, a finding probably linked to a lower vasodilatory response to stress. The incidence of asthma [91] and of type 2 diabetes [92] is also elevated in African Americans. A higher incidence of type 2 diabetes also occurs in Asians and Native Americans, and these groups exhibit impaired vascular responses to vasodilators relative to Caucasians [93]. However, factors other than racial background play a role in the impairment of vascular response to stress. For example, Europeans of African descent exhibit a higher degree of dysfunction in nitric oxide production in endothelial cells than do African Americans [94].

A few studies have examined the mechanisms by which endothelial-dependent vasodilatation in African Americans and European Americans is impaired. Some studies suggest that in African Americans, ENOS has a higher activity than in European Americans [144]. However, in African Americans, production of reactive oxygen species is also elevated. Consequently, nitric oxide is more readily bioconverted to peroxynitrate, which reduces nitric oxide bioavailability in this ethnic group [95].

Other races have gene polymorphisms that affect skin blood flow. Asians, for example, have a genetic polymorphism due to what is called the "thrifty" gene. The gene developed in populations where food supply was limited due to famine. It allows fat to be stored easily when food is available. The thrifty gene controls the production of peroxisome proliferator-activated receptor (PPAR), a nuclear subtransmitter that upregulates carbohydrate metabolism in the cell. This single nucleotide polymorphism plays a role in the development of diabetes by increasing insulin resistance when high-fat to carbohydrate diets are consumed [96, 97]. The defect in this gene may explain why Asians have a lower tolerance for foods that are high in fat. South Asian men exhibit lower brachial artery dilation in response to occlusion, lower vasodilatory responses to acetylcholine, higher levels of insulin resistance, and higher C-reactive protein, an index of endothelial damage, compared to Caucasian men of a similar age with similar anthropometric measurements [98]. Thus, in Asians, the polymorphism in the thrifty gene alters carbohydrate metabolism such that ingesting even a single high-fat meal impairs nitric oxide production and hence tissue blood flow [99, 100]. Typically, an increase in the plasma concentration of free fatty acids after ingesting a high-fat meal induces proinflammatory cytokines [101] and reactive oxygen species within the vascular walls [95]. This in turn activates nuclear factor kappa beta and generates reactive oxygen species [100]. The reactive oxygen species converts nitric oxide to peroxynitrate and other superoxides, reducing the bioavailability of nitric oxide after a high-fat meal [100, 101]. In addition, free fatty acids induce protein kinase C, which inhibits phosphotinol 3 kinase thereby inhibiting the activity and activation of endothelial nitric oxide synthetase especially in Asians compared to Caucasians [102, 103].

Because of genetic polymorphisms, Asians are more susceptible to vascular endothelial impairment. However, the effect of environmental factors should not be discounted. For example, cardiovascular disease and vascular endothelial dysfunction are increasing among native Japanese with Westernized lifestyles and in Japanese men who have moved to the United States [104].

Other minority populations within the United States, such as Pima Indians, also have a higher rate of endothelial dysfunction and a higher incidence of diabetes. Markers of endothelial dysfunction, such as insulin resistance and low-grade inflammation (elevated CRP and other cytokines), are common in Native Americans such as Pima Indians [105]. Other markers of endothelial dysfunction, such as E-selectin, von Willebrand factor, and soluble intracellular adhesion molecule-1 (Sicam-1), are elevated in Pima Indians compared to Caucasians living in a similar area (interestingly, similar markers of endothelial dysfunction have been reported in Koreans) [106, 107]. However, the genesis of endothelial dysfunction in Native Americans populations is poorly understood [105].

Because smoking is more prevalent among Asians, it is likely that smoking-related free radicals block the release of nitric oxide; moreover, free radicals cause oxidative damage in vascular smooth muscle [68]. Children exposed to passive smoking exhibit elevated oxidative markers [108]. The mechanisms by which oxidative stress damages vascular smooth muscle are unknown.

Not all alterations in endothelial nitric oxide synthetase have deleterious effects. For example, in Sherpas, modification of nitric oxide metabolism allows greater vasodilatation in systemic and pulmonary arteries during hypoxia than seen on other races [109]. Thus, this population is more able to tolerate high altitude than people of other races due to a specific polymorphism in the gene for endothelial nitric oxide synthetase [109].

A recent study in populations in the north and south of India described a genetic polymorphism in the gene for endogenous nitric oxide synthetase on chromosome 7q35 through 36, which was associated with an impaired production of nitric oxide in response to stress [110]. This polymorphism resulted in heightened susceptibility to endothelial dysfunction, hypertension, and diabetes. Several other studies have been conducted on south Indian populations [111] and northern Indian populations with similar results [112]. When given large doses of vitamin D or coenzyme Q10 (potent antioxidants), people from India and Korea showed a higher blood flow response to thermal stress and anoxia [102, 107, 113–115].

Aging and Circulation

Aging leads to the natural senescence of organ systems, including the kidney [116], the autonomic nervous system [117], and the heart. It has been stated that man is only as old as his arteries [118]. Certainly, many genes are associated with vascular aging including the forkhead box 0A1, forkhead box 0A3, and many other genes [119]. But many factors as described below are environmental as well. Although many physiologic changes occur as people age, one important factor contributing to decreased tissue function is diminished production of the potent vasodilator, nitric oxide (a) [120]. The sensitivity of beta-adrenergic receptors also diminishes with age [121], which reduces the ability of the sympathetic nervous system to respond to stress. Indeed, damage to the microcirculation is a common denominator for all of the age-related changes in organ function.

Aging principally affects three tissues associated with circulatory control. The first is the vascular endothelial cell. The second is the sympathetic nervous system, which affects control of the peripheral circulation. The third is the dermis of the skin [52].

The function of endothelial cells diminishes gradually, accelerating in the later years. Disorders such as diabetes accelerate endothelial dysfunction [54, 122]. Because diabetes incidence rises with age, the interaction of age and diabetes becomes important clinically. This will be elaborated in the next section.

A major contributing factor to endothelial cell damage with aging is prolonged exposure to angiotensin II [123]. The arterial wall structurally remodels in response to chronic inflammation. Angiotensin II alters both inflammation in the vascular endothelial cell and the surrounding smooth muscle [124]. While angiotensin II is a protective pathway in the young, in the elderly chronic high levels of angiotensin II due to kidney disease cause inflammation that damages nitric oxide production and alters vascular wall stiffness and plaque formation [124–128]. This also increases the incidence of thrombosis [127, 128]. In the elderly, angiotensin II induces proinflammatory factors such as TNF-alpha and MCP-1 and decreases nitric oxide availability [129]. Reactive oxygen species and angiotensin II induce telomere shortening and damage DNA causing endothelial apoptosis [130, 131]. Inflammation also causes remodeling of the media, a region between the elastic laminae of the artery causing erosion in the elasticity [132, 133]. Elastin has been seen to fragment with aging due to angiotensin II [134]. Inflammation also causes intimal cell hyperplasia, a common association with age-related arterial damage [135]. In addition, angiotensin II is associated with small vessel degeneration [136].

In general, both the parasympathetic and sympathetic nervous systems are affected by age. Most studies show only small decreases in blood pressure and diminished heart rate variability during orthostatic stress (e.g., change in body position from sitting to standing) as people age [137]. This might indicate that age has a limited effect on the autonomic nervous system. However, if additional stressors, such as heat exposure during orthostatic stress, are placed on the autonomic nervous system, the reduction in blood pressure is much more pronounced in older people during the same orthostatic stress [138]. Although overall autonomic function diminishes with age [139], a decrease in baroreceptor sensitivity also occurs [140], masking sudden changes in body position not properly detected by the autonomic nervous system.

Specifically, for the vascular endothelial cell and the sympathetic nervous system, there is evidence that age increases vasoconstriction and reduces vasodilation [141]. Therefore, vasoconstrictor muscle tone predominates; the blood flow at rest and during an autonomic stress is lower [141]. The mechanism by which vasodilatation is lost appears due to several factors. First, nitric oxide release from skin blood vessels diminishes with age [141]. Second, beta-adrenergic receptor sensitivity diminishes with age due to structural changes in the receptor that render it insensitive to catecholamines [121]. This further reduces sympathetic activity. Finally, aging also reduces the sensitivity of the parasympathetic nervous system.

Of interest is the effect of exercise on blood vessels and aging. A recent review article conducted a meta-analysis of flow-mediated dilation in arteries [142]. The results showed that while younger athletes do not have better flow-mediated dilation than nonathletes, older athletes do preserve better flow-mediated dilation.

In summary, lifespan has more than doubled in the last 100 years [143]. There is an inverse relationship between aging and endothelial dysfunction. Patients with endothelial dysfunction show accelerated aging [144, 145]. This increase in life is associated with diseases linked to chronic inflammation [146]. Inflammation increases endothelial hyperactivity including overproduction of mediators such as endothelium 1 [147] which in itself mediates vascular smooth muscle contraction and hypertension [148], and some believe it causes more damage than angiotensin II. Medical intervention to reduce inflammation and angiotensin II remains pivotal in reducing morbidity and mortality.

Interaction Between Age and Diabetes

Diabetes, like age, is associated with damage to the autonomic nervous system [149]. Damage to autonomic nerves, causing orthostatic intolerance, can occur before clinical symptoms of diabetes are manifest [150]. Damage to the parasympathetic nervous system results in loss of heart rate control, especially during orthostatic stress [151]. The damage usually occurs at the autonomic ganglia and also at the peripheral nerve endings, where microcirculation is critical. When patients with diabetes are subjected to an orthostatic challenge (e.g., going from sitting to standing) in a thermally neutral environment, 25 % of diabetic patients show a drop of 20 mmHg (0.266 kPa) or more in mean blood pressure [152]. However, as autonomic stressors (such as a greater room temperature) are added, the systolic blood pressure falls in almost all patients with diabetes during standing [153]. The mechanism in these patients appears to be an inability to vasodilate [154]. As with aging, in patients with diabetes the damage appears to be twofold. First, ganglionic damage impairs the ability of the autonomic nerves to generate impulses; secondly, the ability to generate adequate amounts of nitric oxide is impaired [155]. These factors affect both arterial and venous circulations [156].

Thus, diabetes seems to cause damage to the autonomic nervous system and to endothelial cell function similar to that which occurs normally with aging. For this reason, diabetes is thought to accelerate the aging process by causing more severe loss of autonomic function. Neuronal damage can be so pronounced as to cause lesions of the spinal cord [157].

In addition to nerve and circulatory damage, another factor also seems to come into play with both aging and diabetes. This is thickness of the dermal layer of the skin, which decreases with age [158]. In older adults, thinning of the skin is a consequence of a thickening in the stratum corneum and a thinning in the dermal layer. Aging not only reduces skin blood flow but also alters skin structure, including collagen composition and skin thickness [183]. Because the dermal layer is thinner, this implies that the vasculature in the skin in older people is reduced. This is also the case in people with diabetes. Thinner skin would increase susceptibility to injury and, as is the case for people with diabetes, make the skin harder to heal [159]. Vascular smooth muscle is also damaged in type 2 diabetes [159].

For example, as shown in Fig. 4, with both diabetes and age, resting blood flow is less. However, at the same age, diabetes causes a greater reduction in blood flow than age alone. The administration of rosiglitazone for 6 months did reverse the diabetes effect on resting and post-occlusion blood flows (Fig. 5), but not the age effects, pointing to different mechanisms for endothelial damage.

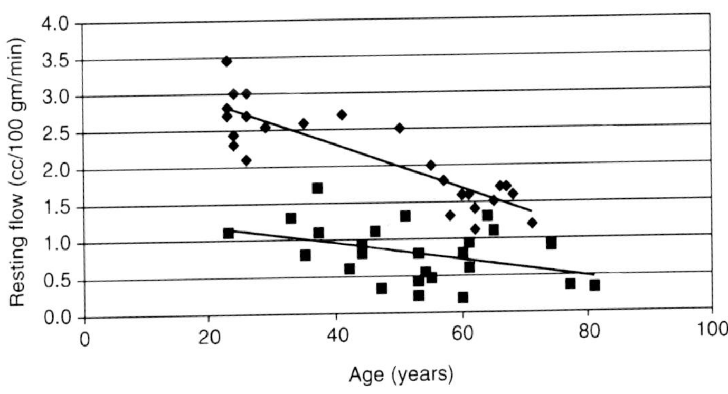

Fig. 4 Illustrated here is the relationship between age and the blood flow in the arm at rest with arm temperature stabilized at 37 °C. In control subjects (*diamonds*) and subjects with diabetes (*squares*), the line through the figure is the regression line calculated by the method of least squares. The regression equation for the control subjects was resting flow = −0.0306age + 3.5106. The regression equation for the subjects with diabetes was resting flow = −0.011age + 1.4087 [168]

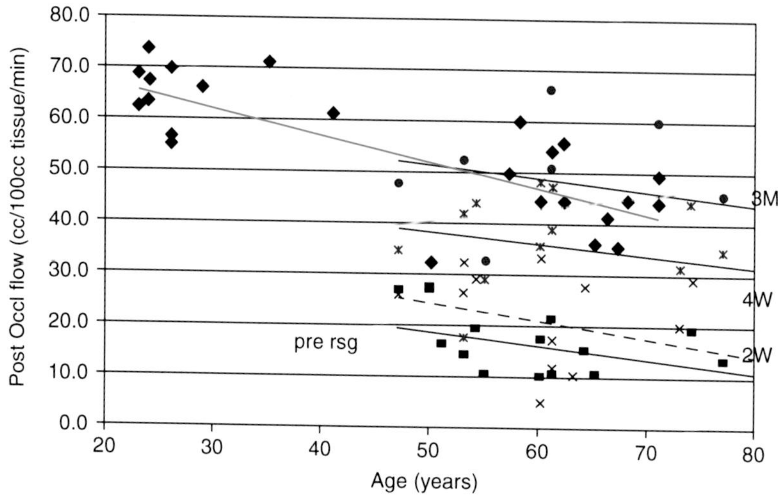

Fig. 5 Illustrated here is the relationship between age and the blood flow in the arm with arm temperature stabilized at 37 °C. The blood flow here is the flow after 4 min of occlusion as the area under the blood flow curve for 2 min. In control subjects (*diamonds*) and subjects with diabetes (*squares*), the *line* through the figure is the regression line calculated by the method of least squares. The *parallel lines* represent the data after 2 weeks (2w), 4 weeks (4w), and 3 months administration of rosiglitazone, a PPAR agonist [160]

Moreover, the layer of subcutaneous fat also becomes thinner with age [158, 161, 162]. The foot becomes particularly susceptible to injury as the reduction in padding over the bone may make the foot more susceptible to lesions during gait. The impact of dermal thinning may be particularly important in people with diabetes. It has been assumed that the reduction in blood flow observed in older people and people with diabetes is solely due to impaired nitric oxide synthesis [14, 50, 158]. However, thinner skin also has a lower density of blood vessels, which may account for some of the reduction in blood flow through the skin. Because people with diabetes have a higher body mass index (BMI) and because BMI correlates with the level of subcutaneous fat, people with diabetes whose weight is normal may have a very thin layer of subcutaneous fat. A thin person with diabetes would be more susceptible to foot injuries caused by gait.

Summary

The vascular endothelial cells mediate the control of circulation in the skin. While they are influenced by anoxia, humoral control, and central neurogenic control, all of these functions are modulated with factors that change during life. In women, beta-estrogen receptors modulate skin blood flow during the menstrual cycle. This is a normal variation that occurs until menopause. But other mediators such as diabetes and high concentrations of free radicals in the blood cause endothelial dysfunction from oxidative damage. Some races are more susceptible than others to free radical damage. Asians including people from India are very susceptible to endothelial damage from high-fat diets. When added to endothelial dysfunction from aging, these factors add in reducing skin blood flow and making the skin susceptible to damage.

References

1. Charkoudian N, Joyner MJ. Physiologic considerations for exercise performance in women. Clin Chest Med. 2004;25(2):247–55.
2. Groupe suisse pour l'étude des trouvailles monétaires. Colloque international (3rd: 2000: Bern Switzerland), et al. Circulation monétaire régionale et supra-régionale: actes du troisième colloque international du Groupe suisse pour l'étude des trouvailles monétaires (Berne, 3-4 mars 2000) = Regionaler

und überregionaler Geldumlauf: Sitzungsbericht des dritten internationalen Kolloquiums der Schweizerischen Arbeitsgemeinschaft für Fundmünzen (Bern, 3.-4. März 2000). Etudes de numismatique et d'histoire monétaire. 2002, Lausanne: Editions du Zèbre. 296 p., 6 leaves of plates.

3. Charkoudian N, Johnson JM. Altered reflex control of cutaneous circulation by female sex steroids is independent of prostaglandins. Am J Physiol. 1999;276 (5 Pt 2):H1634–40.
4. Charkoudian N. Mechanisms and modifiers of reflex induced cutaneous vasodilation and vasoconstriction in humans. J Appl Physiol (1985). 2010;109(4): 1221–8.
5. Petrofsky J, Al Malty A, Suh HJ. Isometric endurance, body and skin temperature and limb and skin blood flow during the menstrual cycle. Med Sci Monit. 2007;13(3):CR111–7.
6. Cankar K, Finderle Z, Strucl M. Gender differences in cutaneous laser doppler flow response to local direct and contralateral cooling. J Vasc Res. 2000;37(3): 183–8.
7. Lee H, et al. Higher sweating rate and skin blood flow during the luteal phase of the menstrual cycle. Tohoku J Exp Med. 2014;234(2):117–22.
8. Bungum L, et al. Laser doppler-recorded reactive hyperaemia in the forearm skin during the menstrual cycle. Br J Obstet Gynaecol. 1996;103(1):70–5.
9. Agner T, Damm P, Skouby SO. Menstrual cycle and skin reactivity. J Am Acad Dermatol. 1991;24(4): 566–70.
10. Kemmett D. Premenstrual exacerbation of atopic dermatitis. Br J Dermatol. 1989;120(5):715.
11. Guo X, et al. Estrogen induces vascular wall dilation: mediation through kinase signaling to nitric oxide and estrogen receptors alpha and beta. J Biol Chem. 2005;280(20):19704–10.
12. Malty AM, Petrofsky J. The effect of electrical stimulation on a normal skin blood flow in active young and older adults. Med Sci Monit. 2007;13(4): CR147–55.
13. Petrofsky J, et al. Effects of contrast baths on skin blood flow on the dorsal and plantar foot in people with type 2 diabetes and age-matched controls. Physiother Theory Pract. 2007;23(4):189–97.
14. Petrofsky JS, et al. The influence of alterations in room temperature on skin blood flow during contrast baths in patients with diabetes. Med Sci Monit. 2006;12(7):CR290–5.
15. Arnal JF, et al. Understanding the controversy about hormonal replacement therapy: insights from estrogen effects on experimental and clinical atherosclerosis. Arch Mal Coeur Vaiss. 2007;100(6–7):554–62.
16. Asahara T, et al. Isolation of putative progenitor endothelial cells for angiogenesis. Science. 1997;275(5302):964–7.
17. Venkov CD, Rankin AB, Vaughan DE. Identification of authentic estrogen receptor in cultured endothelial cells. A potential mechanism for steroid hormone regulation of endothelial function. Circulation. 1996;94(4):727–33.
18. Green S, et al. Cloning of the human oestrogen receptor cDNA. J Steroid Biochem. 1986;24(1):77–83.
19. Walker VR, Korach KS. Estrogen receptor knockout mice as a model for endocrine research. ILAR J. 2004;45(4):455–61.
20. Foresta C, et al. Oestrogen stimulates endothelial progenitor cells via oestrogen receptor-alpha. Clin Endocrinol (Oxf). 2007;67(4):520–5.
21. Hamada H, et al. Estrogen receptors alpha and beta mediate contribution of bone marrow-derived endothelial progenitor cells to functional recovery after myocardial infarction. Circulation. 2006;114(21): 2261–70.
22. Iwakura A, et al. Estrogen-mediated, endothelial nitric oxide synthase-dependent mobilization of bone marrow-derived endothelial progenitor cells contributes to reendothelialization after arterial injury. Circulation. 2003;108(25):3115–21.
23. Strehlow K, et al. Estrogen increases bone marrow-derived endothelial progenitor cell production and diminishes neointima formation. Circulation. 2003;107(24):3059–65.
24. Assmus B, et al. HMG-CoA reductase inhibitors reduce senescence and increase proliferation of endothelial progenitor cells via regulation of cell cycle regulatory genes. Circ Res. 2003;92(9):1049–55.
25. Dimmeler S, et al. HMG-CoA reductase inhibitors (statins) increase endothelial progenitor cells via the PI 3-kinase/Akt pathway. J Clin Invest. 2001;108(3): 391–7.
26. Collado B, et al. Vasoactive intestinal peptide increases vascular endothelial growth factor expression and neuroendocrine differentiation in human prostate cancer LNCaP cells. Regul Pept. 2004;119(1-2):69–75.
27. Ceradini DJ, et al. Progenitor cell trafficking is regulated by hypoxic gradients through HIF-1 induction of SDF-1. Nat Med. 2004;10(8):858–64.
28. Crescioli C, et al. Expression of functional estrogen receptors in human fetal male external genitalia. J Clin Endocrinol Metab. 2003;88(4):1815–24.
29. Dietrich W, et al. Expression of estrogen receptors in human corpus cavernosum and male urethra. J Histochem Cytochem. 2004;52(3):355–60.
30. Goyal HO, et al. Role of estrogen in induction of penile dysmorphogenesis: a review. Reproduction. 2007;134(2):199–208.
31. Mowa CN, et al. Estrogen enhances wound healing in the penis of rats. Biomed Res. 2008;29(5):267–70.
32. Nissen NN, et al. Vascular endothelial growth factor mediates angiogenic activity during the proliferative phase of wound healing. Am J Pathol. 1998;152(6): 1445–52.
33. Lahm T, et al. The effects of estrogen on pulmonary artery vasoreactivity and hypoxic pulmonary vasoconstriction: potential new clinical implications for an old hormone. Crit Care Med. 2008;36 (7):2174–83.

34. English KM, et al. Gender differences in the vasomotor effects of different steroid hormones in rat pulmonary and coronary arteries. Horm Metab Res. 2001;33(11):645–52.
35. McLaughlin VV, McGoon MD. Pulmonary arterial hypertension. Circulation. 2006;114(13):1417–31.
36. Karakitsos D, et al. Androgen deficiency and endothelial dysfunction in men with end-stage kidney disease receiving maintenance hemodialysis. Am J Nephrol. 2006;26(6):536–43.
37. Sokolnicki LA, Khosla S, Charkoudian N. Effects of testosterone and estradiol on cutaneous vasodilation during local warming in older men. Am J Physiol Endocrinol Metab. 2007;293(5):E1426–9.
38. Kenney WL, et al. Decreased active vasodilator sensitivity in aged skin. Am J Physiol. 1997;272(4 Pt 2): H1609–14.
39. Jankovec Z, et al. The influence of insulin pump treatment on metabolic syndrome parameters in type 2 diabetes mellitus. Wien Klin Wochenschr. 2009;121(13–14):459–63.
40. Lacigova S, et al. Influence of cardiovascular autonomic neuropathy on atherogenesis and heart function in patients with type 1 diabetes. Diabetes Res Clin Pract. 2009;83(1):26–31.
41. Comi G, et al. Peripheral nerve abnormalities in newly-diagnosed diabetic children. Acta Diabetol Lat. 1986;23(1):69–75.
42. Vinik AI, Freeman R, Erbas T. Diabetic autonomic neuropathy. Semin Neurol. 2003;23(4):365–72.
43. Pittenger G, Vinik A. Nerve growth factor and diabetic neuropathy. Exp Diabesity Res. 2003;4 (4):271–85.
44. Colberg SR, et al. Cutaneous blood flow in type 2 diabetic individuals after an acute bout of maximal exercise. Diabetes Care. 2003;26(6):1883–8.
45. Maloney-Hinds C, et al. The role of nitric oxide in skin blood flow increases due to vibration in healthy adults and adults with type 2 diabetes. Diabetes Technol Ther. 2009;11(1):39–43.
46. McLellan K, et al. The effects of skin moisture and subcutaneous fat thickness on the ability of the skin to dissipate heat in young and old subjects, with and without diabetes, at three environmental room temperatures. Med Eng Phys. 2009;31(2):165–72.
47. Maloney-Hinds C, Petrofsky JS, Zimmerman G. The effect of 30 Hz *vs.* 50 Hz passive vibration and duration of vibration on skin blood flow in the arm. Med Sci Monit. 2008;14(3):CR112–6.
48. Alemzadeh R, et al. Continuous subcutaneous insulin infusion and multiple dose of insulin regimen display similar patterns of blood glucose excursions in pediatric type 1 diabetes. Diabetes Technol Ther. 2005;7(4):587–96.
49. Peter R, et al. Postprandial glucose – a potential therapeutic target to reduce cardiovascular mortality. Curr Vasc Pharmacol. 2009;7(1):68–74.
50. Petrofsky J, et al. The interrelationships between electrical stimulation, the environment surrounding the vascular endothelial cells of the skin, and the role of nitric oxide in mediating the blood flow response to electrical stimulation. Med Sci Monit. 2007;13(9): CR391–7.
51. Lawson D, Petrofsky JS. A randomized control study on the effect of biphasic electrical stimulation in a warm room on skin blood flow and healing rates in chronic wounds of patients with and without diabetes. Med Sci Monit. 2007;13(6):CR258–63.
52. Petrofsky JS, et al. Skin heat dissipation: the influence of diabetes, skin thickness, and subcutaneous fat thickness. Diabetes Technol Ther. 2008;10(6): 487–93.
53. Langer A, et al. Detection of silent myocardial ischemia in diabetes mellitus. Am J Cardiol. 1991;67 (13):1073–8.
54. Petrofsky J, Lee S, Cuneo M. Effects of aging and type 2 diabetes on resting and post occlusive hyperemia of the forearm; the impact of rosiglitazone. BMC Endocr Disord. 2005;5(1):4.
55. Tabit CE, et al. Endothelial dysfunction in diabetes mellitus: molecular mechanisms and clinical implications. Rev Endocr Metab Disord. 2010;11(1):61–74.
56. Potenza MA, et al. Endothelial dysfunction in diabetes: from mechanisms to therapeutic targets. Curr Med Chem. 2009;16(1):94–112.
57. Toda N, Imamura T, Okamura T. Alteration of nitric oxide-mediated blood flow regulation in diabetes mellitus. Pharmacol Ther. 2010;127(3):189–209.
58. Druhan LJ, et al. Regulation of eNOS-derived superoxide by endogenous methylarginines. Biochemistry. 2008;47(27):7256–63.
59. Holowatz LA, Thompson CS, Kenney WL. L-Arginine supplementation or arginase inhibition augments reflex cutaneous vasodilatation in aged human skin. J Physiol. 2006;574(Pt 2):573–81.
60. Loer CM, et al. Cuticle integrity and biogenic amine synthesis in caenorhabditis elegans require the cofactor tetrahydrobiopterin (BH4). Genetics. 2015;200:237.
61. de Wit C, Boettcher M, Schmidt VJ. Signaling across myoendothelial gap junctions – fact or fiction? Cell Commun Adhes. 2008;15(3):231–45.
62. Schmidt VJ, et al. Gap junctions synchronize vascular tone within the microcirculation. Pharmacol Rep. 2008;60(1):68–74.
63. Gupta PK, et al. Role of voltage-dependent potassium channels and myo-endothelial gap junctions in 4-aminopyridine-induced inhibition of acetylcholine relaxation in rat carotid artery. Eur J Pharmacol. 2008;591(1–3):171–6.
64. Triggle CR, et al. The endothelium in health and disease – a target for therapeutic intervention. J Smooth Muscle Res. 2003;39(6):249–67.
65. Sokolnicki LA, et al. Skin blood flow and nitric oxide during body heating in type 2 diabetes mellitus. J Appl Physiol (1985). 2009;106(2):566–70.
66. Petrofsky J, et al. Effects of a 2-, 3- and 4-electrode stimulator design on current dispersion on the surface

and into the limb during electrical stimulation in controls and patients with wounds. J Med Eng Technol. 2008;32(6):485–97.
67. Petrofsky J, et al. A multi-channel stimulator and electrode array providing a rotating current whirlpool for electrical stimulation of wounds. J Med Eng Technol. 2008;32(5):371–84.
68. Antoniades C, Tousoulis D, Stefanadis C. Smoking in Asians: it doesn't stop at vascular endothelium. Int J Cardiol. 2008;128(2):151–3.
69. Mata-Greenwood E, Chen DB. Racial differences in nitric oxide-dependent vasorelaxation. Reprod Sci. 2008;15(1):9–25.
70. Yudkin JS, et al. Inflammation, obesity, stress and coronary heart disease: is interleukin-6 the link? Atherosclerosis. 2000;148(2):209–14.
71. Heinrich PC, Castell JV, Andus T. Interleukin-6 and the acute phase response. Biochem J. 1990;265(3):621–36.
72. Dahlgren U, et al. Induction of the mucosal immune response. Curr Top Microbiol Immunol. 1989;146:155–60.
73. Mahoney Jr DH, et al. Acquired immune deficiency, myelodysplasia, and acute nonlymphocytic leukemia associated with monosomy 7 and t(3;3) (q21;q26) in a child with Langerhans cell histiocytosis. Am J Pediatr Hematol Oncol. 1989;11(2):153–7.
74. Yokota T, Hansson GK. Immunological mechanisms in atherosclerosis. J Intern Med. 1995;238(6):479–89.
75. Pickup JC, Crook MA. Is type II diabetes mellitus a disease of the innate immune system? Diabetologia. 1998;41(10):1241–8.
76. Hotamisligil GS, et al. Tumor necrosis factor alpha inhibits signaling from the insulin receptor. Proc Natl Acad Sci U S A. 1994;91(11):4854–8.
77. Fichtlscherer S, et al. Elevated C-reactive protein levels and impaired endothelial vasoreactivity in patients with coronary artery disease. Circulation. 2000;102(9):1000–6.
78. Jager A, et al. Increased levels of soluble vascular cell adhesion molecule 1 are associated with risk of cardiovascular mortality in type 2 diabetes: the Hoorn study. Diabetes. 2000;49(3):485–91.
79. Ridker PM, et al. Plasma concentration of soluble intercellular adhesion molecule 1 and risks of future myocardial infarction in apparently healthy men. Lancet. 1998;351(9096):88–92.
80. Hwang SJ, et al. Circulating adhesion molecules VCAM-1, ICAM-1, and E-selectin in carotid atherosclerosis and incident coronary heart disease cases: the Atherosclerosis Risk In Communities (ARIC) study. Circulation. 1997;96(12):4219–25.
81. Thomas GN, et al. Smoking without exception adversely affects vascular structure and function in apparently healthy Chinese: implications in global atherosclerosis prevention. Int J Cardiol. 2008;128(2):172–7.
82. Davis JW, et al. Effects of tobacco and non-tobacco cigarette smoking on endothelium and platelets. Clin Pharmacol Ther. 1985;37(5):529–33.
83. Lam TH, et al. The relationship between fibrinogen and other coronary heart disease risk factors in a Chinese population. Atherosclerosis. 1999;143(2):405–13.
84. Vapaatalo H, Mervaala E. Clinically important factors influencing endothelial function. Med Sci Monit. 2001;7(5):1075–85.
85. Li R, et al. Ultrafine particles from diesel engines induce vascular oxidative stress via JNK activation. Free Radic Biol Med. 2009;46(6):775–82.
86. Fira-Mladinescu O, et al. The effects of chronic exposure to cigarette smoke on vasomotor endothelial function of guinea pig pulmonary arteries. Rev Med Chir Soc Med Nat Iasi. 2008;112(1):213–9.
87. O'Toole TE, Conklin DJ, Bhatnagar A. Environmental risk factors for heart disease. Rev Environ Health. 2008;23(3):167–202.
88. Petrofsky JS, et al. What is more damaging to vascular endothelial function: diabetes, age, high BMI, or all of the above? Med Sci Monit. 2013;19:257–63.
89. Wang SZ, Zhu SZ, el-Fakahany EE. Efficient coupling of m5 muscarinic acetylcholine receptors to activation of nitric oxide synthase. J Pharmacol Exp Ther. 1994;268(2):552–7.
90. Harris MB, et al. Reciprocal phosphorylation and regulation of endothelial nitric-oxide synthase in response to bradykinin stimulation. J Biol Chem. 2001;276(19):16587–91.
91. McDaniel M, Paxson C, Waldfogel J. Racial disparities in childhood asthma in the United States: evidence from the National Health Interview Survey, 1997 to 2003. Pediatrics. 2006;117(5):e868–77.
92. McBean AM, et al. Differences in diabetes prevalence, incidence, and mortality among the elderly of four racial/ethnic groups: whites, blacks, hispanics, and asians. Diabetes Care. 2004;27(10):2317–24.
93. McKeigue PM, Shah B, Marmot MG. Relation of central obesity and insulin resistance with high diabetes prevalence and cardiovascular risk in South Asians. Lancet. 1991;337(8738):382–6.
94. Androne AS, et al. Comparison of metabolic vasodilation in response to exercise and ischemia and endothelium-dependent flow-mediated dilation in African-American versus non-African-American patients with chronic heart failure. Am J Cardiol. 2006;97(5):685–9.
95. Kalinowski L, Dobrucki IT, Malinski T. Race-specific differences in endothelial function: predisposition of African Americans to vascular diseases. Circulation. 2004;109(21):2511–7.
96. Tai ES, et al. Differential effects of the C1431T and Pro12Ala PPARgamma gene variants on plasma lipids and diabetes risk in an Asian population. J Lipid Res. 2004;45(4):674–85.
97. Radha V, et al. Role of genetic polymorphism peroxisome proliferator-activated receptor-gamma2 Pro12Ala on ethnic susceptibility to diabetes in South-Asian and Caucasian subjects: evidence for heterogeneity. Diabetes Care. 2006;29(5):1046–51.

98. Murphy C, et al. Vascular dysfunction and reduced circulating endothelial progenitor cells in young healthy UK South Asian men. Arterioscler Thromb Vasc Biol. 2007;27(4):936–42.
99. Tsai WC, et al. Effects of oxidative stress on endothelial function after a high-fat meal. Clin Sci (Lond). 2004;106(3):315–9.
100. Tripathy D, et al. Elevation of free fatty acids induces inflammation and impairs vascular reactivity in healthy subjects. Diabetes. 2003;52(12):2882–7.
101. Nappo F, et al. Postprandial endothelial activation in healthy subjects and in type 2 diabetic patients: role of fat and carbohydrate meals. J Am Coll Cardiol. 2002;39(7):1145–50.
102. Petrofsky J, et al. The effect of acute administration of vitamin D on micro vascular endothelial function in Caucasians and South Asian Indians. Med Sci Monit. 2013;19:641–7.
103. Bui C, et al. Acute effect of a single high-fat meal on forearm blood flow, blood pressure and heart rate in healthy male Asians and Caucasians: a pilot study. Southeast Asian J Trop Med Public Health. 2010;41(2):490–500.
104. Watanabe H, et al. Influence of westernization of lifestyle on the progression of IMT in Japanese. J Atheroscler Thromb. 2004;11(6):330–4.
105. Weyer C, et al. Humoral markers of inflammation and endothelial dysfunction in relation to adiposity and *in vivo* insulin action in Pima Indians. Atherosclerosis. 2002;161(1):233–42.
106. Kim K, et al. Associations of visceral adiposity and exercise participation with C-reactive protein, insulin resistance, and endothelial dysfunction in Korean healthy adults. Metabolism. 2008;57(9):1181–9.
107. Yim J, et al. Protective effect of anti-oxidants on endothelial function in young Korean-Asians compared to Caucasians. Med Sci Monit. 2012;18(8): CR467–79.
108. Bolukbas C, et al. Increased oxidative stress associated with the severity of the liver disease in various forms of hepatitis B virus infection. BMC Infect Dis. 2005;5:95.
109. Droma Y, et al. Genetic contribution of the endothelial nitric oxide synthase gene to high altitude adaptation in sherpas. High Alt Med Biol. 2006;7(3):209–20.
110. Periaswamy R, et al. Gender specific association of endothelial nitric oxide synthase gene (Glu298Asp) polymorphism with essential hypertension in a south Indian population. Clin Chim Acta. 2008;395(1–2): 134–6.
111. Shoji M, et al. Positive association of endothelial nitric oxide synthase gene polymorphism with hypertension in northern Japan. Life Sci. 2000;66(26): 2557–62.
112. Srivastava K, et al. Association of eNOS Glu298Asp gene polymorphism with essential hypertension in Asian Indians. Clin Chim Acta. 2008;387(1–2):80–3.
113. Petrofsky JS, et al. CoQ10 and endothelial function in Asians from Korea compared to Asians born in the United States and US born Caucasians. Med Sci Monit. 2013;19:339–46.
114. Yim J, et al. Differences in endothelial function between Korean-Asians and Caucasians. Med Sci Monit. 2012;18(6):CR337–43.
115. Petrofsky JS, et al. Reduced endothelial function in the skin in southeast Asians compared to Caucasians. Med Sci Monit. 2012;18(1):CR1–8.
116. Fagard R, Thijs L, Amery A. Age and the hemodynamic response to posture and exercise. Am J Geriatr Cardiol. 1993;2(2):23–40.
117. Cybulski G, Niewiadomski W. Influence of age on the immediate heart rate response to the active orthostatic test. J Physiol Pharmacol. 2003;54(1):65–80.
118. Stein JH. Carotid intima-media thickness and vascular age: you are only as old as your arteries look. J Am Soc Echocardiogr. 2004;17(6):686–9.
119. Tian XL, Li Y. Endothelial cell senescence and age-related vascular diseases. J Genet Genomics. 2014;41(9):485–95.
120. Stadler K, et al. Increased nitric oxide levels as an early sign of premature aging in diabetes. Free Radic Biol Med. 2003;35(10):1240–51.
121. Schutzer WE, Mader SL. Age-related changes in vascular adrenergic signaling: clinical and mechanistic implications. Ageing Res Rev. 2003;2(2):169–90.
122. Petrofsky J, et al. The effect of rosiglitazone on orthostatic tolerance during heat exposure in individuals with type II diabetes. Diabetes Technol Ther. 2007;9(4):377–86.
123. Wang M, Monticone RE, Lakatta EG. Proinflammation of aging central arteries: a mini-review. Gerontology. 2014;60(6):519–29.
124. Wang M, Khazan B, Lakatta EG. Central arterial aging and angiotensin II signaling. Curr Hypertens Rev. 2010;6(4):266–81.
125. Wang M, et al. Proinflammation: the key to arterial aging. Trends Endocrinol Metab. 2014;25(2):72–9.
126. Wang M, Monticone RE, Lakatta EG. Arterial aging: a journey into subclinical arterial disease. Curr Opin Nephrol Hypertens. 2010;19(2):201–7.
127. Go AS, et al. Executive summary: heart disease and stroke statistics – 2014 update: a report from the American Heart Association. Circulation. 2014;129(3):399–410.
128. Go AS, et al. Heart disease and stroke statistics – 2014 update: a report from the American Heart Association. Circulation. 2014;129(3):e28–292.
129. Lakatta EG. The reality of aging viewed from the arterial wall. Artery Res. 2013;7(2):73–80.
130. Brandes RP, Fleming I, Busse R. Endothelial aging. Cardiovasc Res. 2005;66(2):286–94.
131. Yepuri G, et al. Positive crosstalk between arginase-II and S6K1 in vascular endothelial inflammation and aging. Aging Cell. 2012;11(6):1005–16.
132. Wang M, et al. Angiotensin II activates matrix metalloproteinase type II and mimics age-associated carotid arterial remodeling in young rats. Am J Pathol. 2005;167(5):1429–42.

133. McCrann DJ, et al. Upregulation of Nox4 in the aging vasculature and its association with smooth muscle cell polyploidy. Cell Cycle. 2009;8(6):902–8.
134. Wang M, et al. Chronic matrix metalloproteinase inhibition retards age-associated arterial proinflammation and increase in blood pressure. Hypertension. 2012;60(2):459–66.
135. Gennaro G, et al. Role of p44/p42 MAP kinase in the age-dependent increase in vascular smooth muscle cell proliferation and neointimal formation. Arterioscler Thromb Vasc Biol. 2003;23(2):204–10.
136. Sadoun E, Reed MJ. Impaired angiogenesis in aging is associated with alterations in vessel density, matrix composition, inflammatory response, and growth factor expression. J Histochem Cytochem. 2003;51(9):1119–30.
137. Siebert J, et al. Stroke volume variability and heart rate power spectrum in relation to posture changes in healthy subjects. Med Sci Monit. 2004;10(2):MT31–7.
138. Scremin G, Kenney WL. Aging and the skin blood flow response to the unloading of baroreceptors during heat and cold stress. J Appl Physiol (1985). 2004;96(3):1019–25.
139. Ray CA, Monahan KD. Aging attenuates the vestibulosympathetic reflex in humans. Circulation. 2002;105(8):956–61.
140. Guyton AC, Harris JW. Pressoreceptor-autonomic oscillation; a probable cause of vasomotor waves. Am J Physiol. 1951;165(1):158–66.
141. Franzoni F, et al. Effects of age and physical fitness on microcirculatory function. Clin Sci (Lond). 2004;106(3):329–35.
142. Montero D, et al. Flow-mediated dilation in athletes: influence of aging. Med Sci Sports Exerc. 2014;46(11):2148–58.
143. Barton M. Aging and endothelin: determinants of disease. Life Sci. 2014;118(2):97–109.
144. Capell BC, Collins FS, Nabel EG. Mechanisms of cardiovascular disease in accelerated aging syndromes. Circ Res. 2007;101(1):13–26.
145. Merideth MA, et al. Phenotype and course of Hutchinson-Gilford progeria syndrome. N Engl J Med. 2008;358(6):592–604.
146. Franceschi C, et al. Inflamm-aging. An evolutionary perspective on immunosenescence. Ann N Y Acad Sci. 2000;908:244–54.
147. Campia U, et al. The vascular endothelin system in obesity and type 2 diabetes: pathophysiology and therapeutic implications. Life Sci. 2014;118(2):149–55.
148. Meyer MR, et al. Endothelin-1 but not angiotensin II contributes to functional aging in murine carotid arteries. Life Sci. 2014;118(2):213–8.
149. Accurso V, Shamsuzzaman AS, Somers VK. Rhythms, rhymes, and reasons – spectral oscillations in neural cardiovascular control. Auton Neurosci. 2001;90(1–2):41–6.
150. Sagliocco L, et al. Amplitude loss of electrically and magnetically evoked sympathetic skin responses in early stages of type 1 (insulin-dependent) diabetes mellitus without signs of dysautonomia. Clin Auton Res. 1999;9(1):5–10.
151. Ewing DJ, et al. Autonomic neuropathy, QT interval lengthening, and unexpected deaths in male diabetic patients. Diabetologia. 1991;34(3):182–5.
152. Agrawal A, Saran R, Khanna R. Management of orthostatic hypotension from autonomic dysfunction in diabetics on peritoneal dialysis. Perit Dial Int. 1999;19(5):415–7.
153. Petrofsky JS, Besonis C, Rivera D, Schwab E, Lee S. Heat tolerance in patients with diabetes. J Appl Res Clin Exp Ther. 2003;3:28–34.
154. Stansberry KB, et al. Primary nociceptive afferents mediate the blood flow dysfunction in non-glabrous (hairy) skin of type 2 diabetes: a new model for the pathogenesis of microvascular dysfunction. Diabetes Care. 1999;22(9):1549–54.
155. Hsueh WA, Law RE. Cardiovascular risk continuum: implications of insulin resistance and diabetes. Am J Med. 1998;105(1A):4S–14.
156. Winer N, Sowers JR. Vascular compliance in diabetes. Curr Diab Rep. 2003;3(3):230–4.
157. Varsik P, et al. Is the spinal cord lesion rare in diabetes mellitus? Somatosensory evoked potentials and central conduction time in diabetes mellitus. Med Sci Monit. 2001;7(4):712–5.
158. Petrofsky JS, Prowse M, Lohman E. The influence of ageing and diabetes on skin and subcutaneous fat thickness in different regions of the body. J Appl Res Clin Exp Ther. 2008;8:55–61.
159. Montero D, et al. Vascular smooth muscle function in type 2 diabetes mellitus: a systematic review and meta-analysis. Diabetologia. 2013;56(10):2122–33.
160. Petrofsky JS, Bweir S, Lee S, Libarona M. Rosiglitazone improves age related reductions in forearm resting flows and endothelial dysfunction observed in type 2 diabetes. Diabetes. 2004;53:A141.
161. Puig T, et al. Some determinants of body weight, subcutaneous fat, and fat distribution in 25–64 year old Swiss urban men and woman. Soz Praventivmed. 1990;35(6):193–200.
162. Schwartz RS, et al. Body fat distribution in healthy young and older men. J Gerontol. 1990;45(6):M181–5.

Atopic Dermatitis in the Aged

74

Alexandra Katsarou, Melina C. Armenaka, Efterpi Zafiriou, and Efstratios Vakirlis

Contents

A. Katsarou (✉) • M.C. Armenaka
Department of Dermatology and Venereology, University of Athens, A. Sygros Hospital, Athens, Greece
e-mail: alkats.duoa@yahoo.gr; marmenak@auth.gr

E. Zafiriou
Department of Dermatology and Venereology, University of Thessaly, Larissa, Greece
e-mail: zafevi@hotmail.com

E. Vakirlis
Department of Dermatology and Venereology, Aristotle University of Thessaloniki, Thessaloniki, Greece
e-mail: svakirlis@hotmail.com

M.A. Farage et al. (eds.), *Textbook of Aging Skin*,
DOI 10.1007/978-3-662-47398-6_62

Abstract

Atopic dermatitis (AD) is an inflammatory, pruritic, and chronic, or chronically relapsing, skin disease occurring often in families with other atopic diseases. It occurs most frequently in infancy and childhood but also affects adults and elderly population (>65 years old). Over the last decades, the prevalence of AD increased substantially.

Adult AD includes patients with a persistent AD since childhood and those with a late-onset AD. Usually the disease exists for years, compromising quality of life, sex life, and occupational choices. The extrinsic type of AD is more common in adults than in children. Contact allergens and aeroallergens seem to play an important role in exacerbating AD. The disease is more frequent in females during the third decade, although in elderly patients (>65 years old), a male predominance is reported. Clinical features of AD differ characteristically according to the age of patients. In adults and senile patients, the disease (AD) often presents with atypical clinical manifestations, which sometimes make the diagnosis very difficult.

As we might be seeing more adults with AD in the future, there is a need for more studies in older patients, because until today a small number of manuscripts have been published on adult AD compared to the literature devoted to AD in children. In this chapter, the particular characteristics of AD in adult life such as epidemiology, quality of life, diagnostic criteria, clinical features, allergic triggers or irritating factors, pathogenesis, and treatment are discussed.

Introduction

Direct and indirect observations indicate that the prevalence of atopic dermatitis (AD) has increased two- to threefold over the last 30 years [1], especially in adult population. A possible explanation for this increase is a higher susceptibility to sensitization due to environmental factors and the "Western lifestyle." Two main hypotheses have been proposed: the "hygiene hypothesis," which suggests that a reduced exposure to pathogenic microorganisms results in increased susceptibility to atopic diseases [2, 3]. The second hypothesis (hapten-atopy hypothesis) proposes that increased exposure to chemicals generally, and to irritant/haptenic chemicals in particular, during critical periods of life, has also contributed to changes in the prevalence of atopic disease [4].

AD can be a very debilitating, persistent, and costly long-term disease [1]. According to a population-based survey of eczema prevalence in the USA, a substantial proportion of the population has symptoms of eczematous conditions, while 17.8 million met the empirical symptom criteria for AD [5]. Progress in understanding the epidemiology of AD has been slow due to the lack of suitable, uniformly used, simple disease diagnostic criteria that can be used in population surveys among different countries [1].

Atopic dermatitis affects mainly infants and children, but it can also affect adults and elderly subjects, too (>65 years old) [6]. According to many epidemiological studies, in the 1-year period prevalence measure, 5–20 % of children in developed countries are affected [1]. Many differences in the prevalence of AD, between countries and between urban and rural areas within the same country, are noted in the literature [1]. Studies on ethnic groups and migrants found a large increase in the prevalence of AD in immigrant children, as compared to their country of origin [1]. These results suggest that environmental factors and a Western lifestyle are the main causes in the development of AD. Atopic dermatitis also shows an important relationship to social class in children [1]. On the contrary, in adolescents and adults, no differences in social class over time were noted.

In the past 5 years, relatively more information about AD in adults has drawn the attention. Studies from the UK and Norway found that the prevalence in adults over 20 years old is approximately 2 %, and less than 0.2 % of adults over the age of 40 years are affected [1]. The lifetime prevalence of AD is considerably lower in the elderly, compared to younger adults [6]. Adults with a longer duration of school education appear to have a higher risk for atopic diseases [6]. AD in adolescence represents those with AD and/or a personal history of atopy since childhood and those with adult onset of AD or later (onset >18 years) [7]. A study from Thailand concerning adult-onset AD concluded that the disease is not rare in adults and develops mostly during the third decade of life. In 13.6 % of patients, the onset was after the age of 21 [8]. The prevalence of AD in Nigeria was 8.5 %, and 24.5 % of the patients had onset after age 21 years [9]. In another report of 2,604 patients attending a contact dermatitis clinic in Australia, 9 % suffered from AD which began for the first time after age 20, and the main sites were generalized involvement, hands and face [7]. According to a study in Japan [10] on senile-type AD (mean age, 76.5 ± 6.2 years), only 16 subjects were diagnosed with having AD of 66 possible cases from 4,100 hospital attendance cases for various types of eczema and dermatitis. In this age group, AD showed various types of eczematous lesions in the face and neck, extensor and flexure sites of extremities, with predominant clinical presentations of erythroderma (62.5 %) or unclassified chronic eczema (31.5 %). Mean age of onset was 67.7 ± 15.7 years. Fifty percent (8/16) had a personal history of chronic eczema until young adult phase and 18.8 % showed the classical course of child AD [10]. The disease in elderly patients (>65 years old) seems to be more frequent in males, although during the third decade, a female predominance is being reported [7, 10]. Among 259 adult patients with AD, after careful evaluation, only 5.4 % fulfilled the criteria of intrinsic (nonallergic) AD [11]. Lower serum IgE levels and antigen-specific IgE antibodies in healthy people and higher levels in younger AD patients were described. The extrinsic type of AD is more common in adults than in children [11]. Contact allergens and aeroallergens seem to play an important role in exacerbating AD, increasing with age in atopic patients [12, 13]. Based on these figures, the nature and relevance of the nonallergic form of AD in adults deserves further evaluation [11].

Another interesting point is the age distribution of AD. In a study in Japan, the percentage of AD in patients 0–9 years old dropped from 73.9 % in 1967 to 23.4 % by the year 1996. In contrast, the percentage of AD in the ages 20–29 increased remarkably from 3.1 % in 1967 to 38.7 % by the year 1996 [14, 15]. In a nationwide, cross-sectional, multicenter study in Japan (2007–2008), among 67,448 cases in dermatology clinics, AD was the second more frequent skin disorder. The incidence was 9.8 % (6,733). 9.6 % (649/6,733) of those subjects with AD were older than 46 years. In this study, the age distribution was diphasic; two peaks were seen at the ages 0–5 years and 21–35 years [15, 16].

Concerning the natural history of AD, one study suggests that 90 % of affected children will be clear of eczema within 10 years, but other studies noted that only 60 % of the children will be clear after the age of 16 and that 10 % of hospital-based patients suffer from AD in adult life [1]. In a study from Sweden, concerning the prognosis and prognostic factors in adult patients with AD, the majority of adults (59 %) with AD still had the disease after 25–38 years, when they were questioned [17]. The increased prevalence of AD in children and the fact that AD in most adults continues for many years point out that more adult and senile patients with AD are expected in the future [10, 12].

Quality of Life

Atopic dermatitis is one of the commonest chronic relapsing inflammatory dermatoses, with increasing worldwide prevalence and major social and financial implications for patients. The health-related quality of life (HRQOL) in children with chronic skin diseases is at least equal to that caused by many other chronic disorders of childhood, with AD and psoriasis having the greatest impact on HRQOL. In adults, severe chronic inflammatory skin diseases may be considered as severe as angina pectoris, chronic anxiety, rheumatoid arthritis, multiple sclerosis, or regional esophageal cancer [18]. Patients with AD have a significantly lower quality of life than the general population and healthy controls. Patients' mental health, social functioning, and emotional functioning seem to be more affected than physical functioning, and quality of life is compromised because of disturbed sleep and fatigue during the daytime [19]. Quality of life is affected in adult AD patients and relates both to disease severity and to mental components. Among a group of adult dermatology outpatients evaluated using the Dermatology Life Quality Index, those with AD were the highest scoring group compared to those with other skin diseases [20].

Concerning the degree of handicap in relation to the choice of education and occupation, 38 % of the respondents abstained from a specific education or job due to AD, and there were an increased number of sick leave days and early retirement pensions noted. Therefore, there are both personal and social consequences of AD [21]. A recent study has provided evidence that adults with 1-year history of eczema were associated with significantly higher odds of cardiovascular disease ($P \leq 0.02$); angina ($P \leq 0.02$); heart attack ($P \leq 0.047$), ($P < 0.0001$); and stroke ($P \leq 0.02$) [22]. Finally, a decrease in sexual desire due to AD was noted in 57.5 % of patients, while 36.5 % of partners reported that the appearance of eczema had an impact on their sex life.

Disease Subtypes, Clinical Features, Diagnostic Criteria, and Outcome Measurement

Subtypes of Atopic Dermatitis

Atopic dermatitis is an itchy, inflammatory, cutaneous manifestation of a systemic disorder that also includes asthma, allergic rhinitis, and food allergy. AD is an atopic disease, but all symptoms are not related to allergen exposure. Two subtypes of AD are distinguished: the "extrinsic type," associated with polyvalent IgE sensitization against inhalant and/or food allergens, and the "intrinsic type," without elevated IgE levels and no sensitization to inhalant or food allergens. Both forms of AD have the same clinical phenotype and associated eosinophilia. Discrimination between the two types is important, because sensitization correlates with more severe skin disease, and prevention and treatment are more complicated [23].

Intrinsic AD tends to have a late onset in childhood and a female predominance [23]. As previously mentioned, a recent investigation suggests that the intrinsic type of AD is a very rare entity in adults, and this raises the need to clarify the relevance of the intrinsic AD in aged patients [11]. According to a study from Japan involving 16 patients with senile AD, more than 65 years old, 12.5 % had intrinsic AD, based on serum IgE levels and antigen-specific IgE antibodies [10].

Clinical Features

AD usually starts in early childhood. The clinical picture and the distribution of the lesions vary depending on the age of the patient, the duration, and complications of eczema. No single diagnostic criterion exists for AD, but there are a multitude of major and minor features. Dry skin (xerosis) occurs in most atopic patients and is persistent. It is caused by reduced water content capacity of the stratum corneum and frequent irritation.

Pruritus is an important clinical symptom of AD and it is essential for the diagnosis of active disease. It is always present in all phases of AD and in all ages and can be very severe, often disrupting the sleep of patient. The mechanism of pruritus is not completely understood. Several mediators such as neuropeptides, proteases, cytokines, and nerve growth factor are associated with itch in AD.

In most cases of AD, typical, age-related, clinical features exist [24] (Figs. 1, 2, and 3).

Infantile phase (0–2 years). In most cases, AD starts within the first 3–6 months of life and is characterized by dry, erythematous, scaling areas, symmetrically located, on the cheeks, chin, and perioral and paranasal region, whereas infantile eczema tends to spare the diaper area. In more severe disease, vesicular and infiltrated plaques evolve that have a tendency for oozing and crust formation, and secondary infections may complicate the condition. Involvement of the hands, limb folds, upper trunk, arms, and legs is not unusual. The course of AD is relapsing, and, over time, the exudative character of dermatitis is lost.

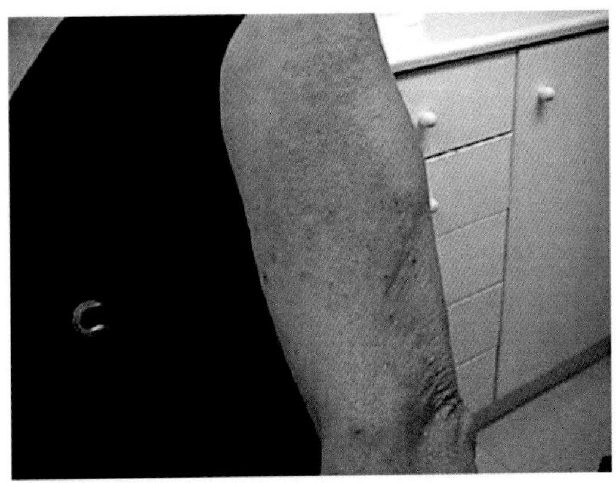

Fig. 1 Case 1. AD in a 62-year-old woman with a history of allergic rhinitis inflammation and lichenification is apparent in the extensor surface of the left arm

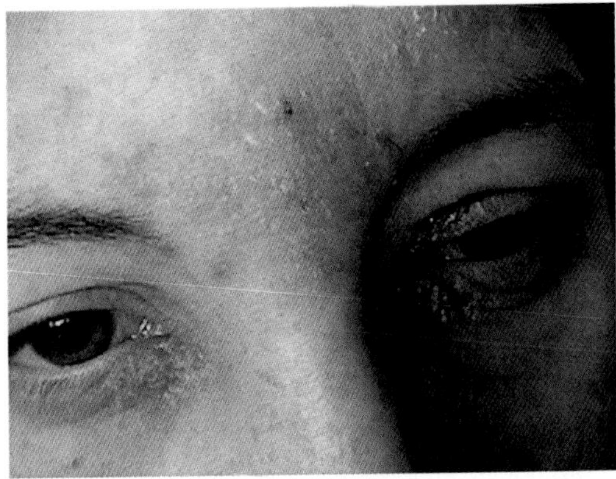

Fig. 2 Case 2. Inflammation around the eyes and face in a 34-year-old woman

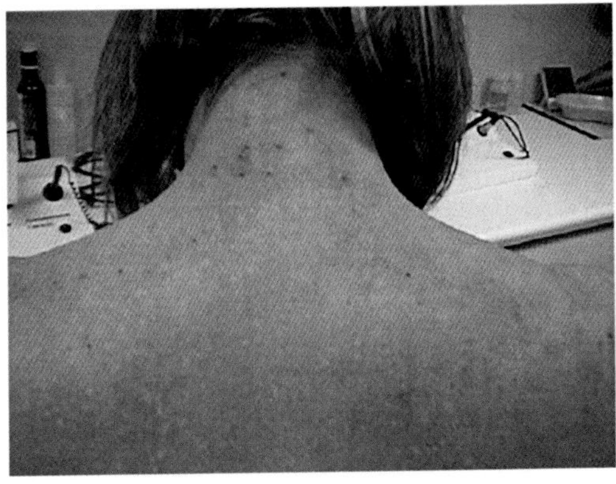

Fig. 3 Case 2. Lichenifications on the neck and upper back with postinflammatory diffuse hypo- and hyperpigmentation

Childhood phase (2–12 years). The inflammatory lesions are characteristically located on flexural areas and signs of lichenification appear. Very often, the clinical picture is polymorphous, due to the coexistence of chronic and acute types of eczema. Skin thickening, lichenification, and scratching due to persistent pruritus, acute erythema, with erosive or infected skin lesions, may affect the same area.

Adolescent and adult phase. The main findings in this age group are dry skin and eczema with lichenification affecting mainly the flexural and extensor areas, but also the face, shoulders, head, and neck, hand and foot dermatitis, and inflammation around the eyes. Especially the head and neck distribution is more commonly seen in adults than in children and occurs often without any history of childhood eczema [7, 12, 13]. A variety of clinical manifestations of acute phase (scaling plaques with vesicular erosive lesions) and chronic phase (lichenification), with persistent itching, coexist in most cases. In addition, a large proportion of adults with sensitive skin and/or irritant contact dermatitis affecting the hands had atopic eczema when they were children. In fact, the hands seem to be the most common site of AD in adulthood. The prevalence of hand dermatitis is two to ten times higher in atopics, and occupational irritants (daily exposure to water, chemicals, detergents) and domestic work favor the development of hand eczema.

Senile phase. Characteristics of AD in the senile phase remain unclear and clinical features resemble the adult phase, except that lichenification in the flexural areas is uncommon [10, 25]. Eczematous erythroderma and chronic unclassified eczema are also important clinical manifestations of AD in elderly subjects [26]. Aged patients showed a male dominance in senile AD with a man to woman ratio of 3:1 [10].

Patients suffering from AD very often present with atypical clinical manifestations that may be site specific (infra-auricular striae, atopic winter feet, cheilitis, hyperlinearity of palms and soles, etc.) or clinical morphology specific (follicular eruption, pityriasis alba, nummular eczema, keratosis pilaris, white dermographism, prurigo-like, etc.).

Several factors influence the course of AD, including climate, textiles, and sweating.

Climate. In most patients, eczema is aggravated during winter, probably due to decreased humidity. Change from a subarctic to a subtropical climate improves skin symptoms and quality of life in patients with AD.

Textiles. Wool and synthetic fabrics cause irritation and itching.

Day care attendance. Patients are also sensitive to irritation from detergents and many chemicals.

Sweating is a cause of itching and exacerbation of eczema.

Unfavorable prognostic factors for AD are persistent dry or itchy skin, widespread dermatitis, associated allergic rhinitis, family history of AD, asthma, early age of onset, and female sex [17]. Follow-up studies in adults with AD showed that the severity of eczema decreases over the years. Poor prognostic factors predicting a persisting eczema for a long time are head and neck eczema, high values of total IgE, and a long duration of eczema [27, 28].

Diagnostic Criteria and Outcome Measurements

No reliable biomarkers are available for the diagnosis of AD. The diagnosis of AD depends on clinical features and personal or family history of the patient concerning atopic disease. As the clinical manifestations are numerous, many diagnostic criteria are used in order to confirm the diagnosis. The Hanifin and Rajka diagnostic criteria have been most extensively validated from 1980, and they propose four major and 23 minor diagnostic criteria for AD [29]. A diagnosis is established if three of the major and three or more of the minor criteria occur in the patient. A refinement of Hanifin and Rajka criteria, these so-called UK diagnostic criteria were introduced in 1997 by Williams et al. The UK criteria for AD consist of one mandatory (pruritus/itching) and three or more minor criteria (*for children* $\geq$*4 years and adults*): (1) history of itchiness in skin creases, (2) personal history of asthma or allergic rhinitis, (3) personal history of general dry skin in the last year, (4) visible flexural dermatitis, and (5) onset under age 2 years [30]. In a systemic review which summarizes the evidence concerning the validity of diagnostic criteria, the authors concluded that the UK diagnostic criteria are the most extensively validated [31].

Although, in many cases, the minor cutaneous atopy signs are not present and atopic mucous manifestations are not associated, these criteria cannot be satisfactory, especially when AD starts after adolescence.

As mentioned before, the presentation of AD may vary widely in adults and elderly subjects, making the diagnosis not often easy (straightforward). Several other conditions can mimic AD in this age group, like other eczematous inflammatory skin diseases (contact dermatitis, seborrheic dermatitis, psoriasis, lichen simplex chronicus, etc.), immunologic disorders (dermatitis herpetiformis, pemphigus foliaceus, etc.), malignant diseases (cutaneous T-cell lymphoma, histiocytosis X, etc.), immunodeficiencies, metabolic diseases (phenylketonuria, zinc deficiency, pyridoxine (vitamin B6) and niacin deficiency, etc.)), infections (*Candida*, dermatophytes, scabies, etc.), nonallergic or allergic reactions to medications, etc. These conditions should be considered or excluded before making a diagnosis of AD [32]. Especially in those subjects with late onset of AD where AD arises de novo, the extension of the lesions is limited and the presentation atypical, but also, in cases of treatment failure, the dermatologist should reconsider and investigate the diagnosis of AD in each patient [28].

A scoring system developed by the European Task Force on Atopic Dermatitis (SCORing Atopic Dermatitis – SCORAD) is one of the best outcome measurements for atopic eczema. While Hanifin's and Rajka's criteria are useful for differential diagnosis, SCORAD is used to evaluate the severity of disease in clinical and epidemiological studies. It takes into account the extent of skin lesions, the severity of the clinical features, and the subjective symptoms [33].

Pathogenesis

Atopic eczema is a multifactorial chronic inflammatory skin disease with a complex background that is characterized by genetic influences, skin barrier dysfunction, and immune deviation with hyperreactivity to environmental stimuli and deficient antimicrobial immunity. Whether skin inflammation is initiated by skin barrier abnormalities (outside-inside hypothesis), or the primary immune dysregulation causes secondary skin barrier defects (inside-outside hypothesis), remains to be elucidated.

Genetics of Atopic Dermatitis

The evolution of atopic dermatitis is influenced by genetic and environmental factors. AD is a complex genetic disorder, and the mode of inheritance and the genes involved are not clear [34, 35]. The evidence for a strong genetic influence in the course of AD comes initially from twin studies. The difference in concordance rates between monozygous and dizygous twins gives an indication of the heritability of the disorder [34]. Segregation analysis indicates that the inheritance of AD does not fit a simple Mendelian pattern, and more than one gene is responsible for the evolution of the disease. The major histocompatibility complex (MHC) has certainly been implicated, and the cluster of interleukins on human chromosome 5 plays an important interactive role in the final expression of atopy, asthma, and atopic eczema [35]. Several genetic studies suggest a linkage between AD and the filaggrin gene, located on the epidermal differentiation complex 1q21 [36]. Loss-of-function mutations in the filaggrin gene FLG are major risk factors for atopic dermatitis. A case-control study reported that FLG mutations were associated with atopic dermatitis occurring at an early age (<8 years), but not with atopic dermatitis developing in late childhood or adulthood [37]. In addition, homozygous FLG mutations appear to be associated with hand and foot dermatitis during adulthood, in patients with history of atopic dermatitis [38]. Many other genes, such as SPINK5 gene, which encodes the protease inhibitor LEKTI, have been found in patients with atopic dermatitis, including genes involved in the formation of the skin barrier or in immune regulation. Recent genetic advances, with high-throughput methods for gene identification, such as DNA microarrays and whole-genome genotyping, will help further dissect this complex trait [34].

Skin Barrier Function in Atopic Dermatitis

The epidermis is the first line of defense between the body and the environment. The human skin consists of two sets of barriers: stratum corneum and tight junctions. The most common symptoms in patients with AD are itching and dry skin, involving both lesional and non-lesional skin. The skin barrier is known to be damaged in patients with AD. There is a four- to eightfold increase in transepidermal water loss (TEWL) in clinically active dermatitis and a two- to fivefold increase in TEWL in clinically uninvolved skin [39]. Since today four causes of xerosis of the skin have been reported: (a) decrease in skin ceramides; (b) alterations of the stratum corneum pH; (c) overexpression of proteases, including kallikreins and chymases; and (d) defect in filaggrin [40].

Many studies have focused on altered content of stratum corneum lipids, as the etiology of barrier permeability dysfunction. Ceramides comprise more than 50 % of the lipids and serve as the major water-retaining molecules in the extracellular space of the cornified envelope. They ensure that the skin barrier is as tight as possible [41]. Reduction of ceramides has been found in lesional and non-lesional skin of patients with AD. In particular, reduction in ceramides 1 and 3 correlated with barrier dysfunction. A possible explanation for this is that sphingomyelin metabolism is altered in AD, resulting in decreased synthesis of ceramides, and/or that the skin of patients with AD is colonized by ceramidase-secreting bacteria, which may contribute to the ceramide deficiency in the stratum corneum [41]. A normal-appearing aged skin is also deficient in ceramide, as compared with that of the younger, healthy controls [42]. These findings indicate that the decrease in stratum corneum lipids, especially ceramides, is a major etiologic factor for atopic dry skin and a primary event in the evolution of aged skin [41, 42].

A deficit of n-6 essential fatty acids (linoleic acid, γ-linolenic acid, columbinic acid) can lead to an inflammatory skin condition [41]. In AD, concentrations of linoleic acid tend to be elevated, but concentrations of linoleic acid metabolites are reduced, due to reduced conversion of linoleic acid to γ-linolenic acid. The oral administration of gamma-linolenic acid seems to improve atopic eczema.

Furthermore, increased skin pH in AD enhances the action of proteases that cause breakdown of the skin barrier [41]. Soaps and detergents also increase the skin pH.

Recent studies have identified mutations in the stratum corneum chymotryptic enzyme (SCCE) protease gene in patients with AD [41]. The most likely consequence of this alteration in the SCCE gene is to produce higher levels of SCCE protease. Proteases cause premature breakdown of corneodesmosomes, basic for the structural integrity of the stratum corneum, leading to a thin skin barrier and increased penetration of irritants, microbes, and allergens [41]. Washing with soap and detergents and long-term application of topical corticosteroids additionally increase production of SCCE.

Several other genetic variations that affect skin barrier function occur in AD [41]. Null mutations in the epidermal barrier protein filaggrin gene, resident in the epidermal differentiation complex, have recently been identified as an important predisposing factor for eczema [36]. This finding has important clinical and therapeutic significance, because it is often the earliest sign of the atopic march and confirms the importance of epidermal barrier disruption as a primary event in the evolution of the disease. Filaggrin mutations are found in more than 50 % of individuals with eczema and may indicate poor prognosis in AD, predisposing to eczema that persists into adulthood and extrinsic eczema [36].

Skin barrier, besides corneocytes, intercellular lipid lamellae, and corneodesmosomes, is also composed of tight junctions in upper stratum granulosum. The role of tight junctions in AD is unknown. The impaired skin barrier function may contribute to the increased penetration of microbes and antigens and to cutaneous hyperreactivity with increased susceptibility to irritants [41]. Genetic abnormalities in skin barrier function are associated with protein allergy in AD patients, because Langerhans cells take up antigen easily from the damaged skin barrier and lead to the release of epidermal-derived mediators, resulting in a T helper type 2 response [43]. Well-documented studies prove that the degree of epidermal barrier disruption correlates with the severity of dermatitis [41]. According to a recent study, the higher the TEWL in AD, the higher is the prevalence of sensitization to environmental airborne allergens. These data suggest the major role of epidermal barrier function in the pathogenesis of AD.

Immune Responses in Atopic Dermatitis

Complex immunologic responses are involved in eczematous skin inflammation, while deficient immunity against microorganisms leads to increased skin infections.

Immune Responses Leading to Skin Inflammation

In atopic dermatitis, complex interactions between immune cells and their products, cytokines and chemokines, lead to a combination of immediate immune responses and delayed cellular immune responses in the inflamed skin [44]. This is reflected in the histopathology of AD.

Histopathology. Acute skin lesions are characterized by epidermal intercellular edema (spongiosis) and an epidermal and dermal perivascular cell infiltrate in which activated memory CD4+ T cells predominate [44]. Antigen-presenting cells bearing IgE molecules are present and mast cell degranulation is evident. Chronic lichenified lesions are characterized by epidermal hyperplasia and dermal infiltration that is dominated by macrophages, IgE-bearing Langerhans cells, activated T cells, and eosinophils [44]. Collagen deposition in the dermis is induced by skin repair cytokines, such as interleukin 11.

The Acute Phase of Inflammation

T-cell deviation and altered cytokine and chemokine levels play an important role in AD [45]. The acute inflammatory phase is dominated by T helper cell type 2 (Th2) cytokine responses. Activated memory Th2 cells that express cutaneous lymphocyte antigen (CLA) are increased in skin lesions and in the peripheral blood of AD patients and correlate with disease severity [44]. CLA is acquired in local lymph nodes after the interaction of skin tissue-draining dendritic cells and enables cells to home in to the skin from the circulation [44, 45]. Activated Th2 cells produce interleukins 4 and 13 (IL4, IL13) that stimulate B cells to produce specific IgE antibodies while downregulating T helper type 1 (Th1) responses. They also produce IL5, an important cytokine for eosinophil development, activation, and survival [44]. The IgE antibodies bind to corresponding receptors in skin immune cells, resulting in the release of histamine and other pro-inflammatory mediators.

Dendritic cells play a pivotal role in the acute sensitization phase. Langerhans cells (LCs) migrate to regional lymph nodes and prime naive T cells to expand the pool of Th2 cells [44]. In addition, LCs expressing the high-affinity IgE receptor (FcεRI) and bearing IgE are increased in AD lesions and must be present in order to provoke eczematous lesions by the topical application of allergen [45].

On the other hand, regulatory T cells (Tregs) that should play a role in suppressing T-cell responses to allergens are absent in the skin and have a reduced suppressive capacity in AD [45]. Despite a "regulatory phenotype," activated CD4 + CD25 + Tregs promote Th2 responses in AD patients.

Environmental airborne allergens, food allergens, products of infectious pathogens, and scratching can induce Th2 immune responses and the production of specific IgE antibodies in patients with AD [44, 45]. Skin damage, caused by scratching, can lead to the production of IgE antibodies against human skin proteins [44, 45]. Such autoantibodies are found in up to 80 % of AD patients during early childhood, as compared to 25 % of adult patients [45].

The Chronic Phase of Inflammation

In chronic AD lesions, T helper type 1 responses are more dominant than T helper type 2 responses, resulting in cellular immune responses or delayed-type hypersensitivity responses. Interferon-γ (IFN-γ), produced by activated Th1 cells, predominates in chronic skin lesions. Levels of IL5, IL12, and granulocyte-macrophage colony-stimulating factor (GM-CSF) are also increased [44]. Keratinocytes, stimulated by IFN-γ, release high levels of chemokines, including RANTES, that lead to further recruitment of T cells, dendritic cells, and eosinophils to the skin [44, 45].

It has been shown that the local production of IL12 in the skin, by antigen-presenting cells and eosinophils, induces differentiation of Th1 cells and causes the phenotype "switch" from Th2 (acute phase) to Th1 (chronic phase) [45]. Moreover, infectious pathogens can directly promote chronic eczema by inducing Th1 immune responses [46].

Antimicrobial Immune Defense

Atopic skin is characterized by decreased ability to eliminate pathogens, as a result of defective innate and acquired immunity. As part innate immunity, keratinocytes and professional antigen-presenting cells in the skin are activated by the recognition of molecular patterns derived from microorganisms [46]. Activation involves action on Toll-like receptors (TLRs) and leads to the production of antimicrobial peptides through a vitamin D-dependent mechanism. Antimicrobial peptides have broad antimicrobial activity against viruses, bacteria, and yeast [45, 46]. In AD, the production of antimicrobial peptides, such as β-defensins and the cathelicidin LL-37, is decreased in the skin [46]. This defect is probably acquired and results from the Th2 cytokine milieu in the skin. Since vitamin D is involved in this defense pathway, it is possible that low vitamin D levels, often found in older populations, might increase susceptibility to infections. Finally, it appears that acquired immunity requires robust Th1 immune responses in order to eliminate microorganisms that come in contact with the skin, whereas Th1 responses to invading microbes are decreased in AD [46].

Skin Microbiome

The skin is not only our first line of defense against foreign invaders, but it is also colonized by a superficial ecosystem composed of nonpathogenic microorganisms, which are known as "skin microbiota" and include bacteria, virus, archaea, and fungi [47]. Skin bacterial microbiome is highly dependent on sampled skin site and the age of the human [48]. Recent findings also suggest a complex interplay between our cutaneous immune system and the microbiome [49].

Atopic dermatitis flares are associated with colonization and infections with *Staphylococcus aureus* and with shifts in the skin microbiome. Kong et al. [50] recently reported that in a pediatric population of AD patients, temporal shifts in the skin microbiota occur over three disease stages, baseline, flare, and after treatment. Lesional skin bacterial diversity decreased during the flare stage, and *S. aureus* was increased during disease flares rather than at baseline or posttreatment and correlated with the deterioration of disease severity. These findings reveal linkages between microbial communities and inflammatory diseases such as AD [50].

Treatments focusing on modulating skin microbiome represent a novel therapeutic strategy of AD. Cutaneous application of an emollient cream containing nonpathogenic bacteria can alleviate inflammation, regulate immune responses, reduce *Staphylococcus* population, and enhance the microbiome biodiversity in lesional skin [51].

Environmental Triggers of Atopic Dermatitis

Important environmental factors that trigger disease exacerbations are food allergens, airborne allergens, microorganisms, skin irritants, contact allergens, and psychological stress.

Foods and Airborne Allergens

Atopic dermatitis is associated with hypersensitivity to foods and/or common airborne allergens. Sensitization increases after early infancy and remains high throughout adult life [45]. According to a study from Japan, allergen-specific IgE antibodies to various inhalant allergens and/or food allergens occur in 87.5 % of elderly patients with senile AD [10].

Food Allergens

In early life, AD is associated with a much higher frequency of food than aeroallergen sensitization [44]. Food allergy causes skin rashes in 40 % of children with eczema, but approximately one third of children outgrow their food allergy after 1–2 years of avoidance [44]. The role of food allergy declines sharply with aging [52, 53]. A large population-based study of adolescents and adults with AD found that food allergy was not clinically important in this age group [52]. However, adult AD patients with persistent, more severe disease are more likely to be sensitized to foods [10, 53].

Sensitized individuals can react to oral food challenges with three clinical patterns: (a) immediate hypersensitivity reactions (urticaria, angioedema, and erythema) occur within a few minutes, (b) soon after ingestion, pruritus leads to exacerbation of eczema, and (c) late eczematous reactions occur after 6–48 h [53]. Combined noneczematous and eczematous reactions may also be seen.

Cow's milk, hen's eggs, wheat, soy, peanuts, tree nuts, and shellfish account for 90 % of food allergic reactions in children and young adults with AD in the USA [53]. Foods cross-reacting to birch pollen (apple, carrot, celery, hazelnut) can trigger AD in adults sensitized to birch, even in the absence of a suspicious history [53]. Studies in German adults documented clinically relevant allergy to pollen-associated foods in a subgroup of birch-sensitized AD patients [52, 53].

In adult AD patients with a positive milk provocation challenge, milk-specific IgE was found in less than half of the patients [53]. Atopy patch tests (APTs), using topically applied food, can elicit late eczematous reactions in some of these patients. A good correlation between positive patch tests and late reactions to ingested foods has been shown in some studies, although other studies show a high rate of false-positive patch test reactions [53].

Finally, certain foods (alcohol, food additives) may cause exacerbations of eczema through nonimmune mechanisms, by acting as irritants or pseudoallergens [54]. Clinical improvement was found in 63 % of adult patient after 6 weeks on a low pseudoallergen diet [54].

Aeroallergens

Sensitization to airborne allergens usually develops at about 3–4 years of age and continues to be important in atopic adults [55]. Adult patients with persisting, severe atopic dermatitis are highly sensitized to aeroallergens, as demonstrated by skin prick tests. The highest amount of serum total IgE and aeroallergen-specific IgE has been found in AD, compared with other atopic diseases, while no significant age-related decrease is observed in aging adults [55, 56].

Important airborne allergens are dust mite, animal dander, grass, birch, molds, and cockroach. Pruritic skin lesions can develop after inhalation or skin exposure to these allergens in sensitized individuals [55]. The eczematous skin reaction that results from topical application of airborne allergens using modified patch testing (atopy patch tests) is similar to atopic eczema and is characterized by skin barrier disruption, cellular infiltration, and cytokine release [55]. Aeroallergens elicit atopy patch tests (APTs) in 30–50 % of AD patients, whereas positive reactions are uncommon in other atopic diseases [35, 55]. In a study involving 115 adults with AD, 54 % demonstrated positive APT to least one aeroallergen, compared to 6 % of healthy controls [57].

Strong evidence favors a causal role of dust mites in atopic dermatitis [55]. In addition to being airborne, they parasitize the skin and release exogenous proteases that can directly damage the epidermal skin barrier [41, 55]. In senile AD, dust mite was found to be the most important allergen, and elevated mite-specific serum IgE levels occurred in 86 % of patients [10]. Furthermore, the positivity of mite atopy patch tests is 45 % in adults with AD [57]. Finally, avoidance of dust mites has been shown to be clinically beneficial in mite-sensitive AD patients [35, 55].

Microorganisms

In AD, skin barrier dysfunction, either resulting from a genetic defect or acquired by scratching and environmental influences, facilitates the increased penetration of microbes and their products [58]. Decreased antimicrobial immunity predisposes patients to develop bacterial skin infections (impetigo, paronychias), localized viral infections (herpes simplex, warts, mollusca contagiosa), or disseminated viral infections (eczema herpeticum, eczema molluscatum, and eczema vaccinatum) and fungal skin infections by *Trichophyton rubrum* and *Candida albicans* [45, 46]. Acute infections can cause AD flares, by several immune mechanisms, including stimulating IL12 production that induces allergen-specific Th2 cells home to the skin [46]. Furthermore, colonization of the skin by *Staphylococcus aureus* and the opportunistic yeast *Malassezia* spp. is very frequently found in AD [59]. Experimental evidence supports the fact that these colonizing skin pathogens can lead to eczematous skin inflammation and may be responsible for treatment failures [59].

Skin colonization with *S. aureus* is detected in more than 90 % of patient with AD and only in 5 % of healthy controls [59]. Colonization rates are high in adults and they are associated with the severity of eczema [59]. Of the strains isolated from skin lesions, 30–60 % secrete *S. aureus* enterotoxins, with superantigen properties, that cause a vigorous immune response and can exacerbate AD by promoting Th2 responses and IgE production [46, 59]. The levels of superantigen-specific IgE antibodies correlate with eczema activity [59]. *S. aureus* superantigens and alpha toxin also promote Th1 responses that contribute to the development of chronic eczema [46, 59]. Finally, proteinases produced by *S. aureus* can directly damage the skin barrier [41, 59].

Skin-colonizing *Malassezia* spp. yeasts (Pityrosporum) are found in up to 90 % of patients with AD, compared to 34 % in healthy controls, and they sensitize 30–80 % of patients with extrinsic and intrinsic types of eczema [59]. In a study of the affects of aging, anti-*Malassezia* IgE antibodies were found more often in adults, compared to children with AD [60]. A high incidence of positive patch test reactions to *Malassezia* is seen in AD, especially in adults with head and neck eczema [59].

Finally, observations support that decreasing skin colonization, with antibiotics or antifungal treatments, decreases the severity of skin lesions [59]. However, this beneficial clinical effect is only short-lived and recolonization occurs.

Water, Skin Irritants, and Contact Allergens

Water hardness may be important in AD. According to an ecological study, water hardness acts on existing dermatitis by exacerbating the disease or prolonging its duration, rather than as a cause of new cases [1].

Atopic skin is known to be prone to react to irritants [35, 41]. In daily life, soaps, detergents, and excessive washing can induce flares of AD and predispose to the development of irritant hand dermatitis [41]. Irritants can act synergistically with allergens to increase skin inflammation in patients with AD [61]. The consecutive application of the irritant sodium lauryl sulfate and aeroallergens on the skin of sensitized atopic adults led to a more severe barrier disruption than the application of each component alone [61].

Due to skin barrier dysfunction, contact allergens can penetrate the skin more easily, and according to a recent study of unselected adults in Norway, AD was a risk factor for allergic contact sensitization [62]. The number of positive contact allergens increases with age in atopic patients [63]. At least one positive patch test to a standard series has been found in approximately 40 % of AD patients [64]. The most common contact allergens were nickel, cobalt, fragrances, and rubber.

Atopic dermatitis is the most common cause of occupational dermatitis and doubles the risk of developing irritant dermatitis in some occupations, particularly those involving wet work, although abrasive hand cleaners and greases also contribute [44, 65]. Occupational exposure to irritants, or to contact allergens, can induce the appearance of widespread eczema in atopic patients in whom eczema was quiescent for years or was never present. Eczema can persist even after removal from the high-risk occupation. Preemployment counseling of adolescents and adults with atopic eczema is crucial, so that they can make correct decisions on their future occupation [65].

Psychological Factors

Patients with AD often suffer from stress-related exacerbations, exhaustion, depression, anxiety, and helplessness [66]. Many studies have explored the personality type of patients. Atopic dermatitis patients have been described as anxious, emotionally unstable, tense, and perfectionist, but, finally, it appears that there is no specific personality type unique to AD, and patients tend to suppress emotions [66].

Neuropeptides, endogenous opioids, and serotonin, released after stress challenge, have also been associated with itching [66]. Neuropeptides in the skin act directly on blood vessel walls and act indirectly, as mediators of inflammation, by inducing release of cytokines from mast cells and endothelial cells, and as immunomodulators via corticotropin-releasing hormone.

Observations that psychological stress may induce AD flares can be explained by studies showing that stress favors a shift in immunity toward a T helper type 2 cell allergic response [66]. Additionally, patients with AD appear to have an inherited hypothalamic deficiency that impairs normal hypothalamic–pituitary–adrenal axis function [66]. Gender differences in response to stress may implicate the hypothalamic–pituitary–gonadal pathway, since female hormones generally enhance inflammation [66]. Skin barrier function is also altered by stress, by means of increased cortisol levels that cause decreased lamellar body secretion and downregulation of epidermal expression of antimicrobial peptides [41]. Psychologic and stress-reduction interventions have shown to improve patient well-being and significantly improve skin manifestations [66].

Table 1 Diagnostic tests for evaluating allergy in AD

IgE mediated (immediate)
Total serum IgE
Specific serum IgE (aeroallergens, foods, human proteins/autoallergens, *S. aureus* enterotoxins, *Malassezia*)
Skin prick tests (aeroallergens, foods)
Oral provocation challenges (foods)
T-cell mediated (delayed)
Atopy patch tests (aeroallergens, foods, *Malassezia*)
Standard patch tests (standard series, occupational series, medicaments)
Modified oral provocation challenges (foods)

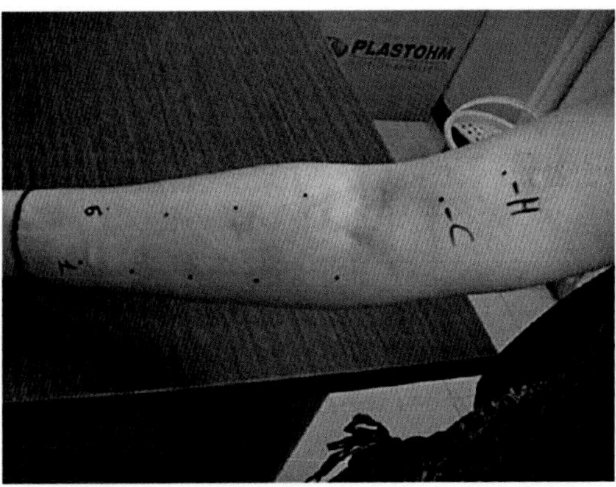

Fig. 4 Prick tests to a panel of aeroallergens applied to the forearm. Positive reactions show a local wheal and flare (*H* histamine, *C* negative control)

Diagnostic Tests

Elevations of eosinophil levels and total and allergen-specific serum IgE levels are common in AD and are associated with more severe dermatitis [41]. Diagnostic tests for evaluating allergy in AD are summarized in Table 1. Sensitization to allergens can be demonstrated by measurement of allergen-specific IgE antibody determination in the serum (RAST, ImmunoCAP) and by skin prick tests [35]. If skin tests are used (Fig. 4), it is important to have in mind that skin reactivity to histamine (a positive control) begins to decrease significantly after the age of 50 and reaches a plateau after the age of 60 [67].

The induction of a local eczematous reaction after application of the allergen using atopy patch tests (APTs) is another important tool for detecting relevant allergens in AD. APTs should be applied to intact, untreated skin of the back for 48 h and read at 48 and 72 h [68]. They have been shown to be reproducible for dust mite and other aeroallergens (Fig. 5), using petrolatum as a vehicle [68]. An aeroallergen panel is now commercially available. APTs can also be used for food allergy testing, preferably using freshly made extracts, since food allergens are often unstable [53]. Recently, *Malassezia* has been used in investigational units [35, 44]. The demonstration of a positive APT reaction can reinforce the need for allergen avoidance and this can lead to significant clinical improvement.

The diagnosis of eczematous reactions to foods in patients with AD requires oral provocation challenges to prove the clinical relevance of history, positive skin prick tests, positive food-specific

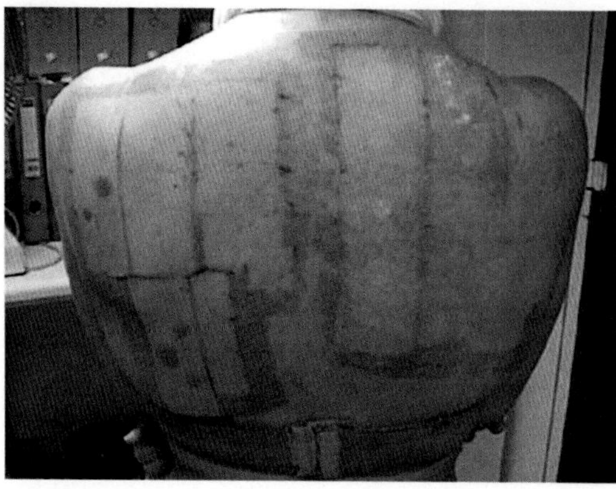

Fig. 5 Patch test results read at 72 h in a patient with AD. An irritant reaction to hypoallergenic adhesive tape is evident. The *right half* of the photo corresponds to the area of the back where aeroallergens (atopy patch tests) were applied and there are no significant reactions. The *left half* corresponds to standard patch tests. The basic European set (*upper left*) showed a (++) reaction to colophony 20 %, while positive reactions to three allergens in the cosmetic panel were also seen (*lower left*)

IgE, or atopy patch tests [53]. Because food-induced eczema usually needs more than 6 h to develop and may require repeated ingestion, oral challenge protocols need to be modified, or else positive reactions may be missed [53]. Patients should be observed for longer than 1 day after each challenge [53]. Furthermore, a diagnostic elimination diet, lasting 4–6 weeks, is often recommended, whereas in older patients, individually tailored diet with foods that rarely cause food allergy or "pseudoallergy" can be used [53, 54].

Finally, patch testing with a standard series of contact allergens and occupational series depending on workplace exposure may be helpful (Fig. 5). Adult patients unresponsive to topical treatment should also be tested for contact sensitization to topical medicaments [34].

Treatment

AD is a chronic relapsing inflammatory skin disease of childhood but also of adult life. The successful approach to the management of AD requires a combination of simultaneous multiple actions and treatments to prevent, identify, and eliminate trigger factors and to improve skin barrier function.

General Measures and Basic Treatment

The education of the patient and/or their families and the communication between the doctor and patient are a very important part of successful management of AD. Recommendations and instructions must be written step by step. The avoidance of specific triggering factors (aeroallergens, foods, contact allergens) and nonspecific triggers (contact irritants, soaps, prolonged hot-water showers, environment with low humidity, wool and synthetic clothing, perfumes, makeup) is indicated for all patients and all types of AD. The prevention of stress, anxiety, and depression is also very important, and the support of a psychologist in many patients is proposed [35].

Topical Treatment

Topical treatment comprises the foundation of AD treatment and is indispensable for all patients suffering from AD.

Emollients

They help restore and preserve the stratum corneum barrier and also decrease itching and the need for topical treatment. Emollients should be applied continuously, even if no active inflammation is evident. Ointments are the most occlusive. Urea-containing moisturizers improve skin barrier function and reduce skin susceptibility to irritants, whereas salicylic acid can be added to an emollient for the treatment of chronic hyperkeratotic lesions. Formulations containing lipids identical to those of stratum corneum, in particular, ceramide supplementation, could better improve the dysfunctional barrier. Emollients must be applied several times daily and should be continued long after other topical treatments have been stopped. Folliculitis is a side effect when the occlusive action is pronounced, and, in this case, the emollient must be changed.

Topical Steroids

Topical steroids have been the cornerstone of treatment of AD for more than 50 years and are still an important tool for the management of AD, especially for acute flares. A large number of topical corticosteroids are in use, ranging from high to low potency of action. Topical steroids should be applied no more than twice daily, as short-time therapy for the acute phase of AD. Many therapeutic schemes are used in order to obtain the optimal therapeutic effect. Intermittent use might be as effective as initial therapy with a high-potency steroid, followed by a time-dependent dose reduction or a change over to a lower potency preparation [24, 35]. Despite their widespread use, side effects are not very frequent for low- to medium-potency topical steroids, although 72.5 % of people worry about using topical corticosteroids on their own or their child's skin [69].

Ultra-high and high-potency topical corticosteroids are used for short-term treatment of lichenified areas in adult patients. To prevent tachyphylaxis, side effects, and rebound phenomena, it is proposed to use them once daily, in combination with frequent application of emollients for the first weeks and then alternate day use is recommended.

Wet-wrap dressings, using diluted steroids and/or emollients, are very effective as a very short-term therapy for acute erythrodermic dermatitis, therapy-resistant AD, and intolerable pruritus [70].

Topical Calcineurin Inhibitors (TCIs)

Pimecrolimus and tacrolimus are the two available calcineurin inhibitors with steroid-free, anti-inflammatory, and immunomodulatory effects [35]. They act by inhibiting inflammatory cytokine transcription in activated T cells and other inflammatory cells via inhibition of calcineurin. Their action is more specific than corticosteroids in the inflammatory process, and they are not associated with skin atrophy and thinning, striae, glaucoma, and other steroid-related side effects. They can be used on the face, eyelids, neck, and any other area with sensitive and thin skin. The most common side effect is a burning sensation of the skin of short duration, related to the skin barrier dysfunction. According to many clinical trials, no evidence of systemic toxicity or local and systemic skin infections has been noted. However, it is recommended to minimize exposure to UVR and to use sun-protective agents. The early use of topical calcineurin inhibitor can lead to better long-term disease control, with fewer flares and less need for topical corticosteroid rescue therapy. Tacrolimus ointment is more effective than pimecrolimus cream in adults with moderate to severe AD, but both agents have a similar safety profile [71].

Finally, combined topical therapy, with corticosteroids and TCI, is proposed by many practitioners, because the two classes have different and possibly complementary mechanisms of action. The recent guidelines of International Consensus Conference on AD recommend corticosteroids for acute control of disease progression and as intermittent treatment in maintenance therapy with TCIs. Proactive, intermittent use of TCIs as maintenance therapy (two to three times per week) is recommended to prevent relapses, reducing the need of corticosteroids, and is more effective than the use of emollients alone [72, 73].

Topical Antimicrobials

To decrease the bacterial and fungal load on involved and uninvolved skin, topical antiseptics, such as triclosan, chlorhexidine, and antifungals, such as ketoconazole shampoo, have been shown to be effective and can be topically used, added to bath water or to bath emollient.

According to many studies, exacerbations of AD are the result of bacterial infections and superinfections, especially to *S. aureus*. Topical antibiotics, alone or in combination with corticosteroids, are effective in mild and localized forms. Fucidin is the most popular topical antimicrobial agent in many countries, with good skin penetration, but long-term therapy results in drug resistance [35]. According to the recommendations of the AAD 2014 about the use of topical antimicrobials and antiseptic for the treatment of AD, except for bleach baths with intranasal mupirocin, no topical antistaphylococcal treatment has been shown to be clinically helpful in patients with AD and is not routinely recommended. Bleach baths and intranasal mupirocin may be recommended to reduce disease activity in patient with moderate to severe AD and clinical signs of secondary bacterial infection [74].

Systemic Treatment

Antihistamines

Sedating antihistamines are effective for reducing itching, and combinations of antihistamines sometimes are needed for better itch control.

Antimicrobial Treatment

Antibiotics are indicated for widespread bacterial infection, especially of *S. aureus*. Clarithromycin, cephalosporins, or semisynthetic penicillins used for 7–10 days are effective, but it has been shown that recolonization occurs soon after treatment [35]. The increased prevalence of antibiotic resistance of *S. aureus* is now recognized as a growing problem in patients with AD [46]. Antimicrobial peptides promise to play an alternative role to conventional antimicrobials. Systemic antiviral agents are very important in the case of herpes simplex viral infections.

Systemic Corticosteroids

Short courses of oral steroids in cases of acute flare-ups are indicated (20–40 mg of prednisolone/adult dose) [24]. Very gradual decrease of the steroid dose may also diminish the possibility of rebound phenomenon. Long-term oral corticosteroid therapy is associated with many well-known side effects.

Cyclosporin A (CyA)

CyA in vivo inhibits calcineurin-dependent pathways and reduces cytokines (IL2, IFN-γ). In cases of severe AD, CyA is effective, but due to possible side effects, particularly renal toxicity and high blood pressure, it should be used in limited patients. Serum creatinine and blood pressure levels must be performed at regular intervals. According to a recent systemic review, concerning systemic treatment in patients with severe AD, in eleven studies CyA effectiveness was shown [75]. These studies demonstrated decreased severity of AD, a dose-related response was found, and effectiveness was similar in adults and children, although tolerability was better in children. The lowest effective dose should be administered for the shortest treatment period, in order to minimize side effects.

Azathioprine

Due to late onset of action and side effects (myelosuppression, hepatotoxicity, immunosuppression), treatment with azathioprine in AD patients is very limited [75].

Phototherapy and Photochemotherapy

Phototherapy is a well-established second-line treatment for adult and adolescent patient with AD [24, 35]. UVB in combination with UVA is more effective, and the addition of topical corticosteroids can improve the favorable response.

Immunotherapy

Allergen-specific immunotherapy for 1 year, in patients with AD and allergic sensitization to house dust mites, is able to improve eczema and to reduce the use of topical steroids [35]. Further studies are needed to this direction, in order to establish the role of immunotherapy for AD.

Biologics

Recent advances in understanding the pathogenesis of AD provide an opportunity for developing biologic therapies. Limited data exist to determine the efficacy of omalizumab (anti-IgE) in the treatment of AD. One double-blind, placebo-controlled study did not show clinical improvement [76]. Another biologic agent dupilumab, a fully human monoclonal antibody that blocks interleukin 4 and interleukin 13, key cytokines of T helper cell type 2 (Th2)-mediated inflammation, showed marked and rapid improvement in all the evaluated measures of atopic dermatitis disease activity in adults [77].

Probiotics

Probiotic bacteria are suggested to reduce eczema symptoms in children with and without food allergy [46]. The probiotic effect is attributed to the normalization of increased intestinal permeability and the improvement of the immunological defense barrier (IgA) of the intestine. In adult patients with moderate AD, food supplementation with probiotic bacteria-rich yogurt was effective, and this effect depended on the recovery of intestinal mucosal barrier function.

Conclusion

The increased prevalence of AD in children and the fact that AD in most adults continues for many years point out that more adult and senile patients with AD are expected in the future.

Cross-References

- ▶ Cutaneous Effects and Sensitive Skin with Incontinence in the Aged
- ▶ The Potential of Probiotics and Prebiotics for Skin Health

References

1. Williams HC. Epidemiology of atopic dermatitis. Clin Exp Dermatol. 2000;25:522–9.
2. Strachan DP. Hay fever, hygiene, and household size. BMJ. 1989;299(6710):1259–60. A systematic review provides evidence for an inverse relationship between atopic dermatitis and exposure to endotoxin, and animals in early life.
3. Flohr C, Pascoe D, Williams HC. Atopic dermatitis and the 'hygiene hypothesis': too clean to be true? Br J Dermatol. 2005;152(2):202–16.
4. McFadden JP, Dearman RJ, White JM, Basketter DA, Kimber I. The Hapten-Atopy hypothesis II: the 'cutaneous hapten paradox'. Clin Exp Allergy. 2011;41(3): 327–37.
5. Hanifin JM, Reed ML. Eczema prevalence in the United States. Dermatitis. 2007;18(2):82–91.
6. Wolkewitz M, Rothenbacher D, Low M, Stegmaier C, Ziegler H, Radulescu M, Brenner H, Diepgen TL. Lifetime prevalence of self-reported atopic diseases in a population-based sample of elderly subjects: results of ESTHER study. Br J Dermatol. 2007;156(4): 693–7.
7. Bannister MJ, Freeman S. Adult-onset atopic dermatitis. Australas J Dermatol. 2000;41(40):225–8.
8. Tay Y, Khoo BP, Goh CL. The profile of atopic dermatitis in a tertiary dermatology outpatient clinic in Singapore. Int J Dermatol. 1999;38:689–92.
9. Nnoruka EN. Current epidemiology of atopic dermatitis in south–eastern Nigeria. Int J Dermatol. 2004;43:739–44.
10. Tanei R, Katsuoko K. Clinical analysis of atopic dermatitis in the aged. J Dermatol. 2008;35(9):562–9.
11. Folster-Holst R, Pape M, Buss YL, Christophers E, Weichenthal M. Low prevalence of the intrinsic form of atopic dermatitis among adult patients. Allergy. 2006;61(5):629–32.
12. Sandström Falk MH, Faergemann J. Atopic dermatitis in adults: does it disappear with age? Acta Derm Venereol. 2006;86(2):135–9.
13. Katsarou A, Armenaka M. Review article. Atopic dermatitis in older patients: particular points. J Eur Acad Dermatol Venereol. 2011;25(1):12–8.
14. Furue M. History of atopic dermatitis. In: Tamaki K, Furue M, Nakagawa H, editors. Atopic dermatitis and topical steroid therapy. Shinjuku: Chugai-Igakusha; 1998. p. 1–19.
15. Masutaka F, Takahito C, Satoshi T. Current status of atopic dermatitis in Japan. Asia Pac Allergy. 2011;1:64–72.
16. Furue M, Yamazaki S, Jimbow K, Tsuchida T, Amagai M, Tanaka T, Matsunaga K, Muto M, Morita E, Akiyama M, Soma Y, Terui T, Manabe M. Prevalence of dermatological disorders in Japan: a nationwide, cross-sectional, seasonal, multicenter, hospital-based study. J Dermatol. 2011;38(4):310–20.
17. Sandström MH, Faergemann J. Prognosis and prognostic factors in adult patients with atopic dermatitis: a long-term follow-up questionnaire study. Br J Dermatol. 2004;1:103–10.
18. Schmitt J, Meurer M, Klon M, Frick KD. Assessment of health state utilities of controlled psoriasis and atopic eczema: a population-based study. Br J Dermatol. 2008;158(2):351–9.
19. Holm EA, Wulf HC, Stegmann H, Jemec GB. Life quality assessment among patients with atopic eczema. Br J Dermatol. 2006;154(4):719–25.

20. Finlay AY, Khan GK. Dermatology Life Quality Index (DLQI)- a simple practical measure for routine clinical use. Clin Exp Dermatol. 1994;19(3):210–6.
21. Holm EA, Esmann S, Jemec GB. The handicap caused by atopic dermatitis- sick leave and job avoidance. J Eur Acad Derm Venereol. 2006;20(3):255–9.
22. Silverberg JI. Association between adult atopic dermatitis, cardiovascular disease and increased heart attacks in 3 population-based studies. Allergy. 2015. doi:10.1111/all.12685. Epub ahead of print.
23. Wüthrich B, Schmid-Grendelmeier P. Definition and diagnosis of intrinsic versus extrinsic atopic dermatitis. In: Bieber T, Leung DYM, editors. Atopic dermatitis. New York: Marcel Dekker; 2002. p. 1–20.
24. Van Leent EJM, Bos JD. Atopic dermatitis. In: Katsambas A, Lotti T, editors. European handbook of dermatological treatments. 2nd ed. Berlin: Springer-Verlag; 2003. p. 54–62.
25. Tanei R. Atopic dermatitis in the elderly. Inflamm Allergy Drug Targets. 2009;8:398–404.
26. Rym BM, Mourad M, Bechir Z, et al. Erythroderma in adults: a report of 80 cases. Int J Dermatol. 2005;44(9):731–5.
27. Katoh N, Hirano S, Kishimoto S. Prognostic factor of adult patients with atopic dermatitis. J Dermatol. 2008;35:477–83.
28. Kanwar AJ, Narang T. Adult onset atopic dermatitis: under-recognized or under-reported? Indian Dermatol Online J. 2013;4(3):167–71.
29. Hanifin JM, Rajka G. Diagnostic features of atopic dermatitis. Acta Derm Venereol (Stockh). 1980; 92(Suppl):44–7.
30. Williams HC, Burney PG, Hay RJ, Archer CB, Shipley MJ, Hunter JJ, Bingham EA, Finlay AY, Pembroke AC, Graham-Brown RA, et al. The U.K. Working Party's diagnostic criteria for atopic dermatitis. I. Derivation of a minimum set of discriminators for atopic dermatitis. Br J Dermatol. 1994;131(3):383–96.
31. Brenninkmeijer EEA, Schram ME, Leeflang MMG, Bos JD, Spuls PI. Diagnostic criteria for atopic dermatitis: a systematic review. Br J Dermatol. 2008;158:754–65.
32. Wedi B, Kapp A. Differential diagnosis of atopic eczema. In: Ring J, Przybilla B, Ruzicka T, editors. Handbook of atopic eczema. 2nd ed. Berlin\Heidelberg: Springer; 2006. p. 100–7.
33. Stalder JF, Taieb A. Severity scoring of atopic dermatitis: the SCORAD index. Consensus report of the European Task Force on atopic dermatitis. Dermatology. 1993;186:23–31.
34. Morar N, Willis-Owen SA, Moffatt MF, Cookson WO. The genetics of atopic dermatitis. J Allergy Clin Immunol. 2006;118:24–34.
35. Akdis CA, Akdis M, Bieber T, Bindslev-Jensen C, Boguniewicz M, et al. Diagnosis and treatment of atopic dermatitis in children and adults: European Academy of Allergology and Clinical Immunology/American Academy of Allergy, Asthma and Immunology/PRAC-TALL Consensus Report. Allergy. 2006;61:969–87.
36. Irvine AD. Fleshing out filaggrin phenotypes. J Invest Dermatol. 2007;127:504–7.
37. Rupnik H, Rijavec M, Korošec P. Filaggrin loss-of-function mutations are not associated with atopic dermatitis that develops in late childhood or adulthood. Br J Dermatol. 2015;172(2):455–61.
38. Heede NG, Thyssen JP, Thuesen BH, Linneberg A, Johansen JD. Anatomical patterns of dermatitis in adult filaggrin mutation carriers. J Am Acad Dermatol. 2015;72(3):440–8.
39. Aalto-Korte K. Improvement of skin barrier function during treatment of atopic dermatitis. J Am Acad Dermatol. 1995;33:969–72.
40. Kabashima K. New concept of the pathogenesis of atopic dermatitis: interplay among the barrier, allergy, and pruritus as a trinity. J Dermatol Sci. 2013;70(1): 3–11.
41. Cork M, Robinson DA, Vassilopoulos Y, Ferguson A, Moustafa M, MacGowan A, Duff GW, Ward SJ, Tazi-Ahnini R. New perspectives on epidermal barrier dysfunction in atopic dermatitis: gene-environmental interactions. J Allergy Clin Immunol. 2006;118:3–21.
42. Jin K, Higaki Y, Tagagi Y, Higuchi K, Yada Y, Kawashima M, Imo-kawa G. Analysis of beta-glucocerebrosidase and ceramidase activities in atopic and aged dry skin. Acta Derm Venereol. 1994;74(5): 337–40.
43. De Benedetto A, Kubo A, Beck L. Skin barrier disruption: a requirement for allergen sensitization? J Invest Dermatol. 2012;132:949–63.
44. Leung DYM, Bieber T. Atopic dermatitis. Lancet. 2003;361:151–60.
45. Bonness S, Bieber T. Molecular basis of atopic dermatitis. Curr Opin Allergy Clin Immunol. 2007;7:382–6.
46. Biedermann T. Dissecting the role of infections in atopic dermatitis. Acta Derm Venereol. 2006;86:99–109.
47. Grice EA, Kong HH, Conlan S, Deming CB, Davis J, Young AC, NISC Comparative Sequencing Program, Bouffard GG, Blakesley RW, Murray PR, Green ED, Turner ML, Segre JA. Topographical and temporal diversity of the human skin microbiome. Science. 2009;324(5931):1190–2.
48. Oh J, Conlan S, Polley EC, Segre JA, Kong HH. Shifts in human skin and nares microbiota of healthy children and adults. Genome Med. 2012;4(10):77.
49. Naik S, Bouladoux N, Wilhelm C, Molloy MJ, Salcedo R, et al. Compartmentalized control of skin immunity by resident commensals. Science. 2012;337:1115–9.
50. Kong HH, Oh J, Deming C, Conlan S, Grice EA, Beatson MA, Nomicos E, Polley EC, Komarow HD, NISC Comparative Sequence Program, Murray PR, Turner ML, Segre JA. Temporal shifts in the skin microbiome associated with disease flares and treatment in children with atopic dermatitis. Genome Res. 2012;22(5):850–9.

51. Gueniche A, Knaudt B, Schuck E, Volz T, Bastien P, Martin R, Röcken M, Breton L, Biedermann T. Effects of nonpathogenic gram-negative bacterium Vitreoscilla filiformis lysate on atopic dermatitis: a prospective, randomized, double-blind, placebo-controlled clinical study. Br J Dermatol. 2008; 159(6):1357–63.
52. Worm M, Forschner K, Lee H-H, Roehr CC, Edenharter G, Niggemann B, Zuberbier T. Frequency of atopic dermatitis and relevance of food allergy in adults in Germany. Acta Derm Venereol. 2006;86:119–22.
53. Werfel T, Ballmer-Weber B, Eigenmann PA, Niggemann B, Rance' F, Turjanmaa K, Worm M. Eczematous reactions to foods in atopic eczema: position paper of the EAACI and GA^{2}LEN. Allergy. 2007;62:723–8.
54. Worm M, Ehlers I, Sterry W, Zuberbier T. Clinical relevance of food additives in adult patients with atopic dermatitis. Clin Exp Allergy. 2000;30:407–14.
55. Erwin EA, Platts-Mills TAE. Aeroallergens. In: Bieber T, Leung D, editors. Atopic dermatitis. New York: Markel Dekker; 2002. p. 357–73.
56. Mediaty A, Neuber K. Total and specific serum IgE decreases with age in patients with allergic rhinitis, asthma and insect sting allergy but not in patients with atopic dermatitis. Immunity Ageing. 2005;2:9.
57. Samochocki Z, Owczarek W, Zabielski S. Can atopy patch tests with aeroallergens be an additional diagnostic criterion for atopic dermatitis? Eur J Dermatol. 2006;16:151–4.
58. Baker BS. The role of microorganisms in atopic dermatitis. Clin Exp Immunol. 2006;144:1–9.
59. Roll A, Cozzio A, Fischer B, Schmid-Grendelmeier P. Microbial colonization and atopic dermatitis. Curr Opin Allergy Clin Immunol. 2004;4:373–8.
60. Takahata Y, Sugita T, Kato H, Nishikawa A, Hiruma M, Muto M. Cutaneous Malassezia flora in atopic dermatitis differ between adults and children. Br J Dermatol. 2007;157:1178–82.
61. Löffler H, Steffes A, Happle R, Effendy I. Allergy and irritation: an adverse association in patients with atopic eczema. Acta Derm Venereol. 2003;83:328–31.
62. Dotterud LK, Smith-Sivertsen T. Allergic contact sensitization in the general adult population: a population-based study from Northern Norway. Contact Dermatitis. 2007;56:10–5.
63. Laminitausta K, Kalimo K, Fagerlund VL. Patch test reactions in atopic patients. Contact Dermatitis. 1992;26:234–40.
64. De Groot AC. The frequency of contact allergy in atopic patients with dermatitis. Contact Dermatitis. 1990;22:273–7.
65. Dickel H, Bruckner TM, Schmidt A, Diepgen TL. Impact of atopic skin diathesis on occupational skin disease incidence in a working population. J Invest Dermatol. 2003;121:37–40.
66. Koblenzer C. The psychological aspects of atopic dermatitis. In: Bieber T, Leung D, editors. Atopic dermatitis. New York: Markel Dekker; 2002. p. 43–66.
67. Skassa-Brociek W, Manderscheid JC, Michel FB, Bousquet J. Skin test reactivity to histamine from infancy to old age. J Allergy Clin Immunol. 1987; 80(5):711–6.
68. Weissenbacher S, Bacon T, Targett D, Behrendt H, Ring J, Darshow U. Atopy patch test- reproducibility and elicitation of itch in different application sites. Acta Derm Venereol. 2005;85:147–51.
69. Charman CR, Morris AD, Williams HC. Topical corticosteroid phobia in patients with atopic eczema. Br J Dermatol. 2000;142:931–6.
70. Oranze AP, Devillers AC, Kunz B, Jones SL, DeRaeve L, Van Gysel D, de Waard-van der Spek FB, Grimalt R, Torrelo A, Stevens J, Harper J. Treatment of patients with atopic dermatitis using wet-wrap dressings with diluted steroids and/or emollients. An expert panel's opinion and review of the literature. J Eur Acad Derm Venereol. 2006;20(10): 1277–86.
71. Reitamo S, Ortonne J-P, Sand C, Bos J, Cambazard F, Bieber T, Grønhøj-Larsen C, Rustin M, Folster-Hölst R, Schuttelaar M. Long term treatment with 0.1% tacrolimus ointment in adults with atopic dermatitis: results of a two-year, multicenter, non-comparative study. Acta Derm Venereol. 2007; 87:406–12.
72. Thaci D, Chambers C, Sidhu M, Dorsch B, Ehlken B, Fuchs S. Twice-weekly treatment with tacrolimus 0.03% ointment in children with atopic dermatitis: clinical efficacy and economic impact over 12 months. J Eur Acad Dermatol Venereol. 2010; 24:1040–6.
73. Luger T, De Raeve L, Gelmetti C, Kakourou T, Kakourou T, Katsarou A, et al. Recommendations for pimecrolimus 1% cream in the treatment of mild-to-moderate atopic dermatitis from medical needs to a new treatment algorithm. Eur J Dermatol. 2013;23(6): 758–66.
74. Eichenfield LF, et al. Guidelines of care for the management of atopic dermatitis. Section 2. Management and treatment of atopic dermatitis with topical therapies. J Am Acad Dermatol. 2014; 71:116–32.
75. Schmitt J, Schäkel K, Schmitt N, Meurer M. Systemic treatment of severe atopic eczema: a systematic review. Acta Derm Venereol. 2007;87:100–11.
76. Heil PM, Maurer D, Klein B, Hultsch T, Stingl G. Omalizumab therapy in atopic dermatitis: depletion of IgE does not improve the clinical course a randomized, placebo-controlled and double blind pilot study. J Dtsch Dermatol Ges. 2010;8:990–8.
77. Beck LA, Thaçi D, Hamilton JD, Graham NM, Bieber T, Rocklin R, Ming JE, et al. Dupilumab treatment in adults with moderate-to-severe atopic dermatitis. N Engl J Med. 2014;371(2):130–9.

Dry Skin in Diabetes Mellitus and in Experimental Models of Diabetes

75

Shingo Sakai and Hachiro Tagami

Contents

Abstract

Diabetic patients often have dry scaly skin. Moreover, diabetes mellitus induces various forms of dermopathy such as bullosis diabeticorum, necrobiosis lipoidica diabeticorum, scleredema diabeticorum, and acanthosis nigricans. Nonhealing ulcers occur in approximately 15 % of patients with diabetes. In general, diabetic atrophy is thought to result from complications such as vasculopathy and neuropathy. Insulin resistance and hyperglycemia contribute to the impaired physiologic function observed in various tissues of these patients. This chapter summarizes how diobetes mellitus induces epidermal changes similar to those observed in aged skin.

Introduction

Patients with diabetes often have dry scaly skin [1–3]. Moreover, diabetes mellitus induces various forms of dermopathy such as bullosis diabeticorum, necrobiosis lipoidica diabeticorum, scleredema diabeticorum, and acanthosis nigricans [4]. Nonhealing ulcers occur in approximately 15 % of patients with diabetes, and therefore, it is imperative to prevent ulcer formation and improve wound healing in these patients [5, 6]. In general, diabetic atrophy is thought to

S. Sakai (✉)
Basic Research Laboratory, Kanebo Cosmetics Inc., Kanagawa, Japan
e-mail: sakai.shingo2@kao.co.jp

H. Tagami
Department of Dermatology, Tohoku University School of Medicine, Sendai, Japan
e-mail: hachitagami@ybb.ne.jp

M.A. Farage et al. (eds.), *Textbook of Aging Skin*,
DOI 10.1007/978-3-662-47398-6_63

result from complications such as vasculopathy and neuropathy. Insulin resistance and hyperglycemia contribute to the impaired physiologic function observed in various tissues of these patients.

Hyperglycemia induces cellular abnormalities via several mechanisms, including nonenzymatic glycosylation, oxidative-reductive stress, aldose reductase activation, activation of diacylglycerol-phosphate kinase C (PKC), etc. [7, 8]. For example, diabetes induces advanced glycosylation end products in the collagen of the dermis [9, 10]. These end products are observed in aged skin also [11] and are postulated to produce the characteristic skin stiffness [12, 13] and delayed wound healing [14, 15] seen in older adults. Reports also indicate that reduced collagen synthesis and increased matrix metalloproteinase production occur in the skin of patients with diabetes [16, 17]. Hence, the dermis of patients with diabetes may share some of the features of the dermis of aged skin [18, 19].

Within the epidermis, insulin acts as an essential growth factor for the proliferation [20] and migration [21, 22] of keratinocytes. The inhibition of keratinocyte proliferation seen in patients with diabetes may contribute to the delayed wound healing. Insulin also regulates keratinocyte differentiation [23]. Interestingly, the surface area of corneocytes is reportedly larger in patients with diabetes than in normal individuals [24], suggesting that diabetes mellitus impairs epidermal turnover. However, it is difficult to distinguish the effects of diabetes on the functional properties of the stratum corneum (SC), because diabetes often accompanies aging. For example, pruritus due to diabetes is difficult to be distinguished clinically from that noted in senile xerosis [4].

A new model of diabetes has been developed in hairless mice by using streptozotocin (STZ) [25], an agent that destroys insulin-secreting pancreatic beta cells [26]. STZ-treated animals serve as a model of type I diabetes. The hairless mouse model exhibits many of the features seen in human patients with uncontrolled diabetes mellitus, including hyperglycemia, polydipsia, and polyuria [27, 28]. The hairless mouse model of STZ-induced diabetes avoids the obstacles to functional and biochemical analysis of the skin posed by the presence and growth of fur. Using this model, the effects of experimentally induced diabetes on SC hydration and barrier function, as well as changes in the SC content of lipids and soluble amino acid, were assessed [25]. These properties of the SC were also examined in patients with diabetes mellitus [29]. As will be detailed herein, the experimental and clinical study results indicate that diabetes mellitus induces epidermal changes similar to those observed in aged skin.

Biophysical Properties of the Stratum Corneum in the Hairless Mouse Model of Diabetes Mellitus

Changes in the Functional Properties of the Stratum Corneum

Streptozotocin (STZ) (150 mg/kg) rapidly induced diabetes symptoms in hairless mice. Blood glucose concentrations increased significantly from the second day after the injection, and the increase continued time dependently for up to 3 weeks.

After the induction of hyperglycemia, high-frequency conductance (HFC) of the skin (a parameter linked to SC hydration) decreased in a time-dependent fashion, relative to that of the untreated mice. Three weeks after the STZ injection, HFC levels in the SC of the diabetic animals were about a half of those of the control group (Fig. 1). In contrast, *no* difference in transepidermal water loss (TEWL), a measure of skin barrier function, was observed. These findings suggest that experimentally induced diabetes in mice impairs water homeostasis in the SC without altering its water barrier function.

Changes of the Amino Acid and Lipid Content of the Stratum Corneum

In mice with STZ-induced diabetes, the amino acid content of the SC increased slightly by 3 weeks after treatment (Fig. 2). Immunoblotting

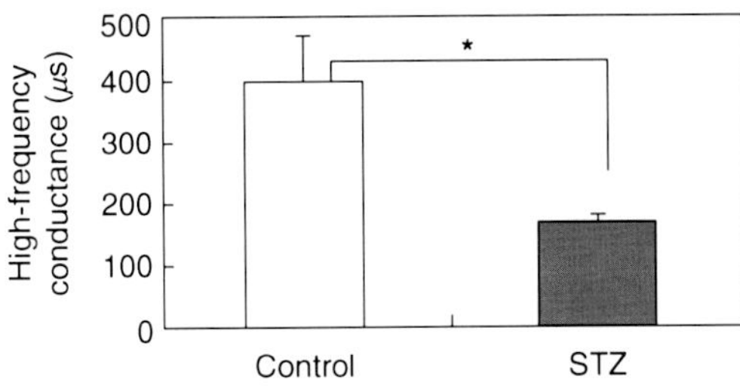

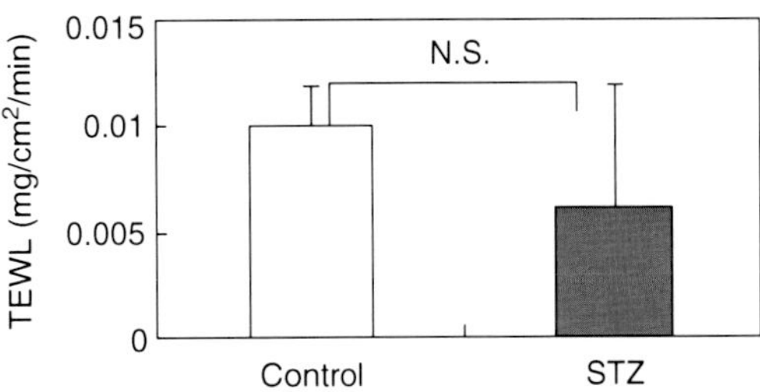

Fig. 1 Mice with streptozotocin-induced diabetes exhibit decreased water content of the stratum corneum without impairment of the water barrier function. CONTROL, buffer-injected group; STZ, streptozotocin-treated group. *Significant ($p < 0.05$); *NS* not significant. Values represent means with SEM from five animals per group

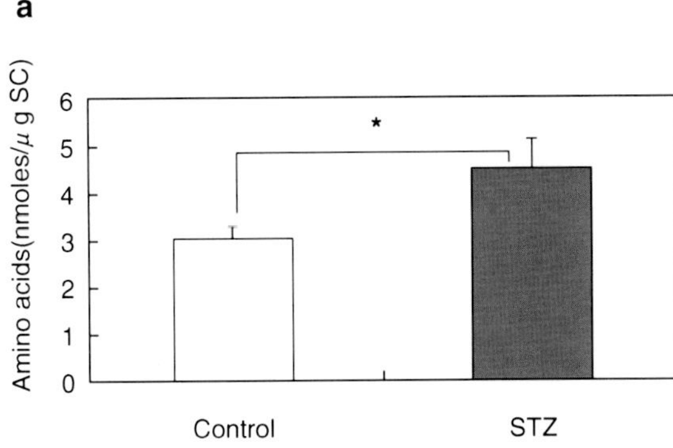

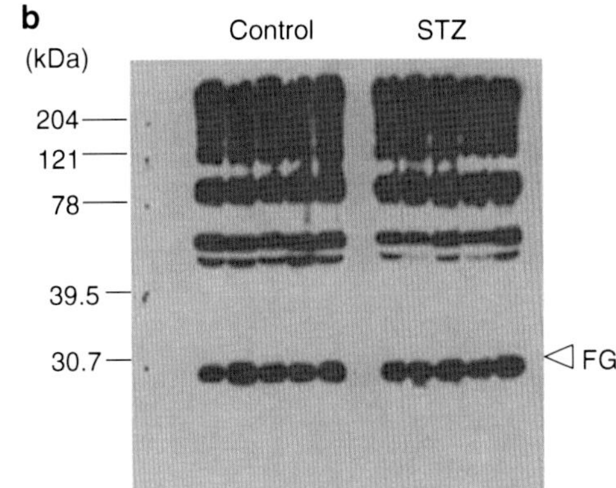

Fig. 2 Mice with streptozotocin-induced diabetes exhibit normal metabolism of amino acids in the stratum corneum. The amino acid content in the SC (**a**) and epidermal (pro) filaggrin content (**b**) were assayed at 3 weeks after a single injection of streptozotocin. *Values represent means with SEM from five animals per group. Significant ($p < 0.05$). FG shows filaggrin monomer protein

analysis demonstrated that the contents of profilaggrin and filaggrin, precursors of the water-soluble amino acids, were almost unchanged in the epidermis of these animals (Fig. 2). This suggests that the normal processing of profilaggrin to amino acids is functional in the epidermis of the mice with STZ-induced diabetes.

The content of the total SC lipids per unit area of the skin was higher in the STZ-treated group than in the control group (Table 1); only the triglyceride content decreased significantly after the induction of diabetes. This result suggests that triglyceride metabolism in the sebaceous glands was impaired in mice with experimentally induced diabetes.

The state of SC hydration is thought to be regulated principally by three factors: the water-soluble natural moisturizing factor (derived mainly from profilaggrin [30]), intercellular lipids [31], and sebum lipids [32]. In the dry skin of patients with atopic dermatitis and in the dry skin of older adults, the levels of both SC amino acids [30, 33] [34] and SC ceramides (the main components of intercellular lipids [35–37]) reportedly decrease. The dry skin of senile xerosis is also characterized by significant decreases in triglycerides [36, 38, 39]. In mice with experimentally induced diabetes, decrease in the water content of the SC was independent of decrease in the content of SC amino acids and ceramides but paralleled a decrease in SC triglycerides. Alterations in triglycerides are similar to the changes seen in older patients with xerosis.

Insulin reportedly stimulates fat synthesis by adipocytes [40, 41]. In rats, STZ treatment stimulated hormone-sensitive lipase activity of the

Table 1 Decreased triglyceride content in the stratum corneum of mice with streptozotocin-induced diabetes

	Content (μg/cm²)	
	STZ-treated Control mice	Control STZ-treated mice
Ceramide I	1.5 ± 0.2	1.9 ± 0.1[a]
Ceramide II–V	9.1 ± 1.1	15.5 ± 1.0[b]
Cholesterol	9.8 ± 1.3	17.2 ± 1.4[b]
Fatty acids	4.5 ± 0.6	8.3 ± 0.3[b]
Triglycerides	20.6 ± 6.9	4.0 ± 4.1[a]
Wax/cholesterol esters	22.6 ± 1.0	41.0 ± 3.3[b]
Total lipids	92.5 ± 3.8	121.6 ± 5.9[b]

Values represent means with SEM from five animals per group (From Ref. [25])
[a]Significant ($p < 0.05$)
[b]Significant ($p < 0.005$)

adipocytes [42]. Reductions in SC triglycerides observed in animals with experimentally induced diabetes may be due to activation of lipolysis in the sebaceous glands. Patients with senile xerosis also have reduced levels of SC triglycerides [38], suggesting that triglycerides play a role in SC moisturization. In general, acetone extraction of skin surface lipids induces a brief but significant reduction in SC hydration. In seborrheic areas, such as the face and scalp, SC hydration returns to pretreatment levels within a few hours as skin surface lipids are replenished by sebum secretion [32].

Glycerol may play a mechanistic role in sebum-induced skin hydration [43]. Studies performed in asebia J1 and 2 J mice (a unique experimental model associated with profound sebaceous gland hypoplasia) showed that these mice exhibit normal homeostasis of the SC permeability barrier and normal extracellular lamellar membrane structures; however, reduced production of sebum-associated lipids resulted in epidermal hyperplasia, inflammation, and a greater than 50 % decrease *in* SC hydration. Application of a mixture of synthetic, sebum-like lipids (sterol/wax esters, triglycerides) failed to restore normal SC hydration: only topical glycerol – the putative product of triglyceride hydrolysis in sebaceous glands – normalized SC hydration. In fact, the glycerol content of the SC of asebia mice was 85 % lower than in normal mice. These findings suggest that glycerol produced by the sebaceous glands may be a major contributor to SC hydration.

Notably, one cannot exclude the possibility that factors besides amino acids, intercellular lipids, and sebum contribute to the reduced water content of the SC in the mouse model of diabetes. A role for other water-soluble moisturizing factors, such as lactate and urea, is speculated; however, few studies have examined the role of water-soluble substances in regulating skin surface hydration.

It has also been speculated that the pathogenesis of diabetic xerosis may involve autonomic, peripheral C fiber neuropathy [1, 3, 44]. Impaired sweating is often observed both in patients with diabetes and in older adults because of the impairment of skin-temperature control [45]. The laboratory showed that lactate, an important component of sweat, plays a role in maintaining SC hydration [46]. Decreased lactate production may be a factor to bring skin dryness in the diabetic patient.

Another possible mechanism of SC hydration is water movement through the epidermis. In mice with experimentally induced diabetes, a chemiosmotic alteration in the SC itself (and/or in keratinocytes beneath the SC layer) may impair the water homeostasis of the SC. Aquaporin, a vital water channel in various tissues such as the kidney, lung, retina, and cornea, may affect epidermal movement of water and glycerol. The author's laboratory showed that aquaporin isoforms are expressed in the keratinocytes and that aquaporin-3 is inducible under hypertonic stress [47]; moreover, other investigators have reported reduced SC hydration in hairless, aquaporin-3-null mice [48]. Aquaporin-3 is also involved in epidermal proliferation [49]. Therefore, the possibility exists that aquaporin modulates epidermal water movement and contributes to SC hydration.

Changes in Epidermal Proliferation and Differentiation

Diabetes also affects epidermal structure, proliferation, and differentiation. The epidermis of mice with STZ-induced diabetes is thinner than that of untreated controls (Fig. 3). The ratio of proliferating cell nuclear antigen (PCNA)-positive basal cells to the total basal cells in the epidermis is significantly lower in STZ-treated mice (Fig. 3); the DNA content of the epidermis is also lower in STZ-treated mice than that in controls (23.4 ± 2.1 μg/cm^2 vs. 29.3 ± 0.6 μg/cm^2, respectively; $n = 5$, $p < 0.05$). These results suggest that diabetes inhibits the epidermal proliferation.

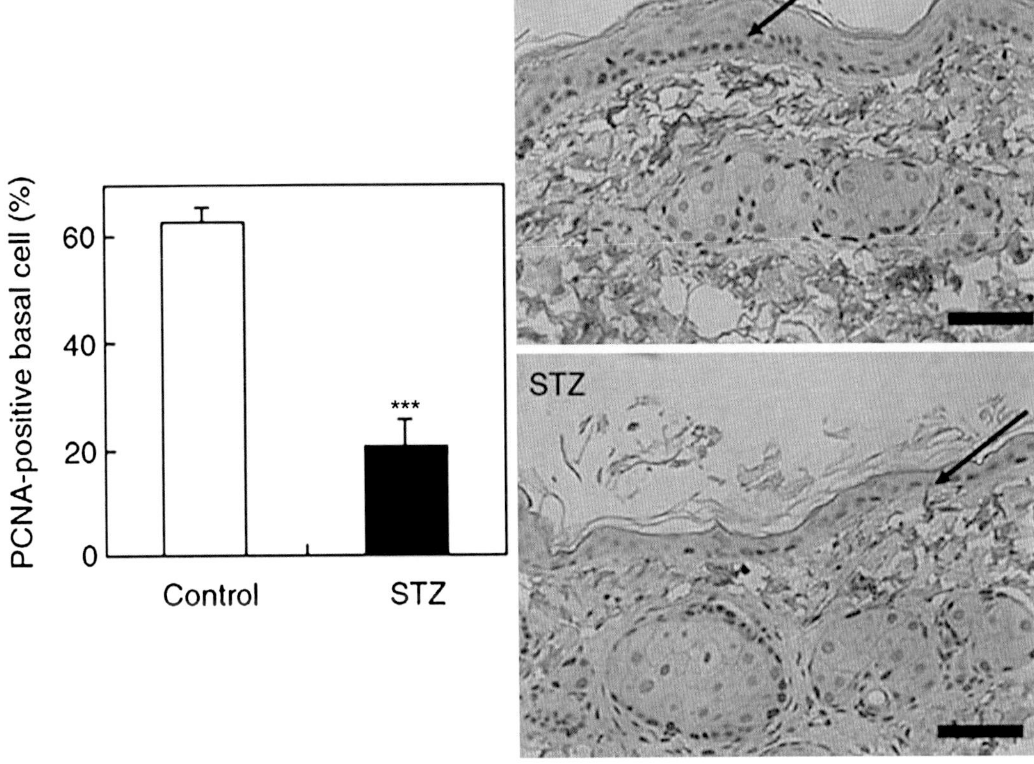

Fig. 3 Mice with streptozotocin-induced diabetes show decreased proliferation of epidermal basal cells at 3 weeks after a single injection of streptozotocin. ***Significant ($p < 0.001$). Values represent means with SEM from four animals per group. *Arrows*: PCNA-positive cells

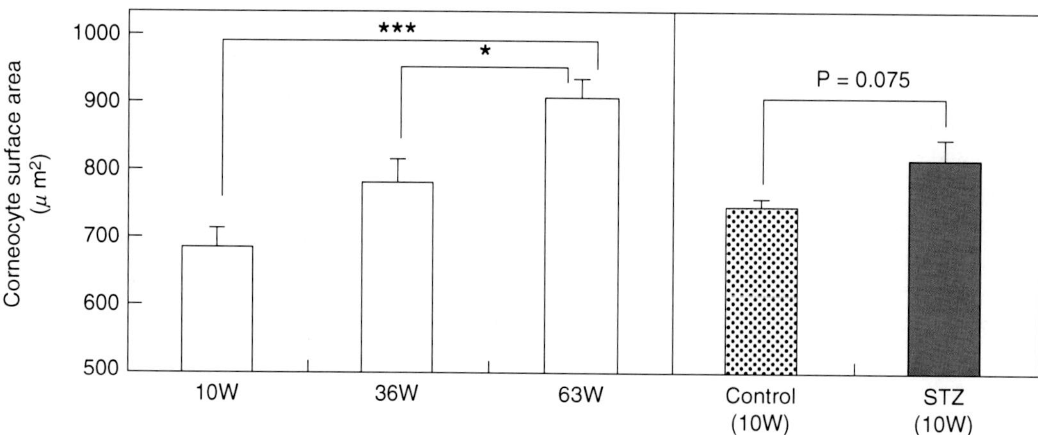

Fig. 4 Surface areas of corneocytes in mice with streptozotocin-induced diabetes. The corneocyte surface areas were measured 3 weeks after a single injection of streptozotocin and also at ages 10, 36, and 63 weeks. Values represent means with SEM from five animals per group. *Significant ($p < 0.05$); ***Significant ($p < 0.001$)

Clinically, the corneocyte surface area is enlarged in both senile xerosis [38, 50] and in patients with diabetes [24], whereas in atopic xerosis corneocyte surface area is reduced [51]. This suggests a slow epidermal turnover rate in senile xerosis and diabetic dry skin and a rapid epidermal turnover in atopic xerosis. Mice with experimentally induced diabetes also had somewhat elevated corneocyte surface areas relative to controls (Fig. 4), which suggests a reduced epidermal cell turnover rate in mice with experimentally induced diabetes, as in aged human skin. Hence, both clinical and experimental diabetes affect corneocytes in a similar manner to the aging process.

Furthermore, epidermal differentiation markers in STZ-treated mice bear some similarities to those in aged skin. For example, the epidermal differentiation markers, keratin 1, keratin 5, keratin 10, and loricrin (58–90 kDa), were normal in STZ-treated animals (Fig. 5). However, three loricrin-derived peptides (with molecular weights 34, 36, and 43 kDa, respectively) were observed in the SC of STZ-treated mice, with a pattern similar to that seen with SC peptides in aged mice (Fig. 5). This suggests that alterations in the processing of the SC proteins that occur in the diabetic state are similar to those observed in aged skin.

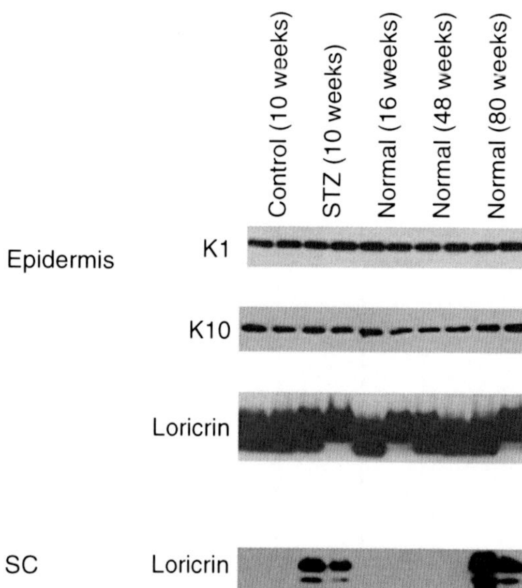

Fig. 5 Effects of streptozotocin on marker proteins of epidermal differentiation. Western blots of epidermal protein extracted 3 weeks after streptozocin treatment. K1, keratin 1; K10, keratin 10. At the same time, the SC protein was extracted and applied to Western blotting using antiloricrin antibody

Loricrin, an insoluble protein of the cornified envelope [52], is produced and cross-linked in the terminal differentiation process. Loricrin-derived peptides were extremely difficult to detect in healthy young mice but were easily solubilized in diabetic and aged mice. Consequently, stages in the maturation, proteolysis, and/or oxidation of loricrin processing were altered in the SC of the diabetic mouse as that of aged ones.

The attenuated insulin signal transduction in diabetic mouse is speculated to be important in the growth and differentiation of keratinocytes. Keratinocytes have constituent insulin receptors [23]; insulin stimulates keratinocyte migration [21] and proliferation [20], and insulin and insulin-like growth factors regulate keratinocyte differentiation [23]. For example, insulin receptor (IR)-null mice exhibited lower epidermal proliferation [53]; similarly, insulin receptor substrate 1 (IRS-1)-null mice had a thin and abnormally differentiated epidermis [54]. In mice with experimentally induced diabetes, insulin signal transduction is attenuated and epidermal proliferation is reduced. Interestingly, these diabetic mice exhibited four features characteristic of senile xerosis: reduced SC hydration, reduced epidermal turnover, accumulated corneocyte layers, and decreased triglyceride content. These observations suggest that in diabetes, hyperglycemia and/or attenuated insulin signaling may promote epidermal aging.

The impact of growth factors on epidermal turnover in diabetes also has been investigated. Expression of nerve growth factor (an autocrine growth factor of keratinocytes [55]) is downregulated in diabetic skin, whereas the expression of nerve growth factor receptors is upregulated [56]. Decreased epidermal turnover in the hairless mouse model of diabetes may be linked to abnormal signal transduction of either insulin or nerve growth factor or both.

Biophysical Properties of the Stratum Corneum in Patients with Diabetes

Hydration, Surface Lipids, and Barrier Function of the Stratum Corneum in Patients with Diabetes

Properties of the stratum corneum were examined in patients with diabetes to determine whether impairments similar to those seen in the hairless mouse model occur [29]. Patients were classified into groups with high- or low-fasting plasma glucose (FPG) (levels above and below 110 mg/dL, respectively) and into groups with high and low HbA_{1C} (levels above and below 5.8 %, respectively). FPG indicates the hyperglycemic state at the time of the measurements, while the HbA_{1C} reflects the average hyperglycemic state in the past 7–8 weeks preceding the measurement. The comparative age ranges of patients in the low- and high-FPG groups and in the low- and high-HbA_{1C} groups were not significantly different.

High-frequency conductance (HFC) of the extensor leg and volar forearm was measured for stratum corneum hydration. The content of skin surface lipids on the forehead was measured using Sebumeter. Measurements were performed in a constant-climate room at 20 °C and at a relative humidity of 50 %. Patients with high FPG exhibited significantly lower SC hydration on the extensor leg and volar forearm than those with low FPG (Fig. 6). The group with high FPG had a significantly lower content of skin surface lipids on the forehead. When patients with high and low HbA_{1C} were compared, those with high HbA_{1C} had a lower content of skin surface lipids on the forehead (Fig. 7). No difference in SC hydration was observed between the low- and high-HbA_{1C} groups. These clinical findings suggest that the state of SC hydration in patients with diabetes is influenced more by the immediate or "real-time" hyperglycemic state rather than by the hyperglycemic state in the preceding weeks.

In contrast with the aforementioned results, patients with high and low FPG exhibited similar levels of TEWL, as measured on the forearm and leg, suggesting that the water barrier function of the skin was not significantly affected. In patients with high HbA_{1C}, TEWL measured on the volar forearm was significantly lower than in patients with low HbA_{1C} (Table 2). Therefore, hyperglycemia does not seem to impair the water barrier function of the SC, as patients with high FPG exhibited lower SC hydration without a consistent change in SC barrier function. These results are consistent with those found in mice with experimentally induced diabetes.

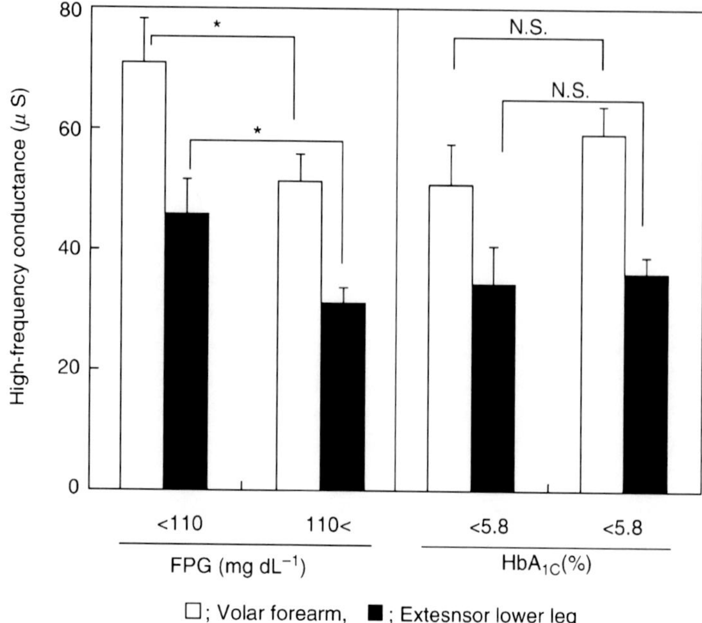

Fig. 6 Decreased SC hydration accompanies the real-time hyperglycemic state. Patients with diabetes were grouped according to above- and below-normal FPG (110 mg/dL) and above- and below-normal HbA_{1C} (5.8 %). Values represent means ± SD $^{*}p < 0.025$, *NS* not significant, □ volar forearm, ▪ extensor lower leg

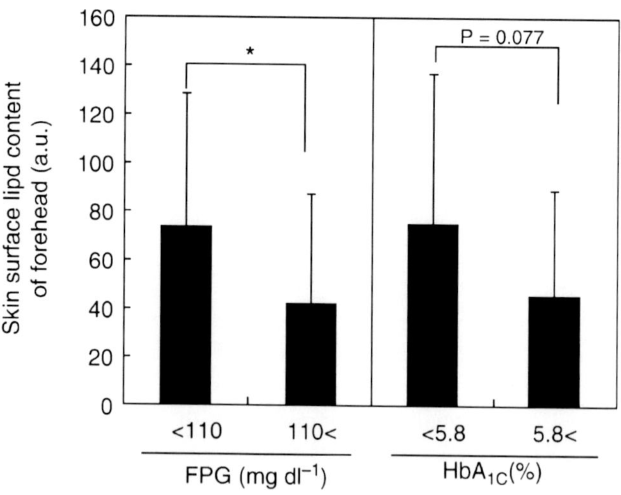

Fig. 7 A hyperglycemic state is associated with reduced surface lipid content of forehead skin in patients with diabetes. Patients with diabetes were grouped according to above- and below-normal FPG (110 mg/dL) and above- and below-normal HbA_{1C} (5.8 %). Values represent means ± SD $^{*}p < 0.05$

Notably, patients with high FPG as well as those with high HbA_{1C} had a low surface lipid content The combination of reduced SC hydration and a low surface lipid content, unaccompanied by impairment of the SC barrier function, is a phenomenon also seen in senile xerosis, a condition characterized by dry scaly skin in older adults [38]. Hence, reduced SC hydration coupled with normal barrier function, as observed in patients with diabetes, mirrors the phenomenon that develops in aged persons.

SC hydration is critical to skin smoothness [57], softness [58], and surface texture [59]. Reduced sebum secretion due to impaired sebaceous gland function also may contribute to reduced SC hydration in patients with diabetes. Sebaceous glands bind insulin, but the level of binding decreases in mice with diabetes [60]. As

Table 2 Comparison of TEWL ($mg/cm^2/h$) in patients with low and high levels of HbA_{1C} g

	TEWL ($mg/cm^2/h$)		
	$HbA_{1C} < 5.8\ \%$ ($n = 11$)	$HbA_{1C} > 5.8\ \%$ ($n = 38$)	p value
Volar forearm	5.8 ± 1.4	3.6 ± 0.3	0.017[a]
Extensor lower leg	3.9 ± 0.8	3.6 ± 0.4	0.702

Values are means ± SEM
[a]Significant (From Ref. [29])

Table 3 Comparison of the functional properties of the stratum corneum between younger and older patients with diabetes

	Age group < 45 years ($n = 23$)	Age group > 45 years ($n = 26$)	p value
Age	19.3 ± 1.7	68.2 ± 1.5	0[a]
FPG (mg/dL)	161.7 ± 17.1	148.8 ± 11.9	0.532
HbA_{1C} (%)	7.13 ± 0.35	6.58 ± 0.15	0.141
Skin surface lipid on forehead (a.u.)	64.7 ± 9.6	40.8 ± 9.9	0.092
TEWL ($mg/cm^2/h$)			
Volar forearm	5.4 ± 0.7	5.0 ± 0.5	0.001[a]
Extensor lower leg	3.0 ± 0.2	2.5 ± 0.3	0.0001[a]
HFC (μS)			
Volar forearm	54.7 ± 4.4	60.0 ± 6.4	0.511
Extensor lower leg	42.3 ± 4.1	29.5 ± 3.5	0.020[a]

Means ± SEM
[a]Significant ($p < 0.025$) (From Ref. [29])

noted earlier, rats with STZ-induced diabetes had lower sebum secretion [61]. Hence, insulin may be required for the homeostasis of the sebaceous gland; impaired insulin secretion may contribute to skin changes observed in diabetes.

Future studies should be geared for assessing the potential role of natural moisturizing factors other than SC amino acids and for characterizing the epidermal chemiosmotic changes.

The Influence of Aging on the Hydration State and Barrier Function of the Skin in Patients with Diabetes

To examine the effect of aging on properties of the SC in abovementioned patients with diabetes, the HFC, TEWL, and skin surface lipids of patients above and below the age of 45 were evaluated. In older patients, HFC was significantly lower only on the extensor surface of the leg; however, TEWL was significantly lower at all of the measured locations (Table 3). A trend to reduced skin surface lipid content on the forehead was also noted in older patients with diabetes. These findings suggest that the age-related changes in the SC properties are promoted by diabetes mellitus. In other words, a diabetic condition might enhance the aging of the SC function.

Conclusion

The problem of xerotic skin is a significant issue for patients with diabetes mellitus, as it is for people with atopic dermatitis, psoriasis, and ichthyosis vulgaris and for most elderly people. Studies in hairless mice with experimentally induced diabetes and in patients with diabetes have shed light on some of the mechanisms that contribute to xerotic skin. Diabetes appears to induce functional changes in the skin similar to those that occur in older people. Indeed, the data strongly suggest that hyperglycemic conditions may promote epidermal aging.

Declining skin hydration has clinical consequences for patients with diabetes [1–3]. For example, plantar xerosis in patients with diabetes is linked to the development of recalcitrant ulcers. Care of the feet in the diabetic patient should include moisturizing the skin of the plantar surface [62].

More research is warranted to develop better skin care approaches for patients with diabetes. Research into the moisturizing mechanisms of substances such sebum, lactate, urea, and other potential natural moisturizing factors may yield valuable insights for skin care in these patients. Moreover, avoiding lifestyle choices that contribute to adult-onset diabetes will not only promote health and well-being but could also be viewed as an antiaging measure to maintain youthful skin.

Cross-References

▶ Influence of Race, Gender, Age, and Diabetes on Blood Flow

References

1. Huntley AC. Cutaneous manifestations of diabetes mellitus. Dermatol Clin. 1989;7:531–46.
2. Yosipovitch G, Hodak E, Vardi P, et al. The prevalence of cutaneous manifestations in IDDM patients and their association with diabetes risk factors and microvascular complications. Diabetes Care. 1998;21:506–9.
3. Pavicic T, Korting HC. Xerosis and callus formation as a key to the diabetic foot syndrome: dermatologic view of the problem and its management. J Dtsch Dermatol Ges. 2006;4:935–41.
4. Jelinek J. The skin in diabetes. Diabet Med. 1993;10:201–13.
5. Reiber GE. The epidemiology of diabetic foot problems. Diabet Med. 1996;13:S6–11.
6. Margolis DJ, Allen-Taylor L, Hoffstad O, et al. Diabetic neuropathic foot ulcers: the association of wound size, wound duration, and wound grade on healing. Diabetes Care. 2002;25:1835–9.
7. Koya D, King GL. Protein kinase C activation and the development of diabetic complications. Diabetes. 1998;47:859–66.
8. Nishikawa T, Edelstein D, Du XL, et al. Normalizing mitochondrial superoxide production blocks three pathways of hyperglycaemic damage. Nature. 2000;404:787–90.
9. Kennedy L, Baynes JW. Non-enzymatic glycosylation and the chronic complications of diabetes: an overview. Diabetologia. 1984;26:93–8.
10. Sternberg M, Cohen Forterre L, Peyroux J. Connective tissue in diabetes mellitus: biochemical alterations of the intercellular matrix with special reference to proteoglycans, collagens and basement membranes. Diabetes Metab. 1985;11:27–50.
11. Schnider SL, Kohn RR. Effects of age and diabetes mellitus on the solubility and nonenzymatic glycosylation of human skin collagen. J Clin Invest. 1981;67:1630–5.
12. Aoki Y, Yazaki K, Shirotori K, et al. Stiffening of connective tissue in elderly patients with diabetes: relevance to diabetic nephropathy and oxidative stress. Diabetologia. 1993;36:79–83.
13. Hashmi F, Malone-Lee J, Hounsell E. Plantar skin in type II diabetes: an investigation of protein glycation and biomechanical properties of plantar epidermis. Eur J Dermatol. 2006;16:23–32.
14. Franzen LE, Roberg K. Impaired connective tissue repair in streptozotocin-induced diabetes shows ultrastructural signs of impaired contraction. J Surg Res. 1995;58:407–14.
15. Bitar MS. Glucocorticoid dynamics and impaired wound healing in diabetes mellitus. Am J Pathol. 1998;152:547–54.
16. Lateef H, Stevens MJ, Varani J. All-trans-retinoic acid suppresses matrix metalloproteinase activity and increases collagen synthesis in diabetic human skin in organ culture. Am J Pathol. 2004;165:167–74.
17. Rodgers KE, Ellefson DD, Espinoza T, et al. Expression of intracellular filament, collagen, and collagenase genes in diabetic and normal skin after injury. Wound Repair Regen. 2006;14:298–305.
18. Johnson BD, Page RC, Narayanan AS, et al. Effects of donor age on protein and collagen synthesis in vitro by human diploid fibroblasts. Lab Invest. 1986;55:490–6.
19. Burke EM, Horton WE, Pearson JD, et al. Altered transcriptional regulation of human interstitial collagenase in cultured skin fibroblasts from older donors. Exp Gerontol. 1994;29:37–53.
20. Tsao M, Walthall B, Ham R. Clonal growth of normal human epidermal keratinocytes in a defined medium. J Cell Physiol. 1982;110:219–29.
21. Benoliel AM, Kahn-Perles B, Imbert J, et al. Insulin stimulates haptotactic migration of human epidermal keratinocytes through activation of NF-kappa B transcription factor. J Cell Sci. 1997;110:2089–97.
22. Ando Y, Jensen PJ. Epidermal growth factor and insulin-like growth factor I enhance keratinocyte migration. J Invest Dermatol. 1993;100:633–9.
23. Wertheimer E, Trebicz M, Eldar T, et al. Differential roles of insulin receptor and insulin-like growth factor-1 receptor in differentiation of murine skin keratinocytes. J Invest Dermatol. 2000;115:24–9.
24. Yajima Y, Sueki H, Fujisawa R. Increased corneocyte surface area in the diabetic skin. Nippon Hifuka Gakkai Zasshi. 1991;101:129–34.
25. Sakai S, Endo Y, Ozawa N, et al. Characteristics of the epidermis and stratum corneum of hairless mice with experimentally induced diabetes mellitus. J Invest Dermatol. 2003;120:79–85.

26. Wilson GL, Leiter EH. Streptozotocin interactions with pancreatic beta cells and the induction of insulin-dependent diabetes. Curr Top Microbiol Immunol. 1990;156:27–54.
27. Tomlinson KC, Gardiner SM, Hebden RA, et al. Functional consequences of streptozotocin-induced diabetes mellitus, with particular reference to the cardiovascular system. Pharmacol Rev. 1992;44:103–50.
28. Cheta D. Animal models of type I (insulin-dependent) diabetes mellitus. J Pediatr Endocrinol Metab. 1998;11:11–9.
29. Sakai S, Kikuchi K, Satoh J, et al. Functional properties of the stratum corneum in patients with diabetes mellitus: similarities to senile xerosis. Br J Dermatol. 2005;153:319–23.
30. Horii I, Nakayama Y, Obata M, et al. Stratum corneum hydration and amino acid content in xerotic skin. Br J Dermatol. 1989;121:587–92.
31. Imokawa G, Kuno H, Kawai M. Stratum corneum lipids serve as a bound-water modulator. J Invest Dermatol. 1991;96:845–51.
32. O'goshi K, Iguchi M, Tagami H. Functional analysis of the stratum corneum of scalp skin: studies in patients with alopecia areata and androgenic alopecia. Arch Dermatol Res. 2000;292:605–11.
33. Denda M, Hori J, Koyama J, et al. Stratum corneum sphingolipids and free amino acids in experimentally-induced scaly skin. Arch Dermatol Res. 1992; 284:363–7.
34. Tanaka M, Okada M, Zhen YX, et al. Decreased hydration state of the stratum corneum and reduced amino acid content of the skin surface in patients with seasonal allergic rhinitis. Br J Dermatol. 1998; 139:618–21.
35. Imokawa G, Abe A, Jin K, et al. Decreased level of ceramides in stratum corneum of atopic dermatitis: an etiologic factor in atopic dry skin? J Invest Dermatol. 1991;96:523–6.
36. Akimoto K, Yoshikawa N, Higaki Y, et al. Quantitative analysis of stratum corneum lipids in xerosis and asteatotic eczema. J Dermatol. 1993;20:1–6.
37. Yoshikawa N, Imokawa G, Akimoto K, et al. Regional analysis of ceramides within the stratum corneum in relation to seasonal changes. Dermatology. 1994; 188:207–14.
38. Hara M, Kikuchi K, Watanabe M, et al. Senile xerosis: functional, morphological, and biochemical studies. J Geriatr Dermatol. 1993;1:111–20.
39. Saint-Leger D, Francois AM, Leveque JL, et al. Stratum corneum lipids in skin xerosis. Dermatologica. 1989;178:151–5.
40. Paulauskis JD, Sul HS. Cloning and expression of mouse fatty acid synthase and other specific mRNAs. Developmental and hormonal regulation in 3T3-L1 cells. J Biol Chem. 1988;263:7049–54.
41. Jensen MD, Caruso M, Heiling V, et al. Insulin regulation of lipolysis in nondiabetic and IDDM subjects. Diabetes. 1989;38:1595–601.
42. Sztalryd C, Kraemer FB. Regulation of hormone-sensitive lipase in streptozotocin-induced diabetic rats. Metabolism. 1995;44:1391–6.
43. Fluhr JW, Mao-Qiang M, Brown BE, et al. Glycerol regulates stratum corneum hydration in sebaceous gland deficient (asebia) mice. J Invest Dermatol. 2003;120:728–37.
44. Navarro X, Kennedy WR, Fries TJ. Small nerve fiber dysfunction in diabetic neuropathy. Muscle Nerve. 1989;12:498–507.
45. McLellan K, Petrofsky JS, Bains G, et al. The effects of skin moisture and subcutaneous fat thickness on the ability of the skin to dissipate heat in young and old subjects, with and without diabetes, at three environmental room temperatures. Med Eng Phys. 2008; 20:20.
46. Nakagawa N, Sakai S, Matsumoto M, et al. Relationship between NMF (lactate and potassium) content and the physical properties of the stratum corneum in healthy subjects. J Invest Dermatol. 2004;122:755–63.
47. Sugiyama Y, Ota Y, Hara M, et al. Osmotic stress up-regulates aquaporin-3 gene expression in cultured human keratinocytes. Biochim Biophys Acta. 2001;1522:82–8.
48. Ma T, Hara M, Sougrat R, et al. Impaired stratum corneum hydration in mice lacking epidermal water channel aquaporin-3. J Biol Chem. 2002;277:17147–53.
49. Hara-Chikuma M, Verkman AS. Prevention of skin tumorigenesis and impairment of epidermal cell proliferation by targeted aquaporin-3 gene disruption. Mol Cell Biol. 2008;28:326–32.
50. Corcuff P, Leveque JL. Size and shape of corneocytes at various body site: influence of age. In: Leveque J-L, Agache PG, editors. Aging skin. New York: Marcel Dekker; 1993. p. 199–216.
51. Watanabe M, Tagami H, Horii I, et al. Functional analyses of the superficial stratum corneum in atopic xerosis. Arch Dermatol. 1991;127:1689–92.
52. Candi E, Melino G, Mei G, et al. Biochemical, structural, and transglutaminase substrate properties of human loricrin, the major epidermal cornified cell envelope protein. J Biol Chem. 1995; 270:26382–90.
53. Wertheimer E, Spravchikov N, Trebicz M, et al. The regulation of skin proliferation and differentiation in the IR null mouse: implications for skin complications of diabetes. Endocrinology. 2001;142:1234–41.
54. Sadagurski M, Nofech-Mozes S, Weingarten G, et al. Insulin receptor substrate 1 (IRS-1) plays a unique role in normal epidermal physiology. J Cell Physiol. 2007;213:519–27.
55. Anand P, Terenghi G, Warner G, et al. The role of endogenous nerve growth factor in human diabetic neuropathy. Nat Med. 1996;2:703–7.
56. Terenghi G, Mann D, Kopelman PG, et al. trkA and trkC expression is increased in human diabetic skin. Neurosci Lett. 1997;228:33–6.

57. Sato J, Denda M, Nakanishi J, et al. Dry condition affects desquamation of stratum corneum in vivo. J Dermatol Sci. 1998;18:163–9.
58. Sakai S, Sasai S, Endo Y, et al. Characterization of the physical properties of the stratum corneum by a new tactile sensor. Skin Res Technol. 2000;6:128–34.
59. Sato J, Yanai M, Hirao T, et al. Water content and thickness of the stratum corneum contribute to skin surface morphology. Arch Dermatol Res. 2000;292:412–7.
60. Jo N, Watanabe M, Kiyokane K, et al. In vivo microradioautographic study of insulin binding in the skin of normal and NIDDM mice: with special reference to acanthosis nigricans. Cell Mol Biol (Noisy-le-Grand). 1997;43:157–64.
61. Toh YC. Effect of streptozotocin-induced diabetes on the activity of the sebaceous glands in rats. Endokrinologie. 1982;80:56–9.
62. Pham HT, Exelbert L, Segal-Owens AC, et al. A prospective, randomized, controlled double-blind study of a moisturizer for xerosis of the feet in patients with diabetes. Ostomy Wound Manage. 2002;48:30–6.

Impaired Wound Repair and Delayed Angiogenesis

76

Megan E. Schrementi, Matthew J. Ranzer, and Luisa A. DiPietro

Contents

Abstract

As the skin ages, the normal signs of aging such as alterations in pigmentation and increased wrinkling become more obvious. Although these changes appear to be mainly cosmetic, under the epidermis there is a gradual change in resident cell populations and loss of function. These changes result in a decreased ability to regulate homeostasis and underlie the delay in skin healing that occurs with age. Changes in hemostasis cause blood clotting to occur slowly and influence the healing progression. Likewise, age-related inflammatory changes in wounds most influence the latter phases of repair, including cellular proliferation and remodeling. Alterations in the stem cell populations that provide new cells to the healing wound occur, since this vital cell population is diminished in aged individuals. Thus, when a wound occurs, the normal stages of wound healing will proceed, although at an altered rate. In unfavorable conditions, this can result in an increased likelihood of infection or ulcer formation. Additionally, diseases associated with aging such as diabetes and vascular disease can amplify the alterations in wound healing, increasing the likelihood of wound complications. As research in the aged skin continues, the changes in the skin that affect wounding will continue to be elucidated, giving rise to new treatments for this growing patient population.

M.E. Schrementi (✉) • M.J. Ranzer • L.A. DiPietro
Center for Wound Healing and Tissue Regeneration, College of Dentistry, University of Illinois at Chicago, Chicago, IL, USA

Department of Biology, DePaul University, Chicago, IL, USA
e-mail: MSCHREME@depaul.edu; mranzermd@gmail.com; ldipiet@uic.edu

M.A. Farage et al. (eds.), *Textbook of Aging Skin*,
DOI 10.1007/978-3-662-47398-6_85

Introduction

Initially, the skin was thought of as a simple barrier to protect our internal organs from the outside world, but now it is understood to be exceptionally more complex than that. The skin serves multiple functions including regulating water loss, thermoregulation, protection from ultraviolet (UV) radiation, and entry of microorganisms and is an integral part of the immune system [1]. The skin ages via two processes, intrinsic aging and extrinsic aging. Intrinsic aging is seen in sun-protected areas of the skin and is subject to the same generalized aging conditions as any other cell or organ system. Extrinsic aging occurs in sun-exposed areas and is the cumulative effect of intrinsic aging plus the effect of environmental exposure to the aging process. The biggest extrinsic factor affecting skin aging is UV radiation encountered from sun exposure, which is also termed photoaging [2]. As the skin ages, it becomes progressively atrophied, dry, and rough, with alterations in pigmentation, decreased turgor, and increased wrinkling. This leads to a progressive loss of function, leaving the aged skin with a decreased ability to regulate homeostasis and more vulnerable to the environment [3].

Traumatic injuries are the fifth leading cause of death for persons over the age of 65 in the United States, and it is estimated that there will be well over 50 million people over the age of 65 by the year 2030 [4, 5]. Understanding the impact of aging on skin wound healing will be vital in dealing with this growing population in the future. Wound healing is a complex process involving multiple concurrent stages, dozens of cell types, and hundreds of mediators. As research on wound repair progresses, we have begun to learn how each of these components changes over time within an individual wound, between different wound conditions, and from wounds of differently aged individuals. Studies dating back almost a century show that wounds from older individuals do not heal as well as younger individuals [6]. More recent studies have provided information on how aging affects the individual components of wound healing including the inflammatory response, deposition of the wound matrix, and angiogenesis [7–9]. In short, the age of an individual has a profound effect on the process of wound healing as nearly any other identifiable condition or disease may have.

Age-Related Changes in the Components of the Skin

Before we can address the issue of how aging affects the wound healing process, we first must examine the changes in the milieu in which this wound healing process is occurring. Skin is a multilayered organ, with each layer's constituents optimized for its function. The outermost layer is the epidermis and is largely composed of squamous epithelial cells called keratinocytes and a smaller population of pigment-producing cells called melanocytes. The epidermis functions as a barrier against moisture loss and water entry. As we age, the thickness of the epidermis does not change although the density of melanocytes decreases and the dermal-epidermal junction becomes flattened giving the appearance of atrophy and cellular heterogeneity [10].

The dermis is composed of multiple cell types, structures, and fibers. Surrounding the hair follicles, sweat glands, and other intradermal glands are various fibers collectively referred to as the extracellular matrix (ECM). The ECM is composed of types I and III collagen, elastin, and glycosaminoglycans. The dermis is divided into two layers, the superficial papillary dermis and the deep reticular dermis. The papillary dermis maintains contact with the epidermis through the formation of papillary ridges. It is these ridges that become flattened as we age resulting in decreased surface contact and the previously mentioned appearance of atrophy, as well as decreased resistance to shear forces with lateral tension in the elderly skin [10]. There is also a decrease in the cellular component of the dermis including fibroblasts, mast cells, macrophages, and other immunologically important cells including Langerhans cells in the epidermis and dendritic cells in the dermis [9, 10]. Senescent cells accumulate in the skin with age and are thought to contribute to damage that accumulates in the skin. Interestingly, though, low levels of transitory senescent cells, which appear in wounds, have been shown to promote optimal wound healing in young animals [11].

The primary structural proteins in the dermis are collagen, fibronectin, and elastic fibers. While there is /a decrease both in the number and diameter of elastin fibers in the papillary dermis with age, in the reticular dermis, the opposite is true with an *increase* in the number and diameter of the elastin fibers [10]. Fibronectin has several functions including regulation of inflammation, cell adhesion, and migration and is closely associated with fibroblast production of collagen [12]. In isolated cell culture, some studies show an increase in fibronectin synthesis with age, but other in vivo studies show an age-related decrease in fibronectin expression with reduced levels of collagen [12, 13]. Collagen, the major protein found in the dermis, may be reduced in quantity in the aging skin, but there still exists some controversy on this point as some studies show a decrease with age, others describe an increase in collagen with age, and others show no change in collagen content with age [12, 14–16]. While there is controversy on the quantity, there is certainly a change in the quality of the collagen in aged skin. Collagen in young skin is typically described as rope-like bundles of dense collagen I fibers, arranged in a lattice or basket weave pattern. In the aged skin, the collagen is coarser, with individual bundles being primarily straight loosely woven fibers, and with an increase in density of the collagen network [10, 12, 17].

Dermal appendages including hair follicles and sweat glands are affected by the aging process as well. Hair follicle numbers are diminished with age but their structure is largely unchanged save for a small decrease in the number of surrounding melanocytes [18]. Sebaceous glands, which produce a waxy substance that coats hair shafts and reduces water evaporation, also decline with age [19]. Sweat glands are also reduced in number and function with age [20]. Microvascular blood flow to the skin decreases with age, with as much as a 40 % reduction in cutaneous blood flow by 70 years of age [21]. Thinning of blood vessel walls and basement membranes, with decreased numbers of perivascular cells, also occurs which promotes extravasation of plasma into the interstitial spaces [22]. Lymphatic drainage in the elderly is reduced, leading to greater edema and increasing the likelihood for ulcers [23].

In summary, at baseline, the aging skin has decreased potential for replication and migration. There is a decrease in the ECM components and a change in ECM architecture, resulting in decreased tensile strength. There is a reduction in dermal skin appendages including sweat glands and hair follicles [18, 19] and a reduction in the nutrient supply in the form of decreased microcirculation. Lastly, there is a greater tendency toward fluid accumulation due to increased permeability of the vasculature coupled with a decrease in lymphatic drainage. Table 1 below lists the age-related changes in the human skin. It is upon this background that we can now introduce the process of the healing wound into this aged skin.

Table 1 Summary of the changes occurring in the human skin with age

Clinical changes
Atrophy
Drying
Roughness
Alterations in pigmentation
Sagging
Wrinkling
Benign and malignant tumors
Histological changes
Flattening of the dermal-epidermal junction
↑ Turnover time
↓ Fibroblasts, mast cells, and macrophages
↓ Collagen content
Disorganized collagen and elastin
↓ Microcirculation
↓ Skin appendages
↓ Lymphatic drainage

↑ = increased, ↓ = decreased

Normal Wound Healing

Generally, wound healing may be described as occurring in four overlapping phases (see Fig. 1) [24]. During the first phase, hemostasis, blood loss is halted by vascular constriction, platelet aggregation, and activation of the clotting cascade. Endothelial cells normally line blood vessels, shielding platelets, and clotting factors from exposure to underlying collagen and basement membrane. After vessel injury and exposure to these normally hidden tissues, platelets are activated and aggregate via a combination of factors including ADP, von Willebrand factor (VWF), collagen, and thromboxane [25]. Activated platelets secrete cytosolic proteins and alpha-granules which contain numerous mediators of clotting and inflammation including transforming growth factor (TGF)-β, TGF-α, platelet-derived growth factor (PDGF), CD-40 ligand, and P-selectin [12, 25]. This leads to the release of fibrin, intracellular granules, and exposure of normally covered extracellular domains, all of which act as potent stimulators for inflammatory cells.

The second phase of wound healing, the inflammatory phase, occurs from time of injury through about the first week or so [26]. This phase is dominated by inflammatory cells beginning with neutrophils which remove invading pathogens and damaged cells and tissue. Although the neutrophil is the first leukocyte to arrive in the wound, when infection is not an issue, neutrophils may be dispensable for normal wound healing to occur [27]. Macrophages are the next inflammatory cell to enter the wound, removing debris and apoptotic cells and coordinating the interaction of other cell types. Unlike neutrophils, the macrophage is a critical mediator of tissue repair [28, 29]. Macrophages are recruited to wounds within a few days of injury by various chemoattractants, including chemokines [30]. Macrophages display a continuum of phenotypes within the wound ranging from highly inflammatory phenotype in the early wound to primarily reparative as healing proceeds. Inflammatory macrophages engulf and phagocytose wound debris and also produce cytokines that further stimulate the inflammatory response. As inflammation subsides, the function of macrophages turns toward supporting the cellular proliferation needed for tissue restitution. Reparative macrophages produce many of the angiogenic and fibrogenic growth factors that promote in the growth phase of repair, a function that is known to be essential for optimal healing [30]. Once the neutrophil and macrophage populations decline in the wound, T lymphocytes become the dominant leukocyte in the later stages of inflammation [31]; the function of these cells in the healing process is not yet well defined. The role of inflammation in wound healing is still an area of active investigation. Excessive inflammation is known to be detrimental to healing, but the exact levels of inflammation and cellular functions

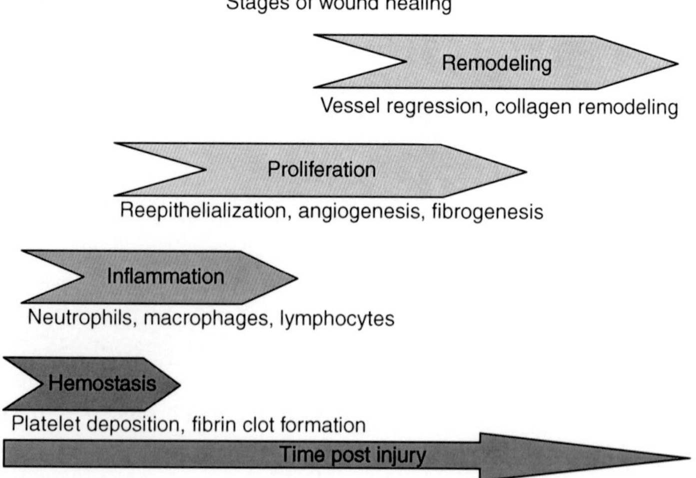

Fig. 1 The four overlapping phases of wound healing

needed for optimal healing are not fully understood [32].

The proliferative phase of wound healing overlaps with inflammation and involves the replacement of missing tissues via cellular proliferation and the production of extracellular matrix. Keratinocytes, fibroblasts, and endothelial cells proliferate and migrate in the wound, laying down new collagen, extracellular matrix, blood vessels, and epithelial covering [33]. During the final remodeling or resolution phase, the tissue undergoes changes that bring it closer to the original architecture. The excessive blood vessels that were initially formed now regress toward normal vascular density, immature collagen is resorbed and replaced with mature collagen, and the epithelium matures. The remodeling phase can last for more than a year, as the tissue is continually modified to approximate normal structure.

Age-Related Alterations in Hemostasis

The activation of platelets occurs quickly after injury, and this initial step is altered with age. During aging, platelets become hyperreactive, with an increase in surface ligands, enhanced aggregation, and an increase in the release of prothrombotic and proinflammatory mediators [34]. Coagulation is also affected by age, including elevated serum concentrations of activated clotting factors, fibrin breakdown products, and inhibitors of clot-destroying enzymes like plasminogen activator inhibitor-1. There are also complimentary decreases in the activity of coagulation inhibitors such as antithrombin III and activated protein C [35]. These changes are summarized in Table 2 below.

Table 2 Summary of age-related changes in hemostasis

↑ Platelet adherence to collagen	↓ Inhibitors of coagulation
↑ Platelet aggregation	↑ Inhibitors of clot lysis inhibitors
↑ Release of mediators	↑ Concentrations of active clotting factors
↑ Concentrations of active clotting factors	

↑ = increased, ↓ = decreased

Age-Related Alterations in the Inflammatory Phase

There are many studies regarding changes seen during the inflammatory phase of wound healing in the aged skin, and multiple perturbations have been noted [36]. Neutrophil function is impaired by aging, as neutrophils isolated from elderly humans have a decreased respiratory burst, diminished capability to phagocytose, and diminished chemotactic ability [37–39]. However, studies demonstrate no difference in wound debridement, cellularity, or connective tissue formation in the wounds of control and neutropenic animals [27]. Although neutrophils may play a role as a first line of defense against bacterial invasion, some studies suggest that the role of neutrophils in uncontaminated wounds is probably minimal or even perhaps detrimental [40, 41]. The macrophage, however, seems to be required for wound healing to occur normally, and age-related changes in this cell type are likely to be important to healing outcomes [30]. Wound repair is accelerated in aged mice that receive ip injections of macrophages harvested from young mice but not from old mice [42], and macrophage-based therapies have been proposed to improve human wound healing. There are many possible explanations for these effects including decreased numbers, diminished chemotaxis, or altered cytokine production in the macrophages with aging. Certain macrophage functions, such as phagocytosis, are well described to diminish with age [43, 44]. The mechanisms to explain this decrease in macrophage function may involve receptor function and signal transduction defects. Several cell surface receptors required for macrophage activation and recognition are decreased including MHC class II [45], and signal transduction pathways in macrophages including the MAP kinases ERK, p38, and JNK are negatively affected by age [46]. Overall, phagocytic activity, cytokine production, infiltration, and antigen presentation are affected in macrophages with age [45, 47]. As

Table 3 Summary of age-related changes during the inflammatory phase

↓ Macrophage function	↓ Neutrophil function
↑ Secretion of inflammatory mediators	↓ Vascular permeability
↓ Secretion of growth factors	↓ Infiltration of macrophages and lymphocytes

↑ = increased, ↓ = decreased

these are all vital components of the wound healing process, the age-related functional deficits displayed by macrophages probably contribute significantly to the healing impairment seen in aging skin. Not surprisingly, aging has been shown to affect the polarization of macrophages from the inflammatory to the regenerative phenotype; this change in the balance of macrophage phenotypes might be critical to the delayed healing that occurs with age [48].

The age-related inflammatory changes that are seen (Table 3) in wounds most probably influence other phases of repair, including cellular proliferation and perhaps remodeling.

Age-Related Changes During the Proliferative Phase

Aging has a high level of impact on the proliferative phase of healing. Delays in reepithelialization and decreases in collagen synthesis and organization have been described in wounds of aged humans and rats [43]. Additional studies establish decreases in wound breaking strength and increases in wound disruption with age [49, 50]. Age-related delays in reepithelialization of wounds have been documented in both animal and human subjects [12, 15, 51] (Fig. 2).

Many studies show that the proliferative capacity of keratinocytes decreases with age and that there is a decline in the rate of normal keratinocyte turnover in the aged skin [52–54]. Additional studies describe a decrease in keratinocyte migration in aged skin as well. Hypoxia is a potent stimulus for keratinocytes from young persons to migrate, but the opposite effect is seen in keratinocytes from aged individuals [55, 56]. This decrease in hypoxia-associated keratinocyte migration in aged skin is partially related to a decrease in MMP production. MMP-1 and MMP-9 which are both associated with keratinocyte migration in wounds are upregulated in young keratinocytes but downregulated in aged keratinocytes [56]. Overall, then, there appears to be a baseline decrease in the proliferation and migration of keratinocytes in aged skin. Once an injury occurs, the normal keratinocyte response to proliferate and migrate across the wound is impaired. The age-related impairment results in a delay of wound closure, increasing the chance for infection or chronic wound development.

Not only are keratinocytes impaired by aging, but the major proliferative cell in the dermis, the fibroblast, displays significant age-related impairments as well [12, 57–59]. A decrease in the number, size, and proliferation rate of fibroblasts in the skin occurs with age. Fibroblasts exhibit age-associated migratory deficiencies, a decline in motility independent of chemotactic stimulus, and a decline in fibronectin-associated migration. Aged fibroblasts also have poorly developed endoplasmic reticulum, suggesting decreased protein synthetic capability [60].

A large number of studies document an age-related decrease in the responsiveness of fibroblasts to a wide variety of cell signaling molecules and cytokines. For example, human fibroblasts have an age-associated decrease in mitogenic response to epidermal growth factor (EGF), insulin, dexamethasone, and transferrin [61]. Human fibroblasts also show decreased responsiveness to FGF-7 (KGF), to PDGF, and to TGFβ1 [12, 62, 63]. Such deficits may be related to receptor function, as a striking difference in EGF receptor (EGFR) number, affinity, and rate of EGF/EGFR internalization is seen in early passage dermal fibroblasts derived from newborn versus young adult versus old adult donors. A decline in insulin receptor levels is also seen in aged fibroblasts [64]. TGF-β receptor types I and II are decreased in hypoxic but not normoxic conditions in aged fibroblasts from human donors, and downstream phosphorylation is also decreased [63]. Some of these receptors are

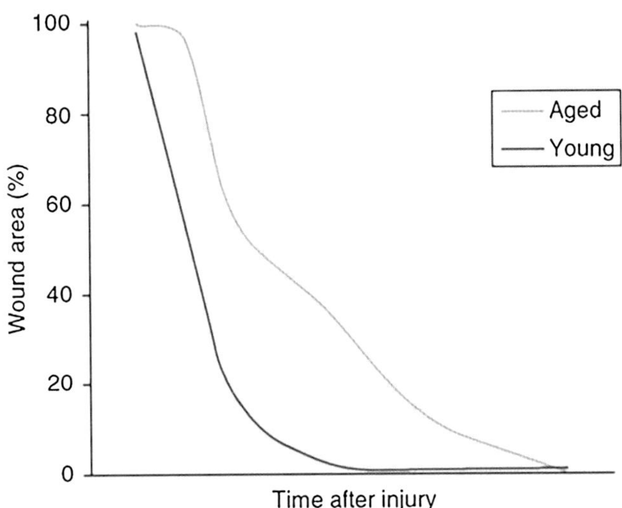

Fig. 2 Representation of the time course of excisional wound reepithelialization in young and aged mice. Young mice have smaller wound areas across all healing times and reach complete closure before aged mice

Table 4 Summary of changes seen during the proliferative phase

↓Collagen deposition	↓ Proliferation of keratinocytes, fibroblasts
↓ Migration of keratinocytes, fibroblasts	→ Reepithelialization
↓ Receptor numbers and response	

↓ = decreased, → = delayed

Table 5 Summary of changes seen during remodeling

→ ↓ Wound strength	↑ Collagen degradation
↓ TIMP	↓ Lysyl oxidase cross-linking

↑ = increased, ↓ = decreased, → = delayed

not only important for proliferation and migration of fibroblasts but are also involved in the production of fibroblast-derived cytokines and fibrogenesis in fibroblasts.

A reduction in the production of cytokines and growth factors by fibroblasts has been described with age. Some of these decreases include FGF-2, FGF-7, VEGF, and TGF-β1 [15, 65]. This reduction in synthetic ability of fibroblasts is not limited to cytokines alone, as declines in fibronectin and collagen production are also described. Although some studies show no age-related changes in collagen production, many studies demonstrate a clear decrease in collagen production with age including reduced collagen production after age 30 in humans, delayed collagen content (but ultimately similar final levels) in wounds of aged mice, and reduced mRNA production of type I collagen with age [8, 15, 66, 67]. Tables 4 and 5 describe the age-related changes seen during the proliferative and remodeling phases of wound healing.

Age-Related Changes During Remodeling

During the remodeling phase of healing, collagen degradation and synthesis both occur, along with maturation of collagen structure, and the dermal architecture moves closer to the original normal structure. In aging, levels of collagen degradation in wounds appear to increase. The enzymes that are most active in collagen degradation are the matrix metalloproteinases (MMPs), a family of proteases that have various functions including acting as intermediary signaling molecules, but are primarily thought to be active as proteolytic degradation enzymes. The MMPs are secreted by various cells including keratinocytes and fibroblasts and collectively are known to degrade collagen, gelatin, and other ECM components. Tissue inhibitors of metalloproteinases (TIMPs) are naturally occurring inhibitors of MMPs, and their presence helps balance the degree of collagen synthesis and breakdown in wound healing. While there are some conflicting reports, the preponderance of evidence currently points toward increased MMP levels and decreased TIMP levels in aging skin [12, 56, 68–70]. As research continues to examine this process, this notion will likely evolve: alterations in protease balance are likely not to be uniform, and depending on the cell types, substrates, and wound conditions being examined, it is quite possible that divergent effects will be seen. It is possible that collagen degradation by MMPs may be enhanced while receptor-mediated interactions with MMPs may be reduced. Divergent effects may also occur over early wound time points versus later wound time points as wound healing is incredibly dynamic requiring appropriate increase and decreases in each element at appropriate times.

The end result of the remodeling phase is a durable dermis, one measure of which is the strength of the wound. Studies demonstrate a decrease in tensile strength in older individuals in a variety of settings including intestinal anastomoses, cutaneous wounds, and abdominal incisions [50, 71]. Tensile strength of wounds is not solely dependent on the amount of collagen present but also relies upon the degree of cross-linking of the collagen fibers and the overall architecture. Collagen can be cross-linked by two mechanisms. In enzymatic cross-linking, collagen is cross-linked by a posttranslational modification via the enzymatic activity of lysyl oxidase (LOX). This enzyme cross-links collagen in a specific pattern and maintains an association with the collagen fibrils preventing nonspecific cross-linking [72]. Enzymatic cross-linking occurs in the normal and wounded skin and contributes to improved collagen architecture and tissue strength. The second method of collagen cross-linking is via a nonspecific chemical modification by cross-link oxidation or nonenzymatic glycosylation [73, 74].

Both enzymatic and nonspecific cross-linking are described to be altered with aging. In regard to enzymatic cross-linking, alterations in LOX activity are described with aging. An age-associated decrease in LOX activity in the skin has been described [75, 76]. Despite this described decrease in LOX activity, increases in collagen insolubility are reported with higher intra- and intermolecular cross-linking in older subjects [72, 77]. This apparent disparity between decreased LOX activity and increased collagen cross-linking may actually go hand in hand. As previously stated, while LOX does cross-link collagen, it also protects it from nonspecific cross-linking. Some studies show that the specific LOX-derived cross-links decrease with age and the nonspecific chemical and glycosylation cross-links increase [72]. This increase in nonspecific collagen cross-links may explain some of the physical changes described in the elderly skin including coarse collagen structure, stiffer ECM, and decreased chemotaxis of inflammatory and proliferative cells such as endothelial cells.

Age-Related Changes in Angiogenesis

While some controversy exists as to whether wound angiogenesis is increased or decreased with age, most studies demonstrate an overall decrease in the angiogenic capacity of the aging skin [13, 15, 78]. Studies on excisional wounds and subcutaneous implant models in aged animals both show a delay in wound capillary ingrowth [15, 79]. This delay may be a function of impaired migration, cellular senescence of endothelial cells, or may be due to decreases in growth factor expression. Many studies have delineated that age-associated impairments in the production and function of proangiogenic factors play a role in the decreased wound angiogenesis [15, 80]. A decrease in capillary density, along with a decrease in the production of the proangiogenic stimuli FGF-2 and VEGF, is demonstrated in excisional wounds from aged mice. In addition, the in vivo response to a defined level of proangiogenic stimulus, implanted subcutaneously, is shown to decrease in aged animals. Other studies demonstrate similar impairments including decreased perfusion and capillary density with decreased VEGF levels in aged animals and a concomitant increase in subsequent vascular density with recombinant VEGF supplementation [81]. The reduction in sprouting of vessels seen in aged mice can be reversed by the addition of growth factors such as IGF-1, VEGF, TGF-β1, or bFGF [82]. An increase in antiangiogenic factors, such as members of the thrombospondin (TSP) family, is found in wounds of aged animals and may provide a second layer of inhibition on endothelial functions beyond the simple deficiency of stimulatory growth factors. Thrombospondin is known to inhibit neovascularization through a variety of mechanisms including limiting vessel density, inducing apoptosis in endothelial cells, and decreasing the response of endothelial cells to various stimulatory signals including VEGF [83]. In one study, TSP-2 expression increases in fibroblasts from wounds of aged mice, and TSP knockout mice have increased angiogenesis compared to wild-type counterparts [7]. Several studies describe an increase in TSP levels with age [7, 13, 84].

SPARC is a multifunctional glycoprotein that modulates cellular-ECM interaction, inhibits cellular proliferation, and regulates the activity of growth factors. SPARC can bind directly to VEGF, inhibit VEGF-receptor interaction, and prevent VEGF-induced phosphorylation of VEGF receptor-1 [85]. SPARC has been shown to inhibit the proliferative and migratory effects of FGF and VEGF on endothelial cells [86, 87]. SPARC expression increases with age in several models both in vivo and in vitro in a variety of studies [87, 88]. This age-related increase in SPARC should contribute to the decrease in VEGF and angiogenesis that is observed in aging. While there are probably many reasons for the decrease in VEGF expression and endothelial cell migration in aging skin and wounds, the increase in inhibitors of angiogenesis like TSP-1 and SPARC provides additional means of inhibition, beyond mere cellular senescence in wounds from aged individuals.

Regardless of the underlying mechanism, endothelial function and angiogenesis are impaired in aging skin (see Table 6). Whether due to an age-related increase in angiogenic inhibitors; a decrease in growth factors like VEGF, EGF, or FGF; a decrease in endothelial migration and proliferation; or an impairment of downstream receptor signaling, the end result is that angiogenesis in wounds from aged individuals is impaired. A significant decrease in angiogenesis can often negatively impact healing. However, the influence of the age-related angiogenic impairment on the healing capacity of any particular wound probably varies due to individual wound conditions.

Table 6 Summary of age-related changes seen in angiogenesis

→ Capillary ingrowth	↓ Migration and proliferation of endothelial cells
↑ Inhibitors of angiogenesis	↓ Angiogenic cytokines
→, ↓ Vascular density	

↑ = increased, ↓ = decreased, → = delayed

Age-Related Changes to Dermal Stem Cells

The constant turnover of cells needed for a proper healing response necessitates reservoirs of stem cells. By classic definition, a stem cell is one that has the ability to differentiate into a specialized cell type and has the ability to self-renew while maintaining an undifferentiated state [89]. Consistent with the link between advanced age and improper healing as described above, stem cells are also susceptible to the aging process [90, 91]. Recent advances have enhanced the identification and isolation of specific cell populations and propagate them successfully in the lab. Thus, several populations of stem cells specific to the healing process have been described. Many groups studying the role of different stem cell populations during the healing process have focused three main stem cell populations: adipose-derived progenitor cells (ADPC), epidermal progenitor cells (EPCs), and mesenchymal stems cells (MSCs). As this continues to be a rapidly growing field of exploration, it can be assumed that additional populations and subpopulations will be defined.

Most stem cells necessary for reepithelialization and remodeling such as the EPC and

ADPC are found at the base of the hair follicle, the base of the sebaceous gland, and within the basal layer of the epidermis [92]. These cells are attracted and activated in the damaged tissue through complex chemokine coordination. Once there, they play a major role in reepithelialization and neovascularization. The hardy and robust EPCs have shown great promise for use in skin grafts in young patients [93]. However, the effect of aging on this stem cell population has yet to be clearly described.

Mesenchymal stem cell (MSC) is found in most adult connective tissues and organs [94]. Thus, they are in abundance and easier to isolate than the EPC. The role of MSCs in wound healing is critical. These include their ability to migrate to the site of injury, induce proliferation of resident cells, secret growth factors, reduce inflammation, and assist in regeneration of damaged tissues [95, 96].

MSCs have been shown to be affected by aging that ultimately impairs the healing process. Aged MSCs show changes in both the proliferative capacity as well as the ability to differentiate properly [90]. MSCs isolated from aged volunteers show a reduced proliferative capacity along with increased in cellular senescence compared to those of younger adults [91]. In rats, aged MSCs have also been shown to have reduced expression of VEGF and TGF-β which is consistent with decreased angiogenesis described in aged individuals [97]. Studies in mice have shown that diminished healing capacity can be attributed to a decrease in the expression of proangiogenic growth factors. Wounds treated with these murine-aged MSCs are unable to improve wound healing or enhance vascularity in aged mice [98]. Thus, MSCs used for autologous transplant in older patients have had limited success as a wound healing treatment. However, more recent studies demonstrate that MSCs harvested from younger mice can improve healing in an aged mouse model [99]. The desirable effects of MSCs in wounds might involve their ability to influence macrophage function. As mentioned earlier, wound macrophage transition from a proinflammatory to a healing or reparative phenotype, and shifts in this transition may be involved in age-related healing deficits. Recent studies have suggested that MSCs can reprogram the proinflammatory macrophage to the pro-regenerative phenotype needed for the final phases of wound repair, providing a mechanism by which MSCs might improve healing of aged skin [100].

Conclusion

Even though angiogenesis and wound healing may be delayed in an aged individual, if they are otherwise healthy and the wound is in optimal condition, no functional detriment might be observed. The wound will close, no infection will set in, and the individual will be none the wiser that it took a few extra hours to close, that there were fewer blood vessels, or that the strength of the skin across the wound will take an extra few weeks to achieve maximal strength. The real impact of the impairment in wound healing and angiogenesis is not on the healthy aged individual, but on the aged individual with baseline impairments: a lower extremity laceration on an elderly woman with peripheral vascular disease or a man with diabetes, for example. For these individuals who already have a baseline deficiency in the maximal potential for wound healing, a slight reduction in angiogenesis or a slight delay in wound closure, cytokines, or growth factor activity could mean the difference between an infection and a clean wound and a chronic ulcer or a healthy scar.

References

1. Harris TJ. The skin. In: Rubin E, Faber J, editors. Pathology. Philadelphia: Lippincott-Raven; 1999. p. 1236–99.
2. Fisher GJ, et al. Pathophysiology of premature skin aging induced by ultraviolet light. N Engl J Med. 1997;337:1419–28.
3. Gilchrest BA, et al. Aging and photoaging affect gene expression in cultured human keratinocytes. Arch Dermatol. 1994;130:82–6.
4. Census Bureau US. Population projections program. Washington, DC: Population Division, U.S. Census Bureau; 2000.

5. McMahon DJ, et al. Comorbidity and the elderly trauma patient. World J Surg. 1996;20:1113–9; discussion 9–20.
6. DuNouy P. Cicatrization of wounds: the relation between the age of the patient, the area of the wound, and the index of cicatrization. J Exp Med. 1916;24:461–70.
7. Agah A, et al. Thrombospondin 2 levels are increased in aged mice: consequences for cutaneous wound healing and angiogenesis. Matrix Biol. 2004;22:539–47.
8. Ashcroft GS, et al. Aging is associated with reduced deposition of specific extracellular matrix components, an upregulation of angiogenesis, and an altered inflammatory response in a murine incisional wound healing model. J Invest Dermatol. 1997;108:430–7.
9. Swift ME, et al. Age-related alterations in the inflammatory response to dermal injury. J Invest Dermatol. 2001;117:1027–35.
10. Kurban RS, Bhawan J. Histologic changes in skin associated with aging. J Dermatol Surg Oncol. 1990;16:908–14.
11. Demaria M, et al. Cell autonomous and non-autonomous effects of senescent cells in the skin. J Invest Dermatol. 2015;135:1722–6.
12. Ashcroft GS, et al. The effects of ageing on cutaneous wound healing in mammals. J Anat. 1995;187 (Pt 1):1–26.
13. Reed MJ, Edelberg JM. Impaired angiogenesis in the aged. Sci Aging Knowledge Environ. 2004;2004:pe7.
14. Clausen B. Influence of age on connective tissue. Hexosamine and hydroxyproline in human aorta, myocardium, and skin. Lab Invest. 1962;11:229–34.
15. Swift ME, et al. Impaired wound repair and delayed angiogenesis in aged mice. Lab Invest. 1999;79:1479–87.
16. Vitellaro-Zuccarello L, et al. Immunocytochemical localization of collagen types I, III, IV, and fibronectin in the human dermis. Modifications with ageing. Cell Tissue Res. 1992;268:505–11.
17. Lavker RM. Structural alterations in exposed and unexposed aged skin. J Invest Dermatol. 1979;73:59–66.
18. Montagna W, Carlisle K. Structural changes in ageing skin. Br J Dermatol. 1990;122 Suppl 35:61–70.
19. Pochi PE, et al. Age-related changes in sebaceous gland activity. J Invest Dermatol. 1979;73:108–11.
20. Silver A. The effect of age on human eccrine sweating. In: Montagna W, editor. Advances in biology of the skin, vol. 6. Oxford: Pergamon; 1965. p. 129–49.
21. Tsuchida Y. The effect of aging and arteriosclerosis on human skin blood flow. J Dermatol Sci. 1993;5:175–81.
22. Braverman IM, Fonferko E. Studies in cutaneous aging: II. The microvasculature. J Invest Dermatol. 1982;78:444–8.
23. Gniadecka M, et al. Age-related diurnal changes of dermal oedema: evaluation by high-frequency ultrasound. Br J Dermatol. 1994;131:849–55.
24. Witte MB, Barbul A. General principles of wound healing. Surg Clin North Am. 1997;77:509–28.
25. Davi G, Patrono C. Platelet activation and atherothrombosis. N Engl J Med. 2007;357:2482–94.
26. Ross R, Benditt EP. Wound healing and collagen formation. II. Fine structure in experimental scurvy. J Cell Biol. 1962;12:533 51.
27. Simpson DM, Ross R. The neutrophilic leukocyte in wound repair a study with antineutrophil serum. J Clin Invest. 1972;51:2009–23.
28. Mirza R, et al. Selective and specific macrophage ablation is detrimental to wound healing in mice. Am J Pathol. 2009;175:2454–62.
29. Leibovich SJ, Ross R. The role of the macrophage in wound repair. A study with hydrocortisone and antimacrophage serum. Am J Pathol. 1975;78: 71–100.
30. Koh TJ, DiPietro LA. Inflammation and wound healing: the role of the macrophage. Expert Rev Mol Med. 2011;13:e23.
31. Ross R, Odland G. Human wound repair. II. Inflammatory cells, epithelial-mesenchymal interrelations, and fibrogenesis. J Cell Biol. 1968;39:152–68.
32. Degen KE, Gourdie RG. Embryonic wound healing: a primer for engineering novel therapies for tissue repair. Birth Defects Res C Embryo Today. 2012;96:258–70.
33. Shaw TJ, Martin P. Wound repair at a glance. J Cell Sci. 2009;122:3209–13.
34. Mohebali D, et al. Alterations in platelet function during aging: clinical correlations with thromboinflammatory disease in older adults. J Am Geriatr Soc. 2014;62:529–35.
35. Hager K, et al. Blood coagulation factors in the elderly. Arch Gerontol Geriatr. 1989;9:277–82.
36. Kovacs EJ. Aging, traumatic injury, and estrogen treatment. Exp Gerontol. 2005;40:549–55.
37. Butcher SK, et al. Senescence in innate immune responses: reduced neutrophil phagocytic capacity and CD16 expression in elderly humans. J Leukoc Biol. 2001;70:881–6.
38. Di Lorenzo G, et al. Granulocyte and natural killer activity in the elderly. Mech Ageing Dev. 1999;108:25–38.
39. Fortin CF, et al. Impairment of SHP-1 down-regulation in the lipid rafts of human neutrophils under GM-CSF stimulation contributes to their age-related, altered functions. J Leukoc Biol. 2006;79:1061–72.
40. Dovi JV, et al. Accelerated wound closure in neutrophil-depleted mice. J Leukoc Biol. 2003;73:448–55.
41. Martin P, et al. Wound healing in the PU.1 null mouse – tissue repair is not dependent on inflammatory cells. Curr Biol. 2003;13:1122–8.
42. Danon D, et al. Promotion of wound repair in old mice by local injection of macrophages. Proc Natl Acad Sci U S A. 1989;86:2018–20.

43. Gosain A, DiPietro LA. Aging and wound healing. World J Surg. 2004;28:321–6.
44. Plowden J, et al. Innate immunity in aging: impact on macrophage function. Aging Cell. 2004;3:161–7.
45. Herrero C, et al. Immunosenescence of macrophages: reduced MHC class II gene expression. Exp Gerontol. 2002;37:389–94.
46. Gomez CR, et al. Innate immunity and aging. Exp Gerontol. 2008;43:718–28.
47. Donnini A, et al. Phenotype, antigen-presenting capacity, and migration of antigen-presenting cells in young and old age. Exp Gerontol. 2002;37:1097–112.
48. Goh J, Ladiges WC. Exercise enhances wound healing and prevents cancer progression during aging by targeting macrophage polarity. Mech Ageing Dev. 2014;139:41–8.
49. Holm-Pedersen P, Viidik A. Tensile properties and morphology of healing wounds in young and old rats. Scand J Plast Reconstr Surg. 1972;6:24–35.
50. Mendoza Jr CB, et al. Veterans Administration cooperative study of surgery for duodenal ulcer. II. Incidence of wound disruption following operation. Arch Surg. 1970;101:396–8.
51. Holt DR, et al. Effect of age on wound healing in healthy human beings. Surgery. 1992;112:293–7; discussion 7–8.
52. Gilchrest BA. In vitro assessment of keratinocyte aging. J Invest Dermatol. 1983;81:184s–9.
53. Rheinwald JG, Green H. Serial cultivation of strains of human epidermal keratinocytes: the formation of keratinizing colonies from single cells. Cell. 1975;6:331–43.
54. Morris GM, et al. The cell kinetics of the epidermis and follicular epithelium of the rat: variations with age and body site. Cell Tissue Kinet. 1989;22:213–22.
55. Ross C, et al. Oxygen tension changes the rate of migration of human skin keratinocytes in an age-related manner. Exp Dermatol. 2011;20:58–63.
56. Xia YP, et al. Differential activation of migration by hypoxia in keratinocytes isolated from donors of increasing age: implication for chronic wounds in the elderly. J Invest Dermatol. 2001;116:50–6.
57. Albini A, et al. Decline of fibroblast chemotaxis with age of donor and cell passage number. Coll Relat Res. 1988;8:23–37.
58. Pienta KJ, Coffey DS. Characterization of the subtypes of cell motility in ageing human skin fibroblasts. Mech Ageing Dev. 1990;56:99–105.
59. Plisko A, Gilchrest BA. Growth factor responsiveness of cultured human fibroblasts declines with age. J Gerontol. 1983;38:513–8.
60. Pieraggi MT, et al. Fibroblast changes in cutaneous ageing. Virchows Arch A Pathol Anat Histopathol. 1984;402:275–87.
61. Phillips PD, et al. Progressive loss of the proliferative response of senescing WI-38 cells to platelet-derived growth factor, epidermal growth factor, insulin, transferrin, and dexamethasone. J Gerontol. 1984;39:11–7.
62. Stanulis-Praeger BM, Gilchrest BA. Growth factor responsiveness declines during adulthood for human skin-derived cells. Mech Ageing Dev. 1986;35:185–98.
63. Mogford JE, et al. Effect of age and hypoxia on TGFbeta1 receptor expression and signal transduction in human dermal fibroblasts: impact on cell migration. J Cell Physiol. 2002;190:259–65.
64. Reenstra WR, et al. Effect of donor age on epidermal growth factor processing in man. Exp Cell Res. 1993;209:118–22.
65. Komi-Kuramochi A, et al. Expression of fibroblast growth factors and their receptors during full-thickness skin wound healing in young and aged mice. J Endocrinol. 2005;186:273–89.
66. Furth JJ. The steady-state levels of type I collagen mRNA are reduced in senescent fibroblasts. J Gerontol. 1991;46:B122–4.
67. Lovell CR, et al. Type I and III collagen content and fibre distribution in normal human skin during ageing. Br J Dermatol. 1987;117:419–28.
68. Burke EM, et al. Altered transcriptional regulation of human interstitial collagenase in cultured skin fibroblasts from older donors. Exp Gerontol. 1994;29:37–53.
69. Hornebeck W. Down-regulation of tissue inhibitor of matrix metalloprotease-1 (TIMP-1) in aged human skin contributes to matrix degradation and impaired cell growth and survival. Pathol Biol (Paris). 2003;51:569–73.
70. Tan EM, et al. Extracellular matrix gene expression by human keratinocytes and fibroblasts from donors of varying ages. Trans Assoc Am Physicians. 1993;106:168–78.
71. Sussman MD. Aging of connective tissue: physical properties of healing wounds in young and old rats. Am J Physiol. 1973;224:1167–71.
72. Szauter KM, et al. Lysyl oxidase in development, aging and pathologies of the skin. Pathol Biol (Paris). 2005;53:448–56.
73. Au V, Madison SA. Effects of singlet oxygen on the extracellular matrix protein collagen: oxidation of the collagen crosslink histidinohydroxylysinonorleucine and histidine. Arch Biochem Biophys. 2000;384:133–42.
74. Ulrich P, Cerami A. Protein glycation, diabetes, and aging. Recent Prog Horm Res. 2001;56:1–21.
75. Quaglino D, et al. Extracellular matrix modifications in rat tissues of different ages. Correlations between elastin and collagen type I mRNA expression and lysyl-oxidase activity. Matrix. 1993;13:481–90.
76. Reiser KM, et al. Analysis of age-associated changes in collagen crosslinking in the skin and lung in monkeys and rats. Biochim Biophys Acta. 1987;926:339–48.
77. Fornieri C, et al. Correlations between age and rat dermis modifications. Ultrastructural-morphometric evaluations and lysyl oxidase activity. Aging (Milano). 1989;1:127–38.

78. Chung JH, Eun HC. Angiogenesis in skin aging and photoaging. J Dermatol. 2007;34:593–600.
79. Yamaura H, Matsuzawa T. Decrease in capillary growth during aging. Exp Gerontol. 1980;15:145–50.
80. Reed MJ, et al. Neovascularization in aged mice: delayed angiogenesis is coincident with decreased levels of transforming growth factor beta1 and type I collagen. Am J Pathol. 1998;152:113–23.
81. Rivard A, et al. Age-dependent impairment of angiogenesis. Circulation. 1999;99:111–20.
82. Arthur WT, et al. Growth factors reverse the impaired sprouting of microvessels from aged mice. Microvasc Res. 1998;55:260–70.
83. Jimenez B, et al. Signals leading to apoptosis-dependent inhibition of neovascularization by thrombospondin-1. Nat Med. 2000;6:41–8.
84. Sadoun E, Reed MJ. Impaired angiogenesis in aging is associated with alterations in vessel density, matrix composition, inflammatory response, and growth factor expression. J Histochem Cytochem. 2003;51:1119–30.
85. Brekken RA, Sage EH. SPARC, a matricellular protein: at the crossroads of cell-matrix communication. Matrix Biol. 2001;19:816–27.
86. Kupprion C, et al. SPARC (BM-40, osteonectin) inhibits the mitogenic effect of vascular endothelial growth factor on microvascular endothelial cells. J Biol Chem. 1998;273:29635–40.
87. Reed MJ, et al. Enhanced angiogenesis characteristic of SPARC-null mice disappears with age. J Cell Physiol. 2005;204:800–7.
88. Shiba H, et al. Effects of ageing on proliferative ability, and the expressions of secreted protein, acidic and rich in cysteine (SPARC) and osteoprotegerin (osteoclastogenesis inhibitory factor) in cultures of human periodontal ligament cells. Mech Ageing Dev. 2000;117:69–77.
89. King A, et al. The role of stem cells in wound angiogenesis. Adv Wound Care (New Rochelle). 2014;3:614–25.
90. Wu W, et al. The effect of age on human adipose-derived stem cells. Plast Reconstr Surg. 2013;131:27–37.
91. Alt EU, et al. Aging alters tissue resident mesenchymal stem cell properties. Stem Cell Res. 2012;8:215–25.
92. Blanpain C, Fuchs E. Epidermal homeostasis: a balancing act of stem cells in the skin. Nat Rev Mol Cell Biol. 2009;10:207–17.
93. Sun BK, et al. Advances in skin grafting and treatment of cutaneous wounds. Science. 2014;346:941–5.
94. da Silva Meirelles L, et al. Mesenchymal stem cells reside in virtually all post-natal organs and tissues. J Cell Sci. 2006;119:2204–13.
95. Hanson SE, et al. Mesenchymal stem cell therapy for nonhealing cutaneous wounds. Plast Reconstr Surg. 2010;125:510–6.
96. Maxson S, et al. Concise review: role of mesenchymal stem cells in wound repair. Stem Cells Transl Med. 2012;1:142–9.
97. Efimenko A, et al. Angiogenic properties of aged adipose derived mesenchymal stem cells after hypoxic conditioning. J Transl Med. 2011;9:10.
98. Madonna R, et al. Age-dependent impairment of number and angiogenic potential of adipose tissue-derived progenitor cells. Eur J Clin Invest. 2011;41:126–33.
99. Duscher D, et al. Aging disrupts cell subpopulation dynamics and diminishes the function of mesenchymal stem cells. Sci Rep. 2014;4:7144.
100. Lee S, et al. Activated mesenchymal stem cells increase wound tensile strength in aged mouse model via macrophages. J Surg Res. 2013;181:20–4.

Hyperpigmentation in Aging Skin

77

Tomohiro Hakozaki, Cheri L. Swanson, and Donald L. Bissett

Contents

T. Hakozaki (✉)
Beauty Technology Division, The Procter & Gamble Company, Mason Business Center, Mason, OH, USA
e-mail: hakozaki.t.1@pg.com

C.L. Swanson
The Procter & Gamble Company, Sharon Woods Innovation Center, Cincinnati, OH, USA
e-mail: swanson.cl@pg.com

D.L. Bissett
Beauty Technology Division, The Procter & Gamble Company, Sharon Woods Innovation Center, Cincinnati, OH, USA
e-mail: donbissett@gmail.com

M.A. Farage et al. (eds.), *Textbook of Aging Skin*,
DOI 10.1007/978-3-662-47398-6_51

Abstract

Hyperpigmentation problems, such as postinflammatory hyperpigmentation, solar lentigos, and melasma, can occur across all skin types with aging. Basic understanding of the pigmentation process and of these skin problems has led to their management by attacking proven targets with proven technologies. To name just a few examples, tyrosinase inhibition, blocking melanosome transfer, inhibition of tyrosinase glycosylation, increasing tyrosinase turnover, and blocking inflammation are clinically demonstrated approaches using, respectively, kojic acid, niacinamide, N-acetyl glucosamine, hexyldecanol, and phytosterol. Yet, because of the complexity of the pigmentation process, changes in skin with aging, and the involvement of a variety of cells (melanocytes, keratinocytes, fibroblasts, and inflammatory cells) in initiation, production, and processing of melanin, there are likely many more potential targets still to be characterized and fully exploited.

This review chapter explores these topics. Also, it briefly discusses other important skin chromophores that likely contribute to the color of aging skin, opening further approaches to understand skin color and to develop approaches for treatment of discoloration. Additionally, investigative tools such as laboratory model systems for understanding the pigmentation process and screening for potential active technologies are presented.

Furthermore, since evaluating the effectiveness of technology on human subjects is a key step in validating any new approach to treatment, clinical methods are also briefly discussed.

Introduction

Human skin color varies greatly around the globe, from very pale Celtic skin to very darkly pigmented skin in sub-Saharan African populations. Yet, all of these skin types can develop hyperpigmentary problems with aging, for example, postinflammatory hyperpigmentation, solar lentigos, and melasma. These problems occur widely in the human population, and control of them is of great interest, with particular desire to achieve uniformity of skin color.

Several proven targets for pigmentation control are known, but recent genomic and proteomic understanding of melanogenesis, the melanocyte, melanocyte-keratinocyte interaction, and melanocyte-fibroblast interaction has revealed potentially hundreds of proteins and other effectors involved in the pigmentation process. This body of knowledge, while complex, should provide the basis for understanding specific aberrations that lead to hyperpigmentary problems. Also available are advanced laboratory screening models and tools for skin color quantification. These are increasing the pace of identification of targets, screening of materials, and clinical evaluation for their effectiveness.

This brief review will focus on problems of hyperpigmentation (particularly as they apply to aging skin), investigative methods to measure and understand the problems, and topical cosmetic treatment approaches.

Pigmentation Process

The pigmentation process has been extensively described in many other documents [1] so will not be discussed in detail here. Briefly, melanocytes are specialized dendritic cells interspersed amongst basal keratinocytes and serve the primary function of producing melanin in intracellular organelles called melanosomes that are then distributed to surrounding keratinocytes. Each melanocyte is in contact with and distributes melanosomes to many keratinocytes via their dendritic processes. Melanins are complex polymers derived from tyrosine and other intermediates, which are converted through a multistep process of oxidative and complex reactions to brown-black eumelanin and yellow-red pheomelanin, which create the diversity of coloration observed across the human population.

The regulation of melanin production is very complex and involves upwards of 80 genes [2, 3]. The synthesis process is regulated by various extracellular signaling components that trigger a signal transduction cascade. There is also evidence that fibroblasts participate in this signaling [4]. While the baseline state of melanin in each individual's skin is dictated by genetic composition, internal and external triggers such as aging and UV exposure can lead to significant alterations in net synthesis of the melanin [5].

Skin Changes with Aging that Are Relevant to Pigmentation

Over the course of an individual's life, skin undergoes many changes [6], and there are many theories regarding causes of the changes. While there is still much to be learned about these and likely other causes, it is clear that key influencers in hyperpigmentation are environmental effects and hormonal changes, which will be discussed below in context with specific hyperpigmentary disorders (see below, section "Hyperpigmentary Disorders and Their Causes").

In general, the number of active melanocytes per unit area of skin decreases with age (10–20 % decline per decade), and there are more active melanocytes in chronically sun-exposed skin than in nonexposed skin [6]. This increased number of active melanocytes in sun-damaged skin indicates the influence of chronic UV exposure (e.g., on face, hands, arms) in stimulating melanogenic potential. Also, since chronic UV exposure also alters dermal fibroblast function in aging skin and since fibroblasts appear to play a regulatory role in melanin production [4], dermal damage from sunlight may contribute to the production of hyperpigmentation in exposed aging skin.

Hyperpigmentary Disorders and Their Causes

Postinflammatory Hyperpigmentation (PIH)

Skin insults that result in inflammation can induce postinflammatory hyperpigmentation [7], which is particularly evident in people with darker skin. Among such insults are acne lesions, ingrown hairs, scratches, insect bites, and surfactant damage. As an example of the latter, exposure of human forearm skin to the harsh surfactant sodium lauryl sulfate (SLS) under patch for a few hours will produce erythema within a day. Over the course of 1–2 weeks after this SLS exposure, hyperpigmentation will result, particularly in relatively darker skin groups, but it will occur even in Caucasian skin. Topical treatment with anti-inflammatory agents such as phytosterol will prevent this (Table 1).

Table 1 Postinflammatory hyperpigmentation (PIH) on the forearm

Test agent	Erythema grade (day 2)	PIH grade (day 11)
Vehicle	2.09	0.93
5 % phytosterol[a]	1.71[b]	0.55[b]

A 20 % solution of SLS (sodium lauryl sulfate) was applied to the forearm skin of Caucasian subjects (n = 19) under occlusive patch (0.2 ml solution in a 19-mm diameter chamber patch). The patch was removed after 1–4 h, depending on the individual subject responsiveness. After washing the site to remove surface SLS, the skin was treated topically twice daily for 5 days with test agent. The skin was graded (0–4 grading scales) daily for erythema and pigmentation (postinflammatory hyperpigmentation; PIH) for 11 days (D. L. Bissett, unpublished work)

[a]Phytosterol is a plant oil-derived mixture of stigmasterol, sitosterol, campesterol, and brassicasterol

[b]Statistically significantly different ($p < 0.05$) versus vehicle

Even the most common cause of hyperpigmentation (sunlight exposure of skin) is likely a postinflammatory response to UV damage to skin [8]. That response may be the result of an obvious acute inflammatory event such as sunburn or of repeated sub-erythemal exposures to UV. While in the latter there may not be visible erythema, histologically, such exposed skin has elevated inflammatory cell content, yielding a "sub-clinical" inflammatory process. It is supported by the fact that topical treatment with anti-inflammatory agents immediately after UVB exposure prevents induction of delayed tanning [9].

Inflammation may result in hyperpigmentation through several mechanisms. Among them is direct stimulation of melanocytes by inflammatory mediators such as IL-1-alpha or ET-1 [10]. Reactive oxygen species such as superoxide and nitric oxide generated in damaged skin (e.g., from UV exposure) or released as by-products from inflammatory cells are also known stimulators of melanocytes. Additionally, damage induced to epidermal cells can lead to release of endocrine inducers of pigmentation such as alpha-MSH [11]. And recently it has been observed that smoking, perhaps through its initiation of oxidative and inflammatory processes, also contributes to initiation of pigmentation [12]. The resulting hyperpigmentation induced by all these effects provides some measure of protection against subsequent insult since melanin has both UV absorption and reactive oxygen species scavenging capacity.

The melanin produced during an inflammatory event also can enter the dermis where it is engulfed by macrophages, producing "melanophages". These cells are often retained in the upper dermis for prolonged periods since removal of dermal melanin apparently is a very slow process. Thus, postinflammatory hyperpigmentation can be a very long-lived problem for the skin [1].

Solar (Actinic) Lentigos

These hyperpigmented spots are also known as lentigines, age spots, and liver spots. They occur on sun-exposed parts of the body (in particular the hands, arms, face, upper chest, and shoulders) and thus occur due to chronic exposure of skin to UV and the resultant chronic inflammation, such as the epidermal endothelin cascade [10]. Their dark appearance certainly results from excessive melanin in the region, and may result from overproduction of melanin in the hyperactive melanocytes [13], longer retention of melanin in aging epidermis due to the slower turnover of this tissue layer [6], longer retention of melanin in keratinocytes within rete ridges [14], and dermal melanin-containing melanophages which have been observed histologically to lie beneath the lentigines [1]. Since with aging, there is reduced wound healing [6, 15] and reduced clearance of materials from dermis apparently due to vascular and lymphatic changes [6], the residence time of melanophages in dermis may be very long.

Within lesional lentigo skin, the rete ridges are greatly exaggerated, extending deeper into the dermis [12]. This deep penetration runs counter to the general observation of flattening of the convoluted dermal-epidermal junction with aging, evidenced by the diminution of the rete ridges [6]. In solar lentigenes, the basement membrane is also perturbed [13], which likely contributes to melanin entering the dermis to result in melanophage formation. These observations suggest there has been a change in the genetic and phenotypic expression of cells (perhaps both epidermal and dermal) within the spot area as compared to cells in the surrounding nonspot skin. The expression levels of several melanogenesis-associated genes are increased in actinic lentigos [16, 17]. There is also an accentuation of the epidermal endothelin inflammatory cascade [10], together with decreased proliferation and differentiation of lesional keratinocytes [18]. Many of these changes appear to be permanent since these spots persist even when further UV exposure is avoided. The details of these apparent genomic expression changes have not been defined.

While lentigos appear to be permanent, their melanin content and thus their intensity will vary seasonally. For example, in evaluation of women with facial hyperpigmented spots in October versus December (in Kobe, Japan or Cincinnati, Ohio, USA), there is a marked reduction in size of spots over that time period, suggesting that the lack of continued exposure to sunlight in winter leads to gradual reduction in melanin production (seasonal fading) even in hyperpigmented spots [19, 20]. Additionally, in a separate examination of facial spots in March versus May (in Cincinnati, Ohio, USA), there was a marked increase in size of spots [20], consistent with the expected increased pigmentation due to increased sun exposure in spring (seasonal darkening).

From a consumer appearance standpoint, hyperpigmented spots and uneven pigmentation are important in the perception of age. In a series of studies [21], facial images were digitally modified to remove all age-defining textural features (e.g., facial furrows, folds, lines, wrinkles), leaving only pigmentation as the variable. Naïve judge evaluation and computer image analysis of the images revealed that pigmentation features can contribute to up to 20 years in perceived age of individuals. And facial hyperpigmentation also contributes to the perceived health of the individual [22]. For this study, subjects were shown digital images of Caucasian facial skin and were allowed to adjust the color to create a more healthy appearance. Subjects increased lightness (reduced darkness) and increased redness to achieve healthier-looking skin. So pigmentation is an important component of age perception.

Melasma

The hyperpigmentary disorder melasma is not well understood [1]. It occurs typically as symmetrical lesions on the face, primarily in darker skin type females at puberty or later in life. Sunlight exposure is likely a factor in the development of melasma since it occurs on the face (a sun-exposed body site) and since the condition worsens in the summer. Most melasma sufferers have a hypersensitivity to ultraviolet radiation, i. e., they display a lower minimum erythemal dose, and even brief exposures to sunlight can stimulate hyperpigmentation. There is also a hormonal component, likely progesterone, since episodes of melasma are often associated with pregnancy and the use of hormonal birth control. There may also be an estrogen component since estrogen receptor expression is increased in melasma [23].

In melasma lesions, there is excess melanin present in both the epidermis and upper dermis, associated with extra-vascular macrophages [1]. Since there is only a slight increase in number of melanocytes, the abnormality appears to be in function of the skin cells, in particular increased expression of factors in keratinocytes, fibroblasts, and melanocytes of the involved skin [24]. In contrast to PIH, there is no apparent inflammatory phase involved in its development. Additionally, there is likely a genetic component predisposing individuals to melasma, although the specific genetic basis for it is not defined.

Genomics and Proteomics of Pigmentation

The pigmentation process is complex as evidenced particularly by recent genomic and proteomic analysis. There are approximately 1500 gene products (proteins) expressed in melanosomes of all developmental stages, with 600 of them being expressed at any given time, and with 100 of them apparently unique to the melanosome [25]. Added to this are many other proteins (membrane-associated, cytoskeletal, transport, etc.) involved in pigmentation in both the melanocyte and the keratinocyte, indicating the complexity of the pigmentary process. While the basic process (e.g., stimulation of melanocytes and conversion of tyrosine to melanin) is well studied, there are many regulatory elements that have emerged from recent research involved in turnover of proteins such as tyrosinase [26], signaling, in the transport of melanosomes within the melanocyte, and the transfer of melanosomes to the keratinocyte [27]. This complexity merely offers a plethora of opportunities to understand the pigmentation process and to control it.

Less well studied are the events that occur in the keratinocyte once melanosomes have been transferred there. In addition to the melanosome engulfment process itself, presumably there are intracellular signals, regulatory elements, and transport mechanisms to distribute the melanosomes within keratinocyte. There is the process of melanin degradation to produce "melanin dust", an apparently enzymatic process which is more active in lighter skin versus darker skin individuals [28–31]. This is an area that is beginning to receive attention in the published literature.

Pigmentation Control Agents

As noted above, since there are many proteins and pathways involved in the pigmentary process, there is a wide array of targets against which to screen for pigmentation control agents. Among the many targets [1] are inhibitors of melanocyte stimulation (e.g., antioxidants, anti-inflammatory agents), cell receptor antagonists (e.g., alpha-MSH antagonists), inhibitors of melanin synthesis enzymes (e.g., tyrosinase, TRP-1, TRP-2), stimulators of protein turnover, inhibition of melanosome transport within the melanocyte and transfer to the keratinocyte (e.g., PAR-2 antagonists), and activators of melanin degradation within the keratinocyte.

While there are several potent drugs (prescription or over-the-counter) and surgical approaches to control of pigmentation (e.g., hydroquinone, trans-retinoic acid, corticosteroid, chemical peel surgery, laser surgery, and combinations of these therapies), the discussion here will focus on agents used in cosmetic formulations [32]. A classic target is inhibition of tyrosinase, the first enzyme in the conversion of tyrosine to melanin. A wide array of compounds, such as kojic acid, arbutin, ascorbic acid, ellagic acid, sulfhydryl compounds, and resorcinols, are effective tyrosinase inhibitors, as is a more recently discussed deoxy-arbutin [33, 34]. However, since several of these materials also have other effects, it is difficult to directly connect a specific mechanism to the observed effect on pigmentation. For example, sulfhydryl compounds are also effective antioxidants. Table 2 overviews a short list of the many possible targets and a few agents effective against them.

Table 2 Pigmentation control targets and some reported effective agents

Pigmentation control target examples	Effective agent examples
Tyrosinase inhibition	Hydroquinone, resorcinols, kojic acid, arbutin, deoxy-arbutin, ascorbic acid (vitamin C)
Tyrosinase copper chelation	Ellagic acid
Inhibition of tyrosinase glycosylation	Glucosamine, *N*-acetyl glucosamine, tunicamycin
Melanosome transfer	Niacinamide, protease inhibitors (soybean trypsin inhibitor, hexamidine, tranexamic acid)
Inhibit binding of alpha-MSH to melanocyte	*N*-undecylenoyl-phenylalanine
Down regulation of tyrosinase	Retinoid (*trans*-retinoic acid, retinol and its esters, retinaldehyde)
Increased protein (tyrosinase) turnover	Hexyl-decanol
Antioxidant	Vitamin C compounds, vitamin E, sulfhydryl compounds
Anti-inflammatory agent	Hydrocortisone, phytosterol, glycyrrhetinic acid, tranexamic acid, chamomile extract, alpha-bisabolol
Increase epidermal turnover	Retinoids, salicylic acid, alpha-hydroxy acids, alpha-keto acids, adenosine monophosphate

In the past several years, niacinamide and glucosamine [in particular its derivative *N*-acetyl glucosamine (NAG)] have been reported to be effective in reducing melanin production in culture. In vitro, glucosamine reduces production of melanin by inhibiting activation of tyrosinase [20], while niacinamide inhibits melanosome transfer from melanocytes to keratinocytes [19]. Cosmetic moisturizer formulations containing niacinamide alone are effective in reducing the appearance of hyperpigmented spots in vivo [19, 35] and the addition of NAG to the formula yields greater effectiveness [20] (Fig. 1). Another new addition to the array of pigmentation control agents is *N*-undecylenoyl-L-phenylalanine which has been reported to inhibit binding of alpha-MSH to the melanocyte in vitro and is effective as a component of cosmetic moisturizer formulations in clinical testing [36], as shown in Fig. 2.

While combinations of materials are definitely an approach to achieve greater effects in controlling pigmentation, even single ingredients can be quite effective. For example, recent clinical testing has shown that niacinamide alone can be nearly as effective as hydroquinone in the treatment of melasma [37], with niacinamide having much better skin tolerance. However, in the quest for increased potency of materials, one must also be mindful of the potential for bleaching and hypo-pigmentation as an unwanted side effect, which has recently been observed with a newly developed technology, rhododendrol [38, 39]. This emphasizes the need for more exhaustive examination of new materials.

Sunscreen is also effective in reducing the appearance of hyperpigmentation by preventing the entrance of UV into skin to stimulate melanocytes. Clinical testing among Japanese females in late summer-fall season (in Kobe, Japan) using SPF 15 sunscreen alone demonstrated acceleration of fading of facial tanning compared to the control [19]. However, even relatively high sunscreen dose (SPF 15) is not completely protective, such as against incidental sunlight exposure. In clinical testing involving daily use of SPF 15 sunscreen [40], there was still a marked increase in size of spots in March versus May (in Cincinnati, Ohio, USA), consistent with increased pigmentation due to increased sun exposure in spring (seasonal darkening). There was greater protection against this seasonal darkening when subjects used a 3-way combination of SPF 15 sunscreen, niacinamide, and NAG, thus indicating the opportunity for greater effectiveness by combining sunscreen with nonsunscreen technologies.

Other Skin Chromophores

While the focus of this review is on hyperpigmentation, it is informative to mention briefly that the appearance of pigmentation likely also

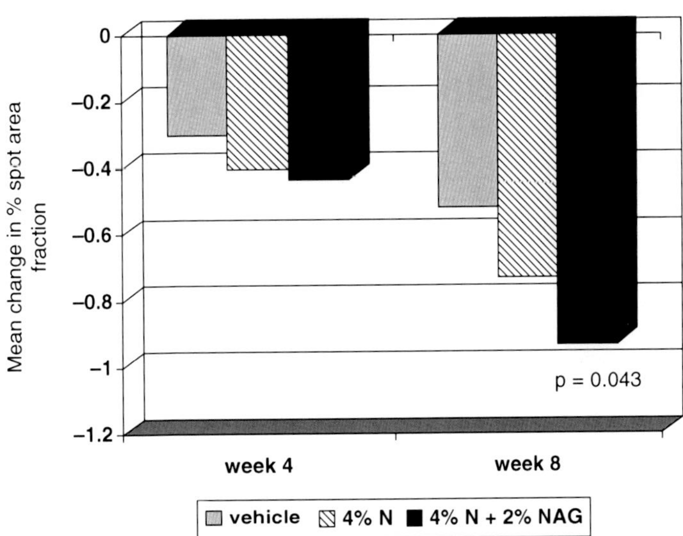

Fig. 1 Hyperpigmented spot reduction by topical treatment with formulas containing niacinamide and *N*-acetyl glucosamine. Spot area fraction was determined by algorithm-based computer image analysis of Caucasian facial digital images ($n = 35$). More negative numbers indicate reduction in hyperpigmentation (improvement). *N* niacinamide, *NAG N*-acetyl glucosamine. The indicated *p* value for N + NAG is versus N

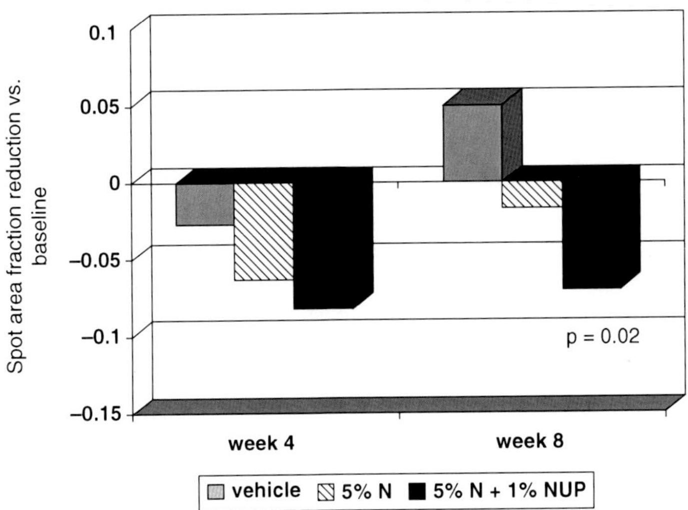

Fig. 2 Hyperpigmented spot reduction by topical treatment with formulas containing niacinamide and *N*-undecyloyl-L-phenylalanine. Spot area fraction was determined by algorithm-based computer image analysis of Japanese facial digital images ($n = 40$). More negative numbers indicate reduction in hyperpigmentation (improvement). *N* niacinamide, *NUP N*-undecylenoyl-L-phenylalanine. The indicated *p* value for N + NUP is versus N

involves other chromophores in the skin. For example, increased vascular content (hemoglobin) associated with hyperpigmentation has been described for melasma [41], and the same may be the case for hyperpigmented spots. Additionally, there is the spontaneous Maillard reaction (glycation; oxidative reactions between protein and sugar that produce Advance Glycation End-products) or carbonylation that yields yellow-brown chromophores [35, 42–44]. When this occurs in proteins with long biological half lives (e.g., structural proteins), the glycation end products or carbonyl modified proteins accumulate with aging, and the yellow-brown color increases and is persistent. Thus, hyperpigmented areas may appear to be darker in part due to other chromophores, opening the opportunity for further understanding of the problem and for additional approaches to treatment.

Investigative Tools

Many of the targets noted above can be investigated in simple mechanism-specific solution assays, melanocyte cell culture, or co-culture systems (e.g., melanocyte-keratinocyte, melanocyte-fibroblast) in the laboratory [19]. These methods permit screening of potentially large numbers of compounds for their inhibitory and stimulatory effects on the specific processes being evaluated. For example, one screening assay involves a simple mixture of tyrosinase and tyrosine in which a brown product (melanin) quickly appears and can be quantified colorimetrically. Tyrosinase inhibitors, of course, reduce the melanin produced. A simple assay of this type can be readily performed in a 96-well plate, allowing rapid robotic high throughput screening of thousands of compounds. Assays involving cells are more complex, but even those can be constructed in a multi-well plate format for moderate throughput screening of potentially hundreds of compounds. Establishing an array of such simple assays permits the screening of a substantial library of compounds through all these assays to identify promising candidates quickly.

Another useful laboratory model that has emerged over the past decade is the skin equivalent culture [4]. These 3-dimensional cultures can contain either or both dermal and epidermal compartments, with fibroblasts, keratinocytes, melanocytes, and potentially other cell types. When they are raised to the air-liquid interface, the keratinocytes will differentiate to form a stratum corneum structure. Also, live human skin organ culture has potential as a useful model [45]. Versus submerged culture of cells, an advantage of both skin equivalent and organ cultures is that they can be treated topically with simple solutions or even complex emulsion formulations or commercial skin care products. Another particular advantage is that they are not mechanism specific – since most or all of the pigmentation machinery are present in the cultures, they potentially can be responsive to materials that affect any of the pigmentation targets. These cultures are available from commercial suppliers. While these are useful tools for material evaluation, they are relatively low throughput due particularly to the high cost of the cultures, but also to the time involved in manipulating the cultures over the course of the multi-day experiments.

There are some in vivo laboratory models that have been used to evaluate pigmentation inhibitory materials. As a recent example, zebra fish have been used in testing topical compounds [46]. Also, a mouse strain develops hyperpigmented spots in response to UV exposure [47], so has potential use as a lentigo model. Other models [1] include live human skin transplanted onto nude mice, Yucatan mini-pig, pigmented SKH-hr/2 mouse, and pigmented guinea pig. Like the skin equivalent cultures, these models will not be mechanism specific and thus are likely to be responsive to a wide range of material mechanisms. While all these models may not be broadly available, there is certainly opportunity to pursue in vivo modeling as a tool in addressing pigmentation problems.

The final proof of value of a technology, of course, requires progressing materials from the laboratory into clinical testing to demonstrate on-skin activity. Clinical methods include live expert grading, chromameter [48], and color image capture and analysis [35]. A new useful clinical measurement tool in assessing effectiveness is based on the principles of noncontact SIAscopy^{TM}, a recently described method to measure skin melanin content and distribution [49]. It rapidly captures facial maps of skin chromophores, permitting determination of the content and distribution of melanin in any spot or any area of the skin. It will also capture maps for any chromophore, and as long as the absorption spectra of the chromophores are known (e.g., hemoglobin, collagen, glycation products), it can differentiate them to yield chromophore-specific distribution maps. And additional methods for evaluating skin chromophores continue to be evaluated, such as confocal microscopy, reflection spectrum resolution, diffuse reflectance spectroscopy, and near-infrared auto-fluorescence imaging [50–53].

Clinical testing on various body sites such as forearm, face, chest, and back [35, 54] have been reported, and all have utility in evaluating technology. Any thoroughly controlled clinical evaluation is expensive and therefore practicality limits testing to only the most promising candidates, several of which (as noted above) have proven to be effective in hyperpigmentation control.

Conclusion

The continually increasing understanding of the pigmentation process and the underlying problems in hyperpigmentary conditions provide bases for establishing targets against which to screen new compounds to identify those that may be effective pigmentation control agents. With the advances in laboratory and clinical methodology, the screening process can occur much faster than in the past. In addition, the consumer desires effective pigmentation control technology, particularly in the cosmetic arena, since hyperpigmentation problems increase perceived aged and even affect perception of health. Advanced pigmentary system understanding and new research capabilities are setting the stage for future technological advancements.

Cross-References

▶ Pigmentation in Ethnic Groups
▶ The New Face of Pigmentation and Aging

References

1. Nordlund JJ, Boissy RE, Hearing VJ, King RA, Ortonne JP. The pigmentary system. New York: Oxford University Press; 1998.
2. Hearing VJ. Biochemical control of melanogenesis and melanosomal organization. J Investig Dermatol Symp Proc. 1999;4:24–8.
3. Schallreuter KU. Advances in melanocyte basic science research. Dermatol Clin. 2007;25:283–91.
4. Cario-Andre M, et al. In vivo and in vitro evidence of dermal fibroblasts influence on human epidermal pigmentation. Pigment Cell Res. 2006;19:434–42.
5. Costin GE, et al. Human skin pigmentation: melanocytes modulate skin color in response to stress. FASEB J. 2007;21:976–94.
6. Gilchrest BA. Skin and aging processes. Boca Raton: CRC Press; 1984.
7. Taylor SC. Cosmetic problems in skin of color. Skin Pharmacol Appl Skin Physiol. 1999;12:139–43.
8. Hachiya A, et al. Biochemical characterization of endothelin-converting enzyme-1 alpha in cultured skin-derived cells and its postulated role in the stimulation of melanogenesis in human epidermis. J Biol Chem. 2002;277:5395–403.
9. Takiwaki H, et al. The degrees of UVB-induced erythema and pigmentation correlate linearly and are reduced in a parallel manner by topical anti-inflammatory agents. J Invest Dermatol. 1994;103:642–6.
10. Kadono S, et al. The role of the epidermal endothelin cascade in the hyperpigmentation mechanism of lentigo senilis. J Invest Dermatol. 2001;116:571–7.
11. Imokawa G. Autocrine and paracrine regulation of melanocytes in human skin and in pigmentary disorders. Pigment Cell Res. 2004;17:96–110.
12. Cho YH, et al. Changes in skin color after smoking cessation. Korean J Fam Med. 2012;33:105–9.
13. Noblesse E, et al. Skin ultrastructure in senile lentigo. Skin Pharmacol Physiol. 2006;19:95–100.
14. Cario-Andre M, et al. Perilesional vs. lesional skin changes in senile lentigo. J Cutan Pathol. 2004;31:441–7.
15. Makrantonaki E, et al. Molecular mechanisms of skin aging: state of the art. Ann N Y Acad Sci. 2007;1119:40–50.
16. Motokawa T, et al. Messenger RNA levels of melanogenesis-associated genes in lentigo senilis lesions. J Dermatol Sci. 2005;37:120–3.
17. Unver N, et al. Alterations in the epidermal-dermal melanin axis and factor XIIIa melanophages in senile lentigo and ageing skin. Br J Dermatol. 2006;155:119–28.
18. Aoki H, et al. Gene expression profiling analysis of solar lentigo in relation to immunohistochemical characteristics. Br J Dermatol. 2007;156:1214–23.
19. Hakozaki T, et al. The effect of niacinamide on reducing cutaneous pigmentation and suppression of melanosome transfer. Br J Dermatol. 2002;147:20–31.
20. Bissett DL, et al. Reduction in the appearance of facial hyperpigmentation by topical N-acetyl glucosamine. J Cosmet Dermatol. 2007;6:20–6.
21. Fink B, et al. The effects of skin colour distribution and topography cues on the perception of female facial age and health. J Eur Acad Dermatol Venereol. 2008;22:493–8.
22. Stephen ID, et al. Facial skin coloration affects perceived health of human faces. Int J Primatol. 2009;30:845–57.
23. Lieberman R, et al. Estrogen receptor expression in melasma: results from facial skin of affected patients. J Drugs Dermatol. 2008;7:463–5.
24. Kang HY, et al. The dermal stem cell factor and c-kit are overexpressed in melasma. Br J Dermatol. 2006;154:1094–9.
25. Chi A, et al. Proteomic and bioinformatic characterization of the biogenesis and function of melanosomes. J Proteome Res. 2006;5:3135–44.

26. Hakozaki T, et al. A regulator of ubiquitin-proteasome activity, 2-hexyldecanol, suppresses melanin synthesis and the appearance of facial hyperpigmented spots. Br J Dermatol. 2013;169S:39–44.
27. Boissy RE. Melanosome transfer to and translocation in the keratinocyte. Exp Dermatol. 2003;12S2:5–12.
28. Chen NN, et al. Cathepsin L2 levels inversely correlate with skin color. J Invest Dermatol. 2006;126:2345–7.
29. Murase D, et al. Autophagy has a significant role in determining skin color by regulating melanosome degradation in keratinocytes. J Invest Dermatol. 2013;133:2416–24.
30. Ebanks JP, et al. Hydrolytic enzymes of the interfollicular epidermis differ in expression and correlate with the phenotypic difference observed between light and dark skin. J Dermatol. 2012;39:1–7.
31. Ebanks JP, et al. Epidermal keratinocytes from light vs. dark skin exhibit differential degradation of melanosomes. J Invest Dermatol. 2011; 131:1226–33.
32. Nakayama H, Ebihara T, Satoh N, Jinnai T. Depigmentation agents. In: Elsner P, Maibach HI, editors. Cosmeceuticals and active cosmetics. Boca Raton: Taylor & Francis; 2005. p. 123–44.
33. Boissy RE, et al. Deoxyarbutin: a nevel reversible tyrosinase inhibitor with effective in vivo skin lightening potency. Exp Dermatol. 2005;14:601–8.
34. Chawla S, et al. Mechanism of tyrosinase inhibition by deoxyarbutin and its second-generation derivatives. Br J Dermatol. 2008;159:1267–74.
35. Bissett DL, et al. Topical niacinamide reduces yellowing, wrinkling, red blotchiness, and hyperpigmented spots in aging facial skin. Int J Cosmet Sci. 2004;26:231–8.
36. Bissett DL, et al. Reduction in the appearance of facial hyperpigmentation by topical N-undecyl-10-enoyl-L-phenylalanine and its combination with niacinamide. J Cosmet Dermatol. 2009;8:260–6.
37. Navarrete-Solis J, et al. A double-blind, randomized clinical trial of niacinamide 4% versus hydroquinone 4% in the treatment of melasma. Dermatol Res Pract. 2011. doi:10.1155/2011/379173.
38. Ito S, et al. Tyrosinase-catalyzed oxidation of rhododendrol produces 2-methylchromane-6,7-dione, the putative ultimate toxic metabolite: implications for melanocyte toxicity. Pigment Cell Melanoma Res. 2014. doi:10.1111/pcmr.12275.
39. Kasamatsu S, et al. Depigmentation caused by application of the active brightening material, rhododendrol, is related to tyrosinase activity at a certain threshold. J Dermatol Sci. 2014;76:16–24.
40. Kimball AB, et al. Reduction in the appearance of facial hyperpigmentation by a combination of topical niacinamide plus N-acetyl glucosamine: results of a randomized, double-blind, placebo-controlled trial. Br J Dermatol. 2010;162:435–41.
41. Kim EH, et al. The vascular characteristics of melasma. J Dermatol Sci. 2007;46:111 6.
42. Dyer DG, et al. Accumulation of maillard reaction products in skin collagen in diabetes and aging. J Clin Invest. 1993;91:2463–9.
43. Ohshima H, et al. Melanin and facial skin fluorescence as markers of yellowish discoloration with aging. Skin Res Technol. 2009;15:496–502.
44. Ogura Y, et al. Dermal carbonyl modification is related to the yellowish color change of photo-aged Japanese facial skin. J Dermatol Sci. 2011;64:45–52.
45. Backvall H, et al. Similar UV responses are seen in a skin organ culture as in human skin in vivo. Exp Dermatol. 2002;11:349–56.
46. Choi T-Y, et al. Zebrafish as a new model for phenotype-based screening of melanogenic regulatory compounds. Pigment Cell Res. 2007;20:120–7.
47. Furuya R, et al. Changes in the proliferative activity of epidermal melanocytes in serum-free primary culture during the development of ultraviolet radiation B-induced pigmented spots in hairless mice. Pigment Cell Res. 2002;15:348–56.
48. Alaluf S, et al. The impact of epidermal melanin on objective measurements of human skin colour. Pigment Cell Res. 2002;15:119–26.
49. Matts PJ, et al. The distribution of melanin in skin determined in vivo. Br J Dermatol. 2007;156:620–8.
50. Nakahima A, et al. Investigation by in vivo reflectance confocal microscopy: melanocytes at the edges of solar lentigenes. Exp Dermatol. 2012;21S1:18–21.
51. Masuda Y, et al. An innovative method to measure skin pigmentation. Skin Res Technol. 2009;15:224–9.
52. Stamatas GN, et al. In vivo measurement of skin erythema and pigmentation: new means of implementation of diffuse reflectance spectroscopy with a commercial instrument. Br J Dermatol. 2008;159:683–90.
53. Han X, et al. Near-infrared autofluorescence imaging of cutaneous melanins and human skin in vivo. J Biomed Opt. 2009;14:024017. doi:10.1117/1.3103310.
54. Ravnbak MH, et al. Skin pigmentation kinetics after UVB exposure. Acta Derm Venereol. 2008;88:223–8.

Pigmentation in Ethnic Groups

78

Howard I. Maibach, Jane Y. Liu, and Ying Zou

Contents

H.I. Maibach (✉)
Department of Dermatology, University of California, San Francisco, CA, USA
e-mail: maibachh@derm.ucsf.edu

J.Y. Liu
Department of Dermatology, University of California, School of Medicine, San Francisco, CA, USA
e-mail: jane.yliu99@gmail.com

Y. Zou
Department of Dermatology, UC San Francisco, San Francisco, CA, USA
e-mail: Ying.Zou@ucsf.edu

M.A. Farage et al. (eds.), *Textbook of Aging Skin*,
DOI 10.1007/978-3-662-47398-6_52

Abstract

While human skin is an important external feature which can distinguish people of different ethnicities, less clear is how variations in human skin pigmentation may contribute to differences in skin structure, function, and pathophysiology. An understanding of differences in pigmentation, skin structure, and function becomes more important for treatment of skin diseases. Many advances have been made in understanding the genetic, molecular, and cellular differences underlying normal variation in human skin pigmentation. Studies have been carried out in order to investigate the complex genetic pathway underlying melanin synthesis and the role of genetic variation in epidermal pigmentation and to elucidate differences in skin pathophysiology among humans from different ethnic backgrounds. As knowledge develops about the intricate process of pigmentation and distinctions between ethnic groups, it can be further understood how pigmentary changes occur with aging, to consequently develop more effective management.

Introduction

To help understand the pigmentary changes which occur throughout the aging process and in the management of aging skin, it is necessary to examine how pigmentation varies among different ethnicities. Skin color among different ethnicities has important social and political connotations, both historically and at the present. While human skin is an important external feature which can distinguish people of different ethnicities, less clear is how variations in human skin pigmentation may contribute to differences in skin structure, function, and pathophysiology. As the demographics of the United States change, the US Census Bureau estimates that by 2050, approximately half of the US resident population will comprise individuals of color [1]. The question of associating race and pigmentation is repeatedly raised, and a recent study demonstrated the need for caution when using pigmentation as a proxy for race or genetic ancestry [2]. Nonetheless, as dermatologists treat more patients of varying ethnic backgrounds and with diverse skin types, an understanding of differences in pigmentation and skin structure and function becomes more important.

Methods

The PubMed database was searched with the specific terms "minority groups," "population groups," and "skin pigmentation" in different combinations. Altogether, 295 results were retrieved, and abstracts were reviewed for relevance. Editorial articles, population-based studies, basic science, and clinical studies were included provided the subject matter was relevant to the topic discussed.

Mechanism of Pigmentation

Human skin color is determined primarily by melanin synthesis. Melanin can act as an effective sunscreen, protecting darker-pigmented individuals from burning and development of skin cancer [3]. Heavy pigmentation in areas of high solar radiation helps protect the skin from carcinogenic effects of ultraviolet light [4]. This might have played a role in selection of darker skin colors evolutionarily in African populations, but how lighter skin was produced as early humans migrated out of Africa and moved into Europe remains controversial. Additionally, there is a correlation between latitude and skin color; skin is lighter in regions toward the north. This correlates with ultraviolet radiation incidence, which is higher near the equator and lower at higher latitudes.

In human skin pigmentation, constitutive skin color refers to genetically determined levels of melanin pigmentation without exposure to ultraviolet radiation or other environmental influences, while facultative skin color refers to increases in melanin pigmentation above the constitutive level induced by exposure to ultraviolet light [5]. Human skin color is dominated by hemoglobin, which provides red color via the network of capillaries in the skin, and melanin, which provides various gradations of brown coloring to the skin surface. There does not appear to be any significant difference in hemoglobin content among various ethnicities, and there is a constant vascular supply under conditions of constant activity and temperature [6]. Furthermore, the effect of hemoglobin in blood flowing in the dermal papillary layer is easily masked by pigments present in the overlying epidermal layers. Thus, it is primarily differences in the amount of melanin which are responsible for normal variation in human skin pigmentation.

Melanin synthesis takes place inside melanosomes, organelles present in the melanocyte. Melanin pigment granules are subsequently transferred to keratinocytes [7]. Specifically, melanosomes are trafficked along dendrites; they are moved along microtubules before being captured at dendrite tips through a molecular complex which includes myosin [8]. Melanosomes are pinched off or released from the melanocyte dendrite and subsequently phagocytosed by adjacent keratinocytes. Suprabasal keratinocytes move upward through epidermal keratinocyte layers where melanocyte dendrites continuously transfer melanosomes to maturing keratinocytes. Eventually, melanin is shed from top layers of stratum corneum with the cornified keratinocytes. The proteinase-activated receptor-2 (PAR-2) is a receptor expressed in keratinocytes and is thought to play a fundamental role in this process of melanosome transfer and skin pigmentation [9].

The overall regulation of melanin formation is complex, and numerous factors affect mammalian melanocytes to regulate melanin synthesis; these include melanotropin, estrogen and progesterone, and agouti signal protein [10]. Further studies must elucidate the complex regulation of melanin formation, the regulation of phagocytosis of melanosomes by keratinocytes, and how signaling intermediates stimulate melanosome transfer. Additionally, it is not clear whether melanosomes are transferred from melanocytes to keratinocytes in membrane-bound clusters or as individual melanosomes or both.

Variations in Pigmentation and Ultrastructural Differences in Skin

Montagna and Carlisle examined the morphology of black and white facial skin among adult women 22–50 years of age [11]. When comparing the epidermis of black skin to white skin, the epidermis of black skin demonstrated more and larger singly distributed melanosomes in corneocytes and keratinocytes. Additionally, the epidermal stratum lucidum was not altered by sunlight exposure in black skin, whereas the stratum lucidum was usually distorted on exposure to the sun in white skin. White skin demonstrated frequent areas of atrophy, while only 1 of 19 black women in the study demonstrated atrophic spots in the epidermis. One of the key indices of dermal photodamage is the presence of elastotic material. Black skin demonstrated minimal elastosis, while white skin showed variable amounts of moderate to extensive elastosis. The authors speculated that the greater numbers of melanosomes and distribution in black skin perhaps protect the epidermis from photodamage. Additionally, the dermis of black skin demonstrated more fiber fragments made of collagen fibrils and glycoproteins, as well as numerous and larger fibroblasts. Finally, black skin showed more mixed apocrine-eccrine sweat glands, as well as more blood and lymphatic vessels, when compared to white skin.

Overall, the most striking difference demonstrated between black skin and white skin appears to be the size of melanosomes and distribution pattern of melanosomes. In darkly pigmented skin, large melanosomes are surrounded by the membrane, whereas smaller melanosomes are grouped or clustered together in a single membrane in lighter skin [12]. Additionally, melanosomal packaging is closer to the basal layer in more darkly pigmented skin as compared to Caucasian skin [13]. Regarding variations in human skin color, the density of pigment-producing melanocytes in the skin (approximately 1,000/mm^2) has not been known to vary with ethnicity [14]. Conversely, the ratio between eumelanin and pheomelanin synthesis was demonstrated to be higher in black compared to white skin [15].

Thong et al. examined the patterns of melanosome distribution in keratinocytes of Asian skin and compared this to light Caucasian skin and dark African-American skin [16]. In this study, the distribution pattern of melanosomes transferred to keratinocytes in the photoprotected skin (volar forearm) from normal Asian individuals was examined. Results demonstrated that melanosomes in keratinocytes of Asian skin are distributed as both individual and clustered melanosomes, with 62.6 % individual and 37.4 % clustered. In dark skin keratinocytes, melanosomes are predominantly individual (88.9 %), and in light Caucasian skin keratinocytes, melanosomes are predominantly clustered (84.5 %). Thus, the melanosome distribution in Asian keratinocytes seems to be intermediate between light Caucasian and dark keratinocytes. When examining the size of melanosomes, there appeared to be a variation in size with ethnicity; melanosomes in dark skin were the largest, followed by melanosomes of Asian and then Caucasian skin. Furthermore, melanosomes which are distributed individually tend to be larger as compared to clustered melanosomes.

Minwalla et al. examined how keratinocytes play a role in regulating the distribution patterns of recipient melanosomes in vitro [17]. Cocultures using melanocytes and keratinocytes from different racial backgrounds were studied with electron microscopy. When keratinocytes from dark skin were cocultured with melanocytes from either dark or light skin, recipient melanosomes were predominantly individual as opposed to clustered. However, when keratinocytes from light skin were cocultured with melanocytes from dark or light skin, recipient melanosomes were predominantly clustered as opposed to individual. Thus, recipient melanosomes overall are predominantly distributed in membrane-bound clusters from light skin keratinocytes and distributed individually by dark skin keratinocytes. Furthermore, melanosome size was not related to how melanosomes were distributed. Authors suggested that keratinocyte regulatory factors may determine how exactly recipient melanosomes are distributed.

Melanin content in photoexposed and photoprotected skin has been examined among varying ethnicities including African, Indian, Mexican, Chinese, and European skin [18]. The lightly pigmented skin types had approximately half as much epidermal melanin as compared to more darkly pigmented skin types. Furthermore, the melanin composition among the lighter skin types (Mexican, Chinese, and European skin) was more enriched with lightly colored, alkali-soluble melanin pigments such as pheomelanin and eumelanin. Epidermal melanin content is greater in chronically photoexposed skin as compared to photoprotected skin, regardless of ethnic background. This analysis, like previous studies, also demonstrated that melanosome size varies with ethnicity: African skin had the largest melanosomes, followed by Indian, Mexican, Chinese, and finally European skin. Thus, the amount of melanin, composition of melanin, and differences in melanosome size may all play roles in determining skin pigmentation.

Halprin et al. reported that glutathione may play a role in the genetically determined differences in skin color among different races [19]. This sulfhydryl-containing epidermal compound plays a role in melanin formation. Halprin described that the tripeptide glutathione (g-glutamyl-cysteinyl-glycine) is present in the human epidermis in sufficient concentrations to be the inhibitor of melanin formation from tyrosine by tyrosinase. Overall, reduced glutathione and the enzyme glutathione reductase, which is needed to maintain glutathione in the reduced state, are found in lower concentrations in African epidermal skin as compared to Caucasian epidermis.

Role of Tyrosinase

Iwata et al. examined the relationship between tyrosinase activity and skin color in human foreskins [20]. Darker skin types appear to have a higher level of melanin production due to the constitutively higher level of activity of tyrosinase, the rate-limiting enzyme in melanin synthesis. Tyrosinase activity was measured with two separate assays, a tyrosinase hydroxylase assay and a [^{14}C] melanin assay, measuring both the hydroxylation of tyrosine to dopa and the conversion of [^{14}C] tyrosine to [^{14}C] melanin. In black foreskin homogenates, tyrosinase activity was measured at nearly three times the activity compared to white skin samples. Tyrosinase activity was generally correlated with melanin content in the skin. Variations in tyrosinase activity may be due to different amounts of enzyme, but also potentially due to differences in catalytic activity of the enzyme in melanocytes.

Tyrosinase is the rate-limiting enzyme in melanin synthesis, and its overall activity is higher in melanocytes of black skin as compared to Caucasian skin [21]. Fuller et al. examined the regulation of tyrosinase in black and Caucasian human melanocyte cell cultures. Their studies showed that variation in enzyme activity is due to differences in the catalytic activity of preexisting tyrosinase rather than differences in tyrosinase abundance or gene activity. In the melanosomes of black melanocytes, tyrosinase has high catalytic activity, while in Caucasian melanocytes, the melanosome-bound enzyme is largely inactive. Furthermore, staining of Caucasian melanocytes with a weak base demonstrated that Caucasian melanosomes are acidic organelles as compared to more neutral in darker skin. Thus, differences in melanosome pH may contribute to variations in pigmentation. Moreover, tyrosinase is inactive in an acidic environment, so it is largely inactive in Caucasian melanosomes as compared to higher activity in melanosomes of black skin.

Maeda et al. compared melanogenesis in human black and light brown melanocytes [22]. Melanin pigment in both human black and light brown melanocytes contains eumelanin and pheomelanin, with black melanocytes containing a larger amount. Tyrosinase activity was higher in the black melanocytes as compared to light brown melanocytes. The differences in pigmentation of the two human melanocyte cell lines (black and light brown) seemed to be derived from differences in activity of tyrosinase, as well as other specific proteins affecting the constitution of melanin polymers. These other proteins include tyrosinase-related protein-1 and dopachrome tautomerase, which modulate distal steps in melanogenesis.

Genetics of Skin Pigmentation

Investigators have begun to develop a better understanding of the complex genetic basis for normal variation in human skin pigmentation. Much of the research investigating the genes playing a role in melanin synthesis have been carried out in animal models. With the help of mouse coat color mutations, many of the biochemical pathways involved in melanin synthesis have been studied and elucidated; over 100 genes have been identified which can affect mouse coat color [23]. Many of these genes have corresponding human phenotypes. One of the genes affecting normal variation in skin pigmentation is the melanocortin 1 receptor (MC1R) gene. Mutations in this gene affect pigmentation in humans, mice, cattle, horses, sheep, pigs, and chickens, among other animals. Specifically, this gene product is in the melanocyte cell membrane and is the receptor for α-melanocyte-stimulating hormone. While polymorphisms in MC1R may play a vital role in shaping human pigmentation, this process is complex, and multiple genes likely determine normal variation in skin pigmentation [24]. Recently, Saternus et al. presented genetic evidence that the activity of pigmentation-related genes including exocyst complex component 2 (EXOC2), tyrosinase (TYR), and TYR-related protein type 1 (TYRP1) can affect serum levels of 25(OH)D in the cohort of 2790 Caucasian patients in Germany. There is a genetic correlation between the melanin-producing system and circulating levels of 25(OH)D3 in the Caucasian population of predominantly German ancestry [25].

In addition, some variation in human skin color is associated with variation in TYR and OCA2, two of the known pigmentation genes [26]. Recent studies have focused on SLC24A5, a putative cation exchanger, which was originally studied in zebra fish and is suggested to play a key role in human skin pigmentation [27]. The SLC24A5 exchanger localizes to an intracellular membrane, likely the melanosome or its precursor; it is thought that variations in this gene may help explain some of the difference in pigmentation between European-Americans and African-Americans. Genes MATP, TYR, and SLC24A5 may play a predominant role in the evolution of lighter skin in Europeans but not East Asians, suggesting that there is a recent convergent evolution of lighter skin pigmentation in East Asians and Europeans [28]. Interestingly, such data also suggest that European skin turned lighter approximately 6,000–12,000 years ago, contradicting a previous hypothesis that European skin grew more pale approximately 40,000 years ago [29].

Response to Ultraviolet Radiation

Tadokoro et al. examined the mechanism of skin tanning in different ethnic groups [30]. The effect of ultraviolet radiation after one minimal erythemal dose exposure was studied. Overall, the density of melanocytes present at the epidermal-dermal junction did not change significantly 1 week following ultraviolet light exposure, and this density was similar among different ethnic skin types. However, the distribution of melanin from the lower layers to middle layers of the skin epidermis was more dramatic in darker skin as compared to lighter skin following ultraviolet exposure.

Erythema responses have also been examined in patients of different complexions [31]. The minimal erythemal dose (MED), defined as the smallest quantity of radiation needed to produce a barely perceptible erythema, was determined in Caucasians and in differing complexions of African-American skin. Among light-, medium-, and dark-complexioned African-Americans, no minimal erythema response was typical. Instead, a spectrum of responses was found which was directly proportional to the degree of pigmentation. Additionally, the average MED of the darker-complexioned African-Americans was 33 times greater than that of Caucasians. Caucasian skin had the smallest amount of pigment and smallest melanosomes, which were mostly contained within melanosome complexes. Further findings included that melanosome size is directly proportional to the intensity of skin pigmentation and darkly pigmented subjects have larger, wider, and denser melanosomes. Generally, with increasing pigmentation, the size of melanosomes, the proportion of singly dispersed melanosomes, and the MED were all shown to increase. Authors suggested that the increased resistance of darker skin to the damaging effects of ultraviolet radiation may be due to larger, more light-absorbing, individually dispersed melanosomes. Furthermore, melanosomes in darkly pigmented skin are degraded less by lysosomes, resulting in more light-absorbing bodies in the stratum corneum [32].

Skin Structure and Function

The skin barrier, made primarily of terminally differentiated keratinocytes in a lipid matrix composed of fatty acids, ceramides, and cholesterols, helps to determine the skin's integrity [33]. When examining the skin barrier and its components, darkly pigmented skin does appear to have some inherent structural and functional differences as compared to lighter skin [34].

One study compared transepidermal water loss and water content among black, white, Latino, and Asian populations [35]. The transepidermal water loss measurements were highest in black, followed by white, Latino, and Asian populations in decreasing order. Furthermore, stratum corneum lipids were significantly lower in black epidermal layers as compared to other races. The skin barrier of more darkly pigmented skin is thought to be more resistant to injury and recover more quickly from injury [36]. Marshall et al. demonstrated that black skin may have decreased susceptibility to cutaneous irritants, suggesting that the black skin barrier may be stronger [37]. Another study by Weigand et al. demonstrated that there may be greater numbers of stratum corneum cell layers in black skin and possibly greater cell cohesiveness as well [38]. However, it has also been suggested that darkly pigmented persons are more susceptible to cold injury as compared to those with lighter pigmentation [39].

One concern about varying levels of pigmentation among human skin of different ethnic backgrounds is the possible effect on cutaneous synthesis of vitamin D. Matsuoka et al. examined this further by testing serum vitamin D levels and levels of active serum metabolites among white, East Asian, South Asian, and black subjects following a fixed dose of ultraviolet B radiation [40]. Because the amount of epidermal melanin determines the number of photons, which reach the lower epidermal layers where vitamin D_3 synthesis takes place, vitamin D formation could be affected by individual characteristics of melanization. However, when assessing vitamin D nutritional status by measuring serum 25-hydroxyvitamin D, ethnic background had only a marginal effect with higher levels in whites compared to blacks. Regarding its active serum metabolite 1,25-dihydroxyvitamin D, levels were similar across all groups. Authors concluded that varying levels of pigmentation do not prevent the generation of normal levels of active vitamin D metabolites, while increasing pigmentation in the epidermis still exerts a strong photoprotective effect.

Objective Measurements of Skin Color

Advances have been made in pigmentation measurement devices, allowing for easy measurement of epidermal melanin using tristimulus reflectometry, narrowband spectroscopy, and diffuse reflectance spectroscopy. The tristimulus chromameter utilizes the L*a*b* color system to determine skin color: L* represents skin reflectance or lightness, a* measures color saturation from red to green, and b* measures color saturation from yellow to blue. The aforementioned measurement devices have been utilized in objectively measuring human skin pigmentation and in examining the impact of melanin on human skin color.

Lee et al. evaluated the Minolta CR-400 chromameter (Tokyo, Japan) as an objective measurement of periocular and facial pigmentation in subjects from different ethnic backgrounds [41]. African-American, Caucasian, and Hispanic subjects had facial and periocular skin color measurements performed. Using the L*a*b* color system, significant differences in L* were observed among all ethnic groups, while a* and b* were less sensitive to pigmentation differences. Additionally, the value L* (i.e., skin reflectance or lightness) demonstrated significant differences between different Fitzpatrick skin types III–VI, the more heavily pigmented groups. The Minolta CR-400 chromameter reliably measures facial pigmentation and can be utilized when evaluating changes in skin pigmentation in studies; the chromameter showed good inter- and intra-instrument reliability as well.

Shriver and Parra compared two methods to measure pigmentation in skin and hair in a group of subjects including European-Americans, African-Americans, South Asians, and East Asians [42]. The tristimulus colorimeter Photovolt ColorWalk (Indianapolis, IN) which uses the L*a*b* color system was compared to the DermaSpectrometer narrowband reflectometer (Hadsund, Denmark) which measures pigment in terms of erythema and melanin indices. Both types of instruments did provide accurate estimates of pigment level in the skin. However, measurements performed by the narrowband reflectometer were less affected by the greater redness of specific body sites due to increased vascularization.

Rigal et al. evaluated the effect of age on skin color and color heterogeneity in four ethnic

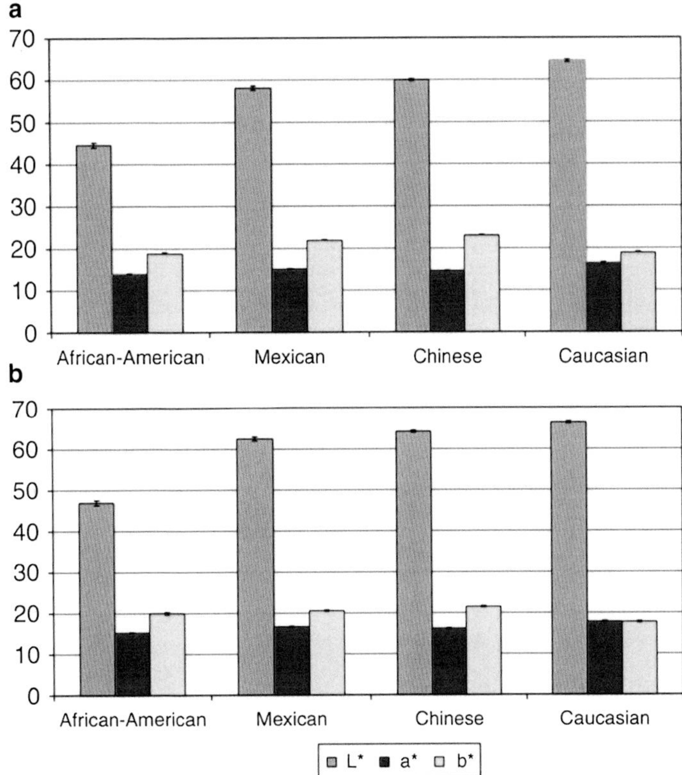

Fig. 1 Skin color versus ethnicity, on the forehead (**a**) and on the cheek (**b**). Results are expressed as mean and standard error of the mean (Figure is reproduced, with permission, from Ref. [43])

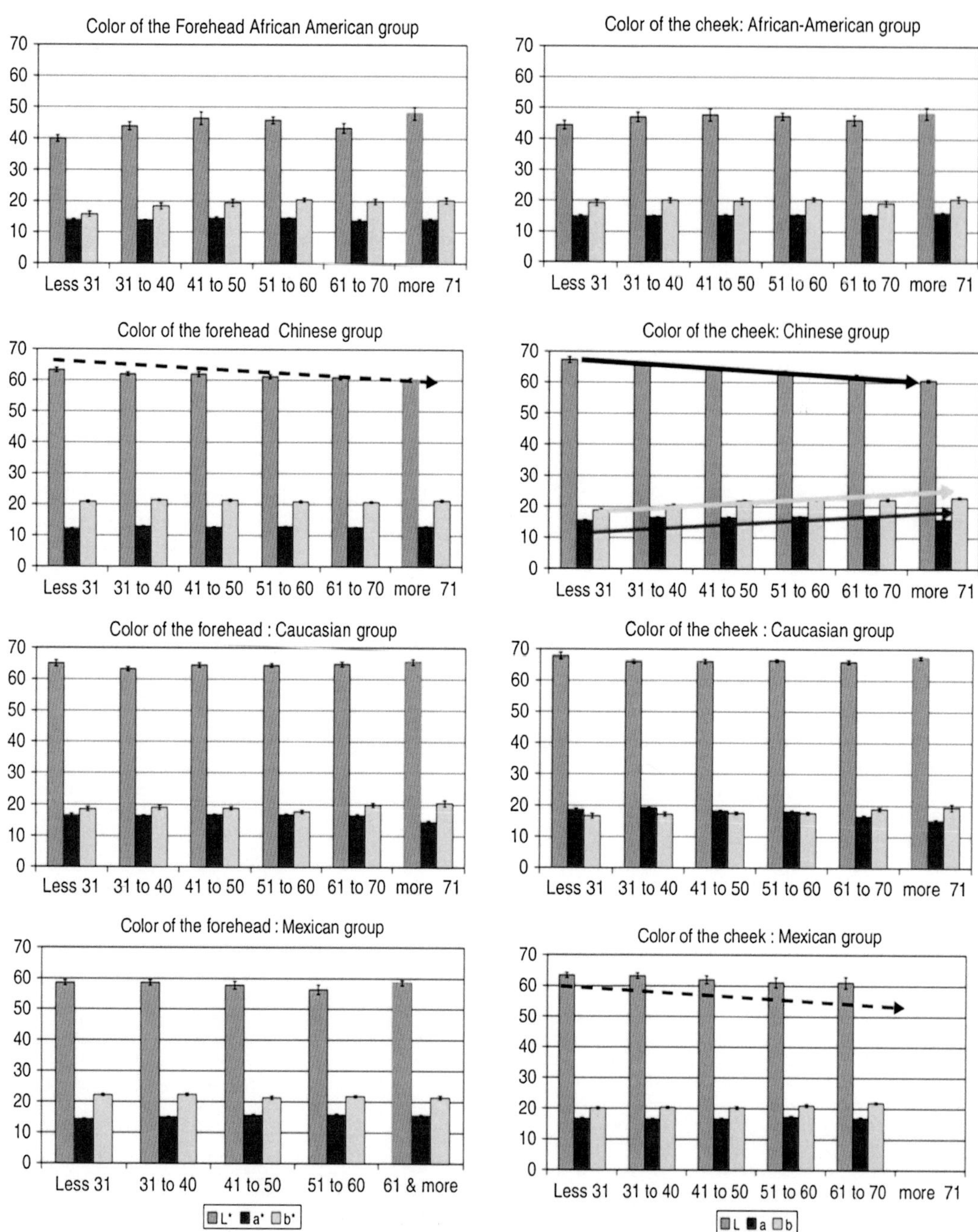

Fig. 2 Age-related changes in skin color on the forehead (*left*) and on the cheek (*right*). Results are expressed as mean and standard error of the mean. *Continuous lines* indicate significant variation and *dotted lines* nonsignificant variations, and the color of the line refers to the parameter (*black* for L* line, *red* for a* line, and *yellow* for b* line) (Figure is reproduced, with permission, from Ref. [43])

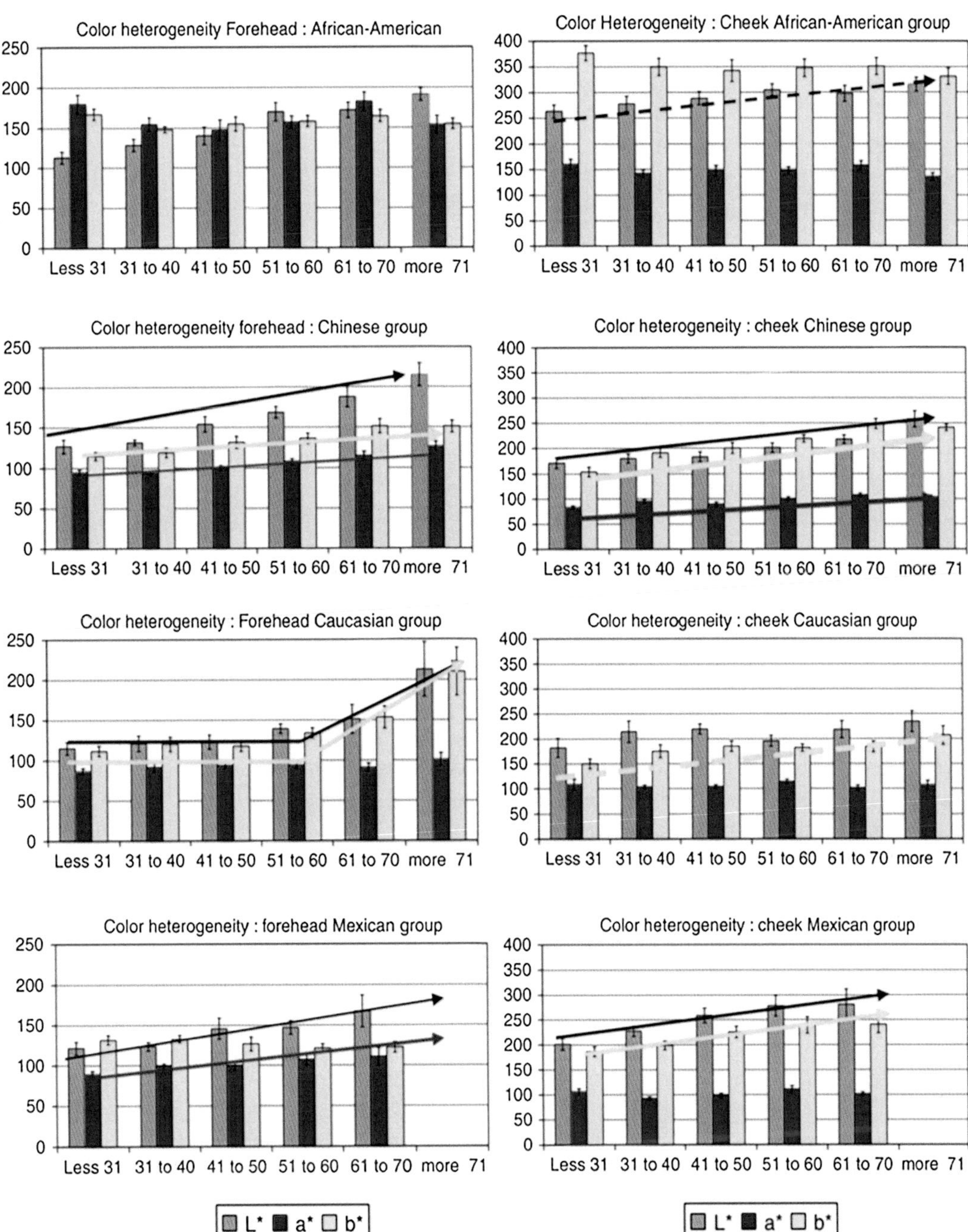

Fig. 3 Age-related changes in skin color heterogeneity on the forehead (*left*) and on the cheek (*right*). Results are expressed as mean and standard error of the mean. *Continuous lines* indicate significant variation and *dotted lines* nonsignificant variation, and the color of the line refers to the parameter (*black* for L* line, *red* for a* line, and *yellow* for b* line) (Figure is reproduced, with permission, from Ref. [43])

groups, including African-American, Caucasian, Chinese, and Mexicans. According to the L*a*b CIE system, clarity (fairness/lightness) was found lower in the African-American group, whereas the hue was lower in Caucasians, which means more red skin. A statistically significant darkening of the skin with age was observed in all ethnic groups, while yellowing of the skin was shown in the Chinese volunteers. Overall, the skin color of the face of African-Americans was more heterogeneous than in the other ethnic groups, but showed the least increase with age [43] (Figs. 1, 2, and 3).

Alaluf et al. examined the impact of epidermal melanin on objective measurements of human skin color [44]. The tristimulus chromameter was used to obtain measurements of human skin color in different ethnic skin types. Tristimulus L*a*b* measurements were made in European, Mexican, Chinese, Indian, and African subjects. Overall, darker skin types tend to have lower L* values, higher a* values, and higher b* values when compared to constitutively lighter skin types. Results demonstrated that total epidermal melanin is the primary determinant of L* values (i.e., skin reflectance or lightness). Melanosome size also has a significant influence on L* values, and larger melanosomes are associated with a darker skin color, as discussed previously. Based on the strength of correlations observed in this study, epidermal melanin content still seems to play a greater role than melanosome size in determining skin color.

Coelho et al. developed a predictive model for the noninvasive determination of ultraviolet radiation (UVR) sensitivity using diffuse reflectance spectroscopy (DR). They analyzed correlations between UVR sensitivity, melanin content, diffuse reflectance spectroscopy (DR), and UVR-induced DNA damage in the skin of subjects from three racial/ethnic groups: Asian, African-American, and white. UVR sensitivity was determined by evaluating each subject's response to one minimal erythemal dose (MED) of UVR 1 day after the exposure. Melanin content was measured using DR and by densitometric analysis of Fontana-Masson staining (FM) in skin biopsies taken from unexposed areas. An individual's UVR sensitivity based on MED highly correlated with melanin content measured by DR and by FM. The MED precision was further improved by taking race/ethnicity into consideration. Predicting UVR sensitivity in humans with the noninvasive DR should be indispensable for determining appropriate UVR doses for therapeutic, clinical, and/or cosmetic devices [45].

Conclusion

Many advances have been made in understanding the genetic, molecular, and cellular differences underlying normal variation in human skin pigmentation. However, further studies must be carried out in order to investigate the complex genetic pathway underlying melanin synthesis and the role of genetic variation in epidermal pigmentation and to elucidate differences in skin pathophysiology among humans from different ethnic backgrounds. As knowledge develops about the intricate process of pigmentation and distinctions between ethnic groups, it can be further understood how pigmentary changes occur with aging and consequently develop more effective management.

Cross-References

▶ Hyperpigmentation in Aging Skin
▶ The New Face of Pigmentation and Aging

References

1. US Census Bureau. Interim projections by age, sex, race, and Hispanic origin. 2004. http://www.census.gov/ipc/www/userinterimproj/. Accessed 22 Sept 2004.
2. Parra EJ, Kittles RA, Shriver MD. Implications of correlations between skin color and genetic ancestry for biomedical research. Nat Genet. 2004;36:S54–60.
3. Jackson IJ. Identifying the genes causing human diversity. Eur J Hum Gen. 2006;14:978–80.
4. Harrison GA. Differences in human pigmentation: measurement, geographic variation, and causes. J Invest Dermatol. 1973;60:418–26.
5. Quevedo Jr WC, Fitzpatrick TB, Pathak MA, Jimbow K. Role of light in human skin color variation. Am J Phys Anthrop. 1975;43:393–408.

6. Kalla AK. Human skin pigmentation, its genetics and variation. Humangenetik. 1974;21:289–300.
7. Westerhof W. A few more grains of melanin. Int J Dermatol. 1997;36:573–4.
8. Scott GA. Melanosome trafficking and transfer. In: Nordlund JJ, Boissy RE, Hearing VJ, King RA, Oetting WS, Ortonne JP, editors. The pigmentary system, physiology and pathophysiology. 2nd ed. Malden: Blackwell; 2006. p. 171–80.
9. Seiberg M. Keratinocyte-melanocyte interactions during melanosome transfer. Pigment Cell Res. 2001;14:236–42.
10. Hearing VJ. The regulation of melanin formation. In: Nordlund JJ, Boissy RE, Hearing VJ, King RA, Oetting WS, Ortonne JP, editors. The pigmentary system, physiology and pathophysiology. 2nd ed. Malden: Blackwell; 2006. p. 191–212.
11. Montagna W, Carlisle K. The architecture of black and white facial skin. J Am Acad Dermatol. 1991;24:929–37.
12. Szabo G, Gerald AB, Pathak MA. Racial differences in human pigmentation on the ultrastructural level. J Cell Biol. 1968;39:132a–3.
13. Toda K, Pathak MA, Parrish JA, Fitzpatrick TB, Quevedo Jr WC. Alteration of racial differences in melanosome distribution in human epidermis after exposure to ultraviolet light. Nat New Biol. 1972;236:143–5.
14. Szabo G. The number of melanocytes in human epidermis. Br Med J. 1954;1:1016–7.
15. Thody AJ, Burchill SA, Ito S. Epidermal eumelanin and phaeomelanin concentrations in different skin types and in response to PUVA. Br J Dermatol. 1990;123:842–5.
16. Thong HY, Jee SH, Sun CC, Boissy RE. The patterns of melanosome distribution in keratinocytes of human skin as one determining factor of skin colour. Br J Dermatol. 2003;149:498–505.
17. Minwalla L, Zhao Y, Le Poole IC, Wicket RR, Boissy RE. J. Keratinocytes play a role in regulating distribution patterns of recipient melanosomes in vitro. Invest Dermatol. 2001;117:341–7.
18. Alaluf S, Atkins D, Barrett K, Blount M, Carter N, Heath A. Ethnic variation in melanin content and composition in photoexposed and photoprotected human skin. Pigment Cell Res. 2002;15:112–8.
19. Halprin KM, Ohkawara A. Glutathione and human pigmentation. Arch Dermatol. 1966;94:355–7.
20. Iwata M, Corn T, Iwata S, Everett MA, Fuller BB. The relationship between tyrosinase activity and skin colour in human foreskins. J Invest Dermatol. 1990;95:9–15.
21. Fuller BB, Spaulding DT, Smith DR. Regulation of the catalytic activity of preexisting tyrosinase in black and Caucasian human melanocyte cell cultures. Exp Cell Res. 2001;262:197–208.
22. Maeda K, Yokokawa Y, Hatao M, Naganuma M, Tomita Y. Comparison of the melanogenesis in human black and light brown melanocytes. J Dermatol Sci. 1997;14:19–206.
23. Westerhof W. Evolutionary, biologic, and social aspects of skin color. Dermatol Clin. 2007;25:293–302.
24. Makova K, Norton H. Worldwide polymorphism at the MC1R locus and normal pigmentation variation in humans. Peptides. 2005;26:1901–8.
25. Saternus R, Pilz S, Gräber S, et al. A closer look at evolution: variants (SNPs) of genes involved in skin pigmentation, including EXOC2, TYR, TYRP1 and DCT, are associated with 25(OH)D serum concentration. Endocrinology. 2015;156:39–47.
26. Shriver MD, Parra EJ, Dios S, Bonilla C, Norton H, Jovel C, et al. Skin pigmentation, biogeographical ancestry and admixture mapping. Hum Genet. 2003;112:387–99.
27. Lamason RL, Mohideen MPK, Mest JR, Wong AC, Norton HL, Aros MC, et al. SLC24A5, a putative cation exchanger, affects pigmentation in zebrafish and humans. Science. 2005;310:1782–6.
28. Norton HL, Kittles RA, Parra E, McKeigue P, Mao X, Cheng K, et al. Genetic evidence for the convergent evolution of light skin in Europeans and East Asians. Mol Biol Evol. 2007;24:710 22.
29. Gibbons A. American Association of physical anthropologists meeting. European skin turned pale only recently, gene suggests. Science. 2007;316:364.
30. Tadokoro T, Yamaguchi Y, Batzer J, Coelho SG, Zmudzka BZ, Miller SA, et al. Mechanisms of skin tanning in different racial/ethnic groups in response to ultraviolet radiation. J Invest Dermatol. 2005;124:1326–32.
31. Olson RL, Gaylor J, Everett MA. Skin color, melanin, and erythema. Arch Dermatol. 1973;108:541–4.
32. Olson RL, Nordquist J, Everett MA. The role of lysosomes in melanin physiology. Br J Dermatol. 1970;83:189–99.
33. Baumann L, Rodriguez D, Taylor SC, Wu J. Natural considerations for skin of color. Cutis. 2006;78(6):2–20.
34. Taylor S, Woolery-Lloyd H. Pigmentation disorders in skin of color: the role of natural substances. Semin Cutan Med Surg. 2008;27:14–5.
35. Sugino K, Imokawa G, Maibach H. Ethnic difference of stratum corneum lipid in relation to stratum corneum function [abstract]. J Invest Dermatol. 1993;100:597.
36. Reed JT, Ghadially R, Elias PM. Effect of race, gender, and skin type of epidermal permeability barrier function. J Invest Dermatol. 1994;102:537. Abstract.
37. Marshall E, Lynch V, Smith H. Variation in the susceptibility of the skin to dichloroethylsulfide. J Pharmacol Exp Ther. 1919;12:291–301.
38. Weigand D, Haygood C, Gaylor J. Cell layers and density of Negro and Caucasian stratum corneum. J Invest Dermatol. 1974;62:563–8.
39. Post PW, Farrington Jr D, Binford Jr RT. Cold injury and the evolution of "white" skin. Hum Biol. 1975;47:65–80.
40. Matsuoka LY, Wortsman J, Haddad JG, Kolm P, Hollis BW. Racial pigmentation and the cutaneous synthesis of vitamin D. Arch Dermatol. 1991;127:536–8.

41. Lee JA, Osmanovic S, Viana MAG, Kapur R, Meghpara B, Edward DP. Objective measurement of periocular pigmentation. Photodermatol Photoimmunol Photomed. 2008;24:285–90.
42. Shriver MD, Parra EJ. Comparison of narrow-band reflectance spectroscopy and tristimulus colorimetry for measurements of skin and hair color in persons of different biological ancestry. Am J Phys Anthropol. 2000;112:17–27.
43. Jd R, Mazis ID, Diridollou S, Querleux B, Yang G, Leroy F, Barbosa VH. The effect of age on skin color and color heterogeneity in four ethnic groups. Skin Res Technol. 2010;16:168–78.
44. Alaluf S, Atkins D, Barrett K, Blount M, Carter N, Heath A. The impact of epidermal melanin on objective measurements of human skin colour. Pigment Cell Res. 2002;15:119–26.
45. Coelho SG, Zmudzka BZ, Yin L, Miller SA, Yamaguchi Y, Tadokoro T, Hearing VJ, Beer JZ. Non-invasive diffuse reflectance measurements of cutaneous melanin content can predict human sensitivity to UVR. Exp Dermatol. 2013;22(4):266–71.

The New Face of Pigmentation and Aging

79

John Nip, S. Brian Potterf, Sheila Rocha, Shilpa Vora, and Carol Bosko

Contents

Abstract

Pigmentation is a universal physiological process that occurs in all organisms from bacteria, fish, and amphibians to birds, mammals, and humans (Bagnara JT, Matsumoto J (2006) Comparative anatomy and physiology of pigment cells in nonmammalian tissues. In: Nordlund JJ, Boissy RE, Hearing VJ, King RA, Oettig WS, Ortonne JP (eds) The pigmentary system. Blackwell, Oxford, pp 11–59). Pigmentation provides camouflage and protection from UV, but also in some lower organisms, pigmentation is involved in wound healing (Sugumaran et al., Pigment Cell Res 12:118–125, 1999; Sugumaran et al., Arch Biochem Biophys 378:393–403, 2000; Sugumaran, Pigment Cell Res 15:2–9, 2002). In humans, the major determinant of skin color is the pigment/complex polymer, melanin. The variation in human skin color is striking and has great physiological and sociological implications. The color of one's skin is a strong predictor of social interactions. That skin color has immense psychosocial impact is evidenced by the billions of dollars spent annually in search of the perfect skin color. Tanning beds and artificial tanners are used to achieve a bronzed glow, while fairness creams and bleaches are used to lighten skin color and achieve even skin tone. The concept of ideal skin color varies across cultures and geographies and has great significance on the perception of beauty. With age, changes in the amount

J. Nip (✉) • S.B. Potterf • S. Rocha • C. Bosko
Unilever Research and Development, Trumbull, CT, USA
e-mail: john.nip@unilever.com; brian.potterf@unilever.com; sheila.rocha@unilever.com; carol.bosko@unilever.com

S. Vora
Unilever Research and Development, Bangalore, India
e-mail: shilpa.vora@unilever.com

M.A. Farage et al. (eds.), *Textbook of Aging Skin*,
DOI 10.1007/978-3-662-47398-6_53

and distribution of melanin are evident. Increases in skin pigmentation as well as the appearance of mottled and discrete hyperpigmented lesions are a hallmark of photoexposure and advancing age. To better understand the changes that may occur in aging skin, a closer look at the pigmentation system and its components is needed. In this chapter, an overview of melanogenesis is provided, from the production of melanin to its transfer to keratinocytes, as well as the genetic and biological pathways that regulate pigment production. Studies on the clinical and biological manifestations of hyperpigmentation in Asian populations will be presented.

Introduction

Melanin is one of the major determinants of human skin color [1–4]. It is produced by neural crest-derived melanocytes, which are found in many sites throughout the body including the skin, hair, eye, ear, and the central nervous system (CNS) [5–7]. Extracutaneous melanocytes do not produce melanin throughout their lifespan, and, unlike epidermal melanocytes, they do not transfer their melanosomes and melanin to neighboring cells [6].

Besides imparting color to our skin, melanin serves many other diverse functions. Undoubtedly, its most important function is protection from the damaging effects of solar UV radiation [8] whose most dire consequence is the development of cancer [9, 10]. The photoprotective properties of melanin have been well documented [11]. Melanin protects the cells of the skin by shielding the cell nuclei, thus preventing DNA damage in the form of cyclobutane pyrimidine dimers and 6-4 DNA photoproducts [12]. In addition to photoprotection, melanin gives the skin, hair, and eyes its color and is also involved in hearing [5–7]. Impaired hearing in individuals with vitiligo may be associated with lack of these melanocytes [13]. Melanins may also serve a unique function in the central nervous system. In fact, neuromelanins found in the dopaminergic neurons in the substantia nigra of the brain have been implicated in the pathology of Parkinson's disease [7].

Melanin Synthesis

Within the melanocyte, melanin is synthesized in specialized organelles called melanosomes, which are subsequently transferred (along with their melanin) to adjacent keratinocytes in the basal epidermal layer, giving rise to skin pigmentation. The type and quantity of melanin produced and the shape, size, and distribution of the melanosomes in basal epidermal keratinocytes affect the final color of an individual's skin.

Human melanin is composed of two distinct polymers, the dark brown/black eumelanin and the yellow/red pheomelanin [14]. Eumelanin and pheomelanin are produced in the eumelanosomes and pheomelanosomes, respectively. Both these types of melanosomes undergo four stages of maturation with the final stages III and IV resulting in synthesis and deposition of melanin. The two types of melanin differ in their composition and physical properties. Due to the incorporation of the sulfur-containing amino acid cysteine in its synthesis, pheomelanin has a higher sulfur and nitrogen content than eumelanin. Eumelanin is made and deposited in ellipsoidal melanosomes which contain lamellar or fibrillar internal structure, whereas pheomelanin is synthesized in spherical melanosomes and is associated with microvesicles [15, 16]. The final melanin composition, and therefore its color, is dependent on the relative amounts of pheo- and eumelanogenesis occurring in the melanocyte.

Eumelanin and pheomelanin are both derived from the common substrate tyrosine. The hydroxylation of tyrosine to dihydroxyphenylalanine (DOPA) and the oxidation of DOPA to dopaquinone are both reactions catalyzed by tyrosinase, the rate-limiting enzyme in melanin synthetic pathway. Evidence has accumulated recently for the requirement of three enzymes for initiation of melanogenesis [17]. Tyrosinase requires millimolar amounts of L-tyrosine that cannot be supplied by facilitated diffusion alone. On the other hand, $6BH_4$-dependent phenylalanine hydroxylase mediates conversion of phenylalanine to tyrosine in amounts sufficient for tyrosinase activity. The third enzyme implicated is tyrosine hydroxylase isoform I which converts tyrosine to L-DOPA. L-DOPA then binds tyrosinase at a site distinct from tyrosine and activates the enzyme. Other enzymes involved in melanogenesis include tyrosinase-related proteins-1 (TYRP1) and -2 (DCT) (Fig. 1).

Clinical studies on human skin have shown that in highly pigmented skin (Fitzpatrick types V and VI) that is chronically photoexposed, the pheomelanin content is only slightly elevated, whereas the eumelanin content is highly elevated [18]. The reflectance or lightness (L*) of human skin, as measured by the chromometer, is correlated with the total melanin content in an exponential manner [18] (Fig. 2).

Lightly pigmented skin types (such as the Chinese and European) have about half as much epidermal melanin as the most darkly pigmented skin types (African and Indian). In all skin types, pheomelanin is a very small part of epidermal melanin. In addition to melanin content, melanosome size, shape, and distribution play a large role in skin color. African skin has the largest

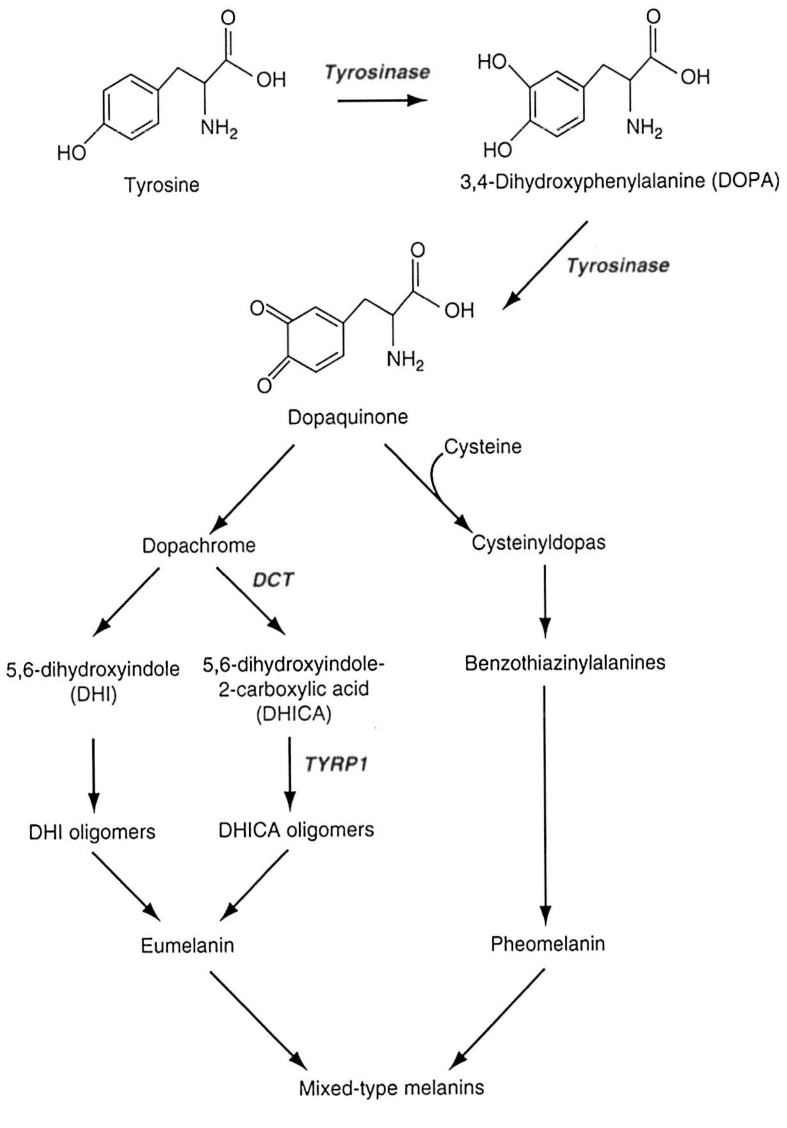

Fig. 1 The melanogenesis pathway. Schematic diagram showing the enzymes involved in melanogenesis and their melanin products

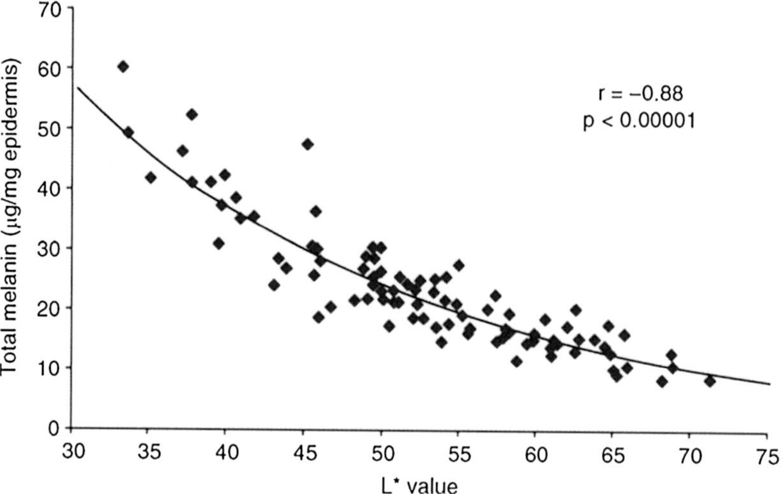

Fig. 2 Exponential relationship between L* and melanin. Graph showing the melanin content of skin from different ethnic donors

melanosome size, and these tend to be deposited singly, while lighter skin types (Chinese, European) have smaller melanosomes that tend to cluster together in the keratinocyte [19, 20].

Boissy et al. have focused on the distribution of melanosomes in the keratinocytes and the role that donor ethnicity plays in this process [19]. In these experiments, keratinocytes and melanocytes from different donors were cocultured, and it was observed that the ethnicity of the keratinocyte donor defined the distribution of the melanosomes. That is, in keratinocytes from Black donors, the melanosomes are distributed individually, regardless of whether Black or Caucasian melanocytes were present in the cocultures. Conversely, when Caucasian keratinocytes were present, melanosomes were distributed in clusters, irrespective of the ethnicity of the melanocyte donor skin. This data points to the importance of the keratinocyte in regulating melanosome distribution and thus may have a relevant role in skin pigmentation in different ethnic skin types.

Human pigmentation variation between different ethnic groups is not due to melanocyte number as there are not any differences between the groups in terms of abundance of melanocytes [21]. The levels of tyrosinase protein, the key enzyme in melanogenesis, are similar across ethnic groups as well. Interestingly, TYRP-1, another important enzyme for melanin production, is more than 2.5-fold elevated in darkly pigmented African and Indian skin types in comparison to more lightly pigmented Chinese and European skin types [21].

Finally, there is evidence from the literature and confirmed recently by Alaluf et al. [21] that chronic hyperpigmentation in sun-exposed body sites (e.g., lateral forearms) is associated with increased melanocyte number. This indicates that melanocyte number (proliferation) may play a role in maintaining long-term, stable changes in skin color on chronically sun-exposed sites.

Melanosome Transfer

The process of melanosome transfer to the keratinocyte is poorly understood. Light and EM studies done on guinea pig skin cultures suggest that melanosome transfer may be due to direct interaction between the melanocyte and keratinocyte, involving phagocytosis of bits of the melanocyte dendrite (containing the melanosomes) by the keratinocytes. Other hypotheses on transfer have been put forth, the most popular being (i) release of melanosomes/melanin by melanocytes followed by their endocytosis into keratinocytes, (ii) direct inoculation (injection) of melanosomes into keratinocytes, and (iii) keratinocyte–melanocyte membrane fusion

[22–24]. Whether melanin itself or the melanosomes are transferred from melanocytes to keratinocyte remains controversial.

The nature of receptors involved in melanocyte–keratinocyte interactions is still speculative. Cadherins are calcium-dependent cell–cell adhesion glycoproteins, of which E-cadherin is expressed by human melanocytes and is thought to be the major mediator of melanocyte–keratinocyte adhesion [25]. Also, lectins and neoglycoproteins inhibit melanin transfer in melanocyte–keratinocyte cocultures [26, 27]. Other cell surface proteins proposed to be involved in the process of melanosome phagocytosis are protease-activated receptor-2 (PAR-2) and keratinocyte growth factor receptor [28–32].

Work from Seiberg et al. [31–33] has shown that the transfer of the melanosomes to the keratinocytes is mediated by a G protein-coupled receptor, the protease-activated receptor 2, on keratinocytes. Activation of the receptor with trypsin or a peptide agonist resulted in pigmentation in skin equivalent models, in human skin xenografted onto SCID mice, and in Yucatan swine [33]. Serine protease inhibitors that prevent activation of the PAR-2 receptors on keratinocytes caused decreased pigmentation in the Yucatan swine model of melanogenesis, presumably by affecting melanosomal transfer to the keratinocytes [33].

Scott et al. [34] showed that UV irradiation (using a xenon arc lamp solar simulator) on human subjects (the buttock skin) altered PAR-2 expression. In UV-irradiated skin, expression of the receptor was localized to the whole epidermis versus just the lower third of the epidermis in a nonirradiated control site on the same individual. They also suggest that there is a delay in upregulation of PAR-2 expression in the skin from phototype I subjects compared to those with type II and III skin.

Our own investigations point to a role for the semaphorin–plexin ligand–receptor system in melanosome transfer. Semaphorins are a class of secreted and membrane-bound proteins that are expressed widely and have been shown to play an important role in a diverse set of biological processes. Semaphorins mediate alterations in cytoskeletal elements, actin filaments, and microtubular networks. Semaphorins were originally identified for their role in neuronal development and play a crucial role in axonal guidance. Semaphorins bind two receptor families, the plexins and the neuropilins. The semaphorin 6 class of proteins are ligands for the plexin receptor family. Semaphorin 6D (Sema6D) is a member of the class 6 of semaphorins and is grouped into six isoforms through differential splicing [35]. The neural crest-derived origin of melanocytes is interesting in light of semaphorins having a role in neuronal axon guidance. It is hypothesized that the semaphorin–plexin system may play a role in keratinocyte–melanocyte interactions. Using RNA-mediated interference, it was demonstrated that knockdown of either the entire semaphorin class, Sema6D specifically, or Plexin A1 protein resulted in a significant inhibition of melanosome transfer. HaCaT keratinocytes transfected with siRNA targeted toward semaphorin 6D specifically or the conserved sema domain resulted in significant decrease in protein and a corresponding decrease in melanosome transfer (Fig. 3). Similarly, a knockdown of Plexin A1 protein in melanocytes inhibited melanosome transfer (data not shown).

Independently, Scott and colleagues reported that semaphorin 7A is expressed on keratinocytes and fibroblasts and is upregulated in fibroblasts in response to UV, and binding of semaphorin 7A to Plexin C1 on melanocytes inhibited dendrite formation. In contrast, binding of semaphorin 7A to β-1-integrin promoted melanocyte dendricity [36]. These results further support a role for the semaphorin–plexin receptor system in keratinocyte–melanocyte communication.

Melanosome transfer is a process regulated by various environmental stimuli and physiological parameters. However, underpinning this it is clear that it is the keratinocyte which regulates this process by paracrine and autocrine factors. Evidence in literature exists for melanocyte–keratinocyte adhesion and interaction as a prelude to transfer of melanosomes to keratinocyte [25, 37]. It has been shown that melanocyte–keratinocyte recognition is a prerequisite to melanosome transfer [38].

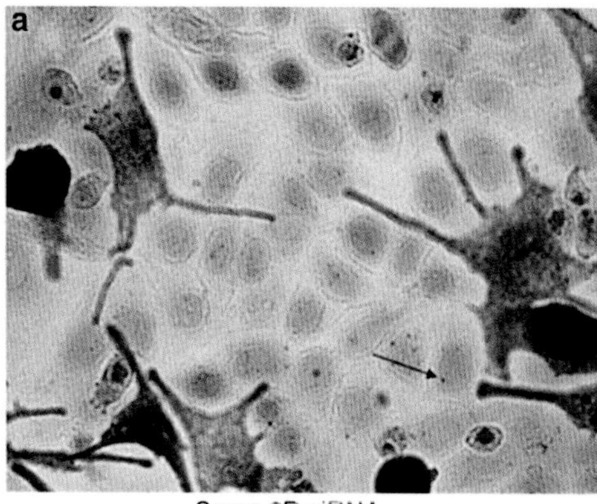

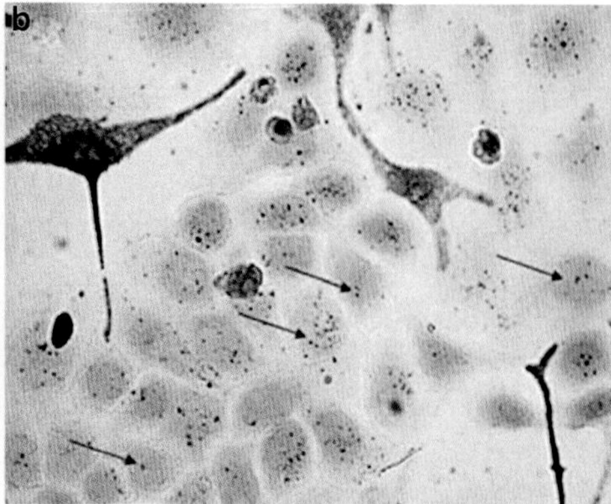

Fig. 3 Semaphorin 6D siRNA knockdown leads to a significant inhibition of melanosome transfer. Coculture of primary human melanocytes and HaCaT keratinocytes transfected with different siRNA. HaCaT keratinocytes were transfected with siRNA for Sema6D (RNAi 1099 (semaphorin 6D-specific) sequence is sense-GCCACACUUU-CUUCAUGCCAUAGAA- and antisense-UUCUAUGGCAUGAA-GAAAGUGUGGC-) (**a**) or scrambled controls (**b**). *Arrows* point to melanosomes within the keratinocytes. 400× magnification

There has been an attempt to decipher some of the melanocyte-induced signaling events in keratinocytes upon melanocyte–keratinocyte interaction. Although melanocytes extend filopodia toward keratinocytes, it is technically not possible to monitor intracellular signaling during the actual event of cell–cell contact. Therefore, it was investigated whether isolated melanocyte cell plasma membrane fraction induced signaling in keratinocytes. When primary human melanocyte plasma membrane fraction was added to HaCaT keratinocytes, a transient increase in $[Ca^{2+}]_i$ was observed in keratinocytes (Fig. 4a).

Further, the calcium signal induced by melanocyte plasma membrane in HaCaT keratinocytes was found to be due to release of Ca^{2+} from intracellular stores (Fig. 4b). It was also noted that calcium might be necessary for pigment transfer, as transfer in melanocyte–keratinocyte cocultures was inhibited when intracellular calcium in keratinocytes was chelated [38]. This led to our hypothesis that a "ligand–receptor"-type interaction exists between melanocytes and keratinocytes, which mediate recognition and eventually melanin transfer.

A technical point in melanosome transfer research is whether the melanosome retains its proteins once transferred to the keratinocyte or does the keratinocyte degrade the melanosomal proteins of the melanosome. The question was indirectly answered in a study done by Virador et al. [39]. They produced a series of melanocyte-specific peptide antibodies to human melanosomal proteins in order to study the distribution of these proteins in the skin from normal individuals and ones with pigmentation disorders. Polyclonal antibodies were synthesized against the peptide sequences of the following human melanosomal proteins – TYR, TYRP-1, DCT, and Pmel17 (gp100). Immunological staining of normal skin (paraffin sections) revealed that TYR, DCT, and to a lesser extent gp100 were not only detected in the melanocytes but were also present in the neighboring keratinocytes and in some keratinocytes higher in the epidermis as well. These findings suggest that it is possible to detect melanosomal proteins in the keratinocytes after transfer; however, the life of these proteins in the keratinocytes may still be limited.

Mutations Affecting Melanosome Transfer

Evidence from three mouse coat color pigmentation mutants revealed that melanosome transport may be a key factor in determining pigmentation

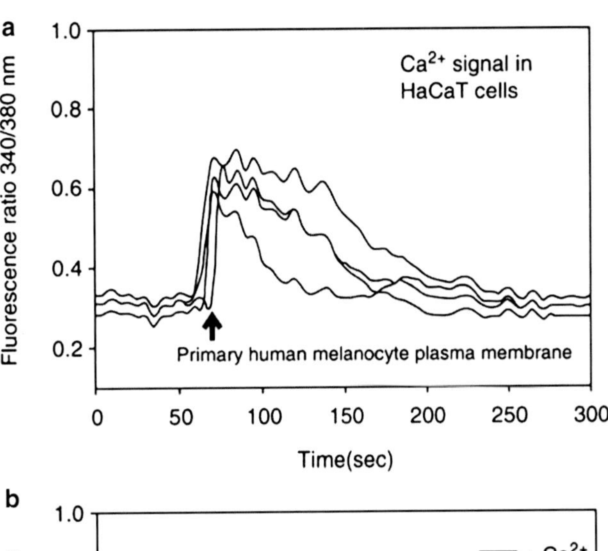

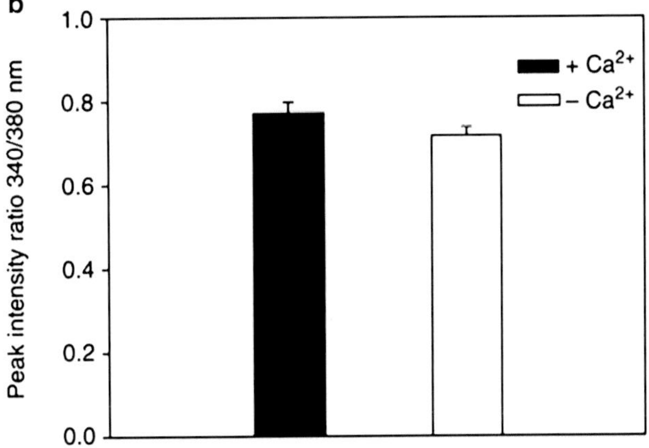

Fig. 4 Primary melanocyte plasma membrane induced calcium signal in HaCaT keratinocytes (**a**). The data shown are representative traces of four cells in a single experiment. Primary melanocyte membrane induced rise in calcium in HaCaT cells in absence or presence (2 mM) of extracellular calcium (**b**). The data are mean+SEM from three separate experiments, $p > 0.1$ [38]

both in the hair and most likely in the skin as well. These three mutations called *ashen*, *dilute*, *and leaden* lead to differences in coat color of the mice by affecting melanosomal transport of melanin and not melanin synthesis itself, as this latter process is not altered in these mouse mutations [40–46]. In fact, the produced melanin is distributed in the perinuclear region of these mutant melanocytes. The genes for these mutants have been discovered, and examination of their function and biochemistry has helped us to better understand the role of melanosome transport in pigmentation. The *ashen* gene encodes a Rab GTPase, Rab27a [46]; the *dilute* gene encodes for myosin Va [41]; and the *leaden* encodes for melanophilin [45].

Alterations at the dilute locus in mice cause a decrease in coat color intensity due to changes in melanosome movement and transfer to the neighboring keratinocytes. Dilute mutant melanocytes were shown to have a perinuclear melanosome distribution and possessed dendrites [47]. However, melanosomes in these mutant melanocytes were less abundant in the dendrites compared to dendrites from wild-type mice. Apparently, the dilute locus encodes the actin-associated motor protein, myosin Va [41]. This protein has been found to be involved in both melanosome transport and dendrite formation [40]. The products of the *ashen*, *dilute*, and *leaden* loci all have been implicated in movement of the melanosomes to the dendrite tips. Rab proteins control movement and transport of intracellular vesicles, including melanosomes, by regulating the interactions between the vesicles and cytoskeletal elements and molecular motors. C-terminal prenylation mediates association of Rab proteins with the cytoplasmic side of the cell membrane, an event which controls Rab activity [48].

Melanosomal movement to the cell periphery involves many different proteins, including the Rab protein, Rab27a, and myosin Va. This transfer of melanosomes from the perinuclear region of the melanocyte to the peripheral areas and concentration at the dendrite tips [49] requires a combination of "long-range," bidirectional movements of the melanosomes along microtubules (along the dendrite) and local myosin Va-dependent capture and local movement of the melanosomes along actin-rich dendrite areas [50, 51]. A closely related family member of Rab27a is Rab27b, which shares over 70 % amino acid sequence identity with each other [52]. The function of this protein has not been as well studied as Rab27a, although its GTPase activity has been shown [53]. In addition, transient expression of dominant-negative forms of Rab27b revealed that the native form of the protein may be involved in the number and length of dendrites as well as movement of melanosomes to the cell periphery in melan-a murine melanocytes [53].

Myosin Va is an actin-based dimeric molecular motor protein that is involved in melanosomal movement along with Rab27a [49, 54–57]. This protein is composed of three different domains including a motor (or the head) domain containing the actin and ATP binding sites, a regulatory (the neck) domain possessing several myosin light chain and calmodulin-binding sites (also called IQ motifs), and the tail domain which consists of an α-helix coil–coil region and a globular region [58]. Alternative splicing in the tail domain can create different tissue-specific forms of myosin Va including a melanocyte form (specifically found in melanocytes) and the brain form (which is present in neural tissues) [59].

Several groups have recently elucidated the interactions of Rab27a, myosin Va, and melanophilin in melanosome transport [40, 44, 60–62]. In fact, these proteins interact with each other in a tripartite complex with the melanophilin protein being the crucial link between the Rab27a and myosin Va [60]. Wu et al. [63] established the sequence of interaction of the three proteins, namely, that Rab27a binds to the melanosome followed by binding of melanophilin to Rab27a and then myosin Va is bound to melanophilin. The alternatively spliced exon-F in myosin Va is required for binding of myosin Va to melanophilin [63].

In human and mouse diseases such as Griscelli syndrome [64, 65], mutation of key proteins involved in the movement of melanosomes in preparation for transfer to the keratinocytes compromises/dilutes the color of the skin. The mutations that cause pigmentation issues in humans are classified into three types: Griscelli syndrome types I, II, and III. Each of these has a mutation in the machinery involved in movement of the melanosomes from the perinuclear region to the tips of the dendrites. For Griscelli syndrome type I, patients present with albinism but also severe neurological defects. The mutation in type I is found on the myosin 5A gene (MYO5A) – which encodes for myosin Va [66].

Albinism in Griscelli syndrome type II is also associated with immunodeficiency and can lead to fatal hemophagocytic syndrome [67]. The defect is caused by mutations in RAB27A gene which encodes Rab27a (a GTPase). This protein is required for T cell cytotoxic granule release, and its defect may explain the immune defects observed [67, 68]. The albinism is a result of the Rab27a defect in transport of the melanosomes in the transfer process.

For Griscelli syndrome type III, the patient displays the characteristic hypopigmentation, but there are no associated neurological or immunological defects. The gene involved is MLPH gene, encoding for melanophilin [69]. As well there have been type III patients which have a deletion in the F-exon of the MYO5A gene [69]. The mutations in both the mouse and human implicate melanosome transfer as crucial for normal expression of the skin and coat color even in the absence of defects in melanin synthesis.

Regulation of Melanogenesis

Human skin color is a heritable, polygenic trait and varies widely across individuals and populations. However, environmental factors such as UVR also have a strong influence on skin color. There is a high correlation between the intensity of incident UV light at the point of anthropological origin and skin color suggesting intense evolutionary selective pressure [70, 71]. UV can degrade folic acid, a critical nutrient for reproductive health. On the other hand, UVB is required for synthesis of vitamin D. It has been speculated that skin color has evolved to maximize the production of these important nutrients while protecting the skin from UV-induced damage.

Much of our knowledge of the genetic regulation of skin color has come from human and animal mutations that result in drastic changes in pigmentation, e.g., albinism. The OMIM lists 18 genes and >100 loci involved in human albinism [72]. However, aside from these rare and extreme changes in color, only a handful of genes are known to influence the normal variation in skin color. Among these, the melanocortin receptor 1 (MCR1) has been strongly correlated with red hair, light skin, and freckling as well as a predisposition to skin cancer [73].

The cloning of the human genome and the development of extensive "hap-maps" of single nucleotide polymorphisms [74] have enabled the study of skin color via genome-wide scans and have facilitated the identification of genes involved in normal skin color variation. Among those identified are SLC24A5, SLC45A2 (MATP), TYR, ASIP, and OCA2 [75, 76].

The role of SLC24A5 in skin color variation was identified in a South Asian population using high-density whole genome array technology [68]. In that population, polymorphisms in three genes, MATP, TYR, and SLC24A5, accounted for a large fraction of the natural variation in skin color, while SLC24A5 alone accounted for >30 % of the variation in skin color. Ginger et al. [77] then demonstrated the role of SLC24A5 in melanogenesis directly. In either B16 or dedifferentiated normal human melanocytes, knockdown of SLC24A5 expression via RNA-mediated interference resulted in a decrease in melanin synthesis.

The hormonal regulation of pigmentation has been reviewed extensively elsewhere [78] and will be only discussed briefly here. It is clear that keratinocytes regulate melanogenesis in a paracrine fashion, and the concept of the epidermal unit comprising 1 melanocyte and 36 keratinocytes is well accepted. However, melanocytes receive paracrine signals from and are regulated by dermal fibroblasts as well.

The importance of the melanocortins in control of pigmentation has been well established. ACTH, α-MSH, and β-MSH stimulate both melanogenesis and the switch from pheo- to eumelanogensis in mammalian systems via the melanocortin receptor (MCR). Injection of MSH peptides in humans stimulates skin pigmentation especially in sun-exposed areas [79]. MCR1, a G protein-coupled receptor, has the highest binding affinity for α-MSH and has received most of the attention. Recently, however, it was observed that β-MSH binding to MCR4 may also stimulate melanogenesis. Moreover, some have proposed a receptor-independent mechanism for the stimulation of tyrosinase activity by α- and β-MSH within the melanosome [17]. The activity of the MCR is antagonized by the agouti signaling protein (ASIP), which binds MCR stimulating a switch to pheomelanogenesis. Ligation of MSH to MCR1 and resultant increase in cAMP induce the microphthalmia transcription factor (MITF), which exerts transcriptional regulation on TYR and TYRP1. Recently, it has been suggested that hepatocyte nuclear factor (HNF)-1alpha also promotes tyrosinase transcription and that p53 is a transcriptional regulator of HNF. Thus, UV, which stimulates p53, may directly affect tyrosinase transcription via HNF in the absence of MITF.

Endothelins 1 and 3, ligands of the G protein-coupled receptor endothelin receptor B, have been implicated in the development of melanocytes and induction of pigmentation [80]. ET-1 is upregulated in keratinocytes exposed to UVB and stimulates tyrosinase expression.

GPCRs signal via cAMP, and it is evident that a number of cAMP receptors may be involved in melanogenesis including histamine, eicosanoids, β2-adrenoceptor, and muscarinic receptors.

The nuclear hormone receptor for estrogen is expressed on human melanocytes, but its role in stimulating pigmentation is the subject of debate. While it is widely believed that circulating sex hormones play a role in the development of melasma, our data suggests that melasma actually increases postmenopausally (see below).

The c-kit ligand stem cell factor (SCF, steel factor) is produced by keratinocytes and influences the proliferation and activity of melanocytes. SCF is a key hormone in embryonic development as it influences migration of melanoblasts from the neural crest [81]. Mutations in either the receptor tyrosine kinase, c-kit, or its ligand result in loss in pigmentation. Human mutations result in the piebaldism phenotype with patchy leukoderma [82]. Basic fibroblast growth factor (bFGF) is another tyrosinase kinase receptor ligand induced by UVB exposure to keratinocytes. In vitro bFGF stimulates melanogenesis although its in vivo role has yet to be established [83].

Age-Related Changes

Age-related changes in pigmentation have been examined in several Asian populations. These studies have identified solar lentigo (SL) lesions to be one of the top pigmented lesions affecting a younger than expected population in Asia (see below). Solar lentigo, also known as senile lentigo or age spot, is a hyperpigmented macule which most often develops on sun-damaged skin of the face, the back of the hands, lateral forearms, the back, and the chest. They are highly symbolic of senescence, as suggested by their common French name "cemetery flowers," and are esthetically unpleasant. SL legions range from 2 to 10+mm and are histologically characterized by a hyperpigmented basal layer, elongated rete ridges, and increased numbers of melanocytes. Aside from the apparent activated state, the melanocytes appear otherwise normal with melanosomes present in all stages of maturation in the cytoplasm and in dendrites. However, the basal keratinocytes have accumulation of numerous melanosome complexes or polymelanosomes [84].

A look at the status of melanogenesis-specific genes reveals increases in POMC, TYR, TYRP-1, DCT, PMEL-17, OCA2, and MITF protein expression which confirms upregulation of melanogenesis in lesional melanocytes and also proposes their involvement in legion formation [85]. However, gene expression involved in cornified envelope formation, such as profilaggrin, and involucrin give weight to the possibility of a malfunctioning cornification process. Increased layers of cells in the stratum corneum point to not only a decrease in cornification but also a slowed desquamation process in the epidermis of SL lesions [86].

SL lesions have fewer Ki67 positive cells as compared to peri-lesional skin, an observation previously made by Unver et al. [87], suggesting that there are fewer dividing keratinocytes in the SL lesions [71]. Endothelin receptor B (ETBR) and stem cell factor (SCF) have been confirmed to be upregulated [88, 89]. Since these same markers, ETBR and SCF, have been shown to be upregulated in other pigmented lesions such as seborrheic keratosis [90, 91], they are not unique to SL lesions.

While concerns about uneven, patchy, and discrete facial hyperpigmentation are present in different ethnicities, these conditions are of particular concern in Asians and appear to be key drivers associated with aging [92, 93]. To further investigate the importance of pigmentation to aging in Asian populations, female subjects, ages 18–65 years, were enrolled in an Institutional Review Board-approved multi-site, facial hyperpigmentation characterization study, with approximately 100 subjects per cell (over 500 total subjects) from China (Shanghai), India (Mumbai), Thailand (Bangkok), Indonesia (Jakarta), and Japan (Tokyo). Subjects were screened for having self-perceived facial hyperpigmentation and a slight to moderate concern for facial hyperpigmentation in general.

Hence, the study does not represent a random sampling of these populations but serves as a clinical baseline under these conditions. Clinical evaluation was performed by a dermatologist of similar ethnic origin from each country to diagnose facial hyperpigmentation across multiple attributes (summarized in Table 1). Additional measures included color measurements with spectrophotometry and digital facial photographs to document clinical facial skin condition. Color measurements on non-lesional, even-toned areas of the face revealed an age-dependent increase cumulative pigmentation, resulting in increasing values of several L* units between women ages 20–60 years old (data not shown). This age-dependent increase in facial pigmentation is presumed to result from chronic, lifelong UV exposure since upper inner arm measurements showed no age dependence on these photo-protected areas. Populations with generally lighter facial skin tones (i.e., Chinese, Japanese) presented with more solar lentigines, while darker toned populations had significantly more post-inflammatory hyperpigmentation (PIH) and melasma that may arise from other, non-UV triggering events. Protective effects of melanin, genetic influences, geography, and habits and attitudes toward sun exposure and face care regimens may account for these differences. It is of interest to investigate facial pigmentation conditions within populations that have wide ranges of basal pigmentation and UV exposure, such as lighter toned Indian and Chinese populations, in more northern latitudes compared to darker toned populations in the south.

Several other differences in hyperpigmentation conditions exist between Asian populations. For example, periocular and periorbital hyperpigmentation were prevalent in the Indian population, but were virtually absent in other populations. The Indian, Thai, and Indonesian populations showed an increased prevalence of PIH due to acne or other reasons, which possibly reflects differences in facial skin care regimes, or more likely due to more exposure to chronic UV and an inherent ability to pigment compared to lighter toned populations. In general the presence of PIH showed an age-dependent decrease in prevalence with sharp reductions as these populations reached age 40–49 range. The incidence of melasma showed an age-dependent increase in both amount and severity in these populations. In general melasma increased and persisted beyond 50 years of age, far beyond childbearing age, which may support factors in addition to hormones as contributing to this disorder. Melanocytic nevi were present in most people by 20 years of age and remained constant throughout the various age ranges. There was an age-dependent increase in solar lentigines in Chinese and Japanese where by ages 40–49 years almost all subjects presented with some type of solar-induced hyperpigmentation. Interestingly, many subjects, ages 20–30 years from these generally sun-avoidance cultures, had significantly accumulated solar lentigines, which contrast with the later age accumulation in sun-seeking Caucasian populations. Additionally, an age-dependent increase in the size and intensity of lentigines was observed. Since lentigo senilis is often recalcitrant to treatment in later stages, early intervention with topical treatment may be beneficial. However, perception of aging in Asian populations may not be solely limited to development and progression of solar lentigines. Therefore, treatment modalities that target differential pathways underlying these disparate hyperpigmented conditions need to be further developed.

Concluding Remarks

Skin color has long been of interest for both its sociological and physiological importance. Despite intense study, many of the mechanisms of melanin production and its regulation, the influence of genetics in skin color, and the mechanisms of melanin distribution remain poorly understood. The melanocortin system is an important positive regulator of pigmentation, but the number of paracrine and autocrine factors implicated in regulation of melanocyte biology and melanogenesis is impressive. It is clear that melanin content as well as its distribution contributes to overall skin color. Naturally occurring mutations in mice and men

Table 1 Dermatological characterization of facial hyperpigmentation in various Asian populations. Dermatologists from each respective region diagnosed facial hyperpigmentation in females in Shanghai, China; Tokyo, Japan; Mumbai, India; Bangkok, Thailand; and Jakarta, Indonesia. Only the most prevalent conditions are contained in the table, and relatively rare disorders (<1–5 %, e.g., nevus of Ota) were excluded. This table is not meant to imply the full complement or extent of facial hyperpigmentation in Asian populations. Dermatologists participating in this study were Dr. Shinichi Watanabe (Tokyo), Dr. Qing-Ping Yang (Shanghai), Dr. Thada Piamphongsant (Bangkok), Dr. Sudhir Medhekar (Mumbai), and Dr. Dwi Retno (Jakarta)

Shanghai, China	Age (years)	All	20–29	30–39	40–49	50–59
N=		106	22	19	43	22
Solar lentigines		76 %	32 %	68 %	91 %	100 %
Freckles (lentigo simplex, other)		62 %	68 %	63 %	56 %	68 %
Melasma		18 %	9 %	16 %	23 %	18 %
PIH due to acne		19 %	55 %	32 %	5 %	0 %
PIH due to other		22 %	32 %	11 %	23 %	18 %
Seborrheic keratoses		19 %	5 %	16 %	21 %	32 %
Melanocytic nevi		82 %	77 %	84 %	86 %	77 %
Tokyo, Japan	Age (years)	All	20–29	30–39	40–49	50–59
N=		102	15	29	38	28
Solar lentigines		94 %	60 %	100 %	100 %	100 %
Bilateral nevus of Ota-like macules		31 %	33 %	45 %	29 %	15 %
Melasma		28 %	0 %	17 %	34 %	50 %
PIH		nd[a]	nd	nd	nd	nd
Seborrheic keratoses		10 %	7 %	0 %	8 %	30 %
Melanocytic nevi		71 %	73 %	62 %	71 %	80 %
Mumbai, India	Age (years)	All	20–29	30–39	40–49	50–59
N=		103	23	30	30	20
Solar lentigines		49 %	30 %	60 %	43 %	60 %
Freckles		11 %	30 %	13 %	0 %	0 %
Melasma		83 %	52 %	87 %	93 %	100 %
PIH due to acne		51 %	74 %	70 %	43 %	10 %
PIH due to other		88 %	91 %	87 %	87 %	90 %
Periocular hyperpigmentation		93 %	96 %	97 %	90 %	90 %
Perioral hyperpigmentation		78 %	78 %	77 %	80 %	75 %
Melanocytic nevi		82 %	77 %	84 %	86 %	77 %
Bangkok, Thailand	Age (years)	All	20–29	30–39	40–49	50–59
N=		109	23	31	33	22
Solar lentigines		17 %	4 %	13 %	9 %	45 %
Freckles		86 %	87 %	98 %	91 %	64 %
Melasma		50 %	13 %	35 %	64 %	86 %
PIH due to acne		31 %	65 %	48 %	6 %	9 %
PIH due to other		12 %	8 %	19 %	9 %	9 %
Melanocytic nevi		80 %	78 %	77 %	82 %	82 %
Jakarta, Indonesia	Age (years)	All	20–29	30–39	40–49	50–59
N=		100	8	31	39	22
Solar lentigines		43 %	13 %	32 %	49 %	59 %
Freckles		23 %	88 %	26 %	18 %	5 %
Melasma		85 %	50 %	84 %	87 %	95 %
PIH due to acne		53 %	38 %	68 %	54 %	36 %
PIH due to other		37 %	38 %	35 %	33 %	45 %
Seborrheic keratoses		53 %	13 %	39 %	59 %	77 %
Melanocytic nevi		63 %	50 %	71 %	67 %	50 %

[a]*nd* not determined

have helped to elucidate pigment biology, but the tools of molecular biology will lead our understanding to new levels. Pigmentary changes are a hallmark of aging in all races and ethnicities and are of growing concern in a world with an aging demographic. Solar lentigines or age spots remain a major concern among individuals globally but are of particular concern in Asian populations. With greater understanding, new therapies to treat dyspigmentations such as age spots will emerge.

Cross-References

- ▶ Hyperpigmentation in Aging Skin
- ▶ Pigmentation in Ethnic Groups

References

1. Bagnara JT, Matsumoto J. Comparative anatomy and physiology of pigment cells in nonmammalian tissues. In: Nordlund JJ, Boissy RE, Hearing VJ, King RA, Oettig WS, Ortonne JP, editors. The pigmentary system. Oxford: Blackwell; 2006. p. 11–59.
2. Sugumaran M, Duggaraju R, Generozova F, Ito S. Insect melanogenesis. II. Inability of Manduca phenoloxidase to act on 5,6-dihydroxyindole-2-carboxylic acid. Pigment Cell Res. 1999;12:118–25.
3. Sugumaran M, Nellaiappan K, Amaratunga C, Cardinale S, Scott T. Insect melanogenesis. III. Metabolon formation in the melanogenic pathway-regulation of phenoloxidase activity by endogenous dopachrome isomerase (decarboxylating) from Manduca sexta. Arch Biochem Biophys. 2000;378:393–403.
4. Sugumaran M. Comparative biochemistry of eumelanogenesis and the protective roles of phenoloxidase and melanin in insects. Pigment Cell Res. 2002;15:2–9.
5. Tachibana M. Sound needs sound melanocytes to be heard. Pigment Cell Res. 1999;12:344–54.
6. Boissy RE. Extracutaneous melanocytes. In: Nordlund JJ, Boissy RE, Hearing VJ, King RA, Ortonne JP, editors. The pigmentary system physiology and pathophysiology. New York: Oxford University Press; 1998. p. 59–72.
7. d'Ischia M, Prota G. Biosynthesis, structure, and function of neuromelanin and its relation to Parkinson's disease: a critical update. Pigment Cell Res. 1997;10:370–6.
8. Li W, Hill HZ. Induced melanin reduces mutations and cell killing in mouse melanoma. Photochem Photobiol. 1997;65:480–5.
9. Black HS, de Gruijl FR, Forbes PD, Cleaver JE, Ananthaswamy HN, de Fabo EC, Ullrich SE, Tyrrell RM. Photocarcinogenesis: an overview. J Photochem Photobiol B. 1997;40:29–47.
10. Pathak MA. Ultraviolet radiation and the development of non-melanoma and melanoma skin cancer: clinical and experimental evidence. Skin Pharmacol. 1991;4 Suppl 1:85–94.
11. Kollias N, Sayre RM, Zeise L, Chedekel MR. Photoprotection by melanin. J Photochem Photobiol B. 1991;9:135–60.
12. Kobayashi N, Muramatsu T, Yamashina Y, Shirai T, Ohnishi T, Mori T. Melanin reduces ultraviolet-induced DNA damage formation and killing rate in cultured human melanoma cells. J Invest Dermatol. 1993;101:685–9.
13. Ardic FN, Aktan S, Kara CO, Sanli B. High-frequency hearing and reflex latency in patients with pigment disorder. Am J Otolaryngol. 1998;19:365–9.
14. Jimbow K, Fitzpatrick TB, Wick MM. Biochemistry and physiology of melanin pigmentation. In: Golsmith LA, editor. Physiology, biology, and molecular biology of the skin. New York: Oxford University Press; 1991. p. 893.
15. Inazu M, Mishima Y. Detection of eumelanogenic and pheomelanogenic melanosomes in the same normal human melanocyte. J Invest Dermatol. 1993;100:172S–5.
16. Jimbow K, Oikawa O, Sugiyama S, Takeuchi T. Comparison of eumelanogenesis and pheomelanogenesis in retinal and follicular melanocytes; role of vesiculo-globular bodies in melanosome differentiation. J Invest Dermatol. 1979;73:278–84.
17. Schallreuter KU, Kothari S, Chavan B, Spencer JD. Regulation of melanogenesis – controversies and new concepts. Exp Dermatol. 2008;17:395–404.
18. Alaluf S, Heath A, Carter N, Atkins D, Mahalingam H, Barrett K, Kolb R, Smit N. Variation in melanin content and composition in type V and VI photoexposed and photoprotected human skin: the dominant role of DHI. Pigment Cell Res. 2001;14:337–47.
19. Thong HY, Jee SH, Sun CC, Boissy RE. The patterns of melanosome distribution in keratinocytes of human skin as one determining factor of skin colour. Br J Dermatol. 2003;149:498–505.
20. Yoshida Y, Hachiya A, Sriwiriyanont P, Ohuchi A, Kitahara T, Takema Y, Visscher MO, Boissy RE. Functional analysis of keratinocytes in skin color using a human skin substitute model composed of cells derived from different skin pigmentation types. FASEB J. 2007;21:2829–39.
21. Alaluf S, Barrett K, Blount M, Carter N. Ethnic variation in tyrosinase and TYRP1 expression in photoexposed and photoprotected human skin. Pigment Cell Res. 2003;16:35–42.
22. Van Den BK, Naeyaert JM, Lambert J. The quest for the mechanism of melanin transfer. Traffic. 2006;7:769–78.
23. Wasmeier C, Hume AN, Bolasco G, Seabra MC. Melanosomes at a glance. J Cell Sci. 2008;121:3995–9.

24. Yamamoto O, Bhawan J. Three modes of melanosome transfers in Caucasian facial skin: hypothesis based on an ultrastructural study. Pigment Cell Res. 1994;7:158–69.
25. Tang A, Eller MS, Hara M, Yaar M, Hirohashi S, Gilchrest BA. E-cadherin is the major mediator of human melanocyte adhesion to keratinocytes in vitro. J Cell Sci. 1994;107(Pt 4):983–92.
26. Greatens A, Hakozaki T, Koshoffer A, Epstein H, Schwemberger S, Babcock G, Bissett D, Takiwaki H, Arase S, Wickett RR, et al. Effective inhibition of melanosome transfer to keratinocytes by lectins and niacinamide is reversible. Exp Dermatol. 2005;14:498–508.
27. Minwalla L, Zhao Y, Cornelius J, Babcock GF, Wickett RR, Le PI, Boissy RE. Inhibition of melanosome transfer from melanocytes to keratinocytes by lectins and neoglycoproteins in an in vitro model system. Pigment Cell Res. 2001;14:185–94.
28. Boissy RE. Melanosome transfer to and translocation in the keratinocyte. Exp Dermatol. 2003;12 Suppl 2:5–12.
29. Cardinali G, Ceccarelli S, Kovacs D, Aspite N, Lotti LV, Torrisi MR, Picardo M. Keratinocyte growth factor promotes melanosome transfer to keratinocytes. J Invest Dermatol. 2005;125:1190–9.
30. Cardinali G, Bolasco G, Aspite N, Lucania G, Lotti LV, Torrisi MR, Picardo M. Melanosome transfer promoted by keratinocyte growth factor in light and dark skin-derived keratinocytes. J Invest Dermatol. 2008;128:558–67.
31. Seiberg M, Paine C, Sharlow E, Andrade-Gordon P, Costanzo M, Eisinger M, Shapiro SS. The protease-activated receptor 2 regulates pigmentation via keratinocyte-melanocyte interactions. Exp Cell Res. 2000;254:25–32.
32. Seiberg M. Keratinocyte-melanocyte interactions during melanosome transfer. Pigment Cell Res. 2001;14:236–42.
33. Seiberg M, Paine C, Sharlow E, Andrade-Gordon P, Costanzo M, Eisinger M, Shapiro SS. Inhibition of melanosome transfer results in skin lightening. J Invest Dermatol. 2000;115:162–7.
34. Scott G, Deng A, Rodriguez-Burford C, Seiberg M, Han R, Babiarz L, Grizzle W, Bell W, Pentland A. Protease-activated receptor 2, a receptor involved in melanosome transfer, is upregulated in human skin by ultraviolet irradiation. J Invest Dermatol. 2001;117:1412–20.
35. Qu X, Wei H, Zhai Y, Que H, Chen Q, Tang F, Wu Y, Xing G, Zhu Y, Liu S, et al. Identification, characterization, and functional study of the two novel human members of the semaphorin gene family. J Biol Chem. 2002;277:35574–85.
36. Scott GA, McClelland LA, Fricke AF. Semaphorin 7a promotes spreading and dendricity in human melanocytes through beta1-integrins. J Invest Dermatol. 2008;128:151–61.
37. Scott G, Leopardi S, Printup S, Madden BC. Filopodia are conduits for melanosome transfer to keratinocytes. J Cell Sci. 2002;115:1441–51.
38. Joshi PG, Nair N, Begum G, Joshi NB, Sinkar VP, Vora S. Melanocyte-keratinocyte interaction induces calcium signalling and melanin transfer to keratinocytes. Pigment Cell Res. 2007;20:380–4.
39. Virador V, Matsunaga N, Matsunaga J, Valencia J, Oldham RJ, Kameyama K, Peck GL, Ferrans VJ, Vieira WD, Bdel-Malek ZA, et al. Production of melanocyte-specific antibodies to human melanosomal proteins: expression patterns in normal human skin and in cutaneous pigmented lesions. Pigment Cell Res. 2001;14:289–97.
40. Hume AN, Collinson LM, Hopkins CR, Strom M, Barral DC, Bossi G, Griffiths GM, Seabra MC. The leaden gene product is required with Rab27a to recruit myosin Va to melanosomes in melanocytes. Traffic. 2002;3:193–202.
41. Mercer JA, Seperack PK, Strobel MC, Copeland NG, Jenkins NA. Novel myosin heavy chain encoded by murine dilute coat colour locus. Nature. 1991;349:709–13.
42. Moore KJ, Swing DA, Rinchik EM, Mucenski ML, Buchberg AM, Copeland NG, Jenkins NA. The murine dilute suppressor gene dsu suppresses the coat-color phenotype of three pigment mutations that alter melanocyte morphology, d, ash and ln. Genetics. 1988;119:933–41.
43. Moore KJ, Swing DA, Copeland NG, Jenkins NA. The murine dilute suppressor gene encodes a cell autonomous suppressor. Genetics. 1994;138:491–7.
44. Nagashima K, Torii S, Yi Z, Igarashi M, Okamoto K, Takeuchi T, Izumi T. Melanophilin directly links Rab27a and myosin Va through its distinct coiled-coil regions. FEBS Lett. 2002;517:233–8.
45. Provance DW, James TL, Mercer JA. Melanophilin, the product of the leaden locus, is required for targeting of myosin-Va to melanosomes. Traffic. 2002;3:124–32.
46. Wilson SM, Yip R, Swing DA, O'Sullivan TN, Zhang Y, Novak EK, Swank RT, Russell LB, Copeland NG, Jenkins NA. A mutation in Rab27a causes the vesicle transport defects observed in ashen mice. Proc Natl Acad Sci U S A. 2000;97:7933–8.
47. Provance Jr DW, Wei M, Ipe V, Mercer JA. Cultured melanocytes from dilute mutant mice exhibit dendritic morphology and altered melanosome distribution. Proc Natl Acad Sci U S A. 1996;93:14554–8.
48. Pereira-Leal JB, Hume AN, Seabra MC. Prenylation of Rab GTPases: molecular mechanisms and involvement in genetic disease. FEBS Lett. 2001;498:197–200.
49. Wu X, Rao K, Bowers MB, Copeland NG, Jenkins NA, Hammer III JA. Rab27a enables myosin Va-dependent melanosome capture by recruiting the myosin to the organelle. J Cell Sci. 2001;114:1091–100.
50. Hammer III JA, Wu XS. Rabs grab motors: defining the connections between Rab GTPases and motor proteins. Curr Opin Cell Biol. 2002;14:69–75.
51. Wu X, Bowers B, Rao K, Wei Q, Hammer III JA. Visualization of melanosome dynamics within wild-type and dilute melanocytes suggests a paradigm

for myosin V function In vivo. J Cell Biol. 1998;143:1899–918.
52. Chen D, Guo J, Miki T, Tachibana M, Gahl WA. Molecular cloning and characterization of rab27a and rab27b, novel human rab proteins shared by melanocytes and platelets. Biochem Mol Med. 1997;60:27–37.
53. Chen Y, Samaraweera P, Sun TT, Kreibich G, Orlow SJ. Rab27b association with melanosomes: dominant negative mutants disrupt melanosomal movement. J Invest Dermatol. 2002;118:933–40.
54. Lambert J, Onderwater J, Vander HY, Vancoillie G, Koerten HK, Mommaas AM, Naeyaert JM. Myosin V colocalizes with melanosomes and subcortical actin bundles not associated with stress fibers in human epidermal melanocytes. J Invest Dermatol. 1998;111:835–40.
55. Nascimento AA, Amaral RG, Bizario JC, Larson RE, Espreafico EM. Subcellular localization of myosin-V in the B16 melanoma cells, a wild-type cell line for the dilute gene. Mol Biol Cell. 1997;8:1971–88.
56. Wei Q, Wu X, Hammer III JA. The predominant defect in dilute melanocytes is in melanosome distribution and not cell shape, supporting a role for myosin V in melanosome transport. J Muscle Res Cell Motil. 1997;18:517–27.
57. Wu X, Bowers B, Wei Q, Kocher B, Hammer III JA. Myosin V associates with melanosomes in mouse melanocytes: evidence that myosin V is an organelle motor. J Cell Sci. 1997;110(Pt 7):847–59.
58. Reck-Peterson SL, Provance Jr DW, Mooseker MS, Mercer JA. Class V myosins. Biochim Biophys Acta. 2000;1496:36–51.
59. Seperack PK, Mercer JA, Strobel MC, Copeland NG, Jenkins NA. Retroviral sequences located within an intron of the dilute gene alter dilute expression in a tissue-specific manner. EMBO J. 1995;14:2326–32.
60. Fukuda M, Kuroda TS, Mikoshiba K. Slac2-a/melanophilin, the missing link between Rab27 and myosin Va: implications of a tripartite protein complex for melanosome transport. J Biol Chem. 2002;277:12432–6.
61. Kuroda TS, Fukuda M, Ariga H, Mikoshiba K. The Slp homology domain of synaptotagmin-like proteins 1-4 and Slac2 functions as a novel Rab27A binding domain. J Biol Chem. 2002;277:9212–8.
62. Strom M, Hume AN, Tarafder AK, Barkagianni E, Seabra MC. A family of Rab27-binding proteins. Melanophilin links Rab27a and myosin Va function in melanosome transport. J Biol Chem. 2002;277:25423–30.
63. Wu XS, Rao K, Zhang H, Wang F, Sellers JR, Matesic LE, Copeland NG, Jenkins NA, Hammer III JA. Identification of an organelle receptor for myosin-Va. Nat Cell Biol. 2002;4:271–8.
64. Griscelli C, Prunieras M. Pigment dilution and immunodeficiency: a new syndrome. Int J Dermatol. 1978;17:788–91.
65. Griscelli C, Durandy A, Guy-Grand D, Daguillard F, Herzog C, Prunieras M. A syndrome associating partial albinism and immunodeficiency. Am J Med. 1978;65:691–702.
66. Pastural E, Barrat FJ, Dufourcq-Lagelouse R, Certain S, Sanal O, Jabado N, Seger R, Griscelli C, Fischer A, de Saint BG. Griscelli disease maps to chromosome 15q21 and is associated with mutations in the myosin-Va gene. Nat Genet. 1997;16:289–92.
67. Menasche G, Pastural E, Feldmann J, Certain S, Ersoy F, Dupuis S, Wulffraat N, Bianchi D, Fischer A, Le DF, et al. Mutations in RAB27A cause Griscelli syndrome associated with haemophagocytic syndrome. Nat Genet. 2000;25:173–6.
68. Stinchcombe JC, Barral DC, Mules EH, Booth S, Hume AN, Machesky LM, Seabra MC, Griffiths GM. Rab27a is required for regulated secretion in cytotoxic T lymphocytes. J Cell Biol. 2001;152:825–34.
69. Menasche G, Ho CH, Sanal O, Feldmann J, Tezcan I, Ersoy F, Houdusse A, Fischer A, de Saint BG. Griscelli syndrome restricted to hypopigmentation results from a melanophilin defect (GS3) or a MYO5A F-exon deletion (GS1). J Clin Invest. 2003;112:450–6.
70. Jablonski NG, Chaplin G. The evolution of human skin coloration. J Hum Evol. 2000;39:57–106.
71. Chaplin G, Jablonski NG. Hemispheric difference in human skin color. Am J Phys Anthropol. 1998;107:221–3.
72. Online Mendelian Inheritance in Man (OMIM). 2009.
73. Schaffer JV, Bolognia JL. The melanocortin-1 receptor: red hair and beyond. Arch Dermatol. 2001;137:1477–85.
74. The international HapMap consortium a haplotype map for the human genome. 2005; 1299–1320.
75. Stokowski RP, Pant PV, Dadd T, Fereday A, Hinds DA, Jarman C, Filsell W, Ginger RS, Green MR, van der Ouderaa FJ, et al. A genomewide association study of skin pigmentation in a South Asian population. Am J Hum Genet. 2007;81:1119–32.
76. Han J, Kraft P, Nan H, Guo Q, Chen C, Qureshi A, Hankinson SE, Hu FB, Duffy DL, Zhao ZZ, et al. A genome-wide association study identifies novel alleles associated with hair color and skin pigmentation. PLoS Genet. 2008;4, e1000074.
77. Ginger RS, Askew SE, Ogborne RM, Wilson S, Ferdinando D, Dadd T, Smith AM, Kazi S, Szerencsei RT, Winkfein RJ, et al. SLC24A5 encodes a trans-Golgi network protein with potassium-dependent sodium-calcium exchange activity that regulates human epidermal melanogenesis. J Biol Chem. 2008;283:5486–95.
78. Slominski A, Tobin DJ, Shibahara S, Wortsman J. Melanin pigmentation in mammalian skin and its hormonal regulation. Physiol Rev. 2004;84:1155–228.
79. Lerner AB, McGuire JS. Effect of alpha- and betamelanocyte stimulating hormones on the skin colour of man. Nature. 1961;189:176–9.
80. Garcia RJ, Ittah A, Mirabal S, Figueroa J, Lopez L, Glick AB, Kos L. Endothelin 3 induces skin

pigmentation in a keratin-driven inducible mouse model. J Invest Dermatol. 2008;128:131–42.
81. Reid K, Nishikawa S, Bartlett PF, Murphy M. Steel factor directs melanocyte development in vitro through selective regulation of the number of c-kit+ progenitors. Dev Biol. 1995;169:568–79.
82. Spritz RA. Piebaldism, Waardenburg syndrome, and related disorders of melanocyte development. Semin Cutan Med Surg. 1997;16:15–23.
83. Imokawa G. Autocrine and paracrine regulation of melanocytes in human skin and in pigmentary disorders. Pigment Cell Res. 2004;17:96–110.
84. Cario-Andre M, Lepreux S, Pain C, Nizard C, Noblesse E, Taieb A. Perilesional vs. lesional skin changes in senile lentigo. J Cutan Pathol. 2004;31:441–7.
85. Motokawa T, Kato T, Katagiri T, Matsunaga J, Takeuchi I, Tomita Y, Suzuki I. Messenger RNA levels of melanogenesis-associated genes in lentigo senilis lesions. J Dermatol Sci. 2005;37:120–3.
86. Aoki H, Moro O, Tagami H, Kishimoto J. Gene expression profiling analysis of solar lentigo in relation to immunohistochemical characteristics. Br J Dermatol. 2007;156:1214–23.
87. Unver N, Freyschmidt-Paul P, Horster S, Wenck H, Stab F, Blatt T, Elsasser HP. Alterations in the epidermal-dermal melanin axis and factor XIIIa melanophages in senile lentigo and ageing skin. Br J Dermatol. 2006;155:119–28.
88. Kadono S, Manaka I, Kawashima M, Kobayashi T, Imokawa G. The role of the epidermal endothelin cascade in the hyperpigmentation mechanism of lentigo senilis. J Invest Dermatol. 2001;116:571–7.
89. Maeda K, Ono T, Matsunaga J. The mechanism of hyperpigmentation in senile lentigo and the efficacy of skin lightening agents. Fragr J. 2006;5:21–9.
90. Manaka L, Kadono S, Kawashima M, Kobayashi T, Imokawa G. The mechanism of hyperpigmentation in seborrhoeic keratosis involves the high expression of endothelin-converting enzyme-1alpha and TNF-alpha, which stimulate secretion of endothelin 1. Br J Dermatol. 2001;145:895–903.
91. Teraki E, Tajima S, Manaka I, Kawashima M, Miyagishi M, Imokawa G. Role of endothelin-1 in hyperpigmentation in seborrhoeic keratosis. Br J Dermatol. 1996;135:918–23.
92. Nouveau-Richard S, Yang Z, Mac-Mary S, Li L, Bastien P, Tardy I, Bouillon C, Humbert P, de Lacharrière O. Skin ageing: a comparison between Chinese and European populations. A pilot study. J Dermatol Sci. 2005;40:187–93.
93. Tsukahara K, Fujimura T, Yoshida Y, Kitahara T, Hotta M, Moriwaki S, Witt PS, Simion FA, Takema Y. Comparison of age-related changes in wrinkling and sagging of the skin in Caucasian females and in Japanese females. J Cosmet Sci. 2004;55:351–71.

Facial Wrinkling: The Marquee Clinical Sign of Aging Skin

80

Greg Hillebrand

Contents

G. Hillebrand (✉)
Amway Corporation, Ada, MI, USA
e-mail: dermscience@yahoo.com

M.A. Farage et al. (eds.), *Textbook of Aging Skin*,
DOI 10.1007/978-3-662-47398-6_86

Abstract

The factors that influence the onset and severity of facial skin wrinkling are many. They include innate factors such as constitutive skin pigmentation and ethnicity, gender, and age. Environmental factors such as acute and chronic sun exposure, diet, smoking history, and exercise are also considered important in facial wrinkling. In this chapter, I review the advances made in our understanding of the epidemiology and etiology of skin wrinkling based on selected publications from 2010 to 2015.

Introduction

Facial wrinkling is indeed the marquee clinical sign of aging skin. Facial wrinkling may also be a clinical sign for certain diseases, a risk factor for hearing impairment, and may even be predictive of life or health span. Wrinkling on body sites other than the face, such as the hands, legs, chest, and knees, has increased in consumer importance, and objective methods are being used to study these kinds of skin wrinkles. Lifetime exposure to solar radiation, especially during childhood, remains the number one environmental factor affecting the severity of skin wrinkles. However, other factors are now gaining attention as having a potential impact on facial wrinkle severity such as indoor and outdoor air pollution, sleeping position, and diet. In this review, I summarize recent work on the epidemiology of skin wrinkling, the etiology of a wrinkle, and wrinkling as surrogate markers for longevity and disease.

Epidemiology

Chronological Age

Chronological age is generally the best predictor of a person's wrinkle severity [1]. However, the age-related changes in wrinkling occur very slowly and are essentially undetectable from one year to the next. To best assess changes in facial skin wrinkles over time, individuals need to be tracked over several years, even decades in a longitudinal study design [2, 3]. Basin and Lévêque [4] followed the crow's feet wrinkles of 20 women and one man over two decades of life (1987–2008) using skin replicas. The skin replicas obtained in 1987 were stored appropriately to prevent any deterioration, and the technician who performed the procedure in 1987 also performed the procedure in 2008. Further, a standard replica was made of a standard metallic plate in 1987 and another one was made of the same standard plate in 2008. The microrelief pattern of the standard replica made in 2008 matched exactly to that of the one made in 1987 confirming there were no artifacts introduced into the experiment. All replicas were imaged under grazing light and wrinkles were quantified by image analysis. With these elegantly derived data, the investigators were able to make strong conclusions about the microscopic changes that occur as a wrinkle first appears and evolves. New wrinkles appeared or ones that were present in 1987 became longer by 2008. In some cases, small wrinkles or lines completely disappeared over the 21-year period (see Fig. 1a, b). Interestingly, the total area of all objects (small, medium, and large) in the crow's feet region did not change over time. Only the distribution of objects changed, at least in the 21 years for the subjects being studied. "Some small objects like pores and lines disappear by merging with pre-existing wrinkles or with other pores or lines. Some short segments of lines also tend to merge with each other to form long thin wrinkles." The authors go on to remark that the aged appearance of people results from the marked increase in the number of large objects. In youth, the skin's microrelief acts as a "deformation reservoir" during facial expression. With age, there is a conversion of this microrelief to visible wrinkles, a model supported by recent in silico experiments [5].

Another remarkable longitudinal study was conducted in Japan by Miyamoto et al. [3] who followed 108 Japanese females over an 11-year period (1999–2010) using both standardized facial imaging and biophysical measurements.

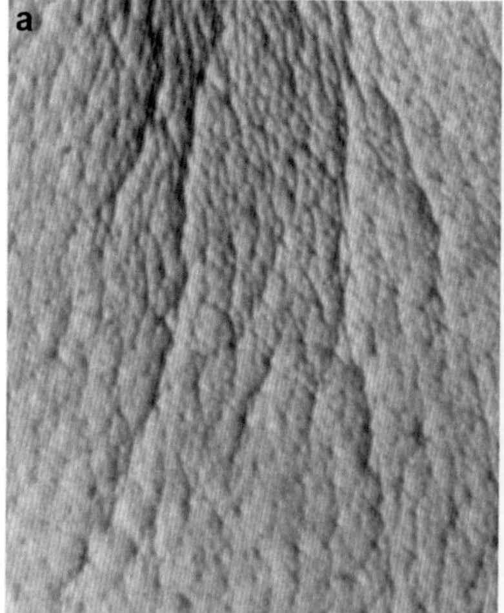

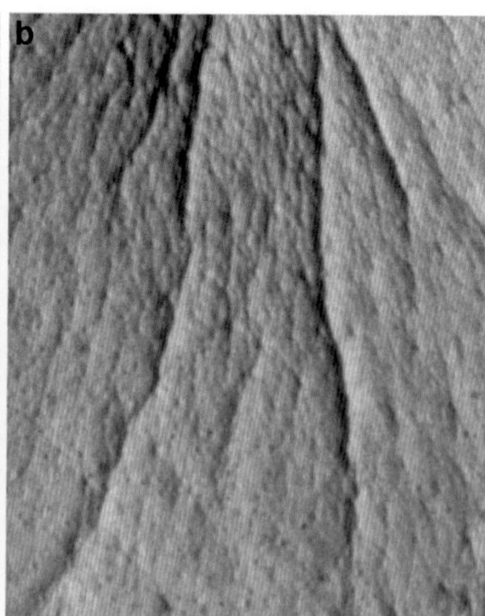

Fig. 1 Wrinkles of the crow's foot of a woman in 1987 (**a**) and 2008 (**b**). In 2008, some small wrinkles have disappeared and microrelief has been slightly smoothed (Reprinted with permission from Ref. [4])

Subjects were classified as having slower or faster rates of perceived aging and the specific facial features that drove perceived age changes were identified. Hyperpigmented spots, skin wrinkling, and overall roughness were the three main drivers of "unsuccessful aging." The authors also noted that the rate of wrinkle formation was faster in the 1930s compared to other decades of life, an observation that was further corroborated using a mechanical compression test in a cross-sectional study of skin wrinkling [6].

Ethnicity

Ethnic differences in facial skin wrinkling have been reported previously. Darker skin types generally show less wrinkling in sun-exposed areas than lighter skin types, due to the photoprotection afforded by more epidermal melanin in the darker skin. Timilshina et al. [7] compared facial skin wrinkling in 240 subjects of either Aryan- (Caucasian) or Mongolian-origin living in the Pokhara Valley of western Nepal, a sunny and hot climate conducive for skin photoaging. Nepal represents a unique environment where different ethnic tribes of different ethnic origin live in the same climate conditions, sharing common eating and lifestyle factors, particularly strong sun exposure. Photos of the subjects were captured and wrinkle severity was graded on a photonumeric scale. The subjects of Aryan-origin skin were more wrinkled than those of Mongolian-origin above 30 years, with significant difference being observed only among subjects over 60 years of age.

Gender

It generally accepted that the age of onset and severity of facial skin wrinkling differ between the sexes with men bearing most of the burden. Both differences in hormonal state, lifestyle, and sun protection habits play a role. Luebberding used 3D imaging combined with clinical grading to compare facial wrinkling in 150 Caucasian men and 50 women aged 20–70 [8]. Wrinkle severity was assessed in the periorbital, glabellar, and forehead regions. Wrinkles manifested earlier and were more severe in men than in women. Forehead lines were evident in the youngest men but did not appear in women before the age of 40; periorbital lines were the first visible wrinkles in women.

Similar gender differences in skin wrinkling have been observed in other ethnic groups [9–11]. In a study of 173 Japanese men and women [11], men showed increased forehead wrinkles compared with women. However, the difference in facial wrinkle severity tended to disappear in the older age groups and there were no gender-related differences at any age for upper eyelid wrinkles. In related work, Tsukahara et al. used a 3D analysis method and found that the depth of eye wrinkles in men showed an annual variation with more wrinkles at the corner of the eye in the fall compared to the spring; no such annual variation was observed in women [10].

Geography

Previous studies have shown that the severity of facial skin wrinkling increases as latitude decreases, presumably reflecting the higher total lifetime sun exposure at lower latitudes [12]. More recently, Gao et al. [13] compared the pattern of lines on the hands of Chinese men and women living in either Sanya (18°N, low latitude) or Shenyang (41°N, high latitude), China. In each age group, the mean skin damage grade for subjects living in the low-latitude region was significantly higher than that subjects living in the high-latitude region subjects ($P < 0.05$).

Kim et al. [14] compared the severity of crow's feet wrinkles in younger (ages 20–35) Chinese women living in either Beijing, Shanghai, Wuhan, or Guangzhou. Interestingly, despite living in a more northern latitude, the Beijing women had the most wrinkles, while the Guangzhou (the southernmost city in the survey) women had the least. The investigators also looked at the area, depth, and length of the wrinkles. Beijing women's wrinkles were deep and large, but Guangzhou women's wrinkles were shallow and

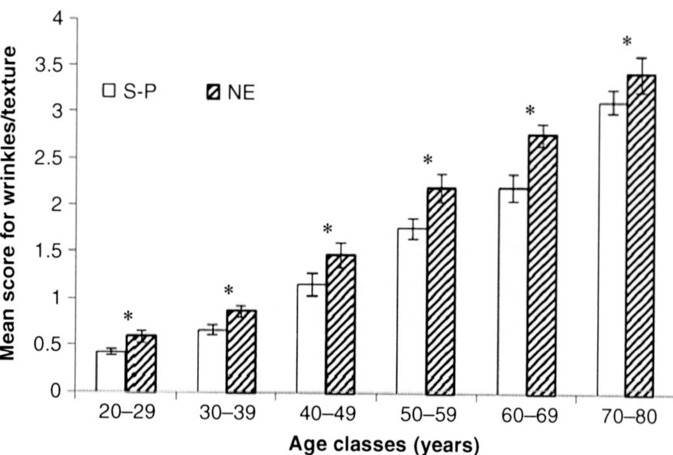

Fig. 2 Comparison of wrinkles and skin texture. Mean scores (±95 % CI) for each age class between normal exposure and sun-phobic. *Statistically significant difference ($P < 0.05$). Abbreviations: S-P sun-phobic, NE normal exposure, CI confidence interval. (Reprinted with permission from Ref. [20])

small. Beijing's dry climate leading to dry skin may have been responsible for the differences in wrinkle severity.

Solar Exposure

Kimlin and Guo [15] captured detailed lifetime sun exposure histories on 180 subjects, both men and women, across a wide age range (18–83). They measured facial wrinkling on every subject using the VISIA Complexion Analysis System®. They observed a nonlinear relationship between lifetime sun exposure and facial skin wrinkling with younger subjects having a higher risk of skin aging compared to elderly subjects.

Ichihashi and Ando [16] theoretically calculated the maximal daily exposure to solar radiation that would allow a person to avoid skin aging until later in life. The mean daily sun exposure time to maintain healthy skin until 80 years of age in the summer was calculated to be only 2.54 min (0.14 MED) for unprotected skin and 127 min with the use of a sunscreen of SPF (sun protection factor) of 50. Chronic UV exposure induces keratinocyte-derived IL-1α and granulocyte macrophage colony stimulating factor both of which induce fibroblast expression of elastase (neprilysin, [17]) activity and subsequent impairment of elastic fiber configuration and skin mechanical properties [18, 19].

Flament et al. [20] evaluated facial wrinkling in a population of Chinese women (n=301) living in Guangzhou, China. The subjects were classified into two subgroups based on their behavior when out in the sun. One group tended to avoid sun exposure ("sun-phobic") by using protective clothing, hats, umbrellas, sunscreens, etc. The other group did not care about sun exposure and went about their daily life without taking any precautions ("normal exposure"). Facial wrinkling increased linearly with age, about 10 % per decade, from age 20–80 years, in both groups. However, the sun-phobic group showed significantly less facial wrinkles than the normal exposure group (see Fig. 2). While the difference was observed across the entire age range of subjects (20–80 years), it was most pronounced in the younger women (+28 % in younger sun-phobic women and +8 % in the older sun-phobic group compared to age-matched normal exposure women).

Seasonal Changes

Several studies have focused on the seasonal and circadian changes in facial wrinkling. A year-long study was conducted to determine the effect of inherent chronologic variation on the appearance of facial wrinkling [21]. The study followed 12 Caucasian females (age 40–65) over a 54-week period with standardized imaging and clinical grading three times per week. During one week in the summer and winter seasons, the subjects endured even more measurements with visits three times per day (morning, midday, and evening) to assess circadian changes. In winter, fine lines, wrinkles, and texture appeared to be less pronounced at noon than in the morning or evening. There was little change across different days during the week. Fine lines and wrinkles were reported to be worse in winter than in summer.

Tsukahara et al. [10] measured facial wrinkling in Japanese men (n = 60) and women (n = 16) in March, June, September, December, and March the following year. Standardized photos were taken at the same time of day to help ensure against any diurnal variation in skin wrinkling. Photos were graded for wrinkle severity at four facial sites (forehead, under eye, crow's feet, and nasolabial fold) on a five-point scale. In addition, silicone replicas were obtained from the same areas and analyzed for 3D profile. The authors reported that the depth of eye wrinkles in men showed an annual variation with slightly more wrinkles at the corner of the eye in the fall compared to the spring. No seasonal intraindividual variation in wrinkle severity was observed in the Japanese women.

Using 3D skin imaging of the crow's feet area, Song et al. [22] did not observe any seasonal variation in skin wrinkling in 100 Korean men despite seeing significant changes in skin hydration. Qiu et al. also noted no significant changes in facial wrinkling of 354 Chinese women in the summer vs. winter [23]. Galzote et al. [24] measured skin wrinkling via live visual grading in the summer and winter on female subjects living in China, Korea, India, and Japan. There was little to no change in wrinkling from summer to winter.

Taken together, these studies suggest that seasonal variation in facial skin wrinkling is likely small and clinically not meaningful.

Air Pollution and Smoking

The effect of indoor and outdoor air pollution on skin aging is a growing concern, especially in urban areas. Polyaromatic hydrocarbons and nano-sized particulates can be inhaled or attached directly to and get absorbed into the skin putting oxidative stress on cells and tissues. Two papers out of Jean Krutman's lab reported results of cross-sectional surveys aimed at understanding the role of air pollution on skin aging [25, 26]. Indoor air pollution resulting from cooking with solid fuels was significantly associated with a 5–8 % more severe wrinkle appearance on the face and a 74 % increased risk of having fine wrinkles on the back of the hands, independent of age and other influences on skin aging [25]. Outdoor air pollution resulting primarily from urban traffic was mostly associated with an increased risk of pigmented spots on the face and to a lesser extent increased severity of the nasolabial fold (but not other wrinkles on the face) [26].

It is generally accepted that cigarette smoking accelerates facial wrinkle formation. Okada et al. [27] compared facial wrinkling in identical twins where one twin had smoked and the other had never smoked. The smoking twins showed significantly more nasolabial folds, upper lip wrinkles, and lower lip vermillion wrinkles than their nonsmoking counterparts (see Fig. 3). Interestingly, there was no significant difference between cohorts in severity of transverse forehead lines, glabellar lines, or crow's feet wrinkles.

Sleeping Position

Does sleeping on one's side or stomach cause sleep creases on the face? Should people sleep on their backs to avoid hours of creasing their face against the pillow? Lateral oblique forehead lines (wrinkles that run vertically on the left and right sides of the forehead) have been thought to be "sleeping lines." However, De Boulle and Turkmani reported case studies of two male subjects presenting with these types of forehead lines [28]. Treatment with onabotulinum toxin A resulted in positive aesthetic improvement suggesting that the wrinkle was the result of muscular contraction, not mechanical creasing of the skin from sleeping on their side or stomach (see Fig. 4). In another report, Kotlus looked at the relationship between sleeping on the right or left side and facial wrinkling. After interviewing

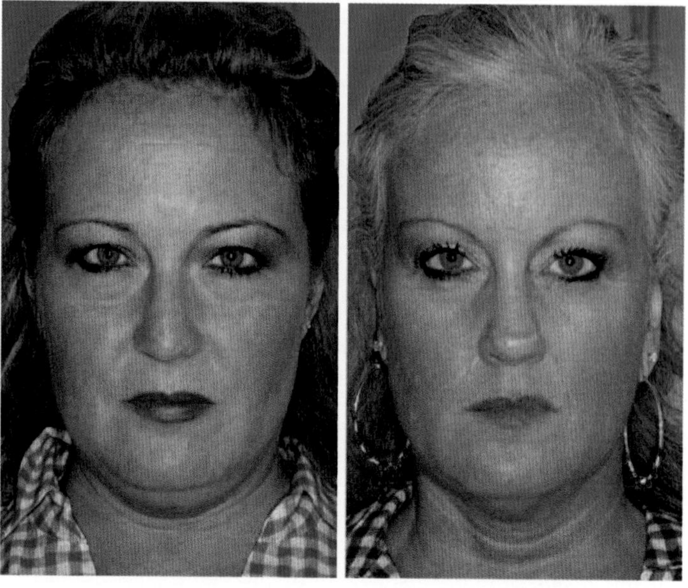

Fig. 3 The twin on the right is a smoker; the twin on the left is a nonsmoker. Notice differences in nasolabial creases (Reprinted with permission from Ref. [27])

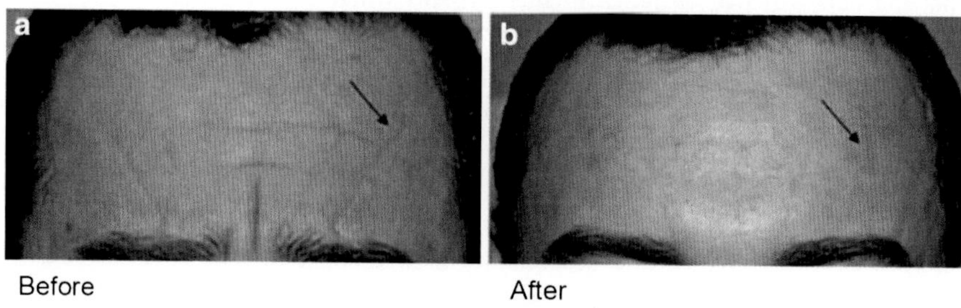

Fig. 4 Lateral oblique forehead lines (a) before and (b) after treatment with BoNT A (Reprinted with permission from Ref. [28])

100 women about their sleeping habits, 41 were found to be right-sided sleepers and 21 left-sided sleepers. Frontal photos of each subject were graded for wrinkling on the left and right sides. No significant correlation was observed between sleep side and the appearance of wrinkles [29]. Thus, sleeping position may not be a significant factor in facial wrinkle formation.

Wrinkling at Body Sites Other than the Face

Much of the focus in skin wrinkling research and treatment intervention has been on facial wrinkles, primarily periorbital or crow's feet wrinkles around the eye. With new consumer understanding on the importance and concern for wrinkling at other body sites, attention is now being given to areas that had previously been largely ignored such as the hands [13], décolletage [30], and even the knees [31]. Treatments originally designed for facial wrinkles are being tested for skin wrinkling at other body sites [32, 33]. Fabi and Bolton [30] have developed a photonumeric grading scale for wrinkles on the décolletage. Yoo et al. [31] looked at the skin on the knee of 38 healthy Korean female volunteers, divided into two groups, young and old. They developed a photonumeric scale of knee wrinkling (see Fig. 5) and used it to show the increase in knee wrinkles with age. Interestingly, the development of wrinkles on the knee correlated highly with development of facial crow's feet wrinkles.

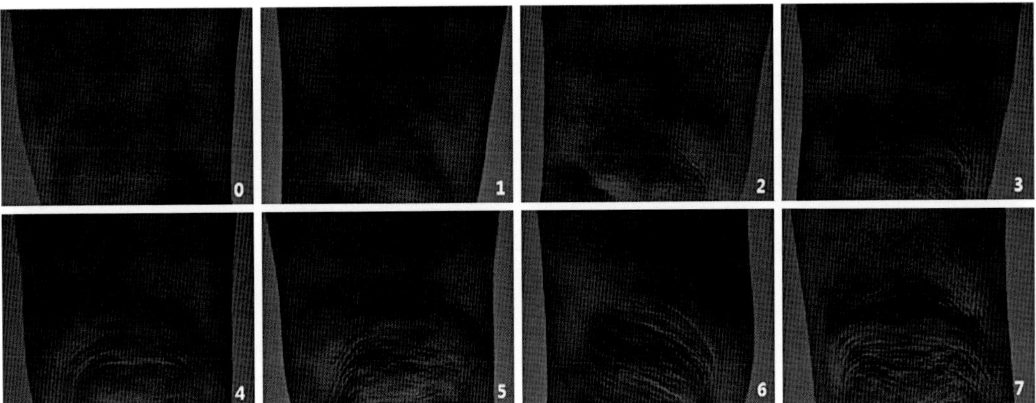

Fig. 5 Skin wrinkle severity scale on the knee (grade 0; no wrinkle ~ grade 7; severe wrinkle). (Reprinted with permission from Ref. [33])

Wrinkle Etiology

The mechanism of skin wrinkle formation is multifaceted with both histological and mechanical components. Mechanical stress during repeated facial expression can cause transient expression wrinkles to progress over time into permanent wrinkles [2, 28, 34]. Kligman explained a wrinkle as a simple configurational change and proposed an "old glove" model for wrinkle formation: "Smooth when new, the fabric develops grooves at sites of long-sustained stress." This model predicts little histological difference between the tissue under the wrinkle and the surrounding non-wrinkled skin [35]. However, some authors report unique histological features specific to the wrinkle while others report essentially identical histology of the wrinkle and the surrounding non-wrinkled skin. The results of Tsukahara et al. [36] may have shed light on the confusion. They studied the elastosis in the skin immediately under forehead and lateral canthus wrinkles of cadaver skin as well as the surrounding non-wrinkled skin. They found that solar elastosis was present both under the wrinkle and in the surrounding skin, but only in shallower wrinkles. In wrinkles greater than 0.6 mm in depth, such as those found on the lateral canthus, elastosis was less evident under the wrinkle compared to the adjacent non-wrinkled skin.

El-Domyati et al. also evaluated the histological and immunohistochemical changes of static forehead wrinkles in relation to surrounding photoaged skin [37]. They evaluated elastin, tropoelastin, and collagen (types I, III, and VII). Slides were evaluated qualitatively by blinded histopathologists and quantitatively using a computer-assisted program. Both methods showed lower amounts of elastin and tropoelastin at the bottom of the wrinkle compared to the adjacent photoaged skin. Interestingly, there was no statistically significant difference in the amount of collagens I and III in the area of the wrinkle compared to the adjacent skin. However, collagen VII was statistically significantly lower at the bottom of the wrinkle in comparison to nearby photoaged skin.

Tamatsu et al. [38] investigated the relationship between wrinkles and sebaceous glands using cadaver skin. Two facial sites were selected: the forehead which is rich in sebaceous glands and the lateral canthus (crow's feet) which is deplete in sebaceous glands. As sebaceous gland density increased, forehead wrinkle depth decreased. No correlation between wrinkle depth and sebaceous gland density was observed in the lateral canthus region, presumably due to the lack of sebaceous glands in that region. Therefore, sebaceous gland density may be an important factor in wrinkle formation. A pilot study in 21 subjects showing a negative correlation between sebum excretion rate and glabellar wrinkles would seem to support this notion [39].

Finally, subdermal changes in the anatomy of the face should be considered in a discussion around the etiology of facial wrinkle formation. Subdermal fat atrophy and changes in the facial skeleton occur in a predictable fashion and most certainly affect the onset and severity of facial skin wrinkling [40, 41].

Wrinkles as a Risk Factor for Longevity and Disease

Several studies have shown associations between the severity of skin wrinkling and systemic aging as well as certain diseases. In a cross-sectional study, Gunn et al. [42] compared the amount of skin wrinkling in the offspring of exceptionally older people (>89 years) vs. partners of their offspring as age-matched controls. They then looked at the risk of cardiovascular disease (CVD) in the same groups using the Framingham CVD risk score. After adjusting for chronological age, smoking, photodamage, and BMI, the female and male offspring had significantly less skin wrinkling on the upper inner arm (a sun-protected site) compared with controls. However, there was no significant difference between offspring of long-lived individuals and age-matched controls for skin wrinkling around the eye and on the cheek (sun-exposed sites). In addition, the male offsprings looked 1.4 years younger for their age than the male controls. Since the offspring of exceptionally older people tend to have long life and health spans, having less skin wrinkling, at least on sun-protected sites, for one's age may be predictive of increased longevity. While skin wrinkling was linked to predicted longevity, skin wrinkling on the arm did not predict risk for CVD, even after controlling for smoking, photodamage, and BMI.

In a prospective study with 35 years of follow-up of 10,885 individuals from the Danish general population, prominent facial wrinkles did not associate with risk of ischemic heart disease or myocardial infarction after adjustment for potential confounders [43]. Thus, there is little evidence for an association between features of skin aging and risk of cardiovascular disease beyond the common association with increasing chronological age [44].

Michikawa et al. hypothesized that chronic sun exposure, as assessed by the severity of facial skin wrinkling, might be associated with hearing impairment through an oxidative stress mechanism. To examine this, they performed a cross-sectional analysis in a total of 805 residents (342 men and 463 women) aged 65 years or older living in Japan. Facial wrinkling was quantified by image analysis of standardized facial images. Hearing impairment was defined as a failure to hear a 30-dB signal at 1 kHz and a 40-dB signal at 4 kHz in the better ear in pure-tone audiometric tests. In men, facial wrinkle was positively associated with hearing impairment. This association was particularly pronounced in men with the low levels of antioxidants and without occupational noise exposure. No apparent association between facial wrinkling and hearing impairment was observed in women [45].

The severity of skin wrinkles in early postmenopausal women correlates with their bone density [46]. The study included 114 women in their late 40s and early 50s who had had their last menstrual period within the past three years and who were not taking hormone therapy. Women were excluded if they had had any cosmetic skin procedures. The investigators found a significant inverse correlation between the wrinkle score and bone density; this relationship was evident at all skeletal sites – hip, lumbar spine, and heel – and was independent of age, body composition, or other factors known to affect bone density [47].

Visible skin wrinkling may be a marker of lung aging. In a study of 697 elderly women, Vierkotter et al. [48] assessed skin wrinkles on a validated scoring system (SCINEXA) and airflow obstruction by spirometry (as a marker of lung aging). As lung obstruction increased, so did wrinkle severity score. The association was statistically significant and independent of smoking or air pollution. The association only occurred in carriers of the matrix metalloproteinase-1 (MMP-1) or the MMP-3 alleles; thus there may be a genetic susceptibility.

Conclusion

Facial wrinkling is one of the most important visible features of aging skin and several advancements have been made in the field of wrinkle research. While wrinkles are inevitable, the age of onset and severity of facial wrinkling is largely under each individual's control. Protecting the skin from acute and chronic sun damage and practicing regular skin care from early childhood will help preserve the skin's health and appearance and slow down the rate of wrinkling over a lifetime.

References

1. Trojahn C et al. Characterizing facial skin ageing in humans: disentangling extrinsic from intrinsic biological phenomena. BioMed Research Int. 2015.
2. Hillebrand GG, et al. New wrinkles on wrinkling: an 8-year longitudinal study on the progression of expression lines into persistent wrinkles. British J Dermatol. 2010;162(6):1233–41.
3. Miyamoto K, et al. Characterization of comprehensive appearances of skin ageing: an 11-year longitudinal study on facial skin ageing in Japanese females at Akita. J Dermatol Sci. 2011;64(3):229–36.
4. Bazin R, Lévêque JL. Longitudinal study of skin aging: from microrelief to wrinkles. Skin Res Technol. 2011;17(2):135–40.
5. Shiihara Y, et al. Microrelief suppresses large wrinkling appearance: an in silico study. Skin Res Technol. 2015;21(2):184–91.
6. Kuwazuru O, et al. Skin wrinkling morphology changes suddenly in the early 30s. Skin Res Technol. 2012;18(4):495–503.
7. Timilshina S, et al. The influence of ethnic origin on the skin photoageing: Nepalese study. Int J Cosmet Sci. 2011;33(6):553–9.
8. Luebberding S, Krueger N, Kerscher M. Quantification of age-related facial wrinkles in men and women using a three-dimensional fringe projection method and validated assessment scales. Dermatol Surg. 2014;40 (1):22–32.
9. Li X, et al. Characterization of Chinese body skin through in vivo instrument assessments, visual evaluations, and questionnaire: influences of body area, inter-generation, season, sex, and skin care habits. Skin Res Technol. 2014;20(1):14–22.
10. Tsukahara K, et al. Seasonal and annual variation in the intensity of facial wrinkles. Skin Res Technol. 2013;19 (3):279–87.
11. Tsukahara K, et al. Gender-dependent differences in degree of facial wrinkles. Skin Res Technol. 2013;19 (1):e65–71.
12. Hillebrand GG, et al. Quantitative evaluation of skin condition in an epidemiological survey of females living in northern versus southern Japan. J Dermatol Sci. 2001;27 Suppl 1:S42–52.
13. Gao Q, et al. An epidemiological survey of skin damage on the dorsal hand in rural populations in northern and southern China. J Photochem Photobiol B. 2013;120:163–70.
14. Kim EJ, et al. Effect of the regional environment on the skin properties and the early wrinkles in young Chinese women. Skin Res Technol. 2014;20(4):498–502.
15. Kimlin MG, Guo Y. Assessing the impacts of lifetime sun exposure on skin damage and skin aging using a non-invasive method. Sci Total Environ. 2012;425:35–41.
16. Ichihashi M, Ando H. The maximal cumulative solar UVB dose allowed to maintain healthy and young skin and prevent premature photoaging. Exp Dermatol. 2014;23 Suppl 1:43–6.
17. Morisaki N, et al. Neprilysin is identical to skin fibroblast elastase: its role in skin aging and UV responses. J Biol Chem. 2010;285(51):39819–27.
18. Imokawa G, Ishida K. Biological mechanisms underlying the ultraviolet radiation-induced formation of skin wrinkling and sagging I: reduced skin elasticity, highly associated with enhanced dermal elastase activity, triggers wrinkling and sagging. Int J Mol Sci. 2015;16(4):7753–75.
19. Imokawa G, Nakajima H, Ishida K. Biological mechanisms underlying the ultraviolet radiation-induced formation of skin wrinkling and sagging II: overexpression of neprilysin plays an essential role. Int J Mol Sci. 2015;16(4):7776–95.
20. Flament F, et al. Solar exposure(s) and facial clinical signs of aging in Chinese women: impacts upon age perception. Clin Cosmet Investig Dermatol. 2015;8:75–84.
21. Osborne R, Li J, Kaczvinsky J, Schnicker M, Marmor M. Chronological changes in facial wrinkles and texture in a longitudinal study. J Am Acad Dermatol. 2014;70(5):AB29.
22. Song EJ, et al. A study on seasonal variation of skin parameters in Korean males. Int J Cosmet Sci. 2015;37 (1):92–7.
23. Qiu H, et al. Influence of season on some skin properties: winter vs. summer, as experienced by 354 Shanghainese women of various ages. Int J Cosmet Sci. 2011;33(4):377–83.
24. Galzote C, et al. Characterization of facial skin of various Asian populations through visual and non-invasive instrumental evaluations: influence of seasons. Skin Res Technol. 2014;20(4):453–62.
25. Li M, et al. Epidemiological evidence that indoor air pollution from cooking with solid fuels accelerates skin

aging in Chinese women. J Dermatol Sci. 2015;79(2): 148–54.
26. Vierkotter A, et al. Airborne particle exposure and extrinsic skin aging. J Invest Dermatol. 2010;130 (12):2719–26.
27. Okada HC, et al. Facial changes caused by smoking: a comparison between smoking and nonsmoking identical twins. Plast Reconstr Surg. 2013;132(5):1085–92.
28. De Boulle K, Turkmani MG. Lateral oblique forehead lines: redefining sleeping lines and treatment with botulinum toxin A. J Cosmet Dermatol. 2013;12(2):163–7.
29. Kotlus BS. Effect of sleep position on perceived facial aging. Dermatol Surg. 2013;39(9):1360–2.
30. Fabi S, et al. The fabi-bolton chest wrinkle scale: a pilot validation study. J Cosmet Dermatol. 2012;11(3):229–34.
31. Yoo MA, et al. How much related to skin wrinkles between facial and body site? Age-related changes in skin wrinkle on the knee assessed by skin bioengineering techniques. Skin Res Technol. 2015;22(1):69–74.
32. Rawlings AV, et al. The effect of a vitamin A palmitate and antioxidant-containing oil-based moisturizer on photodamaged skin of several body sites. J Cosmet Dermatol. 2013;12(1):25–35.
33. Hyun MY, et al. Novel treatment of neck wrinkles with an intradermal radiofrequency device. Ann Dermatol. 2015;27(1):79–81.
34. Fujimura T, Hotta M. The preliminary study of the relationship between facial movements and wrinkle formation. Skin Res Technol. 2012;18(2):219–24.
35. Kligman AM, Zheng P, Lavker RM. The anatomy and pathogenesis of wrinkles. British J Dermatol. 1985;113 (1):37–42.
36. Tsukahara K, et al. Morphological study of the relationship between solar elastosis and the development of wrinkles on the forehead and lateral canthus. Arch Dermatol. 2012;148(8):913–7.
37. El-Domyati M, et al. Forehead wrinkles: a histological and immunohistochemical evaluation. J Cosmet Dermatol. 2014;13(3):188–94.
38. Tamatsu Y, et al. New finding that might explain why the skin wrinkles more on various parts of the face. Clin Anat. 2015;28(6):745–52.
39. Foolad N, et al. The association of the sebum excretion rate with melasma, erythematotelangiectatic rosacea, and rhytides. Dermatol Online J. 2015; 21(6):2.
40. Shaw Jr RB, et al. Aging of the facial skeleton: aesthetic implications and rejuvenation strategies. Plast Reconstr Surg. 2011;127(1):374–83.
41. Mendelson B, Wong CH. Changes in the facial skeleton with aging: implications and clinical applications in facial rejuvenation. Aesthetic Plast Surg. 2012;36 (4):753–60.
42. Gunn DA, et al. Facial appearance reflects human familial longevity and cardiovascular disease risk in healthy individuals. J Gerontol A Biol Sci Med Sci. 2013;68(2):145–52.
43. Christoffersen M, et al. Visible age-related signs and risk of ischemic heart disease in the general population: a prospective cohort study. Circulation. 2014;129 (9):990–8.
44. Christoffersen M, Tybjærg-Hansen A. Visible aging signs as risk markers for ischemic heart disease: epidemiology, pathogenesis and clinical implications. Ageing Res Rev. 2016;25:24–41.
45. Michikawa T, et al. Sunlight exposure may be a risk factor of hearing impairment: a community-based study in Japanese older men and women. J Gerontol A Biol Sci Med Sci. 2013;68(1):96–103.
46. Brown S. IMS updates its recommendations on HRT. Menopause Int. 2011;17(3):75.
47. Wolff E, et al. Skin wrinkles and rigidity in early postmenopausal women vary by race/ethnicity: baseline characteristics of the skin ancillary study of the KEEPS trial. Fertil Steril. 2011;95(2):658–662.e3.
48. Vierkötter A, et al. MMP-1 and −3 promoter variants are indicative of a common susceptibility for skin and lung aging: results from a cohort of elderly women (SALIA). J Invest Dermatol. 2015;135(5):1268–74.

Psoriasis and Aging

81

Paul S. Yamauchi

Contents

Abstract

Psoriasis is the most prevalent immune-mediated disorder when compared to other inflammatory conditions such as rheumatoid arthritis, Crohn's disease, multiple sclerosis, and atopic dermatitis. As the population of people who are 65 years and older in the world continues to increase, the incidence of elderly people suffering from psoriasis will also increase in a proportionate manner. The frequency of comorbidities associated with psoriasis will consequently rise as the psoriasis population continues to age. Despite new advances in the treatment of psoriasis, there is no permanent cure for psoriasis. However, the newer biological agents that are more targeted in the pathogenesis of psoriasis are very efficacious and hold great promise for safely treating elderly psoriatic patients. This article will discuss the epidemiology of psoriasis in the elderly population, the different comorbidities associated with psoriasis that occur during aging, and the various treatments that can be employed to treat psoriasis contingent on the degree of severity as well as patient characteristics.

Epidemiology, Comorbidities, and Quality of Life

While the exact incidence of psoriasis in the elderly population is not certain, psoriasis is prevalent in this age category. In a US population-based study,

P.S. Yamauchi (✉)
Dermatology Institute and Skin Care Center, Santa Monica, CA, USA

David Geffen School of School of Medicine at UCLA, Los Angeles, CA, USA
e-mail: paulyamauchi@yahoo.com

M.A. Farage et al. (eds.), *Textbook of Aging Skin*,
DOI 10.1007/978-3-662-47398-6_156

the highest rate of occurrence of psoriasis occurred in the 60- to 69-year-old age-group (113/100,000 population) [1]. Another study demonstrated that the prevalence of psoriasis was 3.9 % at a tertiary referral center comprised of 16,924 geriatric outpatients [2]. However, the prevalence of psoriasis in another study in patients 60 years of age and older was about 0.1 % (47 of 46,623 cases) [3]. The average age was 67 ± 1 years in this study ranged from 60 to 85 years with a 9:1 male-to-female ratio. The average time course of psoriasis was 25 ± 2 months and associated comorbidities were found in 27 cases (57.5 %). The most observed type of psoriasis in that study was chronic plaque psoriasis and 25.5 % of cases were classified as severe.

As the population of people aged 65 years and older continues to increase, the importance of psoriasis in the elderly is underscored by the fact that the numbers of geriatric patients with this chronic condition and the comorbidities associated with psoriasis will also continue to rise in a comparative manner [4]. Demographic studies have shown that the elderly will constitute up to 25 % of the US population by 2025 [5] and up to 34 % in Europe by 2050 [6].

One study assessed the clinical characteristics of elderly-onset psoriasis (over 60 years) compared to early onset (before 30 years and middle-age onset (between 30 and 60 years) groups [7]). The elderly-onset patients comprised 3.2 % of total patients (129 out of 4049) and showed a lower incidence of family history and the severity of the psoriasis was generally found to be milder compared with early and middle-age onset groups. The proportion of guttate type and generalized pustular psoriasis type was found to be decreased significantly, while the incidence of erythrodermic psoriasis was increased. The location of the psoriasis varied by age-group with the rate of scalp increased in the elderly group but plaque psoriasis on the extensor surfaces of the extremities and the trunk was decreased significantly. There was no significant difference in the degree of pruritus on psoriatic lesions and nail involvement between the three age-groups.

Psoriasis is not simply a chronic skin disease but a condition that is associated with major comorbidities [8]. These include psoriatic arthritis (PsA), cardiovascular disease, metabolic syndrome, lymphomas, malignancies, and depression. PsA occurs in 30 % of patients with psoriasis and tends to occur 10 years after the initiation of the skin symptoms [9]. The onset of PsA typically ranges between the ages of 32 and 60 years, and therefore there is a higher incidence of PsA in the elderly [10]. In a US population-based study, the prevalence of PsA in patients who were older than 65 years was 20 years [11].

Metabolic syndrome has clearly been associated with psoriasis and is defined as the presence of three of the following components: abdominal obesity, insulin-resistant diabetes, decreased HDL cholesterol, hypertriglyceridemia, and hypertension [8, 12, 13]. Psoriasis has been shown to be associated with metabolic syndrome in the elderly, and those patients tend to have had a longer disease duration than those without metabolic syndrome [14]. Patients who develop severe psoriasis at a younger age in their 20s may be at increased risk for the development of multiple cardiovascular risk factors and myocardial infarctions [15, 16]. A European study evaluated the epidemiology and associated comorbidities of 2210 adults with psoriasis with focus on the elderly patients greater than 70 years of age and in patients with very late-onset psoriasis after the age of 70 [17]. The epidemiological and clinical features of early- and late-onset psoriasis with an emphasis on potential outcomes in the comorbidities were evaluated. Out of the total of 2210 adults, 212 (9.5 %) patients were elderly with a higher frequency of females, a later onset of the disease, a lower frequency of family history of psoriasis, but a higher incidence of guttate and inverse psoriasis. Hypertension, diabetes, dyslipidemia, and major cardiovascular events were higher in the elderly group, but not tobacco usage. Fifty eight (2.7 %) patients had late-onset psoriasis which occurred more frequently in women and older. Patients with psoriasis are also at higher risk of developing arrhythmia, particularly if psoriatic arthritis is present that is independent of cardiovascular risk factors [18].

An observational, multicenter study demonstrated there was an increased prevalence of family history of psoriasis, psoriatic arthritis, and depression in patients with early-onset psoriasis

[19]. Conversely, late onset of psoriasis was more frequently associated with obesity and elevated waist circumference compared with the early-onset form. Elderly patients over the age of 75 years with late-onset psoriasis were shown to be at high risk for obesity compared with individuals at the same age with an early-onset disease. The late onset in developing psoriasis may suggest that obesity is an acquired comorbidity that may be a predisposition for the development of psoriasis in the elderly population.

Several case–control studies have demonstrated an increased prevalence of nonalcoholic steatohepatitis in patients with psoriasis, which may be of relevance in the proper selection of a systemic agent [20]. A large prospective population-based cohort study compared the incidence of nonalcoholic steatohepatitis which was diagnosed by ultrasonography in patients with psoriasis versus those without psoriasis [20]. A total of 2292 participants with a mean age 76.2 years were included. Of those, over half were women, the mean body mass index was 27.4, and 118 of the subjects (5.1 %) had psoriasis. The prevalence of nonalcoholic steatohepatitis was 46.2 % in patients with psoriasis compared to 33.3 % of the control group without psoriasis. After adjustment for alcohol consumption, cigarette smoking, and metabolic syndrome, psoriasis remained a significant predictor of nonalcoholic steatohepatitis. The elderly population suffering from psoriasis was 70 % more likely to develop nonalcoholic steatohepatitis than those without psoriasis.

It has clearly been established that patients suffering from psoriasis have lower quality-of-life indices compared to the general population [21, 22]. Psoriasis exhibits higher burdens both physically and mentally when compared to other major medical conditions including cancer, hypertension, arthritis, depression, diabetes, and cardiovascular disease [23]. A cross-sectional study on 305 psoriatic inpatients where the mean age was 71 years was compared based on clinical and social demographic determinants [24]. Psychological distress was higher in psoriatic patients greater than 70 years of age. It is important for health care providers to be cognizant of the specific impact of psoriasis in the elderly group versus the younger-aged patients.

Therapeutic Approaches to Treating Psoriasis in the Elderly

The choice of the various therapeutic options for psoriasis in the elderly is based on the severity of the psoriasis, symptoms such as itching and burning that reduces the quality of their life, prior therapies, and the level to which the appearance of the psoriasis bothers the patient [25]. Drug interactions must be carefully taken into account since elderly patients can be on multiple medications that can potentially interact with systemic agents used to treat psoriasis. In addition, serious medical conditions such as cancer, chronic infections, diabetes, and others may be a contraindication to systemic and biological agents if they are contemplated to treat more severe psoriasis.

Topical agents are frequently prescribed for elderly patients as first-line therapy due to their nonsystemic nature [26]. Because the application of topical agents can be cumbersome, especially in difficult-to-reach areas as well as larger-body-surface areas, compliance may be reduced, especially if the elderly patient requires assistance [27]. The only data for elderly patients with psoriasis are for the topical application of a calcipotriol/betamethasone dipropionate combination product that was found to be effective irrespective of age [27]. Although topical corticosteroids remain widely used for the treatment of psoriasis, the elderly population may be at higher risk of steroid-induced adverse events including atrophy, purpura, telangiectasia, secondary skin infections, rebound phenomenon, and tachyphylaxis [28].

Phototherapy is an appropriate treatment for elderly patients with psoriasis because of its minimally invasive nature (NPF). However, logistical considerations should be taken into account when recommending phototherapy to elderly patients such as the availability of transportation to the phototherapy unit two to three times per week and ensuring that the patient is able to stand adequately during the session without any physical consequence. In addition, any concomitant medications when recommending phototherapy need to be verified to avoid drug-induced photosensitivity, especially in the elderly who might be on a variety of medications.

Traditional systemic agents including methotrexate may be effective to treat psoriasis in the elderly. However, the usage of methotrexate must be carefully considered in the elderly. The dose of methotrexate needed to control severe psoriasis in patients older than 50 years may need to be decreased compared to younger patients due to a reduction of creatinine clearance that is correlated with advanced aging [29]. The clearance of total methotrexate is inversely proportional to age in patients with rheumatoid arthritis and methotrexate clearance due to decreased renal function [30]. Although acute myelosuppression is relatively uncommon with methotrexate, rare deaths may occur as a result. Myelosuppression with methotrexate occurs more commonly in the elderly and diligent monitoring of the complete blood is essential [31]. Although drug interactions are not common with methotrexate; the coadministration of trimethoprim with methotrexate is contraindicated irrespective of age due to a potential serious adverse event of myelosuppression. Care may need to be exercised when nonsteroidal anti-inflammatory agents are prescribed to elderly patients who are on methotrexate due to potential decreased renal clearance [32]. In a retrospective study of 7615 patients with psoriasis and 6707 patients with rheumatoid arthritis, patients given methotrexate had a significantly reduced risk of vascular disease compared with those not given methotrexate after adjusting for age, sex, comorbidities, and other medications [32]. Reduction in vascular disease also was observed among patients who took low to moderate cumulative doses of methotrexate [32].

Although there are no specific outcome studies on the use of oral retinoids such as acitretin to treat psoriasis in the elderly, the risk of elevated triglycerides should be considered but the risk may be acceptable since elevated lipid levels can generally be successfully treated [26]. As the cardiovascular risk of hyperlipidemia generally takes several years to progress, the risk of acitretin-induced hyperlipidemia may be less significant in elderly patients with psoriasis. Xerosis and hair loss are also side effects exhibited by acitretin that the elderly population may not tolerate very well.

Cyclosporine may be warranted in the elderly population for severe flare-ups of psoriasis or the development of erythrodermic or pustular psoriasis. However, because cyclosporine is a powerful immunosuppressant that can induce hypertension, nephrotoxicity, and interacts with several medications, great caution should be exercised in prescribing this medication to elderly patients with psoriasis. The glomerular filtration rate should be measured at baseline before the initiation of cyclosporine [26].

The utilization of biologic agents has revolutionized the treatment of psoriasis and psoriatic arthritis. Their high degree of efficacy, maintenance of response, and long-term safety through selective immunomodulation has made biologics one of the mainstays of therapy. There are a few reports in the literature describing the efficacy and safety of biologic agents specifically in the elderly population.

The safety and efficacy of biological agents as well as oral systemic agents were evaluated in 187 consecutive psoriatic patients greater than 65 years of age [33]. At week 12 of therapy, the Psoriasis Area and Severity Index (PASI) 75 response was achieved by 49 %, 27 %, 46 %, and 31 % of patients who received methotrexate, acitretin, cyclosporine, or PUVA, and 64.1 %, 64.7 %, 93.3 %, 57.1 %, and 100 % of patients who received etanercept, adalimumab, infliximab, and ustekinumab. The rate of adverse events was 0.12, 0.32, 1.4, and 0.5 per patient-year in the methotrexate, acitretin, cyclosporine, and PUVA groups and 0.11, 0.35, 0.19, 0.3, and 0.26 in the etanercept, adalimumab, infliximab, and ustekinumab groups. In this study, the traditional oral systemic agents were less effective than biologics in the elderly population and etanercept was associated with a lower rate of adverse events when compared to other treatments.

A retrospective study was conducted to evaluate the long-term efficacy and safety profile of antitumor necrosis factor (anti-TNF) agents in elderly psoriatic patients [34]. This study included 89 patients aged 65 years and greater with psoriasis and psoriatic arthritis treated with etanercept or adalimumab as monotherapy. The proportion of patients attaining a PASI 50 response was 91.8 and 82.1 % at week 156 with etanercept and adalimumab treatment respectively. The proportion of patients achieving PASI 75 response was 83.6 and 71.4 % at week 156 with etanercept and adalimumab, respectively. The overall safety profile and adherence to treatment was good in this study and long-term treatment with anti-TNF agents was appropriate in the management of psoriasis in the elderly population.

A post hoc analysis of two large phase III randomized placebo trials of etanercept was performed to analyze the effect of etanercept on PASI 50, PASI 75, and Dermatology Life Quality Index (DLQI) in the geriatric and nongeriatric populations [35]. There were no statistically significant differences between the elderly and young with regard to the number of patients attaining a PASI 50 or PASI 75 response with any of the conventional dosing regimens. The baseline DLQI scores were not statistically significant between both groups; the change in DLQI with etanercept was similar in both populations.

A retrospective study evaluated the efficacy and safety profile of ustekinumab for 1 year in elderly patients with psoriasis [36]. The study included 24 psoriatic patients aged over 65 years with a mean of 73.1 years with moderate to severe plaque psoriasis. PASI 75 responses were 56.5 % at week 16, 59.1 % at week 28, and 60.0 % at week 52. None of the patients developed any serious infection during the 1-year treatment. The mean DLQI score at weeks 0, 16, 28, and 52 was 7.8, 2.5, 1.4, and 1.2, respectively. Ustekinumab demonstrated sufficient efficacy for elderly patients with psoriasis without any serious infection over the 1-year treatment.

In general, biologic agents may be associated with a small but significant overall risk of infections. Despite the labeling of these agents to exercise caution when administering these agents to the geriatric population due to higher baseline risk of infections in this population, there is no conclusive evidence that the relative risk of infection with biologic agents increases with age. Current recommendations are to avoid coadministration of live vaccines with biologic agents and to avoid usage of biologic agents during major surgery. Because the elderly population are more apt to receive live vaccines such as zoster or to undergo major surgery such as orthopedic joint replacement or open heart surgery, the timing of the administration of biologic agents needs to be carefully calculated and considered.

Conclusion

The goals of managing psoriasis in the elderly should be no different than treating the younger population. Attaining best possible clearance and improving the quality of life in a safe, efficient, and cost-effective manner are the fundamental objectives. There are a few nuances between the elderly and the young who have psoriasis. The elderly may be more prone to infections, have higher occurrences of malignancies, are on more concomitant medications, undergo major surgeries due to aging, and receive live vaccine such as zoster after the age of 50. These differences must be considered when managing elderly patients, particularly when considering an oral systemic agent or a biologic. Fortunately, the limited data in the published literature seems to suggest the differences may not seem as significant as previously thought.

References

1. Bell LM, Sedlack R, Beard CM, Perry HO, Michet CJ, Kurland LT. Incidence of psoriasis in Rochester, Minn, 1980–1983. Arch Dermatol. 1991;127:1184–7.
2. Liao YH, Chen KH, Tseng MP, Sun CC. Pattern of skin diseases in a geriatric patient groupin Taiwan: a 7-year survey from the outpatient clinic of a university medical center. Dermatology. 2001;203:308–13.
3. Kassi K, Djeha D, Gbery IP, Kouame K, Sangaré A. Psoriasis in elderly patients in the Côte d'Ivoire: socio-demographic, clinical, and therapeutic aspects, and follow-up. Int J Dermatol. 2016;55(2):e83–6.
4. Smith ES, Fleischer Jr AB, Feldman SR. Demographics of aging and skin disease. Clin Geriatr Med. 2001;17:631–41.
5. Projected resident population of the United States as of July 1, 2025, middle series. Population projections program, population division, US Census Bureau, Washington, DC. 20233; 2002.
6. Eurostat. Regional population ageing of the EU at different speeds up to 2025, Statistics in focus. Eurostat. 1999;1999:1–8.
7. Kwon HH, Kwon IH, Youn JI. Clinical study of psoriasis occurring over the age of 60 years: is elderly-onset psoriasis a distinct subtype? Int J Dermatol. 2012;51(1):53–8.
8. Gottlieb AB, Dann F. Comorbidities in patients with psoriasis. Am J Med. 2009;122(1150):e1–9.
9. Gottlieb A, Korman NJ, Gordon KB, Feldman SR, Lebwohl M, Koo JY, et al. Guidelines of care for the management of psoriasis and psoriatic arthritis: section 2. Psoriatic arthritis: overview and guidelines of care

for treatment with an emphasis on the biologics. J Am Acad Dermatol. 2008;58:851–64.
10. Gladman DD, Antoni C, Mease P, Clegg DO, Nash P. Psoriatic arthritis: epidemiology, clinical features, course, and outcome. Ann Rheum Dis. 2005;64(Suppl):ii14–7.
11. Gelfand JM, Gladman DD, Mease PJ, Smith N, Margolis DJ, Nijsten T, et al. Epidemiology of psoriatic arthritis in the population of the United States. J Am Acad Dermatol. 2005;53:573–7.
12. Kimball AB, Gladman D, Gelfand JF, Gordon K, Horn EJ, Korman NJ, et al. National Psoriasis Foundation: clinical consensus on psoriasis comorbidities and recommendations for screening. J Am Acad Dermatol. 2008;58:1031–42.
13. Cohen AD, Gilutz H, Henkin Y, Zahger D, Shapiro J, Bonneh DY, et al. Psoriasis and the metabolic syndrome. Acta Derm Venereol. 2007;87:506–9.
14. Gisondi P, Tessari G, Conti A, Piaserico S, Schianchi S, Peserico A, et al. Prevalence of metabolic syndrome in patients with psoriasis: a hospital-based case–control study. Br J Dermatol. 2007;157:68–73.
15. Neimann A, Shin DB, Wang X, Margolis DJ, Troxel AB, Gelfand JM. Prevalence of cardiovascular risk factor in patients with psoriasis. J Am Acad Dermatol. 2006;55:829–35.
16. Gelfand JM, Neimann AL, Shin DB, Wang X, Margolis DJ, Troxel AB. Risk of myocardial infarction in patients with psoriasis. JAMA. 2006;296(14):1735–41.
17. Phan C, Sigal ML, Estève E, Reguiai Z, Barthélémy H, Beneton N, Maccari F, Lahfa M, Thomas-Beaulieu D, Le Guyadec T, Vermersch-Langlin A, Mery-Bossard L, Pallure V, Kemula M, Labeille B, Beauchet A, Mahé E, GEM RESOPSO. Psoriasis in the elderly: epidemiological and clinical aspects, and evaluation of patients with very late onset psoriasis. J Eur Acad Dermatol Venereol. 2016;30(1):78–82.
18. Chiu HY, Chang WL, Huang WF, Wen YW, Tsai YW, Tsai TF. Increased risk of arrhythmia in patients with psoriatic disease: a nationwide population-based matched cohort study. J Am Acad Dermatol. 2015;73(3):429–38.
19. Herédi E, Csordás A, Clemens M, Adám B, Gáspár K, Törőcsik D, Nagy G, Adány R, Gaál J, Remenyik E, Szegedi A. The prevalence of obesity is increased in patients with late compared with early onset psoriasis. Ann Epidemiol. 2013;23(11):688–92.
20. van der Voort EA, Koehler EM, Dowlatshahi EA, Hofman A, Stricker BH, Janssen HL, Schouten JN, Nijsten T. Psoriasis is independently associated with nonalcoholic fatty liver disease in patients 55 years old or older: results from a population-based study. J Am Acad Dermatol. 2014;70(3):517–24.
21. Finlay AY, Coles EC. The effect of severe psoriasis on the quality of life of 369 patients. Br J Dermatol. 1995;132:236–44.
22. Fortune DG, Main CJ, O'Sullivan TM, Griffiths CE. Quality of life in patients with psoriasis: the contribution of clinical variables and psoriasis-specific stress. Br J Dermatol. 1997;137:755–60.
23. Rapp SR, Feldman SR, Exum ML, Fleischer Jr AB, Reboussin DM. Psoriasis causes as much disability as other major medical diseases. J Am Acad Dermatol. 1999;41:401–7.
24. Sampogna F, Tabolli S, Mastroeni S, Di Pietro C, Fortes C, Abeni D, Italian Multipurpose Psoriasis Research on Vital Experiences (IMPROVE) Study Group. Quality of life impairment and psychological distress in elderly patients with psoriasis. Dermatology. 2007;215(4):341–7.
25. Bonifati C, Carducci M, Mussi A, D'Auria L, Ameglio F. Recognition and treatment of psoriasis: special considerations in elderly patients. Drugs Aging. 1998;12:177–90.
26. Grozdev IS, Van Voorhees AS, Gottlieb AB, Hsu S, Lebwohl MG, Bebo Jr BF, Korman NJ, National Psoriasis Foundation. Psoriasis in the elderly: from the Medical Board of the National Psoriasis Foundation. J Am Acad Dermatol. 2011;65(3):537–45.
27. Parslew R, Trauslen J. Efficacy and local safety of a calcipotriol/betamethasone dipropionate ointment in elderly patients with psoriasis vulgaris. Eur J Dermatol. 2005;15:37–9.
28. Coskey RJ. Adverse effects of corticosteroids, I: topical and intralesional. Clin Dermatol. 1986;4:155–60.
29. Dawn AG, Dawn ME, Yosipovich G. Psoriasis in the elderly. Aging Health. 2007;3:611–23.
30. Collins P, Rogers S. The efficacy of methotrexate in psoriasis – a review of 40 cases. Clin Exp Dermatol. 1992;17:257–60.
31. Boffa M, Chalmers R. Methotrexate for psoriasis. Clin Exp Dermatol. 1996;21:399–408.
32. Ranganath VK, Furst DE. Disease-modifying antirheumatic drug use in elderly rheumatoid patients. Rheum Dis Clin North Am. 2007;33:197–217.
33. Piaserico S, Conti A, Lo Console F, De Simone C, Prestinari F, Mazzotta A, Gualdi G, Guarneri C, Borsari S, Cassano N. Efficacy and safety of systemic treatments for psoriasis in elderly patients. Acta Derm Venereol. 2014;94(3):293–7.
34. Esposito M, Giunta A, Mazzotta A, Zangrilli A, Babino G, Bavetta M, Perricone R, Chimenti S, Chimenti MS. Efficacy and safety of subcutaneous anti-tumor necrosis factor- alpha agents, etanercept and adalimumab, in elderly patients affected by psoriasis and psoriatic arthritis: an observational long-term study. Dermatology. 2012;225(4):312–9.
35. Militello G, Xia A, Stevens SR, Van Voorhees AS. Etanercept for the treatment of psoriasis in the elderly. J Am Acad Dermatol. 2006;55(3):517–9.
36. Hayashi M, Umezawa Y, Fukuchi O, Ito T, Saeki H, Nakagawa H. Efficacy and safety of ustekinumab treatment in elderly patients with psoriasis. J Dermatol. 2014;41(11):974–80.

Skin Aging and Cellulite in Women

82

Márcio Lorencini, Fernanda Camozzato, and Doris Hexsel

Contents

M. Lorencini (✉)
R&D Department, Grupo Boticário, São José dos Pinhais, PR, Brazil
e-mail: marciolo@grupoboticario.com.br; marciolorencini@yahoo.com.br

F. Camozzato
Department of Dermatology, Brazilian Center for Studies in Dermatology, Porto Alegre, RS, Brazil
e-mail: fecamozzato@yahoo.com.br

D. Hexsel
Department of Dermatology, Brazilian Center for Studies in Dermatology, Porto Alegre, RS, Brazil

Department of Dermatology, Pontifícia Universidade Católica do Rio Grande do Sul (PUC-RS), Porto Alegre, RS, Brazil
e-mail: doris@hexsel.com.br

M.A. Farage et al. (eds.), *Textbook of Aging Skin*,
DOI 10.1007/978-3-662-47398-6_160

Abstract

Skin aging is characterized by cumulative molecular and morphological changes that trigger clinical alterations with significant health and aesthetic implications. Disorganization of the original connective tissue architecture in the dermis and subcutaneous compartments is a hallmark of aging and potentially contributes to the appearance of different skin disorders. Cellulite is a distressing condition that originates from changes in the biomechanical and density properties of the cutaneous connective tissue, which affect the skin surface topography. The limited studies that have directly addressed the relationship between cellulite development and skin aging indicate they are potentially correlated. Cellulite tends to worsen with age, and laxity is one of the major skin aggravating factors that may be considered in the efficient diagnosis, treatment, and prevention of this condition.

Introduction

Skin is an exposed organ in which the signs of the aging process become apparent, and it therefore reflects the health and well-being of the individual, as well as numerous aesthetic features [1]. Skin imperfections may result in significant psychosocial issues with a negative influence on self-esteem and considerable emotional distress [2].

Cellulite is characterized by alterations in the skin surface and affects approximately 80–90 % of postpubertal women [3]. It can be a distressing aesthetic condition that may interfere with an individual's quality of life [4]. Among the major age-related changes, those involving alterations in the biomechanical and density properties of the connective tissue have been suggested to play a central role in cellulite development [5, 6].

Considering the multifactorial causes of cellulite and the emergence of new dermatological approaches for the treatment of skin aging, this chapter proposes an overview of these two convergent and potentially interdependent biological processes. An understanding of these processes may represent the key for the development of novel, effective therapeutic opportunities.

Aging-Related Changes in the Fibrous Structure of Skin

As a highly complex biological process that involves cumulative deterioration, aging impairs homeostasis in different tissues and organs over a lifetime [7]. All body parts are subjected to gradual aging, and the skin comprises a marker of this inevitable system. In the process of skin aging, intrinsic and extrinsic factors act synergistically and produce cumulative effects. Intrinsic factors are related to the chronological aging process of the organism and are primarily determined by an individual's genetics, whereas extrinsic factors refer to external components that may contribute to or accelerate natural aging [8]. Aged skin presents several modifications in the architecture of its original layers, which clinically correspond to a more fragile, thinner, relatively flattened, dry, unblemished, hyperdistended, and loose structure. These signs may be even more pronounced in specific areas, including sun-exposed parts of the body, or in individuals with exposure to higher levels of ultraviolet (UV) radiation or other extrinsic factors, such as smoking, pollution, stress, and specific chemicals [6, 9].

Numerous studies have focused on the analysis of skin morphological changes with age, and the majority of these changes are correlated with connective tissue damage in the dermis (Fig. 1). The fibrous structure, which comprises the dermal extracellular matrix, typically represents the most compromised part of this process, with a traditional hallmark of collagen and elastic fiber degeneration [10]. A recent study evaluated 121 skin samples from individuals of different ages (between 2 and 85 years) and observed that as the process of aging advances, both collagen and elastic fibers change their aspect and organization. In the first stage, the thinnest fibers present in the more superficial dermis undergo fragmentation and lysis, whereas they tend to progressively thicken in the deep dermis, which appears

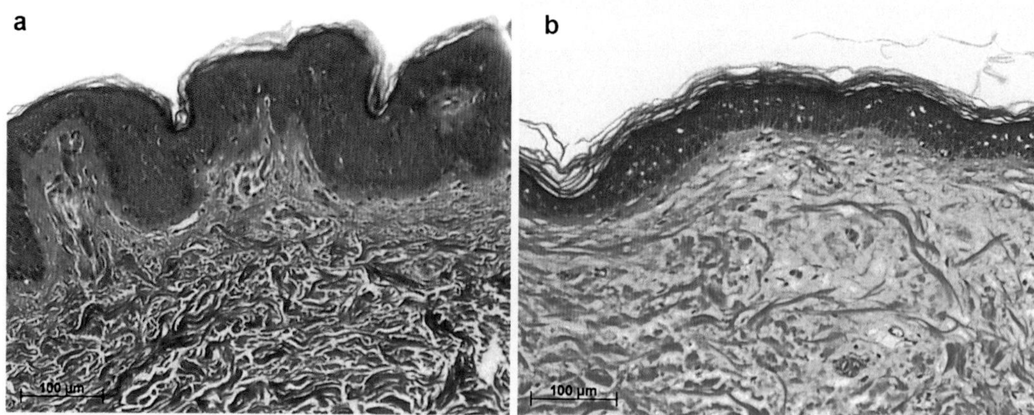

Fig. 1 Aging-related skin morphological changes between a young skin sample from a 30-year-old donor (**a**) and an aged skin sample from a 60-year-old donor (**b**). Masson-Trichrome staining for the evaluation of fibrous architecture

to be a compensatory mechanism to recover the skin resistance that becomes weaker at the surface. This process should start in parallel for distinct types of fibers; however, it occurs faster with elastic ones [11]. In addition to fiber fragmentation, a reduction in total collagen and decreased cell-collagen fiber interactions also characterize chronologically aged skin [12]. Using the innovative and quantitative methodology based on the technique of multiphoton microscopy, Wu et al. [13] demonstrated that collagen exhibits a denser matrix, and the bundles are substantially tighter in younger skin. Moreover, type I collagen fibers have been reported to change their original orientation in aged skin dermis, and the proportion between type I and type III collagen fibers tend to increase in old skin tissues [10, 14].

In addition to the reduced levels of functional collagen and elastin fibers, a reduced number of fibroblasts, which can be accompanied by impaired biological activity, are present in aged dermis. It contributes to the general atrophy of the extracellular matrix primarily because of decreased protein synthesis, which affects type I and III collagen, and increased protein breakdown through the upregulation of enzymes, such as matrix metalloproteinases (MMP) [15]. Thus, a failure to replace damaged collagen with newly synthesized material is also critical to the overall physiology of aging. According to Varani et al. [12], the reduced collagen synthesis in aged skin reflects at least two different underlying mechanisms: cellular fibroblast aging and a lower level of mechanical stimulation. The complexity of aging cannot be reduced to a single process; however, it helps to explain the cumulative effect of aging in the skin. The mechanical structure is compromised by fiber disorganization; thus, fibroblasts are less stimulated to produce new fibers, and a cyclical negative feedback regulation is initiated. It has also been demonstrated that there is a strong correlation between skin collagen loss and estrogen deficiency as a result of menopause, which reinforces the importance of hormonal regulation in skin physiology [16].

Among different molecular theories, some authors support the importance of oxidative stress in the skin aging process and suggest that it may result from a lifetime accumulation of cellular oxidative damage caused by excessive reactive oxygen species (ROS). Although the skin possesses extremely efficient antioxidant activities, ROS levels increase and antioxidant activities decrease with aging, which thereby upregulates MMP expression and provides a plausible mechanism for the increased collagen degradation in aged human skin [15]. ROS may originate from processes such as cell respiration or exogenous agents, such as UV radiation; as a consequence, aged skin exhibits increasing levels of oxidized proteins that become inactive and/or accumulate inside cells [1]. Naturally, the low turnover rate of structural skin proteins makes them more susceptible to the occurrence of cumulative damage. Glycation, the spontaneous chemical reaction of reducing sugars with proteins, is an example of the posttranslational modification involved in the formation of pathological and stable cross-links that affect collagen and elastin fibers with aging [17]. According to Danoux et al. [18], glycation can be linked to oxidative stress in a process that is referred to as glycoxidation, in which the effects potentiate the impairment of proteins and, thus, the age-related stiffening of skin.

Besides the dermis, subcutaneous tissue should also be regarded when discussing skin aging. Located immediately beneath the dermis, it acts as a mattress that provides mechanical protection against trauma and helps to define body contours. Subcutaneous tissue contains cells responsible for fat production and storage, referred to as adipocytes, and represents the connection between the reticular dermis and the deep fascia; it is organized into three layers, including the apical, mantle, and deep compartments, and subdivided into fat sections [19]. Each fat section is filled with fat lobules and defined by a fibrous membrane or fibrous septum, which consists of the intersecting collagenous sheets of fibrous tissue and connects the dermis to fascia, as well as stabilizes the subcutaneous tissue [20] (Fig. 2). Larger blood and lymphatic vessels and sensory nerves follow the fibrous septa [19]. The subcutaneous compartment comprises approximately 85 % of total body fat, and the distribution changes significantly over a lifetime, particularly in the lower body; it also varies among

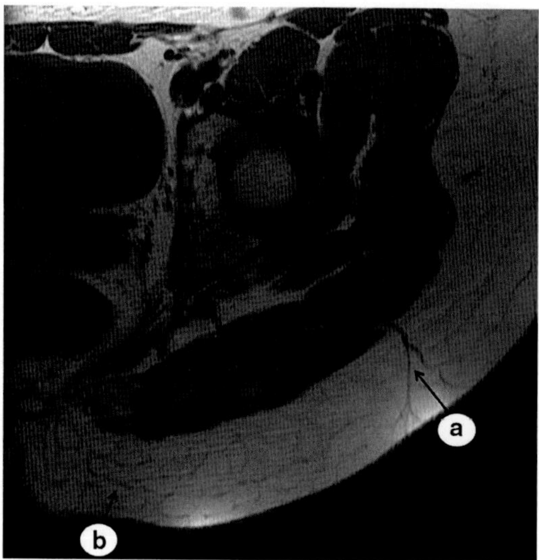

Fig. 2 Magnetic resonance images showing ramified fibrous septum (**a**) and subcutaneous fat lobules (**b**)

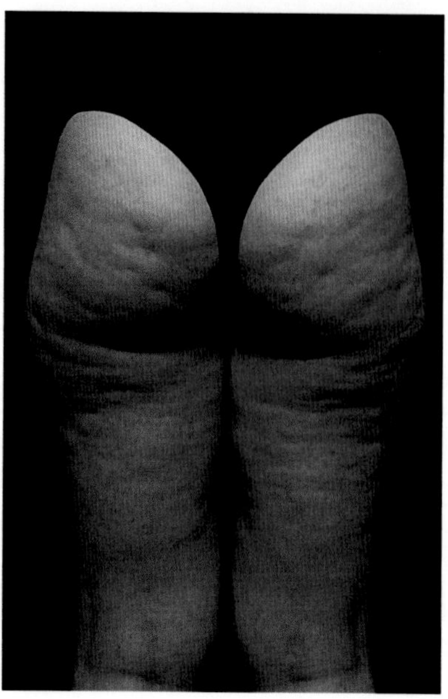

Fig. 3 Typical depressed lesions in areas commonly affected by cellulite. The patient also presents flaccidity, which determines the linear aspect of lesions

races, ethnicities, and sex [21, 22]. According to Kim et al. [22], aging influences both adipocyte number and cell size, and various environmental stimuli that promote skin inflammation, such as UV radiation, heat, or air pollutants, may also affect subcutaneous fat metabolism and accumulation in exposed skin. Aging results in a progressive inability of the human body to maintain an adequate subcutaneous adipose tissue mass, which ultimately may contribute to the development of serious health problems, such as dyslipidemia, insulin resistance, and metabolic syndrome [23]. Certain movements for long periods, such as sitting or reclining, may seriously affect lymphatic drainage and lead to increased fat deposits in certain body regions, such as the female thigh. Additionally, a high concentration of harmful secondary metabolic products can be observed in the interstice that promotes fibrosis and alters properties of the subcutaneous tissue, which gradually hardens with aging [24].

Cellulite

Cellulite is characterized by relief alterations of the skin surface, which have been frequently described as an orange peel, mattress-like, or cottage cheese appearance [25, 26] (Fig. 3). The typical cutaneous surface alterations present in cellulite include raised and depressed lesions, whose number may vary from one to many and shape can be round, oval, or linear. Cellulite is typically present in the lower portion of the buttocks and the upper thigh; however, other areas of the body, such as the abdomen, arms, and back, may also be affected [27].

While the pathophysiology of cellulite is not fully elucidated, several hypotheses have been proposed, including structural, architectural, metabolic, and biochemical alterations; adipose tissue distribution in different parts of the body; tissue vascularity and postinflammatory changes; and effects of body mass index, hormonal, and genetic influences [28–30]. It has been proposed that the cellulite process is initiated with deterioration of the dermal vasculature accompanied by the deposition of glycosaminoglycans in the dermal capillary walls. This phenomenon may cause fluid retention in the dermis, adipocytes, and interlobular septa, which leads to the formation of edema, vascular compression, hypoxia, capillary neoformation, and microhemorrhages [31, 32].

However, there is no consensus regarding the occurrence of these findings in all patients affected with cellulite [33–35]. Inflammation has also been theorized as a potential factor in cellulite pathophysiology [36, 37]. By evaluating cellulite biopsies, Kligman [38] reported the presence of macrophages and lymphocytes in the fibrous septa, which may be the cause of inflammation that results in dermal atrophy, whereas other authors have not identified evidence of inflammation in patients with cellulite [25, 34, 35]. Therefore, it remains controversial whether localized tissue vascularity or inflammation plays a major role in the etiology of cellulite.

Anatomical changes in skin with cellulite result from alterations in the connective tissues in the dermal and subcutaneous compartments [39]. Piérard et al. [34] reported how the spontaneous appearance of dimples is associated with the presence of thin, or even absent, connective tissue in dermo-panniculosis deformans. Mirrashed [37] utilized magnetic resonance imaging (MRI) to demonstrate that women with a major presence of cellulite have weaker and less dense connective tissue. Using the same technology, Hexsel et al. [40] evaluated the subcutaneous tissue structure in areas with and without (control) cellulite on the buttocks of the same subjects and demonstrated that (1) fibrous septa perpendicular to the skin surface were visualized in 96.7 % of the cellulite-affected areas compared with only 16.7 % of the control areas assessed; (2) 73.3 % of septa were ramified in cellulite and 10 % in the control areas; (3) fibrous septa were approximately eight times thicker in areas with cellulite depressions; (4) high-intensity signals on T2 images, which suggest the presence of vascular or lymphatic liquid within the septa, were identified in 70 % of areas with cellulite and 10 % of control areas; and (5) the sensitivity and specificity of fibrous septa were 96.7 % and 83.3 %, respectively, for the diagnosis of cellulite areas.

There is an important difference in the subcutaneous organization between genders, which may indicate why cellulite typically occurs in women. This differentiation occurs by the ninth month of pregnancy and is related to the action of androgens and their effects on fibroblast activity [41]. Nürnberger and Müller [33] reported that fibrous septa are perpendicular to the skin surface in the female subcutaneous tissue, which forms rectangular compartments with protrusions that constitute the papillae adiposae. Under pressure originated from excess weight, water retention, or a sedentary lifestyle, papillae extrude into the dermis interface, which thus imitates the appearance of the skin surface in the so-called mattress phenomenon, a major sign of cellulite in women. In contrast, fibrous septa adopt an oblique zigzag pattern in men, which creates smaller and polygonal compartments that do not favor the development of a womanlike pattern of cellulite; it only occurs in androgen-deficient individuals [33]. Using three-dimensional images, Querleux et al. [35] described in detail the subcutaneous tissue architecture and identified three types of septa, including parallel, perpendicular, and oriented at 45° to the skin surface; these authors also demonstrated that the model originally proposed by Nürnberger and Müller [33] constituted an oversimplification. Moreover, they determined that women with cellulite have a higher percentage of perpendicular fibrous septa compared with women or men without cellulite. By comparing the subcutaneous tissue organization between genders with MRI, Mirrashed [37] demonstrated that (1) men presented thinner adipose tissue, thicker topmost layers, and thicker fibrous septa arranged in oblique planes and smaller capsules; (2) women presented a more radial pattern for septa distribution and larger fat lobules, with their invaginations correlated with the degree of cellulite; and (3) the percentage of adipose tissue relative to connective tissue was similar in men and women with little cellulite.

Although cellulite can affect individuals regardless of their body mass index (BMI), recent studies have demonstrated a correlation between these two factors. Hexsel et al. [42] determined that a higher BMI was associated with more severe cellulite. Smalls et al. [43–45] demonstrated that weight loss decreased the fat percentage and diameter of the thighs but increased the skin laxity, which led to the following consequences: (1) weight loss reduced cellulite severity in patients who initially exhibited higher BMI values and greater cellulite severity; (2) in other patients, weight loss was accompanied by increased cellulite severity induced by a more pronounced skin laxity; and (3) the dimple depth did not necessarily change with weight loss, which may represent a permanent pattern of the structure itself.

Laxity as a Link Between Cellulite and Skin Aging

Despite limited evidence regarding the effects of skin aging on cellulite, some authors state that cellulite visibly worsens with age and is also directly associated with modifications in the skin structure that occur throughout a lifetime [5, 33, 41]. Ortonne et al. [5] reported a premature alteration of retractability and elasticity parameters in the skin of women with cellulite, which indicated that they presented earlier cutaneous aging characteristics compared with a control population (without cellulite). Moreover, the authors demonstrated the existence of two different populations of women according to the grade of cellulite and age: (1) the under 30 age with large dimpled surfaces and normal biomechanical and echogenicity properties and (2) the over 30 age with smaller and numerous dimpled surfaces and altered dermis. Without defining a cause or consequence relationship, they suggested a clear correlation between cellulite and skin aging. The studies of Nürnberger and Müller [33, 41] supported the importance of connective tissue degeneration in the dermis and subcutaneous tissue as part of the normal aging process, which clinically results in flaccidity or loose skin and affects cellulite evolution. Hexsel et al. [40] demonstrated that older patients had higher overall cellulite severity scores, which indicates deeper depressed lesions and more severe raised lesions.

One of the major aging-related aggravating factors in cellulite appears to be skin laxity or flaccidity, which frequently occurs in body regions in which the skin is thinner with potentially less retentive capacity over fat, such as the buttocks, the thighs, the region above the knee, and the inner surface of the arms [27]. Gravity increases the effects of fat on the skin, which increases the laxity and worsens the alterations in the skin surface [27] (Fig. 4a). Together with chronological aging, reduced elasticity caused by UV radiation can aggravate skin laxity, as well as the sudden loss of weight or the diminution in subcutaneous fat as a result of liposuction [46]. Dobke et al. [47] reported that women without cellulite had better skin quality and less laxity

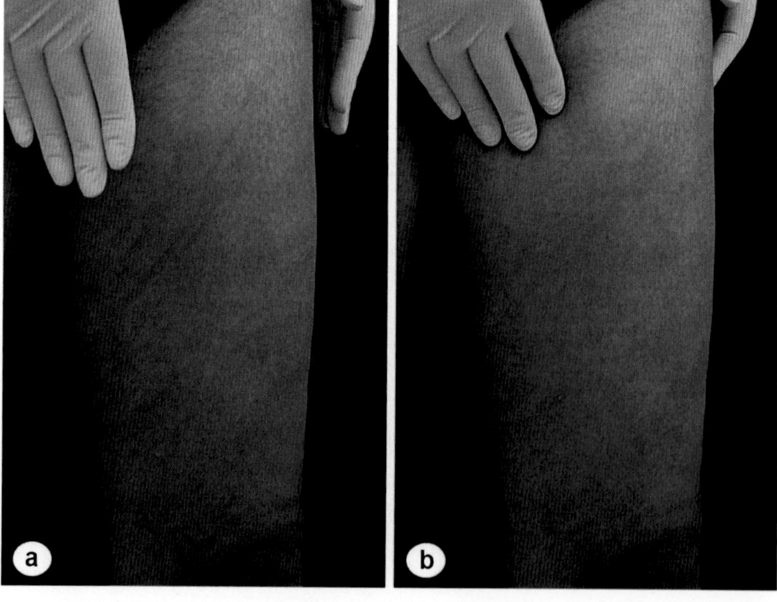

Fig. 4 Patient with skin laxity or flaccidity in standing position (**a**) and an improvement of the draped appearance when the skin is stretched against gravity (distension test) (**b**)

compared with cellulite-affected women, who exhibited weaker connective tissue that extended into the superficial fascia. With increased laxity, cellulite lesions become more evident and can even appear in patients who previously did not present with this aesthetic condition. The lesions tend to be more linear or oval, following the skin lines and providing the skin with a draped appearance. The padded surface is evident, and the skin shakes with movement, thereby changing according to position [48].

To quantify cellulite, Nürnberger and Müller [33] developed a scale that clinically classifies cellulite by four degrees: (1) degree 0 indicates no alteration on the skin surface; (2) degree I indicates the skin of the affected area is smooth while the subject is standing or lying, but skin surface alterations are apparent by pinching the skin or with muscle contraction; (3) degree II indicates the orange skin or mattress appearance is evident when standing without the use of a manipulation (skin pinching or muscle contraction); and (4) degree III indicates the alterations described in degree II are present together with raised areas and nodules. However, this classification is quite imprecise because the different clinical aspects or severities of cellulite may be attributed to the same grade. In addition, other important clinical aspects of cellulite, such as the laxity, number, and depth of the lesions, are not considered. In fact, the clinical evaluation of flaccidity requires a complete medical history, including the aggravating factors and history of surgery. Patients should be evaluated in a standing position, and the clinical assessment of flaccidity may require an additional physical examination. A distension test of the skin and subcutaneous tissue should be performed in the antigravity direction. In the absence of flaccidity, this test tends to not diminish the lesions; however, in the presence of flaccidity, this test leads to the reduction or even disappearance of cellulite lesions (Fig. 4b). With the aim to provide a more comprehensive scale for cellulite evaluation, Hexsel et al. [48] developed the photonumeric cellulite severity scale, which includes different clinical features: (1) number of evident depressions; (2) depth of depressions; (3) morphological appearance of skin surface alterations; (4) grade of laxity, flaccidity, or sagging skin; and (5) classification scale originally described by Nürnberger and Müller [33]. According to this scale, each evaluated item receives a score from 0 to 3, and the total sum grades cellulite as mild (1–5 points), moderate (6–10 points), or severe (11–15 points). The scale enables a qualitative and quantitative assessment of key clinical and morphological aspects related to cellulite severity, as well as attempts to assess laxity, which is one of the most significant effects of skin aging.

Conclusion

With the increased lifetime of the human population, many medical disciplines, including dermatology, are facing a revolution in their approaches to ensure healthcare and quality of life for patients. Cellulite is a challenging condition and commonly affects women from every culture and country. The pathophysiology is indeed controversial. Cellulite diagnosis is essentially clinical, and an evaluation of the morphological aspects is important to determine the degree of cellulite severity. Although few studies have demonstrated a relationship between cellulite and aging, it appears to be important in the treatment and prevention of this condition. Cellulite tends to worsen with aging, with laxity as one of the major skin aggravating factors in this condition.

References

1. Lorencini M, Feferman IHS, Maibach HI. New perspectives in the control of the skin aging process. In: Barel AO, Paye M, Maibach HI, editors. Handbook of cosmetic science and technology. 4th ed. Boca Raton: CRC Press; 2014. p. 245–50.
2. Farage MA, et al. Psychological and social implications of aging skin: normal aging and the effects of cutaneous disease. In: Farage MA, Miller KW, Maibach HI, editors. Textbook of aging skin. 1st ed. Heidelberg: Springer; 2010. p. 949–57.
3. Luebberding S, Krueger N, Sadick NS. Cellulite: an evidence-based review. Am J Clin Dermatol. 2015;16 (4):243–56. doi:10.1007/s40257-015-0129-5.
4. Hexsel DM, et al. Assessment of psychological, psychiatric, and behavioral aspects of patients with

cellulite: a pilot study. Surg Cosmet Dermatol. 2012;4 (2):131–6.

5. Ortonne JP, et al. Cellulite and skin ageing: is there any interaction? J Eur Acad Dermatol Venereol. 2008;22(7):827–34. doi:10.1111/j.1468-3083.2007.02570.x.
6. Hexsel D, Hexsel C. The role of skin tightening in improving cellulite. Dermatol Surg. 2014;40 Suppl 12:180–3. doi:10.1097/DSS.0000000000000204.
7. Kirkwood TBL. Understanding the odd science of aging. Cell. 2005;120(4):437–47. doi:10.1016/j.cell.2005.01.027.
8. Kammeyer A, Luiten RM. Oxidation events and skin aging. Ageing Res Rev. 2015;21:16–29. doi:10.1016/j.arr.2015.01.001.
9. Scharffetter-Kochanek K, et al. Photoaging of the skin from phenotype to mechanisms. Exp Gerontol. 2000;35(3):307–16.
10. Waller JM, Maibach HI. Age and skin structure and function, a quantitative approach (II): protein, glycosaminoglycan, water, and lipid content and structure. Skin Res Technol. 2006;12(3):145–54.
11. Bonta M, Daina L, Muţiu G. The process of ageing reflected by histological changes in the skin. Rom J Morphol Embryol. 2013;54(3):797–804.
12. Varani J, et al. Decreased collagen production in chronologically aged skin: roles of age-dependent alteration in fibroblast function and defective mechanical stimulation. Am J Pathol. 2006;168(6):1861–8.
13. Wu S, et al. Quantitative analysis on collagen morphology in aging skin based on multiphoton microscopy. J Biomed Opt. 2011;16(4):040502. doi:10.1117/1.3565439.
14. Nguyen TT, et al. Changes of skin collagen orientation associated with chronological aging as probed by polarized-FTIR micro-imaging. Analyst. 2014;139 (10):2482–8. doi:10.1039/c3an00353a.
15. Callaghan TM, Wilhelm KP. A review of ageing and an examination of clinical methods in the assessment of ageing skin. Part I: cellular and molecular perspectives of skin ageing. Int J Cosmet Sci. 2008;30(5):313–22. doi:10.1111/j.1468-2494.2008.00454.x.
16. Calleja-Agius J, Muscat-Baron Y, Brincat MP. Skin ageing. Menopause Int. 2007;13(2):60–4.
17. Langton AK, et al. Cross-linking of structural proteins in ageing skin: an in situ assay for the detection of amine oxidase activity. Biogerontology. 2013;14 (1):89–97. doi:10.1007/s10522-012-9394-3.
18. Danoux L, et al. How to help the skin cope with glycoxidation. Clin Chem Lab Med. 2014;52 (1):175–82. doi:10.1515/cclm-2012-0828.
19. Klein JA. Subcutaneous fat: anatomy and histology. In: Klein JA, editor. Tumescent technique: tumescent anesthesia & microcannular liposuction. 1st ed. Saint Louis: Mosby; 2000. p. 213–21.
20. Murphy GF. Histopathology of the skin. In: Elder DE et al., editors. Lever's histopathology of the skin. 1st ed. Philadelphia: Lippincott-Raven; 1997. p. 5–50.
21. Kuk JL, et al. Age-related changes in total and regional fat distribution. Ageing Res Rev. 2009;8(4):339–48. doi:10.1016/j.arr.2009.06.001.
22. Kim EJ, et al. UV modulation of subcutaneous fat metabolism. J Invest Dermatol. 2011;131(8):1720–6. doi:10.1038/jid.2011.106.
23. Krutmann J, Morita A, Chung JH. Sun exposure: what molecular photodermatology tells us about its good and bad sides. J Invest Dermatol. 2012;132(3 Pt 2):976–84. doi:10.1038/jid.2011.394.
24. Christ C, et al. Improvement in skin elasticity in the treatment of cellulite and connective tissue weakness by means of extracorporeal pulse activation therapy. Aesthet Surg J. 2008;28(5):538–44. doi:10.1016/j.asj.2008.07.011.
25. Scherwitz C, Braun-Falco O. So-called cellulite. J Dermatol Surg Oncol. 1978;4(3):230–4.
26. Segers AM, et al. Cellulitis. Histopathologic and histochemical study of 100 cases. Med Cutan Ibero Lat Am. 1984;12(2):167–72.
27. Hexsel DM. Body repair. In: Parish LC, Brenner S, Ramos-e-Silva M, editors. Women's dermatology: from infancy to maturity. 1st ed. New York: Parthenon Publishing Group; 2001. p. 586–95.
28. Hexsel D, Dal'Forno TO, Cignachi S. Definition, clinical aspects, associated conditions, and differential diagnosis. In: Goldman MP et al., editors. Cellulite: pathophysiology and treatment. 1st ed. New York: Taylor & Francis Group; 2006. p. 7–28.
29. Khan MH, et al. Treatment of cellulite: part I. Pathophysiology. J Am Acad Dermatol. 2010;62 (3):361–70. doi:10.1016/j.jaad.2009.10.042.
30. Khan MH, et al. Treatment of cellulite: part II. Advances and controversies. J Am Acad Dermatol. 2010;62(3):373–84. doi:10.1016/j.jaad.2009.10.041.
31. Curri SB. Cellulite and fatty tissue microcirculation. Cosmet Toiletries. 1993;108(4):51–8.
32. Rossi AB, Vergnanini AL. Cellulite: a review. J Eur Acad Dermatol Venereol. 2000;14(4):251–62.
33. Nürnberger F, Müller G. So-called cellulite: an invented disease. J Dermatol Surg Oncol. 1978;4 (3):221–9.
34. Piérard GE, Nizet JL, Piérard-Franchimont C. Cellulite: from standing fat herniation to hypodermal stretch marks. Am J Dermatopathol. 2000;22 (1):34–7.
35. Querleux B, et al. Anatomy and physiology of subcutaneous adipose tissue by in vivo magnetic resonance imaging and spectroscopy: relationships with sex and presence of cellulite. Skin Res Technol. 2002;8 (2):118–24.
36. Draelos ZD, Marenus KD. Cellulite. Etiology and purported treatment. Dermatol Surg. 1997;23 (12):1177–81.
37. Mirrashed F, et al. Pilot study of dermal and subcutaneous fat structures by MRI in individuals who differ in gender, BMI, and cellulite grading. Skin Res Technol. 2004;10(3):161–8.

38. Kligman AM. Cellulite: facts and fiction. J Geriatr Dermatol. 1997;5(4):136–9.
39. Hexsel DM, et al. Lipodistrofia ginóide. In: Kede MPV, Sabatovich O, editors. Dermatologia Estética. 1st ed. São Paulo: Atheneu; 2003. p. 350–9.
40. Hexsel DM, et al. Side-by-side comparison of areas with and without cellulite depressions using magnetic resonance imaging. Dermatol Surg. 2009;35 (10):471–7. doi:10.1111/j.1524-4725.2009.01260.x.
41. Nürnberger F. Practically important diseases of the subcutaneous fatty tissue (including so-called cellulite). Med Welt. 1981;32(18):682–8.
42. Hexsel D, et al. A comparative study of the anatomy of adipose tissue in areas with and without raised lesions of cellulite using magnetic resonance imaging. Dermatol Surg. 2013;39(12):1877–86. doi:10.1111/dsu.12360.
43. Smalls LK, et al. Quantitative model of cellulite: three-dimensional skin surface topography, biophysical characterization, and relationship to human perception. J Cosmet Sci. 2005;56(2):105–20.
44. Smalls LK, Randall Wickett R, Visscher MO. Effect of dermal thickness, tissue composition, and body site on skin biomechanical properties. Skin Res Technol. 2006;12(1):43–9.
45. Smalls LK, et al. Effect of weight loss on cellulite: gynoid lypodystrophy. Plast Reconstr Surg. 2006;118 (2):510–6.
46. Matarasso A, Matarasso SL. When does your liposuction patient require an abdominoplasty? Dermatol Surg. 1997;23(12):1151–60.
47. Dobke MK, et al. Assessment of biomechanical skin properties: is cellulitic skin different? Aesthet Surg J. 2002;22(3):260–6. doi:10.1067/maj.2002.124711.
48. Hexsel DM, Dal'forno T, Hexsel CL. A validated photonumeric cellulite severity scale. J Eur Acad Dermatol Venereol. 2009;23(5):523–8. doi:10.1111/j.1468-3083.2009.03101.x.

Skin Itch in the Elderly

83

Jerrold Scott Petrofsky

Contents

Abstract

Itching is generally known as pruritus. It is a normal reflex and common in the elderly. Aside from causes such as insect stings and contact with certain marine animals, there are other common causes that can be dermatologic, neuropathic, systemic, and psychogenic. The itch reflex is a complex reflex involving separate receptors on sensory neurons that are similar but distinct from pain sensory fibers in the skin. The receptors can be triggered by histamine, G protein receptors, proteases, and toll-like receptors, through TRPV1, TRPV3, and TRPV4 vanilloid receptors on sensory nerves, gastrin, and serotonin, to mention just a few of the stimuli that can trigger itch. The most common of these is histamine. When the skin is inflamed, as histamine is released, it triggers the itch response. In the elderly, chronic itching can interfere with the quality of life. When caused by organ failure or necessary medications such as medications for pain, it offers a quandary – stop the pain medications and increase pain or suffer with chronic itch. This chapter describes the reflex, itching in the elderly, and therapeutic interventions to reduce itch in the elderly.

J.S. Petrofsky (✉)
Department of Physical Therapy, Loma Linda University, Loma Linda, CA, USA

School of Allied Health, Loma Linda University, Loma Linda, CA, USA
e-mail: jpetrofsky@llu.edu

M.A. Farage et al. (eds.), *Textbook of Aging Skin*,
DOI 10.1007/978-3-662-47398-6_126

Introduction

Skin disorders are common in the elderly [1]. Itching is a normal reflex process encountered in daily life [2] and can alter the quality of life in older people [3]. It is a major sensation along with pain, temperature, and other primary senses in the skin [4]. Skin conditions that may cause itching occur in up to 70 % of older people [5], and it is the most common complaint in people over the age of 65 [6]. Itching can be caused by a number of pathologies. It is known generally as pruritus. It was defined over 300 years ago as a reflex that causes a desire to scratch. It can be acute and chronic in nature. The most common cause that people think about is itch due to insect stings or land or marine toxins. Acute itch from these sources can be remedied by scratching. However, chronic itch arises due to skin pathologies and organ inflammation and disease and can be divided into four classes of itch: dermatologic, systemic (e.g., liver failure or end-stage renal disease [7]), neuropathic, and psychogenic [8, 9]. In patients with renal failure, 15–49 % had chronic itch [7, 10]. Neuropathic itch is defined as being caused by a primary lesion in afferent pathways from the skin [9]. Diseases of the skin cause dermatologic itch [11]. Typical examples are eczema, xerosis, and dermatitis. Systemic itch involves disease of an organ other than the skin. One example is uremic pruritus [12, 13]. Neurogenic itch is a type of phantom itch in that the disorder is neuronal damage in either the peripheral or central nervous systems such as is the case for multiple sclerosis. People with obsessive-compulsive disorders are an example of psychopathic itch as well as conditions such as delusional parasitosis [14]. Chronic itch can involve biochemical changes in the body that can alter the skin hydration but the cause is not in the skin itself [15]. Generally, the cause cannot be found. If this is the case, itching in the elderly is classified as idiopathic itching or senile pruritus [11]. Often with systemic diseases that cause itch, there may also be itch from other origins, e.g., neuropathic itch due to nerve fiber damage [7].

The mechanism of the itch reflex takes place from primary afferent sensory nerves from the skin that can be either unmyelinated C fibers or lightly or heavily myelinated nerve fibers. Histamine and non-histamine sources of itch on sensory neurons are both relayed by subsets of C fibers and by the second-order neurons expressing gastrin-releasing peptide receptor (GRPR) and spinothalamic tract (STT) neurons in the spinal cord to the brain [4]. The mechanism is similar to the pain pathways [16, 17]. The cell body is located in the dorsal root ganglia of the spinal cord. Blocking skin myelinated fibers blocks the itch reflex [17, 18]. These sensory nerves synapse with neurons in the dorsal horn of the spinal cord and convey the sensation to the brain [17, 19]. They ascend the lateral spinothalamic tract [20] and transmit information through the thalamus and into the sensory cortex [11]. This chapter will examine mediators of itch, the mechanism of itch, and how this relates to the elderly people. It will also cover some of the treatment that can be used but is not meant to be a comprehensive treatise on pharmacology of itch. A number of reviews cover this topic in more detail [2, 4, 11, 14, 21, 22].

Mediators of Itch

Histamine

Histamine is a cytokine used by the body to mediate the inflammatory process [23] and is released due to noxious stimuli [24]. It is released by numerous cells in the body including mast cells [25]. Synthesized from the amino acid histidine, it activates the itch reflex arc and causes the itch sensation and can also cause pain [2, 26, 27]. It is, therefore, as an inducer of the itch response, classified as a pruritogen [2]. There are four different histamine receptors that mediate the itch response. These are G protein-coupled receptors (GPCR) [25]. The most important in the itch response is the H1R receptor on dorsal root ganglion (DRG) neurons [25]. DRG neurons are the neurons specific to the sensory itch pathway and are unmyelinated C fibers [28]. Activation of the H1 receptor increases intracellular calcium in the nerve endings [29]. There is evidence in rat models that the H1 receptor works through the transient receptor potential vanilloid type 1 (TRPV1) voltage-gated calcium channel as described below. In rats, if the TRPV1 channels are blocked pharmacologically, the H1 receptor response is blocked as well [29]. While the H4R receptor has also been identified as being important to the itch response in humans, complete blockage of the H1R receptor almost completely blocks the itch in response to histamine [30]. Blocking both receptors with antagonists is more effective than the blockage caused by either receptor alone but does not block itch caused by other sources not related to histamine such as uremic pruritus [31]. For this reason, itch has been characterized as either histaminergic or non-histaminergic [31–33]. Treatment with H1 and H4 antagonists has been targeted for future treatment of pruritus [34]. The H4 receptor has been implicated in chronic itch while the H1 in acute itch [35].

G Protein-Coupled Receptors

There is a class of receptors that cause itching called Mas-related G protein-coupled receptors [36, 37]. There are at least 50 members in the class. A number of members of the class are in sensory neurons and mediate non-histamine-related itch [38]. MrgprA3 is a receptor that is the target of the antimalarial drug chloroquine [36]. It can produce a side effect of severe itching when taken by black Americans. MrgprC11 produced strong itching in human skin when the body was injected with bovine adrenal medulla peptide [36]. Another member of the family, MrgprD, is activated by alanine and causes strong itching [39]. Thus, members of this family of receptors are believed to be an important source of non-histamine-related itch on sensory neurons. Many of these receptors are colocated on the same sensory neurons with histamine itch receptors [40]. This suggests that there are specific neurons to sense itch since multiple pharmacological agents can activate the same sensory neuron. The sensory neurons seem to terminate in the superficial skin layer since this is the target of a number of itch-producing chemicals like capsaicin [41].

When the GRPR dorsal horn neurons are blocked by pharmacological intervention, this results in a marked scratching deficit in mice, showing the importance of this pathway in itch [42]. The sensation of pain was still present showing the two separate nerve pathways to the central nervous system, one for pain and one for itch coming from the skin [42].

STT Neurons

Abolition of the GRPR neurons did not totally abolish the scratch reflex. Another set of neurons, the STT neurons, also carry information in the central nervous system about itch [28]. Eighty to 85 % of STT neurons in the spinal cord express a neurokinin-1 receptor. Abolition of this receptor attenuated the itching response to serotonin and pain [43].

Proteases and Protease-Activated Receptors

Protease-activated receptors (PARS) are widely found in different tissues throughout the body [44, 45]. They are part of the GPCR family of receptors but are activated by cleavage of the N-terminus of their own protein structure by proteases [2]. The unmasked N-terminus acts as a tethered ligand to activate the receptor. PAR2 and PAR4 can be activated by many compounds shown to induce itch including cathepsin [46], tryptase [44], and mucunain [47]. For example, a widely found plant in nature is the seedpod of cowhage [47]. If its needle penetrates the skin, it causes a strong itch without a histamine weal.

Antihistamines do not block this itch from this plant. Cathepsin S is an enzyme that is part of the normal immune response of the body [46]. It and cathepsin S are associated with dermatitis and cause itching through the PAR2 and PAR4 receptors [2].

Toll-Like Receptors

Toll-like receptors are proteins that penetrate the plasma membrane of the cell [48]. They are part of the immune system and are the heart of the immune systems response to bacteria. Different toll-like receptors sense different classes of bacteria and viruses [48]. The toll-like receptors are an inherited immune system for protection of the cell [49, 50]. They also recognize molecules released by other cells in response to damage [51, 52]. Once activated, they activate nuclear factor kappa beta (NFKB) which in turn activates the cells in the immune system [49]. NFKB is a nuclear transmitter that penetrates the nuclear membrane and activates DNA transcription of chemokines and cytokines. There are a number of different toll-like receptors on cells. This includes sensory neurons in the skin [53]. One of the toll-like receptors, TLR7, senses ssRNA (immune complexes from viral attacks), antiphospholipid antibodies, adenosine, and guanosine derivatives [54]. TLR7 seems to be involved in the itch reflex since topical application of a TLR7 agonist imiquimod, used to treat warts, causes an itching response [53]. There is some controversial evidence that the action of imiquimod may be on other pathways since the drug also activates adenosine receptors, 1,4,5-trisphosphate receptors, and potassium channels [53, 55]. These may also be involved in the itch sensation. But mice bred genetically without the TLR7 had reduced itch sensation in response to multiple agents known to cause itch [55].

Endothelin-1

One of the small peptides that is secreted from vascular endothelial cells is endothelin-1 [56]. It is classified as a chemokine with paracrine and autocrine effects and whose role is pivotal in maintaining homeostasis as a vasoconstrictor [56]. It is associated in many cases with inflammation. For example, it is suspected to be linked to osteoarthritis and causes destruction of bone cartilage [57, 58]. It is believed to be involved in diabetic kidney disease [59]. It is a marker of whole-body inflammation and endothelial dysfunction in diabetes [60]. It is also involved in the progression of cardiac fibrosis [61].

Intradermal injection of endothelin-1 (ET-1) causes burning and itching [62]. This is accompanied by a flare and weal, linking this response to a coupled histamine reaction [63]. The ET-1 receptor for itching uses two separate GPCR types. These are ET_A and ET_B [64]. Once activated, these receptors raise the concentration intracellularly of cyclic adenosine monophosphate (cAMP). When agonists are applied directly to these receptors, there is a very small response. The response, then, must be mediated by some other pathway to activate the itch response. The weal and flare would suggest that histamine is involved. ET-1 and the ET_A and ET_B receptors may be involved in the itch response to cathepsin E since blocking these receptors diminishes the itch response to this chemical [2]. Recent research has implicated endothelin-converting enzyme as the cause of itch and unrelated to histamine [65]. In chronic itch, this pathway is upregulated [65]. This pathway may be a good therapeutic target for chronic itch.

TRPV1, TRPV3, and TRPV4 Receptors

In mice, the TRPV1 receptor is involved in the itch response. This receptor also mediates the sensation of warmth. It is a voltage-gated calcium channel protein that extends through the plasma membrane. Neuropeptide natriuretic polypeptide b (Nppb) is a primary pruriceptive neurotransmitter secreted by sensory neurons involved in the itch response [66]. It is expressed in a subset of TRPV1 neurons and is involved in the itch response in mice [66]. A later paper found opposite results [67].

TRPV4 voltage-gated calcium channels are involved in temperature, pressure, and osmolarity of the cell [68, 69]. TRPV4 channels in the skin and in vascular endothelial cells regulate cellular osmolarity. In dry skin conditions, vascular endothelial cells reduce their gain for stimuli that cause vasodilation such that skin blood flow is reduced in dry skin [68–71]. Dry skin is associated with itching [72, 73]. Dry skin is common in the elderly and people with diabetes and this response may be mediated by either TRPV1 or TRPV4 channels.

In mice, another member of the TRPV family, TRPV3, has been associated with pruritus. The role of the TRPV3 receptor in itch in humans has not been well investigated and data is from animal studies [74].

Gastrin

In mice, gastrin-releasing peptide and the associated receptor in the spinal cord have a role in the itch reflex. It has not been studied in humans [75].

Serotonin

Serotonin is known to mediate somatosensory transmission in the central nervous system [76]. In the brainstem, injection of 5-HT potentiates the itch response [76]. The effect of serotonin (5-HT) on itch depends on the species [2]. In rats, there is severe itching in response to serotonin injection [77]. In humans, it causes both itch and pain, showing both the itch neurons and pain neurons are activated in the skin [78]. It is secreted naturally from the skin mast cells. The 5-HT receptors are GPCR receptors [79]. The only known exception is the 5-HT1 channels which are gated ion channels. The general feeling is that the 5-HT receptors are important in the itch reflex [80]. Blocking histamine receptors by the H1-antihistamine fexofenadine had no effect on itching due to 5-HT showing a separate pathway [81]. The itch response can be blocked by endocannabinoid type 2 receptor agonists [81].

Interleukin-31 and Other Interleukins

Another cytokine that can be involved in the itch reflex is interleukin-31 [82]. It is part of the interleukin-6 class of cytokines. Interleukin-6 has an important role in the body in mediating metabolism during exercise and during the inflammatory process in the body. The newly discovered interleukin-31 is secreted by lymphocytes and signals via an IL-31 receptor and the oncostatin M receptor [82]. This in turn activates tyrosine kinases which begin a cascade to activate phosphatidylinositol 3-kinase and mitogen-activated protein (MAP) kinase. In mice, overexpression of IL-31 causes severe itching which can lead to lesions resembling atopic dermatitis [82]. In humans with ectopic dermatitis, there are also increased concentrations in the blood of IL-31. IL-31 does not directly activate DRG neurons so the mechanism in causing itch is unknown. IL-31 is also elevated in inflammatory bowel and lung disease [83–85].

There is some evidence that another inflammatory cytokine, IL-2, may also have a role in inducing itch in inflammatory diseases [86].

Substance P

Injection of substance P into the skin causes histamine release and the associated histamine-related itch. The response is blocked by blocking the H1 receptors [16]. The importance of substance P is that it is elevated in patients with contact dermatitis [87]. Like many types of chronic responses to pain or itch, the density of the receptors in the substance P sensory nerves increases with chronic exposure in prurigo nodularis [88]. Using a NK1 antagonist (NK1 is the receptor for substance P) significantly reduces scratching [89].

CQ

CQ is a drug that is used to treat malaria. Its use is associated with systemic pruritus [90]. It is generally not blocked by antihistamines and is triggered by G protein-coupled receptors on DRG sensory neurons [38]. Disruption of this specific

G protein-coupled receptor, called the Mrgrps cluster, causes increased thermal and mechanical pain [91].

Aging and Itch: Causes and Management

The elderly represent the fastest growing part of the population in the United States [21]. Pruritus is a common complaint in the elderly [1, 6]. It is worse at night [7]. Even with such a seemly simple problem, it is a major contributor to a reduction in the quality of life in the elderly [21]. Itching increases with age and is a problematic management problem [92]. In the elderly, with a reduction in the adhesion between the dermal and epidermal layer of skin, itching easily causes lesions in the skin which can be difficult to heal [11, 92]. Secondary skin lesions include excoriations, hyperpigmentation, and scars [7]. Itch can affect the back more than any other area (70 %), followed by the abdomen (46 %), the head (44 %), and the arms (43 %) [93, 94]. With chronic itch, the sensory nerves involved in the pathway for the itch reflex increase and become hypersensitive making the situation even worse [95, 96].

There are obvious causes of itch in the elderly [11]. Chronic itch can lead to emotional distress and a high level of psychological morbidity [97]. It can cause sleep disturbances and fatigue which are common with chronic pruritus [98]. Of patients with atopic dermatitis, 87 % experience daily itch [99]. Between 41 % and 80 % of people with psoriasis experience itching [100]. Liver and kidney failure, and xerosis as cited above, are associated with prurogenic substances that cause itch [2]. Other factors in the skin that may contribute to itch include reduction in skin blood flow with aging [101–103], reduction in skin moisture with aging (xerosis) [5, 68, 71, 104], decreased skin surface lipids [11], reduced sweat production [105] and sebum production, and a reduction in the immune system that causes decreased barrier repair. The reduction in the immune system with aging also is causal to a greater incidence of autoimmune skin disorders [106]. Finally, inflammation in subcutaneous nerves with aging may also contribute to geriatric pruritus [107]. Inflammation is common with aging but also common in cancer, diabetes, and other age-associated diseases [108, 109]. As cited above, chronic inflammation can initiate the itch reflex. Psychological disorders may increase with chronic itching due to fatigue and frustration [9, 14].

In treating elderly patients, a good physical is recommended. Especially if the elderly have dementia, they may not provide a proper history [21]. It has been recommended that there are two major pieces of information that should be answered when looking at the cause of itch in the elderly to narrow the causes. These are (1) is there a rash and (2) is the itch generalized or localized [11]. A sudden onset of itch is uncommon for systemic causes and is frequently due to a drug reaction, contact dermatitis, or infestation of the skin [11]. An important question is the presence of pets at home since the elderly can develop itch from sources such as fleas. A thorough exam of the patient with pruritus in the elderly should look for chronic kidney failure, liver disease, cancer, and endocrine disorders since these are more common with aging and can cause systemic pruritus [6, 21, 109]. A complete listing of causes of itch in the elderly and drugs has been published in a recent review [11]. It has been estimated that one in five patients with generalized pruritus shows no obvious dermatological cause [92]. Chronic itch has been reported in hemodialysis patients [7]. In a study examining 18,801 hemodialysis patients, 42 % had moderate pruritus [20]. Drug-induced pruritus is also common especially in nursing home patients on a variety of medications such as aspirin, opioids, and angiotensin-converting enzyme (ACE) inhibitors, all of which have been shown to induce chemical pruritus [21]. Willan's itch is a generalized pruritus in the elderly in the absence of dry skin [11].

The management first should involve patient education [22]. Patients should become aware of any skin diseases and triggering factors such as itching and scratching and environmental factors. They need to know about daily skin care. They need to know how to inspect their skin and the consequences to their health of continuous itching in geriatric patients. They need to be aware of medical treatment and support groups [22, 110]. In a recent paper, a program of education and nursing care in the Netherlands called "coping with itch" caused significant reduction in itching and skin disorders [22].

To resolve chronic itch, there are multiple measures including moisturizers and barrier creams, keeping fingernails short, wearing light and loose clothing, using a humidifier in the winter, using an air conditioner in the summer, restricting time in the shower or bathtub, avoiding hot water when bathing, and avoiding cleansers and conditioners with a high pH [21]. Topical corticosteroids may also be useful [111]. But excessive use of these compounds can also lead to skin thinning and damage. Topical immunomodulators can also be useful and do not cause skin damage but may cause burning on use [112]. Menthol used topically blocks TRPV1 and TRPV4 channels and may reduce itching [113]. Capsaicin, like menthol, blocks TRPV1 channels and therefore may help itch [114–116]. Topical cannabinoids, salicylic acid, and local anesthetics have also been used to reduce itch in the elderly [117–120]. Opioid agonists and antagonist can also be used to rebalance the pain system [121]. If related to histamine, antihistamines can be used. Finally, for psychological causes, drugs like antidepressants can be used [122]. Serotonin inhibitors that block serotonin reuptake seem to have a positive effect on reducing itch [123]. In a similar manner, selective norepinephrine uptake inhibitors also seem to reduce itch presumably due to their influence on inhibiting both serotonin and catecholamines [9, 124]. A thorough review of many of the drugs that cause and inhibit itch is given in a review by Ward [11]. They seem to work well for night itch [125]. Another treatment is ultraviolet therapy. Ultraviolet B (UV-B) is known to relieve systemic pruritus [94]. Neuropathic and psychogenic itch have not been well studied [9]. Drugs that are commonly used for depression, neuropathic pain, and anxiety seem to help [9].

Conclusion

Itching is a complex reflex process with its own sensory neurons and pathways in the spinal cord. Itching increases in the elderly due to a number of different causes including certain organ disorders and medications such as opioids. It can interfere with the quality of life in the elderly and has complex causes. A number of therapeutic interventions have been examined but itching is still a major problem in the elderly especially when caused by medication necessary to their lives.

References

1. Beauregard S, Gilchrest BA. A survey of skin problems and skin care regimens in the elderly. Arch Dermatol. 1987;123(12):1638–43.
2. Han L, Dong X. Itch mechanisms and circuits. Annu Rev Biophys. 2014;43:331–55.
3. Zachariae R, et al. Dermatology life quality index: data from Danish inpatients and outpatients. Acta Derm Venereol. 2000;80(4):272–6.
4. Jeffry J, Kim S, Chen ZF. Itch signaling in the nervous system. Physiology (Bethesda). 2011;26 (4):286–92.
5. Ward S. Eczema and dry skin in older people: identification and management. Br J Community Nurs. 2005;10(10):453–6.
6. Norman RA. Xerosis and pruritus in the elderly: recognition and management. Dermatol Ther. 2003; 16(3):254–9.
7. Wang H, Yosipovitch G. New insights into the pathophysiology and treatment of chronic itch in patients with end-stage renal disease, chronic liver disease, and lymphoma. Int J Dermatol. 2010;49(1):1–11.
8. Bernhard JD. Itch and pruritus: what are they, and how should itches be classified? Dermatol Ther. 2005;18(4):288–91.
9. Yosipovitch G, Samuel LS. Neuropathic and psychogenic itch. Dermatol Ther. 2008;21(1):32–41.
10. Kurban MS, Boueiz A, Kibbi AG. Cutaneous manifestations of chronic kidney disease. Clin Dermatol. 2008;26(3):255–64.
11. Ward JR, Bernhard JD. Willan's itch and other causes of pruritus in the elderly. Int J Dermatol. 2005; 44(4):267–73.
12. Yosipovitch G, Fleischer A. Itch associated with skin disease: advances in pathophysiology and emerging therapies. Am J Clin Dermatol. 2003;4(9):617–22.
13. Yosipovitch G, Greaves MW, Schmelz M. Itch. Lancet. 2003;361(9358):690–4.
14. Ramirez-Bermudez J, Espinola-Nadurille M, Loza-Taylor N. Delusional parasitosis in neurological patients. Gen Hosp Psychiatry. 2010;32(3):294–9.
15. Kuypers DR. Skin problems in chronic kidney disease. Nat Clin Pract Nephrol. 2009;5(3):157–70.
16. Hosogi M, et al. Bradykinin is a potent pruritogen in atopic dermatitis: a switch from pain to itch. Pain. 2006;126(1–3):16–23.

17. Ikoma A, et al. The neurobiology of itch. Nat Rev Neurosci. 2006;7(7):535–47.
18. Basbaum AI, et al. Cellular and molecular mechanisms of pain. Cell. 2009;139(2):267–84.
19. Ringkamp M, et al. A role for nociceptive, myelinated nerve fibers in itch sensation. J Neurosci. 2011; 31(42):14841–9.
20. Andrew D, Craig AD. Spinothalamic lamina I neurons selectively sensitive to histamine: a central neural pathway for itch. Nat Neurosci. 2001;4(1):72–7.
21. Patel T, Yosipovitch G. The management of chronic pruritus in the elderly. Skin Therapy Lett. 2010; 15(8):5–9.
22. van Os-Medendorp H, et al. Effectiveness of the nursing programme 'Coping with itch': a randomized controlled study in adults with chronic pruritic skin disease. Br J Dermatol. 2007;156(6):1235–44.
23. Volonte C, Parisi C, Apolloni S. New kid on the block: does histamine get along with inflammation in amyotrophic lateral sclerosis? CNS Neurol Disord Drug Targets. 2015;14:168–75.
24. Lewis T, Zotterman Y. Vascular reactions of the skin to injury: part VIII. The resistance of the human skin to constant currents, in relation to injury and vascular response. J Physiol. 1927;62(3):280–8.
25. Simons FE, Simons KJ. Histamine and H1-antihistamines: celebrating a century of progress. J Allergy Clin Immunol. 2011;128(6):1139–50 e4.
26. Hasegawa Y, et al. Intractable itch relieved by 4-phenylbutyrate therapy in patients with progressive familial intrahepatic cholestasis type 1. Orphanet J Rare Dis. 2014;9:89.
27. Broadbent JL. Observations on histamine-induced pruritus and pain. Br J Pharmacol Chemother. 1955;10(2):183–5.
28. Davidson S, Giesler GJ. The multiple pathways for itch and their interactions with pain. Trends Neurosci. 2010;33(12):550–8.
29. Kim BM, et al. Histamine-induced Ca(2+) influx via the PLA(2)/lipoxygenase/TRPV1 pathway in rat sensory neurons. Neurosci Lett. 2004;361(1–3):159–62.
30. Mobarakeh JI, et al. Role of histamine H(1) receptor in pain perception: a study of the receptor gene knockout mice. Eur J Pharmacol. 2000;391(1–2):81–9.
31. Rossbach K, et al. The histamine H receptor as a new target for treatment of canine inflammatory skin diseases. Vet Dermatol. 2009;20(5–6):555–61.
32. Kollmeier A, et al. The histamine H(4) receptor antagonist, JNJ 39758979, is effective in reducing histamine-induced pruritus in a randomized clinical study in healthy subjects. J Pharmacol Exp Ther. 2014;350(1):181–7.
33. Ohsawa Y, Hirasawa N. The antagonism of histamine H1 and H4 receptors ameliorates chronic allergic dermatitis via anti-pruritic and anti-inflammatory effects in NC/Nga mice. Allergy. 2012;67(8):1014–22.
34. Tey HL, Yosipovitch G. Targeted treatment of pruritus: a look into the future. Br J Dermatol. 2011; 165(1):5–17.
35. Thurmond RL, Gelfand EW, Dunford PJ. The role of histamine H1 and H4 receptors in allergic inflammation: the search for new antihistamines. Nat Rev Drug Discov. 2008;7(1):41–53.
36. Dong X, et al. A diverse family of GPCRs expressed in specific subsets of nociceptive sensory neurons. Cell. 2001;106(5):619–32.
37. Lembo PM, et al. Proenkephalin A gene products activate a new family of sensory neuron – specific GPCRs. Nat Neurosci. 2002;5(3):201–9.
38. Liu Q, et al. Sensory neuron-specific GPCR Mrgprs are itch receptors mediating chloroquine-induced pruritus. Cell. 2009;139(7):1353–65.
39. Liu Q, et al. Mechanisms of itch evoked by beta-alanine. J Neurosci. 2012;32(42):14532–7.
40. Han L, et al. A subpopulation of nociceptors specifically linked to itch. Nat Neurosci. 2013;16(2):174–82.
41. Shelley WB, Arthur RP. Mucunain, the active pruritogenic proteinase of cowhage. Science. 1955;122(3167):469–70.
42. Sun YG, et al. Cellular basis of itch sensation. Science. 2009;325(5947):1531–4.
43. Nichols ML, et al. Transmission of chronic nociception by spinal neurons expressing the substance P receptor. Science. 1999;286(5444):1558–61.
44. Soh UJ, et al. Signal transduction by protease-activated receptors. Br J Pharmacol. 2010;160(2):191–203.
45. Zhu WJ, et al. Expression of mRNA for four subtypes of the proteinase-activated receptor in rat dorsal root ganglia. Brain Res. 2005;1041(2):205–11.
46. Reddy VB, et al. Cathepsin S elicits itch and signals via protease-activated receptors. J Invest Dermatol. 2010;130(5):1468–70.
47. Reddy VB, et al. Cowhage-evoked itch is mediated by a novel cysteine protease: a ligand of protease-activated receptors. J Neurosci. 2008;28(17):4331–5.
48. Ratikan JA, et al. Radiation takes its toll. Cancer Lett. 2015;362:122–30.
49. Akira S, Uematsu S, Takeuchi O. Pathogen recognition and innate immunity. Cell. 2006;124(4):783–801.
50. Fischer H, et al. Mechanism of pathogen-specific TLR4 activation in the mucosa: fimbriae, recognition receptors and adaptor protein selection. Eur J Immunol. 2006;36(2):267–77.
51. Matzinger P. An innate sense of danger. Ann N Y Acad Sci. 2002;961:341–2.
52. Matzinger P. The danger model: a renewed sense of self. Science. 2002;296(5566):301–5.
53. Kim SJ, et al. Analysis of cellular and behavioral responses to imiquimod reveals a unique itch pathway in transient receptor potential vanilloid 1 (TRPV1)-expressing neurons. Proc Natl Acad Sci U S A. 2011;108(8):3371–6.
54. Menendez D, et al. The toll-like receptor gene family is integrated into human DNA damage and p53 networks. PLoS Genet. 2011;7(3):e1001360.
55. van den Ancker W, et al. Targeting toll-like receptor 7/8 enhances uptake of apoptotic leukemic cells by monocyte-derived dendritic cells but interferes with

subsequent cytokine-induced maturation. Cancer Immunol Immunother. 2011;60(1):37–47.
56. Davenport AP, Maguire JJ. Endothelin. Handb Exp Pharmacol. 2006;176(Pt 1):295–329.
57. Sin A, et al. The emerging role of endothelin-1 in the pathogenesis of subchondral bone disturbance and osteoarthritis. Osteoarthritis Cartilage. 2015;23(4): 516–24.
58. Kilickesmez KO, et al. Relationship between serum endothelin-1 level and spontaneous reperfusion in patients with acute myocardial infarction. Coron Artery Dis. 2015;26(1):37–41.
59. Fu J, et al. Glomerular endothelial cell injury and cross talk in diabetic kidney disease. Am J Physiol Renal Physiol. 2015;308(4):F287–97.
60. Santi D, et al. Therapy of endocrine disease. Effects of chronic use of phosphodiesterase inhibitors on endothelial markers in type 2 diabetes mellitus: a meta-analysis. Eur J Endocrinol. 2015;172(3):R103–14.
61. Leask A. Getting to the heart of the matter: new insights into cardiac fibrosis. Circ Res. 2015;116(7): 1269–76.
62. Katugampola R, Church MK, Clough GF. The neurogenic vasodilator response to endothelin-1: a study in human skin in vivo. Exp Physiol. 2000;85(6):839–46.
63. McQueen DS, Noble MA, Bond SM. Endothelin-1 activates ETA receptors to cause reflex scratching in BALB/c mice. Br J Pharmacol. 2007;151(2):278–84.
64. Liang J, Kawamata T, Ji W. Molecular signaling of pruritus induced by endothelin-1 in mice. Exp Biol Med (Maywood). 2010;235(11):1300–5.
65. Kido-Nakahara M, et al. Neural peptidase endothelin-converting enzyme 1 regulates endothelin 1-induced pruritus. J Clin Invest. 2014;124(6):2683–95.
66. Mishra SK, Hoon MA. The cells and circuitry for itch responses in mice. Science. 2013;340(6135):968–71.
67. Liu XY, et al. B-type natriuretic peptide is neither itch-specific nor functions upstream of the GRP-GRPR signaling pathway. Mol Pain. 2014;10:4.
68. Petrofsky JS, et al. The interrelationship between air temperature and humidity as applied locally to the skin: the resultant response on skin temperature and blood flow with age differences. Med Sci Monit. 2012;18(4):CR201–8.
69. Petrofsky J, et al. The effect of moist air on skin blood flow and temperature in subjects with and without diabetes. Diabetes Technol Ther. 2012;14(2):105–16.
70. McLellan K, et al. The influence of environmental temperature on the response of the skin to local pressure: the impact of aging and diabetes. Diabetes Technol Ther. 2009;11(12):791–8.
71. Petrofsky J. A method of measuring the interaction between skin temperature and humidity on skin vascular endothelial function in people with diabetes. J Med Eng Technol. 2011;35(6–7):330–7.
72. Akiyama T, Carstens MI, Carstens E. Enhanced scratching evoked by PAR-2 agonist and 5-HT but not histamine in a mouse model of chronic dry skin itch. Pain. 2010;151(2):378–83.
73. Akiyama T, Carstens MI, Carstens E. Spontaneous itch in the absence of hyperalgesia in a mouse hindpaw dry skin model. Neurosci Lett. 2010;484(1):62–5.
74. Yoshioka T, et al. Impact of the Gly573Ser substitution in TRPV3 on the development of allergic and pruritic dermatitis in mice. J Invest Dermatol. 2009;129(3):714–22.
75. Sun YG, Chen ZF. A gastrin-releasing peptide receptor mediates the itch sensation in the spinal cord. Nature. 2007;448(7154):700–3.
76. Zhao ZQ, et al. Descending control of itch transmission by the serotonergic system via 5-HT1A-facilitated GRP-GRPR signaling. Neuron. 2014;84(4):821–34.
77. Schmelz M, et al. Chemical response pattern of different classes of C-nociceptors to pruritogens and algogens. J Neurophysiol. 2003;89(5):2441–8.
78. Akiyama T, Carstens MI, Carstens E. Facial injections of pruritogens and algogens excite partly overlapping populations of primary and second-order trigeminal neurons in mice. J Neurophysiol. 2010;104(5):2442–50.
79. Sommer C. Serotonin in pain and analgesia: actions in the periphery. Mol Neurobiol. 2004;30(2):117–25.
80. Bockaert J, et al. Neuronal 5-HT metabotropic receptors: fine-tuning of their structure, signaling, and roles in synaptic modulation. Cell Tissue Res. 2006; 326(2):553–72.
81. Haruna T, et al. S-777469, a novel cannabinoid type 2 receptor agonist, suppresses itch-associated scratching behavior in rodents through inhibition of itch signal transmission. Pharmacology. 2015;95(1–2):95–103.
82. Dillon SR, et al. Interleukin 31, a cytokine produced by activated T cells, induces dermatitis in mice. Nat Immunol. 2004;5(7):752–60.
83. Neis MM, et al. Enhanced expression levels of IL-31 correlate with IL-4 and IL-13 in atopic and allergic contact dermatitis. J Allergy Clin Immunol. 2006; 118(4):930–7.
84. Szegedi K, et al. Increased frequencies of IL-31-producing T cells are found in chronic atopic dermatitis skin. Exp Dermatol. 2012;21(6):431–6.
85. Takaoka A, et al. Expression of IL-31 gene transcripts in NC/Nga mice with atopic dermatitis. Eur J Pharmacol. 2005;516(2):180–1.
86. Yosipovitch G, Papoiu AD. What causes itch in atopic dermatitis? Curr Allergy Asthma Rep. 2008;8(4): 306–11.
87. Toyoda M, et al. Nerve growth factor and substance P are useful plasma markers of disease activity in atopic dermatitis. Br J Dermatol. 2002;147(1):71–9.
88. Haas S, et al. Low density of sympathetic nerve fibers relative to substance P-positive nerve fibers in lesional skin of chronic pruritus and prurigo nodularis. J Dermatol Sci. 2010;58(3):193–7.
89. Ohmura T, et al. Involvement of substance P in scratching behaviour in an atopic dermatitis model. Eur J Pharmacol. 2004;491(2–3):191–4.
90. Sowunmi A, Walker O, Salako LA. Pruritus and antimalarial drugs in Africans. Lancet. 1989; 2(8656):213.

91. Guan Y, et al. Mas-related G-protein-coupled receptors inhibit pathological pain in mice. Proc Natl Acad Sci U S A. 2010;107(36):15933–8.
92. Fleischer Jr AB. Pruritus in the elderly: management by senior dermatologists. J Am Acad Dermatol. 1993;28(4):603–9.
93. Duque MI, et al. Uremic pruritus is associated with higher kt/V and serum calcium concentration. Clin Nephrol. 2006;66(3):184–91.
94. Patel TS, Freedman BI, Yosipovitch G. An update on pruritus associated with CKD. Am J Kidney Dis. 2007;50(1):11–20.
95. Ward L, Wright E, McMahon SB. A comparison of the effects of noxious and innocuous counter stimuli on experimentally induced itch and pain. Pain. 1996;64(1):129–38.
96. Yosipovitch G, et al. Scratching and noxious heat stimuli inhibit itch in humans: a psychophysical study. Br J Dermatol. 2007;156(4):629–34.
97. van Os-Medendorp H, et al. Prevalence and predictors of psychosocial morbidity in patients with chronic pruritic skin diseases. J Eur Acad Dermatol Venereol. 2006;20(7):810–7.
98. Weiner AA, Sheehan DV. Etiology of dental anxiety: psychological trauma or CNS chemical imbalance? Gen Dent. 1990;38(1):39–43.
99. Harlow D, et al. Impaired quality of life of adults with skin disease in primary care. Br J Dermatol. 2000; 143(5):979–82.
100. Yosipovitch G, et al. The prevalence and clinical characteristics of pruritus among patients with extensive psoriasis. Br J Dermatol. 2000;143(5):969–73.
101. Petrofsky JS. Resting blood flow in the skin: does it exist, and what is the influence of temperature, aging, and diabetes? J Diabetes Sci Technol. 2012; 6(3):674–85.
102. Petrofsky JS, et al. The effect of body fat, aging, and diabetes on vertical and shear pressure in and under a waist belt and its effect on skin blood flow. Diabetes Technol Ther. 2010;12(2):153–60.
103. Petrofsky J, Lee S. The effects of type 2 diabetes and aging on vascular endothelial and autonomic function. Med Sci Monit. 2005;11(6):CR247–54.
104. Petrofsky J, et al. The interrelationship between locally applied heat, ageing and skin blood flow on heat transfer into and from the skin. J Med Eng Technol. 2011;35(5):262–74.
105. Petrofsky JS, et al. Sweat production during global heating and during isometric exercise in people with diabetes. Med Sci Monit. 2005;11(11):CR515–21.
106. Gubbels Bupp MR. Sex, the aging immune system, and chronic disease. Cell Immunol. 2015;294(2):102–10.
107. Bonomini F, Rodella LF, Rezzani R. Metabolic syndrome, aging and involvement of oxidative stress. Aging Dis. 2015;6(2):109–20.
108. Edd SN, Giori NJ, Andriacchi TP. The role of inflammation in the initiation of osteoarthritis after meniscal damage. J Biomech. 2015;48:1420–6.
109. Bessueille L, Magne D. Inflammation: a culprit for vascular calcification in atherosclerosis and diabetes. Cell Mol Life Sci. 2015;72:2475–89.
110. Stangier U, Ehlers A, Gieler U. Predicting long-term outcome in group treatment of atopic dermatitis. Psychother Psychosom. 2004;73(5):293–301.
111. Dykes PJ, Marks R. An appraisal of the methods used in the assessment of atrophy from topical corticosteroids. Br J Dermatol. 1979;101(5):599–609.
112. Stander S, et al. Treatment of pruritic diseases with topical calcineurin inhibitors. Ther Clin Risk Manag. 2006;2(2):213–8.
113. Patel T, Ishiuji Y, Yosipovitch G. Menthol: a refreshing look at this ancient compound. J Am Acad Dermatol. 2007;57(5):873–8.
114. Papoiu AD, Yosipovitch G. Topical capsaicin. The fire of a 'hot' medicine is reignited. Expert Opin Pharmacother. 2010;11(8):1359–71.
115. Wood GJ, et al. An insatiable itch. J Pain. 2009;10(8):792–7.
116. Imamachi N, et al. TRPV1-expressing primary afferents generate behavioral responses to pruritogens via multiple mechanisms. Proc Natl Acad Sci U S A. 2009;106(27):11330–5.
117. Freitag G, Hoppner T. Results of a postmarketing drug monitoring survey with a polidocanol-urea preparation for dry, itching skin. Curr Med Res Opin. 1997;13(9):529–37.
118. Yosipovitch G, et al. The effect of topically applied aspirin on localized circumscribed neurodermatitis. J Am Acad Dermatol. 2001;45(6):910–3.
119. Andoh T, et al. Thromboxane A2 induces itch-associated responses through TP receptors in the skin in mice. J Invest Dermatol. 2007;127(8):2042–7.
120. Szepietowski JC, Szepietowski T, Reich A. Efficacy and tolerance of the cream containing structured physiological lipids with endocannabinoids in the treatment of uremic pruritus: a preliminary study. Acta Dermatovenerol Croat. 2005;13(2): 97–103.
121. Bergasa NV, et al. Oral nalmefene therapy reduces scratching activity due to the pruritus of cholestasis: a controlled study. J Am Acad Dermatol. 1999;41(3 Pt 1):431–4.
122. Davis MP, et al. Mirtazapine for pruritus. J Pain Symptom Manage. 2003;25(3):288–91.
123. Stander S, et al. Treatment of chronic pruritus with the selective serotonin re-uptake inhibitors paroxetine and fluvoxamine: results of an open-labelled, two-arm proof-of-concept study. Acta Derm Venereol. 2009;89(1):45–51.
124. Yosipovitch G, Carstens E, McGlone F. Chronic itch and chronic pain: analogous mechanisms. Pain. 2007;131(1–2):4–7.
125. Hundley JL, Yosipovitch G. Mirtazapine for reducing nocturnal itch in patients with chronic pruritus: a pilot study. J Am Acad Dermatol. 2004;50(6): 889–91.

Control of Skin Blood Flow

84

Jerrold Scott Petrofsky

Contents

Abstract

The circulation of the skin and of other organs is the center of aging and many diseases in the body. The heart of the circulation is the one-cell thick barrier that lines the arteries, capillaries, and veins in the body: the vascular endothelial cell. The smooth muscle surrounding arteries and veins will not, in itself, contract or relax in response to local stimuli and the autonomic nervous system. The processing of environmental, humeral stimuli and the response to sympathetic vasodilators and constrictors in the vascular endothelial cell. These cells respond to heat, osmolarity, pressure, shear forces in arteries, chemokines and cytokines like histamine and bradykinin, and neurotransmitters such as acetylcholine and epinephrine and norepinephrine. Vasodilation and vasoconstriction are accomplished by the release of fat-soluble substances that diffuse from the endothelial cell into the surrounding smooth muscle and either block calcium permeability or enhance it to adjust the contractile state of the smooth muscle. There are also electrical connections between the endothelial cells and the smooth muscle forming electronic synapses. There is some evidence that the main vasodilator substance, nitric oxide, is even released by parasympathetic neurons in the skin. This chapter deals with the control of skin circulation and the various mediators that alter circulation.

J.S. Petrofsky (✉)
Department of Physical Therapy, Loma Linda University, Loma Linda, CA, USA

School of Allied Health, Loma Linda University, Loma Linda, CA, USA
e-mail: jpetrofsky@llu.edu

M.A. Farage et al. (eds.), *Textbook of Aging Skin*,
DOI 10.1007/978-3-662-47398-6_169

Introduction

The circulation to the skin is important both for the skin's nutrition, maintaining it as a live barrier to protect the inner organs, and also to support its role in thermoregulation. Because of this latter role, as much as 99 % of skin circulation may be for thermoregulatory purposes. Thus, the skin has a complex control system allowing it to respond to local stimuli such as pressure, moisture, and heat and also to central sympathetic command to maintain blood pressure with changes in body position and allow for heat loss. Blood vessels in the skin are arranged in two layers, or plexuses [1]. The top of the dermal layer is largely loops (AV shunts) that are used to establish a thermal heat gradient to the upper skin for heat loss in the process of thermoregulation. There are some nutritive vessels in this layer. The blood vessels are innervated and contain two layers of vascular smooth muscle with an inner lining of vascular endothelial cells. The lower dermal layer is at the dermal–subdermal barrier and supplies circulation to the hairs and sweat glands. The lower layer of blood vessels has five layers of smooth muscle. The endothelial cell in the blood vessels has variable permeability depending on the needs of the cells to maintain homeostasis [2]. Endothelial permeability can range from 0.1 to 11.5 nm [3, 4] depending on proinflammatory regulators such as histamine, vascular endothelial growth factor, and other cytokines [5, 6]. Thus, the vasculature is more than a conduit for the blood and serves an important role in the body and is very susceptible to damage from aging.

This chapter will explore how skin circulation is controlled by local and central mechanisms. The companion chapter will review how circulation is altered by age, race, sex hormones, and pathologies such as diabetes.

Normal Skin Circulation

When people are exposed to a thermally neutral environment, skin blood flow averages about 5 % of their cardiac output or about 250–500 ml/min [1, 7]. However, during whole body heating, blood flow through the skin can increase to as high as about 8 l per minute [8, 9].

Measurement of Blood Flow

Although the skin is an easily accessed organ, blood flow measures have been difficult and not one technique gives true results. Early studies examined changes in skin temperature, but the relationship between skin blood flow and skin temperature is nonlinear, making estimates of skin blood flow difficult [1]. Another technique, volume plethysmography, examines whole limb blood flow and does not separate muscle and deep tissue flow from that of the skin. This technique shows resting limb blood flow to be between 2 and 3 ml/100 cc tissue per minute [10]. It has been estimated that about half of this is skin blood flow. During exercise, whole limb blood flows increase to over 50 ml/100 cc tissue per minute due to increases in muscle blood flow [11–13]. The measure is further confounded during heating in that the contribution of muscle blood flow during the heating of the limb has not been determined. Further, even when examining muscle blood flow, it is hard to partition the skin from muscle and understand the dynamics of specific circulations. This was attempted by iontophoresis of the skin with epinephrine in one arm, and muscle and skin blood flows were estimated at about 50 % at rest to the skin [14]. Also, the technique assumes the tissue examined is a cylinder in the calculation and this also introduces some error [10].

Isotope clearance such as xenon 133 clearance has been used but this requires radiation and only shows the results of a small skin area [15, 16]. Many of these isotopes are fat soluble and therefore there is an error in people with greater adiposity. Heat clearance has also been used [17]. The most common technique is to heat one of a pair of thermistors with a small current and then to measure the current required to warm one thermistor to several degrees centigrade above the other. Since higher skin blood flows would cool the heated thermistor, current is proportional to blood flow [18]. This is sometimes called a thermodilution technique. Its problem lies in the fact that local heating in itself increases skin blood flow [19].

Ultrasound Doppler flowmetry is also used to measure skin blood flow. It measures blood flow on a beat-by-beat basis and can provide information as to blood velocity, area of arteries, and estimated blood flow. If the artery is large enough, it corresponds well to venous occlusion plethysmography [1]. Laser Doppler flowmetry offers a different perspective. Ultrasound measures an artery or venous blood flow. With a laser, blood flow is measured in tissue [20]. It provides continuous flow measures and can be adjusted by altering the color and intensity to examine different depths in the dermal layer of the skin [21–23]. Red light penetrates about 50 % of the dermal layer and infrared penetrates most of the dermal layer. Laser Doppler flowmetry can measure a single point, about 1 mm^3 in size, or can scan the skin to create a picture of the skin based on blood flow. The flow measurement comes from measuring the shift in frequency of laser light directed at tissue. The greater the change in frequency, the greater the tissue blood flow [24]. Laser Doppler flowmetry is considered to be highly correlated to actual blood flow. Here, however, the skin must be in view of the laser and movement is not allowed during measurements as it deflects laser light.

Iontophoresis is widely used to indirectly measure the control of blood flow. For example epinephrine can be applied through the skin to cause vasoconstriction by activating adrenergic receptors on vascular endothelial cells [25]. Acetylcholine can also be applied to cause skin vasodilation [26]. In addition blocking agents such as L-NAME can be used to block endothelial nitric oxide synthetase (ENOS) [27].

Control of Circulation

In glabrous (nonhairy) skin (e.g., palms, plantar aspects of the feet, and lips), cutaneous arterioles are innervated by only sympathetic adrenergic vasoconstrictor nerves [1, 28]. Blood flow is also altered in this same skin type by local metabolites and effectors such as temperature and pressure on the skin [1, 29]. In hairy (nonglabrous) skin, which is present in over most of the body, three separate branches of the sympathetic nervous system control skin blood flow: adrenergic vasoconstrictor nerves that reduce (constrict) skin blood vessels and cholinergic and nitrergic nerves that cause vasodilation of blood vessels by releasing the neurotransmitters acetylcholine or nitric oxide, respectively [30, 31]. These neurons play a role in cerebral vasodilation [32]. They are believed to be controlled by the parasympathetic nervous system and enhanced with acetylcholinesterase inhibitors [33]. In other vascular beds such as the heart, it is unclear if nitrergic neurons are involved in the regulation of coronary blood flow [34, 35]. These same types of neurons do seem to play a role in large pulmonary arteries [36] and the kidney [37]. In animals, slow-twitch but not fast-twitch skeletal muscle has nitrergic neurons [38]. In canine skin, there is some evidence for part of the response to local heating is mediated by nitrergic neurons and the vasoconstriction to cold mediated by inhibition of nitric oxide [39]. In humans, evidence is lacking. However, blocking nitric oxide with L-NAME reduces the response of the blood flow to electrical stimulation [40, 41]. Recent evidence shows this response is mediated by nitrergic neurons [42].

In addition, as is the case for glabrous skin, local effectors, such as metabolites and changes in local skin temperature or pressure, may mediate a change in skin blood flow. Thus, the control of the circulation in the skin can be divided into generally two types of control: (1) the local response of vascular endothelial cells to metabolites and other processes (such as local pressure or shear stress on the blood vessel wall) and (2) neurogenic control through the sympathetic nervous system. Both sympathetic synapses and local effectors mediate their effects through the thin layer of cells lining blood vessels, the vascular endothelial cells [9, 19, 43].

Studies conducted in the last 50 years, with drugs that specifically block vasoconstriction (e.g., bretylium tosylate) [44] and agents that inhibit vasodilatation by blocking acetylcholine (cholinergic antagonistic agents), have been used to confirm chemical mediators at neuronal synapses [45]. Sympathetic vasodilator and vasoconstrictor nerves innervate blood vessels by extensive terminal varicosities located on the surface of vascular endothelial cells. The vascular endothelial cell, in turn, releases fat-soluble substances that cause the vascular smooth muscle surrounding it to relax or constrict, thereby mediating a change in skin blood flow. Stripping the inner layer of large conduit arteries (i.e., removing the endothelial layer) eliminates vasodilation and vasoconstriction in vascular smooth muscle [46].

Neuronal Controlled Vasodilatation

Acetylcholine

Acetylcholine, a neurotransmitter that mediates vasodilatation in the skin, is released from the terminal varicosities of sympathetic cholinergic postganglionic neurons and diffuses onto specific acetylcholine receptors on vascular endothelial cells. Therefore, the application of atropine to the skin largely abolishes vasodilatation mediated by the sympathetic nervous system [46]. However, some sympathetic nerves must release co-transmitters in addition to acetylcholine, because a degree of active vasodilator response mediated by sympathetic nerves exists even after atropine is administered. Some studies suggest that a peptide, vasoactive intestinal peptide (VIP), is involved in vasodilatation. For example, when VIP receptors in the skin are blocked, some of the active vasodilatation also is blocked [47]. However, other studies raise doubt as to VIP's true role in active vasodilatation in the skin [48].

Nitric Oxide

A variety of different stressors can elicit an increase or decrease in skin blood flow in hairy skin. The blood flow response is controlled through a range of different mechanisms. In the 1990s, a number of laboratories demonstrated an active role for nitric oxide as a mediator of vasodilatation in the skin [49–51]. Historically, it had been postulated that a substance released from vascular endothelial cells caused vascular smooth muscle to relax [52]. This substance, originally called endothelium-derived relaxing factor, is now known to be several different compounds, one of which is a fat-soluble chemical, nitric oxide [53].

Several lines of evidence indicate that nitric oxide is produced by endothelial cells and in neurons, as cited above, in both human and animal models and over a variety of species. Nitric oxide is produced from the amino acid L-arginine by the enzyme endothelial nitric oxide synthetase (Fig. 1). When L-NAME (N-nitro-L-arginine methyl ester), an inhibitor of nitric oxide

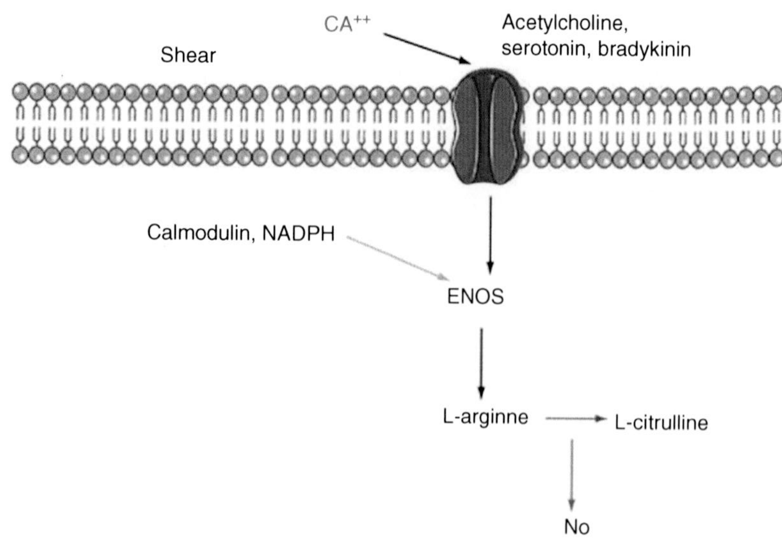

Fig. 1 Synthesis of nitric oxide

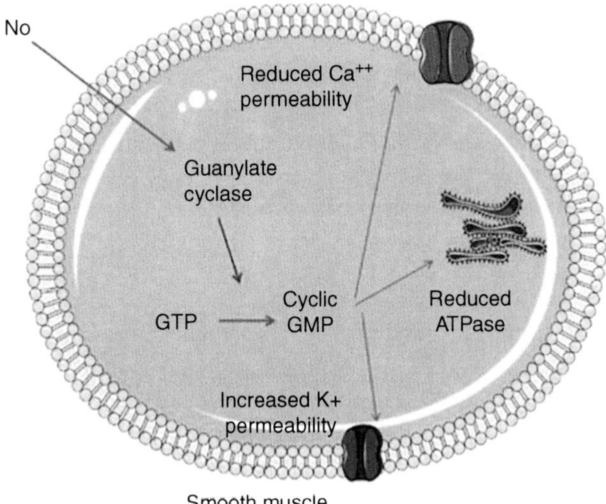

Fig. 2 The effect of nitric oxide on smooth muscle

synthetase, is infused into the skin via microdialysis in both animals and humans, the increase in blood flow due to stressors such as heat is significantly attenuated, although not completely blocked [49]. During whole body heating, the bioavailability of nitric oxide increases in proportion to skin blood flow. Shear forces on the cell and pressure also are associated with an increase in the activation of ENOS [54]. One recent mechanism for shear stress is through the mitogen-activated protein (MAP) kinase pathway which then activates ENOS [55]. There is also evidence that the bradykinin 2 receptor is sensitive to shear stress and causes Ca to enter the endothelial cell and activate ENOS [56].

However, nitric oxide may be generated from sources in addition to endothelial nitric oxide synthetase. For example, evidence exists that H1 histamine receptors on vascular endothelial cells generate nitric oxide during cutaneous active vasodilation [57]. It has also been suggested that the release of histamine from mast cells induced by VIP also could be involved, because histamine increases the bioavailability of nitric oxide in the skin [57, 58].

Nitric oxide, once produced, diffuses both into the blood and into the surrounding vascular smooth muscle. In smooth muscle, nitric oxide activates the soluble enzyme in the cytoplasm, guanylate cyclase, which catalyzes the production of cyclic guanosine monophosphate (cyclic GMP) (Fig. 2) [59].

Cyclic GMP has several biological actions which include decreasing calcium permeability, inhibiting actomyosin ATPase activity, and increasing potassium permeability in vascular smooth muscle. These three functions, taken together, have the combined effect of relaxing vascular smooth muscle [60].

Nitric oxide also has other effects on the endothelial cell and its environment. These autocrine and paracrine effects include nitric oxide being a potent anti-inflammatory agent on blood vessel walls, inhibiting leukocyte adhesion [61], platelet adhesion, and smooth muscle cell proliferation [62], promoting insulin release [63], and mediating the immune response to inflammation [64].

Nitric oxide also is involved in physiologic functions outside of the vascular endothelial cells. These include neuronal transmission [65–67], pulmonary vascular remodeling [68], arterial sclerosis [69], and exercise-induced cardiac protection [70]. Impaired production or bioavailability of nitric oxide leads to endothelial dysfunction and is the root cause of much different cardiovascular pathology including diabetes, hypertension, heart failure, and coronary artery disease [53].

Nitric oxide is derived from the bioconversion of the amino acid, L-arginine, to the amino acid, L-citrulline (Fig. 1). Like all amino acids,

L-arginine and L-citrulline are nitrogen-bearing compounds. The L-arginine molecule has four nitrogens: when bioconverted to L-citrulline, it loses an atom of nitrogen and of oxygen to form nitric oxide and yields another amino acid with three nitrogens, L-citrulline.

A family of enzymes called nitric oxide synthetases produce nitric oxide in various organ systems. The enzymes include neuronal nitric oxide synthetase (NOS), inducible nitric oxide synthetase (INOS), and endothelial nitric oxide synthetase (ENOS) [71]. ENOS is the predominant form of nitric oxide synthetase in the vasculature [72]. There are three subunits in ENOS: a central calmodulin-binding subunit, an oxidative, and reductase end. In vascular endothelial cells, ENOS is normally inactive. It is activated through a complex sequence of chemical reactions that involves the binding of nicotinamide adenine dinucleotide phosphate (NADPH), flavin mononucleotide, and flavin adenosine dinucleotide [72]. Mediated by flavin, electrons are transferred from the carboxylate (COOH) terminal bound to NADPH to the heme of the NH2 terminus. These electrons activate oxygen. L-Arginine is reduced to L-citrulline in two phases. In the first phase, L-arginine binds to ENOS. In the second phase, it is oxidized to L-citrulline and releases nitric oxide [71].

Intracellular calcium modulates the activity of ENOS through the calcium-binding subunit [28]. Intracellular calcium is mobilized through various signaling pathways, and ENOS is ultimately activated by phosphorylation at one of six phosphorylation sites [73]. Calcium-activated calmodulin increases the rate of transfer of electrons from NADPH to ENOS (Fig. 3). (The complex system of reactions used to increase calcium mobility from the extracellular to intracellular space is discussed in another section of this chapter.) Other substances, such as proteins and free fatty acids can also modulate the activation of ENOS [73–75].

Phosphorylation of ENOS via protein kinases is a critical step in its activation [76]. To date, six phosphorylation sites have been identified, including serine 1177, threonine 495, protein kinase B (pkb-akt) 939, adenosine monophosphate-activated kinase, protein kinase A, and protein kinase G [77]. Multiple signaling pathways are associated with different processes in vascular endothelial cells for the activation pathways for ENOS [53, 77]. For example, the ENOS cascade can be activated by receptors

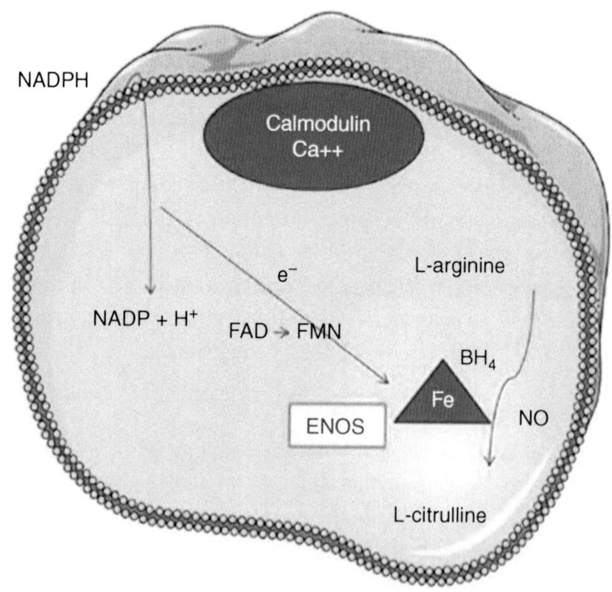

Fig. 3 Reaction and cofactors in ENOS

for estrogen and glucocorticoids [78], insulin and vascular endothelial growth factor (VEGF) [79], blood flow, and laminar shear stress [80, 81].

The balance between nitric oxide production and degradation determines the bioavailability of nitric oxide. When nitric oxide bioavailability is reduced, heightened vasoconstriction occurs, as seen in hypertension, cardiovascular disease, and diabetes [82, 83].

Impairments of ENOS activity can affect nitric oxide production. For example, instability in ENOS may liberate oxygen instead of nitric oxide [79]. Decreased bioavailability of L-arginine may cause ENOS to reduce production of nitric oxide in vivo [84]. Oxidative stress also reduces nitric oxide bioavailability through degradation. Oxides and superoxides degrade nitric oxide, yielding molecules that bear three oxygen atoms, such as peroxynitrate [85]. These reactive oxygen species can in turn cause cellular damage. Oxidative stress potentially can be moderated via activating NADPH oxidases or xanthine oxidases in the vascular wall [86, 87].

Diabetes and cigarette smoking may not alter nitric oxide production via NOS enzymatic pathways, yet still reduce nitric oxide bioavailability by increasing oxidative stress. The result is impaired vasodilatation [85]. This raises cardiac work and blood pressure.

Other Vasodilators

Prostacyclin (PGI_2), a prostaglandin, is another vasodilator released by vascular endothelial cells [88]. In younger people, vasodilation is mediated through the release of both nitric oxide and prostacyclin [88]. However, as people age, prostacyclin production is impaired and nitric oxide becomes the predominant vasodilator [89]. One study of younger subjects revealed that at least 60 % of acetylcholine-mediated vasodilatation was preserved after inhibition of both ENOS and cyclooxygenase (COX) [88]. Although this shows the importance of nitric oxide and prostacyclin in regulating cutaneous circulation, it points to other substances released by vascular endothelial cells, especially in younger individuals, that also mediate an increase in skin blood flow [88].

For example, in studies of chronic inflammation of the skin, neuropeptides such as substance P can be released from sympathetic nerve terminals [90]. Substance P binds to the endothelial cell on the NK-1 receptor [90]. In rats, administration of the NK-1 receptor antagonist, CP-96-345, significantly reduced the blood flow increase which occurred during sympathetic nerve stimulation [90]. Thus, substance P may be responsible for the vasodilation seen with inflammation in rats [91] and in response to electrical stimulation of sympathetic nerves [92] and other conditions such as electrical stimulation of the lumbar sympathetic trunk [90]. Substance P is normally expressed in small dorsal root ganglion neurons and in the skin and is upregulated in inflammatory conditions [93]. Nerve growth factors from inflamed tissue play a role in upregulating the production of substance P [93]. Because sympathetic postganglionic neurons are affected by nerve growth factors from chronic inflammation, it has been hypothesized that upregulation of substance P alters the normal sympathetic combination of neurotransmitters released by sympathetic nerves [90].

Neuronal Controlled Vasoconstriction

Norepinephrine and one or more co-transmitters mediate sympathetic vasoconstriction [94]. Postsynaptic alpha-2-adrenergic receptors on vascular endothelial cells have a high affinity for norepinephrine. Once these receptors bind norepinephrine, vascular endothelial cells release prostaglandin H2, a fat-soluble prostaglandin; this prostaglandin increases the permeability of the surrounding vascular smooth muscle cells to calcium and sodium, causing vasoconstriction.

Other neuropeptides, such as neuropeptides Y and ATP, are colocated in presynaptic storage vesicles with norepinephrine in the nerve terminals. In animal models, these neuropeptides have been shown to participate in altering the speed of response to noradrenergic vasoconstriction [95–97].

Vascular endothelial cells in the skin have both -alpha-1 and alpha-2 adrenergic receptors. However, some adrenergic beta-receptors are also found in the skin vasculature (vasoconstriction) to sympathetic vasoconstrictor stimuli. A complete blockade of alpha-1, alpha-2, and beta adrenergic receptors fails to totally abolish cutaneous vasoconstriction induced by hypothermia. This shows that other substances, such as neuropeptides, are also involved in the vasoconstrictor response. For example, when both alpha- and beta-receptors in the forearm skin of young subjects were blocked, the maximal vasoconstriction at this site induced by whole body cooling was attenuated by only 40 % [98]. However, in subjects over age 61, blocking these receptors eliminated vasoconstriction completely. Thus, as was the case for vasodilation, the number of neurotransmitters and receptors involved in the process of vasoconstriction decreases with age. Said another way, the contribution of co-transmitters to sympathetic vasoconstriction by norepinephrine decreases with age.

Local Effectors of Skin Blood Flow

Anoxia

The smooth muscle response of blood vessels to local pressure, heat, and anoxia is also mediated by the vascular endothelial cell. For example, cutaneous reactive hyperemia occurs when the circulation in the skin is occluded for even a short period of time [99]. The pattern of the transient rise of skin blood flow and the exponential decrease back to baseline blood flow is called a reactive hyperemia. The primary cause is believed to be myogenic relaxation of blood vessels; however, local mediators produced by the ischemic tissues may also play a significant role. One study implicated sensory nerves in this hyperemic response. In healthy adults, blocking sensory nerves with local anesthesia reduced the local reactive hyperemic response of the skin microcirculation.

This raises the possibility of an axon-axon reflex. Mediators of this local response are nitric oxide, prostacyclin, and endothelium-derived hyperpolarizing factors (EDHF). After ischemia, there is an increase in calcium permeability in vascular endothelial cells through a type of voltage-gated calcium channel called a TRPV-4 channel in the endothelial cell membrane. Both sensory nerves and TRPV (transient receptor potential voltage-gated) calcium channels play major roles in the EDHF component of the reactive hyperemia; these contributors to reactive hyperemia work partly independently of nitric oxide and prostaglandin-mediated pathways.

Local Heat

Endothelial cells also mediate the blood flow response of the skin to temperature applied directly to the skin (local heat). When skin temperature rises, cutaneous blood vessels dilate. Maximal skin blood flow is reached when skin temperature is about 42 °C sustained for 30 min. Local vasodilation is a biphasic response, with an initial rapid vasodilation followed by a sustained blood flow response. The biphasic mechanism of local cutaneous vasodilation involves both neuromechanisms (reflexes in axons) as well as generation of nitric oxide. The two mechanisms are independent of each other.

When heat is first applied to the skin, sensory nerves respond with a local reflex which does not involve the spinal cord. Mediated by TRPV-1 sensory receptors, this response causes the release of substance P from nerve endings through a local axon-axon reflex. Substance P causes relaxation in the vascular smooth muscle. But this phase lasts only a few seconds. The sustained response to local temperature is mediated by nitric oxide and is mediated through TRPV-4 calcium channels. This continuous, or plateau, phase is abolished by the nitric oxide inhibitor, L-NAME. Because activation of the enzyme, nitric oxide synthetase, involves heat shock proteins, heat shock protein inhibitors (HSP 90 inhibitors) reduce the magnitude of sustained increase in skin blood flow produced by local heat.

Shear Stress

Shear receptors are present on the surface of vascular endothelial cells sensing shear in blood vessels. These shear receptors activate the enzyme nitric oxide synthetase through a prostaglandin intermediate. The prostaglandin released by shear receptors activates transient receptor potential vanilloid 4 (TRPV-4) voltage-gated calcium channels which then increase calcium permeability of the cell membrane. These are the same TRPV-4 channels that are involved in the prolonged response to elevated skin temperature described above. In both cases, the influx of calcium through TRPV-4 channels activates the enzyme nitric oxide synthetase. Thus, voltage-gated TRPV-4 calcium channels are involved in a number of different processes to activate endothelial nitric oxide synthetase.

Vertical Pressure

Conduit blood vessels as well as blood vessels in the microcirculation are susceptible to local vertical pressures as well as shear forces. Shear receptors detect increases in blood flow downstream; this allows the vascular resistance in these larger blood vessels to be reduced when blood flow rises. Other receptors in blood vessels sense vertical pressure. Vertical pressure, such as standing on the feet or applied pressure against the skin, is sensed by vascular endothelial cells through TRPV-4 voltage-gated calcium channels [100, 101]. Consequently, applying light pressure to the skin (<4 kPa) causes a local increase in circulation. This may be a protective mechanism when skin vessels are constricted by local pressure, causing the vessels to compensate by dilating.

Osmolarity

In many cells in the body, including aortic cells and small vascular endothelial cells, TRPV-4 vanilloid receptor channels also regulate cellular osmolarity. If the cell becomes hyperosmotic, the TRPV-4 calcium channels in the cell are inhibited and calcium influx is reduced. Since the TRPV-4 voltage-gated channel is the same channel that responds to local heat and other stimuli, increased osmolarity can inhibit vasodilation due to other stressors. If there is an increase in blood osmolarity due to dehydration, for example, the normal vasodilatation of skin blood vessels in response to whole body heating is diminished or abolished [102, 103]. The same is true when local heat is applied to the skin. Application of a dry heat pack to the skin causes a smaller increase in skin blood flow than does a moist heat pack at the same skin temperature [41, 104–108]. If the whole body is heated in warm water, the skin blood flow response is greater than that of whole body warming in dry heat [108].

Other Factors that Alter Blood Flow Through Endothelial Cells

Endothelial cells have receptors for adenosine tri phosphate (ATP), histamine, bradykinins, and prostaglandins, which also cause the release of vasodilators and vasoconstrictors by vascular endothelial cells, thereby affecting blood flow. One substance that has a large effect on the endothelial cell is angiotensin II. Endothelial cells in the blood vessels and lungs have an enzyme, angiotensin converting enzyme (ACE). This enzyme converts the inactive forms of angiotensin, angiotensin I, to the vasoactive form, angiotensin II. Binding of angiotensin II on vascular endothelial cells causes the synthesis and release of prostaglandin H2 from endothelial cells. Prostaglandin H2 is derived from arachidonic acid and is fat soluble. It diffuses rapidly to the vascular smooth muscle causing contraction mediated by an increase in smooth muscle cell membrane calcium permeability.

Interaction Between Stimuli on Endothelial Cells

Obviously, a number of stimuli can alter the production of vasodilators and vasoconstrictors released by endothelial cells. There is an interaction that occurs in the vascular smooth muscle between endothelial-released vasoconstrictor to vasodilator compounds. This is in addition to the interaction on the endothelial membrane such as

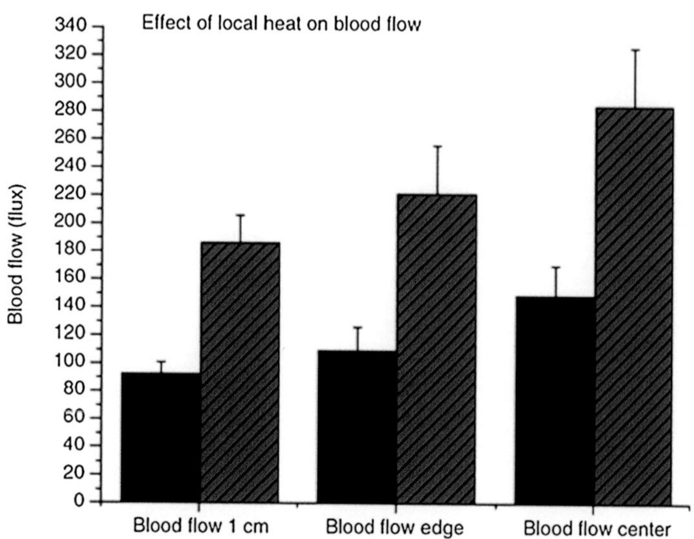

Fig. 4 The effect of local heat on blood flow 1 cm outside and at the edge and inside of wounds in the group of subjects +/− SD. The hatched bars show the post stimulation data

on TRPV-4 channels described above by different stressors. In the sympathetic nervous system, if a greater number of action potentials occur in vasoconstrictor nerves than in vasodilator nerves, in balance, more vasoconstrictors (such as prostaglandin H2) than vasodilators (such as nitric oxide) will be released from endothelial cells. Under these conditions, the smooth muscle is tipped toward vasoconstriction. If, on the other hand, more vasodilatory-inducing compounds are released from endothelial cells than vasoconstrictors, the smooth muscles will dilate on the arteries.

However, when multiple stimuli, such as electric current or heat, are applied simultaneously to vascular endothelial cells, the response is not simply additive but may be synergistic [105]. For example, Fig. 4 shows that in and around a wound, the blood flow in response to inflammatory cytokines such as histamine plus heat has shown a massive increase in blood flow much greater than would be seen by heat alone [109–111]. Another example is heat plus electrical stimulation. If both are applied to the skin at the same time, there is a much greater release of nitric oxide and hence vasodilation of blood vessels than would be due to either stimuli alone or even if added together [41]. Thus, a 1-degree change in skin temperature from 35 to 36 °C causes a much larger increase in blood flow than a 1-degree rise from 34 to 35 °C. If the same current is applied to the skin and local skin temperature is cool (<25 °C), no increase in blood flow occurs at all. A combination of local and global heat also produces synergistic effects. Heating the entire body while using ice to cool skin locally abolishes the local skin blood flow response in that area.

Many of these effects may be caused by interaction of biochemical intermediates in the TRPV-4 calcium channels. For example, raising skin temperature from 25 to 35 °C causes calcium influx into vascular endothelial cells to rise nonlinearly as a function of temperature [107]. Because the receptor channels respond nonlinearly, ENOS activation by temperature is similarly nonlinear. Because of this nonlinearity, the change in blood flow to a complex combination of stimuli (such as global heating of the blood, local heating of the skin, and simultaneous hydration or dehydration of the body) may cause hard-to-predict results on blood flow given the unknown in these biochemical pathways and their receptors. Endothelial agonists and antagonists, such as estrogen, a TRPV agonist, when present, further confound the response. While diabetes, for example, reduces skin blood flow and rest in response to a stressor, the presence of inflammatory mediators associated with obesity also has the same effect making the contribution of metabolic disorders such as diabetes, where obesity is also common, hard to fully distinguish [112].

Conclusion

The control of blood flow is a complex process. The center of the process is the vascular endothelial cell. Normally, it releases a balance between vasodilators and vasoconstrictors. In health, there is a wide margin to increase blood flow to the skin at least 30-fold. Numerous factors can alter blood flow including local pressure, heat, and metabolism as well as control from the autonomic nervous system. It was at one time believed that only the sympathetic nervous system controls blood flow to the skin and organs, but recent research may show a parasympathetic role through neurons that release nitric oxide.

References

1. Johnson JM, Minson CT, Kellogg Jr DL. Cutaneous vasodilator and vasoconstrictor mechanisms in temperature regulation. Compr Physiol. 2014;4 (1):33–89.
2. Sukriti S, et al. Mechanisms regulating endothelial permeability. Pulm Circ. 2014;4(4):535–51.
3. Mehta D, Malik AB. Signaling mechanisms regulating endothelial permeability. Physiol Rev. 2006;86 (1):279–367.
4. Chavez A, Smith M, Mehta D. New insights into the regulation of vascular permeability. Int Rev Cell Mol Biol. 2011;290:205–48.
5. Esser S, et al. Vascular endothelial growth factor induces VE-cadherin tyrosine phosphorylation in endothelial cells. J Cell Sci. 1998;111 (Pt 13):1853–65.
6. Bates DO, Harper SJ. Regulation of vascular permeability by vascular endothelial growth factors. Vasc Pharmacol. 2002;39(4–5):225–37.
7. Farage MA, Miller KW, Ledger WJ. Determining the cause of vulvovaginal symptoms. Obstet Gynecol Surv. 2008;63(7):445–64.
8. Koroxenidis GT, Shepherd JT, Marshall RJ. Cardiovascular response to acute heat stress. J Appl Physiol. 1961;16:869–72.
9. Charkoudian N. Mechanisms and modifiers of reflex induced cutaneous vasodilation and vasoconstriction in humans. J Appl Physiol (1985). 2010;109(4):1221–8.
10. Whitney RJ. The measurement of volume changes in human limbs. J Physiol. 1953;121(1):1–27.
11. Williams CA, Mudd JG, Lind AR. The forearm blood flow during intermittent hand-grip isometric exercise. Circ Res. 1981;48(6 Pt 2):I110–7.
12. Lind AR, et al. Influence of posture on isometric fatigue. J Appl Physiol Respir Environ Exerc Physiol. 1978;45(2):270–4.
13. Lind AR, Williams CA. Changes in the forearm blood flow following brief isometric hand-grip contractions at different tensions [proceedings]. J Physiol. 1977;272(1):97P–8.
14. Edholm OG, Fox RH, Macpherson RK. Vasomotor control of the cutaneous blood vessels in the human forearm. J Physiol. 1957;139(3):455–65.
15. Hagg A, et al. Increase of plasma renin activity at renal blood flow estimations with the xenon133 washout technique in patients with renal artery stenosis. Clin Physiol. 1987;7(1):55–61.
16. Kostuik JP, et al. The measurement of skin blood flow in peripheral vascular disease by epicutaneous application of Xenon133. J Bone Joint Surg Am. 1976;58 (6):833–7.
17. James GW, Paul MH, Wessel HU. Thermal dilution: instrumentation with thermistors. J Appl Physiol. 1965;20(3):547–52.
18. Petrofsky JS. In vivo measurement of brain blood flow in the cat. IEEE Trans Biomed Eng. 1979;26 (8):441–5.
19. Petrofsky JS. Resting blood flow in the skin: does it exist, and what is the influence of temperature, aging, and diabetes? J Diabetes Sci Technol. 2012;6 (3):674–85.
20. Oberg PA. Laser-Doppler flowmetry. Crit Rev Biomed Eng. 1990;18(2):125–63.
21. Lotter O. et al. Utilization of laser Doppler flowmetry and tissue spectrophotometry for burn depth assessment using a miniature swine model. Wound Repair Regen. 2015;23(1):132–6.
22. Mazhar A, et al. Noncontact imaging of burn depth and extent in a porcine model using spatial frequency domain imaging. J Biomed Opt. 2014;19 (8):086019.
23. Ganapathy P, et al. Dual-imaging system for burn depth diagnosis. Burns. 2014;40(1):67–81.
24. Nilsson GE, Tenland T, Oberg PA. Evaluation of a laser Doppler flowmeter for measurement of tissue blood flow. IEEE Trans Biomed Eng. 1980;27 (10):597–604.
25. Lindblad LE, et al. Laser Doppler flow-meter assessment of iontophoretically applied norepinephrine on human finger skin circulation. J Invest Dermatol. 1986;87(5):634–6.
26. Kellogg Jr DL, Johnson JM, Kosiba WA. Selective abolition of adrenergic vasoconstrictor responses in skin by local iontophoresis of bretylium. Am J Physiol. 1989;257(5 Pt 2):H1599–606.
27. Dreyfuss C, et al. L-NAME iontophoresis: a tool to assess NO-mediated vasoreactivity during thermal hyperemic vasodilation in humans. J Cardiovasc Pharmacol. 2013;61(5):361–8.
28. Fox RH, Edholm OG. Nervous control of the cutaneous circulation. Br Med Bull. 1963;19:110–4.
29. Johnson JM, et al. Regulation of the cutaneous circulation. Fed Proc. 1986;45(13):2841–50.
30. Charkoudian N, Johnson JM. Altered reflex control of cutaneous circulation by female sex steroids is

independent of prostaglandins. Am J Physiol. 1999;276(5 Pt 2):H1634–40.
31. Toda N, Okamura T. Recent advances in research on nitrergic nerve-mediated vasodilatation. Pflügers Arch. 2015;467(6):1165–78.
32. Lee TJ, Su C, Bevan JA. Nonsympathetic dilator innervation of cat cerebral arteries. Experientia. 1975;31(12):1424–6.
33. Toda N, Okamura T. Cerebral blood flow regulation by nitric oxide in Alzheimer's disease. J Alzheimers Dis. 2012;32(3):569–78.
34. Toda N, Hayashi S. Responses of canine coronary arteries to transmural electrical stimulation and nicotine. Eur J Pharmacol. 1982;80(1):73–81.
35. Shiraishi S, et al. Differences in adrenergic nerve and receptor function in dog internal thoracic, coronary and mesenteric arteries. Jpn J Pharmacol. 1994;66 (4):481–8.
36. Scott JA, McCormack DG. Nonadrenergic noncholinergic vasodilation of guinea pig pulmonary arteries is mediated by nitric oxide. Can J Physiol Pharmacol. 1999;77(2):89–95.
37. Wang X, Cupples WA. Brown Norway rats show impaired nNOS-mediated information transfer in renal autoregulation. Can J Physiol Pharmacol. 2009;87(1):29–36.
38. Lau KS, et al. nNOS and eNOS modulate cGMP formation and vascular response in contracting fast-twitch skeletal muscle. Physiol Genomics. 2000;2 (1):21–7.
39. Johnson JM, Kellogg Jr DL. Local thermal control of the human cutaneous circulation. J Appl Physiol (1985). 2010;109(4):1229–38.
40. Maloney-Hinds C, et al. The role of nitric oxide in skin blood flow increases due to vibration in healthy adults and adults with type 2 diabetes. Diabetes Technol Ther. 2009;11(1):39–43.
41. Petrofsky J, et al. The interrelationships between electrical stimulation, the environment surrounding the vascular endothelial cells of the skin, and the role of nitric oxide in mediating the blood flow response to electrical stimulation. Med Sci Monit. 2007;13(9): CR391–7.
42. Okamura T, et al. Neurogenic vasodilatation of canine isolated small labial arteries. J Pharmacol Exp Ther. 1999;288(3):1031–6.
43. Rowell LB. Human cardiovascular adjustments to exercise and thermal stress. Physiol Rev. 1974;54 (1):75–159.
44. Del Pozzi AT, Hodges GJ. To reheat, or to not reheat: that is the question: the efficacy of a local reheating protocol on mechanisms of cutaneous vasodilatation. Microvasc Res. 2015;97:47–54.
45. Farrell DM, Bishop VS. Permissive role for nitric oxide in active thermoregulatory vasodilation in rabbit ear. Am J Physiol. 1995;269(5 Pt 2):H1613–8.
46. Kellogg Jr DL, et al. Cutaneous active vasodilation in humans is mediated by cholinergic nerve cotransmission. Circ Res. 1995;77(6):1222–8.
47. Bennett LA, et al. Evidence for a role for vasoactive intestinal peptide in active vasodilatation in the cutaneous vasculature of humans. J Physiol. 2003;552 (Pt 1):223–32.
48. Wilkins BW, et al. Vasoactive intestinal peptide fragment VIP10-28 and active vasodilation in human skin. J Appl Physiol (1985). 2005;99(6):2294–301.
49. Kellogg Jr DL, et al. Nitric oxide and cutaneous active vasodilation during heat stress in humans. J Appl Physiol (1985). 1998;85(3):824–9.
50. Shastry S, et al. Effects of nitric oxide synthase inhibition on cutaneous vasodilation during body heating in humans. J Appl Physiol (1985). 1998;85(3):830–4.
51. Taylor WF, Bishop VS. A role for nitric oxide in active thermoregulatory vasodilation. Am J Physiol. 1993;264(5 Pt 2):H1355–9.
52. Stuart-Smith K. Demystified. Nitric oxide. Mol Pathol. 2002;55(6):360–6.
53. Mata-Greenwood E, Chen DB. Racial differences in nitric oxide-dependent vasorelaxation. Reprod Sci. 2008;15(1):9–25.
54. Quillon A, Fromy B, Debret R. Endothelium microenvironment sensing leading to nitric oxide mediated vasodilation: a review of nervous and biomechanical signals. Nitric Oxide. 2015;45:20–6.
55. Chen KD, et al. Mechanotransduction in response to shear stress. Roles of receptor tyrosine kinases, integrins, and Shc. J Biol Chem. 1999;274 (26):18393–400.
56. Kuhr F, et al. Differential regulation of inducible and endothelial nitric oxide synthase by kinin B1 and B2 receptors. Neuropeptides. 2010;44(2):145–54.
57. Wong BJ, Wilkins BW, Minson CT. H1 but not H2 histamine receptor activation contributes to the rise in skin blood flow during whole body heating in humans. J Physiol. 2004;560(Pt 3):941–8.
58. Kamijo Y, Lee K, Mack GW. Active cutaneous vasodilation in resting humans during mild heat stress. J Appl Physiol (1985). 2005;98(3):829–37.
59. Dupont LL, et al. Role of the nitric oxide-soluble guanylyl cyclase pathway in obstructive airway diseases. Pulm Pharmacol Ther. 2014;29(1):1–6.
60. Harraz OF, Brett SE, Welsh DG. Nitric oxide suppresses vascular voltage-gated T-type Ca2+ channels through cGMP/PKG signaling. Am J Physiol Heart Circ Physiol. 2014;306(2):H279–85.
61. Kubes P, Suzuki M, Granger DN. Nitric oxide: an endogenous modulator of leukocyte adhesion. Proc Natl Acad Sci U S A. 1991;88(11):4651–5.
62. Radomski MW, Palmer RM, Moncada S. The role of nitric oxide and cGMP in platelet adhesion to vascular endothelium. Biochem Biophys Res Commun. 1987;148(3):1482–9.
63. Scherrer U, Sartori C. Defective nitric oxide synthesis: a link between metabolic insulin resistance, sympathetic overactivity and cardiovascular morbidity. Eur J Endocrinol. 2000;142(4):315–23.
64. Keeble JE, Moore PK. Pharmacology and potential therapeutic applications of nitric oxide-releasing

non-steroidal anti-inflammatory and related nitric oxide-donating drugs. Br J Pharmacol. 2002;137(3):295–310.
65. Rauhala P, Andoh T, Chiueh CC. Neuroprotective properties of nitric oxide and S-nitrosoglutathione. Toxicol Appl Pharmacol. 2005;207(2 Suppl):91–5.
66. Vaananen AJ, Kankuri E, Rauhala P. Nitric oxide-related species-induced protein oxidation: reversible, irreversible, and protective effects on enzyme function of papain. Free Radic Biol Med. 2005;38(8):1102–11.
67. de la Torre JC, Aliev G. Inhibition of vascular nitric oxide after rat chronic brain hypoperfusion: spatial memory and immunocytochemical changes. J Cereb Blood Flow Metab. 2005;25(6):663–72.
68. Ricciardolo FL. Multiple roles of nitric oxide in the airways. Thorax. 2003;58(2):175–82.
69. Kawashima S, Yokoyama M. Dysfunction of endothelial nitric oxide synthase and atherosclerosis. Arterioscler Thromb Vasc Biol. 2004;24(6):998–1005.
70. Brunner H, et al. Endothelial function and dysfunction. Part II: association with cardiovascular risk factors and diseases. A statement by the Working Group on Endothelins and Endothelial Factors of the European Society of Hypertension. J Hypertens. 2005;23(2):233–46.
71. Alderton WK, Cooper CE, Knowles RG. Nitric oxide synthases: structure, function and inhibition. Biochem J. 2001;357(Pt 3):593–615.
72. Forstermann U, et al. Isoforms of nitric oxide synthase. Properties, cellular distribution and expressional control. Biochem Pharmacol. 1995;50(9):1321–32.
73. Fulton D, Gratton JP, Sessa WC. Post-translational control of endothelial nitric oxide synthase: why isn't calcium/calmodulin enough? J Pharmacol Exp Ther. 2001;299(3):818–24.
74. Bui C, et al. Acute effect of a single high-fat meal on forearm blood flow, blood pressure and heart rate in healthy male Asians and Caucasians: a pilot study. Southeast Asian J Trop Med Public Health. 2010;41(2):490–500.
75. Yim J, et al. Protective effect of anti-oxidants on endothelial function in young Korean-Asians compared to Caucasians. Med Sci Monit. 2012;18(8):CR467–79.
76. Mount PF, Kemp BE, Power DA. Regulation of endothelial and myocardial NO synthesis by multi-site eNOS phosphorylation. J Mol Cell Cardiol. 2007;42(2):271–9.
77. Chen ZP, et al. AMP-activated protein kinase phosphorylation of endothelial NO synthase. FEBS Lett. 1999;443(3):285–9.
78. Haynes MP, Russell KS, Bender JR. Molecular mechanisms of estrogen actions on the vasculature. J Nucl Cardiol. 2000;7(5):500–8.
79. Montagnani M, et al. Insulin-stimulated activation of eNOS is independent of Ca2+ but requires phosphorylation by Akt at Ser(1179). J Biol Chem. 2001;276(32):30392–8.
80. Dimmeler S, et al. Fluid shear stress stimulates phosphorylation of Akt in human endothelial cells: involvement in suppression of apoptosis. Circ Res. 1998;83(3):334–41.
81. Dimmeler S, et al. Activation of nitric oxide synthase in endothelial cells by Akt-dependent phosphorylation. Nature. 1999;399(6736):601–5.
82. Griendling KK, FitzGerald GA. Oxidative stress and cardiovascular injury: part I: basic mechanisms and in vivo monitoring of ROS. Circulation. 2003;108(16):1912–6.
83. Griendling KK, FitzGerald GA. Oxidative stress and cardiovascular injury: part II: animal and human studies. Circulation. 2003;108(17):2034–40.
84. Forstermann U, et al. Nitric oxide synthase isozymes. Characterization, purification, molecular cloning, and functions. Hypertension. 1994;23(6 Pt 2):1121–31.
85. Rahman I, Biswas SK, Kode A. Oxidant and antioxidant balance in the airways and airway diseases. Eur J Pharmacol. 2006;533(1–3):222–39.
86. Hare JM. Nitroso-redox balance in the cardiovascular system. N Engl J Med. 2004;351(20):2112–4.
87. Kozak AJ, et al. Role of peroxynitrite in the process of vascular tone regulation by nitric oxide and prostanoids–a nanotechnological approach. Prostaglandins Leukot Essent Fat Acids. 2005;72(2):105–13.
88. Lenasi H, Strucl M. The effect of nitric oxide synthase and cyclooxygenase inhibition on cutaneous microvascular reactivity. Eur J Appl Physiol. 2008;103(6):719–26.
89. Malty AM, Petrofsky J. The effect of electrical stimulation on a normal skin blood flow in active young and older adults. Med Sci Monit. 2007;13(4):CR147–55.
90. Koeda T, et al. Substance P is involved in the cutaneous blood flow increase response to sympathetic nerve stimulation in persistently inflamed rats. J Physiol Sci. 2007;57(6):361–6.
91. Lam FY, Ferrell WR. Acute inflammation in the rat knee joint attenuates sympathetic vasoconstriction but enhances neuropeptide-mediated vasodilatation assessed by laser Doppler perfusion imaging. Neuroscience. 1993;52(2):443–9.
92. McDougall JJ, Karimian SM, Ferrell WR. Prolonged alteration of vasoconstrictor and vasodilator responses in rat knee joints by adjuvant monoarthritis. Exp Physiol. 1995;80(3):349–57.
93. Donnerer J, et al. Upregulation, release and axonal transport of substance P and calcitonin gene-related peptide in adjuvant inflammation and regulatory function of nerve growth factor. Regul Pept. 1993;46(1–2):150–4.
94. Stephens DP, et al. Neuropeptide Y antagonism reduces reflex cutaneous vasoconstriction in humans. Am J Physiol Heart Circ Physiol. 2004;287(3):H1404–9.

95. Bradley E, et al. Effects of varying impulse number on cotransmitter contributions to sympathetic vasoconstriction in rat tail artery. Am J Physiol Heart Circ Physiol. 2003;284(6):H2007–14.
96. Hashim MA, Tadepalli AS. Cutaneous vasomotor effects of neuropeptide Y. Neuropeptides. 1995;29(5):263–71.
97. Toba K, et al. Improved skin blood flow and cutaneous temperature in the foot of a patient with arteriosclerosis obliterans by vasopressin V1 antagonist (OPC21268). A case report. Angiology. 1995;46(11):1027–33.
98. Thompson CS, Kenney WL. Altered neurotransmitter control of reflex vasoconstriction in aged human skin. J Physiol. 2004;558(Pt 2):697–704.
99. McLellan K, et al. The effects of skin moisture and subcutaneous fat thickness on the ability of the skin to dissipate heat in young and old subjects, with and without diabetes, at three environmental room temperatures. Med Eng Phys. 2009;31(2):165–72.
100. Fromy B, Abraham P, Saumet JL. Non-nociceptive capsaicin-sensitive nerve terminal stimulation allows for an original vasodilatory reflex in the human skin. Brain Res. 1998;811(1–2):166–8.
101. Garry A, et al. Cellular mechanisms underlying cutaneous pressure-induced vasodilation: in vivo involvement of potassium channels. Am J Physiol Heart Circ Physiol. 2005;289(1):H174–80.
102. Montain SJ, Coyle EF. Fluid ingestion during exercise increases skin blood flow independent of increases in blood volume. J Appl Physiol (1985). 1992;73(3):903–10.
103. Coyle EF, Montain SJ. Benefits of fluid replacement with carbohydrate during exercise. Med Sci Sports Exerc. 1992;24(9 Suppl):S324–30.
104. Petrofsky J, et al. Impact of hydrotherapy on skin blood flow: how much is due to moisture and how much is due to heat? Physiother Theory Pract. 2010;26(2):107–12.
105. Petrofsky J, et al. Does skin moisture influence the blood flow response to local heat? A re-evaluation of the Pennes model. J Med Eng Technol. 2009;33(7):532–7.
106. Petrofsky JS, et al. The effect of the moisture content of a local heat source on the blood flow response of the skin. Arch Dermatol Res. 2009;301(8):581–5.
107. Petrofsky J, et al. The effect of moist air on skin blood flow and temperature in subjects with and without diabetes. Diabetes Technol Ther. 2012;14(2):105–16.
108. Petrofsky J, et al. Dry heat, moist heat and body fat: are heating modalities really effective in people who are overweight? J Med Eng Technol. 2009;33(5):361–9.
109. Lawson D, Petrofsky JS. A randomized control study on the effect of biphasic electrical stimulation in a warm room on skin blood flow and healing rates in chronic wounds of patients with and without diabetes. Med Sci Monit. 2007;13(6):CR258–63.
110. Petrofsky JS, et al. The influence of local versus global heat on the healing of chronic wounds in patients with diabetes. Diabetes Technol Ther. 2007;9(6):535–44.
111. Suh H, et al. A new electrode design to improve outcomes in the treatment of chronic non-healing wounds in diabetes. Diabetes Technol Ther. 2009;11(5):315–22.
112. Petrofsky JS, et al. What is more damaging to vascular endothelial function: diabetes, age, high BMI, or all of the above? Med Sci Monit. 2013;19:257–63.

Part V

Techniques, Methods, and Tools

Bioengineering Methods and Skin Aging

85

Francesca Giusti and Stefania Seidenari

Contents

Abstract

Skin aging is an uneven process characterized by epidermal and dermal disorders, accompanied by many clinical signs such as skin dryness, color changes, loss of elasticity, wrinkles, and risk of developing skin cancers. The elderly appearance of the skin depends on a combination of intrinsic or chronological aging, modulated by genetically predisposing factors and extrinsic aging or photoaging. This chapter reviews data that have emerged from technologies aiming at quantitatively assessing the effects of aging on the skin.

Introduction

During the last decade, skin aging has become an area of increasing research interest, because of the prolongation of life span in modern society.

Skin aging is an uneven process characterized by epidermal and dermal disorders, accompanied by many clinical signs such as skin dryness, color changes, loss of elasticity, wrinkles, and risk of developing skin cancers. The elderly appearance of the skin depends on a combination of intrinsic or chronological aging, modulated by genetically predisposing factors and extrinsic aging or photoaging, due to environmental factors, mainly UV exposure, and also wind, relative humidity, pollution, and so on. The effects of the UV radiations on sun-exposed sites are superimposed on the morphological, biochemical, and functional

F. Giusti (✉) • S. Seidenari
Department of Dermatology, University of Modena and Reggio Emilia, Modena, Italy
e-mail: francesca.giusti@unimore.it; seidenari.stefania@unimore.it

M.A. Farage et al. (eds.), *Textbook of Aging Skin*,
DOI 10.1007/978-3-662-47398-6_65

changes occurring with aging, making distinction between the two phenomena hard.

Besides genetic aspects, all these environmental factors are responsible for the great interindividual and intraindividual variations and the site-dependent variations of the aging process. A precise and noninvasive quantification of aging is of utmost importance for in vivo studies in skin gerontology and for cosmetic research. Several bioengineering methods have been proposed to objectively, precisely, and noninvasively measure skin aging and to detect early skin damage, which is rather difficult to demonstrate clinically.

This chapter reviews the data that have emerged from recently introduced technologies aiming at quantitatively assessing the effects of aging on the skin.

The variations in biophysical parameters such as hydration and trans-epidermal water loss, which have been evidenced in the skin in elderly subjects, will be discussed in detail in other chapters.

To date, high-frequency ultrasonography has been used most extensively to visualize and quantify age-related skin changes. This chapter focuses on ultrasound findings in intrinsic and extrinsic skin aging. In the last decade, a new noninvasive technique has been developed to examine the epidermis and the papillary dermis at a resolution approaching histological detail: confocal scanning laser microscopy. Review literature data on the application of this promising technique for the study of skin aging have also been included at the end of this chapter.

pH

Cutaneous acidity plays a role in skin barrier homeostasis, in stratum corneum desquamation, and in skin defense against microbiological or chemical insults. In order to measure cutaneous pH, instruments like a glass planar electrode are primarily used. They create a potential difference between the two environments separated by the glass slide, that is, the skin surface and the reference solution contained in the electrode. This potential difference is linearly linked to the difference in H^+ concentration.

Limited data are available on skin pH and age. pH is relatively constant from childhood through age 70. Fluhr et al. did not find a significant difference in pH measured on volar forearm between 44 adults aged 21–44 and 44 children aged 1–6 [1]. These data were confirmed on the forehead in 500 female patients aged 20–70 [2]. In contrast, skin acidity decreases significantly in subjects older than 70 [3, 4]. Wilhelm et al. measured pH on 11 skin sites in 14 young volunteers (mean age 27 years) and in 15 aged volunteers (mean age 71 years) and noted significant differences at the ankle and thigh only [4]. Therefore, the authors attributed the higher pH to stasis and reduced oxygen supply frequently observed in the lower limbs in elderly patients.

Sebum

Sebum production is controlled by the levels of circulating hormones and varies according to the anatomical distribution of sebaceous glands. It is generally measured by an instrument allowing a semiquantitative evaluation of sebum excretion (Sebumeter, Courage and Khazaka Electronic, Köln, Germany). This method is based on photometric measurements of light transmission through a transparent plastic film, which is pressed against the skin in order to obtain adhesion of skin lipids. The recorded values are expressed in arbitrary units, which can be converted into microgram per square centimeter, according to the manufacturer's calibration table.

The sebum excretion rate has been demonstrated to decrease with age by different authors [4–7], more markedly at sites of elevated sebum production. When measuring the casual level of sebum in 63 healthy subjects aged 12–60 and in 24 older subjects at 14 body sites [5], a marked decrease in elderly volunteers was observed, with significantly lower values on the forehead and the upper back (Fig. 1).

It has been proposed that changes in sebum excretion during aging reflect the decrease in the endogenous production of androgens occurring in men and women. In menopausal women receiving hormonal replacement therapy, the sebum

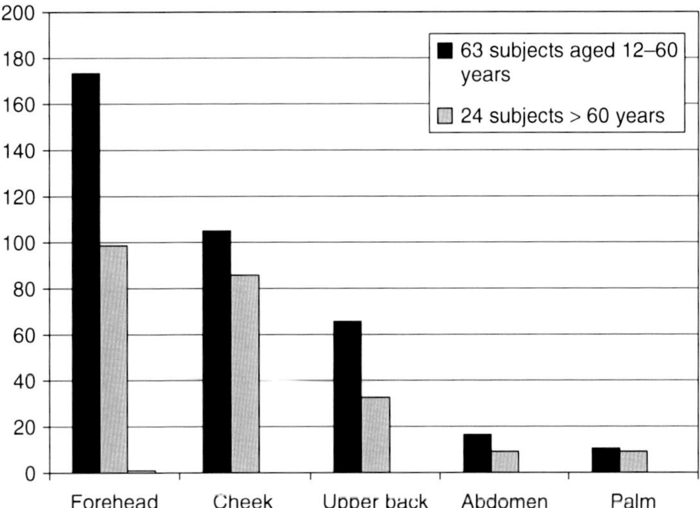

Fig. 1 Casual level of sebum in relation to age ($p < 0.05$ at forehead and upper back)

excretion rate shows a 35 % increase, because of the stimulatory effect of the progestagen component [6]. Caisey et al., by measuring the amount of sebum produced over 1 h on the forehead of 20 young women, 19 premenopausal women, 21 postmenopausal women, and 20 postmenopausal women receiving hormonal replacement therapy, did not find a correlation between age and sebum excretion rate [7]. However, the values in postmenopausal women were significantly lower than in the other groups showing a 35–40 % decrease compared with females receiving estrogen and progesterone. The authors concluded that sebum production is more likely related to hormones than to aging.

Skin Color

Skin color can be determined by a chromameter (Minolta, Osaka, Japan) according to a three-dimensional L* a* b* system. L* represents an attribute on the luminance scale, a* on the red-green color scale, and b* on the yellow-blue one.

Photoaging is clinically characterized by yellowish skin with erythematous areas, associated with telangiectasia and heterogeneity of skin pigmentation. By examining the skin of sun-exposed and adjacent unexposed sites, Richard et al. reported significant differences in L* values and a* values with larger standard deviations at exposed skin sites, indicating a decrease in brightness, an increase in the red component, and color heterogeneity in photodamaged skin in the elderly [8]. In contrast, Warren et al. observed no change in L*a*b* values [9]. In order to study photodamaged skin, Kikuchi-Numagami et al. measured skin color of the dorsum of the hands in 12 middle-aged Japanese golfers, playing golf frequently for the past 4–25 years [10]. By comparing the right hand, exposed to sunlight many hours a day, to the left hand that is protected by a glove from the outer environment, he found that whereas L* value was significantly lower, a* and b* values were significantly higher on the right hand in comparison with the left hand protected by the glove. The differences in L* values were dependent on the length of past golf-playing history.

A negative correlation between L* values and age was found on the lower lips in 80 postmenopausal women, whereas no correspondence was observed between age and the other two color components [7]. L* values were significantly lower in the group of postmenopausal women in comparison with two groups of younger and postmenopausal women receiving hormonal replacement therapy. The authors concluded that menopause may result in a slight darkening of the lip, which could be prevented or corrected by hormonal treatment. Also Guinot et al. reported that menopausal subjects treated with hormonal replacement therapy showed redder lips than untreated menopausal women [11].

Skin Blood Flow

Skin blood perfusion can be quantified by Laser Doppler Flowmetry and Laser Doppler Velocimetry. A helium-neon laser light is transmitted to the skin via an optical fiber to an estimated depth of more than 1 mm. Light reflected from moving erythrocytes is Doppler shifted. The frequency-shifted signal is proportional to blood flow and can be extracted and measured by the instrument in arbitrary units.

Data regarding age-related changes in blood perfusion are often conflicting, probably because of the small sample sizes and the varying age ranges of the studies [1, 3, 12–15]. By using Laser Doppler flowmetry on the volar forearm in 44 children and 44 adults aged 21–44, Fluhr et al. found higher blood flow values in children. On the contrary, Kelly et al. did not observe any significant differences in blood flow perfusion both in ventral forearm and forehead in a small study population comprising ten subjects aged 18–26 and ten subjects aged 65–88 [13]. Likewise, in a study comparing only nine elderly and ten young volunteers, the skin vascular response to heat and cold challenge measured by Laser Doppler Velocimetry was delayed in elderly subjects [14]. This may be due to a reduced vessel density in aged skin. Also in a study population of 201 people aged 10–89, the blood flow measured after immersion in water at 10 °C was lower in subjects over 50 and the restorative ability poorer in subjects over 70 compared with younger ones [15]. The basal blood flow decreased with age in all the areas with high blood flow, such as the lip, finger, nasal tip, and forehead.

In conclusion, trends indicate that aging is associated with a decrease in cutaneous blood perfusion, in particular in photo-exposed areas [1, 3, 12, 14, 15].

Skin Surface Roughness

The morphological study of the skin surface can be performed by optical, mechanical, laser, and transparency profilometry. The first method is based on skin replicas and evaluation of the black-and-white reflections by light irradiation depending on topography of skin furrows. The image is processed using a special image processing software by a CCD camera or a high-resolution black-and-white video and a connected computer. Mechanical profilometry offers a two-dimensional quantification of the absolute height and depth of wrinkles and furrows. Laser profilometry is an optical technique based on the principle of light amplification and reflection from a cutaneous replica. Recently, the visiometer method or transparency profilometry (Skin Visiometer SV600, Courage and Khazaka, Cologne, Germany) has been developed with some advantages, as short processing time and direct visual control of the skin surface topography on the computer monitor. This technique uses a thin silicone gel print of the skin surface, which allows parallel light to pass through and is registered as a change of transparency by a CCD video camera [16].

Aging is characterized by fine and coarse wrinkling, whose estimation is surely of great interest especially in the field of cosmetic research.

By performing laser profilometry on the dorsal surface of the hands in Japanese golfers, Kikuchi-Numagami et al. observed that roughness parameters were increased on the right hand exposed to sun in comparison with the left hand protected by a glove when playing golf [10]. The differences became larger in golfers with lower handicap and longer golf history, probably due to elastogenesis in the dermis of the photoaged skin [9]. Likewise, Quan et al. found significant differences in skin roughness between sun-exposed and sun-protected areas by using mechanical profilometry [17]. However, this difference was significant only in the group of older subjects. To study photodamage and the effect of tretinoin on it, Marks et al. performed optical profilometry on crow's foot areas, associated with other noninvasive and invasive technique, concluding that there is no single method to quantify the degenerative changes due to photodamage [12]. In a study evaluating the crow's feet of 95 women aged 30–50 by transparency profilometry and ultrasonography, an increment of all roughness parameters was observed, as age increases [18]. Moreover, a correlation between skin roughness and dermal density and thickness was found.

Skin Thickness

In order to measure cutaneous thickness under a variety of normal and pathologic, ultrasonography has been widely used for about 30 years. Since penetration depth of the ultrasound waves is inversely related to its frequency, the optimal frequency for achieving a higher resolution for skin examination is 15–20 MHz. The ultrasonic wave (velocity 1,580 m/s) is partially reflected at the boundary between adjacent structures, generating echoes, whose amplitudes are characteristic of the nature of the media. The ultrasonographic image can be evaluated either manually or with computer assistance to quantify skin thickness.

Two forms of ultrasonography, A and B modes, are available. The first gives an unidimensional representation of skin echogenicity and is easier and quicker than the B-mode. However, by A scanning, the determination of the dermis-subcutis interface is based on the observation of a peak corresponding to the impedance jump between adjacent parts of the tissue, making determination of the dermis-subcutaneous tissue interface difficult, whereas B-scan measurement of skin thickness represents the mean of consecutive A-scan lines composing the whole bidimensional image. Thus, the reproducibility of B-mode assessment is higher, enabling the production of bidimensional images of cross sections of the skin. By means of the B-scan method, skin thickness values are approximately 15 % greater than A-scan measurements [19].

Skin thickness has been a widely used parameter to evaluate the influence of different factors on skin aging, but the measurement of age-related changes in skin thickness yielded conflicting results. In fact, depending on the anatomical site, both thinning and thickening are observed. This poor consensus can be explained by differences in the age range and body site of study populations and also in the frequency, mode, and gain curves of the ultrasound technique [20]. Thus, the adhesion to standardized measurements protocols in reproducible conditions is of utmost importance.

Employing A-scan ultrasound on the volar forearm, Tan et al. found that skin thickness increased progressively up to the age of 20 and decreased subsequently [21], whereas Escoffier et al. observed that skin thickness increases up to the age of 20–30 years, remains constant until 65 years, and then gets thinner, being at 90 years significantly thinner than at 5 years [22]. A similar trend was described by de Rigal et al., employing the B-scan method, in a population of 142 females aged from 0 to 90 years [19]. Skin thickness on both the volar and the dorsal aspects of the forearm thickened up to 15 years (maturation phase), did not vary until the seventh decade of life, and diminished thereafter (atrophy phase). These modifications in skin thickness seemed to be correlated with the age-dependent degree of elastosis.

Site-to-site variations in skin thickness related to aging were reported by many authors [23–27].

In 162 volunteers in the age range of 27–90, skin thickness variations were assessed using both A- and B-mode high-frequency ultrasonography at six different anatomical locations (forehead, cheek, volar forearm, dorsal forearm, upper abdomen, and buttocks) [25]. It was found that subjects over 70 years have thinner skin when compared to young volunteers (age *27–31*), but the differences were significant for sun-protected skin sites (abdomen and buttocks) only.

In a study on 90 Danish subjects aged 18–94, skin becomes thicker with age at the forehead and buttocks, but decreases at the extremities (dorsal and ventral forearm, and ankle) significantly [26]. Since these data cannot be explained by differences in sun exposure, the authors concluded that the effect of aging on axial skin could differ from that on extremity skin.

With regard to photoaging, Leveque et al. reported an increase in skin thickness in sun-exposed areas in a study on cyclists in the Tour de France [28]. Likewise, Adhoute et al. observed skin thickening on face and neck sites induced by solar exposure [29]. In 170 women aged from 17 to 76, Takema et al. measured skin thickness on the ventral forearm, forehead, cheeks, and corners of eyes and mouth by employing a 20-MHz A-mode ultrasound scanner [24]. Skin thickness increased with age on all sun-exposed areas of the face, whereas it seemed to decrease on the sun-protected volar forearm. On the contrary, using B-mode ultrasound on the neck of 30 elderly women (age 81 ± 6 years) with high lifetime sun exposure, Richard et al. found that skin thickness was lower on an exposed area in comparison with an adjacent, anatomically equivalent unexposed area [8]. Especially on facial skin, thickness assessment yielded contrasting results. On the forehead, skin thickness appeared both to decrease [23, 30] and to increase [24, 26, 27] with age, in different studies. Employing A-mode ultrasound, Denda et al. measured skin thickness on the forehead and the cheek and observed a decrease with age [23], whereas Takema found an increase in the same areas and also on eye corners [24]. In contrast, using B-mode ultrasound in 95 Korean women aged 30–50, Lee et al. did not observe changes with age on the crow's feet [18]. In a study population of 20 women aged 25–30 and 20 women aged 60–90, skin thickness was assessed at 12 different facial skin sites using a 20-MHz B scanner [27]. Higher values in skin thickness in the elderly were observed on all assessed facial sites except on the infraorbital region. In particular, the increase in skin thickness was statistically significant on the lateral regions of the forehead, the upper and lower lips, and the nose. The fact that facial skin thickness does not show a decreasing trend as at other skin sites can be explained by the observation that on sun-damaged facial skin, the reduction in collagen and ground substance content, which gradually takes place with aging, is counterbalanced by the overall rearrangement of the dermal collagen network and the accumulation of elastotic material [31, 32].

Skin Echogenicity

By providing quantitative data of echogenicity, high-frequency ultrasound permits the noninvasive evaluation of age-dependent modifications in collagen structure, elastosis, and other ultrastructural features of the skin, together with the effects of diurnal and hormonal changes [6, 32–34]. When a B-mode ultrasonographic image of normal skin is generated, a hyperreflective band-like echo is observed between the medium and the skin, the so-called entry echo, corresponding to the epidermis, due to the impedance change from the coupling medium to the stratum corneum. Immediately below the entry echo, there is the corium, rich in collagen fibers, which are the main source of its echogenicity.

In 1989, de Rigal et al. studied 142 females aged 1–90 by B-mode 25-MHz sonography on the volar and dorsal aspects of the forearm [19]. They identified a subepidermal hypoechogenic band, appearing as a relatively homogeneous, echolucent structure, located immediately below the entry echo. This subepidermal low-echogenic band (SLEB), which was invisible in the young, was present in most elderly subjects at the forearm and was located in the upper dermis, in some cases occupying the greater part of the dermis. The thickness of SLEB increased with age progressively and was higher on the dorsal forearm. Comparing two adjacent, anatomically equivalent sites, with and without sun exposure on the neck, Richard et al. noticed that SLEB thickness was greater on sun-exposed sites [8]. The presence of SLEB has been confirmed by many other investigators and was correlated to the severity of photodamage [12, 20, 26, 27, 34]. A Japanese study on 130 women aged 18–83 failed to demonstrate the presence of SLEB on facial areas (forehead, cheeks, and eye corners) probably because of the cultural tendency toward careful facial sun protection [35]. Changes in SLEB have been used to assess the efficacy of antiaging cosmetics [36]. Since the main source of dermal echogenicity is represented by well-arranged collagen bundles, the appearance of SLEB is correlated to the structural changes that occur with age.

In elderly skin, collagen bundles are replaced by a more homogeneously stained material, leading to the dissolution of the regular architecture of the collagen and elastic fibers and to the deposit of a greater amount of hydrated proteoglycans and glycosaminoglycans and of unbound water [37, 38]. Gravitational changes in body water balance throughout the day may explain the diurnal variation in SLEB thickness described by Gniadecka et al. on the volar forearm of 23 subjects aged 75–100 [34]. In 74 % of the study population, a clear diurnal variation in SLEB thickness was found. People who have a thick SLEB in the morning before rising had a thinner SLEB in the afternoon; the opposite was also true. Moreover, a well-developed SLEB was present only in 53 % of cases, and in some volunteers this was irregular with ill-defined borders. In these instances, SLEB thickness measurements were complicated and unreliable. SLEB can be more precisely quantified by image analysis than by visual scoring or thickness measurement. Computer-assisted analysis of the ultrasound image is based on the attribution of arbitrary values by a 0–255 scale to the echoes' amplitudes for each pixel, segments the image by pixel range, and measures regions of echogenicity as specified by the investigators [20]. To calculate echogenicity, the number of low-echogenic pixels, being defined as those with echogenicity 0–30, can be measured and related to the total number of pixels; this ratio is increasing with the decrease in echogenicity.

Ultrasound evaluation of the dermis by means of image segmentation showed that age-related changes are not limited to the upper dermis, characterized by the appearance of SLEB, but also to the lower dermis, which appears more echogenic in elderly subjects at all examined sites [20, 26, 27, 39, 40]. This dermal hyperreflecting band has been reported to become thinner with increasing age on both the volar and the dorsal forearm in 142 females aged 0–90 by de Rigal et al. [19]. In a study population of 90 subjects aged 18–94, Gniadecka et al. studied echogenicity in the different layers of the dermis on regions with different levels of sun exposure (dorsal and volar forearm, forehead, and ankle) and nonexposed buttocks [26]. The echogenicity of the lower dermis increased at all examined sites, including those with little or no sun exposure, suggesting that changes in the dermal echogenic band characterize chronological aging. In contrast, SLEB was present at the sun-exposed dermis alone and, prior to formation of a discernible SLEB a progressive, age-related decrease in echogenicity of the upper dermis was found in sun-exposed areas (dorsal forearm and forehead), but not at moderately exposed sites (ventral forearm and ankle). A significant relationship between skin echogenicity of the upper skin layers, age, and degree of photodamage assessed clinically further indicates that the decrease in subepidermal echogenicity may provide an objective parameter to evaluate solar damage. These results were confirmed in a study on 55 adults aged 18–57, undergoing 20-MHz ultrasonography and image analysis on the volar and the dorsal side of the forearm [40]. The authors demonstrated that skin echogenicity measured as a ratio between the upper and the lower dermis may be used to objectively estimate photoaging.

Evaluating echogenicity of the dermis as a whole, some investigators found that it decreases with increasing age [41]. In contrast, using a 20-MHz B-mode scanner on six skin sites on 24 volunteers aged 27–31 and on 24 volunteers over 60, an increase was found in overall echogenicity of the dermis in the elderly [20].

Depending on different skin areas, nonuniform variations in skin echogenicity from childhood to adulthood were observed [42]. A gradual increase was observed in echogenicity on the limbs with increasing age, whereas on the face and the trunk echogenicity was higher in children than in adults. In ultrasound images, facial skin shows scarce reflectivity, both in the young and the elderly, compared to other skin sites, such as the forearm, where the dermis is highly echogenic and the dermis-hypodermis boundary is well outlined. When evaluating overall skin echogenicity at different facial areas in young and elderly women, an increase with age at all examined sites except the infraorbital regions was found [27]. Moreover, age-related changes in skin echogenicity, consisting in the appearance of a subepidermal band and an enhancement of the lower dermis reflectivity, were present at most facial sites. These findings of increased overall echogenicity in the elderly may be due to an enhancement of the lower dermis echoes, rather than a decreased echogenicity of the upper dermis.

Confocal Scanning Laser Microscopy and Aging

In vivo confocal scanning laser microscopy (CSLM) is a noninvasive technique permitting optical en face sectioning of the skin with good contrast and high resolution, providing cellular and subcellular details. It seems to have a tremendous potential for research and diagnostic purposes in dermatology, since CSLM supplies an open "histological" window to the tissue noninvasively. The commercially available Vivascope microscopes (Lucid, Rochester, NY) use a diode laser source with a wavelength of 830 nm, an illumination power up to 20 mW on the object and water immersion. The penetration depth of imaging allows the visualization of the epidermis and the upper dermis with a good correlation to histologic sections [43, 44].

Sauermann et al. investigated skin aging using CSLM on the volar forearm of 13 young and 13 elderly volunteers [45]. The cells in the granular layer were significantly larger in the older subjects confirming histological findings documenting the increase of corneocytes with age as a result of a lower proliferation rate and turnover of the epidermis. Basal layer thickness decreased significantly, whereas thickness of the epidermis increased in the older volunteers compared to the younger ones. However, the most relevant age-related change in this study was the reduction in the number of dermal papillae per area with age reflecting the flattened epidermal-dermal junction in elderly skin. Histometric measurements by CSLM proved to be a sensitive tool for characterizing histological changes in the epidermis and papillary dermis due to aging and also for cosmetic research. The same authors evaluated the efficacy of a cream containing vitamin C applied twice a day for 4 months on the volar forearm in a study population of 33 women aged 45–67 by using CSLM [46]. Topical vitamin C resulted in a significant increase in the density of dermal papillae and in a reduction of granular layer cell size, indicating relevant effects in correcting the structural changes associated with the aging process.

In CSLM images, Neerken at al. identified a reflecting layer of fibrous structures, whose depth strongly depends on age below the basal layer [47]. In addition, large structural changes, such as the flattening of the dermo-epidermal junction and a thinning of the epidermis, were observed with increasing age.

CLSM was also employed to assess photodamaged skin to study alterations in dermal collagen fibers brought about by long-term sun exposure [48].

Conclusion

Despite the many tools and techniques available for the noninvasive evaluation of age-related changes in skin structure and functions, further work is needed to develop a unified understanding of skin aging. To date, results of some studies on skin aging are often conflicting and difficult to interpret. Instrument and other measurement-related variables can partly explain the differing results. Moreover, the great interindividual and intraindividual variations of the human skin make consensus a challenging objective. Therefore, further studies which include larger study populations and standardized protocols are necessary.

Cross-References

- ▶ Corneocyte Analysis
- ▶ Hydration of the Skin Surface
- ▶ Transepidermal Water Loss in Young and Aged Healthy Humans

References

1. Fluhr JW, Pfistener S, Gloor M. Direct comparison of skin physiology in children and adults with bioengineering methods. Pediatr Dermatol. 2000;17:436–9.

2. Diktein S, Hartzshtark A, Bercovici P. The dependence of low pressure indentation, slackness, and surface pH on age in forehead skin of women. J Soc Cosmet Chem. 1984;35:221–8.
3. Waller JM, Maibach HI. Age and skin structure and function, a quantitative approach (I): blood flow, pH, thickness, and ultrasound echogenicity. Skin Res Technol. 2005;11:221–35.
4. Wilhelm KP, Cua AB, Maibach HI. Skin aging: effect on transepidermal water loss, stratum corneum hydration, skin surface pH and casual sebum content. Arch Dermatol. 1991;127:1806–9.
5. Conti A, Schiavi ME, Seidenari S. Capacitance, transepidermal water loss and casual level of sebum in healthy subjects in relation to site, sex and age. Int J Cosmet Sci. 1995;17:77–85.
6. Callens A et al. Does hormonal aging exist? A study on the influence of different hormone therapy on the skin of postmenopaused women using non-invasive measurement techniques. Dermatology. 1996;193:289–94.
7. Caisey L et al. Influence of age and hormone replacement therapy on the functional properties of the lips. Skin Res Technol. 2008;14:220–5.
8. Richard S, de Rigal J, Lacharriere O, Berardesca E, Leveque JL. Noninvasive measurement of the effect of lifetime exposure to the sun on the aged skin. Photodermatol Photoimmunol Photomed. 1994;10:164–9.
9. Warren R. Age, sunlight, and facial skin: a histologic and quantitative study. J Am Acad Dermatol. 1991;25:751–60.
10. Kikuchi-Numagami K et al. Functional and morphological studies of photodamaged skin on the hands of middle-aged Japanese golfers. Eur J Dermatol. 2000;10(4):277–81.
11. Guinot C et al. Effect of hormonal replacement therapy on cutaneous biophysical properties of menopausal women. Ann Dermatol Venereol. 2002;129:1129–33.
12. Marks R, Edwards C. The measurement of photodamage. Br J Dermatol. 1992;127(41):7–13.
13. Kelly RI et al. The effects of aging on cutaneous microvasculature. J Am Acad Dermatol. 1995;33:749–56.
14. Tolino MA, Wilkin JK. Aging and cutaneous vascular thermoregulation responses. J Invest Dermatol. 1988;90:613.
15. Ishihara M et al. Blood flow. In: Kligman AM, Takase Y, editors. Cutaneous aging. Tokyo: University of Tokyo press; 1988. p. 167–81.
16. Hatzis J. The wrinkle and its measurement-a skin surface profilometric method. Micron. 2004;35:210–9.
17. Quan MB, Edwards C, Marks R. Non-invasive in vivo techniques to differentiate photodamage and ageing in human skin. Acta Dermatol Venereol. 1997;77 (6):416–9.
18. Lee HK, Seo YK, Baek JH, Koh JS. Comparison between ultrasonography (Dermascan C version 3) and transparency profilometry (Skin Visiometer SV600). Skin Res Technol. 2008;14:8–12.
19. de Rigal J et al. Assessment of aging of the human skin by in vivo ultrasonic imaging. J Invest Dermatol. 1989;93:621–5.
20. Seidenari S, Pagnoni A, Di Nardo A, Giannetti A. Echographic evaluation with image analysis of normal skin: variation according to age and sex. Skin Pharmacol. 1995;7:201–9.
21. Tan CY, Stathan B, Marks R, Payne PA. Skin thickness measurement by pulsed ultrasound: its reproducibility, validation and variability. Br J Dermatol. 1982;106:657–67.
22. Escoffier C et al. Age-related mechanical properties of human skin: an in vivo study. J Invest Dermatol. 1989;93:353–7.
23. Denda M, Takahasi M. Measurement of facial skin thickness by ultrasound method. J Soc Cosmet Chem Jpn. 1990;23:316–9.
24. Takema Y, Yorimoto Y, Kawai M, Imokawa G. Age-related changes in the elastic properties and thickness of human facial skin. Br J Dermatol. 1994;131:641–8.
25. Lasagni C, Seidenari S. Echographic assessment of age-dependent variations of skin thickness. A study on 162 subjects. Skin Res Technol. 1995;1:81–5.
26. Gniadecka M, Jemec GBE. Quantitative evaluation of chronological ageing and photoageing in vivo: studies on skin echogenicity and thickness. Br J Dermatol. 1998;139:815–21.
27. Pellacani G, Seidenari S. Variations in facial skin thickness and echogenicity with site and age. Acta Dermatol Venereol. 1999;79:366–9.
28. Leveque JL et al. Influence of chronic sun exposure on some biophysical parameters of the human skin: an in vivo study. J Cutan Aging Cosmet Dermatol. 1989;1:123–7.
29. Adhoute H, de Rigal J, Marchand JP, Privat Y, Leveque JL. Influence of age and sun exposure on the biophysical properties of the human skin: an in vivo study. Photodermatol Photoimmunol Photomed. 1992;9:99–103.
30. Nishimura M, Tuji T. Measurement of skin elasticity with a new suction device. Jpn J Dermatol. 1990;102:1111–7.
31. Shuster S, Black MM, McVitie E. The influence of age and sex on skin thickness, skin collagen and density. Br J Dermatol. 1975;93:639.
32. Pellacani G, Giusti F, Seidenari S. Ultrasound assessment of skin ageing. In: Serup J, Jemec GBE, Grove GL, editors. Non-invasive methods and the skin. Boca Raton: CRC press; 2006. p. 511–4.
33. Altmeyer P, Hoffmann K, Stucker M, Goertz S, El-Gammal S. General phenomena of ultrasound in dermatology. In: Altmeyer P, El-Gammal S, Hoffmann K, editors. Ultrasound in dermatology. Berlin/Heidelberg: Springer; 1992. p. 55–79.
34. Gniadecka M, Serup J, Sondergaard J. Age-related diurnal changes of dermal oedema: evaluation by high frequency ultrasound. Br J Dermatol. 1994;131:849–55.

35. Tsukahara K et al. Age-related alterations of echogenicity in Japanese skin. Dermatology. 2000;200:303–7.
36. Hoffmann K, Dirschka T, El-Gammal S, Altmeyer P. Assessment of actinic elastosis by means of high-frequency sonography. In: Marks R, Plewing G, editors. The Environmental Threat to the Skin. London: Martin Dunitz; 1991. p. 83–90.
37. Richard S et al. Characterization of the skin in vivo by high resolution magnetic resonance imaging: water behaviour and age-related effects. J Invest Dermatol. 1993;100:705–9.
38. Oikarinen A. Aging of the skin connective tissue: how to measure the biochemical and mechanical properties of aging dermis. Photodermatol Photoimmunol Photomed. 1994;10:47–52.
39. Sandby-Moller J, Wulf HC. Ultrasonographic subepidermal low-echogenic band, dependence of age and body site. Skin Res Technol. 2004;10:57–63.
40. Gniadecka M. Effects of ageing on dermal echogenicity. Skin Res Technol. 2001;7:204–7.
41. Nakahigashi N, Sugai T. Assessment of degeneration by sun exposure using ultrasonic imaging with dermascan C. Skin Res. 1996;38:25–30.
42. Seidenari S, Giusti G, Bertoni L, Magnoni C, Pellacani G. Thickness and echogenicity of the skin in children as assessed by 20-MHz ultrasound. Dermatology. 2000;201:218–22.
43. Rajadhyaksha M, Gonzalez S, Avislan JM, Anderson RR, Webb RH. In vivo confocal laser scanning microscopy of human skin II: advances in instrumentation and comparison with histology. J Invest Dermatol. 1999;113:292–303.
44. Branzan AL, Landthaler M, Szeimies RM. In vivo confocal laser scanning microscopy in dermatology. Lasers Med Sci. 2007;22:73–82.
45. Sauermann K et al. Age-related changes in human skin investigated with histometric measurements by confocal laser scanning microscopy in vivo. Skin Res Technol. 2002;8:52–6.
46. Sauermann K, Jaspers S, Koop U, Wenck H. Topically applied vitamin C increases the density of dermal papillae in aged human skin. Dermatology. 2004;4:13–8.
47. Neerken S, Lucassen GW, Bisschop MA, Lenderink E, Nuijs TA. Characterization of age-related effects in human skin: a comparative study that applies confocal laser scanning microscopy and optical coherence tomography. J Biomed Opt. 2004;9:274–81.
48. Bernstein EF et al. Long-term sun exposure alters the collagen of the papillary dermis. Comparison of sun-protected and photoaged skin by northern analysis, immunohistochemical staining and confocal 3laser scanning microscopy. J Am Acad Dermatol. 1996;34:209–18.

Hydration of the Skin Surface

86

Hachiro Tagami

Contents

Abstract

The stratum corneum (SC) samples obtained from dry scaly skin changes such as senile xerosis, ichthyosis, and various inflammatory dermatoses including psoriasis and eczema show very poor content of water-holding substances. Clinically we can quickly assess the hydration state of the skin surface by using the electrical methods that measure either skin conductance or capacitance for high-frequency current. Moreover, we can obtain information about the hygroscopic property as well as the water-holding capacity of such SC within a few minutes by serially measuring the changes occurring in these electrical properties after application of a water droplet on the skin surface just for 10 s. Moreover, studies employing an in vitro simulation model of the SC confirmed that the conductance measurements are suited for the evaluation of the skin after application of topical moisturizing agents, whereas capacitance measurements are suited for the evaluation of dry skin or scaly skin changes. Lastly, by comparing the skin of the same individuals between summer and winter, we can find that there occur seasonal changes in SC hydration showing that the skin surface hydration state is significantly lower in winter than in summer if measured in the identical climate-controlled conditions.

H. Tagami (✉)
Department of Dermatology, Tohoku University School of Medicine, Sendai, Japan
e-mail: hachitagami@ybb.ne.jp

M.A. Farage et al. (eds.), *Textbook of Aging Skin*,
DOI 10.1007/978-3-662-47398-6_66

Introduction

The skin surface is tightly wrapped by an extremely thin but efficient biological barrier membrane, stratum corneum (SC). Since the SC interferes with the permeation of even small molecules, such as those of water, as a skin barrier, it can protect the underlying hydrated living skin tissue from desiccation in this dry atmosphere on the Earth. It is needless to say that the SC also protects the body from the invasion of various external injurious agents. This skin barrier function depends on the structural uniqueness of the SC, which consists of closely overlapped corneocytes, the flattened dead bodies of fully differentiated epidermal keratinocytes, whose narrow intercellular spaces are tightly packed with unique intercellular lipids, the components of which, called hydroxyceramides, tightly bind to the cornified envelope of each corneocyte.

Except for the palmoplantar skin that is covered by more than 50 layers of the corneocytes to withstand a strong physical force such as required to support whole body weight, other bodily regions are covered by SC mostly composed of only 7–15 tightly stacked layers of corneocytes [1]. It is surprising that there exists fully hydrated epidermal tissue just beneath the thin and soft membranous structure of the SC. Then, why does the skin of the elderly tend to become dry and rough in winter?

Dry and Scaly Skin Surface

It was found that more than 95 % of the normal individuals over 60 years of age who live in Sendai, located in the northern part of Honshu Island, present with dry skin, senile xerosis, on their lower backs and lower legs in winter. Furthermore, about half of them complain of pruritus in such skin [2]. Senile xerosis, however, does not indicate lack of water in the whole skin, because the water content of the living skin tissue is rather high in the elderly [3]. The objectively noted dry skin reflects only a decrease in water content in the superficial portion of the SC. In other words, the SC of young individuals efficiently plays another important role in keeping the skin surface soft and smooth.

Almost 60 years ago, Blank [4] made interesting observations in vitro. He found that the isolated fragments of plantar SC became hard and brittle when dehydrated. Attempts to soften them with petrolatum or olive oil, the emollients conventionally used for the treatment of rough and scaly skin, totally failed. Only after absorption of water did they become soft and flexible; thus, water can be regarded as the ultimate moisturizer that improves subjective perception of the mechanical properties of human skin. In contrast to such an in vitro situation, there is always a water supply from the underlying hydrated living tissue in vivo, even in an atmosphere with extremely low relative humidity. However, the SC of the dry skin is not efficient enough to take up water to keep the skin surface soft and supple.

The soft and smooth SC such as that found in young skin is rich in water-holding substances, i.e., amino acids produced by proteolysis of filaggrin that takes place during their slow upward movement in the SC, lactate and potassium derived from sweat, and intercellular lipids, especially their major component ceramides that also play a crucial role in providing barrier function to the SC [5–7]. Moreover, in the locations rich in actively secreting sebaceous glands such as the face and scalp, sebum exerts an occlusive effect by itself [8], and glycerol that results from hydrolysis of triglycerides efficiently binds water in the skin surface [9].

With skin aging, deficiencies develop in these water-binding substances in the superficial portion of the SC [2]. Moreover, there occurs a poor supply of water from the underlying, well-hydrated living tissue, because of an increase in the number of SC cell layers with age, which makes the passage of water through the SC more difficult [1, 2, 10]. Hence, the lesser water supply from the underlying epidermis and poor water-holding capacity of the superficial portion of the

SC itself make the SC of the aged skin less efficient to bind water, leading to the development of dry skin in winter [2].

In the case of commonly observed scaly dermatoses such as chronic eczema, psoriasis, and ichthyosis, their pathologic SC is too deficient in water-binding capacity although the water-barrier deficiency of such SC allows ample water supply from the underlying living tissue [11].

Lack of water in the skin surface produces a dry, rough, or scaly look. Traditionally, various occlusive agents such as petrolatum were applied that slowly exert a softening and smoothing effect on the skin surface by preventing the water loss. Nowadays, various moisturizing agents are available which can directly supply water to the skin surface and quickly change the rough skin surface into a smooth and soft one at least transiently. However, in the case of the treatment of those scaly dermatoses, there is no question about the importance of the medical treatment for the underlying pathologic skin changes.

Thus, one of the most important issues in the field of dermatology and cosmetology is the establishment of the effective method to maintain sufficient skin surface hydration. For such a purpose, it is essential to develop a useful methodology to quantitatively measure the skin surface hydration state that enabled the evaluation of the effectiveness of various topical agents.

Assessment of Skin Surface Hydration with Bioengineering Methods

From the in vitro observation, it has become clear that a decrease in the water concentration in the superficial layers of the SC is known to cause an observable alteration in the physical characteristics of the skin surface, which is noted objectively as dry and scaly skin [12]. Clinical assessment of such dry skin is done in a crude and qualitative fashion, i.e., by simply observing the skin surface and manually palpating it. However, for the quantitative evaluation, more objective and instrumental measurements are needed.

It is not difficult to measure the water content of isolated SC sheets in vitro. Because of the equal distribution of water in such SC samples, it can be expressed as percentage. In contrast, it is difficult to express the amount of water contained in the SC in vivo, because there exists a concentration gradient of water within the SC [12–14] being lowest in the uppermost portion exposed to the dry atmosphere and highest in the lowermost layer facing the viable, moist epidermis. This is due to the fact that the SC is the rate-limiting barrier between the water-saturated viable tissue and the dry outer environment where diffusion of water takes place as a purely passive process through it. As mentioned above, the superficial portion of the SC can remain supple and flexible, as long as its water-holding capacity is intact as noted in the young healthy skin. In contrast, the skin covered by pathologic SC with poor water-holding capacity such as that found in the skin of aged individuals or in that of various skin diseases presents a cracked, scaly appearance.

Despite the urgent demands for the quick and quantitative techniques to assess such hydration state of the exposed portion of the SC, i.e., the skin surface hydration state, there had been a total lack of adequate in vivo methodologies or a practical technique to objectively evaluate the efficacy of moisturizers in vivo until 1980 when a quick and efficient electrical method to measure skin impedance by using high-frequency current was first reported [13]. Thereafter, various commercial instruments have become available.

This electric technique can evaluate the water content at poorly defined portions of the skin surface SC. However, by combining with sequential tape-stripping method, an increasing water concentration gradient from the skin surface can be demonstrated, deep into the viable epidermis as shown with later developed different methodology such as electron probe analysis [14] or just recently introduced confocal Raman spectroscopy that can provide precise information not only about the distribution pattern of the water in the SC but also about the distribution patterns of other functionally important substances in the SC [15]. The confocal Raman spectroscopy can also offer information about the detailed distribution of those substances that are crucial for the barrier as well as hydration of the SC [16].

Electrical Methods for the Evaluation of the Skin Surface

At present, because of the handiness and convenience, the most widely employed techniques to evaluate the hydration state of the skin surface are those involving the measurement of skin impedance. Impedance (Z), the total electrical opposition to the flow of an alternating current, depends on two components, resistance (R) and capacitance (C), and their relationship may be formulated as follows:

$$Z = \left[R^2 + (1/2pfC)^2\right]^{1/2}$$

where f stands for a frequency of an applied alternating current. In old days, many researchers studied the impedance of human skin for reasons of technical simplicity. Tregear [17] speculated that when the skin surface is not deliberately hydrated, the reciprocal of specific impedance should be a measure of the hydration of its surface position. However, because of the high impedance of human skin, which is chiefly due to the properties of the SC, measurements of the skin impedance had to employ damp contact using electrode paste between the electrodes and the skin [18]. Such an approach is not only cumbersome but also has a great influence on the functional properties of the SC.

In 1980, by using high-frequency electric current of 3.5 MHz, it was found that it is possible to evaluate the hydration state of the skin surface quickly and quantitatively in a noninvasive way even with dry electrodes in terms of either conductance ($=1/R$) or capacitance [13]. At that time a circuit developed by Ichijo was used, which enabled the measurement of both conductance and capacitance for a high-frequency current separately. Leveque and de Rigal [19] also reported good sensitivity to the water content of the skin surface with a similar high-frequency instrument developed by them.

With such a method, as soon as the probe is placed on the skin, both conductance and capacitance show a rapid initial increase followed by a gradual increase if the contact is maintained. The level of the initial increase represents the hydration state of the skin surface at the time of application of the probe, and the later slow increase is due to accumulation of water beneath the probe resulting from transepidermal water loss. Thus, the initial value for the evaluation of the hydration of the skin surface is used.

In Vivo Water Sorption–Desorption Test

Information can be easily obtained on the hygroscopic property and water-holding capacity of the SC in a few minutes by conducting an in vivo water sorption–desorption test [20]. This simple test procedure consists of electrical measurements before and after application of a droplet of water on the skin for 10 s to obtain data on the hygroscopic property of the skin surface and later serial measurements at an interval of 30 s for 2 min to evaluate the water-holding capacity. Under usual ambient conditions, normal skin surface shows a high rise in conductance just after the application of water, which is followed by a rapid falloff within 30 s, thereafter by gradual return to the prehydration levels by 2 min (Fig. 1). Such an initial increase measured with capacitance is remarkably smaller than that measured with conductance, indicating rather poor sensitivity of capacitance to a well-hydrated condition of the SC (Fig. 2). This was also the case on the skin occluded by a sheet of polyethylene film. None of these parameters were influenced by the water accumulation of the tissue fluids beneath the epidermis, such as demonstrated on the top of a suction blister.

This test demonstrates that the superficial SC of normal skin is much less hygroscopic and less capable of holding water than the corresponding deeper portions (Fig. 1) and that scaly skin

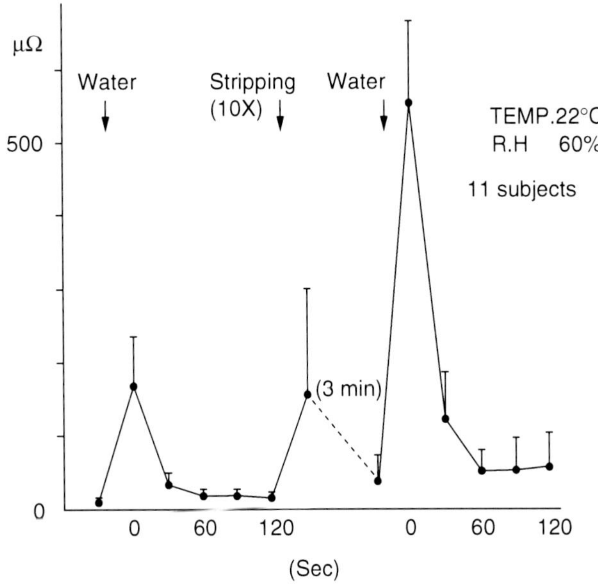

Fig. 1 Water sorption–desorption test on normal skin surface and that repeated 3 min after adhesive tape stripping of the stratum corneum ten times (Reproduced with permission from Tagami et al. [20])

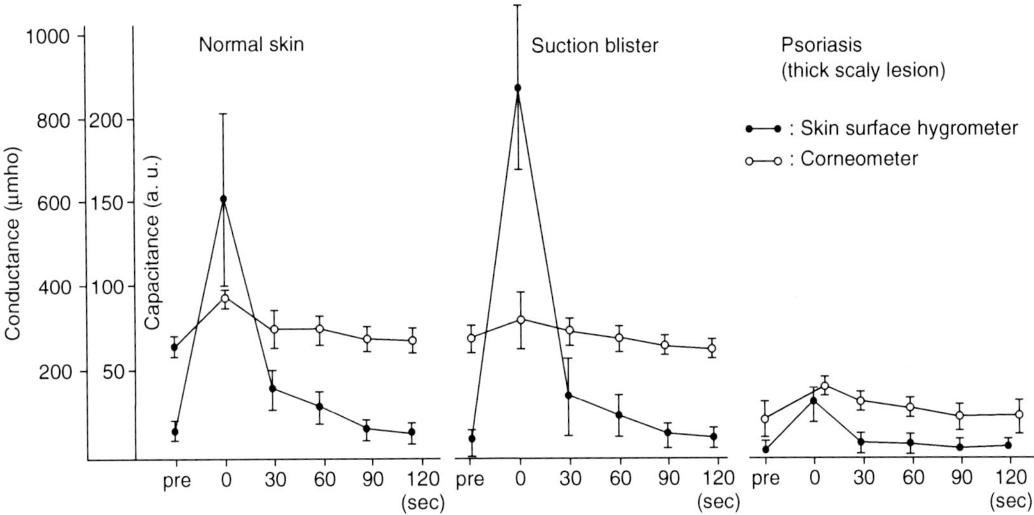

Fig. 2 In vivo water sorption–desorption test measured with Skicon-200EX and Corneometer CM 420 (Reproduced with permission from Hashimoto-Kumasaka et al. [22])

shows a functional defect in both hygroscopicity and water-holding capacity (Fig. 2) between which the former normalizes much faster than the latter after effective treatment of the skin lesions [20].

These findings also indicate that variations in obtained values are much larger with conductance measurement than those with capacitance measurement especially measured on the normal healthy skin surface. It is particularly clear on the well-hydrated skin such as that under occlusion or at such anatomical locations as the face where the recorded values show much greater differences even between closely located sites with the measurement of conductance than with that of capacitance.

Characteristics Observed in the Measurement of Skin Conductance and That of Capacitance

In general, skin conductance and capacitance show a very similar behavior ($r = 0.95$; $P < 0.01$) [13]. However, conductance measured on dry scaly lesional skin or even that on the plantar skin surface of normal individuals appears to be extremely low as compared to capacitance. Thus, it is not easy to compare the grade of the dry state of scaly lesions with conductance measurements, because the obtained values are mostly near zero.

An in vivo simulation model of SC can be constructed to ascertain whether the hydration of the skin surface can actually be evaluated with this electrical method [21]. For this purpose, an intact SC sheet separated from a normal skin edge from surgically obtained skin samples is used. First, an epidermal sheet is obtained, separating it by immersing it in hot water (60 °C) for 2 min. Then, the covering SC is separated from the epidermal sheet by trypsin digestion. Such an isolated SC sheet is mounted on more than five overlapping filter papers saturated with phosphate-buffered saline (PBS), which simulates the well-hydrated living skin tissue, placed on a glass slide, and all the free edges are sealed to a glass with a removable frame of adhesive vinyl tape. Similar to the SC in vivo, this in vitro simulation model of the SC tightly wraps a pad of fully water-saturated filter paper with its lower surface, while the upper surface directly faces the ambient atmosphere. Thus, there takes place water evaporation through the SC sheet just as in vivo. By placing this model in environments with different relative humidities, it was confirmed that the recorded conductance correlated well with the actual water content of the SC ($r = 0.99$). In contrast, the correlation coefficient obtained with capacitance measurement was much less than that with conductance, showing $r = 0.79$ (Fig. 3) [22].

With regard to the electroconductive substances in the SC, it requires soaking of the SC fragment in distilled water for at least 2 weeks for them to be totally depleted, making it unable to measure conductance any more.

Reflecting these differences noted in the in vitro as well as in vivo experiments, it was

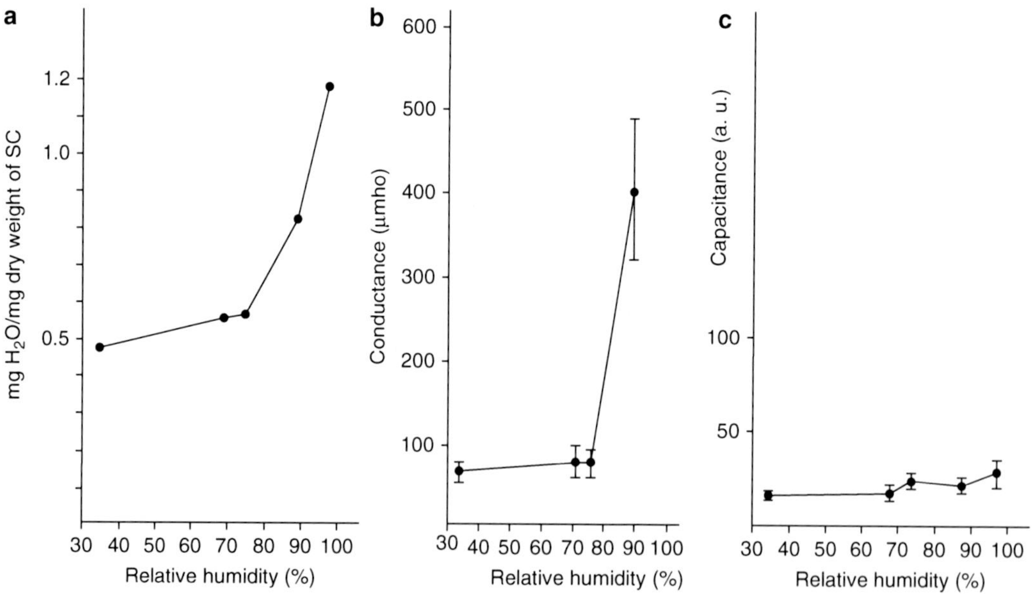

Fig. 3 Relationship between electrical parameters and water content of the stratum corneum sheet placed in various relative humidities. (**a**) Water content by weight determination. (**b**) Conductance measurement. (**c**) Capacitance measurement (Reproduced with permission from Hashimoto-Kumasaka et al. [22])

found that conductance measurement is suited for the evaluation of normal skin and that placed under the influence of topical moisturizing agents [21, 22]. In contrast, the measurement of capacitance seems to be more suited for the evaluation of hydration state in dry skin or clinically scaly skin where conductance cannot clearly detect differences among severely, moderately, and mildly scaly portions [22].

The Thickness of the Underlying Electroconductive Medium

In the devised simple simulation model of an in vivo SC, a concentration gradient of water exists between the surface and the lowermost portion [23], because it consists of an isolated sheet of SC that tightly occludes the underlying water-saturated filter paper. The underlying water-saturated filter paper, like the living cutaneous tissues in vivo, is the water source of overlying SC and is also the conducting medium that allows the formation of an adequate electric field. Conductance values recorded with only one sheet of underlying filter paper were quite low. With an increase in the number of sheets of paper, the conductance value increased until five sheets of filter paper were in place. At this point the readings reached a plateau. The total thickness of five sheets of filter paper saturated with water was approximately 5 mm. Thus, to obtain an optimal reading, the high-frequency current should extend at least 5 mm into the wet and electrically conductive substances [23]. This condition is always attainable in vivo.

A gravimetric determination of water content was performed, together with the high-frequency conductometry, in the simulation model of the SC. As a result, it was confirmed that the recorded conductance values correlated well with the actual water content of the SC ($r = 0.94$). Moreover, by using a model consisting of five overlapped SC sheets simulating that of the palmoplantar SC, it was corroborated that there is a close correlation between the high-frequency conductance values and the water content in the uppermost SC sheet ($r = 0.98$) [23].

Commercially Available Electrical Instruments

There are now many different commercially available instruments for the evaluation of the skin surface hydration which are based on different modes of measurement [24, 25]. Moreover, even cosmetic counters in big stores are now equipped with their own simple instruments, which are constructed by each cosmetic company based on the impedance principle. Thus, the following are the representative instruments that are routinely used for the experimental or clinical purposes worldwide.

Skicon-100, which was manufactured by IBS Ltd., Hamamatsu, Japan, is the initial one among these electrical instruments. There is now a new version, Skicon-200EX, which has built-in computation. The principle is based on conductance method, operating at a single frequency (3.5 MHz). Comparison between the original model 100 and 200EX shows comparable data, although the Skicon-200EX displayed systematically 1.6-fold higher values than the Skicon-100. The two probes measured systematically different levels with the original probe measuring lower values [26].

Corneometer, CM820, and its newer version, CM 825, are manufactured by Courage + Khazaka Electronic GmbH, Cologne, Germany. A resonating system in the instruments measures the shift in frequency of the oscillating system, which results from the changes in the total capacity of the skin surface. In the case of CM 825, the frequency shifts from 0.95 MHz in a hydrated medium to 1.15 MHz for a dry medium.

DermaLab Moisture Unit, manufactured by Cortex Technology, Hadsund, Denmark, is based on impedance measurements operating at single frequency of 100 kHz. It is a combination instrument that allows measurements of elasticity, transepidermal water loss, and hydration.

Nova Dermal Phase Meter, Nova DPM 9003, is manufactured by Nova Technology Corporation, Portsmouth, NH, USA. It measures impedance-based capacitive reactance of the skin at preselected frequencies up to 1 MHz from the observed signal phase delays.

MoistureMeter is manufactured by Delfin Technologies Ltd., Kuopio, Finland. Its SC-4 instrument operates at 1.25 MHz with concentric electrodes. D-3 has larger dimensions of the sensor probe, which increases the effective measuring depth from 0.5 to 5 mm.

Point to Notice Before Conducting In Vivo Measurements

Because the SC is exposed to the atmosphere, its surface hydration state is greatly influenced by the ambient relative humidity. Thus, covered areas such as the trunk show much higher values than the exposed areas in the dry winter season due to the effect of thick, airtight clothes, when the measurement is performed just after removal of the clothes. At least 15 min should be allowed for the skin surface to adapt to the atmosphere.

Measured values sometimes vary greatly even between sites only slightly apart from each other, particularly when the probe is applied to the sites rich in sweat glands such as the palmar surface, axilla, and in some individuals even the forehead. Generally, the highest values are found on the face and the lowest values on the distal portion of the limbs on the body surface [27]. The measurements on the skin areas such as the palmar skin for comparative study should be done carefully, because these areas are always under the influence of mental sweating.

The comparison made between summer and winter in the same subjects at an out-patient clinic with 21–26 °C room temperature showed that high environmental relative humidity of the summer and possibly invisible sweating induced higher conductance values in the summer time [28]. Therefore, the measurements should ideally be conducted in the identical environmental conditions, i.e., by using a climate-controlled chamber. Such a study performed in subjects consisting of different age groups using a climate-controlled chamber maintained at 21 °C and 50 % relative humidity, definitely demonstrated that the skin surface hydration state is significantly lower in winter than in summer whether on the exposed area, the cheek, or on the covered area of the flexor surface of the forearm. These data indicate that the skin surface conditions are greatly influenced by weathering of the skin in the dry and cold winter [28].

An exogenous supply of water on a skin surface results in a remarkable elevation in recorded value. However, this increase is not influenced by the application of either distilled water or a highly concentrated buffer solution; i.e., it is not affected by the presence of other electrolytes in the applied water due to the fact that the skin surface is already rich in various electroconductive substances. As mentioned above, to totally remove such electroconductive substances from a fragment of normal SC, it is necessary to soak it in distilled water for at least 14 days.

Assessment of the Efficacy of Skin Moisturizers

In the dry and cold winter, even normal healthy skin surface becomes much smoother and softer immediately after the application of moisturizing agents. This change can be shown as an increase in conductance depending on the efficacy of the agents. This is followed by a rapid decrease due to evaporation of excess water from the skin surface [29]. Thereafter, the obtained values are maintained at certain increased levels, for several hours, according to the efficacy of the agents, if undisturbed. In contrast, no initial increase is observed after the application of emollients such as petrolatum that does not contain water. However, there is a gradual increase in conductance until reaching a plateau after 2 h due to accumulation of water beneath it. To obtain reproducible results, 20 μL of the agent is applied in a $4 \times 4\ cm^2$ skin area.

Repeated daily applications of moisturizers for several days induce an increase in conductance or capacitance that is demonstrable even several days after the cessation of treatment depending on the efficacy of the moisturizers [30]. Moreover, such repeated applications of a moisturizer not only increase the hydration state of the skin surface but also improve mildly impaired barrier function, as noted in atopic xerosis induced by the dry and cold winter air [31].

Conclusion

Various electrical methods are now available to evaluate the skin surface hydration. Based on the studies conducted in vitro, the high-frequency electrical method is employed to measure quantitatively the skin surface hydration state to estimate the impairment in the water-holding capacity of pathologic SC of various skin lesions or to evaluate the moisturizing effects of various topical agents. The measurement of high-frequency conductance is much more sensitive to the changes in hydration state of the superficial portions of the SC than that of capacitance, but the variations of the obtained values are much greater with the former than the latter reflecting the sensitivity of measurement. For the measurement of dry scaly lesions, the measurement of capacitance appears to be more sensitive to detect differences of severity than that of conductance.

Cross-References

▶ Transepidermal Water Loss in Young and Aged Healthy Humans

References

1. Ya-Xian Z, Suetake T, Tagami H. Number of cell layers of the stratum corneum in normal skin – relationship to the anatomical location on the body, age, sex and physical parameters. Arch Dermatol Res. 1999;291:555–9.
2. Hara M, Kikuchi K, Watanabe M, Denda M, Koyama J, Nomura J, Horii I, Tagami H. Senile xerosis: functional, morphological, and biochemical studies. J Geriatr Dermatol. 1993;1:111–20.
3. Kligman AM. Perspectives and problems in cutaneous gerontology. J Invest Dermatol. 1979;73:39–46.
4. Blank IH. Factors which influence the water content of the stratum corneum. J Invest Dermatol. 1952;18:433–40.
5. Horii I, Nakayama Y, Obata M, Tagami H. Stratum corneum hydration and amino acid content in xerotic skin. Br J Dermatol. 1989;121:587–92.
6. Nakagawa N, Sakai S, Matsumoto M, Yamada K, Nagano M, Yuki T, Sumida Y, Uchiwa H. Relationship between NMF (lactate and potassium) content and the physical properties of the stratum corneum in healthy subjects. J Invest Dermatol. 2004;122:755–63.
7. Imokawa G, Akasaki S, Hattori M, Yoshizuki N. Selective recovery of deranged water-holding properties by stratum corneum lipids. J Invest Dermatol. 1986;87:758–61.
8. O'Goshi K, Iguchi M, Tagami H. Functional analysis of the stratum corneum of scalp skin: studies in patients with alopecia areata and androgenetic alopecia. Arch Dermatol Res. 2000;292:605–11.
9. Fluhr JW, Mao-Qiang M, Brown BE, Wertz PW, Crumrine D, Sundberg JP, Feingold KR, Elias PM. Glycerol regulates stratum corneum hydration in sebaceous gland deficient (asebia) mice. J Invest Dermatol. 2003;120:728–37.
10. Kobayashi H, Tagami H. Distinct locational differences observable in biophysical functions of the facial skin: with special emphasis on the poor functional properties of the stratum corneum of the perioral region. Int J Cosmet Sci. 2004;26:91–101.
11. Tagami H, Yoshikuni K. Interrelationship between water barrier and reservoir functions of pathologic stratum corneum. Arch Dermatol. 1985;181:642–5.
12. Blank IH, Moloney J, Emslie A, Simon I, Apt C. Diffusion of water across the stratum corneum as a function of its water content. J Invest Dermatol. 1984;82:188–94.
13. Tagami H, Ohi M, Iwatsuki K, Kanamaru Y, Yamada M, Ichijo B. Evaluation of the skin surface hydration in vivo by electrical measurement. J Invest Dermatol. 1980;75:500–7.
14. Warner RR, Myers MC, Taylor DA. Electron probe analysis of human skin: determination of the water concentration profile. J Invest Dermatol. 1988;90:218–24.
15. Egawa M, Hirao T, Takahashi M. In vivo estimation of stratum corneum thickness from water concentration profiles obtained with Raman spectroscopy. Acta Derm Venereol (Stockh). 2007;87:4–8.
16. Egawa M, Tagami H. Comparison of the depth profiles of water and water-binding substances in the stratum corneum determined in vivo by Raman spectroscopy between the cheek and volar forearm skin: effects of age, seasonal changes and artificial forced hydration. Br J Dermatol. 2007;158:251–60.
17. Tregear RT. The interpretation of skin impedance measurements. Nature. 1965;205:600–1.
18. Clar EP, Her CP, Sturelle CG. Skin impedance and moisturization. J Cosmet Chem. 1973;26:337–53.
19. Leveque JL, de Rigal J. Impedance methods for studying skin moisturisation. J Soc Cosmet Chem. 1983;34:419–28.
20. Tagami H, Kanamaru Y, Inoue K, Suehisa S, Inoue F, Iwatsuki K, Yoshikuni K, Yamada M. Water sorption–-desorption test of the skin in vivo for functional assessment of the stratum corneum. J Invest Dermatol. 1982;78:425–8.
21. Obata M, Tagami H. Electrical determination of water content and concentration profile in a simulation model

of in vivo stratum corneum. J Invest Dermatol. 1989;92:854–9.

22. Hashimoto-Kumasaka K, Takahashi K, Tagami H. Electrical measurement of water content of the stratum corneum in vivo and in vitro under various conditions: comparison between skin surface hygrometer and corneometer in evaluation of the skin surface hydration state. Acta Derm Venereol. 1993;73:335–9.
23. Blichman CW, Serup J. Assessment of skin moisture. Measurement of electrical conductance, capacitance and transepidermal water loss. Acta Derm Venereol (Stockh). 1988;68:284–90.
24. Barrel AO, Clarys P. Measurement of epidermal capacitance. In: Serup J, Jemec GBE, Grove GL, editors. Handbook of noninvasive methods and the skin. 2nd ed. Boca Raton: Taylor & Francis; 2006. p. 337–44.
25. Gabard B, Clarys P, Barrel AO. Comparison of commercial electrical measurement instruments for assessing the hydration state of the stratum corneum. In: Serup J, Jemec GBE, Grove GL, editors. Handbook of noninvasive methods and the skin. 2nd ed. Boca Raton: Taylor & Francis; 2006. p. 351–8.
26. O'Goshi K, Serup J. Skin conductance; validation of Skicon-200EX compared to the original model, Skicon-100. Skin Res Technol. 2007;13:13–8.
27. O'Goshi K, Okada M, Iguchi M, Tagami H. The predilection sites for chronic atopic dermatitis do not show any special functional uniqueness of the stratum corneum. Exog Dermatol. 2002;1:195–202.
28. Kikuchi K, Kobayashi H, le Fur I, Tschachler E, Tagami H. The winter season affects more severely the facial skin than the forearm skin: comparative biophysical studies conducted in the same Japanese females in later summer and winter. Exog Dermatol. 2002;1:32–8.
29. Tagami H. Impedance measurement for evaluation of the hydration state of the skin surface. In: Leveque J-L, editor. Cutaneous investigation in health and disease. Noninvasive methods and instrumentation. New York: Marcel Dekker; 1989. p. 79–111.
30. Tabata N, O'Goshi K, Zhen YX, Kligman AM, Tagami H. Biophysical assessment of persistent effects of moisturizers after their daily applications: evaluation of corneotherapy. Dermatology. 2000;200:308–13.
31. Kikuchi K, Tagami H. Japanese cosmetic scientist task force for skin care of atopic dermatitis: noninvasive biophysical assessments of the efficacy of a moisturizing cosmetic cream base for patients with atopic dermatitis during different seasons. Br J Dermatol. 2008;158:969–78.

87 Corneocyte Analysis

Tetsuji Hirao

Contents

Abstract

The stratum corneum (SC), the outermost layer of the skin, plays a principal role in maintaining the barrier function and the water holding capacity of the skin. It consists of dead corneocytes and intercellular lipid lamellae. Corneocytes are the final product of terminal differentiation of epidermal keratinocytes, and are continuously renewed. Therefore, the exfoliating superficial SC including corneocytes can be collected easily and noninvasively, as a source of information on the nature of the SC itself, as well as the skin beneath the SC. Morphological observations of flat polygonal corneocytes reflect epidermal turnover rate. Quantitative and qualitative determinations of various constituents of SC, including keratins, intercellular lipids, cornified envelope, and natural moisturizing factors, provide helpful information to understand functional alterations of the SC. Minor but precious factors such as cytokines or biologically active molecules can also be detected by means of highly sensitive biological or immunological assays. Many enzymes involved in processing of SC components within the SC or regulatory system of exfoliation of corneocytes can also be analyzed with small amounts of SC samples. Thus, by applying sophisticated analytical methods, tremendous information related to aging of the skin can be obtained using noninvasively collected SC samples.

T. Hirao
Faculty of Pharmacy, Chiba Institute of Science, Choshi, Japan
e-mail: tetsujihirao@gmail.com

M.A. Farage et al. (eds.), *Textbook of Aging Skin*,
DOI 10.1007/978-3-662-47398-6_68

Introduction

The stratum corneum (SC) forms the outermost layer of the skin and plays a principal role in maintaining the barrier function and the water holding capacity of the skin. It consists of piled up dead corneocytes and intercellular lipid lamellae. Corneocytes are the final product of terminal differentiation of epidermal keratinocytes, and are continuously renewed. Therefore, the superficial SC including corneocytes can be collected easily and noninvasively, as a source of information on the nature of the SC itself, as well as the skin beneath the SC. Extensive morphological observations of corneocytes were performed as long ago as the 1980s [1, 2], and the relationship between corneocyte size and epidermal turnover rate has been well established [3–6]. In the 1990s, biochemical methodologies were applied to analyses of SC components, leading to detailed understandings of SC architecture, organization, and physiological and pathological functions. In this review, analyses of corneocytes and SC collected by noninvasive procedures will be reviewed, focusing especially on studies of skin aging. In this second edition, recent advances applying modern technologies, including LC-MS analysis and proteomics, will be reviewed.

Collecting Procedures

Various procedures have been proposed to collect SC samples. Those that impose the least burden on subjects are preferable, and reproducibility is also an important consideration. Broadly speaking, such collecting procedures applicable to healthy volunteers can be divided into three groups, i.e., tape stripping, polymeric resin, and scrub methods. In addition, SC samples from hyperkeratotic subjects can be spontaneously collected in the form of scales or dandruff, without any special collecting device.

Many kinds of commercially available transparent adhesive tapes, such as Scotch tape and Cellophane tape, can be conveniently used to collect SC samples by tape stripping. However, the amount of SC collected may vary depending on the adhesiveness of the tape and conditions, such as pressure, when it is applied to the skin [7, 8]. To minimize these variations, D-squame has been developed for SC collection [9]. Thus, tape stripping has been widely used for morphological observation of corneocytes. In quantitative analyses with tape-stripped SC samples, normalization of the amount collected on the tape remains an important consideration. Simple optical procedures have been proposed to estimate the amount [10–13], and protein determination is also often used, since the major constituent of the SC is protein [14, 15]. Recently, an optical procedure using infrared absorption measurement to determine the amount of SC collected on a tape has been proposed [16]. These optical methods offer the advantage that protein content can be estimated nondestructively, so the samples remain available for further study. Repeated tape stripping procedures are often used for collection of SC samples of various depths. However, Van der Molen et al. [17] pointed out that tape stripping of SC yields material that originates from various depths because of the presence of furrows in the skin, so care is needed in evaluating parameters whose value varies depending on the depth in the SC.

Cyanoacrylate resin is the most widely used polymeric resin to collect SC samples. This procedure, called skin surface biopsy (SSB), enables us to collect larger amounts of SC samples than tape does stripping, though collection imposes a somewhat greater burden on subjects. This method has the advantages that the two-dimensional distribution of the corneocytes is retained, and that it is applicable to undulating site, such as follicles, where tape stripping is difficult or ineffective.

Collection of exfoliating corneocytes by scrubbing the skin surface with a physiological buffer using a rod is a gentler procedure than tape stripping or SSB with cyanoacrylate resin. Corneocytes can be collected as a suspension in the buffer, and can be concentrated by centrifugation. In some cases, a detergent such as Triton X-100 is added to the buffer to prevent aggregation of corneocytes. This method is suitable for morphological observation of isolated corneocytes, but not for examination of two-dimensional distribution on the skin surface, which can be evaluated by using tape-stripped SC or SSB.

Thus, suitable conditions for collecting SC samples need to be selected case by case, depending on the nature of the analyses to be carried out.

Morphology

Corneocytes have a polygonal, flattened shape, approximately 1 μm thick and 50 μm in diameter, and are piled up in 10–20 layers, depending on the anatomical site, though exceptionally, over 40 layers are stacked at the palm and the sole [18].

Classical microscopic observation of exfoliating corneocytes revealed that healthy corneocytes are anucleated, while nucleated corneocytes, well-known as parakeratotic cells, are detected under pathological conditions such as dermatitis. In addition to the existence or absence of nuclei in corneocytes, the size is a parameter that can be determined easily by microscopy. Several studies have shown that the size of exfoliating corneocytes is well correlated with the turnover rate of the epidermis. Smaller corneocytes are detected in areas with faster epidermal turnover, including sites of dermatitis and tape-stripping-induced rough skin [2, 5, 6]. It is noteworthy that the size of exfoliating corneocytes increases with age in the extremities, suggesting that in these areas, the epidermal turnover rate decreases with aging. Thus, the corneocyte size can provide information about epidermal dynamics.

Electron microscopic observation has enabled more precise morphological characterization of corneocytes. Corneocytes from the deeper layers of the SC exhibit a rough surface with villous projections, while those in the superficial layer have a polygonal shape with a flat surface [19]. However, corneocytes with villous-like projections were detected in the superfical SC of patients with inflammatory disorders [20], as well as in that of normal facial skin [21], as determined by scanning electron-microscopic examination of corneocytes harvested with cyanoacrylate resin or adhesive tape, suggesting that this atypical morphology could reflect irregular maturation of corneocytes. Another approach to examine the surface of corneocytes is the use of scanning electron microscopy to observe freeze-fracture replicas by Simon et al. [22]. They reported a decrease in corneodesmosomal plaques on corneocytes during maturation within the SC. In addition to individual corneocyte morphology, the cellular arrangement has been studied in tape-stripped or cyanoacrylate-collected SC samples from patients with various skin conditions [23, 24].

Kashibuchi et al. [25] performed highly sophisticated three-dimensional analyses of corneocytes using atomic force microscopy. In addition to obtaining two-dimensional data of projected area, which has been widely used as a parameter of corneocyte size, they measured the volume, average thickness, and real surface area of corneocytes, and introduced a flatness index, defined as the projected area divided by its thickness. They found that the flatness index decreased with faster turnover rate, e.g., at the cheek and in skin from patients with inflammatory disorders. The flatness index was also decreased in the deeper layers of the SC as compared with the superficial layer, suggesting morphological change with maturation within the SC. The flatness index of corneocytes isolated from the upper arm increased with increasing age of the subjects, in agreement with previous conventional measurements of the projected area of corneocytes.

Lin et al. [26] carried out TEM observation of the tape-stripped SC and provided over all morphological changes of SC during desquamation processes. Naoe et al. [27] established immunostaining of desmoglein 1 distribution in corneocytes and revealed process of degradation pattern of corneodesmosomes. Interestingly, corneodesmosomes in the periphery of corneocytes still remain in the outermost SC, suggesting contribution via lateral cell-cell contact to generation of characteristic basket weave structure of SC. This method enabled them to show abnormal remnant of corneodesmosomes in the face as well as inflammatory keratinization diseases [27, 28].

Constituents

Major constituents of the corneocytes are keratin intermediate filaments, which fill the inside of the corneocytes. In contrast, cornified envelope (CE) is a thin, insoluble structure surrounding corneocytes, consisting of various kinds of precursor proteins which are cross-linked to each other. The intercellular spaces between corneocytes, outside the CE, contain highly organized lipid lamellae. Free amino acids, which are major components of natural moisturizing factors, can also be analyzed in SC samples.

Keratin intermediate filaments are aggregated in parallel, showing so-called keratin pattern-characteristic bundles, in the SC as observed with transmission electron microscopy [29, 30]. Since the arrangement of keratin filaments is likely to be affected by many conditions, such as water content, simple, noninvasive sampling procedures have not been employed.

Rogers et al. [31] analyzed the intercellular lipid profile in tape-stripped SC samples by high-performance thin-layer chromatography, and examined the effect of aging as well as seasonal variation, finding significantly decreased levels of all major lipid species, in particular ceramides, with increasing age. This age-related alteration is not in agreement with the results of a previous study [32], in which the lipids were collected with solvent directly applied onto the skin surface. Rogers et al. [31] also examined seasonal change, and found that the stratum corneum lipid levels were dramatically depleted in winter compared with spring and summer. They suggested that there might be a relationship between alteration in lipid profile and senile xerosis. Furthermore, intercellular lipid depth profiles were also studied by applying high-performance thin-layer chromatography to sequentially tape-stripped SC, and altered profiles were found in different layers of the SC [33, 34]. Recently, precise characterization of ceramide profiles in the SC has been available using LC/MS technologies [35–37]. Furthermore, van Smeden et al. [38] established analysis of all class of SC lipids including ceramides, free fatty acids, and cholesterol by combination of LC/MS platforms.

The composition of free amino acids in the SC can be analyzed in the water-soluble fraction extracted from SC samples by means of a conventional amino acid analyzer [39]. Free amino acids in the SC are known to be derived from degradation of filaggrin, and some amino acids are further metabolized. For example, glutamine is converted to pyrrolidonecarboxylic acid, and histidine to urocanic acid; the conversion ratio was proposed to be a marker of skin condition [40]. Horii et al. [41] showed that quantity of free amino acids in the SC decreases with increasing severity of dry skin in elderly people. Feng et al. [42] carried out sequential tape strippings of the SC to clarify depth profile of free amino acids and showed that breakdown of fillagrin into amino acids occurred deeper part of the SC. Thus, free amino acids in the SC seem to be closely related with moisturizing function of the skin. To examine amino acid profiles, tape-stripped SC is not necessary; alternatively, direct extraction of amino acids with water from the skin surface can be applied [40, 41]. Recently, confocal Raman spectroscopy has been introduced as a sophisticated in vivo analysis method for constituents in the SC without the need for tape stripping, and has revealed the depth profile of free amino acids in the SC with a resolution of several micrometers [43]. Interestingly, vibrational imaging of isolated corneocytes by infrared and Raman microscopy by Zhang et al. [44] has revealed differences of amino acid concentration between the superficial layer and the deeper layers of the SC. These optical spectroscopic analyses may also be applicable to constituents other than amino acids.

CE can be biochemically isolated as an insoluble envelope-like macromolecular structure by extensive boiling treatment of the epidermis or SC in the presence of sodium dodecyl sulfate (SDS) and a reducing agent, such as β-mercaptoethanol or dithiothreitol; most proteins, including keratins, are solubilized by such treatment. The insolubility of CE is a result of covalent cross-linking between precursor proteins. Typical cross-links are γ-glutamyl-ε-lysine isopeptide bonds, whose formation is mediated by transglutaminases (TGases).

Michel et al. [45] first reported that CE from the deeper SC shows irregular and fragile morphology, while CE from the outer SC has a rigid and polygonal shape, suggesting morphological maturation within the SC. They also reported irregular morphology of CE from psoriatic SC. Reichert et al. [46] characterized CE maturity using tetramethylrhodamine isothiocyanate (TRITC) staining, and noted that rigid CE can be distinguished by strong staining with TRITC as compared with immature CE from the deeper SC. Since TRITC reacts with amino groups, their result may reflect abundant incorporation of precursor proteins into CE during maturation.

Watkinson et al. [47] further characterized differences between rigid CE and fragile CE based on biochemical as well as biophysical approaches. Repetitive tape stripping of the SC revealed that γ-glutamyl-ε-lysine isopeptide content in the CE gradually increases with migration toward the superficial layer in the stratum corneum. Interestingly, a significant difference in maximal compressional force between rigid CE and fragile CE was observed; rigid CE was mechanically stronger than fragile CE, though the rigid CE population showed heterogeneity of maximal compressional force.

We established a novel method to evaluate CE maturity based on the biochemical profile by utilizing the combination of involucrin antigenicity and hydrophobicity recognized by an environment-sensitive fluorescent dye, Nile red [48]. Involucrin is one of the protein components of CE, being located at the exterior surface of CE, and is extensively modified by crosslinking or lipid attachment. Rigid CE from the outermost layer is stained with Nile red and less stained with anti-involucrin. In contrast, fragile CE from the deeper SC is less stained with Nile red, but strongly stained with anti-involucrin. These results suggest that immature CE has less extensively modified involucrin, whose antigenicity might be lost in mature CE as a result of modification by protein cross-linking and/or covalent attachment with lipids. At the same time, these modifications result in acquisition of hydrophobicity in mature CE, leading to intense staining with Nile red. This method of combined Nile red and involucrin staining of CE is a useful tool to study the biochemical maturation process of CE within the SC.

We first applied it to examine regional differences of anatomical sites in healthy subjects, and found that immature and fragile CE is present in the outermost layer of the face SC, while the outermost layer of SC at other sites, including trunk and extremities, shows homogeneously mature phenotype [48]. Interestingly, CE from the deeper layers of the arm, obtained through repetitive tape stripping, exhibits immature phenotype, suggesting that maturation occurs within the SC. It has been demonstrated that the face exhibits particular characteristics, such as higher transepidermal water loss (TEWL) and easier penetration of certain drugs, suggesting some impairment of barrier function [49]. Therefore, a defect in maturation of CE may be one of the factors that impede barrier function of the facial skin. The ratio of immature CE in the face varies among individuals. However, we could not find any significant difference of the ratio with age, gender, or race, though seasonal change was observed. The ratio of immature CE in the face was significantly increased in winter, suggesting a relationship between defective CE maturation and rough skin in winter [50].

Furthermore, CE in the outermost SC of the involved areas of psoriasis vulgaris (PV) and atopic dermatitis (AD), which are typical inflammatory disorders associated with impaired barrier function, showed striking heterogeneity, and consisted of immature CE and mature CE, whereas CE of the corresponding uninvolved areas was relatively homogeneous, exhibiting mature phenotype [51]. The higher ratio of immature CE found in PV and AD suggests that defective CE maturation may, at least in part, account for the impaired barrier function in inflammatory disorders. It is of particular interest that corneocytes with immature CE do not always coincide with parakeratotic cells, indicating that the mechanisms of CE maturation and disappearance of nuclei do not fully overlap, although both of them are closely associated with corneocyte maturation.

This method for evaluation of CE maturity has been applied to characterization of SC of hypertrophic scar [52], as well as to examine the effect of chemical peeling on keratinocyte differentiation [53].

Biochemistry

Corneocytes in the SC are biologically dead cells, but still retain various enzyme activities and biologically active substances.

Various proteases and inhibitors play important roles in physiological functions of the SC. One of the most important events regulated by proteolysis in the SC is degradation of corneodesmosomes, which connect corneocytes. Their degradation leads to a decrease in cohesion of corneocytes in the superficial layer of the SC. In the 1990s, two serine proteases, SC tryptic enzyme (SCTE) and SC chymotryptic enzyme (SCCE), were shown to be involved in desquamation [54–56]. SCTE and SCCE are now called human kallikreins 5 (KLK5) and 7 (KLK7), respectively, according to the new nomenclature for human serine proteases [57]. KLK7 can be activated by partial proteolysis by KLK5, and both proteases coordinately degrade the extracellular portion of corneodesmosomes, consisting of desmoglein 1, desmocollin 1, and corneodesmosin [58, 59]. Proteolysis by these kallikreins is precisely regulated by protease inhibitors during desquamation at the superficial layer of the SC [58–60]. Komatsu et al. [61] used ELISAs for global quantification of human kallikreins in tape-stripped SC samples, finding high levels of KLKs7, 8, and 11, a moderate level of KLK5, and lower levels of KLKs10, 14, 6, and 13. They also reported that levels of KLKs6, 8, and 13 were reduced in aged subjects, whileKLKs5 and 7 did not show any significant change with aging. Although the overall trypsin-like KLKs showed a slight decrease in the aged group, neither trypsin-like nor chymotrypsin-like activities in the SC differed across age groups, whereas Suzuki et al. [62] reported reduced activities of SCCE and SCTE in ichthyotic skin. In addition, no significant regional difference in the quantities of KLKs in the SC was observed among forearm, abdomen, back, and thigh [61]. Komatsu et al. applied these procedures to pathogenic disorders, and found significantly higher levels of human kallikreins in lesional SC of psoriasis [63], atopic dermatitis [64], and peeling skin syndrome type B [65]. Voegeli et al. [66] profiled serine protease activities in the SC, including plasmin-like, urokinase-like, tryptase-like, KLK5-like, and KLK7-like activities, using fluorogenic synthetic substrates, and found elevated serine protease activities in the outer SC as compared with deeper layers, and in the cheek compared with the arm, possibly indicating subclinical inflammation in the cheek, which is exposed to the environment. They expand KLK studies to atopic eczema and showed increased activity of certain serine proteases as well as protein mass in the SC of eczematous atopic skin [67, 68].

In addition to these serine proteases, aspartic proteases are involved in the degradation of corneodesmosomes. Horikoshi et al. [69] described a role of cathepsin D-like activity in desquamation, since the superficial pH is more acidic, around pH 5, than the deeper SC. While in vivo measurement of aspartic protease activities at the surface of animal skin using radio-labeled insulin B-chain as a substrate revealed an age-associated decrease of the activity [70], Horikoshi et al. [71] also measured cathepsin D-like and SCCE-like activities in tape-stripped SC. They showed that treatment with glycolic acid resulted in acute activation of cathepsin D in the lower SC, as well as long-term activation of *de novo* cathepsin D expression.

Caspases are cysteine proteases that play a central role in apoptosis, as well as in the terminal differentiation of epidermal keratinocytes. Among several caspases, activation of caspase-14 is associated with terminal differentiation of human keratinocytes, and its activity is dominant in the SC, while procaspase-14 is detected in incompletely matured SC of parakeratotic skin from psoriasis [72, 73]. Yamamoto et al. [74, 75] established quantification of activated and total caspase-14 and revealed involvement of KLK7 in the activation of caspase-14 during terminal differentiation of keratinocytes [76].

Hibino and his colleagues carried out a series of study on the proteases involved in breakdown of fillagrin into free amino acids, showing that caspases-14 plays a crucial role in breakdown into small peptides followed by final degradation into free amino acids by bleomycin hydrolase, which is a neutral cysteine protease with aminopeptidase activity [77]. Another cysteine protease, cathepsin L, can be detected in the SC by measurement of its activity [78] or by immunochromatographic procedure [79], showing its higher level in the cheek.

Gelatinases are members of the matrix metalloprotease family that degrade various components of the skin, and may be involved in photoaging. Takada et al. [80] detected gelatinase activity in tape-stripped SC of UV-irradiated skin, as well as in that of a sun-exposed area, the face, but not that of unexposed areas. Up-regulation of gelatinases may be an etiological factor in photoaging.

In addition to the proteases described above, other hydrolyzing enzymes have been detected in the SC. Beisson et al. [81] examined esterase activities of tape-stripped SC, towards triacylglycerol, and 4-methylumbelliferyl 7-heptanoate and 7-oleate, suggesting that these esterase activities are involved not only in hydrolysis of endogenous substrates, such as triacylglycerol, but also in that of exogenous substrates, such as some ester-type drugs and ingredients of cosmetics.

Jin et al. [82] examined the activities of enzymes related to ceramide metabolism in the SC. Activities of both β-glucocerebrosidase, which hydrolyzes glucosyl ceramide into ceramide, and ceramidase, which hydrolyzes ceramide into sphingosine and palmitic acid, were detected in the SC. In atopic dermatitis, both enzyme activities are unchanged as compared with healthy subjects. In an aged group, upregulation of ceramidase was observed, while β-glucocerebrosidase activity was unchanged, suggesting a possible involvement of ceramidase in the pathogenesis of aged dry skin. Takagi et al. [83] showed that β-glucocerebrosidase activity is localized in the lower part of the SC, and is involved in conversion of ceramide species within the SC.

Phospholipase A2 (PLA2) catalyzes the release of fatty acids from phospholipids, and has been suggested to play a key role in accumulation of free fatty acids in the SC. Mazereeuw-Hautier et al. [84] detected PLA2 activity in tape-stripped SC samples, and reported that deeper layers exhibited higher activity. Resoules et al. [85] studied five enzyme activities using tape-stripped SC, and reported that SC from atopic dermatitis showed significantly reduced trypsin-like activity, increased phosphatase activity, and no change in the activities of β-glucocerebrosidase, PLA2, and chymotrypsin.

In the SC, protein synthesis no longer occurs, but enzymatic or nonenzymatic modifications of proteins still occur. Enzymes involved in protein modification in the SC include transglutaminase (TGase) and peptidylarginine deiminase (PAD).

TGase mediates formation of γ-glutamyl-ε-lysine isopeptide bonds among CE precursor proteins, and its activity can be measured by using tape-stripped SC samples with labeled cadaverine as a substrate. In addition, maturation of CE was achieved by ex vivo incubation of tape-stripped SC under a humidified condition; this was mediated by TGase [86].

PAD catalyzes conversion of arginine residues in protein into citrulline residues. In the SC, keratins and fillagrin are substrates of PAD, and citrulline residues can be detected in the SC. This conversion seems to alter the isoelectric point of the proteins, and may result in a change in the conformation, but its physiological significance remains to be elucidated. Nachat et al. [87] described detection of PAD1 in extracts of superficial SC, where keratin 1 is deiminated.

The SC at the outermost layer of the skin is exposed various kinds of oxidative stimuli. Both oxidants and antioxidants have been detected in the SC [88, 89]. Measurement of peroxide in the SC using a fluorescent probe, 2′,7′-dichlorofluorescein, have shown that the level varies with the depth [90]. This method can be applied to evaluate the efficacy of antioxidant treatment of the skin.

Carbonylation is a hallmark of oxidatively modified proteins, and is introduced by either direct modification of amino acid residues in the protein or reaction with lipid peroxide-derived aldehydes. Carbonylated proteins in the SC can be easily detected using tape-stripped SC samples by reaction with a labeled hydrazide reagent [91]. Major targets of carbonyl modification are keratins [92], though proteins in the CE are also carbonylated [93]. The carbonyl protein level in the SC is increased under oxidative conditions, e.g., in SC of exposed areas. However, the level in the SC does not change much with age [94, 95], while it is significantly increased in photo-aged dermis [94]. Elevated carbonyl level in sun-exposed areas was confirmed by Fujita et al. using a simpler evaluation procedure [96]. Applying this evaluation method, we have recently studied the effects of carbonyl modification on the biophysical properties of the SC [97–99].

Various antioxidants in the SC, including alpha-tocopherol, ascorbate, uric acid, and glutathione, can also be assessed using tape-stripped SC samples [100, 101]. The levels of these antioxidants gradually decrease near the surface of the SC, and were shown to be depleted under ozone exposure [100, 101]. In addition to antioxidants, endogenous antioxidant enzymes play an important role in protection of the skin from exogenous oxidative stimuli. Hellmans et al. [102] measured the activities of catalase and superoxide dismutase (SOD) in the SC, and showed that the activities decreased near the surface. Sun exposure or UVA irradiation resulted in deactivation of catalase in the SC, which is consistent with reports of low activity of catalase in the SC in summer.

Another important modification is glycation. SC keratins are nonenzymatically glycated in diabetic patients [103, 104], though the effect of glycation on SC function remains to be clarified.

The SC contains bioactive proteins, expressed in epidermal keratinocytes, including cytokines and defensins. Interleukin 1 (IL-1) is a proinflammatory multifunctional cytokine, which had been detected in SC as epidermal thymocyte activating factor produced by epidermal keratinocytes [105]. In addition to IL-1, IL-1 receptor antagonist (IL-1ra) has been detected in SC samples collected by tape stripping. IL-1ra belongs into IL-1 family and can bind IL-1 receptor but cannot activate the receptor, so that it functions as an antagonist of IL-1. We established that both IL-1α and IL-1ra are present in SC as active mature forms, and that the ratio of IL-1ra to IL-1α in the SC is strikingly elevated in a sun-exposed area, the face, as compared with an unexposed area, the inside of the upper arm [106]. The IL-1ra/IL-1α ratio in the SC is elevated not only in UV-induced inflammation, but also in inflammatory disorders, including lesional areas of atopic dermatitis and psoriasis [106, 107]. These results suggest that the face exhibits a profile of subclinical inflammation. Interestingly, the IL-1ra/IL-1α ratio in the SC of the inside of the upper arm decreases with age, while that of the face remains constant [106].

Perkins et al. [108, 109] applied a similar procedure, and showed that levels of IL-1ra and IL-8 were significantly increased in diaper rash, and further, that the IL-1ra/IL-1α ratio and the TNF-α level were higher in seborrheic dermatitis and dandruff-bearing scalp, while the level of IL-1α was not consistent, but depended on the inflammatory skin condition. de Jongh et al. [110, 111] reported that sodium lauryl sulfate-induced irritation resulted in altered cytokine levels in SC; IL-1 decreased and IL-1ra and IL-8 increased with increasing depth. Recently, they carried out an interesting study on the relationship between IL-1 gene polymorphisms, IL-1A-889 (C to T) and IL-1B-31 (T to C), and SC cytokine levels, showing that the IL-1ra/IL-1α ratio was higher in IL-1A-889 C/T and T/T genotypes than that in C/C wild type [112]. This altered expression may be responsible, at least in part, for the interindividual differences in the inflammatory response of the skin.

Yamaguchi et al. [113] reported that SC with atopic dermatitis contains an increased level of nerve growth factor, and the level may reflect the severity of itching and eruptions in atopic dermatitis. Similar approaches have been carried out on thymus and activation-regulated chemokine (TARC) [114] and macrophage migration inhibitory factor (MIF) [115] in the SC, showing correlation with atopic dermatitis severity. Detection of these cytokines in the SC was carried out with

Table 1 Parameters measured by means of noninvasive corneocyte analyses

Categoly	Parameter	Method	References
Morphology	Nuclear remnant	TS, Microscopy	[2, 5, 6]
	Corneocyte size	TS, Microscopy	[19–21]
	Villous-like projection	TS, SEM	[27]
	Corneodesmosome	TS, Microscopy	[25]
	Flatness index	TS, AFM	
Constituents	Intercellular lipids	TS, HPTLC, LC/MS	[31, 33–38]
	Aminoacids	TS, in vivo	[39–42]
	Cornified envelope maturity	TS, Microscopy	[45–53]
Biochemistry			
Protease and hydrolase	Kallikreins	TS, ELISA, Activity	[54–56, 61–68]
	Cathepsin D	TS, Activity	[71]
	Cathepsin L	TS, ELISA	[78, 79]
	Caspases	TS, ELISA	[72–75]
	Bleomycin hydrolase	TS, Activity	[77]
	Gelatinase	TS, Activity	[80]
	Esterase	TS, Activity	[81]
	β-glucocerebrosidase	TS, Activity	[82, 83, 85]
	Ceramidase	TS, Activity	[82]
	Phospholipase	TS, Activity	[84, 85]
Other enzyme	Transglutaminase	TS, Activity	[86]
	Peptidylarginine deiminase	TS, Activity	[87]
Oxidant and antioxidants	Peroxides	TS, Colorimetry	[90]
	Carbonyl proteins	TS, Staining	[91–99]
	Vitamin C, E	TS, HPLC	[100, 101]
	Uric acid	TS, HPLC	[101]
	Glutathione	TS, HPLC	[101]
	Superoxide dismutase	TS, Activity	[102]
Modification	Carbonylation	TS, Staining	[91–99]
	Glycation	TS, Chemical reactn.	[103, 104]
Bioactive molecules	Interleukin 1	TS, ELISA	[106–112]
	Interleukin 1 receptor antagonist	TS, ELISA	[106–112]
	Interleukin 8	TS, ELISA	[108–111]
	Nerve growth factor	TS, ELISA	[113]
	TARC	TS, ELISA	[114]
	MIF	TS, ELISA	[115]
	SCCA1	TS, ELISA	[116]
	Defensin	TS, ELISA	[117]
Nucleic acid	mRNA	TS, RT-PCR	[118, 119]

AFM atomic force microscopy, *ELISA* enzyme-linked immunosorbent assay, *HPLC* high-performance liquid chromatography, *HPTLC* high-performance thin layer chromatography, *LC/MS* liquid chromatography and mass-spectrometry, *SEM* scanning electron microscopy, *TS* tape stripping

highly sensitive immunoassays. Katagiri et al. [116] reported that content of serpin SCCA1 in the SC is closely related with barrier disruption and be an excellent marker to reflect disorganized keratinization.

Antimicrobial peptides, including defensin and cathelicidin, have been reported to play important roles in cutaneous innate immunity to control colonization of microbes. Although expression of β-defensin 2 in the epidermis is down-regulated in atopic dermatitis, Asano et al. [117] reported that the β-defensin 2 level is significantly higher in SC from patients with atopic dermatitis as compared with healthy controls, suggesting a role in defensive response against infection. Gene expression does not occur in SC, but mRNAs can be recovered from tape-stripped SC samples. Wong et al. [118, 119] showed that mRNA can be recovered from tape-stripped SC samples and successfully amplified. Expression of housekeeping gene mRNAs is uniform and reproducible, while the levels of IL-8 and tumor necrosis factor-α mRNAs vary with the anatomical sites and individuals. This technique may be a promising approach to examine gene expression noninvasively, although the origin of the mRNAs remains to be elucidated.

In addition to biology-based technologies, great progress in spectroscopic technologies has been made recently, and constituents of corneocytes can now been analyzed and the distributions of amino acids and lipids imaged [44, 120].

Recent advances in proteomics technologies have been applicable to comprehensive analysis of constituents in the SC. By means of proteomics technologies, characteristic pattern of atopic dermatitis [121, 122], postmenopausal dry skin [123], and several types of ichthyoses [124] have been revealed. These promising technologies will be a powerful tool to understand various skin conditions by combination with noninvasive collection of SC samples.

Conclusion

This chapter reviewed recent studies on corneocytes, as well as SC, collected by means of noninvasive methods. Various useful parameters were listed in Table 1. Evaluation of SC can provide a tremendous amount of information, not only on the nature of SC itself, but also on the properties of the underlying skin.

The most typical alteration in corneocytes associated with physiological aging is a reduction of corneocyte size, reflecting a slower turnover rate. In addition, the intercellular lipid profile and the IL-1ra/IL-1α ratio in SC decrease with aging. However, it is important to note that these age-associated alterations occur in the unexposed areas, and are not directly reflected in sun-exposed areas, such as the face.

Since epidermal turnover is generally rapid, so that physiological age-associated changes are not likely to accumulate, changes in corneocyte parameters reflecting physiological aging are small as compared with those in the dermis. On the other hand, there are many phenotypes of corneocytes reflecting accelerated epidermal turnover, including parakeratic cells (nucleus-retaining corneocytes), smaller cell size, immature CE, villous-like projections, and so on. These phenotypes often appear in skin with accelerated epidermal turnover, such as in inflammatory skin disorders, and in the face. Thus, the age-associated changes in corneocytes in sun-exposed areas are affected by many factors, including exogenous stimuli and intrinsic factors.

Application of more sophisticated analytical technologies, including biochemical, biophysical, and optical procedures, to corneocytes is expected to give further insight into mechanisms of skin aging in the future.

Cross-References

▶ The Stratum Corneum and Aging

References

1. Goldschmidt H, Kligman AM. Exfoliative cytology of human horny layer. Methods of cell removal and microscopic techniques. Arch Dermatol. 1967;96:572–6.
2. Holzle E, Plewig G. Effects of dermatitis, stripping and steroid on the morphology of corneocytes. A new bioassay. J Invest Dermatol. 1977;68:350–6.
3. Plewig G, Marples RR. Regional differences of cell sizes in the human stratum corneum. I. J Invest Dermatol. 1970;54:13–8.
4. Plewig G. Regional differences of cell sizes in the human stratum corneum. II. Effects of sex and age. J Invest Dermatol. 1970;54:19–23.
5. Roberts D, Marks R. The determination of the regional and age variations in the rate of desquamation. A comparison of four techniques. J Invest Dermatol. 1980;74:13–6.
6. Marks R. Measurement of biological ageing in human epidermis. Br J Dermatol. 1981;104:627–33.
7. Bashir SJ, et al. Physical and physiological effects of stratum corneum tape stripping. Skin Res Technol. 2001;7:40–8.
8. Rosado C, Rodrigues LM. *In vivo* study of the physiological impact of stratum corneum sampling methods. Int J Cosmet Sci. 2003;25:37–44.

9. Miller DL. D-squame adhesive discs. In: Wilhelm KP, Elsner P, Berardesca E, Maibach HI, editors. Bioengineering of the skin: skin surface imaging and analysis. Boca Raton: CRC Press; 1997. p. 39–46.
10. Marttin E, et al. A critical comparison of methods to quantify stratum corneum removed by tape stripping. Skin Pharmacol. 1996;9:69–77.
11. Lindemann U, et al. Evaluation of the pseudo-absorption method to quantify human stratum corneum removed by tape stripping using protein absorption. Skin Pharmacol Appl Skin Physiol. 2003;16:228–36.
12. Jacobi U, et al. Estimation of the relative stratum corneum amount removed by tape stripping. Skin Res Technol. 2005;11:91–6.
13. Jacobi U, et al. The number of stratum corneum cell layers correlates with the pseudo-absorption of the corneocytes. Skin Pharmacol Physiol. 2005;18:175–9.
14. Dreher F, et al. Colorimetric method for quantifying human stratum corneum removed by adhesive-tape stripping. Acta Derm Venereol. 1998;78:186–9.
15. Dreher F, et al. Quantification of stratum corneum removal by adhesive tape stripping by total protein assay in 96-well microplates. Skin Res Technol. 2005;11:97–101.
16. Voegeli R, et al. Efficient and simple quantification of stratum corneum proteins on tape strippings by infrared densitometry. Skin Res Technol. 2007;13:242–51.
17. van der Molen RG, et al. Tape stripping of human stratum corneum yields cell layers that originate from various depths because of furrows in the skin. Arch Dermatol Res. 1997;289:514–8.
18. Ya-Xian Z, et al. Number of cell layers of the stratum corneum in normal skin – relationship to the anatomical location on the body, age, sex and physical parameters. Arch Dermatol Res. 1999;291:555–9.
19. King CS, et al. The change in properties of the stratum corneum as a function of depth. Br J Dermatol. 1979;100:165–73.
20. Shukuwa T. Scanning and transmission electron microscopic study of corneocytes: experimental formation of villus-like projections of the corneocytes of human epidermis by keratin layer stripping technique using cyanoacrylate (in Japanese). Nippon Hifuka Gakkai Zasshi. 1988;98:1467–73.
21. Yanagi M, et al. Morphological investigation of desquamated corneocytes from subject with sensitive skin and improvement of their corneocytes by using skin care products (in Japanese). J Jpn Cosmet Sci Soc. 2001;25:203–10.
22. Simon M, et al. Persistence of both peripheral and non-peripheral corneodesmosomes in the upper stratum corneum of winter xerosis skin versus only peripheral in normal skin. J Invest Dermatol. 2001;116:23–30.
23. Kashibuchi N. Improved exfoliative cytology for morphological evaluation of skin (in Japanese). J Soc Cosmet Chem Jpn. 1989;23:143–54.
24. Christophers E. Cellular architecture of the stratum corneum. J Invest Dermatol. 1971;56:165–9.
25. Kashibuchi N, et al. Three-dimensional analyses of individual corneocytes with atomic force microscope: morphological changes related to age, location and to the pathologic skin conditions. Skin Res Technol. 2002;8:203–11.
26. Lin TK, et al. Cellular changes that accompany shedding of human corneocytes. J Invest Dermatol. 2012;132(10):2430–9.
27. Naoe Y, et al. Bidimensional analysis of desmoglein 1 distribution on the outermost corneocytes provides the structural and functional information of the stratum corneum. J Dermatol Sci. 2010;57(3):192–8.
28. Oyama Z, et al. New non-invasive method for evaluation of the stratum corneum structure in diseases with abnormal keratinization by immunofluorescence microscopy of desmoglein 1 distribution in tape-stripped samples. J Dermatol. 2010;37(10):873–81.
29. Norlén L, Al-Amoudi A. Stratum corneum keratin structure, function, and formation: the cubic rod-packing and membrane templating model. J Invest Dermatol. 2004;123:715–32.
30. Norlén L. Stratum corneum keratin structure, function and formation – a comprehensive review. Int J Cosmet Sci. 2006;28:397–425.
31. Rogers J, et al. Stratum corneum lipids: the effect of ageing and the seasons. Arch Dermatol Res. 1996;288:765–70.
32. Denda M, et al. Age- and sex-dependent change in stratum corneum sphingolipids. Arch Dermatol Res. 1993;285:415–7.
33. Bonté F, et al. Existence of a lipid gradient in the upper stratum corneum and its possible biological significance. Arch Dermatol Res. 1997;289:78–82.
34. Weerheim A, Ponec M. Determination of stratum corneum lipid profile by tape stripping in combination with high-performance thin-layer chromatography. Arch Dermatol Res. 2001;293:191–9.
35. Masukawa Y, et al. Comprehensive quantification of ceramide species in human stratum corneum. J Lipid Res. 2009;50(8):1708–19.
36. Masukawa Y, et al. Characterization of overall ceramide species in human stratum corneum. J Lipid Res. 2008;49(7):1466–76.
37. Ishikawa J, et al. Dry skin in the winter is related to the ceramide profile in the stratum corneum and can be improved by treatment with a *Eucalyptus* extract. J Cosmet Dermatol. 2013;12(1):3–11.
38. van Smeden J, et al. Combined LC/MS-platform for analysis of all major stratum corneum lipids, and the profiling of skin substitutes. Biochim Biophys Acta. 2014;1841(1):70–9.
39. Denda M, et al. Stratum corneum sphingolipids and free amino acids in experimentally-induced scaly skin. Arch Dermatol Res. 1992;284:363–7.
40. Koyama J, et al. Free amino acids of stratum corneum as a biochemical marker to evaluate dry skin. J Soc Cosmet Chem. 1984;35:183–95.

41. Horii I, et al. Stratum corneum hydration and amino acid content in xerotic skin. Br J Dermatol. 1989;121:587–92.
42. Feng L, et al. Characteristic differences in barrier and hygroscopic properties between normal and cosmetic dry skin. II. Depth profile of natural moisturizing factor and cohesivity. Int J Cosmet Sci. 2014;36 (3):231–8.
43. Caspers PJ, et al. *In vivo* confocal Raman microspectroscopy of the skin: noninvasive determination of molecular concentration profiles. J Invest Dermatol. 2001;116:434–42.
44. Zhang G, et al. Vibrational microspectroscopy and imaging of molecular composition and structure during human corneocyte maturation. J Invest Dermatol. 2006;126:1088–94.
45. Michel S, et al. Morphological and biochemical characterization of the cornified envelopes from human epidermal keratinocytes of different origin. J Invest Dermatol. 1988;91:11–5.
46. Reichert U, et al. A key structure of terminally differentiating keratinoytes. In: Darmon M, Blumenberg M, editors. Molecular biology of the skin. New York: Academic; 1993. p. 107–50.
47. Watkinson A, et al. Its role in stratum corneum structure and maturation. In: Leyden JJ, Rawlings AV, editors. Skin moisturization. New York: Marcel Decker; 2002. p. 95–117.
48. Hirao T, et al. Identification of immature cornified envelopes in the barrier-impaired epidermis by characterization of their hydrophobicity and antigenicities of the components. Exp Dermatol. 2001;10:35–44.
49. Dupuis D, et al. *In vivo* percutaneous absorption and transepidermal water loss according to anatomic site in man. J Soc Cosmet Chem. 1986;37:351–7.
50. Hirao T, et al. A novel non-invasive evaluation method of cornified envelope maturation in the stratum corneum provides a new insight for skin care cosmetics. IFSCC Mag. 2002;6:103–9.
51. Hirao T, et al. Ratio of immature cornified envelopes does not correlate with parakeratosis in inflammatory skin disorders. Exp Dermatol. 2003;12:591–601.
52. Kunii T, et al. Stratum corneum lipid profile and maturation pattern of corneocytes in the outermost layer of fresh scars: the presence of immature corneocytes plays a much more important role in the barrier dysfunction than do changes in intercellular lipids. Br J Dermatol. 2003;149:749–56.
53. Dainichi T, et al. Chemical peeling by SA-PEG remodels photo-damaged skin: suppressing p53 expression and normalizing keratinocyte differentiation. J Invest Dermatol. 2006;126:416–21.
54. Lundström A, Egelrud T. Stratum corneum chymotryptic enzyme: a proteinase which may be generally present in the stratum corneum and with a possible involvement in desquamation. Acta Derm Venereol. 1991;71:471–4.
55. Suzuki Y, et al. Detection and characterization of endogenous protease associated with desquamation of stratum corneum. Arch Dermatol Res. 1993;285:372–7.
56. Suzuki Y, et al. The role of proteases in stratum corneum: involvement in stratum corneum desquamation. Arch Dermatol Res. 1994;286:249–53.
57. Diamandis EP, et al. New nomenclature for the human tissue kallikrein gene family. Clin Chem. 2000;46:1855–8.
58. Caubet C, et al. Degradation of corneodesmosome proteins by two serine proteases of the kallikrein family, SCTE/KLK5/hK5 and SCCE/KLK7/hK7. J Invest Dermatol. 2004;122:1235–44.
59. Brattsand M, et al. A proteolytic cascade of kallikreins in the stratum corneum. J Invest Dermatol. 2005;124:198–203.
60. Borgoño CA, et al. A potential role for multiple tissue kallikrein serine proteases in epidermal desquamation. J Biol Chem. 2007;282:3640–52.
61. Komatsu N, et al. Quantification of human tissue kallikreins in the stratum corneum: dependence on age and gender. J Invest Dermatol. 2005;125:1182–9.
62. Suzuki Y, et al. The role of two endogenous proteases of the stratum corneum in degradation of desmoglein-1 and their reduced activity in the skin of ichthyotic patients. Br J Dermatol. 1996;134:460–4.
63. Komatsu N, et al. Aberrant human tissue kallikrein levels in the stratum corneum and serum of patients with psoriasis: dependence on phenotype, severity and therapy. Br J Dermatol. 2007;156:875–83.
64. Komatsu N, et al. Human tissue kallikrein expression in the stratum corneum and serum of atopic dermatitis patients. Exp Dermatol. 2007;16:513–9.
65. Komatsu N, et al. Elevated human tissue kallikrein levels in the stratum corneum and serum of peeling skin syndrome-type B patients suggests an over-desquamation of corneocytes. J Invest Dermatol. 2006;126:2338–42.
66. Voegeli R, et al. Profiling of serine protease activities in human stratum corneum and detection of a stratum corneum tryptase-like enzyme. Int J Cosmet Sci. 2007;29:191–200.
67. Voegeli R, et al. Increased stratum corneum serine protease activity in acute eczematous atopic skin. Br J Dermatol. 2009;161:70–7.
68. Voegeli R, et al. Increased mass levels of certain serine proteases in the stratum corneum in acute eczematous atopic skin. Int J Cosmet Sci. 2011;33:560–5.
69. Horikoshi T, et al. Role of endogenous cathepsin D-like and chymotrypsin-like proteolysis in human epidermal desquamation. Br J Dermatol. 1999;141:453–9.
70. Wormser U, et al. Noninvasive procedure for in situ determination of skin surface aspartic proteinase activity in animals; implications for human skin. Arch Dermatol Res. 1997;289:686–91.
71. Horikoshi T, et al. Effects of glycolic acid on desquamation-regulating proteinases in human stratum corneum. Exp Dermatol. 2005;14:34–40.

72. Fischer H, et al. Stratum corneum-derived caspase-14 is catalytically active. FEBS Lett. 2004;577:446–50.
73. Raymond AA, et al. Nine procaspases are expressed in normal human epidermis, but only caspase-14 is fully processed. Br J Dermatol. 2007;156:420–7.
74. Yamamoto M, et al. Quantification of activated and total caspase-14 with newly developed ELISA systems in normal and atopic skin. J Dermatol Sci. 2011;61(2):110–7.
75. Yamamoto-Tanaka M, Hibino T. Caspase-14 protocols. Methods Mol Biol. 2014;1133:89–100.
76. Yamamoto M, et al. Kallikrein-related peptidase-7 regulates caspase-14 maturation during keratinocyte terminal differentiation by generating an intermediate form. J Biol Chem. 2012;287(39):32825–34.
77. Kamata Y, et al. Neutral cysteine protease bleomycin hydrolase is essential for the breakdown of deiminated filaggrin into amino acids. J Biol Chem. 2009;284(19):12829–36.
78. Yamaguchi M, et al. Comparison of cathepsin L activity in cheek and forearm stratum corneum in young female adults. Skin Res Technol. 2009;15:370–5.
79. Yamaguchi M, et al. Noninvasive biosensor for cathepsin L in the stratum corneum. Skin Res Technol. 2012;18:332–8.
80. Takada K, et al. Non-invasive study of gelatinases in sun-exposed and unexposed healthy human skin based on measurements in stratum corneum. Arch Dermatol Res. 2006;298:237–42.
81. Beisson F, et al. Use of the tape stripping technique for directly quantifying esterase activities in human stratum corneum. Anal Biochem. 2001;290:179–85.
82. Jin K, et al. Analysis of beta-glucocerebrosidase and ceramidase activities in atopic and aged dry skin. Acta Derm Venereol. 1994;74:337–40.
83. Takagi Y, et al. Beta-glucocerebrosidase activity in mammalian stratum corneum. J Lipid Res. 1999;40:861–9.
84. Mazereeuw-Hautier J, et al. Identification of pancreatic type I secreted phospholipase A2 in human epidermis and its determination by tape stripping. Br J Dermatol. 2000;142:424–31.
85. Redoules D, et al. Characterisation and assay of five enzymatic activities in the stratum corneum using tape-strippings. Skin Pharmacol Appl Skin Physiol. 1999;12:182–92.
86. Hirao T. Involvement of transglutaminase in *ex vivo* maturation of cornified envelopes in the stratum corneum. Int J Cosmet Sci. 2003;25:245–57.
87. Nachat R, et al. Peptidylarginine deiminase isoforms 1-3 are expressed in the epidermis and involved in the deimination of K1 and filaggrin. J Invest Dermatol. 2005;124:384–93.
88. Thiele JJ. Oxidative targets in the stratum corneum. A new basis for antioxidative strategies. Skin Pharmacol Appl Skin Physiol. 2001;14 Suppl 1:87–91.
89. Thiele JJ, et al. The antioxidant network of the stratum corneum. Curr Probl Dermatol. 2001;29:26–42.
90. Girard P, et al. A new method for assessing, *in vivo* in human subjects, the basal or UV-induced peroxidation of the stratum corneum. Application to test the efficacy of free-radical-scavenging products. Curr Probl Dermatol. 1998;26:99–107.
91. Thiele JJ, et al. Macromolecular carbonyls in human stratum corneum: a biomarker for environmental oxidant exposure? FEBS Lett. 1998;422:403–6.
92. Thiele JJ, et al. Protein oxidation in human stratum corneum: susceptibility of keratins to oxidation in vitro and presence of a keratin oxidation gradient *in vivo*. J Invest Dermatol. 1999;113:335–9.
93. Hirao T, Takahashi M. Carbonylation of cornified envelopes in the stratum corneum. FEBS Lett. 2005;579:6870–4.
94. Sander CS, et al. Photoaging is associated with protein oxidation in human skin *in vivo*. J Invest Dermatol. 2002;118:618–25.
95. Richert S, et al. Assessment of skin carbonyl content as a noninvasive measure of biological age. Arch Biochem Biophys. 2002;397:430–2.
96. Fujita H, et al. A simple and non-invasive visualization for assessment of carbonylated protein in the stratum corneum. Skin Res Technol. 2007;13:84–90.
97. Kobayashi Y, et al. Increased carbonyl protein levels in the stratum corneum of the face during winter. Int J Cosmet Sci. 2008;30:35–40.
98. Iwai I, Hirao T. Protein carbonyls damage the water-holding capacity of the stratum corneum. Skin Pharmacol Physiol. 2008;21:269–73.
99. Iwai I, et al. Change in optical properties of stratum corneum induced by protein carbonylation in vitro. Int J Cosmet Sci. 2008;30:41–6.
100. Thiele JJ, Packer L. Noninvasive measurement of alpha-tocopherol gradients in human stratum corneum by high-performance liquid chromatography analysis of sequential tape strippings. Methods Enzymol. 1999;300:413–9.
101. Weber SU, et al. Vitamin C, uric acid, and glutathione gradients in murine stratum corneum and their susceptibility to ozone exposure. J Invest Dermatol. 1999;113:1128–32.
102. Hellemans L, et al. Antioxidant enzyme activity in human stratum corneum shows seasonal variation with an age-dependent recovery. J Invest Dermatol. 2003;120:434–9.
103. Delbridge L, et al. Non-enzymatic glycosylation of keratin from the stratum corneum of the diabetic foot. Br J Dermatol. 1985;112:547–54.
104. Márová I, et al. Non-enzymatic glycation of epidermal proteins of the stratum corneum in diabetic patients. Acta Diabetol. 1995;32:38–43.
105. Gahring LC, et al. Presence of epidermal-derived thymocyte activating factor/interleukin 1 in normal human stratum corneum. J Clin Invest. 1985;76:1585–91.
106. Hirao T, et al. Elevation of interleukin 1 receptor antagonist in the stratum corneum of sun-exposed

and ultraviolet B-irradiated human skin. J Invest Dermatol. 1996;106:1102–7.
107. Terui T, et al. An increased ratio of interleukin-1 receptor antagonist to interleukin-1alpha in inflammatory skin diseases. Exp Dermatol. 1998;7:327–34.
108. Perkins MA, et al. A noninvasive method to assess skin irritation and compromised skin conditions using simple tape adsorption of molecular markers of inflammation. Skin Res Technol. 2001;7:227–37.
109. Perkins MA, et al. A non-invasive tape absorption method for recovery of inflammatory mediators to differentiate normal from compromised scalp conditions. Skin Res Technol. 2002;8(3):187–93.
110. de Jongh CM, et al. Stratum corneum cytokines and skin irritation response to sodium lauryl sulfate. Contact Dermatitis. 2006;54:325–33.
111. de Jongh CM, et al. Cytokines at different stratum corneum levels in normal and sodium lauryl sulphate-irritated skin. Skin Res Technol. 2007;13:390–8.
112. de Jongh CM, et al. Polymorphisms in the interleukin-1 gene influence the stratum corneum interleukin-1 alpha concentration in uninvolved skin of patients with chronic irritant contact dermatitis. Contact Dermatitis. 2008;58:263–8.
113. Yamaguchi J, et al. Quantitative analysis of nerve growth factor (NGF) in the atopic dermatitis and psoriasis horny layer and effect of treatment on NGF in atopic dermatitis. J Dermatol Sci. 2009;53:48–54.
114. Morita E, et al. Stratum corneum TARC level is a new indicator of lesional skin inflammation in atopic dermatitis. Allergy. 2010;65:1166–72.
115. Yasuda C, et al. Macrophage migration inhibitory factor (MIF) in the stratum corneum: a marker of the local severity of atopic dermatitis. Exp Dermatol. 2014;23:764–6.
116. Katagiri C, et al. Up-regulation of serpin SCCA1 is associated with epidermal barrier disruption. J Dermatol Sci. 2010;57(2):95–101.
117. Asano S, et al. Microanalysis of an antimicrobial peptide, beta-defensin-2, in the stratum corneum from patients with atopic dermatitis. Br J Dermatol. 2008;159:97–104.
118. Wong R, et al. Use of RT-PCR and DNA microarrays to characterize RNA recovered by non-invasive tape harvesting of normal and inflamed skin. J Invest Dermatol. 2004;123:159–67.
119. Wong R, et al. Analysis of RNA recovery and gene expression in the epidermis using non-invasive tape stripping. J Dermatol Sci. 2006;44:81–92.
120. Garidel P. Mid-FTIR-microspectoscopy of stratum corneum single cells and stratum corneum tissue. Phys Chem Chem Phys. 2002;4:5671–7.
121. Broccardo CJ, et al. Peeling off the layers: skin taping and a novel proteomics approach to study atopic dermatitis. J Allergy Clin Immunol. 2009;124 (5):1113–5.
122. Broccardo CJ, et al. Comparative proteomic profiling of patients with atopic dermatitis based on history of eczema herpeticum infection and *Staphylococcus aureus* colonization. J Allergy Clin Immunol. 2011;127(1):186–93.
123. Delattre C, et al. Proteomic analysis identifies new biomarkers for postmenopausal and dry skin. Exp Dermatol. 2012;21(3):205–10.
124. Rice RH, et al. Distinguishing ichthyoses by protein profiling. PLoS One. 2013;8(10):e75355.

The Structural and Functional Development of Skin During the First Year of Life: Investigations Using Noninvasive Methods

88

Georgios N. Stamatas

Contents

G.N. Stamatas (✉)
SkinCare R&D, Johnson & Johnson Santé Beauté France, Issy-les-Moulineaux, France
e-mail: gstamata@its.jnj.com

M.A. Farage et al. (eds.), *Textbook of Aging Skin*,
DOI 10.1007/978-3-662-47398-6_69

Abstract

This chapter is a review of the use of noninvasive methods in studies aiming to understand infant skin structure and function and its relationship to those of adult skin. Investigations on infant skin surface external appearance and three-dimensional structure at the cellular level are based on various types of imaging and microscopy methods. To understand such optical methods, it is important first to examine where the detected signals are coming from and what information we can extract from light–tissue interactions. The same principles are exploited in spectroscopy-based methods used in examining skin function such as water barrier and cell turnover. More emphasis will be given on these optical methods that have expanded dramatically our capabilities beyond the traditionally used electric methods. The application focus in our discussion will be on infant skin maturation and the knowledge that has recently been acquired using such noninvasive methods in clinical studies.

Introduction

The term "skin aging" is usually associated with the changes in skin appearance that occur during one's adult life and their causes, whether biochemical or biophysical. Skin, however, is a dynamic organ that undergoes changes throughout life, including the first years. Moreover, the changes and challenges that the skin faces early in life may affect later developments. A case in point is the relationship between the number of childhood sunburns and the likelihood of developing skin cancer later in life [1]. It is reasonable then to extrapolate the hypothesis that early events in skin's life influence later developments, including photoaging, the capacity of skin to respond to external aggressors, and immune development (e.g., allergic reactions).

Skin ontogenesis begins in utero [2]. During the first trimester, skin barrier development begins with the stratification of the epidermis. While epidermal cell maturation occurs continually during the whole of the pregnancy period, important developments in the third trimester like the formation of *vernix caseosa* are considered to create the right environment for the final steps of barrier maturation. The *stratum corneum* (SC) and the dermoepidermal undulation (early papillae structures) become visible at 34 weeks of gestational age. At this point, the first signs of water barrier function can be measured. However, the older notion that skin development occurs only during pregnancy and that this organ is fully mature and capable of performing all its functions at birth or in a few short weeks thereafter [3] has been recently challenged and revised [4, 5]. New data point to the fact that skin continues to evolve and fine-tune its functions through the first years of life.

Much research has focused on the development of skin functions, in particular, the water barrier, for infants born prematurely; this is because of the danger of dehydration [6, 7]. Nevertheless, even when considering a full-term birth, the cutaneous tissue faces a big transformation in external conditions, from the aqueous environment of the womb to the gaseous environment of the earth's atmosphere. The challenge that it faces is to continue to act as the organ that spatially defines the organism and acts as a barrier against dehydration (keeping water in) and against contamination and infection (keeping pathogens out). Of equal importance is its function as a thermal and immune barrier that also faces a big challenge at birth. The removal of the protective layer of vernix, a common practice at birth, is thought to exacerbate the challenges of the transition [8]. The case of skin adaptation during the first few days to the first month of life has received attention from the scientific community [9–12]. Yet, the continuous evolution of skin function and its underlying causes (structure and composition) during the first years of life have only recently become a subject of research [4, 5].

Finally, there is the obvious interest of the cosmetic value of baby skin in particular, when considering countering the signs and effects of adult skin aging.

The aim of this chapter is to discuss the similarities and differences between infant (1–24 months) and adult skin in terms of function and structure. This undertaking will help shed some light both on the underlying factors that contribute to the better cosmetic quality of baby skin and on the particular skin care needs of infants. The requirement for using noninvasive methods to study infant skin in vivo is obvious. Moreover, the measurement procedure should be comfortable for an infant and the measurement time as rapid as possible, without compromising the accuracy and robustness of the method. The methods that fulfill these requirements and have been used in infant skin studies will be presented and discussed.

Skin Appearance and Structure

Introduction

Skin, like any other biological tissue, is physically and chemically heterogeneous. Its appearance, as well as its mechanical properties (including the way it feels to the touch), depends on its structure at the microscopic level. Documentation of the skin appearance macroscopically can be achieved with the use of high-resolution digital imaging. To better understand the intricacies of this method, the physics of light interaction with the tissue will be discussed.

For many years, the study of skin microstructure was limited to the collection of biopsies followed by histological and microscopic analysis using transmission electron microscopy (TEM) or scanning electron microscopy (SEM). Progress in optics and imaging has allowed for the development of noninvasive alternatives that permit direct observation in vivo. These methods include video microscopy and in vivo confocal laser scanning microscopy (CLSM). The details of these methods and the ways that they have been used in the study of infant skin structure are discussed.

Imaging and Microscopy

Light–Skin Interactions

In any physics handbook, one can read about the double nature of light, which means that it can be considered as either a stream of elementary particles (photons) or as waves of electromagnetic radiation. With the word "light," normally the visible part of the electromagnetic spectrum (400–700 nm) is referred to, though this definition is often extended to the adjacent shorter wavelength region of the ultraviolet (UV) as well as the longer wavelength region of the infrared (IR). These regions are subdivided depending on the energy of the radiation (UVC, UVB, UVA, near-IR, mid-IR, far-IR). Note that the energy is inversely proportional to the wavelength, thus the UV has higher energy than the visible and the visible higher than the IR. Although the applications discussed below are based on visible light, the following discussion about light–tissue interactions can be extended to the UV and IR regions.

Assume that a beam of light is directed toward the skin tissue. No sooner that the light particles hit the skin surface, a small part of them (about 4 %) will bounce back as specular reflection that can be perceived as glare or "shine." The majority of light will penetrate the surface and will be able to travel through the tissue.

Several phenomena can take place during this travel. The energy carried by part of these photons may be absorbed by the electron clouds of specific molecules (such as melanin and hemoglobin) and dissipated in the form of heat. This phenomenon is called light absorption and gives rise to the perception of skin color. For example, hemoglobin molecules are very efficient in absorbing the blue and green regions of the visible spectrum, whereas they absorb red very weakly and therefore blood appears to be red in color.

Light scattering is another phenomenon that relates to the change of direction of the light travel through the tissue. It occurs when light meets the interface of two media with different indices of refraction. In the skin such interfaces include cell membranes, organelles (e.g., melanosomes are strong light scatterers), nuclear membranes, as well as surfaces of large molecular agglomerates such as collagen and elastin fibers in the dermis and compacted keratin structures at the top layers of the tissue.

Skin, like most biological tissues, is considered to be a turbid medium, which means that due to the high likelihood of light scattering events, tissue penetration is limited and a large part of the incident light reemerges back out of the skin surface. Capturing this light is typically performed by means of digital imaging.

Macroscopic Imaging and the Use of Polarizers

A standard macroscopic imaging setup consists of the illumination source or sources (typically flash units) and the detector (typically a high-pixel-count digital camera). Care should be taken for the positioning of the subject to be imaged: in this case a person's skin. Different body sites have different requirements for positioning (e.g., the face vs the arm). The geometry of the imaging setup, including angles of illumination with respect to the subject and the camera, the distance of the camera from the subject, and the selection of the numerical aperture of the lens, is critical for the accurate and reproducible documentation of skin appearance.

As mentioned above, part of the incident light to the skin gets specularly reflected and contributes to the glare in an image. The amount of collected specularly reflected light by the detector can be enhanced or avoided by the proper use of polarizers.

Light waves typically travel in all possible orientations. However, an orientation of preference can be selected by placing a polarizing filter in the path of light travel. Such a filter placed in front of the light source in an imaging setup allows for light traveling only in a preferred plane (polarized light) to be used for imaging. The specularly reflected light will always have the same plane of travel as the incident light, whereas the diffusely reflected light (light that has traveled through the tissue and reemerges at the tissue surface) gets scrambled due to the multiple scattering events it undergoes in the tissue. Therefore, if a second polarizing filter is placed in front of the camera lens at an orientation parallel to the plane of thc filtcr at the light source, it can enhance the contribution of the specularly reflected part, thus enhancing the surface details of the skin. On the other hand, by placing the second filter with its plane orthogonal to the plane of the polarizer at the light source, all specularly reflected light can be blocked, thus enhancing skin color and the inherent information about absorbing structures under the skin surface such as blood vessels and melanin-related structures [13, 14].

Using macroimaging, one can study the overall appearance of skin that closely resembles clinical observations. In the case of infant skin, macroimaging can be used to document the condition of dry skin, diffuse skin erythema, inhomogeneities in skin pigmentation, bruising, ectatic vessels, etc.

In Vivo Video Microscopy

The same principles of physics that govern macroimaging can be applied to light microscopy with the only difference being that of the geometry of the setup (continuous light source, specialized magnifying lens, short lens-to-subject distance due to short depth of field of the lens, etc.). Advancements in electronics and optics have allowed for the commercial availability of instruments equipped with a handheld probe that comes in contact with the skin site of interest and contains in one unit the lens and the detector. Light can be delivered where it is needed by use of fiber optic cables. Fast rate camera detectors permit not only the capture of a high-quality image but also of a time-lapse video.

In vivo video microscopy can be used to document microrelief line density and patterns, hair follicle density, pore size, local diffuse erythema, melanin distribution in lesions, etc.

In Vivo Confocal Microscopy

For the last decade or so, commercial instruments are available that made possible the in vivo use of confocal laser scanning microscopy (CLSM) in reflectance or fluorescence mode. Since the latter typically involves the use of externally applied dyes, its use in infant skin research is limited. This discussion will focus on the reflectance CLSM [15–17].

Reflectance CLSM captures light that has gone through a single scattering event in the tissue. The light source in this case is a beam of laser that is scanned (with the aid of a rotating mirror) in a horizontal plane that optically sections the tissue. Photons that went through a single scattering event are bouncing straight back to the lens that focuses the captured light to the camera detector. By means of moving vertically the objective lens, one is able to optically section the tissue at different depths. The limiting factor for getting a signal from deep in the tissue is that the likelihood of single scattering events decreases almost exponentially with depth. This means that this limits the observation of the whole epidermis, the dermal papillae, and the dermal structures that are found just below them.

The contrast in the image then arises from the areas where a change in index of refraction occurs. As mentioned above, these areas in the skin correspond to the compacted keratin of the SC, keratinocyte cell membranes, nuclei, and melanosomes in the epidermis, as well as collagen and elastin fibers in the dermis. Erythrocytes in the dermal capillaries also give a strong signal in reflectance CLSM, allowing for observations of blood flow in these vessels.

In vivo CLSM can be used in the study of skin organization at the microscopic level. Some of the parameters that can be calculated from confocal images are the cell projected area at different epidermal layers, the thickness of these layers, the depth of microrelief lines, the shape and distribution of dermal papillae, etc.

Other Methods Relating to Skin Structure

High-frequency ultrasound imaging (or ultrasonography) has also been proposed as a noninvasive method for the study of skin structure at the microscopic level. This method provides images that correspond to vertical cross sections through the skin. The resolution is rather low for detecting any structures in the epidermis, and therefore it is best suited for the study of deeper structures. Moreover, the uncertainty of the origin of the signal often renders image interpretation difficult.

Optical coherence tomography (OCT) is another method that has been used in the study of skin structure. Like in ultrasonography, OCT images represent vertical cross sections of the skin. Moreover, similar to in vivo reflectance CLSM, OCT is based on optical properties of the tissue and primarily scattering. Although it was met with big success in the field of ophthalmology, OCT use in dermatology has been limited to research only. One of the reasons is the relatively low resolution and image quality compared to the in vivo CLSM.

Finally, information regarding skin structure can come from sources other than imaging. For example, in vivo Raman microspectroscopy (to be discussed later in this chapter) can be used to extract information about the water concentration profile through the top layers of the skin. The shape of this profile contains inherently information regarding the thickness of the SC [18].

Comparison Between Infant and Adult Skin Structure

Overview of Skin Structure

The structure of interfollicular skin is typically described as being composed of two substantially different layers: the epidermis on top and the dermis below. The epidermis is much thinner (50–100 μm, excluding palms and soles where it is about 1.5 mm) than the dermis (0.3–3 mm). In contrast to the largely noncellular dermis, the epidermis is composed of densely packed specialized epithelial cells, the keratinocytes, with very few and small extracellular domains in between. Other cells that reside in the epidermis in fewer numbers than the keratinocytes are melanocytes (responsible for melanin production), Langerhans cells (cells of the immune system), and Merkel cells (neuronal mechanoreceptor cells). The keratinocytes begin their life at the lower-most layer of the epidermis (the basal layer), where they are attached to the basal lamina, the membrane that separates the epidermis from the dermis. Basal keratinocytes are smaller compared to their counterparts in the upper epidermal layers, and they have the ability to proliferate. At a certain point in its life, the keratinocyte loses its contact with the basal lamina – and with it, the ability to divide – and moves upward toward the skin surface. As it does so, it undergoes several morphologic and metabolic changes that define the epidermal layers (above the basal layer are first, the spinous and later, the granular layer). The last transition for the keratinocyte is to undergo programmed cell death, lose its nucleus, and get compacted by almost doubling its projected area to become a corneocyte, the dead cell that eventually flakes off of the skin surface. Although considered dead, the corneocytes are critical in performing the major task of building the skin barrier. Corneodesmosomes, as well as the extracellular lipid structures and the corneocytes themselves, make up the physical components of the barrier (brick and mortar model) [19].

The skin surface is not however perfectly flat. The superficial SC structures are permeated by lines known as skin microrelief. These lines are thought to give flexibility to the skin surface and are very important as reservoirs of externally applied substances. They are also the preferential location for normal skin microflora.

The hair follicles with the attached sebaceous glands and the sweat ducts are appendages that are lined with cells of epidermal origin. Their secretions (sebum and sweat) are considered to play a

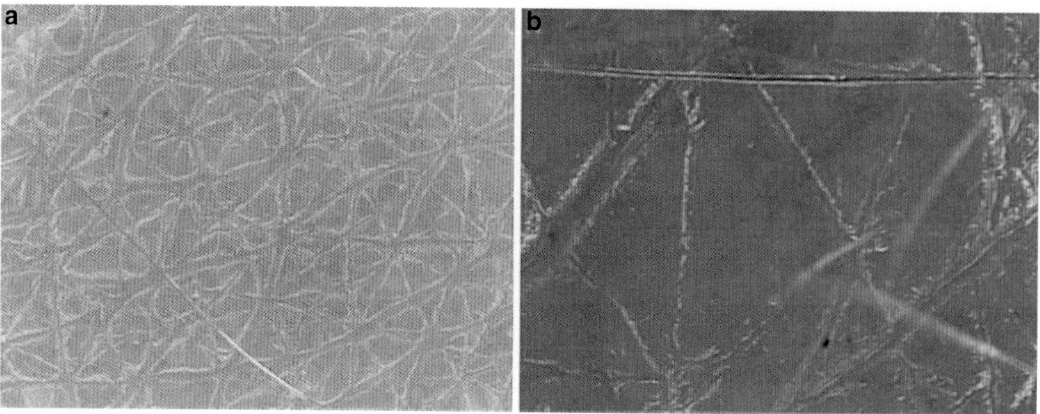

Fig. 1 The infant skin surface shows many differences compared to adult skin. Typical video microscopy images of (**a**) infant and (**b**) adult skin

role in (a) the immune and water barrier through antimicrobial lipids, (b) control of skin surface pH, and (c) production of components of the natural moisturizing factor (NMF).

Underneath the epidermis is the dermis that consists primarily of extracellular matrix material, including collagen and elastin fibers and extrafibrillar matrix (ground substance). The dermis is sparsely populated by fibroblasts. The blood vessels that provide nutrients for the whole skin tissue are found here, along with lymphatic vessels that drain the dermis of excess water. It is common to recognize two distinct layers in the dermis: the papillary layer on top closer to the epidermis and the reticular layer underneath. Each of these layers is characterized by the size of the collagen and elastin fibers (with the reticular dermis having thicker fibers arranged parallel to the skin surface), which give rise to different mechanical properties.

In general, everything that has been described so far regarding skin structure can be observed equally well in adult and infant skin. The following paragraphs focus on the observed differences.

Skin Surface

If healthy infant skin surface is compared to that of adult using video microscopy, it can be readily observed that the microrelief lines and the SC island structures in between look different (Fig. 1). In infant skin, the lines are thinner and more densely arranged than in adult skin. The SC islands are plump and round in infant skin, whereas in adult skin they look larger and flat, with the early signs if flaking at the corners.

In parallel, it is generally accepted that the number of follicles remains constant throughout life. Given their smaller body size, the total skin area in infants is greatly smaller than adults (up to ten times [20]), and therefore the density of hair follicles must be equally larger than adults. This fact needs to be taken into account when considering, for example, the permeability of infant skin to foreign substances.

Epidermal Layer Thickness and Cell Size

As discussed above, the epidermal thickness can be measured using in vivo reflectance CLSM. The SC thickness in infants has been reported to be about 30 % less than in adults, and the overall thickness of the suprapapillary epidermis is 20–30 % less in infants compared to adults [21]. Digital analysis of CLSM images has revealed that infant corneocytes and granular cells are smaller than their adult counterparts. The two observations taken together, along with the fact that infant keratinocytes proliferate at a higher rate than adult (see later in this chapter), may indicate that the residence time of a

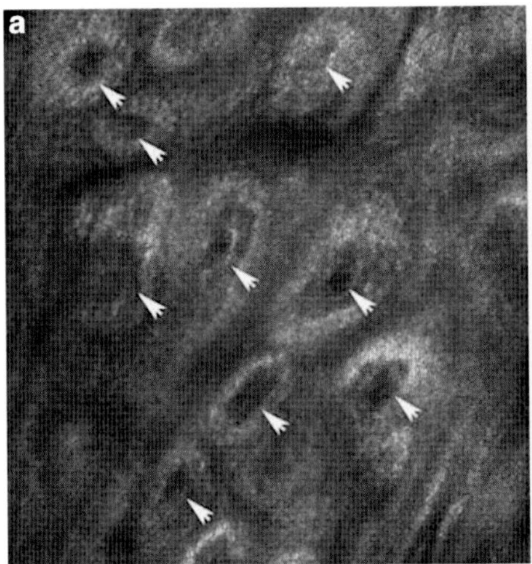

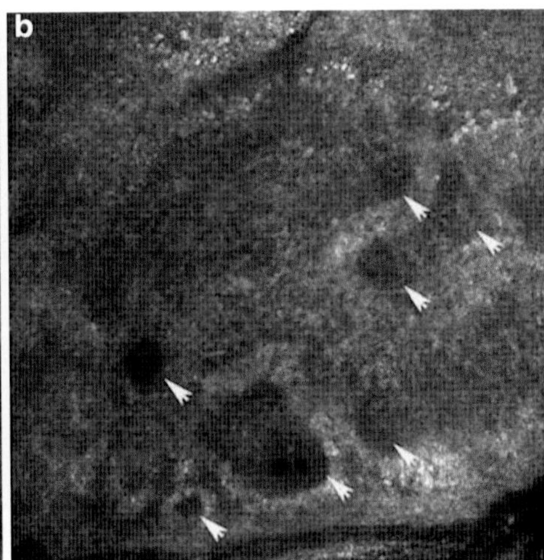

Fig. 2 Infant dermal papillae look different from those of an adult. Typical CLSM images of (**a**) infant and (**b**) adult (biological mother) skin at about 40 mm from the skin surface. The *arrows* point to the lumen of dermal papillae structures. The papillae appear to be denser, and their shape is more uniform in infant skin

keratinocyte in the epidermis is shorter in infant skin compared to adult. Either due to this shorter residence time or possibly due to mechanisms that have not been developed yet in infant skin, adult SC appears to be more cornified and even drier than infant skin (Fig. 1).

Dermal Papillae

The dermal papillae, the undulating structures that characterize the interface between the dermis and the epidermis, appear to be different in infant skin compared to adult when using CLSM (Fig. 2). In infant skin the cross sections of these structures appear to be denser and have more uniform size distribution than in adult.

Considering that the capillaries in the papillae provide the nutrients for the epidermis, the implication of this observation is that the epidermal nourishment may be different in infants compared to adults. One can understand the elevated requirement for nourishment for an epidermis that is proliferating at a higher rate.

Dermis

Beyond the epidermis and its structures, CLSM can be used to extract information about the dermis. When the average image intensity of a CLSM image stack through the skin is plotted against the corresponding depth, the exponential decay of the signal is briefly interrupted by a small maximum at a depth corresponding to a level within the dermis [22]. It has been shown that this maximum occurs due to the increased collagen fiber size in the reticular dermis compared to the smaller fiber size of the papillary dermis.

Interestingly, this maximum can only be observed in adult skin and is not evident in infants [21]. The absence of reticular dermis in babies, observed noninvasively by in vivo CLSM, has been previously observed in histological sections [23]. It can be conjectured that the formation of thicker collagen fibers occurs later in life and possibly requires accumulation of products of cross-linking reactions.

Skin Functions

Introduction

The further skin research progresses, the more the plurality of functions that the skin has to perform is being appreciated. A more obvious function is to provide the interface between the organism and the external world and thus define the shape and volume of the individual in space.

A separate, though not unrelated, function of the skin is to provide a protective barrier from external insults, as well as a barrier that maintains internally the required water content level (about 70 % per weight) that is vital for the survival of internal organs. The water barrier is localized within the uppermost layer of the epidermis, the SC. The notion of comprising a sort of barrier can be applied to skin for a variety of physical and biochemical factors, for example, barrier to external toxic molecules, barrier to UV radiation, barrier to pathogenic microorganisms, immunologic barrier, and thermal barrier.

Maintaining a healthy barrier is a dynamic process, and it requires the epidermal layer to continuously replenish itself as the cells of its top layer, the SC, get continuously sloughed off. Therefore, one of the critical functions of the epidermis is its own self-renewal, which does not cease throughout an individual's life.

Skin has been considered as an extension of the immune system as the first line of defense, but even more astonishingly as an extension of the central nervous system (much recent work has been focused on the skin–brain connection; for a review, see [24]). Furthermore, the psychological aspect of skin appearance should not be underestimated. Finally, in the study of infant skin, it is mandatory to mention the importance of touch stimulation for healthy physiological and psychological development of the infant [25, 26] or even its effect as analgesic [27]. In the interest of this chapter, however, the discussion would be limited to the skin functions that relate to physiology.

Electric and Spectroscopic Methods

Electric Methods Relating to Water Content

The water-handling properties of the SC are implicated in a variety of the skin qualities ranging from its optical and mechanical properties to the plurality of the barrier-related functions. The need for accurate documentation of these properties is evident. The first step is to be able to measure the water content (reservoir) of the SC, based on the idea that although there is a constant flux of water molecules through the SC, there is a value that can be assumed to be relatively constant when the individual is at rest.

Skin water content has traditionally been measured by indirect methods that relate the skin electric properties (impedance, capacitance, and conductance) to the amount of water in the SC [28]. The better hydrated the SC is, the easier an electric current can flow through the top layers of the epidermis due to the higher ionic mobility in an aqueous environment.

There are, however, limitations to electrical methods. Natural skin lipids or externally applied oils may hinder the electric flow and thus may actually decrease the skin conductance values and increase the measured skin capacitance. Moreover, the concentration of total ionic species found in the SC can influence the electric conductivity or equivalently decrease the skin capacitance value.

In spite of these possible artifacts, the portability of electric probes and their ease of use contributed to their general acceptance making them the most commonly used methods in scientific literature regarding skin hydration measurements.

In Vivo Confocal Raman Spectroscopy

Although the electrical methods give an estimation of the SC hydration at the point of measurement, this is an integrated value. To study the actual distribution of water concentration in the SC noninvasively, spectroscopic methods and in particular in vivo confocal Raman microspectroscopy are used.

Raman spectroscopy is based on measuring the energy shift (in wavenumbers) resulting from inelastic scattering of light by electronic vibrations of chemical bonds. Adaptation of this type of spectroscopy on a confocal arrangement allows for the calculation of concentration profiles of certain substances through the SC in vivo [29]. The requirement for a molecule to have a characteristic signal in Raman spectroscopy is that the electronic vibrations of its bonds change their polarizability when encountering an electromagnetic field (typically visible or infrared light). Water is such a molecule, and one can use this method to look at the distribution of water through the first 20–30 μm from the skin surface [30].

The water-holding capacity of SC is thought to depend on certain highly hydroscopic filaggrin breakdown products, such as small amino acids, urea, pyrrolidone carboxylic acid, ornithine, citrulline, urocanic acid, and others. These molecules are considered to be the SC's own humectants and are known in the literature as NMF. Many of these molecules have characteristic signals in Raman spectroscopy, and therefore their concentration profiles through the SC can be monitored using a confocal Raman instrument [29].

Methods Relating to Skin Water Barrier

Arguably, the most studied type of skin barrier is that of keeping water inside and preventing tissue dehydration. The integrity of other types of skin barrier, such as that against the penetration of foreign chemical substances, has been inferred to from measurements of the water barrier [31].

Typically, the quality of the SC water barrier function is assessed by measurements of the transepidermal water loss (TEWL) through the SC, which in turn is inferred to by the measurement of water vapor flux density through a cylindrical chamber that is placed in contact with the skin surface [32]. Low values of TEWL are indicative of good barrier function, whereas high values are associated with compromised or poor barrier, such as in diseases with skin barrier abnormalities (eczema, psoriasis, etc.) [33, 34] or following barrier perturbation (tape stripping, washing by harsh cleansers, occlusion of detergents, etc.) [35].

There have been at least four types of instruments measuring TEWL presented in the literature that differ in the design of the probe: open chamber, closed chamber, closed ventilated chamber, and closed chamber with condenser. Measurements of TEWL may be confounded by factors not relating to water barrier itself, but of other internal (skin temperature, sweat gland activity, and subject stress level) or external (environmental temperature and humidity) factors [36, 37].

Another way to study the water barrier is to measure the skin moisture content over time during a sorption/desorption test [38]. Typically, the protocol involves initial measurement of skin hydration followed by application of a drop of water at the site of interest. The drop is left for 10 s on the skin and then blotted off. Sequential measurements of skin hydration follow at defined time points (typically every 10–15 s) until the value stabilizes. The described method provides at least two pieces of information. The initial rise in measured skin hydration between baseline and immediately following blotting of the externally applied water (sorption) indicates how hydrophilic the SC is. In other words, the lower the sorption part of the skin hydration evolution curve, the better is the water barrier function. The second piece of information relates to the time that it takes for the skin hydration value to return to baseline (desorption). This parameter relates to the water-holding capacity of the SC. Moreover, information relating to the mechanisms involved in water desorption can be inferred from the kinetics of the desorption curve [4].

Recently a method has been proposed for the strength of the water barrier function through the calculation of a parameter corresponding to the "resistance" to water transport through the SC as a function of depth [39]. The method is based on a compartmentalized mathematical model of the SC and requires the TEWL and water concentration profile values as input. The resistance profiles demonstrate clearly that there is a "generation" part that starts at the bottom of the SC, a middle part that is fairly constant, and a decomposition part of the barrier. The method was successfully used to dynamically simulate in silico water sorption/desorption experiments in the presence and absence of a topical occlusive product (petrolatum).

Fluorescence Spectroscopy

It has been mentioned that self-renewal is a critical function of the epidermis. Epidermal stem cells are believed to give rise to transient amplifying cells that reside at the basal layer of the epidermis. These cells are responsible for replenishing the number of cells that are lost due to natural sloughing of the corneocytes at the top of the SC. Moreover, the replicative rate can increase in the case of injury to rapidly repair the damage.

The epidermal cell proliferation rate has been shown to correlate with a signal that can be followed in vivo using fluorescence spectroscopy coupled to a bifurcated fiber optic probe. This signal (295 nm excitation) corresponds to the fluorescence of tryptophan moieties, and it has been shown to be exceedingly high in skin diseases involving abnormally high keratinocyte proliferation rate, like in psoriasis [40]. When the epidermis is induced to increase its replenishing rate (either by mechanical or by chemical means), the tryptophan signal increased accordingly [41]. Finally, this signal has been shown to be inducible following biochemical stimulation [42] or exposure to UV radiation [41].

Interestingly for the study of skin aging, the tryptophan signal decreases with the individual's age (in adults) reflecting the decreased capacity of epidermal cells to proliferate [43]. Moreover, skin sites that are relatively more exposed to environmental factors, such as solar radiation, wind, and cold temperature, are induced to respond by increasing their epidermal proliferation rate, compared to relatively less exposed skin sites. This inducible capacity to respond to external aggressors also decreases with aging [43].

Comparison Between Infant and Adult Skin Functions

Firstly, the activity of skin appendages in infants and adults would be examined, and then the functions of interfollicular skin and in particular the SC water barrier and the keratinocyte proliferation rate would be compared.

Sebaceous and Sweat Gland Activity

The organogenesis of skin appendages like the hair follicles and the sebaceous and sweat glands is complete at birth, which means that the number of these organs remains the same throughout life (or even decreases as in the case of eccrine sweat glands) [44]. However, the smaller total skin surface area relative to body size in infants means that the density of the appendages is higher compared to adults.

The sebaceous glands are well developed and functional in full-term newborns, and it is believed that their production of sebum at levels comparable to those of adult skin is due to the residual influence of maternal hormones [45]. A few days after birth though, they shut down for a long quiescent period that lasts until puberty. Analysis of skin lipids therefore shows differences between infants and adults that can be explained at least in part due to the minimal sebaceous activity for the infants older than 1 month [46].

Although the size and structural maturity of sweat glands are similar in infants and adults, their responses differ. While the sweating that results in response to arousal and pain (palmar–plantar or emotional sweating) is detectable from the early days after birth, the sweating response to overheating (as means of cooling) is minimal [47]. Moreover, during the first year of life, the number of active glands is small, and their function is irregular.

Water Barrier

The water-handling properties of preterm infant and neonatal skin have been studied in extent elsewhere [3]. Here, the properties of infant skin beyond the first month of life would be reviewed.

It has been recently reported that infant skin and adult skin differ in their water-handling properties, which is evidence to the fact that skin continues to develop and fine-tune its functions during the first years of life [4]. Whether measured by TEWL or by the sorption/desorption test, the water barrier function of infant SC was found to be lacking behind the integrity of the adult barrier. Interestingly, the water barrier function is evolving with the age of the infant, tending toward adult values as the infant gets older. A higher variability was also observed in the infant TEWL data compared to the adult data indicating that the homeostatic mechanisms are not yet fully developed. Moreover, the sorption/desorption test showed that infant skin absorbs more water than adult skin but also loses this water following faster kinetics. Interestingly, adult skin appears to involve a single mechanism of desorption, while baby skin apparently involves a second one that is more rapid than the first.

Similar to the TEWL data, using skin conductance measurements, higher values for baseline skin hydration in infants compared to adults [4] were reported. This is important because it distinguishes healthy infant skin water barrier from that of an abnormal condition (e.g., atopic dermatitis or psoriasis). In the case of a barrier impairing skin disease, the TEWL is high and the skin hydration is low. Infant skin on the other hand shows both TEWL and skin hydration to be higher compared to adult skin. This can be an indication that infant skin barrier is not completely compromised but that the involved mechanisms may be different than those in adult skin and that these mechanisms continue to develop during the first years of life.

A further observation that leads to the same conclusion is the fact that although skin hydration is higher in infants compared to adults, the concentration of NMF in infant SC (measured by Raman microspectroscopy) is lower. Therefore, the water-holding capacity of infant SC must rely on a reservoir other than the NMF. Furthermore, the NMF concentration profile through the SC depends on the infant age, with older infants resembling closer the profiles of their mothers.

Raman microspectroscopy measurements moreover confirmed the higher water content of infant SC measured by skin conductance, as well as the higher hydrophilicity following topical application of a drop of water.

The resistance profiles to water transport demonstrate clearly the difference in skin barrier efficacy throughout the SC between infants and adults [39].

Epidermal Cell Proliferation

Infant granular cells and corneocytes are smaller than adult ones. This observation is an evidence to the fact that the turnover rate of epidermal cells in the infant is faster than in the adult skin. Using in vivo fluorescence spectroscopy, it has been confirmed that this is indeed the case [21]. The fluorescence band linked to keratinocyte proliferation is up to ten times higher in young infants (<6 months) than in adults. The high cell turnover rate can explain the improved wound healing properties of infants compared to adults. Moreover, it is in line with published observations that the epidermal cell proliferation rate is decreasing with age throughout lives [43].

Conclusion

In the past, infant skin was believed to be structurally and functionally equivalent to that of adult skin. More recent evidence has been put forward that in many cases this assumption needs to be revised. Facets of skin microstructure (SC cells size, SC and epidermal thickness, skin microrelief line density) as well as elements of skin function (eccrine sweat gland activity, SC water-handling properties, epidermal proliferation rate) have been found to be different when comparing infant and adult skin. Finally, the particular properties that make infant skin different from adult skin continue to persist at least through the first year of life.

References

1. Whiteman DC, Whiteman CA, Green AC. Childhood sun exposure as a risk factor for melanoma: a systematic review of epidemiologic studies. Cancer Causes Control. 2001;12:69–82.
2. Holbrook K. Embryogenesis of the skin. Oxford: Blackwell Science; 2000.
3. Hoath SB, Maibach H, editors. Neonatal skin – structure and function. New York: Marcel Dekker; 2003.
4. Nikolovski J, Stamatas GN, Kollias N, Wiegand BC. Barrier function and water-holding and transport properties of infant stratum corneum are different from adult and continue to develop through the first year of life. J Invest Dermatol. 2008;128:1728–36.
5. Visscher MO, Chatterjee R, Ebel JP, et al. Biomedical assessment and instrumental evaluation of healthy infant skin. Pediatr Dermatol. 2002;19:473–81.
6. Kalia YN, Nonato LB, Lund CH, Guy RH. Development of skin barrier function in premature infants. J Invest Dermatol. 1998;111:320–6.
7. Rutter N, Hull D. Water loss from the skin of term and preterm babies. Arch Dis Child. 1979;54:858–68.

8. Visscher MO, Narendran V, Pickens WL, et al. Vernix caseosa in neonatal adaptation. J Perinatol. 2005;25:440–6.
9. Evans NJ, Rutter N. Development of the epidermis in the newborn. Biol Neonate. 1986;49:74–80.
10. Harpin VA, Rutter N. Barrier properties of the newborn infant's skin. J Pediatr. 1983;102:419–25.
11. Hoath SB. The stickiness of newborn skin: bioadhesion and the epidermal barrier [comment]. J Pediatr. 1997;131:338–40.
12. Yosipovitch G, Maayan-Metzger A, Merlob P, Sirota L. Skin barrier properties in different body areas in neonates. Pediatrics. 2000;106:105–8.
13. Anderson RR. Polarized light examination and photography of the skin. Arch Dermatol. 1991;127:1000–5.
14. Muccini JA, Kollias N, Phillips SB, et al. Polarized light photography in the evaluation of photoaging. J Am Acad Dermatol. 1995;33:765–9.
15. Corcuff P, Bertrand C, Leveque JL. Morphometry of human epidermis in vivo by real-time confocal microscopy. Arch Dermatol Res. 1993;285:475–81.
16. Fink-Puches R, Hofmann-Wellenhof R, Smolle J, Kerl H. Confocal laser scanning microscopy: a new optical microscopic technique for applications in pathology and dermatology. J Cutan Pathol. 1995;22:252–9.
17. Rajadhyaksha M, Gonzalez S, Zavislan JM, et al. In vivo confocal scanning laser microscopy of human skin II: advances in instrumentation and comparison with histology. J Invest Dermatol. 1999;113:293–303.
18. Egawa M, Hirao T, Takahashi M. In vivo estimation of stratum corneum thickness from water concentration profiles obtained with Raman spectroscopy. Acta Derm Venereol. 2007;87:4–8.
19. Nemes Z, Steinert PM. Bricks and mortar of the epidermal barrier. Exp Mol Med. 1999;31:5–19.
20. Haycock GB, Schwartz GJ, Wisotsky DH. Geometric method for measuring body surface area: a height-weight formula validated in infants, children, and adults. J Pediatr. 1978;93:62–6.
21. Stamatas GN, Nikolovski J, Luedtke MA, et al. Infant skin microstructure assessed in vivo differs from adult skin in organization and at the cellular level. Pediatr Dermatol. 2009;27:125–31.
22. Neerken S, Lucassen GW, Bisschop MA, et al. Characterization of age-related effects in human skin: a comparative study that applies confocal laser scanning microscopy and optical coherence tomography. J Biomed Opt. 2004;9:274–81.
23. Holbrook KA. A histological comparison of infant and adult skin. New York: Marcel Dekker; 1982.
24. Tobin DJ. Biochemistry of human skin – our brain on the outside. Chem Soc Rev. 2006;35:52–67.
25. Field TM, Schanberg SM, Scafidi F, et al. Tactile/kinesthetic stimulation effects on preterm neonates. Pediatrics. 1986;77:654–8.
26. Field TM, Grizzle N, Scafidi F, Abrams S. Massage therapy for infants of depressed mothers. Infant Behav Dev. 1996;19:107–12.
27. Gray L, Watt L, Blass EM. Skin-to-skin contact is analgesic in healthy newborns. Pediatrics. 2000;105:e14.
28. Tagami H, Kikuchi K, O'goshi K. Electrical properties of newborn skin. In: Hoath SB, Maibach HI, editors. Neonatal skin structure and function. New York: Mercel Dekker; 2003.
29. Caspers PJ, Lucassen GW, Carter EA, et al. In vivo confocal Raman microspectroscopy of the skin: noninvasive determination of molecular concentration profiles. J Invest Dermatol. 2001;116:434–42.
30. Caspers PJ, Lucassen GW, Bruining HA, Puppels GJ. Automated depth-scanning confocal Raman microspectrometer for rapid in vivo determination of water concentration profiles in human skin. J Raman Spectrosc. 2000;31:813–8.
31. Tupker RA. Prediction of irritancy in the human skin irritancy model and occupational setting. Contact Dermatitis. 2003;49:61–9.
32. Imhof R. TEWL and the skin barrier (invited lecture). In: Sixth annual meeting of the skin forum. Winchester; 2005.
33. Chamlin SL, Kao J, Frieden IJ, et al. Ceramide-dominant barrier repair lipids alleviate childhood atopic dermatitis: changes in barrier function provide a sensitive indicator of disease activity. J Am Acad Dermatol. 2002;47:198–208.
34. Rim JH, Jo SJ, Park JY, et al. Electrical measurement of moisturizing effect on skin hydration and barrier function in psoriasis patients. Clin Exp Dermatol. 2005;30:409–13.
35. Atrux-Tallau N, Huynh NT, Gardette L, et al. Effects of physical and chemical treatments upon biophysical properties and micro-relief of human skin. Arch Dermatol Res. 2008;300:243–51.
36. Chilcott RP, Dalton CH, Emmanuel AJ, et al. Transepidermal water loss does not correlate with skin barrier function in vitro. J Invest Dermatol. 2002;118:871–5.
37. Wilson DR, Maibach H. Transepidermal water loss. New York: Marcel Dekker; 1982.
38. Tagami H, Kanamaru Y, Inoue K, et al. Water sorption–desorption test of the skin in vivo for functional assessment of the stratum corneum. J Invest Dermatol. 1982;78:425–8.
39. van Logtestijn MDA, Domínguez-Hüttinger E, Stamatas GN, Tanaka RJ. Resistance to water diffusion in the stratum corneum is depth-dependent. PLoS One. 2015;10(2):e0117292.
40. Gillies R, Zonios G, Anderson RR, Kollias N. Fluorescence excitation spectroscopy provides information about human skin in vivo. J Invest Dermatol. 2000;115:704–7.
41. Brancaleon L, Lin G, Kollias N. The *in vivo* fluorescence of tryptophan moieties in human skin increases with UV exposure and is a marker for epidermal proliferation. J Invest Dermatol. 1999;113:977–82.
42. Doukas AG, Soukos NS, Babusis S, et al. Fluorescence excitation spectroscopy for the measurement of

epidermal proliferation. Photochem Photobiol. 2001;74:96–102.
43. Stamatas GN, Estanislao RB, Suero M, et al. Facial skin fluorescence as a marker of the skin's response to chronic environmental insults and its dependence on age. Br J Dermatol. 2006;154:125–32.
44. Fenske NA, Lober CW. Structural and functional changes of normal aging skin. J Am Acad Dermatol. 1986;15:571–85.
45. Henderson CA, Taylor J, Cunliffe WJ. Sebum excretion rates in mothers and neonates. Br J Dermatol. 2000;142:110–1.
46. Agache P, Blanc D, Barrand C, Laurent R. Sebum levels during the first year of life. Br J Dermatol. 1980;103:643–9.
47. Rutter N. Eccrine sweating in the newborn. In: Hoath SB, Maibach HI, editors. Neonatal skin structure and function. New York: Mercel Dekker; 2003.

Structure of Stratum Corneum Lipid Studied by Electron Paramagnetic Resonance

89

Kouichi Nakagawa

Contents

K. Nakagawa
Department of Radiological Life Sciences, Graduate School of Health Sciences, Hirosaki University, Hirosaki, Aomori, Japan
e-mail: nakagawa@hirosaki-u.ac.jp

M.A. Farage et al. (eds.), *Textbook of Aging Skin*,
DOI 10.1007/978-3-662-47398-6_70

Abstract

EPR (electron paramagnetic resonance) is useful for elucidating structural aspects of skin. Noninvasive spectroscopic characterization of the outermost layer of the stratum corneum (SC) as well as nail is an important subject in dermatology and cosmetology. However, there is no feasible spectroscopic method to evaluate initial changes of SC and severity of nail with psoriasis. EPR might be feasible for evaluating the conditions in the patients with psoriasis.

A little, broad three-line pattern of the psoriasis vulgaris SC (PV-SC) was observed. The spectral pattern is quite different from those of other SC reported. The spectral pattern suggests that the 5-DSA is mobile or less rigid in the SC. The reasonable agreement between the experimental and simulated spectra was obtained. The S_0 value obtained for 5-DSA in the SC was approximately 0.20. It is noted that the lower value of the S_0 indicates the less rigid (abnormal) structure of the PV-SC. The PV-SC is found to be less rigid of structure than that of the control SC, indicating abnormal architecture of psoriasis vulgaris stratum corneum. The statistical analysis using Student's t-test suggests that the value of PV-SC is significantly smaller than that of the control ($p < 0.01$). In the case of the fingernail, EPR spectra were analyzed using the intensity ratio of the two motions (fast and slow) at the peaks of the lower magnetic field.

The EPR results and the detailed analyses show that there are rigid and fragile sites in the nail. In the case of nail psoriasis, the fragile components are 2 ~ 3 times more than those of the control. Therefore, the EPR assay is of great use for evaluating SC and nail function.

Introduction

Stratum corneum (SC) is the outermost layer of skin and the skin barrier against chemicals, surfactants, UV irradiation, and environmental stresses. The SC has a heterogeneous structure composed of corneocytes embedded in the intercellar lipid lamellae as illustrated in Fig. 1. The morphology of the SC lipids is closely associated with the main epidermal barrier. Knowledge of the lipid structure is important in understanding the mechanism of irritant dermatitis and other SC diseases. The structural information of the SC lipid is obtained by the analysis of aliphatic spin probes incorporated into intercellar lamella lipids using EPR (electron paramagnetic resonance) [1–5]. EPR in conjunction with spin probe method nondistractively measures the ordering of the lipid bilayer of SC.

EPR (or ESR: electron spin resonance) utilizes spectroscopy, which measures an unpaired electron in an atom or molecule. The principles behind magnetic resonance are common to both EPR and nuclear magnetic resonance (NMR), but there are differences in the magnitudes and signs of the magnetic interactions involved. EPR probes an unpaired electron spin, while NMR probes a nuclear spin. EPR can measure 10^{-9} M (moles per liter) concentration of the probe and is one of the most sensitive spectroscopic tools. Therefore, EPR is able to elucidate skin lipid structures as well as dynamics.

It is important to know the composition of SC lipid as well as its structure in relation to depth. The various componentssuch as ceramides, cholesterol, and free fatty acids of SC lipids have been investigated by TLC (thin-layer chromatography) [6, 7]. It was also pointed out that the levels of SC lipids in a group of women aged 41–50 showed a decrease of SC lipid levels [8]. Structural information organized by the components is essential for knowing the detailed functions of SC. The role of the intercellular SC lipid bilayer in relation to barrier function has been investigated by IR (infrared) spectroscopy [9, 10] and X-ray diffraction [11, 12]. IR examination showed that the outer layers were less cohesive and the intercellular lipids are more disordered compared with the deeper membrane, based on the C-H stretching absorbance of the methylene groups of the lipid acyl chains. The X-ray approach is somewhat limited to model lipid membranes containing water or in vitro SC specimens, and it is difficult to obtain information about depth-related changes of the SC. On the other hand, the EPR probe method can provide insight into the SC lipid organization as well as its dynamics. The physicochemical properties of intercellar lipids of SC as a function of various surfactants [1, 2], water contents [3], various kinds of spin probes [4], and ordering (or fluidity) change of the SC lipid [1] were investigated. EPR is a reliable, sensitive, and nondistractive technique to measure the probe in the lipids at any temperature.

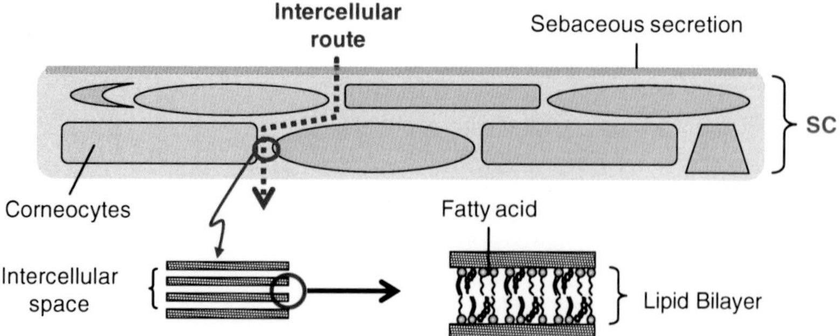

Fig. 1 Schematic representation of the modified "Brick and Mortar" model of the stratum corneum (SC) is shown. Also, there is shown the most likely probe location in the lipid bilayer and pathways of drug (or spin probe) permeation through intact stratum corneum

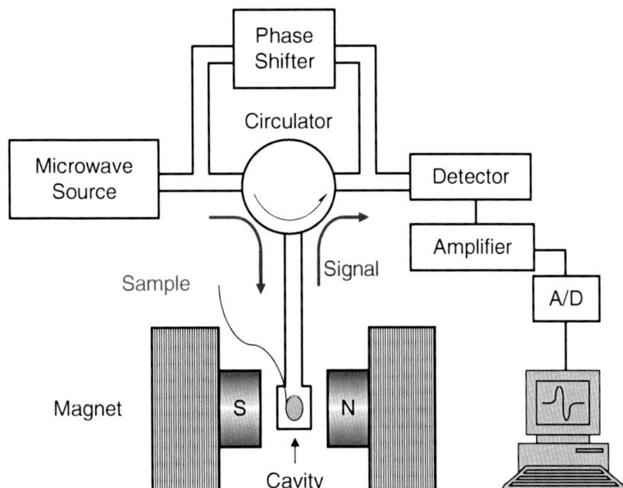

Fig. 2 Block diagram of EPR spectrometer

Apparatus

EPR apparatus consists of a klystron to generate microwaves, electromagnet, resonant cavity, microwave detector, amplifier, A/D converter, and PC as shown in Fig. 2. The microwaves from the klystron have a constant frequency, and those microwaves reflected from the resonant cavity are detected, changed to an electronic signal, amplified, and then recorded.

In contrast to NMR, substances which contain unpaired spin can be observed by EPR. Paramagnetic substances including transition metal complexes, free radicals, macromolecules, and photochemical intermediates are observed. Approximately 10^{-13} unpaired spin number of a substance gives an observable signal, thus EPR has great sensitivity.

Momentum of electron spin in a magnetic field orients only two quantum states: $m_s = ½$ and $-½$.

Application of an oscillating field perpendicular to a steady magnetic field (H) induces transitions between the two states provided the frequency (ν) of the oscillating field satisfies the resonance condition

$$\Delta E = E_{\frac{1}{2}} - E_{-\frac{1}{2}} = g\beta H, \quad (1)$$

Thus,

$$h\nu = \Delta E = g\beta H, \quad (2)$$

where ΔE is the energy level separation, h is Planck's constant, g is a dimensionless constant called the g-value, β is the electron Bohr magneton, and H is the applied magnetic field.

The interaction of an electron spin in resonance with a neighboring nuclear spin in a molecule is called hyperfine coupling. In the case of nitroxide spin probe, ^{14}N of the probe has three quantum states: $m_I = +1, 0,$ and -1. Each quantum state interacts with an electron spin and further splits into two sets of energy states as shown in Fig. 3. The selection rules for transitions in hyperfine coupling are $\Delta m_s = 1$ and $\Delta m_I = 0$.

Thus, one can observe three transition (resonance) lines for fast-tumbling nitroxide spin probe in a spectrum. The interval of the resonance lines is called the hyperfine coupling constant (A). The EPR spectra are usually recorded as the first derivative of the absorption spectrum as shown in the lower part of Fig. 3.

Stratum Corneum Cyanoacrylate Glue Stripping

The sampling method was first utilized by Marks and Dawber [11] to obtain SC sheets. Recently, Yagi, Nakagawa, and Sakamoto developed a process to study SC properties [13]. The SC specimens were successively removed from the

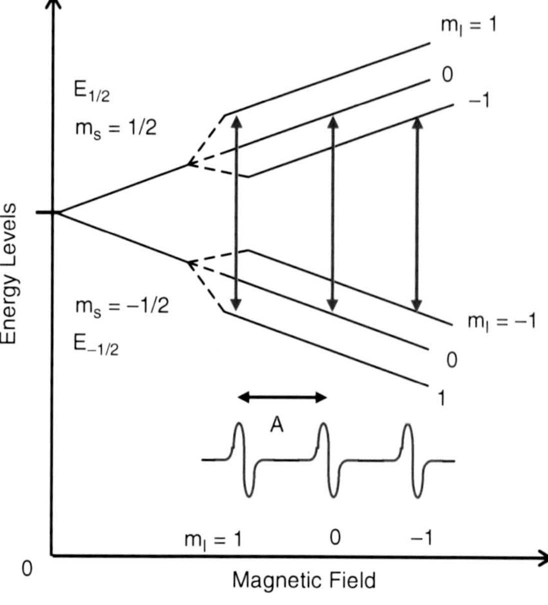

Fig. 3 Hyperfine levels and transitions for a nitroxide nitrogen nucleus (^{14}N) of $I = 1$ with positive coupling constant. An observable EPR observable spectrum is shown

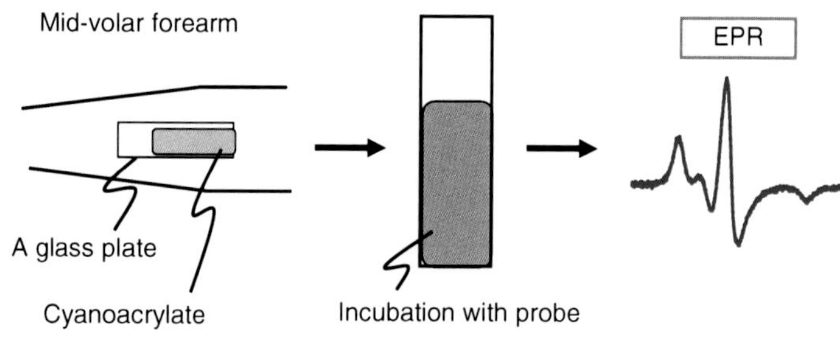

Fig. 4 Schematic representation of SC sample procedures and the EPR spectrum

midvolar forearm and shank of the volunteers, who had given informed consent to the procedure [13]. All subjects had normal skin, as judged by visual assessment. A glass plate (7 mm × 37 mm; Matsunami Glass Ind., Ldt., Tokyo, Japan) on which a single drop (~1.2 mg) of a commercially available cyanoacrylate resin had been uniformly spread was used to strip the SC sheet as depicted in Fig. 4. Only approximately 1 mg of SC sample is required for the studies. Once the glue has solidified, no significant signal arises from the cured resin or from the spin probe dissolved in the resin; the only signal observed arises from the spin probe in the attached SC sheet. This method has the advantage of avoiding prior exposure of the SC to enzymes. EPR intensity slightly depends on how thick a sample is removed by each stripping, but it can be adjusted by the amount and area of glue on the glass plate.

Preparation of SC Sheets for EPR Measurements

One piece of stripped SC (~5 × 22 mm^2) was incubated in ~50 μM of a spin probe (Fig. 5) aqueous solution for about 60 min at 37 °C (Fig. 4). The probe solution was dropped on the SC sheet. The SC sheet repels the aqueous solution, but the probe goes into the lipid phase during the incubation. After rinsing with distilled water to remove excess spin probe, the SC sample was mounted on an EPR cell.

Spin Probes (or Spin Labels)

Organic free radicals containing the nitroxide group are called spin probes or spin labels. The ordering and fluidity of the lipid bilayer is obtained with doxylstearic acid (DSA) which is most commonly used. Commercially available spin probes, 5-doxylstearic acid (5-DSA) and 3β-doxyl-5α-cholestane (CHL), were used to obtain the ordering of the SC lipid. The chemical structures of 5-DSA and CHL are depicted in Fig. 5. Changes of the lipid chain ordering are able to monitor using various probes. The orientation of spin probes reflects the local molecular environment and should serve as indicator of conformational changes in lipid bilayers.

EPR Line Shapes due to Spin Probe Motion

The line shapes and line widths can vary under certain spin probe environments. When line broadening arises from incomplete averaging of the g-value and the hyperfine coupling interactions within the limit of rapid tumbling in a medium, EPR line shape starts changing from the triplet pattern. EPR spectra of nitroxide radicals for different tumbling times as well as different order parameters are presented in Fig. 6. Schematic illustration of lipid bilayer structures and corresponding EPR spectra is also shown in Fig. 7. If a spin probe is oriented (immobilized) in a lipid membrane, EPR spectrum

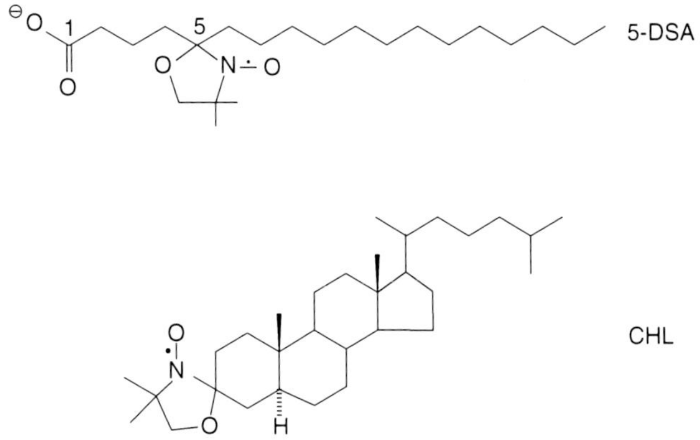

Fig. 5 Chemical structures of 5-doxylstearic acid (5-DSA) and 3β-doxyl-5α-cholestane (CHL) spin probes

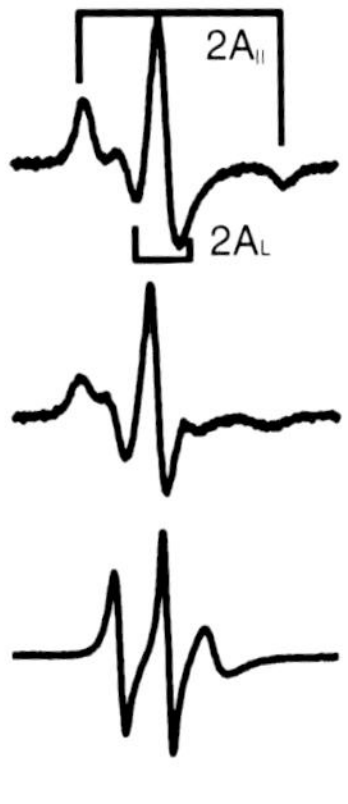

Fig. 6 Nitroxide EPR lineshape as a function of tumbling time and order parameter. The parallel and perpendicular hyperfine couplings, $2A_{\parallel}$ and $2A_{\perp}$, are also indicated for an anisotropic (immobilized) EPR spectrum

Description of spectra	Approx. tumbling time (ns)	Approx. order parameter
Immobilized	0.5	0.7
Moderately Immobilized	2.5	0.3
Weakly Immobilized	5.0	0.1

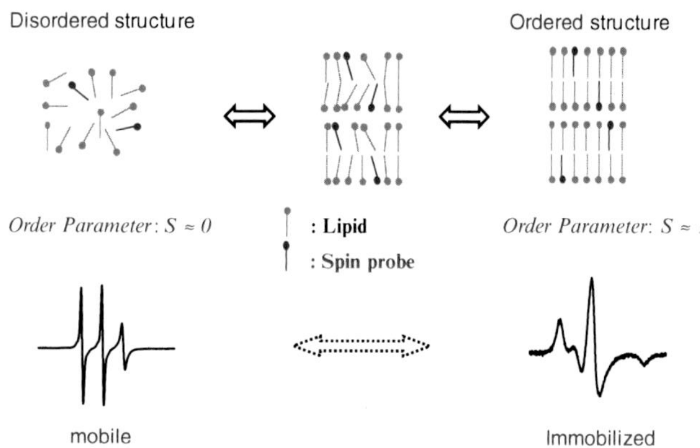

Fig. 7 Schematic representation of lipid bilayer structures as a function of lipid ordering. The corresponding EPR spectral patterns were also indicated

is an anisotropic pattern which clearly shows parallel ($2A_{\parallel}$) and perpendicular ($2A_{\perp}$) hyperfine coupling structures (the top spectrum in Fig. 6). The order parameter is approximately 0.7 or higher. If a spin probe tumbles relatively fast (weakly immobilized) in a lipid membrane, EPR spectrum is a triplet pattern with unequal intensities. The order parameter is usually very small (~0.1).

Qualitative Order Parameter (S_0)

The inclination of the principal axis of the nitroxide radical to the rotational axis of the long-chain probe molecule represents a measure of the order–disorder of the molecular assemblies of a membrane. The order parameter indicates the membrane chain dynamics and microenvironment of the medium in which the spin probe is incorporated.

The conventional order parameter (S) is determined from the hyperfine coupling of the EPR signals according to the following relations [12]:

$$S = \frac{A_{//} - A_{\perp}}{A_{ZZ} - \frac{1}{2}(A_{XX} + A_{YY})} \bullet \frac{a}{a'}, \tag{3}$$

$$a' = \frac{A_{//} + 2A_{\perp}}{3}, \tag{4}$$

where a is the isotropic hyperfine value, $(A_{XX} + A_{YY} + A_{ZZ})/3$; A_{XX}, A_{YY}, and A_{ZZ} are the principal values of the spin probe. The following principal components were used for 5-DSA [14]:

$$A_{XX}, A_{YY}, A_{ZZ} = (0.66,\ 0.55,\ 3.45)\ \text{mT} \tag{5}$$

The experimental hyperfine couplings of $2A_{\parallel}$ and $2A_{\perp}$ are obtained from the experimental spectrum (as shown in Fig. 6). The order parameter indicates that the S value increases with increasing anisotropy of the probe site in the membrane. On the other hand, the S value becomes zero for completely isotropic motion of the nitroxide radical. Since the spin probe is incorporated into the highly oriented intercellular lipid structure in normal skin, in which the probe cannot move freely due to the rigidity of lipid structure, its EPR spectrum represents the microscopically oriented profile as depicted in Fig. 7. When the normal structure is completely destroyed by chemical and/or physical stress, the EPR spectral profile changes to three sharp lines because the probe mobility is unrestricted. Thus, the EPR spectral profile reflects the rigidity of the environment of the probe moiety. However, conventional analysis measuring $2A_{\parallel}$ and $2A_{\perp}$ from the observed spectrum gives limited information concerning the probe moiety in the membrane and may not reveal subtle differences in the overall experimental spectra related to the membrane chain ordering [13].

Quantitative Order Parameter (S_0) by Slow-Tumbling Spectral Simulation

The slow-tumbling motions on the order of 10^{-7} s of the aliphatic spin probes in membranes were evaluated by using the nonlinear least-squares fitting program NLLS to calculate the EPR spectra based on the stochastic Liouville equation [15, 16]. The EPR spectra for spin probes incorporated into the multilamellar lipid bilayer were calculated according to various distributions of the probe in the membrane. The spectrum of a sample can be regarded as the superposition of the spectra of all of the fragments. The lipid and 5-DSA molecules in the lipid bilayer experience ordering (or fluidity) potentials, which restrict the amplitude of the rotational motion. The ordering potential in a lipid bilayer determines the orientational distribution of molecules with respect to the local ordering axis of the bilayer [17]. The overall orientation of the probe can be expressed by the order parameter (S_0), which is defined as follows [16, 18]:

$$S_0\left\langle\frac{1}{2}\left(3\cos^2\gamma-1\right)\right\rangle = \frac{\int d\Omega \exp(-U/kT)D_{00}^2}{\int d\Omega \exp(-U/kT)}, \tag{6}$$

which measures the angular extent of the rotational diffusion of the nitroxide probe moiety. Gamma (γ) is the angle between the rotational diffusion symmetry axis and the z-axis of the nitroxide axis system as shown in Fig. 8. The $\Omega = (\alpha, \beta, \gamma)$ are the Euler angles between the molecular frame of the rotational diffusion tensor, U is the ordering potential, and D is a Winger rotation matrix element. In addition to S_0, the simulation calculates slow-tumbling motions of the probe in the bilayer, providing rotational diffusion coefficients, as described in detail elsewhere [19]. The values of the rotational diffusion coefficients (dynamic values) are in relation to the S_0 values. The $\boldsymbol{A}$ and $\boldsymbol{g}$ of the principal components were used for the simulation of 5-DSA [14]:

$$A_{XX}, A_{YY}, A_{ZZ} = (0.66, 0.55, 3.45)\,\mathrm{mT} \tag{5}$$

$$g_{XX}, g_{YY}, g_{ZZ} = (2.0086, 2.0063, 2.0025). \tag{7}$$

The local or microscopic ordering of the nitroxide probe in the multilamellar lipid bilayer is characterized by the S_0 value. A larger S_0 value indicates highly ordered structure, and a smaller S_0 shows less ordered structure (less rigid or mobile). Changes of the lipid structural ordering of SC are able to be monitored using the aliphatic probes. The orientation of spin probe reflects the local molecular environment and should serve as indicator of conformational changes in lipid bilayers of the SC. The modern simulation takes into account overall experimental intensities, line widths, and hyperfine coupling values and provides the quantitative information regarding the probe environment. Therefore, S_0 value reflects the local ordering of the lipid structure in the membrane. The error of the spectral simulation is a few percent in the case of the dipalmitoylphosphatidylcholine membrane [19]. In the presence of fast motion of the probe in the SC, the simulation may result in the deviation from the experimental spectra.

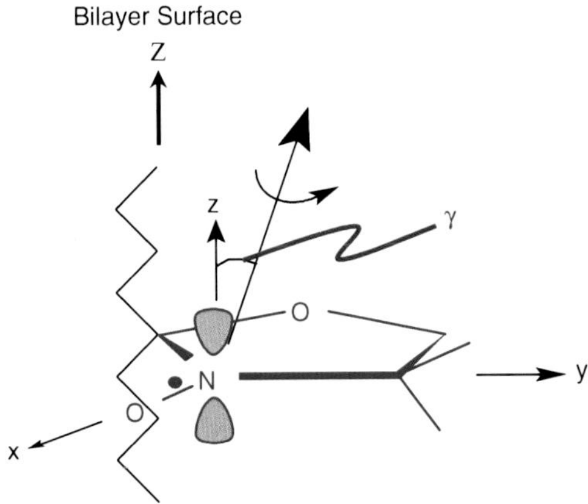

Fig. 8 A schematic representation of a conformation of DSA spin probe in the SC membrane, where Z-axis of the acyl chain is parallel to z-axis of the nitrogen $2P_z$ orbital

Data Analyses: Qualitative Order Parameter (S) and Quantitative Order Parameter (S_0) of SC Lipids

The modified "Brick and Mortar" [20] model of the SC is illustrated in Fig. 1. SC intercellular lipids arrange themselves into bilayers and pack into lamellae. The single-chain 5-DSA normally

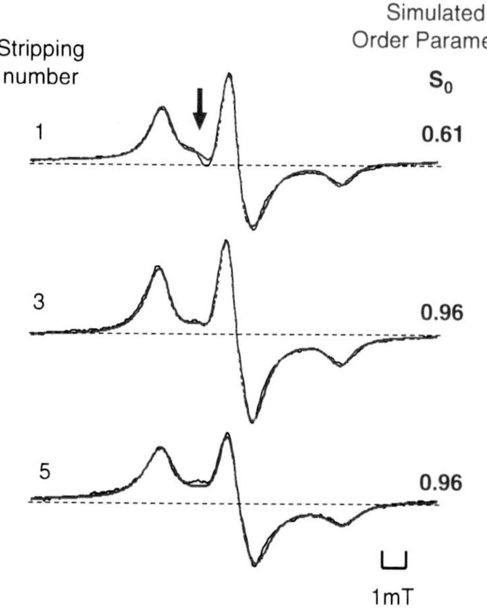

Fig. 9 Experimental (*solid line*) and simulated (*dashed line*) EPR spectra of 5-DSA probe. Stripping numbers show consecutively stripped SC from the surface downwards. The *arrow* of stripping number 1 indicates the characteristic peak. The EPR spectra were obtained with the single scan

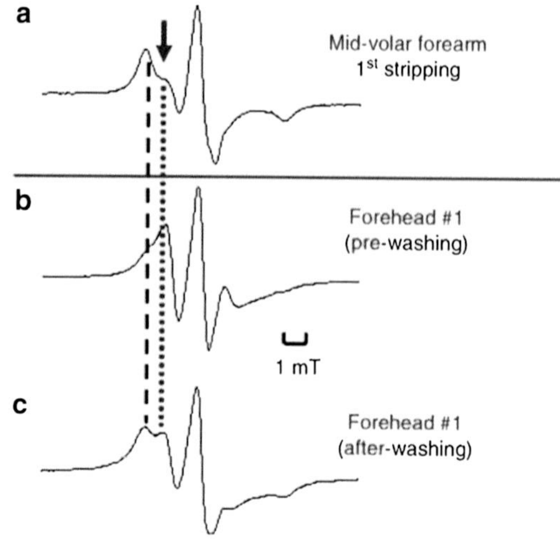

Fig. 10 Experimental EPR spectra of 5-DSA in the first stripped SC from human mid-volar forearm (**a**), the first stripped SC from human forehead pre-washing (**b**), and the first stripped SC from human forehead after-washing (**c**). The *short dashed line* corresponds to the characteristic signal. The *long dashed line* corresponds to the probe incorporated into the SC lipids. The *arrow* indicates the characteristic peak

dissolves into lipids and fat phases. The most likely location of the single-chain probe is the SC. The aliphatic probe will be located in the lipid phase and fat like sebaceous secretion of the SC.

Figure 9 shows the experimental and simulated EPR spectra of 5-DSA in the SC. The reasonable agreement of the experimental and simulated spectra suggests that simulation analysis can provide detailed information regarding the SC lipids. The S_0 value changes from 0.61 to 0.96, while the S value is in the range of 0.56–0.59. The conventional *S* value was obtained by Eq. 3 measuring the hyperfine values from the observed spectrum.

There are significant differences between the conventional and simulated order parameters. Because the slow-tumbling simulation calculates the total line shape of the spectrum, it is able to extract more detailed information about the SC structure than the conventional analysis, which is normally ambiguous in distinguishing the two hyperfine components (parallel and perpendicular) from the experimental spectrum due to the presence of weak and broad signals [5]. Thus, the S_0 values ($0.2 \sim 0.9$) obtained by the simulation suggest that the outermost SC layers are less rigid (or more mobile, $S_0 \sim 0.2$), while the deeper lipid layers ($S_0 \sim 0.9$) have more rigid and oriented structures.

The arrow in the spectrum indicates the characteristic peak, which is prominent only for the first strip (Fig. 9). This peak diminishes in intensity with increasing depth in the SC. The marked peak appears near the center of the spectrum because the probe embedded in the first sample stripped has greater freedom of motion. The other two lines of the nitroxide probe overlaid the central region of the spectrum. Further investigation of the characteristic peak was performed. Figure 10a shows the EPR spectrum of the first strip from SC. The strong and broad peak observed for the SC sheet from the human forehead is shown in Fig. 10b. The peak intensity decreases after washing the SC with soap (Fig. 10c). Thus, the characteristic signal can be attributed to sebaceous secretion [13]. The strength of the signal is considered to reflect the abundant sebaceous secretion at the forehead compared with that of the forearm.

Quantitative Order Parameter (S_0) Related to SC Lipid Structure

One can calculate the angle (γ in Fig. 8) between the rotational diffusion symmetry axis (the lipid in SC) and the z-axis of the nitroxide axis system. Figure 11 represents the schematic illustration of the bilayer distance in relation to the angle. The simulated S_0 value of 0.61 can be the angle of 30°. The value of 0.96 is the angle of 9.4°. The angle suggests that the SC lipids align nearly perpendicularly to the bilayer surface. The larger S_0 value yields larger distance between the lipid bilayers.

The analysis implies that the longer distance of the lipid bilayer can be related to the well-oriented SC structure.

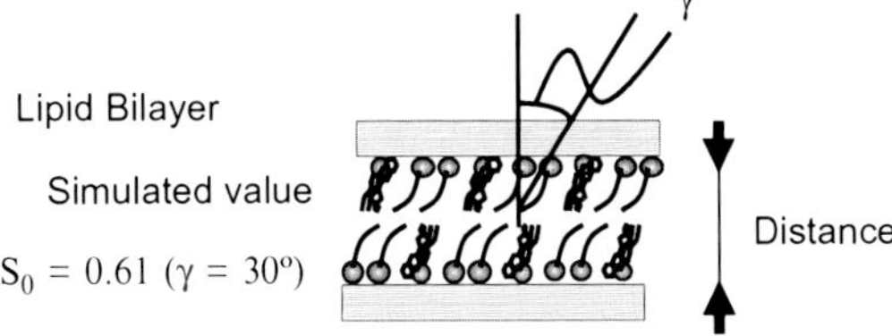

Fig. 11 Schematic illustration of relative lipid bilayer distances and the values of simulated order parameter (S_0) related to the angles (γ) between the bilayer surface and the single-chain probe

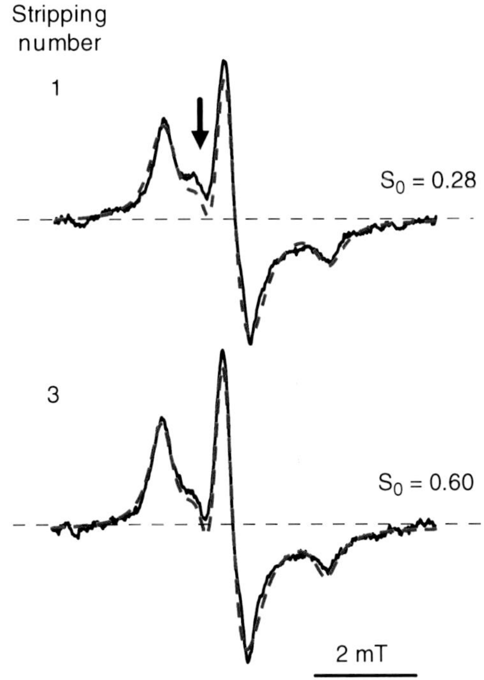

Fig. 12 Experimental (*solid line*) and simulated (*dashed line*) EPR spectra of 5-DSA in the first and the third stripped human SC from lower-leg. The EPR spectrum was obtained with the single scan

Figure 12 shows that human SC stripped from lower leg presents typical EPR spectra of 5-DSA incorporated in the SC lipids. The EPR spectrum about stripping number 1 is slightly different from that of number 3. The characteristic peak indicated by the arrow in the spectrum is prominent for the first strip. The reasonable agreement of the simulated and experimental spectra suggests that simulation analysis can provide comprehensive information regarding the SC lipids. The S_0 value changes from 0.28 to 0.60, while the S value is in the range of 0.63–0.64. The S_0 values of 0.28 and 0.60 are the angles of 44° and 31°, respectively. The higher S_0 value implies that the lower SC lipids have less rigid structure than those of the upper SC lipids. Satisfactory agreement between the experimental and calculated spectra can provide a quantitative S_0, which reveals the microscopic ordering in association with the structure of the SC lipids.

The EPR simulation can potentially provide further insight into skin lipid structures. The order parameter (S_0) of spin probe will provide the useful index about structural dependence as a function of the SC depth. It is notable that the value is not the absolute index for living animals. The value may differ from sample to sample. However, the relative value of the particular SC sample as a function of the depth could provide a useful index of the SC.

Next, interaction between keratin solution from human epidermis and 5-DSA was examined. Figure 13 shows EPR spectra of the keratin/5-DSA and 5-DSA stock solutions. The EPR spectrum of 5-DSA stock solution shows typical nitrogen triplet pattern of the probe in H_2O solution as presented in Fig. 13a.

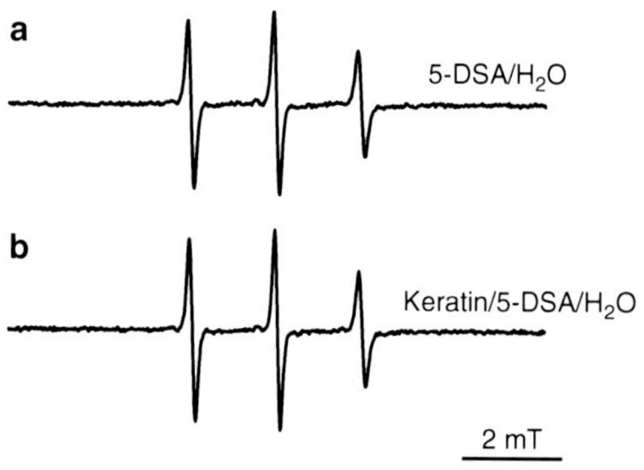

Fig. 13 EPR spectra of (**a**) 5-DSA stock solution and (**b**) keratin/5-DSA solution are shown. EPR spectra were taken at ambient temperature

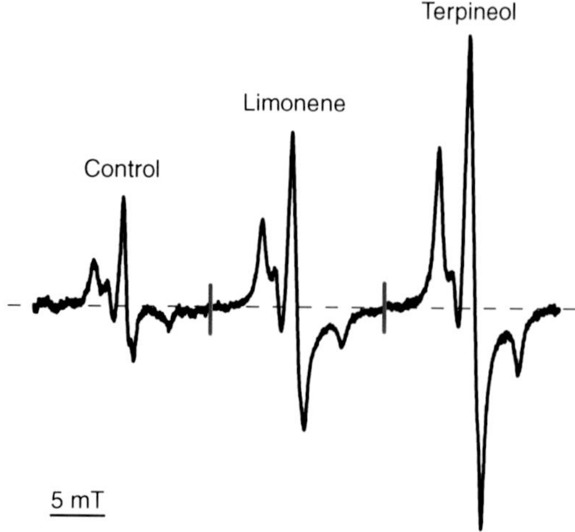

Fig. 14 A comparison of 5-DSA EPR spectra for control, limonene treated, and α-terpineol treated SC is presented. The EPR spectra were obtained for the first stripping of the SC

The EPR spectrum of keratin/5-DSA solution also shows the triplet pattern (Fig. 13b) and stays the same after 1 hour. The similar spectra for both experiments provide that 5-DSA probe does not strongly interact with human keratin in the solution. The results suggest that 5-DSA probes most likely do not permeate keratin in the period [21].

Other Applications of the EPR Method

Effects of Mild Surfactants on SC Lipids

EPR in conjunction with a slow-tumbling simulation was utilized for examining the effect of diluted detergent on stratum corneum (SC) lipid structure. SC from the back of a hairless mouse (HOS:HR-1) was stripped consecutively from one to three times. EPR spectrum of 5-DSA incorporated in the control SC demonstrated a characteristic peak for the first strip. A slow-tumbling simulation for 5-DSA showed slight differences in ordering values (S_0) of the SC for the control and detergent-treated SC. The S_0 values were 0.15 and 0.32, respectively. EPR spectra of the detergent-treated SC showed that the characteristic component was eliminated. Thus, the EPR method along with the simulation analysis revealed the differences in ordering of the detergent-treated SC.

Different types as well as mixtures of surfactants change the SC structure of the lipid bilayer differently. Kawasaki et al. examined the influence of anionic surfactants, sodium lauryl sulfate (SLS) and sodium lauroyl glutamate (SLG), on human SC by the EPR spin label method [1]. The qualitative order parameter obtained by 1.0 % wt SLS-treated cadaver SC was 0.52. On the other hand, the high S value of 0.73 for 1.0 % wt SLG was obtained. The results suggest clear surfactant effects on the ordering of the lipid bilayer. In addition, a reasonable correlation between the qualitative order parameters and human clinical data (visual scores and transepidermal water loss values) was demonstrated.

Effects of Skin Penetration Enhancers on SC Lipids

Interaction of skin penetration enhancer correlates with the fluidity of the intercellular lipid bilayers. Nakagawa and coworkers investigated the effects of terpenes, α-terpineol and (+)-limonene, on SC lipids utilizing the EPR spin probe method [22]. The EPR spectra of α-terpineol-treated SC were totally different from those of untreated SC. The results suggest that α-terpineol increases in the penetration of local bilayers surrounding 5-DSA.

The α-terpineol enhanced permeation of the single chain 5-DSA about three times that of the control as shown in Fig. 14. However, EPR spectra of CHL in the SC did not show a clear difference for each strip, except for the signal intensity. The results imply that CHL permeates SC lipid differently from 5-DSA. The enhancement of the 5-DSA is more significant than that of CHL [22]. Therefore, the present results can be useful for various drug administrations via the skin.

SC with Psoriasis Vulgaris

Psoriasis vulgaris is classified as a disorder of keratinization although its pathogenesis has not been fully elucidated. Tick scale is usually recognized in psoriasis lesions, and hyperkeratosis and parakeratosis are found histologically. Turnover time of psoriatic keratinocytes decreased approximately seven times, and the increase of proliferating cell components in the epidermis may cause differentiation abnormalities of keratinocytes. In fact, many results concerning differentiation abnormalities including increase of K6 and K16 expression and decrease of profilaggrin expression were found in psoriatic epidermis [23–26].

Figure 15a shows 5-DSA in aqueous solution. A sharp three-line signal of the 5-DSA aqueous solution was observed. Figure 15b shows the typical EPR spectrum of 5-DSA in *psoriasis vulgaris* SC (PV-SC). A little, broad three-line pattern was observed. The spectral pattern is quite different from those of other SC reported [4, 5, 13].

The spectral pattern suggests that the 5-DSA is mobile or less rigid in the SC. The red dashed line is the simulated spectrum. The reasonable agreement between the experimental and simulated spectra was obtained as shown in Fig. 15b. The S_0 value obtained for 5-DSA in the SC was approximately 0.20. It is important to note that the lower value of the S_0 indicates the less rigid structure of 5-DSA probe moieties.

One can recognize additional small peaks at lower and higher magnetic fields as indicated by the arrows in Fig. 15b. These peaks can be due to 5-DSA located in the rigid site in the sample. These spectral differences can be related to the structural differences in the PV-SC. Thus, a part of 5-DSA is immobile site in the case of PV-SC.

Figure 15c is EPR spectrum of the midvolar forearm (control). The EPR pattern is very similar to those for the forearm SC previously reported

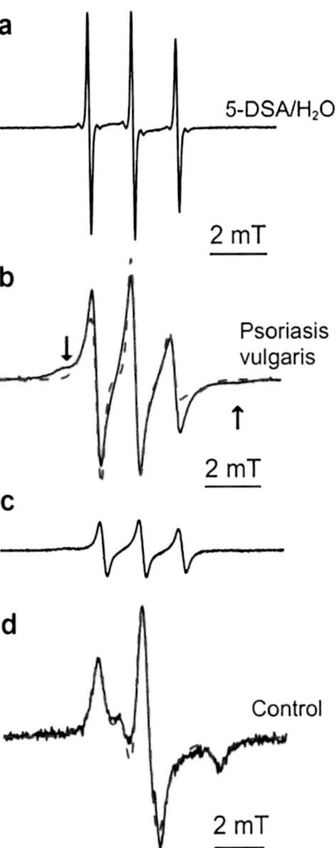

Fig. 15 (**a**) EPR spectrum of aqueous 5-DSA stock solution is presented. (**b**) EPR spectrum of (**b**) *psoriasis vulgaris* SC is presented. Experimental (*solid line*) and simulated (*dash line*) EPR spectra of 5-DSA probe are shown. (**c**) EPR signal due to 5-DSA of the cyanoacrylate on the glass plate. (**d**) EPR spectrum of 5-DSA of the typical mid-volar forearm SC (control) is presented. All EPR spectra were obtained with the single scan. The *arrows* in Fig. 15b indicate rigid components

[4, 5, 13]. The red dashed line is the simulated spectrum. Good agreement between the experimental and simulated spectra was obtained. The S_0 value obtained was 0.42. The quantitative structural ordering (0.42) of the SC lipids also implies that the probe moiety is relatively rigid. In addition, the signal intensity of the control is weaker based on the S/N than that of the PV-SC and does not show the strong three-line pattern. The weak signal demonstrates the low amount permeation of 5-DSA in control SC.

Figure 16 shows the bar chart of the S_0 values corresponding to the control and the PV-SC. The low S_0 value of 0.19 for the PV-SC is associated with irregular structure of the lipids in the

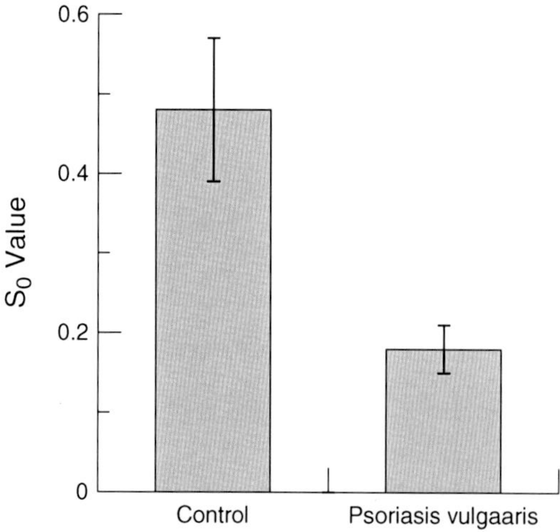

Fig. 16 Plot of simulated or order parameter (S_0) of the control and *psoriasis vulgaris* SC. The statistical results obtained for the control SC and the *psoriasis vulgaris* SC are 4.9 ± 0.90 and 2.0 ± 0.25, respectively. Each value represents mean ± SD three measurements. The S_0 values of the control SC show significantly higher values than those of PV-SC ($p < 0.01$)

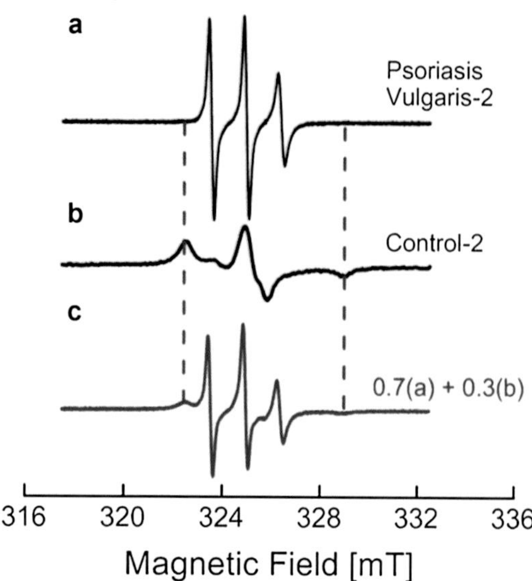

Fig. 17 (**a**) EPR spectrum of *psoriasis vulgaris* SC is presented. (**b**) EPR spectrum of control SC is presented. (**c**) Add EPR spectrum of (0.7 × (a) + 0.3 × (b)) is presented. The *dash lines* indicate immobilized components of the spectrum. The spectrum is re-presentation of the spectrum of Fig. 14 (**b**)

SC. Student's *t*-test analysis suggests that the 0.19 value of PV-SC is significantly smaller than the 0.48 value of the control ($p < 0.01$). The statistical analysis is consistent with those of the experimental spectra obtained.

Figure 17 shows the detailed comparison of PV-SC (a) and control (b). In each case, peak areas (double integral) of the spectrum are normalized to 1. In the case of PV-SC, 5-DSA is in the mobile site of the PV-SC. Figure 17c shows the added spectrum of 0.7 times (a) and 0.3 times (b). The spectrum (c) is very similar to Fig. 15b, except for the broad line width. The line width of Fig. 17a is sharp because 5-DSA is originally mobile in the sample. Contrary in the case of control, 5-DSA is immobile site in the case of control, and EPR spectra show the immobile pattern. These spectral differences can be reflected by the structural differences in the SC samples. Thus, the added spectrum in Fig. 17c suggests that approximately 30 % of 5-DSA in the sample can be in rigid site.

In this study, it was found that the PV-SC is less rigid of structure than that of the control SC, indicating abnormal architecture of *psoriasis vulgaris* stratum corneum. This result is consistent with previous observations [21]. Therefore, it is suggested that this EPR assay is of great use for evaluating SC function and can be extended to other skin diseases with abnormal keratinization.

Psoriatic Nails

Nail lesions are common features of psoriasis and found in almost half of nail psoriatic patients. Clinical manifestations include pitting, onycholysis, hyperkeratosis, splinter hemorrhages, and so on. Nail psoriasis is associated with discomfort and causes significant functional impairments and psychological stress. However, nail involvement is often overlooked, and treatment is focused on cleaning the cutaneous lesions. Furthermore, there is no feasible spectroscopic method to evaluate changes and severity of nail psoriasis. EPR (electron paramagnetic resonance) is also useful for elucidating structural aspects of stratum corneum (SC) [21, 22, 27, 28]. Therefore, it is thought that EPR might be feasible for evaluating nail conditions in the patients with nail psoriasis.

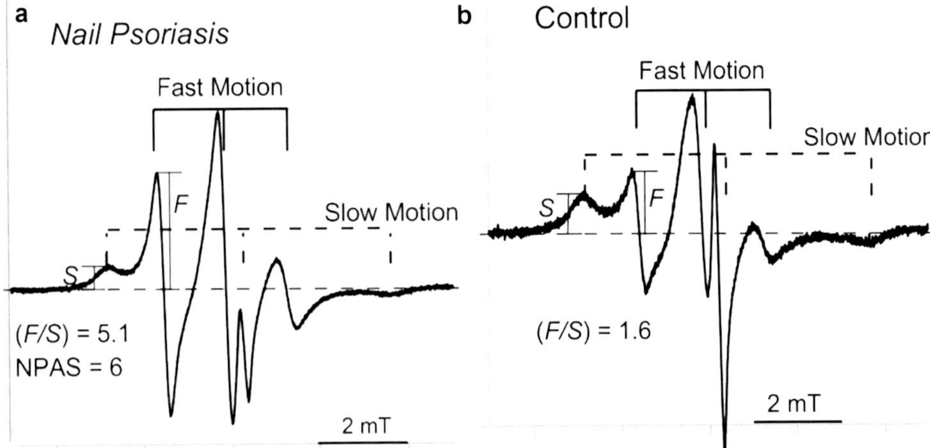

Fig. 18 (**a**) EPR spectrum of finger nail with psoriasis obtained after incubation with 5-DSA aqueous solution is presented. (**b**) EPR spectrum of control nail. Two sites (fast motion (F) and slow motion (S)) three-line pattern in the nails for both (**a**) and (**b**) spectra are presented. The lowest peak intensity of each spectrum was taken for the calculation. The nitrogen hyperfine coupling for the fast motion is smaller than that of the slow motion

EPR spectral changes are due to the molecular motion of the 5-DSA probe, as is discussed in the section of EPR line shape due to spin probe motion. In the fast-motional region, EPR spectrum is a clear three-line pattern. In the slow-motional region, EPR spectrum shows an asymmetric pattern [29]. EPR spectra obtained from the nails are shown in Fig. 18. Both spectra are composed of two components: one is the fast 5-DSA probe motion which indicates smaller hyperfine coupling, and the other is the slow motion in the nail. In order to analyze the spectra obtained, the intensity ratio of the two motions at the peaks of the lower magnetic field can be taken:

$$\frac{F(\text{peak})}{S(\text{peak})} \tag{8}$$

F and S are peak intensities for fast and slow probe motions, respectively. The peaks are indicated in Fig. 18. The fast motion (F) refers to the relatively fast probe molecules in a nail and shows three EPR lines. The nitrogen hyperfine coupling of the 5-DSA is smaller due to the fast probe motion.

The slow motion (S) refers to the relatively slow probe molecules in a nail and shows an anisotropic EPR pattern due to restricted motion in the nail. The spectrum obtained, composed of parallel and perpendicular hyperfine components, shows an asymmetric pattern. This asymmetric EPR pattern is always observed for controlled SC [21, 22, 27, 28]. A stronger asymmetric pattern for the control nails is obtained for those with nail psoriasis. Thus, two distinct motions suggest there are two distinguishable sites in the nails.

The plot of the relative (F/S) values of the fingernails for control and nail psoriasis is shown in Fig. 19. The analyses suggest that the relative intensity of the nails with psoriasis is ~3 times higher than those of the control. The smaller (F/S) values for the control indicate that the rigid site is dominant. In the case of the nail psoriasis, the fast component is more intense than that of the slow component. Student's t-test suggests that the (F/S) value of nail psoriasis is a higher statistical value than those of the control ($p < 0.01$).

Figure 20 shows the calculated EPR spectra for the fast motion (a) and the slow motion (b). Calculation of EPR spectra was performed using EasySpin 4.0.0 version. In the case of fast 5-DSA motion, EPR spectrum shows a three-line pattern. Contrarily, the EPR spectrum shows asymmetric pattern for slow 5-DSA motion. In each case, peak areas (double integral) of the spectrum are normalized to 1. The calculation of the spectra shows that rotational correlation time

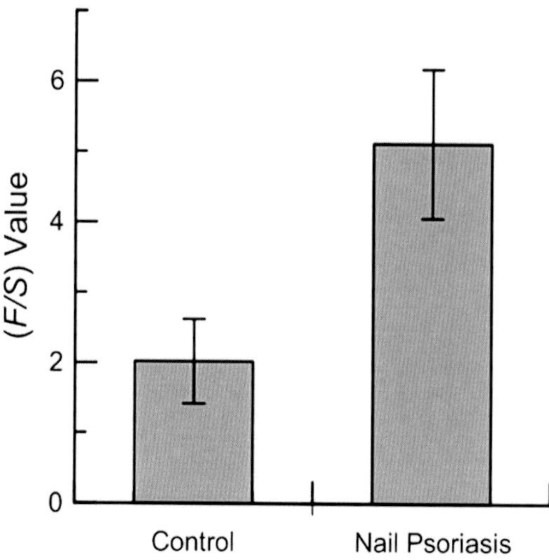

Fig. 19 The bar plot of the relative (F/S) values of the control and nails with psoriasis. The statistical results obtained for the control nails and the psoriasis nails are 2.02 ± 0.606 and 5.12 ± 1.06, respectively. Each value represents mean $\pm$ SD for five individual measurements. The (F/S) values of the control nail show significantly smaller values than those of the psoriasis nails ($p < 0.01$)

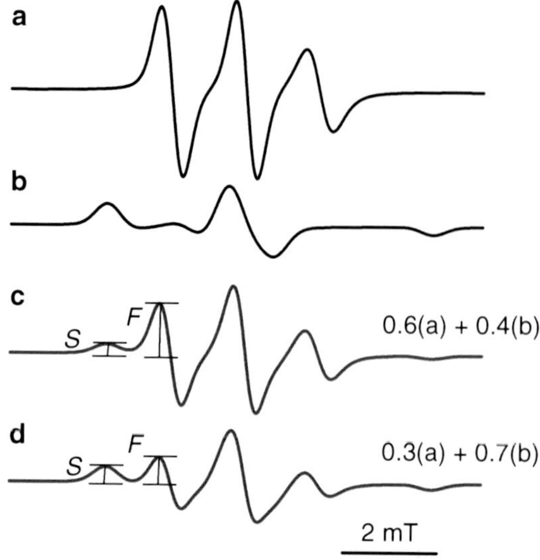

Fig. 20 The calculated EPR spectra for the fast (**a**) and the slow motion (**b**) are presented. In each case, peak areas are normalized to 1. EPR spectrum (**c**) is the result of an addition of 0.6 × (a) and 0.4 × (b). EPR spectrum (**d**) is the result of an addition of 0.3 × (a) and 0.7 × (b)

of the fast motion is approximately 200 times shorter than that of the slow motion.

Figure 20c shows the added spectrum of 0.6 times (a) and 0.4 times (b). The spectrum (c) is very similar to Fig. 15b, except for the central region. The line-width of Fig. 20a is sharp because 5-DSA was originally mobile in the sample. The ordering due to the probe location also reflects g-value difference. The difference can be related to the main spectral discrepancy between the observed and calculated spectra. Contrarily, the 5-DSA motion is slow, and EPR spectrum shows a broad asymmetric pattern. These spectral differences reflect the structural differences in the clipped nail samples. Thus, the added spectrum in Fig. 20c suggests that approximately ~40 % of 5-DSA in the sample can be in rigid site. Figure 20d shows the sum of EPR spectra of 0.3 times (a) and 0.7 times (b). The added spectrum in Fig. 20d suggests that approximately ~70 % of 5-DSA in the sample can be in the rigid site. Most of the 5-DSA is in the rigid site. Thus, these spectral differences reflect the structural differences in the nail samples.

Therefore, the present results show that the structure of the psoriasis nail is less rigid (more fragile) than that of the control. In addition, the NPAS of the examined nails was scored. Although the sample number was small, the NPAS score tended to be correlated with the relative EPR (F/S)) values as well as the calculated spectral values. In the case of nail psoriasis, the fragile components are 2 ~ 3 times more than those of the control. This EPR method is thought to be a novel and reliable method of evaluating the severity of nail psoriasis.

Conclusion

EPR along with a modern computational analysis provides quantitative insight into the various SC and nail structures. The EPR spectral pattern contains important information regarding the probe ordering as well as the SC lipid structure. Satisfactory agreement between the experimental and calculated spectrum can provide the microscopic lipid structure of the SC. The SC lipid structures can be related to the SC barrier functions. In addition, the EPR method recognizes sebaceous exudates [13], detergents [30], penetration enhancers [22], and PV-SC [27]. The 9 GHz surface-type noninvasive detection method which provides new possibilities to study paramagnetic species in fingers and nails was developed by Nakagawa [28]. A topically applied 1.0-mM TEMPOL solution with a commercial lotion (5:1 by weight) on a human finger and nail were investigated. Therefore, the EPR technique could in turn provide more comprehensive information, which would further the understanding of various SC and nails.

Cross-References

▶ The Stratum Corneum and Aging

References

1. Kawasaki Y, Quan D, Sakamoto K, Cooke R, Maibach HI. Influence of surfactant mixtures on intercellular lipid fluidity and skin barrier function. Skin Res Technol. 1999;5:96–101.
2. Mizushima J, Kawasaki Y, Tabohashi T, Maibach HI. Effect of surfactants on human stratum corneum: electron paramagnetic resonance. Int J Pharm. 2000;197:193–202.
3. Alonso A, Meirelles NC, Yushmanov VE, et al. Water increases the fluidity of intercellar membranes of stratum corneum: correlation with water permeability, elastic and electrical resistance properties. J Invest Dermatol. 1996;106:1058–63.
4. Kitagawa S, Ikarashi A. Analysis of electron spin resonance spectra of alkyl spin labels in excised guinea pig dorsal skin, its stratum corneum, delipidized skin and stratum corneum model lipid liposomes. Chem Pharm Bull. 2001;49:165–8.
5. Nakagawa K, Mizushima J, Takino Y, Kawashima T, Maibach HI. Chain ordering of stratum corneum lipids investigated by EPR slow-tumbling simulation. Spectrochim Acta Pt A Mol Biomol Spectrosc. 2006;63:816–20.
6. Bontè F, Saunois A, Pinguet P, Meybeck A. Existence of a lipid gradient in the upper stratum corneum and its possible biological significance. Arch Dermatol Res. 1997;289:78–82.
7. Weerheim A, Ponec M. Determination of stratum corneum lipid profile by tape stripping in combination with high-performance thin-layer chromatography. Arch Dermatol Res. 2001;293:191–9.
8. Rogers J, Harding C, Mayo A, Banks J, Rawlings A. Stratum corneum lipids: the effect of ageing and the seasons. Arch Dermatol Res. 1996;288:765–70.
9. Bommannan D, Potts RO, Guy RH. Examination of stratum corneum barrier function *in vivo* by infrared spectroscopy. J Invest Dermatol. 1990;95: 403–8.
10. Zhang G, Moore DJ, Mendelsohn R, Flach CR. Vibrational microspectroscopy and imaging of molecular composition and structure during human corneocytes maturation. J Invest Dermatol. 2006;126:1088–94.
11. Bouwstra JA, Gooris GS, van der Spek JA, Bras W. Structural investigations of human stratum corneum as determined by small angle X-ray scattering. J Invest Dermatol. 1991;97:1005–12.
12. Pilgram GSK, Engelsma-Van Pelt AM, Bouwstra JA, Koerten HK. Electron diffraction provides new information on human stratum corneum lipid organization studied in relation to depth and temperature. J Invest Dermatol. 1999;113:403–9.
13. Yagi E, Sakamoto K, Nakagawa K. Depth dependence of stratum corneum lipid ordering: a slow-tumbling simulation for electron paramagnetic resonance. J Invest Dermatol. 2007;127:895–9.
14. Marks R, Dawber RP. Skin surface biopsy: an improved technique for the examination of the horny layer. Br J Dermatol. 1999;84:117–23.
15. Hubbell WL, McConnell HM. Molecular motion in spin-labeled phospholipids and membrane. J Am Chem Soc. 1971;93:314–26.
16. Ge M, Rananavare SB, Freed JH. ESR studies of stearic acid binding to bovine serum albumin. Biochim Biophys Acta. 1990;1036:228–326.
17. Schneider DJ, Freed JH. Calculating slow motional magnetic resonance spectra. In: Berliner LJ, Reuben J, editors. Biological magnetic resonance, vol. 8. New York: Plenum; 1989. p. 1–76.
18. Budil DE, Lee S, Saxena S, Freed JH. Nonlinear-least-squares analysis of slow-motion EPR spectra in one and two dimensions using a modified Levenberg-Marquardt algorithm. J Magn Reson Ser A. 1996;120:155–89.
19. Meirovitch E, Igner D, Igner E, Moro G, Freed JH. Electron-spin relaxation and ordering in smectic and supercooled nematic liquid crystals. J Chem Phys. 1982;77:3915–38.
20. Ge M, Freed JH. Polarity profiles in oriented and dispersed phosphatidylcholine bilayers are different. An ESR study. Biophys J. 1998;74:910–7.
21. Crepeau RH, Saxena S, Lee S, Patyal BR, Freed JH. Studies on lipid membranes by two-dimensional Fourier transform ESR: enhancement of resolution to ordering and dynamics. Biophys J. 1994;66:1489–504.
22. Quan D, Maibach HI. An electron paramagnetic resonance study. I. Effect of Azone on 5-doxyl stearic acid-labeled human stratum corneum. Int J Pharm. 1994;104:61–72.
23. Nakagawa K. Elucidated lipid structures of various human stratum corneum investigated by EPR spectroscopy. Skin Res Technol. 2011;17:245–50.

24. Nakagawa K, Anzai K. Stratum corneum lipid of hairless mouse investigated by electron paramagnetic resonance. Appl Magn Reson. 2011;40:557–65.
25. Nakagawa K, Anzai K. Stratum corneum lipid structure investigated by EPR spin-probe method: application of terpenes. Lipids. 2010;45:1081–7.
26. Iizuka H, Takahashi H, Ishida-Yamamoto A. Psoriatic architecture constructed by epidermal remodeling. J Dermatol Sci. 2004;35:93–9.
27. Nakagawa K, Minakawa S, Sawamura D. Spectroscopic evidence of abnormal structure of psoriasis vulgaris stratum corneum. J Dermatol Sci. 2012;65:222–4.
28. Nakagawa K. Development of an innovative 9 GHz EPR surface detection method and its application to non-invasive human fingers and nails investigation. Spectrochim Acta Part A. 2015;150:461–4.
29. Takemoto H, Tamai K, Akasaka E, et al. Relation between the expression levels of the POU transcription factors Skn-1a and Skn-1n and keratinocyte differentiation. J Dermatol Sci. 2010;60:203–5.
30. Elias PM. Epidermal lipids, barrier function and desquamation. J Invest Dermatol. 1983;80(suppl):44–9.

90 Molecular Concentration Profiling in the Skin Using Confocal Raman Spectroscopy

Jonathan M. Crowther and Paul J. Matts

Contents

J.M. Crowther
JMC Scientific Consulting Ltd, Surrey, UK
e-mail: crowther.j.1@pg.com

P.J. Matts (✉)
Procter & Gamble, Greater London Innovation Centre, Egham, Surrey, UK
e-mail: matts.pj@pg.com

M.A. Farage et al. (eds.), *Textbook of Aging Skin*,
DOI 10.1007/978-3-662-47398-6_71

Abstract

The uppermost layer of the skin – the stratum corneum (SC) – plays a vital role in the functioning and protection of the human body. It provides mechanical protection and regulates water movement in and out. Despite the relatively small dimensions of the SC over most of the body parts (its thickness is of the order of 20 μm over a large portion of the body), it is far from a homogeneous structure both physically and chemically. Chemical concentrations change from its surface inward, and these changes are responsible for both the properties it possesses and the processes occurring within it. Furthermore, with the application of topical cosmetic products becoming more popular and widespread, especially in the antiaging market, the monitoring of ingredients that are capable of penetrating into the skin from the outside, which may also influence the processes occurring within and properties of the SC, is now a necessity.

Introduction

The uppermost layer of the skin – the stratum corneum (SC) – plays a vital role in the functioning and protection of the human body. It provides mechanical protection and regulates water movement in and out. Despite the relatively small dimensions of the SC over most of the body parts (its thickness is of the order of 20 μm over a large portion of the body), it is far from a homogeneous structure both physically and chemically. Chemical concentrations change from its surface inward, and these changes are responsible for both the properties it possesses and the processes occurring within it. Furthermore, with the application of topical cosmetic products becoming more popular and widespread, especially in the antiaging market, the monitoring of ingredients that are capable of penetrating into the skin from the outside, which may also influence the processes occurring within and properties of the SC, is now a necessity. To understand the role of all these components within the SC, it is not only necessary to ask "how much is there?" but also "where is it located?" and "how is it distributed?" While many techniques have been developed to analyze concentration gradients within the SC, until recently, it has been impossible to quantitatively assess different chemical components as a function of depth, in vivo.

The aim of this chapter is to present a brief review of research on understanding the role these concentration gradients play within the SC and provide an overview of the use of a relatively new technique, confocal Raman spectroscopy (CRS), for assessing these concentration gradients in vivo. Following this are some of the recent findings demonstrating how water and NMF profiles change throughout the skin using CRS and how this can help bring new understanding.

Measurement of Different Skin Components

The SC itself is not a homogeneous structure and varies greatly across its thickness. From the basal layer, where keratinocytes are born, they mature and differentiate as they transit toward the surface, gradually flattening out to become the familiar flat, "squamous" corneocyte cells of the stratum corneum. Differentiating cells will cause transition through a variety of chemical gradients, including water, natural moisturizing factors (NMFs), lipids, urea, lactic acid, and pH. This section outlines some of these aspects, why they are present, and how they are currently assessed.

Water

The water content of the SC varies across its thickness – at the surface, the SC is constantly losing water to the environment under normal conditions, while at the basal layer, there is a continual replenishment from the viable epidermis. Therefore, across the SC, there exists a water gradient, which decreases toward the outside of the body. Maintenance of a correct state of hydration of the SC has a huge impact on its mechanical and optical properties, helping to maintain skin barrier function and playing an important role in the regulation and activation of both intra- and extracellular enzymes, which control the desquamation process [1, 2]. Deviations in these processes fundamentally affect SC barrier function, and in healthy individuals, the most common expression of this is "dry skin" [3]. Water that is present within the SC can be described as either free or bound [4]. Free water refers to the partially mobile molecules, which can be easily lost if exposed to a dry environment after exposure of the skin to an environment of high water activity. Bound water is held within the corneocytes by both the polar groups within keratin protein molecules and by a blend of so-called natural moisturizing factors (NMFs) that increase the hygroscopicity of these structures.

The first attempt at determining true depth-resolved water profiling in SC was performed by Warner et al. in 1988 [5]. In this experiment, electron probe analysis was carried out on biopsied skin samples, which had been cryo-sectioned and freeze-dried (the local dry mass of a freeze-dried cryo-section of the skin being inversely related to its water content). Further advancements were made to the technique, making it simpler to perform [6]; however, while the technique was able to provide hydration profiles, it still required skin biopsies to be collected, cryo-sectioning to be carried out, and analysis to be performed using a scanning electron microscope (SEM), and as such, it is not a technique that would be possible to deploy easily in a clinical environment.

Cryo-SEM has been used further to understand uptake and loss of water in salt solutions of different strengths within the SC [7]. This demonstrated that the SC does not take up water evenly across its entire thickness but that there are three "zones," which respond differently when hydrated and dehydrated. The behavior of these zones is dependent on the osmotic potential of the hydrating solution. The concept of zones of hydration has also been examined before [8] showing that the central portion of the SC absorbed water strongly under high water activity, while the layers closest to the stratum granulosum showed no swelling under these conditions. The presence of a central zone capable of absorbing and holding water is in excellent agreement with the concentration of natural moisturizing factors (NMFs), known to reach a maximum in the central portion of the SC [9].

Infrared (IR) spectroscopy has been used to examine water as a function of depth in combination with tape stripping [10] and Monte Carlo simulation [11]. However, these methods require compromises to be taken in the collection and analysis of the data. For example, in the work by Brancaleon et al., the tape stripping approach used to sample incrementally into the skin was difficult to correlate with actual depth and, of course, was inherently destructive, thereby making it impossible to repeatedly reassess the same site over the course of a study. The Monte Carlo simulation by Arimoto et al. relies on the assumption that the water content varies linearly from 10 % at the SC surface to 80 % at the interface with the viable epidermis.

NMF and SC Lipids

Two key classes of materials are present within the SC in addition to the corneocyte cellular structure – "natural moisturizing factors" (NMFs) and the intercellular lipid bilayer structure. NMFs comprise a collection of amino acids, salts, and other small hygroscopic molecules that are present within the corneocytes and are derived from the proteolysis of epidermal filaggrin, which initiated a few cell layers above the stratum basale. These hygroscopic NMF components are efficient humectants, helping to bind water and assisting in maintaining skin hydration and flexibility [12].

Confocal Raman spectroscopy has also been used to measure concentration profiles of different NMF components nondestructively and in vivo [13]. The concentration of most NMF components builds gradually from the stratum granulosum, peaking in the midportion of the SC and then showing a characteristic depletion near the surface. This seems to be associated with the water-labile nature of these components and their propensity to be washed out by, for example, daily cleansing. Lactate and urea, as sweat-derived NMF components, are more prevalent at the surface of the SC.

The ability of the SC to control the movement of molecules across it is mediated not only by the physical constraint of the corneocytes themselves but also by the intercellular lipids. These are a mixture of ceramides, cholesterol, and free fatty acids, as well as a small amount of nonpolar liquids and cholesterol sulfates, and are organized along with a small amount of water, into a series of parallel lamellar membranes. However, while some water is trapped in the lipid lamellar structure, most is actually held within the corneocytes themselves [14]. It is this series of lipid bilayer structures, together with the tightly stacked corneocytes, which provide a tight barrier against TEWL, making it difficult for water to transfer across the SC structure. SC lipid content varies both seasonally and as a function of age, and it is generally accepted now that a reduction of approximately 30 % is seen in the elderly [15–17].

Cosmetic Ingredients

With the rapid expansion of the cosmetic product market in recent years, more attention is being focused on understanding how these products partition into and interact with the skin.

Infrared (IR) spectroscopy has been used to monitor the effects of cosmetic ingredients on SC chemical composition [18], and although this technique is capable of detecting changes in lipid packing and organization as a result of using different products, it is not a depth-profiling technique and it is not certain over which depth data is collected. Imhof et al. have used a modified version of IR spectroscopy to assess the delivery of topical components to the skin based on the principle of thermal emission delay from the surface after irradiation with an IR light source [19].

Confocal Raman spectroscopy has been used to monitor penetration of different lipid species into the SC and their corresponding effects on hydration and total skin lipid profiles [20]. Different lipid species were absorbed to different degrees, with petrolatum being most strongly absorbed, most likely due to a combination of its relatively short chain lengths and occlusive properties, resulting in destabilization of SC structure. It was also demonstrated that infant and adult skin behaved similarly in relation to lipid uptake. This is in contradiction to the effect of topical application of water, where infant skin was more capable of uptake than adult skin. Chrit et al. have also used confocal Raman spectroscopy to assess the extent of skin hydration changes after using a glycerol-based moisturizing product in vivo [21] and were able to classify different hydrating products depending on their moisturizing effect on the skin. They showed that a polyphospholipid (poly [2-methacryoyloxylphosphorylcholine] or pMPC) was able to increase water levels in the skin, both in vivo and in vitro, although it should be noted that dosing of the products was not controlled, with any excess product being removed after application and before analysis [22].

Pudney et al. [23] demonstrated the utility of confocal Raman spectroscopy in monitoring the permeation of trans-retinol through the stratum corneum.

In a similar manner, Mohammed et al. [24] showed, in a variety of different vehicles, that the amount of niacinamide which permeated through human skin in an in vitro Franz cell model was linearly proportional to the intensity of the niacinamide signal determined in the stratum corneum by confocal Raman spectroscopy in vivo.

Confocal Raman spectroscopy has also been used to measure (with varying degrees of success) the permeation of a variety of other exogenous species into the stratum corneum including trans-cinnamaldehyde [25], urea [26], caffeine [27], and a variety of oils [28].

pH

While the extracellular fluid within the body is maintained at a pH of approximately 7.4, the surface of the SC is more acidic with a pH between 4.5 and 6 [29, 30]. There is, therefore, a pH gradient across the SC. While this change in pH has been linked with a variety of skin functions, such as barrier function, desquamation, and microbial defense, the mechanism responsible for its presence is not fully understood. However, it has been suggested that a buildup of trans-urocanic acid [31], carbon dioxide diffusion [32], the presence of free fatty acids [33], lactate and lactic acid produced as a by-product of sweating [34], or active regulation by a sodium-hydrogen anti-porter protein [35] is linked with this observed change.

Even though humans are not born with this "acidic mantle," the SC pH at the surface is nearly neutral. Over the first few months of life, the surface becomes more acidic to approach the values seen in adults [36]. This can have significant consequences for newborns as barrier function recovery after acute insult is not as efficient in neutral skin, when compared with acidic skin [37]. It is interesting to note that acidification of neonatal rat SC does not occur from the surface down (so is unlikely to be triggered by microbial colonization occurring after birth) but actually begins deeper down within the skin [38].

A variety of techniques have been used to examine pH as a function of depth. Tape stripping measurements combined with pH assessment has shown the existence of this gradient [30, 36]. Once again, though, it is by nature an inherently destructive technique and is not capable of discriminating between the intra- and intercellular components. Microscopy combined with a pH-sensitive fluorescent marker molecule has been used to determine pH, and the advent of two photons and confocal imaging has pushed resolution to submicron levels [39]. Confocal Raman spectroscopy has also been used to measure concentration profiles of trans-urocanic acid and pyrrolidone carboxylic acid in vivo [13]. As with NMF, the concentration of these species is greatest in the middle portion of the SC, showing a gradual buildup from the stratum granulosum layers and depletion near the surface.

Calcium

Calcium concentration varies across the epidermis, from high levels within the stratum granulosum down to low levels in the basal layer [40]. The calcium concentration is linked with regulation of epidermal keratinocyte proliferation and differentiation and skin structural integrity. It is also strongly linked with rate of barrier recovery after acute insult by detergents, tape stripping, or organic solvents [41]. As with the pH gradient, calcium variation does not exist at birth – it manifests itself concurrently with increasing barrier function in fetal skin [42]. Analysis of calcium concentration as a function of depth has been carried out using scanning electron microscopy of biopsied samples [43].

With quantification of any component in the skin as a function of depth, the ideal solution is determination of concentration in a nondestructive manner, without the need for complex modeling.

Raman Spectroscopy

In 1928, the Indian physicist C.V. Raman first reported the new type of light scattering phenomenon that was eventually to bear his name. Raman reported that when a liquid was irradiated by light of a specific wavelength, while most of the remitted photons were scattered elastically with no change in photon energy, an extremely small proportion of the reflected light had a wavelength different to the incident source. This wavelength shift was related directly to the change in vibrational and rotational energy states of the molecules in the liquid, thereby providing information on the energy levels of the molecules present. As the Raman phenomenon is very weak (occurring approximately once in a million photon interactions), requiring a well-defined monochromatic light source, practical applications were not readily exploited until the development of the laser in the 1960s. Improvements in detection equipment such as photomultiplier tubes further enhanced the appeal and applicability of Raman, and it is now a well-established material analysis technique. Raman spectroscopy is a complimentary technique to IR spectroscopy – molecular vibrations, which are IR active, are not Raman active and vice versa. However, unlike IR spectroscopy, Raman is relatively insensitive to water, which makes it a more considered approach for analyzing the skin (where with IR the intensity of the water signal can mask other chemical species) – and, indeed, a number of researchers in the last 15 years or so have reported varying degrees of success, principally using in vitro models [44–46].

The journey from measurement of in vitro systems to in vivo capture of Raman spectra on the surface of the SC presented many challenges [44, 47], specifically the low signal to noise (based around the safety needs for relatively low laser power when used on live subjects). A huge leap forward in the use of in vivo Raman spectroscopy came with the instrument designs and research of Caspers et al. resulting in very high optical efficiency and enabling rapid, noninvasive collection of Raman spectra [48].

Confocal In Vivo Raman Microspectroscopy

The "Holy Grail" of in vivo SC assessment is the measurement of different components within the skin as a function of depth – a joint measure of chemical composition and location within the skin structure. Recently, confocal Raman spectroscopy (CRS) has been developed to obtain real-time molecular concentration profiles and in vivo [13, 49–51]. Building on the success of their in vivo surface measurements, River Diagnostics designed and marketed the RD3100 in vivo confocal Raman spectrometer, capable of measuring skin chemical profiles by combining the principle of confocal microscopy with Raman spectroscopy. In operation, incident monochromatic laser light is focused to a point on/within the skin tissue, which can be moved by changing the focal point of the microscope. When used to measure the skin, this light enters the SC, most being scattered elastically without a change in energy and wavelength. A small proportion of this incident light, however, becomes Raman-scattered photons. Those scattered photons reaching the skin surface are reemitted with some passing back through the microscope objective lens. Given the confocal nature of the microscope, only light reentering the microscope from the focal plane will pass back through the pinhole – photons reemerging from other depths are excluded. The majority of these collected photons will be elastically scattered and have the same wavelength as the incident light source; however, the small proportion of Raman-scattered photons are isolated and analyzed, enabling the construction of molecular concentration profiles present within the SC.

Using this technique, SC composition can be quantitatively measured by "optically sectioning" skin tissue and expressing the relative chemical content as a function of depth, in a noninvasive, rapid, and nondestructive manner, making it ideal for implementation in a clinical environment. For example, water concentration is calculated from the ratio of the water signal to the combined signal from water and protein within the skin. This method has also been used to estimate differences in SC thickness in vivo at different body sites and during aging [52, 53] and, recently, to evaluate the effects of water and moisturizing ingredients on SC hydration, after short-term treatment [54, 55] and long-term treatment [56].

The majority of current research, using Raman to look at the skin, focuses on the SC and upper layers of the viable epidermis, as light becomes increasingly scattered as it penetrates more deeply, reducing signal strength and making data collection more difficult. However, despite this turbidity, Naito et al. have recently reported using a 1,064-nm light source to probe the dermal chemical structure [57]. The ability to measure deep within the skin opens up the possibility of, for example, probing the development of acne in teenagers and the effects of aging on dermal chemical composition.

All the chemical components of the skin possess different groups with unique vibrational frequencies. Water and protein contain different functional groups in their chemical structure, which vibrate at different frequencies. It is these differences in vibrational frequency that enable the species to be differentiated using Raman spectroscopy. To simplify the analysis of the skin, the Raman spectra can be split into two distinct zones: the "high-wavenumber" and "fingerprint" regions, which can be probed independently depending on what is required. Information regarding water content is contained within the "high-wavenumber" region, while levels of natural moisturizing factors (NMFs), cholesterol, ingredients penetrating into the skin, etc., can be derived from the information in the "fingerprint" spectra. The high-wavenumber spectrum shows characteristic O-H and -CH_3 stretching vibrations at 3,390 and 2,935 cm^{-1}, respectively. Scans in this region are used to calculate percentage hydration values by taking the ratio of the integrated signals of water (i.e., the O-H stretching vibration region between 3,350 and 3,550 cm^{-1}) to that of protein (i.e., the -CH_3 stretching vibration from 2,910 to 2,965 cm^{-1}) [48–51]. Typical skin spectra for the "high-wavenumber" spectral region showing the water and protein peaks, collected at a single scan at an exposure time of 1 s, are given in Fig. 1. During collection of a depth profile, spectra like this are captured at regular intervals from the surface of the SC down into the skin. A correction factor, as determined by Caspers et al. [13], is used to normalize the spectral response of water and protein relative to their mass ratio. Percent hydration is then calculated using the formula (Eq. 1):

$$\text{Percent hydration} = \text{constant} * (\text{water}) \times / [(\text{water}) + (\text{protein})] \quad (1)$$

The normalized water-to-protein ratios obtained from each focal depth are plotted as percent hydration as a function of depth. This, therefore, leads to a direct semiquantitative measure of amount of the water present within the skin as a function of depth. Although the signal intensity drops as the laser penetrates deeper into the skin, the fact that both the water and the protein peaks are derived from the same scan enable quantification throughout the range of analysis.

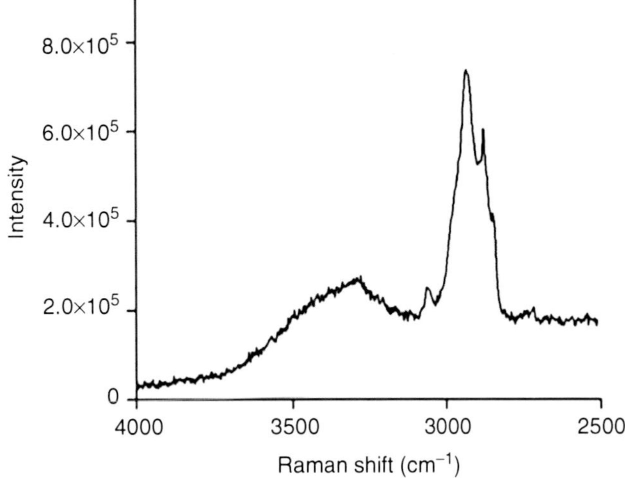

Fig. 1 Typical background-corrected confocal Raman spectra from a single scan of human skin in vivo, collected at ~ 4-μm depth in the high-wavenumber region (671-nm laser excitation, exposure 1 s)

Calculation of SC Thickness

It has been understood for many years that SC thickness varies dynamically with its hydration state and in response to a variety of extrinsic factors. In order to analyze and interpret SC water concentration profiles properly, therefore, it is essential to take into account SC thickness – after all, in a situation where SC thickness is varying dynamically, absolute SC depths are of little meaning. It has recently been demonstrated by the authors that SC thickness can be determined directly from water concentration profiles [56], and this procedure is described below. While the work of Egawa et al. [52, 53] clearly demonstrates the utility of using CRS for deriving SC thickness estimates, these authors offer no formal validation data, establishing a direct relationship between their CRS-derived SC thickness data and values derived from other measurements. It should also be noted that a different (and, it is believed, a more rigorous) approach in calculating SC thickness from the water profile measurements has been used, validating it via correlation with values from a known objective measure of skin thickness (optical coherence tomography [OCT]).

To generate representative Raman hydration profile data for a particular site, multiple, replicate water concentration profiles are derived for each location at each time point. Multiple profiles are collected as this technique is a point measure – a laser spot size in the order of microns – and the inherent biological variability of the skin means that a more accurate measure of thickness and hydration can only be obtained through the use of an average profile. After collection of a set of profiles, obvious outliers (arising, e.g., from scanning through heterogeneous structures, such as skin appendages including hair follicles, sebaceous glands, etc., or profiles recorded while the panelists were moving) are removed. Then, an average hydration profile is fitted through the remaining data, using a customized algorithm based on a four-parameter Weibull curve. The four-parameter Weibull curve is a well-accepted and widely used algorithm capable of accurately modeling a variety of profile shapes with the minimum number of parameters in the equation, producing model curves with very low RMS deviations from the mean data. The upper "leveling-off point" of each profile is determined by a gradient threshold method by calculating the location where the gradient reaches a value of 0.5 moving from the midpoint of the curve (Fig. 2). This point was hypothesized to be the theoretical boundary of the SC (see CRS-OCT comparison below for the test of this hypothesis) and serves as the deeper limit of the SC hydration profile. The area-under-the-curve (AUC) values are determined by integrating each hydration profile from the skin surface ($x = 0$ μm on the profile) to each individual SC boundary (point c in Fig. 2) and used to express the total SC hydration.

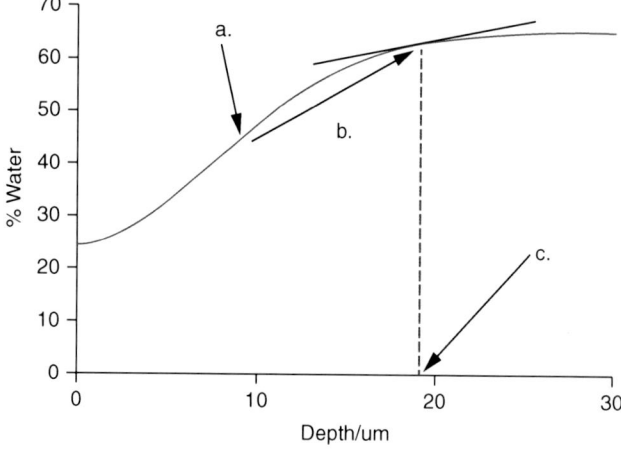

Fig. 2 Calculation of SC thickness using the hydration curve. Working from the middle of the curve (*a*) inward (i.e., deeper in the tissue), the algorithm calculates the point where the gradient equals 0.5 (*b*). The depth at this point corresponds to the base of the SC (*c*)

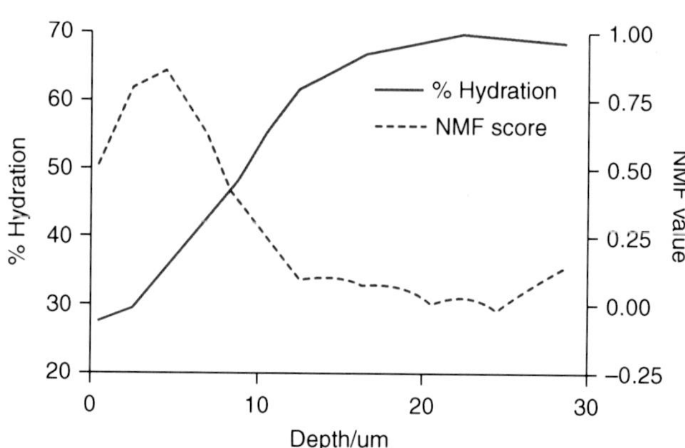

Fig. 3 Comparison of hydration and NMF profiles measured at the same point on the volar forearm

Correlation Between NMF and Hydration Profiles

Using the River Diagnostics RD3100 system, it has been possible to measure hydration and NMF profiles at exactly the same location on the skin, by retaining the volar forearm on the window of the spectrometer and alternating the laser being used from 681 to 785 nm, thereby switching between the "high-wavenumber" and "fingerprint" regions. As can be seen in the example shown in Fig. 3, there is a strong correlation between the leveling-off point location of the hydration profile and the position where the NMF profile starts to rise (profiles presented here are single scans from a specific location on the skin, and that is why they are not smooth curves). This is to be expected, as NMF starts to be expressed a few microns above the base of the SC due to the breakdown of filaggrin, and this correlates well with the behavior of NMF reported by Caspers [13]. While these observations provide increased confidence in the correlation between the leveling-off point in the hydration profile and the location of the lower margin of the SC, it cannot be seen as definitive proof. For example, external environmental variation can also be responsible for changes in the exact location of filaggrin hydrolysis. It was necessary, therefore, to validate empirically the leveling-off point as the SC lower margin, using a separate objective measure of SC thickness.

Correlation Between Optical Coherence Tomography and SC Hydration Profiles

Optical coherence tomography (OCT) is a well-established technique for examining skin structure and thickness [58]. It is based on the principle that photons are backscattered from different structures within the skin. Through the use of interferometry, the depth at which these backscattering events occur can be calculated, providing information on where different structures occur within the skin, for example, boundaries between different layers. In this work, sets of up to eight Raman profiles have been measured from each site, and these are analyzed together, rather than studying each water profile in isolation. Outlying scans were removed in a quality control process before further analysis. Once this was done, the Weibull mathematical model was applied to the data point cloud representing each site, resulting in an "average" hydration profile for that site. The location of the SC boundary as a function of the CRS water concentration profiles was confirmed by comparing SC thicknesses from a number of different body sites obtained directly by OCT and CRS (Figs. 4a, b). Linear regression through the data shows a strong positive correlation between SC thickness derived from CRS and OCT (OCT thickness = 0.9603 × CRS thickness, $r^2 = 0.9339$; $p < 0.0001$). Expanding the area to the lower left of Fig. 4a, corresponding to the thinner skin sites of the body (volar forearm, cheek, and outside of lower leg), shows how the dynamic range for OCT is compressed in this region (Fig. 4b). It can be seen that all of the OCT-derived SC thicknesses are between 9 and 15 μm, while the CRS-derived thicknesses vary between 12 and 30 μm. This is consistent with the expected behavior of the OCT method in areas where the SC is relatively thin – the sensitivity of the OCT is limited by the pixel size of the detector (approximately 5 μm for the system used here). For sites with SC thickness in the region of 10–20 μm, therefore, this corresponds to only a few pixels. For panelists who had cheek, forearm, and leg measures, CRS ranked the sites, in terms of SC thickness, as follows: cheek < forearm < leg (cheek 12.8 ± 0.9 μm, volar forearm 18.0 ± 3.9 μm, and leg 22.0 ± 6.9 μm), whereas OCT gave very similar readings for these three different locations (cheek 11.1 ± 1.8 μm, volar forearm 10.4 ± 0.9 μm, and leg 13.7 ± 1.4 μm). Of note, this ability to rank the sites in the order of thickness gave further confidence that the new CRS method was giving accurate estimates of SC thickness, as it matched exactly with the trends that would be expected, based on known, published values for these sites [59]. The limitations of OCT measurement of thinner skin sites have also been noted recently using in vivo laser scanning fluorescence microscopy [60, 61]. It is believed, therefore, that the results of this work demonstrate convincingly the capability of CRS in providing a new rapid, accurate, and sensitive means of measuring SC thickness in vivo.

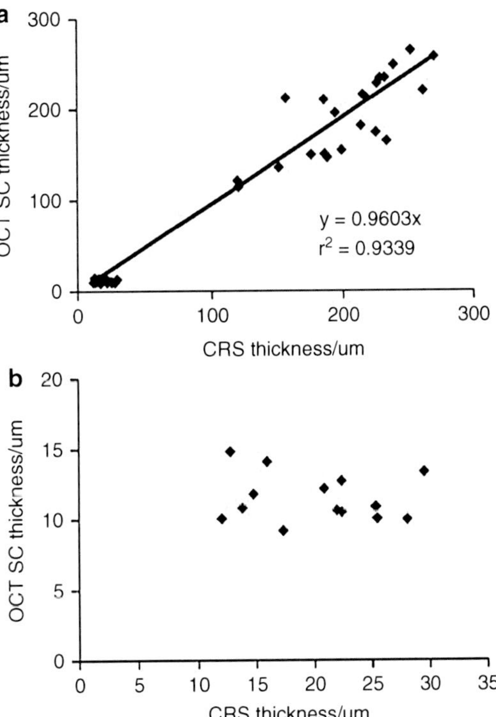

Fig. 4 (**a**) Comparison of OCT- and CRS-derived SC thicknesses at a variety of body sites. (**b**) Comparison of OCT- and CRS-derived SC thicknesses on volar forearm, cheek, and outside of lower leg

Effects of Acute Hydration on SC Water Content and Thickness

A simple study employing forced occlusion to drive maximal short-term acute hydration of the volar forearm was used to demonstrate the ability of the CRS system to measure dynamic, rapid change in SC water profiles. A set of hydration profiles were taken from the volar forearm after equilibration in a standardized environment (Fig. 5a). The forearm was then wrapped in a wet towel soaked in deionized water. The towel was wrapped in Parafilm™ to help ensure complete saturation of the SC by occlusive hydration and the arm left for 90 min. After 90 min, the wrap and towel were removed and any excess surface water removed by gentle patting with a dry towel. Sets of hydration profiles were then measured again using CRS over a time course (Fig. 5b). Given the complex nature of the shape of the hydration curve after this extreme treatment, the profiles here are represented as simple averages of the individual sets of scans rather than Weibull curve-modeled fits. Between measurements, the arm was removed from the CRS optical window and allowed to acclimatize within the measurement room and the window of the CRS cleaned with methanol to remove any residue left behind from the skin. The hydration profiles in Fig. 5b show the changes in SC hydration across its entire thickness, showing significant water uptake over the 90 min. Importantly, the point at which the hydration profile begins to level off after enforced hydration is further from the surface of the SC. From the OCT validation study described above, it can now be confidently said that this is because of SC swelling in the vertical axis, driven by hydration. As observation only, it is interesting to note that the magnitude of this swelling is in the region of 25 %, highly consistent with that noted by Norlen [62] in ex vivo models. It is also interesting that there appears to be a central portion of the SC, which takes up more water than the upper or lower margins.

As the post-occlusion time course is followed and hydration profiles are measured over time, it should also be noted that surface hydration values fall fastest, while the "hump" of hydration in the

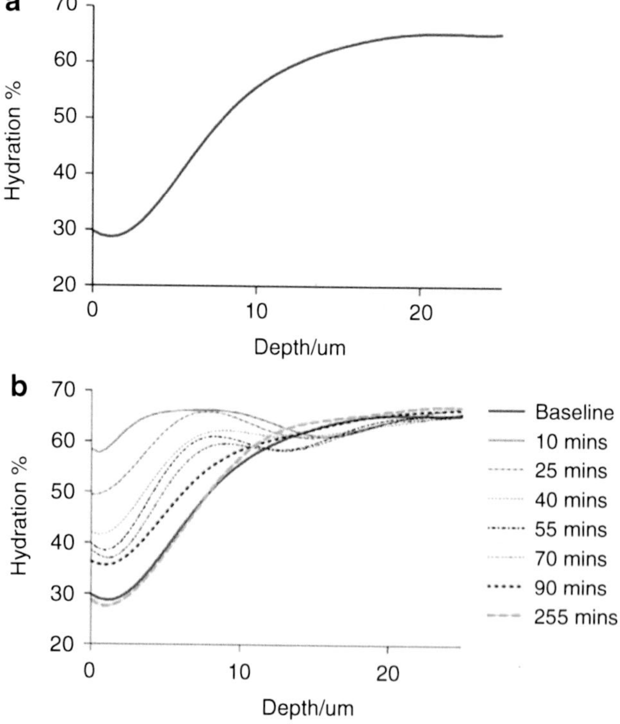

Fig. 5 (**a**) Baseline volar forearm hydration profile. (**b**) Hydration profiles of the volar forearm measured as a function of time after 90-min occlusion with a wet towel

central portion of the SC falls the slowest. These observations are wholly consistent with presence of higher concentrations of hygroscopic NMF components in the central portion of the SC (the lower layers containing less because of the programmed hydrolysis of filaggrin and the upper layers containing less because of an insidious washout of these highly water-labile components by, e.g., daily cleansing). It is also possible that the corneocytes within the central portion of the SC are less physically constrained compared with those closer to the SC-stratum granulosum boundary and, therefore, are potentially more readily capable of swelling and increasing in thickness than those deeper down. This variance in swelling ability of the SC as a function of depth correlates with the work of Bouwstra et al. [8]. Remarkably, baseline conditions are only reestablished after a period of some 4 h, demonstrating the efficient water-binding capacity of native, untreated SC.

Further in vitro validation of CRS has been reported by Wu and Polefka, where they correlated water content as measured using CRS with Karl Fischer assessment, and water content increase for a moisturizing lotion, and decrease in water content after using bar soap [63]. While SC thickness changes as a result of the treatment regimes were not taken into account, and the experiments were carried out on excised pig skin, this does demonstrate further the capability of the technique.

Effect of Long-Term Application of Moisturizers on SC Hydration Profiles

It might be expected that long-term application of moisturizers to the skin would increase SC water content and/or change the shape of the SC hydration profile. A comparison of the effect of long-term application of three moisturizers on SC hydration gradients has recently been reported by Crowther et al. [56]. To examine the effects of moisturizers on SC thickness, water gradients and total SC hydration CRS were used to compare the effects of a formulation containing niacinamide (A), which is known to improve SC barrier function and desquamation better than two other commercially available moisturizers (formulations B and C) [64].

For illustration, average hydration profiles from each treatment from this work are given in Fig. 6. All hydration profiles start at 20–30% hydration at 0-μm depth (i.e., the SC surface) and rise in a "sigmoidal"-type curve to 65–70% hydration, where they plateau. While all hydration profiles at baseline and 1-day treatment show the same shape, differences in shape begin to appear after 1 week of treatment. After 2 weeks, notable differences are observed for formulation A, where a laterally "stretched" profile is evident, which is still present after 1 week of regression. As a result of this stretching, the leveling-off point of the profile has moved deeper in the skin (which indicates an increase in SC thickness).

After 2 weeks of treatment, the increase in SC thickness induced by formulation A was significantly different from the other two products being tested and the untreated control site ($p = 0.0121$), and this difference remained at the 1-week regression time point ($p = 0.0162$). The observed change corresponded to an approximate 10 % increase in SC thickness.

Total hydration in the SC can be calculated from the area under the profile (AUC; integration between $x = 0$ μm and the calculated SC leveling-off point). Concomitant with the increase in SC thickness, total skin hydration increased significantly following treatment with formulation A after 2 weeks of product usage and the 1-week regression ($p = 0.0275$ and 0.0435, respectively).

While all moisturizers have the effect of alleviating dry skin when formulated appropriately, it has become apparent in recent years that different moisturizer formulations can have different effects on the SC and the epidermis (for review, see Loden [65]). Naturally, in the short term, moisturizers will increase SC hydration [51, 54, 55, 64–66] and in the medium term improve desquamation [67, 68]; however, in the longer term, it has become apparent that some can actually compromise SC barrier function [69–73], while others can strengthen it [64, 66, 74–76]. In vitro [7, 8, 77–79] and in vivo [80, 81] studies have also

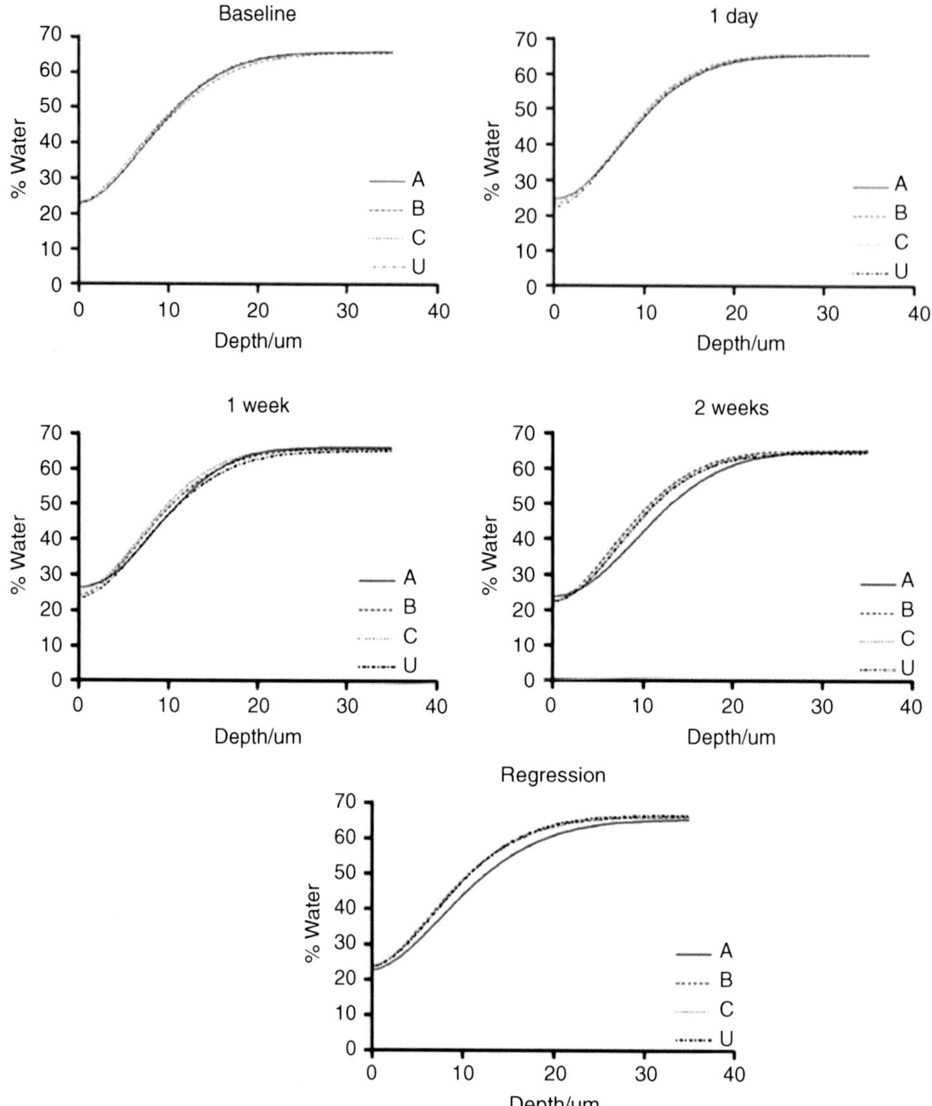

Fig. 6 Average hydration profiles over the course of the study

demonstrated the ability of some moisturizing ingredients to influence SC thickness. Therefore, it is becoming increasingly apparent that not only is there a need for longer-term studies to evaluate the effect of moisturizers but also that the introduction of new measurements in addition to the more "traditional" electrical parameter-based devices is needed to understand their effects more completely [72].

In the moisturizer study presented here, on the first day after starting product application, little difference in CRS-derived hydration profiles is observed between any of the treatments or the untreated control site. After the first week of treatment though, there was a numerical diminution in SC thickness. While not statistically significant, it could have been due to the osmotic effects of glycerol (which was present in all the three formulations). This behavior has been reported before – Caussin et al. [79] reported that changes in SC swelling can occur, when examining the effects of moisturizers on SC hydration and swelling.

Lipophilic moisturizers increased SC thickness, whereas hydrophilic moisturizers tended to reduce SC thickness. This apparent SC thinning may, therefore, be due to osmotic effects of the moisturizing ingredients (used at high concentration), and the work of Fluhr et al. [82] describing the effect of glycerol on reducing corneocyte surface area would tend to support this. However, inconsistencies remain where in vitro [79] and in vivo [80, 81] increased corneocyte swelling has been reported with glycerol solutions. Another possible explanation would be that during the first week of treatment, there was some activation of SC protease activity (simply by elevated water activity), resulting in more efficient desquamation and an ensuing reduction in SC thickness. This effect prompts further investigation.

After the second week of the study, formulation A induced a statistically significant increase in SC thickness (2-μm average increase, corresponding to an approximate 10 % increase in thickness). As already discussed, water content measurements at absolute depths are simply not comparable between time points in a study where SC thickness may change or vary. It is, therefore, more meaningful to extract information from the profiles regarding total SC thickness and express water measurement derivatives as a function of this (e.g., the use of total SC water content). Considering SC thickness first of all, after 2 weeks of treatment, formulation A produced a significantly greater increase in this parameter than the other two treatments and the untreated site ($p = 0.0121$), and this difference remained at the 1-week regression time point ($p = 0.0162$). Of note, increases in SC thickness have also been reported by Jacobson et al. [83] using a lipophilic niacin derivative.

Concomitant with this increase in SC thickness, total SC hydration as measured by CRS increased significantly with the use of formulation A after 2 weeks of treatment. This increase remained at the 1-week regression time point. However, no such effect was observed for treatment with formulations B and C. This data did not, however, correspond with Corneometer measurements taken at the same time points. Significantly, increased Corneometer values were observed for all products even after 1 day of application, and indeed, values remained elevated throughout the 2-week treatment phase. Corneometer values also remained elevated for all treatments at the 1-week regression (although all values were significantly lower than those at the 2-week treatment time point – an effect observed in other regression studies [75, 84]). Considering the ingredients present in all the three formulations, the capacitance effects noted may be attributable partially to the high dielectric constant of glycerol [85, 86]. It therefore appears from the CRS hydration profiles and their relative difference to corresponding Corneometer values, however, that measured changes in capacitance do not directly reflect total SC hydration. This raises the question as to where the capacitance signal is coming from within the skin and what moieties are driving changes in this parameter in the context of treatment with a moisturizer.

While it is not possible here to go into a detailed examination of the role of different ingredients on skin properties (a more complete discussion is given in [56]), it is believed that niacinamide (nicotinamide, vitamin B3), present only in formulation A, was probably the agent responsible for these SC effects. Recent work has been undertaken to further examine the role of niacinamide in SC swelling using freshly prepared biopsy cross sections in a vehicle-controlled study [87].

Other workers have since confirmed this observed effect of niacinamide on SC thickness. Mohammed et al. [88] once again showed that a niacinamide-containing formulation was able to increase SC thickness, as measured by CRS. Significantly, they also demonstrated that skin treated with formulations containing niacinamide were significantly different to pretreatment baseline and untreated/vehicle-control-treated sites in a number of other parameters, with larger and more mature corneocytes, decreased inflammatory process, and decreased TEWL.

Changes in Raman Profiles as a Function of Age

The ability of confocal Raman spectroscopy to rapidly and nondestructively examine large numbers of people in a clinical environment has opened up the possibility to assess changes in skin properties in wide-ranging age groups – from infants to the elderly. Egawa et al. have reported significant differences in NMF levels, lactate, trans-urocanic acid, ceramide, and cholesterol, along with differences in water gradient, and apparent SC thickness, when assessing volar forearm and cheek sites of young (aged 22–40) and older (aged 59–76) female subjects [53]. It should be noted that only two or three Raman spectra were collected for a particular subject, a low number of replicates given the structural heterogeneity of the skin and laser spot size. However, they were able to derive similar forced hydration profiles to the ones described here in Fig. 5b.

Raman profiling of very young skin (3–12 months in age) has shown decreased NMF content and increased water at all depths throughout the SC when compared to adult skin [89]. In their work, Nikolovski et al. also showed that infant skin was more capable of quickly absorbing and desorbing exogenous water when compared to adult skin, which might be expected from the higher TEWL values seen in infants.

More recently, Boireau-Adamezyk et al. [90] used CRS to show (in female subject, Fitzpatrick skin types I–III) an age-dependent increase in SC thickness (in face and arm sites). Other CRS-measured changes were observed in SC lipid-protein ratio, SC lipid compactness, and cholesterol, ceramide, and total water content.

Conclusion

While a number of techniques are currently available to provide information regarding distribution of different components within the skin, until recently none have been capable of determining these, nondestructively, rapidly, and in vivo. As such, it has been difficult to incorporate them into routine clinical test protocols. The recent development of confocal Raman spectroscopy has enabled the assessment of changes in molecular concentration gradients in vivo for the first time for a variety of different chemical species. It is clear that CRS represents a powerful new class of measurement device with significant advantage over traditional measurement techniques through its ability to assess these changes, both rapidly and in a nondestructive manner. The advent of this new technology seems timely as it is considered the development of moisturizers that truly augment SC barrier function.

The capability of in vivo confocal Raman has only been touched upon as the technique is still in its infancy. Even considering its relative youth, Raman spectroscopy of the skin has already provided a valuable new insight into SC behavior and function and demonstrated its potential as a valuable tool for determining chemical concentration gradients in a clinical environment, both in relation to the use of cosmetic products and with regard to the changes associated with the aging process. As the technique becomes more established, its ability to measure these profiles within the skin will provide a deeper understanding of the interaction between chemical composition and location and skin health and function.

Cross-References

▶ Bioengineering Methods and Skin Aging

References

1. Blank IH. Factors which influence the water content of the stratum corneum. J Invest Dermatol. 1952;18:433–40.
2. Grubauer G, Elias PM, Feingold KR. Transepidermal water loss: the signal for recovery of barrier structure and function. J Lipid Res. 1989;30:323–33.
3. Loden M. Biophysical properties of dry atopic and normal skin with special reference to skin care products. Acta Derm Venereol Suppl (Stockh). 1995;192:1–48.
4. Agache P. Stratum corneum histopathology. In: Agache P, Humbert P, editors. Measuring the skin. Berlin: Springer; 2004. p. 95–100.
5. Warner RR, Myers MC, Taylor DA. Electron probe analysis of human skin: determination of the water concentration profile. J Invest Dermatol. 1988;90:218–44.
6. Warner RR, Lilly NA. Correlation of water content with ultrastructure in the stratum corneum. In: Elsner P, Berardesca E, Maibach HI, editors.

Bioengineering of the skin: water and the stratum corneum. Boca Raton: CRC Press; 1994. p. 3–12.
7. Richter T, Peuckert C, Sattler M, et al. Dead but highly dynamic – the stratum corneum is divided into three hydration zones. Skin Pharmacol Physiol. 2004;17:246–57.
8. Bouwstra JA, de Graff A, Gooris GS, et al. Water distribution and related morphology in human stratum corneum at different hydration levels. J Invest Dermatol. 2003;120(5):750–8.
9. Rawlings AV, Scott IR, Harding CR, Bowser P. Stratum corneum moisturization at the molecular level. J Invest Dermatol. 1994;103:731–4.
10. Brancaleon L, Bamberg MP, Sakamaki T, Kollias N. Attenuated total reflection-Fourier transform infrared spectroscopy as a possible method to investigate biophysical parameters of stratum corneum in vivo. J Invest Dermatol. 2001;116:380–6.
11. Arimoto H, Egawa M, Yamada Y. Depth profile of diffuse reflectance near-infrared spectroscopy for measurement of water content in skin. Skin Res Technol. 2005;11:27–35.
12. Rawlings AV, Scott IR, Harding CR, Browser PA. Stratum corneum moisturization at the molecular level. J Invest Dermatol. 1994;17(1):731–40.
13. Caspers PJ, Lucassen GW, Carter EA, et al. In vivo confocal Raman microspectrometer of the skin: noninvasive determination of molecular concentration profiles. J Invest Dermatol. 2001;116:434–42.
14. Wertz PW. Stratum corneum lipids and water. Exog Dermatol. 2004;3:53–6.
15. Rawlings AV, Rogers J, Mayo AM, et al. Changes in lipids in the skin ageing process. Biocosmet Skin Aging. 1993;1:31–45.
16. Rogers J, Harding C, Mayo A, Banks J, Rawlings A. Stratum corneum lipids: the effects of the ageing and the seasons. Arch Dermatol Res. 1996;288:765–70.
17. Imokawa G, Abe A, Jin K, Higaki Y, Kawashima M, Hidano A. Decreased levels of ceramides in stratum corneum of atopic dermatitis: an etiological factor in atopic dry skin? J Invest Dermatol. 1991;96:523–6.
18. Prasch T, Knübel G, Schmidt-Fonk K, Ortanderl S, Nieveler S, Förster T. Infrared spectroscopy of the skin: influencing the stratum corneum with cosmetic products. Int J Cosmet Sci. 2000;22:371–83.
19. Notingher I, Imhof RE. Mid-infrared in vivo depth-profiling of topical chemicals on skin. Skin Res Technol. 2004;10:113–21.
20. Stamatas GN, de Sterke J, Hauser M, von Stetten O, van der Pol A. Lipid uptake and skin occlusion following topical application of oils on adult and infant skin. J Dermatol Sci. 2008;50:135–42.
21. Chrit L, Bastien P, Sockalingum GD, Batisse D, Leroy F, Manfait M, Hadjur C. An in vivo randomized study of human skin moisturization by a new confocal Raman fiber-optic microprobe: assessment of a glycerol-based hydration cream. Skin Pharmacol Physiol. 2006;19:207–15.
22. Chrit L, Bastien P, Biatry B, Simonnet J-T, Potter A, Minondo AM, Flament F, Bazin R, Sockalingum GD, Leroy F, Manfait M, Hadjur C. In vitro and in vivo confocal Raman study of human skin hydration: assessment of anew moisturizing agent, pMPC. Biopolymers. 2006;85:359–69.
23. Pudney PD, Mélot M, Caspers PJ, Van Der Pol A, Puppels GJ. An in vivo confocal Raman study of the delivery of trans retinol to the skin. Appl Spectrosc. 2007;61(8):804–11.
24. Mohammed D, Matts PJ, Hadgraft J, Lane ME. In vitro – in vivo correlation in skin permeation. J Pharm Res. 2014;31(2):394–400.
25. Bonnist EY, Gorce JP, Mackay C, Pendlington RU, Pudney PD. Measuring the penetration of a skin sensitizer and its delivery vehicles simultaneously with confocal Raman spectroscopy. Skin Pharmacol Physiol. 2011;24(5):274–83.
26. Egawa M, Sato Y. In vivo evaluation of two forms of urea in the skin by Raman spectroscopy after application of urea-containing cream. Skin Res Technol. 2015;21(3):259–64.
27. Franzen L, Anderski J, Windbergs M. Quantitative detection of caffeine in human skin by confocal Raman spectroscopy – a systematic in vitro validation study. Eur J Pharm Biopharm. 2015;95(Pt A):110–6.
28. Choe C, Lademann J, Darvin ME. Confocal Raman microscopy for investigating the penetration of various oils into the human skin in vivo. J Dermatol Sci. 2015;79(2):176–8.
29. Dikstein S, Zlotogorski A. Measurement of skin pH. Acta Derm Venereol (Stockh). 1994;185:18–20.
30. Ohman H, Vahlquist A. In vivo studies concerning a pH gradient in human stratum corneum and upper epidermis. Acta Derm Venereol (Stockh). 1994;74:375–9.
31. Krien PM, Kermici M. Evidence for the existence of self regulated enzymatic process within the human stratum corneum: an unexpected role for urocanic acid. J Invest Dermatol. 2000;115:414–20.
32. Aberg C, Wennerstrom H, Sparr E. Transport processes in responding lipid membranes: a possible mechanism for pH gradient in the stratum corneum. Langmuir. 2008;24:8061–70.
33. Lieckfeldt R, Villalain J, Gomez-Fernandez JC, Lee G. Apparent pKa of the fatty acids within ordered mixtures of model human stratum corneum lipids. Pharmacol Res. 1995;12:1614–7.
34. Patterson MJ, Galloway SD, Nimmo NA. Variations in regional sweat composition in normal human males. Exp Physiol. 2000;85:869–75.
35. Behne M, Oda Y, Murata S, Holleran WM, Mauro TM. Functional role of the sodium-hydrogen antiporter, NHE1, in the epidermis: pharmacologic and NHE1 Null-Allele mouse studies. J Invest Dermatol. 2000;114:797.
36. Visscher MO, Chatterjee R, Munson KS, Pickens WL, Hoath SB. Changes in diapered and nondiapered infant skin over the first month of life. Pediatr Dermatol. 2000;17:45–51.
37. Mauro T, Holleran WM, Grayson S, et al. Barrier recovery is impeded at neutral pH, independent of

ionic effects: implications for extracellular lipid processing. Arch Dermatol Res. 1998;290:215–22.
38. Fluhr JW, Behne MJ, Brown BE, Moskowitz DG, Selden C, Mao-Qiang M, Mauro TM, Elias PM, Fiengold KR. Stratum corneum acidification in neonatal skin: secretory Phospholipase A2 and the sodium/hydrogen antiporter-1 acidify neonatal rat stratum corneum. J Invest Dermatol. 2004;122:320–9.
39. Hanson KM, Behne MJ, Barry NP, Mauro TM, Gratton E, Clegg RM. Two-photon fluorescence lifetime imaging of the skin stratum corneum pH gradient. Biophys J. 2002;83:1682–90.
40. Menon GK, Grayson S, Elias PM. Ionic calcium reservoirs in mammalian epidermis: ultrastructural localization by ion-capture cytochemistry. J Invest Dermatol. 1985;84:508–12.
41. Mauro T, Bench G, Sidderas-Haddad E, Fiengold K, Elias PM, Cullander C. Acute barrier perturbation abolishes the Ca2 + and K + gradients in murine epidermis: quantitative measurement using PIXE. J Invest Dermatol. 1998;111:1198–201.
42. Elias PM, Nau P, Hanley K, et al. Formation of the epidermal calcium gradient coincides with key milestones of barrier ontogenesis in the rodent. J Invest Dermatol. 1998;110:399–404.
43. Elias PM, Ahn SK, Brown BE, Crumrine D, Feingold KR. Origin of the epidermal calcium gradient: regulation by barrier status and role of active vs passive mechanisms. J Invest Dermatol. 2002;119:1269–74.
44. Williams AC, Barry BW, Edwards HGM, Farwell DW. A critical comparison of some Raman spectroscopic techniques for studies of human stratum corneum. Pharm Res. 1993;10:1642–7.
45. Williams AC, Edwards HGM, Barry BW. Fourier transform Raman spectroscopy. A novel application for examining human stratum corneum. Int J Pharm. 1992;81:R11–4.
46. Lucassen GW, Caspers PJ, Puppels GJ. In vivo infrared and Raman spectroscopy of human stratum corneum. Proc SPIE. 1998;3257:52–61.
47. Shim MG, Wilson BC. Development of an in vivo Raman spectroscopic system for diagnostic applications. J Raman Spectrosc. 1997;28:131–42.
48. Caspers PJ, Lucassen GW, Wolthuis R, et al. In vitro and in vivo Raman spectroscopy of human skin. Biospectroscopy. 1998;4:S31–9.
49. Caspers PJ, Lucassen GW, Bruining HJ, Puppels GJ. Automated depth-scanning confocal Raman Microspectrometer. For rapid in vivo determination of water concentration profiles in human skin. J Raman Spectrosc. 2000;31:813–8.
50. Caspers PJ, Lucassen GW, Puppels GJ. Combined in vivo confocal Raman spectroscopy and confocal microscopy of human skin. Biophys J. 2003;85:572–80.
51. Chrit L, Hadjur C, Morel S, et al. In vivo chemical investigation of human skin using a confocal Raman fiber optic microprobe. J Biomed Opt. 2005;10 (4):44007.
52. Egawa M, Hirao T, Takahashi M. In vivo estimation of stratum corneum thickness from water concentration profiles obtained with Raman spectroscopy. Acta Derm Venereol. 2007;87(1):4–8.
53. Egawa M, Tagami H. Comparison of the depth profiles of water and water binding substances in the stratum corneum determined by Raman spectroscopy between the cheek and volar forearm: effects of age, seasonal changes and artificial forced hydration. Br J Dermatol. 2008;158:251–60.
54. Chrit L, Bastien P, Sockalingum GD, et al. An in vivo randomized study of human skin moisturization by a new confocal Raman fiber-optic microprobe: assessment of a glycerol-based hydration cream. Skin Pharmacol Physiol. 2006;4:207–15.
55. Chrit L, Bastien P, Biatry B, et al. In vitro and in vivo confocal Raman study of human skin hydration: assessment of a new moisturizing agent, pMPC. Biopolymers. 2007;85(4):359–69.
56. Crowther J, Sieg A, Blenkiron P, et al. Measuring the effects of topical moisturizers on changes in stratum corneum thickness, water gradients and hydration in vivo. Br J Dermatol. 2008;159:567–77.
57. Naito S, Min YK, Osanai O, Kitahara T, Hiruma H, Hamguchi H. In vivo measurement of human dermis by 1064nm-excited fiber Raman spectroscopy. Skin Res Technol. 2008;14:18–25.
58. Welzel J. Optical coherence tomography in dermatology: a review. Skin Res Technol. 2001;7:1–9.
59. Ya-Xian Z, Suetake T, Tagami H. Number of cell layers of the stratum corneum in normal skin – relationship to the anatomical locations on the body, age, sex and physical parameters. Arch Dermatol Res. 1999;291:555–9.
60. Gambichler T, Boms S, Stacker M, et al. Epidermal thickness assessed by optical coherence tomography and routine histology: preliminary results of method comparison. J Eur Acad Dermatol Venereol. 2006;20 (7):791–5.
61. Lademann J, Otberg N, Richter H, et al. Application of optical non-invasive methods in skin physiology: a comparison of laser scanning microscopy and optical coherent tomography with histological analysis. Skin Res Technol. 2007;13(2):119–32.
62. Norlen L. Stratum corneum keratin structure, function and formation – a comprehensive review. Int J Cosmet Sci. 2006;28(6):397–425.
63. Wu J, Polefka TG. Confocal Raman microspectroscopy of stratum corneum: a pre-clinical validation study. Int J Cosmet Sci. 2008;30:47–56.
64. Matts PJ, Gray J, Rawlings AV. The "dry skin cycle" – a new model of dry skin and mechanisms for intervention, International congress and symposium series, vol. 256. London: The Royal Society of Medicine Press; 2005. p. 1–38.
65. Loden M. The clinical benefit of moisturizers. JEADV. 2005;19:672–88.
66. Breternitz M, Kowatski D, Langenauer M, et al. Placebo controlled, double blind, randomized prospective study

of a glycerol-based emollient on eczematous skin in atopic dermatitis: biophysical and clinical evaluation. Skin Pharmacol Physiol. 2008;21:39–45.

67. Summers RS, Summers B, Chandar P, et al. The effect of lipids with and without humectants on skin xerosis. J Soc Cosmet Chem. 1996;47:27–39.
68. Rawlings AV, Watkinson A, Hope J, et al. The effect of glycerol and humidity on desmosome degradation in stratum corneum. Arch Dermatol Res. 1995;287:457–64.
69. Held E, Sveinsdottir S, Agner T. Effect of long term use of moisturizer on skin hydration, barrier function and susceptibility to irritants. Acta Derm Venereol. 1999;79:49–51.
70. Zachariae C, Held E, Johansen JD, et al. Effect of a moisturizer on skin susceptibility to NiCl2. Acta Derm Venereol. 2003;83:93–7.
71. Berardesca E, Distante F, Vignoli GP, et al. Alpha hydroxyacids modulate stratum corneum barrier function. Br J Dermatol. 1997;137:934–8.
72. Buraczewska I, Berne B, Lindberg M, et al. Changes in skin barrier function following long-term treatment with moisturizers, a randomized controlled trial. Br J Dermatol. 2007;156:492–8.
73. Barany E, Lindberg M, Loden M. Unexpected skin barrier influence from non-ionic emulsifiers. Int J Pharm. 2000;195:189–95.
74. Fluhr JW, Gloor M, Lehmann L, et al. Glycerol accelerates recovery of barrier function in vivo. Acta Dermatol Venereol. 1999;79:418–21.
75. Loden M, Andersson AC, Andersson C, et al. Instrumental and dermatologist evaluation of the effect of glycerine and urea on dry skin in atopic dermatitis. Skin Res Technol. 2001;7:209–13.
76. Rawlings AV, Conti A, Verdejo P, et al. The effect of lactic acid isomers on epidermal lipid biosynthesis and stratum corneum barrier function. Arch Dermatol Res. 1996;288:383–90.
77. Norlen L, Emilson A, Forslind B. Stratum corneum swelling. Biophysical and computer assisted quantitative assessments. Arch Dermatol Res. 1997;289:506–13.
78. Richter T, Muller JH, Schwarz UD, et al. Investigation of the swelling of human skin cells in liquid media by tapping mode scanning force microscopy. Appl Phys A. 2001;A72:S125–8.
79. Caussin J, Groenink HWW, de Graaff AM, et al. Lipophilic and hydrophilic moisturizers show different actions on human skin as revealed by cryo-scanning electron microscopy. Exp Dermatol. 2007;16:891–8.
80. Orth DS, Appa Y, Contard P, et al. Effect of high glycerin moisturizers on the ultrastructure of the stratum corneum. In: Poster at the 53rd annual meeting of the American academy of dermatology. Feb 1995.
81. Orth DS, Appa Y. Glycerine: a natural ingredient for moisturizing skin. In: Loden M, Maibach HI, editors. Dry skin and moisturizers: chemistry & function. Boca Raton: CRC Press; 2000. p. 213–28.
82. Fluhr JW, Bornkessel A, Berardesca E. Glycerol-just a moisturizer? Biological and biophysical effects. In: Loden M, Maibach HI, editors. Dry skin and moisturizers. 2nd ed. London: Taylor & Francis; 2006. p. 227–44.
83. Jacobson EL, Kim H, Kim M, et al. A topical lipophilic niacin derivative increases NAD, epidermal differentiation and barrier function in photodamaged skin. Exp Dermatol. 2007;16(6):490–9.
84. Loden M, Wessman C. The influence of a cream containing 20% glycerin and its vehicle on skin barrier properties. Int J Cosmet Sci. 2001;23:115–9.
85. Fluhr JW, Mao-Qiang M, Brown BE, et al. Glycerol regulates stratum corneum hydration in sebaceous gland deficient (Asebia) mice. J Invest Dermatol. 2003;120:728–37.
86. Choi EH, Man MQ, Wang F, et al. Is endogenous glycerol a determinant of stratum corneum hydration in humans? J Invest Dermatol. 2005;125:288–93.
87. Crowther JM, Matts PJ. Publication in preparation.
88. Mohammed D, Crowther JM, Matts PJ, Hadgraft J, Lane ME. Influence of niacinamide containing formulations on the molecular and biophysical properties of the stratum corneum. Int J Pharm. 2013;441 (1–2):192–201.
89. Nikolovski J, Stamatas GN, Kollias N, Wiegand C. Barrier function and water-holding and transport properties of infant stratum corneum are different from adult and continue to develop though the first year of life. J Invest Dermatol. 2008;128:1728–36.
90. Boireau-Adamezyk E, Baillet-Guffroy A, Stamatas GN. Age-dependent changes in stratum corneum barrier function. Skin Res Technol. 2014;20(4):409–15.

The Measurement and Perception of Uneven Coloration in Aging Skin

91

Paul J. Matts

Contents

P.J. Matts (✉)
Procter & Gamble, Greater London Innovation Centre, Egham, Surrey, UK
e-mail: matts.pj@pg.com

M.A. Farage et al. (eds.), *Textbook of Aging Skin*,
DOI 10.1007/978-3-662-47398-6_72

Abstract

While much is known about surface optics and topography, color contrast in skin remains a remarkable unstudied subject. The chapter will review, briefly, recent research in this area that sheds new light on the measurement of the molecular basis of color contrast in skin and its effect on perception of age, health, and attractiveness.

Introduction

Human beings view the world using sensitive light meters that operate on the basis of "contrast sensitivity." "Contrast" can be defined simply as a ratio of adjacent luminance values and "contrast sensitivity" is a measure of how faded or washed-out an image can become before it is indistinguishable from a uniform field. It has been determined experimentally that the minimum discernible difference in grayscale level that the human eye can detect is about 2 % of full brightness [1, 2]. This outstanding contrast sensitivity allows the world around to be perceived in great detail; indeed, without contrast (and a means for achieving this via a variable-focus mechanism), human beings would effectively be rendered blind. The human eye, therefore, is drawn automatically to areas with high ratios of adjacent luminance – in simple terms, the world is viewed through edges created by contrast.

If the human retina responds to only a narrow bandwidth of the electromagnetic spectrum (so-called visible light, a nominal 400–700 nm), the interaction of these wavelengths with skin, therefore, is of utmost importance in understanding the way individuals perceive others and are themselves perceived.

In young skin, reflection from the skin surface is largely diffuse, due to the very large number of reflecting polygonal plateaus that make up "microrelief," and this has been found to be predictive for perception of soft, firm skin [3]. As microrelief is lost with increasing age and cumulative photodamage, so too is this natural "soft-focus" effect, driving low-contrast optics. In aging human skin, contrast is certainly increased by high ratios of adjacent luminance values due to shadowing formed by high-amplitude/low-frequency surface topography – and especially so in the case of linear features such as "lines," "furrows," and "wrinkles."

Color, however, also plays an important role in the perception of age, health, and beauty. It has been firmly established that the processes of intrinsic and, particularly, extrinsic aging drive a steady accumulation of enlarging, localized concentrations of the two colored skin chromophores, melanin, and hemoglobin [4–8]. Contrast can easily be created by color if a homogeneous field is disrupted by colored features of either/both sufficient diameter and ratio of adjacent luminance. In other words, therefore, independent of contrast formed by shape and/or topography, localized concentration of chromophores in aging skin causes a significant increase in contrast, particularly in sun-exposed areas such as the face, neck, and décolletage.

Measurement of the Molecular Basis of Color Contrast in Skin

Human skin coloration is dependent almost exclusively on the concentration and spatial distribution of the chromophores, melanin, and hemoglobin, where melanin plays the dominant role in driving constitutive coloration [9, 10]. Objective approaches to determining skin color in vivo have centered around spectrophotometric or colorimetric approaches and the use of derived color coordinates such as L*a*b*, and various digital imaging/image analysis techniques, reviewed in full by Pierard [11]. While these measures certainly bring objectivity to the measurement of skin color, they still are not able to fully separate the individual contributions of the chromophores responsible for either the measured, integrated remittance spectrum or the final photographic image (no matter how high a quality it may be).

A new measurement capability, SIAscopy™ (spectrophotometric intracutaneous analysis; 12–15), developed by Cotton and Claridge [12] and then Astron Clinica (Cambridge, UK), operates on the principle of "chromophore mapping," that is, the in vivo measurement of the concentration and distribution of eumelanin, oxy-hemoglobin, and dermal collagen, to produce mutually exclusive grayscale concentration maps of these chromophores. The "SIAscope™" is a commercially available instrument (now owned by and available from MedX Health Corporation), and, while it has been shown to have excellent sensitivity and specificity in the early identification of malignant melanoma, the principle of chromophore mapping that it employs can be readily applied to normal, healthy skin [12–15]. The technique is based upon a unique combination of dermatoscopy, contact remittance spectrophotometry, and hyper-spectral imaging. In short, the SIAscope™ is able to obtain a high-resolution composite white-light image of the skin over a defined area and provides four additional, mutually exclusive chromophore maps that display the concentration of epidermal melanin and hemoglobin, collagen and melanin in the papillary dermis, pixel by pixel (Fig. 1). The dermal melanin end point is the key diagnostic criterion used in melanoma diagnosis (not of concern with regard to normal skin).

The contact SIAscope™ comprises a hand-held scanner with a flat glass-fronted probe, placed in contact with the skin using light, but firm, pressure (to avoid blanching). Further research by Astron Clinica yielded "noncontact"

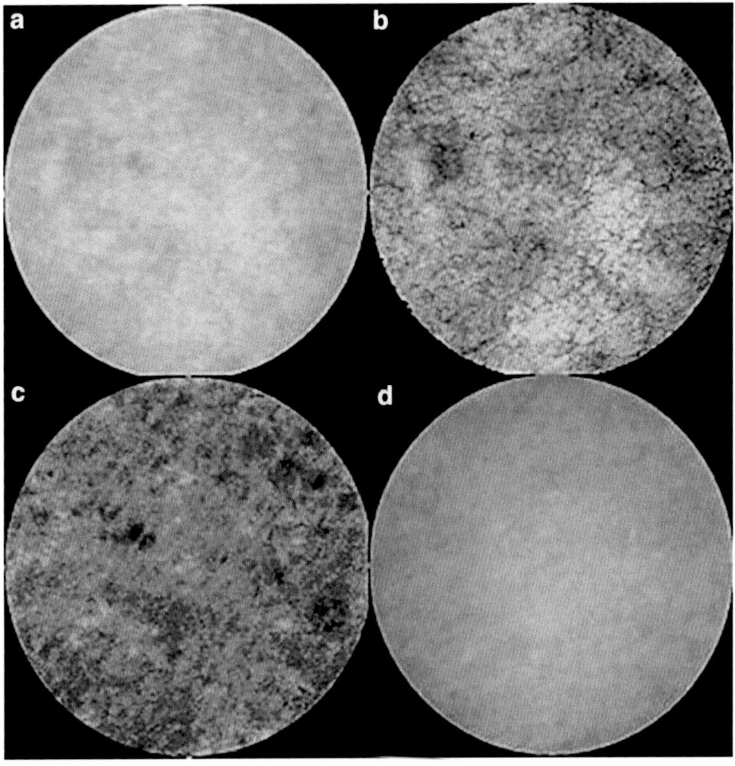

Fig. 1 Example of SIAscope™ II chromophore maps (12 mm diameter). (**a**) Composite white-light image, (**b**) oxyhemoglobin concentration map, (**c**) eumelanin concentration map, (**d**) collagen concentration map

SIAscopy™ (NCS) that overcame the limitations of a skin contact probe. By necessity, this approach needs to be insensitive to local geometry and illumination intensity, in other words, the unavoidable artifacts of measuring 3D objects, rather than flat surfaces.

NCS is implemented [16] using an essentially conventional (although finely calibrated) digital camera and lighting system and may be used to acquire large-field eumelanin and oxyhemoglobin chromophore maps. In deploying NCS, the camera is treated not so much as an imaging device, but more as a three-waveband spectrometer, making use of the RGB Bayer filter over the CCD. The spectral power distribution of the light source and the raw response of the CCD are determined accurately over the visible range (400–700 nm) and are supplied as calibration data to the NCS algorithms, based on the SIA™ mathematical model of light transport within the skin. In short, for every pixel of the original raw image, NCS calculations are performed to yield exclusive concentrations of eumelanin and oxyhemoglobin. When recombined as an array, a parametric gray-scale concentration map is produced, directly analogous to those calculated using the contact technique. It should be noted that a fully cross-polarized lighting system is needed, to eliminate specular reflection (which, by nature, contains no subsurface information). An example of the NCS technique applied to a whole face can be seen in Fig. 2.

The NCS technique now allows routine acquisition of full-face melanin and hemoglobin chromophore maps, and the method has proven an ideal clinical partner. In a recent double-blinded study, NCS was used to provide a quantitative means of measuring the effect of a vehicle containing 2 % N-acetyl glucosamine (NAG) and 4 % niacinamide (N) vs. a vehicle control, applied topically, full face, twice daily for 8 weeks, to two groups of 100 females aged 40–60, respectively, on melanized hyperpigmented spots [17]. Analysis of

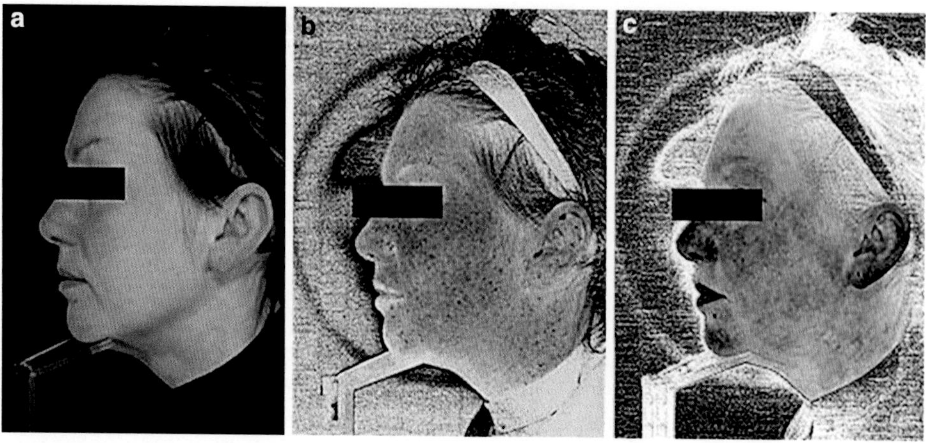

Fig. 2 Example of full-face noncontact SIAscope™ chromophore maps (female subject aged 35). (**a**) Original cross-polarized white-light digital photograph, (**b**) eumelanin concentration map, (**c**) oxyhemoglobin concentration map

the NCS melanin maps demonstrated clear treatment effects for the NAG + N combination vs. vehicle control, resulting in a significant ($p < 0.05$) reduction in melanin spot area fraction and a significant ($p < 0.05$) increase in melanin evenness.

In a separate study [18], an excellent correlation was demonstrated between NCS-derived melanin concentrations and eumelanin concentrations in human skin biopsies, spanning Fitzpatrick skin types I–VI. It must be concluded, therefore, that large-field chromophore mapping by NCS brings a new level of sensitivity and specificity to measurement of human skin color and constitutes a true step forward in the measurement of aging human skin and its treatment.

Color Contrast Plays a Major Role in the Perception of Age, Health, and Attractiveness

Evolutionary psychologists have proposed that preferences for facial characteristics such as symmetry, averageness, and sexual dimorphism may reflect adaptations for "mate choice" because they probably provide visual cues of health and reproductive ability.

Two recent studies found a positive association between homogeneity of skin features and perceived attractiveness. Importantly, however, both studies did not differentiate between visual contrast caused by skin surface topography and skin color distribution. Fink, Grammer, and Thornhill [19] demonstrated that women's facial skin texture affects male judgment of facial attractiveness and found that homogeneous skin (i.e., an even distribution of features relating to both skin color and skin surface topography) is most attractive. Analogous to the manner in which coloration plays a role in mate choice in birds, therefore, visible color and color distribution in human facial skin may provide an indication of the age, health, and attractiveness of the respective individual. More recently, Jones et al. [20] demonstrated that ratings of attractiveness of small areas of skin imaged from the left and right cheeks of male facial images significantly correlated with ratings of facial attractiveness. It was also found that apparent health of skin influences male facial attractiveness, independent of shape information.

Importantly, these studies did *not* differentiate between skin surface topography and skin color distribution. A unique approach was, therefore, used to investigate the single-variable contribution of skin color contrast to perception of biological age, attractiveness, and health [21].

One hundred and sixty-nine Caucasian women aged between 10 and 70 were imaged from front, left, and right views using a custom high-resolution digital imaging system. The use of

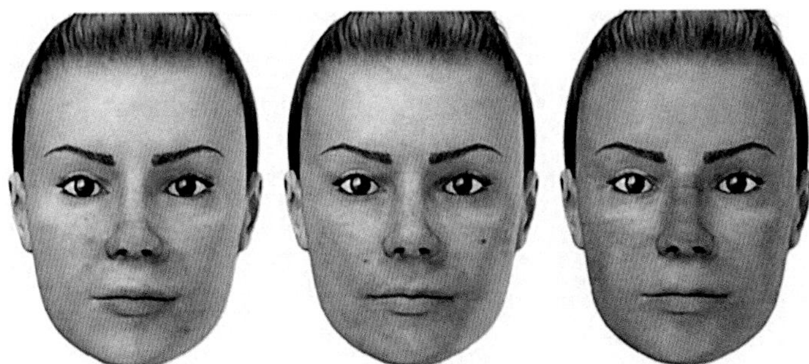

Fig. 3 Examples of three "stimuli" with standardized facial form, feature, and topography with skin color distribution of the original Caucasian female faces as the single-variable difference

cross-polarized lighting eliminated fine surface texture in this imaging stage. The resulting images were processed using a new, unique series of digital manipulations to create "stimulus" heads where skin color distribution was the only remaining variable. Left and right sides were "grafted" onto the frontal image, and then a cloning technique was used to remove any contrast attributable to low-frequency topographical features (lines, furrows, etc.). 2D color maps were then created by fitting the resulting image to a standard 2D template. In this stage, facial features (e.g., pupils, mouth gap, etc.) were standardized geometrically by fitting these to fixed addresses within the 2D template.

To generate 3D facial stimuli from 2D color maps, faces were deformed to match a template grid in order to fit on a shape-standardized wire-frame mesh. In the final rendering process, these corrected 2D maps were fitted to the wire-frame mesh, akin to a virtual skull. In this process, standardized facial features were added (eyes, nose, mouth, ears, hair, etc.) such that the resulting dataset comprised 169 3D head/face stimuli, standard in every respect apart from the subject's original skin color distribution. Examples of the end-result process are shown in Fig. 3.

These stimuli were shown blind to 430 members of the public (aged 13–76), in Germany and Austria, using calibrated monitors. Participants were requested to estimate the biological age of each face using a single-step scale ranging from 10 to 60 years. In addition, participants were asked to rate each face for a total of 15 attributes using a ten-point rating scale combining aspects of perceived attractiveness and health and apparent skin condition.

The estimated biological age (aggregated estimates from all judges for each face) of facial images ranged from 17.8 to 36.7 years, a span of some 20 years, and there was a highly significant positive correlation between the actual biological age of the subjects who provided facial images and the corresponding estimated age of their 3D shape-standardized faces varying only in visible skin color distribution (rho $= .721$, $p < 0.01$, 2-tailed). Significant negative correlations emerged between estimated facial age and the global face attributes (attractive: rho $= -0.527$, $p < 0.01$; healthy: rho $= -0.520$, $p < 0.01$; youthful: rho $= -0.860$, $p < 0.01$).

More recent studies have corroborated and provided more insight into the perception of uneven color in aging skin. [28] investigated visual perception of isolated female facial skin images and compared this with the objectively analyzed homogeneity of these images and corresponding chromophore maps, as assessed using SIAscopy™ technology. Homogeneity of skin images correlated positively with perceived attractiveness, healthiness, and youthfulness, but negatively with estimated age. Homogeneity of hemoglobin and melanin maps was positively correlated with that of skin images and negatively correlated with estimated age. Thus, variation in perceived contrast appears to be an important visual cue for the judgment of age, health, and attractiveness.

Fink and Matts [22] investigated visual perception of female facial images (aged 40 years and older) that varied systematically in skin color distribution and topography. The aim of this study was to investigate (i) whether skin color distribution and skin surface topography cues significantly influence the perception of age and health of female faces and (ii) if they convey differential information concerning the strength of these effects. The results showed that people are sensitive to both skin cues when making judgments of female facial age and health. However, skin color and topography cues differed in the strength of their effect on age and health judgments. Removing skin surface topography cues (such as fine lines and wrinkles) while preserving skin color information, decreased age estimations of female faces by about 10 years compared to unmodified faces. In contrast, digital smoothing of facial discoloration resulted in a decrease of perceived age of only 1–5 years. Female faces were judged the youngest when these image manipulations were combined; when surface topography cues were removed and skin color was smoothed, there was a perceived age decrease of approximately 15 years. This study demonstrated that skin surface topography cues account for a large proportion of variation in facial age perception, whereas skin color distribution appears to be a stronger health cue.

More recent studies that have manipulated skin color distribution and skin surface topography in female faces indicate that both males and females are sensitive to even small changes of these features in female facial images. For example, Samson et al. [23] showed that faces with skin surface topography cues removed were judged significantly younger and more attractive than their original (unmodified) counterparts, with modifications on the forehead and in the periorbital region showing the highest differences. In these areas, participants were able to detect as low as a 20 % change in skin surface topography.

Similar effects have been reported for the manipulation of skin color distribution, showing that a smoothing of inhomogeneity as low as 25 % has a significant effect on facial health perception [24].

While it has been convincingly demonstrated that people have a preference for young- and healthy-looking facial skin in women, signaled by homogenous topography and coloration, the situation in men is less clear. Fink et al. [25], therefore, investigated perception of male skin and related them to objective measures. Perceived age, health, and attractiveness of digitally isolated skin fields from the cheek of male facial cross-polarized images were related to homogeneity measures of corresponding melanin and hemoglobin grayscale concentration maps, as derived using SIAscopy™ technology. It was hypothesized that naive judges would be (i) perceptually sensitive and able to judge images of digitally isolated fields of cheek skin from chronologically older men as older and that (ii) judges would prefer male skin with a higher degree of melanin and hemoglobin homogeneity with correspondingly higher ratings of youth and health. Age, health, and attractiveness perception was strongly related to melanin and hemoglobin distribution, whereby more even distributions led to perception of younger age and greater perceived health and attractiveness. Interestingly, when deconvoluting the visual contributions of each chromophore, melanin distribution was more important for age estimation, whereas hemoglobin distribution was more important for health and attractiveness ratings.

This result underlines the potent signaling role of skin in its own right, independent of shape or other factors, and suggests that visible skin condition, and skin color homogeneity in particular, plays a significant role in the perception of men's faces. In a follow-up work, Fink et al. [26] demonstrated that perceived age, health, and attractiveness in male faces could be predicted by ratings of cheek skin only, such that older men were viewed as older, less healthy, and less attractive. This result underlines, once again, the potent signaling role of skin in its own right, independent of shape or other factors, and suggests strongly that visible skin condition plays a significant role in the perception of men's faces.

Although this study on male skin replicated previous findings on female skin in that overall younger and healthier facial skin is preferred [28], the data were derived from objective measurements and subjective perception of skin coloration only. Thus, the relative impact of male facial skin surface topography and color cues on social perception remains to be demonstrated. The age-related increase of both topography and discoloration can readily explain the decrease of apparent preference for homogeneous melanin and hemoglobin chromophore distribution. However, evolutionary psychologists argue that selection pressure to own and maintain a youthful appearance is acting more strongly on women than on men. Thus, it need not necessarily be the case that age-related changes of skin features in men are considered unhealthy or unattractive, as it has been argued for women [22]. A more realistic scenario lies in an age-appropriate natural balance between skin surface topography and skin coloration. Put differently, looking either too young or too old in relation to one's chronological age may result in less positive social perception.

In summary, therefore, a growing body of studies investigating the perception of visible skin condition supports our assertion that we are remarkably sensitive to subtle age-related changes in skin condition, including skin color evenness. Put another way, evidence continues to mount that, in addition to cues related to face shape, skin color evenness profoundly affects the way in which we judge age, health, and attractiveness. The evidence is strong, consistent, and equally true for both sexes.

It is hypothesized that this is so because color contrast may signal aspects of the underlying physiological condition/health of an individual, relevant for mate choice.

Conclusion

It has been shown that color contrast in human skin, formed by the local distribution and concentration of the chromophores melanin and hemoglobin, plays a major role in perception of age, health, and attractiveness. Strategies to improve the appearance of aging skin, therefore, need to focus not only contrast created by form and topography but also that created by color distribution and the chromophore targets responsible for this.

Cross-References

▶ Hyperpigmentation in Aging Skin
▶ Pigmentation in Ethnic Groups
▶ The New Face of Pigmentation and Aging

References

1. Blackwell HR. Contrast thresholds of the human eye. J Opt Soc Am. 1946;36:42–643.
2. Campbell FW, Robson JG. Application of fourier analysis to the visibility of gratings. J Physiol. 1968;197(3):551–66.
3. Matts PJ, Solechnick ND. Predicting visual perception of human skin surface texture using multiple-angle reflectance spectrophotometry. American Academy of Dermatology 58th annual conference, 2000.
4. American Academy of Dermatology Consensus Conference. Photoaging/Photodamage as a public health concern. Evanston; 1988.
5. National Institutes of Health Consensus Development Conference Statement. Sunlight, ultraviolet radiation, and the skin NIH consens statement. 1989;7(8):1–29.
6. Griffiths CEM. The clinical identification and quantification of photodamage. Br J Dermatol. 1992;127 Suppl 41:37–42.
7. Ryan T. The ageing of the blood supply and the lymphatic drainage of the skin. Micron. 2004;35(3):161–71.
8. Montagna W, Carlisle K. Structural changes in ageing skin. Br J Dermatol. 1990;122 Suppl 35:61–70.
9. Anderson RR, Parrish JA. The optics of human skin. J Invest Dermatol. 1981;77(1):13–9.
10. Bashkatov AA, Genina EA, Kochubey VI, Tuchin VV. Optical properties of human skin, subcutaneous and mucous tissues in the wavelength range from 400 to 2000 nm. J Phys D Appl Phys. 2005;38:2543–55.
11. Pierard GE. EEMCO guidance for the assessment of skin colour. J Eur Acad Dermatol Venereol. 1998;10(1):1–11.
12. Cotton SD, Claridge E. Developing a predictive model of human skin colouring. Proc SPIE. 1996;2708:814–25.
13. Cotton SD, Claridge E, Hall PN. Non-invasive skin imaging. In: Duncan J, Gindi G, editors. Proceedings of information processing in medical imaging, LNCS 1230. New York: Springer; 1997. p. 501–6.
14. Moncrieff M, Cotton SD, Claridge E, Hall PN. Spectrophotometric intracutaneous analysis – a new technique for imaging pigmented skin lesions. Br J Dermatol. 2002;146(3):448–57.
15. Cotton SD. A non-invasive imaging system for assisting in the diagnosis of malignant melanoma. PhD thesis, Birmingham University, Birmingham 1998.
16. Preece S, Cotton SD, Claridge E. Imaging the pigments of skin with a technique which is invariant to changes

in surface geometry and intensity of illuminating light. In: Barber D, editor. Proceedings of medical image understanding and analysis. Sheffield: MIUA; 2003. p. 145–8.

17. Kimball AB, Kaczvinsky JR, Li J, Robinson LR, Matts PJ, Berge CA, Miyamoto K, Bissett DL. Reduction in the appearance of facial hyperpigmentation after use of moisturizers with a combination of topical niacinamide and *N*-acetyl glucosamine: results of a randomized, double-blind, vehicle-controlled trial. Br J Dermatol. 2010;162(2):435–41.
18. Matts PJ, Dykes PJ, Marks R. The distribution of melanin in skin determined in vivo. Br J Dermatol. 2007a;156(4):620–8.
19. Fink B, Grammer K, Thornhill R. Human (Homo sapiens) facial attractiveness in relation to skin texture and colour. J Comp Psychol. 2001;115(1):92–9.
20. Jones BC, Perrett DI, Little AC, Boothroyd L, Cornwell RE, Feinberg DR, Tiddeman BP, Whiten S, Pitman RM, Hillier SG, Burt DM, Stirrat MR, Law-Smith MJ, Moore FR. Menstrual cycle, pregnancy and oral contraceptive use alter attraction to apparent health in faces. Proc Roy Soc Lond B Biol Sci. 2005;272(1561): 347–54.
21. Fink B, Grammer K, Matts PJ. Visible skin colour distribution plays a major role in the perception of age, attractiveness and health in female faces. Evol Hum Behav. 2006;27(6):433–42.
22. Fink B, Matts PJ. The effects of skin colour distribution and topography cues on the perception of female facial age and health. Eur J Dermatol Venereol. 2008;22(4):493–8.
23. Samson N, Fink B, Matts PJ, Dawes NC, Weitz SM. Visible changes of female facial skin surface topography in relation to age and attractiveness perception. J Cosmet Dermatol. 2010;9:79–88.
24. Samson N, Fink B, Matts P. Interaction of skin colour distribution and skin surface topography cues in the perception of female facial age and health. J Cosmet Dermatol. 2011;10(1):78–84.
25. Fink B, Bunse L, Matts PJ, D'Emiliano D. Visible skin colouration predicts perception of male facial age, health and attractiveness. Int J Cosmet Sci. 2012;34(4):307–10.
26. Fink B, Matts PJ, D'Emiliano D, Bunse L, Weege B, Röder S. Colour homogeneity and visual perception of age, health and attractiveness of male facial skin. Eur J Dermatol Venereol. 2012;26(12):1486–92.
27. Matts PJ, Miyamoto K, Bissett DL, Cotton SD. The use of chromophore mapping to measure the effects of a topical *N*-Acetyl glucosamine/niacinamide complex on pigmentation in human skin. American Academy of Dermatology 64th annual conference, 2006.
28. Matts PJ, Fink B, Grammer K, Burquest M. Colour homogeneity and visual perception of age, health and attractiveness of female facial skin. J Am Acad Dermatol. 2007b;57(6):977–84.

Transepidermal Water Loss in Young and Aged Healthy Humans

92

Jan Kottner, Annika Vogt, Andrea Lichterfeld, and Ulrike Blume-Peytavi

Contents

J. Kottner (✉)
Department of Dermatology and Allergy, Clinical Research Center for Hair and Skin Science, Charité-Universitätsmedizin Berlin, Berlin, Germany
e-mail: jan.kottner@charite.de

A. Vogt
Clinical Research Center for Hair and Skin Science, Department of Dermatology and Allergy, Charité-Universitätsmedizin Berlin, Berlin, Germany
e-mail: annika.vogt@charite.de

A. Lichterfeld • U. Blume-Peytavi
Department of Dermatology and Allergy, Clinical Research Center for Hair and Skin Science, Charité-Universitätsmedizin Berlin, Berlin, Germany
e-mail: andrea.lichterfeld@charite.de; ulrike.blume-peytavi@charite.de

M.A. Farage et al. (eds.), *Textbook of Aging Skin*,
DOI 10.1007/978-3-662-47398-6_127

Abstract

The stratum corneum is the most important barrier to a wide range of molecules, irritants, allergens, small particles, and microorganisms. However, small amounts of water continuously diffuse from the inside to the outside which is called transepidermal water loss (TEWL). TEWL is regarded as one of the most important parameters characterizing skin barrier integrity. Elevated TEWL is usually associated with skin barrier impairments, whereas reduced or low TEWL is considered as skin barrier integrity or improvement. Available evidence suggests that the water diffusion through the stratum corneum seems to remain stable and/or to decrease during aging. Possible reasons are the flattening of the corneocytes, altered and reduced intercellular lipids, reduced natural moisturizing factor content, and/or a reduced skin surface temperature. Such a "normal" TEWL masks the decreases of functional capacity of the skin barrier function in intrinsically and extrinsically aged skin.

Introduction

Living human cells and metabolic processes require moist (and usually warm) conditions to function orderly, but we live in a dry (and usually cold) environment. The skin layer that protects us from drying out and thus enabling human life on dry land is the stratum corneum. This small membrane-like structure is composed of interconnected flat corneocytes and densely packed intercellular lipids. It separates the last layer of living epidermal cells – the stratum granulosum – from the outer environment. The stratum corneum is extremely effective in forming an inside-out but also an outside-in barrier to a wide range of lipophilic and hydrophilic molecules, irritants, allergens, small particles, and microorganisms. However, despite the impermeability of a wide range of substances, some molecules are able to penetrate. Among others there is a constant inside-out diffusion of water from the highly hydrated epidermal and dermal layers toward the stratum corneum surface where these water molecules eventually evaporate. This continuous inside-out diffusion of water through the stratum corneum was first proposed by Loewy and Wechselmann in 1911 [1]. Later, in 1955, the US American dermatologist Stephen Rothman introduced the term "transepidermal water loss" (TEWL) into the dermatological literature [2].

Transepidermal Water Loss

TEWL is the flux density of water which diffuses through the stratum corneum and it is expressed in $g/m^2/h$. It is generally assumed that the main diffusion route of water is intercellular through the lipid bilayers [3], but evidence suggests that a substantial amount of water molecules take a transcellular way through the corneocytes [4].

TEWL cannot be observed directly. Instead the flux density of the condensed water from the skin surface can be measured by commercially available evaporimetry devices [5, 6]. However, this flux density is identical with TEWL only if other sources of water and concurrent evaporation from skin surface (e.g., sweating, free surface water) are excluded [7]. Therefore, to enhance measurement accuracy standardization is necessary, e.g., acclimatization to standardized ambient temperature and relative humidity prior measurements, probe placement on the horizontal skin surface, etc. Different instrumental devices for TEWL measurements are available. They might be broadly classified into open- and closed-chamber methods using different measurement technologies [8]. Consequently, different devices produce (slightly) different TEWL values [5, 8]. However, available evidence suggests that TEWL estimates are comparable and at least they are highly correlated [5]. Recommendations how to standardize TEWL measurements are available and should be followed [9, 10]. Unfortunately, there are many circumstances where these recommended levels of standardization are not possible, e.g., TEWL measurements in workplace or other nonclinical settings. Guidance of how to measure in these more variable settings is also available [6], but the comparability of TEWL estimates is limited.

TEWL is regarded as one of the most important parameters characterizing skin barrier integrity [9–11]. Elevated TEWL is usually associated with skin barrier impairments, whereas reduced or low TEWL is considered as skin barrier integrity or improvement. However, despite extensive research during the last decades in this area, it seems that a "normal" TEWL does not exist [6]. Irrespective from measurement devices and conditions observed, TEWL values are affected by ethnicity, skin area, skin temperature, day time, body mass index, smoking status, and possibly other factors like gender [5, 6, 12, 13] not directly associated with skin barrier health. Therefore, TEWL should be interpreted cautiously and not in absolute terms. Baseline TEWL estimates contain important information but are of limited clinical value for distinguishing between "normal" and "abnormal" skin barrier [14]. More meaningful are changes of TEWL, for instance, during the course of a disease, an experiment or treatment. In this context, TEWL is, for instance, widely used as an epidermal recovery parameter after artificial removal and/or damage of the stratum corneum [15], in epidermal wound healing studies [16], or after chemical irritation [17].

TEWL During Skin Aging

Skin aging is associated with a continuous change in skin structure and function. Because also the anatomy and physiology of the stratum corneum change during aging [18, 19], changes in TEWL

Table 1 Comparison of transepidermal water (TEWL) loss between young and aged subjects according to Kottner et al. [5]

	TEWL	
Skin area	18–64 years	65+ years
Forehead right[a]	Higher	Lower
Upper eyelid[a]	Similar	
Nose[a]	Similar	
Cheek right[a]	Higher	Lower
Nasolabial right[a]	Similar	
Perioral[a]	Similar	
Postauricular	Similar	
Chin[a]	Similar	
Neck[a]	Similar	
Upper arm	Similar	
Midvolar left	Higher	Lower
Midvolar right	Higher	Lower
Forearm left dorsal[a]	Higher	Lower
Forearm right dorsal[a]	Similar	
Palm right	Higher	Lower
Abdomen	Higher	Lower
Upper back right	Higher	Lower
Lower back right	Higher	Lower
Thigh	Higher	Lower
Leg lateral	Similar	
Ankle	Higher	Lower

[a]Skin areas influenced by photodamage

are to be expected. Worldwide, numerous studies have been published comparing TEWL estimates of different age groups. Results are conflicting, but the majority of published research seems to indicate a TEWL decrease during aging [20, 21]. Available TEWL estimates in healthy skin reported until June 2012 have been summarized recently in a systematic review and meta-analysis providing TEWL reference values for 50 skin areas [5]. Using a cutoff of 65 years, pooled results indicate that TEWL is either similar (e.g., postauricular, upper arm) or statistically significantly lower (e.g., forehead, midvolar forearm, abdomen, back) (Table 1).

Results of latest studies in this field indicate again either no associations between TEWL and age [12, 13, 22, 23] or that TEWL in the aged is lower compared to mid-aged humans [18, 24]. Until today, there is no single study demonstrating (baseline) TEWL increases during aging. Taken together, these findings clearly indicate that the water diffusion through the stratum corneum seems to remain stable and/or to decrease during aging.

Possible Reasons for Reduced TEWL in the Aged

Reduced TEWL in old-aged compared to mid-aged indicates an increased stratum corneum water diffusion resistance and a decreased water diffusion coefficient. The exact reasons for these phenomena are not known, but the following factors are discussed in the literature:

- Corneocytes become thinner but longer with age (flattening). Thus, the intercellular lipid pathway is longer and more "tortuous," and with increasing corneocyte size, the water diffusion resistance increases [3, 4, 19, 20, 25].
- Stratum corneum thickness either increases or remains unchanged, but there is a mild increase of the number of corneocyte layers. Similarly to the abovementioned "flattening," this increases the path length of water molecules [11, 18, 20].
- Epidermal lipid synthesis is changed and reduced. This might lower the water diffusion coefficient increasing the resistance [18–20].
- Natural moisturizing factors and stratum corneum hydration are reduced. Thus, the ability of corneocytes to attract and to transport water might be reduced [19, 20].
- Skin temperature is decreased. The density of dermal capillaries reduces with age [26] possibly decreasing the skin temperature leading to decreased water diffusion [20, 21].

Probably all of the abovementioned mechanisms contribute to reduce TEWL [27].

Intrinsic Versus Extrinsic Skin Aging

There is a substantial amount of literature covering intrinsic and extrinsic aspects of skin aging. Intrinsic aging is considered to be caused by chronological aging per se and is often regarded as the "normal" course of functional decline. In addition, extrinsic skin aging might be primarily caused by external environmental influences whereby ultraviolet radiation is by far the most important factor ("photoaging"). However, both concepts are interrelated, and skin aging might rather be conceptualized as a composite and complex interaction of intrinsic and extrinsic mechanisms [23, 28].

Despite the extensive knowledge in the skin aging field, little is known about intrinsic and extrinsic aging effects on the stratum corneum and specifically on skin barrier function in terms of TEWL. Histologically, photo exposed stratum corneum appears to be more compact [29], but how this morphological characteristic translates into changed barrier function is unclear. Some authors assume decreased TEWL in photoaged skin compared to intrinsically aged skin [30]. However, the majority of studies suggest that there seem to be no difference in (baseline) TEWL between both [31–33]. In Table 1, the skin areas supposed to be affected by photodamage are marked. Also these comparisons indicate no obvious systematic difference between skin areas affected by intrinsic or extrinsic skin aging.

Discussion

Despite possible biophysical explanations of unchanged and/or reduced TEWL in aged skin, the clinical relevance of this phenomenon is unclear. Aged stratum corneum is clearly more vulnerable, less resistant to external threats, and dryer, and xerosis cutis is one of the most prevalent skin conditions in aged populations [19, 21, 34]. Therefore, a "normal" or decreased TEWL in aging skin should not be interpreted as a competent skin barrier or even as a barrier improvement [18, 35, 36]. Instead, the larger corneocytes might lower the permeation possibly to compensate the reduced lipid synthesis in order to maintain the barrier function [19]. Such mechanisms are well known from other organs and functional body systems to compensate physiologically acute or low-level challenges in order to maintain function and to limit decline [37]. Such a mechanism might also exist for maintaining the skin barrier function during the life course. This supports the aforementioned recommendation to interpret seemingly "normal" or decreased TEWL values cautiously in terms of barrier function. Baseline TEWL represents the overall resistance of the stratum corneum to passive water diffusion.

Barrier insufficiencies become especially apparent in aged skin following barrier disruption [34, 36]. Compared to younger populations, the reactivity patterns to irritation or skin barrier disruption are usually delayed and less pronounced. In epidermal irritation tests, TEWL changes (Δ) after the experimental insults are often lower and delayed, and skin barrier repair processes are slower compared to younger skin [17, 38]. However, even if delayed, the biological processes involved in skin barrier recovery and the end result – an intact epidermis – are similar between healthy young and aged individuals [38, 39].

Conclusions

TEWL is considered to be the most important inside-out water skin barrier parameter indicating the integrity of the stratum corneum. During skin aging, TEWL seems to either remain stable or to decrease. Flattening of the corneocytes, changed epidermal lipid synthesis, and reduced proportions of natural moisturizing factors in the stratum corneum are likely to contribute to these observations. A normal TEWL should not be interpreted as skin barrier improvement. The aged epidermal barrier is less efficient, and therefore TEWL might not be the best candidate to indicate functional capacity.

References

1. Loewy A, Wechselmann W. The physiology and pathology of water changing and heat regulation on the part of the skin organs. (After tests on three people who are related by blood and have ectodermal inhibition cultivation, especially of the skin gland systems).

Virchows Arch Pathol Anat Physiol Klin Med. 1911;206(1):79–121.

2. Rothman S. Insensible water loss. In: Rothman S, editor. Physiology and biochemistry of the skin. Chicago: The University of Chicago; 1955. p. 233–43.
3. Hadgraft J, Lane ME. Transepidermal water loss and skin site: a hypothesis. Int J Pharm. 2009;373 (1–2):1–3.
4. Xiao P, Imhof RE. Two dimensional finite element modelling for dynamic water diffusion through stratum corneum. Int J Pharm. 2012;435(1):88–92.
5. Kottner J, Lichterfeld A, Blume-Peytavi U. Transepidermal water loss in young and aged healthy humans: a systematic review and meta-analysis. Arch Dermatol Res. 2013;305(4):315–23.
6. du Plessis J, et al. International guidelines for the in vivo assessment of skin properties in non-clinical settings: part 2. Transepidermal water loss and skin hydration. Skin Res Technol. 2013;19(3):265–78.
7. Imhof B, McFeat G. Evaluation of the barrier function of skin using transepidermal water loss (TEWL): a critical overview. In: Barel AO, Paye M, Maibach HI, editors. Handbook of cosmetic science and technology. Boca Raton: CRC Press; 2014. p. 131–9.
8. Imhof RE, et al. Closed-chamber transepidermal water loss measurement: microclimate, calibration and performance. Int J Cosmet Sci. 2009;31(2):97–118.
9. Rogiers V. EEMCO guidance for the assessment of transepidermal water loss in cosmetic sciences. Skin Pharmacol Appl Skin Physiol. 2001;14(2):117–28.
10. Pinnagoda J, et al. Guidelines for transepidermal water loss (TEWL) measurement. A report from the standardization group of the European Society of Contact Dermatitis. Contact Dermatitis. 1990;22(3):164–78.
11. Tagami H. Location-related differences in structure and function of the stratum corneum with special emphasis on those of the facial skin. Int J Cosmet Sci. 2008;30 (6):413–34.
12. Firooz A, et al. Variation of biophysical parameters of the skin with age, gender, and body region. Sci World J. 2012;2012:386936.
13. Luebberding S, Krueger N, Kerscher M. Skin physiology in men and women: in vivo evaluation of 300 people including TEWL, SC hydration, sebum content and skin surface pH. Int J Cosmet Sci. 2013;35(5):477–83.
14. Lu N, et al. Characteristic differences in barrier and hygroscopic properties between normal and cosmetic dry skin. I. Enhanced barrier analysis with sequential tape-stripping. Int J Cosmet Sci. 2014;36(2):167–74.
15. Sextius P, et al. Large scale study of epidermal recovery after stratum corneum removal: dynamics of genomic response. Exp Dermatol. 2010;19(3):259–68.
16. Kottner J, et al. Characterisation of epidermal regeneration in vivo: a 60-day follow-up study. J Wound Care. 2013;22(8):395–400.
17. Angelova-Fischer I, et al. Tandem repeated irritation in aged skin induces distinct barrier perturbation and cytokine profile in vivo. Br J Dermatol. 2012;167 (4):787–93.
18. Boireau-Adamezyk E, Baillet-Guffroy A, Stamatas GN. Age-dependent changes in stratum corneum barrier function. Skin Res Technol. 2014;20(4):409–15.
19. Rawlings AV. The stratum corneum and aging. In: Farage MA, Miller KW, Maibach HI, editors. Textbook of aging skin. Berlin/Heidelberg: Springer; 2010. p. 55–75.
20. Alikhan A. Transepidermal water loss and aging. In: Farage MA, Miller KW, Maibach HI, editors. Textbook of aging skin. Berlin/Heidelberg: Springer; 2010. p. 696–703.
21. Wilhelm K-P, Brandt M, Maibach HI. Transepidermal water loss and barrier function of aging human skin. In: Fluhr J et al., editors. Bioengineering of the skin: water and the stratum corneum. New York/London: Informa Healthcare; 2005. p. 143–58.
22. Sato N, Kitahara T, Fujimura T. Age-related changes of stratum corneum functions of skin on the trunk and the limbs. Skin Pharmacol Physiol. 2014;27(4):181.
23. Trojahn C, et al. Characterizing facial skin ageing in humans: disentangling extrinsic from intrinsic biological phenomena. Biomed Res Int. 2015;2015:318586.
24. Kottner J, et al. Do repeated skin barrier measurements influence each other's results? An explorative study. Skin Pharmacol Physiol. 2014;27(2):90–6.
25. Marks R. Measurement of biological ageing in human epidermis. Br J Dermatol. 1981;104(6):627–33.
26. Helmbold P, et al. Detection of a physiological juvenile phase and the central role of pericytes in human dermal microvascular aging. J Invest Dermatol. 2006;126 (6):1419–21.
27. Ghadially R. Aging and the epidermal permeability barrier: implications for contact dermatitis. Am J Contact Dermat. 1998;9(3):162–9.
28. Pierard GE. The quandary of climacteric skin ageing. Dermatology. 1996;193(4):273–4.
29. Bhawan J, et al. Photoaging versus intrinsic aging: a morphologic assessment of facial skin. J Cutan Pathol. 1995;22(2):154–9.
30. Zheng Y, et al. Cathepsin d repairing role in photodamaged skin barrier. Skin Pharmacol Physiol. 2015;28(2):97–102.
31. Reed JT, Elias PM, Ghadially R. Integrity and permeability barrier function of photoaged human epidermis. Arch Dermatol. 1997;133(3):395–6.
32. Kikuchi-Numagami K, et al. Functional and morphological studies of photodamaged skin on the hands of middle-aged Japanese golfers. Eur J Dermatol. 2000;10(4):277–81.
33. Blaak J, et al. Irritability of skin barrier: a comparison of chronologically aged and photo-aged skin in elderly and young adults. Eur Geriatr Med. 2011;2:208–11.
34. Ghadially R, et al. The aged epidermal permeability barrier. Structural, functional, and lipid biochemical abnormalities in humans and a senescent murine model. J Clin Invest. 1995;95(5):2281–90.
35. Tagami H, et al. Environmental effects on the functions of the stratum corneum. J Investig Dermatol Symp Proc. 2001;6(1):87–94.

36. Jia Q, Nash F. Pathology of aging skin. In: Farage MA, Miller KW, Maibach HI, editors. Textbook of aging skin. Berlin/Heidelberg: Springer; 2010. p. 277–91.
37. Kuh D, et al. Life course epidemiology, ageing research, and maturing cohort studies: a dynamic combination for understanding healthy ageing. In: Kuh D et al., editors. A life course approach to healthy ageing. Oxford: Oxford University Press; 2014. p. 3–15.
38. Sextius P, et al. Analysis of gene expression dynamics revealed delayed and abnormal epidermal repair process in aged compared to young skin. Arch Dermatol Res. 2015;307:351–64.
39. Ranzer MJ, DiPietro LA. Impaired wound repair and delayed angiogenesis. In: Farage MA, Miller KW, Maibach HI, editors. Textbook of aging skin. Berlin: Springer; 2010. p. 897–906.

Reconstructed Skin to Create In Vitro Flexible Models of Skin Aging: New Results and Prospects

93

Daniel Asselineau, Sylvie Ricois, Herve Pageon, Helene Zucchi, Sarah Girardeau-Hubert, Céline Deneuville, Valerie Haydont, Véronique Neiveyans, and Isabelle Lorthois

Contents

Dedication: In Memoriam Jean-François Grollier (1944–2015), L'Oréal former Vice-President and General Director Research and Development.

D. Asselineau (✉) • S. Ricois • H. Pageon • H. Zucchi • S. Girardeau-Hubert • C. Deneuville • V. Haydont • V. Neiveyans
L'Oreal, Research and Innovation, Aulnay-sous-bois, France
e-mail: dasselineau@rd.loreal.com; sricois@rd.loreal.com; hpageon@rd.loreal.com; hzucchi@rd.loreal.com; shubert@rd.loreal.com; crabot@rd.loreal.com; vhaydont@rd.loreal.com; vneiveyans@rd.loreal.com

I. Lorthois
Centre LOEX de l'Université Laval, Québec, QC, Canada
e-mail: isabelle.lorthois.1@ulaval.ca

M.A. Farage et al. (eds.), *Textbook of Aging Skin*,
DOI 10.1007/978-3-662-47398-6_48

Abstract

Despite the fact that a fully differentiated and keratinized epidermis can be produced at the air-liquid interface on acellular dermal substrates or even on membranes it appeared necessary in order to investigate adequately skin physiology and skin aging to deal with a full thickness skin construct made with a living dermis which contains fibroblasts. Based on the pioneering work of Bell and coworkers we have developed such a system in our laboratory which allowed us to investigate skin aging with two separate but complementary approaches. One way was to look at modifications occurring in the dermal matrix like collagen glycation which allowed us to propose for the first time a model of skin aging. Another way was to look at the actual actors of the dermis which are the fibroblasts and to study their destiny during aging which led us to show the key evolution of the papillary fibroblast population during skin aging. In addition to these important findings we have created a skin model for dermal filler studies and we are on the way to create ethnic specific models of skin in vitro.

Combining several parameters like the type of the fibroblast population, the age of the donors, the glycation status, and UV exposure, we now look forward to obtaining more complex but more realistic models of skin aging closer to the in vivo situation. An example of this is shown in which the glycation status, the nature of the fibroblast population used, and the age of the donors were combined.

Moreover, based on a new way to prepare dermal equivalents, we show that it becomes possible to make them with more than two layers which allows to add hypodermis to dermis in our system. Finally in order to escape from the current flat dermal-epidermal junction of our reconstructed skin this method allows us to start investigating the possibility to create reliefs like rete ridge-like or wrinkle-like structures.

Introduction: Aging

Aging has gained a lot more interest considering that human life expectancy has considerably increased during recent decades. Aging is a complex phenomenon in which several mechanisms operate together. These include accumulation of mutations in the genetic material, accumulation of toxic metabolites, formation of free radicals to produce oxidative damage, chemical modifications, and cross-linking of macromolecules by glycation (Table 1).

Skin is a unique model for aging studies because it is exposed to both extrinsic influences from the environment mostly sun exposure and intrinsic factors mostly of genetic origin. Intrinsic aging also termed chronological aging is a time-dependant process which leads to gradual changes which affect the structure and function of all organs and tissues of the organism.

Skin represents a useful model to study aging in humans not only because it is affected by this

Table 1 Aging: theories and mechanisms

Classical theories	Oxidative stress Alteration of the genome/ mutations "Error catastrophe" (L.E Orgel 1963) Programmed aging-genetic clock: Limited replicative protential (Hayflick 1966) Auto immune responses, deterioration of the immune system Accumulation of toxic metabolites Formation of cross links
Proposed interpretation of "old theories"	Oxidative stress: DNA, Proteins, Lipids, Mitochondria DNA – repair (mutations) Function (expression) Replication (telomere length) Proteins: structure and function – post translational modifications Glycation (AGE, cross-links) Transglutaminase (cross-links) Farnesylation Methylation etc. . . .

process but also because it is easily accessible. Clinical signs due to aging include wrinkles, laxity, dryness, and heterogeneity in pigmentation [1–3]. Histologically the dermal-epidermal junction becomes flat; atrophy develops associated with reduction in epidermal thickness. However, major changes also take place in the dermis characterized by modification and disorganization of extracellular matrix components like collagen, elastic tissue, and proteoglycans.

An attractive characteristic of skin and skin cells is that it is possible to isolate, cultivate, and use these cells to reproduce in vitro the three-dimensional architecture of skin by serially reconstructing the dermal and epidermal compartments. Those constructs are named organotypic cultures or skin equivalents or reconstructed skins. In this chapter we prefer to use "reconstructed skin" to designate them.

The Reconstruction of Skin

The reconstruction of skin represents a well-recognized alternative to in vivo studies. Historically mainly four authors published their respective approaches almost at the same time: Prunieras proposed the reconstruction of epidermis on de-epidermized dermis or DED [4]; Green introduced the culture of epidermal keratinocytes in the presence of feeder layers which resulted in epidermal sheets in vitro suitable for grafting [5]; Bell created the collagen fibroblast contracted lattice [6]; and Yannas and Burke engineered a synthetic dermal matrix based on the association of collagen and glycoseaminoglycans [7]. Many different ways have been proposed to produce skin equivalents [8]. However, because of the extensive use of membranes [9, 10] or other dermal substitutes [11] which appeared to be sufficient to obtain a fully differentiated epidermis only a few of them took in account the full thickness of skin, a crucial prerequisite to appropriately investigate skin physiology in vitro. This needs to include both a dermal compartment containing living cells like fibroblasts and the epidermal

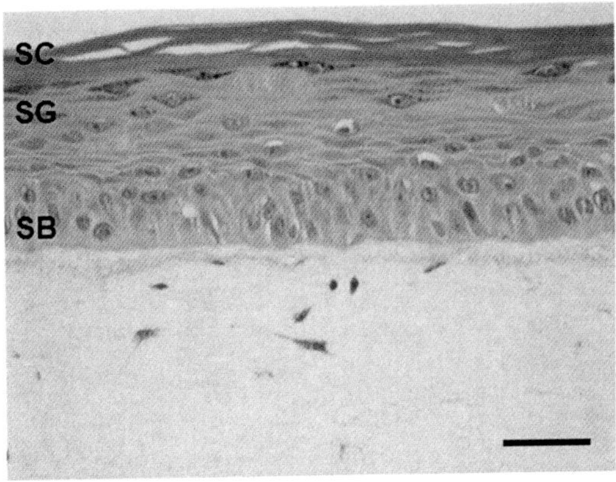

Fig. 1 Histology of reconstructed skin grown at the air-liquid interphase. Complete differentiation and keratinization was observed when keratinocytes were classically grown on the surface of the dermal equivalent in order to form epidermis (*SB* stratum basale, *SG* stratum granulosum, *SC* stratum corneum). Bar, 25 μm

compartment made with keratinocytes [12, 13]. In our laboratory based on the pioneering work of Bell and coworkers [14] this was achieved by producing dermal equivalents made by mixing collagen and fibroblasts in conditions leading to the formation of a firm dermal tissue in the Petri dish [15]. This initial step was then followed by the reconstruction of epidermis by growing keratinocytes on this substrate and raising [16] the culture at the air-liquid interphase. As shown in Fig. 1 the final result is a full thickness skin model. The success came from the use of a two step procedure to uncouple keratinocyte proliferation and differentiation which since then became a universal method. It consisted in keeping the culture first submerged to allow full coverage of the dermal substrate by proliferating keratinocytes before lifting the culture at the air-liquid interphase to trigger keratinocyte stratification and differentiation instead of using a single step procedure consisting of seeding directly keratinocytes on the lifted dermal substrate.

The signals involved in the morphogenesis of the epidermis are of interest. First, surprisingly we found that the contact with air is not mandatory since we showed that a liquid-oil interphase does not prevent the morphogenesis of a fully stratified and keratinized epidermis containing granular and horny layers (see Fig. 2). Secondly, the air-liquid interphase clearly results in a filtering effect of the medium through the dermis since increasing the thickness of the dermis or piling up several dermal equivalents leads to influence the differentiation pattern (see Fig. 3). More interestingly in addition to the classical filtering effect also mentioned previously [17] it is likely that an internal gradient inside the epidermis also takes place. This could possibly be explained by the distribution of cellular retinoic acid binding proteins in epidermis [18], a concept which is supported by the observation that folding the dermal equivalent or adding a second dermal equivalent upside down on top of the first one when the culture is raised at the air-liquid interphase also results in both cases in the formation of a second differentiated epidermis upside down on top of the first one. As shown in Fig. 4 the morphogenesis of the top-down epidermis is completely normal as evidenced by the presence of granular and horny layers.

An interesting feature of the model is the fact that the fully formed epidermis results from the stratification and differentiation of a monolayer epithelium formed by undifferentiated epidermal keratinocytes. This raises the possibility to perform kinetic studies of epidermal morphogenesis. This is shown by means of immunofluorescence (see Fig. 5) and by means of western blots (see Fig. 6) for the appearance of the classical differentiation markers K1 and K10 keratins and the appearance and maturation of profilaggrin/filaggrin. Such possibility can also be exploited for the identification and classification of new differentiation markers (early vs late) by means of 2D gel electrophoresis (Pommes and Asselineau, unpublished results).

Reconstructed skin has been successfully used for many studies especially upon the effect of soluble factors that can be added to the tissue culture medium. For instance, the effect of retinoic acid, the acidic and active form of vitamin A or retinol, has been extensively investigated in this system [19] and more recently the effect of vitamin C [20]. This 3D system has the advantage to allow a very precise description of the effect of such compounds both on epidermis and dermis as well as the dermal-epidermal junction. Moreover, the possibility to use samples in which dermal fibroblasts have been eliminated allows studies of the relative roles of these two tissues.

In vitro studies of reconstructed skins are mostly concentrated on skin physiology and/or the differentiated state of the incorporated cells; for instance, it has been shown that fibroblasts in the dermal equivalent share common properties with fibroblasts in in vivo skin [21] and are also quiescent like in the in vivo normal steady-state situation [22]; however, the flexibility of the system is also of high interest for mechanical purposes. In addition to the mechanics of the dermal equivalent on which previous studies have been concentrated [23], considerations related to the type of epidermal morphogenesis which can be obtained by varying experimental conditions are also of interest and potentially useful in a mechanobiological context. For instance, when keratinocytes are seeded on the dermal equivalent, as previously shown the dermal equivalent is kept not only submerged but also attached to the bottom of the dish [24] to provide a firm substrate to keratinocytes in order to favor the formation of an epidermal sheet which at this stage (before being lifted on a grid at the air-liquid interphase) is a confluent monolayer, but interestingly if this dermal substrate is detached from the dish the epidermal sheet becomes stratified (but remains undifferentiated) whereas if the dermal equivalent is detached and raised at the air-liquid interphase the epidermal sheet formed as a monolayer in the submerged condition becomes stratified (and differentiated) as opposed to a condition in which the dermal equivalent is raised and attached to the grid which prevents partially stratification (without altering differentiation).

These observations (see Fig. 7) suggest that the quality of the dermal substrate (degree of stiffness) closely controls epidermal stratification (without influencing differentiation). As explained above

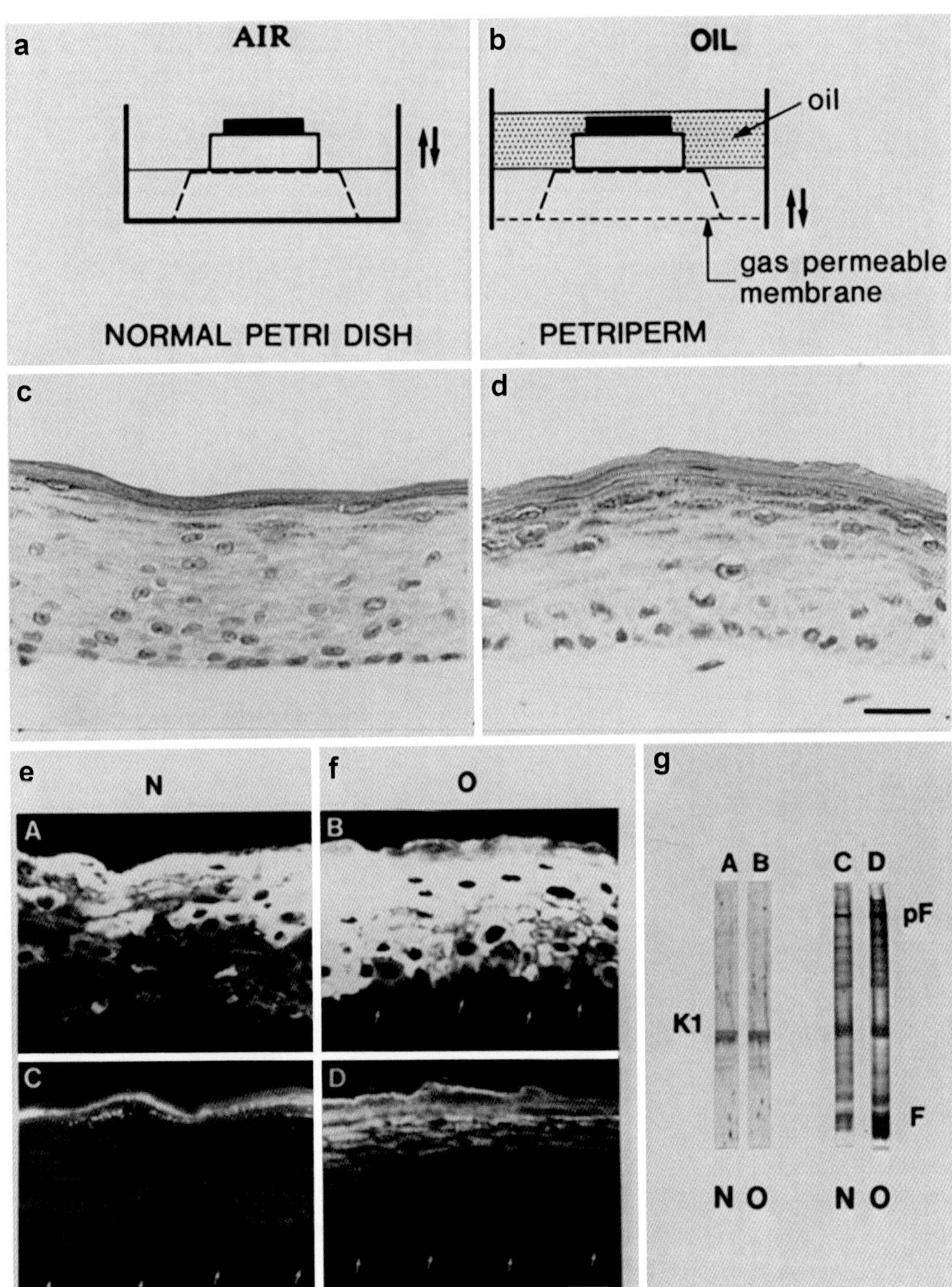

Fig. 2 Comparison of the results obtained when the epidermis formed by human keratinocytes on dermal equivalents was grown at the air-liquid interface (**a**, **c**, **e**) or at an oil-liquid interface (**b**, **d**, **f**). Schematic representation **a**, **b**., histology **c**, **d**. profilaggrin/filaggrin immunohistolabelling (**e**, **f**), and profilaggrin/filaggrin immunoblots (**g**). Note that normal epidermal stratification and complete differentiation occurs in both experimental situations

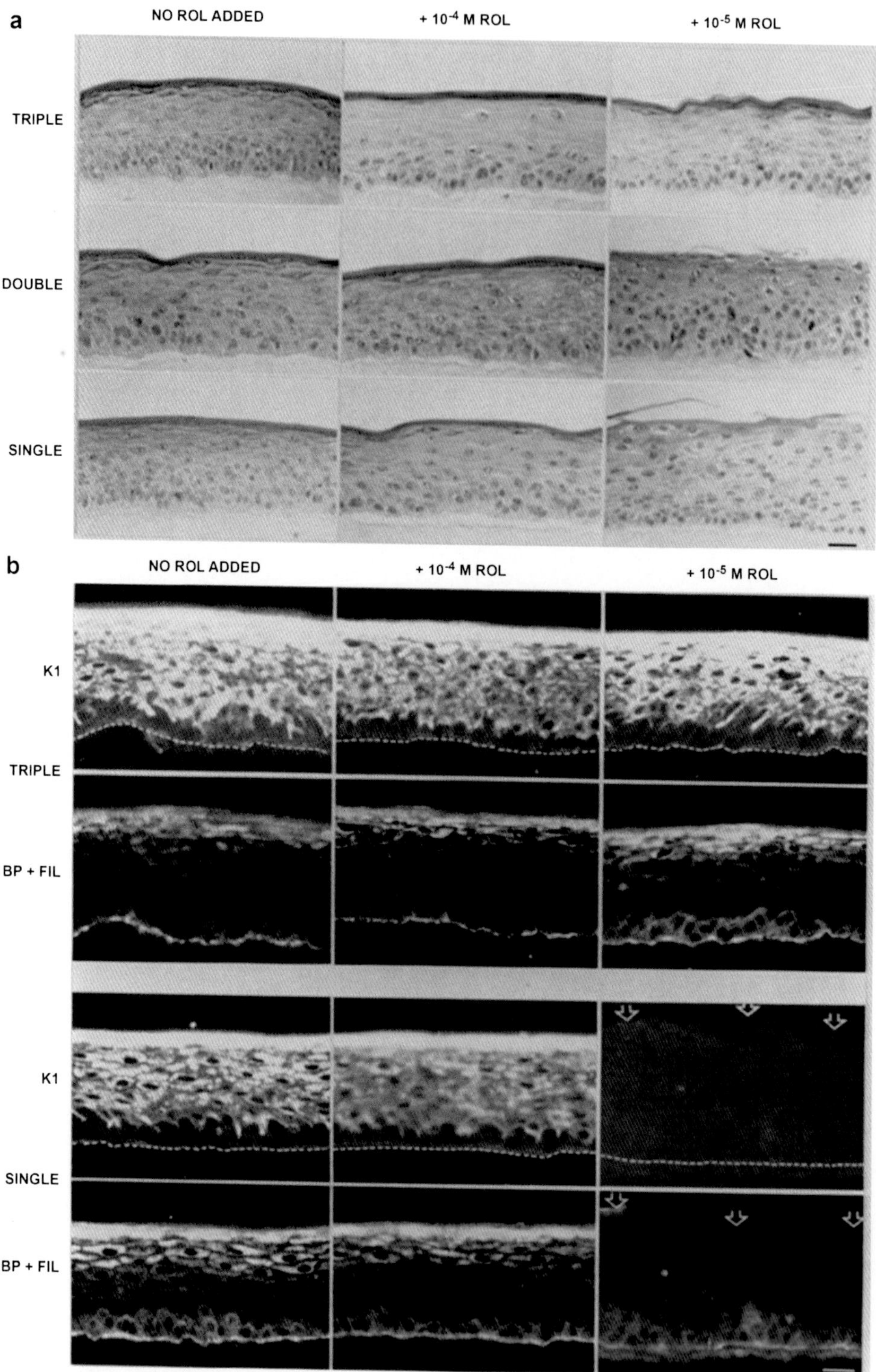

Fig. 3 Morphology (**a**) of the epidermis formed by human keratinocytes grown on dermal equivalents at the air-liquid interface in absence of retinol, or 10-6 M or 10-5 M retinol added when a single (standard) dermal equivalent was used as a substrate or two dermal equivalents piled up or three dermal equivalent piled up in order to increase the thickness of the dermal substrate. Note that the thicker the dermal substrate is the later the inhibitory effect of retinol

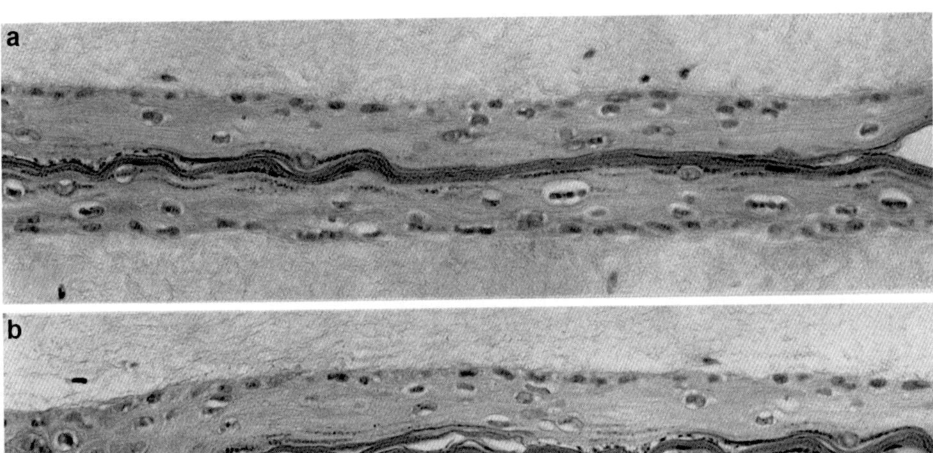

Fig. 4 Morphogy of the epidermis formed by human keratinocytes grown on dermal equivalents when two dermal equivalents were lifted together at the air-liquid interface the second one upside down on top of the first one (**a**) or when the dermal equivalent was folded at the time it was raised at the air-liquid interface (**b**). Note that a fully stratified and differentiated epidermis was formed on both dermal substrates (**a**) or on the total length of the dermal equivalent (**b**) resulting in epidermal mirror images (**a, b**)

epidermal differentiation is controlled by other factors; however, these observations seem of interest if related to skin aging during which a reduction of epidermal thickness is observed and consequently also of potential interest to develop new antiaging strategies.

Strategic Considerations for Skin Aging Studies Using Reconstructed Skin

As previously mentioned aging is a complex phenomenon. Regardless of much progress made in the field of reconstructed skin during the two or three previous decades, the development of models of skin aging by means of reconstructed skin remains a difficult challenge.

In fact there were two main ways to approach this question. First reconstructed skin can be made “as usual” and then submitted to a mechanism presumably leading to skin aging or involved in skin aging. The advantage of this strategy is to provide information about early events of aging. The disadvantage is that it is unlikely that aging has actually occurred because aging is a long-term phenomenon due to chronic exposure to adverse effects while in vitro cultures are strongly limited in time. We have, however, successfully followed this strategy in the context of UV light studies

Fig. 3 (continued) appears on epidermal differentiation as defined by the presence of granular and horny layers. Triple immunolabelling (**b**) of Bullous Pemphigoid antigen and filaggrin or K1 keratin detected in the epidermis formed by human keratinocytes grown on dermal equivalents at the air-liquid interface in absence of retinol, 10-6 M or 10-5 M retinol when a single (standard) dermal equivalent was used as a substrate or three dermal equivalents piled up to increase the thickness of the dermal substrate. Note that in the presence of the thickest dermal substrate the inhibitory effect of retinol is no longer observed as evidenced by the detection of both K1 keratin (early differentiation marker) and filaggrin (late differentiation marker)

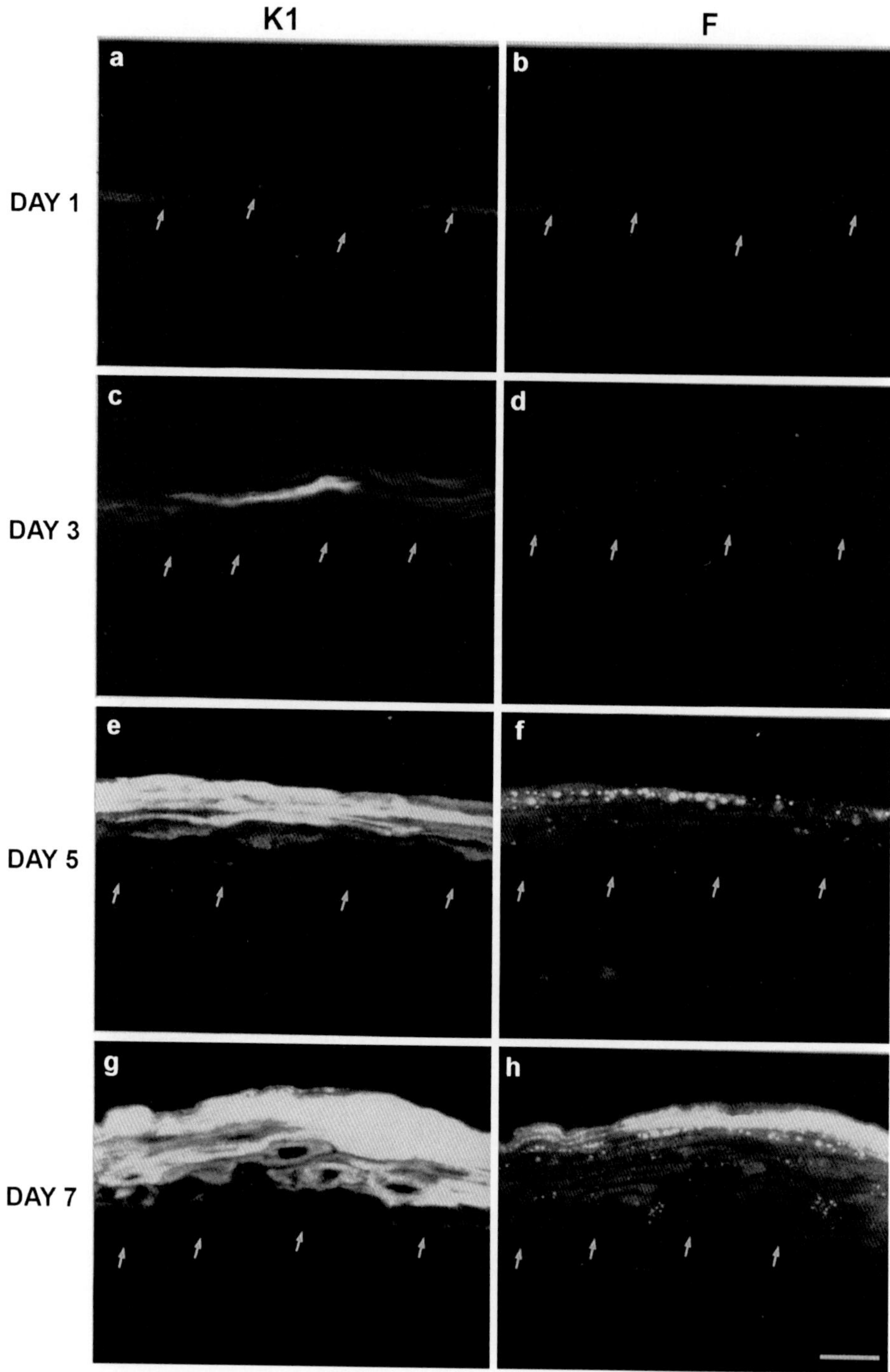

Fig. 5 Immunolabelling of K1 keratin (**a**, **c**, **e**, **g**) and profilaggrin/filaggrin (**b**, **d**, **f**, **h**) in the epidermis formed by human keratinocytes grown on dermal equivalents at the air_liquid interface after 1 day (**a**, **b**), 3 days (**c**, **d**), 5 days (**e**, **f**), and 7 days (**g**, **h**). Note the sequential sequence of appearance of K1 keratin at day 3, profilaggrin at day 5 and filaggrin at day 7

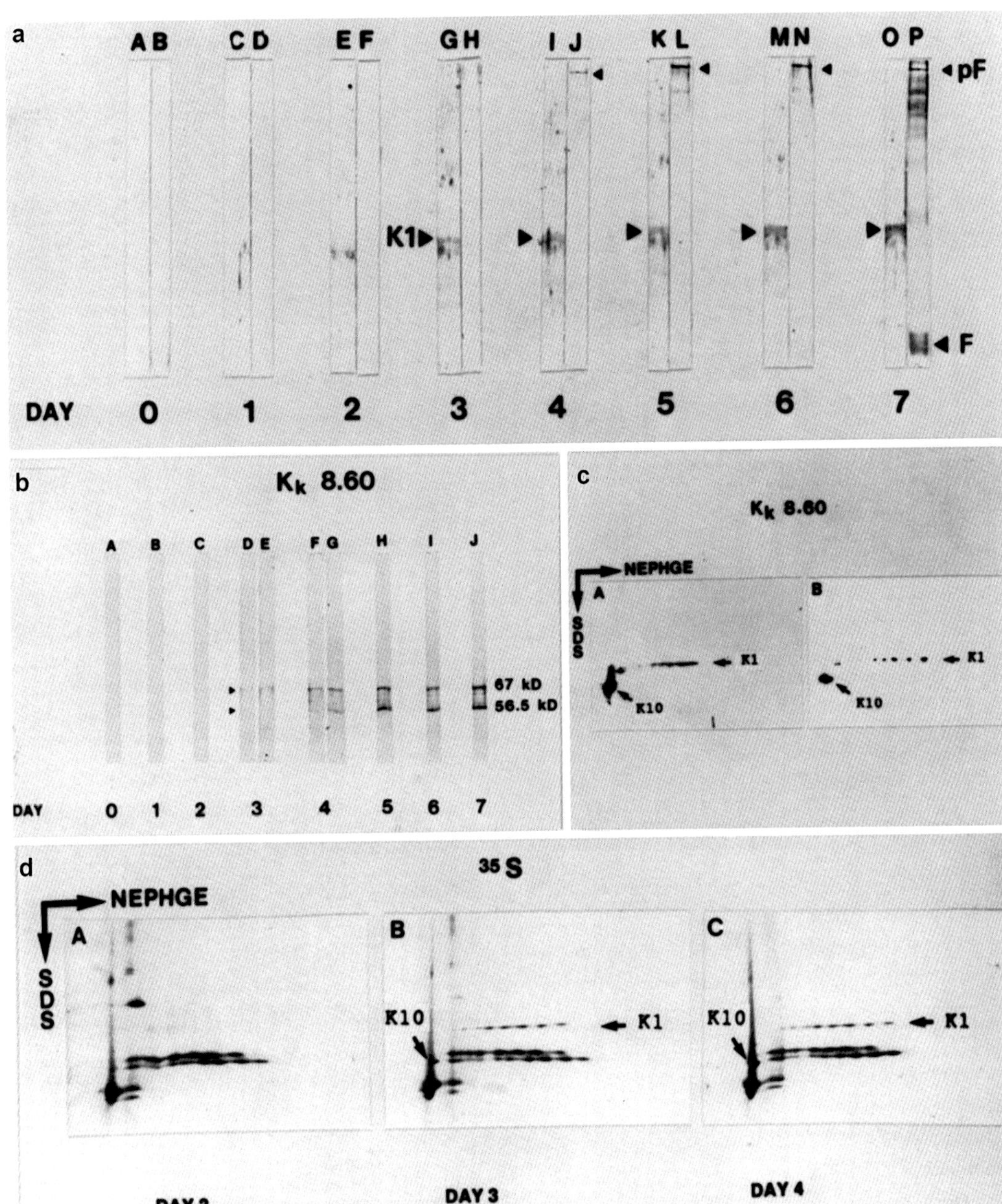

Fig. 6 Day by day up to 7 days immunodetection of both K1 keratin, profilaggrin/filaggrin (**a**), and both K1 (67 kD) and K 10 (56. 5 kD) keratins (**b**) in the epidermis formed by human keratinocytes grown on dermal equivalents at the air-liquid interface. Note the sequential appearance of coupled K1 and K10 keratins at day 3, profilaggrin at day 4 and filaggrin at day 7. 2D immunoelectrophoretic detection and characterization of K1 and K10 keratins (c) and 2D 35S labelling of these keratins at day 2, 3, 4 (d) confirming their coupled appearance at day 3

aimed at approaching photoaging. Secondly and alternatively it is also possible to reproduce a given mechanism responsible for chronological skin aging in order to mimic established aging in reconstructed skin. The advantage of this approach is that the effect of a given mechanism

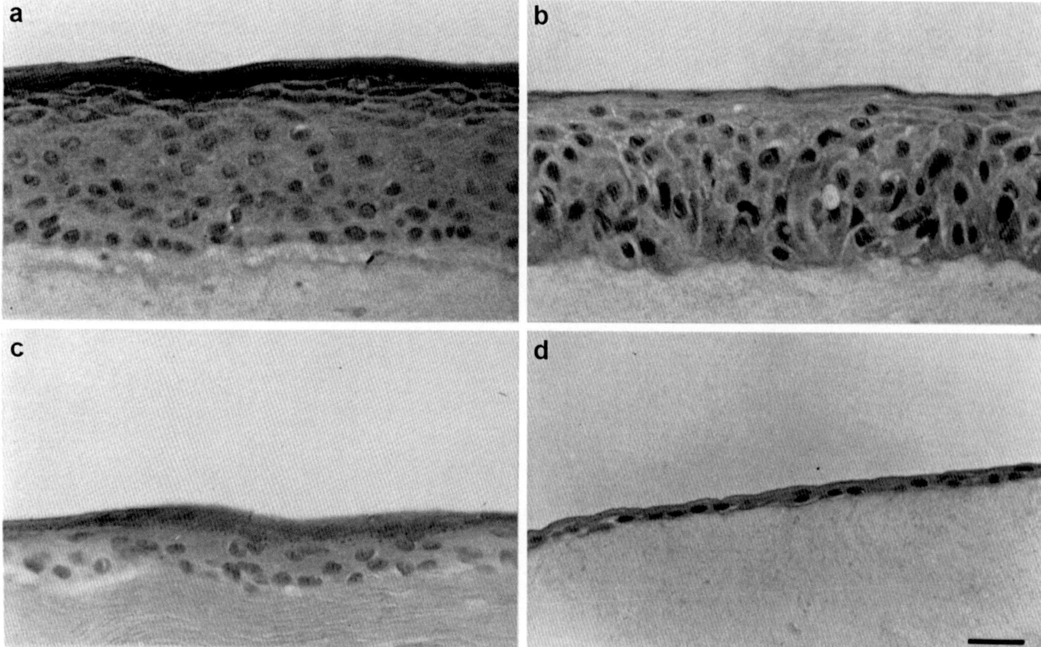

Fig. 7 Morphology the epidermis formed by human keratinocytes grown on a dermal equivalent at the air liquid interface (**a**, **c**) loose on the grid –our standard condition- (**a**) or attached (**c**) or kept submerged by the culyure medium (**b**, **d**) with the dermal equivalent attached to the dish –our standard condition- (**d**) or detached from the dish (**c**). Note that optimal differentiation and keratinization (granular and horny layers) was seen in (**a**) and (**c**) while optimal stratification was seen in (**a**) and (**b**)

of skin aging will be actually reproduced and its consequences evaluated in vitro while the disadvantage of this approach is that a single mechanism of aging will be used although aging is a complex multifactorial phenomenon. We have, however, also successfully followed this strategy in order to mimic chronological aging in vitro using the glycation reaction and, as mentioned later in this chapter, interesting results were obtained.

These two complementary strategies and their respective advantages are summarized in Table 2.

We will see, however, that there is a different way to look at aging which was recently developed in our laboratory. It consists of considering distinct cellular populations and their changes as a function of aging in vivo in order to reproduce these changes in the reconstructed skin system. Because the dermis is key in skin aging we have done this by studying fibroblast subpopulations and this will also be discussed later in this chapter.

Current Models of Skin Aging

UV Exposure as an Approach of Photo Aging

Photoaging is due to solar exposure. The effects of photoaging have been well described [25]. The UV domains seem to be the key domains of solar light involved in skin aging, especially UVB and UVA which correspond to the two wavelength domains reaching human beings on earth. It is also well known that UVB radiations are more energetic but less penetrating than UVA radiations. Therefore, it is likely that in real life UVB will affect preferentially the surface of skin including epidermis while UVA will affect skin in its depth.

Table 2 Strategies used in reconstruction of skin to create in vitro models of skin aging

	Method 1 Initiation	Method 2 Reproduction
Photoaging: UV exposure	Description of the effects of UV light on the reconstructed skin system at equilibrium (= epidermal differentition completed) - CHOSEN -	Collagen is pre exposed to UV radiations for the induction of dermal modifications potentially relevant to photoaging - NOT TESTED -
Chronological aging: glycation	Induction of glycation by culturing the dermal equivalent in the presence of sugar (in excess) - TESTED BUT NOT CHOSEN (toxic effects)	Collagen is pre-incubated with sugar (ribose or glucose) prior use for preparing reconstructed skin - TESTED AND CHOSEN -
Benefit obtained in the selected strategy	This strategy allows: A description of precocious effects of UV radiations but not established photoaging The complete reconstructed skin is UV exposed	This strategy allows: An approach of established chronological aging but only one mechanism is involved
Application for anti-aging studies	In vitro photoprotection studies: Solar filter studies by topical application on reconstructed skin	Anti-glycation molecules can be tested as an approach to select new anti-aging agents

To approach these questions we manufactured reconstructed skins and submitted them to either UVB or UVA single exposures for performing dose–response and kinetic experiments.

We found that UVB preferentially affects the epidermal compartment where it produces complex alterations involving both DNA lesions and modifications of the epidermal differentiation pathway [26]. The most obvious effect of UVB exposure was the production of histologically easily recognized apoptotic keratinocytes also called sunburn cells in the in vivo situation and constitute obvious markers of the effect of UVB in real life.

Similarly we found that UVA preferentially affects the dermal compartment by inducing apoptosis of the most superficial fibroblasts at doses at which keratinocytes seemed to be unaffected suggesting differential resistance of these two cell types to UVA radiations [27].

Interestingly our kinetic experiments showed that these effects were reversible since epidermal differentiation was rapidly normalized while the dermal compartment also recovered its fibroblast content after a few days. However, as opposed to the cellular recovery we noticed a slight irreversible reduction of the dermal thickness after UVA exposure due to collagen degradation by collagenase production. These observations provided the basis of the approach of the mechanisms of photoaging using the reconstructed skin system. As an example a very complete description of the effect of long wave UVA has been recently undertaken using the reconstructed skin approach [28].

These findings allowed to define markers of the specific effects of both UVB and UVA domains -schematically sunburn cells or fibroblast disappearance; they were historically very useful for the first in vitro studies of solar filters applied on the surface of reconstructed skins thus demonstrating the relevance of in vitro photoprotection studies [29]. For instance, the broad-spectrum protection (which means both UVB and UVA protection) provided by the mexoryl filter as opposed to the initially restricted identified protection in the UVA domain was demonstrated this way [30].

In conclusion it is important to emphasize that these in vitro data were at the origin of new and very accurate strategies for photoprotection strategies relevant in real life.

Glycation of the Collagen as an Approach of Chronological Aging

Glycation is a one enzymatically driven reaction between free amine groups like those of amino acids like lysine and arginine and circulating reducing sugars like glucose. This reaction also known as the Maillard reaction leads to so-called Advanced Glycation End products (AGEs) which are terminal products of the reaction eventually involved in the formation of cross-links between macromolecules.

This chemical reaction preferentially affects tissues characterized by poor renewal and is therefore thought to play an important role in aging [31]. In skin glycation is thought to affect dermal macromolecules especially those known for having a very slow turnover like collagen and elastin and hence the formation of cross-links may play a role in the alteration of mechanical properties of skin like stiffness appearing as a function of age (see a specific glycation review in ► Chap. 96, "Glycation and Skin Aging" in this book).

We have therefore investigated the effect of glycation in the reconstructed skin model.

Preglycation of collagen was used in order to avoid possible toxic effects on cultured skin cells due to prolonged exposure to high concentrations of sugar. The morphology of reconstructed skin was found to be altered [32]. In addition several skin markers of interest were found to be modified in a way recalling aging in vivo. For instance, we found that Matrix Metalloproteinase 1 (MMP1) as well as the distribution of specific integrins like β1 integrin were modified in epidermis in a way similar to aged skin in vivo [32]. At first sight it was surprising to find modifications in epidermis but we were able to show that diffusible factors were involved suggesting that dermal-epidermal interactions were modified when fibroblasts were in contact with glycated collagen. This also suggests that crosstalks between the two tissues can be affected during aging. We have previously described these results in detail [33].

Another way currently under investigation is to induce glycation by adding transiently the sugar to the culture medium. This approach may be useful for kinetic studies aiming at following the sequential appearance of the various glycation products and also to fabricate a more homogeneously glycated dermal equivalent.

Another aspect of this work is that by the use of reconstructed skin and specific preparations of glycated collagen in which one particular AGE is at least predominant, if not specifically cross-linked to the collagen, we were able to show that the different AGEs are not equal in terms of their biological effects [34]. Recent in vivo studies are also in favor of such findings [35]. Moreover, addition of specific AGEs in solution in the culture medium confirmed this important finding (Pageon and coll, this edition, in press).

In addition to the effects of glycation on biological markers, mechanical and optical measurements suggest that physical properties of the dermal equivalent are also modified by glycation in a way which can be related to skin aging (Pageon and coll. unpublished observations).

Our current findings are schematically summarized in Fig. 8. The main conclusions are that glycation of collagen (and the use of preglycated collagen) is sufficient to reproduce some manifestations of skin aging in the reconstructed skin approach. This shows that glycation is probably an important phenomenon involved in skin aging and that the modified reconstructed skin obtained by glycation does indeed represent a model of skin aging [36]. It is also of interest to note that this system would allow to investigate the antiglycation effect of various molecules or extracts suspected to potentially represent antiaging candidates [37].

Major Role of Papillary Fibroblasts in Skin Aging

The dermal part of skin is histologically heterogeneous. The superficial dermis or papillary dermis which is subjacent to epidermis is rather thin as opposed to the deep dermis or reticular dermis which constitutes the vast majority of this tissue. The reticular dermis is characterized by the accumulation of thick fibers which are thought to be responsible for the mechanical properties of the dermis. It is now known that the fibroblast populations of these two regions are different. However, during the two last decades only a small number of laboratories have investigated their respective properties including their growth potential [38]. Only during recent years numerous new findings have been published so that at present a number of important data exist [39]

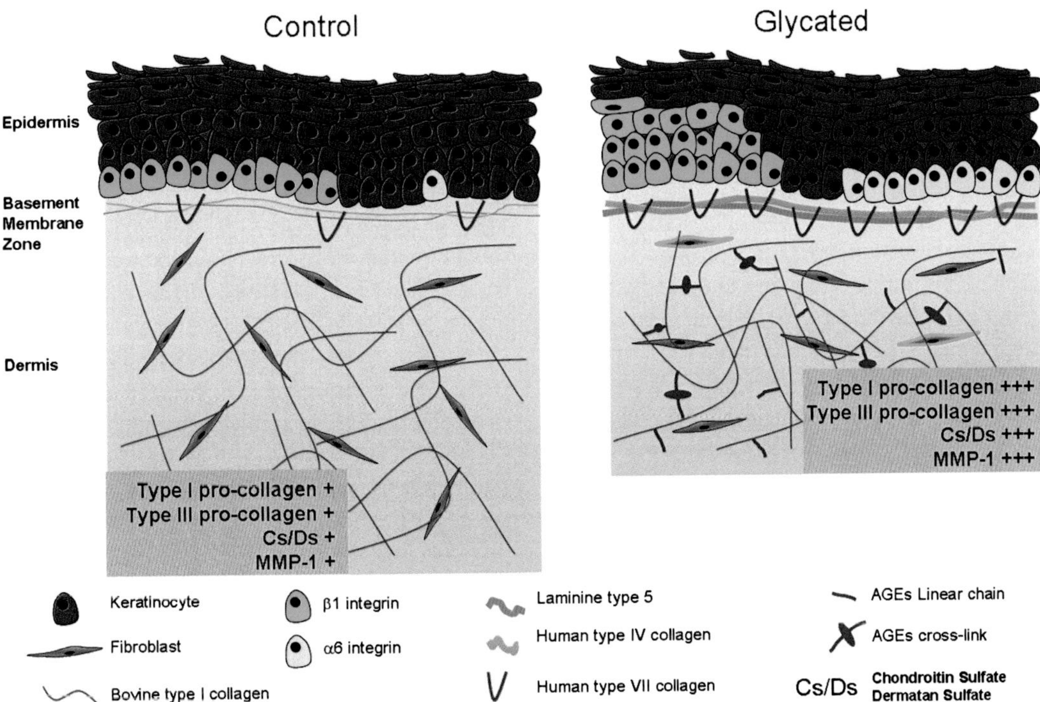

Fig. 8 Schematic representation of reconstructed skin produced either in absence of pre glycated collagen (*left*) or when preglycated collagen was used (*right*). Note that basement membrane components (in *brown* and *dark green*) are more abundant when pre glycated collagen was used together with other extracellular matrix molecules of the dermis (as mentioned). As indicated also note increased distribution of both β1 (in *green*) and α6 (in *yellow*) integrins in epidermis

although their role and fate during aging still remains to be elucidated. We have isolated and characterized these two populations and we investigated their properties and their behavior during aging. In a first attempt we investigated their potential role in the morphogenesis of reconstructed skins containing one population or the other in the dermal compartment. We noticed an important role of papillary fibroblasts in the cross talk with epidermis and a more pronounced role of reticular fibroblasts in the production of matrix elements [39]. Secondly we investigated the evolution of these populations as a function of aging. This was made possible by isolation of numerous site-matched pairs of papillary and reticular fibroblasts from donors of increasing age. Their growth characteristics, cytokine, and other diffusible factor production were studied by cell sorting and by performing cloning experiments. Reconstructed skins with dermal compartments containing one population or the other were compared by means of dermal contraction and the ability to contribute to skin reconstruction in terms of capacity to promote epidermal morphogenesis [40]. To summarize a large body of data we found that the reticular fibroblast population does not seem to be modified by aging as opposed to the papillary fibroblast population. The latter seems to disappear during aging under conditions that still remain to be fully elucidated yet which, in addition to possible modifications of the population itself, comprise various other possibilities such as apoptosis of papillary fibroblast or replacement of papillary fibroblasts by upward migration of reticular fibroblasts or differentiation of papillary fibroblasts into reticular fibroblasts during aging.

Our findings were recently published in detail and schematically represented in detail [41]. In this context it is important to note that as opposed to the work of Janson et al. suggesting differentiation of papillary fibroblasts [42] recent work of the group of Watt [43] suggests that superficial fibroblasts and fibroblasts from the deepest layers of skin derive from two separate lines during development which suggests that differentiation of papillary fibroblasts into reticular fibroblasts seems unlikely. Detailed transcriptomic studies performed in our laboratory aim at better understanding the nature and fate of the two fibroblast populations during aging and to investigate these opposite possibilities (Haydont et al. in preparation).

In terms of fibroblast populations a simplified way to take into account our conclusions would be to consider that a model of reconstructed skin with a dermal compartment containing only reticular fibroblasts is a reasonable approach of a reconstructed skin model of aged skin (see Fig. 9).

Flexibility of the Reconstructed Skin Model

Flexibility is a very attractive property of our reconstructed skin model. For instance, we know how to vary its shape [32] and dermal thickness [32], how to make several – at least two – dermal compartments, and to manipulate the cell population content of this or these dermal compartment (s) including destruction of the fibroblast population by osmotic shock to provide a negative control if necessary [13].

Being able to make different dermal compartments is of potential interest for the incorporation of different fibroblast populations in different layers. This also opens the possibility to create different adjacent dermal compartments underlying the epidermis to investigate the consequences of dermal regional differences on epidermis. In the long run, this may open the way to create a model for wrinkled skin in vitro (see Fig. 10).

Collagen glycation has already been mentioned as an example of the possibility to modify the extracellular matrix. The use of different fibroblast populations is an additional illustration of the possibility to change the content of reconstructed skin at the cellular level especially if combined with the possibility to create several dermal or regional dermal compartments. Such flexibility is critical in our hands to create new in vitro aging models.

In view of the growing interest in aesthetic methods in dermatology like the injection of collagen or hyaluronic acid, we became interested in this issue and wondered about the possibility to set up a 3D model. To approach this goal we have created a new model of reconstructed skin which contains a dermal inclusion of hyaluronic acid (HA) thus mimicking the injection performed in vivo (see Fig. 11). Examining the properties of our model we have evidenced the stimulation of the biological activity of the fibroblasts close to the inclusion such as collagen I and III and MMP1 production [44]. We have shown that this was due to both direct effects via the HA CD44 receptor and indirect effects (fibroblast stretching).

RealSkin: A Successful Standardization of Full Thickness Reconstructed Skin

In addition it is also possible to standardize the fabrication of the reconstructed skin system to adapt it to production. This was achieved in our laboratory by casting the fibroblast contracted collagen gel or dermal equivalent directly into inserts placed in multiwell plates (see Fig. 12). This system which is a full thickness reconstructed skin system was recently named RealSkin and is very close to the "historical" reconstructed skin system produced classically in individual Petri dishes with the help of stainless steel rings (epidermal cell seeding) and stainless steel grids (air-liquid interphase), albeit that using this system, tension is generated in the dermis. However, the tension is accompanied by the presence of more abundant Extra Cellular Matrix (ECM) macromolecules (Fig. 13).

All these different types of construction are obtained with dermal equivalents obtained by contraction. Recently we have started using a new approach to make dermal equivalent by compression instead of contraction as proposed by

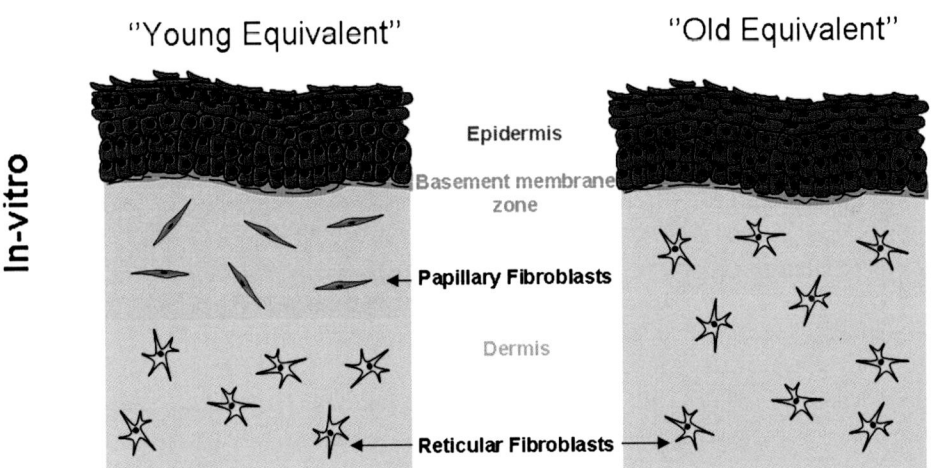

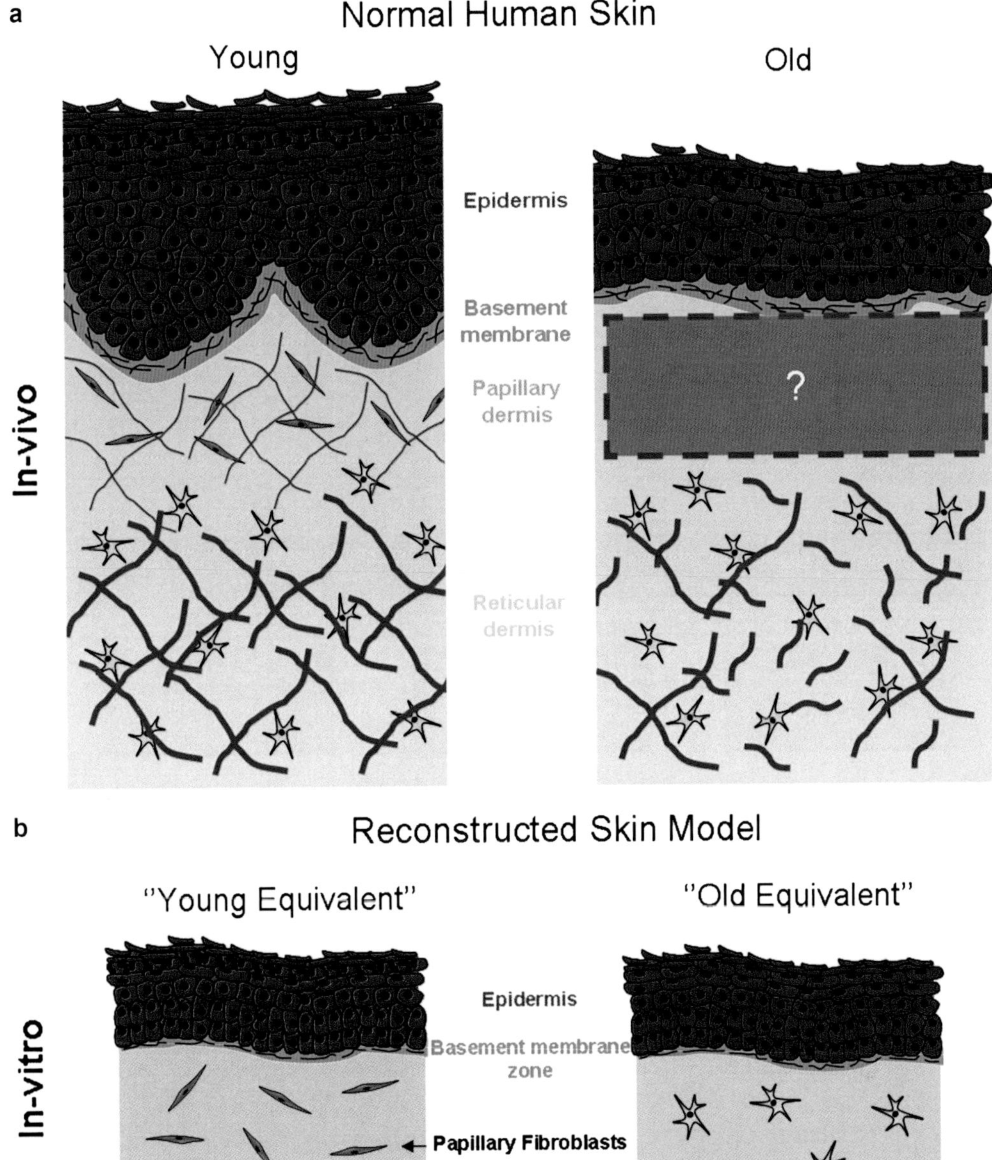

Fig. 9 Schematic representation of both young human skin (*top left*) and old human skin (*top right*) emphasizing the so far not completely elucidated modification occurring in the papillary dermis and corresponding schematic representation of both young-like skin equivalent (*down left*) or old-like skin equivalent (*down right*). These schematic representations were made to emphasize the idea that a reconstructed skin lacking the papillary dermal component is an easy first approximation of old skin

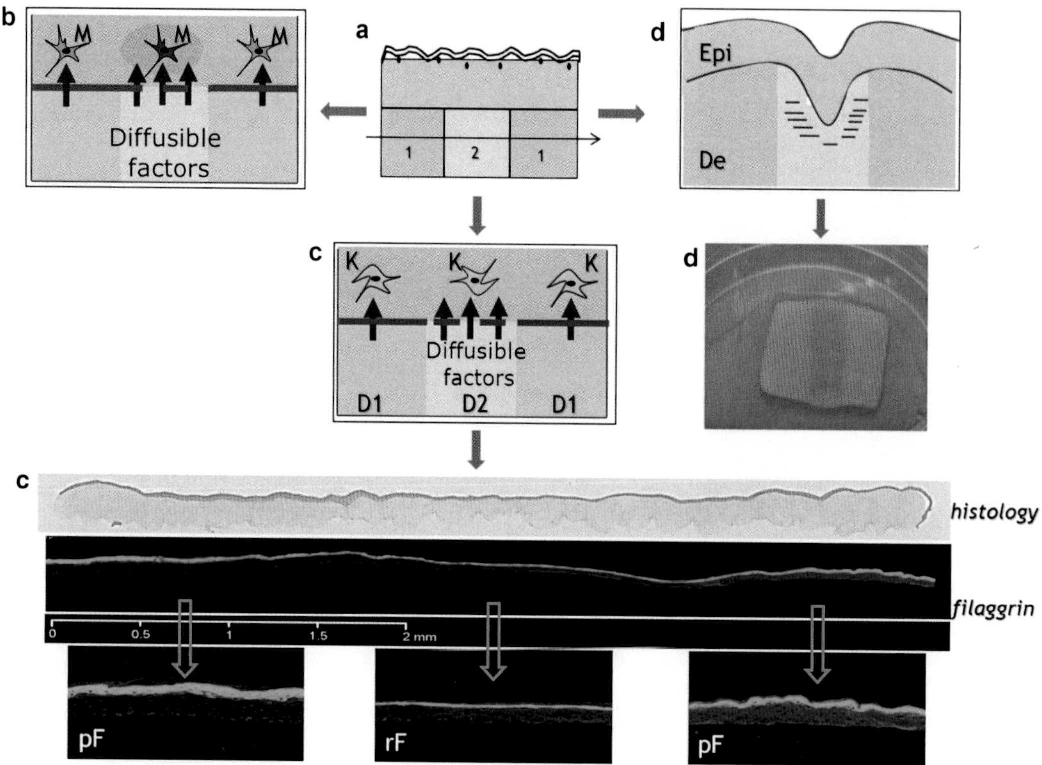

Fig. 10 Schematic representation (**a**) of the construction of different regions in the dermal equivalent in order to manipulate the dermal-epidermal zone aiming at obtaining different epidermal regions in terms of pigmentation: schematic representation (**b**), or in terms of keratinization: schematic representation, histology and filaggrin staining (**c**) of a representative example obtained by manipulating the fibroblast content as indicated: papillary (*pF*) – reticular (*rF*) – papillary (*pF*), or in terms of relief: schematic representation and corresponding example (**d**)

Brown and colleagues to provide a new way in tissue engineering [45]. In our hands this was obtained by loading the collagen gel with a defined weight placed on top of it. No obvious differences were noted in the dermal equivalents made that way by comparison with those made by contraction (see Fig. 13). This allows a faster preparation of the reconstructed skin, and opens new possibilities to obtain more than two compartments by making sequentially several dermal compartments containing different populations of cells (Fig. 14). For instance, this will be very useful in the future to prepare full thickness skin constructs with hypodermis included in addition to the compartments with papillary and reticular fibroblasts. It is worth mentioning that so far attempts at making reconstructed skin containing adipocytes are limited to a single compartment containing those cells [46]. The compression method also opens new possibilities to create a relief at the dermal-epidermal junction thus mimicking rete ridges or representing a new way to create wrinkle-like structures.

Future Models of Reconstructed Skin with Special Emphasis on Skin Aging

It is important to recall that adult human skin cells cultured in vitro completely keep their potential since skin constructs made with these cells after grafting onto the nude mouse can form a fully differentiated epidermis [47] as well as a dermis progressively resembling actual dermis in vivo through a vascularization process [48].

Modifications of classically reconstructed skin comprise the incorporation of new cell types generally present in epidermis such as melanocytes in

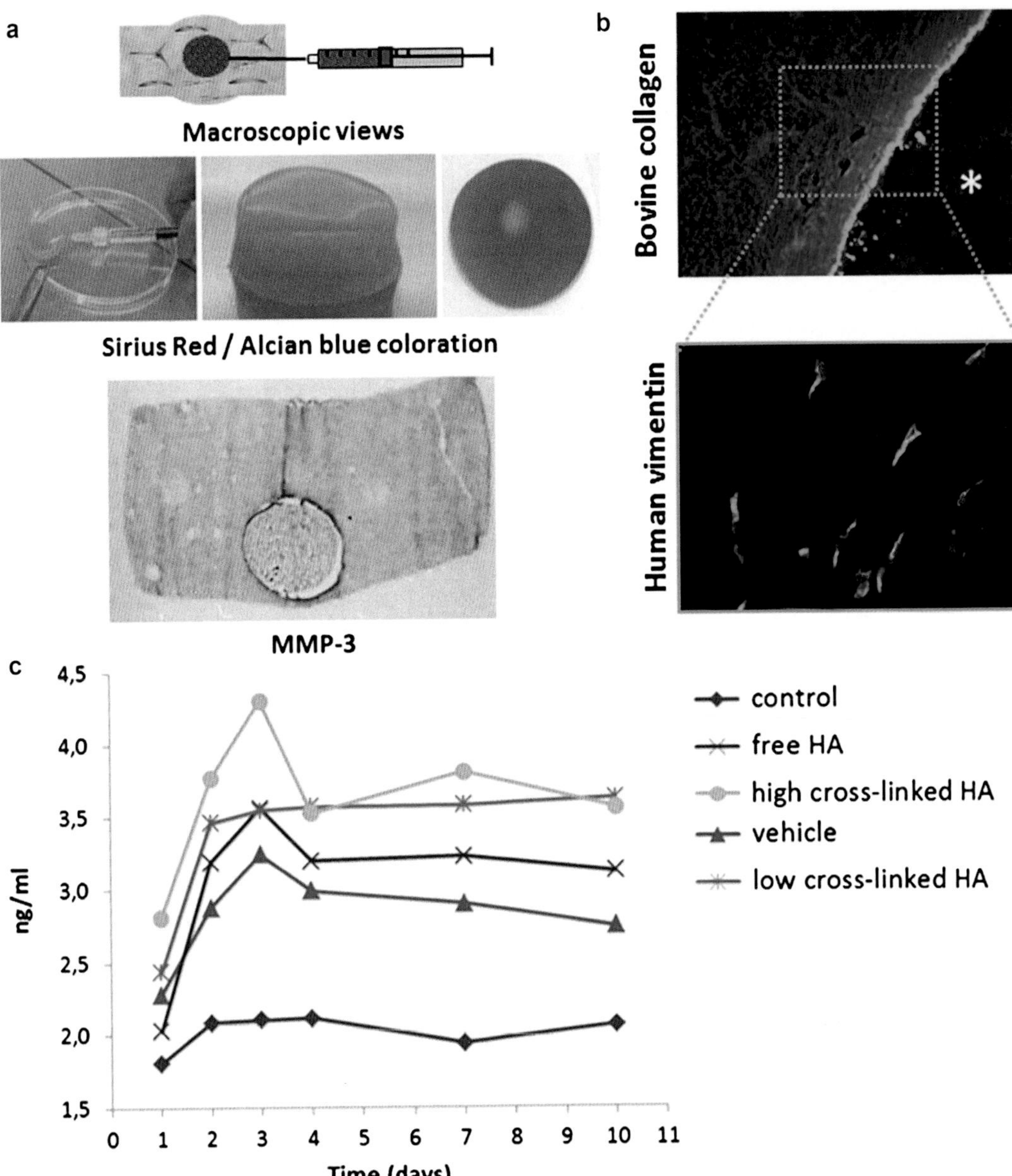

Fig. 11 Injection of products in an in vitro thick dermal equivalent (**a**). The product (50 μl) was injected in the middle of the dermal equivalent and can be visualized as a transparent zone on a macroscopic view. A combined staining of cryosections was performed namely Sirius red for the collagen fibers of the dermal equivalent and Alcian blue for the exogenous cross-linked HA based filler injected. Injection of the cross-linked HA dermal filler appeared to induce morphological and cytosqueletton related changes in the fibroblasts of the local surrounding environment (**b**). Immunostaining of the bovine collagen used to prepare the dermal equivalents shows a compaction of the fibers around the injection of the dermal filler (*) while detection of vimentin showed that the human fibroblasts incorporated adopted preferentially a spindle shape form. Nuclei were counterstained with propidium iodure. Increased expression of metalloproteinase 3 (MMP-3) in the presence of injected cross-linked HA dermal filler (**c**). Effects of both highly cross-linked HA and mildly cross-linked HA on MMP-3 secretion in the culture medium of the dermal equivalent were compared to vehicle, free HA and control (no injection) during 10 days. The maximum effects were observed at day 2–3 in the presence of the highly cross-linked HA. Means are reported for each time points

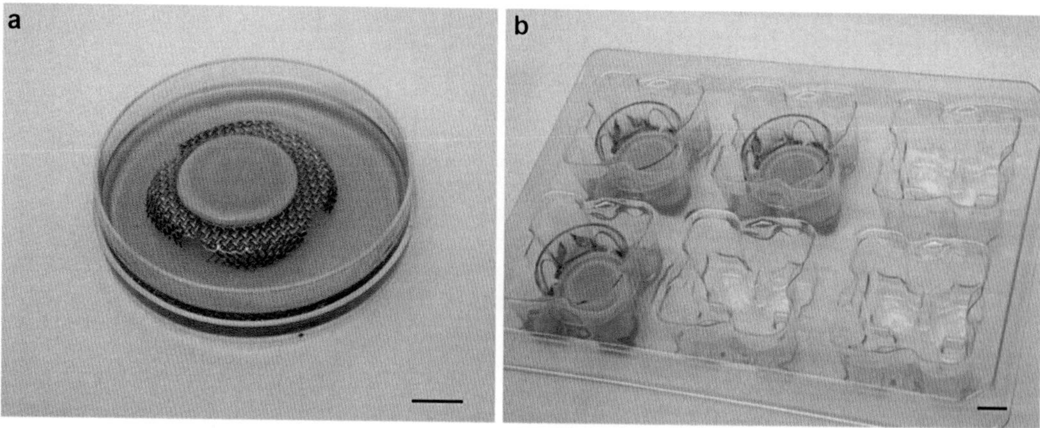

Fig. 12 Macroscopic view of classical reconstructed skin (**a**) made in individual petri dishes and reconstructed skins made in multiwell plates (**b**). Bar, 1 cm

order to achieve pigmentation in the reconstructed skin. Our point of view is that it would also be of high interest especially in the context of creating new models of skin aging to add new dermal cells, especially endothelial cells, as already done by others [49] in order to create blood vessel structures. This possibility is of particular interest because of the fact that endothelial cells seem to interact preferentially with papillary fibroblasts [50]. Moreover we have shown that dermal papillae or rete ridges which probably result from skin vasculature form preferentially in the presence of papillary fibroblasts after grafting onto the nude mouse [51]. We have shown it was possible to make dermal constructs containing both papillary fibroblasts and reticular fibroblasts. By making serially two gels containing first reticular fibroblasts and then papillary fibroblasts it is quite possible to lay down endothelial cells on top of the first gel before casting the second gel.

Another expected modification of reconstructed skin of interest would be to introduce changes in the content of extracellular matrix molecules in dermal equivalents. Little has been done in that area with the exception of combining collagen with glycosaminoglycans [52]. It would be of interest of course to introduce molecules other than collagen in dermal equivalent like elastin; for instance, it would also be of high interest to introduce various types of collagens specific from the different regions of the dermis like adding collagen III to better reproduce the papillary dermis. Other strategies in that area would also consist of replacing collagen classically provided by animal species like bovine collagen by human collagen [53] or by replacing the collagen classically provided in individual molecules in solution by preparations in which the organization of collagen in fibers is better preserved in order to be closer to the actual structure and organization of collagen in skin (Pageon, unpublished observations).

In the context of creating new models of reconstructed skin for skin aging studies it would be quite interesting to investigate human genetic diseases by creating in vitro models of these diseases through incorporation of skin cells isolated and amplified from small biopsies provided by patients. For instance, we have successfully reproduced the Xeroderma pigmentosum (XP) phenotype by showing lack of repair of DNA lesions in XP reconstructed skin after UV exposure [54] in a way strikingly recalling the in vivo situation. Similarly in the future it would be of high interest to create new in vitro models of accelerated aging by incorporating human skin cells corresponding to other genetic diseases like Progeria or the Werner syndrome. Reconstructed skins with a dermal compartment containing Werner fibroblasts are currently being made in our laboratory. Another exciting way to obtain accelerated aging would be to approach situations in which accelerated aging is induced by the environnement.

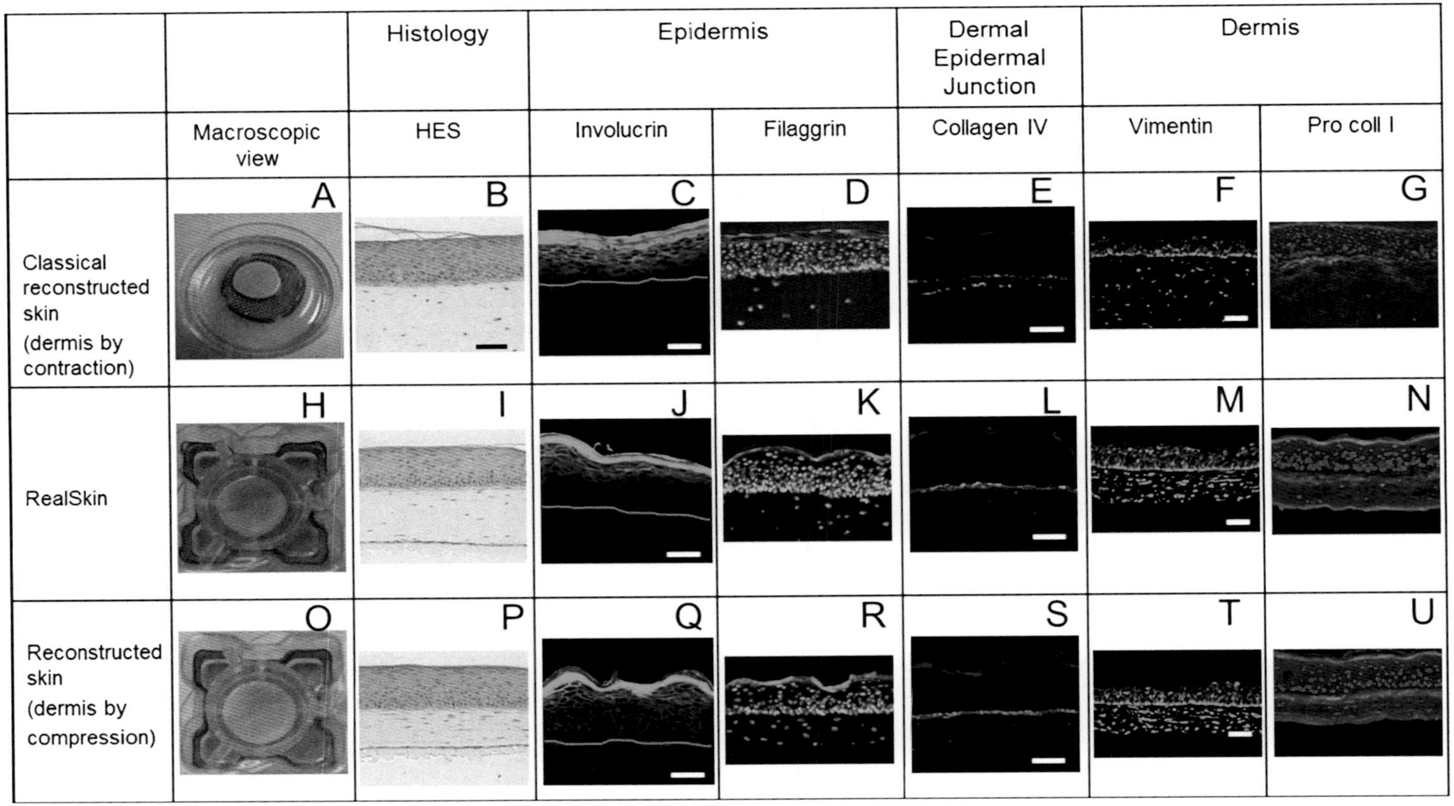

		Histology	Epidermis		Dermal Epidermal Junction	Dermis	
	Macroscopic view	HES	Involucrin	Filaggrin	Collagen IV	Vimentin	Pro coll I
Classical reconstructed skin (dermis by contraction)	A	B	C	D	E	F	G
RealSkin	H	I	J	K	L	M	N
Reconstructed skin (dermis by compression)	O	P	Q	R	S	T	U

Fig. 13 Classical reconstructed skin (**a**–**g**) and reconstructed skin produced in multiwell plates with dermal equivalent obtained by contraction (**h**–**n**) or by compression (**o**–**u**). Macroscopic view (**a**,**h**,**o**) Histology (**b**, **i**, **p**), Involucrin (**c**, **j**, **q**), Filaggrin (**d**, **k**, **r**), Collagen IV (**e**, **l**, **s**), Vimentin (**f**, **m**, **t**), Procollagen I (**g**, **n**, **u**) immunostainings. Note increased presence of extracellular matrix material in reconstructed skin produced in multiwell plates as compared to classical reconstructed skin. Also note that vimentin labeling which shows orientation of fibroblasts in the dermal equivalent shows no tension in the dermis of classical reconstructed skin (random orientation) as opposed to tension visible in reconstructed skin produced in multiwell plates (horizontal orientation). Bar, 25 μm

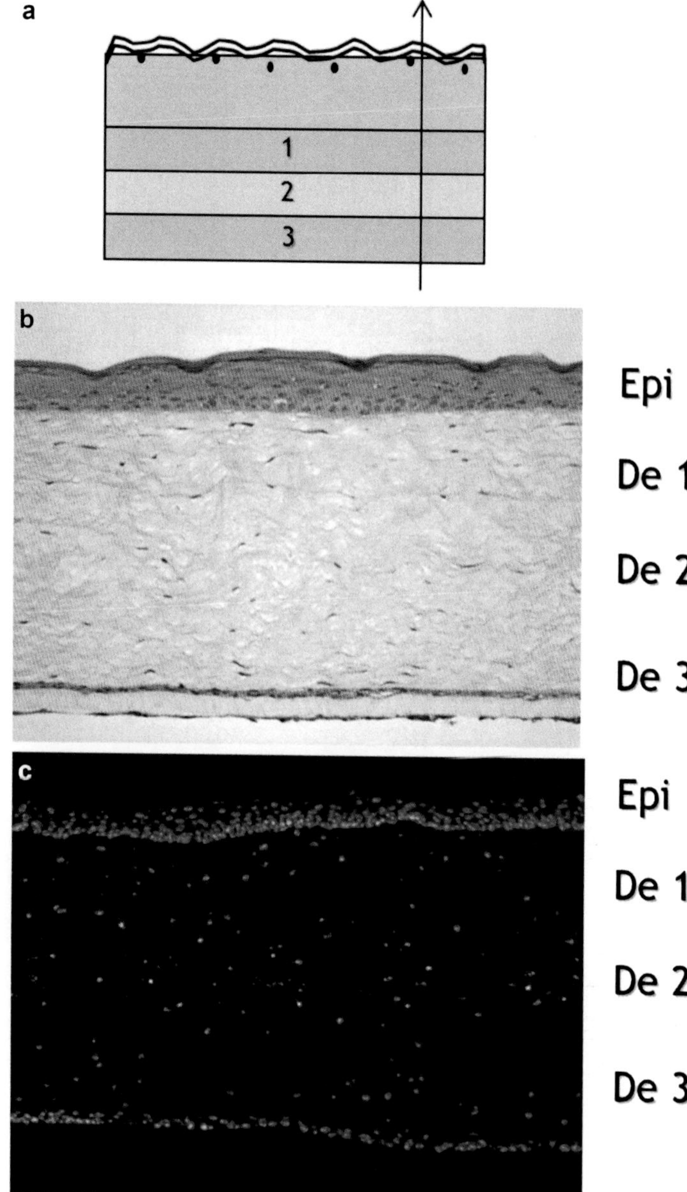

Fig. 14 Schematic representation (**a**) of the construction of up to three dermal compartments corresponding to different dermal layers obtained by successive compressions of three different collagen gels casted sequentially containing independant fibroblast populations. Histology (**b**), nuclei labellings (**c**). Note that this new procedure allows the formation of a much thicker dermal compartment (as compared with our standard conditions) and that the different fibroblast populations stay in their layers evidenced by the nuclei labellings (**c**)

For instance this situation can result from the absence of gravity undergone by humans in space. Experimentally it is possible to explore it by submitting cultured cells to simulated microgravity in random positioning machines.

An interesting point refers to different function of skin depending on the anatomic site. For instance, in the epidermis of distinct regions of the body specific keratins are expressed which are not seen elsewhere. It is well known that palm of foot sole epidermis contains keratin 9. There are certainly many regional differences which remain to be discovered but could become the subject of specific models based on skin of different body regions, in order to investigate whether they age the same way. Obviously those skin models would be relevant especially in the context of cosmetic purposes.

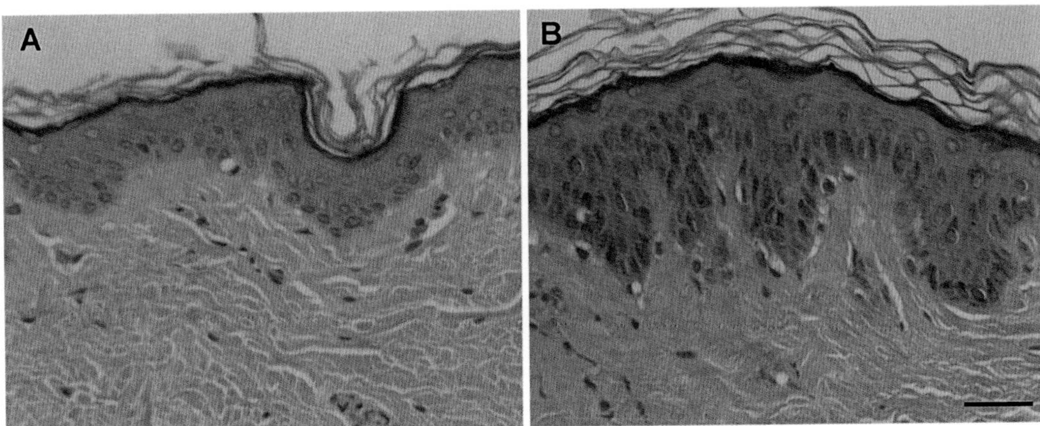

Fig. 15 Histology of respectively Caucasian human skin (**a**) and African human skin (**b**). Note pronounced dermal-epidermal invaginations in African skin. Bar, 25 μm

Another striking observation is that skin is obviously different as a function of ethnic origin. Beyond obvious differences related to pigmentation we have recently shown that the Caucasian skin type versus the African skin type differ morphologically in their depth since the dermal-epidermal junction is more invaginated in African skin relative to Caucasian skin (see Fig. 15). Moreover the production of certain factors like MCP1 and KGF from papillary fibroblasts is different between the two types of skin [55] suggesting that not only epidermis but also dermis could be different. Such results raise the question of whether the two types of skin age the same way and how since it was suggested that aging affects preferentially the dermal component of Caucasian skin. To address this question we have undertaken making reconstructed skins containing either Caucasian or African skin types keratinocytes and fibroblasts in order to look for differences. Beyond our preliminary results [56], this strategy appears extremely promising (Girardeau-Hubert et al. in preparation). This is therefore a very interesting first step prior to comparative aging studies which means making reconstructed skins both age and ethnic origin dependent.

Skin aging is not only the result of chronologically related intrinsic factors like in all other organs of the body but it has the property to be submitted to external influences especially sun exposure leading to photoaging. Therefore it was of interest to combine these two types of aging in our system in order to create a more realistic model of skin aging. For instance, we have made glycated reconstructed skins exposed to UVA and observed some manifestations of the elastosis phenomenon which could not be observed previously either in unglycated reconstructed skins exposed to UVA or glycated but UVA-unexposed skins (Pageon et al. in preparation).

Finally there are many other possibilities which are not mentioned in this review. We have seen in this updated review that in the near future not only classical antiaging studies involving topical application of formulations will be developed but also so-called aesthetic approaches of antiaging will expand.

Using reconstructed skin it seems possible in the future to evaluate in vitro the effect produced by dermal fillers in order to determine their specific effects (beneficial versus adverse) as a function of the type of filler used and the way it is distributed.

Toward More Complex and "Ideal" Models of Reconstructed Skin

It therefore goes without saying that in the future even more complex reconstructed skin systems will be manufactured by varying simultaneously several parameters. For instance, thanks to the

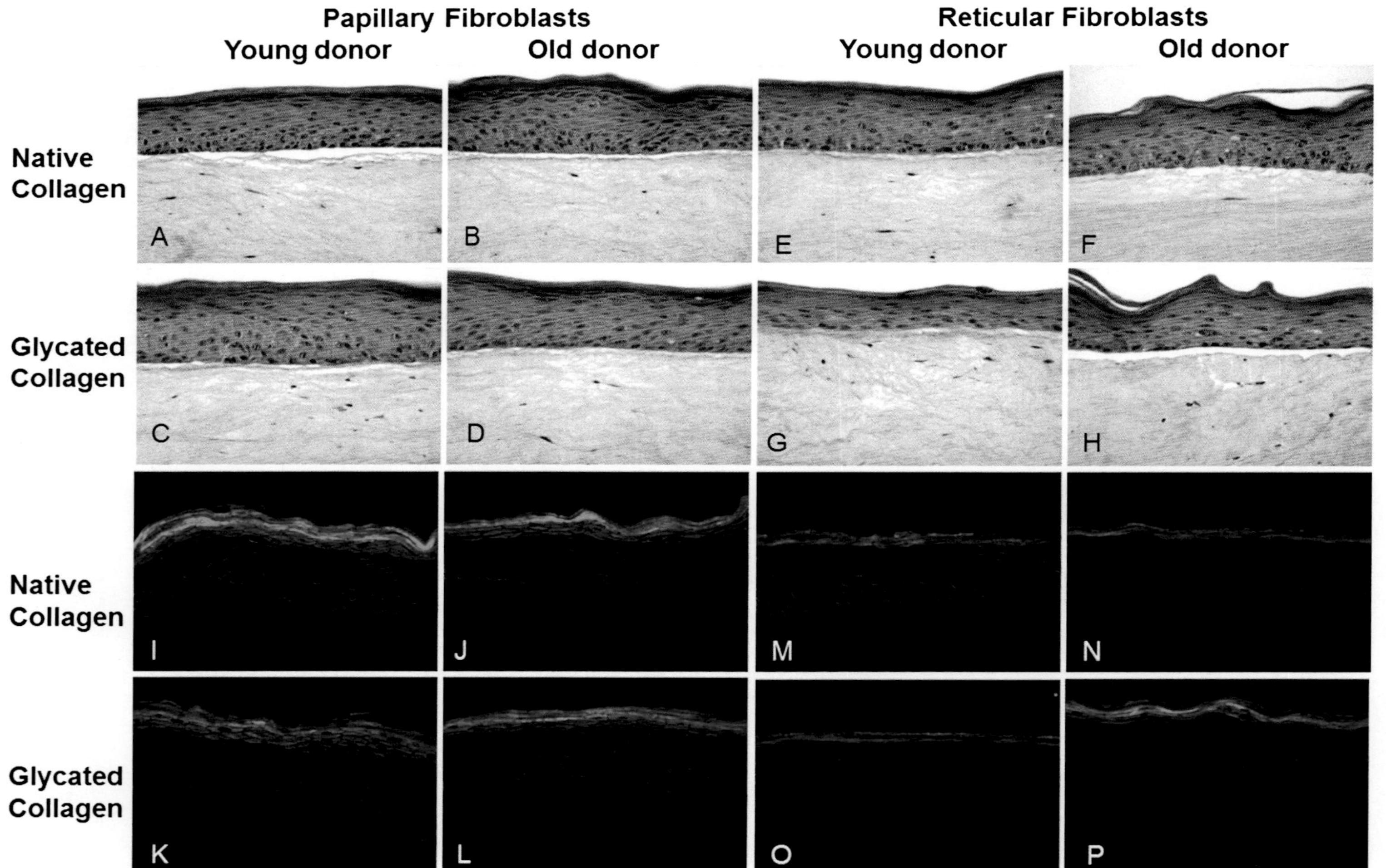

Fig. 16 (continued)

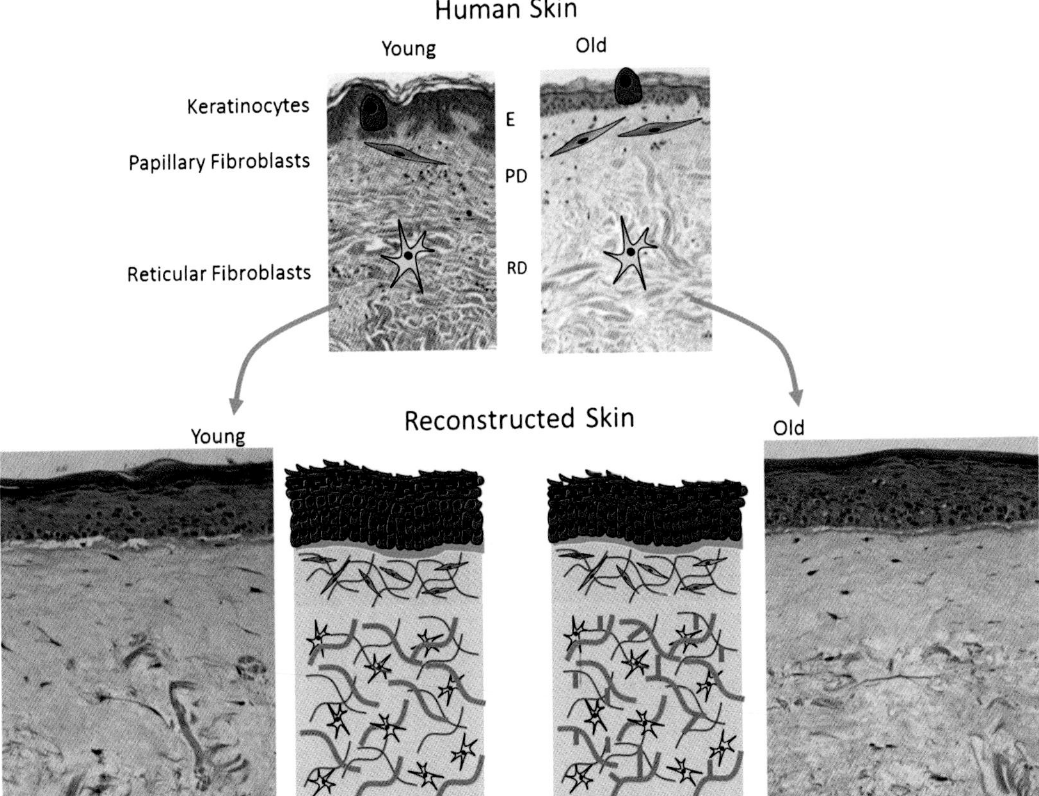

Fig. 17 Histology of both young and old skin is shown for comparison with schematic representation and histology of both young and old reconstructed skin models from our laboratory. These models are the closest to skin in vivo that can be obtained so far. They comprise the use of cells isolated from young or old donors and the fabrication of both papillary and reticular dermal compartments containing respectively papillary and reticular fibroblasts in the presence of a preglycated collagen characterized by thick fibers for the reticular dermis of the "old" equivalent while normal unglycated thick fibered collagen would be used for the papillary dermal compartment of the "young" equivalent. Note that, by means of histology, the two different dermal compartments mimicking both papillary and reticular dermis can be evidenced in the reconstructed skins

Fig. 16 Morphology of the epidermis formed on dermal equivalents raised at the air-liquid interface when not glycated (**a**, **b**, **e**, **f**) or glycated collagen (**c**, **d**, **g**, **h**),, papillary (**a**, **b**, **c**, **d**) or reticular fibroblasts (**e**, **f**, **g**, **h**), fibroblasts from young (**a**, **c**, **e**, **g**) or old donors (**b**, **d**, **f**, **h**) were used. Note that epidermal differentiation was optimal when papillary fibroblasts were used (**a**–**d**) as compared to reticular fibroblasts where it was slightly delayed (**e**–**h**) regardless of the glycation status. Also note that when reticular fibroblasts were used epidermal differentiation was better in the presence of native collagen (**e**, **f**) as compared to glycated collagen when reticular fibroblasts were isolated from young donors (**g**) while no effect of glycation on differentiation could be detected when reticular fibroblasts were isolated from old donors (**h**). Immunostaining of filaggrin in epidermis formed on dermal equivalents raised at the air-liquid interface when not glycated (**i**, **j**, **m**, **n**) or glycated collagen (**k**, **l**, **o**, **p**),, papillary (**i**, **j**, **k**, **l**) or reticular fibroblasts (**m**, **n**, **o**, **p**), fibroblasts from young (**i**, **k**, **m**, **o**) or old donors (**j**, **l**, **n**, **p**) were used. Note that filaggrin staining was optimal when papillary (**i**, **j**, **k**, **l**) as compared to reticular fibroblasts where it was weaker (**m**, **n**, **o**, **p**) regardless of the glycation status. Also note that when reticular fibroblasts were used filaggrin staining was more pronounced in the presence of native collagen (**m**, **n**) as compared to glycated collagen when reticular fibroblasts were isolated from young donors (**o**) while no effect of glycation on filaggrin staining could be detected when reticular fibroblasts were isolated from old donors (**p**)

knowledge and fibroblast collection of our laboratory parameters like the type of fibroblasts (papillary versus reticular), the age of the donors (young versus old), and the glycation status of the collagen used (preglycated versus normal) can be appropriately varied.

A good example of this is a combination of the age of the donor (young vs. old) with the presence or absence of glycation and the type of fibroblast (papillary vs. reticular) incorporated in the dermal compartments. Our results (see Fig. 16) show the sensitivity of young papillary fibroblasts to the glycation of the matrix. This type of experiment and model suggests the possibility to manipulate the phenotype of the fibroblast by modification of the quality of the matrix which represents an interesting direction for the future for attempting rejuvenation of the dermal fibroblast population through matrix manipulation.

Conclusion

It is possible to move toward improved aged skin models made in vitro closer to the in vivo situation. For instance, such constructs would comprise in the case of "young" (normal) skin a thick reticular-like dermis containing reticular fibroblasts and made with a thick fibered collagen and a thin papillary dermis containing papillary fibroblasts and made with classical collagen on which keratinocytes would be grown while the corresponding "old" skin would be made the same way except that the thick collagen of the reticular dermal compartment would be glycated and that the papillary dermal compartment would be almost absent. This is schematically represented in Fig. 17 and an example of reconstructed skins made that way is shown. The range of possibilities to improve such models looks important and very promising for the future. The long-run future will also include new revolutionary strategies in biology like the manipulation of stem cells or precursor cells (for instance we already know that cultured adult human epidermal keratinocytes have kept the potential to differentiate into other epithelial cells [57]) and tissue engineering like bioprinting which will permit to address in more detail the complexity of skin and the fabrication of skin appendages.

Cross-References

▶ Aging and Senescence of Skin Cells in Culture

References

1. Yaar M, Eller MS, Gilchrest BA, et al. Fifty years of skin aging. J Investig Dermatol Symp Proc. 2002;7:51–8.
2. Farage MA, Miller KW, Elsner P, et al. Intrinsic and extrinsic factors in skin ageing: a review. Int J Cosmet Sci. 2008;30:87–95.
3. Zouboulis CC, Makrantonaki E. Clinical aspects and molecular diagnostics of skin aging. Clin Dermatol. 2011;29:3–14.
4. Prunieras M, Regnier M, Schlotterer M. New procedure for culturing human epidermal cells on allogenic or xenogenic skin: preparation of recombined grafts. Ann Chir Plast. 1979;24:357–62.
5. Green H, Kehinde O, Thomas J. Growth of cultured human epidermal cells into multiple epithelia suitable for grafting. Proc Natl Acad Sci U S A. 1979;76:5665–8.
6. Bell E, Ivarsson B, Merrill C. Production of a tissue-like structure by contraction of collagen lattices by human fibroblasts of different proliferative potential in vitro. Proc Natl Acad Sci U S A. 1979;76:1274–8.
7. Yannas IV, Burke JF. Design of an artificial skin. I. Basic design principles. J Biomed Mater Res. 1980;14:65–81.
8. Boyce ST. Cultured skin substitutes: a review. Tissue Eng. 1996;2:255–66.
9. Bernstam LI, Vaughan FL, Bernstein IA. Keratinocytes grown at the air-liquid interface. In Vitro Cell Dev Biol. 1986;22:695–705.
10. Rosdy M, Clauss LC. Terminal epidermal differentiation of human keratinocytes grown in chemically defined medium on inert filter substrates at the air-liquid interface. J Invest Dermatol. 1990;95:409–14.
11. Lillie JH, MacCallum DK, Jepsen A. Growth of stratified squamous epithelium on reconstituted extracellular matrices: long-term culture. J Invest Dermatol. 1988;90:100–9.
12. Coulomb B, Saiag P, Bell E, Breitburd F, Lebreton C, Heslan M, Dubertret L. A new method for studying epidermalization in vitro. Br J Dermatol. 1986; 114:91–101.
13. Coulomb B, Lebreton C, Dubertret L. Influence of human dermal fibroblasts on epidermalization. J Invest Dermatol. 1989;92:122–5.
14. Bell E, Sher S, Hull B, et al. The reconstitution of living skin. J Invest Dermatol. 1983;81:2S–10.

15. Asselineau D, Prunieras M. Reconstruction of 'simplified' skin: control of fabrication. Br J Dermatol. 1984;111:219–21.
16. Asselineau D, Bernhard B, Bailly C, et al. Epidermal morphogenesis and induction of the 67 kD keratin polypeptide by culture of human keratinocytes at the liquid-air interface. Exp Cell Res. 1985;159:536–9.
17. Regnier M, Prunieras M. Growth and differentiation of adult human epidermal cells on dermal substrates. Front Matrix Biol. 1981;9:4–35.
18. Siegenthaler G, Saurat JH, Ponec M. Terminal differentiation in cultured human keratinocytes is associated with increased levels of cellular retinoic acid-binding protein. Exp Cell Res. 1988;178:114–26.
19. Asselineau D, Bernard B, Bailly C, et al. Retinoic acid improves epidermal morphogenesis. Dev Biol. 1989;133:322–35.
20. Marionnet C, Vioux-Chagnoleau C, Pierrard C, et al. Morphogenesis of dermo-epidermal junction in a model of reconstructed skin: beneficial effects of vitamin C. Exp Dermatol. 2006;15:625–33.
21. Coulomb B, Dubertret L, Bell E, Merrill C, Fosse M, Breton-Gorius J, Prost C, Touraine R. Endogenous peroxidases in normal human dermis: a marker of fibroblast differentiation. J Invest Dermatol. 1983;81:75–8.
22. Sarber R, Hull B, Merrill C, Soranno T, Bell E. Regulation of proliferation of fibroblasts of low and high population doubling levels. Mech Ageing Dev. 1981;17:107–17.
23. Rhee S, Grinnell F. Fibroblast mechanics in 3D collagen matrices. Adv Drug Deliv Rev. 2007;59:1299–305.
24. Asselineau D, Bernard BA, Darmon M. Three dimensional culture of human keratinocytes on a dermal equivalent: a model system to study epidermal morphogenesis and differentiation in vitro. In: Lowe N, Maibach HI, editors. Models of dermatology, vol. 3. Basel: Karger; 1987. p. 1–17.
25. Oikarinen A, Karvonen J, Uitto J, et al. Connective tissue alterations in skin exposed to natural and therapeutic UV-radiation. Photodermatol. 1985;2:15–26.
26. Bernerd F, Asselineau D. Successive alteration and recovery of epidermal differentiation and morphogenesis after specific UVB-damages in skin reconstructed in vitro. Dev Biol. 1997;183:123–38.
27. Bernerd F, Asselineau D. UVA exposure of human skin reconstructed in vitro induces apoptosis of dermal fibroblasts: subsequent connective tissue repair and implications in photoaging. Cell Death Differ. 1998;5:792–802.
28. Marionnet C, Pierrard C, Golebiewski C, et al. Diversity of biological effects induced by longwave UVA rays (UVA1) in reconstructed skin. PLoS One. 2014;9, e105263.
29. Bernerd F, Asselineau D. An organotypic model of skin to study photodamage and photoprotection in vitro. J Am Acad Dermatol. 2008;58:S155–9.
30. Bernerd F, Vioux C, Asselineau D. Evaluation of the protective effect of sunscreens on in vitro reconstructed human skin exposed to UVB or UVA irradiation. Photochem Photobiol. 2000;71:314–20.
31. Frye EB, Degenhardt TP, Thorpe SR, et al. Role of the maillard reaction in aging of tissue proteins. J Biol Chem. 1998;273:18714–9.
32. Asselineau D, Ricois S, Pageon H, et al. The use of reconstructed skin to create new in vitro models of skin aging with special emphasis on the flexibility of reconstructed skin. In: Farage MA, Miller W, Maibach HI, editors. Text book of aging skin. 1st ed. Berlin/Heidelberg: Springer; 2010. p. 461–75.
33. Pageon H, Bakala H, Monnier VM, et al. Collagen glycation triggers the formation of aged skin in vitro. Eur J Dermatol. 2007;17:12–20.
34. Pageon H, Zucchi H, Dai Z, et al. Biological effects induced by specific advanced glycation end products in the reconstructed skin model of aging. Biores Open Access. 2015;4:54–64.
35. Pageon H, Poumes-Ballihaut C, Zucchi H, et al. Aged human skin is more susceptible than young skin to accumulate advanced glycoxidation products induced by sun exposure. J Aging Sci. 2013;1:1–5.
36. Pageon H, Zucchi H, Rousset F, et al. Skin aging by glycation: lessons from the reconstructed skin model. Clin Chem Lab Med. 2014;52:169–74.
37. Pageon H, Técher MP, Asselineau D, et al. Reconstructed skin modified by glycation of the dermal equivalent as a model for skin aging and its potential use to evaluate anti-glycation molecules. Exp Gerontol. 2008;43:584–8.
38. Harper RA, Grove G. Human skin fibroblasts derived from papillary and reticular dermis: differences in growth potential in vitro. Science. 1979;204:526–7.
39. Sriram G, Bigliardi PL, Bigliardi-Qi M. Fibroblast heterogeneity and its implications for engineering organotypic skin models in vitro. Eur J Cell Biol. 2015;94:483–512.
40. Pageon H, Zucchi H, Asselineau D. Distinct and complementary roles of papillary and reticular fibroblasts in skin morphogenesis and homeostasis. Eur J Dermatol. 2012;22:324–32.
41. Mine S, Fortunel NO, Pageon H, et al. Aging alters functionally human dermal papillary fibroblasts but not reticular fibroblasts: a new view of skin morphogenesis and ageing. PLoS One. 2008;3, e4066.
42. Janson D, Saintigny G, Mahé C, et al. Papillary fibroblasts differentiate into reticular fibroblasts after prolonged in vitro culture. Exp Dermatol. 2013;22:48–53.
43. Driskell RR, Lichtenberger BM, Hoste E, et al. Distinct fibroblast lineages determine dermal architecture in skin development and repair. Nature. 2013;504:277–81.
44. Girardeau-Hubert S, Teluob S, Pageon H, et al. The reconstructed skin model as a new tool for investigating in vitro dermal fillers: increased fibroblast activity by hyaluronic acid. Eur J Dermatol. 2015;25:312–22.
45. Brown RA, Wiseman M, Chuo C, et al. Ultra rapid engineering of biomimetic materials and tissues:

fabrication of nano- and microstructures by plastic compression. Adv Funct Mater. 2005;15:1762–70.
46. Labbé B, Marceau-Fortier G, Fradette J. Cell sheet technology for tissue engineering: the self-assembly approach using adipose-derived stromal cells. Methods Mol Biol. 2011;702:429–41.
47. Bosca AR, Tinois E, Faure M, et al. Epithelial differentiation of human skin equivalents after grafting onto nude mice. J Invest Dermatol. 1988;91:136–41.
48. Demarchez M, Hartmann DJ, Regnier M, et al. The role of fibroblasts in dermal vascularization and remodeling of reconstructed human skin after transplantation onto the nude mouse. Transplantation. 1992;54:317–26.
49. Black AF, Berthod F, L'heureux N, et al. In vitro reconstruction of a human capillary-like network in a tissue-engineered skin equivalent. FASEB J. 1998;12:1331–40.
50. Sorrell JM, Baber MA, Caplan AI. Human dermal fibroblast subpopulations; differential interactions with vascular endothelial cells in coculture: nonsoluble factors in the extracellular matrix influence interactions. Wound Repair Regen. 2008;16:300–9.
51. Asselineau D, Técher MP, Caplan AI, et al. Complex reconstructed skin equivalents made with papillary and reticular fibroblast populations incorporated in distinct layers: re-expression of papillary and reticular fibroblast characteristics after grafting onto nude mice. J Invest Dermatol. 2000;114:863.
52. Boyce ST, Hansbrough JF. Biologic attachment, growth, and differentiation of cultured human epidermal keratinocytes on a graftable collagen and chondroitin-6-sulfate substrate. Surgery. 1988;103:421–31.
53. Yang C, Hillas PJ, Báez JA, Nokelainen M, Balan J, et al. The application of recombinant human collagen in tissue engineering. BioDrugs. 2004;104:103–19.
54. Bernerd F, Asselineau D, Vioux C, et al. Clues to epidermal cancer proneness revealed by reconstruction of DNA repair-deficient xeroderma pigmentosum skin in vitro. Proc Natl Acad Sci U S A. 2001;93:7817–22.
55. Girardeau S, Mine S, Pageon H, et al. The Caucasian and African skin types differ morphologically and functionally in their dermal component. Exp Dermatol. 2009;18:704–11.
56. Girardeau-Hubert S, Pageon H, Asselineau D. In vivo and in vitro approaches in understanding the differences between Caucasian and African skin types: specific involvement of the papillary dermis. Int J Dermatol. 2012;51:1–4.
57. Asselineau D, Darmon M. Retinoic acid provokes metaplasia of epithelium formed in vitro by adult human epidermal keratinocytes. Differentiation. 1995; 58:297–306.

In Vitro Method to Visualize UV-Induced Reactive Oxygen Species in a Skin Equivalent Model

94

Tomohiro Hakozaki

Contents

T. Hakozaki (✉)
Beauty Technology Division, The Procter & Gamble Company, Mason Business Center, Mason, OH, USA
e-mail: hakozaki.t.1@pg.com

M.A. Farage et al. (eds.), *Textbook of Aging Skin*,
DOI 10.1007/978-3-662-47398-6_49

Abstract

The skin is the only organ directly exposed to ultraviolet (UV) light from the sun. Oxidative cellular stress and DNA damage caused by UV exposure have been recognized to participate in various photogenesis of the skin. Among several oxidative stressors, reactive oxygen species (ROS) is well known to play important roles in the process of UV-induced skin damage including photoaging, immunomodulation, melanogenesis, and ultimately photo-carcinogenesis. To examine the impact of UV-induced ROS in the skin, it is critical to observe the ROS changes quantitatively in real time, while it has been challenging because ROS are extremely short-lived and essentially non-emissive. For this purpose, in the past two decades, several evaluation methods such as chemiluminescence, photoemission, fluorescence, or ESR spectroscopy using spin probes have been developed. With the advance of technologies, more and more methods became available not only to detect and quantify but also to visualize free radicals and ROS under much closer conditions to the actual human skin by utilizing the human skin equivalent models. These advanced in vitro visualization methods especially using human skin equivalent models enable us to more precisely characterize the ROS-related responses in human skin as a substitute for animal model and identify protective compounds against oxidative stress and its antiaging effect.

Introduction

When the skin is exposed to ultraviolet (UV) light consisting of UVA (320–400 nm) and UVB (290–320 nm), reactive oxygen species (ROS) such as superoxide anion radical ($^{\bullet}O_2^{-}$), hydrogen peroxide ($^{\bullet}H_2O_2$), hydroxyl radical (OH), singlet oxygen ($^1O_2$), as well as lipid peroxides and their radicals (LOOH and LOO$^{\bullet}$) are formed [1, 2]. It is well documented that these free radicals and ROS cause oxidative cellular stress, cell injury, and DNA damage in the epidermis [3, 4] and eventually induce inflammation, skin photoaging, phototoxicity, or malignant tumors [5–8]. To protect skin from these radical species, there are multiple natural defense mechanisms in the skin. For instance, antioxidant enzymes such as superoxide dismutase (SOD), catalase (CAT), and glutathione peroxidase (GSH-Px) play important roles in protecting the skin against degenerative changes by free radicals or ROS [9, 10].

In order to examine the impact and role of UV-induced free radicals or ROS in the skin, it is essential to detect and visualize them in a real time. However, due to extremely short-lived and essentially non-emissive nature, free radicals and ROS are difficult to detect directly. Several evaluation methods such as chemiluminescence (CL) probe [1, 11], photon emission detection [12–15], fluorescence detection [16, 17], and electron spin resonance (ESR) spectroscopy using spin probes [18–21] have been developed to detect ROS and investigate their species and behaviors.

Meanwhile, in the past two decades, human skin equivalent models have been developed for multiple purposes, such as a replacement of animal models for compound safety evaluation. Now several models have become commercially available and are used not only for safety assessment but also to investigate biological functions of the skin or responses against various stimulations such as compound treatment or UV exposure.

This chapter introduces recent research and methods to detect and visualize oxidative stress or ROS utilizing human skin equivalent models.

Oxidative Stress Measurement for the Evaluation of UV-Induced DNA Damage in a Human Skin Equivalent Model

Several techniques were developed for assessing skin damages in human skin equivalent models. Among them, an oxidatively modified DNA base, 8-hydroxy-2'-deoxyguanosine (8-OHdG), is induced by hydroxyl radical ($^{\bullet}$OH), singlet oxygen ($^1O_2$), photodynamic reaction, or peroxynitrite ($ONOO^{-}$). It is also mutagenic when present during DNA replication [22]. In 2006, a combination of a human skin equivalent model and 8-OHdG immunohistochemistry was proposed by Toyokuni et al. [23]. UVB-induced DNA modification was evaluated by utilizing produced 8-OHdG level as a biomarker. Specifically, the human skin equivalent model was exposed to UVB radiation, and the induction of 8-OHdG was examined by immunohistochemical analysis with catalyzed signal amplification on formalin-fixed paraffin sections. The immunohistochemical images were processed with ImageJ (National Institutes of Health [NIH] image software) to qualify 8-OHdG by multiplying positively stained area and density (8-OHdG index) [4, 24]. Formation of 8-OHdG in the skin equivalent model by UVB exposure was demonstrated, and it is produced in a UV-dose-dependent manner (Fig. 1). Interestingly, little nuclear staining of 8-OHdG was observed in the negative control samples without UVB exposure, but the increase of 8-OHdG staining was clearly observed in the UVB-exposed samples.

The effect of pretreatment of several antioxidants was also examined. The formation of 8-OHdG was effectively suppressed by the treatment of anti-oxidative compounds (Fig. 2). It provides evidence to the fact that the combination of human skin equivalent model and 8-OHdG immunohistochemistry is considered as a distinct screening strategy for identifying active compounds, which prevent UV-induced skin damage with the following three characteristics: (1) alternative to animal experiments; (2) expensive instruments are not required; and (3) higher sensitivity compared with the animal model.

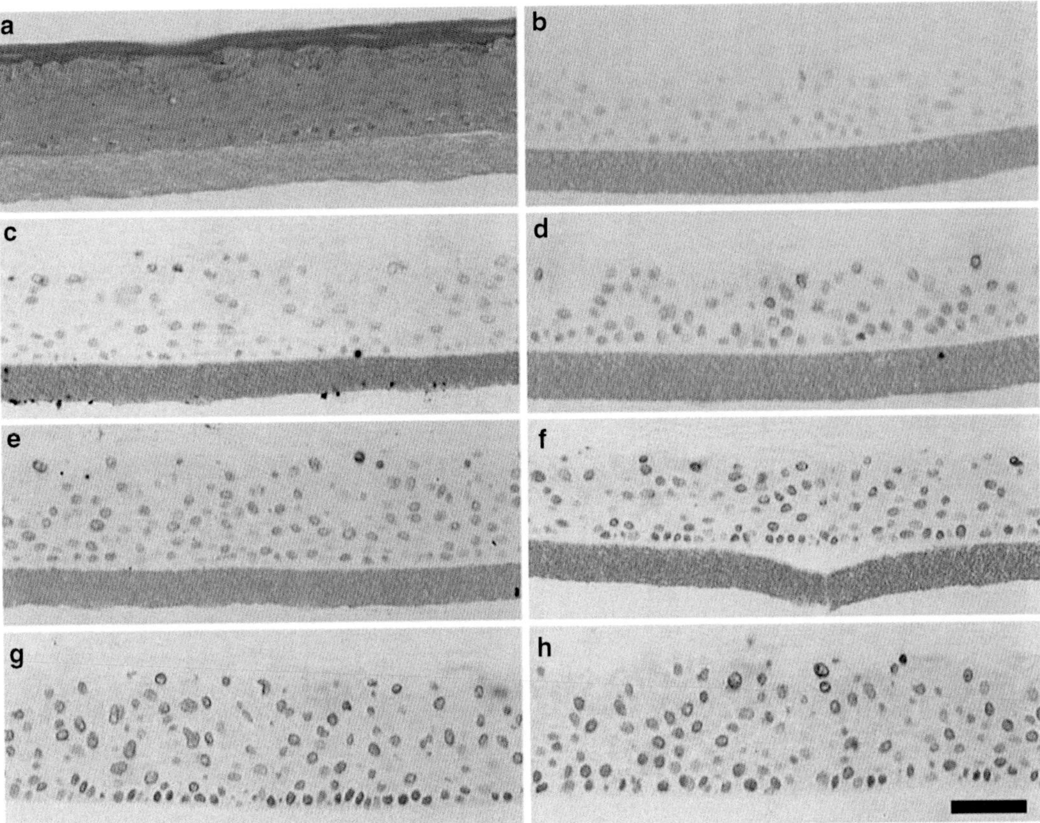

Fig. 1 Localization of 8-OHdG in a human skin equivalent model. (**a**) Hematoxylin and eosin staining of an untreated specimen. Immunostaining of 8-OHdG after UVB exposure (2.25 mJ/cm^2/min) at various time periods. (**b**) 0 min, (**c**) 12 min, (**d**) 18 min, (**e**) 24 min, (**f**) 36 min, (**g**) 48 min, and (**h**) 60 min. Bar = 100 μm

In 2008, new research was reported by Bernerd and Asselineau utilizing a skin reconstructed model containing a dermal equivalent and a fully differentiated epidermis [25]. The authors investigated the effects of UV light (UVB and UVA) on photodamage by employing the sunburn cell formation, which is linked to the presence of DNA lesions, such as pyrimidine dimers and (6,4) photoproducts being a direct chromophore for UVB radiation. They found that UVB-induced damage was essentially epidermal, with the typical sunburn cells and DNA lesions, whereas UVA-induced damage was mostly located within the dermal compartment. The model and end points used for UVB- and UVA-induced damages appeared to be very useful for the in vitro evaluation of sunscreens or compounds, in particular to investigate their protective effects against the effects of UV radiation. It will also allow distinguishing the efficiency of UV absorbers depending on their absorption spectrum [25, 26].

Currently, there is an emerging concept that there are fragile genomic sites to oxidative stress as well as UV-specific DNA base modifications. In the future, human skin equivalent models will be further applied to the investigation of skin damages at molecular or cellular level by combining with the emerging new technologies such as

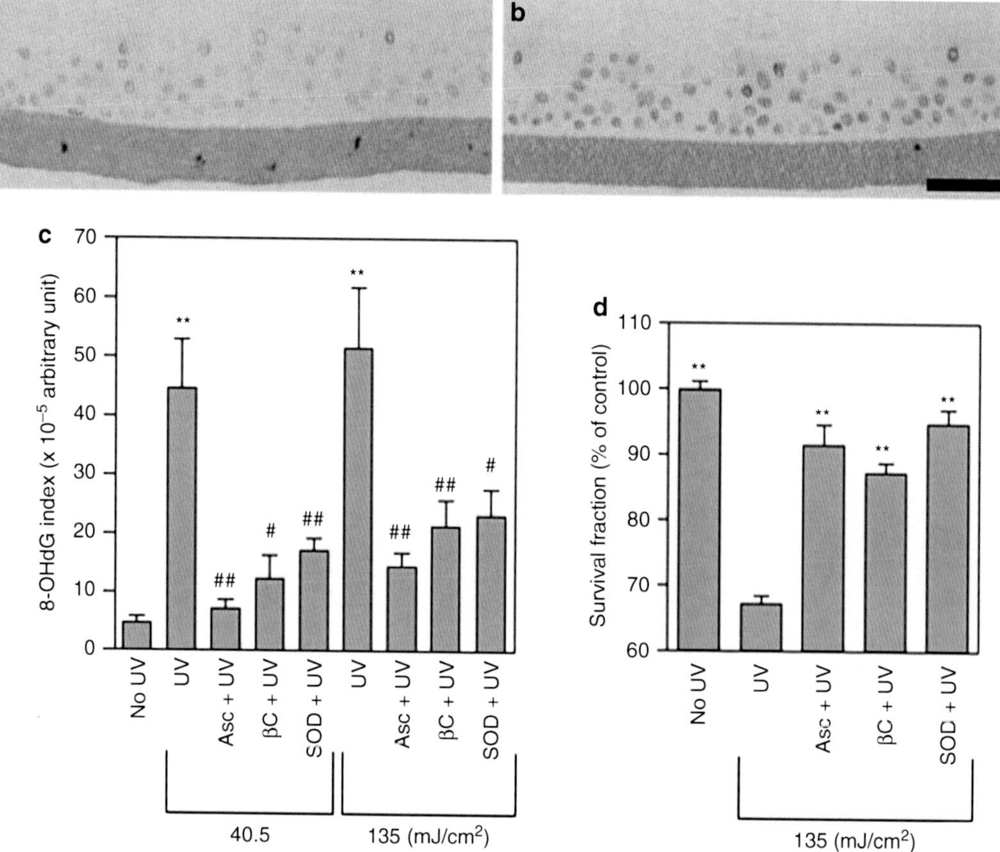

Fig. 2 Amelioration of UVB-induced 8-OHdG in a human skin equivalent model by various agents. Immunohistochemistry of 8-OHdG after UVB exposure of 40.5 mJ/cm^2 (18 min) (**a**) with or (**b**) without prior treatment of 10 mM ascorbate. (**c**) Quantitation of 8-OHdG immunostaining by NIH image freeware. *Asc* ascorbate, *βC* β-carotene, *SOD* Cu-Zn superoxide dismutase. Means ± SEM, $N = 5$; $^{**}p < 0.01$ versus untreated control (no UV); $^{\#}p < 0.05$, $^{\#\#}p < 0.01$ versus UVB exposure alone. (**d**) Cell viability determined by MTT assay after UVB exposure of 135 mJ/cm^2 (60 min). Means ± SEM, $N = 4 - 6$; $^{**}p < 0.01$ versus UVB exposure alone. Bar = 100 μm

laser capture microdissection (LCM), which is a new method for isolating specific cells of interest from microscopic regions of tissue that has been sectioned [27]. Especially, the application of LCM is rapidly expanding to mass spectrometry, DNA genotyping and loss of heterozygosity analysis, RNA transcript profiling, cDNA library generation, proteomics discovery, and signal kinase pathway profiling [28]. These emerging techniques will enable deeper understanding in skin aging not only utilizing human skin equivalent models but also utilizing human explant model or biopsy samples.

Photon Emission and Fluorescence Technique to Detect ROS in Human Skin Equivalent Models

Photons participate in many atomic and molecular interactions and processes. Recent biophysical research has discovered ultraweak radiation emitted from the biological tissues. Several physical or chemical environmental stressors generate ROS, which trigger oxidative reactions in/around the cells or tissues and thereby induce a correlated ultraweak photon emission (UPE) signal. Several works on photon emission detection and imaging in the skin have been documented. Khabiri and Hangen reported a highly sensitive method to assess oxidative processes in biological molecules using weak photon emission generated due to oxidation of proteins or amino acids. For instance, strong UPE signals are detected by the oxidation of Phe, Trp, His, and Cys and weak UPE signals from Lys and Thr. They proposed the noninvasive method for monitoring of UVA-induced oxidative skin stress by UPE measurement to assess the potency of topical antioxidants in ex vivo porcine skin and in vivo human skin [12, 13].

Niggli et al. reported an improved UPE measurement from UVA laser-induced biophotonic emission of different cultured cells to detect biophysical changes between young and adult fibroblasts, as well as the changes between fibroblasts and keratinocytes [14]. Van Wijk et al. reviewed the current status of human photon emission techniques and the protocols for recording the human oxidative status. Systematic studies on human emission have presented information on: (a) procedures for reliable measurements and spectral analysis, (b) anatomic intensity of emission and left-right symmetries, (c) biological rhythms in emission, (d) physical and psychological influences on emission, (e) novel physical characteristics of emission, and (f) the identification of UPE with the staging of ROS-related damage and disease. It is concluded that both patterns and physical properties of UPE hold considerable promise as measure for the oxidative status [15]. Rastoqi and Pospísil also applied UPE measurement to assess oxidative metabolic processes in the human hand skin [29]. They tested various antioxidants and concluded spontaneous UPE can be used as a noninvasive tool for the temporal and spatial monitoring of the oxidative metabolic processes and intrinsic antioxidant system in the human skin.

While UPE detection is one promising technique, fluorescence techniques with chemical probes for detection and visualization of ROS are also useful tools. Fluorescence as well as chemiluminescence can offer high detection sensitivity. There are several research studies on the detection and imaging of ROS in the UV-exposed human skin equivalent models by using fluorescent techniques. Hanson and Clegg reported the method to observe and quantify UV-induced ROS in the ex vivo human skin [16, 17]. Their proposed method consists of two-photon fluorescence microscopy to detect UV-induced ROS. They observed ROS by using a human skin equivalent model and the epidermis and the dermis of the ex vivo human skin. In their study, the human epidermal skin model was incubated with the nonfluorescent ROS probe dihydrorhodamine (DHR), which reacted with ROS such as O_2^- and H_2O_2 to form fluorescent rhodamine 123. They reported that the two-photon excitation provides a depth penetration through the skin unlike confocal microscopic techniques. Thus, this method can provide submicron spatial resolution such that subcellular areas where ROS are generated could be detected. This would enable the monitoring of UV-induced ROS at different depths within the skin. In the future, the method might be applicable to evaluate the ability of sunscreens or antioxidants to prevent ROS generation and photodamage at targeted depth or the region in the skin.

Electron Spin Resonance Technique to Detect ROS in a Human Skin Equivalent Model

Electron spin resonance (ESR) techniques have been widely used to study ROS and oxidative stress in biological systems in vitro. However, the limited number of research studies has been documented by using human skin equivalent models, the ex vivo human skin, and even less for in vivo human skin.

In 2000, Togachi et al. reported a spin-trapping detection of ROS using X-band ESR spectroscopy and described the detection of ROS such as singlet oxygen ($^1O_2$) and hydroxyl radical ($^{\bullet}OH$) by the spin trap 5,5-dimethyl-1-pyrroline-*N*-oxide (DMPO) and ESR spectroscopy in vitro. They also did in vivo ESR detection of ROS using a nitroxide spin probe, 3-carbamoyl-2,2,5,5-tetramethylpyrrolidine-1-oxyl (PCM), for noninvasive imaging of oxidative stress in living animals [18].

In 2003, Herrling et al. reported the detection of UV-induced free radicals and ROS generated in the ex vivo human skin (skin biopsies) by ESR spectroscopy using several nitroxides such as 2,2,6,6-tetramethylpiperidine-1-oxyl (TEMPO), 3-carbamoyl-2,2,5,5-tetramethylpyrrolidine-1-oxyl (PCM), and 3-carboxy-2,2,5,5-tetramethyl pyrrolidine-1-oxyl (PCA) [19]. The authors found that the reduction rates were different among the nitroxides. TEMPO was decreased due to both UV radiation and enzymatic activity in the skin, while PCM and PCA were sufficiently stable in the skin and solely reduced by UV-generated free radicals/ ROS. They also imaged the spatial distribution of UV-induced free radicals and ROS by using the PCA probe. By assuming the homogeneous distribution of PCA in the skin, they estimated the penetration profile of UVA and UVB irradiation, as the UV irradiation decreases the PCA intensity corresponding to its irradiance and penetration into the skin. Interestingly, this reduction was caused mainly by UVA radiation (320–400 nm), suggesting the importance of UVA protection.

In 2006, they reported their further work on detection and imaging of UVA-induced ROS in the human skin biopsies by the combination of the nitroxide spin probe PCA and an L-band ESR spectrometer. The main parts of ROS were generated by UVA (320–400 nm) so that the spatial distribution of free radicals reaches up to the lower side of the dermis. In addition, they proposed a new radical sun protection factor (RSF) to assess antioxidant compounds and UV filters on how much they can protect against UV-induced ROS [20].

As another application of ESR techniques, Date et al. recently reported ESR spin-trapping method with new probes to detect ROS in a human epidermal skin model [21]. 5,5-Dimethyl-1-pyrroline-1-oxide (DMPO) probe, which is known to detect superoxide anion radical ($^{\bullet}O_2^-$) and hydroxyl radical ($^{\bullet}OH$) selectively, was used. The combination of 2,2,6,6-tetramethyl-4-piperidone (TMPD) and $K_3Fe(CN)_6$ for the detection of singlet oxygen ($^1O_2$) was also examined. The model was verified by testing the application of the antioxidants known to scavenge specific ROS such as mannitol ($^{\bullet}OH$ scavenger), SOD ($^{\bullet}O_2^-$ scavenger), ascorbate ($^{\bullet}O_2^-$, $^{\bullet}OH$, and $^1O_2$ scavenger), and β-carotene ($^1O_2$ quencher). It demonstrated diminishing of the ESR signal of DMPO-OH (to detect $^{\bullet}O_2^-$ and $^{\bullet}OH$) by mannitol ($^{\bullet}OH$ scavenger) or SOD ($^{\bullet}O_2^-$ scavenger), as well as suppression of the ESR signal of 4-oxo-TEMPO (TMPD-$^1O_2$) to detect $^1O_2$ by β-carotene ($^1O_2$ quencher) compared with UVB-exposed control samples, as expected (Figs. 3 and 4). This technique will be a useful tool not only to predict UV-induced ROS-related responses in human skin but also to find the protective compounds against UV-induced oxidative stress in the human skin.

Chemiluminescent Technique to Detect or Visualize ROS in a Human Skin Equivalent Model

Chemiluminescent (CL) techniques have been widely used to study oxidative stress in biological systems in vitro; however, several methods are reported using human skin equivalent models, explant organ skin, or in vivo skin. In 2000, a unique technique using an in vivo real-time chemiluminescent (RT-CL) detection and two-dimensional ultralow-light imaging of endogenously generated ROS in the skin of living animals after UVA light exposure was proposed by Yasui and Sakurai [1]. They used a CL probe, Cypridina luciferin analog (CLA), and an ultralow-light imaging apparatus equipped with a charge-coupled device (CCD) camera (NightOWL™). CLA reacts specifically with superoxide anion radical ($^{\bullet}O_2^-$) or singlet oxygen ($^1O_2$) and emits chemiluminescence at 380 nm according to the consecutive reaction through the intermediate dioxetane (Fig. 5). The CL emissions are measured using the high-performance ultralow-light imaging luminograph system. The authors applied this CL method to measure the rate constants of $^{\bullet}O_2^-$ or $^1O_2$ and also demonstrated that it is useful not only in characterizing the ROS but also in finding protective compounds against UV-induced skin damage and in characterizing ROS generated in the UV (UVA and UVB) light-exposed skin [2, 30]. With this

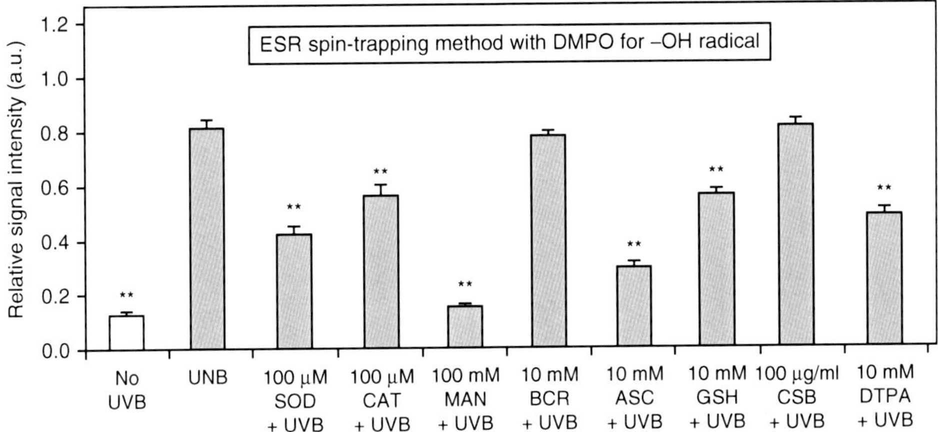

Fig. 3 Effect of antioxidants to suppress $^{\bullet}O_2^-$ and $^{\bullet}OH$ by ESR with DMPO. The human skin equivalent model was treated with 1 M DMPO and exposed to UVB at a dose of 27 mJ/cm^2. 10 mM mannitol, 10 mM ascorbate, and 100 μM SOD pretreatments significantly scavenged the ESR signal of DMPO-OH, and 100 μM catalase (*CAT*), 10 mM glutathione (*GSH*), and 10 mM diethylenetriamine-*N,N,N′,N″,N″*-pentaacetic acid (*DTPA*) pretreatments slightly scavenged its ESR signal. While, 10 mMβ -carotene (*BCA*) and 10 βμg/mL chondroitin sulfate B (*CSB*) pretreatments did not scavenge its ESR signal $^{**}p < 0.01$ versus UVB exposure ($n = 3$/each group)

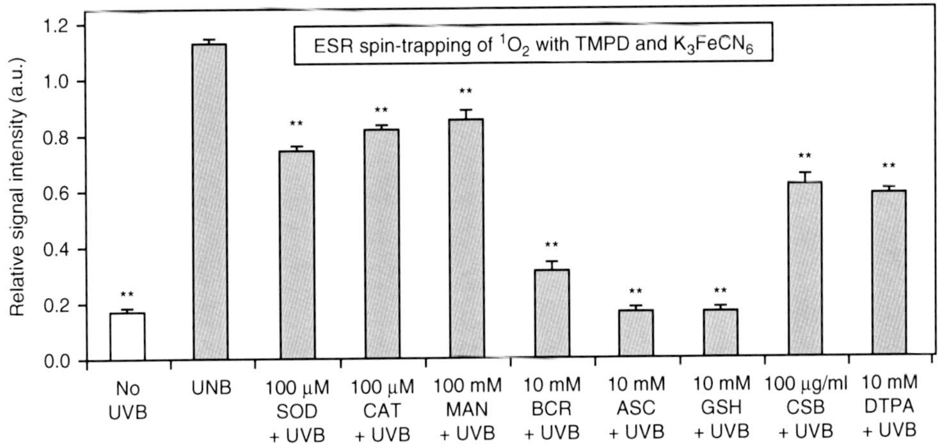

Fig. 4 Effect of antioxidants to suppress $^1O_2$ measured by ESR with TMPD/ $K_3Fe(CN)_6$. The human skin equivalent model was treated with 200 mM TMPD and exposed to UVB at a dose of 27 mJ/cm^2, and then 100 mM $K_3Fe(CN)_6$ was added to the system. The ESR signal of 4-oxo-TEMPO due to the reaction between $^1O_2$ and TMPD was considerably observed. 10 mM ascorbate (*ASC*), 10 mM β-carotene (*BCR*), and 10 mM glutathione pretreatments significantly scavenged the ESR signal of 4-oxo-TEMPO (TMPD-$^1O_2$), and 100 μM catalase (*CAT*), 10 μg/mL chondroitin sulfate B (*CSB*),10 mM diethylene-triamine-*N,N,N′,N″,N″*-pentaacetic acid (*DTPA*), 10 mM mannitol, and 100 μM SOD pretreatments slightly scavenged its ESR signal $^{**}p < 0.01$ versus UVB exposure ($n = 3$/each group)

method, they identified that superoxide anion radical was formed intrinsically, and superoxide anion radical and singlet oxygen were generated by UVA exposure to the living animal skin. In addition, they indicated that anti-oxidative ability against ROS in the skin decreases by aging [2].

The former method is informative and useful; however, it uses live animals. In 2006, the combination of a human skin equivalent model (EpiDerm™ skin model EPI-200, MatTek) and the RT-CL method consisting of a sensitive CL probe, CLA, and an ultralow-light imaging

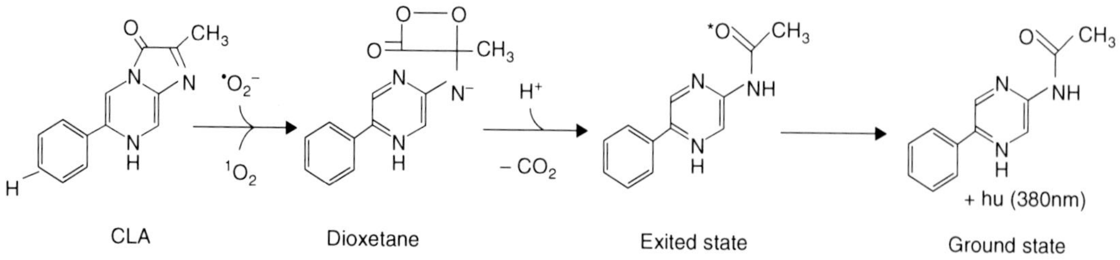

Fig. 5 Principle of CLA probe. Cypridina luciferin analog (*CLA*) reacts specifically with superoxide anion radical ($O_2^{\bullet -}$) or singlet oxygen ($^1O_2$) and emits chemiluminescence at 380 nm according to the consecutive reaction through the intermediate dioxetane

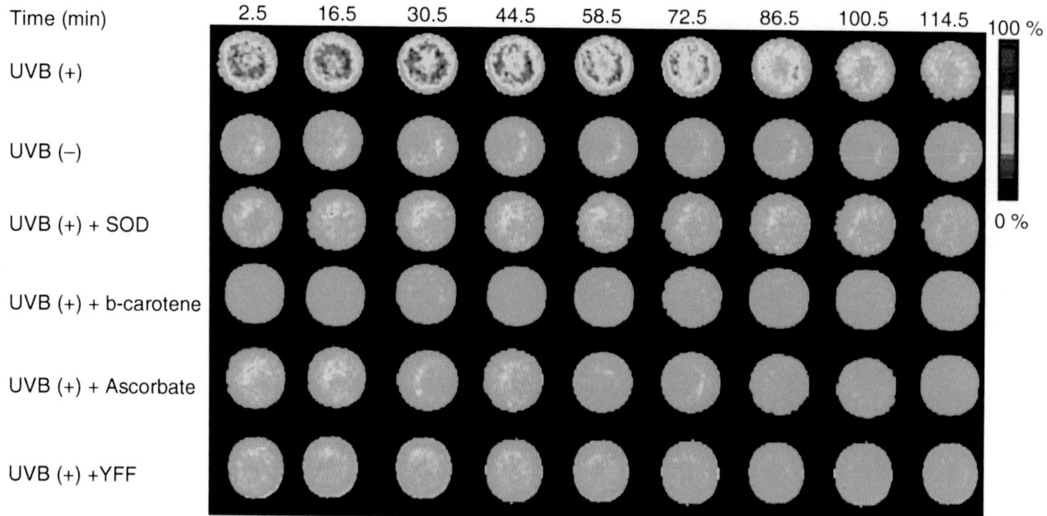

Fig. 6 Typical visualization of the chemiluminescent signals in the human skin equivalent model due to ROS generation. The highest level (*red* color) of ROS generation in the skin was found 44.5 min after UVB exposure at the dose of 27 mJ/cm^2. The low chemiluminescence (*green-yellow* color) was also observed in the human skin equivalent model without UVB exposure, suggesting that live epidermal cells produce ROS intrinsically. ROS-reducing effects of anti-oxidative compounds such SOD, β-carotene, ascorbate, and YFF were clearly demonstrated

apparatus was proposed by Yasui et al. as a new novel tool to detect and visualize UVB-induced ROS generation [31]. With this system, CL emission due to the reaction of CLA with endogenously generated ROS increased significantly in the UVB-exposed skin compared with that in the intact skin, maximum level being observed at a dose of 27 mJ/cm^2. The treatment of SOD ($^{\bullet}O_2^-$ scavenger) and β-carotene ($^1O_2$ quencher) effectively suppressed UVB-induced CL intensities, indicating the generation of $^{\bullet}O_2^-$ and $^1O_2$ in the skin equivalent model under UVB exposure. These results were consistent with those observed in the skin of living animals, thus supporting the relevancy of usage of skin equivalent model for the purpose.

Hakozaki et al. have further evaluated various anti-oxidative compounds such as ascorbate, β-carotene, SOD, and yeast ferment filtrate (YFF), which was reported to suppress superoxide anion and hydroxyl radical [21]. A typical visualization of CL from the human skin equivalent model with and without UVB exposure is shown in Fig. 6 [32]. The UVB-exposed skin samples exhibited significantly higher CL levels (red color) than did the intact skin samples (green-

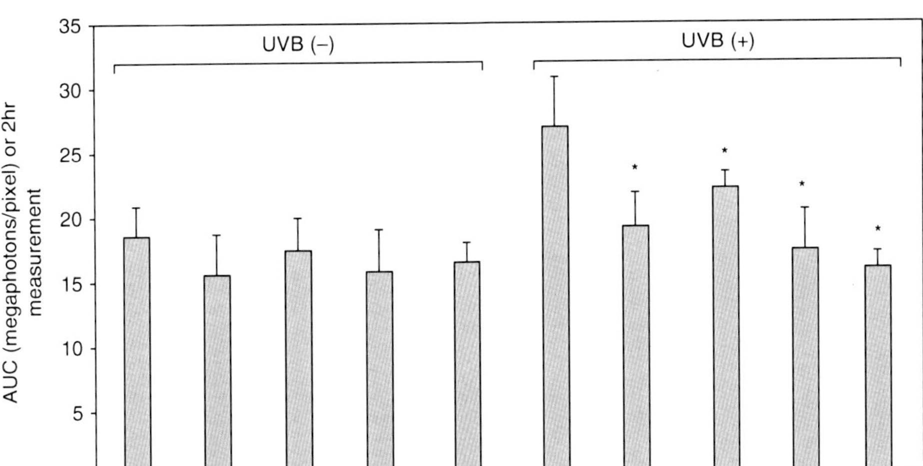

Fig. 7 Semi-quantification of UVB-induced ROS and effect of antioxidants. Suppressive effects of SOD, β-carotene (*BCR*), ascorbate (*ASC*), and YFF on the UVB-induced ROS in the human skin equivalent model. Data are expressed as the means ± SD for 8–10 samples in each experiment. Significant suppressions versus control [UVB(+)] were observed in all treatments in UVB-exposed group (*$p < 0.05$), while no significant differences versus control [UVB(−)] were found in all treatments in non-UVB-exposed group ($p > 0.05$)

yellow color), indicating the increased generation of ROS in the epidermal skin model. The tested compounds greatly reduced UVB-induced CL intensities immediately after the measurement. For semiquantitative comparison, the areas under the curve of CL intensities (AUC) were calculated for all tested compounds as shown in Fig. 7. Compared with the UVB-induced control group, the treatment with anti-oxidative compounds exhibited statistically significantly lower CL intensities. This unique method will be an effective tool for (1) investigating the impact of ROS in human skin damage and photoaging and (2) screening protective compounds to suppress ROS generation against UVB-induced skin damage with a powerful visualization ability.

Conclusion

With the advance of technology, more and more methods are available to detect and visualize free radicals and ROS in the skin and its equivalent models. In the future, these in vitro methods using human skin equivalent models will be considered to be a relevant and handy tool to identify protective compounds against oxidative stress and its aging effect and predict ROS-related responses in the human skin as a substitute for animal model.

Cross-References

- ▶ Cutaneous Responses to Tropospheric Ozone Exposure
- ▶ Environmental and Genetic Factors in Facial Aging in Twins
- ▶ Climate Change and Its Dermatologic Impact on Aging Skin
- ▶ Skin Photodamage Prevention: State of the Art and New Prospects

References

1. Yasui H, Sakurai H. Chemiluminescent detection and imaging of reactive oxygen species in live mouse skin exposed to UVA. Biochem Biophys Res Commun. 2000;269:131–6.
2. Yasui H, Sakurai H. Age-dependent generation of reactive oxygen species in the skin of live hairless rats

exposed to UVA light. Exp Dermatol. 2003;12:655–61.
3. Chen Q, et al. Oxidative DNA damage and senescence of human diploid fibroblast cells. Proc Natl Acad Sci U S A. 1995;92:4337–41.
4. Hattori Y, et al. 8-Hydroxy-2'-deoxyguanosine is increased in epidermal cells of hairless mice after chronic UVB exposure. J Invest Dermatol. 1996;107:733–7.
5. Kligman LH. The ultraviolet-irradiated hairless mouse: a model for photoaging. J Am Acad Dermatol. 1989;21:623–31.
6. Ichihashi M, et al. UV-induced skin damage. Toxicology. 2003;189:21–39.
7. Bech-Thomsen N, Wulf HC. Carcinogenic and melanogenic effects of a filtered metal halide UVA source and a tubular fluorescent UVA tanning source with or without additional solar-simulated UV radiation in hairless mice. Photochem Photobiol. 1995;62:773–9.
8. Kripke ML, et al. Pyrimidine dimers in DNA initiate systemic immunosuppression in UV-irradiated mice. Proc Natl Acad Sci U S A. 1992;89:7516–20.
9. Sasaki H, Akamatsu H, Horio T. Protective role of copper, zinc superoxide dismutase against UVB-induced injury of the human keratinocyte cell line HaCaT. J Invest Dermatol. 2000;114:502–7.
10. Hellemans L, et al. Antioxidant enzyme activity in human stratum corneum shows seasonal variation with an age-dependent recovery. J Invest Dermatol. 2003;120:434–9.
11. Ou-Yang H. A chemiluminescence study of UVA-induced oxidative stress in human skin *in-vivo*. J Invest Dermatol. 2004;122:1020–9.
12. Khabiri F, et al. Non-invasive monitoring of oxidative skin stress by ultraweak photon emission (UPE)-measurement. I: mechanisms of UPE of biological materials. Skin Res Technol. 2008;14:103–11.
13. Hagens R, et al. Non-invasive monitoring of oxidative skin stress by ultraweak photon emission measurement. II: biological validation on ultraviolet A-stressed skin. Skin Res Technol. 2008;14:112–20.
14. Niggli HJ, et al. Laser-ultraviolet-A induced ultra weak photon emission in human skin cells: a biophotonic comparison between keratinocytes and fibroblasts. Indian J Exp Biol. 2008;46:358–63.
15. Van Wijk R, et al. Free radicals and low-level photon emission in human pathogenesis: state of the art. Indian J Exp Biol. 2008;46:273–309.
16. Hanson KM, Clegg RM. Observation and quantification of ultraviolet-induced reactive oxygen species in ex vivo human skin. Photochem Photobiol. 2002;76:7–63.
17. Hanson KM, Clegg RM. Two-photon fluorescence imaging and reactive oxygen species detection within the epidermis. Methods Mol Biol. 2005;289:413–22.
18. Togashi H, et al. Analysis of hepatic oxidative stress status by electron spin resonance spectroscopy and imaging. Free Radic Biol Med. 2000;28:846–53.
19. Herrling T, et al. UV-induced free radicals in the skin detected by ESR spectroscopy and imaging using nitroxides. Free Radic Biol Med. 2003;35:59–67.
20. Herrling T, Jung K, Fuchs J. Measurements of UV-generated free radicals/reactive oxygen species (ROS) in skin. Spectrochim Acta A Mol Biomol Spectrosc. 2006;63:840–5.
21. Date A. et al. Detection and identification of reactive oxygen species and followed free radicals generated in the UVB-exposed three dimensional human epidermal cells- Epiderm ™ as measured by ESR spin-trapping method. In: 126th annual meeting of pharmaceutical society of Japan, Sendai, vol 174; 2006. pp. 28.
22. Kasai H. Analysis of a form of oxidative DNA damage, 8-hydroxy-2'-deoxyguanosine, as a marker of cellular oxidative stress during carcinogenesis. Mutat Res. 1997;387:147–63.
23. Toyokuni S, et al. Novel screening method for ultraviolet protection: combination of a human skin-equivalent model and 8-hydroxy-2'-deoxyguanosine. Pathol Int. 2006;56:760–2.
24. Toyokuni S, et al. Quantitative immunohistochemical determination of 8-hydroxy-2'-deoxyguanosine by a monoclonal antibody N45.1: its application to ferric nitrilotriacetate-induced renal carcinogenesis model. Lab Invest. 1997;76:365–74.
25. Bernerd F, Asselineau D. An organotypic model of skin to study photodamage and photoprotection *in-vitro*. J Am Acad Dermatol. 2008;58:155–9.
26. Fourtanier A, Moyal D, Seité S. Sunscreens containing the broad-spectrum UVA absorber, Mexoryl® SX, prevent the cutaneous detrimental effects of UV exposure: a review of clinical study results. Photodermatol Photoimmunol Photomed. 2008;24:164–74.
27. Espina V, et al. Laser capture microdissection technology. Expert Rev Mol Diagn. 2007;7:647–57.
28. Golubeva Y, et al. Laser capture microdissection for protein and NanoString RNA analysis. Methods Mol Biol. 2013;931:213–57.
29. Rastogi A, Pospísil P. Spontaneous ultraweak photon emission imaging of oxidative metabolic processes in human skin: effect of molecular oxygen and antioxidant defense system. J Biomed Opt. 2011;16:096005. doi:10.1117/1.3616135.
30. Nishimura H, Yasui H, Sakurai H. Generation and distribution of reactive oxygen species in the skin of hairless mice under UVA: studies on *in-vivo* chemiluminescent detection and tape stripping methods. Exp Dermatol. 2006;15:891–9.
31. Yasui H, et al. Real-time chemiluminescent imaging and detection of reactive oxygen species in the UVB-exposed human skin equivalent model. Biochem Biophys Res Commun. 2006;347:83–8.
32. Hakozaki T, et al. Visualization and characterization of UVB-induced reactive oxygen species in a human skin equivalent model. Arch Dermatol Res. 2008;300: S51–6.

Aging and Senescence of Skin Cells in Culture

95

Suresh I. S. Rattan

Contents

Abstract

Studying age-related changes in the physiology, biochemistry, and molecular biology of isolated skin cell populations in culture has greatly expanded the understanding of the fundamental aspects of skin aging. The three main cell types that have been studied extensively with respect to cellular aging in vitro are dermal fibroblasts, epidermal keratinocytes, and melanocytes. Serial subcultivation of normal diploid skin cells can be performed only a limited number of times, and the emerging senescent phenotype can be categorized into structural, physiological, biochemical, and molecular phenotypes, which can be used as biomarkers of cellular aging in vitro. The rate and phenotype of aging are different in different cell types. There are both common features and specific features of aging of skin fibroblasts, keratinocytes, melanocytes, and other cell types. A progressive accumulation of damage in all types of macromolecules is a universal feature of cellular aging in all cell types. A progressive failure of molecular maintenance and repair pathways is the ultimate cause of cellular aging in vitro and in vivo.

Introduction

In modern biogerontology, the terms "cellular aging," "cell senescence," and "replicative senescence" most commonly imply the study of normal

S.I.S. Rattan (✉)
Laboratory of Cellular Ageing, Department of Molecular Biology and Genetics, Aarhus University, Aarhus C, Denmark
e-mail: rattan@mb.au.dk

M.A. Farage et al. (eds.), *Textbook of Aging Skin*,
DOI 10.1007/978-3-662-47398-6_50

diploid cells in culture, which during serial subcultivation undergo a multitude of changes culminating in the permanent cessation of cell division. This process of cellular aging in vitro is generally known as the Hayflick phenomenon, and the limited division potential of normal cells is called the Hayflick limit, in recognition of the observations first reported by Leonard Hayflick in 1961 [1–4]. The study of age-related changes in the physiology, biochemistry, and molecular biology of isolated skin cell populations in culture has greatly expanded the understanding of the fundamental aspects of skin aging. The three main cell types that have been studied extensively with respect to cellular aging in vitro are dermal fibroblasts, epidermal keratinocytes, and melanocytes [5–11].

The aim of this article is to describe the experimental system of aging of skin cells in culture; to provide an overview of the age-related changes in the structural and functional aspects of cells including physiological, biochemical, and molecular changes; and to evaluate the use of such a system in testing and developing effective interventions for maintaining and/or re-achieving a healthy skin during aging.

Experimental Model System of Cellular Aging in Culture

Once the primary culture of normal cells is established in culture from the normal tissue (e.g., a skin biopsy), by using any of the standard methods such as the explant growth and enzymic dissociation of cells, the primary culture can then be subcultivated repeatedly each time it becomes confluent. This repeated subculturing of cells is also known as serial passaging [4]. In a description of the Hayflick phenomenon, Phase I is the period of the establishment of the primary culture from the normal tissue, Phase II is a relatively long period of serial passaging, growth, and cell proliferation at a constant rate, and Phase III is the final period of slowing-down of growth, which results in the cessation of cell division and end of replicative life span of cells. The whole duration of serial passaging is considered as the process of cellular aging, and the end-stage irreversible growth arrest in G_1 is termed as replicative senescence [1, 2].

After reaching a state of replicative senescence, some cells can still stay alive and be metabolically active at a minimal level for sometime and generally resist undergoing apoptosis [3, 4]. Although the exact culturing conditions, such as the type of the culture medium, the source of growth factors, the use of antibiotics, and the incubation temperature, humidity, and gaseous composition, may vary for different cell types, serial subcultivation of normal diploid cells can be performed only a limited number of times. This is in contrast to the high proliferative capacity of transformed, cancerous, and immortalized cells, whose cultures can be subcultivated and maintained indefinitely [3, 4].

The total number of cell divisions, measured as the cumulative population doublings (CPD), which can be achieved by a specific cell type in vitro, depends upon several biological factors. These include the maximum life span of the species, the developmental and adult age of the donor of the tissue biopsy, the site of the biopsy, and the health status of the donor [12]. For example, for human fibroblasts, the range of CPD for the cell strains originating from embryonic tissues is between 50 and 70, whereas for those originating from adult biopsies, it is generally less than 50 CPD. A similar range for CPD attained by human keratinocytes and melanocytes has been reported [5–10]. Additionally, gaseous composition, especially oxygen levels, and the quality of the nutritional serum and growth factors added to the culture medium can significantly affect the proliferative life span of cells in vitro. For example, culturing of fibroblasts in vitro in the air with about 20 % oxygen levels reduces their replicative life span which could be otherwise achieved at low-level (2 %) concentration akin to in vivo conditions [13, 14]. Furthermore, the site of the skin biopsy, for example, sun-exposed versus sun-protected area, has a significant effect on the CPD levels achieved by cells in culture [4, 15].

The Phenotype of Aging Skin Cells

Serial passaging of normal diploid skin cells is accompanied by a progressive and accumulative occurrence of a wide variety of changes before the final cessation of cell replication occurs. The emerging senescent phenotype of serially passaged normal diploid skin cells can be categorized into the structural, physiological, biochemical, and molecular phenotypes, which can be used as biomarkers of cellular aging in vitro, as summarized in Tables 1, 2, and 3. There are more than 200 such structural, physiological, biochemical, and molecular characteristics that have been studied during cellular aging, and a list of major characteristics that appear progressively in cell cultures and distinguish between young and senescent cells, generally before the end of proliferative life span and their irreversible arrest in the G_1 phase of the cell cycle, can be found in several publications [3, 4]. Here a summary of such phenotypic changes is given below.

(A) *Structural phenotype of aging skin cells*: Table 1 lists the major structural changes observed in aging skin cells in culture. Most commonly, a progressive increase in cell size and the loss of homogenous morphological pattern are the most dramatic and easily identifiable differences in early-passage young and late-passage old or senescent skin cells (Fig. 1).

Other structural changes during aging of skin cells include cytoskeletal and membrane rigidity, altered extracellular matrix, accumulation of intracellular debris, and incomplete cytokinesis leading to multinucleation.

In addition to the gross structural alterations listed in Table 1, there are several ultrastructural changes reported by using electron microscopic methods. These include the presence of distorted mitochondria,

Table 1 Structural phenotype of skin cells undergoing aging in vitro

Increased cell size
Change of shape from thin, long, and spindle-like to flattened and irregular
Loss of whorl-like arrangement in parallel arrays on the cell culture substrate
Rodlike polymerization of the cytoskeletal actin filaments and disorganized microtubules
Increased membrane rigidity
Increased multi-nucleation
Increased number of vacuoles and dense lysosomal autophagous bodies

Table 2 Physiological phenotype of skin cells undergoing aging in vitro

Altered calcium flux, pH, viscosity, and membrane potential
Reduced activity of ionic pumps
Reduced mobility
Reduced respiration and energy production
Reduced response to growth factors and other mitogens
Increased sensitivity to toxins, drugs, irradiation, and other stresses
Increased basal levels of autophagy
Increased basal levels of stress proteins

Table 3 Biochemical and molecular phenotype of skin cells undergoing aging in vitro

Permanent growth arrest in late G_1 phase of the cell cycle near the S phase boundary
Increased mRNA and protein levels of cell cycle inhibitors
Increased mRNA and protein levels of inhibitors of proteases
Decreased expression, levels, and activities of numerous housekeeping enzymes
Decreased expression, levels, and activities of macromolecular turnover pathways
Reduced levels of methylated cytosines in the DNA
Reduced length of telomeres
Increased levels of damage in nuclear and mitochondrial DNAs
Altered profiles of micro-RNAs
Increased levels of damaged and abnormal proteins
Increased levels of macromolecular cross-linking
Increased levels of reactive oxygen species
Altered profile of secreted proteins

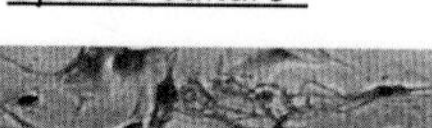

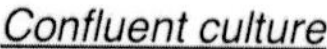

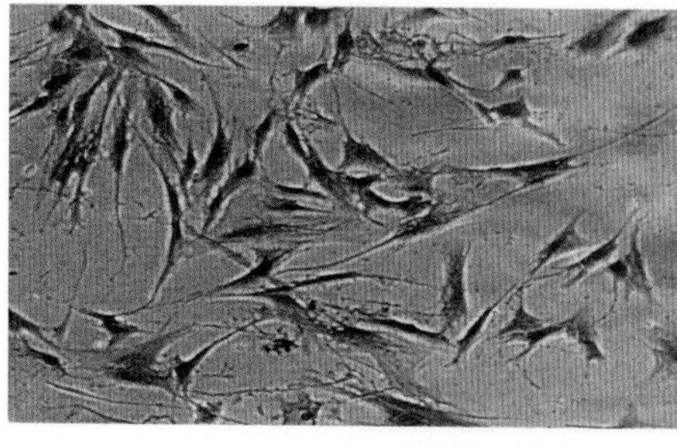
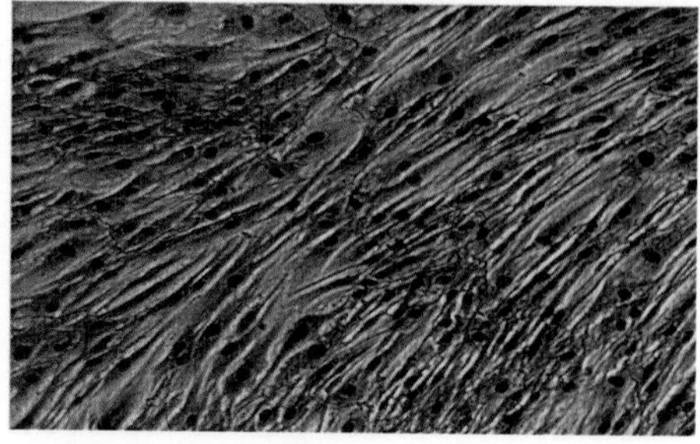

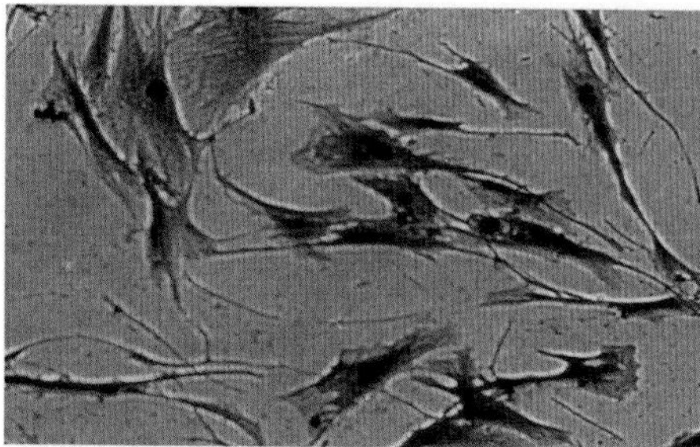
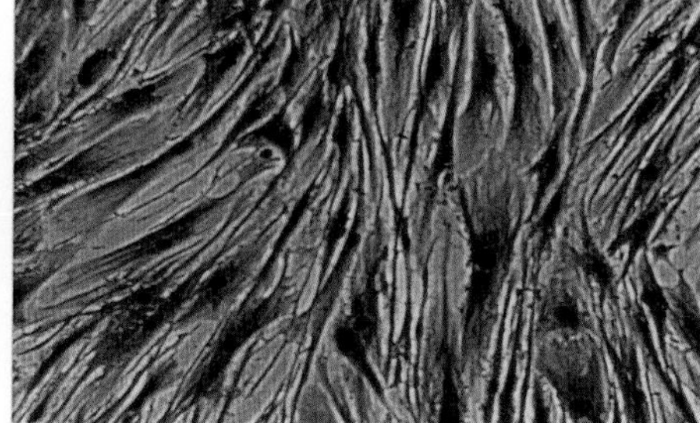

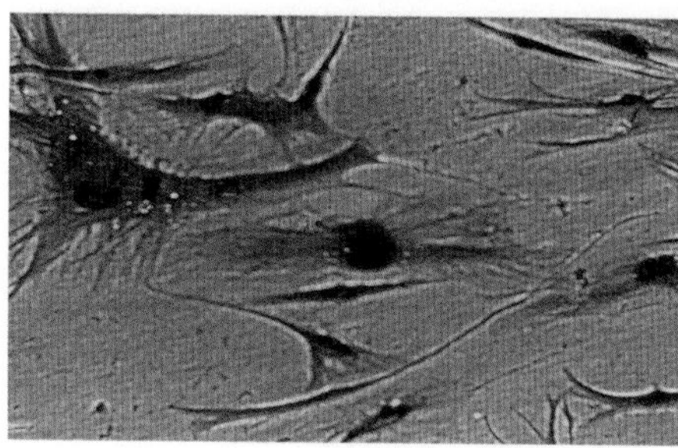
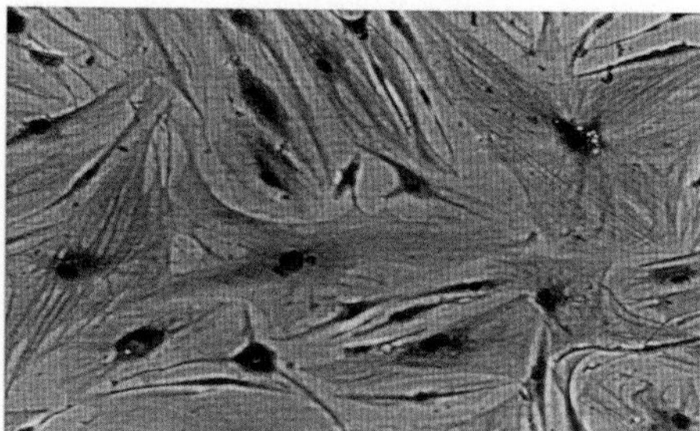

Fig. 1 Figure shows Giemsa-stained light microscopic phase contrast pictures of serially passaged human skin fibroblasts at various points in their in vitro life span. Sparse and confluent cultures at three stages during replicative life span are compared: (1) early-passage young adult skin fibroblasts with less than 30 % life span completed, (2) middle-aged cells with 60–80 % replicative life span completed, and (3) late-passage senescent cells with more than 95 % life span completed

increased level of chromosomal aberrations, overcondensation of chromatin, increased nucleolar fragmentation, and the accumulation of lipid-protein conjugate lipofuscin in lysosomes [16–18].

(B) *Physiological phenotype of aging skin cells*: Numerous studies have been performed elucidating changes in various functional and physiological parameters of skin cells undergoing aging. Table 2 lists some of the main such changes, which clearly indicate that almost all aspects of cellular function and physiology become impaired during aging. Collectively, these data show that aging skin cells progressively become less active, have reduced the ability to maintain various physiological functions, and become more prone to the negative effects of harmful substances.

Altered responsiveness of cells during aging is one of the most significant age-related changes, which can be a rate-limiting factor for the use of any potential modulators of aging. Several studies have been performed in order to understand the mechanisms for age-related alteration of responsiveness, and the pathways include unaltered receptor numbers and affinities, ineffective signal transduction, and interrupted networks [12]. Furthermore, increased levels of intracellular stress as manifested in increased basal levels of stress proteins and autophagy in serially passaged senescent skin cells are a hallmark of cellular aging [19].

(C) *Biochemical and molecular phenotype of aging skin cells*: At the biochemical and molecular levels, a large body of data is available which indicates that skin cells undergo a plethora of changes, which form the mechanistic bases of structural and physiological alterations. Table 3 gives a list of main categories of biochemical and molecular changes that have been reported in aging skin cells in culture.

Depending on the available technologies and the prevailing trends, changes in the amounts and activities of thousands of proteins and in the levels of thousands of mRNAs have been reported for aging skin cells. Recently, data are beginning to be collected for age-related changes in the so-called epigenome, micro-RNAs, metabolome, secretome, and proteome, including posttranslational modifications [15, 20]. All such data will further strengthen the descriptive understanding of the phenomenon of aging of skin cells.

Although every single piece of descriptive data for aging skin cells is yet to be collected, a generalized picture of the aging phenomenon has emerged, Therefore, based on the large amount of data collected so far, important inferences and generalizations can already be made, which have implications with respect to developing effective interventions for a healthy skin. These are as follows:

1. The rate and phenotype of aging are different in different cell types. There are both common features and specific features of aging of skin fibroblasts, keratinocytes, melanocytes, and other cell types.
2. A progressive accumulation of damage in all types of macromolecules is a universal feature of cellular aging in all cell types.
3. Replicative senescence of cells in culture is not due to the activation of any aging-specific genes but is an indirect consequence of occurrence and accumulation of molecular damage and molecular heterogeneity.
4. A progressive failure of molecular maintenance and repair pathways is the ultimate cause of cellular aging.

From Cellular Aging In Vitro to Understanding Aging In Vivo

The Hayflick system of aging of skin cells in culture has proved to be very useful in developing the cellular and molecular understanding of the overall process of aging. A loss of proliferative capacity of any of the cell types has a deteriorative impact on the functioning and survival of the entire organism. A loss or slowing-down of proliferation of osteoblasts, glial cells, myoblasts, epithelial cells, lymphocytes, and fibroblasts can lead to the onset of many age-related diseases and impairments including osteoporosis, arthritis, immune deficiency, altered drug clearance, delayed wound healing, and altered functioning of the brain. Furthermore, the occurrence of fully senescent or near-senescent heterogenous cells in vivo can promote dysfunctioning of the other tissues by producing harmful signals and can also promote and stimulate the growth of other precancerous and cancerous cells [21, 22].

However, the existence of the Hayflick-type senescent cells in vivo is not very well established so far. A commonly used biomarker of senescent cells is the so-called senescence-associated beta-galactosidase (SABG), which has been used to demonstrate the presence of senescent cells in the human skin and some other tissues [23]. However, there are several limitations regarding the use of SABG as a marker of cellular aging in vitro, since SABG can also be detected in immortal cells under various conditions [24]. More and multiple independent markers of senescent cells are needed for this purpose.

The correlation between cellular aging in vitro and in vivo is often based on the evidence gathered from studies on the effects of donor age, species life span, and premature aging syndromes on cellular proliferative capacity in culture. These studies indicate that the genetic and intrinsic Hayflick limit of diploid cell strains in culture is a true reflection of what is going on during aging of an organism. However, there are some recent critiques of this based on the replicative potential of stem cells, which in the case of the skin appear to be maintained throughout the life span [25, 26]. Similarly, some changes observed in the Hayflick system in vitro, such as increased basal levels of autophagy, may not be present in the aging skin tissues [19]. In contrast to this, there is evidence showing that the stem cell population in the skin also undergoes aging and the number of stem cells declines as a function of donor age and during aging of the skin equivalents in vitro [27].

Modulators of Aging Skin Cells

The Hayflick system of cellular aging in culture is primarily a model for the study of slow and progressive accumulation of damage resulting in the arrest of cells in a non-proliferative state [4]. This system has been proved to be very useful for testing various physical, chemical, and biological conditions for their harmful or beneficial effects and for understanding other aspects of cellular aging with implications in the origin of age-related diseases. For example, irradiation; severe oxidative stress by UV, hydrogen peroxide, or dicarbonyls; and gene transfection have been used to induce a sudden and rapid increase in molecular damage, resulting in premature appearance of the senescent phenotype [28]. On the other hand, insertion of catalytically active component of the telomerase gene can completely bypass the Hayflick limit in many cell types including skin cells, and such cells can proliferate indefinitely with or without becoming transformed [29]. Similarly, normal diploid cells can be transformed and immortalized by chemical carcinogens, irradiation, and viral genes. Such approaches are helpful for unraveling the molecular details of cell cycle regulation in normal cells and its dysregulation in cancer cells [29].

The Hayflick system of cellular aging in culture has also been very useful for testing various natural and synthetic molecules as potential antiaging and health-promoting compounds for the skin. Some of the well-tested examples are cytokinins kinetin and zeatin [30], a dipeptide carnosine [31], curcumin which is a component of the spice turmeric [32, 33], and extracts from medicinal plants and sea algae [34]. Several of these tests have resulted in the successful development, production, and marketing of various products with pharmaceutical, cosmeceutical, and nutritional applications [34].

Another use of the model system of cellular aging in culture has been to test the principle of mild stress-induced beneficial and antiaging effects, which is the phenomenon of hormesis [35]. For example, human skin fibroblasts and keratinocytes exposed to repeated mild heat stress (41 °C, 1 h, twice a week) show several hormetic effects, such as improved protein degradation pathways, higher levels of chaperones, increased resistance to other stresses, improved differentiation, and increased proliferative life span [10]. Such studies can form the basis of testing novel hormetic agents, including potential hormetins of natural or synthetic origin, for improved skin care during aging [10, 35, 36].

Conclusion

It could be reemphasized that the present understanding of the cellular and molecular basis of aging of the skin owes a lot to the use of the

Hayflick system of aging of skin cells in culture. Most importantly, studies performed by using this model system have demonstrated that aging of cells is characterized by the accumulation of damage in various molecules that results in the failure of maintenance and repair systems. Detailed genomic, proteomic, and metabolomic studies using this system can further identify the interacting networks of regulatory pathways, which will then be accessible to modulation for the maintenance of the structural and functional integrity of the skin.

References

1. Hayflick L, Moorhead PS. The serial cultivation of human diploid strains. Exp Cell Res. 1961;25:585–621.
2. Hayflick L. The limited in vitro lifetime of human diploid cell strains. Exp Cell Res. 1965;37:614–36.
3. Campisi J, d'Adda di Fagagna F. Cellular senescence: when bad things happen to good cells. Nat Rev Mol Cell Biol. 2007;8:729–40.
4. Rattan SIS. Cellular senescence in vitro. In: Encyclopedia of life sciences. John Wiley & Sons; 2008. p. 1–3. doi:10.1002/9780470015902.a0002567.pub2
5. Norsgaard H, et al. Distinction between differentiation and senescence and the absence of increased apoptosis in human keratinocytes undergoing cellular aging in vitro. Exp Gerontol. 1996;31:563–70.
6. Yaar M, Gilchrest BA. Ageing and photoageing of keratinocytes and melanocytes. Clin Exp Dermatol. 2001;26:583–91.
7. Lin JY, Fisher DE. Melanocyte biology and skin pigmentation. Nature. 2007;445:843–50.
8. Berge U, et al. Sugar-induced premature aging and altered differentiation in human epidermal keratinocytes. Ann NY Acad Sci. 2007;1100:524–9.
9. Berge U, et al. Kinetin-induced differentiation of normal human keratinocytes undergoing aging in vitro. Ann NY Acad Sci. 2006;1067:332–6.
10. Berge U, et al. Hormetic modulation of differentiation of normal human epidermal keratinocytes undergoing replicative senescence in vitro. Exp Gerontol. 2008;43:658–62.
11. Tran SL, et al. Absence of distinguishing senescence traits in human melanocytic nevi. J Invest Dermatol. 2012;132:2226–34.
12. Cristofalo VJ, et al. Replicative senescence: a critical review. Mech Ageing Dev. 2004;125:827–48.
13. Packer L, Fuehr K. Low oxygen concentration extends the lifespan of cultured human diploid cells. Nature. 1977;267:423–5.
14. Chen Q, et al. Oxidative DNA damage and senescence of human diploid fibroblast cells. Proc Natl Acad Sci U S A. 1995;92:4337–41.
15. Holly AC, et al. Comparison of senescence-associated miRNAs in primary skin and lung fibroblasts. Biogerontology. 2015;16(4):423–34.
16. Macieira-Coelho A. Ups and downs of aging studies in vitro: the crooked path of science. Gerontology. 2000;46:55–63.
17. Terman A, et al. Autophagy, organelles and ageing. J Pathol. 2007;211:134–43.
18. Swanson EC, et al. Higher-order unfolding of satellite heterochromatin is a consistent and early event in cell senescence. J Cell Biol. 2013;203:929–42.
19. Demirovic D, et al. Basal level of autophagy is increased in aging human skin fibroblasts in vitro, but not in old skin. PLoS One. 2015;10:e0126546.
20. Waldera Lupa DM, et al. Characterization of skin aging-associated secreted proteins (SAASP) produced by dermal fibroblasts isolated from intrinsically aged human skin. J Invest Dermatol. 2015;135:1954–68.
21. Campisi J. Senescent cells, tumor suppression, and organismal aging: good citizens, bad neighbors. Cell. 2005;120:513–22.
22. Blagosklonny MV, Campisi J. Cancer and aging: more puzzles, more promises? Cell Cycle. 2008;7:2615–8.
23. Dimri GP, et al. A biomarker that identifies senescent human cells in culture and in aging skin in vivo. Proc Natl Acad Sci U S A. 1995;92:9363–7.
24. Yang NC, Hu ML. The limitations and validities of senescence associated-b-galactosidase activity as an aging marker for human foreskin fibroblast Hs68 cells. Exp Gerontol. 2005;40:813–9.
25. Rubin H. The disparity between human cell senescence in vitro and lifelong replication in vivo. Nat Biotechnol. 2002;20:675–81.
26. Giangreco A, et al. Epidermal stem cells are retained in vivo throughout skin aging. Aging Cell. 2008;7:250–9.
27. Youn SW, et al. Cellular senescence induced loss of stem cell proportion in the skin in vitro. J Dermatol Sci. 2005;35:113–23.
28. Sejersen H, Rattan SIS. Dicarbonyl-induced accelerated aging in vitro in human skin fibroblasts. Biogerontology. 2009;10:203–11.
29. Collado M, et al. Cellular senescence in cancer and aging. Cell. 2007;130:223–33.
30. Rattan SIS, Clark BFC. Kinetin delays the onset of ageing characteristics in human fibroblasts. Biochem Biophys Res Commun. 1994;201:665–72.
31. McFarland GA, Holliday R. Retardation of the senescence of cultured human diploid fibroblasts by carnosine. Exp Cell Res. 1994;212:167–75.
32. Lima CF, et al. Curcumin induces heme oxygenase-1 in normal human skin fibroblasts through redox signaling: relevance for anti-aging intervention. Mol Nutr Food Res. 2011;55:430–42.

33. Demirovic D, Rattan SIS. Curcumin induces stress response and hormetically modulates wound healing ability of human skin fibroblasts undergoing ageing in vitro. Biogerontology. 2011;12:437–44.
34. Rattan SIS, et al. Hormesis-based anti-aging products: a case study of a novel cosmetic. Dose Response. 2013;11:99–108.
35. Rattan SIS. Hormesis in aging. Ageing Res Rev. 2008;7:63–78.
36. Rattan SIS. Hormetic modulation of aging in human cells. In: Le Bourg E, Rattan SIS, editors. Mild stress and healthy aging: applying hormesis in aging research and interventions. Dordrecht: Springer; 2008. p. 81–96.

Glycation and Skin Aging

96

Herve Pageon, Helene Zucchi, Paula C. Pennacchi, and
Daniel Asselineau

Contents

H. Pageon (✉) • H. Zucchi • D. Asselineau
L'Oreal, Research and Innovation, Aulnay-sous-bois, France
e-mail: hpageon@rd.loreal.com; hzucchi@rd.loreal.com; dasselineau@rd.loreal.com

P.C. Pennacchi
Department of Clinical Chemistry and Toxicology, School of Pharmaceutical Sciences, University of Sao Paulo, Sao Paulo, Brazil
e-mail: paulapennacchi@gmail.com

M.A. Farage et al. (eds.), *Textbook of Aging Skin*,
DOI 10.1007/978-3-662-47398-6_128

Abstract

Our skin, just like our whole body is submitted to aging. Important changes occur: skin gets dryer, thinner, age spots appear. It becomes less elastic and more rigid, fine lines and wrinkles appear, and complexion changes. Skin aging is characterized by all these visible signs, which depend on many factors. One of them has been studied for many years and is known to be one of the mechanisms involved in body aging: the glycation reaction.

One of the causes of skin aging is the appearance of AGEs (advanced glycosylation end roducts). AGEs cause biomecanics properties alterations and biological changes involving activation of synthesis of molecules (macromolecules of the extracellular matrix, cytokines) and the activation of the matrix metalloproteinases or MMPs (matrix-degrading enzymes). The effect of UV on some AGEs (e.g., pentosidine) generates reactive oxygen species (ROS) in the matrix with induced additional deleterious effects. AGEs can be formed intracellularly also and consequently change the biological homeostasis of the cell. Taken together, these modifications induced by AGEs stress the importance of glycation in skin aging.

Introduction

Our skin, just like our whole body, is submitted to aging. Important changes occur: skin gets dryer, thinner, age spots appear. It becomes less elastic and more rigid, fine lines and wrinkles appear, and complexion changes. Skin aging is characterized by all these visible signs, which depend on many factors. One of them has been studied for many years and is known to be one of the mechanisms involved in body aging: the glycation reaction. Indeed, the glycation reaction leads to products called AGEs (advanced glycosylation end products) known to form crosslinks and to accumulate in tissues. The nonenzymatic glycation of proteins is a common factor in the pathophysiology related to aging disorders and diseases such as diabetes mellitus (DM). In elderly subjects, the nonenzymatic glycation is high, not only because of possible hyperglycemia but also due to long-term exposure to normoglycemic conditions. The glycation of proteins has been described at a cutaneous level [1] and in organs such as the kidney, blood vessels, and lens [2].

The Glycation Reaction

This reaction is also known as the Maillard reaction described in the early 1900s by Louis Camille Maillard. Maillard discovered that amino acids heated in the presence of reducing sugars developed a yellow-brown coloration [3].

The reaction of glycation is a nonenzymatic reaction between sugar and free amine function of amino acids (lysine, arginine) in proteins. This reaction occurs not only in the skin. Indeed, AGEs (advanced glycation end products) are also found in the kidney, lens, vessels, etc. This reaction takes place in proteins with long half-life and/or low renewal.

In 1981, Monnier and Cerami connect the browning reaction in nonenzymatic glycosylation of proteins (for the reaction occurring between glucose and the amino groups of proteins without intervention of enzyme) with glycation in aging of the lens, collagen, and more generally of the extracellular matrix [4].

There are several factors that can modulate the accumulation of AGEs: renewal of proteins, concentration and type of molecule, availability and reactivity of amino acids on protein to initiate the reaction, degradation of AGEs, and their removal by the body [5].

Mechanism of the Glycation Reaction

The aldehydic group of the reducing sugar such as glucose reacts with a free amino group of amino acid (lysine, arginine) proteins. This reaction leads to unstable Schiff base which turns into Amadori product (which will undergo rearrangements and fragmentation) to eventually

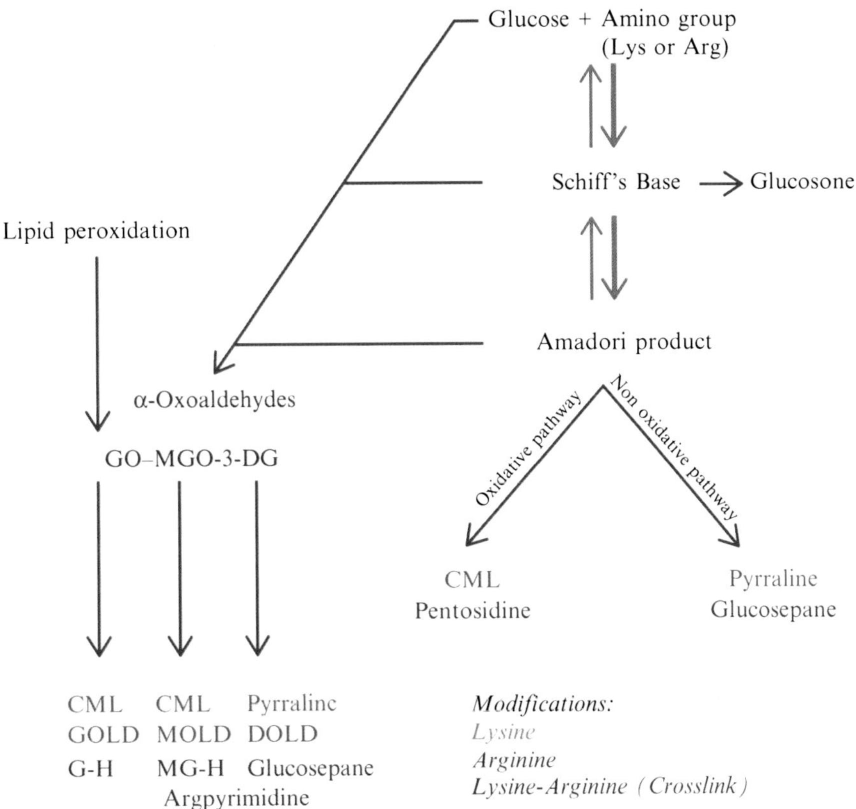

Fig. 1 Schematic representation of glycation reaction. *CML* carboxymethyl-lysine, *CEL* carboxyethyl-lysine, *GOLD* glyoxal-lysine dimer, *MOLD* methylglyoxal- lysine dimer, *DOLD* 3-deoxyglucosone-lysine dimer, *G-H* G-hyydroimidazolone, *MG-H* MG-hydroimidazolone, *GO* glyoxal, *MGO* methylglyoxal, *3-DG* 3-deoxyglucosone (Adapted from Singh [28, 29])

produce advanced glycosylation end products or AGEs.

There are different metabolic pathways that can lead to the appearance of AGEs. Briefly, there are three steps in the glycation reaction: an early stage which consists in the formation of a Schiff base, an intermediate step in which are found intermediate molecules known as "propagators," and at the end the formation of AGEs (Fig. 1).

Many AGEs have been identified to date. Structures are varied, forming linear chains or cyclic structures on the surface of proteins or even crosslinks between two protein chains (Fig. 2). The same AGE and intermediate product can be produced from various metabolites. The intermediate products such as glyoxal, methylglyoxal, and 3-deoxyglucosone (3 DG) are known as the dicarbonyl compounds or oxoaldehydes [6–8]. Methylglyoxal (MGO) can be generated by glycolysis, oxidation of threonine, ketone groups [9] or ascorbic acid [10]. 3-DG is formed by a nonoxidative rearrangement and hydrolysis of the product of Amadori [8] and by the fructose-3-phosphate, which is a metabolite of the polyols pathway [11]. CML appears from the oxidation of the Amadori product (fructose-lysine) catalyzed by transition metals or peroxynitrite, ascorbic acid, lipid peroxidation, and different pathways involving the formation of glyoxal and glycoaldehyde [12]. The pentosidine is formed with pentose, ascorbic acid, or by oxidation and fragmentation of the fructose-lysine [13, 14]. The nature of the

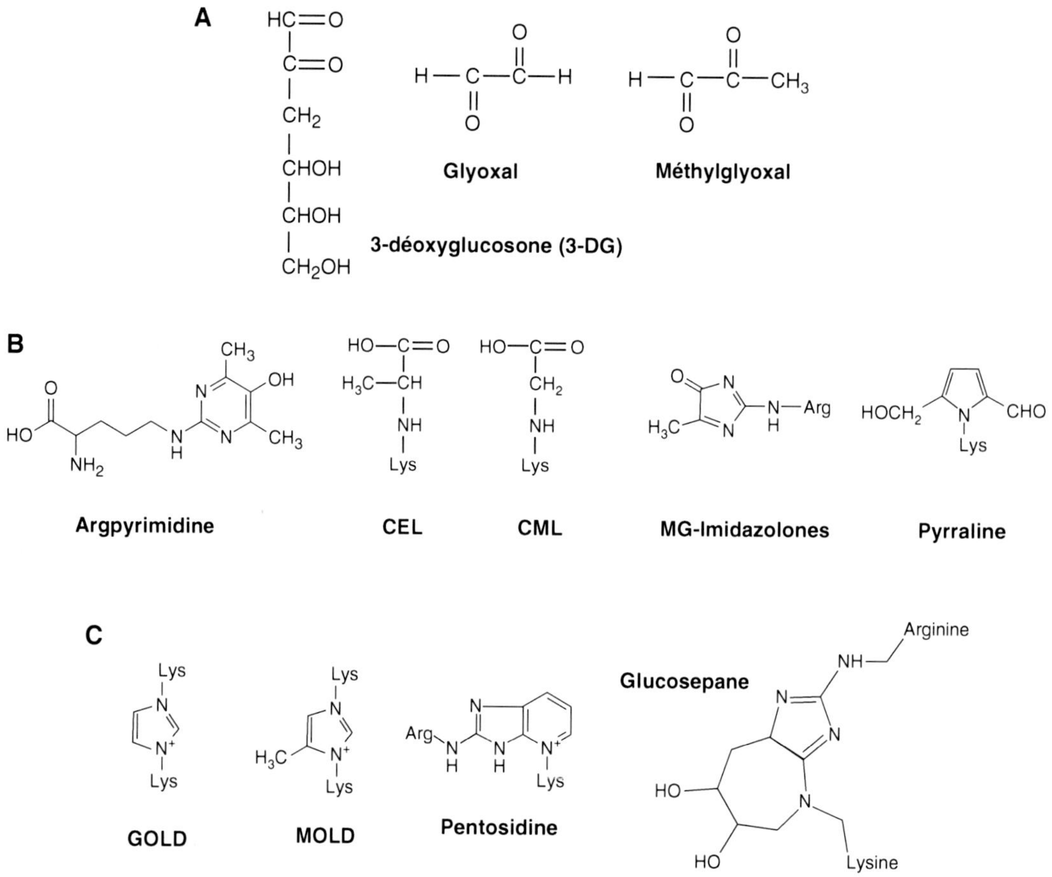

Fig. 2 **Chemical structure of α-oxoaldehydes and AGEs identified in skin.** (**a**) Carbonyls group or α-oxoaldehydes which lead to AGEs. (**b**) AGEs without crosslinks. (**c**) AGEs with crosslinks

metabolite and the oxidative environment is an important parameter to be considered in the development of the glycation end products. The formation of AGEs can be catalyzed by metals of transitions [15].

In addition, it should be noted that compounds such as methylglyoxal or deoxyglucosone derivatives in interaction with lysine can produce the allysine which in the presence of hydrogen peroxide (H_2O_2) leads to 2-aminoadipic acid stable by oxidation [16] and the decarbamylation of arginine product form ornithine which accumulates with age [17]. Ornithine is the deguanidinylation product of arginine resulting from the reaction with oxoaldehydes including methylglyoxal, glyoxal, and also the glucosepane. Ornithine can be produced from different AGEs involving arginine [18].

Glycation Modulation by Oxidative Stress

The majority of the steps leading to glycation end products is accompanied by an oxidative stress (except apparently the pathway leading to glucosepane [19]) and often referred to as glycoxidation [20]. The glycation reaction generates oxygen radicals in the initial, intermediate, and advanced steps. The Amadori product and glycated proteins can react with oxygen to form superoxide ion [21] or hydrogen peroxide [22]. Namiki described unstable imine formed in the initial steps of the reaction likely to be oxidized and to lead to the appearance of oxoaldehydes [23] such as glyoxal, methylglyoxal, and 3-deoxyglucosone. Oxidation of glucose (catalyzed by transition metals) can generate hydrogen peroxide and cetoaldehydes [24].

Glycation pathways lead to AGE compounds some of which are common to those derived from lipid peroxidation and especially polyunsaturated fatty acids (named ALEs for advanced lipoxydation products) [25, 26]. CML may serve as a biomarker of general oxidative stress resulting from both carbohydrate and lipid oxidation reactions [27].

The RAGE Receptor (Advanced Glycation End-Products Receptor)

AGEs have the ability to bind to specific membrane proteins [28]. There are several types of receptors for AGEs: AGE receptor 1 or AGE-R1 (protein OST-48, complex oligosaccharyl transferase). AGE-R1 is able to bind AGEs, remove oxidative stress [30] and the induced inflammatory response [31]. Copurified with AGE-R1, AGE-R2 (protein 80 K - H, membrane substrate of protein kinase) has been described as a protein involved in intracellular signaling of multiple receptors [32]. AGE-R2 was found associated with another protein that can bind AGEs: AGE-R3 (Galectin 3). AGE-R3 performs different functions including the internalization and degradation of AGEs [33]. Recently, an inverse correlation between Galectin 3 and AGEs localization in human skin was described, suggesting a protection against accumulation of AGEs in wound healing [34]. AGE-R3 is colocalized with AGE-R1 and AGE-R2 and are overexpressed in contact with AGEs [35]. Macrophage scavenger receptor (MSR) enables macrophagic cells to internalize and degrade the AGEs. The MSR are of two types: MSR-AII (macrophage scavenger receptor class A type II) [36] and MSR-BI (class B scavenger receptor type I), or CD36 [37].

However, the well-known receptor and probably the most studied is RAGE, the receptor for AGEs (Fig. 3). RAGE is a member of the immunoglobulin superfamily. The extracellular domain of RAGE is composed by one variable part (V) and two constant parts (C). The RAGE is a multiligand receptor: CML, AGE peptides, AOPPs (advanced oxidation protein products), HMGB1, S100A12/B/A6, amyloid β products [38]. The cytoplasmic domain of RAGE is linked to the extracellular domain by a simple membrane domain. The intracellular domain is short (< amino acids 50) and highly charged. This cytoplasmic domain binds to diaphanous-1 (mDia-1 or mammalian diaphanous-1), a binding which is required for cell activation after binding AGEs-RAGE [38] (Fig. 3a). The extracellular domain of the RAGE can be cleaved via the action of ADAM10 (A Disintegrine And Metallopeptidase 10) and releases the soluble receptor (sRAGE). A second soluble receptor, esRAGE (endogenous secretory RAGE), can be released resulting from alternative splicing of mRNA coding for the RAGE (Fig. 3b). sRAGE and esRAGE are supposed to act as a decoy receptor for AGEs (competitive binding of AGEs) and could facilitate their elimination. sRAGE would decrease the binding between AGEs and the cell surface, therefore preventing the activation of the cell. The binding AGEs-RAGE leads to a loop of activation, in which inflammatory stimuli activate NFκB, which induces the expression of RAGE, followed again by NFκB activation. NFκB stimulates multiple cell signaling pathways that lead to increased production of many growth factors and cytokines, influence cell growing, gene expression, inflammation, and extracellular matrix synthesis [38–40] (Fig. 3c). RAGE activation induces also oxidative stress by activating NADPH-oxidase, decreasing SOD, catalase activity, and also GSH (intracellular antioxidative systems) which by consequence reduces Glo1 activity [41–42]. The stimulation of esRAGE, the increasing of sRAGE, and blocking of mDia-1 link could be opportunities to inhibit the response of the cell to AGEs. Recently it has been shown that high levels of sRAGE were correlated with longevity of humans [43].

Glycation in Skin

One of the causes of skin aging is the appearance of AGEs (advanced glycosylation end products). AGEs cause biological changes involving activation of synthesis of molecules (macromolecules of

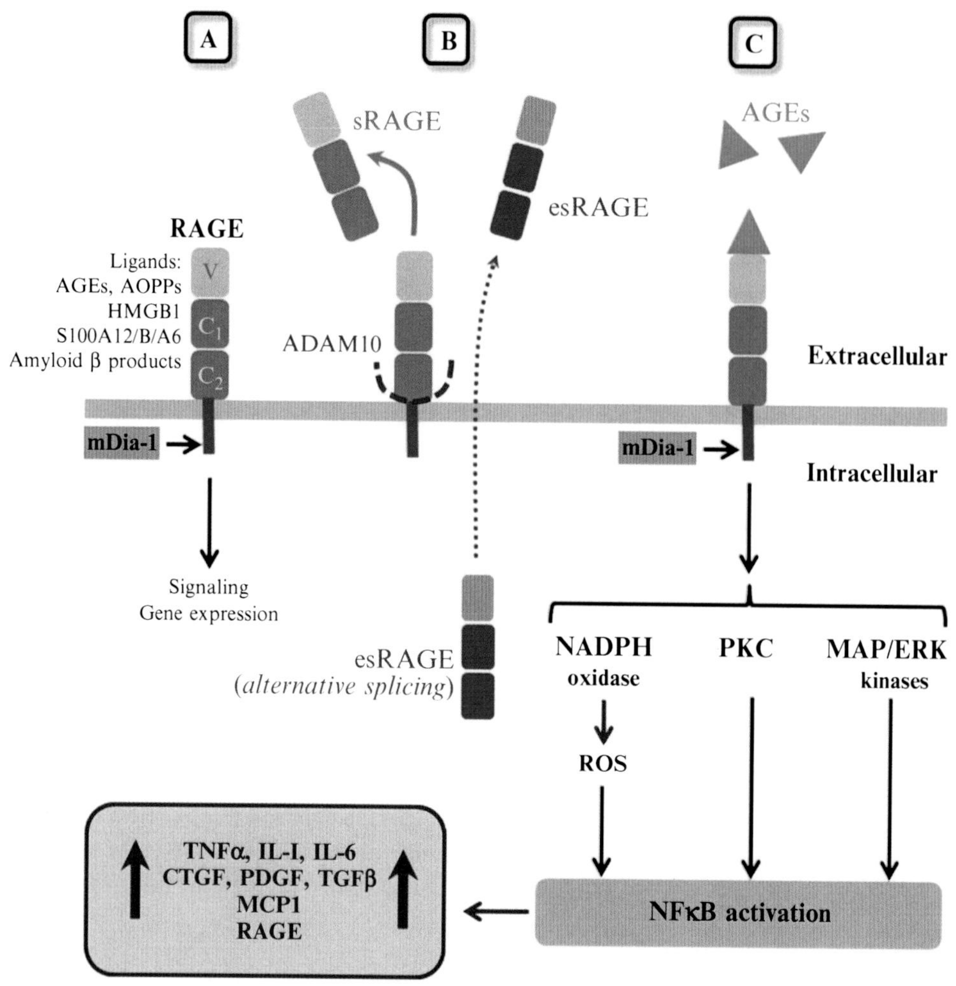

Fig. 3 Schematic representation of Advanced Glycation End Products Receptor: RAGE. Modulation, signaling pathways, and consequences. (**a**) RAGE structure. (**b**) Soluble RAGE. (**c**)Signaling pathways and consequences (Adapted from Yan [38] and Barlovic [40])

the extracellular matrix, cytokines) and the activation of the matrix metalloproteinases or MMPs (matrix-degrading enzymes). The effect of UV on some AGEs (e.g., pentosidine) generates reactive oxygen species (ROS) in the matrix with induced additional deleterious effects. AGEs can be formed intracellularly also and consequently change the biological homeostasis of the cell.

Accumulation of AGEs in Skin

AGEs are known to accumulate in human skin during chronological aging [44]. This accumulation of AGEs in tissues may also be dependent of the protein turnover. Thus in human skin, the fact that collagen has a half-life of 15 years makes it a potential target for the reaction of glycation and accordingly for the accumulation of AGEs [45]. Verzijl has shown using HPLC analysis that the appearance of AGEs in skin seems to be linear during chronological aging. This observation has been confirmed using AGEs immunostaining [46] and by autofluorescence measurement of skin using AGE-Reader which is correlated with the amount of pentosidine [47].

Previously, Sell showed that the accumulation of AGEs (pentosidine) in the skin was inversely proportional to longevity of the species, suggesting that the alteration of the processes controlling the speed of the collagen glycoxidation may be under genetic control, and within the same species according to the considered tissue (and renewal) the rate of accumulation of pentosidine is different [48]. In the skin, the quantities of CML, CEL, or pentosidine are increased by a factor of 3–4 between 20 and 80 years [45]. Glycation collagen accumulates at the rate of 3.7 % annually [49].

However, if the accumulation is linear, structures and levels may be different. All the structures identified as AGEs do not coexist in human skin. For example, the identification of the AGEs in human skin of subject aged 80 years allowed to highlight various structures (linear or crosslinking forming bonds between protein) [50]. The most important AGEs in concentration in skin (from the most highly concentrated to the least concentrated) are: glucosepane, fructosyl-lysine, CML, pentosidine, and CEL. If some AGEs are in significant quantities like glucosepane (on average 1000 pmol/mg protein), others on the contrary are in low concentrations, less than 10 pmol/mg protein (e.g., GOLD = glyoxal-lysine dimer).

If AGEs have been strongly evidenced in the dermis, they were recently observed in epidermis of human skin [51]. In addition to the chronobiological accumulation of AGEs, solar irradiation accelerates their formation [46, 52] (see section "Modulation of glycation by UV light").

AGES Alter Physical Parameters of Skin

Glycation is known to change the organization of collagen fibers and to induce expansion of the molecular packing of collagen [53]. The presence of AGEs in skin changes the mechanical properties thereof in part through the formation of crosslinks. It has been shown that mechanical parameters, using the multiaxial test mode, were altered in elderly diabetic (noninsulin-dependent diabetes mellitus) subjects compared to nondiabetic subjects of the same age (>74-year-old age group) [54]. This modification of the mechanical parameters is equivalent to that obtained in vitro by incubation for 4 weeks of normal human skin with 0.5 M glucose-6-phosphate [54]. The intermolecular crosslinks of adjacent collagen fibers changes its biomechanical properties [55]. More recently, Wilson et al. described that age-related intermolecular and intramolecular collagen crosslinks interfere with fibrillogenesis, change collagen monomer structure and macroscopic properties. Indeed, these modifications influence the ability of the cells to contract and remodel the collagen constructs [56]. This result was obtained with collagen from rat tail tendon; however, the process with human skin collagen should be similar. In 2008, Corstjens has suggested that the accumulation of AGEs in human skin of elderly subjects and/or overweight could contribute to loss of elasticity [49]. In dermal equivalents containing collagen modified by glycation and fibroblasts used in reconstructed skin models, the properties of contraction are also altered. Dermal equivalents containing collagen modified by glycation show a reduction of contraction as compared to control without glycation [57, 58]. In addition, intracellular glycation has also been shown to reduce collagen gel contraction [59]. In diabetic subjects of type 2, with an increase in the concentrations of fructose-lysine and pentosidine, the plantar skin shows an increase of its thickness and its elastic property is reduced compared to nondiabetic control group [60].

The formations of AGEs on chains of collagen change the global charge. In consequence, the contact with cells and proteins is altered and affect the structure reactivity [61].

Yoshinaga et al. show by optical microscopy that aggregates of CML-modified α-elastin are larger than the unmodified α-elastin. Comparison of the elastic modulus and rupture elongation between unmodified and CML-modified elastic fiber sheets reveals decreased elastic modulus and rupture elongation of the glycated sheets [62].

AGEs could also increase the yellowish change in the skin. In acellular dermis model only a slight yellowish change was produced by the treatment with 200 mM ribose or 10 mM glyoxal. [63].

If changes in the mechanical properties are essentially observed for the dermis or its equivalent, there are also changes in the epidermis. Indeed, the presence of AGEs has been reported in epidermis. Pentosidine identified in the stratum corneum modifies the viscoelasticity properties and could be implicated in the ulceration pathology [60]. Glycated stratum corneum and epidermis-dermis differentially regulate the permeability of hydrophilic molecules [64].

The mechanical changes of skin induced by AGEs thus participate in alterations in elastic properties of skin observed during aging.

Effects of AGEs on Skin Cell Viability

The CML-collagen injection into mouse skin (scalp site) triggers a process of apoptosis of fibroblasts at the site of injection [65]. The same authors also obtained this result with human dermal fibroblasts cultured in the presence of CML-collagen. A time course experiment determined that CML-induced apoptosis was not detected before 6 hours and increased after this time. In addition CML-collagen induced a dose dependent increase in fibroblast apoptosis mediated by RAGE. The CML-collagen-induced apoptosis is highly dependent on the presence of caspases 3, 8, and 9. In addition, after extraction of the fibroblasts cultured in the presence of CML-collagen, the level of mRNA coding for genes involved in apoptosis was altered (P53 gene was upregulated six-fold while Bcl-2 gene was downregulated by two-fold). The proapoptotic FOXO1 transcription factor induced by CML-collagen stimulated the fibroblast apoptosis and reduced by 75 % if FOXO1 is silenced [66]. The use of inhibitors helped to highlight that the CML-collagen-induced apoptosis was dependent on reactive oxygen species (ROS), of nitric oxide (NO), ceramide, p38, and JNK MAP kinase activation, inducing FOXO1 and caspase 3. Similar results involving the effect of the ROS inducing changes of proliferation and cell death have been reported [67]. In the culture medium of cultured fibroblasts in the presence of glyoxal and methylglyoxal, the concentration of hydrogen peroxide increases by a factor of 2 causing a growth arrest without apoptotic process [68]. The involvement of receptor RAGE and growth factor receptors (EGFR, FGFR-1, and FGFR-2) were likely to be involved in apoptosis and also in maintaining the effect after exposure to AGEs [67]. This is correlated with the results of Ravelojaona and colleagues that demonstrate a cytotoxic effect when fibroblasts are cultured in the presence of AGEs. This effect persisted when fibroblasts were transferred into a new medium devoid of glycation end products. The authors suggest that the persistence of the toxicity is maintained by RAGE [69]. However, recent results show that apoptosis is not necessarily due to the presence of RAGE. Indeed, 3-deoxyglucosone (3DG), a highly reactive precursor α-dicarbonyl of AGEs, induces oxidative stress and activation of caspase 3 without the intervention of the RAGE. Apoptosis induced by the 3DG would be via integrin $\alpha1\beta1$ [41].

AGEs could provoke cellular senescence. Indeed, as a function of passages, fibroblasts accumulate pentosidine and the number of cells decreases. These results suggest an alteration of antiglycoxidation defense systems of the cell when the passages increase allowing accumulation of pentosidine and altering the properties of fibroblasts [70]. When fibroblasts are submitted to AGEs and perform successive passages, β-galactosidase positive cells increase as compared to fibroblasts which were not in contact with the AGEs. The increase in the number of fibroblasts with a senescent phenotype is a function of the AGE contact time [71]. We showed in our laboratory that the type of AGEs can be important also in the cellular senescence process. Indeed, the exposure of fibroblasts to CML or MG-H1 during one week caused an increase in β-galactosidase positive cells after successive passages. The number of senescent cells increase according to the time spent in culture, as expected, and this increase is higher when the cells are preexposed to AGE products. It seems that the senescent potential effect was higher with MG-H1 as compared with CML (Fig. 4). Incubation of fibroblasts with glyoxal or methylglyoxal also causes this increase in senescence. The

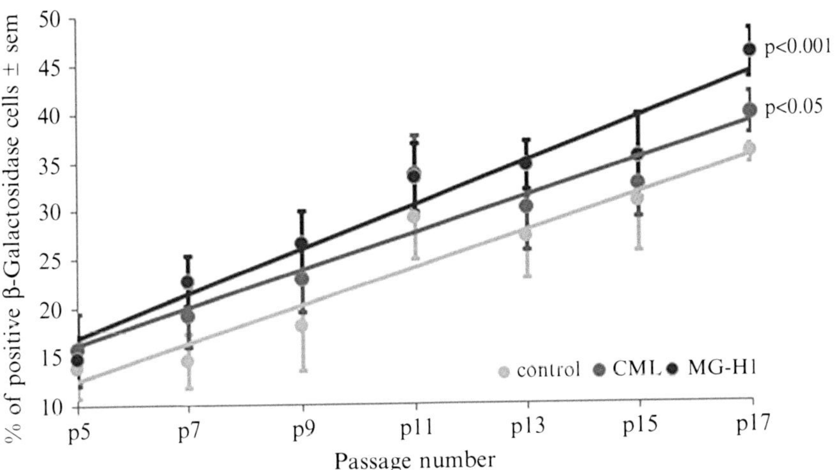

Fig. 4 Percentage of senescent cells (positive β-galactosidase cells) in function of passage number. Each point represents the mean of human skin fibroblasts cultures from four donors treated or not with CML (600 μM) or MG-H1 (600 μM) during 1 week before the successive passages

reversion of the phenomenon does not appear before 72 h after replacing fibroblasts in a new culture medium without AGEs [68]. Like fibroblasts, normal human keratinocytes show a decrease of viability in presence of glucose or glyoxal. The proportion of β-galactosidase-positive cells increased significantly in number by 52 % in 100 mM glucose and by 44 % in 100 μM glyoxal-treated keratinocytes and in the same time glycoxidation level of total proteins was 58 and 68 % higher, respectively [72]. The AGEs effect on the keratinocyte viability has also been reported and associated to loss of their migratory and proliferation abilities [73].

Solar irradiation can affect the viability also. The viability of dermal fibroblasts cultured in presence of AGEs and exposed to UVA is reduced [74].

This effect of AGEs on cell viability (senescence and apoptosis) is particularly important because it could contribute to cell loss observed during aging of the skin.

Effect of AGEs on the Synthesis of the Dermal Matrix and Epidermal Cells

The bibliography described essentially the glycation modifications on the collagens and elastin; however, any protein is susceptible to be modified and in consequence to participate to dermal dysfunction [46, 55, 62, 75]. Glycation end products affect the physiology of fibroblasts in terms of mRNA and protein expression. Indeed when fibroblasts are cultured in the presence of AGEs, the synthesis of extracellular matrix proteins is altered. Thus, the synthesis of collagen type I is increased by 28 % and synthesis of hyaluronic acid is reduced by 40–50 %. Modulation of this synthesis is based on the concentration of AGEs in the culture medium [76]. Unlike Okano et al. it has been observed a decrease in the synthesis of type I procollagen. The same authors also observed alteration of type I procollagen mRNA expression in the presence of β2 microglobulin or bovine serum albumin (BSA) as amended by glycation [77]. More recently, other authors have described other changes on the extracellular matrix mRNA expression using microarrays: downregulation of fibronectin, chain α2 of type I collagen, chain α1 of type III collagen, and decorin [78]. If Molinari described a reduction of these mRNAs, however, other authors observed overexpression of mRNA for the chain α2 of type I procollagen and chain α1 of type III procollagen [79]. Using a reconstructed skin system modified by glycation, an increase of type I procollagen [80], type III procollagen, and type VII collagen [81, 82] synthesis was also observed.

In addition, specific AGEs influence soluble factor releasing like growth factor or proinflammatory molecules [80]. VEGF (vascular endothelial growth factor) was reduced which could lead to the increasing scarcity of vessels reported in skin aging [83] or enhanced MCP1 (monocytes chemoattractant protein type I) known to be involved in matrix protein synthesis [84] or in inflammatory response [85, 86].

Indirectly, glycation in the dermis could modify the biology of epidermis. Indeed, a persistence of β1 integrin subunit was observed in the suprabasal layer of epidermis and an increase of α6 expression in the basal layer mediated by soluble factor synthesis from fibroblasts [58, 81]. These integrin subunits have been reported to be associated with epidermal stem cells [87], or a dedifferentiation process [88] or a hyperproliferative process [89].

Recently CML was detected in human epidermis associated with keratin 10 [51] and probably with other members of the keratin family [90]. Other authors identified previously the presence of glycated proteins in the stratum corneum of diabetic subject [91] and more specifically pentosidine in the stratum corneum of plantar epidermis [60]. As a consequence, AGEs could modify the epidermal physiology like keratinocyte migration [73]: by increasing MMP9 expression [92, 93], by induction of terminal differentiation markers [92], or by reducing the synthesis of antimicrobial peptides like defensin β2 and β3 [94, 95]. These modifications could be involved in wound-healing defect or infection in diabetic subjects.

It has been recently reported that changes in the dermal matrix caused by collagen I glycation also affects the epidermal compartment. Indeed, glycation of collagen induces the synthesis of carboxymethyllysine in both dermal and epidermal compartments. The aging phenotype consisting of poor stratification of epidermal layers and vacuolization of keratinocyte cytoplasm, increasing expression of cell–cell adhesion markers, such as desmoglein and E-cadherin or upregulation of keratin 10 and 14 were observed in glycated skins [96]. Recently, a system of reconstructed skin treated by glyoxal to induce CML showed an alteration of capillary and nerve networks associated with a lack of both loricirin and filaggrin in epidermis reflected an epidermal terminal differentiation defect [97].

If all experiments show that the AGEs alter the expression and synthesis of extracellular matrix molecules, the results are not necessarily the same (either increased or decreased). This can be explained by the different AGEs structures generated in protein solutions modified by glycation. All these extracellular matrix molecules are essential actors in the stability of the dermal matrix and their alteration can change the balance and have a role in aging of the skin.

Effect of AGEs on the Degradation of the Dermal Matrix

AGEs can also modify the expression and synthesis of enzymes which are responsible for ECM degradation. AGEs has been showed to alter the elastase-type matrix metalloproteinase (ET-MMT) activity in human fibroblasts: ET-MMT activity was reduced in a dose-dependent manner (by −27 % and −41 % for 1.25 and 10 mg of AGEs per ml) while no effect was detected on the secretion of MMP1 in the culture medium. Dysfunctions of dermal fibroblasts are induced by AGEs [76]. The modulation of MMPs (matrix metalloproteinases) by AGEs in fibroblasts cultures was observed in another study. Indeed, Molinari et al. have observed an upregulation of mRNA coding for MMP8 and 9 (202 % and 160 %, respectively, as compared to the control) [78]. A decrease of mRNA MMP3 expression in fibroblasts has been observed after contact with CML [98] and also the MMP3 expression in in vitro skin 3D model containing CML in the dermis [80]. Using a 3D system, containing collagen modified by glycation and fibroblasts without keratinocytes, MMP1 synthetized by fibroblasts was decreased but no modification of pro-MMP2. However, MMP2 activation (observed by zymography method) was strongly inhibited by AGEs without modification of tissue inhibitors of metalloproteinase (TIMP-1 and 2) production [57]. In a full thickness reconstructed skin system, AGEs induced overexpression of MMPs synthesis and activity which could be correlated with a decrease of the thickness dermis probably degraded by these MMPs [81].

Concept of AGE's Biological Specificity in Skin

The AGEs family is characterized by different chemical structure like linear chain or cyclic structure or crosslinks between proteins. AGEs bound to lysine or arginine residues could have opposite effects concerning the expression of biological markers (blocking of Lys or Arg and/or leading to modifications of charge). Indeed, it seems that AGEs-crosslinks (like pentosidine) induce a downregulation of mRNA coding for matrix molecules [80] which could explain in part the volume reduction of dermal molecules which is observed during aging skin like collagen [99], proteoglycans, and glycosaminoglycans [100]. This concept of specific reactivity has been previously notified without structure identification. Indeed, Ohashi et al. described with monocytes a response depending on the BSA-AGE preparation. BSA-AGEs obtained after incubation with D-glyceraldehyde or D-glycoladehyde stimulate the RAGE expression and increase cytokine production while with BSA-AGEs obtained by methylglyoxal or glyoxal no effect are detected [101]. In the same way, fibroblasts cultivated in presence of methylglyoxal induce an upregulation of mRNA Col1A1, Col3A1, TGFβ1, and β1 integrin as opposed to incubation with 3-deoxyglucosone which provoke a downregulation of these mRNA [102]. In addition, Abe et al. demonstrated a different invasive potential with tumoral melanocytes in function of the AGEs preparation type [103]. In addition, our results seem to show a different effect concerning the senescence intensity when human dermal fibroblasts were cultivated in presence of CML or MG-H1 (Fig. 4).

Glycation and the Monocyte Lineage in Skin

The effect of AGEs on monocytes and macrophages has been studied; the most important effects are proliferation, apoptosis, and differentiation. Hou et al. reported that AGEs delayed apoptosis of monocytes and induced monocytic differentiation into macrophage morphology [104]. Also, dendritic cell maturation of monocyte-derived cells by AGEs was reported [105]. AGES could affect the number of monocyte-derived cells ($CD45^+$, CD14+) in the dermis and lead to dendritic cells/macrophages differentiation [106]. Interestingly, Gunin et al. observed a monocyte cell increase in the dermis with aging [107]. AGEs exert a chemotactic effect toward the monocytes [108] and endothelial cells in contact with AGEs released the chemokines MCP-1 – monocyte chemoattractant protein type 1 [109–111]. AGEs stimulate the synthesis of factors or proinflammatory cytokines by monocytes and macrophages [104, 111–114] or increase the extracellular matrix degradation induced by metalloproteinase, e.g., MMP-9 [115, 116]. Both receptors, SRA and RAGE were expressed by $CD14^+$ cells [106]. RAGE was reported to induce the secretion of MMPs [116, 117] and inflammatory factors by monocytes or macrophages [113, 114]. Overexpression of SRA suppressed RAGE-induced MAPK signaling, whereas RAGE activation in macrophages favors a proinflammatory phenotype in absence of SRA [118]. As a consequence, the accumulation of these cells in skin could favor an inflammation process, a loss of dermal matrix balance, and skin homeostasis.

Interaction of AGEs with Cell Membranes

AGEs seem to have an important interaction with cell membranes. After incubation of fibroblasts in the presence of AGEs, a level of AGEs in the cellular lysate associated to liposomes and an increase in membrane fluidity was observed [76]. In addition, the lactate dehydrogenase

(LDH) release from fibroblasts measured in the culture media in the presence of AGEs was found to be increased in a dose-dependent manner without affecting cell viability corresponding to a loss of membrane permeability.

AGEs and Intracellular Activity

If AGEs alter extracellular matrix in skin, also intracellular proteins are modified by AGEs products. Kueper et al. reported that vimentin (intermediate filament) was the major target for CML in human skin fibroblasts. Crosslinked by AGEs, vimentin was redistributed into a perinuclear aggregate. This rearrangement of CML-vimentin was identified as an "aggresome". The consequence was a reduction of contraction properties on collagen gel by fibroblasts. A treatment of fibroblasts by glyoxal exhibited CML modification in vimentin. Like this, the contractile capacity of three-dimensional collagen gel as compared to untreated fibroblasts was decreased [59]. In another study, the same author demonstrated that methylglyoxal induced also the aggregation of vimentin. Vimentin could be modified, not only by CML and CEL but also by pentosidine and pyrraline [119]. The accumulation of modified vimentin is observed in fibroblasts from human facial skin biopsies of aged donors [59]. The skin of the face being exposed to UV, we can hypothesize that these "aggresome" formations could be directly related to the oxidative stress induced by them via the generation of α-dicarbonyl compounds such as glyoxal. Interestingly, Shin et al. reported that expression of CML-vimentin increased in HDMEC (human dermal microvascular endothelial cells) during culture and passage, an effect which was reversed by intense pulsed light treatment [120].

AGEs can also modify other constituents of the cell. Indeed, the enzymatic activity of proteasome (intracellular proteolytic system involved in the removal of altered proteins) can be reduced by glycation after glyoxal treatment on dermal fibroblasts [121]. Also, the proteinase activities of the proteasome decline during aging, probably due to posttranslational modifications of the subunits forming the proteasome complex. An age-related increase in glycated α7 subunit of the proteasome was observed after serial passing of human skin fibroblasts [122]. Glycation of the proteasome has also been reported for keratinocytes. After glucose treatment, proteasome glycation increased by +61 % with a synchronous decrease of its activity (−44 %) [72]. AGE-modified proteins, with a decrease in proteasome activity and content, were found in keratinocytes from old donors [123].

Also alterations of antioxidant (SOD and Catalase) enzyme activities were observed [68, 124] with increased oxidative reactions in the cells.

In addition, HScP 70 (heat shock cognate protein 70) is a target for AGE modification in senescent human dermal fibroblasts [125].

DNA of the cells is also sensitive to glycation. To mimic the cellular carbonyl stress, keratinocytes and fibroblasts from human skin were cultivated in presence of glyoxal or methylglyoxal. Both dicarbonyl compounds caused growth inhibition of cells (concentration dependent) and in addition this treatment provoked CML accumulation in histones (<0.10 mmol CML/mol lysine from untreated and 1.3 mmol CML/mol lysine from glyoxal treated keratinocytes) and DNA strand cleavage. Interestingly, at the molecular level the effects of α-dicarbonyl compounds were different. Indeed, glyoxal caused DNA strand breaks, while methylglyoxal produced extensive DNA-protein crosslinking [126].

Modulation of Glycation by UV Light

It is now well known that ultraviolet radiations and especially UVA have a deleterious effect on dermis and fibroblasts [127]. The dermal extracellular matrix is sensitive to UVA. UVA induces an oxidant stress in the dermis environment which could be related to existing crosslinking on collagen [128]. In vitro, the viability of dermal fibroblasts cultured in the presence of AGEs and exposed to UVA decreases and the rate of lipid peroxides in fibroblasts and liposomes increases [74]. This loss of viability can be explained by the production of radical oxygen species like superoxide anion radicals ($\cdot O^-_2$) and hydroxyl radicals ($\cdot OH$) after AGEs irradiation. The hydroxyl radical is derived from the production of hydrogen peroxide after irradiation of AGEs via the Fenton reaction. Hydrogen peroxide (H_2O_2) increases in an AGEs concentration-dependent and UVA dose-dependent manner. Pentosidine-rich compounds exposed to UVA release H_2O_2 [129] and provoke cellular deleterious effects like cell damage leading to LDH accumulation outside the cell. In addition, the enzymatic system able to eliminate H_2O_2 declines with age. The activity of catalase in stratum corneum declines in an age-dependent manner on sun-exposed sites and the creatine kinase activity decreases after in vitro glycation by methylglyoxal [130], and in addition the inactivations of catalase and superoxide dismutase by sugars of different glycating abilities have been described [124].

Pentosidine is established as photosensitizer-AGEs because associated to UVA it leads to the formation of $_1O^2$. Consequently, AGE sensitization can be implicated in photodamage of glycated lens proteins and chronologically aged human skin. Photosensitization of skin cell as photooxidative stress by UVA-irradiation of AGE modified proteins has been demonstrated in cultured human skin fibroblasts and keratinocytes [131]. Due to accumulation of skin AGEs during aging, involvement of AGE photosensitization in skin photooxidative stress may contribute to UVA-induced photoaging and carcinogenesis. Accumulation of AGEs was enhanced with UV preirradiated DED and incubated with sugar [46]. In vivo, CML and pentosidine accumulation in sun-exposed skin especially in the aged group has been described. A vicious circle is envisioned in which the presence of AGEs in a tissue accelerates the formation of additional glycoxidation products following UV exposure [52]. Another study shows that AGE staining was increased in UV-exposed dermis as compared to UV-protected skin [132]. In the dermis of sun-exposed skin, the number and the intensity of CML positive cells in both fibroblasts and endothelial cells was higher compared to sun-protected site and significantly enhanced in older subjects [2]. Interestingly, low dose of UVA associated with the presence of AGEs in skin in vitro could provoke inflammation and matrix degradation by synthesis of IL1α and upregulation of mRNA MMPs [133].

In solar elastosis, a colocalization of elastin and CML has been observed [75]. The oxidation induced via ultraviolet could promote the emergence of CML (a glycoxidation product) at this particular zone. This accumulation of AGEs which correlates with the presence of elastin was also observed by Jeanmaire et al. [46]. The CML-modified elastin is more resistant to degradation by elastase [62]. After irradiation of in vitro skin containing AGEs, upregulations of mRNA coding for tropoelastin, elastase, and MMP12 were observed emphasizing the possible direct implication in the elastosis process [133]. In addition, in monolayer culture of fibroblasts we showed an increase of tropoelastin synthesis after stimulation by MG-H1. No effect was observed after CML stimulation (Fig. 5).

Also CML was detected in human epidermis associated with different members of the keratin family after UVB exposition [90]. AGEs were enhanced in the stratum corneum and in the nuclear of epidermal cells of UV-exposed as compared to UV-protected skin [132]. An age-dependent adaption and protective mechanisms of the epidermis has been suggested against sunlight-associated oxidative stress like CML formation [134].

RAGE in Skin Aging

The distribution pattern of AGEs receptor (RAGE) is modified in epidermis and dermis in function of chronological aging and photo-aging (sun-protected or sun-exposed site). In young skin from breast (sun-protected), RAGE was more expressed in the upper part of the epidermis and dermis as opposed to old donor where RAGE was preferentially expressed in lower parts. In the sun-exposed face (old donor) the distribution of

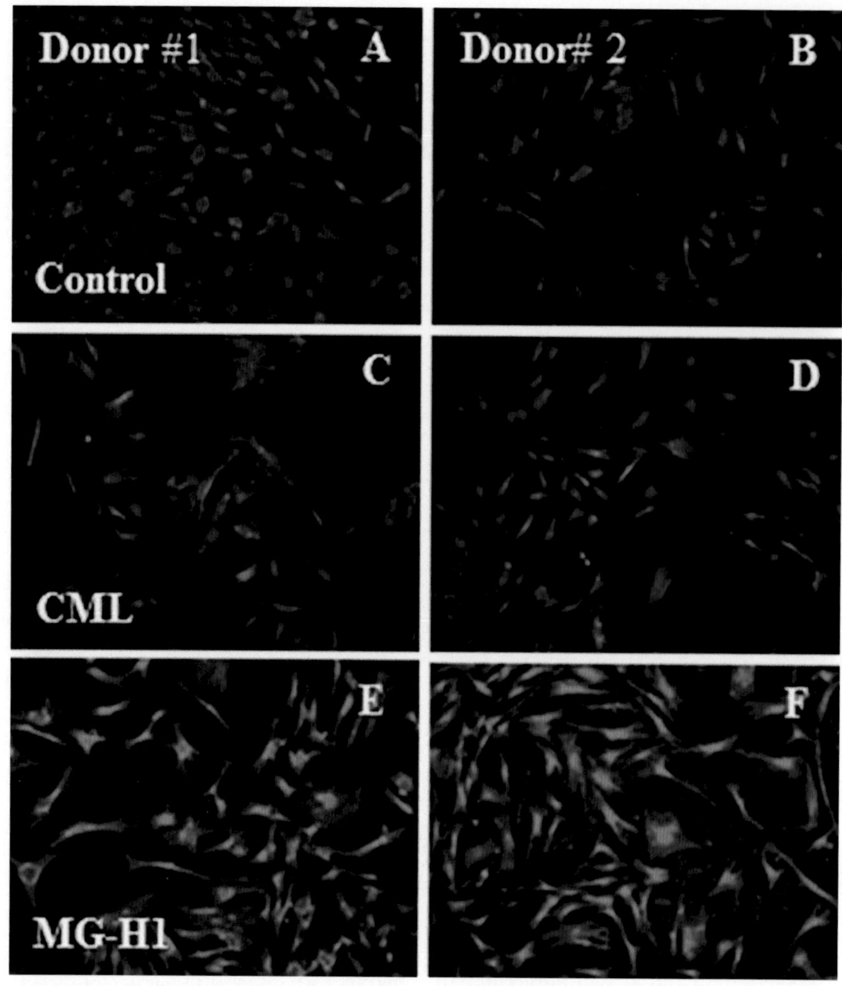

Fig. 5 Stimulation of the tropoelastin synthesis by AGEs. Immunostaining of tropoelastin (**a**–**f**) on human dermal fibroblasts from two different donors – donor#1 (**a**, **c**, **e**) and donor#2 (**b**, **d**, **f**) treated with CML (**c**, **d**) or MG-H1 (**e**, **f**) or without treatment (**a**, **b**). 100× magnification

RAGE was almost similar to old skin from breast except for the upper dermis where RAGE was more expressed which can be attributed to photo-aging. RAGE is highly expressed in skin and upregulated in sun-exposed sites [98]. Interestingly, human foreskin fibroblasts stimulated by CML and tumor necrosis factor-alpha (TNFα) resulted in upregulation of RAGE expression and CML induced profibrogenic markers like connective tissue growth factor (CTGF), transforming growth factor-beta 1 (TGFβ1), and chain α1 of type I procollagen. CML could not be the only AGEs structure responsible for the induction of RAGE. Indeed, Buetler et al. demonstrated that CML do not form the necessary structure to interact with RAGE. This could be explained by the method of CML preparation which would generate other structures which can react with RAGE [135]. Such observation was previously reported by Twigg et al. since CTGF was induced by AGE-BSA stimulated human dermal fibroblasts but not by the RAGE-specific ligand CML-BSA [136]. However, it was interesting to note that a weak expression of RAGE in fibroblasts [137] and absence of induction in the expression of mRNA RAGE in keratinocytes have been reported [92].

It was highlighted that the presence of AGEs could induce the differentiation of normal human keratinocytes (increase of keratin 10 and involucrin) and increases the expression of MMP9 via CD36 receptor expression (but not other types of receptors). This interaction could contribute to explain the mechanism involved in some pathologies related to diabetes such as perforating dermatosis (biopsies of these patients express strongly the CD36 and MMP9) [92]. A more recent study has also shown the involvement of AGEs in wound-healing defects related to diabetes via an increase in the rate of MMP9 (protein and mRNA) as shown on cultures of keratinocytes [73] mediated by RAGE, ERK1/2, p38MAPK pathways, and also activation of NFκB. In the mouse model, RAGE expression in keratinocytes is involved in acute inflammation and supports the role of RAGE in paracrine communication between keratinocytes and stromal immune cells like monocytes and macrophages [138]. Also RAGE was described to be involved in skin pathologies. Indeed, e.g., RAGE is involved in tumoral pathology like melanoma [103] or promoted the development of immune mediated disorders, like psoriasis, through the regulation of many proinflammatory genes [139]. Recently, the implication of RAGE in squamous cell carcinoma (SCC) has been described. The proliferation and migratory activity of normal keratinocytes and SCC was induced by S100A8/A9 and abolished by blocking RAGE [140].

Particular Case of Melanocyte/ Melanoma

AGEs could also influence melanocyte physiology. Indeed, an indirect effect mediated by MCP1 released by fibroblasts in contact with AGEs has been reported. Melanocyte MCP1 receptor could induce tyrosinase expression and increase activity [141]. In addition, upregulation of MCP1 mRNA [110] and MCP1 protein [142] is induced by endothelial cells after contact with AGEs. Previously, it has been described that in parallel with AGEs inhibition, a reduction of tyrosinase activity was observed, suggesting a possible relationship between them [143]. However, in the Japanese population, the AGEs index does not seem to indicate an alteration in the melanin amount [144]. More recently, Leblanc-Noblesse et al. described the correlation between AGEs and solar lentigo. In this study, CML was enhanced in the dermis of solar lentigo as compared to the adjacent photoexposed zone. Autofluorescence measurement (AGE Reader) of the skin was linked to depigmentation [145].

In pathologies such as melanoma (described in the mouse model), overexpression of RAGE might be responsible for the development of tumors and the metastatic ability of cells; the use of anti-RAGE antibodies reduces this effect [103]. This observation has been reported more recently in humans in the case of melanoma where the expression of the RAGE and S100 ligand are strongly increased [146]. Also, binding extracellular S100P to RAGE or coupling the intracellular S100P with ezrin (a cytoskeletal protein) was involved in tumor growth, invasion, and metastasis. The coordinate upregulation of S100P, RAGE, and ezrin may provoke the malignant transformation of melanoma [147].

How to Fight Against AGEs?

Since AGEs are known to have an impact on aging and certain diseases (including diabetes-related), work has been undertaken in order to find ways to reduce the reaction of glycation, accumulation of AGEs, and its effects on tissues. Many dedicated publications [148–150] have detailed various molecules and strategies to protect from glycation. The main possibilities to protect from glycation with some examples are described below:

Prevention

Different types of strategies [149] or molecules [148] already exist to prevent glycation: (i) competition with protein amino groups (for example, aspirin can react with the amino group by acetylation, anti-inflammatory molecules like ibuprofen and diclofenac have a protective effect against glycation by protecting the enzymes from inactivation via the glycation as catalase for example); (ii) binding to the protein to reduce the accessibility of the amino group, the elimination of the open form of the sugar in the reaction of glycation (amino acids, polyamines, peptides as carnosine which can also react with the protein carbonylated and prevent the formation of crosslinks) and (iii) binding to a reactive intermediate to prevent the appearance of the terminal product (aminoguanidine can react with the product of Amadori thus blocking the following reactions. However, the aminoguanidine can also react directly with the sugar, to eliminate methylglyoxal and other dicarbonyls and to act as a chelator of metals. Another example is the metformin which could act by removing the intermediate reagents).

The use of plant extracts is also a source of glycation inhibitors, most often associated with antioxidant activities of the molecule families contained in extracts like blueberry. Using blueberry extract in reconstructed skin as glycation inhibitor, a return to a normal pattern concerning the biological markers previously modified by the presence of AGEs has been observed [58]. Flavonoids (antioxidants present in vegetal foods) at micromolar concentrations are very potent inhibitors of pentosidine formation in collagens [151]. Other vegetable substances containing the puerarine and chlorogenic acid have also inhibitory activity [152]. Consumable plants are also sources of AGEs inhibition (in vitro) like ginger, cumin, black pepper, green tea [153]. Tea polyphenols like epicatechin and theaflavin can also trap the methylglyoxal and reduce the accumulation of AGEs [154].

Crosslinks Breakers

Thiazolium salts have been studied and the first results suggested they were able to break crosslinks (especially of the di-ketone crosslinks) [155, 156]. If the exact mechanism of action remains disputed [157], experimental results showed a restoration of the flexibility of arteries after administration of thiazolium salts to animals characterized by experimentally induced diabetes [158].

Prevention of the Consequences of Glycation

Modulation of RAGE expression could be a means to reduce the incidence of AGEs [159]. For instance, nifedipine can inhibit overexpression of RAGE by removing the appearance of reactive oxygen species [160].

Intracellular Defense Systems

Several systems of defense against glycation are described in the literature. This role is played by several enzymes: the fructosylamine oxidase (amadoriases), fructosamine 3 kinase (FN3K), and the glyoxalase system.

Fructosylamine Oxidase or Amadoriases: Horiuchi has isolated fructosylamine oxidase (FAO) from *Corynebacterium* sp. [161]. Subsequently various FAO have been isolated and cloned from different microorganisms. It may be noted that two enzymes have been isolated from *Aspergillus* sp. (amadoriase I and amadoriase II). FAO oxidizes the Amadori product and generates H_2O_2. The Amadori product obtained after oxidation breaks down spontaneously through hydrolysis. The result is a free amine, glucosone, and H_2O_2. In higher organisms the FAO has not been identified. FAO can remove AGEs only from products with low molecular weight but is not active on the BSA glycated proteins as example. Two hypotheses can explain this activity: (i) small PM products can be easily placed near the active site of the enzyme and (ii) the charges brought by the protein affect the protein enzyme interaction [162].

Fructosamine 3-Kinase (***FN3K***): Szwergold identified 3-phosphate fructose in the lens of diabetic rats [163]. Then the fructoamine 3-kinase was identified from a lysate of erythrocytes [164]. Fructosamine 3 kinase phosphorylates Amadori products and generates 3-phosphate fructose which breaks down into a residue lysine, a phosphate and 3-deoxyglucosone (3DG). The fructosamine 3 kinase (FN3K) gene is expressed in all tissues. The enzyme was intracellular and ATP dependent; the deglycation of the product of

Amadori in the extracellular matrix is, therefore, not possible. The existence of a fructosamine 3-kinase-related-protein (FN3KRP) has been described in addition to the FN3K with a similar mechanism [165]. It can be assumed that the use of assets protecting these enzymes or their disappearance during the aging process (if this is the case) would be beneficial for the cell.

Glyoxalase: The glyoxalase system present in the cytosol of cells catalyzes the conversion of methylglyoxal in D-lactate via an intermediary S-D-lactoylglutathione [42]. The system consists of two enzymes, glyoxalase I (Glo1) and glyoxalase II (Glo2) and the GSH (glutathione). The main substrate of Glo1 is the methylglyoxal, but glyoxal(the hydroxypyrivaldehyde) and 4, 5-doxovalerate are also potential substrates. Glo1 and the glyoxalase system prevent the α-oxoaldehydes formation inside the cells. Enzymatic defense (glyoxalase) decreases during aging (particularly Glo1). Oxidative stress is closely linked with glycation because GSH depletion in oxidative stress also decreases activity in situ of Glo1 and thus increases the concentrations of glyoxal and methylglyoxal and therefore accumulation of AGEs as well as possible increase of radical oxygen.

In the aging of *C. elegans*, an accumulation of MG-H1 (methylglyoxal hydroimidazolone) in the mitochondria was observed. If Glo1 is stimulated, MG-H1 appearance is prevented and the life of *C. elegans* increases. If Glo1 is silenced the lifespan of *C. elegans* decreases. The decline of Glo1 with aging has been also highlighted in rodents and humans. The Glo1 activity is directly proportional to the concentration of GSH. In lens, the concentration of GSH decreases with age while MG-H1 increases, thus the protective role of GSH in aging is not only related to its antioxidant function but also its role as cofactor in the glyoxalase system. Recent results suggest that hyperglycemia could decrease the expression of Glo1 by increased activity and activation of RAGE [166, 167]. It was reported that the genomic expression of Glo1 is variable; therefore, the significance of the expression of Glo1 could be an important factor to be considered in research on aging.

DJ-1/PARK7

Recently has been reported a new antiglycating enzyme activity. This enzyme is DJ-1/PARK7. The Parkinsonism-associated protein DJ-1/Park7 is described as a multifunctional oxidative stress response protein. DJ-1 is a protein deglycase that repairs methylglyoxal- and glyoxal-glycated amino acids and proteins by acting on early glycation intermediates and releases deglycated proteins and lactate or glycolate, respectively [168].

Diet

It is established that the origin of AGEs in the body is not only endogenous but also exogenous. Glycation reagents (named glycotoxines) are present in aqueous tobacco extract and smoke in a form that can quickly react with proteins to form AGEs and this reaction is inhibited by aminoguanidine [169]. It is also known that food and the way used for cooking can be a source of exogenous AGEs by ingestion. Recently, Uribarri has published a list of foods with AGEs, named dAGEs for dietary AGEs. Heat (cooking mode) increases the formation of new dAGEs by ten- to hundredfold as compared to the raw food. The cooking mode or the use of acidic ingredients (e.g., lemon juice) can reduce the formation of the dAGEs [170].

If the cooking mode affects the appearance of AGEs, caloric restriction can also regulate the concentration of AGEs [171]. Animal caloric restriction studies have shown an increase in life expectancy, a decline in the rate of insulin and glucose [172], or even a reduction of oxidative damage [173]. In addition, some caloric restriction studies have been conducted in humans in whom a decrease of atherosclerosis risk, diabetes, and a reduction of inflammatory processes were observed [174]. Most of these changes can be linked to the reduction of the rate of glycation.

Taken together, these findings suggest that healthy diet associated with selected cooking modes could limit the addition of an exogenous supply of AGEs.

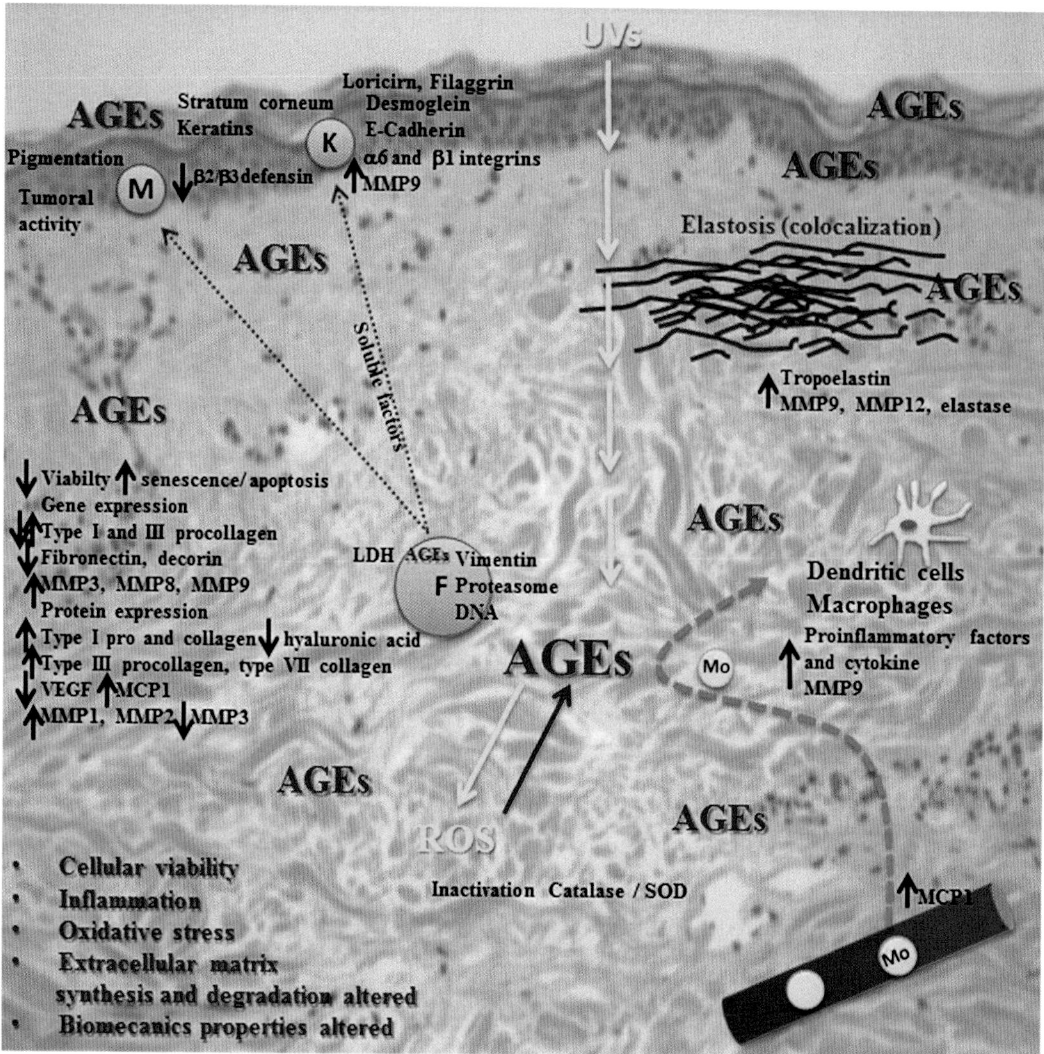

Fig. 6 **Schematic effects of AGEs in the skin**. *F* fibroblasts, *K* feratinocytes, *M* melanocyte, *Mo* monocytes, *LDH* lactate deshydrogenase, *MMP* matrix metalloproteinase, *VEGF* vascular endothelial growth factor, *MCP1* monocyte chemoattractan protein type 1, *ROS* reactive oxygen species

Conclusion

Taken together, these reports brought together in this chapter allow us to stress the importance of glycation in skin aging. Most skin alterations caused by AGEs (Fig. 6) are correlated with the major biochemical changes and signaling pathways involved in the generation of intrinsically and extrinsically aged skin [175]. Skin aging is characterized by the progressive degradation of skin components, the development of an inflammatory environment, and it's self-maintaining due to the progressive accumulation of AGE products.

References

1. Hofmann B, Adam AC, Jacobs K, et al. Advanced glycation end product associated skin autofluorescence: a mirror of vascular function? Exp Gerontol. 2013;48(1):38–44.
2. Crisan M, Taulescu M, Crisan D, et al. Expression of advanced glycation end-products on sun-exposed and

non-exposed cutaneous sites during the ageing process in humans. PLoS One. 2013;8(10):1–8. e75003.
3. Maillard LC. Action des acides aminés sur les sucres: formation des mélanoïdines par voie méthodique. C R Acad Sci. 1912;154:66–8.
4. Monnier VM, Cerami A. Nonenzymatic browning in vivo: possible process for aging of long-lived proteins. Science. 1981;211(4481):491–3.
5. Tessier FJ. The Maillard reaction in the human body. The main discoveries and factors that affect glycation. Pathol Biol (Paris). 2010;58(3):214–9.
6. Skovsted IC, Christensen M, Breinholt J, et al. Characterisation of a novel AGE-compound derived from lysine and 3-deoxyglucosone. Cell Mol Biol (Noisy-le-Grand). 1998;44(7):1159–63.
7. Wells-Knecht KJ, Brinkmann E, Wells-Knecht MC, et al. New biomarkers of Maillard reaction damage to proteins. Nephrol Dial Transplant. 1996;11 Suppl 5:41–7.
8. Baynes JW, Thorpe SR. Role of oxidative stress in diabetic complications: a new perspective on an old paradigm. Diabetes. 1999;48(1):1–9.
9. Thornalley PJ. Dicarbonyl intermediates in the maillard reaction. Ann N Y Acad Sci. 2005;1043:111–7.
10. Reihl O, Lederer MO, Schwack W. Characterization and detection of lysine-arginine cross-links derived from dehydroascorbic acid. Carbohydr Res. 2004;339 (3):483–91.
11. Sima AA, Sugimoto K. Experimental diabetic neuropathy: an update. Diabetologia. 1999;42(7):773–88.
12. Glomb MA, Monnier VM. Mechanism of protein modification by glyoxal and glycolaldehyde, reactive intermediates of the Maillard reaction. J Biol Chem. 1995;270(17):10017–26.
13. Grandhee SK, Monnier VM. Mechanism of formation of the Maillard protein cross-link pentosidine. Glucose, fructose, and ascorbate as pentosidine precursors. J Biol Chem. 1991;266(18):11649–53.
14. Dyer DG, Blackledge JA, Thorpe SR, et al. Formation of pentosidine during nonenzymatic browning of proteins by glucose. Identification of glucose and other carbohydrates as possible precursors of pentosidine in vivo. J Biol Chem. 1991;266 (18):11654–60.
15. Chappey O, Dosquet C, Wautier MP, et al. Advanced glycation end products, oxidant stress and vascular lesions. Eur J Clin Invest. 1997;27(2):97–108.
16. Sell DR, Strauch CM, Shen W, et al. 2-aminoadipic acid is a marker of protein carbonyl oxidation in the aging human skin: effects of diabetes, renal failure and sepsis. Biochem J. 2007;404(2):269–77.
17. Sell DR, Monnier VM. Ornithine is a novel amino acid and a marker of arginine damage by oxoaldehydes in senescent proteins. Ann N Y Acad Sci. 2005;1043:118–28.
18. Monnier VM, Sell DR. Prevention and repair of protein damage by the Maillard reaction in vivo. Rejuvenation Res. 2006;9(2):264–73.
19. Fan X, Sell DR, Zhang J, et al. Anaerobic vs aerobic pathways of carbonyl and oxidant stress in human lens and skin during aging and in diabetes: a comparative analysis. Free Radic Biol Med. 2010;49(5):847–56.
20. Dyer DG, Blackledge JA, Katz BM, et al. The Maillard reaction in vivo. Z Ernahrungswiss. 1991;30(1):29–45.
21. Gillery P, Monboisse JC, Maquart FX, et al. Glycation of proteins as a source of superoxide. Diabete Metab. 1988;14(1):25–30.
22. Jiang ZY, Woollard AC, Wolff SP. Hydrogen peroxide production during experimental protein glycation. FEBS Lett. 1990;268(1):69–71.
23. Namiki M, Hayashi T. A new mechanism of the Maillard reaction involving sugar fragmentation and free radical formation. In: Waller GR, Feather MS, editors. The Maillard reaction in foods and nutrition, ACS symposium, series 215. Washington DC: American Chemical Society; 1983.
24. Wolff SP, Jiang ZY, Hunt JV. Protein glycation and oxidative stress in diabetes mellitus and ageing. Free Radic Biol Med. 1991;10(5):339–52.
25. Baynes JW, Thorpe SR. Glycoxidation and lipoxidation in atherogenesis. Free Radic Biol Med. 2000;28(12):1708–16.
26. Fu MX, Requena JR, Jenkins AJ, et al. The advanced glycation end product, Nepsilon-(carboxymethyl) lysine, is a product of both lipid peroxidation and glycoxidation reactions. J Biol Chem. 1996;271 (17):9982–6.
27. Requena JR, Fu MX, Ahmed MU, et al. Lipoxidation products as biomarkers of oxidative damage to proteins during lipid peroxidation reactions. Nephrol Dial Transplant. 1996;11 Suppl 5:48–53.
28. Singh R, Barden A, Mori T, et al. Advanced glycation end-products: a review. Diabetologia. 2001;44 (2):129–46. Review. Erratum in: Diabetologia 2002; 45(2):293.
29. Sell DR, Monnier VM. Molecular basis of arterial stiffening: role of glycation - a mini review. Gerontology. 2012;58(3):227–237.
30. Cai W, He JC, Zhu L, et al. Advanced glycation end product (AGE) receptor 1 suppresses cell oxidant stress and activation signaling via EGF receptor. Proc Natl Acad Sci U S A. 2006;103(37):13801–6.
31. Lu C, He JC, Cai W, et al. Advanced glycation endproduct (AGE) receptor 1 is a negative regulator of the inflammatory response to AGE in mesangial cells. Proc Natl Acad Sci U S A. 2004;101 (32):11767–72.
32. Goh KC, Lim YP, Ong SH, et al. Identification of p90, a prominent tyrosine-phosphorylated protein in fibroblast growth factor-stimulated cells, as 80K-H. J Biol Chem. 1996;271(10):5832–8.
33. Vlassara H, Li YM, et al. Identification of galectin-3 as a high-affinity binding protein for advanced glycation end products (AGE): a new member of the AGE-receptor complex. Mol Med. 1995;1 (6):634–46.

34. Pepe D, Elliott CG, Forbes TL, et al. Detection of galectin-3 and localization of advanced glycation end products (AGE) in human chronic skin wounds. Histol Histopathol. 2014;29(2):251–8.
35. Stitt AW, He C, Vlassara H. Characterization of the advanced glycation end-product receptor complex in human vascular endothelial cells. Biochem Biophys Res Commun. 1999;256(3):549–56.
36. Matsumoto K, Sano H, Nagai R, et al. Endocytic uptake of advanced glycation end products by mouse liver sinusoidal endothelial cells is mediated by a scavenger receptor distinct from the macrophage scavenger receptor class A. Biochem J. 2000;352 (Pt 1):233–40.
37. Ohgami N, Nagai R, Ikemoto M, et al. Cd36, a member of the class b scavenger receptor family, as a receptor for advanced glycation end products. J Biol Chem. 2001;276(5):3195–202.
38. Yan SF, Ramasamy R, Schmidt AM. Soluble RAGE: therapy and biomarker in unraveling the RAGE axis in chronic disease and aging. Biochem Pharmacol. 2010;79(10):1379–86.
39. Bierhaus A, Humpert PM, Morcos M, et al. Understanding RAGE, the receptor for advanced glycation end products. J Mol Med (Berl). 2005;83 (11):876–86.
40. Barlovic DP, Soro-Paavonen A, Jandeleit-Dahm KA. RAGE biology, atherosclerosis and diabetes. Clin Sci (Lond). 2011;121(2):43–55.
41. Loughlin DT, Artlett CM. Precursor of advanced glycation end products mediates ER-stress-induced caspase-3 activation of human dermal fibroblasts through NAD(P)H oxidase 4. PLoS One. 2010;5 (6):1–15. e11093.
42. Xue M, Rabbani N, Thornalley PJ. Glyoxalase in ageing. Semin Cell Dev Biol. 2011;22(3):293–301.
43. Geroldi D, Falcone C, Minoretti P, et al. High levels of soluble receptor for advanced glycation end products may be a marker of extreme longevity in humans. J Am Geriatr Soc. 2006;54(7):1149–50.
44. Hipkiss AR. Accumulation of altered proteins and ageing: causes and effects. Exp Gerontol. 2006;41:464–73.
45. Verzijl N, DeGroot J, Thorpe SR, et al. Effect of collagen turnover on the accumulation of advanced glycation end products. J Biol Chem. 2000;275 (50):39027–31.
46. Jeanmaire C, Danoux L, Pauly G. Glycation during human dermal intrinsic and actinic ageing: an in vivo and in vitro model study. Br J Dermatol. 2001;145:10–8.
47. Meerwaldt R, Graaff R, Oomen PH, et al. Simple non-invasive assessment of advanced glycationendproduct accumulation. Diabetologia. 2004;47 (7):1324–30.
48. Sell DR, Lane MA, Johnson WA, et al. Longevity and the genetic determination of collagen glycoxidation kinetics in mammalian senescence. Proc Natl Acad Sci U S A. 1996;93(1):485–90.
49. Corstjens H, Dicanio D, Muizzuddin N, et al. Glycation associated skin autofluorescence and skin elasticity are related to chronological age and body mass index of healthy subjects. Exp Gerontol. 2008;43:663–7.
50. Monnier VM, Mustata GT, Biemel KL, et al. Cross-linking of the extracellular matrix by the maillard reaction in aging and diabetes: an update on "a puzzle nearing resolution". Ann N Y Acad Sci. 2005;1043:533–44.
51. Kawabata K, Yoshikawa H, Saruwatari K, et al. The presence of N(ε) (Carboxymethyl) lysine in the human epidermis. Biochim Biophys Acta. 2011;1814(10):1246–52.
52. Pageon H, Poumès-Ballihaut C, Zucchi H, Bastien P, Tancrede E, Asselineau D. Aged human skin is more susceptible than young skin to accumulate advanced glycoxidation products induced by sun exposure. J Aging Sci. 2013;1(3):1–5.
53. Tanaka S, Avigad G, Brodsky B, et al. Glycation induces expansion of the molecular packing of collagen. J Mol Biol. 1988;203(2):495–505.
54. Reihsner R, Melling M, Pfeiler W, et al. Alterations of biochemical and two-dimensional biomechanical properties of human skin in diabetes mellitus as compared to effects of in vitro non-enzymatic glycation. Clin Biomech (Bristol, Avon). 2000;15:379–86.
55. Avery NC, Bailey AJ. The effects of the Maillard reaction on the physical properties and cell interactions of collagen. Pathol Biol (Paris). 2006;54 (7):387–95.
56. Wilson SL, Guilbert M, Sulé-Suso J, et al. A microscopic and macroscopic study of aging collagen on its molecular structure, mechanical properties, and cellular response. FASEB J. 2014;28(1):14–25.
57. Rittié L, Berton A, Monboisse JC, et al. Decreased contraction of glycated collagen lattices coincides with impaired matrix metalloproteinase production. Biochem Biophys Res Commun. 1999;264:488–92.
58. Pageon H, Técher MP, Asselineau D. Reconstructed skin modified by glycation of the dermal equivalent as a model for skin aging and its potential use to evaluate anti-glycation molecules. Exp Gerontol. 2008;43:584–8.
59. Kueper T, Grune T, Prahl S, et al. Vimentin is the specific target in skin glycation. Structural prerequisites, functional consequences, and role in skin aging. J Biol Chem. 2007;282:23427–36.
60. Hashmi F, Malone-Lee J, Hounsell E. Plantar skin in type II diabetes: an investigation of protein glycation and biomechanical properties of plantar epidermis. Eur J Dermatol. 2006;16(1):23–32.
61. Haitoglou CS, Tsilibary EC, Brownlee M, et al. Altered cellular interactions between endothelial cells and nonenzymatically glucosylated laminin/type IV collagen. J Biol Chem. 1992;267(18):12404–7.
62. Yoshinaga E, Kawada A, Ono K, et al. N(ε)-(carboxymethyl)lysine modification of elastin alters

its biological properties: implications for the accumulation of abnormal elastic fibers in actinic elastosis. J Invest Dermatol. 2012;132(2):315–23.
63. Ogura Y, Kuwahara T, Akiyama M, et al. Dermal carbonyl modification is related to the yellowish color change of photo-aged Japanese facial skin. J Dermatol Sci. 2011;64(1):45–52.
64. Yokota M, Tokudome Y. Permeation of hydrophilic molecules across glycated skin is differentially regulated by the stratum corneum and epidermis-dermis. Biol Pharm Bull. 2015;38(9):1383–8.
65. Alikhani Z, Alikhani M, Boyd CM, et al. Advanced glycation end products enhance expression of pro-apoptotic genes and stimulate fibroblast apoptosis through cytoplasmic and mitochondrial pathways. J Biol Chem. 2005;280(13):12087–95.
66. Alikhani M, Alikhani Z, Boyd C, et al. Advanced glycation end products stimulate osteoblast apoptosis via the MAP kinase and cytosolic apoptotic pathways. Bone. 2007;40(2):345–53.
67. Peterszegi G, Molinari J, Ravelojaona V, et al. Effect of advanced glycation end-products on cell proliferation and cell death. Pathol Biol (Paris). 2006;54 (7):396–404.
68. Sejersen H, Rattan SI. Dicarbonyl-induced accelerated aging in vitro in human skin fibroblasts. Biogerontology. 2009;10(2):203–11.
69. Ravelojaona V, Péterszegi G, Molinari J, et al. Demonstration of the cytotoxic effect of Advanced Glycation Endproducts (AGE-s). J Soc Biol. 2007;201(2):185–8.
70. Sell DR, Primc M, Schafer IA, et al. Cell-associated pentosidine as a marker of aging in human diploid cells in vitro and in vivo. Mech Ageing Dev. 1998;105(3):221–40.
71. Ravelojaona V, Robert AM, Robert L. Expression of senescence-associated beta-galactosidase (SA-beta-Gal) by human skin fibroblasts, effect of advanced glycation end-products and fucose or rhamnose-rich polysaccharides. Arch Gerontol Geriatr. 2009;48(2):151–4.
72. Berge U, Behrens J, Rattan SI. Sugar-induced premature aging and altered differentiation in human epidermal keratinocytes. Ann N Y Acad Sci. 2007;1100:524–9.
73. Zhu P, Yang C, Chen LH, et al. Impairment of human keratinocyte mobility and proliferation by advanced glycation end products-modified BSA. Arch Dermatol Res. 2011;303(5):339–50.
74. Masaki H, Okano Y, Sakurai H. Generation of active oxygen species from advanced glycation end-products (AGEs) during ultraviolet light A (UVA) irradiation and a possible mechanism for cell damaging. Biochim Biophys Acta. 1999;1428:45–56.
75. Mizutari K, Ono T, Ikeda K, et al. Photo-enhanced modification of human skin elastin in actinic elastosis by N(epsilon)-(carboxymethyl)lysine, one of the glycoxidation products of the Maillard reaction. J Invest Dermatol. 1997;108(5):797–802.
76. Okano Y, Masaki H, Sakurai H. Dysfunction of dermal fibroblasts induced by advancedglycation end-products (AGEs) and the contribution of a nonspecific interaction with cell membrane and AGEs. J Dermatol Sci. 2002;29:171–80.
77. Owen Jr WF, Hou FF, Stuart RO, et al. Beta 2-microglobulin modified with advanced glycation end products modulates collagen synthesis by human fibroblasts. Kidney Int. 1998;53(5):1365–73.
78. Molinari J, Ruszova E, Velebny V, et al. Effect of advanced glycation endproducts on gene expression profiles of human dermal fibroblasts. Biogerontology. 2008;9:177–82.
79. Andreea SI, Marieta C, Anca D. AGEs and glucose levels modulate type I and III procollagen mRNA synthesis in dermal fibroblasts cells culture. Exp Diabetes Res. 2008;2008(473603):1–7.
80. Pageon H, Zucchi H, Dai Z, et al. Biological effects induced by specific advanced glycation end products in the reconstructed skin model of aging. Biores Open Access. 2015;4(1):54–64.
81. Pageon H, Bakala H, Monnier VM, et al. Collagen glycation triggers the formation of aged skin in vitro. Eur J Dermatol. 2007;17(1):12–20.
82. Pageon H, Zucchi H, Rousset F, et al. Skin aging by glycation: lessons from the reconstructed skin model. Clin Chem Lab Med. 2014;52(1):169–74.
83. Ranzer MJ, Dipietro LA. Impaired wound repair and delayed angiogenesis. In: Farage MA, Miller KW, Maibach HI, editors. Text book of aging skin. Berlin/Heidelberg: Springer; 2010. p. 897–907.
84. Gharaee-Kermani M, Denholm EM, Phan SH. Costimulation of fibroblast collagen and transforming growth factor beta1 gene expression by monocyte chemoattractant protein-1 via specific receptors. J Biol Chem. 1996;271(30):17779–84.
85. Goto M. Inflammaging (inflammation + aging): a driving force for human aging based on an evolutionarily antagonistic pleiotropy theory? Biosci Trends. 2008;2(6):218–30.
86. Latil A, Libon C, Templier M, et al. Hexanic lipidosterolic extract of Serenoa repens inhibits the expression of two key inflammatory mediators, MCP1/CCL2 and VCAM-1, in vitro. BJU Int. 2012;110(6 Pt B):E301–7.
87. Fortunel NO, Chadli L, Bourreau E, et al. Cellular adhesion on collagen: a simple method to select human basal keratinocytes which preserves their high growth capacity. Eur J Dermatol. 2011;21 Suppl 2:12–20.
88. Asselineau D, Bernard BA, Bailly C, et al. Retinoic acid improves epidermal morphogenesis. Dev Biol. 1989;133(2):322–35.
89. Bernerd F, Asselineau D, Vioux C, et al. Clues to epidermal cancer proneness revealed by reconstruction of DNA repair-deficient xeroderma pigmentosum skin in vitro. Proc Natl Acad Sci U S A. 2001;98 (14):7817–22.
90. Mori Y, Aki K, Kuge K, et al. UV B-irradiation enhances the racemization and isomerizaiton of

aspartyl residues and production of N-ε-carboxymethyl lysine (CML) in keratin of skin. J Chromatogr B Analyt Technol Biomed Life Sci. 2011;879(29):3303–9.

91. Márová I, Záhejský J, Sehnalová H. Non-enzymatic glycation of epidermal proteins of the stratum corneum in diabetic patients. Acta Diabetol. 1995;32(1):38–43.
92. Fujimoto E, Kobayashi T, Fujimoto N, et al. AGE-modified collagens I and III induce keratinocyte terminal differentiation through AGE receptor CD36: epidermal-dermal interaction in acquired perforating dermatosis. J Invest Dermatol. 2010;130(2):405–14.
93. Zhu P, Ren M, Yang C, et al. Involvement of RAGE, MAPK and NF-κB pathways in AGEs-induced MMP-9 activation in HaCaT keratinocytes. Exp Dermatol. 2012;21(2):123–9.
94. Lan CC, Wu CS, Huang SM, et al. High-glucose environment inhibits p38MAPK signaling and reduces human β-defensin-3 expression [corrected] in keratinocytes. Mol Med. 2011;17(7–8):771–9.
95. Lan CC, Wu CS, Huang SM, et al. High glucose environment reduces human beta-defensin 2 expressions in human keratinocytes: implications for poor diabetic wound healing. Br J Dermatol. 2012;166:1221–9.
96. Pennacchi PC, de Almeida ME, Gomes OL, et al. Glycated reconstructed human skin as a platform to study the pathogenesis of skin aging. Tissue Eng Part A. 2015;21(17–18):2417–25.
97. Cadau S, Leoty-Okombi S, Pain S, et al. In vitro glycation of an endothelialized and innervated tissue-engineered skin to screen anti-AGE molecules. Biomaterials. 2015;51:216–25.
98. Lohwasser C, Neureiter D, Weigle B, et al. The receptor for advanced glycation end products is highly expressed in the skin and upregulated by advanced glycation end products and tumor necrosis factor-alpha. J Invest Dermatol. 2006;126:291–9.
99. Varani J, Dame MK, Rittie L, et al. Decreased collagen production in chronologically aged skin: roles of age-dependent alteration in fibroblast function and defective mechanical stimulation. Am J Pathol. 2006;168(6):1861–8.
100. Oh JH, Kim YK, Jung JY, et al. Changes in glycosaminoglycans and related proteoglycans in intrinsically aged human skin in vivo. Exp Dermatol. 2011;20(5):454–6.
101. Ohashi K, Takahashi HK, Mori S, et al. Advanced glycation end products enhance monocyte activation during human mixed lymphocyte reaction. Clin Immunol. 2010;134(3):345–53.
102. Sassi-Gaha S, Loughlin DT, Kappler F, et al. Two dicarbonyl compounds, 3-deoxyglucosone and methylglyoxal, differentially modulate dermal fibroblasts. Matrix Biol. 2010;29(2):127–34.
103. Abe R, Shimizu T, Sugawara H, et al. Regulation of human melanoma growth and metastasis by AGE-AGE receptor interactions. J Invest Dermatol. 2004;122(2):461–7.
104. Hou FF, Miyata T, Boyce J, et al. beta(2)-Microglobulin modified with advanced glycation end products delays monocyte apoptosis. Kidney Int. 2001;59(3):990–1002.
105. Buttari B, Profumo E, Capozzi A, et al. Advanced glycation end products of human β_2 glycoprotein I modulate the maturation and function of DCs. Blood. 2011;117(23):6152–61.
106. Pageon H, Hubert S, Zucchi H, et al. Can glycation be involved in skin inflamm-aging? First elements of proof in reconstructed skin. 11th International symposium on the maillard reaction; 2012. p. 287.
107. Gunin AG, Kornilova NK, Vasilieva OV, et al. Age-related changes in proliferation, the numbers of mast cells, eosinophils, and cd45-positive cells in human dermis. J Gerontol A Biol Sci Med Sci. 2011;66(4):385–92.
108. Miyata T, Iida Y, Ueda Y, et al. Monocyte/macrophage response to beta 2-microglobulin modified with advanced glycation end products. Kidney Int. 1996;49(2):538–50.
109. Guo ZJ, Hou FF, Liang M, et al. Advanced glycation end products stimulate human endothelial cells to produce monocyte chemoattractant protein-1. Zhonghua Yi Xue Za Zhi. 2003;83(12):1075–9.
110. Xu SH, Wang KF, Xu CS, et al. Effect of atorvastatin on advanced glycation end products induced monocyte chemoattractant protein-1 expression in cultured human endothelial cells. Zhonghua Xin Xue Guan Bing Za Zhi. 2011;39(6):512–7.
111. Xu Y, Feng L, Wang S, et al. Calycosin protects HUVECs from advanced glycation end products-induced macrophage infiltration. J Ethnopharmacol. 2011;137(1):359–70.
112. Pertyńska-Marczewska M, Kiriakidis S, Wait R, et al. Advanced glycation end products upregulate angiogenic and pro-inflammatory cytokine production in human monocyte/macrophages. Cytokine. 2004;28(1):35–47.
113. Rashid G, Luzon AA, Korzets Z, et al. The effect of advanced glycation end-products and aminoguanidine on TNFalpha production by rat peritoneal macrophages. Perit Dial Int. 2001;21(2):122–9.
114. Sasaki T, Horiuchi S, Yamazaki M, et al. Induction of GM-CSF production of macrophages by advanced glycation end products of the Maillard reaction. Biosci Biotechnol Biochem. 1999;63(11):2011–3.
115. Poitevin S, Garnotel R, Antonicelli F, et al. Type I collagen induces tissue factor expression and matrix metalloproteinase 9 production in human primary monocytes through a redox-sensitive pathway. J Thromb Haemost. 2008;6(9):1586–94.
116. Zhang F, Banker G, Liu X, et al. The novel function of advanced glycation end products in regulation of MMP-9 production. J Surg Res. 2011;171(2):871–6.
117. Bao W, Min D, Twigg SM, et al. Monocyte CD147 is induced by advanced glycation end products and high glucose concentration: possible role in diabetic

complications. Am J Physiol Cell Physiol. 2010;299 (5):C1212–19.

118. Ma K, Xu Y, Wang C, et al. A cross talk between class A scavenger receptor and receptor for advanced glycation end-products contributes to diabetic retinopathy. Am J Physiol Endocrinol Metab. 2014;307 (12):E1153–65.
119. Kueper T, Grune T, Muhr GM, et al. Modification of vimentin: a general mechanism of nonenzymatic glycation in human skin. Ann N Y Acad Sci. 2008;1126:328–32.
120. Shin JU, Lee WJ, Oh SH, et al. Altered vimentin protein expression in human dermal microvascular endothelial cells after ultraviolet or intense pulsed light treatment. Lasers Surg Med. 2014;46(5):431–8.
121. Bulteau AL, Verbeke P, Petropoulos I, et al. Proteasome inhibition in glyoxal-treated fibroblasts and resistance of glycated glucose-6-phosphate dehydrogenase to 20S proteasome degradation in vitro. J Biol Chem. 2001;276:45662–8.
122. Gonzalez-Dosal R, Sørensen MD, Clark BF, et al. Phage-displayed antibodies for the detection of glycated proteasome in aging cells. Ann N Y Acad Sci. 2006;1067:474–8.
123. Petropoulos I, Conconi M, Wang X, et al. Increase of oxidatively modified protein is associated with a decrease of proteasome activity and content in aging epidermal cells. J Gerontol A Biol Sci Med Sci. 2000;55(5):B220–7.
124. Yan H, Harding JJ. Glycation-induced inactivation and loss of antigenicity of catalase and superoxide dismutase. Biochem J. 1997;328:599–605.
125. Unterluggauer H, Micutkova L, Lindner H, et al. Identification of Hsc70 as target for AGE modification in senescent human fibroblasts. Biogerontology. 2009;10(3):299–309.
126. Roberts MJ, Wondrak GT, Laurean DC, et al. DNA damage by carbonyl stress in human skin cells. Mutat Res. 2003;522:45–56.
127. Bernerd F, Asselineau D. UVA exposure of human skin reconstructed in vitro induces apoptosis of dermal fibroblasts: subsequent connective tissue repair and implications in photoaging. Cell Death Differ. 1998;5(9):792–802.
128. Ou-Yang H, Stamatas G, Kollias N. Dermal contributions to UVA-induced oxidative stress in skin. Photodermatol Photoimmunol Photomed. 2009;25:65–70.
129. Okano Y, Masaki H, Sakurai H. Pentosidine in advanced glycation end-products (AGEs) during UVA irradiation generates active oxygen species and impairs human dermal fibroblasts. J Dermatol Sci. 2001;27 Suppl 1:S11–8.
130. Corstjens H, Declercq L, Hellemans L, et al. Prevention of oxidative damage that contributes to the loss of bioenergetic capacity in ageing skin. Exp Gerontol. 2007;42:924–9.
131. Wondrak GT, Jacobson MK, Jacobson EL. Endogenous UVA-photosensitizers: mediators of skin photodamage and novel targets for skin photoprotection. Photochem Photobiol Sci. 2006;5 (2):215–37.
132. Mamalis A, Fiadorchanka N, Adams L, et al. An immunohistochemical panel to assess ultraviolet radiation-associated oxidative skin injury. J Drugs Dermatol. 2014;13(5):574–8.
133. Pageon H, Zucchi H, Asselineau D. Glycation combined with UVA exposure leads to a new model of skin aging in-vitro. 11th International symposium on the maillard reaction; 2012. p. 99.
134. Toyokuni S, Hirao A, Wada T, et al. Age- and sun exposure-dependent differences in 8-hydroxy-2'-deoxyguanosine and N-(carboxymethyl)lysine in human epidermis. J Clin Biochem Nutr. 2011;49 (2):121–4.
135. Buetler TM, Leclerc E, Baumeyer A, et al. N(epsilon) carboxymethyllysine-modified proteins are unable to bind to RAGE and activate an inflammatory response. Mol Nutr Food Res. 2008;52:370–8.
136. Twigg SM, Chen MM, Joly AH, et al. Advanced glycosylation end products up-regulate connective tissue growth factor (insulin-like growth factor-binding protein-related protein 2) in human fibroblasts: a potential mechanism for expansion of extracellular matrix in diabetes mellitus. Endocrinology. 2001;142:1760–9.
137. Sunahori K, Yamamura M, Yamana J, et al. Increased expression of receptor for advanced glycation end products by synovial tissue macrophages in rheumatoid arthritis. Arthritis Rheum. 2006;54(1):97–104.
138. Leibold JS, Riehl A, Hettinger J, et al. Keratinocyte-specific deletion of the receptor RAGE modulates the kinetics of skin inflammation in vivo. J Invest Dermatol. 2013;133(10):2400–6.
139. Mezentsev AV, Bruskin SA, Soboleva AG, et al. Pharmacological control of receptor of advanced glycation end-products and its biological effects in psoriasis. Int J Biomed Sci. 2013;9(3):112–22.
140. Iotzova-Weiss G, Dziunycz PJ, Freiberger SN, et al. S100A8/A9 stimulates keratinocyte proliferation in the development of squamous cell carcinoma of the skin via the receptor for advanced glycation-end products. PLoS One. 2015;10(3):18.
141. Yahagi S. Advanced glycation end products (AGEs) in the dermis trigger melanogenesis in epidermal melanocytes. Poster from 10th ASCS Korean; 2011.
142. Ishibashi Y, Matsui T, Takeuchi M, et al. Vardenafil, an inhibitor of phosphodiesterase-5, blocks advanced glycation end product (AGE)-induced up-regulation of monocyte chemoattractant protein-1 mRNA levels in endothelial cells by suppressing AGE receptor (RAGE) expression via elevation of cGMP. Clin Exp Med. 2011;11(2):131–5.
143. Rout S, Banerjee R. Free radical scavenging, anti-glycation and tyrosinase inhibition properties of a polysaccharide fraction isolated from the rind from Punica granatum. Bioresour Technol. 2007;98(16):3159–63.
144. Ohshima H, Oyobikawa M, Tada A, Maeda T, Takiwaki H, Itoh M, Kanto H. Melanin and facial

skin fluorescence as markers of yellowish discoloration with aging. Skin Res Technol. 2009;15(4):496–502.
145. Leblanc-Noblesse E, Juan M, Loubens V, et al. Dermal compartment and solar lentigo: focus on glycation. IFSCC. 2014.
146. Leclerc E, Heizmann CW, Vetter SW. RAGE and S100 protein transcription levels are highly variable in human melanoma tumors and cells. Gen Physiol Biophys. 2009; 28 Spec No Focus:F65–75.
147. Zhu L, Ito T, Nakahara T, Nagae K, et al. Upregulation of S100P, receptor for advanced glycation end products and ezrin in malignant melanoma. J Dermatol. 2013;40(12):973–9.
148. Monnier VM. Intervention against the Maillard reaction in vivo. Arch Biochem Biophys. 2003;419(1):1–15.
149. Ahmed N. Advanced glycation endproducts–role in pathology of diabetic complications. Diabetes Res Clin Pract. 2005;67(1):3–21.
150. Harding JJ, Ganea E. Protection against glycation and similar post-translational modifications of proteins. Biochim Biophys Acta. 2006;1764(9):1436–46.
151. Urios P, Grigorova-Borsos AM, Sternberg M. Flavonoids inhibit the formation of the cross-linking AGE pentosidine in collagen incubated with glucose, according to their structure. Eur J Nutr. 2007;46(3):139–46.
152. Gasser P, Arnold F, Peno-Mazzarino L, et al. Glycation induction and antiglycation activity of skin care ingredients on living human skin explants. Int J Cosmet Sci. 2011;33(4):366–70.
153. Saraswat M, Reddy PY, Muthenna P, et al. Prevention of non-enzymic glycation of proteins by dietary agents: prospects for alleviating diabetic complications. Br J Nutr. 2009;101(11):1714–21.
154. Lo CY, Li S, Tan D, et al. Trapping reactions of reactive carbonyl species with tea polyphenols in simulated physiological conditions. Mol Nutr Food Res. 2006;50(12):1118–28.
155. Asif M, Egan J, Vasan S, et al. An advanced glycation end product cross-link breaker can reverse age-related increases in myocardial stiffness. Proc Natl Acad Sci U S A. 2000;97(6):2809–13.
156. Vasan S, Foiles P, Founds H. Therapeutic potential of breakers of advanced glycation end product-protein crosslinks. Arch Biochem Biophys. 2003;419 (1):89–96.
157. Yang S, Litchfield JE, Baynes JW. AGE-breakers cleave model compounds, but do not break Maillard crosslinks in skin and tail collagen from diabetic rats. Arch Biochem Biophys. 2003;412(1):42–6.
158. Candido R, Forbes JM, Thomas MC, et al. A breaker of advanced glycation end products attenuates diabetes-induced myocardial structural changes. Circ Res. 2003;92(7):785–92.
159. Grossin N, Boulanger E, Wautier MP, et al. The different isoforms of the receptor for advanced glycation end products are modulated by pharmacological agents. Clin Hemorheol Microcirc. 2010;45(2):143–153.
160. Yamagishi S, Takeuchi M. Nifedipine inhibits gene expression of receptor for advanced glycation end products (RAGE) in endothelial cells by suppressing reactive oxygen species generation. Drugs Exp Clin Res. 2004;30(4):169–175.
161. Horiuchi T, Kurokawa T, Saito N. Purification and properties of fructosyl-amino acid oxidase from *Corynebacterium* sp. 2-4-1. Agric Biol Chem. 1989;53:103–10.
162. Wu X, Monnier VM. Enzymatic deglycation of proteins. Arch Biochem Biophys. 2003;419:16–24.
163. Szwergold BS, Kappler F, Brown TR. Identification of fructose 3-phosphate in the lens of diabetic rats. Science. 1990;247(4941):451–4.
164. Delpierre G, Rider MH, Collard F, et al. Identification, cloning, and heterologous expression of a mammalian fructosamine-3-kinase. Diabetes. 2000;49 (10):1627–34.
165. Szwergold B, Manevich Y, Payne L, et al. Fructosamine-3-kinase-related-protein phosphorylates glucitolamines on the C-4 hydroxyl: novel substrate specificity of an enigmatic enzyme. Biochem Biophys Res Commun. 2007;361(4):870–5.
166. Thornalley PJ. Dietary AGEs and ALEs and risk to human health by their interaction with the receptor for advanced glycation endproducts (RAGE)—an introduction. Mol Nutr Food Res. 2007;51(9):1107–10.
167. Rabbani N, Thornalley PJ. Glyoxalase in diabetes, obesity and related disorders. Semin Cell Dev Biol. 2011;22(3):309–17.
168. Richarme G, Mihoub M, Dairou J, et al. Parkinsonism-associated protein DJ1/Park7 is a major protein deglycase that repairs methylglyoxal- and glyoxal-glycated cysteine, arginine, and lysine residues. J Biol Chem. 2015;290(3):1885–97.
169. Cerami C, Founds H, Nicholl I, et al. Tobacco smoke is a source of toxic reactive glycation products. Proc Natl Acad Sci U S A. 1997;94(25):13915–20.
170. Uribarri J, Woodruff S, Goodman S, et al. Advanced glycation end products in foods and a practical guide to their reduction in the diet. J Am Diet Assoc. 2010;110(6):911–6.
171. Sell DR, Lane MA, Obrenovich ME, et al. The effect of caloric restriction on glycation and glycoxidation in skin collagen of nonhuman primates. J Gerontol A Biol Sci Med Sci. 2003;58(6):508–16.
172. Bodkin NL, Alexander TM, Ortmeyer HK, et al. Mortality and morbidity in laboratory-maintained Rhesus monkeys and effects of long-term dietary restriction. J Gerontol A Biol Sci Med Sci. 2003;58(3):212–9.
173. Zainal TA, Oberley TD, Allison DB, et al. Caloric restriction of rhesus monkeys lowers oxidative damage in skeletal muscle. FASEB J. 2000;14(12):1825–36.
174. Holloszy JO, Fontana L. Caloric restriction in humans. Exp Gerontol. 2007;42(8):709–12.
175. Zouboulis CC, Makrantonaki E. Clinical aspects and molecular diagnostics of skin aging. Clin Dermatol. 2011;29(1):3–14.

Assessing Quality of Life in Older Adult Patients with Skin Disorders

97

Miranda A. Farage, Kenneth W. Miller, Susan N. Sherman, and Joel Tsevat

Contents

M.A. Farage (✉)
Winton Hill Business Center, The Procter & Gamble Company, Cincinnati, OH, USA
e-mail: farage.m@pg.com

K.W. Miller
Margoshes-Miller Consulting, LLC, Cincinnati, OH, USA
e-mail: 822mbb@gmail.com; bbbns2@fuse.net

S.N. Sherman
SNS Research, Cincinnati, OH, USA
e-mail: sns@cinci.rr.com

J. Tsevat
Division of General Internal Medicine, Department of Internal Medicine, University of Cincinnati College of Medicine and Cincinnati VA Medical Center, Cincinnati, OH, USA
e-mail: tsevatj@ucmail.uc.edu

M.A. Farage et al. (eds.), *Textbook of Aging Skin*,
DOI 10.1007/978-3-662-47398-6_73

Abstract

Older adults experience a number of skin diseases and age-related changes that substantially affect quality of life. This review of available literature briefly describes skin conditions associated with aging that affect the skin's appearance (e.g., age spots, wrinkles, and prominent veins), function (e.g., decreases in skin barrier function, mechanical protection, sensory perception, wound-healing capability), and structure (e.g., dryness, roughness, and skin laxity). Summaries are provided for a number of quality of life instruments that can be used for adult dermatology patients to assess the effects of treatment and disease progression, perceptions of well-being, and the value that patients place on their dermatologic state of health. These include instruments assessing the effect of dermatology on overall health-related quality of life (e.g., Dermatology Life Quality Index, Family Dermatology Life Quality Index, and Skindex), an instrument assessing the impact on health-related quality of life of various consumer products (the Farage Quality of Life Questionnaire), and condition-specific measures (e.g., the Quality of Life Index for Atopic Dermatitis, Charing Cross Venous Ulcer Questionnaire, Pressure Ulcer Quality of Life, Psoriasis Disability Index, and Rosacea-Specific Quality of Life). Although a number of such validated dermatology-related instruments are available, an opportunity exists for developing and validating health-related quality of life measures specifically for older patients and the dermatologic conditions most pertinent to them.

Introduction

What Is Health-Related Quality of Life?

Quality of life (QoL) is a broad concept that can touch on many aspects of life, including fulfillment of basic needs, social and emotional well-being, and physical well-being [1]. Health-related quality of life (HRQoL) is a subset of the broad definition of QoL and has become an important component of health surveillance. Self-assessed health status has proven to be a powerful predictor of mortality and morbidity [2]. While HRQoL instruments tend to focus on perceived physical and mental health and function, they are intimately connected to the broader aspects of life. To paraphrase the World Health Organization, health is not merely the absence of disease, it is the state of complete physical, mental, and social well-being [1].

Why Is It Important to Measure Health-Related Quality of Life?

Patient's histories, clinical examination, and diagnostic testing provide information about patients' health and the progression (or regression) of disease. Assessments of HRQoL provide a measure of the integration of the disease and its treatment into daily living and the ability of a person to lead an enjoyable and productive life [3]. Further, it involves patients in their care by allowing them to express their opinions about the value they place on health and how their illness and its treatment affect them (Fig. 1). For patients with chronic illness, HRQoL assessment measures the changes in their well-being throughout the course of the disease. At the community level, HRQoL enables health agencies to address broader areas of public policy pertaining to health-care providers and social services [2].

How to Measure Quality of Life?

QoL is at once a simple yet complex paradigm, with philosophers, sociologists, psychologists, economists, theologians, clinicians, and lay persons all having different conceptualizations [4–7]. While a consensus exists that HRQoL is important to patient care, there is no absolute agreement among researchers on how to assess either HRQoL or QoL in general [8]. Nevertheless, two fundamentally different approaches are commonly applied: (1) health status measurement and (2) utility/value/preference assessment.

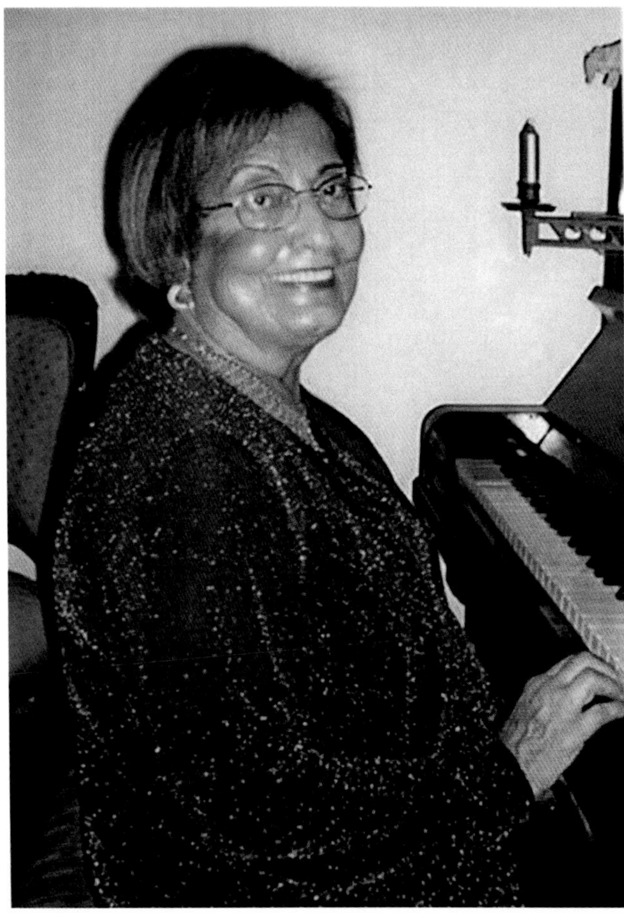

Fig. 1 A woman in her golden years still enjoying playing music on the piano

Health status measures assess various domains of a person's physical, physiological, or mental health. Health status measures can be either generic (applicable to any disease or health state) or disease-specific (applicable to a single condition or disease) [8]. One of the most commonly used generic health status instruments is the SF-12 Health Survey, a 12-item measure encompassing eight domains: physical functioning, social functioning, mental health, role limitations due to physical problems, role limitations due to emotional problems, vitality (energy and fatigue), pain, and general health perceptions. Each domain is scored separately from 0 (worst) to 100 (best), and Physical Component Summary and Mental Component Summary scores can be calculated [9]. State-of-the-art health status measurement is based on item response theory, which draws from a bank of validated questionnaire items covering the spectrum of a domain of HRQoL, such as depression or fatigue. Item response theory is conducive to computerized HRQoL assessment with but a limited number of questions and to developing short forms of measures [10, 11]. Besides such generic measures, a wide variety of disease-specific measures have been developed. Health status measures specific to dermatology are reviewed in detail later in this chapter.

Utility/value/preference measures of HRQoL, in contrast to health status measures, assess the value or desirability of a state of health against an external metric such as risk, time, or money [8, 12, 13]. The most common instruments used to measure utility/value/preference, hereafter referred to as utility measures, are (1) the standard gamble, (2) time trade-off, and (3) the rating scale. The standard gamble determines the risk of (usually) death that one would be willing to take to improve a state of health. Scores on the standard gamble can range from 0 to 1, where 0 usually represents dead and 1 represents excellent or perfect health. The time trade-off technique asks how many months or years of life one would be willing to give up in exchange for a better health state. The rating scale is not strictly a measure of utility because it does not involve comparison against an external metric. Instead, the rating scale asks the subject to rate his or her health on a scale, e.g., from 0 (dead) to 100 (perfect health). This instrument is the simplest of the three utility measures of HRQoL.

A less common utility measure, known as willingness to pay (WTP), assesses the amount of money, in the form of either cash or insurance premiums, one is willing to pay for a cure [14]. This instrument is particularly germane to nonlife-threatening conditions and, hence, can be applied to many dermatologic diseases.

Applicability of Health Status Measures and Utility Measures of HRQoL

Health status or utility measures of HRQoL are applicable to different forms of health monitoring. For example, health status measures can be used (1) to interpret and monitor outcomes in clinical treatment programs, (2) as end points in clinical trials, (3) to monitor population health, and (4) to estimate the burden of different disease conditions. Utility measures are used primarily to calculate quality-adjusted life years in decision and cost-effectiveness analyses. Although not as sensitive to changes in health as health status measures, particularly disease-specific health status measures, utility measures can be used to supplement measures of health status. For example, if a particular therapy in a clinical trial is found to be superior in several aspects of health status, but inferior in others, utility measures could "break the tie" and determine the optimal therapy.

Direct and Indirect HRQoL Measures

Health status measures are generally ascertained directly, from either patients, their surrogate decision makers, or their health-care providers. Utility measures can be ascertained directly from either patients, their decision makers, or health-care providers or indirectly by surveying the general population. For example, the direct assessment of utility may involve asking a respondent to make trade-offs between a particular state of health and a hypothetical gamble involving some chance of a better or worse outcome [15]. The indirect assessment of utility involves first assessing the patient's health status and then mapping a previously derived utility to that particular state of health. The indirectly derived utility measure is obtained by surveying a sample from the general population that has been given descriptions of various health states and asked to assess their value [8]. Examples of indirect utility measures, also known as health state classification systems, include the EQ-5D [16], the SF-6D [17], the Health Utilities Index [18], and the Quality of Well-Being Scale [19].

Dermatologic Changes in Older People and Their Impact on Health

As the population ages, managing older dermatology patients will become increasingly important [20]. Older adults experience a number of skin diseases and disorders that substantially affect QoL [21]. Chang and colleagues reported that approximately one-quarter of dermatology visits in 2011 at Stanford Hospital and Clinics were by patients aged 65 years or older [22].

The aging process differs among individuals based on genetic variability, the toxicity of by-products of metabolic processes, and the sufficiency of physiologic resources available for somatic maintenance and repair [23]. Guinot and coauthors [23] identified four categories of factors that contribute to the skin aging process: (1) biological (genetically predetermined and unalterable), (2) environmental (e.g., damage from exposure to sunlight, pollutants, and/or nicotine), (3) mechanical (e.g., repetitive muscle movements such as squinting or frowning), and (4) miscellaneous (e.g., sleep patterns, dietary intake, comorbid conditions, and mental health and well-being).

Skin changes associated with aging are readily apparent: thin, dry skin, age spots, wrinkles, prominent veins, etc. Such changes can be classified broadly as either age-related changes or photoaging [24]. Age-related skin changes are further classified as (1) functional or (2) structural. Functional changes include decreases in skin barrier function, mechanical protection, sensory perception, wound-healing capability, immunologic responsiveness, thermoregulation, and vitamin D production [24] (Table 1). Structural changes lead to dryness, roughness, wrinkling, skin laxity, and decreased skin elasticity [22]. Structural changes emerge as the skin becomes progressively thinner during adulthood (Fig. 2) [25]. Those changes include a reduction in the number of cells comprising the epidermis, changes in cellular shape, uneven pigmentation, reduced cutaneous immunity, reduced sebum production, and lower water content causing drier skin, even xerosis [25].

Older adults are more likely to experience skin irritation or dermatologic disease than younger adults. In fact, most persons over the age of 65 have two or more skin diseases/disorders that could require medical treatment [26]. Urinary and fecal incontinence, for example, are common among older people, and because aging skin is vulnerable to prolonged moisture, dermatologic complications associated with incontinence are frequent [27]. Untreated incontinence can lead to incontinence dermatitis, dermatological infections, intertrigo, vulvar folliculitis, and pruritus ani. Chronic incontinence can produce a continuing cycle of skin damage, irritation, and inflammation.

Skin cancer is also more prevalent among older persons. In recent years, public education about skin cancer prevention has raised awareness about strategies such as using sunscreen and reducing sun exposure. However, people over the age of 65 have greater morbidity and mortality from skin cancer. The National Cancer Institute reported on data collected from 2007 to 2011. During that time, 44.4 % of new cases of melanoma were diagnosed among people aged 65 and over, and 59.3 % of deaths were due to melanoma [28].

Health-Related Quality of Life Instruments for Skin Diseases

HRQoL instruments that measure either patients' health status or the utility and value that patients place on their state of health may be validated for

Table 1 Age-related changes in the skin

Physiologic decrement	Clinical consequence(s)
Barrier function	Increased skin dryness
	Increased itch
	Slower return to full barrier function after perturbation
Cell replacement	Delayed wound healing
	Rougher skin surface
Lipogenesis	Skin thinning due to decreased subcutaneous fat
	Increased skin dryness
DNA repair	Increased photocarcinogenesis
Elasticity	Lax skin
Immunologic responsiveness	Chronic low-grade skin infections
Inflammatory responsiveness	Inapparent injuries and infections
Mechanical protection	Frequent injuries
Sensory perception	Frequent injuries
Sweating	Tendency for hypothermia
Thermoregulation (vascular)	Vulnerability to heat and cold
Vitamin D production	Suboptimal vitamin D stores, osteomalacia, muscle weakness
Wound healing	Persistent wounds, weak scars

From Chang AL et al. [22] and The Merck Manual of Geriatrics [24]

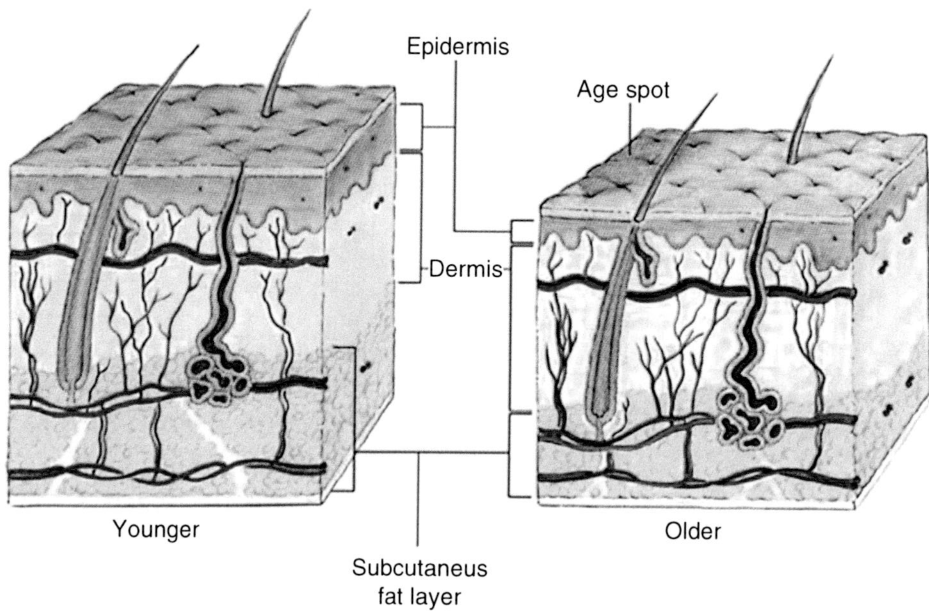

Fig. 2 Changes of aging skin (From Farage MA et al. [25], with permission from Informa Healthcare)

use in particular populations or validated in a wide variety of cultures, regions, and languages. Constructing and validating a new HRQoL instrument entails both qualitative and quantitative methods [3, 29]. HRQoL instruments should be evaluated for validity, reliability, and responsiveness [30, 31].

The validity of a questionnaire refers to whether the questionnaire or survey measures what it intends to measure. Validity can be assessed with regard to content, criterion or predictive ability, and construct. *Content validity* can be determined qualitatively through literature review, expert reviews, or cognitive interviews in which people are asked to describe and define what individual questions mean to them, as well as how they arrived at their answers [32]. *Criterion validity* refers to the extent to which survey items predict or agree with an objective assessment of the particular criterion (e.g., in clinical evaluations, patient reports are compared with physician reports or medical records). *Construct validity* examines the assumption that items in the survey that are hypothesized to measure the same concept (e.g., two indicators of emotional well-being) do, in fact, agree. Conversely, items hypothesized to be unrelated should not agree (discriminant validity). Correlation analysis and factor analysis are quantitative techniques used to assess whether variables are measuring the same underlying construct [33].

The reliability of a measure refers to its stability over time, that is, the consistency of answers given by the same individual to the same item. The reliability of survey items can be assessed using statistical methods, such as calculating mean absolute differences in scores on repeat measurement, coefficients of variation, kappa statistics, or correlation coefficients appropriate for the type of data (nominal, ordinal, or interval) [34]. Several types of reliability can be assessed. *Test–retest reliability* examines the correspondence between answers given by an individual when the item(s) is readministered over a brief interval (sufficiently brief so that an underlying change in health status is not anticipated to occur between administrations). *Inter-rater reliability* assesses how closely data obtained by different interviewers match. Cronbach's alpha is commonly calculated as a measure of internal consistency, that is, how closely related a set of items are as a group [35, 36].

The interpretability of the questionnaire refers to the ability to compare data from the survey to other available information [31]. For example, responses of a patient population cannot be interpreted without some understanding of the responses of a healthy population. A related concept is the minimal clinically important difference (MCID) [37], i.e., the minimal change in score considered to be clinically meaningful, as opposed to just statistically significant. As an example, Basra and colleagues published results of a longitudinal study among patients with inflammatory skin disorders. Patients ($n = 107$) were asked to complete the 10-item *Dermatology Life Quality Index* (DLQI) prior to starting a new treatment regimen. After 1–3 months of treatment, the questionnaires were administered a second time. Based on responses, patients were grouped into 4 categories: those having experienced "no change" ($n = 23$) showed a mean improvement of 2.7 points in the DLQI score, a "small change" ($n = 31$) showed a mean improvement of 3.3 points, a "moderate change" ($n = 25$) showed a mean improvement of 4.4 points, and a "large change" ($n = 28$) showed a mean improvement of 6 points. The authors recommended that 4 points be considered the MCID for the DLQI.

HRQoL Instruments Applicable to Older Adults

A number of HRQoL instruments have been developed to assess skin-related effects. Most of these instruments have been developed for the general population. However, since older adults were included in the development and validation process, many are applicable to older individuals. Table 2 shows a list of available instruments developed to measure HRQoL for skin-related conditions. Selected ones are discussed in greater detail below.

Instruments for General Well-being and Appearance

Farage Quality of Life Questionnaire

Despite the existence of numerous HRQoL measures, few if any are geared to evaluating the impact of consumer products on HRQoL. A general measure, the *Farage Quality of Life Questionnaire* (FQoL), was developed to assess the impact of products use on various aspects of HRQoL [38]. The self-administered general FQoL consists of 27 general items scored on a Likert scale and covering overall QoL (1 item), well-being (12 items), and energy and vitality (14 items). The Well-Being domain has 3 subscales: Emotion, Self-Image, and Self-Competence. The Energy and Vitality domains also have 3 subscales: Personal Pleasure, Physical State, and Routine Activity. A recent publication described the translation of the FQoL into Chinese [39].

BeautyQoL Questionnaire

An improvement in facial attractiveness is associated with positive changes in self-esteem and in the emotional and social dimensions of one's life [40]. The *BeautyQoL* questionnaire was developed specifically to assess QoL relevant to cosmetic products and physical appearance [41]. This instrument was developed in 13 countries representing 16 different languages. Development of the BeautyQoL questionnaire followed a 3-phase validation process. Initial items were generated via face-to-face interviews of 309 subjects in 10 different countries. The second phase was an acceptability study performed on 874 subjects from 13 countries. In the final phase, 3231 subjects were recruited in those countries to complete the questionnaire. A retest was performed 8 days later on a subgroup of 652 subjects. The resulting questionnaire consists of 42 items in 5 dimensions: social life, self-confidence, mood, energy, and attractiveness. The measure has been translated into 16 languages.

Table 2 Examples of skin-related health-related quality of life measures for adults

Disease(s)	Measure	Abbreviation	References
General well-being and appearance			
	Farage Quality of Life Questionnaire	FQoL	[38]
	BeautyQoL Questionnaire	BeautyQoL	[41]
Generic for dermatology			
	Dermatology Life Quality Index	DLQI	[42, 79]
	Dermatology Quality of Life Scales	DQoLS	[43, 79]
	Family Dermatology Life Quality Index	FDLQI	[44, 79]
	Skindex/Skindex-29/Skindex-16	Skindex	[45, 79, 80]
	Impact of Chronic Skin Disease on Daily Life	ISDL	[49]
Specific dermatologic conditions			
Acne	Acne Quality of Life Questionnaire	Acne-QoL	[79, 81]
	Acne Disability Index	ADI	[79, 82]
	Dermatology-Specific Quality of Life Instrument for Acne	DSQL-Acne	[50, 79]
Alopecia	Kingsley Alopecia Profile	KPA	[79, 83]
	Alopecia Areata Symptom Impact Scale	AASIS	[84]
Atopic dermatitis	Quality of Life Index for Atopic Dermatitis	QoLIAD	[79, 85]
Contact dermatitis	Dermatology-Specific Quality of Life Instrument for Contact Dermatitis	DSQL-CD	[50, 79]
Eczema	Dermatitis Family Impact Questionnaire	DFI	[42, 79]
	Patient-Oriented Eczema Measure	POEM	[79, 86]
Itch/pruritus	Itch Severity Scale	ISS	[52]
	Pruritus-specific	*ItchyQoL*	[54]
	Scalp dermatitis	*Scalpdex*	[55]
	Pruritus-related Life Quality Index	PLQI	[87]
Leg ulcer	Charing Cross Venous Ulcer Questionnaire	CCVUQ	[56, 79]
	Leg and Foot Ulcer Questionnaire	LFUQ	[79, 88]
	Diabetic Foot Ulcer Scale	DFS	[58, 79]
	Diabetic Foot Ulcer Scale – Short Form	DFS-SF	[59, 79]
Pressure ulcer	Pressure Ulcer Quality of Life	PU-QOL	[61]
Psoriasis	Psoriasis Disability Index	PDI	[76, 79]
	12-Item Psoriasis Quality of Life Questionnaire	PQOL-12	[79, 89]
	Psoriatic Arthritis Quality of Life Instrument	PsAQoL	[79, 90]
	REFlective evaLuation of psoriasis Efficacy of Treatment and Severity	REFLETS	[79, 91]
	Psoriasis Area and Severity Index	PASI	[79, 92]
Onychomycosis	Onychomycosis Quality of Life Questionnaire	ONYCHO	[93]
Rosacea	Rosacea-Specific Quality of Life	RosaQoL	[65]
Systemic lupus erythematosus	Lupus Patient-Reported Outcome tool	LupusPRO	[79, 94]
	Systemic Lupus Erythematosus Quality of Life Questionnaire	SLEQoL	[79, 95]
	British Isles Lupus Assessment Group Index	BILAG Index	[79, 96]
	European Consensus Lupus Activity Measurement	ECLAM	[79, 97]
	Systemic Lupus Erythematosus Disease Activity Index	SLEDAI	[79, 98]
Vitiligo	Vitiligo-specific quality-of-life instrument	VitiQoL	[99]

Instruments Suitable for Dermatologic Conditions in General

The Dermatology Life Quality Index (DLQI)

The DLQI is a simple, 10-question, validated questionnaire used widely in clinical settings and available in more than 40 languages [42]. The DLQI was developed based on the responses of 120 patients with various skin diseases who were asked how their disease and its treatment affected their life. For further validation, the DLQI was subsequently administered to 200 consecutive patients attending a dermatology clinic. Analysis of the responses revealed that atopic eczema, psoriasis, and generalized pruritus have a greater impact on HRQoL than do acne, basal cell carcinoma, and viral warts. When the instrument was administered to 100 healthy volunteers (i.e., no apparent dermatologic disease), mean scores were very low (better), supporting the validity of the instrument. A 1-week, test–retest reliability analysis in 53 patients found that the DLQI instrument was highly reliable [42].

Dermatology Quality of Life Scales

The *Dermatology Quality of Life Scales* (DQoLS) was developed to assess the impact of skin conditions on patients' psychosocial state and everyday activities [43]. The instrument was developed using written input from 50 dermatology outpatients who were asked about all the ways in which their skin condition affected them. Responses were distilled into a list of 17 psychosocial items, 12 physical activity items, and 12 symptom items. The resulting questionnaire was completed by 118 patients, and responses were used to evaluate internal consistency, test–retest reliability, and construct validity. Factor analysis grouped the psychosocial and physical activity items into four subscales each. The 12 questions on symptoms did not cluster and were, therefore, treated as an overall symptom score. The DQoLS can be completed quickly by patients to provide measures of patient-perceived impacts to complement traditional clinical indicators.

The Family Dermatology Life Quality Index

The *Family Dermatology Life Quality Index* (FDLQI) is a 10-item questionnaire administered to patients' family members to measure the indirect impact of skin disease on the family [44]. The FDLQI is responsive to changes in the patient: family members' scores changed in association with improvement or worsening of the patient's condition. There were strong statistical associations between FDLQI scores and the patients' DLQI scores, FDLQI scores and inflammatory versus noninflammatory disease, and FDLQI scores and the severity of the patient's disease. There was a positive relationship between FDLQI scores of the family members and the patient's disease severity, as measured by the DLQI. Thus, the FDLQI has been shown to be a simple and practical additional outcome measure in clinical practice and evaluation research.

Skindex

The *Skindex* instrument is widely used to evaluate dermatological HRQoL. The original 61-item, self-administered *Skindex* questionnaire was first developed in the mid-1990s [45] and focused on skin diseases and the frequency and severity of their impact on QoL: cognitive effects, social effects, depression, fear, embarrassment, anger, physical discomfort, and physical limitations. Several revised versions of the instrument have been developed to improve upon discriminative and evaluative capability and administration time. The 29-item Skindex-29 [46], which takes about 5 min to complete, has since been translated into eleven languages. The even shorter, single-page

Table 3 Skindex-16 (Reprinted with permission from Chren MM et al. [47])

During the past week, how often have you been bothered by		Never Bothered ↓						Always Bothered ↓
1	Your skin condition **itching**	□$_0$	□$_1$	□$_2$	□$_3$	□$_4$	□$_5$	□$_6$
2	Your skin condition **burning** or **stinging**	□$_0$	□$_1$	□$_2$	□$_3$	□$_4$	□$_5$	□$_6$
3	Your skin condition **hurting**	□$_0$	□$_1$	□$_2$	□$_3$	□$_4$	□$_5$	□$_6$
4	Your skin condition **being irritated**	□$_0$	□$_1$	□$_2$	□$_3$	□$_4$	□$_5$	□$_6$
5	The **persistence/reoccurrence** of your skin condition	□$_0$	□$_1$	□$_2$	□$_3$	□$_4$	□$_5$	□$_6$
6	**Worry** about your skin condition (e.g., that it will spread, get worse, scar, and be unpredictable)	□$_0$	□$_1$	□$_2$	□$_3$	□$_4$	□$_5$	□$_6$
7	The **appearance** of your skin condition	□$_0$	□$_1$	□$_2$	□$_3$	□$_4$	□$_5$	□$_6$
8	**Frustration** about your skin condition	□$_0$	□$_1$	□$_2$	□$_3$	□$_4$	□$_5$	□$_6$
9	**Embarrassment** about your skin condition	□$_0$	□$_1$	□$_2$	□$_3$	□$_4$	□$_5$	□$_6$
10	**Being annoyed** about your skin condition	□$_0$	□$_1$	□$_2$	□$_3$	□$_4$	□$_5$	□$_6$
11	**Feeling depressed** about your skin condition	□$_0$	□$_1$	□$_2$	□$_3$	□$_4$	□$_5$	□$_6$
12	The effects of your skin condition on your **interactions with others** (e.g., interactions with family, friends, and close relationships)	□$_0$	□$_1$	□$_2$	□$_3$	□$_4$	□$_5$	□$_6$
13	The effects of your skin condition on your **desire to be with people**	□$_0$	□$_1$	□$_2$	□$_3$	□$_4$	□$_5$	□$_6$
14	Your skin condition making it hard to **show affection**	□$_0$	□$_1$	□$_2$	□$_3$	□$_4$	□$_5$	□$_6$
15	The effects of your skin condition on your **daily activities**	□$_0$	□$_1$	□$_2$	□$_3$	□$_4$	□$_5$	□$_6$
16	Your skin condition making it hard to **work or do what you enjoy**	□$_0$	□$_1$	□$_2$	□$_3$	□$_4$	□$_5$	□$_6$

Skindex-16 scoring	
Scale	Items
Symptoms	1–4
Emotion	5–11
Functioning	12–16
Item scores transformed to 0–100 scale	
Scale score: average of items in given scale	
Total score: average of all 16 items	

Skindex-16 is copyrighted and used with permission from both Dr. Chren and Springer Publishing Co.

16-item Skindex-16 (Table 3) [47] has been translated into 16 languages. At the time of writing this chapter, a Chinese translation is being validated [48].

The Impact of Chronic Skin Disease on Daily Life

The *Impact of Chronic Skin Disease on Daily Life* (ISDL) instrument assesses the effect of chronic skin diseases and their treatments on both dermatology-specific and generic aspects of HRQoL [49]. Specifically, the ISDL assesses physical functioning, itching/scratching, pain, fatigue, stigmatization, psychological functioning, illness cognitions, and social support. The reliability and validity of the instrument were assessed in patients with psoriasis or atopic dermatitis. The authors demonstrated reliability and high test–retest reliability. In addition, the ISDL was sensitive to changes in health status resulting from ultraviolet B radiation therapy or cognitive behavioral therapy for itching [49].

Measures Suitable for Specific Dermatologic Conditions

Contact Dermatitis

Dermatology-Specific Quality of Life Instrument for Contact Dermatitis

The *Dermatology-Specific Quality of Life Instrument for Contact Dermatitis* (DSQL-CD) was created to quantify the effect of skin disease on physical discomfort and symptoms, psychological well-being, social functioning, self-care activities, performance at work or school, and self-perceptions [50]. Reliability and validity were assessed in patients with contact dermatitis or acne vulgaris. The validity of the instrument was assessed by correlating DSQL scores with global ratings of bothersome symptoms and their perceived severity and by the instrument's ability to discriminate among clinically defined severity-of-illness groups. Test–retest reliability was assessed at 3 and 7 days. The instrument's domains had good internal consistency and test–retest reliability. The subscale scores were also moderately to highly correlated with globally validated ratings of symptoms of distress and with overall disease severity. As expected, patients with severe contact dermatitis or scarring from acne vulgaris had worse DSQL scores than those with milder disease.

Pruritus and Itch

Chronic pruritus is a common condition among older adults. The most common cause of chronic pruritus or itch is dry skin, which is a natural consequence of skin aging [22]. In addition, a number of medications commonly taken by older individuals can induce pruritus, such as antihypertensive drugs, anticoagulants, and lipid-lowering drugs [51]. A number of instruments have been developed to evaluate the impact of pruritus.

Itch Severity Scale

The *Itch Severity Scale* (ISS) is a self-administered questionnaire to measure the severity of pruritus [52]. To develop the instrument, an existing pruritus instrument was modified and administered to patients with psoriasis-associated pruritus, along with the RAND-36 Health Status Inventory [53] (a generic health status measure), and the DLQI. The resulting ISS instrument contains just seven questions and was demonstrated to be a valid and reliable means of assessing the severity of pruritus as well as the effectiveness of treatments [52].

ItchyQoL

ItchyQoL is another pruritus-specific HRQoL instrument [54]. It includes 22 pruritus-specific questions covering three major domains: symptoms, functional limitations, and emotions. Initially, two versions of the instrument were created based on patient interviews and items from Skindex-16 and Skindex-29, one with "frequency" questions and the other with "bother" questions. Eighty-nine patients took part in the validation phase and 101 patients participated in the clinical application phase. The final instrument contains 27 questions: 18 capture both frequency and bother and the remaining nine items pertaining to emotion assess frequency only. Although the authors cited lack of generalizability and potential selection bias as possible limitations, they found this initial pruritus-specific questionnaire to be reliable, valid, and responsive [54].

Scalpdex

Scalpdex [55] is the first HRQoL instrument specific for scalp dermatitis. Scalpdex is based on three major domains of quality of life: symptoms, functioning, and emotions. The 23-question instrument was demonstrated to be reliable, valid, and responsive. Scalpdex can be used by clinicians to determine which aspect of the disease bothers the patient the most so as to choose treatment options for maximum benefit [55].

Leg and Foot Ulcers

Charing Cross Venous Ulcer Questionnaire

The *Charing Cross Venous Ulcer Questionnaire* (CCVUQ) [56] is a 21-item self-administered instrument to assess patients' perceptions of their health when venous ulceration is present. Items for the questionnaire were selected from patient interviews and a literature review. The resulting questionnaire was administered to 98 patients with venous ulcers. Concurrently, patients were asked to complete an established HRQoL instrument (the 36-Item Short Form Health Survey (SF-36) [57]) for comparison. The CCVUQ instrument showed good reliability and internal consistency and good test–retest reliability. Results correlated well with the SF-36.

Diabetic Foot Ulcer Scale

The *Diabetic Foot Ulcer Scale* (DFS) [58] is a 64-item self-administered instrument developed to assess the impact of diabetic foot ulcers and their treatment on patients' QoL in a broad range of areas, including physical health, leisure and daily activities, attitudes and emotions, and social interactions. Items for inclusion were based on interviews and focus group discussions with patients. The resulting instrument was initially tested on 173 patients with diabetes: 48 with current foot ulcers, 54 with healed foot ulcers, and 71 with no history of foot ulcers. The results demonstrated good internal consistency and adequate test–retest reliability. In addition, the instrument was responsive to changes in wound status over time. A shorter instrument, the *Diabetic Foot Ulcer Scale – Short Form* (DFS-SF) [59] was developed in conjunction with clinical trials of treatments for leg ulcers. This 29-item self-administered questionnaire showed good internal consistency, reliability, and construct validity and demonstrated responsiveness to ulcer healing.

Pressure Ulcers

Pressure (decubitus) ulcers are localized areas of tissue necrosis involving the skin and underlying tissue, usually over a bony prominence [60]. The sacrum, buttocks, and heels are particularly vulnerable [61]. Pressure ulcers are common in elderly patients with limited mobility. As reviewed by Farage and coauthors [60], the prevalence of pressure ulcers among patients has been reported to be 25 % in skilled nursing home facilities, 14 % in acute care facilities, and 12 % in home care. People aged 70–75 have double the risk of pressure ulcers compared with those aged 55–69 years. Many affected patients have a variety of concomitant health and function problems.

Pressure Ulcer Quality of Life

A *Pressure Ulcer Quality of Life* (PU-QoL) measure is being developed to evaluate the impact on HRQoL of the pressure ulcers and of interventions for preventing and treating them [61]. The most recent PU-QOL version consists of 13 scales (87 items): pain, exudate, odor, sleep, vitality, mobility, daily activities, mood, anxiety, self-consciousness and appearance, autonomy, isolation, and participation [62]. It can be self-administered or administered with the assistance of an interviewer. At the time of writing of this chapter, further development work is still needed on the PU-QoL to ensure that questions and approaches to administration meet the needs of the broad range of individuals with pressure ulcers. Nevertheless, this is a promising approach to developing of a patient-reported outcome measure for pressure ulcers.

Rosacea

Rosacea is a chronic dermatologic condition that increases in prevalence with age. In men, the prevalence of rosacea increases abruptly after age 50 and reaches a peak of 3.9 % in the 76- to 80-year age group [63]. In women, the increase in prevalence occurs earlier, i.e., after 35 years of age, and peaks at 2.8 % in the 61- to 65-year age group [63]. Its clinical appearance varies, but rosacea most recognizably manifests as erythema on the central area of the face or as phymatoid changes around the nose. Pharmacological treatments are often inadequate [64]; thus, a rosacea-specific instrument could be beneficial in assessing the patient's perspective on treatment effectiveness.

Rosacea-Specific Quality of Life Instrument

Based on in-depth patient interviews [65], three domains pertinent to HRQoL were identified: symptoms, functioning, and emotions. To validate the instrument, patients with rosacea were randomly selected from dermatology clinics, and the Skindex-29 questionnaire, 21 rosacea-specific questions, and five questions about general health were administered by telephone. Because rosacea severity can vary throughout the year, the interviews were performed over a 4-year period. The patients answered all questions at baseline, at 72 h (allowable range: 3–7 days), and at 4–6 months. Follow-up interviews allowed inconsequential or insensitive questions to be eliminated. The process yielded the 21-item *Rosacea-Specific Quality of Life* (RosaQoL) instrument [65] (Table 4). The RosaQoL's reliability, validity, and responsiveness were assessed by psychometric and statistical analyses. The developers believe it to be a promising, practical instrument for use in both clinical and research settings [65].

Utility/Value/Preference Measures for Dermatologic Conditions

Utility measures can provide important information for assessing cost-effectiveness of treatment approaches and the desirability for certain health outcomes. Instruments have been developed to evaluate WTP for control or cure of a medical condition and/or willingness to live a shorter life without the current medical condition (time trade-off) [66]. Perceived utility or value varies not only from condition to condition but also from patient to patient with a given condition, by assessment method, and by respondent type [13, 67–70]. For example, utility measures for controlled atopic eczema, uncontrolled atopic eczema, controlled psoriasis, and uncontrolled

Table 4 The Rosacea-Specific Quality of Life (RosaQoL) instrument (Reprinted with permission from Nicholson K et al. [65])

RosaQoL item	Hypothesized construct
1. I worry that my rosacea may be serious	Emotion
2. My rosacea burns or stings	Symptom
3. I worry about scars from my rosacea	Emotion
4. I worry that my rosacea may get worse	Emotion
5. I worry about side effects from rosacea medications	Emotion
6. My rosacea is irritated	Symptom
7. I am embarrassed by my rosacea	Emotion
8. I am frustrated by my rosacea	Emotion
9. My rosacea makes my skin sensitive	Symptom
10. I am annoyed by my rosacea	Emotion
11. I am bothered by the appearance of my skin (redness, blotchiness)	Emotion
12. My rosacea makes me feel self-conscious	Emotion
13. I try to cover up my rosacea (with makeup)	Functioning
14. I am bothered by the persistence/recurrence of my rosacea	Emotion
15. I avoid certain foods or drinks because of my rosacea	Functioning
16. My skin feels bumpy (uneven, not smooth, irregular)	Symptom
17. My skin flushes	Symptom
18. My skin gets irritated easily (cosmetics, aftershaves, cleansers)	Symptom
19. My eyes bother me (feel dry or gritty)	Symptom
20. I think about my rosacea	Emotion
21. I avoid certain environments (heat, humidity, cold) because of my rosacea	Functioning

Used with permission from both Dr. Nicholson and Elsevier Publishing Co.

psoriasis have been evaluated in a 2006 study in the general population in Germany and in German patients with atopic eczema or psoriasis [67]. On the time trade-off, the median score for controlled atopic eczema was 0.97, indicating that respondents were willing to give up a median of 3 % of their life expectancy (=[1.0 − 0.97] × 100 %) in order to have perfect health (no atopic eczema). For controlled psoriasis, the median utility was 0.93. By contrast, median utilities were much lower for uncontrolled atopic eczema (0.64) and uncontrolled psoriasis (0.56). The study also asked people about WTP. People from the general population would be willing to pay a median of €50/month for an effective treatment (with no side effects) for controlled atopic eczema, €150/month for uncontrolled atopic eczema, €75/month for a treatment for controlled psoriasis, and €200/month for uncontrolled psoriasis. Another study reported that patients with psoriasis would be willing to pay on average 14 % of their monthly income to get rid of their psoriasis [71].

Seidler and colleagues evaluated WTP among dermatology patients diagnosed with a variety of skin diseases [72]. These investigators reported patients were willing to pay a median of 2 % of their annual income for a cure of their condition or 1.6 % for control of their condition. A group of investigators in Germany conducted studies of utility measures for several dermatologic conditions. In a study of 1,023 patients with vitiligo [73], they reported that 32.9 % of patients would pay a median of €3,000 in order to achieve complete disease remission. In a 2013 study among patients with rosacea (n = 475), subjects were willing to pay a median of €500 for complete healing [74]. Finally, in a study of patients with atopic dermatitis (n = 384), the median WTP for complete healing was €1,000 [75].

Several researchers have modified the time trade-off method by asking patients how many hours each day they would be willing to devote to treating their skin condition if the treatment was curative [71, 76, 77]. Patients with psoriasis would be willing to spend a mean (SD) of 2.8 (3.7) hours each day to be relieved of their psoriasis [71], whereas patients with port wine stains would be willing to devote 1.2 (0.9) hours each day to be rid of their port wine stains [77].

In a particularly comprehensive study of utility measures for dermatologic conditions, life expectancy time trade-off utilities for 20 different skin conditions were evaluated in 236 patients [78]. The mean (SD) utility for all skin conditions was 0.943 (0.124), but varied depending on the disorder in question. For example, pruritus and related conditions had a utility of 0.915 (0.145), and ulcers had a utility of 0.923 (0.154).

Conclusion

Older adults experience a number of skin diseases and disorders that adversely affect quality of life. In the past several years, a number of disease-specific HRQoL measures have been developed for the general dermatology patient to assess the effects of treatment and disease progression, perceptions of well-being, and the value that patients place on their dermatologic state of health. Some instruments have been validated and further refined over time, while others are in earlier stages of development. Opportunity exists for developing and validating HRQoL specifically for dermatologic conditions most pertinent to older patients. Dermatology-specific HRQoL instruments will continue to be investigated with the common goal of increasing understanding of how skin diseases and their treatment affect HRQoL in people of all ages.

Cross-References

▶ Aging Skin: Some Psychosomatic Aspects
▶ Psychological and Social Implications of Aging Skin: Normal Aging and the Effects of Cutaneous Disease

References

1. World Health Organization. WHOQOL: measuring quality of life. World Health Organization CH-1211 Geneva 27. 1997. Switzerland.

2. Centers for Disease Control and Prevention. Health-Related Quality of Life (HRQOL). Centers for Disease Control and Prevention Atlanta, GA, USA. 2011.
3. Chwalow AJ. Cross-cultural validation of existing quality of life scales. Patient Educ Couns. 1995;26:313–8.
4. Wilson IB, Cleary PD. Linking clinical variables with health-related quality of life. A conceptual model of patient outcomes. JAMA. 1995;273:59–65.
5. Johnson RJ, Wolinsky FD. The structure of health status among older adults: disease, disability, functional limitation, and perceived health. J Health Soc Behav. 1993;34:105–21.
6. Calman KC. Quality of life in cancer patients – an hypothesis. J Med Ethics. 1984;10:124–7.
7. Michalos AC. Multiple discrepancies theory (MDT). Soc Indic Res. 1985;16:347–413.
8. Tsevat J, Weeks JC, Guadagnoli E, Tosteson AN, et al. Using health-related quality-of-life information: clinical encounters, clinical trials, and health policy. J Gen Intern Med. 1994;9:576–82.
9. Ware JJ, Kosinski M, Keller SD. A 12-Item Short-Form Health Survey: construction of scales and preliminary tests of reliability and validity. Med Care. 1996;34:220–33.
10. Cella D, Yount S, Rothrock N, Gershon R, et al. The Patient-Reported Outcomes Measurement Information System (PROMIS): progress of an NIH Roadmap cooperative group during its first two years. Med Care. 2007;45:S3–11.
11. Embretson SE, Reise SP. Item response theory for psychologists. Mahwah, NJ: Lawrence Erlbaum Associates; 2000.
12. Torrance GW. Measurement of health state utilities for economic appraisal. J Health Econ. 1986;5:1–30.
13. McCombs K, Chen SC. Patient preference quality of life measures in dermatology. Dermatol Ther. 2007;20:102–9.
14. Khanna D, Ahmed M, Yontz D, Ginsburg SS, et al. Willingness to pay for a cure in patients with chronic gout. Med Decis Making. 2008;28:606–13.
15. Tengs TO, Yu M, Luistro E. Health-related quality of life after stroke a comprehensive review. Stroke. 2001;32:964–72.
16. Rabin R, de Charro F. EQ-5D: a measure of health status from the EuroQol Group. Ann Med. 2001;33:337–43.
17. Brazier J, Roberts J, Deverill M. The estimation of a preference-based measure of health from the SF-36. J Health Econ. 2002;21:271–92.
18. Furlong WJ, Feeny DH, Torrance GW, Barr RD. The Health Utilities Index (HUI) system for assessing health-related quality of life in clinical studies. Ann Med. 2001;33:375–84.
19. Kaplan R, Anderson JP, Ganiats GG. The quality of Well-Being Scale: rationale for a single quality of life index. In: Walker SR, Rosser RM, editors. Quality of Life assessment: key issues in the 1990s. Dordrecht: Kluwer Academic Publishers; 1993. p. 65–94.
20. Farage MA, Miller KW, Elsner P, Maibach HI. Intrinsic and extrinsic factors in skin ageing: a review. Int J Cosmet Sci. 2008;30:87–95.
21. Farage MA, Miller KW, Sherman SN, Tsevat J. Assessing quality of life in older adult patients with skin disorders. Glob J Health Sci. 2012;4:119–31.
22. Chang AL, Wong JW, Endo JO, Norman RA. Geriatric dermatology review: major changes in skin function in older patients and their contribution to common clinical challenges. J Am Med Dir Assoc. 2013;14:724–30.
23. Guinot C, Malvy DJ, Ambroisine L, Latreille J, et al. Relative contribution of intrinsic vs extrinsic factors to skin aging as determined by a validated skin age score. Arch Dermatol. 2002;138:1454–60.
24. The Merck Manual of Geriatrics. Section 15, Dermatologic and sensory organ disorders. Chapter 122, Aging and the skin. Age-related changes in skin structure and function; photoaging. 2015 Merck Sharp & Dohme Corp., a subsidiary of Merck & Co., Inc., Kenilworth, NJ., USA.
25. Farage MA, Miller KW, Elsner P, Maibach HI. Structural characteristics of the aging skin: a review. Cutan Ocul Toxicol. 2007;26:343–57.
26. Kligman AM, Koblenzer C. Demographics and psychological implications for the aging population. Dermatol Clin. 1997;15:549–53.
27. Farage MA, Miller KW, Berardesca E, Maibach HI. Incontinence in the aged: contact dermatitis and other cutaneous consequences. Contact Dermatitis. 2007;57:211–7.
28. National Cancer Institute. SEER Stat Fact Sheets: melanoma of the skin. Surveillance, Epidemiology, and End Results Program. 2014. NCI; Rockville, MD-USA. http://seer.cancer.gov/statfacts/html/melan.html
29. Elasy TA, Gaddy G. Measuring subjective outcomes: rethinking reliability and validity. J Gen Intern Med. 1998;13:757–61.
30. Chen SC. Dermatology Quality of Life instruments: sorting out the quagmire. J Invest Dermatol. 2007;127:2695–6.
31. Both H, Essink-Bot ML, Busschbach J, Nijsten T. Critical review of generic and dermatology-specific health-related quality of life instruments. J Invest Dermatol. 2007;127:2726–39.
32. Willis GB. Cognitive interviewing: a tool for improving questionnaire design. Thousand Oaks: Sage Publications; 2005.
33. Aday LA, Cornelius LJ. Designing and conducting health surveys: a comprehensive guide. 2nd ed. San Francisco: Jossey-Bass; 1996.
34. Littenberg B, Partilo S, Licata A, Kattan MW. Paper Standard Gamble: the reliability of a paper questionnaire to assess utility. Med Decis Making. 2003;23:480–8.
35. Cronbach LJ. Coefficient alpha and the internal structure of tests. Psychometrika. 1951;16:297–334.
36. Bland JM, Altman DG. Cronbach's alpha. BMJ. 1997;314:572.

37. Basra MK, Salek MS, Camilleri L, Sturkey R, et al. Determining the minimal clinically important difference and responsiveness of the Dermatology Life Quality Index (DLQI): further data. Dermatology. 2015;230:27–33.
38. Farage MA, Nusair TL, Hanseman D, Sherman SN, et al. The Farage Quality of Life measure for consumer products: development and initial implementation. Appl Res Qual Life. 2010;5:1–25.
39. Farage MA, Rodenberg C, Chen J. Translation and Validation of the Farage Quality of Life (FQoL) instrument for consumer products into traditional Chinese. Glob J Health Sci. 2013;5:1–12.
40. Sadick NS. The impact of cosmetic interventions on quality of life. Dermatol Online J. 2008;14:2.
41. Beresniak A, de Linares Y, Krueger GG, Talarico S, et al. Validation of a new international quality-of-life instrument specific to cosmetics and physical appearance: BeautyQoL questionnaire. Arch Dermatol. 2012;148:1275–82.
42. Finlay AY, Khan GK. Dermatology Life Quality Index (DLQI) – a simple practical measure for routine clinical use. Clin Exp Dermatol. 1994;19:210–6.
43. Morgan M, McCreedy R, Simpson J, Hay RJ. Dermatology quality of life scales – a measure of the impact of skin diseases. Br J Dermatol. 1997;136:202–6.
44. Basra MK, Sue-Ho R, Finlay AY. The Family Dermatology Life Quality Index: measuring the secondary impact of skin disease. Br J Dermatol. 2007;156:528–38.
45. Chren MM, Lasek RJ, Quinn LM, Mostow EN, et al. Skindex, a quality-of-life measure for patients with skin disease: reliability, validity, and responsiveness. J Invest Dermatol. 1996;107:707–13.
46. Chren MM, Lasek RJ, Flocke SA, Zyzanski SJ. Improved discriminative and evaluative capability of a refined version of Skindex, a quality-of-life instrument for patients with skin diseases. Arch Dermatol. 1997;133:1433–40.
47. Chren MM, Lasek RJ, Sahay AP, Sands LP. Measurement properties of Skindex-16: a brief quality-of-life measure for patients with skin diseases. J Cutan Med Surg. 2001;5:105–10.
48. He Z, Lu C, Chren MM, Zhang Z, et al. Development and psychometric validation of the Chinese version of Skindex-29 and Skindex-16. Health Qual Life Outcomes. 2014;12:4.
49. Evers AW, Duller P, van de Kerkhof PC, van der Valk PG, et al. The Impact of Chronic Skin Disease on Daily Life (ISDL): a generic and dermatology-specific health instrument. Br J Dermatol. 2008;158:101–8.
50. Anderson RT, Rajagopalan R. Development and validation of a quality of life instrument for cutaneous diseases. J Am Acad Dermatol. 1997;37:41–50.
51. Reich A, Stander S, Szepietowski JC. Drug-induced pruritus: a review. Acta Derm Venereol. 2009;89:236–44.
52. Majeski CJ, Johnson JA, Davison SN, Lauzon CJ. Itch Severity Scale: a self-report instrument for the measurement of pruritus severity. Br J Dermatol. 2007;156:667–73.
53. Hays RD, Morales LS. The RAND-36 measure of health-related quality of life. Ann Med. 2001;33:350–7.
54. Desai NS, Poindexter GB, Monthrope YM, Bendeck SE, et al. A pilot quality-of-life instrument for pruritus. J Am Acad Dermatol. 2008;59:234–44.
55. Chen SC, Yeung J, Chren MM. Scalpdex: a quality-of-life instrument for scalp dermatitis. Arch Dermatol. 2002;138:803–7.
56. Smith JJ, Guest MG, Greenhalgh RM, Davies AH. Measuring the quality of life in patients with venous ulcers. J Vasc Surg. 2000;31:642–9.
57. Brazier JE, Harper R, Jones NM, O'Cathain A, et al. Validating the SF-36 health survey questionnaire: new outcome measure for primary care. BMJ. 1992;305:160–4.
58. Abetz L, Sutton M, Brady L, McNulty P, et al. The Diabetic Foot Ulcer Scale (DFS): a quality of life instrument for use in clinical trials. Pract Diabet Int. 2002;19:167–75.
59. Bann CM, Fehnel SE, Gagnon DD. Development and validation of the Diabetic Foot Ulcer Scale-Short Form (DFS-SF). Pharmacoeconomics. 2003;21:1277–90.
60. Farage MA, Miller KW, Berardesca E, Maibach HI. Clinical implications of aging skin: cutaneous disorders in the elderly. Am J Clin Dermatol. 2009;10:73–86.
61. Gorecki C, Brown JM, Cano S, Lamping DL, et al. Development and validation of a new patient-reported outcome measure for patients with pressure ulcers: the PU-QOL instrument. Health Qual Life Outcomes. 2013;11:95.
62. Rutherford C, Nixon J, Brown JM, Lamping DL, et al. Using mixed methods to select optimal mode of administration for a patient-reported outcome instrument for people with pressure ulcers. BMC Med Res Methodol. 2014;14:22.
63. Wollina U. Rosacea and rhinophyma in the elderly. Clin Dermatol. 2011;29:61–8.
64. Powell FC. Clinical practice. Rosacea. N Engl J Med. 2005;352:793–803.
65. Nicholson K, Abramova L, Chren MM, Yeung J, et al. A pilot quality-of-life instrument for acne rosacea. J Am Acad Dermatol. 2007;57:213–21.
66. Seidler AM, Kini SP, DeLong LK, Veledar E, et al. Preference-based measures in dermatology: an overview of utilities and willingness to pay. Dermatol Clin. 2012;30:223–9. xiii.
67. Schmitt J, Meurer M, Klon M, Frick KD. Assessment of health state utilities of controlled and uncontrolled psoriasis and atopic eczema: a population-based study. Br J Dermatol. 2008;158:351–9.
68. Lundberg L, Johannesson M, Silverdahl M, Hermansson C, et al. Quality of life, health-state

utilities and willingness to pay in patients with psoriasis and atopic eczema. Br J Dermatol. 1999;141:1067–75.
69. Chen S, Shaheen A, Garber A. Cost-effectiveness and cost-benefit analysis of using methotrexate vs Goeckerman therapy for psoriasis. A pilot study. Arch Dermatol. 1998;134:1602–8.
70. Zug KA, Littenberg B, Baughman RD, Kneeland T, et al. Assessing the preferences of patients with psoriasis. A quantitative, utility approach. Arch Dermatol. 1995;131:561–8.
71. Schiffner R, Schiffner-Rohe J, Gerstenhauer M, Hofstadter F, et al. Willingness to pay and time trade-off: sensitive to changes of quality of life in psoriasis patients? Br J Dermatol. 2003;148:1153–60.
72. Seidler AM, Bayoumi AM, Goldstein MK, Cruz PDJ, et al. Willingness to pay in dermatology: assessment of the burden of skin diseases. J Invest Dermatol. 2012;132:1785–90.
73. Radtke MA, Schafer I, Gajur A, Langenbruch A, et al. Willingness-to-pay and quality of life in patients with vitiligo. Br J Dermatol. 2009;161:134–9.
74. Beikert FC, Langenbruch AK, Radtke MA, Augustin M. Willingness to pay and quality of life in patients with rosacea. J Eur Acad Dermatol Venereol. 2013;27:734–8.
75. Beikert FC, Langenbruch AK, Radtke MA, Kornek T, et al. Willingness to pay and quality of life in patients with atopic dermatitis. Arch Dermatol Res. 2014;306:279–86.
76. Finlay AY, Coles EC. The effect of severe psoriasis on the quality of life of 369 patients. Br J Dermatol. 1995;132:236–44.
77. Schiffner R, Brunnberg S, Hohenleutner U, Stolz W, et al. Willingness to pay and time trade-off: useful utility indicators for the assessment of quality of life and patient satisfaction in patients with port wine stains. Br J Dermatol. 2002;146:440–7.
78. Chen SC, Bayoumi AM, Soon SL, Aftergut K, et al. A catalog of dermatology utilities: a measure of the burden of skin diseases. J Investig Dermatol Symp Proc. 2004;9:160–8.
79. Caron M, Perrier LL, Emery MP. In 2012, the Patient-Reported Outcomes and Quality of Life Instruments Database (PROQOLID) Celebrates a Major Feat: Its 10th Anniversary! Patient Reported Outcomes Newsletter. Spring Issue 2012; 47, pp.26–27.
80. Chren MM. The Skindex instruments to measure the effects of skin disease on quality of life. Dermatol Clin. 2012;30:231–6. xiii.
81. Martin AR, Lookingbill DP, Botek A, Light J, et al. Health-related quality of life among patients with facial acne – assessment of a new acne-specific questionnaire. Clin Exp Dermatol. 2001;26:380–5.
82. Motley RJ, Finlay AY. How much disability is caused by acne? Clin Exp Dermatol. 1989;14:194–8.
83. Kingsley DH. The development and validation of a quality of life measure for the impact of androgen-dependent alopecia [dissertation]. Portsmouth: Portsmouth University; 1999.
84. Mendoza TR, Osei JS, Shi Q, Duvic M. Development of the alopecia areata symptom impact scale. J Investig Dermatol Symp Proc. 2013;16:S51–2.
85. Whalley D, McKenna SP, Dewar AL, Erdman RA, et al. A new instrument for assessing quality of life in atopic dermatitis: international development of the Quality of Life Index for Atopic Dermatitis (QoLIAD). Br J Dermatol. 2004;150:274–83.
86. Charman CR, Venn AJ, Williams HC. The patient-oriented eczema measure: development and initial validation of a new tool for measuring atopic eczema severity from the patients' perspective. Arch Dermatol. 2004;140:1513–9.
87. Erturk IE, Arican O, Omurlu IK, Sut N. Effect of the pruritus on the quality of life: a preliminary study. Ann Dermatol. 2012;24:406–12.
88. Hyland ME, Lay A, Thomson B. Quality of life of leg ulcer patients: questionnaire and preliminary findings. J Wound Care. 1994;3:294–8.
89. Koo J. Population-based epidemiologic study of psoriasis with emphasis on quality of life assessment. Dermatol Clin. 1996;14:485–96.
90. McKenna SP, Doward LC, Whalley D, Tennant A, et al. Development of the PsAQoL: a quality of life instrument specific to psoriatic arthritis. Ann Rheum Dis. 2004;63:162–9.
91. Roborel de Climens A, Bachelez H, Bagot M et al. Development of a unique tool reflecting patient and physician perceptions of psoriasis severity and treatment efficacy. Presented at: 20th Congress of the European Academy of Dermatology and Venereology (EADV); October 20 2011; Lisbon, Portugal.
92. Fredriksson T, Pettersson U. Severe psoriasis – oral therapy with a new retinoid. Dermatologica. 1978;157:238–44.
93. Drake LA, Patrick DL, Fleckman P, Andr J, et al. The impact of onychomycosis on quality of life: development of an international onychomycosis-specific questionnaire to measure patient quality of life. J Am Acad Dermatol. 1999;41:189–96.
94. Jolly M, Pickard AS, Block JA, Kumar RB, et al. Disease-specific patient reported outcome tools for systemic lupus erythematosus. Semin Arthritis Rheum. 2012;42:56–65.
95. Doward LC, McKenna SP, Whalley D, Tennant A, et al. The development of the L-QoL: a quality-of-life instrument specific to systemic lupus erythematosus. Ann Rheum Dis. 2009;68:196–200.
96. Symmons DP, Coppock JS, Bacon PA, Bresnihan B, et al. Development and assessment of a computerized index of clinical disease activity in systemic lupus erythematosus. Members of the British Isles Lupus Assessment Group (BILAG). Q J Med. 1988;69:927–37.

97. Vitali C, Bencivelli W, Isenberg DA, Smolen JS, et al. Disease activity in systemic lupus erythematosus: report of the Consensus Study Group of the European Workshop for Rheumatology Research. II. Identification of the variables indicative of disease activity and their use in the development of an activity score. The European Consensus Study Group for Disease Activity in SLE. Clin Exp Rheumatol. 1992;10:541–7.
98. Bombardier C, Gladman DD, Urowitz MB, Caron D, et al. Derivation of the SLEDAI. A disease activity index for lupus patients. The Committee on Prognosis Studies in SLE. Arthritis Rheum. 1992;35:630–40.
99. Lilly E, Lu PD, Borovicka JH, Victorson D, et al. Development and validation of a vitiligo-specific quality-of-life instrument (VitiQoL). J Am Acad Dermatol. 2013;69:e11–8.

Skin Aging: A Generalization of the Microinflammatory Hypothesis

98

Paolo U. Giacomoni and Glen Rein

Contents

P.U. Giacomoni (✉)
Elan Rose Int., Tustin, CA, USA
e-mail: paologiac@gmail.com

G. Rein
Innovative Biophysical Technologies, Ridgway, CO, USA
e-mail: glenrein@ymail.com

M.A. Farage et al. (eds.), *Textbook of Aging Skin*,
DOI 10.1007/978-3-662-47398-6_76

Abstract

The micro-inflammatory hypothesis of skin aging can be represented as a cyclic phenomenon as follows. A cell is damaged by endogenous or exogenous factors. The damaged cell releases proinflammatory signals (prostaglandins, leukotrienes, etc.). Inflammatory signals bind to resident mast cells and induce the release of histamine and TNF-α that diffuse to blood vessels lined by endothelial cells. Stimulated by histamine and TNF-α, endothelial cells synthesize and mobilize ICAM-1. ICAM-1 synthesis can also be stimulated by anoxia, glycated proteins, neuropeptides, hormonal imbalance, or other signals not originating from damaged cells, which all are factors of skin aging. Circulating immune cells bind to ICAM-1, roll over, release hydrogen peroxide, and perform diapedesis. In the presence of chemotactic signals from damaged cell, immune cells fray a path across the dermis by releasing singlet oxygen and matrix metalloproteinases. In the absence of chemotactic signals, immune cells damage the connective tissue surrounding the blood vessels. When the damaged cell is reached, immune cells release an oxidative burst to destroy the damaged cell, engulf the debris, and proceed to the lymphatic system. In these steps, innocent bystander cells can be damaged, thus triggering another round of release of proinflammatory signals, and the cycle is repeated.

Introduction

If "eternal youth" can be achieved by restoring, to the *status quo ante*, molecular changes as soon as they occur, then aging can be defined as the accumulation of damage, where damage is understood as molecular change [1]. This chapter describes how the micro-inflammatory hypothesis of skin aging has been induced upon analyzing the clinical, biophysical, histological, electron microscopy, cellular, and macromolecular aspects of skin aging. It points out environmental and lifestyle factors that accelerate the rate of aging. In addition, it explores metabolic and genetic factors participating in the process of accumulating damage.

Factors of aging provoke physiological responses that share common mechanistic features. For an example, let us consider the pathways to the onset of two visible signs of aging as diverse as solar elastosis and varicose vein.

Ultraviolet (UV) radiation damages epidermal cells. Damaged cells trigger the arachidonic acid cascade and the release of prostaglandins and leukotrienes. Upon binding these molecules, resident mast cells release histamine and tumor necrosis factor α (TNF-α), which promote synthesis and mobilization of intercellular adhesion molecule 1 (ICAM-1) in nearby endothelial cells. Circulating monocytes and macrophages bind ICAM-1, roll over, enter the dermis, and chemotactically migrate to reach the UV-damaged cell. Evidence for this phenomenon is provided by the histology-documented inflammatory infiltration [2]. In so doing, immune cells release proteases and damage the extracellular matrix (ECM), thus accelerating the rate of damage formation and accumulation, that is, aging process, which can be defined as accumulation of damage versus time [1, 3, 4]. Damaged elastic fibers are slowly replaced by new, disorganized ones [5, 6] and, with chronic exposure to solar radiation, the elastic properties of the skin are lost and solar elastosis is observed.

Varicose veins are visible under the skin. They appear as if they were no longer maintained in the socket of the vein-surrounding smooth muscle. When constrained to a static standing position over time, a person develops anoxia in the veins of the lower legs. Anoxia provokes the synthesis and the mobilization of ICAM-1 in the endothelial cells lining the vein walls [7], and monocytes and macrophage bind ICAM-1, roll over, perform diapedesis, and infiltrate the surrounding extracellular matrix (ECM). Not having chemotactic signals to follow, monocytes and macrophages release oxidative bursts and proteases in the proximity of the smooth muscle cells surrounding the vein. With chronic exposure to anoxia, the inflammatory infiltration persists, the smooth muscle cells are heavily damaged, the vein walls collapse, and varicose veins appear as a sign of accelerated vascular aging.

It thus appears that two totally unrelated phenomena such as solar elastosis and varicose vein, which are the effect of causes as different as ultraviolet radiation and anoxia, do result from the same mechanism, that is, the synthesis and mobilization of ICAM-1. The comparison of the onset of solar elastosis and of varicose vein led to the proposal of the micro-inflammatory model for skin aging [4]. Due to accumulating evidence that environmental, lifestyle, and metabolic factors can also trigger the synthesis of ICAM-1 and the onset of the inflammatory process, the micro-inflammatory model can be now considered more of a testable hypothesis than a simple mechanistic model.

The Micro-inflammatory Hypothesis of Skin Aging

The aging of the skin is the consequence of the three oxidative steps subsequent to the synthesis and mobilization of intercellular adhesion molecule 1 within the endothelium of cutaneous vessels. Agents able to provoke this synthesis and mobilization contribute to skin aging [4].

First oxidative step. Vascular cell adhesion molecule-1 (VCAM-1) activates endothelial cell Nicotinamide Adenosine Dinncletide Phosphate Reduced (NADPH) oxidase, which catalyzes the production of reactive oxygen species (ROS).

This activity is required for VCAM-1-dependent lymphocyte migration [8]. Upon binding ICAM-1 and rolling over, circulating inflammatory cells release hydrogen peroxide [9], and endothelial cells lose intercellular contact, round up, and allow monocytes and macrophages to perform diapedesis across the vascular wall.

Second oxidative step. In the extracellular matrix, inflammatory cells can either follow chemotactic signals to reach damaged somatic cells or agents of infection or just exert their lytic functions randomly. In both cases, reactive oxygen species are released, together with specific matrix metalloproteinases.

Third oxidative step. In the presence of cells to destroy, engulf, and remove (such as damaged somatic cells, foreign bacteria, or molds), inflammatory cells release H_2O_2. By-standing resident cells can be damaged by this oxidative burst and trigger the arachidonic acid cascade and the release of prostaglandins and leukotrienes which will be relayed by the secretion of histamine and TNF-α from resident mast cells, and these cytokines and autacoids will induce synthesis and mobilization of ICAM-1, thus perpetuating the inflammatory process.

The accumulation of oxidative and proteolytic damage experienced over time by the extracellular matrix, together with the remodeling of fibers in a disorganized mode, leads to skin aging. The micro-inflammatory hypothesis emphasizes the aging of the cutaneous connective tissue and of the extracellular matrix. Macroscopic consequences of this hypothesis are verified by experiment. The recognition that post-UV repair and wound healing share ECM remodeling as a common feature has allowed one to understand why blood vessels are deeper down in aged skin than in young skin. The sagging of the dermis is the consequence of a modified ECM and is accompanied by an overall increase in the surface area of the skin, particularly of the face. With time, under the action of gravitational pull, the surface of the skin increases. It can be surmised that in order to keep the skin around the skull, nerves and muscles act and pull the skin. Facial wrinkles form along the sites of attachment of the skin to muscles. Wrinkles have a neuromuscular cause and that is evidenced by their disappearance in hemiplegics, when the individual is under general anesthesia, or when wrinkled skin is treated with Botox. The increase of skin surface area and the reduction of total body volume can be invoked to explain the observation that, notwithstanding a nearly constant rate of turnover of the keratinocytes through the life span, the thickness of the epidermis is diminished with aging. This is more the consequence of the stretching of the skin than the consequence of a modification of the turnover rate of the keratinocytes. Indeed, the turnover of the keratinocytes does not change with aging, and this is confirmed by the fact that the thickness of the **stratum corneum** is, in fact, constant with aging [10].

Early Justification of the Micro-inflammatory Hypothesis

Environmental and lifestyle factors capable of accelerating skin aging were recognized by biomedical investigations in the course of the twentieth century, and, as a consequence of the work of the European Network for the Biology of Aging, it was pointed out in 1996 that several factors of skin aging share as a common feature, the capability of inducing the synthesis and the mobilization of ICAM-1 in the endothelium [4]. The factors first recognized as having this capability were ultraviolet radiation, tractions, wounds, infections, trauma, anoxia, cigarette smoke, and specific hormonal imbalances. A cause–effect relationship was later inferred between ICAM-1 synthesis and mobilization and protein glycation, stretching, electromagnetic fields, psychological stressors, and neuropeptides [11].

Some of the factors of skin aging are also direct cell- or tissue-damaging factors. When damage to cells or tissue is generated (e.g., by UV radiation, smoke-related free radicals, infectious agents, or wounds and traumas), a number of modifications are provoked to the ECM, to resident cells, and to vessel walls by the free radicals and lytic enzymes which are released in the course of the inflammatory response, consequent to the diffusion of cytokines produced via the arachidonic acid cascade. What about other factors of aging which are not directly damaging agents? Traction and gravitational forces provoke the activation of phospholipase A2, an enzyme involved in the arachidonic acid cascade. Anoxia induces ICAM-1 synthesis and diapedesis of macrophages, which start digesting the ECM around veins or other blood vessels. Glucose binds to proteins in a nonenzymatic glycation process, and glycated proteins are inducers of ICAM-1 synthesis. Electromagnetic fields associated with computers provoke the release of histamine, IL-1, and IL-6. Neuropeptides regulate the expression of cell adhesion molecules on both leukocytes and endothelial cells in a coordinated effort to control neurogenic inflammation. These phenomena trigger a cycle of self-maintained inflammatory responses, which comprises the induction of mobilization and neosynthesis of ICAM-1, and are summarized in [4, 5, 11].

Extension of the Validity of the Micro-inflammatory Hypothesis

Recent investigations have generated further results indicating that other factors of skin aging, the mode of action of which was not previously understood, induce physiological responses consistent with the micro-inflammatory hypothesis. Exposure to low temperatures, consumption of specific nutritional elements, neuromediators, physical exercise, and sleep deprivation are discussed.

Cold

Epidemiological evidence indicates that exposure to low temperatures is associated with visible signs of skin aging, from type I and type II rosacea to the appearance of spider veins. Exposure to low temperatures provokes a vasoconstriction, which is mediated by endothelin-1. Indeed, levels of circulating endothelin-1 increase sevenfold in venous plasma from a hand immersed in ice water and threefold in venous plasma from the non-immersed, contralateral hand [12]. The levels of circulating adhesion soluble molecules, such as sICAM-1, sVCAM-1, and sE-selectin, are indicators of an existing inflammatory reaction and were found to increase within an hour after healthy individuals were subjected to a cold pressor test [13].

Remarkably enough, endothelin-1 increased the expression of E-selectin and ICAM-1 on Human Coronary Artery Endothelial Cells (HCAEC) [14]. Endothelin-1 was also reported to mediate the induction of ICAM-1 and VCAM-1 by C-reactive protein in human saphenous vein endothelial cells [15]. All these results are consistent with the conclusion that endothelin-1 regulates cell surface adhesion molecules including ICAM-1, which is key to cell–cell and cell–matrix adhesion and leukocyte infiltration [16].

From these studies one can expect that, upon chronic exposure to cold, the vasoconstriction provoked by endothelin-1 will be associated with a moderate increase in the levels of adhesion molecules with consequent diapedesis of circulating inflammatory cells. These could damage the smooth muscle cells surrounding the cutaneous blood vessels, thus maintaining a mild vasodilation, which can provoke a persistent erythema sometimes diagnosed as type I or type II rosacea. When the damage to smooth muscle cells causes the collapse of the capillary walls, the erythema can become permanent and be accompanied by broken capillaries, visible as spider veins.

Ethanol

The physiological effects of ethanol consumption are known to differ according to the dose and the frequency of ingestion. Moderate drinkers, with an intake of 20–40 g ethanol/day, have lower serum ICAM-1 and VCAM-1 levels than teetotalers, whereas heavy drinkers display much higher levels of adhesion molecules than moderate drinkers or abstinent controls [17]. Furthermore, moderate consumption of sparkling wine, red wine, or white wine in healthy individuals promotes the decrease of serum level of circulating VCAM-1, E-selectin, and P-selectin [18, 19]. These results suggest that moderate alcohol intake has anti-inflammatory effects on the cardiovascular system, but at higher doses ethanol can exert a proinflammatory effect. Indeed, chronic alcoholics exhibit significantly higher serum levels of endothelial adhesion molecules than abstainers or moderate drinkers [20]. It can therefore be surmised that the smooth muscle surrounding the blood vessels of heavy drinkers is subjected to the persistent damaging effect of the inflammatory infiltrate, which can cause the collapse of the walls of the vessels and the appearance of spider veins.

Neuromediators

The skin is innervated by peripheral sensory nerves, which can form direct synapses with epidermal and dermal cells. These sensory neurons contain and release a variety of neuropeptides and neurohormones, which regulate a wide variety of biochemical processes and cell functions of keratinocytes, Langerhans cells, mast cells, dermal microvascular endothelial cells, and infiltrating leukocytes under physiological and pathological conditions. Furthermore, many of these cell types can act as a source of neuropeptides and in turn affect the survival, regeneration, and functional capacity of sensory neurons.

Expression and regulation of receptors for neuromodulators that are synthesized on a variety of skin cells determine the cellular responses mediated by these peptides. A majority of studies address diseased human skin, but in most cases these phenomena are universal across most species and tissues and the results from these studies can be extrapolated to normal skin. Of particular interest here are the vasoactive effects of cutaneous neuropeptides resulting in inflammatory processes, previously proposed as a hallmark of skin aging [11]. However, other proinflammatory neuromodulators are also discussed.

In addition to its well-known cardiovascular effects, serotonin can activate neuronal cells to release Calcitonin gene Releated Peptide (CGRP) and endothelial cells to secrete NO [21]. Recent research has focused on characterizing the different 5-HT receptor subtypes. Activation of nociceptor type 1D is associated with inflammatory pain which is mediated by trigeminal neurons [22]. Serotonin receptor agonists (including 1D) block neurogenic inflammation [23] by inhibiting the release of substance P and CGRP from peptidergic afferents [24]. Some serotonin receptor agonists are currently being used in the treatment of migraine pain [25].

Substance P and CGRP are co-localized in sensory cutaneous neurons and are released locally in response to injury and induce neurogenic inflammation [26]. These neuropeptides increase microvascular permeability, enhance leukocyte extravasation, and increase cellular migration [27] resulting in wheal and flare [28] and pain [29].

There is strong evidence that cell adhesion molecules play a major role in neurogenic inflammation [11]. The role of substance P and CGRP in increasing the expression of ICAM-1, VCAM-1, and P- and E-selectins is well established.

In patients with atopic eczema, a single intracutaneous injection of Vasoactive Intestinal Polypeptide (VIP) increased local blood flow in a dose-dependent manner, induced a wheal-and-flare reaction, and increased pruritus [30]. These results have been corroborated in in vivo animal studies where subcutaneous injections of VIP caused concentration-dependent plasma extravasation in rat skin, although this was significantly less effective than identical concentrations of substance P [31].

The proinflammatory activity of VIP in human skin is also mediated by a direct action on inflammatory mediators: the addition of VIP to human keratinocytes in culture increases in the intracellular expressions of IL-1α, IL-8, and TNF-α mRNA [32]. IL-1 and IL-8 protein levels were also increased in culture medium of VIP-treated cells. A similar effect of VIP was observed on human mast cells where it induced the release of IL-8, TNF-α, and monocyte chemoattractant protein-1 [33].

Bradykinin (BK) and other kinins are produced at sites of tissue injury and contribute to inflammatory processes including edema formation, vasodilatation, and pain [34]. BK receptors have been found on vascular endothelial cells, smooth muscles, mast cells, and sensory neurons [34]. In the case of sensory nerve activation, BK causes the release of proinflammatory peptides including substance P and CGRP. Thus, the response to BK is mediated indirectly by neuropeptides including substance P and CGRP [35]. Furthermore, at least with respect to edema, BK and CGRP are synergistic [36].

Furthermore, BK increases plasma extravasation in knee joints, although in this case no edema was observed [37]. Its actions are mediated through BK receptors and indirectly by release or amplification of inflammatory mediators including neuropeptides. More recently, the role of ectoenzymes kininasc and metalloendopeptidase, which metabolize BK, has been shown to regulate active BK receptors on peripheral sensory neurons [38].

Physical Exercise

Psychological stress triggers the release of proinflammatory mediators [11]. In at least one study, similar phenomena were observed with both psychological stress and physical exercise [39], suggesting that both factors mediate age-accelerating inflammatory processes. Several studies indicate that moderate-intensity exercise is associated with a reduction in inflammatory mediators (perhaps by reducing the risk of anoxia) [40–42]. It has therefore been suggested that the health benefits associated with physical exercise are due to this anti-inflammatory response. This conclusion is supported by a recent study measuring the expression of hundreds of neutrophil genes before and after a single 30-min cycling exercise at 80 % peak oxygen uptake. Both proinflammatory and anti-inflammatory genes showed increased expression immediately following this exercise regime [43].

However, the beneficial anti-inflammatory effects of exercise are critically dependent on the type of exercise, its duration and intensity, the level of fitness, and the time when the markers of inflammation are measured after the exercise regime. Since these factors vary from one study to another, results reported in the scientific literature are sometimes difficult to compare. Typically, studies which employ more intense exercise regimes use more fit individuals. One interesting study measured the inflammatory response to 20 min of treadmill exercise (65–70 % VO_2 maximum) in younger/fit versus older/unfit individuals. This regime increased leukocyte adhesion to endothelial cells in vitro only in younger and fitter subjects [44].

Other studies, using different exercise programs, however, have shown proinflammatory changes immediately after relatively intense resistive exercise. In an attempt to use real-life exercises, wrestling matches are often used as an acute, intense, resistive form of exercise for adolescents, as they are known to induce muscle injury. This form of exercise was used to study the change in the number and type of circulating leukocytes. Using Fluorescence Activated Cell Sorter (FACS) flow cytometry, an increase in the density of lymphocytes expressing ICAM-1 and LFA-1 was observed immediately after a single 1.5-h wrestling practice session [45]. Furthermore, results from the redistribution of other lymphocyte subsets indicate an increase in memory T cells. These lymphocytes are intimately involved with inflammation since they preferentially adhere to endothelial cells and are selectively recruited into inflammatory sites [46] and express IL-6 [47].

In addition to leukocyte cell numbers, other studies have measured circulating levels of proinflammatory markers following physical exercise in healthy individuals using a variety of regimes. These studies report increases in ICAM-1/VCAM [48], IL-6 [49], TNF-α [50], PGE2 and substance P [51], iNOS and *NF*-κβ [52], and C-reactive protein [53]. The acute phase inflammatory response typically occurs within the first 48 h but can be maintained for several days [54], depending on which inflammatory marker is measured. These inflammatory responses occur in both young and old healthy individuals.

Sleep Deprivation

A lifestyle factor known to promote apparent skin fatigue and perhaps to accelerate aging, and which has been proven to trigger inflammatory responses in healthy individuals, is sleep deprivation. Like extensive physical exercise, sleep deprivation is associated with poor quality of life, mood changes, higher psychological stress levels, and increased susceptibility to a variety of diseases (notably cardiovascular disease). Both sleep deprivation and extensive physical exercise increase serum concentrations of proinflammatory cytokines, circulating leukocytes, and soluble cell adhesion molecules. In a study where volunteers were subjected to both 7 days of semicontinuous strenuous exercise and sleep deprivation (1 h/night), plasma levels of IL-6, TNF-α, and IL-1β were increased and isolated leukocytes showed enhanced release of these proinflammatory markers when stimulated with Lipo Poly saccharides (LPS) [55]. Similar results were obtained by numerous other investigators examining sleep deprivation alone, although severe sleep deprivation protocols often keep subjects awake for extended periods of time with no sleep at all. In these studies, sleep is typically monitored using polysomnography, and sleep quality is usually assessed by subjective reports using the Pittsburgh Sleep Quality Index (PSQI). Results from these studies reveal that in addition to the proinflammatory cytokines [55], increased plasma levels of ICAM-1 and E-selectin [56], endothelin-1 [57], and PGE2 [58] were observed in healthy individuals.

Results from these studies are often complicated by the fact that circadian fluctuations in levels of proinflammatory cytokines are known to exist. However, several studies have taken these circadian variations into account and reached the same conclusions. In the case of IL-6, for example, sleep deprivation leads to daytime oversecretion and nighttime undersecretion [59]. In general, similar proinflammatory changes are reported in both young and old subjects, although it is worth considering that chronic sleep impairment can contribute to age-related changes in inflammatory responses [60].

Conclusion

The micro-inflammatory hypothesis of skin aging was proposed as a mechanistic model [4]. The original model showed that skin aging is accelerated by agents or treatments able to induce the synthesis and mobilization of ICAM-1 in endothelial cells. Other factors induce the synthesis and the mobilization of ICAM-1 in endothelial cells and/or in circulating leukocytes. These factors are now believed to be accelerators of skin aging.

Thus, the micro-inflammatory mechanistic model of skin aging is a testable hypothesis open for experimental challenge and experimental confirmation.

In recent years further experimental evidence supported the micro-inflammatory hypothesis of skin aging, and inflammatory contribution to the aging of organs as diverse as the brain and articular joints has been pointed out [61, 62].

References

1. Giacomoni PU. Aging and cellular defence mechanisms. In: Franceschi C, Crepaldi G, Cristofalo VJ, Vijg J, editors. Aging and cellular defence mechanisms, Annals of the New York Academy of Sciences, vol. 663. New York: New York Academy of Sciences; 1992. p. 1–3.
2. Hawk JLM, Murphy GM, Holden GA. The presence of neutrophils in human cutaneous ultraviolet-B inflammation. Br J Dermatol. 1988;118:27–30.
3. Novoltsev VN, Novoltseva J, Yashin A. A homeostatic model of oxidative damage explains paradoxes observed in the earlier aging experiments: a fusion and extension of older theories of aging. Biogerontology. 2001;2:127–38.
4. Giacomoni PU, D'Alessio P. Skin ageing: the relevance of antioxidants. In: Rattan SIS, Toussaint O, editors. Molecular gerontology: research status and strategies. New York: Plenum Press; 1996. p. 177–92.
5. Giacomoni PU, Rein G. A mechanistic model for the aging of human skin. Micron. 2004;35:179–84.
6. Wlaschek M, Schneider LA, Kohn M, Nüßeler E, Treiber N, Scharffetter-Kochanek K. Aging after solar

radiation. In: Giacomoni PU, editor. Biophysical and Physiological Effects of Solar Radiation on Human Skin. Cambridge: RSC Publishing; 2007. p. 191–210.

7. Arnould T, Michiels C, Janssens D, Delaive E, Remacle J. Hypoxia induces PMN adherence to umbilical vein endothelium. Cardiovasc Res. 1995;30:1009–16.
8. Tudor KS, Hess KL, Cook-Mills JM. Cytokines modulate endothelial cell intracellular signal transduction required for VCAM-1-dependent lymphocyte transendothelial migration. Cytokine. 2001;15:196–211.
9. Goldman G, Welbourn R, Klausner JM, Kobzik L, Valeri CR, Shepro D, Hechtman HB. Intravascular chemoattractants inhibit diapedesis by selective receptor occupancy. Am J Physiol. 1991;260:H465–72.
10. Gilchrest B. Aging of skin. In: Fitzpatrick TB, Zur Hausen A, Wolff K, Freedberg IM, Austen KF, editors. Dermatology in General Medicine. New York: McGraw-Hill; 1993. p. 150–7.
11. Giacomoni PU, Rein G. Factors of skin aging share common mechanisms. Biogerontology. 2001;2:219–29.
12. Fyhrquist F, Saijonmaa O, Metsärinne K, Tikkanen I, Rosenlöf K, Tikkanen T. Raised plasma endothelin-1 concentration following cold pressor test. Biochem Biophys Res Commun. 1990;169:217–21.
13. Coppolino G, Bolignano D, Campo S, Loddo S, Teti D, Buemi M. Circulating progenitor cells after cold pressor test in hypertensive and uremic patients. Hypertens Res. 2008;31:717–24.
14. Zouki C, Baron C, Fournier A, Filep JG. Endothelin-1 enhances neutrophil adhesion to human coronary artery endothelial cells: role of ET(A) receptors and platelet-activating factor. Br J Pharmacol. 1999;127:969–79.
15. Verma S, Li SH, Badiwala MV, Weisel RD, Fedak PW, Li RK, Dhillon B, Mickle DA. Endothelin antagonism and interleukin-6 inhibition attenuate the proatherogenic effects of C-reactive protein. Circulation. 2002;105:1890–6.
16. Waters CE, Shi-Wen X, Denton CP, Abraham DJ, Pearson JD. Signaling pathways regulating intercellular adhesion molecule 1 expression by endothelin 1: comparison with interleukin-1 ß in normal and scleroderma dermal fibroblasts. Arthritis Rheum. 2006;54:649–60.
17. Sacanella E, Badia E, Nicolas JM, Fernandez-Sola J, Antunez E, Urbano-Marquez A, Estruch R. Differential effects of moderate or heavy alcohol consumption on circulating adhesion molecule levels. Thromb Haemost. 2002;88:52–5.
18. Vazquez-Agell M, Sacanella E, Tobias E, Monagas M, Antunez E, Zamora-Ros R, Andres-Lacueva C, Lamuel-Raventos RM, Fernandez-Sola J, Nicolas JM, Estruch R. Inflammatory markers of atherosclerosis are decreased after moderate consumption of cava (sparkling wine) in men with low cardiovascular risk. J Nutr. 2007;137:2279–84.
19. Sacanella E, Vazquez-Agell M, Mena MP, Antunez E, Fernandez-Sola J, Nicolas JM, Lamuela-Raventos RM, Ros E, Estruch R. Down-regulation of adhesion molecules and other inflammatory biomarkers after moderate wine consumption in healthy women: a randomized trial. Am J Clin Nutr. 2007;86:1463–9.
20. Sacanella E, Estruch R. The effect of alcohol consumption on endothelial adhesion molecule expression. Addict Biol. 2003;8:371–8.
21. Cocks TM, Arnold PJ. 5-Hydroxytryptamine (5-HT) mediates potent relaxation in the sheep isolated pulmonary vein via activation of 5-HT4 receptors. Br J Pharmacol. 1992;107:591–6.
22. Ahn AH, Basbaur AI. Tissue injury regulates serotonin 1D receptor expression: implications for the control of migraine and inflammatory pain. J Neurosci. 2006;26:8332–8.
23. Bolay H, Reuter U, Dunn AK, Huang Z, Boas DA. Moskowitz MA Intrinsic brain activity triggers trigeminal meningeal afferents in a migraine model. Nat Med. 2002;8:136–42.
24. Buzzi MG, Carter WB, Shimizu T, Heath 3rd H, Moskowitz MA. Dihydroergotamine and sumatriptan attenuate levels of CGRP in plasma in rat superior sagittal sinus during electrical stimulation of the trigeminal ganglion. Neuropharmacology. 1991;30:1193–200.
25. Ahn AH, Basbaum AI. Where do triptans act in the treatment of migraine? Pain. 2005;115:1–4.
26. Ansel JC, Armstrong CA, Song I, Quinlan KL, Olerud JE, Caughman SW, Bunnett NW. Interactions of the skin and nervous system. J Investig Dermatol Symp Proc. 1997;2:23–6.
27. Björklund H, Dalsgaard CJ, Jonsson CE, Hermansson A. Sensory and autonomic innervation of non-hairy and hairy human skin. An immunohistochemical study. Cell Tissue Res. 1986;243:51–7.
28. Jensen K, Tuxen C, Pedersen-Bjergaard U, Jansen I. Pain, tenderness, wheal and flare induced by substance-P, bradykinin and 5-hydroxytryptamine in humans. Cephalalgia. 1991;11:175–82.
29. Birklein F, Schmelz M. Neuropeptides, neurogenic inflammation and complex regional pain syndrome (CRPS). Neurosci Lett. 2008;437:199–202.
30. Rukwied R, Heyer G. Cutaneous reactions and sensations after intracutaneous injection of vasoactive intestinal polypeptide and acetylcholine in atopic eczema patients and healthy controls. Arch Dermatol Res. 1998;290:198–204.
31. Cardell LO, Stjärne P, Wagstaff SJ, Agustí C, Nadel JA. PACAP-induced plasma extravasation in rat skin. Regul Pept. 1997;71:67–71.
32. Dallos A, Kiss M, Polyánka H, Dobozy A, Kemény L, Husz S. Effects of the neuropeptides substance P, calcitonin gene-related peptide, vasoactive intestinal

polypeptide and galanin on the production of nerve growth factor and inflammatory cytokines in cultured human keratinocytes. Neuropeptides. 2006;40:251–63.
33. Kulka M, Sheen CH, Tancowny BP, Grammer LC, Schleimer RP. Neuropeptides activate human mast cell degranulation and chemokine production. Immunology. 2008;123:398–410.
34. Hall JM. Bradykinin receptors: pharmacological properties and biological roles. Pharmacol Ther. 1992;56:131–90.
35. Wahlestedt C, Bynke G, Hakanson R. Pupillary constriction by bradykinin and capsaicin: mode of action. Eur J Pharmacol. 1985;106:577–83.
36. Brain SD, Williams TJ. Inflammatory oedema induced by synergism between calcitonin gene-related peptide (CGRP) and mediators of increased vascular permeability. Br J Pharmacol. 1985;86:855–60.
37. Cambridge H, Brain SD. Calcitonin gene-related peptide increases blood flow and potentiates plasma protein extravasation in the rat knee joint. Br J Pharmacol. 1992;106:746–50.
38. Petho G, Reeh PW. Sensory and signaling mechanisms of bradykinin, eicosanoids, platelet-activating factor and nitric oxide in peripheral nociceptors. Physiol Rev. 2012;92:1699–775.
39. Goebel MU, Mills PJ. Acute psychological stress and exercise and changes in peripheral leukocyte adhesion molecule expression and density. Psychosom Med. 2000;62:664–70.
40. Chung HY, Cesari M, Anton S, Marzetti E, Giovannini S, Seo AY, Carter C, Yu BP, Leeuwenburgh C. Molecular inflammation: underpinnings of aging and age-related diseases. Ageing Res Rev. 2009;8:18–30.
41. Thomas NE, Williams DR. Inflammatory factors, physical activity, and physical fitness in young people Scand J Med Sci Sports. 2008;18:543–556.
42. Nielsen AR, Pedersen BK. The biological roles of exercise-induced cytokines: IL-6, IL-8 and IL-15. Appl Physiol Nutr Metab. 2007;32:833–9.
43. Radom-Aizik S, Zaldivar Jr F, Leu SY, Galassetti P, Cooper DM. Effects of 30 min of aerobic exercise on gene expression in human neutrophils. J Appl Physiol. 2008;104:236–43.
44. Mills PJ, Hong S, Redwine L, Carter SM, Chiu A, Ziegler MG, Dimsdale JE, Maisel AS. Physical fitness attenuates leukocyte endothelial adhesion in response to acute exercise. J Appl Physiol. 2006;101:785–8.
45. Nemet D, Mills PJ, Cooper DM. Effect of intense wrestling exercise on leucocytes and adhesion molecules in adolescent boys. Br J Sports Med. 2004;38:154–8.
46. Newman I, Wilkinson PC. Locomotor responses of human CD45 lymphocyte subsets: preferential locomotion of CD45RO + lymphocytes in response to attractants and mitogens. Immunology. 1993;78:92–8.
47. Hamann D, Baars PA, Rep MH, Hooibrink B, Kerkhof-Garde SR, Klein MR, van Lier RA. Phenotypic and functional separation of memory and effector human CD8 T cells. J Exp Med. 1997;186(9):1407–18.
48. Bartzeliotou AI, Margeli AP, Tsironi M, Skenderi K, Bacoula C, Chrousos GP, Papassotiriou I. Circulating levels of adhesion molecules and markers of endothelial activation in acute inflammation induced by prolonged brisk exercise. Clin Biochem. 2007;40:765–70.
49. Fischer CP. Interleukin-6 in acute exercise and training: what is the biological relevance? Exerc Immunol Rev. 2006;12:6–33.
50. Silva LA, Silveira PC, Pinho CA, Tuon T, Dal Pizzol F, Pinho RA. *N*-acetylcysteine supplementation and oxidative damage and inflammatory response after eccentric exercise. Int J Sport Nutr Exerc Metab. 2008;18:379–88.
51. Dousset F, Avela J, Ishikawa M, Kallio J, Kuitunen S, Kyroelainen H, Linnamo V, Komi PV. Bimodal recovery pattern in human skeletal muscle induced by exhaustive stretch-shortening exercise. Med Sci Sports Exerc. 2007;39:453–60.
52. Jimenez-Jimenez R, Cuevas MJ, Almar M, Lima E, Garcia-Lopez D, De Paz JA, Gonzalez-Gallego J. Eccentric training impairs NF-kappaB activation and overexpression of inflammation-related genes induced by acute eccentric exercise in the elderly. Mech Ageing Dev. 2008;129:313–21.
53. Ispirlidis I, Fatouros IG, Jamurtas AZ, Nikolaidis MG, Michailidis I, Douroudos I, Margonis K, Chatzinikolaou A, Kalistratos E, Katrabasas I, Alexiou V, Taxildaris K. Time-course of changes in inflammatory and performance responses following a soccer game. Clin J Sport Med. 2008;18(5):423–31.
54. Neubauer O, Koenig D, Wagner KH. Recovery after an Ironman triathlon: sustained inflammatory responses and muscular stress. Eur J Appl Physiol. 2008;104:417–26.
55. Gundersen Y, Opstad PK, Reistad T, Thrane I, Vaagenes P. Seven days' around the clock exhaustive physical exertion combined with energy depletion and sleep deprivation primes circulating leukocytes. Eur J Appl Physiol. 2006;97:151–7.
56. Frey DJ, Fleshner M, Wright Jr KP. The effects of 40 hours of total sleep deprivation on inflammatory markers in healthy young adults. Brain Behav Immun. 2007;21:1050–7.
57. Mills PJ, von Kaenel R, Norman D, Natarajan L, Ziegler MG, Dimsdale JE. Inflammation and sleep in healthy individuals. Sleep. 2007;30:729–35.
58. Haack M, Sanchez E, Mullington JM. Elevated inflammatory markers in response to prolonged sleep restriction are associated with increased pain experience in healthy volunteers. Sleep. 2007;30:1145–52.
59. Vgontzas AN, Papanicolaou DA, Bixler EO, Lotsikas A, Zachman K, Kales A, Prolo P, Wong ML,

Licinio J, Gold PW, Hermida RC, Mastorakos G, Chrousos GP. Circadian Interleukin-6 secretion and quantity and depth of sleep. J Clin Endocrinol Metab. 1999;84:2603–7.

60. Prinz PN. Age impairments in sleep, metabolic and immune functions. Exp Gerontol. 2004;39: 1739–43.

61. Wyss-Coray T, Rogers J. Inflammation in Alzheimer disease-A brief Review of the basic Science and Clinical Literature. Cold Spring Harb Perspect Med. 2012;2:1–23.

62. Yudoh K, Karasawa R. Statin prevents chondrocyte aging and degeneration of articular cartilage in osteoarthritis (OA). Aging. 2010;2:990–8.

The Potential of Probiotics and Prebiotics for Skin Health

99

A. C. Ouwehand, S. Lahtinen, and Kirsti Tiihonen

Contents

A.C. Ouwehand (✉) • S. Lahtinen • K. Tiihonen
Active Nutrition, DuPont Nutrition and Health, Kantvik, Finland
e-mail: arthur.ouwehand@dupont.com; sampo.lahtinen@dupont.com; kirsti.tiihonen@dupont.com

M.A. Farage et al. (eds.), *Textbook of Aging Skin*,
DOI 10.1007/978-3-662-47398-6_77

Abstract

The skin is one of the body's main barriers to the outside world. Similar to many other such barriers, the skin is colonized by a variety of microbes; their composition appears to depend on the place of the skin but is also influenced by age. Furthermore, a number of skin diseases are associated with an altered skin microbiota; cause and effect of the different skin microbiota and the disease/condition may not always be clear. There may, thus, be a benefit in changing the composition of the skin microbiota. Some immunological conditions, however, such as atopic dermatitis may actually benefit from a change in the intestinal microbiota through the consumption of probiotics and prebiotics. Also UV induced immune suppression seems to benefit from the consumption of specific probiotics. Furthermore, in animals probiotics have been reported to improve fur health. There are thus opportunities for topical and oral probiotics in improving skin health.

Introduction

Microbes are ubiquitous in our environment, and despite last century's improvement in hygiene, we are continuously exposed to them. We are not only exposed to microbes, we are also hosting them. An adult human being consists of an estimated 10^{13} eukaryotic cells. At the same time, we are hosting an estimated 10^{14} microbes, most of them in the large intestine but also appreciable amounts on the various sites of the skin. The composition of this microbiota (formerly known as "microflora") is complex and influenced by various environmental factors. It is therefore not surprising that different parts of the human body, which are exposed to the outside environment, will have a different microbiota. The composition and activity of the skin microbiota will be discussed in further detail below.

Aberrancies in the skin microbiota, and also in the intestinal microbiota (as will be discussed below), may contribute to disease. It may therefore be desirable to modulate the composition and/or activity of this microbiota. The most widely used method to modulate a microbiota is by the use of antibiotics. Antibiotics, although very powerful and sometimes reasonably selective, have the risk of inducing antibiotic resistance and unintentionally modifying other parts of the microbiota, as is evidenced by the induction of, for example, antibiotic-associated diarrhea. Also the skin microbiota has been observed to be influenced by oral antibiotic therapy and has been observed to slow down wound healing [1]. Although antibiotics are likely to remain essential therapeutics, alternative or complementary treatments to modify a microbiota exist: probiotics and prebiotics.

According to a generally accepted definition of a FAO/WHO work group, which was recently slightly adapted, probiotics are "live microorganisms that, when administered in adequate amounts, confer a health benefit on the host" [2, 3]. The most common probiotics are members of the genera *Lactobacillus* and *Bifidobacterium*, but probiotics of other genera exist as well (Table 1). It is important to note that only specific strains are probiotic, not the species. Furthermore, different strains may have different probiotic properties, and properties from one strain cannot be extrapolated to another strain, not even of the same species.

Prebiotics are commonly defined as "nondigestible food ingredients that, when consumed in sufficient amounts, selectively stimulate the growth and/or activity of one or a limited number of microbes in the colon resulting in documented health benefits" [4]. Although prebiotics are nondigestible and in many cases would fall under the definition of dietary fiber, they are not synonymous; not all fibers are prebiotic as they may not always be selectively utilized by a limited (and beneficial) part of the microbiota. The most widely investigated prebiotics are the fructo-oligosaccharides (FOS), inulin, and galacto-oligosaccharides (GOS). But there is a wide range of other (potential)

Table 1 Examples of microorganisms commonly used as probiotics. Note that not the species but specific strains within these species may be probiotic

Lactobacilli	Bifidobacteria	Other lactic acid bacteria	Nonlactic acid bacteria
L. acidophilus	*B. adolescentis*	*Enterococcus faecalis*	*Bacillus subtilis*
L. casei	*B. animalis* ssp. *lactis*	*Enterococcus faecium*	*Bacillus cereus*
L. crispatus	*B. bifidum*	*Lactococcus lactis*	*Bacillus coagulans*
L. delbrueckii ssp. *bulgaricus*	*B. breve*	*Streptococcus thermophilus*	*Clostridium butyricum*
L. fermentum	*B. longum* ssp. *infantis*		*Escherichia coli*
L. johnsonii	*B. longum* ssp. *longum*		*Propionibacterium freudenreichii*
L. paracasei			*Saccharomyces cerevisiae* (boulardii)
L. plantarum			
L. reuteri			
L. rhamnosus			
L. salivarius			

Table 2 Examples of substances commonly used for their prebiotic properties

Prebiotic (candidate)	Abbreviation	Main monomer(s)	Degree of polymerization	Linkage
Fructo-oligosaccharide (Oligofructose)	FOS	Fructose	1–7	β-(1,2)[a]
Galacto-oligosaccharide (Trans galacto-oligosaccharide)	GOS (TOS)	Galactose		β-(1,4)[a]
Inulin	–	Fructose	10–60	β-(1,2)
Lactitol	–	Galactose, Glucitol,	2	α-(1,4)
Lactulose	–	Galactose, Fructose	2	β-(1,4)
Partially hydrolysed guar gum	PHGG	Mannose, Galactose	10–300	β-(1,4) α-(1,6)
Polydextrose	PDX	Glucose	12–30	(1,6)
Xylo-oligosaccharide	XOS	Xylose	2–7	β-(1,4)
Resistant starch	RS	Glucose	10–100	α-(1,4) α-(1,6)

[a]Depending on the enzyme used in manufacture

prebiotics, see Table 2. Also different prebiotics have their specific health benefits that cannot be extrapolated to others. What is, however, currently not clear is whether prebiotics of the same "class," for example, GOS, but produced by different processes (different process conditions, different enzymes, etc.) and therefore with different degree of polymerization and type of glycosidic linkages will have the same health benefits or should these different types of the same prebiotic "class" be regarded as separate prebiotics in analogy to probiotic strains?

Probiotics and prebiotics are typically included in a variety of functional foods; the definition of the latter does not even consider nonfood applications. Normally administered orally, they may, nevertheless, have beneficial effects on the skin. The intestine is the body's main immune organ, and the mucosal immune system of the gut is linked to the immune system of the skin (and other mucosae) through migration of immune cells. Probiotics, and to a lesser extend prebiotics, have been documented to modulate the immune system. They may therefore indirectly also affect the functionality of the skin, as will be discussed further on. Pre- and probiotics may also influence the bioavailability of nutrients and that way affect the condition of for example, the skin. Functional foods targeting this "beauty from within" are already on the market, and some do have limited scientific evidence suggesting their efficacy. Unfortunately, many such products do not have documentation and their efficacy remains speculative. Topical application of probiotics and especially prebiotics has received limited attention to date. Topical products on the market do usually not contain live bacteria but fermentates or extracts. The topical application of live microbes may seem unusual; however, the skin has its own microbiota, which thus may be influenced similar as the intestinal microbiota. Concerning prebiotics, also sweat contains small amounts of glycogen which is likely to function as an endogenous prebiotic.

Skin Structure and Function

The human skin is the largest organ in a human body and has an average surface area of about 2 m^2. Skin structure and function varies between different anatomical sites. The thickness of the skin epidermis varies substantially from eyelids to soles of the feet. Moreover, the skin secretions mixed with the dead cells vary from one anatomical site to another and provide different environments for skin microbes. Secretions of sweat and sebaceous glands as well as detached cells from the epidermis are highest on the forehead and upper back. Palms, lips, and soles of the feet do

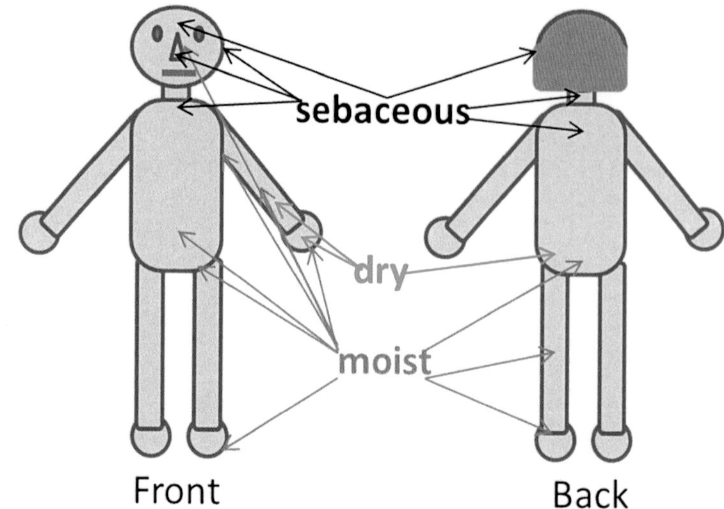

Fig. 1 Distribution of microenvironments of the human skin (sebaceous, dry, or moist)

not have sebum-producing glands. Hair follicles and associated sebaceous glands are also part of skin. The different distribution of sebaceous and sweat glands divides the skin in three types of environments: sebaceous, moist, and dry (Fig. 1). This, of course, influences the skin microbiota as will be discussed below.

The human skin has two main layers: the inner dermis and the outer epidermis. The epidermis and its secretions provide the primary protective barrier against external UV radiation, toxins, pathogens, dehydration, and mechanical disturbances. Although the epidermis is continuously replacing itself within 30–40 days, it does not contain blood vessels. Its nutrient and oxygen supply is dependent on diffusion from the dermal blood circulation. The regulation of balanced epidermal turnover is crucial for skin health. As an example, psoriasis is considered a skin disease with a markedly increased rate of epidermal turnover.

The epidermis can be divided into various sublayers with different functional characteristics: basal cell, spinous cell, granular cell, and cornified cell layers. The principle cells in the epidermis are keratinocytes. Other cell types in the epidermis are pigment-producing melanocytes, immunogenic Langerhans cells, and Merkel cells which act as mechanoreceptors. Langerhans cells, part of the dendritic cell family, play an important role in the skin immune system, which protects the body from environmental stressors and pathogens. Hyaluronan is the principal extra cellular matrix protein in the epidermis, facilitating tissue remodeling and other cellular and metabolic processes. The dermis consists mainly of collagen and elastin fibers with fibroblast, blood and lymph vessels, muscles, nerves, and glands. Below the dermis is hypodermis, containing adipocytes.

During normal differentiation, keratinocytes originating in the basal layer of the epidermis move toward the skin surface and change their function and composition. At the surface, the keratinocytes undergo apoptosis and become filled with keratin protein. This outermost layer of skin, the so-called stratum corneum, functions as the main barrier against water loss and external disturbances. The special lipid/water lamellar structure in the stratum corneum is important to maintain the permeability barrier of the skin. Natural moisturizing factor (NMF), which is mainly composed of water-soluble amino acids, prevents water loss from corneocytes.

The water content in deeper keratinocyte layers is important for the maturation of the skin cells. Hyaluronan is the most important extracellular matrix regulating tissue remodeling and water balance in the living keratinocyte layers. In addition to extracellular matrix, also organic osmolytes such as inositol, betaine, and taurine are known to participate in osmoregulation of keratinocytes during hyperosmotic stress and

UV radiation [5]. Recent findings indicate also that epidermal tight junctions have an important role in regulating the skin barrier and thereby water balance of skin [6]. Cells of different layers in the epidermis express only selected types of cellular junctions. Granular cells are interconnected with tight junctions whose structural proteins are zonula occludens-1 (ZO-1), occludin, and claudin-1 and -4. Abnormal distribution of occludin and ZO-1 occurs in psoriasis plaques.

Below the epidermis lies the dermis which mainly consists of connective tissue, collagen fibers, elastin, fibroblasts, blood vessels, and cells with immune activity. Fibroblasts are responsible of the collagen synthesis in dermis and they have also important role in wound healing.

Clinical Alterations in Skin Aging

Typical age-related changes of the skin are wrinkles, dryness, and changes in color and structure. The skin structure is mainly dependent on the collagen and elastin fibers which undergo changes during aging. The dryness of the aging skin is caused by decreased blood circulation in the dermis and a decreased lipid content in the stratum corneum as well as decreases in sweat and oil secretion by glands. Moreover, thinness of the skin can be caused by loss of underlying fat and increased loss of water. The impaired barrier function of stratum corneum in aged skin has recently been shown to be compensated by improved tight junction functionality, for review see Svoboda et al. [7]. Thin skin also makes small dilated blood vessels near the skin surface (telangiectasias) more visible. The fragile blood vessels increase blood leakage to skin. Free radicals may accelerate the age-related alterations in skin. Abnormalities of the expression of tight junction-associated proteins (occludin, ZO-1, claudin-1, and claudin-4) have been identified in malignant disorders of keratinization. Seborrheic keratoses are noncancerous growths of the outer layer of skin which are more common in elderly people.

Typical changes in aging skin are decrease in keratinocyte proliferation and differentiation, which cause thickening and drying of the stratum corneum. In the aging process, collagen and elastin fibers are not produced correctly by fibroblast or the fibers are degraded enzymatically. Also numbers of melanocytes and Langerhans cells decrease. Thus, changes in extracellular matrix such as decreases in elastin, collagen, and hyaluronan biosynthesis cause decrease in skin elasticity. Moreover, blood circulation in the dermis layer slows down, decreasing the delivery of nutrients and oxygen to skin cells. In addition, also endocrinological changes and fat redistribution in subcutaneous layer cause loss of skin structure.

In addition to chronological aging, environmental stressors and diet can cause premature skin aging. Free radicals produced by smoking, dehydration, pollution, and UV radiation are the primary source of premature aging of cell membranes, mitochondria, elastin, and collagen fibers as well as DNA damage. Decrease of collagen fibers and formation of abnormal elastin fibers speed up the structural aging and premature apoptosis and inflammation, the functional disturbances in skin.

Skin Microbiota

Human skin is covered with a continuous layer of microbes, which reside within epidermis, dermis, and the skin-associated glands and follicles, forming a diverse multicellular community known as the normal skin microbiota. The skin microbiota constitutes mainly of different bacteria but also of fungal species. The total number of microbes on the skin surface is typically within the range of 10^4 to 10^6 cells cm^{-2}. The healthy skin microbiota contributes to skin homeostasis and plays a role in both health and disease. The composition of the normal microbiota of the human skin is diverse and differences between the skin microbiota of different individuals are high [8], although some studies suggest relatively low interpersonal variation [9]. Notably, the composition of skin microbiota also varies between different anatomical sites, which provide different environmental conditions (e.g., moisture, temperature, pH, presence of hairs, follicles and other microbes, sweat, nutrients, and exposure to light and oxygen; see Fig. 1) for microbes to proliferate [9] and even in the same anatomical site due to altering host-related and environmental factors (e.g., host genotype, age, skin pigmentation) [10]. Normal skin bacterial microbiota is dynamic over time [11], while the fungal skin microbiota is thought to be more stable [12].

The recent expansion in the use of modern molecular techniques in the characterization of skin microbiota has facilitated the research in this field and has provided knowledge on the complexity of the skin microbiota. Most common new methods allow the determination of skin microbiota based on various sequencing techniques.

A recent study sampled two volunteers at 400 body surface sites, each. The most commonly detected taxa were from the phyla *Actinobacteria, Firmicutes, Proteobacteria, Cyanobacteria,* and *Bacteroidetes*. Members of the family *Staphylococcaceae* were found in moist areas, such as on the foot, under the breast, in the neck, and around the nose. *Staphylococcus* was mainly detected on the foot and around the nose. Members of the genus *Propionibacterium* were found in sebaceous regions, such as the head, face, upper back, and upper chest. The genus *Corynebacterium* was most commonly detected on the head, groin, and toe regions. Organisms such as *Pseudomonas* and *Lactobacillus* were detected over the entire skin surface of the volunteers. Interestingly, *Streptococcus, Haemophilus*, and *Rothia*, members of the normal oral microbiota, were detected on the skin, primarily around the mouth [13].

Earlier studies using molecular techniques have sampled fewer sites, but larger numbers of volunteers. Also in those studies, the topological difference between microbiota in different skin sites has been clear. Assessing 14 skin sites on ten healthy adult volunteers, Findley and coworkers [14] observed that *Propionibacterium* was the dominant genus on the forehead, ear, upper chest, fore arm, hand palm, upper back, and back of the head, but appears to be almost absent from the foot. *Corynebacterium* was most commonly detected on the nares, groin, toe web, and toenail. *Staphylococcus* was observed to be the predominant genus in the groin, toe web, toenail, and heel, though it is also a prominent member of the forearm, nares, ear, and back of the head. Fungi appear to be only minor components but are present at each tested skin site. The dominant member is usually a member of the genus *Malassezia*; only on the foot other fungal species may be present and even dominate (toe web and heel). Viruses are also commonly detected on each tested site, but especially on the nares, fore arm, and groin. The foot was observed to have the greatest microbial diversity: heel (median 80 genera), toe web (median 60 genera), and toenail (median 40 genera). The arm and hand were found to have intermediate diversity (18–32 genera) while the various sites on the head, chest, and back and low diversity (2–10 genera).

Skin Infections

Not surprisingly, the composition of the skin microbiota influences disease risk. Pathogenic microbes associated with various skin diseases are numerous, but an extensive review of these is not within the scope of the current chapter.

An interesting recent finding is that the presence and absence of certain groups increases or reduces the risk of the formation of pustules by *Haemophilus ducreyi*. Skin sites that had a greater abundance of *Proteobacteria, Bacteroidetes, Micrococcus, Corynebacterium, Paracoccus,* and *Staphylococcus* species were more likely to support the formation of pustules by *H. ducreyi*, whereas sites that had higher levels of *Actinobacteria* and *Propionibacterium* species were less likely to yield pustules in volunteers when challenged [15]. Various microbes and their metabolites have been shown to modulate the tight junctions in cultured epidermis [16, 17], indicating the important role of the skin microbiota in epidermal barrier formation. Such findings open up possibilities for the identification of new probiotic or microbiota modulating strategies.

Acne

Healthy skin follicles have been suggested to be almost exclusively colonized by *Propionibacterium acnes*, while follicles of acne patients also include other microbes such as *Staphylococcus epidermidis* [18]. *P. acnes* has been proposed as the causative agent of acne, but current evidence of the causative role of *P. acnes* in the disease is conflicting. This can be explained by the fact that the pathogenicity appears to be strain specific and not dependent on the relative abundance of *P. acnes* [19].

Psoriasis

Psoriasis and other inflammatory skin disorders are associated with alterations in skin microbiota. In psoriatic lesions, bacteria belonging to the phylum *Firmicutes* and genus *Streptococcus* have been reported to be overrepresented, while bacteria typical of healthy skin such as phyla *Actinobacteria* and *Proteobacteria* and genus *Propionibacterium* and *Staphylococcus* are underrepresented compared to skin microbiota of healthy persons or uninvolved skin of patients with psoriasis [20, 21]. Another study observed that the combined relative abundance of the genera *Corynebacterium*, *Streptococcus*, and *Staphylococcus* was associated with psoriatic lesions [22]. Skin fungal microbiota does not appear to be altered in psoriatic lesions, although there is an increased skin fungal diversity in psoriasis patients as compared to health controls, there does not appear to be a difference in composition [23]. In contrast to healthy adults, who are mainly colonized by *Malassezia sympodialis*, psoriasis patients appear to be typically colonized by the *Malassezia furfur* [24].

Atopic Dermatitis

Aberrant skin microbiota has also been linked with atopic dermatitis (AD) [25]. Presence of *Staphylococcus aureus* has been suggested to be one of the driving forces behind the eczema. Treatment with antibiotics reversed skin dysbiosis and skin inflammation in mice [26].

S. aureus on inflamed skin of AD patients was associated with a high IgE response, increased expression of inflammatory and Th2/Th22 transcripts, and the prevalence of a peripheral allergic response. Exposure to *Staphylococcus epidermidis* metabolites, however, promoted the activity of regulatory T cells in suppressing the allergic response [27]. Flare up of AD has indeed been observed to be associated with an increase in *S. aureus* but also *S. epidermidis* and a concomitant reduction in nonStaphylococcus skin organisms. A reduction in these two staphylococci coincided with a reduction in atopic disease [28].

While healthy adults are colonized by *M. sympodialis*, AD patients appear to be more frequently and exclusively colonized by the species [24]. Another study, however, observed that AD was in particular associated with *Malassezia restricta* [29].

Body Odor

Body odor is to a large extent caused by the metabolism of sweat and sebaceous excretions by the skin microbiota. Various species of *Staphylococcus* such as *S. hominis, S. haemolyticus*, and *S. lugdunensis* have been observed to metabolize dipeptide-conjugated thioalcohols such as *S*-[1-(2-hydroxyethyl)-1-methylbutyl]-(L)-cysteinylglycine. *S. epidermidis* and *Corynebacterium tuberculostearicum*, which are numerically dominant in the armpit, have only a minor ability to perform this transformation and are therefore less likely to contribute to body odor [30]. Nevertheless, Troccaz and coworkers [31] identified that the genus *Corynebacterium* was positively correlated to armpit odor, also *C. tuberculostearicum*, while the genus *Propionibacterium* was reverse correlated. *S. hominis* was indeed found to positively correlate with body odor as predicted by Bawdon and coworkers [30]; also *Anaerococcus* was observed to correlate with armpit odor.

Dandruff

Dandruff is characterized by scaling of the scalp and is considered to be a form of mild seborrheic dermatitis. The skin microbiota is thought to play a role in the etiology of dandruff. Traditionally, *Malassezia* is thought to be associated with dandruff, and indeed a recent study using molecular techniques observed an increased colonization with *Malassezia restricta*, but also of

Staphylococcus species in dandruff as compared to healthy scalps [32]; however, the picture may be more complex than this. While Malassezia was detected more frequently in dandruff patients than in healthy subjects, it was not a major component. Dandruff patients were mainly colonized by Basidiomycota, in particular *Filobasidium floriforme*; healthy subjects exhibited a smaller but more diverse Basidiomycota population with a dominance of *Cryptococcus* spp. Dandruff patients were less colonized by Ascomycota, but mainly *Acremonium* spp. Healthy subjects were more colonized by Ascomycota, and although also *Acremonium* spp. were detected, the population was smaller while a larger fraction of Didymella bryoniae was detected [33]. It should be noted that many of these studies were performed with relatively small numbers of subjects.

Aging

Few studies have compared the skin microbiota between different age groups. Comparing the forearm microbiota between young and older adults did not indicate a difference in diversity of the skin microbial community. However, the intragroup similarity of both age groups was notably higher than that of the intergroups, which suggests a difference in the dominant microbiota between the older and the younger group. The counts of total bacteria and *Corynebacterium* spp. were significantly less in the young group. Counts of *Staphylococcus* spp. and *S. epidermidis* were not different between the age groups [34]. However, Si and colleagues [10] observed that when comparing the subjects younger and older than 35 years of age, there was an increased diversity in the older cohort.

Middle aged and older adults (>50 years of age) have been observed to be more commonly colonized by *Malassezia globosa* and *M. sympodialis* on the trunk and to a lesser extent on the scalp by *M. globosa* compared to younger adults [35].

From the above, it becomes evident that certain members of the skin microbiota are more often associated with certain health conditions than others, though cause and effect may not always be clear. Correlation can, however, be more complex, involving reduced diversity or the absence or reduction of certain organisms that are eclipsed by the new dominant microbiota members. Furthermore, many of the studies have used relatively small numbers of volunteers or few sampling sites, suggesting caution with the interpretation of the results. Nevertheless, the role of skin microbes in skin health and disease does provide a rationale for therapies aiming at maintenance or restoration of a healthy skin microbiota. Probiotics and prebiotics have been suggested as potential applications of such therapies. It has been suggested that probiotics could also be used to promote skin cell development. Many of the current probiotic strains are also known for their potential to modify host immune responses, providing an additional possible mechanism for probiotics aimed at skin health. Modulation of host immune system function could be achieved locally (topical applications) or through systemic immune functions (e.g., oral applications). Most probiotics currently used are microbes typical for what is considered a healthy gastrointestinal microbiota, such as strains of *Lactobacillus* and *Bifidobacterium*. These are usually administered orally and are most commonly aimed at promotion of gut health and improvement of immune system function. The currently established probiotic strains may also have potential for being used as probiotics for skin health, and indeed some probiotic strains are already being used to prevent or treat allergic skin diseases particularly eczema as will be described below. An alternative approach is to select potential probiotics which are species typical of healthy skin microbiota, specifically targeted for maintenance of skin health. Such strains could be isolated from the normal skin microbiota of healthy individuals and used as topical probiotic applications.

Probiotic Applications for Skin Health

Eczema

The mucosae and skin form a common immunological entity, connected by systemic and lymphatic immune functions. Hence, immune effects elicited in the gastrointestinal tract also influence immune responses in the oral cavity, mammary glands, urogenital tract, and skin. B-cells that are activated in the Peyer's patches in the intestine may travel to other sites of the body. Also the production of cytokines by immune cells in the gut may have influences in peripheral sites like the skin. It is therefore not so surprising that oral consumption of immunoactive components, such as probiotics or allergens, may have an influence on immune responses of the skin. Indeed, mouse studies have suggested that orally administered probiotic extracts may influence skin immune abnormalities [36].

Probiotics, and to a lesser extend prebiotics, have been investigated for their ability to treat or prevent atopic eczema. These investigations have been mainly performed in infants and young children. Allergy-related immune benefits in children above the age of 2 years and adults appear to be difficult to obtain as the immune system has matured and is difficult to influence. The elderly, however, may have reduced immune function and have been found to be responsive to immune modulating probiotics. Consumption of probiotic bacteria *Bifidobacterium lactis* HN019 and *Lactobacillus rhamnosus* HN001 has been observed to improve natural killer cell and phagocytic activity [37]. It would therefore not be unreasonable to hypothesize that specific probiotic strains might also positively influence immunological disorders of the skin in elderly. Though, to date this has not been investigated. As an example, the influence of probiotics and prebiotics on atopic dermatitis in infants will be discussed.

Under natural circumstances, humans are exposed to an abundance of microbes. Affluent societies have gradually eliminated this exposure through an improvement in hygiene. This has led to a dramatic reduction in the incidence of infectious diseases but has been accompanied by an increase in allergic and autoimmune diseases. For proper development of the immune system, microbial exposure is essential. Probiotics might form a safe alternative for microbial exposure. Studies have therefore been performed where at-risk children (i.e., children with a first degree family member with allergic disease) were prophylactically treated with specific strains of probiotics. Although some strain-dependent differences are observed, the main indication is that for a successful intervention, consumption of probiotics has to start by the mother before delivery [38]. Also an infant formula containing a prebiotic mixture of 90 % GOS and 10 % long chain FOS has been observed to reduce the incidence of atopic eczema in at-risk children [39].

Probiotics have, with varying success, also been used in the treatment of atopic disease in infants. A recent meta-analysis of studies concludes however that the results for treatment are less convincing than for prevention [40]. Inclusion of selected probiotic strains into extensively hydrolysed formula has in some cases been shown to speed up the reduction of eczema. Similarly, inclusion of certain probiotic strains into exclusion diets has been observed to improve eczema.

To what extend these observations in, sometimes very young, children can be used to prevent immune-related skin disorders in elderly remains to be determined. In addition to eczema-related skin inflammation, mouse studies have suggested that immune modulation by orally administered probiotics or prebiotics [41] may reduce contact-induced skin inflammation.

Treatment Options for Premature Aging of Skin

The changes in skin by aging are dependent on genetics but also nutrition, UV light, environmental pollutants, and stress. The primary treatment for photoaging is photoprotection and secondary antioxidants as well as other novel compounds such as osmolytes, polyphenols, probiotics, and prebiotics may have potential here.

Traditionally, products targeted to skin health are applied topically and are therefore likely to affect the uppermost skin layers. The skin barrier prevents most compounds and practically all microbes penetrating deeper layers. However, external compounds, microbes, and/or microbial metabolites may have an effect on the function of the skin barrier. Oral applications have different treatment options, as they can affect skin functions via the immune system and vasculature from inside the body.

Current applications for antiaging are targeted to prevent UV damages and to increase the skin elasticity, cell renewal, and hydration. Current knowledge on the effects of probiotics and prebiotics in skin care are quite limited. However, some studies on the effects of microbes or their metabolites on skin hydrating and inflammation, UV protection, as well as atopic dermatitis in children exist, see below.

Photoaging

The clinical alterations caused by UV light include freckles, lentigo solaris, and squamous cell carcinoma. Although freckles have a genetic background, the formation of freckles is triggered by UVB radiation, which activates melanocytes to increase the melanin production. Lentigines are freckles that may not fade in the winter. Typically they form after years of exposure to the sun, becoming more common in older people. Solar keratosis is a premalignant condition of skin that may be accompanied by the UV damage.

Exposure of skin to solar UV radiation can cause skin cancer, photoaging, and other cellular and immunological changes. As a defense against UV radiation, melanocytes produce melanin that blocks damage caused by UV. UVB radiation causes direct DNA damage by the free radicals, while UVA causes indirect damage penetrating deeper layers. Immunosuppression caused by UV exposure is mediated by interleukin (IL)-10 released by keratinocytes and immune cells.

Probiotics and Protection from Sun Burn

Protection and recovery from sunburn has been one of the early research targets of probiotics for the skin. These early studies were carried out with fractions of bifidobacteria applied to the skin. The results of these early studies were contradictory, which may relate to the use of different fractions and *Bifidobacterium* strains, a common complication in probiotic research.

Animal studies have shown that oral administration of *Lactobacillus johnsonii* La1 reduced UV-induced immune suppression. Feeding of the strain was also found to counteract UV-induced Langerhans cell depletion and IL-10 induction. Nonirradiated mice did not show any change in these immune markers, indicating that the strain contributes to maintaining skin immunity homeostasis. Subsequent human studies showed that consumption of this strain 56 days prior to experimental UV exposure did not protect the skin from UV-induced damage, but facilitated the recovery, most likely by stimulating the UV-depleted immune function of the skin. This effect was seen only in UV-sensitive subjects, not in UV tolerant subjects, about half of the volunteers [42]. Similarly, in a study with light-sensitive patients, consumption of a combination of *L. johnsonii* La-1, lycopene, and β-carotene was found to improve the condition and was accompanied by an increase in intercellular adhesion molecule-1 (ICAM-1), suggesting an immunological response [43]. Such observations are in agreement with what has been described above for the skin immunity modulating potential of certain probiotic strains.

Oral administration of *Lactobacillus plantarum* HY7714 to hairless mice was found to inhibit the number, depth, and area of wrinkles in skin. Furthermore, histological data showed that administration of the strain inhibited UVB-induced epidermal thickness in mice [44]. Also *Bifidobacterium breve* B-3 administration to hairless mice suppressed the changes of transepidermal water loss, skin hydration, and epidermal thickening and attenuated the damage to the tight junction structure and basement membrane induced by chronic UVB irradiation [45].

In extension to this, one could consider the use of microbes that produce carotenoids; carotenoids are known to protect the skin from UV damage. Many microbes are known to produce carotenoids, such as the yeast genus *Rhodotorula* which is present on certain surface-ripened cheeses. They could possibly function as a skin protective probiotic of known safe use. In fact, the skin of frequent sunbathers has been observed to be more colonized with carotenoid-containing bacteria than infrequent sunbathers. In addition to providing protection from UV irradiation, the carotenoids would have a potential cosmetic benefit as they might contribute to improved tanning. Interestingly, carotenoids-producing *Bacillus indicus* has been isolated from human feces and could be considered an endogenous source of these compounds. Microbial carotenoid supplementation does therefore seem to be feasible.

Probiotics for Cosmetic Applications

The use of probiotics in cosmetic applications has been proposed. Although controlled scientific trials are scarce, several patent applications have been filed in this field. Some in vitro and animal studies relating to potential cosmetic applications of probiotics have been carried out.

Probiotics or their metabolites may have a role as moisturizing agents, although other compounds such as betaine are likely to be much more effective in this respect. Baba and coworkers [46] showed that in an in vitro skin cell model, *Lactobacillus helveticus*-fermented milk whey enhanced the expression of profilaggrin mRNA, a precursor of filaggrin, a protein which binds to keratin fibers in epithelial cells and contributes to skin moisture retention. In the same study, *L. helveticus*-fermented milk was observed to induce keratinocyte differentiation in vitro. Hyaluronic acid, a major component of body extracellular matrix, is widely distributed throughout the epithelial tissue and is commonly used in cosmetic applications. Soy milk fermented with *Bifidobacterium* has been shown to induce hyaluronic acid production by skin cells in vitro and in an animal model [47]. In vitro exposure of HaCaT cells to *Lactobacillus plantarum* K8 lysates was found to increase hyaluronic acid content in the cells. Oral administration of *L. plantarum* K8 lysates to hairless mice attenuated horny layer formation and decreased epidermal thickening, while skin barrier function was improved after oral administration of *L. plantarum* K8 lysates in a mouse model of atopic dermatitis. Human volunteers consuming *L. plantarum* K8 lysates experienced significant increase in hydration of the face and forearm compared to control. Decreases in horny layer thickness and TEWL value were also observed on the face and forearm of the experimental group, suggesting that *L. plantarum* K8 lysates have a moisturizing potential [48].

Reinforcing subjects' own *S. epidermidis* population has been observed to increase the skin water content and reduce water evaporation. For this, *S. epidermidis* was isolated from volunteers, cultured, and applied to the skin of the same volunteer (i.e., each volunteer received her own strain back). As long as the bacteria were applied, an increase in *S. epidermidis* skin levels was observed, which returned to base line when application was stopped. The *S. epidermidis* increase coincided with the increase in water and lipid content of the skin as well as increased levels of glycerine, lactic acid, and propionic acid [49].

Interestingly, a recent study observed that administration of *Lactobacillus reuteri* ATCC 6475 to aged mice increased subcuticular folliculogenesis yielding a more lustrous fur. The animals also exhibited a quicker regrowth of their fur after shaving [50]. The mechanism behind this is thought to be the induction of interleukin-10 and oxytocin [51], again suggesting an immunological response.

Potential Forms of Probiotics for Skin

Probiotics are usually consumed as live microbes. It is commonly thought that viable probiotics are more likely to be biologically active than inactivated probiotics, since they maintain metabolic activity, may colonize the host at least transiently, may be more likely to attach to host mucosa and cells than inactivated cells, and are likely to possess better antimicrobial activity against harmful microorganisms. In the case of skin probiotics, it may be speculated that viable probiotics could remain viable on the skin and thereby colonize the skin. It is likely that this would require specifically selected species of probiotics, most likely from members of the normal skin microbiota. Nevertheless, permanent colonization of probiotics aimed at skin health may be considered unlikely, as in the case of orally administered probiotics, it is known that these microbes do not colonize the host permanently and that the effects of probiotics typically last only through the period of administration.

While in general viable probiotics are considered to be more active than nonviable probiotics, the latter are not without an effect [52]. In addition, in certain cases the health benefit of a probiotic is attributed to a metabolite produced by the bacteria, not to the cell itself. Inactivated skin probiotics, cell components of inactivated bacteria, or probiotic metabolites may be the preferred choice in cases in which safety and adverse effects are of concern. For example, in the case of wounds, the application of viable probiotics could lead to translocation of bacteria into the bloodstream with the risk of bacteraemia. Moreover, inactivated probiotics are likely to be more stable at room temperature than viable microbes, as the latter in liquid solutions usually require cold storage, which may not be feasible for skin applications. Indeed, inactivated forms of probiotics, components of probiotics, and cell-free extracts of probiotics have already been assessed for different skin applications [48]. Nevertheless, the demonstration of the health benefit is of utmost importance when selecting probiotics for skin application. If a health benefit is demonstrated for a probiotic strain in viable form, the same health benefit cannot be directly assumed for inactivated form of the same strain (and vice versa).

New Skin Targets for Probiotics and Prebiotics

The most potential target for the oral probiotics could be regulating abnormal immune responses in skin. As described above, probiotics have already indicated to have beneficial effects on allergy, eczema, and psoriasis. They have also shown to protect from UV-induced immune suppression in vitro. In addition to immune cells, oral probiotics may influence the dermal fibroblasts via blood circulation. Fibroblasts are responsible of the collagen synthesis and they have important role in wound healing.

Antiaging

Probiotics, and especially their metabolites, may have an important role in epidermal dynamics. The balance of skin renewal and repair requires optimal water, oxygen, and nutrient balance as well as growth factors which are typically decreased with aging.

New targets for probiotic use in antiaging could be to inhibit the formation of fragmented elastin fibers, scavenge free radicals, and activate dermal microcirculation. The role of probiotics in the function of epidermal tight junctions and lipid lamellae between corneocytes may provide new skin applications to probiotics.

Topically applied probiotics and their metabolites have shown to increase hyaluronic acid production. Topical probiotics or prebiotics may also resist pathogen invasion to mechanically or chemically irritated skin areas. Furthermore, topical probiotics and their metabolites may also be protective against environmental toxins by binding or degrading them. The permeation barrier of the skin may limit the use of the topically applied prebiotics, probiotics, or their metabolites in skin care. However, novel techniques such as liposomes may facilitate the permeation of these products across the skin barrier. Moreover, the effect of living probiotics on technical properties of topical skin care products may need more developmental work.

Wound and Burn Care

The use of probiotics in wound and burn care has been proposed. Inflammation and injuries activate keratinocytes to produce growth factors which are important for wound healing but also in diseases such as skin cancer and psoriasis. In cultured keratinocytes, probiotics have shown to increase filaggrin production which in turn may promote their differentiation. A more thorough understanding of the role probiotics can play in regulating cell renewal and skin barrier repair is needed to evaluate their potential for skin healing. The efficacy of *Lactobacillus plantarum* and its metabolites against *Pseudomonas aeruginosa*, a common pathogen of burns and wounds, has been demonstrated [53], suggesting that probiotic metabolites may be useful in topical treatment of burns and wounds. Moreover, topical application of kefir (a fermented dairy product) gel has been shown to enhance wound healing and reduce scar tissue in an animal model [54]. The efficacy of probiotics in the care of severe wounds (gunshot wounds) has been assessed in animal model using both topical application (irrigation of the wound with probiotic suspension) and oral application [55]. The oral application is based on the hypothesis that in the case of serious trauma, the intestinal barrier function is dysfunctioning and significant translocation of intestinal bacteria into the body occurs, and this translocation is used as a route for probiotics to enter the deep wounds, where they inhibit the proliferation of pathogenic organisms causing wound infection. It should be noted that application of live bacteria to wounds involves a risk of bacteria entering the blood stream and causing bacteraemia and increasing the risk of infections. Inactivated microbial cells, isolated cell components, or microbial metabolites may offer a safer alternative, free of the risk of bacteremia. Indeed, germ-free animals that have been observed exhibit quicker wound healing with less scar tissue compared to conventional animals [56]. Nevertheless, extensive safety testing of probiotics and related compounds aimed at wound care is required.

Conclusion

Pre- and probiotics have been shown to influence parameters of the skin immune system and contribute to relief of atopic eczema and UV-induced immune suppression. Other immune-related skin conditions could be considered. For topical application of pre- or probiotics, a better understanding of the different skin microbiota is necessary. This would open the way for the selection of new potential probiotic candidates and novel therapeutic targets.

Cross-References

▶ Atopic Dermatitis in the Aged
▶ Probiotics in Aging Skin

References

1. Zhang M, Jiang Z, Li D, Jiang D, Wu Y, Ren H, et al. Oral antibiotic treatment induces skin microbiota dysbiosis and influences wound healing. Microb Ecol. 2015;69(2):415–21. Epub 2014/10/11.
2. FAO/WHO, editor. Guidelines for the evaluation of probiotics in food. 2002. http://www.who.int/foodsafety/publications/fs_management/probiotics2/en/
3. Hill C, Guarner F, Reid G, Gibson GR, Merenstein DJ, Pot B, et al. Expert consensus document: the International Scientific Association for probiotics and prebiotics consensus statement on the scope and appropriate use of the term probiotic. Nat Rev Gastroenterol Hepatol. 2014;11(8):506–14. Epub 2014/06/11.
4. Ouwehand AC, Mäkeläinen H, Tiihonen K, Rautonen N. Digestive health. In: Mitchell H, editor. Sweeteners and sugar alternatives in food technology. Oxford: Blackwell; 2006. p. 44–53.
5. Warskulat U, Flogel U, Jacoby C, Hartwig HG, Thewissen M, Merx MW, et al. Taurine transporter knockout depletes muscle taurine levels and results in severe skeletal muscle impairment but leaves cardiac function uncompromised. FASEB J. 2004;18(3):577–9. Epub 2004/01/22.
6. Brandner JM, Haftek M, Niessen CM. Adherens junctions, desmosomes and tight junctions in epidermal barrier function. Open Dermatol J. 2010;4(1):14–20.
7. Svoboda M, Bilkova Z, Muthny T. Could tight junctions regulate the barrier function of the aged skin? J Dermatol Sci. 2016;81(3):147–152. Epub 2015/12/08.
8. Grice EA, Kong HH, Conlan S, Deming CB, Davis J, Young AC, et al. Topographical and temporal diversity of the human skin microbiome. Science. 2009;324(5931):1190–2. Epub 2009/05/30.
9. Grice EA, Kong HH, Renaud G, Young AC, Bouffard GG, Blakesley RW, et al. A diversity profile of the human skin microbiota. Genome Res. 2008;18(7):1043–50.
10. Si J, Lee S, Park JM, Sung J, Ko G. Genetic associations and shared environmental effects on the skin microbiome of Korean twins. BMC Genomics. 2015;16(1):992. Epub 2015/11/26.
11. Gao Z, Tseng CH, Strober BE, Pei Z, Blaser MJ. Substantial alterations of the cutaneous bacterial biota in psoriatic lesions. PLoS One. 2008;3(7):e2719.
12. Paulino LC, Tseng CH, Strober BE, Blaser MJ. Molecular analysis of fungal microbiota in samples from healthy human skin and psoriatic lesions. J Clin Microbiol. 2006;44(8):2933–41. Epub 2006/08/08.

13. Bouslimani A, Porto C, Rath CM, Wang M, Guo Y, Gonzalez A, et al. Molecular cartography of the human skin surface in 3D. Proc Natl Acad Sci U S A. 2015;112 (17):E2120–9. Epub 2015/04/01.
14. Findley K, Oh J, Yang J, Conlan S, Deming C, Meyer JA, et al. Topographic diversity of fungal and bacterial communities in human skin. Nature. 2013;498 (7454):367–70. Epub 2013/05/24.
15. van Rensburg JJ, Lin H, Gao X, Toh E, Fortney KR, Ellinger S, et al. The human skin microbiome associates with the outcome of and is influenced by bacterial infection. mBio. 2015;6(5):e01315–15. Epub 2015/09/17.
16. Putaala H, Tiihonen K, Ouwehand AC, Rautonen N. Probiotics modulate tight junction integrity and expression of junctional proteins in cultured normal human epidermal keratinocytes. J Probiot. 2012;7 (2):81–90.
17. Sonoda N, Furuse M, Sasaki H, Yonemura S, Katahira J, Horiguchi Y, et al. *Clostridium perfringens* enterotoxin fragment removes specific claudins from tight junction strands: evidence for direct involvement of claudins in tight junction barrier. J Cell Biol. 1999;147(1):195–204. Epub 1999/10/06.
18. Bek-Thomsen M, Lomholt HB, Kilian M. Acne is not associated with yet-uncultured bacteria. J Clin Microbiol. 2008;46(10):3355–60. Epub 2008/08/22.
19. Fitz-Gibbon S, Tomida S, Chiu BH, Nguyen L, Du C, Liu M, et al. *Propionibacterium acnes* strain populations in the human skin microbiome associated with acne. J Invest Dermatol. 2013;133(9):2152–60. Epub 2013/01/23.
20. Gao Z, Tseng CH, Pei Z, Blaser MJ. Molecular analysis of human forearm superficial skin bacterial biota. Proc Natl Acad Sci U S A. 2007;104(8):2927–32. Epub 2007/02/13.
21. Fahlen A, Engstrand L, Baker BS, Powles A, Fry L. Comparison of bacterial microbiota in skin biopsies from normal and psoriatic skin. Arch Dermatol Res. 2012;304(1):15–22. Epub 2011/11/09.
22. Alekseyenko AV, Perez-Perez GI, De Souza A, Strober B, Gao Z, Bihan M, et al. Community differentiation of the cutaneous microbiota in psoriasis. Microbiome. 2013;1(1):31. Epub 2014/01/24.
23. Takemoto A, Cho O, Morohoshi Y, Sugita T, Muto M. Molecular characterization of the skin fungal microbiome in patients with psoriasis. J Dermatol. 2015;42(2):166–70. Epub 2014/12/17.
24. Jagielski T, Rup E, Ziolkowska A, Roeske K, Macura AB, Bielecki J. Distribution of *Malassezia* species on the skin of patients with atopic dermatitis, psoriasis, and healthy volunteers assessed by conventional and molecular identification methods. BMC Dermatol. 2014;14:3. Epub 2014/03/08.
25. Dekio I, Sakamoto M, Hayashi H, Amagai M, Suematsu M, Benno Y. Characterization of skin microbiota in patients with atopic dermatitis and in normal subjects using 16S rRNA gene-based comprehensive analysis. J Med Microbiol. 2007;56 (Pt 12):1675–83. Epub 2007/11/24.
26. Kobayashi T, Glatz M, Horiuchi K, Kawasaki H, Akiyama H, Kaplan DH, et al. Dysbiosis and *Staphylococcus aureus* colonization drives inflammation in atopic dermatitis. Immunity. 2015;42(4):756–66. Epub 2015/04/23.
27. Laborel-Preneron E, Bianchi P, Boralevi F, Lehours P, Fraysse F, Morice-Picard F, et al. Effects of the *Staphylococcus aureus* and *Staphylococcus epidermidis* secretomes isolated from the skin microbiota of atopic children on CD^{4+} T cell activation. PLoS One. 2015;10 (10):e0141067. Epub 2015/10/29.
28. Kong HH, Oh J, Deming C, Conlan S, Grice EA, Beatson MA, et al. Temporal shifts in the skin microbiome associated with disease flares and treatment in children with atopic dermatitis. Genome Res. 2012;22(5):850–9. Epub 2012/02/09.
29. Zhang E, Tanaka T, Tajima M, Tsuboi R, Nishikawa A, Sugita T. Characterization of the skin fungal microbiota in patients with atopic dermatitis and in healthy subjects. Microbiol Immunol. 2011;55 (9):625–32. Epub 2011/06/28.
30. Bawdon D, Cox DS, Ashford D, James AG, Thomas GH. Identification of axillary Staphylococcus sp. involved in the production of the malodorous thioalcohol 3-methyl-3-sufanylhexan-1-ol. FEMS Microbiol Lett. 2015;362(16). Epub 2015/07/15.
31. Troccaz M, Gaia N, Beccucci S, Schrenzel J, Cayeux I, Starkenmann C, et al. Mapping axillary microbiota responsible for body odours using a culture-independent approach. Microbiome. 2015;3(1):3. Epub 2015/02/06.
32. Wang L, Clavaud C, Bar-Hen A, Cui M, Gao J, Liu Y, et al. Characterization of the major bacterial-fungal populations colonizing dandruff scalps in Shanghai, China, shows microbial disequilibrium. Exp Dermatol. 2015;24(5):398–400. Epub 2015/03/06.
33. Park HK, Ha MH, Park SG, Kim MN, Kim BJ, Kim W. Characterization of the fungal microbiota (mycobiome) in healthy and dandruff-afflicted human scalps. PLoS One. 2012;7(2):e32847. Epub 2012/03/07.
34. Li W, Han L, Yu P, Ma C, Wu X, Moore JE, et al. Molecular characterization of skin microbiota between cancer cachexia patients and healthy volunteers. Microb Ecol. 2014;67(3):679–89. Epub 2014/01/10.
35. Prohic A, Simic D, Sadikovic TJ, Krupalija-Fazlic M. Distribution of *Malassezia* species on healthy human skin in Bosnia and Herzegovina: correlation with body part, age and gender. Iranian J Microbiol. 2014;6(4):253–62. Epub 2015/03/25.
36. Cinque B, Di Marzio L, Della Riccia DN, Bizzini F, Giuliani M, Fanini D, et al. Effect of *Bifidobacterium infantis* on Interferon- gamma- induced keratinocyte apoptosis: a potential therapeutic approach to skin immune abnormalities. Int J Immunopathol Pharmacol. 2006;19(4):775–86. Epub 2006/12/15.
37. Ouwehand A, Lahtinen S, Nurminen P. Lactobacillus rhamnosus HN001 and *Bifidobacterium lactis* HN019. In: Lee YK, Salminen S, editors. Handbook of

probiotics and prebiotics. Hoboken: Wiley; 2009. p. 473–7.

38. Mansfield JA, Bergin SW, Cooper JR, Olsen CH. Comparative probiotic strain efficacy in the prevention of eczema in infants and children: a systematic review and meta-analysis. Mil Med. 2014;179 (6):580–92. Epub 2014/06/06.
39. Foolad N, Armstrong AW. Prebiotics and probiotics: the prevention and reduction in severity of atopic dermatitis in children. Benefic Microbes. 2014;5 (2):151–60. Epub 2014/01/28.
40. Kim SO, Ah YM, Yu YM, Choi KH, Shin WG, Lee JY. Effects of probiotics for the treatment of atopic dermatitis: a meta-analysis of randomized controlled trials. Ann Allergy Asthma Immunol. 2014;113 (2):217–26. Epub 2014/06/24.
41. Sasajima N, Ogasawara T, Takemura N, Fujiwara R, Watanabe J, Sonoyama K. Role of intestinal *Bifidobacterium pseudolongum* in dietary fructo-oligosaccharide inhibition of 2,4-dinitrofluorobenzene-induced contact hypersensitivity in mice. Br J Nutr. 2010;103(4):539–48. Epub 2009/12/17.
42. Peguet-Navarro J, Dezutter-Dambuyant C, Buetler T, Leclaire J, Smola H, Blum S, et al. Supplementation with oral probiotic bacteria protects human cutaneous immune homeostasis after UV exposure-double blind, randomized, placebo controlled clinical trial. Eur J Dermatol. 2008;18(5):504–11.
43. Marini A, Jaenicke T, Grether-Beck S, Le Floc'h C, Cheniti A, Piccardi N, et al. Prevention of polymorphic light eruption by oral administration of a nutritional supplement containing lycopene, beta-carotene, and *Lactobacillus johnsonii*: results from a randomized, placebo-controlled, double-blinded study. Photodermatol Photoimmunol Photomed. 2014;30 (4):189–94. Epub 2013/11/29.
44. Kim HM, Lee DE, Park SD, Kim YT, Kim YJ, Jeong JW, et al. Oral administration of *Lactobacillus plantarum* HY7714 protects hairless mouse against ultraviolet B-induced photoaging. J Microbiol Biotechnol. 2014;24(11):1583–91. Epub 2014/08/13.
45. Satoh T, Murata M, Iwabuchi N, Odamaki T, Wakabayashi H, Yamauchi K, et al. Effect of *Bifidobacterium breve* B-3 on skin photoaging induced by chronic UV irradiation in mice. Benefic Microbes. 2015;6(4):497–504. Epub 2015/03/27.
46. Baba H, Masuyama A, Takano T. Effects of *Lactobacillus helveticus* -fermented milk on the differentiation of cultured normal human epidermal keratinocytes. J Dairy Sci. 2006;89(6):2072–5.
47. Miyazaki K, Hanamizu T, Iizuka R, Chiba K. *Bifidobacterium*-fermented soy milk extract stimulates hyaluronic acid production in human skin cells and hairless mouse skin. Skin Pharmacol Appl Skin Physiol. 2003;16(2):108–16.
48. Kim H, Kim HR, Jeong BJ, Lee SS, Kim TR, Jeong JH, et al. Effects of oral intake of kimchi-derived *Lactobacillus plantarum* K8 lysates on skin moisturizing. J Microbiol Biotechnol. 2015;25(1):74–80. Epub 2014/09/03.
49. Nodake Y, Matsumoto S, Miura R, Honda H, Ishibashi G, Matsumoto S, et al. Pilot study on novel skin care method by augmentation with *Staphylococcus epidermidis*, an autologous skin microbe – a blinded randomized clinical trial. J Dermatol Sci. 2015;79(2):119–26. Epub 2015/05/28.
50. Levkovich T, Poutahidis T, Smillie C, Varian BJ, Ibrahim YM, Lakritz JR, et al. Probiotic bacteria induce a "glow of health". PLoS One. 2013;8(1): e53867. Epub 2013/01/24.
51. Erdman SE, Poutahidis T. Probiotic "glow of health": it's more than skin deep. Benefic Microbes. 2014;5 (2):109–19. Epub 2014/03/29.
52. Ouwehand AC, Salminen SJ. The health effects of viable and non-viable cultured milks. Int Dairy J. 1998;8:749–758.
53. Brachkova MI, Marques P, Rocha J, Sepodes B, Duarte MA, Pinto JF. Alginate films containing *Lactobacillus plantarum* as wound dressing for prevention of burn infection. J Hosp Infect. 2011;79(4):375–7. Epub 2011/10/18.
54. Huseini HF, Rahimzadeh G, Fazeli MR, Mehrazma M, Salehi M. Evaluation of wound healing activities of kefir products. Burns. 2012;38(5):719–23. Epub 2012/01/13.
55. Nikitenko VI. Infection prophylaxis of gunshot wounds using probiotics. J Wound Care. 2004;13 (9):363–6. Epub 2004/11/03.
56. Canesso MC, Vieira AT, Castro TB, Schirmer BG, Cisalpino D, Martins FS, et al. Skin wound healing is accelerated and scarless in the absence of commensal microbiota. J Immunol. 2014;193(10):5171–80. Epub 2014/10/19.

Probiotics in Aging Skin

100

Benedetta Cinque, Paola Palumbo, Cristina La Torre, Esterina Melchiorre, Daniele Corridoni, Gianfranca Miconi, Luisa Di Marzio, Maria Grazia Cifone, and Maurizio Giuliani

Contents

B. Cinque (✉) • P. Palumbo • C. La Torre • E. Melchiorre • G. Miconi • M.G. Cifone • M. Giuliani
Life, Health and Environmental Sciences, University of L'Aquila, L'Aquila, Italy
e-mail: benedetta.cinque@univaq.it; paolapalumbo.gtca@gmail.com; crix_latorre@libero.it; este.melchiorre@libero.it; gianfranca.miconi@gmail.com; cifone@univaq.it; maurizio.giuliani@cc.univaq.it

D. Corridoni
Division of Gastroenterology and Liver Disease, Department of Medicine, Case Western Reserve University School of Medicine, Cleveland, Ohio, USA
e-mail: corridoni@hotmail.com

L. Di Marzio
Department of Pharmacy, University of Chieti - Pescara "G d'Annunzio", Chieti - Pescara, Italy
e-mail: l.dimarzio@unich.it

M.A. Farage et al. (eds.), *Textbook of Aging Skin*,
DOI 10.1007/978-3-662-47398-6_78

Abstract

Health benefits of probiotics have been established recently and the scientific literature shows that the clinical uses of probiotics are broad and are open to continuing evaluation. The most common microorganisms used as probiotics are strains of lactic acid bacteria (LAB) including *Lactobacilli* and *Bifidobacteria*, which are part of the intestinal microbiota. Most probiotics are included in foods or dietary supplements and are aimed at functioning in the intestine. However, even if gastrointestinal tract has been the primary target, it is becoming evident that other conditions not initially associated with the gut microbiota might also be affected by probiotics.

Introduction

Health benefits of probiotics have been established by several studies in animals and humans, and the scientific literature shows that the clinical uses of probiotics are broad and are open to continuing evaluation. The most common microorganisms used as probiotics are strains of lactic acid bacteria (LAB), which are gram-positive, nonsporing, catalase-negative organisms that are devoid of cytochromes and of nonaerobic habit but are aerotolerant, acid-tolerant, and strictly fermentative; lactic acid is the major end product of sugar fermentation. Particular attention is paid to specific species of lactic acid bacteria (LAB), including *Lactobacilli* and *Bifidobacteria*, which are part of the intestinal microbiota. Most probiotics are included in foods or dietary supplements and are aimed at functioning in the intestine. However, even if gastrointestinal tract has been the primary target, it is becoming evident that other conditions not initially associated with the gut microbiota might also be affected by probiotics. It was speculated that the skin status could benefit from reinforced gut homeostasis. Nutritional intervention, particularly with dietary antioxidants, has been proposed to protect against UV-induced skin damage, and an increasing interest has been shown for new nutritional approaches using live microorganisms as probiotics. Moreover, the capacity of probiotics to modulate the systemic immune status, including the release of regulatory cytokines, might influence skin homeostasis. In addition, reports showing the efficacy of a selected probiotic extract in increasing ceramide levels in vivo, on stratum corneum (SC) of healthy young and old subjects, as well as in atopic dermatitis patients, thus reducing dryness, loss of tone, fullness, and water loss, opened new potential probiotic-based strategies against those pathophysiological skin alterations, including aging, associated with a reduced amount of the ceramide, major water-holding molecule in the extracellular space of the horny layer.

Overall, even if the potential use of probiotics for the skin has been hardly considered in the past, more recent experimental studies have suggested interesting, potential, new applications. The aim of the present review is to outline the main challenges associated with accumulating evidence in support of skin health claims for probiotics and to give a perspective of the scientific gaps that need to be addressed to advance the probiotic-based preventive or therapeutic approaches in aging skin, which is one of the most common dermatologic concerns.

Probiotic Microorganisms and Health Benefits

The history and evolution of the definition of "probiotic microorganism" has been extensively reviewed by Fioramonti et al. [1]. The concept of probiotics was most likely derived from a theory first proposed by Nobel Prize-winning Russian scientist Elia Metchnikoff, who suggested in 1908 that long life of Bulgarian peasants resulted from their consumption of fermented milk products. The term "probiotic," which literally means "for life," was first used by Lilly and Stillwell (1965) [1] to describe "substances secreted by one microorganism, which stimulate the growth of another." A powerful evolution of this definition was coined by Parker (1974), who proposed that probiotics are "organisms and substances which contribute to intestinal microbial balance [1]." Fuller (1989), then modified the definition in 1989 to "a live microbial feed supplement, which beneficially affects the host animal by improving its microbial balance [1]." Afterwards, Salminen et al. in 1998 defined probiotics as "foods which contain live bacteria, which are beneficial to health," whereas Marteau et al. in 2002 defined them as "microbial cell preparations or components of microbial cells that have a beneficial effect on the health and well-being." In these definitions, the concept of an action on the gut microflora, and even that of live microorganisms disappeared. In 2001, a new and complete definition of probiotic has been presented by the Food and Agriculture Organization of the United Nations-World Health Organization (FAO-WHO) and approved by the International Scientific Association for Probiotics and Prebiotics and best exemplifies the breadth and scope of probiotics as they are known today: "*Live microorganisms, which when administered in adequate amounts, confer a health benefit on the host.*" This definition retains the historical elements of the use of living organisms for health purposes but does not restrict the application of the term only to oral probiotics with intestinal outcomes [2]. Probiotics represent a large variety of bacterial genera, species, and strains. Several criteria have been proposed for considering a given microorganism as probiotic. These include the ability to adhere to cells; exclude or reduce pathogenic adherence; persist and multiply; produce acids, hydrogen peroxide, and bacteriocins antagonistic to pathogen growth; be safe, noninvasive, noncarcinogenic, and nonpathogenic; and coaggregate to form a normal balanced flora. Different strains have different actions in different clinical situations, and moreover, it is important to stress that each probiotic microrganism displays its own properties and so data obtained from one strain cannot be extrapolated to another. The most common microorganisms used as probiotics are strains of lactic acid bacteria such as *Lactobacillus*, *Bifidobacterium* genera, other bacterial genera including *Enterococcus* and *Streptococcus*. Moreover, VSL#3, a patented bacterial preparation including four strains of *Lactobacilli*, three strains of *Bifidobacteria*, and one strain of *Streptococcus salivarius* subsp. *thermophilus*, also possesses properties that make it a probiotic agent.

With the first publication in 1987 on the general properties of the *Lactobacillus GG* and its antimicrobial substance [3], a new era was initiated in which research laboratories from many countries began serious investigations on a variety of probiotic strains.

Probiotics provide an attractive alternative to antibiotics in the treatment of inflammatory bowel disease (IBD) [4]. In addition, there is considerable evidence that the highly concentrated cocktail of probiotics, VSL#3 is efficacious in preventing onset and relapse of pouchitis, a nonspecific inflammation of the ileal reservoir after ileo-anal anastomosis, which appears to be associated with bacterial overgrowth and dysbiosis [5]. Probiotics have also been implicated in the prevention and decreased recurrence of colon and bladder cancer [6, 7]. Antitumoral effects of selected strains of probiotics in vitro and in vivo have also been reported [8–10].

Probiotics have been demonstrated to have an adjuvant effect on immunological responses; their interaction with mesenteric lymph nodes can result in an up-regulation of pIgA against intestinal pathogens and food antigens [11].

Promising applications include the prevention of respiratory infections in children, prevention of dental caries, elimination of nasal pathogen carriage, prevention of relapsing *Clostridium difficile*-induced gastroenteritis. Proposed future applications include the treatment of rheumatoid arthritis, treatment of irritable bowel syndrome, prevention of ethanol-induced liver disease, treatment of diabetes, and prevention or treatment of graft versus host disease [10].

Probiotics in Aging Skin

Aging has been defined as the accumulation of molecular modifications, which manifest as macroscopic clinical changes. Human skin, unique among mammalians insofar as it is deprived of fur, is particularly sensitive to environmental stress. Major environmental factors have been recognized to induce modifications of the morphological and biophysical properties of the skin. Factors as diverse as ultraviolet radiation, atmospheric pollution, wounds, infections, traumatisms, anoxya, cigarette smoke, and hormonal status have a role in increasing the rate of accumulation of molecular modifications and have, therefore, been termed "factors of aging." Aging of the skin is commonly associated with increased wrinkling, sagging, and increased laxity, but when considering the underlying reasons for these changes, it is important to distinguish between the effects of true biological aging (intrinsic aging) and environmental factors, such as exposure to the sun (extrinsic aging). Generally, the molecular changes of photoaging are considered to be as augmentation and amplification of the molecular changes associated with chronological skin aging [12]. In terms of biochemical and molecular mechanisms, skin aging is a really complex process, which involves a variety of changes and a lot of molecules. This section highlights certain aspects of the properties of probiotics that could have interesting implications in the skin aging treatment, even if future investigations will be indispensable. In Fig. 1, a scheme is reported, which summarizes the main biochemical, molecular, and cellular changes underlying skin aging process that include alterations of skin-associated microflora, skin pH increase, reduced stratum corneum lipid levels, abnormal oxidative stress, collagen level reduction, and altered immune responsiveness. The possible sites of action of probiotics useful to slow down or inhibit the process of cutaneous aging are also highlighted.

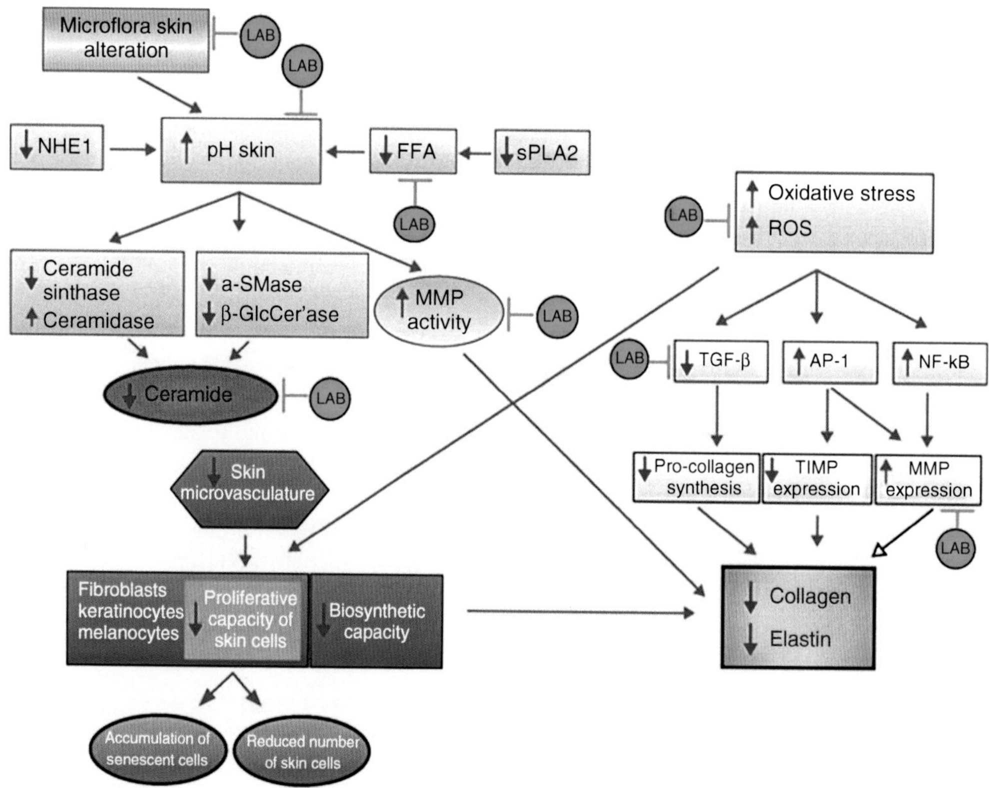

Fig. 1 Skin aging-associated biochemical, molecular, and cellular changes and possible sites of action of probiotics

Probiotics and Skin Aging-Associated Microflora Changes

The probiotic principle is likely to be applicable to any environment where a normal microflora exists. The skin also has a normal microflora [13], albeit less complex than the intestinal microflora because of the harsh environment provided by the human skin. The normal microflora of the skin is composed of a limited number of microbial types, mainly gram-positive species. A number of physiological conditions such as hydration, pH, O_2, and growth substrates are the major factors in determining the limited number of microbial species that colonize human skin. Cutaneous microflora defends the skin against premature aging, inflammation, and dehydration and is involved in competitive exclusion of pathogens and increases the acidic nature of the skin, thereby making it even more inhospitable to many pathogens [14]. Some microflora are able to breakdown the fatty acid molecules (from the natural oils) in the skin and thereby increase its acidity. Skin microflora is different depending on the site of the body. The most common genera found in the microflora of the skin are *Propionibacteria*, *Staphylococcus*, *Micrococcus*, *Corynebacterium*, and the yeast *Malassezia* [13]. Based on the proposed probiotic therapy to positively modulate the intestinal microflora, the use of probiotics is postulated to also change the composition of the skin microflora from a potentially harmful composition towards a microflora that would be beneficial for the host [15]. Due to competition for adhesion sites and nutrients, and possibly the production of antimicrobial substances, levels of certain less desirable genera can decrease. However, because the skin has an entirely different environment than the intestine, some different selection criteria for probiotics would be applied. Acid and bile resistance are prime selection criteria for intestinal probiotics, obviously these are not relevant for application to the skin. On the other hand, adhesion is important for the skin as well, to improve transient colonization and colonization resistance toward potential pathogens. Also, production of antimicrobial substances is important for an application on the skin, which, together with inhibition of pathogen adhesion, provides colonization resistance. Of interest, Ouwehand et al. [15] have investigated the possibility of applying probiotics to the skin [15]. Propionic acid bacteria (PAB) were chosen as potential probiotics because they are members of the normal microbiota [16] and have been observed to exhibit antifungal activity [17]. All tested probiotic strains were found to inhibit the growth of some of the target strains, the *Candida albicans* strains being mainly sensitive. All of the tested potential probiotic strains were found to exhibit some adhesion to keratin, the main protein of the skin. Two of the tested strains were, in fact, found to adhere well: 16 % and 20 % of the applied cells, *Propionibacterium freudenreichii* ssp. *freudenreichii* 20271 and *Lactobacillus rhamnosus* 5·5a, respectively. The results of this study strongly encourage the use of skin probiotics even if further studies are needed and should focus on the identification and assessment of strains that also exhibit activity in vivo against potential skin pathogens and will indeed persist on the skin in vivo and be active there.

Probiotics and Skin Aging-Associated pH Changes

Normal skin pH is somewhat acidic and in the range of 4.2–5.6 and has been attributed largely to endogenous agents including the Na^+/H^+ antiporter, NHE1, and one or more secretory phospholipase/s A2 ($sPLA_2$) enzymes, which hydrolyses membrane phospholipids, thereby generating free fatty acids (FFAs) that contribute to the acidification of the stratum corneum [18, 19]. The acid mantle, the combination of sebum (oil) and perspiration, on the skin's surface protects and renders the skin less vulnerable to damage. It also protects from attack by environmental factors, such as the sun and wind, and leaves it less prone to dehydration. The acidic skin pH keeps the resident bacterial flora (see above) attached to the skin, whereas an alkaline pH promotes its dispersal from the skin [20]. The natural pH varies from one part of the body to the other and, in general, the pH of a man's skin is lower than a woman's skin. This acidic environment is very important, as it discourages bacterial colonization and provides a moisture barrier through absorption of moisture by amino acids, salts, and other substances in the acid mantle and in addition regulates the activity of many of the enzymes in the stratum corneum [21]. For example, the activities of both β-glucocerebrosidase and acidic sphingomyelinase are optimal at or below pH 5.5. If the pH of the stratum corneum is increased, the activities of β-glucocerebrosidase and acidic sphingomyelinase are reduced and the extracellular processing of glucosylceramides and sphingomyelins to ceramides is impaired, leading to abnormalities in the structure of the extracellular lipid membranes and decreased permeability barrier function [22–24]. On the other hand, many of the proteases in the stratum corneum have, instead, an optimum pH of 7 or higher; therefore, their activity is low at the usual stratum corneum pH. Thus, increases in stratum corneum pH stimulate protease activity, resulting in increased corneocyte desquamation [22–24]. Skin pH is relatively constant from childhood to approximately age 70 and then rises significantly, the increase being especially pronounced in lower limbs, possibly related to impaired circulation and, consequently, to stasis and reduced oxygen supply [25]. Recently, a decreased NHE1 expression that accounts for the pH abnormality in moderately aged epidermis in mice and human has been reported [26]. The reduced NHE1 expression could account the impairment of lipid processing and epidermal barrier homeostasis in aged skin even if further studies will be required to delineate whether altered $sPLA_2$ activity also contributes to the functional abnormalities in moderately aged epidermis. An interesting property of probiotics is the fermentative metabolism that involves the production of acid molecule, thus acidifying the surrounding environment. Moreover, Yadav and Sinha [27] have recently reported the ability of probiotic *Lactobacilli* to increase the production of free fatty acids (FFAs) by lipolysis of milk fat and to produce conjugated linoleic acid (CLA) by using internal linoleic acid, which may confer nutritional and therapeutical value to probiotic treatment [27].

These evidences suggest that the oral assumption and/or the topical application of probiotic preparation on the aged skin could cause a pH decrease thus coming back near the physiological acid pH. Consequently, the most important cutaneous enzymes that have been impaired by aging could again function.

Probiotics and Skin Aging-Associated Altered Stratum Corneum Lipid Composition

Several studies have demonstrated that ceramides play an essential role in both the barrier and water-holding functions of healthy stratum corneum (SC), suggesting that the dysfunction of the stratum corneum associated with aging as well as that observed in patients with several skin diseases could result from a ceramide deficiency [28]. A previous study reported a significant increase in skin ceramide levels in healthy subjects, after a treatment in vivo with a cream containing sonicated *S. salivarium* ssp. *thermophilus* [29]. The presence of high levels of neutral sphingomyelinase activity in this organism was responsible for the observed increase of stratum corneum ceramide levels, thus leading to an improvement in barrier function and maintenance of stratum corneum flexibility. There is also evidence that the treatment with a sonicated preparation of a *S. salivarium* ssp. *thermophilus* S244 was able to induce an increasing ceramide levels in vivo, on stratum corneum of atopic dermatitis patients [30]. Considering the role of the ceramides in regulating the water-holding capacity and in maintaining skin integrity, the possibility that the topical application of a probiotic formulation, representing a source of exogenous SMase able to hydrolyze skin SM and consequently to generate ceramides, may lead to reduce dryness, loss of tone, fullness, and water loss, thus slowing the process of skin aging [31], has been recently investigated. The skin barrier and the water-holding capacity are the other most important functions of the SC and these functions are related to the composition and structure of SC intercellular lipids [32, 33], including cholesterol, ceramides, and fatty acid. Therefore, the capacitance and ceramide levels as markers of epidermal hydration were determined. The findings indicated that the barrier improvement, resulting in a prompt increase in the water-holding capacity, was observed when the aged subjects were applied *S. thermophilus*-containing cream. In fact, at the end of the treatment a statistically significant increase in hydration values was shown when compared with the values observed at the beginning. An amelioration in hydration skin could be attributed to the increase of the stratum corneum ceramides levels. Topical application of a sonicated *S. salivarium* ssp. *thermophilus* preparation lead to increased nonhydroxy and hydroxy fatty acid ceramides levels in stratum corneum. These results could be again explained with the presence of high levels of neutral SMase in *S. thermophilus*. Altogether, the findings suggest that there are two eventual possibilities by which topical application of a sonicated *S. thermophilus* preparation may contribute to the improvement of lipid barrier and a more effective resistance against aging-associated skin xerosis. One possibility would be that the presence of high levels of neutral SMase in *S. thermophilus* hydrolyses skin SM thus generating ceramides, with structural function in the stratum corneum lipid bilayers. The other eventuality is that *S. thermophilus* SMase-produced ceramides are involved in epidermal differentiation and proliferation signaling pathway as important second messenger, as previously described [34]. Thus, although the mechanism of action of topical application of a sonicated *S. thermophilus* preparation needs to be further elucidated, the results obtained with this experimental cream consist in a relevant increase of skin ceramide levels, which was associated to a more effective resistance against aging-associated skin xerosis.

Probiotics and Skin Aging-Associated Oxidative Stress

The epidermis of skin possesses an extremely efficient antioxidant activity that is superior to most tissues [35], and it has been proposed that the reduction in efficiency of this system during aging is an important factor in skin aging. There are many reports describing the reduction of antioxidant enzymes in skin with age, while others suggest that skin aging is not due to a general decline in antioxidant capacity. However, all agree that the accumulation of free radicals throughout life most likely promotes cellular aging. Generation of reactive oxide species (ROS) is thought to play a major role in skin aging. All the biological structures, as human skin, undergo the detrimental action of ROS. The free radical theory of aging proposes that aging results from accumulation of oxidative damage over a lifetime due to excess ROS, which result from aerobic metabolism [36]. ROS generation is increased in aged skin and represents a key step in molecular pathways, which eventually lead to increased collagen breakdown. ROS cause damage to lipids, proteins, and DNA and also influence cellular senescence [37]. In addition, free radicals also cause damage to connective tissue components of the dermis, particularly collagen [38], which again is likely to influence cell behavior via cell-matrix interactions. Indeed, poorly maintained cellular redox levels lead to elevated activation of nuclear transcription factors such as NF-κB and AP-1, which are involved in several aging-associated degenerating processes, including extracellular matrix degradation [39]. Probiotics have been demonstrated extracellularly to produce effective bioactive molecules exerting several beneficial effects as antioxidative effects by different mechanisms, including the release of exopolysaccharides (EPSs), a class of such effective biomolecules that probiotic bacteria release into the surroundings to protect themselves under starvation conditions and also at extreme pH and temperature conditions [40]. These EPSs are long-chain, high-molecular-mass polymers, which are used in food and dairy industries as texturizers, viscosifiers, and syneresis-lowering agents [41, 42]. They have also been reported to show antiulcer, immunomodulatory, antiviral, antioxidant, and various other biological activities. Recently, studies have demonstrated that microbial EPS has significant antioxidant and free radical scavenging activities, and also have numerous potential applications as pharmaceutical formulations [43].

A widespread mechanism for protection against oxidative stress is provided by the antioxidant enzyme superoxide dismutase (SOD). Bruno-Bàrcena et al. [44] showed that heterologous expression of an SOD gene in intestinal *Lactobacilli* provides protection against peroxide toxicity [44]. Indeed, the authors suggest that it may be possible to use these SOD-rich species in the biotherapy for treatment of peptic ulcers or ulcerative colitis. Using a similar approach, the cumulative oxidative damage could also be reduced in the aged skin.

Probiotics and Skin Aging-Associated Collagen Level Reduction

The processes associated with intrinsic skin aging are thought to result from a combination of events including decreased proliferative capacity of skin-derived cells, decreased matrix synthesis in the dermis, and increased expression of enzymes that degrade the collagenous matrix. Collagen is one of the main building blocks of human skin, providing much of the skin's strength. Dermal fibroblasts make precursor molecules called procollagen, which is converted into collagen. There are two important regulators of collagen production: transforming growth factor (TGF)-β, a cytokine that promotes collagen production, and activator protein (AP)-1, a transcription factor that inhibits collagen production and up-regulates collagen breakdown by up-regulating enzymes called matrix metalloproteinases (MMPs) [45, 46]. In aged skin, there is elevation of AP-1 as compared to young skin [47]. MMP activity is increased in aged human skin and is associated with dramatic increased levels of degraded collagen [12]. In addition, synthesis of types I and III procollagen is reduced in aged human skin [48]. The combination of increased breakdown of collagen and decreased synthesis of new collagen results in an overall decrease in collagen levels in the dermis. The MMPs are a large family of degradative enzymes and four in particular are thought to be important in matrix degradation in the skin. The combined actions of collagenase (MMP1), 92 kDa gelatinase (MMP2), 72 kDa gelatinase (MMP9), and stromelysin 1 (MMP3) can fully degrade skin collagen and components of the elastic network. Coupled with these changes, elastin gene expression is markedly reduced after the age of 40–50, as determined by mRNA steady state levels in cultured fibroblasts, and there is a progressive disappearance of elastic tissue in the dermis. In aged skin there is an increase of MMP activity and reduced collagen I expression. Moreover, an irradiation of human skin with just a single dose of UV light has been shown to increase the activities of MMPs, and this has been associated with significant degradation of collagen fibers. In presenescent dermal fibroblasts, metalloproteinase activity is relatively low with MMP1 and MMP3 shown to be expressed at very low levels. In contrast, levels of matrix metalloproteinase inhibitors TIMP1 and TIMP3 are high, further reducing degradative capacity. In senescent fibroblasts, however, this is reversed with an increase in matrix metalloproteinase expression and a reduction in the expression of tissue inhibitors of metalloproteinase (as a review, see [49]). Ulisse et al. [50] demonstrated the capacity of an oral VSL#3 treatment to decrease MMP activity at the tissue level in the maintenance treatment of patients with pouchitis [50]. Further insights into the molecular basis of periodontitis have identified the potential clinical significance, giving the experimental ground for a new innovative, simple, and efficacious therapeutical approach of periodontal disease [51]. In particular, the anti-inflammatory effects of *L. brevis* extracts on periodontitis patients, which were associated to a significant decrease of MMP levels in saliva samples, were assayed by zymogram and Western blotting. Moorthy et al. [52] evaluated the effect of *L. rhamnosus* and *L. acidophilus* on neutrophil infiltration and lipid peroxidation during *Shigella dysenteriae 1*-induced diarrhea in rats demonstrating a reduction of levels of myeloperoxidase, lipid peroxidation, alkaline phosphatase, and the expression of MMP2 and MMP9 [52]. Together, these data suggest that probiotic treatment could decrease skin aging-associated MMP activity and may represent a new, promising, and inexpensive approach to treat the cutaneous laxity.

Probiotics and Skin Aging-Associated Altered Immune Response

Aging is accompanied by a reduction in the functional capacity of all the organs in the body, and accordingly, the activity of the immune system also declines with age (as a review, see [53]). The senescence of the immune system especially affects cell-mediated as well as humoral immunity. A decrease has also been observed in the ratio of mature to immature T lymphocytes and an increase in proinflammatory cytokine and ROS production [54]. Age-related alterations in immune function also affect the skin and may account for the increased susceptibility in the elderly to cutaneous infections and malignancies and decreased or variable contact hypersensitivity reactions [55]. Perhaps associated with these immunological changes and certainly with other physiological and environmental factors, the bifidobacteria numbers in the gut decrease markedly after 55–60 years of age [56]. The immune system of the elderly is a potential target for probiotics, as it is known to be affected adversely by the aging process, leading to decreasing resistance to diseases [56]. Several studies have reported the capacity of probiotics to counteract the immunosenescence process and to protect against infection [57, 58]. Probiotics have been demonstrated to induce an adjuvant effect on immunological responses, and this evidence suggests that the use of probiotics could also be effective in enhancing the skin barrier function, even if not all probiotics have the same immunological properties (as a review, see [59]). Immune regulation by probiotics is thought to be mediated through the balancing control of pro- and anti-inflammatory cytokines. Some strains of the genus *Bifidobacterium* exhibit powerful anti-inflammatory properties and thus may be able to restore an unbalanced cytokine production [60]. The efficacy of probiotic organisms in the treatment of pouchitis is also reported, an effect that could be in part attributed to nitric oxide synthase (NOS)-II activity decrease [50]. Nitric oxide (NO) is a paracrine regulator of various biological functions and is known to be involved in the physiology and pathophysiology of many systems, including the skin. It is synthesized from l-arginine by NOS. Of interest, the expression of NOS-II is also strongly implicated in several inflammatory skin conditions [61]. A recent study aimed to investigate the beneficial effects of *L. brevis* extracts on periodontitis patients reported that the relevant anti-inflammatory effects of *L. brevis* extracts could be attributed to the presence of high levels of arginine deiminase, which, also in this inflammatory model, metabolizing arginine to citrulline and ammonia, indirectly leads to nitric oxide (NO) generation inhibition, by competing with NOS for the same substrate, arginine [51]. The association between the composition of the *Bifidobacterium* microbiota and the different levels of proinflammatory cytokine TNF-α as well as anti-inflammatory cytokine TGF-β and regulatory cytokine IL-10 has been recently investigated [62]. The results showed that *Bifidobacterium* microbiota of the elderly may be modified through a probiotic intervention, and that even modest changes in the levels of specific *Bifidobacterium* species may be associated with changes in the cytokine levels, indicating that modulation of the intestinal *Bifidobacterium* microbiota may provide a means of influencing the inflammatory responses in the elderly. Nutritional intervention, particularly with dietary antioxidants, has been proposed to protect against UV-induced skin damage, and during recent years, an increasing interest has been shown for new nutritional approaches using live microorganisms as probiotics. UV radiation is known to alter the cutaneous and systemic immune systems implicated in the development of skin tumors. Of note, findings suggest that ingested probiotic bacteria (*L. johnsonii* La1) can maintain in a mouse model as well as in humans a normal cutaneous immune capacity after UV exposure [63, 64]. The presented evidence would suggest that La1, via priming the immune system in the gut, may be considered an immunoprotector against the predicted

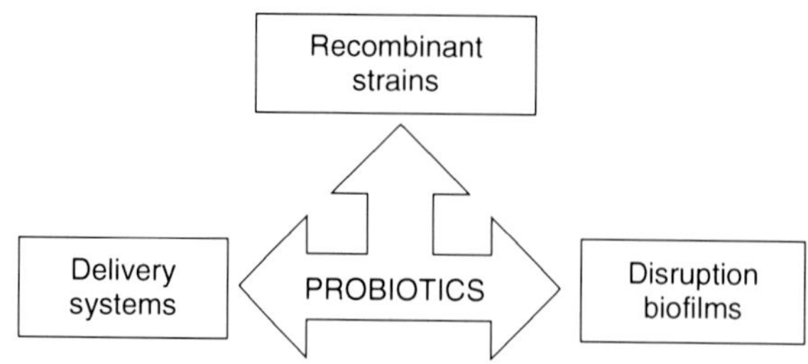

Fig. 2 New frontiers in probiotic research

immunosuppressive effect of UV on the skin immune system. In particular, probiotic ingestion was able to allow a protective cutaneous hypersensitivity reaction, a normal epidermal Langerhans cell density, as well as to maintain or restore the systemic IL-10 production to levels equivalent to non-UV-exposed conditions, thus confirming the ability of La1 to preserve the capacity of the organism to respond to immunological changes.

Of note, the ingestion of probiotics has been associated with a diminution in the severity of autoimmune, particularly intestinal inflammatory, diseases as well as allergic disorders [65, 66].

In conclusion, the scientific literature strongly supports the ability of probiotics to modulate the immune response as well as their capacity to counteract the immunosenescence process and to protect against infection [57, 58].

New Frontiers in Probiotic Research and Concluding Remarks

As the elderly population increases, the prevalence of aging-related diseases will increase and functional foods that provide health benefits to control aging and prolong health span will become more desirable. The experimental evidences summarized in the present review strongly encourage the treatment with selected probiotic strains as sun protector, in ameliorating the aging skin condition, in improving dermocosmetic treatments, in recovering skin properties after an injury, as well in preparing skin to cutaneous laser resurfacing. Laser procedures for the aging face are numerous and emerging rapidly. Ablative laser resurfacing is considered to be the gold standard to improve clinical features of the aging face and generally refers to treatment with a carbon dioxide laser (10,600 nm) [67]. It improves fine and some coarse wrinkles and overall dyspigmentation, lightens dark under-eye circles, and generally improves the texture of skin; it can also be used to ameliorate old acne scarring. Side effects include increased erythema immediately following the treatment, slight discomfort, swelling, and potential bruising. Pretreatment clinical assessment and consultation are critical before prescribing or performing the treatments and procedures to review the risks and complications [39]. The potent anti-inflammatory effects exerted by selected strains of probiotics could render them good candidates to prevent or reduce, at least partially, the side effects associated to ablative laser resurfacing. Moreover, considering that most of the topically applied cosmetic products have only a short-term effect on superficial structures, the oral supplementation can be integrated with topical products to obtain an even more effective result.

Since probiotics are intrinsically benign bacteria and they appear to implant, at least temporarily, in the gastrointestinal tract of nearly everyone who consumes them, they can be used as vehicles for transporting genes of medical importance to the host [68]. This approach is also helpful to slow the process of skin aging.

Advances in the field of probiotic research provide new delivery systems, creation of disease-targeted recombinant strains, and isolation and characterization of signaling molecules that can modulate microbial biofilms and infectious processes [2] (Fig. 2). Moreover, the development of new delivery mechanisms could provide encapsulating probiotics, such that they rehydrate at specific sites, and encasing prebiotics in nanoaggragates that could protect against stomach acid and deliver their payload when the pH reaches 7.4 [69]. Potentially, such nanoencapsulation will also allow probiotic delivery in foods, such as biscuits [2]. At the macromolecular level, it will be possible to coat capsules with biosensors that detect the optimal conditions for release of probiotic contents as suggested by Hopper [70]. An alternative approach to improving probiotic efficacy is to enhance a strain's ability to cope with stress at the genetic level. This approach has been successfully employed to increase the stress tolerance profile of two probiotic strains: *L. salivarium* UCC118 and *Bifidobacterium breve* UCC [71, 72]. Cloning the *betL* gene into *L. salivarium* resulted in a significant increase in the ability of the transformed strain to accumulate betaine, which confer increased salt tolerance and osmotolerance, thus improving the clinical efficacy of the probiotic.

The growing rates of antibiotic resistance and the realization that biofilm formation makes it more difficult for antibiotics to eradicate infections have led to studies of new approaches for managing infectious biofilms using probiotics. These include disruption or penetration of biofilms by beneficial microbes or alteration of the environment to restore a noninfectious biofilm. An in vitro study has shown that *Gardnella vaginalis* species biofilms can be penetrated by *L. rhamnosus* GR-1, leading to rapid disruption and death of the pathogens [73]. Other studies have shown that this *Lactobacillus* strain can also prevent the formation of *C. albicans* biofilms, and it can kill the yeast in vitro [2]. Moreover, fluorescent in situ hybridization and confocal laser microscopy, used successfully to study complex oral biofilms, could be used to better understand how gram-negative and gram-positive bacteria interact in biofilms and are affected by different nutrients, as suggested by Thurnheer [74]. In summary, biotechnology holds the key to future advances in the clinical application of probiotic product.

An additional message, supported by scientific evidence, strongly emerges that probiotics can enhance health in a more holistic manner, by improving the balance of the intestinal flora, preventing disease, reducing allergic events, interdicting the introduction of harmful microorganisms, and suppressing intestinal enzyme activity that could have detrimental effects. Probiotics must be viewed as healthy additions to everyone's diet. The discovery of new probiotics has been based on a calculated strategy of considering the characteristics of an ideal strain and then asking nature to provide it within the diversity of the microbial world. Now the objective should be to define the appropriate uses of probiotics and to discover new applications, which will bring benefit to human health including ameliorating the aging skin condition.

Cross-References

▶ The Potential of Probiotics and Prebiotics for Skin Health

References

1. Fioramonti J, et al. Probiotics: what are they? What are their effects on gut physiology? Best Pract Res Clin Gastroenterol. 2003;17(5):711–24.
2. Reid G. How science will help shape future clinical applications of probiotics. Clin Infect Dis. 2008;46 Suppl 2:S62–6.
3. Silva M, et al. Antimicrobial substance from a human *Lactobacillus* strain. Antimicrob Agents Chemother. 1987;31:1231–3.
4. Heczko PB, et al. Critical evaluation of probiotic activity of lactic acid bacteria and their effects. J Physiol Pharmacol. 2006;57 Suppl 9:S5–12.
5. Gionchetti P, et al. Antibiotics and probiotics in treatment of inflammatory bowel disease. World J Gastroenterol. 2006;12:3306–13.
6. Farnworth ER. The evidence to support health claims for probiotics. J Nutr. 2008;138(6):1250S–4.
7. Sleator RD, et al. New frontiers in probiotic research. Lett Appl Microbiol. 2008;46(2):143–7.
8. Di Marzio L, et al. Apoptotic effects of selected strains of lactic acid bacteria on a human T leukemia cell line are associated with bacterial arginine deiminase and/or sphingomyelinase activities. Nutr Cancer. 2001;40 (2):185–96.
9. de Moreno de LeBlanc A, et al. The application of probiotics in cancer. Br J Nutr. 2007;98 Suppl 1: S105–10.
10. Goldin BR. Clinical indications for probiotics: an overview. Clin Infect Dis. 2008;46 Suppl 2:S96–100.

11. Macpherson AJ, et al. Induction of protective IgA by intestinal dendritic cells carrying commensal bacteria. Science. 2004;303:1662–5.
12. Fisher GJ, et al. Mechanisms of photoaging and chronological skin aging. Arch Dermatol. 2002;138 (11):1462–70.
13. Bojar RA, et al. Review: the human cutaneous microflora and factors controlling colonisation. World J Microbiol Biotechnol. 2002;18(9):889–903.
14. Cogen AL, et al. Skin microbiota: a source of disease or defence? Br J Dermatol. 2008;158(3):442–55.
15. Ouwehand AC, et al. Probiotics for the skin: a new area of potential application? Lett Appl Microbiol. 2003;36 (5):327–31.
16. Tannock GW. Normal microflora. An introduction to microbes inhabiting the human body. London: Chapman & Hall; 1995.
17. Suomalainen R, et al. Propionic acid bacteria as protective cultures in fermented milks and breads. Lait. 1999;79:165–74.
18. Fluhr JW, et al. Generation of free fatty acids from phospholipids regulates stratum corneum acidification and integrity. J Invest Dermatol. 2001;117:44–51.
19. Fluhr JW, et al. Stratum corneum acidification in neonatal skin: secretory phospholipase A2 and the sodium/hydrogen antiporter-1 acidify neonatal rat stratum corneum. J Invest Dermatol. 2004;122:320–9.
20. Lambers H, et al. Natural skin surface pH is on average below 5, which is beneficial for its resident flora. Int J Cosmet Sci. 2006;28(5):359–70.
21. Mauro T. SC pH: measurement, origins, and functions. In: Elias P, Feingold K, editors. Skin barrier. New York: Taylor & Francis; 2006. p. 223–9.
22. Fluhr JW, et al. Functional consequences of a neutral pH in neonatal rat stratum corneum. J Invest Dermatol. 2004;123:140–51.
23. Hachem JP, et al. pH directly regulates epidermal permeability barrier homeostasis, and stratum corneum integrity/cohesion. J Invest Dermatol. 2003;121:345–53.
24. Hachem JP, et al. Sustained serine proteases activity by prolonged increase in pH leads to degradation of lipid processing enzymes and profound alterations of barrier function and stratum corneum integrity. J Invest Dermatol. 2005;125:510–20.
25. Waller JM, et al. Age and skin structure and function, a quantitative approach (I): blood flow, pH, thickness, and ultrasound echogenicity. Skin Res Technol. 2005;11(4):221–35.
26. Choi EH, et al. Stratum corneum acidification is impaired in moderately aged human and murine skin. J Invest Dermatol. 2007;127(12):2847–56.
27. Yadav H, et al. Production of free fatty acids and conjugated linoleic acid in probiotic dahi containing *Lactobacillus acidophilus* and *Lactobacillus casei* during fermentation and storage. Int Dairy J. 2007;17 (8):1006–10.
28. Holleran WM, et al. Epidermal sphingolipids: metabolism, function, and roles in skin disorders. FEBS Lett. 2006;580(23):5456–66.
29. Di Marzio L, et al. Effect of the lactic acid bacterium *Streptococcus thermophilus* on ceramide levels in human keratinocytes in vitro and stratum corneum in vivo. J Invest Dermatol. 1999;113(1):98–106.
30. Di Marzio L, et al. Effect of the lactic acid bacterium *Streptococcus thermophilus* on stratum corneum ceramide levels and signs and symptoms of atopic dermatitis patients. Exp Dermatol. 2003;12(5):615–20.
31. Di Marzio L, et al. Increase of skin-ceramide levels in aged subjects following a short-term topical application of bacterial sphingomyelinase from *Streptococcus thermophilus*. Int J Immunopathol Pharmacol. 2008;21 (1):137–43.
32. Denda M, et al. Age- and sex-dependent change in stratum corneum sphingolipids. Arch Dermatol Res. 1993;285(7):415–7.
33. Motta S, et al. Abnormality of water barrier function in psoriasis. Role of ceramide fractions. Arch Dermatol. 1994;130(4):452–6.
34. Jensen JM, et al. Acid and neutral sphingomyelinase, ceramide synthase, and acid ceramidase activities in cutaneous aging. Exp Dermatol. 2005;14(8): 609–18.
35. Kohen R, et al. Skin low molecular weight antioxidants and their role in aging and in oxidative stress. Toxicology. 2000;148(2–3):149–57.
36. Hensley K, et al. Reactive oxygen species and protein oxidation in aging: a look back, a look ahead. Arch Biochem Biophys. 2002;397(2):377–83.
37. Tzaphlidou M. The role of collagen and elastin in aged skin: an image processing approach. Micron. 2004;35 (3):73–177.
38. Dalle Carbonare M, et al. Skin photosensitizing agents and the role of reactive oxygen species in photoaging. J Photochem Photobiol. 1992;14(1–2):105–24.
39. Helfrich YR, et al. Overview of skin aging and photoaging. Dermatol Nurs. 2008;20(3):177–83.
40. Kodali VP, et al. Antioxidant and free radical scavenging activities of an exopolysaccharide from a probiotic bacterium. Biotechnol J. 2008;3(2):245–51.
41. Cerning J. Exocellular polysaccharides produced by lactic acid bacteria. FEMS Microbiol Rev. 1990;7 (1–2):113–30.
42. Welman AD, et al. Exopolysaccharides from lactic acid bacteria: perspectives and challenges. Trends Biotechnol. 2003;21(6):269–74.
43. Kishk YFM, et al. Free-radical scavenging and antioxidative activities of some polysaccharides in emulsions. LWT- Food Sci Technol. 2007;40(2):270–7.
44. Bruno-Bárcena JM, et al. Expression of a heterologous manganese superoxide dismutase gene in intestinal lactobacilli provides protection against hydrogen peroxide toxicity. Appl Environ Microbiol. 2004;70 (8):4702–10.
45. Kang S, et al. Photoaging and topical tretinoin: therapy, pathogenesis, and prevention. Arch Dermatol. 1997;133(10):1280–4.
46. Massagué J. TGF-β signal transduction. Annu Rev Biochem. 1998;67:753–91.

47. Chung JH, et al. Decreased extracellular-signal-regulated kinase and increased stress-activated MAP kinase activities in aged human skin in vivo. J Invest Dermatol. 2000;115(2):177–82.
48. Varani J, et al. Vitamin A antagonizes decreased cell growth and elevated collagen-degrading matrix metalloproteinases and stimulates collagen accumulation in naturally aged human skin. J Invest Dermatol. 2000;114(3):480–6.
49. Jenkins G. Molecular mechanisms of skin ageing. Mech Ageing Dev. 2002;123(7):801–10.
50. Ulisse S, et al. Expression of cytokines, inducible nitric oxide synthase, and matrix metalloproteinases in pouchitis: effects of probiotic treatment. Am J Gastroenterol. 2001;96(9):2691–9.
51. Riccia DN, et al. Anti-inflammatory effects of *Lactobacillus brevis* (CD2) on periodontal disease. Oral Dis. 2007;13(4):376–85.
52. Moorthy G, et al. Protective role of lactobacilli in *Shigella dysenteriae 1*-induced diarrhea in rats. Nutrition. 2007;23(5):424–33.
53. Dorshkind K. The ageing immune system: is it ever too old to become young again? Nat Rev Immunol. 2009;9(1):57–62.
54. Victor VM, et al. *N*-acetylcysteine improves in vitro the function of macrophages from mice with endotoxininduced oxidative stress. Free Radic Res. 2002;36:33–45.
55. Dewberry C, et al. Skin cancer in elderly patients. Dermatol Clin North Am. 2004;22:93–6.
56. Nova E, et al. Immunomodulatory effects of probiotics in different stages of life. Br J Nutr. 2007;98 Suppl 1: S90–5.
57. Chiang BL, et al. Enhancing immunity by dietary consumption of a probiotic lactic acid bacterium (*Bifidobacterium lactis* HN019): optimization and definition of cellular immune responses. Eur J Clin Nutr. 2000;54:849–55.
58. Gill HS, et al. Optimizing immunity and gut function in the elderly. J Nutr Health Aging. 2001;5:80–91.
59. Caramia G, et al. Probiotics and the skin. Clin Dermatol. 2008;26(1):4–11.
60. Isolauri E. Probiotics in human disease. Am J Clin Nutr. 2001;73:S1142–6.
61. Cals-Grierson MM, et al. Nitric oxide function in the skin. Nitric Oxide. 2004;10(4):179–93.
62. Ouwehand AC, et al. *Bifidobacterium* microbiota and parameters of immune function in elderly subjects. FEMS Immunol Med Microbiol. 2008;53(1):18–25.
63. Guéniche A, et al. Supplementation with oral probiotic bacteria maintains cutaneous immune homeostasis after UV exposure. Eur J Dermatol. 2006;16:511–7.
64. Peguet-Navarro J, et al. Supplementation with oral probiotic bacteria protects human cutaneous immune homeostasis after UV exposure-double blind, randomized, placebo controlled clinical trial. Eur J Dermatol. 2008;18:504–11.
65. Canche-Pool EB, et al. Probiotics and autoimmunity: an evolutionary perspective. Med Hypotheses. 2008;70:657–60.
66. Hsu CJ, et al. Emerging treatment of atopic dermatitis. Clin Rev Allergy Immunol. 2007;33:199–203.
67. Railan D, et al. Ablative treatment of photoaging. Dermatol Ther. 2005;18:227–41.
68. Gorbach SL. Probiotics in the third millennium. Dig Liver Dis. 2002;34 Suppl 2:2–7.
69. Fan YF, et al. Preparation of insulin nanoparticles and their encapsulation with biodegradable polyelectrolytes via the layer-by-layer adsorption. Int J Pharm. 2006;324:158–67.
70. Hooper LV, et al. A molecular sensor that allows a gut commensal to control its nutrient foundation in a competitive ecosystem. Proc Natl Acad Sci U S A. 1999;17(96):9833–8.
71. Sheehan VM, et al. Heterologous expression of BetL, a betaine uptake system, enhances the stress tolerance of *Lactobacillus salivarium* UCC118. Appl Environ Microbiol. 2006;72(3):2170–7.
72. Sheehan VM, et al. Improving gastric transit, gastrointestinal persistence and therapeutic efficacy of the probiotic strain *Bifidobacterium breve* UCC2003. Microbiol. 2007;153(10):3563–71.
73. Saunders S, et al. Effect of *Lactobacillus* challenge on *Gardnerella vaginalis* biofilms. Colloids Surf B Biointerfaces. 2007;55(2):138–42.
74. Thurnheer T, et al. Multiplex FISH analysis of a six-species bacterial biofilm. J Microbiol Methods. 2004;56:37–47.

Animal Models

101

Shalini Krishnasamy, Sara Flores, Farzam Gorouhi, and Howard I. Maibach

Contents

S. Krishnasamy
University of California, Los Angeles, CA, USA
e-mail: SKrishnasamy@mednet.ucla.edu

S. Flores
Department of Dermatology, University of Cincinnati, Cincinnati, OH, USA
e-mail: primaragazza1@yahoo.com

F. Gorouhi (✉)
Department of Dermatology, University of California, Davis, CA, USA
e-mail: gorouhif@gmail.com

H.I. Maibach
Department of Dermatology, University of California, San Francisco, CA, USA
e-mail: maibachh@derm.ucsf.edu

M.A. Farage et al. (eds.), *Textbook of Aging Skin*,
DOI 10.1007/978-3-662-47398-6_75

Abstract

Skin aging is a complex process that is categorized into either intrinsic or extrinsic actinic aging. Extrinsic actinic aging results from environmental factors, namely ultraviolet (UV) radiation, which is commonly referred to as photoaging, and is characterized by wrinkles and dryness. In contrast to extrinsic aging, intrinsic aging is gene dependent and occurs over time due to variety of physiological factors (ex/ hormonal changes). Numerous studies have been performed in an attempt to understand how the architecture of the skin changes with age and to uncover the mechanism by which this occurs [1]. There is also a large body of studies focused on determining how to prevent and reverse the effects of photoaging. As such, providing an in-depth review of the literature would not be possible in a single chapter. Therefore, the aim of this chapter is to lay a general framework of the various studies that have been performed in animal models regarding skin aging and to highlight what conclusions can be drawn from them and what has yet to be uncovered.

Introduction

Aging is influenced by a combination of biological, physiological, and environmental factors. Skin aging in particular can be divided into actinic aging and intrinsic aging. Actinic aging refers to ultraviolet (UV) radiation-induced changes, whereas intrinsic aging refers to changes that occur independent of the environment and are influenced by biologic and physiologic factors. In an attempt to understand age-related changes that occur within the skin, numerous in vivo studies using model organisms have been performed. Since human and mouse genomes are ninety-nine percent conserved, rodents are great animal models to study human disease. Moreover, the ability to genetically engineer rodents enables us to study the relationship between genetics and the pathophysiology of various diseases. Here we present a basic framework of the leading in vivo studies that have been performed which have shaped what we currently know about aging.

Actinic Aging

In an attempt to understand the relationship between long-term UV exposure and the development of elastosis, studies were initially performed using the Dublin Imprinting Control Region (ICR) Albino Random Bred mouse, which contains a mutation in the gene encoding tyrosinase, an enzyme needed to produce melanin. In 1964, Sams et al. reported that exposing the shave back of these mice to long-term UV radiation resulted in solar elastosis [2]. While the study recapitulated the effects of long-term exposure to UV radiation, the dose applied greatly exceeded normal levels of UV radiation. Moreover, the mice developed tumors that were thought to be different from those produced in humans; thus, scientists were in search of a more appropriate mouse model to study the effects UV radiation has on humans.

The hairless mouse became the model of choice after Winkelmann et al. observed that an engineered hairless mouse possessing mutant alleles of the hairless gene (hr gene) produced tumors in response to UV radiation that were similar to human tumors [3, 4]. Since then, the hairless mouse has been used to study various photobiologic phenomena including phototoxicity, photoimmune effects, carcinogenesis, and UV-induced DNA damage [5]. Subsequent investigation reveled that the UV-induced connective tissue damage in these mice is analogous to that in humans and that the acute edema that develops in response to UV radiation is comparable to the erythema humans develop when they get a sunburn [6, 7]. Although pigmented and albino hairless mice can be engineered, the most commonly used hairless mouse model to study photoaging is the albino Skh hairless mouse [8].

Elastosis has been the most common measure for assessing the long-term effects of UV exposure. In 1980, Berger et al. used the naked (Ng/-) albino strain to produce elastosis in a hairless mouse [9]. Since then, numerous studies have demonstrated ultraviolet-induced elastosis. Johnston et al. demonstrated that the levels of cross-linked elastin in the skin of mice treated with UVA or UVB were decreased, while the levels of collagen remained unchanged. Biological assays reveled that collagen synthesis via prolyl hydroxylase (PH) was impaired with UVA exposure and thus may lead to decreases in collagen synthesis and subsequent dermal atrophy over time [10]. Further studies using immunohistochemistry, electron microscopy, and biochemical experiments showed UV radiation-induced elastosis [7, 11].

While the former studies emphasized the impact of UV light on elasticity, a dermal component, other studies have demonstrated the effect of UV light on the viscosity of the skin, an epidermal component. In order to assess the influence 1,25-dihydroxyvitamin D_3 has on photo-wrinkling, Fujimura et al. treated female HR/ICR hairless mice topically with 1,25-dihydroxyvitamin D_3, which in humans is produced in the kidneys [12]. The mice were treated once daily, 5 days per week with 1.00 μg, 0.20 μg, or 0.05 μg of 1,25-dihydroxyvitamin D_3. Skin sagging was assessed using a scale described by Bisset et al. [13]. Four grades were used, with the fourth being the most severe. After 6 weeks of treatment with 1.0 μg/day of 1,25-dihydroxyvitamin D_3, the skin on the backs of these mice developed coarse, deep wrinkles. While this suggested that 1,25-dihydroxyvitamin D_3 may promote degeneration of skins architecture, it was unclear if it was due to changes in the epidermis or dermis. This led to further experiments investigating the effect of topical 1,25-dihydroxyvitamin D_3 on the immediate distension (U_e) and the delayed distension (U_v), which are parameters of skin elasticity and viscosity, respectively. While topical application of high levels of 1,25-dihydroxyvitamin D_3 did not influence U_e, it did lead to a decrease in U_v. Since U_e is largely a measure of the dermal component and U_v an epidermal component, this study suggests that changes in the mechanical properties of the skin after topical 1,25-dihydroxyvitamin D_3 are due to physical changes in the epidermis [12].

Fujimura et al. also compared immediate retraction (U_r) and final distension (U_f) before and after topical application of 1,25-dihydroxyvitamin D_3 and found that the ratio of U_r/U_f decreased after application of 1,25-dihydroxyvitamin D_3, as is expected with normal aging. Interestingly, the decrease that resulted from application of 1,25-dihydroxyvitamin D_3 was a result of a decrease in U_r, instead of an increase in U_f which usually occurs with age-related skin changes. Further studies are needed to elucidate the reason for this difference. Together these experiments by Fujimara et al. suggest that although vitamin D is recommended to prevent osteoporosis, vitamin D may have damaging effects on other organs. Therefore, it may be worthwhile to investigate if vitamin D causes accelerated degradation of organs other than the skin.

The degradation of collagen and other components of the dermal extracellular matrix in part is due to upregulation of matrix metalloproteinases (MMPs). Matrix metalloproteinases are a family of endopeptidases that cleave the constituents of the extracellular matrix in connective tissues [14]. MMPs have been implicated in the pathogenesis of various conditions including atherosclerosis and emphysema. Their association with photoaging has been revealed in studies showing the upregulation of MMPs in irradiated cultured fibroblasts [15]. UVB induces expression of MMP-1, MMP-3, and MMP-9, whereas UVA induces expression of MMP-1, MMP-2, and MMP-3 [16, 17]. Further experiments revealed that in addition to MMPS, expression of matrix metalloelastase changed in response to UV exposure. Immunohistochemistry of samples of skin from of hairless mice exposed to UV radiation for increasing periods of time reveled that the longer the mice were exposed to radiation, the higher the level of expression of MME in the dermis. This suggests that photoaging may be attributed to UV-induced degeneration of the dermal extracellular matrix by both MMPs and MMEs.

Since UVB rays induce expression of MMP-1, MMP-3, MMP-9, via Cathepsin G, a serine protease, Son et al. hypothesized that inhibition of Cathepsin G may prevent UVB-induced photoaging [18]. Comparison of the skin of hairless mice before and after exposure to UVB radiation revealed that the mice treated with topical Cathepsin G had less of a decrease in collagen and an attenuated upregulation of MMP compared to mice that did not have Cathepsin applied to their skin. Thus, topical application of Cathepsin G inhibitors may be useful for the prevention of UVB-induced photoaging in humans by attenuating upregulation of MMP, thereby minimizing damage to the extracellular matrix.

Since UV radiation is oxidizing, Hwang et al. postulated that topical application of Gallic acid (GA), a substance that possesses antioxidant and anti-inflammatory properties, would prevent UVB-induced photoaging [19]. To test this hypothesis, hairless mice were randomly divided into three groups of six mice that received varying amounts of GA following UVB irradiation and two control groups, one that received no UVB exposure and no GA and the other that received UVB exposure without topical GA. For 3 weeks, the mice received 1 h of UVB radiation followed by topical application of GA. Comparison of skin from mice exposed to UVB with and without GA showed that GA-treated mice had less prominent wrinkles, less dryness, decreased skin thickness, and lower levels of MMP-1. Thus, topical application of GA may be useful in preventing UVB-induced photoaging by negatively modulating levels of MMP-1.

Since UV-induced photoaging is mediated by reactive oxygen species that in turn generate lipid peroxidation carbonyl-containing products, such as acrolein (4HNE), Larroque-Cardoso et al. hypothesized that 4HNE mediates photoaging through formation of adducts with elastin and therefore topical application of a carbonyl scavenger like carnosine should reverse UV-induced photoaging [20]. Using immunofluorescence, Hwang et al. showed that the dermis of hairless mice exposed to UVA daily exhibited an increase in 4HNE and 4HNE-elastin adducts and demonstrated that daily application of carnosine completely reversed the development of photoaging alternations including 4-HNE-adduct formation on elastin. In summary, this study highlights the role of 4HNE-elastin adducts in photoaging and suggests that application of topical carbonyl scavengers has a protective effect against photoaging.

All-*trans*-retinoic acid (RA) is another topical treatment for repairing UV-induced skin damage that has been well studied. Klingman et al. for example used the Skh *hairless*-1 albino mouse model to determine if topical all-*trans*-retinoic acid (RA) could reverse UV-induced skin damage using the Skh *hairless*-1 albino mouse model. The mice were irradiated three times a week for 10 weeks to produce UV-induced changes in the skin, and RA was subsequently applied in varying concentrations. Histology and electron microscopy were used to assess structural changes in the skin before and after the use of RA. The study revealed that RA could repair UV-induced dermal damage in mice by hyperactivating fibroblasts, which in turn leads to increased collagen synthesis [21]. Soon Park et al. performed another study regarding reversing photoaging. Since prior wound repair studies demonstrated that adipose-derived stem cells (ADSCs) could stimulate fibroblast migration and collagen synthesis [22], Soon Park et al. hypothesized that ADSCs could be used as a cosmetic treatment to reverse collagen degradation and deceleration of collagen synthesis resulting from photodamage. To test this hypothesis, ADSCs were injected intradermally into the backs of three micropigs twice over a 14-day interval. Histologic and western blot analysis revealed that there was an increase in collagen in skin 1 month after injection of ADSCs, suggesting that ADSCs may be a potential treatment to reverse skin aging.

Apart from UV radiation, there are many other environmental oxidizing agents that are damaging to the skin. Tobacco smoke, for example, has been shown in in vitro studies to have particularly deleterious effects on the extracellular matrix of the skin [23]. There is evidence from in vivo studies that tobacco smoke induces premature skin aging [24]. In 2007, Tanaka et al. was the first to examine the effects of cigarette smoke on the connective tissue matrix of hairless mice. An aqueous smoke solution prepared by dissolving cigarette smoke in phosphate buffered saline was either applied topically or administered intracutaneously to the backs of the hairless mice three times a week over a 6-month period. Immunohistochemistry revealed that there was a loss of discernable collagen bundles in the dermis of the mice treated with the aqueous smoke solution as compared to the control. This was the first of many studies to show that tobacco smoke directly induces premature aging of the skin using an in vivo model [24]. Subsequently, many groups studied the influence cigarette smoke has on blood flow to the skin. According to *Leow and Maibach's* review of the literature, all studies showed a consistent decrease in blood flow during the first two minutes of smoking cigarettes [25]. A later study by Manfrecola et al. reported a 38.1 % reduction in cutaneous blood flow in smokers and 28.1 % reduction in nonsmokers, with smokers having a shorter recovery time than for smokers [26].

Intrinsic Aging

Our understanding of intrinsic aging is limited in comparison with that of actinic aging. Since UV radiation is a quantitative external variable, the consequences of actinic damage can be observed more readily. Intrinsic aging however occurs over many years due to various biologic or physiologic influences, independent of any environmental factors. It is therefore more difficult to experimentally design studies to investigate intrinsic aging. Scientists have yet to understand why different individuals age at different rates. The experiments reviewed below are just the beginning of our attempt to elucidate the various factors responsible for intrinsic aging.

Hiromi Kimoto-Nira et al. used senescence-accelerated mice (SAM) to observe various physical changes associated with aging, including those in the skin. As their name implies, SAK develop normally, but show an early onset of aging. It is therefore a great mouse model to study how age alone effects various organs in the body. Hiromi Kimoto-Nira et al. examined how probiotics influence aging by orally administering *Lactococcus lactic* subsp. *cremoris* H61(strain H61), a probiotic to SAM for 5–9 months [27]. Using a grading system developed by Hosokawa et al. in 1984, Hiromi Kimoto-Nira et al. observed that the mice receiving probiotics had a lower incidence of skin ulcers and diminished rate of hair loss [27, 28], suggesting that probiotics may be able to slow the progression of intrinsic aging.

In 1975, Murai et al. attempted to understand how collagen changes on a molecular level with age, by examining the levels of hydroxylysine-linked carbohydrates units in collagen molecules at various ages. Since glycosylation renders molecules to be more insoluble, Murai et al. examined how the ratio of soluble to insoluble fractions obtained from skin of rats changed with age. Examination of the degree of glycosylation in the insoluble fraction revealed an absolute decrease in levels of glycosylated hydroxylysine in collagen with age in addition to a gradual increase in ratio insoluble : soluble collagen with age [27]. While the role of glycosylation in formation of collagen had yet to be understood at the time this experiment was performed, this was among the first experiments to use an animal model to examine molecular changes in collagen with age.

Another model that has been employed to study changes in skin attributed to intrinsic aging is the Ishibashi (IS) rat. Interestingly, their skin develops wrinkles and furrows at 12 weeks of age independent of UV radiation; thus, Sakuraoka et al. compared how the skin composition of elastin and collagen of IS rats changed over time compared to control Sprague–Dawley (SD) rats [28, 29]. Using the method described by Prockop et al., collagen content was determined by measuring levels of hydoxyproline, while high performance liquid chromatography was used to estimate elastin content by measuring isodesmosine, a lysine derivative in elastin molecules [30]. No significant difference in the amount of collagen was observed between aged skin of IS and SD rats and their younger counterparts. This suggests that the intrinsic aging observed in the skin of IS rats is unlikely related to collagen. Subsequent comparison of levels of isodesmosine between aged and young counterparts of IS and SD rats revealed that while aged IS rats had a notable reduction in isodesmosine content, aged SD rats did not. This decrease in isodesmosine content in the skin of IS rats coupled with the lack of changes in isodesmosine levels in skin of SD rats suggests that intrinsic aging of skin in IS rats may be related to changes in elastin content. Thus, the IS rat may be a good model to understand intrinsic aging in humans.

Although a majority of in vivo studies related to skin aging have been performed in rodents, there are few studies that have been performed using dogs. In one study, Mexican hairless dogs with spotty pigmentation were used to study the effects of kinetin (KN) on reversing hyperpigmentation. After 50 days of topical application of one side of the body, the KN-treated sites showed normalization of pigmentation and a more rejuvenated appearance of the skin. Thus, the authors proposed that kinetin may be a safe treatment in humans to reverse age-associated hyperpigmentation [31].

Fgf23 and Klotho as Future Models

Fibroblast growth factor 23 (FGF-23) null mice and *klotho* mice are two transgenic strains that have a premature aging phenotype characterized by early onset arteriosclerosis, osteopenia, ectopic calcifications, pulmonary emphysema, diminished hearing, and senile atrophy of the skin [32]. Thus, these mice may be good models to understand the various factors influencing intrinsic aging. The similar phenotypes of these mice are likely a result of both strains of mice possessing mutations in genes encoding proteins linked via a common pathway [33].

Preliminary studies with these mice reveal that *Klotho* and *FGF-23* null mice have high increased vitamin D activity in their serum, suggesting that there may be a correlation between vitamin D and premature aging in various organs including the skin, as suggested previously by Fujimara et al. More recent data from Yamashita et al. showing that klotho mice exhibit significant phenotypic similarities with aged skin such as atrophy and delayed wound healing suggest that the Klotho mouse may be a good model to investigate wound healing in the elderly [34].

Conclusion

The examples discussed here are just a few of the studies investigating changes associated with skin aging. Furthermore, this chapter only reviews studies using animal models and does not include any examples of studies performed in humans or in xenografts. It is our hope that this text allows one to familiarize themselves with the various models available and the methods employed to study skin aging. As our understanding of the aging mechanism becomes more intricate, new models more closely resembling processes in humans will be needed to further our understanding of aging.

While the number of studies investigating actinic aging greatly outweigh those on intrinsic aging, the *Klotho and FGF-23* mice are two models provide us with a means to better characterize how systemic processes influence the structure, function, and appearance of skin over time. In addition to broadening our understanding of how the skin is influenced by systemic factors, it is our hope that future studies regarding skin aging will also able to shed light on how various organs change with age.

Acknowledgment We would like to thank Dr. John Epstein for his generous assistance.

References

1. Hedrick H. ed. The laboratory mouse. In: G.a.P. Bullock P. The handbook of experimental animals. San Diego: Elsevier; 2004.
2. Sams WM, Smith JG, Burke PG. The experimental production of elastosis with ultraviolet light. J Invest Dermatol. 1964;43:467–71.
3. Winkelmann RK, Blades EJ, Zollman PE. Squamous cell tumors induced in hairless mice with ultraviolet light. J Invest Dermatol. 1960;34:131–8.
4. Benavides F, Oberyszyn T, VanBuskirk A, Reeve V. The hairless mouse in skin research. J Dermatol Sci. 2009;53:10–8.
5. Maibach H, Lowe NJ, editors. Models in dermatology, vol. 1. Basel: Karger; 1985.
6. Cole CA, Davies RE, Forbes PD, D'Aloisio LC. Comparison of action spectra for acute cutaneous responses to ultraviolet radiation: man and albino hairless mouse. Photochem Photobiol. 1983;37: 623–31.
7. Kligman LH, Akin FJ, Kligman AM. Prevention of ultraviolet damage to the dermis of hairless mice by sunscreens. J Invest Dermatol. 1982;78:181–9.
8. Kligman L. The hairless mouse model for photoaging. Clin Dermatol. 1996;14:183–95.
9. Berger H, Tsambaos D, Mahrle G. Experimental elastosis induced by chronic ultraviolet expotal elastosis induced by chronic ultraviolet exposure. Arch Dermatol Res. 1980;269:39–49.
10. Johnston KH, Oikarinen AI, Lowe NJ, Clark JG, Uitto J. Ultraviolet radiation-induced connective tissue changes in the skin of hairless mice. J Invest Dermatol. 1984;82:587–90.
11. Hirose R, Kligman LH. An ultrastructural study of ultraviolet-induced elastic fiber damage in hairless mouse skin. J Invest Dermat. 1988;90:697–702.
12. Fujimura T, Moriwaki S, Takema Y, Imokawa G. Epidermal change can alter mechanical properties of hairless mouse skin topically treated with 1α, 25 – dihydroxyvitamin D_3. J Dermatol Sci. 2000;24:105–11.
13. Bisset DL, Hannon D, Orr TV. An animal model of solar-aged skin: histological, physical, and visible changes in UV-irradiated hairless mouse skin. Photochem Photobiol. 1987;46:367–78.
14. Birkedal-Hansen H, et al. Matrix Metalloproteinases: a review. Crit Rev Oral Biol Med. 1993;4(2):197–250.
15. Herrmann G, et al. UVA irradiation stimulates the synthesis of various matrix-metalloproteinases (MMP) in cultured human fibroblasts. Exp Dermatol. 1993;2:92–7.
16. Scharfetter K, Wlaschek M, Hogg A, et al. UVA irradiation induces collagenase in human dermal fibroblasts in vitro and in vivo. Arch Dermatol Res. 1991;283:506–11.
17. Koivukangas V, Kallioinen K, Autio-Harmainen H, Oikarinen AI. UV irradiation induces the expression of gelatinases in human skin in vivo. Acta Derm Venereol. 1994;74:279–82.
18. Son EDL, Shim JH, Choic H. Cathepsin G inhibitor prevents ultraviolet B-induced photoaginig in hairless mice via inhibition of fibronectin fragmentation. Dermatology. 2012;224:352–60.

19. Hwang E, Park S-Y, Lee HJ. Galic acid regulates skin photoaging in UVB-exposed fibroblast and hairless mice. Phytother Res. 2014;28:1778–88.
20. Larroque-Cardoso P, Camare C, Nadal-Wollbold F. Elastin modification by 4-hydroxynonenal in hairless mice exposed to UV-A. Role in photoaging and actinic elastosis. Soc Invest Dermatol. 2015;135:1873–81.
21. Kligman LH, Chen HD, Kligman AM. Topical retinoic acid enhances the repair of ultraviolet damaged dermal connective tissue. Connect Tissue Res. 1984;12:139–50.
22. Park B-S, et al. Adipose-derived stem cells and their secretory factors as a promising therapy for skin aging. Dermatol Surg. 2008;34:1323–6.
23. Morita A. Tobacco smoke causes premature aging. J Dermatol Sci. 2007;48:169–75.
24. Tanaka H, Ono Y, Nakata S, Shintani Y, Sakakibara N, Morita A. Tobacco smoke extract induces premature skin aging in mouse. J Dermatol Sci. 2007;46:69–71.
25. Leow Y-HM, Howard I. Cigarette smoking, cutaneous vasculature and tissue oxygen. Clin Dermatol. 1998;16 (5):579–84.
26. Monfrecola G, Riccio G, Savarese C, Posteraro G, Procaccini EM. The acute effect of smoking on cutaneous microcirculation blood flow in habitual smokers and nonsmokers. Dermatology. 1998;197 (2):115–8.
27. Kimoto-Nira H, Suzuki C, Kobayashi M, Sasaki K, Kurisaki J, Mizumachi K. Anti-ageing effect of a lactococcal strain: analysis using senescence-accelerated mice. Br J Nutr. 2007;98:1178–86.
28. Hosokawa M, Kasai R, Kiguchi K, et al. Grading score system: a method for evaluation of the degree of senescence in senescence accelerated mouse (SAM). Mech Ageing Dev. 1984;26:91–102.
29. Sakuraoka K, Tajima S, Seyama Y, Teramoto K, Ishibashi M. Analysis of connective tissue macromolecular components in Ishibashi rat skin: Role of collagen and elastin in cutaneous aging. J Dermatol Sci. 1996;12:232–7.
30. Prockop DJ, Udenfriend S. A specific method for the analysis of hydroxyproline in tissue and urine. Anal Biochem. 1960;1:228–39.
31. Kimura T, Doi K. Depigmentation and rejuvenation effects of kinetin on the aged skin of hairless descendants of Mexican hairless dogs. Rejuvenation Res. 2004;7(1):32–9.
32. Nabeshima Y-i. Klotho: a fundamental regulator of aging. Ageing Res Rev. 2002;1:627–38.
33. Lanske B, Razzaque MS. Premature aging in klotho mutant mice: cause or consequence? Ageing Res Rev. 2007;6:73–9.
34. Yamashit K, Yotsuyanagi T, Yamauchi M. Klotho mice: a novel woulnd model of aged skin. Plast Reconstr Surger Glob Open. 2014;2, e101.

New Insights in Photoaging Process Revealed by In Vitro Reconstructed Skin Models

102

Claire Marionnet, Christine Duval, and Françoise Bernerd

Contents

C. Marionnet (✉) • C. Duval • F. Bernerd
L'Oreal Research and Innovation, Aulnay-sous-bois, France
e-mail: cmarionnet@rd.loreal.com; cduval@rd.loreal.com; fbernerd@rd.loreal.com

M.A. Farage et al. (eds.), *Textbook of Aging Skin*, DOI 10.1007/978-3-662-47398-6_163

Abstract

Photoaging, clinically characterized by wrinkles, sagging, and age spots, mostly results from chronic impacts of solar ultraviolet (UV) rays affecting the whole skin, from surface to deep dermis. Three-dimensional (3-D) organotypic skin models represent useful in vitro tools to better understand the early UV-induced biological events. Such systems not only allow to reproduce in vitro well-known biomarkers for sunburn reaction but also to identify new key biological alterations induced by UVA exposure and involved in dermal photoaging process. Based upon new scientific proofs of the harmful role of chronic suberythemal UV exposures, the effects of exposures to nonextreme daily UV spectrum, mimicking more realistic everyday life conditions, have revealed a true biological impact upon skin with a strong oxidative stress and a major contribution of UVA rays. More recent data have demonstrated the damaging effects of long UVA wavelengths (UVA1), although less energetic than UVB or UVA2. UVA1 exposure could actually induce the production of reactive oxygen species (ROS) and DNA lesions but also impair several major biological functions and pathways in both epidermis and dermis. These data are in line with recent in vivo data, altogether strongly supporting the need for an adequate UVA1 photoprotection. Finally, the development of a full-thickness pigmented skin model allows to prove the role of dermal fibroblasts on the pigmentary function, showing that the photoaging of dermal fibroblasts can stimulate skin pigmentation. A link between photoaging-induced dermal alterations and pigmentary changes could then be established thanks to an appropriate in vitro skin model.

Introduction

Characteristics of Photoaging

Skin represents the main organ of our body to ensure the protective function against solar UV exposures. This role is played in a coordinate manner by the two compartments, epidermis and dermis. Epidermis represents the first line of defense of the skin, and the underlying dermal compartment, mostly composed of ECM (extracellular matrix) proteins synthesized by dermal fibroblasts, provides a mechanical and thermal protective layer and is absolutely required for providing nutriments to all skin cells. The integrity of the whole skin structure is therefore a key element for maintaining its homeostasis and normal functions.

Exposure to environmental aggressions is one of the major factors involved in skin aging process. Acute and chronic sun exposures have been shown to highly contribute to the development and exaggeration of clinical signs of aging. The resulting effect of such chronic photodamage, called photoaging, leads to an apparent or perceived age often above the chronological age [1]. Convincing data have been recently published from comparative studies in cohorts of twins or hemifacial dermatoheliosis cases [2, 3]. The most frequent clinical signs related to photoaging process are formation of coarse wrinkles often associated with a leathery appearance of the skin, rough skin, telangiectasia, and various pigmentary disorders such as mottled pigmentation, dyschromia, loss of skin tone, and the development of pigmented spots, the most frequent being actinic lentigines also called age spots [4]. Chronic UV exposures could also lead to the development of precancerous lesions, actinic keratosis, as well as basal or squamous cell carcinomas that are also considered as signs of photoaging.

At the histological level, similarly to what could be observed in intrinsic aging, severe photoaged epidermis appeared thinner with a flattening of the dermal-epidermal junction (DEJ). Apart from mutagenic events resulting from UV-induced DNA lesions, very little is known about photoaging of the epidermis. Some abnormalities have been found in keratinocyte differentiation process, with a decrease in the normal cornified envelope formation and a significant impairment of the water-binding capacity of the stratum corneum (SC) [5]. The loss of epidermal rete ridges is also associated with abnormal basement membrane and extensive reduplication of lamina densa [6]. However, the most characteristic features of photoaged skin are predominantly observed within dermis with major changes in the composition and organization of ECM. Total collagen content is decreased together with alterations of the biochemical properties of collagen proteins such as solubility or the production of advanced glycation end products [7, 8]. Fragmentation of the dermal ECM has been associated with the decrease in skin mechanical properties and the progressive formation of a permissive environment toward wrinkle formation and tumor development. The amount of sulfated glycosaminoglycans (GAGs) is increased, but some proteoglycans associated with collagen fibers such as decorin appear decreased [9]. However, the major histological trait of photoaged skin is the accumulation of material with the staining characteristics of elastin, called solar elastosis, that corresponds to an accumulation in the mid-dermis of elastotic material composed of abnormal elastic fibers, fibronectin, and other extracellular matrix proteins or proteoglycans, such as versican [9, 10]. The accumulation of sun-induced elastotic material has been linked to the loss of elasticity and the leathery appearance of skin.

From a molecular point of view, several teams have demonstrated a change in ECM synthesis and degradation, with a decrease in collagen gene expression and synthesis [11] and an increase in the production of matrix-degrading enzymes such as various matrix metalloproteinases (MMPs) [12, 13]. MMPs increase and activation can be triggered directly by UV exposure through stimulation of AP1 or NFkB transcription factors [14], induction of mitochondrial DNA deletion [13], but also indirectly by various soluble factors including cytokines produced by skin cells including dermal fibroblasts [15]. Elastotic material was also found to be more resistant to elastases due to lysozyme deposition leading to its progressive accumulation [16]. Increased activity of matrix-degrading enzymes can also be attributed to many other cell types than dermal fibroblasts, e.g., mast cells, endothelial cells, and infiltrating inflammatory cells. Analysis of photoaged skin has shown the presence of perivascular and perifollicular histiocytic–lymphocytic infiltrates including high numbers of mast cells, macrophages, T cells, especially in elastosis areas, leading to the appearance of chronic inflammation [17]. UV exposure is also responsible for decorin degradation by neutrophil elastase leading collagen fibers more susceptible to MMPs [18].

Considering pigmentary disorders, actinic (senilis) lentigines are the most undisputed lesions associated with chronic solar exposure [4]. However, although very frequent, their pathogenesis remains unclear. Morphological alterations have been identified with various degrees of cutaneous alterations, such as frequent elongations of epidermal rete ridges associated with an accumulation of melanin mostly in the basal layer of the epidermis [19, 20]. Change in the melanocyte number, which has been reported either increased [19] or unchanged [21], still remains inconclusive. Chen et al., suggested a role of Keratinocyte Growth Factor (KGF) in the molecular pathology of actinic lentigos, as a result of chronic UV-induced signaling cascade [22]. It has been proposed that loss of heparan sulfate at the DEJ of lentigo could enhance the transfer of this factor from the dermis to melanocytes, hence promoting melanogenesis [23].

UV Radiation Exposures and Photoaging

Among environmental factors involved in photoaging, solar ultraviolet (UV) exposures are paramount. Solar UV rays that reach the Earth's surface are a combination of UVB (290–320 nm) and UVA (320–400 nm). The latter comprise shortwave range UVA2 (320–340 nm) and longwave range UVA1 (340–400 nm). UVB rays have beneficial effects with vitamin D production but due to their high energy can directly damage the DNA of epidermal cells, provoke the sunburn reaction, and, in the long term, largely contribute to UV-induced carcinogenesis. Although UVB wavelengths have poor penetrating capacity, mostly targeting epidermal cells, they have been shown to contribute to dermal alterations observed during photoaging through the activation of MMPs [12]. UVB rays are also involved in the release of several proinflammatory cytokines able to activate MMPs via a paracrine mechanism [24, 25]. On the other hand, UVA photons are, in average, 1000 times less energetic than UVB photons but penetrate much deeper into skin, reaching deep dermis. The major mode of action of UVA rays relates to the production of reactive oxygen species (ROS) and subsequent activation of various signaling pathways [26]. ROS, leading to oxidative stress are well-known activators of inflammatory responses and matrix remodeling processes, evidencing their involvement in skin photoaging. The contribution of UVA to dermal alterations and solar elastosis has been supported both at the biological and clinical levels [3, 27].

Sun exposure conditions can vary according to geo-orbital and environmental factors including latitude, season, and hour of the day or to environmental factors such as clouds, thickness of the ozone layer, or aerial pollutants. This results in changes in UVA/UVB ratio due to the differences in penetration properties of UVB and UVA wavelengths [28, 29], UVAs being less affected by these factors, as compared to UVBs [30, 31]. It is now admitted that beyond acute erythemal sun exposure often associated with a sunburn reaction, the chronic exposure to low doses of UV are even more effective at inducing biological responses [32]. This implies that photoaging process takes place progressively – and silently – in everyday life and outdoor activities even when unaware of and not alerted to the level of daily UV exposure we may face [33].

Reconstructed Skin Models as Tools for Studying Photoaging

As previously mentioned, both acute and chronic UV exposures lead to damage in the whole skin, affecting both epidermis and dermis. The knowledge of early events occurring post UV exposure is crucial for a better understanding of events responsible for photoaging process. In vivo studies in human volunteers are often difficult to set up for practical and ethical reasons. In contrast, in vitro classical two-dimensional (2-D) skin cell cultures poorly reproduce physiological conditions and tissue organization, such as a correct epidermal differentiation, cell-cell, and cell-matrix interactions. In vitro three-dimensional (3-D) engineered skin models have therefore been developed in the last 30 years to come much closer to cutaneous physiology and organization [34]. In addition, the 3-D architecture of organotypic models allow to take into account penetration properties of UV wavelengths, a major parameter regarding responses to UV exposure.

Although some studies have been performed using reconstructed epidermis only, it appears that the most appropriate 3-D skin models for characterizing UV-induced skin damage comprise both epidermis and dermis leading to a fully differentiated epidermis cultured on a fibroblast-populated dermal equivalent.

UVB or UVA-induced damage can then be studied in reconstructed skin models to determine the nature and location of specific impacts of each wavelength range. Combination of UVB and UVA can also be used to simulate more realistic solar exposure. The main biological effects identified after such UV exposure conditions in 3-D skin models are summarized in Fig. 1 and further detailed.

UVB Exposure of Reconstructed Skin Allows to Reproduce Epidermal Sunburn-Related Biomarkers and to Identify an Indirect Contribution to Dermal Alterations

The UVB part of the solar spectrum does not penetrate skin in depth, but, due to its high energy, it does contribute to significant acute sun damage, clinically revealed by the sunburn reaction. It was therefore of interest to verify that the corresponding biomarkers could be induced in the in vitro 3-D skin models.

Following UVB exposure of reconstructed human skin, major epidermal changes were observed, similar to those observed in human

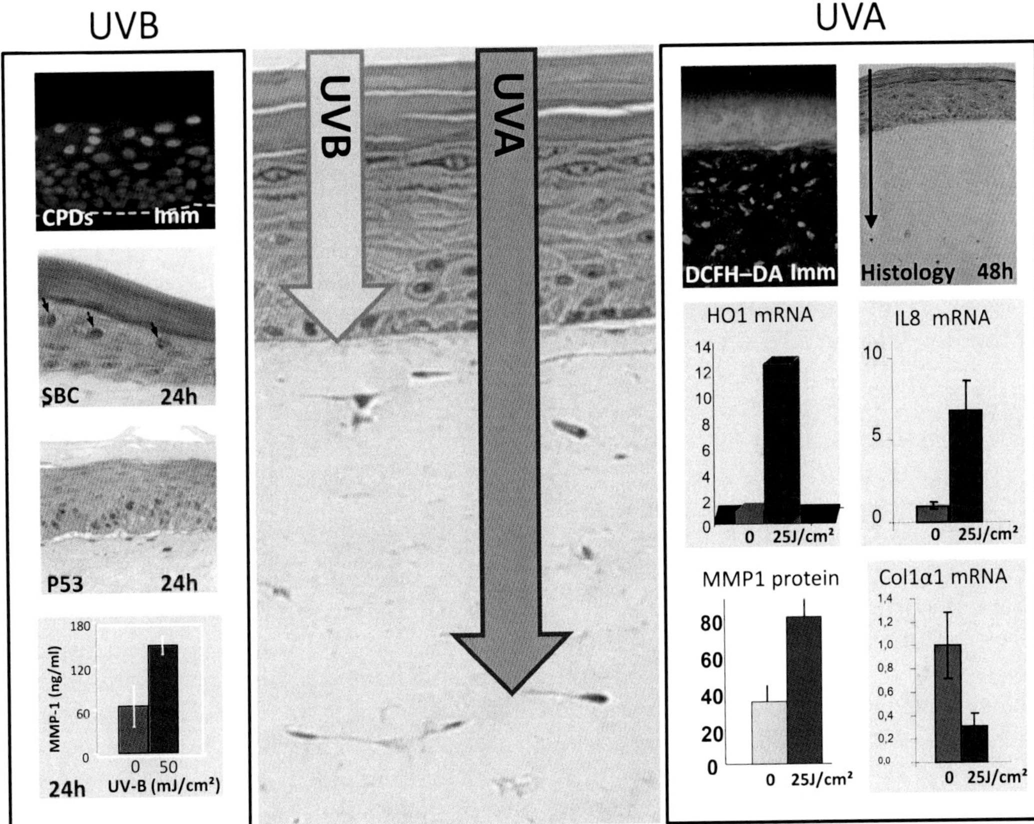

Fig. 1 Major biological damage induced by UVB or UVA in reconstructed skin model. UVB-induced effects are mostly related to sunburn reaction (*CPDs* cyclobutane pyrimidine dimers, *SBC* sunburn cells, p53 protein accumulation, MMP1 secretion). UVA-induced effects are characterized by ROS generation (DCFH-DA probe), alterations within the dermal compartment (disappearance of superficial fibroblasts, histology), and modulation of well-known biomarkers of photoaging process (up-regulation of HO1, IL8 gene expression, MMP1 secretion, and down-regulation of COL1A1 gene expression)

skin, in vivo. Several events representing the biological signature of a moderate sunburn reaction can be detected in reconstructed skin after UVB exposure, such as DNA damage formation, p53 accumulation, sunburn cells (SBC), and apoptotic features.

The direct absorption of UVB photons by DNA leads to DNA lesions such as pyrimidine dimers that could be evidenced immediately following UVB exposure in epidermal keratinocytes of reconstructed skin and persisted 24 h later in the nuclei of keratinocytes of epidermal upper suprabasal and granular layers. These lesions were completely removed within the next few days by the nucleotide excision repair mechanism [35]. Twenty four hours post UVB exposure, a direct consequence of such DNA lesions is the formation of SBC with typical histological features (round shape, loss of connection with surrounding keratinocytes, condensed pycnotic nucleus, eosinophilic cytoplasm, and suprabasal location), representing the biological hallmarks of a sunburn reaction. Colocated with SBC, apoptotic keratinocytes could be detected mostly in the deeper epidermal layers as revealed by the TUNEL reaction, while actors or markers of apoptotic pathways had their expression altered by UVB exposure, such as p53 protein that accumulated and BCl2 with a decreased level or cleavage of Caspase 3 [36–39].

In addition to the multiple direct effects of UVB on human epidermis, dermal compartment can also be impacted via indirect mechanisms: following UVB exposure of reconstructed skin, keratinocytes release diffusible IL1 and IL6 cytokines, leading to an increase in matrix metalloproteinase 1 (MMP-1) protein expression in fibroblasts [24, 25].

A Major Impact of UVA Exposure is Induced in the Deeper Layers of the Reconstructed Skin

In contrast to UVBs, major histological features of UVA effects were located in the dermal compartment of reconstructed skin in vitro, in correlation with previous human in vivo studies showing that repetitive exposures to low UVA doses induced early morphological and biochemical alterations in the dermis [40, 41]. Forty-eight hours post UVA exposure of reconstructed skin, the dermal fibroblasts located in the superficial part of the dermal equivalent disappeared, underlining the significant biological impact of UVA upon deeper layers of skin. The cytotoxicity of UVA toward fibroblasts was shown straight and mostly due to apoptosis [42]. This particular impact upon dermis was emphasized by the upregulation of several MMP gene and protein expressions (e.g., MMP-1, MMP-9, MMP-3) [43]. In contrast to UVB exposure, UVA exposure directly induces the production of MMP-1 by fibroblasts, since the removal of epidermis immediately after UVA exposure did not alter this effect [38]. The expression of COL1A1 gene was downregulated in fibroblasts of reconstructed skin exposed to UVA rays [44]. The epidermal structure and organization were, to a lesser extent, impacted by exposure to UVA, with a slight impact upon the upper layers and parakeratosis [42].

The analysis of earlier events occurring after such UVA exposure in reconstructed human skin showed that, as observed in vivo, the immediate damage following UVA exposure was the generation of reactive oxygen species (ROS) in both fibroblasts and keratinocytes, leading to oxidative stress [38]. In addition to ROS generation, UVA exposure leads to DNA damage, especially pyrimidine dimers albeit in a much lower amount than post UVB exposure, and 8-oxo-7,8-dihydro-2′-deoxyguanosine (8-OHdG) accumulating in basal keratinocytes [45, 46]. Moreover, repeated UVA exposures can lead to p53 mutations in reconstructed skin [47] suggesting that UVA may have a role in photocarcinogenesis but also favor the formation of p53 mutated keratinocyte patches that are observed in chronically sun-exposed skin [48].

Altogether these results illustrate the penetration properties of UVA rays as shown by the direct UVA-induced biological damage in dermis and the particular vulnerability to UVA rays of the deepest epidermal layer, where epidermal stem cells, proliferative keratinocytes, and melanocytes reside [31]. The particular impact of UVA on the dermal compartment observed in vivo and in 3-D models in vitro may be involved in early events occurring during photoaging leading to drastic alterations of dermal structure and formation of solar elastosis [10]. Analysis of the repair process occurring after UVA-induced fibroblast alterations revealed that a progressive repair process occurred within the next two weeks, with a recolonization of the dermal equivalent by activated fibroblasts located in the deeper part of dermis [42]. These fibroblasts display an activated phenotype during the regeneration phase with a high synthesis activity of several ECM proteins, such as fibronectin. The thickness of the dermal equivalent was also found reduced at the end of the process. This phenomenon has to be considered with regard to in vivo solar elastosis formation and accumulation of several ECM proteins in the mid-dermis [10]. This sequence of events is very similar to the model of pathophysiology of dermal photoaging described by J Voorhees and G Fisher assimilated to a "solar scar" resulting from repetitive dermal degradation and abnormal repair events [49].

Effects of Exposures to Solar Simulated UV

To study the effects of combined UVB-UVA radiation using solar simulation, the "UV-solar simulated radiation" (UV-SSR) irradiance spectrum has been widely used (Fig. 2). This spectrum

Exposure type	Extreme – zenithal	Non extreme – non zenithal
Real life situations	Sun bathing Summer global sunlight Clear sky Zenithal sun, around noon	Every day life; outdoors activities Latitudes 60S-60N All the year SEA <45, morning and evening sun Spring-Autumn daylight
Ratio UVA/UVB	UVA/UVB <18	UVA/UVB = 27
Induction of erythema in real life conditions	YES	NO
Simulated spectrum	Solar Simulated Radiation (UV-SSR)	Daily UV Radiation (DUVR)

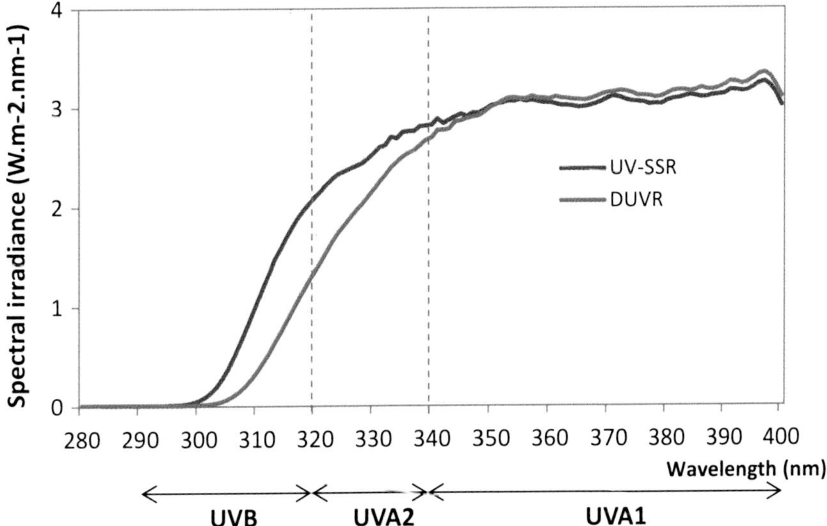

Fig. 2 Characteristics and spectra of UV-SSR and DUVR exposure conditions. SEA, solar elevation angle, in degrees

including UVA and UVB wavelengths reproduces summer zenithal sunlight, with a UVA/UVB ratio close to 10. Corresponding exposure conditions occur in summer, around noon, at low latitudes, under clear sky, and represent the "worst-case scenario" for the human skin. Such type of exposure condition can lead to erythema, predominantly induced by the high UVB erythemogenic spectral part [50, 51].

Consequences of UV-SSR exposure on reconstructed skin closely resemble those observed after UVB exposure. UV-SSR exposure leads to DNA damage in keratinocytes of reconstructed skin, such as pyrimidine dimers and (6–4) photoproducts [52, 53]. This is followed by an accumulation of p53 and upregulation of genes involved in DNA repair and in cell cycle regulation, under p53 control.

Histological changes induced by UV-SSR exposure of reconstructed skin were mostly observed in epidermis, similar to those observed in vivo, with the induction of epidermal SBC formation. In addition to these epidermal direct effects, UV-SSR exposure of reconstructed human skin leads to the increased production of MMP-1 by fibroblasts [53, 25].

Since photoaging process seems to be more associated with chronic sun exposures, experiments were also performed following repeated exposures to lower UV doses that do not induce the formation of sunburn biomarkers. In such conditions, major alterations were observed in the dermal compartment with alterations of fibroblasts. These results strongly suggest that, in nonerythemal conditions, the UVA part of solar UV spectrum does induce harmful dermal effects. These results are in agreement with in vivo data showing that many biological and clinical effects could be induced by suberythemal doses of UV [32].

New Insights into Daily UV Exposure Effects to Mimic More Realistic Everyday Life Conditions

As stressed in the previous parts, photoaging process is not fully correlated with intense sun exposures that only concern a very limited part of the world population in everyday life. However, the wide majority of photobiology studies used UV-SSR spectrum (UVA/UVB ratio around 10) that mimics a summer zenithal sun exposure, i.e., sunbathing on a beach in summer under a clear sky, that may rapidly lead to erythema in human skin in vivo.

Daily UV Radiation Spectrum

Therefore a new UV spectrum called "daily UV radiation" spectrum (DUVR) has been defined (Fig. 2). It simulates "nonextreme" conditions of sun exposure corresponding to a western spring or autumn sunlight, with a solar elevation angle lower than 45°, which does not give rise to any visible immediate clinical damage. Such types of exposure conditions exhibit a UVA/UVB ratio around 27, corresponding to 96.5 % UVA and 3.5 % UVB, a twofold higher ratio than that found in zenithal conditions of exposure. Consequently, DUVR spectrum exhibits a UVA/UVB irradiance ratio comprised between 23 and 32 [54].

In parallel with in vivo studies, in vitro studies have been performed using a 3-D reconstructed human skin model composed of a dermal equivalent including living adult fibroblasts recovered by a fully differentiated epidermis, for characterizing the cellular and molecular impacts and the early events induced by "nonextreme" exposure conditions [55].

Histological Changes Induced by DUVR

First, histological analysis of the reconstructed skin model exposed to increasing doses of DUVR have been performed to establish the DUVR biological efficient dose (BED), previously defined as the minimal dose able to induce morphological alterations following acute UV exposure [37, 42]. The determined DUVR BED was 13 J/cm^2 and corresponded to a realistic dose since representing 20 % of the daily dose of UV received in Paris in mid-April. Moreover, it correlates with human in vivo average minimal erythema dose (MED) of 12 J/cm^2 DUVR for skin phototypes II and III [56].

Following exposure of reconstructed skin to this BED of DUVR, alterations were mostly located in the dermal compartment and were characterized by the disappearance of fibroblasts. Such changes have also been observed following exposure to UVA alone. In addition, some alterations were detected within epidermis such as slight alterations in the granular layer similar to those observed following UVA exposure and epidermis thinning together with a thickening of the cornified layer. Moreover only a few SBC and p53 positive keratinocytes could be detected. The histological damage induced by DUVR was accompanied by the release of MMP-1 in the culture medium [57].

DUVR Generates Oxidative Stress

Immediately post DUVR exposure, ROS were detected in both basal keratinocytes and fibroblasts of the reconstructed skin, in a dose-dependent manner. A dose as low as 7 J/cm^2 DUVR that neither led to any detectable histological changes nor induction of any sunburn-related biomarkers was sufficient to generate ROS, even within deep dermis, reflecting the high penetration properties of UVA wavelengths included in high proportion in the DUVR spectrum [57].

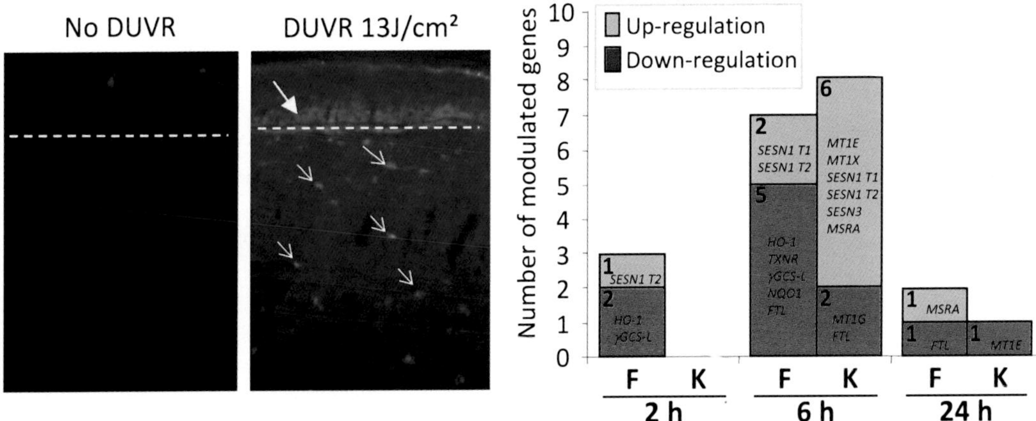

Fig. 3 DUVR- induced oxidative stress in reconstructed skin. (**a**) Generation of reactive oxygen species (*ROS*) immediately after exposure to DUVR in keratinocytes and fibroblasts, followed by (**b**) modulation of numerous genes involved in oxidative stress response in fibroblasts (*F*) and keratinocytes (*K*), at 2, 6 and 24 h after exposure of reconstructed skin to 13 J/cm^2 DUVR

Since DUVR induced immediate ROS formation, cell responses to oxidative stress induced by physiological doses of DUVR were carefully studied in the reconstructed human skin model. The expression of 24 genes encoding proteins involved in oxidative stress response was studied in both fibroblasts and keratinocytes of reconstructed skin exposed to DUVR [57] (Fig. 3). The expression of four gene families was particularly altered by DUVR, i.e., the cytoprotective to oxidative and electrophilic stress NF-E2-related factor 2 (Nrf2) pathway, sestrins that participate in the regeneration of overoxidized peroxiredoxins, metallothioneins that scavenge ROS and metal ions, and methionine sulfoxide reductase (MSRA), a protein involved in the maintenance of protein structure and function. In addition, fibroblasts and keratinocytes showed a differential response to oxidative stress. For instance, in fibroblasts, oxidative stress response occurred as early as 2 h post exposure, with a majority of upregulated gene expressions, whereas in keratinocytes gene modulations were mostly detected 6 h post DUVR exposure, with a higher proportion of downregulations (Fig. 3). Different genes were modulated in fibroblasts as compared to keratinocytes: Nrf2 target genes were significantly upregulated in dermal fibroblasts by DUVR, while in keratinocytes, only NQO1 gene expression was significantly induced. Genes encoding metallothioneins were also differently modulated in fibroblasts versus keratinocytes, with a downregulation by DUVR of MT1X, MT1E, and MTE2A found only in keratinocytes. For other genes or gene families, such as sestrins and MSRA, gene modulation induced by DUVR was quite similar between fibroblasts and keratinocytes [57]. The discrepancy of response to oxidative stress between keratinocytes and fibroblasts can be explained by differences in basal antioxidant defense equipment [58] and can also be attributed to wavelength penetration, considering that only UVA can reach dermal fibroblasts.

DUVR Alters Gene Expression, Impacting Diverse Functional Families

Gene expression alteration by DUVR was not restricted to genes involved in response to oxidative stress. The expression of more than 200 genes related to skin biology and stress response in fibroblasts and keratinocytes of reconstructed skin exposed to DUVR was studied, showing that, in both cell types, DUVR induced modulation of expression of numerous genes related to diverse functional families. Again, the low dose of 7 J/cm^2 DUVR that did not lead to any detectable histological changes was sufficient to modulate gene expression.

Response to stress, with the DUVR-induced expression of genes encoding heat shock proteins (HSP), was a particularly enriched pathway following DUVR exposure. UV-induction of HSP has already been described and is considered to be part of a natural defense mechanism against UV exposure, and some of them such as HSP70, play a particular role in photoaging [59].

In addition, in the epidermis, DUVR affects the expression of keratinocyte markers involved in the differentiation/proliferation balance, such as numerous members of the epidermal differentiation complex (e.g., filaggrin, loricrin, involucrin, SPPR genes, etc.) and other markers of differentiation (CDSN, calmodulin-like 5, TGM1, stratifin, serpinB2). DUVR also alters the expression of markers related to epidermal proliferation and markers expressed in basal keratinocytes (K5, K6B, Ki67, and ODC1) [60]. These modulations could be linked to in vivo skin surface alterations observed following DUVR exposure such as perturbations in skin hydration and microtopography, as well as epidermal proliferation and thickening [56].

In line with in vivo data underlying the role of low DUVR doses in the development of photoaging clinical signs [56], DUVR exposure affects the expression of genes encoding components of ECM and DEJ as well as genes encoding proteins involved in ECM maturation and remodeling. The expression of collagens and fibronectin was downregulated, while the expression of remodeling genes MMP1, MMP3, and members of the plasminogen activator system serpin1, serpinB2, and plasminogen activator tissue PLAT was upregulated [60].

DUVR exposure also altered the expression of genes encoding growth factors, receptors, and hormones. For example, the expression of Heparin-Binding EGF-like Growth Factor (HBEGF), Growth Differentiation Factor 15 (GDF15), Transforming Growth Factor alpha (TGFA), granulocyte/macrophage colony-stimulating factor (GMCSF/CSF2), and Fibroblast Growth Factor 7 (FGF7/KGF) was strongly upregulated [60]. Interestingly, FGF7/KGF and CSF2 proteins were shown to be positive regulators of skin pigmentation.

Skin immunity-related markers were also impacted by DUVR exposure: genes encoding cytokines and inflammation markers such as interleukins and chemokines (e.g., IL6, IL8, ICAM1, CSF2, TNF, PTGS2/COX2) were strongly upregulated. In contrast, DUVR downregulated the expression of genes encoding members of innate immunity such as TLR1, TLR3, or TNFSF10. This data reinforced the fact that daily and moderate UV exposure may be involved in the UV-induced immunological response of skin [61].

Biological Contribution of UVA Wavelengths in Cell Response to DUVR

Since i/ DUVR induces immediate ROS formation, ii/ DUVR spectrum includes a high and constant proportion of UVA wavelengths, well-known stimulators of ROS production, and iii/ histological changes induced by DUVR closely resemble those induced by UVA, the molecular biological contribution of the UVA wavelengths included in the DUVR spectrum was investigated. Accordingly, gene expression profiles were performed in reconstructed skins exposed either to UVA alone or to DUVR. Comparisons of modulated genes between both types of exposure strikingly revealed the massive biological contribution of the UVA part included in DUVR spectrum, especially for dermal fibroblasts, located deeper in skin. Indeed, among genes found modulated in fibroblasts, 92 % were common to DUVR and UVA. In keratinocytes, the vast majority (80 %) of the modulated genes were also identical in DUVR or UVA exposure conditions. These results showed that both types of exposures share in common many biological targets [62] (Fig. 4).

In keratinocytes, 20 % of genes were specifically modulated by DUVR and not by UVA, suggesting that the modulation of these genes is imputable to UVB wavelengths comprised within

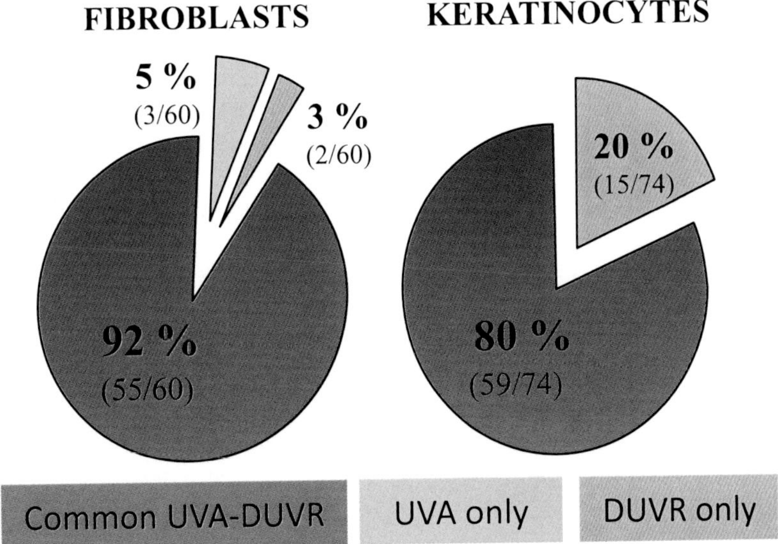

Fig. 4 Number of modulated genes in fibroblasts and keratinocytes exposed to DUVR or to UVA. In fibroblasts, among the 225 studied genes, UVA (25 J/cm^2) and DUVR (13 J/cm^2) exposures modulated the expression of 60. In keratinocytes, among the 241 studied genes, UVA and DUVR exposures modulated the expression of 74. Some genes were modulated by both DUVR and UVA (*red portion*), some were modulated post UVA but not DUVR exposure (*yellow portion*), others were modulated post DUVR but not UVA exposure (*grey portion*)

the DUVR spectrum. Due to their upper location, keratinocytes are exposed to photons of the whole DUVR spectrum (UVB + UVA), while in contrast, fibroblasts, in dermis, are mostly exposed to UVA wavelengths of the DUVR spectrum, leading to only 3 % of modulated genes specific to DUVR exposure [62].

Altogether, these results revealed the insidious impact of "nonextreme" daily exposure to solar UV, at various skin depths, the dermal compartment being highly susceptible to such type of exposure. Most of the DUVR alterations, like histological changes and gene expression modulations, could be attributable to the highly prevailing UVA part in the DUVR spectrum.

The Biological Contribution of UVA1: More Important and Detrimental Than Previously Thought

UVA rays (320–400 nm), highly represented in daily UV radiation spectrum, were greatly responsible for DUVR effects in reconstructed human skin. Within the UVA part, long-wave UVA1 rays (340–400 nm) can make up to 80 % of DUVR. Due to their lowest energy among UV photons, little attention has been paid, until recently, upon their precise biological contribution.

From a physical point of view, UVA1 not only exhibit high skin penetration properties but are less impacted than UVB or UVA2 by geo-orbital and environmental parameters such as latitude, time of the year, hour of the day, meteorological conditions, and ozone layer thickness. With increasing latitudes, the intensity of UVA1 rays exhibits low variation: in more temperate latitudes, UVA1 irradiance is less affected by seasons, with a more uniform irradiance throughout the year. Moreover, UVA1 are not blocked by glass or cloudy sky [31].

From a biological point of view, due to their low energy, the contribution of UVA1 to skin damage has long been neglected. However, a recent growing body of information showed harmful impact of UVA1 [31]. In vivo studies demonstrated UVA1 contribution to photoaging, carcinogenesis, and photoimmunosuppression [63–65].

In order to deepen the knowledge on the biological impact of UVA1, their tissue, cellular, and molecular effects were investigated using an in vitro reconstructed skin model.

Early Skin Damage Induced by UVA1 and Subsequent Morphological Alterations

Immediately after UVA1 exposure, ROS were detected in deeper skin layers, especially in basal keratinocytes and dermal fibroblasts even at the very low dose of 10 J/cm^2 UVA1. A UVA1 dose response (10–40 J/cm^2) showed a progressive higher amount of ROS but also an increase in the depth of their detection up to 400 μm at 40 J/cm^2, in relation to the ability of such wavelengths to target the deep dermis. The UVA1-induced ROS production was followed 24 h later by lipid peroxidation in reconstructed skin, as revealed by the increase in arachidonic acid derivative, 8-isoprostane, in culture medium. Meanwhile, UVA1 also induced thymine dimers specifically located in the nuclei of basal keratinocytes [66]. These DNA lesions were also found in vivo post UVA1 exposure and reflect the potential role of such wavelengths in photocarcinogenesis [67]. These events were induced at physiological doses, since the highest dose of 40 J/cm^2 can be attained in a few hours (e.g., in about 2 h in Hawaï). Within the 2 days following such immediate oxidative stress injury and DNA damage, morphological alterations could be detected especially in the dermal compartment, with induction of superficial fibroblast apoptosis leading to their disappearance at 48 h. The epidermis was impacted to a much lesser extent by UVA1 exposure, with alterations of granular layers and occasionnal parakeratosis [66].

A Wide Panel of Genes Have Their Expression Altered Following Exposure to UVA1

To go deeper into the description of UVA1 impact, especially at molecular level, and to describe an overall view of molecular early events occurring following UVA1 exposure, without any a priori, a transcriptomic study was performed. It aimed at analyzing the level of expression of every known human gene, using a whole transcript Affymetrix array, in keratinocytes and fibroblasts of reconstructed skin exposed to 40 J/cm^2 UVA1 [66].

Hierarchical clustering of whole gene expression data revealed a UVA1 gene expression signature, implying that UVA1 exposure leads to a true biological impact in both skin compartments. The number of modulated genes was similar in dermal fibroblasts (461 probe sets) and in epidermal keratinocytes (502 probe sets), strongly supporting the fact that the intensity of the stress is comparable from the surface to the deeper part of the skin. However, although similar in quantity, the nature of modulated genes differed between fibroblasts and keratinocytes. In addition, UVA1 induced more downregulations than upregulations in fibroblasts, while in keratinocytes an opposite trend was found.

Analysis of distribution of UVA1 modulated genes in functional families and pathways using Gene Ontology, KEGG, and a detailed bibliographic study focusing on skin biology revealed the wide panel of functions impacted by UVA1 exposure (Fig. 5).

Although fibroblasts and keratinocytes showed different gene modulation profiles after UVA1, both cell types shared similar altered functions. Gene ontology analysis revealed that the most enriched functional families following UVA1 exposure were related to response to stimulus, signaling, and cell communication, attesting that UVA1 exposure was a true stress for both cell types of reconstructed skin. Particularly, skin cells exhibited a defense response to oxidative stress, with the upregulation of the expression of Nrf2 pathway genes and the strong upregulation of the expression of genes encoding heat shock proteins, especially in fibroblasts of reconstructed skin.

The detailed bibliographic study revealed that, apart from response to stress, two major functional families were altered by UVA1 exposure. Genes related to cellular homeostasis including development, proliferation, apoptosis, and cancer represent about one quarter of the modulated genes. For instance, numerous oncogenes had an increased gene expression such as FOS, FOSB,

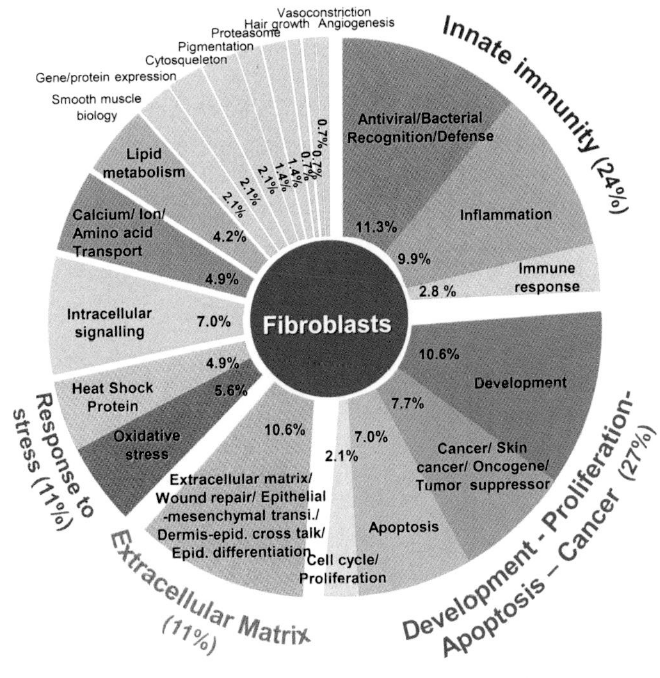

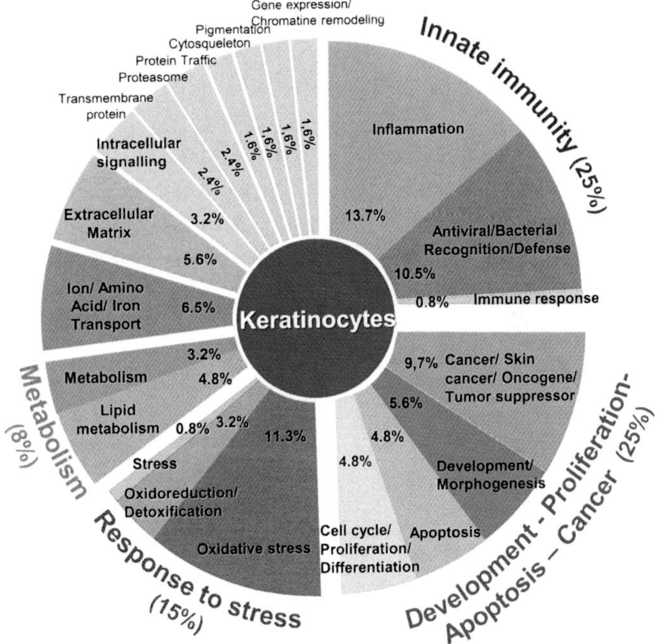

Fig. 5 UVA1- modulated expression of genes related to various functional families. The most UVA1-modulated genes (fold change >2 for up-regulation or <0.5 for downregulation and adjusted p value < 0.001), in fibroblasts and keratinocytes of reconstructed skin, were distributed in functional families by performing an extensive bibliographic study that included skin and dermatology literature [66]

JUN whereas two tumor suppressors (FETB, RARRES1) were downregulated. Most of these genes had been shown to be modulated by UV, and we showed that UVA1 per se modulate these markers [66].

Another quarter of modulated genes in both cell types were genes involved in innate immunity (Fig. 5), with a strong upregulation of proinflammatory markers. As said in the introduction, the inflammatory environment is a key feature of photoaging, and these data confirmed that the UVA1 part of the solar spectrum may actively contribute to it. Meanwhile, a striking downregulation of genes related to antiviral innate immunity, such as numerous interferon inducible genes (SAMD9, IFIT1,2,3, MX1, 2, OAS1, 2, CXCL10, etc.), and genes encoding receptors to double-stranded RNA (TLR3, DDX58) [66]. This UVA1-driven downregulation of antiviral defense gene expression could be correlated with the reactivation of herpes simplex virus observed in humans following UVA1 phototherapy, and more generally after the first solar exposure of summer [68]. In addition to deficiency in antiviral response, this downregulation may have harmful consequences on antitumoral defense since the type I interferon response is also involved in tumor suppression [69]. These results also emphasized and confirmed the essential role of keratinocytes and fibroblasts in the immune function of skin.

In fibroblasts, 11 % of modulated genes were genes encoding extracellular matrix components and actors, such as growth factors (FGF1, FIGF, HGF) that were downregulated and members of the TGF pathway, e.g., BMP2 and GDF15, that were strongly upregulated 6 h post UVA1 exposure. In addition, 24–48 h post UVA1 exposure, MMP genes and expressed proteins (MMP1 and MMP3) were upregulated while COL1A1 gene, encoding one of the major dermal component, was strongly repressed [66]. These early gene modulations reinforced the knowledge on the contribution of UVA1 exposure to the photoaging process and clinical signs such as dermatoheliosis and solar elastosis.

In fibroblasts and in keratinocytes, the transcriptomic study revealed that 4–5 % of the modulated genes were related to lipid metabolism. These results were particularly interesting since recent studies showed that, during photoaging, the process of lipid metabolism was altered and that, in sun-exposed skin, the degradation of triglycerides was increased [70, 71]. In addition to lipid metabolism, glucose metabolism was also impacted after UVA1 exposure, especially in keratinocytes, with modulation of genes involved in regulation of energy production and in the balance glycolysis/gluconeogenesis attesting an alteration in energy production. Again these results appear correlated with a recent in vivo study showing that, in sun-exposed skin, glucose, lactate, and other metabolites are upregulated [71].

In conclusion, early events that occur following exposure to a moderate and physiological dose of UVA1 have been characterized in reconstructed skin. UVA1 can generate oxidative stress and does impact the expression of genes and proteins related to a wide variety of functions, from skin surface (epidermal keratinocytes) to deep dermis (fibroblasts embedded in ECM). Altogether, they evidence that UVA1-induced damage actively contributes to significant alterations of a variety of cutaneous functions that may be linked ultimately to in vivo clinical consequences of chronic UV exposure, such as photoaging, photoimmunosuppression, and skin cancers and plea for an efficient photoprotection against UVA1. These in vitro results may also emphasize the predictivity of such 3-D skin models regarding their clinical relevance since they are in line with in vivo results obtained after experimental UVA1 exposure but also with reported clinical side effects of UVA1 phototherapy.

Pigmented Full-Thickness Reconstructed Skin to Assess the Role of Photoaging in Pigmentation

As previously mentioned, some clinical features of photoaging are closely linked to the pigmentary function of the skin, UV exposure being the major inducer of melanogenesis and pigmentation.

To better understand regulation and dysregulation of skin pigmentation, in vitro systems that reproduce the physiology of the pigmentary system as close as in the native skin are required. Hence, several parameters, from the organization of melanocytes within the epidermis to the interactions with the surrounding environment, have to be taken into account.

Skin pigmentation results from the production of melanin by melanocytes located at the DEJ, the boundary structure between epidermis and dermis. Melanocytes synthesize melanin within specific organelles called melanosomes that are transferred through dendrites to surrounding keratinocytes. The association that involves 1 melanocyte and about 40 keratinocytes receiving and processing its melanin-containing melanosomes is called the epidermal melanin unit (EMU). Following the keratinocyte differentiation program, melanin and melanosomes migrate up to the outermost epidermal layers and are further eliminated by the natural desquamation of corneocytes.

Constitutive pigmentation depends on the amount of melanins, their quality (eu/pheomelanin), the mode of transfer and processing of melanosomes inside the keratinocytes, and not on the number of melanocytes along the basal layer, which is relatively constant in a given skin site, irrespective of the color skin type. In epidermis, the tight contact between melanocytes and keratinocytes is not only essential for melanin transfer but also for intensive cross-talk occurring between these two cell types. These interactions are involved in the control of pigmentation, through the release of paracrine factors and the direct connections mediated by E-cadherin. The contribution of keratinocytes is of particular importance in the UV-induced melanogenesis [72, 73].

In the development of physiological pigmented skin models, a first significant advance was achieved with the successful integration of normal human melanocytes into reconstructed human epidermis which made possible the study of pigmentation in a 3-D epidermal structure. Coseeding normal human melanocytes and keratinocytes onto an inert human dermal support or dead de-epidermized human dermis (DED) gives rise to a stratified, pigmented epidermis reproducing the melanin epidermal unit and thus allowing the natural interaction between melanocytes and keratinocytes [72, 74–76]. The ability of melanocytes to respond to UV radiation resulting in an increased pigmentation was evidenced after UV exposure and corresponds to the so-called tanning observed in vivo. Indeed, repeated UVB exposures lead to increased proliferation, dendricity and activity of melanocytes, increased melanin production, and melanosome transfer from melanocytes to keratinocytes, resulting in a noticeable tanning of the reconstructed epidermis [72, 77, 78]. UVA and UV-SSR also lead to an increased pigmentation in epidermal reconstructs [72, 76].

Development of a Full-Thickness Pigmented Reconstructed Skin

However, besides epidermal keratinocytes, the mesenchymal compartment including fibroblasts and fibroblast-derived ECM proteins is currently recognized to contribute to the regulation of melanocyte homeostasis. Rising from the mid-1990s, first findings showed that ECM proteins modulate melanocyte proliferation, apoptosis resistance, and melanogenic activity [79–81]. More recently, the role of dermal fibroblasts, through the secretion of specific soluble factors, has been increasingly underlined in regulating constitutive pigmentation and development of pigmentary disorders. A major finding was the identification of Dikkopf-1 (DKK-1), a soluble factor, specifically produced by dermal fibroblasts located in palms and soles and thought to be responsible for the very low pigmentation of these anatomical sites via a repressive effect upon melanocyte growth and melanogenesis [82]. Few years later, another factor secreted by fibroblasts from dark skin, neuregulin-1 (NGR-1), has been shown possessing a propigmenting effect potentially involved in highly pigmented skin color type [83]. Other factors such as stem cell factor (SCF), hepatocyte growth factor (HGF), or keratinocyte growth factor (KGF), known for their promelanogenic action, have also been shown to be highly produced in congenital hyperpigmented disorders such as systemic scleroderma, dermatofibroma, café-au-lait macules of neurofibromatosis, and generalized progressive dyschromatosis [84–87].

Tight reciprocal interactions and regulatory loops between epidermal and mesenchymal compartments may also play a role in melanocyte homeostasis and pigmentation. It has been shown that laminin 332, a major component of the epidermal basement membrane, contributes to melanin production by regulating L-tyrosine uptake [88]. An example of growth factor/cytokine

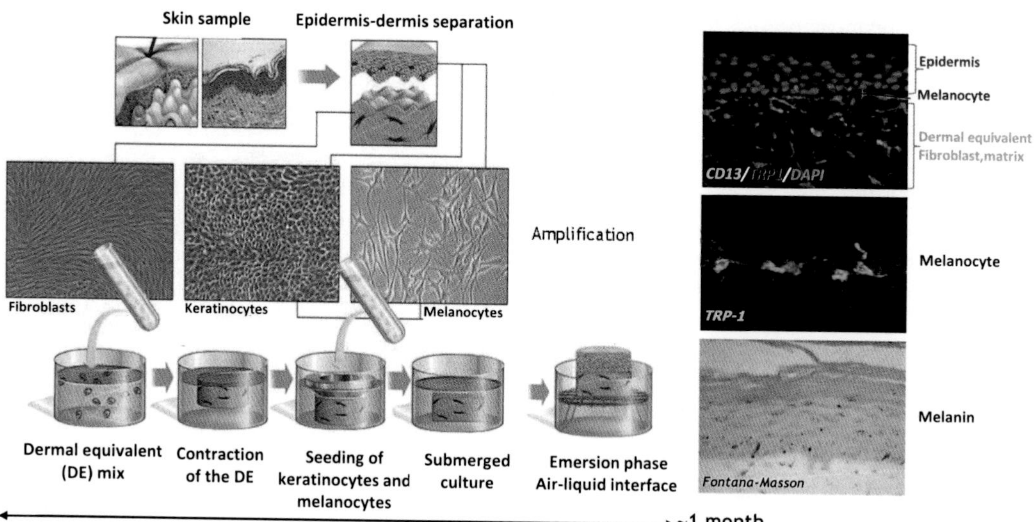

Fig. 6 Full thickness pigmented reconstructed skin model. Schematic representation of the reconstruction protocol and culture phases. Histological sections of pigmented reconstructed skin showing the epidermis containing functional melanocytes (TRP-1) and the fibroblasts-populated dermal equivalent (CD13)

feedback loop is given by the fact that some keratinocyte-produced cytokines, such as interleukin 1 alpha or tumor necrosis factor alpha, may stimulate fibroblasts which in turn release melanocyte-stimulating factors such as hepatocyte growth factor or stem cell factor [89, 90].

Interestingly, FGF7/KGF and CSF2/GM-CSF were found upregulated following DUVR exposure. Upregulation of genes related to skin pigmentation by DUVR suggested a potential contribution of such "nonextreme" exposures to some pigmentary disorders associated with chronic sun exposure [22, 91].

Based upon these converging elements that indicate a role of the dermal compartment in the pigmentation process, an in vitro full-thickness pigmented skin model that allows interactions to take place between the melanocyte-containing epidermis and the dermal compartment including living fibroblasts becomes necessary for studying skin pigmentation in more physiological conditions. However, such a 3-D skin model is not commonly available. The only pigmented skin models comprising a living dermal equivalent developed by different teams reported drawbacks especially the limited survival or the lack of functionality of normal melanocytes [92–94].

By combining experience of (i) reconstructing skin models comprising collagen gel with embeded fibroblasts [37] and (ii) reconstructing pigmented epidermis [72], a functional pigmented skin model comprising a melanocyte-containing epidermis cultured on a fibrobast-populated dermal equivalent was successfully developed (Fig. 6). This was achieved by adjusting various culture conditions, notably adding KGF during the air-liquid interface culture phase [95].

Melanocytes were correctly integrated at the basal layer of the epidermis and displayed a physiological differentiation, as revealed by melanin production and transfer into keratinocytes (constitutive pigmentation). Using melanocytes from more or less pigmented skins, various pigmentation phenotypes could be obtained. Validation of the functionality of the model was checked by stimulating pigmentation with known propigmenting agents, αMSH and forskolin, or reducing it with a depigmenting agent.

One advantage of this skin model reproducing the 3-D architecture of the melanocyte environment is the possibility to modify the source of the epidermal cells or dermal cells, and thus to analyze the respective role of each cell type on skin pigmentation. Particularly, it represents a powerful and unique tool to analyze the overall impact of dermal fibroblasts on pigmentation, which can occur through the secretion of soluble factors and the production of ECM proteins.

Pigmented Full-Thickness Skin Model as a Model to Study the Involvement of the Dermal Compartment in Pigmentation Process: Proof of Concept

In vitro studies, aimed at demonstrating the regulatory role of dermal fibroblast on pigmentation, assessed the effects of fibroblastic soluble factors or fibroblast-conditioned medium directly on 2-D or 3-D cell cultures (melanocytes alone or cocultured with keratinocytes, pigmented reconstructed epidermis) [83, 92, 96–98]. Other approaches consist in using living fibroblasts either (i) as a proliferating monolayer cultured underneath a pigmented reconstructed epidermis [83] or (ii) embedded in collagen gel put underneath an insert containing melanocytes growing on [82]. However, these systems are restrictive to the contribution of potential soluble factors and do not integrate the structural and functional influence of the dermal extracellular matrix on epidermal cells nor the tissue architecture that ensures the necessary physiological interplay between melanocytes, keratinocytes, and fibroblasts.

A more relevant pigmented full-thickness skin model was set up to clarify the link between pigmentation and dermal fibroblasts. At first, its responsiveness was assessed with regard to variations in fibroblast's component to demonstrate that changes in fibroblastic parameters do modulate the skin pigmentation level [99]. Hence, a first experiment was performed to highlight the overall role of fibroblasts by reconstructing skins with or without living fibroblasts in the dermal equivalent. Results showed drastic differences in the level of pigmentation at the macroscopic level (visually). This was confirmed by measuring the Luminance L*, a colorimetric parameter from the L*a*b* system that expresses the lightness/darkness of the sample and by quantifying melanin content on Fontana Masson stained skin sections. Actually, the absence of dermal fibroblasts led to a substantial increase in pigmentation as shown by a strong decrease of L* and a tenfold increase in melanin content. An increase in melanocyte number, although more modest, was also revealed (factor of 3.3). The intense increase in pigmentation level associated with the higher melanocyte pool in the fibroblast-deprived skin model suggest that the presence of dermal cells results in a slowing down of both melanogenesis and melanocyte population.

After having demonstrated the overall impact of dermal fibroblasts upon skin model pigmentation, functional validation of the model was extended by determining the influence of the phenotype of dermal fibroblasts on pigmentation. Accordingly, fibroblasts from fetal and adult origins known to have different characteristics were chosen. Actually, fetal fibroblasts differ from adult fibroblasts with regard to their physiological effect (rapid healing and scar-free wound repair) and to their biological intrinsic properties in terms of ECM, growth factors, and inflammatory cytokine production [100, 101].

Interestingly, the pigmentation of skin sample containing fetal fibroblasts was significantly increased, macroscopically and on histological sections, as compared to that with adult fibroblasts (Fig. 7). The difference of pigmentation was confirmed by a substantial decrease of L* and an increase in melanin content by a factor of 6.6. Although the melanocyte population also increased (3.3 fold), the melanin content still remained twofold higher, indicating that the melanogenesis process (per melanocyte) was definitely stimulated. This pigmentation variation observed when using fibroblasts with different intrinsic characteristics shows that the model does respond to changes in the nature of the fibroblasts integrated within the dermal equivalent.

As a result, this proof of principle shows that dermal fibroblasts do impact skin pigmentation and that the pigmented reconstructed skin can detect such impact at both microscopic and macroscopic levels. This validated the relevance of the model to further investigate the influence of fibroblasts from various real-life conditions on skin pigmentation.

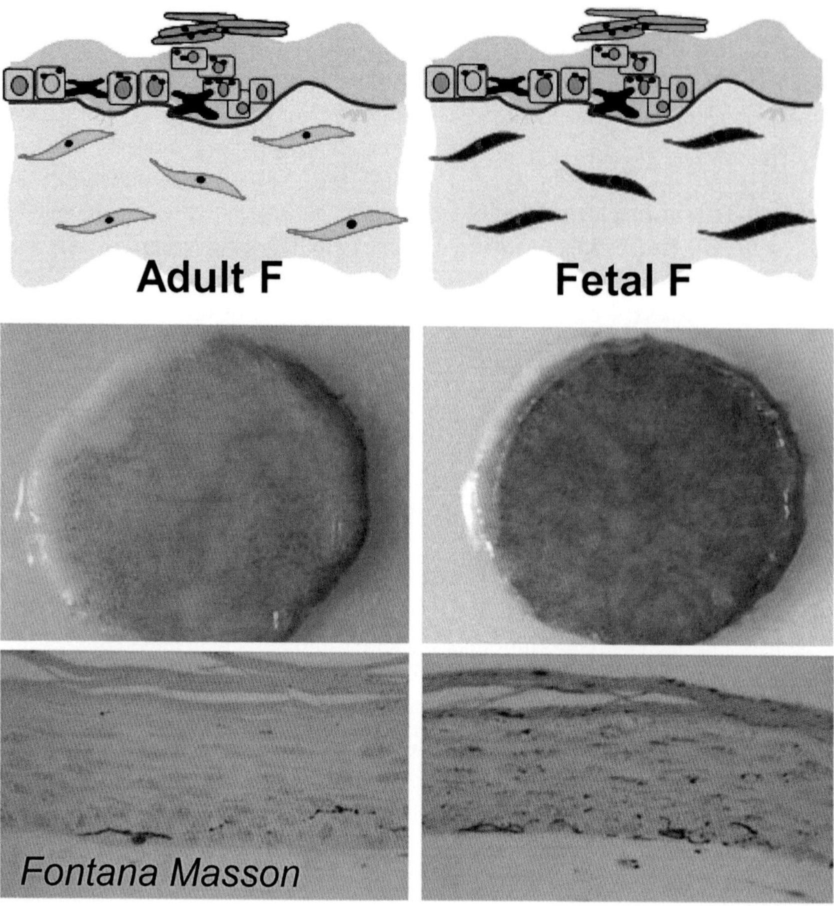

Fig. 7 Role of dermal fibroblast origin on skin pigmentation. Pigmented reconstructed skin containing different fibroblast strains, either adult or fetal, within the dermal equivalent. Difference in level of pigmentation shows that the model is responsive to change in the nature of the integrated fibroblasts

Impact of Photoaging Upon Skin Pigmentation: Evidence Given Using the Pigmented Full-Thickness Skin Model

Pigmentary alterations represent characteristic features of skin photoaging, and especially hyperpigmented spots such as actinic lentigines in sun-exposed areas are considered to be a hallmark of photoaged skin. It is also well known that skin photoaging is associated with profound structural dermal alterations and severe biological changes in dermal fibroblasts. These elements led to hypothetize that functional alterations of dermal fibroblasts acquired over time may play a role in the photoaging-associated hyperpigmentations.

This issue was therefore addressed by studying the influence of fibroblasts obtained from naturally photoaged skins on the pigmentation of the full-thickness skin model [99]. Three different strains of fibroblasts from photoaged skin (facial area, caucasian donors older than 70 years) were compared to three strains of fibroblasts isolated from Caucasian young donors <20 years. Cells from photoaged skin in monolayer displayed characteristic features of senescence such as decrease in proliferation (e.g., increase in doubling population time) and beta-galactosidase staining (Fig. 8a). The six strains were used individually to make dermal equivalents, and epidermis was reconstructed using similar keratinocyte and melanocyte strains onto the respective dermal substrates. Morphologically,

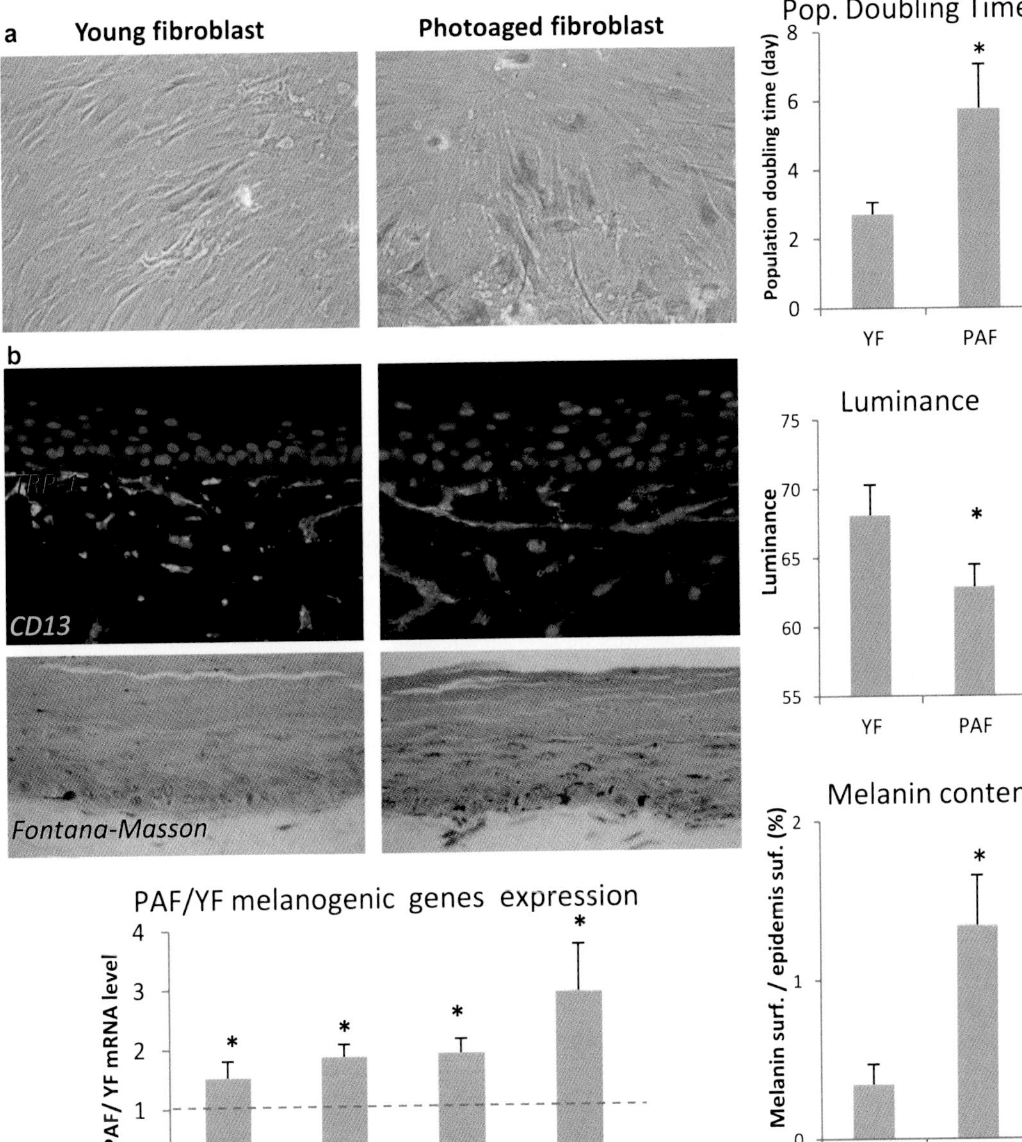

Fig. 8 Impact of photoaged fibroblasts on skin pigmentation. (**a**) Fibroblasts isolated from photoaged skin (*PAF*) or young non-exposed skin (*YF*) before their integration within dermal equivalent: beta galactosidase staining and population doubling time show the senescence trait of PAF. (**b**) Pigmented reconstructed skin containing either photoaged fibroblasts or young fibroblasts. Histological sections show melanocytes (*red*) at the DEJ, fibroblasts (*green*) within the dermal equivalent (nuclei in *blue*), and melanin pigment colored by Fontana-Masson staining. Bar graphs: quantification of Luminance L*, melanin content and variation in the expression of melanogenic genes (mRNA fold change in PAF vs. YF skins) demonstrate the increased pigmentation and melanogenic activity of melanocytes in the pigmented reconstructed skin containing PAF versus YF

the skin reconstructed with photoaged fibroblasts displayed correct differentiation of the epidermis and contained well-integrated fibroblasts but showing elongated shape, a characteristic feature of photoaging [102] (Fig. 8b). However, melanocyte activity and pigmentation showed a significant difference between the two dermal conditions (photoaged vs. young) even though melanocyte number, location, and morphology remained comparable. Actually, melanocyte activity was found stimulated by the presence of photoaged fibroblasts as compared to younger ones, and a higher level of epidermal pigmentation, quantified by a decrease of L* and an increase in melanin content, was found in the presence of photoaged (PAF) fibroblasts (Fig. 8b). Thus, these results demonstrated, for the first time, a direct link between dermal photoaging and skin pigmentation.

Previous studies have attempted to investigate the effect of "photoaged" fibroblasts on pigmentation by using fibroblasts grown in monolayer and artificially induced senescent [91, 96, 98]. However, these 2-D cultures never gave a clear demonstration nor a visualization of the modulation of pigmentation. Using naturally photoaged fibroblasts integrated in a 3-D model was more relevant for at least three reasons: (i) isolated from photoaged skin, these cells have retained their long history of chronic sun exposures, (ii) residing within a 3-D equivalent, fibroblasts have kept their natural quiescent status, conditioning physiological cellular metabolism and secretory activity, and (iii) the influence of fibroblasts occurring through their secretion of soluble factors or the production of various extracellular matrix proteins could be globally assessed.

To understand the mechanisms that underlie the induction of pigmentation by photoaged fibroblasts, 18 soluble factors known to modulate pigmentation were determined in the supernatants of dermal equivalent containing either photoaged or young fibroblasts [99]. The results did not however reveal significant or consistent modulation of any of these factors that could be related to a hyperpigmented phenotype as observed in photoaged condition. Additional broad proteomic investigations or ECM studies would be necessary for identifying the molecular actors involved.

Altogether, these data demonstrated that the presence, the nature and the history of dermal fibroblasts are key factors in regulating skin pigmentation and that fibroblasts from chronically sun-exposed skin may contribute to the pigmentation disorder which is associated with photoaging.

Conclusion

Major difficulties arise when studying the photoaging process through in 2-D vitro models, due to (i) the complexity of the solar UV spectrum and exposure conditions (wavelengths' characteristics, "extreme" vs. daily exposure conditions, exposure regimen, ...), (ii) the diversity of the biological effects and their cutaneous locations and (iii) the heterogeneity of clinical consequences arising from short to long term (wrinkles, sagging, immune response, photocancers, pigmentary disorders). Significant advances were made by the development of appropriate 3-D skin models comprising different cell types organized in a physiological architecture. They reproduce cellular interactions and allow responses to being obtained taking into account the penetration of UV rays through the whole skin structure. Historically based upon the analysis of sunburn related biomarkers, recent data summarized in this review brought new insights in the biological and the molecular events involved in photoaging process occurring after more realistic daily UV exposures while highlighting the contribution of wavelengths often neglected due to their lower energy, such as UVA1. In addition, thanks to the combination of 3-D models with a global approach such as transcriptomic, the diversity of biological alterations have been described and revealed that essential functions are indeed impaired by moderate solar exposures. The development of the 3-D full thickness pigmented skin has allowed a link for the first time to being brought out between the dermal alterations occurring during photoaging and the pigmentary function. This has been possible thanks to the flexibility of the system and the ability to modulate the cell origin and history. Altogether, the data here shows the added value of such 3-D skin models for a better understanding of biological events related to photoaging process, offering in addition a very precise description of the underlying molecular mechanisms.

Finally, the in vitro data often appears predictive to the in vivo situation.

References

1. Flament F, Bazin R, Laquieze S, Rubert V, Simonpietri E, Piot B. Effect of the sun on visible clinical signs of aging in Caucasian skin. Clin Cosmet Invest Dermatol. 2013;6:221–32.
2. Gunn DA, Rexbye H, Griffiths CE, Murray PG, Fereday A, Catt SD, Tomlin CC, Strongitharm BH, Perrett DI, Catt M, Mayes AE, Messenger AG, Green MR, van der Ouderaa F, Vaupel JW, Christensen K. Why some women look young for their age. PLoS One. 2009;4:e8021.
3. Gordon JR, Brieva JC. Images in clinical medicine. Unilateral dermatoheliosis. N Engl J Med. 2012;366: e25.
4. Ortonne JP, Bissett DL. Latest insights into skin hyperpigmentation. J Invest Dermatol Symp Proc. 2008;13:10–4.
5. Tagami H. Functional characteristics of the stratum corneum in photoaged skin in comparison with those found in intrinsic aging. Arch Dermatol Res. 2008;300 Suppl 1:S1–6.
6. Lavker RM. Cutaneous aging: chronologic versus photoaging. In: Gilchrest BA, editor. Photodamage. Cambridge, MA: Blackwell; 1995. p. 123–35.
7. Talwar HS, Griffiths CE, Fisher GJ, Hamilton TA, Voorhees JJ. Reduced type I and type III procollagens in photodamaged adult human skin. J Invest Dermatol. 1995;105:285–90.
8. Jeanmaire C, Danoux L, Pauly G. Glycation during human dermal intrinsic and actinic ageing: an in vivo and in vitro model study. Br J Dermatol. 2001;145:10–8.
9. Bernstein EF, Fisher LW, Li K, LeBaron RG, Tan EM, Uitto J. Differential expression of the versican and decorin genes in photoaged and sun-protected skin. Comparison by immunohistochemical and northern analyses. Lab Invest. 1995;72:662–9.
10. Chen VL, Fleischmajer R, Schwartz E, Palaia M, Timpl R. Immunochemistry of elastotic material in sun-damaged skin. J Invest Dermatol. 1986;87:334–7.
11. Chung JH, Seo JY, Choi HR, Lee MK, Youn CS, Rhie G, Cho KH, Kim KH, Park KC, Eun HC. Modulation of skin collagen metabolism in aged and photoaged human skin in vivo. J Invest Dermatol. 2001;117:1218–24.
12. Fisher GJ, Datta SC, Talwar HS, Wang ZQ, Varani J, Kang S, Voorhees JJ. Molecular basis of sun-induced premature skin ageing and retinoid antagonism. Nature. 1996;379:335–9.
13. Berneburg M, Plettenberg H, Krutmann J. Photoaging of human skin. Photodermatol Photoimmunol Photomed. 2000;16:239–44.
14. Fisher GJ, Voorhees JJ. Molecular mechanisms of photoaging and its prevention by retinoic acid: ultraviolet irradiation induces MAP kinase signal transduction cascades that induce Ap-1-regulated matrix metalloproteinases that degrade human skin in vivo. J Invest Dermatol Symp Proc. 1998;3:61–8.
15. Ma W, Wlaschek M, Tantcheva-Poor I, Schneider LA, Naderi L, Razi-Wolf Z, Schuller J, Scharffetter-Kochanek K. Chronological ageing and photoageing of the fibroblasts and the dermal connective tissue. Clin Exp Dermatol. 2001;26:592–9.
16. Seite S, Zucchi H, Septier D, Igondjo-Tchen S, Senni K, Godeau G. Elastin changes during chronological and photo-ageing: the important role of lysozyme. J Eur Acad Dermatol Venereol. 2006;20:980–7.
17. Hase T, Shinta K, Murase T, Tokimitsu I, Hattori M, Takimoto R, Tsuboi R, Ogawa H. Histological increase in inflammatory infiltrate in sun-exposed skin of female subjects: the possible involvement of matrix metalloproteinase-1 produced by inflammatory infiltrate on collagen degradation. Br J Dermatol. 2000;142:267–73.
18. Li Y, Xia W, Liu Y, Remmer HA, Voorhees J, Fisher GJ. Solar ultraviolet irradiation induces decorin degradation in human skin likely via neutrophil elastase. PLoS One. 2013;8:e72563.
19. Cario-Andre M, Lepreux S, Pain C, Nizard C, Noblesse E, Taieb A. Perilesional vs. lesional skin changes in senile lentigo. J Cutan Pathol. 2004;31:441–7.
20. Andersen WK, Labadie RR, Bhawan J. Histopathology of solar lentigines of the face: a quantitative study. J Am Acad Dermatol. 1997;36:444–7.
21. Unver N, Freyschmidt-Paul P, Horster S, Wenck H, Stab F, Blatt T, Elsasser HP. Alterations in the epidermal-dermal melanin axis and factor XIIIa melanophages in senile lentigo and ageing skin. Br J Dermatol. 2006;155:119–28.
22. Chen N, Hu Y, Li WH, Eisinger M, Seiberg M, Lin CB. The role of keratinocyte growth factor in melanogenesis: a possible mechanism for the initiation of solar lentigines. Exp Dermatol. 2010;19:865–72.
23. Iriyama S, Ono T, Aoki H, Amano S. Hyperpigmentation in human solar lentigo is promoted by heparanase-induced loss of heparan sulfate chains at the dermal-epidermal junction. J Dermatol Sci. 2011;64:223–8.
24. Fagot D, Asselineau D, Bernerd F. Direct role of human dermal fibroblasts and indirect participation of epidermal keratinocytes in MMP-1 production after UV-B irradiation. Arch Dermatol Res. 2002;293:576–83.
25. Fagot D, Asselineau D, Bernerd F. Matrix metalloproteinase-1 production observed after solar-simulated radiation exposure is assumed by dermal fibroblasts but involves a paracrine activation through

epidermal keratinocytes. Photochem Photobiol. 2004;79:499–505.
26. Wlaschek M, Tantcheva-Poor I, Naderi L, Ma W, Schneider LA, Razi-Wolf Z, Schuller J, Scharffetter-Kochanek K. Solar UV irradiation and dermal photoaging. J Photochem Photobiol B. 2001;63:41–51.
27. Krutmann J. Ultraviolet A radiation-induced biological effects in human skin: relevance for photoaging and photodermatosis. J Dermatol Sci. 2000;23 Suppl 1: S22–6.
28. Commission Internationale de l'Éclairage (CIE). Solar spectral irradiance. Technical report, CIE 085–1989, www.cie.co.at, Vienna; 1989.
29. Lubin D, Jensen EH. Effects of clouds and stratospheric ozone depletion on ultraviolet radiation trends. Nature. 1995;377:710–3.
30. Sabziparvar AA, Shine KP, Forster PMD. A model-derived global climatology of UV irradiation at the Earth's surface. Photochem Photobiol. 1999;69:193–202.
31. Tewari A, Grage MM, Harrison GI, Sarkany R, Young AR. UVA1 is skin deep: molecular and clinical implications. Photochem Photobiol Sci. 2013;12:95–103.
32. Seite S, Fourtanier A, Moyal D, Young AR. Photodamage to human skin by suberythemal exposure to solar ultraviolet radiation can be attenuated by sunscreens: a review. Br J Dermatol. 2010;163:903–14.
33. Mahe E, Correa MP, Godin-Beekmann S, Haeffelin M, Jegou F, Saiag P, Beauchet A. Evaluation of tourists' UV exposure in Paris. J Eur Acad Dermatol Venereol. 2013;27:e294–304.
34. Eungdamrong NJ, Higgins C, Guo Z, Lee WH, Gillette B, Sia S, Christiano AM. Challenges and promises in modeling dermatologic disorders with bioengineered skin. Exp Biol Med (Maywood). 2014;239:1215–24.
35. Bernerd F, Asselineau D, Vioux C, Chevallier-Lagente O, Bouadjar B, Sarasin A, Magnaldo T. Clues to epidermal cancer proneness revealed by reconstruction of DNA repair-deficient xeroderma pigmentosum skin in vitro. Proc Natl Acad Sci U S A. 2001;98:7817–22.
36. Haake AR, Polakowska RR. UV-induced apoptosis in skin equivalents: inhibition by phorbol ester and Bcl-2 overexpression. Cell Death Differ. 1995;2:183–93.
37. Bernerd F, Asselineau D. Successive alteration and recovery of epidermal differentiation and morphogenesis after specific UVB-damages in skin reconstructed in vitro. Dev Biol. 1997;183:123–38.
38. Vioux-Chagnoleau C, Lejeune F, Sok J, Pierrard C, Marionnet C, Bernerd F. Reconstructed human skin: from photodamage to sunscreen photoprotection and anti-aging molecules. J Dermatol Sci. 2006;2(Suppl): S1–12.
39. Fernandez TL, Van Lonkhuyzen DR, Dawson RA, Kimlin MG, Upton Z. Characterization of a human skin equivalent model to study the effects of ultraviolet B radiation on keratinocytes. Tissue Eng Part C Methods. 2014;20:588–98.
40. Lavker RM, Veres DA, Irwin CJ, Kaidbey KH. Quantitative assessment of cumulative damage from repetitive exposures to suberythemogenic doses of UVA in human skin. Photochem Photobiol. 1995;62:348–52.
41. Berneburg M, Krutmann J. Mitochondrial DNA deletions in human skin reflect photo- rather than chronologic aging. J Invest Dermatol. 1998;111:709–10.
42. Bernerd F, Asselineau D. UVA exposure of human skin reconstructed in vitro induces apoptosis of dermal fibroblasts: subsequent connective tissue repair and implications in photoaging. Cell Death Differ. 1998;5:792–802.
43. Marionnet C, Grether-Beck S, Seite S, Marini A, Jaenicke T, Lejeune F, Bastien P, Rougier A, Bernerd F, Krutmann J. A broad-spectrum sunscreen prevents UVA radiation-induced gene expression in reconstructed skin in vitro and in human skin in vivo. Exp Dermatol. 2011;20:477–82.
44. Meloni M, Farina A, de Servi B. Molecular modifications of dermal and epidermal biomarkers following UVA exposures on reconstructed full-thickness human skin. Photochem Photobiol Sci. 2010;9:439–47.
45. Dekker P, Parish WE, Green MR. Protection by food-derived antioxidants from UV-A1-induced photodamage, measured using living skin equivalents. Photochem Photobiol. 2005;81:837–42.
46. Tewari A, Sarkany RP, Young AR. UVA1 induces cyclobutane pyrimidine dimers but not 6–4 photoproducts in human skin in vivo. J Invest Dermatol. 2012;132:394–400.
47. Huang XX, Bernerd F, Halliday GM. Ultraviolet A within sunlight induces mutations in the epidermal basal layer of engineered human skin. Am J Pathol. 2009;174:1534–43.
48. Jonason AS, Kunala S, Price GJ, Restifo RJ, Spinelli HM, Persing JA, Leffell DJ, Tarone RE, Brash DE. Frequent clones of p53-mutated keratinocytes in normal human skin. Proc Natl Acad Sci U S A. 1996;93:14025–9.
49. Fisher GJ, Wang ZQ, Datta SC, Varani J, Kang S, Voorhees JJ. Pathophysiology of premature skin aging induced by ultraviolet light. N Engl J Med. 1997;337:1419–28.
50. Deutsches Institut für Normung e.V.(DIN). Experimentelle Bewertung des Erythemschutzes von externen Sonnenschutzmitteln für die menschliche Haut (Experimental evaluation of the protection from erythema by external sunscreen products for the human skin). Berlin; 1999.
51. Commission Internationale de l'Eclairage (CIE). Spectral weighting of solar ultraviolet radiation. 2003. www.cie.co.at. CIE 151, Vienna. Ref Type: Report.
52. Bissonauth V, Drouin R, Mitchell DL, Rhainds M, Claveau J, Rouabhia M. The efficacy of a broad-

spectrum sunscreen to protect engineered human skin from tissue and DNA damage induced by solar ultraviolet exposure. Clin Cancer Res. 2000;6:4128–35.

53. Bernerd F, Vioux C, Lejeune F, Asselineau D. The sun protection factor (SPF) inadequately defines broad spectrum photoprotection: demonstration using skin reconstructed in vitro exposed to UVA, UVBor UV-solar simulated radiation. Eur J Dermatol. 2003;13:242–9.
54. Christiaens FJ, Chardon A, Fourtanier A, Frederick JE. Standard ultraviolet daylight for nonextreme exposure conditions. Photochem Photobiol. 2005;81:874–8.
55. Marionnet C, Tricaud C, Bernerd F. Exposure to non-extreme solar UV daylight: spectral characterization, effects on skin and photoprotection. Int J Mol Sci. 2014;16:68–90.
56. Seite S, Medaisko C, Christiaens F, Bredoux C, Compan D, Zucchi H, Lombard D, Fourtanier A. Biological effects of simulated ultraviolet daylight: a new approach to investigate daily photoprotection. Photodermatol Photoimmunol Photomed. 2006;22:67–77.
57. Marionnet C, Pierrard C, Lejeune F, Sok J, Thomas M, Bernerd F. Different oxidative stress response in keratinocytes and fibroblasts of reconstructed skin exposed to non extreme daily-ultraviolet radiation. PLoS One. 2010;5:e12059.
58. Leccia MT, Richard MJ, Joanny-Crisci F, Beani JC. UV-A1 cytotoxicity and antioxidant defence in keratinocytes and fibroblasts. Eur J Dermatol. 1998;8:478–82.
59. Matsuda M, Hoshino T, Yamakawa N, Tahara K, Adachi H, Sobue G, Maji D, Ihn H, Mizushima T. Suppression of UV-induced wrinkle formation by induction of HSP70 expression in mice. J Invest Dermatol. 2013;133:919–28.
60. Marionnet C, Pierrard C, Lejeune F, Bernerd F. Modulations of gene expression induced by daily ultraviolet light can be prevented by a broad spectrum sunscreen. J Photochem Photobiol B. 2012;116:37–47.
61. Norval M, Halliday GM. The consequences of UV-induced immunosuppression for human health. Photochem Photobiol. 2011;87:965–77.
62. Marionnet C, Lejeune F, Pierrard C, Vioux-Chagnoleau C, Bernerd F. Biological contribution of UVA wavelengths in non extreme daily UV exposure. J Dermatol Sci. 2012;66:238–40.
63. de Laat A, van der Leun JC, de Gruijl FR. Carcinogenesis induced by UVA (365-nm) radiation: the dose-time dependence of tumor formation in hairless mice. Carcinogenesis. 1997;18(5):1013–20.
64. Damian DL, Matthews YJ, Phan TA, Halliday GM. An action spectrum for ultraviolet radiation-induced immunosuppression in humans. Br J Dermatol. 2011;164:657–9.
65. Wang F, Smith NR, Tran BA, Kang S, Voorhees JJ, Fisher GJ. Dermal damage promoted by repeated low-level UV-A1 exposure despite tanning response in human skin. JAMA Dermatol. 2014;150:401–6.
66. Marionnet C, Pierrard C, Golebiewski C, Bernerd F. Diversity of biological effects induced by longwave UVA rays (UVA1) in reconstructed skin. PLoS One. 2014;9:e105263.
67. Tewari A, Sarkany RP, Young AR. UVA1 induces cyclobutane pyrimidine dimers but not 6-4 photoproducts in human skin in vivo. J Invest Dermatol. 2012; 132:394–400.
68. York NR, Jacobe HT. UVA1 phototherapy: a review of mechanism and therapeutic application. Int J Dermatol. 2010;49:623–30.
69. Takaoka A, Hayakawa S, Yanai H, Stoiber D, Negishi H, Kikuchi H, Sasaki S, Imai K, Shibue T, Honda K, Taniguchi T. Integration of interferon-alpha/beta signalling to p53 responses in tumour suppression and antiviral defence. Nature. 2003;424:516–23.
70. Kim EJ, Jin XJ, Kim YK, Oh IK, Kim JE, Park CH, Chung JH. UV decreases the synthesis of free fatty acids and triglycerides in the epidermis of human skin in vivo, contributing to development of skin photoaging. J Dermatol Sci. 2010;57:19–26.
71. Randhawa M, Southall M, Samaras ST. Metabolomic analysis of sun exposed skin. Mol Biosyst. 2013;9:2045–50.
72. Duval C, Regnier M, Schmidt R. Distinct melanogenic response of human melanocytes in mono-culture, in co-culture with keratinocytes and in reconstructed epidermis, to UV exposure. Pigment Cell Res. 2001;14:348–55.
73. Imokawa G. Autocrine and paracrine regulation of melanocytes in human skin and in pigmentary disorders. Pigment Cell Res. 2004;17:96–110.
74. Regnier M, Duval C, Galey JB, Philippe M, Lagrange A, Tuloup R, Schmidt R. Keratinocyte-melanocyte co-cultures and pigmented reconstructed human epidermis: models to study modulation of melanogenesis. Cell Mol Biol. 1999; 45:969–80.
75. Duval C, Smit NP, Kolb AM, Regnier M, Pavel S, Schmidt R. Keratinocytes control the pheo/eumelanin ratio in cultured normal human melanocytes. Pigment Cell Res. 2002;15:440–6.
76. Duval C, Schmidt R, Regnier M, Facy V, Asselineau D, Bernerd F. The use of reconstructed human skin to evaluate UV-induced modifications and sunscreen efficacy. Exp Dermatol. 2003;12 (Suppl):64–70.
77. Gibbs S, Murli S, De BG, Mulder A, Mommaas AM, Ponec M. Melanosome capping of keratinocytes in pigmented reconstructed epidermis–effect of ultraviolet radiation and 3-isobutyl-1-methyl-xanthine on melanogenesis. Pigment Cell Res. 2000;13: 458–66.
78. Bessou S, Surleve-Bazeille JE, Sorbier E, Taieb A. Ex vivo reconstruction of the epidermis with melanocytes and the influence of UVB. Pigment Cell Res. 1995; 8:241–9.

79. Buffey JA, Messenger AG, Taylor M, Ashcroft AT, Westgate GE, MacNeil S. Extracellular matrix derived from hair and skin fibroblasts stimulates human skin melanocyte tyrosinase activity. Br J Dermatol. 1994;131:836–42.
80. Hedley SJ, Wagner M, Bielby S, Smith-Thomas L, Gawkrodger DJ, Mac Neil S. The influence of extracellular matrix proteins on cutaneous and uveal melanocytes. Pigment Cell Res. 1997;10:54–9.
81. Scott G, Cassidy L, Busacco A. Fibronectin suppresses apoptosis in normal human melanocytes through an integrin-dependent mechanism. J Invest Dermatol. 1997;108:147–53.
82. Yamaguchi Y, Itami S, Watabe H, Yasumoto K, Abdel-Malek ZA, Kubo T, Rouzaud F, Tanemura A, Yoshikawa K, Hearing VJ. Mesenchymal-epithelial interactions in the skin: increased expression of dickkopf1 by palmoplantar fibroblasts inhibits melanocyte growth and differentiation. J Cell Biol. 2004;165:275–85.
83. Choi W, Wolber R, Gerwat W, Mann T, Batzer J, Smuda C, Liu H, Kolbe L, Hearing VJ. The fibroblast-derived paracrine factor neuregulin-1 has a novel role in regulating the constitutive color and melanocyte function in human skin. J Cell Sci. 2010;123:3102–11.
84. Yamamoto T, Sawada Y, Katayama I, Nishioka K. Local expression and systemic release of stem cell factor in systemic sclerosis with diffuse hyperpigmentation. Br J Dermatol. 2001;144:199–200.
85. Shishido E, Kadono S, Manaka I, Kawashima M, Imokawa G. The mechanism of epidermal hyperpigmentation in dermatofibroma is associated with stem cell factor and hepatocyte growth factor expression. J Invest Dermatol. 2001;117:627–33.
86. Okazaki M, Yoshimura K, Suzuki Y, Uchida G, Kitano Y, Harii K, Imokawa G. The mechanism of epidermal hyperpigmentation in cafe-au-lait macules of neurofibromatosis type 1 (von Recklinghausen's disease) may be associated with dermal fibroblast-derived stem cell factor and hepatocyte growth factor. Br J Dermatol. 2003;148:689–97.
87. Cardinali G, Kovacs D, Giglio MD, Cota C, Aspite N, Mantea A, Girolomoni G, Picardo M. A kindred with familial progressive hyperpigmentation-like disorder: implication of fibroblast-derived growth factors in pigmentation. Eur J Dermatol. 2009;19:469–73.
88. Chung H, Jung H, Lee JH, Oh HY, Kim OB, Han IO, Oh ES. Keratinocyte-derived Laminin-332 protein promotes melanin synthesis via regulation of tyrosine uptake. J Biol Chem. 2014;289:21751–9.
89. Imokawa G, Yada Y, Morisaki N, Kimura M. Biological characterization of human fibroblast-derived mitogenic factors for human melanocytes. Biochem J. 1998;330:1235–9.
90. Mildner M, Mlitz V, Gruber F, Wojta J, Tschachler E. Hepatocyte growth factor establishes autocrine and paracrine feedback loops for the protection of skin cells after UV irradiation. J Invest Dermatol. 2007;127:2637–44.
91. Kovacs D, Cardinali G, Aspite N, Cota C, Luzi F, Bellei B, Briganti S, Amantea A, Torrisi MR, Picardo M. Role of fibroblast-derived growth factors in regulating hyperpigmentation of solar lentigo. Br J Dermatol. 2010;163:1020–7.
92. Cario-Andre M, Pain C, Gauthier Y, Casoli V, Taieb A. In vivo and in vitro evidence of dermal fibroblasts influence on human epidermal pigmentation. Pigment Cell Res. 2006;19:434–42.
93. Souto LR, Rehder J, Vassallo J, Cintra ML, Kraemer MH, Puzzi MB. Model for human skin reconstructed in vitro composed of associated dermis and epidermis. Sao Paulo Med J. 2006;124:71–6.
94. Okazaki M, Suzuki Y, Yoshimura K, Harii K. Construction of pigmented skin equivalent and its application to the study of congenital disorders of pigmentation. Scand J Plast Reconstr Surg Hand Surg. 2005;39:339–43.
95. Duval C, Chagnoleau C, Pouradier F, Sextius P, Condom E, Bernerd F. Human skin model containing melanocytes: essential role of keratinocyte growth factor for constitutive pigmentation-functional response to alpha-melanocyte stimulating hormone and forskolin. Tissue Eng Part C Methods. 2012;18:947–57.
96. Shin J, Kim JH, Kim EK. Repeated exposure of human fibroblasts to UVR induces secretion of stem cell factor and senescence. J Eur Acad Dermatol Venereol. 2012;26:1577–80.
97. Hirobe T, Hasegawa K, Furuya R, Fujiwara R, Sato K. Effects of fibroblast-derived factors on the proliferation and differentiation of human melanocytes in culture. J Dermatol Sci. 2013;71:45–57.
98. Salducci M, Andre N, Guere C, Martin M, Fitoussi R, Vie K, Cario-Andre M. Factors secreted by irradiated aged fibroblasts induce solar lentigo in pigmented reconstructed epidermis. Pigment Cell Melanoma Res. 2014;27:502–4.
99. Duval C, Cohen C, Chagnoleau C, Flouret V, Bourreau E, Bernerd F. Key regulatory role of dermal fibroblasts in pigmentation as demonstrated using a reconstructed skin model: impact of photo-aging. PLoS One. 2014;9:e114182.
100. Pouyani T, Papp S, Schaffer L. Tissue-engineered fetal dermal matrices. In Vitro Cell Dev Biol Anim. 2012;48:493–506.
101. Namazi MR, Fallahzadeh MK, Schwartz RA. Strategies for prevention of scars: what can we learn from fetal skin? Int J Dermatol. 2011;50:85–93.
102. Varani J, Schuger L, Dame MK, Leonard C, Fligiel SE, Kang S, Fisher GJ, Voorhees JJ. Reduced fibroblast interaction with intact collagen as a mechanism for depressed collagen synthesis in photodamaged skin. J Invest Dermatol. 2004;122:1471–9.

Skinomics: A New Toolbox to Understand Skin Aging

103

Sidra Younis, Mayumi Komine, Marjana Tomic-Canic, and Miroslav Blumenberg

Contents

Dr. Blumenberg's research is supported by the Ronald O. Perelman Department of Dermatology, NYU Langone Medical Center.

S. Younis
The R.O. Perelman Department of Dermatology, and Department of Biochemistry and Molecular Pharmacology, NYU Langone Medical Center, New York, NY, USA

Department of Biochemistry, Quaid-i-Azam University, Islamabad, Pakistan
e-mail: sidra.younis@gmail.com

M. Komine
Department of Dermatology, Jichi Medical University, Shimotsuke, Tochigi, Japan
e-mail: mkomine12@jichi.ac.jp

M. Tomic-Canic
Wound Healing and Regenerative Medicine Research Program, Department of Dermatology and Cutaneous Surgery and Hussman Institute of Human Genomics, University of Miami Miller Medical School, Miami, FL, USA
e-mail: mtcanic@med.miami.edu

M. Blumenberg (✉)
The R.O. Perelman Department of Dermatology, NYU Langone Medical Center, New York, NY, USA

Department of Biochemistry and Molecular Pharmacology, NYU Langone Medical Center, New York, NY, USA
e-mail: Miroslav.Blumenberg@nyumc.org

M.A. Farage et al. (eds.), *Textbook of Aging Skin*,
DOI 10.1007/978-3-662-47398-6_164

Abstract

In recent years, we have witnessed the dawn of "omics" technologies, approaches that comprehensively deal with the entire genome, transcriptome, proteome, microbiome, etc. Because of its ease of access and direct visibility, the skin was among the first targets of analysis using DNA microarrays, and dermatology was one of the first medical specialties to embrace the omics approaches, giving rise to the term "skinomics" or the use of omics techniques in dermatology and skin biology. Microarrays have been used to identify loci associated with predisposition to, e.g., psoriasis, to define skin disease markers in melanoma, and even to follow the progress and efficacy of treatment of dermatologic conditions. The aging process has been studied using omics technology in many tissues and organs, notably the brain, especially in the context of Alzheimer's disease. Several groups studied skin aging using microarrays and related high data content methodologies. The skinomics techniques involve highly sophisticated and complex procedures. They start with sample acquisition, its processing to retrieve a complete set of DNA, RNA, protein, metabolites, etc., and then analysis using microarrays or next-generation sequencing. An essential part of skinomics is the computer-based processing of large amount of data. The bioinformaticians have assembled an impressive and continuously growing and improving tool set for data analysis. Alas, this aspect of skinomics is not yet user-friendly enough for use in clinic. Soon, however, microarrays and related "skinomics" techniques will be mature to become applicable to the personalized dermatology practice of the future.

Skinomics

Recent developments of bioinformatic technologies advanced our research capabilities for acquiring, managing, and processing large volumes of biological information [1]. Such information can include medical, genetic, imaging, biochemical, and biophysical data and requires computer-based resources, including data repositories, algorithms, and theoretical approaches to deal with the sheer volume of the data [1, 2]. "Omics" refers to studies of an entire biological system, e.g., genomics for all the genes of an organism, microbiomics for all microorganisms in a given habitat, etc. Similar to, e.g., "microscopy," bioinformatics is defined by its methodology rather than the object of its study. The bioinformatic community has developed Bioconductor, a set of computer programs, freely accessible and communally and cooperatively maintained and expanded [3]. A recent review of various bioinformatic tools is given in reference [4].

Skinomics, then, is a field of bioinformatics applied for studies of large-scale data in dermatology and skin biology. Skinomics technologies include acquiring, managing, and processing large amounts of medical, genetic, biochemical, and biophysical data related to the integument.

Paradoxically, skinomics studies enable us to see both the forest and the trees: they allow a broad and, at the same time, a detailed insight into properties, functions, and diseases of the skin. Skinomics studies can define both the global molecular pathways involved in a given process, such as aging, as well as identify a handful of genes whose expression can provide specific markers for diagnosis.

Historic roots of skinomics are at Stanford University, where Dr. Pat Brown and his group developed the first DNA microarrays [5]. Soon thereafter this methodology was applied to skin biology, when Iyer et al., using standard model for cell cycle synchronization, found that dermal fibroblasts respond to serum by inducing the wound healing responses [6]. Dr. Paul Khavari, also at Stanford, was the first to apply microarrays in dermatology to analyze replacement gene therapy for junctional epidermolysis bullosa. In dermatology, wound healing, skin cancers, and inflammatory diseases, such as psoriasis and eczema, have been the target of numerous skinomics studies and so have been studies of skin aging, as recorded below. The large agglomeration of skinomics data is now ready for to meta-analysis studies; Dr. Noh and his group were among the first to use meta-analysis of microarray data in dermatology [7].

DNA Microarrays

A microarray is an ordered arrangement of proteins, nucleic acids, carbohydrates, small molecules, etc., on solid supports, allowing large-scale analysis of complex biochemical samples. A DNA microarray consists of thousands of different genes, essentially the entire protein-coding genome, which has made possible comprehensive and systematic comparisons of all genes expressed in a given tissue or cell type. Development of DNA microarrays for transcriptional profiling provided a large impetus in bioinformatics [5]. The use of microarrays, and more recently next-generation DNA sequencing, constitutes a steadily growing segment of biomedical knowledge (Fig. 1). The mechanics and protocols for the use of microarrays have been described by us and others, and here we list some of the references to help interested readers get acquainted with the particulars [8–13].

Oligonucleotide microarrays are commercially available from several companies including Affymetrix (Fig. 2), Illumina, Agilent, etc. While the commercial microarrays come with a significant price tag, $500 or more, they go through extensive quality control and suppliers provide data analysis software. The data analysis tools have been largely developed as academic freeware, although a few commercial companies also provide proprietary algorithms and even databases. Microarray results are usually very large and difficult to interpret spreadsheets that require expert analysis. Unfortunately, the results are often presented as simplified multicolored graphs, which tend to be even more confusing and ambiguous (Fig. 3). The lack of meaningful, simple, and intuitive illustration of the microarray results is currently a major obstacle to their widespread use.

Microarray data are usually deposited into annotated and curated databases, such as the Gene Expression Omnibus (GEO), available at http://ncbi.nlm.nih.gov/geo [14]. This databank contains close to 1,000,000 gene expression profiles and grows by 150 % annually. Most journals nowadays require deposition of the raw data into a publicly accessible format. This enables meta-

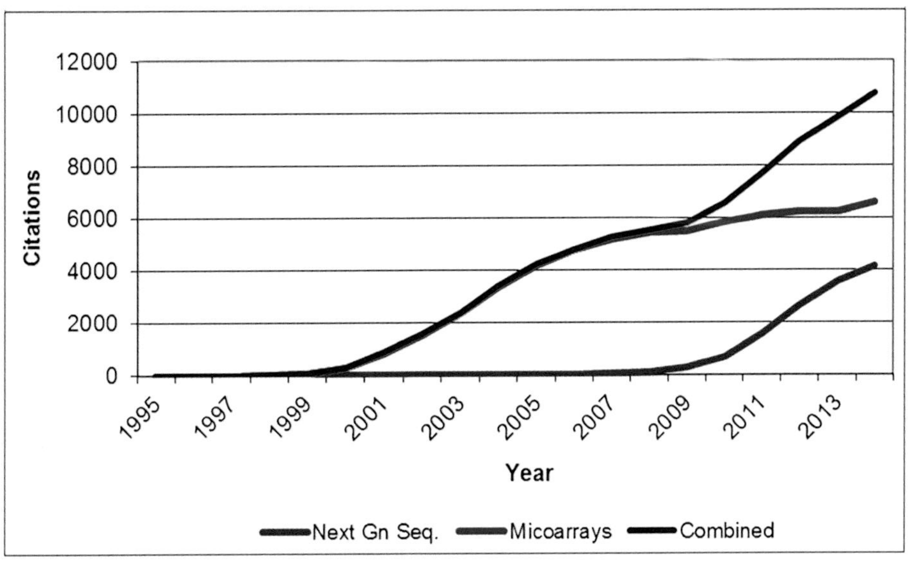

Fig. 1 Growth of transcriptomics analysis. The yearly number of PubMed articles involving DNA microarray or next-generation sequencing studies of transcriptional profiling

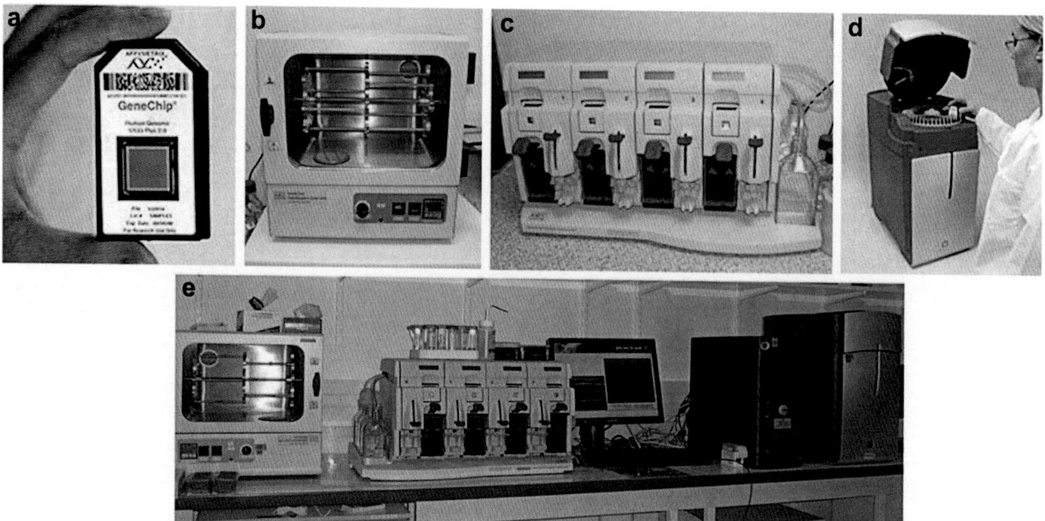

Fig. 2 Affymetrix DNA microarray equipment. (**a**) An example of microarray chips. (**b**) Hybridization oven. (**c**) Fluidic station for microarray washing, processing, etc. (**d**) Microarray scanner with a carousel for loading multiple microarrays at once. (**e**) The entire setup, with its associated computer, fits atop an ordinary lab bench

	Treated				Control				Treated					Control				Treated				
GSE11792	MCF7H	MCF7H	MCF7H	MCF7H	MCF7H	MCF7H	MCF7H	MCF7H	Wt Tam	Wt Tam	Wt Tam	Wt Tam	Wt Tam	Wt Tam	Wt Tam	Wt Tam	Wt Tam	MCF C	MCF Co	MCF C	MCF	
ID																						
Probesets	GSM20	GSM20	GSM20	GSM20	GSM20	GSM20	GSM20	GSM20	GSM20	GSM20	GSM20	GSM20	GSM20	GSM20	GSM20	GSM20	GSM20	GSM20	GSM20	GSM20	GSM2	EZ_
1007_s_at	9.214	9.329	9.464	9.554	9.214	9.23	9.037	9.187	9.336	9.512	9.388	9.422	9.55	9.503	9.282	9.65	9.594	10.26	10.09	10.39	10.6	780
1053_at	6.927	7.188	6.729	6.849	7.003	6.974	6.817	7.144	6.814	6.906	7.293	7.069	6.942	7.006	7	6.795	7.024	7.549	7.362	7.241	7.25	982
117_at	5.751	5.432	5.703	5.697	5.445	5.43	5.585	5.662	5.477	5.633	5.395	5.509	5.598	5.529	5.573	5.942	5.677	5.357	5.707	5.438	5.6	310
121_at	7.029	6.971	6.964	6.991	6.983	7.021	6.779	6.83	6.89	6.837	6.822	6.704	6.946	6.97	6.753	6.936	6.915	6.912	7.005	6.934	7.04	849
1255_g_at	4.386	4.186	4.254	4.26	4.284	4.175	4.254	4.292	4.346	4.346	4.222	4.335	4.288	4.169	4.253	4.347	4.347	4.284	4.503	4.401	4.18	978
1294_at	6.524	6.583	6.644	6.743	6.576	6.674	6.389	6.272	6.503	6.595	6.388	6.452	6.473	6.825	6.571	6.61	6.996	6.147	6.195	6.053	6.28	318
1316_at	5.827	5.636	5.683	5.784	5.795	5.651	5.671	5.41	5.758	5.602	5.429	5.617	5.825	5.799	5.696	5.857	5.551	5.621	5.728	5.644	5.79	067
1320_at	4.652	4.66	4.816	4.674	4.514	4.704	4.866	4.68	4.694	4.474	4.465	4.707	4.761	4.593	4.446	4.638	4.706	4.637	4.86	4.722	4.9	099
1405_i_at	4.364	4.758	3.925	4.326	4.446	3.843	3.963	4.122	4.242	4.364	4.352	4.626	4.684	4.753	5.183	4.849	4.804	3.693	3.679	3.485	4.68	352
1431_at	4.079	4.003	4.23	4.127	4.046	4.256	3.953	4.216	3.985	4.007	3.834	4.317	3.837	4.382	3.904	4.003	3.876	4.279	4.308	4.046	4.26	571
1438_at	5.583	5.751	5.914	6.038	5.096	5.328	5.258	5.506	5.6	5.912	5.646	5.696	5.739	5.561	5.196	5.472	5.878	5.572	5.214	5.614	6.13	049
1487_at	7.501	7.631	7.505	7.357	7.641	7.496	7.596	7.554	7.629	7.507	7.543	7.537	7.551	7.437	7.387	7.457	7.46	7.349	7.222	7.16	7.58	101
1494_f_at	5.21	5.157	5.34	4.765	5.105	4.909	4.935	4.892	4.964	4.989	4.826	4.829	5.335	4.789	4.927	5	5.054	5.184	5.104	5.02	4.95	548
1552256_a_at	6.832	7.183	6.881	6.42	7.306	7.337	6.932	7.105	6.568	6.399	6.683	6.7	6.614	6.667	6.907	6.787	6.939	7.545	7.376	7.654	8.21	949
1552257_a_at	7.651	7.966	7.637	7.51	7.715	7.618	7.554	7.848	7.54	7.505	7.422	7.471	7.533	7.411	7.568	7.599	7.611	7.622	7.671	7.881	7.91	170
1552258_at	4.69	4.587	4.737	4.459	4.596	4.473	4.626	4.463	4.491	4.466	4.592	4.799	4.729	4.625	4.37	4.519	4.656	4.84	4.69	4.781	4.9	597
1552261_at	5.245	5.172	5.537	5.248	5.367	5.411	5.11	5.305	5.187	5.209	5.198	5.151	5.442	5.161	5.055	5.388	5.379	5.092	5.264	5.448	5.41	406
1552263_at	4.409	4.139	4.18	4.219	4.471	3.91	4.093	4.174	4.469	4.253	4.079	4.283	4.217	4.555	4.258	4.418	4.027	4.267	4.699	4.507	4.76	594
1552264_a_at	5.988	6.145	5.869	5.653	5.718	6.006	5.872	5.89	5.618	5.834	6.091	5.66	5.894	5.767	5.755	5.924	6.077	6.583	6.366	6.43	6.3	594
1552266_at	4.479	4.279	4.015	4.166	4.332	4.288	4.381	4.243	4.422	4.092	4.011	4.153	3.983	4.41	4.165	4.457	4.372	4.521	4.511	4.641	4.42	102
1552269_at	4.43	4.198	4.396	5.33	4.474	4.47	5.013	4.712	5.377	6.118	6.244	6.308	6.541	6.031	6.238	6.178	5.607	5.454	5.497	5.255	5.58	153
1552271_at	5.557	5.565	5.637	5.49	5.452	5.76	5.518	5.584	5.577	5.735	5.611	5.609	5.588	5.72	5.365	5.676	5.554	5.523	5.672	5.475	5.5	154
1552272_a_at	5.113	5.072	5.151	4.826	5.194	5.299	5.086	4.856	4.874	4.947	5.048	5.015	5.208	4.87	5.315	5.103	5.337	5.116	5.089	5.213	5.16	154
1552274_at	4.985	4.931	4.855	4.977	4.507	4.761	5.29	4.706	4.689	5.513	5.239	5.203	5.394	4.649	5.431	4.763	5.019	4.807	4.407	4.756	4.82	899
1552275_s_at	4.81	4.859	4.838	4.505	4.582	4.646	4.457	4.547	4.859	4.54	4.746	4.618	4.678	4.626	4.48	4.64	4.862	4.488	4.705	4.741	4.63	899
1552276_a_at	5.596	5.704	5.903	5.856	5.675	5.941	5.972	5.746	5.832	5.985	5.551	5.738	5.798	5.811	5.897	5.68	5.777	5.465	5.685	5.562	5.32	617
1552277_a_at	7.564	7.772	7.502	6.972	7.464	7.358	6.891	7.298	6.942	6.902	7.263	7.095	7.117	6.832	7.003	6.871	6.946	6.781	6.584	6.576	6.86	283
1552278_a_at	5.006	4.866	4.917	4.976	5.129	4.779	4.732	4.73	4.619	4.887	4.825	5.019	4.945	4.605	4.843	4.867	5.031	4.757	4.923	4.875	4.83	235
1552279_a_at	5.943	5.97	6.057	5.911	5.68	5.834	5.782	5.815	6.055	5.985	5.809	5.902	6.212	5.765	5.91	6.111	5.938	5.494	5.763	5.615	5.59	235
1552280_at	3.838	4.083	3.973	4.119	4.057	4.17	3.94	4.021	4.063	4.039	3.898	4.084	4.395	4.056	3.776	4.014	4.269	3.894	4.08	4.083	3.85	937
1552281_at	6.365	6.231	6.454	6.383	6.321	6.393	6.392	6.276	6.458	6.114	6.302	6.368	6.306	6.295	6.448	6.323	6.458	6.264	6.529	6.475	6.28	375
1552283_s_at	4.708	4.376	4.476	4.478	4.411	4.33	4.405	4.456	4.723	4.389	4.322	4.288	4.278	4.55	4.646	4.446	4.29	4.145	4.489	4.134	4.17	844
1552286_at	5.95	5.352	5.566	5.632	5.982	5.645	6.108	5.679	5.962	5.623	5.309	5.659	5.673	5.524	5.799	5.82	5.759	5.832	6.18	5.879	5.94	423
1552287_s_at	7.251	7.196	7.072	6.766	7.467	6.958	7.363	7.201	7.041	6.867	7.308	7.636	7.591	7.222	7.259	6.903	7.499	7.813	7.52	7.945	8.15	172
1552288_at	4.607	4.766	4.65	4.557	4.63	4.86	4.257	4.543	4.574	4.557	4.597	4.193	4.314	4.723	4.426	4.447	4.611	4.734	4.771	4.731	4.48	113
1552289_a_at	4.677	4.607	4.941	4.65	4.703	4.817	5.005	4.97	4.526	4.722	4.519	5.046	4.918	4.878	4.757	4.963	5.132	4.575	4.81	4.566	4.54	113
1552291_at	6.42	6.322	6.013	6.333	6.572	6.31	6.198	6.371	6.581	6.365	6.739	6.555	6.331	6.525	6.886	6.38	6.172	6.417	6.429	6.511	6.46	965
1552293_at	5.073	4.843	5.003	4.732	4.86	4.891	4.967	4.91	5.104	5.016	4.661	4.724	4.844	4.878	5.015	5.111	4.868	4.956	5.142	5.043	5.23	130

3

Fig. 3 Microarray analysis output. A spreadsheet of raw data is on the *left*, a color diagram representation on the *right*

analysis approaches leveraging the enormous amount of publicly available data [15].

Microarrays in Skin Biology

Because of its accessibility, the skin was one of the first tissues analyzed using "omics" and dermatology one of the first medical disciplines to embrace the approach. Omics methodology has made great progress: (1) genome-wide association studies, (2) transcriptional profiling, and (3) the microbiome. These have been used to identify and describe disease markers and even follow the course of treatment of skin diseases. Melanomas, basal and squamous cell carcinomas psoriasis, keloid formation, etc. have been intensely investigated using gene profiling. Unlike any other medical specialty, dermatology allows for noninvasive and easy tissue sampling using tape stripping, based on early work of Morhenn et al. [16] and developed by Dr. Benson and collaborators at DermTech International. It was demonstrated that simple tape stripping provides adequate quality and quantity of RNA samples, useful in analysis of psoriasis and in melanoma transcriptomes [17, 18]. Dermatology promises to lead advance toward "omics" techniques directly applied to personalized medicine.

On the other hand, patient's skin samples have problems relating to differences in proportions of various cell types, age and body sites of the sample origin, and other issues difficult to standardize, such as history of sun exposure, lifestyle, nutrition, presence of underlying disease, etc. [19].

One of the most active fields of skinomics involves epidermal stem cells, pioneered by Dr. E. Fuchs and her coworkers [20]. Dr. Vogel's team at the N.I.H. used laser capture to compare the transcriptomes of human stem cells with the neighboring keratinocytes, identifying several novel stem cell markers. In the epidermis, when the basal cells were separated from suprabasal ones, the specific transcriptional program of epidermal differentiation was defined. These studies identified novel markers of epidermal differentiation and indicated the signaling mechanisms involved in this process.

Because epidermal keratinocytes are programmed to respond to a very wide variety of physical, chemical, and biological influences, epidermal keratinocytes have been a popular target for related studies. DNA microarrays have been used to define the transcriptional responses of epidermal keratinocytes to UV light, hormones, vitamins, inflammatory and immunomodulating cytokines, toxins, and physical injury [21–24]. Our team focused on the transcriptional effects of proinflammatory and immunomodulatory cytokines and growth factors, such as IL-1, IL-12, IFNγ, TNFα, TGFβ, oncostatin M, etc. [25–29].

Skinomics Genome-Wide Association Studies

Genome-wide association studies, GWAS, comprise examination of many common single-nucleotide polymorphisms to see if any are associated with a given disease. They compare the DNA of people with the disease with controls to determine if any of the polymorphisms are statistically associated with the disease. Such polymorphisms can serve as powerful pointers to the DNA region where the disease-causing mutations map. The approach relies on the Human Genome Project and the International HapMap Project, which include computerized databases that contain the map of human genetic polymorphisms and methodologies to analyze quickly and accurately the potential associations between the polymorphisms and a disease. An archive of GWAS data is available through an NCBI Web site at: http://www.ncbi.nlm.nih.gov/entrez/query.fcgi?db=gap. GWAS are particularly useful in the analysis of common but multifactorial diseases with a strong genetic component, such as psoriasis.

Psoriasis, a common, hyperproliferative autoimmune skin disease, affects approximately 2 % of the population and involves keratinocytes and T cells; it has both genetic and environmental causes [30]. A paradigm of successful GWAS has been the tour-de-force success of skinomics microarray analysis of the psoriasis susceptibility loci, accomplished by a multinational effort from many countries (Fig. 4) and reported in an elegant

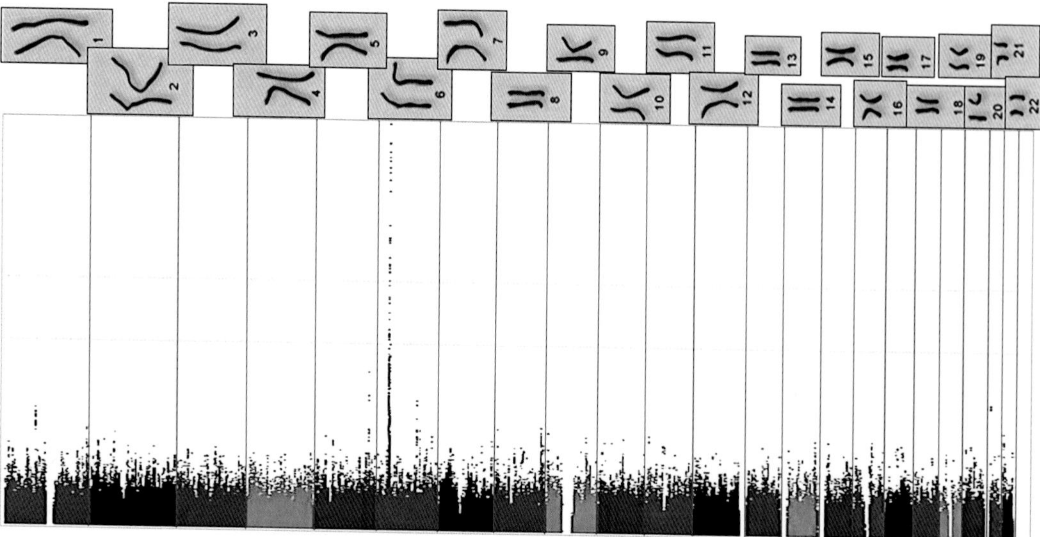

Fig. 4 GWAS results for psoriasis susceptibility loci. The complement of human chromosomes is shown on the *top*, with the known psoriasis susceptibility loci associated with their chromosomes on the *bottom*. The *dots* above the background show association of psoriasis with a DNA polymorphism at the mapped locus. Note the particularly high association with the HLA locus on chromosome 6, but also additional associations, e.g., on chromosomes 1 and 5

series or interrelated manuscripts [31–38]. More recently, additional loci have been identified [39, 40], bringing the total to 36 loci associated with psoriasis in European individuals, with additional ones in the Chinese populations. Other skin diseases have also received considerable GWAS attention. Specifically, eczema was followed in a study including 5,600 cases and 20,500 controls. Several loci were associated with this disease, including MHC on chromosome 6 and epidermal differentiation complex (EDC) on chromosome 1, which includes the filaggrin gene.

Carcinomas and melanoma were also analyzed using GWAS. For example, basal and squamous cell carcinomas have both common and individual susceptibility loci [41]; these are not associated with melanoma risks. GWAS also identified several loci important for skin pigmentation [42].

Skinomics of the Cutaneous Microbiome

Perhaps the most exciting new frontier in skinomics is the analysis of the skin microbiome pioneered by Dr. Blaser at NYU Langone Medical Center and Dr. Segre at the NIH. The human skin is populated by a wide variety of microorganisms, bacterial, viral, and fungal, mostly commensal, many beneficial, and a few pathogens. Because vast majority of skin-resident microorganisms have never been cultured, the NYU and NIH groups used the next-generation sequencing of the ribosomal RNAs to identify the skin-resident bacteria [43, 44]. The skin on our forearm contains some 300 different bacteria, predominantly Actinobacteria, Proteobacteria, and Firmicutes (Fig. 5). Importantly, the microbiomes differ between healthy and psoriatic epidermis, the overall microbial diversity apparently reduced in psoriatics [45, 46]. The microbiomes from different human body sites can be characterized as “dry,” “wet,” and “oily” [47].

Transcriptomic Profiling Studies in the Skin

Transcriptomics are the studies of the complete set of RNA transcripts expressed in a specific tissue, using either microarray analysis or, more recently, next-generation sequencing. Comparison of

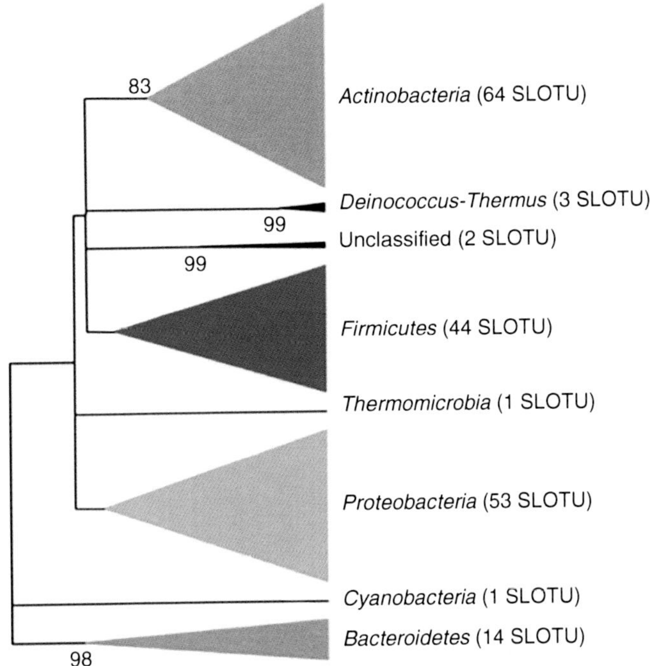

Fig. 5 Microbiome of the human skin. The bacterial microbiome is dominated by three phyla

transcriptomes allows the identification of genes that are differentially expressed, e.g., in young versus aged skin, as described below.

The transcriptional profiling in psoriasis is led by Dr. Krueger and collaborators at Rockefeller U., who studied the activation of T cells, integrated the molecular effects of several cytokines, correlated the transcriptional and genetic data, and used skinomics to follow the effects of treatment in psoriatic patients [48–52]. In two large independent studies, the groups of Drs. Krueger and Gudjonsson (U. Michigan) compared the transcriptomes of 350 (!) biopsies of healthy, lesional, and non-lesional psoriasis samples [53, 54]. The availability of such a large data collection led to meta-analysis of the psoriatic transcriptome [55]. As mentioned, noninvasive skin sampling has been applied to psoriasis [17], and interestingly, psoriasis-associated markers can be also found in the serum of patients [54].

Several cytokines and growth factors have been linked with psoriasis, including IL-1, IL-12, TNFα, interferon-γ, and oncostatin M, and the effects of these signaling proteins on epidermal keratinocytes in culture have been extensively studied [25–29, 51, 56]. The transcriptional profiling studies focused on the effects of anti-inflammatory agents, corticosteroids, revealed that in addition to the known inhibitory effects on TNFa and IL-1, corticosteroids also block activation of IFN-γ pathway [23]. Furthermore, the anti-inflammatory effects of corticosteroids have timed responses: anti-TNFα is the earliest (first hour), followed by anti-IL1 (24–48 h) and anti-IFN-γ (72 h).

Eczema and psoriasis were compared using microarrays in a series of studies, which showed that the expression of many antimicrobial proteins of the innate immune response genes is decreased in eczema compared with psoriasis [57–61]. These results could explain the increased susceptibility to infection in eczematous skin.

Because of its lethalness, melanoma was included in one of the earliest microarray studies of transcriptomes of human neoplasms, merely 1 year after the first report of cDNA microarrays [5, 62]. Melanoma diagnosis and its natural history have received a great amount of attention by the microarray researchers [62–73]. Several groups used laser capture microdissection to compare the transcriptomes of pigmented moles, primary melanomas and melanoma metastases

[65]. More recently, epigenetic characteristics of melanomas, including the differences in the DNA genome [74] and its methylation [75, 76], came into focus. Several research groups addressed the role of miRNAs in melanoma comparing samples from melanoblasts, melanocytes, congenital nevi, and acral, mucosal, cutaneous, and uveal melanomas to detect 539 known miRNAs and predicted 279 novel miRNA candidates [77–79]. The wealth of skinomics data relevant to melanoma enabled meta-analysis approaches consolidating results from many studies [80–82] and identified a "melanoma signature" gene sets [83].

Another currently very active area of skinomics research concerns wound healing [84–86]. A complex, multistep process involving highly coordinated, interacting regulatory pathways, wound healing is well suited for study using microarray technology [84]. For example, we have shown that microarrays can be utilized to guide surgical debridement of nonhealing wounds [19]. Specifically, the healing edges of ulcers express keratinocyte markers, such as KRT16 and KRT17, filaggrin, and SPRR psoriasin, whereas the nonhealing ones express specifically dermal and inflammatory markers [87]. Chronic venous ulcers and diabetic foot ulcers have different transcriptional profiles [87, 88]. Infection represents a significant danger in nonhealing wounds, and therefore, the microbiomes of chronic wounds and wound healing have also been examined [89].

The epidermis being our first line of defense from ultraviolet light, its responses to UV have been the focus of extensive studies [22, 90–95]. Keratinocytes in response to UV induce a cell repair program and also act to protect the underlying organism (Fig. 6). Importantly, the results from several laboratories were highly congruent, despite the differences in experimental conditions. Using DNA sequencing technologies, it was shown that the mutations in the p53 tumor suppressor gene are very frequent in sun-exposed human skin [96].

Currently, the microarray studies in skin biology and dermatology are expanding to deal with

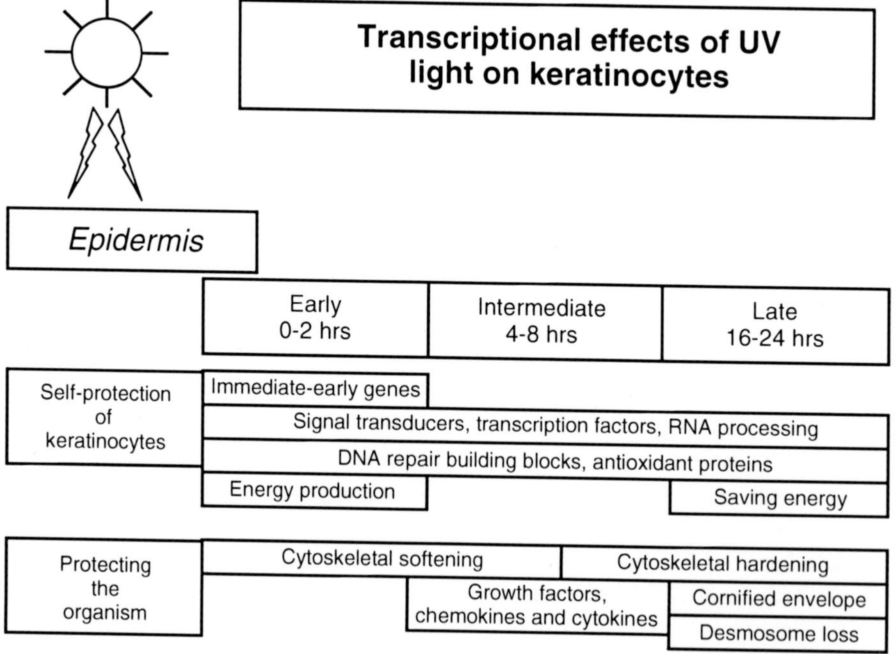

Fig. 6 Skinomics studies of the molecular effects of UV light on human epidermal keratinocytes. The keratinocytes protect themselves, as well as the underlying tissues, and alert the organism to the damage

many other diseases including alopecia [97], vitiligo [98], cutaneous T-cell lymphoma (CTCL) [99], Merkel cell carcinoma [100, 101], etc.

Omics Studies of Aging (Not in the Skin)

Currently, the omics studies of aging are proceeding in several directions (including extensively in analysis of skin aging; see below). This topic has been reviewed [102, 103]. The methodology of using microarrays in studies of aging has been described [104], and even specific conferences on the microarrays in aging have been convened [105]. Several animal models of aging exist and bioinformatic comparisons have been made among them [106]. This analysis identified shared regulation patterns across orthologous genes. Even two highly diverged animals, the nematode *Caenorhabditis elegans* and the fruit fly *Drosophila melanogaster*, share age-associated regulation of genes involved in mitochondrial metabolism, DNA repair, catabolism, etc. The National Institute on Aging has established a dedicated Aging Microarray Facility [107], and interested researchers have established a specific database and data mining platform "Gene Aging Nexus" (GAN), set aside specifically for the studies of aging accessible at http://gan.usc.edu [108].

Omics of aging has been studied in several organs and tissues other than the skin. For example, the aging in the brain has received significant attention due to focus on Alzheimer's disease and other age-related neurological infirmities identifying genes and biological processes common to Alzheimer's disease and chronological aging [109]. Postmortem studies associated age-related changes in the brain to hypoxia [110]. Musculoskeletal system aging has also been explored [111–114].

Particularly useful have been omics studies of progeria, a rare genetic mutation causing symptoms of aging being manifested at an early age in multiple organs. Comparisons of transcription profiles in fibroblasts from progeria patients with fibroblasts from young, middle-aged, and elderly donors clearly indicated that progeria resembles accelerated aging at the molecular level [115]. On the other hand, cellular senescence, studied in cells in vitro, while recapitulating several aspects of chronological aging, was associated with certain notable differences, indicating that senescence is not the same as aging [116, 117]. Cellular senescence has been specifically addressed in keratinocytes [118]. Comparison of epidermal and oral human keratinocytes, serially passaged to induce senescence, using an array of over 3,000 genes, revealed 37 and 55 differentially expressed genes, of which 16 genes were common to the two cell types. Interestingly, dysbiosis, an imbalance or disruption of the healthy, normal microbiome in humans, is also associated with aging, which may open new avenues to treatment of the symptoms of aging by using probiotics agents [119].

The above studies have identified several molecular mechanisms that seem to play important roles in the aging process. Prominent among these is the Wnt signaling pathway, which has been found induced during aging in several tissues, including the skin, but also in muscle and in blood vessels [120]. Two transcription factors apparently play a role in aging, and their inhibition may slow down or potentially reverse the aging process; these are the NFkB and the BACH2 transcription factors [121, 122]. Large dataset of age-related omics studies made possible initial meta-analysis studies as well [123]. Age-related gene expression changes tend to involve overexpression of inflammation and immune response genes and underexpression of genes associated with energy metabolism, particularly mitochondrial genes; importantly for the aging of the skin, collagen genes are generally underexpressed [124].

Human Skinomics Studies of Aging Using Microarrays

The skin is, of course, the most obvious sentinel, display, and gauge of aging. The features, symptoms, and potential treatments have been extensively examined, and we note several recent reviews [125–127]. The skinomics approaches to the skin, i.e., the use of transcriptional profiling to compare youthful and aged skin, illuminated and clarified important molecular aspects of the process. Importantly, the large number of different studies, using different conceptual approaches, different subject populations, and different methodologies, arrived at a fairly congruent, overlapping set of genes and ontological processes associated with skin aging. The consistent results are due to the fact that the basic process of aging seems common to all or most cells [128]. The use of microarray gene chip technology led to translational application of pharmacogenomics to develop framework of metabolic pathways in the skin with a potential to modulate therapeutic efficacy of treatments for aging [129]. Molecular comparisons of transcriptional profiles of young versus aged and sunprotected versus sunexposed skin indicate that photoaging and chronical aging, while overlapping to a large extent, also show characteristic features. The effects common to photoaging and chronological aging tend to be more severe in photoaging [130].

The early studies of gene expression in aging and photoaging [131] received a significant boost with the advent of omics techniques. Specifically, serial analysis of gene expression was used to compare preauricular and postauricular skin, representatives of photoaged and sun-protected skin, which identified several photoaging-associated genes [132]. Using microarrays containing over 2,000 genes to compare patterns of gene expression in naturally aged skin of 3–4-year-olds with that of 68–72-year-olds, it was found that approximately 5 % of the genes are differentially expressed [133]. The regulated genes are associated with cell cycle, inflammation, metabolism, and the cytoskeleton. Complementing the transcriptional arrays that measure RNAs, the proteomic profiling using two-dimensional gel electrophoresis, again comparing young and old foreskin samples, identified additional markers of intrinsic aging, including aging-related posttranslational modified proteins [134].

Photoaging was analyzed by comparing pre- and postauricular skin in Chinese population using large-capacity Illumina microarrays that cover, essentially, the entire human protein-coding genome [135]. This substantially more comprehensive approach identified over 1,600 differentially expressed genes. Ontological analysis showed that in the sunexposed skin the TGF-beta signaling pathway and extracellular matrix receptor interaction are induced, while the metabolic enzymes are suppressed.

Several research laboratories, ours included, have used microarrays to define the in vitro transcriptional effects of UV light on epidermal keratinocytes [22, 90, 93]. The lists of UV-regulated genes were remarkably congruent in all studies, considering the differences in experimental approaches and sampling times between different laboratories. Unexpectedly, like in the parable of the blind men and the elephant, different researchers emphasized different aspects of the results: we focused on the metabolic effects and epidermal differentiation, Sesto et al. on DNA repair, Murakami et al. on oncogenes, while Howell et al. on angiogenesis [22, 90, 93]. In keratinocytes exposed to γ-irradiation or X-rays, the transcriptional changes were similar to those in the UV-treated cells; specifically, the genes involved in energy metabolism were induced [136, 137]. These in vitro studies led to in vivo microarray analysis of UV-irradiated skin of human volunteers [94, 95].

Focusing on the effects of long-wave ultraviolet, UVA, on miRNA expression in dermal fibroblasts, it was found that photoaging is associated with five upregulated and seven downregulated miRNAs [138]. The predicted targets of the miRNAs were associated with cancer-related pathways, and the TGFb pathway may be specifically targeted.

A very interesting study compared in vivo samples of lentigines with adjacent sun-exposed skin and matched samples of sun-protected buttocks skin [139]. Sixty-five genes were specifically upregulated in solar lentigo, including melanocyte-related genes, as well as genes related to fatty acid metabolism, and genes related to inflammation.

Besides UV light, hormones are known to play a crucial role in skin aging. Indeed, the skin is known to produce and metabolize steroids [140], which can affect the rate of intrinsic skin aging.

One of the major hormonal influences on skin aging is estrogen. For example, it was found that in Chinese women, some 240 genes were significantly related to estrogen-associated intrinsic skin aging [141]. Specifically in sebocytes, hormonal influences seem important, and the comparison of these cells grown in vitro under culture conditions approximating young versus aged hormonal levels identified closely to a 1,000 differentially expressed genes [142]. These genes are related to cell cycle, oxidative stress, mitochondrial function, proteolysis, immune responses, and steroid biosynthesis, processes characteristics of aging.

Impaired wound healing is one of the hallmarks of aging. Using Affymetrix microarrays to compare gene expression between male elderly versus young human wounds, it was found that the differences are to a large degree related to regulation by estrogen. Over 80 % of genes found differentially expressed in aged skin were regulated by estrogen [143]. These results suggest that in the context of wound healing, and perhaps aging in general, estrogen has a more profound influence than previously thought.

Graying is another hallmark of aging and an analysis of differential gene expressions between pigmented, gray, and white human scalp skin hair follicles identified close to 200 upregulated genes and as many downregulated in gray hair. As expected, melanogenesis melanosome structure genes are overrepresented; genes associated with energy metabolism were also altered [144].

Pharmacological interventions for aging skin have been studied using skinomics approaches. For example, *Terminalia arjuna* bark extract, containing pentacyclic triterpenoids, improves the appearance of aging skin, and its effects were demonstrated using microarray analysis [145]. Similarly, equol, a polyphenolic isoflavonoid, regulated expression of extracellular matrix proteins and inflammatory genes [146].

In addition to transcriptional profiling, skinomics studies of aging include epigenetic analyses, such as DNA methylation, but exploration of epigenetics of aging is in its infancy [147] and, to our knowledge, has not been reported relating to aging. Epigenetic changes may constitute an important, if barely beginning to be explored, component of aging.

Murine models are not suitable for studies of skin aging because in mice the principal protective layer is their hair and not the epidermis. However, dietary collagen hydrolysate, hypothesized to improve skin barrier function, did cause significant cutaneous changes with 135 upregulated and 448 downregulated genes [148].

Murine models of organismal aging have made great progress in understanding of the aging process. It was shown, for example, that "heterochronic parabionts" in which the circulatory systems of young and aged animals are directly connected can alleviate effects of brain aging in the older animals at the molecular and cognitive level [149]. The mechanism may include, in part, activation of the CREB transcription factor in the aged hippocampus. Murine models using microarrays also demonstrated life and healthspanextending effects of caloric restriction [150]. Caloric restriction shifted the genomic profile of old control mice toward the "slow-aging" profile.

Conclusions

In summary, great strides have been achieved in omics technology and especially in skinomics, as the technology is applied in dermatology and skin biology. Application of skinomics to the process of aging is already making significant progress. We can expect, in the near future, to understand the skin aging process much better, to a greater detail as well as in whole, both the trees and the forest, which should lead to novel, better targeted therapies. Skinomics techniques will eventually lead to individualized treatments and to personalized medicine for our aging patients. Great and wonderful times are ahead.

References

1. Brown SM. Bioinformatics becomes respectable. Biotechniques. 2003;34(6):1124–7.

2. Hubbard T. Biological information: making it accessible and integrated (and trying to make sense of it). Bioinformatics. 2002;18 Suppl 2:S140.
3. Reimers M, Carey VJ. Bioconductor: an open source framework for bioinformatics and computational biology. Methods Enzymol. 2006;411:119–34.
4. Kouskoumvekaki I, Shublaq N, Brunak S. Facilitating the use of large-scale biological data and tools in the era of translational bioinformatics. Brief Bioinform. 2013;1:1.
5. Schena M, Shalon D, Davis RW, Brown PO. Quantitative monitoring of gene expression patterns with a complementary DNA microarray. Science. 1995;270(5235):467–70.
6. Iyer VR, Eisen MB, Ross DT, Schuler G, Moore T, Lee JC, Trent JM, Staudt LM, Hudson Jr J, Boguski MS, Lashkari D, Shalon D, Botstein D, Brown PO. The transcriptional program in the response of human fibroblasts to serum. Science. 1999;283 (5398):83–7.
7. Noh M, Yeo H, Ko J, Kim HK, Lee CH. MAP17 is associated with the T-helper cell cytokine-induced down-regulation of filaggrin transcription in human keratinocytes. Exp Dermatol. 2010;19(4):355–62. Epub 2009 Jul 8.
8. Bilitewski U. DNA microarrays: an introduction to the technology. Methods Mol Biol. 2009;509:1–14. doi:10.1007/978-1-59745-372-1_1.
9. Auer H, Newsom DL, Kornacker K. Expression profiling using affymetrix GeneChip microarrays. Methods Mol Biol. 2009;509:35–46. doi:10.1007/978-1-59745-372-1_3.
10. Dong Z, Chen Y. Transcriptomics: advances and approaches. Sci China Life Sci. 2013;56(10):960–7. doi:10.1007/s11427-013-4557-2. Epub 2013 Oct 5.
11. Mimoso C, Lee DD, Zavadil J, Tomic-Canic M, Blumenberg M. Analysis and meta-analysis of transcriptional profiling in human epidermis. Methods Mol Biol. 2014;1195:61–97. doi:10.1007/7651_2013_60.
12. Blumenberg M. Skinomics: past, present and future for diagnostic microarray studies in dermatology. Expert Rev Mol Diagn. 2013;13(8):885–94. doi:10.1586/14737159.2013.846827.
13. Lee DD, Zavadil J, Tomic-Canic M, Blumenberg M. Comprehensive transcriptional profiling of human epidermis, reconstituted epidermal equivalents, and cultured keratinocytes using DNA microarray chips. Methods Mol Biol. 2010;585:193–223.
14. Barrett T, Suzek TO, Troup DB, Wilhite SE, Ngau WC, Ledoux P, Rudnev D, Lash AE, Fujibuchi W, Edgar R. NCBI GEO: mining millions of expression profiles – database and tools. Nucleic Acids Res. 2005;33(Database issue):D562–6.
15. Irizarry RA, Warren D, Spencer F, Kim IF, Biswal S, Frank BC, Gabrielson E, Garcia JG, Geoghegan J, Germino G, Griffin C, Hilmer SC, Hoffman E, Jedlicka AE, Kawasaki E, Martinez-Murillo F, Morsberger L, Lee H, Petersen D, Quackenbush J, Scott A, Wilson M, Yang Y, Ye SQ, Yu W. Multiple-laboratory comparison of microarray platforms. Nat Methods. 2005;2(5):345–50. Epub 2005 Apr 21.
16. Morhenn VB, Chang EY, Rheins LA. A noninvasive method for quantifying and distinguishing inflammatory skin reactions. J Am Acad Dermatol. 1999;41 (5 Pt 1):687–92.
17. Benson NR, Papenfuss J, Wong R, Motaal A, Tran V, Panko J, Krueger GG. An analysis of select pathogenic messages in lesional and non-lesional psoriatic skin using non-invasive tape harvesting. J Invest Dermatol. 2006;126(10):2234–41. Epub 006 Jun 1.
18. Wachsman W, Morhenn V, Palmer T, Walls L, Hata T, Zalla J, Scheinberg R, Sofen H, Mraz S, Gross K, Rabinovitz H, Polsky D, Chang S. Noninvasive genomic detection of melanoma. Br J Dermatol. 2011;164 (4):797–806. doi:10.1111/j.365-2133.011.10239.x. Epub 2011 Mar 25.
19. Brem H, Stojadinovic O, Diegelmann RF, Entero H, Lee B, Pastar I, Golinko M, Rosenberg H, Tomic-Canic M. Molecular markers in patients with chronic wounds to guide surgical debridement. Mol Med. 2007;13(1–2):30–9.
20. Kaufman CK, Zhou P, Pasolli HA, Rendl M, Bolotin D, Lim KC, Dai X, Alegre ML, Fuchs E, Sinha S, Fan J. GATA-3: an unexpected regulator of cell lineage determination in skin dissection of a complex enhancer element: maintenance of keratinocyte specificity but loss of differentiation specificity. Genes Dev. 2003;17(17):2108–22. Epub 003 Aug 15.
21. Lee DD, Stojadinovic O, Krzyzanowska A, Vouthounis C, Blumenberg M, Tomic-Canic M. Retinoid-responsive transcriptional changes in epidermal keratinocytes. J Cell Physiol. 2009;220 (2):427–39.
22. Li D, Turi TG, Schuck A, Freedberg IM, Khitrov G, Blumenberg M. Rays and arrays: the transcriptional program in the response of human epidermal keratinocytes to UVB illumination. FASEB J. 2001;15(13):2533–5.
23. Stojadinovic O, Lee B, Vouthounis C, Vukelic S, Pastar I, Blumenberg M, Brem H, Tomic-Canic M. Novel genomic effects of glucocorticoids in epidermal keratinocytes: inhibition of apoptosis, interferon-gamma pathway, and wound healing along with promotion of terminal differentiation. J Biol Chem. 2007;282(6):4021–34. Epub 2006 Nov 9.
24. Tomic-Canic M, Stojadinovic O, Lee B, Walsh R, Blumenberg M. Nexus between epidermolysis bullosa and transcriptional regulation by thyroid hormone in epidermal keratinocytes. Clin Transl Sci. 2008;1(1):45–9.
25. Banno T, Adachi M, Mukkamala L, Blumenberg M. Unique keratinocyte-specific effects of interferon-gamma that protect skin from viruses, identified using transcriptional profiling. Antivir Ther. 2003;8(6):541–54.
26. Banno T, Gazel A, Blumenberg M. Effects of tumor necrosis factor-alpha (TNF alpha) in epidermal

keratinocytes revealed using global transcriptional profiling. J Biol Chem. 2004;279(31):32633–42. Epub 2004 May 15.

27. Finelt N, Gazel A, Gorelick S, Blumenberg M. Transcriptional responses of human epidermal keratinocytes to Oncostatin-M. Cytokine. 2005;31 (4):305–13.
28. Gazel A, Rosdy M, Bertino B, Tornier C, Sahuc F, Blumenberg M. A characteristic subset of psoriasis-associated genes is induced by oncostatin-M in reconstituted epidermis. J Invest Dermatol. 2006;17:17.
29. Molenda M, Mukkamala L, Blumenberg M. Interleukin IL-12 blocks a specific subset of the transcriptional profile responsive to UVB in epidermal keratinocytes. Mol Immunol. 2006;43 (12):1933–40. Epub 2006 Feb 8.
30. Bowcock AM, Krueger JG. Getting under the skin: the immunogenetics of psoriasis. Nat Rev Immunol. 2005;5(9):699–711.
31. Nair RP, Duffin KC, Helms C, Ding J, Stuart PE, Goldgar D, Gudjonsson JE, Li Y, Tejasvi T, Feng BJ, Ruether A, Schreiber S, Weichenthal M, Gladman D, Rahman P, Schrodi SJ, Prahalad S, Guthery SL, Fischer J, Liao W, Kwok PY, Menter A, Lathrop GM, Wise CA, Begovich AB, Voorhees JJ, Elder JT, Krueger GG, Bowcock AM, Abecasis GR. Genome-wide scan reveals association of psoriasis with IL-23 and NF-kappaB pathways. Nat Genet. 2009;41(2):199–204. Epub 2009 Jan 25.
32. Zhang XJ, Huang W, Yang S, Sun LD, Zhang FY, Zhu QX, Zhang FR, Zhang C, Du WH, Pu XM, Li H, Xiao FL, Wang ZX, Cui Y, Hao F, Zheng J, Yang XQ, Cheng H, He CD, Liu XM, Xu LM, Zheng HF, Zhang SM, Zhang JZ, Wang HY, Cheng YL, Ji BH, Fang QY, Li YZ, Zhou FS, Han JW, Quan C, Chen B, Liu JL, Lin D, Fan L, Zhang AP, Liu SX, Yang CJ, Wang PG, Zhou WM, Lin GS, Wu WD, Fan X, Gao M, Yang BQ, Lu WS, Zhang Z, Zhu KJ, Shen SK, Li M, Zhang XY, Cao TT, Ren W, Zhang X, He J, Tang XF, Lu S, Yang JQ, Zhang L, Wang DN, Yuan F, Yin XY, Huang HJ, Wang HF, Lin XY, Liu JJ. Psoriasis genome-wide association study identifies susceptibility variants within LCE gene cluster at 1q21. Nat Genet. 2009;41(2):205–10. doi:10.1038/ng.310. Epub 2009 Jan 25.
33. de Cid R, Riveira-Munoz E, Zeeuwen PL, Robarge J, Liao W, Dannhauser EN, Giardina E, Stuart PE, Nair R, Helms C, Escaramis G, Ballana E, Martin-Ezquerra G, den Heijer M, Kamsteeg M, Joosten I, Eichler EE, Lazaro C, Pujol RM, Armengol L, Abecasis G, Elder JT, Novelli G, Armour JA, Kwok PY, Bowcock A, Schalkwijk J, Estivill X. Deletion of the late cornified envelope LCE3B and LCE3C genes as a susceptibility factor for psoriasis. Nat Genet. 2009;41(2):211–5. Epub 2009 Jan 25.
34. Strange A, Capon F, Spencer CC, Knight J, Weale ME, Allen MH, Barton A, Band G, Bellenguez C, Bergboer JG, Blackwell JM, Bramon E, Bumpstead SJ, Casas JP, Cork MJ, Corvin A, Deloukas P, Dilthey A, Duncanson A, Edkins S, Estivill X, Fitzgerald O, Freeman C, Giardina E, Gray E, Hofer A, Huffmeier U, Hunt SE, Irvine AD, Jankowski J, Kirby B, Langford C, Lascorz J, Leman J, Leslie S, Mallbris L, Markus HS, Mathew CG, McLean WH, McManus R, Mossner R, Moutsianas L, Naluai AT, Nestle FO, Novelli G, Onoufriadis A, Palmer CN, Perricone C, Pirinen M, Plomin R, Potter SC, Pujol RM, Rautanen A, Riveira-Munoz E, Ryan AW, Salmhofer W, Samuelsson L, Sawcer SJ, Schalkwijk J, Smith CH, Stahle M, Su Z, Tazi-Ahnini R, Traupe H, Viswanathan AC, Warren RB, Weger W, Wolk K, Wood N, Worthington J, Young HS, Zeeuwen PL, Hayday A, Burden AD, Griffiths CE, Kere J, Reis A, McVean G, Evans DM, Brown MA, Barker JN, Peltonen L, Donnelly P, Trembath RC. A genome-wide association study identifies new psoriasis susceptibility loci and an interaction between HLA-C and ERAP1. Nat Genet. 2010;42(11):985–90. Epub 2010 Oct 17.
35. Stuart PE, Nair RP, Ellinghaus E, Ding J, Tejasvi T, Gudjonsson JE, Li Y, Weidinger S, Eberlein B, Gieger C, Wichmann HE, Kunz M, Ike R, Krueger GG, Bowcock AM, Mrowietz U, Lim HW, Voorhees JJ, Abecasis GR, Weichenthal M, Franke A, Rahman P, Gladman DD, Elder JT. Genome-wide association analysis identifies three psoriasis susceptibility loci. Nat Genet. 2010;42(11):1000–4. Epub 2010 Oct 17.
36. Ellinghaus E, Ellinghaus D, Stuart PE, Nair RP, Debrus S, Raelson JV, Belouchi M, Fournier H, Reinhard C, Ding J, Li Y, Tejasvi T, Gudjonsson J, Stoll SW, Voorhees JJ, Lambert S, Weidinger S, Eberlein B, Kunz M, Rahman P, Gladman DD, Gieger C, Wichmann HE, Karlsen TH, Mayr G, Albrecht M, Kabelitz D, Mrowietz U, Abecasis GR, Elder JT, Schreiber S, Weichenthal M, Franke A. Genome-wide association study identifies a psoriasis susceptibility locus at TRAF3IP2. Nat Genet. 2010;42(11):991–5. Epub 2010 Oct 17.
37. Sun LD, Cheng H, Wang ZX, Zhang AP, Wang PG, Xu JH, Zhu QX, Zhou HS, Ellinghaus E, Zhang FR, Pu XM, Yang XQ, Zhang JZ, Xu AE, Wu RN, Xu LM, Peng L, Helms CA, Ren YQ, Zhang C, Zhang SM, Nair RP, Wang HY, Lin GS, Stuart PE, Fan X, Chen G, Tejasvi T, Li P, Zhu J, Li ZM, Ge HM, Weichenthal M, Ye WZ, Shen SK, Yang BQ, Sun YY, Li SS, Lin Y, Jiang JH, Li CT, Chen RX, Cheng J, Jiang X, Zhang P, Song WM, Tang J, Zhang HQ, Sun L, Cui J, Zhang LJ, Tang B, Huang F, Qin Q, Pei XP, Zhou AM, Shao LM, Liu JL, Zhang FY, Du WD, Franke A, Bowcock AM, Elder JT, Liu JJ, Yang S, Zhang XJ. Association analyses identify six new psoriasis susceptibility loci in the Chinese population. Nat Genet. 2010;42 (11):1005–9. Epub 2010 Oct 17.
38. Huffmeier U, Uebe S, Ekici AB, Bowes J, Giardina E, Korendowych E, Juneblad K, Apel M, McManus R,

Ho P, Bruce IN, Ryan AW, Behrens F, Lascorz J, Bohm B, Traupe H, Lohmann J, Gieger C, Wichmann HE, Herold C, Steffens M, Klareskog L, Wienker TF, Fitzgerald O, Alenius GM, McHugh NJ, Novelli G, Burkhardt H, Barton A, Reis A. Common variants at TRAF3IP2 are associated with susceptibility to psoriatic arthritis and psoriasis. Nat Genet. 2010;42(11):996–9. Epub 2010 Oct 17.

39. Tsoi LC, Spain SL, Knight J, Ellinghaus E, Stuart PE, Capon F, Ding J, Li Y, Tejasvi T, Gudjonsson JE, Kang HM, Allen MH, McManus R, Novelli G, Samuelsson L, Schalkwijk J, Stahle M, Burden AD, Smith CH, Cork MJ, Estivill X, Bowcock AM, Krueger GG, Weger W, Worthington J, Tazi-Ahnini R, Nestle FO, Hayday A, Hoffmann P, Winkelmann J, Wijmenga C, Langford C, Edkins S, Andrews R, Blackburn H, Strange A, Band G, Pearson RD, Vukcevic D, Spencer CC, Deloukas P, Mrowietz U, Schreiber S, Weidinger S, Koks S, Kingo K, Esko T, Metspalu A, Lim HW, Voorhees JJ, Weichenthal M, Wichmann HE, Chandran V, Rosen CF, Rahman P, Gladman DD, Griffiths CE, Reis A, Kere J, Nair RP, Franke A, Barker JN, Abecasis GR, Elder JT, Trembath RC. Identification of 15 new psoriasis susceptibility loci highlights the role of innate immunity. Nat Genet. 2012;44(12):1341–8. doi:10.038/ng.2467. Epub 012 Nov 11.

40. Julia A, Tortosa R, Hernanz JM, Canete JD, Fonseca E, Ferrandiz C, Unamuno P, Puig L, Fernandez-Sueiro JL, Sanmarti R, Rodriguez J, Gratacos J, Dauden E, Sanchez-Carazo JL, Lopez-Estebaranz JL, Moreno-Ramirez D, Queiro R, Montilla C, Torre-Alonso JC, Perez-Venegas JJ, Vanaclocha F, Herrera E, Munoz-Fernandez S, Gonzalez C, Roig D, Erra A, Acosta I, Fernandez-Nebro A, Zarco P, Alonso A, Lopez-Lasanta M, Garcia-Montero A, Gelpi JL, Absher D, Marsal S. Risk variants for psoriasis vulgaris in a large case-control collection and association with clinical subphenotypes. Hum Mol Genet. 2012;21(20):4549–57. Epub 2012 Jul 19.

41. Nan H, Xu M, Kraft P, Qureshi AA, Chen C, Guo Q, Hu FB, Curhan G, Amos CI, Wang LE, Lee JE, Wei Q, Hunter DJ, Han J. Genome-wide association study identifies novel alleles associated with risk of cutaneous basal cell carcinoma and squamous cell carcinoma. Hum Mol Genet. 2011;20(18):3718–24. doi:10.1093/hmg/ddr287. Epub 2011 Jun 23.

42. Nan H, Kraft P, Qureshi AA, Guo Q, Chen C, Hankinson SE, Hu FB, Thomas G, Hoover RN, Chanock S, Hunter DJ, Han J. Genome-wide association study of tanning phenotype in a population of European ancestry. J Invest Dermatol. 2009;129(9):2250–7. doi:10.1038/jid.2009.62.EpubApr2.

43. Gao Z, Tseng CH, Pei Z, Blaser MJ. Molecular analysis of human forearm superficial skin bacterial biota. Proc Natl Acad Sci U S A. 2007;104(8):2927–32. Epub 007 Feb 9.

44. Grice EA, Kong HH, Renaud G, Young AC, Bouffard GG, Blakesley RW, Wolfsberg TG, Turner ML, Segre JA. A diversity profile of the human skin microbiota. Genome Res. 2008;18(7):1043–50. Epub 2008 May 23.

45. Gao Z, Tseng CH, Strober BE, Pei Z, Blaser MJ. Substantial alterations of the cutaneous bacterial biota in psoriatic lesions. PLoS One. 2008;3(7), e2719.

46. Paulino LC, Tseng CH, Blaser MJ. Analysis of Malassezia microbiota in healthy superficial human skin and in psoriatic lesions by multiplex real-time PCR. FEMS Yeast Res. 2008;8(3):460–71. Epub 2008 Feb 20.

47. Grice EA, Kong HH, Conlan S, Deming CB, Davis J, Young AC, Bouffard GG, Blakesley RW, Murray PR, Green ED, Turner ML, Segre JA. Topographical and temporal diversity of the human skin microbiome. Science. 2009;324(5931):1190–2.

48. Oestreicher JL, Walters IB, Kikuchi T, Gilleaudeau P, Surette J, Schwertschlag U, Dorner AJ, Krueger JG, Trepicchio WL. Molecular classification of psoriasis disease-associated genes through pharmacogenomic expression profiling. Pharmacogenomics J. 2001;1(4):272–87.

49. Bowcock AM, Shannon W, Du F, Duncan J, Cao K, Aftergut K, Catier J, Fernandez-Vina MA, Menter A. Insights into psoriasis and other inflammatory diseases from large-scale gene expression studies. Hum Mol Genet. 2001;10(17):1793–805.

50. Zhou X, Krueger JG, Kao MC, Lee E, Du F, Menter A, Wong WH, Bowcock AM. Novel mechanisms of T-cell and dendritic cell activation revealed by profiling of psoriasis on the 63,100-element oligonucleotide array. Physiol Genomics. 2003;13(1):69–78.

51. Haider AS, Peters SB, Kaporis H, Cardinale I, Fei J, Ott J, Blumenberg M, Bowcock AM, Krueger JG, Carucci JA. Genomic analysis defines a cancer-specific gene expression signature for human squamous cell carcinoma and distinguishes malignant hyperproliferation from benign hyperplasia. J Invest Dermatol. 2006;126(4):869–81.

52. Hochberg M, Zeligson S, Amariglio N, Rechavi G, Ingber A, Enk CD. Genomic-scale analysis of psoriatic skin reveals differentially expressed insulin-like growth factor-binding protein-7 after phototherapy. Br J Dermatol. 2007;156(2):289–300. PubMed.

53. Gudjonsson JE, Ding J, Johnston A, Tejasvi T, Guzman AM, Nair RP, Voorhees JJ, Abecasis GR, Elder JT. Assessment of the psoriatic transcriptome in a large sample: additional regulated genes and comparisons with in vitro models. J Invest Dermatol. 2010;130(7):1829–40. Epub 2010 Mar 11.

54. Suarez-Farinas M, Li K, Fuentes-Duculan J, Hayden K, Brodmerkel C, Krueger JG. Expanding the psoriasis disease profile: interrogation of the skin and serum of patients with moderate-to-severe psoriasis. J Invest Dermatol. 2012;132(11):2552–64. doi:10.1038/jid.2012.184.EpubJul5.

55. Tian S, Krueger JG, Li K, Jabbari A, Brodmerkel C, Lowes MA, Suarez-Farinas M. Meta-analysis derived (MAD) transcriptome of psoriasis defines the "Core" pathogenesis of disease. PLoS One. 2012;7(9), e44274. Epub 2012 Sep 5.
56. Banno T, Gazel A, Blumenberg M. The use of DNA microarrays in dermatology research. Retinoids. 2004;20(3):1–4.
57. Nomura I, Goleva E, Howell MD, Hamid QA, Ong PY, Hall CF, Darst MA, Gao B, Boguniewicz M, Travers JB, Leung DY. Cytokine milieu of atopic dermatitis, as compared to psoriasis, skin prevents induction of innate immune response genes. J Immunol. 2003;171(6):3262–9.
58. Nomura I, Gao B, Boguniewicz M, Darst MA, Travers JB, Leung DY. Distinct patterns of gene expression in the skin lesions of atopic dermatitis and psoriasis: a gene microarray analysis. J Allergy Clin Immunol. 2003;112(6):1195–202.
59. de Jongh GJ, Zeeuwen PL, Kucharekova M, Pfundt R, van der Valk PG, Blokx W, Dogan A, Hiemstra PS, van de Kerkhof PC, Schalkwijk J. High expression levels of keratinocyte antimicrobial proteins in psoriasis compared with atopic dermatitis. J Invest Dermatol. 2005;125(6):1163–73.
60. Ogawa K, Ito M, Takeuchi K, Nakada A, Heishi M, Suto H, Mitsuishi K, Sugita Y, Ogawa H, Ra C. Tenascin-C is upregulated in the skin lesions of patients with atopic dermatitis. J Dermatol Sci. 2005;40(1):35–41.
61. Guttman-Yassky E, Lowes MA, Fuentes-Duculan J, Whynot J, Novitskaya I, Cardinale I, Haider A, Khatcherian A, Carucci JA, Bergman R, Krueger JG. Major differences in inflammatory dendritic cells and their products distinguish atopic dermatitis from psoriasis. J Allergy Clin Immunol. 2007;119 (5):1210–7. PubMed.
62. DeRisi J, Penland L, Brown PO, Bittner ML, Meltzer PS, Ray M, Chen Y, Su YA, Trent JM. Use of a cDNA microarray to analyse gene expression patterns in human cancer. Nat Genet. 1996;14(4):457–60.
63. Dooley TP, Curto EV, Davis RL, Grammatico P, Robinson ES, Wilborn TW. DNA microarrays and likelihood ratio bioinformatic methods: discovery of human melanocyte biomarkers. Pigment Cell Res. 2003;16(3):245–53.
64. Hoek K, Rimm DL, Williams KR, Zhao H, Ariyan S, Lin A, Kluger HM, Berger AJ, Cheng E, Trombetta ES, Wu T, Niinobe M, Yoshikawa K, Hannigan GE, Halaban R. Expression profiling reveals novel pathways in the transformation of melanocytes to melanomas. Cancer Res. 2004;64(15):5270–82.
65. Haqq C, Nosrati M, Sudilovsky D, Crothers J, Khodabakhsh D, Pulliam BL, Federman S, Miller 3rd JR, Allen RE, Singer MI, Leong SP, Ljung BM, Sagebiel RW, Kashani-Sabet M. The gene expression signatures of melanoma progression. Proc Natl Acad Sci U S A. 2005;102(17):6092–7. Epub 2005 Apr 15.
66. Becker B, Roesch A, Hafner C, Stolz W, Dugas M, Landthaler M, Vogt T. Discrimination of melanocytic tumors by cDNA array hybridization of tissues prepared by laser pressure catapulting. J Invest Dermatol. 2004;122(2):361–8.
67. Gallagher WM, Bergin OE, Rafferty M, Kelly ZD, Nolan IM, Fox EJ, Culhane AC, McArdle L, Fraga MF, Hughes L, Currid CA, O'Mahony F, Byrne A, Murphy AA, Moss C, McDonnell S, Stallings RL, Plumb JA, Esteller M, Brown R, Dervan PA, Easty DJ. Multiple markers for melanoma progression regulated by DNA methylation: insights from transcriptomic studies. Carcinogenesis. 2005;26 (11):1856–67. Epub 2005 Jun 15.
68. Nambiar S, Mirmohammadsadegh A, Doroudi R, Gustrau A, Marini A, Roeder G, Ruzicka T, Hengge UR. Signaling networks in cutaneous melanoma metastasis identified by complementary DNA microarrays. Arch Dermatol. 2005;141(2):165–73.
69. Busam KJ, Zhao H, Coit DG, Kucukgol D, Jungbluth AA, Nobrega J, Viale A. Distinction of desmoplastic melanoma from non-desmoplastic melanoma by gene expression profiling. J Invest Dermatol. 2005;124 (2):412–8.
70. Talantov D, Mazumder A, Yu JX, Briggs T, Jiang Y, Backus J, Atkins D, Wang Y. Novel genes associated with malignant melanoma but not benign melanocytic lesions. Clin Cancer Res. 2005;11(20):7234–42.
71. Zhou Y, Dai DL, Martinka M, Su M, Zhang Y, Campos EI, Dorocicz I, Tang L, Huntsman D, Nelson C, Ho V, Li G. Osteopontin expression correlates with melanoma invasion. J Invest Dermatol. 2005;124 (5):1044–52.
72. Winnepenninckx V, Van den Oord JJ. Gene expression profiling of primary cutaneous melanoma. Verh K Acad Geneeskd Belg. 2007;69(1):23–45. PubMed.
73. Winnepenninckx V, Lazar V, Michiels S, Dessen P, Stas M, Alonso SR, Avril MF, Ortiz Romero PL, Robert T, Balacescu O, Eggermont AM, Lenoir G, Sarasin A, Tursz T, van den Oord JJ, Spatz A. Gene expression profiling of primary cutaneous melanoma and clinical outcome. J Natl Cancer Inst. 2006;98 (7):472–82. PubMed.
74. Gast A, Scherer D, Chen B, Bloethner S, Melchert S, Sucker A, Hemminki K, Schadendorf D, Kumar R. Somatic alterations in the melanoma genome: a high-resolution array-based comparative genomic hybridization study. Genes Chromosomes Cancer. 2010;49(8):733–45. doi:10.1002/gcc.20785.
75. Conway K, Edmiston SN, Khondker ZS, Groben PA, Zhou X, Chu H, Kuan PF, Hao H, Carson C, Berwick M, Olilla DW, Thomas NE. DNA-methylation profiling distinguishes malignant melanomas from benign nevi. Pigment Cell Melanoma Res. 2011;24(2):352–60. doi:10.1111/j.755-148X.2011.00828.x. Epub 2011 Feb 18.
76. Hou P, Liu D, Dong J, Xing M. The BRAF(V600E) causes widespread alterations in gene methylation in the genome of melanoma cells. Cell Cycle. 2012;11

(2):286–95. doi:10.4161/cc.11.2.18707. Epub 2012 Jan 15.

77. Stark MS, Tyagi S, Nancarrow DJ, Boyle GM, Cook AL, Whiteman DC, Parsons PG, Schmidt C, Sturm RA, Hayward NK. Characterization of the melanoma miRNAome by deep sequencing. PLoS One. 2010;5 (3), e9685.
78. Couts KL, Anderson EM, Gross MM, Sullivan K, Ahn NG. Oncogenic B-Raf signaling in melanoma cells controls a network of microRNAs with combinatorial functions. Oncogene. 2013;32(15):1959–70. doi:10.038/onc.2012.209. Epub Jul 2.
79. Sand M, Skrygan M, Sand D, Georgas D, Gambichler T, Hahn SA, Altmeyer P, Bechara FG. Comparative microarray analysis of microRNA expression profiles in primary cutaneous malignant melanoma, cutaneous malignant melanoma metastases, and benign melanocytic nevi. Cell Tissue Res. 2013;351(1):85–98. doi:10.1007/s00441-012-1514-5. Epub 2012 Oct 31.
80. Widmer DS, Cheng PF, Eichhoff OM, Belloni BC, Zipser MC, Schlegel NC, Javelaud D, Mauviel A, Dummer R, Hoek KS. Systematic classification of melanoma cells by phenotype-specific gene expression mapping. Pigment Cell Melanoma Res. 2012;25 (3):343–53. doi:10.1111/j.755-148X.2012.00986.x. Epub 2012 Mar 2.
81. Schramm SJ, Campain AE, Scolyer RA, Yang YH, Mann GJ. Review and cross-validation of gene expression signatures and melanoma prognosis. J Invest Dermatol. 2012;132(2):274–83. doi:10.1038/jid.2011.305.EpubSep29.
82. Mithani SK, Smith IM, Califano JA. Use of integrative epigenetic and cytogenetic analyses to identify novel tumor-suppressor genes in malignant melanoma. Melanoma Res. 2011;21(4):298–307. doi:10.1097/CMR.0b013e328344a003.
83. Liu W, Peng Y, Tobin DJ. A new 12-gene diagnostic biomarker signature of melanoma revealed by integrated microarray analysis. Peer J. 2013;1, e49. doi:10.7717/peerj.49. Print 2013.
84. Tomic-Canic M, Brem H. Gene array technology and pathogenesis of chronic wounds. Am J Surg. 2004;188(1A Suppl):67–72.
85. Nuutila K, Siltanen A, Peura M, Bizik J, Kaartinen I, Kuokkanen H, Nieminen T, Harjula A, Aarnio P, Vuola J, Kankuri E. Human skin transcriptome during superficial cutaneous wound healing. Wound Repair Regen. 2012;20 (6):830–9. doi:10.1111/j.524-475X.2012.00831.x. Epub 2012 Oct 19.
86. Deonarine K, Panelli MC, Stashower ME, Jin P, Smith K, Slade HB, Norwood C, Wang E, Marincola FM, Stroncek DF. Gene expression profiling of cutaneous wound healing. J Transl Med. 2007;5:11.
87. Charles CA, Tomic-Canic M, Vincek V, Nassiri M, Stojadinovic O, Eaglstein WH, Kirsner RS. A gene signature of nonhealing venous ulcers: potential diagnostic markers. J Am Acad Dermatol. 2008;59 (5):758–71. doi:10.1016/j.jaad.2008.07.018. EpubAug20.
88. Brem H, Tomic-Canic M. Cellular and molecular basis of wound healing in diabetes. J Clin Invest. 2007;117(5):1219–22.
89. Grice EA, Segre JA. Interaction of the microbiome with the innate immune response in chronic wounds. Adv Exp Med Biol. 2012;946:55–68.
90. Sesto A, Navarro M, Burslem F, Jorcano JL. Analysis of the ultraviolet B response in primary human keratinocytes using oligonucleotide microarrays. Proc Natl Acad Sci U S A. 2002;99(5):2965–70.
91. Murakami T, Fujimoto M, Ohtsuki M, Nakagawa H. Expression profiling of cancer-related genes in human keratinocytes following non-lethal ultraviolet B irradiation. J Dermatol Sci. 2001;27(2):121–9.
92. Takao J, Ariizumi K, Dougherty II, Cruz Jr PD. Genomic scale analysis of the human keratinocyte response to broad-band ultraviolet-B irradiation. Photodermatol Photoimmunol Photomed. 2002;18(1):5–13.
93. Howell BG, Wang B, Freed I, Mamelak AJ, Watanabe H, Sauder DN. Microarray analysis of UVB-regulated genes in keratinocytes: downregulation of angiogenesis inhibitor thrombospondin-1. J Dermatol Sci. 2004;34 (3):185–94.
94. Enk CD, Shahar I, Amariglio N, Rechavi G, Kaminski N, Hochberg M. Gene expression profiling of in vivo UVB-irradiated human epidermis. Photodermatol Photoimmunol Photomed. 2004;20 (3):129–37.
95. Enk CD, Jacob-Hirsch J, Gal H, Verbovetski I, Amariglio N, Mevorach D, Ingber A, Givol D, Rechavi G, Hochberg M. The UVB-induced gene expression profile of human epidermis in vivo is different from that of cultured keratinocytes. Oncogene. 2006;25(18):2601–14.
96. Stahl PL, Stranneheim H, Asplund A, Berglund L, Ponten F, Lundeberg J. Sun-induced nonsynonymous p53 mutations are extensively accumulated and tolerated in normal appearing human skin. J Invest Dermatol. 2011;131(2):504–8. Epub 2010 Oct 14.
97. Coda AB, Sinha AA. Integration of genome-wide transcriptional and genetic profiles provides insights into disease development and clinical heterogeneity in alopecia areata. Genomics. 2011;98(6):431–9. doi:10.1016/j.ygeno.2011.08.009.EpubSep17.
98. Yu R, Broady R, Huang Y, Wang Y, Yu J, Gao M, Levings M, Wei S, Zhang S, Xu A, Su M, Dutz J, Zhang X, Zhou Y. Transcriptome analysis reveals markers of aberrantly activated innate immunity in vitiligo lesional and non-lesional skin. PLoS One. 2012;7(12), e51040. doi:10.1371/journal.pone.0051040. Epub 2012 Dec 10.
99. Ralfkiaer U, Hagedorn PH, Bangsgaard N, Lovendorf MB, Ahler CB, Svensson L, Kopp KL, Vennegaard MT, Lauenborg B, Zibert JR, Krejsgaard T, Bonefeld CM, Sokilde R, Gjerdrum LM, Labuda T, Mathiesen

AM, Gronbaek K, Wasik MA, Sokolowska-Wojdylo-M, Queille-Roussel C, Gniadecki R, Ralfkiaer E, Geisler C, Litman T, Woetmann A, Glue C, Ropke MA, Skov L, Odum N. Diagnostic microRNA profiling in cutaneous T-cell lymphoma (CTCL). Blood. 2011;118(22):5891–900. doi:10.1182/blood-2011-06-358382. Epub 2011 Aug 24.

100. Shuda M, Arora R, Kwun HJ, Feng H, Sarid R, Fernandez-Figueras MT, Tolstov Y, Gjoerup O, Mansukhani MM, Swerdlow SH, Chaudhary PM, Kirkwood JM, Nalesnik MA, Kant JA, Weiss LM, Moore PS, Chang Y. Human Merkel cell polyomavirus infection I. MCV T antigen expression in Merkel cell carcinoma, lymphoid tissues and lymphoid tumors. Int J Cancer. 2009;125(6):1243–9. doi:10.002/ijc.24510.
101. Harms PW, Patel RM, Verhaegen ME, Giordano TJ, Nash KT, Johnson CN, Daignault S, Thomas DG, Gudjonsson JE, Elder JT, Dlugosz AA, Johnson TM, Fullen DR, Bichakjian CK. Distinct gene expression profiles of viral- and nonviral-associated merkel cell carcinoma revealed by transcriptome analysis. J Invest Dermatol. 2013;133(4):936–45. doi:10.1038/jid.2012.445.EpubDec6.
102. Melov S, Hubbard A. Microarrays as a tool to investigate the biology of aging: a retrospective and a look to the future. Sci Aging Knowledge Environ. 2004;2004(42), re7.
103. Helmberg A. DNA-microarrays: novel techniques to study aging and guide gerontologic medicine. Exp Gerontol. 2001;36(7):1189–98.
104. Masuda K, Kuwano Y, Nishida K, Rokutan K. Application of DNA microarray technology to gerontological studies. Methods Mol Biol. 2013;1048:285–308. doi:10.1007/978-1-62703-556-9_19.
105. Nair PN, Golden T, Melov S. Microarray workshop on aging. Mech Ageing Dev. 2003;124(1):133–8.
106. McCarroll SA, Murphy CT, Zou S, Pletcher SD, Chin CS, Jan YN, Kenyon C, Bargmann CI, Li H. Comparing genomic expression patterns across species identifies shared transcriptional profile in aging. Nat Genet. 2004;36(2):197–204. Epub 2004 Jan 18.
107. Nadon NL, Mohr D, Becker KG. National Institute on Aging microarray facility – resources for gerontology research. J Gerontol A Biol Sci Med Sci. 2005;60 (4):413–5.
108. Pan F, Chiu CH, Pulapura S, Mehan MR, Nunez-Iglesias J, Zhang K, Kamath K, Waterman MS, Finch CE, Zhou XJ. Gene aging nexus: a web database and data mining platform for microarray data on aging. Nucleic Acids Res. 2007;35(Database issue): D756–9. Epub 2006 Nov 7.
109. Panigrahi PP, Singh TR. Computational studies on Alzheimer's disease associated pathways and regulatory patterns using microarray gene expression and network data: revealed association with aging and other diseases. J Theor Biol. 2013;334:109–21. doi:10.1016/j.jtbi.2013.06.013. Epub Jun 26.
110. Wharton SB, Simpson JE, Brayne C, Ince PG. Age-associated white matter lesions: the MRC cognitive function and ageing study. Brain Pathol. 2015;25(1):35–43. doi:10.1111/bpa.12219.
111. Rai MF, Patra D, Sandell LJ, Brophy RH. Transcriptome analysis of injured human meniscus reveals a distinct phenotype of meniscus degeneration with aging. Arthritis Rheum. 2013;65 (8):2090–101. doi:10.1002/art.37984.
112. Kohler J, Popov C, Klotz B, Alberton P, Prall WC, Haasters F, Muller-Deubert S, Ebert R, Klein-Hitpass-L, Jakob F, Schieker M, Docheva D. Uncovering the cellular and molecular changes in tendon stem/progenitor cells attributed to tendon aging and degeneration. Aging Cell. 2013;12(6):988–99. doi:10.1111/acel.12124. Epub 2013 Jul 22.
113. Remondini D, Salvioli S, Francesconi M, Pierini M, Mazzatti DJ, Powell JR, Zironi I, Bersani F, Castellani G, Franceschi C. Complex patterns of gene expression in human T cells during in vivo aging. Mol Biosyst. 2010;6(10):1983–92. doi:10.039/c004635c. Epub 2010 Aug 5.
114. Alves H, van Ginkel J, Groen N, Hulsman M, Mentink A, Reinders M, van Blitterswijk C, de Boer J. A mesenchymal stromal cell gene signature for donor age. PLoS One. 2012;7(8), e42908. doi:10.1371/journal.pone.0042908. Epub 2012 Aug 23.
115. Aliper AM, Csoka AB, Buzdin A, Jetka T, Roumiantsev S, Moskalev A, Zhavoronkov A. Signaling pathway activation drift during aging: Hutchinson-Gilford Progeria Syndrome fibroblasts are comparable to normal middle-age and old-age cells. Aging (Albany NY). 2015;7(1):26–37.
116. da Jang H, Bhawal UK, Min HK, Kang HK, Abiko Y, Min BM. A transcriptional roadmap to the senescence and differentiation of human oral keratinocytes. J Gerontol A Biol Sci Med Sci. 2015;70(1):20–32. doi:10.1093/gerona/glt212. Epub 2014 Jan 7.
117. Liesenfeld M, Mosig S, Funke H, Jansen L, Runnebaum IB, Durst M, Backsch C. SORBS2 and TLR3 induce premature senescence in primary human fibroblasts and keratinocytes. BMC Cancer. 2013;13:507. doi:10.1186/471-2407-13-507.
118. Baek JH, Lee G, Kim SN, Kim JM, Kim M, Chung SC, Min BM. Common genes responsible for differentiation and senescence of human mucosal and epidermal keratinocytes. Int J Mol Med. 2003;12 (3):319–25.
119. Rampelli S, Candela M, Severgnini M, Biagi E, Turroni S, Roselli M, Carnevali P, Donini L, Brigidi P. A probiotics-containing biscuit modulates the intestinal microbiota in the elderly. J Nutr Health Aging. 2013;17(2):166–72. doi:10.1007/s12603-012-0372-x.
120. Marchand A, Atassi F, Gaaya A, Leprince P, Le Feuvre C, Soubrier F, Lompre AM, Nadaud S. The Wnt/beta-catenin pathway is activated during advanced arterial aging in humans. Aging Cell.

2011;10(2):220–32. doi:10.1111/j.474-9726.2010.00661.x. Epub 2010 Dec 29.

121. Adler AS, Kawahara TL, Segal E, Chang HY. Reversal of aging by NFkappaB blockade. Cell Cycle. 2008;7(5):556–9. Epub 2007 Dec 26.
122. Uittenboogaard LM, Payan-Gomez C, Pothof J, van Ijcken W, Mastroberardino PG, van der Pluijm I, Hoeijmakers JH, Tresini M. BACH2: a marker of DNA damage and ageing. DNA Repair (Amst). 2013;12(11):982–92. doi:10.1016/j.dnarep.2013.08.016.EpubSep24.
123. van Dam S, Cordeiro R, Craig T, van Dam J, Wood SH, de Magalhaes JP. GeneFriends: an online co-expression analysis tool to identify novel gene targets for aging and complex diseases. BMC Genomics. 2012;13:535. doi:10.1186/471-2164-13-535.
124. de Magalhaes JP, Curado J, Church GM. Meta-analysis of age-related gene expression profiles identifies common signatures of aging. Bioinformatics. 2009;25(7):875–81. doi:10.1093/bioinformatics/btp073. Epub 2009 Feb 2.
125. Lorencini M, Brohem CA, Dieamant GC, Zanchin NI, Maibach HI. Active ingredients against human epidermal aging. Ageing Res Rev. 2014;15:100–15. doi:10.1016/j.arr.2014.03.002. Epub Mar 25.
126. Rittie L, Fisher GJ. Natural and sun-induced aging of human skin. Cold Spring Harb Perspect Med. 2015;5(1):a015370. doi:10.1101/cshperspect.a.
127. Monnat Jr RJ. "…Rewritten in the skin": clues to skin biology and aging from inherited disease. J Invest Dermatol. 2015;135(6):1484–90. doi:10.038/jid.2015.88. Epub Mar 26.
128. Benech PD, Patatian A. From experimental design to functional gene networks: DNA microarray contribution to skin ageing research. Int J Cosmet Sci. 2014;36(6):516–26. doi:10.1111/ics.12155. Epub 2014 Sep 18.
129. Rizzo AE, Maibach HI. Personalizing dermatology: the future of genomic expression profiling to individualize dermatologic therapy. J Dermatolog Treat. 2012;23(3):161–7. doi:10.3109/09546634.2010.535806. Epub 2011 Jan 22.
130. Robinson MK, Binder RL, Griffiths CE. Genomic-driven insights into changes in aging skin. J Drugs Dermatol. 2009;8(7 Suppl):s8–11.
131. Gilchrest BA, Garmyn M, Yaar M. Aging and photoaging affect gene expression in cultured human keratinocytes. Arch Dermatol. 1994;130(1):82–6.
132. Urschitz J, Iobst S, Urban Z, Granda C, Souza KA, Lupp C, Schilling K, Scott I, Csiszar K, Boyd CD. A serial analysis of gene expression in sun-damaged human skin. J Invest Dermatol. 2002;119(1):3–13.
133. Lener T, Moll PR, Rinnerthaler M, Bauer J, Aberger F, Richter K. Expression profiling of aging in the human skin. Exp Gerontol. 2006;41(4):387–97. Epub 2006 Mar 10.
134. Laimer M, Kocher T, Chiocchetti A, Trost A, Lottspeich F, Richter K, Hintner H, Bauer JW, Onder K. Proteomic profiling reveals a catalogue of new candidate proteins for human skin aging. Exp Dermatol. 2010;19(10):912–8. doi:10.1111/j.600-0625.2010.01144.x.
135. Yan W, Zhang LL, Yan L, Zhang F, Yin NB, Lin HB, Huang CY, Wang L, Yu J, Wang DM, Zhao ZM. Transcriptome analysis of skin photoaging in Chinese females reveals the involvement of skin homeostasis and metabolic changes. PLoS One. 2013;8(4), e61946. doi:10.1371/journal.pone.0061946.Print2013.
136. Koike M, Shiomi T, Koike A. Identification of Skin injury-related genes induced by ionizing radiation in human keratinocytes using cDNA microarray. J Radiat Res (Tokyo). 2005;46(2):173–84.
137. Lamartine J, Franco N, Le Minter P, Soularue P, Alibert O, Leplat JJ, Gidrol X, Waksman G, Martin MT. Activation of an energy providing response in human keratinocytes after gamma irradiation. J Cell Biochem. 2005;95(3):620–31.
138. Li W, Zhou BR, Hua LJ, Guo Z, Luo D. Differential miRNA profile on photoaged primary human fibroblasts irradiated with ultraviolet A. Tumour Biol. 2013;34(6):3491–500. doi:10.1007/s13277-013-0927-4. Epub 2013 Jul 7.
139. Aoki H, Moro O, Tagami H, Kishimoto J. Gene expression profiling analysis of solar lentigo in relation to immunohistochemical characteristics. Br J Dermatol. 2007;156(6):1214–23. Epub 2007 Apr 5.
140. Jozic I, Stojadinovic O, Kirsner RS, Tomic-Canic M. Stressing the steroids in skin: paradox or fine-tuning? J Invest Dermatol. 2014;134(12):2869–72. doi:10.1038/jid.2014.363.
141. Yan W, Zhao Z, Zhang L, Wang D, Yan L, Yin N, Wu D, Zhang F. Identification of estrogen-associated intrinsic aging genes in Chinese Han female skin by cDNA microarray technology. Biomed Environ Sci. 2011;24(4):364–73. doi:10.3967/0895-3988.2011.04.007.
142. Makrantonaki E, Adjaye J, Herwig R, Brink TC, Groth D, Hultschig C, Lehrach H, Zouboulis CC. Age-specific hormonal decline is accompanied by transcriptional changes in human sebocytes in vitro. Aging Cell. 2006;5(4):331–44. Epub 2006 Jun 29.
143. Hardman MJ, Ashcroft GS. Estrogen, not intrinsic aging, is the major regulator of delayed human wound healing in the elderly. Genome Biol. 2008;9(5):R80. doi:10.1186/gb-2008-9-5-r80.EpubMay13.
144. Peters EM, Liezmann C, Spatz K, Ungethum U, Kuban RJ, Daniltchenko M, Kruse J, Imfeld D, Klapp BF, Campiche R. Profiling mRNA of the graying human hair follicle constitutes a promising state-of-the-art tool to assess its aging: an exemplary report. J Invest Dermatol. 2013;133(5):1150–60. doi:10.038/jid.2012.462. Epub Dec 13.
145. Farwick M, Kohler T, Schild J, Mentel M, Maczkiewitz U, Pagani V, Bonfigli A, Rigano L, Bureik D, Gauglitz GG. Pentacyclic triterpenes from Terminalia arjuna show multiple benefits on aged and

dry skin. Skin Pharmacol Physiol. 2014;27(2):71–81. doi:10.1159/000351387. Epub 2013 Sep 5.

146. Lephart ED. Protective effects of equol and their polyphenolic isomers against dermal aging: microarray/protein evidence with clinical implications and unique delivery into human skin. Pharm Biol. 2013;51(11):1393–400. doi:10.3109/13880209.2013.793720. Epub 2013 Jul 18.

147. Jones MJ, Goodman SJ, Kobor MS. DNA methylation and healthy human aging. Aging Cell. 2015;25(10):12349.

148. Oba C, Ito K, Ichikawa S, Morifuji M, Nakai Y, Ishijima T, Abe K, Kawahata K. Effect of orally administered collagen hydrolysate on gene expression profiles in mouse skin: a DNA microarray analysis. Physiol Genomics. 2015;47(8):355–63. doi:10.1152/physiolgenomics.00009.2015. Epub 2015 Jun 9.

149. Villeda SA, Plambeck KE, Middeldorp J, Castellano JM, Mosher KI, Luo J, Smith LK, Bieri G, Lin K, Berdnik D, Wabl R, Udeochu J, Wheatley EG, Zou B, Simmons DA, Xie XS, Longo FM, Wyss-Coray T. Young blood reverses age-related impairments in cognitive function and synaptic plasticity in mice. Nat Med. 2014;20(6):659–63. doi:10.1038/nm.3569. Epub 2014 May 4.

150. Cao SX, Dhahbi JM, Mote PL, Spindler SR. Genomic profiling of short- and long-term caloric restriction effects in the liver of aging mice. Proc Natl Acad Sci U S A. 2001;98(19):10630–5. Epub 2001 Sep 4.

Reflectance Confocal Microscopy and Aging

104

Anthony P. Raphael, Danielle Tokarz, Marco Ardigò, and Tarl W. Prow

Contents

A.P. Raphael (✉)
Dermatology Research Centre, School of Medicine, The University of Queensland, Princess Alexandra Hospital, Translational Research Institute, Brisbane, QLD, Australia

Wellman Center for Photomedicine, Massachusetts General Hospital, Harvard Medical School, Boston, MA, USA
e-mail: a.raphael1@uq.edu.au

D. Tokarz
Wellman Center for Photomedicine, Massachusetts General Hospital, Harvard Medical School, Boston, MA, USA

Princess Margaret Cancer Centre, University Health Network, Toronto, ON, Canada
e-mail: dtokarz@mgh.harvard.edu

M. Ardigò
Clinical Dermatology, IFO San Gallicano Dermatological Institute, Rome, Italy
e-mail: ardigo@ifo.it

T.W. Prow
Dermatology Research Centre, School of Medicine, The University of Queensland, Princess Alexandra Hospital, Translational Research Institute, Brisbane, QLD, Australia
e-mail: t.prow@uq.edu.au

M.A. Farage et al. (eds.), *Textbook of Aging Skin*,
DOI 10.1007/978-3-662-47398-6_161

Abstract

Limitations in conventional clinical and histopathological assessment of chronological aging and photoaging have seen interest grow in noninvasive microscopy techniques. At the forefront is the use of reflectance confocal microscopy (RCM). Typically referred to as RCM, it results in quasi-histological resolution of the cellular and subcellular structures within the stratum corneum down to the epidermal-dermal junction and upper papillary dermis. RCM can be used for en face serial imaging of the same site over time resulting in unique features that provide a mechanistic understanding of the aging process. This chapter discusses these features in relation to conventional approaches and how computational analysis can be used for automated objective assessment of skin aging. Lastly, advancements in RCM and alternative microscopy techniques are introduced, providing insight into the pathways for clinical integration of noninvasive microscopy.

Introduction

Skin aging is a complex biological process resulting from intrinsic and extrinsic factors that alter skin morphology at both the macroscopic and microscopic levels. The intrinsic factors associated with natural aging progression result in decreased elasticity and increased fine wrinkling of the skin predominantly due to degradation of the underlying dermal collagen matrix. External environmental factors, in particular excessive UV exposure, significantly exaggerate these skin changes in a dose-dependent manner. Photodamaged skin presents with coarse wrinkling and skin thickening, disruption to the cellular packing within the epidermis, and accumulation of elastotic material within the upper to mid-dermis, known as solar elastosis. Severely photoaged skin has a high microscopic and biological correlation with the development of actinic keratosis lesions and their progression to nonmelanoma skin cancers. Therefore, longitudinal assessment of photoaging skin for preventive risk management is of great interest. For the purpose of this chapter, skin aging will be discussed in the context of photoaging and its downstream pathological consequences.

A benefit of the diverse range of morphological changes to the skin during aging is that there are multiple techniques that can be used to assess and quantify the disruption. These include clinical observation, noninvasive microscopy, and molecular assays. The current gold-standard approach is a combination of clinical observation followed by histological assessment of collagen degradation and epidermal involvement. However, the need for a skin biopsy limits the practicality of this approach due to photoaged skin presenting as relatively large discreet or continuous lesions across multiple anatomical sites (e.g., face, arms, legs).

The above limitations have resulted in a shift toward noninvasive procedures suitable for large-area skin assessment. This has resulted in the development and increased utilization of reflectance confocal microscopy (RCM), nonlinear multiphoton microscopy (MPM), optical coherence tomography (OCT), and ultrasound approaches.

In particular, RCM has shown great promise as a clinical tool. RCM results in quasi-histological resolution of the cellular and subcellular structures within the stratum corneum down to the epidermal-dermal junction and upper papillary dermis (approximately 200 μm in depth). Unlike histological hematoxylin and eosin (H&E) assessment, RCM enables serial imaging of the same site over time via gray-scale en face 3D image stacks stitched over large areas.

The introduction of such microscopic systems into the clinic is not straightforward. Effort must be made to ensure practitioners can benchmark and standardize new assessment approaches in an objective manner with standard techniques. The systems need to be made compatible within current infrastructural restrictions in a cost-effective and user-friendly manner. These limitations are being addressed from both scientific and commercial communities in the area of noninvasive clinical imaging techniques. There is little doubt that advanced microscopy systems will become standard practice for preventative risk management of skin aging.

Clinical and Histopathological Features of Skin Aging

To place in context the need for noninvasive microscopy techniques such as RCM, it is useful to have an understanding of the features being used to characterize photoaging through conventional clinical observation and histopathology. Clinical features include, but are not limited to, fine and coarse wrinkling, mottled pigmentation, telangiectasia, surface roughness, and neoplastic growths [1, 2]. Although clinical observation is technically the least challenging approach, it is relatively subjective with variability in interobserver agreement and intra-observer repeatability. In order to improve objectivity and obtain statistically significant information, several scoring systems have been developed based on descriptive, visual analogue and photographic grading scales. Although they all vary with the amount and type of features assessed, it has been suggested that at the very least fine wrinkles, coarse wrinkles, and pigmentation be included due to their noticeable correlation with photoaging [3].

For example, in 2011 McKenzie et al. published a photographic scoring method consisting of the above three features in addition to a global feature (overall impression of sun exposure) [2]. Each criterion was assessed on a 0–9 point scale (0 = absent) with the remaining numerical scale classified as mild (1–3), moderate (4–6), and severe (7–9). One academic clinician and five dermatologists ranked the photographs of the volunteers' dorsal forearms. The academic clinician's score was used as the reference score and it was calculated that the other five assessors were in agreement 71–92 % of the time.

With the focus of the study on inter-observational agreement, there was no information on photographic score and volunteer age. However, it has been observed by others that due to the limited grading scale, a relatively binary outcome (young or old) is achieved when scoring large cohorts [4]. This is due to difficulty in distinguishing subtle changes within the skin during aging. Furthermore, the approach does not account for lesional hyperkeratosis and overall skin thickness. This is less of an issue for undamaged skin; however, for photoaged skin where there is increased risk of nonmelanoma skin cancer, it is important to have early diagnostic information of individuals in high-risk groups.

On the other side of the spectrum, a 2009 study by Vierkotter and colleagues introduced a more comprehensive 23 feature scoring system for the assessment and distinction of intrinsic and extrinsic aging (SCINEXA) [5]. Each feature was graded on a scale of 0–3. The study population consisted of 74 volunteers aged between 19 and 72 years of age. To assess their grading scale, the volunteers were divided into two groups based on either weekly sunbed use over the last 10 years or minimal use with none in the last 18 months. The intrinsic features consisted of uneven pigmentation, fine wrinkles, lax appearance, benign tumors, and reduced subcutaneous adipose tissue. The extrinsic factors also assessed pigmentation and wrinkling in addition to skin discoloration, dryness, scarring, erythema, telangiectasia, melanoma, and nonmelanoma skin cancers in addition to several other benign growths. The grading system successfully categorized 92 % of the volunteers based on sunbed use. The deviation in clinical score of sunbed users was much tighter than what was observed for nonusers. Without assessing the raw data, it can be inferred that there is a threshold in photodamage to the skin, with the severity equalizing among individuals. However, with improved imaging modalities such as RCM and improved histopathology grading schemes, there is a general consensus that photoaging and its transition to nonmelanoma skin cancers consist of a continuous spectrum.

The previous studies inferred that photographic assessment is potentially less subjective than person-to-person assessment due to standardization of the images. However, maintaining consistent imaging parameters (e.g., external lighting, body positioning, color levels) is challenging and a major barrier for translating the photographic approach to the clinic. A lesional-focused approach with consistent imaging that has garnered much interest within the clinic is dermoscopy [6, 7]. The imaging device consists of small handheld instrument consisting of a polarized light source and simple lens for magnification up to a 100-fold. In 2013, Isik and colleagues introduced a dermoscopic photoaging scale based on the following features – yellowish discoloration and yellow papules, white linear scarring, freckling, mottled pigmentation, telangiectasia, actinic keratosis, senile comedones, and wrinkling [6]. These features can also be seen clinically with the naked eye. However, only once they become more pronounced. However, as photoaging becomes severe, dermoscopy is limited in differentiating between actinic keratosis and early stage squamous cell carcinoma.

The gold-standard approach for characterizing intrinsic and extrinsic aging is histopathology. When assessing chronic UV exposure, the accumulation of elastotic material in replacement of collagen within the dermis is the primary feature (solar elastosis). With severely photoaged skin, histopathology is capable of distinguishing the transition from actinic keratosis to squamous cell carcinoma. However, the technique does not come without challenges, with subjectivity, and interobserver variability. The relatively high complexity of the images and variability makes it difficult to define grading systems for histopathology assessment of aging. Therefore, the technique is more suited for later-stage aging in relation to grading early onset of aging.

Overall, the above techniques present a group of features that aid in distinguishing the degree and type of aging within skin. In summary, Fig. 1 shows a comparison of the clinical photography, dermoscopy, and histopathology, in addition to RCM, outlining the main features observed for the diagnosis of a pigmented actinic keratosis lesion [8]. Being limited to viewing the top of the skin, the predominant features of clinical assessment are wrinkling and pigmentation. Although clear-cut lesions such as actinic keratosis can be identified based on skin texture and erythema, misdiagnosis is possible as the lesions progress to nonmelanoma skin cancer. Histopathology provides accurate insight into epidermal and dermal changes. However, it is time consuming and laborious, and the need for many biopsies prevents its suitability for assessment of large areas of sun-exposed skin. Therefore, there is a technological and clinical need for noninvasive microscopy techniques that can build on current clinical features, in addition to providing their own unique set of criteria.

Technical Aspects of Reflectance Confocal Microscopy

In its most basic form, RCM consists of a small laser focal spot where scattering and reflection occurs by epidermal and dermal microstructures directing the light back through the microscope where it is focused through a pinhole-sized spatial filter placed in front of a photodetector (Fig. 2). The pinhole-sized spatial filter prevents out-of-focus light from reaching the photodetector in order to achieve optical sectioning. Contrast is obtained by local refractive index variations within the skin as well as scattering from structures, which are similar in size to the illumination wavelength. Background noise is limited by stray reflections of particles in the focusing light cone and limiting depth penetration of the technique. A 3D tomography of the skin is built by scanning the light spot across the region of interest followed by a stepwise change in the axial position.

In 1957, Marvin Minsky described the general principles of reflectance confocal microscopy [9]. A decade later, one of the first reflectance confocal microscopes was developed for imaging dorsal root ganglia of frogs. The instrument consisted of a mercury lamp as the excitation source with scanning achieved by a spinning disk [10]. With advancements in light sources, scanning techniques, and computers, several research groups further developed RCM in the early 1990s to image animal and human eyes, kidney, liver, adrenal, thyroid, epididymis, muscle, and connective tissue [11–14] in vivo. It was not until 1995 that one of the first RCMs used to image human skin in vivo was developed by Rajadhyaksha et al. Their RCM consisted of a

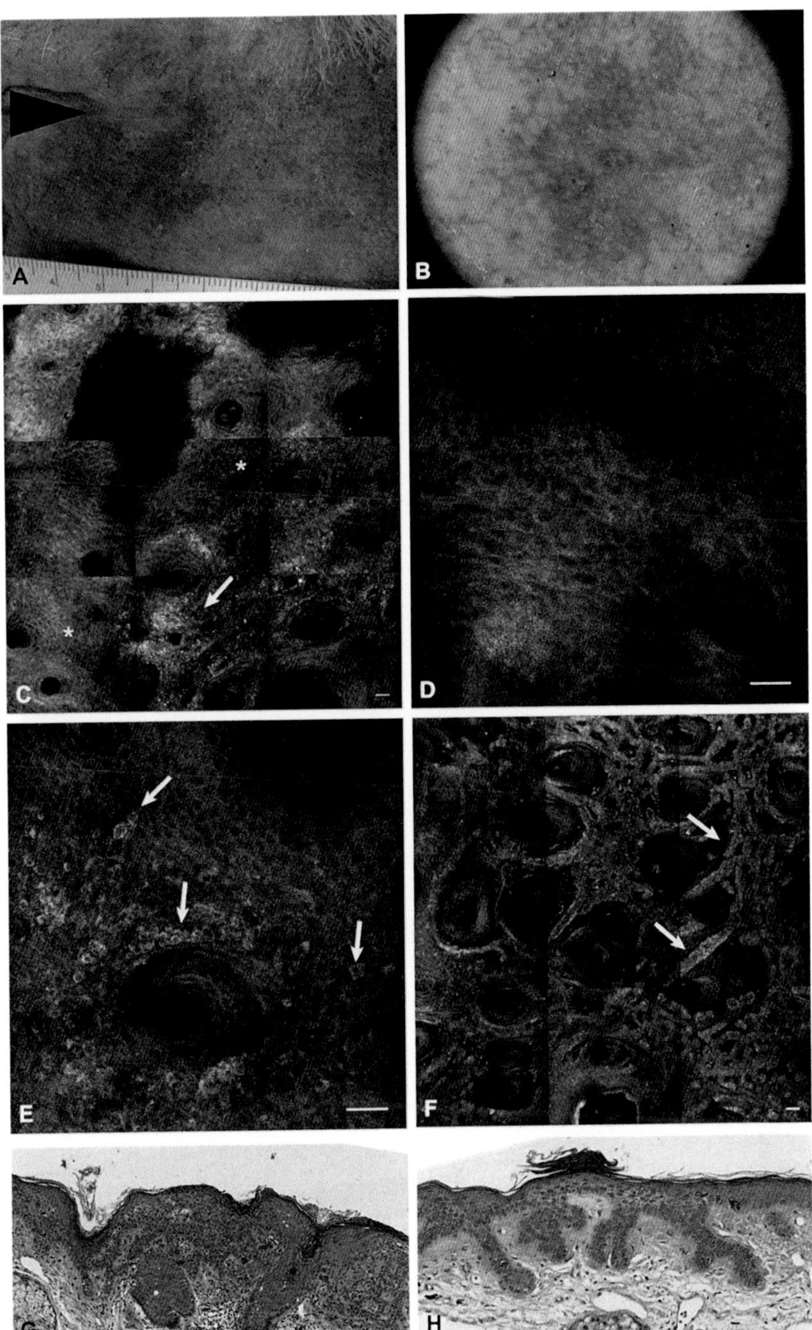

Fig. 1 Comparison of clinical, dermoscopy, and reflectance confocal microscopy and histopathology of a pigmented actinic keratosis. (**a**) Clinical photograph of 1.5–3.2-cm reddish brown lesion. (**b**) Dermatoscopy features resulted in brown and grayish interlacing. (**c**–**f**) Reflectance confocal microscopy (*RCM*) features showed atypical honeycomb pattern (*asterisks*), small bright nucleated cells (*arrow*), irregular size and shape of keratinocytes with broadened intracellular spaces, and anastomosing cords of epithelial cells (RCM scale bars 50 μm). (**g**–**h**) Histopathology features result in morphology similar to superficial reticular seborrheic keratosis; however, atypical keratinocytes and parakeratosis led to the diagnosis of pigmented actinic keratosis. (Original magnification: 35 and 310, respectively) (Reprinted from Wurm et al. [8], Copyright (2012), with permission from Elsevier)

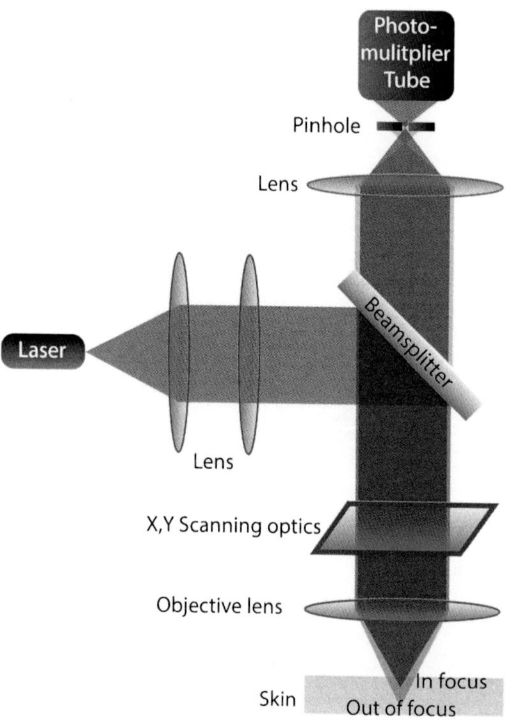

Fig. 2 Schematic illustration of reflectance confocal microscopy. A focused laser beam is scanned across the tissue. A photomultiplier tube then detects the reflected back-scattered light. The pinhole spatial filter blocks out-of-focus light

laser light source in the visible and near-infrared spectrum (488–800 nm), and laser scanning was achieved with a polygon mirror and a galvanometric mirror [15]. The integration of a laser light source instead of mercury lamp had the advantage of a narrow bandwidth for specific wavelength selection and increased power of illumination [15], which is important for skin imaging, where the tissue is highly scattering and contains a large amount of endogenous fluorophores.

Since then, the cost, size, and practicality of lasers for medical purposes have improved. Combined with an increase in the understanding of light and tissue interaction, biological imaging has seen a shift toward near-infrared light sources. This is due in part to longer wavelengths scattering less and as a result are capable of deeper tissue imaging. Rajadhyaksha et al. demonstrated that the stratum corneum all the way to the dermal-epidermal junction could be imaged with a 647 nm Krypton laser, while imaging with an 800 nm Titanium Sapphire laser allowed further penetration to the papillary dermis [15]. Currently, typical RCM systems consist of near-infrared light ranging from 700 to 1400 nm with less than 20 to 40 mW laser power to avoid tissue damage [16, 17]. While the depth of penetration that can be reached in the dermis varies due to wavelength-dependent scattering and absorption of the laser, RCM imaging at depths between 200 and 300 μm can be achieved with near-infrared lasers [17].

The resolution of RCM depends on a number of factors including the size of the pinhole, the numerical aperture (NA) of the objective lens, and the wavelength of the light source. For example, Rajadhyaksha et al. achieved a lateral resolution of ~1 μm and an axial resolution of ~3 μm with an RCM using a 1.32 NA objective lens and 50 μm pinhole [15]. This resolution was suitable for discrimination of discrete cells, in addition to subcellular and extracellular components. Typically, water or oil immersion objective lenses are used for focusing the laser light, as the refractive index of water is similar to the refractive index of the epidermis. Matching lens and tissue refractive indices minimizes spherical aberrations which result when light passes through an air-tissue interface [17].

Data acquired by RCM consist of gray-scale en face images, either as a single image, a 3D stack, wide area mosaic, or a 3D mosaic. The detailed reflective signal comes from the local differences in refractive index of the components within the skin. For example, individual cells can be detected due to large differences in refractive index between the membrane and the extracellular environment. In particular, high contrast is seen from cells containing melanin such as basal keratinocytes, melanocytes, and melanophages due to melanin having a high refractive index (1.7) [17]. This is also true for collagen, keratin, and lipids. Further, high contrast is observed from microstructures which are similar in size to the laser illumination wavelength such as melanosomes, which are similar in size to the near-infrared wavelength as well as organelles or granules present in the cytoplasm of Langerhans cells, lymphocytes, or keratinocytes [17].

Reflectance Confocal Microscopy Features of Skin Aging

With its ability to image the skin's cellular and subcellular components at a quasi-histological resolution, RCM is a complementary if not comparable approach to histopathology assessment [18]. Initial studies focused on the utilization of RCM for characterizing melanoma and nonmelanoma skin cancers [19] and skin disease including psoriasis [20], contact dermatitis [21], and folliculitis [22]. Although accepted early on that RCM provides significant contrast of pigmented cells, it was not until the mid-2000s that researchers started reporting the use of RCM as a tool for monitoring UV-related changes in the skin [23]. These studies combined with RCM characterization of actinic keratosis helped to establish a foundation for the technique to be used as a tool for characterizing photoaging.

In the last few years, several papers have been published systematically assessing a large range of potential features of intrinsic and extrinsic aging (Fig. 3). A study in 2012 by Wurm and colleagues compared the RCM features related to chronological aging and photoaging [24]. The authors assessed 21 criteria from the stratum corneum down to the upper dermis. However, only the following 15 resulted in significant correlation: subsurface epidermis (small, large, and disarranged rhomboidal furrowing, linear furrowing, and furrow width), the middle epidermis (regular, irregular, and disarray of keratinocyte packing (honeycomb pattern) and mottled pigmentation), dermo-epidermal junction (DEJ) (regularity and irregularity of papillary rings and whether they were polycyclic (elongated and partially anastomosing forming ring-like structures) and effacement), and upper dermis (thin collagen fibers and collagen clods). In an effort to correlate their findings with other grading techniques, the features were graded on a semiquantitative scale from 1 (small) to 3 (large). Additionally several features were graded based on overall presence within the image area: 0 = absent; 1 < 10 % of the imaged area; 2, 10–50 % of the imaged area; and 3, > 50 % of the imaged area. Using this method the three assessors resulted in strong agreement for furrow pattern, furrow width, mottled pigmentation, and papillary ring structure. However, smaller features such as sunburn cells resulted in poor agreement.

Kutlu Haytoglu et al. (2014) observed a similar pattern in agreement between assessors [25]. The larger high signal structures such as number of dermal papillary and furrow depth resulted in high agreement. These were two features not explored in the Wurm et al., yet were shown to be significant features for aging. The smaller more discreet signals attributed to cells (e.g., honeycomb pattern) also showed positive agreement but lower (Cohen's kappa value of >0.614 compared to >0.941). Other features have also been explored such as sebaceous gland number and morphology [26].

Two significant RCM features for characterizing aging were the same as those observed clinically – furrow morphology (wrinkles) and pigmentation. An important RCM structure not observable in the clinic is the dermal papillary rings. In relation to histopathology, the major feature used for characterizing photoaging is the deformation of the dermal collagen and elastin. Although collagen features are used for assessment within RCM, due to limited penetration depth of the technology, these features are not as significant and resulted in lower interobserver agreement. These three components are used in the majority of RCM studies for the assessment of chronological and photoaged skin. However, as the severity in photodamage increases and the lesional areas transition toward actinic keratosis, it has been observed that epidermal cellular features such as the regularity of the honeycomb pattern and immune cell infiltration begin to play a more important role [27]. Therefore, it is recommended that the minimal features that should be used for assessing intrinsic and extrinsic aging are furrow morphology, keratinocyte

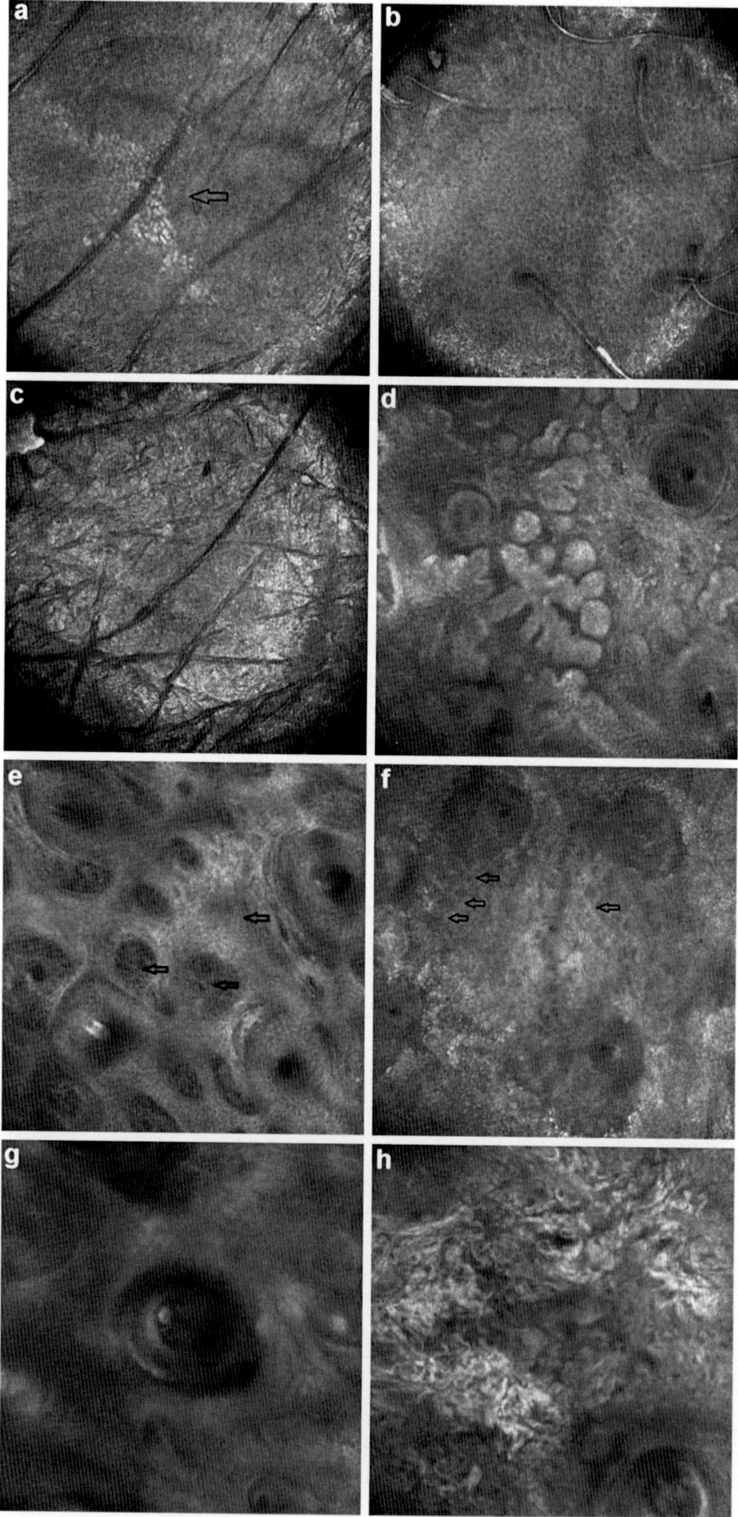

Fig. 3 Overview of reflectance microscopy features. (**a**) Mottled pigmentation shown by bright signal in clustered cells (*arrow*). (**b**) Irregular honeycomb pattern of keratinocytes with variation in size, shape, and cell borders. (**c**) Dark regions associated with furrows. (**d**) Irregular dermal papillary rings with polycyclic (elongated and partially anastomosing forming ring-like structures) morphology and effacement. (**e**) Thin reticulated collagen (*arrows*). (**f**) Coarse collagen (*arrows*). (**g**) Huddled collagen shown by hyporefractive regions. (**h**) Solar elastosis, as shown by curled wavy bright structures (Reprinted from Kutlu Haytoglu et al. [25], Copyright (2014), with permission from John Wiley and Sons)

honeycomb pattern, and dermal papillary morphology.

Utility of Reflectance Confocal Microscopy as an Objective Grading Tool

RCM is emerging as a promising technique for characterizing skin aging. However, clinical translation is not trivial. Conventional histopathology consists of colored H&E stained 2D cross-sectional tissue slices. This is in contrast to RCM, which consist of en face gray-scale image slices that can be viewed as 3D blocks. Additionally RCM data can be obtained in real time, in contrast with the longer time needed by histology, resulting in large datasets across multiple body sites and time. For accurate and reliable diagnostic characterization of such large amounts of information, it is essential that clinicians be trained and that RCM data be benchmarked with current routine histopathology. However, with current reports showing variation among assessors and difficulty in standardizing the same features across studies, researchers have been investigating automated imaging approaches to improve objectivity and throughput.

To validate the utility of computational analysis of RCM, Raphael et al. compared the results with clinical assessment (SCINEXA), clinical photography, and observer-graded RCM [4]. The authors utilized a blinded approach, whereby the mathematical descriptors were based on unknown RCM features, independent of the features selected in the morphological RCM score (observer assessment). Four computational techniques were utilized – intensity, segmentation, 2D wavelet transform, and 2D Fourier transform. Within each technique, there were several analytic approaches used for the characterization of the intensity, segmentation, or transformation (e.g., standard deviation, kurtosis, skewness, ordering [for full details refer to [4]]).

Only four mathematical descriptors were found to correlate with the clinician assessment of the RCM images. These were particle circularity and length following segmentation within the stratum corneum and viable epidermis, respectively. These features related to the degree and morphology of furrowing. The other two descriptors were the ratio between the maximum and minimum order direction and the minimum order direction following Fourier transform. Again, these descriptors were only significant within the stratum corneum and viable epidermis, respectively. They related to how regular the ordering of the tissue is and how aligned that order is to a direction. The authors then combined their descriptors into a single normalized feature score for each volunteer's RCM data. When comparing their method to the photographic, SCINEXA, and assessor RCM score, it was observed that computational grading resulted in an almost continuous spectrum from least to most photoaged. SCINEXA resulted in a spread of scores for the older volunteers but was less effective at distinguishing differences in the younger volunteers. This was reversed for the assessor-graded RCM scores. Although the photography scoring showed a relatively continuous grading profile, there was obvious separation between the two age groups of the volunteers with little overlap (20–30 and 50–60 years old). Representations of clinical photographs and RCM images for a single 20–30-year-old and 50–60-year-old, in addition to the overall grading scores, are shown in Fig. 4.

The study by Raphael and colleagues showed that computational assessment could produce clinically relevant unbiased results. However, a potential limitation of the study was that for a mathematical descriptor to be chosen, it had to result in significant correlation with at least one feature defined by the assessor RCM grading. Even when blinded against which feature was being correlated with the descriptor, there is an inherent limitation in that the approach relies on the assessor RCM grading to be 100 % accurate and without bias. This could result in certain computational descriptors not resulting in strong correlation. For example, no descriptors were related to the dermal-epidermal junction (dermal

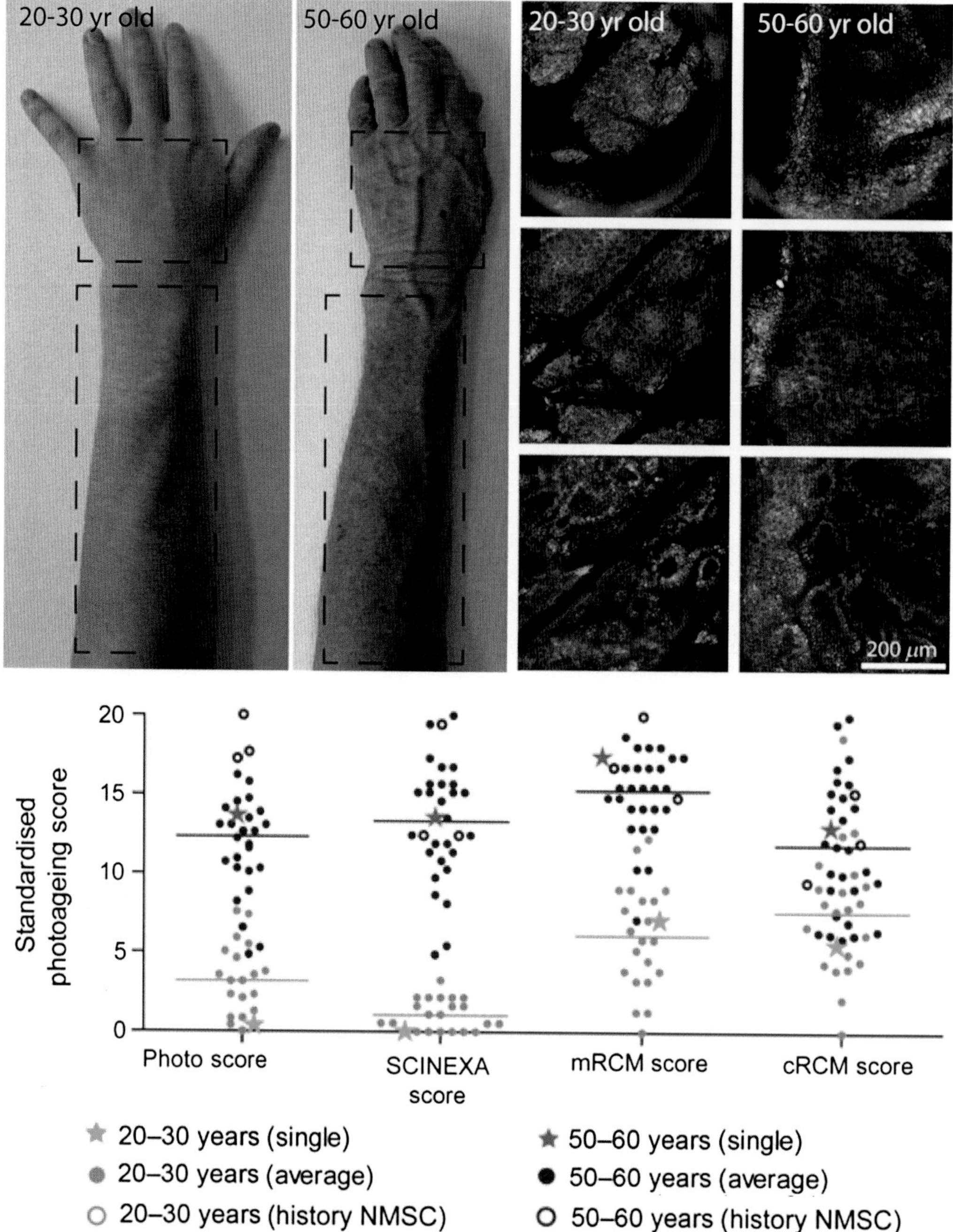

Fig. 4 Comparison of computational scoring with photography, clinical assessment, and manual RCM grading. *Top panels*: representative clinical photographs of a single volunteer from the two age groups investigated. The outlined regions correspond to the site assessed for photoaging. The combined forearm and hand were also scored. The volunteers' respective RCM images are shown to the right for the stratum corneum, stratum spinosum, and dermo-epidermal junction. *Bottom panel*: comparison of the overall scores from the four methods (clinical photography, SCINEXA, manual RCM assessment [*mRCM*], and computational [*cRCM*]). The *green* and *orange stars* represent the 20–30- and 50–60-year-old volunteers shown above (Reprinted from Raphael et al. [4], Copyright (2013), with permission from John Wiley and Sons)

papillary). Yet, this is a common feature utilized in the majority of user-assessed RCM analysis. The difficulty with automated analysis of the dermal-epidermal junction is the reliance of an intact, highly reflective stratum basale. Although with increased photoaging the dermal-epidermal junction becomes less regular, individuals with fairer skin (Fitzpatrick scales I–III) do not have highly reflective melanin-rich cells. Combined with less resolved imaging ability due to increased penetration, depth further compounds the difficulty of computational assessment. However, there is still much interest in automated characterization of the dermal-epidermal junction with a report by Kurugol and colleagues introducing an algorithm for localization of the dermal-epidermal junction [28–30]. The method utilized similar image analysis features described in Raphael et al. (segmentation, pixel intensity depth profiles, 2D texture analysis, and image transformations). The defining feature that contributed to locating the dermal-epidermal junction was the high level of reflectance from melanin-rich cells within the stratum basale.

In parallel, researchers are also exploring automated computational techniques for keratinocyte identification and morphological characterization [31]. In the context of photoaging, variation in the honeycomb pattern of the keratinocytes is a significant feature used for characterizing later-stage photodamage and progression of actinic keratosis to squamous cell carcinoma. Gareau exploited the regularity of the viable epidermal cells and their uniformity in RCM signal where each keratinocyte has a bright periphery and a dark nucleus [31]. The discrepancy in signal intensity was used to distinguish the keratinocyte nuclei and segmentation used to identify cell boundaries.

A benefit of RCM imaging over clinical photography and to an extent histopathology is that the data can be acquired with relatively little training and for the most part are uniform between patients. This advantage aids in the development of computational algorithms with two main approaches taking the forefront. The first is to mimic the methods utilized by trained assessors to identity features related to intrinsic and extrinsic aging. Alternatively, an untargeted approach can be developed similar to Raphael et al., whereby mathematical descriptors are identified in an unbiased manner. These approaches can be defined as a data-driven process versus an expert-driven process. However, with much of this research still in the pioneering stage, it is expected that the path forward will be a decision support system combining expert knowledge and data-driven software.

Looking Forward: Clinical Advances in Reflectance Confocal Microscopy and Alternate/Complementary Technologies

Overcoming Limitations in RCM

RCM is a reliable alternative to conventional histopathology assessment. However, it has several technical limitations one of which is poor penetration depth. Penetration depth is dependent on a number of factors including laser wavelength, laser power, and the scattering properties of skin. Therefore, this limitation could be surmounted by the use of lasers with longer infrared wavelengths that penetrate deeper into the skin than the common Titanium Sapphire laser used for RCM imaging at the expense of resolution or increase laser power at the risk of laser-mediated thermal tissue damage.

RCM typically uses high NA objective lenses (0.7–1.4) with high magnifications (20× to 100×) resulting in a small field of view between 200 and 1000 μm [32]. To create a larger field of view, software is used to stitch a sequence of captured RCM images creating a mosaic. Two different algorithms can be used for stitching RCM images. One of the algorithms includes cropping the overlap region between adjacent images and merging the resultant images [32]. This method is quick but leaves seams at the edges of the stitched images [32]. The second algorithm involves matching features in the overlapping regions and averaging these regions [32]. This method is not as quick as the first method but creates mosaics without seams [32]. Alternatively, RCM can be combined with dermoscopy to select regions of interest [33].

Another limitation to RCM is specificity which can be overcome by the development of contrast agents to enhance the identification of different cell populations as well as their subcellular structures [33]. Acetic acid and aluminum chloride have been found to be potential contrast agents for RCM imaging. Aluminum chloride [34] and acetic acid [35] enhance nuclear contrast for improved tumor visibility in RCM images. In particular, Scope et al. also showed that aluminum chloride enhances the nuclear morphology of keratinocytes [36]. Increased backscattering of the nuclei is seen in RCM with these agents as both acetic acid and aluminum chloride cause chromatin to compress [35, 36].

From a logistical standpoint, one that is applicable to many optical systems is their relatively large size and complex components. A major advancement that has helped to address this is the utilization of an optical fiber for both laser illumination and photodetection. In this scheme, a single-mode optical fiber acts as the spatial filter [9]. The elimination of the confocal pinhole and large optical components in this system has enabled the development of fiber-optic RCMs as handheld devices allowing flexibility and mobility [9]. This has been critical in facilitating the use of RCM assessment for difficult to access body sites.

As RCM becomes more routinely used in clinical studies, another challenge that will have to be overcome is the interpretation of gray-scale en face RCM images [33]. Dermatologists and pathologists will require training before becoming confident with their analysis of these images [33]. An interesting approach to potentially overcome this limitation has been proposed. Working with histology sections, Gareau stained them with a single dye (acridine orange) followed by RCM scanning [37]. The images were "digitally stained" to mimic conventional H&E histopathology resulting in remarkably similar H&E pseudo-colored images. There were still discrepancies between the techniques, and the need of acridine orange limits the digital staining to ex vivo samples. However, the work sets the foundation for the development of RCM techniques resulting in 3D "H&E"-like images that would be well accepted into current clinical analysis.

In parallel to RCM development, there is several alternative skin imaging techniques such as nonlinear optical microscopy and optical coherence tomography that are being explored. The use of these techniques either in combination or separately to RCM could aid the improved identification of biomarkers for aging skin, photoaged skin, and actinic keratosis.

Nonlinear Optical Microscopy

Nonlinear optical microscopy is a novel technique, which can be used to complement confocal reflectance in order to obtain additional contrast of the dermis and epidermis. A nonlinear optical microscope operates in a similar way to RCM. One important difference is the utilization of pulsed ultrafast (femtosecond and picosecond) lasers that are necessary in order to achieve high peak power without inducing damage to the sample. By utilizing longer wavelengths in the IR spectrum (700–1700 nm), tissue damage can be further reduced, facilitating in vivo applications. An added benefit of the higher infrared excitation wavelengths is that in nonlinear microscopy deeper penetration of light into the skin is achieved [38].

In contrast to RCM, nonlinear optical microscopy has inherent confocality, and therefore, the confocal pinhole is not necessary to obtain optical sectioning. The nonlinear optical processes are naturally confined to the focal volume because the intensity of second-order and third-order nonlinear optical processes is proportional to the second or third power of the incident laser intensity. Typical nonlinear optical microscopy setups are similar to RCM setups, and images of 2D optical sections are obtained by raster scanning the laser beam along two orthogonal directions, while 3D data is obtained by translating the sample along the optical axis. Since both techniques are so similar, hybrid systems have been constructed by the addition of a pinhole for backward confocal microscopy in nonlinear optical microscopes [39].

Several nonlinear optical processes have shown potential for imaging skin including multiphoton excitation fluorescence (MPF), second harmonic generation (SHG), and third harmonic generation (THG).

Multiphoton Excitation Fluorescence Microscopy

Multiphoton excitation fluorescence occurs when a fluorophore simultaneously absorbs multiple photons. MPF can be detected from a number of endogenous fluorophores including NAD(P)H, flavoproteins, keratin, lipofuscin, elastin, collagen, and melanin. Consequently, MPF microscopy has become a valuable tool in dermatological research.

Recently, MPF microscopy has been used to morphologically characterize changes in keratinocytes in actinic keratosis. Koehler et al. imaged keratinocytes in the human epidermis of volunteers at 760 and 820 nm with MPF microscopy and found strong fluorescence from in the stratum granulosum resulting from keratohyalin in the cytoplasm of cells [40]. In the stratum spinosum, MPF signal was also observed in the cytoplasm due to cell organelles containing NAD(P)H, while in the stratum basale, MPF signal originates from melanin deposits [40]. MPF microscopy has been used to explore differences between patients with actinic keratosis versus control. In patients with actinic keratosis, Koehler et al. observed larger nuclei, increased intercellular spacing as well as heterogeneity in cell shape, and cellular MPF signal in the stratum granulosum, the stratum spinosum, and the stratum basale [40]. The two features unique to MPF that are not capable with current RCM resolution are the ratio of nuclear to cell size and accurate characterization of intercellular spacing. Although unique, it is yet to be known whether these features provide more relevant clinical information on early detection of actinic keratosis progression.

Second Harmonic Generation Microscopy

The SHG signal from collagen is particularly informative in dermatology. Previously, SHG microscopy was combined with MPF modality to study the photoaging process in skin. With 760 nm excitation in an ex vivo study, Lin et al. found SHG signal decreases with age, while MPF signal increases with age suggesting that collagen is being replaced by elastin [41]. Consistent findings were also found by Koehler et al. in vivo [42].

Often used as a complementary technique to multiphoton excitation fluorescence microscopy, second harmonic generation occurs when two photons of wavelength λ combine to produce one photon of wavelength $\lambda/2$ [43]. Unlike MPF, the SHG process itself does not deposit energy into the sample; however, other nontargeted pigments sometimes occur in tissues that undergo MPF and induce sample damage; therefore, power has to be limited. An important property of SHG is that only structures that contain noncentrosymmetric material induce SHG, allowing the technique to have inherent specificity. In biological samples, muscle [44, 45], microtubules [46], and collagen [47, 48] give rise to intense SHG signals.

In the context of photoaging, the benefit of SHG over the RCM and MPF is that it not only can provide images of dermal collagen but also detailed structural information. In harmonic generation processes, the tensorial relationship between signal intensity and polarization as a function of the laser polarization can be used to extract structural parameters of the collagen in the focal volume. The application of polarization SHG microscopy has been recently demonstrated on the skin, by Yasui et al., who demonstrated that detectable changes in collagen orientation with UVB-exposed skin could be shown with polarization-dependent SHG [49]. Further information could be obtained using the more accurate polarization-in, polarization-out SHG microscopy [50], as well as double-stokes Mueller SHG microscopy

[51]. These features coincide with the assessment of solar elastosis observed via histopathology, thereby allowing SHG to be benchmarked with conventional assessment.

Third Harmonic Generation Microscopy

Similar to second harmonic generation, third harmonic generation occurs when three photons combine to produce a single photon having wavelength λ/3 [43]. THG is mathematically restricted to occur at the interface of two materials where there is a difference in the refractive index or third-order nonlinear optical susceptibility (third-order nonlinear optical property of materials). In biological samples, THG signals have been observed from biological membranes [52], cell walls [53], lipid bodies [54], erythrocytes [55], myocytes [44], leukocytes [56], and adipocytes [57].

In 2005, Tai et al. demonstrated simultaneous epi-collection of SHG and THG signals from fixed skin tissue with 1230 nm chromium forsterite laser where THG signal from keratinocytes was detected [58]. Their optical system consisted of galvanometric mirrors for scanning and a 0.9 NA objective lens resulting in a lateral resolution of 410 nm, an axial resolution of 1 μm, and 300 μm penetrability [58, 59].

Four years later, simultaneous in vivo SHG and THG imaging were performed on the ventral forearm skin of humans to demonstrate the potential use of harmonic generation microscopy in clinical applications [60]. Total exposure time to the laser was limited to 30 min, and two different scanning modes were applied referred to as slow (90 mW and 0.37 Hz) and fast (120 mW and 2 Hz) [60]. A dermatologist evaluated the exposed skin at several time points after the experiment and found no changes in skin color and pigmentation as well as no presence of wound, blister, or ulceration [60]. In this study, THG signal revealed the multilayered stratum corneum as well as cells in the stratum granulosum, stratum spinosum, and straum basale [59]. In particular, strong THG signal was seen from subcellular organelles in the cytoplasm of keratinocytes [59]. In the dermis, THG signal from fibroblasts, erythrocytes, collagen fiber bundles, and elastin fibers was observed [59].

Morphological changes in keratinocytes in human skin with THG microscopy in vivo at 1230 nm was explored by Liao et al. who observed an increase in the intercellular spacing and an increase in cellular and nuclear size of keratinocytes in the stratum basale with aging skin [59]. In patients with actinic keratosis, an increase in the total nuclear area to the total cytoplasmic area of keratinocytes was observed as compared to control [59].

Similar to SHG microscopy, structural information can be obtained with polarization-dependent THG microscopy [61]. Such a technique could be applied to study protein aggregates within cells that form as a result of photoaging.

There are a number of advantages to using SHG and THG microscopy in comparison to RCM. One of the key advantages of harmonic generation microscopy is its high signal-to-noise ratio which is achieved because SHG and THG intensities scale quadratically with the number density of molecules within the focal volume [43]; therefore, signal-to-noise is limited by integration time due to the low noise. RCM in contrast is limited by the noise from other structures, which scatter the beam before the focal spot; hence, RCM is limited because the intensity scales linearly with the number density of molecules the same as the noise, and therefore, higher contrast cannot be obtained by higher integration times. Lastly, THG imaging has an increased penetration depth, and so far 956 μm penetration has been achieved [38] in mouse brain.

Although nonlinear systems are resulting in unique features that can be used to characterize the aging process, the technology is still in its infancy. Instead of looking for correlation and comparison with current techniques, reports are focused predominantly on what can be observed. Furthermore, systems are large and costly limiting their use in routine clinical settings. However, its ability to resolve subcellular components in greater detail and high resolution of collagen results in unique features related to nuclear/cytoplasm ratios, intercellular distances, cellular infiltration, and solar elastosis. Therefore, nonlinear microscopy will continue to grow as an important assessment technique for intrinsic and extrinsic aging.

Optical Coherence Tomography

Optical coherence tomography is another complementary technique to RCM. The setup is similar to RCM, where a laser beam is directed to a small spot on the sample, and reflected light is collected; however, in OCT the incident beam is split before the sample, and then the reflected beam and the reference beam are combined with the resulting interfere pattern analyzed. OCT generates 2D vertical cross-sectional images of tissue analogous to histology, and more specialized systems can create 3D images [62]. OCT offers larger scan areas as well as deeper penetration imaging compared with RCM and nonlinear optical microscopy. However, this comes at a cost of lower resolution. The axial resolution of OCT is dependent upon the coherence length and bandwidth of light, while the lateral resolution is determined by the numerical aperture of the focusing objective lens [61].

In human skin, an axial resolution of 7 μm and a lateral resolution of 4 μm were achieved with OCT at 1300 nm [63]. Although RCM has better axial and lateral resolution than OCT, penetration depths of 1 mm or greater can be achieved with OCT [63]. There have also been new advances in OCT which include the development of high-definition optical coherence tomography (HD-OCT) which has greater resolution than OCT. HD-OCT has achieved an axial and lateral resolution of 3 μm [64]. In this setup, the movement of the mirror used for the reference beam path is synchronized with the movement of the focal plane, and a two-dimensional infrared (1000–1700 nm) imaging array is used for photodetection. Boone et al. demonstrated intrinsic aging changes in volunteers using HD-OCT [64]. The authors utilized many of the same features as RCM, and due to comparable resolution, there were not any obvious unique features like what can be achieved with harmonic generation and multiphoton fluorescence.

Although the resolution of RCM is greater than the resolution of OCT and HD-OCT, OCT and RCM can be used to resolve cells in the epidermis. The major benefit of OCT is that it provides a greater imaging depth than RCM as well, a wide field of view of 5–10 mm. Therefore, the two techniques combined may generate complementary information [65].

Conclusion

Skin aging consists of both intrinsic and extrinsic factors that result in a diverse range of morphological changes to both cellular and extracellular components. The high correlation of severely photoaged skin with the development of actinic keratosis and its progression to nonmelanoma skin cancers warrants the development of noninvasive longitudinal assessment. Reflectance confocal microscopy is at the forefront of advanced microscopy techniques with commercial systems being developed for clinical use. Its ability to produce images with quasi-histological resolution of the cellular and subcellular structures in addition to serial imaging of the same site over time makes it a powerful clinical tool.

However, standardized RCM features are yet to be established, and with continual improvements in imaging, researchers are being overwhelmed with a wealth of information that needs to be sifted through to determine what is significant for photoaging. That being said, RCM has shown strong correlation with conventional histopathology and clinical grading, in many ways bridging the benefits between the two approaches. The major RCM features related to skin aging are furrowing otherwise known as fine/coarse wrinkling, which is an important feature in clinical grading; keratinocyte morphology and packing arrangement, which can be observed in histopathology; changes in dermal fibers; and regularity of the dermal papillae, which is unique to en face imaging such as RCM.

Like all techniques, there is a need for standardization and objectivity. A benefit of RCM data is that it can be readily utilized for computational assessment. As clinical features and computational descriptors are integrated and validated, it is envisioned that the future of noninvasive microscopy will shift toward automated and objective data-driven analysis. This will result in unique and powerful tools for preventative risk management of skin aging.

References

1. Kappes UP, Elsner P. Clinical and photographic scoring of skin aging. Skin Pharmacol Appl Skin Physiol. 2003;16:100–7.
2. McKenzie NE, et al. Development of a photographic scale for consistency and guidance in dermatologic assessment of forearm sun damage. Arch Dermatol. 2011;147:31–6. doi:10.1001/archdermatol.2010.392.
3. Weiss JS, et al. Tretinoin therapy: practical aspects of evaluation and treatment. J Int Med Res. 1990;18 Suppl 3:41C–8.
4. Raphael AP, et al. Computational characterization of reflectance confocal microscopy features reveals potential for automated photoageing assessment. Exp Dermatol. 2013;22:458–63. doi:10.1111/exd.12176.
5. Vierkotter A, et al. The scinexa: a novel, validated score to simultaneously assess and differentiate between intrinsic and extrinsic skin ageing. J Dermatol Sci. 2009;53:207–11. doi:10.1016/j.jdermsci.2008.10.001.
6. Isik B, et al. Development of skin aging scale by using dermoscopy. Skin Res Technol. 2013;19:69–74. doi:10.1111/srt.12033.
7. Argenziano G, et al. Dermoscopy of pigmented skin lesions: results of a consensus meeting via the internet. J Am Acad Dermatol. 2003;48:679–93. doi:10.1067/mjd.2003.281.
8. Wurm EM, et al. Confocal features of equivocal facial lesions on severely sun-damaged skin: four case studies with dermatoscopic, confocal, and histopathologic correlation. J Am Acad Dermatol. 2012;66:463–73. doi:10.1016/j.jaad.2011.02.040.
9. Minsky M. Microscopy apparatus. International Patent USA 1957.
10. Egger MD, Petran M. New reflected-light microscope for viewing unstained brain and ganglion cells. Science. 1967;157(305):305–7.
11. Cavanagh HD, et al. Confocal microscopy of the living eye. Contact Lens Assoc Ophthalmol. 1990;16 (65):65–73.
12. Jester JV, et al. In vivo, real-time confocal imaging. J Electron Microsc Tech. 1991;18:50–60.
13. Andrews PM, et al. Tandem scanning confocal microscopy (tscm) of normal and ischemic living kidneys. Am J Anat. 1991;191:95–102.
14. Masters BR, Thaer AA. In vivo human corneal confocal microscopy of identical fields of subepithelial nerve plexus, basal epithelial, and wing cells at different times. Microsc Res Tech. 1994;29:350–6.
15. Rajadhyaksha M, et al. In vivo confocal scanning laser microscopy of human skin: melanin provides strong contrast. J Invest Dermatol. 1995;104:946–52.
16. Anderson RR, Parrish JA. The optics of human skin. J Invest Dermatol. 1981;77:13–9.
17. Sanchez-Mateos JLS, et al. Reflectance-mode confocal microscopy in dermatological oncology. In: Nouri K, editor. Lasers in dermatology and medicine/lasers in dermatology and medicine. New York: Springer London Limited; 2011. p. 285–308.
18. Kawasaki K, et al. Age-related morphometric changes of inner structures of the skin assessed by in vivo reflectance confocal microscopy. Int J Dermatol. 2015;54:295–301. doi:10.1111/ijd.12220.
19. Aghassi D, et al. Confocal laser microscopic imaging of actinic keratoses in vivo: a preliminary report. J Am Acad Dermatol. 2000;43:42–8. doi:10.1067/mjd.2000.105565.
20. Gonzalez S, et al. Characterization of psoriasis in vivo by reflectance confocal microscopy. J Med. 1999;30:337–56.
21. Gonzalez S, et al. Allergic contact dermatitis: correlation of in vivo confocal imaging to routine histology. J Am Acad Dermatol. 1999;40:708–13.
22. Gonzalez S, et al. Confocal reflectance imaging of folliculitis in vivo: correlation with routine histology. J Cutan Pathol. 1999;26:201–5.
23. Middelkamp-Hup MA, et al. Detection of uv-induced pigmentary and epidermal changes over time using in vivo reflectance confocal microscopy. J Invest Dermatol. 2006;126:402–7. doi:10.1038/sj.jid.5700055.
24. Wurm EM, et al. In vivo assessment of chronological ageing and photoageing in forearm skin using reflectance confocal microscopy. Br J Dermatol. 2012;167:270–9. doi:10.1111/j.1365-2133.2012.10943.x.
25. Haytoglu NS, et al. Assessment of skin photoaging with reflectance confocal microscopy. Skin Res Technol. 2014;20:363–72. doi:10.1111/srt.12127.
26. Longo C, et al. Skin aging: in vivo microscopic assessment of epidermal and dermal changes by means of confocal microscopy. J Am Acad Dermatol. 2013;68: e73–82. doi:10.1016/j.jaad.2011.08.021.
27. Prow TW, et al. Reflectance confocal microscopy: hallmarks of keratinocyte cancer and its precursors. Curr Probl Dermatol. 2015;46:85–94. doi:10.1159/000366541.
28. Kurugol S, et al. Automated delineation of dermal-epidermal junction in reflectance confocal microscopy image stacks of human skin. J Invest Dermatol. 2015;135:710–7. doi:10.1038/jid.2014.379.
29. Kurugol S, et al. Validation study of automated dermal/epidermal junction localization algorithm in reflectance confocal microscopy images of skin. Proc SPIE Int Soc Opt Eng. 2012;8207. doi:10.1117/12.909227.

30. Kurugol S, et al. Pilot study of semiautomated localization of the dermal/epidermal junction in reflectance confocal microscopy images of skin. J Biomed Opt. 2011;16:036005. doi:10.1117/1.3549740.
31. Gareau D. Automated identification of epidermal keratinocytes in reflectance confocal microscopy. J Biomed Opt. 2011;16:030502. doi:10.1117/1.3552639.
32. Gareau DS, et al. Confocal mosaicing microscopy in skin excisions: feasibility of cancer margin screening at the bedside to guide mohs. J Biomed Opt. 2008;13:054001. doi:10.1117/1.2981828.
33. Calzavara-Pinto P, et al. Reflectance confocal microscopy for in vivo skin imaging. Photochem Photobiol. 2008;84:1421–30.
34. Tannous Z, et al. In vivo real-time confocal reflectance microscopy: a noninvasive guide for mohs micrographic surgery facilitated by aluminum chloride, an excellent contrast enhancer. Dermatol Surg. 2003;29:839–46.
35. Rajadhyaksha M, et al. Detectability of contrast agents for confocal reflectance imaging of skin and microcirculation. J Biomed Opt. 2004;9:323–31.
36. Scope A, et al. In vivo reflectance confocal microscopy of shave biopsy wounds: feasibility of intra-operative mapping of cancer margins. Br J Dermatol. 2010;163:1218–28.
37. Gareau DS. Feasibility of digitally stained multimodal confocal mosaics to simulate histopathology. J Biomed Opt. 2009;14:034050. doi:10.1117/1.3149853.
38. Horton NG, et al. In vivo three-photon microscopy of subcortical structures within an intact mouse brain. Nat Photonics. 2013;7(205):205–9.
39. Wang H, et al. Perfectly registered multiphoton and reflectance confocal video rate imaging of in vivo human skin. J Biophotonics. 2013;6:305–9.
40. Koehler MJ, et al. Keratinocyte morphology of human skin evaluated by in vivo multiphoton laser tomography. Skin Res Technol. 2011;17:479–86.
41. Lin S-J, et al. Evaluating cutaneous photoaging by use of multiphoton fluorescence and second-harmonic generation microscopy. Opt Lett. 2005;30:2275–7.
42. Koehler MJ, et al. In vivo assessment of human skin aging by multiphoton laser scanning tomography. Opt Lett. 2006;31:2879–81.
43. Boyd RW. Nonlinear optics. 3rd ed. Amsterdam: Academic; 2008.
44. Chu SW, et al. Studies of x((2))/x((3)) tensors in submicron-scaled bio-tissues by polarization harmonics optical microscopy. Biophys J. 2004;86:3914–22. doi:10.1529/biophysj.103.034595.
45. Greenhalgh C, et al. Influence of semicrystalline order on the second-harmonic generation efficiency in the anisotropic bands of myocytes. Appl Opt. 2007; 46:1852–9.
46. Dombeck DA, et al. Uniform polarity microtubule assemblies imaged in native brain tissue by second-harmonic generation microscopy. Proc Natl Acad Sci U S A. 2003;100:7081–6.
47. Freund I, Deutsch M. Second-harmonic microscopy of biological tissue. Opt Lett. 1986;11:94–6.
48. Stoller P, et al. Polarization-modulated second harmonic generation in collagen. Biophys J. 2002;82:3330–42.
49. Yasui T, et al. Observation of dermal collagen fiber in wrinkled skin using polarization-resolved second-harmonic-generation microscopy. Opt Express. 2009;17:912–23.
50. Tuer AE, et al. Hierarchical model of fibrillar collagen organization for interpreting the second-order susceptibility tensors in biological tissue. Biophys. 2012;103:2093–105. doi:10.1016/j.bpj.2012.10.019.
51. Samim M, et al. Double stokes mueller polarimetry of second-harmonic generation in ordered molecular structures. J Opt Soc Am B. 2015;32:451–61.
52. Muller M, et al. 3d microscopy of transparent objects using third-harmonic generation. J Microsc (Oxf). 1998;191:266–74.
53. Squier JA, et al. Third harmonic generation microscopy. Opt Express. 1998;3:315–24.
54. Debarre D, et al. Imaging lipid bodies in cells and tissues using third-harmonic generation microscopy. Nat Methods. 2006;3:47–53. doi:10.1038/Nmeth813.
55. Millard AC, et al. Third-harmonic generation microscopy by use of a compact, femtosecond fiber laser source. Appl Opt. 1999;38:7393–7.
56. Tsai C-K, et al. Imaging granularity of leukocytes with third harmonic generation microscopy. Biomed Opt Express. 2012;3:2234–43.
57. Tsai C-K, et al. Virtual optical biopsy of human adipocytes with third harmonic generation microscopy. Biomed Opt Express. 2013;4:178–86.
58. Tai S-P, et al. Optical biopsy of fixed human skin with backward-collected optical harmonics signals. Opt Express. 2005;13:8231–42.
59. Liao Y-H, et al. Determination of chronological aging parameters in epidermal keratinocytes by in vivo harmonic generation microscopy. Biomed Opt Express. 2013;4:77–88.
60. Chen S-Y, et al. In vivo harmonic generation biopsy of human skin. J Biomed Opt Let. 2009;14:0605051–3.
61. Tokarz D, et al. Molecular organization of crystalline beta-carotene in carrots determined with polarization-dependent second and third harmonic generation microscopy. J Phys Chem B. 2014;118:3814–22.
62. Babalola O, et al. Optical coherence tomography (OCT) of collagen in normal skin and skin fibrosis. Arch Dermatol Res. 2014;306:1–9.
63. Pagnoni A, et al. Optical coherence tomography in dermatology. Skin Res Technol. 1999;5:83–7.
64. Boone MA, et al. High-definition optical coherence tomography intrinsic skin ageing assessment in women: a pilot study. Arch Dermatol Res. 2015;307:705–20. doi:10.1007/s00403-015-1575-x.
65. Malvehy J. A new vision of actinic keratosis beyond visible clinical lesions. J Eur Acad Dermatol Venereol. 2015;29:3–8.

Part VI

Toxicology/Safety and Microbiology

Susceptibility to Irritation in the Elderly

105

Miranda A. Farage, Kenneth W. Miller, G. Frank Gerberick, Cindy A. Ryan, and Howard I. Maibach

Contents

M.A. Farage (✉)
Winton Hill Business Center, The Procter & Gamble Company, Cincinnati, OH, USA
e-mail: farage.m@pg.com

K.W. Miller
Margoshes-Miller Consulting, LLC, , Cincinnati, OH, USA
e-mail: miller.kw.1@pg.com; bbbns2@fuse.net

G.F. Gerberick
Human Safety Department, Procter and Gamble Company, Cincinnati, OH, USA
e-mail: gerberick.gf@pg.com

C.A. Ryan
The Procter and Gamble Company, Cincinnati, OH, USA
e-mail: ryan.ca@pg.com

H.I. Maibach
Department of Dermatology, University of California, San Francisco, CA, USA
e-mail: maibachh@derm.ucsf.edu

M.A. Farage et al. (eds.), *Textbook of Aging Skin*,
DOI 10.1007/978-3-662-47398-6_80

Abstract

Numerous changes in the structure of the skin occur as the skin ages and modulate cutaneous function in a variety of ways. Exactly how, and to what extent, structural changes in the aging skin influence its ability to act as a barrier to exogenous agents is a matter of ongoing research. Skin irritation in the elderly can result from many factors including impaired percutaneous absorption, diminished barrier function (measured by transepidermal water loss), and compromised microcirculation. Environmental factors, such as very cold or dry conditions, can exacerbate irritation. Thus there are numerous factors that can influence skin testing results. Several testing approaches increase the ability to define differences in irritant potential among even the mildest of consumer products, as well as providing some correlation between subclinical skin changes and discomfort that has been formerly considered purely sensory in nature. Included in this chapter are brief discussions of the behind-the-knee (BTK) method employing mechanical friction; the modified forearm-controlled application test (mFCAT), patch testing that includes chemical exposure as well as repeated wiping; the use of cross-polarized light which facilitates subsurface visualization; measurement of cytokine mediators of inflammation; and infrared thermographic scanning to measure skin surface temperature.

Introduction

Numerous changes in the structure of the skin occur as the skin ages [1]; these structural changes modulate cutaneous function in a variety of ways [2, 3]. A critical role of the skin is to protect the vulnerable internal tissues from a multitude of potentially harmful exogenous agents [4]. Exactly how, and to what extent, structural changes in the aging skin influence its ability to act as a barrier to exogenous agents is a matter of ongoing research [5]. Definitive differences in skin structure and physiology between younger and older subjects are difficult to establish due to interpersonal variation in populations and methodological approaches and statistical difficulties inherent in sampling.

One factor that can influence a substance's skin irritation potential is its ability to penetrate the skin. Both skin barrier and the capacity of the microvasculature play a role in percutaneous absorption which is, by definition, a functional concept describing the process by which external substances (including both toxins and drugs) pass from the skin surface into the internal physiological milieu [6].

The first step in percutaneous absorption is the penetration of the chemical agent [4], dependent primarily upon the competency and hydration of the stratum corneum (SC) barrier [4, 5].

The SC is a two-component structure consisting of lipid-depleted corneocytes embedded in a continuous, lipid-enriched, extracellular matrix [7]. The barrier thickness varies substantially at different anatomical sites, about 15 stacked cell layers (roughly 10 μm) at most body sites, although areas such as the face and genitalia can be less than 10 cell layers, while the soles of the feet may be as many as 50 [8]. The structure of the SC prohibits permeability through organization into a lamellar membrane structure, the composition of the lipid component (including very long-chain fatty acids but no polar lipids), and the extracellular location of the lipid fraction, as well as a critical balance (1:1:1 in molar ratio, although ceramides are about 50 % by weight) [9] of three key lipids: ceramides, cholesterol, and free fatty acid [7] which form a barrier to diffusion [10]. Stratum corneum competence determines the diffusion of compounds across the skin and is dependent on functional biogenesis of corneocytes as well as the proper synthesis and processing of intracellular lipids [10]. Penetration is the limiting step in the formation of cutaneous reactions to chemicals and is always by passive diffusion [10]. A penetrating chemical may, however, cause structural and functional damage to the barrier, resulting in facilitation of increased penetration by the offending agent [11]. Some well-characterized skin irritants such as sodium lauryl sulfate, hydrochloric acid, and nonanoic acid are capable of causing such types of damage.

The second step in percutaneous absorption is diffusion through the viable epidermis and the dermis [12], a large sink (compared to the SC) where compounds are significantly diluted and may undergo significant changes in composition and structure [10]. The third step is successful uptake of the compound by the microcirculation so that it comes in contact with internal physiology [4].

Factors in Skin Irritation in the Elderly

Percutaneous Absorption

Structural alterations that occur as the skin ages have the potential to alter the process of percutaneous absorption. The aged epidermis displays several functional abnormalities possibly related to impaired percutaneous absorption, including altered drug permeability [7], a decreased tendency to exhibit irritant contact dermatitis [13], and decreased immunocompetence [14–16].

A definitive understanding of the effects of age on percutaneous absorption is elusive. Animal data are conflicting, and in vitro experiments have demonstrated little difference between younger and older skin [17]. Percutaneous penetration would appear to be largely impaired in older patients as compared to younger patients, as most compounds studied have been observed to be less efficiently absorbed by aged individuals (Table 1). One study investigated the percutaneous absorption of six different compounds as follows: testosterone, estradiol, hydrocortisone, benzoic acid, acetylsalicylic acid, and caffeine. Testosterone and estradiol absorption in patients older than 65 were slightly suppressed (16.6 ± 2.5 vs. 19.0 ± 4.4 and 5.4 ± 0.4 vs. 7.1 ± 1.1, respectively), neither significant, as compared to subjects aged 22–40 years, while benzoic acid, acetylsalicylic acid, hydrocortisone, and caffeine absorption were dramatically decreased [22]. To date, no observation of increased absorption in aged has occurred, despite a presupposition that older skin would display diminished barrier function [20].

It has been suggested that observed differences in absorption of different compounds may relate to the hydrophobic or hydrophilic nature of the penetrant itself. The biophysical characteristics of aged skin (reduced hydration levels and reduced

Table 1 Cutaneous absorption in the elderly

Percutaneous absorption	Test parameters	Definition of aged population	Effect of age	Reference
Water soluble-dye fluorescein	In vitro, forearm	61–90 years	Increased diffusion	Tagami [12]
Tetrachlorosalicylanilide (1.5 % in ethylene glycol)	In vivo, forearm	62–82 years	Greater time for penetration	Tagami [8]
Testosterone	In vitro	>75 years	Increased absorption	Roskos et al. [18]
Estradiol	In vitro	>75 years	Decreased absorption	Roskos et al. [18]
Hydrocortisone	In vitro	>75 years	Decreased absorption	Roskos et al. [18]
Benzoic acid	In vitro	>75 years	Decreased absorption	Roskos et al. [18]
Methyl nicotinate	In vitro	64–86 years	No difference	Roskokos et al. [19]
Testosterone 1.0 $\mu Ci/cm^2$	In vivo, forearm	Menopause (mean age 55)	No difference	Oriba et al. [20]
Fluorescein	In vitro	Cadavers 67–78 years	Decreased penetration	Christopher and Kligman [21]
Testosterone	In vivo, back	71–82 years	Decreased absorption	Christopher and Kligman [21]
Sodium chloride	In vivo	71–82 years	Reduced intradermal clearance rate	Christopher and Kligman [21]

lipid content) would predict facilitated penetration of hydrophobic compounds and relatively poor penetration of hydrophilic compounds [17], and a striking relationship between the hydrophobicity of a compound and its permeability coefficient has been observed [10]. In the evaluation of six compounds above, lipophilic compounds exhibited the same absorption in younger versus older subjects, while hydrophilic compounds (hydrocortisone, benzoic acid, acetylsalicylic acid, and caffeine) exhibited decreased absorption in older subjects [4], with relative absorption of each compound consistent to its permeability coefficient [17].

Barrier Function

Many components of healthy barrier function are known to decline with age (Table 2), casting suspicion on the efficacy of barrier function in the elderly. Stratum corneum thickness remains constant with age [41], but a global decrease in lipid content (as much as 68 %) leads to alterations in lamellar bilayer morphology [27]. Water-holding capacity, which is a function of the ceramide fraction of the intercellular lipid component of the SC, is diminished in aged skin [13]. An additional age-associated decrease in the sterol ester and triglyceride fraction of the SC lipids [4] contributes to the decrease in water-binding capacity, producing decreased hydration of the SC in aged individuals. It is known that skin barrier function is impaired in many dermatoses, including psoriasis, atopic dermatitis, and contact dermatitis [8, 10]. Characteristics of aged skin with the potential to influence barrier function are displayed in Table 2.

Transepidermal water loss (TEWL) is considered a measurement of the integrity of the horny layer, as one of the primary functions of the SC is to impede passive loss of water from the body [18]. Much research effort has evaluated whether or not baseline TEWL is significantly affected by aging [4]. The evaporation process was demonstrated to be slower in aged skin as compared to younger skin in vitro [42]. Also, aging enhances skin maceration. Considering that maceration is a risk factor for the skin damage, the development of technology to promote skin barrier recovery after maceration in the elderly is warranted [43].

Although several studies have observed a decreased TEWL in older patients, most studies have observed no impact or only slight decreases [4]. Importantly, TEWL measurements have been observed to be highly variable, with 8 % variation within individual by site and 21 % within the same individual from day to day and up to 48 % variation between healthy individuals [10]. The tendency for many substances to be less well absorbed in older skin has led some authors to suggest a slight enhancement of barrier function in the elderly [7, 8]. Despite the deterioration of the skin on many levels (with regard to the SC, most importantly the global loss of lipids), baseline TEWL in older patients appears to be normal [8]. Under normal conditions, barrier function is preserved, with lipid deficits compensated for by an increase in the thickness of the SC, larger corneocytes, and a decrease in the rate of desquamation [8].

Further investigation, however, has revealed that the apparently normal TEWL in the geriatric population masks substantial impairment of barrier function; obvious differences in permeability support the hypothesis that a barrier abnormality may, in fact, exist [27]. The functional pathology of the SC is revealed only after active insult [7].

In younger patients, barrier disruption stimulates the release of numerous cellular messengers which stimulate epidermal lipid synthesis and effect rapid restoration of barrier integrity [44]. The skin of aged individuals exhibits normal baseline barrier function, but recovery of barrier activity after perturbation is markedly reduced [10, 45]. TEWL measurements in vivo in both aged (greater than 80 years) and young (20–30 years) patients before and after disturbance of the barrier by tape stripping demonstrated a dramatic delay in recovery times in the older patients as compared to the younger. Younger subjects had recovered 50 % of barrier function by 24 h, whereas older patients had only recovered 15 % of barrier function; 90 % recovery was achieved within 4 days in younger patients, while older

Table 2 Components of barrier function in the aged

Skin parameter	Effect of aging	Reference
pH of skin surface	Elevated	Summers and Hunn [23]
SC water content	Normal	Elsner et al. [24], Thune [25], and Wilhelm et al. [26]
	Slightly decreased Decreased (4.43 ± 0.16 g/m^2 vs. 6.41 ± 0.93 g/m^2 ($p < 0.05$)	Ghadially et al. [27] and Potts et al. [28]
Total lipid content of SC	Decreased 65 %	Akomoto et al. [29]
Corneocyte surface area	Increased	Lévêque et al. [30]
Delivery of secreted lipids to SC	Reduced	Ghadially et al. [27]
Number of extracellular lamellar bilayers in the SC as visualized by electron microscopy with ruthenium tetroxide postfixation	Decreased	Ghadially et al. [27]
Reduction in global lipid content	1/3 less by weight	Elias and Ghadially [7]
Interleukin-1alpha	Reduced	Ye et al. [31]
Amphiregulin	Reduced	Ye et al. [31]
Upregulation of lipid synthesis after barrier disruption	Reduced	Ghadially et al. [32]
Mitotic response to glucosylceramide	Reduced	Marchell et al. [33]
Epidermal proliferation and differentiation	Significantly decreased in older individuals	Engelke et al. [34]
Barrier function	Less stable (18 ± 2 tape strippings required for perturbation in older skin (volar forearm) vs. 31 ± 5 in young	Ghadially et al. [27]
	Less cohesive (disrupted with fewer strippings)	Reed et al. [35]
Barrier recovery	Compromised 15 % recovery at 24 h in older patients, 50 % at 24 h in younger 90 % recovery seen at 7 days in older vs. 4 days in younger	Ghadially et al. [27]
TEWL	Normal	Ghadially et al. [27]
	Subnormal	Wilhelm et al. [26], Cua et al. [36], and Thune et al. [37]
	Decreased significantly after the age of 60	Lévêque et al. [38]
Mitotic activity and turnover time	Decreased	Baker and Blair [39]
Capacity for repair	Impaired (aged 65–75 years) compared to 18–25 years	Grove et al. [40]

SC stratum corneum, *TEWL* transepidermal water loss

patients required a full week. Erosion of barrier function was shown to be correlated to lipid content of the skin and thus likely related to a deficiency of key SC lipids in old age [27]. A similar experiment showed that delayed recovery times in the aged are extended by 20 % in aged skin when characterized by superimposed photoaging [35].

Microcirculation

Absorption into the blood stream depends on the integrity of the microcirculation. The microvasculature in elderly skin appears to be compromised [46]. Histological observations show structural impairment, with a decrease in the number of dermal capillary loops and flattening of the dermoepidermal junctions, creating a decreased area for absorption [47, 48].

In addition, functional deficits have been observed. Perfusion in the dorsum of the foot by capillary blood flow amplitude has been found to be significantly decreased in older patients [49]. Blood flow at multiple body sites evaluated by laser Doppler velocimetry showed significant decreases in areas of high blood flow [50]. A recent study showed that cryotherapy improved blood flow by slowing movement within the microcirculation and thus might potentially provide a therapeutic benefit to prevent leg ulcers [51].

Age-associated decreases in the sensitivity of the microvasculature have been linked to autonomic control. A significant time delay in expected blood flow changes after the Valsalva maneuver (in which exhalation is performed against resistance) as well as after postural changes was observed in aged patients [52]; similar impairments in vascular response were observed after body cooling [53], cold-arm challenge [53, 54], and inspiratory gasp [53].

Clearance experiments are a more specific measure of the ability of the cutaneous microvasculature to absorb penetrants into the systemic pool [18]. There is substantial evidence that drug clearance is impaired in elderly patients; reduced drug elimination due to compromised blood flow in elderly patients is an integral pharmaceutical consideration in determining doses in the elderly, with an approximately 40 % cumulative blood flow decline in a person 70 years of age [55]. The comparative permeability of aged skin, as well as the functional status of the stratum corneum and the skin's microcirculation, impacts both contact irritation and contact sensitivity in aged skin. The effects of aging on skin sensitization are reviewed elsewhere in this work [56]. This review will focus on aging and skin irritation, particularly new techniques being used to increase sensitivity in irritation testing.

Irritant Response

An inflammatory reaction in the skin due to a single exposure to an offending chemical is termed acute irritant dermatitis [57–59]. Cumulative contact irritation, more common, is the result of ongoing contact with low-level irritants. Clinical irritation depends primarily on the irritant potential of the substance, as well as the chronological and anatomical extent of exposure [60]. Threshold concentrations in viable tissue are also dependent on the surface concentration, degree of occlusion, number of exposures, and vehicle of delivery [10]. Individual predictors of the degree of irritation achieved include the integrity of the SC, the quality of the epidermal repair response, and the ability to mount an inflammatory response to the irritant [7]. Irritation is more commonly associated with formulations than with individual substances [60]. Certain individuals experience more intense and frequent adverse sensory effects than the normal population when exposed to certain substances, even substances that are benign in the majority of the population [61]. This phenomenon, termed "sensitive skin," is a subject of focused research, as subjective irritation often occurs in the absence of any objective signs [61]. Environmental factors, such as very cold or dry conditions, can also exacerbate irritation [62, 63]. Skin dryness and irritability in the elderly are enhanced in photoaged skin [45].

Numerous authors have observed a decreased susceptibility to cutaneous irritation in the aged. Irritation is less likely to develop, positive reactions are slower to develop, and, where irritation does occur, reactions are less intense. The aged also have a diminished capacity for recovery [13, 64, 65]. Irritant reactions are also more prolonged in older groups [56, 66].

Initial research into the effect of age on irritant response found decreased reactivity in the elderly to substances like soap [67] and croton oil [68]. Primary irritant response in both younger and older patients after application of a 1:1 solution of ammonium hydroxide in water demonstrated that although the time to raise a blister was reduced in older subjects, the time to fully fill the blister was significantly extended [40].

Further research evaluated a variety of irritants with different mechanistic actions as follows: dimethyl sulfoxide and ethyl nicotinate

Table 3 Effects of age on irritant reactions

Irritant	Criteria of aged population	Characteristics of older skin as compared to younger	Reference
Aqueous solution of ammonium hydroxide (1:1)	Over 75	Initial response time faster in older subjects, time to fully tense blister slower	Grove et al. [40]
Dimethyl sulfoxide, histamine, ethyl nicotinate, chloroform-methanol, lactic acid	Over 75	Reduction in visual scores of inflammation	Grove et al. [69]
SLS (0.25 %) with occlusion, 24 h	Over 65	Older: lower visual score, lower percentage or responders	Cua et al. [36]
		TEWL lower in older (indicative of decrease in inflammatory response)	
Soap	Over 50	Lower prevalence of positive tests	Bettley et al. [67]
SLS	Postmenopausal	Slower reaction, less intense, 9 visual score	Elsner et al. [78]
SLS	Mean age 74.6	Less intensity of response (visual score, TEWL)	Cua et al. [70]
		Reduction in SC 0.3 water content	
Croton oil		Decreased prevalence of positive reactions	Coenraads et al. [68]
SLS (0.1 %, 0.5 %, 1 %) applied to forearm	$N = 20$ (premenopausal 32.2 mean age, postmenopausal 63.2 mean age	Less prevalence of erythema in postmenopausal women (5/10 vs. 9/10), lower degree of TEWL induction, smaller increase in relative capacitance	Elsner et al. [73]
SLS (2, 3, 5 %) applied to forearm	$N = 20$ (premenopausal 32.2 mean age, postmenopausal 63.2 mean age	Less prevalence of erythema in postmenopausal women (6/10 vs. 8/10), lower degree of TEWL induction, smaller increase in relative capacitance	Elsner et al. [73]
SLS (2 %) applied to face and neck	$N = 20$, younger group average age 25.2, older group average 73.7	Less prevalence of erythema in older group, lower degree of TEWL	Marrakchi and Maibach [71]

SC stratum corneum, *SLS* sodium lauryl sulfate, *TEWL* transepidermal water loss

(nonimmunologic contact urticants), histamine (a mediator of immunological contact urticaria), chloroform-methanol (a stinging irritant), and lactic acid. All substances tested, despite having widely disparate mechanisms of irritation, produce much less irritation, quantified by visual inflammatory scores, in older patients as compared to younger [69].

Numerous authors have looked at differences in response to sodium lauryl sulfate between older and younger skin, at a variety of anatomical sites and concentrations, and have uniformly found a decrease in reactivity in older patients, including both prevalence of positivity and strength of reaction when present [70–77]. Less irritant reactivity was observed, both in visual scoring by erythema and by lesser increases in TEWL in response to application of irritant to older skin [4]. Inflammatory reactions in elderly are less intense in causing scaly, dry eczematous response, less vesicular, and less erythema than in younger patients [72]. A summary of the effects of age on the irritant response is found in Table 3.

Vulvar Susceptibility to Dermatitis

The unique characteristics of the epithelium of the vulvar area may make this region of the body more susceptible to irritation caused by topical medicaments and hygiene products [79]. The vulvar epithelium is derived from two different embryological layers. The mons pubis and labia majora, derived from embryonic ectoderm, physiologically resemble exposed skin: It is keratinized and stratified, with sweat glands, sebaceous glands, and hair. In contrast to exposed keratinized skin, however, it is occluded, more hydrated than exposed tissues, and subject to more frictional stress. The keratinized areas of the vulva have been shown to be seven times more permeable than forearm skin, determined by application of radiolabeled hydrocortisone in benzene: ethanol or acetone solution [20, 74, 80], although permeability varies with skin thickness [80].

The nonkeratinized area, from the inner third of the labia minora through the vulvar vestibule (derived from embryonic endoderm), is thinner and more loosely packed. It is also known to be significantly more permeable than keratinized skin [81, 82].

Vulvar symptoms are often related to irritant contact dermatitis [46]. In fact, prevalence rates as high as 54 % for vulvar dermatitis have been reported in vulvar clinic patients [83].

Extrinsic factors often exacerbate the intrinsic susceptibility to irritation produced by friction and occlusion in the vulvar area. Personal hygiene habits, characterized by excessive cleansing routines and use of soaps and other hygiene products with surfactants, alcohols, and antiseptics, are the most common causes of contact dermatitis in the vulvar area [46]. It should be noted, however, that self-medication of vaginal itch with over-the-counter products is often the source of secondary sensitization to topical medicaments.

Approaches in Skin Irritant Testing

Numerous factors can influence skin testing results. Best practice in skin testing of irritant response would ensure standardization of protocols in choice of irritant, test site, environmental controls, batch volume and concentration, delivery vehicle, use of occlusive dressing, time to evaluation, assessment tools, and, in females, menstrual cycle phase [84].

Skin testing which evaluates consumer products tests, by definition, substances intended to have no irritant potential. Such testing often utilizes an approach which seeks to exaggerate exposure conditions in a controlled manner and typically proceeds through patch testing followed by visual scoring. Such testing, however, is not practical for some products or anatomical areas (e.g., genital area) and may not be robust enough to detect irritation which may nonetheless cause consumer discomfort [85].

The Behind-the-Knee (BTK) Test

The behind-the-knee (BTK) approach was developed specifically to test frictional and chemical irritation [86] and employs the popliteal fossa as a test site, applying samples to the back of the knee with an elastic knee band (Fig. 1a–d). The BTK test more closely simulates real-world exposures, as mechanical friction is supplied in addition to the chemical exposure provided by traditional testing [87]. The test has now been utilized in testing of more than 25 different materials, including topsheets, interlabial pads, pantiliners, tampons, and lotion coatings on products such as facial tissues, producing reproducible data of equivalent quality to traditional clinical testing [85].

The BTK test offers other advantages to traditional testing in that it provides a controlled environment in which solid products like catamenial pads and diapers may be tested under convenient and controlled conditions [88] as well as the opportunity to independently evaluate different test conditions (e.g., wet vs. dry product) or do side-by-side comparisons of two different products. In addition, BTK testing can employ any healthy adult (i.e., does not require menstruating or incontinent patients), exposure can be controlled, and grading is not intrusive and is relatively inexpensive and productive of rapid results.

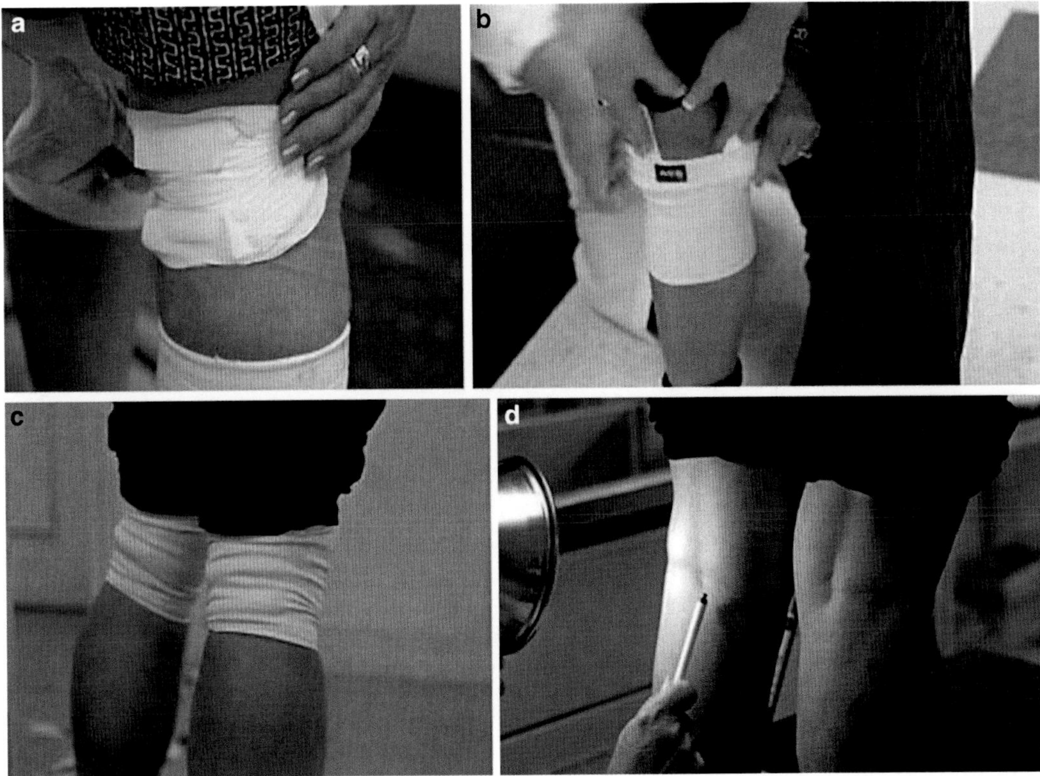

Fig. 1 The behind-the-knee (BTK) method: test material is placed horizontally and held in place behind the knee by an elastic knee band of appropriate size (**a-c**). Skin irritation grading is then performed by an expert grader (**d**)

In addition, the BTK method facilitated shorter exposure periods, allowing the traditional 24-h patch test (consisting of four applications) to be shortened to a 6-h, two-application method while producing equivalent results [87].

BTK testing has demonstrated utility beyond irritation testing, in one study being used in quantifying subject exposure to a lotion component added to sanitary pads [89]. Three different lotions were evaluated side-by-side in 54 healthy females by applying products (feminine pads containing lotion) to the popliteal fossa and comparing data obtained to that of traditional clinical testing. BTK data was found to be more consistent than that obtained with traditional testing, as well as being obtained at a fraction of the cost [89].

BTK testing has been used in concert with other newly developed techniques, as discussed below, with additional potential to enhance the sensitivity of current testing procedures. Despite extensive testing of consumer products, which document the absence of irritant potential in manufactured products, consumers often develop product preference on the basis of perceived sensory effects that were not revealed during testing [85]. Sensory data has recently been added to BTK irritant testing with the objective of correlating subjective sensory effects produced by different irritants with the development of objective signs of irritation. BTK testing was able to detect subtle differences between two products, consistent across a variety of test conditions; in addition, subjective data gathered with regard to sensory discomfort demonstrated product preference identical to that predicted by irritation observed through BTK testing [86].

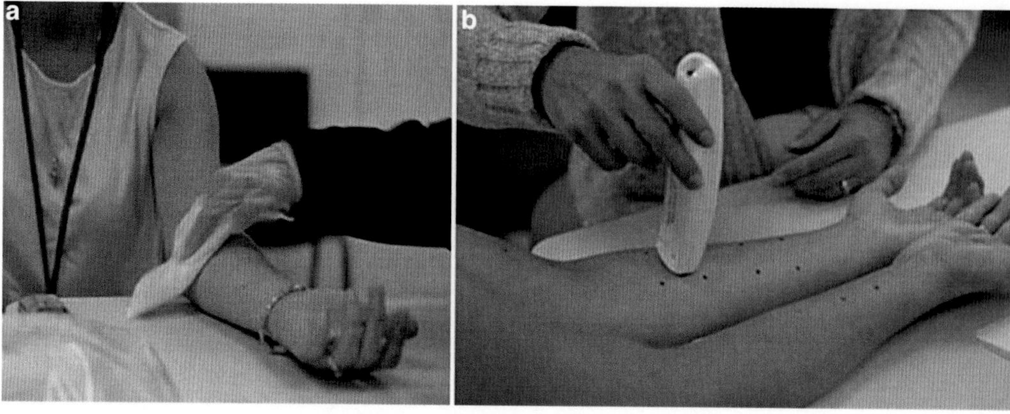

Fig. 2 Modified forearm-controlled application test (mFCAT)

Modified Forearm-Controlled Application Test (mFCAT)

Additional methodology which combined a mechanical friction component to patch testing in order to simulate real-world exposures was designed to distinguish among products intended to be extremely mild, such as facial tissues and baby wipes [85]. The forearm-controlled application test (FCAT), in which several products are tested on adjacent sites on the volar forearm (Fig. 2), was modified by the addition of repeated wiping in order to simulate the use of lotion-infused facial tissues in cold sufferers. Testing evaluated seven different lotions on SLS-treated skin (added to simulate underlying irritation common in skin around the nostril in cold sufferers); each test site was wiped 400 times and irritation evaluated by visual scoring [2]. The technique was successful in demonstrating consistent product differences, supporting its benefit in skin testing in irritancy that results from more than just simple chemical exposure [90]. Visual scoring has been the foundation of skin irritation testing, producing excellent reproducibility with trained graders [85, 91]. Optimal testing, however, would have the ability to detect subclinical skin alterations which occur before frank visibility occurs, an improvement in testing sensitivity which would facilitate future product-development efforts and may prove instrumental in understanding the currently elusive connection between and irritancy and skin sensitivity (which often occurs without objective signs).

There are several investigative approaches designed to increase the sensitivity of scoring. Methods include enhancement of visual scoring, measurement of inflammatory components, and use of novel instrumentation.

Cross-Polarization

One promising approach focuses on the improvement of visualization through the use of polarized light, a technique which has previously demonstrated improved visualization of various dermatological conditions. The use of cross-polarized light (which facilitates subsurface visualization) (Fig. 3) was more effective than unaided visual grading in detecting very minor irritation (upper arm testing) and more effective than unaided scoring in the differentiation of two specific products (BTK) [92]. Results of enhanced grading in the BTK test were also consistent with data collected on subjective sensory effects (Fig. 4) [92].

Enhanced visualization through polarized light was recently employed in the evaluation of dryness and irritation in women with unexplained vulvovaginal pain [93]. Subsurface visualization through cross-polarized light was more sensitive in detecting genital erythema and dryness at all sites regardless of whether or not clinical

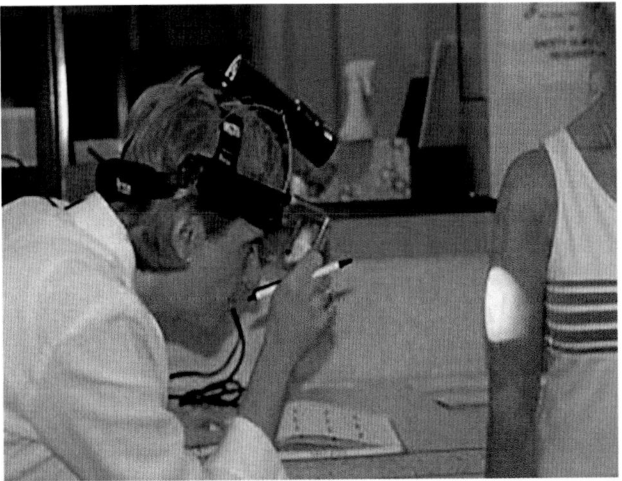

Fig. 3 Enhancing visual grading by using cross-polarization techniques such as the v600™ instrument

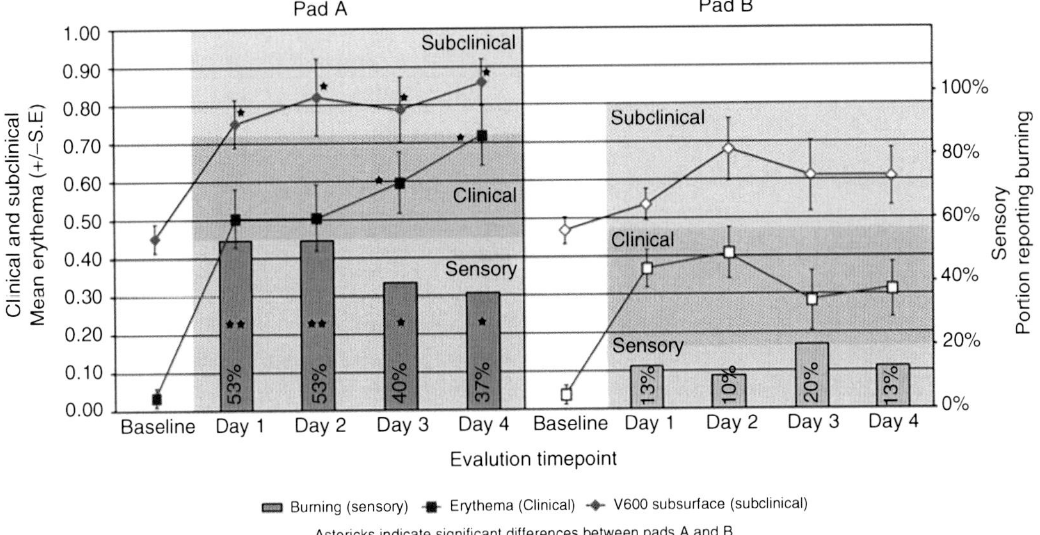

Fig. 4 The percentage of panelists who experienced burning sensations at the test sites is shown. With every sample application, there was a significantly higher number of individuals reporting burning sensations with Pad A compared with Pad B. In addition, a significantly higher number of individuals reported pain with Pad A during the third sample application and the sensation of the sample sticking to the skin during the second and third application. Enhanced visual scoring (subclinical changes) enables detection of physiological changes that are not apparent using standard visual scoring. This current investigation confirms that sensory effects correlate with visual scoring in the BTK and confirms that sensory effects enable the differentiation between two very similar products shown in this figure. *Significantly different than pad B ($p < 0.05$). **Significantly different than pad B ($p \leq 0.001$)

symptoms were present. In addition, subsurface inflammation of specific anatomical sites was observed to be specific to women with vulvar vestibulitis syndrome, demonstrating physical signs in a condition heretofore believed to be of sensory origin [93].

Cytokine Mediators

Skin irritation testing has also been recently performed through measurement of cytokine mediators of inflammation. Cytokine levels were measured in uncompromised skin as well as skin experiencing diaper or heat rash, skin which was SLS treated, and skin that was sun exposed through the use of an adhesive tape which absorbs oils. Tape was applied to skin and then processed to quantify levels of Il-1α, Il-1RA, and IL-8.

Il-1 levels were demonstrated to be higher in diaper rash, heat rash, and SLS-treated samples than in normal controls [94].

Infrared Thermographic

Another approach to assessing irritation through quantification of inflammation involves measuring skin surface temperature via an infrared thermographic scanner (Fig. 5). Skin temperature changes were consistent and proportional to visual signs of irritation but were less consistently associated with subjective sensory effects than were visual scoring of erythema [95].

Increasing Clinical Sensitivity for the Elderly

Improved sensitivity of testing methods, with enhanced ability to detect subclinical changes in the structure and physiological function of the skin, is profoundly relevant to the burgeoning population of older individuals in industrialized societies. Visible signs of irritation in older individuals are delayed and less intense than in younger people, despite the fact that older people are far more affected by skin irritation in general in the form of dryness and chronic itch. A recent, comprehensive evaluation of the results of irritant testing which specifically utilized BTK testing and compared younger and older individuals observed a consistent trend toward decreased erythema but increased skin irritation with age [96, 97].

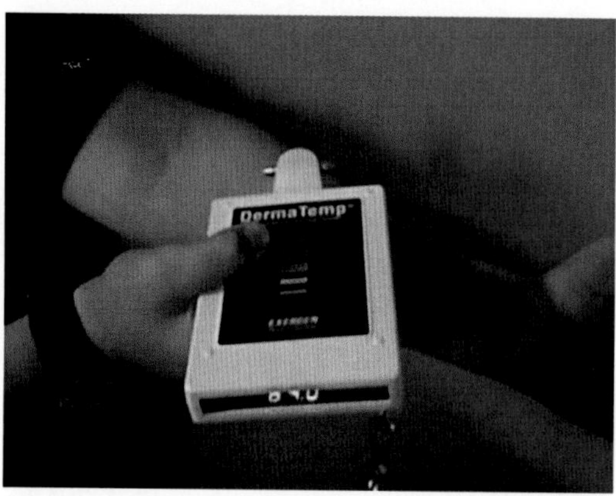

Fig. 5 Infrared thermographic scanner using the DermaTemp™

Conclusion

The skin of older subjects is compromised both structurally and functionally by the intrinsic and extrinsic effects of aging and may therefore be less effective at providing a barrier between the vulnerable internal tissues and the environment outside. Contact irritation is a potential sequela to a comprised barrier. Surprisingly, with age, structural changes which produce attenuation of barrier function, impacting absorption, permeability, and vascular health, appear to be compensated for by increased SC thickness and a retardation of the desquamation process. The elderly thus appear to be less susceptible to irritant responses. Traditional irritant testing, however, relies on visual scoring of erythema and other physical signs of irritation, while patients often report sensory discomfort in the absence of physical signs. Increasing the sensitivity of current skin testing methods, through intensifying exposure or by increasing sensitivity of scoring, is needed.

Several new testing approaches are increasing the ability to define differences in irritant potential among even the mildest of consumer products, as well as providing some correlation between subclinical skin changes and discomfort that has been formerly considered purely sensory in nature. In addition, results from these recently developed techniques that provide correlation between objective and subjective data suggest that although objective signs of irritation decrease with age, sensory discomfort from dry, defective, and pruritic skin increases.

It is also important to recognize that the decrease in inflammatory response in the elderly has the potential to negatively affect patient health. Elderly patients are at higher risk of serious injury, for example, from burns, because early warning signs do not as rapidly appear. Medicaments or other treatments may cause irritation or even skin damage yet be continued because objective signs of irritation are absent [13].

In addition, impairment in percutaneous absorption discourages penetration of toxins, as well as potentially therapeutic topical medicines. The reduction in clearance of penetrants also means that both toxins and medicines remain in skin tissues for a longer amount of time. An understanding of the ramifications of differences of penetration, absorption, and clearance of contact irritants in aged skin, as well as the unique presentation of contact irritation in older patients, is necessary for optimal therapeutic choices and efficacious dosing in the treatment of dermatological conditions in the aged patient [13].

Cross-References

- ▶ Bioengineering Methods and Skin Aging
- ▶ Cutaneous Effects and Sensitive Skin with Incontinence in the Aged
- ▶ Irritant Contact Dermatitis
- ▶ Percutaneous Penetration of Chemicals and Aging Skin

References

1. Farage MA, Miller KW, Elsner P, et al. Structural characteristics of the aging skin: a review. Cutan Ocul Toxicol. 2007;26:343–57.
2. Farage MA, Miller KW, Elsner P, et al. Functional and physiological characteristics of the aging skin. Aging Clin Exp Res. 2008;20:195–200.
3. Jafferany M, Huynh TV, Silverman MA, et al. Geriatric dermatoses: a clinical review of skin diseases in an aging population. Int J Dermatol. 2012;51:509–22.
4. Harvell JD, Maibach HI. Percutaneous absorption and inflammation in aged skin: a review. J Am Acad Dermatol. 1994;31:1015–21.
5. Marks R. The stratum corneum barrier: the final frontier. J Nutr. 2004;134:2017S–21.
6. Blood D, Studder V, Gay C, editors. Saunders comprehensive veterinary dictionary. New York: Elsevier Saunders; 2007.
7. Elias PM, Ghadially R. The aged epidermal permeability barrier: basis for functional abnormalities. Clin Geriatr Med. 2002;18:103–20. vii.
8. Tagami H. Functional characteristics of the stratum corneum in photoaged skin in comparison with those found in intrinsic aging. Arch Dermatol Res. 2008;300 Suppl 1:S1–6.
9. Schurer NY, Elias PM. The biochemistry and function of stratum corneum lipids. Adv Lipid Res. 1991;24:27–56.
10. Schaefer H, Redelmeier T. Skin penetration. In: Frosch P, Menne T, Lepoittevin J, editors. Contact dermatitis. New York: Springer; 2006.
11. Wilhelm KP, Freitag G, Wolff HH. Surfactant-induced skin irritation and skin repair. Evaluation of the acute human irritation model by noninvasive techniques. J Am Acad Dermatol. 1994;30:944–9.
12. Tagami H. Functional characteristics of aged skin. I. Percutaneous absorption. Acta Dermatol Kyoto Engl Ed. 1971;67:19–21.
13. Suter-Widmer JElsner P. Age and irritation. In: Agner T, Maibah H, editors. The irritant contact dermatitis syndrome. Boca Raton: CRC Press; 1996.
14. Thivolet J, Nicolas JF. Skin ageing and immune competence. Br J Dermatol. 1990;122 Suppl 35:77–81.
15. Corsini E, Racchi M, Lucchi L, et al. Skin immunosenescence: decreased receptor for activated C kinase-1 expression correlates with defective tumour necrosis factor-alpha production in epidermal cells. Br J Dermatol. 2009;160:16–25.
16. Newton SJR, Cook JMP. Considerations for percutaneous absorption. Int J Pharm Comp. 2010;14:301–4.
17. Brain K, Walters K, Watkinson A. Methods for studying percutaneous absorption. In: Walters K, editor. Dermatological and transdermal formulations. New York: Informa Health Care; 2007.
18. Roskos KV, Guy RH, Maibach HI. Percutaneous absorption in the aged. Dermatol Clin. 1986;4:455–65.
19. Roskos KV, Bircher AJ, Maibach HI, et al. Pharmacodynamic measurements of methyl nicotinate percutaneous absorption: the effect of aging on microcirculation. Br J Dermatol. 1990;122:165–71.
20. Oriba HA, Bucks DA, Maibach HI. Percutaneous absorption of hydrocortisone and testosterone on the vulva and forearm: effect of the menopause and site. Br J Dermatol. 1996;134:229–33.
21. Christopher E, Kligman A. Percutaneous absorption in aged skin. In: Montagna W, editor. Advances in biology of the skin. Oxford, UK: Oxford University Press; 1965.
22. Roskos KV, Maibach HI, Guy RH. The effect of aging on percutaneous absorption in man. J Pharmacokinet Biopharm. 1989;17:617–30.
23. Summers PR, Hunn J. Unique dermatologic aspects of the postmenopausal vulva. Clin Obstet Gynecol. 2007;50:745–51.

24. Elsner P, Wilhelm D, Maibach HI. Frictional properties of human forearm and vulvar skin: influence of age and correlation with transepidermal water loss and capacitance. Dermatologica. 1990;181:88–91.
25. Thune P. Evaluation of the hydration and the water-holding capacity in atopic skin and so-called dry skin. Acta Derm Venereol Suppl (Stockh). 1989;144:133–5.
26. Wilhelm KP, Cua AB, Maibach HI. Skin aging. Effect on transepidermal water loss, stratum corneum hydration, skin surface pH, and casual sebum content. Arch Dermatol. 1991;127:1806–9.
27. Ghadially R, Brown BE, Sequeira-Martin SM, et al. The aged epidermal permeability barrier. Structural, functional, and lipid biochemical abnormalities in humans and a senescent murine model. J Clin Invest. 1995;95:2281–90.
28. Potts RO, Buras EMJ, Chrisman DAJ. Changes with age in the moisture content of human skin. J Invest Dermatol. 1984;82:97–100.
29. Akimoto K, Yoshikawa N, Higaki Y, et al. Quantitative analysis of stratum corneum lipids in xerosis and asteatotic eczema. J Dermatol. 1993;20:1–6.
30. Lévêque JL, François G, Sojic N, et al. A new technique to in vivo study the corneocyte features at the surface of the skin. Skin Res Technol. 2008;14:468–71.
31. Ye J, Calhoun C, Feingold K, et al. Age-related changes in the IL-1 gene family and their receptors before and after barrier abrogation. J Invest Dermatol. 1999;112:543 [Abstract 125].
32. Ghadially R, Brown BE, Hanley K, et al. Decreased epidermal lipid synthesis accounts for altered barrier function in aged mice. J Invest Dermatol. 1996;106:1064–9.
33. Marchell NL, Uchida Y, Brown BE, et al. Glucosylceramides stimulate mitogenesis in aged murine epidermis. J Invest Dermatol. 1998;110:383–7.
34. Engelke M, Jensen JM, Ekanayake-Mudiyanselage S, et al. Effects of xerosis and ageing on epidermal proliferation and differentiation. Br J Dermatol. 1997;137:219–25.
35. Reed JT, Elias PM, Ghadially R. Integrity and permeability barrier function of photoaged human epidermis. Arch Dermatol. 1997;133:395–6.
36. Cua AB, Wilhelm KP, Maibach HI. Frictional properties of human skin: relation to age, sex and anatomical region, stratum corneum hydration and transepidermal water loss. Br J Dermatol. 1990;123:473–9.
37. Thune P, Nilsen T, Hanstad IK, et al. The water barrier function of the skin in relation to the water content of stratum corneum, pH and skin lipids. The effect of alkaline soap and syndet on dry skin in elderly, non-atopic patients. Acta Derm Venereol. 1988;68:277–83.
38. Leveque JL, Corcuff P, de Rigal J, et al. In vivo studies of the evolution of physical properties of the human skin with age. Int J Dermatol. 1984;23:322–9.
39. Baker H, Blair CP. Cell replacement in the human stratum corneum in old age. Br J Dermatol. 1968;80:367–72.
40. Grove GL, Duncan S, Kligman AM. Effect of ageing on the blistering of human skin with ammonium hydroxide. Br J Dermatol. 1982;107:393–400.
41. Lavker RM, Zheng PS, Dong G. Aged skin: a study by light, transmission electron, and scanning electron microscopy. J Invest Dermatol. 1987;88:44s–51.
42. Oriba HA, Maibach HI. Vulvar transepidermal water loss (TEWL) decay curves. Effect of occlusion, delipidation, and age. Acta Derm Venereol. 1989;69:461–5.
43. Miniszewska J, Juczyński Z, Ograczyk A, et al. Health-related quality of life in psoriasis: important role of personal resources. Acta Derm Venereol. 2013;93:551–6.
44. Menon GK, Feingold KR, Moser AH, et al. De novo sterologenesis in the skin. II. Regulation by cutaneous barrier requirements. J Lipid Res. 1985;26:418–27.
45. Blaak J, Luttje D, John SM, et al. Irritability of the skin barrier: a comparison of chronologically aged and photo-aged skin in elderly and young adults. Eur Geriatr Med. 2011;2:208–11.
46. Farage MA. Vulvar susceptibility to contact irritants and allergens: a review. Arch Gynecol Obstet. 2005;272:167–72.
47. Ryan T. Cutaneous circulation. In: Goldsmith L, editor. Biochemistry and physiology of the skin. New York: Oxford University Press; 1983.
48. Roustit M, Cracowski J. Assessment of endothelial and neurovascular function in human skin microcirculation. Trends Pharmacol Sci. 2013;34:373–84.
49. Weiss M, Milman B, Rosen B, et al. Analysis of the diminished skin perfusion in elderly people by laser Doppler flowmetry. Age Ageing. 1992;21:237–41.
50. Ishihara M, Itoh M, Ohsawa K, et al. Cutaneous blood flow. In: Kligman A, Takase Y, editors. Cutaneous aging. Tokyo: University of Tokyo Press; 1988.
51. Kelechi TJ, Mueller M, Zapka JG, et al. The effect of a cryotherapy gel wrap on the microcirculation of skin affected by chronic venous disorders. J Adv Nurs. 2011;67:2337–49.
52. Oimomi M, Hatanaka H, Maeda Y, et al. Autonomic nervous function determined by changes of periflux blood flow in the aged. Arch Gerontol Geriatr. 1986;5:159–63.
53. Khan F, Spence VA, Belch JJ. Cutaneous vascular responses and thermoregulation in relation to age. Clin Sci (Lond). 1992;82:521–8.
54. Richardson D, Tyra J, McCray A. Attenuation of the cutaneous vasoconstrictor response to cold in elderly men. J Gerontol. 1992;47:M211–4.
55. Ansel H, Stoklosa M. Pharmaceutical calculations. Philadelphia: Lippincott Williams & Wilkins; 2005.
56. Robinson M. Aging and skin sensitivity. In: Farage MA, Miller K, Maibach H, editors. Textbook of aging skin. Berlin/Heidelberg: Springer; 2010.
57. Modjtahedi B, Toro J, Engasser P, et al. Cosmetic reactions. In: Zhai H, Wilhelm K, Maibach H, editors. Marzulli and Maibach's dermatotoxicology. Boca Raton: CRC Press; 2008.

58. Frosch PJ, John SM. Clinical aspects of irritant contact dermatitis. In: Johansen JD, Frosch PJ, Lepoittevin J, editors. Contact dermatitis. Berlin/Heidelberg: Springer; 2011.
59. Zhai H, Meier-Davis SR, Cayme B, et al. Irritant contact dermatitis: effect of age. Cutan Ocul Toxicol. 2012;31:138–43.
60. Basketter D, Kimber I. Predictive tests for irritants and allergens and their use in quantitative risk assessment. In: Frosch P, Menne T, Lepoittevin J, editors. Contact dermatitis. New York: Springer; 2006.
61. Farage MA, Katsarou A, Maibach HI. Sensory, clinical and physiological factors in sensitive skin: a review. Contact Dermatitis. 2006;55:1–14.
62. Farage MA. Perceptions of sensitive skin: changes in perceived severity and associations with environmental causes. Contact Dermatitis. 2008;59:226–32.
63. Antonov D, Schliemann S, Elsner P. Therapy and rehabilitation of allergic and irritant contact dermatitis. In: Johansen JD, Frosch PJ, Lepoittevin J, editors. Contact dermatitis. Berlin/Heidelberg: Springer; 2011.
64. Agner T, Menne T. Individual predisposition to irritant and contact dermatitis. In: Frosch P, Menne T, Lepoittevin J, editors. Contact dermatitis. New York: Springer; 2006.
65. Kleinsmith DM, Perricone NV. Common skin problems in the elderly. Dermatol Clin. 1986;4:485–99.
66. Patil S, Maibach HI. Effect of age and sex on the elicitation of irritant contact dermatitis. Contact Dermatitis. 1994;30:257–64.
67. Bettley FR, Donoghue E. The irritant effect of soap upon the normal skin. Br J Dermatol. 1960;72:67–76.
68. Coenraads PJ, Bleumink E, Nater JP. Susceptibility to primary irritants: age dependence and relation to contact allergic reactions. Contact Dermatitis. 1975;1:377–81.
69. Grove G, Lavker R, Hoelzle E, et al. Use of non-intrusive tests to monitor age-associated changes in human skin. J Soc Cosmet Chem. 1981;32:15–26.
70. Cua AB, Wilhelm KP, Maibach HI. Cutaneous sodium lauryl sulphate irritation potential: age and regional variability. Br J Dermatol. 1990;123:607–13.
71. Marrakchi S, Maibach HI. Sodium lauryl sulfate-induced irritation in the human face: regional and age-related differences. Skin Pharmacol Physiol. 2006;19:177–80.
72. Nedorost ST, Stevens SR. Diagnosis and treatment of allergic skin disorders in the elderly. Drugs Aging. 2001;18:827–35.
73. Elsner P, Wilhelm D, Maibach HI. Irritant effect of a model surfactant on the human vulva and forearm. Age-related differences. J Reprod Med. 1990;35:1035–9.
74. Britz MB, Maibach HI, Anjo DM. Human percutaneous penetration of hydrocortisone: the vulva. Arch Dermatol Res. 1980;267:313–6.
75. Angelova-Fischer I, Becker V, Fischer TW, et al. Tandem repeated irritation in aged skin induces distinct barrier perturbation and cytokine profile in vivo. Br J Dermatol. 2012;167:787–93.
76. White EA, Orazem ME, Bunge AL. Characterization of damaged skin by impedance spectroscopy: chemical damage by dimethyl sulfoxide. Pharm Res. 2013;30:2607–24.
77. Elsner P, Seyfarth F, Antonov D, et al. Development of a standardized testing procedure for assessing the irritation potential of occupational skin cleansers. Contact Dermatitis. 2014;70:151–7.
78. Elsner P, Wilhelm D, Maibach HI. Sodium lauryl sulfate-induced irritant contact dermatitis in vulvar and forearm skin of premenopausal and postmenopausal women. J Am Acad Dermatol. 1990;23:648–52.
79. Pullen SK, Warshaw EM. Vulvar allergic contact dermatitis from clotrimazole. Dermatitis. 2010;21:59–60.
80. Feldmann RJ, Maibach HI. Regional variation in percutaneous penetration of 14C cortisol in man. J Invest Dermatol. 1967;48:181–3.
81. Lesch CA, Squier CA, Cruchley A, et al. The permeability of human oral mucosa and skin to water. J Dent Res. 1989;68:1345–9.
82. van der Bijl P, Thompson IO, Squier CA. Comparative permeability of human vaginal and buccal mucosa to water. Eur J Oral Sci. 1997;105:571–5.
83. Fisher G. The commonest causes of symptomatic vulvar disease: a dermatologist's perspective. Australas J Dermatol. 1996;37:12–8.
84. Ong MWS, Simion FA, Maibach HI. Methods for testing irritation potential. In: Alikhan A, Lachapelle J, Maibach HI, editors. Textbook of hand eczema. Berlin/Heidelberg: Spring; 2014.
85. Farage MA. Evaluating mechanical and chemical irritation using the behind-the-knee test: review. In: Zhai H, Wilhelm K, Maibach H, editors. Marzulli and Maibach's dermatotoxicology. Boca Raton: CRC Press; 2008.
86. Farage MA. The behind-the-knee test: an efficient model for evaluating mechanical and chemical irritation. Skin Res Technol. 2006;12:73–82.
87. Farage MA, Meyer S, Walter D. Evaluation of modifications of the traditional patch test in assessing the chemical irritation potential of feminine hygiene products. Skin Res Technol. 2004;10:73–84.
88. Farage MA, Maibach H. Dermatotoxicology of specialized epithelia: adapting cutaneous test methods to assess topical effects on vulva. In: Zhai H, Wilhelm K, Maibach H, editors. Marzulli and Maibach's dermatotoxicology. Boca Raton: CRC Press; 2008.
89. Farage MA. Evaluating lotion transfer to skin from feminine protection products. Skin Res Technol. 2008;14:35–44.
90. Farage MA, Ebrahimpour A, Steimle B, et al. Evaluation of lotion formulations on irritation using the modified forearm-controlled application test method. Skin Res Technol. 2007;13:268–79.
91. Farage MA. Are we reaching the limits or our ability to detect skin effects with our current testing and

measuring methods for consumer products. Contact Dermatitis. 2005;52:297–303.
92. Farage MA. Enhancement of visual scoring of skin irritant reactions using cross-polarized light and parallel-polarized light. Contact Dermatitis. 2008;58:147–55.
93. Farage MA, Singh M, Ledger WJ. Investigation of the sensitivity of a cross-polarized light visualization system to detect subclinical erythema and dryness in women with vulvovaginitis. Am J Obstet Gynecol. 2009;201:20.e1–6.
94. Perkins MA, Osterhues MA, Farage MA, et al. A non-invasive method to assess skin irritation and compromised skin conditions using simple tape adsorption of molecular markers of inflammation. Skin Res Technol. 2001;7:227–37.
95. Farage MA, Wang B, Miller KW. Surface skin temperature in tests for irritant dermatitis. In: Berardesca E, Maibach H, Wilhelm K, editors. Non invasive diagnostic techniques in clinical dermatology. Berlin/Heidelberg: Springer; 2013.
96. Farage MA, Miller KW, Gerberick GF, et al. Susceptibility to irritation in the elderly: new techniques. In: Farage MA, Miller KW, Maibach HI, editors. Textbook of aging skin. Berlin/Heidelberg: Springer; 2010.
97. Bjerke D. Considerations for thermal injury: the elderly as a sensitive population. In: Farage MA, Miller KW, Maibach HI, editors. Textbook of aging skin. Berlin/Heidelberg: Springer; 2010.

The Vaginal Microbiota in Menopause

106

Miranda A. Farage, Kenneth. W. Miller, Yuli Song, and Jack Sobel

Contents

M.A. Farage (✉)
Winton Hill Business Center, The Procter & Gamble Company, Cincinnati, OH, USA
e-mail: farage.m@pg.com

K.W. Miller
Margoshes-Miller Consulting, LLC, Cincinnati, OH, USA
e-mail: miller.kw.1@pg.com; 822mbb@gmail.com

Y. Song
The Procter & Gamble Company, Mason Business Center, Mason, OH, USA
e-mail: song.y.7@pg.com

J. Sobel
Infectious Diseases, Wayne State University, Detroit, MI, USA
e-mail: jsobel@med.wayne.edu

M.A. Farage et al. (eds.), *Textbook of Aging Skin*,
DOI 10.1007/978-3-662-47398-6_84

Abstract

Over a woman's life span, the vagina microbiota will be in constant flux as the ecosystem is buffeted by a variety of both internal and external insults that have the potential to modulate the vaginal milieu. Hormonal changes are a major influence, ethnicity influences the microbiota, and many external factors may affect the composition of the microbiota including the use of personal hygiene products or medications. After menopause, the vagina is likely to harbor more commensal species than during the reproductive years; the vaginal flora of postmenopausal women is altered, often being colonized by potentially pathogenic organisms. Hormone replacement therapy (HRT) can provide benefits to the ecosystem of the lower genital tract. After menopause, estrogen depletion elevates vaginal pH, reduces vaginal colonization by lactic acid-producing microbes, and facilitates colonization by enteric organisms. This increases the risk of urinary tract infections (UTIs), a factor that contributes to incontinence in elderly women. HRT restores vaginal pH and reestablishes normal vaginal microbiota in postmenopausal women, thereby promoting a more healthful vaginal ecosystem. By better understanding the dynamics of vaginal environment in all stages of life and by identifying those events that promote disease, there is hope that more effective therapies can be developed to promote vaginal health throughout a woman's life.

Introduction

The adult human is colonized by more than 100 trillion microbes [1], with an estimated 10^{12} bacteria on the skin, 10^{10} in the oral cavity, 10^{14} in the gastrointestinal tract, and 10^{9} in the vaginal vault [2]. In any specific anatomical habitat, colonization is determined by pH, temperature, redox potential, endogenous secretions of lysozyme and immunoglobulins, and levels of nutrients, including oxygen and water [3]. Colonization of an anatomical area by a specific microorganism also depends on the ability of the bacterium to adhere to the tissue [2]. Moist interior tissues, protected from the harsh external environment, are ideal habitats; the vaginal vault is colonized within 24 h of a female child's birth and remains colonized until death [4].

Together, the human vagina and its resident microbiota comprise a dynamic yet fine-tuned ecosystem. Historically, culture-based and biochemical methods have attempted to define the composition of "normal" vaginal microbiota; guidelines based on these methods have been used to distinguish "normal" from "pathogenic" biota for more than two decades [5]. Nugent criteria have defined the "normal" microbiota as that which is dominated by *Lactobacillus* species [5] and the "diseased" microbiota (bacterial vaginosis or BV) as that lacking *Lactobacillus* dominance but displaying a preponderance of anaerobes and the presence of microorganisms believed to be pathogenic (e.g., *Gardnerella* and *Bacteroides*) [6]. However, recent studies using molecular-based approach indicated that even though approximately 70–80 % of asymptomatic women have microbiota dominated by *Lactobacillus* spp., about 20–30 % of asymptomatic, healthy women have vaginal microbiota dominated by a diverse group of anaerobic and facultative bacteria [7, 8].

In the past several years, with the advance of high-throughput pyro-sequencing methodology, as well as NIH Human Microbiome Program, our knowledge of vaginal microbiota has significantly broadened [8, 9]. 16S rDNA gene-based analysis has conclusively shown that the vagina is colonized by a temporally and spatially dynamic microbial community; its composition and stability varies by race and age and even temporally within an individual. Studies also revealed that vaginal microbiota dysbiosis is consistently associated with vaginal infection such as HIV, human papillomavirus (HPV), and *Trichomonas vaginalis* infection. Bacterial vaginosis can be best described as a poly-bacterial dysbiosis, with reduced *Lactobacillus* and increased bacterial diversity (anaerobic and facultative bacteria) [10, 11]. There are still knowledge gaps in vaginal microbiota, such as we do not fully understand how the vaginal microbiome is established and maintained and how bacterial dysbiosis develops and resolves, but there are studies under way to understand the functional role of vaginal microbiota in vaginal health and diseases.

In a clinical setting, Nugent system is still considered as the gold standard for the diagnosis of bacterial vaginosis. However, the usefulness of the Nugent system is limited by the fact that the onset of clinical symptoms does not correlate tightly with the types and numbers of bacteria identified and by the fact that BV is often asymptomatic, regressing spontaneously in about 50 % of cases [12].

Asymptomatic cases of BV (as identified by Nugent criteria) may represent vaginal flora with functionally sufficient levels of *Lactobacillus*, although these may be undetectable by Gram stain. Moreover, other acid-producing bacteria may confer the necessary functionality to create an asymptomatic condition. From another aspect, whether bacterial dysbiosis is symptomatic or not most likely depends on the degree and nature of the dysbiosis, bacterial loads, type and quantity of virulence factors expressed by bacteria, and the intensity and nature of the host's immune responses. These observations suggest that the normal vaginal microbiota cannot be rigidly and permanently defined for all women, but instead represents a spectrum of mutualistic and functional interrelationships. The spectrum of species in normal microbiota may vary among women (depending on host and environmental variables) and even vary over time within an individual woman. For example, as will be discussed in this chapter, hormonal changes of a female lifecycle produce predictable variations in the vaginal microbiota.

Over a woman's life span, the vagina microbiota will be in constant flux [13] – changing daily and even hourly [14] – as the ecosystem is buffeted by a variety of both internal and external insults that have the potential to modulate the vaginal milieu [13, 15]. Hormonal changes that mark the stages of a human female's life – puberty, the menstrual cycle, pregnancy, and menopause – are in themselves a major influence [13, 16]; ethnicity influences the microbiota as well [17]. External factors that may affect the composition of the microbiota include methods of contraception [13], sexual behaviors (including the age of first sexual experience, the frequency of sex, number of sexual partners, and sexual practices), the presence of sexually transmitted infections, and even the introduction of semen [13, 18]. The use of personal hygiene products or medications may also play a role [19], as may cultural practices [20] and even diet [21]. The normal vaginal microbiota cannot be viewed as static or universal but is a dynamic equilibrium dependent on both microbial and host characteristics.

Changes in the Vaginal Microbiota Over a Woman's Life Span

Normal Microbiota During Childhood and Puberty

During birth and shortly after, maternal estrogens in the newborn's circulatory system produce a high glycogen level in the vaginal epithelium, producing an environment in which lactic acid-producing microbes can thrive [4]. Because adrenal or gonadal hormones are inactive at this age, as maternal estrogen depletes, the prevalence of lactic acid-producing microbes present in neonates also decreases [16]. Vaginal pH during early childhood is neutral or slightly alkaline [16].

The morphology and physiology of the vulva and vagina change at puberty [22]. With adrenal and gonadal maturation, cyclic hormonal patterns are established and menstruation begins. Mid-cycle estrogen levels produce peaks in the glycogen content of the vaginal epithelium, increasing the prevalence of lactic acid-producing microbes in the vaginal microbiota [16]. By adulthood, the morphology of the vulva is mature, and the menstrual cycle has become well established [16].

Normal Microbiota During the Reproductive Years

Lactic acid-producing microbes are numerically dominant in most healthy adult women [16, 23] at levels of approximately 10^7 lactobacilli per gram of vaginal secretion, as estimated from culture-based techniques [24]. Generally, only a single strain of *Lactobacillus* is cultured from any one individual; [25] in one report, 92 % of individuals cultured had a single strain [26]. The most common *Lactobacillus* species identified by traditional culture techniques are *L. crispatus* and *L. fermentum*, although *L. brevis*, *L. jensenii*, *L. casei*, *L. delbrueckii*, and *L. salivarius* also are isolated [24]. Generally, levels of *Lactobacillus* spp. in the vagina rise and fall in parallel with circulating levels of estrogen [24] (see Table 1). Differences in the composition and stability of the microbial community between pregnant and nonpregnant women are also observed [27–30]. Antibiotic administration during pregnancy also alters vaginal microbiota ecology with potential long-term effects on the early microbial colonization of the neonate [31]. Other bacteria commonly identified by traditional methods, but at lower population numbers, include *Staphylococcus* species and *Ureaplasma*, *Corynebacterium*, *Streptococcus*,

Table 1 *Lactobacillus* species recovered from the human vagina

Most common
L. crispatus
L. fermentum
L. casei
L. jensenii
L. delbrueckii
Less common
L. iners[a]
L. minutus
L. brevis
L. leichmannii
L. plantarum
L. salivarius
L. gallinarum
L. gasseri
L. johnsonii
L. paracasei
L. rhamnosus
L. reuteri
L. vaginalis

Table compiled from References [24, 35, 68, 82–84]
[a]*L. iners* is more often recovered via molecular techniques

Peptostreptococcus, *Gardnerella*, *Bacteroides*, *Mycoplasma*, *Enterococcus*, *Escherichia*, *Veillonella*, *Bifidobacterium*, and *Candida* spp. [24] (see Table 2).

The use of molecular techniques to evaluate the normal microbiota has confirmed that the vaginal ecosystems of most healthy fertile women are dominated by *Lactobacillus* species [13, 32]. However, novel *Lactobacillus* species that do not grow readily on standard media also have been identified, as have other acid-producing species not formerly detected at numerically significant levels [13]. The culture-independent techniques are providing a much clearer understanding of the vaginal microbiota community and the dynamic interrelationship of several.

During the reproductive years, estrogen production stimulates vaginal epithelial cells to proliferate, producing a mid-cycle peak in intracellular glycogen levels in the vaginal mucosa [33] and a subsequent increase in lactic acid-producing microbes in the vaginal milieu [16]. By virtue of metabolizing glycogen, lactobacilli acidify the vaginal environment: pH in the vaginal vault of fertile women ranges generally from 3.8 to 4.5 [34]. The acidity of the vaginal environment appears to be the principal inhibitor of secondary bacterial infection [35]; H_2O_2 produced by some *Lactobacillus* species also may assist in inhibiting colonization by other vaginal flora [36]. In addition, some H_2O_2-producing lactobacilli appear to have viricidal activity [36].

It has been widely accepted that maintaining vaginal acidity through the production of lactic acid by *Lactobacillus* species is critical to vaginal health. However, up to 42 % of women who do not exhibit lactobacillus-dominant microbiota are nonetheless able to maintain normal vaginal ecosystems [24, 37, 38]. Molecular techniques have detected other species capable of producing lactic acid in their microbiota, which indicates that although a community of lactic acid producers is maintained in healthy women, the composition of that community can vary.

Lactobacillus species and other lactic acid producers have the ability to inhibit growth of numerous other bacterial species in vitro [24]. Many factors contribute to this effect (see Table 3). Communities dominated by lactic acid producers can serve as a barrier to colonization by potentially pathogenic organisms and to overgrowth of organisms that are otherwise commensal. Such communities inhibit the transmission of sexually transmitted infections [19], including heterosexual transmission of HIV (human immunodeficiency virus) [39–44].

BV, a noninflammatory condition in which the vaginal microbiota exhibits a paucity of lactobacilli and a preponderance of anaerobes, has long been an enigma. The chain of events which tips the scales from a functional ecosystem to the development of BV is still a mystery [24]; the phenomenon seems to involve changes in the interplay between

Table 2 Commensal and pathogenic organisms of the human vagina

Organism	Facultative and aerobic	Prevalence	Anaerobic	Prevalence
Gram-positive cocci	*Staphylococcus* epidermis	+++	*Peptostreptococcus*	+++
	Staphylococcus aureus	+	*Streptococcus**	+++
	Streptococcus spp. (α-hemolytic, nonhemolytic, groups B, D, S)*	+++		
	Micrococcus	++~		
	*Enterococcus faecalis**	+		
Gram-positive bacilli	*Lactobacillus*	+++	*Lactobacillus*	+++
	Corynebacteria	+++	Propionibacteria	++~
			Clostridium	
			Eubacteria	+++
			Bifidobacteria	
			Actinomyces	
Gram-negative cocci	*Neisseria**	+	*Veillonella*	++~
Gram-negative bacilli	*Escherichia coli*	+	*Bacteroides**	+++
	Klebsiella		*Fusobacterium*	
	*Ureaplasma urealyticum**	+		
	Enterobacteria	+		
Gram-variable bacillus	*G. vaginalis**	+		
Other organisms	*Candida**	+		
	*Mycoplasma hominis**	+		
	Mycoplasma fermentans	+		

Table compiled from References [2, 24, 85]
+++ very common, ++~ common but only occur in low numbers, ++ occasional, + rare
*Potentially pathogenic organism

Table 3 Role of *Lactobacillus* in stabilizing normal vaginal microbiota

	Reference
Production of hydrogen peroxide	[25, 86]
Production of bacteriocins	[87]
Lactic acid depression of vaginal pH	[88]
Inhibition of *E. coli* adherence	[89]
Penetration of *E coli* biofilms	[87]
Augmentation of host immunity	[90]

factors both endogenous and exogenous to the vagina that allow potentially pathogenic organisms to gain dominance [10, 19, 24, 45–49]. However, healthy women with normal vaginal flora regularly experience transient yet significant changes dramatic enough to shift normal flora into a potentially pathogenic state [50], and substantial perturbation in the microbiota is often a prelude to vaginal disease [51, 52].

Normal Microbiota During Menopausal and Postmenopausal Years

Functionally, menopause begins when the numbers of primordial follicles (which decline steadily from birth on) hit a critical predetermined low [53]. The age at which women enter menopause has a genetic component, as demonstrated by solid patterns with regard to time of onset in individual families [54]. The genetic contribution to age of onset is estimated by several studies to approach 50 % [55]. Onset of menopause in women of European extraction has remained at about the current average of age 50 for at least the

Table 4 Changes in vaginal structure and function due to estrogen depletion after menopause

	Change	Reference
Structural changes		
Vaginal epithelium	Loses rugae, thins	[16]
	Pales, develops fine petechial hemorrhages	[91]
	Atrophy	[92]
Dermis	Collagen bundles fuse and undergo hyalinization	[91]
	Elastin fibers fragment	[91]
Vascular system	Progressive avascularization	[93]
Functional changes		
Dyspareunia		[94]
Loss of elasticity		[93]
Dryness		[94]
Decreased blood flow		[95]

last thousand years [53]. However, both epidemiological and prospective studies have revealed a slightly but significantly earlier age of onset of menopause in black women in both the USA [56] and Africa [57] and a slightly but significantly later onset in both ethnic Asian populations [58]. Moreover, the onset of the menopause is also influenced by the timing and number of pregnancies [53], nutrition [58], and smoking [58].

The plasma content of estrogen drops from about 129 ng/L in the reproductive years to about 18 ng/L after menopause [59], dramatically affecting the vagina [60] (see Table 4). The vaginal epithelium contains estrogen-alpha receptors: as estrogen levels drop, the vaginal epithelium atrophies and its glycogen content fall; this in turn depletes cell densities of lactobacilli [61], diminishes the production of lactic acid from glucose [62], and causes the vaginal pH to rise to about 6.0–8.0 [61]. This rise in vaginal pH, absent BV or other vaginal pathology, is a reliable indicator of menopausal status [63].

Vaginal pH appears to depend not only on constituents of the microbiota, but also on hydrogen ion secretion by ectocervical epithelial cells in the human vagina [64]. In postmenopausal women, these cells become atrophied and secretion of hydrogen ion (H+) is attenuated: postmenopausal estrogen treatment restores cell function. In premenopausal women with estrogen deprivation, estrogen treatment fully reactivates H+ secretion; this implies that treating perimenopausal women with estrogen early, before intracellular estrogen is depleted, would be advantageous [65].

Microbial constituents of the vaginal ecosystem adapt to changing pH and hormone levels [3]. After menopause, the prevalence and cell density of *Lactobacillu* s drops [61, 63, 66], which is considered a normal maturational change: prevalence in postmenopausal women was zero in some studies [67]. *Lactobacillus* species confer considerable stability on the vaginal ecosystem [68], an assertion supported by the observation that *Lactobacillus* -dominant vaginal microbiota retain a normal balance of flora for months, despite the presence of known pathogens [35]. In the perimenopause, depletion of the numbers of vaginal lactobacilli erodes the functional barrier to colonization by other bacteria. Consequently, after menopause, the vagina is likely to harbor more commensal species than during the reproductive years, which produces a more complex microbial community in the vaginal vault (see Table 5).

The vaginal flora of postmenopausal women is altered, often being colonized by potentially pathogenic organisms [34]. The shift of the vaginal pH from a normal acidity (pH 3.8–4.5 in the estrogenized vagina [69]) to a state of alkalinity allows potentially pathogenic bacteria, particularly enteric bacteria [16], to invade or expand their colonization of the vagina. Culture-based techniques indicate that the alkaline vagina is often colonized primarily with fecal flora such as *Enterobacteriaceae* [70, 71], which rarely occurs when vaginal pH is less than 4.5 [72]. Other organisms isolated in substantial numbers from postmenopausal patients (by selective culture techniques) are *G. vaginalis* (27 %), *U. urealyticum* (13 %), *Prevotella* (33 %), and

Table 5 Comparison of normal vaginal flora in healthy postmenopausal women with and without hormone replacement therapy

Organism	Prevalence in non-HRT-treated women	Prevalence in HRT-treated women	Reference
Lactobacilli	41 %	81 %	[73]
	20 %	95 %	[62]
	49 %	NA	[63]
	NA	100 %[a]	[35]
Escherichia coli	40 %	38 %	[73]
	35 %	10 %	[62]
	40 %	NA	[63]
Gardnerella	10 %	33.3 %	[62]
	27 %	NA	[63]
Mobiluncus	30 %	16.7 %	[62]
Bacteroides	40 %	8.3 %	[62]
Group B *Streptococcus*	5 %	16.7 %	[62]
	23 %	NA	[63]
Coryneforms	15 %	16.7 %	[62]
	58 %	NA	[63]
Candida	0	23.3 %	[62]
	1 %	NA	[63]
	NA	25 %[a]	[35]
Ureaplasma urealyticum	13 %	NA	[63]

HRT hormone replacement therapy, *NA* not available
[a]Prevalence rates determined by molecular methodology

coliforms (41 %) [63]. *Bacteroides* has been isolated from 40 % and *E. coli* from 35 % of postmenopausal subjects not treated with hormone replacement therapy (HRT) [62]. In postmenopausal women, vaginal colonization with *E. coli* was inversely associated with the presence of lactobacilli: relatively heavier growth of lactobacilli being associated with a lower frequency of *E coli* colonization [73]. Table 6 shows a summary of studies on the makeup of the postmenopausal vaginal microbiota.

Interestingly, in a study of 48 postmenopausal women, molecular techniques demonstrated the presence of vaginal lactobacilli in every subject, yielding a technical (and actual) prevalence rate of BV of zero, in contrast to the 10.5 % prevalence rate ascertained by Nugent methodology at baseline [60]. It has been noted that the Nugent system of scoring was developed for pregnant women [74] and may not be suitable or appropriate for evaluating women in menopause. This is underscored by the frequency of null flora – the absence of significant numbers of lactobacilli in postmenopausal women – yet without BV-associated microorganisms [75, 76]. Such a state is extremely rare in fertile women [61]. Null flora becomes more common with advancing age and increasing atrophy of the vaginal epithelium [75, 77]. Null flora, representing a nearly sterile environment, meets the criteria for a Nugent score of 4, which is interpreted as an intermediate state between normal flora and BV. Yet, in postmenopausal women, this state is natural and nonpathogenic [74]. Additional research in postmenopausal women using culture-independent molecular techniques will provide much greater clarity as to the vaginal microbiota community and what is "normal" for postmenopausal women.

Table 6 Studies on vaginal microbiota in postmenopausal women not using HRT

Study population	How menopause defined	Experimental parameters	Results	Reference
25 healthy women	NA	Culture	Increase in Gram-negative bacteria	[96]
50 postmenopausal women, aged 55–73, mean 63.7	None described	Culture	No significant differences	[71]
14 HRT users, 36 HRT nonusers				
28 healthy women, mean age 59	Greater than 2 years since last period	Culture	29 % cultures sterile, 19 % of cultures contained anaerobes[a]	[97]
46 postmenopausal women	NA	Culture	65 % *Lactobacillus* positive	[98]
171 healthy women in cancer prevention program	NA	Culture	Increase in *G. vaginalis*	[99]
350 menopausal UTI patients, aged 65–84 (mean 72.3), > 3 months since any HRT therapy	Advanced age	Culture	20 % *Lactobacillus* dominant, most subjects characterized by very sparse growth fecal bacteria dominant average KPI 3.0 ± 0.9, only 16.3 % greater than 10 pH 6.5 ± 0.1	[66]
73 healthy postmenopausal women, no HRT use for ≥1 year	≥5 years since last period, FSH level	Culture Gram stain/ Nugent lactic acid production, H_2O_2 production	13 % *Lactobacillus* dominant, 87 % intermediate, 49 % *Lactobacillus* positive	[63]
100 healthy postmenopausal women	FSH	Gram stain/ modified Nugent score	44 % normal flora, 17 % intermediate, 18 % BV, 21 % null flora	[75]
20 healthy postmenopausal women, aged 44–72, mean age 58.9	None described	Culture Gram stain/ Nugent score	95 % *Lactobacillus* positive	[79]
		PCR/DGGE	30 % normal, 30 % intermediate, 40 % BV	

BV bacterial vaginosis, *DGGE* denaturing gradient gel electrophoresis, *FSH* follicle-stimulating hormone, H_2O_2 hydrogen peroxide, *HRT* hormone replacement therapy, *KPI* karyopyknotic index, *NA* not available, *PCR* polymerase chain reaction, *UTI* urinary tract infection

[a]Anaerobes appeared only in the presence of aerobic bacteria

Vaginal Microbiota and Hormone Replacement Therapy in the Postmenopausal Woman

In postmenopausal women, replacement estrogens can be successfully administered orally, intravaginally, and transdermally (see Table 7). Several decades ago, it was first demonstrated that estrogen therapy lowered vaginal pH and increased the presence of lactobacilli in the vagina [78]. Since then, studies have demonstrated convincingly that HRT normalizes vaginal pH and vaginal microbiota in postmenopausal women [35, 62, 63, 67]. For example, in a group of postmenopausal women who were all devoid of vaginal *Lactobacillus* at baseline, intravaginal administration of estriol resulted in a 61 % colonization rate by lactobacilli after just 1 month, with a concurrent decline in vaginal pH from 5.5 to 3.8 [67]. In addition, the prevalence of colonization by *Enterobacteriaceae*, which was 67 % at baseline, fell to 31 % in the same time period [67].

In the postmenopausal stage of life, it is considered a paradox that despite the depletion of protective *Lactobacillus* in the vagina and the accompanying increase in colonization by fecal bacteria, the prevalence of clinically diagnosed BV remains low. Interestingly, although HRT

Table 7 Effects of hormone replacement therapy on vaginal environment in menopausal women

Population	Definition of menopause	Experimental parameters	Results	Reference
15 menopausal women (natural)	FSH levels	Estradiol (dermal patch) 0.1 mg/day	Percentage of cultures in which anaerobes were isolated dropped from 47 % to 13 %	[100]
	Serum estrogen levels		Post-HRT; vaginal pH in subjects with *Lactobacillus*-dominant flora was 4.4 compared to 5.2 in subjects with non-*Lactobacillus*-dominant flora	
60 postmenopausal women, aged 51–81, mean age 65.0 years	None described	36 treated, 24 placebo, 8 months culture, pH	No *Lactobacillus* is detected in any patient at baseline; after 1 month *Lactobacillus* species are detected in 61 % of treated subjects	[67]
59 postmenopausal women with vaginal dryness or discharge	NA	Oral estriol, 14 days	*Enterobacteriaceae* in treated group fell from 67 % to 33.1 % after 1 month	[101]
		Culture	Detection of lactobacilli in vaginal flora increased from 9 % at baseline to 42 % after treatment	
258 institutionalized menopausal women with UTIs	Advanced age (mean age 83 years)	Intravaginal estrogen, 0.5 g/day, 3 times per week	Vaginal pH	[92]
			Baseline: 7.4 ± 0.71	
			At 6 weeks: 6.8 ± 0.70	
			At 12 weeks: 6.7[a]	
921 healthy postmenopausal women, 590 HRT users, 331 HRT nonusers	Greater than 1 year since last menses	Oral and transdermal estrogen	Users: 84.9 % normal flora, 5.4 % BV, 68.9 % with full *Lactobacillus* colonization	[74]
		Culture	Nonusers: 46.3 % normal flora,	
		Gram stain/Nugent score	6.3 % BV, 34.1 % with full *Lactobacillus* colonization	
40 healthy postmenopausal women, aged 41–82	None described	Gram stain/Nugent score	HRT users	[68]
		PCR/DGGE history of HRT (Premarin® – a conjugated equine estrogen with progesterone) >2 years	100 % *Lactobacillus* +	
			54 % only one organism (90 % of these *Lactobacillus*), 87 % three or less, 5.6 % BV	
			Nonusers: 91 % colonized by more than one organism, 31 % BV	
			Bacteria associated with BV and/or UTI tenfold higher than in HRT users	

(*continued*)

Table 7 (continued)

Population	Definition of menopause	Experimental parameters	Results	Reference
89 healthy postmenopausal women, 30 natural menopause with estrogen and progestin, 30 surgical menopause with estrogen replacement only, 20 natural menopause, untreated controls	Greater than 1 year since last period	HRT 2–24 months	Vaginal microbiota: HRT nonusers vs. users	[62]
		Culture/g stain with Schroder's score	*Lactobacillus* 20 % vs. 90 %	
		pH	*G. vaginalis* 10 % vs. 33.3 %	
			Mobiluncus 30 % vs. 17 %	
			Bacteroides 40 % vs. 8 %	
			Group B *Strep.* 5 % vs. 16.7 %	
			E. coli 35 % vs. 10 %	
			pH average 5.35 among nonusers, 4 among users	
48 menopausal women with vaginal complaints, 58–75 years of age	Greater than 5 years since last period	CEE at 0.625 for 90 days	Baseline 0 % Nugent score type I (100 % type III)	[60]
		Gram stain with Nugent score	30 days 46 % type I	
		pH	90 days 74 % type I	
		Transvaginal sonography	pH dropped from 7.0 at baseline to 4.5 at 90 days	

BV bacterial vaginosis, *CEE* conjugated equine estrogens, *DGGE* denaturing gradient gel electrophoresis, *FSH* follicle-stimulating hormone, *HRT* hormone replacement therapy, *NA* not available, *PCR* polymerase chain reaction, *UTI* urinary tract infection

[a]pH still depressed at 6 weeks after estrogen therapy discontinued

reestablishes the *Lactobacillus*-dominated vaginal microbiota of the reproductive years, BV prevalence rates do not return to the levels seen in premenopausal women. Although the potential protective mechanisms in women undergoing hormone replacement therapy are not yet understood, HRT must induce changes beyond establishing a *Lactobacillus*-dominant flora that lower the risk of acquiring BV.

Normal Flora in Menopause and Urinary Tract Infection

HRT provides other benefits to the ecosystem of the lower genital tract. Molecular profiles of the vaginal microbiota in untreated menopausal women sometimes reveal either colonization with a single type of pathogenic organism or the presence of an unstable vaginal microbial environment [79].

As noted earlier, the alkaline vaginal environment that exists after menopause may allow uropathogenic *E. coli* and other enterobacteria to displace vaginal lactobacilli. Molecular methods demonstrate that such *E. coli* infections can persist, creating a stable but abnormal vaginal microbiota that places these women at higher risk for urinary tract infection (UTI) [79, 80]. Urinary tract infections, in turn, contribute significantly to urinary incontinence in older women [81]. Orally or intravaginally administered HRT reduces the frequency of UTIs in postmenopausal women: the treatment restores an acidic vaginal pH and reestablishes normal vaginal flora, which improves vaginal health [67] and reduces the risk of UTI (see Table 8).

Conclusion

The vaginal ecosystem changes continually over a woman's lifetime, as both intrinsic and extrinsic factors assail the fragile balance between competing organisms, sometimes on a daily basis. *Lactobacillus* and other lactic acid-

Table 8 Effects of hormone replacement therapy on urinary tract infections

Population	Study design	Length of HRT use	Results	Reference
3,616 patients with first UTI, ages 50–69	Case-control, observational	HRT use ≥1 year	Increased risk of UTI (odds ratio 1.9, 95 % CI 1.5–2.2)	[102]
Patients with UTI, USA and Israel, aged 40–64	Case-control, observational	HRT use in recent past	Cases less likely than controls to report HRT use, but significant only in the USA	[103]
40 healthy women, aged 66–91 years	Randomized, placebo-controlled clinical trial	Oral estriol vs. placebo for 8 weeks: 1 mg/day for 4 weeks then 1 mg/day for 8 weeks	Estriol significantly reduced UTI frequency as compared to placebo over the last 8 weeks of the study period	[104]
93 postmenopausal women with history of recurrent UTIs	Randomized, double-blind placebo-controlled clinical trial	Intravaginal estriol, 8-month study period	Incidence of UTI in estriol group significantly reduced (0.5 vs. 5.9 episodes per patient year, $p <$ 0.001)	[67]
53 postmenopausal women	Multicenter randomized controlled open clinical trial	Intravaginal estriol (vaginal rings) for 36 weeks	45 % of treated group remained UTI over study period compared to 20 % controls	[105]
72 postmenopausal women 60 years of age	Randomized, double-blind, placebo-controlled trial	Oral estriol (3 mg/day) vs. placebo	No significant differences between groups (authors concluded that problems with study design failed to elicit clear differences)	[106]

HRT hormone replacement therapy, *USA* United States of America, *UTI* urinary tract infection

producing microbes form the foundation of a healthy vaginal microbiota during the reproductive years. Vaginal lactobacilli depend on the presence of estrogen; after menopause, estrogen depletion elevates vaginal pH, reduces vaginal colonization by lactic acid-producing microbes, and facilitates colonization by enteric organisms. This increases the risk of UTIs, a factor that contributes to incontinence in elderly women. HRT restores vaginal pH and reestablishes normal vaginal microbiota in postmenopausal women, thereby promoting a more healthful vaginal ecosystem.

Because women in industrialized countries will spend one third of their lives in menopause, disorders of the aging vagina will continue to be a significant medical concern. A more comprehensive understanding is needed of the spectrum of microbes that constitute the normal vaginal microbiota and of the complex interplay of intrinsic and extrinsic factors that either maintain a healthy vaginal microbiota or promote disease. Molecular tools are shedding light on the array of microbiota that constitute healthy vaginal ecosystems and may eventually yield insights on changes in the microbiota that could signal the potential for pathogenesis. By better understanding the dynamics of vaginal environment in all stages of life and by identifying those events that promote disease, there is hope that more effective therapies can be developed to promote vaginal health throughout a woman's life.

Cross-References

▶ Aging Skin Microbiology

References

1. Sousa T, Paterson R, Moore V, et al. The gastrointestinal microbiota as a site for the biotransformation of drugs. Int J Pharm. 2008;363:1–25.

2. Todar K. The bacterial flora of humans. http://textbookofbacteriology.net/normalflora.html
3. Davis C. Normal Flora. In: Baron S editor. Medical microbiology. 4th ed. http://gsbs.utmb.edu/microbook/ch006.htm
4. Marshall W, Tanner J. Puberty. In: Davis J, Dobbing J, editors. Puberty. London: Heinemann; 1981.
5. Nugent RP, Krohn MA, Hillier SL. Reliability of diagnosing bacterial vaginosis is improved by a standardized method of gram stain interpretation. J Clin Microbiol. 1991;29:297–301.
6. Hillier SL, Krohn MA, Nugent RP, et al. Characteristics of three vaginal flora patterns assessed by gram stain among pregnant women. Vaginal Infections and Prematurity Study Group. Am J Obstet Gynecol. 1992;166:938–44.
7. Ma B, Forney LJ, Ravel J. Vaginal microbiome: rethinking health and disease. Annu Rev Microbiol. 2012;66:371–38. See comment in PubMed Commons below.
8. van de Wijgert JHHM, Borgdorff H, Verhelst R, et al. The vaginal microbiota: what have we learned after a decade of molecular characterization? PLoS One. 2014;9(8):e105998.
9. Petrova MI, Lievens E, Malik S, et al. Lactobacillus species as biomarkers and agents that can promote various aspects of vaginal health. Front Physiol. 2015;6:81.
10. Nardis C, Mosca L, Mastromarino P. Vaginal microbiota and viral sexually transmitted diseases. Ann Ig. 2013;25:443–56.
11. Cone RA. Vaginal microbiota and sexually transmitted infections that may influence transmission of cell-associated HIV. J Infect Dis. 2014;210 Suppl 3: S616–21.
12. Bump RC, Zuspan FP, Buesching WJ, et al. The prevalence, six-month persistence, and predictive values of laboratory indicators of bacterial vaginosis (nonspecific vaginitis) in asymptomatic women. Am J Obstet Gynecol. 1984;150:917–24.
13. Zhou X, Bent SJ, Schneider MG, et al. Characterization of vaginal microbial communities in adult healthy women using cultivation-independent methods. Microbiology. 2004;150:2565–73.
14. Seddon JM, Bruce AW, Chadwick P, et al. Introital bacterial flora – effect of increased frequency of micturition. Br J Urol. 1976;48:211–8.
15. Fredricks DN. Molecular methods to describe the spectrum and dynamics of the vaginal microbiota. Anaerobe. 2011;17:191–5.
16. Farage M, Maibach H. Lifetime changes in the vulva and vagina. Arch Gynecol Obstet. 2006;273:195–202.
17. Zhou X, Brown CJ, Abdo Z, et al. Differences in the composition of vaginal microbial communities found in healthy Caucasian and black women. ISME J. 2007;1:121–33.
18. Priestley CJ, Jones BM, Dhar J, et al. What is normal vaginal flora? Genitourin Med. 1997;73:23–8.
19. Newton ER, Piper JM, Shain RN, et al. Predictors of the vaginal microflora. Am J Obstet Gynecol. 2001;184:845–53; discussion 853–5.
20. Nam H, Whang K, Lee Y. Analysis of vaginal lactic acid producing bacteria in healthy women. J Microbiol. 2007;45:515–20.
21. Neggers YH, Nansel TR, Andrews WW, et al. Dietary intake of selected nutrients affects bacterial vaginosis in women. J Nutr. 2007;137:2128–33.
22. Jones IS. A histological assessment of normal vulval skin. Clin Exp Dermatol. 1983;8:513–21.
23. Eschenbach DA, Thwin SS, Patton DL, et al. Influence of the normal menstrual cycle on vaginal tissue, discharge, and microflora. Clin Infect Dis. 2000;30:901–7.
24. Larsen B, Monif GR. Understanding the bacterial flora of the female genital tract. Clin Infect Dis. 2001;32:e69–77.
25. Hillier SL, Krohn MA, Rabe LK, et al. The normal vaginal flora, H_2O_2-producing lactobacilli, and bacterial vaginosis in pregnant women. Clin Infect Dis. 1993;16 Suppl 4:S273–81.
26. Antonio MA, Hawes SE, Hillier SL. The identification of vaginal *Lactobacillus* species and the demographic and microbiologic characteristics of women colonized by these species. J Infect Dis. 1999;180:1950–6.
27. Romero R, Hassan SS, Gajer P, et al. The composition and stability of the vaginal microbiota of normal pregnant women is different from that of non-pregnant women. Microbiome. 2014;2:4.
28. Petricevic L, Domig KJ, Nierscher FJ, et al. Characterisation of the vaginal *Lactobacillus* microbiota associated with preterm delivery. Sci Rep. 2014;4:5136.
29. Vitali B, Cruciani F, Baldassarre ME, et al. Dietary supplementation with probiotics during late pregnancy: outcome on vaginal microbiota and cytokine secretion. BMC Microbiol. 2012;12:236.
30. Galiñanes S, Coppolillo E, Cifarelli M, et al. Vaginal inflammatory status in pregnant women with normal and pathogenic microbiota in lower genital tract. ISRN Obstet Gynecol. 2011;2011:835926.
31. Stokholm J, Schjørring S, Eskildsen CE, et al. Antibiotic use during pregnancy alters the commensal vaginal microbiota. Clin Microbiol Infect. 2014;20:629–35.
32. Shipitsyna E, Roos A, Datcu R, et al. Composition of the vaginal microbiota in women of reproductive age – sensitive and specific molecular diagnosis of bacterial vaginosis is possible? PLoS One. 2013;8: e60670.
33. Shafer MA, Sweet RL, Ohm-Smith MJ, et al. Microbiology of the lower genital tract in postmenarchal adolescent girls: differences by sexual

activity, contraception, and presence of nonspecific vaginitis. J Pediatr. 1985;107:974–81.
34. Boskey ER, Telsch KM, Whaley KJ, et al. Acid production by vaginal flora in vitro is consistent with the rate and extent of vaginal acidification. Infect Immun. 1999;67:5170–5.
35. Devillard E, Burton JP, Hammond J, et al. Novel insight into the vaginal microflora in postmenopausal women under hormone replacement therapy as analyzed by PCR-denaturing gradient gel electrophoresis. Eur J Obstet Gynecol Reprod Biol. 2004;117:76–81.
36. Eschenbach DA, Patton DL, Meier A, et al. Effects of oral contraceptive pill use on vaginal flora and vaginal epithelium. Contraception. 2000;62:107–12.
37. Hiller S. Normal vaginal flora. In: Holmes K, Sparkling P, March P, Lemon S, Stamm W, Piot P, Wasserhelt J, editors. Normal vaginal flora. New York: McGraw-Hill; 1999.
38. Redondo-Lopez V, Cook RL, Sobel JD. Emerging role of lactobacilli in the control and maintenance of the vaginal bacterial microflora. Rev Infect Dis. 1990;12:856–72.
39. Schwebke JR, Weiss H. Influence of the normal menstrual cycle on vaginal microflora. Clin Infect Dis. 2001;32:325.
40. Petrova MI, van den Broek M, Balzarini J, et al. Vaginal microbiota and its role in HIV transmission and infection. FEMS Microbiol Rev. 2013;37:762–92.
41. O'Hanlon DE, Moench TR, Cone RA. Vaginal pH and microbicidal lactic acid when lactobacilli dominate the microbiota. PLoS One. 2013;8:e80074.
42. Frank DN, Manigart O, Leroy V, et al. Altered vaginal microbiota are associated with perinatal mother-to-child transmission of HIV in African women from Burkina Faso. J Acquir Immune Defic Syndr. 2012;60:299–306.
43. Mitchell C, Hitti J, Paul K, et al. Cervicovaginal shedding of HIV type 1 is related to genital tract inflammation independent of changes in vaginal microbiota. AIDS Res Hum Retroviruses. 2011;27:35–9.
44. Hummelen R, Fernandes AD, Macklaim JM, et al. Deep sequencing of the vaginal microbiota of women with HIV. PLoS One. 2010;5:e12078.
45. King AE, Critchley HOD, Kelly RW. Innate immune defences in the human endometrium. Reprod Biol Endocrinol. 2003;1:116.
46. Ravel J, Brotman RM, Gajer P, et al. Daily temporal dynamics of vaginal microbiota before, during and after episodes of bacterial vaginosis. Microbiome. 2013;1:29.
47. Ling Z, Liu X, Chen W, et al. The restoration of the vaginal microbiota after treatment for bacterial vaginosis with metronidazole or probiotics. Microb Ecol. 2013;65:773–80.
48. Cruciani F, Brigidi P, Calanni F, et al. Efficacy of rifaximin vaginal tablets in treatment of bacterial vaginosis: a molecular characterization of the vaginal microbiota. Antimicrob Agents Chemother. 2012;56:4062–70.
49. Ling Z, Kong J, Liu F, et al. Molecular analysis of the diversity of vaginal microbiota associated with bacterial vaginosis. BMC Genomics. 2010;11:488.
50. Sullivan A, Fianu-Jonasson A, Landgren B, et al. Ecological effects of perorally administered pivmecillinam on the normal vaginal microflora. Antimicrob Agents Chemother. 2005;49:170–5.
51. Zhou X, Westman R, Hickey R, et al. Vaginal microbiota of women with frequent vulvovaginal candidiasis. Infect Immun. 2009;77:4130–5.
52. Gao W, Weng J, Gao Y, et al. Comparison of the vaginal microbiota diversity of women with and without human papillomavirus infection: a cross-sectional study. BMC Infect Dis. 2013;13:271.
53. Ginsberg J. What determines the age at the menopause? BMJ. 1991;302:1288–9.
54. de Bruin JP, Bovenhuis H, van Noord PA, et al. The role of genetic factors in age at natural menopause. Hum Reprod. 2001;16:2014–8.
55. Murabito JM, Yang Q, Fox C, et al. Heritability of age at natural menopause in the Framingham Heart Study. J Clin Endocrinol Metab. 2005;90:3427–30.
56. Bromberger JT, Matthews KA, Kuller LH, et al. Prospective study of the determinants of age at menopause. Am J Epidemiol. 1997;145:124–33.
57. Noreh J, Sekadde-Kigondu C, Karanja JG, et al. Median age at menopause in a rural population of western Kenya. East Afr Med J. 1997;74:634–8.
58. Henderson KD, Bernstein L, Henderson B, et al. Predictors of the timing of natural menopause in the Multiethnic Cohort Study. Am J Epidemiol. 2008;167:1287–94.
59. Chen GD, Oliver RH, Leung BS, et al. Estrogen receptor alpha and beta expression in the vaginal walls and uterosacral ligaments of premenopausal and postmenopausal women. Fertil Steril. 1999;71:1099–102.
60. Galhardo CL, Soares JMJ, Simões RS, et al. Estrogen effects on the vaginal pH, flora and cytology in late postmenopause after a long period without hormone therapy. Clin Exp Obstet Gynecol. 2006;33:85–9.
61. Caillouette JC, Sharp CFJ, Zimmerman GJ, et al. Vaginal pH as a marker for bacterial pathogens and menopausal status. Am J Obstet Gynecol. 1997;176:1270–5; discussion 1275–7.
62. Gupta S, Kumar N, Singhal N, et al. Vaginal microflora in postmenopausal women on hormone replacement therapy. Indian J Pathol Microbiol. 2006;49:457–61.
63. Hillier SL, Lau RJ. Vaginal microflora in postmenopausal women who have not received estrogen replacement therapy. Clin Infect Dis. 1997;25 Suppl 2:S123–6.

64. Gorodeski GI. Effects of estrogen on proton secretion via the apical membrane in vaginal-ectocervical epithelial cells of postmenopausal women. Menopause. 2005;12:679–84.
65. Bachmann G. Quantifying estrogen treatment effect on vagina tissue: cellular age matters. Menopause. 2005;12:656–7.
66. Milsom I, Arvidsson L, Ekelund P, et al. Factors influencing vaginal cytology, pH and bacterial flora in elderly women. Acta Obstet Gynecol Scand. 1993;72:286–91.
67. Raz R, Stamm WE. A controlled trial of intravaginal estriol in postmenopausal women with recurrent urinary tract infections. N Engl J Med. 1993;329:753–6.
68. Heinemann C, Reid G. Vaginal microbial diversity among postmenopausal women with and without hormone replacement therapy. Can J Microbiol. 2005;51:777–81.
69. Meltzer R. Vulvovaginitis. In: Sciarra J, editor. Vulvovaginitis. Philadelphia: JB Lippincott; 1987.
70. Bartlett JG, Onderdonk AB, Drude E, et al. Quantitative bacteriology of the vaginal flora. J Infect Dis. 1977;136:271–7.
71. Osborne NG, Wright RC, Grubin L. Genital bacteriology: a comparative study of premenopausal women with postmenopausal women. Am J Obstet Gynecol. 1979;135:195–8.
72. Stamey TA, Sexton CC. The role of vaginal colonization with enterobacteriaceae in recurrent urinary infections. J Urol. 1975;113:214–7.
73. Pabich WL, Fihn SD, Stamm WE, et al. Prevalence and determinants of vaginal flora alterations in postmenopausal women. J Infect Dis. 2003;188:1054–8.
74. Cauci S, Driussi S, De Santo D, et al. Prevalence of bacterial vaginosis and vaginal flora changes in peri- and postmenopausal women. J Clin Microbiol. 2002;40:2147–52.
75. Taylor-Robinson D, McCaffrey M, Pitkin J, et al. Bacterial vaginosis in climacteric and menopausal women. Int J STD AIDS. 2002;13:449–52.
76. Blum M, Elian I. The vaginal flora after natural or surgical menopause. J Am Geriatr Soc. 1979;27:395–7.
77. Brotman RM, Shardell MD, Gajer P, et al. Association between the vaginal microbiota, menopause status, and signs of vulvovaginal atrophy. Menopause. 2014;21:450–8.
78. Molander U, Milsom I, Ekelund P, et al. Effect of oral oestriol on vaginal flora and cytology and urogenital symptoms in the post-menopause. Maturitas. 1990;12:113–20.
79. Burton JP, Reid G. Evaluation of the bacterial vaginal flora of 20 postmenopausal women by direct (Nugent score) and molecular (polymerase chain reaction and denaturing gradient gel electrophoresis) techniques. J Infect Dis. 2002;186:1770–80.
80. Kirjavainen PV, Pautler S, Baroja ML, et al. Abnormal immunological profile and vaginal microbiota in women prone to urinary tract infections. Clin Vaccine Immunol. 2009;16:29–36.
81. Fantl J, Newman K, Coiling J, et al. Urinary incontinence in adults: acute and chronic management. Washington, DC: US Department of Health and Human Services, Public Health Service, Agency for Health Care Policy and Research (AHCPR); 1996.
82. Burton JP, Cadieux PA, Reid G. Improved understanding of the bacterial vaginal microbiota of women before and after probiotic instillation. Appl Environ Microbiol. 2003;69:97–101.
83. Ison CA, Hill MJ, Marsh PD, et al. Factors affecting the microflora of the lower genital tract of healthy women. In: Factors affecting the microflora of the lower genital tract of healthy women. Boca Raton: CRC Press; 1990.
84. Pascual LM, Daniele MB, Pájaro C, et al. Lactobacillus species isolated from the vagina: identification, hydrogen peroxide production and nonoxynol-9 resistance. Contraception. 2006;73:78–81.
85. Onderdonk A, Wisseman K. Normal vaginal microflora. In: Elsner P, Martius J, editors. Normal vaginal microflora. New York: Marcel Dekker; 1993.
86. Strus M, Brzychczy-Włoch M, Gosiewski T, et al. The in vitro effect of hydrogen peroxide on vaginal microbial communities. FEMS Immunol Med Microbiol. 2006;48:56–63.
87. Reid G, Jass J, Sebulsky MT, et al. Potential uses of probiotics in clinical practice. Clin Microbiol Rev. 2003;16:658–72.
88. Rönnqvist PDJ, Forsgren-Brusk UB, Grahn-Håkansson EE. Lactobacilli in the female genital tract in relation to other genital microbes and vaginal pH. Acta Obstet Gynecol Scand. 2006;85:726–35.
89. Mack DR, Michail S, Wei S, et al. Probiotics inhibit enteropathogenic *E. coli* adherence in vitro by inducing intestinal mucin gene expression. Am J Physiol. 1999;276:G941–50.
90. Kim Y, Ohta T, Takahashi T, et al. Probiotic Lactobacillus casei activates innate immunity via NF-kappaB and p38 MAP kinase signaling pathways. Microbes Infect. 2006;8:994–1005.
91. Pandit L, Ouslander JG. Postmenopausal vaginal atrophy and atrophic vaginitis. Am J Med Sci. 1997;314:228–31.
92. Maloney C, Oliver ML. Effect of local conjugated estrogens on vaginal pH in elderly women. J Am Med Dir Assoc. 2001;2:51–5.
93. Long C, Liu C, Hsu S, et al. A randomized comparative study of the effects of oral and topical estrogen therapy on the vaginal vascularization and sexual function in hysterectomized postmenopausal women. Menopause. 2006;13:737–43.
94. Robinson D, Cardozo L. The menopause and HRT. Urogenital effects of hormone therapy. Best Pract Res Clin Endocrinol Metab. 2003;17:91–104.
95. Tsai CC, Semmens JP, Semmens EC, et al. Vaginal physiology in postmenopausal women: pH value,

transvaginal electropotential difference, and estimated blood flow. South Med J. 1987;80:987–90.
96. Tashjian JH, Coulam CB, Washington JA. Vaginal flora in asymptomatic women. Mayo Clin Proc. 1976;51:557–61.
97. Blum M, Elian I. The upper vaginal and cervical anaerobic flora in menopausal women. Eur J Obstet Gynecol Reprod Biol. 1981;12:183–7.
98. Larsen B, Goplerud CP, Petzold CR, et al. Effect of estrogen treatment on the genital tract flora of postmenopausal women. Obstet Gynecol. 1982;60:20–4.
99. Ceddia T, Cappa F, Cialfi R, et al. Prevalence of non-specific vaginitis and correlation with isolation of *Gardnerella vaginalis* in Italian outpatients. Eur J Epidemiol. 1989;5:529–31.
100. Ginkel PD, Soper DE, Bump RC, et al. Vaginal flora in postmenopausal women: the effect of estrogen replacement. Infect Dis Obstet Gynecol. 1993;1:94–7.
101. Yoshimura T, Okamura H. Short term oral estriol treatment restores normal premenopausal vaginal flora to elderly women. Maturitas. 2001;39:253–7.
102. Orlander JD, Jick SS, Dean AD, et al. Urinary tract infections and estrogen use in older women. J Am Geriatr Soc. 1992;40:817–20.
103. Foxman B, Somsel P, Tallman P, et al. Urinary tract infection among women aged 40 to 65: behavioral and sexual risk factors. J Clin Epidemiol. 2001;54:710–8.
104. Kirkengen AL, Andersen P, Gjersøe E, et al. Oestriol in the prophylactic treatment of recurrent urinary tract infections in postmenopausal women. Scand J Prim Health Care. 1992;10:139–42.
105. Eriksen B. A randomized, open, parallel-group study on the preventive effect of an estradiol-releasing vaginal ring (Estring) on recurrent urinary tract infections in postmenopausal women. Am J Obstet Gynecol. 1999;180:1072–9.
106. Cardozo L, Bachmann G, McClish D, et al. Meta-analysis of estrogen therapy in the management of urogenital atrophy in postmenopausal women: second report of the Hormones and Urogenital Therapy Committee. Obstet Gynecol. 1998;92:722–7.

Irritant Contact Dermatitis

107

Judit Lukács and Peter Elsner

Contents

Abstract

Both irritant contact dermatitis (ICD) and allergic contact dermatitis (ACD) are the results of the exposure to external agents, which cause inflammation of the skin. Both show a similar histopathological and immunohistochemical pattern [1]. Exposure to irritants causes an unspecific impairment of keratinocytes and leads to expression of integrin receptors and the intracellular adhesion molecule 1 (ICAM-1) [3, 4]. Consequently, production of proinflammatory cytokines (especially interleukin-6, interleukin-8, interleukin-2, tumor necrosis factor α, granulocyte-macrophage colony-stimulating factor (GM-CSF), and interleukin-1b) becomes enhanced [5, 6].

An age dependence of irritation is only to be seen if very young people are compared with very old people. Within the subgroup of adult individuals younger than 50, there is no relation between age and severity of irritation [12, 13]. On the other hand, children are more susceptible to irritation. Investigations of recent years provided some information about the influence of age on regulation of the epidermal barrier after disruption (Fig. 1) [20]. Different biochemical pathways have been elucidated, which are enhanced after barrier disruption and affect its stabilization. The epidermal barrier is represented mainly by the hydrophobic stratum corneum lipid structures (very-long-chain saturated fatty acids, cholesterol, and ceramides in equimolar proportion)

J. Lukács (✉)
Klinik für Hautkrankheiten, Universitätsklinikum Jena, Jena, Germany
e-mail: Judit.Lukacs@med.uni-jena.de

P. Elsner
Department of Dermatology and Dermatological Allergology, Universitätsklinikum Jena, Jena, Germany
e-mail: elsner@derma-jena.de

M.A. Farage et al. (eds.), *Textbook of Aging Skin*,
DOI 10.1007/978-3-662-47398-6_79

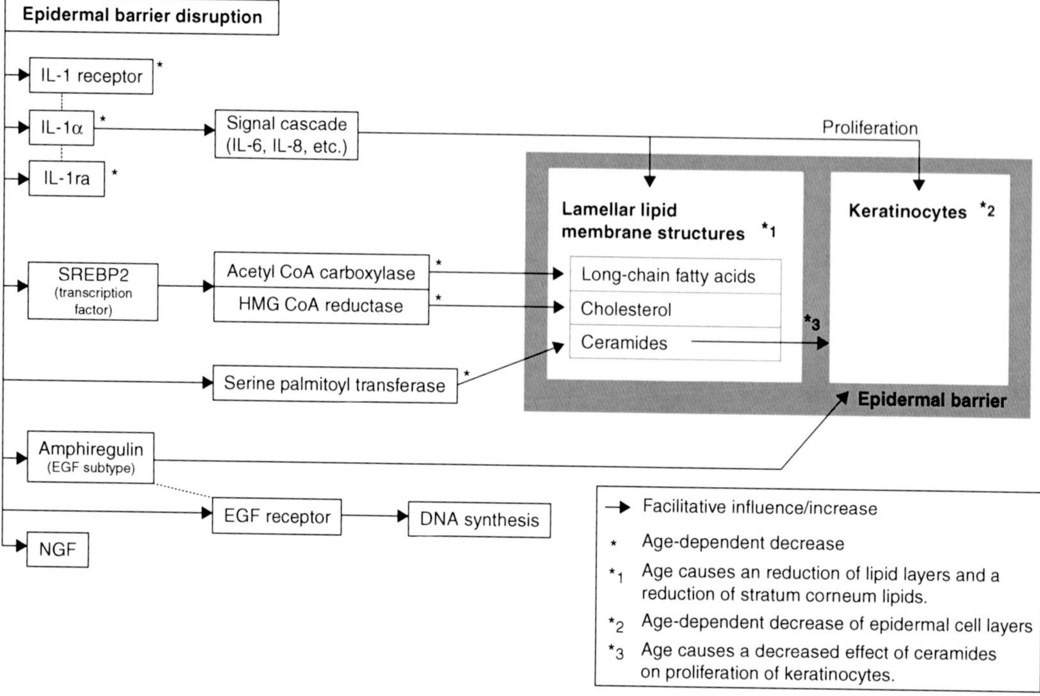

Fig. 1 The influence of age on epidermal barrier recovery by Elias and Ghadially [20]. *IL-1 ra* IL-1 receptor antagonist, *SREBP2* sterol regulatory element-binding protein 2, *NGF* nerve growth factor, *EGF* epidermal growth factor

and the upper layer of nucleated keratinocytes. The skin irritation depends on the body area exposed to the irritant. The most sensitive areas are the face, the upper back, and the retroauricular as well as the genital skin [3]. Some authors showed a higher sensitivity in the face compared to the back. Within the face, the chin and nasolabial folds are the most vulnerable regions [4]. The clinical picture is characterized by dryness, erythema, lichenification, and hyperkeratosis ("xerotic dermatitis"). While occupational cumulative irritant contact dermatitis is especially a problem in younger people [41], older persons show another distribution of clinical subtypes of ICD. The term "irritant contact dermatitis" includes various subtypes, each one with its own age distribution [40]. The perineal or "incontinence" dermatitis is typical for older individuals. The clinical presentation of ICD in older people is more discrete than in younger, with the TEWL increase being less pronounced. On the other hand, older skin regenerates more slowly.

Introduction

Both irritant contact dermatitis (ICD) and allergic contact dermatitis (ACD) are the results of the exposure to external agents, which cause inflammation of the skin. Both show a similar histopathological and immunohistochemical pattern [1].

The clinical picture of ICD differs in dependence from the duration of disease. Acute forms feature erythema, edema, vesicles (in part coalescing), bullae, oozing, and, in severe cases, after contact to corrosive substances, necrosis and/or ulceration. Chronic forms are characterized by erythema, lichenification, excoriations, scaling, and hyperkeratosis.

In acute ICD, intraepidermally located vesicles or bullae dominate the histological picture, surrounded by a variably pronounced spongiosis. An inflammatory infiltrate may be present, consisting of mononucleated cells. Parakeratosis of the stratum corneum is sometimes described. The upper dermis is characterized by edematous alterations. In contrast, chronic ICD shows acanthosis, marked hyper- and parakeratosis, and slight spongiosis. Vesicles are absent. The inflammatory infiltrate generally has a perivascular distribution in the upper dermis [2].

Since morphological criteria are insufficient for differentiation of ICD from ACD, one has to rely on anamnestic and exposure data, patch test results, and the location of the dermatitis. ICD is often found on the hands; in older incontinent patients, it can also be found in the perineal region.

Pathophysiology of ICD in Aged Skin

For a long time, the pathophysiology of the irritant contact dermatitis (ICD) was considered to be very different from allergic contact dermatitis. While ACD is associated with hapten-specific lymphocytes, ICD was explained as a completely nonimmunological reaction to exogenous irritants [3]. Utilizing the scientific progress of the last few years, immune response to irritants was investigated, which led to a more complex view on ICD [4]. Exposure to irritants causes an unspecific impairment of keratinocytes and leads to expression of integrin receptors and the intracellular adhesion molecule 1 (ICAM-1) [3, 4]. Consequently, production of proinflammatory cytokines (especially interleukin-6, interleukin-8, interleukin-2, tumor necrosis factor α, granulocyte-macrophage colony-stimulating factor (GM-CSF), and interleukin-1b) becomes enhanced [5, 6].

Interestingly, the same cytokines, which are also found in allergic contact dermatitis, are detected in ICD. Additionally, activation of CCL21, a chemokine of lymphatic tissues, was described [4].

Irritation and the activation of the inflammation cascade are linked to the damage of the stratum corneum lipid barrier, which is associated with loss of cohesion of corneocytes and desquamation causing an increased transepidermal water loss (TEWL) [7]. Thus, TEWL is used as a marker for irritation and epidermal barrier disruption.

The basal TEWL decreases with age, suggesting a lower irritability of aged skin. In this context, Thune et al. showed a TEWL decrease in aged patients suffering from dry skin (median age, 65 years) compared with a younger control group (median age, 29 years), while the hydration showed no significant differences between the groups [8]. This was confirmed by Cua et al. [9], who found a lower TEWL increase and attenuated patch test results ("visual score") after irritation with Sodium laureth sulfate (SLS) in elderly subjects. Schnichels and Elsner performed an acute irritation by patch testing with SLS in an older (50–70 years) and a younger (20–40 years) age group. The baseline TEWL level before exposure was generally lower in the old age group. After acute irritation, twice as many older persons showed no erythema compared with the young group, which presented more intense clinical signs and a more increased TEWL after irritation [7]. However, when irritation by SLS is terminated, TEWL decreases faster to normal values in younger persons, suggesting faster barrier recovery in this age group.

In another study, Elsner et al. [10] compared the reactivity of premenopausal women with postmenopausal women by SLS irritation on the forearm. The older group showed a slower and less intense reaction than the younger women (visual score, TEWL).

Coenraads et al. [11] found less susceptibility in aged people for croton oil but not for thymoquinone and crotonaldehyde.

An age dependence of irritation is only to be seen if very young people are compared with very old people. Within the subgroup of adult individuals younger than 50, there is no relation between age and severity of irritation [12, 13]. On the other hand, children are more susceptible to irritation. For example, there is more irritation after exposure to DMSO and SLS in children [9], while older people show a milder, but persistent skin reaction [14].

The most studies presented here draw their conclusions from SLS exposure and determination of the TEWL, which may be a point of criticism.

On the one side, it is difficult to determine if the study results are transferable to other irritants than SLS; on the other side, some authors consider that TEWL decrease in aged skin does not reflect less irritability. Thune et al. [8] attributed this effect to a generally decreased hydration of aged skin, possibly due to decreased ceramide levels [7]. Other studies could not affirm decreased water content due to age [9, 15–18]. Ghadially et al. interpreted the decreased TEWL in the older skin as a result of reduced sweating rates, decreased microcirculation, and decreased temperature in old subjects [19]. Starting from the observation of decreased permeability of lipophilic drugs in aged skin, the authors emphasized a decrease of the epidermal lipid content in old people. This hypothesis is supported by electron microscopic analysis, which revealed a decreased number of lamellar bodies in the stratum granulosum–stratum corneum interface, as well as a reduced lipid content in a mouse model. Additionally, tape stripping experiments resulted in a faster-occurring TEWL increase in old subjects compared with young ones. Finally, the time which was needed for normalization of TEWL after acetone exposure was longer in older test persons. The authors conclude that "the aged epidermal permeability barrier is both easier to perturb and slower to repair" [19].

Investigations of recent years provided some information about the influence of age on regulation of the epidermal barrier after disruption (Fig. 1) [20]. Different biochemical pathways have been elucidated, which are enhanced after barrier disruption and affect its stabilization. The epidermal barrier is represented mainly by the hydrophobic stratum corneum lipid structures (very-long-chain saturated fatty acids, cholesterol, and ceramides in equimolar proportion) and the upper layer of nucleated keratinocytes. Lipid synthesis and the proliferation of keratinocytes are enhanced after activation of the interleukin-1α cascade due to barrier disruption, which is accompanied by an increase of interleukin-1 receptor type 2 (T2 IL-1 R) and the interleukin-1 receptor antagonist (IL-1 ra) [21]. Interestingly, concentrations of interleukin-1α, T2 interleukin-1 R, and interleukin-1 ra in old mice show a reduced increase after irritation, compared with young mice. Moreover, aged interleukin-1α knockout mice show a notably impaired barrier reconstitution compared with the wild type [21, 22].

Angelova-Fischer et al. found that the alterations in the in vivo cytokine profile as a result of the application of the irritant tandems (SLS and undiluted toluene) were characterized by decreased amounts of IL-1 ra as well as lower IL-1 ra/IL-1α ratio [22]. These findings were independent of the age or the irritant exposure [22].

Another important molecule more expressed after barrier disruption is the transcription factor SREBP2 (sterol regulatory element-binding protein 2), which induces expression of β-hydroxy-β methylglutaryl-coenzyme A (HMG-CoA) reductase and acetyl coenzyme A carboxylase. Both enzymes play a key role in the synthesis of long-chain fatty acids and cholesterol and, thus, in barrier recovery.

The expression of the enzyme serine palmitoyl transferase is directly enhanced by barrier disruption and facilitates synthesis of ceramides, which – for their part – stimulate proliferation of keratinocytes.

In aged skin, there are lower levels of all three enzymes for lipid synthesis to be found, supporting the thesis of a reduced barrier recovery in age.

Next to cytokines and lipid synthesis, nerve growth factor (NGF) and epidermal growth factors (EGF) are upregulated after disruption. The EGF subtype amphiregulin shows elevated levels especially in aged skin [20].

Irritants

Studies in occupational dermatology emphasize wet work as a crucial influencing factor on ICD. Wet work thereby is characterized by a repetitive exposure to water and detergents, especially under occlusive conditions. Hereunder, water increases erythema, pH, cutaneous blood flow, TEWL, and the permeability to low-molecular-weight irritants [23]. Additionally, the frictional coefficient as a predictor of skin vulnerability also increases. Consecutively, there is a higher risk for pressure ulcers and increased susceptibility for bacterial infection [23].

Important chemical irritants, arranged in order of frequency, are detergents (e.g., soap), solvents, oil, dusts and fibers, and, last but not least, acids and alkalis. Important physical irritants are heat, sweating, friction, pressure, vibration, UV irradiation, and occlusion [4]. Occlusion increases the signs of inflammation, pH, TEWL, stratum corneum hydration, skin surface temperature, and skin permeability [23]. Furthermore, lipid organization and metabolism, as well as cellular function (e.g., DNA synthesis, mitosis), are inhibited [23].

Other common exogenous factors on irritation are the temperature of detergents [24] and climatic conditions, especially dry air [3, 4].

Predisposing Factors for ICD

ICD is not only dependent on the irritant, but there is also a high number of endogenous factors predisposing for ICD, such as concomitant atopic eczema [4, 25–29] or any other concomitant dermatitis [30]. Although experimental studies concerning irritability in atopic and nonatopic skin did not support this hypothesis unanimously [31, 32], determination of an atypical filaggrin gene as a marker of atopy is also assumed as predictor for ICD [33]. The protein filaggrin is involved in the formation of the skin barrier. Independent from atopic diathesis, tumor necrosis factor α polymorphism was recommended as a genetic marker for ICD [4]. Other factors are structural properties of the skin, a deficient hardening phenomenon of the skin, and an increased sensitivity to UV irradiation [3], especially in subjects with skin type I [34]. Concerning sex, the influence on irritation is ambiguous [9]. While experimental studies did not support a correlation between sex and irritability [35, 36], epidemiological studies emphasize a higher incidence of ICD in women [26, 37, 38]. Additionally, skin irritation depends on the body area exposed to the irritant. The most sensitive areas are the face, the upper back, and the retroauricular as well as the genital skin [3]. Some authors showed a higher sensitivity in the face compared to the back. Within the face, the chin and nasolabial folds are the most vulnerable regions [4]. Several investigations with ammonium hydroxide [39], dimethylsulfoxide (DMSO), and SLS [9] showed a higher sensitivity at the forearms and hands compared to the legs and feet.

Clinical Types of ICD

The term irritant contact dermatitis includes various subtypes, each one with its own age distribution [40]. The most common type is *cumulative irritant contact dermatitis* [4], which is important in occupational dermatology and is found mainly in young adults [41]. The disease is caused by repetitive irritation of the skin over the years with mild symptoms, which are often neglected by the patient. Thus, irritation continues unnoticed, until a threshold is reached and a severe ICD develops [3]. The clinical picture is characterized by dryness, erythema, lichenification, and hyperkeratosis ("xerotic dermatitis"). The prognosis is poor. Meding et al. found that after 15 years of follow-up, 44 % of patients still had hand eczema within the past year [42]. Veien et al. confirm these findings reporting a persistent or intermittent hand eczema 5 years after the initial diagnosis in 65 % of all cases [43]. For persistent ICD in spite of changing the workplace, the term *post-occupational dermatitis* was introduced [44].

The so-called non-erythematous ICD, which shows changes in skin-physiological parameters without any visible inflammation, and the *irritant reaction* can be regarded as a pre-stage of cumulative ICD. *Non-erythematous ICD* is also seen after exposure to cocamidopropyl betaine, coconut diethanolamide, etc. [45]. The *irritant reaction* displays only one or few clinical signs, for example, dryness, scaling, redness, vesicles, pustules, and erosions. These reactions mostly appear after a period of intense contact to water, especially in young professionals. Their ability for an intrinsic skin hardening determines whether the irritant reaction disappears or a cumulative ICD develops.

Acute ICD develops within minutes or hours after accidental contact to potent irritants. Thereafter, the symptoms such as burning, itching, algesia, and formation of erythema, edema, bullae, or necrosis rise quickly. After the symptoms have exceeded a maximum and the irritant stimuli were eradicated, the process of healing starts and is marked by a good prognosis.

The clinical course of *delayed acute ICD* is different from *acute ICD*, whereas the clinical picture is identical. Inflammation becomes visible not before 8–24 h after contact to the irritants (e.g., anthralin/dithranol, benzalkonium chloride, and tretinoin).

Traumatic ICD develops after traumata like burns or severe acute ICD and displays erythema, vesicles/papulovesicles, and scaling instead of healing of the trauma. It resembles nummular dermatitis [46].

Another type of ICD is *pustular dermatitis* due to contact to metals, tars, oils, chlorinated agents, and naphthalene.

Sensory irritation, characterized by stinging, burning, tightness, itching, or painful sensations occurring immediately or delayed after contact to mainly cosmetic products, seems to be a problem mostly in middle-aged, Caucasian, and Asian women [47]. In contrast, aged people seldom show this form of ICD, which is addressed to the lower content of nerve fibers in aged skin [48].

Asteatotic irritant dermatitis (synonyms, *exsiccation eczematoid*, *winter eczema*, or *eczema craquele*, Fig. 2) is found mainly in older patients [49] with a maximum in the winter depending on a decreased air moisture [50]. Another contributing factor is misbehavior in personal care (frequent bathing/showering and extensive usage of soaps and cleansing products), which is assumed to be a common problem in older people [51]. Intensive care practices learned in the youth are missed to become adapted to the aged skin with its special properties (decreased stratum corneum hydration and decreased levels of stratum corneum lipids and ceramides) [52–54]. Patients with *asteatotic irritant dermatitis* show dry skin with ichthyosiform scaling and fissuring, especially on the extremities. TEWL and pH are increased [8], and keratinosomes are disturbed [55]. The most compromising symptom is intensive itching, wherefore this disease has to be considered as differential diagnosis in patients with pruritus senilis (see Table 1). Interestingly, xerosis cutis induced by HMG-CoA reductase inhibitors mimics asteatotic irritant dermatitis [57].

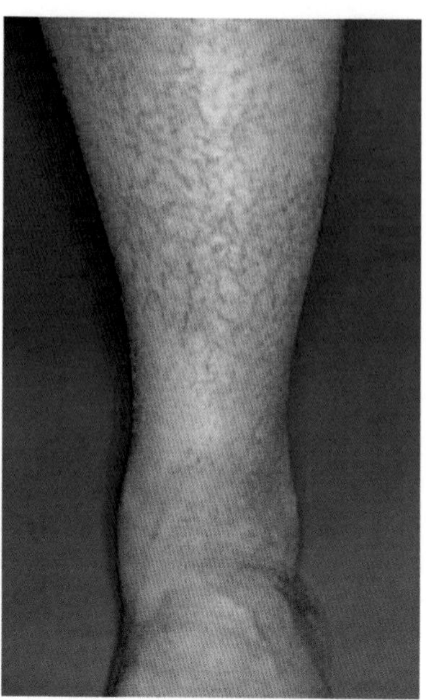

Fig. 2 Exsiccation eczema (Courtesy: Department of Dermatology, Jena)

Table 1 List of differential diagnosis of generalized pruritus by Elewski et al. [56]

Pruritus	
Xerosis cutis/asteatotic ICD	Malign tumors (lymphomas, leukemia, etc.)
Diabetes mellitus	Polycythemia
Hepatic and biliary diseases	Hypothyreosis, hyperthyreosis
Nephrological diseases	Dermatitis herpetiformis
Iron deficiency	Psychogeneous
Drugs	Parasite infestation

For treatment of ICD, avoiding irritants, topical corticosteroids, moisturizers, rich oil-based creams, cold compresses and cold water for washing, and UV radiation and training programs are recommended [3].

Perineal and Genital ICD in the Aged Skin

While occupational cumulative irritant contact dermatitis is especially a problem in younger people [41], older persons show another distribution of clinical subtypes of ICD.

The perineal or "incontinence" dermatitis is typical for older individuals. In the USA, 48.4 % of the women older than 50 years suffer from urinary incontinence, 15.2 % from fecal incontinence, and 9.4 % from both [23]. The clinical picture is characterized by an initially mild and sometimes pruritic erythema, which becomes complicated by the development of small vesicles and erosions, with a tendency to superinfection (*Staphylococcus aureus*, candidiasis, tinea). In severe cases, pressure ulcers develop. Depending on the type of incontinence, the disease begins in the perianal (fecal incontinence) or vulvar region (urine incontinence) [23], which is more irritable and permeable than the skin from body areas [58]. Perineal ICD is related to typical irritants, primarily to urine or stool as chemical irritants.

Urine, as cause of a humid environment under occlusive conditions in the perineal region, is an equivalent to wet work in the younger patient, who has to wear gloves permanently on his hands, which provokes ICD of the hands. Additionally, urine is characterized by a high amount of ammonia, which causes a skin pH increase to 8. Thus, synthesis of lipid barrier components and keratinization is inhibited and repair functions of the skin are impaired [23]. Next to urine, there is a high amount of other potential vulvar irritants like sweat, secretions, cosmetics, disinfectants, vaginal douches (especially in younger women [59]), lubricants, spermicides, antifungal creams and other topical medicaments, depilatory cream, and semen [60]. Physical irritants might be sanitary pads, tampon strings, tight clothing, synthetic underwear, toilet paper, overzealous cleansing, scrubbing, shaving, plucking hair, and prolonged sitting [60]. Occlusion caused by the use of diapers is an essential contributing factor in perineal ICD [23], especially in older individuals and also in neonates.

Vulvar ICD is generally the most frequent vulvar disease with a high impact on genital pruritus [60]. In contrast, genital allergic contact dermatitis against "applied medicaments, contraceptives, lubricants, or feminine hygiene deodorant spray" seems to be less frequent [61].

Relevant irritants in feces are lipases and proteases. Andersen et al. performed occlusive irritation tests with fecal enzymes and different bile mixtures on dorsal skin of individuals aged between 21 and 66 years. The influence on visual score, TEWL, and pH was investigated. After 21 days, "severe skin erythema and epidermal barrier disruption" were observed [62]. Furthermore, specific endogenous factors in aged people play an important role in the pathogenesis of perineal ICD, for example, lower immune function, inadequate care, impaired cognition, and less mobility [23]. Farage and Maibach reviewed characteristics of vulvar skin in aged women [63]. A decrease of vaginal secretion, a reduction of lubrication, and a higher susceptibility to infective agents, for example, enteric organisms, were concluded. Contrary to the statement that aged vulvar skin "is intrinsically less hydrated, less elastic, more permeable, and more susceptible to irritation" [63], no significant differences accrued from skin-physiological studies (water barrier function, friction coefficient) of vulvar skin from premenopausal and postmenopausal women [17]. On the other hand, 47 % of postmenopausal women suffer from vaginal dryness [64], which is interpreted as manifestation of atrophic vulvovaginitis [65]. This disease is characterized by dryness, itching, and dyspareunia and depends on low estrogen levels, causing vaginal atrophy, increase of pH, and enforcement of susceptibility to microbial pathogens [65].

Compared with senile female perineal and genital ICD, this genital ICD is rarely investigated in elderly men. In Fritsch's Textbook of Dermatology [66], the term "Reinlichkeitsbalanitis" (balanitis of neatness) is used and stated to be coincident with high age. Birley et al. report irritant balanitis according to excessive washing as most frequent subtype in nonspecific balanitis [67], while other authors assume an infectious balanitis as most important [68].

Occupational Dermatology in Aged Employees

The knowledge about the influence of age on occupational hand dermatitis is limited, since generally few epidemiological data are available concerning occupational dermatology [69]. Thus, the influence of age may be underestimated, which is problematic, especially within the scope of an aging society and an increase of aged workers. However, age-adapted training programs on the basis of secondary and tertiary prevention of occupational ICD are still missing.

In general, incidences of hand ICD and atopic hand dermatitis are assumed to be higher than allergic contact dermatitis, whereas nonoccupational hand dermatitis is more frequent than occupational ICD [26, 37, 70]. In 1990, Meding estimated a point prevalence of 5.4 % for hand eczema (hereof 35 % ICD, 19 % ACD, 22 % atopic eczema). Risk factors were history of childhood eczema, female sex, occupational exposure, a history of asthma and/or hay fever, and a service occupation (multiple logistic regression analysis) [26]. However, the age as influencing factor was not considered.

The few epidemiological data concerning age are ambiguous. Soder et al. detected a decrease of quality of life, especially in older patients with occupational hand dermatitis [71]. While older works point out a positive influence of age on development of occupational ICD [72, 73], Diepgen and Kanerva emphasize that neither sex nor age is a risk factor for the manifestation of this disease [69]. Thus, conditions at the workplace, atopic diathesis, and xerosis cutis are the leading risk factors [69]. Another study by Diepgen and Coenraads deals with the mean age of employees at the beginning of their occupational skin diseases [41]. According to these data, the beginning of occupational dermatitis is associated with an early age (haircutter, 19 years; food worker, 22 years; medical personnel, 24 years; metal worker, 33 years) [41]. In contrast, the mean age of construction and cement workers with occupational ICD is relatively high (~39 years) [74, 75].

Conclusion

Irritant contact dermatitis is an underestimated problem in aged people. Epidemiological data are scarce. In spite of this, immunological studies have contributed to the preliminary understanding of the pathophysiological processes in ICD of the aged.

The clinical presentation of ICD in older people is more discrete than in younger, with the TEWL increase being less pronounced. On the other hand, older skin regenerates more slowly.

Although occupational hand dermatitis manifests itself mainly in young professionals, the requirements of older patients have to be studied more intensively, considering the increasing percentage of aged employees due to the demographic change.

The demographic change will also cause an increased need for sufficient geriatric care, which has to regard the irritant potential of personal hygiene products especially in aged people. Thereby, perineal ICD claims specific attention, since it has to be considered as preliminary stage of decubital ulcers.

Cross-References

- ▶ Bioengineering Methods and Skin Aging
- ▶ Cutaneous Effects and Sensitive Skin with Incontinence in the Aged
- ▶ Susceptibility to Irritation in the Elderly

References

1. Brasch J, Burgard J, Sterry W. Common pathogenetic pathways in allergic and irritant contact dermatitis. J Invest Dermatol. 1992;98:166–70.
2. Le TK, Schalkwijk J, van de Kerkhof PC, van Haelst U, van der Valk PG. A histological and immunohistochemical study on chronic irritant contact dermatitis. Am J Contact Dermat. 1998;9:23–8.
3. Loffler H, Effendy I, Happle R. Irritant contact dermatitis. Hautarzt. 2000;51:203–15.
4. Slodownik D, Lee A, Nixon R. Irritant contact dermatitis: a review. Australas J Dermatol. 2008;49:1–9, quiz 10–11.
5. Hunziker T, Brand CU, Kapp A, Waelti ER, Braathen LR. Increased levels of inflammatory cytokines in human skin lymph derived from sodium lauryl sulphate-induced contact dermatitis. Br J Dermatol. 1992;127:254–7.
6. Enk AH, Katz SI. Early molecular events in the induction phase of contact sensitivity. Proc Natl Acad Sci U S A. 1992;89:1398–402.

7. Suter-Widmer J, Elsner P. In: van der Valk PGM, Maibach H, editors. The irritant contact dermatitis syndrome. Boca Raton: CRC Press; 1996. p. 257–61.
8. Thune P, Nilsen T, Hanstad IK, Gustavsen T, Lovig Dahl H. The water barrier function of the skin in relation to the water content of stratum corneum, pH and skin lipids. The effect of alkaline soap and syndet on dry skin in elderly, non-atopic patients. Acta Derm Venereol. 1988;68:277–83.
9. Cua AB, Wilhelm KP, Maibach HI. Cutaneous sodium lauryl sulphate irritation potential: age and regional variability. Br J Dermatol. 1990;123:607–13.
10. Elsner P, Wilhelm D, Maibach HI. Sodium lauryl sulfate-induced irritant contact dermatitis in vulvar and forearm skin of premenopausal and postmenopausal women. J Am Acad Dermatol. 1990;23:648–52.
11. Coenraads PJ, Bleumink E, Nater JP. Susceptibility to primary irritants: age dependence and relation to contact allergic reactions. Contact Dermatitis. 1975;1:377–81.
12. Agner T. Noninvasive measuring methods for the investigation of irritant patch test reactions. A study of patients with hand eczema, atopic dermatitis and controls. Acta Derm Venereol Suppl (Stockh). 1992;173:1–26.
13. Tupker RA, Coenraads PJ, Pinnagoda J, Nater JP. Baseline transepidermal water loss (TEWL) as a prediction of susceptibility to sodium lauryl sulphate. Contact Dermatitis. 1989;20:265–9.
14. Elsner P, Wilhelm D, Maibach HI. Irritant dermatitis and aging. Contact Dermatitis. 1990;23:275.
15. Wilhelm KP, Cua AB, Maibach HI. Skin aging. Effect on transepidermal water loss, stratum corneum hydration, skin surface pH, and casual sebum content. Arch Dermatol. 1991;127:1806–9.
16. Thune P. Evaluation of the hydration and the water-holding capacity in atopic skin and so-called dry skin. Acta Derm Venereol Suppl (Stockh). 1989;144:133–5.
17. Elsner P, Wilhelm D, Maibach HI. Frictional properties of human forearm and vulvar skin: influence of age and correlation with transepidermal water loss and capacitance. Dermatologica. 1990;181:88–91.
18. Cua AB, Wilhelm KP, Maibach HI. Frictional properties of human skin: relation to age, sex and anatomical region, stratum corneum hydration and transepidermal water loss. Br J Dermatol. 1990;123:473–9.
19. Ghadially R, Brown BE, Sequeira-Martin SM, Feingold KR, Elias PM. The aged epidermal permeability barrier. Structural, functional, and lipid biochemical abnormalities in humans and a senescent murine model. J Clin Invest. 1995;95:2281–90.
20. Elias PM, Ghadially R. The aged epidermal permeability barrier: basis for functional abnormalities. Clin Geriatr Med. 2002;18:103–20, vii.
21. Ye J, Garg A, Calhoun C, Feingold KR, et al. Alterations in cytokine regulation in aged epidermis: implications for permeability barrier homeostasis and inflammation. I. IL-1 gene family. Exp Dermatol. 2002;11:209–16.
22. Angelova-Fischer I, Becker V, Fischer TW, Zillikens D, Wigger-Alberti W, Kezic S. Tandem repeated irritation in aged skin induces distinct barrier perturbation and cytokine profile in vivo. Br J Dermatol. 2012;167(4):787–93. PubMed.
23. Farage MA, Miller KW, Berardesca E, Maibach HI. Incontinence in the aged: contact dermatitis and other cutaneous consequences. Contact Dermatitis. 2007;57:211–7.
24. Rothenborg HW, Menne T, Sjolin KE. Temperature dependent primary irritant dermatitis from lemon perfume. Contact Dermatitis. 1977;3:37–48.
25. Shahidullah M, Raffle EJ, Rimmer AR, Frain-Bell W. Transepidermal water loss in patients with dermatitis. Br J Dermatol. 1969;81:722–30.
26. Meding B. Epidemiology of hand eczema in an industrial city. Acta Derm Venereol Suppl (Stockh). 1990;153:1–43.
27. Wilhelm KP, Maibach HI. Factors predisposing to cutaneous irritation. Dermatol Clin. 1990;8:17–22.
28. Coenraads PJ, Diepgen TL. Risk for hand eczema in employees with past or present atopic dermatitis. Int Arch Occup Environ Health. 1998;71:7–13.
29. Berndt U, Hinnen U, Iliev D, Elsner P. Role of the atopy score and of single atopic features as risk factors for the development of hand eczema in trainee metal workers. Br J Dermatol. 1999;140:922–4.
30. Tupker RA. Prediction of irritancy in the human skin irritancy model and occupational setting. Contact Dermatitis. 2003;49:61–9.
31. Gallacher G, Maibach HI. Is atopic dermatitis a predisposing factor for experimental acute irritant contact dermatitis? Contact Dermatitis. 1998;38:1–4.
32. Basketter DA, Miettinen J, Lahti A. Acute irritant reactivity to sodium lauryl sulfate in atopics and non-atopics. Contact Dermatitis. 1998;38:253–7.
33. Palmer CN, Irvine AD, Terron-Kwiatkowski A, Zhao Y, et al. Common loss-of-function variants of the epidermal barrier protein filaggrin are a major predisposing factor for atopic dermatitis. Nat Genet. 2006;38:441–6.
34. Lammintausta K, Maibach HI, Wilson D. Susceptibility to cumulative and acute irritant dermatitis. An experimental approach in human volunteers. Contact Dermatitis. 1988;19:84–90.
35. Bjornberg A. Skin reactions to primary irritants in men and women. Acta Derm Venereol. 1975;55:191–4.
36. Hogan DJ, Dannaker CJ, Maibach HI. The prognosis of contact dermatitis. J Am Acad Dermatol. 1990;23:300–7.
37. Sertoli A, Francalanci S, Acciai MC, Gola M. Epidemiological survey of contact dermatitis in Italy (1984–1993) by GIRDCA (Gruppo Italiano Ricerca Dermatiti da Contatto e Ambientali). Am J Contact Dermat. 1999;10:18–30.
38. Nilsson E. Individual and environmental risk factors for hand eczema in hospital workers. Acta Derm Venereol Suppl (Stockh). 1986;128:1–63.

39. Frosch PJ, Kligman AM. Rapid blister formation in human skin with ammonium hydroxide. Br J Dermatol. 1977;96:461–73.
40. Wigger-Alberti W, Elsner P. In: Kanerva L, Elsner P, Wahlberg J, Maibach HI, editors. Handbook of occupational dermatology. New York: Springer; 2000. p. 99–110.
41. Diepgen TL, Coenraads PJ. The epidemiology of occupational contact dermatitis. Int Arch Occup Environ Health. 1999;72:496–506.
42. Meding B, Wrangsjo K, Jarvholm B. Fifteen-year follow-up of hand eczema: persistence and consequences. Br J Dermatol. 2005;152:975–80.
43. Veien NK, Hattel T, Laurberg G. Hand eczema: causes, course, and prognosis II. Contact Dermatitis. 2008;58:335–9.
44. Sajjachareonpong P, Cahill J, Keegel T, Saunders H, Nixon R. Persistent post-occupational dermatitis. Contact Dermatitis. 2004;51:278–83.
45. Charbonnier V, Morrison Jr BM, Paye M, Maibach HI. Subclinical, non-erythematous irritation with an open assay model (washing): sodium lauryl sulfate (SLS) versus sodium laureth sulfate (SLES). Food Chem Toxicol. 2001;39:279–86.
46. Lammintausta K, Maibach H. In: Adams RM, editor. Occupational skin disease. Philadelphia: W.B. Saunders; 1990. p. 1–15.
47. Farage MA, Katsarou A, Maibach HI. Sensory, clinical and physiological factors in sensitive skin: a review. Contact Dermatitis. 2006;55:1–14.
48. Besne I, Descombes C, Breton L. Effect of age and anatomical site on density of sensory innervation in human epidermis. Arch Dermatol. 2002;138:1445–50.
49. Simon M, Bernard D, Minondo AM, Camus C, et al. Persistence of both peripheral and non-peripheral corneodesmosomes in the upper stratum corneum of winter xerosis skin versus only peripheral in normal skin. J Invest Dermatol. 2001;116:23–30.
50. Melnik B, Braun-Falco O. The value of oil baths for adjuvant basic therapy of inflammatory dermatoses with dry, barrier-disrupted skin. Hautarzt. 1996;47:665–72.
51. Effendy I, Kerscher M. Haut und Alter. Stuttgart/New York: Thieme; 2005.
52. Raab WP. The skin surface and stratum corneum. Br J Dermatol. 1990;122(35):37–41.
53. Rogers J, Harding C, Mayo A, Banks J, Rawlings A. Stratum corneum lipids: the effect of ageing and the seasons. Arch Dermatol Res. 1996;288:765–70.
54. Jin K, Higaki Y, Takagi Y, Higuchi K, et al. Analysis of betaglucocerebrosidase and ceramidase activities in atopic and aged dry skin. Acta Derm Venereol. 1994;74:337–40.
55. Tezuka T. Electron-microscopic changes in xerosis senilis epidermis. Its abnormal membrane-coating granule formation. Dermatologica. 1983;166:57–61.
56. Elewski BE, Hughey LC, Parsons ME. Dermatologische Differentialdiagnose. München: Elsevier Urban & Fischer Verlag; 2007.
57. Krasovec M, Elsner P, Burg G. Generalized eczematous skin rash possibly due to HMG-CoA reductase inhibitors. Dermatology. 1993;186:248–52.
58. Elsner P, Maibach HI. The effect of prolonged drying on transepidermal water loss, capacitance and ph of human vulvar and forearm skin. Acta Derm Venereol. 1990;70:105–9.
59. Brotman RM, Klebanoff MA, Nansel T, Zhang J, et al. Why do women douche? A longitudinal study with two analytic approaches. Ann Epidemiol. 2008;18:65–73.
60. Welsh B, Howard A, Cook K. Vulval itch. Aust Fam Physician. 2004;33:505–10.
61. Buechner SA. Common skin disorders of the penis. BJU Int. 2002;90:498–506.
62. Andersen PH, Bucher AP, Saeed I, Lee PC, et al. Faecal enzymes: in vivo human skin irritation. Contact Dermatitis. 1994;30:152–8.
63. Farage M, Maibach H. Lifetime changes in the vulva and vagina. Arch Gynecol Obstet. 2006;273:195–202.
64. Dennerstein L, Dudley EC, Hopper JL, Guthrie JR, Burger HG. A prospective population-based study of menopausal symptoms. Obstet Gynecol. 2000;96:351–8.
65. Van Voorhis BJ. Genitourinary symptoms in the menopausal transition. Am J Med. 2005;118(12B):47–53.
66. Fritsch P. Dermatologie, Venerologie. Heidelberg: Springer; 2004.
67. Birley HD, Walker MM, Luzzi GA, Bell R, et al. Clinical features and management of recurrent balanitis; association with atopy and genital washing. Genitourin Med. 1993;69:400–3.
68. Edwards S. Balanitis and balanoposthitis: a review. Genitourin Med. 1996;72:155–9.
69. Diepgen TL, Kanerva L. Occupational skin diseases. Eur J Dermatol. 2006;16:324–30.
70. Kühner-Piplack B. [Klinik und Differentialdiagnose des Handekzems. Eine retrospektive Studie am Krankengut der Universitätshautklinik Heidelberg 1982–1985.] Thesis. Universität Heidelberg, Heidelberg, 1987.
71. Soder S, Diepgen TL, Radulescu M, Apfelbacher CJ, et al. Occupational skin diseases in cleaning and kitchen employees: course and quality of life after measures of secondary individual prevention. J Dtsch Dermatol Ges. 2007;5:670–6.
72. Coenraads PJ, Nater JP, van der Lende R. Prevalence of eczema and other dermatoses of the hands and arms in the Netherlands. Association with age and occupation. Clin Exp Dermatol. 1983;8:495–503.
73. Varigos GA, Dunt DR. Occupational dermatitis. An epidemiological study in the rubber and cement industries. Contact Dermatitis. 1981;7:105–10.
74. Bock M, Schmidt A, Bruckner T, Diepgen TL. Occupational skin disease in the construction industry. Br J Dermatol. 2003;149:1165–71.
75. Conde-Salazar L, Guimaraens D, Villegas C, Romero A, Gonzalez MA. Occupational allergic contact dermatitis in construction workers. Contact Dermatitis. 1995;33:226–30.

108 Safety Evaluation in the Elderly via Dermatological Exposure

Mario Bramante

Contents

Abstract

This chapter discusses the relevance of advanced age in the human safety risk assessment of substances that may come in contact with the skin through use of consumer products for personal use. Susceptibility of the elderly to chemical toxicity is reviewed in the context of current risk assessment practices for the general population and default assumptions for human variability.

Introduction

The relevance of advanced age in the human safety risk assessment of substances that may come in contact with the skin through use of consumer products for personal use are discussed in this chapter. Susceptibility of the elderly to chemical toxicity is reviewed in the context of current risk assessment practices for the general population and default assumptions for human variability.

Consumer products for personal use, ranging from solid manufactured items such as absorbent hygiene devices to cosmetics, may contain a broad range of substances that are not formulated to penetrate inside the human body to have any active function beyond the skin nor to have a pharmacological action. Avoidance of hazardous constituents is either enforced by regulations (e.g., for cosmetics) or a basic expectation, in recognition of the close contact of these products with the

M. Bramante (✉)
Product Safety and Regulatory Affairs, Procter & Gamble Service GmbH, Schwalbach am Taunus, Germany
e-mail: bramante.m@pg.com

M.A. Farage et al. (eds.), *Textbook of Aging Skin*,
DOI 10.1007/978-3-662-47398-6_81

consumer, and their wide accessibility by the general population. Because of these characteristics, consumer products tend to have a low potential for toxicity, confirmation of good skin compatibility being often the key focus of their safety evaluations.

The proportion of elderly people in the general population continues to grow rapidly [1] driven by a steep increase in life expectancy. This trend has heightened the interest of researchers, risk assessors, and safety decision makers in better understanding of age-related changes and their potential impact on chemical toxicity.

Most of the knowledge on elderly-related physiological changes is derived from medical research on pharmaceutical agents, driven by the need to optimize drug dosage regimens, to account for concomitant illnesses and comedications that are frequent in the aged patient. Already in 1989, guidelines for the study of drugs to be used by the elderly were published by the US Food and Drug Administration, and today's international guidelines on drug development strongly recommend inclusion of older adults in clinical trials [2].

Beyond pharmaceuticals, regulatory guidelines for risk assessment of chemicals stress the importance to identify sensitive subpopulations and characterize their specific risk, age being recognized an important variable [3, 4]. In 2002, the US Environmental Protection Agency announced a coordinated effort to study and prioritize environmental health threats to the elderly [5].

Physiological changes associated with aging can alter the processes of absorption, distribution, metabolism, and elimination of substances [6], and the aged skin progressively looses structural integrity and physiological function [7]. The significance of these changes for risk assessment is discussed in the following paragraphs.

Elderly Skin Susceptibility to Irritation

A number of skin structures decline with age with a progressive reduction in skin thickness, dermal vascularization, number of hair follicles, epidermal turnover rate, and sensory nerve endings, the latter associated with an increase in pain threshold [8]. Alterations in collagen and elastin organization produce a less stretchable and resilient dermis with a reduced resistance to shearing forces [9].

As aged skin tends to be drier and easier to crack due to loss of elasticity, mechanical damage is more likely to occur. A diminished repair capacity prolongs wound healing, general skin recovery from damage, and restoration of skin barrier [10].

Despite the thin and fragile appearance of older skin, the inflammatory response is delayed and less intense [11], and older subjects react to skin irritants less sharply and more slowly than younger individuals [12, 13]. The reduction in basal transepidermal water loss (TEWL) observed in the elderly indicates that skin barrier is not compromised and is indicative of a decreased susceptibility to irritants with advancing age [14].

Several studies based on in vivo human test methods could be quoted in support of a decreased sensitivity of aged skin to irritants. A human 4-h patch test, developed as a valid and predictable alternative to animal testing [15], was used in a series of investigations on population differences in acute skin irritation response to common chemical irritants [13]. These investigations demonstrated a significantly reduced irritation in the oldest 56–74 age cluster, with only directional reduction for weaker irritants. Milder reactions with advancing age were also reported in clinical studies performed with a variety of substances like dimethyl sulfoxide, histamine, ethyl nicotinate, chloroform-methanol, and lactic acid [16], with fewer studies reporting no significant differences.

Compared to younger individuals, irritant response to sodium lauryl sulfate (SLS), evaluated via TEWL and visual scores, decreases in the elderly on various body sites [12]. For example, TEWL value of upper arm and abdomen was three to four times lower in the aged. The forearm skin of premenopausal women also produced more erythema when exposed to 0.1 % SLS solution as compared to postmenopausal women [17].

Overall, the body of evidence supports that aged skin is generally less susceptible to irritant insults: test methods and irritation risk assessment practices that are adequate for the general adult population would also cover the elderly.

In addition to chemical irritation, depending on the nature of the product being assessed, mechanical irritation could be an additional endpoint to consider due to higher susceptibility of aged skin to damage caused by friction and shearing forces. Simulated in-use clinical testing or specific test methods can be used to evaluate the mechanical irritation potential of a whole product [18].

Elderly Skin Susceptibility to Sensitization

Allergic contact dermatitis differs from skin irritation in its requirement for initial recognition by the immune system of allergenic, low molecular weight molecules (induction). A secondary exposure to the allergen can elicit a dermatitis response with clinical manifestations very similar to irritant dermatitis. The attention of safety assessors is primarily devoted towards the prevention of the onset of a sensitization via induction.

The induction of sensitization is recognized to be a threshold phenomenon which depends on allergens' intrinsic allergenic potency, amount of allergen on exposed skin surface, and duration of exposure. The quantitative skin sensitization risk assessment approach is based on the determination of a no observed adverse effect level (NOAEL) for the contact allergen in humans, specifically the unexpected sensitization induction level (NESIL) determined as dose per unit area, and is compared to the estimated human skin exposure to that allergen [19]. Accordingly to this approach, three areas of variability (also referred as uncertainty factors) have to be properly weighted and accounted for in risk assessment. These areas of variability cover for interindividual susceptibility to a given allergen (genetic variability and other population differences), for the effect of a vehicle or product matrix (e.g., concomitant presence of irritants or skin penetration enhancers could lower the nonsensitizing exposure threshold), and for skin-site exposure considerations (dermal integrity, site of body exposed, effect of occlusion) [20]. Age-related susceptibility is included in the tenfolds interindividual variability factor, which is considered appropriate to cover for human population differences in susceptibility to sensitizers.

An overall decline in immune function in the aged is reported as compared to young individuals, including a reduction in epidermal Langerhans cells [21] that are necessary during the induction phase of the immune response, the critical initial step in the onset of allergic contact dermatitis. This is suggestive of a lower susceptibility of the aged subject to develop an allergic contact dermatitis.

Most studies on skin sensitization as a function of age are retrospective and describe the incidences of elicitation responses through diagnostic patch testing. These studies are not considered useful for evaluation of age susceptibility to the development of a new sensitization as no insight is provided, e.g., on the impact of age on the NESIL.

There are few studies available on population differences in susceptibility to the induction of a skin sensitization. Ability to acquire a sensitivity to poison ivy [22] and the capacity of potent sensitizer 2,4-dinitrochlorobenzene for developing an allergic contact dermatitis was reported to decrease with increasing age. In a study involving 116 elderly subjects, 69 % of individuals over 70 years of age developed a sensitization to 2,4-dinitrochlorobenzene versus 96 % in the population under 70 years [23]. In another study, about only one fourth of population greater than 65 years became sensitized by 2,4-dinitrochlorobenzene as compared to subjects aged 20–40 years [24].

Other studies failed to demonstrate a difference in the ability to sensitize the adult and the elderly. Exposure of naive subjects to 2,4-dinitrochlorobenzene resulted in no significant differences in the incidence of sensitization in three age cohorts: 21–59 years, 60–79 years, and greater than 80 years [25].

Kwangsukstith and Maibach reviewed the effect of age and gender on induction and elicitation of contact dermatitis [26]. They concluded that in the elderly there is an age-dependent decrease of delayed hypersensitivity reactions, a decreased ability to be sensitized to new allergens, and a reduced elicitation response in presensitized individuals.

In a subsequent review by Robinson on population differences and their implication for skin irritation and sensitization, the author concluded that standard risk assessment procedures and safety testing can be considered relatively conservative to cover age, gender, and racial differences [27], recognizing that there is very little age-related difference in sensitization susceptibility.

In conclusion, the elderly appears to be less or at maximum equally susceptible to sensitization than younger ages. Risk assessments incorporating default human population variability assumptions are adequate to protect the elderly population. The likelihood for predisposed individuals to acquire a sensitization from exposure to a contact allergen is dependent on occasions and level of exposure to a much larger extent than any age-related population difference.

Risk Assessment Approach for Systemic Toxicity

The risk assessment process for substances with a threshold for toxicity was described by the US National Academy of Sciences in 1983 [28] (Fig. 1). The approach has been applied widely by regulatory agencies and institutions to assess health endpoints related to exposure to chemicals present in food, air, or drinking water, sometimes with slight modifications and different terminology [29, 30]. The initial step of risk assessment (hazard identification) evaluates the inherent toxicity of a substance, and whether it can cause an adverse health effect, given the relevant route of exposure, considering all potential safety endpoints. The second step is a dose–response evaluation to assess the relationship between the dose of a chemical and the incidence and severity of an adverse health effect in the exposure population. The third step is the accurate and robust assessment of exposure to the substance taking into account all relevant exposure scenarios and routes. Finally, the risk characterization and final assessment step integrates hazard, dose–response, and exposure considerations into advise suitable for use in decision making or risk management. All relevant areas of data extrapolations and uncertainty are accounted for including, e.g., interspecies variability, allowing extrapolations from animal to man, and human variability, to account for sensitive individuals of the population. The term margin of safety (MOS) is commonly used to compare estimated human exposure to a risk value for which the risk of causing adverse effects in humans is considered to be none-to-minimal such as a reference dose (RfD, used, e.g., by the US Environmental Protection Agency to describe an acceptable daily exposure to an environmental substance) or an acceptable daily intake (ADI, typically used by the WHO/FAO for chemicals in food).

An essentially similar sequence of steps is followed for nonthreshold effects (such as cancer from a genotoxic mechanism), where according to

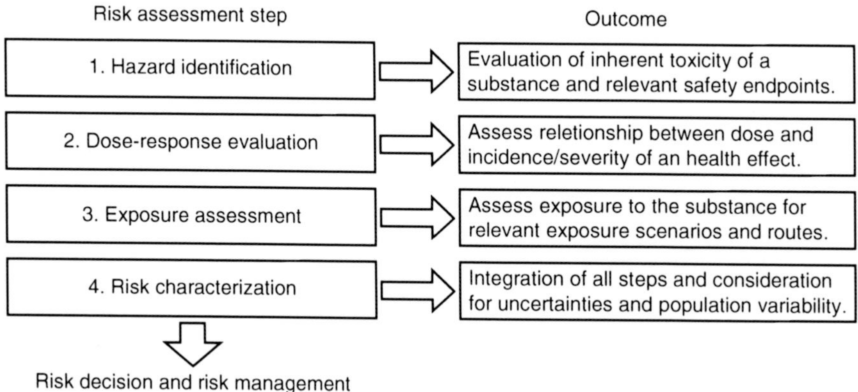

Fig. 1 Schematic representation of quantitative risk assessment process for substances with threshold toxicity

the current paradigm, low level of exposure or even a single molecule could hypothetically increase the probability of genetic mutation. For nonthreshold effects, however, the outcome of risk assessment is the quantification of the risk to human health associated with a particular level of exposure.

Human Variability in Susceptibility to Chemical Toxicity

It is an integral part of risk assessment to account for human population variability in susceptibility to toxicants, including potential for age differences. Risk assessors and health agencies worldwide, for many years, have adopted a standard default uncertainty factor (or safety factor) of 100-fold to derive acceptable exposure levels for compounds with threshold toxicity. This uncertainty factor comprises a tenfold factor for interspecies differences and a tenfold factor for human variability, which can be further subdivided into a $10^{0.5}$ (3.16) factor for toxicokinetic (absorption, distribution, metabolism, elimination), and in another $10^{0.5}$ (3.16) factor for toxicodynamic (how the target tissue responds to a given target tissue dose) [30]. This subdivision allows for chemical-specific toxicokinetic and mechanistic data to be considered allowing for substance-specific risk assessment refinement [31] (Fig. 2).

Renwick and Lazarus [32] developed a model to evaluate impact of human variability on risk assessment of chemicals based on toxicokinetics data from 60 therapeutic drugs metabolized and eliminated through a variety of pathways and on toxicodynamic data from 49 different effects.

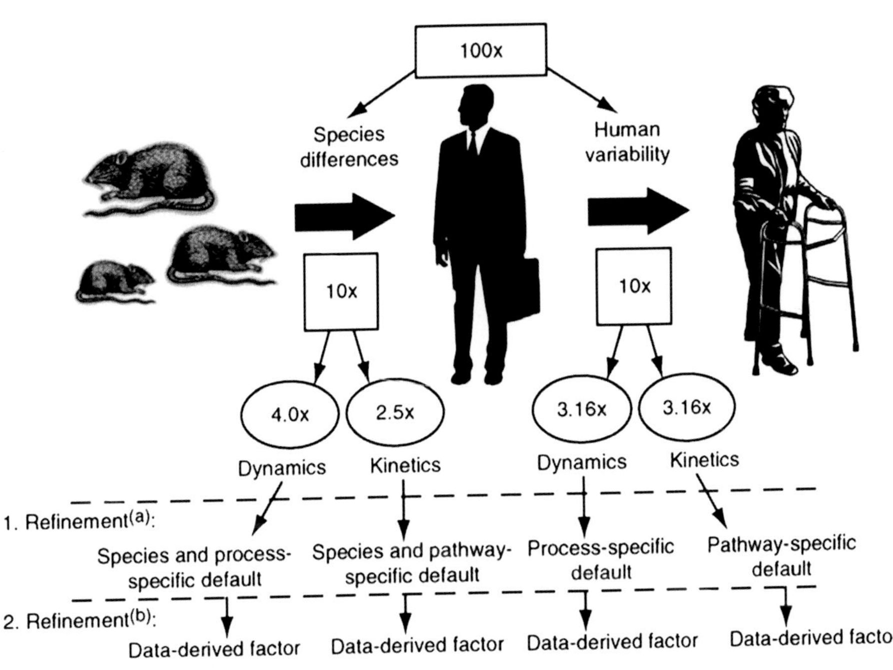

Fig. 2 Use of uncertainty factors in risk assessment and approaches for their refinement. The 100-fold uncertainty factor can be considered the product of two separate tenfold factors for interspecies differences and human variability. These tenfold factors can be further subdivided into toxicokinetic and toxicodynamic differences (World Health Organization [30]). (**a**) If data are available on population variability on the major route of elimination or on a mode of action for a chemical, default kinetic, and dynamics values could be replaced by categorical factors such as pathway-related factors (Dorne et al. [33]). (**b**) If chemical-specific data on toxicokinetic or toxicodynamic are available for a compound under assessment, such data can be used instead of defaults World Health Organization [31]

Based on the model, they concluded that the general 3.16 toxicokinetic uncertainty factor would cover on average the 99.1 % of total human population, although no specific break out was made for the elderly. When accounting for combined toxicokinetics and toxicodynamics, the default cumulative tenfold uncertainty factor for human variability would cover on average more than >99.9 % of human population. It was acknowledged by the authors that genetic polymorphisms can influence the universal validity of a 3.16-folds kinetic uncertainty factor. From a risk assessment impact point of view, polymorphisms may pose a greater risk when genetic mutations inactivate or reduce the activity of an enzyme involved in detoxification. Subjects with these mutations are defined poor metabolizers, if enzymatic activity is reduced, or nonphenotyped if completely missing. A greater risk is also associated to polymorphic metabolic pathways when multiple copies of a gene overexpress an enzyme responsible for bioactivation of a parent compound into a toxic metabolite (fast metabolizers). For many compounds, however, the presence of alternative or multiple pathways of elimination would not necessarily invalidate the validity of default uncertainty factors for human variability.

Dermal Absorption in the Elderly

Dermally applied substances that penetrate the skin barrier and become systemically bioavailable can potentially cause an adverse health effect if a sufficiently high concentration reaches the relevant target organ.

Default risk assessments often start with the assumption of 100 % dermal penetration, but there are many factors influencing the actual penetrant fraction of the substance.

Effectiveness of skin barrier function is the key factor influencing skin permeability, which largely depends on integrity and hydration of stratum corneum and its lipid content and the hydrophilicity of the substance in question. Aged skin is drier, thinner, and has lower lipid content as compared to the young [34]. Although reduction in both water and lipids may suggest compromising of the skin barrier, the decline in TEWL with age [14, 35] signals that barrier function is not impaired, and reduced skin hydration indicates a lower dermal penetration potential for hydrophilic compounds in the aged human skin. Furthermore, the reduced cutaneous vascularization in the skin of older individuals also suggests a poorer absorption capability due to reduced removal of permeable compounds from dermal compartment by impaired microcirculation [34].

An in vivo percutaneous penetration study with both lipophilic (testosterone, estradiol) and hydrophilic (hydrocortisone, benzoic acid) compounds indeed demonstrated a reduced absorption of hydrophilic substances in older skin, while no age relationship was found for the two lipid-soluble compounds [34]. Other studies have confirmed the slower percutaneous absorption in the aged of hydrocortisone and benzoic acid and no age difference for estradiol and testosterone [36]. Hydrocortisone and testosterone penetration through both vulva and forearm skin were also directionally reduced in postmenopausal versus premenopausal women, with significant reduction only for hydrocortisone applied to the vulva of postmenopausal women [37]. Significantly, lower skin permeation in the older was also reported for water-soluble compounds methyl nicotinate, methyl salicyclic acid, caffeine [34], and tetrachlorosalicylanilide [38]. The extent of the reduction for water-soluble compounds ranged from 36 % to 52 % in the older ages (greater than 65 years) versus the young adults (22–40 years) [34].

These data are consistent with outcomes from previous studies, which imply that the barrier function of human skin in vivo increases with increasing age [39], with a general decrease in skin permeability especially for compounds with low solubility in lipids. Highly lipid-soluble chemicals may still dissolve readily in the stratum corneum of aged skin, even if lipid medium is reduced to the same extent of younger skin.

Distribution, Metabolism, and Elimination in the Elderly

Body weight, total body water, and lean body mass decrease with advancing age. The average percent body fat in young adults is about 1/3 and

1/5 of total body mass in women and men, respectively. Between the ages of 25 and 65–70 years body fat percentage increases on average by +48 % in women and by +79 % in men [40]. By the age of 70 years, body fat reaches approximately 36 % and 48 % of total body weight of males and females, respectively [41]. The consequence of these changes is that hydrophilic compounds have smaller volumes of distribution, resulting in higher serum levels, while lipophilic compounds have higher volumes of distribution with increasing age.

The kidney is the main route of excretion of water-soluble compounds and for the water-soluble metabolites of lipophilic compounds. Renal mass, blood flow, tubular excretory capacity, glomerular filtration rate, and general function decline with age. Glomerular filtration rate, quantitatively the most important parameter for renal excretory function, declines by approximately 30 % between 30 and 80 years in many elderly subjects [42]. Decreased renal function can result in a prolongation of the half-life of metabolites.

Liver is by far the most important organ for metabolism of drugs and xenobiotics. Advancing age is associated with a 20–40 % reduction in liver size [43] and liver blood flow [44] that may reduce hepatic first-pass metabolism and clearance of substances. Alteration of hepatic structure and enzymatic functions with aging, however, is moderate: in the elderly healthy person, routine tests for liver function involving the metabolism and elimination of specific dyes, radioisotopes, and protein synthesis do not show significant differences between 50–69 years and 70–89 years [45–47]. Studies on human liver tissue showed that monooxygenase activities are maintained even in advanced old age [48]. In general, phase I metabolic function (hydrolysis, reduction, oxidation) is reduced in the elderly while phase II functions (glucoronidation, sulfation, acetylation, methylation, conjugation with glutathione or amino acids) are not affected by aging [49].

The cytochrome P450 family is the primary enzyme system involved in phase I metabolic reactions. In an investigation of microsomal enzyme activity of human liver, a reduction of about 30 % of CYP-450-linked drug metabolism was reported after 70 years of age [50], while other studies found no significant differences in the level and activity of human liver microsomal enzymes [51].

Table 1 Toxicokinetics in the elderly: Difference in absorption, distribution, metabolism, and elimination in the older individual versus the younger adult

Dermal absorption in the elderly
Water-soluble substances: reduced absorption versus young adults
Lipid-soluble substances: no difference versus younger adults
Skin barrier function increases with increasing age
Distribution in the elderly
Water-soluble substances: Smaller volumes of distribution, higher serum levels
Lipid-soluble substances: Higher volumes of distribution
Reduction in total body weight
Metabolism in the elderly
Decrease in liver size and blood flow
Generally reduced phase I metabolic functions
Generally unaffected phase II metabolic functions
Elimination in the elderly
Decline in glomerular filtration rate (by ~30 %)
Decline in renal mass, renal blood flow, tubular excretory capacity

See Table 1 for a summary of kinetic differences in the elderly.

Toxicokinetics Variability in the Elderly and Significance for Risk Assessment

Age-related human variability in toxicokinetics and toxicodynamics is embedded in default human variability factor in standard risk assessments.

Clewell et al. [52] conducted a comprehensive review on age- and gender-related differences in physiological, biochemical, and kinetic parameters based on data sets from 70 substances with different physicochemical characteristics. A few differences were found between young adults and the elderly in estimates of target tissue exposure, related to the declined capacities of some enzyme systems and renal elimination.

Clinical data for specific therapeutic drugs have been used to characterize human variability in pharmacokinetics within a therapeutic class [53, 54]. The resulting chemical-specific kinetic factors ranged from 1.2 to 3.2 for unimodal population distribution, and a kinetic factor of 3.0 was specifically calculated for the elderly.

The adequacy of default uncertainty factor to cover the human variability in toxicokinetics, including the elderly, was the subject of a recent review by Dorne and Renwick [33]. The authors conducted a meta-analysis of metabolism and pharmacokinetic data for probe substrates of a number of phase I and phase II metabolic and renal excretion pathways, including seven major isozymes of the cytochrome P450 superfamily (CYP) that constitutes the major oxidative hepatic system for metabolism of xenobiotics. Despite the impairment of hepatic and renal function in the elderly subpopulation, the default 3.16 kinetic factor was found to be adequate for most monomorphic pathways, except for renal excretion and CYP3A4 metabolism, for which specific pathway-related kinetic factors for the elderly were calculated as 4.2 and 4.9, respectively, covering the ninety-ninth percentile of the elderly population. Uncertainty factors were above default kinetic factor for nonphenotyped elderly subjects for CYP2D6 and CYP2C19 metabolism (8.4 and 4.3 pathway-related kinetic factor, respectively) and for slow acetylators (7.6 factor).

The majority of kinetics data have been obtained with pharmaceuticals, which tend to have physiochemical and biochemical properties that may differ from many compounds of relevance for consumer product assessments, such as environmental contaminants. While several chemicals of toxicological concern are lipohilic, pharmaceuticals tend to be water soluble and can be preferentially metabolized by specific enzyme subsystems, such as the CYP3A4, which are less relevant, e.g., for environmental substances [55].

In a study aimed to investigate age- and gender-related differences in physiological and biochemical processes that affect tissue dosimetry for the purpose of development of a predictive physiologically based pharmacokinetic life-stage model, two water-soluble chemicals (isopropanol and nicotine) and four lipophilic chemicals (vinyl chloride, methylene chloride, perchloroethylene, and 2,3,7,8-terachlorodibenyo-p-dioxin) were analyzed [55]. The choice of substances reflected the need to better represent the variety of physiochemical, biochemical, and mode of action properties of nonpharmaceuticals, including CYP2E1 metabolism which is relevant for many environmental toxicants. The model was based on a number of simplifications and approximations, and authors cautioned that model predictions should be regarded as reasonable expectations not as validated predictive extrapolations. Nonetheless, their results were based on reasonable descriptions of age-dependent physiological and biochemical processes, and provide useful insights on the potential differences in toxicokinetics across life stages, and how these differences may impact internal dose metrics. Overall, the results of the simulations indicated that variations of toxicokinetic dose metrics associated with aging are relatively modest. In the 75 year old, the average internal daily dose was slightly higher as compared to the 25 year old only for perchloroethylene (+20 %), for its metabolite trichloroacetic acid (+40 %), and for the reactive metabolite of methylene chloride (+30 %). For all other compounds and their metabolites, the average internal daily dose was generally comparable or slightly lower in the 75 year old as compared to the 25 years old (−17 % as maximum reduction). In all cases, the magnitude of the resulting human toxicokinetic factor was significantly lower than default kinetic factor of 3.16 used in standard assessments, reaching at maximum a factor of 1.4 for trichloroacetic acid. In the same study, blood concentrations of isopropanol and of its metabolite acetone were assessed for cross-route internal exposure comparison [55]. Specifically for the dermal exposure route, higher peak concentrations of isopropanol in arterial blood were predicted by the model to occur in advanced age, with an approximate increase of +25 % by the age of 75 years versus the age of 25 years. Blood concentration of isopropanol metabolite acetone did not vary much between these two ages. Again the magnitude of the resulting human toxicokinetic factor was 1.1, significantly lower than default value of 3.16 (Table 2).

Table 2 Studies on toxicokinetic variability in the elderly and correlated toxicokinetic factors

Data source	Derived toxicokinetic factor
Default uncertainty/safety factor for human variability in toxicokinetics, elderly implicitly included (World Health Organization [30])	3.16 → Default factor for human variability
Study objective: To characterize interindividual differences and derive acceptable daily intake values. *Data type*: Pharmacokinetic clinical data on therapeutic agents representative of various classes (antidepressants, ACE-inhibitors, nonsteroidal anti-inflammatory drugs, cholesterol lowering agents, antibiotics) (Silverman et al. [53], Naumann et al. [54])	3.0 → Chemical-specific adjustment factor for elderly patients, accounting for interindividual differents in kinetic for drugs in one therapeutic class
Study objective: To derive pathway-related uncertainty factors associated with variability in kinetics. *Data type*: Meta-analysis of metabolism and kinetic data for pharmaceutical probe substances, including elderly-specific data for seven phase I (CYP1A2, CYP2A6, CYP2C9, CYP2E1, CYP3A4, alcohol dehydrogenase, hydrolis) and three phase II enzymatic monomorphic pathways (glucuronidation, glycine conjugation, sulfate conjugation) plus renal excretion pathway. Analysis considered polymorphism for some pathways (nonphenotyped subjects for CYP2C19 and CYP2D6, fast metabolizers for CYP2D6, fast and slow acetylators) (Dorne et al. [33])	*Monomorphic Pathways*: (ninety-ninth population) 1.5–3.16 → Elderly-specific factor for nine pathways 4.9 → Elderly-specific factor for CYP3A4 metabolism 4.2 → Elderly-specific factor for renal excretion *Polymorphic Pathways*: (ninety-ninth population) 2.3–2.9 → Elderly-specific factor for fast metabolizers; 4.3–8.4 → Elderly-specific factors for nonphenotyped 7.6 → Elderly-specific factor for slow acetylators
Study objective: To develop a life-stage, physiologically based pharmacokinetic life-stage model. *Data type*: Chemical-specific adjustment factor based on metabolism data of two water-soluble (isopropanol and nicotine) and four lipid-soluble (vinyl chloride, methylene chloride, perchloroethylene, and 2,3,7,8-terachlorodibenyo-p-dioxin) probe substances selected to represent differences in physicochemical properties and in metabolic characteristics of environmental chemicals (Clewell et al. [55])	0.83–1.4 → Range of elderly-related chemical-specific adjustment factors 1.1 → Elderly-related, isopropanol-specific adjustment factor, specific to the dermal exposure route

Exposure Considerations for the Elderly

A robust exposure assessment should be based on accurate, product-specific data on frequency, extent, and duration of an exposure as well as on proper characterization of anatomical site in contact with the substance, skin conditions (occlusion or compromise), and dimensions of skin-contact area.

Skin permeability potential differs by anatomical site and can be amplified by occlusion, abraded, or otherwise damaged skin. The prevalence of these conditions may increase with older age and in particular subgroups (e.g., perineal dermatitis in subjects with fecal or urine incontinence, occluded skin, and pressure sores of immobilized patients).

Age-related patterns may exist in type of product used as well as in frequency and amount of product used per exposure event, collectively referred as habits and practices. Products like incontinence absorbent aids or antiwinkles treatments are predominantly used by the senior population. Elderly subjects, especially women, may use hair products such as dyes, permanent waves, and others more regularly because of the hair graying and loss [56]. Cosmetics and toiletry products may be equally appealing, for different reasons, to the younger as well as the older who wants to protect his fragile and dry skin.

On the other side of the spectrum, a number of products may not be used in the elderly or not used to the same extent of younger ages. Self-reported oral hygiene habits among institutionalized elderly subjects identified inadequate oral hygiene practices, with 26 % of dentate population reporting no tooth brushing [57] hence, virtually no exposure to common oral care products (dentifrices, toothbrushes) should be expected in a quarter of the surveyed population, without accounting for prevalence of denture wearers.

The amount of published data on habits and practices for consumer products is limited. Existing data does not include detailed segmentations for age, and the elderly tend to be inadequately represented in the surveyed populations. Building on an internal database of habits and practices, an experimental probabilistic exposure assessment model was developed for various consumer products. The model was used to investigate exposure variability and its dependency from age, gender, ethnic, and geographic origin among other factors (unpublished data). Hair-care data analysis, for example, revealed that frequency of hair washing significantly decreases with advancing age, with a parallel reduction in the use of shampoo and conditioners and related exposures. The magnitude of exposure reduction to these products for the population older than 65 years, versus teenagers, was bigger than default uncertainty factor for human kinetics. This example illustrates the importance of accurate exposure estimate in risk assessments for the elderly: for shampoos and conditioners, use of exposure data obtained from the general population inclusive of younger consumers would lead to a significant overestimation of the actual risk for the elderly.

Beyond exposure assessment, a proper characterization of exposed elderly population is important for risk management considerations. The aged population undergoes progressive sensory deficits (in vision, hearing, taste, smell), decreased short-term memory, and other cognitive changes which can make the older adult more inclined to err when using pharmaceuticals, cleaning agents, and personal care products [58]. These changes may reduce the ability to recognize and interpret warnings, cues, and product instructions that might render risk reduction measures ineffective. Proper consideration should be given to these aspects when designing products for the elderly, including their packaging and use instructions.

Conclusion

This chapter evaluated the adequacy of current risk assessment practices and default human variability factors when assessing consumer product substances for the elderly.

Research has started to elucidate the variability of human response to toxic insults and the specific risk for susceptible populations. Risk assessment approaches are under constant refinement to incorporate emerging knowledge into more accurate risk predictions and models. Some of these refinement options are based on inclusion in the assessment of chemical-specific metabolism and toxicokinetic data. However, available data are limited to a restricted number of substances, mainly therapeutic agents. This limits routine applicability of refined approaches to common constituents of consumer products, and the use of default uncertainty factors to account for human variability in the elderly remains an important option for routine assessments.

The risk assessment for consumer products is an iterative process that progresses via successive refinements. An initial assessment is often based on a number of worst-case assumptions, upper estimates, or extreme product uses such as 100 % dermal penetration, complete release of a substance from a product, highest theoretical frequency of product use that, when taken together, lead to a significant overestimation of the real risk. In the risk characterization step, an expert professional estimates if the available data are adequate to protect the most sensitive individuals of a target population at the light of latest knowledge and evolution of risk assessment concepts. This includes considerations for special subpopulation that might not be adequately covered by default variability factors, such as genetic polymorphism in the elderly. If the outcome of an initial assessment is favorable, then the assessment can be stopped at this stage. If the outcome of risk characterization is that a substance is of potential concern in the most sensitive subpopulation, further refinement of the default assessment parameters is needed that may require additional data to reduce the level of conservatism.

A number of age-related differences have been highlighted in this chapter, and their relevance for the safety evaluation of substances in the elderly has been reviewed in the light of current risk assessment practices.

Dermatological effects, specifically skin irritation and skin sensitization, are often the most relevant toxicological endpoints in the risk assessment of substances contained in consumer products. Available evidence suggests that the elderly does not constitute a specific risk population for skin irritation or the induction of contact sensitization. Current safety assessment approaches, built-in conservatism, and test methods appear to adequately cover the older segment of the population. Because of the increased susceptibility of elderly skin to mechanical insults and diminished repair capacity, mechanical irritation may be an additional endpoint to consider, depending on the type of product being assessed.

Elderly skin does not constitute an easier barrier for substances to cross than younger skin. Dermal penetration in the elderly is either reduced for hydrophilic compounds or unchanged for lipophilic ones, which also have higher volumes of distribution in the aged body. Despite specific physiological and functional differences have been highlighted in the elderly that affect the systemic distribution, metabolism, and excretion of substances, these tend to be relatively modest in their contribution to the final risk level when default uncertainty factors for human variability in sensitivity to chemicals is incorporated in risk assessment. Default uncertainty factors appear to be overconservative for the majority of the population but generally protective for the elderly.

Regardless of age, further research is needed to better understand the contribution of genetic polymorphism in individual susceptibility to chemicals. However, older age does not seem to be an important aggravating factor. The limited data available mainly for drugs on genetic polymorphism indicate that elderly-specific, kinetics-driven susceptibility to toxicants might be increased by a factor of 2–3 versus the human default factor applied in standard risk assessments. This is a considerable difference, e.g., in a risk assessment of a therapeutic agent with a low therapeutic index but is a modest factor in the context of an initial, favorable consumer product risk assessment built on conservative assumptions and high-end use scenarios. In fact, it might be sufficient to refine those initial conservative assumptions, e.g., via generation of more accurate exposure data, to demonstrate an adequate margin of safety also for those highly susceptible individuals. Methods for refinement of an assessment via incorporation of chemical-specific kinetic or dynamic data are also available that could be used if needed.

A proper characterization of the exposed population and a precise estimate of the dose of substance reaching the skin are particularly important aspects in the context of the exposure assessment step, with exposure being a potential source of significant variability in final risk estimate. Therefore, it should be considered that older age may determine the product of choice (ranging from almost no use to exclusive use) and that it can influence how products are used, how often, and how much.

Cross-References

▶ Dermal Safety Evaluation: Use of Disposable Diaper Products in the Elderly
▶ Susceptibility to Irritation in the Elderly

References

1. Population Division, Department of Economic and Social Affairs, United Nations Secretariat. Proceedings of the UN expert group meeting on social and economic implications of changing population age structure. Mexico City; 31 Aug–2 Sept 2005. Available from http://www.unpopulation.org
2. European Medicines Agency. Studies in support of special populations: geriatrics. In: ICH harmonized tripartite guideline. London: EMEA; 1994.
3. Agency US-Environmental Protection. Science policy council: risk characterization handbook. Washington, DC; 2000. p. 3809. http://www.epa.gov/osa/spc/pdfs/rchandbk.pdf
4. European Commission, Institute for health and Consumer Protection. Technical guidance document on

risk assessment. 2nd ed. Ispra: European Chemicals Bureau; 2003. p. 46, 74 and 180. http://ecb.jrc.ec.europa.eu/tgd/

5. Environmental Protection Agency; 2016. Aging initiative website: http://www.epa.gov/aging/index.htm
6. Williams L, Lowenthal DT. Drug therapy in the elderly. South Med J. 1992;85(2):127–31.
7. Farage MA, Miller KW, Elsner P, Maibach HI. Functional and physiological characteristics of the aging skin. Aging Clin Exp Res. 2007;20(3):195–200.
8. Kaminer MS, Gilchrest BA. Aging of the skin. In: Hazzard WR, Bierman EL, editors. Principles of geriatric medicine and gerontology. 3rd ed. New York: McGraw-Hill; 1994. p. 411–29.
9. Lavker RM, Zheng P, Dong G. Morphology of aged skin. Clin Geriatr Med. 1989;5:53–67.
10. Grove GL, Klingman AM. Age-associated changes in human epidermal cell renewal. J Gerontol. 1983;38:137–42.
11. Harvell JD, Maibach HI. Percutaneous absorption and inflammation in aged skin: a review. J Am Acad Dermatol. 1994;194:1015–21.
12. Martini F. Fundamentals of anatomy and physiology. San Francisco: Benjamin-Cummings; 2004.
13. Robinson MK. Population differences in acute skin irritation responses. Contact Dermatitis. 2002;46:86–93.
14. Suter-Widmer J, Elsner P. Age and Irritation. In: Agner T, Maibach H, editors. The irritant contact dermatitis syndrome. Boca Raton: CRC Press; 1999. p. 275–65.
15. Basketter DA, Whittle EG, Griffiths HA, York M. The identification and classification of skin irritation hazard by a human patch test. Food Chem Toxicol. 1994;32:769–75.
16. Grove GL, Lavker RM, Haelzle E. Use of non intrusive tests to monitor age-associated changes in human skin. J Soc Cosmet Chem. 1981;32:15–26.
17. Elsner P, Wilhelm D, Maibach HI. Effect of low-concentration sodium lauryl sulfate on human vulvar and forearm skin. Age-related differences. J Reprod Med. 1991;36:77–81.
18. Farage MA, Gilpin DA, Enane NA, Baldwin S. Development of a new test for mechanical irritation: behind the knee as a test site. Skin Res Technol. 2001;7:193.
19. Gerberick GF, Robinson MK. A skin sensitization risk assessment approach for evaluation of new ingredients and products. Am J Contact Dermatitis. 2000;11:65–73.
20. Felter SP, Robinson MK, Basketter DA, Gerberick GF. A review of the scientific basis for uncertainty factors for use in quantitative risk assessment for the induction of allergic contact dermatitis. Contact Dermatitis. 2002;47:257–66.
21. Gilchrest BA, Murphy G, Soter NA. Effect of chronologic aging and ultraviolet irradiation on Langerhans cells in human epidermis. J Invest Dermatol. 1982;79:85–58.
22. Lejman E, Stoudemayer T, Grove G, Klingman AM. Age differences in poison ivy dermatitis. Contact Dermatitis. 1984;11:163–7.
23. Waldorf D, Willkens R, Decker J. Impaired delayed hypersensitivity in an aging population. JAMA. 1986;203:111–4.
24. Girard JP, Paychere M, Cuevas M, Fernandes B. Cell-mediated immunity in an aging population. Clin Exp Immunol. 1977;27:85–91.
25. Schwartz M. Eczematous sensitization in various age groups. J Allergy. 1952;24:143–8.
26. Kwangsukstith C, Maibach HI. Effect of age and sex on the induction and elicitation of allergic contact dermatitis. Contact Dermatitis. 1995;33:289–98.
27. Robinson MK. Population differences in skin structure and physiology and the susceptibility to irritants and allergic contact dermatitis: implications for skin safety testing and risk assessment. Contact Dermatitis. 1999;41:65–79.
28. National Academy of Sciences. Risk assessment in the federal government. Washington, DC: National Research Council/ National Academy Press; 1983.
29. U.S. Environmental Protection Agency. A review of the reference dose and reference concentration process. EPA/630/P-02/002F, 2002.
30. World Health Organization. International program on chemical safety: principles for the assessment of risks to human health from exposure to chemicals. Environmental Health Criteria 210. Geneva: World Health Organization; 1999.
31. World Health Organization. International program on chemical safety: chemical-specific adjustment factors for interspecies differences and human variability: guidance document for use data in dose/concentration-response assessment. Geneva: World Health Organization; 2005. http://whqlibdoc.who.int/publications/2005/9241546786_eng.pdf
32. Renwick AG, Lazarous NR. Human variability and noncancer risk assessment. An analysis of the default uncertainty factor. Regul Toxicol Pharmacol. 1998;27:3–20.
33. Dorne JLCM, Walton K, Renwick AG. Human variability in xenobiotic metabolism and pathway-related uncertainty factors for chemical risk assessment: a review. Food Chem Toxicol. 2005;43:203–16.
34. Roskos KV, Maibach HI, Guy RH. The effect of aging on percutaneous absorption in man. J Pharmacokinet Biopharm. 1989;17(6):617–30.
35. Roskos KV, Maibach HI. Percutaneous absorption and age-implications for therapy. Drugs Aging. 1992;2:432–49.
36. Ghadially R. Aging and epidermal permeability barrier: implications for contact dermatitis. Am J Contact Dermatitis. 1998;9:162–9.
37. Oriba HA, Bucks DA, Maibach HI. Percutaneous absorption of hydrocortisone and testosterone on the vulva and forearm: effect of the menopause and site. Br J Dermatol. 1996;134:229–33.

38. Grove GL. Physiologic changes in older skin. Clin Geriatr Med. 1989;5:115–25.
39. Christophers E, Kligman AM. Percutaneous absorption in aged skin. In: Montagna W, editor. Advances in biology of skin VI. New York: Pergamon Press; 1965. p. 163–75.
40. Mayersohn M. Pharmacokinetics in the elderly. Environ Health Perspect. 1994;112(S11):119–24.
41. DeVane CL. Metabolism and pharmacokinetics of selective serotonin reuptake inhibitors. Cell Mol Neurobiol. 1999;19(4):443–66.
42. Lindeman RD, Tobin J, Shock NW. Longitudinal studies on the rate of decline in renal function with age. J Am Geriatr Soc. 1985;33(4):278–85.
43. Woodhouse KW, James OF. Hepatic drug metabolism and ageing. Br Med Bull. 1990;46(1):22–35.
44. Wynne HA, Goudevenos J, Rawlins MD, James OF, Adams PC, Woodhouse KW. Hepatic drug clearance: the effect of age using indocyanine green as a model compound. Br J Clin Pharmacol. 1990;30(4):634–7.
45. Koff RS, Garvey AJ, Burney SW, Bell B. Absence of an age effect on sulfobromophtalein retention in healthy men. Gastroenterology. 1973;65:300–2.
46. Kampmann JP, Sinding J, Moller-Joergensen I. Effect of age on liver function. Geriatrics. 1975;30:91–5.
47. Fu A, Sreekumaran NK. Age effect on fibrinogen and albumin synthesis in humans. Am J Physiol. 1998;275: E1023–30.
48. Hunt CM, Westerkam WR, Stave GM. Effect of age and gender on the activity of human hepatic CYP3A. Biochem Pharmacol. 1992;44:275–83.
49. Eddington ND. Pharmacokinetics. In: Roberts J, Snyder DL, Friedman E, editors. Handbook of pharmacology and aging. Boca Raton: CRC Press; 1996. p. 1–22.
50. Sotaniemi EA, Arranto AJ, Pelkonen O, Pasanen M. Age and cytochrome P450-linked drug metabolism in humans: an analysis of 226 subjects with equal histopathologic conditions. Clin Pharmacol Ther. 1997;61(3):331–9.
51. Schmucker DL, Woodhouse KW, Wang RK. Effects of age and gender on in vitro properties of human liver microsomal monooxygenases. Clin Pharmacol Ther. 1990;48(4):365–74.
52. Clewell H, Teeguarden J, McDonald T, Sarangapani R, Lawrence G, Covington T, Gentry R, Shipp A. Review and evaluation of the potential impact of age and gender-specific pharmacokinetic differences on tissue dosimetry. Crit Rev Toxicol. 2002;32(5):329–89.
53. Silverman KC, Naumann BD, Holder DJ, Dixit R, Faria E, Sargent E, Gallo M. Establishing data-derived adjustment factors from published pharmaceutical clinical trial data. Human Ecol Risk Assess. 1999;5 (5):1059–89.
54. Naumann BD, Silverman KC, Dixit R, Faria E, Sargent EV. Case studies of categorical data-derived adjustment factors. Human Ecol Risk Assess. 2001;7 (1):61–105.
55. Clewell HJ, Gentry PR, Covington TR, Sarangapani R, Teeguarden JG. Evaluation of the potential impact of age- and gender-specific pharmacokinetic differences on tissue dosimetry. Toxicol Sci. 2004;79:381–93.
56. Ramos-E-Silva M, Coelho D, Iva S, Carneiro S. Cosmetics for the elderly. Clin Dermatol. 2001;19:413–23.
57. Marchini L, Vieira PC, Bossan TP, Montenegro FLB, Cunha VPP. Self-reported oral hygiene habits among institutionalized elderly and their relationship to the condition of oral tissues in Taubaté, Brazil. Gerodontology. 2006;3(1):33–7.
58. Blair KA. Aging: physiological aspects and clinical implications. Nurse Pract. 1990;15(2):14–28.

Dermal Safety Evaluation: Use of Disposable Diaper Products in the Elderly

109

Daniel S. Marsman, Prashant Rai, and Susan P. Felter

Contents

D.S. Marsman (✉) • S.P. Felter
The Procter & Gamble Company, Cincinnati, OH, USA
e-mail: marsman.ds@pg.com; felter.sp@pg.com

P. Rai
L'Oreal China, Shanghai, China
e-mail: drprashantrai@hotmail.com

M.A. Farage et al. (eds.), *Textbook of Aging Skin*,
DOI 10.1007/978-3-662-47398-6_82

Abstract

Disposable diapers for adults are widely used in many parts of the developed world to safely and effectively manage urinary and fecal incontinence. Their usage is relatively uncommon in the developing world, although adult diapers are manufactured and exported from and used in India and China, to a limited extent. It is estimated that 90–95 % of adult incontinence diapers that are used in developed nations are of the disposable kind. These products are in direct contact with the skin of the individual when worn, and given that adult diapers are changed three times a day on average, an incontinent adult may be exposed to approximately a thousand disposable diapers per year. This manuscript provides an overview of the application of quantitative risk assessment principles to the safety evaluation of adult care disposable diapers.

Introduction

Disposable diapers for adults are widely used in many parts of the developed world, to safely and effectively manage urinary and fecal incontinence. Their usage is relatively uncommon in the developing world, although adult diapers are manufactured and exported from and used in India and China, to a limited extent. It is estimated that 90–95 % of adult incontinence diapers that are used in developed nations are of the disposable kind. These products are in direct contact with the skin of the individual when worn, and given that adult diapers are changed three times a day on average, an incontinent adult may be exposed to approximately a thousand disposable diapers per year.

The significant exposure of incontinent adults to disposable diapers necessitated the development of robust and practical methods for assessing the safe and effective use of these important products. A generalized risk assessment (RA) paradigm was established by the National Academy of Sciences in 1983 [1], which consists of a four-step process: hazard identification, dose–response assessment, exposure assessment, and risk characterization. Although the application of this process varies slightly and is described using different terminologies by different organizations and institutions, the basic principles are the same [2–4]. Kosemund et al. [5] have described the use of this paradigm for the safety evaluation of baby diaper products.

Design and Use of Disposable Diapers: Implications for Safety Assessment

The modern adult care disposable diaper benefits from a number of innovations in design and materials. These improvements have resulted in products that are highly absorbent and ensure a snug, comfortable, and discreet fit. These improvements also allow for the manufacture of a product that promotes improved skin health and hygiene in the elderly by effectively containing urine and excreta and thus maintaining skin health by reducing direct exposure to these bodily wastes [6–8].

Adult Incontinence Diaper Design

A number of different material layers are employed in the construction of a typical adult care disposable diaper. In general, these diapers consist of absorbent layers in the diaper core, contained within an outer structure or chassis that ensures proper fit (Fig. 1). These adult diapers are also available in the form of insert pads, which are worn inside the larger outer disposable diaper. These insert pads (which are quite similar to, but larger than, feminine protection pads that are used by women for menstrual fluid management) are commonly used by care institutions that provide adult care facilities and by individuals who do not wish to change the more expensive outer diaper at every instance of soiling.

Components of a typical diaper include a polypropylene topsheet that is in direct contact with the skin, cellulose pulp, superabsorbent polyacrylate granules contained within the adult diaper core away from direct skin contact, and barrier leg cuffs that ensure fit and prevent leakage, as illustrated in Fig. 1. Different kinds of

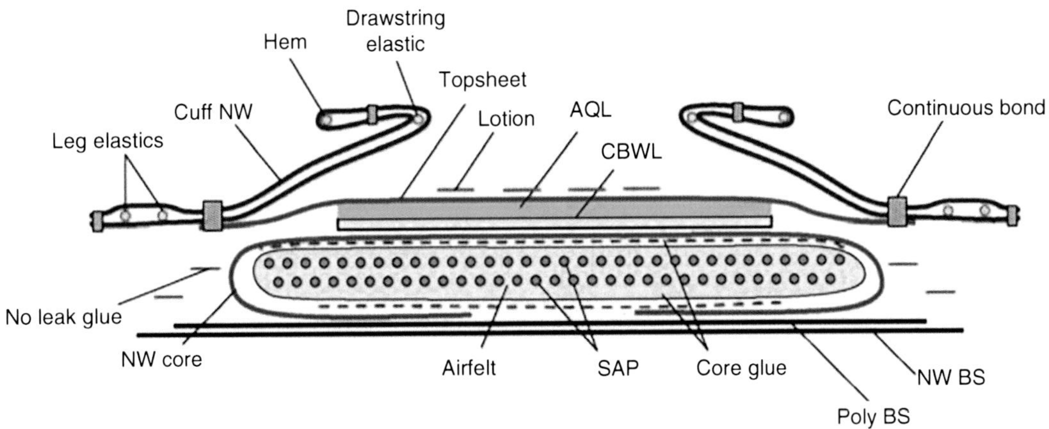

Fig. 1 Cross section of a typical adult care disposable diaper. *NW* nonwoven, *SAP* superabsorbent polymer, *AQL* acquisition layer, *BS* backsheet, *CBWL* cellulose-based wicking layer

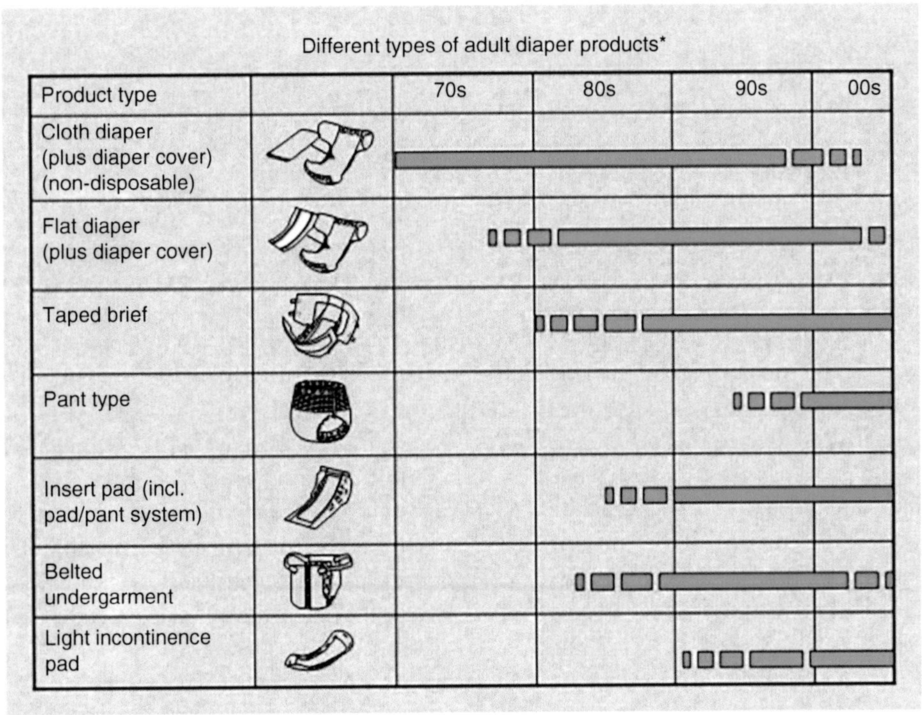

Different types of adult diaper products*

Product type		70s	80s	90s	00s
Cloth diaper (plus diaper cover) (non-disposable)					
Flat diaper (plus diaper cover)					
Taped brief					
Pant type					
Insert pad (incl. pad/pant system)					
Belted undergarment					
Light incontinence pad					

Fig. 2 Types of adult diaper products
*Presented at the 5th International Society of Gerontology Meeting, Nagoya, Japan, 2005 by Mr. Yukio Heki, P&G Japan (Courtesy of Mr. Yukio Heki, Principal Scientist, Procter & Gamble Japan K.K.)

adult incontinence management products are illustrated in Fig. 2. Additional components include an outer protective barrier layer of polyethylene film, elastic materials that improve fit, and adhesive or loop tapes for fastening the diaper. Adhesives are commonly used throughout the diaper to hold the layers in proper position. Some diaper variants may also feature lotion on the topsheet, which helps to improve the softness/smoothness properties of diapered skin and reduces the incidences of adverse skin reactions. Additionally, the topsheet may also be treated with very low levels of mild surfactants to overcome the otherwise hydrophobic nature of the polymer topsheet, allowing urine to pass through more readily. Most of the diaper weight is made up of large molecular weight polymers of natural or synthetic origin.

Raw materials used in diaper construction, including the topsheet and superabsorbent materials, have all shown low irritancy and no evidence of sensitization potential in standard skin testing. Because these polymeric materials are solid materials that are biologically inert and have low bioavailability, they enjoy a highly favorable human safety profile. Diapers may also contain small quantities of low molecular weight ingredients or residual materials that are part of the manufacturing process. These materials may come into contact with the skin, either through direct exposure or as a result of urine extraction, and therefore are relevant to the assessment of diaper safety.

Overall, the safety assessment of an adult disposable diaper involves the identification of ingredients of toxicological relevance in individual raw materials (including impurities and manufacturing aids) and their evaluation via the quantitative risk assessment (QRA) process. Given the potential for skin contact and dermal absorption, the hazard evaluation process involves confirmation of safety for both dermal and systemic toxicological end points.

Adult Disposable Diaper Choice and Effects on Skin

A 1999 NAFC (National Association for Continence) [4] [23] survey showed that about 60 % of incontinent individuals used some type of disposable liner or pad or underwear. It is noteworthy that, at that time, 26.8 % of all women with incontinence mentioned that they used sanitary napkins and 17.4 % of all women used tissues, paper towels, or toilet paper in lieu of any specially designed absorbent product. Similarly, 26.5 % of all men who responded said they used reusable pads, diapers, or other reusable briefs.

Adult diaper manufacturers have designed several types of disposable diapers to suit varying needs. Choice of an adult diaper product type is largely dependent upon the severity and type of incontinent symptoms suffered by an individual. The age of the incontinent individual is often not a major consideration in this case. The mobility of an incontinent individual also is a significant factor when choosing an adult incontinence management product. Younger, normally mobile, lightly incontinent individuals (30–50 years of age) typically tend to choose more discreet products, like thin insert pads, light incontinence pads, or pull-up pants-type diapers for management of urinary incontinence. Typically, these lighter and thinner products are changed frequently, and as a result prolonged skin contact with the same (wet) product is often reduced. However, if the volume of incontinent urine in these individuals is high, a heavier, thicker pad or diaper may be the product of choice. In contrast, for older, less mobile, moderate to severely incontinent individuals (60–90 years of age), where the volume of incontinent urine may be high, the choice of product may be restricted only to thicker and heavier types of diapers/pads. The use of a thicker, highly absorbent product also does not necessitate frequent change, a condition which is well suited to less mobile or bedridden individuals.

Separately, incontinent individuals may also be cared for by other family members at home or professional caregivers/nurses in senior-citizen institutions, where the choice of incontinence management product may be made by the caregiver. Here too, depending on the mobility of the individual and the extent of incontinence, the caregiver may choose to use a lighter, thinner product if symptoms of incontinence are mild and a heavier/thicker product if the extent of incontinence is moderate to severe.

With regard to adult incontinence-related skin problems, it is very important to apply a holistic perspective to understand the influences due to the individual's extent of incontinence and skin

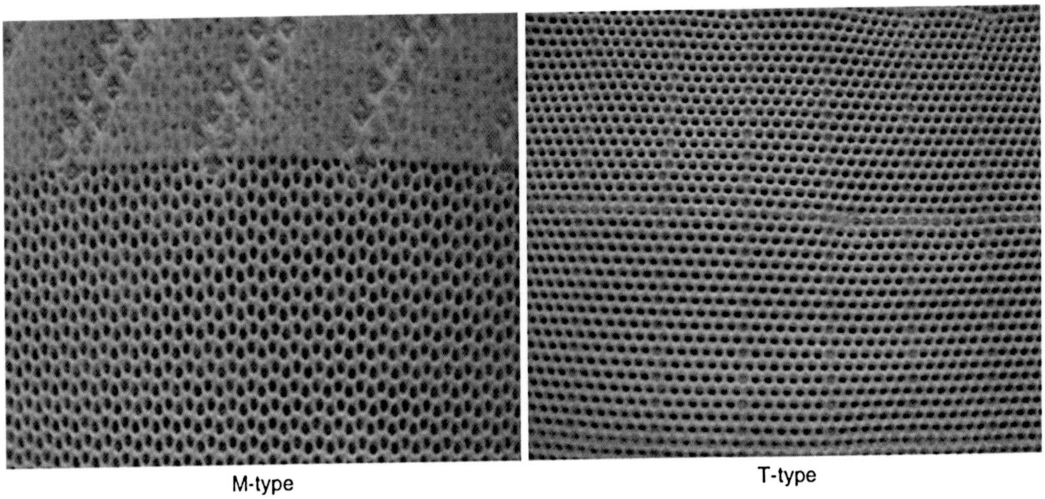

M-type T-type

Fig. 3 Aperture formed film M and T types of product topsheets (Courtesy of Mr. Yukio Heki, Principal Scientist, Procter & Gamble Japan K.K.)

condition, as well as the hygiene and skin care measures practiced at home, or provided professionally. Individuals with frail, sensitive skin or with pre-existing skin diseases may preferably have to use high-absorbency, lotion-containing, thicker diaper products (with superabsorbent polymers and moisture-permeable backsheets) to minimize the risk of skin complications. Also, diaper topsheets have been engineered creatively by manufacturers, to minimize the risk of skin conditions. For example, immobile incontinent individuals have benefited greatly from products that contain the high-performance aperture formed film (T type) type of topsheet, which helps to quickly wick away incontinent fluids (due to larger pore size), thus keeping the skin clean and dry for longer periods of time (Fig. 3). In contrast, products engineered with the common aperture formed film (M type) type of topsheet exhibit slower wicking speeds (due to reduced pore size) and hence are known to provide reduced skin management benefits. In contrast, adult diapers that are manufactured with more conventional nonwoven topsheets are known to provide better long-term skin comfort benefits when compared to aperture formed film types of topsheets, which are excellent for absorption, but do not perform well in regions with high temperatures and high humidity.

Exposure Parameters

Being a complex, layered product, with each layer having a different function, the exposure potential for various diaper components ranges from continual direct skin contact for some materials (e.g., the topsheet) to materials with transient or very minimal/negligible skin contact (e.g., the fasteners). As noted above, the majority of chemical components in a diaper are large, inert polymers that are not absorbed through the skin. These materials are of little concern when evaluating diaper safety. In contrast, low molecular weight materials that may be present in the topsheet need to be thoroughly assessed. Ingredients/monomers may also be released from diaper core components, solubilize in urine, and become bioavailable at the surface of the adult diaper and become relevant for exposure analysis.

Materials in Direct Skin Contact

Adult diaper raw materials that are in direct contact with the skin include the topsheet, the lotion ingredients, the barrier leg cuffs, and the waistband. Skin transfer of chemicals or materials from hese components does not necessarily require solubilization in body fluids that may be loaded onto the diaper. Chemicals may be deposited or transferred onto the skin directly, or via solubilization in sweat, urine, or sebum. However, even with materials in direct contact with the skin, only a fractional amount of topsheet ingredients are expected to be transferred onto the skin. This is due to the integration of the raw materials/chemicals within the polymeric matrix resin of the topsheet. Typically, obtaining precise analytical data on the leachability of the chemical/raw material from the topsheet is recommended, in order to calculate exposure.

Studies have shown that only approximately 10 % of a typical topsheet coating material, such as a lotion, is actually transferred to the skin of the adult diaper wearer (P&G unpublished data). Thus, this lotion transfer factor can be used as a reasonable and conservative estimate for transfer of all other topsheet ingredients. Residual monomers and contaminants incorporated into the substrate of the topsheet are presumed to be transferred in substantially less quantities than this worst-case estimate.

Materials Not in Direct Skin Contact

Diaper components beneath the topsheet are not in direct contact with the skin. These materials include the acquisition layer, the superabsorbent polymer, nonwoven core wrap material, core, and chassis glues. These materials may contain ingredients with the potential to migrate to the skin, typically being carried toward the skin via urine. Exposure to these materials can occur via extraction or solubilization in urine and other body fluids, followed by these fluids resurfacing to the skin.

Therefore, urine that resurfaces to the skin may be assumed to be the key carrier for these ingredients. In the absence of experimental data from which to estimate the migration of low molecular weight materials from the diaper interior to the skin surface, a highly conservative default assumption of 100 % migration may be used for exposure calculations. A refined exposure evaluation would include actual quantification of the extractable ingredient from the fluid matrix.

The Reflux Approach

Reflux (also known as rewet or retention of wetness) is a relevant factor for quantifying exposure to non-skin-contact materials. Reflux is defined as the amount of liquid (i.e., urine) that resurfaces to the top of a diaper and has the potential to come into contact with the skin. Diaper core ingredients that are not in direct skin contact require urine as an aqueous vehicle or carrier to resurface to the skin. This urine that resurfaces to the topsheet is assumed to be the most relevant carrier for ingredients that may be located deep within the diaper. Current diaper risk assessments are based upon the presence and use of highly absorbent core technologies, such as superabsorbent polymer (SAP), which have reduced the reflux level of adult care disposable diapers. No default reflux values are recommended for exposure calculations for these types of raw material ingredients. Taped adult diapers show the highest actual reflux value (1.6 %), whereas a reflux value of 0.1 % is measured for all other types and variants of adult care disposable diapers. The difference between these values reflects the difference in construction of the core of these diapers. All taped diaper variants typically contain an additional blue-colored cellulose-based wicking layer placed just above the absorbent core. Due to the presence of this layer, the core is constructed with slightly reduced amounts of SAP, thus resulting in higher rewet values.

The reflux factor has been measured, typically using an absorbing filter paper or a collagen sheet, under pressure, on top of a moist diaper. The diaper is typically loaded with synthetic urine or other aqueous solvents. The filter paper/collagen sheet utilizes the high capillary forces of cellulose fibers to identify very small differences in absorbency between different products.

Reflux values measured by using filter paper are more conservative and in the range of 2–2.5 %. Reflux values obtained by using the collagen method (Post Acquisition Collagen Reflux Method; PACORM) are generally considered more realistic and are similar to actual diaper in-use conditions, as collagen closely mimics the re-absorbency characteristics of the upper epidermal layers of the skin. The PACORM uses a stretched diaper on a fastening plate [9]. Following diaper loading (typically, four large gushes of 150 mL each of synthetic urine or saline, depending on diaper size), four circular collagen sheets (diameter 9 cm each, area 64 cm^2 each) are stacked onto the topsheet and pressure is applied (approximately 236 g/cm^2). Reflux is calculated as the weight difference of the collagen sheets before and after exposure to the topsheet. One limitation of this method is that reflux is measured only under the 64 cm^2 collagen sheet area and not from the entire diaper core surface which is in direct skin contact (1,660 cm^2). However, the reflux number obtained is still considered reasonably conservative, as collagen sheets are placed on the central loading area with the highest liquid concentration in the diaper core.

Consumer Usage Data and Assumptions for Quantitative Risk Assessment

Different diaper usage habits are relevant parameters when determining overall exposure to diaper raw materials and chemicals. Normal consumer habits and practices for diaper usage are varied across different geographies. Procter & Gamble consumer research (unpublished data) indicates that the highest number of adult care disposable diapers used per day is observed in Japan, while fewer diapers are used per day in countries such as Italy, Spain, and Portugal. Adult care disposable diaper usage in the USA shows that numbers are slightly higher than those observed in Europe.

For adult care diaper exposure assessments, the following parameters are particularly relevant:

- The adult body weight is assumed to be 60 kg, to account for differences in sex and global diversity.
- The *number of adult diapers used per day* (diaper change frequency) differs in different geographies. The consumer data from Japan suggests that the highest change frequency is observed with insert pads (3.5–4.0 times per day), whereas outer taped briefs or pull-on diapers are changed less frequently (1.5–1.75 times per day). Italy, Spain, and Portugal demonstrate similar diaper change frequencies, with approximately 2–3 pads being worn per day, irrespective of type. Approximately 3–5 disposable briefs are worn by consumers in the USA in institutional and home care settings. For simplification, a conservative average diaper changing frequency of 3 is assumed in the calculations to account for change frequencies and usage of all adult disposable diaper types.
- The *topsheet transfer factor* (10 %) is the amount of an ingredient that is transferred from the topsheet of the diaper to the skin of the adult. As noted earlier, this is a conservative default value of direct contact ingredient transfer from data generated in support of diaper topsheet lotions, where the intention is to transfer components to the skin during adult diaper wear as a skin health benefit. This value is based upon measurements of actual lotion transfer observed during clinical studies with adult diapers in Europe (P&G, unpublished data). It is assumed that transfer of any substance from the topsheet will not be greater than the transfer of an intentionally added-on ingredient such as lotion.
- The *reflux factor* is 1.6 % for taped diapers and 0.1 % for all other diaper types. The superabsorbent core of adult diapers is not in direct contact with the skin of the individual and is made up of a polymeric gelling material that quickly soaks up urine and contains it within the core. This core technology is specifically engineered to minimize/eliminate any re-exposure of the skin to urine. However, minute amounts of urine might still resurface to the skin, via the phenomenon of reflux (Fig. 4). Thus resurfacing of ingredients from the lower layers of the diaper, albeit remote, is still possible, and resurfacing urine may be assumed to be the carrier of any chemicals

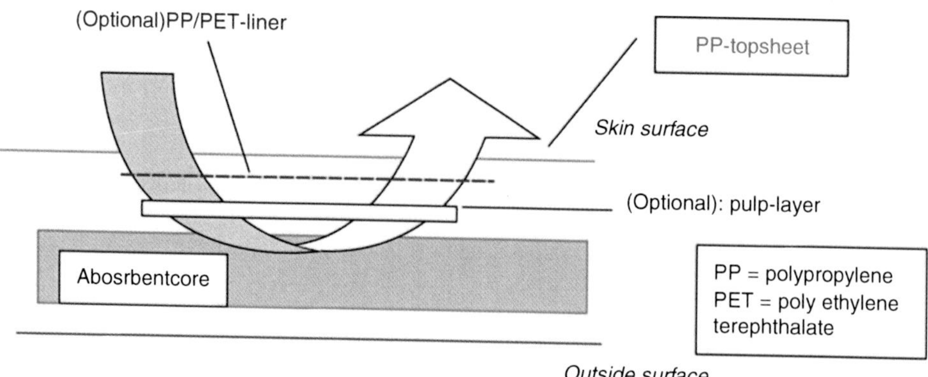

Fig. 4 Illustration of adult care disposable diaper reflux measurement

that might reside in these core lower-layer materials that are not in direct skin contact.

Materials with Negligible Skin Contact

Several diaper materials used on the outside of the diaper chassis (e.g., outer polypropylene liners, graphic printed surfaces, fastening tapes, disposal tapes) have negligible or very minimal direct skin contact. In terms of exposure assessment, these materials are generally judged to have negligible exposure and can often be considered to contribute insignificantly toward overall exposure to materials during diaper wear.

Principles of Quantitative Risk Assessment (QRA) Examples

Adult care disposable diapers are mainly constructed of inert, polymeric materials. In general, these materials are considered safe, and no inherent toxicity issues are anticipated. However, low levels of non-polymeric components or monomers may be present in the product, or these may be residuals from the diaper raw material manufacturing process, or they could be components of aesthetic materials such as perfumes or lotions that are added to the diaper at low levels.

The following section provides examples of exposure-based QRAs for materials in adult care

$$CH_3\underset{\displaystyle CH_3}{\underset{|}{C}}{=}CHCH_2CH_2\underset{\displaystyle CH_3}{\underset{|}{C}}{=}CH\overset{\displaystyle O}{\overset{||}{C}}H$$

Fig. 5 Citral ($C_{10}H_{16}O$)

disposable diapers. Citral, a perfume raw material, and acrylic acid, a residual monomer in superabsorbent polymers that form the core of the diaper, serve as case studies to showcase the principles of QRA as applied to an adult diaper during consumer use.

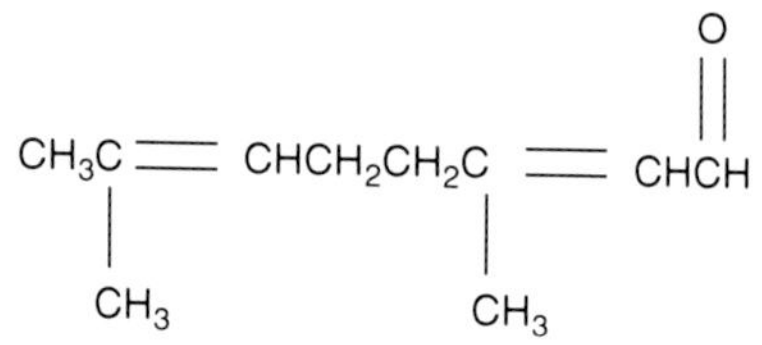

Risk Assessment for Citral

Citral (CAS # 5392-40-5) (Fig. 5) is a well-known flavoring agent and is the main constituent of lemon and orange oils. It is commonly used in perfumes and may be a low-level component of the overall complex perfume formula that may be added in a diaper. Perfumes may be added to diapers, typically between the absorbent core and the backsheet, to enhance the overall aesthetics of the diaper. Given the deep-layer application of the perfume in a diaper, it is recommended to use a reflux level of 1.6 % for determining potential exposure. Citral is classified as a weak sensitizer, but exposure to low levels does not pose any health risk.

Table 1 Identification of weight-of-evidence no-expected-sensitization-induction level (WoE NESIL) for citral (International Fragrance Association, 2006 [12], Lalko J, Api AM 2008 [13], Scientific Committee on Cosmetic Products and non-Food Products Intended for Consumers, 1999 [14])

Name of raw material	CAS #	IFRA standard limit (skin contact products)	LLNA weighted mean EC3 values (μg/cm^2)	NOEL-HRIPT (induction) (μg/cm^2)	NOEL-MAX (induction) (μg/cm^2)	LOEL (induction) (μg/cm^2)	Potency classification	WoE NESIL
Citral	5392-40-5	NA	5.7 % (1,414)	1,400	NA	3,876	Weak	1,400

LLNA local lymph node assay, *NOEL* no-observed-effect level, *HRIPT* human repeat insult patch test, *LOEL* lowest-observed-effect level

The identification of such a safe level is achieved through the sensitization QRA approach for fragrance ingredients. This approach follows the same four basic steps of the risk assessment paradigm defined by the National Academy of Sciences: hazard identification, dose–response assessment, exposure assessment, and risk characterization [1].

Recently, a common recommended methodology has been adopted for the QRA of fragrance ingredients by Api et al. [10] and by the European Cosmetics, Toiletry, and Perfumery Association (COLIPA) Toxicology Advisory Group and the Joint COLIPA/International Association for Soaps, Detergents and Maintenance Products (AISE)/European Flavor and Fragrance Association (EFFA)/International Fragrance Association (IFRA) Perfume Safety group [11].

Clear guidance on different elements of the dermal sensitization QRA process (e.g., uncertainty factors or sensitization assessment factors) is also offered in these references. A weight-of-evidence (WoE) approach is used to determine a no-expected-sensitization-induction level (NESIL), which introduces a more robust approach to allergen potency evaluation for use in risk assessment. Additionally, sensitization assessment factors (SAFs) within the exposure-based QRA process are based on published data. The SAFs take into account three parameters: interindividual variability (the same as in general toxicology), vehicle/product matrix effects, and use considerations (specific for dermal sensitization). A consumer exposure level (CEL) is determined for the perfume raw material, and it is essential to express this entity in units of dose/cm^2 of the skin. This updated process of QRA for perfume ingredients represents an important step forward in skin sensitization risk assessment.

Once the NESIL, SAF, and CEL for citral are defined, it is possible to confirm its safety via quantitative risk assessment and specifically a lack of sensitization hazard, as a result of exposure to citral. There are two key elements involved in this process of risk characterization:

- The establishment of an acceptable exposure level (AEL): The AEL is determined by dividing the WoE NESIL by the SAF, i.e., AEL = WoE NESIL/SAF. Identification of the WoE NESIL is shown in Table 1.
- Comparison of the AEL to the CEL: This is determined by dividing the AEL by the CEL, which is an indication of the acceptability of the CEL relative to the AEL. The percent concentration of the fragrance ingredient, citral, in a diaper is acceptable if the ratio of AEL to CEL is favorable to support safe use of citral.

Assumptions to calculate CEL for citral as a result of diaper wear are:

- Diaper = 0.01/diaper = 0.019 g = 19 mg
- Amount of citral in perfume = 0.026 %
- Amount of citral/diaper = 0.005 mg
- Three diapers worn/day (based on habits and practices data)
- Reflux factor = 1.6 % (or alternatively 0.1 %)

Table 2 Application of QRA for citral in perfumes used in adult care disposable diaper products

Citral	
WoE NESIL	1,400 μg/cm^2
SAF[a]	100 (10 × 1 × 10)
AEL	1,400/100 = 14 μg/cm^2
CEL	0.00024 μg/cm^2
AEL/CEL	14/0.00024 = 60,000
Risk assessment for citral	Acceptable, since AEL > CEL

[a]SAF: Interindividual variability = 10; this is based upon well-established principles of general toxicology and is meant to provide protection for susceptible subpopulations. Vehicle matrix = 1; matrix is very different from the experimental test conditions under which the WOE NESIL was determined. However, it is not expected to be more irritating, and the diaper matrix is an inert material and not skin impactful. Use considerations = 10; in this case, the skin areas being considered are the buttocks, groin, lower stomach, and upper thighs. Skin integrity may be compromised in some cases. Mucus membrane exposure may occur, along with somewhat occlusive diaper-wearing conditions

Fig. 6 Acrylic acid

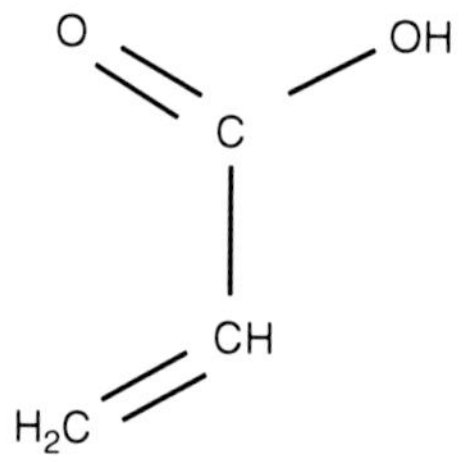

- Skin contact area = 1,000 cm^2 (surface area of smallest adult care disposable diaper)

Therefore, CEL for citral = 0.005 mg × 0.016 × 3/1,000 cm^2 = 0.00000024 mg/cm^2/day = 0.00024 μg/cm^2/day

The QRA for citral in adult diapers is summarized in Table 2. It is observed that the AEL is greater than the actual CEL by a factor of 60,000, indicating that use of citral as a perfume ingredient in adult care disposable diapers is safe. A margin of safety of 60,000, while providing overwhelming safety assurance, also indicates that citral as a perfume ingredient may be safely used at much higher levels in adult care disposable diapers, without the risk of skin sensitization.

Exposure to a Diaper Absorbent Core Raw Material: Acrylic Acid

Although adult disposable diapers are mostly composed of large molecular weight polymeric materials, there may be unreacted, low molecular weight monomers, or other small molecular weight components (e.g., processing aids or impurities) present in these polymeric materials. Minimal exposure to absorbent core raw materials of diapers may also occur under various conditions. One route of exposure is via the skin, where small molecular weight components of direct/indirect skin contact materials might be absorbed into the skin. These monomers or small molecular weight compounds may reach the skin via the phenomenon of reflux in the diaper and, depending on the material and molecular weight, may also be absorbed through the skin [15].

The SAP in diapers comprises one of two main components that make up the absorbent core of a diaper, the other being an absorbent fluff pulp, comprised of cellulose fibers. The most important function of SAP is to take up urine and lock it away, which in turn renders the urine non-available to the skin, thus reducing potential incidences of diaper rash. Typically, SAP is made by polymerization of acrylic acid (Fig. 6) in an aqueous solution. During polymerization, the carboxylic acid groups are partially neutralized (75 %) with sodium hydroxide. Therefore, a major component of SAP is the neutralized, salt form of acrylic acid, namely, sodium acrylate, and a very small component is pure acrylic acid. The large molecular weight polyacrylates are generally not a cause for toxicological concern, because they are not bioavailable.

Free acrylic acid monomers are expected to be available, although in very limited quantities. Furthermore, under physiological conditions in a

Table 3 Hazard profile of acrylic acid

Acute toxicity	Irritation – oral and dermal
Irritation/ corrosion	Corrosion – dermal, eyes, and respiratory tract
Sensitization	Not sensitizing
Repeated dose toxicity	Irritation, unspecific
Mutagenicity	Non-mutagenic – Acrylic acid is non-mutagenic in *Salmonella* and CHO cells, but positive in the mouse lymphoma assay and in the in vitro chromosomal aberration test. However, in vivo acrylic acid did not produce mutagenic effects in either rat bone marrow cells or mouse germ cells after oral administration. Based on these results and considering data from structurally related acrylic compounds, it is concluded that acrylic acid is not mutagenic in vivo
Carcinogenicity	Noncarcinogenic – Studies on animals indicate that acrylic acid is not carcinogenic
Reproductive toxicity	Not a reproductive toxin – In oral reproductive toxicity studies (rats), no effects on reproductive function (fertility) were observed, but some signs of postnatal developmental toxicity (retarded body weight gain of the pups) were seen following exposure of the parental generation. No gross abnormalities were observed in the offspring. No prenatal developmental toxicity was observed (rats and rabbits, inhalation)

diaper, most of the carboxylic groups will be present as the salt form, i.e., sodium acrylate, which does not penetrate the skin as easily as does the acidic form. A 2002 CIR report on the "Safety of Acrylates Copolymer and 33 Related Cosmetic Ingredients" [16] indicates that linear polymers of acrylic acid may contain unreacted starting materials and catalysts, with residual monomer concentrations typically between 10 ppm and 1,000 ppm, with an upper limit of 1,500 ppm. SAP raw material suppliers for disposable diapers are currently required to maintain an upper specification limit of 500 ppm for free acrylic acid monomers (*P&G specification to suppliers*). Thus, the presence of unreacted acrylic acid monomers in SAP is limited but likely, and the main route of exposure to this residual acrylic acid is dermal, via the phenomenon of reflux.

Acrylic Acid: Hazard Characterization

Acrylic acid has been evaluated for safety as part of the European Risk Assessment Program (EEC 793/93) [17] and as part of the CIR report on the "Final Report on the Safety Assessment of Acrylates Copolymer and 33 Related Cosmetic Ingredients" [16]. It has also been evaluated by the US EPA [18]. The hazard profile of acrylic acid as described in these references is summarized in Table 3.

At low levels, however, acrylic acid is not irritating. Irritation or corrosivity is concentration dependent. Acrylic acid at 1 % in acetone shows signs of minimal irritation and is well tolerated by animals in dermal carcinogenicity studies.

Systemic Risk Assessment for Acrylic Acid

- The US EPA Integrated Risk Information System (IRIS) oral reference dose (RfD) for acrylic acid [18] is 0.5 mg/kg/day, which is based on a two-generation reproductive study in rats, with supporting data from a chronic drinking water study in rats, developmental studies by the inhalation route in rats and rabbits, and an inhalation/dermal/oral/IV bioavailability study in rats and mice. It is based on a no-observed-adverse-effect level of 53 mg/kg/day and an uncertainty factor of 100, which includes a factor of 10 for interspecies extrapolation and a factor of 10 to protect sensitive individuals. This RfD represents a daily exposure level that is considered to be safe for a lifetime of exposure, including sensitive subpopulations.
- A default reflux value of 1.6 % is recommended for exposure calculations for materials that are not in direct skin contact,

Table 4 Application of QRA to available acrylic acid in diaper absorbent cores

Acrylic acid	
RfD of acrylic acid (US EPA)	0.5 mg/kg/day
Total amt of SAP/pad	22 g
Amt of extractable monomer (RM specs)[a]	500 ppm (conservative)
Number of diapers/day	3
Total available acrylic acid/day	500 ppm × 22 g = 11 mg/day × 3 = 33 mg/day
Weight of adult	60 kg
Total available acrylic acid/kg body weight	33/60 = 0.55 mg/kg/day
Reflux factor	1.6 % = 0.016
Dermal absorption	100 % (conservative)
Potential consumer exposure	0.55 mg/kg/day × 0.016 × 1 = 0.009 mg/kg/day
Margin of safety	
(MOS) = RfD/consumer exposure	0.5/0.009 mg/kg/day = 55

[a]500 ppm is the maximum limit of available acrylic acid monomers that suppliers of SAP are currently required to meet, for use in adult diapers

and this value may be used for acrylic acid, as a conservative approach.

Exposure Assessment of Acrylic Acid

The QRA for acrylic acid in diaper cores is summarized in Table 4.

It is noted that this exposure assessment is highly conservative and assumes that 100 % of the ingredient is represented as free acrylic acid in the entire diaper and that this chemical is available for reflux and fully penetrates the skin for each of the three diapers used, on a daily basis.

Based on the risk assessment and exposure evaluation and a margin of safety (MOS) that is greater than 1, it can be concluded that for systemic toxicological end points, residual acrylic acid that may be present in the SAP core of adult diapers does not present any systemic human safety risk.

Threshold of Toxicological Concern (TTC)

The absence of chemical-specific safety data for some chemicals found at very low levels in diapers may be encountered during the process of safety evaluation. Many of the materials used in the construction of adult care disposable diapers are complex materials that may contain many different chemicals or may have low-level impurities. For example, low levels of unreacted monomers may be present in a high molecular weight polymer, or a low level of a solvent may be present in an adhesive. Traditional risk assessment approaches are generally used to confirm safety, based on evaluating the potential for these chemicals to migrate out of the diaper and reach the skin. However, there may be very low residual levels of chemicals/contaminants that do not have a robust safety dataset. To confirm safety for such low-level residuals, an assessment based on the concept of threshold of toxicological concern (TTC) can be used. This approach is based on the fundamental premise that there is an exposure to chemicals below which adverse effects will be negligible or absent. This TTC framework provides a conservative estimate of an acceptable chronic exposure, in the absence of chemical-specific data. Although originally developed by the US FDA [19, 22] to support low-level exposures to indirect food additives (e.g., packaging materials), this framework has since been expanded for application to materials that may be used in consumer and personal care products [20, 21]. The TTC approach has been described in the literature in some detail [5]. For a chemical that does not have structural alerts for genotoxicity, an acceptable exposure limit is generally accepted to be 1.5 μg/day for an adult.

Exposure Assessment of Adhesive Contaminant

An example of the application of TTC to determine an acceptable level of a residual level of a chemical contaminant in an adhesive used in the construction of an adult care disposable diaper is shown below. Total exposure to the adhesive itself is determined to be 192 mg/day.

$$(Cp^{*}F^{*}Rf/100^{*}Rw/100^{*}Ab/100^{*}ED/100)$$

$$\text{Exposure} = 4{,}000^{*}3^{*}1^{*}0.016^{*}1^{*}1 = 192 \text{ mg/day}$$

Cp	Amount of adhesive in the diaper in g = 4.0 = 4,000 mg *(Maximum level. This can range from 1 g to 4 g/diaper)*
F	Number of diapers used per day = 3
Rf	Release factor = 100 (very conservative)
Rw	Reflux Factor = 1.6 %
Ab	Absorption of the adhesive through skin = (default 100 %)
ED	Exposure duration, percent of lifetime = (default 100 %)

Assuming a body weight of 60 kg, this exposure is equivalent to 192 mg/day divided by 60 kg = 3.2 mg/kg/day (3,200 μg/kg/day). Therefore, an acceptable upper limit of the contaminant in this adhesive can be established:

$$\frac{\text{Acceptable exposure to contaminant } 1.5 \ \mu\text{g/day}}{\text{Exposure to entire adhesive } 192 \ \text{mg/kg/day}} = 0.0000078 = 8 \ \text{ppm}$$

In this example, it can be established that a level of up to 8 ppm of a contaminant (without structural alerts for genotoxicity) in the adhesive can be supported using the TTC method. Similarly, if the exact level of the potential adhesive contaminant is known in advance, the TTC method can be used to confirm its safety. In this case, any level below 8 ppm would be considered to be acceptable using this method. It is noted that the TTC method is highly conservative, and if the exposure is determined to be *above* a TTC-based limit, then generally there are opportunities to refine the assessment with more realistic assumptions before determining that the level of the contaminant is unacceptably high.

Conclusion

The conduct of scientifically sound risk assessments for establishing safety of raw materials used in the manufacture of personal care products, such as adult care disposable diapers, is achieved by using established methods of QRA. QRA is currently used to support the safe introduction of new products and their ingredients into the market for almost all classes of personal care products. Kosemund et al. [5] have previously described details of this method, with reference to baby diapers.

Being complex, multilayered products, adult care disposable diapers are composed of various raw materials that may or may not directly contact the skin. Most of the components of adult care disposable diapers are large molecular weight, inert polymers that have low bioavailability and are therefore not absorbed through the skin (even though there may be direct skin contact). On the other hand, exposure evaluation of low molecular weight ingredients, such as lotion components, perfume ingredients, residual contaminants, residual monomers, or residual process aids, is relevant to ensure overall safety of the raw material and of the diaper as a whole.

Skin exposure to deeper diaper materials may be possible via the phenomenon of reflux, where an aqueous vehicle such as urine may help to carry these materials toward the surface of the diaper and hence toward the skin. This is particularly relevant when diapers are worn all night long, with a very high urine load. Reflux of a diaper is typically determined by one of two currently existing methods, and these methods provide a worst-case estimation of the amount of chemical that may be carried toward the skin.

For the purposes of evaluation of exposure to adult disposable diaper raw materials, various parameters such as consumer usage habits (number of diapers used per day), surface area of the diaper, topsheet transfer factor, weight of the individual, and reflux factor are taken into account. These parameters are the foundation for characterizing exposure to a particular diaper raw material. Each of these is evaluated in detail, and, depending on the parameter, conservative default assumptions are made, or the actual values of the parameter are used for risk assessment. Default assumptions may be replaced with actual values: a process that helps to refine the overall exposure assessment. Familiarity with both the product and the consumer is also required for a robust assessment of safety. Disposable diapers today have substantial holding and performance capacity, and, as such, skin health is generally substantially better than when using cloth diapers. However, broken skin, especially in geriatric patients, can be a serious clinical concern. As such, the use of a 100 % dermal penetration factor is a highly conservative assumption but, as mentioned earlier, a more realistic or exact skin penetration factor is also a usable option, whenever it is available.

Two examples are used to demonstrate the principles of QRA for adult diapers: citral, a common ingredient in perfumes, is evaluated for its sensitizing potential, and acrylic acid, a constituent ingredient of SAP, is evaluated for its systemic toxicity potential.

QRA of citral for allergen potency demonstrated that a higher AEL of citral versus the calculated CEL did not pose an increased risk for sensitization when it is used as a perfume constituent in an adult disposable diaper. The wide MOS of the AEL versus the CEL (60,000) provides overwhelming safety assurance that use of citral in diaper products does not pose a risk of sensitization.

Similarly, QRA for acrylic acid showed that it enjoys a wide MOS (55) versus actual exposure when residual monomers of acrylic acid are evaluated for systemic toxicity potential.

The safety of low residual levels of chemicals or contaminants whose toxicological profiles are not known or do not exist can be confirmed by using the concept of threshold of toxicological concern (TTC). Use of TTC is based on the fundamental premise that there is an exposure to contaminants or chemicals below which adverse effects will be negligible or absent. The TTC method can be used to drive the establishment of safe levels of residuals or contaminants that may be present in diaper raw materials.

Despite variations in diaper usage habits and practices across various countries (and tiers of consumers), and despite the diversity of different diaper raw materials used to construct a diaper, the consistent use of the QRA method for the evaluation of diaper raw materials has demonstrated the robustness of the method. The use of QRA helps to ensure that all raw materials that are used in adult disposable diapers globally are safe. Thus, the safe introduction of new materials and cutting-edge technologies in adult disposable diapers are ensured by this process. This allows consumer goods companies to be able to innovate with newer and emerging materials and provide the latest diaper designs and technologies to consumers around the world.

Cross-References

▶ Safety Evaluation in the Elderly via Dermatological Exposure

References

1. National Academy of Science. Risk assessment in the federal government. National Research Council. Washington: National Academy Press; 1983.
2. Hopper LD, Oehme FW. Chemical risk assessment: a review. Vet Hum Toxicol. 1989;31(6):543–54.
3. International Programme on Chemical Safety. Environmental health criteria 210: principles for the assessment of risks to human health from exposure to chemicals. 1999. http://www.inchem.org/documents/ehc/ehc/ehc210.htm. Accessed Apr 2007.
4. Organisation for Economic Co-operation and Development (OECD). About chemicals hazard/risk assessment. 2007. http://www.oecd.org/about/0,2337,en_2649_34373_1_1_1_1_1,00.html. Accessed May 2008.
5. Kosemund K, Schlatter H, Ochsenhirt J, Krause E, Marsman D, Erasala G. Safety evaluation of superabsorbent baby diapers. Regul Toxicol Pharmacol. 2009;53:81–9.
6. Farage MA, Miller KW, Berardesca E, Maibach HI. Cutaneous effects and sensitive skin with incontinence in the aged. In: Farage MA, Miller KW, Maibach HI, editors. Textbook of aging skin. Berlin/Heidelberg: Springer; 2010. p. 663–71.
7. Farage MA, Miller KW, Berardesca E, Nabil AM, Tzeghai GE, Maibach H. Changes to skin with aging and the effects of menopause and incontinence. In:

Skin, mucosa and menopause: management of clinical issues. Berlin/Heidelberg: Springer; 2015.

8. Farage MA, Tzeghai G, Miller KW, Tepper B, O'Connor B, Qin W, Odio M. Dermatologic effects and management of urine and feces on infants and incontinent adults. Br J Med Med Res. 2014;4: 3671–88.
9. Herrlein MK. European patent EP0797967 A1. 1996.
10. Api AM, Basketter DA, Cadby PA, Cano M-F, Ellis G, Gerberick GF, Griem P, McNamee PM, Ryan CA, Safford R. Dermal sensitization quantitative risk assessment for fragrance ingredients. Regul Toxicol Pharmacol. 2008;52(1):3–23.
11. QRA Expert Group, Api AM, Basketter DA, Cadby PA, Cano M-F, Ellis G, Gerberick GF, Griem P, McNamee PM, Ryan CA, Safford R. Dermal sensitization quantitative risk assessment (QRA) for fragrance ingredients, Technical Dossier. 2006. http://www.rifm.org/doc/QRA_Technical%20Dossier%20FINAL%20REV%202006%206%2022_1.pdf. Accessed May 2008.
12. International Fragrance Association. IFRA standard, 40th amendment: citral. 2006. http://www.ifraorg.org/Home/Publications/Download-the-IFRA-Amendments/page.aspx/134. Accessed May 2008.
13. Lalko J, Api AM. Citral: identifying a threshold for induction of dermal sensitization. Regul Toxicol Pharmacol. 2008;52(1):62–73. Accessed at via Science Direct, May 2008.
14. Scientific Committee on Cosmetic Products and non-Food Products Intended for Consumers. Opinion concerning fragrance allergy in consumers, SCCNFP/0017/98 Final. 1999.
15. Bos JD, Meinardi MHM. The 500-dalton rule for the skin penetration of chemical compounds and drugs. Exp Dermatol. 2000;9:165–9.
16. Fiume MZ. Final report on the safety of assessment of acrylates copolymer and 33 related cosmetic ingredients. Int J Toxicol. 2002;21(S3):1–50.
17. Institute for Health and Consumer Protection, European Chemicals Bureau. Acrylic acid European Union Risk Assessment Report, 28: EUR 19836. Luxembourg: Office for Official Publications of the European Communities; 2002.
18. US Environmental Protection Agency. Acrylic acid integrated risk information systems (IRIS). 1994. http://cfpub.epa.gov/ncea/iris/index.cfm?fuseaction=iris.showQuickView&substance_nmbr=0002. Accessed May 2008.
19. US Food and Drug Administration. Food additives: threshold of regulation of substances used in food-contact articles: final rule. Fed Regist. 1995;60: 36582–96.
20. Blackburn KL, Stickney JA, Carlson-Lynch HL, Mc Ginnis PM, Chappell L, Felter SP. Application of the threshold of toxicological concern approach to ingredients in personal and household care products. Regul Toxicol Pharmacol. 2005;43:249–59.
21. Kroes R, Renwick AG, Feron V, Galli CL, Gioney M, Greim H, Guy RH, Lhuguenot JC, Vande Sandt JJ. Application of the threshold of toxicological concern to the safety evaluation of cosmetic ingredients. Food Chem Toxicol. 2007;45(12): 2533–62.
22. Kroes R, Renwick AG, Cheeseman M, et al. Structure-based thresholds of toxicological concern (TTC): guidance for application to substances present at low levels in the diet. Food Chem Toxicol. 2004;42: 65–83.
23. National Association for Continence. 1999. http://www.nafc.org/

Aging Skin Microbiology

110

Duane L. Charbonneau, Yuli Song, and Chengxu Liu

Contents

D.L. Charbonneau (✉) • C. Liu
The Procter & Gamble Company, Cincinnati, OH, USA
e-mail: charbonneau.dl@pg.com; liu.c.34@pg.com

Y. Song
The Procter & Gamble Company, Mason Business Center, Mason, OH, USA
e-mail: song.y.7@pg.com

M.A. Farage et al. (eds.), *Textbook of Aging Skin*,
DOI 10.1007/978-3-662-47398-6_83

Abstract

Our skin is colonized with large numbers of microbes and provides selective niches for various microbial communities. The analysis of 16S and/or 18S rRNA gene sequences revealed that, similar to the other parts of our body, the skin hosts highly diverse microbial communities that are not only site specific but also differ among different individuals. Furthermore, studies have also begun to bring to light the intimate relationships shared between host and resident microbes and to reveal the role of skin microbiota in skin health and diseases. Studies also show that as the skin ages, changes in skin physiology alter the associated microbiota, with implications for skin integrity and susceptibility to infection. In this chapter, the present understanding of the microbiota associated with human skin and its role in skin health and disease is described, and what is currently known about changes to such communities as the skin ages is reviewed.

Introduction

The skin, the largest organ of the body, was initially perceived as a passive barrier between the host and the environment. It is now clear that the skin is more than just a physical barrier that prevents penetration of undesirable environmental materials; it is also an immunological barrier. Skin is equipped with a highly sophisticated immune system: when operating optimally, the skin immune system manages the innate and adaptive immunity in a dialogue with the microbes living on it to select, calibrate, and terminate responses in the most appropriate manner to ensure effective host defense and also to maintain or restore tissue homeostasis and overall health.

Like any other part of our body that is exposed to external environment, our skin is colonized with large numbers of microbes and provides selective niches for various microbial communities. Historically, microbiota associated with the skin was characterized by techniques that identified only those organisms amenable to culturing. However, advances in genomic analysis yield a more comprehensive and complex picture of the microbial inhabitants of our skin. Furthermore, studies have also begun to bring to light the intimate relationships shared between host and resident microbes. In this chapter, the present understanding of the microbiota associated with human skin and its role in skin health and disease is described, and what is currently known about changes to such communities as the skin ages is reviewed. These changes in microbial communities may be related to environmental changes within the various skin environments that are natural consequences of the aging process such as changes in pH, moisture, and nutrients within the skin matrix.

Skin Microbiota

The skin harbors large numbers of microbes: cell densities of bacteria on forehead skin, for example, range from 10^4 to 10^6 cfu/cm^2, as assessed by culture [1]. Microbes that inhabit the skin are considered to be either transient or resident biota [2]. Transient biota becomes attached to the skin as a result of contact with contaminated items or environmental surfaces, for example, by handling raw foods or by resting the forearms on a table. Such microbes are inconsistently isolated from the skin surfaces. The transfer of transient biota to and from fomites and from person to person plays a critical role in infectious disease transmission. Studies have documented transfer of such organisms from an individual's hands to other parts of the body as well as transfer between individuals. The classic example is the work of Gwaltney and colleagues [3] which demonstrated the importance of hand-to-hand transmission of the common cold virus. In contrast, resident skin biota is the complex communities of microbes that consistently inhabit the skin and are not routinely removed by washing with non-medicated soaps. Resident bacteria include *Staphylococcus*, *Micrococcus*, *Corynebacterium*, *Rhodococcus*, *Propionibacterium*, *Brevibacterium*, *Dermabacter*, and *Acinetobacter* [2]. The community composition of resident skin biota is believed to be as essential to the health of the skin as gut microorganisms are to the overall health of the individual [4]. Resident microbiota promote health through pathogen inhibition, immune modulation, and by sustaining the integrity of the skin barrier; however, under the right conditions, certain constituents of the skin biota, such as *Staphylococcus aureus*, *Staphylococcus epidermidis*, *Streptococcus pyogenes*, *Candida* spp., and *Acinetobacter* spp., may become opportunistic pathogens [2, 5]. Additionally, constant exposure to particular microbiota that are transient in nature may result in a transition of a microorganism from transient to resident.

Diversity of the Skin Microbiota

Historically, the skin was considered to harbor rather simple microbial communities, based on the culturing-based analysis. However, with the advances of next-generation sequencing technologies, combined with NIH Human Microbiome program [6], our knowledge on skin microbiome and its contributions to our skin health is significantly broadened. The analysis of 16S and/or 18S rRNA gene sequences revealed that, similar to the other parts of our body, the skin hosts highly diverse microbial communities that are not only site specific but also differ among different individuals [7–12]. Studies show that the bacterial community of the skin includes a vast array of anaerobic and aerobic communities; among the fungal biota, yeasts of the genus *Malassezia* appear to predominate [11, 12]. Moreover, bacteria were also detected in subepidermal compartments of the skin [13] though it is unclear if these or any microorganisms identified by sequencing approaches are metabolically active, as these techniques are unable to distinguish viable from nonviable microorganisms. Different skin environmental surfaces also harbor unique resident microbiota which may occur because of the unique conditions at that skin site.

There are at least 19 bacterial phyla detected from the skin using 16S rRNA gene analysis, but most sequences are assigned to four phyla: *Actinobacteria*, *Firmicutes*, *Proteobacteria*, and *Bacteroidetes*. Although all subjects bear diverse communities of skin microbiota, only a few species were consistently found on the skin of every subject. Consequently, it has been suggested that the skin microbiota form a scaffold that rests on a small number of resident genera and species but supports a high frequency of diverse and variable transients [14].

Variation by sites: The complexity and stability of the microbial community are determined primarily by the specific physiological characteristics of the skin sites; different distribution of hair follicles, eccrine and apocrine glands, and sebaceous glands contribute to the variable cutaneous microenvironments and likely select for subsets of bacteria that can thrive in those specialized conditions. The studies showed that the microbiota is more similar to the same site on another individual than to any other site on the same individual, indicating that the host physiology of a site is a greater determinant of the microbiota composition than the individual genetic variation among healthy subjects. At the sebaceous sites, such as the forehead, retroauricular crease (behind the ear), the back, and the alar crease (side of the nostril), lipophilic microorganisms (e.g., *Propionibacterium* spp. and *Malassezia* spp.) are found to be the dominant organisms. In these sites, bacterial diversity seems to be lowest, suggesting that there is selection for specific subsets of organisms that can tolerate conditions in these areas. In contrast, the dry areas, such as the forearm, buttock, and various parts of the hand, harbor the most diverse bacterial phylogenetic types, with a greater prevalence of β-*Proteobacteria* and *Flavobacteriales*. Costello et al. [9] found that in these dry skin areas, the bacterial diversity is greater than communities in the gut and oral cavity. At the moist sites including the umbilicus (navel), the axillary vault, the inguinal crease (side of the groin), the gluteal crease (topmost part of the fold between the buttocks), the sole of the foot, the popliteal fossa (behind the knee), and the antecubital fossa (inner elbow), the microorganisms that thrive in moist condition (e.g., *Staphylococcus* and *Corynebacterium* spp.) are the most abundant. In a recent study [11] on fungal microbial communities, analysis showed that 11 core body and arm sites were dominated by fungi of the genus *Malassezia*, with only species-level classifications revealing fungal-community composition differences between sites. By contrast, 3 ft sites – plantar heel, toenail, and toe web – showed high fungal diversity.

Interpersonal variations: The interpersonal variation of microbiota at various body sites is different. High level of microbial variability among individuals is observed at dry skin areas. Studies show that the volar forearm of different individuals was found to only share 2 % of species-level OTUs (operational taxonomic units) [14], while the hands share 13 % of OTUs [15]. Comparisons of male and female skin microbiota suggest that females harbor a greater diversity of bacteria on their hands, but it remains unclear whether this observed difference is due to physiological factors or differences in hygiene and cosmetic usage [15]. In Grice et al.'s study [8], they demonstrated that interpersonal variation is lowest in sebaceous areas such as the alar crease, the back, and the manubrium (upper chest). These studies depict the skin microbiota as predominately composed of a handful of stable inhabitants (such as *Propionibacterium* and *Staphylococcus* spp.). Rare and/or transient species make up the balance and account for interpersonal variation. Factors driving the variability are unclear, but it is postulated that they may include external environmental factors (e.g., climate and geography), host immune status, host pathophysiology, and/or historical exposures.

Temporary variations: Variation between human body sites in adults is relatively stable over time, even though it is site dependent. In the Grice study [8], they found that the most consistent sites over time were the external auditory canal (inside the ear), the nare (inside the nostril), and the inguinal crease, whereas there were appreciable variation at the popliteal fossa, volar forearm, and buttock. In general, sites that harbor a greater diversity of microorganisms tend to be less stable over time; these sites include the volar forearm (forearm), the popliteal fossa, the antecubital fossa, the plantar heel (the bottom of the heel of the foot), and the interdigital web space (between the fingers). Compared with the microbiome of the gut and the mouth, these skin sites' microbiome had the greatest variability over time which may be a reflection of interactions with the environment or the overall stability of the particular skin site [16].

Important Constituents of the Skin Microbiota

Gram-Positive Bacteria

Staphylococcus spp. on the skin are considered commensals that may, in some cases, become opportunistic pathogens [17]. The most common *Staphylococcus* species on the skin are distinguished by their inability to produce coagulase, an enzyme that plays a role in virulence. There are 32 species of coagulase-negative staphylococci, of which 15 are exclusive to humans, and 10 routinely isolated from normal glabrous skin. *S. epidermidis* and *Staphylococcus hominis* are the species most frequently isolated from the skin by culture-dependent techniques. *S. epidermidis* colonizes the upper part of the body preferentially and constitutes over 50 % of the resident staphylococci identified with these methods. Occasionally, these organisms cause nosocomial infections in patients with indwelling foreign bodies such as heart valves and intravenous catheters. Staphylococci also can spread from one person to another in patient care settings, setting off a cascade of infection among susceptible individuals. Such has been the case in several hospital outbreaks, where improper hand washing by care providers facilitates transmission of staphylococcus infection.

For as long as microorganisms have been cultured from the skin and from sites of infection, *S. aureus*, a coagulase-positive *Staphylococcus*, has been identified as a constituent of the skin biota. This microorganism is considered transient because it is not routinely isolated from all skin sites. However, it is often found on the hands and perineum and in the vaginal biota and, as noted earlier, is considered a normal constituent of the biota of the nasal cavity [18, 19]. An estimate shows that 86.9 million people in the USA are colonized with *S. aureus* in the nares, where the organisms appear to be acting as a commensal [20]. *S. aureus* are important human pathogens, particularly those strains that produce superantigenic toxins. The organism causes clinical outcomes ranging from minor and self-limited skin infections to invasive and life-threatening diseases. *S. aureus* expresses many virulence factors (both secreted and cell surface associated) that contribute to evasion. At present, *S. aureus* infections are treated with antibiotics; unfortunately, many antibiotic-resistant strains have arisen, including methicillin-resistant *S. aureus* (MRSA), now found in both hospital and community settings [21]. Vancomycin-intermediate and vancomycin-resistant *S. aureus* strains (VISA and VRSA) have also been documented [22–24], a critical development as vancomycin has been regarded an antibiotic of last resort.

Two other ubiquitous members of the skin microbiota, *S. epidermidis* and *Propionibacterium acnes*, are predominant on human epithelia and in sebaceous follicles, respectively. Some bacterial physiological properties suggest they can help to keep transient, potential pathogens at bay. For examples, *S. epidermidis* is able to produce antimicrobials and *P. acnes* can produce short-chain fatty acids that inhibit the proliferation of various bacterial and fungal species. These features can function together with host-derived components of the innate host defense to establish and maintain the composition of a health-associated skin microbiota. However, depending largely on the host status, the relationship between the human host and *S. epidermidis* and *P. acnes* can also be parasitic features as well.

Other gram-positive bacteria are worthy of mention. Although less frequently detected by culture-dependent techniques than the staphylococci, at least eight different *Micrococcus* species have been identified from human skin [2]. *Micrococcus luteus* is by far the most common of the micrococci detected by culture, followed by *Micrococcus varians*. Coryneforms are gram-positive pleomorphic bacilli included in the classification of skin commensals. This group includes the *Corynebacterium* spp., *Propionibacterium* spp., *Dermabacter* spp., and *Brevibacterium* spp. *P. acnes*, abundant on the skin of the scalp, forehead, and back, is by far the most predominant coryneform.

Gram-Negative Bacteria

Gram-negative rods are not commonly isolated from normal healthy adult skin, probably because the skin is too dry as an environment. Gram-negative bacterial species on the skin often derive from the gastrointestinal system and contaminate other areas of the body. These microbes occasionally become resident flora in moist intertriginous areas such as the axilla and toe webs and also may become established on mucosal surfaces of the nose. In addition, *Acinetobacter* and *Pseudomonas* species are Gram-negative constituents of the skin biota; as noted earlier, their presence seems to be site dependent [7].

Mycobiota

Fungi and yeast are often detected in the skin microbiota of healthy people, particularly *Malassezia*, which inhabit the hair follicles. Pityrosporum species are most numerous on the back and chest, with highest numbers paralleling areas of highest sebum excretion. Yeasts such as *Candida* species, normally found on up to 40 % of mucous membranes, seldom colonize healthy skin. Increased skin colonization by these yeasts is seen in immunosuppressed patients, diabetics, and patients with psoriasis or atopic dermatitis [11, 12].

Tables 1 and 2 show the skin microorganisms by culture-based and molecular-based methods.

Table 1 The resident skin microflora identified by culture-based methods

I. Gram-positive bacteria	
Micrococcaceae	
Staphylococcus	Coagulase-positive *Staphylococcus*
	S. aureus
	Coagulase-negative *Staphylococcus*
	S. epidermidis
	S. hominis
	S. haemolyticus
	S. capitis
	S. midis
	S. warneri
	S. pyogenes
	S. saprophyticus
	S. simulans
	S. xylosus
	S. cohnii
	S. saccharolyticus
	S. sciuri
Micrococcus	*M. luteus*
	M. varians
	M. lylae
	M. kristinae
	M. sedentarius
	M. roseus
	M. nishinomiyaensis
	M. agieis
Coryneforms	
Corynebacterium	*C. diphtheriae*
	C. diphtheriae gravis
	C. diphtheriae mitis
	C. diphtheriae belfanti
	C. diphtheriae intermedius
	Nondiphtheriae corynebacteria (diphtheroids)
	C. minutissimum
	C. tenuis
	C. xerosis
	C. jeikeium (CDC group JK)
	C. striatum
	C. afermentans

(*continued*)

Table 1 (continued)

Propionibacterium	*P. acnes*
	P. granulosum
	P. avidum
Brevibacterium	
Dermabacter	
II. Gram-negative bacteria	
Acinetobacter	*A. calcoaceticus*
	A. johnsonii
	S. junii
Pseudomonas	*P. aeruginosa*
III. Mycoflora	
Pityrosporum	*P. ovale*
	P. orbiculare
Malassezia	*M. furfur*
	M. sympodialis
	M. globosa
	M. slooffiae
	M. restricta
	M. robusta
	M. pachydermatis
Candida	*C. albicans*
	C. tropicalis
	C. parapsilosis

Contributions of Skin Microbiota to a Healthy Host

The manner in which the skin microbiota contributes to the health of the host is not fully defined, but the existence of microcolonies and biofilms on the skin may imply the existence of consortia of microbial symbionts and commensals that function in concert with the host to assure homeostasis. Some mechanisms by which the microbiota contribute to the health of the host are discussed below.

Direct Pathogen Inhibition Through Production of Antimicrobial Substances

Pathogen inhibition by symbionts and commensals is accomplished by various mechanisms. The first is a passive mechanism – competitive exclusion – whereby resident microbiota occupy skin sites that could be inhabited by pathogenic

Table 2 Skin microflora bacteria species only detected by 16S gene clone library

Phyla/genus	Genus/species
Actinobacteria	
Corynebacterium	*C. coyleae*
	C. mucifaciens
	C. lipophiloflavum
	C. appendicis
	C. imitans
	C. sundsvallense
	C. glaucum
	C. glucuronolyticum
	C. matruchotii
	C. durum
	C. pseudotuberculosis
	C. pseudogenitalium
	C. tuberculostearicum
	C. accolens
	C. simulans
	C. aurimucosum
	C. nigricans
	C. singulare
	C. amycolatum
	C. kroppenstedtii
Mycobacterium	*M. chlorophenolicum*
	M. obuense
Tsukamurella	*T. tyrosinosolvens*
Rhodococcus	*R. erythropolis*
	R. corynebacterioides
Dietzia	*D. maris*
Gordonia	*G. sputi*
	G. bronchialis
	G. terrae
Mobiluncus	*M. curtisii* subsp. *holmesii*
Actinomyces	*A. neuii*
	A. naeslundii
Gardnerella	*G. vaginalis*
Brevibacterium	*B. paucivorans*
Janibacter	*J. melonis*
Tetrasphaera	*T. elongata*
Kocuria	*K. marina*
	K. palustris
	K. rhizophila
Rothia	*R. aeria*
	R. nasimurium
	R. mucilaginosa
	R. dentocariosa
Nakamurella	*N. multipartita*
Microlunatus	*M. phosphovorus*

(*continued*)

Table 2 (continued)

Phyla/genus	Genus/species
Atopobium	*A. vaginae*
Firmicutes	
Anaerococcus	*A. prevotii*
Peptoniphilus	*P. harei*
Peptostreptococcus	*P. anaerobius*
Veillonella	*V. dispar*
	V. parvula
Lactobacillus	*L. crispatus*
	L. jensenii
Leuconostoc	*L. argentinum*
Streptococcus	*S. infantis*
	S. gordonii
	S. parasanguinis
	S. sanguinis
	S. cristatus
	S. salivarius
	S. intermedius
	S. agalactiae
Gemella	*G. haemolysans*
	G. morbillorum
	G. sanguinis
Facklamia	*F. hominis*
	F. languida
Eremococcus	*E. coleocola*
Granulicatella	*G. elegans*
Enterococcus	*E. faecalis*
Bacillus	*B. licheniformis*
	B. subtilis
Proteobacteria	
Methylobacterium	*M. extorquens*
	M. mesophilicum
Bradyrhizobiaceae	*Bradyrhizobiaceae* spp.
Rhizobiales	*Rhizobiales* spp.
Pedomicrobium	*P. australicum*
Hyphomicrobium	*H. facile*
Paracoccus	*Paracoccus* spp.
Sphingopyxis	*Sphingopyxis* spp.
Sphingobium	*S. amiense*
Caulobacteraceae	*Caulobacteraceae* spp.
Paracraurococcus	*Paracraurococcus* spp.
Brevundimonas	*B. aurantiaca*
	B. vesicularis
Pasteurellaceae	*Pasteurellaceae* spp.
Haemophilus	*Haemophilus* spp.
Serratia	*S. marcescens* subsp. *sakuensis*
Diaphorobacter	*D. nitroreducens*

(*continued*)

Table 2 (continued)

Phyla/genus	Genus/species
Acidovorax	*A. temperans*
Aquabacterium	*Aquabacterium* spp.
Pseudomonas	*P. saccharophila*
Burkholderiales	*Burkholderiales* spp.
Neisseria	*Neisseria subflava*
Neisseriaceae	*Neisseriaceae* spp.
Betaproteobacteria	*Betaproteobacteria* spp.
Stenotrophomonas	*S. maltophilia*
Xanthomonadaceae	*Xanthomonadaceae* spp.
Acinetobacter	*A. ursingii*
	A. haemolyticus
Alkanindiges	*Alkanindiges* spp.
Enhydrobacter	*E. aerosaccus*
Gammaproteobacteria	*Gammaproteobacteria* spp.
Pseudomonas	*P. stutzeri*
	P. tremae
Bacteroidetes	
Hymenobacter	*Hymenobacter* spp.
Chitinophaga	*Chitinophaga* spp.
Flavobacteriaceae	*Flavobacteriaceae* spp.
Porphyromonas	*Porphyromonas* spp
Prevotella	*P. corporis*
	P. disiens
	P. bivia
	P. melaninogenica
Cyanobacteria	
Deinococcus-Thermus	
Thermomicrobia	

Cited data from Gao et al. [14], Dekio et al. [25]

microorganisms. For example, *S. epidermidis* occupies receptors on the host cell that also can be recognized by more virulent bacteria such as *S. aureus*. A second mechanism is the scavenging of nutrients essential for the growth and proliferation of pathogenic bacteria. For example, *Corynebacterium jeikeium* produces siderophores that sequester iron and also has specialized mechanisms for acquiring of manganese. Manganese acquisition is essential for protecting this bacterium from superoxide radicals. Superoxide dismutase, a manganese-dependent enzyme, may protect both the resident bacterium and the host from oxidative damage. The sequestering of iron and manganese by resident bacteria robs potential pathogens of these growth-limiting substrates.

Table 3 Antimicrobial substances produced by *S. epidermidis*

Factor	Function	Reference
Esp, an extracellular serine protease	Destroys preexisting *S. aureus* biofilms and enhances the bactericidal activity of β-defensin 2 toward *S. aureus* in biofilms	[26, 27]
Phenol-soluble modulins (PSMs)	Selectively kill skin pathogens like *S. aureus* via disruption of lipid membrane and enhance the antimicrobial activity of host-derived antimicrobial peptides	[28]
Epidermin, epilancin K7 and 15X, epicidin 280 and Pep5	Lanthionine-containing antibacterial peptides, effective against *S. aureus*, group A streptococcus, and *Streptococcus pyogenes*	[29–31]
Autoinducing peptides	Suppress the expression of virulence factors in *S. aureus* via cross inhibition of *S. aureus* quorum-sensing system	[32]
Succinic acid (fermentation of S. epidermidis of glycerol)	Antimicrobial efficacy against *P. acnes*	[33]

A third mechanism is the production by resident microbiota of secondary metabolites with antimicrobial and/or antibiofilm properties. Table 3 shows the examples of antimicrobial substances produced by *S. epidermidis*.

In addition to *S. epidermidis*, other skin commensals also show the properties of antimicrobial effects. For example, *S. aureus* can be a commensal inhabitant of the skin, especially in the nasal area. It is estimated that 32 % of the US population carries *S. aureus* without infection [16]. Certain strains of *S. aureus* produce bacteriocins (e.g., staphylococcin 462 peptide) that inhibit the growth of other *S. aureus* strains. Thus, colonization by *S. aureus* can result in a positive benefit for the host. Propionibacteria also produce bacteriocins and bacteriocin-like compounds. These compounds include propionicin PLG-1; jenseniin G; propionicins SM1, SM2, and T1; and acnecin, which are inhibitory toward lactic acid-producing bacteria, gram-negative bacteria, yeasts, and molds. *Pseudomonas aeruginosa* is a member of the resident skin microbiota in certain moist areas of the skin. These bacteria produce potent compounds that inhibit the growth of other microorganisms. *P. aeruginosa* has been shown to suppress the growth of fungal species such as *Candida krusei*, *C. kefir*, *C. guilliermondii*, *C. tropicalis*, *C. lusitaniae*, *C. parapsilosis*, *C. pseudotropicalis*, *C. albicans*, *Saccharomyces cerevisiae*, *Torulopsis glabrata*, and *Aspergillus fumigatus*. A classic example is the production of pseudomonic acid A by *P. fluorescens*. Pseudomonic acid A is the active ingredient in the commercial topical antibiotic, Mupirocin®, commonly used in the treatment and prevention of streptococcal and staphylococcal infections [17].

Immune Modulation of Host Defense Function

Growing evidence suggests cross talk between the microbiota and the skin immune system. The skin microbes control the production of antimicrobial peptides by keratinocytes through Toll-like receptor (TLR) signaling. Li et al. [34] found that Lipopeptide LP01 produced by *S. epidermidis* increases the expression of β-defensin 2 and β-defensin 3 in neonate human epidermal keratinocytes via activation of TLR2/CD36-p38 MAPK. Wanke et al. [35] showed that *S. epidermidis* triggers TLR2 and thus NF-κB activation in primary human keratinocytes, whereas *S. aureus* activates the mitogen-activated protein kinase and phosphatidylinositol 3-kinase/AKT signaling pathways, suggesting that *S. epidermidis* sensitizes human keratinocytes toward pathogenic bacteria and amplifies the innate immune response. The skin microbiota also promotes the expression of other potent and highly conserved pathways of host defense. For instance, skin-resident microbes can increase expression of components of the complement system. This system is composed of a large number of proteins that react with one another to opsonize pathogens and induce inflammatory responses that promote clearance of pathogens. The skin microbiota also controls the level of expression of interleukin-1 (IL-1), a cytokine involved in the initiation and amplification of immune responses. Most recently, a study showed that the colonization with *S. epidermidis* induces IL-17A(+) CD8(+) T cells, enhances innate barrier immunity, and limits pathogen invasion. Commensal-specific T-cell responses result from the coordinated action of skin-resident dendritic cell subsets and are not associated with inflammation, revealing that tissue-resident cells are poised to sense and respond to alterations in microbial communities [36]. Collectively, these results reveal their capacity to promote various aspects of innate and adaptive responses [37].

Maintaining Skin Tissue Homeostasis

Group A streptococci produce a cytolytic toxin known as streptolysin O (SO) that is considered part of the pathogenic arsenal of this organism. Despite its toxigenic effects, SO also plays a role in wound healing by stimulating keratinocyte migration. Low concentrations of SO induce the cell adhesion molecule, CD44, and subsequently increase the production of collagen, hyaluronate, and other extracellular matrix components that facilitate wound healing [38]. The cytotoxin, streptokinase, also derived from streptococcal species, is now used clinically for fibrinolysis. Consequently, it is becoming apparent that certain virulence factors produced by group A streptococci also may be an asset to the host. A more recent study demonstrated for the first time a mutually beneficial relationship between *S. epidermidis* and keratinocyte inflammatory responses; a unique lipoteichoic acid (LTA) produced by *S. epidermidis* inhibits uncontrolled skin inflammation during skin injury through its capacity to bind to the innate immune receptor TLR 2 [39]. Another study [40] showed preliminary data suggesting that protective immunity to a cutaneous pathogen is critically dependent on the skin microbiota. It showed that germ-free mice could not mount an appropriate immune response against intradermal *Leishmania* major infection; however, immunity could be rescued by allowing *S. epidermidis* colonization on the skin of germ-free mice. IL-1α production was significantly reduced in GF and monoassociation of GF mice with *S. epidermidis* restored the production of this cytokine, suggesting resident commensals are required for optimal IL-1 signaling in the skin, which in turn promotes local effector responses (IL-17 production).

Skin Microbiota and Skin Disease

Although the resident skin microbiota typically may play a role in protecting the host, under certain circumstances, constituents of the resident biota may themselves be pathogenic [2]. When the potential role of the microbiota in health or disease is explored, it has to be put in the context of host states. The capacity of a given microbe to trigger or promote disease is highly dependent on the state of activation of the host's genetic predisposition, the localization of the particular microbe, or the coexistence of other microbial members as well as environmental factors of the environment. Many studies have suggested that microbes not only contribute to skin infections but also may contribute to noninfectious pathologies, such as atopic dermatitis, psoriasis, rosacea, and acne [41–45].

Breaches in skin integrity provide opportunities for infection by cutaneous biota. *S. aureus* and *S. pyogenes* are the two major organisms responsible for common skin and soft tissue infections [46]. Similarly, CA-MRSA infections are commonly associated with breaches in the skin integrity [47]. *S. epidermidis*, long considered an important member of the resident skin biota, is a nosocomial pathogen associated with infections of surgical wounds and medical implants [5, 48]. Other resident microbiota, such as *S. warneri*, *Corynebacterium* spp., and *Pseudomonas* spp., have also been demonstrated to cause infections. Yeast vulvovaginitis is a common example of pathogenesis by constituents of skin and mucosal biota. *Candida albicans* and other *Candida* species commonly colonize the vagina and external genitalia of healthy women without frank infection, but disruptions to the community composition of the vulvovaginal microbiota can lead to overgrowth of these organisms and the development of yeast vulvovaginitis [49].

There is emerging evidence indicating the association of skin disease with an imbalance of microbiome, known as dysbiosis. *P. acnes* is a common skin commensal microorganism, but it is also the primary disease-associated bacterium of acne. Studies indicate only certain strains of *P. acnes* are highly associated with acne [50, 51]. Atopic dermatitis (AD) has long been associated with increased *S. aureus*, but a recent metagenomic study showed that *Staphylococcus* species increased during flares, but, surprisingly, both *S. aureus* and *S. epidermidis* increased. Clinical effectiveness of AD treatments does not rely on the total elimination of *S. aureus*, suggesting that therapeutic modalities may act to recalibrate the diversity of the skin microbiome [52–54]. The yeasts of the genus *Malassezia* are also believed to contribute to and exacerbate the development of atopic dermatitis, seborrheic dermatitis, and dandruff [55]. Patients with atopic dermatitis or atopic eczema are more likely to raise *Malassezia*-specific IgE antibodies than healthy controls [56]. Furthermore, the higher cutaneous pH of patients with atopic dermatitis may enhance the release of allergens from some *Malassezia* species [57]. Interestingly, although certain *Malassezia* species (e.g., *M. globosa* and *M. restricta*) are found in both AD patients and healthy subjects, specific genotypes are more highly associated both with AD [58] and with seborrheic dermatitis [59]. In the case of psoriasis, no clear dichotomy in fungal microbiota has been found between patients and healthy subjects [60], but significant alterations have been observed in the bacterial composition: bacterial diversity was higher in psoriatic lesions than on healthy skin of the same patient or on the skin of disease-free subjects, with overrepresentation of the *Firmicutes* phylum and underrepresentation of the *Actinobacteria* and *Proteobacteria* phyla [61]. Most strikingly, the genus *Propionibacterium*, including the major cutaneous species *P. acnes*, was highly underrepresented on affected skin. Hence, psoriasis lesions are accompanied by a significant ecological shift in associated skin microbiota, but the mechanisms underlying this shift remain to be determined.

Skin microbiota also play a role in disease transmission. Differentiating between transient and resident biota has shed light particularly on the role that skin biota on the hands play in the transmission of infectious disease. Frequent exposure to certain transient microbes may lead to their becoming established constituents of the resident skin biota. For example, nurses performing similar tasks within a hospital exhibit similarities among their resident microbiota, but the skin microbiota of those assigned to different tasks have distinct constituents [62]. Similarly, bacterial constituents of the resident skin microbiota of homemakers often are identical to those of isolates identified within the home environment [63]. Multiple studies have established an association of skin biota on the hands with hospital-acquired and community-acquired infections [64–66].

Microbiology of Skin Aging

Intrinsic and Extrinsic Aging

Two primary processes, known as intrinsic and extrinsic aging, contribute to aging skin. Intrinsic aging is the result of genetically programmed cellular aging processes that occur naturally. Extrinsic aging, also known as premature aging, refers to degeneration associated with exogenous causes, some of which include sun exposure, poor nutrition, smoking, alcohol consumption, and pollution. The best-studied extrinsic aging process is caused by solar UV radiation, resulting in wrinkling, altered pigmentation, and, potentially, neoplasia. Prematurely damaged or aged skin also presents challenges to the attendant microbiota, with consequences for the health of the host.

Studies on human microbiota have shown the links that exist between the microbiota and a variety of clinical problems plaguing older adults such as *Clostridium colitis*, vulvovaginal atrophy, colorectal carcinoma, and atherosclerotic disease. There is also growing evidence that microbes also affect the rate of aging itself [67, 68]. A study in invertebrate systems indicates microbes extend their effects beyond host pathology, to systemic modulation of the rate of aging. Data indicates that beyond their role as a nutrient source and potential pathogen, *E. coli* secreted diffusible molecules including metabolites and small RNAs that directly impacted *Caenorhabditis elegans* aging [67]. In the skin, studies also show that as the skin ages, changes in skin physiology alter the associated microbiota, with implications for skin integrity and susceptibility to infection; however, the role of microbiome in skin aging is unknown.

Skin Microbiota in Childhood Through Adolescence

The time of birth marks a significant change for the skin of the newborn as it undergoes transitions from an aqueous and mostly sterile environment of the womb to a gaseous one with constant microbial interaction. During this time of development, infant skin has been shown to differ from adult skin in structure, function, and biochemical composition [69]. It has been reported by both of culture-based and molecular-based analysis that skin microbiota of newborns within 24 h after birth correlates strongly with the model of delivery; the microbiome of infants delivered vaginally is close to the one of mother's vagina dominated by *Lactobacillus*, *Prevotella*, or *Sneathia* spp., and C-section infants harbored bacterial communities similar to those found on the skin surface, dominated by *Staphylococcus*, *Corynebacterium*, and *Propionibacterium* spp. [70]. However, a latter study [71] did not show any significant difference in microbiome with regard to model of delivery. The data from this study [71] indicates the microbiota of newborns is not fully established within the first few weeks or even months of life but rather evolves over the first year and likely beyond. It is dynamic enough that initial differences (within 24 h of delivery) arising from model of delivery disappear within a month of life. 16S rDNA sequencing analysis showed that in contrast to adult skin where *Proteobacteria*, *Actinobacteria*, and *Firmicutes* dominated in that order, the infants are colonized predominantly by *Firmicutes* (*Staphylococcus* and *Streptococcus*), followed in abundance by *Actinobacteria*, *Proteobacteria*, and *Bacteroidetes*. It also demonstrates that although the number of genera in an area does not significantly change over the first year, the relative abundance of the community significantly increases with age. The microbial colonization during this early period could affect the long-term stability of microbiome and is expected to critically affect the development of the skin immune function and perhaps the maturation of other skin barrier functions as well as the development of the systemic immune system.

Yeast components of the skin microbiota in children are predominantly *Candida* species (non-lipophilic yeasts) and *Malassezia* species (lipophilic yeasts) [72]. In preterm infants, staphylococci colonize the skin earlier than *Propionibacterium* and *Malassezia* species, as latter have a slower growth rate and might require greater maturation of epidermal structures [73]. In babies, most skin infections are associated with *S. aureus* (which colonizes the umbilicus and nasopharynx of many infants) or with either *S. epidermidis*, coliforms, *Pseudomonas*, or yeasts [74]. *Malassezia* species are significant in that they have been implicated in certain systemic neonatal infections [75].

Progression from infancy to adulthood encompasses major biological changes with significant physiologic skin alterations that in turn influence the host-microbiome relationship. In the 1970s, changes in facial skin biota with age were studied. The levels of resident aerobic and anaerobic bacteria on the face depend on age [76], and changes seem to be related to sebum production. For example, concentrations of anaerobic diphtheroids and surface aerobic micrococci were higher in the infants than in young children. At puberty, cell densities of microorganisms on facial skin increased, especially during late adolescence. The observed changes in skin microbiota may be the result of hormonal or physiological changes that alter the skin environments as the skin matures. An obvious example is the increased incidence of acne and other skin infections in adolescents compared to prepubertal children. Moreover, host factors can also affect the types of metabolites produced by the skin microbiota. For example, sex hormones have been shown to have an impact on the compositions of gingival biota [77]. A more recent study [78] using 16S rDNA sequence analysis showed that the microbiome of young children and adolescent/post-adolescent individuals clustered into two distinct groups. A greater diversity of bacteria including *Streptococcus* and gram-negatives *Moraxella*, *Haemophilus*, and *Neisseria* dominated the young children; in contrast, the adolescent/post-adolescent individuals were dominated by lipophilic bacteria including *Propionibacterium*, *Corynebacterium*, and *Turicella*.

Skin Microbiota in Adults

As discussed extensively in the previous sections, the microbiota of adult human are both complex and variable based on site, age, sex, and ethnicity. Within the inhabitant microbial communities, the relationship with the host ranges from mutualistic to parasitic. The resident skin microbiota is thought to play a critical role in establishing homeostasis within the host. However, the balance between the host and the microbiota is delicate and can change rapidly following breaches in skin integrity, leading to infection. Bacterial and fungal species and strains on the skin vary considerably depending on the skin environment and immune status. With the advent of culture-independent molecular techniques, the range of microorganisms identified from human skin has expanded significantly, and understanding of the composition of the skin microbiota will likely continue to increase as these techniques become routine. Recent studies have shown that there is a core set of microorganisms that comprise most of the resident skin microbiota, but less common bacteria comprising the balance of the population may be transients that differ significantly among individuals and between sample times.

Skin Microbiota in the Aged

Several structural and functional changes in the skin occur intrinsically as the skin ages. The skin becomes drier, barrier function is reduced, skin turnover rates diminish, and structural proteins, such as collagen, become more disorganized. These, as well as other cellular changes, are a natural consequence of passing time. Other physiological effects, such as hormonal changes, changes in immune function, and lower rates of wound healing, affect the skin's ability to function as the interface between internal and external environments [79]. Aged skin has a higher pH, is less hydrated, less elastic, more permeable, and more susceptible to infection. A dysregulation of immune function and a possible decline in cell-mediated immunity (signaled by reduced numbers of epidermal Langerhans cells that process and present antigen to T cells) likely affects host resistance to infections. In some populations, malnutrition, obesity, institutional care, and dementia also become risk factors for infection. Consequently, the skin of older adults is structurally and functionally different from that of younger age groups. For example, a study showed that the prevalence of skin colonization by *Proteus mirabilis* and *Pseudomonas aeruginosa* in people over 65 is 25 % higher than that in younger people [80]. Yeasts are also recovered more often encountered in the flora of the skin of the elderly [81].

The microbiota of aged populations has not been completely characterized. However, older adults are more susceptible to a number of skin infections. For example, cellulitis, a bacterial infection of the lower dermis and subcutaneous tissue, is more common among the aged. Breaches in skin integrity from various causes can be precipitating factors for this infection. *S. pyogenes* (β-hemolytic streptococci belonging to Lancefield group A) and *S. aureus* are the most common pathogens associated with cellulitis [79].

Infections causing deep tissue necrosis, which can lead to sepsis, also are more commonly associated with elderly patients. They can be attributed to a dysbiosis, or imbalance, that occurs between the microbiota and the host. Polymicrobial necrotizing infections (type I necrotizing fasciitis) are typically associated with combinations of gram-positive organisms such as streptococci and either staphylococci, enterococci, enteric gram-negative bacteria, or anaerobes. In contrast, monomicrobial necrotizing infections (type II necrotizing fasciitis) are predominately associated with either a group A streptococci or *S. aureus*. Fungal infections, which usually are not serious, can occur in older adults when there is trauma, chaffing, or poor hygiene. Candidiasis develops in moist, intertriginous areas such as the groin, perineum, and axillae. Ringworm (dermatophytosis) and tinea versicolor are also seen in this population.

Conclusion

The skin is the first line of defense against environmental insults and pathogenic microbes. The resident skin microbiota plays a critical role in maintaining the health of the skin by inhibiting pathogen invasion, stimulating host innate immunity, and maintaining skin barrier function. The intrinsic and extrinsic processes that contribute to skin aging are well understood, but the impact of these changes on the composition and function of skin microbiota has not been studied extensively.

Recent studies have begun to bring to light the intimate relationships shared between host and resident microbes. There is accumulating data that show potential benefit of the resident bacteria on the skin; they do not only coexist despite our immune defense network but actually modify immunity, and the potential negative consequences of complete depletion microbiota from the skin by indiscriminate use of topical and systemic antibiotics. As knowledge of the characteristics and functionality of the skin microbiota expands and lifetime changes in the skin biota are better understood, it may become possible to develop probiotic or other targeted forms of therapy to reduce skin infections in the aged and to help maintain skin health throughout a lifetime.

Cross-References

▶ The Vaginal Microbiota in Menopause

References

1. Evans CA. Persistent individual differences in the bacterial flora of the skin of the forehead: numbers of propionibacteria. J Invest Dermatol. 1975;64:42–6.
2. Chiller K, Selkin BA, Murakawa GJ. Skin microflora and bacterial infections of the skin. J Invest Dermatol. 2001;6:170–4.
3. Gwaltney JM, Moskalski Jr PB, Hendley JO. Hand-to-hand transmission of rhinovirus colds. Ann Intern Med. 1978;88:463–7.
4. Christensen GJ, Brüggemann H. Bacterial skin commensals and their role as host guardians. Benefic Microbes. 2014;5:201–15.
5. Dong Y, Speer CP. The role of *Staphylococcus epidermidis* in neonatal sepsis: guarding angel or pathogenic devil? Int J Med Microbiol. 2014;304:513–20.
6. Collaborators, Human Microbiome Project Consortium. A framework for human microbiome research. Nature. 2012;486:215–21.
7. Grice EA, Kong HH, Renaud G, et al. A diversity profile of the human skin microbiota. Genome Res. 2008;18:1043–50.
8. Grice EA, Kong HH, Conlan S, Deming CB, Davis J, Young AC. Topographical and temporal diversity of the human skin microbiome. Science. 2009;324:1190–2.
9. Costello EK, Lauber CL, Hamady M, Fierer N, Gordon JI, Knight R. Bacterial community variation in human body habitats across space and time. Science. 2009;326:1694–7.
10. Ursell LK, Clemente JC, Rideout JR, Gevers D, Caporaso JG, Knight R. The interpersonal and intrapersonal diversity of human-associated microbiota in key body sites. J Allergy Clin Immunol. 2012;129:1204–8.
11. Findley K, Oh J, Yang J, Conlan S, Deming C, Meyer JA, Schoenfeld D, Nomicos E, Park M, NIH Intramural Sequencing Center Comparative Sequencing Program, Kong HH, Segre JA. Topographic diversity of fungal and bacterial communities in human skin. Nature. 2013;498:367–70.
12. Paulino LC, Tseng CH, Blaser MJ. Analysis of *Malassezia* microbiota in healthy superficial human skin and in psoriatic lesions by multiplex real-time PCR. FEMS Yeast Res. 2008;8:460–71.
13. Nakatsuji T, Chiang HI, Jiang SB, Nagarajan H, Zengler K, Gallo RL. The microbiome extends to subepidermal compartments of normal skin. Nat Commun. 2013;4:1431.
14. Gao Z, Tseng CH, Pei Z, Blaser MJ. Molecular analysis of human forearm superficial skin bacterial biota. Proc Natl Acad Sci U S A. 2007;104:2927–32.
15. Fierer N, Hamady M, Lauber CL, Knight R. The influence of sex, handedness, and washing on the diversity of hand surface bacteria. Proc Natl Acad Sci U S A. 2008;105:17994–9.
16. Caporaso JG, Lauber CL, Costello EK, Berg-Lyons D, Gonzalez A, Stombaugh J, Knights D, Gajer P, Ravel J,

Fierer N, Gordon JI, Knight R. Moving pictures of the human microbiome. Genome Biol. 2011;12:R 50.
17. Cogen AL, Nizet V, Gallo RL. Skin microbiota: a source of disease or defence? Br J Dermatol. 2008;158:442–55.
18. Peacock SJ, de Silva I, Lowy FD. What determines nasal carriage of *Staphylococcus aureus*? Trends Microbiol. 2001;9:605–10.
19. von Eiff C, Becker K, Machka K, Stammer H, Peters G. Nasal carriage as a source of *Staphylococcus aureus* bacteremia. Study Group. N Engl J Med. 2001;344:11–6.
20. Mainous 3rd AG, Hueston WJ, Everett CJ, Diaz VA. Nasal carriage of *Staphylococcus aureus* and methicillin-resistant S aureus in the United States, 2001–2002. Ann Fam Med. 2006;4:132–7.
21. Goetghebeur M, Landry PA, Han D, Vicente C. Methicillin-resistant *Staphylococcus aureus*: a public health issue with economic consequences. Can J Infect Dis Med Microbiol. 2007;18:27–34.
22. Aligholi M, Emaneini M, Jabalameli F, Shahsavan S, Dabiri H, Sedaght H. Emergence of high-level vancomycin-resistant *Staphylococcus aureus* in the Imam Khomeini Hospital in Tehran. Med Princ Pract. 2008;17:432–4.
23. Oliveira GA, Dell'Aquila AM, Masiero RL, et al. Isolation in Brazil of nosocomial *Staphylococcus aureus* with reduced susceptibility to vancomycin. Infect Control Hosp Epidemiol. 2001;22:443–8.
24. Tiwari HK, Sen MR. Emergence of vancomycin resistant *Staphylococcus aureus* (VRSA) from a tertiary care hospital from northern part of India. BMC Infect Dis. 2006;6:156.
25. Dekio I, Sakamoto M, Hayashi H, Amagai M, Suematsu M, Benno Y. Characterization of skin microbiota in patients with atopic dermatitis and in normal subjects using 16S rRNA gene-based comprehensive analysis. J Med Microbiol. 2007;56:1675–83.
26. Iwase T, Uehara Y, Shinji H, Tajima A, Seo H, Takada K, Agata T, Mizunoe Y. *Staphylococcus epidermidis* Esp inhibits *Staphylococcus aureus* biofilm formation and nasal colonization. Nature (London). 2010;465:346–9.
27. Vengadesan K, Macon K, Sugumoto S, Mizunoe Y, Iwase T, Narayana SVL. Purification, crystallization and preliminary X-ray diffraction analysis of the *Staphylococcus epidermidis* extracellular serine protease Esp. Acta Crystallogr Sect F Struct Biol Cryst Commun. 2013;69:49–52.
28. Cogen AL, Yamasaki K, Muto J, Sanchez KM, Crotty Alexander L, Tanios J, Lai Y, Kim JE, Nizet V, Gallo RL. *Staphylococcus epidermidis* antimicrobial delta-toxin (phenol-soluble modulin-gamma) cooperates with host antimicrobial peptides to kill group A *Streptococcus*. PLoS One. 2010;5(1):e8557.
29. Bierbaum G, Gotz F, Peschel A, et al. The biosynthesis of the lantibiotics epidermin, gallidermin, Pep5 and epilancin K7. Antonie Van Leeuwenhoek. 1996;69:119–27.
30. Ekkelenkamp MB, Hanssen M, Danny Hsu ST, et al. Isolation and structural characterization of epilancin 15X, a novel lantibiotic from a clinical strain of *Staphylococcus epidermidis*. FEBS Lett. 2005;579:1917–22.
31. Sahl HG. Staphylococcin 1580 is identical to the lantibiotic epidermin: implications for the nature of bacteriocins from Gram-positive bacteria. Appl Environ Microbiol. 1994;60:752–5.
32. Otto M. *Staphylococcus aureus* and *Staphylococcus epidermidis* peptide pheromones produced by the accessory gene regulator *agr* system. Peptides. 2001;22:1603–8.
33. Wang Y, Kuo S, Shu M, Yu J, Huang S, Dai A, Two A, Gallo RL, Huang C-M. *Staphylococcus epidermidis* in the human skin microbiome mediates fermentation to inhibit the growth of Propionibacterium acnes: implications of probiotics in acne vulgaris. Appl Microbiol Biotechnol. 2014;98:411–24.
34. Dongqing L, Hu L, Zhiheng L, Hongquan L, Yue W, Yuping L. A novel lipopeptide from skin commensal activates TLR2/CD36-p38 MAPK signaling to increase antibacterial defense against bacterial infection. PLoS One. 2013;8(3):e58288.
35. Wanke I, Steffen H, Christ C, Krismer B, Gotz F, Peschel A, et al. Skin commensals amplify the innate immune response to pathogens by activation of distinct signaling pathways. J Invest Dermatol. 2011;131:382–90.
36. Naik S, Bouladoux N, Linehan JL, Han SJ, Harrison OJ, Wilhelm C, Conlan S, Himmelfarb S, Byrd AL, Deming C, Quinones M, Brenchley JM, Kong HH, Tussiwand R, Murphy KM, Merad M, Segre JA, Belkaid Y. Commensal-dendritic-cell interaction specifies a unique protective skin immune signature. Nature. 2015;520:104–8.
37. Nakamizo S, Egawa G, Honda T, Nakajima S, Belkaid Y, Kabashima K. Commensal bacteria and cutaneous immunity. Semin Immunopathol. 2015;37:73–80.
38. Tomic-Canic M, Mamber SW, Stojadinovic O, Lee B, Radoja N, McMichael J. Streptolysin O enhances keratinocyte migration and proliferation and promotes skin organ culture wound healing in vitro. Wound Repair Regen. 2007;15:71–9.
39. Lai Y, Di Nardo A, Nakatsuji T, Leichtle A, Yang Y, Cogen AL, Wu ZR, Hooper LV, Schmidt RR, von Aulock S, Radek KA, Huang CM, Ryan AF, Gallo RL. Commensal bacteria regulate Toll-like receptor 3-dependent inflammation after skin injury. Nat Med. 2009;15:1377–82.
40. Naik S, Bouladoux N, Wilhelm C, Molloy MJ, Salcedo R, Kastenmuller W, Deming C, Quinones M, Koo L, Conlan S, Spencer S, Hall JA, Dzutsev A, Kong H, Campbell DJ, Trinchieri G, Segre JA, Belkaid Y. Compartmentalized control of skin immunity by resident commensals. Science. 2012;337:1115–9.
41. Weyrich LS, Dixit S, Farrer AG, Cooper AJ, Cooper AJ. The skin microbiome: associations between altered

microbial communities and disease. Australas J Dermatol. 2015 PubMed 25715969.
42. SanMiguel A, Grice EA. Interactions between host factors and the skin microbiome. Cell Mol Life Sci. 2015;72:1499–515.
43. Belkaid Y, Segre JA. Dialogue between skin microbiota and immunity. Science. 2014;346:954–9.
44. Grice EA. The skin microbiome: potential for novel diagnostic and therapeutic approaches to cutaneous disease. Semin Cutan Med Surg. 2014;33:98–103.
45. Sanford JA, Gallo RL. Functions of the skin microbiota in health and disease. Semin Immunol. 2013;25:370–7.
46. Elston DM. Epidemiology and prevention of skin and soft tissue infections. Cutis. 2004;73:3–7.
47. Redziniak DE, Diduch DR, Turman K, et al. Methicillin-resistant *Staphylococcus aureus* (MRSA) in the Athlete. Int J Sports Med. 2009;30 (8):557–62.
48. O'Gara JP, Humphreys H. *Staphylococcus epidermidis* biofilms: importance and implications. J Med Microbiol. 2001;50:582–7.
49. Sobel JD. Vulvovaginal candidosis. Lancet. 2007;369:1961–71.
50. Lomholt HB, Kilian M. Population genetic analysis of *Propionibacterium acnes* identifies a subpopulation and epidemic clones associated with acne. PLoS One. 2010;5:e12277.
51. Yu Y, Champer J, Garbán H, Kim J. Typing of Propionibacterium acnes: a review of methods and comparative analysis. Br J Dermatol. 2015;172:1204–9.
52. Kong HH, Oh J, Deming C, Conlan S, Grice EA, Beatson MA, Nomicos E, Polley EC, Komarow HD, NISC Comparative Sequence Program, Murray PR, Turner ML, Segre JA. Temporal shifts in the skin microbiome associated with disease flares and treatment in children with atopic dermatitis. Genome Res. 2012;22:850–9.
53. Sanchez DA, Nosanchuk JD, Friedman AJ. The skin microbiome: is there a role in pathogenesis of atopic dermatitis and psoriasis? J Drugs Dermatol. 2015;14 (2):127–30.
54. Salava A, Lauerma A. Role of the skin microbiome in atopic dermatitis. Clin Transl Allergy. 2014;4:33.
55. Harada K, Saito M, Sugita T, Tsuboi R. *Malassezia* species and their associated skin diseases. J Dermatol. 2015;42:250–7.
56. Brodská P, Panzner P, Pizinger K, Schmid-Grendelmeier P. IgE-mediated sensitization to *malassezia* in atopic dermatitis: more common in male patients and in head and neck type. Dermatitis. 2014;25:120–6.
57. Selander C, Zargari A, Mollby R, Rasool O, Scheynius A. Higher pH level, corresponding to that on the skin of patients with atopic eczema, stimulates the release of *Malassezia* sympodialis allergens. Allergy. 2006;61:1002–8.
58. Sugita T, Tajima M, Amaya M, Tsuboi R, Nishikawa A. Genotype analysis of *Malassezia* restricta as the major cutaneous flora in patients with atopic dermatitis and healthy subjects. Microbiol Immunol. 2004;48:755–9.
59. Tajima M, Sugita T, Nishikawa A, Tsuboi R. Molecular analysis of *Malassezia* microflora in seborrheic dermatitis patients: comparison with other diseases and healthy subjects. J Invest Dermatol. 2008;128:345–51.
60. Takemoto A, Cho O, Morohoshi Y, Sugita T, Muto M. Molecular characterization of the skin fungal microbiome in patients with psoriasis. J Dermatol. 2015;42:166–70.
61. Gao Z, Tseng CH, Strober BE, Pei Z, Blaser MJ. Substantial alterations of the cutaneous bacterial biota in psoriatic lesions. PLoS One. 2008;3:e2719.
62. Aiello AE, Cimiotti J, Della-Latta P, Larson EL. A comparison of the bacteria found on the hands of 'homemakers' and neonatal intensive care unit nurses. J Hosp Infect. 2003;54:310–5.
63. Larson EL, Gomez-Duarte C, Lee LV, Della-Latta P, Kain DJ, Keswick BH. Microbial flora of hands of homemakers. Am J Infect Control. 2003;31:72–9.
64. Bloomfield SF, Aiello AE, Cookson B, O'Boyle C, Larson EL. The effectiveness of hand hygiene procedures in reducing the risks of infections in home and community settings including handwashing and alcohol-based hand sanitizer. Am J Infect Control. 2007;35(10 Suppl 1):S27–64.
65. Hadaway LC. Skin flora and infection. J Infus Nurs. 2003;26:44–8.
66. Larson E. Skin hygiene and infection prevention: more of the same or different approaches? Clin Infect Dis. 1999;29:1287–94.
67. Heintz C, Mair W. You are what you host: microbiome modulation of the aging process. Cell. 2014;156:408–11.
68. Zapata HJ, Quagliarello VJ. The microbiota and microbiome in aging: potential implications in health and age-related diseases. J Am Geriatr Soc. 2015;63:776–81.
69. Stamatas GN, Nikolovski J, Luedtke MA, Kollias N, Wiegand BC. Infant skin microstructure assessed in vivo differs from adult skin in organization and at the cellular level. Pediatr Dermatol. 2010;27:125–31.
70. Dominguez-Bello MG, Costello EK, Contreras M, Magris M, Hidalgo G, Fierer N, Knight R. Delivery mode shapes the acquisition and structure of the initial microbiota across multiple body habitats in newborns. Proc Natl Acad Sci U S A. 2010;107:11971–5.
71. Capone KA, Dowd SE, Stamatas GN, Nikolovski J. Diversity of the human skin microbiome early in life. J Invest Dermatol. 2011;131:2026–32.
72. Nobel WC. Microbiology of human skin. 2nd ed. - London: Lloyd Luke Medical Books; 1981.
73. Bernier V, Weill FX, Hirigoyen V, et al. Skin colonization by *Malassezia* species in neonates: a prospective study and relationship with neonatal cephalic pustulosis. Arch Dermatol. 2002;138:215–8.
74. Venkatesh MP, Placencia F, Weisman LE. Coagulase-negative staphylococcal infections in the neonate and

child: an update. Semin Pediatr Infect Dis. 2006;17:120–7.
75. Juncosa Morros T, Gonzalez-Cuevas A, Alayeto Ortega J, et al. Cutaneous colonization by *Malassezia* spp. in neonates. An Esp Pediatr. 2002;57:452–6.
76. Leyden JJ, McGinley KJ, Mills OH, Kligman AM. Age-related changes in the resident bacterial flora of the human face. J Invest Dermatol. 1975;65:379–81.
77. Klinger G, Eick S, Klinger G, et al. Influence of hormonal contraceptives on microbial flora of gingival sulcus. Contraception. 1998;57:381–4.
78. Oh J, Conlan S, Polley EC, Segre JA, Kong HH. Shifts in human skin and nares microbiota of healthy children and adults. Genome Med. 2012;10:4–77.
79. Klein NC, Cunha BA. Skin and soft tissue infections. In: Yoshikawa TT, Norman DC, editors. Infectious disease in the aging. Totowa: Human Press; 2001. p. 139–45.
80. Lertzman BH, Gaspari AA. Drug treatment of skin and soft tissue infections in elderly long-term care residents. Drugs Aging. 1996;9:109–21.
81. Somerville DA. The normal flora of the skin in different age groups. Br J Dermatol. 1969;81:248–58.

Percutaneous Penetration of Chemicals and Aging Skin

111

Michael F. Hughes

Contents

M.F. Hughes
U.S. Environmental Protection Agency, Office of Research and Development, National Health and Environmental Effects Research Laboratory, Research Triangle Park, NC, USA
e-mail: hughes.michaelf@epa.gov

M.A. Farage et al. (eds.), *Textbook of Aging Skin*,
DOI 10.1007/978-3-662-47398-6_74

Abstract

Human skin undergoes several changes as a person ages. Physiological changes within the body have a major influence on intrinsic aging, and exposure to ultraviolet radiation has a dominant role in extrinsic aging. Changes that occur in aging skin include dryness, reduction of sebaceous gland activity, decreased amount of skin surface lipid, and others. Several human and animal studies have examined the effect of age on chemical penetration of skin. This potential effect of age on chemical penetration is important as humans are living longer now than 20–30 years ago. Animal studies show skin penetration of chemicals is related to the hair growth cycle in hairless mice. This strain is born hairless, rapidly grows hair, and becomes hairless again around 25 days of age. The in vitro penetration of several alkanols increased up to 25 days of age in hairless mice and then started to decline out to 60 days of age. The skin penetration of the alkanols then remained constant. Other animal studies using older age groups report no or limited age effects on chemical skin penetration. The results of a human in vivo study suggest that age affects the dermal absorption of chemicals that are hydrophilic (e.g., benzoic acid). Penetration of these type of chemicals was greater in a younger (<41 years old) than older (65–86 years old) age group. The penetration of hydrophobic chemicals (e.g., testosterone) was not affected by age. Overall, more studies are needed to assess the effect of age on chemical penetration of skin.

Introduction

The human body undergoes changes, for better or worse, from infancy to the elderly stages of life. These changes are observed from the biochemical level within cells to the morphology and function of whole organs. The skin is an organ that changes with age from both intrinsic and extrinsic factors. Intrinsic aging of the skin is primarily determined by genetics. Extrinsic aging of the skin is principally caused by environmental exposure to ultraviolet light. This is also termed photoaging. In areas of the skin that are sun exposed, these two processes of aging may be superimposed upon one another [1]. In the industrialized world, humans are living longer because of advancements in agriculture, medicine, and public health. In the United States, the Census Bureau projects the percentage of the population 65 years of age or older will increase from 13 % in 2010 to 20 % in 2040 [2]. Because of the increasing age of the population, it is important to know how age-related changes in organs, such as skin, will impact overall health, particularly with exposure to environmental chemicals and the administration of drugs using transdermal delivery systems.

Changes occur in the epidermis and dermis with increasing age [3–5]. Within the stratum corneum, the outermost layer of the epidermis, alterations with increasing age include decreased content of moisture [6] and skin surface lipids [7]. However, Luebberding et al. [8] recently examined the skin barrier function of 150 healthy women of 18–80 years of age by measuring transepidermal water loss (TEWL), stratum corneum hydration, sebum content, and pH value. They examined several skin regions such as the forehead and forearm. Overall, the age of the subject was not related to TEWL and stratum corneum hydration. Sebum production decreased significantly with age and the pH of the skin surface significantly increased in women of ages 50–59 years. The epidermis becomes thinner and more flattened with age, although the thickness of the stratum corneum is not altered [9, 10]. The area of contact and adherence between the epidermis and the underlying dermis is decreased. Thus, in the elderly, simple trauma to the skin may remove the epidermis more easily than in younger adults. Within the dermis, the vasculature, principally the capillaries that supply blood to the viable epidermis, is diminished. The decreased blood flow in the skin of the aged appears to be affected by autonomic influences and may be site dependent [11]. This reduced blood supply can result in a longer time for wounds to heal, decreases in inflammatory response, and altered thermal regulation.

Humans are exposed to chemicals throughout their life span. Exposure to chemicals, including drugs, environmental contaminants, industrial and household chemicals, agrochemicals, personal care products, and others, can be intentional or accidental. Exposure to chemicals occurs by the oral, pulmonary, or percutaneous routes and can result in their systemic absorption. The amount of chemical absorbed and potential effects that may result are dependent on the route of exposure as well as other factors.

In order for a chemical to be systemically absorbed following dermal exposure, it must undergo a series of partitioning steps through the epidermis [12]. Active and facilitated transport mechanisms, such as those that occur in oral absorption, are not involved in dermal absorption. Dermal absorption is a process of passive diffusion. First, the chemical on the skin surface partitions into the stratum corneum. This may require partitioning of the chemical from a vehicle or formulation. The chemical then diffuses across the stratum corneum and partitions into the underlying viable epidermis. Diffusion of the chemical across the viable layers of the epidermis occurs, followed by partitioning into the dermis. The final steps are diffusion across the dermis and partitioning into the circulatory or lymphatic system. The main driver in dermal absorption is the concentration of the chemical on the surface of the stratum corneum. Upon dermal exposure to a chemical, a concentration gradient is produced and results in a mass transfer of chemical from

Table 1 Exposure-, skin-, and chemical-related factors that can affect dermal absorption of chemicals

Exposure related	Skin related	Chemical related
Chemical concentration	Age	Molecular weight
Duration	Thickness	Lipid solubility
Use of protective equipment	Blood flow	Water solubility
Climate (temperature and humidity)	Damage	Irritancy
Matrix (e.g., soil)	Metabolism	Other chemicals (e.g., enhancers)
Surface area	Occlusion	
Vehicle	Anatomical site of exposure	
	Hair and pore density	

Adapted from Semple [13]

the surface of the skin, through the epidermis, and into the dermis.

There are three proposed routes of dermal absorption [12]. These include the intercellular, transcellular, and appendageal routes. It is generally thought that the intercellular route predominates in dermal absorption, while the other two routes have a minor role. The mechanism by the intercellular route involves partitioning of the chemical into the lipid-rich extracellular regions of the stratum corneum cells, the corneocytes. The chemical then diffuses around the corneocytes. Lipophilic chemicals diffuse through the lamellar acyl chains of the lipid, while hydrophilic chemicals diffuse through the polar head groups of the lipid. For the transcellular route, the chemical goes through the keratin-filled corneocytes by partitioning into and out of the extracellular lipid. For the appendageal route, the chemical bypasses the stratum corneum by entering the shunts of the hair follicles and sebaceous and sweat glands.

Many but not all chemicals are able to penetrate the skin and are absorbed into the systemic circulation; the extent and rate of absorption vary between chemicals and are affected by many variables (Table 1). The main barrier is the stratum corneum, which is lipid-rich and impedes the absorption of many compounds, particularly those with hydrophilic properties. Because of its lipid-rich nature, the stratum corneum can be a reservoir for lipophilic chemicals [14]. Lipophilic chemicals partition into the stratum corneum but diffuse no further or to a limited extent because of their physical and chemical properties. The more aqueous environment of the lower layers of the viable epidermis and dermis relative to the stratum corneum also has an impact on the penetration of lipophilic compounds, adding to this reservoir effect. Over time, these chemicals may eventually be systemically absorbed or lost when the stratum corneum is sloughed off.

Dermal absorption of chemicals can be affected by exposure-, skin-, and chemical-related factors (Table 1). These include anatomical site of exposure, species, vehicle, and age. A classic example of the effect of age on dermal absorption is the toxicity that occurred following the use of hexachlorophene as a disinfectant on the skin of preterm infants [15]. Preterm infants are susceptible to the effects of chemicals and drugs applied to the skin, because their stratum corneum is not fully developed at birth [16]. These exposed preterm infants later developed neurological deficiencies because hexachlorophene, a neurotoxicant, was absorbed through their skin that had not fully matured. Skin that has fully developed can retard the absorption of many chemicals.

Whether aging skin maintains its barrier properties to the absorption of chemicals has been questioned and is still being investigated. From microscopic examination, the barrier of the stratum corneum does not appear to be compromised in aged skin [10]. Nevertheless, this alone does not indicate the barrier properties of aged skin are intact. Studies in the 1960s by Christophers and Kligman [17] suggested that the permeability of skin from the elderly (>66 years old) was different from that of younger adults (<29 years old). In vitro experiments using human cadaver skin showed the permeability of fluorescein was about seven times greater in the skin from the older than the younger subjects [17]. However, in another in vitro experiment using skin from living subjects, there was no difference in the permeability of water between the two age groups [17]. Christophers and Kligman [17] also conducted an in vivo experiment with radiolabeled testosterone applied to the backs of young and old subjects. In contrast to the in vitro study with fluorescein, the penetration of testosterone over 24 h was greater in the younger than in the older group. It should be noted that this experiment was done by measuring the loss of radioactivity on the skin, which is not the most reliable measurement for assessing the penetration of a chemical through the skin. In a final experiment by Christophers and Kligman [17], intradermally injected radiolabeled sodium and non-labeled fluorescein were cleared at a more rapid rate in the younger than the elderly group. This suggested changes in the microcirculation occurred in the dermis of the latter group. However, DeSalva and Thompson [18] reported contrasting results in a similar study. They observed similar clearance rates of radiolabeled sodium administered intradermally in the face and hands of subjects 50 years of age or older, but the rates were slower in subjects 30 years of age or younger. However, when administered into the hand, the clearance of radiolabeled sodium was slower in subjects aged 71 years or older than subjects 60 years of age or younger. Studies by Tagami [19] suggested that the barrier of the stratum corneum to absorption of chemicals was increased in the elderly. In one in vivo study with young (21–35 years old) and old (52–81 years old) subjects, fewer older subjects developed erythema following a 2-min exposure on the forearm to 0.1 % tetrahydrofurfuryl nicotinic acid ester. In another in vivo study [19], it took 2–2.5 h for tetrachlorosalicylanilide (TSCA) (1.5 % in ethylene glycol) to penetrate the stratum corneum of the forearms of older subjects (62–82 years old). In younger subjects (22–39 years old), the TSCA penetration time was about 1.5 h. Tagami [19] also conducted a study of the clearance of intradermally injected fluorescein and radiolabeled sodium in the mid-back and forearm of young (<36 years old) and older (>60 years old) subjects. The tissue clearance of the substances was lower in the older than in the younger group. The studies from these three laboratories indicate there are age-related differences in the dermal absorption of chemicals as well as their clearance after intradermal administration. However, there were discrepancies in their results. Some suggested greater absorption in the elderly, while some suggested greater absorption in younger subjects. Thus, at the time of completion of these studies, it was difficult to determine if an age group of adults was at potential risk from altered dermal absorption of chemicals due to age-related changes in skin.

Whether the changes in skin that occur in the elderly put them at risk for altered dermal absorption (enhanced or reduced) and potentially increased adverse health effects are not firmly established. Because it is unlikely that many of the elderly are employed, the potential for occupational dermal exposure to chemicals is low. However, environmental exposure is a reality as well as the use of chemicals (e.g., paint) in the home, health-care facilities, and other places an elderly person may reside. Changes in the skin with age could also impact the use of transdermal drug delivery in the elderly [20]. Transdermal drug delivery can be beneficial to those that are polymedicated, such as in the elderly. In addition, transdermal drug delivery has several advantages over oral and parenteral administration. In comparison to oral administration, transdermal administration bypasses hepatic first-pass metabolism and minimizes potential adverse effects that may arise from peak plasma drug concentrations and improves patient compliance. There is also a decreased risk of infection with transdermal delivery compared with parenteral administration. Health-care providers who prescribe drugs that are delivered transdermally should be aware of the issue of damaged skin in the incontinent and dependent elderly patient [21]. Dermal absorption of chemicals is generally increased when the integrity of the skin is damaged. In these types of patients, more drugs may be absorbed than intended if the transdermal patch is applied to damaged skin. Konda et al. [22] have summarized age-related pharmacokinetic data from new drug application submissions and drug labels of marketed transdermal products in the United States. Of the 15 drugs presented, 14 had age groups of adult and aged or elderly tested. There were no age-related relationships reported.

There has been a continued but somewhat limited effort in the laboratory setting to assess how the aging process affects dermal absorption. Several investigators have used animal models, generally mice and rats, and in vitro and in vivo techniques in their studies. The investigators have also taken a more systematic approach, examining the dermal absorption of chemicals that have similar structure (e.g., alkanols, phenols) and taking into account their physical and chemical properties (e.g., hydrophobic, hydrophilic). In vitro dermal absorption studies have advantages over in vivo studies in that more chemicals can be tested in a controlled setting, they can be less costly, and there is no direct testing of chemicals on animals. One drawback to the in vitro studies is that the vasculature in the dermis is not functional, which is important for dermal absorption in vivo. Although in vitro studies have become more acceptable to risk assessors, the results still need to be regarded carefully because the experimental technique cannot completely capture the events that occur in an in vivo exposure. The extrapolation from in vitro experiments using animal skin to human skin in vivo does include several uncertainties and makes meaningful predictions challenging.

Studies in Animals

Animal skin is commonly used as a model for human skin in dermal absorption studies of chemicals either used (e.g., pesticides) or found in the environment (e.g., arsenic). Reasons for this include that animal skin is more readily available than human skin for in vitro studies and that sample size can be increased for both in vitro and in vivo animal studies. Another benefit of the use of animals is that chemicals can be more easily tested in a controlled environment. Several studies have used animals that could be considered elderly. One drawback for the use of animals in these types of studies is that rodent skin tends to be more permeable to chemicals than human skin [23]. Thus, absorption values obtained from the use of animals in a controlled setting would most likely overestimate absorption in humans. This would need to be considered when assessing the potential risk to humans from dermal exposure to chemicals.

Behl et al. [24] examined the in vitro dermal absorption of radiolabeled alkanols using skin from male SKH/hr (hairless) mice ranging from 4 to 360 days of age. The mean life span of this mouse strain ranges from about 420 to 560 days. This strain is born hairless and rapidly grows hair, and they become fully hairless around 25 days of age. The alkanols varied from polar, moderately nonpolar to nonpolar solutes (methanol to n-octanol). The infinite dosing technique was used, which maintains a constant concentration gradient across the skin. Full-thickness skin from the abdomen and mid-back were used. If hair was present, it was removed with surgical scissors before placing the skin between two glass diffusion cells. The diffusion cells consisted of a donor cell and receptor cell, which were filled with physiological saline. A high concentration of chemical is placed in the donor cell. Aliquots of saline are removed over time from the receptor cell and analyzed for chemical. From this data, a permeability rate can be determined.

The permeability rates of the alkanols followed the same trend. Starting at 4 days of age, the permeability rates of the alkanols increased to a peak around 25 days of age. At this time of peak permeability, methanol had the lowest rate and n-octanol the highest. The rates for all of the alkanols then declined until the mice were about 60 days of age. From this age onward, the rates remained similar. The dorsal skin was more permeable to the alkanols than the abdominal skin. This difference lasted up to about 60 days, and then the permeability rates of the alkanols through the abdominal and dorsal skin were similar. The only exception was for n-octanol. The permeation rate for this alkanol was the same for either site at all ages. The increased permeability appeared to be related to the hair growth cycle of this mouse strain. Other than this time period, the barrier properties of the skin of this strain of mouse do not appear to be dependent on age. This laboratory reported similar in vitro results using hydrocortisone and the skin from even older SKR/hr mice than used with the alkanols [25]. The results from these studies provide useful information on the relationship between the physical and chemical properties of chemicals and dermal absorption. They also show that age can affect dermal absorption, although this effect in the mice was related to their hair growth cycle. This effect would most likely not be of relevance in humans, because the density of hair follicles in humans is less than in mice.

Hughes et al. [26] examined the in vitro dermal absorption of radiolabeled para-substituted phenols in male C57Bl/6 mice of ages 3, 15, and 27 months. The median life span of the female C57Bl/6 mouse is about 29–30 months. The chemicals were acetamidophenol, phenol, cyanophenol, and heptyloxyphenol. Hair from the dorsal surface was removed the day before the experiment. Full-thickness dorsal skin from the mice was placed in flow-through diffusion cells. The finite dosing technique was used, whereby chemical is applied onto the epidermal surface of the skin in a small volume of volatile vehicle. In this technique, the chemical is depleted from the surface over time as it penetrated the skin, and thus the concentration gradient is diminished. However, unlike the infinite dosing technique, the epidermal surface is open to the environment, as normally occurs. In this flow-through system, an aqueous-based receptor fluid was pumped below the skin into vials placed in a fraction collector. The chemicals were applied in ethanol at a dosage of 4 $\mu g/cm^2$. The experiment lasted 72 h and then the skin was washed with 70 % ethanol to remove unabsorbed chemical. Wash, skin, and receptor fluid were analyzed for chemical-derived radioactivity.

Significant age effects were detected in the absorption of phenol and heptyloxyphenol (Fig. 1). There was a significantly greater percent of the dose of these two compounds in the receptor fluid of the 27-month-old mice than of mice of the younger age groups. Conversely, there was a significantly greater percent of the dose of these two compounds in the skin of the two younger age groups. Also, there was a significantly greater percent of the dose of phenol in the receptor fluid of the 15-month- than of the 3-month-old mice. Overall, these age-dependent differences were <5 % for phenol detected in receptor fluid but were >40 % for heptyloxyphenol. There was no difference in the absorption of cyanophenol among the three age groups. For acetamidophenol, there was a significantly greater percent of the dose in the skin of the 15- and 27-month-old mice than in the 3-month-old mice. Although not significantly different, the skin wash removed about twice as much acetamidophenol from the 3-month-old mice than from the skin of the two older groups. The phenols tested differed in lipophilicity, with acetamidophenol the least lipid-soluble (Log octanol/water partition coefficient (Log P) 0.32) and heptyloxyphenol the most lipid soluble (Log P 4.75). The thickness of the dermis in this strain of mouse decreases with age [27]. Thus, the chemicals have a shorter distance to completely diffuse through the skin of the older than the younger mice in the in vitro setting. This change in mouse skin thickness may result in increased in vitro absorption of lipophilic compounds that can penetrate into the skin but are unable to efficiently partition out of it into the receptor fluid as observed with heptyloxyphenol in the 3- and 15-month-old mice. In this study, the mouse skin was a reservoir for heptyloxyphenol. However, the composition of the lipids in the skin of the 27-month-old mice may have changed that increased the ability of heptyloxyphenol to partition from the skin into the receptor fluid. This study indicates that, in addition to aging skin, the physical and chemical properties of a chemical can alter the extent of dermal absorption.

Banks et al. [28] examined the in vivo dermal absorption of radiolabeled 2,3,7,8-tetrachlorodibenzo-ρ-dioxin (TCDD) and 2,3,4,7,8-pentachlorodibenzofuran (4PeCDF) in male Fischer 344 rats of various ages (10, 36, and 96 weeks for TCDD; 10, 36, 64, 96, and

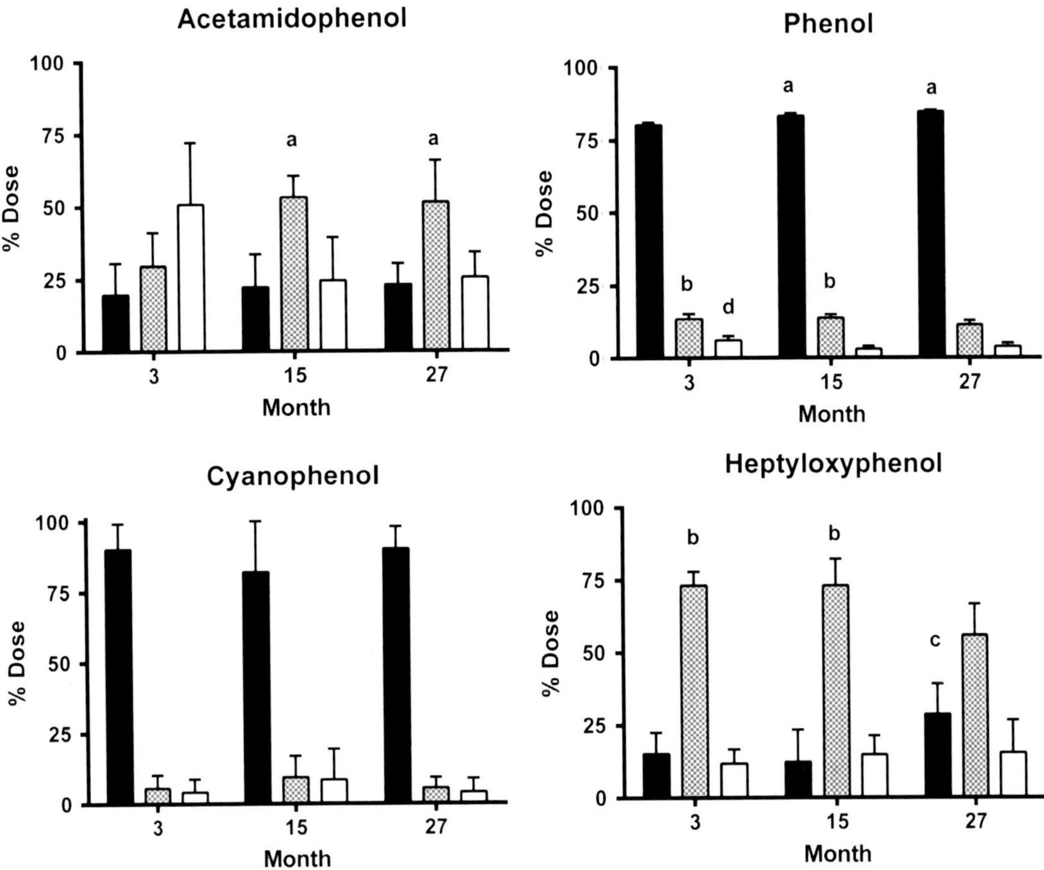

Fig. 1 Distribution of acetamidophenol-, phenol-, cyanophenol-, and heptyloxyphenol-derived radioactivity in receptor fluid (■), skin (▒), and skin wash (□) 72 h after exposure to mouse skin of different age groups [26]. Data represents mean ± standard deviation, $N = 4–9$. [a]Significantly greater than 3-month-old mice; [b]significantly greater than 27-month-old mice; [c]significantly greater than 3- and 15-month-old mice; [d]significantly greater than 15- and 27-month-old mice

120 weeks for 4PeCDF). The life span of this rat strain ranges from 120 to 160 weeks. The chemicals were applied in acetone at a dose of 0.1 μmole/kg over 1.8 cm^2 on the back of a shaved animal. The dose site was then covered with a non-occluding stainless steel cap. The animals were housed in individual metabolism cages for 3 days following exposure. Urine and feces were collected over the 3-day period. At the end of the experiment, the animals were sacrificed and tissues and the skin dosing site were removed. The excreta, tissues, and skin were analyzed for chemical-derived radioactivity. Chemical-derived radioactivity detected in excreta and tissues was considered absorbed. The treated skin was not washed to remove unabsorbed chemical. A previous study from this laboratory [29] reported that 80 % or more of the dose of TCDD and 4PeCDF was removed by an acetone swab wash 3 days after application. Thus, the authors considered chemical-derived radioactivity detected in the skin not absorbed.

In the treated skin, 80–94 % and 66–87 % of the dose of TCDD and 4PeCDF, respectively, were detected. Absorption of TCDD and 4PeCDF decreased with increasing age of the animals (Fig. 2). The changes were primarily between the 10- and 36-week-old rats. After 36 weeks, there were no significant age-related changes in absorption of TCDD. There was a significant difference in the tissue levels of 4PeCDF between the 64- and 96-week-old rats,

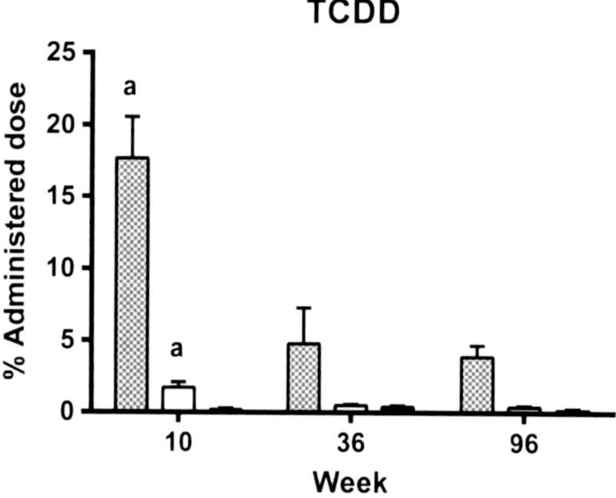

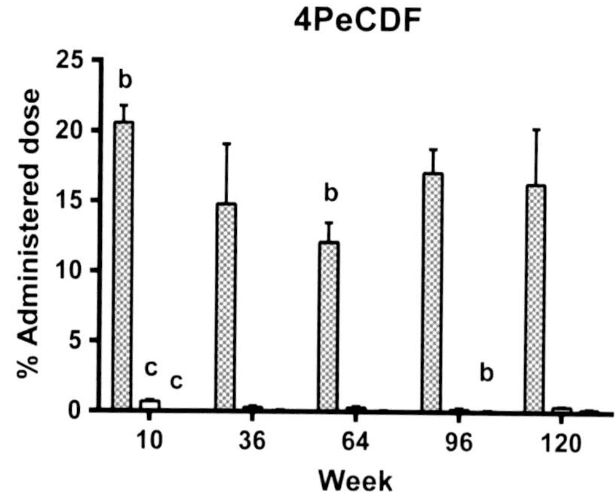

Fig. 2 Percent of the administered dose (0.1 μmol/kg) of TCDD- and 4PeCDF-derived radioactivity in tissues (▒), feces (□), and urine (■) of rats of different ages following a 3-day dermal exposure [28]. Data represents mean ± standard deviation, $N = 3–4$. [a]Significantly different ($p < 0.05$) versus 36- and 96-week-old TCDD-treated rats; [b]significantly different ($p < 0.05$) versus next age group of 4PeCDF-treated rats; [c]significantly different ($p < 0.05$) versus 36-, 64-, 96-, and 120-week-old 4PeCDF-treated rats

but the authors suggested this difference was due to experimental variability. Thus, this age-related decrease in the dermal absorption of these two lipophilic compounds occurred at an age when the rats would not be considered elderly but approaching midlife.

Lehman and Franz [30] examined the effect of age and caloric-restricted diet on the in vitro dermal absorption of water (tritiated), lidocaine, and hydrocortisone (tritated) in female Fischer 344 rat skin. Rodents on a caloric-restricted diet live longer and the age-related changes in the body are delayed compared to rodents fed ad libitum. The ages of the rats tested were from 11 to 144 weeks old. They used full-thickness skin and the finite dosing technique with Franz static diffusion cells. The hair on the dorsal surface of the rats was carefully clipped before placing the skin on the cells. In static cell studies, the receptor fluid remains below the skin and is directly sampled over time. The aliquots are then analyzed for chemical.

In the case of water, with the exception of the 144-week-old group of the ad libitum animals, neither age nor diet had an effect on its penetration (Fig. 3). (Note: there were only two surviving ad libitum animals in the last age group, out of the original 50.) With lidocaine in the ad libitum group, its permeability increased starting at 44 weeks and continued up to the last age group tested. In the caloric-restricted animals, lidocaine permeability increased at 44 weeks but then decreased with increasing age. For hydrocortisone, the penetration followed the same course as lidocaine, increasing at 44 weeks for both groups and continuing to increase in the ad libitum group, but decreasing in the caloric-restricted group. Thus, the penetration of the lipophilic compounds lidocaine and hydrocortisone increased with age in both dietary groups, relative to the ad libitum 11-week-old animals. This suggested that the innate aging of the skin was independent of dietary factors. The difference between the dietary groups was that, in the ad libitum animals, the total penetration of lidocaine and hydrocortisone kept increasing with age, whereas it decreased for both from the peak at 44 weeks in the caloric-restricted animals (but still remained higher than the ad libitum 11-week-old animals). The caloric-restricted animals were most likely not deficient in essential fatty acids, because they received 10 % corn oil in their diet. For an unknown reason, the skin of the caloric-restricted animals became more impervious to the lipophilic chemicals relative to the age-matched ad libitum animals. The age-related changes in the skin of the rat resulted in increased in vitro dermal absorption of lidocaine and

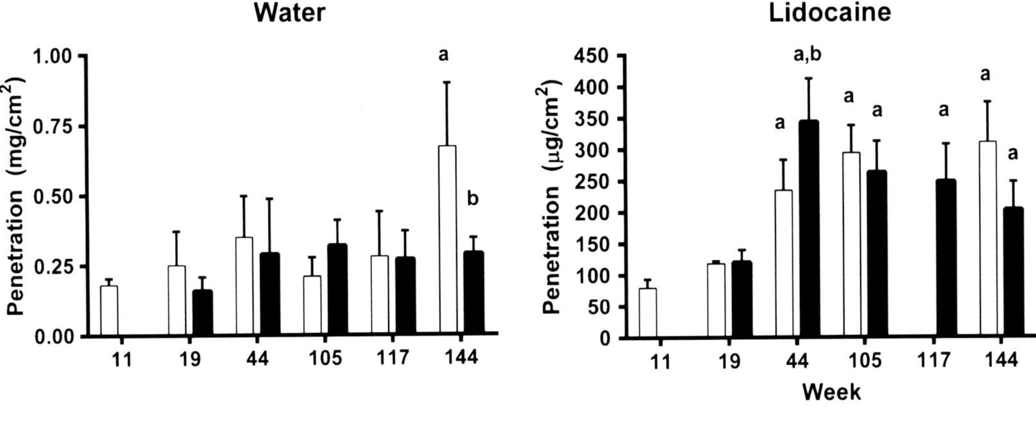

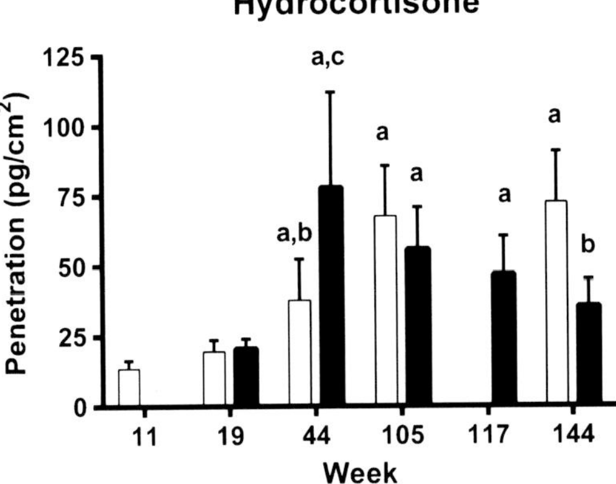

Fig. 3 Total in vitro penetration of water, lidocaine, and hydrocortisone through rat skin of different ages and diets (□, ad libitum; ■, caloric restricted) [30]. Data represents mean ± standard error of the mean, $N = 2$–6. [a]Significantly different from 11-week-old ad libitum animals; [b]significantly different from age-matched diet cohort; [c]significantly from 144-week-old diet-matched animals

hydrocortisone. This effect on the dermal absorption can be modified with the diet. The different result from the Banks et al. [28] study could be from the techniques used (in vitro vs. in vivo) and the chemical and physical properties of the chemicals used in these two studies.

The effect of photoaging from exposure to ultraviolet (UV) radiation and ovariectomy on dermal absorption was examined by Hung et al. [31]. As females enter the life stage of menopause, hormone deficiency begins to develop and as a result aging of the skin progresses [32]. The normal function of the skin is dependent on sex hormones; estrogen deficiency leads to loss of skin collagen. Collagen provides strength and elasticity to the skin. With loss of collagen, the skin becomes more fragile and can more easily be damaged. This damage may lead to increased dermal absorption to chemicals. Using the female nude mouse, there were four groups: (1) control, (2) UV light (separated into UVA and UVB) exposure, (3) ovariectomized, and (4) ovariectomized and exposed to UV light.

The stratum corneum was disrupted by UVB exposure and ovariectomy, as evidenced by increased transepidermal water loss in these two groups. Using Franz static diffusion cells, Hung et al. [31] assessed the in vitro dermal absorption of tretinoin, a lipophilic topical drug (Log P = 6.3) in the different groups. The skin accumulation and flux across the skin of tretinoin increased in UVA and UVB alone and ovariectomized plus UV light-exposed mice relative to control and ovariectomized alone mice. Uptake of tretinoin by the follicles was also increased in ovariectomized and ovariectomized plus UV light-exposed mice. The in vitro dermal absorption of estradiol was also assessed in this study. Skin deposition of estradiol (Log $P = 4.01$) was not affected by UV light alone or in any of the ovariectomized mice with and without UV light exposure. The flux of estradiol in the ovariectomy plus UVA-exposed mice was significantly increased. For follicular uptake, UVA alone and the ovariectomy plus UV light group were significantly elevated for estradiol. The high molecular weight compound dextran (4 kDa) was also examined in this same system with similarly pre-treated mice. The dermal absorption of high molecular weight compounds is generally low. Dextran was not detected in the media of any of the samples. Skin accumulation was significantly increased for UVA and UVB alone and in ovariectomy plus UVA-exposed mice. Dextran was not detected in the skin of ovariectomy plus UVB-exposed mice. In this same group, dextran was not detected in the follicles. There were no differences in the follicular amount of dextran in any of the other groups.

Studies in Humans

Roskos et al. [33] examined the in vivo percutaneous absorption of a select group of chemicals in humans of two age groups. A young group consisted of males and females of ages 22–40 years. An old group consisted of males and females of ages 65–86 years. All subjects were Caucasian and had no history of dermatologic disease. The test compounds were radiolabeled and included testosterone, estradiol, hydrocortisone, benzoic acid, acetylsalicylic acid, and caffeine. The chemicals were applied (4 μg/cm^2) in acetone onto the ventral surface of the forearm. Following evaporation of the acetone, a non-occluding patch was placed over the dosing site. Urine was collected at several time points up to 7 days postexposure. At 24 h postexposure, the patch was removed and the dosing site was washed to remove unabsorbed chemical. Following this wash, the dosing site was covered with a non-occluding patch. At 7 days postexposure, the patch was removed and the dosing site was washed again. To account for incomplete urinary excretion of chemical, each subject was administered the chemical intravenously. Urine was collected for 7 days after intravenous administration of chemical. The washes, patches, and urine were analyzed for chemical-derived radioactivity. The percent of the dose in the urine following dermal administration was corrected for incomplete urinary excretion by dividing this value by the percent of the dose in urine collected after intravenous administration. The adjusted value for percent of the dose in urine following dermal exposure to the chemicals was considered the absorbed dose.

The chemicals tested were divergent with respect to their water and lipid solubility. Testosterone is insoluble in water and the most lipophilic of the chemicals tested (Log P 3.32). Caffeine is the most water soluble (21.7 g/L) and the least lipid soluble (Log P 0.01). Roskos et al. [33] reported that there were no differences between the young and old groups in the urinary excretion of chemical-derived radioactivity of the six chemicals administered intravenously. This suggests that, once any of these chemicals is absorbed, for the two age groups, the chemicals are excreted similarly. The urine was not analyzed for metabolites of these chemicals, so the effect of age on their metabolism could not be determined. Nevertheless, if there were age differences in the metabolism, it did not affect the urinary elimination of the chemicals or their metabolites.

For the two most lipid-soluble compounds (and least water soluble), testosterone and estradiol, there was no difference in the cumulative percent dose absorbed between the two age groups (Fig. 4). However, an age difference was observed in the dermal absorption for the more hydrophilic compounds. Significant differences were noted in the absorption of benzoic acid, acetylsalicylic acid, and caffeine, with a greater cumulative percent of dose absorbed in the young than in the old age group. For hydrocortisone, the cumulative percent of dose absorbed in the young age group was about three times greater than in the old age group. However, no statistical difference was detected. The reason may have been a low sample size ($n = 3$ for young; $n = 7$ for old), the

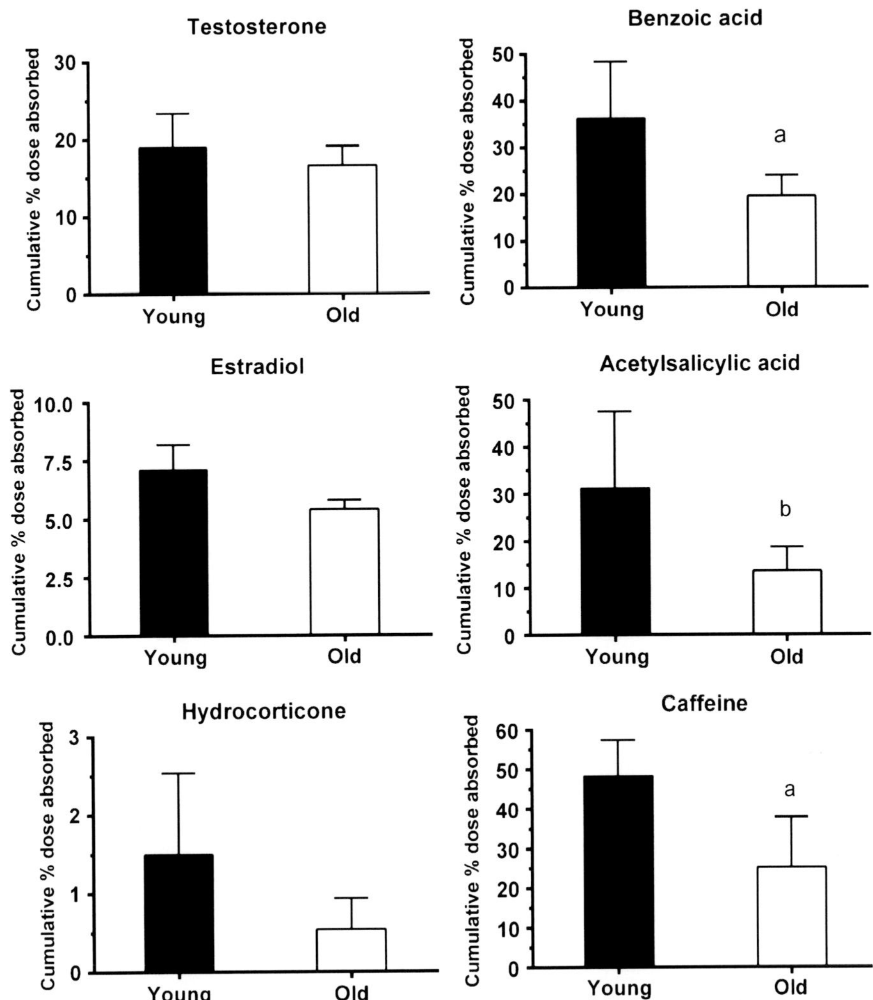

Fig. 4 Cumulative % dose absorbed of ^{14}C-labeled testosterone, estradiol, hydrocortisone, benzoic acid, acetylsalicylic acid, and caffeine in vivo in young (18–40 years, ■) and old (65–86 years, □) humans following dermal exposure [33]. Absorption was determined by collecting urine of treated subjects for 7 days and analyzing for chemical-derived radioactivity. The absorption data was adjusted for incomplete elimination of radioactivity following intravenous administration of radiolabeled chemical and collection of urine for 7 days. Data represents mean ± standard deviation, N = 3–8. [a]Significantly different from young group, $p < 0.05$. [b]Significantly different from young group, $p < 0.01$

observed variability within groups, or that the overall absorption of hydrocortisone was low (<2 %) in both groups.

The results of this study suggest that in humans, age affects the dermal absorption of chemicals that are more hydrophilic and less lipophilic. As a person ages, the skin becomes more dry [6], sebaceous gland activity is reduced, and there is a decreased amount of skin surface lipid [34]. Roskos et al. [33] suggested that with the lower hydration, there is less of a medium for hydrophilic compounds to traverse through the skin. In addition, with a lower amount of lipid available to solubilize chemicals before penetration into and through the skin, the less lipophilic compounds (benzoic acid, acetylsalicylic acid, caffeine) are impacted the greatest extent.

Thompson et al. [35] compared the dermal absorption of fentanyl in young (18–40 years) and old (>60 years) patients who had undergone lower abdominal surgery. The fentanyl was administered to relieve the pain from the surgery. The patients were treated with a transdermal patch of fentanyl for 72 h following surgery. Blood was withdrawn from the patients over time following application of the patch and after its removal. The blood was centrifuged and the resulting plasma was analyzed for fentanyl.

Between the two age groups, there was no difference in the maximal plasma concentration of fentanyl, the time this occurred, the plasma area under the curve, and the elimination half-life after the patch was removed. The only significant difference was in the half time for the plasma concentration of fentanyl to double. In the older group, this half time was 11.1 h, and in the younger group, it was 4.2 h. This lag in fentanyl absorption could be due to changes in the lipid composition of the skin as it ages. It could also be due to the alteration of the microcirculation in the dermis. Fentanyl is a lipophilic compound (Log P $\approx$ 4.0) and may be retained in the skin because of the decreased circulation. Also, the elderly may react differently than the younger patients to the surgery. This could impact cardiac output, circulatory volume, and body temperature.

Holmgaard et al. [36] have recently examined the effect of age on the in vitro dermal absorption of fentanyl citrate. Full-thickness skin from the breast of female donors was mounted on to static diffusion cells. The donors were divided into three groups based on age: $<$30 years of age, $\geq$30 years and $<$60 years of age, and $\geq$60 years of age. Fentanyl citrate in water was applied to the epidermal surface. The receptor chamber contained phosphate buffer. Samples from the receptor chamber were collected over time to 48 h and analyzed for fentanyl. In vitro absorption of fentanyl citrate in the skin of the youngest group was greater in amount and rate than in the middle and oldest age groups.

Conclusion

It is well known that the skin of preterm infants is more permeable to chemicals than full-term infants. Dermal absorption of chemicals through adulthood appears to be stable. Questions have been raised if dermal absorption is altered in the elderly as it is known that there are age-related changes that occur in the biochemistry, physiology, and morphology of the skin. Since the age of the population is increasing, knowledge of an age-dependent change in dermal absorption would be beneficial for the elderly that use transdermal drug delivery systems or exposed residentially or environmentally to chemicals.

The results from the animal studies are somewhat conflicting. In one in vitro study [25], the age-related change in absorption occurred when the animals were young and appeared to be related to their hair growth cycle. So the relevance of this study to human exposure can be questioned. In the two other in vitro studies [26, 30], there was an increase in absorption of lipophilic compounds as the animals aged beyond young adulthood. In an in vivo rat study [28], the absorption of the lipophilic compounds decreased. The differences in results could potentially be due to technique (in vitro vs. in vivo) as well as disparities in the physical and chemical properties of the chemicals studied. It has not been adequately established whether animal skin, particularly rodents, can adequately predict permeability of chemicals in humans. There are also questions about the in vitro technique, because it only tests the barrier property of the skin, not the removal of absorbed chemicals by the vasculature in the dermis. The study with ovariectomized mice and UV light (photoaging) was interesting but also provided no definitive trend on alterations in dermal absorption with "induced" aging.

The limited number of rigorous studies in humans suggests that age affects the dermal absorption of hydrophilic compounds, but not lipophilic compounds to the same extent. The data from Thompson et al. [35] are consistent with the Roskos et al. [33] study. The extent of the lipophilic compound fentanyl was not affected by age in vivo [35], as observed with testosterone and estradiol [28]. However, the in vitro study [36] with fentanyl citrate showed that dermal absorption decreased with age.

What is needed for a better understanding of the age-related changes in dermal absorption are more complete studies, with a greater number of subjects and chemicals that vary in physical and chemical properties. Certainly, Roskos et al. [33] did this with the chemicals that varied in water and lipid solubility. One of the limitations of this study was the low number of subjects. However, it is difficult to conduct laboratory studies in humans for ethical, monetary, and logistical reasons. The animal studies presented looked at a wide range of ages and included very old mice and rats. However, the results were not consistent with the human data [33, 35], although only a few of the same chemicals were tested. An approach that could be taken is for a laboratory to test the same set of chemicals, in animals and humans, using in vitro and in vivo techniques. The chemicals should be carefully selected, so that the physical and chemical properties are well known.

Because the age of the population is increasing in many parts of the world, it is important to understand their risk for potential dermal absorption of the chemicals that surround everyone. Understanding whether age-related changes in skin alters the dermal absorption of chemicals will ultimately lead to reduced risk for the development of adverse health effects from exposure to these chemicals in the elderly population.

Disclaimer This article has been reviewed in accordance with the policy of the National Health and Environmental Effects Research Laboratory, US Environmental Protection Agency, and approved for publication. Approval does not signify that the contents necessarily reflect the views and policies of the Agency nor does mention of trade names or commercial products constitute endorsement or recommendation for use.

Cross-References

▶ Susceptibility to Irritation in the Elderly

References

1. Jenkins G. Molecular mechanisms of skin ageing. Mech Ageing Dev. 2002;123:801–10.
2. U.S. Census Bureau. The next four decades. The older population in the United States: 2010 to 2050. 2010; U.S. Department of Commerce. https://www.census.gov/prod/2010pubs/p25-1138.pdf. Accessed 17 June 2015.
3. Montagna W, Carlisle K. Structural changes in aging human skin. J Invest Dermatol. 1979;73:47–53.
4. Cerimele D, Celleno L, Serri F. Physiological changes in ageing skin. Br J Dermatol. 1990;122 Suppl 35:13–20.
5. Balin AK, Pratt LA. Physiological consequences of human skin aging. Cutis. 1989;43:431–6.
6. Potts RO, Buras EM, Chrisman DA. Changes with age in the moisture content of human skin. J Invest Dermatol. 1984;82:92–100.
7. Nazzaro-Porro M, Passi S, Boniforti L, et al. Effects of aging on fatty acids in skin surface lipids. J Biol Chem. 1979;73:112–7.
8. Luebberding S, Krueger N, Kerscher M. Age-related changes in skin barrier function – quantitative evaluation of 150 female subjects. Int J Cosmet Sci. 2013;34:183–90.
9. Fenske NA, Lober CW. Structural and functional changes of normal aging skin. J Am Acad Dermatol. 1987;14:571–85.
10. Lavker RM, Zheng P, Dong G. Aged skin: a study by light, transmission electron, and scanning electron microscopy. J Invest Dermatol. 1987;88:44S–51.
11. Harvell JD, Maibach HI. Percutaneous absorption and inflammation in aged skin: a review. J Am Acad Dermatol. 1994;31:1015–21.
12. Hotchkiss SAM. Cutaneous toxicity: kinetic and metabolic determinants. Toxicol Ecotoxicol News. 1995;2:10–8.
13. Semple S. Dermal exposure to chemicals in the workplace: just how important is skin absorption? Occup Environ Med. 2008;61:376–82.
14. Poet TS, McDougal JN. Skin absorption and human risk assessment. Chem Biol Interact. 2002;140:19–34.
15. Anderson JM, Kilshaw BH, Harkness RA, et al. Spongioform myelinopathy in premature infants. Br Med J. 1975;2:175–6.
16. Harpin VA, Rutter N. Barrier properties of the newborn infant's skin. J Pediatr. 1983;102:419–25.
17. Christophers E, Kligman AM. Percutaneous absorption in aged skin. In: Montagna W, editor. Advances in biology of the skin. Permagon Press, Oxford, England, vol. 6: Aging; 1965. p. 163–75.
18. DeSalva SJ, Thompson G. $Na^{22}Cl$ skin clearance in humans and its relation to skin age. J Invest Dermatol. 1965;45:315–8.
19. Tagami H. Functional characteristics of aged skin. Acta Dermatol (Kyoto). 1972;67:131–8.
20. Kaestli L-Z, Wasilewski-Rasca A-F, Bonnabry P, et al. Use of transdermal drug formulations in the elderly. Drugs Aging. 2008;25:269–80.
21. Jeter KF, Lutz JB. Skin care in the frail, elderly, dependent, incontinent patient. Adv Wound Care. 1996;9:29–34.
22. Konda S, Meier-Davis SR, Cayme B, et al. Age-related percutaneous penetration part 2: effect of age on dermatopharmacokinetics and overview of transdermal products. Skin Therapy Lett. 2012;17:5–7.

23. Bronaugh RL, Stewart RF, Congdon ER. Methods for in vitro percutaneous absorption studies. II. Animal models for human skin. Toxicol Appl Pharmacol. 1982;62:481–8.
24. Behl CR, Flynn GL, Kurihara T, et al. Age and anatomical site influences on alkanol permeation of skin of the male hairless mouse. J Soc Cosmet Chem. 1984;35:237–52.
25. Behl CR, Flynn GL, Linn EE, et al. Percutaneous absorption of corticosteroids: age, site, and skin-sectioning influences on rates of permeation of hairless mouse skin by hydrocortisone. J Pharm Sci. 1984;73:1287–90.
26. Hughes MF, Fisher HL, Birnbaum LS, et al. Effect of age on the in vitro percutaneous absorption of phenols in mice. Toxicol In Vitro. 1994;8:221–7.
27. Monteiro-Riviere NA, Banks YB, Birnbaum LS. Laser Doppler measurements of cutaneous blood flow in ageing mice and rats. Toxicol Lett. 1991;57:329–38.
28. Banks YB, Brewster DW, Birnbaum LS. Age-related changes in dermal absorption of 2,3,7,8-tetrachlorodibenzo-ρ-dioxin and 2,3,4,7,8-pentachlorodibenzofuran. Fundam Appl Toxicol. 1990;15:163–73.
29. Brewster DW, Banks YB, Clark A-M, et al. Comparative dermal absorption of 2,3,7,8-tetrachlorodibenzo-ρ-dioxin and three polychlorinated dibenzofurans. Toxicol Appl Pharmacol. 1989;90:243–52.
30. Lehman PA, Franz TJ. Effect of age and diet on stratum corneum barrier function in the Fischer 344 female rat. J Invest Dermatol. 1993;100:200–4.
31. Hung E-F, Chen W-Y, Aljuffali IA, et al. Skin aging modulates percutaneous drug absorption: the impaction of ultraviolet irradiation and ovariectomy. Age. 2015;37:21.
32. Calleja-Agius J, Muscat-Baron Y, Brincat MP. Skin ageing. Menopause Int. 2007;13:60–4.
33. Roskos KV, Maibach HI, Guy RH. The effect of aging on percutaneous absorption in man. J Pharmacokinet Biopharm. 1989;17:617–30.
34. Pochi PE, Strauss JS, Downing DT. Age-related changes in sebaceous gland activity. J Invest Dermatol. 1979;73:103–11.
35. Thompson JP, Bower S, Liddle AM, et al. Perioperative pharmacokinetics of transdermal fentanyl in elderly and young adult patients. Br J Anaesth. 1998;81:152–4.
36. Holmgaard R, Benfeldt E, Sorensen JA, et al. Chronological age affects the permeation of fentanyl through human skin in vitro. Skin Pharmacol Physiol. 2013;26:155–9.

112 Application of In Vitro Methods in Preclinical Safety Assessment of Skin Care Products

Gertrude-Emilia Costin and Kimberly G. Norman

Contents

Abstract

One of the critical responsibilities of cosmetic and personal care industry is to determine the safety profile of the ingredients and/or formulations before launching new products on the market for consumers' use. While products manufactured by other industries are thoroughly regulated (pharmaceuticals, pesticides, etc.), the safety assessment of cosmetic and personal care products seems to be less strictly integrated in the regulatory framework, despite the fact that the type of testing methods allowed for use became more restrictive in recent years. As such, a ban on animal testing of cosmetic ingredients and final formulations in the European Union (EU) took effect between 2009 and 2013. Thereon, industry used testing strategies based on nonanimal methods that were often designed to assess the safety profile of specific product lines. A diverse range of in vitro methods is now available and considered suitable to provide reliable interpretation of the safety data regarding ingredients used in finished cosmetic and personal care products. These methods range from simple cell monoculture test systems to more complex such as explants or three-dimensional reconstructed organotypic tissue models. This chapter discusses the use of several in vitro methods in the preclinical safety assessment of skin care products with special emphasis on skin irritation and sensitization endpoints.

G.-E. Costin (✉)
The Institute for In Vitro Sciences, Inc. (IIVS), Gaithersburg, MD, USA
e-mail: ecostin@iivs.org

K.G. Norman
Norman Institute for In Vitro Sciences, Gaithersburg, MD, USA
e-mail: knorman@iivs.org

M.A. Farage et al. (eds.), *Textbook of Aging Skin*,
DOI 10.1007/978-3-662-47398-6_130

Introduction

Cosmetic industry faces nowadays a significant increase in the consumers' demand for safe, efficacious, novel, and organic products. The consumers also became more conscious of the means industry uses to assess the safety and efficacy of such products. Thus, claims of using green chemistry or nonanimal testing methods are now noticed on the products labels. Skin care formulations represent a large percentage of the personal care industry's production, and antiaging products seem to be situated at the luxury end of the cosmetics line. Regardless of the intended use, complexity of the formulation process, or consumer demand, industry is responsible of assessing the safety of all products launched to the public using the most modern available laboratory techniques.

The current EU legislation bans all types of animal testing for cosmetic ingredients, final formulations, and also the marketing of animal-tested cosmetics [1]. Therefore, their safety profile should be assessed using appropriate alternative methods that replace animal testing. Consequently, there is an increasing interest in using in vitro methods because they are scientifically more relevant to consumer exposure (particularly when based on cells of human origin), less time consuming, and more cost-effective and contribute to reducing the participation of human volunteers in the safety assessment process.

In general, the safety assessment of cosmetic products is not necessarily integrated into a well-defined, strict regulatory framework. This is in part due to the wide diversity of the products manufactured in terms of composition, intended use, targeted population, etc. In time it became necessary to generate a "checklist" of endpoints that are critical for the safety assessment of cosmetic products. Of these endpoints, skin irritation and sensitization occupy a central place and are one of the first to be addressed. This chapter discusses in chemico, in vitro cell- and tissue-based test systems that are currently used for these endpoints in the preclinical safety assessment of skin care products. The critical positioning of these in vitro methods in the larger context of the manufacturing process is also analyzed. Besides their use for safety assessment, modern in vitro methods provide relevant and reliable biological data that bring a strong scientific added value to the products (e.g., mechanistic insights). This added value further supports the decision-making processes in the research and development and/or marketing phase of the complex process that leads to the launching of a new product for consumers' use.

Preclinical Safety Assessment Framework for Skin Care Products: Integrating In Vitro Testing Strategies

Testing strategies addressing multiple endpoints are often used for the safety assessment of skin care products before launching in order to limit the risks associated with human exposure. Although it may often be viewed as a generic endpoint checklist, it is this absolute need to have confidence in moving forward with an ingredient or formulation that actually positions the safety assessment on a central place in the complex manufacturing process of skin care products. Furthermore, it is always a crossing point in any project considering new ingredients or innovative formulation processes if those are not determined by testing to be safe. In the production continuum initiated with an innovative idea and progressing up to the post-market follow-up studies, ensuring the safety is a constant requirement throughout the life of a product and plays a critical role in the decision-making process, often providing insights useful to efficacy and clinical testing in a matrix approach (Fig. 1).

For cosmetic and personal care products (including skin care lines), there is no formal, strictly regulated approach for the safety assessment. This evaluation often varies based on the type of product, concentration of the ingredient (s), novelty of the composition, population targeted, intended use, frequency and duration of contact, normal conditions of use, and any foreseeable misuse. In general, the toxicological profile of a cosmetic ingredient/formulation is obtained by analyzing data provided by in vitro

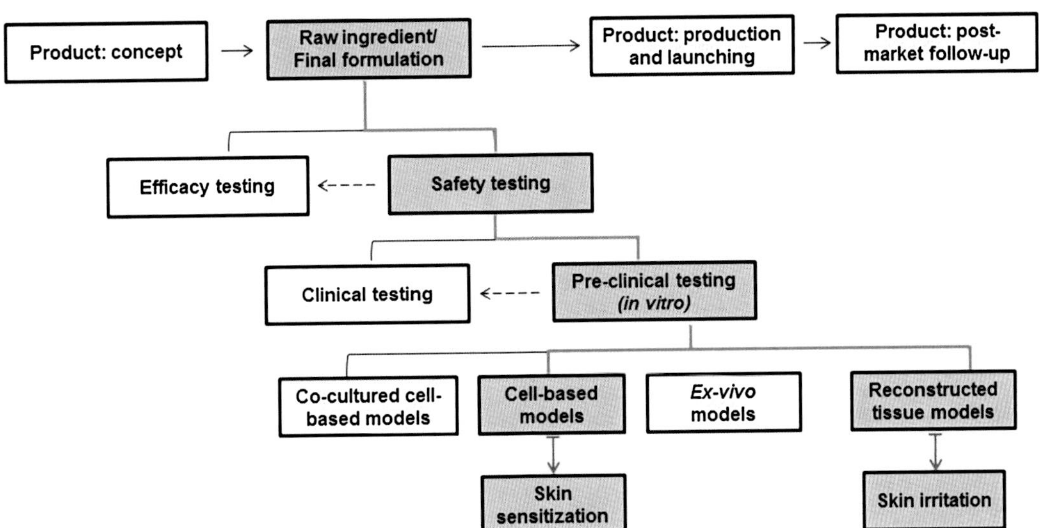

Fig. 1 Integration of the in vitro preclinical safety testing methods in the skin care products manufacturing framework. In *gray*: concepts and methods discussed in the chapter. *Dashed lines* indicate indirect contribution to other components of the framework

and clinical testing, as well as results of epidemiological studies or reports of intended or accidental human exposure experience (market follow-up studies, input from factory workers, beauticians, etc.) where available.

Despite an apparent loosely regulated environment, it remains industry's utmost responsibility toward the consumer to conduct safety testing of the formulations and ingredients contained therein in order to avoid adverse reactions with general use. While animals are still used particularly in the pharmaceutical industry for the preclinical safety testing, the personal care and cosmetic industry was open to rapidly adopt alternative in vitro methods, which reduce, refine, and replace the use of animals. The use of validated in vitro assays is of particular interest in the effort to comply with the most recent legislative measures banning the marketing of the products that contain ingredients tested in animal models (i.e., Regulation (EC) No 1223/2009). Furthermore, industry was the initiator and driver of the development of a wide array of in vitro assays routinely used for internal safety evaluations. Thus, industry created cutoff values of relevant endpoints for specific lines of products and immediately acknowledged the need to qualify through repeated testing benchmark (reference) materials that could be used for prototype exploration. It became the companies' decision as of how to design custom-made testing strategies to ensure the safety of their products and to optimize the effectiveness of the process. Some companies may use in vitro assays as a screening tool before initiating a clinical test, while others may use a single assay or a tiered testing strategy to assess a single or multiple endpoints without further clinical confirmation (often used to address reformulations). The strategy of choice often depends on historical data available for the ingredients or formulations, company's general approach as far as the production timeline is concerned, sequence of steps leading to launching, on budget and experience with available in vitro assays, and data interpretation (Fig. 1).

Safety testing strategies based on validated regulatory or non-regulatory in vitro assays serve a multitude of purposes within the cosmetic and personal care industry and are flexible enough to address a large variety of questions. For example, complex in vitro methods are often used by R&D, New Technology, and Discovery groups very early in the products' design process to gain knowledge on certain ingredients' mechanisms of action, synergistic effects, and new pathways to explore for cosmetic use. Product Development and Innovation groups use in vitro assays as a tool for screening libraries of compounds that may have been previously considered of interest to another industry (e.g., pharmaceuticals). Following this approach, often used when the ingredients are novel and never used for cosmetic purposes, a so-called short list of ingredients that are determined to be safe for consumer's use can be generated and can advance to further testing as necessary. In this case, the in vitro assays are used upstream in the production framework as a first informative step that provides not only safety information but also insights regarding any restrictions (concentration, skin area of interest) that could support the efficacy or clinical testing employed downstream for further confirmatory testing (Fig. 1). Often times, industry may decide to bypass the clinical testing entirely and to rely on data provided by in vitro assays for ingredients that have a relatively known, well-characterized safety profile or when considering minor changes of basic formulations that may have been previously tested. Since the in vitro tests used for safety assessment are usually performed during the early phases of new product development, the results are generated relatively fast and allow performing (re)formulation(s) and ingredient characteristic screening within ranges that could not be otherwise accommodated by clinical studies.

For cosmetic product manufacturers, various in vitro test systems of increasing complexity can be used to address numerous endpoints of interest as part of an integrated testing strategy. For example, cocultures of different cell types or ex vivo and/or three-dimensional (3D) organotypic tissue models can be used for confirmation or further in-depth assessment of effects initially identified in monolayer cell culture systems. The following sections will focus on in chemico and in vitro assays that can be used for skin irritation and sensitization assessment. The advantages and limitations of the in vitro methods detailed in the chapter will be analyzed, and guidance on data interpretation and subsequent use in the decision-making process will be provided.

In Vitro Methods Used in the Preclinical Safety Assessment of Skin Care Products

Skin Irritation

The safety assessment for skin corrosion/irritation potential of ingredients and finished products is an essential part of the toxicological evaluation prior to manufacture, transport, or marketing. The intent is to protect consumers from toxicity associated with normal product use and reasonably foreseeable misuse exposures in the marketplace.

Traditionally, the in vivo corrosion/irritation test using rabbits introduced by Draize in the 1940s has been used to predict hazardous effects of substances coming in contact with human skin [2]. Throughout years of use, it was recognized that the visual grading of the effects is highly subjective and that the test overpredicts irritating effects of substances in relation to human skin [3–6]. Furthermore, the use of animals to assess skin safety has been criticized on inhumane grounds and unnecessary suffering. Thus, the combined needs to protect humans without exposing volunteers to potentially irritating products, to comply with regulations, and to reduce animal testing have led to significant efforts to develop alternative test methods that are predictive, rapid, and reproducible.

Over the years, a variety of cell culture systems have been developed and evaluated for prediction of skin corrosion and irritation potential. Simple monolayer keratinocyte cultures were investigated for their capacity to predict skin irritation using cell viability endpoints. They are useful in large-scale, first-line screening tests and are informative for potential hazards and to eliminate materials that are significantly cytotoxic. However, the monolayer systems are limited by materials' solubility in the cell culture medium and lack the 3D architecture and epidermal–dermal interactions that are critical for skin homeostasis. This limitation was addressed by the use of explants (skin organ cultures) and, most importantly, by terminally differentiated in vitro reconstructed human skin equivalents (epidermal and full thickness) [7].

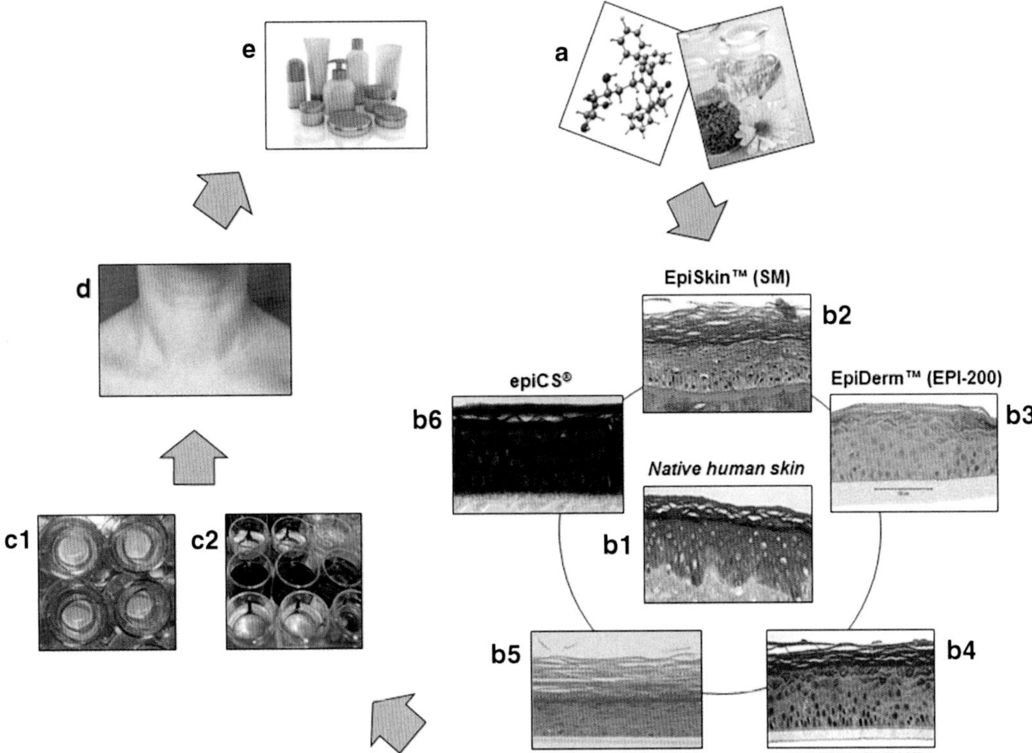

Fig. 2 Skin safety assessment cycle using in vitro methods and clinical tests: from ingredients to finished products. (*a*) Ingredients or chemicals of interest are selected and tested using in vitro methods (*b*) in order to predict the human clinical response (*d*); (*b1*) structure of native human skin (*center*) and reconstructed tissue models (satellites: *b2*-EpiSkin™ (SM) from Episkin, Lyon, France; *b3*-EpiDerm™ from MatTek Corporation, Ashland, MA, USA; *b4*-SkinEthic™ RHE from Episkin, Lyon, France; *b5*-LabCyte EPI-MODEL from Japan Tissue Engineering Co., Ltd., Gamagori City, Aichi, Japan; *b6*-epiCS® from CellSystems Biotechnologie Vertrieb GmbH, Troisdorf, Germany); (*c1*) example of a reconstructed tissue model as received for testing; (*c2*) assessment of reconstructed tissues' viability (as a measure of toxicity and subsequent irritation potential) using a colorimetric method: *purple* color is indicative of a viable tissue (not affected by a potential irritant); (*e*) finished product ready to be used by a consumer after the safety assessment is complete. Images *b2–b6* are available online at http://www.episkin.com; http://www.mattek.com; http://www.jpte.co.jp; http://cellsystems.de, respectively

The 3D skin models can be designed to have only an epidermal compartment (containing mainly keratinocytes but also melanocytes or Langerhans cells) or can gain complexity by addition of a dermal compartment (containing fibroblasts and endothelial cells). The models are generated by growing the cultures at the air–liquid interface on de-epidermized dermis, acellular or fibroblast-populated dermal substrates such as inert filters, or collagen matrix. The cultures exhibit a stratified and cornified epidermis, with basal, spinous, and granular layers along with a functional *stratum corneum*, mimicking the architecture of the normal human skin (Figs. 2b1 and 3a) and allowing the direct topical application of ingredients or formulations. Although they reached a high level of architectural complexity, the models are yet to exhibit the degree of competency found in native human skin (Fig. 2b2–b6) [7–9].

Variability in the reconstructed human skin equivalents' response to irritants and other insults is expected and may be influence, for example, by the source of the keratinocytes used to develop the

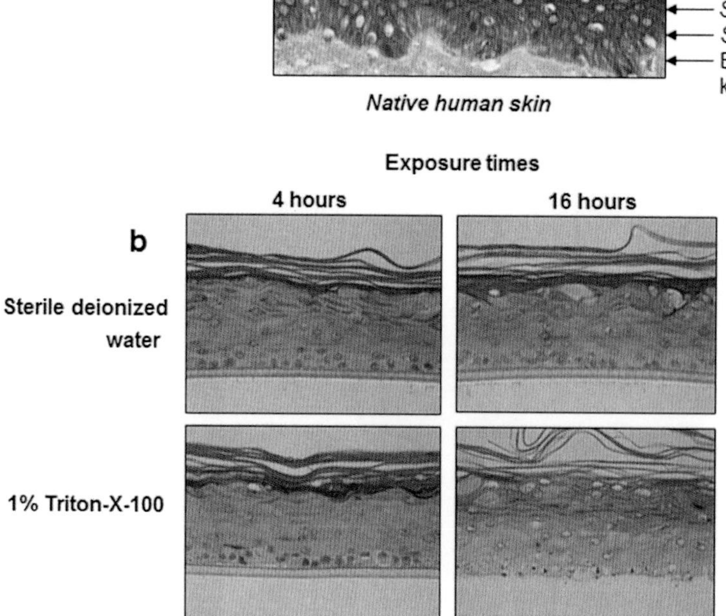

Fig. 3 Use of the EpiDerm™ model for in vitro toxicity tests: the irritation effect of different materials was examined histologically after topical application on the surface of the tissues for various exposure times. The tissues have been fixed and stained with hematoxylin and eosin (*H&E*), and pictures were taken (400x magnification) (**b**), analyzed, and compared to the structure of the native human skin (**a**). Sterile, deionized water was used as the negative control, and it showed no adverse effect on the tissue's architecture at either the short (4 h) or the long exposure time used (16 h). One surfactant, Triton X-100, with known irritation potential was also tested as a 1 % (w/v) dilution prepared in sterile, deionized water. The tissues treated with the surfactant showed early signs of toxicity at the short exposure time (4 h) as demonstrated by the disorganized structure of the tissue layers, sloughing of the *stratum corneum* and decreased thickness of the tissue. The long exposure time (16 h) to the 1 % Triton X-100 induced a progressive degradation of the tissues

models (neonatal foreskin or adult skin) [10, 11] or by variations in the barrier function. The models have been determined to have a higher permeability [12] compared to the native human skin. While this could be an advantage when testing mild formulations (typical for cosmetic industry), it could also result in overpredictions due to an increased penetration rate and thus higher availability to the viable keratinocytes [12].

The reconstructed human skin equivalents offer a relevant model to study basic skin biology processes such as wound repair, regulation of melanogenesis, phototoxicity, drug transfer, metabolism of topically applied products, pathogenesis of skin diseases, etc. [11, 13]. The 3D skin models also found clinical applications as grafts. The models gained regulatory recognition through validations and can therefore be used to address the demands of regulatory authorities, animal welfare organizations, and consumers. Thus, one immediate use of the in vitro methods based on 3D models was in the regulatory setting for hazard identification and labeling of chemicals, transport of dangerous substances, and occupational safety/industrial hygiene. The methods used for these purposes usually employ a single exposure time/dose and endpoint to address a specific regulatory query (e.g., skin corrosion/irritation) rather than to provide the possibility for a comparative analysis of irritation potential between ingredients or formulations, which is more relevant for cosmetic products [14].

Cosmetic and personal care products frequently undergo reformulations in order to improve performance or to adjust concentrations of ingredients to levels that can be tolerated by the skin without adverse effects. Skin irritation that can be induced by minor formulation adjustments is reflected in effects of a range of severity, from near corrosive to cumulative or only sensory irritation or inflammatory reaction [15]. As a result, the assays using test systems based on 3D skin models and developed initially to examine corrosion or severe degrees of irritation were later optimized to be able to capture more subtle effects that are typical to cosmetic and personal care products of low cytotoxicity profiles. Since the current legislation imposes increasing measures of safety as well as the limitation of animal use for such testing [16], the in vitro methods based on available 3D models became almost the default test system to use as a cautious, convenient, and efficient alternative before considering the conduct of human clinical testing.

The primary goal of safety testing is to predict the results of human exposure to ingredients or formulations that is ultimately addressed in clinical studies using human volunteers (panelists). As an inherent variability exists for in vitro models, the same stands true for clinical studies, and thus a direct comparison of safety testing results may prove challenging. For example, in clinical testing the degree of response to a given substance may vary with the age of the subject as well as the location of the test site even if from the same individual [17]. The results of the clinical studies may also be affected by the mode of application (patch, occlusive or nonocclusive, rinse-off, etc.), the frequency of the application or implement used to apply the test material, the test material's physical properties (solubility, melt point, etc.), and its concentration (tested at the full strength of dilution) [18]. As with in vivo studies, one criticism of the human skin irritation test resides with the subjective nature of visual grading of the endpoints (erythema and edema) and a high degree of inter-subject variability. Most importantly, clinical irritation studies can result in unforeseen, dangerous reactions for the individuals tested.

The human skin irritation test methods range from short, graduated skin patch tests (up to 4 h) developed to meet the regulatory labeling requirements [19, 20] to 14-day (or longer) cumulative irritation skin patch tests for assessing the irritancy of very mild products (e.g., cosmetics). Of the many clinical protocols available, the 4-h human patch test (4-h HPT) seems to be better developed and described in the literature to obtain controlled human acute skin irritation information and to further correlate with the in vitro skin irritation test data [19, 21–23]. The 4-h HPT provides the opportunity to identify single substances, mixtures, or formulations with significant skin irritation potential without recourse to the use of animals [24]. The method also provides gold standard data for future validations of alternative in vitro methods to replace the in vivo rabbit test for classification and labeling purposes in regulatory toxicology. The 14-day cumulative irritation patch test is used to assess and rank-order the skin irritation potential of milder cosmetics after repetitive exposure. For assessment of the skin sensitization potential of cosmetics, the human repeat insult patch test (HRIPT) is commonly used. Skin sensitization assessment differs from skin irritation due to the involvement of an immune response. The substance is applied to the skin, and then there is a rest period, followed by a repeated exposure to the substance after which skin reactions are scored by a dermatologist. There are different HRIPT protocols available, but the general principles of the assay remain the same.

Given the wide range of irritation potential of cosmetic ingredients or the more narrow irritation potential of final formulations, the clinical tests and in vitro methods developed for preclinical screening purposes became highly customized to specifically address effects of human exposure. Subsequently, the correlation of these data became necessary and proved rather challenging given the limited sets of data publicly available. This is the first attempt to an extended analysis that intends to provide a platform for future similar studies and to increase confidence in the capability of in vitro methods to predict human responses to ingredients and finished products of cosmetic and personal care industry.

In Vitro Assays Validated for Regulatory Purposes

The Skin Irritation Test (SIT)

Assays using 3D skin models represent one of the most promising alternatives to animal testing for regulatory labeling purposes of potential skin corrosives and irritants. Several commercially developed 3D models have been validated by the European Centre for the Validation of Alternative Methods (ECVAM) for this purpose (Fig. 2b2–b6). The validated SIT (OECD TG 439) is based on the measurement of mitochondrial activity using the 3-[4,5-dimethylthiazol-2-yl]-2,5-diphenyltetrazolium bromide (MTT) endpoint as a measure of tissue viability (Fig. 2c2). While this method can separate an irritant substance from a nonirritant, one of its major limitations is that it cannot rank the potency of an irritant chemical [25]. Despite this limitation, the SIT found its applications in the assessment of skin irritation for cosmetic products.

The study by Jirova et al. [16] analyzed paired skin irritation data generated in in vivo, in vitro, and clinically for 25 substances (from the ECVAM validation study and several other commercially available chemicals) [16]. Among the 15 substances predicted as skin irritants by the in vivo test, only five were found to be irritating by the 4 h HPT. These results confirmed the findings of an extensive study published previously by Basketter et al. [6] showing that about 40 % of the substances classified as skin irritants by the rabbit test did not trigger skin irritation when tested in the 4 h HPT. The in vitro EpiDerm™-based SIT using a 15-min exposure correlated better with the clinical data (four of the five irritants were correctly classified), while the optimized (60 min) version reached higher concordance with the rabbit test. This study was the first to advance the concept of using 4-h HPT data for the validation of alternative methods because of its relevance in detecting acute skin irritation potential to humans. While the substances analyzed in this study may not be immediately relevant to cosmetic formulations, the study provided an introductory view of the possibility to use the SIT to predict irritation in humans.

The study by Hoffmann et al. [26] investigated how in silico, in vitro (EpiDerm™- and EpiSkin-based SIT), and in vivo data could be used in a combined fashion for the assessment of skin irritation hazard relevant to human exposure. The authors analyzed a database of 100 chemicals of which only 31 had 4-h HPT data available (2 irritants and 29 nonirritants). The data showed that the EpiSkin™-based SIT correctly predicted 19 chemicals as nonirritants and overpredicted 12, while the EpiDerm™-based SIT correctly predicted 22 nonirritants, overpredicted 8, and underpredicted 1 skin irritant. The results of this study further advanced the in vitro-clinical correlation that encouraged the industry to consider alternative assays for the prediction of skin irritation potential of ingredients and formulations.

A recent study [27] took the data analysis one step further by performing a comparative analysis of in vitro (EpiDerm™-based SIT), clinical (exaggerated human occlusive patch test), and controlled consumer usage data for whole-body, leave-on skin care products containing 1–5 % behentrimonium chloride (BTC). The BTC-containing formulations were predicted to be nonirritant to skin by the in vitro method, and these results were confirmed by clinical and postmarketing data.

In a study published last year [28], a new in vitro method using human viable skin obtained during surgery was reported. The results obtained for four chemicals (and based on histology analysis) were compared to the in vitro (EpiDerm™- and EpiSkin™-based SIT, 15-min exposure) and 4-h HPT results. The data analysis revealed an accuracy of 100 % compared to the human test, and a 75 % accuracy with the other validated in vitro methods. This study advanced yet another in vitro method to be considered and further investigated for the safety assessment of ingredients and formulations.

Even though still limited in their predictivity for irritation induced by complex cosmetic products particularly when of reduced irritation potential, the regulatory assays are occasionally used as a preclinical screening tool to assess acute skin irritation and to avoid unnecessary animal and clinical tests.

In Vitro Assays Not Validated for Regulatory Purposes

The Time-to-Toxicity Assay

Contact irritants vary significantly with regard to the relative potency to induce skin irritation. To address the irritancy ranking and to meet the typical needs of product development groups charged with the design of increasingly milder cosmetic and personal care products, the in vitro methods have been adapted to use multiple endpoints and exposure times and to allow for interpretation of potency. The assays are based on the effective time (ET_{50} value) representing the exposure time that decreases the tissue viability by 50 % as measured by the tissue's ability to reduce MTT (time-to-toxicity methods). While this method has not yet been validated for regulatory purposes, it is frequently used as a rapid screening tool able to rank-order the irritation potential of mild cosmetic formulations.

The time-to-toxicity method was the first one to be investigated for its potential to predict the acute skin irritation in humans, with the goal of validating an in vitro assay for such purposes [29]. A pre-validation study was performed for ten known skin irritants and ten nonirritants tested on three different tissue models: EpiSkin™, EpiDerm™, and PREDISKIN. The data were analyzed in comparison to unambiguous skin irritation classifications derived from the rabbit data included in the ECETOC (European Centre for Ecotoxicology and Toxicology of Chemicals) database [15, 30]. Of the 20 chemicals investigated, 4 h HPT human data were found only for four (dl-citronellol; 10-undecenoic acid; methylpalmitate; hydroxycitronellal) and allowed for a limited analysis of the predictive capacity when correlating the data with the human test results. All four chemicals were predicted as nonirritant to skin (nonclassified) by the 4-h HPT; hydroxycitronellal was the only one correctly predicted by the animal model, while the other three were overpredicted. The in vitro assays based on the EpiSkin™- and EpiDerm™ models correctly predicted only methylpalmitate as nonirritant and overpredicted the other three chemicals; hydroxycitronellal and dl-citronellol were correctly predicted as nonirritants to the skin even though intra-lab and inter-lab variability was reported. While the pre-validation study concluded that the method investigated was not ready for inclusion in a large-scale formal validation study, the assay was appealing to industry for preclinical screening purposes and started to be used quite frequently.

Despite not advancing through validation, the time-to-toxicity assay was used in several studies that investigated the capacity of various reconstructed tissue models to predict the irritation potential of a wide variety of cosmetic and personal care products. One such model was Skin$^{2®}$ ZK1301 (ATS; La Jolla, CA, USA), comprised of human dermal fibroblasts cocultured on a nylon mesh with partially stratified epidermal keratinocytes; the model is not produced anymore. Developed originally for autologous grafting in burned patients and diabetics, the Skin$^{2®}$ ZK1301 model was also used in two separate studies to analyze the skin irritation potential of surfactants used to formulate household cleaning products, laundry products, shampoos, and other personal care and cosmetic products [31, 32]. Both studies considered a wide range of exposure times (from 30 min to 24 h) and correlated the data with the 24-h human clinical patch test [31] and a human clinical modified repeat application soap chamber test [32], respectively. In both studies, the percentage tissue viability results obtained for the 30-min exposure correlated best with the clinical data, thus supporting the use of a relatively short exposure time for rinse-off products.

The study by Doyle et al. [32] also investigated the EpiDerm™ model and used the ET_{50} value for correlation with the clinical data and for further comparison with results generated using the Skin$^{2®}$ ZK1301 model [32]. The EpiDerm™ model is a human tissue model comprised of human-derived epidermal keratinocytes cultured on permeable cell culture inserts, which allows for differentiation and formation of a multilayered, highly differentiated model of the human epidermis (Fig. 2b3). The complexity of the EpiDerm™ model was reflected in higher percentage viability values of the tissues treated with eight complex shampoo formulations and when compared to those obtained for the Skin$^{2®}$ ZK1301 after 1 h exposure. Furthermore, the data from the EpiDerm™-based test system resulted into a better correlation with relevant human clinical data.

The EpiDerm™ model is also sensitive enough to capture effects of surfactants applied topically for multiple exposure times (Costin, unpublished data and Fig. 3b). These results and the studies by Demetrulias et al. [31] and Doyle et al. [32] are very encouraging and demonstrate that the in vitro test systems based on reconstructed tissue models can serve as reliable screening tools prior to clinical studies.

The Fixed Exposure(s) Assays Using Cytokine Endpoints

Personal care and cosmetic products are often purposely formulated to be mild or extremely mild to the skin while preserving their efficacy for the intended end result. To address subtle formulation modifications, the in vitro assays based on 3D skin models have been adapted to address multiple biological inquiries by assessing additional endpoints besides the tissue viability.

The skin is a fully immunocompetent organ, capable of initiating an inflammatory reaction in response to irritants primarily driven by the release of primary cytokines such as interleukin (IL)-1α and tumor necrosis factor (TNF)-α from keratinocytes [33]. The inflammatory cascade further involves multifunctional secondary and chemotactic cytokines, growth factors, etc. that either escalate and drive the inflammatory cascade or repress the reaction through negative feedback [33–35]. IL-1α was routinely used in addition to MTT as a secondary (but more revealing) endpoint in in vitro assays based on 3D tissue models, particularly to provide insights on the irritation potential of materials that otherwise would be considered nonirritants based on simple viability assays. When using in vitro assays based on 3D skin models, the culture media can be collected and analyzed for the IL-1α released by the tissues following exposure to various materials. IL-1α can result either from an active secretion from viable cells (de novo synthesis or activated by irritants) or a passive release from damaged cells [36]. By far, the best-described mechanism by which chemicals induce skin irritation is that triggered by surfactants which can disrupt the cell membrane resulting in the release of IL-1α into the cytoplasm [37, 38].

The in vitro assays based on 3D skin models and using cytokine analysis as a secondary endpoint tend to vary widely regarding the exposure time, dosing volume, cytokines analyzed, etc. The variations are necessary for the assessment of the irritation potential of a large variety of products (leave-on or wash-off, surfactants or other complex formulations, etc.). The correlation with clinical data thus becomes even more challenging as the clinical tests are also adapted to address the respective classes of products investigated and their effect on consumers. Table 1 provides an overview of the in vitro and clinical methods analyzed in this section of the chapter for correlation purposes and captures all the variations of these methods.

In most of the studies reported thus far and using IL-1α as a skin irritation indicator (Table 1), the 3D tissues were exposed to the test materials for long exposure times (up to 24 h or longer) thus extending the detection limits of the in vitro test system to make it capable to capture irritation events induced by very mild products [12, 22, 38–42]. In these studies, the culture media was collected immediately after the completion of the exposure time(s). This strategy intends to mimic the effects of leave-on products on the skin and seems to provide a better correlation with the clinical tests that address either long human exposures or repeated applications of the test materials (24- or 48-h patch test, or 14-day or longer tests, respectively) [12, 38–40].

For example, the study by Roguet et al. [39] showed that the concordance between the in vitro tissue viability results and the associated IL-1α release data and the human irritation data was 74 %. Overall, only one out of six oils tested was overpredicted by the in vitro assay, while from the 17 emulsions tested, three were underpredicted and one was overpredicted. Of the tested mascaras, four out of nine were underpredicted and one was overpredicted as irritant to the skin. The IL-1α levels obtained from

Table 1 Overview of reports correlating in vitro and clinical data – focus on inflammatory cytokines

In vitro test system								Clinical test	References
		Test material			Endpoint				
3D tissue model	Exposure time (h)	Type	Number (total)	Dosing volume/ weight	Tissue viability	IL-1α	Others (specify)		
[b]EpiSkin™	18	Gel, oil, emulsion, mascara	38	150 μl or 150 mg	√[d]	√[a]	–	48-h occlusion test	[39]
[c]Skin equivalent	24	Lotion, mascara, shower gel, deodorant, cream, serum, toothpaste, bath oil, lip stick, makeup, shower cream	14	10 μl	√[d]	√[a]	–	48-h patch test (occlusive or semiocclusive)	[40]
[e]EpiDerm™; EpiDerm™ cocultured with human dermal fibroblasts; [f]SKIN^2™ model ZK1350	1	Raw materials representing the major classes of surfactants used in consumer products; prototype facial creams	16	100 μl	√[g]	√[h]	IL-6, IL-8, IL-10, SCF, c-Kit, GM-CSF, TNF-α, TNF-R1, IFN-γ, TGFβ, ICAM-1	Modified human cumulative irritation test (48-h patch test – semiocclusive;) Human clinical closed patch test (24 h)	[43]
[e]EpiDerm™	1	Facial cleansing bar formulations, liquid facial cleansers	6	100 μl	√[g]	√[h]	IL-1ra	Exaggerated human arm wash test	[44]
[e]EpiDerm™	1–24	Surfactants, cosmetics, antiperspirants, deodorants	7	100 μl	√[d]	√[a]	AST, histology	24-h patch test (surfactants); human 14-day cumulative irritation test (cosmetics)	[12]
[i]SkinEthic	72	Vaseline; SDS (0.2 %, 0.4 %, 0.8 %); calcipotriol; all-*trans*-retinoic acid	7	10 mg/cm^2	√[d]	√[a]	IL-8, RNA, histology	Repeated 24-h application over 3 weeks under Finn chamber patches	[38]

(*continued*)

Table 1 (continued)

In vitro test system									
		Test material			Endpoint				
3D tissue model	Exposure time (h)	Type	Number (total)	Dosing volume/ weight	Tissue viability	IL-1α	Others (specify)	Clinical test	References
[e]EpiDerm™	3	Soaps (commercially available or experimental)	5	100 μl	√[d]	√[a]	-	Forearm-controlled application technique	[41]
[e]EpiDerm™	Up to 24	Antiperspirants, deodorants	11	NP	√[d]	√[a]	AST	Reported incidence (in subject diaries)	[22]
[e]EpiDerm™; [j]EpiSkin™; [k]Cosmital	1–16	Surfactant-based formulations, shampoos, mascaras, emulsions, gels, oils, creams	22	26 μl; 50 μl (EpiSkin only)	√[d]	√[a]	–	Modified Frosch-Kligman soap chamber patch test with repetitive occlusive application	[42]
[i]SkinEthic	4	Chemicals from ECVAM pre-validation	50	100 μl	√[d]	√[a]	Histology	4-h patch test	[46]

AST aspartate aminotransferase, *ECVAM* European Centre for the Validation of Alternative Methods, *GM-CSF* granulocyte-macrophage colony-stimulating factor, *ICAM* intercellular adhesion molecule, *IFN* interferon, *IL* interleukin, *LDH* lactate dehydrogenase, *MTT* 3-[4,5-dimethylthiazol-2-yl]-2,5-diphenyltetrazolium bromide, *MTS* 3-(4,5-dimethylthiazol-2-yl)-5-(3-carboxymethoxyphenyl)-2-(4-sulfophenyl)-2H-tetrazolium, inner salt, *NP* not provided, *RNA* ribonucleic acid, *SCF* stem cell factor, *SDS* sodium dodecyl sulfate, *TGF* transforming growth factor, *TNF* tumor necrosis factor, *TNF-R* tumor necrosis factor receptor

[a]Culture media collected immediately after exposure

[b]IMEDEX (Chaponost, France)

[c]Laboratoire des Susbstitus Cutanés

[d]MTT and/or LDH assessment

[e]MatTek Corporation (Ashland, MA, USA)

[f]Advanced Tissue Sciences (ATS; La Jolla, CA, USA)

[g]MTS and/or Alamar Blue

[h]Culture media collected 24 h post-exposure

[i]SkinEthic, Nice, France

[j]Episkin SNC (L'Oréal, Chaponost, France)

[k]Wella/Cosmital SA (Research Company of Wella AG, Germany), Marly, Switzerland

the tissues exposed to the test materials included in this study (Table 1) varied widely for correctly predicted irritants (111.6–565.1 μg/ml), overpredicted materials (72.0–188.1 μg/ml), or underpredicted materials (15.8–215.1 μg/ml), while the range was tighter for correctly predicted nonirritants to human skin (1.65–38.4 μg/ml). The wide range of IL-1α response likely resides with the nature of the ingredient or formulation, bioavailability, kinetics of penetration, etc. and makes the correlation with human clinical data difficult for some of the products tested.

The study by Augustin et al. [40] used an in vitro test system based on the skin equivalent (SE) which mimics the skin architecture better than the dermal equivalent (DE) model. The results obtained for the SE test system and using the tissue viability endpoint for the prediction model with a single cutoff value of 80 % (and no apparent cutoff values established for IL-1α) had a 79 % concordance with the human data (Table 1). The materials tested covered clinically five irritation categories (eight nonirritants, one very slightly irritating, three slightly irritating, one moderately irritating, and one strong irritant). When based on the single cutoff viability value used for the data analysis, the in vitro method had a mixed predictive capacity for the materials with intermediate irritation potential. The method was however capable of predicting correctly seven out of the eight nonirritating materials and the single strong irritant. The difficulty to address the materials with intermediate irritation potential by the in vitro assays revealed the need to either introduce more cutoff values for the viability endpoint, create cutoff values for the IL-1α endpoint, or further refine the assay to address the middle-range potential.

The study by Perkins et al. [12] correlated the in vitro response of 3D tissues to human skin data for a variety of materials (Table 1). Of particular interest were the antiperspirants and deodorants for which the IL-1α release data showed the greatest capacity to distinguish irritancy over a broad range and correlated well with consumer reported irritation (14-day cumulative irritancy test). A single study analyzed the IL-1α production by tissues exposed to antiperspirants and deodorants in comparison to reported incidence (in subject diaries) data of adverse skin effects. Despite the semiquantitative nature of this analysis, a remarkable correlation between the IL-1α data and adverse responses reported with human use was observed across the entire range of clinical responses [22].

The design of the in vitro methods described thus far revealed technical aspects that could be improved to further increase the predictive capacity of the test system when relying on the IL-1α endpoint. As such, the analysis of the IL-1α after long exposure times may not be particularly relevant to certain classes of materials (surfactants) [42] or may have limited reliability for other classes, especially those of mild irritant profile [20]. Addressing the middle irritation range is critical for comparison and ranking purposes as correctly isolating nonirritants can be achieved by many other assays without the need for a secondary endpoint.

To address the ranking of very mild, wash-off products, the in vitro methods based on 3D skin models were further refined in two studies published by Bernhofer et al. [43, 44] (Table 1) by introducing a short exposure time (1 h) and a postexposure period (24 h) to allow the secretion of IL-1α. The first study showed that the full thickness model used (Skin^{2}™ Model ZK1350, containing fibroblasts) separated irritating formulations (facial creams) from milder ones based on the expression of several cytokines [IL-1 receptor antagonist (ra), granulocyte-macrophage colony-stimulating factor (GM-CSF), and IL-8] [43]. However, these endpoints were not as efficient in identifying differences between mild irritants of this category. To address this issue, the EpiDerm™ model (without fibroblasts) was used and the IL-1α and IL-1ra responses were analyzed for the tissues with >80 % viability. The data showed that the lack of fibroblasts increased the sensitivity of the test system and enabled the detection of differences between surfactants of mild irritation potential [44]. This was particularly relevant for the IL-1ra endpoint which is part of a negative feedback system protecting against potential damage from an excess of IL-1α secretion. IL-1ra is secreted in response to topically applied irritants but is otherwise suppressed in the presence of fibroblasts. The reliability and relevance of the test system was confirmed in the second study [44] that analyzed cleansing bars and cleansing lotions that exhibited varying degrees of irritation potential in the mild range and correlated well with clinical data (Table 1).

A recent study [45] used a similar protocol to investigate the correlation of IL-1α release and clinical skin irritation results for various classes of surfactants. The manuscript advances the field significantly by analyzing the data from the structure/toxicity relationship perspective and introduces several new parameters specific to surfactants in the attempt to explain the cytotoxicity of this class of ingredients very frequently used in the cosmetic industry. The manuscript opens the door to similar investigations that could address other chemistries used for personal care and skin care products.

The efforts to model the in vitro methods to best predict human exposure continued by introducing an in vitro patch test to correlate with the similar clinical test [46]. The study showed that the in vitro patch test met the specificity, sensitivity, and overall accuracy performance criteria defined for the ECVAM pre-validation study [29] and even proposed a prediction model for the data analysis. This in vitro protocol was very promising for the advancement through a formal pre-validation; however, no progress was reported in recent years.

In an effort to allow for better correlations between in vitro and clinical data, attempts have been made to refine the clinical tests as well. For example, cytokine profiling of different skin layers was investigated in hopes of providing a mechanistic view of toxicity induced by various materials. Noninvasive methods to collect samples directly from human skin in clinical studies and using simple dermal tape adsorption technique were investigated [12, 47]. This procedure has been used to investigate baseline cytokine levels in the skin, to assess normal skin condition, and to evaluate changes due to chemical insult, existing dermatitis, or sun exposure by direct comparison between cytokines (IL-1α, IL-1ra, IL-8) and classic clinical endpoints such as erythema or transepidermal water loss (TEWL) [48–50]. It is of consideration to further compare the cytokine expression in the stripped human skin and in the culture media collected from 3D skin models treated with various materials and to generate relevant and reliable prediction models.

In conclusion, multiple in vitro assays are available for the preclinical safety assessment of skin care products. They are relied upon by industry before performing clinical studies or as standalone; some became validated, while others are undergoing further improvements to best address the safety testing needs of cosmetic and personal care products.

Skin Sensitization

Determination of skin sensitization potential is a critical toxicological endpoint in the safety assessment of cosmetic ingredients and formulations. Preservatives, hair dyes, and natural extracts are the most commonly implicated cosmetic ingredients in inducing an allergic reaction. These low-molecular-weight chemicals are known to cause a type IV delayed hypersensitivity reaction in the skin, also known as allergic contact dermatitis (ACD). ACD is the most prevalent form of immunotoxicity in humans with an occupational health-related adverse response cost of up to one billion per year estimated by NIOSH in 2009. Although in vivo tests including the guinea pig maximization test (GPMT) and the local lymph node assay (LLNA) have traditionally been used to assess skin sensitization, recent activity has focused on the development of novel nonanimal assays for the endpoint. European legislation and US research activities toward "twenty-first-century toxicology" are setting the standards for animal-free toxicological assessments, and the cosmetics industry has been the first to feel the effects. As per EU Regulation 1223/2009, animal testing of cosmetic ingredients and finished products is currently banned in the EU, as is the marketing of finished cosmetic products and the ingredients contained therein which were tested on animals for cosmetic safety assessment purposes. The marketing ban is creating a global ripple effect as non-EU-based companies that employ animal testing are no longer able to sell their cosmetics in the EU. The ban on animal testing does not imply that safety testing is unnecessary but rather that scientifically sound, proven methods using cellular and computational models serve as a replacement.

Hundreds of skin sensitizers have been identified, and research has accordingly focused on the mechanistic understanding of allergic contact dermatitis and the development of assays for detection of skin sensitizers. The adverse outcome pathway (AOP) for skin sensitization describes each key event in the complex cascade leading to allergic contact dermatitis [51]. The AOP concept supports a toxicity testing paradigm focused on toxicity pathways. The molecular initiating event (MIE) and the cellular, organ, and organism responses are defined, and assays which address each of these key responses are considered for inclusion in a testing strategy for that endpoint. Specifically for skin sensitization, a chemical must first penetrate into the viable epidermis and covalently interact with proteins in the skin (MIE), leading to cellular activation and the expression of genes, cell surface markers and cytokines (cellular response), then proliferation of T cells in lymph nodes (organ response), and ultimately the clinical manifestation of ACD (organism response). Three methods, each modeling a key event in the AOP, have reached an advanced regulatory status: the direct peptide reactivity assay (DPRA) modeling protein reactivity, the KeratinoSens^{TM} assay modeling keratinocyte activation, and the human cell line activation test (h-CLAT) modeling Langerhans cell activation and expression of related cell surface markers. Each assay has been evaluated for transferability, reproducibility, and accuracy, and following successful interlaboratory investigations has been endorsed by EURL ECVAM (European Union Reference Union Reference Laboratory for Alternatives to Animal Testing) as part of an integrated testing strategy to assess skin sensitization potential. As a culmination of these efforts, the Organisation for Economic Co-operation and Development (OECD) published the following test guidelines for nonanimal skin sensitization testing on 5 February 2015: direct peptide reactivity assay (DPRA) (OECD TG 442C) [52] and ARE-Nrf2 luciferase test method (also referred to as the KeratinoSens^{TM} Assay) (OECD TG 442D) [53]. The human cell line activation test (h-CLAT) has reached an advanced stage of pre-validation, and OECD TG is expected to be published soon. Although each assay was initially designed for the assessment of pure substances, ongoing research aims to understand how they may also be used for assessing formulations.

A common characteristic of all chemical allergens is their covalent modification of proteins followed by immune activation. Chemical allergens are intrinsically electrophilic, or may be transformed into electrophiles, and react with nucleophilic amino acids within proteins. Therefore, research has focused on the ability to identify chemical allergens, specifically skin sensitizers, based on their reactivity with peptides/proteins. The direct peptide reactivity assay (DPRA) is an in chemico assay that identifies dermal sensitizers based on their reactivity with synthetic peptides containing either lysine (Lys) or cysteine (Cys) [54]. The assay models the first key event, protein reactivity, in the skin sensitization AOP. In the DPRA method, the test chemical is incubated with two peptides, one containing Cys and one containing Lys, for 24 h. Following this reaction period, peptide depletion is analyzed by HPLC-UV. Depletion of the peptide is then used as a quantitative measure of reactivity and may be correlated with skin sensitization potential, with minimal reactivity indicating a non-sensitizer and mean peptide depletion of the Cys- and Lys peptides of >6.38 % indicating skin sensitization potential.

The KeratinoSens^{TM} assay is a cell-based reporter gene assay which identifies skin sensitizers by measuring the induction of a luciferase gene under the control of the antioxidant response element (ARE) derived from the human AKR1C2 gene [55]. Electrophilic chemicals are detected by inducing conformational changes in the Keap1 target protein, which in turn activates the ARE and leads to an upregulation of the luciferase reporter. The degree of upregulation is measured by relative luminescence, and cell viability is measured in parallel. In the adverse outcome pathway (AOP) leading to skin sensitization, this method addresses the second key event, gene expression in keratinocytes associated with the antioxidant/electrophile response element (ARE)-dependent pathway. In the KeratinoSens^{TM} assay, cells are grown for 24 h in 96-well plates, then the medium is replaced with medium containing the test chemical at 12 dilutions ranging from 0.98 to 2000 μM, and cells are incubated for 48 h followed by measurement of luciferase activity and cell viability. The assay includes a full dose–response analysis for each chemical and is performed in three independent experiments, with each experiment being performed in triplicate. Luciferase gene induction and cell viability relative to the solvent controls included on each plate are calculated, and chemicals can be rated as positive or negative using the prediction model for the assay. A chemical is positive if it meets the following criteria: (1) it produces a statistically significant induction of luciferase activity >1.5-fold in at least 2/3 experiments, (2) the concentration where this induction is observed (EC1.5 value) is below 1000 μM, and (3) the viability at the EC1.5 value-determining concentration is greater than 70 %. Alternatively, a chemical is rated as negative if it fails to meet these criteria.

The human cell line activation test (h-CLAT) is a cell-based skin sensitization assay which identifies skin sensitizers based on increased expression of CD86 and CD54 in THP-1 cells (a human leukemia cell line) in response to treatment with test chemical [56]. The h-CLAT method is proposed to address the third key event (dendritic cell activation) in the skin sensitization AOP. It is well known that dendritic cells in the skin, Langerhans cells, play a critical role in the induction of skin sensitization. Upon antigen capture, the Langerhans cells undergo maturations and migrate to the draining lymph nodes. This Langerhans cells maturation is characterized by the upregulation of cell surface markers, CD86 and CD54. In the assay, THP-1 cells are grown in 24-well plates and treated with eight concentrations of test chemical for 24 h, then cell staining with CD86 and CD54 antibodies is performed, and expression of cell surface antigens and cell viability (using propidium iodide) is analyzed by flow cytometry. Each chemical is evaluated in three independent experiments. For a test chemical to be rated as positive, the relative fluorescence intensity (RFI) of CD86 and CD54 should be greater than 150 or 200, respectively, for at least one concentration.

Thus far, over 100 chemicals have been evaluated using these assays, and the results indicate a good predictive value for each assay as compared to the available correlative in vivo and human clinical data. Data suggest that each assay may serve as a valuable preclinical screening tool to assess the skin sensitization potential of a wide range of ingredients. However, due to the complex cascade of events leading to skin sensitization, it is generally thought that an integrated testing approach combining multiple assays and in silico predictive tools will be needed to fully replace the animal-based methods. There is a significant effort underway to ascertain how the nonanimal assays may be combined to both qualitatively and quantitatively assess skin sensitization most effectively.

Conclusions

Although there has been significant focus on the regulatory applicability of nonanimal methods, the most routine use of the assays is screening during product development and evaluating products which do not require pre-market approval. Since cosmetics fall in this category, companies may choose how to design their testing strategies to ensure the safety of their products. Some companies may use the assays as a screening tool before initiating a clinical test, while others may use a single in vitro assay or a combination of assays to assess a single endpoint without further clinical confirmation. The in vitro assays presented herein address the first critical endpoints, skin irritation and skin sensitization, for assessing the safety of cosmetics and personal care ingredients and formulations. Use of these assays will be essential for understanding the skin toxicity profile of novel ingredients and formulations before progressing into clinical testing or consumer use.

Beyond cosmetics, other industries not required by law to replace animal methods have proactively developed programs to phase out animal testing and only test on animals when required for regulatory purposes. Developing an in vitro program may be spurred by the changing regulatory landscape, ethical considerations for the reduction of animal use for safety assessments, the need for quicker and relatively inexpensive screening tools, or a combination of the above.

References

1. Morganti P, Paglialunga S. EU borderline cosmetic products review of current regulatory status. Clin Dermatol. 2008;26:392–7.
2. Draize J, Woodard G, Calvery H. Methods for the study of irritation and toxicity of substances applied topically to the skin and mucous membranes. J Pharmacol Exp Ther. 1944;82:377–90.
3. Weil CS, Scala RA. Study of intra- and interlaboratory variability in the results of rabbit eye and skin irritation tests. Toxicol Appl Pharmacol. 1971;19:276–360.
4. Phillips 2nd L, Steinberg M, Maibach HI, Akers WA. A comparison of rabbit and human skin response to certain irritants. Toxicol Appl Pharmacol. 1972;21:369–82.
5. Nixon GA, Tyson CA, Wertz WC. Interspecies comparisons of skin irritancy. Toxicol Appl Pharmacol. 1975;31:481–90.
6. Basketter DA, York M, McFadden JP, Robinson MK. Determination of skin irritation potential in the human 4-h patch test. Contact Dermatitis. 2004;51:1–4.
7. Netzlaff F, Lehr CM, Wertz PW, Schaefer UF. The human epidermis models EpiSkin, SkinEthic and EpiDerm: an evaluation of morphology and their suitability for testing phototoxicity, irritancy, corrosivity, and substance transport. Eur J Pharm Biopharm. 2005;60:167–78.
8. Gibbs S, Vicanova J, Bouwstra J, Valstar D, Kempenaar J, Ponec M. Culture of reconstructed epidermis in a defined medium at 33 degrees C shows a delayed epidermal maturation, prolonged lifespan and improved stratum corneum. Arch Dermatol Res. 1997;289:585–95.
9. Gibbs S, Vietsch H, Meier U, Ponec M. Effect of skin barrier competence on SLS and water-induced IL-1alpha expression. Exp Dermatol. 2002;11:217–23.
10. Boelsma E, Gibbs S, Faller C, Ponec M. Characterization and comparison of reconstructed skin models: morphological and immunohistochemical evaluation. Acta Derm Venereol. 2000;80:82–8.
11. Ponec M, Boelsma E, Weerheim A, Mulder A, Bouwstra J, Mommaas M. Lipid and ultrastructural characterization of reconstructed skin models. Int J Pharm. 2000;203:211–25.
12. Perkins MA, Osborne R, Rana FR, Ghassemi A, Robinson MK. Comparison of in vitro and in vivo human skin responses to consumer products and ingredients with a range of irritation potential. Toxicol Sci. 1999;48:218–29.
13. Wells T, Basketter DA, Schröder KR. In vitro skin irritation: facts and future. State of the art review of mechanisms and models. Toxicol In Vitro. 2004;18:231–43.
14. Costin G-E, Raabe H, Curren R. In vitro safety testing strategy for skin irritation using the 3D reconstructed human epidermis. Rom J Biochem. 2009;46:165–86.
15. ECETOC. Technical report No. 66. Skin irritation and corrosion: referenced chemicals data bank. 1995.
16. Jirova D, Liebsch M, Basketter D, Spiller E, Kejlova K, Bendova H, Marriott M, Kandarova H. Comparison of human skin irritation and photo-irritation patch test data with cellular in vitro assays and animal in vivo data. AATEX. 2007;14:359–65.
17. Cua AB, Wilhelm K-P, Maibach HI. Cutaneous sodium lauryl sulfate irritation potential: age and regional variability. Br J Dermatol. 1990;123:607–13.
18. Dillarstone A, Paye M. Antagonism in concentrated surfactant system. Contact Dermatitis. 1993;28:198.
19. Basketter DA, Whittle E, Griffiths HA, York M. The identification and classification of skin irritation hazard by a human patch test. Food Chem Toxicol. 1994;32:769–75.
20. Robinson MK, Perkins MA, Basketter DA. Application of a 4-h human patch test method for comparative and investigative assessment of skin irritation. Contact Dermatitis. 1998;38:194–202.
21. Basketter DA, Chamberlain M, Griffiths HA, Rowson M, Whittle E, York M. The classification of skin irritants by human patch test. Food Chem Toxicol. 1997;35:845–52.
22. Robinson MK, Osborne R, Perkins MA. In vitro and human testing strategies for skin irritation. Ann N Y Acad Sci. 2000;919:192–204.
23. Robinson MK, McFadden JP, Basketter DA. Validity and ethics of the human 4-h patch test as an alternative method to assess acute skin irritation potential. Contact Dermatitis. 2001;45:1–12.
24. Robinson MK, Kruszewski FH, Al-Atrash J, Blazka ME, Gingell R, Heitfeld FA, Mallon D, Snyder NK, Swanson JE, Casterton PL. Comparative assessment of acute skin irritation potential of detergent formulations using a novel human 4-h patch test method. Food Chem Toxicol. 2005;43:1703–12.
25. Spielmann H, Hoffmann S, Liebsch M, Botham P, Fentem JH, Eskes C, Roguet R, Cotovio J, Cole T, Worth A, Heylings J, Jones P, Robles C, Kandarova H, Gamer A, Remmele M, Curren R,

Raabe H, Cockshott A, Gerner I, Zuang V. The ECVAM international validation study on in vitro tests for acute skin irritation: report on the validity of the EPISKIN and EpiDerm assays and on the Skin Integrity Function Test. Altern Lab Anim. 2007;35:559–601.
26. Hoffmann S, Saliner AG, Patlewicz G, Eskes C, Zuang V, Worth AP. A feasibility study developing an integrated testing strategy assessing skin irritation potential of chemicals. Toxicol Lett. 2008;180:9–20.
27. Cameron DM, Donahue DA, Costin GE, Kaufman LE, Avalos J, Downey ME, Billhimer WL, Gilpin S, Wilt N, Simion FA. Confirmation of in vitro and clinical safety assessment of behentrimonium chloride-containing leave-on body lotions using post-marketing adverse event data. Toxicol In Vitro. 2013;27:2203–12.
28. Miles A, Berthet A, Hopf NB, Gilliet M, Raffoul W, Vernez D, Spring P. A new alternative method for testing skin irritation using a human skin model: a pilot study. Toxicol In Vitro. 2014;28:240–7.
29. Fentem JH, Briggs D, Chesne C, Elliott GR, Harbell JW, Heylings JR, Portes P, Roguet R, van de Sandt JJ, Botham PA. A prevalidation study on in vitro tests for acute skin irritation. Results and evaluation by the management team. Toxicol In Vitro. 2001;15:57–93.
30. Bagley DM, Gardner JR, Holland G, Lewis RW, Regnier JF, Stringer DA, Walker AP. Skin irritation: reference chemicals data bank. Toxicol In Vitro. 1996;10:1–6.
31. Demetrulias J, Donnelly T, Morhenn V, Jessee B, Hainsworth S, Casterton P, Bernhofer L, Martin K, Decker D. Skin$^{2®}$ – and in vitro human skin model: the correlation between in vivo and in vitro skin testing of surfactants. Exp Dermatol. 1998;7:18–26.
32. Doyle JM, Dressler WE, Rachui SR. Evaluation of two in vitro human skin equivalents (EpiDERM™ and SKIN^{2}™ model ZK13000 for assessing the skin irritation potential of personal care products and chemicals. In: Salem H, Katz SA, editors. Advances in animal alternatives for safety and efficacy testing. Washington, DC: Taylor & Francis; 1998. p. 285–91.
33. Sauder D, Pastore S. Cytokines in contact dermatitis. Am J Contact Dermat. 1994;4:215–24.
34. Kimber I, Dearman RJ, Cumberbatch M. Epidermal cytokines and the induction of allergic and non-allergic contact dermatitis. Arch Toxicol Suppl. 1997;19:229–38.
35. McKenzie RC, Sauder DN. The role of keratinocyte cytokines in inflammation and immunity. J Invest Dermatol. 1990;95:105S–7.
36. Broeckx A, Blondeel A, Boom-Gossens A, Achten G. Cosmetic intolerance. Contact Dermat. 1987;16:189–94.
37. Osborne R, Perkins MA. An approach for development of alternative test methods based on mechanisms of skin irritation. Food Chem Toxicol. 1994;32:133–42.
38. de Brugerolle de Fraissinette A, Picarles V, Chibout S, Kolopp M, Medina J, Burtin P, Ebelin ME, Osborne S, Mayer FK, Spake A, Rosdy M, De Wever B, Ettlin RA, Cordier A. Predictivity of an in vitro model for acute and chronic skin irritation (SkinEthic) applied to the testing of topical vehicles. Cell Biol Toxicol. 1999;15:121–35.
39. Roguet R, Cohen C, Robles C, Courtellemont P, Tolle M, Guillot JP, Pouradier DX. An interlaboratory study of the reproducibility and relevance of EpiSkin, a reconstructed human epidermis, in the assessment of cosmetics irritancy. Toxicol In Vitro. 1998;12:295–304.
40. Augustin C, Collombel C, Damour O. Use of dermal equivalent and skin equivalent models for in vitro cutaneous irritation testing of cosmetic products: comparison with in vivo human data. J Toxicol Cutan Ocul Toxicol. 1998;17:5–17.
41. Warren R, Sanders LM, Curtis SL, Wong LF, Zhu C, Tollens FR, Otte TE. Human in vitro and in vivo cutaneous responses to soap suspension: role of solution behavior in predicting potential irritant contact dermatitis. In Vitr Mol Toxicol. 1999;12:97–107.
42. Faller C, Bracher M. Reconstructed skin kits: reproducibility of cutaneous irritancy testing. Skin Parmacol Appl Skin Physiol. 2002;15:74–91.
43. Bernhofer LP, Seiberg M, Martin KM. The influence of the response of skin equivalent systems to topically applied consumer products by epithelial-mesenchymal interactions. Toxicol In Vitro. 1999;13:219–29.
44. Bernhofer LP, Bakovic S, Appa Y, Martin KM. IL-1alpha and IL-1ra secretion from epidermal equivalents and the prediction of the irritation potential of mild soap and surfactant-based consumer products. Toxicol In Vitro. 1999;13:231–9.
45. Lémery E, Briançon S, Chevalier Y, Border C, Oddos T, Gohier A, Molzinger MA. Skin toxicity of surfactants: structure/toxicity relationships. Colloids Surf A Physicochem Eng Asp. 2015;469:166–79.
46. Tornier C, Rosdy M, Maibach HI. In vitro skin irritation testing on reconstituted human epidermis: reproducibility for 50 chemicals tested in two protocols. Toxicol In Vitro. 2006;20:401–16.
47. Perkins MA, Osterhues MA, Farage MA, Robinson MK. A noninvasive method to assess skin irritation and compromised skin conditions using simple tape adsorption of molecular markers of inflammation. Skin Res Technol. 2001;7:227–37.
48. de Jongh CM, Verberk MM, Withagen CE, Jacobs JJ, Rustemeyer T, Kezic S. Stratum corneum cytokines and skin irritation response to sodium lauryl sulfate. Contact Dermatitis. 2006;54:325–33.
49. de Jongh CM, Lutter R, Verberk MM, Kezic C. Differential cytokine expression in skin after single and repeated irritation by sodium lauryl sulfate. Exp Dermatol. 2007;16:1032–40.
50. de Jongh CM, Verberk MM, Spiekstra SW, Gibbs S, Kezic S. Cytokines at different stratum corneum levels in normal and sodium lauryl sulfate-irritated skin. Skin Res Technol. 2007;13:390–8.

51. Mackay C, Davies M, Summerfield V, Maxwell G. From pathways to people: applying the adverse outcome pathway (AOP) for skin sensitization to risk assessment. ALTEX. 2013;30:473–86.
52. OECD. Test No. 442C: In chemico skin sensitisation: Direct Peptide Reactivity Assay (DPRA), OECD guidelines for the testing of chemicals, Section 4. Paris: OECD Publishing; 2015. doi:10.1787/9789264229709-en.
53. OECD. Test No. 442D: In vitro skin sensitisation: ARE-Nrf2 Luciferase Test Method, OECD guidelines for the testing of chemicals, Section 4. Paris: OECD Publishing; 2015. doi:10.1787/9789264229822-en.
54. Gerberick FG, Vassallo JD, Bailey RE, Chaney JG, Morrall SW, Lepoittevin JP. Development of a peptide reactivity assay for screening contact allergens. Toxicol Sci. 2004;81:332–43.
55. Emter R, Ellis G, Natsch A. Performance of a novel keratinocyte-based reporter cell line to screen skin sensitizers in vitro. Toxicol Appl Pharmacol. 2010;245:281–90.
56. Ashikaga T, Yoshida Y, Hirota M, Yoneyama K, Itagaki H, Sakaguchi H, Miyazawa Y, Ito Y, Suzuki H, Toyoda H. Development of an in vitro skin sensitization test using human cell lines: human cell line activation test (h-CLAT). I. Optimization of the h-CLAT protocol. Toxicol In Vitro. 2006;20:767–73.

Textbook of Aging Skin

Miranda A. Farage • Kenneth W. Miller
Howard I. Maibach
Editors

Textbook of Aging Skin

Second Edition

Volume 3

With 574 Figures and 224 Tables

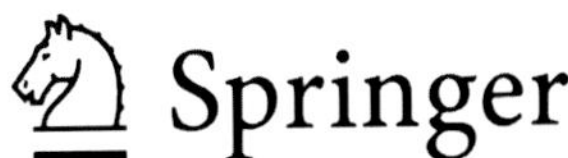

Editors
Miranda A. Farage
Winton Hill Business Center
The Procter and Gamble Company
Cincinnati, OH, USA

Kenneth W. Miller
Margoshes-Miller
Consulting, LLC
Cincinnati, OH, USA

Howard I. Maibach
Department of Dermatology
University of California
San Francisco, CA, USA

ISBN 978-3-662-47397-9 ISBN 978-3-662-47398-6 (eBook)
ISBN 978-3-662-47399-3 (print and electronic bundle)
DOI 10.1007/978-3-662-47398-6

Library of Congress Control Number: 2009938632

Printed on acid-free paper

This Springer imprint is published by Springer Nature
The registered company is Springer-Verlag GmbH Germany
The registered company address is: Heidelberger Platz 3, 14197 Berlin, Germany

Dedication

To a forgotten and sometimes lonely and scary aging journey – Much more dignity and respect are deserved for all of you. MAF, KWM, and *HIM*

When things go wrong as they sometimes will,
When the road you're trudging seems all uphill,
When the funds are low and the debts are high,
And you want to smile but you have to sigh,
When care is pressing you down a bit
Rest if you must, but don't you quit.
Success is failure turned inside out,
The silver tint on the clouds of doubt,
And you can never tell how close you are,
It may be near when it seems afar.
So, stick to the fight when you're hardest hit
It's when things go wrong that you mustn't quit.

—Unknown

Foreword

We mourn the loss of Professor Albert Kligman – a man whose energy, enthusiasm and intelligence benefited the specialty and many of us. His remarks below are as cogent today – as when written for the first Edition in December 2009.

Editors
MAF, KWM and HIM

The population is aging rapidly. Centenarians are no longer a rarity. The fastest growing segment of the population in the United States is people over 80. In the next 25 years, half of the population in the United States will be aged over 50.

These shifts will have a tremendous impact on the delivery of healthcare to the elderly and will require a new awareness of how cutaneous disorders affect the quality of life, comprising a heavy burden on health and wellbeing.

Physicians and healthcare workers are woefully ignorant of the distress, discomfort, and anxieties of people afflicted by disorders of the skin. There exists a widespread misconception that skin disorders are simply cosmetic nuisances that can be self-treated by a great assortment of anti-aging creams and lotions available at the local drug store. Most of these include high-sounding ingredients such as antioxidants, vitamins, nutrients, botanicals, and ancient folkloristic remedies, the efficacy and safety of which have never been tested. They offer little more than hope in a bottle. The fact is that common skin diseases may not often be lethal but can ruin enjoyment of life. Chronic itchy rashes can be maddening, lowering one's self-esteem, embarrassing, interfering with sleep, and often accompanied by depression, social isolation, and deterioration of appearance; they can also be uncomfortable, and, not least, costly to treat.

The elderly commonly take 15–20 oral supplements daily to fight the ailments of old age. These are generally useless and may be harmful, often interacting adversely with prescription drugs. The elderly often resort to alternative medicines instead of seeing their doctor to obtain FDA-approved drugs, and also often skip their daily doses to save money. Noncompliance is common. Misdiagnosis and mistreatment of the elderly by health-care workers are common. National surveys show that skin diseases increase steadily throughout our life-span. Old people may have as many as 5–10 coexistent cutaneous problems that are worthy of medical attention. Moreover, the clinical manifestations of skin diseases in the aged often have different

appearances than in the young, confounding diagnosis. Importantly, healing of chronic lesions, especially ulcers, is impaired in the elderly. Immunity is weakened, increasing susceptibility to infections. Response to treatment is slower, leading to noncompliance. Adverse drug reactions are common and too commonly not suspected. Management of chronic conditions is difficult and frustrating.

The above litany of problems makes this textbook edited by Farage, Miller, and Maibach a welcome addition to the literature. It is invaluable as a reference resource covering exhaustively an enormous number of clinical conditions. No topic is neglected including cosmetic treatments. The numerous contributions are by highly qualified experts who have a published record of expertise.

This comprehensive volume is also practical and relevant to the everyday world of clinical practice. The information will be useful to physicians, manufacturers of drugs and skincare products, educators, investigators, nursing home personnel, estheticians, and federal regulators.

This first edition is up to date, including much new material that belongs to the shelves of every library, which deals with geriatric problems. Dermatologists especially will be remiss if they do not put this volume within easy reach for consultation as they encounter a swelling clientele of aging patients.

University of Pennsylvania
Philadelphia, PA, USA

Albert M. Kligman M.D., Ph.D.
Professor Emeritus

Preface

The skin is a portal of knowledge on aging. From its softness and smoothness in infancy, through its suppleness in youth, to its wrinkled texture in elders, the skin displays the most visible and accessible manifestations of aging.

Due to falling birth rates and rising life expectancies in industrialized countries, the average age of the population is increasing. People are more preoccupied with looking and "staying" young, and research into the process of aging has expanded.

Although excellent compendia exist on the subject of aging skin, the body of knowledge is burgeoning and we still have more to learn. The purposes of this textbook are: (1) to compile the most current information into one comprehensive reference (it covers a range of topics, from the basics of skin structure and function to the cellular and molecular mechanisms of aging, to the latest bioengineering instruments used to assess age-related changes in the skin); (2) to guide on how to utilize skin as a tool for insights into the remainder of organs; and (3) to encourage the rapidly expanding universe of aging research in a more holistic aspect (heart, lung, brain, etc., as well as laboratories and investigators/foundations/government agencies) to utilize the readily available skin as an entry/surrogate for research on other organs.

Contributors are internationally recognized experts from multiple disciplines germane to this topic. We gratefully acknowledge all contributors for sharing their time and expertise.

We expect this second edition of the textbook to be valuable to researchers and students with an interest in aging skin, and the aging process in general. Because research progress in this area is rapid, we hope to update this compendium periodically as advances in the field dictate.

The editors welcome suggestions for the third edition.

Miranda A. Farage
Kenneth W. Miller
Howard I. Maibach

Acknowledgments

Deep appreciation and grateful thank yous are extended to the many experts who contributed both knowingly and indirectly to this book.

A special thank you to Drs. N. Enane-Anderson, G. Collier, P. Schofield, R. Leboeuf, Mr. Ron Visscher, and Mr. John Cooper, who generously offered their time and expertise to peer-review relevant chapters and for their support of this book. No praise is excessive for their efforts, and they have our heartfelt gratitude.

Many thanks go to the significant efforts of all the contributors of this book and the valuable time they dedicated preparing their chapters. This book represents the fruits of a jointly conceived and executed venture and has benefited from global and diverse partners.

We would also like to single out Ms. Sunali Mull (Springer Editorial-India) for a special recognition. Her great efforts, time, discipline, and dedication helped moved this book forward on a timely and organized manner. In addition, we would like to thank Mr. S. Klemp, Mr. A. Baroi, Ms. R. Amos, Ms. A. Singh, Ms. S. Friedrichsen, and Ms. S. Westendorf (Springer Office) for their help in moving this book forward. We acknowledge the usefulness of the new "SpringerMeteor" system which helped contributors and editors get the first glance of the future of electronic information/submission/editing.

In addition, Dr. D. A. Hutchins, Ms. Z. Schwen, Ms. W. Wippel, Ms. G. Entrup, Dr. T. L. Nusair, and Ms. P. Fifth (Rest in Peace our dear friend; your memories will always be with us) have all assisted with this book.

Above all, our everlasting gratitude, thanks, and love go to our parents who inspired us and to our families and children who supported, helped, and encouraged us all the way with their incredible patience. Your continuous care, unconditional love, and sacrifice made all this possible and easier to achieve.

MAF, *KWM*, and *HIM*

Contents

Volume 1

About the Editors

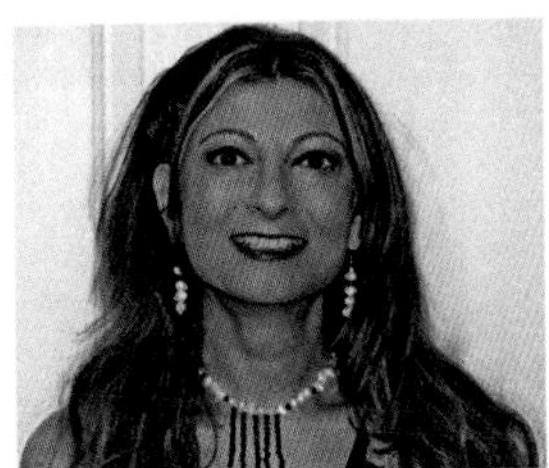

Miranda A. Farage is a Research Fellow in the Global Clinical Sciences Innovation at the Procter & Gamble Company, Cincinnati, Ohio. Dr. Farage leads global research on genital health, dermatological testing and claims, new clinical methods development, sensitive skin, physiology, clinical toxicology, women's health, quality of life, and related fields. Dr. Farage has invented novel state-of-the-art clinical test methods that have resulted in efficient ways of assessing new technologies and products as well as the filing of 15 patent applications. She has published more than 200 manuscripts and chapters in peer-reviewed journals and medical books. She is the Editor-in-Chief of several books such as *The Vulva*; *Textbook of Aging Skin*, first edition; *Topical Application and the Mucosa*; and *Skin, Mucosa and Menopause: Management of Clinical Issues*.

Dr. Farage is a member of many scientific societies including the American Academy of Dermatology, the European College of Society of Vulva Diseases, the National Vulvodynia Association, the American Society for Testing and Materials (ASTM) International, and the Science Advisory Board. Currently, she is serving on the editorial boards of more than a dozen scientific, dermatology, and medical journals. She received a Ph.D. in Medical Sciences and a master degree (MS) in Biology from the University of Illinois, Urbana-Champaign. Before joining Procter & Gamble, she was a faculty member at the Virginia Polytechnic Institute and State University (Virginia Tech).

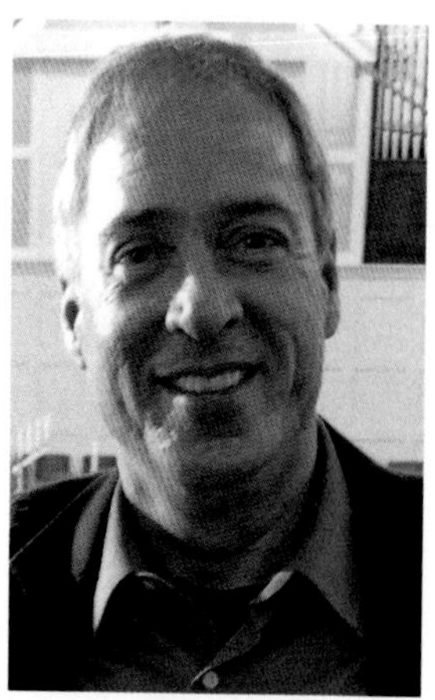

Kenneth W. Miller

- Principal Consultant, Margoshes Miller Consulting LLC, for Product Safety, Toxicology, and Regulatory Strategy (June 2015 to present).
- Associate Director, The Procter & Gamble Company (July 1984–June 2015), with global safety and regulatory experience in medical devices, OTC health care products, and food products.
- Diplomate, American Board of Toxicology (1986–2006).
- Postdoctoral Fellow, University of Medicine and Dentistry of New Jersey (June 1982–July 1984), Nutritional Biochemistry.
- Doctoral degree (Ph.D.): Cornell University, 1982, Toxicology and Food Chemistry.
- Master's degree (M.S.): Cornell University, 1979, Toxicology and Food Chemistry.
- Bachelor's degree (B.S.): Iowa State University, 1977, Biology.
- Dr. Miller has published over 50 manuscripts in the area of toxicology in peer-reviewed journals plus numerous abstracts, book chapters, and presentations at meetings of scientific societies. He is a member of several scientific and professional societies.

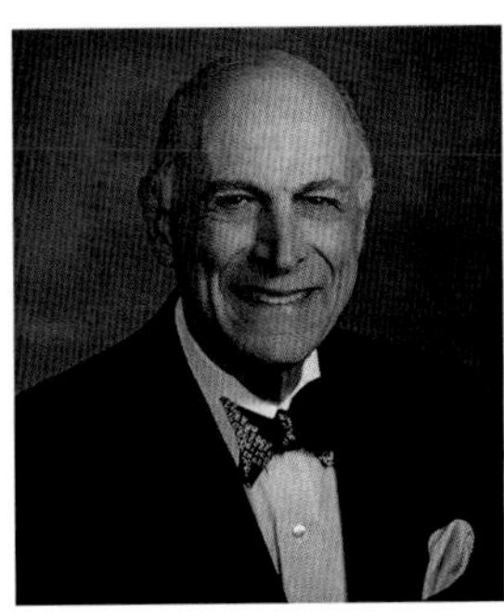

Howard I. Maibach
Present Title: Professor

Education	Degree
Tulane University, New Orleans, LA	A.B.
Tulane University, New Orleans, LA	M.D.
USPHS, Hospital of the University of Pennsylvania	Resident/Fellow

Honorary degrees	Degree	Year
L'Universite de Paris-Sud, France	Ph.D.	1985
Université Claude Bernard Lyon 1, France	Ph.D.	2008
University of Southern Denmark	M.D.	2010

Dr. Howard Maibach joined the University of California Faculty as Assistant Professor and is currently Professor of Dermatology.

Dr. Maibach, an expert in contact and occupational dermatitis, sees patients at the Environmental Dermatoses Clinic, which is part of the Dermatology Clinic at UCSF. His most active fields of research are in dermatopharmacology, dermatotoxicology, and environmental dermatoses. He has been doing human subject research for 45 years.

He has been on the editorial board of more than 30 scientific journals. His bibliography includes more than 2790 publications and 100 books.

He is member of 19 professional societies including the American Academy of Dermatology (AAD), San Francisco Dermatological Society (SFDS), North American Contact Dermatitis Group (NACDG), American Contact Dermatitis Society (ACDS), International Contact Dermatitis Research Group (ICDRG), Society of Toxicology (SOT), European Environmental and Contact Dermatitis Research Group (EECDRG), and the Internal Commission on Occupational Health. He is a consultant to government, academia, and industry worldwide.

Dr. Howard Maibach was honored as the 2013 recipient of The Master Dermatologist Award by The American Academy of Dermatology's 71st Annual Conference held in Miami, Florida. This prestigious award recognizes an Academy member's significant contributions to the field of dermatology and to the American Academy of Dermatology.

In March 2015, The International League of Dermatological Societies (ILDS) awarded Dr. Maibach their 2014 ILDS Certificate of Appreciation in recognition of his outstanding contribution to dermatology, both nationally and internationally, through his work, research, publications, and teaching in the USA and over 60 countries.

Contributors

Rami Abadi Department of Dermatology, American University of Beirut Medical Center, Beirut, Lebanon

Ossama Abbas Department of Dermatology, American University of Beirut Medical Center, Beirut, Lebanon

Jihane Abou Rahal Department of Dermatology, American University of Beirut Medical Center, Beirut, Lebanon

Jean Adamus Unilever Research and Development, Trumbull, CT, USA

Mohamed A. Adly Department of Zoology, Faculty of Science, Sohag University, Sohag, Egypt

Avani Ahuja Department of Biotechnology, Jaypee Institute of Information Technology, Noida, UP, India

Denize Ainbinder Institute of Drug Research, School of Pharmacy, The Hebrew University of Jerusalem, Jerusalem, Israel

A. Deniz Akkaya Department of Dermatology, Koç University Hospital, Istanbul, Turkey

Department of Dermatology, V.K. Foundation, American Hospital of Istanbul, Istanbul, Turkey

Ali Alikhan Department of Dermatology, University of Cincinnati, Cincinnati, OH, USA

Satoshi Amano Shiseido Research Center, Yokohama, Japan

Marco Ardigò Clinical Dermatology, IFO San Gallicano Dermatological Institute, Rome, Italy

Melina C. Armenaka Department of Dermatology and Venereology, University of Athens, A. Sygros Hospital, Athens, Greece

Hanan Assaf Department of Dermatology, Saudi German Hospital, Jeddah, Saudi Arabia

Daniel Asselineau L'Oreal, Research and Innovation, Aulnay-sous-bois, France

Carmela Rita Balistreri Department of Pathobiology and Medical Biotechnologies, University of Palermo, Immunosenescence Unit, Palermo, Italy

Elma Baron Department of Dermatology, Case Western Reserve University, Cleveland, OH, USA

Leslie S. Baumann Baumann Cosmetic and Research Institute, Miami, FL, USA

Enzo Berardesca San Gallicano Dermatological Institute, Rome, Italy

Françoise Bernerd L'Oreal Research and Innovation, Aulnay-sous-bois, France

Christiane Bertin SkinCare R&D, Johnson & Johnson Santé Beauté France, Issy-les-Moulineaux, France

Marianne Berwick Internal Medicine, Division of Epidemiology, University of New Mexico, Albuquerque, NM, USA

Tapan K. Bhattacharyya Otolaryngology-Head and Neck Surgery, University of Illinois, Chicago, IL, USA

Emil Bisaccia Columbia University College of Physicians and Surgeons, New York, NY, USA

Johannes Bischof Department of Cell Biology, Division of Genetics, University of Salzburg, Salzburg, Austria

Donald L. Bissett Beauty Technology Division, The Procter & Gamble Company, Sharon Woods Innovation Center, Cincinnati, OH, USA

Donald L. Bjerke The Procter & Gamble Company, Central Product Safety, Cincinnati, OH, USA

Thomas Blatt The Beiersdorf Research Center, Hamburg, Germany

Miroslav Blumenberg The R.O. Perelman Department of Dermatology, NYU Langone Medical Center, New York, NY, USA

Department of Biochemistry and Molecular Pharmacology, NYU Langone Medical Center, New York, NY, USA

Ulrike Blume-Peytavi Department of Dermatology and Allergy, Clinical Research Center for Hair and Skin Science, Charité-Universitätsmedizin Berlin, Berlin, Germany

Markus Böhm Department of Dermatology, Laboratory for Neuroendocrinology of the Skin and Interdisciplinary Endocrinology, University of Münster, Münster, Germany

Carol Bosko Unilever Research and Development, Trumbull, CT, USA

Mario Bramante Product Safety and Regulatory Affairs, Procter & Gamble Service GmbH, Schwalbach am Taunus, Germany

Douglas E. Brash Departments of Therapeutic Radiology, Genetics, and Dermatology, Yale School of Medicine, New Haven, CT, USA

Stéphane Brézillon Laboratoire de Biochimie, CNRS UMR 7369, Faculté de Médecine, Université de Reims-Champagne-Ardenne, Reims, France

Centre National de la Recherche Scientifique, CNRS UMR 7369, Reims, France

Carla Abdo Brohem R&D Department, Grupo Boticário, São José dos Pinhais, PR, Brazil

Robert L. Bronaugh Office of Cosmetics and Colors, Center for Food Safety and Applied Nutrition, Food and Drug Administration, College Park, MD, USA

John Jay P. Cadavona Department of Dermatology, University of California, San Francisco, CA, USA

Fernanda Camozzato Department of Dermatology, Brazilian Center for Studies in Dermatology, Porto Alegre, RS, Brazil

Giuseppina Candore Department of Pathobiology and Medical Biotechnologies, University of Palermo, Immunosenescence Unit, Palermo, Italy

Calogero Caruso Department of Pathobiology and Medical Biotechnologies, University of Palermo, Immunosenescence Unit, Palermo, Italy

Anne Lynn S. Chang Department of Dermatology, Stanford University School of Medicine, Redwood City, CA, USA

Duane L. Charbonneau The Procter & Gamble Company, Cincinnati, OH, USA

Alexandra Charruyer Department of Dermatology and Eli and Edythe Broad, Center of Regeneration Medicine and Stem Cell Research, University of California, Veterans Affairs Medical Center, San Francisco, CA, USA

Adele Chedraoui Department of Dermatology, Lebanese American University, Beirut, Lebanon

Ying Chen Global R&D, Equity and Claims, Reckitt Benckiser, Montvale, NJ, USA

Shujiang (Suzie) Cheng Colgate-Palmolive Company, Piscataway, NJ, USA

Raymond J. Cho Department of Dermatology, University of California, San Francisco, CA, USA

Yun-Hee Choi Anti-aging Research Institute of BIO-FD&C Co. Ltd., Incheon, Republic of Korea

Departments of Pharmacology and Global Medical Science, Institute of Lifestyle Medicine and Nuclear Receptor Research Consortium, Wonju College of Medicine, Yonsei University, Wonju, Republic of Korea

Kaare Christensen The Danish Twin Registry and The Danish Aging Research Center, Department of Public Health, University of Southern Denmark, Odense C, Denmark

Jin Ho Chung Department of Dermatology, Seoul National University College of Medicine, Seoul, Korea

Maria Grazia Cifone Life, Health and Environmental Sciences, University of L'Aquila, L'Aquila, Italy

Benedetta Cinque Life, Health and Environmental Sciences, University of L'Aquila, L'Aquila, Italy

Daniele Corridoni Division of Gastroenterology and Liver Disease, Department of Medicine, Case Western Reserve University School of Medicine, Cleveland, OH, USA

Giovanni Corsetti Department of Clinical and Experimental Sciences, Division of Human Anatomy and Physiopathology, University of Brescia, Brescia, Italy

Gertrude-Emilia Costin The Institute for In Vitro Sciences, Inc. (IIVS), Gaithersburg, MD, USA

Justine Courtois Laboratory of Skin Bioengineering and Imaging, Department of Dermatopathology, University Hospital of Liège, Liège, Belgium

Jonathan M. Crowther JMC Scientific Consulting Ltd, Surrey, UK

Shweta Dang Department of Biotechnology, Jaypee Institute of Information Technology, Noida, UP, India

Razvigor Darlenski Department of Dermatology and Venereology, Tokuda Hospital Sofia, Sofia, Bulgaria

Nancy C. Dawes The Procter and Gamble Company, Cincinnati, OH, USA

Philippe Delvenne Department of Dermatopathology, University Hospital of Liège, Liège, Belgium

Céline Deneuville L'Oreal, Research and Innovation, Aulnay-sous-bois, France

Luisa Di Marzio Department of Pharmacy, University of Chieti - Pescara "G d'Annunzio", Chieti - Pescara, Italy

Francesco S. Dioguardi Department of Internal Medicine and Community Health, University of Milan, Milan, Italy

Luisa A. DiPietro Center for Wound Healing and Tissue Regeneration, College of Dentistry, University of Illinois at Chicago, Chicago, IL, USA

Department of Biology, DePaul University, Chicago, IL, USA

Alexander S. Donath Cincinnati Facial Plastic Surgery, Cincinnati, OH, USA

Frank Dreher MERZ North America, Inc., San Mateo, CA, USA

Laurence Du-Thumm Colgate-Palmolive Company, Piscataway, NJ, USA

Christine Duval L'Oreal Research and Innovation, Aulnay-sous-bois, France

Kimberly M. Eickhorst Dermatology Associates Of W CT, Danbury, CT, USA

Moetaz El-Domyati Department of Dermatology, Al-Minya University, Al-Minya, Egypt

Akram Elmahdy Department of Dermatology, University of California, San Francisco, CA, USA

Peter Elsner Department of Dermatology and Dermatological Allergology, Universitätsklinikum Jena, Jena, Germany

Alex Eshaghian AE Skin, Encino, CA, USA

Khaled Ezzedine Department of Dermatology, CHU Saint-André, Bordeaux, France

Miranda A. Farage Winton Hill Business Center, The Procter & Gamble Company, Cincinnati, OH, USA

Susan P. Felter The Procter & Gamble Company, Cincinnati, OH, USA

Vincenzo Flati Department of Biotechnological and Applied Clinical Sciences, University of L'Aquila, L'Aquila, Italy

Sara Flores Department of Dermatology, University of Cincinnati, Cincinnati, OH, USA

Joachim W. Fluhr Department of Dermatology, Charité University Clinic, Berlin, Germany

Reema Gabrani Department of Biotechnology, Jaypee Institute of Information Technology, Noida, UP, India

Mary Carmen Gasco-Buisson P&G Brand Creation and Innovation, Procter & Gamble, Cincinnati, OH, USA

Licia Genovese Minerva Research Labs Ltd, London, UK

G. Frank Gerberick Human Safety Department, Procter and Gamble Company, Cincinnati, OH, USA

Ruby Ghadially Department of Dermatology and Eli and Edythe Broad, Center of Regeneration Medicine and Stem Cell Research, University of California, Veterans Affairs Medical Center, San Francisco, CA, USA

Paolo U. Giacomoni Elan Rose Int., Tustin, CA, USA

Sarah Girardeau-Hubert L'Oreal, Research and Innovation, Aulnay-sous-bois, France

Maurizio Giuliani Life, Health and Environmental Sciences, University of L'Aquila, L'Aquila, Italy

Francesca Giusti Department of Dermatology, University of Modena and Reggio Emilia, Modena, Italy

Paraskevi Gkogkolou Department of Dermatology, Laboratory for Neuroendocrinology of the Skin and Interdisciplinary Endocrinology, University of Münster, Münster, Germany

Farzam Gorouhi Department of Dermatology, University of California, Davis, CA, USA

James C. Grotting Department of Plastic Surgery, University of Alabama, Birmingham, AL, USA

Linna Guan Department of Dermatology, Case Western Reserve University, Cleveland, OH, USA

Christiane Guinot Biometrics and Epidemiology Unit, CE.R.I.E.S., Neuilly-sur-Seine, France

David A. Gunn Unilever Research and Development, Colworth Science Park, Sharnbrook, Bedfordshire, UK

Madhulika A. Gupta Department of Psychiatry, Schulich School of Medicine and Dentistry, University of Western Ontario, London, ON, Canada

Prashant Gupta Department of Biotechnology, Jaypee Institute of Information Technology, Noida, UP, India

Sanjay Gupta Department of Biotechnology, Jaypee Institute of Information Technology, Noida, UP, India

Varun Gupta Department of Plastic Surgery, Vanderbilt University, Nashville, TN, USA

Bahman Guyuron Department of Plastic Surgery, University Hospitals of Cleveland, Case Western Reserve University, Cleveland, OH, USA

Elisabeth Hahnel Department of Dermatology and Allergy, Clinical Research Center for Hair and Skin Science, Charité-Universitätsmedizin Berlin, Berlin, Germany

Tomohiro Hakozaki Beauty Technology Division, The Procter & Gamble Company, Mason Business Center, Mason, OH, USA

Stacy S. Hawkins Unilever Research and Development, Trumbull, CT, USA

Valerie Haydont L'Oreal, Research and Innovation, Aulnay-sous-bois, France

Timothy P. Heffernan Departments of Therapeutic Radiology, Genetics, and Dermatology, Yale School of Medicine, New Haven, CT, USA

Peter Helmbold Department of Dermatology, University of Heidelberg, Heidelberg, Germany

Trinh Hermanns-Lê Laboratory of Skin Bioengineering and Imaging, Department of Dermatopathology, University Hospital of Liège, Liège, Belgium

Electron Microscopy Unit, Department of Dermatopathology, Unilab Lg, University Hospital of Liège, Liège, Belgium

Doris Hexsel Department of Dermatology, Brazilian Center for Studies in Dermatology, Porto Alegre, RS, Brazil

Department of Dermatology, Pontificia Universidade Católica do Rio Grande do Sul (PUC-RS), Porto Alegre, RS, Brazil

K. Kye Higdon Department of Plastic Surgery, Vanderbilt University, Nashville, TN, USA

Greg Hillebrand Amway Corporation, Ada, MI, USA

Tetsuji Hirao Faculty of Pharmacy, Chiba Institute of Science, Choshi, Japan

Regina Hourigan Colgate-Palmolive Company, Piscataway, NJ, USA

Christopher R. Hughes Internal Medicine, Division of Epidemiology, University of New Mexico, Albuquerque, NM, USA

Michael F. Hughes U.S. Environmental Protection Agency, Office of Research and Development, National Health and Environmental Effects Research Laboratory, Research Triangle Park, NC, USA

Young Hui University of California, San Diego, CA, USA

Mahmoud R. Hussein Department of Pathology, Assir Central Hospital, and Assuit University, Assuit, Egypt

Qunshan Jia The Procter & Gamble Company, Central Product Safety, Cincinnati, OH, USA

Mary B. Johnson Beauty Technology Division, The Procter & Gamble Company, Sharon Woods Innovation Center, Cincinnati, OH, USA

Nancy Karapasha The Procter & Gamble Company, Cincinnati, OH, USA

Alexandra Katsarou Department of Dermatology and Venereology, University of Athens, A. Sygros Hospital, Athens, Greece

Linda M. Katz Office of Cosmetics and Colors, Center for Food Safety and Applied Nutrition, Food and Drug Administration, College Park, MD, USA

Abdul Ghani Kibbi Department of Dermatology, American University of Beirut Medical Center, Beirut, Lebanon

Christine C. Kim Dermatology Institute and Skin Care Center, Santa Monica, CA, USA

Hyeong-Sik Kim Anti-aging Research Institute of BIO-FD&C Co. Ltd., Incheon, Republic of Korea

Ki Woo Kim Departments of Pharmacology and Global Medical Science, Wonju College of Medicine, Yonsei University, Wonju, Republic of Korea

Institute of Lifestyle Medicine and Nuclear Receptor Research Consortium, Wonju College of Medicine, Yonsei University, Wonju, Republic of Korea

Won-Serk Kim Department of Dermatology, Kangbuk Samsung Hospital, Sungkyunkwan University College of Medicine, Seoul, South Korea

Mayumi Komine Department of Dermatology, Jichi Medical University, Shimotsuke, Tochigi, Japan

Jan Kottner Department of Dermatology and Allergy, Clinical Research Center for Hair and Skin Science, Charité-Universitätsmedizin Berlin, Berlin, Germany

Aleksandar Krbanjevic Department of Dermatology, Indiana University School of Medicine, Indianapolis, IN, USA

Shalini Krishnasamy University of California, Los Angeles, CA, USA

Nils Krueger Rosenpark Research, Darmstadt, Germany

Jean Krutmann Environmental Health Research Institute (IUF), Heinrich-Heine-University, Duesseldorf, Germany

Atul Kulkarni Anti-aging Research Institute of BIO-FD&C Co. Ltd., Incheon, Republic of Korea

School of Mechanical Engineering, Sungkyunkwan University, Suwon, South Korea

Mazen Kurban Department of Dermatology, American University of Beirut Medical Center, Beirut, Lebanon

Department of Biochemistry and Molecular Genetics, American University of Beirut Medical Center, Beirut, Lebanon

Department of Dermatology, Columbia University, New York, NY, USA

Cristina La Torre Life, Health and Environmental Sciences, University of L'Aquila, L'Aquila, Italy

S. Lahtinen Active Nutrition, DuPont Nutrition and Health, Kantvik, Finland

Samuel M. Lam Willow Bend Wellness Center, Lam Facial Plastic Surgery Center and Hair Restoration Institute, Plano, TX, USA

William J. Ledger Department of Obstetrics and Gynecology, The New York-Presbyterian Hospital, Weill Medical College of Cornell University, New York, NY, USA

Jeong Hun Lee Anti-aging Research Institute of BIO-FD&C Co. Ltd., Incheon, Republic of Korea

Marianne Lesuisse Department of Dermatology, Unilab Lg, Regional Hospital Citadelle, Liège, Belgium

Department of Dermatology, Regional Hospital of Huy, Huy, Belgium

Jacquelyn Levin West Dermatology, Rancho Santa Margarita, CA, USA

Davina A. Lewis Department of Anatomic Pathology and Histology, Covance CLS, Indianapolis, IN, USA

Aikaterini I. Liakou Departments of Dermatology, Venereology, Allergology and Immunology, Dessau Medical Center, Dessau, Germany

University of Athens Medical School, Athens, Greece

Andrea Lichterfeld Department of Dermatology and Allergy, Clinical Research Center for Hair and Skin Science, Charité-Universitätsmedizin Berlin, Berlin, Germany

Low Chai Ling The Sloane Clinic, Singapore, Singapore

Chengxu Liu The Procter & Gamble Company, Cincinnati, OH, USA

Jane Y. Liu Department of Dermatology, University of California, School of Medicine, San Francisco, CA, USA

Márcio Lorencini R&D Department, Grupo Boticário, São José dos Pinhais, PR, Brazil

Isabelle Lorthois Centre LOEX de l'Université Laval, Québec, QC, Canada

Stefanie Luebberding Rosenpark Research, Darmstadt, Germany

Judit Lukács Klinik für Hautkrankheiten, Universitätsklinikum Jena, Jena, Germany

John Lyga Avon Global R&D, Suffern, NY, USA

Howard I. Maibach Department of Dermatology, University of California, San Francisco, CA, USA

Robert Maidof Avon Global R&D, Suffern, NY, USA

Evgenia Makrantonaki Departments of Dermatology, Venereology, Allergology and Immunology, Dessau Medical Center, Dessau, Germany

Geriatry Research Group, Charité Universitaetsmedizin Berlin, Berlin, Germany

Department of Dermatology and Allergology, University Medical Center Ulm, Ulm, Germany

Denis Malvy EA 3677 and Centre René-Labusquière, Université Victor Segalen, Bordeaux, France

Department of Internal Medicine and Tropical Diseases, University Hospital Center, Bordeaux, France

Valéria Maria Di Mambro R&D Department, Grupo Boticário, São José dos Pinhais, PR, Brazil

François-Xavier Maquart Laboratoire de Biochimie, CNRS UMR 7369, Faculté de Médecine, Université de Reims-Champagne-Ardenne, Reims, France

Centre National de la Recherche Scientifique, CNRS UMR 7369, Reims, France

Centre Hospitalier et Universitaire (CHU) de Reims, Reims, France

Anna Margolina Research and Development, Skin Biology, Bellevue, WA, USA

Claire Marionnet L'Oreal Research and Innovation, Aulnay-sous-bois, France

Slaheddine Marrakchi Department of Dermatology, Hedi Chaker Hospital, Sfax, Tunisia

Daniel S. Marsman The Procter & Gamble Company, Cincinnati, OH, USA

Jean-Yves Mary INSERM U717, Biostatistics and Clinical Epidemiology, DBIM, Saint-Louis Hospital, University Paris 7, Paris, France

Paul J. Matts Procter & Gamble, Greater London Innovation Centre, Egham, Surrey, UK

Walid Medhat Department of Dermatology, Al-Minya University, Al-Minya, Egypt

Reena Mehra Sleep Medicine Center, The Cleveland Clinic, Cleveland, OH, USA

Esterina Melchiorre Life, Health and Environmental Sciences, University of L'Aquila, L'Aquila, Italy

Helen Meldrum Unilever Research and Development, Trumbull, CT, USA

Joseph Merregaert Laboratory of Molecular Biotechnology, Department of Biomedical Sciences, University of Antwerp, Antwerp, Belgium

Afton Metkowski Department of Dermatology and Itch Center, Temple University School of Medicine, Philadelphia, PA, USA

Thomas A. Meyer Bayer Healthcare, Memphis, TN, USA

Gianfranca Miconi Life, Health and Environmental Sciences, University of L'Aquila, L'Aquila, Italy

Kenneth W. Miller Margoshes-Miller Consulting, LLC, Cincinnati, OH, USA

Jillian Wong Millsop Department of Dermatology, University of California, Davis, Sacramento, CA, USA

Shivangi Mishra Department of Biotechnology, Jaypee Institute of Information Technology, Noida, UP, India

Sang Hyun Moh Anti-aging Research Institute of BIO-FD&C Co. Ltd., Incheon, Republic of Korea

Akimichi Morita Department of Geriatric and Environmental Dermatology, Nagoya City University Graduate School of Medical Sciences, Nagoya, Japan

D. James Morré MorNuCo, Inc, West Lafayette, IN, USA

Dorothy M. Morré MorNuCo, Inc, West Lafayette, IN, USA

Zeenat Nabi Colgate-Palmolive Company, Piscataway, NJ, USA

Kouichi Nakagawa Department of Radiological Life Sciences, Graduate School of Health Sciences, Hirosaki University, Hirosaki, Aomori, Japan

J. Frank Nash The Procter & Gamble Company, Central Product Safety, Cincinnati, OH, USA

Dany Nassar Department of Dermatology, American University of Beirut Medical Center, Beirut, Lebanon

Department of Anatomy, Cell Biology and Physiological Sciences, American University of Beirut Medical Center, Beirut, Lebanon

Véronique Neiveyans L'Oreal, Research and Innovation, Aulnay-sous-bois, France

Isaac M. Neuhaus Department of Dermatology, University of California, San Francisco, CA, USA

Paul Nghiem Departments of Therapeutic Radiology, Genetics, and Dermatology, Yale School of Medicine, New Haven, CT, USA

Kasra Soltani Nia Department of Dermatology, University of California, School of Medicine, San Francisco, CA, USA

Georgios Nikolakis Departments of Dermatology, Venereology, Allergology and Immunology, Dessau Medical Center, Dessau, Germany

John Nip Unilever Research and Development, Trumbull, CT, USA

Jean-Luc Nizet Department of Plastic Surgery, University Hospital of Liège, Liège, Belgium

Alex Nkengne Clarins Laboratories, Pontoise, France

Kimberly G. Norman Institute for In Vitro Sciences, Gaithersburg, MD, USA

John Oblong Beauty Technology Division, The Procter & Gamble Company, Sharon Woods Innovation Center, Cincinnati, OH, USA

Mutsumi Okazaki Department of Plastic and Reconstructive Surgery, Graduate School of Science, Tokyo Medical and Dental University, Bunkyo-ku, Tokyo, Japan

Yasemin Oram Department of Dermatology, V.K. Foundation, American Hospital of Istanbul, Istanbul, Turkey

A. C. Ouwehand Active Nutrition, DuPont Nutrition and Health, Kantvik, Finland

Noritaka Oyama Dermatology and Dermato-Allergology, Matsuda General Hospital, Ohno, Fukui, Japan

Department of Dermatology, Fukui University, Fukui, Japan

Herve Pageon L'Oreal, Research and Innovation, Aulnay-sous-bois, France

Paola Palumbo Life, Health and Environmental Sciences, University of L'Aquila, L'Aquila, Italy

Apostolos Pappas The Johnson & Johnson Skin Research Center, CPPW, a Division of Johnson & Johnson Consumer Companies, Inc, Skillman, NJ, USA

Byung-Soon Park Cellpark Dermatology Clinic, Seoul, South Korea

Evasio Pasini "S. Maugeri Foundation", IRCCS, Cardiology Rehabilitative Division, Medical Centre of Lumezzane, Brescia, Italy

Paula C. Pennacchi Department of Clinical Chemistry and Toxicology, School of Pharmaceutical Sciences, University of Sao Paulo, Sao Paulo, Brazil

Jerrold Scott Petrofsky Department of Physical Therapy, Loma Linda University, Loma Linda, CA, USA

School of Allied Health, Loma Linda University, Loma Linda, CA, USA

Christina Phuong Department of Dermatology, University of California San Francisco, San Francisco, CA, USA

Loren Pickart Research and Development, Skin Biology, Bellevue, WA, USA

Gérald E. Piérard Laboratory of Skin Bioengineering and Imaging, Department of Dermatopathology, University Hospital of Liège, Liège, Belgium

Sébastien L. Piérard Telecommunication and Imaging Laboratory, INTELSIG, Montefiore Institute, University of Liège, Liège, Belgium

Claudine Piérard-Franchimont Laboratory of Skin Bioengineering and Imaging, Department of Dermatopathology, University Hospital of Liège, Liège, Belgium

Department of Dermatology, Regional Hospital of Huy, Huy, Belgium

Raimondo Pinna Plastic and Reconstructive Surgery and Burns Centre, Brotzu Hospital, Cagliari, Italy

Thomas G. Polefka Life Science Solutions, LLC, Somerset, NJ, USA

S. Brian Potterf Unilever Research and Development, Trumbull, CT, USA

Tarl W. Prow Dermatology Research Centre, School of Medicine, The University of Queensland, Princess Alexandra Hospital, Translational Research Institute, Brisbane, QLD, Australia

Prashant Rai L'Oreal China, Shanghai, China

Utkrishta L. Raj Department of Biotechnology, Jaypee Institute of Information Technology, Noida, UP, India

Vibha Rani Department of Biotechnology, Jaypee Institute of Information Technology, Noida, UP, India

Matthew J. Ranzer Center for Wound Healing and Tissue Regeneration, College of Dentistry, University of Illinois at Chicago, Chicago, IL, USA

Department of Biology, DePaul University, Chicago, IL, USA

Anthony P. Raphael Dermatology Research Centre, School of Medicine, The University of Queensland, Princess Alexandra Hospital, Translational Research Institute, Brisbane, QLD, Australia

Wellman Center for Photomedicine, Massachusetts General Hospital, Harvard Medical School, Boston, MA, USA

Christina Raschke Department of Dermatology, University Hospital Jena, Jena, Germany

Suresh I. S. Rattan Laboratory of Cellular Ageing, Department of Molecular Biology and Genetics, Aarhus University, Aarhus C, Denmark

Anthony V. Rawlings AVR Consulting Ltd, Cheshire, UK

Glen Rein Innovative Biophysical Technologies, Ridgway, CO, USA

Klaus Richter Department of Cell Biology, Division of Genetics, University of Salzburg, Salzburg, Austria

Sylvie Ricois L'Oreal, Research and Innovation, Aulnay-sous-bois, France

Mark Rinnerthaler Department of Cell Biology, Division of Genetics, University of Salzburg, Salzburg, Austria

Caroline Ritacco Laboratory of Skin Bioengineering and Imaging, Department of Dermatopathology, University Hospital of Liège, Liège, Belgium

Diana Alyce Rivers The Department of Basic Biomedical Sciences, Touro College of Osteopathic Medicine, New York, NY, USA

Michael K. Robinson Global Biotechnology and Life Sciences Technology Platform, The Procter & Gamble Company, Mason Business Center, Mason, OH, USA

Sheila Rocha Unilever Research and Development, Trumbull, CT, USA

Igor Roganin DAO Clinic, Moscow, Russia

Claudia Romano Department of Clinical and Experimental Sciences, Division of Human Anatomy and Physiopathology, University of Brescia, Brescia, Italy

David J. Rowe University Hospitals, Case Western Reserve University, Cleveland, OH, USA

Nelly Rubeiz Department of Dermatology, American University of Beirut Medical Center, Beirut, Lebanon

Anna Rufo Department of Biotechnological and Applied Clinical Sciences, University of L'Aquila, L'Aquila, Italy

Cindy A. Ryan The Procter and Gamble Company, Cincinnati, OH, USA

Shingo Sakai Basic Research Laboratory, Kanebo Cosmetics Inc., Kanagawa, Japan

Salah Salman Department of Dermatology, American University of Beirut Medical Center, Beirut, Lebanon

Preamjit Saonanon Department of Ophthalmology, King Chulalongkorn Memorial Hospital, The Thai Red Cross Society, Chulalongkorn University, Bangkok, Thailand

Giovanni Scapagnini Department of Health Sciences, University of Molise, Campobasso, Italy

Richard Scarborough University Hospitals Case Medical Center, Cleveland, OH, USA

Dwight Scarborough Clinical Assistant Professor of Medicine, Division of Dermatology, The Ohio State University Wexner Medical Center, Columbus, OH, USA

Megan E. Schrementi Center for Wound Healing and Tissue Regeneration, College of Dentistry, University of Illinois at Chicago, Chicago, IL, USA

Department of Biology, DePaul University, Chicago, IL, USA

Peter Schroeder Environmental Health Research Institute (IUF), Heinrich-Heine-University, Duesseldorf, Germany

Miri Seiberg Seiberg Consulting, LLC, Princeton, NJ, USA

Stefania Seidenari Department of Dermatology, University of Modena and Reggio Emilia, Modena, Italy

Hyo Hyun Seo Anti-aging Research Institute of BIO-FD&C Co. Ltd., Incheon, Republic of Korea

Garima Sharma Department of Biotechnology, Jaypee Institute of Information Technology, Noida, UP, India

Susan N. Sherman SNS Research, Cincinnati, OH, USA

Shuichi Shibuya Department of Advanced Aging Medicine, Chiba University Graduate School of Medicine, Chiba, Japan

Takahiko Shimizu Department of Advanced Aging Medicine, Chiba University Graduate School of Medicine, Chiba, Japan

William Shingleton General Electric Company, Cardiff, UK

Sara Sibilla Minerva Research Labs Ltd, London, UK

Neha Singh Department of Biotechnology, Jaypee Institute of Information Technology, Noida, UP, India

James E. Sligh Medicine, Dermatology, The University of Arizona, Tucson, AZ, USA

Jack Sobel Infectious Diseases, Wayne State University, Detroit, MI, USA

Mi Young Song Anti-aging Research Institute of BIO-FD&C Co. Ltd., Incheon, Republic of Korea

Yuli Song The Procter & Gamble Company, Mason Business Center, Mason, OH, USA

Dan F. Spandau Departments of Dermatology and Biochemistry and Molecular Biology, Indiana University School of Medicine, Indianapolis, IN, USA

Georgios N. Stamatas SkinCare R&D, Johnson & Johnson Santé Beauté France, Issy-les-Moulineaux, France

Robert Stern The Department of Basic Biomedical Sciences, Touro College of Osteopathic Medicine, New York, NY, USA

Maria Karolin Streubel Department of Cell Biology, Division of Genetics, University of Salzburg, Salzburg, Austria

Paul R. Summers University of Utah School of Medicine, Salt Lake City, UT, USA

Cheri L. Swanson The Procter & Gamble Company, Sharon Woods Innovation Center, Cincinnati, OH, USA

Hachiro Tagami Department of Dermatology, Tohoku University School of Medicine, Sendai, Japan

Haw-Yueh Thong Department of Dermatology, University of California, San Francisco, CA, USA

Kirsti Tiihonen Active Nutrition, DuPont Nutrition and Health, Kantvik, Finland

Danielle Tokarz Wellman Center for Photomedicine, Massachusetts General Hospital, Harvard Medical School, Boston, MA, USA

Princess Margaret Cancer Centre, University Health Network, Toronto, ON, Canada

Marjana Tomic-Canic Wound Healing and Regenerative Medicine Research Program, Department of Dermatology and Cutaneous Surgery and Hussman Institute of Human Genomics, University of Miami Miller Medical School, Miami, FL, USA

Salina M. Torres Department of Pathology, Center for HPV Prevention, University of New Mexico, Albuquerque, NM, USA

Elka Touitou Institute of Drug Research, School of Pharmacy, The Hebrew University of Jerusalem, Jerusalem, Israel

Jeffrey B. Travers Departments of Pharmacology and Toxicology and Dermatology, Boonshoft School of Medicine at Wright State University, Dayton, OH, USA

Joel Tsevat Division of General Internal Medicine, Department of Internal Medicine, University of Cincinnati College of Medicine and Cincinnati VA Medical Center, Cincinnati, OH, USA

Katsuhiko Tsuchida Research and Development Department, Naris Cosmetics Co. Ltd., Osaka, Japan

Gabe Tzeghai Wyoming, OH, USA

Efstratios Vakirlis Department of Dermatology and Venereology, Aristotle University of Thessaloniki, Thessaloniki, Greece

Giuseppe Valacchi Department of Life Sciences and Biotechnology, University of Ferrara, Ferrara (FE), Italy

Department of Food and Nutrition, Kyung Hee University, Seoul, South Korea

Rodrigo Valdes-Rodriguez Department of Dermatology and Itch Center, Temple University School of Medicine, Philadelphia, PA, USA

Fabien Valet Biostatistics Department, Institut Curie, Paris, France

Jessica Michelle Vasquez-Soltero Research and Development, Skin Biology, Bellevue, WA, USA

Annika Vogt Clinical Research Center for Hair and Skin Science, Department of Dermatology and Allergy, Charité-Universitätsmedizin Berlin, Berlin, Germany

Shilpa Vora Unilever Research and Development, Bangalore, India

Kenji Watanabe Department of Advanced Aging Medicine, Chiba University Graduate School of Medicine, Chiba, Japan

Yanusz Wegrowski Laboratoire de Biochimie, CNRS UMR 7369, Faculté de Médecine, Université de Reims-Champagne-Ardenne, Reims, France

Centre National de la Recherche Scientifique, CNRS UMR 7369, Reims, France

Horst Wenck The Beiersdorf Research Center, Hamburg, Germany

Katherine M. Whipple Envision Eye and Aesthetics, Fairport, NY, USA

Cornelia Wiegand Department of Dermatology, University Hospital Jena, Jena, Germany

Julian Winocour Department of Plastic Surgery, Vanderbilt University, Nashville, TN, USA

Klaus-Peter Wittern The Beiersdorf Research Center, Hamburg, Germany

Hidekazu Yamada Department of Dermatology of Kinki University, Faculty of Medicine Nara Hospital, Kinki University Antiaging Center, Higashiosaka, Osaka Prefecture, Japan

Paul S. Yamauchi Dermatology Institute and Skin Care Center, Santa Monica, CA, USA

David Geffen School of School of Medicine at UCLA, Los Angeles, CA, USA

Daniel B. Yarosh The Estee Lauder Companies, Inc., Melville, NY, USA

Max Yeslev Department of Plastic Surgery, Vanderbilt University, Nashville, TN, USA

Koutaro Yokote Department of Clinical Cell Biology and Medicine, Chiba University Graduate School of Medicine, Chiba, Japan

Hyun Sun Yoon Department of Dermatology, Seoul National University Boramae Hospital, Seoul, Korea

Gil Yosipovitch Department of Dermatology and Itch Center, Temple University School of Medicine, Philadelphia, PA, USA

Sidra Younis The R.O. Perelman Department of Dermatology, and Department of Biochemistry and Molecular Pharmacology, NYU Langone Medical Center, New York, NY, USA

Department of Biochemistry, Quaid-i-Azam University, Islamabad, Pakistan

Efterpi Zafiriou Department of Dermatology and Venereology, University of Thessaly, Larissa, Greece

Hanjiang Zhu Department of Dermatology, UC San Francisco, San Francisco, CA, USA

Ying Zou Department of Dermatology, UC San Francisco, San Francisco, CA, USA

Christos C. Zouboulis Departments of Dermatology, Venereology, Allergology and Immunology, Dessau Medical Center, Dessau, Germany

Helene Zucchi L'Oreal, Research and Innovation, Aulnay-sous-bois, France

Part VII

Genomics

Genetic Basis of Healthy Skin Aging 113

Anne Lynn S. Chang

Contents

Abstract

While much is known about environmental factors that contribute to skin aging, little is known about genetic or intrinsic factors that promote healthy-appearing skin. This chapter discusses insights from rare genetic syndromes that reveal the pathways important for maintaining healthy-appearing skin and highlights recent data exploring gene variants that control skin youthfulness. In addition, technologies such as broadband light and fractionated ablative lasers and their potential to reverse aging pathways, not just improve appearance, will be discussed. Finally, the connection between skin aging, photoaging, and age-associated disease such as skin cancer will be covered.

Introduction: Insights on Skin Aging from Rare Genetic Syndromes

We are only beginning to understand the important genetic and epigenetic pathways that control the basis of healthy skin aging. With age, human skin exhibits a number of visible changes including fine wrinkling and sagging. Examples of the role of genes in maintaining skin health are revealed through rare genetic diseases that display phenotypes similar to aging skin. For instance, individuals with premature sagging of the skin can carry a variety of genetic mutations including

A.L.S. Chang (✉)
Department of Dermatology, Stanford University School of Medicine, Redwood City, CA, USA
e-mail: alschang@stanford.edu

M.A. Farage et al. (eds.), *Textbook of Aging Skin*,
DOI 10.1007/978-3-662-47398-6_131

in genes such as fibulin, as seen in autosomal dominant cutis laxa, or ATP7A, which can lead to X-linked cutis laxa [1]. Individuals with mutations in lamin A manifest with accelerated aging and shortened lifespan, termed progeria [2], and display markedly wrinkled and thin-appearing skin. These examples involving different molecular pathways that go awry and the skin phenotypes observed are hints to the variety of ways that skin appearance and skin health may be controlled.

This chapter highlights some of the data currently in the literature on the genetic control of healthy human skin aging.

Insights on the Genetic Basis of Skin Aging from Twin Studies

To date, the strongest data on the role of genetics in skin appearance are from monozygotic versus dizygotic twin studies, in which heritability analysis indicates approximately 50 % of skin appearance is genetic [3]. Specifically, perceived age, pigmented age spots, skin wrinkles, and the appearance of sun damage were due to both genetic and environmental factors. Hair graying, recession of hair from the forehead, and lip height were mostly due to genetic factors.

Recently, a genome-wide association study in an Ashkenazi population with extreme longevity found that skin youthfulness is not due to the same genetic variants as longevity [4]. Gene variants that were associated with skin that appeared younger than chronological age were close to KCND2, EDEM1, and DIAPH2. KCND2 is found on Langerhans cells of the epidermis, although the exact function of this gene variant and its contribution to the antiaging phenotype remain to be determined. The other two genetic variants associate with genes with known aging roles, for instance, EDEM1 associates with lifespan in animal models [5] and DIAPH2 associates with premature ovarian insufficiency [6, 7, 8]. Whether these variants also associate with skin youthfulness in non-Ashkenazi populations remains to be studied. Nevertheless, these genes represent new candidates to study the molecular basis of healthy skin aging.

Plasticity of Molecular Pathways Influencing Skin Aging

Nevertheless, the skin phenotype from a person's genes can be altered in a way that reverses the aging process. Histologically, the epidermis thins with age, and the phenomenon is also seen in animal models such as mice. This change can be reversed with inducible blockade of the transcription factor NFkB including global changes in gene expression to resemble young skin [9]. This reversibility of age-related molecular pathways is also possible in humans. In humans, a commonly used FDA-approved device in clinics called broadband light or intense pulse light can reduce redness and dyspigmentation [10, 11]. Off label, it is used for "rejuvenation" effects [12]. In a recent study, three treatments of this technology led to significant changes in molecular pathways that were detectable 6 weeks after the last treatment. The pathways that became more similar to younger skin after treatment included NFkB-related genes and long noncoding RNAs [13]. Other gene pathways with known aging function that were significantly altered include ZMPSTE24, a metalloproteinase that processes lamin A, the gene defective in the dramatic premature aging syndrome, Hutchinson-Gilford progeria. In addition, IGF-1R was also altered after treatment, and this gene product is linked to aging and longevity [14, 15] as well as other model organisms. Future studies may determine how long these effects last and whether combination with other treatment modalities may enhance the antiaging effects.

Genetics of Healthy Skin Aging, Photoaging, and Skin Cancer

In general, chronological aging strongly associates with sporadic skin cancers such as melanoma (see http://seer.cancer.gov/statfacts/html/melan.html), basal cell carcinoma, and squamous cell carcinoma. This association between chronological aging and skin cancers is even stronger in the presence of substantial ultraviolet radiation exposure, which accumulates with increasing age. While ultraviolet radiation exposure promotes the phenotype known as "photoaging," which can manifest as coarse wrinkling, sagging, and dyspigmentation, genetic factors such as skin type [16] or race modify the effect of ultraviolet radiation exposure.

Although skin cancer is associated with chronological aging, its association with photoaging may depend on the skin cancer type. While there is a strong connection between increased ultraviolet radiation exposure and skin cancer such as squamous cell carcinoma, the association between ultraviolet radiation exposure and basal cell carcinoma may be more complex. For instance, facial photoaging as assessed through wrinkling in 118 successive white patients with basal cell and 121 controls without skin cancer demonstrated that individuals with basal cell carcinoma had decreased wrinkling than controls [17]. Although the reasons for this discordance are not well studied, one possibility is that intermittent ultraviolet radiation exposure which is thought to underlie basal cell formation may lead to a more fibrotic dermal response that preserves collagen than a non-fibrotic response from chronic lower grade ultraviolet radiation exposure that leads to squamous cell carcinoma formation. Another possibility is that intermittent sun exposure does not deplete Langerhans cells of the epidermis like chronic sun exposure does [18], and the presence of Langerhans cells promotes improved skin appearance.

Ultraviolet radiation exposure is known to activate matrix metalloproteinases [19] and collagen breakdown and thus lead to photoaged phenotype. However, other pathways are involved in photoaging as well. For instance, ultraviolet radiation can alter aging-related pathways such as NFkB and IGF-1/IGF-1R [20, 21, 22]. Furthermore, procedures such as fractional ablative laser (used in the clinical setting to reduce some visible signs of skin aging) may correct some of the aberrant responses by dermal fibroblasts to ultraviolet B that is found in geriatric skin, namely, the ability of fibroblasts to produce IGF-1 [23]. Whether this correction can decrease skin cancer susceptibility remains to be determined.

Conclusion

Much more research is needed to better identify the pathways controlling healthy skin appearance. These insights will likely help us to better prevent or treat age-associated conditions of the skin, such as cutaneous malignancies.

References

1. Berk DR, Bentley DD, Bayliss SJ, et al. Cutis laxa: a review. J Am Acad Dermatol. 2012;66(5):842. e1–e17.
2. Conneely KN, Capell BC, Erdos MR, et al. Human longevity and common variations in the LMNA gene: a meta-analysis. Aging Cell. 2012;11:475–81.
3. Gunn D, Rexbye H, Griffiths C, et al. Why some women look young for their age. PLoS One. 2009. doi:10.1371/journal.pone.0008021.
4. Chang ALS, Atzmon G, Bergman A, Atwood S, Brugmann S, Chang HY, Barzilai N. Identification of genes promoting skin youthfulness. J Invest Dermatol. 2014;3(1):40–5.
5. Shenkman M, Groisman B, Ron E, et al. A shared endoplasmic reticulum-associated degradation pathway involving the EDEM1 protein for glycosylated and nonglycosylated proteins. J Biol Chem. 2013;288:2167–78.
6. Bione S, Sala C, Manzini C, et al. A human homologue of the *Drosophila melanogaster* diaphanous gene is disrupted in a patient with premature ovarian failure: evidence for conserved function in oogenesis and implications for human sterility. Am J Hum Genet. 1998;62:533–41.
7. Marozzi A, Manfredini E, Tibiletti MG, et al. Molecular definition of Xq common-deleted region in patients affected by premature ovarian failure. Hum Genet. 2000;107:304–11.
8. Marozzi A, Vegetti W, Manfredini E, et al. Association between idiopathic premature ovarian failure and fragile X premutation. Hum Reprod. 2000;15:197–202.
9. Adler AS, Sinha S, Kawahara TLA, et al. Motif module map reveals enforcement of aging by continual NFKB activity. Genes Dev. 2007;21:3244–57.
10. Negishi K, Tezuka Y, Kushikata N, et al. Photorejuvenation for Asian Skin by Intense pulsed light. Dermatol Surg. 2001;27:627–31.
11. Prieto VG, Sadick NS, Lloreta J, et al. Effects of intense pulsed light on sun-damaged human skin, routine, and ultra-structural analysis. Lasers Surg Med. 2002;30:82–5.
12. Bitter PH. Noninvasive rejuvenation of photodamaged skin using serial, full-face intense pulse light. Derm Surg 2000;26(9):835–42. Discussion 843.
13. Chang ALS, Bitter PH, Qu K, Lin M, Rapicavoli NA, Chang HY. Rejuvenation of gene expression pattern of

aged human skin by broadband light treatment. J Invest Dermatol. 2013;133(2):394–402.
14. Tazearslan C, Huang J, Barzilai N, et al. Impaired IGF1R signaling in cells expressing longevity-associated human IGF1R alleles. Aging Cell. 2011;10:551–4.
15. van Heemst D, Beekman M, Mooijaart SP, et al. Reduced insulin/IGF-1 signalling and human longevity. Aging Cell. 2005;4:79–85.
16. Elfakir A, Ezzedine K, Latreille J, et al. Functional MC1R-gene variants are associated with increased risk for severe photoaging of facial skin. J Invest Dermatol. 2010;130:1107–15.
17. Brooke RC, Newbold SA, Telfer NR, Griffiths CE. Discordance between facial wrinkling and the presence of basal cell carcinoma. Arch Dermatol. 2001;137(6):751–4
18. Thiers BH, Maize JC, Spicer SS, et al. The effect of aging and chronic sun exposure on human Langerhans cell populations. J Invest Dermatol. 1984;82:223–6.
19. Quan T, Qin A, Xia W, et al. Matrix-degrading metalloproteinases in photoaging. J Invest Dermatol. 2009;14:20–4.
20. Lewis DA, Spandau DF. UVB-induced activation of NF-kB is regulated by the IGF-1R and dependent on p38 MAPK. J Invest Dermatol. 2008;128:1002–29.
21. Lewis DA, Travers JB, Somani AK, et al. The IGF-1/IGF-1R signaling axis in the skin: a new role for the dermis in age-associated skin cancer. Oncogene. 2010;29:1475–85.
22. Lee Y, Kim H, Kim S, et al. Activation of toll-like receptors 2, 3, or 5 induces matrix metalloproteinase-1 and -9 expression with the involvement of MAPKs and NFkB in human epidermal keratinocytes. Exp Dermatol. 2009;19:e44–9.
23. Spandau D, Lewis DA, Somani A, Travers JB. Fractionated laser resurfacing corrects the inappropriate UVB response in geriatric skin. J Invest Dermatol. 2012;132:1591–6.

Genodermatoses with Premature Aging/Syndromes

114

Adele Chedraoui, Abdul Ghani Kibbi, and Mazen Kurban

Contents

A. Chedraoui
Department of Dermatology, Lebanese American University, Beirut, Lebanon
e-mail: adele_chedraoui@hotmail.com

A.G. Kibbi
Department of Dermatology, American University of Beirut Medical Center, Beirut, Lebanon
e-mail: agkibbi@aub.edu.lb

M. Kurban (✉)
Department of Dermatology, American University of Beirut Medical Center, Beirut, Lebanon

Department of Biochemistry and Molecular Genetics, American University of Beirut Medical Center, Beirut, Lebanon

Department of Dermatology, Columbia University, New York, NY, USA
e-mail: mk104@aub.edu.lb

M.A. Farage et al. (eds.), *Textbook of Aging Skin*,
DOI 10.1007/978-3-662-47398-6_132

Abstract

The aging process is a very complex one, affected by both genetic and environmental factors. This chapter will discuss in depth intrinsic factors affecting the aging process, namely DNA damage and DNA repair mechanisms. Continuous DNA damage in all replicating cells occurs constantly whether due to endogenous errors in DNA replication or exogenous factors such as ultraviolet radiation, smoking, etc. Nature, however, has provided us with an intricate system of repair tools in order to maintain genetic stability and continuous DNA replication necessary for life. DNA repair mechanisms are highly conserved in nature indicating the importance of such mechanisms in maintaining cell survival despite genetic instability.

Inherited disorders with characteristic premature aging will be discussed. A greater understanding of the genetic basis of these disorders and their contribution to the aging process may help elucidate the different aspects of the aging process and improve the ability to increase human lifespan.

Introduction

Aging is a multifactorial mechanism that is affected both by intrinsic and extrinsic factors that determine the lifespan and the quality of life. A lot of work has aimed to understand the main genetic factors which determine lifespan in an attempt to treat neurodegenerative disorders, to end the life of cancerous cells, and to prevent aging in humans.

Several theories have been hypothesized to explain the aging process:

1. Programmed cell death: This theory explains cellular senescence as a built in program aimed at preventing the accumulation of cellular damage but at the extent of decreased regeneration capacity [1].
2. Genetic instability: This theory is explained by the accumulation of nuclear and mitochondrial DNA damage coupled to a tightly controlled repair mechanism in every cell. This theory is illustrated by the fact that actively dividing cells and animals with a high basal metabolic rate overuse their repair mechanism and subsequently have a short lifespan [1, 2].
3. Free radicals theory: Free radicals generated by oxidative stress affect the stability/degradation of proteins and cause lipid peroxidation resulting in disruption of membranes and mitochondrial dysfunction resulting in cell death [1, 2].
4. Redundancy failure for critical genes: This theory explains aging as an inability of survival of the cell due to an improper transcription or translation of critical genes that are necessary for survival and a failure of a compensatory mechanism [3].
5. Telomere shortening: This theory is exemplified by the fact that cells manifest decreased telomere length with normal aging and telomerase knockout mouse models are prone to accelerated aging [1, 4].
6. Stem cell exhaustion: This theory attributes aging and death to a decreased production or depletion of stem cells. In favor of this theory is the evidence provided by simplest animals such as sponges and cnidarians. Sponges can live up to several hundreds or even thousands of years, and some cnidarians can potentially be immortal. These longest living animals have a great regenerative potential ability and a highly malleable potential to cycle between an adult stage and a relatively simpler stage due to their characteristic large number of pluripotent stem cells [4, 5].
7. Deregulated nutrient sensing: This theory relies on experiments on mice showing that their lifespan can be improved by giving these mice a diet containing all nutrients and minerals but with the least total caloric intake [6]. In line with this theory, studies showed a direct

Table 1 Genes associated with human longevity

Chrom	Gene	Protein	Function	Association
19q13.2	APO E gene	Apolipoprotein E	Part of lipoproteins	APOE e4 allele is related to the risk of Alzheimer disease and cardiovascular diseases
6q21	FOXO3A gene	Forkhead box O3 transcription factor	A trigger for apoptosis sensor and regulator of oxidative stress regulates the insulin receptor/insulin-like growth factor-I signaling pathway	FOX O3 is associated with acute leukemia and rhabdomyosarcoma
1q43	EXO1 gene	Exonuclease 1	5′ to 3′ exonuclease RNase H activity involved in mismatch repair and recombination	Gene polymorphism in EXO1 gene associated with cancer susceptibility
4q24	CISD2 gene		Regulating cellular Ca++ homeostasis and mitochondrial integrity	Mutation associated with Wolfram syndrome-2

role of the insulin/insulin-like growth factor (IGF1) signaling in longevity [7].

Aging Studies in Animals

Researchers have identified animal models that can be used to study human aging. An example is the Klotho mutant mouse (kl/kl) characterized by decreased wound healing ability. Klotho mice exhibit a progeric phenotype with dry, atrophic, and wrinkled skin. They are characterized by infertility, emphysema, atherosclerosis, osteoporosis, and short life span. Therefore, the Klotho mouse is regarded as the first laboratory animal model for human aging that is caused by a single gene mutation. Other studies revealed that mice which are deficient in Sirt6 display genomic instability and premature aging phenotypes [8]. In addition, transgenic mice with p 16 induction showed features of physiologic aging: reduced and lightened hair, kyphosis, skin wrinkling, reduced body weight and subcutaneous fat, an increased myeloid fraction in peripheral blood, poor dentition, and cataracts. These aging features were reversed with de-induction of p 16 [9]. In fact, it was shown that p16 accumulates in aging tissues of mice and humans. Therefore, p 16 is regarded as a useful biomarker for cellular senescence, both in vitro and in vivo.

Human Studies

The current belief is that aging as an intrinsic process is the result of a number of genes, contributing each, to a certain extent to the whole genetic makeup that determines lifespan. A study of over 10,000 genes across 30 mammalian species has identified genes that are conserved among long-lived species. These genes are referred to as longevity-associated genes (LAGs). LAGs include growth hormone receptor (GHR), early onset breast cancer (BRCA1), FANCB, FBXO6, CD3EAP, CD8B, and IL7R genes [10]. In humans, studies aimed at identifying specific genes that most closely correlate with a longer lifespan are ongoing. Comparing the genetic makeup of older individuals to that of younger individuals can help to identify genes most closely related to longer lifespan. A genome wide linkage study performed on 308 centenarians and near-centenarians found a statistically significant linkage within chromosome 4 [11].

So far, data has pointed to two groups of genes affecting longevity:

1. Lipid metabolism genes
2. Genes involved in maintenance of genome integrity

Genes that are most closely associated with human lifespan (see Table 1) include:

- E4 allele of the apolipoprotein E (ApoE) gene: ApoE is the most important genetic factor influencing human longevity. A genome wide linkage study has so far only found statistical significance with respect to ApoE gene [11, 12]. The ApoE gene is associated with the likelihood of reaching exceptional longevity (reaching >100 years old) [12].
- Human forkhead box O3A (FOXO3A) gene: FOXO3A is associated with the ability to live long [12]. FOXO3A has been found to be particularly active in centenarians [12, 13]. In mammals, the only family member directly linked to aging is FOXO3A. FOXO3A is a negative regulator of autophagy in multiple cancer cell lines. FOXO3 negatively regulates autophagy in human cancer cells by inhibiting forkhead box protein O1 expression and cytosolic accumulation. FOXO3A activation contributes to the increase of autophagy activity in senescent cells via blocking ATP synthesis.
- Exonuclease 1 (EXO1) gene: Exonucleases are key enzymes involved in many aspects of cellular metabolism and maintenance and are essential to genome stability [14].
- CISD2 gene: CISD2 is a recently identified gene located within the candidate region on chromosome 4q. Mutations in CISD2, however, were found to cause type 2 Wolfram syndrome, a rare neurodegenerative and metabolic disorder associated with a shortened lifespan. CISD2 expression was recently shown to affect lifespan in mammals [15].

Others genes, including mitochondrial Fas, FasL, MHC class I, microsomal transfer protein, were investigated in several studies as factors potentially modulating lifespan with different degrees of success [16].

Another approach to the study of genes involved in human aging is the classical approach whereby functional analysis of genes in which naturally occurring polymorphisms or mutations result in a change in the aging process. Although Hutchinson–Gilford and Werner syndromes are the two syndromes that most closely mimic physiological aging, genetic analysis failed to show any association between polymorphisms affecting the WRN gene and longevity. Nonetheless, the association of disorders with defective DNA repair mechanisms and precocious aging highlights the importance of DNA repair pathway in the maintenance of life [17].

DNA repair mechanisms are the ways through which the cell is capable of survival despite the continuous DNA damage caused by endogenous and exogenous factors. DNA repair mechanisms can be divided in two categories: nucleotide excision repair and translesional synthesis.

Nucleotide Excision Repair (NER)

Nucleotide excision repair (NER): The NER pathway directly participates in the repair of all DNA lesions generated either through endogenous oxidative stress. NER can be divided into two major categories: Global genome repair and transcription coupled repair [18].

- Global genome repair (GGR) depends on a series of proteins involved in recognizing damaged DNA (XPC/HR23B protein complex as the primary DNA damage detector and XPE), unwinding the double helix (helicases), removing the damaged strand (XPG proteins and the XPF/ER+CC1 complex are the main endonucleases that nick DNA at both sides), and filling the gap (DNA polymerases and DNA Ligase1) [17, 18].

  Global genome repair is the main mechanism responsible for repair of ultraviolet radiation (UVR) induced DNA damage and maintenance of genetic stability. A defect in this mechanism will result in photosensitivity, genetic instability, increased mutagenesis, and cancer.
- Transcription coupled repair (TCR) involves the action of RNA polymerases. CSA and CSB proteins play a crucial role in the recognition of DNA lesions in the TCR pathway. An inability of TCR to repair transcription blockage caused by endogenous oxidative stress and reactive oxygen will result in an increased rate of cell death manifested clinically by more

severe neural and developmental problems in addition to premature aging [17, 18].

Therefore, inabilities to repair DNA damage caused by oxidative stress will most likely result in a severe phenotype and premature aging, whereas a defect limited to the ability to repair UVR induced damaged DNA will result only in photosensitivity [19].

Translesional Synthesis (TLS)

This process allows the DNA replication machinery to replicate despite DNA damage. It relies on specialized translesion polymerases among which DNA polymerase eta and polymerase η. It is through natural evolution that same cells acquired TLS to bypass the damaged DNA part and to continue replication of the remaining DNA strand [17, 19].

Premature Aging Syndromes

Premature aging syndromes also known as progeroid syndromes are a class of rarely occurring genetic disorders with premature aging. They can be broadly classified into unimodal progeroid syndromes such as Alzheimer and Parkinson's disease (aging affecting only one tissue) and segmental progeroid syndromes (aging of several tissues similar to physiological aging). This Chapter discusses segmental progeroid syndromes arising from single gene mutations in the affected individuals. These disorders may provide a clue to researchers as to the genetic basis of human aging. Correlation of the clinical manifestations of these genodermatoses with the genetic mutation gives insight into the function of the gene involved and the role of this particular gene in DNA damage and cell death. Different mutations within the same gene lead to different clinical manifestations and variable severity giving rise to a multitude of phenotypes within the same genetic disorder [20]. Disorders with premature aging can be divided in two broad categories: disorders with defect in DNA repair mechanism (see Table 2) and disorders not involving DNA repair pathways.

Disorders Related to Defects in DNA Repair Mechanism

Xeroderma Pigmentosum

Xeroderma pigmentosum (XP) is the first described genetic disorder associated with premature aging and defect in NER. The dermatologists Moritz Kaposi and Ferdinand Ritter von Hebra provided the first clinical description of XP patients. The disease was referred to as XP from the Greek words xero and derma; and Latin word pigmentosum because patients manifested dry and pigmented skin. XP affects one to four per million live births and has an autosomal recessive pattern of inheritance. The carrier frequency is estimated to be 0.2–0.4 % in the general population [21].

Clinical Manifestations

XP patients present with variable degree of photosensitivity, and with repeated sun exposure during early life severe sunburn occurs, resulting in an abnormal freckle-like pigmentation over sun-exposed areas. Subsequently, multiple nonmelanoma skin cancer (NMSC) may arise; the risk being 10,000 times higher than healthy individuals. The median age of first NMSC is around 8 years. XP patients have also a 2,000-fold higher risk of MM than the general population [20, 21]. In addition, ocular abnormalities are observed in up to 40 % of patients. Ocular symptoms include photophobia, keratitis, corneal opacification, loss of eyelashes, and ectropion. Cheilitis and SCC of the tip of tongue may also be seen. Neurological abnormalities occur in 30–60 % of patients with XP. Progressive central and peripheral neurological degeneration result in microcephaly, mental retardation, retarded growth, deafness, seizures, ataxia, and paresis. XP patients with the most severe neurologic manifestation are referred to as De Sanctis-Cacchione syndrome. XP Variant (XPV) do not present with

Table 2 Diseases associated with DNA repair mechanisms

Complementation group	Gene	Chromosome	Function	Defect	Photosensitivity	Cancer
XPA	XPA gene	Chrom 9q34.1	Position of the DNA repair machinery	Defect in NER	++	++
XPB	ERCC3 gene	Chrom 2q14.3	Helicase 3′-5′, TFIIH subunit	Defect in NER	++	++
XPC	XPC gene	Chrom 3p25.1	DNA damage recognition	Defect in NER (GGR)	−−	++
XPD	ERCC2	Chrom 19q13.3	Helicase 5′-3′, TFIIH subunit	Defect in NER	++	++
XPE	DDB2	Chrom 11p11.2	DNA damage recognition	Defect in NER (GGR)	−−	++
XPF	ERCC4	Chrom 16p13.12	Endonuclease 5′-incision	Defect in NER	++	++
XPG	ERCC5	Chrom 13q33.1	Base excision repair	Defect in NER	++	++
XPV	POLH	Chrom 6p21.1	Bypass polymerase η	Defect in TLS	−−	++
	ERCC1 gene	Chrom 19q13.32	Endonuclease 5′-incision	Defect in NER		
CSA	ERCC8	Chrom 5q12.1	RNA Pol II cofactor	Defect in NER (TCR)	+	−−
CSB	ERCC6 gene	Chrom 10q11.21	RNA Pol II cofactor	Defect in NER (TCR)	+	−−
UVSS	UVSSA gene	Chrom 4p16.6	RNA Pol II cofactor	Defect in NER	+++	−−
TTD		Chrom 6p25.3	TFIIH subunit	Defect in NER	++	−−

neurologic manifestations. XP patients are at increased risk of internal malignancies including tumors of the brain, lung, gastrointestinal, and hematopoietic system.

XP patients die at a median age of 32 years, 38 years younger than that for the general population. The most frequent causes of death are metastatic skin cancer and neurological degeneration (34.5 % and 31 %, respectively). In general, XP patients with neurodegeneration had poor survival compared to patients without neurological involvement.

XP can be classified into seven different complementation groups (XP-A to XP-G), depending on the underlying genetic defect (Table 2). It is well established that clinical heterogeneity is associated with the mutational site even within the same complementation group. XPA, XPD, and XPG usually have a prominent neurodegenerative features. All patients with XPB and some patients with XPG have associated Cokayne syndrome (CS). XPD patients may have both CS and trichothiodystrophy (TTD). All XP patients have mutations in the genes coding for enzymes involved in NER. In XP variants (XPV), the NER mechanism functions properly, but there is a defect involving the post-replication repair system namely TLS associated with DNA polymerase activity.

XPA: Patients with typical XPA phenotype exhibit both severe neurological abnormalities (De Sanctis-Cacchione syndrome) and extreme photosensitivity. XPA gene is localized on chromosome 9q34.1. Mutations within exons 3, 4, and 5 of the XPA gene result in an alteration of XPA protein. XPA acts as the main coordinator of the NER complex because of its diverse functions. XPA interacts with almost all other NER proteins. XPA protein has a preferential ability to recognize and bind to damaged DNA. In addition, XPA maintains an intricate network of contact with the core repair complex and has a crucial role in NER. XPA variant is the most complementation group of XP in Japan and around 1 % of the Japanese population carries a mutation in the XPA gene [21].

XPC represents the most common XP complementation group. The XPC complex includes two proteins: RAD23 homologue B (RAD23B), which is a UV excision repair protein, and centrin 2 (CETN2), which recognizes damaged DNA. XPC plays a key role in the initiation of GG-NER.

XPE represents a group of XP patients who harbor a mutation in XPE gene coding for DNA damage-binding protein DDB2 which increases the affinity of XPC to damaged DNA. Patients of XPC and XPE exhibit only mild photosensitivity but have the highest incidence of cancer of all the XP complementation groups.

Unlike the previously described XP patients with the complementation group mutations, XPV has a normal NER. It is caused by mutations in the gene that encodes DNA polymerase η gene (also known as Pol H or hRad30A). This enzyme is responsible for bypassing damaged DNA during replication. XPV represents approximately 10 % of all XP patients and is primarily found in Europe and the USA [21].

Treatment

Management relies on early and strict sun protection. With extreme sun protection measures, XP patients should be supplemented with calcium and vitamin D. Treatment of premalignant and malignant skin tumors includes cryotherapy, curettage, electrodessication, and surgery. Other therapies include topical imiquimod, topical 5 Flouuracil, and oral retinoids. Chemoprevention of malignant lesions with topical application of bacterial DNA repair enzyme, T4 endonuclease V, has been tried with some success. In an attempt to delay or stop the progression of neurodegenerative symptoms, clinical trials are currently testing NF-kb inhibitors in the treatment of XP since NF-kb is known to regulate cell survival in response to stress [19, 21].

Cockayne Syndrome

Cockayne syndrome is a rare autosomal recessive progeroid syndrome, first described by Cockayne in 1936. There is a great variation in the manifestations and severity of the disease. Cockayne syndrome can occur alone or in association with xeroderma pigmentosum (XPB-CS, XPD-CS, XPG-CS). CS type A is considered to be a mild type and CS type B a severe type manifesting even before birth.

Clinical Manifestations

Patients with CS typically present with characteristic facies known as "bird-like" (sunken eyes, prominent ears). Clinical manifestations of premature aging include growth retardation, kyphosis, cachectic dwarfism, atrophic skin, thin hair, osteoporosis, and loss of subcutaneous fat. Ocular abnormalities include retinal atrophy and cataract. The occurrence of cataract during the first 3 years of life is a marker of CS type B and predicts early death. Neurodevelopmental abnormalities include microcephaly, diffuse dysmyelination, and calcium deposits in the cortex and basal ganglia. Calcification of the brain can be observed on head computed tomography (CT) and is highly valuable in establishing the diagnosis. Other features include progressive hearing and visual loss, progressive ataxia, delayed psychomotor development, mental retardation, and arrested sexual development. Patients with CS exhibit photosensitivity, but in contrast to XP patients do not have a freckled face, and lack skin cancer susceptibility. CSA patients die at a mean age of 12.5 years whereas CSB die at a younger age (6–7 years of life); the most common cause of death being deterioration of the central nervous system and respiratory tract infections [22].

CSA and CSB patients are characterized by defects of TCR-NER. The genetic makeup of patients with CS revealed a defect in RNA synthesis after ultraviolet radiation induced DNA damage. Studies have identified two different complementation groups for CS cells. CSA (ERCC8) gene defective in CSA is located on chromosome 5 (locus 5q12.3) and encodes CSA protein belonging to the family of WD-repeat proteins. CSB (ERCC6) gene characteristic of CSB is located on chromosome 10 (locus 10q11) and encodes another member of the helicase family. CSA and CSB proteins are key components of TCR sub pathway of the NER system [23]. Both CSA and CSB interact with p44 subunit of TFIIH and help in the recruitment of TFIIH to the site of DNA damage and are part of RNA polymerase II-associated complexes involved in RNA synthesis [24]. In addition, CSB also plays a pivotal role in maintaining mitochondrial function against oxidative stress. Therefore, the severity of CS type B is attributed to a vicious cycle of impaired mitochondrial DNA repair resulting in increased ROS production which in turn leads to more DNA damage in nucleus and mitochondria. This will result in defective or insufficient transcription, senescence, and cell death, leading to tissue-specific defects, degenerative changes, and accelerated aging. In contrast to XP patients who have a fundamental defect in GG-NER, CS patients are not at an increased risk of cutaneous or internal malignancies, highlighting the importance of GG-NER in the prevention of carcinogenesis.

Treatment

Treatment is only symptomatic since there is no effective therapy to halt the progression of the disease.

XP/CS Group of Patients

CS may occur in conjunction with XPB-CS, XPD-CS, and XPG-CS. This category of patients combines features of XP (lentigines and cutaneous cancers) and CS (pigmentary retinal degeneration and basal ganglia calcification).

Similar to all XP patients, XP-CS patients have up to a 10,000-fold increase in skin cancers, including squamous cell carcinomas, basal cell carcinomas, and melanomas, all of which occur at sun-exposed sites. The defective global genome nucleotide excision repair in those patients is the main cause of mutagenesis and carcinogenesis [21, 22].

Cerebro-Oculo-Facio-Skeletal Syndrome

Cerebro-oculo-facio-skeletal syndrome (COFS) is considered to be a severe form of CS. Patients present at birth with congenital microcephaly, congenital cataract, and microphthalmia. They progressively develop arthrogryposis and severe growth failure. Mutations in COFS occur in the CSB gene (coding for ERCC6 protein which functions in base excision repair), ERCC1 gene (protein functions in interstrand crosslink repair (ICLR), single-strand annealing (SSA) and gene conversion), and XPD gene (ERCC2 gene encoding for TFIIH basal transcription factor complex XPD subunit) [21, 23, 24].

Trichothiodystrophy

TTD is a group of autosomal recessive disorders with characteristic short and brittle hair due to decreased number of cysteine cross-links in hair proteins.

Clinical Manifestations

TTD present with mental retardation (86 %), short stature (73 %), ichthyosis (65 %), photosensitivity, and infertility (40 %). Typical facies include microcephaly, a receding chin, protruding ears, and abnormal nail and teeth. Light microscopy reveals trichorrhexis nodosa or trichoschisis. Diagnosis can be made by polarized microscopy which shows "Tiger-tail" banding of hair shafts.

Children with TTD have a significantly increased risk of infections and a 20-fold higher than normal rate of infection-related deaths in the first 10 years of age. Mothers of TTD fetuses are also at a higher risk of pregnancy-related complications. In addition, exacerbations of TTD symptoms during febrile episodes were reported to be due to a temperature sensitive XPD allele [24].

TTD associated with XPD mutation is the most common type of TTD accounting for 85 % of cases. TTD may also be associated with mutations in the genes encoding XPB, XPG, or subunits of transcription factor II H (TFIIH), namely TFB5 or GTF2H5 [23, 24]. Mutations in chromosome 7 open reading frame 11 were found to cause a nonphotosensitive form of TTD. TTD mutations affect the stability and repair function of TFIIH thereby interfering with its transcription function during the final stages of terminal differentiation of hair, nail, and skin cells. In addition, different mutations of TFIIH subunits have a widely variable effect over the TCR-NER and the GG-NER pathways accounting for the clinical heterogeneity of patients with TTD.

Treatment

No specific treatment is available.

UV-Sensitive Syndrome

UV-Sensitive syndrome (UVSS) is a relatively newly described disorder of the Japanese population. Patients with UVSS have photosensitivity and lentigines (similar to XP), but since they have a normal GG-NER, they do not develop skin cancers. Mutations in UVSS have been described to occur in the ERCC6 gene. Recently, mutations in the UVSSA gene were also identified [21, 23, 24]. UVSS can be considered the mildest form of TCR deficiency. The defect in UVSS is limited to UVB-induced photoproducts, whereas repair of oxidative damage remains intact. Therefore, UVSS patients demonstrate a high degree of photosensitivity without the risk of XP cancers and CS neurologic abnormalities. Therefore, UVSS patients have a normal lifespan.

Progeroid Syndromes Due to Defective Lamin A Production

A group of diseases with progeroid features and reduced lifespan are referred to as laminopathies because they are caused by lamin mutations. Lamins are proteins located in the nuclear lamina and play a major role in chromatin organization.

Hutchinson-Gilford Progeria Syndrome

Hutchinson-Gilford syndrome (HGPS) is a very rare autosomal dominant sporadic syndrome first described by Hutchinson and Gilford in 1886. The term progeria originates from the Greek word "geras" which means old age.

Clinical Manifestations

HGPS patients present with premature aging that typically starts within the first year of life. Patients have a short lifespan with a median of 13.4 years. They have characteristic phenotypic features, known as plucked bird appearance. They exhibit midface hypoplasia, micrognathia, prominent eyes, protruding ears with absent earlobes, delayed closure of fontanelles and sutures, and delayed dentition. The appearance of facial features occurs at the age of 2–3 years and marks the onset of growth failure. The skin shows atrophy, decreased subcutaneous fat, sclerodermoid features, and mottled hyperpigmentation. Diffuse alopecia develops starting the first year of life, and prominent veins over the scalp are observed. HGPS have a short stature and lack sexual maturation. Examination shows thin limbs, prominent abdomen, pyriform (pear shaped) thorax, stiff joints, prominent kyphosis, generalized osteodysplasia with osteolysis and pathologic fractures, dystrophic nails, and high-pitched voice. Death usually occurs as a result of myocardial infection or stroke. Interestingly, Hutchinson-Gilford syndrome is not characterized by precocious brain aging or metabolic abnormalities and does not have an increased risk of cancer. Therefore, Hutchinson-Gilford syndrome is considered the progeroid syndrome that most closely mimics physiological human aging [25].

The exact mechanism that underlies the pathophysiology of Hutchinson-Gilford syndrome is not fully understood. More than 90 % of HGPS subjects have the same C > T substitution at codon 608, a site considered a "hotspot" for recurring point mutations in the lamin gene, LMNA, located on chromosome 1q. Mutations in the LMNA gene lead to an aberrantly spliced, truncated form of lamin A, called progerin. It is a major part of the nuclear lamina and has an essential role in the maintenance of nuclear structure, gene expression, chromatin organization, cell cycle regulation, and apoptosis. Progerin was shown to have a direct p53-mediated effect on telomeres, causing early senescence of cells. In fact, fibroblasts from HGPS patients exhibit DNA damage and short telomeres, a defect that can be repaired by telomerase [26]. The lack of neurodevelopmental delay in HGPS can be explained by the presence of brain specific expression of miR-9 which was shown to inhibit progerin expression [27]. In addition, resistance of the immune system to a defective progerin was demonstrated in a study which found median telomere length of hematopoietic cells comparable to that of age-matched controls [28].

Evidence of similarities between physiologic human aging and premature aging in HGPS is illustrated by increased progerin levels in coronary arteries with gradual aging [29].

Treatment

Treatment is symptomatic and aims at treating diabetes mellitus and cardiovascular complications. Genetic counseling is done for affected families. Some patients may benefit from growth hormone treatment.

In an attempt to halt the aging process, more targeted therapies are currently being developed in order to target the different aspects of HGPS ranging from telomere dysfunction, altered gene–protein interaction, disturbed epigenetic regulation, and chromatin remodeling defects. Based on evidence form HGPS showing abnormal progerin protein permanently anchored to nuclear membrane, farnesyltransferase inhibitors (FTIs) and N-acetyltransferase inhibitors (e.g., remodelin) were investigated. These drugs inhibit farnesylation of prelamin A preventing its abnormal anchoring to nuclear membrane. The mechanism of action of FTIs and remodelin involves a downstream common pathway for microtubule maintenance of the nucleus shape. Restoring nuclear shape was achieved by FTIs in lamin-A-depleted cells of HGPS. Attempts to treat progeria patients with FTIs showed promising results in reducing the incidence of nuclear deformities associated with HGPS [30]. Other drugs able to block the farnesyl pyrophosphate pathway, such as statins and bisphosphonates, are also explored as potential treatment. For example, Mevinoline, an inhibitor of the synthesis of precursors of the farnesyl group, works synergistically with trichostatin A (histone deacetylase inhibitor) to reestablish the correct chromatin organization in cells from HGPS patients.

Other available therapies include telomerase treatment which was shown to extend cellular lifespan by toning down the DNA damage signaling triggered by progerin. Treating mutant mice with HDAC inhibitor (Sodium Butyrate) restored the acetylation level of H4 and reversed the progeroid features. Small interfering RNAs (siRNAs) designed to target lamin A mRNA were also shown to effectively downregulate lamin A production. In addition, studies showed a promising role for the chromatin modifiers (enhancers of mTOR signaling: mammalian sirtuin (SIRT1), resveratrol) in delaying senescence [31, 32].

Metageria

Metageria is an autosomal recessive disorder with an equal female to male ratio. There is a great overlap between HGPS and metageria symptoms. Features present in both include beaked nose, prominent eyes, alopecia, and loss of subcutaneous fat. In addition to atherosclerosis, metageria is also characterized by the onset of diabetes mellitus. However, in contrast to HGPS, metageria patients are usually tall and thin and show poikilodermatous changes, mottled hyperpigmentation with prominent cutaneous leg ulcers [25].

Acrogeria

Acrogeria, also known as Gottron syndrome, is inherited as autosomal dominant or recessive and has a female predominance. In acrogeria, symptoms start at birth with poikiloderma, thin nose with atrophic tip, and micrognathia. Cutaneous atrophy of hands and feet with dystrophic nails are observed along with prominent veins of the trunk. However, in contrast to HGPS, these patients have a normal stature and a normal lifespan [25].

Neonatal Progeroid Syndrome (Wiedemann–Rautenstrauch Syndrome)

Neonatal progeroid syndrome, also known as Wiedemann–Rautenstrauch syndrome, is a rare autosomal recessive disorder characterized by intrauterine growth retardation, failure to thrive, short stature, a progeroid appearance, hypotonia, subcutaneous lipoatrophy, variable mental impairment, and death in childhood. There are few individuals who have lived well in to the teens and very few still live in their 20s [25].

LMNA-Associated Cardiocutaneous Progeria Syndrome

LMNA-associated cardiocutaneous progeria syndrome is an "atypical" progeria syndrome (APS) with a less severe disease, late onset, and prominent cutaneous and cardiovascular manifestations. Patients develop cardiac valve calcification and dysfunction, prominent atherosclerosis, and cardiomyopathy, leading to death in the fourth decade of life.

Néstor–Guillermo Progeria Syndrome (NGPS)

Néstor–Guillermo progeria syndrome (NGPS) is a recently described progeroid syndrome caused by BANF (barrier to autointegration factor 1) gene mutation. These patients manifest premature aging but lack signs of ischemia or atherosclerosis present in HGPS. BANF1 protein is localized to the nuclear envelope and interacts with lamin and histone H3 and plays a crucial role in tethering the chromatin to the nuclear envelope [33].

Other Progeroid Syndromes

Different point mutations in the same LMNA gene can result in a variety of progeroid phenotypes. Substitutions at the 527 coding site in LMNA gene may cause different disorders such as Emery–Dreifuss muscular dystrophy and mandibuloacral dysplasia. Mutations in the gene coding for FACE-1/ZMPSTE24 (metalloprotease involved in posttranslational processing of lamin) were established as primary events leading to other laminopathies such as restrictive dermopathy, lipodystrophies, neuropathies, muscular dystrophies, and dilated cardiomyopathies. Since the amount of progerin produced is the main determinant of phenotype severity, ZMPSTE24/FACE1-linked phenotypes represent the most severe phenotype, with total enzyme inactivation and extreme prelamin A accumulation [33].

The diverse function of lamins explains in part the different phenotypic manifestations of laminopathies. Syndromes such as Emery–Dreifuss, limb girdle muscular dystrophies, dilated cardiomyopathy with conduction disease, autosomal recessive axonal neuropathy, mandibuloacral dysplasia, familial partial lipodystrophy, Greenberg skeletal dysplasia, and Pelger–Huet anomaly are characterized by LMNA mutations that simultaneously affect both lamin A and lamin C, which are alternatively spliced isoforms of the same LMNA gene. The preferential expression of lamin C in neural tissues accounts for the presence of brain and developmental abnormalities in these laminopathies.

Whereas expression of A-type lamins is limited to most somatic lineages, B-type lamins are expressed in pluripotent stem cells and in their differentiated progeny. No point mutations in lamin B1 have been linked to any specific disease, but loss of lamin B1 can be used as a marker to identify senescent cells in vitro and in vivo [34]. For example, lamin-B1-deficient mouse embryonic fibroblasts exhibit nuclear abnormalities, impaired proliferation, and premature senescence. It is suggested that lamin B1 deficiency impairs cellular function which, in conjunction with additional stress, can trigger senescence. On the other hand, elevated levels of lamin B1 have been observed in cells from patients with ataxia telangiectasia (AT) and adult-onset autosomal dominant leukodystrophy (ADLD), pointing to a link between lamin B1 overexpression and myelin abnormalities.

Disorders Due to Defective DNA Helicases

Werner Syndrome (WS)

Werner syndrome is an autosomal recessive inherited disease first described by Werner in 1904. To date, it is the most common progeroid syndrome. Most of the patients with WS come from Japan. It affects one in one million births with an equal female to male ratio.

Clinical Manifestations

WS typically presents at puberty with short stature and absence of pubertal spur. Signs of aging similar to physiological aging appear during the second decade of life. Typical facies include manifest a beaked nose, micrognathia, protuberant teeth, prominent veins, premature graying, loss of hair, skin atrophy, osteoporosis of the lower extremities, and central obesity. During the third decade of life, diabetes mellitus type II, juvenile bilateral cataract, atherosclerotic changes of arterioles, and calcifications of cardiac valves develop. In contrast to physiological aging, however, WS is characterized by the development of sclerodermoid changes, keratoses over bony prominences, and trophic ulcerations around the elbows and ankles. Patients typically die at an average of 47 years of age from myocardial infarction or cancer. WS is associated with an increased risk of cancers, particularly soft tissue sarcomas, osteosarcomas of the lower extremities, myeloid disorders, thyroid cancers, and melanomas occurring in non-sun-exposed sites.

WS is considered a lineage-specific aging phenomenon whereby mesenchymal tissues are severely affected whereas neural lineage is spared. In fact, one study found that telomere length in pluripotent WS cells is initially normal but premature senescence occurs with differentiation, preferentially affecting mesenchymal stem cells (MSCs). This aging discrepancy is regulated by telomerase which protects neural progenitor cells from DNA damage [35].

The hallmark of WS is genetic instability. Mutations affecting WRN (RECQL2) gene have been identified on chromosome 8p11–12 locus. WRN gene encodes for a protein from the RecQ subfamily helicases acting both as $3' \rightarrow 5'$ DNA helicase and as a $3' \rightarrow 5'$ exonuclease. WRN interacts with several protein components of the DNA replication complex, such as proliferating cell nuclear antigen (PCNA), topoisomerase I, DNA polymerase, and Bloom syndrome helicase (BLM). Moreover, WRN protein has been found on telomeres where it is recruited by TRF2, a telomeric repeat binding factor, essential to maintain telomere structure [36]. Therefore, WRN protein plays a major role in genetic stability, and the absence of WRN protein leads to the accumulation of genetic aberrations and an increased risk of neoplastic transformation. Interestingly, a direct relationship exists between WRN protein and p53-dependant apoptosis. The increased rate of soft tissue sarcomas in WS is attributed to upregulation of MYC protooncogene.

Atypical Werner Syndrome

A subset of patients has an earlier onset of symptoms with severe age-related symptoms. Atypical Werner is inherited as autosomal dominant with missense mutations in the LMNA gene. It is considered as a late onset HGPS.

SPRTN Syndrome

SPRTN syndrome is an atypical Werner-like progeroid syndrome presenting with features of Werner syndrome such as short stature, graying hair, muscular atrophy, and cataracts but without mutations in WRN gene. Patients develop hepatocellular carcinoma in their teens. Investigators identified mutations in both alleles of a single gene called SPRTN implicated in translesional DNA synthesis and acting as an important factor to prevent replication stress.

Treatment

Genetic counseling and identification of heterozygotes in affected families is very helpful to initiate early prevention of diabetes mellitus and cardiovascular complications and allows regular screening for internal malignancies. Inhibition of p38 mitogen-activated protein kinase (MAPK) with SB203580 significantly increased the replicative lifespan and growth rate of WS cells [37]. This treatment supports the role of MAPK p38 in senescence induced by oxidative stress, Ras activation, and telomere shortening. Consequently, there is currently a phase 2 clinical trial exploring p38 inhibitors as candidate therapeutic agents for WS.

Bloom Syndrome

Bloom syndrome is an autosomal recessive genodermatosis first described by Bloom in 1954. It is most commonly present in Ashkenazi Jews due to inbreeding.

Clinical Manifestations

Growth retardation starts prenatally and patients with Bloom syndrome are born with narrow, bird-like face, small mandible, prominent nose, and big ears. Patients are found to have disproportionately big hands. During childhood, photosensitivity, facial telangiectasia, hyper- and hypopigmented lesions start to appear. An SLE like butterfly rash appears during the first or second year of life and sometimes the dorsa of the hands and forearms may be involved. Associated decrease in the levels of immunoglobulin (IgA and IgM) predisposes patients to respiratory and gastrointestinal tract infections. In addition, Bloom syndrome patients may suffer from diabetes mellitus and decreased fertility. Bloom syndrome patients have a near normal lifespan, and the most common cause of death in these patients is cancer. They have up to 300-fold increased risk of a wide variety of malignancies, mostly leukemias, which occur at an early age and solid tumors during the fourth decade of life [38].

The defective gene in Bloom syndrome is located on chromosome 15 (locus 15q26.1) and encodes a BLM protein (RECQL3) homologous to RecQ helicases. Similar to WRN protein, BLM protein is a 3′→5′ DNA helicase involved in the suppression of hyper recombination events. BLM protein interacts with a number of other enzymes such as topoisomerase IIIα, replication protein A, RAD51, 5′-flap endonuclease/5′–3′ exonuclease (FEN-1), and BRCA1-associated genome surveillance complex [38]. All of these interactions are necessary for the proper functioning of BLM protein in the recognition and repair of defective DNA. The absence of the BLM protein leads to high frequency of chromosomal aberrations and sister chromatid exchange (SCE) due to excessive recombination events. In addition, BLM protein works in conjunction with p53 at DNA replication forks explaining the abnormal rate of malignancies in Bloom syndrome.

Interestingly, studies in yeast showed that restoring BLM function can prevent premature aging in yeast. However, the role of this protein in ordinary human aging remains to be elucidated.

Rothmund–Thomson Syndrome (RTS)

Rothmund–Thomson syndrome is an autosomal recessive inherited disorder first described in 1868.

Clinical Manifestations

Patients initially present at 3–6 months of age with blistering on the face, edematous, and erythematous plaques over the cheeks. Photosensitivity starts on the face and subsequently spreads to the extremities and buttock sparing the trunk. Characteristic facies include a prominent forehead; sparse or absent scalp hair, eyelashes, and eyebrows; prognathism; and saddle nose. All patients have poikiloderma as a characteristic feature. Poikilodermatous changes including telangiectasia, hypo- and hyperpigmentation, and skin atrophy develop with time. Additional features include with small or absent thumbs and/or underdeveloped forearm bones, palmoplantar hyperkeratotic lesions, dystrophic nails, dental abnormalities, growth delay, low birth weight, short stature, hypogonadism, and reduced fertility. Despite these precocious aging symptoms and signs, patients with RTS usually have a normal lifespan. The cancers that are mostly associated with Rothmund–Thomson syndrome are osteosarcomas and skin cancers [39].

Clinically RTS can be divided into two types: Type I manifest ectodermal dysplasia and bilateral juvenile cataracts in addition to poikiloderma. Type II RTS is more associated with congenital bone defects and an increased risk of osteosarcomas.

The genetic etiology of RTSI remains unknown. The gene responsible for RTSII is RECQL4 gene. RECQL4 gene has been localized on chromosome 8 (locus 8q24.3) and codes for a protein similar to RecQ helicases. The exact function of RECQL4 is not fully elucidated. RECQL4 is a multifunctional protein and each specific function may require different domains explaining the heterogeneity of RTS phenotypes. Unlike WRN and BLM, RECQL4 lacks DNA helicase activity. RECQL4 plays a role in the initiation of DNA replication enabling cells to recover from oxidative stress. RECQL4 interacts with the telomere shelterin proteins, TRF1 and TRF2, and functions in telomere maintenance. Therefore, the absence of BLM results in greater DNA damage due to replication stress and explains the development of premature aging in RTS [40]. Mutations in RECQL4 gene have been linked to the development of associated osteosarcomas. All RECQL4-negative RTS patients are not at an increased risk of cancer.

Treatment

Genetic counseling should be provided for RTS patients and their families. Screening of all patients with RTSII should be done to detect osteosarcomas. Patients are treated by pulsed dye laser to address telangiectasia. Cataracts are managed by surgery.

Progeroid Syndromes Due to an Unknown Defect

Ataxia telangiectasia

Ataxia telangiectasia (AT), also known as Louis–Bar syndrome, is an autosomal recessive progeroid syndrome caused by a defect in ATM kinase. Patients with AT present with progressive cerebellar degeneration, severe ataxia, oculocutaneous telangiectasia, and immunological defects. Telangiectasias develop over the face, neck, dorsa of the hands and feet, antecubital, and popliteal areas. AT patients are characterized by an extreme sensitivity to ionizing radiation and have an increased risk of cancer particularly leukemia and Hodgkin lymphoma [41].

AT is caused by mutations in the ATM gene coding for an ATM kinase which regulates downstream targets involved in the cellular response to DNA damage. ATM kinase interacts with the insulin-like growth factor-1 receptor pointing to the presence of mechanisms other than DNA repair enzymes and laminopathies involved in the aging processes [42].

Dyskeratosis Congenita (DC)

Dyskeratosis congenita (DC) is a disorder of telomere dysfunction. The X-linked form is caused by mutations in the DKC1 gene which encodes the protein dyskerin, a highly conserved nucleolar protein essential for human telomerase RNA stability. Dyskerin catalyzes conversion of uridines into pseudouridine in ribosomal rRNAs. DC may be also inherited as autosomal dominant, autosomal recessive, and sporadic autosomal and may be due to mutations in other genes regulating telomerase or telomere function [43].

Clinical Manifestations

Dyskeratosis congenita presents with severe nail dystrophy and leukoplakia. Skin involvement includes poikilodermatous changes which occur during childhood, at a later age than RTS. The skin manifests with hypo, hyper, or reticulate pigmentation over the face, neck, trunk, and thighs. Other abnormalities include teeth and mental retardation. About 80–90 % of patients develop bone marrow failure by the age of 30, and this is the main cause of early death in these patients.

The exact pathophysiology of premature aging in DC is not known. The manifestations of DC are mostly in tissues with high proliferative index. A growing body of evidence suggests that absent dyskerin protein leads to increased DNA damage response, telomere shortening and p53 induction, causing senescence and death. Studies have also shown that programmed −1 ribosomal frame shifting signal, a mechanism involved in telomere maintenance and cell cycle control, is implicated in DC. Therefore, aging is at least in part affected by − 1 PRF signaling [44].

Kindler Syndrome (Bullous Acrokeratotic Poikiloderma)

Kindler syndrome was first described by Kindler in 1954 when he reported a patient with acral blisters and photosensitivity. Similar cases were subsequently described with both autosomal dominant and recessive inheritance pattern.

Clinical Manifestations

Clinical manifestations of Kindler syndrome may appear at birth with skin fragility and acral bullae. Congenital erosions are frequently observed on the shins and forearms. Bullae usually appear on the trauma prone areas of arms and legs, hands and feet. Scarring is not a consistent feature. Photosensitivity starts in early childhood, with pigmentary changes and telangiectasia appearing at puberty. The hallmark of Kindler syndrome, however, is poikiloderma and cigarette paper like atrophy of the skin mostly over hands and feet. Poikiloderma is mostly pronounced over the face and neck and may involve sun-protected areas. Other features include acral hyperkeratosis, nail dystrophy, and mucosal involvement. Ectropion, stenosis of the urethral meatus, gingival fragility, erosions, and poor dentition may also be observed. A slightly increased risk of malignancies is reported, namely SCC of the lip and palate and bladder cancer [45].

Kindler syndrome is cause by mutations in KIND1 gene coding for kindling-1 protein. This protein plays a role in linking the actin cytoskeleton to the extracellular matrix. Kindlin is expressed in basal keratinocytes, and when absent leads to the formation of bullae over trauma prone sites. Absence of immunostaining of skin biopsies from Kindler syndrome with anti-kindklin-1 antibodies may be an additional clue to the diagnosis.

Treatment

Treatment is symptomatic and aims at addressing the bullae and providing appropriate wound care.

Poikiloderma with Neutropenia (Clericuzio Type Poikiloderma)

Clericuzio type poikiloderma with neutropenia is an autosomal recessive disorder characterized by poikiloderma over the face and limbs starting in infancy and short stature. Those features are in common with RTS. However, unlike RTS, photosensitivity is lacking, and poikiloderma affects the rest of the body, including flexural areas and trunk. Neutropenia causes recurrent pulmonary infections. Other features include hyperkeratotic nails, especially of the toes. The gene for Clericuzio type poikiloderma with neutropenia (PN) has been recently identified confirming the distinct genetic control of PN and RTS [46].

Wolfram Syndrome (WFS)

Wolfram syndrome (WFS) is an autosomal recessive disease also known as the DIDMOAD syndrome. Patients present with symptoms of diabetes insipidus, diabetes mellitus, optic atrophy, and deafness. Type 1 WFS and type 2 WFS are caused respectively by WFS1 and CISD2 genes [47]. The WFS1 gene encodes wolframin, a transmembrane protein located in the endoplasmic reticulum (ER), whereas Cisd2 has been shown to be expressed at different subcellular localizations (in the mitochondrial outer membrane (MOM) fraction, the ER, and the mitochondria-associated ER membranes (MAMs) in various cell types [48]. CISD2 protein functions in the regulation of Ca++ transmission between ER and mitochondria. In addition, Cisd2 interacts with Gimap5 and helps preserving the maintenance of mitochondrial integrity. Similarly, Cisd2 interacts with Bcl-2 and is directly involved in the Bcl-2 mediated regulation of autophagy.

Interestingly, CISD2 gene is located within the candidate region on chromosome 4q where a genetic component for human longevity has been identified. Moreover, CISD2 gene is an evolutionarily conserved gene present in nematodes, insects, chordates, fish, amphibians, reptiles, birds, and mammals [49]. Studies in mice have shown the importance of Cisd2 in determining lifespan. Knockout mice have a short lifespan and demonstrate premature aging phenotypes, whereas transgenic (gain-of-function) mice have a long-lived phenotype and a delay in age-associated diseases [50].

The role of CISD2 in determining longevity in humans in not known. It would be of great importance to compare the gene activity of CISD2 between normal populations and long-lived centenarian groups and to determine the role of CISD2 in other genodermatoses with premature aging.

Cutis Laxa

Cutis laxa is a multisystemic disorder characterized clinically by skeletal, cardiovascular, pulmonary, and central nervous system disease. Cutis laxa can be inherited as an autosomal dominant, X-linked, or autosomal recessive disorder and is characterized by a heterogeneous genetic defect.

Clinical Manifestations

The clinical phenotype is highly variable and patients might have a normal phenotype during the first months of life. Characteristic features such as a triangular face, short nose, long philtrum, and large ears are sometimes visible. Skin laxity is observed in some but not all patients, mostly over the abdomen and hands and feet. With age, a sagging face is sometimes present and the chin becomes very prominent resulting in prognathism.

Wrinkly skin syndrome is a type of autosomal recessive cutis laxa (Debré type) (ARCL2A) characterized by generalized cutis laxa, delayed closure of the enlarged anterior fontanel, developmental delay, cobblestone-like brain malformations, and occasionally a neurodegenerative phenotype with seizures and dementia. The genetic mutation responsible for this phenotype lies in ATP6V0A2 gene which encodes a V-type H + -ATPase subunit a2 responsible for Golgi membrane trafficking of skin fibroblasts [51].

A more severe form of cutis laxa is De Barsy syndrome (DBS), which has been also referred to as ARCL type III (ARCL3). The clinical hallmarks of this type are a progeroid appearance, short stature, corneal clouding, hypotonia, and pronounced intellectual disability. Recently, two genes have been identified: PYCR1 gene which encodes for a protein in mitochondria and functions mostly in the development of skeletal, fat, and connective tissues but is not crucial for CNS. Therefore, patients with a deletion of the entire PYCR1 locus do not show intellectual disability [52]. ALDH18A1 is another gene that is identified in patients with severe ARCL phenotype with marked intellectual disability.

The role of PYCR1 gene is crucial early in life and becomes less important with age explaining why the progeroid appearance and growth delay get milder with age in PYCR1-related ARCL.

Future Perspectives in Treatment

A lot of work is being dedicated to development of antiaging substances, addressing aging-related diseases, and improving human lifespan through regenerative therapy, modulation of energy metabolism, genetics, and immunotherapy.

Therapies based on stem cells are currently a promising strategy thought to reverse or slow the process of tissue aging. Reprogramming of human adult cells using six genetic factors (OCT4, SOX2, C MYC, KLF4, NANOG, and LIN28) have allowed researchers to obtain induced pluripotent cells (iPSC), with characteristics and potential similar to human embryonic stem cells (hESC) capable into differentiation into any specialized cell without the ethical restrictions related to using embryonic stem cells [53].

Other potential targets for antiaging therapy include hormone modulation with estrogen through its inhibition of lipid peroxidation, neutralizing reactive oxygen species, and activating a number of antiapoptotic signaling pathways [54].

Targeting the respiratory chain affecting energy and metabolism is also considered a critical factor for preventing cellular senescence. Recent findings suggest that a decrease in intracellular NAD+ levels is clinically related to the progression of age-associated disorders. NAD+ is known to serve as a substrate for some longevity-associated maintenance enzymes, such as the histone-deacetylating Sirtuins (SIRT) [55]. A well-known stimulant of Sirtuins is Resveratrol, a polyphenolic compound found in red wine. One study found that rats receiving Resveratrol exhibited enhanced expression of genes vital for learning and memory function, such as SIRT1 and FOXO3, the latter being highly associated with longevity. SIRT1 is considered as a key mediator of metabolism, positioned at the cross road of cancer, metabolism, and aging. In line with this, lifespan-extending effects of Ginseng berries extracts were demonstrated and thought to be mediated by polyphenol syringaresinol via enhanced SIRT expression [56].

Based on the caloric restriction theory, studies are exploring the potential role of Rapamycin, a known inhibitor of mTOR which induces upregulation of mitochondrial antioxidative enzymes [57]. In response to caloric restriction, Mafl (a protein involved in transfer RNA synthesis) plays a key role in mitochondrial antioxidative response which promotes longevity. Studies on mice showed that chronic treatment with Rapamycin extended lifespan, and delayed aging, and reversed Alzheimer's disease (AD)-like memory deficits [58]. Age-associated mitochondrial defects can also be targeted by the so-called epigenetic regulation. Epigenetic regulation refers to addition of chemical structures or proteins, which alter the physical structure of the DNA, without changing the DNA sequence itself resulting in genes turning on or off. For example, researchers showed that regulation of the genes CGAT and SHMT2 involved with the production of glycine can reverse the age-associated respiration defects in the elderly human fibroblasts [59].

Immunotherapy as an antiaging is based on the intimate relation between the immune function, the micro environment, and age-related chronic inflammatory conditions.

Genetic modalities used to increase lifespan include the use of modified messenger RNA to extend the telomeres. The RNA used in these experiments contains the coding sequence for TERT, the active component of telomerase [60]. Statins were also shown to reduce the rate at which telomeres shorten and patients on statins had higher telomerase activity in their white blood cells, compared to the control group [61]. Therefore, chronic statin treatment may extend human lifespan beyond lowering cholesterol levels and reducing the cardiovascular risk.

References

1. Tower J. Programmed cell death in aging. Ageing Res Rev. 2015;23:90–100.
2. Jin K. Modern biological theories of aging. Aging Dis. 2010;1(2):72–4.
3. Afanas'ev I. Signaling and damaging functions of free radicals in aging – free radical theory, Hormesis, and TOR. Aging Dis. 2010;1(2):75–88.
4. Clay Montier LL, Deng JJ, Bai Y. Number matters: control of mammalian mitochondrial DNA copy number. J Genet Genomics. 2009;36(3):125–31.
5. Petralia RS, Mattson MP, Yao PJ. Aging and longevity in the simplest animals and the quest for immortality. Ageing Res. 2014;16:66–82.
6. Shimokawa I, Trindade LS. Dietary restriction and aging in rodents: a current view on its molecular mechanisms. Aging Dis. 2010;1(2):89–104.

7. Van Heemst D. Insulin, IGF-1 and longevity. Aging Dis. 2010;1(2):147–57.
8. Kuro-o M, Matsumura Y, Aizawa H, et al. Mutation of the mouse klotho gene leads to a syndrome resembling ageing. Nature. 1997;390:45–51.
9. Sato S, Kawamata Y, Takahashi A, et al. Ablation of the p16 (INK4a) tumour suppressor reverses ageing phenotypes of klotho mice. Nat Commun. 2015;6:7035.
10. Linborg CM, Propert KJ, Pignolo RJ. Conservation of pro longevity genes among mammals. Mech Ageing Dev. 2015;146:146–8-23.
11. Nebel A, Kleindorp R, Caliebe A, et al. A genome-wide association study confirms APOE as the major gene influencing survival in long-lived individuals. Mech Ageing Dev. 2011;132:324–30.
12. Garatachea N, Marín PJ, Santos-Lozano A, et al. The ApoE gene is related with exceptional longevity: a systematic review and meta-analysis. Rejuvenation Res. 2015;18(1):3–13.
13. Flachsbart F, Caliebe A, Kleindorp R, et al. Association of FOXO3A variation with human longevity confirmed in German centenarians. Proc Natl Acad Sci U S A. 2009;106(8):2700–5.
14. Nebel A, Flachsbart F, Till A, et al. A functional EXO1 promoter variant is associated with prolonged life expectancy in centenarians. Mech Ageing Dev. 2009;130(10):691–9.
15. Chen YF, Kao CH, Kirby R et al. Cisd2 mediates mitochondrial integrity and lifespan in mammals. Autophagy. 2009;5(7):1043–45.
16. Geesaman BJ, Benson E, Brewster SJ, et al. Haplotype-based identification of a microsomal transfer protein marker associated with the human lifespan. Proc Natl Acad Sci U S A. 2003;100 (24):14115–20.
17. Moriwaki S. Hereditary disorders with defective repair of UV-induced DNA damage. Jpn Clin Med. 2013;4:29–35.
18. Menck CFM, Munford V. DNA repair diseases: what do they tell us about cancer and aging? Genet Mol Biol. 2014;37(1 suppl):220–33.
19. Kraemer KH, Patronas NJ, Schiffmann R, et al. Xeroderma pigmentosum, trichothiodystrophy and Cockayne syndrome: a complex genotype-phenotype relationship. Neuroscience. 2007;145(4):1388–96.
20. Amr K, Messaoud O, El Darouti M, et al. Mutational spectrum of Xeroderma pigmentosum group A in Egyptian patients. Gene. 2014;533(1):52–6.
21. Niedernhofer LJ, Bohr VA, Sander M, et al. Xeroderma pigmentosum and other diseases of human premature aging and DNA repair: molecules to patients. Mech Ageing Dev. 2011;132(6–7):340–7.
22. Schärer OD. Nucleotide excision repair in eukaryotes. Cockayne syndrome: the expanding clinical and mutational spectrum. Cold Spring Harb Perspect Biol. 2013;5:161–70.
23. Kamenisch Y, Berneburg M. Mitochondrial CSA and CSB: protein interactions and protection from ageing associated DNA mutations. Mech Ageing Dev. 2013;134(5–6):270–4.
24. Giglia-Mari G, Coin F, Ranish JA. A new, tenth subunit of TFIIH is responsible for the DNA repair syndrome trichothiodystrophy group. Genet. 2004;36(7):714–9.
25. Pollex RL, Hegele RA. Hutchinson–Gilford progeria syndrome. Clin Genet. 2004;66(5):375–81.
26. Musich PR, Zou Y. Genomic instability and DNA damage responses in progeria arising from defective maturation of prelamin A. Aging. 2009;1(1):28–37.
27. Jung HJ, Tu Y, Yang SH, et al. New Lmna knock-in mice provide a molecular mechanism for the 'segmental aging' in Hutchinson-Gilford progeria syndrome. Hum Mol Genet. 2014;23(6):1506–15.
28. Decker ML, Chavez E, Vulto I, Lansdorp PM. Telomere length in Hutchinson-Gilford progeria syndrome. Mech Ageing Dev. 2009;130(6):377–83.
29. Olive M, Harten I, Mitchell R, et al. Cardiovascular pathology in Hutchinson–Gilford progeria: correlation with the vascular pathology of aging. Arterioscler Thromb Vasc Biol. 2010;30(11):2301–9.
30. Gordon LB, Massaro J, D'Agostino Sr RB, et al. Impact of farnesylation inhibitors on survival in Hutchinson-Gilford progeria syndrome. Circulation. 2014;130(1):27–34.
31. Liu B, Ghosh S, Yang X, et al. Resveratrol rescues SIRT1-dependent adult stem cell decline and alleviates progeroid features in laminopathy-based progeria. Cell Metabol. 2012;16(6):738–50.
32. Ibrahim MX, Sayin VI, Akula MK, et al. Targeting isoprenylcysteine methylation ameliorates disease in a mouse model of progeria. Science. 2013;340 (6138):1330–3.
33. Xiong Z, Lu Y, Xue J, et al. Hutchinson–Gilford progeria syndrome accompanied by severe skeletal abnormalities in two Chinese siblings: two case reports. J Med Case Rep. 2013;7:63.
34. Shimi T, Butin-Israeli V, Adam SA, et al. The role of nuclear lamin B1 in cell proliferation and senescence. Genes Dev. 2011;25(24):2579–93.
35. Cheung HH, Liu X, Canterel-Thouennon L, et al. Telomerase protects Werner syndrome lineage-specific stem cells from premature aging. Stem Cell Rep. 2014;2(4):534–46.
36. Machwe A, Xiao L, Orren DK. TRF2 recruits the Werner syndrome (WRN) exonuclease for processing of telomeric DNA. Oncogene. 2004;23(1):149–56.
37. Davis T, Baird DM, Haughton MF, et al. Prevention of accelerated cell aging in Werner syndrome using a p38 mitogen-activated protein kinase inhibitor. J Gerontol A Biol Sci Med Sci. 2005;60(11):1386–93.
38. Wu L, Davies SL, Levitt NC, et al. Potential role for the BLM helicase in recombinational repair via a conserved interaction with RAD51. J Biol Chem. 2001;276(22):19375–81.
39. Larizza, et al. Rothmund-Thomson syndrome. Orphanet J Rare Dis. 2010;5:2.
40. Macris MA, Krejci L, Bussen W, et al. Biochemical characterization of the RECQ4 protein, mutated in

Rothmund-Thomson syndrome. DNA Repair. 2006;5 (2):172–80.
41. Teive HA, Moro A, Moscovich M, et al. Ataxia-telangiectasia – a historical review and a proposal for a new designation: ATM syndrome. J Neurol Sci. 2015;355(1–2):3–6.
42. Shiloh Y. ATM and related protein kinases: safeguarding genome integrity. Nat Rev Cancer. 2003;3(3):155–68.
43. Brault ME, Lauzon C, Autexier C. Dyskeratosis congenita mutations in dyskerin SUMOylation consensus sites lead to impaired telomerase RNA accumulation and telomere defects. Hum Mol Genet. 2013;122 (17):3498–507.
44. Lai-Cheong JE, McGrath JA. Kindler syndrome. Dermatol Clin. 2010;28(1):119–24.
45. Koparir A, Gezdirici A, Koparir E, et al. Poikiloderma with neutropenia: genotype-ethnic origin correlation, expanding phenotype and literature review. Am J Med Genet A. 2014;164A(10):2535–40.
46. Blanco-Aguirre ME, la Parra DR, Tapia-Garcia H, et al. Identification of unsuspected Wolfram syndrome cases through clinical assessment and WFS1 gene screening in type 1 diabetes mellitus patients. Gene. 2015;566(1):63–7.
47. Wang CH, Chen YF, Wu CY, et al. Cisd2 modulates the differentiation and functioning of adipocytes by regulating intracellular Ca 2++ homeostasis. Hum Mol Genet. 2014;23(18):4770–85.
48. Wang C-H, Kao C-H, Chen Y-F, et al. Cisd2 mediates lifespan. Free Radic Res. 2014;48(9):1109–14.
49. Chen YF, Kao CH, Chen YT, et al. Cisd2 deficiency drives premature aging and causes mitochondria-mediated defects in mice. Genes Dev. 2009;23 (10):1183–94.
50. Fischer B, Dimopoulou A, Egerer J, et al. Further characterization of ATP6V0A2-related autosomal recessive cutis laxa. Hum Genet. 2012;131(11):1761–73.
51. Dimopoulou A, Fischer B, Gardeitchik T, et al. Genotype-Phenotype spectrum of PYCR1-related autosomal recessive cutis laxa. Mol Genet Metab. 2013;110(3):352–61.
52. Stambler I. Stop Aging Disease! Aging Dis. 2015;6 (2):76–94.
53. Lapasset L, Milhavet O, Prieur A, et al. Rejuvenating senescent and centenarian human cells by reprogramming through the pluripotent state. Genes Dev. 2011;25(21):2248–53.
54. Cen J, Zhang H, Liu Y, et al. Anti-aging effect of estrogen on telomerase activity in ovariectomised rats – animal model for menopause. Gynecol Endocrinol. 2015;31(7):582–5.
55. Labat-Robert J, Ladislas R. Longevity and aging. Mechanisms and perspectives. Pathol Biol. 2015; pii: S0369-8114(15)00069-3. doi:10.1016/j.patbio.2015.08.001.
56. Ramis MR, Esteban S, Miralles A, et al. Caloric restriction, resveratrol and melatonin: role of SIRT1 and implications for aging and related-diseases. Mech Ageing Dev. 2015;146:28–41.
57. Mazucanti CH, Cabral-Costa JV, Vasconcelos AR, et al. Longevity pathways (mTOR, SIRT, Insulin/IGF-1) as key modulatory targets on aging and neurodegeneration. Curr Top Med Chem. 2015;15 (21):2116–38.
58. Caccamo A, De Pinto V, Messina A, Branca C, Oddo S. Genetic reduction of mammalian target of rapamycin ameliorates Alzheimer's disease-like cognitive and pathological deficits by restoring hippocampal gene expression signature. J Neurosci. 2014;34 (23):7988–98.
59. Hashizume O, Ohnishi S, Mito T, et al. Epigenetic regulation of the nuclear-coded GCAT and SHMT2 genes confers human age-associated mitochondrial respiration defects. Sci Rep. 2015;5: 10434.
60. Ramunas J, Yakubov E, Brady JJ, et al. Transient delivery of modified mRNA encoding TERT rapidly extends telomeres in human cells. FASEB J. 2015. doi:10.1096/fj.14-259531.
61. Boccardi V, Barbieri M, Rizzo MR, et al. A new pleiotropic effect of statins in elderly: modulation of telomerase activity. The. FASEB J. 2013;27:3879. doi:10.1096/fj.13-232066.

Resetting Skin Genome Back to Health Naturally with GHK

115

Loren Pickart, Jessica Michelle Vasquez-Soltero, and Anna Margolina

Contents

L. Pickart (✉) • J.M. Vasquez-Soltero • A. Margolina
Research and Development, Skin Biology, Bellevue, WA, USA
e-mail: lorenpickart@skinbiology.com; jessie16@uw.edu; anna@amargolina.com

M.A. Farage et al. (eds.), *Textbook of Aging Skin*,
DOI 10.1007/978-3-662-47398-6_162

Abstract

The copper-binding tripeptide GHK (glycyl-L-histidyl-L-lysine) is a naturally occurring plasma peptide widely used in skin care products. It is especially popular in antiaging cosmetic formulations due to its various and well-established positive biological effects on aging skin. It has been established that GHK-Cu improves wound healing and tissue regeneration and stimulates collagen and decorin production. GHK-Cu also supports angiogenesis and nerve outgrowth, improves the biological condition of aging skin and hair and possesses DNA repair, antioxidant, and anti-inflammatory effects. In addition, it increases cellular stemness and secretion of trophic factors by mesenchymal stem cells. GHK's antioxidant actions have been demonstrated in vitro and in animal studies. They include blocking the formation of reactive oxygen and carbonyl species, detoxifying toxic products of lipid peroxidation such as acrolein, protecting keratinocytes from lethal UVB radiation, and blocking hepatic damage by dichloromethane radicals. In recent studies, GHK has also been found to switch cellular gene expression from a diseased state to a healthier state for certain cancers and for chronic obstructive pulmonary disease (COPD). The human gene expression actions provide a unique view of the complex and intricate gene actions underlying visible changes in human skin. This chapter reviews biological and gene data related to the positive antiaging effects of GHK on human skin.

Introduction

Since the dawn of time, people have aspired to find a way to reverse aging. Among the most popular ingredients of the elusive elixir of youth sought by ancient mages and alchemists were herbs, powdered gems, gold, silver, and mercury as well as animal parts and extracts. The most powerful magic has been attributed to human blood – it was believed that blood contained the "essence of youth," which can be transferred from young to old people. Today, it is known that plasma and other body fluids (such as saliva) indeed contain soluble activities that can enhance reparative and renewing activity of various cells and tissues [1].

Some of the human "youth essence" may reside in the copper-binding tripeptide GHK (glycyl-L-histidyl-L-lysine) that naturally occurs in blood plasma but significantly declines during human aging. Today, there is a wealth of data confirming the diverse positive effects of GHK on aging skin; however, the exact mechanism of GHK's action remains to be established. Recently, it has been discovered that GHK can modulate expression of a great number of human genes related to aging.

Discovery of GHK

The GHK activity was discovered by Loren Pickart during studies from 1962 to 1967, as a graduate student at the University of Minnesota and later at the Sansum Foundation in Santa Barbara, California, on the relationship between human aging, cardiovascular disease, free fatty acids (FFA), and the plasma protein fibrinogen [2, 3]. Fibrinogen rises with age and more so in heart patients, forms the polymer protein in blood clots, inhibits blood flow through the microcirculation, and is an excellent predictor of mortality [4].

Blood plasma from young, male medical students of ages 20–25, when tested on a human liver biopsies obtained during surgery, produced less fibrinogen and more albumin than plasma from male heart patients over age 60. During these studies, it was discovered that certain albumin fractions, such as Cohn Fraction 5 albumin, possessed an activity more like that of the young medical students. However, crystalline albumin lacked this activity. Thus, an impurity in the albumin fraction was thought to be responsible for these actions. What is even more impressive is when plasma taken from young subjects was added to liver biopsy tissue of older heart patients, it made old liver cells produce proteins in a pattern similar to that produced by younger cells [5]. It seemed as if young blood contained some "youth essence" just as ancient alchemists believed.

Later (1969–1973), during PhD thesis work at the University of California at San Francisco,

Fig. 1 GHK-Cu

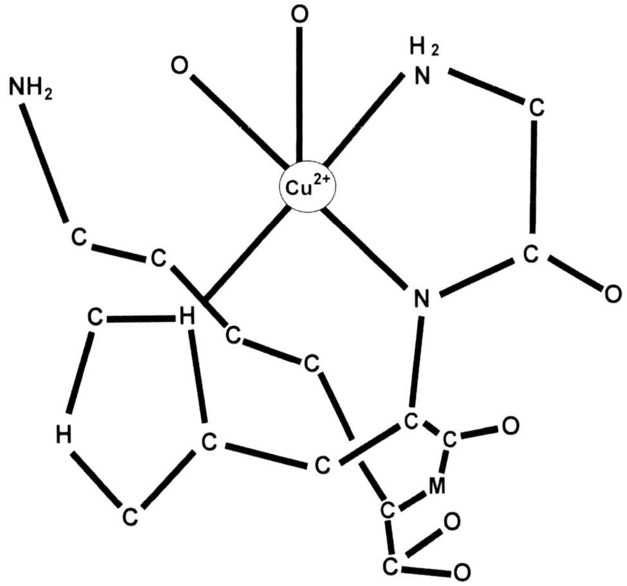

Pickart isolated GHK from albumin as the active factor contaminant associated with albumin. It was a tripeptide with the amino acid sequence glycyl-L-histidyl-L-lysine which possessed a very high affinity for copper (II), thus forming GHK-Cu (Fig. 1).

Today, GHK-Cu is a widely used cosmetic ingredient, which can be found in antiaging skin products, hair products, as well as skin protective formulations. Even though the cosmetic industry now produces hundreds of biologically active peptides every year and each of them has an impressive list of biological effects, none of them has been studied in such depth with such an impressive yield of scientific discoveries as the human tripeptide GHK-Cu. It has been shown to improve wound healing in experimental animals, stimulate the production of collagen, elastin, and glycosaminoglycans, stimulate hair growth, DNA repair in damaged fibroblasts, better antioxidant defense and blood vessel growth, possess anti-inflammatory effects, and much more [6].

GHK and Copper 2+

During wound healing studies in rats, mice, and pigs, copper-free GHK produced a very mild stimulation of healing, but the addition of copper 2+ to GHK strongly enhanced repair. The interaction of GHK with copper 2+ is important, and it is likely that a mixture of GHK and GHK-copper 2+ exists in cell culture and in vivo experiments. GHK has an extraordinary affinity for copper 2+ (pK of association is 16.4) and can obtain copper 2+ from albumin (pK of association is 16.2) [7].

Since many of GHK's cellular effects occur at about 1 nM, it is possible that even copper-free systems act through GHK-Cu action as GHK binds to trace copper 2+.

GHK Data Sources and Effects

By human aging, in this chapter, we mean the loss of the younger attributes of skin such as elasticity and thickness, fewer senescent or cancerous cells, but not an extension of the maximum lifespan.

There are three types of evidence on GHK actions:

1. In vivo mammalian data, including human clinical studies.

   These data relate to the elasticity, thickness, acceleration of dermal wound healing, enlargement of hair follicles, and so on.

2. In vitro cell culture and organ culture results.

   Culture results give evidence about the effect of GHK on cellular production of collagen and other structural proteins, the effect on stem cell function, the recovery of cellular function after anticancer radiation, ultraviolet radiation, and sensitivity of cells to oxidative molecules.
3. Gene expression data.

   This information on GHK was first available in 2010 from the Broad Institute in Boston. The Broad's Connectivity Map is used to acquire GHK's human gene expression data. The Connectivity Map is a large database that contains more than 7,000 gene expression profiles of five human cell lines treated with 1,309 distinct small molecules [8, 9]. Three GHK profiles are contained in this repository. Due to multiple probe sets mapping to the same gene, the fold changes in mRNA production produced are converted to percentages, then averaged for all probe sets representing the same gene. It was determined that the 22,277 probe sets in the Broad data represent 13,424 genes.

Biological Effects of GHK-Cu in Aging Skin

The primary goal of our skin is to be a protective barrier between our tender inner organs and the hostile environment. Since the day we are born and to the day we die, the skin shields us against harmful microorganisms, UV-rays, toxins, and moisture loss. As any fortress that withstands continuous aggression, our skin often gets damaged and needs to be constantly repaired. As we age, our skin's ability to repair itself declines, which results in accumulation of visible damage and many skin cells sink into senescence or become cancerous.

Many studies are focused on factors that lead to premature skin aging resulting from excessive damage. Among those factors are free radicals, UV-radiation, mechanical damage, and recreational toxins such as tobacco smoke and alcohol [10]. Consequently, the cosmetic industry offers a multitude of skin protective ingredients, such as plant antioxidants, UV-filters, and antibacterial ingredients. However, in addition to protecting skin from damage, it is important to restore its natural ability to repair and renew itself. There is abundant evidence that GHK-Cu plays an essential role in the natural skin repair process.

GHK Supports Skin Remodeling and Repair

In 1988, Maquart et al. from Université de Reims Champagne-Ardenne (France) found that GHK was able to stimulate the synthesis of collagen in fibroblasts at low concentrations beginning at 0.01 nM and maximizing at 1 nM. The authors noted that the GHK sequence is present in the alpha 2(I) chain of type I collagen. They proposed a mechanism by which skin stimulates its own repair – when skin is wounded, proteolytic enzymes break down collagen, releasing GHK into the site of injury [11]. It was also demonstrated that GHK-Cu helps prevent excessive skin damage during wound healing by regulating the activity of metalloproteinases – enzymes that facilitate breakdown of proteins of extracellular matrix [12, 13].

In other studies, GHK increased the production of collagen I, glycosaminoglycans (dermatan sulfate and chondroitin sulfate), and the small proteoglycan, decorin [14, 15]. Also, GHK was found to attract immune and endothelial cells to the site of injury [16].

A series of in vivo experiments confirmed the wound healing activity of GHK-Cu. In rabbits, GHK facilitated wound healing, causing better wound contraction, faster development of granular tissue, and improved vessel growth [17]. Also, GHK alone and in combination with a high dose helium neon laser stimulated granulation, increased the formation of new blood vessels and elevated the level of antioxidant enzymes in the dermal wounds in rabbits [18].

GHK-Cu was also used to create a novel wound dressing – collagen membrane with incorporated biotinylated GHK. This material has been shown to significantly improve wound healing processes in rats when compared to nontreated wounds and to wounds treated with collagen matrix alone. Collagen dressing with incorporated GHK stimulated wound contraction and cell proliferation, as well as increased the expression of antioxidant enzymes [19]. The most important finding was GHK's ability to improve wound healing in difficult-to-heal wounds, such as diabetic wounds in rats. GHK treatment resulted in faster wound contraction and epithelization, higher level of antioxidants such as glutathione and ascorbic acid, increased synthesis of collagen, and activation of fibroblasts and mast cells [20]. Also GHK-Cu improved healing of ischemic open wounds in rats. Wounds displayed faster healing, decreased concentration of metalloproteinases 2 and 9, as well as of TNF-beta (a major inflammatory cytokine) compared with vehicle alone or with untreated wounds [21].

Animal experiments confirmed that GHK has great potential to improve skin conditions. It speeds up skin repair, improves circulation, strengthens antioxidant defense, and increases production of skin proteins. All these qualities are highly desirable in cosmetics. The ability of GHK-Cu to improve difficult-to-heal wounds can be helpful in managing skin healing after plastic surgery, especially in advanced age patients and in patients with underlying health conditions.

GHK Supports Fibroblasts

GHK has been found to have positive effect on fibroblasts – the key cells in skin reparative and renewal processes. Huang et al. evaluated the effect of GHK alone or in combination with LED irradiation (light-emitting diode irradiation, 625–635 nm) on human fibroblasts. Combined GHK and LED treatment resulted in 12.5-fold increase in cell viability, 230 % increase in basic fibroblast growth factor (bFGF) production, and 70 % increase in collagen I mRNA production compared with the LED irradiation alone [22].

GHK was also able to restore normal function in cultured human fibroblasts exposed to radioactive treatment (5,000 rad). The irradiated fibroblasts treated with GHK showed much faster growth, similar to the normal (nonirradiated control) cells. In addition, GHK-treated irradiated fibroblasts showed increased production of important growth factors [23].

Fibroblasts are central cells in both wound healing and tissue renewal processes. They not only synthesize different components of the dermal matrix but also produce a number of growth factors that regulate cell growth and migration. The fact that GHK-Cu restored damaged fibroblast activity to that of normal, nonirradiated fibroblasts, opens new possibilities in enhancing fibroblasts' function in aged skin.

GHK's Effect on Skin Stem Cells

Stem cells for the skin are thought to arise from enlarged hair follicles [24]. The first indication that GHK affects stem cells came from mouse studies where GHK:Copper(2+) produced a very strong amplification of hair follicle size. A similar peptide, Ala-His-Lys-copper 2+ produced even stronger actions.

The mouse in Fig. 2 was shaved, then treated in three spots with GHK:Copper(2+). The result is a much more rapid hair growth (the three circular patches of hair) in the spots treated with copper peptides.

In the microscopic images in Fig. 3, the magnifications are identical. The top photo is the untreated mouse skin – the control. The bottom photo is mouse skin treated with copper peptides. Note the larger hair follicles (elongated purple columns) in the lower photo, the increased content

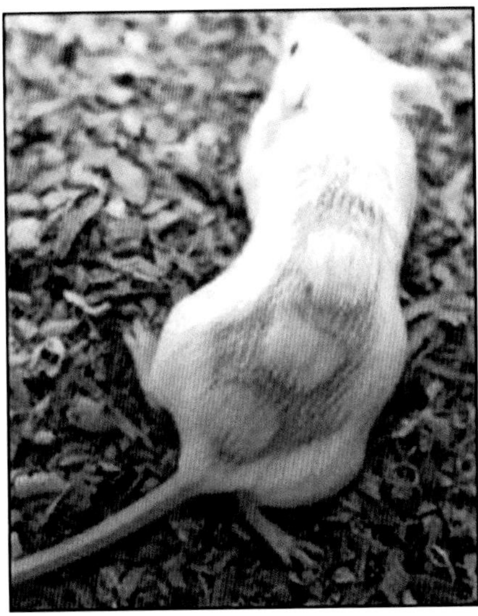

Fig. 2 GHK-treated mouse

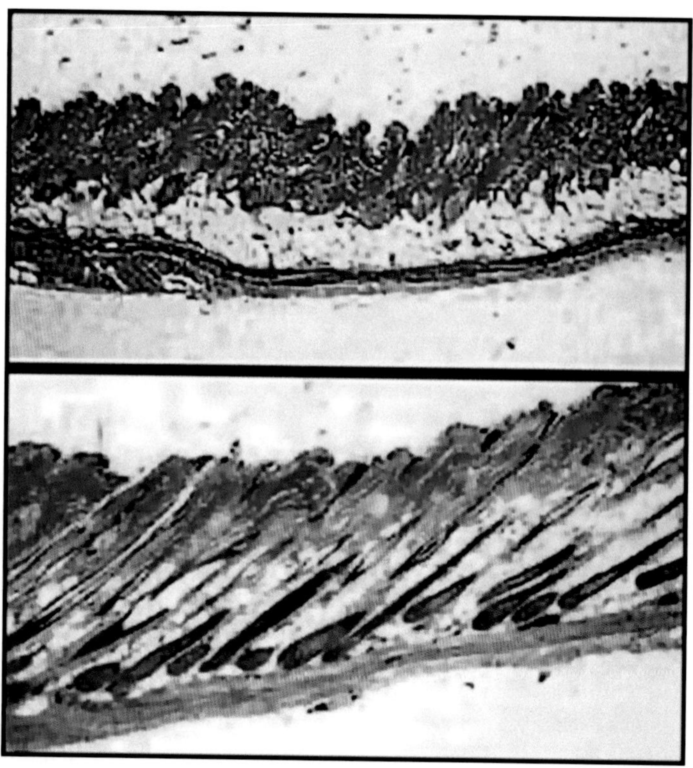

Fig. 3 Microscopic images of untreated mouse (*top*) versus GHK-treated mouse (*bottom*)

of subcutaneous fat in the skin (white material in the center of the skin), and the increased thickness of the skin. Hair researchers have noted the accumulation of this fat around healthy follicles that are vigorously growing hair and its relative lack around dormant follicles. They have postulated that these cells serve a supportive function for the hair follicle. It must be emphasized that effects in humans on hair follicle health are not as dramatic [25].

In 1995, Godet and Marie reported that GHK: Copper(2+) stimulated the growth of human marrow stromal cells. Today, these are called mesenchymal stem cells [26].

In 2005, Peled and colleagues claimed that copper-free GHK maintained the clonogenic potential of stem cells while GHK-Cu increased cell copper by 2,162 % above the control value and caused stem cell differentiation [27].

In 2009, researchers from Seoul National University (Republic of Korea) demonstrated that GHK-Cu (0.1–10 μM) in a skin equivalent culture system stimulated the proliferation of keratinocytes in a dose dependent manner. Additional GHK-Cu resulted in noticeable changes in epidermal basal cells. Their integrins and p63 expression markedly increased, and their shape became more cuboidal, as is characteristic for stem cells. The authors concluded that GHK-Cu is able to maintain "stemness" of basal keratinocytes as well as to revive their proliferative potential [28].

In 2015, Jose et al. reported that GHK added to cultured mesenchymal cells caused a dose-dependent increases in vascular endothelial growth factor (VEGF), alpha-6 and beta-1 integrins. It was suggested that GHK could increase their clinical potential when used for tissue repair [29].

Stimulation of Hair Growth

GHK's ability to stimulate hair growth was confirmed in animal experiments. In fuzzy rats a copper-binding peptide PC1031, a structural analog of GHK (ghkvfv-copper complex), produced effects comparable to that of minoxidil. Both 5 % minoxidil and 5 % PC1031 almost doubled follicle size after 3–4 months of treatment, and caused 80 % increase in the number of actively growing hair follicles. In addition, hair follicles became more robust and displayed increased DNA synthesis and cell proliferation [30].

Today, analogs of GHK-Cu with hydrophobic amino acids are used to enhance hair growth in the commercial product Tricomin (Procyte Corp). Also, a product GraftCyte (Procyte Corp) is used to increase success of hair transplants with clinically confirmed efficiency [31].

Antioxidant Activity of GHK-Cu

Every time skin is exposed to UV-radiation, it has to deal with reactive oxygen species (ROS) – highly damaging free radicals, which can impair skin barrier, damage proteins, and even damage DNA. Even though skin contains numerous antioxidants, which promptly neutralize ROS before they can do any damage, there are many situations in which the antioxidant system becomes overwhelmed. In this case, a condition known as oxidative stress can occur. Repeated oxidative stress in skin is the main cause of premature skin aging or photoaging.

GHK's antioxidant actions have been demonstrated in vitro and in animal wound healing studies. They include blocking the formation of reactive carbonyl species, detoxifying toxic products of lipid peroxidation such as acrolein, protection of keratinocytes from lethal UVB radiation, and blocking hepatic damage by dichloromethane radicals.

GHK blocked the extent of in vitro Cu(2+)-dependent oxidation of low-density lipoproteins (LDL). Treatment of LDL with 5 μM Cu(2+) for 18 h in either phosphate buffered saline (PBS) or Ham's F-10 medium resulted in extensive oxidation as determined by the content of thiobarbituric acid reactive substances (TBARs). In PBS, oxidation was entirely blocked by histidine and GHK. In comparison, superoxide dismutase (SOD1) provided only 20 % protection [32].

Acrolein, a well-known carbonyl toxin, is produced by lipid peroxidation of polyunsaturated fatty acids. GHK directly blocks the formation of 4-hydroxynonenal and acrolein toxins created by carbonyl radicals that cause fatty acid decomposition [33, 34].

GHK also blocks lethal ultraviolet radiation damage to cultured skin keratinocytes by binding and inactivating reactive carbonyl species such as 4-hydroxynonenal, acrolein, malondialdehyde, and glyoxal. This protection was found at a relatively high level of GHK, 20 mg/ml or 0.2 %, but this concentration can be easily added to protective sunscreens [35].

The intraperitoneal injection of 1.5 mg/kg of GHK into rats for 5 days before dichloromethane poisoning and 5 days thereafter provided protection of the functional activity of hepatocytes and immunological responsiveness. Dichloromethane is toxic to hepatic tissue via the formation of a dichloromethane free radical that induces acute toxic damage [36].

It has been established that the intraperitoneal injections of peptides in equimolar doses – Gly-His-Lys (0.5 μg/kg), dalargin (1.2 μg/kg), and thymogen (0.5 μg/kg) – during 10 days in rats with experimental bone fractures produced a decrease of malonic dialdehyde concentration and increase of catalase activity in blood as well as increase of reparative activity. The combination of peptides was more potent than any of the studied peptides injected separately. The synergetic action of peptides Gly-His-Lys, thymogen, and dalargin was proposed for the stimulation of reparative osteogenesis [37].

GHK-Cu produced an 87 % inhibition of iron release from ferritin by apparently blocking iron's exit channels from the protein. Iron has also been shown to have a direct role in the initiation of lipid peroxidation. An Fe(2+)/Fe(3+) complex can serve as an initiator of lipid oxidation. In addition, many iron complexes can catalyze the decomposition of lipid hydroperoxides to the corresponding lipid alkoxy radicals. The major storage site for iron in serum and tissue is ferritin.

Ferritin in blood plasma can store up to 4,500 atoms of iron per protein molecule and superoxide anion can promote the mobilization of iron from ferritin. This free iron may then catalyze lipid peroxidation and the conversion of superoxide anion to the more damaging hydroxyl radical [38].

GHK and Gene Expression: From Cancer to Emphysema

In 2010, Hong et al. identified a metastasis-prone signature for aggressive early stage mismatch-repair colorectal cancer consisting of a 54 gene set yielded by the best classification model. The Broad Institute's Connectivity Map, a compendium of transcriptional responses to compounds, which contains data on 1,309 bioactive molecules, was used to find compounds that reverse the differential expressions of these genes, suggesting they may have a therapeutic effect on the metastasis-prone patients. The results indicated that two wound healing and skin remodeling bioactive molecules, GHK at 1 μM and securinine at 18 μM, could significantly reverse the differential expression of these genes [39].

Further evidence for the validity of the Broad Institute's computer predictions came in 2012 when Campbell et al. identified 127 genes whose expression levels were associated with regional severity of chronic obstructive pulmonary disease (COPD), a disease consisting of emphysema, small airway obstruction, and/or chronic bronchitis that results in significant loss of lung function over time. Due to the ineffective therapeutic strategies for COPD, Campbell et al. sought to use computational methods to identify compounds that might modulate molecular processes associated with emphysema pathogenesis. The Connectivity Map predicted that GHK would reverse the aberrant gene-expression signature associated with emphysematous destruction and induce expression patterns consistent with healing and repair. When GHK, at 10 nM, was added to cultured fibroblasts from the affected lung areas of patients, the peptide changed gene expression patterns from tissue destruction to tissue repair. This led to the organization of the actin cytoskeleton, elevated the expression of integrin beta 1, and restored collagen contraction [40].

Table 1 Estimate of number of genes affected by GHK

Percent change (%)	Genes stimulated	Genes suppressed
50–99	1,569	583
100–199	646	469
200–299	227	196
300–599	196	207
600–899	39	42
900–1,199	8	7
1,200 or more	2	4

An estimate of the number of genes affected by GHK at various cutoff points can be seen in Table 1. The number of genes stimulated or suppressed by GHK with a change greater than or equal to 50 % is 31.2 %. GHK increases gene expression in 59 % of the genes while suppressing it in 41 %. Most discussions of gene expression, especially by cosmetic companies, focus on "turning genes on." Yet, suppressing genes may be just as important to health. Conditions such as pregnancy, acute stress, exposure to low temperatures, and so on, may activate many genes unnecessary for normal bodily functions [41].

Resetting Human Genes to Better Health

Most gene research in the past has focused on various gene mutations that impair the function of an animal. However, the major cause of human diseases appears to be a loss of proper gene controls. Regular physical exercise of older humans (as little as 30 min daily, three times a week) can reset mitochondrial human DNA to a gene expression more like that of a younger person. Other things such as healthy diet, wine consumption, and flavonoid supplements are able to modify the activity of certain genes, as well [42, 43]. Various types of meditation and antistress methods are also recommended to improve gene expression.

In studies at the University of California at San Francisco, young (age 20–25), male medical students were found to have about 200 ng/mL of GHK in their blood, while the healthy, male medical school faculty (average age of 60) had 80 ng/mL of GHK. One could argue that the young medical students are among the healthiest humans in terms of mental and physical attributes. The medical school faculty is another very healthy group that tends to strongly adhere to a "health conscious lifestyle"; however, they still show a sharp drop in GHK levels. Thus, this argues that stronger methods such as resetting genes are needed [7].

Tuning the Piano Keys of Health

Unlike mutations, which are mostly undesirable, GHK induced changes do not include modification of the genetic code and involve only up- or down-regulation of gene activity. You can imagine this as a series of on/off (up/down) switches in the DNA, which can be used to regulate protein synthesis to increase or decrease the level of a certain protein. Since many proteins are involved in intricate biochemical pathways, up- or down-regulation of such genes can have profound effect on a cell's biochemistry.

Such ability is well established for GHK-Cu. Recent discoveries on the actions of the human plasma tripeptide GHK suggest that this simple and safe molecule may be able to reset the human genome to a healthier state. One could think of human genes as piano keys. In the young students, the gene piano keys are well tuned and produce the beautiful music of good health and the fires of life burn brightly. However, in the aging faculty GHK is already in sharp decline despite their deep knowledge of health. Their song is less pure, and smoke is beginning to replace the fire.

GHK Gene Expression Data, Diseases of Aging, and Postulated Theories of Human Aging

There are many theories postulated as causative factors in the development of diseases of aging. Interestingly, GHK affects gene expression in a manner that might be considered antiaging or at least disease ameliorating. It is also possible that common diseases and maximum human lifespan are controlled by separate systems since telomerase activation is a factor in cancerous growths. See Table 2.

GHK Suppresses Expression of Fibrinogen Genes

As expected, based on biological data, GHK strongly suppresses the gene for the beta chain of fibrinogen. See Table 3. A suppression of the fibrinogen beta chain will effectively inhibit fibrinogen synthesis since equal amounts of all three polypeptide chains are needed to produce fibrinogen.

Fibrinogen, the protein which is used to make blood clots, is also a strong predictor of mortality in cardiovascular patients. After vascular incidents, such as myocardial infarction, fibrinogen concentrations increase sharply. When fibrinogen is increased, it decreases blood flow through microcirculation, preventing oxygen and nutrient flow to the tissues. Decreased circulation contributes to skin aging by impairing skin repair and renewal, since these processes are dependent on adequate nutrition and oxygenation [44].

GHK also suppresses the production of the inflammatory cytokine interleukin-6 (IL-6), which is a main positive regulator of fibrinogen synthesis through its interaction with fibrinogen genes [45].

In summary, the effects of GHK on the FGB gene plus its effects on IL-6 production should suppress overall fibrinogen production.

GHK and Antioxidant Gene Expression

A search of antioxidant associated genes effected by GHK yielded 17 genes with significant antioxidant activity [46]. Interleukin-17A and TNF are inflammatory factors that are strongly suppressed and in this sense GHK has an antioxidant effect. See Table 4.

Table 2 GHK's effect on systems associated with human aging

System	Effect of system	Effect of GHK	GHK in vivo mammalian data	GHK cell culture data	GHK gene expression data
Fibrinogen	Increases mortality	Suppresses fibrinogen synthesis	Yes	Yes	Yes Strongly suppresses fibrinogen beta chain
Antioxidants	Prevents damage to DNA and cells	Primarily antioxidant	Yes	Yes	Yes 15 genes up 2 genes down
DNA repair	Repairs damaged DNA	Strongly increases	No	Yes	Yes 47 genes up 5 genes down
Cancer	Increases aberrant cell growth	Suppresses mouse sarcoma	Yes, in mice	Yes	Yes 9 caspase system genes up 80 growth-controlling genes altered for antigrowth effect
Insulin and insulin-like system	High levels reduce lifespan	Decreases insulin and insulin-like gene expression	Suppression of system increases lifespan of nematodes up to tenfold	Yes	2 genes up 6 genes down
COPD	Causes rigidity in lungs	Resets genes to healthy state	No	Yes	Suppresses tissue destructive genes, increases repair genes
Ubiquitin/ proteosome system	Removes damaged proteins from cells High in human centenarians	Strongly increases	No	No	Yes 41 genes up 1 gene down

Table 3 GHK and fibrinogen

Gene title	Percent change in gene expression
Fibrinogen chain alpha, FGA	121
Fibrinogen chain beta, FGB	−475

DNA Repair Genes

GHK was primarily stimulatory for DNA Repair genes (47 UP, 5 DOWN) suggesting an increased DNA repair activity. This can explain its ability to restore cells damaged by radiation as discussed above. Many beneficial effects observed in cosmetic studies, where GHK was found to greatly improve aging skin's condition, can be also explained through its ability to help cells repair their own DNA. See Tables 5 and 6.

GHK May Help Prevent Cancer Growth

As it was mentioned above, the first study that established GHK's ability to modulate a number of human genes demonstrated its ability to suppress genes related to an aggressive growth of colon cancer. Further evidence of GHK's potential

Table 4 Gene expression related to antioxidant activity

Genes	Percent change in gene expression	Comments
TLE1	762	Inhibits the oxidative/inflammatory gene NF-κB
SPRR2C	721	This proline-rich, antioxidant protein protects outer skin cells from oxidative damage from ROS. When the ROS level is low, the protein remains in the outer cell membrane, but when the ROS level is high, the protein clusters around the cell's DNA to protect it
ITGB4	609	Up-regulation of ITGB4 promotes wound repair ability and antioxidative ability
APOM	403	Binds oxidized phospholipids and increases the antioxidant effect of high-density lipoproteins (HDL)
PON3	319	Absence of PON3 (paraoxonase 3) in mice resulted in increased rates of early fetal and neonatal death. Knockdown of PON3 in human cells reduced cell proliferation and total antioxidant capacity
IL18BP	295	The protein encoded by this gene is an inhibitor of the pro-inflammatory cytokine IL18. IL18BP abolished IL18 induction of interferon-gamma (IFNgamma), IL8, and activation of NF-κB in vitro. Blocks neutrophil oxidase activity
HEPH	217	Inhibits the conversion of Fe(2+) to Fe(3+). HEPH increases iron efflux, lowers cellular iron levels, suppresses reactive oxygen species production, and restores mitochondrial transmembrane potential
GPSM3	193	Acts as a direct negative regulator of NLRP3. NLRP3 triggers the maturation of the pro-inflammatory cytokines IL-1β and IL-18
FABP1	186	Reduces intracellular ROS level. Plays a significant role in reduction of oxidative stress
PON1	149	PON1 (paraoxonase 1) is a potent antioxidant and a major anti-atherosclerotic component of HDL
MT3	142	Metallothioneins (MTs) display in vitro free radical scavenging capacity, suggesting that they may specifically neutralize hydroxyl radicals. Metallothioneins and metallothionein-like proteins isolated from mouse brain act as neuroprotective agents by scavenging superoxide radicals
PTGS2	120	Produces cyclooxygenase-II (COX-II), which has antioxidant activities
SLC2A9	117	The p53-SLC2A9 pathway is a novel antioxidant mechanism. During oxidative stress, SLC2A9 undergoes p53-dependent induction and functions as an antioxidant by suppressing ROS, DNA damage, and cell death
NFE2L2	56	Helps activate antioxidant responsive element-regulated genes which contribute to the regulation of the cellular antioxidant defense systems
PTGS1	50	Produces cyclooxygenase-I (COX-I), which has antioxidant activity
TNF	−115	GHK suppresses this pro-oxidant TNF gene
IL17A	−1,018	This cytokine can stimulate the expression of IL6 and cyclooxygenase-2 (PTGS2/COX-2), as well as enhance the production of nitric oxide (NO). High levels of this cytokine are associated with several chronic inflammatory diseases including rheumatoid arthritis, psoriasis, and multiple sclerosis (http://www.ncbi.nlm.nih.gov/gene/3605)

ability to suppress cancer can be found in its ability to reactivate the natural apoptosis system. Normal healthy cells have checkpoint systems to self-destruct if they are synthesizing DNA incorrectly through programmed cell death or the apoptosis system.

Matalka et al. demonstrated that GHK, at 1–10 nM, reactivated the apoptosis system, as measured by the caspases 3 and 7, and inhibited the growth of human SH-SY5Y neuroblastoma cells and human U937 histiocytic lymphoma cells. In contrast, the GHK accelerated the growth of healthy human NIH-3T3 fibroblasts [47].

Following this Pickart et al. determined the effect of GHK on genes important to cancer growth using the Broad Institute data [48].

Table 5 GHK and DNA repair gene expression

Percent change in gene expression (%)	Genes up	Genes down
50–100	41	4
100–150	2	1
150–200	1	0
200–250	2	0
250–300	1	0

Table 6 Most affected DNA repair genes

	Gene title	Percent change in gene expression
Up		
1	Poly (ADP-ribose) polymerase family, member 3, PARP3	253
2	Polymerase (DNA directed), mu, POLM	225
3	MRE11 meiotic recombination 11 homolog A MRE11A	212
4	RAD50 homolog (*S. cerevisiae*), RAD50	175
5	Eyes absent homolog 3 (*Drosophila*), EYA3	128
6	Retinoic acid receptor, alpha, RARA	123
Down		
1	Cholinergic receptor, nicotinic, alpha 4, CHRNA4	−105

The results suggest that GHK acts in a manner which may help to slow cancer growth. It was found that GHK enhanced the expression of ten caspases and caspase-associated genes and also affected 84 other genes (general and DNA repair) that may help control abnormal cancerous growths. While it is known that cancer growth controls are often uncertain, these results suggest that a variety of genes may serve to inhibit cancerous cell replication, at least early in life. During wound healing, GHK has tissue remodeling actions, the phase of healing in which cell migration into the wound area is stopped and cellular debris removed. The antitumor actions of the molecule may be related to these types of GHK effects. See Tables 7, 8, and 9. GHK's combination of tissue regenerative and anticancer actions are similar to retinoic acid, which is widely used both for skin care and as a cancer treatment [49].

Table 7 GHK and gene expression of apoptosis protein genes

Genes	Percent change in gene expression	Comment
CASP 1	432	Caspase proteins activate programmed cell death
CASP 3	65	
CASP 6	23	
CASP 7	48	
CASP 8	399	
CASP 10	195	
NLRP1	249	Apoptosis caspase recruitment domain
CARD10	173	Apoptosis signaling gene
BCL2L14	153	Apoptosis facilitator

GHK Suppresses the Insulin and Insulin-Like Systems

Suppression of insulin and insulin-like genes is a major theory on animal lifespan. Suppression of the insulin family by modification of the genes on the *C. elegans* roundworm has extended the lifespan of the worms from three- to tenfold. Insulin/IGF-1-like signaling is conserved from worms to humans. In vitro experiments show that mutations that reduce insulin/IGF-1 signaling have been shown to decelerate the degenerative aging process and extend lifespan in many organisms, including fruit flies, mice, and possibly humans. Reduced IGF-1 signaling is also thought to contribute to the "antiaging" effects of calorie restriction [50].

GHK stimulates two genes in this system and suppresses six genes. The insulin/IGF-1-like receptor pathway is a contributor to the biological aging process in many organisms. The gene

Table 8 GHK and gene expression in cancer suppressors

Genes	Percent change in gene expression	Comment
USP29	1,056	Ubiquitin specific peptidase 29 May stabilize P53 tumor suppressor
IFNA21	955	Combined treatment of IFN-alpha and IL-21 increases anticancer effects
TP73	938	Tumor suppressor
TP63	Uncertain	Tumor suppressor Gene probes are inconsistent; however, TP63 was induced by GHK in keratinocyte cells in skin equivalent organ culture
LEFTY2	935	Inhibition of pancreatic cancer cells
IL25	891	Inhibits breast cancer cell growth
IL15	875	Induces natural killer cells Antitumor and antiviral
D4S234E	731	p53-responsive gene, induces apoptosis in response to DNA damage
MTUS2	474	Microtubule-associated tumor suppressor
C13orf18	352	Inhibits cervical cancer cells
ING2	337	Functions in DNA repair and apoptosis
CTNNA1	336	Suppresses cancer invasion of tissues
CDKN1C	277	Breast cancer inhibitor
PAWR	199	Induces apoptosis in cancer cells
APC	195	Suppresses colon cancer
PTEN	165	Cancer suppressor
NRG1	164	Cancer suppressor
NF1	143	Neurofibromin 1
ATM	107	Senses DNA damage
ING4	107	Cancer suppressor
DCN	44	Suppresses cancer growth and metastasis In rat wound chamber experiments GHK increased mRNA for decorin 302 %
BRCA1	44	Cancer suppressor

Table 9 GHK and gene expression in cancer enhancers

Genes	Percent change in gene expression	Comment
ABCB1	−1,537	Increases drug resistance in cancer cells
STAT5	−982	Signals cancer cells to grow
FGFR2	−904	FGFR2 inhibitors reduce some cancers
FAIM2	−749	Prevents apoptosis
IGF1	−522	Risk factor for cancer
TNF	−115	May promote cell cancer invasion

expression data suggests that GHK suppresses this system as six of eight affected insulin/IGF-1 genes are suppressed. See Table 10.

GHK Strongly Increases Expression of Genes Within the Ubiquitin/Proteasome System

The ubiquitin proteasome system (UPS) functions in the removal of damaged or misfolded proteins. Aging is a natural process that is characterized by a progressive accumulation of unfolded, misfolded, or aggregated proteins. In particular, the proteasome is responsible for the removal of normal as well as damaged or misfolded proteins. Maintenance of the ubiquitin/proteasome system activity correlates with visible skin benefits. Recent work has demonstrated that proteasome activation by either genetic means or use of compounds retards aging [51].

Table 10 GHK and insulin/insulin-like genes

	Gene title	Percent change in gene expression
Up		
1	Insulin-like 6, INSL6	188
2	Insulin-like growth factor binding protein 3, IGFBP3	62
Down		
1	Insulin receptor-related receptor, INSRR	−437
2	Insulin, INS	−289
3	Insulin-like 3 (Leydig cell), INSL3	−188
4	Insulin-like growth factor 1 (somatomedin C), IGF1	−147
5	Insulin-like growth factor binding protein 7, IGFBP7	−110
6	Insulin-like 5, INSL5	−101

According to the Broad Institute's data GHK increases gene expression in 41 UPS genes while suppressing one UPS gene [41]. Thus, GHK should have a positive effect on this system. See Table 11.

GHK as a Cosmetic Ingredient

Today, peptide-based cosmetic products continue gaining popularity. However, not all peptides that are used in today's cosmetic products have enough scientific data confirming their efficacy. Also, the main problem with peptide-based cosmetics is that most peptides cannot pass through the stratum corneum and therefore cannot reach the viable layers of the epidermis. Since peptides are used for their cell regulatory activity, inability to permeate the stratum corneum is a serious handicap.

Mazurowska et al. demonstrated that GHK-Cu is able to pass through the lipid barrier of the stratum corneum and reach epidermal cells [52]. Moreover, the GHK-Cu complex appears to be the only peptide-copper complex that can penetrate the stratum corneum membranes [53]. By transdermal delivery GHK was delivered in potentially anti-inflammatory amounts [54, 55].

At present, GHK-Cu undoubtedly has more scientific data than any peptide used in today's cosmetic practice [56]. Its efficacy was confirmed in several placebo-controlled independent trials.

A study of 20 women compared the skin's production of collagen after applying creams containing GHK-Cu, vitamin C, or retinoic acid to thighs daily for 1 month. New collagen production was determined by skin biopsy samples using immunohistological techniques. After 1 month, GHK-Cu increased collagen in 70 % of those treated versus 50 % treated with vitamin C and 40 % treated with retinoic acid [57].

Another study found that GHK-Cu facial cream reduced visible signs of aging after 12 weeks of application to the facial skin of 71 women with mild to advanced signs of photoaging. The cream improved skin laxity, clarity, and appearance, reduced fine lines and the depth of wrinkles, and increased skin density and thickness comparing with the placebo [58].

A GHK-Cu eye cream, tested on 41 women for 12 weeks with mild to advanced photodamage, was compared to a placebo control and an eye cream containing vitamin K. The GHK-Cu cream performed better than both controls in terms of reducing lines and wrinkles, improving overall appearance, and increasing skin density and thickness [59].

In another 12-week facial study of 67 women between 50 and 59 years of age with mild to advanced photodamage, a GHK-Cu cream was applied twice daily and improved skin laxity, clarity, firmness and appearance, reduced fine lines, coarse wrinkles and mottled hyperpigmentation, and increased skin density and thickness. The result was assessed visually by a trained technician (wrinkles, pigmentation, laxity, roughness, and overall appearance) as well as a ballistometer (firmness of the skin) and ultrasound (skin density). The GHK cream also strongly stimulated dermal keratinocyte proliferation as determined by histological analysis of biopsies. At the same time, GHK-containing cream has proved to be very safe. The GHK-Cu complex was proven to be nonallergenic even at its 20x recommended use level. It also did not produce eye irritation [60].

Table 11 Ubiquitin/proteasome system and GHK

	Gene title	Percent change
Up		
1	Ubiquitin specific peptidase 29, USP29	1,056
2	Ubiquitin protein ligase E3 component *n*-recognin 2, UBR2	455
3	Gamma-aminobutyric acid (GABA) B receptor, 1 /// ubiquitin D, GABBR1 /// UBD	310
4	Ubiquitin specific peptidase 34, USP34	195
5	Parkinson protein 2, E3 ubiquitin protein ligase (parkin), PARK2	169
6	Ubiquitin-conjugating enzyme E2I (UBC9 homolog, yeast), UBE2I	150
7	Ubiquitin protein ligase E3 component *n*-recognin 4, UBR4	146
8	Ubiquitin protein ligase E3B, UBE3B	116
9	Ubiquitin specific peptidase 2, USP2	104
10	Ubiquitin-like modifier activating enzyme 6, UBA6	104
11	Ubiquitination factor E4B (UFD2 homolog, yeast), UBE4B	99
12	Ubiquitin-conjugating enzyme E2M (UBC12 homolog, yeast), UBE2M	92
13	Ubiquitin-like modifier activating enzyme 7, UBA7	88
14	HECT, C2, and WW domain containing E3 ubiquitin protein ligase 1, HECW1	81
15	Proteasome (prosome, macropain) 26S subunit, ATPase, 3, PSMC3	81
16	Ubiquitin-conjugating enzyme E2D 1 (UBC4/5 homolog, yeast), UBE2D1	79
17	Proteasome (prosome, macropain) subunit, beta type, 2, PSMB2	79
18	Ubiquitin protein ligase E3 component *n*-recognin 5, UBR5	77
19	Ubiquitin specific peptidase 21, USP21	76
20	OTU domain, ubiquitin aldehyde binding 2, OTUB2	76
21	Proteasome (prosome, macropain) inhibitor subunit 1 (PI31), PSMF1	75
22	Ubiquitin-conjugating enzyme E2H (UBC8 homolog, yeast), UBE2H	73
23	Ubiquitin-conjugating enzyme E2N (UBC13 homolog, yeast), UBE2N	72
24	Ubiquitin carboxy-terminal hydrolase L5, UCHL5	71
25	Proteasome (prosome, macropain) 26S subunit, non-ATPase, 13, PSMD13	70
26	Ubiquitin-associated protein 1, UBAP1	70
27	Ubiquitin-conjugating enzyme E2B (RAD6 homolog), UBE2B	69
28	TMEM189-UBE2V1 readthrough /// ubiquitin-conjugating enzyme E2 variant 1, TMEM189-UBE2V1 /// UBE2V1	67
29	Proteasome (prosome, macropain) 26S subunit, non-ATPase, 1, PSMD1	64
30	Proteasome (prosome, macropain) 26S subunit, non-ATPase, 3, PSMD3	64
31	Ariadne homolog, ubiquitin-conjugating enzyme E2 binding protein, 1 (Drosophila), ARIH1	61
32	BRCA1-associated protein-1 (ubiquitin carboxy-terminal hydrolase), BAP1	60
33	Ubiquitin interaction motif containing 1, UIMC1	60
34	Ubiquitin-associated protein 2-like, UBAP2L	57
35	Ubiquitin protein ligase E3 component *n*-recognin 7 (putative), UBR7	56
36	Ubiquitin-conjugating enzyme E2G 1 (UBC7 homolog, yeast), UBE2G1	54
37	Itchy E3 ubiquitin protein ligase homolog (mouse), ITCH	54
38	Ubiquitin-conjugating enzyme E2D 4 (putative), UBE2D4	51
39	Proteasome (prosome, macropain) 26S subunit, non-ATPase, 10, PSMD10	50
40	WW domain containing E3 ubiquitin protein ligase 1, WWP1	50
41	Ubiquitin-like 3, UBL3	50
Down		
1	Ubiquitin associated and SH3 domain containing A, UBASH3A	−89

These results are not at all surprising considering GHK-Cu's remarkable ability to reset the human genome back to health.

Conclusion

To date, the exact mechanism of action of the GHK-Cu peptide remains to be established. However, modern genetic profiling technology allows us to take a glimpse into an exciting new field of the future GHK-Cu research. As more and more researchers become interested in the pleiotropic effects of the GHK-Cu peptide and its ability to modify gene expression, we should expect more understanding of how this simple molecule acts in the human body. Based on animal and cell research as well as human cosmetic studies, we can already conclude that so far all effects of GHK-Cu are beneficial, and this molecule is able to help skin balance and restore its natural functions, such as wound repair, antioxidant defense, and collagen synthesis among others.

GHK is readily available at low cost and can be easily incorporated into a wide range of skin products, such as sunscreens and protective cosmetic creams as well as medicated ointments. It penetrates the stratum corneum and can be incorporated in liposomes or skin patches [54, 55, 61]. The molecule appears to have low toxicity, and no issues have ever arisen during its use as a skin cosmetic or in human wound healing studies.

GHK-Cu can be incorporated into sunscreens and daytime creams and serums due to its ability to enhance antioxidant defense and prevent skin damage from UV-radiation. It is also very useful for nighttime regenerative creams and serums due to its ability to stimulate skin regeneration and renewal. Another possible area for GHK-Cu application is before and after plastic surgery or aggressive cosmetic procedures, such as chemical peels and dermabrasion, to help skin reduce inflammation and speed up the recovery process. Hair growth products especially those used before and after hair transplantation is another area where the GHK-Cu peptide is extremely useful.

Someday, we can also see dietary supplements containing the liposomal form of the GHK-Cu peptide, which can enhance and support the actions of skin care products [62].

References

1. Zelles T, Purushotham KR, Macauley SP, Oxford GE, Humphreys-Beher MG. Saliva and growth factors: the fountain of youth resides in us all. J Dent Res. 1995;74:1826–32.
2. Pilgeram LO, Pickart L, Bandi Z, Bell O. FFA/Albumin – a function of thrombogenesis and aging. Fed Proc. 1966;25:619.
3. Pilgeram LO, Pickart LR. Control of fibrinogen biosynthesis: the role of free fatty acid. J Atheroscler Res. 1968;8:155–66.
4. Pickart L. Fat metabolism, the fibrinogen/fibrinolytic system and blood flow: new potentials for the pharmacological treatment of coronary heart disease. Pharmacology. 1981;23:271–80.
5. Pickart L. A tripeptide from human serum which enhances the growth of neoplastic hepatocytes and the survival of normal hepatocytes. San Francisco: University of California; 1973.
6. Pickart L, Margolina A. Anti-aging activity of the GHK peptide – the skin and beyond. J Aging Res Clin Pract. 2012;1:13–6.
7. Pickart L. The human tri-peptide GHK and tissue remodeling. J Biomater Sci Polym Ed. 2008;19:969–88. doi:10.1163/156856208784909435.
8. Lamb J. The Connectivity Map: a new tool for biomedical research. Nat Rev Cancer. 2007;7:54–60. doi:10.1038/nrc2044.
9. Iorio F, Bosotti R, Scacheri E, Belcastro V, Mithbaokar P, Ferriero R, Murino L, Tagliaferri R, Brunetti-Pierri N, Isacchi A, di Bernardo D. Discovery of drug mode of action and drug repositioning from transcriptional responses. Proc Natl Acad Sci U S A. 2010;107:14621–6. doi:10.1073/pnas.1000138107.
10. Farage MA, Miller KW, Elsner P, Maibach HI. Intrinsic and extrinsic factors in skin ageing: a review. Int J Cosmet Sci. 2008;30:87–95. doi:10.1111/j.1468-2494.2007.00415.x.
11. Maquart F, Pickart L, Laurent M, Gillery P, Monboisse J, Borel J. Stimulation of collagen synthesis in fibroblast cultures by the tripeptide-copper complex glycyl-L-histidyl-L-lysine-Cu2+. FEBS Lett. 1988;238:343–6.
12. Simeon A, Monier F, Emonard H, Gillery P, Birembaut P, Hornebeck W, Maquart F. Expression and activation of matrix metalloproteinases in wounds:

modulation by the tripeptide-copper complex glycyl-L-histidyl-L-lysine-Cu2+. J Invest Dermatol. 1999;112:957–64. doi:10.1046/j.1523-1747.1999.00606.x.

13. Simeon A, Emonard H, Hornebeck W, Maquart F. The tripeptide-copper complex glycyl-L-histidyl-L-lysine-Cu2+ stimulates matrix metalloproteinase-2 expression by fibroblast cultures. Life Sci. 2000;67:2257–65.
14. Simeon A, Wegrowski Y, Bontemps Y, Maquart F. Expression of glycosaminoglycans and small proteoglycans in wounds: modulation by the tripeptide-copper complex glycyl-L-histidyl-L-lysine-Cu(2+). J Invest Dermatol. 2000;115:962–8. doi:10.1046/j.1523-1747.2000.00166.x.
15. Wegrowski Y, Maquart F, Borel J. Stimulation of sulfated glycosaminoglycan synthesis by the tripeptide-copper complex glycyl-L-histidyl-L-lysine-Cu2+. Life Sci. 1992;51:1049–56.
16. Buffoni F, Pino R, Dal Pozzo A. Effect of tripeptide-copper complexes on the process of skin wound healing and on cultured fibroblasts. Arch Int Pharmacodyn Ther. 1995;330:345–60.
17. Cangul IT, Gul NY, Topal A, Yilmaz R. Evaluation of the effects of topical tripeptide-copper complex and zinc oxide on open-wound healing in rabbits. Vet Dermatol. 2006;17:417–23. doi:10.1111/j.1365-3164.2006.00551.x.
18. Gul NY, Topal A, Cangul IT, Yanik K. The effects of topical tripeptide copper complex and helium-neon laser on wound healing in rabbits. Vet Dermatol. 2008;19:7–14. doi:10.1111/j.1365-3164.2007.00647.x.
19. Arul V, Gopinath D, Gomathi K, Jayakumar R. Biotinylated GHK peptide incorporated collagenous matrix: a novel biomaterial for dermal wound healing in rats. J Biomed Mater Res B Appl Biomater. 2005;73:383–91. doi:10.1002/jbm.b.30246.
20. Arul V, Kartha R, Jayakumar R. A therapeutic approach for diabetic wound healing using biotinylated GHK incorporated collagen matrices. Life Sci. 2007;80:275–84. doi:10.1016/j.lfs.2006.09.018.
21. Canapp SJ, Farese J, Schultz G, Gowda S, Ishak A, Swaim S, Vangilder J, Lee-Ambrose L, Martin F. The effect of topical tripeptide-copper complex on healing of ischemic open wounds. Vet Surg. 2003;32:515–23. doi:10.1053/jvet.2003.50070.
22. Huang P, Huang Y, Su M, Yang T, Huang J, Jiang C. In vitro observations on the influence of copper peptide aids for the LED photoirradiation of fibroblast collagen synthesis. Photomed Laser Surg. 2007;25:183–90. doi:10.1089/pho.2007.2062.
23. Pollard J, Quan S, Kang T, Koch R. Effects of copper tripeptide on the growth and expression of growth factors by normal and irradiated fibroblasts. Arch Facial Plast Surg. 2005;7:27–31. doi:10.1001/archfaci.7.1.27.
24. Ohyama M. Hair follicle bulge: a fascinating reservoir of epithelial stem cells. J Dermatol Sci. 2007;46:81–9. doi:10.1016/j.jdermsci.2006.12.002.
25. Trachy R, Fors T, Pickart L, Uno H. The hair follicle-stimulating properties of peptide copper complexes. Results in C3H mice. Ann N Y Acad Sci. 1991;642:468–9.
26. Godet D, Marie P. Effects of the tripeptide glycyl-L-histidyl-L-lysine copper complex on osteoblastic cell spreading, attachment and phenotype. Cell Mol Biol (Noisy-le-Grand). 1995;41:1081–91.
27. Peled T, Fibach E, Treves A (2005) Methods of controlling proliferation and differentiation of stem and progenitor cells. This is U.S. Patent 6,962,698.
28. Kang Y, Choi H, Na J, Huh C, Kim M, Youn S, Kim K, Park K. Copper-GHK increases integrin expression and p63 positivity by keratinocytes. Arch Dermatol Res. 2009;301:301–6. doi:10.1007/s00403-009-0942-x.
29. Jose S, Hughbanks ML, Binder BY, Ingavle GC, Leach JK. Enhanced trophic factor secretion by mesenchymal stem/stromal cells with Glycine-Histidine-Lysine (GHK)-modified alginate hydrogels. Acta Biomater. 2014;10:1955–64. doi:10.1016/j.actbio.2014.01.020.
30. Uno H, Kurata S. Chemical agents and peptides affect hair growth. J Invest Dermatol. 1993;101:143S–7.
31. Perez-Meza D, Leavitt M, Trachy R. Clinical evaluation of GraftCyte moist dressings on hair graft viability and quality of healing. Int J Cosmetic Surg. 1998;6:80–4.
32. Thomas CE. The influence of medium components on Cu(2+)-dependent oxidation of low-density lipoproteins and its sensitivity to superoxide dismutase. Biochim Biophys Acta. 1992;1128:50–7.
33. Beretta G, Arlandini E, Artali R, Anton JM, Maffei Facino R. Acrolein sequestering ability of the endogenous tripeptide glycyl-histidyl-lysine (GHK): characterization of conjugation products by ESI-MSn and theoretical calculations. J Pharm Biomed Anal. 2008;47:596–602. doi:10.1016/j.jpba.2008.02.012.
34. Beretta G, Artali R, Regazzoni L, Panigati M, Facino RM. Glycyl-histidyl-lysine (GHK) is a quencher of alpha, beta-4-hydroxy-*trans*-2-nonenal: a comparison with carnosine. insights into the mechanism of reaction by electrospray ionization mass spectrometry, 1H NMR, and computational techniques. Chem Res Toxicol. 2007;20:1309–14. doi:10.1021/tx700185s.
35. Cebrian J, Messeguer A, Facino R, Garcia Anton J. New anti-RNS and -RCS products for cosmetic treatment. Int J Cosmet Sci. 2005;27:271–8. doi:10.1111/j.1467-2494.2005.00279.x.
36. Smakhtin Mi, Konoplia A, Sever'ianova L, Shveinov I. Pharmacological correction of immuno-metabolic disorders with the peptide Gly-His-Lys in hepatic damage induced by tetrachloromethane. Patol Fiziol Eksp Ter Russ. 2003:19–21. http://www.ncbi.nlm.nih.gov/pubmed/12838768.
37. Cherdakov VY, Smakhtin MY, Dubrovin GM, Dudka VT, Bobyntsev II. Synergetic antioxidant and reparative action of thymogen, dalargin and peptide Gly-His-Lys in tubular bone fractures. Exp Biol Med. 2010;4:15–20.

38. Miller DM, DeSilva D, Pickart L, Aust SD. Effects of glycyl-histidyl-lysyl chelated Cu(II) on ferritin dependent lipid peroxidation. Adv Exp Med Biol. 1990;264:79–84.
39. Hong Y, Downey T, Eu K, Koh P, Cheah P. A "metastasis-prone" signature for early-stage mismatch-repair proficient sporadic colorectal cancer patients and its implications for possible therapeutics. Clin Exp Metastasis. 2010;27:83–90.
40. Campbell JD, McDonough JE, Zeskind JE, Hackett TL, Pechkovsky DV, Brandsma CA, Suzuki M, Gosselink JV, Liu G, Alekseyev YO, Xiao J, Zhang X, Hayashi S, Cooper JD, Timens W, Postma DS, Knight DA, Marc LE, James HC, Avrum S. A gene expression signature of emphysema-related lung destruction and its reversal by the tripeptide GHK. Genome Med. 2012;4:67. doi:10.1186/gm368.
41. Pickart L, Vasquez-Soltero JM, Margolina A. GHK and DNA: resetting the human genome to health. BioMed Res Int. 2014;2014:151479. doi:10.1155/2014/151479.
42. Szarc vel Szic K, Declerck K, Vidakovic M, Vanden Berghe W. From inflammaging to healthy aging by dietary lifestyle choices: is epigenetics the key to personalized nutrition? Clin Epigenetics. 2015;7:33. doi:10.1186/s13148-015-0068-2.
43. Kaliman P, Alvarez-Lopez MJ, Cosin-Tomas M, Rosenkranz MA, Lutz A, Davidson RJ. Rapid changes in histone deacetylases and inflammatory gene expression in expert meditators. Psychoneuroendocrinology. 2014;40:96–107. doi:10.1016/j.psyneuen.2013.11.004.
44. Pickart LR, Thaler MM. Fatty acids, fibrinogen and blood flow: a general mechanism for hyperfibrinogenemia and its pathologic consequences. Med Hypotheses. 1980;6:545–57.
45. Carty CL, Heagerty P, Heckbert SR, Jarvik GP, Lange LA, Cushman M, Tracy RP, Reiner AP. Interaction between fibrinogen and IL-6 genetic variants and associations with cardiovascular disease risk in the Cardiovascular Health Study. Ann Hum Genet. 2010;74:1–10. doi:10.1111/j.1469-1809.2009.00551.x.
46. Pickart L, Vasquez-Soltero JM, Margolina A. GHK-Cu may prevent oxidative stress in skin by regulating copper and modifying expression of numerous antioxidant genes. Cosmetics. 2015;2:236–47.
47. Matalka LE, Ford A, Unlap MT. The tripeptide, GHK, induces programmed cell death in SH-SY5Y neuroblastoma cells. J Biotechnol Biomater. 2012;2:1–4. doi:10.4172/2155-952X.1000144.
48. Pickart L, Vasquez-Soltero JM, Pickart FD, Majnarich J. GHK, the human skin remodeling peptide, induces anti-cancer expression of numerous caspase, growth regulatory, and DNA repair genes. J Anal Oncol. 2014;3:79–87.
49. Tang XH, Gudas LJ. Retinoids, retinoic acid receptors, and cancer. Annu Rev Pathol. 2011;6:345–64. doi:10.1146/annurev-pathol-011110-130303.
50. Xie L, Wang W. Weight control and cancer preventive mechanisms: role of insulin growth factor-1-mediated signaling pathways. Exp Biol Med (Maywood). 2013;238:127–32. doi:10.1177/1535370213477602.
51. Imbert I, Gondran C, Oberto G, Cucumel K, Dal Farra C, Domloge N. Maintenance of the ubiquitin-proteasome system activity correlates with visible skin benefits. Int J Cosmet Sci. 2010;32:446–57. doi:10.1111/j.1468-2494.2010.00575.x.
52. Mazurowska L, Mojski M. Biological activities of selected peptides: skin penetration ability of copper complexes with peptides. J Cosmet Sci. 2008;59:59–69.
53. Mazurowska L, Mojski M. ESI-MS study of the mechanism of glycyl-L-histidyl-L-lysine-Cu(II) complex transport through model membrane of stratum corneum. Talanta. 2007;72:650–4. doi:10.1016/j.talanta.2006.11.034.
54. Hostynek J, Dreher F, Maibach H. Human skin penetration of a copper tripeptide in vitro as a function of skin layer. Inflamm Res. 2011;60:79–86.
55. Hostynek J, Dreher F, Maibach H. Human skin retention and penetration of a copper tripeptide in vitro as function of skin layer towards anti-inflammatory therapy. Inflamm Res. 2010;59:983–8.
56. Gorouhi F, Maibach HI. Role of topical peptides in preventing or treating aged skin. Int J Cosmet Sci. 2009;31:327–45. doi:10.1111/j.1468-2494.2009.00490.x.
57. Abdulghani A, Sherr A, Shirin S, Solodkina G, Tapia E, Wolf B, Gottlieb A. Effects of topical creams containing vitamin C, a copper-binding peptide cream and melatonin compared with tretinoin on the ultrastructure of normal skin – a pilot clinical, histologic, and ultrastructural study. Disease Manag Clin Outcomes. 1998;1:136–41.
58. Leyden J, Stephens T, Finkey M, Appa Y, Barkovic S. Skin care benefits of copper peptide containing facial cream. New Orleans, LA: American Academy of Dermatology; 2002.
59. Leyden J, Stephens T, Finkey M, Barkovic S. Skin care benefits of copper peptide containing eye creams. New Orleans, LA: American Academy of Dermatology; 2002.
60. Finkley M, Appa Y, Bhandarkar S. Copper peptide and skin. In: Elsner P, Maibach H, editors. Cosmeceuticals and active cosmetics. Drugs versus cosmetics. 2nd ed. - New York: Marcel Dekker; 2005. p. 549–63.
61. Swaminathan J, Ehrhardt C. Liposomal delivery of proteins and peptides. Expert Opin Drug Deliv. 2012;9:1489–503. doi:10.1517/17425247.2012.735658.
62. Li P, Nielsen HM, Mullertz A. Oral delivery of peptides and proteins using lipid-based drug delivery systems. Expert Opin Drug Deliv. 2012;9:1289–304. doi:10.1517/17425247.2012.717068.

Part VIII

Skin Scales and Typing System

Assessing Quality of Ordinal Scales Depicting Skin Aging Severity

116

Fabien Valet, Khaled Ezzedine, Denis Malvy, Jean-Yves Mary, and Christiane Guinot

Contents

F. Valet (✉)
Biostatistics Department, Institut Curie, Paris, France
e-mail: fabien.valet@paris7.jussieu.fr

K. Ezzedine
Department of Dermatology, CHU Saint-André, Bordeaux, France
e-mail: khaled.ezzedine@chu-bordeaux.fr

D. Malvy
EA 3677 and Centre René-Labusquière, Université Victor Segalen, Bordeaux, France

Department of Internal Medicine and Tropical Diseases, University Hospital Center, Bordeaux, France
e-mail: denis.malvy@chu-bordeaux.fr

J.-Y. Mary
INSERM U717, Biostatistics and Clinical Epidemiology, DBIM, Saint-Louis Hospital, University Paris 7, Paris, France
e-mail: jean-yves.mary@paris7.jussieu.fr

C. Guinot
Biometrics and Epidemiology Unit, CE.R.I.E.S., Neuilly-sur-Seine, France
e-mail: christiane.Guinot@ceries-lab.com

M.A. Farage et al. (eds.), *Textbook of Aging Skin*,
DOI 10.1007/978-3-662-47398-6_87

Abstract

Severity rating scales have been extensively used in dermatology and in plastic surgery to describe and quantify the severity of skin disorders. With the development of esthetic procedures, assessment of severity before and after treatment of skin aging features as well as the identification of significant determinants of skin aging (UV exposure, smoking, genetic polymorphisms) are increasingly reported. Among these scales, ordinal severity scales illustrated by photographs have been widely developed to help plastic surgeons and dermatologists in more objective assessments.

Introduction

In dermatology and in plastic surgery, severity rating scales have been extensively used to describe and quantify the severity of skin disorders [1–4], to assess treatment outcomes, efficacy of cosmetic surgical procedures, and even patients' concern and satisfaction [5–7]. With the development of esthetic procedures, assessment of severity before and after treatment of skin aging features [8] as well as the identification of significant determinants of skin aging [9, 10] (UV exposure, smoking, genetic polymorphisms) are increasingly reported. Among these scales, ordinal severity scales illustrated by photographs have been widely developed to help plastic surgeons and dermatologists in more objective assessments [1, 9].

For the use of ordinal rating scales, in addition to validity and sensitivity to changes, reproducibility is also required [11]. Reproducibility can be defined as the ability to obtain similar results when several measurements of the same objects are performed. In particular for patients, the reproducibility of ratings is a major issue, because their classification into one of the different categories of an ordinal scale may have important consequences on their therapeutic follow-up and possibly on their quality of life. Therefore, it is of prime importance to analyze the variability of ratings resulting from the use of such scales and to investigate the reproducibility of these ratings as a major component of the quality of this scale. With this aim, the same signs are usually rated independently by the same observer at two distant times (intraobserver ratings) and also by several observers (interobserver ratings). The reproducibility evaluation of the intra- and interobserver variations is usually performed through the weighted Kappa statistic [12]. This method provides a global evaluation of the degree of agreement between two observers but gives no information on the quality of the scale and the possible defects within its structure. In 2007, Valet et al. proposed a method to estimate distinguishabilities between all adjacent categories of the scale [13]. This method is able to highlight difficulties in distinguishing some of the categories of the scale among observers, that is, any specific reproducibility defect in the scale.

Skin aging results from a number of processes including intrinsic factors, such as chronological age, and extrinsic or environmental factors, such as chronic ultraviolet (UV) exposure and smoking habits. Aging is accelerated in the areas exposed to UV radiation, a process known as photoaging. Sun-induced cutaneous changes (photoaging) are superimposed on intrinsic aging and are characterized clinically by wrinkles, roughness, laxity, irregular pigmentation (lentigines), elastosis, and telangiectasia [14]. To assess the effects of chronic sun exposure on the skin, different photographic scales have been proposed [15–18]. Standardized grading systems for photodamage are mandatory, in particular because they can improve the quality of related clinical studies and can be used in large epidemiologic surveys [19].

In this chapter, two methods proposed for the assessment of the quality of an ordinal rating scale are described: the weighted Kappa statistic and Valet's method. The properties of both methods are illustrated using intradermatologist and interdermatologists ratings resulting from the use of Larnier's photoaging scale [15]. Through this example, the benefits of the use of each statistical method for the analysis of the quality of ordinal scales are highlighted.

Study Population

In the context of the SU.VI.MAX study – a randomized placebo-controlled trial, conducted on French middle-aged adult volunteers, that focused on the effects of vitamin and mineral supplementation on health [20, 21] – an ancillary cross-sectional study was undertaken to investigate the expression of facial skin aging features. This study was conducted on a subsample of 567 females (age range 44–70 years), who lived in the Paris area and who agreed to participate in this ancillary protocol.

Collection of Digital Images

The digital images database was collected in 2002. Standardized images of the whole face were taken from the 567 volunteers. The women had to follow specific skin care instructions: no application of detergent or cosmetic products on the facial skin for at least 12 h before the photograph was captured. The digital images were taken with a Kodak DSC 760 camera, which provides high-resolution images (2,036 × 3,060 pixels), combined with a 105 mm camera lens. The camera was mounted on a monopod to allow standardized positions of the camera. A specifically designed chair was used to allow standardized positions of the women's faces. Lighting conditions were also standardized by using two symmetrical lamps, placed at a 45° angle to each side of the volunteer's face, which provided a continuous daylight spectrum.

Study Design and Assessment of Severity of Photoaging

Larnier's scale is a 6-grade ordinal scale of photodamage, each grade being depicted by three reference photographs that illustrate the diversity and range of pigmentation disorders, wrinkling, and looseness [15]. Due to logistic planification, among the 567 photographs, a first set of 314 was rated by a trained dermatologist (D) twice (D_1 and D_2), at a one-year interval (Table 1). Following this, four experimented dermatologists (A, B, C, and D) independently rated the remaining 253 photographs (Table 2). All ratings were made independently using the reference photographs responding to each grade of the scale.

Methods

Estimating Degree of Agreement: Kappa Statistic

To estimate the degree of agreement between two ordinal ratings – made by two independent observers or by the same observer at two different times – the weighted Kappa statistic is generally used [12]. The Kappa statistic measures the percentage of data values in the main diagonal (percentage of agreement) of the table and then adjusts these values for the amount of agreement that could be expected due to chance only (percentage of agreement due to chance). For ordinal ratings, the weighted Kappa statistic is an improvement on the classical Kappa statistic, as it can attribute different weights to each possible combination of discordant observations. In this study, equal-spacing weights as defined by Cicchetti and Alisson [22] were used. Kappa values range from −1 to 1, 0 indicating null agreement, 1 and −1 accounting for perfect agreement and perfect disagreement, respectively. To interpret the level of agreement, the five-level nomenclature proposed by Landis and Koch [23] was used: kappa values of 0–0.2, 0.21–0.40, 0.41–0.60, 0.61–0.80, and 0.80–1.00 can be interpreted as poor, fair, moderate, substantial, and perfect agreement, respectively.

Estimating Degree of Distinguishability Between Adjacent Categories: Valet's Method

The degree of distinguishability (DD) between two categories of an ordinal scale is the raters' ability to distinguish between these two categories. In other words, it expresses the distance between these categories on the scale. Defined

Table 1 Ratings of the first set of 314 photographs of women faces, by one dermatologist at two successive times, D_1 and D_2, using Larnier's scale

		D_1					
		1	2	3	4	5	6
D_2	1	19	9	6	1	0	0
	2	5	15	19	5	0	0
	3	1	11	40	26	2	0
	4	0	1	22	75	16	0
	5	0	0	1	9	28	2
	6	0	0	0	0	0	1

by Darroch and McCloud [24], the DD between two categories ranges from 0 to 1:1 indicates a perfect distinguishability between these categories, whereas a value of 0 indicates that these categories are not distinguishable. Recently, Valet et al. proposed a new method to estimate DD between adjacent categories [13]. The authors argued that the DD between different pairs of adjacent categories of an ordinal scale (i.e., 1 and 2, 2 and 3, and so on) are not necessarily equal and may vary all along the scale. Therefore, the analysis of the DD variations may reveal heterogeneity within the structure of the scale and can indicate where agreement failed. For this reason, estimation of DD is of prime interest to analyze the structure of agreement and hence the quality of the scale. The structure of the scale can be easily illustrated through the graphical display of its DD estimates. For example, an almost perfect scale would have all its DD estimates close to 1 (Fig. 1a). In a less perfect scale, DD estimates between adjacent categories would be identical but with a lower value, stressing that these adjacent categories are equal but difficult to distinguish (Fig. 1b). In problematic scales, DD estimates would appear heterogeneous, highlighting the observers' difficulties in distinguishing between some adjacent categories, compared to others (Figs. 1c–e).

Computation and Expression of the Results

The weighted Kappa statistic and the DD estimates have been computed using SAS© software release 9.1.3 (SAS Institute Inc., SAS Campus Drive, Cary NC 27513, USA, *FREQ* procedure option AGREE, and *GENMOD* procedure, respectively), and R software release 8 (R Development Core Team, R Foundation for Statistical Computing, Vienna, Austria, *Kappa* function package *vcd*, and *glm* function, respectively). Both software programs provided identical results (codes are available on request). For each time of assessment (D_1 and D_2 of the intradermatologist ratings) and for each of the six pairs of dermatologists (interdermatologists ratings), the Kappa and DD estimates were expressed with their 95% confidence intervals.

Results

Due to the age range of the sample, category 6 was pooled with category 5 (Tables 1 and 2). Table 3 shows estimates of weighted Kappa (Kw) and degrees of distinguishability (DD) for each pair of ratings in intradermatologist and interdermatologists studies. Furthermore, to illustrate the heterogeneity of DD values all along the scale, a

Table 2 Ratings of the second set of 253 photographs of women faces, by four dermatologists (A, B, C, and D) using Larnier's scale

B \ A	1	2	3	4	5	6
1	14	9	3	0	0	0
2	5	26	13	1	0	0
3	1	11	35	3	0	0
4	0	4	58	30	6	0
5	0	0	6	21	6	0
6	0	0	0	0	1	0

C \ A	1	2	3	4	5	6
1	1	0	0	0	0	0
2	11	11	2	0	0	0
3	8	33	33	2	0	0
4	0	6	71	33	2	0
5	0	0	9	20	11	0
6	0	0	0	0	0	0

D \ A	1	2	3	4	5	6
1	12	14	4	0	0	0
2	5	19	17	0	0	0
3	3	16	52	8	2	0
4	0	1	42	40	3	0
5	0	0	0	7	8	0
6	0	0	0	0	0	0

C \ B	1	2	3	4	5	6
1	1	0	0	0	0	0
2	14	8	1	1	0	0
3	10	28	25	13	0	0
4	1	9	24	64	14	0
5	0	0	0	20	19	1
6	0	0	0	0	0	0

D \ B	1	2	3	4	5	6
1	20	9	1	0	0	0
2	5	16	13	7	0	0
3	1	19	27	31	3	0
4	0	1	9	56	20	0
5	0	0	0	4	10	1
6	0	0	0	0	0	0

D \ C	1	2	3	4	5	6
1	1	14	14	1	0	0
2	0	7	26	8	0	0
3	0	3	33	42	3	0
4	0	0	3	59	24	0
5	0	0	0	2	13	0
6	0	0	0	0	0	0

graphical display of the DD estimates from Table 3 is proposed in Fig. 2.

Intradermatologist Study

The weighted Kappa estimate was equal to 0.62 (i.e., a substantial agreement according to the Landis and Koch nomenclature). Moreover, the estimate of the degree of distinguishability between categories 4 and 5 (0.92) was much larger than that for adjacent categories from 1 to 4 (0.70). These results, illustrated in Fig. 2, suggested that the dermatologist distinguished adjacent categories 4 and 5 more easily than the other adjacent ones.

Interdermatologists Study

The Kappa statistic estimates ranged from 0.35 to 0.58 (fair to moderate agreement). The DD

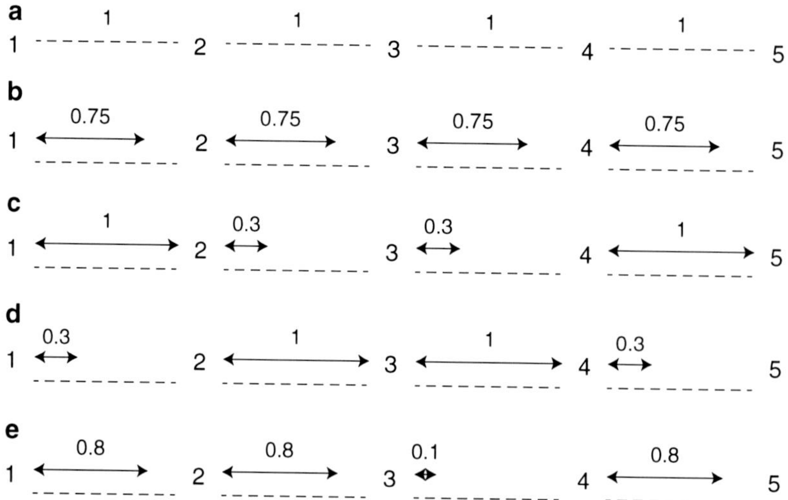

Fig. 1 Examples of DD variations for five-grade severity scales. Scale (*a*): Depicts a perfect scale. In this case, the DD values are equal to 1 all along the scale, which is indicated by *dashed lines* of similar length. The other scales illustrate four examples of unperfected scales. For these scales, distinguishabilities are indicated by *black arrows* with lengths proportional to DD values. Scale (*b*): Distinguishability smaller than 1, but homogeneous all along the scale. Scale (*c*): Perfect distinguishability between the extreme adjacent grades, but low distinguishability between intermediate adjacent ones. Scale (*d*): Perfect distinguishability between the intermediate adjacent grades, but low distinguishability between extreme adjacent ones. Scale (*e*): Distinguishability smaller than 1 but nonhomogeneous all along the scale, with a very low distinguishability between two adjacent intermediate grades

Table 3 Estimates of weighted Kappa (*Kw*) and degrees of distinguishability (*DD*) between successive adjacent categories *i* & *i* + 1, for each pair of ratings. Standards errors (s.e.) are given for each estimate

		DD (s.e.) between adjacent categories			
Ratings	*Kw (s.e.)*	1 & 2	2 & 3	3 & 4	4 & 5
D_1 & D_2[a]	0.62 (0.07)	0.70 (0.08)	0.70 (0.08)	0.70 (0.08)	0.92 (0.07)
A & B	0.43 (0.07)	0.68 (0.20)	0.68 (0.20)	0.90 (0.07)	0.90 (0.07)
A & C	0.54 (0.07)	0.69 (0.12)	0.69 (0.12)	0.86 (0.09)	0.86 (0.09)
A & D	0.58 (0.08)	0.84 (0.08)	0.47 (0.33)	0.84 (0.08)	0.84 (0.08)
B & C	0.35 (0.07)	0.85 (0.06)	0.85 (0.06)	0.85 (0.06)	0.85 (0.06)
B & D	0.47 (0.07)	0.78 (0.08)	0.78 (0.08)	0.78 (0.08)	0.78 (0.08)
C & D	0.51 (0.07)	0.77 (0.08)	0.77 (0.08)	0.77 (0.08)	0.77 (0.08)

[a]D_1 and D_2 are ratings from dermatologist D at two different times

estimates between all adjacent categories were equal all along the scale and greater than 0.60, except for the pairs involving dermatologist A. In these particular cases, DD estimates were found to be lower between the first three adjacent categories (adjacent categories 1 and 2, and 2 and 3) than between the others adjacent ones (adjacent categories 3 and 4, and 4 and 5). These results are illustrated in Fig. 2.

Discussion

From the perspective of evidenced-based medicine, it is of prime importance to provide measurement tools that allow the detection of clinically relevant changes that are due to disease evolution or therapeutic responses, rather than measurement errors [25]. The primary objective of an ordinal

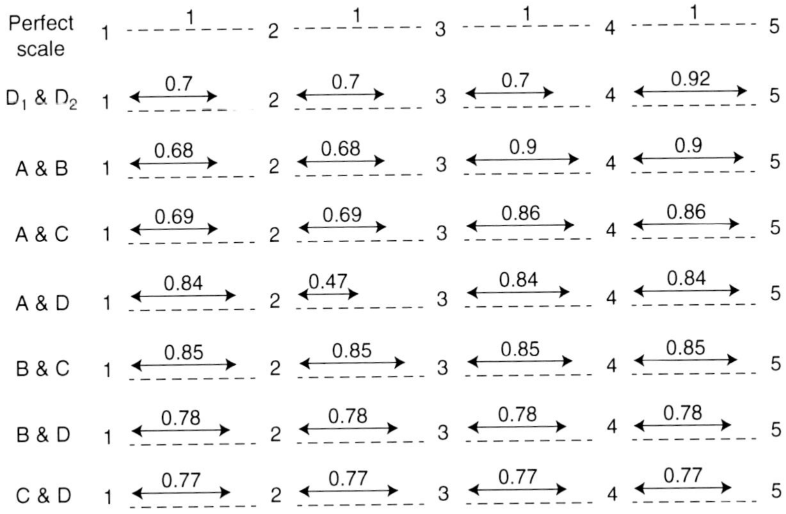

Fig. 2 DD estimates for each pair of ratings. Lengths of *black arrows* are proportional to the DD values. The first scale depicts a perfect scale, with DD values equal to 1 all along the scale, which are indicated by *dashed lines* of similar lengths. The other scales illustrate DD estimates between adjacent categories for each pair of ratings indicated by *black arrows* with lengths proportional to DD estimates

	1–2	2–3	3–4	4–5
Perfect scale	1	1	1	1
D_1 & D_2	0.7	0.7	0.7	0.92
A & B	0.68	0.68	0.9	0.9
A & C	0.69	0.69	0.86	0.86
A & D	0.84	0.47	0.84	0.84
B & C	0.85	0.85	0.85	0.85
B & D	0.78	0.78	0.78	0.78
C & D	0.77	0.77	0.77	0.77

scale is to produce an efficient, valuable, and practical tool. In this context, the reproducibility of ratings is the main component of its quality. To date, a number of dermatological rating scales (with or without photograph standards) have been developed to accurately evaluate skin aging features [26–30]. However, despite the wide use of ordinal scales for skin aging assessment, only a very few have been investigated for their reproducibility, and most of them have been stated as "validated" with a Kappa threshold greater than 0.60. Nevertheless, none of them has been investigated for reproducibility using tools that provide some information on the structure of the scale.

In this study, the intradermatologist degree of agreement reached 0.62; this value is similar to those found in the original paper [15] (median Kappa value = 0.63, calculated from eight intradermatologist ratings). Both values correspond to substantial degrees of agreement. Concerning the interdermatologists results, the Kappa estimates ranged from 0.35 to 0.58 (fair to moderate degrees of agreement). Moreover, the degrees of agreement between ratings involving dermatologist B were systematically lower than the others (0.35–0.47), highlighting that this investigator had some difficulties in using this scale. In the original paper [15], the ratings of each dermatologist were compared to the ratings of a consensus panel on two different occasions (median Kappa values = 0.58 and 0.61). Therefore, these last results cannot be compared to the results of this study, as the study designs are definitely different. Using Valet's method, differences within the degrees of distinguishability between adjacent categories were evidenced, suggesting that dermatologist D experienced some difficulties in distinguishing between the three first adjacent grades. In the interdermatologists variation study, the DD estimates were all lower than 1 but homogeneous all along the scale, except for comparisons involving dermatologist A. Indeed, dermatologist A experienced some difficulties in distinguishing between the three first adjacent grades. Except for this dermatologist, the DD estimates between adjacent categories are identical all along the scale but with lower values than a perfect scale.

The experimental conditions of the reproducibility study were fairly suitable. Indeed, the raters were well-trained, experienced dermatologists. In addition, one of the strengths of this study is that the sample size was rather large (314 individuals in the intradermatologist study and 253 in the interdermatologists study) in comparison to similar published studies [26–30]. Nevertheless, due to the women's characteristics, in particular the age range (44–70 years), the last category of the scale was almost unused. For that reason, the extreme adjacent categories were not tested. An additional limitation should be underlined, which concern both methods in the case of more than two observers. Indeed, for Valet's method, the DD estimates between the scale categories must be calculated for each possible pair of observers. No method has yet been developed that can estimate a "global" DD between the scale categories for more than two observers. Similarly, the estimate of the degree of agreement using the Kappa statistic method can also be calculated between each possible pair of observers. A global Kappa statistic has been proposed to deal with more than two observers, corresponding roughly to an average Kappa [31]. However, as the contingency tables associated to each pair of dermatologists are not independent, the interpretation of this global statistic is problematic.

The method developed by Valet et al. provides estimates of the DD between each pair of adjacent categories of an ordinal scale. Therefore, this method also provides an indication of the degree of agreement through the DD estimates between adjacent categories. Indeed, an equal and high DD value between all adjacent categories of the scale would clearly lead to a lower variability within ratings and hence a better agreement between them. In addition, contrary to the Kappa statistic method, this method can highlight DD heterogeneities between adjacent categories and may suggest some modifications to improve the quality of the scale. For example, a low DD between two adjacent categories would clearly suggest that they should be pooled or redefined in order to improve the reproducibility – and hence the quality – of the scale in forthcoming studies. The Kappa statistic is useful for rapid tests and has widespread use, even though its interpretation using the nomenclature of Landis and Koch is questionable. Several authors have pointed out the limits of this global index of agreement [32, 33], and for weighted Kappa statistics, the choice of weights may be arbitrary and may strongly influence the Kappa level estimates. When using the squared error weights on this data set, as proposed by Fleiss [34, 35], the weighted Kappa levels would be higher (indicating substantial or almost perfect agreements) than those estimated with equal-spacing weights (linear error). In addition, as highlighted by Valet et al. [36], the Kappa statistic may indicate an almost perfect degree of agreement even if a major scale defect exists. Indeed, this method does not provide any indication that could be used for scale improvement.

Conclusion

According to the present findings, the reproducibility of Larnier's scale appears to be questionable. It appears that some dermatologists had difficulties in distinguishing between some adjacent categories, highlighting some major scale defects. Consequently, the quality of this scale could be improved. Among suggestions for these improvements, the reference photographs should be discussed in order to redefine the three first categories and illustrate the concerned categories using new reference photographs.

Acknowledgments The authors gratefully acknowledge the dedicated efforts of the SU.VI.MAX participants and the investigators and staff involved in this study, in particular Dr. Raymonde Danila and Dr. Randa Jdid. The authors wish also to gratefully acknowledge Dr. Catherine Larnier for her kind interest in this research.

References

1. Coenraads PJ, et al. Construction and validation of a photographic guide for assessing severity of chronic hand dermatitis. Br J Dermatol. 2005;152(2):296–301.
2. Berth-Jones J, et al. A study examining inter- and intrarater reliability of three scales for measuring severity of psoriasis: psoriasis area and severity index, physician's global assessment and lattice system physician's global assessment. Br J Dermatol. 2006;155(4):707–13.
3. Hanifin JM, et al. The eczema area and severity index (EASI): assessment of reliability in atopic dermatitis. EASI Evaluator Group Exp Dermatol. 2001;10 (1):11–8.
4. Witkowski JA, Parish LC. The assessment of acne: an evaluation of grading and lesion counting in the measurement of acne. Clin Dermatol. 2004;22(5):394–7.
5. Ching S, et al. Measuring outcomes in aesthetic surgery: a comprehensive review of the literature. Plast Reconstr Surg. 2003;111(1):469–80.
6. Most SP, Alsarraf R, Larrabee WF. Outcomes of facial cosmetic procedures. Facial Plast Surg. 2002;18 (2):119–24.
7. Heckmann M, Schon-Hupka G. Quantification of the efficacy of botulinum toxin type A by digital image analysis. J Am Acad Dermatol. 2001;45(4):508–14.

8. Alsarraf R, et al. Measuring cosmetic facial plastic surgery outcomes: a pilot study. Arch Facial Plast Surg. 2001;3(3):198–201.
9. Chung JH, et al. Cutaneous photodamage in Koreans: influence of sex, sun exposure, smoking, and skin color. Arch Dermatol. 2001;137(8):1043–51.
10. Guinot C, et al. Relative contribution of intrinsic vs extrinsic factors to skin aging as determined by a validated skin age score. Arch Dermatol. 2002;138 (11):1454–60.
11. Shoukri MM. Measures of interobserver agreement. Boca Raton: Chapman & Hall/CRC; 2004.
12. Cohen J. Weighted kappa: nominal scale agreement with provision for scaled disagreement or partial credit. Psychol Bull. 1968;70:213–20.
13. Valet F, et al. Log-linear non-uniform association models for agreement between two ratings on an ordinal scale. Stat Med. 2007;26(3):647–62.
14. Rabe JH, et al. Photoaging: mechanisms and repair. J Am Acad Dermatol. 2006;55(1):1–19.
15. Larnier C, et al. Evaluation of cutaneous photodamage using a photographic scale. Br J Dermatol. 1994;130 (2):167–73.
16. Griffiths CE, et al. A photonumeric scale for the assessment of cutaneous photodamage. Arch Dermatol. 1992;128(3):347–51.
17. Helfrich YR, et al. Effect of smoking on aging of photoprotected skin: evidence gathered using a new photonumeric scale. Arch Dermatol. 2007;143 (5):397–402.
18. Carruthers A, et al. A validated grading scale for crow's feet. Dermatol Surg. 2008;34 Suppl 2:S173–8.
19. Malvy D, et al. Epidemiologic determinants of skin photoaging: baseline data of the SU.VI.MAX cohort. J Am Acad Dermatol. 2000;42(1 Pt 1):47–55.
20. Hercberg S, et al. A primary prevention trial using nutritional doses of antioxidant vitamins and minerals in cardiovascular diseases and cancers in a general population: the SU.VI.MAX study-design, methods, and participant characteristics. SUpplementation en VItamines et Mineraux AntioXydants. Control Clin Trials. 1998;19(4):36–351.
21. Hercberg S, et al. The SU.VI.MAX Study: a randomized, placebo-controlled trial of the health effects of antioxidant vitamins and minerals. Arch Intern Med. 2004;164(21):2335–42.
22. Cicchetti DV, Allison T. A new procedure for assessing reliability of scoring EEG sleep recordings. Am J EEG Technol. 1971;11:101–9.
23. Landis JR, Koch GG. The measurement of observer agreement for categorical data. Biometrics. 1977;33 (1):159–74.
24. Darroch JN, McCloud PI. Category distinguishability and observer agreement. Aust J Stat. 1986;28:371–88.
25. Weyers W. The 21st century – time for a reliable method for diagnosis in clinical dermatology. Arch Dermatol. 2000;136(1):103–5.
26. Lemperle G, et al. A classification of facial wrinkles. Plast Reconstr Surg. 2001;108(6):1735–50.
27. Ryu JS, et al. Improving lip wrinkles: lipstick-related image analysis. Skin Res Technol. 2005;11(3):157–64.
28. Day DJ, et al. The wrinkle severity rating scale: a validation study. Am J Clin Dermatol. 2004;5 (1):49–52.
29. Kim EJ, Reeck JB, Maas CS. A validated rating scale for hyperkinetic facial lines. Arch Facial Plast Surg. 2004;6(4):253–6.
30. Morizot F, et al. Development of photographic scales documenting features of skin aging based on digital images. Ann Dermatol Venereol. 2002;129(10 Pt 1):1s402.
31. Fleiss JL. Measuring nominal scale agreement among many raters. Psychol Bull. 1971;76:378–82.
32. Feinstein AR, Cicchetti DV. High agreement but low kappa: I. The problems of two paradoxes. J Clin Epidemiol. 1990;43(6):543–9.
33. Cicchetti DV, Feinstein AR. Feinstein AR. High agreement but low kappa: II. Resolving the paradoxes. J Clin Epidemiol. 1990;43(6):551–8.
34. Fleiss JL, Cohen J. The equivalence of weighted kappa and the intraclass correlation coefficient as measures of reliability. Educ Psychol Meas. 1973;33:613–9.
35. Fleiss JL. Statistical methods for rates and proportions. New York: Wiley; 1981.
36. Valet F, et al. Quality assessment of ordinal scale reproducibility: log-linear models provided useful information on scale structure. J Clin Epidemiol. 2008;61 (10):983–90.

The Baumann Skin Typing System 117

Leslie S. Baumann

Contents

L.S. Baumann (✉)
Baumann Cosmetic and Research Institute, Miami, FL, USA
e-mail: DrB@derm.net; lbwork@derm.net

M.A. Farage et al. (eds.), *Textbook of Aging Skin*,
DOI 10.1007/978-3-662-47398-6_88

Abstract

The biology of various skin phenotypes, such as oily, dry, acne-prone, rosacea-prone, dyschromia, and photoaged, affects the interaction and efficacy of cosmeceutical ingredients. This chapter will review how cosmeceuticals influence basic skin biology and how they interact with each other in various patient phenotypes, as characterized by the Baumann Skin Typing System (BSTS). Developed in 2004, the BSTS, derived from a scientifically validated questionnaire, offers specific guidance for physicians and patients/consumers in identifying the most suitable ingredients and skin products as it takes into account multiple concurrent cutaneous characteristics and gathers historical data. The reader will be provided with knowledge of the basic science of different skin issues and will obtain a scientific perspective on how to design skin care regimens, combine cosmeceuticals with prescription medications, educate staff and patients on their proper use, and ethically prescribe skin care products using this standardized methodology.

Introduction

As of 2011, the cosmeceutical industry was considered to be a \$6.5 billion business [1], and global sales of topical cosmeceuticals surpassed \$33 billion in 2012, with projected sales exceeding \$42 billion by 2017 [2]. The promise of financial success has resulted in the discovery of many new cosmeceutical technologies and significant advances in understanding skin science and the effects on skin by topically applied substances. The emergence of many new ingredients and topical formulations has manifested in an abundance of products on the market, exaggerated marketing claims, and confusion on the part of consumers, aestheticians, and physicians. The major current challenge is to sift through the copious technologies and formulations and match cosmeceutical technologies to the appropriate type of skin. As new genetic data lead to advances in skin care technologies, the importance of the genotype as well as the phenotype cannot be overstated. An ingredient is only efficacious when it is placed on the correct skin phenotype. Combining ingredients affects their chemical structure, efficacy, and penetration; therefore, the order in which products are placed on the skin is important. The phenotype of the skin will also affect how ingredients penetrate into the skin and react with each other. In order to maximize outcomes with cosmeceuticals, there are many steps that should be taken to properly match a skin care regimen with the proper skin phenotype (Table 1).

The Baumann Skin Typing System (BSTS) was developed in 2004 and classifies skin according to four dichotomous parameters: dry or oily, sensitive or resistant, pigmented or nonpigmented, and wrinkled or unwrinkled. Simultaneously assessing the skin based on these four non-mutually exclusive parameters yields 16 potential and distinct skin phenotypes (Table 2). The Baumann Skin Type® designations for each phenotype are derived from a scientifically validated questionnaire known as the Baumann Skin Type Indicator (BSTI). The Baumann Skin Type can change after significant alterations in lifestyle habits, hormones, medical condition, and environment and therefore should be retaken annually or when the current skin care regimen seems insufficient [3, 4].

Table 1 How to maximize outcomes from cosmeceuticals

1. Know ingredient science
2. Understand cosmeceutical formulation
3. Understand manufacturing and packaging
4. Understand ingredient interactions
5. Choose the best products from each brand
6. Combine products from various brands to form set regimens
7. Diagnose the patient's Baumann Skin Type® using the validated BSTI (5)
8. Match the regimen to the correct skin type
9. Test the regimens on each individual skin type
10. Take baseline photographs and standardized measurements
11. Educate your patients (clients) to increase compliance
12. Schedule regular follow-up visits to adjust the regimen
13. Ensure proper use of the correct products

The BSTS, by nature, offers specific guidance for physicians and patients/consumers in identifying the most suitable ingredients and skin products as it takes into account multiple concurrent cutaneous characteristics and gathers historical data. The questionnaire probes how the skin reacts in various situations, allowing the collection of historical data and the current skin condition.

Each of the distinct Baumann Skin Types display characteristics that determine which ingredients are beneficial and which are deleterious. For example, a person with dry, sensitive, pigmented, wrinkle-prone skin (DSPW) would require significantly different skin care products than a person with oily, resistant, nonpigmented, "tight" (not wrinkle-prone) skin (ORNT). Oily-resistant skin types have a strong skin barrier with an extra layer of sebum to prevent penetration of ingredients; therefore, individuals with this skin type require an increased concentration of active ingredients or penetration enhancers to demonstrate efficacy. Dry, sensitive skin types, on the other hand, have an impaired barrier that allows increased penetration of ingredients; these individuals are more prone to inflammation. In the DSPW type, the skin-lightening ingredients and antiaging ingredients that are required should not be ones that will incite inflammation. Lower concentrations can be used because of the defect in the skin barrier.More than 300,000 people worldwide have taken the BSTI, and it is used by multiple dermatologists around the world to diagnose patient skin phenotype. It has been shown to be valid for all ethnicities, ages, and genders. The most recent version

Table 2 **The BSTS skin type paradigm.** Each of the Baumann Skin Types® is assigned a color and a number

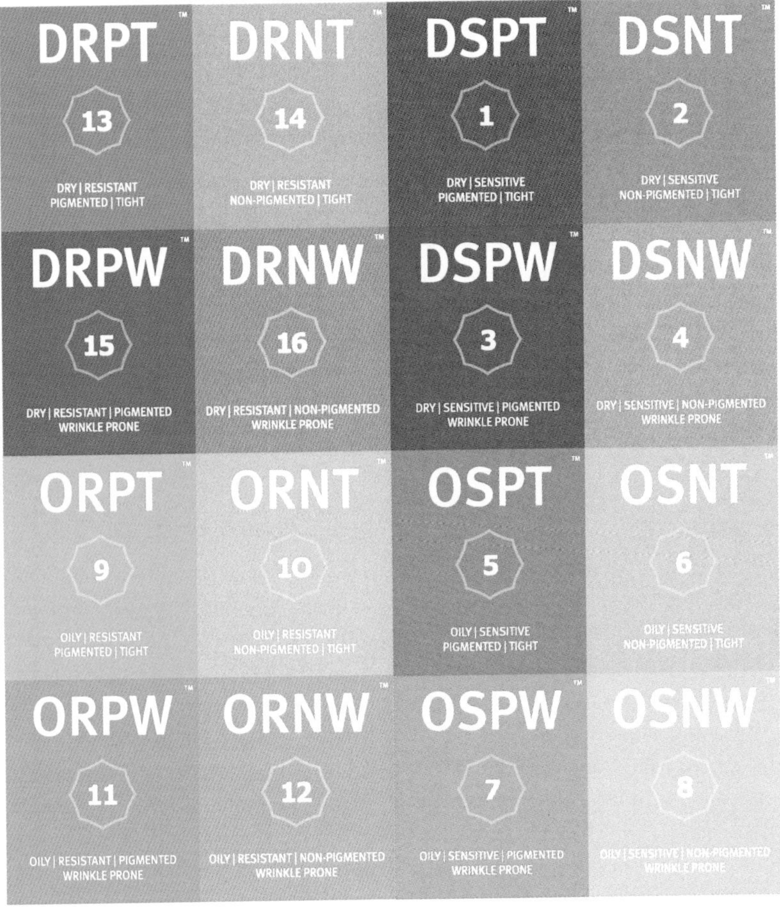

<table>
<tr><td>DRPT™
13
DRY | RESISTANT
PIGMENTED | TIGHT</td><td>DRNT™
14
DRY | RESISTANT
NON-PIGMENTED | TIGHT</td><td>DSPT™
1
DRY | SENSITIVE
PIGMENTED | TIGHT</td><td>DSNT™
2
DRY | SENSITIVE
NON-PIGMENTED | TIGHT</td></tr>
<tr><td>DRPW™
15
DRY | RESISTANT | PIGMENTED
WRINKLE PRONE</td><td>DRNW™
16
DRY | RESISTANT | NON-PIGMENTED
WRINKLE PRONE</td><td>DSPW™
3
DRY | SENSITIVE | PIGMENTED
WRINKLE PRONE</td><td>DSNW™
4
DRY | SENSITIVE | NON-PIGMENTED
WRINKLE PRONE</td></tr>
<tr><td>ORPT™
9
OILY | RESISTANT
PIGMENTED | TIGHT</td><td>ORNT™
10
OILY | RESISTANT
NON-PIGMENTED | TIGHT</td><td>OSPT™
5
OILY | SENSITIVE
PIGMENTED | TIGHT</td><td>OSNT™
6
OILY | SENSITIVE
NON-PIGMENTED | TIGHT</td></tr>
<tr><td>ORPW™
11
OILY | RESISTANT | PIGMENTED
WRINKLE PRONE</td><td>ORNW™
12
OILY | RESISTANT | NON-PIGMENTED
WRINKLE PRONE</td><td>OSPW™
7
OILY | SENSITIVE | PIGMENTED
WRINKLE PRONE</td><td>OSNW™
8
OILY | SENSITIVE | NON-PIGMENTED
WRINKLE PRONE</td></tr>
</table>

of the BSTI questionnaire is only accessible online to physicians who have met various criteria and completed a training program to ensure the proper use of ingredients [5]. The BSTI is instrumental in diagnosing skin type and helping the doctor or designee prescribe the proper cosmeceuticals, over-the-counter and prescription medications, and procedures that are most appropriate for the patient's Baumann Skin Type®. The non-identifying data culled from the BSTI has the potential to broaden our knowledge of skin types, their prevalence around the world, and how to improve patient outcomes. It also allows standardization in study subject recruitment so that only certain skin phenotypes are included in research studies. The BSTI and its use are beyond the scope of this chapter; however, information on how to apply to be chosen to use this system can be found at STSFranchise.com. The program is designed to be used under the guidance of a physician and incorporates prescription and nonprescription products and in-office therapies.

The four parameters on which the BSTI is based will guide the discussion in this chapter. Emphasis will be placed on defining the characteristics of these dichotomies and focusing on pertinent basic science. Various aspects of the 16 skin phenotype variations will be described in the process. Cutaneous aging is explained in the context of the wrinkled (W) to tight (T) continuum. Approaches to skin care or treatment options that follow from the BSTS will also be cited, with noninvasive, mostly topical therapies addressed.

Skin Hydration: The Oily (O) To Dry (D) Continuum

Oily skin is caused by the excess production of sebum; dry skin, also known as xerosis, is associated with a complex, multifactorial etiology including an impaired barrier. Individuals with oily skin often are unable to find a sunscreen that they can tolerate due to greasiness, while people with dry skin types are more easily irritated by retinoids and acne medications. The most important factors that regulate the degree of dryness/oiliness are stratum corneum lipids, sebum, natural moisturizing factor, and aquaporin, a discussion of which follows [6].

Stratum Corneum (SC)

The role of the stratum corneum (SC), particularly its ability to maintain skin hydration, is the most significant factor in preventing or setting the stage for xerosis. The SC is composed of keratinocytes surrounded by a coating of ceramides, cholesterol, and fatty acids, among other constituents. These primary components of the SC, when present in the appropriate amount and balance, assist in protecting the skin and keeping it watertight. The stimulation of lipid synthesis and keratinocyte proliferation by multiple factors, including diet, medications, hormones, and immunomodulators such as cytokines, contributes to maintaining SC equilibrium [7].

When ceramides, cholesterol, and fatty acids are imbalanced, the SC endures a cascade of interrelated events, resulting in a reduced capacity to maintain water and increased susceptibility to exogenous elements, thereby elevating susceptibility to skin surface sensitivity and xerosis. Such an impairment in the SC is measurable as an increase in transepidermal water loss (TEWL). When the skin becomes dehydrated, the desquamation of corneocytes is adversely affected because the enzymes necessary for desmosome metabolism require water [8]. The abnormal or compromised desquamation leads to a visible collection of keratinocytes manifesting in skin surface irregularities that result in skin that feels rough and loses radiance because it poorly reflects light [9]. This is a common complaint of patients that say that their skin "looks old" or "is no longer glowing." Many skin care companies take advantage of this imbalance by offering demonstrations of their products that exfoliate, resulting in an instant glow to the skin that often prompts the customer to purchase the product. However, these exfoliating products are treating the symptom of roughness but not the underlying cause, which is dehydration.

Not all moisturizers that contain ceramides, cholesterol, and fatty acids are effective at repairing the skin barrier because the ceramides and fatty acids must mimic the naturally occurring three-dimensional structure of the multilamellar bilayer of lipids known as the skin barrier. For example, a moisturizer that contains increased fatty acid levels and decreased ceramide levels causes a perturbation in the lipid bilayer of the SC, which is also linked to xerosis [10]. For this reason, moisturizers designed to repair the skin barrier must contain the proper ratio of fatty acids, ceramides, and cholesterol. In addition, the type of fatty acid is important. Oleic acid, because of the structure of its fatty acid chains, causes tiny holes in the skin barrier, while other fatty acids such as stearic acid are able to pack in closer together, thereby strengthening the skin barrier [11]. There are synthetic "multilamellar emulsions" such as MLE technology (myristoyl/palmitoyl oxostearamide/arachamide MEA) that utilize fatty acids and ceramides that mimic the same three-dimensional structure as the native bilayer membrane [12].

The skin's protective lipid bilayer needs constant replenishment in those whose underlying mechanisms are insufficient to produce adequate amounts of ceramides, fatty acids, and cholesterol because this lipid bilayer is susceptible to deleterious effects induced by exogenous factors such as ultraviolet (UV) radiation, detergents, acetone, chlorine, and prolonged water exposure. Changes in temperature, humidity, and pH affect cohesion and desquamation of corneocytes from the SC by activating numerous extracellular proteases [13], which in turn can impact the skin's protective layer by thinning or thickening the SC.

Improving skin hydration by strengthening the skin barrier in dry skin types begins with the selection of a nonfoaming cleanser. Foaming cleansers should be avoided because they often have detergents (surfactants) that surround and remove the lipids from the SC. A barrier repair moisturizer should be used twice a day and should contain a 1:1:1 ratio of ceramides, fatty acids, and cholesterol. The optimal fatty acids are linoleic, palmitic, and stearic acids, which have been shown to repair the skin barrier within 2 h when applied exogenously [14]. These fatty acids are found in large amounts in some natural ingredients such as almond oil, argan oil, shea butter, sunflower oil, safflower oil, grape seed extract, and macadamia oil, as well as in synthetic ingredients such as glyceryl stearate and myristoyl/palmitoyl oxostearamide/arachamide MEA.

Natural Moisturizing Factor (NMF)

Natural moisturizing factor (NMF) is an intracellular, hygroscopic substance present only in the SC. Low NMF levels are correlated with xerosis and ichthyosis vulgaris. NMF is produced by lamellar bodies via the breakdown of the protein filaggrin (or filament-aggregating protein). Filaggrin is composed of lactic acid, urea, citrate, and sugars and is broken down into free amino acids, such as arginine, glutamine (glutamic acid), and histidine by a cytosolic protease in the outer layer of the SC [15]. These water-soluble free amino acids remain inside the keratinocytes as NMF and play an integral intracellular humectant role by maintaining water within skin cells. The process of NMF production is elegantly controlled by ambient humidity levels. Aspartate protease (cathepsin), the enzyme responsible for the rate of filaggrin decomposition, has been shown to be susceptible to changes in ambient humidity, allowing fluctuations in NMF production [16]. After an individual enters a low-humidity environment, NMF synthesis usually increases over the course of several days [17]. UV radiation as well as surfactants (detergents) can suppress the development of NMF.

As of yet, no products or procedures have been developed that have the capacity to artificially influence or regulate NMF synthesis because its intracellular location makes it difficult to replace topically. The best course of action is to avoid foaming cleansers (detergents) and UV exposure to preserve native NMF.

Aquaporin-3

Aquaporin (AQP)-3 is member of a subclass of aquaporins labeled aquaglyceroporins, which selectively transport water, glycerol, urea, and other small solutes through a water channel protein. AQP-3 exerts an influential role in skin hydration by regulating this water channel [18]. AQP-3 is found in the kidney, lungs, and GI tract and in human epidermal keratinocytes [19]. The water conduction function in the skin occurs along an osmotic gradient beneath the SC, thereby facilitating the hydration of skin layers below the SC.

In the superficial SC, a high concentration of solutes (Na^+, K^+, and Cl^-) and a low concentration of water (13–35 %) [20] generate in the steady-state gradients of solutes and water from the skin surface to the viable epidermal keratinocytes [21–23]. The molecular mechanisms of fluid transport across epidermal keratinocyte layers and the relationship between keratinocyte fluid transport and SC hydration have not been elucidated. It is hypothesized that AQP-3 enhances transepidermal water movement to protect the SC from evaporation from the skin surface and/or to spread water gradients throughout the epidermal keratinocyte layer [19]. In one study, researchers noted that the water permeability of human epidermal keratinocytes was inhibited by mercurials and low pH, which was consistent with AQP-3 involvement [19]. Another study found significantly lower water and glycerol permeability, and conductance measurements revealed much lower SC water content in AQP-3 null mice, supporting previous evidence that AQP-3 functions as a plasma membrane water/glycerol transporter in the epidermis [24]. Water transport across AQP-3 was found to be slower in skin than in other tissues [25].

Despite the fact that some cosmeceutical manufacturers boast of aquaporin on their ingredient lists, it is not possible to exogenously insert AQP-3 into the keratinocyte membrane. At this time, the only way to affect aquaporin function with a topical formulation is with extracts that stimulate AQP-3 function. A solitary example is an extract of the herb *Ajuga turkestanica*, which has been shown to enhance the activity of AQP-3 [26]. At the time of publication of this chapter, no other ingredients have been able to mimic this activity.

Sebum

Sebum is the oily secretion of the sebaceous glands that contains wax esters, sterol esters, cholesterol, di- and triglycerides, and squalene. Sebum imparts an oily protective film on the surface of the skin but also plays a causal role in the formation of comedones and acne [27]. The exact composition of sebum is determined by genetics, diet, medications, and other poorly understood factors. Sebum, which is an important source of the antioxidant vitamin E, confers cutaneous protection from exogenous factors such as UV light. It also functions as an occlusive moisturizer on the skin's surface, impeding TEWL. Subjects with an impairment in the lipid bilayer surrounding the keratinocytes in the SC skin may suffer less from dehydration and irritant (or allergen)-mediated inflammation when a higher level of protective sebum is present. When sebum production is below the normal range, it is thought by some to play a role in the development of dry skin, especially when it coincides with an impaired skin barrier [28]. It is important to note that low sebaceous gland activity has not been shown to cause xerosis in the absence of an impaired skin barrier. In fact, the protective role that sebum plays in preventing skin xerosis seems to be independent of skin barrier function because skin with few sebaceous glands, as in prepubertal children, can manifest normal skin barrier function [29]. In addition, barrier function or SC lamellar membranes are not impacted by the pharmacologic involution of sebaceous glands with supraphysiologic isotretinoin doses resulting in dry skin [30–32].

Sebum likely exerts its skin-hydrating effect through occlusive activity rather than an influence on barrier function. The protective effect of glandular lipids is demonstrated by the meibomian glands, which are modified sebaceous glands located in the eyes that have the capacity to stave off dryness by preventing tear evaporation [33, 34]. The separate role of sebum in skin hydration was demonstrated in a study that assessed permeability barrier homeostasis and SC hydration in asebia J1 mice with sebaceous gland hypoplasia [35]. The asebia mice had consistent levels of the three primary barrier lipids (ceramides, free sterols, and free fatty acids) and normal barrier function but were sebum deficient. The researchers demonstrated that the asebia J1 mice manifested reduced SC hydration, implying that while an intact intercellular membrane bilayer system suffices for permeability barrier homeostasis, the presence of sebum is necessary for normal SC hydration.

The investigators in the asebia J1 study noted that the topical application of glycerol restored normal SC hydration to the sebum-deficient mice. Glycerol is a humectant that helps bind water to the skin's surface. Sebaceous gland-derived triglycerides (TG) are hydrolyzed to glycerol before transport to the skin surface in normal skin. In fact, the use of glycerol has also been demonstrated to be effective in accelerating SC recovery [36]. For this reason, sebum has both an occlusive and a humectant effect on the skin's surface and, through hydrolyzation of its triglycerides to glycerol, has the ability to hasten barrier repair.

Many factors contribute to sebum production rates. The age-related trajectory of sebum production levels is well understood. During childhood, sebum levels are usually low, then rise in the middle-to-late teens, and remain relatively stable for decades until declining in the 7th and 8th decades as endogenous androgen production falls

[37]. Sebum production is also affected by diet and stress, but the influence of these is not well understood. Androgenic hormones are well known to increase sebaceous gland activity. Genetic predisposition to sebum production was demonstrated in a fascinating study of 20 pairs each of identical and nonidentical like-sex twins. Almost equivalent sebum excretion rates were observed in the identical twins, but there were significant variations in sebum production among the nonidentical twins, demonstrating the strong genetic influence on sebum secretion rates [38].

Differences in Skin Care for Oily and Dry Skin

An intact SC and skin barrier, normal levels of NMF and hyaluronic acid (HA), normal AQP-3 activity, and balanced sebum secretion together characterize an ideal cutaneous state. The goal of a properly designed skin care regimen is to achieve this idealized state by removing excess sebum in oily skin types and repairing the skin barrier in dry skin types.

Oily Skin Care

Treatment of individuals with oily skin should be aimed at decreasing surface sebum levels with surfactant-containing foaming cleansers because there are no topical ingredients that have convincingly demonstrated the ability to decrease sebum production, despite manufacturer claims to the contrary. Oral retinoids, oral spironolactone, and oral contraceptives have been well established as effective in reducing sebaceous gland activity, but topical retinoids and topical antiandrogens have not yet been demonstrated to exhibit this capacity. Oily skin types should avoid lipid-laden moisturizers such as heavy creams and oils. Gels, serums, and light lotions are a better choice for oily skin types. Oily types often omit sunscreen because of the greasiness associated with chemical sunscreen ingredients and dimethicone, which is often found in SPF preparations. Choosing an SPF that does not have oily components will increase sunscreen compliance in oily types. Omitting a moisturizer in the morning and using a sunscreen instead is one way to increase sunscreen compliance in oily skin types. Oily skin types must cleanse the face completely at night to remove make up, sunscreen, dimethicone, dirt, and other debris that can contribute to comedone formation.

Dry Skin Care

An impaired skin barrier and diminished NMF characterize xerotic skin. Skin care should aim to preserve and replace skin lipids. Harsh foaming detergents (present in hand, body, and facial cleansers) strip lipids and NMF from the skin and should be avoided by all patients with dry skin. Individuals with dry skin should also be advised to abstain from protracted bathing, especially in hot or chlorinated water. People with extremely dry skin use humidifiers in low-humidity environments and apply moisturizers two to three times daily and after bathing. Moisturizers should include barrier repair ingredients in a 1:1:1 ratio of ceramides, fatty acids, and cholesterol. In addition, occlusive and humectant ingredients can be added to boost skin hydration. Dry skin is very prevalent, especially in the winter as evidenced by the fact that of all the OTC topical skin care product types, moisturizers are the third most frequently recommended [39]. It is important to remember that sebaceous glands are only found on the face, back, and chest. Therefore, some patients who demonstrate oily facial skin that is masking an impaired skin barrier will exhibit dry skin on the limbs and body.

Moisturizers are typically packaged as water-in-oil emulsions or oil-in-water emulsions or as an oil. A brief discussion follows of the differences among moisturizer types, which is important to a practitioner's knowledge base in terms of offering appropriate product selection recommendations to patients.

Occlusives

Occlusive agents are lipid-filled compounds that mimic the effects of sebum and are incorporated into skin care formulations in order to coat the SC and prevent TEWL. In addition to inhibiting TEWL, occlusives exhibit emollient properties and are therefore appropriate products for smoothing the roughness associated with dry skin.

Petrolatum and mineral oil were once thought to be the most effective occlusive ingredients. Used as a skin care product since 1872, petrolatum was considered one of the best moisturizers and is still the gold standard by which other occlusive agents are measured [40]. For example, petrolatum displays a resistance to water vapor loss that is 170 times that of olive oil [41]. Many consumers deem petrolatum to be cosmetically unacceptable because of its greasy texture, and prefer a more "environmentally friendly" option, but efficacy of moisturizers is still often compared to that of petrolatum. Other frequently used occlusive ingredients include paraffin, squalene, silicone derivatives (dimethicone, cyclomethicone), almond oil, argan oil, soybean oil, grape seed oil, macadamia nut oil, propylene glycol, lanolin, lecithin, stearyl stearate, and beeswax [42, 43].

Lanolin, which is derived from the sebaceous secretions of sheep, warrants special mention. It contains the important SC lipid cholesterol and can coexist with SC lipids as solids and liquids at physiologic temperatures. However, lanolin has been identified as an allergen [44] and is derived from animals, which has greatly lessened its popularity. Functioning as both a humectant and an occlusive agent, propylene glycol (PG) is an odorless liquid that also exhibits antimicrobial and keratolytic activity. In addition, PG has been demonstrated to contribute to the cellular penetration of some drugs, such as minoxidil and steroids. Although believed to be a weak sensitizer, PG may provoke or factor into contact dermatitis by facilitating allergen penetration into the epidermis [45].

Occlusive ingredients are a temporary solution for smoothing skin and helping prevent TEWL, but they are not a replacement for barrier repair ingredients, and they do not confer long-lasting benefits. Once an occlusive product is removed from the skin, TEWL returns to its previous level. The reduction of TEWL by more than 40 %, which can result from overuse of occlusive agents, poses a risk of maceration with increased bacteria levels; therefore, occlusive agents are typically used in combination with humectant ingredients to decrease the amount of occlusion needed to restore hydration [46].

Humectants

Humectants are hygroscopic, water-soluble substances that strongly bind water. In conditions with at least 80 % humidity, humectants applied to the skin exhibit the capacity to attract water from the external environment to the skin surface. In low-humidity conditions, however, humectants applied to the skin can absorb water from the deeper epidermis and dermis, thus contributing to TEWL and exacerbating xerosis [47]. Combining humectants with occlusive products decreases TEWL and skin dehydration in a low-humidity environment. Cosmetic moisturizers are often formulated with humectants in order to prevent product evaporation and thickening, thus extending the product's shelf-life. By drawing water into the skin, humectants engender a minor swelling of the SC, leaving a perception of smoother skin with fewer wrinkles, but these effects are temporary. Some humectants impart other benefits such as emollient and bacteriostatic properties [48]. Glycerin and glycerol are considered the most effective humectant ingredients found in skin care products. Alpha hydroxy acids, carboxylic acid, gelatin, honey and other sugars, panthenol, propylene glycol, sodium hyaluronate, sodium and ammonium lactate, sodium pyrrolidine carboxylic acid, sorbitol, and urea are among other substances that function as active humectant ingredients [43]. Moisturizers typically incorporate occlusive as well as humectant ingredients, but the benefits of these are short lived. Some barrier repair moisturizers incorporate occlusives and humectants so that the preparation will have both long-term and short-term benefits.

Glycerin

Glycerin is a potent humectant [49]. Using ultrastructural analyses of skin treated with high-glycerin formulations, investigators have demonstrated that this humectant expands the SC by enhancing corneocyte thickness and creating greater distance between corneocyte layers [50]. In addition, after a 5-year study that compared two high-glycerin moisturizers with 16 other popular moisturizers, including petrolatum preparations, used by 394 patients with severe xerosis, researchers reported that the high-glycerin products were the most effective, rapidly restoring dry skin to normal hydration with longer-lasting results than the other products [9]. Glycerin has also been shown to stabilize and hydrate cell membranes along with the enzymes essential for desmosome degradation [9]. Glycerin is another name for glycerol. Glycerol forms the backbone of fatty acids and is therefore released when fatty acids are digested [51].

Urea

Also known as carbamide, urea is an end product of mammalian protein metabolism as well as an NMF constituent. This versatile compound exhibits humectant and mild antipruritic activity [52]. Urea has been included as an ingredient in several hand cream formulations since the 1940s [53]. In addition, it has been successfully used in combination with hydrocortisone, retinoic acid, and other ingredients to facilitate the cutaneous penetration of these agents [54, 55]. However, despite such findings in the mid-to-late 1980s, skepticism lingered regarding the ability of urea to promote such action. In 2005, the Cosmetic Ingredient Review (CIR) Expert Panel declared that urea does indeed have the capacity to enhance the percutaneous absorption of other chemicals and, further, that urea is safe for use in cosmetic products [56]. Regarding its humectant activity, a 3-week double-blind study comparing 3–10 % urea cream revealed the study formulations to be more effective in ameliorating clinical signs of dry skin than the vehicle control. Both creams successfully reduced scaling and enhanced hydration. The 3 % cream caused the skin to appear gold or yellow and had no impact on TEWL, whereas the 10 % cream reduced TEWL, although subjects reported the creams to be equally effective [57].

Hydroxy Acids

Alpha hydroxy acids (AHAs) are naturally occurring organic acids that have been discovered to display humectant and exfoliant activity. Glycolic and lactic acids, respectively derived from sugar cane and sour milk, are the AHAs most often used in moisturizing products and were the first ones to become commercially available. Citric, malic, and tartaric acids are among the other AHAs. Topical preparations that contain AHAs were demonstrated more than 40 years ago to confer significant effects on epidermal keratinization [58]. Nearly 20 years ago, glycolic acid was shown to act as a photoprotective agent [59]. Salicylic acid, the only beta hydroxy acid (BHA), is derived from willow bark, wintergreen leaves, and sweet birch. BHA functions as a chemical exfoliant and is found in synthetic form in several topical formulations [60]. At the lowest levels of the SC, corneocyte cohesiveness is attacked and eroded by AHAs and BHA, influencing pH in the process, as these ingredients break down desmosomes, thus contributing to desquamation [61, 62].

Lactic acid is an AHA as well as a component of NMF. Lactic acid was first used as part of the dermatologic armamentarium in 1943 for the treatment of ichthyosis [63]. Since then, in vitro and in vivo experiments have demonstrated that lactic acid can augment ceramide synthesis by keratinocytes [53, 64]. This moisturizing AHA ingredient has also been shown to combat signs of photoaging. Specifically, 8 % L-lactic acid was found to be superior to the vehicle in a double-blind vehicle-controlled study, with statistically significant improvements measured in sallowness, skin coarseness, and blotchiness [65].

Emollients

Emollients are substances that fill in the gaps between desquamating corneocytes, yielding a smooth skin surface [42]. In addition, emollient formulations improve cohesion, flattening out the curled edges of individual corneocytes [43]. A smoother skin surface, in turn, lessens friction while enhancing light refraction. Emollients are composed primarily of lipids and oils and may also fall into the categories of occlusives or humectants. Emollients are included in cosmetics to hydrate, soften, and smooth the skin. Emollient ingredients are divided into classes of compounds, including those that exhibit astringent, desiccating, fatting, protective, and protein-rejuvenating activity [49].

Reports of adverse effects linked to moisturizing agents are very rare; reactions are more likely to be due to other ingredients added to the formula. There have been reports of allergic contact dermatitis associated with products that contain preservatives, perfumes, solubilizers, sunscreens, and some other classes of compounds. Specifically, cases of contact dermatitis associated with lanolin, propylene glycol, vitamin E, and Kathon CG have been reported [66, 67].

Collagen and Polypeptide Ingredients

It is important for physicians and patients to know that the preponderance of collagen "extracts" contained in the host of expensive moisturizers touted for the capacity to restore collagen lost due to aging has a molecular weight of 15,000–50,000 Da, but only compounds with a molecular weight of 5000 Da or less can actually penetrate the SC [46]. In other words, these products cannot deliver on their advertised claims of replacing collagen. However, the collagen and other hydrolyzed proteins and polypeptides yield a temporary film on the epidermis that, upon drying, fills in surface depressions and other irregularities. Essentially, the film generated by these products provides a subtle stretching out of fine skin wrinkles. Using a humectant product can further enhance the fuller or somewhat plumper appearance created by collagen and polypeptide ingredients. Formulations that contain collagen and polypeptide ingredients have little or no effect on TEWL but are usually labeled as moisturizers and firming creams.

Skin Sensitivity: The Sensitive (S) to Resistant (R) Continuum

Sensitive skin is defined as skin that is susceptible to inflammation, while resistant skin is not. Individuals with resistant skin rarely experience acne, rosacea, stinging skin, or contact/irritant dermatitis. Although resistant skin is as likely to sunburn as other skin types, it has less of a chance of inflammation due to other causes (such as allergens, irritants, and friction) as compared to sensitive skin types. In terms of skin care product usage, resistant skin might be considered a double-edged sword, because individuals with resistant skin can use most skin care products without experiencing inflammation or irritation, but products may demonstrate less efficacy because of less ingredient penetration through resistant skin. Individuals with resistant skin will achieve better efficacy when hydroxy acids or penetration-enhancing ingredients are added to the skin care regimen.

Sensitive skin is an increasingly common complaint, which may be due in part to the popularity of botanical ingredients and fragrances that can incite an allergic response [68]. Sensitive skin can be accurately categorized into four discrete subtypes: Type 1 (acne type) exhibits the proclivity to develop acne; Type 2 (rosacea type) has the propensity to experience facial redness; Type 3 (stinging type) suffers from episodes of stinging or burning sensations; and Type 4 (allergic type) is prone to allergic and irritant reactions resulting in erythema, pruritus, and skin flaking. Such variations in sensitive skin characteristics present treatment challenges to the consumer as products marketed for "sensitive skin" are not specific about which subtype they are formulated for and therefore not suitable for all sensitive skin subtypes. The four subtypes of sensitive skin share one salient quality: inflammation. Consequently, any sensitive skin treatment program must focus on reducing and eradicating inflammation and should be undertaken under the care of a physician who is knowledgeable about the underlying etiology of the sensitive skin subtypes. Patients may suffer simultaneously from more than one sensitive subtype, thus requiring more complex treatment regimens.

Acne Type

Acne is estimated to affect 40–50 million people in the USA annually [69] and is easily the most common skin disease [70]. Teenagers and adult women are particularly susceptible. The confluence of four primary factors has been implicated in the pathogenesis of acne including elevated sebum production, a buildup of incompletely desquamated keratinocytes inside the hair follicles, the presence of *Propionibacterium acnes* bacteria, and inflammation. The characteristic cycle of acne is the adherence of dead keratinocytes in the hair follicles due to augmented sebum production, leading to comedones and increased levels of *P. acnes*, followed by initiation of inflammatory cascades by toll-like receptors and other cell signaling mechanisms. Initiation of the inflammatory response results in the development of papules and pustules. The acne cycle from buildup of keratinocytes in the hair follicle to the resulting pustule typically takes 8 weeks. For this reason, acne treatment regimens must include continuous preventative measures in order to break the acne cycle.

Acne therapy targets the four primary etiologic factors: decreasing sebum production (with retinoids or oral contraceptives), unclogging pores (with retinoids or hydroxy acids), stabilizing keratinization (with retinoids and hydroxy acids), eliminating bacteria (with benzoyl peroxide, antibiotics, antimicrobials, blue light, or silver), and reducing inflammation.

Rosacea Type

Approximately 16 million Americans, usually adults between 25 and 60 years of age, are affected by rosacea [71]. Rosacea overlaps with acne because many rosacea sufferers also exhibit papules and pustules in addition to characteristic facial redness, flushing, and the formation of prominent telangiectasias. Although the pathophysiology of rosacea remains to be elucidated, there are many unproven hypotheses about the cause(s). Recent topical vasoconstrictive medications have been used to successfully treat the facial flushing of rosacea through alpha-agonist activity; however, these treat the symptoms rather than the underlying cause of rosacea. In addition to vasoconstrictive topical medications, rosacea therapy should focus on addition of anti-inflammatory ingredients to the diet and skin care regimen. Triggers such as spicy and hot food and/or alcohol should also be avoided. Moisturizers, serums, and oils used on the face in these patients should include anti-inflammatory ingredients such as aloe vera, argan oil, arnica, chamomile, colloidal oatmeal, cucumber extract, feverfew, grape seed extract, licochalcone, licorice extract, niacinamide, salicylic acid, sulfacetamide, sulfur, and zinc [72]. These should be combined with oral and topical prescription medications and vascular laser therapies to slow progression of this bothersome disorder.

Stinging Type

In reaction to various triggers, some people experience a stinging sensation, which is a nonallergic neural sensitivity. The stinging propensity, or patients characterized as "stingers," can be identified through various available tests. In particular, the lactic acid stinging test is well regarded and established as a method for assessing patients who report invisible and subjective cutaneous irritation. The problem is that not all patients sting in response to the same substance. For example, one patient might sting to lactic acid, while another stings when in contact with benzoic acid. For this reason, historical data are more accurate at identifying a "stinger" than any physical test. It is worth noting that the stinging response seen in these patients is not necessarily associated with erythema; many patients experience stinging without exhibiting redness or other visible skin changes [73]. However, rosacea patients often associate facial flushing with a sensation of stinging or burning, especially when exposed to lactic acid [74]. Patients that are confirmed to have the stinging subtype of sensitive skin should be advised to avoid topical products containing the following ingredients: AHAs (particularly glycolic acid), ascorbic acid, benzoic acid, bronopol, cinnamic acid compounds, Dowicil 200, formaldehyde, lactic acid, propylene glycol, quaternary ammonium compounds, sodium lauryl sulfate, sorbic acid, or urea. When patients desire a form of vitamin C, they can tolerate ascorbyl phosphate much better than ascorbic acid because ascorbic acid is formulated at a low pH, which leads to stinging in susceptible patients. It is worth noting that any patient who is beginning a retinoid may exhibit stinging to almost all ingredients including water during the first few weeks of retinoid therapy initiation, but this is transient and will resolve once the skin has acclimated to the retinoid.

Allergic Type

An epidemiologic survey in the UK published in 2004 reported that 23 % of women and 13.8 % of men displayed adverse reactions to a personal care product (e.g., deodorants and perfumes, skin care products, hair care products, and nail cosmetics) over the course of 1 year [75]. More recently, in a 1999–2006 Brazilian study of 176 patients (154 women and 22 men) who were seen in a private office and complained of dermatoses resulting from cosmetics, 45 % had dermatoses linked to cosmetics, and 14 % had skin lesions that were found to be caused by inappropriate use of cosmetics [76]. In addition, several studies have demonstrated that about 10 % of dermatologic patients who are patch tested for 20–100 ingredients exhibit allergic sensitivity to at least one ingredient common in cosmetic products [75]. Fragrances and preservatives are the most common allergens, and women aged 20–60 years old represent the demographic group that experiences the majority of these reactions [77]. Individuals that are overexposed to skin care products and patients with an impaired SC, as manifested by dry skin, reportedly have increased susceptibility to allergic reactions [78]. These findings underscore both the significance of the allergic subtype as well as the need for matching skin type and skin care products, which the BSTI facilitates.

Treatment Approaches for Sensitive Skin

The treatment of sensitive skin depends on the underlying subtype. It is crucial that the type of sensitive skin be identified and that the patient be referred to a physician who can offer a prescription medication combined with the proper skin care regimen to treat the particular type of sensitive skin. Those patients that suffer from acne will require antimicrobial ingredients and retinoids, while those that suffer from redness will need to avoid causative agents and add prescription rosacea medications, anti-inflammatory foods, supplements, and skin care products to their daily regimen. Patients undergoing procedures such as surgery or laser treatments need to discuss pre- and postoperative skin care measures with their physicians to avoid complications from their sensitive skin. In some cases, silver-containing pillowcases and other textiles in combination with skin care products can be used to reduce symptoms.

Skin Pigmentation: The Pigmented (P) to Nonpigmented (N) Continuum

This skin type parameter refers not to skin color but to the tendency to develop dyschromia (hyperpigmentation), mainly on the face or chest. Within the BSTS, pigmentary conditions that can be ameliorated using topical formulations or minor dermatologic procedures include ephelides, melasma, post-inflammatory hyperpigmentation, and solar lentigos. Congenital nevi, seborrheic keratoses, and other skin lesions that require excision or treatment beyond topical skin care are outside the scope of the BSTS system. The mechanisms of pigmentation should be clearly understood in order to prepare physicians to prevent and treat these anxiety-producing pigmentary conditions.

The enzymatic breakdown of tyrosine by tyrosinase into dihydroxyphenylalanine (DOPA) and then dopaquinone ultimately results in the production of the skin pigment melanin, specifically the two melanin types eumelanin and pheomelanin [79]. Melanin is produced by melanocytes utilizing the enzyme tyrosinase and then transferred via melanosomes to keratinocytes. Melanogenesis can be induced by UV exposure and infrared heat. Melanin production represents the cutaneous defense against the insult of UV and infrared irradiation because when melanocytes accelerate melanin synthesis and transfer it to keratinocytes [80], the melanin surrounds and protects cellular DNA from damage. This is visually noted as skin darkening or tanning [81].

The melanocytes, each of which are typically attached to about 30 keratinocytes, load melanin into melanosomes and then transfer the melanosomes into keratinocytes through the PAR-2 receptor [82]. PAR-2 is believed to regulate melanosome transfer and thus pigmentation, through interactions between keratinocytes and melanocytes [83].

Cutaneous pigmentation can be hindered via three primary pathways: inhibition of tyrosinase, blocking of the PAR-2 receptor, or exfoliation of the melanin-containing keratinocytes. Hydroquinone, vitamin C, kojic acid, arbutin, mulberry extract, and licorice extract are examples of ingredients that inhibit tyrosinase. Soybean trypsin inhibitor (STI) and Bowman-Birk inhibitor (BBI), which are proteins contained in natural soy, have been found to suppress skin pigmentation development. STI and BBI have also been shown, in vitro and in vivo, to prevent UV-induced pigmentation [84]. Melanosome transfer into keratinocytes is influenced by STI and BBI by dint of their inhibition of the cleavage of PAR-2. The introduction of niacinamide, a vitamin B_3 derivative, has also been demonstrated to impede the transfer of melanosomes to keratinocytes [85]. Soy and niacinamide, which are considered the most effective PAR-2 blockers, are the most commonly used topical agents for inhibiting melanin transfer to keratinocytes. Not all soy is able to block PAR-2, but a complete discussion of soy is beyond the scope of this chapter [86].

In addition to the tyrosinase inhibitors and PAR-2 blockers, exfoliating agents such as AHAs, BHA, and retinoids can sufficiently accelerate cell turnover to outpace melanin synthesis. A broad-spectrum sunscreen and sun-protective clothing should also be included in any skin care regimen intended to diminish or eliminate the development of undesired dyschromias. The most effective way to prevent pigmentary and other harmful changes to the skin is to practice sun and heat avoidance, within reason. A "P" skin type designation in the BSTS correlates with the presence of dyschromia and the need for skin-lightening ingredients, while the "N" designation implies that the skin is even toned.

Skin Aging: The Wrinkled (W) to Tight (T) Continuum

Exogenous and endogenous factors play considerable roles in the complex, multifactorial process of cutaneous aging. Extrinsic aging, which results from chronic exposure to various environmental insults, particularly UV radiation, is affected by lifestyle choices such as tanning or smoking. Natural intrinsic aging is genetically driven, or cellularly programmed, and is thus inevitable until the genes responsible are identified and understood. Both pathways ultimately manifest in visible skin alterations, particularly wrinkles, lost elasticity, and skin fragility and thinning.

The BSTI questionnaire identifies "W" or wrinkle-prone individuals based on their habits and chronological age. Individuals with the following habits are more likely to develop wrinkles because of the cellular damage that these habits cause: excessive sugar intake, smoking, exposure to pollution, poor nutrition, tanning bed use, increased stress, lack of sleep, and – the biggest culprit – solar exposure. The diverse mechanisms through which UV radiation results in damage to the skin include the development of sunburn cells, as well as pyrimidine and thymine dimers, collagenase synthesis, loss of elastin, and the promotion of an inflammatory response. Aging and photodamage, in particular, have been associated with signaling through the p53 pathway after UV (especially UVB)-induced telomere disruption [87, 88]. Although much remains to be learned regarding the mechanisms by which UV irradiation initiates and promotes deleterious effects, UV (particularly UVA) irradiation is well known as the cause of photoaging, photocarcinogenesis, and photo-immunosuppression [89]. Insofar as UV irradiation impairs DNA and accelerates telomere shortening, this chief cause of extrinsic aging can be thought of as exerting an impact on the natural course of intrinsic aging.

The primary evidence of cutaneous aging is the development of rhytides (wrinkles), the formation of which is initiated in the lower dermal layers. It is important to note that few skin care formulations can actually penetrate far enough into the dermis or the deeper epidermis to reverse deep wrinkles, despite the multitude of products that tout such a capacity. Preventing loss of collagen, HA, and skin elasticity and at the same time coercing fibroblasts into increasing collagen and HA production is the primary focus of antiaging skin care [90]. Accordingly, topical products are formulated to prevent the degradation or promote the synthesis of the three primary skin constituents – collagen, elastin, and HA. Specifically, collagen production has been demonstrated to be promoted by topical preparations of retinoids, vitamin C, and copper peptides, as well as oral vitamin C [91–93]. The synthesis of HA has been shown in animal models to be stimulated by retinoids [94, 95], and HA levels are also thought to be enhanced through glucosamine supplementation [96]. Currently, no products have been shown to be effective, or approved, for spurring elastin synthesis.

Inflammation reduction is also a significant target for wrinkle prevention, because inflammation is known to influence the degradation of collagen, elastin, and HA. Antioxidants, which protect the skin through several mechanisms, are used in this approach to mitigate ROS activity. This is important because ROS act directly on growth factor and cytokine receptors in keratinocytes, and cutaneous inflammation can be initiated in these epidermal cells [97]. ROS can also contribute to glycation, a process by which a sugar is bound to a protein causing damage to the protein.

UV irradiation is the biggest culprit in aging, and it causes its harmful effects by initiating a cascade of events that result in downstream signal transduction by activating mitogen-activated protein (MAP) kinase pathways (extracellular signal-regulated kinase, c-jun N-terminal protein kinase, and p38). These then amass in cell nuclei, forming c-Fos/c-Jun complexes of transcription factor activator protein 1, and provoking the matrix metalloproteinases collagenase, 92 kDa gelatinase, and stromelysin to degrade collagen and other cutaneous connective tissue [98, 99].

The direct effects of ROS on cutaneous aging and the overall aging process are less clearly understood. In 2003, Kang et al. demonstrated that ROS activation of MAP kinase pathways induces collagenase production, thus contributing to collagen degradation [99]. The use of antioxidants is believed to block these pathways, thus inhibiting the process of photoaging by preventing collagenase synthesis and its ensuing deleterious impact on collagen. Specifically, Kang et al. found that the pretreatment of human skin with the antioxidants genistein and N-acetyl cysteine hindered UV induction of the cJun-driven enzyme collagenase.

The vast array of topical skin care products include antioxidants such as vitamins C and E, coenzyme Q_{10}, argan oil, caffeine, coffeeberry, ferulic acid, feverfew, ginger, grape seed extract, green tea, idebenone, mushrooms, phloretin, polypodium leucotomos, pomegranate, pycnogenol, resveratrol, rosemary, and silymarin [100]. The antioxidant capacity of these compounds is well established in the literature; however, their efficacy in topical formulations designed to reverse or diminish the cutaneous signs of aging is unclear because long-term aging prevention is difficult to prove. Antioxidant use should be combined with several practical measures including avoiding/limiting solar exposure (especially from 10 am to 4 pm), using broad-spectrum sunscreen on a daily basis, avoiding cigarette smoke and pollution, eating a diet high in fruits and vegetables, taking oral antioxidant supplements and topical antioxidant formulations, regular use of topical retinoids, reduction of sugar in the diet, and averaging 7 h of sleep per night in addition to stress reduction activities. In the near future, technological innovations in tissue engineering and gene therapy may lead to breakthroughs in the therapeutic uses of growth factors, cytokines, and telomerase [101], including dermatologic applications. At this time, stem cells and peptides are not associated with sufficient scientific data to support their use in topical skin care geared to treat wrinkle-prone skin.

Skin Care Regimens Based on Baumann Skin Type

Assessing the four skin type dichotomies together, as discussed above, provides insight into the simultaneous state or tendencies of an individual's skin along four different spectra, yielding 16 different possible skin type phenotypes (Table 2). Each of the individual Baumann Skin Types requires a regimen designed specifically for its needs. For example, formulations containing ingredients with the capacity to repair the skin barrier and provide anti-inflammatory activity would be appropriate selections for a person with dry, sensitive, nonpigmented, tight skin (DSNT). In addition to barrier repair and anti-inflammatory ingredients, DSNW (dry, sensitive, nonpigmented, wrinkle-prone) skin would require antiaging ingredients such as ascorbic acid and retinol. However, ascorbic acid and retinol can cause stinging and retinoid dermatitis in the susceptible DSNW skin types; therefore, the order of delivery of the agents is essential. In this example, retinoids should be applied after a moisturizer that contains both occlusive and barrier repair ingredients, which will decrease retinol penetration and minimize side effects. The moisturizer should also contain anti-inflammatory ingredients. In each skin type, the regimen steps are adjusted to maximize efficacy and decrease adverse events. Particular care is taken in choosing the order in which products are applied so that the ingredient interactions are maximized. The actions of ingredients can be greatly altered by pH, exposure to oxidizing agents, interaction with other ingredients, and exposure to penetration inhibitors or enhancers. All of these effects must be taken into account when choosing the steps of the skin care regimen.

Environmental conditions, diet, exercise, sleep, and stress can impact skin type by affecting the barrier, cortisol levels, and inflammatory cascades. For this reason, it is recommended that individuals take a baseline BSTI questionnaire and retake the test when stress, significant life changes, or cutaneous symptoms are present. Specifically, stress, pregnancy, menopause, exposure to variable climates or moving to a different climate, and various other significant exogenous or endogenous alterations can manifest in skin type changes. Essentially, if the skin care regimen stops working, it is time to retake the BSTI questionnaire. With baseline and updated BSTI scores, a physician is better equipped to arrive at a more holistic, integrated, or informed skin type assessment and treatment approach.

Summary

The use of the Baumann Skin Typing System (BSTS), based on the results of the Baumann Skin Type Indicator (BSTI), a self-administered questionnaire, allows for the evaluation of skin according to four dichotomous spectra – dry or oily, sensitive or resistant, pigmented or nonpigmented, and wrinkled or tight (unwrinkled). The BSTI is only available through physicians and is used to develop preset regimens for patients. By developing the regimens ahead of time and using a consistent methodology to diagnose skin type and prescribe skin care, outcomes are improved through staff and patient education. The discussion that arises from the use of the BSTI can also improve the physician–patient relationship, with such communication serving also to educate the patient about the importance of proper skin care. The BSTS is also used in research trials to select what types of patients are most likely to benefit from a cosmeceutical ingredient. The Fitzpatrick skin typing system is another skin type classification system that categorizes skin according to the skin's response to ultraviolet light. The Glogau photoaging scale classifies skin according to the level of skin aging. Patients self-classify their skin as dry, oily, combination, or sensitive, but there is much disparity about the meaning of each of these. Studies show that patients self-classify incorrectly, especially along the realms of oily versus dry [102]. Researchers and cosmetic scientists should take the time to properly categorize the skin type of the subjects used in cosmeceutical research studies so that the efficacy of ingredients can be properly evaluated. Scientific advances are happening rapidly, and more advanced ingredients are expected to enter the market in the next 5 years. These may include ingredients designed to address genetic deficiencies, the immune system, or organelles such as lysosomes or mitochondria.

References

1. Freedonia. Cosmeceuticals to 2015 – Demand and sales forecasts, market share, market size, market leaders. Available at: http://www.freedoniagroup.com/Cosmeceuticals.html. Accessed 11 May 2015.
2. PR Newswire. Cosmeceuticals: products and global markets. Business Week online, 12 Aug 2013. Available at: http://www.prnewswire.com/news-releases/cosmeceuticals-products-and-global-markets-219303311.html. Accessed 11 May 2015.
3. Baumann L. The skin type solution. New York: Bantam Dell; 2006.
4. Baumann LS, Penfield RD, Clarke JL, Duque DK. A validated questionnaire for quantifying skin oiliness. J Cosmet Dermatol Sci App. 2014;4:78–84.
5. Baumann L. Understanding and treating various skin types: the Baumann skin type indicator. Dermatol Clin. 2008;26:359–73.
6. Baumann L. Dry skin. In: Baumann L, Saghari S, Weisberg E, editors. Cosmetic dermatology: principles and practice. 2nd ed. New York: McGraw-Hill; 2009. p. 83–93.
7. Elias PM. Stratum corneum defensive functions: an integrated view. J Invest Dermatol. 2005;125(2):183–200.
8. Wildnauer RH, Bothwell JW, Douglass A. Stratum corneum biomechanical properties. I. Influence of relative humidity on normal and extracted human stratum corneum. J Invest Dermatol. 1971;56(1):72–8.
9. Orth D, Appa Y. Glycerine: a natural ingredient for moisturizing skin. In: Loden M, Maibach H, editors. Dry skin and moisturizers. Boca Raton: CRC Press; 2000. p. 214–7.
10. Rawlings A, Hope J, Rogers J, et al. Skin dryness-what is it? J Invest Dermatol. 1993;100:510.
11. Baumann L. Barrier repair ingredients. In: Cosmeceuticals and cosmetic ingredients. New York: McGraw-Hill; 2014. p. 54–6.
12. Park BD, Youm JK, Jeong SK, Choi EH, Ahn SK, Lee SH. The characterization of molecular organization of multilamellar emulsions containing pseudoceramide and type III synthetic ceramide. J Invest Dermatol. 2003;121:794–801.
13. Ekholm IE, Brattsand M, Egelrud T. Stratum corneum tryptic enzyme in normal epidermis: a missing link in the desquamation process? J Invest Dermatol. 2000;114(1):56–63.
14. Man MQM, Feingold KR, Thornfeldt CR, Elias PM. Optimization of physiological lipid mixtures of barrier repair. J Invest Dermatol. 1996;106:1096–101.
15. Elias PM. The epidermal permeability barrier: from the early days at Harvard to emerging concepts. J Invest Dermatol. 2004;122(2):xxxvi–ix.
16. Scott IR, Harding CR. Filaggrin breakdown to water binding compounds during development of the rat stratum corneum is controlled by the water activity of the environment. Dev Biol. 1986;115(1):84–92.
17. Sato J, Denda M, Chang S, Elias PM, Feingold KR. Abrupt decreases in environmental humidity induce abnormalities in permeability barrier homeostasis. J Invest Dermatol. 2002;119(4):900–4.
18. Wang F, Feng XC, Li YM, Yang H, Ma TH. Aquaporins as potential drug targets. Acta Pharmacol Sin. 2006;27(4):395–401.
19. Sougrat R, Morand M, Gondran C, Barre P, Gobin R, Bonte F, Dumas M, Verbavatz JM. Functional expression of AQP3 in human skin epidermis and reconstructed epidermis. J Invest Dermatol. 2002;118(4):678–85.
20. Takenouchi M, Suzuki H, Tagami H. Hydration characteristics of pathologic stratum corneum – evaluation of bound water. J Invest Dermatol. 1986;87(5):574–6.
21. Warner RR, Bush RD, Ruebusch NA. Corneocytes undergo systematic changes in element concentrations across the human inner stratum corneum. J Invest Dermatol. 1995;104(4):530–6.
22. Warner RR, Myers MC, Taylor DA. Electron probe analysis of human skin: element concentration profiles. J Invest Dermatol. 1988;90(1):78–85.
23. Warner RR, Myers MC, Taylor DA. Electron probe analysis of human skin: determination of the water concentration profile. J Invest Dermatol. 1988;90(2):218–24.
24. Ma T, Hara M, Sougrat R, Verbavatz J, Verkman AS. Impaired stratum corneum hydration in mice lacking epidermal water channel aquaporin-3. J Biol Chem. 2002;277(19):17147–53.
25. Yang B, Verkman AS. Water and glycerol permeabilities of aquaporins 1–5 and MIP determined quantitatively by expression of epitope-tagged constructs in Xenopus oocytes. J Biol Chem. 1997;272(26):16140–6.
26. Baumann L. Cosmetics and skin care in dermatology. In: Goldsmith LA, Katz SI, Gilchrest BA, et al., editors. Fitzpatrick's dermatology in general medicine, vol. 2. 8th ed. New York: McGraw-Hill; 2012. p. 3010.

27. Thiboutot D. Regulation of human sebaceous glands. J Invest Dermatol. 2004;123(1):1–12.
28. Clarys P, Barel A. Quantitative evaluation of skin surface lipids. Clin Dermatol. 1995;13 (4):307–21.
29. Thody AJ, Shuster S. Control and function of sebaceous glands. Physiol Rev. 1989;69(2):383–416.
30. Elias PM, Fritsch PO, Lampe M, Williams ML, Brown BE, Nemanic M, Grayson S. Retinoid effects on epidermal structure, differentiation, and permeability. Lab Invest. 1981;44(6):531–40.
31. Gomez EC. Differential effect of 13-cis-retinoic acid and an aromatic retinoid (Ro 10–9359) on the sebaceous glands of the hamster flank organ. J Invest Dermatol. 1981;76(1):68–9.
32. Geiger JM. Retinoids and sebaceous gland activity. Dermatology. 1995;191(4):305–10.
33. Mathers WD, Lane JA. Meibomian gland lipids, evaporation, and tear film stability. Adv Exp Med Biol. 1998;438:349–60.
34. Tiffany JM. The role of meibomian secretion in the tears. Trans Ophthalmol Soc UK. 1985;104 (Pt 4):396–401.
35. Fluhr JW, Mao-Qiang M, Brown BE, Wertz PW, Crumrine D, Sundberg JP, Feingold KR, Elias PM. Glycerol regulates stratum corneum hydration in sebaceous gland deficient (asebia) mice. J Invest Dermatol. 2003;120(5):728–37.
36. Fluhr JW, Gloor M, Lehmann L, Lazzerini S, Distante F, Berardesca E. Glycerol accelerates recovery of barrier function in vivo. Acta Derm Venereol. 1999;79(6):418–21.
37. Pochi PE, Strauss JS, Downing DT. Age-related changes in sebaceous gland activity. J Invest Dermatol. 1979;73(1):108–11.
38. Walton S, Wyatt EH, Cunliffe WJ. Genetic control of sebum excretion and acne – a twin study. Br J Dermatol. 1988;118(3):393–6.
39. Vogel CA, Balkrishnan R, Fleischer AB, Cayce KA, Feldman SR. Over-the-counter topical skin care products – a common component of skin disease management. Cutis. 2004;74(1):55.
40. Morrison D. Petrolatum. In: Loden M, Maibach H, editors. Dry skin and moisturizers. Boca Raton: CRC Press; 2000. p. 251.
41. Spruit D. The interference of some substances with the water vapour loss of human skin. Dermatologica. 1971;142(2):89–92.
42. Draelos Z. Moisturizers. In: Draelos Z, editor. Atlas of cosmetic dermatology. New York: Churchill Livingstone; 2000. p. 83–5.
43. Kraft JN, Lynde CW. Moisturizers: what they are and a practical approach to product selection. Skin Therapy Lett. 2005;10(5):1–8.
44. Kligman AM. The myth of lanolin allergy. Contact Dermatitis. 1998;39(3):103–7.
45. Hannuksela M. Glycols. In: Loden M, Maibach H, editors. Dry skin and moisturizers. Boca Raton: CRC Press; 2000. p. 413–5.
46. Wehr RF, Krochmal L. Considerations in selecting a moisturizer. Cutis. 1987;39(6):512–5.
47. Idson B. Dry skin: moisturizing and emolliency. Cosmet Toiletr. 1992;107:69.
48. Mitsui T, editor. New cosmetic science. New York: Elsevier; 1997. p. 134.
49. Chernosky ME. Clinical aspects of dry skin. J Soc Cosmet Chem. 1976;65:376.
50. Orth D, Appa Y, Contard E, et al. Effect of high glycerin therapeutic moisturizers on the ultrastructure of the stratum corneum. Poster presentation at the 53rd annual meeting of the American Academy of Dermatology, New Orleans Feb 1995.
51. Baumann L. Glycerin. In: Cosmeceuticals and cosmetic ingredients. New York: McGraw-Hill; 2014. p. 74.
52. Kligman AM. Dermatologic uses of urea. Acta Derm Venereol. 1957;37(2):155–9.
53. Harding C, Bartolone J, Rawlings A. Effects of natural moisturizing factor and lactic acid isomers on skin function. In: Loden M, Maibach H, editors. Dry skin and moisturizers. Boca Raton: CRC Press; 2000. p. 217–36.
54. Wohlrab W. The influence of urea on the penetration kinetics of topically applied corticosteroids. Acta Derm Venereol. 1984;64(3):233–8.
55. Wohlrab W. Effect of urea on the penetration kinetics of vitamin A acid in human skin. Z Hautkr. 1990;65 (9):803–5.
56. The Cosmetic Ingredient Review (CIR) Expert Panel. Final report of the safety assessment of Urea. Int J Toxicol. 2005;24 Suppl 3:1–56.
57. Serup J. A double-blind comparison of two creams containing urea as the active ingredient. Assessment of efficacy and side-effects by non-invasive techniques and a clinical scoring scheme. Acta Derm Venereol Suppl (Stockh). 1992;177:34–43.
58. Van Scott EJ, Yu RJ. Control of keratinization with alpha hydroxy acids and related compounds. I. Topical treatment of ichthyotic disorders. Arch Dermatol. 1974;110(4):586–90.
59. Perricone NV, Dinardo JC. Photoprotective and antiinflammatory effects of topical glycolic acid. Dermatol Surg. 1996;22(5):435–7.
60. Draelos ZD. Rediscovering the cutaneous benefits of salicylic acid. Cosm Derm Suppl. 1997;10(4).
61. Van Scott EJ, Yu R. Hyperkeratinization, corneocyte cohesion, and alpha hydroxy acids. J Am Acad Dermatol. 1984;11(5 Pt 1):867–79.
62. Berardesca E, Distante F, Vignoli GP, et al. Alpha hydroxyacids modulate stratum corneum barrier function. Br J Dermatol. 1997;137(6):934–8.
63. Stern E. Topical application of lactic acid in the treatment and prevention of certain disorders of the skin. Urol Cutaneous Rev. 1943;50:106.
64. Rawlings AV, Davies V, Carlomusto M, et al. Effect of lactic acid isomers on keratinocyte ceramide synthesis, stratum corneum lipid levels and stratum corneum barrier function. Arch Dermatol Res. 1996;288 (7):383–90.

65. Stiller MJ, Bartolone J, Stern R, et al. Topical 8 % glycolic acid and 8 % L-lactic acid creams for the treatment of photodamaged skin. A double-blind vehicle-controlled clinical trial. Arch Dermatol. 1996;132(6):631–6.
66. Gonzalo MA, de Argila D, Garcia JM, et al. Allergic contact dermatitis to propylene glycol. Allergy. 1999;54(1):82–3.
67. Baumann LS, Spencer J. The effects of topical vitamin E on the cosmetic appearance of scars. Dermatol Surg. 1999;25(4):311–5.
68. Draelos ZD. Cosmetic selection in the sensitive-skin patient. Dermatol Ther. 2001;14:194.
69. http://www.wrongdiagnosis.com/a/acne/prevalence.htm#prevalence_intro. Accessed 16 May 2015.
70. National Institute of Arthritis and Musculoskeletal and Skin Diseases. Available at http://www.niams.nih.gov/Health_Info/Acne/default.asp. Accessed 16 May 2015.
71. National Rosacea Society. Available at: http://www.rosacea.org/index.php. Accessed 16 May 2015.
72. Brown DJ, Dattner AM. Phytotherapeutic approaches to common dermatologic conditions. Arch Dermatol. 1998;134(11):1401–4.
73. Basketter DA, Griffiths HA. A study of the relationship between susceptibility to skin stinging and skin irritation. Contact Dermatitis. 1993;29(4):185–8.
74. Lonne-Rahm SB, Fischer T, Berg M. Stinging and rosacea. Acta Derm Venereol. 1999;79(6):460–1.
75. Orton DI, Wilkinson JD. Cosmetic allergy: incidence, diagnosis, and management. Am J Clin Dermatol. 2004;5(5):327–37.
76. Duarte I, Campos Lage AC. Frequency of dermatoses associated with cosmetics. Contact Dermatitis. 2007;56(4):211–3.
77. Mehta SS, Reddy BS. Cosmetic dermatitis – current perspectives. Int J Dermatol. 2003;42(7):533–42.
78. Jovanovic M, Poljacki M, Duran V, Vujanovic L, Sente R, Stojanovic S. Contact allergy to compositae plants in patients with atopic dermatitis. Med Pregl. 2004;57(5–6):209–18.
79. Freedberg IM, Eisen AZ, Wolff K, et al., editors. Fitzpatrick's dermatology in general medicine. 5th ed. New York: McGraw-Hill; 1999. p. 996.
80. Hermanns JF, Petit L, Martalo O, Pierard-Franchimont C, Cauwenbergh G, Pierard GE. Unraveling the patterns of subclinical pheomelanin-enriched facial hyperpigmentation: effect of depigmenting agents. Dermatology. 2000;201(2):118–22.
81. Wakamatsu K, Kavanagh R, Kadekaro AL, Terzieva S, Sturm RA, Leachman S, Abdel-Malek Z, Ito S. Diversity of pigmentation in cultured human melanocytes is due to differences in the type as well as quantity of melanin. Pigment Cell Res. 2006;19(2):154–62.
82. Jimbow K, Sugiyama S. Melanosomal translocation and transfer. In: Nordlund JJ et al., editors. The pigmentary system. Physiology and pathophysiology. New York: Oxford University Press; 1998.
83. Seiberg M, Paine C, Sharlow E, Andrade-Gordon P, Costanzo M, Eisinger M, Shapiro SS. Inhibition of melanosome transfer results in skin lightening. J Invest Dermatol. 2000;115(2):162–7.
84. Paine C, Sharlow E, Liebel F, Eisinger M, Shapiro S, Seiberg M. An alternative approach to depigmentation by soybean extracts via inhibition of the PAR-2 pathway. J Invest Dermatol. 2001;116(4):587–95.
85. Hakozaki T, Minwalla L, Zhuang J, Chhoa M, Matsubara A, Miyamoto K, Greatens A, Hillebrand GG, Bissett DL, Boissy RE. The effect of niacinamide on reducing cutaneous pigmentation and suppression of melanosome transfer. Br J Dermatol. 2002;147(1):20–31.
86. Baumann L. Soy. In: Cosmeceuticals and cosmetic ingredients. New York: McGraw-Hill; 2014. p. 129–34.
87. Kosmadaki MG, Gilchrest BA. The role of telomeres in skin aging/photoaging. Micron. 2004;35(3):155–9.
88. Kappes UP, Luo D, Potter M, Schulmeister K, Runger TM. Short- and long-wave UV light (UVB and UVA) induce similar mutations in human skin cells. J Invest Dermatol. 2006;126(3):667–75.
89. Marrot L, Belaïdi JP, Meunier JR. Importance of UVA photoprotection as shown by genotoxic related endpoints: DNA damage and p53 status. Mutat Res. 2005;571(1–2):175–84.
90. Baumann L. How to prevent photoaging? J Invest Dermatol. 2005;125(4):xii–xiii.
91. Varani J, Warner RL, Gharaee-Kermani M, Phan SH, Kang S, Chung JH, Wang ZQ, Datta SC, Fisher GJ, Voorhees JJ. Vitamin A antagonizes decreased cell growth and elevated collagen-degrading matrix metalloproteinases and stimulates collagen accumulation in naturally aged human skin. J Invest Dermatol. 2000;114(3):480–6.
92. Nusgens BV, Humbert P, Rougier A, Colige AC, Haftek M, Lambert CA, Richard A, Creidi P, Lapiere CM. Topically applied vitamin C enhances the mRNA level of collagens I and III, their processing enzymes and tissue inhibitor of matrix metalloproteinase 1 in the human dermis. J Invest Dermatol. 2001;116(6):853–9.
93. Kockaert M, Neumann M. Systemic and topical drugs for aging skin. J Drugs Dermatol. 2003;2(4):435–41.
94. Margelin D, Medaisko C, Lombard D, Picard J, Fourtanier A. Hyaluronic acid and dermatan sulfate are selectively stimulated by retinoic acid in irradiated and nonirradiated hairless mouse skin. J Invest Dermatol. 1996;106(3):505–9.
95. Tajima S, Hayashi A, Suzuki T. Elastin expression is up-regulated by retinoic acid but not by retinol in chick embryonic skin fibroblasts. J Dermatol Sci. 1997;15(3):166–72.
96. Matheson AJ, Perry CM. Glucosamine: a review of its use in the management of osteoarthritis. Drugs Aging. 2003;20(14):1041–60.

97. Fitzpatrick RE. Endogenous growth factors as cosmeceuticals. Dermatol Surg. 2005;31(7 Pt 2):827–31.
98. Fisher GJ, Voorhees JJ. Molecular mechanisms of photoaging and its prevention by retinoic acid: ultraviolet irradiation induces MAP kinase signal transduction cascades that induce Ap-1-regulated matrix metalloproteinases that degrade human skin in vivo. J Investig Dermatol Symp Proc. 1998;3(1):61–8.
99. Kang S, Chung JH, Lee JH, Fisher GJ, Wan YS, Duell EA, Voorhees JJ. Topical N-acetyl cysteine and genistein prevent ultraviolet-light-induced signaling that leads to photoaging in human skin in vivo. J Invest Dermatol. 2003;120(5):835–41.
100. Baumann L, Allemann IB. Antioxidants. In: Baumann L, Saghari S, Weisberg E, editors. Cosmetic dermatology: principles and practice. 2nd ed. New York: McGraw-Hill; 2009. p. 292–311.
101. Ostler EL, Wallis CV, Aboalchamat B, Faragher RG. Telomerase and the cellular lifespan: implications of the aging process. J Pediatr Endocrinol Metab. 2000;13 Suppl 6:1467–76.
102. Youn SW, Kim SJ, Hwang IA, Park KC. Evaluation of facial skin type by sebum secretion: discrepancies between subjective descriptions and sebum secretion. Skin Res Technol. 2002;8:168–72.

Part IX

Skin Health, Nutrition, Resilience, Rejuvenation, and Management of Aging Skin

Preventive Skin Care During Skin Aging

118

Andrea Lichterfeld, Elisabeth Hahnel, Ulrike Blume-Peytavi, and Jan Kottner

Contents

A. Lichterfeld (✉) • E. Hahnel • U. Blume-Peytavi • J. Kottner
Department of Dermatology and Allergy, Clinical Research Center for Hair and Skin Science, Charité-Universitätsmedizin Berlin, Berlin, Germany
e-mail: andrea.lichterfeld@charite.de; elisabeth.hahnel@charite.de; ulrike.blume-peytavi@charite.de; jan.kottner@charite.de

M.A. Farage et al. (eds.), *Textbook of Aging Skin*,
DOI 10.1007/978-3-662-47398-6_133

Abstract

Aging causes various anatomical, physiological, and psychological changes. Skin aging can be broadly conceptualized into intrinsic and extrinsic aging. The geriatric population is particularly vulnerable for developing certain skin diseases. The prevalence of pathological skin diseases increases substantially with age. The most prevalent skin diseases in aged populations are fungal infections including onychomycosis and tinea pedis, various forms of dermatitis and xerosis cutis with pruritus, as well as actinic keratosis, benign skin tumors, and pressure ulcers. Prevention is a powerful strategy to avoid, to delay, and/or to treat diseases at first clinical signs. Prevention of skin health can be defined as interventions to support skin barrier function and to restore or increase immune function and protection of the skin across the life span. This concept includes primary, secondary, and tertiary prevention. Primary skin health prevention includes activities to protect healthy individuals from skin diseases. Lifelong sun protection, for example, reduces the risk for the development of accelerated extrinsic skin aging and cancer. Secondary skin prevention is the early diagnosis and treatment of existing skin diseases, e.g., skin cancer screenings. Targeted interventions and therapies for the stabilization and avoidance of deterioration of skin diseases is tertiary skin health prevention, e.g., treatment of incontinence associated dermatitis. A formal and well-implemented skin health preventive approach across the life span might reduce the frequency and severity of cutaneous problems and diseases.

Introduction

The world population is growing and aging. Nearly 12.3 % of the world population are aged over 60 years and this proportion will grow up to 17.6 % in 2050 [1]. Associated with these demographic changes, the prevalence of chronic diseases and functional limitations is increasing [2, 3]. Aging causes various anatomical, physiological, and psychological changes. Morphological alterations become especially visible on the skin in terms of wrinkles, sagging, or dyspigmentation [4]. Skin aging can be broadly conceptualized into intrinsic and extrinsic aging. Extrinsic factors are, for instance, excessive sun exposure, smoking, or environmental influences. Intrinsic skin aging can be regarded as natural biological changes occurring over time leading to thinning of the epidermis, increase of skin surface pH, and vascular changes. Aged skin with reduced elasticity, increased fragility, and altered immune response may have a substantial impact on psychosocial well-being besides the primarily perceived "cosmetic" problems of "looking old" [5–7].

The prevalence of skin diseases like fungal infections, xerosis cutis with pruritus, dermatitis, skin cancer, pressure ulcers, and skin tears increases substantially with age [2, 8]. Age-related skin diseases are an upcoming health issue in the future, especially in the light of increasing numbers of multimorbid patients and the growing complexity of care [9]. The geriatric population is particularly vulnerable for skin diseases [10–12].

Prevention is a powerful strategy to avoid, to delay, and/or to treat diseases at first clinical signs [13]. This concept includes primary, secondary, and tertiary prevention. Primary prevention focuses on the avoidance and reduction of risks for the development of diseases in healthy individuals (e.g., vaccination). Secondary prevention is the early diagnosis and therapy of diseases that already occurred with the aim to stop the process early and to prevent deterioration (e.g., cancer screening). Therapies and interventions for the improvement and stabilization of diseases are dedicated to tertiary prevention with the aim to prevent degradation and loss of function [14, 15]. This approach is well established, for instance, in the management of chronic diseases like heart failure [16, 17]. In dermatology, such formal preventive approaches are applied in occupational dermatology (e.g., [18]) or in skin cancer management (e.g., [19]). However, a comprehensive skin health preventive approach across the human life course has not been developed so far.

Functional Capacity

Besides morphological changes, skin and tissue aging leads to the loss of functional capacity [20]. Functional capacity is the ability of complex biological systems to cope with external stress. A decline and the ultimate loss of functional capacity is a common feature of (complex) aging biological systems. The concept of functional capacity or vitality goes back to Ruiz-Torres et al. [21] and it can be applied to human aging in general and specifically to skin aging. Figure 1 describes the development of the functional capacity of the skin during the life course. After birth, individuals are more or less comparable in terms of skin structure and function. Immediately after birth, the skin adapts, grows, and matures (e.g., [22]) to achieve its biological optimum. After this optimum follows a period of decline leading eventually to "skin failure" [23]. Based on this simplified model several conclusions can be drawn: (1) Aging and skin aging are not diseases. They are normal biological processes occurring nearly everywhere in nature. Because skin aging is not a disease, it must not be treated. (2) Due to the reduced functional capacity, very young and aged skin is at increased risk to develop cutaneous problems. (3) Intrinsic and extrinsic factors may increase the vitality and prolong the period of optimal functioning or accelerate the functional decline (e.g., due to accumulation of risks).

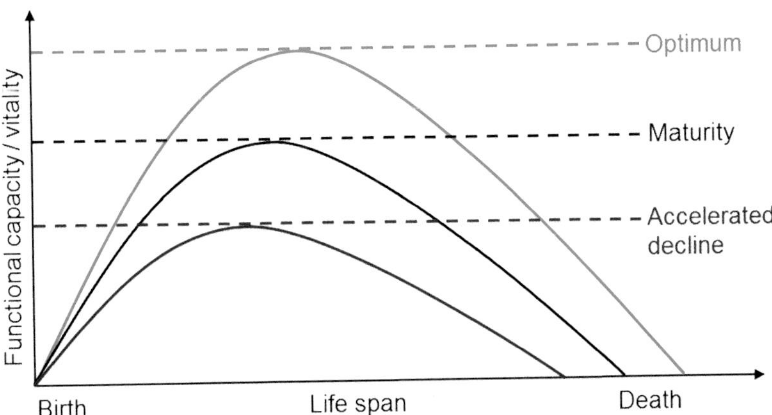

Fig. 1 Variance of skin aging

Table 1 Selected age-related skin and subcutaneous tissue changes and clinical relevance (e.g., [27, 28])

	Changes	Risks and conditions
Skin surface	Increase of pH	Pathologic colonization and infection Reduced cohesion of the corneocytes within the stratum corneum
Epidermis	Reduced stratum corneum hydration Altered intercellular lipid composition and corneocyte morphology Reduced barrier function Reduced number and function of melanocytes and Langerhans cells Dysregulation of cytokine function Change of number and function of antimicrobial peptides Reduced activity of basal cells and reduced epidermal turnover	Xerosis cutis, itch Increased susceptibility against physical, chemical, and biological insults ("immunosenescence") Increased risks for actinic keratosis and tumors Delayed epithelialization and barrier recovery
Dermoepidermal junction	Flattening	Increased risk for shear-type injuries (skin tears) and blister development
Dermis	Reduced number of dermal papillae Reduced sensory perception Reduced dermal circulation and PIV Reduced collagen production	Increased risk for injuries (e.g., due to heat) and ulceration Delayed wound healing Altered thermoregulation
Subcutis	Atrophy	Increased risk for injuries and pressure ulcers

Nevertheless, skin aging is a biological process exhibiting a wide range of variability.

Clinical Relevance of Skin Aging

Based on the age-related changes of the skin and underlying soft tissues there is an increased risk to develop adverse skin diseases. In Table 1, selected examples are given for the clinical relevance of skin aging. For instance, there is an age-associated increase of the skin surface pH. This leads to decreased stratum corneum cohesion, disturbed skin barrier recovery, and to an increased susceptibility to pathologic colonization and infection [24, 25]. Other examples are the reduced water and altered lipid content, reduced sebum production, and a decrease of natural moisturizing factors of the stratum corneum causing dry skin and itch [12]. Due to diminished immune responses, aged skin reacts more slowly to irritants and allergens but is more susceptible to infections [26].

The Epidemiology of Skin Diseases in the Aged

The epidemiological prevalence and incidence figures are useful parameters to indicate disease risks and frequencies. Prevalence is defined as "the number of affected persons present in the population at a specific time divided by the number of persons in the population at that specific time" [29]. Incidence is defined as "the number of new cases of a disease that occur during a specific time period divided by the number of cases who are at risk in the defined time period" [29]. Both concepts are relevant for obtaining information about frequencies and impact of diseases, for example, for public health decisions.

Table 2 provides a brief overview of selected prevalence and incidence figures of the most common skin diseases in aged populations. Based on the available epidemiological literature, the following skin diseases are most prevalent in aged populations: fungal infections including onychomycosis and tinea pedis, various forms of dermatitis and xerosis, as well as actinic keratosis, benign skin cancer, and pressure ulcers.

Fungal Infections

Fungal infections of the skin and nails are usually caused by two groups of yeasts (pityrosporum and candida), one group of dermatophytes [30], and rarely nondermatophyte molds [31]. Reported prevalence of fungal skin infections ranges from 10.4 % [32] to 49.7 % [2].

Tinea pedis and onychomycosis (Figs. 2 and 3) are the most common fungal infections. The current literature shows that these mainly dermatophytic infections range from 3.7 % [33] to 33 % [2] for tinea pedis and from 17.9 % [33] to 47.7 % [34] for onychomycosis.

Dermatitis and Eczema

Generally, dermatitis is an umbrella term for various eczematous skin changes. In aged populations, contact dermatitis, atopic dermatitis, and eczema are especially relevant [9, 11]. The prevalence of dermatitis in general ranges from 14.4 % [35] to 58.7 % [36] in clinical settings. The prevalence of atopic dermatitis is lower ranging from 0.4 % [37] to 4.4 % [8]. The current literature shows prevalences up to 19.8 % [38] for contact dermatitis and up to 39 % [39] for eczema in hospitals in aged populations.

Xerosis Cutis

The available evidence suggests that dry skin (Xerosis cutis L85.3, Figs. 4 and 5) is one of the most frequent skin diseases in the elderly. In ambulatory and outpatient settings, the prevalence of xerosis cutis ranges from 5.4 % [32] to 77 % [40]. The proportions of care receivers in hospitals and long-term care with xerosis cutis are higher ranging between 30 % [41], 50 % [42], and 85 % [43].

A higher severity of xerosis cutis is associated with older age and, for example, related to polypharmacy [12]. Xerosis cutis is the primary cause of pruritus [44]. There is a clear association between dry skin and pruritus, which is one of the most distressing and burdensome skin symptoms in the aged [9]. In community and outpatient care settings, the prevalence of pruritus ranges from 1 % [45] to 36 % [46]. The prevalence of pruritus in long-term care ranges between 10 % [2], 29 % [43], and 70 % [47]. The severity and duration of chronic pruritus is also associated with quality of life and emotional well-being [48].

Skin Tumors

The current evidence of neoplastic changes like benign or malignant tumors in the elderly shows prevalence rates from 1.7 % [8] to 18.6 % [49]. This wide range includes seborrheic keratosis (Fig. 6) and soft fibromas as benign tumors. For malignant tumors, basal cell carcinomas (Figs. 7 and 8), squamous cell carcinoma, malignant melanoma, and cutaneous T-cell lymphoma are common. Less often are B-cell lymphomas

Table 2 Overview of most common skin diseases in the aged (65+ years)

Disease	Prevalence (%)	Incidence (%)	Source
Fungal infections	49.7	–	Kiliç et al., 2008
	38.0	–	Liao et al., 2001
	15.8	–	Yalçin et al., 2006
	14.3	–	Perera et al., 2000
	10.4	–	Bilgili et al., 2012
Onychomycosis	47.7	–	Gunduz et al., 2013
	40.0	–	Nkjondo Minkoumou et al., 2012
	36.6	–	Kiliç et al., 2008
	36.3	–	Liao et al., 2001
	17.9	25.7	Piérard et al., 2001
Tinea pedis	33.0	–	Kiliç et al., 2008
	11.4	–	Djeridane et al., 2006
	3.7	–	Piérard et al., 2001
Dermatitis	58.7	–	Liao et al., 2001
	22.9	–	Perera et al., 2000
	20.4	–	Yalçin et al., 2006
	14.4	–	Rubegni et al., 2012
Xerosis	77.0	–	Tindall and Smith, 1963
	55.6	–	Paul et al., 2011
	45.3	–	Kiliç et al., 2008
	5.4	–	Bilgili et al., 2012
Pruritus	18.9	–	Rubegni et al., 2012
	14.4	–	Liao et al., 2001
	11.5	–	Yalçin et al., 2006
	10.3	–	Kiliç, 2008
	8.8	–	Bilgili, 2012
Actinic keratosis	32.8	–	Templier et al., 2015
	29.3	–	Kiliçet al., 2008
	28.7	–	Memon et al., 2000
	4.7–24.2	–	Flohil et al., 2013
Benign tumors	18.6	–	Perera et al., 2000
	13.5	–	Rubegni et al., 2012
	12.8	–	Liao et al., 2001
	1.7	–	Yalçin et al., 2006
Malignant tumors	13.2	–	Rubegni et al., 2012
	5.2	–	Yalçin et al., 2006
	2.1	–	Liao et al., 2001
Pressure ulcer	46	–	Davis and Caseby, 2001
	15.6	–	Bours et al., 2002
	13.6	6.2	Baumgarten et al., 2006
	10.3	–	Baumgarten et al., 2003
	8.1	28.9	Kwong et al., 2009
	1	–	Kiliç et al., 2008
IAD	22.6	–	Long et al., 2012
	–	3.4	Zimmaro-Bliss et al., 2006
Skin tears	19.8	–	Lopez et al., 2011
	–	43.1	Carville et al., 2014
	–	29	Alessi et al., 2002

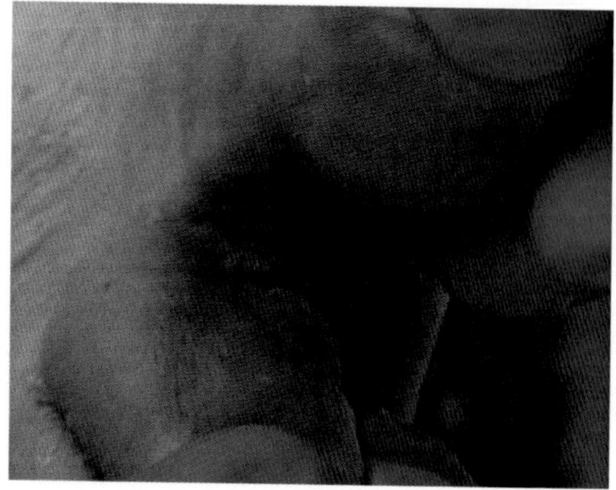

Fig. 2 Interdigital mycosis

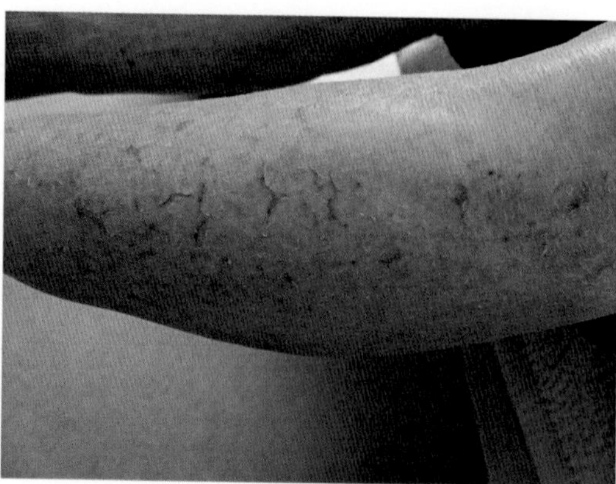

Fig. 4 Xerosis cutis and eczema craquelé

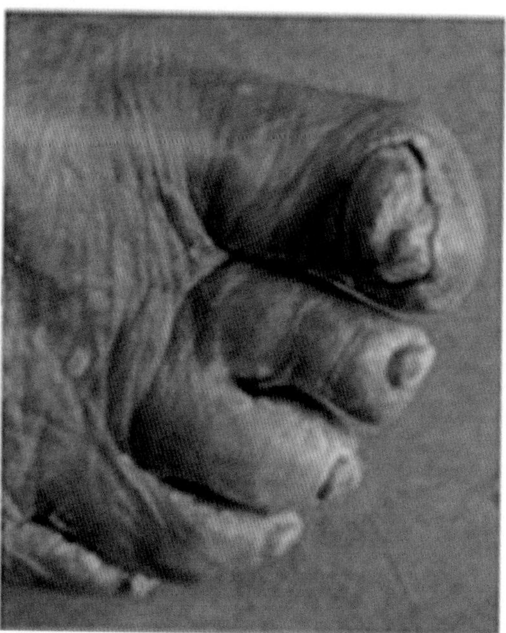

Fig. 3 Onychomycosis

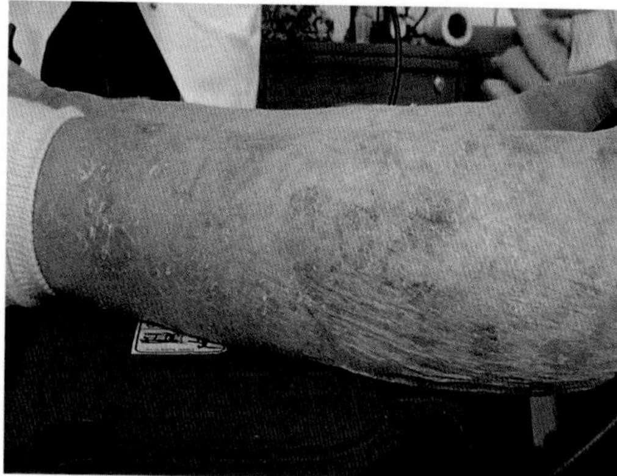

Fig. 5 Xerosis cutis and eczematous changes

with a prevalence of 2.1 % [36] or cutaneous metastases with a prevalence of 1.4 % [35].

Evidence indicates that the prevalence of actinic keratosis, a chronic damage of the epidermis, which is mainly caused by prolonged UV radiation, increases significantly above the age of 54 years [50]. The prevalence of this in situ squamous cell carcinoma of the skin ranges from 4.7 % [51] to 32.8 % [52] in domesticity and

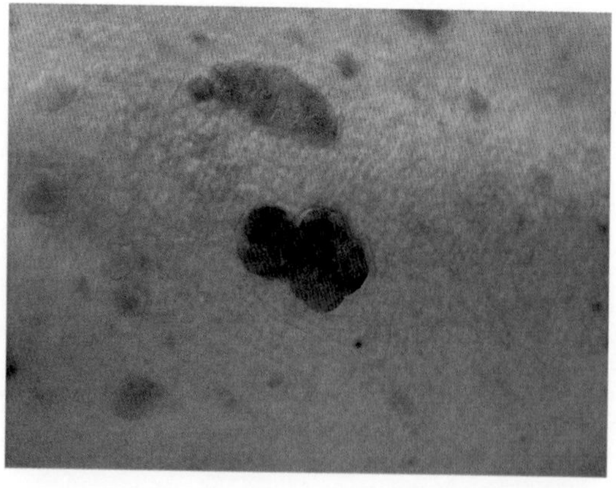

Fig. 6 Seborrheic keratosis

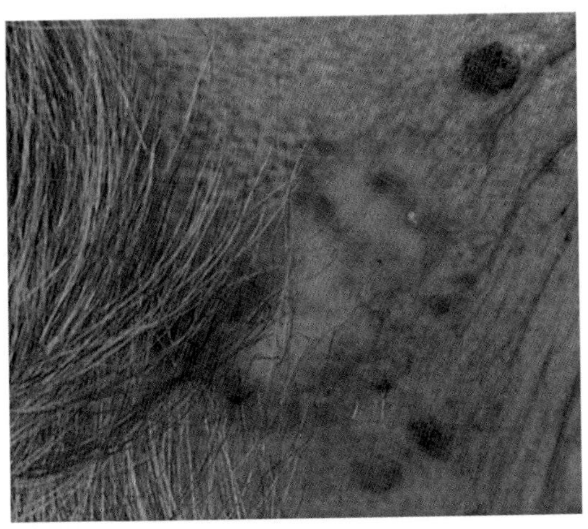

Fig. 7 Superficial basal cell carcinoma (BCC) in the temporal region

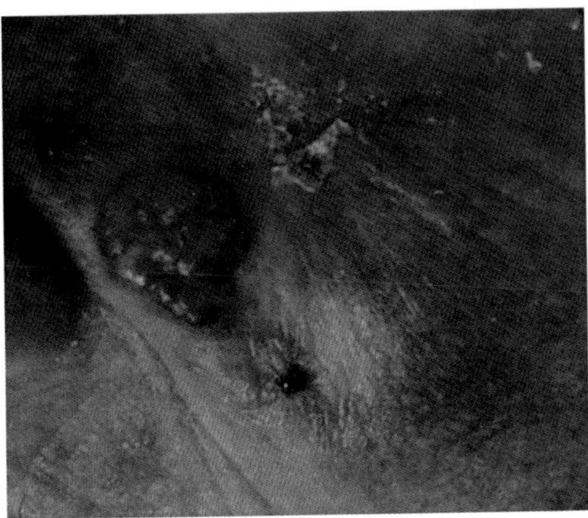

Fig. 8 BCC of the nodular type on the cheek

hospital settings. In institutional long-term care, the prevalence was reported to be 29.3 % [2].

Pressure Ulcers, Skin Tears, and Incontinence Associated Dermatitis

Advanced age, functional and cognitive impairments, and impaired mobility are the key risk factors for the so-called geriatric syndromes like delirium or falls [53] which may be associated with skin diseases like incontinence associated dermatitis (Fig. 9), intertrigo (Figs. 10 and 11), skin tears, or pressure ulcers [54, 55].

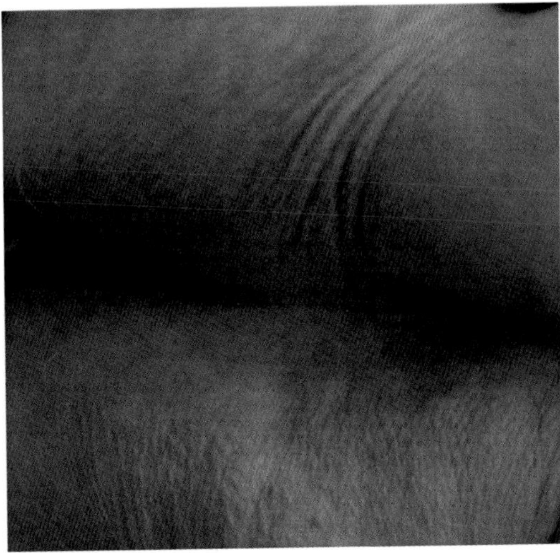

Fig. 9 Incontinence associated dermatitis

Pressure ulcers are usually categorized into four categories ranging from nonblanchable erythema, to full thickness tissue loss [56]. Reported prevalence ranges from 1 % [2] to 46 % [57] in long-term care settings. Prevalence figures for hospital settings are lower ranging from 1.8 % [58] to 30 % [59]. Incidence figures range from 6.2 % [60] to 28.9 % [61]. Up to 47 % of pressure ulcer sites are at the sacrum and 16.5 % at the heels [60].

Prevalence and incidence figures of incontinence associated dermatitis and skin tears are rare. Reported prevalence in institutional long-term care for incontinence associated dermatitis is 22.6 % [62] and 19.8 % [63] for skin tears. The current evidence shows incidence rates from 29 % [64] to 43.1 % [65] for skin tears and 3.4 % [66] for incontinence associated dermatitis.

Preventive Skin Care

The selected epidemiological figures presented above clearly indicate the high burden of skin disease in the elderly. Therefore, skin health prevention might be an option, to decrease the frequencies and severity of cutaneous problems in the elderly. There is an overlap between the concepts

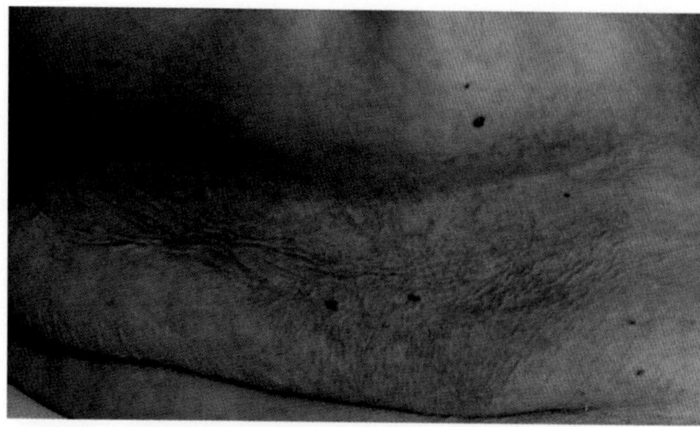

Fig. 10 Manifestation of intertrigo in the submammary fold

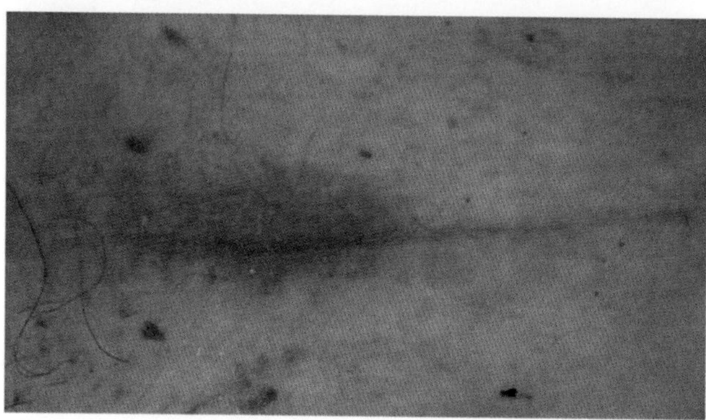

Fig. 11 Manifestation of intertrigo in the groin

of health promotion and prevention. Health promotion has the overall aim to promote and strengthen resources to maintain health. Prevention is primarily considered to reduce the risk of disease manifestation. Applying these general considerations to the skin, prevention can be defined as interventions to support skin barrier function and to restore or increase immune function and protection of the skin. In this context, skin care is defined as skin cleansing and caring in order to maintain and improve the skin barrier function and integrity of healthy skin or skin deemed at risk for damage. Skin care practices include washing, bathing, showering with or without cleansing products, and application of leave-on products such as lotions, creams, or ointments [3, 67, 68].

Primary Preventive Skin Care

Primary skin prevention activities aims to protect healthy individuals against skin diseases. Lifelong sun protection, for example, reduces the risk for the development of skin cancers (e.g., [69]). The avoidance of excessive personal hygiene and skin-damaging soaps reduces the risk for occurrence of xerosis cutis and skin infections. Skin care is regarded as a major strategy, especially for children and aged or geriatric persons, for maintaining skin barrier function, skin integrity, and skin health.

Secondary Preventive Skin Care

Secondary skin prevention is the early diagnosis and treatment of existing skin diseases. Skin cancer screening services help to detect cancers in the early development. In dry skin, frequent washing and bathing should be avoided. The bathing duration should be no more than 5 min once daily in lukewarm water [3, 67]. A general advice is that cleansing the skin with traditional soap and water should be avoided. Traditional alkaline soap should be replaced by syndet soaps. Syndets contain milder synthetic surfactants compared to traditional soaps and have pH-values of 4–5 that is more compatible with the acid mantle of healthy skin. Cleansers containing humectants like urea or glycerin should be preferred. Skin care products should be used after consideration of the individual skin condition. Lipid and humectant containing leave-on products should be applied to dry skin areas at least twice a day. In severe dry skin, the application should be more frequent [3]. Skin in "humid" areas (e.g., between the toes) should be dried carefully but thoroughly after cleaning. In special cases, moisture absorbent deposits can be used (e.g., under the breasts or in skin folds). In humid skin (e.g., urine or fecal incontinence) or areas (e.g., skin folds, under the breasts) a protectant should be applied. Barrier creams including occlusive ingredients like dimethicone or petrolatum have protective effects especially in prevention of incontinence associated dermatitis and skin tears. The skin of incontinent patients should be cleaned after every incontinent episode and protected with a barrier cream before and after exposure to urine and/or feces [68].

Tertiary Preventive Skin Care

Adequate interventions and therapies for stabilization and avoidance of deterioration of skin diseases are performed by tertiary skin prevention activities, e.g., treatment of incontinence associated dermatitis, skin tears, or present wounds (e.g., [70, 71]). Table 3 and Fig. 12 provide an overview of the three preventive categories, possible interventions, and settings in relation to the model of functional capacity of the skin during life course.

The levels of prevention are not static [15]. Preventive skin care strategies are important across the entire life span. However, skin diseases get greater emphasis in older age and the sense of urgency increases in later stages of life.

Conclusion

The skin undergoes numerous morphological changes during aging. The risk of developing skin diseases increases with age. The prevalence of, e.g., xerosis cutis, benign skin cancers, or fungal infections significantly increases in the aged population. Epidemiological data indicate

Table 3 Preventive skin care: levels of prevention

Prevention stage	Primary	Secondary	Tertiary
Definition	Protection for healthy individuals from developing skin problems/ diseases	Interventions for early diagnosis and treatment of existing skin problems; self-examination and screening visits by a dermatologist for early detection of skin cancers; skin protection against lesions and wounds (e.g., skin tears, superficial pressure ulcers, and incontinence associated dermatitis in frail elderly patients)	Therapeutic and rehabilitative interventions if skin diseases are established
Intervention (examples)	UVR protection, skin protection, mild skin care practices, and healthy life style (e.g., no smoking)	Early screening services (e.g., skin cancer screening), dry skin management	Interventions and treatment of skin diseases (e.g., wound therapy, emollient therapy for dry skin control and maintaining skin integrity)
Settings (examples)	Kindergarten, school	Dermatological practices	Nursing homes, hospitals

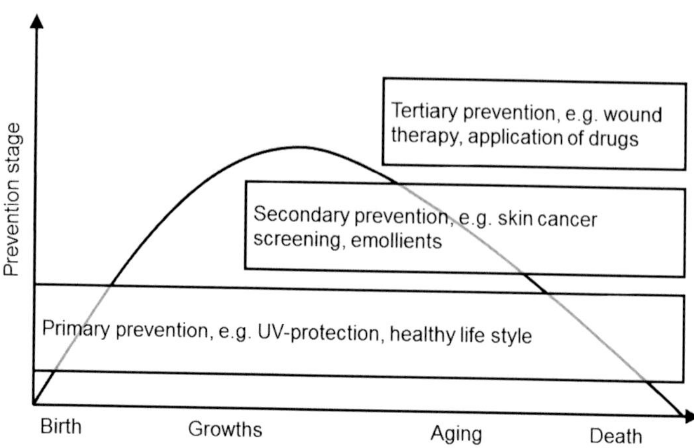

Fig. 12 Skin prevention during life course: Prevention stages

that there is an urgent need for preventive skin health strategies. Preventive approaches are well established for the management of chronic diseases like heart failure. A preventive approach for skin care does not exist so far. The empirical evidence supporting certain skin health preventive activities is heterogeneous. A preventive approach for skin health from birth to death is first formally described in this chapter. It consists of primary, secondary, and tertiary prevention. This approach can enhance the functional capacity of the skin during life span. The aim of this preventive approach is to reduce the frequency and severity of cutaneous problems and diseases during life span.

References

1. United Nations, World population prospects, the 2015 revision. 2015. http://esa.un.org/unpd/wpp/. Accessed 25 Sept 2015.
2. Kilic A, et al. Dermatological findings in the senior population of nursing homes in Turkey. Arch Gerontol Geriatr. 2008;47(1):93–8.
3. Kottner J, et al. Maintaining skin integrity in the aged: a systematic review. Br J Dermatol. 2013;169 (3):528–42.
4. Dobos G, et al. Evaluation of skin ageing: a systematic review of clinical scales. Br J Dermatol. 2015;172 (5):1249–61.
5. Kligman AM. Psychological aspects of skin disorders in the elderly. Cutis. 1989;43(5):498–501.
6. Kligman AM, Koblenzer C. Demographics and psychological implications for the aging population. Dermatol Clin. 1997;15(4):549–53.
7. Farage MA, et al. Intrinsic and extrinsic factors in skin ageing: a review. Int J Cosmet Sci. 2008;30(2):87–95.
8. Yalcin B, et al. The prevalence of skin diseases in the elderly: analysis of 4099 geriatric patients. Int J Dermatol. 2006;45(6):672–6.
9. Hay RJ, et al. The global burden of skin disease in 2010: an analysis of the prevalence and impact of skin conditions. J Invest Dermatol. 2014;134(6):1527–34.
10. Diepgen TL. Demographic changes in Germany. Consequences in health policy and dermatology. Hautarzt. 2003;54(9):804–8.
11. Jafferany M, et al. Geriatric dermatoses: a clinical review of skin diseases in an aging population. Int J Dermatol. 2012;51(5):509–22.
12. White-Chu EF, Reddy M. Dry skin in the elderly: complexities of a common problem. Clin Dermatol. 2011;29(1):37–42.
13. National Public Health Partnership. The language of prevention. Melbourne: NPHP; 2006.
14. Brandes I, Walter U. Health in older age: cost of illness and cost-effectiveness of prevention. Z Gerontol Geriatr. 2007;40(4):217–25.
15. Kottner J, et al. Skin health promotion in the elderly. Z Gerontol Geriatr. 2015;48(3):231–6.
16. Grodin JL, Tang WH. Treatment strategies for the prevention of heart failure. Curr Heart Fail Rep. 2013;10(4):331–40.
17. Houston BA, et al. Volume overload in heart failure: an evidence-based review of strategies for treatment and prevention. Mayo Clin Proc. 2015;90(9):1247–61.
18. Mollerup A, et al. Effectiveness of the Healthy Skin Clinic – a randomized clinical trial of nurse-led patient counselling in hand eczema. Contact Dermatitis. 2014;71(4):202–14.
19. Holm RP, et al. Skin cancer prevention and screening. S D Med. 2015;Spec No:75–7, 79–81.
20. Ghadially R, et al. The aged epidermal permeability barrier. Structural, functional, and lipid biochemical abnormalities in humans and a senescent murine model. J Clin Invest. 1995;95(5):2281–90.

21. Ruiz-Torres A, et al. Measuring human aging using a two-compartmental mathematical model and the vitality concept. Arch Gerontol Geriatr. 1990;10(1):69–76.
22. Ludriksone L, et al. Skin barrier function in infancy: a systematic review. Arch Dermatol Res. 2014;306 (7):591–9.
23. Irvine C. 'Skin failure' – a real entity: discussion paper. J R Soc Med. 1991;84(7):412–3.
24. Behne MJ, et al. NHE1 regulates the stratum corneum permeability barrier homeostasis. Microenvironment acidification assessed with fluorescence lifetime imaging. J Biol Chem. 2002;277(49):47399–406.
25. Hachem JP, et al. pH directly regulates epidermal permeability barrier homeostasis, and stratum corneum integrity/cohesion. J Invest Dermatol. 2003;121 (2):345–53.
26. Castelo-Branco C, Soveral I. The immune system and aging: a review. Gynecol Endocrinol. 2014;30(1):16–22.
27. Al-Nuaimi Y, et al. Skin health in older age. Maturitas. 2014;79(3):256–64.
28. Farage MA, et al. Functional and physiological characteristics of the aging skin. Aging Clin Exp Res. 2008;20(3):195–200.
29. Gordis L. Epidemiology. 4th ed., Philadelphia: Elsevier Saunders; 2008. p. 466.
30. Martin ES, Elewski BE. Cutaneous fungal infections in the elderly. Clin Geriatr Med. 2002;18(1):59–75.
31. Loo DS. Cutaneous fungal infections in the elderly. Dermatol Clin. 2004;22(1):33–50.
32. Bilgili SG, et al. The prevalence of skin diseases among the geriatric patients in Eastern Turkey. J Pak Med Assoc. 2012;62(8):535–9.
33. Pierard G. Onychomycosis and other superficial fungal infections of the foot in the elderly: a pan-European survey. Dermatology. 2001;202(3):220–4.
34. Gunduz T, et al. Epidemiological profile of onychomycosis in the elderly living in the nursing homes European. Geriatr Med. 2013;5:172–4.
35. Rubegni P, et al. Skin diseases in geriatric patients: our experience from a public skin outpatient clinic in Siena. G Ital Dermatol Venereol. 2012;147(6):631–6.
36. Liao YH, et al. Pattern of skin diseases in a geriatric patient group in Taiwan: a 7-year survey from the outpatient clinic of a University Medical Center. Dermatology. 2001;203(4):308–13.
37. Furue M, et al. Prevalence of dermatological disorders in Japan: a nationwide, cross-sectional, seasonal, multicenter, hospital-based study. J Dermatol. 2011;38 (4):310–20.
38. Bilgili ME, et al. Prevalence of skin diseases in a dermatology outpatient clinic in Turkey. A cross-sectional, retrospective study. J Dermatol Case Rep. 2013;7(4):108–12.
39. Grover S, Narasimhalu CR. A clinical study of skin changes in geriatric population. Indian J Dermatol Venereol Leprol. 2009;75(3):305–6.
40. Tindall JP, Smith JG. Skin lesions of the aged and their association with internal changes. JAMA. 1963;186: 1039–42.
41. Weismann K, et al. Prevalence of skin diseases in old age. Acta Derm Venereol. 1980;60(4):352–3.
42. Lichterfeld A, Kottner J. Hautpflege. In: Dassen T, editor. Pflegeprobleme in Deutschland, Ergebnisse von 14 Jahren Forschung in Pflegeheimen und Kliniken 2001–2014. Berlin: Charité- Universitätsmedizin Berlin, Institute für Gesundheits- und Pflegewissenschaften; 2014. p. 30–8.
43. Beauregard S, Gilchrest BA. A survey of skin problems and skin care regimens in the elderly. Arch Dermatol. 1987;123(12):1638–43.
44. Berger TG, et al. Pruritus in the older patient: a clinical review. JAMA. 2013;310(22):2443–50.
45. Siragusa M, et al. Skin pathology findings in a cohort of 1500 adult and elderly subjects. Int J Dermatol. 1999;38(5):361–6.
46. Adam JE, Reilly S. The prevalence of skin disease in the geriatric age group. Australas J Dermatol. 1987;28 (2):72–6.
47. Fleischer AB, et al. Skin conditions and symptoms are common in the elderly: the prevalence of skin symptoms and conditions in an elderly population. J Geriatr Dermatol. 1996;4:78–87.
48. Matterne U, et al. Prevalence, correlates and characteristics of chronic pruritus: a population-based cross-sectional study. Acta Derm Venereol. 2011;91 (6):674–9.
49. Perera A, et al. Prevalence of skin diseases in suburban Sri Lanka. Ceylon Med J. 2000;5(3):123–8.
50. Schafer T, et al. The epidemiology of nevi and signs of skin aging in the adult general population: results of the KORA-survey 2000. J Invest Dermatol. 2006;126 (7):1490–6.
51. Flohil SC, et al. Prevalence of actinic keratosis and its risk factors in the general population: the Rotterdam Study. J Invest Dermatol. 2013;133(8):1971–8.
52. Templier C, et al. Systematic skin examination in an acute geriatric unit: skin cancer prevalence. Clin Exp Dermatol. 2015;40(4):356–60.
53. Inouye SK, et al. Geriatric syndromes: clinical, research, and policy implications of a core geriatric concept. J Am Geriatr Soc. 2007;55(5):780–91.
54. Kottner J, et al. Pressure ulcers: a critical review of definitions and classifications. Ostomy Wound Manage. 2009;55(9):22–9.
55. Gray M. Optimal management of incontinence-associated dermatitis in the elderly. Am J Clin Dermatol. 2010;11(3):201–10.
56. European Pressure Ulcer Advisory Panel, Pan Pacific Pressure Injury Alliance, National Pressure Ulcer Advisory Panel, Prevention and treatment of pressure ulcers: quick reference guide. Haesler E, editor. Osborne Park: Cambridge Media; 2014.
57. Davis CM, Caseby NG. Prevalence and incidence studies of pressure ulcers in two long-term care facilities in Canada. Ostomy Wound Manage. 2001;47 (11):28–34.
58. Eberlein-Gonska M, et al. The incidence and determinants of decubitus ulcers in hospital care: an analysis of

routine quality management data at a university hospital. Dtsch Arztebl Int. 2013;110(33–34):550–6.

59. Amlung SR, et al. The 1999 national pressure ulcer prevalence survey: a benchmarking approach. Adv Skin Wound Care. 2001;14(6):297–301.
60. Baumgarten M, et al. Pressure ulcers among elderly patients early in the hospital stay. J Gerontol A Biol Sci Med Sci. 2006;61(7):749–54.
61. Kwong EW, et al. Pressure ulcer development in older residents in nursing homes: influencing factors. J Adv Nurs. 2009;65(12):2608–20.
62. Long MA, et al. Incontinence-associated dermatitis in a long-term acute care facility. J Wound Ostomy Continence Nurs. 2012;39(3):318–27.
63. Lopez V, et al. Skin tear prevention and management among patients in the acute aged care and rehabilitation units in the Australian Capital Territory: a best practice implementation project. Int J Evid Based Healthc. 2011;9(4):429–34.
64. Alessi CA, et al. Incidence and costs of acute medical conditions in long-stay incontinent nursing home residents. J Am Med Dir Assoc. 2002;3(4):229–42.
65. Carville K, et al. The effectiveness of a twice-daily skin-moisturising regimen for reducing the incidence of skin tears. Int Wound J. 2014;11(4):446–53.
66. Zimmaro Bliss D, et al. Incontinence-associated skin damage in nursing home residents: a secondary analysis of a prospective, multicenter study. Ostomy Wound Manage. 2006;52(12):46–55.
67. Guenther L, et al. Pathway to dry skin prevention and treatment. J Cutan Med Surg. 2012;16(1):23–31.
68. Lichterfeld A, et al. Evidence-based skin care: a systematic literature review and the development of a basic skin care algorithm. J Wound Ostomy Continence Nurs. 2015;42(5):501–24.
69. Seite S, et al. Photodamage to human skin by suberythemal exposure to solar ultraviolet radiation can be attenuated by sunscreens: a review. Br J Dermatol. 2010;163(5):903–14.
70. Holroyd S, Graham K. Prevention and management of incontinence-associated dermatitis using a barrier cream. Br J Community Nurs. 2014; Dec; Suppl Wound Care:32–8.
71. Moradian S, Klapper AM. A novel way to treat skin tears. Int Wound J. 2015;[Epub ahead of print]. doi: 10.1111/iwj

119 Discovering the Link Between Nutrition and Skin Aging

Aikaterini I. Liakou, Apostolos Pappas, and Christos C. Zouboulis

Contents

Abstract

Current consumer trends have brought the nutritional supplements, among other antiaging products, into a high-profit enterprise. The main pillar of the marketing campaign is the pharmacological activity of nutrients that are called "nutraceuticals." Nutrition has long been associated with skin health, beauty, and aging. Although the frequency of nutritional deficiencies is low in the developed countries, incomplete diets could influence health and affect skin health. Oral supplementation with vitamins, trace minerals, and fatty acids has been shown in clinical studies to modulate skin function and possibly hair health. Vitamin, carotenoid, and fatty acid supplementation may prevent skin diseases. Vegetables, legumes, and olive oil may be protective against cutaneous actinic damage and skin wrinkling. Oral fish polysaccharide supplementation may improve dermal thickness, skin wrinkling, color, and viscoelasticity. Benefits on hydration, skin barrier, defense against inflammation, and skin roughness were reported under intake of essential fatty acids. Carotenoids (pro-vitamin A) as well as the vitamins C and E have been extensively associated with the protection of the skin against photodamage (sunburn, tanning) and subsequently photoaging, as well as precancerous conditions and cancers.

A.I. Liakou
Departments of Dermatology, Venereology, Allergology and Immunology, Dessau Medical Center, Dessau, Germany

University of Athens Medical School, Athens, Greece
e-mail: a.i.liakou@googlemail.com

A. Pappas
The Johnson & Johnson Skin Research Center, CPPW, a Division of Johnson & Johnson Consumer Companies, Inc, Skillman, NJ, USA
e-mail: apostolos_pappas@yahoo.com

C.C. Zouboulis (✉)
Departments of Dermatology, Venereology, Allergology and Immunology, Dessau Medical Center, Dessau, Germany
e-mail: christos.zouboulis@klinikum-dessau.de

M.A. Farage et al. (eds.), *Textbook of Aging Skin*,
DOI 10.1007/978-3-662-47398-6_134

Introduction

Current consumer trends have brought the antiaging industry and the consumer product companies (from nutritional supplements to skin care) into a billion dollar profit range that previously only drugs used to reach. Most of these products are tightly connected with the health, wellness, and needs of the twenty-first-century consumer. The main pillars of the marketing campaign and power behind these products are the pharmacological activity of a series of nutrients that are called "nutraceuticals." These nutrients do not include only vitamins but a variety of nonvitamin classified antioxidants as well.

Nutrition and Skin Health

Nutrition has long been associated with skin health, beauty, and aging, through multiple mechanisms and roles that yet have to be explored especially at a clinical setting. Health status, medications, drug abuse, stress, and malnutrition could have a tremendous impact in the pathophysiology of skin abnormalities and aging. Deficiencies in vitamins and essential fatty acids clearly result in cutaneous manifestations. Although the frequency of nutritional deficiencies is low in the western developed countries, unbalanced and incomplete diets could result from disease, aging, and chemical substance abuse that would certainly influence health and thereby affect the skin health [1, 2]. Correcting and optimizing a diet may not only prevent skin and hair problems but certainly also correct any potentially underlying condition. Studies investigating the effects of oral supplementation with relatively high doses of vitamins, trace minerals, and fatty acids have showed the possibility that diet components can modulate skin function and possibly hair health [1, 3]. Reviews on the effect of vitamin, carotenoid, and fatty acid supplementation for improving the skin condition and preventing skin diseases have been published outlining the nutritional factors that bring potential benefits on the skin [4]. Reports on food and nutrient intake that could influence skin aging have been published on actinic damage as well [5]. It was outlined that skin wrinkling could be associated with poor food habits and the high intake of vegetables, legumes, and olive oil seemed to be protective against cutaneous actinic damage.

A study with oral fish polysaccharides supplementation in an antioxidant mix has been shown to improve dermal thickness, skin wrinkling, color, and viscoelasticity after 8 weeks of supplementation [6]. When lycopene (6 mg), vitamin C (60 mg), and soy isoflavones (50 mg) were combined in a clinical setting benefits on skin density, skin firmness, and microrelief, hydration, and tone were reported in menopausal women [7, 8].

In addition, a study that introduced higher intake of vitamin C and linoleic acid, as well as lowered the intake of fat and carbohydrate, demonstrated an association with a general better skin appearance [9]. Green tea polyphenols applied topically have been shown to protect DNA and prevent other damaging effects of ultraviolet (UV) light such as sunburn response, immunosuppression, and photoaging of the skin [10]. Perhaps consumption of dietary flavonoids from tea may confer photoprotection and improve skin quality. Another set of nutritional promising studies are around the consumption of flavanol-rich cocoa that has a potential for photoprotection and therefore could certainly act against the UV-induced aging process [11–15].

Another important class of nutrients that could alter skin appearance and health is the essential fatty acids linoleic acid (LA) and α-linolenic acid (ALA) which are called essential since they are literally like vitamins, where they are solely acquired by the diet and our human cells lack their synthesis mechanism. The liver can biotransform LA to γ-linoleic acid (GLA); however, this rate of transformation can be reduced with aging or in subjects under psychological stress [16]. Human skin seems unable to synthesize GLA from its precursor LA since there is a lack of the δ-6 desaturase [17, 18] in epidermis and therefore we can speculate sensitivity to changes in the blood levels of GLA. The δ-5 and δ-6 desaturases are the rate-limiting enzymes in the formation of the long-chain polyunsaturated fatty acid metabolites (PUFAs) [19–21]. The genes fatty acid desaturase (FADS)1 and FADS2 [22] are respectively responsible for these activities and convert LA to GLA, which through a series of elongations and desaturations becomes arachidonic acid (AA). A human clinical study has demonstrated a profound effect of ingested LA and ALA, from borage and flaxseed oil respectively, in healthy women for 12 weeks [23]. Benefits on hydration, skin barrier, defense against inflammation, and skin roughness were reported in this study that allows us to consider that there are potential skin antiaging benefits from the ingestion of vegetable oils rich in these essential fatty acids. In addition, interesting epidemiological studies suggested that there is a link between multivitamin use and longer telomere length (a marker of biological aging) in women [24].

Vitamins with Antioxidant Activity (proA, C, E) Act Against Photoaging

One of the most studied in the world of dermatology vitamins with antioxidant activity are the carotenoids (pro-vitamin A) as well as the vitamins C and E, which have been extensively associated with the protection of the skin against photodamage (sunburn, tanning) and subsequently photoaging, as well as precancerous conditions and cancers.

Many reports have recently outlined the synergistic enhancement of oxidative damage to the skin when the skin is exposed to UVA and environmental irritants, including cigarette smoke [25, 26]. This cumulative damage could be responsible for unattractive premature aging of the skin, and more seriously to precancers and cancers of the skin. Visible signs of the premature skin aging are attributed to the repeated exposure of the skin to solar UV radiation, leading to the generation of oxidative free-radical molecules, which can damage cellular lipids, proteins, and DNA, thereby influencing cell survival or death [27]. Therefore UV radiation and the skin type of the individual exposed are important parameters for premature aging of the skin called photoaging [28]. Sunburn is also a phenomenon related to exposure to UV radiation. If the concentration of free radicals in the body exceeds a critical threshold elastic fibers in elastin and collagen can be damaged [29, 30]. Thus, enhancement of the antioxidative network of human skin is recommended [31–33].

Photoaging could compromise the skin appearance at an aged individual since it has been associated with mottled dark spots, wrinkles, and sagging skin. Since the majority of skin cancers and all photoaging are caused by sun exposure, effective sun protection can prevent this damage. Apparently less than 33 % of the population applies sunscreen regularly despite the current increased publicity promoting the need for protection [34].

The challenge with the vitamins C and E is that they could be in much higher concentrations in skin when applied topically rather than orally [35, 36]. Topical application of these vitamins over time is promising for repair and against photodamage. This could possibly happen either by enhancing collagen synthesis since vitamin C can directly correct the collagen loss that causes wrinkles [37] or by possible inhibition of the elastin biosynthesis by fibroblasts [38], which are hypothesis formulated by the cited in vitro studies.

Topical vitamin C has also been shown to enhance collagen production in human skin in vivo. Clinically, a significant decrease was observed in deep furrows which were further substantiated by silicone replicas and histology demonstrated elastic tissue repair. Possibly this happens via the enhanced synthesis of collagen and inhibition of metalloproteinase (MMP)-I decreases wrinkles [39]. In addition few controlled studies have directly compared the topical efficacy of the various forms of vitamin E for photoprotection against UV-induced erythema in rabbits [40, 41] and against UV-induced photoaging in mice [42]. In a long-term, 44-week, mouse study, two vitamin E forms, d-α-tocopherol and d-α-tocopheryl succinate, were proven effective in protecting against all acute and chronic UV-induced damage, with d-α-tocopherol most effective for all parameters (i.e., decreasing sunburn, tanning, skin cancer incidence) [36]. Some clinical evidence also has been published with registered benefits on skin tone and on the periorbital wrinkles besides the histological improvements but again for the topical d-α-tocopherol [43].

The literature on the effect of the various carotenoids on skin photoprotection is vaster than the aforementioned nutrients. The effects of dietary carotenoids in protecting the skin against the damaging effects of the UV exposure have been recently summarized by Thakkar et al. and certainly their efficacy in scavenging the UV-reactive oxygen species has been more extensively described. Therefore it is fair to assume that their proven presence in various skin components protects the skin from the photodamaged induced aging [44]. In addition, vitamin A and its natural metabolites have been approved for topical and systemic treatment of mild, moderate, and severe recalcitrant acne, as well as photoaging and biological skin aging [45].

Heinrich et al. demonstrated that skin roughness is reduced after systemic application of antioxidants [15]. In that study the ingestion of a nutritional supplement with various natural carotenoids, combined with selenium and vitamin E, over a period of 12 weeks resulted in a significant increase in skin density and thickness assessed by ultrasonography examination. The surface structure of the skin was positively influenced in general [46].

Long-Term Effects of Nutrition on Skin Aging Via Glycation

Proteins, such as collagen and elastin molecules, which apparently have long structures and residence in the dermis, in the presence of sugars undergo a series of nonenzymatic glycation and oxidation reactions that result in intra- and intermolecular cross-links.

Advanced glycation end products (AGEs) accumulate in the dermis as a function of chronological aging [47, 48]. Moreover, the rate of the AGE accumulation is higher in individuals with diabetes [49, 50], which is attributed to be the result of chronically high levels of glucose in the blood. This has been proven by fluorescence spectroscopy, which demonstrated AGE accumulation in the skin with aging [47, 48, 51].

Although it is well accepted that AGEs increase with aging and are in higher levels in diabetic patients, it remains controversial whether a diet high in carbohydrates could potentially accelerate the accumulation of AGEs in dermal collagen [52–54]. In experimental animal models, studies outlined that certain nutrients may prevent high rates of dermal AGE formation in animals [55–58].

Although there is not a proper double-blinded placebo-controlled nutritional clinical study of a sensible length that looks at the skin aging in a universal way and in depth, we could only hypothesize that the individual antiaging benefits that are captured in the short-term clinical studies with all the above vitamins and antioxidants could potentially extend to long-term antiaging benefits.

Conclusion

Nutrition may play an important role to the maintenance of skin health and beauty. Photoaging may be prevented by the intake of vitamin C, vitamin E, or carotenoids (pro-vitamin A). Skin wrinkling and actinic damage may be prevented by oral fish polysaccharide supplementation. The intake of essential fatty acids has benefits on hydration of the skin, skin barrier, and skin roughness. In conclusion, dietary products may benefit or damage skin quality and should be chosen very carefully in everyday life.

References

1. Prendiville JS. Skin signs of nutritional disorders. Semin Dermatol. 1992;11:88–97.
2. Smith KE. Cutaneous manifestations of alcohol abuse. J Am Acad Dermatol. 2000;43:1–16.
3. McLaren DS. Fat soluble vitamins. In: Garrow JS, James WPT, editors. Human nutrition, dietetics. 9th

ed. Edinburgh: Churchill Livingstone; 1993. p. 208–38.
4. Boelsma E, Hendriks HFJ, Roza L. Nutritional skin care: health effects of micronutrients and fatty acids. Am J Clin Nutr. 2001;73:853–64.
5. Purba M, Kouris-Blazos A, Wattanapenpaiboon N, Lukito W, Rothenberg EM, Steen BC, et al. Skin wrinkling: can food make a difference? J Am Coll Nutr. 2001;1:71–80.
6. Distante F, Scalise F, Rona C, Bonfigli A, Fluhr JW, Berardesca E. Oral fish cartilage polysaccharides in the treatment of photoageing: biophysical findings. Int J Cosmet Sci. 2002;24:81–7.
7. Dréno B. New assessment methods applied to a patented lacto-lycopene, soy isoflavones and vitamin C in the correction of skin aging. Les Nouvelles Dermatol. 2003;22:1–6.
8. Piccardi N, Manissier P. Nutrition and nutritional supplementation: impact on skin health and beauty. Dermatoendocrinology. 2009;1:271–4.
9. Cosgrove MC, Franco OH, Granger SP, Murray PG, Mayes AE. Dietary nutrient intakes and skin-aging appearance among middle-aged women. Am J Clin Nutr. 2007;86:1225–31.
10. Yusuf N, Irby C, Katiyar SK, Elmets CA. Photoprotective effects of green tea polyphenols. Photodermatol Photoimmunol Photomed. 2007;23(1):48–56.
11. Scapagnini G, Davinelli S, Di Renzo L, De Lorenzo A, Olarte HH, Micali G, Cicero AF, Gonzalez S. Cocoa bioactive compounds: significance and potential for the maintenance of skin health. Nutrients. 2014;6 (8):3202–13.
12. Mogollon JA, Boivin C, Lemieux S, Blanchet C, Claveau J, Dodin S. Chocolate flavanols and skin photoprotection: a parallel, double-blind, randomized clinical trial. Nutr J. 2014;13:66.
13. Williams S, Tamburic S, Lally C. Eating chocolate can significantly protect the skin from UV light. J Cosmet Dermatol. 2009;8(3):169–73.
14. Neukam K, Stahl W, Tronnier H, Sies H, Heinrich U. Consumption of flavanol-rich cocoa acutely increases microcirculation in human skin. Eur J Nutr. 2007;46(1):53–6.
15. Heinrich U, Neukam K, Tronnier H, Sies H, Stahl W. Long-term ingestion of high flavanol cocoa provides photoprotection against UV-induced erythema and improves skin condition in women. J Nutr. 2006;136(6):1565–9.
16. Fan YY, Chapkin RS. Importance of dietary gamma-linolenic acid in human health and nutrition. J Nutr. 1998;128:1411–4.
17. Saaf AM, Tengvall-Linder M, Chang HY, et al. Global expression profiling in atopic eczema reveals reciprocal expression of inflammatory and lipid genes. PLoS One. 2008;3:e4017.
18. Ziboh VA, Cho Y, Mani I, et al. Biological significance of essential fatty acids/prostanoids/lipoxygenase-derived monohydroxy fatty acids in the skin. Arch Pharm Res. 2002;25:747–58.
19. Innis SM. Perinatal biochemistry and physiology of long-chain polyunsaturated fatty acids. J Pediatr. 2003;143:S1–8.
20. Nakamura MT, Nara TY. Structure, function, and dietary regulation of delta6, delta5, and delta9 desaturases. Annu Rev Nutr. 2004;24:345–76.
21. Sprecher H, Luthria DL, Mohammed BS, et al. Reevaluation of the pathways for the biosynthesis of polyunsaturated fatty acids. J Lipid Res. 1995;36:2471–7.
22. Marquardt A, Stohr H, White K, et al. CDNA cloning, genomic structure, and chromosomal localization of three members of the human fatty acid desaturase family. Genomics. 2000;66:175–83.
23. De Spirt S, Stahl W, Tronnier H, Sies H, Bejot M, Maurette JM, Heinrich U. Intervention with flaxseed and borage oil supplements modulates skin condition in women. Br J Nutr. 2009;101(3):440–524.
24. Xu Q, Parks CG, De Roo LA, Cawthon RM, Sandler DP, Chen H. Multivitamin use and telomere length in women. Am J Clin Nutr. 2009;89:1–7.
25. Burke KE, Wei H. Synergistic damage by UVA radiation and pollutants. Toxicol Ind Health. 2009; 25:219–24.
26. Wang Y, Saladi R, Wei H. Synergistic carcinogenesis of chemical carcinogens and long wavelength UVA radiation. Trends Photochem Photobiol. 2003;10:31–45.
27. Fisher GJ, et al. Mechanisms of photoaging and chronological skin aging. Arch Dermatol. 2002;138 (11):1462–70.
28. Helfrich YR, Sachs DL, Voorhees JJ. Overview of skin aging and photoaging. Dermatol Nurs. 2008;20 (3):177–83.
29. Monboisse JC, Borel JP. Oxidative damage to collagen. EXS. 1992;62:323–7.
30. Kawaguchi Y, Tanaka H, Okada T, Konishi H, Takahashi M, Ito M, et al. Effect of reactive oxygen species on the elastin mRNA expression in cultured human dermal fibroblasts. Free Radic Biol Med. 1997;23:162–5.
31. Darvin M, Patzelt A, Gehse S, Schanzer S, Benderoth C, Sterry W, et al. Cutaneous concentration of lycopene correlates significantly with the roughness of the skin. Eur J Pharm Biopharm. 2008;69:943–7.
32. Schroeder P, Lademann J, Darvin ME, Stege H, Marks C, Bruhnke S, et al. Infrared radiationinduced matrix metalloproteinase in human skin: implications for protection. J Invest Dermatol. 2008;128: 2491–7.
33. Schroeder P, Calles C, Benesova T, Macaluso F, Krutmann J. Photoprotection beyond ultraviolet radiation–effective sun protection has to include protection against infrared A radiation-induced skin damage. Skin Pharmacol Physiol. 2010;23:15–7.

34. The Skin Cancer Foundation – Guidelines. http://www.skincancer.org/Guidelines/ (2010). Accessed July 2010.
35. Darr D, Combs S, Dunsten S, et al. Topical vitamin C protects porcine skin from ultraviolet radiationinduced damage. Br J Dermatol. 1992;127:247–53.
36. Burke DE, Clive J, Combs Jr GF, et al. The effects of topical and oral vitamin E on pigmentation and skin cancer induced by ultraviolet irradiation in Skh:2 hairless mice. Nutr Cancer. 2000;38:87–97. Published by Taylor and Francis, Ltd. www.informaworld.com.
37. Phillips CL, Combs SB, Pinnell SR. Effects of ascorbic acid on proliferation and collagen synthesis in relation to donor age of human dermal fibroblasts. J Invest Dermatol. 1994;103:228–32.
38. Davidson JM, Luvalle PA, Zoia O, et al. Ascorbate differentially regulates elastin and collagen biosynthesis in vascular smooth muscle cells and skin fibroblasts by pretranslational mechanisms. J Biol Chem. 1997;272:345–52.
39. Humbert PG, Haftek M, Creidi P, et al. Topical ascorbic acid in photoaged skin. Clinical topographical and ultrastructural evaluation: double-blind study vs. placebo. Exp Dermatol. 2003;12:237–44.
40. Gensler HL, Aickin M, Peng YM, Xu M. Importance of the form of topical vitamin E for prevention of photocarcinogenesis. Nutr Cancer. 1996;26:183–91.
41. Roshchupkin D, Pistsov MY, Potapenko AY. Inhibition of ultraviolet light-induced erythema by antioxidants. Arch Dermatol Res. 1979;266:91–4.
42. Bissett DL, Chatterjee R, Hannon DP. Photoprotective effect of superoxide-scavenging antioxidants against ultraviolet radiation-induced chronic skin damage in the hairless mouse. Photodermatol Photoimmunol Photomed. 1990;7:56–62.
43. Burke KE. Photoprotection of the skin with vitamins C and E: antioxidants and synergies. In Pappas A (ed) Nutrition and skin: lessons for anti-aging, beauty and healthy skin. New York: Springer; 2011:43–58.
44. Thakkar SK et al. Carotenoids and skin. In Pappas A (ed) Nutrition and skin: lessons for anti-aging, beauty and healthy skin. New York: Springer; 2011:59–78.
45. Reichrath J, Lehmann B, Carlberg C, Varani J, Zouboulis CC. Vitamins as hormones. Horm Metab Res. 2007;39(2):71–84. Review.
46. Heinrich U, Tronnier H, Stahl W, Bejot M, Maurette JM. Antioxidant supplements improve parameters related to skin structure in humans. Skin Pharmacol Physiol. 2006;19:224–31.
47. Odetti PR, Borgoglio A, et al. Age-related increase of collagen fluorescence in human subcutaneous tissue. Metabolism. 1992;41(6):655–8.
48. Stamatas GN, Estanislao RB, et al. Facial skin fluorescence as a marker of the skin's response to chronic environmental insults and its dependence on age. Br J Dermatol. 2006;154(1):125–32.
49. Dyer DG, Dunn JA, et al. Accumulation of Maillard reaction products in skin collagen in diabetes and aging. J Clin Invest. 1993;91(6):2463–9.
50. Ediger MN, Olson BP, et al. Noninvasive optical screening for diabetes. J Diabetes Sci Technol. 2009;3(4):776–80.
51. Corstjens H, Dicanio D, et al. Glycation associated skin autofluorescence and skin elasticity are related to chronological age and body mass index of healthy subjects. Exp Gerontol. 2008;43(7):663–7. Epub 2008 Feb 9.
52. Cefalu WT, Bell-Farrow AD, et al. Caloric restriction decreases age-dependent accumulation of the glycoxidation products, N epsilon-(carboxymethyl) lysine and pentosidine, in rat skin collagen. J Gerontol A Biol Sci Med Sci. 1995;50(6):B337–41.
53. Novelli M, Masiello P, et al. Protein glycation in the aging male Sprague-Dawley rat: effects of antiaging diet restrictions. J Gerontol A Biol Sci Med Sci. 1998;53(2):B94–101.
54. Lingelbach LB, Mitchell AE, et al. Accumulation of advanced glycation endproducts in aging male Fischer 344 rats during long-term feeding of various dietary carbohydrates. J Nutr. 2000;130(5):1247–55.
55. Sajithlal GB, Chithra P, et al. Effect of curcumin on the advanced glycation and cross-linking of collagen in diabetic rats. Biochem Pharmacol. 1998;56(12):1607–14.
56. Rutter K, Sell DR, et al. Green tea extract suppresses the age-related increase in collagen crosslinking and fluorescent products in C57BL/6 mice. Int J Vitam Nutr Res. 2003;73(6):453–60.
57. Thirunavukkarasu V, Nandhini AT, et al. Fructose diet-induced skin collagen abnormalities are prevented by lipoic acid. Exp Diabesity Res. 2004;5(4):237–44.
58. Nandhini TA, Thirunavukkarasu V, et al. Taurine prevents fructose-diet induced collagen abnormalities in rat skin. J Diabetes Complications. 2005;19(5):305–11.

120 Aging Skin: Nourishing from the Inside Out – Effects of Good Versus Poor Nitrogen Intake on Skin Health and Healing

Giovanni Corsetti, Evasio Pasini, Vincenzo Flati, Claudia Romano, Anna Rufo, and Francesco S. Dioguardi

Contents

G. Corsetti • C. Romano
Department of Clinical and Experimental Sciences, Division of Human Anatomy and Physiopathology, University of Brescia, Brescia, Italy
e-mail: giovanni.corsetti@unibs.it

E. Pasini
"S. Maugeri Foundation", IRCCS, Cardiology Rehabilitative Division, Medical Centre of Lumezzane, Brescia, Italy

V. Flati • A. Rufo
Department of Biotechnological and Applied Clinical Sciences, University of L'Aquila, L'Aquila, Italy
e-mail: vincenzo.flati@univaq.it

F.S. Dioguardi (✉)
Department of Internal Medicine and Community Health, University of Milan, Milan, Italy
e-mail: fsdioguardi@gmail.com

M.A. Farage et al. (eds.), *Textbook of Aging Skin*,
DOI 10.1007/978-3-662-47398-6_135

Abstract

Skin is the outermost defense organ which protects us from the environment, constituting around 8 % of an adult's body weight. Healthy skin contains one-eighth of the body's total proteins. The balance of turnover and synthesis of skin proteins is primarily dependent on the availability of sufficient nitrogen-containing substrates, namely, amino acids, essential for protein metabolism in any other tissue and body organs. The turnover of skin proteins has been shown to be rapid, and the mobilization of amino acids at the expense of skin proteins is relevant in experimental models of protein malnutrition. As a result, alterations in nutritional status should be suspected, diagnosed, and eventually treated for any skin lesions. Protein malnutrition has a dramatic prevalence in patients aged >70 or more, independent of the reason for hospitalization. The quality of nutrition and content of essential amino acids are strictly connected to skin health and integrity of its protein components. Collagen fiber deposition is highly and rapidly influenced by alterations in the essential to nonessential amino acid ratios. The most relevant nutritional factor of skin health is the prevalence of essential amino acids.

Introduction

Skin is an organ consisting of around 8 % of an adult's body weight and is the outermost defense organ that protects us from environment. The skin is composed of the dermis and epidermis. The dermis is the inner layer and it has a mesodermic origin. The epidermis (epi = over) is the outermost layer of the skin, and it has an ectodermic origin [1]. The dermis provides all nutrients and oxygen to the epidermis through blood and lymph vessels. Thus, the oxygen and nutrition of the epidermis are provided from the internal to the external environment of the body (from the *inside out*), which should be borne in mind when considering skin health and its relationship with nutrition.

Collagen is ubiquitous in all organs and the most abundant protein in the human body (30 % of all body proteins) and represents around 50 % of skin weight. Functionally, collagen maintains skin integrity by continuous remodeling stressed structures, so consuming a high amount of both energy and substrates for protein metabolism [2]. Indeed, collagen synthesis requires around four high-energy bonds (~ATP equivalents) for each amino acid inserted into the molecule [3]. Similar costs have been calculated for protein synthesis only in bacteria [4]. Therefore, the costs and complexity of wound healing (lesions of the epidermis and dermis from outside in) are an enormous metabolic problem, as discussed in ▶ Chap. 121, "Aging Skin: Nourishing from Out-In – Lessons from Wound Healing" in this textbook.

Consequently, the relationship between body protein and skin protein metabolism should be considered closely interlinked. The impairment of body protein metabolism would reflect similar impairment of skin health particularly in aged patients as will be discussed later. This is why treatment of wounds, especially chronic ones, solely by topical treatment, is only marginally effective. Therefore, before any procedure, dermatologists should assure that the patient's nitrogen/protein metabolism is supported adequately; otherwise, its local care, although potentially beneficial, could be ineffective.

Although alterations of skin structure are visible features of aging, there is only incomplete knowledge about the relation between normal or altered diet and skin aging, in particular when compared with the huge amount of published literature dealing with aging, diet, and peripheral muscle maintenance [5–7].

Healthy skin contains one-eighth of the body's total proteins. In addition, it contains collagen, constituting 70 % of the total nitrogen content of the skin. So, the hypothesis that alterations of protein synthesis linked to malnutrition may drive alterations of the skin's extracellular matrix structure [8], as observed in many other organs, also makes sense in humans. As such, the collagen anabolic/catabolic ratios and balances may be strictly linked, and both skin and bone collagen health is coordinated by the whole-body protein synthesis balance, particularly in the elderly.

Simple Steps and Methodology for Detecting and Monitoring Protein Malnutrition: The First Step to Therapeutic Success

Early identification and evaluation of protein metabolic impairment are fundamental steps for better patient care, avoiding additional and independent damage and allowing traditional therapy to work properly. Assessment by specific biomarkers of early changes in body protein metabolism may be fundamental in identifying and monitoring initial damage and protein metabolic-related abnormalities before they are irreversible [9].

The first step in assessing global metabolic impairment is to evaluate body mass index (BMI). However, BMI cannot distinguish lean muscular from fatty tissues separately, and it is also influenced by fluid retention. Thus, body global protein metabolism can be more reliably measured by static, functional, and dynamic biomarkers. Indeed, we believe that a single ideal biomarker of protein metabolism impairment does not exist at this time. Each measurement has certain advantages, disadvantages, and/or limitations. It is recommended to use an integrated critical evaluation for best therapeutic success.

Static Biomarkers

These include: *(1)* anthropometric measurements, which distinguish muscular lean mass from fatty mass, and *(2)* visceral blood proteins, which provide information on visceral protein synthesis:

1. ***Anthropometric Measurements***. The gold standard equipment for anthropometric measurements of body composition is the dual-energy X-ray absorptiometry (DEXA or DXA). However, DXA scanners are expensive equipment, and although DXA uses low-energy X-ray, patients are still exposed to radiation.

   Skinfold thickness and *arm muscle area* are simpler methods for analyzing body composition and indirectly evaluating general protein metabolism. These biomarkers can be routinely evaluated at the patient's bedside, so specific training is not needed [10, 11]:
   - *Skinfold Thickness*. This is an index of fatty mass. It should be measured using a plicometer in specific body sites such as the *triceps (TSF)*, measuring along the midline on the back of the triceps of the right arm pinching the skin so that the fold is running vertically; *pectoral*, using a line from the fold of the axillary to the nipple, determining the midpoint; *abdominal*, measuring about 1 in. laterally to the right side, from 0.5 in. below the umbilicus lifting a horizontal fold of skin; *supra-iliac*, measuring the top of the iliac crest; and *thigh*, using a midline of the front of the thigh and measuring midway between the inguinal crest.
   - *Arm Muscle Area (AMA)*. This is an index of lean muscular mass. First, we have to measure the mid-arm muscle circumference (MAMC). Then, the AMA can be calculated also using TSF according to the following formula:

$$\mathrm{MAMC(cm)} = \mathrm{MAC(cm)} - 3.14 \times \mathrm{TSF(mm)}/10 - [3.14 \times \mathrm{TSF(mm)}/10].$$

   TSF and AMA can be used in patients with fluid retention [12].

2. ***Blood Visceral Protein Assessment***. Albumin, transferrin, prealbumin (or TTR), and retinol-binding proteins (RBP) are the most commonly used serum proteins. They have different blood half-lives with different turnovers [13].
   - *Albumin*. Serum level of albumin <3.5 g/l is considered a biomarker of highly reduced protein metabolism. Concentrations less than 3.2 g/l should be considered a biomarker of severe impairment, possibly

associated with the onset of cachexia. Albumin has a blood half-life of about 20 days; consequently, it is not a rapid biomarker of successful protein synthesis after nutritional intervention, and it can be influenced by several diseases, such as severe nephrosis, protein-losing enteropathy, liver insufficiency, and fluid retention.

- *Transferrin*. This correlates with a mortality risk in hospitalized patients. It has a blood half-life of about 8 days, and this makes transferrin useful also for monitoring the medium-term effects of specific nutritional therapies.
- *Prealbumin* (Transthyretin, TTR). This has a plasma half-life of only about 24–36 h, so it responds quickly to changes in protein metabolism.
- *Retinol-Binding Protein*. This has a turnover of about 12 h. Therefore, it is used to monitor rapid changes of protein metabolism. It is commonly available only in specialized laboratories.

A Functional Biomarker

The lymphocyte blood count is an indirect functional biomarker of cell proliferation, protein synthesis, and energy availability. Reduced lymphocyte protein metabolism causes cell-cycle loss with consequent low counts of circulating lymphocytes. Scarce circulating lymphocytes induce the malfunction of systemic immunity with an increased risk of infection [14]. This biomarker is easy to monitor but it should be interpreted together with other information.

Dynamic Biomarkers

1. ***Nitrogen Balance*** (NB). NB is the ratio of nitrogen introduced into an organism from consumed food AAs to the quantity of nitrogen excreted in the urine. NB is expressed as g/day according to the formula:

$$\begin{aligned} NB = {} & \text{Nitrogen intake (NI)} \\ & - \text{Nitrogen output by urine (NV)} \\ & + 2\,\text{g} \end{aligned}$$

where:

NI = nitrogen intake/supply in g/day^{-1} evaluated by protein intake (g/day) where g of N is equal to intact protein/6.25 g.

NV = urinary nitrogen excretion as urea in g/day^{-1} + 20 % NV for non-urea N excretion.

2 g is the nitrogen lost in feces and sweat.

If NB >1 g/day^{-1} indicates the prevalence of protein synthesis, then NB <1 g/day^{-1} suggests the prevalence of protein degradation [15].

NB is neither easy to obtain or to calculate. Moreover, NB depends mostly on urea concentrations as has recently been indicated. Urea concentrations in plasma and urine critically depend on the arginine content of diets, as arginine is the precursor of urea synthesis, cleaved by arginases forming urea and ornithine mostly but not exclusively by the liver. Arginase-1 (in the liver and erythrocytes) is rapidly inducible by high arginine content in diets. These modifications have multiple consequences; the misleading achievement of sufficient essential amino acid intake by a positive NB due to rapid elevation of plasma and urinary urea is just a part of this very complex clinical picture [16].

2. ***3-Methylhistidine*** (3-MeH). 3-MeH is an index of proteolysis. 3-MeH originates from methylation of histidine. This process is stimulated by catabolic hormones, inflammatory molecules, and/or insufficient qualitative and quantitative nutrient intake including AAs [17]. Therefore, the massive presence of 3-MeH in the blood or urine would suggest protein degradation. 3-MeH measurement is not easy to perform, and its value should be integrated with other biomarkers and indicators.

Skin Aging, Collagen, and the Effects of Malnutrition

The worst is not/ so long as we can say 'This is the worst'. (W. Shakespeare, *King Lear*, 4.1.29–30 Edgar)

Collagen makes up for 70 % of the total nitrogen content of the skin, and its fractional synthesis rate is relatively high in both animals and humans. Indeed, the collagen synthesis rate is superior to 56–72 % a day in the epidermis and 2.6–2.9 % in the dermis [18]. Furthermore, rapid transportation of nutrients between the dermis and epidermis has been found in healthy well-fed patients, able to maintain epidermal integrity.

With the progression of age, the skin undergoes a series of events that gradually reduce its structural integrity and function with changes of appearance and structure. As already observed, the dermis owes its structural stability and resilience to collagen, so the reduction and/or alteration of collagen proteins leads to changes of the appearance and function of the skin. The quality of the collagen that remains is altered by greater disorder. Like collagen, elastin displays morphology alterations, which decreases the elasticity of the skin in the aged dermis [19]. It is interesting to note that skin collagen and bones as well as connective tissue of most body organs have similar amino acid sequences typical of collagen type I.

The functional, age-related, changes of the skin include slowing of reepithelialization. Thus, the skin becomes more fragile and thin, and in the elderly, skin wounds need more time to complete healing. However, the clinical impact of these changes in acute wound healing of healthy people seems to be small. On the contrary, poor healing in chronic wounds is largely seen in the elderly with comorbidities [20].

Histological analysis of skin thickness shows that the dermis of malnourished animals is significantly thinner compared to well-nourished animals [8]. This observation is concomitant with compromised collagen synthesis in other organs such as the intestinal wall [21]. These findings indicate that skin collagen integrity is strictly entangled with protein malnutrition. Clinically, this has been proven by the impaired growth in malnourished children [22] and the importance of implementing an adequate protein intake in the elderly to maintain bone health [23].

It is also interesting to note that malnutrition impairs skin vitamin D_3 production. Interestingly, vitamin D_3 is involved in anabolic processes reducing other aspects of body metabolic efficiency [24, 25]. Therefore, the skin of aging people may pay debts that are shared with all other body organs, so the skilled dermatologist should be able both to detect protein malnutrition and to solicit adequate nutrition protocol. If not, the topical therapeutic approach will not be efficient. Finally, there are many different molecular mechanisms connected with skin aging [26]; the most representative are described below.

Molecular Biologist's View of Skin Aging: Intrinsic and Extrinsic Factors at Play

It is well known that skin aging is a consequence of genetically determined biological factors influenced by oxidative stress [27, 28] and environmental (such as sunlight ultraviolet radiation) factors [29]. The first type of skin aging is called intrinsic aging, while the second is called extrinsic aging [30, 31]. Nevertheless, it is reasonable to think that extrinsic aging works on the same basis as the intrinsic mechanisms of aging.

The intrinsic aging process is thought to be similar to that occurring in internal organs. The external *stratum corneum* seems to be unaffected, while the epidermis and dermis lose their function and structure. Indeed, a reduced number of fibroblasts and a reduction of their biosynthetic capacity have been observed. Furthermore, there is an increase in the density of collagen fibers that are also randomly oriented [26].

The main molecular determinants of the skin aging process include reduced skin cell proliferation capacity, reduced collagen type I synthesis, and increased collagen breakdown mediated by matrix metalloproteinase (MMP) activity, further promoted by a concomitant decrease of MMP inhibitors. The result is the alteration, structural and compositional, of the long-lived collagen types I and II, which are the main structural components of the extracellular matrix proteins of the dermis [32]. Indeed, it has been shown that changes of the epidermis are minimally involved with skin aging, while in major alterations involving the dermis, there can be seen damaged and disorganized collagen fibrils.

Furthermore, a reduced proliferative rate of skin cells (fibroblasts, keratinocytes, melanocytes) is also found with aging. These changes tip the balance from matrix-producing to matrix-degrading phenotype, so determining atrophy of the dermis and so the occurrence of wrinkles. Nevertheless, the molecular mechanisms underlining the intrinsic and the extrinsic skin aging, although sharing similarities, are different with MMP activity, particularly on photoaged skin.

At the molecular level, it has been shown [33] that ultraviolet radiation (probably the most important factor responsible for extrinsic skin aging) is capable of modulating MMP induction through the activation of growth factor receptors on fibroblasts and keratinocytes. The activated epidermal growth factor receptor (EGFR), through the GTP-binding regulatory protein p21Ras, mediates the activation of the MAP kinase signal transduction, which activates ERK, JNK, and p38MAPK. Both JNK and p38MAPK phosphorylate and activate the activating transcription factor 2 (ATF2) that upregulate c-Jun expression. This associates with the constitutively expressed c-Fos to form the activator protein (AP) 1 transcription factor which is necessary for the transcription of MMP genes. c-Jun expression is elevated in the old skin. Indeed, in human skin, the AP-1 transcription factor activity is limited by the expression of c-Jun being c-Fos expressed at the same rate in the young and in the old skin.

Other growth factor receptors, such as interleukin-1 receptor, tumor necrosis factor receptor, and platelet-derived growth factor receptor, also share this action mechanism. The common endpoint is the loss of collagen in the skin with a remodeling of elastic fibers. This event is modulated differently in extrinsic and intrinsic aging and is associated with the loss of tissue compliance and resilience and the formation of wrinkles. It therefore seems that there is a causative link between elastic fiber remodeling and functional changes (loss of elasticity) in aging skin.

Studies conducted by several groups have revealed that UV radiation mainly increases three MMPs, that is, the collagenase MMP1, the stromelysin-1 MMP3, and the gelatinase MMP9. All of these are regulated at the transcriptional level by the AP-1 transcription factor. These MMPs are induced in the epidermis (epidermal keratinocytes) and are secreted in the dermis where they degrade collagen. It has been hypothesized that dermal cells might also be involved with MMP production through a paracrine mechanism mediated by the release of growth factors or cytokines, which in turn modulate MMP production in epidermal keratinocytes [34, 35].

Fragments of elastin and fibrillin-1 deriving from elastic fiber remodeling are capable of influencing the expression of MMPs and, as a consequence, promoting the degradation of most dermal proteins such as collagen. Furthermore, fibrillin may play a role in mediating homeostasis of the tissue by mediating the sequestration of TGFβ [36–38]. TGFβ is a tightly regulated growth factor that controls cell proliferation, survival, differentiation, and migration. Its latent and inactive form is non-covalently bound to other proteins such as the latency-associated pro-peptide (LAP) to form the small latent complex (SLC), and when bound by latent TGFβ-binding protein (LTBP), it forms a large latent complex (LLC).

LTBPs are proteins structurally related to fibrillins that regulate TGFβ activity. It has been suggested that the activation of the latent TGFβ is mediated by its proteolytic release from the inactive latent complex, by the competition of thrombospondin-1 with SLC, by pH changes, or by the action of reactive oxygen species. The active TGFβ then binds to the TGFβ-R1 and TGFβ-R2 heterodimer, which leads to the phosphorylation of the TGFβ-R1, which in turn phosphorylates the intracellular signaling proteins SMAD2 and SMAD3. Their phosphorylation allows the binding of another intracellular protein called SMAD4, which in turn allows the translocation of the complex into the nucleus where it acts as a transcription factor (in association with cofactors) for the regulation of target-gene expression. Fibrillin-1 has been shown to mediate TGFβ release from the inactive latent complex, thus promoting its activity. The impairment of the TGFβ pathway is therefore probably responsible for the reduction of procollagen synthesis in aged skin.

Since dryness and the associated loss of elasticity are also associated with skin aging, a further important mediator is the skin's capacity to retain water in order to maintain skin moisture. The key molecular mediator involved with skin moisture maintenance is hyaluronic acid (HA). This is a glycosaminoglycan mainly expressed in the extracellular matrix of the skin. It is synthesized by HA synthases (HAS), while it is degraded by hyaluronidases. The rate of HA turnover is dynamic, and in the skin, it has a half-life less than a day. TGFβ is an important stimulator of HA synthesis since the expression of HAS1 and HAS2 is regulated by TGFβ, although differentially in the dermis and epidermis. The marked reduction of HA in aging skin is associated with its loss in the epidermis, while it is conserved in the dermis. Furthermore, a reduction in size of the HA polymers in the skin [39] has also been observed.

Extrinsic skin aging is also characterized by a distinct homeostasis of HA [40]. Photo-exposed skin shows an increased amount of degraded (lower molecular weight) HA compared with the photo-protected skin, and this degradation is associated with an increase of hyaluronidases 1, 2, and 3 and with a decreased expression of HAS1. This underlines differences at a molecular level which distinguish photoaging (extrinsic) from natural aging (intrinsic).

Evidence from Experimental Models of Essential Amino Acids in the Diet as a Key Factor in Maintaining the Integrity of Aged Skin and Accelerating Wound Closure

Amino acids (AAs) are known to regulate protein metabolism, and they have been tested in order to establish their effect on the dermal tropocollagen synthesis rate. It has been observed that a combination of branched-chain AA (BCAA) and glutamine or proline derived from glutamine metabolism is important for restoring the impaired dermal collagen protein synthesis in malnourished animals [41].

It is accepted that protein malnutrition is a well-established factor damaging skin health. However, the role and relevance of peculiar amino acids in skin health and improvement of wound-healing processes are not clear. Indeed, previous results showed that the excess of nonessential AA (NEAA) provokes negative effects on protein synthesis and cannot be considered "nonbelligerent" in protein metabolism. Indeed, an excess of NEAA impairs wound health and healing (see also ▶ Chap. 121, "Aging Skin: Nourishing from Out-In – Lessons from Wound Healing"). Thus, in order to study the role and effects of the availability of different percentages of EAA and NEAA, an experimental pilot study in healthy middle-aged rats (12 months) compared the effects of three different feeds on wound healing, each of which contained a different ratio of EAA to NEAA, while nitrogen content remained strictly the same. The three groups (identified in images as A, E, and D) had the following percentage of AA as components of nitrogen intake: (1) diet A contained exclusively EAA (100 %); (2) diet E contained 45 % of EAA and 55 % of NEAA, which is the same ratio found in casein (used as control group); and (3) diet D contained predominantly NEAA (85 %) while EAAs were only 15 %.

Preliminary data showed that already after 15 days, there was a marked difference in body weight (b.w.) between the three groups. In particular, the tendency to reduce b.w. in group D compared to an increase in group E. After 15 and 60 days of treatment, b.w. difference between animals fed with different diets varied significantly. In particular, diet D caused a steady and rapid decrease of weight, reaching 28 % after 60 days. By contrast, with diet E, there was an increase of about 12.5 % in b.w., while diet A did not lead to any significant changes in b.w., although growth in length was not affected and there was evident loss of abdominal fat, with only 6 % of increases in b.w. after 60 days. Curiously, the animals fed with the diet D, although they had a considerably reduced b.w., ate about 23 % more than the control group and drank about 50 % more than diet E-fed animals.

The physical impairment of the animals was also accompanied by early alteration of skin structure. Feeding with diet D reduced the thickness of the epidermis and altered cellular organization. The basal layer was formed by abnormal cells with flattened and elongated nuclei, while the granular layer was absent or very reduced (Fig. 1a–c). Moreover, a diet deficient in EAA also changes the organization of the dermis. In fact, with diet D the collagen fibers became thinner and more spaced and tended to arrange themselves in a more disorganized manner (Fig. 1d–f).

The effect of the different relations between EAA and NEAA was also observed in the time needed to heal identical wounds. The wounds produced in animals fed with diet A, composed mainly of EAA, healed quicker compared to the standard diet E, based on casein and therefore containing about 55 % of NEA. In contrast, the wounds of the animals fed with diet D, poorest in EAA (85 % of NEA), had significantly greater healing times (Fig. 2).

The different timespans of wound closure also seem to be due to the fact that the availability of

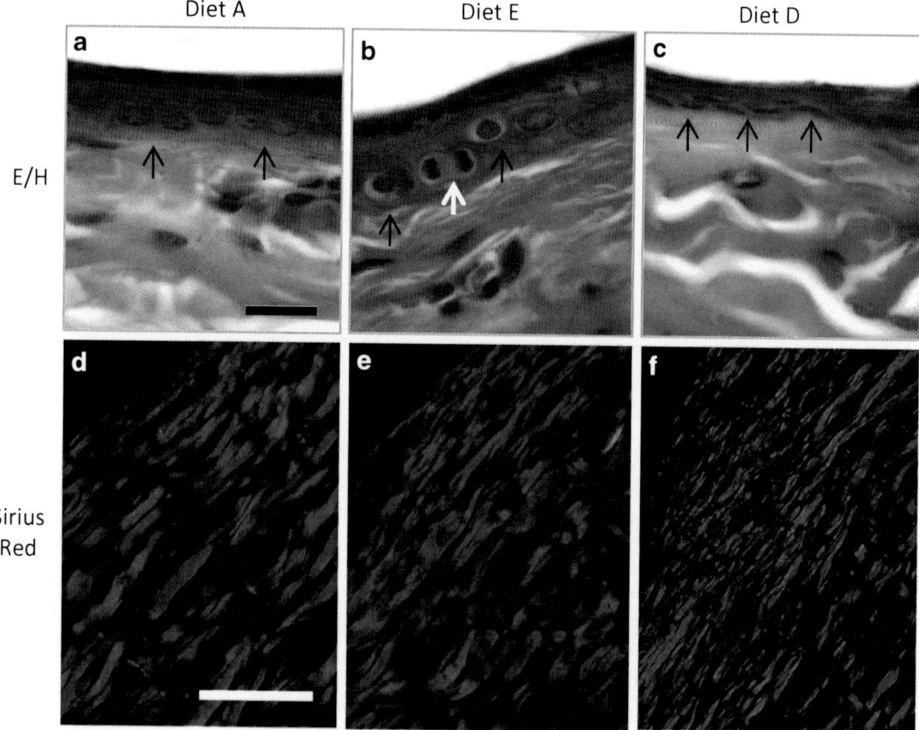

Fig. 1 (**a, b**). Eosin-hematoxylin staining. Epidermis after 60 days of treatment with the diets. (**a**) With diet A, the organization of the epidermis and cell morphology of basal layer (*arrows*) are regular. (**b**) With diet E, the organization of the epidermis does not undergo significant changes; the basal layer frequently shows duplicating cells (*white arrow*) and more mature cells without cytoplasm (*black arrows*). (**c**) Diet D reduces the thickness of the epidermis and alters the cellular organization. The basal layer is formed by abnormal cells with flattened and elongated nuclei (*arrows*), while the granular layer is absent or very reduced. Scale bar 150 um. (**d, e**). Sirius red stain for collagen (polarized light). The organization of collagen in the dermis changes with the type of diet. (**d**) With diet A, the collagen fibers are thicker and more compact. (**e**) With diet E, the collagen fibers do not seem to vary significantly; however, the tendency to thinning is observed. (**f**) With diet D, the collagen fibers become thinner and more spaced and tend to arrange themselves in a more disorganized manner. Scale bar 300 um (Corsetti et al.)

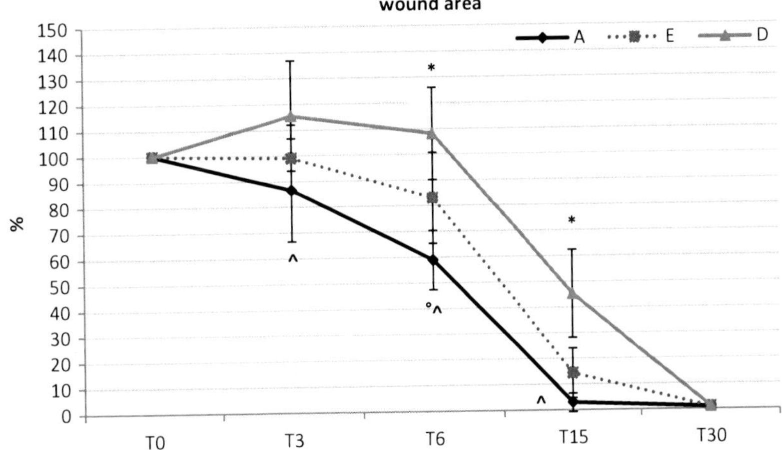

Fig. 2 Wound area according to diet. All wound areas were converted to 100 % on the day of wounding (day 0). On subsequent days (3, 6, 15, and 30), the areas were expressed as a percentage of original area on day zero. * and ° = $p > 0.05$ versus diet E. ^ = $p > 0.05$ versus diet D (Corsetti et al.)

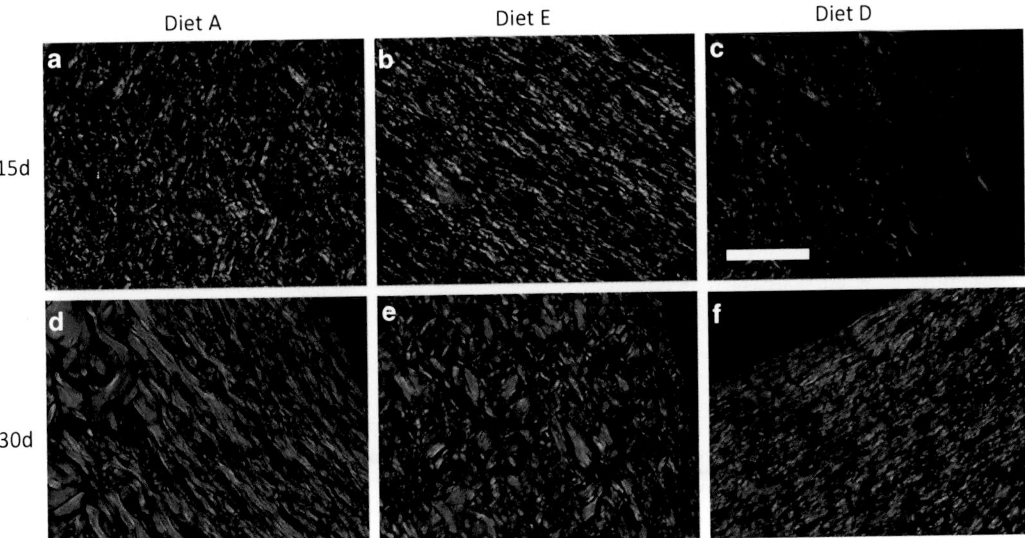

Fig. 3 Wound area. Sirius red stain – polarized light. Collagen fibers in the upper layers of the newly formed tissue in the wound area after 15 (**a–c**) and 30 days (**d–f**) according to diets. The different thickness and quantity of the collagen fibers in the diet D were observed compared to the other diets, as well as the disorganization of fibers after 15 and 30 days from the wound. Scale bar 100 um (Corsetti et al.)

EAA affects the production and organization of collagen fibers. Indeed, already after 15 days from the wound, with diet A, abundant production of thick and well-oriented collagen fibers was observed. On the contrary, diet D produced scarce and thin collagen fibers with random orientation (Fig. 3a–c).

Similarly, after 30 days from wounding, although wounds were healed for all groups, the organization and thickness of the collagen fibers were largely different (Fig. 3d–f). These observations suggest that it is not the amount of nitrogen, but the quality of the nitrogen sources that affects the physical condition. Although the study is still preliminary, physical exhaustion and morphological and structural changes of the skin seem comparable with those observed during senescence. It is therefore possible that the prevalence of EAA in the diet may be a key to prevent or slow tissue aging, confirming the observations by D'Antona et al. [42] in muscles and the heart. However, preliminary data also provide another aspect until recently little known, i.e., that NEAA significantly hinders the normal cell physiology in a dose-dependent manner. This was particularly evident in influencing the timing of wound healing. In accordance with this, as reported in another ▶ Chap. 121, "Aging Skin: Nourishing from Out-In – Lessons from Wound Healing," NEAA significantly hinders the normal cell physiology in a dose-dependent manner since they are particularly efficient in influencing the timespan of wound healing.

We believe that these findings may open new scenarios in understanding the causes that lead to the impairment of health of aging skin, as well as suggesting procedures for the prevention or treatment of related pathologies.

Conclusion

Collagen metabolism is fundamental for maintaining skin integrity as it makes up 70 % of total nitrogen content of skin proteins. However, skin collagen metabolism is negatively altered in protein-malnourished states often present in aged people. The alterations of skin linked to protein metabolism impairment are an aspect of human pathophysiology, although not easily evaluable, this is worth attention and the development of the specific procedures of assessment of damages and success of therapies. Indeed, insufficient amino acids or altered balance between EAA and NEAA modifies the balance of collagen protein turnover and resynthesis. Although there is debate about which is the best formulation of amino acids suitable for maintaining and promoting skin collagen health, certainly a primary role is linked to sufficient essential amino acid availability. This is not an isolated requirement of skin, but an obliged requirement of skin in a complex balance ruled by metabolism requirements of the whole body's tissues and organs. Consequently, matching the needs of sufficient essential AA intakes is important for the body's organ metabolism and the skin's needs should be included in these total requirements.

References

1. Xua Z, et al. Teleost skin, an ancient mucosal surface that elicits gut-like immune responses. Proc Natl Acad Sci U S A. 2013;110(32):13097–102.
2. Xiao-Jun Z, et al. Measurement of protein metabolism in epidermis and dermis. Am J Physiol Endocrinol Metab. 2003;284:1191–201. doi:10.1152/ajpendo.00460.2002.
3. Browne GJ, Proud CG. Regulation of peptide-chain elongation in mammalian cells. Eur J Biochem. 2002;269:5360–8. doi:10.1046/j.1432-1033.2002.03290.x.
4. Kaleta C, et al. Metabolic costs of amino acid and protein production in *Escherichia coli*. Biotechnol J. 2013;8:1105–14. doi:10.1002/biot.201200267.
5. Kim J, et al. Association between healthy diet and exercise and greater muscle mass in older adults. J Am Geriatr Soc. 2015;63(5):886–92. doi:10.1111/jgs.13386.
6. Paddon-Jones D, et al. Protein and healthy aging. Am J Clin Nutr. 2015;101:1339S–45. doi:10.3945/ajcn.114.084061.
7. Murphy CH, et al. Hypoenergetic diet-induced reductions in myofibrillar protein synthesis are restored with resistance training and balanced daily protein ingestion in older men. Am J Physiol Endocrinol Metab. 2015;308:E734–43. doi:10.1152/ajpendo.00550.2014.
8. Leite SN, et al. Experimental models of malnutrition and its effect on skin trophism. An Bras Dermatol. 2011;86(4):681–8.
9. Pasini E, et al. The enemy within. How to identify chronic diseases induced-protein metabolism impairment and its possible pharmacological treatment. Pharmacol Res. 2013;76:28–33.
10. Cogill B. Anthropometric indicators measurement guide. Washington, DC: Food and Nutrition Technical Assistance Project, Academy for Educational Development; 2001.
11. Magnani R. Sampling guide. Arlington: Food Security and Nutrition Monitoring (IMPACT) Project, ISTI, Inc., for the U.S. Agency for International Development; 1999.
12. Frisancho AR. Anthropometric standard for assessment of growth and nutritional status. Ann Arbor: University of Michigan Press; 2004. p. 38–62. ISBN 0-472-10146-3.
13. Watson RR. Nutritional stresses: levels of complement proteins and their functions. In: Watson RR, editor. Nutrition, disease resistance and immune function. New York: Marcel Dekker; 1984. p. 175–88.

14. Acanfora D, et al. Relative lymphocyte count: a prognostic indicator of mortality in elderly patients with congestive heart failure. Am Heart J. 2001;142 (1):167–73.
15. Aquilani R, et al. Is nutritional intake adequate in chronic heart failure patients? J Am Coll Cardiol. 2003;42:1218–23.
16. Dioguardi FS. Nutrition and skin. Collagen integrity: a dominant role for amino acids. Clin Dermatol. 2008;26 (6):636–40.
17. Ferrari F, et al. A rapid method for simultaneous determination of creatinine, 1- and 3 methylhistidine in human urine. Electrophoresis. 2009;30:1–3.
18. Zhang XJ, et al. Measurement of protein metabolism in epidermis and dermis. Am J Physiol Endocrinol Metab. 2003;284:1191–201.
19. Lavker RM, et al. Aged skin: a study by light, transmission electron, and scanning electron microscopy. J Invest Dermatol. 1987;88:44S–51.
20. Thomas DR, Burkemper NM. Aging skin and wound healing. Clin Geriatr Med. 2013;29(2):xi–xx. doi:10.1016/j.cger.2013.02.001
21. Nakajima V, et al. Alterations in the intestinal wall due to protein malnutrition in rats: evaluation of the rupture strength and the tissue's collagen. Acta Cir Bras. 2008;23(5):435–40.
22. Allison SP. Malnutrition, disease, and outcome. Nutrition. 2000;16(7/8):590–3.
23. Beasley JM, et al. Biomarker-calibrated protein intake and bone health in the Women's Health Initiative clinical trials and observational study. Am J Clin Nutr. 2014;99:934–40.
24. MacLaughlin J, Holick MF. Aging decreases the capacity of human skin to produce Vitamin D_3. J Clin Invest. 1985;76:1536–8.
25. Bikram S, et al. Nutritional deficiencies after bariatric surgery. Nat Rev Endocrinol. 2012;8:544–56.
26. Jenkins G. Molecular mechanisms of skin ageing. Mech Ageing Dev. 2002;7:801–10.
27. Poljsak B, et al. Intrinsic skin aging: the role of oxidative stress. Acta Dermatovenerol Alp Pannonica Adriat. 2012;21:33–6.
28. Rinnerthaler M, et al. Oxidative stress in aging human skin. Biomolecules. 2015;5:545–89.
29. Farage MA, et al. Characteristics of the aging skin. Adv Wound Care. 2013;2:5–10.
30. Farage MA, et al. Intrinsic and extrinsic factors in skin ageing: a review. Int J Cosmet Sci. 2008;30:87–95.
31. Vierkotter A, Krutmann J. Environmental influences on skin aging and ethnic-specific manifestations. Dermatoendocrinol. 2012;4:227–31.
32. Fisher GJ, et al. Mechanisms of photoaging and chronological skin aging. Arch Dermatol. 2002;138:462–70.
33. Fisher GJ, et al. Retinoic acid inhibits induction of c-June protein by ultraviolet irradiation that occurs subsequent to activation of mitogen activated protein kinase pathways in human skin in vivo. J Clin Invest. 1998;101:1432–40.
34. Quan T, et al. Matrix-degrading metalloproteinases in photoaging. J Investig Dermatol Symp Proc. 2009;14:20–4.
35. Chauhan P, Shakya M. Modeling signaling pathways leading to wrinkle formation: identification of the skin aging target. Indian J Dermatol Venereol Leprol. 2009;75:463–8.
36. Ashworth JL, et al. Fibrillin degradation by matrix metalloproteinases: implications for connective tissue remodelling. Biochem J. 1999;340:171–81.
37. Kaartinen V, Warburton D. Fibrillin controls TGF-beta activation. Nat Genet. 2003;33:331–2.
38. Chaudhry SS, et al. Fibrillin-1 regulates the bioavailability of TGFbeta1. J Cell Biol. 2007;176:355–67.
39. Papakonstantinou E, et al. Hyaluronic acid: a key molecule in skin aging. Dermatoendocrinol. 2012;4:253–8.
40. Tzellos TG, et al. Extrinsic ageing in the human skin is associated with alterations in the expression of hyaluronic acid and its metabolizing enzymes. Exp Dermatol. 2009;18:1028–35.
41. Murakami H, et al. Combination of BCAAs and glutamine enhances dermal collagen protein synthesis in protein-malnourished rats. Amino Acids. 2013;44:969–76.
42. D'Antona G, et al. Branched-chain amino acid supplementation promotes survival and supports cardiac and skeletal muscle mitochondrial biogenesis in middle-aged mice. Cell Metab. 2010;12:362–72.

Aging Skin: Nourishing from Out-In – Lessons from Wound Healing 121

Giovanni Corsetti, Vincenzo Flati, Evasio Pasini, Claudia Romano, Anna Rufo, Raimondo Pinna, and Francesco S. Dioguardi

Contents

G. Corsetti • C. Romano
Department of Clinical and Experimental Sciences, Division of Human Anatomy and Physiopathology, University of Brescia, Brescia, Italy
e-mail: giovanni.corsetti@unibs.it

V. Flati • A. Rufo
Department of Biotechnological and Applied Clinical Sciences, University of L'Aquila, L'Aquila, Italy
e-mail: vincenzo.flati@univaq.it

E. Pasini
"S. Maugeri Foundation", IRCCS, Cardiology Rehabilitative Division, Medical Centre of Lumezzane, Brescia, Italy

R. Pinna
Plastic and Reconstructive Surgery and Burns Centre, Brotzu Hospital, Cagliari, Italy

F.S. Dioguardi (✉)
Department of Internal Medicine and Community Health, University of Milan, Milan, Italy
e-mail: fsdioguardi@gmail.com

M.A. Farage et al. (eds.), *Textbook of Aging Skin*,
DOI 10.1007/978-3-662-47398-6_136

Abstract

Skin lesion therapy, peculiarly in the elderly, cannot be isolated from understanding that the skin is an important organ consisting of different tissues. Furthermore, dermis health is fundamental for epidermis integrity, and so adequate nourishment is mandatory in maintaining skin integrity. The dermis nourishes the epidermis, and a healthy epidermis protects the dermis from the environment, so nourishing the dermis through the epidermal barrier is a technical problem yet to be resolved. This is also a consequence of the laws and regulations restricting cosmetics, which cannot have properties that pass the epidermal layer. There is higher investment in cosmetics than in the pharmaceutical industry dealing with skin therapies, because the costs of drug registration are enormous and the field is unprofitable. Still, wound healing may be seen as an opportunity to "feed" the dermis directly. It could also verify whether providing substrates could promote efficient healing and test optimal skin integrity maintenance, if not skin rejuvenation, in an ever aging population.

Introduction

The skin is the outermost defense organ protecting us from the environment. Wounds are probably the most ancient threat faced by living beings. Mammal skin is an evolution of the skin mucosal surface present in extremely ancient bony vertebrates, living in the sea. The epidermis (epi = over), the outermost layer of the skin, has an ectodermic origin. This is unlike the dermis, the inner skin layer, with a mesodermic origin, which provides oxygen and nutrition to the epidermis through blood and lymph vessels [1].

Therefore, the dermis nourishes the epidermis and not vice versa, which should be borne in mind when considering health maintenance of the skin from out-in. As a result epidermis health and healing require primarily dermis health and healing. Wounds allow the dermis to be in contact with the environment, and both are active in the healing process. As a result, the balance between the severity of environmental aggression and the efficiency of dermis cells mediates the degree and quality of the healing process.

As the skin is the outermost environmental defense, when it is broken, environmental threats (e.g., chemicals, viruses, or bacteria) have to be faced. However, the loss of liquids and proteins from wounds extending to the dermis has also to be faced. This insight should be taken into account as a possible threat to the integrity of the whole organism and not of the skin alone.

The energy costs of wound healing are enormous, but as shown by studies on the dynamics of collagen in the dermis, it is also expensive to maintain skin integrity. This is because continuous remodeling of stressed structures that consume a large amount of body energy and substrates needed for protein metabolism [1] is required. For example, collagen, the most abundant protein in the human body, represents around 50 % of skin weight and 30 % of all body proteins. Synthesis of any individual collagen molecule requires around four high-energy bonds (~ATP equivalents) for each amino acid inserted into the molecule [2]. Similar energy costs have also been calculated for protein synthesis in bacteria [3].

An analysis of recent literature shows that there is consensus that for best healing, the wound microenvironment should be protected with moist or wet medication [4]. There is a continuous flow of literature which discusses different materials potentially useful for wounds treatment [5].

However, the wounds are considered almost exclusively as a loss of tissue integrity, so there is far less documentation concerning another pivotal question, i.e., is it useful to look at wounds as active sites for the refueling of cells involved in the management of tissue regeneration to improve the efficiency of healing?

Previously, it has been shown that shortening healing time can be promoted by feeding fibroblasts with a peculiar amino acid formulation. This formulation should be based on synthetic requirements suggested by the highly peculiar and repetitive composition of the collagen molecule [6].

Previous research has demonstrated that the major repair agents of wounds (TGF-β, eNOs and iNOs, VEGF) are highly modulated by medications providing the specific stoichiometric ratios between amino acids found in procollagen (glycine, proline, and lysine) when compared with untreated lesions in healthy animals [7]. Presently, further current research has explored how different nitrogen inputs could influence the wounds healing process in experimental models, testing a large variety of different substrates containing different ratios of amino acids.

Characteristic Age-Related Changes of Normal Skin

The skin is the outermost defense organ of the body, which protects us from the environment. It is composed of three layers: the epidermis, the dermis, and subcutaneous tissue. The epidermis (epi = over) is the outermost layer of the skin. It consists predominantly of squamous epithelial cells (keratinocytes), and it produces cutaneous appendages, including the sebaceous glands, apocrine and eccrine sweat glands, hair follicles, and nails. The *stratum corneum*, the external surface layer, gives the skin its waterproofing barrier properties. This property depends on skin lipids (ceramides, cholesterol, and fatty acids) and on the mixture of natural moisturizing molecules, such as amino acids, organic acids, urea, and inorganic ions [8, 9], which can absorb large amounts of water.

The dermis lies between the epidermis and subcutaneous fat. The dermis, comprised of fibroblasts and the extracellular matrix (ECM) (formed by types I and III collagen, elastin, and glycosaminoglycans), is divided into the superficial papillary dermis and the deep reticular dermis. The papillary dermis forms ridges which maintain contact with the epidermis [1]. The dermis is the main contributor to skin thickness and provides oxygen and nutrition to the epidermis through blood and lymph vessels; as such it is very important for the skin's cosmetic appearance. Collagen gives the dermis its structural stability and resilience [9]. Therefore, the dermis nourishes the epidermis and not vice versa, as already mentioned. How nutrition affects the skin and dermis health is discussed in details in a later chapter of this textbook (please refer to "▶ Chap. 120, Aging Skin: Nourishing from the Inside Out – Effects of Good Versus Poor Nitrogen Intake on Skin Health and Healing").

Progressively, the aging skin undergoes a series of events that gradually reduce its structural integrity and its function. The thickness of the epidermis remains fairly constant with age [10], but there is a flattening of the dermal-epidermal junction, which allows the appearance of atrophy [11]. In addition, the time taken by the keratinocytes to migrate from the basal layer to the skin surface, a key process in repair, increases by 50 % in the elderly [12]. Aging, the dermis loses its thickness, elasticity, and water content also as a consequence of the reduction of lipids and amino acids in the *stratum corneum*, moreover dermis loses the melanocyte and Langerhans cell density, the sebum production, and the number of dermal blood vessels. As a result blood flow decreases, reducing the supply of nutrients and altering thermoregulation [9]. In addition, there is a flattening of the papillary dermis, decreasing surface contact between the dermis and epidermis [13]. This predisposes separation of the dermal-epidermal junction with laterally applied tension [11]. Furthermore, the cellular content of the dermis (fibroblasts, mast cells, Langerhans cells, and macrophages) also decreases with age [14]. Finally, the functional characteristics of the skin are compromised.

Moreover, there is a decrease of the dermis proteins content, primarily collagen with age. This is the result of both decreased production and increased collagen degradation [15]. The quality of the remaining collagen is altered, with fewer organized fibers, ropelike bundles, and a greater degree of disorganization. The quantity of elastin, a determinant of skin elasticity, is fairly constant with age. However, like collagen, elastin in the aged dermis has a disorganized morphology, resulting in decreased skin elasticity [16, 17].

Wound and Wound Healing

Wounds allow the environment to contact the dermis directly; thus, an efficient wound healing process must be activated quickly in order to protect the whole organism from environmental threats. Therefore, tissue repair and regeneration are important topics in aging. The main protein involved with the repair of the injured tissue is collagen. This is the most abundant protein in the animal kingdom, accounting for 30 % of total protein in the human body [18].

In normal tissues collagen provides strength, integrity, and structure. When tissues are disrupted, collagen is needed to repair the defect and restore the normal structure and function of the skin. Collagen mass in normal tissues is dependent on the balance between the rates of synthesis and degradation. A rapid increase of collagen production in wounds is indicative of higher rates of granulation tissue formation, resulting in faster reepithelialization.

The cells responsible for collagen deposition are the fibroblasts of the connective tissue. Within the wound bed, fibroblasts also produce two other important components of the ECM, glycosaminoglycans and proteoglycans, which play a fundamental role in the organization of collagen fibers and subsequently in wound closure. However, if too much collagen is deposited in the wound site, anatomical structure is lost, function is compromised, and fibrosis and scars occur. On the contrary, if an insufficient amount of collagen is deposited, the wound is weak and may dehisce [19].

A lot of interest has been generated by the observation that increased amounts of TGF-β are found in wounds that heal by scar formation as opposed to tissue regeneration. TGF-β is a negative regulator of wound reepithelialization. This finding has led to clinical efforts to block scar formation with antibodies and small molecules directed against TGF-β and other pro-inflammatory mediators. Recent evidence also suggests that changes in the wound physical environment might result in over-healing, by affecting the wound mechanical environment [20].

The healing of acute wounds is a very complex regenerative process. It is controlled by temporal interactions between cells, extracellular matrix components, and signaling molecules, and it is of great importance in clinical medicine. Acute wounds normally heal in an orderly and efficient manner characterized by distinct phases called hemostasis/inflammation, proliferation, and remodeling, which all overlap. Each healing phase depends on various factors such as tissue type, age, infections, health status, and, very importantly, nutritional status [20–28].

The first phase begins immediately after injury and is characterized by hemostasis and inflammation as a response to the injury. This phase usually lasts about 4–6 days after injury. During coagulation, the platelet releases several growth factors (PDGF, PF4, TGF-α, and TGF-β) and pro-inflammatory cytokines (TNF-α, iNOs, IL1) which initiate the inflammatory response [29]. These substances also act as chemoattractants for neutrophils and monocytes that clean the wound from foreign substances, increase vascular permeability, and promote fibroblast activity. In this phase the neutrophils elaborate ROS, protease, and metalloprotease (MMP) to kill bacteria and clear the extracellular matrix.

About 2–4 days after injury, monocytes transform into macrophages, which replace the predominant neutrophils and phagocytize debris product, bacteria, and apoptotic cells. Macrophages also release many chemoattractant molecules to recruit more macrophages and fibroblasts. Furthermore, macrophages initiate provisional matrix formation through the activation of TGF-β, which stimulates fibroblast proliferation and collagen synthesis [29]. The activation of macrophages and the balanced modulation of growth factors and cytokines during the inflammation phase direct the quality of tissue repair and are fundamental for the transition to the second step of wound repair, i.e., the proliferative phase.

The second stage of wound repair occurs 2–10 days after injury and is characterized by cellular proliferation (new tissue formation) and the migration of different cell types that overlap with the inflammatory phase. The new provisional matrix (the granulation tissue) invades the wound space. Fibroblasts and macrophages move into this space and provide a source of growth factors necessary to stimulate fibroplasia and angiogenesis. Macrophages and fibroblasts release protease that activates the TGF-β, which in turn stimulates fibroblast proliferation and collagen synthesis. The fibroblasts are responsible for the synthesis, deposition, and remodeling of the extracellular matrix [30].

The third stage of wound repair, remodeling, begins 2–3 weeks after injury and lasts for a year or more. During this stage, all processes activated after injury wind down and cease. Most of the endothelial cells, macrophages, and myofibroblasts undergo apoptosis (programmed cell death) or exit the wound, leaving a mass that contains few cells and consists mostly of collagen and other extracellular matrix proteins. This phase consists of the maturation and remodeling of new tissues inside the wounded area. The main feature of this phase is the deposition of collagen in an organized and well-mannered network, and so the fibroblasts play a pivotal role [29]. Epithelial-mesenchymal interactions probably continuously regulate skin integrity and homeostasis [20]. However, the tissue never regains the properties of uninjured skin [31].

The rate of wound healing is dependent on effective synchronization of these phases [32]. The biological and/or chemical agent with the ability to influence the repair process could improve their synchronization, thus lowering healing time.

Fibroblasts are cells that play a major role in the synthesis and reorganization of the extracellular matrix during all phases of wound repair. It is logical to think that maintaining the ideal nutritional environment for the fibroblasts is fundamental to facilitate the proper wound repair.

Alterations of the ECM that occur with advancing age, although less than in disease, may be linked to the altered functionality of fibroblasts, which decrease in number and size, slow their function, and fail to produce adequate amounts of molecules necessary to adjust wound repair. These age-related changes slow down the regeneration of tissue and wound closure in animal models as well as in human wounds [17]. However, the response of dermal fibroblast cultures derived from young and elderly subjects and stimulated with cytokines such as TGF-β1, EGF, TNF-α, and PDGF does not vary with the age of the donor [33]. They have also both demonstrated a significant increase in production of collagen-I and of other extracellular matrix proteins [34]. This suggests that proper nutrition and stimulation of cells may play a key role in the repair of skin lesions.

Dressing and Wound Nutrition

The main goal in the management of surgical and nonsurgical skin wounds is to obtain the physiological wound closure in the shortest period of time, in particular in the case of aged skin. Furthermore, the modulation of the synthesis and degradation of collagen during the phases of the repair process is of particular importance.

Presently, there are a wide variety of dressings available for wound care. The aim of wound dressing is to apply compression for hemorrhage or venous stasis, to immobilize an injured body part, to reduce pain, and to protect the wound and surrounding tissue. But dressings are also important because they are capable of promoting healing. Indeed, the aim of all care products is to create an aseptic environment preventing infection and moisturizing the wound tissue, enhancing epithelization and granulation tissue formation [35]. So, the ideal dressing material has to maintain a moist environment, act as a bacterial barrier, and act as a medium for free exchange of gases while providing a barrier against toxic contaminants. Furthermore, logically, it should also contain all the nutrients needed for proteins synthesis and tissue regeneration. But since it is assumed that nutrients are transported to the site of injury through the bloodstream, products for wound dressing rarely take into account this nutritional component.

At present we are still far from an ideal dressing. This is demonstrated by the large amount of medications available on the market. Unfortunately, a very small number of the products most widely used to treat wounds take into account the strong demand of nutrients by the cells to regenerate tissue and close the wound. However, many other natural substances such as honey, plant extracts, vitamins, amino acids, etc., have been used as adjuvants of wound closure [36]. For example, honey, one of the oldest known wound dressings, is a bee-derived supersaturated solution composed mainly of fructose and glucose, also containing proteins and amino acids, vitamins, enzymes, minerals, antibiotics, and other minor components. The renewed interest in the use of honey for topical wound care is probably because it combines low-cost antimicrobial properties with the maintenance of hydration and the presence of nutrients useful in tissue protection and regeneration [37]. More recently it has been suggested that beneficial action of honey in wound care could be explained, at least tentatively, by the production of lactic acid by microbiota and by the presence of active compounds such as proteins, fatty acids, anesthetics, organic acids, volatiles, and hydrogen peroxide [38, 39]. All these substances could modulate the microenvironment of the wound.

Topical wound dressings based on plant extracts may also act by modulating the inflammatory and oxidative stress responses. For example, the flavonoid fraction and luteolin from *Martynia annua* leaves when used for diabetic rats may have potential benefit in enhancing wound healing [40]. In another clinical trial in patients with neuropathic diabetic foot ulcers, the natural compounds contained in the kiwi fruit improved various aspects of the wound healing process [41]. More recently, treatment of excision wounds with papaya extract reduced inflammation-associated oxidative damage apparently via cyclooxygenase-specific inhibition, improved arginine metabolism, and induced the upregulation of antioxidant enzymes, thus improving wound healing [42].

Topical vitamin application is another approach to wound care. Vitamins should normally be present in the human skin as cofactors of enzymatic activities and because they are part of a system of antioxidants that protect the skin from oxidative stress. Vitamins, mainly A, C, E, K, and B_3, have been shown to have potent antioxidant and anti-inflammatory properties demonstrating wound healing potential in full-thickness wound models and under diabetic conditions [43–45].

All these topical therapeutic "natural" approaches show obvious benefits aiding wound repair. They act mainly in the initial step of healing, by reducing inflammation and oxidative stress response. Indeed inflammation has been shown to delay healing and so increasing scarring and predisposition to cancer development [46]. Conversely, scar-free wounds are characterized by reduced inflammation [47]. Numerous publications have highlighted the link between aging and inflammation [48]; therefore, the containment of chronic systemic and/or local inflammatory phenomena could help to slow the aging of tissues and promote wound healing.

A more fashionable molecular approach of wound repair in the last decade is the topical administration of growth factors and hormones. However, these approaches have not led to substantial advances in patient care. Indeed, they have only a moderate impact on wound repair in a clinical setting, probably due to the high plasticity and redundancy of the components of the wound repair process or because of their rapid degradation at the wound site [20].

Recently, a number of bioactive therapeutic peptides with significant in vitro activity have been identified from a wide variety of proteins, including collagen. Unfortunately, their action in vivo was often scarce or absent, probably because of rapid degradation. More recently, the multifunctional cryptic peptide E1 has been isolated from bovine tendon collagen type I and administered topically. However, being derived from a heterologous protein, it has been proposed as effective in accelerating the closure of wounds by lowering oxidative stress and promoting the rapid production of the ECM in excision and incision wound experimental models. This confirms the key role played by collagen peptides in accelerating the healing process and justifies their use as a pharmaceutical agent [49]. Although collagen-based dressing materials like hydrocolloids and hydrogels have been proven to be beneficial [50], topical applications of bioactive molecules such as the one derived from bovine tendon could be an effective way to sustain wound repair.

Over 30 years ago, a simple, safe, and effective method to improve repair and control of infection of human wounds from several causes has been proposed. This consists of debridement daily and application topically of a balanced solution of salts, amino acids, a high molecular weight D-glucose polysaccharide, and ascorbic acid [51]. In practice, the author tried to recreate the nutritional conditions and molecular setting suitable for tissue regeneration and for the containment of infection and oxidative stress.

The availability of adequate amounts of nutrients, in particular proteins, is essential for proper wound healing. This is probably due to the increased protein request needed for tissue regeneration and repair. Indeed, protein depletion appears to delay wound healing by prolonging the inflammatory phase; inhibiting fibroplasia, collagen and proteoglycan synthesis, and neo-angiogenesis (proliferation phase); and inhibiting wound remodeling [47]. However, proteins are formed from amino acids, and as such it seems logical to think that the availability of amino acids in the wound can accelerate and improve healing.

Researchers have investigated the effects of specific amino acids on the healing process and determined that arginine and glutamine appear to be necessary for proper wound healing [36, 52–55]. Recent data reveal that age-associated delay in acute healing is accompanied by a local reduction of arginase in wound granulation tissue associated with increased inflammation (increased iNOs expression) and defects in matrix deposition [56]. Glutamine accounts for about

60 % of the intracellular amino acid pool. It is considered to be conditionally essential, as a deficiency can occur rapidly after injury [54]. However, arginine and glutamine, although they may play a possible role in wound healing, are not the only amino acids needed by cells to activate the complex biosynthetic processes required for regeneration of the tissues.

In the past, the importance of the influence of nitrogen balance in the production of collagen for repair of skin wounds has been shown in weanling and young adult rats. This therefore demonstrates that age in itself is not necessarily a limiting factor for the speed of wound closure, which is, however, strongly influenced by the mix of nutrients available to the cells [57]. The importance of an optimal nutritional status of the patients with wounds is of fundamental importance for the right and rapid wound healing and is discussed in a separate chapter of this volume. Nevertheless, in addition to nutrition, the availability of medications that can adequately feed the tissues in injured area by maintaining the right nitrogen balance could be a readily available source of nutrients essential for the sustenance of cells during tissue regeneration.

Nourishing Fibroblasts Based on Analysis of Collagen Composition

Following the immediate vessel constriction needed to promote hemostasis, all steps of the wound healing process are primarily oriented toward providing the energy and materials necessary for the proliferative state. Oxygen is the most necessary substrate, but metabolism of the cells involved in the repairing process should also be replenished adequately. Thus, angiogenesis triggered by TGF-β1, platelet-derived growth factor (PDGF), and FGFs cooperates with hypoxia for VEGF-mediated neovascularization and repair of damaged blood vessels. The outer area of the wound is relatively avascular at the beginning, and diffusion from capillaries at the wound edge is the sole way of substrates to be provided. Thus, is medical intervention from out-in helpful to provide substrates and so help reduce the wound healing span and possible other related damage?

It was shown that lesion dressing of chronic human wounds of various etiologies, with a patented mixture of four specific amino acids (AAs) needed for collagen synthesis [glycine (29,28 %), L-proline (46,22 %), L-lysine (5,55 %), L-leucine (3,54 %)] plus Na hyaluronate (15,41 %), identified as GPLL-NaHy [according to US Patent n° 5,198,465, released on March 1993], induces rapid tissue regeneration and wound closure, thus opening new perspectives in chronic ulcer treatment [58]. The rationale for treating wounds by hydrocolloidal medications enriched with the formulation of AA by providing the peculiar stoichiometric composition of the AA most contained in collagen was carefully discussed by the author [6].

Subsequently, it was experimentally demonstrated that the topical therapy of wounds in aged rats by using a gel containing a specific formulation of four AAs required for collagen production shortens wound healing time and effectively reduces inflammation modulating the expression of the major controlling players of wound repair (TGF-β, eNOs and iNOs, VEGF). Furthermore, eNOs expression was found both to parallel TGF-β1 immuno-localization and to be associated with the increase density of fibroblasts and thus the promoted synthesis of collagen fibers. This was associated with a shorter healing time, when compared with the gel containing NaHy but AA free, used in control wounds. Also, TGF-β1 expression and suppression patterns were more precocious than in controls [7], providing support to the rationale that feeding wounds from out-in is an efficient approach promoting a more efficient dynamic homeostasis of wound healing. How changes in nitrogen content provided by nutrition affect skin and dermis health has been discussed in detail in a specific chapter of this textbook (please refer to "▸ Chap. 120, Aging Skin: Nourishing from the Inside Out – Effects of Good Versus Poor Nitrogen Intake on Skin Health and Healing").

There is a question concerning the use of NaHy to improve wound closure physiology. That is, are the formulations of proline, glycine, and lysine in the stoichiometric ratios used (25:50:25) the sole agents responsible for success, or is there also a role for L-leucine (a neutral branched chain AA), even if present in smaller amounts compared to other AAs?

To try to answer this question, an experimental study on an excisional wound model in healthy aged rats to test and compare a full set of different AA formulations (Table 1) as topical dressing has recently been launched. The control wounds did not receive any medication. Preliminary data had shown that dressing wounds with balanced mixture of essential AA (EAAs), branched chain AA (BCAA) alone, and a formulation containing all EAAs plus proline and glycine, identified by the letter T, significantly shortens the closure of wounds compared to other formulations. Wounds medicated with placebocream (vehicle of all cream dressing), NaHy, GPLL, and GPLL-NaHy and obviously undressed wound closed slower (Fig. 1). Interestingly, the topical dressing with the only essential non-BCAA (NBCAA) had longer wound closure times. Conversely, the only BCAA dressing had the same effect on the closure timing of the wound shown by the complete EAA mixture. However, it should be considered that the aged animals used in these experiments were healthy and they had food and water ad libitum. So, the proper amount of NBCAA needed for optimal wound closure could presumably derive from the diet. The NaHy dressing seemed to favor wound closure when compared to placebo, but when compared to any of the blends of AA, its effectiveness was poor.

Therefore, although the addition of amino acids specific to collagen synthesis has been demonstrated to be a promising approach to wound dressing, the cells at wound margins, such as newly formed cells, need the right amount of all EAAs in each phase of the healing process in order to proliferate efficaciously, regenerate tissues, and then quickly promote wound closure.

Conclusions

While laboratory studies are still in progress and will be reported elsewhere when accomplished, it can be concluded that wound healing in healthy living mammals is a naturally successful process, which may be favorably influenced by wet medications providing substrates from out-in. Wet medications are a simple and efficient medical aid and should be recommended in wound therapy. There are numerous approaches to skin wound treatment, both acute and chronic, which are helping to gradually understand mechanisms

Table 1 AA mixture composition of dress cream. *EAA* essential amino acid mixture, *BCAAs* branched chain amino acids, *T* EAA + proline + glycine, *GPLL* glycine + L-proline + L-lysine + L-leucine, *Plac* placebo, *NaHy* sodium hyaluronate

	EAA	BCAA	NBCAA	T	GPLL	GPLL + NaHy	NaHy	Plac
L-Leucine	x	x		x	x	x		
L-Lysine	x		x	x	x	x		
L-Isoleucine	x	x		x				
L-Valine	x	x		x				
L-Threonine	x		x	x				
L-Cysteine	x		x	x				
L-Histidine	x		x	x				
L-Phenylalanine	x		x	x				
L-Methionine	x		x	x				
L-Tyrosine	x		x	x				
L-Tryptophan	x		x	x				
L-Proline				x	x	x		
Glycine				x	x	x		
Na hyaluronate						x	x	
Vehicle *(water, glucomannane, vegetal glycerin)*	x	x	x	x	x	x	x	x

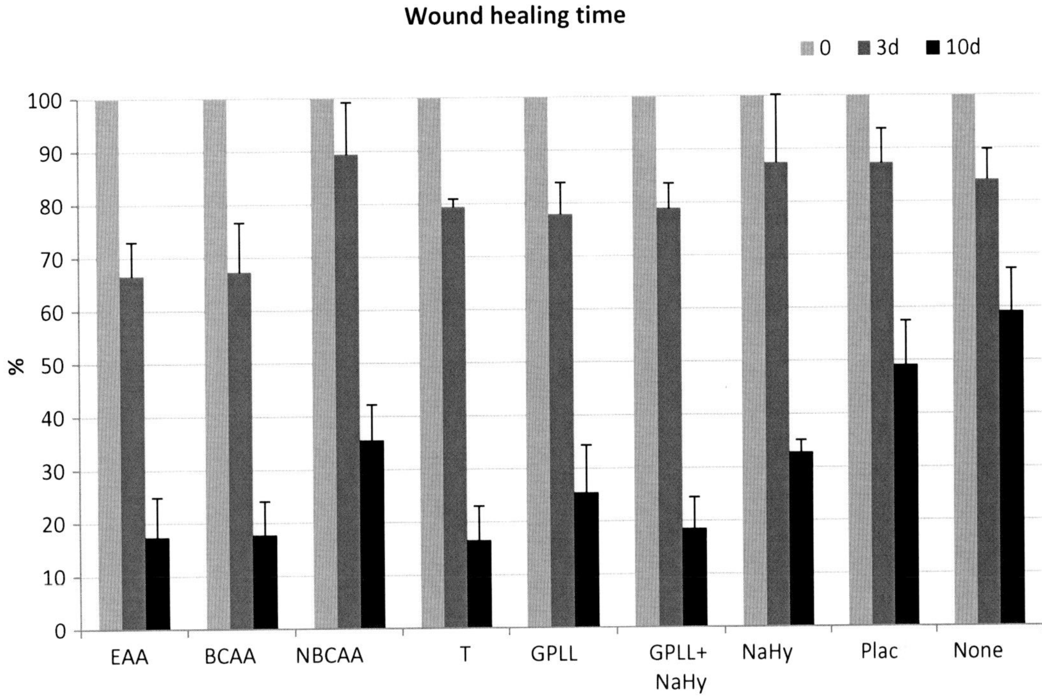

Fig. 1 Percentage of wound area from the original wound (day 0, pale grey column) and after 3 and 10 post-wounding days according to dressing composition. See also Table 1 for cream composition (Source Corsetti et al. [7])

that drive wound repair. Although all potentially promising, an ideal dressing is still far from being identified.

However, an important aspect that should be taken into account and should accompany all other approaches to wound care is the proper nutrition of patients as a preliminary approach to the success of any topical wound medication. This is particularly important in the elderly, where protein malnutrition is too often present and underestimated as a comorbidity of skin aging, as discussed in "▶ Chap. 121, Aging Skin: Nourishing from Out-In – Lessons from Wound Healing" of this textbook. Thus, creating a microenvironment where cells can constantly find the right amount of all necessary substances, particularly AA in the proper ratios, may be a safe and efficient therapeutic approach. This is particularly important in the elderly, where the prevalence of chronic inflammation, as well as altered nutrient availability, can slow or prevent complete healing of wounds. In conclusion, the proper nutrition of all tissues and particularly in injured areas appears to be a key factor that physicians should consider for the success of wound repair therapy.

References

1. Xua Z, et al. Teleost skin, an ancient mucosal surface that elicits gut-like immune responses. Proc Natl Acad Sci U S A. 2013;110(32):13097–102.
2. Browne GJ, Proud CG. Regulation of peptide-chain elongation in mammalian cells. Eur J Biochem. 2002;269:5360–8. doi:10.1046/j.1432-1033.2002.03290.
3. Kaleta C, et al. Metabolic costs of amino acid and protein production in *Escherichia coli*. Biotechnol J. 2013;8:1105–14. doi:10.1002/biot.201200267.
4. Junker JPE, et al. Clinical impact upon wound healing and inflammation in moist, wet, and dry environments. Adv Wound Care. 2013;2(7):348–56. doi:10.1089/wound.2012.0412.
5. Chandika P, et al. Marine-derived biological macromolecule-based biomaterials for wound healing and skin tissue regeneration. Int J Biol Macromol. 2015;14(77):24–35. doi:10.1016/j.ijbiomac.2015.02.050.

6. Dioguardi FS. Collagen synthesis: a determinant role for amino acids. J Clin Dermatol. 2008;26:636–40.
7. Corsetti G, et al. Topical application of dressing with amino acids improves cutaneous wound healing in aged rats. Acta Histochem. 2010;112(5):497–507. doi:10.1016/j.acthis.2009.05.003.
8. Segre JA. Epidermal barrier function and recovery in skin disorders. Clin Invest. 2006;116:1150–8.
9. Thomas DR, Burkemper NM. Aging skin and wound healing. Clin Geriatr Med. 2013;29(2):xi–xx. doi:10.1016/j.cger.2013.02.001.
10. Whitton JT, Everall JD. The thickness of the epidermis. Br J Dermatol. 1973;89:467–76.
11. Kurban RS, Bhawan J. Histologic changes in skin associated with aging. J Dermatol Surg Oncol. 1990;16:908–14.
12. Gilchrest BA, et al. Effect of chronologic aging and ultraviolet irradiation on Langerhans cells in human epidermis. J Invest Dermatol. 1982;79:85–8.
13. Montagna W, Carlisle K. Structural changes in aging human skin. J Invest Dermatol. 1979;73:47–53.
14. Swift ME, et al. Age-related alterations in the inflammatory response to dermal injury. J Invest Dermatol. 2001;117:1027–35.
15. Bernstein EF, et al. Long-term sun exposure alters the collagen of the papillary dermis. Comparison of sun-protected and photoaged skin by northern analysis, immunohistochemical staining, and confocal laser scanning microscopy. J Am Acad Dermatol. 1996;34:209–18.
16. Lavker RM, et al. Aged skin: a study by light, transmission electron, and scanning electron microscopy. J Invest Dermatol. 1987;88:44S–51.
17. Gosain A, Di Pietro LA. Aging and wound healing. World J Surg. 2004;28:321–6.
18. Prockop DJ, Kivirikko KI. Collagens: molecular biology, diseases, and potentials for therapy. Ann Rev Biochem. 1995;64:403–34.
19. Lazarus GS, et al. Definitions and guidelines for assessment of wounds and evaluation of healing. Arch Dermatol. 1994;130(4):489–93.
20. Gurtner GC, et al. Wound repair and regeneration. Nature. 2008;453:314–21.
21. Werner S, Grose R. Regulation of wound healing by growth factors and cytokines. Physiol Rev. 2003;83 (3):835–70.
22. Lau K, et al. Exploring the role of stem cells in cutaneous wound healing. Exp Dermatol. 2009;18 (11):921–33.
23. Martin P. Wound healing-aiming for perfect skin regeneration. Science. 1997;276(5309):75–81.
24. Rahban SR, Garner WL. Fibroproliferative scars. Clin Plast Surg. 2003;30(1):77–89.
25. McDaniel JC, et al. Omega-3 fatty acids effect on wound healing. Wound Repair Regen. 2008;16 (3):337–45.
26. Novotný MT, et al. ER-agonist induces conversion of fibroblasts into myofibroblasts, while ER-agonist increases ECM production and wound tensile strength of healing skin wounds in ovariectomised rats. Exp Dermatol. 2011;20(9):703–8.
27. Cardoso CR, et al. Influence of topical administration of n-3 and n-6 essential and n-9 nonessential fatty acids on the healing of cutaneous wounds. Wound Repair Regen. 2004;12(2):235–43.
28. Araujo LU, et al. Profile of wound healing process induced by allantoin1. Acta Cir Bras. 2010;25(5):460–6.
29. Broughton G, et al. The basic science of wound healing. Plast Reconstr Surg. 2006;117(7S):12S–34.
30. Singer AJ, Clark RAF. Cutaneous wound healing. N Engl J Med. 1999;341(10):738–46.
31. Levenson SM, et al. The healing of rat skin wounds. Ann Surg. 1965;161:293–308.
32. Schultz GS, Wysocki A. Interactions between extracellular matrix and growth factors in wound healing. Wound Repair Regen. 2009;17:153–62.
33. Freedland M, et al. Fibroblast responses to cytokines are maintained during aging. Ann Plast Surg. 1995;35:290–6.
34. Reed MJ, et al. TGF-beta 1 induces the expression of type I collagen and SPARC, and enhances contraction of collagen gels, by fibroblasts from young and aged donors. J Cell Physiol. 1994;158:169–79.
35. Sarabahi S. Recent advances in topical wound care. Indian J Plast Surg. 2012;45(2):379–87. doi:10.4103/0970-0358.101321.
36. MacKay D, Miller AL. Nutritional support for wound healing. Altern Med Rev. 2003;8(4):359–77.
37. Burlando B, Cornara L. Honey in dermatology and skin care: a review. J Cosmet Dermatol. 2013;12(4):306–13.
38. Olofsson TC, et al. Lactic acid bacterial symbionts in honeybees – an unknown key to honey's antimicrobial and therapeutic activities. Int Wound J. 2014. doi:10.1111/iwj.12345.
39. Butler É, et al. A pilot study investigating lactic acid bacterial symbionts from the honeybee in inhibiting human chronic wound pathogens. Int Wound J. 2014. doi:10.1111/iwj.12360.
40. Lodhi S, Singhai AK. Wound healing effect of flavonoid rich fraction and luteolin isolated from *Martynia annua* Linn. on streptozotocin induced diabetic rats. Asian Pac J Trop Med. 2013;6(4):253–9.
41. Mohajeri G, et al. Effects of topical Kiwifruit on healing of neuropathic diabetic foot ulcer. J Res Med Sci. 2014;19(6):520–4.
42. Nafiu AB, Rahman MT. Anti-inflammatory and antioxidant properties of unripe papaya extract in an excision wound model. Pharm Biol. 2015;53 (5):662–71.
43. Lima CC, et al. Ascorbic acid for the healing of skin wounds in rats. Braz J Biol. 2009;69(4):1195–201.
44. Lin TS, et al. Evaluation of topical tocopherol cream on cutaneous wound healing in streptozotocin-induced diabetic rats. Evid Based Complement Alternat Med. 2012;2012:491027.
45. Hemmati AA, et al. Topical vitamin K1 promotes repair of full thickness wound in rat. Indian J Pharmacol. 2014;46(4):409–12.

46. Eming SA, et al. Inflammation in wound repair: molecular and cellular mechanisms. J Invest Dermatol. 2007;127:514–26.
47. Wild T, et al. Basic in nutrition and wound healing. Nutrition. 2010;26(9):862–6.
48. Jurk D, et al. Chronic inflammation induces telomere dysfunction and accelerates ageing in mice. Nat Commun. 2014;5:4172. doi:10.1038/ncomms5172.
49. Banerjee P, et al. Wound healing activity of a collagen IV derived cryptic peptide. Amino Acids. 2015;47:317–28.
50. Pielesz A, Paluch J. Therapeutically active dressings--biomaterials in a study of collagen glycation. Polim Med. 2012;42:115–20.
51. Silvetti AN. An effective method of treating long-enduring wounds and ulcers by topical applications of solutions of nutrients. J Dermatol Surg Oncol. 1981;7(6):501–8.
52. Shi HP, et al. Supplemental L-arginine enhances wound following trauma/hemorrhagic shock. Wound Repair Regen. 2007;15:66–70.
53. Gould A, et al. Arginine metabolism and wound healing. Wound Heal S Afr. 2008;1(1):48–50.
54. Demling RH. Nutrition, anabolism, and the wound healing process: an overview. ePlasty. 2009;9:65–94.
55. Raynaud-Simon A, et al. Arginine plus proline supplementation elicits metabolic adaptation that favors wound healing in diabetic rats. Am J Physiol Regul Integr Comp Physiol. 2012;303(10):1053–61.
56. Campbell L, et al. Local arginase 1 activity is required for cutaneous wound healing. J Invest Dermatol. 2013;133:2461–70.
57. Hennessey PJ, et al. The effects of age and various fat/carbohydrate caloric ratios on nitrogen retention and wound healing in rats. J Pediatr Surg. 1991;26(4):367–73.
58. Cassino R, Ricci E. Amino acids and wound bed: a possible interaction for a topic and general treatment in the chronic skin lesion repair. Acta Vulnol. 2005;3:111–5.

Part X

Psychosocial Implications

Psychological and Social Implications of Aging Skin: Normal Aging and the Effects of Cutaneous Disease

122

Miranda A. Farage, Kenneth W. Miller, Enzo Berardesca, and Howard I. Maibach

Contents

M.A. Farage (✉)
Winton Hill Business Center, The Procter & Gamble Company, Cincinnati, OH, USA
e-mail: farage.m@pg.com

K.W. Miller
Margoshes-Miller Consulting, LLC, Cincinnati, OH, USA
e-mail: bbbns2@fuse.net

E. Berardesca
San Gallicano Dermatological Institute, Rome, Italy
e-mail: berardesca@berardesca.it

H.I. Maibach
Department of Dermatology, University of California, San Francisco, CA, USA
e-mail: maibachh@derm.ucsf.edu

M.A. Farage et al. (eds.), *Textbook of Aging Skin*,
DOI 10.1007/978-3-662-47398-6_89

Abstract

Although much of gerontological research in dermatology has focused on an esthetic abeyance of the signs of aging, little real medical attention has been paid to the psychosocial effects of aging skin. Patients with skin disease, including elderly patients, have a substantial burden of psychosocial suffering. The high visibility of skin diseases, particularly when superimposed on the already compromised aged skin, induces both unconscious and intentional stigmatization of the patient. The awareness of one's compromised appearance makes interpersonal relationships uncomfortable and promotes social withdrawal. Having a rough, itchy, aged skin is associated with a significant level of both physical and psychological discomfort. Dermatologists and patients differ in their assessment of the psychosocial impact of dermatological conditions. Patient health should be measured not only by physical symptoms but also by the likely psychological and social sequelae, all having impact on the quality of life.

Introduction

Aging, by definition, is a progressive deterioration of body structure and function [1, 2]. All organs age, skin included. The skin wrinkles, sags, and thins, becoming drier, rougher, and less elastic [1]. Successful aging transcends the inevitable physical decline and is characterized by adaptive psychosocial functioning that facilitates the maintenance of good mental health and satisfaction in daily life [3]. Although much of gerontological research in dermatology has focused on an esthetic abeyance of the signs of aging, little real medical attention has been paid to the psychosocial effects of an aging integument [4]. The skin is the envelope of the self and therefore the visible manifestation of personal identity [4]. It displays emotion, blanching, blushing, and sweating in response to internal feelings [5]. The "social" skin and its gerontological issues, then, must be contrasted to the merely biological skin [5].

Even in the absence of frank disease, the aged skin no longer looks or feels good, a subjective evaluation whose currency is not biology, but psychology [6, 7]. Skin that does not look or feel good is emotionally burdensome [6]. Skin that is rough and itchy is uncomfortable, with the potential to cause considerable emotional distress [6]. Skin that becomes discolored, blemished, or loose, or is obviously oozing or crusting over, is unappealing, eroding the self-esteem of its owner, and causing anxiety, depression, and social withdrawal [8].

In addition, the prevalence of skin disease increases steadily throughout life [9]. Most people over 65 have at least two skin diseases worthy of treatment [5]; 10 % of those over 70 years of age have more than ten concurrent complaints [6]. Dry skin and pruritus affect virtually everybody by the eighth decade of life [6]. The view is widespread even among medical personnel that skin disorders in old age are trivial, with largely cosmetic ramifications [5]. In fact, skin disorders in the elderly are often the bane of their existence, the source of a significant amount of discomfort and distress [10], and having an adverse effect on almost every area of life [11].

The impact of cutaneous disorders in the elderly on the "social skin" has been largely ignored until recently [4]. Skin disease can be disfiguring, adding to the psychological burden of the already aged skin and causing further embarrassment and loss of self-confidence [8, 12]. Skin diseases can repel physical contact by others, leading to social withdrawal and obstruction of interpersonal relationships [6]. Skin diseases can also disrupt daily life activities and interfere with both work and leisure pursuits [13]. Decreasing quality of life (QoL) due to cutaneous disease in the elderly leads frequently to depression, anxiety, and other psychological dysfunctions, robbing many older people of QoL in their later years [13].

Beauty and the Aged Skin

An attractive appearance is a very valuable commodity [4]. Those deemed physically attractive by their fellow members of society have been shown to reap personal, educational, occupational, and social rewards [14]. Social reinforcement of physical attractiveness begins early: babies with a pleasing appearance receive more attention than more homely babies [15]. Esthetically pleasing children get better grades and less punishment in school [16].

Those endowed with pleasing looks are believed to have equally appealing personalities [17], to have positive life experiences [17], and to be smarter, more successful, and more capable of emotional intimacy [18]. The physically blessed draw higher salaries and more rapid promotions than their more homely colleagues [19].

Youthfulness is very much considered a component of attractiveness in the twenty-first century Western society [4]. The elderly are dismissed as unimportant or even inconvenient [4] and inevitably judged as unattractive simply because they are aged [4]. The skin is a primary contributor to the evaluation of age [20], a fact instinctively appreciated by those with aged skin. People with photodamaged skin exhibited high anxiety and a high level of discomfort in interpersonal relationships, an issue which normalized after treatment ameliorated the cutaneous manifestations of photodamage [21, 22].

Advanced age is viewed increasingly as a negative thing [23] and interestingly no longer something which must be stoically endured; the social culture that has developed over the last few generations carries an expectation that signs of age must be staved off whenever possible [23], putting perhaps more psychological pressure on the aging individual. Ameliorating the physical signs of aging, when possible, however, is medically advisable. Attractive older people are more favorably perceived by others [6].

In addition, being deemed "attractive," and therefore successful, competent, and pleasant, is to some extent a self-fulfilling label [4, 24]. An "attractive" group of older people was observed to be actually happier, more satisfied with life, and socially more active than an age-matched group of more unattractive seniors [5, 20], a finding with long-term implications. In a longitudinal study which evaluated 24 age-related functions, the most attractive 15 % of a senior study population had better functional scores than did the most unattractive 15 %. More importantly, the more attractive 15 % had significantly longer lifespans [25].

Factors in Individual Adaption to Aging

There is a diversity in how people age. Some age more successfully than others [3, 4]. Individual physiological aging is determined by the effects of lifestyle choices on a genetic foundation [1, 2]. Personal psychosocial adaptation is also based on a genetically determined personality, modulated by early developmental influences as well as later-life experiences [4].

There are numerous factors that go into the psychosocial burden that cutaneous disease in old age will represent to any particular individual. The severity and location of the lesions, the nature of the lesions, and the nature and severity of pain or itching play a major role in determining the extent of psychological distress [26]. In studies of psoriasis patients, plaques on visible skin were, predictably, more disabling than plaques located only in occulted areas [27], although, surprisingly, even plaques in invisible areas could cause substantial psychosocial disturbance [28]. Indeed, resistant psoriasis, even in non-visible areas, can be an indication to systemic treatment. Contagious diseases cause more social withdrawal than noncontagious [26] and life-threatening diseases more distress than nonthreatening disorders [26].

Whether the disease is self-limiting or chronic is also an important consideration. With chronic skin diseases, where alleviation of symptoms is not expected, physical symptoms and emotional symptoms can synergistically spiral downward. For example, intense itching will often disrupt sleep patterns, causing emotional distress. As the intensity of physical symptoms increases, the cycle may deteriorate until significant impairments in emotional health, social functioning, and sleep patterns are experienced, causing increasing fatigue and depression [29]. As attention to hygiene and grooming wanes with waxing psychosocial dysfunction, an aversion and/or rejection of the subject may also occur, accelerating the downward spiral [28].

Existing psychological health is also an important component to coping with a debilitating skin disease. The strongest single predictor of later psychosocial adjustment in early psychiatric history – tranquilizer use before the age of 50 – predicts less favorable mental health in old age [30].

A foundational self-esteem is a critical determinant of psychological health, sowed largely in early months of life as the mother positively responds to her baby's needs. Self-esteem thus established in the early months of life lays down positive body image, emotional stability, a sense of personal security, and a conviction of personal ability to determine life events [4]. The person who develops self-esteem in childhood will, as an adult, find ways to reinforce that self-esteem [4]. Self-esteem, which endows these individuals with a basic belief that they can change negative circumstances, also helps a negative life circumstance to be eventually accepted, integrated, and used as a springboard for personal growth [5]. People whose body image and self-esteem are less stable have been observed to exhibit dysmorphic tendencies, an obsession with personal appearance, and depression as a reaction to skin disease [31].

Many other personality characteristics have been associated with difficulty in accepting and coping with a skin disease. Patients with high levels of perceived helplessness have demonstrably worse physical and psychological functioning [32]. A high need for approval, an elevated fear of negative evaluation, and difficulty expressing anger also correlated to an increased psychological burden and an increased level of disability in psoriasis patients [33]. Individuals with narcissistic personalities have demonstrated more difficulty in handling signs of aging and/or cutaneous disease [34]. Finally, a high internal need for control (obsessive-compulsive personality) increases distress with regard to skin aging or disease [8].

In addition, the level of social support available plays a role in how an individual adapts to the psychosocial ramifications of skin disease. The perceived level of specific support and the size of the available social network influence psychosocial functioning [32].

Psychosocial Effects of Skin Disease in Old Age

It has been demonstrated that physical attractiveness influences social acceptance: more attractive individuals enjoy preferential treatment in social interactions [17, 35]. Throughout history, those with skin disease have been social outcasts [4]. Skin diseases have been assumed to be contagious [26] or to be a punishment for some type of wrongdoing [6] and have been responded to by revulsion and aversive behaviors [5]. Today, caregivers in nursing homes and hospital have been shown to be more distant and less nurturing when patients are aged or otherwise unattractive [34].

Patients with skin disease are familiar with being asked to leave swimming pools, gyms, parties, beaches, and other public places because of their affliction [26]: for example, 40 % of psoriasis patients have been asked to leave public swimming pools or hair salons [27]. Such stigmatization can understandably cause profound psychological distress [36], with sufferers feeling rejected, humiliated, embarrassed, and singled out [28, 37]. Many patients, particularly those who have been rejected previously, anticipate rejection and withdraw, avoiding parties, sports, meeting new people, being photographed, or unnecessarily exposing skin [38]. One survey of psoriasis sufferers found that 64 % avoid short-sleeved clothes, 57 % felt stared at, 55 % felt that people believed psoriasis to be contagious, 55 % felt untouchable, 50 % felt sexual relationships affected, and 34 % avoided hair salons; notably, 12 % avoided public contact altogether [39]. Chronic dermatological diseases are also known to impact male sexual dysfunction [40, 41].

Skin disease can also have a substantial effect on the sufferer's livelihood. The presence of a chronic skin disease can quite often limit the choice and the progression of a career [38], but even when established in a career, 20 % of those with cutaneous disease reported interference with work performance. Indeed, 31 % of psoriasis sufferers report some degree of financial difficulty related to the disease [27, 42].

Older people with skin disease in general feel less stigmatized than younger individuals [26], with anticipation of rejection, sensitivity to the opinion of others, and feelings of guilt and shame being less pronounced in older patients at the onset of psoriasis [43]. Older patients experience distress equal to their younger counterparts when manifestations of psoriasis and other disfiguring skin diseases are severe [32]. The attitudes of the people closest to the patient proved to be the most important determinant in the impact that the disease had with regard to social functioning [26].

An important consideration in social interaction for skin disease patients, particularly the aged, relates to the human emotional need for touch. It has been demonstrated that a broad area of tactile stimulation increases self-esteem in children [4]; the benefits of touch are at least as important in the aged [44]. However, as a human being ages, the skin becomes rougher, less attractive, and less pleasant to touch [5], while at the same time the pool of potential touchers typically becomes smaller [4]. Less attractive residents of nursing homes have been observed to be less likely to elicit touching by caregivers than more attractive residents [44].

Touching interventions, however, in nursing home populations have demonstrated that residents who receive regular touch through massages, hugs, and hand squeezes are more alert and less confused than those who are not touched [44, 45]. Conversely, 26 % of psoriasis patients in one study had experienced in the previous month an event in which someone made a conscious effort to avoid touching them, thus setting the stage for psychological distress. The Carroll rating scale for depression correlates depression with a lack of recent touch [46].

Psychological Effects

Skin imperfections have a negative influence on self-esteem [6], often in dramatic disproportion to the physical severity of the disease. A survey of 236 dermatology patients by a general health questionnaire found a higher prevalence of psychiatric disorder among patients with skin disease (i.e., acne, eczema, psoriasis, alopecia); patients severely affected with psoriasis exhibited the highest level of depression scores (using the Carroll rating scale for depression), equivalent to clinical depression [47]. Psychological effects related to depression are displayed in Table 1.

Certain diseases (e.g., vitiligo) that involve a change in skin pigmentation, but no health consequences whatsoever, have the potential to create a significant psychosocial burden [48]. As the skin represents the interface between the internal self and the external world, patients take skin disease personally. Skin disease makes the patient feel anomalous and out of control [26]. Even modern patients often attribute their own skin disease to some personal wrongdoing [6]. There is therefore often an inherent sense of guilt; the patient feels that he or she must have done something to deserve the affliction [26], and the disease engenders feelings of helplessness, anger, shame, embarrassment, and frustration [49, 50].

In a group of patients with a variety of skin disease, specific contributors to psychological stress were identified as fatigue, a perceived lack of control, feelings of alienation, and a perceived lack of social support [32, 51]. In a study focused on patients with atopic dermatitis, itching was the biggest component to psychological distress, with 63.2 % stating that it was very or extremely bothersome, followed by occasional sleep disturbances (57 %), dryness (52.3 %), rashes (47.2 %), and open sores (21.2 %) [29]. One percent of the patients reported continual sleep disruption [29]. In atopic dermatitis, severe itching was also strongly related to psychological distress [32]. Itching is far less tolerable than pain, as well as more intractable to treatment [6]. Psychosocial factors likely contribute to the development and exacerbation of chronic spontaneous urticaria (CSU) [52, 53]. Generalized, intractable pruritus is the most common dermatological cause of suicide [6]. In an evaluation of the psychosocial burden of venous ulcers using the *Skindex-29* index, older patients displayed worse QoL scores than younger patients [54]. In venous ulcer patients, 80.5 % reported pain, 69.4 % itching, 66.7 % altered appearance, 66.6 % sleep deficit, and 58.3 % functional limitations [54]. Venous ulcers have also been shown to produce embarrassment [55] and social isolation [56] (Tables 2 and 3).

The effects of psychological stress include an increased risk of destructive behaviors such as alcohol and tobacco abuse, the use of tranquilizers, sleeping medications, and the use of antidepressants [64, 65], particularly in men [66, 67].

Table 1 The prevalence of psychological effects in psoriasis and atopic dermatitis

	Depression	Anxiety	Despair	Suicidal ideation	Distress
Psoriasis	46 %[a] [32]	33 %[a] [32]	26 % [37]	2.5 % [32] in outpatients	21 % [37]
	20 %[b] [32]	13 %[b] [32]		7.5 % (in inpatients) [32]	
Atopic dermatitis	45 %[a] [32]	30 %[a] [32]		2.1 % [32]	

[a]Identified as depressed or anxious by virtue of scoring equal to or higher than the mean average of psychiatric outpatients on the depressed mood and anxiety scale

[b]Identified as depressed or anxious by virtue of scoring equal to or higher than patients with a diagnosis of clinical depression or clinical anxiety

Table 2 Common disorders in the aged and their psychosocial implications

Disorder	Prevalence	Sources of psychosocial suffering	Reference
Xerosis	Nearly 100 % by eighth decade of life [57]	Skin becomes dry and itchy and cracks	[58]
Pruritus	Up to 29 % [57]	Intense itching, sleep disturbances, can be a significant psychosocial stress	[59]
Fungal infections, primarily of feet	38 % [57]	Unsightly, discomfort, may be disabling	[57]
Seborrheic dermatitis	6 % [57]	Unsightly, itchy	[60]
Benign neoplasms	12.8 % [57]	Unsightly	[57]
Pigment disorders	4.4 % [57]	Unsightly	[57]
Malignant tumors	2.1 % [57]	Unsightly, anxiety	[57]

Patients with acne, psoriasis, and facial conditions are more likely to have reactive depression and be at risk of suicide [68–71].

Elderly patients were found to suffer at least as much psychological distress as younger patients as the result of both psoriasis and atopic dermatitis [32]. Severe psychological distress suffered by victims of vitiligo was also determined to be as pronounced in the aged as in younger patients [72]. In general, suicide is attempted less often but is successful more often in older patients, and suicide rates rise significantly after the age of 75 [73]. It is not unlikely that the psychosocial ramifications of aged skin and its attendant disfiguring and disabling disorders contribute to the increased risk of suicide in the aged population [8].

Quality of Life

Numerous indexes have been validated for the measuring of QoL in skin conditions: *Dermatology Life Quality Index*, *Dermatology Quality of Life Scales*, *Dermatology-Specific Quality of Life*, *Psoriasis Disability Index*, and *Skindex-29*. Studies using these indices routinely demonstrate that skin diseases have a profound effect on the patient's quality of life. QoL indices attempt to measure the various ways in which skin disease impacts the patient's life: psychological stress, social function, and functional limitations with regard to work, daily life, or leisure activities.

Many patients feel they have been discriminated socially, economically, and by medical insurers [38, 74]. They report intense psychological upheaval and strong feelings of alienation and rejection, using words like *mortified*, *unspeakable*, *hideous*, *gruesome*, and *hateful* [26, 75]. In a study of 100 patients (diseases represented included eczema, psoriasis, and acne), 40 % reported social isolation, 74 % reported interference with work, 80 % reported shame, 60 % reported anxiety, and 30 % reported experiencing depression [76]. Photodermatoses, a group of skin disorders caused or exacerbated by ultraviolet and/or visible radiation, collectively affect a high proportion of the population and substantially affect QoL [22].

Several studies have compared the quality of life for skin disease patients with that of other serious diseases. The impact of psoriasis on QoL was found to be as pronounced as that of cancer, heart attacks, or chronic pulmonary diseases [77]. A full 46 % of psoriasis patients felt it at least as bad to have psoriasis as diabetes [66]. In addition, patients with psoriasis were observed to have both physical and mental function reduced to a level comparable to arthritis, cancer, depression, and heart disease [77, 78]. The only group with higher risk of mental illness than psoriasis was those who experience major depression [77]. A large British survey found the disability impact of skin diseases to be equivalent to that of angina, asthma, bronchitis, arthritis, diabetes, hypertension, and back pain [38].

Table 3 Less common dermatological complaints of the aged with a high psychosocial burden

	Visible manifestations	Sensory manifestations	Natural history	Impact on QoL	Prognosis	Reference
Psoriasis	Typically, thick keratin salmon-colored plaques covered with silvery scales of dead skin	Severe itching, irritation	Chronic, relapsing	Affects self-image, discomfort, high cost in time and money to treat, social withdrawal	Idiosyncratic	[32]
Eczema	Erythema, can excoriate, crust, ooze	Itching, pain if scratching produces excoriation	Chronic	Unsightly, causes discomfort, causes self-image disturbances, social withdrawal	Tends to be chronic, some forms increase with old age	[61]
Atopic dermatitis	Cycle of itching and scratching results in erythema, exudation, excoriation, dryness, cracking, lichenification	Pain, itching	Chronic	Unsightly, causes discomfort	Improves throughout lifespan but can persist into old age	[29]
Leg ulcers	Ulcerated open wound	Pain, itching	Chronic	Unsightly, requires bulky dressings, exudes embarrassing odor	Onset typically in old age, some resolve but many chronic	[55]
Rosacea	Reddened, inflamed cheeks with or without presence of papules or pustules	Irritation, burning	Chronic	Unsightly, negative effect on self-image, social withdrawal, occupational effects	Onset in early maturity, persists	[62]
Urticaria	Erythema, cutaneous swellings accompanied by pruritus	Pain, itching	Less than 48 h	Affects self-image, discomfort, activity limitation, social withdrawal		[63]
Contact dermatitis	Erythema, possible exudation, excoriation	Pain, itching	Related to exposure	Unsightly, causes discomfort	Possible at any life stage	[62]

In a comparison of QoL between younger and older psoriasis patients, those younger than 54 had more difficulty with psychosocial issues, while those 55 and up had more disability and limitation on life activities. Older patients had more trouble sleeping (22 %), using hands (19 %), walking (14 %), and sitting (15 %) or standing (15 %) for long periods of time [27].

Studies Which Have Evaluated Psychosocial Burden of Skin Disease in Older People

Studies that looked specifically at the psychosocial effects of skin disease on older patients have been very limited [79].

One study observed that older people with rashes had significantly poorer quality of life than patients with lesions (including skin cancer), with the extent of disease inversely associated with the QoL [80]. Patients enrolled in the study had a variety of cutaneous diseases, including basal cell carcinoma (BCC), squamous cell carcinoma (SCC), malignant melanoma (MM), actinic keratoses, Bowen's disease, basal cell papilloma, granuloma annulare, eczema, xerosis, psoriasis, venous ulceration, lichenoid eruptions, extensive actinic damage, and urticarial reactions [80].

Older psoriasis patients have been observed to have relatively fewer issues with socialization than younger psoriasis patients [64]. Nevertheless, QoL in older patients suffers. A hospital-based, cross-sectional study evaluated the effect of age on QoL in psoriasis patients, using *Skindex-29*, the *Dermatology Life Quality Index* (*DLQI*), the *Psoriasis Disability Index*, the *General Health Questionnaire*, and the *Psoriasis Life Stress Inventory*. QoL was observed to be significantly worse in older patients and the psychological distress higher. Older women suffering from anxiety or depression had greatest impairment of quality of life [81]. In another study on psoriasis in ambulatory psoriasis patients, psychological distress was higher in the aged [82]. Psychological stress in the elderly patient is largely the result of pruritus and functional limitation [27].

Quality of life was also evaluated in vitiligo patients using the *Skindex-29* index. QoL impairment was very pronounced, with 39 % of all patients probably with depression. QoL effects were equally pronounced in aged patients as in younger ones [83].

Pemphigus, an autoimmune blistering disease, related to QoL was also evaluated in older patients. Pemphigus was observed to induce a markedly impaired QoL, with decreases in positive emotions and functioning. Depression and/or anxiety was observed in 39.7 % of patients. Older patients were more significantly affected than younger patients [84].

Therapeutic Options

First of all, the dermatologists must consciously monitor their elderly patients for indications of psychiatric pathology related to dermatological disease, which was often missed in the past [13]. It was observed that dermatologists consistently underestimated the level of psychological suffering related to dermatological disorders, often assuming the severity of psychosocial suffering to be determined by the clinical severity of disease [13]. Once the emotional ramifications of skin disease are recognized, there should be a plan of intervention [85].

Physicians must work to optimize doctor-patient relationship [26]. This is critical in order for the patient with skin disease to overcome overwhelming feelings of alienation and isolation. The physician must acknowledge the feelings of their patients with skin issues, remove embarrassment as much as possible, and provide complete and appropriate information [4], because a well-educated patient feels more in control and appropriately emotionally distanced from the disorder [26, 86]. In a recent clinical study, adalimumab treatment reduced psoriasis symptoms, reduced depression symptoms, and improved health-related QoL in patients with moderate to severe psoriasis [87]. Propylthiouracil is another therapeutic option in psoriasis, especially when the standard drugs cannot be used due to their toxicities or prohibitive costs [88, 89]. A recent study evaluated the effect of oral isotretinoin, an effective treatment in the clinical control of acne, on symptoms of anxiety and/or depression and improving QoL. At the end of the study, there was a significant reduction in the negative impact on QoL, in which the mean level of patient satisfaction with improvement of symptoms was 84.4 % [90].

The health-care provider must also be cognizant of the deep need for touch in these patients [4] and encourage the use of sunscreening agents, retinoids, alpha hydroxy acids, adequate moisturizers, and emollients to improve the appearance and texture of skin [4]. For example, appropriate use of commercial cosmetics and dermatological concealers is to be encouraged; the use of the dermatological covering makeup (Unifiance® [La Roche-Posay]) to conceal discolorations, lesions, rosacea, vitiligo, and acne improved the mean DLQI score from 9.2 to 5.5. Maximizing physical attractiveness is to be encouraged in order to reduce stereotypical responses to the elderly [4]. Enhanced understanding of the molecular pathways that lead to aged appearance will also help design drugs and devices to treat aging skin [91]. Tumors and other blemishes should be destroyed or removed, as well as wrinkles, scars, and pigmentation issues in order to optimize appearance [6]. More involved procedures should be pursued as appropriate, keeping in mind the very real psychological and physical benefits of improved appearance [4, 6]. Esthetic procedures often are viewed as vain or frivolous: the patient may need to be convinced of the very real medical benefits to be gained from optimizing appearance [6]. The physician should encourage participation in support groups [26, 92], which increases confidence, decreases the sense of isolation, provides a relief from embarrassment, and provides a safe haven to share the emotional burden of the disease [85]. Significant improvements in healing rates have been observed in support group for leg ulcers [55]. Education of patients earlier in life will help put them on paths to a healthy and successful old age [4]. Social support for patients with psoriasis can help reduce the debilitating skin disorder-related emotional disorders such as anxiety and depression [93]. Treatment regimens for psoriasis patients should also include stress-reduction strategies, such as biofeedback, meditation, yoga, and self-help approaches [75].

Beyond patient care, there is a need for social change. Physicians when possible should act to change societal dehumanization of the elderly [4, 92]. In addition, third-party insurers currently do not typically recognize the psychosocial ramifications of skin disease in the elderly. Because relatively inexpensive procedures could potentially avert much more serious psychological illness [4], the fact that these procedures are often disallowed by insurers responsible [5] is a false economy [4]. Patients who feel attractive and comfortable in their skin and socially at ease will seek interaction more and are more active; this will boost to overall health [94], which is ultimately the goal of every patient-provider encounter.

Conclusion

Patients with skin disease, including elderly patients, have a substantial burden of psychosocial suffering. The high visibility of skin diseases, particularly when superimposed on the already compromised aged skin, induces both unconscious and intentional stigmatization of the patient. The awareness of one's compromised appearance makes interpersonal relationships uncomfortable and promotes social withdrawal. Having a rough, itchy, aged skin is associated with a significant level of both physical and psychological discomfort.

Dermatologists and patients differ in their assessment of the psychosocial impact of dermatological conditions: dermatologists consistently underestimated the degree of psychological distress that their patients suffered, a misconception that may impede the recognition of psychiatric disorders in their patients [95]. Dermatologists tend to estimate the psychological burden by the severity of the physical disease, while in fact, it is not uncommon (particularly with psoriasis) for a patient with less severe disease to have impairment in psychosocial function equivalent to that in a patient with much more severe physical symptoms [96]. The psychosocial effect of skin disease on patients' lives, in fact, has been shown to be comparable to the impact of several diseases considered much more serious [49]. The effect of skin disease on psychosocial functioning, therefore, is underappreciated [49].

Patient health should be measured not only by physical symptoms but also by the likely psychological and social sequelae. Patients should be asked how they are coping and how much of a burden their disease is to them [97]. Health policy should be aimed not only at the management of symptoms of skin disease but also at QoL issues [38]. The high rate of clinical depression and suicidal ideation among patients with disfiguring and disabling dermatological diseases highlights the importance of evaluating the presence of psychosocial morbidity associated with these disorders [47]. No one dies of old skin [5]; skin diseases in the elderly will not generally end life or even shorten it, but can certainly greatly reduce quality of life in the last years [5]. Physicians who seek to treat both the biological and the social skins will improve their patients' lives as well as earn their gratitude [49].

Cross-References

▸ Aging Skin: Some Psychosomatic Aspects
▸ Assessing Quality of Life in Older Adult Patients with Skin Disorders

References

1. Farage MA, Miller KW, Elsner P, et al. Structural characteristics of the aging skin: a review. Cutan Ocul Toxicol. 2007;26:343–57.
2. Farage MA, Miller KW, Elsner P, et al. Functional and physiological characteristics of the aging skin. Aging Clin Exp Res. 2008;20:195–200.
3. Bowling A. The concepts of successful and positive ageing. Fam Pract. 1993;10:449–53.
4. Koblenzer CS. Psychologic aspects of aging and the skin. Clin Dermatol. 1996;14:171–7.
5. Kligman AM, Koblenzer C. Demographics and psychological implications for the aging population. Dermatol Clin. 1997;15:549–53.
6. Kligman AM. Psychological aspects of skin disorders in the elderly. Cutis. 1989;43:498–501.
7. Özmen M. Importance of psychosomatic approach for dermatological diseases. Turkderm. 2010;4:7–9.
8. Gupta MA, Gilchrest BA. Psychosocial aspects of aging skin. Dermatol Clin. 2005;23:643–8.
9. Johnson M. Relevance of dermatologic disease among persons 1–74 years of age, vol. 4. Bethesda: Vital Health Statistics of the National Center for Health Statistics; 1977.
10. Fleischer A, McFarlane M, Hinds M, et al. Skin conditions are common in the elderly; the prevalence of skin symptoms and conditions in an elderly population. J Geriatr Dermatol. 1996;4:78–87.
11. Clark A. The psychological impact of living with skin disease. Prof Nurse. 2003;18:689.
12. Ghosh S, Behere RV, Sharma P, et al. Psychiatric evaluation in dermatology: an overview. Indian J Dermatol. 2013;58:39–43.
13. Sampogna F, Picardi A, Melchi CF, et al. The impact of skin diseases on patients: comparing dermatologists' opinions with research data collected on their patients. Br J Dermatol. 2003;148:989–95.
14. Hatfield E. Physical attractiveness in social interaction. In: Graham J, Kligman A, editors. The psychology of cosmetic treatments. New York: Praeger; 1985.
15. Researchers show parents give unattractive children less attention. http://www.sciencedaily.com/releases/2005/04/050412213412.htm. Accessed 3 Sept 2014.
16. Dion K, Berscheid E, Walster E. What is beautiful is good. J Pers Soc Psychol. 1972;24:285–90.
17. Johnson D. Appearance and the elderly. In: Graham J, Kligman A, editors. The psychology of cosmetic treatments. New York: Praeger; 1985.
18. Adams G. Attractiveness through the ages: implication of facial attractiveness over the life cycle. In: Graham J, Kligman A, editors. The psychology of cosmetic treatments. New York: Praeger; 1985.
19. Cash T, Kilcullen R. The eye of the beholder: susceptibility to sexism and beautyism in the evaluation of managerial applicants. J Appl Soc Psychol. 1985;15:591–605.
20. Graham J, Kligman A. Physical attractiveness, cosmetic use and self-perception in the elderly. Int J Cosmet Sci. 1985;77:85–97.
21. Gupta MA, Goldfarb MT, Schork NJ, et al. Treatment of mildly to moderately photoaged skin with topical tretinoin has a favorable psychosocial effect: a prospective study. J Am Acad Dermatol. 1991;24:780–1.
22. Rizwan M, Reddick CL, Bundy C, et al. Photodermatoses: environmentally induced conditions with high psychological impact. Photochem Photobiol Sci. 2013;12:182–9.
23. Hirshbein LD. Popular views of old age in America, 1900–1950. J Am Geriatr Soc. 2001;49:1555–60.
24. Koblenzer C. Psychologic aspects of skin disease. In: Fitzpatrick T, Eisen A, Wolff K, Wolff K, Freedburg I, Austen K, editors. Dermatology in general medicine. New York: McGraw-Hill; 1993.
25. Borkan GA, Norris AH. Assessment of biological age using a profile of physical parameters. J Gerontol. 1980;35:177–84.
26. Ginsburg IH. The psychosocial impact of skin disease. An overview. Dermatol Clin. 1996;14:473–84.
27. Krueger G, Koo J, Lebwohl M, et al. The impact of psoriasis on quality of life: results of a 1998 National Psoriasis Foundation patient-membership survey. Arch Dermatol. 2001;137:280–4.
28. Schmid-Ott G, Schallmayer S, Calliess IT. Quality of life in patients with psoriasis and psoriasis arthritis with a special focus on stigmatization experience. Clin Dermatol. 2007;25:547–54.

29. Anderson RT, Rajagopalan R. Effects of allergic dermatosis on health-related quality of life. Curr Allergy Asthma Rep. 2001;1:309–15.
30. Vaillant GE, DiRago AC, Mukamal K. Natural history of male psychological health, XV: retirement satisfaction. Am J Psychiatry. 2006;163:682–8.
31. Gupta MA, Gupta AK, Ellis CN, et al. Some psychosomatic aspects of psoriasis. Adv Dermatol. 1990;5:21–30; discussion 31.
32. Evers AWM, Lu Y, Duller P, et al. Common burden of chronic skin diseases? Contributors to psychological distress in adults with psoriasis and atopic dermatitis. Br J Dermatol. 2005;152:1275–81.
33. Weiss SC, Bergstrom KG, Weiss SA, et al. Quality of life considerations in psoriasis treatment. Dermatol Nurs. 2003;15(120):123–7; quiz 128.
34. Gupta M, Gupta A. Psychological impact of aging and the skin. In: Koo J, Lee C, editors. Psychocutaneous medicine. New York: Marcel Dekker; 2003.
35. Magin P, Adams J, Heading G, et al. 'Perfect skin', the media and patients with skin disease: a qualitative study of patients with acne, psoriasis and atopic eczema. Aust J Prim Health. 2011;17:181–5.
36. Ginsburg IH, Link BG. Psychosocial consequences of rejection and stigma feelings in psoriasis patients. Int J Dermatol. 1993;32:587–91.
37. Morgan M, McCreedy R, Simpson J, et al. Dermatology quality of life scales – a measure of the impact of skin diseases. Br J Dermatol. 1997;136:202–6.
38. Report on the enquiry into the impact of skin disease on people's lives. London: All Party Parliamentary Group on Skin; 2003.
39. Ramsay B, O'Reagan M. A survey of the social and psychological effects of psoriasis. Br J Dermatol. 1988;118:195–201.
40. Ermertcan AT. Sexual dysfunction in dermatological diseases. J Eur Acad Dermatol Venereol. 2009;23:999–1007.
41. Ermertcan AT, Temeltaş G. Dermatologic diseases and their effects on male sexual functions. J Dtsch Dermatol Ges. 2010;8:592–7.
42. Menter A. The effect of psoriasis on patients' quality of life and improvements associated with alefacept therapy. J Cutan Med Surg. 2004;8 Suppl 2:20–5.
43. Ginsburg IH, Link BG. Feelings of stigmatization in patients with psoriasis. J Am Acad Dermatol. 1989;20:53–63.
44. Field T. Touch. Cambridge, MA: MIT Press; 2001.
45. Cowdell F, Garrett D. Older people and skin: challenging perceptions. Br J Nurs. 2014;23:S4–8.
46. Gupta MA, Gupta AK, Watteel GN. Perceived deprivation of social touch in psoriasis is associated with greater psychologic morbidity: an index of the stigma experience in dermatologic disorders. Cutis. 1998;61:339–42.
47. Gupta MA, Gupta AK. Depression and suicidal ideation in dermatology patients with acne, alopecia areata, atopic dermatitis and psoriasis. Br J Dermatol. 1998;139:846–50.
48. Porter J, Beuf A, Nordlund JJ, et al. Personal responses of patients to vitiligo: the importance of the patient-physician interaction. Arch Dermatol. 1978;114:1384–5.
49. Barankin B, DeKoven J. Psychosocial effect of common skin diseases. Can Fam Physician. 2002;48:712–6.
50. Gupta MA, Gupta AK. Evaluation of cutaneous body image dissatisfaction in the dermatology patient. Clin Dermatol. 2013;31:72–9.
51. Ograczyk A, Malec J, Miniszewska J, et al. Psychological aspects of atopic dermatitis and contact dermatitis: stress coping strategies and stigmatization. Post Dermatol Alergol. 2012;1:14–8.
52. Ben-Shoshan M, Blinderman I, Raz A. Psychosocial factors and chronic spontaneous urticaria: a systematic review. Allergy. 2013;68:131–41.
53. O'Donnell BF. Urticaria: impact on quality of life and economic cost. Immunol Allergy Clin North Am. 2014;34:89–104.
54. Hareendran A, Bradbury A, Budd J, et al. Measuring the impact of venous leg ulcers on quality of life. J Wound Care. 2005;14:53–7.
55. Morris P, Sander R. Leg ulcers. Nurs Older People. 2007;19:33–7.
56. Brown A. Does social support impact on venous ulcer healing or recurrence? Br J Community Nurs. 2008;13: S6–8. S10 passim.
57. Liao YH, Chen KH, Tseng MP, et al. Pattern of skin diseases in a geriatric patient group in Taiwan: a 7-year survey from the outpatient clinic of a university medical center. Dermatology. 2001;203:308–13.
58. Lim SPR, Abdullah A. Managing skin disease in elderly patients. Practitioner. 2004;248:100–4. 106, 108-9.
59. Fleischer ABJ. Pruritus in the elderly: management by senior dermatologists. J Am Acad Dermatol. 1993;28:603–9.
60. Gupta AK, Nicol KA. Seborrheic dermatitis of the scalp: etiology and treatment. J Drugs Dermatol. 2004;3:155–8.
61. Davies A. Management of dry skin conditions in older people. Br J Community Nurs. 2008;13:250–2. 254–7.
62. Farage MA, Miller KW, Berardesca E, et al. Clinical implications of aging skin: cutaneous disorders in the elderly. Am J Clin Dermatol. 2009;10:73–86.
63. O'Donnell BF, Lawlor F, Simpson J, et al. The impact of chronic urticaria on the quality of life. Br J Dermatol. 1997;136:197–201.
64. Gupta MA, Gupta AK. The psoriasis life stress inventory: a preliminary index of psoriasis-related stress. Acta Derm Venereol. 1995;75:240–3.
65. Hayes J, Koo J. Psoriasis: depression, anxiety, smoking, and drinking habits. Dermatol Ther. 2010;23:174–80.

66. Finlay AY, Coles EC. The effect of severe psoriasis on the quality of life of 369 patients. Br J Dermatol. 1995;132:236–44.
67. Uhlenhake E, Yentzer BA, Feldman SR. Acne vulgaris and depression: a retrospective examination. J Cosmet Dermatol. 2010;9:59–63.
68. Cotterill JA, Cunliffe WJ. Suicide in dermatological patients. Br J Dermatol. 1997;137:246–50.
69. Halvorsen JA, Stern RS, Dalgard F, et al. Suicidal ideation, mental health problems, and social impairment are increased in adolescents with acne: a population-based study. J Invest Dermatol. 2011;131:363–70.
70. Gupta MA, Gupta AK. Cutaneous body image dissatisfaction and suicidal ideation: mediation by interpersonal sensitivity. J Psychosom Res. 2013;75:55–9.
71. Picardi A, Lega I, Tarolla E. Suicide risk in skin disorders. Clin Dermatol. 2013;31:47–56.
72. Kent G, al-Abadie M. Factors affecting responses on dermatology life quality index items among vitiligo sufferers. Clin Exp Dermatol. 1996;21:330–3.
73. Sadock B, Sadock V. Suicide, violence and other psychiatric emergencies. In: Sadock B, Sadock V, editors. Kaplan & Sadock's pocket handbook of clinical psychiatry. Philadelphia: Lippincott, Williams & Wilkins; 2001.
74. Hrehorów E, Salomon J, Matusiak L, et al. Patients with psoriasis feel stigmatized. Acta Derm Venereol. 2012;92:67–72.
75. Basavaraj KH, Navya MA, Rashmi R. Stress and quality of life in psoriasis: an update. Int J Dermatol. 2011;50:783–92.
76. Jowett S, Ryan T. Skin disease and handicap: an analysis of the impact of skin conditions. Soc Sci Med. 1985;20:425–9.
77. Rapp SR, Feldman SR, Exum ML, et al. Psoriasis causes as much disability as other major medical diseases. J Am Acad Dermatol. 1999;41:401–7.
78. Miniszewska J, Juczyński Z, Ograczyk A, et al. Health-related quality of life in psoriasis: important role of personal resources. Acta Derm Venereol. 2013;93:551–6.
79. Jafferany M, Huynh TV, Silverman MA, et al. Geriatric dermatoses: a clinical review of skin diseases in an aging population. Int J Dermatol. 2012;51:509–22.
80. Shah M, Coates M. An assessment of the quality of life in older patients with skin disease. Br J Dermatol. 2006;154:150–3.
81. Sampogna F, Tabolli S, Mastroeni S, et al. Quality of life impairment and psychological distress in elderly patients with psoriasis. Dermatology. 2007;215:341–7.
82. Sampogna F, Chren MM, Melchi CF, et al. Age, gender, quality of life and psychological distress in patients hospitalized with psoriasis. Br J Dermatol. 2006;154:325–31.
83. Sampogna F, Raskovic D, Guerra L, et al. Identification of categories at risk for high quality of life impairment in patients with vitiligo. Br J Dermatol. 2008;159:351–9.
84. Paradisi A, Sampogna F, Di Pietro C, et al. Quality-of-life assessment in patients with pemphigus using a minimum set of evaluation tools. J Am Acad Dermatol. 2009;60:261–9.
85. Burr S, Gradwell C. The psychosocial effects of skin diseases: need for support groups. Br J Nurs. 1996;5:1177–82.
86. Lanigan SW, Farber EM. Patients' knowledge of psoriasis: pilot study. Cutis. 1990;46:359–62.
87. Menter A, Augustin M, Signorovitch J, et al. The effect of adalimumab on reducing depression symptoms in patients with moderate to severe psoriasis: a randomized clinical trial. J Am Acad Dermatol. 2010;62:812–8.
88. Gnanaraj P, Malligarjunan H, Dayalan H, et al. Therapeutic efficacy and safety of propylthiouracil in psoriasis: an open-label study. Indian J Dermatol Venereol Leprol. 2011;77:673–6.
89. Malligarjunan H, Dayalan H, Gnanaraj P, et al. Impact of propylthiouracil on quality of life in psoriasis patients. Indian J Med Sci. 2011;65:331–6.
90. Marron SE, Tomas-Aragones L, Boira S. Anxiety, depression, quality of life and patient satisfaction in acne patients treated with oral isotretinoin. Acta Derm Venereol. 2013;93:701–6.
91. Sachs DL, Voorhees JJ. Age-reversing drugs and devices in dermatology. Clin Pharmacol Ther. 2011;89:34–43.
92. Yadav S, Narang T, Kumaran MS. Psychodermatology: a comprehensive review. Indian J Dermatol Venereol Leprol. 2013;79:176–92.
93. Dowling VL. The psychological impact of psoriasis: a review of short-term psychotherapy group participation for psoriasis patients. J Dermatol Nurses Assoc. 2010;2:163–7.
94. Bailis DS, Chipperfield JG. Compensating for losses in perceived personal control over health: a role for collective self-esteem in healthy aging. J Gerontol B Psychol Sci Soc Sci. 2002;57:P531–9.
95. Chuh A, Wong W, Zawar V. The skin and the mind. Aust Fam Physician. 2006;35:723–5.
96. Kirby B, Richards HL, Woo P, et al. Physical and psychologic measures are necessary to assess overall psoriasis severity. J Am Acad Dermatol. 2001;45:72–6.
97. Finlay AY. Dowling Oration 2000. Dermatology patients: what do they really need? Clin Exp Dermatol. 2000;25:444–50.

Aging Skin: Some Psychosomatic Aspects

123

Madhulika A. Gupta

Contents

Abstract

A request for cosmetic procedures for aging skin is typically emotionally or psychosocially motivated as such procedures are usually life enhancing versus life saving. The primary responsibility of the clinician is to ensure that (i) he or she can accomplish what the patient desires and that (ii) the patient is satisfied with treatment outcome. Both of these points can be significantly influenced by psychosomatic factors. Overall trends indicate an increasing number of younger individuals in the 13–29 years age group, and mainly women are seeking cosmetic treatments for facial rejuvenation, especially the minimally invasive procedures. This has important implications as two-thirds of patients with body dysmorphic disorder (BDD), which is considered a contraindication for cosmetic procedures, experience symptoms prior age 18 years. In addition to BDD, younger age, male gender, minimal deformities, unrealistic expectations, and narcissistic and obsessional personality traits are some of the major negative predictors for patient satisfaction with outcome of cosmetic procedures. A slim and well-toned body is typically a feature of a youthful appearance, and in some individuals fear of aging can culminate in excessive drive for thinness and an eating disorder. Several studies suggest that patients seeking cosmetic procedures should be screened for depressive symptoms with a special focus on recent significant losses such as bereavement

M.A. Gupta (✉)
Department of Psychiatry, Schulich School of Medicine and Dentistry, University of Western Ontario, London, ON, Canada
e-mail: magupta@uwo.ca

M.A. Farage et al. (eds.), *Textbook of Aging Skin*,
DOI 10.1007/978-3-662-47398-6_90

and divorce. A direct enquiry about abuse history can be psychiatrically destabilizing and heighten suicide risk in patients who may seek cosmetic procedures as an unconscious attempt to "fix" a body that is perceived as tainted by childhood sexual abuse.

Introduction

The skin, especially the facial skin, is a powerful organ of communication and one of the most easily visible indicators of age, health, and disease, and of various socially important attributes such as social status, wealth, and sexual attractiveness [1]. The face is the part of the body invested with the greatest interpersonal meaning and is the focus of attention during communication. The aging of the facial skin secondary to both intrinsic and extrinsic factors (e.g., photodamage and smoking) and the development of hyperfunctional facial lines due to repeated expression of emotion over time can lead to aging of the appearance. Over the last several decades, the cultural and social meanings of growing old have changed and old age has started to acquire increasingly negative connotations. Often normal intrinsic aging is viewed as a medical and social problem that needs to be addressed by health-care professionals. The idea that chronological age itself does not signal the beginning of old age, and that one can get older without the signs of aging, has become increasingly prevalent, with a high value placed by the society on the maintenance of a youthful appearance [1].

Facial appearance and expressions, for example, as a result of the corrugator muscle activity of the forehead (resulting in a frown), play a substantial role in the expression of emotions in addition to signaling attributes such as age [2]. From a Darwinian evolutionary perspective [3], the interpretation of facial expression is an integral component of interpersonal communication and tends to be universal and constant across time and cultures [2]. The face is the focus of human communication, and facial expressions have evolved as a means of nonverbal communication and as a way of enhancing verbal communication [2]. The repeated expression of emotion over time produces hyperfunctional facial lines. The presence of these lines when the face is at repose may give the person an aged appearance or give an erroneous impression of emotions or personality characteristics. As the skin ages and the support of the underlying cutaneous structures is lost, more wrinkles and folds develop, and gradually the dynamic lines that communicate emotion change to static lines ingrained on the face at rest. The orientation and depth of these folds is greatly influenced by the underlying activity of the facial muscles. These hyperfunctional lines are common in the forehead, between the brows, around the eyes, and in the area of the mouth. For example, hyperfunctional forehead lines may give an impression of aging, and frown lines or deep vertical creases in the glabellar region give the impression of anger or dissatisfaction. It has been observed that these hyperfunctional lines can result in a "malfunction of the facial organ of communication" [2, 4]. With aging, the corner of the mouth will often droop creating an appearance that may be misinterpreted as displeasure or sadness, or the drooping of the brow or sagging of the upper eyelid may result in the appearance of drowsiness and exhaustion [2]. Therefore, the internal emotion may be quite different from the message received by others, and the disparity between the internal mood and the external appearance can be a significant source of anxiety and may culminate in a feeling of disconnect between the inner self and the face that the individual sees in the mirror. This incongruity may be confirmed in social interactions, resulting in a sense of alienation. These social miscues may further affect reciprocal behavior; for example, a frown is more likely to elicit a frown rather than a smile from another person, and negative responses usually reinforce negative behavior, resulting in greater social alienation. The increasing presence of hyperfunctional facial lines with age therefore has implications far beyond considerations of attractiveness, as they affect the perception of emotions and perceived personality traits of the individual, and treatments to smooth the hyperfunctional facial lines may be warranted because of their positive social ramifications [2].

Cutaneous body-image dissatisfaction has been associated with suicidal ideation when the individual experiences increased interpersonal sensitivity and social alienation during interpersonal interactions [5].

Data from the American Society of Plastic Surgeons [6] report 15.6 million cosmetic procedures in 2014; just under two million of these treatments were traditional cosmetic surgical procedures such as facelift, liposuction, rhinoplasty, and breast augmentation, and 13.9 million procedures involved minimally invasive procedures such as botulinum toxin A injections, soft tissue fillers, laser hair removal, microdermabrasion, and chemical peels, which are largely used to rejuvenate the appearance. It is reported [6] that from 2000 to 2014 the overall frequency of cosmetic surgical procedures has decreased by 12 %, while the overall frequency of cosmetic minimally invasive procedures has increased by 154 %. Similar trends are reported for facial rejuvenation procedures over the 1-year period from 2013 to 2014; for example, the frequency of facelift (rhytidectomy) decreased by 4 % from 2013 to 2014, while the frequency of botulinum toxin type A injections has increased by 6 % over this period. It is noteworthy that from 2000 to 2014, the frequency of cosmetic botulinum toxin A injections has increased almost eightfold (748 %) and use of soft tissue fillers increased 2.5-fold (253 %) [6]. The numbers for cosmetic minimally invasive procedures reported by the American Society of Plastic Surgeons [6] are likely a gross underestimate of the total number of procedures to rejuvenate the appearance, since a large number of the minimally invasive procedures are being performed by nonplastic surgeons.

The gender difference in the experience of the aging of the appearance or the "double standard of aging" [7] between men and women is a very important factor when considering the psychosomatic dimension of aging skin. The gender bias is likely a confounding factor in the psychiatric presentation of individuals with concerns about aging skin, for example, major depressive disorder and eating disorders are more common in women and are also encountered in individuals with concerns about aging skin. In men, cutaneous signs of aging, such as graying hair, wrinkles, and a weathered appearance, are typically considered features of a "distinguished" look [8]. The same signs of aging in women are seen as a sign of "defeat" [7], wherein the woman has somehow lost the battle against the ravages of time, and women are pressured to fight the natural process of aging with creams, antiaging products, nonsurgical or minimally invasive procedures, and cosmetic surgery. For example, American Society of Plastic Surgeons data from 2014 report that in 2014, women underwent 87 % of all cosmetic surgical procedures and 92 % of all cosmetic minimally invasive procedures [6]; women were recipients of 94 % of botulinum toxin A injections and 96 % of procedures involving soft tissue fillers [6].

Another aging-related phenomenon is that a greater number of individuals are becoming concerned about aging-related changes at a much younger age. For example, in a telephone survey of 1406 American women, after controlling for demographic and psychosocial factors, aging anxiety related to loss of attractiveness was higher among the 25–35-year-old women (odds ratio or OR $\pm$ SE = 6.924 $\pm$ 2.709) versus the 56–65 age group (OR $\pm$ SE = 3.504 $\pm$ 1.321) [9]. A study of nonclinical subjects reports that over 50 % of women under the age of 30 reported dissatisfaction with the appearance of their skin, and some of the attributes they were dissatisfied with such as wrinkles and "bags" and "darkness" under the eyes are the signs of aging of the skin [10]. It is noteworthy that the American Society of Plastic Surgeons data reports an increase from 2013 to 2014 of 7 % in cosmetic botulinum toxin A injections in the 13–19 years age group and 6 % in the 20–29 years age group, versus a 5 % increase in botulinum toxin A use in the 40–54 years age group. This emerging trend, wherein younger individuals may be seeking treatments for cutaneous rejuvenation, further emphasizes the importance of the psychosocial dimension in the overall assessment and management of these patients.

This chapter reviews some of the psychosomatic aspects of aging skin that may be of importance in the clinical management of patients seeking treatment for rejuvenation of their appearance using surgical, minimally invasive procedures and topical therapies.

Review of Literature

Cosmetic Surgical Treatments

An earlier (1964) comprehensive study [11, 12] of 106 consecutive patients seen at the Johns Hopkins Hospital over a period of 12 years for the surgical correction of facial evidences of aging evaluated the preoperative and postoperative psychiatric state of 46 of the 64 patients (mean age 48.5 years, seven males) who qualified for the surgery. Forty-two of the 106 patients that were excluded had a higher incidence of previous psychiatric treatment and suffered from a much higher incidence of family disruption during childhood. Among the patients that received surgery, "two patterns of interpersonal relationships" were observed; 43 % were "emotionally distant or mistrustful" and were "diagnosed psychiatrically as manifesting hysterical tendencies," and "two-thirds of them described an unhappy marriage"; the remaining 57 % were described as having "passive-dependent" personalities. Edgerton et al. [12] further observe that "over 74 % (of the 46 patients who were psychiatrically evaluated) were diagnosed as having some associated but not primary psychiatric disorder" and "only four patients had been previously hospitalized for mental illness" and "only one of these had been found psychotic." The psychiatric diagnoses among the 46 patients who were evaluated psychiatrically were as follows: "neurotic depressive reaction (often after husband's death)" in 15 of 46 or 32.6 %, "personality trait disturbance" in 12 out of 46 or 26.1 %, "schizoid personality" in six patients (three of whom were men), and "anxiety reaction" in one patient; the remaining 12 patients had "no psychiatric disorder." The motivations for patients coming for facelifts differed by age groups: the "emotionally dependent group" (age 29–39 years) represented 22 % of patients who "tended to be insecure and dependent on their spouses," reported significantly more family disruption during childhood than the older patients, and demonstrated "problems of adjustment to adult responsibilities"; the "worker group" (age 40–49 years) constituted 37 % of patients whose "major motivation for surgery was to meet vocational requirements for a youthful attractive appearance"; and the "grief group" (age 50 years and older) who comprised 40 % of the sample, and "two-thirds of these were suffering grief over the death of a spouse or separation from children" and sought surgery to give them "self-confidence," "self-esteem," and "a new chance to make friends," but "underlying depression was very common in this group." Examination of the gender differences revealed that in contrast to the female patients, all the seven male patients had a history of emotional illness and all received a psychiatric diagnosis. As for their reason for seeking surgery, none of the men cited the loss of a loved one as principal motivation. All male patients were reported as facing "a critical life decision at the time of their first visit" and wished to look "less stern" and "not so old and tired" and "to adjust to American living" (in the case of an immigrant). The authors caution that "plastic surgeons should seek to uncover the nature of the decision and determine whether rhytidectomy will realistically aid the outcome."

The early postoperative course [11, 12] was "generally mild and without serious emotional disturbance": nine patients showed "mild depression or transient tears" usually on the third or fourth postoperative day, and "some reexperienced the grief previously suffered at the loss of a loved one"; paresthesia and numbness of the facial skin after operation were common and "sometimes augmented the patient's feeling of unreality." If blepharoplasty was performed, the blindfolding resulting from pressure bandages over the eyes during the first 48 h postoperatively was associated with heightened anxiety in some patients. This was in contrast with other procedures such as rhinoplasty and augmentation mammaplasty where up to 40 % of patients have been reported to experience significant short-term emotional disturbances. Patients were followed up psychiatrically between 6 months and 12 years postoperatively, and "over 85 % of patients reported significant improvement" in each of the following areas: "personal comfort," "less self-critical," "better satisfied with their lives," "less self-conscious," "more social ease," "more self-esteem," and "happier." Furthermore, 55 % had obtained one or more of the following: "a new job," "marriage," "a promotion or raise," "a merit award," "formation of other new, close relationships," or "termination of an old, detrimental relationship without emotional upset." No patients reported "guilt feelings" or "having any feelings of deception about her age." The authors conclude that "satisfactory psychologic result of facelifting depends on several variables" such as "how the patient approaches surgery, with confidence or mistrustful attitudes," "a genuine and personal interest on part of the surgeon and whether the surgery constitutes a therapeutic or 'rebirth' experience," "the potential for realistic improvement in the patient's personal environment as a result of the surgical experience," "how much positive feedback the patient receives from their friends and associates regarding an improvement in their appearance," and finally "the actual anatomic improvement that the facial skin and subcutaneous tissue permit"; contraindications to surgery where "basically good procedures may produce poor results" included "unresolved emotional conflicts"; and "the effectiveness of a psychiatrist in helping the plastic surgery patient is directly proportional to his interest and experience with the problems of deformity."

Goin et al. [13] evaluated 50 female facelift patients preoperatively and postoperatively for up to 6 months with semistructured psychiatric interviews and psychological tests. The 50 patients were chosen from 117 consecutive facelift consultations; 20 % of patients were rejected by the surgeon for psychological reasons, which were as follows: patients were "unable or unwilling to listen, were excessively fearful, idealized the surgeon (believing he could accomplish what others had failed to do), or had a history of severe psychological disturbance following other operations." Preoperatively, psychological testing, e.g., with the Minnesota Multiphasic Personality Inventory (MMPI), revealed "a relatively normal group," and "there were no clear diagnostic groupings." Only one patient showed neurotic pathology with high scores on several MMPI scales and none were psychotic. Four patients were "in the midst of grieving over dead loved ones" at the time of surgery. Clinical evaluation revealed "some evidence of clinical depression," rated as mild to moderate, in seven or 14 % of patients. Postoperatively, 27 or 54 % of patients "displayed clinical evidence of psychological disturbance," and 30 % of these patients experienced depression 6 months postoperatively. The patients with depression reactions were divided into four categories [13]: six patients or 12 % described "feelings of depression or anxiety occurring sometime within the first 5 days," and these symptoms were gone by the end of the first week; and another 12 % had "transient episodes of depression occurring around the second or third week, which lasted 3–5 days," and "the depression was related to some new stress in the patient's life" such as divorce and illness in the family. Thirty percent of patients reported more prolonged depression, which was present up to 6 months postoperatively; among these 16 % "were depressed within the first 5 days and continued to be depressed for several weeks" and 14 % "developed a clinical depression in the second or third postoperative week, which lasted for several weeks." This group with prolonged clinical depression was reported preoperatively to have "either a preexisting and clinically detectable depression or a high depression score on the MMPI," and the authors conclude that the surgery either "intensified" or "unmasked" their depression. No other preoperative factors were associated with postoperative depression. The subgroup that became depressed within the first 5 days were more "independent and self-reliant and wanted to control their lives," "did not anticipate any changes in their self-esteem," and "had hoped that the facelift would slow down the aging process." In contrast, the subgroup with later onset depression comprised "passive-dependent women who wished to be cared for and did not want to be in charge of their lives." This group also had less favorable surgical results. Therefore, overall decrease in the support from the immediate postoperative period and disappointment with results of surgery contributed to the depressive reaction in this last group of women. Postoperatively, improvement was noted in other areas including "increased self-esteem" (28 %), "better able to cope with life" (8 %), "more assertive and comfortable at work" (8 %), and "diminished grief reactions" (8 %). Some of the factors associated with a postoperative improvement in psychological state were as follows: preoperatively, the desire for an improved self-image; a higher-than-average score on the paranoid subscale of the MMPI preoperatively and greater reinvolvement of these patients with friends and colleagues after surgery, which reduced the intensity of their previous distorted perceptions about people; and the patient's desire preoperatively to improve the chances of retaining a job or advancing her career, or if she had previous cosmetic operations.

A French study [14, 15] measured psychosocial factors in 103 facial cosmetic surgery patients using standardized rating scales and semistructured interviews, both presurgery and 9 months after facial cosmetic surgery. In presurgery, 50 % of patients reported that they had used a psychotropic therapy of which 27 % were antidepressants, 20 % were seeking employment, and 59 % were "motivated by a search for well-being." The patients had high depression scores presurgery and this did not change significantly after the surgery. Presurgery patients had high scores on measures of social anxiety, especially fear of speaking in public rather than a fear of social interaction, and this decreased significantly postsurgery. Of several psychological motives studied, a lack of self-confidence associated with a desire to create and enhance interpersonal relationships predicted the greatest improvement on postsurgical scores.

In a Brazilian study [16] 32 female Caucasian patients, aged 46–68 years, undergoing rhytidoplasty, were examined preoperatively and 2 and 6 months postoperatively. Measures of health perception, energy, and social function were significantly improved at 6 months postoperatively, while measures of mental health which were related to anxiety and depression, and self-esteem, showed improvement both at 2 and 6 months postoperatively. The authors discuss the improvement in the patients' overall sense of well-being and not just their psychological health, after the surgery for facial rejuvenation.

A Canadian study [17] examined 93 patients (82 females and 11 males) who had undergone rhinoplasty (49 %) and surgery for the aging face (51 %). All patients were administered the 59-item Derriford Appearance Scale (DAS59), a validated instrument that measures body image-related distress and dysfunction, preoperatively and 3 months after surgery. Patients were routinely screened for psychiatric disorders, and patients with body dysmorphic disorder (BDD) or related psychiatric disorders were excluded from participation. Facial aging patients and patients in the highest age category ($\geq$51 years) had the lowest baseline DAS59 scores indicating the least amount of appearance-related emotional concern. Postoperatively, there was a significant reduction in all dimensions of the DAS59, with the greatest mean reduction in the factor measuring "general self-consciousness of appearance," whereas the least improvement was noted for "self-consciousness of sexual and bodily appearance." Men had higher preoperative levels of distress in contrast to women, especially the males undergoing rhinoplasty; men also exhibited a greater overall percentage decrease in scores postsurgery. The greatest mean percentage improvement in presurgery or postsurgery DAS59 scores was noted in the >50 years age group. Therefore, while the $\geq$ 51 years age group showed a decline in appearance-related concerns presurgery according to their DAS59 scores, the greatest relative benefits postsurgery were derived for the oldest subgroup of patients.

A prospective American study [18] examining patient satisfaction among individuals undergoing deep plane facelift and other facial rejuvenation procedures ($n = 93$; mean $\pm$ SD age 56.6 $\pm$ 9.2 years, age range 35.3–82.8 years; 88.2 % female) found that following surgery (1–43-month follow-up), 96.7 % (89/93) reported a more youthful appearance, 87.1 % reported a positive reaction by others, 82.8 % reported improved self-esteem, and 69.6 % reported improved quality of life after the surgery. There were no reports of depressed mood following surgery, although this was not directly assessed; overall, 50.5 % of patients (47/93) reported a large psychological benefit of surgery, 38.7 % reported a little benefit, and only 10.8 % reported no psychological benefit. No significant effect of age on the above variables was reported. Sarwer et al. [19, 20] examined changes in body image, appearance evaluation, self-esteem, and depressive symptoms among 100 participants (mean age 42.59 ± 13.44) over the course of 2 years following surgery. Of the 127 surgeries conducted, 40.9 % were directly aging- related (29 blepharoplasties and 23 facelifts). Three months following surgery, significant improvements were seen in appearance evaluation and evaluation of body area of concern as well as negative emotion-associated appearance; these improvements were maintained for 24 months postsurgery. Improvements were seen in depressive symptoms and self-esteem, although these did not reach significance at any of the time points assessed.

A similar prospective Norwegian study was conducted by von Soest and colleagues [21, 22] in which women ($n = 130$; mean ± SD age 37.7 ± 11.2 years) were followed over the course of 5 years after surgery. Of the 154 surgeries performed, only 14 were directly aging related (blepharoplasties). Significant improvements were seen in appearance evaluation and evaluation of area of concern both 6 months and 5 years following surgery, although in comparison to the general population, individuals were still significantly less satisfied with the appearance of the area of concern. In contrast to the Sarwer study, a significant improvement in self-esteem was also observed after 6 months and was maintained at the 5-year time point. Interestingly, psychological problems prior to surgery were predictive of regretting the surgery and reporting that they would not choose the surgery again.

Although not commonly considered a procedure to combat facial aging, recent publications [23] have considered rhinoplasty as a possible means to rejuvenate the facial appearance. There is some evidence that older individuals undergoing rhinoplasty may have greater difficulty integrating their new nose with their body image. Individuals who have only recently started to dislike their nose may be at greater risk to be dissatisfied with the surgical results, although others have reported that individuals who have disliked their nose for a large portion of their life may hold unrealistic expectations of the possible surgical results.

The literature suggests that, overall, patients tend to be satisfied with the results of facial cosmetic surgery. A systematic review of the literature [24] revealed the following factors (in addition to body dysmorphic disorder) tended to be negative predictors, for patient satisfaction with facial cosmetic surgery: male gender, younger age, minimal deformities, unrealistic expectations, "demanding patients," "surgiholics," relational or family disturbances, an "obsessive personality," and a "narcissistic personality."

Nonsurgical or Minimally Invasive Treatments

A study of 20 patients with mild to moderately photodamaged skin [25] who had entered a study to evaluate the efficacy of topical tretinoin for the treatment of photodamaged skin reported that at baseline the subjects had high scores on the interpersonal sensitivity and phobic anxiety subscales of the Brief Symptom Inventory (BSI). The interpersonal sensitivity (BSI) subscale measures a lack of ease during interpersonal interactions, and the phobic anxiety (BSI) subscale provides an index of a persistent fear response to certain situations including social situations that lead to avoidance of the situations that provoke anxiety. High scores on these BSI subscales therefore suggest that the subjects with photodamage, who were concerned enough about the photodamage-related skin changes to seek treatment, were experiencing uneasiness during their interpersonal interactions [25]. After 24 weeks of therapy, both the interpersonal sensitivity (BSI) and phobic anxiety (BSI) scores decreased significantly ($p < 0.05$) in the topical tretinoin, but not in the control group that was receiving the inactive vehicle [25]. These findings were confirmed in another study [26] involving 40 additional subjects with moderate to severe photodamage. In this study

[26] a significant decrease in phobic anxiety (BSI) ($p < 0.05$) was observed after 24 weeks of therapy with topical tretinoin, while an increase in phobic anxiety (BSI) ($p < 0.05$) was noted in the group receiving the inactive vehicle. General body-image concerns related to body weight and shape were measured with the Eating Disorder Inventory (EDI) pretreatment and posttreatment with topical tretinoin. The patients receiving the active treatment with topical tretinoin and not the control group reported a significant decline ($p < 0.01$) in drive for thinness (EDI) and body dissatisfaction (EDI), which measure an excessive concern about thinness, body shape, and body weight. These findings indicate that aging-related changes affecting the skin caused increased social anxiety and concerns about general aspects of body image related to body weight and shape, and this anxiety and general dissatisfaction with body image decreased with the treatment of some of the cutaneous changes of photodamage [26].

Carbon dioxide (CO_2) laser skin resurfacing is increasingly used for treating wrinkles and photoaged skin because of its favorable risk-benefit ratio, and patients report high satisfaction with the procedure including improvements with self-esteem and self-satisfaction and an overall improvement with skin-specific quality of life [27]. However, satisfaction with the outcome depends on expectations of minimal to moderate improvement in appearance and health of skin [28]. Interestingly, predictors of dissatisfaction with CO_2 laser skin resurfacing included ideas that the procedure would improve self-esteem as well as a belief of previous facial disfigurement [28]. Treatment of glabellar frown lines with botulinum toxin A has been associated with a favorable psychosocial outcome. In one study [29] 20 women between 35 and 60 years of age, assessed as having moderate to severe glabellar rhytids, received botulinum toxin A treatment to the forehead and crow's feet area and had standardized frontal and lateral view photographs taken, which were rated for "first impressions" on the following domains: social skills, academic performance, dating success, occupational success, attractiveness, financial success, relationship success, and athletic success. Botulinum toxin A improved first impression scores for dating success, attractiveness, and athletic success ratings; the first impressions on academic performance and occupational success demonstrated a significantly lower (i.e., lower degree of agreement with the descriptive statement associated with the domains) rating after treatment with botulinum toxin A, and this effect was no longer observed when a "smile/relax" variable was added to the model. Another preliminary study [30] used botulinum toxin A to treat glabellar frown lines in ten female patients, ranging in age between 36 and 63 years, diagnosed with DSM-IV [31] criteria for major depressive disorder (MDD) despite treatment with psychotropic drugs and psychotherapy. The time period for which the patients had been depressed ranged from 2 to 17 years, and 7 out of 10 patients had been tried on two or more antidepressant medications. The patients were evaluated 2 months later, and 9 out of 10 patients were no longer depressed both by clinical criteria and scores on standardized rating scales, and the remaining patient who had an improvement in her mood had bipolar disorder. The authors [30] discuss the Darwinian notion that "the free expression, by outward signs of an emotion intensifies it. On the other hand, repression, as far as this is possible, of all outward signs softens our emotions." Increased frown muscle activity has been associated with depression, and patients that have their frown lines treated with botulinum toxin A appear to be happier, and enhancement of the facial expression of happiness may also make the treated individuals feel happier [30]. Other studies have found similar results and reported that depressed individuals had significant reduction in depressive symptoms, as assessed by the Beck Depression Inventory following botulinum toxin A injections into glabellar frown lines [32]. Patients who received botulinum toxin injections to the forehead had significantly more positive mood than those who did not, which mainly reflected in lower anxiety and depression scores [33]. It is hypothesized that the paralysis of the corrugator muscles from the botulinum toxin therapy results in the lack of negative mood feedback which makes it harder to maintain negative facial expressions and a negative mood [33]. Similarly, a double-blind randomized controlled trial, examining the effect of botulinum toxin A on quality of life and self-esteem, determined that 3 months post-botulinum toxin A administration, patients scored higher on measures of body appearance, satisfaction with weight, and overall life satisfaction and contentment, whereas the placebo group only reported improvements in self-consciousness and ability to understand things [34].

Psychosomatic Assessment of the Patient

The request for cosmetic procedures is typically emotionally or psychosocially motivated. Cosmetic procedures are supposed to be life enhancing, not life saving. The primary responsibility of the clinician who is performing an aesthetic procedure is to ensure that (1) he or she can accomplish what the patient desires and (2) the patient is satisfied with the outcome of the procedure. An acceptable indication for an aesthetic procedure is that the procedure will improve the patient's quality of life. The most common psychiatric comorbidities that can be associated with an unfavorable treatment outcome (Table 1) are discussed below in detail; the presence of body dysmorphic disorder is generally considered to be a contraindication for cosmetic procedures. Edgerton et al. [35] have reported the course of 87 severely psychologically disturbed patients "ranging from moderate degrees of neurosis to frank psychosis" who underwent aesthetic plastic surgery and were followed up for an average of 6.2 years. As many as 82.8 % of patients had a "positive psychological outcome," 13.8 % experienced "minimal improvement" from surgery, and three patients or 3.4 % were "negatively affected"; among the "negatively affected," the first patient who had rhinoplasty said that "she had expected to erase the emotional scars from an early childhood trauma," the second patient with blepharoplasty had a poor surgical outcome, and the third patient who had rhinoplasty was identified as having untreated body-image issues. The authors [35] report that there were no suicides, psychotic decompensations, or lawsuits and further observe that patients with severe psychological disturbances benefited from a "combined surgical-psychiatric treatment designed to address the patient's profound sense of deformity."

Some general demographic considerations include the fact that male patients seeking cosmetic procedures tend to have more severe psychopathology than their female counterparts and individuals in their late 40s tend to have the maximum concern about aging of their appearance as at this life stage for the first time "losses are uncompensated by new gains" [11]. Other considerations during assessment include other life stresses, especially bereavement. During the clinical evaluation, the clinician should assess gender identity concerns which may be covert and a history of abuse. When abuse is suspected, it may be prudent to refer the patient to a mental health specialist, as direct enquiry about the abuse can lead to psychiatric decompensation in patients who are excessively somatically focused. The clinician should be aware of the two to three times higher suicide rate among women who have received cosmetic breast implants [36], as these patients may also seek treatments for facial rejuvenation.

Psychiatric Disorders Encountered in Patients Requesting Treatments for Aging Skin

The diagnostic criteria [37] for some of the most clinically important psychiatric comorbidities are summarized in Table 1.

Body Dysmorphic Disorder (BDD)

BDD is classified under "Obsessive-compulsive and related disorders" (DSM-5) [37]. The prevalence of BDD (Table 1) is 9–15 % among dermatology patients, 7–8 % among US cosmetic surgery patients, and, according to most studies, 3–16 % among international cosmetic surgery patients [37]. The mean age of onset of BDD is 16–17 years, the median age of onset is 15 years,

Table 1 Some clinical features (Diagnostic and Statistical Manual for Mental Disorders, Fifth Edition) (DSM-5) [37] of psychiatric disorders commonly encountered in patients seeking cosmetic procedures

Body image pathologies
1. **Body dysmorphic disorder** (BDD) (also referred to as "dysmorphophobia") (classified under obsessive-compulsive and related disorders in DSM-5):
(a) The patient is preoccupied with one or more perceived defects or flaws in their physical appearance that are not observable or appear slight to others. The degree of insight regarding the BDD beliefs can range from good or fair to complete absence of insight where the individual is completely convinced that the BDD beliefs are true
(b) At some point during the course of the disorder performs repetitive behaviors (e.g., excessive grooming, skin picking) or mental acts (e.g., comparing the appearance with that of others), in response to the appearance concerns
(c) There is marked distress or impairment in social, occupational, or other areas of functioning resulting from the preoccupation about the appearance, and the preoccupation is not attributable to another psychiatric disorder, such body fat or weight concerns in patients who have comorbid eating disorders
(d) Common complaints in BDD can include imagined or slight flaws affecting many body areas, most commonly the skin (e.g., perceived acne, scars, lines, wrinkles, paleness), hair (e.g., perceived thinning or excessive body or facial hair), or size and/or shape of the nose. Any body region can be the focus of concern (e.g., eyes, teeth, size or shape of face, lips, chin, eyebrows)
(e) Common repetitive behaviors include excessive grooming (e.g., excessive combing, styling, shaving, plucking, or pulling hair), camouflaging (repeated use of makeup, covering of disliked regions with clothing, etc.), excessive tanning, or compulsive shopping for beauty products. Other body parts such as the genitals, breasts, buttocks, abdomen, upper and lower extremities, overall body size, body build, and muscularity can also be the focus of concern, and several attributes may be the focus of concern simultaneously. Body dysmorphia, presenting with a preoccupation that the body is too small or not sufficiently lean or muscular, is a form of BDD encountered almost exclusively in males
(f) BDD is most commonly comorbid with major depressive disorder and may be associated with repeated psychiatric hospitalizations, suicidal ideation, suicide attempts, and completed suicide. Eating disorders and BDD can be comorbid. Other emergencies may be associated with the BDD patients' attempts to correct their perceived flaws by, for example, self-surgery and other self-administered remedies
2. **Eating disorders** (anorexia nervosa and bulimia nervosa)
(a) **Anorexia nervosa** (AN) is characterized by a refusal to maintain a minimally normal body weight (<85 % of expected weight). The patient has an intense fear of gaining weight or becoming fat even though underweight, and there is a disturbance in the way in which one's body weight or shape is experienced, undue influence of body weight or shape on self-evaluation, or denial of the seriousness of the current low body weight. Secondary amenorrhea (absence of at least three consecutive menstrual periods) is present when onset is postmenarcheal. AN can be of the restricting type, where the patient simply restricts her food intake or of the binge eating/purge type, where the patient engages in binge eating and purging behavior
(b) **Bulimia nervosa** (BN) is characterized by repeated episodes of binge eating, which consists of eating an abnormally large amount of food over a discrete period of time (within a 2-h period) when the patient experiences a sense of lack of control over the eating behavior. Patients may engage in recurrent inappropriate compensatory behaviors to prevent weight gain, e.g., self-induced vomiting, fasting, or excessive exercise, and abuse of laxatives, diuretics, emetics, and diet pills. The binge eating and inappropriate compensatory behaviors have to occur at least twice weekly for a period of 3 months for the diagnosis of BN. The self-evaluation of the patient is unduly influenced by body weight and shape. BN can be purging type and nonpurging type
Mood disorders
1. **Major depressive disorder** (MDD) is characterized by one or more major depressive episodes. The essential feature of major depressive episode is a period of at least 2 weeks during which the patient experiences either a depressed mood or loss of interest and pleasure in nearly all activities that they had previously found pleasurable. The patient must also experience at least four of the following vegetative symptoms of depression during this period: significant weight loss when not dieting or weight gain or decrease or increase in appetite, insomnia or hypersomnia, psychomotor agitation or retardation, fatigue or loss of energy, feelings of worthlessness or excessive or inappropriate guilt, diminished ability to think or concentrate or indecisiveness, and recurrent thoughts of death and suicidal ideation with or without a specific plan for committing suicide. These symptoms cause significant distress or impairment in social, occupational, or other important areas of functioning. The symptoms are not attributable to the physiological effects of a substance or to another medical condition
2. **Bipolar disorder** is typically characterized by one or more manic (Bipolar I) or hypomanic (Bipolar II) episodes, in patients who also have a history of major depressive episodes. As the symptoms of mania are usually obviously pathological, the patient with Bipolar I disorder is less likely to be overlooked than the patient with Bipolar II disorder

(*continued*)

Table 1 (continued)

where the symptoms can be more subtle. Mania is characterized by a distinct period of abnormally and persistently elevated, expansive, or irritable mood and abnormally or persistently increased goal-directed activity or energy, lasting at least 1 week, associated with at least three of the following: inflated self-esteem or grandiosity; decreased need for sleep; increased talkativeness or pressure to keep talking; flight of ideas or subjective experience that thoughts are racing; distractibility; increase in goal-directed activity socially, at work, or sexually, e.g., patient may take on multiple new business ventures without regard to the risk, and almost always there is increased sociability and increased involvement in pleasurable activities that have a high potential for painful consequences, e.g., unrestrained buying sprees; and sexual indiscretions. Hypomania is similar to mania with a shorter duration of 4 days and, unlike mania, is typically not severe enough to cause a marked impairment in social or occupational functioning or require hospitalization.
Personality disorders
1. **Narcissistic personality disorder** presents as a pervasive pattern of grandiosity, need for admiration, lack of empathy beginning by early adulthood, and present in a variety of contexts as indicated by at least five of the following: grandiose sense of self-importance (e.g., exaggeration of achievements, expectation to be recognized as superior without commensurate achievements), preoccupation with fantasies of unlimited success, belief that one is "special" and can only be understood by people or institutions who are special or of high status, need for excessive admiration, sense of entitlement, tendency to be interpersonally exploitative, lack of empathy, envy of others and belief that others are envious of the patient, and arrogant attitude
2. **Histrionic personality disorder** presents as a pervasive pattern of excessive emotionality and attention seeking beginning by early adulthood and present in a variety of contexts as indicated by at least five of the following: lack of comfort in situations where the patient is not the center of attention, interpersonal inactions often characterized by inappropriate sexually seductive or provocative behavior, rapidly shifting or shallow expression of emotions, consistent use of physical appearance to draw attention to oneself, style of speech that is excessively impressionistic and lacking in detail, self-dramatization and exaggerated expression of emotion, easily influenced by others, and tendency to consider relationships to be more intimate than they really are
3. **Obsessive-compulsive personality disorder** presents as a pervasive pattern of preoccupation with perfectionism, orderliness, and mental and interpersonal control, at the expense of flexibility and efficiency, beginning in early adulthood, and presents in a variety of contexts indicated by at least four of the following: preoccupation with details, rules, order, and organization to the extent that the major point of the activity is lost, perfectionism that interferes with task completion, excessive devotion to work and productivity to the exclusion of leisure, overconscientiousness and inflexibility about matters of morality and ethics, inability to discard worn out objects even when they have no value, reluctance to delegate tasks to others, miserly spending style toward self and others, and tendency for rigidity and stubbornness

and the most common age at onset is 12–13 years [37]. Subclinical BDD symptoms usually emerge, on average, at age 12–13 years, and the subclinical concerns usually evolve into the full syndrome, although some individuals experience abrupt onset of BDD [37]. Two-thirds of BDD patients have their disorder before age 18 years [37]. Rates of suicidal ideation and suicide attempts are high in both children/adolescents and adults with BDD [37]; suicide risk is reported to be high in adolescents, and BDD onset before age 18 years is more likely to be associated with suicide attempts and greater comorbidity [37]. The preoccupation about a perceived defect or flaw in the appearance in BDD can focus on one or many body areas, most commonly the skin, with some of the common preoccupations consisting of complaints about lines, wrinkles, paleness, and thinning hair [37], concerns that are all typically associated with aging. These have important implications as current trends indicate that an increasing number of individuals are becoming concerned about and seeking treatments for aging-related changes of the skin at a much younger age [6]. Various studies have suggested that patients with BDD who undergo cosmetic procedures experience no change or worsening of their symptom or develop a preoccupation with another imagined flaw [38–40]. BDD patients have been known to become violent toward their cosmetic surgeons when they are dissatisfied with the outcome of surgery. BDD is a contraindication for cosmetic procedures, and these patients require psychiatric management of their disorder.

The patient seeking treatment for aging skin who also has BDD is not likely to have a typical presentation. Preoccupation with an imagined or slight defect in appearance (Table 1), the first diagnostic criterion of BDD, describes the presentation of the majority of cosmetic surgery patients with body-image pathology [38]. When assessing the patient presenting with concerns about aging of the appearance the clinician needs to have a greater index of suspicion for underlying BDD, as it may be difficult to assess, for example, whether the concerns of a 35-year-old woman about some wrinkles or sagging of facial muscles is out of proportion to the clinical severity of the problem. BDD usually begins during adolescence [37]; however, the disorder may not be diagnosed for many years often because the patient may be reluctant to reveal their symptoms, or a major life event such as bereavement or divorce may bring underlying BDD symptoms to the forefront. BDD is usually chronic, although improvement may occur with appropriate treatments; BDD presents with similar clinical features in children, adolescents, and adults, and while BDD occurs in the elderly, little is known about the disorder in this age group [37]. Patients with BDD tend to be significantly younger than other psychiatric inpatients [41]; however, it is difficult to determine whether this indicates to an overall younger demographic or whether younger individuals tend to have more severe BDD requiring treatment. Therefore, the clinician should obtain a history of body-image concerns starting in early adolescence and enquire about a history of other cosmetic procedures which initially may appear to be unrelated to the presenting concern. Secondly, the clinician should enquire about the degree of distress and impairment in functioning caused by the current aging-related problem or other body-image problem with a question like "What does your concern (i.e., the body-image problem) stop you from doing?" For example, if the patient reports that their appearance-related concern has prevented them from maintaining a job or significantly impaired their social functioning, diagnosis of BDD should be considered.

Eating Disorders (ED)

Anorexia nervosa (AN) and bulimia nervosa (BN) (Table 1) usually start during adolescence and young adulthood [37], and among some patients can have a relapsing course with exacerbations and remissions, and persist into late life [42]. A youthful look is typically associated with a slim and well-toned body, and some individuals may become excessively preoccupied with diet and exercise as their appearance ages [43]. In a small group of individuals who have other risk factors for the development of an eating disorder, the fear of aging precipitated by the cutaneous changes of aging can culminate in eating disorder-related symptoms including anorexia nervosa [44, 45]. Both AN and BN commonly begin during adolescence and young adulthood, and late onset (after age 40 years) AN or BN is considered to be rare for AN and uncommon for BN [37].

It has been noted that ED tend to be underdiagnosed in midlife and beyond because of the prevailing assumption that ED are only disorders of adolescence and early adulthood [46]. ED in midlife can be triggered by midlife transitions such as loss of parents, siblings, or children, divorce, and "empty nest" in conjunction with the loss of a youthful appearance [46, 47]. A study of women who developed first onset ED at age 40 or older (age range 40–65) showed a mean onset of ED at age 45 years (range 40–62 years), with mean $\pm$ SD duration of 4 $\pm$ 4.7 years [47]. Depression was a commonly observed psychiatric comorbidity (seen in 86 % of women), and history of sexual abuse (present in 64 % of women) presented as a major risk factor for the development of disordered eating pathology after the age of 40 [47]. Menopausal transition can also be a factor in the development of eating pathology, where exit from the reproductive age is a particularly vulnerable period, analogous to the increased risk for ED observed at the entrance into reproductive life in puberty [48, 49]. Additionally, age-associated changes in appearance, such as emergence of wrinkles, loss of hair, and redistribution of body fat, can be associated with a negative impact on physical appearance in the menopausal woman [50]. In older women, aging anxiety and menopause were predictive of disordered eating and body dissatisfaction [51]. A study on body satisfaction in women aged 50 years and older found that only 12.2 % endorsed satisfaction with their body size and that these women had significantly lower BMI [52]. Patients often do not disclose the fact that they have an eating disorder and are ashamed of their chaotic eating patterns, which can range from severe dietary restriction to bingeing and purging, which is often carried out in secrecy. Some patients can experience significant fluctuations in body weight, which can in turn lead to redundant skinfolds, and premature aging of the appearance. In some eating-disordered patients, the concern about cutaneous body image may be grossly inconsistent with the norms for their age [10]. In a cross-sectional study [10] examining concerns about various aspects of skin appearance among under 30-year-old eating-disordered patients ($n = 32$) and nonclinical controls ($n = 34$), it was observed that 81 % of the eating-disordered patients versus 56 % of controls reported dissatisfaction with the appearance of their skin ($p = 0.03$). Some of the cutaneous attributes that were of the greatest concern to the eating-disordered patients were those that are also associated with aging and photodamage, e.g., "darkness" under the eyes, freckles, fine wrinkles, and patchy hyperpigmentation.

One of the central psychopathological factors underlying eating disorders, which have a peak incidence during the teenage years, is difficulties in dealing with the developmental tasks of adolescence and young adulthood. It is possible that the greater concern about aging skin in the eating-disordered sample is an index of the overall difficulties experienced by these patients in dealing with "growing up and growing old," which may lead this group of patients to seek treatments for their aging face. It is also interesting to note that a study of psychosocial factors among facelift patients [11, 12] identified that 22 % of their patients between the age of 29 and 39 years were "emotionally dependent" and demonstrated "many problems of adjustment to adult responsibilities." The association between concerns about aging of the appearance and drive for thinness has been studied in nonclinical samples. In a survey of 71 men and 102 women who were all nonclinical subjects attending a shopping mall [53], it was observed that concerns about the effect of aging on the appearance correlated directly ($r = 0.4$; $p < 0.05$) with the drive for thinness subscale of the Eating Disorder Inventory (EDI) even after the possible confounding effect of body mass index and chronological age were partialled out statistically. This correlation was significant among both men and women. The drive for thinness (EDI) subscale measures an excessive preoccupation with dieting and exercise and an ardent desire to lose weight. Furthermore, among the women the belief that having younger-looking skin is a prerequisite to good looks correlated with drive for thinness (EDI) ($r = 0.3$; $p < 0.01$) and body dissatisfaction (EDI) ($r = 0.4$; $p < 0.01$) after the effects of age and body mass index were partialled out statistically. The body dissatisfaction (EDI) subscale measures dissatisfaction with body shape and weight and the concern that certain body regions such as the abdomen, hips, and thighs are too fat. This finding has been replicated among another randomly selected sample of nonclinical subjects [45]. These findings highlight the impact of aging skin on satisfaction with overall body image that is not necessarily related to aging, and this relation was observed independent of chronological age. In clinical samples of patients undergoing the treatment of aging skin with topical tretinoin [25, 26] (discussed under "Nonsurgical or Minimally Invasive Treatments" above), ED-related concerns were measured with the Eating Disorder Inventory (EDI) subscales pre- and posttreatment with topical tretinoin. The patients receiving the active treatment with topical tretinoin (who demonstrated objective improvement in their aging-related cutaneous changes) and not the control group reported a significant decline ($p < 0.01$) in drive for thinness (EDI) and body dissatisfaction (EDI), which measure an excessive concern about thinness, body shape, and body weight.

Mood Disorders

Most of the psychosocial studies on the treatment of aging skin observed the importance of depressive symptoms of some type; around 14 % [13] to 33 % [11, 12] of patients were described as having depressive symptoms prior to their facelift surgery; during the early postoperative course, up to 24 % of patients [13] were observed to experience a transient flare-up of depressive symptoms which were partly related to the emergence of feeling about the recent death of a loved one and other psychosocial stressors; 30 % [13] of patients experienced a more prolonged course of depression and this group also had more depressive symptoms preoperatively. In one study [14, 15], the depression scores did not change significantly presurgery to postsurgery. In nonsurgical studies, patients seeking treatment for photodamaged skin with topical tretinoin [25, 26] did not have high depression scores at baseline; and a preliminary study indicates treatment of glabellar frown lines with botulinum toxin A, in patients with major depressive disorder, was associated with remission of depression, which was previously treatment resistant in all patients except one who turned out to have bipolar disorder [30]. More recent studies [32–34] have found similar results, which are discussed above under "Nonsurgical or Minimally Invasive Treatments." These findings from a wide range of studies suggest that patients seeking cosmetic procedures should be screened for depressive disease with a special focus on recent bereavement or other significant losses (e.g., children leaving home); management of depressive illness prior to therapy is likely to be associated with a more favorable postoperative course.

The clinician should specifically assess for bipolar disorder (Table 1) because a patient who presents with depressive symptoms may in fact be bipolar. The bipolar patients who are most likely to be overlooked are those with more subtle symptoms, i.e., patients with Bipolar II disorder. The patient with Bipolar II disorder who is hypomanic may present as a social, extroverted individual who is highly motivated to improve her appearance, or she may have a grandiose and unrealistic view of how the cosmetic procedure can further improve her appearance. Hypomanic patients can be very pleasant and complimentary, or they may be irritable, in which case they are more likely to get psychiatric attention. The patient's motivation for surgery or desire to have a cosmetic procedure may totally change once the patient is no longer hypomanic. A hypomanic patient may be on a spending spree and not be able to afford procedures that they have signed up for. Some bipolar patients may "overcompensate" psychologically and have a hypomanic reaction after major bereavement, e.g., death of a spouse. It is important to identify such situations, especially as the literature [11–13] suggests that a significant number of patients seeking treatments for aging skin have recently suffered the loss of their spouse.

Anxiety Disorders

The literature suggests that patients seeking treatment for aging skin suffer from a range of anxiety-related symptoms, but generally do not meet all the criteria for an anxiety disorder [31]. Prior to treatment, some patients reported anxiety during interpersonal interactions and increased self-consciousness [11–13, 25, 26]. These represent some features of social phobia or social anxiety disorder [31], which is characterized by clinically significant anxiety provoked by exposure to certain types of social or performance situations, often leading to avoidance behavior. Overall, there was an improvement in social anxiety-related symptoms post-treatment.

Trauma and Stress-Related Disorders

The clinician should be aware that some patients seeking body-image surgery are survivors of childhood sexual abuse [54] and may be suffering from posttraumatic stress disorder (PTSD) [31, 37]. It has been observed that "plastic surgeons treat child sexual abuse survivors without being aware of it." Such patients often appear well adjusted and may become symptomatic under the specific stresses of surgery [54]; for example, they may start having flashbacks of their trauma. For some patients, the decision to have cosmetic procedures is their attempt, albeit unconscious, to "fix" a body that is tainted by abuse. A commentary by Summit [54] notes that the abused child "will tend to blame his or her body for causing the abuse and will tend to search for the idealized authority figures who might both redeem the body and undo the abuse." Some patients may have a history of multiple cosmetic procedures [54] which they may not have found to be satisfactory; many patients with histories of childhood sexual abuse may not have conscious recollection of the their traumatic experiences. Summit [54] cautions against being too intrusive as a direct enquiry regarding a history of abuse can seriously psychiatrically destabilize some patients with chronic PTSD; he observes that "walking the fine line between support and intrusion requires experience and deserves consultation with specialist colleagues." Several epidemiologic studies have reported that the suicide rate among women with cosmetic breast implants is two to three times the expected rate [36]; it is not difficult to speculate that this may be related to the fact that patients with childhood sexual abuse and PTSD who are at a much greater risk for suicide are also more likely to seek body-image surgeries.

Dissociative Disorders

Patients with dissociative disorders may experience psychiatric decompensation after body-image surgery. Depersonalization disorder following massive weight loss has been reported, with a male patient aged 44 reporting emotional numbing and estrangement from his body 4 weeks following bariatric surgery; these symptoms lessened but persisted even in the face of individualized therapy sessions [55]. Cosmetic procedures for facial rejuvenation can theoretically trigger dissociation in patient with dissociative disorders. If the clinician suspects an underlying dissociative disorder, it is advisable that a mental health clinician be involved when informed consent is being obtained to carry out the procedure; as in cases of severe dissociative disorders such as dissociative identity disorder (or multiple personality disorder), all dissociated parts may not consent to the procedure.

Psychotic Disorders

Cosmetic procedures for facial rejuvenation have generally not been associated with psychotic decompensation [35]; this is in contrast to aesthetic rhinoplasty patients who, for example, have been shown to develop psychotic disorders such as schizophrenia years after the surgery. Schweitzer et al. [56] have described the case of a woman who underwent routine rhytidectomy with satisfactory aesthetic results. The patient had no past psychiatric history. Twenty-four hours postsurgery, she became delusional; however, her sensorium was clear. Her symptoms cleared within 2 weeks after antipsychotic drug therapy was started. The patient had a history of severe abuse and neglect during her childhood; appearance was of overriding importance for the female family members, and the patient's mother used to be very critical of the patient's appearance. It is possible that the patient's decision to seek surgery was related to some unresolved issues from her childhood which surfaced after surgery and resulted in a psychotic decompensation. In such cases, it is helpful to ascertain the symbolic significance of the procedure for the patient.

Personality Disorders

Patients seeking procedures for rejuvenation of their appearance have been identified as having some "Cluster B" (narcissistic and histrionic) and "Cluster C" (obsessive-compulsive and dependent) personality traits [31, 37]. Both narcissistic and obsessional personality traits have been associated with patient dissatisfaction with cosmetic facial plastic surgery [24]. Individuals with severely narcissistic personalities may develop a major adjustment disorder in reaction to the cutaneous signs of aging. Among such narcissistic individuals who typically have pervasive pattern of grandiosity and need for admiration, having a youthful appearance is often a precondition for self-acceptance and trusting that they will be accepted by others; and an aging appearance can result in a significant emotional crisis, including a severe depressive reaction. A patient with severe narcissistic personality traits is therefore more likely to have unreasonable expectations of cosmetic procedures for facial rejuvenation [57]. The patient with histrionic personality traits tends to be excessively emotional and attention seeking, may use her physical appearance to draw attention to herself, and will tend to react negatively to decreased attention from others as a result of aging-related changes; such patients are also likely to have unrealistic expectations of what treatment has to offer. Several studies have shown that patients seeking cosmetic procedures have a greater need to be in control of their lives and have obsessive-compulsive personality traits [13], and the younger group of patients seeking facelifts [11, 12] tended to have dependent personality traits. Some of these patients experienced short-term depressive reactions postsurgery; however, generally they were satisfied with the outcome of the cosmetic procedures.

Patients with borderline personality disorder (BPD) (also classified under "Cluster B") [37] may seek treatment from plastic surgeons in two different situations: for treatment of self-inflicted injury or as a feature of their insatiable requests for aesthetic procedures [58]. BPD patients' preoccupation with appearance tends to shift from one body part to another over time, and BPD patients may request corrections involving multiple body regions to avoid perceived abandonment by the surgeon or because of their impulsivity [58]. BPD patients tend to have unrealistic expectations of treatment outcome, and it is important that the clinician remain inflexible to any unrealistic requests. BPD may express disappointment or anger toward the surgeon by externalizing behaviors, changing doctors or intentional self-mutilation [58]. In a study of 133 plastic surgery patients over a 1.5-year period, BPD patients had on average 4.5 requests for operating sites and were the most dissatisfied personality type [57]. Because of the fluctuating concerns with appearance and tendency for unrealistic expectations, it is recommended that plastic surgery on individuals with BPD be avoided [58].

Goin et al. [13] have further observed that a patient with paranoid personality traits improved after surgery for a facelift even though "ordinarily psychiatrists are quite wary about recommending elective operations for patients known to be paranoid." They observe that the paranoid patient had a favorable adjustment as the alterations produced by a facelift are not drastic body alterations and the changes do not necessitate "extreme personality organization." The paranoid patient became more socially interactive following her facelift, and this reduced her paranoid thinking.

Conclusion

Cosmetic procedures for aging skin are typically life enhancing versus life saving and tend to be primarily emotionally or psychosocially motivated. Psychosomatic aspects of aging skin should therefore be taken into consideration in the patient seeking treatment for rejuvenation of their appearance (using surgical, minimally invasive procedures or topical therapies), as they can play an important role in the clinical management and patient satisfaction with treatment outcome.

Cross-References

- ▶ Assessing Quality of Life in Older Adult Patients with Skin Disorders
- ▶ Psychological and Social Implications of Aging Skin: Normal Aging and the Effects of Cutaneous Disease

References

1. Gupta MA, Gilchrest BA. Psychosocial aspects of aging skin. Dermatol Clin. 2005;23:643–8.
2. Finn JC, Cox SE, Earl ML. Social implications of hyperfunctional facial lines. Dermatol Surg. 2003;29:450–5.
3. Heckmann M, Ceballos-Baumann A. Botulinum toxin overrides depression: not surprising, yet sensational. Dermatol Surg. 2007;33:765.

4. Khan JA. Aesthetic surgery: diagnosing and healing the miscues of human facial expression. Ophthal Plast Reconstr Surg. 2001;17:4–6.
5. Gupta MA, Gupta AK. Cutaneous body image dissatisfaction and suicidal ideation: mediation by interpersonal sensitivity. J Psychosom Res. 2013;75:55–9.
6. American Society of Plastic Surgeons. 2014 Plastic Surgery Statistics Report. 2015; Accessed on: June 1, 2015. Available at: http://www.plasticsurgery.org/Documents/news-resources/statistics/2014-statistics/cosmetic-procedure-trends-2014.pdf.
7. Sontag S. The double standard of aging. Saturday Rev Soc. 1972;23:29–38.
8. Saucier MG. Midlife and Beyond: Issues for Aging Women. J Couns Dev. 2004;82:420–5.
9. Barrett AE, Robbins C. The multiple sources of women's aging anxiety and their relationship with psychological distress. J Aging Health. 2008;20:32–65.
10. Gupta MA, Gupta AK. Dissatisfaction with skin appearance among patients with eating disorders and non-clinical controls. Br J Dermatol. 2001;145:110–3.
11. Webb WL, Slaughter R, Meyer E, Edgerton M. Mechanisms of psychosocial adjustment in patients seeking "face-lift" operation. Psychosom Med. 1965;27:183–92.
12. Edgerton MT, Webb WL, Slaughter R, Meyer E. Surgical results and psychosocial changes following rhytidectomy; an evaluation of face-lifting. Plast Reconstr Surg. 1964;33:503–21.
13. Goin MK, Burgoyne RW, Goin JM, Staples FR. A prospective psychological study of 50 female face-lift patients. Plast Reconstr Surg. 1980;65:436–42.
14. Meningaud JP, Benadiba L, Servant JM, Herve C, Bertrand JC, Pelicie Y. Depression, anxiety and quality of life among scheduled cosmetic surgery patients: multicentre prospective study. J Craniomaxillofac Surg. 2001;29:177–80.
15. Meningaud JP, Benadiba L, Servant JM, Herve C, Bertrand JC, Pelicier Y. Depression, anxiety and quality of life: outcome 9 months after facial cosmetic surgery. J Craniomaxillofac Surg. 2003;31:46–50.
16. Alves MC, Abla LE, Santos Rde A, Ferreira LM. Quality of life and self-esteem outcomes following rhytidoplasty. Ann Plast Surg. 2005;54:511–4; discussion 515–6.
17. Litner JA, Rotenberg BW, Dennis M, Adamson PA. Impact of cosmetic facial surgery on satisfaction with appearance and quality of life. Arch Facial Plast Surg. 2008;10:79–83.
18. Swanson E. Outcome analysis in 93 facial rejuvenation patients treated with a deep-plane face lift. Plast Reconstr Surg. 2011;127:823–34.
19. Sarwer DB, Gibbons LM, Magee L, Baker JL, Casas LA, Glat PM, et al. A prospective, multi-site investigation of patient satisfaction and psychosocial status following cosmetic surgery. Aesthet Surg J. 2005;25:263–9.
20. Sarwer DB, Infield AL, Baker JL, Casas LA, Glat PM, Gold AH, et al. Two-year results of a prospective, multi-site investigation of patient satisfaction and psychosocial status following cosmetic surgery. Aesthet Surg J. 2008;28:245–50.
21. von Soest T, Kvalem IL, Roald HE, Skolleborg KC. The effects of cosmetic surgery on body image, self-esteem, and psychological problems. J Plast Reconstr Aesthet Surg. 2009;62:1238–44.
22. von Soest T, Kvalem IL, Skolleborg KC, Roald HE. Psychosocial changes after cosmetic surgery: a 5-year follow-up study. Plast Reconstr Surg. 2011;128:765–72.
23. Rainsbury JW. The place of rhinoplasty in the ageing face. J Laryngol Otol. 2010;124:115–8.
24. Herruer JM, Prins JB, van Heerbeek N, Verhage-Damen GW, Ingels KJ. Negative predictors for satisfaction in patients seeking facial cosmetic surgery: a systematic review. Plast Reconstr Surg. 2015;135:1596–605.
25. Gupta MA, Goldfarb MT, Schork NJ, Weiss JS, Gupta AK, Ellis CN, et al. Treatment of mildly to moderately photoaged skin with topical tretinoin has a favorable psychosocial effect: a prospective study. J Am Acad Dermatol. 1991;24:780–1.
26. Gupta MA, Schork NJ, Ellis CN. Psychosocial correlates of the treatment of photodamaged skin with topical retinoic acid: a prospective controlled study. J Am Acad Dermatol. 1994;30:969–72.
27. Kohl E, Meierhofer J, Koller M, Zeman F, Groesser L, Karrer S, et al. Fractional carbon dioxide laser resurfacing of rhytides and photoaged skin – a prospective clinical study on patient expectation and satisfaction. Lasers Surg Med. 2015;47:111–9.
28. Koch RJ, Newman JP, Safer DL. Psychological predictors of patient satisfaction with laser skin resurfacing. Arch Facial Plast Surg. 2003;5:445–6.
29. Dayan SH, Lieberman ED, Thakkar NN, Larimer KA, Anstead A. Botulinum toxin a can positively impact first impression. Dermatol Surg. 2008;34 Suppl 1: S40–7.
30. Finzi E, Wasserman E. Treatment of depression with botulinum toxin A: a case series. Dermatol Surg. 2006;32:645–9; discussion 649–50.
31. American Psychiatric Association. Diagnostic and statistical manual for mental disorders (DSM IV-TR). Washington, DC: American Psychiatric Association; 2000.
32. Hexsel D, Brum C, Siega C, Schilling-Souza J, Dal'Forno T, Heckmann M, et al. Evaluation of self-esteem and depression symptoms in depressed and nondepressed subjects treated with onabotulinumtoxinA for glabellar lines. Dermatol Surg. 2013;39:1088–96.
33. Lewis MB, Bowler PJ. Botulinum toxin cosmetic therapy correlates with a more positive mood. J Cosmet Dermatol. 2009;8:24–6.
34. Dayan SH, Arkins JP, Patel AB, Gal TJ. A double-blind, randomized, placebo-controlled health-outcomes survey of the effect of botulinum toxin type a

injections on quality of life and self-esteem. Dermatol Surg. 2010;36 Suppl 4:2088–97.
35. Edgerton MT, Langman MW, Pruzinsky T. Plastic surgery and psychotherapy in the treatment of 100 psychologically disturbed patients. Plast Reconstr Surg. 1991;88:594–608.
36. Sarwer DB, Brown GK, Evans DL. Cosmetic breast augmentation and suicide. Am J Psychiatry. 2007;164:1006–13.
37. American Psychiatric Association. Diagnostic and statistical manual of mental disorders. 5th ed. Arlington: American Psychiatric Association; 2013.
38. Crerand CE, Franklin ME, Sarwer DB. Body dysmorphic disorder and cosmetic surgery. Plast Reconstr Surg. 2006;118:167–80.
39. Crerand CE, Menard W, Phillips KA. Surgical and minimally invasive cosmetic procedures among persons with body dysmorphic disorder. Ann Plast Surg. 2010;65:11–6.
40. Sarwer DB, Crerand CE. Body dysmorphic disorder and appearance enhancing medical treatments. Body Image. 2008;5:50–8.
41. van der Meer J, van Rood YR, van der Wee NJ, den Hollander-Gijsman M, van Noorden MS, Giltay EJ, et al. Prevalence, demographic and clinical characteristics of body dysmorphic disorder among psychiatric outpatients with mood, anxiety or somatoform disorders. Nord J Psychiatry. 2012;66:232–8.
42. Keel PK, Gravener JA, Joiner Jr TE, Haedt AA. Twenty-year follow-up of bulimia nervosa and related eating disorders not otherwise specified. Int J Eat Disord. 2010;43:492–7.
43. Gupta MA. Concerns about aging skin and eating disorders. In: Strumia R, editor. Eating disorders and the skin. Berlin/Heidelberg: Springer; 2013. p. 97–102.
44. Gupta MA. Fear of aging: a precipitating factor in late onset anorexia nervosa. Int J Eat Disord. 1990;9:221–4.
45. Gupta MA. Concerns about aging and a drive for thinness: a factor in the biopsychosocial model of eating disorders? Int J Eat Disord. 1995;18:351–7.
46. Brandsma L. Eating disorders across the lifespan. J Women Aging. 2007;19:155–72.
47. Cumella EJ, Kally Z. Profile of 50 women with midlife-onset eating disorders. Eat Disord. 2008;16:193–203.
48. Mangweth-Matzek B, Hoek HW, Pope Jr HG. Pathological eating and body dissatisfaction in middle-aged and older women. Curr Opin Psychiatry. 2014;27:431–5.
49. Mangweth-Matzek B, Hoek HW, Rupp CI, Kemmler G, Pope Jr HG, Kinzl J. The menopausal transition – a possible window of vulnerability for eating pathology. Int J Eat Disord. 2013;46:609–16.
50. McQuaide S. Women at midlife. Social Work. 1998;43:21–31.
51. Slevec JH, Tiggemann M. Predictors of body dissatisfaction and disordered eating in middle-aged women. Clin Psychol Rev. 2011;31:515–24.
52. Runfola CD, Von Holle A, Peat CM, Gagne DA, Brownley KA, Hofmeier SM, et al. Characteristics of women with body size satisfaction at midlife: results of the Gender and Body Image (GABI) Study. J Women Aging. 2013;25:287–304.
53. Gupta MA, Schork NJ. Aging-related concerns and body image: possible future implications for eating disorders. Int J Eat Disord. 1993;14:481–6.
54. Morgan E, Froning ML. Child sexual abuse sequelae and body-image surgery. Plast Reconstr Surg. 1990;86:475–8; discussion 479–80.
55. Hunnemeyer K, Hain B, Wild B. Who is the man in the mirror? Depersonalization disorder after obesity surgery. Surg Obes Relat Dis. 2012;8:43–5.
56. Schweitzer I, Hirschfeld JJ. Postrhytidectomy psychosis: a rare complication. Plast Reconstr Surg. 1984;74:419–22.
57. Napoleon A. The presentation of personalities in plastic surgery. Ann Plast Surg. 1993;31:193–208.
58. Morioka D, Ohkubo F. Borderline personality disorder and aesthetic plastic surgery. Aesthetic Plast Surg. 2014;38:1169–76.

Advanced Glycation End Products (AGEs): Emerging Mediators of Skin Aging

124

Paraskevi Gkogkolou and Markus Böhm

Contents

P. Gkogkolou • M. Böhm (✉)
Department of Dermatology, Laboratory for Neuroendocrinology of the Skin and Interdisciplinary Endocrinology, University of Münster, Münster, Germany
e-mail: paraskevi.gkogkolou@ukmuenster.de; bohmm@uni-muenster.de

M.A. Farage et al. (eds.), *Textbook of Aging Skin*,
DOI 10.1007/978-3-662-47398-6_137

Abstract

Advanced glycation end products (AGEs) derive from nonenzymatic reactions between reducing sugars and proteins, lipids or nucleic acids. In this chapter, we highlight the role of AGEs as an emerging class of mediators of skin aging. After a short section on the biochemistry and biology of AGEs we will put these molecules into the context of skin aging. Evidence will be provided that: (1) AGEs are detectable in skin, (2) that they accumulate over time in aged skin, and (3) that they act via diverse mechanisms (receptor and nonreceptor-mediated) on various cellular and noncellular targets of the skin. Special emphasis will be devoted to the connections between AGEs and reactive oxygen species, the latter established players of cutaneous aging. Finally, current and future strategies are described by which the impact of AGEs on skin aging may be counteracted.

Introduction

Advanced glycation end products (AGEs) derive from nonenzymatic reactions between reducing sugars, such as glucose and proteins, lipids or nucleic acids. This process is called glycation [1] and is distinguished from glycosylation, which is an enzymatic procedure. Glycation was first described by Maillard in 1912 [2] but its role in food browning during thermal processing was disclosed by Hodge only 50 years later [3].

Since then, AGEs have been detected in various tissues during aging but especially in patients with diabetes where elevated glucose levels exist. Moreover, deposition of AGEs has been implicated in a number of diabetes- and age-associated complications such as diabetic angiopathy [4], neurodegenerative disorders, and osteoarthritis [5].

In the last years, the potential role of AGEs in skin aging has attracted many scientists. Targeting AGE-mediated pathways could become a novel strategy to prevent not only diabetes-related complications but also to promote healthier aging in general and to prevent aging of the skin.

A Brief Biochemistry of AGEs

AGEs are nonenzymatic reaction products between reactive sugars such as glucose and various other molecules. During the formation of AGEs simple and complicated multistep reactions are involved. During the classical Maillard reaction strong, reactive, electrophilic carbonyl groups of glucose or other sugars (fructose, ribose) react with free amine groups of neutrophilic amino acids (usually lysine or arginine), nucleic acids, or lipids, leading to formation of a nonstable Schiff base [1]. In a second rearrangement reaction, a more stable ketoamine (Amadori product) is formed. Schiff bases and Amadori products are reversible reaction products. These can further irreversibly react with amino acid residues of peptides and proteins leading to formation of stable protein adducts or protein crosslinks [1]. Various oxidation, dehydration, polymerization, and oxidative breakdown reactions can give rise to numerous other AGEs. Oxygen, reactive oxygen species (ROS), and redox active transition metals accelerate these nonenzymatic reactions. If an oxidation process is involved, these products are called advanced glycoxidation end products.

Biochemically, AGEs are a heterogeneous group of molecules. Since discovery of the first glycated protein, glycated hemoglobin in diabetes patients, numerous other AGEs have been identified. Some of them have characteristic autofluorescent properties, which facilitates their identification in situ after tissue sampling but may also allow in vivo detection by noninvasive methods. Table 1 highlights the most commonly found AGEs in the skin.

N-ε-(Carboxymethyl)lysine (CML) is the most common AGE in vivo and the major epitope of

Table 1 Detected AGEs in skin[a]

AGE	Skin compartments involved	Targets of glycation	Methods of detection	References
CML	Epidermis	Epidermis (SC -CK10, SS, SG)	LC-ESI-TOF-MS, IF, IB	[6]
	Aged and diabetic dermis Photoaging – actinic elastosis	Collagen Vimentin Elastin	SIM/GC-MS IHC ELISA, confocal microscopy	[7, 8] [9, 10]
Pentosidin	Aged and diabetic dermis	Collagen	Reversed-phase HPLC	[8]
GO	Aged dermis	Collagen	LC/MS	[11]
MGO	Aged dermis	Collagen	LC/MS	[11]
Glucosepane	Aged dermis	Collagen	LC/MS	[11]
Fructoselysine	Aged dermis	Collagen	LC/MS	[11]
CEL	Aged dermis	Collagen	SIM/GC-MS	[11]
GOLD	Aged dermis	Collagen	LC/MS	[12]
MOLD	Aged dermis	Collagen	LC/MS	[12]

[a]Abbreviations: *ELISA* enzyme-linked immunosorbent assay, *GO* glyoxal, *HPLC* high performance liquid chromatography, *IHC* immunohistochemistry, *IB* immunoblotting, *IF* immunofluorescence, *LC-ESI-TOF-MS* liquid chromatography–electrospray ionization time-of-flight mass spectrometry, *LC/MS* liquid chromatography/mass spectrometry, *MGO* methylglyoxal, *SIM/GC-MS* selected ion monitoring gas chromatography-mass spectrometry, *SC stratum corneum*, *SG stratum granulosum*, *SS stratum spinosum*; all other abbreviations are already explained in the text

many commercially available anti-AGE antibodies [13]. It is a nonfluorescent protein adduct and formed via oxidative degradation of Amadori products or direct addition of glyoxal to lysine.

Pentosidine is composed of an arginine and a lysine residue crosslinked to a pentose [14]. It is a fluorescent glycoxidation product and represents the major AGE involved in protein-protein crosslinks.

3-Deoxyglucosome (3GO), methylglyoxal (MG), and glyoxal (GO) are very reactive dicarbonyl compounds which mainly derive from oxidative degradation or autoxidation of Amadori products and typically lead to molecular crosslinking [1, 15].

Other in vivo detected AGEs include glucosepane, carboxymethyl-hydroxy-lysine, carboxyethyllysine (CEL), fructoselysine, methylglyoxal-derived hydroimidazolones, and pyrraline. They form nonfluorescent protein adducts while glyoxal-lysine dimer (GOLD) and methylglyoxal-lysine dimer (MOLD) form nonfluorescent protein crosslinks [1].

AGEs are generated at low rates as endogenous by-products during normal metabolic processes. As expected, increased bioavailability of glucose as found in diabetes but also smoking and ultraviolet (UV) irradiation increase formation of AGEs [9, 16]. AGEs may be also exogenously inserted into the organism via diet, with approximately 10–30 % of ingested AGEs reaching the circulation [17]. The content of AGEs in food depends on the method of preparation, i.e., especially cooking and temperature, with fried food containing higher amounts of AGEs than boiled or steamed food [18]. Finally, it seems that the level of circulating AGEs is genetically determined [19].

Once formed, AGEs can be removed from the organism via intrinsic detoxifying mechanisms. Two isoforms of glyoxalase (Glo) utilize reduced glutathione to catalyze the conversion of glyoxal, methylglyoxal, and other α-oxoaldehydes to the less toxic D-lactate [20]. The intracellular fructosamine kinases phosphorylate and destabilize Amadori products leading to their spontaneous breakdown [21]. Fructosamine-3-kinase (FN3K), one of the most studied enzymes in this system, is almost ubiquitously expressed in human tissues including the skin and plays an important role on the intracellular breakdown of Amadori products [21]. The fructosyl-amine oxidases (FAOXs) or "amadoriases" also recognize and oxidatively break Amadori products; however, these are expressed in bacteria, yeast, and fungi but not in mammals [21]. Finally, cathepsins D and L are capable of degrading endocytosed AGE-modified proteins [22].

Receptors of AGEs

Various receptors and binding proteins for AGEs have been identified. The most thoroughly investigated one is RAGE (receptor for AGEs). It belongs to the immunoglobulin superfamily of cell surface receptors and is encoded by a gene on chromosome 6 near the major histocompatibility complex III. RAGE is a pattern recognition receptor and binds in addition to AGEs other molecules such as S-100/calgranulins, high motility group protein B1 (amphoterine), amyloid β-peptides, and beta-sheet fibrils [23]. Mitogen-activated protein kinases (MAPKs), extracellular signal-related kinases (ERK) 1 and 2, p38, stress-activated protein kinase-c/Jun-N-terminal kinase (SAPK/JNK), phosphatidyl-inositol 3 kinase (PI-3K), the janus kinases, and protein kinase C are activated in a cell type-specific manner upon engagement of RAGE with a ligand. RAGE stimulation leads to sustained and self-perpetuating activation of NF-κB and transcription of many proinflammatory genes like tumor necrosis factor-α, interleukin (IL)-6, and C-reactive protein (CRP). Furthermore, RAGE activation directly increases oxidative stress via activation of nicotinamide adenine dinucleotide phosphate (NADPH) oxidase, inactivation of antioxidant enzymes like superoxide dismutase (SOD) and catalase, as well as via reduction of glutathione (GSH), the latter a coenzyme of the major AGE-degrading enzyme Glo I [24].

In addition to the cell-bound RAGE, soluble RAGE (sRAGE) and endogenous secretory RAGE have been identified as binding partners for AGEs. Both are extracellular truncated forms of RAGE containing the ligand-binding domain but not the transmembrane domain. They are formed via alternative gene splicing and post-translational proteolysis of RAGE. Due to the lack of the transmembrane domain they do not elicit signaling and are considered as decoy receptors of AGEs which counteract RAGE-mediated signaling [25].

Another group of AGE-receptors include macrophage scavenger receptor types I and II, oligosaccharyl transferase-48 (AGE-R1), 80K-H phosphoprotein (AGE-R2), and galectin-3 (AGE-R3) which are thought to regulate endocytosis and degradation of AGEs and counteract the effects of RAGE. AGE-R1 has been further shown to counteract AGE-induced oxidative stress via inhibition of RAGE signaling [26].

RAGEs are almost ubiquitously expressed in the organism, typically in low numbers. Expression of RAGE is upregulated in response to pathologic conditions [23, 27]. In skin, RAGE is expressed within epidermis and dermis, and its expression is higher in sun-exposed sites. A wide variety of human cell types including keratinocytes, fibroblasts, endothelial cells, and immune cells (dendritic cells, monocytes) express RAGE in vitro and in vivo.

Detection of AGEs in Aged Skin

Skin, due to its direct accessibility, offers excellent opportunities for direct detection of glycation using minimal invasive techniques in skin biopsies or even noninvasive techniques which take advantage of the autofluorescent properties of AGEs. Initially, AGEs deposition in the skin was studied with Western blots or autofluorescence in skin biopsies. Recently, AGE-Readers (DiagnOptics™ B.V., Groningen, The Netherlands; TrūAge Scanner™ Morinda, Orem, UT, USA) were introduced in the market as a noninvasive method for in vivo measurements of AGEs accumulation based on their characteristic autofluorescence [28].

Skin glycation has been thoroughly investigated not only in diabetic skin but also in intrinsically and extrinsically aged skin. Glycation-associated autofluorescence correlated with chronological aging in a large number of nondiabetic subjects [29]. Moreover, AGEs are more abundant in sun-exposed skin in sites of solar elastosis [7]. Smoking has been shown to enhance formation of AGEs and increase their deposition in various tissues including skin [9]. Although a correlation of dietary AGEs with serum levels of AGEs has been shown, a possible correlation with skin AGEs has not been investigated yet.

Since most AGEs are formed via slow, nonenzymatic reactions it was initially believed that their accumulation depends on protein turnover rate, with long-lived proteins like collagen as well as elastin and fibronectin being the major targets of glycation [8]. Accordingly, presence of glycated collagen is first observed at the age of 20, with a yearly accumulation rate of about 3.7 % and reaching a 30–50 % increase at 80 years of age [7, 30]. However, CML was recently identified in keratin 10 of the upper epidermal layers of healthy subjects, suggesting a potential involvement of short-lived proteins in glycation [6]. In accordance with this, both epidermis and dermis were modified by glycation in an in vitro reconstructed skin organ model [31].

Interestingly, skin glycation has been shown to correlate with various systemic diabetes- and age-related complications such as angiopathy and chronic renal disease [32].

These findings indicate that skin glycation is not only a marker for diabetic monitoring but also – at least in nondiabetic individuals – a read-out for the extent of skin aging.

Cellular and Noncellular Targets of AGEs Within the Skin

Advanced glycation can directly act on a variety of biomolecules including proteins, lipids, and nucleic acids in the intracellular and extracellular compartments. These modifications can alter enzyme-substrate interactions, protein-DNA interactions, and protein-protein interactions, affecting numerous physiological functions of the organism. Moreover, AGEs react with RAGE to elicit genomic and nongenomic effects that modulate cell homeostasis, metabolism, redox balance, matrix protein turnover, and immune and inflammatory responses.

Extracellular Matrix Proteins

Extracellular matrix (ECM) proteins not only create a supportive framework for skin cells but also directly interact with them regulating important cellular functions such as migration, differentiation, and proliferation. Due to their long lifetime before degradation they represent the molecules which mainly suffer from glycation.

Crosslinking of adjacent *collagen* results in increased stiffness and decreased resistance to mechanical forces [33]. AGE-mediated changes on side chains of collagen affect its contact sites with cells and other matrix proteins and consequently its ability to react with them [34]. For example, actin polymerization and migration of immune cells is subsequently impaired [35]. The precise aggregation of monomers into the triple helix and the association of collagen IV with laminin in the basal membrane are affected. Moreover, degradation by matrix metalloproteinases (MMPs) is impaired, thus inhibiting removal of modified collagen and replacement by newly synthesized and functional one [5]. Accordingly, tissue permeability and turnover is impaired.

Other ECM proteins suffering from advanced glycation are *elastin* [7, 9] and *fibronectin* [8]. CML-modified elastin assembles in large and irregular structures, has decreased elasticity, and is resistant to proteolytic degradation [36]. CML-modified elastin is found almost exclusively in sites of actinic elastosis and not in sun-protected skin. UV irradiation stimulates glycation of elastin in the presence of sugars in vitro. Glycation of fibronectin impairs its interaction with integrin $\alpha\nu\beta1$ and delays wound healing [37].

In vitro glycated skin samples have impaired biomechanical properties [38]. In vivo, decreased skin elasticity characterizes diabetic subjects in comparison to healthy controls [39].

Intracellular Proteins

AGEs modify and lead to aggregation and poor assembly of intermediate filaments such as *keratin 10* in keratinocytes [6] and *vimentin* in fibroblasts [10]. As a result, instability of the cytoskeleton, cell shape and defects in migration, cellular division, and contraction occur. Various other intracellular proteins including *enzymes* may be targeted by glycation. Moreover, glycation of enzymes of the *ubiquitin proteasome system* and of the *lysosomal proteolytic* system has been shown to inhibit their function [40]. Antioxidant and other protective enzymes such as Cu-Zn-superoxide dismutase (Cu-Zn-SOD) can be inactivated [41]. Other intracellular components, such as DNA and lipids can be glycated with detrimental effects on their function [42].

Growth Factors and Growth Factor Receptors

AGE-adducts of growth and their receptors can alter their binding affinities and impair their signal transduction properties. Glycated basic fibroblast growth factor (bFGF) displays impaired mitogenic activity in endothelial cells [43]. Dicarbonyls such as glyoxal and methylglyoxal also alter signaling of epidermal growth factor receptor (EGFR), a receptor controlling various cellular functions such as proliferation, differentiation, motility and survival, by formation of EGFR crosslinks, blocking of phosphorylation and impaired activation of ERKs and phospholipase C (PLC) [44].

Cutaneous Cell Types Responding to AGEs

RAGE is expressed by various cell types of human skin including keratinocytes, dermal fibroblasts, and endothelial cells as shown by in vitro cell culture studies. In situ RAGE expression is abundant in sites of solar elastosis and its expression is enhanced by AGEs and proinflammatory cytokines such as TNF-α [27].

AGEs have been shown to affect various cellular functions in vitro (Table 2). In keratinocytes, AGEs impair cell differentiation [46], induce senescence [46], decrease cell viability [46] and

Table 2 Effects of AGEs on skin morphology and physiology[a]

Keratinocytes	Proliferation ↓ Viability ↓ ROS ↑ MMP-9 ↑, TIPM ↓ β-galactosidase ↑- Senescence ↑ Involucrin ↓- differentiation ↓ NF-κB ↑ $\alpha_2\beta1$-integrin ↓ - Migration ↓	Cell renewal ↓ Epidermal homeostasis ↓	[45] [46] [47] [45, 48] [46] [46] [48] [46]
Fibroblasts	Proliferation ↓ Apoptosis ↑ ECM synthesis ↓ MMP ↑ Senescence ↑ NF-κB ↑ ROS ↑ Contractile properties ↓	Cell renewal ↓ Dermal homeostasis ↓ Skin contractile function ↓	[49] [49] [50] [50] [51] [49] [47, 51] [10]
Melanocytes	?	?	
Extracellular matrix proteins (collagen, fibronectin, elastin)	Crosslinking Resistance to MMP degradation Impaired assembly of macromolecules to normal 3D structures Defect cross-talking to cells	Elasticity ↓ Stiffness ↑ Resistance to repair mechanisms Tissue permeability ↓	[7–9] [5] [5, 33] [5, 34]
Vascular endothelial cells	VCAM, ICAM, E-selectin ↑ Permeability ↑ TNF-α, IL-6 ↑ MCP-1 ↑	Induction of proinflammatory mediators and recruitment of immune cells	[52] [52] [52] [52]

[a]Abbreviations: *ICAM* intercellular adhesion molecule, *MCP-1* monocyte chemotactic protein-1, *TIPM* tissue inhibitor of MMP, *VCAM* vascular cell adhesion molecule; all other abbreviations are already explained in the text

migration [45], and induce MMP expression [45], partly via enhanced NF-κB signaling [48]. Furthermore, they decrease expression of β-defensin-2 and -3 leading to increased susceptibility to infections [53]. Recently, S100 A8/A9-RAGE interaction has been implicated in the pathogenesis of squamous cell carcinomas in human skin [54].

AGEs furthermore decrease proliferation and induce apoptosis of human dermal fibroblasts, an effect which is mediated via RAGE-signaling and leads to transcription of various proapoptotic genes and activation of NF-κB and caspases-3, -8, and -9 [49]. Expression of beta-galactosidase, a marker of senescence, is induced [51]. Collagen and ECM protein synthesis have been also found to be decreased, while the expression of MMPs is induced by AGEs [50].

In endothelial cells, AGEs increase expression of proinflammatory cytokines and chemokines like TNF-α, IL-6, and MCP-1 [52]. Moreover, they increase expression of adhesion molecules like VCAM-1 and increase vascular permeability [52]. Furthermore, AGE-modification of bFGF decreases mitogenic activity of these cells [43].

In the context of photoaging, UVA irradiation in the presence of AGEs increases ROS production and decreases viability of both epidermal keratinocytes [47] and dermal fibroblasts [55].

AGEs and ROS

ROS – generated during normal cell metabolism throughout lifetime and also increasingly propagated via UV exposure (photoaging) and other noxious stimuli – are central mediators of intrinsic and extrinsic skin aging. Importantly, in vitro exposure of AGEs to UVA leads to ROS formation such as superoxide anion, hydrogen peroxide, and hydroxyl radicals [55]. AGEs can lead to ROS formation within cells by various pathways. Firstly, they can stimulate NADPH oxidase in various cell types including human dermal fibroblasts, endothelial cells, and in immune cells at least partly via interaction with RAGE [24]. Activation of the catalytic subunits NOX1 [56], NOX2 [57], NOX 4 [58] as well as of the regulatory subunit p47phox [59] in a cell-specific manner has been reported. Secondly, AGEs can suppress antioxidative defense systems including Cu-Zn-SOD which is inactivated by crosslinking and site-specific fragmentation of the Cu-ZnSOD molecule [41]. During these crosslinking reactions, AGEs can directly act as electron donors leading to formation of superoxide anion [60]. Finally, AGEs with chromophores can act as endogenous photosensitizers leading to increased ROS formation after UVA irradiation of human skin.

Anti-AGEs Strategies as a Perspective Against Skin Aging

Since AGEs play an important pathogenetic role in aging, substances able to inhibit formation of AGEs, to break already formed AGEs, or to antagonize their signaling could have a beneficial effect on skin aging as well as on age-related skin diseases. Until now various substances have been proposed and some of them are already being tested in clinical trials [61].

Aminoguanidine, one of the first identified substances, is a nucleophilic hydrazine which traps and inactivates early glycation products like dicarbonyl compounds. Although it showed promising results in various in vivo animal models, further drug development was stopped after a phase III clinical trial showed significant toxicity [62]. Notably, the anti-AGE properties of aminoguanidine have been demonstrated in in vitro and tissue-engineered skin models but in vivo data of this chemical on human skin are lacking [31, 63].

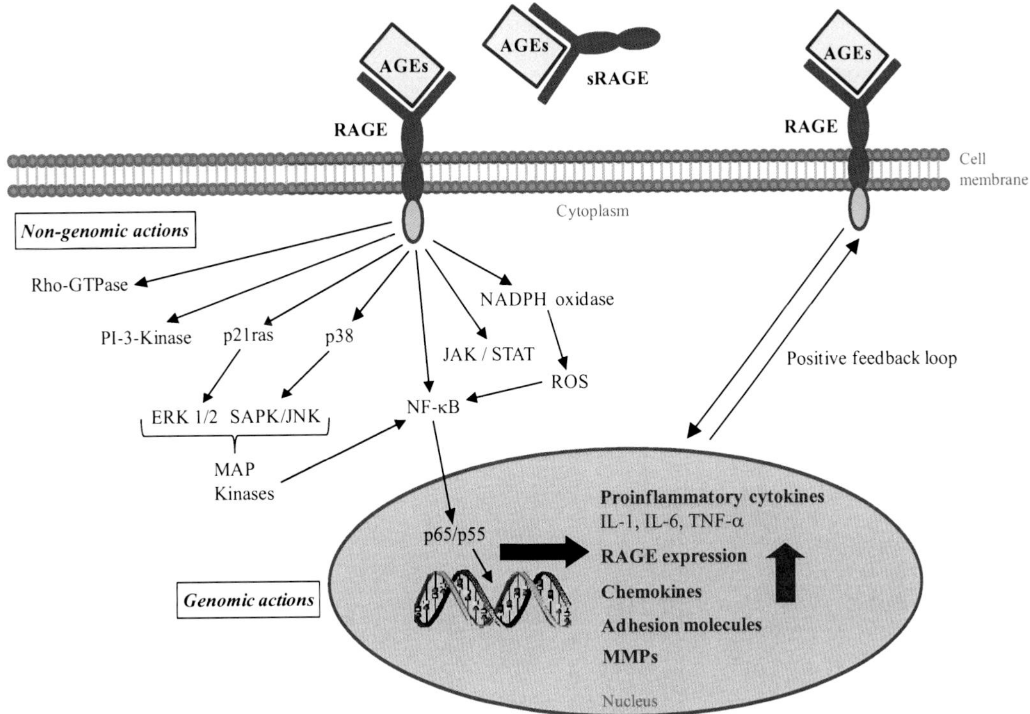

Fig. 1 Genomic and nongenomic actions of RAGE

Pyridoxamine is a naturally occurring vitamin B6 isoform which traps reactive carbonyl intermediates and scavenges ROS. Oral intake of pyridoxamine inhibited CML formation in skin collagen of diabetic rats [64]. However, its potential against skin aging remains to be shown.

"AGE-breakers" are chemical substances which recognize and break the Maillard reaction crosslink via a thiazolium structure like dimethyl-3-phenayl-thiazolium chloride (ALT-711), *N*-phenacylthiazolium, and N-phenacyl-4,5-dimethylthiazolium [65]. Of note, topical ALT-711 application improved skin hydration in a rat aging model [65].

Interference with intrinsic AGE-detoxification enzymes like Glo I and II, fructosamine kinases, and FAOXs could be a further strategy against AGEs as these enzymes recognize specific substrates and their inhibition may be associated with fewer side effects compared with the above chemicals. Interestingly, it has been shown that Glo I is transcriptionally controlled by Nrf2 and that pharmacological Nrf2 activators increase Glo I mRNA and protein levels as well as its activity [66]. Therefore, pharmacological activation of the Nrf2 pathway, e.g., by electrophils or other compounds, may lead to increased expression of Glo I and could have beneficial effects on skin aging by reducing the amounts of deposited AGEs.

Since oxidation reactions are involved in many steps of AGEs formation, substances with antioxidative or metal chelating properties may act as AGE-inhibitors. A lot of interest has been therefore directed to nutrients and vitamins, so-called nutraceuticals, as natural weapons against AGEs [61]. The list of such substances is

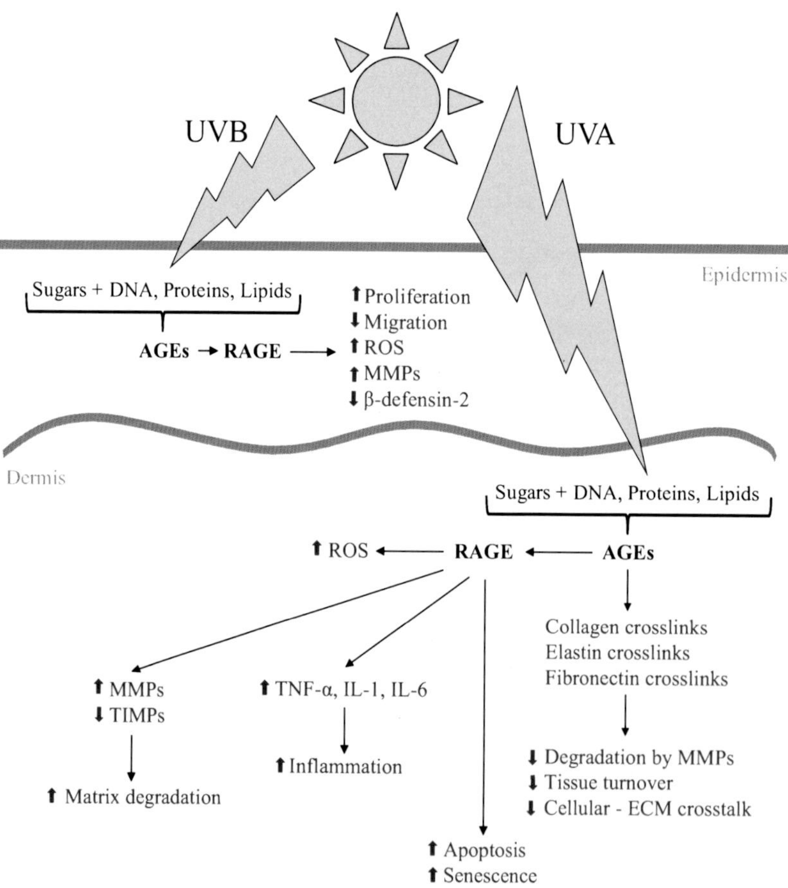

Fig. 2 Effects of AGEs in skin

long: ascorbic acid, α-tocopherol, niacinamide, pyridoxal, rivoflavin, zinc, α-lipoic acid, green tea, vitamins C and E, *N*-acetylcysteine, taurine, spices and herbs like ginger, cinnamon, cloves, and marjoram, and naturally occurring flavonoids such as luteolin, quercetin, and rutin have all shown antiglycating properties mostly in vitro but also in animal models [67, 68]. A blueberry extract, an AGE-inhibitor and C-xyloside, a glycosaminoglycan (GAG) synthesis stimulator, was tested in female diabetic subjects for 12 weeks and showed significant improvement on firmness, wrinkles, and hydration of skin although they failed to show a significant decrease in the cutaneous content of AGEs [69]. Recently, oral intake of a mangosteen extract showed some reduction in AGE-related skin autofluorescence and improved skin hydration as well as elasticity in healthy volunteers [70].

Restriction of intake of dietary AGEs may be perhaps the simplest strategy to prevent accumulation of AGEs in the body and to limit their deleterious effect. Dietary glycotoxins significantly increase concentrations of systemic inflammatory mediators like TNF-α, IL-6, and CRP [4]. A diet with a low content in AGEs was shown to reduce circulating AGEs and inflammatory biomarkers in patients with diabetes and renal failure [71]. In mice, low dietary AGEs had beneficial effects on wound healing [72]. There are no studies investigating the effects of AGE-poor diets on skin aging in humans. However, it has been shown that skin collagen glycation positively correlates with blood glucose levels in diabetes and that intensive treatment can reduce the levels of skin glycation [73], implicating that a diet low in AGEs may have a beneficial effect on skin glycation.

Antagonism of AGEs at the receptor level would be another potential strategy against AGEs. Interesting effects in various systems have been shown in vitro *and* in vivo by neutralizing RAGE or with small-molecule RAGE inhibitors [74]. Moreover, protective effects of sRAGE, the natural soluble decoy receptor of AGE, have been reported in diabetes and inflammatory models [23, 24]. Accordingly, sRAGE attenuates impaired wound healing in diabetic mice [75]. Further studies will be needed to investigate if these antibodies and small molecules have also promising effects in preclinical models of skin aging.

Finally, topical application of molecular chaperones such as carnosine and carnitine has shown an improvement of skin appearance which appeared to be at least in part mediated by lowering cutaneous accumulation of AGEs [76].

Conclusion

There is clear evidence that AGEs affect many targets in the skin via receptor- and nonreceptor-mediated pathways (Figs. 1 and 2). These cellular and noncellular targets are important players in the context of skin aging. In light of the intimate connection between ROS and AGEs glycation therefore appears to be an important contributor to cutaneous aging. Until now, there are several studies that assessed the value of anti-AGE strategies in patients with diabetes. As clinical trials on the effects of these anti-AGE strategies on skin aging are still missing, this could be a promising field in the future to further promote healthier skin aging.

References

1. Ahmed N. Advanced glycation endproducts-role in pathology of diabetic complications. Diabetes Res Clin Pract. 2005;67:3–21.
2. Maillard LC. Action des acides amines sur les sucres: formation des melanoidines par voie methodique. C R Acad Sci (Paris). 1912;154:66–8.
3. Hodge JE. Dehydrated foods, chemistry of browning reactions in model systems. J Agric Food Chem. 1953;1:928–43.
4. Vlassara H, Cai W, Crandall J, Goldberg T, Oberstein R, Dardaine V, et al. Inflammatory mediators are induced by dietary glycotoxins, a major risk factor for diabetic angiopathy. Proc Natl Acad Sci U S A. 2002;99:15596–601.
5. DeGroot J, Verzijl N, Wenting-Van Wijk MJ, Bank RA, Lafeber FP, Bijlsma JW, et al. Age-related decrease in susceptibility of human articular cartilage to matrix metalloproteinase-mediated degradation: the role of advanced glycation end products. Arthritis Rheum. 2001;44:2562–71.
6. Kawabata K, Yoshikawa H, Saruwatari K, Akazawa Y, Inoue T, Kuze T, et al. The presence of N(ε)-

(carboxymethyl) lysine in the human epidermis. Biochim Biophys Acta. 2011;1814:1246–52.

7. Jeanmaire C, Danoux L, Pauly G. Glycation during human dermal intrinsic and actinic ageing: an in vivo and in vitro model study. Br J Dermatol. 2001;145:10–8.
8. Dyer DG, Dunn JA, Thorpe SR, Bailie KE, Lyons TJ, McCance DR, et al. Accumulation of Maillard reaction products in skin collagen in diabetes and aging. J Clin Invest. 1993;91:2463–9.
9. Mizutari K, Ono T, Ikeda K, Kayashima K, Horiuchi S. Photo-enhanced modification of human skin elastin in actinic elastosis by N(epsilon)-(carboxymethyl) lysine, one of the glycoxidation products of the Maillard reaction. J Invest Dermatol. 1997;108:797–802.
10. Kueper T, Grune T, Prahl S, Lenz H, Welge V, Biernoth T, et al. Vimentin is the specific target in skin glycation. Structural prerequisites, functional consequences, and role in skin aging. J Biol Chem. 2007;282:23427–36.
11. Fan X, Sell DR, Zhang J, Nemet I, Theves M, Lu J, et al. Anaerobic vs aerobic pathways of carbonyl and oxidant stress in human lens and skin during aging and in diabetes: a comparative analysis. Free Radic Biol Med. 2010;49:847–56.
12. Frye EB, Degenhardt TP, Thorpe SR, Baynes JW. Role of the Maillard reaction in aging of tissue proteins. Advanced glycation end product-dependent increase in imidazolium cross-links in human lens proteins. J Biol Chem. 1998;273:18714–9.
13. Reddy S, Bichler J, Wells-Knecht KJ, Thorpe SR, Baynes JW. N epsilon-(carboxymethyl) lysine is a dominant advanced glycation end product (AGE) antigen in tissue proteins. Biochemistry. 1995;34:10872–8.
14. Sell DR, Monnier VM. Isolation, purification and partial characterization of novel fluorophores from aging human insoluble collagen-rich tissue. Connect Tissue Res. 1989;19:77–92.
15. Thornalley PJ, Langborg A, Minhas HS. Formation of glyoxal, methylglyoxal and 3-deoxyglucosone in the glycation of proteins by glucose. Biochem J. 1999;344:109–16.
16. Cerami C, Founds H, Nicholl I, Mitsuhashi T, Giordano D, Vanpatten S, et al. Tobacco smoke is a source of toxic reactive glycation products. Proc Natl Acad Sci U S A. 1997;94:13915–20.
17. Uribarri J, Cai W, Peppa M, Goodman S, Ferrucci L, Striker G, et al. Circulating glycotoxins and dietary advanced glycation endproducts: two links to inflammatory response, oxidative stress, and aging. J Gerontol A Biol Sci Med Sci. 2007;62:427–33.
18. Goldberg T, Cai W, Peppa M, Dardaine V, Baliga BS, Uribarri J, et al. Advanced glycoxidation end products in commonly consumed foods. J Am Diet Assoc. 2004;104:1287–91.
19. Leslie RD, Beyan H, Sawtell P, Boehm BO, Spector TD, Snieder H. Level of an advanced glycated end product is genetically determined: a study of normal twins. Diabetes. 2003;52:2441–4.
20. Xue M, Rabbani N, Thornalley PJ. Glyoxalase in ageing. Semin Cell Dev Biol. 2011;22:293–301.
21. Van Schaftingen E, Collard F, Wiame E, Veiga-da-Cunha M. Enzymatic repair of Amadori products. Amino Acids. 2012;42:1143–50.
22. Grimm S, Horlacher M, Catalgol B, et al. Cathepsins D and L reduce the toxicity of advanced glycation end products. Free Radic Biol Med. 2012;52:1011–23. doi:10.1016/j.freeradbiomed.2011.12.021.
23. Bierhaus A, Humpert PM, Morcos M, Wendt T, Chavakis T, Arnold B, et al. Understanding RAGE, the receptor for advanced glycation end products. J Mol Med (Berl). 2005;83:876–86.
24. Ramasamy R, Vannucci SJ, Yan SS, Herold K, Yan SF, Schmidt AM. Advanced glycation end products and RAGE: a common thread in aging, diabetes, neurodegeneration, and inflammation. Glycobiology. 2005;15:16R–28.
25. Vazzana N, Santilli F, Cuccurullo C, et al. Soluble forms of RAGE in internal medicine. Intern Emerg Med. 2009;4:389–401. doi:10.1007/s11739-009-0300-1.
26. Lu C, He JC, Cai W, Liu H, Zhu L, Vlassara H. Advanced glycation endproduct (AGE) receptor 1 is a negative regulator of the inflammatory response to AGE in mesangial cells. Proc Natl Acad Sci U S A. 2004;101:11767–72.
27. Lohwasser C, Neureiter D, Weigle B, Kirchner T, Schuppanm D. The receptor for advanced glycation end products is highly expressed in the skin and upregulated by advanced glycation end products and tumor necrosis factor-alpha. J Invest Dermatol. 2006;126:291–9.
28. Meerwaldt R, Links T, Graaff R, Thorpe SR, Baynes JW, Hartog J, et al. Simple noninvasive measurement of skin autofluorescence. Ann N Y Acad Sci. 2005;1043:290–8.
29. Corstjens HM, Dicanio D, Muizzuddin N, Neven A, Sparacio R, Declercq L, et al. Glycation associated skin autofluorescence and skin elasticity are related to chronological age and body mass index of healthy subjects. Exp Gerontol. 2008;43:663–7.
30. Dunn JA, McCance DR, Thorpe SR, Lyons TJ, Baynes JW. Age-dependent accumulation of N epsilon-(carboxymethyl)lysine and N epsilon-(carboxymethyl)hydroxylysine in human skin collagen. Biochemistry. 1991;30:1205–10.
31. Pageon H. Reaction of glycation and human skin: the effects on the skin and its components, reconstructed skin as a model. Pathol Biol (Paris). 2010;58:226–31.
32. Smit AJ, Gerrits EG. Skin autofluorescence as a measure of advanced glycation endproduct deposition: a novel risk marker in chronic kidney disease. Curr Opin Nephrol Hypertens. 2010;19:527–33.
33. Avery NC, Bailey AJ. The effects of the Maillard reaction on the physical properties and cell interactions of collagen. Pathol Biol (Paris). 2006;54:387–95.

34. Haitoglou CS, Tsilibary EC, Brownlee M, Charonis AS. Altered cellular interactions between endothelial cells and nonenzymatically glucosylated laminin/type IV collagen. J Biol Chem. 1992;267:12404–7.
35. Haucke E, Navarrete-Santos A, Simm A, et al. Glycation of extracellular matrix proteins impairs migration of immune cells. Wound Repair Regen. 2014;22:239–45. doi:10.1111/wrr.12144.
36. Yoshinaga E, Kawada A, Ono K, Fujimoto E, Wachi H, Harumiya S, et al. N(ϵ)-(carboxymethyl)lysine modification of elastin alters its biological properties: implications for the accumulation of abnormal elastic fibers in actinic elastosis. J Invest Dermatol. 2012;132:315–23.
37. Jacobsen JN, Steffensen B, Häkkinen L, et al. Skin wound healing in diabetic β6 integrin-deficient mice. APMIS. 2010;118:753–64. doi:10.1111/j.1600-0463.2010.02654.x.
38. Reihsner R, Melling M, Pfeiler W, Menzel EJ. Alterations of biochemical and two-dimensional biomechanical properties of human skin in diabetes mellitus as compared to effects of in vitro non-enzymatic glycation. Clin Biomech. 2000;15:379–86.
39. Yoon HS, Baik SH, Oh CH. Quantitative measurement of desquamation and skin elasticity in diabetic patients. Skin Res Technol. 2002;8:250–4.
40. Uchiki T, Weikel KA, Jiao W, Shang F, Caceres A, Pawlak D, et al. Glycation-altered proteolysis as a pathobiologic mechanism that links dietary glycemic index, aging, and age-related disease (in non diabetics). Aging Cell. 2012;11:1–13.
41. Ukeda H, Hasegawa Y, Ishi T, Sawamiura M. Inactivation of Cu, Zn-superoxide dismutase by intermediates of Maillard reaction and glycolytic pathway and some sugars. Biosci Biotechnol Biochem. 1997;61:2039–42.
42. Baynes JW. The Maillard hypothesis on aging: time to focus on DNA. Ann N Y Acad Sci. 2002;959:360–7.
43. Giardino I, Edelstein D, Brownlee M. Nonenzymatic glycosylation in vitro and in bovine endothelial cells alters basic fibroblast growth factor activity. A model for intracellular glycosylation in diabetes. J Clin Invest. 1994;94:110–7.
44. Portero-Otín M, Pamplona R, Bellmunt MJ, Ruiz MC, Prat J, Salvayre R, et al. Advanced glycation end product precursors impair epidermal growth factor receptor signaling. Diabetes. 2002;51:1535–42.
45. Zhu P, Yang C, Chen LH, Ren M, Lao GJ, Yan L. Impairment of human keratinocyte mobility and proliferation by advanced glycation end products-modified BSA. Arch Dermatol Res. 2011;303:339–50.
46. Berge U, Behrens J, Rattan SI. Sugar-induced premature aging and altered differentiation in human epidermal keratinocytes. Ann N Y Acad Sci. 2007;1100:524–9.
47. Wondrak GT, Roberts MJ, Jacobson MK, Jacobson EL. Photosensitized growth inhibition of cultured human skin cells: mechanism and suppression of oxidative stress from solar irradiation of glycated proteins. J Invest Dermatol. 2002;119:489–98.
48. Zhu P, Ren M, Yang C, Hu YX, Ran JM, Yan L. Involvement of RAGE, MAPK and NF-κB pathways in AGEs-induced MMP-9 activation in HaCaT keratinocytes. Exp Dermatol. 2012;21:123–9.
49. Alikhani Z, Alikhani M, Boyd CM, Nagao K, Trackman PC, Graves DT. Advanced glycation end products enhance expression of pro-apoptotic genes and stimulate fibroblast apoptosis through cytoplasmic and mitochondrial pathways. J Biol Chem. 2005;280:12087–95.
50. Molinari J, Ruszova E, Velebny V, Robert L. Effect of advanced glycation endproducts on gene expression profiles of human dermal fibroblasts. Biogerontology. 2008;9:177–82.
51. Sejersen H, Rattan SI. Dicarbonyl-induced accelerated aging in vitro in human skin fibroblasts. Biogerontology. 2009;10:203–11.
52. Schmidt AM, Hori O, Chen J, Li JF, Crandall J, Zhang J, et al. Advanced glycation endproducts interacting with their endothelial receptor induce expression of vascular cell adhesion molecule-1 (VCAM-1): a potential mechanism for the accelerated vasculopathy of diabetes. J Clin Invest. 1995;96:1395–403.
53. Lan CC, Wu CS, Huang SM, et al. High-glucose environment reduces human β-defensin-2 expression in human keratinocytes: implications for poor diabetic wound healing. Br J Dermatol. 2012;166:1221–9. doi:10.1111/j.1365-2133.2012.10847.x.
54. Iotzova-Weiss G, Dziunycz PJ, Freiberger SN, et al. S100A8/A9 stimulates keratinocyte proliferation in the development of squamous cell carcinoma of the skin via the receptor for advanced glycation-end products. PLoS One. 2015;10, e0120971. doi:10.1371/journal.pone.0120971.
55. Masaki H, Okano Y, Sakurai H. Generation of active oxygen species from advanced glycation end-products (AGE) under ultraviolet light A (UVA) irradiation. Biochem Biophys Res Commun. 1997;235:306–10.
56. San Martin A, Foncea R, Laurindo FR, Ebensperger R, Griendling KK, Leighton F. Nox1-based NADPH oxidase-derived superoxide is required for VSMC activation by advanced glycation end-products. Free Radic Biol Med. 2007;42(11):1671–9. Epub 2007 Feb 12.
57. Zhang M, Kho AL, Anilkumar N, Chibber R, Pagano PJ, Shah AM, Cave AC. Glycated proteins stimulate reactive oxygen species production in cardiac myocytes: involvement of Nox2 (gp91phox)-containing NADPH oxidase. Circulation. 2006;113(9):1235–43. Epub 2006 Feb 27.
58. Loughlin DT, Artlett CM. Precursor of advanced glycation end products mediates ER-stress-induced caspase-3 activation of human dermal fibroblasts through NAD(P)H oxidase 4. PLoS One. 2010;5(6), e11093. doi:10.1371/journal.pone.0011093.

59. Omori K, Ohira T, Uchida Y, Ayilavarapu S, Batista Jr EL, Yagi M, et al. Priming of neutrophil oxidative burst in diabetes requires preassembly of the NADPH oxidase. J Leukoc Biol. 2008;84(1):292–301. doi:10.1189/jlb.1207832. Epub 2008 Apr 7.
60. Yim MB, Yim HS, Lee C, Kang SO, Chock PB. Protein glycation: creation of catalytic sites for free radical generation. Ann N Y Acad Sci. 2001;928:48–53.
61. Elosta A, Ghous T, Ahmed N. Natural products as antiglycation agents: possible therapeutic potential for diabetic complications. Curr Diabetes Rev. 2012;8:92–108.
62. Reddy VP, Beyaz A. Inhibitors of the Maillard reaction and AGE breakers as therapeutics for multiple diseases. Drug Discov Today. 2006;11:646–54.
63. Cadau S, Leoty-Okombi S, Pain S, et al. In vitro glycation of an endothelialized and innervated tissue-engineered skin to screen anti-AGE molecules. Biomaterials. 2015;51:216–25. doi:10.1016/j.biomaterials.2015.01.066.
64. Degenhardt TP, Alderson NL, Arrington DD, Beattie RJ, Basgen JM, Steffes MW, et al. Pyridoxamine inhibits early renal disease and dyslipidemia in the streptozotocin-diabetic rat. Kidney Int. 2002;61:939–50.
65. Vasan S, Foiles P, Founds H. Therapeutic potential of breakers of advanced glycation end product-protein crosslinks. Arch Biochem Biophys. 2003;419:89–96.
66. Xue M, Rabbani N, Momiji H, Imbasi P, Anwar MM, Kitteringham N, et al. Transcriptional control of glyoxalase 1 by Nrf2 provides a stress-responsive defence against dicarbonyl glycation. Biochem J. 2012;443:213–22.
67. Dearlove RP, Greenspan P, Hartle DK, Swanson RB, Hargrove JL. Inhibition of protein glycation by extracts of culinary herbs and spices. J Med Food. 2008;11:275–81.
68. Wu CH, Yen GC. Inhibitory effect of naturally occurring flavonoids on the formation of advanced glycation endproducts. J Agric Food Chem. 2005;53:3167–73.
69. Draelos ZD, Yatskayer M, Raab S, Oresajo C. An evaluation of the effect of a topical product containing C-xyloside and blueberry extract on the appearance of type II diabetic skin. J Cosmet Dermatol. 2009;8:147–51.
70. Ohno R, Moroishi N, Sugawa H, et al. Mangosteen pericarp extract inhibits the formation of pentosidine and ameliorates skin elasticity. J Clin Biochem Nutr. 2015;57:27–32. doi:10.3164/jcbn.15-13.
71. Yamagishi S, Ueda S, Okuda S. Food-derived advanced glycation end products (AGEs): a novel therapeutic target for various disorders. Curr Pharm Des. 2007;13:2832–6.
72. Peppa M, Brem H, Ehrlich P, Zhang JG, Cai W, Li Z, et al. Adverse effects of glycotoxins on wound healing in genetically diabetic mice. Diabetes. 2003;52:2805–13.
73. Monnier VM, Bautista O, Kenny D, Sell DR, Fogarty J, Dahms W, et al. Skin collagen glycation, glycoxidation, and crosslinking are lower in subjects with long-term intensive versus conventional therapy of type 1 diabetes: relevance of glycated collagen products versus HbA1c as markers of diabetic complications. DCCT Skin Collagen Ancillary Study Group. Diabetes Control and Complications Trial. Diabetes. 1999;48:870–80.
74. Hudson BI, Bucciarelli LG, Wendt T, Sakaguchi T, Lalla E, Qu W, et al. Blockade of receptor for advanced glycation endproducts: a new target for therapeutic intervention in diabetic complications and inflammatory disorders. Arch Biochem Biophys. 2003;419:80–8.
75. Goova MT, Li J, Kislinger T, Qu W, Lu Y, Bucciarelli LG, et al. Blockade of receptor for advanced glycation end-products restores effective wound healing in diabetic mice. Am J Pathol. 2001;159:513–25.
76. Babizhayev MA, Nikolayev GM, Nikolayeva JG, Yegorov YE. Biologic activities of molecular chaperones and pharmacologic chaperone imidazole-containing dipeptide-based compounds: natural skin care help and the ultimate challenge. Implication for adaptive responses in the skin. Am J Ther. 2012;19:69–89.

Part XI

Aging Perception

Facial Skin Attributes and Age Perception

125

Alex Nkengne, Georgios N. Stamatas, and Christiane Bertin

Contents

A. Nkengne (✉)
Clarins Laboratories, Pontoise, France
e-mail: alex.nkengne@clarins.com

G.N. Stamatas • C. Bertin
SkinCare R&D, Johnson & Johnson Santé Beauté France, Issy-les-Moulineaux, France
e-mail: gstamata@its.jnj.com; cbertin@its.jnj.com

M.A. Farage et al. (eds.), *Textbook of Aging Skin*,
DOI 10.1007/978-3-662-47398-6_91

Abstract
The quest for a youthful appearance has been a major segment of cosmetics and surgical procedures over the last decades. The age perception appears as a driver of social interactions, and it is therefore important to understand the link between physiological changes affecting the face with age and their impact on the way one is perceived. Several studies, ranging from psychological-based approaches to statistical ones, have tried to determine the facial cues that are mainly affecting the age perception. Taken as a whole, the results of these studies suggest that the perception of aging is highly influenced by the appearance of the lip area (volume and upper lip wrinkles) and the eye area (crow's feet and under-eye wrinkles, dark circles, bags under the eyes) and the skin tone uniformity (brown spots, skin color uniformity).

Introduction

The age of a person is an important factor of social interactions. The way one acts, the verbal and body language one chooses to address someone else, depends on age. Therefore, people since childhood develop a capacity to estimate age based on physical attributes. These attributes can be related to dress code or body gesture, but they are primarily linked to facial appearance. It is obvious that anyone can distinguish the face of a baby from a young adult and from a senior one since some evident characteristics such as the size of the head and the number of wrinkles are affected dramatically by age.

As people get older the entire body is altered by chronological and environmental aging factors, with facial appearance often showing the most pronounced changes due to increased exposure to the outside environment. Chronological aging or intrinsic aging refers to the ongoing natural physiological changes in tissues. Environmental factors, such as sun exposure or life-related stress, affect the apparent or perceived age of an individual by modifying the aspect and the properties of his/her skin. In the case of excessive sun exposure, photoaging can lead to an increased gap between chronological and apparent age.

Consequently, facial appearance of a person does not always reflect his/her chronological age. Some people look younger or older than their real age, depending on several factors including genetic disposition, sun exposure, smoking habits, lifestyle choices, and mood. Some events in life like the death of a loved one or a long-lasting disease can accelerate the process of apparent aging. Makeup, antiaging creams, exercise, diet, and surgery are a few of the methods people use to reduce their apparent age.

In fact, the perceived idea of a person's age is a subjective judgment that is influenced by the skin aspect. To better understand the factors affecting a person's apparent age, the following questions need to be addressed:

- Since apparent age is subjectively perceived by observers, is there a consensus on the apparent age that would be given to an individual? If not, will the observer be influenced by their own experience?
- What are the main facial skin attributes that drive age perception?

Many studies have described the changes in facial attributes (skin color, wrinkles, sagging, microrelief, etc.) with age, but few have analyzed their influence on the perceived age. The objectives of this chapter are to analyze the contribution of individual skin attributes of the face on the perceived age and to assess the influence of age and gender of observers with regard to the age perception. Firstly, the different biases that affect the estimation of age are presented. Secondly, how the facial skin attributes have an effect on the perception of age has been evaluated.

What Is Perceived Age?

The human capacity to estimate age has probably been developed through the evolutionary process since age is a key point for social interaction.

It is generally claimed that "Humans can easily categorize a person's age group and are often precise in this estimation" [1]. However, it can also be noticed that some people are easier to categorize than others. In fact, there is no strict consensus among observers when guessing someone else's age. Thus, the factors of variability need to be explored that lead to the differences among observers and to build a consensus on how the "perceived age" will be defined.

Accuracy in Age Perception

An experiment was conducted, asking 48 "graders" (20 men and 28 women, from 20 to 64 years of age) recruited from a Caucasian population living in Paris and its suburbs to assess the age of 173 female subjects based on their "en face" facial images [2]. The age of these women was uniformly distributed between 20 and 74 years. Photographs were randomly presented to the graders on a computer screen. They were requested to estimate the subject's age using a computer interface that featured a slider bar spanning from 0 to 100 for age estimation. There was no time limit for the grading.

For 77.6 % of the subjects, the given age follows a normal distribution (Jarque-Bera test of normality; significance = 95 %) with no outlier. Therefore for each subject, the apparent age could be defined as the mean value from the age given by all graders. Figure 1 displays the correlation between perceived age and real age. They

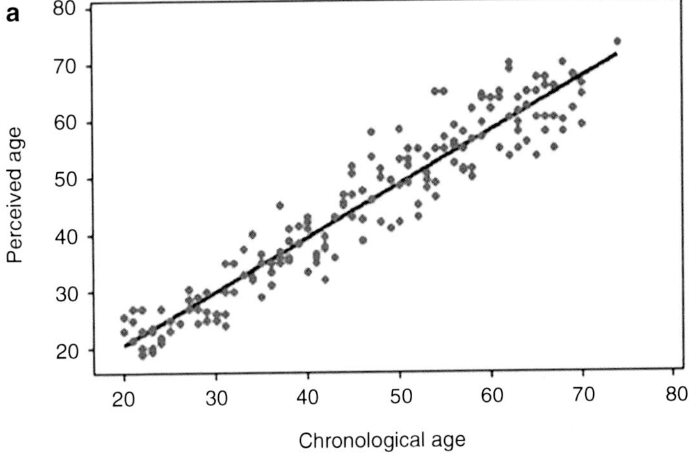

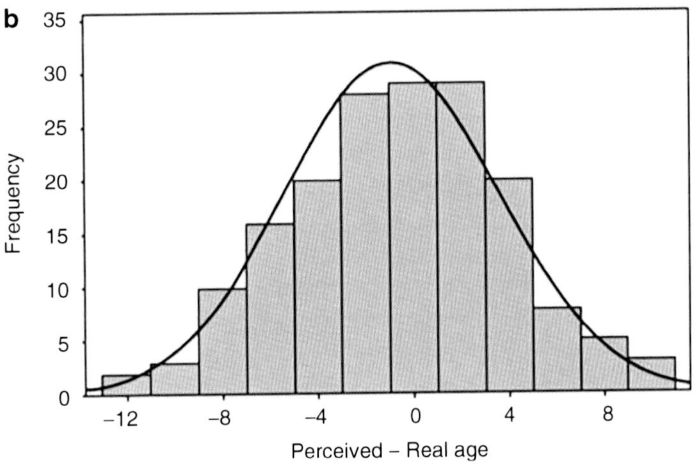

Fig. 1 Mean age versus perceived age

are highly correlated ($R = 0.95, p < 0.001$), and the residual follows a Gaussian distribution with a mean of 0.9 years and a standard deviation of 4.49 years. Even if the difference between real age and perceived one is not high (0.9), a pair-wise t-test shows that the perceived age is significantly lower than the real age ($p < 0.01$). This would mean that overall, the women of the dataset were perceived as 1 year younger than they are in reality.

Biases Affecting the Perception

The ability to recognize and therefore to classify faces has been demonstrated to be plagued by several "own-group" biases. People are generally better at recognizing, remembering, and classifying individuals belonging to their own group. The own-group bias effect has been found for such characteristics as age, race, and gender; but the reasons underlying these biases are not clear yet [3]. One possible explanation is that people tend to interact more with others in their own racial, age, and gender group and thus are more trained (and efficient) with these categories of faces.

Own-Race Bias

The visible signs of facial aging do not occur at the same trends for the different ethnicities. Consequently, the perception of age is both influenced by the observers and the subjects' ethnicity. The own-race bias is known as the capacity for people to better recognize faces from their own race [4]. A meta-analysis [5] involving 35 articles with around 5,000 participants clearly highlights this bias, which is now taken into account for testimonies in New Jersey Courts. In fact it seems that face recognition, in general, and age estimation, in particular, involves learning processes through which people are trained by their environment.

Dehon et al. [4] specifically studied the own-race bias in age estimation. They asked Caucasian and African participants to estimate the age of Caucasians and Africans from their facial pictures. Caucasian participants were better at estimating Caucasian faces than Africans'. However, Africans had the same performance for the two groups. Since the study was run in Belgium, the authors suggest that Africans had been trained during their daily life to recognize and to classify Caucasian faces. This hypothesis is in line with Wright et al. [6] who stated that the ability to recognize other-group faces depends on the degree of exposure and contact with people from these groups.

Porcheron et al. [7] asked a group of Chinese women to rate the age and attractiveness of manipulated pictures of Chinese and Caucasian women over 60 years of age. The picture modifications included reduction of wrinkles, dark spots, dark circles, and sagging. The reduction of dark spots was considered as the most important change whatever the population, while the reduction of wrinkles had a more important impact on the age estimation of Caucasian women.

Own-Gender Bias

Rehnman [3] has recently published a state-of-the-art review about the own-gender bias in face recognition. He concluded that women have greater accuracy in face recognition and could more easily recognize female faces than men. On the contrary, men did not show any difference in recognizing women's or men's faces.

Looking at gender bias in age prediction, it has also been demonstrated that women and men do not estimate age the same way [6]. A hypothesis to explain these differences is that, depending on one's age or gender, different facial attributes are focused on when estimating someone's age.

In evaluating the own-gender bias from the experiment mentioned above, the population of imaged volunteers included only females, while the graders were males ($N = 20$) and females ($N = 28$). If an own-gender bias existed, the female graders should be more accurate in age prediction than men. To test this hypothesis, the perceived age given by women and men was compared: the perceived age given by women versus the real age and the perceived age given by men versus the real age using a pair-wise t-test. The mean perceived age within male graders (mean = 44.93) was significantly different from real age

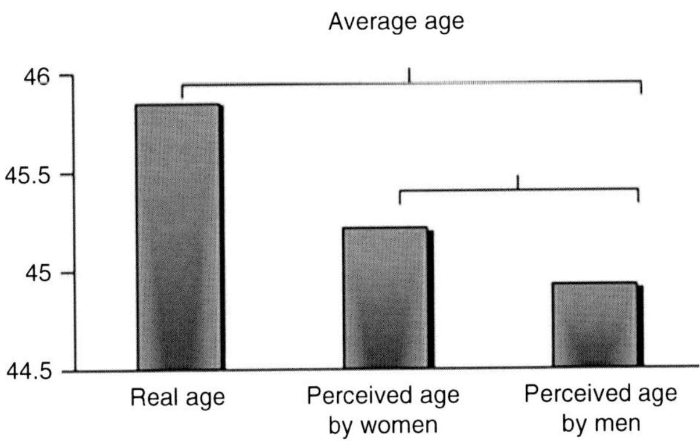

Fig. 2 Women are more accurate than men when predicting women's age. *The mean perceived age within male graders (mean = 44.93) is significantly different from the real age (mean = 45.85, p < 0.01) and from perceived age within female graders (mean = 45.21, p < 0.05).* (**a**) Correlation curve between real age and perceived age. (**b**) Histogram of the differences between real age and perceived age (residual)

(mean = 45.85, $p < 0.010$) and from perceived age within female graders (mean = 45.21, $p < 0.05$). The difference between perceived age by female graders and real age was not significant ($p = 0.06$). Male graders perceived that the imaged subjects look younger than they really were, and female graders were more accurate in age prediction than male graders (Fig. 2).

Own-Age Bias

Own-age bias has been documented by several authors [8–12], with most of them evaluating the confidence that could be given to eyewitness testimony. A literature review by Anastasi and Rhodes [11] showed mixed and inconclusive results for own-age bias.

The underlying assumption in own-age bias is that people are judging another person's age relative to themselves and should therefore be more accurate in judging their age range. An own-age bias has been reported by George and Hole [9]. They asked two groups (25 young adults and 25 old adults) to assess the age of faces aged between 5 and 70 years. In addition, the volunteers were asked to judge three images per age group. It appears that young people overestimate the age of older people, older people overestimate the age of younger people, and finally people are more accurate when estimating age within their own age group. Based on these results, Sörqvist tried to evaluate the own-age bias and improved age estimation accuracy by training. They asked two groups of people, young (15–24 years) and middle age (34–46 years), to evaluate 78 facial images from people in the three groups of age (young, middle age, old). They found that young participants were better with their age groups than with older people, but the middle age group was not significantly better when judging people from their group of age. Thus, the own-age bias hypothesis was not totally confirmed.

In exploring own-age bias using the experiment described earlier, the populations of graders and evaluated subjects were divided into three groups: young (under 35 years), middle age (35–50 years), and senior (over 50 years). This segmentation is relevant to what is reported in the literature.

Table 1 shows the mean absolute error and the standard deviation for each age group of subjects and graders. The highest error and standard deviation are observed for the senior group of subjects. The youngest group of graders (less than 35 years) has smaller errors with a narrow distribution, being more accurate and having a better agreement than the other age groups. The smallest error and standard deviation are obtained when young graders judge young subjects. Thus, the results confirmed, in part, the own-age bias.

The means and standard deviations are calculated from the absolute values of the differences

Table 1 Means and standard deviations of absolute values of errors in age prediction

Subjects' age				
Graders' age		Under 35	35–50	Over 50
	Under 35	4.55 (3.50)	5.98 (4.82)	6.21 (4.78)
	35–50	4.98 (3.78)	6.43 (4.71)	7.52 (5.75)
	Over 50	5.40 (4.70)	6.65 (5.02)	6.42 (4.92)
	All graders	5.01 (4.06)	6.57 (4.95)	6.78 (5.33)

between real age and perceived age. Each cell corresponds to the mean and standard deviation of the errors from all the graders of an age group on subjects of an age group.

Facial Skin Attributes Influencing Age Perception

The estimation of age is not only based on facial attributes but also on hair, voice, body movement, and posture [13]. When looking at a face to predict someone's age, a 3D stimulus is being processed. This stimulus includes information related to shape, texture, and color [14]. The aging process affects the following groups of attributes:

- Changes in shape: They occur in the spatial dimensions with a centimetric range. They may be caused by the growth of bones or loss of bones due to osteoporosis, changes in muscle and fat distributions, and skin sagging caused by the loss of elasticity and gravity.
- Changes in texture: They happen in the spatial dimensions at a millimetric range. They are linked with skin aging and can affect wrinkles, pores, and microrelief.
- Changes in color: They are also linked with skin aging. They involve a more yellowish tone and color unevenness with the appearance of brown spots, freckles, and scars.
- Changes in contrast: The main facial contrasts correspond to the morphological or color difference between the facial features (lips, eyes, eyebrows, nose, etc.) and the surrounding skin. Facial contrasts are affected by changes in the facial shape, texture, and color.

Consequently, skin transformation will have an important influence in the perceived age.

Two kinds of approaches have been used to understand the influence of facial attributes on perceived age. Mono-dimensional approaches focus on a specific group of attributes such as wrinkles or color and evaluate its impact on global perception. Multidimensional methods have recently been proposed. They employ a multidimensional statistical model to depict the relative importance of each facial attribute (including shape, texture, and color attributes) in the overall perception.

Mono-Dimensional Approaches

The principle of mono-dimensional approaches is to present stimuli of faces on which one specific attribute has been enhanced or reduced by image processing manipulations. These manipulations may include stretching the images to simulate the growth of bones, blurring to remove wrinkles, applying a round mask to remove information about jawline drawing, or changing the pigmentation of the skin. Using image processing manipulations, one can separately investigate the influence of the shape, the texture, and the color of the face/skin on the perceived age.

Influence of Shape

One way to explore the impact of shape transformations is to distort the facial images to mimic the cranium growth. However, the effect of the cranium on age perception only enables to distinguish children from adults [15].

The second way to study the impact of shape information on perception is to present inverted faces to observers (the mouth on the top and the eyes down). These kinds of stimuli enable to capture the importance of spatial interrelationship of facial features, such as the relative position of the nose, eyes, and mouth. One can also use negative pictures, with inverted bright and dark areas. These stimuli distort 3D perception of volumes, making the faces look flatter. George and Hole [15] have presented original, inverted, negative, and negative-inverted images of 27 faces from people aged between 0 and 80 years to 80 observers aged between 18 and 40 years. They found that negation and inversion do not affect the estimation of age, while their combination does it for subjects under 50. Negative and inverted images were considerably overestimated, with a poor agreement among the graders. George and Hole (the role of spatial cues) suggested that observers were able to pick up the spatial cues left by the inversion or the negation. The combination of these two transformations disrupted too many cues, making it hard to guess the real age.

Probably, none has explicitly focused on the influence of the sagging of the face (jawline and chin). The stimuli of faces [9] with the shape altered by a rounded mask, meaning without jawline information, have also been presented. They notice that the spatial configuration of facial features, the color, and the textural information were used successfully in that case.

Influence of Texture

Textural information is related to the skin wrinkling aspect. Wrinkles are generally considered as the most visible signs of facial aging. Their importance on the perception of age was confirmed by several authors [9, 15–17].

Burt and Perrett [16] presented 28 blended faces and 40 normal faces as stimuli to 40 observers (20 young persons and 20 older persons, half male and female). The blended faces did not capture textural information. They found that blended faces were rated younger than they were and the error increased with the age. This experiment suggested that textural information is important for the perception of age.

George and Scaife [15] focused on children's ability to predict age on unfamiliar faces. They presented four different versions of facial photographs to 134 children between 4 and 6 years old. The photographs were taken from volunteers ranging in age from 1 to 80 years. The different versions of the face presented were original image, internal facial features only (eyes-nose-mouth), skin blur only, and overall blur (skin + features). Performances with the four sets of images were comparable, meaning that no conclusion could be drawn about the relative contribution of each facial feature. George concluded that the facial information related to the facial features and the skin texture were alternatively used for age prediction. However, his blur image also contained color information, meaning that one cannot really conclude on the importance of the texture only.

Influence of Color

Skin color is affected by chronological aging and photoaging, resulting in some changes in its hue, brightness, and homogeneity.

The impact of color changes has been explored by Burt and Perrett [16]. They captured 147 Caucasian male faces, from volunteers aged between 20 and 62 years. They defined an algorithm to modify the shape or the color of the face to simulate the aging process. This algorithm caricatures differences between older faces and younger ones. Their methods modified the red, blue, and green intensity distribution of the images, thus encompassing hue, saturation, and lightness. The pictures were then presented to 40 observers for age estimation, and the impact of color and shape transformation was analyzed. Burt and Perrett found that each transformation increased the age significantly; their combination was even more effective.

Fink et al. [18] studied the influence of the color homogeneity on the perceived age. They collected front and side pictures from 169 Caucasian women aged between 11 and 79 years of age. Facial features (mouth, eyes) and textural details such as wrinkles were removed to only keep information related to the skin color, leading to 2D skin color maps. The 2D skin color maps were then applied on a 3D standardized model of face. As a result, they obtained similar faces in terms of shape and texture, the only difference being the color hue and homogeneity. Four hundred and thirty observers were asked to give an age to the generated facial stimuli. The perceived age spanned from 17.8 to 36.7 years and was correlated with the chronological age ($r = 0.708$, $p < 0.01$). Fink et al. consequently concluded that the perceived age is influenced by the skin color distribution.

Influence of Contrast

The main facial contrast is the result of horizontal lines such as the eyebrows, the eyes, and the lips. With aging, the lips tend to become thinner, and the eyebrows disappeared, while the upper eyelids slope down and the bags become more visible. Porcheron et al. [19] mainly studied the evolution of eyebrow, eye, and lip contrast with age and their impact on the perception. Contrast was defined as the luminance and color difference (in L*a*b*) between the given facial feature and the surrounding skin. They found that the contrast between the features and the skin decreases with age. They also demonstrated that increasing facial contrasts would reduce perceived age.

Multidimensional Approaches

Few attempts have been made to comparatively assess the facial signs of aging and to rank them according to their influence on age perception [2, 7, 13, 20].

The multidimensional approaches have been proposed to study the influence of a large number of facial attributes on the perceived age. They differ from the mono-dimensional approaches because the facial stimuli are not altered as in that method.

In general, facial images are presented to observers who are asked to grade for age. Then, an assessment is done to link the visual age to the facial characteristics of each face. This step can be done by describing the facial attributes qualitatively (open questionnaire) or quantitatively (clinical grading).

Qualitative Analysis

Rexbye and Povlsen [13] asked 40 graders to evaluate the age of 74 subjects older than 70 years old from their facial photographs. Then the graders were interviewed to report the main features that have driven their perception.

Rexbye and Povlsen found that age was assessed stepwise. First, the given picture would be classified over or under 80. After that, age would be refined first by decades, then by 5 years, and finally by single year. Almost all informants used information related to biological attributes. The main biological markers were eyes and skin. In the eye area, the graders would have focused on wrinkles, bags under the eyes, sunken and "watery" eyes, and finally the vitality of the gaze. Concerning the skin, the graders would have focused on wrinkles on the face and the neck and second on pigmentation, color, and sagging.

Finally, the authors suggested that age estimation is more difficult on subjects with contradictory signs of aging such as a healthy skin but with an old-fashioned hairstyle. However, their method does not allow precisely evaluation of the weight of each attribute to the overall perception.

Quantitative Analysis

A statistical approach was proposed [2] to link the facial attributes and the perceived age. This approach enables to compare the influence of the different attributes and to rank them using a linear regression model.

Regression methods can be used to study the dependence of the perceived age on several facial attributes. When the attributes are highly correlated, partial least squares (PLS) regression is the appropriate tool to understand the role of each attribute in the regression [21]. This regression model handles both highly correlated variables (facial attributes) and relatively small sample size [22] (173 subjects). The more important is an attribute, the highest is its weight in the model [23].

A trained grader was asked to evaluate 20 facial skin attributes from the 173 women whose pictures were taken (section "Accuracy in Age Perception"). The attributes related to the shape of the face were evaluated (nasolabial fold, jawline, lip volume, bags under the eyes, eye opening, sloping upper eyelid), as well as its color (overall color, brown spots, border lip definition, dark circles under the eyes, color uniformity) and its texture (wrinkles: crow's feet [wrinkles and fine lines], frown line, upper lip, cheek, forehead, under the eyes, microtexture).

Seven PLS models were built to predict age from these facial attributes. The first two models allowed to predict the chronological and the perceived age. The three other models were used to predict the perceived age as given by the three groups of graders: young, middle age, and seniors. The last two models were built to predict perceived age as estimated by men only and by women only.

The weight of the facial attributes for each model was expressed as a percentage (the sum of the weight being set to 1), making it possible to compare the relative contribution of each attribute for different models.

Perceived Versus Chronological Age

The model built when predicting the chronological age and the one built for the perceived age were put side by side. Some statistically significant differences were detected with a certain number of attributes (Fig. 3). "Eye opening" and

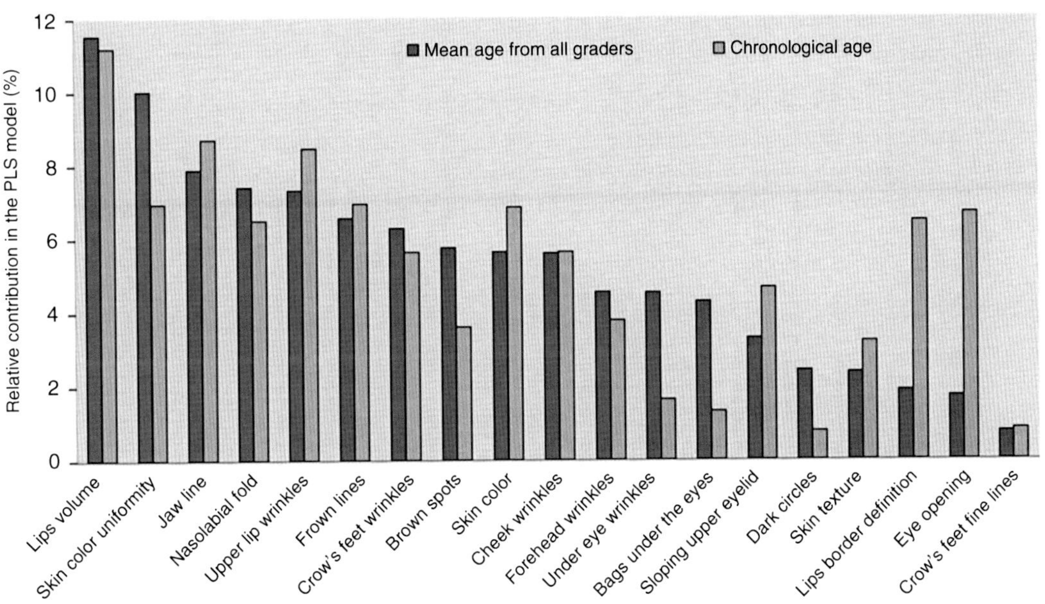

Fig. 3 Comparison between PLS models of real age and perceived age. Each bar chart represents the relative contribution of the facial attributes while building the PLS model for age prediction. The higher is the value, the more important is the attribute for the given model. The attributes are ranked from the most important to the least important for chronological age. The parameters of which the contribution differs the most between the two models are skin color uniformity (p = 1.14E-59), lip border definition (p = 6.46E-69), under-eye wrinkles (p = 7.43E-68), eye opening, and bags under the eyes (p = 2.12E-42)

"lip border definition" play an important role for chronological age, while "under-eye wrinkles," "dark circles," "bags under the eyes," "skin color uniformity," and "brown spots" play a more significant role on the perceived age. These results suggest that the eye area and the skin color uniformity are overused when looking at a face for age assessment.

Influence of Age and Gender

The models of the three age groups also presented some differences as shown in Fig. 4. Particularly, the oldest group overused the attributes "eye opening," "lip border definition," and "lip volume." In contrast, they disregarded the attributes "nasolabial fold," "dark circles," and "brown spots."

The comparison between the PLS models of perceived ages by men and women did not show any statistical significant difference. The study did not highlight any difference in terms of interpretation of attributes between men and women.

Conclusion

In this chapter, the influence of different facial attributes on the perceived age has been discussed. The studies reviewed and the results presented are mainly focusing on the Caucasian population. All the studies reported were done on facial pictures which are static stimuli. In reality, faces are dynamic and expressions and emotions may also contribute to the perceived age. In addition, people also use hair, clothes, and body posture information when available [13]. While focusing on skin facial attributes, an attempt has been made to list all types of clinical changes with age and to review their incidence on age perception. The attributes were divided into three categories (shape, texture, color) for easier understanding. Two different methodologies were also described.

The mono-dimensional approach enables to focus on a specific attribute and to evaluate its influence. The related works give interesting insights about the importance of the attributes. However, the method has two main drawbacks. First, this is in agreement with George et al. [15] who concluded that facial attributes are always

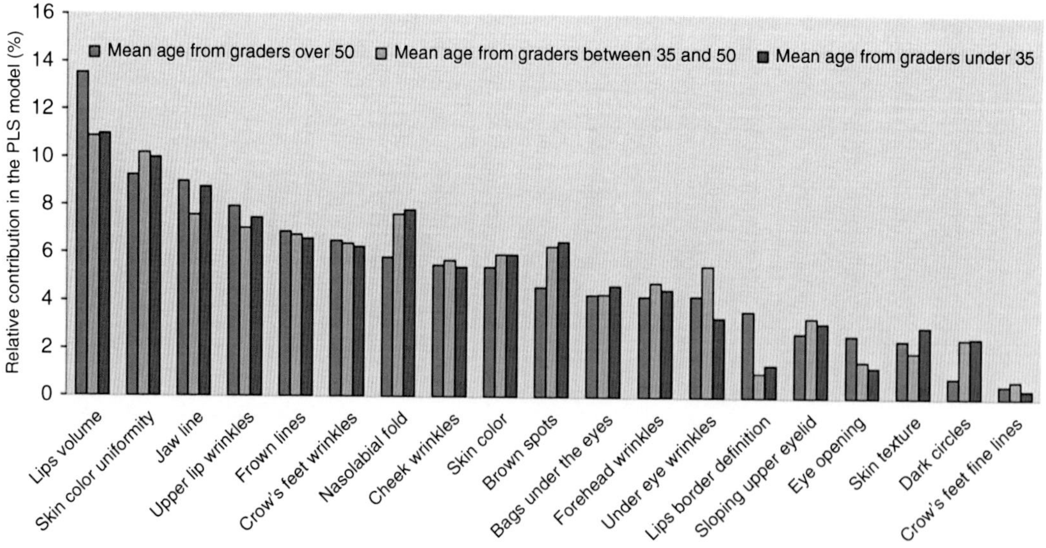

Fig. 4 Comparison between PLS models of perceived ages for different age groups of graders. Each bar chart represents the relative contribution (in %) of the facial attributes while building the PLS model for age prediction. The higher is the value, the more important is the attribute for a given model. Attributes are ranked from the most important to the least important to predict perceived age by the youngest group of graders

used in combination. Therefore, a missing attribute from a modified stimulus may be replaced by another when guessing the age. For subjects with contradictory signs of aging [13], the results may be meaningless. Second, a facial stimulus which has been modified is no more a face and thus does not correspond to the regular experience of observers.

The multidimensional approach uses facial pictures, which have not been transformed to avoid the bias. Multiple regression models enable to rank the facial attributes according to their weight in the perception.

It is found that the importance of the nasolabial fold, dark circles, bags under the eyes, skin color, and uniformity as well as brown spots decreases with graders' age. In contrast, the importance of the lip area increases with graders' age.

Taken as a whole, the results suggest that the perception of aging is highly influenced by the appearance of the lip area (volume and upper lip wrinkles), the eye area (crow's feet and under-eye wrinkles, dark circles, bags under the eyes), and the skin tone uniformity (brown spots, skin color uniformity). The importance of the eye area confirms the finding of Lanitis [24] and Rexbye [13] who also found skin wrinkling and color as important factors in perception. Compared with the two previous authors, the results also draw attention to the lip area, and this finding might justify the recent popularity of fillers for lips.

Cross-References

▶ Assessing Quality of Ordinal Scales Depicting Skin Aging Severity

References

1. Gandhi M. A method for automatic synthesis of aged human facial images. Montreal: McGill University; 2004.
2. Nkengne A, Bertin C, Stamatas G, et al. Influence of facial skin attributes on the perceived age of Caucasian women. J Eur Acad Dermatol Venereol. 2008;22: 982–91.
3. Rehnman J, Herlitz A. Women remember more faces than men do. Acta Psychol. 2007;124:344–55.
4. Dehon HBS. An "other-race" effect in age estimation from faces. Perception. 2001;30:1107–13.
5. Meissner C, Brigham J. Thirty years of investigating the own-race bias in memory for faces. Psychol Public Policy Law. 2001;7:3–35.
6. Daniel B, Wright BS. An own gender bias and the importance of hair in face recognition. Acta Psychol. 2003;114:101–14.
7. Porcheron A, Latreille J, Jdid R, et al. Influence of skin ageing features on Chinese women's perception of facial age and attractiveness. Int J Cosmet Sci. 2014;36(4):312–20.
8. Daniel B, Wright JNS. Age differences in lineup identification accuracy: people are better with their own age. Law Hum Behav. 2002;26:614–54.
9. George PA, Hole G. Factors influencing the accuracy of age estimates of unfamiliar faces. Perception. 1995;24:1059–73.
10. Paul Willner GR. Alcohol servers' estimates of young people's ages. Drugs Educ Prev Policy. 2001;8 (4):375–83.
11. Anastasi J, Rhodes M. Evidence for an own-age bias in face recognition. N Am J Psychol. 2006;8:237–52.
12. Sorqvist P, Eriksson M. Effects of training on age estimation. Appl Cogn Psychol. 2007;21:131.
13. Rexbye H, Povlsen J. Visual signs of ageing: what are we looking at? Int J Ageing Later Life. 2007;2:61–83.
14. Nkengne A. Predicting people's age from their facial image: a study based on the characterization and the analysis of the signs of aging. In: ED 393 – SANTE PUBLIQUE: Epidémiologie et sciences de l'Information Biomédicale University Pierre et Marie Curie. Paris: Paris VI; 2008. p. 137.
15. George PA, Hole GJ. The role of spatial and surface cues in the age-processing of unfamiliar faces. Vis Cogn. 2000;7:485–509.
16. Burt D, Perrett D. Perception of age in adult caucasian male faces: computer graphic manipulation of shape and colour information. Proc R Soc Lond B. 1995;259:137–43.
17. Montepare JM, McArthur LZ. The influence of facial characteristics on children's age perceptions. J Exp Child Psychol. 1986;42:303–14.
18. Fink B, Grammer K, Matts P. Visible skin color distribution plays a role in the perception of age, attractiveness, and health in female faces. Evol Hum Behav. 2006;27:433–42.
19. Porcheron A, Mauger E, Russel R. Aspects of facial contrast decrease with age and are cues for age perception. PLoS One. 2013;8(3):e57985.
20. Guinot C, Malvy D, Ambroisine L, et al. Relative contribution of intrinsic vs extrinsic factors to skin aging as determined by a validated skin age score. Arch Dermatol. 2002;138:1454–60.
21. Tenenhaus M, La Régression P. Théorie et Pratique. Paris: Technip; 1998.

22. Wold S, Sjöström M, Eriksson L. PLS-regression: a basic tool of chemometrics. Chemom Intell Lab Syst. 2001;58:109–30.
23. Burnham A, MacGregor J, Viveros R. Interpretation of regression coefficients under a latent variable regression model. J Chemom. 2001;15:265–84.
24. Lanitis A. Digital signal processing, 2002. DSP 2002. In: 2002 14th International Conference on the significance of different facial parts for automatic age estimation. Nicosia: Department of Computer Science and Engineering; 2002.

The Neuroscience of Age Perception 126

Daniel B. Yarosh

Contents

Abstract

The appearance of aging skin is important to us because people judge our social standing and reproductive fitness by its signals. The brain uses dedicated complex neural circuits to accurately assess age, some of which are not available to our consciousness. It focuses on specific signs that change with intrinsic and extrinsic aging, many of which are driven by sex hormones that decline with age. People make efforts to deceive each other regarding their age by masking these signs and in fact deceive themselves regarding age judgments when it is to their advantage.

Introduction

Skin aging is important not only because the biological functions of the skin decline with time but also the *appearance* of aging past the prime of life is an assault on self-esteem and confidence [1]. The desire to reduce the signs of skin aging fuels a multibillion dollar cosmetic industry, which is separate from, but often overlaps, the dermatology and plastic surgery medical treatments designed to correct the underlying causes of skin aging.

The *appearance* of aged skin is as important as its function because it helps highly social humans reach accurate judgments about each other's status and success potential. In particular, age is used, along with other skin and body signs, to

D.B. Yarosh (✉)
The Estee Lauder Companies, Inc., Melville, NY, USA
e-mail: dyarosh@danyarosh.com

M.A. Farage et al. (eds.), *Textbook of Aging Skin*,
DOI 10.1007/978-3-662-47398-6_138

assess attractiveness [2, 3], which includes standing in the community, desirability as a partner, and reproductive potential.

Age Perception Skill

People are extremely accurate at judging the age of others just by viewing their faces, with a correlation coefficient of 95 % [4]. By viewing only a swatch of skin, people are able to correctly judge age, with a correlation coefficient of more than 60 % [5]. Women are slightly more accurate than men, who tend to perceive women as younger than they are [4]. This is an interesting characteristic that will be discussed later in the section on Deception and Self-Deception.

While people are conscious of the obvious characteristics of age such as pigment spots, wrinkles, and gray hair, they are also able to discern signs of age in others using subtler clues, even though they are not able to verbalize how they reached their judgments [6]. This is a skill performed in an instant that is not willfully taught to children and probably has components genetically programmed into neural circuitry.

Brain Activity in Assessing Age

The brain devotes an isolated and specialized region, the fusiform face area (FFA) of the fusiform gyrus, specifically to facial recognition [7]. Damage to the FFA causes prosopagnosia, in which patients are unable to recognize faces by sight, although they can recognize the same people by voice [7]. The FFA recognizes and processes the location of facial features (especially the eyes, nose, and mouth) and their spacing [8] and passes the representation to other brain regions, such as the occipital face area (OFA) and the ventral anterior temporal lobes (vATLs) for feature abstraction and assessment [9].

People have distinct eye movement patterns, called scanpath routines, when they judge the age of unfamiliar faces [10], and they simultaneously engage the FFA region during this routine [11]. Research on the downstream processing of age assessments is very limited. One study implicated the anterior insula, inferior parietal cortex, and dorsolateral prefrontal cortex, the later region closely associated with value judgments [12].

Age and Inclusive Reproductive Fitness

The reason that age is of such interest to people is that youth is a major component of facial attractiveness [13] and underlies most of the specific characteristics people look for in judging attractiveness. Older faces are judged as less attractive, less likeable, less distinctive, and less energetic [14]. Assessments of attractiveness are surprisingly similar both within and across cultures [15].

Judgments of attractiveness have real consequences because they are cues of a person's health and fitness, which indicate the ability to donate good genes and successfully raise children. Attractiveness is the most important predictor of who gets the preferred choice in mates [16]. In fact, in the modern world, physical attractiveness is significantly associated with reproductive success [17]. This means that attractiveness *and the ability to accurately detect attractiveness* are under evolutionary selective pressure. Therefore, it is not surprising that the brain has developed specialized systems to accurately assess age, as well as other attractiveness characteristics.

Men and women have different strategies for reproductive success that were honed during tens of thousands of prehistoric years. Women seek men who will contribute material resources as well as good genes to her children, while men seek one or more partners with good genes, some of whom they may provide resources. As a consequence male and female consistently differ in their judgments of the effect of age on attractiveness. The sharp decline in attractiveness with women's age after menopause is largely driven by male perception, while the perception of increased power of men with age is predominantly due to female opinions [18].

Perception of Age

A detailed analysis of individual facial features concluded that the most important factors in judging age are the size of the eyes and the lips and the evenness of skin tone, regardless of what that tone might be [2]. Both eyes and lips become smaller with age, so they are reliable indicators of intrinsic age. Skin tone gradually becomes uneven with sun exposure, so this is an indicator of environmental exposure over time.

Eyes become smaller (top to bottom) with age, and the larger size of eyes is positively correlated with perception of youth [19]. As the size of eyes in real or schematic pictures is increased, the perception of age by observers decreases [20]. Lip height also declines with age and is an independent predictor of how old people appear to others [21]. In another study, lip volume was one of the strongest factors used by observers to judge age [4].

Uneven skin texture caused by wrinkling is responsible for a large fraction of how people perceive the age of others [22]. Smiling accentuates wrinkles, particularly periorbital wrinkles, and people perceive smiling faces as older [23]. Sun exposure contributes to wrinkles that people detect as signs of aging [21].

Sun exposure also causes unevenness of skin tone, due to deposition of pigment and change in subcutaneous vascularization. A strong correlation was found between judging someone as older and unevenness of hemoglobin and melanin distribution in the skin, independent of other signs of aging [5]. Pigmented spots, which are often related to sun exposure, are strongly correlated with the perception of older age [21]. Homogeneity of skin tone was correlated with people perceiving increased attractiveness and healthiness [24], while uneven skin color distribution was perceived as a sign of poor health [22].

People also use the color and thickness of hair to judge age. Hair graying and thinning is a visual clue of age [21]. The contrast of hair color to face tone declines with age as hair grays and skin tone darkens, particularly in most Caucasians. People with greater contrast from the top of the head down are perceived as younger [25].

In summary, people use several facial features as reliable indicators of chronological age, because they change with time intrinsically or with environmental exposure. These include eye and lip size, homogeneity of skin tone and texture, and contrast between hair and face tone.

Biological Drivers of Age Signs

Many of these facial features used in assessing age are strongly influenced by the sex hormones testosterone and estrogen, which build up subcutaneous bone and fat to deepen periorbital and plump perioral structures, stretch out and soften wrinkles, and thicken and darken hair. For women, facial features considered most attractive are correlated with circulating levels of estrogen [26]. For men, testosterone increases the appearance of dominance, but the highest levels of testosterone are less attractive than moderate levels [27]. Both in men and women, bioavailable testosterone and estrogen levels are highest at ages of peak fertility and decline with age [28, 29]. Therefore, the facial features people use to assess age are strongly associated with sex hormones, and they may be judging the underlying reproductive potential. For women, youth and peak fertility are the most attractive. For men, who contribute resources as well as genes, testosterone levels below the peak may indicate a mature age, reduced aggression, and accumulation of material goods and therefore are more attractive.

Deception and Self-Deception

With so much at stake, it is not surprising that people may try to deceive each other regarding their age. Women may try to look younger, and men may try to look mature. For centuries people have used nonsurgical methods to conceal signs of aging and mislead others as to their real age. These efforts focus on the very facial features the brain uses to assess age.

Female Disguises

The most widely used makeup products by women are intended to increase the appearance of eye and lip size (e.g., eye and lip liner, eye shadow, lipstick, false eyelashes), as well as to even out skin tone and enhance contrast (e.g., foundation, concealer, face powder, and blush). Women use makeup to estrogenize their appearance, compensate for changes in facial appearance brought on by age, and thereby make themselves more attractive [6].

Eye makeup has the greatest effect on attractiveness as judged by both men and women [30]. Observers look at the eyes of women with eye makeup 40 % longer than women without it, and if the rest of the face is made up, the attention to the eyes increased 80 % [31]. Lipstick increases attention to the lips by 26 % [32]. For people shown pictures of both made-up and no makeup faces, the number of eye fixations and dwell time were positively correlated with skin color homogeneity [31]. Cosmetics create a deceptively youthful look by increasing facial contrast, which is interpreted by the brain as reduced age [32].

Where makeup is not used is just as telling as where it is used. There are no makeup products that accentuate the appearance of the nose or ears. The reason is that the length of both the ears [33] and nose [34] relative to the face continue to increase with age. Instead, makeup, jewelry, and hair styles are often used to diminish and draw attention away from these features.

Male Disguises

Men use far fewer cosmetic products, but they are concerned with youthful appearance. While some signs of maturity are attractive, loss of the frontal hairline is perceived as a significant sign of aging because it reduces facial contrast and has been a male concern for centuries [35]. Although testosterone increases facial hair, it reduces scalp hair in androgenic alopecia, in what is called the "androgen paradox" [36]. Men may make various efforts to disguise balding, such as comb-overs, hair transplant and hair coloring, or even wearing a hat.

Men have darker pigmentation than women in all cultures, likely under the influence of testosterone [37]. While skin-lightening products are popular among women because they increase facial contrast, they are unlikely to ever be popular among men because they signal reduced testosterone.

Self-Deception

While people are very good at judging others, they have trouble making accurate self-assessments. Correlations between self-ratings and objective measures of individual attractiveness are remarkably low: 24 % for men and 25 % for women [38]. When people are shown a full array of computer-morphed photos of themselves, from 50 % more attractive to 50 % less attractive, they choose the 20 % better-looking photo as the one they like the most and think they most resemble [39]. They are also quicker to recognize the more attractive photo than their actual photo, a revealing result considering that people recognize objects more quickly when they match their mental representations. Both Western Europeans and Asians show this preference for enhanced self-image. This self-deception is part of a larger optimism bias that behavioral economists call the "superiority illusion" [40]. People tend to think of themselves as better than their peers. The rationale is that we are better able to deceive others when we believe the lie ourselves, and this is evolutionarily beneficial when the costs of errors in judgment are low and the benefits of self-deception are high [41].

Recall now that women are very accurate in judging other people's age, while men systematically underestimate the age of women [4]. This is a form of bias wherein men deceive themselves into attraction for some women by reporting to themselves they are younger than they actually appear to be. This is a classic case where the cost of error is relatively small for men and the benefits are great.

Conclusion

The neuroscience of age and attractiveness perception is at its infancy. A few key brain regions have been identified, but much more research is needed to understand how the brain extracts information from faces and processes it to reach its judgments. Accurate age perception provides a selective advantage in identifying potential collaborators, competitors, and mates who have the greatest potential to impact our own reproductive fitness. This evolutionary perspective helps explain many of the factors that are most important in perceiving age and why so much time and money is spent on concealing age. It also helps explain why people might systematically err in their age judgments. This perspective implies that current attitudes about youth and age are not fads of our modern culture, but hardwired characteristics of human behavior.

References

1. Gupta M, Gilchrest BA. Psychosocial aspects of aging skin. Dermatol Clin. 2005;23:643–8.
2. Korthase K, Trenholme I. Perceived age and perceived physical attractiveness. Percept Mot Skills. 1982;54:1251–8.
3. Kwart DG, et al. Age and beauty are in the eye of the beholder. Perception. 2012;41:925–38.
4. Nkenge A, et al. Influence of facial skin attributes on the perceived age of Caucasian women. J Eur Acad Dermatol Venerol. 2008;22:982–91.
5. Matts P, Fink B, Grammer K, Burquest B. Color homogeneity and visual perception of age, health, and attractiveness of female facial skin. J Am Acad Dermatol. 2007;57:977–84.
6. Perrett D. In your face. Palgrave Macmillan; 2010 London.
7. Kanwisher N, Yovel G. The fusiform face area: a cortical region specialized for the perception of faces. Phil Trans Roy Soc B. 2006;361:2109–28.
8. Liu J, et al. Perception of face parts and face configurations: an fMRI study. J Cogn Neurosci. 2010;22:203–11.
9. Collins JA, Olson IR. Beyond FFA: the role of the ventral anterior temporal lobes in face processing. Neuropsychologia. 2014;61:65–79.
10. Kanan C, et al. Humans have idiosyncratic and task-specific scanpaths for judging faces. Vision Res. 2015;108:67–76.
11. Wiese H, et al. Perceiving age and gender in unfamiliar faces: an fMRI study on face categorization. Brain Cogn. 2012;78:163–8.
12. Bzdok D, et al. The modular neuroarchitecture of social judgments. Cereb Cortex. 2012;22:951–61.
13. Tatarunaite E, et al. Facial attractiveness: a longitudinal study. Am J Orthod Dentofacial Orthop. 2005;127:676–82.
14. Ebner NC. Age of face matters: age-group differences in ratings of young and old faces. Behav Res Methods. 2008;40:130–6.
15. Langlois JH, et al. Maxims or myths of beauty? A meta-analytic and theoretical review. Psych Bull. 2000;126:390–423.
16. Halberstadt J. Proximate and ultimate origins of a bias for prototypical faces. In: Forgas J, Haselton G, von Hippel W, editors. Evolution and the social mind. Sydney: Psychology Press; 2007.
17. Jokela M. Physical attractiveness and reproductive success in humans: evidence from the late 20th century United States. Evol Hum Behav. 2009;30:342–50.
18. Maestripieri D, et al. A greater decline in female facial attractiveness during middle age reflects women's loss of reproductive value. Front Psych. 2014. doi:10.3389/fpsyg.2014.00179.
19. Berry DS, McArthur LZ. Some components and consequences of a babyface. J Pers Soc Psychol. 1985;48:312–23.
20. McArthur LZ, Apatow K. Impressions of babyfaced adults. Soc Cogn. 1984;2:315–42.
21. Gunn DA, et al. Why some women look young for their age. PLoS One. 2009;4(12), e8021. doi:10.1371/journal.pone.0008021.
22. Fink B, Matts PJ. The effect of skin color distribution and topography cues on the perception of female facial age and health. J Eur Acad Dermatol Veneral. 2008;22:493–8.
23. Ganel T. Smiling makes you look older. Psychon Bull Rev. 2015; doi:10.3758/s13423-015-0822-7.
24. Fink B, et al. Visible skin color distribution plays a role in the perception of age, attractiveness, and health in female faces. Evol Hum Behav. 2006;27:433–42.
25. Porcheron A, et al. Aspects of facial contrast decrease with age and are cues for age perception. PLoS One. 2013;8(3), e57985. doi10.1371/journal.pone.0057985.
26. Smith, et al. Facial appearance is a cue to oestrogen levels in women. Proc Biol Sci. 2006;22:135–40.
27. Swaddle JP, Reierson GW. Testosterone increases perceived dominance but not attractiveness in human males. Royal Soc. 2002;269:2285–9.
28. Ferrini RL, Barrett-Connor E. Sex hormones and age: a cross-sectional study of testosterone and estradiol and their bioavailable fractions in community dwelling men. Am J Epidemiol. 1998;147:750–4.
29. Thornhill R, Gangestad S. The evolutionary biology of human female sexuality. New York: Oxford University Press; 2008. p. 129.

30. Samson N, Fink B, Matts P. Visible skin condition and perception of human facial appearance. Intl J Cosmet Sci. 2010;32:167–84.
31. Cula G, Wu I-T, Barkovic S, Appa Y. Quantifying the effect of makeup on facial attractiveness. J Am Acad Dermatol. 2010;62:AB58.
32. Porcheron A, Mauger E, Russel R. Aspects of facial contrast decrease with age and are cues for age perception. PLoS One. 2013;8, e57985.
33. Tan R, Osman V, Tan G. Ear size as a predictor of chronological age. Arch Gerontol Geriatr. 1997;25:187–91.
34. Edelstein D. Aging of the normal nose in adults. Laryngoscope. 1996;106:1–25.
35. Rawnsley D. Hair restoration. Facial Plast Surg Clin North Am. 2008;16:289–97.
36. Inui S, Itami S. Androgen action on the human hair follicle: perspectives. Exp Dermatol. 2013;22:168–71.
37. Jablonski N. Skin: a natural history. Berkeley: University of California Press; 2006.
38. Alam M, Dover J. On beauty: evolution, psychosocial considerations, and surgical enhancement. Arch Dermatol. 2001;137:795–807.
39. Epley N, Whitchurch E. Mirror, mirror on the wall: enhancement in self-recognition. Pers Soc Psychol Bull. 2008;34:1159–70.
40. Shalot T. The optimism bias. New York: Vintage Books; 2012.
41. Kurzban R. Why everyone else is a hypocrite. Princeton: Princeton University Press; 2012.

Part XII

Gender, Ethnicity, and Lifestyle Differences

127 Determinants in the Rate of Skin Aging: Ethnicity, Gender, and Lifestyle Influences

Miranda A. Farage, Kenneth W. Miller, and Howard I. Maibach

Contents

Abstract

This chapter discusses in detail all the various factors that affect the process of skin aging. Skin aging depends upon a combination of intrinsic and extrinsic factors. Intrinsic factors include gender, ethnicity, and anatomical variations, which are genetically determined. Extrinsic factors such as lifestyle, nutrition, smoking, and sun exposure can also accelerate skin aging. Most intrinsic factors cannot be avoided, but extrinsic factors, such as sun exposure and smoking, can be reduced or eliminated, with substantial impact on the visible appearance of the skin. Lifestyle factors such as smoking or nutritional choices can modulate the effects of both genetic and environmental aging. Exposure to solar ultraviolet light initiates a flurry of molecular and cellular responses that promote rapid and dynamic changes in the skin. Greater understanding of the molecular processes which contribute to skin aging, as well as how lifestyle choices accelerate or impede those changes, may help improve both physical and psychological health for the increasing percentage of the population in the latter years of their lives.

M.A. Farage (✉)
Winton Hill Business Center, The Procter & Gamble Company, Cincinnati, OH, USA
e-mail: farage.m@pg.com

K.W. Miller
Margoshes-Miller Consulting, LLC, Cincinnati, OH, USA

H.I. Maibach
Department of Dermatology, University of California, San Francisco, CA, USA
e-mail: maibachh@derm.ucsf.edu

M.A. Farage et al. (eds.), *Textbook of Aging Skin*,
DOI 10.1007/978-3-662-47398-6_92

Introduction

The population of those in the USA over the age of 60 is expected to nearly double by 2025 [1], with half the US population predicted to be older than 65 by 2030 [2].

Aging is a complex, multifactorial process characterized by a deterioration of the ability of the body to maintain homeostasis, an increase in vulnerability to environmental insults, and a progressive loss of both structural integrity and physiological function [3]. Obviously, however, the process of physiological aging does not occur in all individuals at the same rate.

Aging involves both intrinsic and extrinsic processes, occurring in parallel [4], that individually affect the pace at which the integument ages [5]. Intrinsic aging, the inevitable natural deterioration of body structure and function with age, is genetically determined and proceeds at a fairly predictable rate, affected by the inherent toxicity of certain by-products of metabolism and a lack of sufficient physiological resources dedicated to somatic maintenance and repair [6]. Estrogen depletion after menopause drives gender differences in the rate at which skin ages [7]. Significant differences in skin structure and lipid content at different anatomical sites also have the potential to influence the process of intrinsic aging [8, 9].

Extrinsic aging is the result of exogenous insults such as infectious agents, environmental toxins, and ultraviolet (UV) radiation [10] which attack skin integrity daily, causing thousands of DNA alterations per cell each day [10, 11]. UV exposure, in particular, creates cumulative skin damage which accentuates the results of chronological aging [12]. More than 90 % of deleterious age-related changes in the appearance of skin, particularly facial skin, result from UV damage [13] (Fig. 1). In addition, lifestyle factors like smoking or nutritional choices can modulate the effects of both genetic and environmental aging [6, 14].

Although hormone replacement therapy can delay the effects of intrinsic aging in estrogen-deficient older women [15], intrinsic aging is inevitable. Many of the components of extrinsic aging, however, can be avoided, with substantial decreasing of both morbidity and premature mortality in older individuals [5].

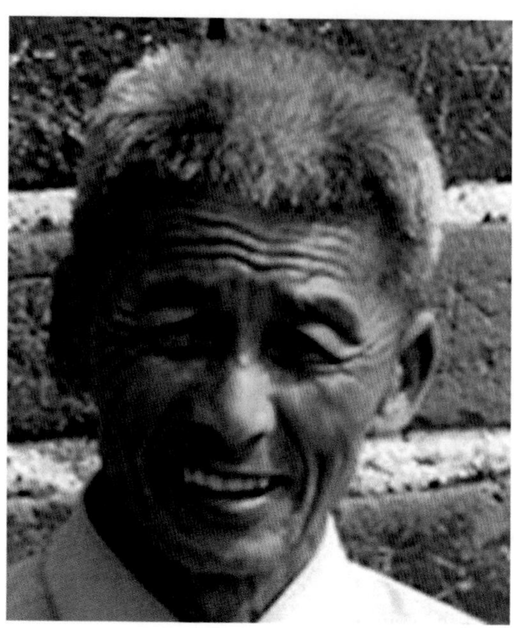

Fig. 1 The deep wrinkles, age spots, and leathery skin indicate premature aging caused by years of unprotected exposure to the sun (Thank you to Dr. Brian Gray)

Factors That Contribute to Skin Aging

Intrinsic Factors

Gender

Estrogen and other sex steroids have a significant influence on skin biology and structure and are known to affect epidermal keratinocytes, dermal fibroblasts, melanocytes, hair follicles, and sebaceous glands [16].

Women have more estrogen receptors than men. Skin thickness has been observed to increase over the menstrual cycle with rising levels of estrogen [17]. Estrogen increases DNA repair capacity by 25 % [18]. A woman's skin contains numerous estrogen receptors; nearly every structural and functional change which accompanies the menopause in women has been demonstrated to be at least partially reversible with estrogen replacement therapy. It is believed that threshold levels of estrogen are required to maintain skin integrity [19]. Skin aging can be significantly delayed by the administration of estrogen at menopause [16].

Estrogens may be involved in regulating the inflammatory response, as improvements in inflammatory skin disorders such as psoriasis have been reported during pregnancy [20]. It also appears to offer some protection against skin photoaging [16, 21].

Numerous differences between the skin of men and women have been observed. In young women the skin has less collagen content than in men; collagen content decreases dramatically after menopause, which makes older women's skin age rapidly [18]. In men, skin thins gradually, about 1 % per year; the thickness of women's skin remains relatively constant until menopause and then thins dramatically in a fairly short time [22]. Women experience a substantial decrease in skin elasticity after menopause, a drop which does not occur to the same degree in men [18]. Skin roughness, however, increases with age at a lesser rate in women [23]. Dermal wounds heal more quickly in women than men [24]; but mucosal wounds heal more rapidly in men than women, probably due to relatively high levels of testosterone in saliva [24]. A direct relationship exists in men between skin thickness and collagen content, a correlation which is absent in women of reproductive age [22]. Mortality rates for all skin cancers are significantly lower in women [25].

The distinct impact that the hormonal deficiency of menopause has on the skin has recently begun to be recognized [18]. Many women report a sudden onset of skin aging – thinner skin, wrinkling, dryness, and decreasing firmness and elasticity – several months after onset of menopause, as estrogen levels plummet [15]. In arguably the clearest evidence of a genuine gender difference in the rate of skin aging, noninvasive laser imaging of collagen and elastin revealed that the ratio of collagen to elastin fibers in the dermis decreased with age at a faster rate in women [7]. In general, skin changes in women were correlated more strongly with the estrogen deficit of menopause than with chronological age.

Ethnicity

Differences in skin pigmentation have the greatest effect on skin aging related to ethnicity, as this property lends the skin differing abilities to respond to UV-light insult [26]. High levels of pigmentation offer protection from the cumulative effects of photoaging, with blacks showing little cutaneous difference in signs of aging between exposed and unexposed sites [27]. In addition, pigmentation provides black skin up to a 500-fold level of protection over white skin from UV radiation (based on skin cancer rates) [28]. Basal cell carcinoma and squamous cell carcinoma occur almost exclusively on sun-exposed skin of light-skinned people [29].

Studies of ethnic differences in skin aging have been confounded by nonuniformity in various investigational parameters, particularly by varying definitions of race versus skin type. Often, small numbers of people were investigated. Most studies have focused on white, black, or Asian skin, with Hispanic or Native Americans less often included, with little attempt to delineate among the significant variety of skin types that each category may contain [30]. For example, American blacks are now considered racially distinct from African blacks [31]. Other factors which need standardization are anatomical site, season, and hormonal status. For example, very substantial differences in desquamation have been found by anatomical site [26].

Despite methodological issues, however, some distinct racial differences in the aging of skin have been observed. Caucasian skin wrinkles and sags, with a much higher risk of skin cancers. Darker skin wrinkles at a much slower pace [32]. Aging Asian and black skin experiences hyperpigmentation and uneven skin tone [33, 34].

Understanding ethnic differences in skin biochemistry would provide foundation for more effective skin care products and treatments targeted to ethnically diverse populations [35]. A comparison of structural and functional

Table 1 Comparison of racial differences in structural skin properties

Parameter	Comparison	Reference
Stratum corneum		
Thickness	Equal in blacks and whites	[146, 147]
Number of cell layers	Higher in blacks than whites	[148]
	Higher in whites than Asians	
Resistance to tape stripping	Higher in blacks than whites	[148]
Lipid content	Higher in blacks than whites (> twofold)	[149]
Electrical resistance	Higher in blacks than whites (twofold)	[150]
Desquamation	Higher in blacks than whites (twofold)	[151, 152]
	Lower in blacks than whites	
Corneocyte size	Equal in blacks, whites, and Asians	[151]
Ceramide content	Asians > Hispanics > Caucasians > blacks[a]	[153]
Variability in skin structure	Higher in blacks than whites	[148]
Water content	Higher in blacks than whites	[43, 152, 153]
	Higher in Asians than blacks	
	Higher in Hispanics than blacks	
NMF levels	Lower in Asians than in blacks or Caucasians	[26]
Dermis		
Dermal thickness	Higher in Asians than Caucasians	[154]
Collagen content	Higher in Asians than Caucasians	[154]
Melanin content	Higher in Asians than Caucasians	[154]
Melanosome size and distribution	Black skin: large, uniform size, single units with membrane	[155]
	Asian skin: small, uniform size, clustered in groups of up to 10	[155]
	White skin: melanocyte size and shape highly variable, clustered in groups of up to 10	[155]
Melanosome stage in keratinocytes	Black skin: keratinocytes contain mainly stage IV melanosomes	[155]
	Asian skin: keratinocytes contain stage II, III, and IV melaosomes, stage IV predominates	[155]
	White skin: keratinocytes contain mainly stage II and III melano	[156]
Melanosome induction	Black skin: UV induces all stage melanosomes	[156]
	Asian skin: UV induces primarily stage II and III melanosomes	[156]
	White skin: UV induces primarily stage IV melanosomes	[156]
Ground substance	Less in Asians than Caucasians	[155]
Sebaceous glands		
Sebum production	Glands bigger; sebum production higher in blacks than in East Asians and East Asians higher than Hispanics	[26]

[a]50 % lower in blacks compared to Caucasians or Hispanics

differences in skin of different races is displayed in Tables 1 and 2.

Anatomical Variations

Huge variations in some skin parameters have been observed with respect to the body site studied, underscoring a need to standardize both the study site and the age range of the population in order to obtain meaningful comparative results [36]. Large differences in skin SC thickness exist at different body sites: about 3 stratum corneum cell layers on the eyelid and 5 layers in most

Table 2 Comparison of racial differences in functional skin properties

Permeability	In vitro penetration of fluocinolone acetonide	Lower in blacks than Caucasians	[157]
	In vitro penetration of water	No difference	[157, 158]
		Differences	
	Topical application of anesthetic mixture	Less efficacy in blacks than Caucasians	[159]
	In vivo penetration of C-labeled dipyrithione	Lower in blacks (34 % lower) than Caucasians	[160]
	Methylnicotinate-induced vasodilation	Time to peak response equal than Caucasians	[161–163]
		Slower in blacks	
Transepidermal water loss	Baseline TEWL (in vitro)	Higher in blacks	[163, 164]
		Higher in blacks (in vitro)	
	TEWL in response to SLS irritation (in vivo)	Higher in blacks and Hispanics	[165]
	Baseline TEWL (in vivo)	Blacks > Caucasians > Asians	[153]
	Return to baseline TEWL after tape stripping	Blacks faster than whites	[166]
	Reactivity to SLS (measured by TEWL)	Higher in blacks than Caucasians	[164]
Skin irritant reactivity	Reactivity to dichlorethyl sulfide (1 %)	Lower in blacks (measured by erythema, 15 % vs. 58 %) than Caucasians	[167]
	Reactivity to 0-chlorobenzylidene malononitrile	Lower, longer time to response in blacks than Caucasians	[168]
	Reactivity to dinitrochlorobenzene	Lower in blacks, but trend toward equalization after removal of stratum corneum than Caucasians	[148]
	Reactivity to octanoic acid, 20 % SLS, 100 % decanol, 10 % acetic acid	Asians more reactive than Caucasians (react more quickly)	[169]
	Stinging response	Lower in blacks than whites	[12, 170–172]
		Equal in blacks and whites	
		Higher in Asians than whites	
Stinging response	UV protection factor of stratum corneum	Higher in blacks (about 50 % higher) than Caucasians	[136]
Skin transparency	UVB transmission in stratum corneum	Lower in blacks (about 50 % lower	[136]
	Spectral emittance	Lower in blacks (above 300 nm: two- to threefold)	[173]
	UV protection factor of epidermis	Higher in blacks (fourfold)	[136]
	UVA transmission through epidermis	Lower in blacks (almost fourfold)	[136]
	UVB transmission through epidermis	Lower in blacks (fourfold)	[136]
	Contribution of malpighian layer	Black skin: twice as effective in absorbing UVB as white skin	[136]
Photoprotection of epidermis	Skin extensibility on dorsal (sun exposed) and volar (sun protected) forearms	Black skin maintains extensibility on sun-exposed sites, but Hispanic skin extensibility is reduced on sun-exposed sites	[43]

(*continued*)

Table 2 (continued)

Consequence of photoaging	Elastic recovery	Black skin maintains recovery on sun-exposed sites, white and Hispanic skins reduced	[43]
	Drying	Higher in Caucasians and Asians than in Hispanics and blacks	[35]
	Hypertrophic scarring	Higher in Asians than Caucasians	[174]
Response to insult	Pigmented dermatoses	Higher in Asians than Caucasians	[174, 175]
	Wrinkling	Average onset is 10 years later in Asians than Caucasians	[175]
	Wrinkling	Average onset is 20 years later in blacks than Caucasians	[155]
	Thermal tolerance	Blacks have a lower threshold than whites	[176]
Somatosensory function	Elastic recovery (tested on the cheek)	1.5 times greater in black as compared with white subjects	[26, 152]

SLS sodium lauryl sulfate, *TEWL* transepidermal water loss, *UV* ultraviolet, *UVA* UV band A, *UVB* UV band B

nonexposed areas of the body, but up to 50 layers on the soles of feet [37]. The decrease in epidermal thickness with aging was found to be smaller at the temple than at the volar forearm [38, 39] – which may be the effect of cumulative photoaging.

The lipid composition of human stratum corneum displays striking regional variation in both content and compositional profile [40]. There is a much higher proportion of sphingolipids and cholesterol in palmoplantar stratum corneum than on extensor surfaces of the extremities, abdominal, or facial stratum corneum [40]. There is also an inverse relationship between the lipid weight percentage of a particular body site and its permeability [40]. Subcutaneous tissue with age depletes selectively in the face as well as the dorsal aspects of hands and shins [41].

Skin rigidity is much higher at the forehead than at the cheek in postmenopausal women [42]. In areas of the body with high blood flow (e.g., lip, finger, nasal tip, forehead), blood flow decreased with age [36]; in areas with normally low blood flow, no difference was observed [36]. In all races, significant differences in conductance exist between the volar and dorsal forearms [43]. The decrease in sensory perception with aging is more pronounced in the nasolabial fold and cheek, than in the chin and forehead [40, 44].

It is commonly assumed that aged skin is intrinsically less hydrated, less elastic, more permeable, and more susceptible to irritation [38, 45] due to an apparently impaired functional barrier [46] as measured by higher TEWL [38, 46]. The highest TEWL in all phases of life is measured on the lips, a value three times higher than that of the surrounding face, which is also higher than most other body sites [47]. Interestingly, the upper lip is more hydrated than the lower [48].

A high density of estrogen receptors is present on the genitalia, as well as on the face and lower limbs. Estrogen acts on both epidermis and dermis [18]. Estrogen receptors alpha and beta are found in varying densities by anatomic site and have different affinities for specific estrogen types, so that the potency of specific estrogens varies from tissue to tissue [18].

The morphology and the physiology of the vulva and vagina undergo numerous changes associated with hormonal changes at menopause [45]. Skin in the vulvar area derives from three different embryonic layers. The cutaneous epithelia of the mons pubis, labia, and clitoris originate from the embryonic ectoderm and exhibit a keratinized, stratified structure similar to the keratinized, stratified skin at other sites [49]. The mucosa of the vulvar vestibule originates from the embryonic ectoderm and is nonkeratinized. The vagina is derived from the embryonic mesoderm and is responsive to estrogen cycling [38, 45]. There are fewer estrogen receptors on the vulva than on the vagina [18].

After menopause the following changes occur: vaginal epithelium atrophies, cervicovaginal secretions become sparse, vaginal pH rises, atrophic vaginitis becomes more common [38, 45], collagen and water content decreases, pubic hair grays and becomes sparse, the labia majora loses subcutaneous fat, and also the labia (labia minora, vestibule, and vaginal mucosa) atrophy [38, 45]. In addition, vaginal secretions decrease, and the thinned tissue is more easily irritated and susceptible to infection [38, 45]. The cumulative effect of estrogen deficiency contributes to poor wound healing [50]. Skin collagen content and thickness also decrease as a consequence of hormonal decline after removal of the ovaries [51]. Also, dramatic hormonal changes, particularly thyroid, testosterone, and estrogen, alter epidermal lipid synthesis [40]. In people with limited mobility, atrophied genital tissue is more susceptible to shear forces and may be more susceptible to the pH changes and enzymatic action associated with incontinence [38, 45].

Vulvar skin is more resistant to tape stripping and recovers more quickly in younger subjects than in older ones [52]. Also, vulvar skin has an increased rate of epidermal turnover [38, 52] and increased basal cutaneous blood flow [38, 52]. Although aged forearm skin has a less frequent and slower reaction to sodium lauryl sulfate (SLS) irritation than younger forearm skin, no age-related differences were observed in the vulvar area [53].

Elderly patients are susceptible to contact dermatitis in the vulvar area, principally due to urinary moisture under occlusion. Urinary ammonia elevates local pH, which alters barrier function, further compromising skin integrity thereby increasing risk of infection [38, 45].

The vulvar area is more susceptible to persistent vulval itch and irritation in old age [54, 55]. A combination of factors contributes to this, including sweating, occlusion, vaginal discharge, friction, use of hygiene products, and incontinence. There is a significant decrease in the size and number of free nerve endings in aged skin in genital mucous membranes, with a corresponding decrease in sensory perception in the genital area [38, 41].

Extrinsic Factors

Lifestyle Influences

The skin is at high risk of damage from reactive oxygen species because its high level of vascularity creates a high degree of exposure to oxygen and because its exterior surface is exposed to atmospheric oxygen. The skin is also exposed to reactive oxygen species generated by UV light. Damage to epidermal cells and subcutaneous tissues caused by the reactive oxygen species manifests as skin aging [56]. The skin is particularly susceptible to oxidative damage because of its high lipid content. Skin proteins and DNA are also sensitive to oxidation [57].

Nutrition

Over the last decade, fruits, vegetables, legumes, herbs, and teas have been found to contain antioxidative compounds [56, 58, 59]. In a study evaluating 4,025 middle-aged American women, higher vitamin C intakes were associated with a decreased risk of wrinkles (odds ratio 0.89; 95 % confidence interval [CI] 0.82–0.96) and a decreased risk of senile dryness (odds ratio 0.93; 95 % CI 0.87–0.99) [60]. Higher linoleic acid intakes were associated with a decreased risk of senile dryness (odds ratio 0.75; 95 % CI 0.64–0.88) and a lower likelihood of skin atrophy (odds ratio 0.78; 95 % CI 0.65–0.95) [60].

In a study of the protective effects of nutrition among Greek, Australian, and Swedish subjects, resilience to photoaging was associated with a higher intake of vegetables ($p < 0.0001$), olive oil ($p < 0.0001$), fish ($p < 0.0001$), and legumes (p & 0.0001) and with a lower intake of butter ($p < 0.0001$), margarine ($p < 0.001$), sugar ($p < 0.01$), or dairy products (p & 0.01). Vegetables, legumes, and olive oil appeared to be particularly protective, collectively explaining 20 % of the variance in resistance to photoaging. Among Australian Anglo-Celtics, prunes, apples, and tea explained 34 % of protective variance [56]. Another recent clinical study investigated the association between the risk of photoaging, monounsaturated fatty acid intake, and the sources of monounsaturated fatty acids. The findings support the beneficial effect of dietary olive

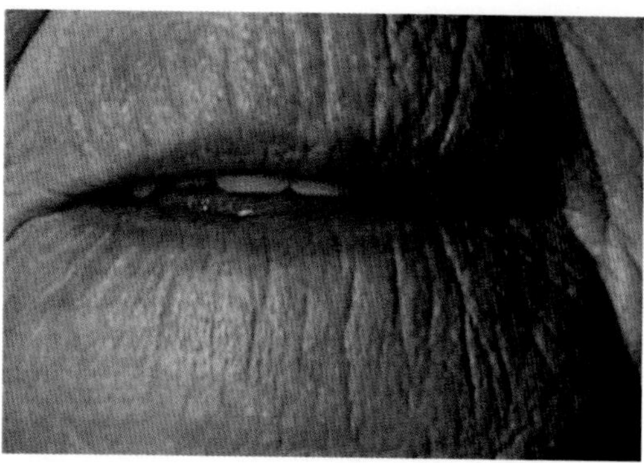

Fig. 2 Smoking effect and wrinkles (With kind permission from the Procter and Gamble Co.)

oil or healthy diet habits associated with olive oil consumption on the severity of facial photoaging [61].

In another study, higher fat intake was associated with an increased risk of wrinkles and skin atrophy. Higher carbohydrate intake was associated with increased risk of skin atrophy, with findings independent of age, race, social status, UV exposure, menopausal status, body mass index, exercise, or energy intake [60]. Vitamin A has also been observed to decrease production of matrix metalloproteinases (MMPs), associated with degradation of the extracellular matrix [62, 63]. Fish oil consumption can confer an SPF as high as 4 [64]. Vitamin C deficiency delays healing [65].

Ambient conditions such as temperature and humidity also affect the skin. An increase in skin temperature of 7–8 °F doubles the evaporative water loss [8]. Low temperature stiffens the skin and decreases evaporative water loss even with plenty of humidity in the air, as structural proteins and lipids in the skin are critically dependent on temperature for appropriate conformation [8]. Extreme changes in ambient humidity in either direction lower skin hydration [8]. Some medications affect the skin as well, particularly hypocholesterolemic drugs, which may induce abnormal increased desquamation [66].

By far, however, the two exogenous factors that exact a heaviest toll on the skin are smoking [67] and exposure to UV light. Cigarette smoking is strongly associated with elastosis in both sexes and with telangiectasia (red spots on skin) in men [68, 69]. Smoke causes damage to collagen and elastin in lung tissue and may do so in skin as well [68]. Nicotine constricts the vasculature [68], causing a decrease in capillary blood flow in the skin, which may contribute to wrinkling [51]. Smoking significantly affects the ability of the skin to repair itself, most likely related to effects on the vasculature [70–72]. Smoking increases the risk of poor outcomes such as skin necrosis after facial cosmetic surgeries (including rhytidectomies and face lifts) [73]. Frequent smokers (defined as greater than one pack/day) were observed to have three times the risk of skin necrosis after facial skin procedures than former smokers, those who had never smoked, and those who smoked at a much less frequent level [74].

Smoking increases keratinocyte dysplasia and skin roughness [75]. A clear dose-response relationship between wrinkling and smoking has been demonstrated [67] (Fig. 2); smoking contributes more to facial wrinkling than sun exposure [68]. In fact, smoking was shown to be an independent risk factor for premature wrinkling when age, sun exposure, and pigmentation were controlled [68, 76]. Moreover, although hormone replacement therapy reverses wrinkling in older patients, the skin of longtime smokers did not respond [51]. In one study, the relative risk for moderate to severe wrinkling for current smokers compared to that of lifelong nonsmokers was 2.57 (CI 1.83–3.06; $p < 0.0005$) [51]. Wrinkle scores were three times greater in smokers than in nonsmokers, with a significant increase in the risk of wrinkles after 10 pack-years [77]. (Pack-years are calculated by multiplying the number of packs of cigarettes smoked per day by the number of years the person has smoked; e.g., 10 pack-years is the equivalent of smoking one pack a day for 10 years or two packs a day for 5 years [77].) Smoking is an important risk factor in cutaneous squamous cell carcinoma [68]. Specific effects of smoking on the skin are shown in Table 3.

Exposure to Ultraviolet Light (Photoaging)

As people age, intrinsic changes occur in the skin, such as decreases in skin cell turnover, chemical clearance, thickness and cellularity, thermoregulation, mechanical protection, immune responsiveness, sensory perception, sweat and sebum production, and vascular reactivity [38, 78]. These changes manifest as generalized skin atrophy with few structural alterations up to the age of 50, which is followed by slow deterioration in skin condition [8, 79].

In contrast, exposure to solar UV light initiates a flurry of molecular and cellular responses that promote rapid and dynamic changes in the skin [8]. Photodamage is damage produced in tissue by single or repeated exposure to UV light (Figs. 3 and 4). This is believed to account for the vast majority of the skin's age-related cosmetic changes as well as certain clinical problems [38, 78]. UV light induces photochemical changes that can lead to either acute effects (e.g., erythema or sunburn) or chronic effects (e.g., premature skin aging, neoplasms) [38, 80]. UV band B ([UVB] 290–320 nm) is considered the primary causative agent of UV effect on skin, causing modification gene expression as well as mutations in DNA [38]. Ultraviolet radiation is a complete carcinogen in that it both initiates cancers through DNA mutations and promotes cancer growth through the inflammatory processes inherent in cumulative UV exposure [38, 81, 82]. Modern Western culture has promoted tanned skin as healthy, resulting in steadily increasing rates of skin cancer and prematurely aged skin [38, 54] (Fig. 5). Senescence in aged cells creates an extended window of time in which DNA mutations can accumulate and eventually result in carcinogenesis.

Table 3 Effects of smoking on skin structure and function

Increased appearance of age	[177, 178]
Decreased collagen production	[179]
Induction of MMPs	[180]
Degradation of collagen by MMPs	[179]
Degradation of elastin fibers by MMPs	[179]
Increased reduction of elastotic material	[181]
Degradation of proteoglycans by MMPs	[179]
Increase in circulating free radicals	[179]
Increased sallowness	[90, 182]
Increased wrinkling	[183]
Increased roughness	[183]
Decreased cutaneous blood flow	[184, 185]
Decreased skin temperature	[185]
Reactive hyperemia	[186]
Subcutaneous oxygen saturation	[187]

MMPs matrix metalloproteinases

UV exposure is the largest contributor to the detrimental aging of the skin [38, 54]. It is believed to account for more than 80 % of facial aging [83]. It has recently been reported that it may be UV band A (UVA) that is responsible for the bulk of epidermal skin damage (Figs. 3 and 4). UVA excitation of trans-urocanic acid initiates chemical processes that result in photoaging of the skin [84].

Virtually all Caucasian Westerners with normal recreational practices have subclinical signs of skin damage on exposed skin by the time they are 15 years old [81], whereas changes become discernible in unexposed skin in the early 30s [38, 85]. In Caucasians, as little as one minimal erythema dose of UV radiation is sufficient to disrupt production of natural moisturizing factor (NMF) amino acids [86]. UV exposure which causes moderate pinkness but not sunburn in Caucasians increases MMP levels in the irradiated tissue by hundreds of times [87]. The same level of exposure also reduces collagen production by 80 % [87].

The clinical signs of cutaneous photoaging include changes in visible skin color and surface texture [38, 54], including the early appearance of

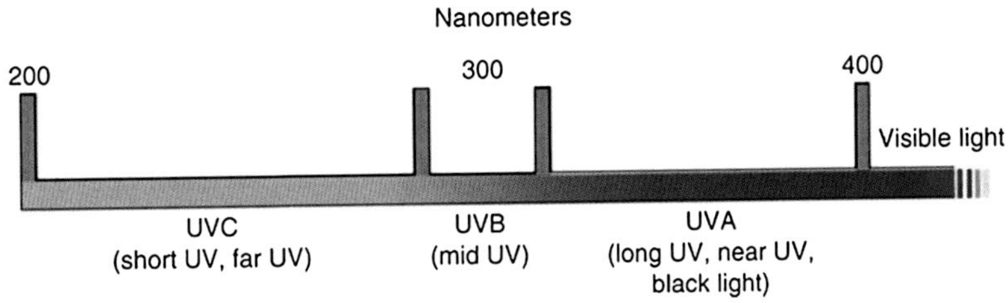

Fig. 3 The spectrum of ultraviolet radiation

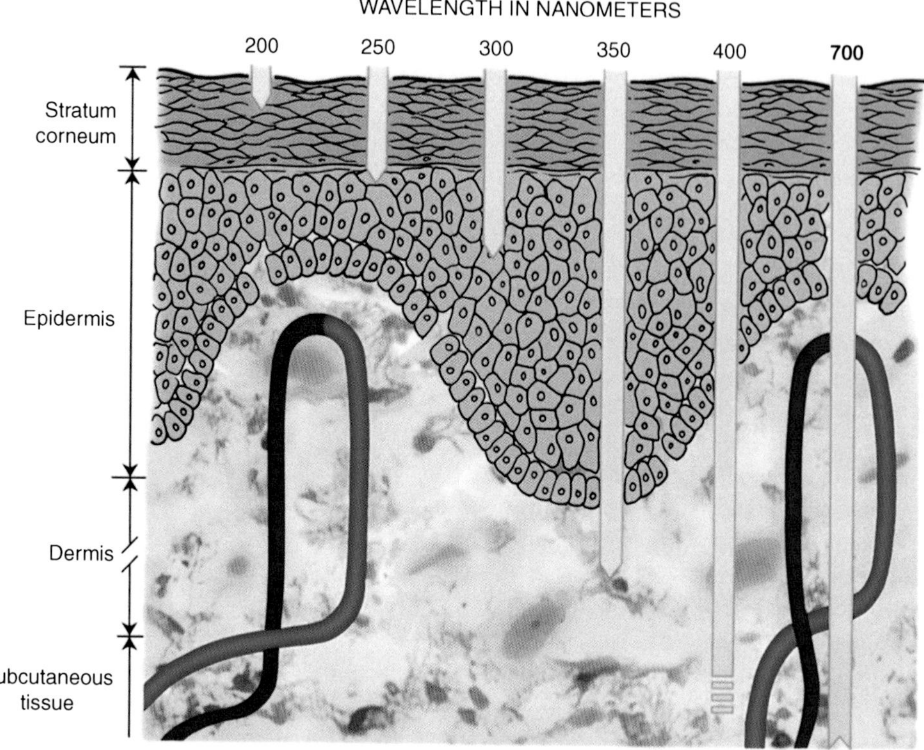

Fig. 4 The depth of penetration of UV radiation of different wavelengths into the skin: UVB mainly affects the epidermis, while UVA penetrates deeper into the dermis

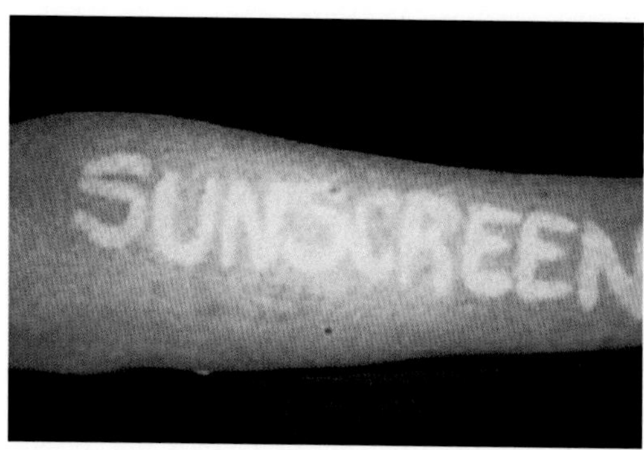

Fig. 5 Sun tan is a defense against the sun which arises as a result of UV-induced skin damage. Sunscreens protect the skin from burning rays (Reproduced with permission from the American Academy of Dermatology© 2008. All rights reserved)

dyschromia and lentigines, loss of normal translucency or pink glow, sallowness, and the gradual appearance of telangiectasia and purpura [38, 54]. Textural changes include increased roughness, frank keratoses, and the development of fine rhytides which progress to deeper folds and creases [38, 54]. Although plasma concentration of retinol increases with age, within the epidermis, vitamin A is destroyed by sun exposure [88].

Although one primary effect of photodamage is skin thickening, severe UV exposure results in dramatic thinning [29, 38]. Sun damage creates a state of chronic inflammation, with ongoing release of proteolytic enzymes by inflammatory cells that disrupts the dermal matrix [29, 38]. Epidermal thickness increases; then decreases, with an eventual loss of epidermal polarity (orderly maturation); and increased atypically among individual keratinocytes [29, 38, 89]. Another observed change is the decrease in perfusion in aged skin, which is more pronounced in photo-exposed areas [8]. Physical responses to UV exposure are displayed in Table 4.

UV radiation of the skin produces both local and distant effects [29, 38] (Fig. 4). Irradiated skin

Table 4 Response of human skin to UV exposure

Acute surge in induction of MMP	[90, 188, 189]
Procollagen depleted	[90]
Procollagen synthesis upregulated, degradation of collagen by MMPs more significantly upregulated, net collagen decreased	[90]
Inflammation (acute)	[93]
Thickening of stratum corneum (acute)	[93]
Decrease in NMF and amino acid production	[86]
Induction of elafin, which binds to elastic fibers creating increase in elastotic material	[92]
Accumulation of elastic fibers	[190]
Accumulation of proteoglycans	[190]
Induction of *c-fos*, causing cellular proliferation	[4]
Downregulation of *c-myc*, causing cellular division	[4]
Induction of GADD, response to injury	[4]
Induction of Il-1α, keratinocyte mitogen, fibroblast mitogen	[4]
Induction of Il-1β, keratinocyte mitogen	[4]
Induction of SRP2, involved in differentiation	[4]
Decreased HA levels	[83]
Increased chondroitin sulfate proteoglycans	[83]

GADD growth arrest and DNA damage protein, *HA* hyaluronic acid, *Il-1α* interleukin-1 alpha, *Il-1β* interleukin-1 beta, *MMP* matrix metalloproteinase, *NMF* natural moisturizing factor, *SRP* serine/arginine-rich protein

was observed to have a decreased capacity for inflammatory response [38, 41]. UV light reduced the quantity of epidermal Langerhans cells and induced proliferation of suppressor T cells, facilitating tumor induction [38, 41].

Histologically, corneocytes in sun-exposed areas become pleomorphic with increasing anomalies that include retention of nuclear remnants, loss of overlapping lines, and roughening of border edges [12, 85]. However, the most dramatic histological differences between photoaging and chronological aging occur in the dermis [90, 91]. UVA light penetrates more deeply (Fig. 4). Although it does not cause pronounced erythema, it may damage the dermis more than UVB light, as UVA radiation induces elafin expression in fibroblast, which inhibits proteolytic breakdown and leads to an accumulation of elastotic material in photodamaged skin [92]. The most prominent microscopic alteration in the structure of photodamaged dermis is the replacement of normal collagen fibers with large quantities of abnormal, thickened, tangled, nonfunctional elastic fibers, which finally degenerate into a nonfibrous, amorphous mass [93]. Damaged dermal tissue provides less support to its vasculature, causing vessels to widen and become visible at the skin surface as telangiectasia [8].

At the genetic level, UV exposure modulates expression of Collagen I, III, and VI genes, heat shock protein 47 (Hsp47) genes, and matrix metalloproteinase 1 (MMP 1), contributing to the general disruption of skin structure. Collagen I is time- and age-dependently reduced after single UV exposure in human skin in vivo [38, 80, 94]. Photoaging is associated with increased expression of MMP 1, MMP 9, as well as COX-2, all involved in degradation of skin structure [38, 95–105].

With acute sun exposure, genes with reparative, protective, or apoptotic functions, as well as stress communication genes, are rapidly activated [28, 106–109]. Aging strikingly increases the expression of these genes when exposed to UV [110].

Skin repair processes can repair UV damage as long as chronic exposure is avoided. With chronic ongoing insult, however, acute reversible effects become chronic degenerative changes that accumulate in the tissue over time [111–114].

Over the past several years, many advances in attempts to combat photoaging have been undertaken [108, 115–134]. For example, the combination of adipose-derived stem cells (ADSCs) and fractional CO_2 laser treatment improves healing of photoaging skin [130]. Also, red-orange extract intake can strengthen physiological antioxidant skin defenses, protecting skin from the damaging processes involved in photoaging and leading to an improvement in skin appearance and pigmentation [127]. Recent evidence from a randomized clinical trial showed that the application of retinoids might not only clinically and biochemically repair photoaged skin, but their use might also prevent photoaging [135].

Table 5 Comparing photoaging to intrinsic aging

Characteristic	Photoaging	Intrinsic aging	Reference
Overall			
Metabolic processes	Pronounced increase	Slow down	[191]
Clinical appearance	Nodular, leathery, blotchy	Smooth, unblemished	[54]
	Coarse wrinkles, furrows	Loss of elasticity, fine wrinkles	[54]
Skin color	Irregular pigmentation	Pigment diminishes to pallor	[28]
Skin surface marking	Markedly altered, often effaced	Maintains youthful geometric patterns	[29]
Onset	As early as late teens	Typically 50s–60s (women earlier than men)	[192]
Severity	Strongly associated with degree of pigmentation	Only slightly associated with degree of pigmentation	[28]
Gene expression			
SPR-2 (differentiation-associated protein)	Decreased	Dramatically increased	[193]
Interleukin-1 antagonist receptor	Decreased	Dramatically increased	[193]
Epidermis			
Thickness	Acanthropic in early stages	Thins with aging	[194]
	Atrophy in end stages		[195]
Proliferative rate	Higher than normal	Lower than normal	[195]
Keratinocytes	Atopic, with polarity loss and numerous dyskeratoses	Modest cellular irregularity	[196]
Dermo-epidermal junction	Extensive reduplication of lamina dense	Modest reduplication of lamina dense	[29]
Vitamin A content	Destroyed by sun exposure	Retinol content of plasma increases	[107]
Dermis			
Elastin	Marked elastogenesis followed by massive degeneration, dense accumulations on fibers	Elastogenesis followed by elastolysis – "moth-eaten fibers"	[196]
Elastin matrix	Massive increase in elastic fibers, replacing the collagenated dermal matrix	Gradual decline in production of dermal matrix, only modest increase in the number and thickness of elastic fibers in the reticular dermis	[88]
Lysozyme deposition on elastic fibers	Increased	Modest	[29]
Collagen production	Decrease in amounts of mature collagen	Mature collagen more stable to degradation	[195]
Glycosaminoglycan production	Great increase	No change	[195]
Grenz zone	Prominent	Absent	[195]
Microvasculature	Abnormal deposition of basement membrane-like material	Normal	[29]
Microcirculation	Vessels become dilated, deranged	Microvessels decrease, remaining vessels do not change	[29]
	Horizontal superficial plexus virtually destroyed	Horizontal superficial plexus largely undisturbed	[29]
Inflammatory response	Pronounced inflammation, perivenular, histiocytic-lymphocytic infiltrate	No inflammatory response observed	[29]

SRP serine/arginine-rich protein

One caveat to this discussion is that separating the effects of actinic damage from normal chronological degeneration of the skin over a lifetime can be difficult, as actinic effects are always superimposed on intrinsic changes [93]. The most common approach has been to compare exposed skin to unexposed skin at a different anatomic site, but constitutive anatomic differences may exist.

Pigmentation levels of black skin are photoprotective at all wavelengths of light [136], but white skin is transparent to both UV and visible wavelengths [137]. More UVA and UVB are reaching the dermal layer in white skin more than in black (Fig. 4). Consequently, racial differences in skin structure become more easily discerned as a result of photoaging. In whites, damage to the dermis is much more pronounced than in blacks, with focal areas of atrophy and necrosis [26]. The number of melanocytes decreases by as much as 20 % per decade after the age of 30 in all races, but whites, with limited melanin-based protection, become increasingly susceptible with age to photodamage. What is more, melanin distribution also becomes patchy, with some areas eventually having little or no protection [93, 138, 139].

Characteristics of photoaging as compared with intrinsic aging are in Table 5.

Pollution

Chemicals in smog created by fossil fuel emissions are chemically altered in sunlight, creating ozone [6, 140]. Ozone attacks the outer layers of the epidermis, depleting antioxidants like vitamin E and ascorbic acid (vitamin C) [141]. With the skin's endogenous antioxidants compromised, the skin is susceptible to oxidative damage [142, 143]. Cutaneous exposure to common chemical components of pollution has been demonstrated to induce morphological changes to epidermal structure [144, 145].

Conclusion

In barely more than 20 years, half of the population is expected to be older than 65 [86]. Patients in this age group typically have multiple dermatological disorders that require treatment [2]. The field of gerontological dermatology, therefore, will inevitably grow in size and importance. The challenge at the present time is not only to optimize treatment of the variety of dermatological disorders associated with old age but to gain understanding of the intrinsic and extrinsic mechanisms of skin aging in order to preserve the function and appearance of the integument into old age.

Skin aging depends on a combination of intrinsic and extrinsic factors. Most intrinsic factors cannot be avoided, but extrinsic factors, such as sun exposure and smoking, can be reduced or eliminated, with substantial impact on the visible appearance of the skin.

Greater understanding of the molecular processes which contribute to skin aging, as well as how lifestyle choices accelerate or impede those changes, may enable physicians in the future to prevent the underlying biological processes, improving both physical and psychological health for the increasing percentage of the population in the latter years of their lives.

In addition, because of the association between solar UV exposure and skin cancer, encouraging people to avoid detrimental behaviors such as sun tanning would promote a youthful appearance and reduce cancer-related mortality. This would be an important goal of patient education.

Cross-References

▸ Aging in Asian Skin
▸ Gender Differences in Skin

References

1. Arias E. United States life tables, 2002. Natl Vital Stat Rep. 2004; 53(6):1–38.
2. Kligman AM, Koblenzer C. Demographics and psychological implications for the aging population. Dermatol Clin. 1997;15:549–53.
3. Farage MA, Miller KW, Elsner P, et al. Structural characteristics of the aging skin: a review. Cutan Ocul Toxicol. 2007;26:343–57.
4. Ghersetich I, Troiano M, De Giorgi V, et al. Receptors in skin ageing and antiageing agents. Dermatol Clin. 2007;25:655–62.

5. Farage MA, Miller KW, Elsner P, et al. Intrinsic and extrinsic factors in skin ageing: a review. Int J Cosmet Sci. 2008;30:87–95.
6. Puizina-Ivić N. Skin aging. Acta Dermatovenerol Alp Panonica Adriat. 2008;17:47–54.
7. Koehler MJ, König K, Elsner P, et al. In vivo assessment of human skin aging by multiphoton laser scanning tomography. Opt Lett. 2006;31:2879–81.
8. McCallion R, Li Wan Po A. Dry and photo-aged skin: manifestations and management. J Clin Pharm Ther. 1993;18:15–32.
9. Helfrich YR, Sachs DL, Voorhees JJ. Overview of skin aging and photoaging. Dermatol Nurs. 2008;20:177–83. quiz 184.
10. Menon G, Ghadially R. Morphology of lipid alterations in the epidermis: a review. Microsc Res Tech. 1997;37:180–92.
11. Sjerobabski Masnec I, Poduje S. Photoaging. Coll Antropol. 2008;32 Suppl 2:177–80.
12. Grove GL. Physiologic changes in older skin. Clin Geriatr Med. 1989;5:115–25.
13. Gilchrest BA. The UV-induced SOS response: importance to aging skin. J Dermatol. 1998;25:775–7.
14. Landau M. Exogenous factors in skin aging. Curr Probl Dermatol. 2007;35:1–13.
15. Brincat MP. Hormone replacement therapy and the skin. Maturitas. 2000;35:107–17.
16. Stevenson S, Thornton J. Effect of estrogens on skin aging and the potential role of SERMs. Clin Interv Aging. 2007;2:283–97.
17. Eisenbeiss C, Welzel J, Schmeller W. The influence of female sex hormones on skin thickness: evaluation using 20 MHz sonography. Br J Dermatol. 1998;139:462–7.
18. Wines N, Willsteed E. Menopause and the skin. Australas J Dermatol. 2001;42:149–8. quiz 159.
19. Piérard GE. Ageing across the life span: time to think again. J Cosmet Dermatol. 2004;3:50–3.
20. Boyd AS, Morris LF, Phillips CM, et al. Psoriasis and pregnancy: hormone and immune system interaction. Int J Dermatol. 1996;35:169–72.
21. Weinstock MA. Epidemiologic investigation of nonmelanoma skin cancer mortality: the Rhode Island Follow-Back Study. J Invest Dermatol. 1994;102:6S–9.
22. Dao H Jr.; Kazin R. Gender differences in skin: a review of the literature. Gender Medicine 2007;4 (4):308–328.
23. Lagarde JM, Rouvrais C, Black D. Topography and anisotropy of the skin surface with ageing. Skin Res Technol. 2005;11:110–9.
24. Engeland CG, Bosch JA, Cacioppo JT, et al. Mucosal wound healing: the roles of age and sex. Arch Surg. 2006;141:1193–7. discussion 1198.
25. Miller JG, Mac Neil S. Gender and cutaneous melanoma. Br J Dermatol. 1997;136:657–65.
26. Rawlings AV. Ethnic skin types: are there differences in skin structure and function? Int J Cosmet Sci. 2006;28:79–93.
27. Robinson MK. Population differences in skin structure and physiology and the susceptibility to irritant and allergic contact dermatitis: implications for skin safety testing and risk assessment. Contact Dermatitis. 1999;41:65–79.
28. Rees JL. The genetics of sun sensitivity in humans. Am J Hum Genet. 2004;75:739–51.
29. Gilchrest BA. A review of skin ageing and its medical therapy. Br J Dermatol. 1996;135:867–75.
30. Asakura K, Nishiwaki Y, Milojevic A, et al. Lifestyle factors and visible skin aging in a population of Japanese elders. J Epidemiol. 2009;19:251–9.
31. Taylor SC. Skin of color: biology, structure, function, and implications for dermatologic disease. J Am Acad Dermatol. 2002;46:S41–62.
32. Tsukahara K, Fujimura T, Yoshida Y, et al. Comparison of age-related changes in wrinkling and sagging of the skin in Caucasian females and in Japanese females. J Cosmet Sci. 2004;55:351–71.
33. Chung JH. Photoaging in Asians. Photodermatol Photoimmunol Photomed. 2003;19:109–21.
34. Taylor SC. Utilizing combination therapy for ethnic skin. Cutis. 2007;80:15–20.
35. Diridollou S, de Rigal J, Querleux B, et al. Comparative study of the hydration of the stratum corneum between four ethnic groups: influence of age. Int J Dermatol. 2007;46 Suppl 1:11–4.
36. Waller JM, Maibach HI. Age and skin structure and function, a quantitative approach (I): blood flow, pH, thickness, and ultrasound echogenicity. Skin Res Technol. 2005;11:221–35.
37. Tagami H. Functional characteristics of the stratum corneum in photoaged skin in comparison with those found in intrinsic aging. Arch Dermatol Res. 2008;300 Suppl 1:S1–6.
38. Martini F. Fundamentals of anatomy and physiology. San Francisco: Benjamin-Cummings; 2004.
39. Neerken S, Lucassen GW, Bisschop MA, et al. Characterization of age-related effects in human skin: a comparative study that applies confocal laser scanning microscopy and optical coherence tomography. J Biomed Opt. 2004;9:274–81.
40. Elias PM. Stratum corneum architecture, metabolic activity and interactivity with subjacent cell layers. Exp Dermatol. 1996;5:191–201.
41. Fenske NA, Lober CW. Structural and functional changes of normal aging skin. J Am Acad Dermatol. 1986;15:571–85.
42. Wolff EF, Narayan D, Taylor HS. Long-term effects of hormone therapy on skin rigidity and wrinkles. Fertil Steril. 2005;84:285–8.
43. Berardesca E, de Rigal J, Leveque JL, et al. In vivo biophysical characterization of skin physiological differences in races. Dermatologica. 1991;182:89–93.
44. Stoebner P, Meunier L. Photoaging of face. Ann Dermatol Venereol. 2008;135:1S21–6.
45. Farage M, Maibach H. Lifetime changes in the vulva and vagina. Arch Gynecol Obstet. 2006;273: 195–202.

46. Elsner P, Wilhelm D, Maibach HI. Effect of low-concentration sodium lauryl sulfate on human vulvar and forearm skin. Age-related differences. J Reprod Med. 1991;36:77–81.
47. Kobayashi H, Tagami H. Distinct locational differences observable in biophysical functions of the facial skin: with special emphasis on the poor functional properties of the stratum corneum of the perioral region. Int J Cosmet Sci. 2004;26:91–101.
48. Caisey L, Gubanova E, Camus C, et al. Influence of age and hormone replacement therapy on the functional properties of the lips. Skin Res Technol. 2008;14:220–5.
49. Farage MA, Miller KW, Berardesca E, et al. Incontinence in the aged: contact dermatitis and other cutaneous consequences. Contact Dermatitis. 2007;57:211–7.
50. Brincat MP, Baron YM, Galea R. Estrogens and the skin. Climacteric. 2005;8:110–23.
51. Castelo-Branco C, Figueras F, Martínez de Osaba MJ, et al. Facial wrinkling in postmenopausal women. Effects of smoking status and hormone replacement therapy. Maturitas. 1998;29:75–86.
52. Wilhelm D, Elsner P, Maibach HI. Standardized trauma (tape stripping) in human vulvar and forearm skin. Effects on transepidermal water loss, capacitance and pH. Acta Derm Venereol. 1991;71:123–6.
53. Elsner P, Wilhelm D, Maibach HI. Sodium lauryl sulfate-induced irritant contact dermatitis in vulvar and forearm skin of premenopausal and postmenopausal women. J Am Acad Dermatol. 1990;23:648–52.
54. Glogau RG. Physiologic and structural changes associated with aging skin. Dermatol Clin. 1997;15:555–9.
55. Marren P, Wojnarowska F, Powell S. Allergic contact dermatitis and vulvar dermatoses. Br J Dermatol. 1992;126:52–6.
56. Purba MB, Kouris-Blazos A, Wattanapenpaiboon N, et al. Skin wrinkling: can food make a difference? J Am Coll Nutr. 2001;20:71–80.
57. Kohen R. Skin antioxidants: their role in aging and in oxidative stress – new approaches for their evaluation. Biomed Pharmacother. 1999;53:181–92.
58. Cimino F, Cristani M, Saija A, et al. Protective effects of a red orange extract on UVB-induced damage in human keratinocytes. Biofactors. 2007;30:129–38.
59. Schagen SK, Zampeli VA, Makrantonaki E, et al. Discovering the link between nutrition and skin aging. Dermatoendocrinol. 2012;4:298–307.
60. Cosgrove MC, Franco OH, Granger SP, et al. Dietary nutrient intakes and skin-aging appearance among middle-aged American women. Am J Clin Nutr. 2007;86:1225–31.
61. Latreille J, Kesse-Guyot E, Malvy D, et al. Dietary monounsaturated fatty acids intake and risk of skin photoaging. PLoS One. 2012;7, e44490.
62. Varani J, Warner RL, Gharaee-Kermani M, et al. Vitamin A antagonizes decreased cell growth and elevated collagen-degrading matrix metalloproteinases and stimulates collagen accumulation in naturally aged human skin. J Invest Dermatol. 2000;114:480–6.
63. Cho S, Lee DH, Won C, et al. Differential effects of low-dose and high-dose beta-carotene supplementation on the signs of photoaging and type I procollagen gene expression in human skin in vivo. Dermatology. 2010;221:160–71.
64. Rhodes LE, Durham BH, Fraser WD, et al. Dietary fish oil reduces basal and ultraviolet B-generated PGE2 levels in skin and increases the threshold to provocation of polymorphic light eruption. J Invest Dermatol. 1995;105:532–5.
65. Goode HF, Burns E, Walker BE. Vitamin C depletion and pressure sores in elderly patients with femoral neck fracture. BMJ. 1992;305:925–7.
66. Jackson SM, Williams ML, Feingold KR, et al. Pathobiology of the stratum corneum. West J Med. 1993;158:279–85.
67. Kennedy C, Bastiaens MT, Bajdik CD, et al. Effect of smoking and sun on the aging skin. J Invest Dermatol. 2003;120:548–54.
68. Leow YH, Maibach HI. Cigarette smoking, cutaneous vasculature, and tissue oxygen. Clin Dermatol. 1998;16:579–84.
69. Helfrich YR, Yu L, Ofori A, et al. Effect of smoking on aging of photoprotected skin: evidence gathered using a new photonumeric scale. Arch Dermatol. 2007;143:397–402.
70. Mosely LH, Finseth F. Cigarette smoking: impairment of digital blood flow and wound healing in the hand. Hand. 1977;9:97–101.
71. Wilson GR, Jones BM. The damaging effect of smoking on digital revascularisation: two further case reports. Br J Plast Surg. 1984;37:613–4.
72. Harris GD, Finseth F, Buncke HJ. The hazard of cigarette smoking following digital replantation. J Microsurg. 1980;1:403–4.
73. Riefkohl R, Wolfe JA, Cox EB, et al. Association between cutaneous occlusive vascular disease, cigarette smoking, and skin slough after rhytidectomy. Plast Reconstr Surg. 1986;77:592–5.
74. Goldminz D, Bennett RG. Cigarette smoking and flap and full-thickness graft necrosis. Arch Dermatol. 1991;127:1012–5.
75. Friedman O. Changes associated with the aging face. Facial Plast Surg Clin North Am. 2005;13:371–80.
76. Urbańska M, Nowak G, Florek E. Cigarette smoking and its influence on skin aging. Przegl Lek. 2012;69:1111–4.
77. WebRef.org. http://www.webref.org/cancer/p/pack_year.htm
78. Barland CO, Zettersten E, Brown BS, et al. Imiquimod-induced interleukin-1 alpha stimulation improves barrier homeostasis in aged murine epidermis. J Invest Dermatol. 2004;122:330–6.
79. Montagner S, Costa A. Molecular basis of photoaging. An Bras Dermatol. 2009;84:263–9.

80. Südel KM, Venzke K, Mielke H, et al. Novel aspects of intrinsic and extrinsic aging of human skin: beneficial effects of soy extract. Photochem Photobiol. 2005;81:581–7.
81. Green B, Bluth J. Measuring the chemosensory irritability of human skin. J Toxicol-Cutan Ocul Toxicol. 1995;14:23–48.
82. Chang KCN, Shen Q, Oh IG, et al. Liver X receptor is a therapeutic target for photoaging and chronological skin aging. Mol Endocrinol. 2008;22:2407–19.
83. Baumann L. Skin ageing and its treatment. J Pathol. 2007;211:241–51.
84. Reed JT, Elias PM, Ghadially R. Integrity and permeability barrier function of photoaged human epidermis. Arch Dermatol. 1997;133:395–6.
85. Bergfeld WF. The aging skin. Int J Fertil Womens Med. 1997;42:57–66.
86. Verdier-Sévrain S, Bonté F. Skin hydration: a review on its molecular mechanisms. J Cosmet Dermatol. 2007;6:75–82.
87. Fisher GJ, Varani J, Voorhees JJ. Looking older: fibroblast collapse and therapeutic implications. Arch Dermatol. 2008;144:666–72.
88. Hanson KM, Simon JD. Epidermal trans-urocanic acid and the UV-A-induced photoaging of the skin. Proc Natl Acad Sci U S A. 1998;95:10576–8.
89. Wu S, Li H, Zhang X, et al. Optical features for chronological aging and photoaging skin by optical coherence tomography. Lasers Med Sci. 2013;28:445–50.
90. Chung JH, Lee SH, Youn CS, et al. Cutaneous photodamage in Koreans: influence of sex, sun exposure, smoking, and skin color. Arch Dermatol. 2001;137:1043–51.
91. Amano S. Possible involvement of basement membrane damage in skin photoaging. J Investig Dermatol Symp Proc. 2009;14:2–7.
92. Schalkwijk J. Cross-linking of elafin/SKALP to elastic fibers in photodamaged skin: too much of a good thing? J Invest Dermatol. 2007;127:1286–7.
93. Wulf HC, Sandby-Møller J, Kobayasi T, et al. Skin aging and natural photoprotection. Micron. 2004;35:185–91.
94. Zhuo S, Zhu X, Chen J, et al. Quantitative biomarkers of human skin photoaging based on intrinsic second harmonic generation signal. Scanning. 2013;35:273–6.
95. Bernstein IA, Vaughan FL. Cultured keratinocytes in in vitro dermatotoxicological investigation: a review. J Toxicol Environ Health B Crit Rev. 1999;2:1–30.
96. Habib MA, Salem SAM, Hakim SA, et al. Comparative immunohistochemical assessment of cutaneous cyclooxygenase-2 enzyme expression in chronological aging and photoaging. Photodermatol Photoimmunol Photomed. 2014;30:43–51.
97. Latreille J, Ezzedine K, Elfakir A, et al. MC1R polymorphisms and facial photoaging. Ann Dermatol Venereol. 2011;138:385–9.
98. Hughes MC, Bredoux C, Salas F, et al. Comparison of histological measures of skin photoaging. Dermatology. 2011;223:140–51.
99. Elfakir A, Ezzedine K, Latreille J, et al. Functional MC1R-gene variants are associated with increased risk for severe photoaging of facial skin. J Invest Dermatol. 2010;130:1107–15.
100. Chang KCN, Wang Y, Oh IG, et al. Estrogen receptor beta is a novel therapeutic target for photoaging. Mol Pharmacol. 2010;77:744–50.
101. Rijken F, Bruijnzeel PLB. The pathogenesis of photoaging: the role of neutrophils and neutrophil-derived enzymes. J Investig Dermatol Symp Proc. 2009;14:67–72.
102. Quan T, Qin Z, Xia W, et al. Matrix-degrading metalloproteinases in photoaging. J Investig Dermatol Symp Proc. 2009;14:20–4.
103. Codriansky KA, Quintanilla-Dieck MJ, Gan S, et al. Intracellular degradation of elastin by cathepsin K in skin fibroblasts – a possible role in photoaging. Photochem Photobiol. 2009;85:1356–63.
104. Moriwaki S, Takahashi Y. Photoaging and DNA repair. J Dermatol Sci. 2008;50:169–76.
105. Iddamalgoda A, Le QT, Ito K, et al. Mast cell tryptase and photoaging: possible involvement in the degradation of extra cellular matrix and basement membrane proteins. Arch Dermatol Res. 2008;300 Suppl 1:S69–76.
106. Sauermann K, Jaspers S, Koop U, et al. Topically applied vitamin C increases the density of dermal papillae in aged human skin. BMC Dermatol. 2004;4:13.
107. Seité S, Bredoux C, Compan D, et al. Histological evaluation of a topically applied retinol-vitamin C combination. Skin Pharmacol Physiol. 2005;18:81–7.
108. Tewari A, Grys K, Kollet J, et al. Upregulation of MMP12 and its activity by UVA1 in human skin: potential implications for photoaging. J Invest Dermatol. 2014;134:2598.
109. Reimann V, Krämer U, Sugiri D, et al. Sunbed use induces the photoaging-associated mitochondrial common deletion. J Invest Dermatol. 2008;128:1294–7.
110. Sesto A, Navarro M, Burslem F, et al. Analysis of the ultraviolet B response in primary human keratinocytes using oligonucleotide microarrays. Proc Natl Acad Sci U S A. 2002;99:2965–70.
111. Ortonne J, Marks R. Photodamaged skin: clinical signs, causes and management. London: Martin Dunitz; 1999.
112. Oh J, Kim YK, Jung J, et al. Intrinsic aging- and photoaging-dependent level changes of glycosaminoglycans and their correlation with water content in human skin. J Dermatol Sci. 2011;62:192–201.
113. Green AC, Hughes MCB, McBride P, et al. Factors associated with premature skin aging (photoaging) before the age of 55: a population-based study. Dermatology. 2011;222:74–80.

114. Kim EJ, Kim M, Jin X, et al. Skin aging and photoaging alter fatty acids composition, including 11,14,17-cicosatrienoic acid, in the epidermis of human skin. J Korean Med Sci. 2010;25:980–3.
115. Guimarães COZ, Miot HA, Bagatin E. Five percent 5-fluorouracil in a cream or for superficial peels in the treatment of advanced photoaging of the forearms: a randomized comparative study. Dermatol Surg. 2014;40:610–7.
116. Han A, Chien AL, Kang S. Photoaging. Dermatol Clin. 2014;32:291–9.
117. Herane MI, Orlandi C, Zegpi E, et al. Clinical efficacy of adapalene (differin(®)) 0.3% gel in Chilean women with cutaneous photoaging. J Dermatolog Treat. 2012;23:57–64.
118. Iannacone MR, Hughes MC, Green AC. Effects of sunscreen on skin cancer and photoaging. Photodermatol Photoimmunol Photomed. 2014;30:55–61.
119. Ji J, Zhang L, Ding H, et al. Comparison of 5-aminolevulinic acid photodynamic therapy and red light for treatment of photoaging. Photodiagnosis Photodyn Ther. 2014;11:118–21.
120. Lin R, Feng X, Li C, et al. Prevention of UV radiation-induced cutaneous photoaging in mice by topical administration of patchouli oil. J Ethnopharmacol. 2014;154:408–18.
121. Permatasari F, Hu Y, Zhang J, et al. Anti-photoaging potential of Botulinum Toxin Type A in UVB-induced premature senescence of human dermal fibroblasts in vitro through decreasing senescence-related proteins. J Photochem Photobiol B. 2014;133:115–23.
122. Tanaka YT, Tanaka K, Kojima H, et al. Cynaropicrin from Cynara scolymus L. suppresses photoaging of skin by inhibiting the transcription activity of nuclear factor-kappa B. Bioorg Med Chem Lett. 2013;23:518–23.
123. Asadamongkol B, Zhang JH. The development of hyperbaric oxygen therapy for skin rejuvenation and treatment of photoaging. Med Gas Res. 2014;4:7.
124. Chen C, Chiang A, Liu H, et al. EGb-761 prevents ultraviolet B-induced photoaging via inactivation of mitogen-activated protein kinases and proinflammatory cytokine expression. J Dermatol Sci. 2014;75:55–62.
125. Fabi SG, Goldman MP. Comparative study of hydroquinone-free and hydroquinone-based hyperpigmentation regimens in treating facial hyperpigmentation and photoaging. J Drugs Dermatol. 2013;12:S32–7.
126. Pickett A. Comments on "Anti-photoaging potential of Botulinum Toxin Type A in UVB-induced premature senescence of human dermal fibroblasts in vitro through decreasing senescence-related proteins". J Photochem Photobiol B. 2014;138:355.
127. Puglia C, Offerta A, Saija A, et al. Protective effect of red orange extract supplementation against UV-induced skin damages: photoaging and solar lentigines. J Cosmet Dermatol. 2014;13:151–7.
128. Rabello-Fonseca RM, Azulay DR, Luiz RR, et al. Oral isotretinoin in photoaging: clinical and histopathological evidence of efficacy of an off-label indication. J Eur Acad Dermatol Venereol. 2009;23:115–23.
129. Sachs DL, Kang S, Hammerberg C, et al. Topical fluorouracil for actinic keratoses and photoaging: a clinical and molecular analysis. Arch Dermatol. 2009;145:659–66.
130. Xu X, Wang H, Zhang Y, et al. Adipose-derived stem cells cooperate with fractional carbon dioxide laser in antagonizing photoaging: a potential role of Wnt and β-catenin signaling. Cell Biosci. 2014;4:24.
131. Mezzana P. "Multi Light and Drugs": a new technique to treat face photoaging. Comparative study with photorejuvenation. Lasers Med Sci. 2008;23:149–54.
132. Tanaka K, Asamitsu K, Uranishi H, et al. Protecting skin photoaging by NF-kappaB inhibitor. Curr Drug Metab. 2010;11:431–5.
133. Li Y, Wu Y, Wei H, et al. Protective effects of green tea extracts on photoaging and photommunosuppression. Skin Res Technol. 2009;15:338–45.
134. Kim W, Park B, Sung J. Protective role of adipose-derived stem cells and their soluble factors in photoaging. Arch Dermatol Res. 2009;301:329–36.
135. Serri R, Iorizzo M. Cosmeceuticals: focus on topical retinoids in photoaging. Clin Dermatol. 2008;26:633–5.
136. Kaidbey KH, Agin PP, Sayre RM, et al. Photoprotection by melanin – a comparison of black and Caucasian skin. J Am Acad Dermatol. 1979;1:249–60.
137. Pathak M, Fitzpatrick T. The role of natural photoprotective agent in human skin. In: Fitzpatrick T, Pathak MA, Harver LC, Seiji M, Kukita A, editors. The role of natural photoprotective agent in human skin. Tokyo: University of Tokyo Press; 1974.
138. Peres PS, Terra VA, Guarnier FA, et al. Photoaging and chronological aging profile: understanding oxidation of the skin. J Photochem Photobiol B. 2011;103:93–7.
139. Shin M, Jeong K, Oh I, et al. Clinical features of idiopathic guttate hypomelanosis in 646 subjects and association with other aspects of photoaging. Int J Dermatol. 2011;50:798–805.
140. Lanuti EL, Kirsner RS. Effects of pollution on skin aging. J Invest Dermatol. 2010;130:2696.
141. Xu F, Yan S, Wu M, et al. Ambient ozone pollution as a risk factor for skin disorders. Br J Dermatol. 2011;165:224–5.
142. Romieu I, Castro-Giner F, Kunzli N, et al. Air pollution, oxidative stress and dietary supplementation: a review. Eur Respir J. 2008;31:179–97.
143. Zussman J, Ahdout J, Kim J. Vitamins and photoaging: do scientific data support their use? J Am Acad Dermatol. 2010;63:507–25.

144. Giacomoni PU, Rein G. Factors of skin ageing share common mechanisms. Biogerontology. 2001;2:219–29.
145. Vierkötter A. Environmental pollution and skin aging. Hautarzt. 2011;62:577–8.
146. Freeman R, Cockerell E, Armstrong J, et al. Sunlight as a factor influencing the thickness of epidermis. J Invest Dermatol. 1962;39:295–8.
147. Thomson ML. Relative efficiency of pigment and horny layer thickness in protecting the skin of Europeans and Africans against solar ultraviolet radiation. J Physiol. 1955;127:236–46.
148. Weigand DA, Gaylor JR. Irritant reaction in Negro and Caucasian skin. South Med J. 1974;67:548–51.
149. Reinertson RP, Wheatley VR. Studies on the chemical composition of human epidermal lipids. J Invest Dermatol. 1959;32:49–59.
150. Johnson LC, Corah NL. Racial differences in skin resistance. Science. 1963;139:766–7.
151. Corcuff P, Lotte C, Rougier A, et al. Racial differences in corneocytes. A comparison between black, white and oriental skin. Acta Derm Venereol. 1991;71:146–8.
152. Warrier A, Kligman AM, Harpert R, et al. A comparison of black and white skin using noninvasive methods. J Soc Cosmet Chem. 1996;47:229–40.
153. Sugino K, Imokawa G, Maibach H. Ethnic difference of stratum corneum lipid in prelation to stratum corneum function. J Invest Dermatol. 1993;100:587. [Abstract 594].
154. Kim MM, Byrne PJ. Facial skin rejuvenation in the Asian patient. Facial Plast Surg Clin North Am. 2007;15:381–6.
155. Kelly AP. Aesthetic considerations in patients of color. Dermatol Clin. 1997;15:687–93.
156. Szabo G, Gerald A. The ultrastructure of facial color difference in man. In: Riley V, editor. The ultrastructure of facial color difference in man. New York: Appleton-Century Crofts; 1972.
157. Berardesca E, Maibach H. Racial differences in skin pathophysiology. J Am Acad Dermatol. 1996;34:667–72.
158. Bronaugh RL, Stewart RF, Simon M. Methods for in vitro percutaneous absorption studies. VII: use of excised human skin. J Pharm Sci. 1986;75:1094–7.
159. Hymes J, Spraker M. Racial differences in the effectiveness of a topically applied mixture of local anesthetics. Reg Anesth. 1986;11:11–3.
160. Wedig JH, Maibach HI. Percutaneous penetration of dipyrithione in man: effect of skin color (race). J Am Acad Dermatol. 1981;5:433–8.
161. Guy RH, Tur E, Bjerke S, et al. Are there age and racial differences to methyl nicotinate-induced vasodilatation in human skin? J Am Acad Dermatol. 1985;12:1001–6.
162. Berardesca E, Maibach HI. Racial differences in pharmacodynamic response to nicotinates in vivo in human skin: black and white. Acta Derm Venereol. 1990;70:63–6.
163. Kompaore F, Marty JP, Dupont C. In vivo evaluation of the stratum corneum barrier function in blacks, Caucasians and Asians with two noninvasive methods. Skin Pharmacol. 1993;6:200–7.
164. Wilson D, Berardesca E, Maibach HI. In vitro transepidermal water loss: differences between black and white human skin. Br J Dermatol. 1988;119:647–52.
165. Berardesca E, Maibach HI. Racial differences in sodium lauryl sulphate induced cutaneous irritation: black and white. Contact Dermatitis. 1988;18: 65–70.
166. Reed JT, Ghadially R, Elias PM. Skin type, but neither race nor gender, influence epidermal permeability barrier function. Arch Dermatol. 1995;131: 1134–8.
167. Marshall E, Lynch V, Smith H. Variation in susceptibility of the skin to dichlorethylsulfide. J Pharmacol Exp Ther. 1919;12:291–301.
168. Weigand D, Mershon M. The cutaneous irritant reaction to agent O-chlorobenzylidene malonitrile (CS); quantitation and racial influence in human subjects. 1970.
169. Robinson MK. Population differences in acute skin irritation responses. Race, sex, age, sensitive skin and repeat subject comparisons. Contact Dermatitis. 2002;46:86–93.
170. Frosch P, Kligman A. A method for appraising the stinging capacity of topically applied substances. J Soc Cosmet Chem. 1981;28:197–209.
171. Aramaki J, Kawana S, Effendy I, et al. Differences of skin irritation between Japanese and European women. Br J Dermatol. 2002;146:1052–6.
172. Foy V, Weinkauf R, Whittle E, et al. Ethnic variation in the skin irritation response. Contact Dermatitis. 2001;45:346–9.
173. Anderson RR, Parrish JA. The optics of human skin. J Invest Dermatol. 1981;77:13–9.
174. McCurdy J. Cosmetic surgery of the Asian face. In: Paper I, editor. Cosmetic surgery of the Asian face. New York: Thieme; 2002.
175. Nouveau-Richard S, Yang Z, Mac-Mary S, et al. Skin ageing: a comparison between Chinese and European populations. A pilot study. J Dermatol Sci. 2005;40:187–93.
176. Edwards RR, Fillingim RB. Ethnic differences in thermal pain responses. Psychosom Med. 1999;61:346–54.
177. Doshi DN, Hanneman KK, Cooper KD. Smoking and skin aging in identical twins. Arch Dermatol. 2007;143:1543–6.
178. Rexbye H, Petersen I, Johansens M, et al. Influence of environmental factors on facial ageing. Age Ageing. 2006;35:110–5.
179. Morita A. Tobacco smoke causes premature skin aging. J Dermatol Sci. 2007;48:169–75.
180. Lahmann C, Bergemann J, Harrison G, et al. Matrix metalloproteinase-1 and skin ageing in smokers. Lancet. 2001;357:935–6.

181. Boyd AS, Stasko T, King LEJ, et al. Cigarette smoking-associated elastotic changes in the skin. J Am Acad Dermatol. 1999;41:23–6.
182. Smith JB, Fenske NA. Cutaneous manifestations and consequences of smoking. J Am Acad Dermatol. 1996;34:717–32. quiz 733–4.
183. Koh JS, Kang H, Choi SW, et al. Cigarette smoking associated with premature facial wrinkling: image analysis of facial skin replicas. Int J Dermatol. 2002;41:21–7.
184. van Adrichem LN, Hovius SE, van Strik R, et al. Acute effects of cigarette smoking on microcirculation of the thumb. Br J Plast Surg. 1992;45:9–11.
185. Bornmyr S, Svensson H. Thermography and laser-Doppler flowmetry for monitoring changes in finger skin blood flow upon cigarette smoking. Clin Physiol. 1991;11:135–41.
186. Richardson DR. Effects of habitual tobacco smoking on reactive hyperemia in the human hand. Arch Environ Health. 1985;40:114–9.
187. Jensen JA, Goodson WH, Hopf HW, et al. Cigarette smoking decreases tissue oxygen. Arch Surg. 1991;126:1131–4.
188. Fiers SA. Breaking the cycle: the etiology of incontinence dermatitis and evaluating and using skin care products. Ostomy Wound Manage. 1996;42:32–4. 36, 38–40, passim.
189. Fisher GJ, Wang ZQ, Datta SC, et al. Pathophysiology of premature skin aging induced by ultraviolet light. N Engl J Med. 1997;337:1419–28.
190. Yin L, Morita AT, Suji T. Skin aging induced by ultraviolet exposure and tobacco smoking: evidence from epidemiological and molecular studies. Photodermatol Photoimmunol Photomed. 2001;17:178–83.
191. Soter NA. Acute effects of ultraviolet radiation on the skin. Semin Dermatol. 1990;9:11–5.
192. Kligman AM. The treatment of photoaged human skin by topical tretinoin. Drugs. 1989;38:1–8.
193. Garmyn M, Yaar M, Boileau N, et al. Effect of aging and habitual sun exposure on the genetic response of cultured human keratinocytes to solar-simulated irradiation. J Invest Dermatol. 1992;99:743–8.
194. Takema Y, Yorimoto Y, Kawai M, et al. Age-related changes in the elastic properties and thickness of human facial skin. Br J Dermatol. 1994;131:641–8.
195. Lavker RM. Cutaneous aging: chronologic versus photoaging. In: Gilchrest B, editor. Cutaneous aging: chronologic versus photoaging. Cambridge: Blackwell Science; 1995.
196. Kligman A, Lavker R. Cutaneous aging: the differences between intrinsic aging and photoaging. J Cutan Aging Cosmet Dermatol. 1988;1:5–12.

Gender Differences in Skin

128

Christina Phuong and Howard I. Maibach

Contents

C. Phuong (✉)
Department of Dermatology, University of California San Francisco, San Francisco, CA, USA
e-mail: cphuong49@gmail.com

H.I. Maibach
Department of Dermatology, University of California, San Francisco, CA, USA
e-mail: maibachh@derm.ucsf.edu

M.A. Farage et al. (eds.), *Textbook of Aging Skin*,
DOI 10.1007/978-3-662-47398-6_93

Abstract

Genetic differences between men and women are the cause of many phenotypic and functional differences. In addition, men and women generally lead different lifestyles. How this affects various aspects of aging skin is an extensive area of study. Analyzing gender's influence in characteristics of the skin, including structural and anatomical characteristics, biochemical composition, mechanical properties, and skin color, has been a primary topic. Homeostatic and functional variations such as in sweat rate, blood flow, pH, sensory response, response to irritants, and reparative abilities affect the integrity of the skin. In addition, there are many hormone-dependent mechanisms related to the skin, thereby suggesting sex-based differences of these mechanisms. Seasonal variation, also, alters skin physiology. Taken together, research suggests gender does, indeed, affect skin properties. However, some studies report no difference or contradicting results. This is likely due to varied experimental designs. Thus, emphasis should be placed on maintaining standard methods for results to be comparable and taking note of parameters such as types of population, age, lifestyle, and environment. Overall, elucidating which aspects of aging skin are affected and how they are affected will improve sex-specific approaches toward skin care treatment.

Introduction

In order to intervene in skin aging, one must first have knowledge of the intricacies of gender-related skin differences. That men and women are genetically different goes without saying. How this affects phenotypic and functional differences between the sexes has been a topic much researched. In studying the skin, consideration is warranted as to the role that genetic and sex-specific environmental exposures may play in cutaneous appearance and structure. Environmental and occupational exposures are likely dictated by the social culture and biases therein that characterize each sex's experience. These differences are biologically important as they can affect the interpretation of various skin examinations and the therapeutic decision-making process. The importance of sex-specific treatment of aging skin continues to be elucidated.

Structural and Anatomical Characteristics

Skin thickness has been measured using echographic evaluation, ultrasonic echography, optical coherence tomography, X-ray, and histological analysis. Men have thicker skin than women across all age ranges [1–4], but no difference exists between men and women regarding the thickness of the stratum corneum [3, 5] or of the epidermis [6, 7]. Both men and women experience thinning of the epidermis and dermis with increasing age [4, 7, 8]. Hormone treatment in postmenopausal women increases dermal thickness [9, 10] as well as the number of collagen fibers [10, 11]. Both sexes show decreasing collagen content of the skin with age with the same rate of collagen loss, but total skin collagen content is less in women than men at all ages [8]. The evolutionary significance of these differences requires explanation.

The distribution of body fat differs between sexes for both obese and nonobese individuals [12]. Men tend to accumulate fat in the upper body and abdomen whereas women tend to accumulate fat in the lower body, particularly in the gluteal and upper portions of the legs [13]. In a cohort of more than 2,000 subjects aged 6–18, there was no difference between the sexes up to age 12 in fat distribution. After age 12, the relative mass of the subcutaneous fat continued to increase only in females [14]. In addition to the distribution, the amount of fat differs between men and women. Japanese women aged 18–22 had greater subcutaneous fat thickness than men [15]. Regarding skin fold thickness, the use of a caliper demonstrated that forearm measurements were thinner in women than men starting at age 35 [16], whereas another study found women to have thinner skin fold thickness at the forearm, thigh, and calf in a younger age range of 17–24 years [17]. The evolutionary significance and mechanism remain elusive (Table 1).

Biochemical Composition

Past studies found no difference in casual sebum levels between men and women measured at multiple anatomical locations [18–20]. However, in 2006, casual sebum levels, determined with a sebumeter in 46 Korean women and 37 Korean men, were higher in men at five facial sites sampled [21]. Again, in a study of 60 Korean participants, males had significantly higher casual sebum secretion at all facial sites tested [22]. Further, in a larger study of 713 subjects, males tended to have higher sebum content than females at both the forehead and, less dramatically, at the forearm. Sebum levels increased significantly in both genders after the age of 12 and reached comparable peak values. However, women reached their peak about a decade earlier, around the age of 40 [23]. In another study with 300 participants, sebum levels at the forehead were significantly higher in males compared with females at every age group. At the cheek, levels were significantly higher for those over 50 years of age. In males, sebum levels at the forehead increased slightly with age and stayed the same at the cheek. In females, sebum levels at both sites decreased with age after 40 [24]. Thus, it seems that age affects sebum secretion differently at different anatomical sites in males and females but data indicates generally higher sebum content in males than females.

Stratum corneum sphingolipid composition had significant age-related differences in women but not men. Ceramides 3 and 6 decreased from prepuberty to adulthood along with an increase in ceramides 1 and 2. Ceramide 2 decreased and ceramide 3 increased following maturity [25]. The total skin surface lipid content was lower on the forehead, postauricular area, and dorsal forearm in women as compared to men [26].

Sex was demonstrated to be a factor in the quantity and population characteristics of the normal flora of the skin. Women carried fewer organisms than men and the prevalence of specific organisms differed between the sexes [27, 28].

Metal content of human hair was found to differ in women but not men in regard to age. Women's hair had a greater copper concentration than men's which increased with age in women only [29]. Again, the evolutionary significance of these differences mandates explanation, as they might have functional and mechanistic significance (Table 2).

Mechanical Properties

Results have been diverse from studies seeking to determine if sex is a primary determinant in the barrier function of the skin. Men had greater transepidermal water loss (TEWL) values than women [20, 30–33], or no difference existed between sexes [18, 19, 34]. Following 5 days of topical caffeine application, 6 of 9 men experienced decreased TEWL values whereas 0 of the 7 women studied did [32]. It was hypothesized that androgens are damaging to barrier function through their ability to increase cAMP levels. Because caffeine antagonizes the effects that androgens have on cAMP, its application decreased the negative effects of androgens, demonstrated by decreased TEWL measurements. Another study showed men had significantly lower TEWL than women between the ages of 20–49, but differences assimilated after 50 at all locations except the forearm [24]. Gender has been reported to have varying results on TEWL, if any. Thus, a more systematic method is necessary to reduce the number of variables affecting results.

In the past, a difference in skin hydration and moisture has not been demonstrated between the sexes [19, 35, 36]. A study in 2009 showed that there was no generalized difference between sexes; however, differences existed at certain age groups and at certain locations. In both sexes, hydration typically increased with age and peaks around the age of 40–50 before decreasing. On the forehead, males had significantly higher hydration levels than women. Males also showed more variation with age at the forearm [23]. This study showed that both sexes typically follow the same

Table 1 Structure and anatomy (Adapted with permission from Tur E [12])

Findings [reference]	Obtained by	Subjects	Conclusions
Significant differences			
Women with thinner skin than men, except for the lower back of young subjects [1]	Echographic evaluation	24 women, 24 men; half 27–31 years, half 60–90 years	
Women's skin thinner than men's across entire age range of 5–90 years [2]	Ultrasonic echography	69 women, 54 men; 5–90 years	
Cellular epidermis thicker in men than women [3]	Histologic analysis	37 women, 34 men; 20–68 years. Skin types II–IV. Smoking status: 32 never, 27 previous, 12 current	
Men with thicker epidermis than women in the age group 50–60 years; men with thicker dermis in the age groups 20–30 and 70–80 years [4]	Histologic analysis	34 women, 30 men; 20–80 years	
Men and women with decreasing epidermal thickness with increasing age between 20–50 years. Men and women with decreasing dermal thickness between 20–40 years [4]	Histologic analysis	34 women, 30 men; 20–80 years	
Skin thickness constant in women up to the fifth decade then decreased with advancing age. Skin thickness of men decreased steadily with increasing age [8]	Chemical and histological analysis of skin collagen, skin thickness, and collagen density	Collagen: 80 women, 79 men; 15–93 years. Thickness: 107 women, 90 men; 12–93 years. Density: 26 women, 27 men; 15–93 years	Total skin collagen content is greater in men than women at all ages, though the rate of collagen loss is the same in men and women
Dermal thickening after 12 months estrogen therapy [9]	Conjugated estrogen therapy	28 estrogen, 26 placebo; women 51–71 years	Skin thickness affected by estrogens
Greater collagen content in hormone-treated women vs. non-treated women. Inverse relationship between collagen content and increasing years since menopause in the untreated group. Greater skin thickness in hormone-treated group vs. non-treated group [10]	Histologic analysis X-ray	108 postmenopausal women; 52 treated with estradiol and testosterone for 2–10 years, 66 no treatment	
Increased number of collagen fibers in the hormone-treated group 6 months posttreatment, no change in the placebo group. No change in epidermal thickness, keratin thickness, and elastic fiber content for both groups [11]	Histological analysis	41 postmenopausal women: 21 estradiol and cyproterone acetate treatment, 20 placebo	Hormone treatment increases collagen fiber content in postmenopausal women

(*continued*)

Table 1 (continued)

Findings [reference]	Obtained by	Subjects	Conclusions
Women with greater lipoprotein lipase activity. Women with greater values in the gluteus; men with greater values in the abdomen [13]	Hybridization and Northern blot of lipoprotein lipase activity and mRNA levels	8 women, 11 men; 33–41 years	Fat distribution and total fat content might be affected by regional sex differences in lipoprotein lipase activity. Variation at mRNA and post-translational level
Up to 12 years of age boys and girls both with greater than threefold increase in subcutaneous fat and less than doubling of internal fat mass. Girls only with increased relative mass of subcutaneous fat after the age of 12 [14]	Caliper	1,292 women, 1,008 men; 6–18 years	
Women's subcutaneous fat thicker than men's [15]	Caliper, ultrasound	45 women, 41 men; Japanese. 18–22 years	
Starting at age 35 women have thinner forearm skin than men. Forearm skinfold thickness decreases starting at age 35 in women and age 45 in men [16]	Caliper	145 women and men; 8–89 years	
Lower skinfold thickness in women at the thigh, calf and forearm [17]	Caliper	42 women, 37 men; 17–24 years	
No significant differences			
No difference between men and women in thickness of stratum corneum [3]	Histologic analysis	37 women, 34 men; 20–68 years. Skin types II–IV. Smoking status: 32 never, 27 previous, 12 current	
No difference in the number of cell layers in the stratum corneum between men and women. Both men and women with slightly increasing numbers of cell layers in the stratum corneum with increasing age [5]	Histologic analysis	158 men, 143 women; Japanese. 1–97 years	
No difference in the thickness of the epidermis between men and women [6]	Ultrasound	29 men, 61 women; Caucasian. 18–94 years. Skin type I–III	
No difference in skin thickness between men and women at five anatomic sites, except for women's skin thinner on the forehead than men in the older group. Thinner epidermal thickness at all six sampled sites in the older group of both men and women compared to the younger group [7]	Optical coherence tomography	Young: 13 women, 17 men; 20–40 years; Caucasian. Old: 17 women, 24 men; 60–80 years, Caucasian. "Ethnic group": 6 women, 6 men; 20–40 years. Skin types IV–VI	

Table 2 Biochemical composition (Adapted with permission from Tur E [12])

Findings	Obtained by	Subjects	Conclusions
Significant differences			
Casual sebum levels higher in men than women at five facial sites [21]	Sebumeter	46 women, 21–37 years; 37 men, 23–39 years; Korean	
Sebum levels higher in men than women at five facial sites tested [22]	Sebumeter	30 women, 30 men	
Sebum levels higher in men than women on the forehead and forearm [23]	Sebum Cassette	385 women, 328 men; age ranges 0–12, 13–35, 36–50, 51–70, over 70	Changes in sebum content reached comparable maximums but at different ranges – 40s in women, 50s in men
Sebum levels higher in men than women. Sebum levels in women decrease with age and increases or remains the same in men as they age [24]	Sebumeter	150 women, 150 men; age range 20–74	
In women but not men, stratum corneum sphingolipid composition differs with age [25]	Ethanolic extracts, biochemical methods of lipid identification	27 women, 26 men; 10–79 years	Stratum corneum sphingolipids influenced by female hormones
Women with lower skin surface lipid on the forehead and forearm and postauricularly [26]	Sebumeter	7 women, 23–26 years; 7 women, 72–77 years. 7 men, 28–29 years; 8 men 71–75 years	
Greater metal concentration in women's hair. Copper concentrations increase in women with increasing age but not in men [27]	Liquid chromatography, trace metal determination	60 women, 72 men; 6–40 years	
Prevalence of specific microorganisms considered to be normal flora different for men and women [28]	Microorganism culture of biologic samples	50 premature infants. 51 healthy babies; 4–7 days old. 80 children; 3–12 years. 166 healthy adults; 18–45 years. 63 adults; >60 years	Age and sex affect composition of skin normal flora
Women with fewer microorganisms than men in the the groin, axilla, and thigh [29]	Microorganism culture of biologic samples	8 men, 8 women	Sex affects composition of skin flora
No significant differences			
No difference between men and women in casual sebum level [18]	Sebumeter	7 men, 7 women; mean 27 years. 7 men, 8 women; mean 70.5 years	
No difference between men and women in sebum rate [19]	Sebumeter	6 women, 6 men; 23–25 years. Skin types II–III	
Although slightly higher, sebum levels in males were not significantly higher than females [20]	Sebumeter	5 women and 5 men in each age group:10–20, 20–30, 30–40, 40–50, 50–60 years old	

trend with age; however, absolute level values in each age group and at different locations differ depending on gender. This group also found that on the forehead, there was a significant positive correlation between sebum content and SC hydration only in females [23]. Thus, more investigation into the relation between sebum content and SC hydration is necessary, as well as how gender may affect these properties. A study in 2013 showed that SC hydration is stable or increasing with age in women but is decreasing with age in men at most locations. Further, aside from the hands, SC hydration was significantly higher in males from 20 to 39 years of age than females of the same age. Women displayed highest hydration levels at the cheek while men displayed highest levels at the neck [24]. While these data indicate phenotypic differences in SC hydration based on gender and age, the differences vary depending on location tested; therefore, conclusive trends cannot be made and much remains to be understood.

Tissue dielectric constant (TDC) provides an indicator of tissue water content. TDC values at the forearm were about 13 % greater for men than women [37]. TDC values at the forehead, cheek, and forearm were significantly higher in males than females [38]. Because TDC values are likely to be related to skin thickness, which is widely accepted to be thicker in men than women, these absolute TDC values cannot be directly correlated with relative local skin tissue water differences and must be corrected for.

In vivo and in vitro data, respectively, found adhesion of the stratum corneum greater in women than in men [39], or no difference existed [40]. In vivo adhesion properties were assessed by measuring the speed of blister formation induced by controlled suction [39]. Women exhibited longer blistering times than men in the age range of 15–69, after which the difference dissipated. In vitro analysis of skin biopsies from multiple sites did not reveal any difference in stratum corneum adhesion between men and women [40].

Frictional properties as measured by a friction meter [34], skin elasticity as measured by two suction cup methods [41], and torsional extensibility as measured by a twistometer, did not produce differing results between men and women [2]. In general accordance with these data, skin elasticity measured by a handheld probe demonstrated that at 9 of 11 sampled anatomical sites, no difference exists between the sexes, except at the volar forearm and forehead. The ratio between viscoelastic properties of the skin and immediate distention was greater in men at the forearm at a load of 500 mbar. The ability of the skin to return to its original position after deformation, as estimated by the ratio between immediate retraction and total distention, was greater in men than in women at the forehead [42]. Firooz et al. reported higher skin elasticity in females measured with a cutometer, although results were not statistically significant [20].

Another study accessed skin elasticity by measuring cutaneous resonance running time (CRRT) in various directions on the left dorsal hand, forehead, and left canthus using a reviscometer. On the hand and canthus, CRRTs were shorter, longer, or had no difference in females compared to males depending on age group, direction, and location. Further, while CRRT values generally decrease with age, some directions measured on the hand and canthus showed more significant reductions in one sex; on the forehead, no significant differences between genders were observed [43]. This study demonstrated directional differences in skin elasticity due to age, gender, and site.

Measurements of the foot demonstrated that the rate of stretch on traction, estimated from the series elastic element (SEE), was greater in women than in men. Conversely, the SEE on retraction was greater for men than for women on the foot. Skin plasticity of the foot was greater in women than in men [44]. Likewise, following hydration, skin extensibility found to be identical at baseline between the sexes increased in women only. It is inferred that hydration softens the stratum corneum, allowing the thickness of the dermis to be the primary determinant in extensibility. In this situation, the thinner dermis of women allowed for a rapid extensibility of female skin [45].

Venkatesan and Barlow combined a reflection-dependent fiber-optic displacement sensor with a pneumatic stimulator for real-time investigation of mechanical properties of glabrous skin.

Women demonstrated greater skin displacement than men in response to TAC-Cell stimulus pressure, further confirmed by power spectrum analysis [46] (Table 3).

Functional Differences

Eccrine Sweating

Men have greater sweat rates compared to women [35, 47–49]. This has been found to be true across all age ranges and stages of sexual maturity [48]. Prepubertal and pubertal boys as well as adult men were found to have higher mean sweat rates when compared to girls and adult women in like age groups. For males, sweat rate increased with increasing age whereas in females, adult women had lower mean sweat rates than pubertal and prepubertal girls. This is challenged by one study, which found that when anthropometric variables were accounted for, the greater sweat rate for men no longer existed [50]. This same study concluded that a greater overall sweat production for men was associated with a greater total sweat lactate production, but the lactate concentration did not differ between the sexes as it was proportional in both men and women to total sweat production. A more recent study using methacholine (MCh) and acetylcholine (ACh) as sweat stimuli showed that given higher concentrations, men have increased sweat rates than women. However, females had greater active sweat glands, thereby suggesting that their sweat gland output rate was lower compared to men. Further, as mean body temperature increased, men exhibited greater sweat rate and sweat gland output than women, while the number of active sweat glands was similar [51]. The log concentrations of the agonist causing 50 % of the maximal response were similar between the sexes. Taken together, these results suggest that sex differences in sweating are a result of lower maximum sweating capacity of female sweat glands and not a difference in cholinergic sensitivity of the sweat gland [51]. Evolutionary mechanisms and significance have not been explored.

pH

The pH of the skin has been measured at multiple different sites in men and women with varying results in regard to gender differences. Measurements taken from the volar forearm have revealed no difference between men and women [18], men with lower mean pH values than women [19, 52], and women with lower mean pH values than men [53]. Similarly, measurements from the axilla have produced results of no difference between the sexes [54] or women with lower baseline pH values than men [55]. Men were also found to have lower pH values at five different facial sites sampled as compared to women. In a study of 713 participants, no significant differences in pH were found with age for women at the forearm and forehead, except pH values were significantly lower at the forehead in the 0–12 age group. Overall, there was a positive linear correlation between skin surface pH and age in both sexes. In addition, pH levels on the forehead of females aged 13–70 and at the forearm of those aged 0–12, 36–50, and 51–70 were significantly higher than that in males in the same age group [23]. Another study showed that the pH of men was significantly lower than that of women and generally increased with age, whereas women's pH generally decreased with age [24]. In acne patients, males showed a decrease in pH with increasing age (lacking statistical significance though), while females showed a statistically significant increase in pH with increasing age. Overall, women had higher pH values than men [56]. These results highlight the significance that sampling different locations can have and also again emphasize the need for further elucidation regarding the existence and significance of sex differences. There remains no consensus on how age and gender affect skin surface pH.

Wound Healing

In mice, plasmin plays an important role in wound healing to varying extents in males compared to females. Healing in wild-type mice was comparable. Healing in plasmin-deficient mice was markedly delayed in both genders, but gender-specific

Table 3 Mechanical properties (Adapted with permission from Tur E [12])

Findings	Obtained by	Subjects	Conclusions
Significant differences			
Men with greater TEWL values [30]	Evaporimeter	8 men, 10 women; Caucasian. 18–28 years	
Lower TEWL values in young women than young men at 10/10 sites sampled. Lower TEWL values in elderly women than elderly men except at chest. Young women with greater TEWL than elderly men at 6/10 sites. Young men with greater TEWL than elderly women at 8/10 sites [31]	Evaporimeter	34 young men; 23–33 years. 34 young women; 25–35 years. 28 elderly men; 66–74 years. 35 elderly women; 64–76 years	
Men with slightly higher basal TEWL than women. Men with decreased TEWL values 7 days post-HEC gel or 0.5 % caffeine in HEC but not women [32]	Tewameter	7 women, 26–50 years; 9 men, 28–45 years	Androgens are damaging to skin barrier function. Topical caffeine may be reparative to skin barrier dysfunction
Lower baseline TEWL in women than men; similar values in men and women after irritation [33]	Sodium lauryl sulfate irritation. Evaporimeter	15 women, 23 men; 18–39 years	Female skin more irritable based on irritation index defined as the difference between irritated and unirritated values over irritated
Men had greater TEWL than women [20]	Tewameter	5 women and 5 men in each age group:10–20, 20–30, 30–40, 40–50, 50–60 years old	
Men had significantly lower TEWL than women between the ages of 20–49, but differences assimilated after 50 at all locations except the forearm [24]	Tewameter	150 women, 150 men; age range 20–74	TEWL values assimilate among men and women at all locations except at the forearm
TDC values at the forearm was about 13 % greater for men than women [37]	MoistureMeter-D	30 women with mean age 25±2.5 years, 30 men with mean age 27.4±6.6 years	
TDC values at the forehead, cheek, and forearm were significantly higher in males than females [38]	MoistureMeter-D	30 women with mean age 25.6±2.9 years, 30 men with mean age 26.3±4.4 years	TDC values on the forehead, cheek, and forearm skin differed significantly
Blistering times longer in women than men ages 15–69. No difference in older ages [39]	Time required for blisters to form by controlled suction. Speed of dermal-epidermal separation measured	178 women, 15–101 years; 209 men, 16–96 years	
The ratio between the viscoelastic properties of the skin and immediate distention at a load of 500 mbar was greater in men at the volar forearm	Cutometer	8 women, mean age 25; 9 women mean age 75; 8 men, mean age 28; 8 men, mean age 75	

(*continued*)

Table 3 (continued)

Findings	Obtained by	Subjects	Conclusions
than for women. The ratio between immediate retraction and total distention greater in men than women at the forehead [42]			
Series elastic element (rate of stretch) on traction greater in women than men. Series elastic element greater for retraction in men than women at three locations on the foot. Women with greater foot skin plasticity than men [44]	Cutometer	38 men, 49 women; 35–81 years	
Women with greater cutaneous extensibility only after hydration [45]	Bioengineering methods	15 women, 14 men; 23–49 years and 60–93 years	The thinner dermis of women can be made more extensible once hydrated
Women demonstrated greater skin displacement than men in response to TAC-Cell stimulus pressure, further confirmed by power spectrum analysis [46]	Fiber-optic sensor	9 women mean age 23.11, 9 men mean age 24.44	
No significant differences			
No difference in TEWL between men and women [18]	Evaporimeter	7 men, 7 women; 23–29 years. 7 men, 8 women; 56–84 years	
No difference in TEWL or stratum corneum hydration between men and women [19]	Tewameter	6 women, 6 men; 23–25 years. Skin types II–III	
No difference in TEWL, moisture, or friction between men and women [34]	Bioengineering measurement	7 women, 25 years (mean); 7 men, 29 years. 7 women, 75 years; 8 men, 74 years	
No difference in moisture between men and women [35]	Bioengineering; chronic renal insufficiency and healthy subjects	Healthy: 24 women, 21 men Patients: 30 women, 50 men	
No difference between men and women in stratum corneum hydration or scaling [36]	Clinical assessment and bioengineering measurement	50 women, 22 men; 21–61 years.	
Hydration increases with age and peaks at around 40–50 years old but varied in specific age ranges and locations [23]	Corneometer	385 women, 328 men; age ranges 0–12, 13–35, 36–50, 51–70, over 70	
No sex-related difference in stratum corneum adhesion [40]	Biopsy; force needed to separate cells measured in vitro	9–34 women and men; number varied based on site sampled. 20–40 years	

(*continued*)

Table 3 (continued)

Findings	Obtained by	Subjects	Conclusions
Capacitance, dynamic skin friction coefficient, or transepidermal water loss did not differ between men and women at 11 different anatomical locations [34]	Capacitance meter; friction meter; evaporimeter; thermistor	7 women, 23–26 years; 7 women, 72–77 years. 7 men, 28–29 years; 8 men, 71–75 years	
No difference in skin elasticity between men and women [41]	In vivo suction device	Young: 8 women, 26 years; 8 men, 28 years. Old: 9 women, 75 years; 8 men, 75 years	
Females had slightly higher skin elasticity but results were insignificant [20]	Cutometer	5 women and 5 men in each age group:10–20, 20–30, 30–40, 40–50, 50–60 years old	
CRRT values generally decreased with age and had no overall differences between genders; however, certain directional CRRT values and certain locations were significantly different [43]	Reviscometer	398 women, 408 men, age range 2.5–94 years	
No difference in torsional extensibility between men and women [2]	Twistometer	69 women, 54 men; 5–90 years	

healing curves differed; females displayed accelerated wound healing. Female sex hormones may play a role in the initial healing process but did not contribute to overall difference in wound healing between genders [57]. This study suggests that plasmin influences tissue remodeling efficiency, and female mice may have a mechanism to better compensate for plasmin deficiency than males. Studies in humans are necessary to determine if these conclusions are translatable to humans (Table 4).

Differences in Response to Irritants

The reported incidence of irritant dermatitis is greater in women than in men [58], though there has been no consensus from experimental results as to which sex experiences more irritant dermatitis [12]. A review on gender differences in allergic contact dermatitis (ACD) concluded that sex was much less likely an endogenous factor predisposing to ACD but more likely a factor that influences environmental exposure to allergens. It was concluded that exposure history played the central role in determining a predisposition to ACD, with sex being a factor in determining exposure patterns, as opposed to sex determining intrinsic skin characteristics [59]. That sex is not a primary factor in determining response to irritants was highlighted by a study in which neither sex had a tendency toward stronger reactions to 11 different irritants in two groups of men and women, one with and one without hand eczema [60]. What has been shown in experimental results as well as anecdotal reports is that the decreased barrier function of the skin and a subjective increase in the severity of symptoms related to skin diseases such as eczema occur in the time period just prior to the onset of or during menstruation [61, 62]. This would imply that hormonal factors related to sex do play a role in the reactivity of skin.

Experimental results of skin prick testing in over 600 subjects found a small but significant difference with men having an increased response to

Table 4 Functional differences (Adapted with permission from Tur E [12])

Findings	Obtained by	Subjects	Conclusions
Significant differences			
Women sweat less than men [35]	Pilocarpine iontophoresis; chronic renal insufficiency and healthy subjects	Healthy: 24 women, 21 men; patients: 30 women, 50 men; 18–75 years	
Men with greater sweat rate than women [47]	Scale weight pre- and posttest; two separate experiments	Study 1: 40 women, 58 men. Study 2: 56 women, 56 men	
Prepubertal boys, pubertal boys, and adult men sweat more than girls and adult women of the same age group. Both sexes with increasing sweat secretion rate with increasing age. Adult men sweat more than prepubertal and pubertal boys; adult women sweat less than prepubertal and pubertal girls [48]	Pilocarpine iontophoresis	Prepubertal: 67 girls, 68 boys; 6–13 years. Pubertal: 80 girls, 39 boys; 9–19 years. Adults: 34 women, 24 men; 20–75 years	Sweat secretion rate dependent on sex and age. Change with age different for men and women
Women in both the luteal and follicular phases sweat less than men. Local sweat production less in women than men except at the thigh. Cutaneous blood flow similar in men and women except at the thigh where it is greater in women [49]	Ventilated capsule method; scale weight pre- and posttest. Laser Doppler	10 women, 20–22 years; 6 men, 20–26 years	
Men had greater sweat rates than women, but women had the same number or increased number of active sweat glands. The log concentration of the agonist causing 50 % of the maximal response were similar between the sexes [51]	Laser Doppler flow probe, iodine-paper technique	12 women, 12 men	Results suggest women have lower sweat gland output rate and not a difference in cholinergic sensitivity of the sweat gland
Women with higher mean pH than men at the forearm [19]	pH meter	6 women, 6 men; 23–25 years. Skin types II–III	
Women with higher pH than men at the forearm [52]	Glass electrode and pH meter	12 men, 8 women; 25–49 years	
Women with lower mean pH than men at the forearm [53]	pH meter	6 men, 31–59 years; 6 women, 26–54 years	
Women with lower pH than men in the axilla at baseline [46]	pH meter	10 men, 19–29 years; 10 women, 26–55 years	
pH levels on the forehead of females aged 13–70 and at the forearm of those aged 0–12, 36–50, and 51–70 were significantly higher than that in males in the same age group [23]	pH meter	385 women, 328 men; age ranges 0–12, 13–35, 36–50, 51–70, over 70	

(*continued*)

Table 4 (continued)

Findings	Obtained by	Subjects	Conclusions
pH of men was significantly lower than that of women and generally increased with age, whereas women's pH generally decreased with age [24]	pH meter	150 women, 150 men; age range 20–74	
In acne patients, males showed a decrease in pH with increasing age (lacking statistical significance though), while females showed a statistically significant increase in pH with increasing age [56]	pH meter	Acne patients: 270 women, 270 men	
In plasmin-deficient mice, gender-specific healing curves differed; females displayed accelerated wound healing compared to males [57]	Digital calipers	Mice about 5 and 6 weeks old	Study suggests plasmin influences tissue remodeling efficiency, and female mice may have a mechanism to better compensate for plasmin deficiency than males
No significant differences			
No difference between men and women in mean sweat rate when sweat rate expressed per unit surface area. Blood and sweat lactate concentrations not different between the sexes [50]	Capillary blood sampling; capillary tube sampling	6 men, 6 women; college aged	Men with greater overall sweat rate than women but difference no longer significant when body surface area accounted for. Greater overall sweat production associated with greater total sweat lactate secretion; no difference in sweat lactate concentration
No difference between men and women in pH [18]	pH meter	7 men, 7 women; 23–29 years. 7 men, 8 women; 56–84 years	
No difference in skin surface pH in the axilla between men and women. No gender difference in sweat pH of axilla [54]	pH meter; pH glass probe; microprocessor pH meter	81 women, 105 men; 18–55 years	

histamine compared to women, determined by resultant wheel size [63]. This is in contrast to a study of just over 70 subjects in which women produced larger wheels than men following histamine administration by iontophoresis [64]. Sodium lauryl sulfate (SLS) applied daily for 5 days followed by patch testing of the upper back did not demonstrate sex-related susceptibility to developing irritant dermatitis [65]. The use of SLS in this experiment produced results that have been interpreted differently by separate groups due to opposing definitions of what constitutes the irritation index. The group who performed the study concluded that women had more irritable skin following SLS application as indicated by having a higher irritation index determined from TEWL values. At baseline women showed lower TEWL values than men, but following irritation with SLS, both sexes had similar TEWL values. The irritation index defined by the authors of the study was the ratio of the difference of the values of irritated and unirritated skin to the value of unirritated skin. Despite the values for irritated skin not differing between men and women, the index was higher in women given the lower baseline unirritated values. The authors concluded this to mean that women had more irritable skin, whereas a review article later challenged that the study showed no sex-related differences in SLS irritation if the absolute end value of irritation was used to define the irritation index [12].

Sensitive Skin

Sensitive skin is a physiologic complaint of both sexes (although commonly associated with women), to which there remains an undefined etiology. Perceived sensitivity of the skin in general and on the body was comparable between sexes. However, women reported more sensitive skin on the face and genital area than men. Further, men and women had some different opinions regarding reasons for their sensitive skin [66]. Differences in sensitivity may be partially affected by different lifestyles of men and women. For example, increased use of cosmetics and facial products may cause irritation [66] (Table 5).

Cutaneous Microvasculature

The difference in skin blood flow between men and women is hormone dependent [12]. Differences between men and women depend on sexual maturation and, for women, the phase of the menstrual cycle [67]. Basal blood flow was lowest in the luteal phase and highest in the preovulatory phase. Compared to the other phases of the menstrual cycle, it was demonstrated that during the luteal phase, finger skin perfusion had the greatest cold-induced constriction and the least recovery following [67]. Supporting evidence that female sex hormones influence skin circulation includes an increased occurrence of vasospastic diseases such as Raynaud's phenomenon in women, an increased prevalence during the reproductive years, and that these conditions improve during pregnancy [12, 67]. Sex hormones may be directly influencing the blood vessel wall or may be indirectly acting systemically causing a cyclical pattern in women [12].

The sympathetic nervous system is influenced by estrogen. In the presence of estrogen, alpha-2 adrenoceptors are upregulated [12]. Consequently, laser Doppler flowmetry has shown a decreased basal cutaneous blood flow in women as compared to men provided age is under 50 [68–71]. Administration of an alpha 2 antagonist decreased the local response to cooling in women only, supporting the sex difference in alpha-2 adrenoceptors [72]. Administration of an alpha 1 antagonist decreased the response to cooling in both men and women. Following local heating both men and women experienced an increase in perfusion, though men continued to have a greater tissue blood flow than women [69]. In contrast to the aforementioned difference, laser Doppler has also shown no difference in baseline flux between the sexes measured at the hand [73].

In women, vasodilation in response to local heating occurred at a lower temperature [51, 74]. Women had a greater decrease in laser Doppler flux ipsilaterally and contralaterally to local cooling as compared to men [73]. Additionally, young women when compared to older women and young men had a prolonged response to cooling [71]. However, the maximum cutaneous blood flow subsequent to heating the skin was not different between the sexes, nor was the postocclusive reactive hyperemia response in a study of women aged 20–59 [51, 68]. On the contrary, one study that separated women according to age demonstrated both women over 50 and young men to have greater reactive hyperemia response than young women [71].

Skin blood flow is, in part, regulated by nitric oxide (NO)-dependent mechanisms [75]. At the forearm but not the calf, women exhibited decreased reliance on these mechanisms to increase blood flow compared to men [76].

Based on the difference demonstrated between sexes in over 300 subjects, one group went so far as to propose that the accepted upper limit of normal capillary refill time be specified based on sex and age. This study was divided into three groups composed of males and females: children, adults 20–49 years, and elderly adults 62–95 years. Pediatric females, pediatric males, and adult males had

Table 5 Response to irritants (Adapted with permission from Tur E [12])

Findings	Obtained by	Subjects	Conclusions
Significant differences			
Women with higher incidence of irritant dermatitis than men [58]			Likely role of occupational factors
Women with more frequent contact dermatitis to nickel than men; prevalence of piercing greater in women than men [59]	Literature review		Exposure risk a greater factor than sex in developing contact dermatitis
Transepidermal water loss higher on the day of minimal estrogen/progesterone secretion compared to the day of maximal secretion. TEWL greater with maximal progesterone secretion than maximal estrogen secretion [61]	Evaporimeter	9 women, 19–46 years	Just prior to the onset of menses, skin barrier function is impaired as compared to the days just prior to ovulation
Eczema worsens in the time period immediately preceding or during menstruation [62]	Literature review		Cyclical patterns of skin disease symptoms related to the menstrual cycle
Larger wheels produced in women secondary to histamine [63]	Histamine administered by iontophoresis	33 women, 38 men; 15–52 years	Sex differences in the stratum corneum affect reactivity
Men with greater response than women to skin prick test with histamine. Increasing reactivity with increasing age [64]	Skin prick, forearm	307 men, 313 women; mean age 24 years	
Women reported more sensitive skin on the face and genital area than men [66]	Survey	869 women, mean age 35.1; 163 men, mean age 38.6	Different lifestyle and product usage may contribute to sensitive skin
No significant differences			
No significant differences between the sexes regardless of having or not having hand eczema [60]	Irritation tested for 11 irritants at several concentrations	21 women, 21 men, with hand eczema; 21 women, 21 men, without hand eczema. 20–60 years	Neither sex with stronger tendency to reactions. Occupational exposure may lead to greater irritant exposure
Men and women with same incidence of cumulative irritant dermatitis [65]	Repeated once daily application of three concentrations of sodium lauryl sulfate, 5 days, followed by patch testing. Bioengineering measurements	7 women, 7 men; 16–65 years	

significantly shorter capillary refill times than adult females, elderly females, and elderly males [77].

Mapping skin blood perfusion using laser Doppler imagery was done following iontophoresis of acetylcholine, an endothelium-dependent vasodilator, as well as nitroprusside and isoprenaline, two different endothelium-independent vasodilators with different modes of action. Premenopausal women had a greater response to nitroprusside, and to a lesser extent acetylcholine, than postmenopausal women, reflecting a change in skin vasculature with aging [78].

No difference could be demonstrated between men and women in cutaneous blood flow response to topical and intradermal histamine administration on the back, volar forearm, and ankle [79]. It was secondarily deduced that no functional difference exists between the sexes in the skin microvascular response to histamine [12].

Changes in oxygen pressure at the skin surface primarily determined by skin blood flow have been measured by assessing alterations in transcutaneous oxygen pressure [12]. Skin surface measurements have demonstrated that women have higher transcutaneous oxygen pressure than men [80, 81]. Supposing women have a thinner epidermis than men, this difference may be accounted for [12]. Transcutaneous oxygen pressure measurements revealed age-related sex differences during postocclusive reactive hyperemia. No difference existed between the younger sexes but adult women had greater values than adult men [82] (Table 6).

Sensory Functions

Thermoregulatory Response

A difference between the sexes was demonstrated in a study of the physiological response to heat stress. However, when accounting for differences in anthropometric variables, such as percent body fat and the ratio of body surface to mass, the effect of gender did not hold [83]. This highlights the impact sex-specific variables can have on thermoregulation and the need to account for these when interpreting results [12].

In contrast, despite similar body surface area-to-mass ratios in a cohort of young Japanese subjects, women's tolerance to cold was superior to men's in the winter [84]. Differences in the distribution of body fat may have contributed to the difference in cold tolerance despite similar body surface area-to-mass ratios [12].

In opposition to results that women tolerate temperature change better, other studies found women to be more sensitive to thermal stimuli. One study demonstrated that women reported perceived stimulus to both warm and cold at a lower threshold. This thermosensitivity difference was not affected by the phase of the menstrual cycle women were in [85]. Secondly, women exhibited a greater fast cooling time than men. Fast cooling was taken to represent cooling of the superficial epidermal layers. A thicker male stratum corneum may account for this difference. No difference existed between the sexes for slow cooling, a representation of the deeper epidermis and dermal layers [86]. Experiments using whole-body cryotherapy, again, showed women had higher levels of skin cooling than men, which is likely to be, in part, attributed to anthropometric and thermoregulatory differences [87].

Thermal Response to Stimulation

Women had a greater decrease in finger temperature in response to musical stimulus [88]. It was suggested that a difference in the sensitivity or density of peripheral vascular adrenergic receptors creates a difference between men and women in vascular autonomic sensitivity to music [12].

Women and men may also have a different hemispheric response to auditory stimuli. Electrodermal asymmetry has been likened to an index of hemispheric specialization [12]. Right-handed men displayed more asymmetry in the frequency and magnitude of skin conductance between hands, with larger responses on the left hand after hearing tones [89].

Thermal and Pain Sensation and Pressure Sensitivity

Mechanical, electrical, chemical, and thermal pain stimuli have all been used to study skin sensation in relation to pain. Women had a lower threshold of pricking pain sensation at the forearm. The pressure threshold was lower in women than men on the palm and sole, but not at the forearm [90]. No difference existed between men and women in the thermal pain threshold [91]. Possible explanations for the differences in pain sensations between the sexes include anatomical differences in skin thickness, differences in blood flow,

Table 6 Cutaneous microvasculature (Adapted with permission from Tur E [12])

Findings	Obtained by	Subjects	Conclusions
Significant differences			
Skin circulation differed with phases of the menstrual cycle: basal flow lowest in the luteal phase, highest in the pre-ovulatory phase. In the luteal phase, greatest cold-induced constriction and lowest recovery [67]	Bioengineering measurements at four times during the menstrual cycle	31 women, 15–45 years	Hormone changes during the menstrual cycle affect skin blood flow and its response to cold
Basal skin blood flow reduced in women [68]	Bioengineering measurements	56 women, 44 men; 20–59 years	
Facial basal skin blood flow reduced in women [69]	Laser Doppler	5 women, 5 men; 25–52 years	
Basal skin blood flow reduced in women [70]	Bioengineering measurements, cooling and warming to change sympathetic tone	26 women, 23 men; 22–38 years	Sympathetic tone is increased
Young women with lower reactive hyperemia response compared to women over 50oryoung men. Young women with extended response to cooling compared to older women and younger men [71]	Bioengineering measurement. Postocclusive reactive hyperemia and direct and indirect cooling	12 women, 19–39 years; 13 women, 51–67 years; 13 men, 22–47 years	
Men with greater mean tissue blood flow and red cell circulating volume at the face as compared to women at baseline. When heated, men continued to have a greater tissue blood flow than women [69]	Laser Doppler	5 men, 5 women, 25–52 years	Difference between the sexes in the number of perfused microvessels may account for findings
Direct and indirect cooling caused a greater decrease in cutaneous LD flux in women as compared to men. Injection of an alpha-2 adrenoreceptor antagonist decreased the direct response to cold in women only. Injection of an alpha-1 adrenoreceptor antagonist reduced the indirect response to cooling in men only [72]	Laser Doppler	6 men, 38–46 years; 6 women, 32–40 years	A sex-specific response to cooling exists for alpha-2 adrenoreceptors at the level of cutaneous microvasculature
Greater ipsilateral and contralateral decrease in LD flux in response to local cooling in women [73]	Laser Doppler	10 men, mean age 33; 10 women, mean age 35	
Skin temperature at which local heating produced vasodilation lower in women [74]	Bioengineering measurement	9 women, 6 men; age not specified	
At the forearm but not the calf, women exhibited decreased reliance on these	Doppler flowmetry probe	9 women, 10 men; age 23±1 year	

(*continued*)

Table 6 (continued)

Findings	Obtained by	Subjects	Conclusions
NO-dependent mechanisms to increase blood flow compared to men [76]			
Capillary refill times shorter for pediatric females, pediatric males, and adult males as compared to adult women, adult elderly women, and adult elderly men [77]	Time to return of baseline distal phalanx color after 5 s of applied pressure was released	100 children, 2–12 years; 104 adults, 20–49 years; 100 elderly adults, 62–95 years	The currently accepted upper limit of capillary refill time for men and women of all ages should be adjusted according to sex and age
Premenopausal women with a greater response to nitroprusside than postmenopausal women [78]	Laser Doppler perfusion imager, iontophoresis	21 women, 13 men; 18–80 years	Functional and structural changes in skin vasculature occur in women with aging
No significant differences			
No difference in baseline flux between men and women [73]	Laser Doppler	10 men, mean age 33 years; 10 women, mean age 35 years	
Transcutaneous oxygen pressure			
Significant differences			
Women with higher values of transcutaneous oxygen pressure [80]	Bioengineering; 23 sites on face, extremities and trunk	7 women, 12 men; 21–36 years	
Women with higher values of transcutaneous oxygen pressure [81]	Bioengineering; anterior chest, forearm	18 women, 42 men; 22–88 years	
Adult women with greater transcutaneous oxygen pressure during postocclusive reactive hyperemia than adult men; no difference between boys and girls [82]	Bioengineering measurement; postocclusive reactive hyperemia	Adults: 30 women, 37 men; 22–60 years. Children before puberty: 34	Indication of hormonal influence
No significant differences			
Histamine caused no change in cutaneous blood flow response [79]	Topical and intradermal administration; bioengineering methods	10 women, 10 men; 24–34 years	

cutaneous vasculature that absorbs heat transmitted to skin, and variations in nervous structure or function [12].

Autonomic Function

Neonate girls had greater cutaneous conduction than boys [92]. Skin conductance is one measure of autonomic function. This difference may represent dissimilarity in maturation [12] (Table 7).

Skin Color

Skin color differs between the sexes and between different age groups. Studies from Iran [93], India [94], and Australia [95] have demonstrated women have lighter skin. Differences in melanin, hemoglobin, carotene, hormonal influence, and environmental sun exposure may all be involved [12]. The change in skin color that occurs with aging is both similar and different for men and

Table 7 Sensory functions (Adapted with permission from Tur E [12])

Findings	Obtained by	Subjects	Conclusions
Significant differences			
Women with a greater tolerance to cold in the winter than men [84]	Cold exposure to 12 °C for 1 h at rest in the winter and summer; skin and body temperature	7 women, 8 men; Japanese. 18–26 years	Despite similar body surface area-to-mass ratios, differences in fat distribution between men and women may have contributed to differing tolerance to cold
Women with lower thresholds for warm and cold sensation as compared to men. Results not affected by phase of menstrual cycle [85]	Middlesex Thermal Testing System; reported perceived stimulus produced by thermode	10 men, mean age 31 years; 10 women, mean age 28 years	Women had greater thermosensitivity than men
Fast cooling (representative of superficial epidermal layers) longer in men than women. No difference in cooling time between the sexes for slow cooling (representative of the deeper epidermal and dermal layers) [86]	Skin temperature; time to cool	7 men, mean age 25 years; 7 women, mean age 24 years	The thicker stratum corneum of men caused a longer fast cooling time as compared to women
Women had higher levels of skin cooling than men, which is likely to be, in part, attributed to anthropometric and thermoregulatory differences [87]	Scales, stadiometer, FLIR Thermal Imaging Camera, liquid nitrogen-cooled cryogenic chamber	14 women, mean age 28.3±6.4; 18 men, mean age 29.5±4.4	
Women with a greater decrease in finger temperature in response to musical stimulus [88]	Auditory stimulation: music; skin temperature	60 women, 60 men; young students	Results may be due to a difference between the sexes in autonomic sensitivity to music
Men with more asymmetry between hands than women. Women with larger skin conductance responses on right hand; men with large responses on left hand [89]	Auditory stimulus; magnitude and frequency of skin conductance responses	15 women, 15 men; 19–27 years. Right-handed	Auditory stimuli may cause a differing hemispheric response in men and women
The palm and sole are more sensitive to stimulus in women, but not on the forearm [90]	Pressure threshold measurement	68 women, 68 men; 17–30 years	
Higher conductance in neonate girls as compared to boys [92]	Skin conductance (autonomic function)	20 women, 20 men; neonates: 60–100 h	Difference in maturation may account for differences in conductance
No significant differences			
Men and women have different physiological responses to heat stress but depend on body surface area and fat content [83]	Heat stress, ergometer; oxygen uptake, body and skin temperature, sweat rate	12 women, 12 men; 20–28 years	When percent body fat and ratio of body surface area to mass were accounted for, sex differences no longer existed
No difference in thermal pain threshold between men and women [91]	Thermal sensory analyzer	19 men, 30 women; 19–59 years. Skin types III–VI	

Table 8 Skin color (Adapted with permission from Tur E [12])

Findings	Obtained by	Subjects	Conclusions
Significant differences			
Lighter skin in women [93]	Spectrophotometry	33 women, 68 men; 8–24 years	Vascular dissimilarity, differences in tanning
Lighter skin in women [94]	Spectrophotometry	566 women, 578 men; 1–50 years	Female skin lightens during puberty; male skin darkens. Varying MSH levels differ. Role for environmental and hereditary variables
Women's skin lighter. Skin color darkens in both sexes with age [95]	Spectrophotometry	461 women, 346 men; 20–69 years	History of sun exposure and MSH levels differ
Boys' foreheads darker than girls'. Medial upper arms of girls darker than boys in early adolescence, not different in middle adolescence, and lighter during late adolescence [96]	Skin color reflectance	105 women, 10–16 years; 105 men, 12–18 years	Different physiologic changes between the sexes may account for results
Men's skin darker and redder than women's in the elderly, not in the young [97]	Colorimetric measurements	8 women, 5 men, 65–88 years; 9 women, 4 men, 18–26 years	
Men with redder skin as compared to women at the upper back and forearm. Women 36–73 years with greater luminance of skin on upper back than men of the same age [98]	Colorimetric measurements	21 men, 31 women, 19–35 years; 22 men, 23 women, 36–50 years; 22 men, 30 women, 51–65 years; 10 men, 7 women, 66–73 years	

women. In general, both sexes darken with increasing age [95]. Following the onset of puberty, both men and women lighten, though females more so [94]. It is hypothesized that hormonal influence alone cannot explain this difference since both estrogen and testosterone cause skin darkening [12]. A difference in environmental exposure to UV light has also been proposed as an explanation, though results of a study of adolescent medial upper-arm skin (less sun exposure) challenge this.

The aforementioned study found that the forehead (sun exposed) pigmentation of boys was darker than of girls. The medial upper arm (less sun exposed) of girls was darker than boys during early adolescence, similar for the sexes during adolescence, and significantly lighter for girls than boys in late adolescence [96].

Colorimetric measurements demonstrated elderly men to have redder skin than elderly women, though this did not hold true in a younger population [97]. A separate study of colorimetry also found men to have more red skin than women and found this across all ages 19–73 [98]. Additionally, women had less regional variation in reflectance spectrophotometry and, as such, were more homogeneous in color than men [99] (Table 8).

Hormonal Influence

It has already been mentioned that hormones increased the thickness of the skin in postmenopausal women [9, 10], are implicated in the change in skin blood flow and transepidermal water loss that occurs during the menstrual cycle [61, 67], and affect the severity of symptoms associated with pathologic skin conditions, such as eczema [62]. Hormone replacement also limited the age-related skin extensibility in menopausal women, whereas women without

Table 9 Hormonal influence (Adapted with permission from Tur E [12])

Findings	Obtained by	Subjects	Conclusions
Significant differences			
Decreased age-related extensibility in skin in hormone replacement-treated women [100]	Computerized suction device measuring skin deformability and viscoelasticity	43 nonmenopausal women, 19–50 years; 25 menopausal not treated, 46–76 years; 46 on hormonal replacement since the onset of menopause, 38–73 years	Skin slackness can be limited by hormone replacement therapy
Hormone replacement-treated women had 48 % increased collagen content as compared to non-treated subjects [101]	Hydroxyproline and collagen content; biopsies	Postmenopausal women, 35–62 years: 29 untreated, 26 estradiol + testosterone	The decreased content of collagen in skin that occurs with aging can be prevented with hormone treatment
Postmenopausal women receiving hormone replacement therapy had an increased proportion of type III collagen [102]	Analysis of collagen types; biopsies	Postmenopausal women, 41–66 years: 14 untreated, 11 estradiol + testosterone	Total collagen increased by hormone replacement therapy. Ratio of type III to type I collagen by hormone treatment
Vmax for17β-estradiol formation 1.7 times larger than for estrone formation in women. Vmax for estrone formation 2.5 times larger than for17β- estradiol formation in men [103]	High-performance liquid chromatography	7 women, 40–72 years; 9 men, 21–75 years; cadavers	Sex differences exist in the affinity of the cutaneous enzyme17β-hydroxysteroid dehydrogenase to interconvert hormones

hormone replacement demonstrated an increase in extensibility [100].

Loss of collagen has been associated with the occurrence of skin thinning post-menopause. Two separate studies demonstrated that collagen content increased 48 % [101] and 34 % [10] following hormone treatment as compared to non-treated subjects. Additionally, the ratio of type III to type I collagen in the skin decreased with aging [12]. Postmenopausal women receiving hormone replacement therapy had an increased proportion of type III collagen cutaneously [102].

The cutaneous enzyme 17β-hydroxysteroid dehydrogenase (17β-HSD) was found, in vivo, to have a different affinity in men and women for interconverting estrone (E1) and 17β-estradiol (E2) in the skin. 17β-HSD catalyzes the reduction of weak steroids to strong ones, e.g., E1 to E2. The skin of women had a tendency to activate estrogen – Vmax for E2 formation 1.7 times larger than for E1 formation. The skin of men tended to deactivate estrogen – Vmax for E1 formation 2.5 times larger than for E2 formation [103] (Table 9).

Pilosebaceous Unit

Sebaceous glands are hormone dependent. Androgenic steroids of both adrenal and gonadal origin can directly stimulate sebaceous gland activity. Administration of the appropriate hormone during puberty can cause an increase in their activity [12]. Thyroid-stimulating hormone (TSH), corticotrophin (ACTH), follicle-stimulating hormone (FSH), and luteinizing hormone (LH) act indirectly by stimulating their respective endocrine tissues. Other hormones such as growth hormone (GH) act synergistically with another hormone that the sebaceous gland is sensitive to [12]. For the age range 20–69 years, the average values for sebum secretion were higher in men than women. This was not true for the age range 15–19 years [104]. In the age range 50–70 years, secretion in men remained unaltered, whereas women had a significant decrease in sebum secretion likely secondary to decreased ovarian activity [12]. Additionally, the composition of sebum is affected by hormonal influence as an age-related decline in the secretion of wax ester starting in young adulthood has been demonstrated [12].

Hair distribution in men and women is one of the more obvious attributes that differs between the sexes. Systemic factors, e.g., hormones, and external factors play an important role in the evolution and phases of follicular growth. This is in addition to mechanisms inherent to the follicles themselves [12]. The evaluation of one study found that in the month of January, women's hair was denser and the percentage of telogen hair was lower as compared to men [12, 105]. This seasonal effect exemplified one difference between men and women in regard to environmental conditions. The hormonally stimulated transformation of vellus to terminal hair and racial and genetic factors are all components in the diversity of hair patterns of men and women [12].

Body site is also important in the effect of androgens on hair growth. At puberty men's vellus hair on the face transforms to terminal hair whereas on the scalp the reverse occurs. Despite the same exposure to circulatory hormones, the activity of hair follicles depends on anatomical location. Targets such as the eyelashes have no response to hormonal stimulation, whereas the face, scalp, axilla, and pubic follicles are main androgenic targets [12]. Melanocyte-stimulating hormone, prolactin, thyroid hormone, pregnancy, and nutritional state also affect cells targeted by androgens [106] (Table 10).

Single-Gender Studies

In a study of Korean males, skin hydration, TEWL levels, elasticity, sebum content, and number of pores were higher in the summer compared to the winter. Skin sensitivity and pH levels were higher in the winter. Skin brightness and wrinkles were unaffected [107].

A separate study also found sebum levels and water content to be lowest in the winter. However, TEWL levels were lowest in the summer and highest in the winter, contrary to the previous study. Corneocyte-projected area showed a parabolic trend peaking in the summer. This study also suggested that excess sebum led men to perceive a tacky feeling. Excess sebum correlated with lower TEWL levels, indicating SC barrier function impairment [108].

In a study of Korean females, hydration, elasticity, and sebum levels also were higher in the winter; however, statistical significance in this study was not calculated. Skin brightness was lowest in the fall, following a parabolic trend. Scaliness was higher in the winter than summer [109]. The effect of environmental factors on skin biophysical parameters has not been studied much; however, these data suggest they may be important.

Environmental conditions vary year to year; thus, these studies on individual genders cannot be directly compared to analyze gender differences in response to seasonal changes. Different seasons indicate differences in factors such as

Table 10 Pilosebaceous unit (Adapted with permission from Tur E [12])

Findings	Obtained by	Subjects	Conclusions
Significant differences			
No difference between the sexes in sebum secretion ages 15–19. Greater sebum secretion in men than women ages 20–69. Men 50–70 years with no change in secretion; women with significantly decreased sebum output [104]	Sebum production	330 women, 458 men; 15–>69 years	Sebum secretion may change in elderly women due to decreased ovarian activity
Plasma testosterone did not correlate with sebum production [104]	Sebum production and plasma androgen levels	8 women, 28 men	
Women's hair more dense and with a lower percentage of telogen hair in January as compared to men [105]	Phototrichogram, hair count after washing	7 women, 29–49 years; 7 men, 25–47 years	

Table 11 Single-gender studies

Findings	Obtained by	Subjects	Conclusions
Men			
Skin hydration, TEWL levels, elasticity, sebum content, and number of pores were higher in the summer compared to the winter. Skin sensitivity and pH levels were higher in the winter. Skin brightness and wrinkles were unaffected [107]	Corneometer, pH meter, tewameter, sebumeter, cutometer, 3D skin measurement system, facial analysis system	100 Korean men, age range 20–59 years	Extrinsic environmental factors such as temperature and humidity affect skin physiology
Sebum levels and water content to be lowest in the winter, TEWL levels were lowest in the summer and highest in the winter, men perceive a tacky feeling due to excess sebum [108]	Tewameter, SKICON 200, sebumeter, tape stripping, questionnaire	45 Japanese men, ages from the 20s to 50s	
Women			
Hydration, elasticity, and sebum levels were higher in the winter, skin brightness was lowest in the fall, following a parabolic trend, scaliness was higher in the winter than summer [109]	Corneometer, sebumeter, UVA-light video camera, spectrophotometer, cutometer	89 Korean women aged 29.7±6.2 years	

temperature, humidity, and precipitation. Thus, more studies are necessary to elucidate how they affect skin as well as how they may affect males and females differently (Table 11).

Conclusion

Interpreting the findings in the studies reveals a need for developing a systematic approach to study the inherent structure and pathophysiology of the skin. The relatively small subject number that characterizes many of the studies results in a lack of power to support findings. In this day and age, a large number of instruments exist to sample the various functional, mechanical, and structural properties of the skin. This is both advantageous and detrimental. Direct comparison between different studies is complicated by the different instruments and methods used to evaluate the same topic. Multiple studies have not only interindividual variability but also intraindividual variability secondary to the different anatomical sites sampled. Additionally, comparison of in vivo and in vitro testing requires extrapolation in reasoning to make a conclusion based on both methods of experimentation. These fundamental techniques of experimentation are further complicated by hormonal factors in many cases, but to what extent, continues to need to be elucidated and scientifically, not merely anecdotally, proven. These confounding variables leave much room for further study in larger sample populations and with as stringent experimental protocols as possible. Taken together, the data totality can be interpreted to suggest that the differences are more important than the similarities, indicating that exploring the mechanisms and significance will provide a better understanding of skin- and gender-related skin management.

Cross-References

▶ Determinants in the Rate of Skin Aging: Ethnicity, Gender, and Lifestyle Influences

References

1. Seidenari S, Pagnoni A, Di Nardo A, et al. Echographic evaluation with image analysis of normal skin: variations according to age and sex. Skin Pharmacol. 1994;7:201–9.

2. Escoffier C, de Rigal J, Rochefort A, et al. Age-related mechanical properties of human skin: an in vivo study. J Invest Dermatol. 1989;93:353–7.
3. Sandby-Moller J, Poulsen T, Wulf HC. Epidermal thickness at different body sites: relationship to age, gender, pigmentation, blood content, skin type and smoking habits. Acta Derm Venereol. 2003;83:410–3.
4. Branchet MC, Boisnic S, Frances C, et al. Skin thickness changes in normal aging skin. Gerontology. 1990;36:28–35.
5. Ya-Xian Z, Suetake T, Tagami H. Number of cell layers of the stratum corneum in normal skin-relationship to the anatomical location on the body, age, sex and physical parameters. Arch Dermatol Res. 1999;291:555–9.
6. Gniadecka M, Jemec GBE. Quantitative evaluation of chronological ageing and photoageing in vivo: studies on skin echogenicity and thickness. Br J Dermatol. 1998;139:815–21.
7. Gambichler T, Matip R, Moussa G, et al. In vivo data of epidermal thickness evaluated by optical coherence tomography: effects of age, gender, skin type, and anatomic site. J Dermatol Sci. 2006;44:145–52.
8. Shuster S, Black MM, McVitie E. The influence of age and sex on skin thickness, skin collagen and density. Br J Dermatol. 1975;93:639–43.
9. Maheux R, Naud F, Rioux M, et al. A randomized, double-blind placebo-controlled study on the effect of conjugated estrogens on skin thickness. Am J Obstet Gynecol. 1994;170:642–3.
10. Brincat M, Moniz CJ, Studd JW, et al. Long-term effects of the menopause and sex hormones on skin thickness. Br J Obstet Gynaecol. 1985;92:256–9.
11. Sauerbronn AV, Fonseca AM, Bagnoli VR, et al. The effects of systemic hormonal replacement therapy on the skin of postmenopausal women. Int J Gynaecol Obstet. 2000;68:35–41.
12. Tur E. Physiology of the skin – differences between women and men. Clin Dermatol. 1997;15:5–16.
13. Arner P, Lithell H, Wahrenberg H, Bronnegard M. Expression of lipoprotein lipase in different human subcutaneous adipose tissue regions. J Lipid Res. 1991;32:423–9.
14. Malyarenko TN, ANtonyuk SD, Malyarenko YE. Changes in the human fat mass at the age of 6–18 years. Arkh Anat Gistol Embriol. 1988;94:43–7.
15. Hattori K, Okamoto W. Skinfold compressibility in Japanese university students. Okajimas Folia Anat Jpn. 1993;70:69–78.
16. Leveque J, Corcuff P, de Rigal J, et al. In vivo studies of the evolution of physical properties of the human skin with age. Int J Dermatol. 1984;18:322–9.
17. Davies BN, Greenwood EJ, Jones SR. Gender difference in the relationship of performance in the handgrip and standing long jump tests to lean limb volume in young adults. Eur J Appl Physiol. 1988;58:315–20.
18. Wilhelm KP, Cua AB, Maibach HI. Skin aging. Effect on transepidermal water loss, stratum corneum hydration, skin surface pH, and casual sebum content. Arch Dermatol. 1991;127:1806–9.
19. Jacobi U, Gautier J, Sterry W, Lademann J. Gender-related differences in the physiology of the stratum corneum. Dermatology. 2005;211:312–7.
20. Firooz A, Sadr B, Babakoohi S, et al. Variation of biophysical parameters of the skin with age, gender, and body region. Sci World J. 2012
21. Kim MK, Patel RA, Shinn AH, et al. Evaluation of gender difference in skin type and pH. J Dermatol Sci. 2006;41:153–6.
22. Kim BY, Choi JW, Park KC, Youn SW. Sebum, acne, skin elasticity, and gender differences - which is the major influencing factor for facial pores? Skin Res Technol. 2013;19(1):e45–53.
23. Man MQ, Xin SJ, Song SP, Cho SY, Zhang XJ, Tu CX, Feingold KR, Elias PM. Variation of skin surface pH, sebum content and stratum corneum hydration with age and gender in a large Chinese population. Skin Pharmacol Physiol. 2009;22(4):190–9.
24. Luebberding S, Krueger N, Kerscher M. Skin physiology in men and women: in vivo evaluation of 300 people including TEWL, SC hydration, sebum content and skin surface pH. Int J Cosmet Sci. 2013;35(5):477–83.
25. Denda M, Koyama J, Hori J, et al. Age and sex-dependent change in stratum corneum sphingolipids. Arch Dermatol Res. 1993;285:415–7.
26. Cua AB, Wilhelm KP, Maibach HI. Skin surface lipid and skin friction: relation to age, sex and anatomical region. Skin Pharmacol. 1995;8:246–51.
27. Somerville DA. The normal flora of the skin in different age groups. Br J Dermatol. 1969;81:248–58.
28. Marples R. Sex, constancy, and skin bacteria. Arch Dermatol Res. 1982;272:317–20.
29. Sturado A, Parvoli G, Doretti L, et al. The influence of color, age and sex on the content of zinc, copper, nickel, manganese, and lead in human hair. Biol Trace Elem Res. 1994;40:1–8.
30. Chilcott RP, Farrar R. Biophysical measurements of human forearm skin in vivo: effects of site, gender, chirality and time. Skin Res Technol. 2000;6:64–9.
31. Nicander I, Nyren M, Emtestam L, et al. Baseline electrical impedance measurements at various skin sites- related to age and sex. Skin Res Technol. 1997;3:252–8.
32. Brandner JM, Behne MJ, Huesing B, Moll I. Caffeine improves barrier function in male skin. Int J Cosmet Sci. 2006;28:343–7.
33. Goh CL, Chia SE. Skin irritability to sodium lauryl sulphate-as measured by skin water vapor loss-by sex and race. Clin Exp Dermatol. 1988;13:16–8.
34. Cua AB, Wilhelm KP, Maibach HI. Frictional properties of human skin: relation to age, sex and anatomical region, stratum corneum hydration and transepidermal water loss. Br J Dermatol. 1990;123:473–9.
35. Yosipovitch G, Reis J, Tur E, et al. Sweat secretion, stratum corneum hydration, small nerve function and

pruritus in patients with advanced chronic renal failure. Br J Dermatol. 1995;133:561–4.
36. Jemec GBE, Serup J. Scaling, dry skin and gender. Acta Derm Venereol (Stockh). 1992;177:26–8.
37. Mayrovitz HN, Carson S, Luis M. Male–female differences in forearm skin tissue dielectric constant. Clin Physiol Funct Imaging. 2010;30:328–32.
38. Mayrovitz HN, Bernal M, Carson S. Gender differences in facial skin dielectric constant measured at 300 MHz. Skin Res Technol. 2012;18(4):504–10.
39. Kiistala U. Dermal-epidermal separation. Ann Clin Res. 1972;4:10–22.
40. Chernova TA, Melikyants IG, Mordovtsev VN, et al. Mechanical properties of the skin in normal subjects. Vestn Dermatol Venereol. 1984;2:12–5.
41. Pedersen L, Hansen B, Jemec GB. Mecahnical properties of the skin: a comparison between two suction cup methods. Skin Res Technol. 2003;2:111–5.
42. Cua AB, Wilhelm KP, Maibach HI. Elastic properties of human skin: relation to age, sex, and anatomical region. Arch Dermatol Res. 1990;282:283–8.
43. Xin S, Man W, Fluhr JW, Song S, Elias P, Man MQ. Cutaneous resonance running time varies with age, body site and gender in a normal Chinese population. Skin Res Technol. 2010;16(4):413–21.
44. Hashmi F, Malone-Lee J. Measurement of skin elasticity on the foot. Skin Res Technol. 2007;13:252–8.
45. Auriol F, Vaillant L, Machet L, et al. Effects of short time hydration on skin extensibility. Acta Derm Venereol (Stockh). 1993;73:344–7.
46. Venkatesan L, Barlow SM. Characterization of sex-based differences in the mechanical properties of human finger glabrous tissue using a fiberoptic sensor. J Biomech. 2014;47(10):2257–62.
47. Mehnert P, Brode P, Griefahn B. Gender-related difference in sweat loss and its impact on exposure limits to heat stress. Int J Ind Ergon. 2002;29:343–51.
48. Main K, Nilsson KO, Skakkebaek NE. Influence of sex and growth hormone deficiency on sweating. Scand J Clin Lab Invest. 1991;51:475–80.
49. Inoue Y, Tanaka Y, Omori K, et al. Sex- and menstrual cycle-related differences in sweating and cutaneous blood flow in response to passive heat exposure. Eur J Appl Physiol. 2005;94:323–32.
50. Green JM, Bishop PA, Muir IH, Lomax RG. Gender differences in sweat lactate. Eur J Appl Physiol. 2000;82:230–5.
51. Gagnon D, Crandall CG, Kenny GP. Sex differences in postsynaptic sweating and cutaneous vasodilation. J Appl Physiol. 2013;114(3):394–401.
52. Ohman H, Vahlquist A. In vivo studies concerning a pH gradient in human stratum corneum and upper epidermis. Acta Derm Venereol. 1994;74:375–9.
53. Ehlers C, Ivens UI, Moller ML, et al. Females have lower skin surface pH than men. A study on the surface of gender, forearm site variation, right/left difference and time of the day on the skin surface pH. Skin Res Technol. 2001;7:90–4.
54. Burry JS, Coulson HF, Esser I, et al. Erroneous gender differences in axillary skin surface/sweat pH. Int J Cosmet Sci. 2001;23:99–107.
55. Williams S, Davids M, Reuther T, et al. Gender difference of in vivo skin surface pH in the axilla and the effect of a standardized washing procedure with tap water. Skin Pharmacol Physiol. 2005;18:247–52.
56. Youn SH, Choi CW, Choi JW, Youn SW. The skin surface pH and its different influence on the development of acne lesion according to gender and age. Skin Res Technol. 2013;19(2):131–6.
57. Rono B, Engelholm LH, Lund LR, Hald A. Gender affects skin wound healing in plasminogen deficient mice. PLoS One. 2013;8(3), e59942.
58. Wilhelm KP, Maibach HI. Factors predisposing to cutaneous irritation. Dermatol Clin. 1990;8:17–22.
59. Modjtahedi BS, Modjtahedi SP, Maibach HI. The sex of the individual as a factor in allergic contact dermatitis. Contact Dermatitis. 2004;50:53–9.
60. Bjornberg A. Skin reactions to primary irritants. Acta Derm Venereol (Stockh). 1975;55:191–4.
61. Harvell J, Hussona-Safed I, Maibach HI. Changes in transepidermal water loss and cutaneous blood flow during the menstrual cycle. Contact Dermatitis. 1992;27:294–301.
62. Farage MA, Berardesca E, Maibach HI. The effect of sex hormones on irritant and allergic response: possible relevance for skin testing. Br J Dermatol. 2009;160:450–1.
63. Bordignon V, Burastero SE. Age, gender and reactivity to allergens independently influence skin reactivity to histamine. J Investig Allergol Clin Immunol. 2006;16:129–35.
64. Magerl W, Westerman RA, Mohner B, et al. Properties of transepidermal histamine iontophoresis: differential effects of season, gender, and body region. J Invest Dermatol. 1990;94:347–52.
65. Lammintausta K, Maibach HI, Wilson D. Irritant reactivity in males and females. Contact Dermatitis. 1987;17:276–80.
66. Farage MA. Does sensitive skin differ between men and women? Cutan Ocul Toxicol. 2010;29 (3):153–63.
67. Bartelink ML, WOllersheim A, Theeuwes A, et al. Changes in skin blood flow during the menstrual cycle: the influence of the menstrual cycle on the peripheral circulation in healthy female volunteers. Clin Sci. 1990;78:527–32.
68. Maurel A, Hamon P, Macquin-mavier I, et al. Flux microcirculatoire cutane etude par laser-doppler. Presse Med. 1991;20:1205–9.
69. Mayrovitz HN, Regan MB. Gender differences in facial skin blood perfusion during basal and heated conditions determined by laser Doppler flowmetry. Microvasc Res. 1993;45:211–8.
70. Cooke JP, Creager MA, Osmundson PJ, et al. Sex differences in control of cutaneous blood flow. Circulation. 1990;82:1607–15.

71. Bollinger A, Schlumpf M. Finger blood flow in healthy subjects of different age and sex in patients with primary Raynaud's disease. Acta Chir Scand. 1975;465(Suppl):42–7.
72. Cankar K, Finderle Z, Strucl M. The role of alpha1- and alpha2- adrenoceptors in gender differences in cutaneous LD flux response to local cooling. Microvasc Res. 2004;68:126–31.
73. Cankar K, Finderle Z. Gender differences in cutaneous vascular and autonomic nervous response to local cooling. Clin Auton Res. 2003;13:214–20.
74. Walmsley D, Goodfield MJD. Evidence for an abnormal peripherally mediated vascular response to temperature in Raynaud's phenomenon. Br J Rheumatol. 1990;29:181–4.
75. Warren JB. Nitric oxide and human skin blood flow responses to acetylcholine and ultraviolet light. FASEB J. 1994;8(2):247–51.
76. Stanhewicz AE, Greaney JL, Kenney WL, Alexander LM. Sex- and limb-specific differences in the nitric oxide-dependent cutaneous vasodilation in response to local heating. Am J Physiol Regul Integr Comp Physiol. 2014;307(7):R914–9.
77. Schriger DL, Baraff L. Defining normal capillary refill: variation with age, sex, and temperature. Ann Emerg Med. 1988;17:932–5.
78. Algotsson A, Nordberg A, Winblad B. Influence of age and gender on skin vessel reactivity to endothelium-dependent and endothelium-independent vasodilators tested with iontophoresis and a laser Doppler perfusion imager. J Gerontol A Biol Sci Med Sci. 1995;50:121–7.
79. Tur E, Aviram G, Zeltser D, et al. Histamine effect on human cutaneous blood flow: regional variations. Acta Derm Venereol (Stockh). 1994;74:113–6.
80. Orenstein A, Mazkereth R, Tsur H. Mapping of the human body skin with transcutaneous oxygen pressure method. Ann Plast Surg. 1988;64:546–50.
81. Glenski JA, Cucchiara RF. Transcutaneous O_2 and CO_2 monitoring of neurosurgical patients: detection of air embolism. Anesthesiology. 1986;64:546–50.
82. Ewald U. Evaluation of the transcutaneous oxygen method used at 37-C for measurement of reactive hyperaemia in the skin. Clin Physiol. 1984;4:413–23.
83. Havenith G, van Middendorp H. The relative influence of physical fitness, acclimatization state, anthropometric measures and gender on individual reactions to heat stress. Eur J Appl Physiol. 1990;61:419–27.
84. Sato H, Yamasaki K, Yasukouchi A, et al. Sex differences in human thermoregulatory response to cold. J Hum Ergol. 1988;17:57–65.
85. Golja P, Tipton MJ, Mekjavic IB. Cutaneous thermal thresholds - the reproducibility of their measurements and the effect of gender. J Therm Biol. 2003;28:341–6.
86. Jay O, Havenith G. Finger skin cooling on contact with cold materials: an investigation of male and female responses during short-term exposures with a view on hand and finger size. Eur J Appl Physiol. 2004;93:1–8.
87. Hammond LE, Cuttell S, Nunley CP, Meyler J. Anthropometric characteristics and sex influence magnitude of skin cooling following exposure to whole body cryotherapy. Biomed Res Int. 2014.
88. McFarland RA, Kadish R. Sex differences in finger temperature response to music. Int J Psychophysiol. 1991;11:295–8.
89. Martinez-Selva JM, Roman F, Garcia-Sanchez FA, et al. Sex differences and the asymmetry of specific and non-specific electrodermal responses. Int J Psychophysiol. 1987;5:155–60.
90. Weinstein S, Sersen E. Tactual sensitivity as a function of handedness and laterality. J Comp Physiol Psychol. 1961;54:665–9.
91. Yosipovitch G, Meredith G, Chan YH, et al. Do ethnicity and gender have an impact on pain thresholds in minor dermatologic procedures? A study on thermal pain perception thresholds in Asian ethnic groups. Skin Res Technol. 2004;10:38–42.
92. Weller G, Bell RQ. Basal skin conductance and neonatal state. Child Dev. 1965;36:647–57.
93. Mehrai H, Sunderland E. Skin colour data from Nowshahr City, Northern Iran. Ann Hum Biol. 1990;17:115–20.
94. Banerjee S. Pigmentary fluctuation and hormonal changes. J Genet Hum. 1984;32:345–9.
95. Green A, Martin NG. Measurement and perception of skin colour in a skin cancer survey. Br J Dermatol. 1990;123:77–84.
96. Kalla AK, Tiwari SC. Sex differences in skin color in man. Acta Genet Med Gemellol. 1970;19:472–6.
97. Kelly RI, Pearse R, Bull RH, et al. The effects of aging on the cutaneous microvasculature. J Am Acad Dermatol. 1995;33:749–56.
98. Fullerton A, Serup J. Site, gender and age variation in normal skin colour on the back and the forearm: tristimulus colorimeter measurements. Skin Res Technol. 1997;3:49–52.
99. Frost P. Human skin color: a possible relationship between its sexual dimorphism and its social perception. Perspect Biol Med. 1988;32:38–58.
100. Pierard GE, Letawe C, Dowlati A, et al. Effect of hormone replacement therapy for menopause on the mechanical properties of skin. J Am Geriatr Soc. 1995;43:662–5.
101. Brincat M, Moniz CF, Studd JWW, et al. Sex hormones and skin collagen content in postmenopausal women. Br Med J. 1983;287:1337–8.
102. Savvas M, Bishop J, Bishop J, Lauent G, et al. Type III collagen content in the skin of postmenopausal women receiving oestradiol and testosterone implants. Br J Obstet Gynaecol. 1993;100:154–6.
103. Hikima T, Maibach HI. Gender differences of enzymatic activity and distribution of 17beta-hydroxysteroid dehydrogenase in human skin in vitro. Skin Pharmacol Physiol. 2007;20:168–74.

104. Pochi PE, Strauss JS. Endocrinologic control of the development and activity of the human sebaceous gland. J Invest Dermatol. 1974;62:191–201.
105. Courtois M, Loussouarn G, Hourseau S, et al. Periodicity in the growth and shedding of hair. Br J Dermatol. 1996;134:47–54.
106. Randall VA, Thornton MJ, Messenger AG, et al. Hormones and hair growth: variations in androgen receptor content of dermal papilla cells cultured from human and red deer (Cervus Elaphus) hair follicles. J Invest Dermatol. 1993;101: 114S–20.
107. Song EJ, Lee JA, Park JJ, Kim HJ, Kim NS, Byun KS, Choi GS, Moon TK. A study on seasonal variation of skin parameters in Korean males. Int J Cosmet Sci. 2015;37(1):92–7.
108. Mizukoshi K, Akamatsu H. The investigation of the skin characteristics of males focusing on gender differences, skin perception, and skin care habits. Skin Res Technol. 2013;19(2):91–9.
109. Nam GW, Baek JH, Koh JS, Hwang JK. The seasonal variation in skin hydration, sebum, scaliness, brightness and elasticity in Korean females. Skin Res Technol. 2015;21:1–8.

Aging in Asian Skin

129

Low Chai Ling

Contents

L.C. Ling (✉)
The Sloane Clinic, Singapore, Singapore
e-mail: soul@sloaneclinic.com

M.A. Farage et al. (eds.), *Textbook of Aging Skin*,
DOI 10.1007/978-3-662-47398-6_94

Abstract

Asian skin differs from Caucasian skin in both structure and physiology. As a result of these distinctions, Asian skins with their darker pigmentation respond differently when exposed to ultraviolet light, lasers, and other light devices. This needs to be recognized by cosmetic surgeons and laser practitioners. Asian skins also exhibit alternate clinical manifestations of photoaging. Asian skins may benefit from skin treatments targeting different aging issues as compared to those affecting Caucasian skins. This chapter will review the biology of Asian skin and discuss a clinical approach to the aesthetic management of Asian skin.

Introduction

Asian skin differs from Caucasian skin in both structure and physiology (Fig. 1). As a result of these distinctions, Asian skins with their darker pigmentation respond differently when exposed to ultraviolet light, lasers, and other light devices. This needs to be recognized by cosmetic surgeons and laser practitioners. Asian skins also exhibit alternate clinical manifestations of photoaging. As a result, Asian skins may benefit from skin treatments targeting different aging issues as compared to those affecting Caucasian skins. This chapter will review the biology of Asian skin and discuss a clinical approach to the aesthetic management of Asian skin.

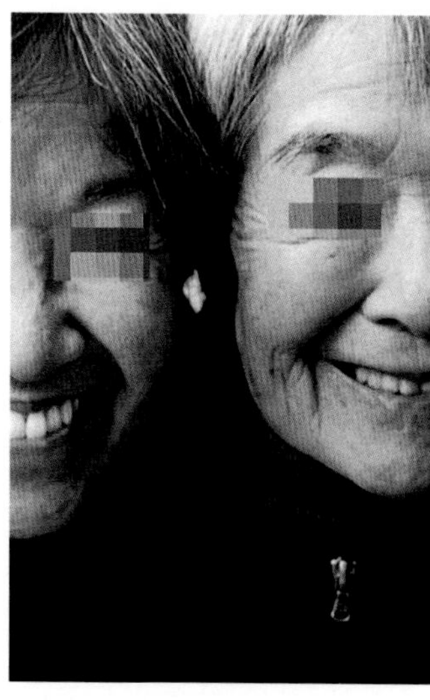

Fig. 1 Asian skins exhibit different manifestations of aging from their Caucasian counterparts

Structural Differences Between Asian and Caucasian Skin

Skin Structure

There have been no firm conclusions to suggest clear racial differences in the structure of skin. Some studies do suggest that heavily pigmented skin is more compact and may have more cell layers compared with lightly pigmented skin. Changes in skin biophysical properties with age demonstrate that the darker skin types retain younger skin properties compared with the fair skin types. There seems to be ethnic variability in the structure of dermal collagen and the abundance of surface lipids. Darker skin types found in certain Asian groups seem to have larger fibroblasts and varying structure of collagen bundles. Stratum corneum lipid content is higher in Asian patients compared with other ethnicities [1]. Asian skins are reported to have an overall weaker skin barrier function. Several studies indicate that Asian skin may be more sensitive to exogenous chemicals probably due to a thinner stratum corneum and higher eccrine gland density [2].

Clearly, this is an area which needs to be studied in depth as there is more to uncover in the differences in skin structure between Asian skins and the other skin types.

Melanin

There are no clear differences in the overall number of melanocytes between the races [3]. Differences in skin color between the races are mainly attributed to variations in melanosomes.

Melanosomes are tissue-specific lysosome-related organelles of pigment cells in which melanins are synthesized and stored. The main determinants of skin color have been attributed to (1) the quantity and type of melanin within the epidermis and (2) the number, size, aggregation pattern, and distribution of melanosomes [4]. In fact, it has been well documented that African-Americans and Caucasians exhibit different distribution patterns of melanosomes, thereby accounting for the differences in their skin color.

The skin's response to UV irradiation is dependent on the epidermal content of melanin as well as the distribution of melanosomes. Melanin confers some degree of photoprotection on the skin. This inherent photoprotection influences the rate of the skin aging changes between the different racial groups. As a result of the higher melanin content in Asian skin compared with white skin, Asian skins generally manifest the classic signs of photoaging later in life, typically beyond the fifth decade [5].

Despite a degree of photoprotection conferred by melanin, pigmented Asian skins can still experience significant photodamage if inadequate sun protection is used [6]. In fact, because Asian skin is less susceptible to the immediate deleterious effects from UV light exposure (sunburn), patients may not be aware that their skin is reactive to the long-term, cumulative effects of unprotected exposure. Photodamage is present histologically as epidermal atypia and atrophy, dermal collagen and elastin damage, and marked hyperpigmentation [6].

Apart from pigmentation from photodamage, Asian patients are most susceptible to post-

Table 1 Fitzpatrick skin phototype

Skin phototype	Skin color	Features
I	Ivory white	Always burns, never tans
II	Fair white	Usually burns, tans poorly
III	White	Sometimes burns, average tan
IV	Beige to olive, lightly tanned	Rarely burns, tans easily
V	Moderate brown or tanned	Very rarely burns, profuse tan
VI	Dark brown to black	Never burns, always tans darkly

inflammatory hyperpigmentation as a direct consequence of cutaneous inflammation or injury due to the increased melanin content.

Skin Phototype

The Fitzpatrick skin phototype system is used to categorize skin types in people of all skin color [7]. The classification depends on the amount of melanin pigment in the skin. Melanin, along with water and hemoglobin, is the target chromophore in skin for lasers and light devices. This is an important consideration because laser energy intended for deeper targets can be absorbed by melanin in the basal layer of the epidermis and can cause unintended epidermal damage, risking blistering, permanent dyspigmentation, textural changes, focal atrophy, and scarring in darker skin types.

Patients are categorized from very fair skin types (Fitzpatrick skin type I) to very dark skin types (VI) based on two parameters: constitutive skin color and response to sunlight and UV radiation (Table 1). The Fitzpatrick classification describes the propensity for sun reactivity. In general, all skin types are susceptible to photoaging but of different degrees. Pale or white skin burns easily and tans slowly and poorly: it needs more protection against sun exposure. Higher Fitzpatrick phototypes are less susceptible to sunburns, likely due to the protective role of melanin. However, higher skin phototypes are more prone to develop post-inflammatory pigmentation after cutaneous injury (brown marks). Asians generally fall into categories IV–VI, with Chinese subjects showing the predominant skin type to be type III, followed by type II and then type IV [8].

It is worth noting that in Asian patients, constitutive skin color does not always correlate with skin response to UV radiation [9]. It is important to assess specifically for Fitzpatrick skin phototype when evaluating a patient before laser or light therapies, because their constitutive skin color alone may not predict response to such melanin-targeted therapies. Patients with higher Fitzpatrick skin types are extremely prone to post-inflammatory hyperpigmentation. When treating such patients with light and laser therapies, practitioners are advised to proceed with caution, and a conservative approach may be appropriate. For example, an ablative laser treatment may also be replaced by a fractionated resurfacing laser or a non-ablative laser treatment to minimize the risk of post-inflammatory hyperpigmentation in such individuals. Such patients may also benefit from pretreatment and posttreatment topical skin lightening regimens to minimize this undesired result. Common skin lightening regimens include hydroquinone 2–4 %, kojic acid 1–4 %, azelaic acid 20 %, and arbutin 1 %. Hydroquinone is banned in the European Union, Australia, and Japan due to its carcinoma-inducing concerns.

With topical hydroquinone, there is still a small risk of contact dermatitis though this usually responds promptly to topical steroids. An uncommon, yet important, adverse effect of hydroquinone is exogenous ochronosis. Ochronosis is characterized by progressive bluish black darkening of the skin area exposed to hydroquinone. Histologically, degeneration of collagen and elastic fibers occurs, followed by the appearance of characteristic ochronotic deposits consisting of crescent-shaped, ochre-colored fibers in the dermis. Carbon dioxide lasers and dermabrasion have been reported to be helpful in the treatment of exogenous ochronosis. Reports have also described effective therapy with the Q-switched alexandrite 755-nm laser.

Aging Processes

Anatomy of Aging Skin

Aging skin exhibits progressive changes such as thinning, skin laxity, fragility, and wrinkles. Sun-exposed areas demonstrate additional skin changes, including dyschromia, premature wrinkling, actinic elastosis, and telangiectasias [10].

When a cell stops replicating, it enters into a period of decline known as "cell senescence." Aging at the cellular level is thought to be related to cellular senescence. This refers specifically to the shortening of telomeres (the terminal portions of chromosomes) with each cell cycle. Telomere shortening ultimately results in apoptosis once a critical length is reached.

Histopathologically, photoaging is characterized by disorganized collagen fibrils, decreased normal collagen, and increased abnormal elastic fibers termed solar elastosis at the upper dermis, as well as flattening of the dermal-epidermal junction with elongated and collapsed fibroblasts [11].

Intrinsic Versus Extrinsic Skin Aging

Cutaneous aging is an interplay of intrinsic and extrinsic aging processes. Intrinsic aging occurs naturally and can be exacerbated by extrinsic aging. Most of the efforts in facial rejuvenation are targeted toward counteracting the effects of extrinsic aging.

Intrinsic Aging

Intrinsic or chronologic aging is a genetically determined process of aging which occurs in the skin; this type of aging also occurs in photoprotected skin. Additional contributing factors include the effects of gravity, expression, and hormones. Intrinsic aging is characterized by dryness, laxity, and skin atrophy, affecting both sun-exposed and non-sun-exposed skin. In Asian patients, intrinsic aging predominantly results in a decrease in skin elasticity.

Extrinsic Aging

Extrinsic aging is environmentally induced. It has been established that chronic inflammation at the cellular level is the cause of extrinsic aging [12]. The two most important factors in Asian patients that contribute to the extrinsic aging process are a history of smoking and chronic UV light exposure. As in white-skinned patients, the effects of cigarette smoking and excessive chronic sun exposure seem multiplicative [13]. In Asian patients, extrinsic aging manifests as pigmentary changes, rhytides, laxity, and coarseness of skin texture with pigmentary changes predominating as the initial signs of the extrinsic aging process.

Ultraviolet irradiation leads to dermal damage with histologic evidence of disorganized collagen fibrils and abnormal solar elastotic material. Elevated matrix metalloproteinases and collagen degeneration lead to dermal breakdown [14]. This manifests clinically as progressive skin laxity and the formation of rhytides.

Aging Skin

There are numerous factors that contribute to aging skin. Even among patients of Asian heritage, these factors appear in varying degrees in each individual resulting in great discrepancies in the aging process even among individuals of the same ethnicity. The clinical signs of aging include dyschromia, loss of smooth surface skin texture, loss of translucency, skin volume loss, and functional loss [15]. By accurately identifying the relative contributing factors to an aged appearance, individual-specific skin treatment can be selected, and the risk-benefit ratios of the possible therapies weighed. This is an essential part of a

Table 2 Photoaging scale (Glocau RG [18])

Skin type	Age in years	Clinical findings
I (mild)	20–30	Little or no photoaging, little or no wrinkling, no keratoses
II (moderate)	30–50	Early to moderate photoaging, wrinkles present with motion
III (advanced)	50–60	Advanced photoaging, wrinkles with rest, visible keratoses, noticeable discolorations
IV (severe)	60 and over	Severe photoaging, deep wrinkles – both dynamic and gravitational wrinkling, actinic keratoses

comprehensive cosmetic consultation and, ultimately, a successful and safe skin rejuvenation treatment process.

Photoaging

Ethnic and genetic differences in skin structure and function mean that the clinical manifestations of photoaging in Asian skin differ from those of white skin. Asian skins have different natural defense mechanisms against chronic UV exposure. In addition, different cultural habits related to UV exposure should also be taken into consideration. While photoaging in white individuals manifests as premature and progressive development of fine lines and rhytides, the primary manifestation of photoaging in Asian skin is pigmentary changes, with rhytides being less conspicuous and usually not noticeable until after the fifth decade [16, 17].

Photoaging Scale

A photoaging scale was devised by Glogau (Table 2) to aid in assessing severity of skin photodamage [18]. This can be helpful in discussing potential results of facial cosmetic procedures with patients. Although initially used to describe white skin, the Glogau photoaging scale, with slight alteration, is also very useful in analysis of Asian skin and has the advantage of practical clinical application.

In type I or early photoaging, no wrinkles are present. There is little or no visible pigmentary changes present. Female patients in this category usually require no makeup. Asian patients may not be aware that their skin is reactive to the long-term, cumulative effects of unprotected exposure because Asian skin is less susceptible to the immediate deleterious effects from UV light exposure (sunburn). Daily sun protection should nonetheless be advocated.

In type II photoaging, pigmentary changes become more prevalent, with development of mottled skin tone and solar lentigo. Superficial brown pigmentation and freckling can be accentuated with Wood's lamp illumination. These mild and flat pigmentary changes respond readily to topical agents, such as retinoids, ascorbic acid (vitamin c), hydroquinone, and alpha hydroxy acids [19]. Superficial chemical peels, microdermabrasion, and intense pulsed light therapies also yield results at this early stage [20]. Lasers such as the Q-switched Nd:YAG laser can also be considered for more resistant pigmented lesions. Although no obvious wrinkles appear when facial musculature is at rest, dynamic wrinkles appear when the face is in motion. These rhytides often first appear on the upper third of the face along the lateral orbits as "crow's feet," the glabella as "frown lines," and the forehead as "horizontal lines" [21]. Chemical muscle denervation with botulinum toxin can also be considered to relax dynamic wrinkles and to improve the appearance of the face in motion.

In patients exhibiting type III photoaging, pigmentary changes are advanced. Deeper pigmentary disorders, such as melasma and Hori's nevus, may manifest. These lesions are more difficult to treat. Raised brown lesions, such as seborrheic keratoses, further disrupt the surface texture of the skin. Laser treatment of pigmentary disorders of this type is challenging. Patients in this stage also display obvious static wrinkles. The skin no longer has a smooth texture and exhibits reduced reflectance. In addition to chemical denervation, soft tissue augmentation is indicated to replace volume loss and to plump up static wrinkles such as the nasolabial lines. Fractional ablative lasers in addition to the above light therapies listed for type II photoaging can be considered to improve skin texture and skin dyschromia. However because of increased risk for post-inflammatory hyperpigmentation, these techniques must be used with caution and with adequate counseling and preparation of patient expectations.

Finally, in patients with type IV photoaging, wrinkles predominate, while numerous severe pigmentary lesions are also present. Hardly any normal skin remains. Topical therapy does not effect a significant benefit, and noninvasive aesthetic treatments may only give limited improvements. Surgical correction in addition to skin rejuvenation measures may be considered.

Pigmentary Changes

In Asian patients, photodamage predominantly presents as pigmentary changes rather than wrinkling. This difference is partially due to the higher epidermal melanin content, which can predispose these patients to a higher risk for hyperpigmentation from light source treatment. Long-term UV light damage to the skin is the most common trigger of dyschromia. Visible color changes include early appearance of uneven skin tone, followed by various pigmented growths. The most common pigmentary disorders seen in chronically UV-exposed skin include ephelides (freckling), solar lentigo, melasma, and seborrheic keratosis [16]. The development of seborrheic keratosis seems to be more prevalent in Asian men, whereas hyperpigmented maculae are more prominent in women [13]. Each of these pigmentary disorders is caused by pathology in varying levels of the epidermis and dermis. To differentiate epidermal from dermal lesions, one can use a Wood's lamp in the examination of a patient with dyspigmentation. Superficial (epidermal) melanin is accentuated with Wood's lamp illumination, whereas deeper (dermal) melanin does not appear enhanced.

Accurate diagnosis of the etiology of pigment alteration allows for targeted, more effective treatment. For epidermal pigmented lesions, IPL can be effective [20]. Q-switched laser and fractional resurfacing laser are options used to remove dermal pigment.

Textural Changes

Textural changes begin with a loss of smoothness and reflectance, gradually progressing to the development of raised growths, such as seborrheic keratoses. Yellow thickened bumps (*elastosis* or *heliosis*) appear and are due to tangled masses of damaged elastin protein in the dermis. There is also increased dermal collagen due to scarring from repeated inflammation. This thick dermis loses elasticity and is weaker than normal, putting aging skin at higher risk for injury. Rubbing or pulling on the skin can cause skin tears. The skin appears sallow and dull. Visible coarseness of the skin may also develop because of sebaceous hyperplasia, enlarged pore size, and thickening of unwanted facial hair [22].

As the skin and underlying supporting structures lose elasticity over time, it becomes less resistant to the cumulative effects of gravity and underlying musculature. With early aging, wrinkles appear only when the face is in motion, usually at the expression lines around the eyes and mouth. Over time, as elasticity of the skin further diminished, wrinkles are visible even when the face is at rest.

Volume Loss

Facial aging is associated with loss of soft tissue fullness in certain areas and descent or hypertrophy in others [23]. An overall loss of volume occurs in the periorbital, forehead, malar, temple, mandibular, mental, glabellar, and perioral sites, while hypertrophy of fat occurs in the submental, lateral nasolabial folds and labiomental crease, jowls, infraorbital pouches, and malar fat pad. Gradual relaxation of the ligamentous support leads to descent and separation of the fat pads.

Remodeling of the craniofacial skeleton leads to a reduction in facial height [23]. This decreases the space available to support the overlying soft tissues causing the face to collapse in on itself. The orbits increase in diameter as the orbital shelf descends, resulting in the malposition of the lower eyelid which presents as lateral bowing and scleral show.

Maxillary resorption causes loss of support in the upper lip, and this contributes to perioral wrinkling, thinning, and inversion of the lips.

Assessment of the aging face should include an analysis of the quality and position of the underlying fat.

Functional Loss

The main functional losses experienced by aging skin are a decrease in cell replacement, barrier function, chemical clearance, mechanical protection, immune responsiveness, wound healing, thermoregulation, and vitamin D production.

With aging, the barrier function is compromised. There are some differences in barrier function between Caucasian and Asian skins. Barrier function relates to the total architecture of the stratum corneum as well as its lipid levels. Asian skin is reported to possess a similar basal transepidermal water loss (TEWL) to Caucasian skin and similar ceramide levels but reduced stratum corneum natural moisturizing factors [2]. Upon mechanical challenge it has weaker barrier function compared to Caucasian skins. Both skin types also exhibit differences in intercellular cohesion. The frequency of skin sensitivity is quite similar across different racial groups, but the stimuli for its induction show subtle differences. Nevertheless, several studies indicate that Asian skin may be more sensitive to exogenous chemicals probably due to a thinner stratum corneum and higher eccrine gland density [2].

Due to decreases especially in melanocytes and the dermis, there is a disruption in the mechanical protection served by the skin. This results in increased UV penetration and damage as well as decreased nutrient transfer.

With aging, wound healing is impaired with increased breakdown in tissue. This explains why the elderly has a predisposition to chronic wounds.

Immune responsiveness is impaired in aging skin as Langerhans cells exhibit a reduction in number as well as an impairment of their antigen-presenting capacity with age. Acute inflammatory reactions are less noticeable.

Aging skin shows a decrease in sweat glands, vasculature, nerves, sweat glands, and sebaceous secretions. These changes result in an overall reduction in thermoregulation and a lower threshold for pain perception and reaction.

Vitamin D production decreases with age. This may in turn decrease calcium levels and predispose the elderly to osteomalacia. The melanin in darker skin types acts as a sunscreen and may slow down production of vitamin D3. However, race had only a marginal effect on the production of active vitamin D metabolites. While racial pigmentation has a photoprotective effect, it does not prevent the generation of normal levels of active vitamin D metabolites [24].

Conclusion

Recognizing the unique characteristics of Asian skin allows physicians to optimize cosmetic results and ultimately to a successful facial rejuvenation for an aging Asian skin. Differences in the structure and physiology of Asian skin, particularly in melanin content, account for variations in response to UV light exposure and alternate clinical manifestations of photoaging. Cosmetic surgeons and laser practitioners should be aware of the distinct presentations of photodamage in Asians and understand the increased risk of post-inflammatory hyperpigmentation associated with various therapeutic modalities.

Cross-References

▶ Determinants in the Rate of Skin Aging: Ethnicity, Gender, and Lifestyle Influences

References

1. Richards GM, Oresajo CO, Halder RM. Structure and function of ethnic skin and hair. Dermatol Clin. 2003;21(4):595–600.
2. Rawlings AV. Ethnic skin types: are there differences in skin structure and function? Int J Cosmet Sci. 2006;28 (2):79–93.
3. Staricco RJ, Pinkus H. Quantitative and qualitative data on the pigment cells of adult human epidermis. J Invest Dermatol. 1957;28(1):33–45.
4. Goldschmidt H, Raymond JZ. Quantitative analysis of skin color from melanin content of superficial skin cells. J Forensic Sci. 1972;17(1):124–31.
5. Siegrid SY, Grekin RC. Aesthetic analysis of Asian skin. Facial Plast Surg Clin North Am. 2007;15 (3):361–5.
6. Kotrajaras R, Kligman AM. The effect of topical tretinoin on photodamaged facial skin: the Thai experience. Br J Dermatol. 1993;129(3):302–9.
7. Fitzpatrick TB. The validity and practicality of sun reactive skin type I through VI. Arch Dermatol. 1988;124:869–71.
8. Liu W, Lai W, Wang XM, et al. Skin phototyping in a Chinese female population: analysis of four hundred and four cases from four major cities of China. Photodermatol Photoimmunol Photomed. 2006;22 (4):184–8.
9. Choe YB, Jang SJ, Jo SJ, et al. The difference between the constitutive and facultative skin color does not reflect skin phototype in Asian skin. Skin Res Technol. 2006;12(1):68–72.
10. Gilchrest BA, Yaar M. Ageing and photoageing of the skin: observations at the cellular and molecular level. Br J Dermatol. 1992;127 Suppl 41:25–30.
11. Bernstein EF, Chen YQ, Kopp JB, et al. Long-term sun exposure alters the collagen of the papillary dermis: comparison of sun-protected and photoaged skin by northern analysis, immunohistochemical staining, and confocal laser scanning microscopy. J Am Acad Dermatol. 1996;34(2 Pt 1):209–18.
12. Thornfeldt CR. Chronic inflammation is the etiology of extrinsic aging. J Cosmet Dermatol. 2008;7:78–82.
13. Chung JH, Lee SH, Youn CS, et al. Cutaneous photodamage in Koreans: influence of sex, sun exposure, smoking, and skin color. Arch Dermatol. 2001;137(8):1043–51.
14. Fisher GJ, Wang ZQ, Datta SC, et al. Pathophysiology of premature skin aging induced by ultraviolet light. N Engl J Med. 1997;337:1419–28.
15. Calderone DC, Fenske NA. The clinical spectrum of actinic elastosis. J Am Acad Dermatol. 1995;32 (6):1016–24.
16. Chung JH. Photoaging in Asians. Photodermatol Photoimmunol Photomed. 2003;19(3):109–21.
17. Nouveau-Richard S, Yang Z, Mac-Mary S, et al. Skin ageing: a comparison between Chinese and European populations. A pilot study. J Dermatol Sci. 2005;40 (3):187–93.
18. Glocau RG. Aesthetic and anatomic analysis of the aging skin. Semin Cutan Med Surg. 1996;15 (3):134–8.
19. Griffiths CE, Goldfarb MT, Finkel LJ, et al. Topical tretinoin (retinoic acid) treatment of hyperpigmented lesions associated with photoaging in Chinese and Japanese patients: a vehicle-controlled trial. J Am Acad Dermatol. 1994;30(1):76–84.
20. Feng Y, Zhao J, Gold MH. Skin rejuvenation in Asian skin: the analysis of clinical effects and basic mechanisms of intense pulsed light. J Drugs Dermatol. 2008;7(3):273–9.
21. Glogau RG. Physiologic and structural changes associated with aging skin. Dermatol Clin. 1997;15 (4):555–9.
22. Bolognia JL. Aging skin. Am J Med. 1995;98 (1A):99S–103.
23. Sydney R. Coleman, Rajiv Grover. The anatomy of the aging face: volume loss and changes in 3-dimensional topography. Aesthet Surg J. 2006;26(1):S4–9.
24. Matsuoka LY, Wortsman J, Haddad JG, Kolm P, Hollis BW. Racial pigmentation and the cutaneous synthesis of vitamin D. Arch Dermatol. 1991;127(4):536–8.

Part XIII

Sensitive Skin and Aging

Perceptions of Sensitive Skin with Age

130

Miranda A. Farage

Contents

M.A. Farage (✉)
Winton Hill Business Center, The Procter & Gamble Company, Cincinnati, OH, USA
e-mail: farage.m@pg.com

M.A. Farage et al. (eds.), *Textbook of Aging Skin*,
DOI 10.1007/978-3-662-47398-6_95

Abstract

Sensitive skin is generally agreed to describe unpleasant subjective sensory reactions in response to common external factors and intrinsic stressors. It is commonly assumed that physiological changes that occur as skin ages leave skin more sensitive to irritation and discomfort. However, a comprehensive review of clinical assessments of the erythematous response in older people suggests that susceptibility to skin irritation generally decreases with age. We used an epidemiological approach to compare perceptions of skin sensitivity among older and younger adults through a questionnaire-based survey of 1,039 people. Data were evaluated based on age group: ≤ 30 ($n = 295$), 31–39 ($n = 492$), 40–49 ($n = 128$), and ≥ 50 ($n = 101$). There were no significant differences between age groups in perceived sensitive skin overall or of the face or body. Sensitivity of genital skin was significantly ($p = 0.01$) more likely to be reported by those aged 50 or older, and the perception of skin sensitivity at this site rose directionally with age ($\leq 30 = 53$ %, 31–39 = 55 %, 40–49 = 58 %, and $\geq 50 = 66$ %). A significantly higher proportion of women specifically perceived their genital skin to be sensitive (58 % of females and 44 % of males) ($p < 0.03$), and within age groups, the association of age and perceived genital skin sensitivity was significant only for women ($p = 0.01$). Surprisingly, women were no more likely than men to perceive their facial skin to be sensitive, regardless of age. Older adults also reported that their skin had become more sensitive over time and had a higher frequency of medically diagnosed skin allergies than younger people. Additional comparisons between age groups, ethnicities, and gender are also reported.

Introduction

Sensitive skin is generally agreed to describe unpleasant subjective sensory reactions (such as prickling, burning, tingling, or pain) in response to common external factors (such as ultraviolet light, heat, cold, wind, cosmetics, cleaning products, etc.) and intrinsic stressors (such as stress or hormones) [1]. The etiology of sensitive skin is unknown, but the disorder is believed to be the product of multiple etiologies with multiple components, including deficiencies in barrier function, neurosensory dysfunction, compound-specific irritancy, and cultural influences [2, 3].

The sensory effects that are the hallmark of sensitive skin are only occasionally accompanied by erythema or other demonstrable irritation or immunological responses [1]. In fact, little correlation exists between individuals' perceptions of the sensitivity of their skin and objective clinical assessments of skin reactivity to irritants [4]. Individuals who exhibit a low threshold of response to a particular irritant may not be susceptible to all other types of irritant stimuli.

A sizeable proportion of people in the general population claim some degree of skin sensitivity (recently reviewed in [2, 5]). A number of studies have been conducted in Europe. Overall, some degree of skin sensitivity was claimed by 50–90 % of responders in several studies in France [1, 6–11], 75 % of responders in Germany [12], over 50 % in Italy [13], and 64 % in Greece [14]. In the UK, 38.2 % of the men and 51.4 % of the women claimed to have sensitive skin [15]. In the USA, the prevalence of self-declared sensitive skin has been reported at 44–83 % [16–21].

The reported prevalence of sensitive skin in China is much lower than that in Europe and the USA. In a survey of 9,154 subjects in three cities in China, the mean prevalence of self-proclaimed sensitive skin was 13 % (8.62 % in men and 15.93 % in women) [22]. In another study conducted among 408 women in China, some degree of skin sensitivity was claimed by 94 (23 %) of respondents [5].

In a study conducted in Mexico using 246 subjects self-diagnosed sensitive skin was found in 36.2 % subjects [23]. This study indicated a higher prevalence of sensitive skin in subjects with lighter skin phototypes (types II and III) compared to darker ones (types IV and V).

Compared to the overall population, less information is available on perceptions of skin sensitivity among older adults, specifically. In a phone survey conducted in the USA among 994 subjects, 44.6 % declared having "sensitive" or "very sensitive" skin [20]. However, there were no significant differences in the prevalence when the data were considered based on subgroups of 18–24 years, 25–34 years, 35–44 years, 45–54 years, 55–64 years, and ≥65 years. In contrast, in the survey conducted in China [22], there was a statistically significant difference among three age groups in the study, younger group (<25 years), middle group (25–49 years), and older group (≥50 years), with the reported prevalence decreasing inversely with age.

Susceptibility of Aging Skin to Irritants

The physiological changes that occur as skin ages might lead one to conclude that older skin is more susceptible to irritant effects. Such changes (reviewed in [24, 25]) include:

- Reduced epidermal thickness and reduced epidermal turnover
- Lower sensory perception
- Reduced hydration
- Increased permeability
- Flattening of the dermal-epidermal junction
- Lower elasticity and diminished tensile strength, due to changes in the architecture of the collagen and elastin networks
- Reduced dermal thickness (~20 %)

- Reduced cellularity and vascularity of the dermis
- Slower wound healing

Although it is commonly assumed that aging skin is more sensitive to irritation and discomfort, a comprehensive review of clinical assessments of the erythematous response in older people suggests that susceptibility to skin irritation generally decreases with age [26]. For example, a compilation of results of skin patch tests conducted among older people over a period of 4 years demonstrated a trend toward lower reactivity to four common irritants with age [27]. Specifically, older people exhibited significantly lower reactivity to two strong irritants (20 % sodium dodecyl sulfate and 100 % octanoic acid) and directionally lower reactivity (approaching statistical significance) to two milder irritants (100 % decanol and 10 % acetic acid); however, the severity of the observed irritant responses was unrelated to people's perception of the sensitivity of their skin. People aged 65–84 years were less reactive to stinging caused by 5 % sodium lauryl sulfate (SLS) than people aged 18–25 years [28]. Pretreatment with 0.25 % SLS also had less of an effect on skin barrier function and susceptibility to irritants in elderly people (mean age, 74.6 years) than in younger adults (mean age, 25.9 years) [29]. Lastly, elderly adults were less reactive to a range of irritants (histamine, DMSO, 48/80 mixture of chloroform-methanol, lactic acid, ethyl nicotinate, and the blistering agent, ammonium hydrazide) [30].

Perceptions of Sensitive Skin Among Older Adults

The conclusion that elderly skin is less susceptible to skin irritation is based on objective assessments in patch tests and sting tests. However, because little correlation exists between objective and subjective assessments of skin sensitivity, objective tests provide little insight on individuals' perceptions about the sensitivity of their skin. Our research group compared perceptions of skin sensitivity among older and younger adults through a questionnaire-based survey of 1,039 people conducted in 2006 in the Midwestern USA. Results for the entire group have been reported previously [18, 19, 31].

Population Demographics

The population was recruited from among people participating in consumer product preference tests. Consequently, the surveyed population was predominantly female, and 76 % were under the age of 40 (Table 1). The analyses were performed on the following age subgroup years: $\leq$30 years, 31–39 years, 40–49 years, and $\geq$50 years. The two older age groups each comprised over 100 subjects, enabling valid statistical comparisons.

One consumer product test was related to urinary incontinence products. This subset of women was used to evaluate the potential differences in perceptions of sensitive skin among individuals with urinary incontinence compared to age- and gender-matched subjects without this condition.

No criteria related to skin sensitivity (e.g., hyper-reactivity to consumer products, a history of skin or respiratory allergies) were used in recruitment. Ethnic representation within the population reflected that of the location where the study was conducted [32]. The small number of Latinos and Asians did not produce valid conclusions to be drawn for these demographic groups.

Perceptions of Skin Sensitivity at Different Anatomical Sites Among Age Groups

Sixty-eight percent of the study population described themselves as having sensitive skin to some degree (Table 2): 77 % perceived their facial skin to be sensitive, 61 % perceived their overall body, and 56 % their genital area to be sensitive. The most frequent single cause of skin sensitivity claimed by all age groups was extreme weather conditions (Table 3). About half of each age group also claimed adverse reactions to products.

Table 1 Breakdown of the test population by age, gender, and ethnicity

	All ages		≤30		31–39		40–49		≥50	
	Number	%	Number	%	Number	%	Number	%	Number	%
Both genders, all ethnicities	1,039[a]	100 %	295	28 %	492	48 %	128	12 %	101	10 %
Females	869	84 %	261	25 %	421	41 %	83	8 %	84	8 %
Males	163	16 %	30	3 %	70	7 %	44	4 %	17	2 %
Females ($n = 869$)	Number	%[b]	Number	%	Number	%	Number	%	Number	%
Caucasian	684	77 %	213	25 %	344	40 %	58	7 %	54	6 %
African-American	108	12 %	35	4 %	42	5 %	10	1 %	17	2 %
Hispanic	10	1 %	2	0 %	8	1 %	0	0 %	0	0 %
Asian	13	1 %	2	0 %	8	1 %	1	0 %	1	0 %
Not given	54	6 %	9	1 %	19	2 %	14	2 %	12	1 %
Males ($n = 163$)	Number	%[c]	Number	%	Number	%	Number	%	Number	%
Caucasian	118	72 %	21	13 %	54	33 %	28	17 %	15	9 %
African-American	20	12 %	3	2 %	8	5 %	7	4 %	1	1 %
Hispanic	8	4 %	2	1 %	2	1 %	3	2 %	0	0 %
Asian	5	3 %	1	1 %	3	2 %	1	1 %	0	0 %
Not given	12	7 %	3	2 %	3	2 %	5	3 %	1	1 %

A total of 1,039 individuals filled out sensitive skin questionnaires. Demographic data are summarized for all responders. The percentage of ethnicity subgroups was calculated separately for each gender

[a]7 subjects did not provide their gender. An additional 22 subjects did not provide their age (20 females and 2 males)

[b]% of females

[c]% of males

Table 2 Perceptions of sensitive skin

	Question: Some people have skin that is more sensitive than others. How would you describe your skin?		Question: Please rate your skin in each of the following areas:	
	Overall rating of skin sensitivity	Facial area	Body area	Genital area
Total number of subjects responding	1,039	1,033	1,035	1,031
Very sensitive	51 (5 %)	111 (11 %)	19 (2 %)	88 (9 %)
Moderately sensitive	239 (23 %)	245 (24 %)	189 (18 %)	140 (14 %)
Slightly sensitive	421 (41 %)	443 (43 %)	420 (41 %)	352 (34 %)
Not sensitive	328 (32 %)	234 (23 %)	407 (39 %)	451 (44 %)
Sensitive (any degree)	711 (68 %)	799 (77 %)	628 (61 %)	580 (56 %)

Participants were questioned about how they would describe their skin (very sensitive, moderately sensitive, slightly sensitive, not sensitive). On a subsequent page of the questionnaire, participants were asked to rate the skin of three anatomical sites: facial area, body area, and genital area. Responses are shown above for the overall rating (number followed by percentage) and for the ratings at the three anatomical sites

Table 3 Most common reason given for perceiving sensitive skin

Question: Select one of the following statements that *best* describes why you think you have sensitive skin					
I have sensitive skin because....	All	≤30	31–39	40–49	≥50
1. Some products cause my skin to break out in a rash (redness and/or swelling)	25 %	27 %	25 %	27 %	21 %
2. Some products cause burning, stinging, itching, or other unpleasant sensations	25 %	23 %	27 %	23 %	29 %
3. My skin is sensitive to extreme weather conditions (hot, cold, dry, humid)	36 %	34 %	37 %	35 %	33 %
4. Items that rub against my skin (such as washcloths, clothing, etc.) cause my skin to become sensitive	7 %	7 %	6 %	8 %	7 %
5. I have sensitive skin due to another reason	7 %	9 %	6 %	7 %	10 %
Relationship to age group is not significant		$p = 0.9015$			

Participants were asked to choose the one reason why they perceived their skin to be sensitive. Analysis for a significant relationship between the response and age were done using Cochran-Mantel-Haenszel statistics

Sensitivity of genital skin was significantly more likely to be reported by those aged 50 or older and the perception of skin sensitivity at this site rose directionally with age (Fig. 1d). A lower percentage of people aged 40–49 years reported facial skin sensitivity compared to those aged 31–39, respectively (Fig. 1b).

Analysis of the results by gender yielded additional insights. In the population as a whole, gender was not associated with overall claims of skin sensitivity (data not shown). However, a significantly higher proportion of women specifically perceived their genital skin to be sensitive (58 % of females and 44 % of males) ($p < 0.03$). Moreover, within age groups, the association of age and perceived genital skin sensitivity was significant only for women ($p = 0.01$) (Fig. 2d). Surprisingly, women were not more likely than men in any age group to report facial skin sensitivity.

Ethnic Differences in Perceptions of Sensitive Skin at Different Anatomical Sites by Age

Among Caucasians, people aged 50 and over were more likely to report facial skin sensitivity than those aged 40–49; those aged 30–39 reported more body skin sensitivity than those 30 and under; and, as previously noted, those 50 and over were more likely than all other age groups to report genital skin sensitivity (Fig. 3). Among African-Americans, a slightly higher frequency of skin sensitivity was reported among people aged 50 and older at all anatomical sites, but the differences were not statistically significant, probably because of the smaller sample size. Within age groups, no statistically significant differences in perceived skin sensitivity were found between Caucasians and African-Americans at any body site.

Differences in Diagnosed Skin Allergies by Age

The proportion of people reporting a medically diagnosed skin allergy increased significantly with age ($p = 0.002$) (Fig. 4a), but only among those who perceived their skin to be sensitive ($p = 0.0006$) (Fig. 4b, c). The age-related increase in medically diagnosed skin allergies among those with sensitive skin held true for each specific anatomical site (face, body, or genitalia). Among people who perceived their skin to be sensitive at any site, those aged 50 or older reported a higher frequency of medically diagnosed skin allergies than any other age group (Fig. 4b).

Other investigators have reported associations between sensitive skin and dermatologist consultations [8] and between sensitive skin and nickel contact allergy [12]. Possibly, the perception of "sensitive skin" may be part of a syndrome of skin hyper-reactivity that includes a higher propensity to developing contact allergy.

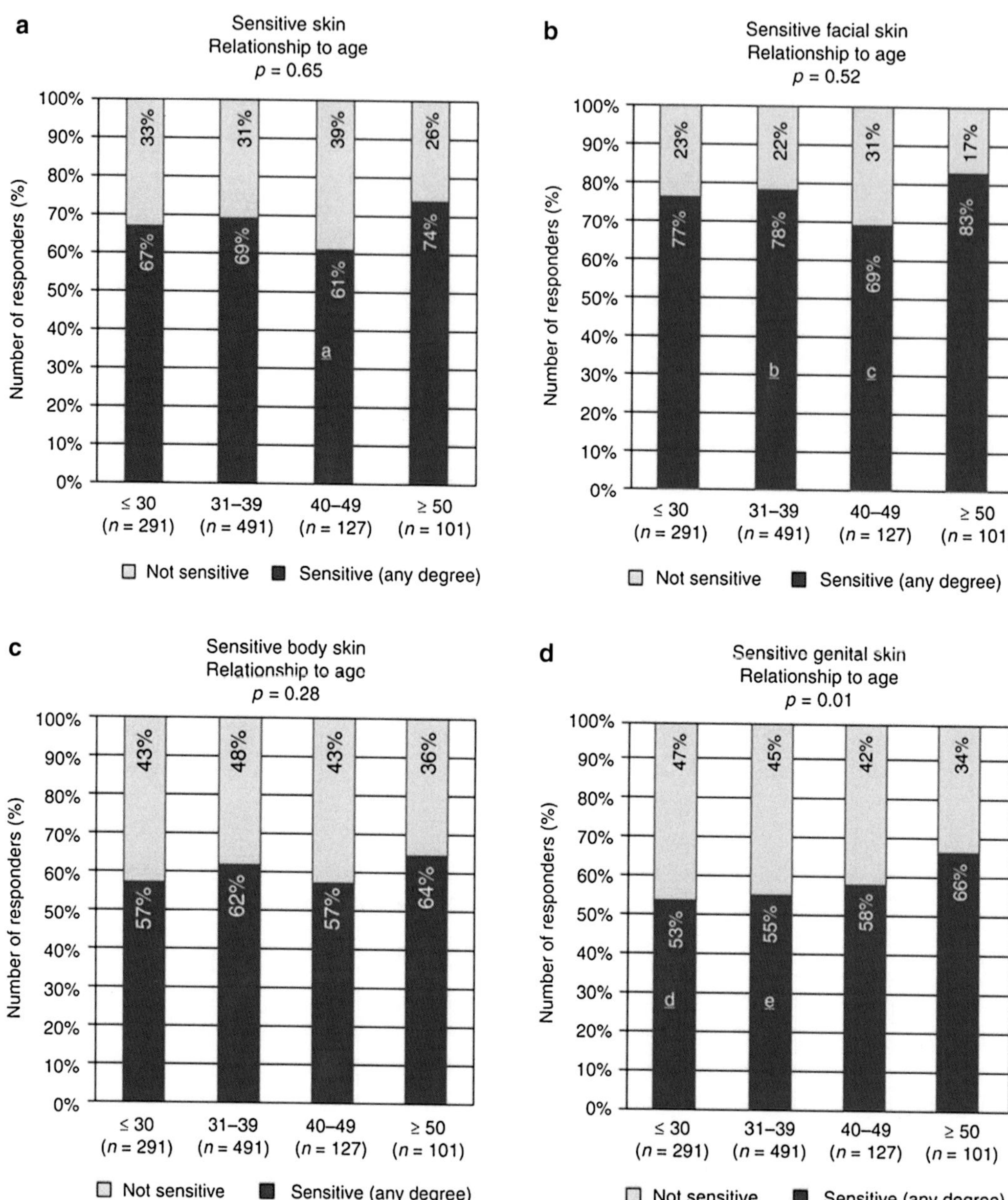

Fig. 1 Age group differences in perceptions of sensitive skin. The percentage of participants who claimed some degree of sensitivity overall (**a**) or sensitivity of the facial, body, or genital areas (**b**–**d**). Correlations between perceptions of sensitive skin and age were assessed by MH chi-square. Paired age group comparisons were performed by chi-square analysis. (**a**) On the bar of figure 1 a – 40–49 group significantly lower than 50 group ($p = 0.04$). (**b**) On the bar of figure 1b – 31–39 group significantly higher than 40–49 group ($p = 0.03$). (**c**) On the bar of figure 1b – 40–49 group significantly lower than 50 group ($p = 0.02$). (**d**) On the bar of figure 1d –30 group significantly lower than 50 group ($p = 0.02$). (**e**) On the bar of figure 1d – 31–39 group significantly lower than 50 group ($p = 0.04$)

Alternatively, the need to seek medical treatment for allergic reactions may heighten patients' awareness of skin sensations and reactions, causing them to perceive their skin to be sensitive. Although the perception of sensitive skin is subjective, these associations suggest that there may be a biological basis for some claims of sensitivity.

Changes in Perceived Skin Sensitivity Over Time

As stated in the beginning of this chapter, of the entire test population, 68 % claimed sensitive skin to some degree. Among those who claimed sensitive skin, over 62 % of the total population stated that their skin has been sensitive for more than 10 years and 16 % claimed their skin has been sensitive 6–10 years (Fig. 5a). As expected, there was a significant relationship between the duration of perceived sensitive

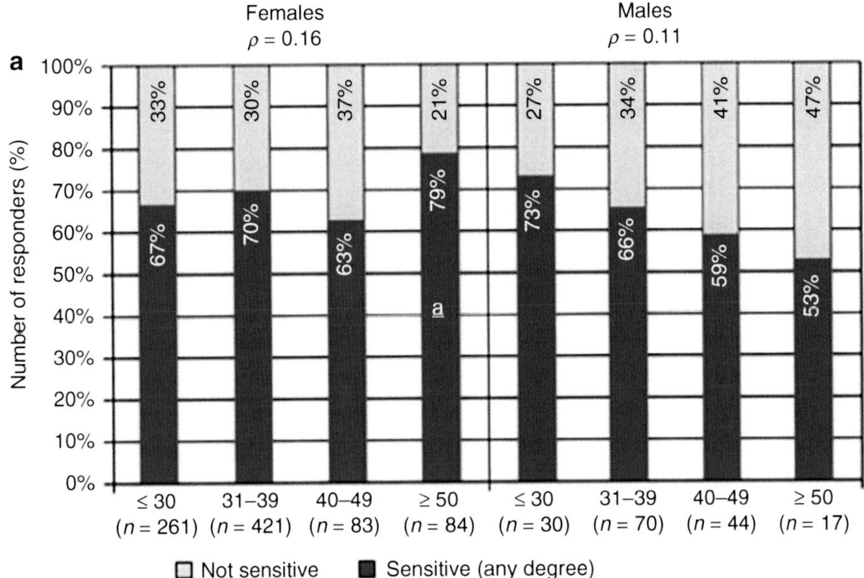

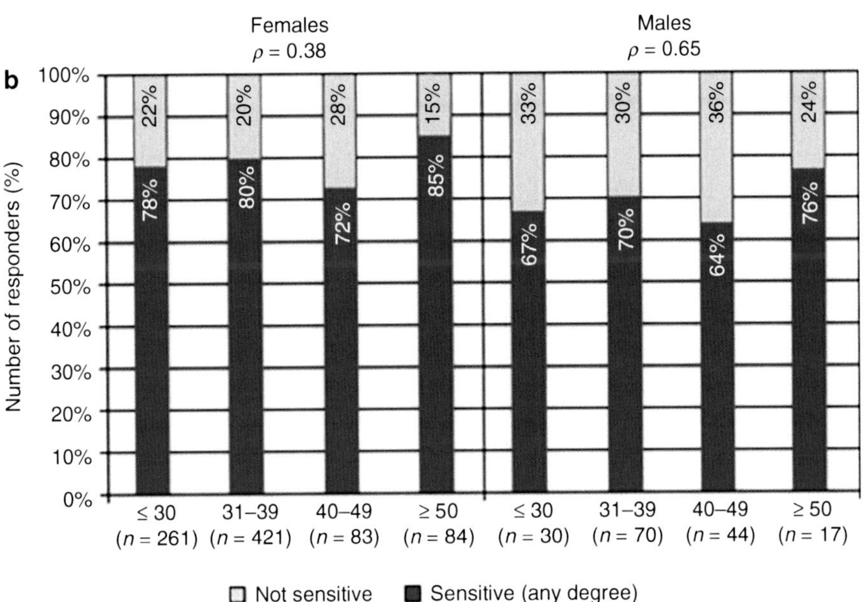

Fig. 2 (continued)

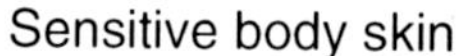

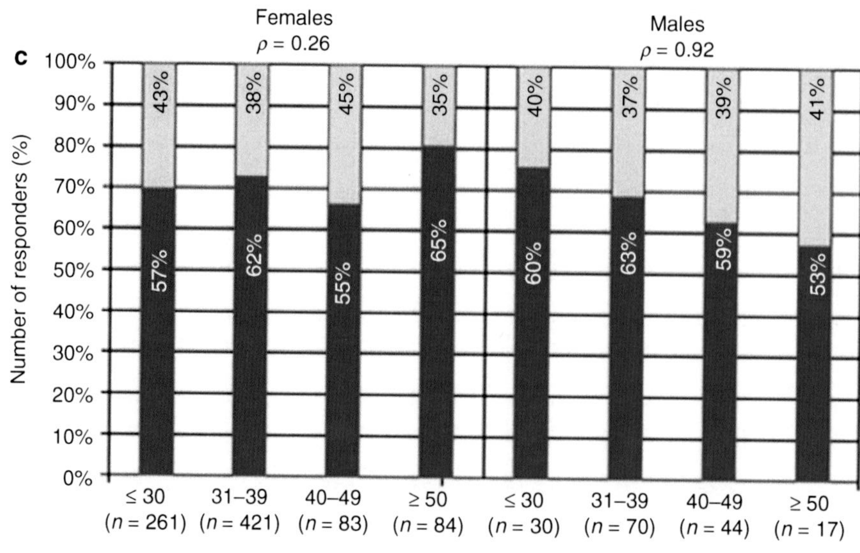

Sensitive genital skin

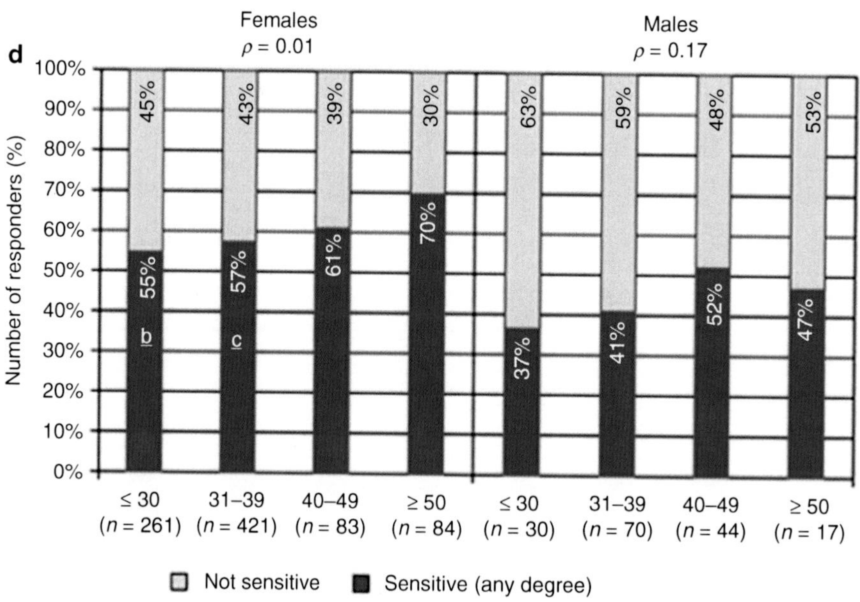

Fig. 2 Age group differences in perceptions of sensitive skin among males and females. MH chi-square was used to test for correlations between perceptions of sensitive skin and age for each gender (shown above the chart). Differences by gender within age groups were tested by chi-square. (**a**) On the bar of figure 2a – women ≥ 50 significantly higher than men ≥ 50 ($p = 0.04$). (**b**) On the bar of figure 2d – women ≤ 30 significantly higher than men ≤ 30 ($p = 0.05$). (**c**) On the bar of figure 2d – women 31–39 significantly higher than men 31–39 ($p = 0.01$)

skin and age, with an increased proportion of older subjects responding that their skin has been sensitive longer ($p = 0.001$). Among the ≥50 age group, 69 % claimed their skin had been sensitive for more than 10 years and 20 % for 6–10 years.

Forty-six percent (46 %) of people who considered their skin to be sensitive reported that their skin sensitivity increased over time: 37 % claimed their skin to be slightly more sensitive than in the past, and 9 % claimed their skin to be much more sensitive than in the past (Fig. 5b). People aged 50 and older were more likely to claim that their skin was presently "much more sensitive" (16 % frequency) ($p = 0.003$).

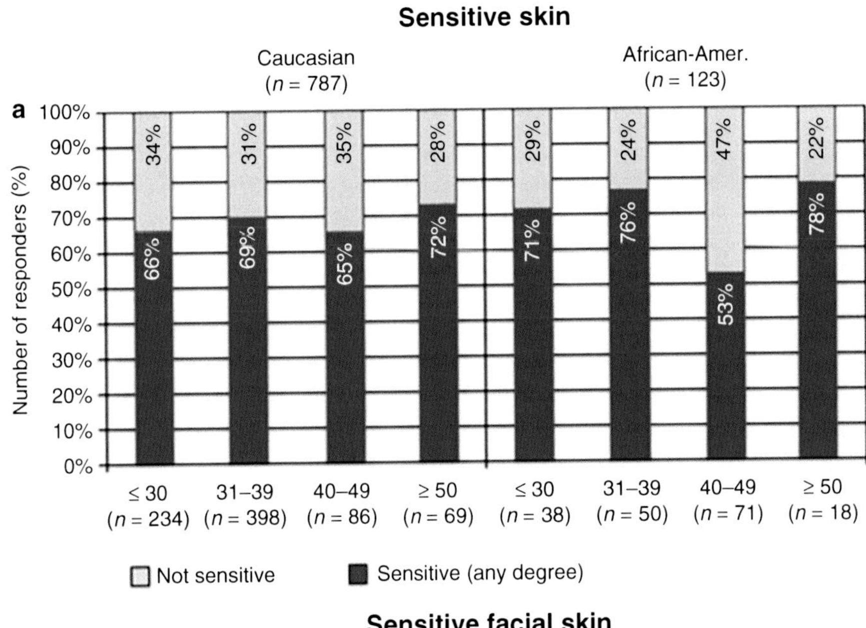

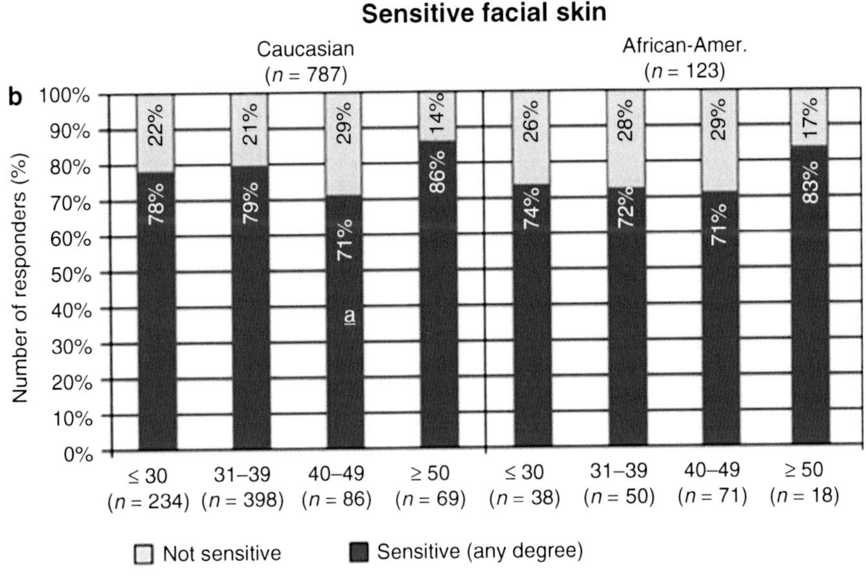

Fig. 3 (continued)

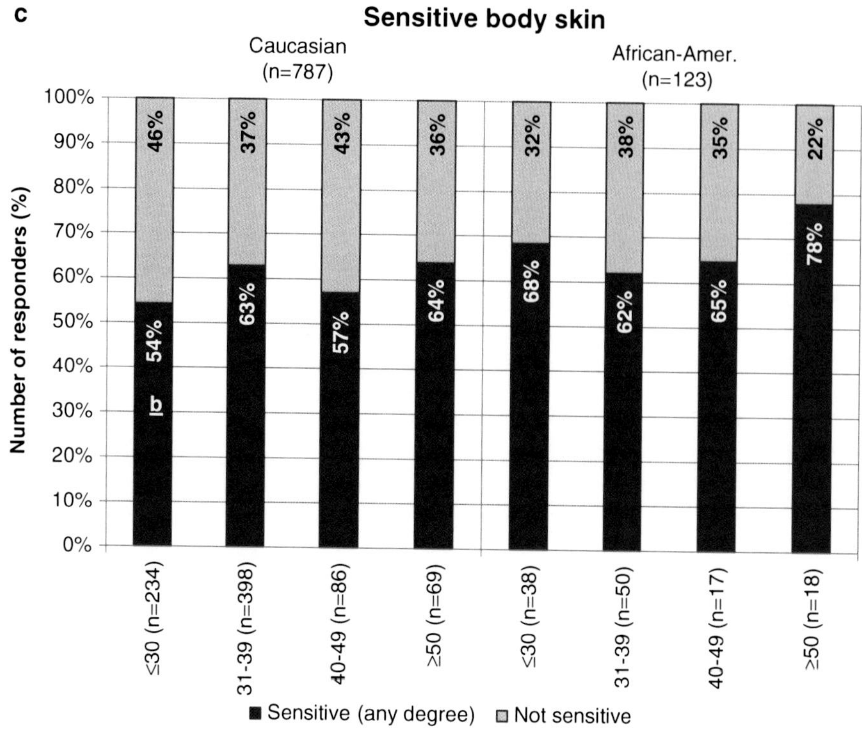

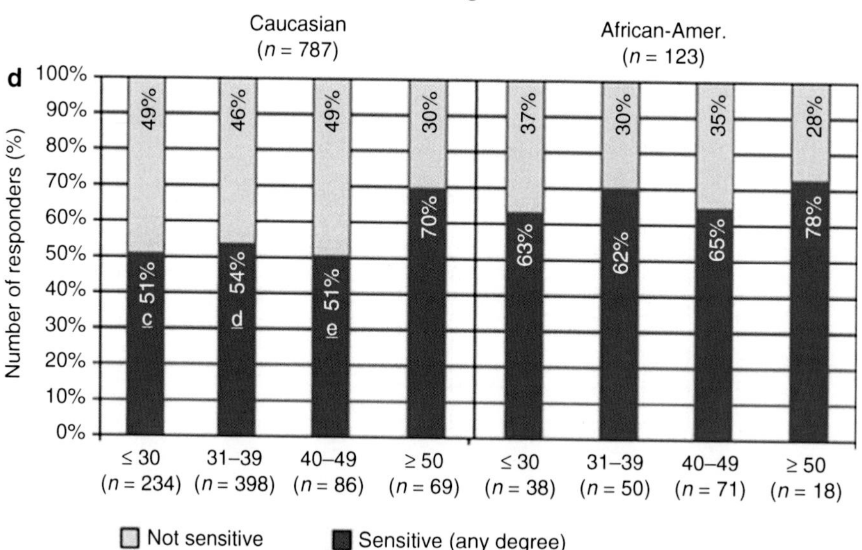

Fig. 3 Age group differences in perceptions of sensitive skin among different ethnic groups. Participants who claimed some degree of sensitivity are summarized for each ethnic group. Within each ethnic group, paired comparisons of age groups were conducted by chi-square analysis. (**a**) On the bar of figure 3b – among Caucasians, 40–49 group significantly lower than ≥50 group (p = 0.03). (**b**) On the bar of figure 3 c – among Caucasians ≤30 group significantly lower than 31–39 group (p = 0.03). (**c**) On the bar of figure 3d – among Caucasians ≤30 group significantly lower than ≥50 group (p = 0.006). (**d**) On the bar of figure 3d – among Caucasians 31–39 group significantly lower than ≥50 group (p = 0.02). (**e**) On the bar of figure 3d – among Caucasians, 40–49 group significantly lower than ≥50 group (p = 0.02)

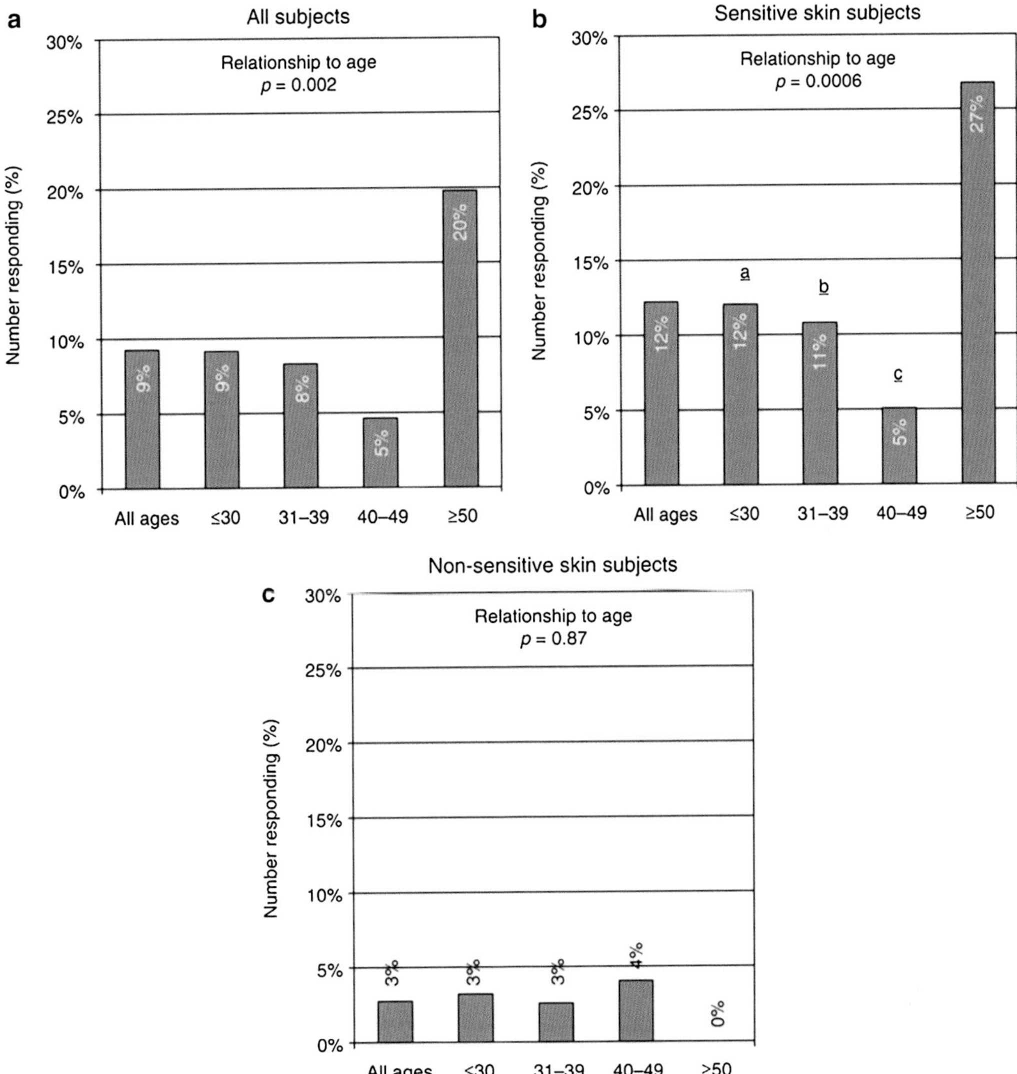

Fig. 4 Medically diagnosed skin allergies diagnosed by age group. (**a**) The percentage of participants who responded affirmatively to the question: "Do you have any known skin allergies that have been confirmed by a doctor?" (**b**) The percentage of affirmative responses among those who did claim to have sensitive skin. (**c**) The percentage of affirmative responses among those who did not claim to have sensitive skin. In (**b**), correlations between confirmed skin allergies and age and differences in confirmed allergies between age groups were assessed by Fisher's exact test. (**a**) On b – ≤30 group significantly lower than ≥50 group ($p = 0.005$). (**b**) On b – 31–39 group significantly lower than ≥50 group ($p = 0.0006$). (**c**) On b – 40–49 group significantly lower than ≥50 group ($p = 0.0002$)

Sensitive Skin and Family History

Individuals who have perceived their skin to be sensitive were significantly more likely to report that someone in the family also had sensitive skin (Fig. 6); this was significant for all age groups. A child was the relatively most likely identified as also having sensitive skin (reported previously in [31]).

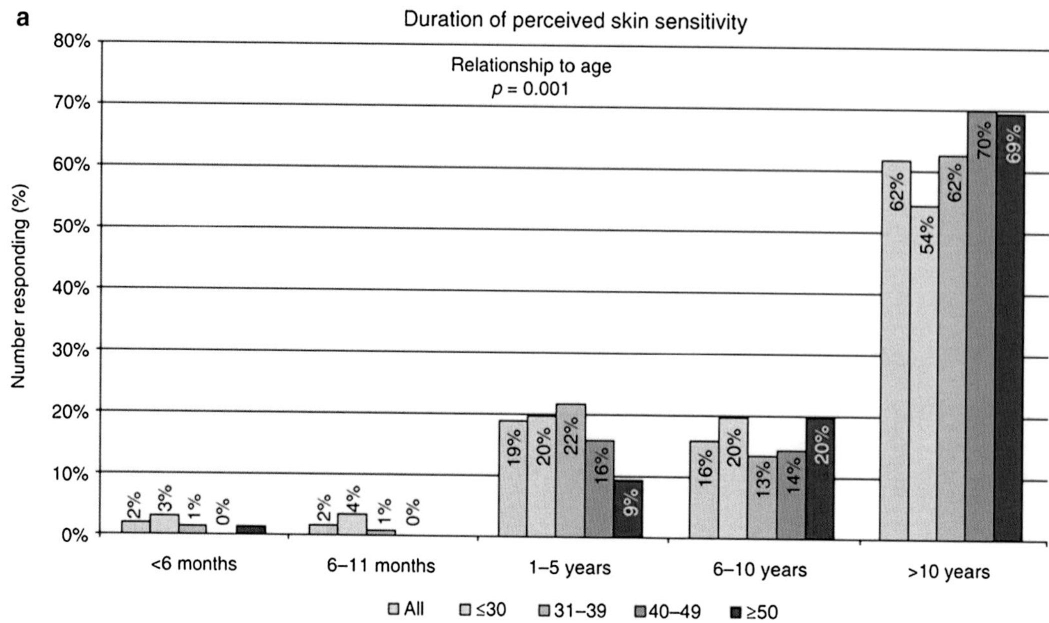

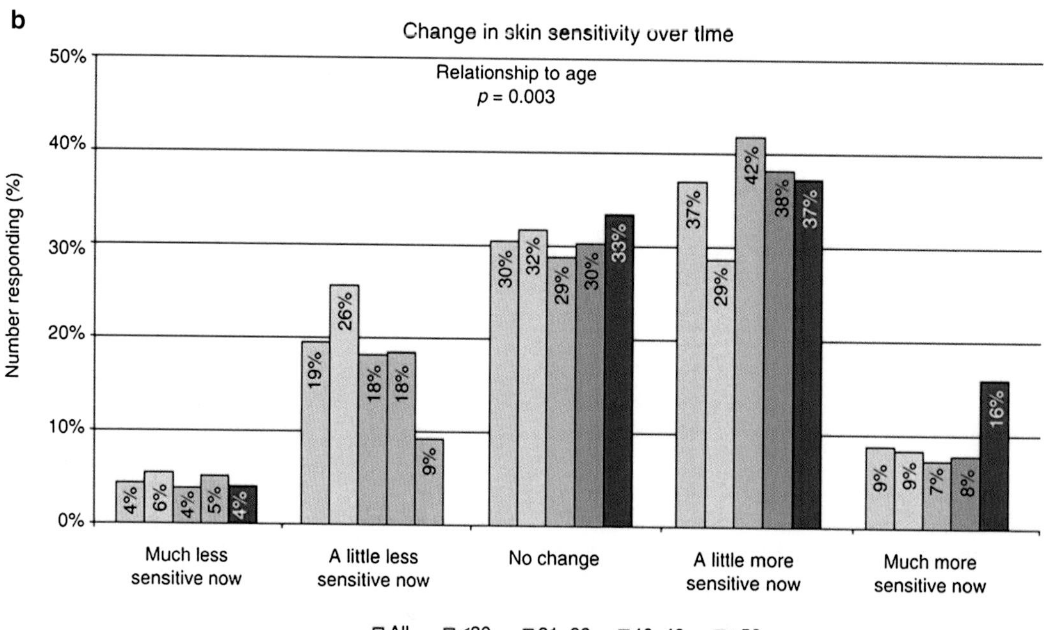

Fig. 5 Duration of skin sensitivity and change in skin sensitivity over time. (**a**) Participants were asked: "How long have you had sensitive skin?" (**b**) Responses to the question "How has your skin sensitivity changed over the years?" for the whole population and by age group. Correlations of responses to age were assessed by the Cochran-Mantel-Haenszel statistic (shown above the chart)

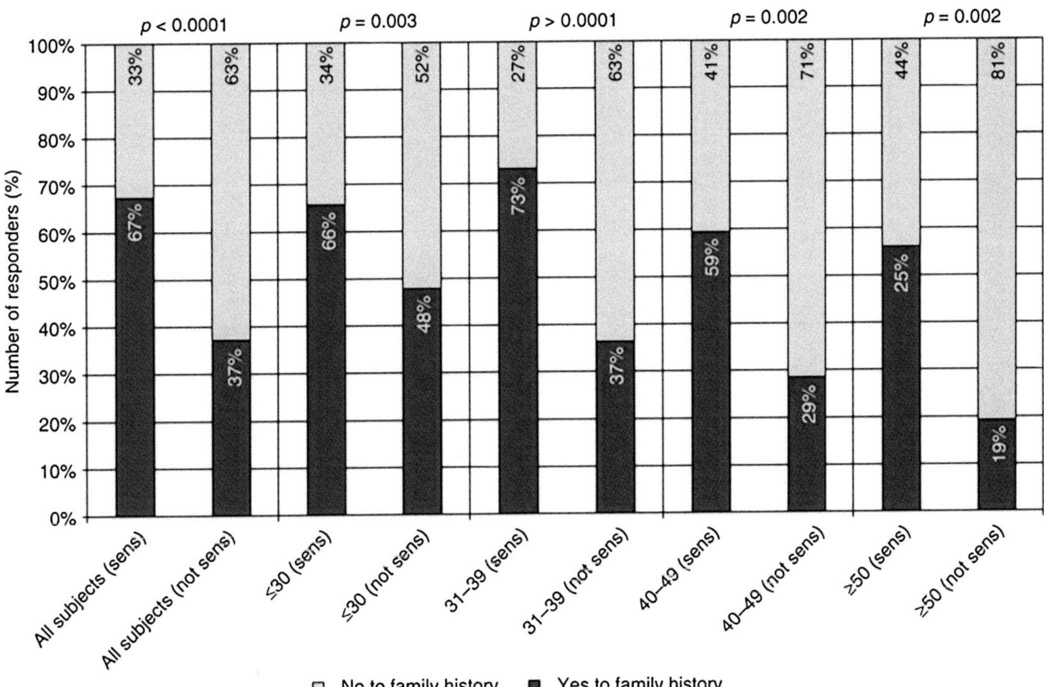

Fig. 6 Family history of sensitive skin. The percentage of subjects responding yes and no to the question "Does any member of your family have sensitive skin?" The relationship between the perceived skin sensitivity and a family history of sensitive skin was tested by chi-square analysis

Irritation Due to Environmental Factors

It has been reported that environmental factors such as dry air, cold, and wind are perceived to contribute to skin sensitivity [10]. Table 4 summarizes results for the environmental factors for each of the age groups, including the number of subjects who gave a response to the question, and the percentage who claimed that the environmental factor caused skin irritation. In the present investigation, all environmental factors were significantly more likely to be perceived to contribute to skin reactivity by those who claimed to have sensitive skin, regardless of age. Among those who claimed to have sensitive skin, hot weather was more frequently identified as a contributing factor by people aged 50 or older (91 % of respondents) than by other age groups (62–67 % of respondents). For each environmental factor, paired comparisons were done for each age group (Table 5). Hot weather and rough fabrics were factors most strongly associated with skin sensitivity among the oldest adults (aged 50 and over) and were specifically associated with genital skin sensitivity in this group; cold weather was most strongly associated with skin sensitivity in mid-life (40–49 age group); and stress was the most important factor cited by younger adults. The menstrual cycle was perceived to contribute to skin sensitivity by women of all age groups except those aged 50 or older.

Perceived Contribution of Household and Personal Products to Skin Sensitivity

Table 6 describes perceptions of irritation attributed to household, facial, and personal care products. In all age groups, those who claimed to have

Table 4 Perceptions about irritation due to certain environmental factors for sensitive skin and nonsensitive skin subjects

	Hot weather	Cold weather	Sun	Rough fabric	Wind	Dry weather	Stress	Humid weather	Menstrual cycle[a]
≥50									
Total sensitive responders	65	66	69	69	67	65	67	66	24
Factor causes irritation (%)	91 %	89 %	88 %	81 %	81 %	77 %	57 %	53 %	33 %
Total nonsensitive responders	19	22	23	24	21	22	22	23	9
Factor causes irritation (%)	47 %	73 %	74 %	67 %	57 %	45 %	23 %	26 %	0 %
p value (sensitive vs. nonsensitive)	0.0005	0.03	0.005	0.01	0.01	0.003	0.007	0.03	0.07
40–49									
Total sensitive responders	70	74	71	71	72	68	70	66	42
Factor causes irritation (%)	67 %	88 %	83 %	72 %	76 %	82 %	56 %	48 %	57 %
Total nonsensitive responders	46	45	46	46	44	46	46	44	24
Factor causes irritation (%)	28 %	62 %	63 %	54 %	52 %	54 %	20 %	7 %	25 %
p value (sensitive vs. nonsensitive)	0.0001	<0.0001	0.005	0.0001	0.0002	0.0002	0.0002	<0.0001	0.002
31–39									
Total sensitive responders	321	328	328	323	316	322	324	309	280
Factor causes irritation (%)	62 %	86 %	81 %	70 %	72 %	79 %	62 %	45 %	62 %

Total nonsensitive responders	137		142		140		131		135		136		131		136		111	
Factor causes irritation (%)		31%		73%		66%		37%		53%		54%		23%		10%		35%
p value (sensitive vs. nonsensitive)	<0.0001		<0.0001		<0.0001		<0.0001		<0.0001		<0.0001		<0.0001		<0.0001		<0.0001	
≤30																		
Total sensitive responders	187		191		189		187		185		193		188		184		161	
Factor causes irritation (%)		63%		86%		79%		68%		65%		78%		67%		48%		62%
Total nonsensitive responders	88		89		92		87		88		88		86		87		79	
Factor causes irritation (%)		28%		66%		66%		38%		53%		53%		27%		15%		34%
p value (sensitive vs. nonsensitive)	<0.0001		<0.0001		0.0004		<0.0001		0.004		<0.0001		<0.0001		<0.0001		<0.0001	

Participants were asked: "Please indicate how often the following factors cause irritation (redness, burning, itching) to your skin." Responses are summarized above for each of the four age groups. Total sensitive responders refers to the total number of subjects who claimed some degree of overall skin sensitivity who responded to the question about each environmental factor. The percentage of these responders who claimed the environmental factor caused some degree of skin irritation (i.e., "sometimes," "frequently," or "always") is given in the following line. Analyses were conducted using MH chi-square using *all four levels* of potential irritation reaction frequency (never, sometimes, frequently, or always) (data not shown) vs. two levels of sensitivity (sensitive to any degree or not sensitive)

[a]Women only

Table 5 Perceptions about irritation due to environmental factors for those claiming genital skin sensitivity

Sensitive skin in the genital area	Hot weather		Cold weather		Rough fabric		Dry weather		Stress		Humid weather		Menstrual cycle[a]	
≥50														
Total sensitive responders	59		59		64		60		62		60		23	
Factor causes irritation (%)		88 %[b]		86 %		86 %[c]		72 %		58 %		47 %		30 %[d]
40–49														
Total sensitive responders	68		70		70		67		68		66		42	
Factor causes irritation (%)		57 %		79 %		71 %		73 %		44 %[e]		39 %		52 %
31–39														
Total sensitive responders	256		261		255		257		256		245		229	
Factor causes irritation (%)		64 %		86 %		71 %		79 %		62 %		44 %		62 %
≤30														
Total sensitive responders	151		151		150		152		150		147		137	
Factor causes irritation (%)		59 %		82 %		75 %		76 %		65 %		45 %		65 %

Responses to the question summarized in Table 4 were evaluated for those who claimed some degree of skin sensitivity of the genital area. Total sensitive responders refers to the number of subjects with skin sensitivity of the genital area who responded to this question. The percentage of these responders who claimed the environmental factor caused some degree of skin irritation (i.e., "sometimes," "frequently," or "always") is given in the following line. Paired comparisons of age groups were done using the MH chi-square test

[a]Women only

[b]≥50 age group significantly higher than 40–49, 31–39, and ≤30 age groups ($p \leq 0.001$)

[c]≥50 age group significantly higher than 40–49, 31–39, and ≤30 age groups ($p \leq 0.03$)

[d]≥50 age group significantly lower than 31–39 and ≤30 age groups ($p < 0.02$)

[e]40–49 age group significantly lower than 31–39 and ≤30 age groups ($p < 0.02$)

sensitive skin were significantly more likely than those who did not claim sensitive skin to connect a wide variety of household and facial products to skin irritation with one exception, antiaging products. Among people aged 50 and older, those who believed their skin to be sensitive were not significantly more likely to report that antiaging products (specifically alpha-hydroxy products) caused skin irritation. Spearman coefficients were calculated to determine the strength of the association between perceived sensitive skin and the products listed in Table 6 (data not shown). Among household products, those with scent or fragrance were most strongly associated with irritation by all age groups. Among facial products, facial cosmetics were most strongly associated with irritation by sensitive skin individuals aged 50 and over and by those aged 30 and under. Facial cleansers were most strongly associated with irritation in the 40–49 and 31–39 age groups.

In contrast to the household product category, there were several personal care products, such as soaps, shampoos and conditioners, and other hair products, where sensitive skin people were *not* significantly more likely to report perceived irritation in the ≥50 age group (Table 6 part c). Results were similar for the 40–49 group, with no significant difference for soaps, antiperspirants, hair colorants, deodorants, body lotions, shampoos and conditioners, sunscreens, and powders. In the two younger age groups, perceived

Table 6 Perceptions about irritation due to certain household and personal products for different age groups

	a. Household products					b. Facial products					
	Laundry detergents	Fragranced or scented products	Dishwashing liquids	Fabric softener (liquid or dryer sheets)	Household cleaners	Facial cleansers	Facial astringents	Eye cosmetics[a]	Facial cosmetics[a]	Facial moisturizers/ lotions	Antiaging products (α-hydroxy acids)
≥50											
Total sensitive responders	70	63	70	66	70	61	52	50	34	66	51
Product causes irritation (%)	69 %	65 %	49 %	47 %	0 %	75 %	73 %	72 %	71 %	56 %	53 %
Total nonsensitive responders	24	22	22	23	23	16	16	16	10	22	13
Product causes irritation (%)	33 %	23 %	9 %	13 %	43 %	38 %	25 %	38 %	0 %	14 %	23 %
p value (sensitive vs. nonsensitive)	0.006	0.002	0.02	0.006	0.02	0.004	0.003	0.006	0.001	0.003	0.08
40–49											
Total sensitive responders	73	71	69	71	76	59	55	44	39	60	43
Product causes irritation (%)	49 %	59 %	32 %	37 %	67 %	53 %	62 %	43 %	56 %	48 %	40 %
Total nonsensitive responders	46	44	45	43	48	41	36	28	28	43	30
Product causes irritation (%)	26 %	14 %	4 %	5 %	38 %	5 %	22 %	29 %	7 %	7 %	13 %
p value (sensitive vs. nonsensitive)	<0.0001	<0.0001	<0.0001	<0.0001	0.0002	<0.0001	0.002	<0.0001	<0.0001	<0.0001	0.01

(*continued*)

Table 6 (continued)

31–39											
Total sensitive responders	334	323	330	324	333	315	259	269	274	313	209
Product causes irritation (%)	48 %	59 %	28 %	35 %	64 %	63 %	67 %	41 %	57 %	58 %	39 %
Total nonsensitive responders	145	140	143	140	143	129	116	114	115	131	107
Product causes irritation (%)	14 %	15 %	6 %	9 %	28 %	20 %	27 %	15 %	15 %	18 %	12 %
p value (sensitive vs. nonsensitive)	<0.0001	<0.0001	<0.0001	<0.0001	<0.0001	<0.0001	<0.0001	<0.0001	<0.0001	<0.0001	<0.0001
≤30											
Total sensitive responders	193	189	191	194	195	188	162	157	162	189	115
Product causes irritation (%)	56 %	56 %	24 %	41 %	53 %	68 %	65 %	39 %	63 %	58 %	33 %
Total nonsensitive responders	91	91	91	91	92	88	76	77	76	87	66
Product causes irritation (%)	23 %	16 %	11 %	15 %	33 %	23 %	25 %	22 %	17 %	16 %	8 %
p value (sensitive vs. nonsensitive)	<0.0001	<0.0001	0.01	0.0002	0.0004	<0.0001	<0.0001	0.004	<0.0001	<0.0001	0.0002

	c. Personal care products									
	Soaps (bar or liquid)	Antiperspirants	Hair colorants/ dyes	Deodorants	Perfumes/ colognes	Body lotions/ moisturizers	Shampoos or conditioners	Hair products (sprays, gels, mousse)	Sunscreens	Powders/ talc
≥50										
Total sensitive responders	70	63	50	66	64	71	66	60	60	56
Product causes irritation (%)	74 %	68 %	66 %	65 %	63 %	61 %	50 %	45 %	40 %	32 %
Total nonsensitive responders	23	21	14	23	23	22	22	17	22	21
Product causes irritation (%)	30 %	24 %	21 %	30 %	26 %	14 %	5 %	6 %	14 %	10 %
p value (sensitive vs. nonsensitive)	0.57	0.001	0.007	0.004	0.001	0.007	0.57	0.57	0.001	0.001
40–49										
Total sensitive responders	77	70	49	70	69	73	75	61	69	62
Product causes irritation (%)	75 %	56 %	45 %	63 %	54 %	56 %	27 %	33 %	32 %	23 %
Total nonsensitive responders	47	45	28	46	44	43	46	41	44	37
Product causes irritation (%)	23 %	29 %	36 %	33 %	14 %	7 %	13 %	12 %	14 %	3 %
p value (sensitive vs. nonsensitive)	0.15	0.14	0.14	0.14	<0.0001	0.14	0.15	0.008	0.14	0.14
31–39										
Total sensitive responders	335	311	252	326	304	325	334	315	318	252
Product causes irritation (%)	72 %	50 %	37 %	51 %	45 %	60 %	27 %	30 %	48 %	22 %

(*continued*)

Table 6 (continued)

Total nonsensitive responders	145	138	112	140	138	143	145	140	144	127
Product causes irritation (%)	26 %	17 %	13 %	19 %	12 %	12 %	10 %	11 %	13 %	5 %
p value (sensitive vs. nonsensitive)	<0.0001	<0.0001	<0.0001	<0.0001	<0.0001	<0.0001	<0.0001	<0.0001	<0.0001	<0.0001
≤30										
Total sensitive responders	198	189	150	195	186	189	194	184	186	158
Product causes irritation (%)	69 %	50 %	35 %	56 %	44 %	60 %	28 %	23 %	36 %	27 %
Total nonsensitive responders	92	88	80	89	89	90	91	89	89	79
Product causes irritation (%)	26 %	20 %	16 %	26 %	17 %	14 %	14 %	15 %	12 %	9 %
p value (sensitive vs. nonsensitive)	<0.0001	<0.0001	0.003	<0.0001	<0.0001	<0.0001	0.02	0.05	0.00004	0.001

Participants were asked: "Please indicate how often each of the following products cause irritation (redness, burning, itching) to your skin – "never," "sometimes," "frequently," or "always"." Responses are summarized above for each of the four age groups, and analyses were conducted in a manner identical to Table 4. Analyses were conducted using MH chi-square using *all four levels* of potential irritation reaction frequency (never, sometimes, frequently, or always) (data not shown) vs. two levels of sensitivity (sensitive to any degree or not sensitive)

[a]Women only

Table 7 Shopping choices for different age groups

Question: When shopping for skin care products, do you look for claims such as "safe for sensitive skin," "hypoallergenic," etc.? (yes or no)					
			"Yes" responses		
		Total	Number	Percent	p value
All ($n = 1{,}010$)	Women	849	575	68 %	**<0.0001**
	Men	161	77	48 %	
≥50 ($n = 101$)	Women	84	63	75 %	**0.02**
	Men	17	8	47 %	
40–49 ($n = 127$)	Women	83	53	64 %	0.15
	Men	44	22	50 %	
31–39 ($n = 491$)	Women	421	293	70 %	**<0.0001**
	Men	70	30	43 %	
≤30 ($n = 291$)	Women	261	166	64 %	0.5
	Men	30	17	57 %	

Participants were asked about whether or not they shop specifically for skin-related claims. Responses are summarized above for all responders and each of the four age groups. Analyses were conducted using chi-square

irritation due to the personal care products was significantly different for all products. Personal care products most strongly associated with perceived irritation in sensitive skin individuals were antiperspirants (≥50 age group), perfumes and colognes (40–49 age group), and body lotions (ages 39 and under) (data not shown).

The influence of skin benefit claims on product choices was also assessed. Overall, women were significantly more likely to look for skin benefit claims than are men (Table 7); this difference was primarily attributable to responses of women aged 31–39 and women aged 50 or older.

Contribution of Products to Perceived Skin Sensitivity of the Genital Area

Among individuals claiming sensitive genital skin in all age groups, all products used in the genital area were perceived to contribute to genital irritation, with the exception of tampons, which were not significantly associated with genital irritation in women aged 50 or older (likely because usage falls in postmenopausal women) (Table 8). The products most frequently identified as causing irritation by all age groups were undergarments and clothing (men and women) and menstrual pads (women only). For women, menstrual pads were most strongly associated with genital irritation, regardless of age; both men and women aged 39 and under, undergarments were most strongly associated with irritation, whereas in men and women 50 or over, incontinence products were most significantly associated with irritation at this anatomical site.

Perceptions of Women with Urinary Incontinence

Urinary incontinence is extremely common among women. There are varying reports of the precise percentage of the female population who suffer from this condition, from 16 % to over 48 % [33]. Our study included a subset of 29 women aged 50 and older who experienced urinary incontinence. Responses of these individuals were compared to 42 age- and gender-matched controls. Those who experienced urinary incontinence were significantly more likely to perceive their skin to be sensitive, but, surprisingly, these individuals were not more likely to report sensitivity of the genitalia (the expected site to be affected) or of the face or other body site (Table 9).

Table 8 Perceptions about sensitive genital skin and irritation due to personal products for each age group

	Products used by women and men			Products used by women only				
	Undergarments/ clothing	Toilet paper	Incontinence pads	Menstrual pads	Feminine wipes	Panty liners	Douching products	Tampons
≥50								
Total sensitive responders	61	58	20	34	41	44	31	19
Product causes irritation (%)	61 %	41 %	40 %	68 %	56 %	48 %	42 %	32 %
Total nonsensitive responders	28	28	10	12	12	15	12	8
Product causes irritation (%)	21 %	11 %	30 %	17 %	17 %	7 %	0 %	0 %
p value (sensitive vs. nonsensitive)	0.01	0.01	0.001	0.001	0.02	0.001	0.02	0.13
40–49								
Total sensitive responders	68	64	17	43	30	46	26	39
Product causes irritation (%)	65 %	33 %	6 %	65 %	33 %	52 %	23 %	49 %
Total nonsensitive responders	49	49	13	29	24	30	17	25
Product causes irritation (%)	6 %	6 %	0 %	7 %	13 %	13 %	0 %	4 %
p value (sensitive vs. nonsensitive)	0.006	0.006	0.0005	<0.0001	0.001	0.0005	0.005	0.001
31–39								
Total sensitive responders	257	253	57	228	118	223	74	194
Product causes irritation (%)	58 %	31 %	12 %	58 %	44 %	47 %	37 %	35 %
Total nonsensitive responders	204	196	83	166	102	167	84	155
Product causes irritation (%)	12 %	8 %	4 %	13 %	8 %	9 %	5 %	5 %
p value (sensitive vs. nonsensitive)	<0.0001	<0.0001	0.04	<0.0001	<0.0001	<0.0001	<0.0001	<0.0001
≤30								
Total sensitive responders	154	150	55	137	90	133	59	127
Product causes irritation (%)	53 %	26 %	22 %	54 %	39 %	39 %	32 %	42 %
Total nonsensitive responders	126	130	66	109	82	107	61	102
Product causes irritation (%)	9 %	5 %	0 %	13 %	4 %	7 %	2 %	3 %
p value (sensitive vs. nonsensitive)	<0.0001	<0.0001	<0.0001	<0.0001	<0.0001	<0.0001	<0.0001	<0.0001

Participants were asked: "Please indicate how often you have experienced irritation (redness, burning, itching) in the genital area after use of the following products – "never," "sometimes," "frequently," or "always"." Responses were evaluated for those who claimed some degree of skin sensitivity of the genital area. Total sensitive responders refer to the number of subjects with skin sensitivity of the genital area who responded to this question. The percentage of these responders who claimed the product caused some degree of skin irritation (i.e., "sometimes," "frequently," or "always") is given in the following line. Analyses were done using MH chi-square using *all four levels* of potential irritation reaction frequency (never, sometimes, frequently, or always) (data not shown) vs. two levels of sensitivity (sensitive to any degree or not sensitive)

Table 9 Comparison of perceived skin sensitivity for the incontinent subgroup and matched controls

		General		Face		Body		Genital area	
		Number	Percentage	Number	Percentage	Number	Percentage	Number	Percentage
Control ≥50	Total	42		41		41		41	
	Very sensitive	1	2 %	2	5 %	1	2 %	5	12 %
	Moderately	10	24 %	13	32 %	9	22 %	6	15 %
	Slightly sensitive	21	50 %	19	46 %	17	42 %	17	42 %
	Not sensitive	10	24 %	7	17 %	14	34 %	13	32 %
Incontinent ≥50	Total	29		29		29		29	
	Very sensitive	5	17 %	3	10 %	1	3 %	2	7 %
	Moderately	12	41 %	12	41 %	9	31 %	8	28 %
	Slightly sensitive	7	24 %	10	35 %	10	35 %	15	52 %
	Not sensitive	5	17 %	4	14 %	9	31 %	4	14 %
p value			0.01		0.25		0.57		0.43

A subset of participants in this study consisted of 29 women in the ≥50 age group who suffer from urinary incontinence. Responses were compared to a control group consisting of 42 women in the ≥50 age group who were not suffering from incontinence. Analyses were conducted using MH chi-square

Conclusion

Objective clinical assessments have generally shown older people to be less susceptible to irritant effects, but little correlation exists between clinical assessments and individuals' perceptions of the sensitivity of their skin. Most of the research on skin sensitivity has been conducted among populations composed of individuals of wide-ranging ages [8, 10, 15, 16]. Our research surveyed adults in the Midwestern USA ranging in age from 18 to over 50 years, with the ability to evaluate subgroups of individuals within specific age groups. People aged 50 or older were more likely to claim to have sensitive skin than younger adults and to perceive skin in the genital area (but not the face or other body sites) to be more sensitive to irritation. Among these older adults, women were more likely than men to claim genital skin sensitivity. Surprisingly, women were no more likely than men to perceive their facial skin to be sensitive, regardless of age. Older adults also reported that their skin had become more sensitive over time.

Medically diagnosed skin allergies were more common among those who claimed to have sensitive skin; moreover, older people with sensitive skin had a higher frequency of medically diagnosed skin allergies than younger people who claimed skin sensitivity. People who perceived their skin to be sensitive were also more likely to report a family member (most often a child) with sensitive skin.

People who perceived their skin to be sensitive were also more likely to associate skin irritation with environmental factors, personal products, or household products. Older adults believed hot weather can exacerbate their skin sensitivity, whereas younger adults deemed cold weather and stress to be more crucial factors to their skin sensitivity. Older adults also were more likely to associate antiperspirants with skin irritation, whereas younger adults were more likely to attribute skin irritation to fragrances and body lotions. Overall, a significantly higher proportion of people who believed their skin to be sensitive looked for skin-related claims when shopping.

Despite the fact that older women in particular were more likely to perceive genital skin to be sensitive to irritation, all age groups attributed genital irritation to the same types of products. Both men and women in all age groups attributed genital skin irritation to undergarments and clothing; women considered menstrual products were the most important contributing factor to genital irritation.

A significantly higher proportion of women aged 50 and over who experienced urinary incontinence considered their skin to be sensitive compared to age- and gender-matched controls; nevertheless, women with incontinence did not differ from other women in this age group with respect to the anatomical sites they considered to be sensitive.

In summary, elderly adults from the Midwestern USA are more likely to perceive their skin to be sensitive than younger adults, with genital sensitivity being of particular concern to elderly women. Elderly women with incontinence also were more likely than women of a similar age to consider their skin to be sensitive. Hot weather was perceived to exacerbate overall skin sensitivity and genital sensitivity among older adults.

Cross-References

► Effects of Aging on skin reactivity
► Cutaneous Effects and Sensitive Skin with Incontinence in the Aged

References

1. Saint-Martory C, Roguedas-Contios AM, Sibaud V, Degouy A, Schmitt AM, Misery L. Sensitive skin is not limited to the face. Br J Dermatol. 2008;158:130–3. doi:10.1111/j.1365-2133.2007.08280.x [PMID:17986305].
2. Farage MA, Berardesca E, Maibach HI. Sensitive skin: a valid syndrome of multiple origins. In: Wilhelm K-P, Zhai H, Maibach HI, editors. Marzulli and Maibach's dermatotoxicology. 8th ed. London: Informa Healthcare; 2012. p. 238–47.
3. Berardesca E, Farage MA, Maibach HI. Sensitive skin: an overview. Int J Cosmet Sci. 2013;35:2–8. doi:10.1111/j.1468-2494.2012.00754.x [PMID:22928591].
4. Marriott M, Holmes J, Peters L, Cooper K, Rowson M, Basketter DA. The complex problem of sensitive skin. Contact Dermatitis. 2005;53:93–9. doi:10.1111/j.0105-1873.2005.00653.x [PMID: 16033403].
5. Farage MA, Mandl CP, Berardesca E, Maibach HI. Sensitive skin in China. J Cosmet Dermatol Sci Appl. 2012;2:184–95. doi:10.4236/jcdsa.2012.23035
6. Morizot F, Guinot C, Lopez S, Le Fur I, Tschachler E, Wood C. Sensitive skin: analysis of symptoms, perceived causes and possible mechanisms. Cosmet Toiletries. 2000;115:83–9.
7. Misery L, Myon E, Martin N, Verriere F, Nocera T, Taieb C. [Sensitive skin in France: an epidemiological approach]. Ann Dermatol Venereol. 2005;132:425–9 [PMID:15988353].
8. Misery L, Myon E, Martin N, Consoli S, Nocera T, Taieb C. Sensitive skin: epidemiological approach and impact on quality of life in France. In: Berardesca E, Fluhr JW, Maibach HI, editors. Sensitive skin syndrome. New York: Taylor & Francis; 2006. p. 181–91.
9. Guinot C, Malvy D, Mauger E, Ezzedine K, Latreille J, Ambroisine L, Tenenhaus M, Preziosi P, Morizot F, Galan P, Hercberg S, Tschachler E. Self-reported skin sensitivity in a general adult population in France: data of the SU.VI.MAX cohort. J Eur Acad Dermatol Venereol. 2006;20:380–90. doi:10.1111/j.1468-3083.2006.01455.x [PMID:16643133].
10. Misery L, Myon E, Martin N, Consoli S, Boussetta S, Nocera T, Taieb C. Sensitive skin: psychological effects and seasonal changes. J Eur Acad Dermatol Venereol. 2007;21:620–8. doi:10.1111/j.1468-3083.2006.02027.x [PMID:17447975].
11. Querleux B, Dauchot K, Jourdain R, Bastien P, Bittoun J, Anton JL, Burnod Y, de Lacharriere O. Neural basis of sensitive skin: an fMRI study. Skin Res Technol. 2008;14:454–61. doi:10.1111/j.1600-0846.2008.00312.x [PMID:18937781].
12. Loffler H, Dickel H, Kuss O, Diepgen TL, Effendy I. Characteristics of self-estimated enhanced skin susceptibility. Acta Derm Venereol. 2001;81:343–6 [PMID:11800141].
13. Sparavigna A, Di Pietro A, Setaro M. 'Healthy skin': significance and results of an Italian study on healthy population with particular regard to 'sensitive' skin. Int J Cosmet Sci. 2005;27:327–31. doi:10.1111/j.1467-2494.2005.00287.x [PMID:18492170].
14. Farage MA, Bowtell P, Katsarou A. Self-diagnosed sensitive skin in women with clinically diagnosed atopic dermatitis. Clin Med Dermatol. 2008;2:21–8. doi:10.4137/CMD.S902.
15. Willis CM, Shaw S, De Lacharriere O, Baverel M, Reiche L, Jourdain R, Bastien P, Wilkinson JD. Sensitive skin: an epidemiological study. Br J Dermatol. 2001;145:258–63 [PMID:11531788].
16. Jourdain R, de Lacharriere O, Bastien P, Maibach HI. Ethnic variations in self-perceived sensitive skin: epidemiological survey. Contact Dermatitis. 2002;46:162–9 [PMID:12000326].
17. Farage MA, Katsarou A, Maibach HI. Sensory, clinical and physiological factors in sensitive skin: a review.

Contact Dermatitis. 2006;55:1–14. doi:10.1111/j.0105-1873.2006.00886.x [PMID:16842547].
18. Farage MA. How do perceptions of sensitive skin differ at different anatomical sites? An epidemiological study. Clin Exp Dermatol. 2009;34:e521–30. doi:10.1111/j.1365-2230.2009.03487.x [PMID:19719761].
19. Farage MA. Perceptions of sensitive skin: women with urinary incontinence. Arch Gynecol Obstet. 2009;280:49–57. doi:10.1007/s00404-008-0870-6 [PMID:19083008].
20. Misery L, Sibaud V, Merial-Kieny C, Taieb C. Sensitive skin in the American population: prevalence, clinical data, and role of the dermatologist. Int J Dermatol. 2011;50:961–7. doi:10.1111/j.1365-4632.2011.04884.x [PMID:21781068].
21. Farage MA, Miller KW, Wippel AM, Berardesca E, Misery L. Sensitive skin in the United States: survey of regional differences. Fam Med Sci Res. 2013;2:1–8. doi:10.4172/2327-4972.1000112.
22. Xu F, Yan S, Wu M, Li F, Sun Q, Lai W, Shen X, Rahhali N, Taieb C, Xu J. Self-declared sensitive skin in China: a community-based study in three top metropolises. J Eur Acad Dermatol Venereol. 2013;27:370–5. doi:10.1111/j.1468-3083.2012.04648.x [PMID:22844976].
23. Hernández-Blanco D, Castanedo-Cázares JP, Ehnis-Pérez A, Jasso-Ávila I, Conde-Salazar L, Torres-Á lvarez B. Prevalence of sensitive skin and its biophysical response in a Mexican population. World J Dermatol. 2013;2:1–7. doi:10.5314/wjd.v2.i1.1.
24. Farage MA, Miller KW, Elsner P, Maibach HI. Intrinsic and extrinsic factors in skin ageing: a review. Int J Cosmet Sci. 2008;30:87–95. doi:10.1111/j.1468-2494.2007.00415.x [PMID:18377617].
25. Runeman B. Skin interaction with absorbent hygiene products. Clin Dermatol. 2008;26:45–51. doi:10.1016/j.clindermatol.2007.10.002 [PMID:18280904].
26. Robinson MK. Age and gender as influencing factors in skin sensitivity. In: Berardesca E, Fluhr JW, Maibach HI, editors. Sensitive skin syndrome. New York: Taylor & Francis; 2006. p. 169–80.
27. Robinson MK. Population differences in acute skin irritation responses. Race, sex, age, sensitive skin and repeat subject comparisons. Contact Dermatitis. 2002;46:86–93 [PMID:11918601].
28. Lejman E, Stoudemayer T, Grove G, Kligman AM. Age differences in poison ivy dermatitis. Contact Dermatitis. 1984;11:163–7 [PMID:6238788].
29. Cua AB, Wilhelm KP, Maibach HI. Cutaneous sodium lauryl sulphate irritation potential: age and regional variability. Br J Dermatol. 1990;123:607–13 [PMID:2248890].
30. Grove GL, Duncan S, Kligman AM. Effect of ageing on the blistering of human skin with ammonium hydroxide. Br J Dermatol. 1982;107:393–400 [PMID:7126450].
31. Farage MA. Self-reported immunological and familial links in individuals who perceive they have sensitive skin. Br J Dermatol. 2008;159(1):237–8. doi:10.1111/j.1365-2133.2008.08585.x [PMID:18476961].
32. U.S. Census Bureau: Census 2000 Data for the State of Ohio. 2011 https://www.census.gov/census2000/states/oh.html
33. Brown JS, Grady D, Ouslander JG, Herzog AR, Varner RE, Posner SF. Prevalence of urinary incontinence and associated risk factors in postmenopausal women. Heart & Estrogen/Progestin Replacement Study (HERS) Research Group. Obstet Gynecol. 1999;94:66–70 [PMID:10389720].

Effects of Aging on Skin Reactivity

131

Michael K. Robinson

Contents

M.K. Robinson (✉)
Global Biotechnology and Life Sciences Technology Platform, The Procter & Gamble Company, Mason Business Center, Mason, OH, USA
e-mail: robinson.mk@pg.com

M.A. Farage et al. (eds.), *Textbook of Aging Skin*,
DOI 10.1007/978-3-662-47398-6_96

Abstract

There is a general caution that needs to be applied to studies that report population differences in skin biology, reactivity, or symptoms. The caution simply relates to the fact that known intra- and interindividual differences in skin reactivity and the potential breadth of reactivity across large population clusters makes it difficult to draw definitive conclusions from studies on limited numbers of subjects. Age-related differences in skin reactivity tend to be more consistent in the response patterns that have emerged from individual studies than studies of other population comparisons (e.g., gender or ethnicity). A trend toward reduced skin irritation responsiveness in elderly subjects is a fairly common observation. Self-perception of skin sensitivity and sensory skin responses, as a function of age, have not been studied well enough to draw firm conclusions, though the limited data available also supports an age-related reduction in responsiveness. The situation is a bit more complicated with allergic responses. Here, except for the very young developing immune system, sensitivity may be as much related to exposure history as to inherent differences in susceptibility per se, although the prevalence and severity of elicitation responses can show some decline with age. This is likely due to the known age-related general decline in immune function.

Introduction

Any attempt to assess and understand skin sensitivity or reactivity differences within and between human subpopulations is complicated by a variety of factors. Perhaps the most important of these is a simple statistical reality of the inherent difficulty in making population-level assertions on the basis of studies conducted with relatively small numbers of subjects. Figure 1 illustrates the dilemma by providing two different scenarios: one in which two sample populations with very different reactivity profiles are drawn from two relatively nonoverlapping parent populations (A) and a second in which the sample populations (again with different reactivity) are drawn from virtually indistinguishable parent populations (B). In the first instance, measured (and statistically significant) differences between the two sample populations would be representative of the actual populations from which the samples were drawn, whereas in the second case, one would only be sampling within the overall reactivity ranges of the parent populations.

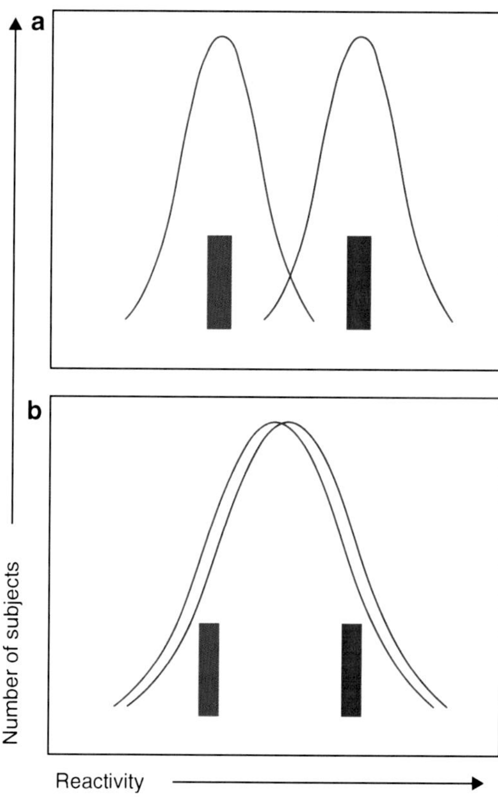

Fig. 1 Schematic representation of the two small study populations with different reactivity profiles, but drawn from (**a**) two parent populations with distinctly different profiles or (**b**) two parent populations with virtually identical reactivity profiles (Source: from [45] (with permission))

In the case of population differences in skin reactivity, we are, of course, completely uncertain of the exact nature of the parent populations or the dynamics of those populations over time. We are only able to test a limited number of subjects of the representative groups and, based on the results obtained, make presumptions about the global nature of populations from which those subjects were drawn. Observations of differences in reactivity among subsets of any population must be tempered by this uncertainty. This explains why the literature on population differences in fundamental skin biology or skin responsiveness is so often conflicted [1].

Skin aging is a dynamic process involving both intrinsic biological changes and the chronic strain imposed by environmental stressors such as UV irradiation [2]. Within the past two decades, the term "inflammaging" has been coined to describe the cascade of proinflammatory responses that accumulate with age and that lead to a variety of chronic inflammation-related disease states [3]. Inflammaging of the skin is one such state. It is central to the dichotomy of aging skin function that the inflammatory and immune responses act as both protector of the skin (from harmful agents like bacteria, viruses, and cancer cells), and restoration of the skin (wound healing), while also promoting the skin aging process [4]. Inflammation has long been known to accompany skin aging; however, it has been difficult to determine whether it is a driving force in the aging process or an epiphenomenon [5]. Recent genome-wide assessment of changes in gene expression associated with chronological aging and photoaging has clearly demonstrated that inflammation is a central theme in both processes, but exacerbated in photoaging [6, 7]. It is on top of this ever-changing proinflammatory milieu that we attempt to ascribe true differences in skin reactivity and their underlying mechanistic bases.

Effect of Age on Basic Parameters of Skin Biology and Physiology

Although beyond the scope of this chapter, it is pertinent to at least briefly consider differences in some of the basic characteristics of skin that may be influenced by age. Characteristics such as skin thickness, barrier function, elasticity, wound repair potential, etc. can certainly influence overall skin reactivity profiles. A selection of published studies and reviews has indicated the following:

1. Reduced forearm skin elasticity with age (comparing pre- and postmenopausal women) [8]
2. Lack of differences in epidermal thickness with age [9]
3. Likely reduction in barrier function and delayed recovery after barrier insult in photoaged skin [10, 11]
4. Qualitatively similar wound healing response in elderly versus young subjects, but delayed response in the elderly [12]
5. Other literature disparity on effects of aging on wound healing rates [13]
6. Defective removal of UV-induced pyrimidine dimers from epidermis of older (age 70–78) versus younger (age 22–26) subjects [14]
7. Reduced noradrenalin-induced vasoconstriction during skin cooling in older (age 62–76 years) versus younger (age 8–30 years) subjects [15]
8. Reduced wheal response to histamine skin prick test challenge in very elderly (age >90 years) versus younger (age 65–75 years). Note, however, that this was restricted to female subjects [16]

In general, there is a tendency toward a gradual diminution in skin structure and function with age, although the variability in results across these studies makes it difficult to make very definitive conclusions around specific endpoints. In fact, there is a fairly extensive literature on the above topics and individual research studies commonly report alternative findings, particularly when different assessment methods are used. Again, this points to the difficulty in extrapolating from small-scale studies to the population as a whole.

Effect of Age on Objective Skin Irritation Responses

If aging skin is subjected to even low-level chronic inflammation, one might expect that the response to acute irritant exposure would be heightened due to the known priming effect of underlying skin irritation on other types of skin reactivity, like allergic contact dermatitis [17]. In contrast, the literature on age-related susceptibility to skin irritation generally shows a reduced sensitivity in older (i.e., >60 years) versus younger adults. A comparison of two widely different age-groups (18–25 and 65–84) for reactivity to a strong irritant stimulus [24-h patch exposure to 5 % sodium lauryl sulfate (SLS)] showed greater mean reactivity in the young versus old subjects (4.57 vs. 2.62 on a 0–5 visual grading scale) [18]. A similar study using a 20-fold lower SLS concentration gave comparable results [19]. The mean response and percent positive responders were greater in young (average age 25.9) versus older (average age 74.6) test subjects. In some areas of the body (e.g., thighs), the response difference was quite dramatic. The lower visual grades in the older subjects were matched by a decrease in the magnitude of SLS-induced changes in barrier function.

Grove et al. [20] studied different types of chemical-induced skin irritation in young and old subjects. Using ammonium-hydroxide-induced blistering responses, they saw a more rapid initiation of blistering in older (65–75) versus younger (18–30) subjects, but a much slower development of the full blister response. They also examined the response to a variety of irritants (e.g., histamine, DMSO, 48/80, chloroform–methanol, lactic acid, and ethyl nicotinate). In all cases, the visual grades were greater in the younger subjects. The decline in histamine reactivity with advancing age was, in fact, a confirmation of a much earlier study which showed a trend of decreasing skin reactivity to intracutaneous injection of various concentrations of histamine across 10-year age cohorts from 0–10 to >70 years of age [21]. Elderly subjects also showed reduced reactivity to ultraviolet irradiation [22]. Very few studies have shown the

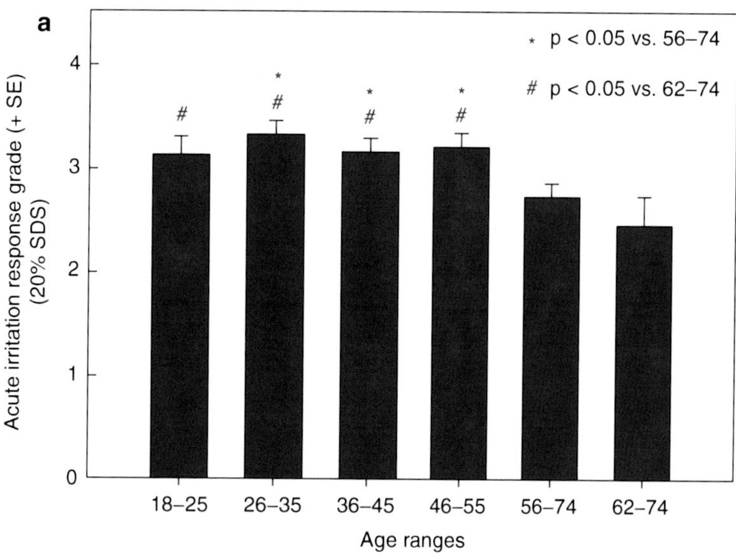

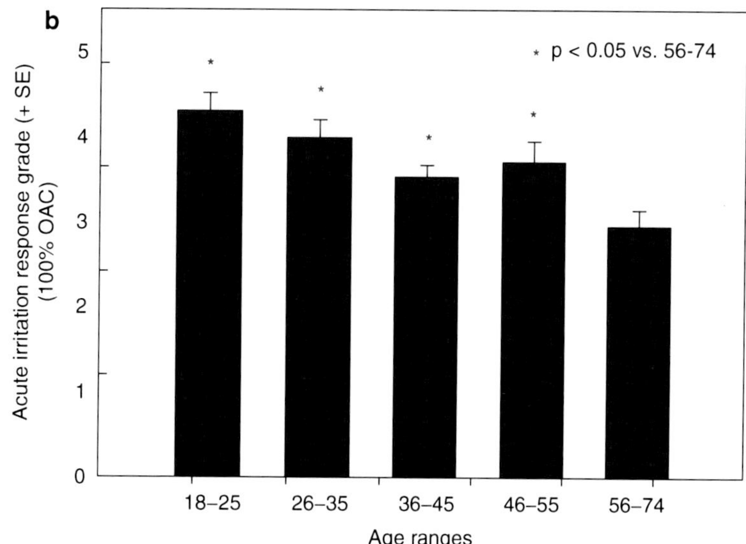

Fig. 2 (**a**, **b**) The mean (+SE) acute irritation response grades for the indicated age group clusters to 20 % SDS (2a) and 100 % OAc (2b). For SDS, the numbers of test subjects in each age cluster were: 18–25 years (44), 26–35 years (77), 36–45 years (118), 46–55 years (80), 56–74 years (64), and 62–74 years (22) (one subject did not have his/her age recorded and was omitted from the analysis). For OAc, the numbers of test subjects in each age cluster were 18–25 (21), 26–35 (21), 36–45 (29), 46–55 (30), and 56–74 (34). The mean grades for each age cluster were cross-compared by statistical analysis. Abbreviations: *SDS* sodium dodecyl sulfate, *OAc* octanoic acid (Source: from [24] (with permission))

opposite effect (increased irritation in the elderly), although some exist [23]. Barrier function can also be more susceptible to the compromising effects of UV treatment among older subjects, even though visible skin reactivity is diminished [22].

In a recent survey of acute patch-test reactions to common irritants [24], results from multiple studies conducted over a period of 4 years were combined. In comparing response profiles across different age clusters, the oldest cohort of study subjects showed significantly reduced reactivity to two strong irritants (Fig. 2). Responses to weaker irritants were directionally, but not significantly, reduced in these subjects (data not shown). Therefore, this larger population analysis supported the conclusions from smaller base size studies that elderly subjects are somewhat less susceptible to common skin irritants. It should be noted that the reduction in susceptibility shown in Fig. 2 is a statistical distinction, and may reflect minimal biological response distinction especially given the overall subject-to-subject and intrasubject variation seen in these types of clinical response patterns [25, 26]. Still, the results of all of these acute irritation studies would

suggest that the underlying proinflammatory state of photoaged skin [5, 7] does not appear to prime the skin for increased reactivity to acute chemical irritants.

Effect of Age on the Subjective (Sensory) Skin Irritation Response

In addition to objective skin irritation responses, there are many parameters of skin reactivity that are purely subjective or symptomatic in nature. These include the self-assessed quality of "sensitive" versus "normal" skin. They also include the various severities (e.g., mild, moderate, severe) and qualities (e.g., sting, burn, itch) of skin sensitizations to physical, chemical, or thermal insult. There are ways to quantify these symptomatic responses, but such measurements must be carefully controlled to avoid artifacts [27]. Also, the type of scales used to measure such responses can greatly influence the utility of the data for comparative analyses [27] like population response patterns or differences.

Direct testing of sensory irritation involves application of chemical (e.g., lactic acid, capsaicin, histamine), thermal (heat, cold), or mechanical (tactile) stimuli to various parts of the body and capture of the resulting sensation by symptom grading. Examples include the lactic acid, chloroform/methanol, and capsaicin stinging/burning tests [28–31]. Although studies of this type are plentiful, few have directly addressed age-related differences in response profiles. One study of noxious and thermal stimulation of different areas of the face indicated disparate findings on age-related effects, although a slight reduction in response thresholds was observed with increased age (age range 20–89) [32] consistent with results on objective skin irritation described above. A histological study showed reduced expression of nerve growth factor in the epidermis of older (51–81) versus younger (6–18 and 19–50) subjects [33]. There has also been a reported decrease, with aging, of the epidermal nerve density (at least in the face) [34]. These observations may provide a mechanistic explanation for a reduced sensory response threshold in older adults.

Itch is a fairly unique symptom of skin disease, and it has been reported to be the single most bothersome symptom of dermatologic disease in the elderly. The incidence is high and may be correlated with other parameters of skin dysfunction (e.g., dry skin, reduced barrier function) described above [35].

Effect of Age on the Skin Sensitization Response

Skin sensitization differs from skin irritation in its requirement for initial immune recognition of cutaneously encountered low molecular weight allergens. However, the allergic contact dermatitis that is elicited after a secondary exposure to the same allergen can be very similar in visual appearance to primary irritant contact dermatitis. The requirement for immune recognition and response introduces an additional factor into the consideration of age-related differences in skin reactivity, i.e., immune competence. This is particularly noteworthy given the commonly accepted notion of reduced immune competence with advancing age [36].

Age-related studies of skin sensitization are mainly limited to retrospective analysis of elicitation patterns and incidences across patch testing cohorts. Here the data are mixed and, because of the nature of the testing approach, it is difficult to separate age-related inherent susceptibility from age-related patterns of exposure. An early study [37] showed no age-related differences in the incidence of allergic patch test reactions across four common contact allergens (nickel, neomycin, ethylenediamine, and benzocaine). However, other investigators have seen different trends. Goh [38] studied the response incidence to common patch test tray allergens and saw a general increase in incidence in subjects >40 versus those <40. The trend was even greater when he compared subjects >59 versus those <20. Since these totals were cumulative, they may just represent a greater tendency to become sensitized to different allergens as one advances in age, due to possible repetitive exposures and the fact that the sensitized state is generally permanent. Young [39] looked at the incidence on a per allergen basis and observed different patterns depending on the allergen; cobalt and nickel sensitivity was greater in those <30 versus those >50, but the reverse was true for wood tar. Again, this could be related to the exposure opportunities but may also be a reflection of some diminution in response in older subjects assuming that they would have had the potential to be sensitized as younger adults.

A study of the elicitation of Rhus reactivity in presensitized young and older subjects showed temporal differences in onset and resolution of skin reactions [18]. Young subjects showed a quick onset of reactivity and resolution by 9–15 days. Older subjects responded more slowly and the reaction resolved more slowly (12–26 days). This suggests that the grading period for allergic skin reactions might need to be extended in older patients to account for a delayed evolution of the positive patch response [40].

Examination of sensitization to standard allergens as a function of age (from birth to >70 years of age) showed similar incidence of response across 0–7, 8–14, and 20–50 age groups but a reduced incidence in the oldest (>70) age group [41]. Kwangsukstith and Maibach [42] have suggested that the incidence of allergic contact dermatitis gradually increases from birth to 14 years of age, then holds steady in overall incidence but greatly varies by allergen based on exposure patterns. The actual incidence of allergic responses can show considerable ranges from study to study as well [40]. The incidence declines with advancing age in terms of both the severity of response (possibly related to similar reduction in irritation responses discussed above) and a waning of the allergic response in previously sensitized individuals [42].

The only way to truly assess allergic sensitivity is to evaluate the induction of allergic contact sensitization in previously naive subjects. Studies of this type are not generally done today, but studies from the earlier literature do shed some light on age-related susceptibility. Back in the early 1950s, Schwartz [43] studied the induction of sensitization to dinitrochlorobenzene (DNCB) in previously naive subjects of different ages. Approximately half of 174 subjects became sensitized. Among three age cohorts (21–59, 60–79, >80) there was no significant difference in the incidence of sensitization. Thus, for very potent sensitizers, there appears to be little age-related difference in allergic sensitivity. Although focused on the very young, a different result was obtained more recently using DNCB induction and challenge in infants from birth to 9 months of age [44]. Using a set DNCB dose for induction and one-tenth of that dose for challenge, sensitization rates increased from approximately 7 % at birth (up to 15 days of age) to 26 % at the end of the first month to 63 % by the third month and 91 % by the ninth month of life. These results are consistent with the understanding of the fact that the immune system is still maturing in the first months of life.

Looking at a different type of immune response, immediate skin hypersensitivity (an IgE mediated response), there is also "historical" evidence of an age-related decline in skin immune reactivity [21]. In this study, the investigators simply analyzed intracutaneous skin testing records for reactivity to both common and uncommon food allergens from among 100 subjects from their allergy practice in each 10 year age cluster by decade (0–10, 11–20, 21–30, etc.) to >70 years of age. For the common allergens there was a dramatic age-related decline in the number of positive skin reactions (both slight positive and moderate to marked positive reactions). They showed a fairly progressive linear decline in % responses with each advancing decade of patient age. The % positive reactions to uncommon allergens were decidedly fewer, but a similar age-related decline was observed. Hence, the prevailing evidence on skin reactivity (for both immediate and delayed skin hypersensitivity responses) supports the notion of some degree of senescence in skin immune competence with advancing age.

Summary

The unique dichotomy of our skin, as it ages, is that (at least in sun-exposed areas) there is a continual stimulation of at least a subclinical level of inflammation that is now thought to be a contributing factor in the skin aging process. In spite of this continual priming of the inflammatory response infrastructure, the actual immune and inflammatory reactivity of the skin to typical irritants and (perhaps) allergens is somewhat diminished. This goes along with findings of various other structural/functional and physiological declines in the skin with age. Some of this diminished structural and functional response capability likely contributes to observed increases in age-related susceptibility to different skin conditions. The interest in evaluating and understanding inherent patterns of skin reactivity and significant differences in reactivity across populations continues to grow. Much of this is due to the current trend in development of products with improved tolerance profiles for all consumers, especially those with heightened skin sensitivity. It may also reflect the interest in marketing to specifically targeted segments of the population, the development of skin antiaging products being one example. Regardless of the driving forces, clinical research on this topic is likely to continue and this should enhance our understanding of this complex skin physiology in the years ahead.

Cross-References

- ▶ Cutaneous Effects and Sensitive Skin with Incontinence in the Aged
- ▶ Perceptions of Sensitive Skin with Age

References

1. Robinson MK. Population differences in skin structure and physiology and the susceptibility to irritant and allergic contact dermatitis: implications for skin safety testing and risk assessment. Contact Dermatitis. 1999;41:65–79.
2. Uitto J. The role of elastin and collagen in cutaneous aging: intrinsic aging versus photoexposure. J Drugs Dermatol. 2008;7(2s):12–16.
3. Franceschi C, Bonafè M, Valensin S, Olivieri F, De Luca M, Ottaviani E, et al. Inflamm-aging. An evolutionary perspective on immunosenescence. Ann N Y Acad Sci. 2000;908:244–54.
4. Bennett MF, Robinson MK, Baron ED, Cooper KD. Skin immune systems and inflammation: protector of the skin or promoter of aging? J Investig Dermatol Symp Proc. 2008;13:15–9.
5. Krutmann J, Gilchrest BA. Photoaging of skin. In: Krutmann J, Gilchrest BA, editors. Skin aging. Berlin: Springer; 2006. p. 33–44.
6. Robinson MK, Tiesman JP, Binder RL, Juhlin KD. Immune and inflammatory gene expression profiles of chronological skin aging and photoaging. J Am Acad Dermatol. 2008;58:408.
7. Robinson MK, Binder RL, Griffiths CE. Genomic-driven insights into changes in aging skin. J Drugs Dermatol. 2009;8(7s):8–11.
8. Sumino H, Ichikawa S, Abe M, Endo Y, Ishikawa O, Kurabayashi M. Effects of aging, menopause, and hormone replacement therapy on forearm skin elasticity in women. J Am Geriatr Soc. 2004;52:945–9.
9. Sandby-Moller J, Poulsen T, Wulf HC. Epidermal thickness at different body sites: relationship to age, gender, pigmentation, blood content, skin type and smoking habits. Acta Derm Venereol. 2003;83: 410–3.
10. Ghadially R. Aging and the epidermal permeability barrier: implications for contact dermatitis. Am J Contact Dermatol. 1998;9:162–9.
11. Reed JT, Ghadially R, Elias PM. Skin type, but neither race nor gender, influence epidermal permeability barrier function. Arch Dermatol. 1995;131:1134–8.
12. Gosain A, Luisa MD, DiPietro A. Aging and wound healing. World J Surg. 2004;28:321–6.
13. Norman D. The effects of age-related skin changes on wound healing rates. J Wound Care. 2004;13: 199–201.
14. Yamada M, Udono MU, Hori M, Hirose R, Sato S, Mori T, et al. Aged human skin removes UVB-induced pyrimidine dimers from the epidermis more slowly than younger adult skin in vivo. Arch Dermatol Res. 2006;297:294–302.
15. Thompson CS, Holowatz LA, Lost D. Attenuated noradrenergic sensitivity during local cooling in aged human skin. J Physiol. 2005;564:313–9.
16. Song WJ, Lee SM, Kim MH, Kim SH, Kim KW, Cho SH, et al. Histamine and allergen skin reactivity in the elderly population: results from the Korean Longitudinal Study on Health and Aging. Ann Allergy Asthma Immunol. 2011;107:344–52.
17. Agner T, Johansen JD, Overgaard L, Volund A, Basketter D, Menne T. Combined effects of irritants and allergens. Contact Dermatitis. 2002;47:21–6.
18. Lejman E, Stoudemayer T, Grove G, Kligman AM. Age differences in poison ivy dermatitis. Contact Dermatitis. 1984;11:163–7.
19. Cua AB, Wilhelm KP, Maibach HI. Cutaneous sodium lauryl sulphate irritation potential: age and regional variability. Br J Dermatol. 1990;123:607–13.
20. Grove GL, Duncan S, Kligman AM. Effect of ageing on the blistering of human skin with ammonium hydroxide. Br J Dermatol. 1982;107:393–400.

21. Tuft L, Heck VM, Gregory DC. Studies in sensitization as applied to skin test reactions. III. Influence of age upon skin reactivity. J Allergy. 1955;26:359–66.
22. Gilchrest BA, Stoff JS, Soter NA. Chronologic aging alters the response to ultraviolet-induced inflammation in human-skin. J Invest Dermatol. 1982;79:11–5.
23. Nilzen A, Voss Lagerlund K. Epicutaneous tests with detergents and a number of other common allergens. Dermatologica. 1962;124:42–52.
24. Robinson MK. Population differences in acute skin irritation responses – race, sex, age, sensitive skin and repeat subject comparisons. Contact Dermatitis. 2002;46:86–93.
25. Robinson MK. Racial differences in acute and cumulative skin irritation responses between Caucasian and Asian populations. Contact Dermatitis. 2000;42:134–43.
26. Robinson MK. Intra-individual variations in acute and cumulative skin irritation responses. Contact Dermatitis. 2001;45:75–83.
27. Green BG. Measurement of sensory irritation of the skin. Am J Contact Dermat. 2000;11:170–80.
28. Frosch PJ, Kligman AM. A method for appraising the stinging capacity of topically applied substances. J Soc Cosmet Chem. 1977;28:197–209.
29. Soschin D, Kligman AM. Adverse subjective responses. In: Kligman AM, Leyden JJ, editors. Safety and efficacy of topical drugs and cosmetics. New York: Grune & Stratton; 1982. p. 377–88.
30. Christensen M, Kligman AM. An improved procedure for conducting lactic acid stinging tests on facial skin. J Cosmet Sci. 1996;47:1–11.
31. Green BG, Bluth J. Measuring the chemosensory irritability of human skin. J Toxicol-Cutan Ocul Toxicol. 1995;14:23–48.
32. Heft MW, Cooper BY, Obrien KK, Hemp E, Obrien R. Aging effects on the perception of noxious and non-noxious thermal stimuli applied to the face. Aging-Clin Exp Res. 1996;8:35–41.
33. Adly MA, Assaf H, Hussein MR. Age-associated decrease of the nerve growth factor protein expression in the human skin: preliminary findings. J Dermatol Sci. 2006;42:268–71.
34. Besné I, Descombes C, Breton L. Effect of age and anatomical site on density of sensory innervation in human epidermis. Arch Dermatol. 2002;138:1445–50.
35. Garibyan L, Chiou AS, Elmariah SB. Advanced aging skin and itch: addressing an unmet need. Dermatol Ther. 2013;26:92–103.
36. Oyeyinka GO. Age and sex differences in immunocompetence. Gerontology. 1984;30:188–95.
37. Prystowsky SD, Allen AM, Smith RW, Nonomura JH, Odom RB, Akers WA. Allergic contact hypersensitivity to nickel, neomycin, ethylenediamine, and benzocaine. Relationships between age, sex, history of exposure, and reactivity to standard patch tests and use tests in a general population. Arch Dermatol. 1979;115:959–62.
38. Goh CL. Prevalence of contact allergy by sex, race and age. Contact Dermatitis. 1986;14:237–40.
39. Young E, van Weelden H, van Osch L. Age and sex distribution of the incidence of contact sensitivity tostandard allergens. Contact Dermatitis. 1988;19:307–8.
40. Balato A, Balato N, Di Costanzo L, Ayala F. Contact sensitization in the elderly. Clin Dermatol. 2011;29:24–30.
41. Wantke F, Hemmer W, Jarisch R, Gotz M. Patch test reactions in children, adults and the elderly – a comparative study in patients with suspected allergic contact dermatitis. Contact Dermatitis. 1996;34:316–9.
42. Kwangsukstith C, Maibach HI. Effect of age and sex on the induction and elicitation of allergic contact dermatitis. Contact Dermatitis. 1995;33:289–98.
43. Schwartz M. Eczematous sensitization in various age groups. J Allergy. 1952;24:143–8.
44. Cassimos C, Kanakoudi-Tsakalidis F, Spyroglou K, Ladianos M, Tzaphi R. Skin sensitization to 2, 4 dinitrochlorobenzene (DNCB) in the first months of life. J Clin Lab Immunol. 1980;3:111–3.
45. Robinson MK. Age and gender as influencing factors in skin sensitivity. In: Berardesca E, Fluhr JW, Maibach HI, editors. Sensitive skin syndrome. New York: Taylor & Francis; 2006. p. 169–80.

Skin Reactivity of the Human Face: Functional Map and Age Related Differences

132

John Jay P. Cadavona, Slaheddine Marrakchi, and Howard I. Maibach

Contents

J.J.P. Cadavona (✉) • H.I. Maibach
Department of Dermatology, University of California, San Francisco, CA, USA
e-mail: jcadavona@medicine.nevada.edu; maibachh@derm.ucsf.edu

S. Marrakchi
Department of Dermatology, Hedi Chaker Hospital, Sfax, Tunisia
e-mail: slaheddine.marrakchi@tunet.tn

M.A. Farage et al. (eds.), *Textbook of Aging Skin*,
DOI 10.1007/978-3-662-47398-6_17

Abstract

The skin of the human face is much more complex and diverse, physiologically, than to be expected. It is imperative to observe and understand the variation that exists among the various regions of face skin. The aim of this chapter was to discuss the findings of studies that assess these regions in terms of biophysical parameters: upper dermis vascularization, stratum corneum turnover, transepidermal water loss, stratum corneum hydration, skin temperature, skin sebum content, and pH. The nasolabial region showed highest values for stratum corneum turnover (in the younger group), transepidermal water loss, skin temperature, and sebum content. Laser Doppler flowmeter (LDF) revealed that upper dermis vascularization was highest in the nasal region. Hydration was highest in the neck, and pH was highest (most alkaline) in the chin. Additionally, this chapter examines studies that evaluated reactivity of the skin of various facial regions in response to hexyl nicotinate and sodium lauryl sulfate. In terms of skin reactivity, induction of nonimmunologic contact urticaria by hexyl nicotinate showed highest values in the chin (of aged group), while sodium lauryl sulfate was nonreactive in the forearm.

Introduction

An early report of age- and anatomical-related variations in percutaneous absorption was presented by Feldmann and Maibach [1] more than 40 years ago.

Additionally, in a series of articles, Montagna described anatomical variations in the histological structure of various sites of the face [2]. More recently, bioengineering methods allowed accurate and objective measurements of skin reactivity to chemicals in order to establish a map of the human face by focusing on regional variation, age-related differences in terms of biophysical parameters, and reactivity to chemicals [3–7]. Among these bioengineering tools, capacitance meters usually evaluate stratum corneum (SC) hydration. Transepidermal water loss (TEWL), which evaluates the SC water barrier function, is measured by tewameters. Skin pH, skin temperature, and lipid content of the skin surface are measured by appropriate instruments. Laser blood flow monitors are used to evaluate dermal blood flow.

Aging skin is under the influence of various factors. Intrinsic influences on skin aging might include genetic (i.e., racial) and hormonal factors and normally involve the entire integument. Extrinsic influences, including environmental and ultraviolet (UV) exposure, alcohol, and smoking, involve mainly the exposed facial skin, but also less studied other sites. This area has to be better studied in order to try to explain the various modifications that occur with aging. Furthermore, only a few reports in the literature extensively evaluated the effect of various chemicals on the areas of the face. Some of these studies focused on age and regional differences of reactivity to chemicals between different areas of the face. Correlation studies were also undertaken to understand how the skin reacts to chemicals and which intrinsic and extrinsic factors could influence reactivity [3–5, 7].

This chapter focuses on the few studies that establish a map of the human face based on the objectively measured biophysical parameters. These studies demonstrated regional and age-related differences and correlations between some measured parameters. Various chemicals experimentally used to induce irritant dermatitis or contact urticaria also showed age- and region-related differences as well as significant correlations in aged persons, between reactivity of the skin and some measured biophysical parameters.

Biophysical Parameters of Skin: Map of the Human Face

As anatomical variations have been reported in facial skin, an attempt was made to establish a map of the human face for six biophysical parameters used to explore various components of the skin: transepidermal water loss (TEWL), skin hydration (capacitance), upper dermis vascularization by laser Doppler flowmeter (LDF), skin surface temperature, skin surface pH, and lipid content of the skin surface (sebum). Stratum corneum turnover (dansyl chloride test) was also studied.

These parameters were studied in ten aged (66–83 years) Caucasian and Hispanic men and women volunteers. This group was compared to a young group, aged 29.8 ± 3.9 years, ranging from 24 to 34 years. Nine regions – the forehead (FH), upper eyelid (UE), nasolabial area (NL), perioral area (PO), nose, cheek, chin, neck, and volar forearm (FA) – were studied. TEWL was measured using an evaporimeter. Results were expressed as gram per square meter per hour. Electrical capacitance of the SC was measured with a capacitance meter. Results were expressed in arbitrary units. An infrared pyrometer was used to measure skin temperature. Skin pH was recorded using a skin surface pH meter. Lipid content of the skin surface (sebum) was determined with a Sebumeter. The measurements were expressed in microgram per square centimeter. Stratum corneum turnover was studied in all the areas cited except the UE. A concentration of 5 % dansyl chloride in petrolatum was applied on the eight studied skin sites for 16 h, using patch tests. Stratum corneum turnover was determined by detecting fluorescence on each skin site every day, using a UV lamp. The time for the disappearance of fluorescence was considered the SC turnover.

All parameters were correlated with each other without considering the regions separately.

Anatomical Variations in the Human Face: SC Turnover

SC turnover, as determined by the disappearance time of dansyl chloride, was slower in the FA (18.3 ± 3.6 days) and NL areas (15.5 ± 3.9 days) than in the chin (10.4 ± 2.8 days), the FH (11.1 ± 2.4 days), the cheek (11.2 ± 2.6 days), the PO areas (11.2 ± 3.8 days), the neck (11.5 ± 2.3 days), and the nose (11.8 ± 2.7 days) [5]. Compared with the young group, aged individuals showed a trend to a faster SC turnover in almost all the areas studied, with statistically significant values in the nose and the neck (Fig. 1). Grove and Kligman found a significant correlation between SC transit time and corneocyte size in the volar forearm [8]. Plewig and Jansen [9] found face corneocytes to be larger than those of extremities, suggesting that epidermal proliferation in the face was more active than in the extremities. They found corneocyte size in the aged subjects larger than in the young people, suggesting that proliferation activity in aged people diminishes with age, and this was confirmed by Kobayashi and Tagami [7]. The authors focused on the perioral area and demonstrated that corneocyte size increases with age in the cheek, the nasolabial fold, and the chin. It is likely that deuterated H_2O technology will further refine this metric [10].

LDF Measurements

Blood flow in the nose area was significantly higher than in all the other areas except the chin [6] (Table 1). This was followed by volume of blood flow in the chin, PO and NL areas, and cheek. These areas showed higher blood flow values than the neck and forearm. FH and neck blood flow was higher than only the FA. Correlation between sebum and LDF was relatively strong ($r = 0.65, p < 0.01$).

In concordance with the Shriner classification [3], the nose area showed the highest blood flow

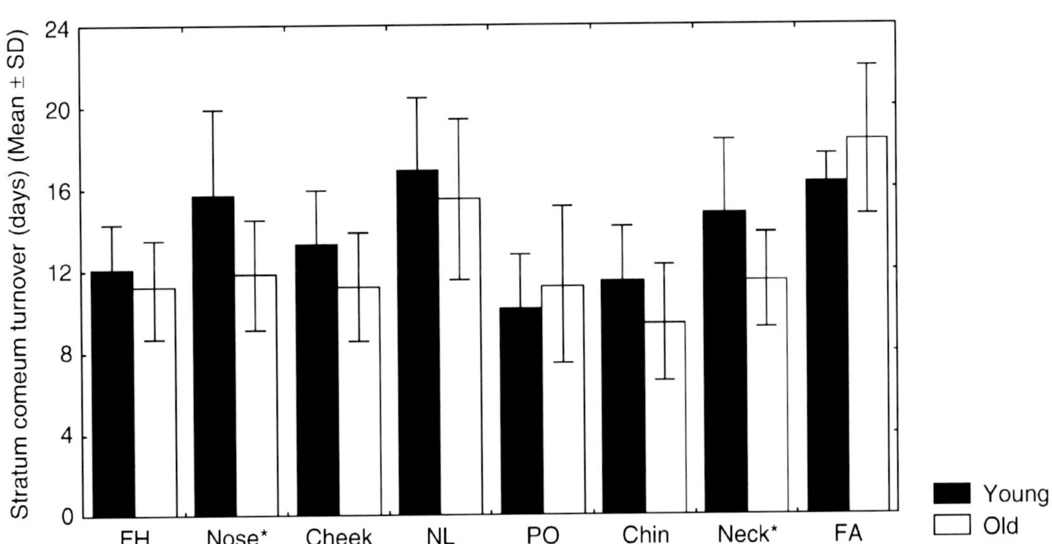

Fig. 1 Stratum corneum turnover. Regional variation in the young and aged groups and age-related differences *FH* forehead, *NL* nasolabial area, *PO* perioral area, *FA* forearm (*Regions where the difference between the two age groups was significant ($p < 0.05$))

Table 1 LDF (expressed in arbitrary units) (Marrakchi et al. [6])

	Young group	Aged group
Area	Mean ± SD	Mean ± SD
Forehead	96.50 ± 115.18	98.60 ± 37.70
Nose	147.87 ± 78.87	204.57 ± 80.07
Cheek	132.96 ± 145.96	129.77 ± 80.81
Nasolabial	94.71 ± 45.66	118.78 ± 54.38
Perioral	136.14 ± 87.99	127.59 ± 75.03
Chin	134.94 ± 69.53	167.71 ± 121.69
Neck	75.51 ± 86.36	73.88 ± 25.89
Forearm	18.13 ± 11.66	24.51 ± 24.95

Table 2 TEWL (expressed as g/m^2h) by regions of the face and age group (Firooz et al. [13])

	TEWL		
Area	Mean ± SD		Age
Forehead	12.27 ± 10.05	9.18 ± 6.46	Age 10–20
Cheek	9.57 ± 7.22	14.90 ± 12.59	Age 20–30
Nasolabial fold	14.05 ± 8.25	13.67 ± 8.99	Age 30–40
Neck	10.47 ± 9.23	14.64 ± 11.08	Age 40–50
Forearm	10.12 ± 9.54	9.87 ± 8.50	Age 50–60

levels. A great spatial and temporal intraindividual heterogeneity of LDF measurements was demonstrated by Braverman [11]. This variation could be related to anatomical organization of the microcirculation units of the upper dermis. The vascular unit was compared to an umbrella, with the handle representing ascending arterioles, and the umbrella proper representing the arteriolar and venular branches forming the upper vascular plexus. Ascending arterioles are spaced at intervals of 1.5–7 mm and give high erythrocytes flux and high concentration of moving red blood cells. The areas of relative avascularity give low erythrocytes flux and low concentration of moving red blood cells. Thus, LDF depends upon the position of the LDF probe on the skin. The moderate correlation found between LDF and sebum content is not surprising, since arterioles and capillaries are organized in vascular units around the appendages of the face, and an increase in sebaceous gland number and sebum production might require more vascularization [12].

Transepidermal Water Loss (TEWL)

The highest values were found in the NL fold, while the lowest were in the cheek [12] (Table 2). Marrakchi [6] further measures TEWL to be significantly higher in the PO, the chin, and the UE areas than in the FH, cheek, FA, and neck areas. Thus, water retention is less efficient in the areas surrounding the mouth and nose. Lopez [13] divided three areas of the face (the cheek, forehead, and chin) into 90 small segments, measured TEWL in each segment, and established a map for these three areas. Conclusions were that locations surrounding the orifices (mouth and nose) showed higher TEWL values. Although the study evaluated five young women, it reinforces the results of regional variations of TEWL in the human face.

Firooz [12] further compared TEWL among age groups. Table 2 presents this data as the average of all measured areas (the FH, cheek, NL, neck, FA, dorsal hand, palm, and leg), with five males and five females per age group. No statistical differences were found between the groups. However, conflicting results were published concerning the effect of aging on TEWL. Some studies reported a significant decrease in TEWL with age, mainly after the sixth decade [7, 15]. Others reported a trend to decrease in TEWL with age, without reaching statistical significance [3, 16]. The results reported in the literature are difficult to compare, because only a few studies involving various areas of the face in aged people have been published [3, 7]. Nevertheless, a careful meta-analysis supports the earlier Wilhelm analysis [17, 15]. Therefore, more studies are needed to evaluate age-related changes in TEWL. In the future, the studied groups should be more homogeneous as race, gender, exposure to sunlight, and other environmental factors could induce the SC changes that usually occur with age.

Various factors could influence water retention in the SC. In the same study [6], TEWL was found moderately correlated to skin temperature ($r = 0.44$, $p < 0.01$) in aged individuals. NL and PO areas showed the highest skin temperature values. This could partly explain the high TEWL values in these areas. As described earlier [16, 18], skin temperature and TEWL are correlated when sweat glands are inactivated.

Corneocyte size correlates to stratum corneum renewal [8] and inversely correlates to TEWL [19]. Plewig [9] found that the corneocytes of the face were smaller than those of the extremities, and corneocytes in the aged were much larger than in young individuals, which could partly explain the tendency to higher TEWL in aged individuals. However, the influence of various factors on TEWL in aged people should be considered as a complex phenomenon, with the intervention of various factors that could interact with each other to determine a final TEWL value.

Stratum Corneum Hydration (Capacitance)

The neck was the most hydrated area, followed by the cheek, then FH, FA, and finally NL area [13] (Table 3). Marrakchi [6] found that the UE, FH, PO, and NL had higher capacitance values than the nose, but without reaching statistical significance. As reported by Shriner [3] and Tagami [20], the neck has to be considered as the most hydrated area of the skin, independent of the age.

Firooz [13] further compared capacitance among various age groups. Table 3 presents this data as the average of all measured areas (the FH, cheek, NL, neck, FA, dorsal hand, palm, and leg), with five males and five females per age group. Adults aged 40–50 showed the highest SC hydration, while those 50–60 showed the lowest. No statistical differences were found between each age group. However, conflicting results were published with regard to the influence of age on facial skin hydration. Tagami [20] reported that only the perioral areas (nasolabial fold and the chin) are influenced by aging or photoaging. These areas showed an increased hydration state with age. The author related the hydration state to lipid content of the skin. Therefore, more data are needed to determine the influence of age on skin hydration. Study of more homogeneous groups should be considered in order to reduce the influence of race and gender on the hydration state of the facial skin.

Considering two parameters (capacitance and TEWL), the facial skin may be subdivided into three areas based on the dynamic characteristics of water motion within the epidermis:

(i) Areas with a lack of influx of water in the epidermis: low capacitance and low TEWL values (nose and FH areas)
(ii) Areas with excess of water evaporation: high TEWL and low capacitance (NL and PO areas)
(iii) Areas with high water-holding capacity: high capacitance and low TEWL (neck area)

Table 3 Capacitance (expressed in arbitrary units) by regions of the face and by age group (Firooz et al. [13])

	Capacitance		
Area	Mean ± SD		Age
Forehead	53.54 ± 16.49	49.74 ± 19.25	Age 10–20
Cheek	62.12 ± 15.63	47.08 ± 16.61	Age 20–30
Nasolabial fold	38.19 ± 18.02	50.53 ± 17.69	Age 30–40
Neck	62.88 ± 15.28	53.34 ± 20.78	Age 40–50
Forearm	51.00 ± 15.92	43.04 ± 20.58	Age 50–60

Skin Temperature

The NL area, followed by the PO area and the chin, showed the highest skin temperature [6] (Table 4).

Skin temperature of the NL area was significantly higher than the skin temperature in three areas (the FH, UE, and FA areas). The PO area

Table 4 Skin temperature (expressed in degrees Celsius) (Marrakchi et al. [6])

Area	Young group Mean ± SD	Aged group Mean ± SD
Forehead	33.6 ± 0.9	34.0 ± 1.1
Upper eyelid	33.6 ± 1.1	34.0 ± 1.3
Nose	32.7 ± 2.9	33.5 ± 3.6
Cheek	32.9 ± 2.0	34.1 ± 1.3
Nasolabial	34.6 ± 1.7	35.3 ± 1.4
Perioral	34.1 ± 1.7	35.2 ± 1.3
Chin	34.1 ± 1.6	35.0 ± 1.5
Neck	34.6 ± 1.1	34.8 ± 1.5
Forearm	32.8 ± 1.7	33.6 ± 1.5

Table 5 Sebum content (expressed in g/cm^2) by regions of the face and by age group (Firooz et al. [13])

	Sebum		
Area	Mean ± SD		Age
Forehead	95.65 ± 51.38	53.75 ± 77.94	Age 10–20
Cheek	73.39 ± 64.05	50.10 ± 51.81	Age 20–30
Nasolabial fold	136.98 ± 72.33	42.06 ± 60.42	Age 30–40
Neck	64.41 ± 64.51	66.71 ± 73.42	Age 40–50
Forearm	18.45 ± 37.88	41.77 ± 57.72	Age 50–60

temperature was higher than that of the FH and FA areas. Skin temperature in the chin area was almost significantly higher than the temperature in the FH and FA areas. Temperature was similar in the remaining six areas: the neck, cheek, FH, UE, FA, and nose areas.

As reported previously [3], skin temperature in the aged people was higher than in the young, although statistical significance was not reached.

As reported by Kobayashi [7], moderate to weak correlations were found between skin surface temperature and TEWL ($r = 0.44, p < 0.01$) and between skin temperature and surface sebum content ($r = 0.29$, $p < 0.01$). Correlation with TEWL has already been discussed (TEWL section). Correlation between sebum levels and skin temperature was confirmed by the previous report demonstrating that increase in skin temperature by 1 °C increases sebum excretion by 10 % [21]. Also, as reported by Lopez [14], (using young subjects, however) sebum levels and skin temperature showed comparable patterns, the distribution occurring in a T-shaped pattern, with highest values in the FH area and central part of the face for both parameters.

Sebum Skin Content

Sebum production follows a T-shaped pattern in the human face [6, 14] (Table 5). However, few studies investigated facial sebum excretion in aged individuals in detail. According to Firooz [13], sebum content was found to be highest in the NL area, followed by the forehead, cheek, and neck. The mean sebum content for FA is considerably lower.

Firooz [13] further compared sebum content among age groups. Table 5 presents this data as the average of all measured areas (the FH, cheek, NL, neck, FA, dorsal hand, palm, and leg), with five males and five females per age group. No statistical differences were found between the groups. Correlation with LDF has been previously discussed (LDF measurements section) as has correlation with temperature (skin temperature section). Correlation with TEWL could be an indirect relationship, linked to the well-known and demonstrated correlation between TEWL and skin temperature.

However, sebum excretion could be a more complicated process than expected. Le Fur [22] showed chronological variation in sebum production in the human face. Other factors beside age (hormonal, gender, and race) could influence sebum secretion, rendering the need for standardized protocols and experimental conditions mandatory.

pH

Skin pH in the chin area was higher than the pH in four areas: the FH, UE, nose, and PO areas [6] (Table 6). In the FA, neck, and NL areas, skin pH was higher than the pH in the FH and UE areas. The FH and UE areas demonstrated the most

Table 6 Skin pH (Marrakchi et al. [6])

Area	Young group Mean ± SD	Aged group Mean ± SD
Forehead	4.43 ± 0.44	5.19 ± 0.44
Upper eyelid	4.62 ± 0.40	5.13 ± 0.49
Nose	5.23 ± 0.55	5.39 ± 0.50
Cheek	5.07 ± 0.45	5.47 ± 0.52
Nasolabial	5.17 ± 0.58	5.59 ± 0.51
Perioral	5.05 ± 0.48	5.35 ± 0.56
Chin	5.55 ± 0.57	5.86 ± 0.31
Neck	5.20 ± 0.43	5.67 ± 0.49
Forearm	5.30 ± 0.32	5.75 ± 0.43

acidic skin pH in the face. Compared to the young group, skin pH was significantly higher in the aged individuals in four areas: the FH, UE, neck, and FA.

In concordance with these data, Wilhelm's [15] comparison of the skin pH of the FA and FH areas with nine other skin areas in two age groups found that the pH in the FH area was among the most acidic, while the pH of the FA area was among the most alkaline. In the same study, the pH of the FH area was higher in the elderly compared to young individuals.

Zlotogorski [23], who studied the skin pH distribution in the FH and cheek areas, found that the pH was lower in the FH area in 89 % of the subjects and that the pH in these two areas was significantly higher in individuals more than 80 years of age.

In a chronobiologic study of biophysical parameters of the skin, Le Fur [22] found a circadian rhythm of pH in the facial skin, but not in the FA skin, suggesting that structural specificities of the epidermis might account for the area-related variability of skin pH measurements.

Although few studies focused on the skin pH in terms of regional variations and age-related differences [15, 23], Marrakchi and Maibach confirmed that facial skin pH is more alkaline in aged subjects and that regional differences exist among the various areas of the face.

A moderate and negative correlation was found between skin pH and sebum content in two areas (which is not surprising with regard to the fatty acid content of sebum): the chin ($r = -0.49$, $p =-0.03$) and the neck ($r = -0.53, p = 0.02$).

Skin Reactivity

Nonimmunologic Contact Urticaria Induced by Hexyl Nicotinate: Functional Map of the Human Face and Age-Related Differences

Beside age-related and regional variation studies of the biophysical parameters of the human face, a few studies evaluated the effect of chemicals on the facial skin [3–5]. Data of skin reactivity, obtained after hexyl nicotinate (HN) was applied to eight areas of the skin (the FH, nose, cheek, NL, PO, chin, neck, and FA areas), is reported here. Hexyl nicotinate, a lipophilic compound used in cosmetic products, is known to induce nonimmunologic contact urticaria in the skin. The regional and age-related blood flow changes induced by HN were investigated. The vasodilation induced by HN was recorded by a laser Doppler flowmeter. Two age groups were studied: ten healthy young volunteers, aged 29.8 ± 3.9 years, ranging from 24 to 34 years, and ten older volunteers, aged 73.6 ± 17.4 years, ranging from 66 to 83 years.

Baseline cutaneous blood flow was monitored at one measurement per second for 30 s, and the values were averaged. Subsequently, using a saturated absorbent filter paper disc (0.8 cm diameter) (Finn Chamber[1]; Epitest Ltd Oy), 5 mM HN in ethanol was applied on the eight skin areas for 15 s to elicit NICU. Following this, the blood flow measurements were taken every 10 min for 1 h in order to detect the maximum vascular response of the skin to HN (peak value, considered as the response of the skin to HN).

In the aged group, the chin, followed by the cheek and the NL areas, showed higher mean peak values (Fig. 2). However, no statistically significant differences were found between the various areas of the face. The FA was found to be the less-sensitive area.

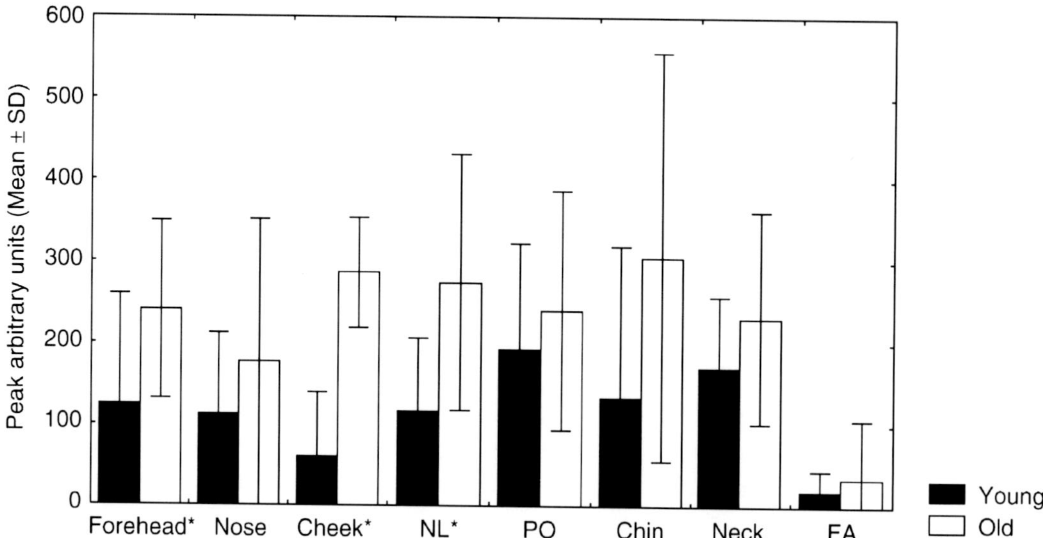

Fig. 2 Baseline LDF to peak changes. Regional variation in the young and aged groups and age-related differences *FH* forehead, *NL* nasolabial area, *PO* perioral area, *FA* forearm (*Regions where the difference between the two age groups was significant ($p < 0.05$))

Peak values were higher in the aged group in three areas: the FH ($p = 0.047$), cheek ($p < 0.001$), and NL ($p = 0.012$) areas. The higher reactivity in the aged group could be explained by the enlargement of sebaceous glands in the elderly [24]. UVA light has been reported to induce sebaceous gland hyperplasia [24], which may lead to the enlargement of sebaceous glands of the face when compared to other areas [2] and in the elderly when compared to the younger subjects [24, 25]. Appendages may be an important factor in HN absorption, because the areas in the aged group where peak values were significantly higher than those in the young group are known to have a high appendage density [26]. Hueber [27] demonstrated that the appendageal route accounts for the transport of hydrocortisone and testosterone, but it is more important for the latter, which is the more lipophilic compound. Vellus hair follicle density has been measured at different body sites: the back, the thorax, the upper arm, the forearm, the thigh, and the calf [28]. The highest density was found in facial skin, the forehead showing an average follicular density of 292 follicles/cm^2. The diameters of the follicular orifices showed great variations on the forehead. The authors estimated that this could be explained by the seborrheic nature of this area as compared to the other areas.

Another aspect could explain the variations in skin penetration of chemicals: the lipid contents of the skin. Morganti [29] estimated that a lipophilic vehicle can easily penetrate the facial skin where the SC is lipid rich (10–20 % by weight), compared to palmoplantar skin (2 % by weight).

In a similar study, Shriner [3] found regional and age-related differences in facial skin reactivity to benzoic acid. The neck was the most reactive area, and the young individuals reacted more than the aged group.

Based on these conflicting results, one should consider that skin penetration might be dependent on the nature of the compound (more or less lipophilic), which penetrates more or less easier in some specific areas of the skin, depending on hydration status, density of follicles, and the composition of the lipids.

Moreover, reactivity of the skin to chemicals depends not only upon their transcutaneous penetration but could be the expression of variability in the vascularization of the epidermis. Vascular anatomy of the facial skin was reported to change with age [30]. Chung studied 21 healthy volunteers age-distributed from the third to ninth decade finding that the intrinsically aged skin (buttock) and photoaged skin (face) showed a reduction in the cutaneous vessel size, with a diminished dermal area covered by the vessels. However, only photoaged skin showed significantly reduced density of dermal vessels. Thus age-related variability of the facial skin to HN could be due to a combination of multiple factors that need more extensive studies, which should take into account racial and gender differences, as well as environmental influences.

Sodium Lauryl Sulfate-Induced Irritation in the Human Face: Regional and Age-Related Differences

Sodium lauryl sulfate (SLS) ($C_{12}H_{25}SO_4Na$) is an anionic surfactant used for its thickening effect in toothpastes, shampoos, and shaving foams [4]. However, it has a potential irritant effect on the skin. It has been extensively studied in dermatological research. TEWL was considered a predictive parameter for skin susceptibility to SLS [31]. With regard to the lack of investigations exploring its irritant action on human facial skin, a study that investigated regional and age-related differences in skin reactivity to SLS when applied to various areas of the human face was conducted [4]. The potential role of TEWL as a predictive parameter of skin response to SLS was also investigated.

Various protocols (concentration, application time) used SLS in a water solution to induce skin irritation. In this study, as the face was suspected to be more sensitive to irritants than the remaining integuments of the human body, SLS 2 % was only applied for 1 h, under occlusion. This protocol was sufficient to induce subclinical irritation in most of the areas of the face, but not in the FA area, confirming that the face is more sensitive than the FA area.

Two age groups were included: ten young subjects, aged 25.2 ± 4.7 years (range 19–30 years) and ten elderly subjects, aged 73.7 ± 3.9 years (range 70–81 years). Twelve Caucasian and eight Hispanic volunteers of both sexes were included in the study. Eight areas of the skin (the FH, nose, cheek, NL, and PO; chin, neck, and volar FA) were studied. Baseline TEWL and capacitance were measured before a 2 % SLS w/v solution was applied for 1 h under occlusion to each of the eight areas. On the contralateral side, water was applied in the same condition as control. To evaluate skin irritation, TEWL was measured 23 h after removal of SLS.

TEWL values of the areas tested were corrected according to the changes in the control areas:

$$\begin{aligned}\mathrm{DTEWL} = {} & \mathrm{TEWL}_{23\,h} \\ & - (\mathrm{TEWL}_{H2O\ 23h} - \mathrm{TEWL}_{H2O\ 0h}) \\ & - \mathrm{TEWL}_{0h}\end{aligned}$$

where TEWL_{23h} is the measured TEWL in the tested area at 23 h, TEWL_{0h} is the baseline TEWL in the tested area, $\mathrm{TEWL}_{H2O\ 23h}$ is the measured TEWL in the control area at 23 h, and $\mathrm{TEWL}_{H2O\ 0h}$ is the baseline TEWL in the control area. DTEWL expresses the skin reactivity to SLS.

Little is known about susceptibility of the facial skin to the irritant potential of SLS [32].

With age, there is a decrease of irritation induced by SLS in at least some areas of the facial skin, as demonstrated earlier. This is in concordance with the overall decrease in sensitivity in the elderly [32, 33].

Skin reactivity to SLS is summarized in Table 7. In the young group, all the areas except the FA area reacted to SLS. In the aged group, all regions reacted except the nose, PO, and FA areas. The cheek and chin showed the highest DTEWL mean values in the aged group. These two areas showed significantly higher reactivity when compared to the FA area, and the chin area demonstrated higher reactivity when compared to the FH area.

Although the cheek and chin areas showed the highest DTEWL mean values, statistically significant regional differences in facial skin reactivity to SLS were not detected. This is probably related to the high SD observed in DTEWL values (Table 7).

Skin sensitivity to water-soluble irritants has also been explored by the stinging test [34, 35]. Marked regional variation in the intensity of stinging was found [34]: the nasolabial fold area > cheek area > chin area > retroauricular area > forehead. A stinging test probably expresses more than just percutaneous diffusion of the irritant compound; it may also express the magnitude of sensory nerve response, which may depend upon nerve density in the skin, which was found to be variable in human epidermis [36]. This was a regional variability, with a higher number of epidermal nerves in the facial skin (upper eyelid and preauricular areas) compared to truncal skin. The authors also demonstrated a trend toward the decrease of innervation of the facial skin with increase in age [36]. Skin irritation expressed by DTEWL is the result of percutaneous penetration of the compound and the changes made to the skin barrier. This could explain why both methods (stinging test and SLS-induced irritation) might give different results in regional variation of sensitivity in the human face, although the cheek and the chin areas were demonstrated as among the most sensitive by both methods.

Table 7 Reactivity of regions in the young and aged groups (Marrakchi et al. [4])

Area	ΔTEWL (mean ± SD) g/m^{2}h		p value
	Young group	Aged group	
Cheek	15.1 ± 12.8	6.8 ± 7.3	0.093
Chin[a]	13.5 ± 9.9	6.0 ± 3.3	0.035
Forcarm	1.9 ± 2.1	1.1 ± 1.5	0.354
Forehead	10.4 ± 13.9	2.3 ± 2.3	0.086
Neck	6.8 ± 6.0	3.6 ± 3.7	0.165
Nasolabial area[a]	12.4 ± 6.3	4.4 ± 4.8	0.005
Nose	8.6 ± 7.6	5.0 ± 6.0	0.251
Perioral area	10.7 ± 10.0	4.2 ± 4.1	0.074

ΔTEWL = TEWL 23 h after patch test removal corrected to the control – baseline TEWL
[a]Difference between the young and aged group statistically significant ($p < 0.05$)

Comparison between both groups showed that facial skin reactivity to SLS in the young group was higher, but the differences were significant only in the chin area ($p = 0.035$) and the NL area ($p = 0.005$).

Correlation between baseline TEWL and DTEWL revealed that baseline TEWL is a predictive factor of facial skin reactivity to SLS in five areas: the cheek, FH, neck, NL, and PO areas (Table 8).

Table 8 Correlations in each area between baseline TEWL (BTEWL) and reactivity of the skin to SLS, 23 h after patch removal (ΔTEWL) (Marrakchi et al. [4])

Area	BTEWL (Mean ± SD)	TEWL 23 h (Mean ± SD)	ΔTEWL (Mean ± SD)	r	p
Cheek[a]	15.63 ± 6.70	26.63 ± 15.30	10.96 ± 11.01	0.4616	0.04
Chin[a]	20.87 ± 6.37	30.47 ± 12.08	9.77 ± 8.13	0.3535	0.126
Forearm	8.64 ± 3.97	9.70 ± 4.92	1.51 ± 1.83	–	–
Forehead[a]	14.10 ± 5.71	20.40 ± 14.96	6.39 ± 10.53	0.6474	0.002
Neck[a]	11.55 ± 4.35	16.63 ± 8.54	5.18 ± 5.12	0.6273	0.003
Nasolabial area[a]	28.74 ± 8.56	36.93 ± 13.44	8.40 ± 6.78	0.4831	0.031
Nose[a]	19.04 ± 6.03	25.27 ± 11.15	6.77 ± 6.92	0.3218	0.166
Perioral	24.25 ± 8.93	29.98 ± 14.6	7.47 ± 8.17	0.4547	0.044

r = coefficient of correlation
p = significance (significant correlation when $p < 0.05$)
[a]Areas which reacted to SLS: statistically significant ($p > 0.05$) difference baseline TEWL and TEWL 23 h after patch removal

This comparative study used SLS to induce an acute irritation. However, repeated or cumulatively induced irritation should better reflect the common use of potential irritants on the skin. This was done by Schwindt, who compared the effect of SLS on the skin of the back in young and aged humans [37]. In the skin of the aged group, repeated application of SLS induced less pronounced irritation than in the young group. This was believed to be related to a decrease in percutaneous absorption and an altered inflammatory skin reaction. The process by which irritants induce skin modifications is complex and still under investigation. Several mechanisms seem to be implicated. SLS induces modification in the proteins of the SC [38] as well as in the lipid bilayers [39], leading to modifications in the skin barrier function. There are also inflammatory changes secondary to the toxic effect of SLS on keratinocytes. These changes involve cytokines that induce infiltration of the epidermis by inflammatory cells and vasodilation in the dermis [40].

Correlation study showed that skin reactivity to SLS (DTEWL) and baseline TEWL values were correlated in five facial areas (Table 8). The correlations between baseline TEWL and TEWL measured 23 h after SLS removal were stronger. The facial areas that reacted to SLS showed strong correlation coefficients, varying from 0.76 to 0.88, with a high significance ($p < 0.001$). However, correlation between basal TEWL and the absolute value measured after irritation ($TEWL_{23h}$) does not imply that higher basal TEWL values predispose to higher skin sensitivity, but that only the correlation between baseline TEWL and the changes in TEWL after irritation (DTEWL) may have this significance. Conflicting results have been published with regard to this aspect. Some authors correlated absolute TEWL values before and after induction of irritation [31], while others [41] correlated basal TEWL and changes to TEWL (DTEWL). Agner [41], studying healthy and atopic subjects, reported a positive correlation between baseline TEWL and the increase in TEWL induced by SLS only in the healthy group. Although basal TEWL was significantly higher in the atopic group, the changes in TEWL detected after exposure to the irritant were not significantly different between the two groups. These findings are in concordance with Marrakchi and Maibach's results, where some areas of the face (NL area) showed higher basal TEWL values than others (the cheek), but failed to induce higher sensitivity (Table 8). Therefore, beside basal TEWL, each region of the skin face probably has its own characteristics that influence the skin sensitivity to irritants. Using a tape-stripping method, de Jongh [42] evaluated penetration parameters of SLS in the SC. The partition coefficient of SLS between water and SC, K, determines the amount of SLS that enters the SC. Diffusion coefficient, D, gives the rate by which SLS moves into the SC. Both parameters, K and D, constitute the penetration parameters of SLS. When associated with baseline TEWL and SC thickness, the penetration parameters demonstrated a better predictive value of impairment of the skin water barrier function induced by SLS than baseline TEWL and SC thickness alone [42].

Conclusion

A map of the human face based on objectively measured biophysical parameters was established. Various chemicals experimentally used to induce irritant dermatitis or contact urticaria also showed age- and region-related differences as well as significant correlations in aged persons, between reactivity of the skin and some measured biophysical parameters.

References

1. Feldman RJ, Maibach HI. Regional variation in percutaneous penetration of ^{14}C cortisol in man. J Invest Dermatol. 1967;48:181–3.
2. Dimond RL, Montagna W. Histology and cytochemistry of human skin. XXXVI. The nose and lips. Arch Dermatol. 1976;112:1235–44.
3. Shriner DL, Maibach HI. Regional variation of nonimmunologic contact urticaria: functional map of the human face. Skin Pharmacol. 1996;9:312–21.

4. Marrakchi S, Maibach HI. Sodium lauryl sulfate-induced irritation in the human face: regional and age-related differences. Skin Pharmacol Physiol. 2006;19:177–80.
5. Marrakchi S, Maibach HI. Functional map and age-related differences in the human face: nonimmunologic contact urticaria induced by hexyl nicotinate. Contact Dermatitis. 2006;55:15–9.
6. Marrakchi S, Maibach HI. Biophysical parameters of skin: map of human face, regional and age-related differences. Contact Dermatitis. 2007;57:28–34.
7. Kobayashi H, Tagami H. Distinct location differences observable in biophysical functions of the facial skin: with special emphasis on the poor functional properties of the stratum corneum of the perioral region. Int J Cosmet Sci. 2004;26:91–101.
8. Grove GL, Kligman AM. Corneocytes size as an indirect measure of epidermal proliferative activity. In: Marks R, Plewig G, editors. Stratum corneum. Berlin: Springer; 1983. p. 191–5.
9. Plewig G, Jansen T. Size and shape of corneocytes: variation with anatomical site and age. In: Wilhelm KP, Elsner P, Berardesca E, Maibach HI, editors. Bioengineering of the skin: skin surface imaging and analysis. Boca Raton: CRC Press; 1997. p. 181–96.
10. Emson CL, Fitzmaurice S, Lindwall G, Li KW, Hellerstein MK, Maibach HI, Liao W, Turner SM. Pilot study demonstrating non-invasive measurement of protein turnover in skin disorders: application to psoriasis. Clin Transl Med. 2013;2:12.
11. Braverman IM. The cutaneous microcirculation. J Investig Dermatol Symp Proc. 2000;5:3–9.
12. Moretti G, Elis RA, Mescon H. Vascular patterns in the skin of the face. J Invest Dermatol. 1959;33:103–12.
13. Firooz A, Sadr B, Babakoohi S, Sarraf-Yazdy M, Fanian F, Kazerouni-Timsar A, Nassiri-Kashani M, Naghizadeh MM, Dowlati Y. Variations of biophysical parameters of the skin with age, gender, and body region. Sci World J. 2012;2012:386936.
14. Lopez S, Le Fur I, Morizot F, Heuvin G, Guinot C, Tschachler E. Transepidermal water loss, temperature and sebum levels on women's facial skin follow characteristic patterns. Skin Res Technol. 2000;6:31–6.
15. Wilhelm K-P, Cua AB, Maibach HI. Skin aging: effect on transepidermal water loss, stratum corneum hydration, skin surface pH, and casual sebum content. Arch Dermatol. 1991;127:1806–9.
16. Roskos KV, Guy RH. Assessment of skin barrier function using transepidermal water loss: effect of age. Pharmacol Res. 1989;6:949–53.
17. Lamel SA, Myer KA, Younes N, Zhou JA, Maibach H, Maibach HI. Placebo response in relation to clinical trial design: a systemic review and meta-analysis of randomized controlled trials for determining biologic efficacy in psoriasis treatment. Arch Dermatol Res. 2012;304:707–17.
18. Mathias CGT, Wilson DM, Maibach HI. Transepidermal water loss as a function of skin surface temperature. J Invest Dermatol. 1981;77:219–20.
19. Marks R, Nicholls S, King CS. Studies on isolated corneocytes. Int J Cosmet Sci. 1994;3:251–8.
20. Tagami H. Location-related differences in structure and function of the stratum corneum with special emphasis on those of the facial skin. Int J Cosmet Sci. 2008;30:413–34.
21. Cunliff WJ, Burton JL, Shuster S. The effect of local temperature variations on the sebum excretion rate. Br J Dermatol. 1970;83:650–4.
22. Le Fur I, Reinberg A, Lopez S, Morizot F, Mechkouri M, Tschachler E. Analysis of circadian and ultradian rhythms of skin surface properties of face and forearm of healthy women. J Invest Dermatol. 2001;117:718–24.
23. Zlotogorski A. Distribution of skin surface pH on the forehead and cheek of adults. Arch Dermatol Res. 1987;279:398–401.
24. Kligman AM, Balin AK. Aging of human skin. In: Balin AK, Kligman AM, editors. Aging and the skin. New York: Raven; 1989. p. 1–42.
25. Smith L. Histopathologic characteristics and ultrastructure of aging skin. Cutis. 1989;43:419–24.
26. Blume U, Ferracin I, Verschoore M, Czernielewski JM, Schaefer H. Physiology of the vellus hair follicle: hair growth and sebum excretion. Br J Dermatol. 1991;124:21–8.
27. Hueber F, Wepierre J, Schaefer H. Role of transepidermal and transfollicular routes in percutaneous absorption of hydrocortisone and testosterone: in vivo study in the hairless rat. Skin Pharmacol. 1992;5:99–107.
28. Otberg N, Richter H, Schaefer H, Blume-Peytavi U, Sterry W, Lademann J. Variations of hair follicle size and distribution in different body sites. J Invest Dermatol. 2004;122:14–9.
29. Morganti P, Ruocco E, Wolf R, Ruocco V. Percutaneous absorption and delivery system. Clin Dermatol. 2001;19:489–501.
30. Chung JH, Yano K, Lee MK, Youn CS, Seo JY, Kim KH, Cho KH, Eun HC, Detmar M. Differential effects of photoaging vs intrinsic aging on the vascularization of human skin. Arch Dermatol. 2002;138:1437–42.
31. Tupker RA, Coenraads P-R, Pinnagoda J, Nater JP. Baseline transepidermal water loss (TEWL) as a prediction of susceptibility to sodium lauryl sulfate. Contact Dermatitis. 1989;20:265–9.
32. Cua AB, Wilhelm KP, Maibach HI. Cutaneous sodium lauryl sulfate irritation potential: age and regional variability. Br J Dermatol. 1990;123:607–13.
33. Elsner P, Wilhelm D, Maibach HI. Irritant effect of a model surfactant on the human vulva and forearm. J Reprod Med. 1990;35:1035–9.

34. Frosch PJ, Kligman AM. A method for appraising the stinging capacity of topically applied substances. J Soc Cosmet Chem. 1977;28:197–209.
35. Seidenari S, Francomano M, Mantovani L. Baseline biophysical parameters in subjects with sensitive skin. Contact Dermatitis. 1998;38:311–5.
36. Besné I, Descombes C, Breton L. Effect of age and anatomical site on density of sensory innervation in human epidermis. Arch Dermatol. 2002;138:1445–50.
37. Schwindt D, Wilhelm K-P, Miller DL, Maibach HI. Cumulative irritation in older and younger skin: a comparison. Acta Derm Venereol. 1998;78:279–83.
38. Faucher JA, Goddard ED. Interaction of keratinous substrates with sodium lauryl sulfate. J Soc Cosmet Chem. 1978;29:323–37.
39. Jiang SJ, Zhou XJ, Sun GQ, Zhang Y. Morphological alterations of the stratum corneum lipids induced by sodium lauryl sulfate treat- ment in hairless mice. J Dermatol Sci. 2003;32:243–6.
40. de Jongh CM, Verberk MM, Spiekstra SW, Gibbs S, Kezic S. Cytokines at different stratum corneum levels in normal and sodium lauryl sulphate-irritated skin. Skin Res Technol. 2007;13:390–8.
41. Agner T. Susceptibility of atopic dermatitis patients to irritant dermatitis caused by sodium lauryl sulphate. Acta Derm Venereol. 1990;70:296–300.
42. de Jongh CM, Jakasa I, Verberk MM, Kesic S. Variation in barrier impairment and inflammation of human skin as determined by sodium lauryl sulphate penetration rate. Br J Dermatol. 2006;154:651–7.

Part XIV

Ingredients, Products, and Cosmetics for Aging Skin Beauty

133 Aging and Antiaging Strategies

Carmela Rita Balistreri, Giuseppina Candore, Giovanni Scapagnini, and Calogero Caruso

Contents

C.R. Balistreri (✉) • G. Candore • C. Caruso
Department of Pathobiology and Medical Biotechnologies, University of Palermo, Immunosenescence Unit, Palermo, Italy
e-mail: carmelarita.balistreri@unipa.it; gcandore@unipa.it; calogero.caruso@unipa.it

G. Scapagnini
Department of Health Sciences, University of Molise, Campobasso, Italy
e-mail: giovanni.scapagnini@unimol.it

M.A. Farage et al. (eds.), *Textbook of Aging Skin*,
DOI 10.1007/978-3-662-47398-6_97

Abstract

Ageing of human skin may result from both the passage of time (intrinsic ageing) and from cumulative exposure to external influences (extrinsic ageing) such as ultraviolet radiation (UVR) which promotes wrinkle formation and loss of tissue elasticity. Whilst both ageing processes are associated with phenotypic changes in cutaneous cells, we summarize, in this chapter, related mechanisms involved, discuss on potentential treatment until now disposable, and suggest preventive measures.

Introduction

During the last century, life expectancy at birth rose by a remarkable 30 years in Western countries and in Japan, initially because of reductions in infant, child, and maternal mortality and then because of declining mortality in middle and old age. So, during the past century, humans have gained more years of average life expectancy than in the last 10,000 years: we are now living in a rapidly ageing world [1]. Accordingly, the extraordinary increase of the elderly in developed countries underscore the importance of studies on ageing and longevity and the need for the prompt spread of knowledge about ageing in order to satisfactorily decrease the medical, economic and social problems associated to advancing years for the increase of the subjects which are not autonomous and are affected by invalidating pathologies [2].

Ageing is a complex process, induced by an intricate interaction of genetic, epigenetic, stochastic and environmental factors. They determine the lost of molecular fidelity followed by an increased entropy [3, 4]. As result, loss complexity and random accumulation of damages (i.e., particularly damages to nuclear and mitochondrial DNA) at cellular, tissue, organ levels and/or of whole body arise, compatibly with the disposable soma theory of ageing [5]. Thus, it establishes a condition, which modifies both architecture and functioning of physiological processes and regulatory systems. This determines a deterioration of the homeostasis. Accordingly, it becomes more easily vulnerable to internal and external stressors, with frailty, disability and disease. On the other hand, the loss of DNA integrity, the principal random damages able in modifying cellular fidelity and inducing cellular and whole body senescence, determines the decline of the functionality of stress resistance and survival pathways (i.e., autophagic uptake mechanisms, chaperone systems, DNA repair mechanisms, apoptotic process, immune/inflammatory response), involved in cellular and organism defense to environmental stress and maintaining homeostasis.

As above mentioned, it is generally accepted that ageing has two principal determinants: the intrinsic disposition (genetic makeup, somatic capacity and composition) delineating what is maximally possible, and extrinsic factors (life style, nutrition, environmental influences) determining how the pre-set frame of opportunity is exploited in the course of the individual ageing trajectory. Extrinsic ageing is thus closely related to the quality, with which life-supportive tasks are adjusted to the environmental condition, and inseparably linked to mechanisms of stress response and adaptation. Insufficient adaptation and/or collateral maladaptation due to trade-offs with other probiotic or species-protective processes (e.g., fertility or tumour suppression) are thought to be major principles of extrinsic ageing [6].

As a result, it generates an imbalance between inflammatory and anti-inflammatory networks, which results in the low chronic grade of ageing pro-inflammatory status, "*inflamm-ageing*." Such chronic inflammatory response could build up with time and gradually causes tissue damage. It is, indeed, considered as one of the driving forces for age-related diseases such as diabetes, atherosclerosis, Alzheimer's disease and cancer (i.e., skin cancer) [7].

Augment of age-related body fat and consequent increase of visceral adiposity, age-related decline of sex hormones, oxidative and genotoxic stress, cellular and tissue damage, nutrition, alterations of physical condition of gut microbiota, other organs (brain, liver) and *immune and endocrine* systems have been associated with inflamm-ageing [8–10]. In addition, factors linking to physiological stress, such a long-term smoking and depression, seem also to contribute to inflammageing [8–10]. However, the most important factor for age related inflammation is the long-life pathogen burden [11]. Some recent studies have, indeed, evidenced associations between past infections and levels of chronic inflammation and increased risk of heart attack, stroke, and cancer [8, 10].

In line with these observations, it is possible to underline that a low grade of systemic inflammation characterizes ageing and inflammatory markers are significant predictors of mortality in old humans [12]. One the other hand, it has been recently proposed that during evolution the host defense and the ageing process have become linked together [4]. Host defense and ageing mechanisms seem to be overlapping. In particular, host defences seem to be involved in ageing process, to active inflammatory network and also to evocate the release of so-called *senescence associated secretory phenotype* (SASP), represented by a myriad of factors, such as the pro-inflammatory cytokines, chemokines, adhesion molecules, eicosanoids, growth factors, metallo-proteinases, nitric oxide, etc. [13, 14]. A large range of defense factors and mechanisms are involved in inducing of inflammatory network and related release of SASP, and they are all (or the major number) linked to the NF-κB pathway, an ancient signaling pathway specialized to the host defense [15, 16]. Namely, its induction is linked to several recognition pathway, i.e., Toll-like receptors (TLRs) and inflammasome, as well as through different upstream kinase cascades via canonical or non-canonical pathways [9]. SASP occurs in several cells, such as fibroblasts and epithelial cells, and it participates, together the phenomenon of inflammageing, in the low chronic inflammation, improving both entropic ageing process and onset risk for age-related degenerative diseases, i.e., skin cancer. Several pathways and factors in the different cellular types induce the release of SASP [13]. On the other hand, ageing of different cell types, tissues and organs is associated with distinct patterns of altered gene expression and tissue function, whereas isolated genetic defects in ageing-relevant pathways give rise to segmental, tissue-selective ageing phenotypes. For most tissues it remains, however, unclear, which age-related alterations play a leading and causative role in the ageing process, and which ones are just epiphenomena. In this chapter, particular emphasis is given in describing skin ageing, related mechanisms and factors involved and potential anti-ageing strategies.

Skin Ageing

The ageing process is noticeable within all organs of the body, and manifests itself visibly in the skin. So, skin ageing is particularly important because of its social impact, and also represents an ideal model organ for investigating the ageing process. In skin, as well as in all organs, ageing is caused by a combination of factors. Metabolic processes and mitochondria cause increases in the levels of reactive oxygen species (ROS), which cause damage to all cellular macromolecules, including lipids, proteins and nucleic acids [17]. In addition, environmental factors such as smoke, pollution and ultraviolet (UV) radiation exposure (photo-ageing) make important contributions to skin ageing [18]. Aged human skin shows peculiar features that mirror the physiological decrement of its functions with time. With age, the skin becomes thinner, more transparent, flattened and fragile. Fine wrinkles appear, desquamation and wound healing are delayed, and skin appendages and their functions are reduced; thus, the skinis dry, and hair loss is common. Skin pigmentation produces typical age spots; occasionally, seborrhoeic keratosis, a benign neoplastic condition, appears [19].

In order to elucidate the related mechanisms, we briefly report the structure of skin and its function. As well recognized, skin is the physical barrier between the body's internal organs and the environment, and its failure causes loss of body temperature control; percutaneous loss of fluid, electrolytes and proteins; inability to prevent penetration of infective agents and dangerous substances; and inability to respond to tissue in curie [20, 21]. Three stratified regions compose normal skin: the hypodermis, which is the inner subcutaneous tissue and consists mostly of adipose cells supporting the upper connective tissue; the dermis; and the external and more complex layer, the epidermis. The dermis consists of fibroblasts that are able to synthesise and secrete several matrix proteins (different types of collagen, fibronectin, elastin, and glycans) into the extracellular space, conferring elasticity and resilience as well as resistance and strength to skin. The epidermis, which is the real protective barrier, continuously self-renews. It is rich in stratified cells called keratinocytes that proliferate in the basal layer and are committed to terminal differentiation through the upper spinous, granular and corneous layers. Epidermal stem cells, located in the basal layer and in the hair follicle bulge, are responsible for the continuous renewal of this organ, giving rise to transient amplifying cells that are able to undergo a specific number of divisions (clonal expansion) before ascending through the upper layers and terminally differentiating over a period of 2–3 weeks [20, 21]. Other cellular types are present in the epidermis such as pigment-producing melanocytes, antigen-presenting Langerhans cells and sensorial cells. All of these cells are subject to age-related changes and contribute to the acquisition of an aged skin phenotype. Precisely, epidermal stem cells are maintained at normal levels throughout life. Consequently, it supposes that skin ageing is rather due to their impaired mobilization or reduced capacity to respond to proliferative signals, likely limited to very low number of stem cells with advancing age. In the skin, existence of several distinct stem cell populations has been reported. The self-renewal and multi-lineage differentiation of skin stem cells make these cells attractive for ageing process studies, but also for regenerative medicine, tissue repair, gene therapy, and cell-based therapy with autologous adult stem cells not only in dermatology. In addition, they provide in vitro models to study epidermal lineage selection and its role in the ageing process [19]. However, cutaneous ageing consists of distinct processes due to either intrinsic or extrinsic factors [20, 21]. Ageing of non-exposed skin areas is mainly due to intrinsic genetic or metabolic factors, while exposed areas of the body, such as the face and hands, are also influenced by extrinsic factors, particularly sunlight [20–22].

Intrinsic skin ageing is a physiological process that occurs as a result of chronological changes in tissue. A 10–50 % thinning of the epidermis between ages 30 and 80 years is the result of gradual tissue atrophy. In tissues with high turnover, such as the epidermis, stem cells and their transient amplifying progeny undergo an additional process, replicative senescence, which is a progressive reduction in their proliferative potential accompanied by the accumulation of senescent cells and a decline in tissue regenerative capability. All diploid cells undergo a finite number of successive divisions (Hayflick limit). The phenomenon of telomere shortening provides an explanation for this limit: the repetitive DNA sequences at the end of linear telomeric DNA shorten by approximately 50–200 bp per cell division; when they reach a minimal length, further cell divisions are prohibited. This phenomenon is probably not the only cause of cellular senescence, as demonstrated by the fact that non-dividing tissues, such as the brain, also age [22]. The balance between damage and repair ability appears to be the most accredited principle associated with cellular senescence theories. The metabolic rate is directly correlated with an increase in oxidative DNA damage and damage to other macromolecules, a cumulative effect that, together with an impaired cellular response and a specific gene expression signature, produces a senescent phenotype under these stress conditions [22]. Senescent cultured keratinocytes appear enlarged, flattened and vacuolised; they are arrested in the G1 phase of the cell cycle, positive for senescence-associated (SA) – β-gal staining and express senescence markers such as $p16^{INK4A}$ and hypo-phosphorylated retinoblastoma protein (Rb) [22]. In older subjects, a reduced cell number is also evident in dermal fibroblasts, melanocytes, other skin cell types and populations of hypodermic adipocytes. These events, together with a decreased cutaneous microvasculature, also lead to dermal atrophy, which is characterised by disaggregation and disintegration of collagen and elastic fibres.

The extrinsic ageing, also known as photo ageing, is clinically, biologically, and molecularly distinct from intrinsic ageing. Photoageing is typically characterized by prominent alterations of the cellular components and the extracellular matrix of the connective tissue. Photoageing primarily depends on the degree of sun exposure and skin pigment. Individuals who have outdoor lifestyles, live in sunny climates, and are lightly pigmented will experience the greatest degree of photoageing [22]. Solar UV radiations hurt epidermal and connective tissues, activating complex molecular cascades able to accelerate physiological ageing [22]. Photoageing is characterized by specific and peculiar clinical and histopathological features. The former include deep wrinkles, roughness and dryness, laxity, atrophy, yellowish complexion, hyper-chromic areas (solar lentigo, flat seborrheic keratoses, and freckles) and hypochromic areas, telangectasie, purpura, cutaneous fragility and pseudostellate scars, finally resulting in preneoplastic and neoplastic lesion development on chronically photo-exposed areas. UV damages can be linked mostly to the photochemical overproduction of ROS and reactive nitrogen species (RNS). ROS and RNS UV-generated can directly alter cellular components (DNA, proteins, lipids), and also affect regulation of gene expression of signalling molecules/cascades such as mitogen activated protein kinases (MAPKs) and interrelated inflammatory cytokines as well as NF-kB and activator protein-1 (AP-1) [22]. It is also well documented that photoexposure induces the activation of the enzymatic systems, e.g., lipoxygenase (LOX) and cyclooxygenase (COX), which are responsible for the production of inflammatory mediators. Of particular interest is gene regulation and oxidative activation of matrix metalloproteinase (MMP), a family of Zn-dependent endopeptidases which are produced by different cell types and taken together are capable of degrading all the components of the intercellular matrix of the connective tissue. MMPs take part in the development of the alterations, typical of photoageing. Even limited exposure to solar light may induce MMP synthesis beyond the control of specific inhibitors [22]. The role played by ROS in controlling MMP activity has been largely documented, and a critical role is due to the activation of the transcription factor AP-1 [22].

The adverse acute and long-term effects of solar exposure are well established, and in general, are related to skin type. It is widely assumed that sensitivity to UV is directly related to pigmentation or tanning ability and this assumption is primarily based on epidemiological evidence that shows that skin cancer and photoageing are much less common in people who tan well or who have high levels of constitutive pigmentation [22]. Furthermore, studies comparing dark-skinned peoples with related albinos [22] show the latter to have a higher incidence of photoageing. Pigmentation, whether constitutive (i. e., base skin colour) or induced by UV, depends on the balance between two classes of melanins: the eumelanins that are insoluble black or brown nitrogenous pigments and phaeomelanins that are alkali-soluble yellow to reddish-brown pigments that usually contain sulphur as well as nitrogen [22]. Unlike eumelanins, which are mainly protective, phaeomelanins are considerably photolabile, and may produce highly cytotoxic and mutagenic free radical species on photoexcitation, which would account for the greater proclivity of red-haired Celtic-type population to photoageing, skin cancer, and sunburn [22].

In addition, individual ability to counteract noxious molecular events induced by UV, depends by the activation of a complex defence system against oxidative stress. Among the numerous defensive genes expressed during cellular stress response to UV exposure, a critical role seems to be played by a heterogeneous family of proteins, the heat shock proteins (HSPs) [22]. This family includes the HSP70, an inducible protein able to refold damaged proteins, and Heme Oxygenase 1 (HO-1), a redox sensitive enzyme with strong cytoprotective effects in several tissues, including skin [22]. Cellular ability to maintain adequate expression levels of protective genes such as HSP70 and HO-1, in response to a stressful insult, such as UV exposure, seems to be essential to preserve cellular homeostasis, and to delay ageing related degenerative processes [22]. Individual variability in the efficacy to activate these defensive genes is due to mechanisms not completely understood that include genetic makeup, responsible also for different phototypes and age. At molecular level post trascriptional regulation might represent a putative mechanism to modulate individual efficiency in the activation of cellular stress response. Post transcriptional regulation is fundamental to modify the half-life of some messenger RNAs [22]. Both HSP70 and HO-1 have been shown to be post transcriptionally regulated in various cell lines [22], and this process is thought to be altered during ageing. This evidence has been proposed as a possible cause for the impaired efficacy of defensive genes such as HSPs [22]. In recent years, natural derived polyphenols have attracted considerable attention because of their skin photoprotection effects [22]. Many of these substances have been shown to activate specifically the expression of some HSPs and in general genes involved in cellular stress response [22]. Having a better understanding of the protective role played by HSPs in photoageing processes and mechanisms, regulating their activation, will allow identifying the novel pharmaceutical strategies to prevent photoageing.

The immune system may either have a protective role against sunburn and skin cancer, or conversely, promote solar damage. The skin is poised to react to infections and injury, such as sunburn, with rapidly acting mechanisms (innate immunity) that precede the development of acquired immunity and serve as an immediate defense system. Some of these mechanisms, including activation of defensins and complement, modify subsequent acquired immunity. An array of induced immune-regulatory and pro-inflammatory mediators is evident, at the gene expression level, from the microarray analysis of both intrinsically aged and photoaged skin. Thus, inflammatory mechanisms may accentuate the effect of UV radiation to amplify direct damageing effects on molecules and cells, including DNA, proteins, and lipids, which cause immunosuppression, cancer, and photoageing. A greater understanding of the cutaneous immune system's response to photo-skin interactions is essential to comprehensively protect the skin from adverse solar effects. Sunscreen product protection, measured only as reduction in redness (current "sun" protection factor) may no longer be sufficient, as it is becoming clear that protection against UV-induced immune changes is of equal if not of greater importance [23].

However, both intrinsic and extrinsic mechanisms, in a vicious circle, through ROS production and telomere shortening, are responsible of a skin pro inflammatory status, hence worsening skin ageing.

MicroRNA in Skin Ageing

MicroRNAs (miRNAs) are small noncoding RNAs that take part in post-transcriptional regulation either by arresting the translation or by cleavage (degradation) of mRNA targets. MiRNA regulation is performed by pairing the miRNA to sites in the messenger RNA of protein coding genes. miRNAs have been thought to be involved in many pathobiological processes (i.e., cell proliferation, death, differentiation, tissue degeneration, cancer, age-related diseases) and are believed to regulate the expression of approximately one-third of all human genes. Mature miRNAs bind to their target mRNAs by complete or incomplete complementation of their 50-end nucleotides 1–8 (seed sequences) with a binding site in the 30- or 50-untranslated regions of target transcripts or in the coding sequences. This process results in direct cleavage of the targeted mRNAs or inhibition of translation. Currently, nearly 1700 human miRNAs have been identified [24].

Recent findings demonstrate that microRNAs play key roles in regulating the balance between a cell's proliferative capacity and replicative senescence. Here, we focus on the molecular mechanisms regulated by senescence-associated microRNAs and their validated targets in both keratinocytes and dermal fibroblasts. In particular, we aim to highlight the contribution of miRNAs as modulators and regulators of cellular replicative senescence, focusing on keratinocytes and dermal fibroblasts [25].

The first study to identify senescence-associated miRNAs (SA-miRNAs) in human epidermal keratinocytes revealed a set of regulated miRNAs. In particular, miR-137 and miR-668 are upregulated during replicative cellular senescence and organismal ageing and they are able to induce senescence in proliferating human keratinocytes with a concomitant induction of the senescence markers p53 and p16^{INK4A} [26]. However, the direct targets that are important for the described phenotype have not yet been identified. Rivetti di Val Cervo and colleagues determined that miR-138, miR-181a, miR-181b and miR-130b were upregulated during replicative senescence in keratinocytes [27]. These authors found that upregulation of these miRNAs (also singularly) in proliferating cells is sufficient per se to induce SA-β-galactosidase activity, suggesting that they interfere with important pathways involved in cell proliferation and maintenance. It is interesting that three of the miRNAs identified in this study, miR-138, miR-181a and miR-181b, target *SIRT1* mRNA, suggesting that Sirt1 activity is crucial for keratinocyte replicative senescence. In fact, *SIRT1* knockdown in proliferating keratinocytes induces cellular senescence [27]. Sirt1 is a member of the NAD$^+$-dependent deacetylase family. By the deacetylation of proteins, which regulates cellular stress responses, replicative senescence, immune responses and metabolism, Sirt1 protects cells and organisms against age-related diseases [28].

On the other hand, miR-130a targets *p63*mRNA. p63, which is a transcription factor and member of the p53 family, is known as the master gene of epithelia development [25]. P63 is strongly involved in counteracting ageing/senescence both in vitro and in vivo. Indeed, p63- and p63 isoform-specific depletion induces premature ageing in different mouse models [25]. In human keratinocytes, *p63* knockdown is sufficient to induce cellular senescence, again suggesting an important role for p63 in counteracting cellular senescence and ageing in general. This potential role is strongly supported by the finding that p63 directly inhibits the expression of the senescence-inducing miRNAs miRNA-138, miRNA-181a, miR-181b and miR-130b [27]. The importance of miR-181a, miR181, miR138 and miR-130a, as well as their targets *p63* and *SIRT1*, has also been examined in a study of human skin ageing in vivo that was performed on a cohort of healthy young (<10 years) and older (>60 years) subjects. In this study, the SA-miRNAs were significantly upregulated in aged skin, in parallel with a significant downregulation of their targets *p63* and *SIRT1* [27]. The studies described thus far clearly demonstrate that modulation of SA-miRNA expression affects the execution of many gene expression programmes in human keratinocytes, resulting in the promotion or counteraction of cellular senescence. Many of the target genes identified (e.g., *p63*, *SIRT1*) are also strongly associated with organismal ageing.

In aged skin, human dermal fibroblasts (HDFs) lose the ability to remodel and organise the extracellular matrix (ECM), and evidence has shown that these features could also be mediated by miRNAs. In particular, this effect is due to decreased expression of transmembrane receptors, such as integrins, and components of the ECM, such as collagens, in senescent dermal fibroblasts. In a recent study, miR-152 and miR-181a were shown to induce senescence in proliferating human dermal fibroblasts. Interestingly, miR-152 has a specific role in ECM remodelling; in fact, its direct target is integrin alpha 5 (*ITGA5*). Integrin-α5 promotes cell adhesion and migration on fibronectin through activation of focal adhesion kinases; thus, it plays an important role in enhancing cell adhesion and migration. Through the downregulation of *ITGA5*, miR-152 is able to significantly reduce dermal fibroblast adhesion, suggesting an important role in the aged dermis. In addition, in senescent fibroblasts, the expression of collagen XVI (*COL16A1*) is downregulated, and it has been demonstrated that *COL16A1*mRNA is a direct target of miR-181a, which in turn is upregulated. Collagen XVI is a minor component of the skin ECM; it is expressed in the dermal-epidermal junction zone of the papillary dermis and connects ECM proteins to cells, ensuring mechanical anchoring. These findings suggest that miR-152 and miR-181a may have a complex role in the dermal ECM remodelling that is typical of aged skin [25].

The importance of miRNAs in inducing the replicative senescence of fibroblasts was highlighted by another study, in which it was shown that the expression of miR-29a and miR-30 increases during fibroblast senescence. miR-29a and miR-30 induce senescence by directly repressing the expression of *BMYB*. B-Myb is a transcription factor, and it regulates cellular senescence by controlling the expression of a variety of genes involved in cell proliferation; therefore, inhibition of *BMYB* expression by siRNA or exogenous overexpression of miR-29a and miR-30 results in senescence [25].

By contrast, the miR-17-92 cluster and miR-106 were found to be downregulated during dermal fibroblast senescence [25]. Many studies indicate that the miR-17-92 cluster contributes to the transcriptional regulation of genes involved in cell cycle control and tumorigenesis, such as *BCL2L11* (*BIM*), *p63*, *p57*, *p27* and *p21*, thus suggesting that these miRNAs counteract senescence by promoting proliferation [25]. Transcription of the miR-17-92 cluster is activated by the transcription factors e2f1 and e2f3 and repressed by p53 [25]. These transcriptional regulators account for the decreased expression of the miR-17-92 cluster in senescent cells. Fewer e2f family members have been observed in senescent cells, whereas p53, which is a decisive switch in ageing and tumorigenesis, is increasingly active in senescence [25]. Thus, miR-17-92 is actively, although it remains unclear how and why miR-17-92 is downregulated during ageing and senescence.

Microarray studies have also identified miRNAs involved in premature cellular senescence after exposing cells to UVB irradiation and examining expression changes [25]. MiR-34c-5p is upregulated in irradiated cells and targets the 3′-UTR of *E2F3*. E2f3 plays an essential role in cell cycle progression, proliferation and development and protects dermal fibroblasts from UVB-induced premature senescence via the regulation of the senescence-related genes *p53* and *p21WAF-1* [25]. MiR-101 is also upregulated upon UVB irradiation and targets the 3′-UTR of *EZH2*. There is evidence that the functional interaction of miR-101 and *EZH2* is implicated in UVB-induced senescence of human dermal fibroblasts; however, the upregulation of miR-101 and the concomitant downregulation of Ezh2 are not sufficient to block the UVB-induced senescence phenotype, thus suggesting redundancy in this system [25].

All the evidence obtained by studying UV-induced senescence in vitro strongly suggests that miRNAs also have an important role in extrinsic skin ageing.

Finally, several studies on keratinocyte and fibroblast senescence have identified many miRNAs that target components of the conserved signalling pathways involved in ageing. In particular, senescence-associated miRNAs affect cell cycle regulators, chromatin modifiers, cell metabolism and cell adhesion. Additional studies on the skin senescence-associated miRNAs, including the identification of additional targets and their functions, will provide insight into how ageing mechanisms are regulated at the cell, tissue and organismal levels. Furthermore, it will be crucial to understand the upstream factors that control the differential expression of miRNAs during skin senescence and ageing.

Potentetial Anti-Ageing Interventions

The clinical treatment of choice, or "gold standard," to benefit both intrinsically aged and photoaged skin is the topical application of a class of molecules, the retinoids, which are derivatives of vitamin A [29]. Their positive effects on UV-damaged, photoaged skin are well characterised and influence both the collagenous and elastic dermal matrices. Clinically, the skin appears "rejuvenated," with significant reductions in the appearance of fine lines and wrinkles [30]. This is in part explained by the induction and deposition of newly synthesised collagens I and III [30] coupled with a significant increase in the number of anchoring fibrils [30]. More recent work has identified that retinoids can also induce deposition of fibrillin-rich microfibrils in the upmost papillary dermis, adjacent to the the dermal–epidermal junction [30], so potentially re-establishing a physical link between superficial skin layers and mature elastic fibres in the deep dermis. In an in vivo system, it has been shown that induction of fibrillin-1 expression occurs prior to that of the collagens, so making this elastic fibre component a useful biomarker of skin repair [30]. This system has now been used to assess the potential for repair of over-the-counter cosmetic products [30]. However, whilst the deposition of fibrillin in the dermal matrix following the application of both retionoids and over-the-counter cosmetic products is promising, it is still unclear whether the resultant newly formed fibrillin-rich microfibrils are structurally and functionally analogous to those thatthey seek to replenish. Finally, the effects of systemic treatments, such as the TGF antagonist losartan [30], on the structure and function of the ageing elastic fibre system remain to be determined.

Several anti-oxidants are also incorporated into topical skin care products, including vitamins C and E, co-enzyme Q10, ferulic acid, green tea, idebenone, pycnogenol and silymarin. Resurfacing procedures have been shown to sometimes spur the formation of new collagen with a normal staining pattern, as opposed to the basophilic elastotic masses of collagen characteristic of photo-aged skin [30]. It is possible that the potential of growth factors, cytokines and telomerase will eventually be harnessed via technological advancement and innovation in the burgeoning fields of tissue engineering and gene therapy [30].

Although there are several treatments available for aged skin, prevention of extrinsic ageing remains the best approach and should be encouraged to all patients. Of course, this entails avoiding exposure to the sun, using sun-screen when sun avoidance is impossible, avoiding cigarette smoke and pollution, eating a diet high in fruits and vegetables, and taking oral anti-oxidant supplements or topical anti-oxidant formulations. The regular use of prescription retinoids can also help prevent or treat wrinkles.

Prevention

The formation of rhytides is considered the most conspicuous and common manifestation, and nearly a *sine qua non* feature, of skin ageing. Wrinkles appear as a result of changes in the lower, dermal layers of the skin. It might come as a surprise to many consumers, given the ubiquity of advertising that touts the newest topical formulations to eliminate wrinkles and the related expenditure of millions of dollars by consumers on these "anti-ageing" products, that few skin care product ingredients have the capacity to penetrate far enough into the dermis to ameliorate deep wrinkles. Prevention of wrinkle development, therefore, has assumed a fundamental status in anti-ageing skin care [30]. To prevent the formation of wrinkles, it is necessary to halt the degradation of the skin's three primary structural constituents, collagen, elastin and hyaluronic acid (HA), since all three components are known to decline with age. Consequently, most anti-ageing procedures and products are designed or formulated with the intention of salvaging at least one of these basic cutaneous substances. Because the technology required to suitably deliver these compounds into the skin has not yet been developed, topical products containing collagen, elastin or HA are unable to serve as adequate replacements for what is lost from the skin through ageing. Although no products replenish these key skin components, some products do promote the natural synthesis of these substances. For example, collagen production has been shown to be stimulated by the use of retinoids, vitamin C and copper peptide [30]. Collagen synthesis may also be brought about through the use of oral vitamin C. In animal models, retinoids have been shown to increase production of HA and elastin. HA levels are also thought to be augmented with glucosamine supplementation. There are no products yet approved for increasing the production of, or enhancing, elastin [30].

Because inflammation is a known contributor to the degradation of collagen, elastin and HA, reducing inflammation is another integral approach to preventing wrinkle formation. Anti-oxidants, all of which display various distinguishing characteristics and activities, are believed to be an important focus in this endeavour, as these free radical scavengers protect the skin via several mechanisms that are just beginning to be elucidated [30].

In terms of preventing the effects of photo-ageing, it is not yet known which anti-oxidants are the most effective. Using topical and oral anti-oxidants in combination will likely be the favoured recommendation in the near future. Anti-oxidants should also be used in combination with sunscreens and retinoids to enhance their protective effects. Indeed, it is worth remembering that not all sunscreens have an anti-oxidant effect and not all anti-oxidants have a sunscreen effect. However, a recent study has demonstrated that vitamins C and E combined with ferulic acid impart both a sunscreen effect and an anti-oxidant effect [30].

Conclusion

Skin ageing is a dynamic, multifactorial process, best characterized and understood in dichotomous expressions: intrinsic or natural ageing is cellularly determined, is inevitable and results in cutaneous alterations; extrinsic ageing, which also manifests in cutaneous changes, originates from exogenous sources and is avoidable. In other words, intrinsic ageing is a natural result of the passage of time, and not subject to the realm or whims of human control or behaviour. Extrinsic ageing results from various factors, but exposure to the sun is the primary source. Therefore, photo-ageing is roughly synonymous with, although technically a subset of, extrinsic ageing.

The American Academy of Dermatology, practicing dermatologists and other clinicians have been preaching the mantra that "there is no such thing as a healthy tan," with some portion of the populace absorbing this message. Citing the attendant wrinkling and pigmentary changes associated with photo-ageing and the potentially more serious consequences of chronic sun exposure can be effective approaches for doctors, as this method appeals to an individual's strong concern about appearance. The clinical appearance of photoageing is characterized by rough, dry skin, mottled pigmentation and wrinkling. Such cutaneous manifestations, particularly when extensive or severe, can be harbingers of skin cancer. It is important for physicians to impress upon patients that photodamage represents the cutaneous signs of premature ageing. A summary of the role of telomeres in cellular ageing and cancer and/or a brief discussion of the differences between intrinsic and extrinsic ageing might prove useful in altering the behaviour of patients and stemming the tide of photodamage, photo-ageing, and photo-induced skin cancers.

The only known defences against photo-ageing beyond sun avoidance are using sunscreens to block or reduce the amount of UV reaching the skin, using retinoids to inhibit collagenase synthesis and to promote collagen production, and using anti-oxidants, particularly in combination, to reduce and neutralize free radicals.

Cross-References

► Cosmetic Antiaging Ingredients
► Cosmetics and Aging Skin
► Topical Growth Factors for Skin Rejuvenation
► Topical Peptides and Proteins for Aging Skin

References

1. Caruso C, Passarino G, Puca A, Scapagnini G. "Positive biology": the centenarian lesson. Immun Ageing. 2012;9:5.
2. Christensen K, McGue M, Petersen I, Jeune B, Vaupel JW. Exceptional longevity does not result in excessive levels of disability. Proc Natl Acad Sci U S A. 2008;105:13274–9.
3. Hayflick L. Entropy explains aging, genetic determinism explains longevity, and undefined terminology explains misunderstanding both. PLoS Genet. 2007;3:e220.
4. Salminen A, Kaarniranta K. Genetics vs. entropy: longevity factors suppress the NF-kappaB-driven entropic aging process. Ageing Res Rev. 2010;9:298–314.
5. Kirkwood TB, Holliday R. The evolution of ageing and longevity. Proc R Soc Lond B Biol Sci. 1979;205:531–46.
6. Kirkwood TB, Melov S. On the programmed/non-programmed nature of ageing within the life history. Curr Biol. 2011;21:R701–7.
7. Franceschi C, Campisi J. Chronic inflammation (inflammaging) and its potential contribution to age-associated diseases. J Gerontol A Biol Sci Med Sci. 2014;69 Suppl 1:S4–9.
8. Licastro F, Candore G, Lio D, Porcellini E, Colonna-Romano G, Franceschi C, Caruso C. Innate immunity and inflammation in ageing: a key for understanding age-related diseases. Immun Ageing. 2005;2:8.
9. Balistreri CR, Caruso C, Candore G. The role of adipose tissue and adipokines in obesity-related inflammatory diseases. Mediators Inflamm. 2010;2010:1–19.
10. Balistreri CR, Colonna-Romano G, Lio D, Candore G, Caruso C. TLR4 polymorphisms and ageing: implications for the pathophysiology of age-related diseases. J Clin Immunol. 2009;29:406–15.
11. Candore G, Caruso C, Colonna-Romano G. Inflammation, genetic background and longevity. Biogerontology. 2010;11:565–73.
12. Balistreri CR, Candore G, Accardi G, Colonna-Romano G, Lio D. NF-κB pathway activators as potential ageing biomarkers: targets for new therapeutic strategies. Immun Ageing. 2013;10:24.
13. Salminen A, Kauppinen A, Kaarniranta K. Emerging role of NF-κB signaling in the induction of senescence-associated secretory phenotype (SASP). Cell Signal. 2012;24:835–45.
14. Tchkonia T, Zhu Y, van Deursen J, Campisi J, Kirkland JL. Cellular senescence and the senescent secretory phenotype: therapeutic opportunities. J Clin Invest. 2013;123:966–72.
15. Gilmore TD, Wolenski FS. NF-κB: where did it come from and why? Immunol Rev. 2012;246:14–35.
16. Newton K, Dixit VM. Signaling in innate immunity and inflammation. Cold Spring Harb Perspect Biol. 2012;4:1–19.
17. Rattan SI. Theories of biological aging: genes, proteins, and free radicals. Free Radic Res. 2006;40:1230–8.
18. Yaar M, Gilchrest BA. Photoageing: mechanism, prevention and therapy. Br J Dermatol. 2007;157:874–87.
19. Zouboulis CC, Makrantonaki E. Clinical aspects and molecular diagnostics of skin aging. Clin Dermatol. 2011;29:3–14.
20. Proksch E, Brandner JM, Jensen JM. The skin: an indispensable barrier. Exp Dermatol. 2008;17:1063–72.
21. Farage MA, Miller KW, Elsner P, Maibach HI. Characteristics of the Aging Skin. Adv Wound Care (New Rochelle). 2013;2(1):5–10.

22. Naylor EC, Watson RE, Sherratt MJ. Molecular aspects of skin ageing. Maturitas. 2011;69:249–56.
23. Zhuang Y, Lyga J. Inflammaging in skin and other tissues – the roles of complement system and macrophage. Inflamm Allergy Drug Targets. 2014;13:153–61.
24. Bartel DP. MicroRNAs: genomics, biogenesis, mechanism, and function. Cell. 2004;116:281–97.
25. Mancini M, Lena AM, Saintigny G, Mahé C, Di Daniele N, Melino G, Candi E. MicroRNAs in human skin ageing. Ageing Res Rev. 2014;17:9–15.
26. Shin KH, Pucar A, Kim RH, Bae SD, Chen W, Kang MK, Park NH. Identification of senescence-inducing microRNAs in normal human keratinocytes. Int J Oncol. 2011;39:1205–11.
27. Rivetti di Val Cervo P, Lena AM, Nicoloso M, Rossi S, Mancini M, Zhou H, Saintigny G, Dellambra E, Odorisio T, Mahé C, Calin GA, Candi E, Melino G. p63-microRNA feedback in keratinocyte senescence. Proc Natl Acad Sci U S A. 2012;109:1133–8.
28. Donmez G, Guarente L. Aging and disease: connections to sirtuins. Aging Cell. 2010;9:285–90.
29. Kafi R, Kwak HSR, Schumacher WE, et al. Improvement of naturally aged skin with vitamin A (retinol). Arch Dermatol. 2007;143:606–12.
30. Baumann L. Skin ageing and its treatment. J Pathol. 2007;211:241–51.

Cosmetics and Aging Skin

134

Robert L. Bronaugh and Linda M. Katz

Contents

Abstract

Cosmetics, a category of consumer products that are sold worldwide, are often referred to as personal care products by industry, to account for some of the diversity of these consumer products. However, not all personal care products marketed in the USA are regulated as cosmetics. This chapter will focus on the use of some categories of personal care products currently marketed to improve the appearance of aging while at the same time discussing the process of how the skin ages, and interventions (not including surgical) by which the appearance of wrinkles may be altered, prevented, or reduced are discussed under more than one regulatory oversight within the USA, such as cosmetics, drugs, or devices. The regulatory authority that has jurisdiction over the specific product categories marketed within the USA is identified and discussed. Specific focus is given to alpha hydroxy acids (AHAs), retinoids, collagen synthesis, moisturizers and skin hydration, sunscreens, hydroquinone, and peels or scrubs, which will embrace the bulk of the products available over the counter (OTC) to consumers. Some products, such as Botox, which are available only through a physician, are also briefly discussed.

R.L. Bronaugh • L.M. Katz (✉)
Office of Cosmetics and Colors, Center for Food Safety and Applied Nutrition, Food and Drug Administration, College Park, MD, USA
e-mail: linda.katz@fda.hhs.gov

M.A. Farage et al. (eds.), *Textbook of Aging Skin*,
DOI 10.1007/978-3-662-47398-6_98

Introduction

Cosmetics are a category of consumer products that are sold worldwide. Many trade and regulatory agencies now refer to cosmetics as personal care products to try and better account for some of the diversity of these products; however, not all personal care products marketed in the USA are regulated as cosmetics. For the 12-month period up to December 2008, the personal care products industry worldwide sales grew by 4 % to 247 billion [1]. The use of some categories of personal care products to improve the appearance of aging is discussed here.

As the skin ages, it loses its natural elasticity and becomes thinner, more fragile, and lax, taking on a wrinkled appearance [2]. Aging of the skin has been attributed to two processes referred to as intrinsic or extrinsic processes [3]. The intrinsic process occurs through the passage of time and appears as fine wrinkles on the skin. The extrinsic process is often referred to as the effects that the environment (such as sun) and other exposures (such as weather) have on the skin. These changes often appear as deeper or coarser wrinkles, crevices, scaling or skin dryness, and age spots. In addition, wrinkles have been classified into three different types based on morphology [4] and are influenced by environmental and genetic factors. Crinkles are defined as fine wrinkles that occur as a result of the loss of elastin and may be accelerated by exposure to sun. These changes are particularly apparent on the face and other sun-exposed areas. Glyphic wrinkles are creases that accentuate normal skin markings and occur in prematurely aged skin, again accelerated by exposure to sun. The third type is linear furrows, which are long, straight, or curved grooves usually seen on the face. An example would be "crow's feet," which is also accelerated by sun exposure.

The interventions (not including surgical) by which the appearance of wrinkles may be altered, prevented, or reduced are discussed under more than one regulatory oversight within the USA, such as cosmetics, drugs, or devices. The regulatory authority that has jurisdiction over the specific product categories marketed within the USA is identified. Specific focus is given to alpha hydroxy acids (AHAs), retinoids, collagen synthesis, moisturizers and skin hydration, sunscreens, hydroquinone, and peels or scrubs, which will embrace the bulk of the products available over the counter (OTC) to consumers. Some products, such as Botox, which is available only through a physician, are also briefly discussed.

Drug Versus Cosmetic

Cosmetics have been used worldwide for over thousands of years to enhance appearance. In addition to improving appearance, they are also used to cover up flaws. However, as labeling claims have become more creative, consumers also have greater expectations from their cosmetic products, to the point that they are often looking for a quick fix from a bottle.

The Federal Food, Drug, and Cosmetic Act (the Act) broadly defines a drug and a cosmetic and specifies requirements that need to be followed to market these products. In the Act a cosmetic is defined as: "(i) articles intended to be rubbed, poured, sprinkled, or sprayed on, introduced into, or otherwise applied to the human body or any part thereof for cleansing, beautifying, promoting attractiveness, or altering the appearance, and (ii) articles intended for use as a component of any such articles, except that such term shall not include soap" [5]. Soaps are generally exempt from the cosmetic provisions of the Act and are often classified as consumer care products regulated either by the Consumer Product Safety Commission or as a drug, depending on the nature of the product and its claims. In other words, cosmetics in the USA are intended to make the user look better, without affecting the structure or function of the body.

A drug, on other hand, is defined in the Act as "(B) articles intended for use in the diagnosis, cure, mitigation, treatment, or prevention of disease in man.. (C) articles (other than food) intended to affect the structure or any function of the body..and (D) articles intended for use as a component of any [such] articles" [6]. In other words, drugs are intended to be used to prevent, mitigate, treat, or cure a problem. Thus, in the USA, products such as sunscreens, which are used to prevent exposure to harmful rays from the sun, are regulated as drugs. In addition, several other agents that will be discussed may also be regulated as drugs, because their intended purpose is either to affect the structure and function of the body or to treat or prevent a condition.

Sunscreens

Sunscreens in the USA are regulated as drugs, because their intended purpose is to prevent the effects of harmful exposure to the sun, such as sunburn, which may ultimately lead to accelerated wrinkling, thickening of the skin, and cancer. Currently, marketed sunscreens are rated by their sun protection factor (SPF) and more recently have added UVA protection. SPF is a measure of how much solar energy (UV radiation or UVB) may be required to produce sunburn on protected skin [2]. A common misunderstanding is that the number on the product implies the amount of time a person can be in the sun and not develop sunburn. SPF, however, is a measure of exposure to the amount of solar energy, not the time. It is commonly known that there are multiple factors influencing whether or not a person will develop sunburn. These include amount of solar exposure, which is influenced by time of day, geographic location (latitude), weather, skin type, amount of sunscreen applied and reapplication frequency, and activities being carried out.

In May 1999, the US Food and Drug Administration (FDA) published a final rule that set standards for formatting, testing, and labeling of OTC sunscreen products that protect against UVB, which is responsible for causing sunburn. In August 2007, the FDA proposed new sunscreen regulations that focused on sunscreen protection from UVA exposure. In this proposal, sunscreen rating was proposed via two tests: one would be used to determine a sunscreen's ability to reduce the amount of UVA light that passes through it; the other would determine a sunscreen's ability to prevent tanning [7]. Further, this proposed rule would require manufacturers to print a warning statement advising consumers of risk from sun exposure and ways to limit exposure.

Thus, the importance of sunscreens is their use in the prevention of harmful consequences of sun exposure, rather than being able to reduce or eliminate wrinkles and other signs once they have occurred.

Botox and Other Injectable

This category consists of a wide range of products that can either be used alone or in combination with other products, most commonly peels. The products in this category are regulated in the USA as drugs or biologics.

Botox, the oldest injectable in use to decrease wrinkling, was approved by the FDA in 2002. Botox is injected into multiple sites and causes the reduction of wrinkles by the temporary paralysis of the cutaneous nerves, usually wearing off within 3–6 months. As the Botox wears off, patients are again able to wrinkle their foreheads and the facial lines gradually begin to reappear.

Bovine collagen has also been used to improve facial scars and wrinkles. Like Botox, the effects are also temporary, with wrinkling reappearing within approximately 6 months. Glutaraldehyde cross-linked collagen was introduced as a way to extend the effect, but this has not been found to be the case [8]. Approximately 3 % of patients react to test doses, but late allergic reactions appear to be less common.

Injection with silicon, gelatin matrix implant, and polytetrafluoroethylene has gone out of favor. These substances were felt to give permanent results. However, with their permanence also came reports of unexpected and imperfect consequences. In addition, their use has been associated with the development of inflammatory reactions [9].

Hydroquinone

Hydroquinone has been used in cosmetic and drug products. The latter use has usually been for higher doses and for longer duration, as a skin bleaching product, especially to remove the dark ("age") spots that have been caused by sun exposure. The mechanism of action of hydroquinone is unknown but it has been hypothesized that it may affect the cellular processes of melanogenesis [10].

Over the past decade, much research has been done to evaluate the safety and toxicity from recurrent use. The FDA, in addition to the NDMA (Nonprescription Drug Manufacturer's Association, now known as CHPA), has evaluated the carcinogenic risk from topically applied hydroquinone, as well as the risk for ochronosis. Because of these potential risks, the FDA has proposed [11] that the use of skin bleaching drug products should be restricted to prescription use, so that individuals can be closely monitored by a physician. Further, the FDA has concluded that the actual benefits from use of OTC skin bleaching drug products are insignificant when compared to the relative benefit. It appears from research that the benefit is directly related to the absorption of the product, which also increases the potential for harm.

Moisturizers

Moisturizers are formulations designed to maintain the water content of the skin between 10 % and 30 % [12]. Creams and lotions are the most popular moisturizers for consumers, and these are emulsions of oil- and water-soluble ingredients [13]. The ingredients in moisturizers that cause hydration of the skin are humectants and emollients. Humectants are ingredients that attract moisture into the stratum corneum, resulting in increased hydration of the skin [13]. Examples of humectant ingredients in cosmetics are glycerin, urea, and propylene glycol. Emollients are lipid-based ingredients that form a barrier on the surface of the skin to trap moisture in the skin to prevent its evaporation [13]. Examples of emollients in cosmetics are octyldodecanol, oleyl oleate, and isopropyl myristate.

Moisturizers are designed to mimic the function of epidermal lipids in the skin barrier [12]. The lipid composing the intercellular space in the stratum corneum is composed of a mixture of ceramides, cholesterol, and fatty acids. The barrier properties of the stratum corneum are related to the organizational arrangement of these lipids into lamellar granules within the intercellular space [14]. Extraction of these lipids from the skin with solvents leads to xerosis (dry skin), directly in proportion to the amount of lipid removed [12]. This mixture of lipids also contains natural moisturizing factors consisting of amino acids, lactic acid, pyrrolidone carboxylic acids, and urea. Due to the hydroscopic properties of this mixture, water can be maintained within the stratum corneum even under very extreme conditions [15].

The water content within the skin is also essential for normal desquamation and barrier integrity [15]. Normal plasticity of the tissue depends on water content [12]. Low content of water in the tissue inhibits enzyme activity of the proteinases, glycosidase, and lipases essential for shedding of the corneocytes. Skin aging occurs based on the sum of its two components – intrinsic or chronological aging and photoaging [13, 15]. Intrinsic skin aging occurs from the normal physiological changes in the body as people age. Photoaging is due to the damage caused by UV irradiation on sun-exposed areas of the body. Photoaging therefore results in premature aging of the skin. Dry skin is the result of a decreased ability of aged skin to retain water in the stratum corneum. Low moisture content in the skin can result in abnormal desquamation by inhibiting the enzymatic activity of proteases responsible for corneodesmosomal degradation [15]. The corneodesmosomes are the principal cohesive linkage between the corneocytes that make up the stratum corneum.

Relative humidity was shown to affect the water content of the stratum corneum, with a dramatic decrease in the normal process of desquamation when the relative humidity was below 80 %. A glycerol-containing moisturizing lotion increased desquamation of freshly obtained pig skin in vitro, demonstrating that water content of the stratum corneum was the rate-limiting factor in the final stages of desquamation [16].

Visual observations of the skin are often used to assess its dryness. However, different bioengineering methods have been developed to assess the dryness of the skin more objectively. A measurement of the capacitance of the skin is most commonly used to assess water content. Transepidermal water loss (TEWL) can measure a compromised stratum corneum, as the passage of water from beneath the stratum corneum to outside the body is rapidly increased. The use of adhesive tape to obtain samples of the surface stratum corneum can be used to measure the extent and thickness of skin scaling [13].

Safety Studies on Alpha Hydroxy Acids

Hydroxy acids are thought to act by reducing cohesion between newly formed corneocytes in the newly formed stratum corneum, thereby enhancing desquamation of skin [17, 18]. The ability of these chemicals to penetrate into the stratum corneum, and possibly deeper into the skin, likely affects the activity of hydroxy acids on skin. The pH of the formulation was determined to markedly affect the absorption of hydroxy acids into the different layers of the skin [19]. A comparison of absorption values from oil-in-water (O/W) emulsions at pH 3 and pH 7 showed that stratum corneum concentrations of glycolic acid and lactic acid were greater at the lower pH by 4.8-fold and 2.0-fold, respectively. Because the AHAs were unionized at pH 3.0 and therefore more lipophilic, they penetrated into the skin much more readily. Reducing the pH of the formulation to the pKa (or below) greatly increases the activity of AHAs in eliciting desquamation. The p*K*a of glycolic acid is 3.8.

Dermal Effects of AHAs and UV Light

The effect of glycolic acid pretreatment of skin on UV light irradiation has been examined in several studies. In one study, a formulation containing 10 % glycolic acid at pH 3.5 was applied once daily for 4 days to 15 volunteers with skin types suggesting increased sensitivity to sun (Fitzpatrick skin types I and II) [20]. Other sites on the skin of the volunteers were treated daily either by rubbing with a moistened mechanical sponge for 15 s or applying 8 % glycerin. The test sites were irradiated with one minimal erythema dose (MED) of primarily UVB light 15 min after the last dosing of the treatments applied each day. Biopsies were taken from the test sites to evaluate the formation of sunburn cells. The glycolic acid formulation did not statistically increase sunburn cell formation when compared to untreated skin, the 8 % glycerin, or the mechanical exfoliating sponge.

Another study was conducted using similar procedures, except that the skin test areas were treated for a much longer period of time – 12 weeks [20]. Two groups were examined in this study with 16 subjects each and with different glycolic acid formulations. Group A used 10 % glycolic acid in a thickened aqueous vehicle at pH 4.0. Group B used a 10 % formulation of glycolic acid at pH 3.5. Treatment of both groups with glycolic acid for 12 weeks, followed by UV irradiation, resulted in a significant increase in sunburn cells compared to untreated skin and control vehicles.

A clinical study conducted by other investigators evaluated the effects of daily glycolic acid treatment (6 days per week) on the MED, sunburn cells, and cyclobutyl pyrimidine dimers (CPDs). Treatment lasted for 4 weeks, followed by exposure to UV light [21]. Either a 10 % glycolic acid formulation (pH 3.5) or a placebo (formulation without glycolic acid) was applied to the backs of 29 Caucasian volunteers. Subjects were primarily Fitzpatrick skin type III and were placed in either Group 1 or Group 2.

After the 4 weeks of treatment, subjects in Group 1 were irradiated with a solar simulator. One week later, they were irradiated again to determine recovery. Biopsies were removed from the test sites to determine both the MED and sunburn cell formation. There was a statistically significant decrease in the MED of the treated skin after 4 weeks of treatment with the glycolic acid formulation compared to the placebo or untreated skin. The MED on the treated site returned to normal after glycolic acid treatment was discontinued for 1 week. Compared to sunburn cells formed in the sites treated with the placebo, the number of sunburn cells induced by UV light following 4 weeks of glycolic acid treatment increased 1.9-fold. However, the number of sunburn cells at the glycolic acid-treated sites and the placebo sites were not significantly different after 1 week of discontinued treatment.

The 12 subjects in Group 2 received 4 weeks of treatment with glycolic acid and placebo, followed by 1.5 MED irradiation with UV light. The difference in CPDs measured in the glycolic acid-treated sites compared to placebo was not significant.

The FDA issued a Guidance for Industry document in January 2005 entitled "Labeling for Topically Applied Cosmetic Products Containing Alpha Hydroxy Acids as Ingredients." Because of evidence suggesting that topically applied cosmetic products containing AHAs might increase the sensitivity of skin to sunlight, the FDA recommends that the following statement appear on the labels of these products:

> Sunburn Alert: This product contains an alpha hydroxy acid (AHA) that may increase your skin's sensitivity to the sun and particularly the possibility of sunburn. Use a sunscreen, wear protective clothing, and limit sun expo- sure while using this product and for a week afterwards.

Alpha hydroxy acids are often found in cosmetic products formulated to improve the appearance of skin. Care should be taken when using these products and spending time under the sun.

Retinoids

Retinoic acid (tretinoin) seems to have some effectiveness in treating the appearance of photoaging [22]. The mechanisms responsible for this activity may include the shedding of corneocytes due to the proliferation of keratinocytes [23] and may also be associated with new collagen produced in the upper dermis [24]. The action of retinoic acid in the skin may be ultimately associated with activation of retinoid receptors [25]. The application of retinol to skin has been reported to induce expression of cellular binding proteins and to cause other molecular changes that are the same as those observed after treatment with retinoic acid [26].

Retinol and its ester retinyl palmitate are frequently used in cosmetic products. In vitro skin penetration techniques that maintained skin viability demonstrated that retinyl palmitate could be absorbed into human and hairless guinea pig skin [27]. Only 0.2 % of the applied dose was absorbed through human skin, but 18 % of the dose was found in the skin at the end of a 24-h study. Approximately half of the retinyl palmitate remaining in the skin had been metabolized to retinol. No further biotransformation of retinol to retinoic acid was observed at the level of detection in this in vitro system.

Retinol penetration through excised human skin has been measured following application of cosmetic formulations to skin assembled in diffusion cells [28]. Penetration through the skin into the receptor fluid was 1.3 % of the applied dose from an emulsion vehicle and 0.3 % of the dose from a gel vehicle in 24-h studies. Retinol and retinoic acid skin penetration were found in vivo in human subjects, with induction of retinoic acid 4-hydroxylase activity used as an endpoint for making the comparison [29]. Significant induction of enzyme activity was observed when retinoic acid was applied to skin (under occlusion) in concentrations as low as 0.001 %. Retinol (also applied under occlusion) required a concentration of 0.025 % to produce significant effects on induction of 4-hydroxylase enzyme activity.

Liposomes have been reported to enhance the penetration of retinol through human skin assembled in diffusion cells [30]. The skin penetration rates following infinite dosing of retinol were compared following application of retinol in either a control vehicle without liposomes or in deformable (flexible) liposomes made with Tween 20. At the end of 24 h, control retinol absorption was found to be approximately 1 ug/cm^2, while approximately 30 mg/cm^2 skin of retinol had penetrated through the skin from the flexible liposomes.

Enhanced penetration of retinol was found from solid lipid nanoparticles contained in an oil-in-water cream as compared to a conventional cosmetic formulation [31]. Highest retinol levels were found in the stratum corneum and the upper viable epidermal region. The absorption of retinyl palmitate was influenced even more by delivery with the solid lipid nanoparticles.

Certain retinoids (retinol, retinyl palmitate) are frequently found in cosmetic products formulated to improve the appearance of skin. Additional studies are needed to completely clarify the mechanisms of action of these retinoids. As with AHAs, irritation of the skin can be caused by higher dosage levels of these ingredients, especially with exposure to the sun.

Collagen Synthesis and Aging Skin

Many of the skin changes associated with aging, including changes in pigmentation and deep wrinkling, are the result of overexposure to the sun [32]. Chronologic aging is characterized by changes in skin, such as fine wrinkling and skin laxity. Both chronologic aging and photoaging are associated with decreased collagen levels in the dermis. As collagen fibers serve as the primary structural support of the skin, it follows logically that a reduction in skin collagen levels would be associated with the formation of skin wrinkles. Photoeffects on aging include the formation of activator proteins that inhibit the production of collagen and the formation of reactive oxygen species (ROS), leading to increased breakdown of collagen. Similar mechanisms seem to be involved, but at a reduced level, in the chronologic aging of skin [32, 33]. Recent work has focused on the dermal collagen matrix and resultant fragmentation by matrix metalloproteinases. Fragmentation of collagen in the matrix prevents the activity of fibroblasts (where collagen is synthesized), resulting in low levels of collagen in the dermis [34].

Topical drug products such as retinoic acid appear to have antiaging effects based on their ability to increase collagen levels in skin. A recent study has shown that retinoic acid (in vitro) and retinol (in vivo) significantly reduced cysteine-rich protein 61 (CCN1) expression in skin [35]. CCN1 has previously been shown to be an important chemical regulator resulting in lower collagen levels in aged and photoaged human skin [36]. Topical products other than retinoic acid that affect collagen synthesis may be drug or cosmetic products, depending on the claims that are made. Several commercially available products were evaluated for their effects on extracellular matrix proteins, using a 12-day occluded patch test in nine volunteers. One product contained 2 % of a lipopentapeptide, and another product contained the same peptide at a 6 % concentration and retinyl palmitate in a basic moisturizer cream. A third product contained retinoic acid as a positive control for collagen increase, and a fourth product was the moisturizer lotion. Retinoic acid treatment produced a significant increase in fibrillin-1, a biomarker for connective tissue. And the 6 % lipopeptide and retinyl palmitate formulation produced significant increases in fibrillin-1 and procollagen 1 levels in the dermis. It was suggested that these levels indicated partial repair of photoaged human skin [37]. A human tripeptide GHK (glycyl-L-histidyl-L-lysine) complexed with copper has been reported to increase skin collagen and to reduce fine lines and depth of wrinkles in clinical studies [38].

Conclusion

In conclusion, several approaches for reducing the appearance of wrinkles have been used in various cosmetic products. In some cases, such as with sunscreens and Botox, the products are not cosmetics and are regulated by other FDA centers. AHAs and retinoids can be irritating to the skin, particularly when users are exposed to the sun. Moisturizers and sunscreens can be used with fewer side effects.

Cross-References

▶ Aging and Antiaging Strategies
▶ Cosmetic Antiaging Ingredients

▶ Topical Growth Factors for Skin Rejuvenation
▶ Topical Peptides and Proteins for Aging Skin

References

1. Pitman S. Personal care products buck downward retail sales trend (2009) Cosmeticsdesign.com. http://www.cosmeticsdesign.com/financial/personal-care-bucks-downward-retail-sales-trend. Accessed 30 Jan 2009.
2. Kligman AM, Lavker RM. Cutaneous aging. The difference between intrinsic aging and photoaging. J Cutan Aging Cosmet Dermatol. 1988;1:5–12.
3. Watson REB, Long SP, Bowden JJ, et al. Repair of photoaged dermal matrix by topical application of a cosmetic "antiageing" product. Br J Dermatol. 2008;158:472–7.
4. Kligman AM, Zheng P, Lavker RM. The anatomy and pathogenesis of wrinkles. Br J Dermatol. 1985;113:37–42.
5. Federal Food, Drug, and Cosmetic Act, Section 201 (i).
6. Federal Food, Drug, and Cosmetic Act, Section 201 (g).
7. FDA – CDER web. Summary of key points on over-the-counter sunscreen products. 23 Aug 2007.
8. Walker NPJ, Lawrence CM, Barlow RJ. Physical and laser therapies. In: Burns T, Breathnach S, Cox N, Griffiths C, editors. Rook's textbook of dermatology, vol. 77. 7th ed. Oxford: Blackwell Publishing; 2004. p. 1–24.
9. Clark DP, Hanke CW, Swanson NA. Dermal implants: safety of products injected for soft tissue augmentation. J Dermatol Surg Oncol. 1989;21:992–8.
10. Le Palumbo A, d'Ischia M, Misuraca G, et al. Mechanism of inhibition of melanogenesis by hydroquinone. Biochim Biophys Acta. 1991;1073:85–90.
11. Skin bleaching drug products for over-the-counter human use; Proposed rule. Federal Register. 71 (167):51146–55, 29 Aug 2006.
12. Draelos D. Therapeutic moisturizers. Dermatol Clin. 2000;18:597–607.
13. Bikowski J. The use of therapeutic moisturizers in various dermatologic disorders. Cutis. 2001;68:3–11.
14. Wertz P. Lipids and barrier function of the skin. Acta Derm Venerol. 2000;208(Suppl):7–11.
15. Hashizume H. Skin aging and dry skin. J Dermatol. 2004;31:603–9.
16. Watkinson A, Harding C, Moore A, et al. Water modulation of stratum corneum chymotryptic enzyme activity and desquamation. Arch Dermatol Res. 2001;293:470–6.
17. Van Scott E, Yu R. Alpha hydroxy acids: procedures for use in clinical practice. Cutis. 1989;43:222–8.
18. Van Scott E, Yu R. Actions of alpha hydroxy acids on skin compartments. J Geriatr Dermatol. 1995;3(Suppl A):19A–24.
19. Kraeling M, Bronaugh R. In vitro percutaneous absorption of alpha hydroxy acids in human skin. J Soc Cosmet Chem. 1997;48:187–97.
20. Anderson F (ed). Final report on the safety assessment of glycolic acid, ammonium, calcium, potassium, and sodium glycolates, methyl, ethyl, propyl, and butyl glycolates, and lactic acid, ammonium, calcium, potassium, sodium, and TEA-lactates, methyl, ethyl, isopropyl, and butyl lactates, and lauryl, myristyl, and cetyl lactates. Int J Toxicol. 1998;17(Suppl 1):1–241.
21. Kaidbey K, Sutherland B, Bennett P, Wamer W, Barton C, Dennis D, Kornhauser A. Topical glycolic acid enhances photodamage by ultraviolet light. Photodermatol Photoimmunol Photomed. 2003;19:21–7.
22. Kang S, Leyden J, Lowe N, Ortonne J-P, Phillips T, Weinstein G, Bhawah J, Lew-Kaya D, Matsunoto R, Sefton J, Walker P, Gibson J. Tazarotene cream for the treatment of facial photodamage: a multicenter, investigator-masked, randomized, vehicle-controlled, parallel comparison of 0.01%, 0.025%, 0.05% and 0.1% Tazarotene creams with 0.05% Tretinoin emollient cream applied once daily for 24 weeks. Arch Dermatol. 2001;137:1597–604.
23. Baumann L, Vujevich J, Halern M, Martin L, Kerdel F, Lazarus M, Pacheco H, Black L, Bryde J. Open-label pilot study of Alitretinoin Gel 0.1% in the treatment of photoaging. Cutis. 2005;76:69–73.
24. Gilchrest B. Treatment of photodamage with topical Tretinoin: an overview. J Am Acad Dermatol. 1997;36: S27–36.
25. Elder J, Astrom A, Pettersson U, Tavakkol A, Griffiths C, Krust A, Kastner P, Chambon P, Vorhees J. Differential regulation of retinoic acid receptors and binding proteins in human skin. J Invest Dermatol. 1992;98:673–9.
26. Kang S, Duell E, Fisher G, Datta S, Wang Z-Q, Reddy A, Tavakkol A, Yi J, Griffiths C, Elder J, Vorhees J. Application of retinol to human skin in vivo induces epidermal hyperplasia and cellular retinoid binding proteins characteristic of retinoic acid but without measurable retinoic acid levels or irritation. J Invest Dermatol. 1995;105:549–56.
27. Boehnlein J, Sakr A, Lichtin J, Bronaugh R. Characterization of esterase and alcohol dehydrogenase activity in skin. Metabolism of retinyl palmitate to retinol (vitamin A) during percutaneous absorption. Pharm Res. 1994;11:1155–9.
28. Yourick J, Jung C, Bronaugh R. In vitro and in vivo percutaneous absorption of retinol from cosmetic formulations: Significance of the skin reservoir and prediction of systemic absorption. Toxicol Appl Pharmacol. 2008;231:117–21.
29. Duell E, Kang S, Voorhees J. Unoccluded retinol penetrates human skin in vivo more effectively than unoccluded retinyl palmitate or retinoic acid. J Invest Dermatol. 1997;109:301–5.
30. Oh Y-K, Kim M, Shin J-Y, Kim T, Yun M-O, Yang S, Choi S, Jing W-W, Kim J, Choi H-G. Skin permeation

of retinol in tween 20- based deformable liposomes: In vitro evaluation in human skin and keratinocyte models. J Pharm Pharmacol. 2006;58:161–6.
31. Jenning V, Gysler A, Schafer-Korting M, Gohla S. Vitamin A loaded solid lipid nanoparticles for topical use: occlusive properties and drug targeting to the upper skin. Eur J Pharm Biopharm. 2000;49:211–8.
32. Helfrich Y, Sachs D, Voorhees J. Overview of skin aging and photoaging. Dermatol Nurs. 2008;20:177–83.
33. Callaghan TW. A review of ageing and an examination of clinical methods in the assessment of ageing skin. Part 1: cellular and molecular perspectives of skin ageing. Int J Cosmet Sci. 2008;30:313–22.
34. Fisher G, Varani J, Vorhees J. Looking older: fibroblast collapse and therapeutic implications. Arch Dermatol. 2008;144:666–72.
35. Quan T, Qin Z, Shao Y, Xu Y, Voorhees JJ, Fisher G. Retinoids suppress cysteine-rich protein 61 (CCN1), a negative regulator of collagen homeostasis, in skin equivalent cultures and aged human skin in vivo. Exp Dermatol. 2011;20:572–6.
36. Quan T, He T, Shao Y, Lin L, Kang S, Vorhees J, Fisher G. Elevated cysteine-rich 61 mediates aberrant collagen homeostasis in chronologically aged and photoaged human skin. Am J Pathol. 2006;169:482–90.
37. Watson R, Long S, Bowden J, et al. Repair of photoaged dermal matrix by topical application of a cosmetic "antiaging" product. Br J Dermatol. 2008;158:472–7.
38. Pickart L. The human tri-peptide GHK and tissue remodeling. J Biomater Sci Polym Ed. 2008;19:969–88.

Cosmetic Antiaging Ingredients

135

Donald L. Bissett, Mary B. Johnson, and John Oblong

Contents

D.L. Bissett (✉) • M.B. Johnson • J. Oblong
Beauty Technology Division, The Procter & Gamble Company, Sharon Woods Innovation Center, Cincinnati, OH, USA
e-mail: donbissett@gmail.com; johnson.mb.3@pg.com; oblong.je@pg.com

M.A. Farage et al. (eds.), *Textbook of Aging Skin*,
DOI 10.1007/978-3-662-47398-6_99

Abstract

Several topical cosmetic materials claim to have antiaging effects. As there are many such materials and also because "antiaging" encompasses many definitions, this chapter focuses on a few classes of cosmetic agents that are reported to provide improvement in the wrinkling, firming, and/or sagging appearance of the skin. Particular attention will be directed to those materials within these classes for which there are readily available or published clinical data to support the reported benefits in improving skin appearance.

Introduction

Many cosmetic materials claim to have antiaging effects when applied topically. As there are many such materials and also because "antiaging" encompasses many definitions (e.g., prevention vs. improvement; wide array of benefit areas such as wrinkling, sagging, texture, sallowness, and hyperpigmentation), this relatively short chapter must be very selective regarding the materials discussed. Thus, the focus will be on only a few classes of cosmetic agents that are reported to provide improvement in the wrinkling, firming, and/or sagging appearance of the skin. Particular attention will be directed to those materials within these classes for which there are readily available or published clinical data to support the reported benefits in improving skin appearance.

Vitamin A

Forms

There are several forms of vitamin A used cosmetically, in particular retinol, retinyl esters (e.g., retinyl acetate, retinyl propionate, and retinyl palmitate), and retinaldehyde. Through endogenous enzymatic reactions in the skin, these forms are all converted ultimately to trans-retinoic acid, which is the active form of vitamin A in the skin. Specifically, retinyl esters are converted to retinol via esterases. Retinol is then converted to retinaldehyde by retinol dehydrogenase. Finally, retinaldehyde is oxidized to retinoic acid by retinaldehyde oxidase [1].

Mechanisms

The active form of vitamin A in the skin is trans-retinoic acid (t-RA). t-RA interacts with nuclear receptor proteins, which then interact with specific DNA sequences to either increase or decrease expression of many specific proteins/enzymes [1]. Some specific changes that could be relevant to skin antiaging effects are those that result in thicker skin (epidermis and dermis) to diminish the appearance of fine lines and wrinkles, such as increased epidermal proliferation and differentiation, increased production of epidermal ground substance (glycosaminoglycans or GAGs, which bind water), and increased dermal production of extracellular matrix components such as collagen.

On the inhibitory side, retinoids are reported to inhibit production of collagenase [2] to reduce loss of dermal collagen. While retinoid will stimulate production of GAGs in epidermis, it will inhibit production of excess ground substance in photoaged dermis. Excess dermal GAGs are associated with altered dermal collagen structure and wrinkled skin appearance [3, 4].

As at least some of the epidermal effects of topical retinoid (e.g., epidermal thickening) [5] occur relatively rapidly (days) after initiation of treatment, diminution of appearance of fine lines may be realized quickly. The dermal effects likely occur on a much longer time frame (weeks to months), so that reduction in appearance of deep wrinkles requires much longer time frames.

Efficacy

While much of the substantial literature on the improvement in the appearance of skin wrinkles by topical retinoids is focused on t-RA, data is also available on the vitamin A compounds that are used cosmetically. As retinoids are irritating to

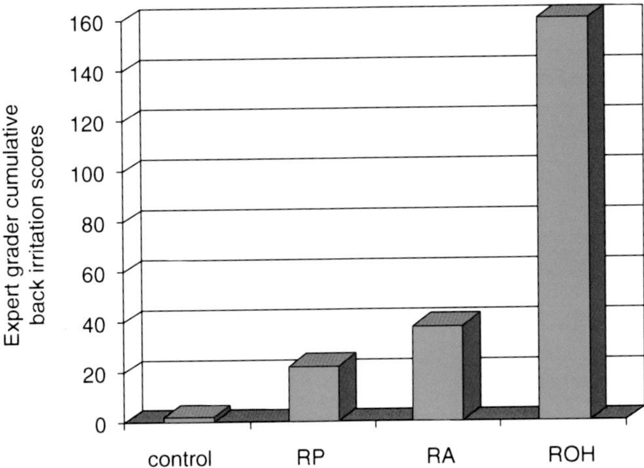

Fig. 1 Retinoid irritation in cumulative human back irritation testing (double-blind, vehicle-controlled, randomized study; daily patching for 20 days, under semi-occluded patch, $n = 45$; 0–3 irritation grading). Doses and abbreviations used were 0.09 % RP (retinyl propionate), 0.086 % RA (retinyl acetate), and 0.075 % ROH (retinol). RP and RA were significantly ($p < 0.05$) less irritating than ROH, and RP was less irritating than RA ($p < 0.10$)

the skin, defining skin-tolerated doses clinically is a key step in working effectively with these materials. Retinol is better tolerated by the skin than t-RA [2], and the ester retinyl propionate is milder to the skin than retinol and retinyl acetate (Fig. 1).

As retinoids in general tend to be fairly potent, cosmetic moisturizer formulations containing less than 1 % are generally sufficient to obtain significant improvement in appearance. At low levels, both retinol and retinyl propionate have been shown [1] to be significantly effective in reducing the appearance of facial wrinkles (Fig. 2). The effectiveness of 0.05 % retinaldehyde on facial skin has also been reported [6], although it has irritation potential similar to retinol [7]. Retinyl palmitate has very low irritation potential and is effective if tested at a high dose, such as at 2 % [8].

Product/Formulation Challenges

A challenge in working with retinoids is their tendency to induce skin irritation, which negatively affects skin barrier properties and consumer acceptance. Mitigation of the irritation may be managed to some extent with appropriate formulation to meter delivery into the skin, use of retinyl esters that are less irritating than retinol, or inclusion of other moisturizing ingredients to counter this issue.

Retinoids are unstable to oxygen and light. Thus, formulation and packaging should be done in an environment that minimizes exposure to oxygen and light. The final product packaging should be opaque and oxygen-impermeable and should also include the use of a small package orifice to reduce oxygen exposure once the container is opened. In addition, other strategies can be employed, such as encapsulation of the retinoid and inclusion of stabilizing antioxidants.

Vitamin B3

Forms

There are three primary forms of vitamin B3 that have found utility in skin care products: niacinamide (*aka* nicotinamide), nicotinic acid, and nicotinate esters (e.g., myristyl nicotinate, benzyl nicotinate).

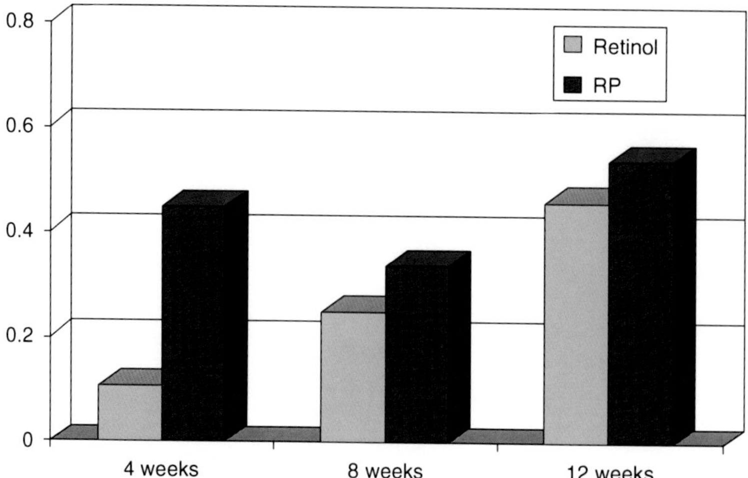

Fig. 2 Reduction in the appearance of wrinkles in a 12-week clinical study (double-blind, left-right randomized, split-face, placebo vehicle-controlled study with once daily application, $n = 52–56$ per product). Evaluation for reduction versus baseline in wrinkling and hyperpigmentation was done by three independent expert graders (0–4 grading scale) on blind-coded images after 4, 8, and 12 weeks of treatment. The grader scores at each time point were averaged. There were significant effects for both treatments across the study. The data presented here are averages for all three time points. S indicates significant at $p \leq 0.05$. The low irritation of retinyl propionate (*RP*) versus retinol (ROH) permits use of higher levels to achieve greater effects without significant negative aesthetic issues

Mechanisms

Vitamin B3 serves as a precursor to a family of endogenous enzyme cofactors, specifically nicotinamide adenine dinucleotide (NAD), its phosphorylated derivative (NADP), and their reduced forms (NADH, NADPH), which have antioxidant properties. These cofactors are involved in many enzymatic reactions in the skin and thus have potential to influence many skin processes [9]. This precursor role of vitamin B3 may be the mechanistic basis for the diversity of clinical effects observed for niacinamide [10]. The antiaging effects relevant to this discussion include:

- Inhibition of sebum production, specifically affecting the content of triglycerides and fatty acids, likely contributing to reduction in appearance of skin pore size and thus improved skin texture
- Increase in epidermal production of skin barrier lipids (e.g., ceramides) and also skin barrier layer proteins and their precursors (keratin, involucrin, filaggrin), leading to the observed enhancement of barrier function as determined by reduced transepidermal water loss (TEWL)
- Increase in production of collagen, based on in vitro measurements, which may contribute to the observed reduction in the appearance of fine lines/wrinkling
- Reduced production of excess dermal GAGs (glycosaminoglycans) in culture

As nicotinic acid and its esters are also precursors to NAD(P), they would be expected to provide these same benefits to the skin. Nicotinic acid and many (if not all) of its esters (following in-skin hydrolysis to free nicotinic acid) also stimulate blood flow, leading to increased skin redness or a flush response [11].

Efficacy

As representative of the vitamin B3 family of compounds, topical niacinamide [10] reduces the appearance of fine lines/wrinkling (Fig. 3). The effect increases over time and is significant after

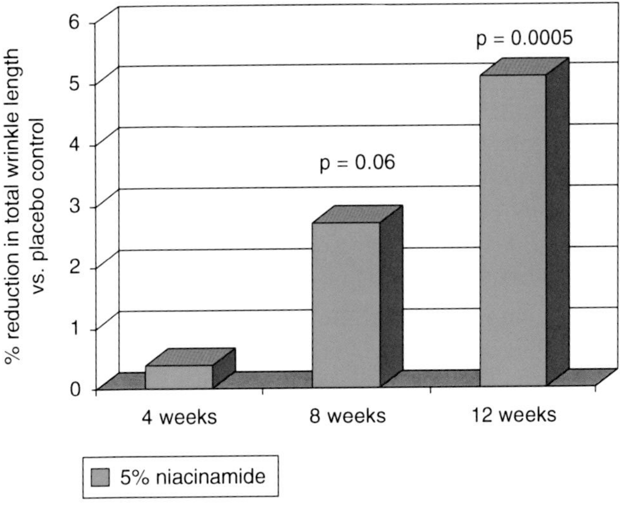

Fig. 3 Topical moisturizer formulation containing 5 % niacinamide reduces appearance of fine lines/wrinkling in facial skin. Subjects were female Caucasians ($n = 50$) who applied placebo control versus 5 % niacinamide formulations to their faces (12-week, double-blind, split-face, left-right randomized clinical trial)

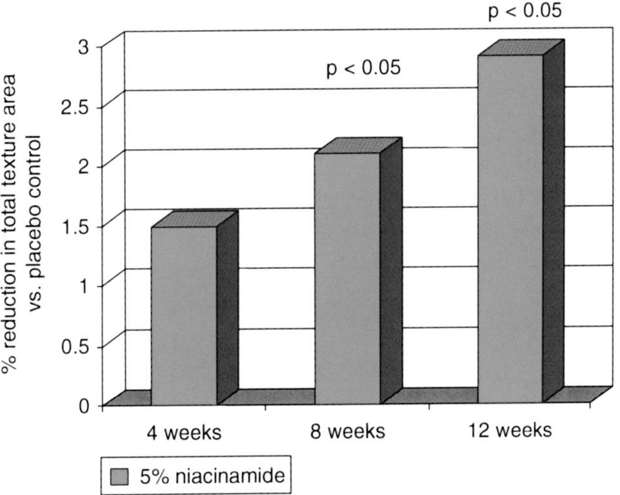

Fig. 4 Topical moisturizer formulation containing niacinamide improves skin surface texture. Subjects were female Caucasians ($n = 50$) who applied placebo control versus 5 % niacinamide formulations to their faces (12-week, double-blind, split-face, left-right randomized clinical trial)

8–12 weeks of treatment. Topical niacinamide also improves other aspects of aging skin, such as reduction in sebaceous lipids (oil control) and pore size, which likely contribute at least in part to improved skin texture (Fig. 4). Fairly high doses (2–5 %) of vitamin B3 have been used to achieve desired benefits. However, since there is very high tolerance of the skin to niacinamide even with chronic usage, high doses can be used acceptably.

Some data on myristyl nicotinate has been presented [12] to suggest that a similar broad array of benefits occurs with this agent when used topically (1–5 % doses). Clinical antiaging data for topical nicotinic acid and other esters is not available.

Product/Formulation Challenges

The key challenge for formulating with niacinamide and nicotinate esters is avoiding hydrolysis to nicotinic acid. Nicotinic acid, even at low doses, can induce an intense skin reddening (flushing) response [11]. While a little skin redness (increased skin "pinkness") may be a desired effect, the flushing response among individuals is highly variable in terms of dose to induce it, time to onset of the response, and duration of response. Additionally, the flushing can also have associated issues such as burning, stinging, and itching, particularly under cold and/or dry conditions. To avoid hydrolysis, formulating in the pH range of

5–7 is preferred. This flushing issue also requires that the purity of the raw material (e.g., niacinamide) should be very high to minimize any contaminating free acid.

There are many commercial options for nicotinate esters. Unfortunately, many of them are readily hydrolyzed to nicotinic acid on or in the skin, such that flushing responses occur rapidly (within seconds to minutes) even at very low concentrations ($\ll$1 %). The longer chain esters (e.g., myristyl nicotinate) are apparently more resistant to this hydrolysis and thus appear to be more suitable for topical use.

Vitamin C

Forms

There are many forms of this vitamin as incorporated into cosmetic products, with some of the more commonly used ones being ascorbic acid, ascorbyl phosphate (magnesium or sodium salts), ascorbyl palmitate, and ascorbyl glucoside.

Mechanisms

Vitamin C is well known to be an antioxidant. Particularly relevant to antiaging use is the in vitro observation that ascorbic acid serves as an essential cofactor for the enzymes lysyl hydroxylase and prolyl hydroxylase, both of which are required for posttranslational processing in collagen (Types I and III) biosynthesis [13, 14]. Thus, by stimulating these biosynthetic steps, ascorbic acid will increase the production of collagen in vitro, which has the potential to lead to reduction in the appearance of wrinkles, as discussed above.

Hydrolysis of the derivatives to free ascorbic acid is likely required for optimal effectiveness as an antioxidant and for the increased collagen production effect. Demonstration of the hydrolysis of all these derivatives in the skin has not been well documented in the literature.

Efficacy

Topical ascorbic acid, typically at low pH, has been reported to prevent oxidative damage to skin [15] and to reduce appearance of facial fine lines/wrinkles [15–18] (Fig. 5). The doses employed were fairly high (3–10 %). At the high dose, there may be skin irritation issues, as evidenced by the high subject dropout rate in such testing [18]. Ascorbyl phosphate [15] and tetrahexyldecyl ascorbate [18] have also been reported to be effective.

Product/Formulation Challenges

The key challenge with vitamin C compounds in general is stability (oxygen sensitivity), particularly with ascorbic acid. Not only does oxidation lead to loss of the active material, there is also rapid product yellowing (a likely aesthetic negative for the cosmetic user). Various stabilization strategies can be attempted to address the issue, such as exclusion of oxygen during formulation, oxygen-impermeable packaging, encapsulation, low pH, minimization of water, and inclusion of other antioxidants. In spite of all these approaches, in general ascorbate stability remains a challenge, and some of these approaches (e.g., very low pH) can lead to unwanted effects of skin irritation.

For the ascorbyl phosphates (Mg and Na salts), the resulting high content of salt in the product can dramatically impact the thickener system, requiring increased thickener ingredient concentration. These ascorbate derivatives are also considerably more expensive than other ascorbate compounds.

Peptides

Forms

There is a limitless array of possible peptides, based on amino acid sequence, number of amino acids, use of amino acids not normally found in proteins, and use of derivatives/isomers of amino

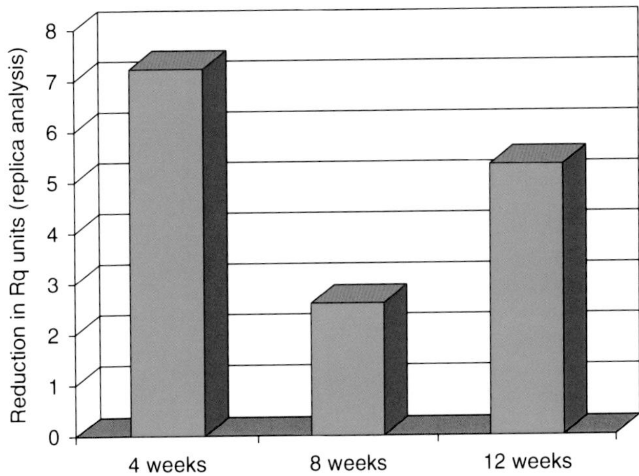

Fig. 5 Reduction in the appearance of facial wrinkles (skin replica analysis) by topical application of 3 % ascorbic acid. In a double-blind, placebo-controlled, split-face 12-week study [37], stabilized 3 % ascorbic acid applied topically ($n = 23$) was found to be well tolerated by the skin and reduced facial wrinkles as determined by skin replica analysis

acids. A few pure peptides with well-characterized sequences that have received particular focus in the cosmetic industry are palmitoyl-lysine-threonine-threonine-lysine-serine (pal-KTTKS; Matrixyl®), acetyl-glutamate-glutamate-methionine-glutamine-arginine-arginine (Ac-EEMQRR; Argireline®), and the tripeptide copper-glycine-histidine-lysine (Cu-GHK).

Mechanisms

KTTKS is a fragment of dermal collagen and has been shown to stimulate production of collagen in vitro and has thus been discussed with regard to wound healing [19]. Incorporation of long-chain lipophilic residues such as palmitoyl onto peptides can dramatically improve their delivery into the skin [20]. Thus, palmitoyl-KTTKS was synthesized for topical use. Like the underivatized peptide, the palmitate derivative (pal-KTTKS) is also active in stimulating collagen production in vitro [21, 22]. In addition, at extremely low levels (ppb) in culture, pal-KTTKS reduces excess dermal GAGs (Fig. 6). As discussed above, this effect may also contribute to an improvement in the appearance of wrinkles.

Like KTTKS, GHK is also a fragment of dermal collagen [23]. Copper is a required factor for activity of lysyl oxidase, an enzyme involved in collagen synthesis [24]. The complex of these two (Cu-GHK) has been shown to stimulate wound-healing processes by increasing production of dermal matrix components such as collagen and specific matrix remodeling MMPs (matrix metalloproteinases) [25, 26]. Ac-EEMQRR is described as a mimic of botulinum neurotoxin (Botox®), which functions by inhibiting neurotransmitter release, thus "relaxing" the muscles involved in defining facial wrinkles [27].

As the reported mechanisms of pal-KTTKS and Cu-GHK involve matrix production and remodeling, their appearance benefits would be expected to require chronic treatment. In contrast, Ac-EEMQRR should have acute benefit effects based on its reported Botox®-like mechanism.

Efficacy

The peptide pal-KTTKS has been shown to be quite potent clinically, providing a significant improvement in the appearance of wrinkles from the very low topical dose of 3 ppm (Fig. 7) [21]. This low dose for clinical activity is consistent with the very low concentration (as low as ppb) required to observe in vitro effects (Fig. 6). This topical peptide was extremely well tolerated by test subjects, i.e., it did not induce skin irritation responses (no redness, dryness, burning, stinging, or itching responses) and did not affect skin barrier function [21]. In contrast to the potency of pal-KTTKS, the reported skin antiaging effects of other peptides require much

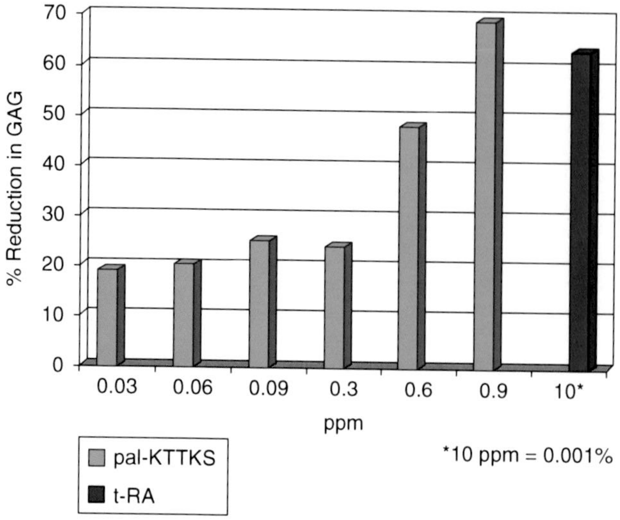

Fig. 6 Pal-KTTKS reduces excess dermal GAGs. In cell culture fibroblasts from an old donor (57 years old), there was a two- to threefold increase in GAGs (measured as hyaluronic acid) versus from a young donor (neonatal). Pal-KTTKS was effective in reducing the excess GAG level in old fibroblasts. Abbreviation: *t-RA* trans-retinoic acid

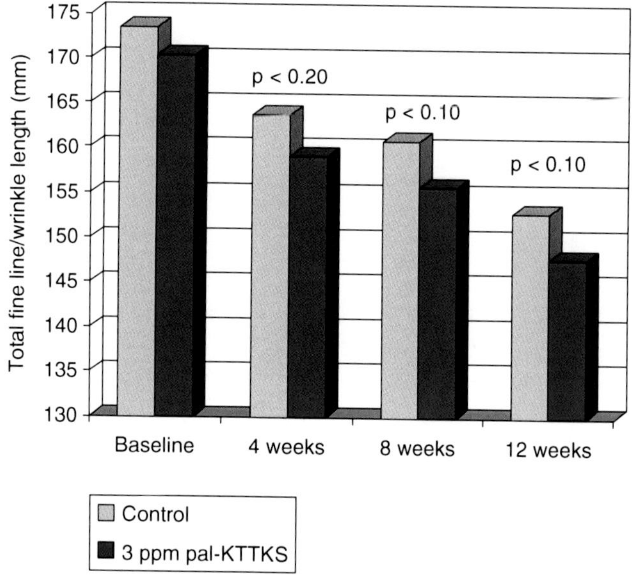

Fig. 7 Topical moisturizer formulation containing pal-KTTKS improves the appearance of facial skin wrinkles (quantitative computer image analysis; female Caucasian subjects, $n = 93$). Smaller numbers indicate fewer fine lines/wrinkles

higher doses, such as 2 % for Cu-GHK [28] and as high as 10 % for Ac-EEMQRR [27].

Product/Formulation Challenges

An important challenge is delivery into the skin, as peptides are poorly penetrating, especially as the number of amino acid residues, and thus peptide size, increases. An approach to this problem is addition of a lipophilic chain (e.g., palmitate), which, in the case of KTTKS, increases peptide skin penetration severalfold over the underivatized version.

An additional challenge is cost. As the number of amino acid residues increases, the cost of peptide synthesis can increase dramatically. The consequences are that only low levels of peptide can be used in a product (which is acceptable if the peptide is potent, as in the case of pal-KTTKS), or the finished product cost to the consumer must be high.

Dimethylaminoethanol (DMAE)

Mechanism

DMAE (also known as deanol) is a precursor to acetylcholine, a neurotransmitter involved in increased muscle tone. There could thus be firming of the skin via effects on the facial musculature. In addition, acetylcholine may affect the keratinocytes (specifically their proliferation, adhesion, and motility), leading to "epidermal contractility," resulting in a firming/tightening/anti-sagging effect on the skin [29]. DMAE also has antioxidant properties, which may contribute to its antiaging effects [30]. This agent additionally has been shown to induce vacuolar cell expansion, which may contribute to a skin tightening or fullness effect [31].

Efficacy

Several topical studies have been discussed and overviewed [29–32]. Significant improvements were reported in the appearance of skin lifting and skin firming (e.g., under-eye firming, cheek area firming, jaw line lifting and firming, increased elasticity). The topical treatment (3 % DMAE) was well tolerated by test subjects. The interesting aspect of the clinical effects is that while some testing has been for a duration of weeks to months, the onset of the benefit was reported to be very rapid, within minutes of topical application [29–32]. This seems consistent with the suggested mechanisms.

Product/Formulation Challenge

DMAE, a base, has historically been used as a formula pH adjusting agent. In the unneutralized state, its pH is approximately 10. Thus, pH adjustment to the desired value appears to be sufficient for its use in formulation.

Plant Growth Factors

Forms

There are three forms discussed in the literature: kinetin (N_6-furfuryladenine), zeatin, and pyratine 6.

Mechanisms

These materials are plant growth hormones. While their specific mechanisms have not been elucidated, they have been observed to promote growth and have anti-senescence effects in plants. They have powerful natural antioxidant effects in protecting DNA and protein from oxidative damage. In human fibroblast cell culture, even very low levels (ppm) delay the onset of changes associated with cell aging, such as appearance of lipofuscin, appearance of multinucleate cells, microtubule disorganization, and more youthful phenotype [33, 34].

Efficacy

In clinical tests, topical 0.1 % kinetin was reported to improve the appearance of several problems associated with aging skin, such as wrinkling and poor texture [33, 35]. The 0.1 % dose is well tolerated by the skin, with no significant irritation issues described. Zeatin and pyratine-6 have similarly been shown to provide antiaging effects [34, 36], including improved appearance of facial skin wrinkling.

Product/Formulation Challenge

The limitation with these materials is their fairly low solubility in formulation, thus restricting the upper dose to a low level (e.g., 0.1 %) for an aesthetically elegant formulation. This also impacts delivery into skin, although even from this relatively low dose sufficient material does enter skin to provide beneficial skin effects.

Triterpenoids

Forms

There are numerous plant-derived triterpenoid compounds and derivatives of them, with a few receiving attention in the cosmetic area, e.g., asiatic acid, ursolic acid, madecassic acid, oleanolic acid, betulinic acid, and boswellic acid. There are also naturally occurring saccharide esters of these, such as asiaticoside, which is the ester of asiatic acid.

Mechanisms

There are many reported mechanisms for triterpenoids, for example, antioxidant, anti-inflammatory, elastase inhibition, wound healing, and promotion of collagen and ceramide production [37, 38]. As triterpenoids share some structural similarity to steroidal compounds such as hydrocortisone, that is consistent with the reported mechanistic properties and potency of such compounds (e.g., anti-inflammatory effects).

Efficacy

There is little published information to illustrate the clinical effects of triterpenoids causing improvement in appearance. Topical triterpenoid (asiatic acid) has been described as providing increased ceramides to improve skin barrier and improving the appearance of skin extensibility and firmness [38, 39]. There were no reported skin issues from use of triterpenoids. The doses used were apparently very low (<0.1 %).

Product/Formulation Challenge

The key issue with triterpenoids is poor solubility, which also results in limited skin delivery. Formulation in liposomes has been employed to improve both delivery and formula solubility, although the resulting increase in oil content of the formulations may negatively impact aesthetics.

Ubiquinone (Coenzyme Q10)

Mechanism

Ubiquinone is an endogenous antioxidant present throughout the body, including the skin. The levels decrease with age. Topical ubiquinone replenishes the level and increases the antioxidant capacity of the skin [40, 41].

Efficacy

In a brief summary [42], topical treatment of facial skin with 0.3 % ubiquinone was observed to reduce apparent wrinkle depth in the eye area. The corneocyte area, which increases with aging due at least in part to slower stratum corneum turnover, was also reported to be reduced by this topical treatment of skin, suggesting increased turnover. In this testing, topical ubiquinone was well tolerated by the skin.

Product/Formulation Challenge

Ubiquinone is yellow-orange in color. Thus, only relatively low doses (<1 %) can be used in topical cosmetic skin care products to avoid aesthetic color concerns.

Other Technologies

Hydroxy and Keto Acids

This older technology has been in use cosmetically for a couple of decades. There are many compounds within this group: alpha-hydroxy acids such as glycolic acid and lactic acid, alpha-keto acids such as pyruvic acid, and beta-hydroxy acids such as salicylic acid. A key mechanism involves accelerated exfoliation of the stratum corneum, leading to improvement in skin surface texture. They have been described extensively elsewhere [43].

Flavonoids

This family of plant-derived and synthetically prepared chemicals encompasses a huge variety of compounds. They are beginning to appear in cosmetic products and are a fertile area for identification of materials active in improving aging skin.

Plant Extract Components

In addition to flavonoids, plant extracts are a rich source of diverse compounds. Extracts themselves, or new materials isolated from them, hold promise as an ongoing source of novel skin care ingredients.

Conclusion

It is clear that several ingredients that are used cosmetically do provide benefits by improving the appearance of aging skin. While the benefits may be small, they are significant and do meaningfully improve skin appearance with continued use of the materials. It is difficult to quantitatively compare the magnitude of the effects among the various technologies because there are many variables across studies: the specific end points measured are often different (e.g., surface replicas vs. facial image analysis); equipment and method sensitivities vary; formulation types vary, which can impact active delivery into skin; different body sites are used (e.g., forearm vs. face); clinical base sizes range from very small to large; and controls are different (e.g., vehicle-controlled, no treatment-controlled, baseline-controlled), among others. Also, extensive data for all compounds is not readily available for evaluation to judge comparative effectiveness (Table 1, although even this tabular assessment does not reveal the depth and breadth of clinical assessment). For example, vitamin A and vitamin B3 have been extensively studied clinically, with many publications describing their variety of on-skin effects. In contrast, some other technologies are only sparsely described in the literature. Regardless, it is reasonable to state that they are all probably less effective than an Rx technology such as trans-retinoic acid.

Table 1 Summary of data availability for cosmetic agents discussed in this chapter

		Availability of cosmetic antiaging human skin testing data set[a]		
Cosmetic agent	Single-variable, placebo-controlled study?	Technical meeting presentation	Review chapter	Peer-reviewed journal article
Retinol	Yes	Yes	Yes	Yes
Retinyl esters	Yes	Yes	Yes	Yes
Retinaldehyde	Yes	Yes	Yes	Yes
Niacinamide	Yes	Yes	Yes	Yes
Myristyl nicotinate	Yes	Yes	No	No
Ascorbic acid	Yes	Yes	Yes	Yes
Ascorbate esters	No	No	No	No
Pal-KTTKS	Yes	Yes	Yes	Yes
Ac-EEMQRR	No	Yes	No	No
Cu-GHK	Yes	Yes	Yes	No
DMAE	Yes	Yes	Yes	Yes
Plant growth factors	Yes	Yes	Yes	Yes
Triterpenoids	No	Yes	Yes	No
Ubiquinone	Yes	Yes	Yes	Yes

[a]At the time of writing of this antiaging review chapter

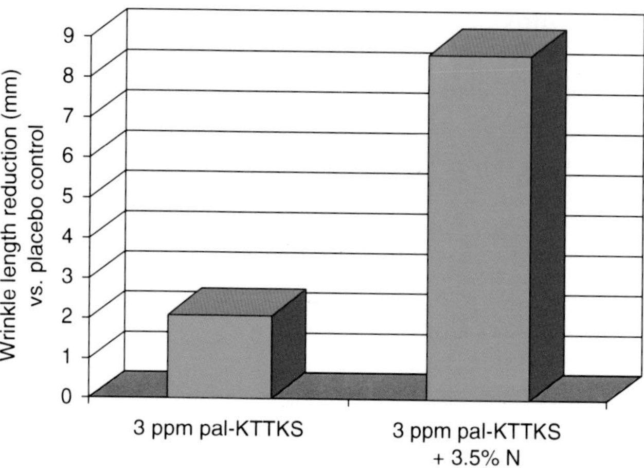

Fig. 8 Topical moisturizer formulation combining niacinamide (*N*) with pal-KTTKS improves skin appearance

While the benefits of individual current technologies may be small, the magnitude can, in some instances, increase by combining materials, especially those with different mechanisms of action. For example, combining a vitamin B3 with a vitamin A or with a peptide (Fig. 8) leads to greater benefits than the individual materials. As a further example, the combination of kinetin with niacinamide has also recently been shown to provide what the authors described as synergistic effects above what niacinamide alone provided [35]. Thus, combinations of ingredients have great potential to drive cosmetic effects higher.

Cross-References

- ▶ Aging and Antiaging Strategies
- ▶ Cosmetics and Aging Skin
- ▶ Topical Growth Factors for Skin Rejuvenation
- ▶ Topical Peptides and Proteins for Aging Skin

References

1. Oblong JE, Bissett DL. Retinoids. In: Draelos ZD, editor. Procedures in cosmetic dermatology, cosmeceuticals. Philadelphia: Elsevier Saunders; 2005. p. 35–42.
2. Kang S, Duell EA, Fisher GJ, et al. Application of retinol to human skin in vivo induces epidermal hyperplasia and cellular retinoid binding proteins characteristic of retinoic acid but without measurable retinoic acid levels of irritation. J Invest Dermatol. 1995;105:549–56.
3. Dunstan RW, Kennis RA. Selected heritable skin diseases of domesticated animals. In: Sundberg JP, editor. Handbook of mouse mutations with skin and hair abnormalities. Boca Raton: CRC Press; 1994. p. 524–5.
4. Kligman AM, Baker TJ, Gordon HL. Long-term histologic follow-up of phenol face peels. Plast Reconstructr Surg. 1975;75:652–9.
5. Griffiths CE, Finkel LJ, Tranfaglia MG, et al. An in vivo experimental model for effects of topical retinoic acid in human skin. Br J Dermatol. 1993;129:389–94.
6. Creidi P, Humbert P. Clinical use of topical retinaldehyde on photoaged skin. Dermatology. 1999;199S:49–52.
7. Fluhr JW, Vienne MP, Lauze C, et al. Tolerance profile of retinol, retinaldehyde, and retinoic acid under maximized and long-term clinical conditions. Dermatology. 1999;199S:57–60.
8. Erling T. Skin treatment with two different galenical formulations of retinyl palmitate in humans. J Appl Cosmetol. 1993;11:71–6.
9. Matts PJ, Oblong JE, Bissett DL. A review of the range of effects of niacinamide in human skin. Int Fed Soc Cosmet Chem Mag. 2002;5:285–9.
10. Bissett DL, Miyamoto K, Sun P, et al. Topical niacinamide reduces yellowing, wrinkling, red blotchiness, and hyperpigmented spots in aging facial skin. Int J Cosmet Sci. 2004;26:231–8.
11. Andersson RG, Aberg G, Brattsand R, et al. Studies on the mechanism of flush induced by nicotinic acid. Acta Pharmacol Toxicol. 1977;41:1–10.
12. Jacobson MK, Kim H, Kim M, et al. Modulating NAD-dependent DNA repair and transcription regulated pathways of skin homeostasis: evaluation in human subjects. Poster, 60th annual meeting of the American Academy of Dermatology, New Orleans, 2002, 22–27 Feb.
13. Tajima S, Pinnell SR. Ascorbic acid preferentially enhances type I and III collagen gene transcription in

human skin fibroblasts. J Dermatol Sci. 1996;11:250–3.
14. Geesin JC, Darr D, Kaufman R, et al. Ascorbic acid specifically increases type I and type III pro-collagen messenger RNA levels in human skin fibroblasts. J Invest Dermatol. 1988;90:420–4.
15. Raschke T, Koop U, Dusing HJ, et al. Topical activity of ascorbic acid: From in vitro optimization to in vivo efficacy. Skin Pharmacol Physiol. 2004;17:200–6.
16. Fitzpatrick RE, Rostan EF. Double-blind, half-face study comparing topical vitamin C and vehicle for rejuvenation of photodamage. Dermatol Surg. 2002;28:231–6.
17. Humbert PG, Haftek M, Creidi P, et al. Topical ascorbic acid on photoaged skin: clinical, topographical and ultrastructural evaluation: double-blind study vs. placebo. Exp Dermatol. 2003;12:237–44.
18. Traikovich SS. Use of topical ascorbic acid and its effects on photodamaged skin topography. Arch Otolaryngol Head Neck Surg. 1999;125:1091–8.
19. Katayama K, Armendariz-Borunda J, Raghow R, et al. A pentapeptide from type procollagen promotes extracellular matrix production. J Biol Chem. 1999;268:9941–4.
20. Foldvari M, Attah-Poku S, Hu J, et al. Palmitoyl derivatives of interferon alpha: potent for cutaneous delivery. J Pharm Sci. 1998;87:1203–8.
21. Robinson L, Fitzgerald N, Doughty DG, et al. Topical Palmitoyl Pentapeptide provides improvement in photoaged human facial skin. Int J Cosmet Sci. 2005;27:155–60.
22. Lintner K, Mas-Chamberlin C, Mondon P. Pentapeptide facilitates matrix regeneration of photoaged skin. Ann Dermatol Venereol. 2002;129:1S401.
23. Pickart L. Copperceuticals and the skin. Cosmet Toilet. 2003;118:24–8.
24. Smith-Mungo LL, Kagan HM. Lysyl oxidase: properties, regulation and multiple functions in biology. Matrix Biol. 1998;16:387–98.
25. Canapp SO, Farese JP, Schulz GS, et al. The effect of topical tripeptide-copper complex on healing of ischemic open wounds. Vet Surg. 2003;32:515–23.
26. Buffoni F, Pino R, Dal Pozzo A. Effect of tripeptide-copper complexes on the process of skin wound healing and on cultured fibroblasts. Arch Int Pharmacodyn Ther. 1995;330:345–60.
27. Blanes-Mira C, Clemente J, Jodas G, et al. A synthetic hexapeptide (Argireline) with antiwrinkle activity. Presentation, 37th annual conference of the Australian Society of Cosmetic Chemists, Queensland, 13–16 Mar 2003.
28. Kruger N, Fiegert L, Becker D, et al. For the treatment of skin aging: trace elements in form of a complex of copper tripeptide. Cosmet Med. 2003;24:31–3.
29. Cole CA, Bertin C. Dimethylaminoethanol: a new skin-care ingredient for aging skin. In: Baran R, Maibch HI, editors. Textbook of cosmetic dermatology. 3rd ed. Abingdon: Taylor & Francis; 2005. p. 95–101.
30. Nagy I, Floyd RA. Electron spin resonance spectroscopic demonstration of the hydroxyl free radical scavenger properties of dimethylaminoethanol in spin trapping experiments confirming the molecular basis for the biological effects of centrophenoxine. Arch Gerontol Geriatr. 1984;3:297–310.
31. Morissette G, Germain L, Marceau F. The antiwrinkle effect of topical concentrated 2-dimethylaminoethanol involves a vacuolar cytopathology. Br J Derm. 2007;156:433–9.
32. Uhoda L, Faska N, Robert C, et al. Split-face study on the cutaneous tensile effect of 2-dimethylaminoethanol (deanol) gel. Skin Res Technol. 2002;8:164–7.
33. Levy SB. Kinetin. In: Baran R, Maibach HI, editors. Textbook of cosmetic dermatology. 3rd ed. Abingdon: Taylor & Francis; 2005. p. 129–32.
34. Rattan SI, Sodagam L. Gerontomodulatory and youth-preserving effects of zeatin on human skin fibroblasts undergoing aging in vitro. Rejuvenation Res. 2005;8:46–57.
35. Chiu P-C, Chan C-C, Lin H-M, et al. The clinical anti-aging effects of topical kinetin and niacinamide in Asians: a randomized double-blind, placebo-controlled, split-face comparative trial. J Cosmet Derm. 2007;6:243–9.
36. McCullough JL, Garcia RL, Reece B. A clinical study of topical pyratine 6 for improving the appearance of photodamaged skin. J Drugs Dermatol. 2008;7:131–5.
37. Lu L, Ying K, Wie SM, et al. Asiaticoside induction for cell-cycle progression, proliferation and collagen synthesis in human dermal fibroblasts. Int J Dermatol. 2004;43:801–7.
38. Yarosh DB, Both D, Brown D. Liposomal ursolic acid (Merotaine) increases ceramides and collagen in human skin. Horm Res. 2000;54:318–21.
39. Martelli L, Berardesca E, Martelli M. Topical formulation of a new plant extract complex with refirming properties: clinical and non-invasive evaluation in a double-blind trial. Int J Cosmet Sci. 2000;22:201–6.
40. Passi S, DePita O, Grandinetti M, et al. The combined use of oral and topical lipophilic antioxidants increases their levels both in sebum and stratum corneum. Biofactors. 2003;18:289–97.
41. Stab F, Wolber R, Blatt T, et al. Topically applied antioxidants in skin protection. Methods Enzymol. 2000;319:465–78.
42. Hoppe U, Bergemann J, Diembeck W, et al. Coenzyme Q10, a cutaneous antioxidant and energizer. Biofactors. 1999;9:371–8.
43. Yu RJ, Van Scott EJ. Alpha-hydroxyacids, polyhydroxyacids, aldobionic acids and their topical actions. In: Baran R, Maibach HI, editors. Textbook of cosmetic dermatology. 3rd ed. Abingdon: Taylor & Francis; 2005. p. 77–93.

Topical Growth Factors for Skin Rejuvenation

136

Frank Dreher

Contents

Abstract

Growth factors play a key role in the regulation of numerous cell processes including wound healing. More recently, they have been recognized also for use in skin rejuvenation. Aged skin reveals a similarly altered growth factor response as a chronic wound. Growth factors may reduce signs of skin aging due to their capacity to promote dermal fibroblast proliferation and to stimulate extracellular matrix formation. Growth factor products for skin rejuvenation can contain either recombinant growth factors, growth factors as part of conditioned cell culture media, or growth factors as part of cell lysates. Numerous randomized controlled clinical trials demonstrated the good tolerability and efficacy of those products. Today, there is evidence that the signs of aging skin may be best improved with a balanced mixture of growth factors.

Introduction

Growth factors are polypeptides or proteins that play a key role in the regulation of numerous cell processes [1]. Together with cytokines, they help regulate division, differentiation, chemotaxis and adhesion, trafficking, activation, apoptosis, survival, and transformation of cells. Growth factors are able to mediate activities within a specific

F. Dreher (✉)
MERZ North America, Inc., San Mateo, CA, USA
e-mail: frank.dreher@merz.com

M.A. Farage et al. (eds.), *Textbook of Aging Skin*,
DOI 10.1007/978-3-662-47398-6_100

tissue microenvironment at extremely low concentrations. The growth factor binds to its corresponding receptor, located on the outer surface of the target cell, and ultimately, through a complex cascade of events, elicits a response.

Growth factors are key regulators of the wound healing process [2], and their topical use for cutaneous wound healing has been extensively described [3–5]. Clinical trials have indicated that the topical administration of certain growth factors reduces healing time and improves the rate of wound closure. These particular growth factors include epidermal growth factor (EGF), fibroblast growth factor-2 (FGF-2), transforming growth factor-beta (TGF-β), and platelet-derived growth factor (PDGF).

While for the most part, adult cutaneous wounds heal with scar formation to restore tissue integrity after wounding, in utero, rapid and perfect skin repair occurs [6]. Although complex and not fully understood, current research indicates that at specific ratios, several growth factors and cytokines participate in the scarless wound repair that is observed in fetal skin.

Richard E. Fitzpatrick first demonstrated that topical growth factors help improve such signs of skin aging as wrinkles [7]. In fact, it is recognized that aged and photodamaged skin, related to an altered growth factor response, reveals attributes similar to a chronic wound [8]. Growth factors may reduce signs of skin aging due to their capacity to promote dermal fibroblast proliferation and to stimulate extracellular matrix formation, including that of collagen and hyaluronic acid.

A study on the role of growth factors in human skin aging revealed that TGF-β1 and its downstream target, connective tissue growth factor (CTGF), are significantly reduced in aged human skin in vivo [9]. Moreover, it was shown that in a serum, a higher ratio of insulin-like growth factor-1 (IGF-1) to its binding protein (insulin-like growth factor binding protein-3 or IGFBP-3) was associated with a lower perceived age. This association was established because of its connection with reduced skin wrinkling [10]. However, whether or not high levels of IGF-1 delay the onset of skin wrinkles remains to be investigated.

This chapter provides a brief overview of growth factors and wound healing including their role in scarless skin repair and focuses on the review of clinical studies of topical growth factors for skin rejuvenation.

Growth Factors in Wound Healing

Wound healing is a regulated process consisting of distinct phases: hemostasis, inflammation, granulation tissue formation, and remodeling [3]. It is well recognized that growth factors are one of the key regulators of the wound healing process [2]. After skin injury occurs, platelets arrive and release several growth factors and cytokines. Once released, these proteins initiate the wound healing process by attracting neutrophils and monocytes. The result is an acute inflammatory phase that lasts between 1 and 2 days in normal wounds. After that, the growth factors (which include FGF-2, PDGF, and TGF-β) promote cell proliferation and new tissue formation that also includes fibroblast-initiated extracellular matrix production. During this time, the number of inflammatory cells decreases and the number of fibroblasts in the wound area increases. Stimulated by EGF, epithelial cells from the wound margins and dermal appendages migrate under the scab for re-epithelialization. During the final phase of wound healing, the extracellular matrix is reorganized. Over time, collagen type III, which was initially produced by fibroblasts, is gradually replaced with collagen type I. This type I collagen has a higher mechanical strength than its type III counterpart because of a higher degree of cross-linking. Several growth factors participate in the remodeling phase, which can take up to 2 years to complete, and often results in scarring. High levels of TGF-β1 and TGF-β2 are associated with scar formation [11].

As in the case of chronic wounds, sometimes healing can be significantly impaired. In contrast to acute wounds, pressure and non-healing dermal ulcers produce reduced levels of growth factors EGF, FGF-2, TGF-β, PDGF, and VEGF (vascular endothelial growth factor) [4]. It would seem evident, therefore, that topical applications of a mixture of growth factors would help patients with chronic wounds: for example, those growth factors that have been well studied in chronic wound healing such as EGF, FGF-2, TGF-β, PDGF-BB, VEGF, or KGF-2 (keratinocyte growth factor) [3]. In fact, recombinant human PDGF-BB (at a concentration of 0.01 % in a hydrogel vehicle) was the first topical growth factor formulation to be approved in the United States for the treatment of deep neuropathic diabetic foot ulcers.

Wounds heal slower with age [12]. In the elderly, re-epithelialization is significantly delayed as the rate of collagen formation decreases. Wound healing becomes impaired as dermal fibroblasts decrease and as the proliferative capacity of keratinocytes, dermal fibroblasts, and vascular endothelial cells is reduced. Animal experiments reveal that reduced productions of growth factors and their receptors may be responsible for impaired wound repair in aged mice [13, 14].

While cutaneous wound healing may result in scar formation in adults, wound healing in utero (fetal wound healing) is scarless [6]. Early gestation fetuses in both animals and humans have the remarkable ability to heal skin wounds without forming a scar. It has been established that scarless wound repair is independent of the obvious environmental differences (i.e., amniotic fluid) between fetus and adult and can progress outside the uterus [6]. In fact, the fetal fibroblast was found to be the main effector cell for scarless wound healing [15]. Fetal fibroblasts have the ability to deposit collagen in a fine, highly organized pattern during fetal skin wound repair that is indistinguishable from the surrounding uninjured dermal collagen. This is in contrast to the coarse pattern of collagen deposition observed during wound healing in adults. Skin is primarily composed of collagen types III and I. The former is smaller and finer than the latter, and although type I is the predominant form in both fetal and adult skin, collagen type III is more abundant in fetal skin. In humans, collagen type III comprises 30–60 % of the total fetal skin. In adults, it comprises only 10–20 % [6]. As the fetus develops, the ratio of skin collagen types I to type III approaches that of adults, correlating with the transition from scarless wound repair to scar formation. TGF-β is believed to be one of the most implicated growth factors in regulating scar formation and for this purpose has been widely studied [6, 14]. Three highly homologous isoforms are known in humans: β1, β2, and β3. In fetal wounds, low levels of TGF-β1 and TGF-β2 and high levels of TGF-β3 are associated with scarless repair. Conversely, in the wounds of adults, predominantly TGF-β1 and TGF-β2 are present, which is linked to fibrosis and ultimately scarring. As TGF-β1 and β2 neutralizing antibodies, or exogenous TGF-β3, have in part been shown to prevent scarring [16, 17], so too should growth factors, and cytokines other than TGF-β participate in scarless wound repair. For example, PDGF, VEGF, and FGF isoforms were implicated in the transition from scarless to scar-forming wound repair [6]. Despite an increase over the past decades in our knowledge of the mechanisms of wound healing, that of fetal wound healing remains only partially understood.

Skin Aging

Skin's mechanistic, protective, and restorative properties are impaired with age. Skin aging occurs through two biologically distinct processes: intrinsic and extrinsic aging [18]. Intrinsic skin aging is a naturally occurring process caused by an accumulation of age-associated degenerative changes, such as progressive telomere shortening and oxidative damage as a result of aerobic cellular metabolism [19]. In human skin, intrinsic aging is characterized by dermal atrophy (thinning), flattening of the rete ridges, and a reduction in dermal fibroblasts. A loss of vascular network or a weakening of blood vessels also causes intrinsic aging. Intrinsic aging has a significant effect on the dermal collagen fiber network. Collagen biosynthesis steadily declines toward the third and fourth decades of life. Subsequently, it remains at levels too low to permit mature skin to repair and replace the collagen it loses as part of the degenerative, age-associated process [18]. Collagen depletion is the age-related consequence of a decrease in collagen formation and an increase in collagen-degrading enzymes (such as matrix-metalloproteases-1 or MMP-1). Elastin provides skin with elasticity and resilience. Until around 50 years of age, elastin biosynthesis remains constant. After that, it declines sharply [18, 20]. Although it is established that both elastase and also MMP-2 play a role in elastin degradation, the underlying etiology of age-related changes in elastin is not well understood.

Extrinsic or premature skin aging is interconnected with the intrinsic components of skin aging. Premature skin aging is primarily caused by photodamage – the exposure of unprotected skin to ultraviolet irradiation from the sun. Sun exposure is thought to account for up to 80 % of facial aging [19]. Smoking, air pollution, and poor nutrition are other causes of premature skin aging. Chronic sun exposure promotes degradation of collagen and elastin, resulting in the accumulation of abnormal amorphous elastic material in the dermis (solar elastosis). The increased degradation of extracellular matrix proteins caused by sun exposure, combined with the decreased regenerative capacity of dermal fibroblasts caused by aging, lead to the characteristic signs of photoaged skin (deep wrinkling, furrowing, and the loss of skin elasticity).

Skin Rejuvenation with Growth Factors

A large variety of antiaging ingredients and sunscreens are used today in an attempt to slow or reverse skin aging [19, 21]. One such ingredient that has recently emerged is the growth factor. The following paragraphs review growth factors and their role in skin rejuvenation.

There are three distinguishable categories of skincare products that contain growth factors:

- Products that contain single or multiple recombinant growth factors
- Products that contain a combination of growth factors as part of conditioned cell culture media
- Products containing a mixture of growth factors as part of cell lysates

Skincare Products with Recombinant Growth Factors

Several products available today are marketed as containing one or more recombinant growth factors – usually TGF-ß1 or EGF. Regrettably, limited studies exist that report on the efficacy of such products for skin rejuvenation. These particular recombinant growth factors are often obtained from yeasts or plants that are altered to produce the desired growth factor proteins. This process, which involves genetic engineering, is known as "recombinant DNA technology." In wound healing, TGF-ß1 and EGF are two of the more widely studied growth factors. So predictably, several antiaging products are marketed as containing those growth factors.

A study investigated the efficacy of an antiaging formulation containing TGF-ß1 and ascorbic acid in a silicon base [22]. In the study, 7 of the 12 (58 %) female participants indicated that they saw a visible improvement in their wrinkles and skin texture after 3 months of twice-daily use. This perception was confirmed by a panel of four dermatologists who used a five-point facial wrinkle visual scale to assess the high-quality digital photographs taken before and after the treatments. A later study [23] reported that for reducing wrinkles, the same TGF-ß1-containing product was superior to a similar cream that did not contain TGF-ß1. In the study, 4 of the 12 (33 %) participants noticed an improvement when using the product free of TGF-ß1. Both products were well tolerated.

More recently, a study in 29 female subjects demonstrated that serum containing barley-bioengineered EGF [24] improved visible signs of aging in the facial skin when used twice a day for 3 months. Clinical evaluations showed statistically significant improvements within the first month of use in the appearance of pore size, skin texture, fine lines, rhytids, and various dyschromatic conditions. These trends continued to improvement for the duration of the study. The serum was well tolerated with minimal treatment-related complications.

A study of a preparation comprising recombinant EGF, bFGF, KGF-2, IGF-1, and hyaluronic acid [25] demonstrated that the formula significantly improved periorbital wrinkles after 4 and 8 weeks of twice-daily use. An investigator assessed the subjects using a skin roughness analysis.

Because the particular skin functions that are affected by aging are responsive to growth factors, it would make sense that a skincare product containing more than one growth factor would be efficacious in reducing the visual signs of skin aging. However, limited clinical data exist that report on skincare products comprising more than one recombinant growth factor. The majority of skincare products that contain multiple growth factors obtain these proteins using technologies other than recombinant DNA technology. These product types are further described in the following paragraph.

Skincare Products with Growth Factors as Part of Conditioned Cell Culture Media

Currently, there are several lines of skincare products that contain a mixture of natural (nonrecombinant) growth factors as a part of the conditioned media. These growth factor ingredients are manufactured in a biotechnology process that involves collecting the cell culture media after the cells have been cultured. The cell culture media, also known as conditioned media, consists of growth factors and cytokines, as well as remnants of the original medium that was used to culture the cells. It does not, however, contain cells.

The first growth factor ingredient used for skin aging that was obtained from conditioned media (Tissue Nutrient Solution; TNS®) is collected after culturing neonatal human dermal fibroblasts [7]. It is reported to contain over 110 growth factors, cytokines, and soluble matrix proteins [22]. Since its introduction, several scientific articles have reported on the efficacy of TNS for skin rejuvenation.

One journal article described a study involving 14 subjects that used TNS in a hydrogel formulation [7]. The study reported that after 2 months of twice-daily application, an improvement of 12.2 % ($p \leq 0.05$) was observed in the periorbital area and 8.5 % ($p = 0.09$) in the perioral area. Photodamage was clinically graded using a nine-point visual wrinkle scale. At the beginning and end of each treatment session, photodamage and skin roughness of the lateral cheek area were assessed using silicon replica technology and punch biopsy.

In a 3-month split-face study of the hydrogel, 14 of the 19 (74 %) subjects completing the study showed improved or no worsening of their averaged wrinkle scores [21]. The severity of wrinkles was assessed by four dermatologists using a five-point visual scale and high-quality digital photographs taken before and after each treatment. The same study included a comparison of a TGF-β formulation and the TNS hydrogel. Twenty-seven of the 31 (87 %) participants showed improved or no worsening of their average wrinkle scores after treatment with the single growth factor formulation. On average, the wrinkle scores of all 31 subjects improved by 12 % [23]. Using a selected statistical model, the investigators concluded that there was no statistically significant difference between the hydrogel formulation with the growth factor mixture and the formulation with the single growth factor. Both products were well tolerated.

The antiaging benefit of TNS hydrogel was confirmed in a double-blind, placebo-controlled study of 60 subjects [26]. For at least 4 weeks after enrollment, each subject used a basic skincare regimen consisting of a gentle skin cleanser and a daily facial moisturizer, which provided a sun protection factor (SPF 15). After that, subjects were randomized into two groups and instructed to apply to their skin either the active hydrogel or the vehicle twice a day for 6 months. They were instructed to apply the respective hydrogel formulation after skin cleansing and before application of the SPF15 moisturizer. The investigator clinically assessed treatment efficacy by using a five-point visual scale and silicon replica technology. An independent panel of three dermatologists reviewed photodamage from photographs using an 11-point comparative scale. Assessments were conducted at the baseline visit at 3 months and again at the 6-month visit. As assessed by the investigator after 6 months, in the active group (27 subjects), photodamage parameters, namely fine wrinkling (0.33 ± 0.55), mottled pigmentation (0.48 ± 0.58), and tactile roughness (0.52 ± 0.85) score units significantly decreased from baseline. In the vehicle group (26 subjects), mottled pigmentation (0.65 ± 0.69) and tactile roughness (0.58 ± 0.81) also decreased. Fine wrinkling, however, did not significantly decrease (0.15 ± 0.46). In the vehicle group, photographic evaluation showed a worsening of photodamage indicated by a negative change in the photodamage scores. The active group showed either a slight improvement or a substantial prevention of worsening in photodamage as indicated by a smaller change from baseline at 6 months. Whereas the difference between active and vehicle group was not statistically significant ($p = 0.323$) after 3 months, there was a leaning toward a statistically significant difference ($p = 0.083$) after 6 months. When analyzing the data from only those with severe photodamage, the five subjects who used the active hydrogel for 6 months showed a statistically significant improvement (by 0.4 points). The six subjects in the vehicle group, however, showed a statistically significant worsening (by 1 point) in photodamage scores. The study showed that after 3 and 6 months of treatment, the active hydrogel reduced fine lines and wrinkles better than the vehicle, when a silicon replica technology was used to assess roughness and shadow parameters of the periorbital area. After 3 months of treatment, no significant differences between the active and vehicle groups were noticed in either the reduction of deep lines or in skin roughness ($p = 0.290$). In the reduction of fine line shadows ($p = 0.045$), the differences were either significant or tended toward statistical significance. After 6 months, the differences were either significant or tended toward statistical significance in the reduction of deep lines and roughness ($p = 0.06$) and in the reduction of fine line shadows ($p = 0.072$). Although one subject treated with active gel discontinued because of dislike of the cosmetic attributes of the product, overall the active hydrogel was well tolerated.

In a 3-month study of 37 subjects, a serum containing TNS hydrogel, combined in situ with collagen-building peptides, antioxidants, and depigmenting agents, was evaluated for the improvement of the visible signs of facial photodamage [27]. After 1 month of treatment, the clinical evaluations showed statistically significant reductions in coarse and fine wrinkles and improvements in skin tone, texture, and radiance with continued improvements after 2 and 3 months. Decreased skin extensibility and increased resiliency were further measured. The serum was well tolerated with no treatment-related adverse events reported during the study period.

Recently, another company introduced a product containing growth factors derived from human cell-conditioned media. The growth factors were obtained from neonatal cells cultured under conditions of low oxygen tension. Although the so-obtained conditioned media contain a variety of growth factors and cytokines (including VEGF, KGF, and IL-8), it is devoid of TGF-β proteins [28]. In a proof of concept study, two products with this conditioned media were tested over 3 months in 21 female subjects with mild to moderate photodamage, fine lines, and wrinkles [29]. The study results showed that after 2 weeks, tactile roughness, texture, and wrinkles significantly improved ($p < 0.05$) from baseline and continued to improve. At 12 weeks, an improvement over baseline reached 44.9 %, 46.2 %, and 29.9 %, respectively. No treatment-related adverse events were recorded during the study.

Skincare Products with Growth Factors as Part of Cell Lysates

Inspired by the scarless wound healing properties of fetal skin cells, another company developed a skincare product with the cell lysate of fibroblasts (Processed Skin Cell Proteins; PSP®). The cells are obtained from a dedicated cell bank of cultured human fetal fibroblasts. The cell bank, which originated from a single biopsy of donated skin tissue, was established for the purpose of developing wound healing products. PSP is produced from cultured fibroblasts that are harvested by centrifugation. The conditioned culture liquid (or spent culture media) produced during the process is removed and discarded as it consists of cellular waste, red dye, and remnants of unwanted culture media. The collected fibroblasts are washed with a physiological buffer to help remove any lingering traces of culture media, and the cell walls are freeze-thawed. This freeze-thaw process ruptures the cell membranes, leading to cell lysis, and allows the fetal fibroblast cell lysate to be obtained.

PSP is made up of a combination of proteins and other cytokines that include human growth factors. Proteomic analysis of the formula detected more than 100 growth factors and cytokines, including those growth factors most studied in the regulation of cutaneous wound healing [2]. Additionally, PSP was shown to contain several anti-inflammatory cytokines, including the interleukin-1 receptor antagonist (IL-1RA). In their study, Kupper and Groves demonstrated that IL-1RA exerts an anti-inflammatory response by competitively binding the IL-1 receptors without triggering a signal [30]. Other cytokines such as tumor necrosis factor α (TNF-α), interferon γ (INF-γ), and the tissue inhibitors of metalloproteinases 1 and 2 (TIMP-1, TIMP-2) were also detected in PSP.

In an 8-week study to evaluate the antiaging benefits of the first cream with PSP, doctors Gold and Goldman assessed 20 female subjects between the ages of 35 and 65 years with demonstrable facial wrinkles [31]. Investigators determined improvements using a five-point visual score of both clinical assessments and photographs of perioral and periorbital wrinkles. Subjects determined improvements using a questionnaire. After 1 month of treatment, a statistically significant ($p \leq 0.05$) reduction in periorbital and perioral wrinkles was observed. After 2 months, the periorbital wrinkles decreased by an additional 17 % and the perioral wrinkles by 13 %. After the full 8-week study period, of all the subjects who completed the study, 83 % showed an improved average wrinkle score of at least 0.5 units around the eye area and 50 % around the mouth.

PRIMOS, or Phase shift Rapid In-vivo Measurement of Skin (PRIMOS, GFM, Tetlow, Germany), is an optical three-dimensional (3D) in vivo skin-measuring device that allows contact-free, direct, and fast measurement of skin surface topography at high resolution. PRIMOS measurements are based on a digital parallel stripe pattern-imaging technique that is projected onto the surface of the skin and depicted in the charge-coupled device (CCD) chip of a high-resolution camera. The light patterns are created by a digital micromirror projector (Texas Instruments, Irving, Texas) that is valuable when applied to optical 3D in vivo skin measurements because exposure times are short, and the high light intensity can be controlled point- and pixel-wise, or both. Because the device is contact-free, it is less prone to artifact buildup and, therefore, more reliable than the silicon replica technology commonly used for topography purposes [33, 34]. Complex mathematical algorithms embedded in the analytical software reconstruct the data into highly precise 3D skin surface images, which allow accurate measurements of the depth of fine lines and wrinkles. Additionally, the short exposure time guarantees that the involuntary movements of the subject do not influence the captured data. Finally, PRIMOS allows the recorded data (i.e., the precisely located skin wrinkles) to be matched and thus accurately compared from the before- and after-treatment images (See Fig. 1a, b).

In a study by Gold and colleagues, subjects treated with PSP cream were assessed after quantitatively measuring skin surface topography using the PRIMOS device [32]. Eighteen female subjects completed a double-blind, placebo-controlled split-face study aimed at assessing skin topography after 2 months of twice-daily Bio-Cream application. The study revealed significant improvements in periorbital skin topography. When the after-treatment was compared to the before-treatment images, skin surface roughness was shown to have decreased between 10 % and 18 % ($p \leq 0.05$), depending on the roughness parameters. The roughness parameters for maximum depths R_{zmax}, R_{3zmax}, and R_{zISO}, in particular, decreased by 15 % or more after the

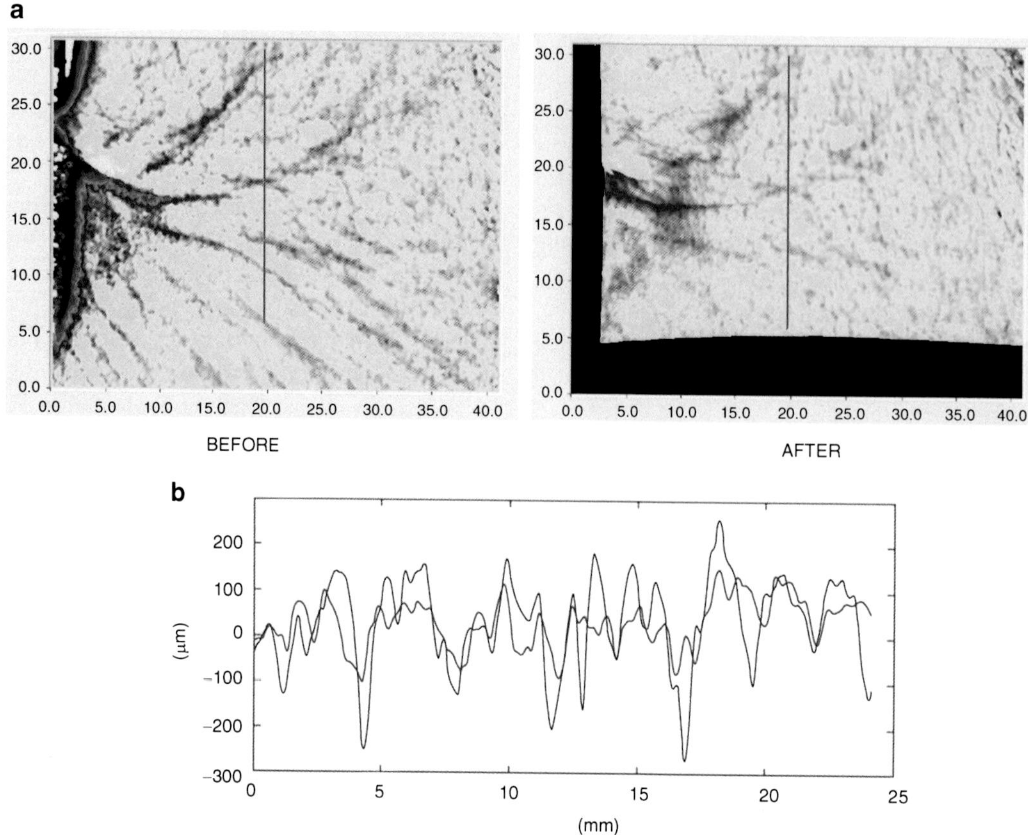

Fig. 1 Example of PRIMOS-3D color-coded skin topography picture of 40 × 30 mm periorbital skin measurement area before (**a**, *left*) and after (**b**, *right*) 2 months of twice-daily use of the human growth factor and cytokine skin cream. The color-coded scale for skin depth is in millimeters (mm). The pictures were matched in order to overlap the periorbital surfaces of the before and the after measurement. This allows analysis of structural changes caused by the treatment along cut lines. The skin profile along the vertical cut lines of major periorbital wrinkles including the crow's feet is shown in (**b**). As compared to the baseline profile (**b**, *black profile*), a significantly smoother profile representative for decreased skin roughness or a reduction in the depth of fine lines and moderate and deep wrinkles was obtained after the treatment (**b**, *blue profile*)

study period. The "extreme" roughness parameters described such pronounced signs of periorbital facial skin aging as moderate and deep wrinkles, including those of crow's feet. In contrast to the cream, twice-daily treatments for 2 months with the placebo formula (which was identical to the PSP cream) did not result in significant changes to the roughness parameters R_{zmax}, R_{3z}, R_{3zmax}, and R_{zISO}. Only R_a and R_z significantly decreased (by about 10 %). After the study period, the differences between active and placebo groups for Rz_{max}, R_{3z}, and R_{zISO} were statistically significant ($p \leq 0.05$). The differences between active and placebo for R_a (Remark: Although the average roughness R_a is one of the most frequently used parameters in surface measurement, this parameter does not inform about all aspects of the surface. Surfaces with the same Ra may differ significantly in shape. In order to distinguish surfaces, other parameters about peaks and valleys and profile shapes and spacing are commonly used.), R_z (Remark: R_z is a mean parameter; here, it is the average of five single roughness depths over the entire sample length. This parameter has some advantages in finding extremes in the roughness, but it is not sensitive to single unusual features of the surface. R_{zmax}, which corresponds to the maximal R_z within the five measuring length, seems a better descriptor for unusual features of the surface. In the present case, deep wrinkles such as crow's feet can be regarded as such an unusual feature. R_{zISO} is another parameter which helps to further describe rather extreme and unusual skin surface patterns), and R_{3zmax} did not reach statistical significance. The difference, however, for R_{3zmax} was close to significant ($p = 0.06$) and may have reached statistical significance if more subjects had participated in the study. The baseline values for the roughness parameters did not differ significantly between the active and placebo groups. The cream was well tolerated.

The antiaging benefits of skin cream with PSP were confirmed in an additional study investigating improvements of signs of facial skin aging when used for a prolonged period (6 months) [35]. The 11 female subjects who completed the study all underwent a punch biopsy for light and electron microscopy evaluation at the beginning and end of the treatment periods. Further evaluations included photographic and clinical assessment of skin for signs of facial wrinkles using the same five-point visual wrinkle scale as was used in the 2-month IL-1RA study by Kupper and Groves [30]. After the 6-month treatment period, signs of periorbital wrinkles were reduced by 33 % and perioral wrinkles by 25 %. Furthermore, chin texture improved by 21 % and cheek by 39 %. All subjects tolerated the cream well without the occurrence of adverse events.

An eye cream with PSP was evaluated in a multicenter study investigating periorbital skin rejuvenation [36]. Thirty-seven female subjects between the ages of 36 and 65 years completed the study. Results revealed that on average, signs of wrinkles – lower eyelid bags, sagging, and dark circles – and skin texture were significantly reduced ($p \leq 0.05$) by between 14 % and 28 % after 6 weeks of twice-daily application. A subject questionnaire further confirmed the clinical improvements. The subjects reported that their "tired look" improved on average by 32 %. The eye cream was well tolerated and all subjects "liked the way it felt." The formulation's efficacy, excellent tolerability in the delicate periorbital skin area, and pleasant sensory properties explain why a large majority (78 %) of the subjects indicated that they would continue regular use with the eye cream. In addition to PSP®, Lumière Bio-restorative Eye Cream contains caffeine, bisabolol, and glycyrrhetinic acid, which may contribute to the cream's observed efficacy.

Discussion

Even though the crucial role of growth factors in cutaneous wound healing is extensively studied and well recognized, the beneficial use of growth factors for skin rejuvenation has only been confirmed in the last few years. About a dozen clinical studies and articles describing the safety and efficacy of topical growth factor products for skin rejuvenation in humans exist in professional medical and scientific journals today. While a few articles report on recombinant growth factor products, the majority of articles describe antiaging studies with skincare products that contain natural mixtures of growth factors and other cytokines that are obtained by either collecting the conditioned cell culture medium or by cell lysis. All of the articles, however, demonstrate that growth factor products are effective at improving the signs of facial skin aging. Some studies indicate that efficacy is a function of time, with signs of significant wrinkle reduction seen only after prolonged product use (i.e., after 6 months or more). These observations seem comparable to those of some retinoic acid studies [37], where the severity of photodamage improves only after prolonged topical treatments. Placebo-controlled studies on skincare products that contain growth factors, such as TGF-β, TNS, and PSP, report that when compared, the signs of skin aging of the active groups are significantly more reduced than those of their vehicle counterparts. It is worth noting that vehicles are not completely "inactive," since they do contain moisturizers, and the effects of moisturizing can produce some improvements in fine lines and wrinkles. Even with that being the case, placebo-controlled studies clearly demonstrate that topical growth factors are superior in reducing the signs of skin aging than moisturizers alone.

In theory, growth factors can participate in skin rejuvenation at various levels due to their multifunctional activities. However, to be effective, growth factors must penetrate the skin to reach their respective cell surface receptors (keratinocytes, fibroblasts, or endothelial cells). Despite their relatively large size (>5 kDa), growth factors are able to penetrate intact skin. In this, they are not alone, as other large proteins have the same ability, for example, latex protein allergens (3–26 kDa) and botulinum toxin type A (900 kDa) – although to a lesser extent [38, 39]. Growth factors are also effective at very low concentrations (10^{-9}–10^{-12} of a mole). Thus, a low level of penetration is more than sufficient to induce a response. Proteins such as growth factors predominantly penetrate the skin through a vertical pathway, also known as the skin's "natural imperfections." These imperfections include the follicular apparatus of hair follicles, sweat glands, and microlesions in the interfollicular stratum corneum [40].

Those cutaneous functions that are impaired by the aging process seem to respond well to growth factors. Thus, the signs of aging skin may be improved with the topical use of an appropriate mixture of growth factors. However, due to the complexity and enormous expense associated with the development and manufacture of growth factor-containing products, only a limited number of skincare products are currently available that incorporate a mixture of growth factors. The question, therefore, of what combinations of growth factors and cytokines are most effective for skin rejuvenation remains to be further investigated.

Most recently, a novel peptide mixture consisting of matrikine and matrikine-like peptides was shown to provide statistically non-distinguishable anti-wrinkle benefits as compared to PSP and TNS [41]. A matrikine is a matrix-originating peptide with cytokine activity that is generated from the degradation of connective tissue proteins. The mixture (Micro-Protein Complex; MPC™), which comprises capryloyl carnosine (a dipeptide), palmitoyl tripetide-1 acetate, and tetrapeptide-21, demonstrated an ability to stimulate in vitro the formation of collagens I, III, and VII, elastin, and hyaluronic acid – all of which deplete considerably as skin ages. This indicates that matrikines, in particular MPC, may be valuable growth factor alternatives for skin rejuvenation.

Conclusion

In the last decade, topical growth factor products have become well accepted for use in skin rejuvenation. Numerous randomized controlled clinical trials demonstrated their good tolerability and efficacy. Today, there is evidence that the signs of aging skin may be best improved with a mixture of growth factors. Yet, what combinations of growth factors are most optimal for skin rejuvenation by topical application remains to be further investigated.

Cross-References

- ▶ Aging and Antiaging Strategies
- ▶ Cosmetics and Aging Skin
- ▶ Cosmetic Antiaging Ingredients
- ▶ Topical Peptides and Proteins for Aging Skin

References

1. Taub DD. Cytokine, growth factor, and chemokine ligand database. Curr Protoc Immunol. 2004 Sep; Chapter 6: Unit 6.29.
2. Werner S, Grose R. Regulation of wound healing by growth factors and cytokines. Physiol Rev. 2003;83 (3):835–70.
3. Braund R, Hook S, Medlicott NJ. The role of topical growth factors in chronic wounds. Curr Drug Deliv. 2007;4(3):195–204.
4. Barrientos S, Stojadinovic O, Golinko MS, Brem H, Tomic-Canic M. Growth factors and cytokines in wound healing. Wound Repair Regen. 2008;16 (5):585–601.

5. Leahy PJ, Lawrence WT. Biologic enhancement of wound healing. Clin Plast Surg. 2007;34(4):659–71.
6. Bullard KM, Longaker MT, Lorenz HP. Fetal wound healing: current biology. World J Surg. 2003;27 (1):54–61.
7. Fitzpatrick RE, Rostan EF. Reversal of photodamage with topical growth factors: a pilot study. J Cosmet Laser Ther. 2003;5(1):25–34.
8. Fitzpatrick RE. Endogenous growth factors as cosmeceuticals. Dermatol Surg. 2005;31(7 Pt 2): 827–31. discussion 831.
9. Quan TH, Shao Y, He T, Voorhees JJ, Fisher G. Reduced expression of Connective Tissue Growth Factor (CTGF/CCN2) mediates collagen loss in chronologically aged human skin. J Invest Dermatol. 2010;130:415–24.
10. Noordam R, Gunn DA, Tomlin CC, Maier AB, Griffiths T, Ogden S, et al. Serum insulin-like growth factor 1 and facial ageing: high levels associate with reduced skin wrinkling in a cross-sectional study. Br J Dermatol. 2013;168(3):533–8.
11. Beanes SR, Dang C, Soo C, Ting K. Skin repair and scar formation: the central role of TGF-beta. Expert Rev Mol Med. 2003;5(8):1–22.
12. Gosain A, DiPietro LA. Aging and wound healing. World J Surg. 2004;28(3):321–6.
13. Swift ME, Kleinman HK, DiPietro LA. Impaired wound repair and delayed angiogenesis in aged mice. Lab Invest. 1999;79(12):1479–87.
14. Komi-Kuramochi A, Kawano M, Oda Y, Asada M, Suzuki M, Oki J, et al. Expression of fibroblast growth factors and their receptors during full-thickness skin wound healing in young and aged mice. J Endocrinol. 2005;186(2):273–89.
15. Lorenz HP, Lin RY, Longaker MT, Whitby DJ, Adzick NS. The fetal fibroblast: the effector cell of scarless fetal skin repair. Plast Reconstr Surg. 1995;96 (6):1251–9. discussion 1260–1261.
16. Ferguson MWJ, O'Kane S. Scar-free healing: from embryonic mechanisms to adult therapeutic intervention. Philos Trans R Soc Lond B Biol Sci. 2004;359 (1445):839–50.
17. Wu L, Siddiqui A, Morris DE, Cox DA, Roth SI, Mustoe TA. Transforming growth factor beta 3 (TGF beta 3) accelerates wound healing without alteration of scar prominence. Histologic and competitive reverse-transcription-polymerase chain reaction studies. Arch Surg. 1997;132(7):753–60.
18. Uitto J. The role of elastin and collagen in cutaneous aging: intrinsic aging versus photoexposure. J Drugs Dermatol. 2008;7(2 Suppl):s12–6.
19. Baumann L. Skin ageing and its treatment. J Pathol. 2007;211(2):241–51.
20. Seite S, Zucchi H, Septier D, Igondjo-Tchen S, Senni K, Godeau G. Elastin changes during chronological and photo-ageing: the important role of lysozyme. J Eur Acad Dermatol Venereol. 2006;20 (8):980–7.
21. Yaar M, Gilchrest BA. Photoageing: mechanism, prevention and therapy. Br J Dermatol. 2007;157(5):874–87.
22. Rao J, Ehrlich M, Goldman MP. Facial skin rejuvenation with a novel topical compound containing transforming growth factor β1 and vitamin C. Cosmet Dermatol. 2004;17:705–13.
23. Ehrlich M, Rao J, Pabby A, Mitchel P. Improvement in the appearance of wrinkles with topical transforming growth factor β_1 and L-ascorbic acid. Dermatol Surg. 2006;32(5):618–25.
24. Schouest JM, Luu TK, Moy RL. Improved texture and appearance of human facial skin after daily topical application of barley produced, synthetic, human-like Epidermal Growth Factor (EGF) serum. J Drugs Dermatol. 2012;11(5):613–20.
25. Lee DH, Oh IY, Koo KT, Suk JM, Jung SW, Park JO, et al. Improvement in skin wrinkles using a preparation containing human growth factors and hyaluronic acid serum. J Cosmet Laser Ther. 2015;17(1):20–3.
26. Mehta RC, Smith SR, Grove GL, Ford RO, Canfield W, Donofrio LM, et al. Reduction in facial photodamage by a tropical growth factor product. J Drugs Dermatol. 2008;7(9):864–71.
27. Atkin DH, Trookan NS, Rizer RL, Schreck LE, Ho ET. Combination of physiologically balanced growth factors with antioxidants for reversal of facial photodamage. J Cosmet Laser Ther. 2010;12(1):14–20.
28. Zimber MP, Mansbridge JN, Taylor M, Stockton T, Hubka M, Baumgartner M, et al. Human cell-conditioned media produced under embryonic-like conditions result in improved healing time after laser resurfacing. Aesthet Plast Surg. 2012;36(2):431–7.
29. Bruce S, Karnik J, Dryer L, Burkholder D. Anti-aging proof of concept study: results and summary. J Drugs Dermatol. 2014;13(9):1074–81.
30. Kupper TS, Groves RW. The interleukin-1 axis and cutaneous inflammation. J Invest Dermatol. 1995;105 (1 Suppl):62S–6.
31. Gold MH, Goldman MP, Biron J. Efficacy of novel skin cream containing mixture of human growth factors and cytokines for skin rejuvenation. J Drugs Dermatol. 2007;6(2):197–201.
32. Gold MH, Goldman MP, Biron J. Human growth factor and cytokine skin cream for facial skin rejuvenation as assessed by 3D in vivo optical skin imaging. J Drugs Dermatol. 2007;6(10):1018–23.
33. Lévêque JL. EEMCO guidance for the assessment of skin topography. J Eur Acad Dermatol Venereol. 1999;12(2):103–14.
34. Friedman PM, Skover GR, Payonk G, Kauvar AN, Geronemus RG. 3D in-vivo optical skin imaging for topographical quantitative assessment of non-ablative laser technology. Dermatol Surg. 2002;28 (3):199–204.

35. Hussain M, Phelps R, Goldberg DJ. Clinical, histologic, and ultrastructural changes after use of human growth factor and cytokine skin cream for the treatment of skin rejuvenation. J Cosmet Laser Ther. 2008;10 (2):104–9.
36. Lupo ML, Cohen JL, Rendon MI. Novel eye cream containing a mixture of human growth factors and cytokines for periorbital skin rejuvenation. J Drugs Dermatol. 2007;6(7):725–9.
37. Gilchrest BA. Treatment of photodamage with topical tretinoin: an overview. J Am Acad Dermatol. 1997;36 (3 Pt 2):S27–36.
38. Hayes BB, Afsahri A, Millecchia L, Willard PA, Povoski SP, Meade BJ. Evaluation of percutaneous penetration of natural rubber latex proteins. Toxicol Sci. 2000;56(2):262–70.
39. Glogau RG. Topically applied botulinum toxin type A for the treatment of primary axillary hyperhidrosis: results of a randomized, blinded, vehicle-controlled study. Dermatol Surg. 2007;33(1 Spec No):S76–80.
40. Schaefer H, Lademann J. The role of follicular penetration. A differential view. Skin Pharmacol Appl Skin Physiol. 2001;14 Suppl 1:23–7.
41. Dreher F, Gold M. Matrikine-based micro-protein complex technology for topical skin rejuvenation. 73rd Annual Meeting of the American Academy of Dermatology Poster 1822. 20–24 Mar 2015. San Francisco.

Topical Peptides and Proteins for Aging Skin

137

Farzam Gorouhi and Howard I. Maibach

Contents

F. Gorouhi (✉)
Department of Dermatology, University of California, Davis, CA, USA
e-mail: gorouhif@gmail.com

H.I. Maibach
Department of Dermatology, University of California, San Francisco, CA, USA
e-mail: maibachh@derm.ucsf.edu

M.A. Farage et al. (eds.), *Textbook of Aging Skin*,
DOI 10.1007/978-3-662-47398-6_101

Abstract

By 2030, the preponderance of older individuals over younger ones will transform the shape of the age distribution graph into a rectangle rather than the current pyramid observed. This chapter summarizes the characteristics and in vitro and in vivo studies on effect of peptides and proteins on aging skin.

Introduction

In the year 2000, individuals over the age of 65 represented 13 % of the US population; this is expected to increase to 20 % by 2030. This preponderance of older individuals over younger ones will transform the shape of the age distribution graph into a rectangle rather than the current pyramid observed [1].

This demographic shift calls for increased efforts to prevent the aging process and develop safe and effective drugs for the elderly. In cosmetic dermatology, experts are exploring better antisolar, antiaging, antiwrinkle, and firming products. Pharmaceutical companies frequently use peptides as active ingredients in their creams.

Peptides have different effects on the skin, especially for cosmetics purposes, but the most important concern to use them topically is their permeability to penetrate the skin.

Generally, permeation ability depends on different factors: physicochemical properties of the substance (acid dissociation constant [p*K*a], molecular size, stability, binding affinity, solubility, and partition coefficient); the timescale of permeation; integrity, thickness, and components of the skin, cutaneous metabolism; site, area, and duration of application; properties of the transdermal device; and the creation of a local depot at the site of application [2, 3].

In summary, it is ideal to have a topical drug with parameters within the belowmentioned listed range:

1. Molecular weight less than 500 Da
2. Moderate log of partition coefficient octanol/water between 1 and 3
3. Melting point less than 200 °C
4. Reasonable aqueous solubility (>1 mg/ml)
5. No or few polar centers [4, 5]

Diffusivity of the molecules in stratum corneum is related to the number of hydrogen-bonding groups on a molecule, being maximal for small non-hydrogen-bonding molecules and reaching a low minimum with about four hydrogen-bonding groups [6].

Since peptides and proteins contain many amide bonds (as hydrogen-bond donor and acceptor groups), and because of their large molecular size, they have low diffusivity in the skin. Furthermore, as they are often charged at physiological pH, they are intrinsically hydrophilic. Hence, the lipophilic stratum corneum is a significant barrier to penetration [7].

Overall, topical peptides and proteins have been successfully and widely used. Patch test of PPD tuberculin protein and more specific derivatives like MPB64 have been effectively addressed for active tuberculosis diagnosis [8, 9]. Tacrolimus and pimecrolimus (with lower permeability) penetrate through the skin to treat atopic dermatitis patients [10, 11].

Frech et al. [12] found a safe and protective vaccine patch containing heat-labile protein enterotoxin to prevent diarrhea in travelers to Mexico and Guatemala. Even topical cyclosporine A with molecular weight more than 1,200 Da could be delivered into the skin with delivery-enhancing methods [13].

The main barrier for topical drugs is stratum corneum, the outermost layer of the epidermis. Several techniques overcome such a barricade. Chemical penetration enhancer might be useful for peptide dermal delivery [14].

One study [15] addressed usefulness of iontophoresis for topical insulin application. Other mechanisms like sonophoresis in liposomal peptides [16] and colloidal carrier systems [17] are considered helpful in this regard. Carrier peptides can increase and accelerate the permeation process. Chen and colleagues [18] reported that a short synthetic peptide (ACSSSPSKHCG) identified by in vivo phage display facilitated efficient transdermal insulin delivery through intact skin. Although topical use of a peptide has potential to be effective, delivery across skin can be difficult due to the ionic nature of such materials. An approach to improving delivery is use of fatty acid derivatives to increase the lipophilic property of the peptide. For example, the palmitoyl derivative of the polypeptide interferon α penetrates across human skin fivefold to sixfold greater than the simple peptide [19] and also, facial skin improvement has been reported after topical pal-KTTKS (palmitoyl pentapeptide-4) therapy [20].

Many peptides and proteins are used for cosmetic indications; GHK-Cu is most widely utilized for wound healing and antiaging indications. Abdulghani et al. [21] revealed its enhanced but insignificant antiaging effects when compared to tretinoin, vitamin C, and melatonin.

Palmitoyl KTTKS is another frequently used peptide that was shown to have better significant results than placebo and an active comparator [20, 22]. Acetyl hexapeptide-3 (Argireline®) had promising results. The depth of wrinkles was reduced more than 30 % for Argireline® versus 10 % for placebo after 30 days [23].

All of the aforementioned examples of peptides can suggest that these agents may be effective.

Note that in the only published systematic review [24] on interventions for photodamaged skin no peptide therapy was included.

Here, published peptides and proteins – classified into four categories – their characteristics, in vitro studies, and in vivo efficacy data are examined.

Materials and Methods

Pubmed, EMBASE, and Scopus were systematically searched from 1974 to June 15, 2008 (Table 1). Different words have been used to locate any known peptides or proteins, find all possible topical therapies, locate all cosmeceutical-related papers, and rule out irrelevant papers. All references of relevant articles were screened to find other eligible resources. In addition, some in vitro and in vivo data were collected from pharmaceutical companies' web sites. For efficacy data, only randomized trials were included.

Results and Discussions

Surprisingly, there were scarce data about permeation abilities of these topical peptides. Only permeation coefficients for three widely used topical cosmeceutical peptides (GHK [25], GSH [25], and MSH [26, 27]) and some monopeptides [28, 29] as well as their copper complexes were reported (Table 2).

Braun et al. [30] reported relative superoxide dismutase content that has been absorbed in the epidermis and the dermis after penetration over 8 h. The ratios of total concentration for epidermis and dermis were 0.009 % and 0.010 % after 4 h and 0.031 % and 0.010 % after 8 h, respectively.

The characteristics of included substances are in Table 3. Eligible in vivo efficacy studies are summarized in Table 4.

Topical peptides and proteins are classified into four categories:

1. Signal peptide
2. Enzyme inhibitor peptide
3. Neurotransmitter-inhibitor peptide
4. Carrier peptide

Signal Peptides

Signal peptides stimulate matrix protein production in general and collagen synthesis in specific. They may be accomplished by stimulation and growth of different skin cells like human skin fibroblasts. Signal peptides can also increase elastin, proteoglycan, glycosaminoglycans, and fibronectin proliferation. By increasing matrix cell activities and consequently collagen production, the skin looks firmer and younger.

The tripeptide-1 (glycyl-L-histadyl-L-lysine or GHK) is primarily known as carrier peptides. It mainly helps to stabilize and deliver copper. Carrier peptides are discussed later. GHK was originally isolated from human plasma in 1973 by Pickart and Thaler [31] and its wound repair properties observed in 1985 by Maquart et al. [32]. In 1999, Maquart et al. concluded that GHK or its copper complex functioned as an activator of tissue remodeling [32]. It is also a signal peptide that promotes extra-large collagen aggregates degradation in scars; regular collagen synthesis in normal skin; elastin, proteoglycans, and glycosaminoglycans production; growth rate and migration of different cell types; and anti-inflammatory and antioxidant responses [33–37]. In a controlled ex vivo study [38], biotinyl-GHK and vehicle were investigated. Biotinyl-GHK, but not vehicle solution, showed stimulation of collagen IV, laminin production, and keratinocyte mitosis.

Tripeptide-1 can be also conjugated with palmitic acid and form pal-tripeptide-1 (Biopeptide-CL). In vitro and in vivo studies approved that Biopeptide-CL stimulates collagen and gylcosaminoglycans synthesis [39].

Palmitoyl tripeptide-3/5 (Syn®-Coll) is a synthetic signal peptide. Thrombospondin-I is a protein that binds to tissue growth factor beta (TGF-β) and makes it biologically inactive. Syn®-Coll mimics Thrombospondin-I tripeptide sequence to activate TGF-β. Therefore, it promotes collagen formation via TGF-β [40]. In a

Table 1 Search strategy

Target of search	Search strategy
To locate all potentially used topical peptides for this indication	("peptide"/exp OR "decapeptide" OR "tripeptide"/exp OR "octapeptide"/exp OR "oligopeptide"/exp OR "pentapeptide"/exp OR "ghk" OR "ghk cu" OR "iamin" OR "ghl" OR "gsh"/exp OR "gsh cu" OR "neova" OR "complex cu3" OR "biopeptide" OR "collagen pentapeptide" OR "manganese tripeptide" OR "egf" OR "igf 1" OR "fgf" OR "growth factor"/exp OR "thiorexidin" OR "growth hormone"/exp OR "hgh"/exp OR "vegf"/exp OR "kgf" OR "tgf" OR "ahk" OR "Argireline" OR "hexapeptide"/exp OR "pal kttks" OR "matrixyl" OR "lipospondin" OR "elaidyl kfk" OR "syn coll" OR "syn ake" OR "syn tacks" OR "tetrapeptide"/exp OR "vialox" OR "fvapfp" OR "vgvapg" OR "leuphasyl" OR "dipeptide"/exp OR "serilesine" OR "decorinyl" OR "eyeseryl" OR "saccharomyces lysate extract" OR "oxy 229-bt" OR "pepha timp" OR "placentol" OR "kinetin"/exp OR "neuropeptide"/exp OR "algae extract"/exp OR "amaranth protein" OR "fnk protein" OR "gelatin protein" OR "keratin protein" OR "elastin protein" OR "collagen protein" OR "rh sod" OR "superoxide dismutase"/exp OR "bovine albumin"/exp OR "pep-1 ribosomal protein" OR "pl 14736" OR "skin respiratory factor" OR "becaplermin"/exp OR "psp"/exp OR "etaf" OR "tns" OR "glutathione"/exp OR "secma" OR "ctp complex" OR "soy protein"/exp OR "wheat protein" OR "oat protein" OR "rice protein" OR "corn protein" OR "vegetable protein"/exp OR "milk protein"/exp OR "silk protein" OR "yeast extract"/exp OR "honey protein" OR "revitalin" OR "immucell" OR "sericin"/exp OR "lipeptide" OR "elhibin" OR "colhibin" OR Hsp70 OR "heat shock protein" OR melatonin OR MSH OR "aquaporin" OR "pyratine 6" OR "AcTP" OR "pal kt" OR "snap 8")
To locate all topical therapies	AND ("topical"/exp OR "skin"/exp OR cutaneous)
To locate all cosmeceutical indications	AND (cosmetic* OR cosmeceutical* OR hydrat* OR ("hair growth"/exp OR "hair growth") OR ("hair loss"/exp OR "hair loss") OR moistur* OR ("aged"/exp OR "aged") OR ("aging"/exp OR "aging") OR ("elderly"/exp OR "elderly") OR senile OR photoaged OR photodamaged OR firm* OR lift* OR "conditioner" OR "hair conditioning" OR "skin repair" OR ("rejuvenation"/exp OR "rejuvenation") OR "antiwrinkle" OR "hair remover" OR tightening OR "hair care" OR "scalp care" OR lightening)
Alternative search strategy obtained from EMBASE EMTREE	OR (("skin"/exp OR "skin") OR ("skin care"/exp OR "skin care") OR ("cutaneous parameters"/exp OR "cutaneous parameters") OR ("cosmetic"/exp OR "cosmetic") AND (("proteomics"/exp OR "proteomics") OR ("peptide"/exp OR "peptide")))
To rule out all irrelevant articles	NOT (melanoma*:ti,ab OR cancer*:ti,ab OR carcino*:ti,ab OR malignan*:ti,ab OR onco*:ti,ab OR neoplas*:ti,ab OR tumor*:ti,ab OR tumor*:ti,ab OR sarcoma*:ti,ab OR lymphoma*:ti,ab OR "c-reactive":ti,ab OR vaccine:ti,ab OR vaccines:ti,ab OR infectio*:ti,ab OR antimicrobial:ti,ab OR psoria*:ti,ab OR pemphig*:ti,ab OR *menopaus*:ti,ab OR replacement:ti,ab OR asthma*:ti,ab OR allerg*:ti OR sclerosis:ti,ab OR vasculitis:ti,ab OR arthritis:ti,ab OR obesity:ti,ab OR tuberculosis:ti,ab OR aortic:ti,ab OR lupus:ti,ab OR scleroderma:ti,ab OR alzheimer*:ti,ab OR "sezary syndrome":ti,ab OR "mycosis fungoides":ti,ab OR hypertens*:ti,ab OR bullous:ti OR onchocerc*:ti,ab OR polyneuropath*:ti,ab OR dialysis:ti,ab OR renal:ti OR kidney:ti OR apoptosis:ti,ab OR orthop*:ti,ab)

controlled trial, 60 healthy volunteers received 2.5 % Syn®-Coll cream versus 10 % palmitoyl pentapeptide-3 cream versus placebo cream twice daily for 84 days. Syn®-Coll significantly decreased average and maximum relief by −22 and −36 μm, respectively, when compared to pal-pentapeptide-3; it showed better significant results for Ra, Rz, and Rt parameters [40].

Tripeptide-10 Citrulline (Decorinyl™) is a peptide with firming effects and mimics the

Table 2 Permeation coefficients (*Kp*) of available relevant peptides

Peptide	Permeation coefficient (cm/s^{-1})
GHK[a]	1.36×10^{-9} [25]
GHK-Cu[a]	1.35×10^{-9} [25]
GSH[a]	8.63×10^{-10} [25]
GSH-Cu[a]	1.5×10^{-9} [25]
Histidine[b]	4.44×10^{-9}, pH = 7.6 [29]
	5.55×10^{-9}, pH = 7.4
Histidine-Cu[a]	$2.72 \times 10^{-6} \pm 0.05 \times 10^{-6}$ [28]
Alanine[b]	1.03×10^{-8}, pH = 6.0 [29]
	1.53×10^{-8}, pH = 7.4
Alanine-Cu[a]	$1.90 \times 10^{-6} \pm 0.16 \times 10^{-6}$ [28]
Lysine[b]	1.08×10^{-7}, pH = 9.8 [29]
	5.83×10^{-9}, pH = 7.4
Lysine-Cu[a]	$1.66 \times 10^{-6} \pm 0.07 \times 10^{-6}$ [28]
Glycine[b]	3.30×10^{-8}, pH = 6.0 [29]
	1.05×10^{-8}, pH = 7.4
Glycine-Cu[a]	$1.62 \times 10^{-6} \pm 0.06 \times 10^{-6}$ [28]
Valine[b]	1.25×10^{-8}, pH = 6.0 [29]
	3.61×10^{-9}, pH = 7.4
Valine-Cu[a]	$1.59 \times 10^{-6} \pm 0.07 \times 10^{-6}$ [28]
α-MSH (hisetal)[b]	1.55×10^{-8} [27]
α-MSH (hisetal)[c]	2.58×10^{-9} [26]
Methionine[b]	4.72×10^{-9}, pH = 5.6 [29]
	8.61×10^{-9}, pH = 7.4
Proline[b]	9.16×10^{-9}, pH = 6.3 [29]
	7.50×10^{-9}, pH = 7.4
Serine[b]	1.00×10^{-8}, pH = 5.6 [29]
	8.33×10^{-9}, pH = 7.4
Threonine[b]	3.27×10^{-8}, pH = 6.2 [29]
	3.61×10^{-9}, pH = 7.4
Isoleucine[b]	1.44×10^{-8}, pH = 6.0 [29]
	3.61×10^{-9}, pH = 7.4
Leucine[b]	4.44×10^{-9}, pH = 6.0 [29]
	8.05×10^{-9}, pH = 7.4
Asparagine[b]	1.14×10^{-8}, pH = 5.4 [29]
	9.72×10^{-9}, pH = 7.4
Aspartic acid[b]	2.38×10^{-8}, pH = 2.8 [29]
	2.22×10^{-9}, pH = 7.4
Glutamine[b]	8.88×10^{-9}, pH = 5.6 [29]
	1.39×10^{-8}, pH = 7.4
Glutamic acid[b]	1.36×10^{-8}, pH = 7.4 [29]
	2.78×10^{-9}, pH = 7.4
Phenylalanine[b]	6.78×10^{-8}, pH = 5.4 [29]
	8.33×10^{-9}, pH = 7.4
Arginine[b]	9.05×10^{-8}, pH = 10.8 [29]
	2.77×10^{-8}, pH = 7.4
Tyrosine[b]	7.22×10^{-9}, pH = 5.6 [29]
	4.44×10^{-9}, pH = 7.4
Tryptophan[b]	5.28×10^{-9}, pH = 5.7 [29]
	4.17×10^{-9}, pH = 7.4
Cysteine[b]	9.44×10^{-9}, pH = 5.2 [29]
	5.28×10^{-9}, pH = 7.4

References given in parenthesis next to the equation
[a]Liposome model membranes were used
[b]Hairless mouse skins were used
[c]Human skin was used

sequences of decorin that binds to collagen fibrils. It also regulates fibrillogenesis and controls fibril growth and their uniformity [41]. Puig et al. [42] presented a single-blind parallel-group-controlled trial comparing 0.01 % liposomal Decorinyl™ and placebo creams. Tripeptide-10 induced a 54 % increase in skin suppleness ($p < 0.001$). No significant changes were seen in placebo group.

Biopeptide-EL, a hydroglycolic solution of pal-val-gly-val-ala-pro-gly, is another peptide with firming effects that upregulates TGF-β expression and increases collagen production [43].

Peptamide-6 (FVAPFP), a firming peptide that is biotechnologically derived from *Saccharomyces* yeast fermentation, increases collagen synthesis and upregulates growth factors, transmembrane, matrix, and cell shock proteins [44]. This peptide was applied onto half-face (periorbital and cheek) of 25 healthy subjects twice daily for 4 weeks. Initial skin elasticity and deformation response were improved at week 4 [44].

Pal-KTTKS (palmitoyl pentapeptide-4), a synthetic signal peptide from procollagen-I fragment, stimulates collagen I, III, and VI, and also fibronectin, elastin, and glycosaminoglycan production [38] and has been frequently used as topical antiaging or antiwrinkle agents. In a study [20] on 93 Caucasian females, Pal-KTTKS had significantly better scores than placebo for expert grader assessment and subject self-assessment of age hyperpigmented spots. Osborne et al. [22] showed a robust result for this peptide in reducing bumpy texture and fine wrinkles compared to other baseline and comparators.

Pal-KT, a palmitoyl dipeptide and shorter form of pal-KTTKS, stimulates collagen I, III, IV, fibronectin, elastin, and glycosaminoglycans proliferation [45].

Palmitoyl VGVAPG is an elastin-derived hexapeptide (pal-val-gly-val-ala-pro-gly) and used as the antiaging agent and moisturizer. It stimulates angiogenesis, skin fibroblast proliferation, and downregulates elastin expression. In addition, it increases DOPA-positive cell number and enhances dendrite formation [46–49].

Hexapeptide-11, synthesized from yeast fermentation and used mainly for antiaging and hair conditioning purposes, upregulates key genes, which are responsible for collagen and important extracellular matrix components production such as hyaluronic acid [50].

SECMA 1® is another synthetic hexapeptide extracted from *green algae of Ulva* and modulates the production of proteoglycans and glycosaminoglycans in human fibroblasts [51].

Aquaporin is a natural peptide that is extracted from *Ajuga turkestanica*. One study [52] showed a significant transepidermal water loss (TEWL) decrease in aquaporin-treated forearms versus untreated forearms (4.8 ± 0.4 vs. 5.4 ± 0.3).

Pauly et al. [53] evaluated two new synthetic peptides: acetyl tetrapeptide-9 (AcTP1) and acetyl tetrapeptide-11 (AcTP2). In vitro study revealed an increase in collagen I and lumican synthesis for AcTP1 and stimulation of keratinocyte cell growth and syndecan-1 synthesis for AcTP2. In vivo study showed significant increase in skin thickness (5 %) and skin firmness (Ur/Uf = 7.5 %) for AcTP1 cream. AcTP1 was also more effective than placebo. AcTP2 had significant effect on biomechanical parameters of the superficial layers of epidermis and 5–10 % better effect than placebo [53].

Growth factors play important role in reversing the aging process on the skin caused by extrinsic and intrinsic factors, although main use of growth factors is in wound healing. Recombinant human growth hormone has mitogenic effect on keratinocytes and fibroblasts [54] and increases IGF-1 and sebum production [55]. Cutaneous wound healing properties were confirmed by two trials on acute wounds [56, 57].

Kinetin (N6-furfuryladenine), first isolated from autoclaved Herring sperm DNA in 1955, was the first identified cytokinin [58, 59]. It is a major signal peptidic growth factor that is naturally derived from plants and has antioxidant properties. Kinetin delays the onset of aging characteristics in human fibroblasts and also inhibits keratinocyte growth [60–62]. It may act directly to be involved in signal transduction and stimulates defense pathways such as DNA repair [63]. Kinetin also acts indirectly as antioxidants [64], preventing the formation of reactive oxygen species, or as a direct free radical scavenger [65]. It increases superoxide dismutase activity in plants [64]. Kinetin's multipotency makes it more appropriate for antiaging purposes [66]. In an in vitro aging study, kinetin solution was applied to young and old human skin fibroblast cell cultures. Cell enlargement, presence of multinucleated giant cells, accumulation of cellular debris and lipofuscin, and changes in actin filaments and microtubules were all attenuated by kinetin [62]. Kinetin's cosmeceutical indication mainly limits to antiaging/antiwrinkle and antisolar purposes. Dorsum of three 10-year-old male hairless hybrid dogs was used to compare 10, 100, 1,000, and 10,000 μM and 2 % kinetin solutions. All concentrations showed significant improvement in skin color, decrease in the thickness of corneal layers, and increase in epidermal thickness [67].

In an uncontrolled study, Katz and Bruck [68] applied 0.1 % kinetin cream on the face and neck of 18 volunteers. At week 24, 55 % of subjects noted mild to moderate improvement. Average number of UV spots decreased from 69 to 43. Mean porphyrin count decreased from 262 to 101. In another uncontrolled study [69], 0.1 % kinetin lotion significantly improved the appearance of skin texture, mottled hyperpigmentation, fine wrinkles, and TEWL parameter.

Ninety-eight volunteers with mild to moderate photodamaged facial skin applied kinetin-containing lotion and creams for 10 weeks in an uncontrolled study. All subjects were evaluated for photodamage parameters. All parameters had

Table 3 Characteristics of peptides and proteins

Peptides and proteins	Alternate/generic names	Source	Peptide type	Mechanism of action	Cosmeceutical uses
Copper tripeptide complex	Copper tripeptide-1 or GHK-Cu or Iamin®	Synthetic	Signal and carrier peptide	Promotes 1. "Extra-large" collagen aggregates degradation – found in scars 2. The more regular collagen synthesis – found in normal skin 3. Elastin, proteoglycans, glycosaminoglycans production 4. Growth rate and migration of different cell types 5. Anti-inflammatory responses 6. Antioxidant responses	Antiaging, antiwrinkle, After-sun products, after skin resurfacing, Skin moisturizer, hair growth stimulator
Manganese tripeptide complex	Manganese tripeptide-1 or GHK-Mn	Synthetic	Signal and carrier peptide	Stimulates 1. matrix protein growth 2. Antioxidant responses 3. Manganese-superoxide dismutase pathway	Antiaging, antiwrinkle
Biopeptide-CL	Pal-GHK	Synthetic	Signal peptide	Stimulates collagen and gylcosaminoglycans synthesis	Antiaging, antiwrinkle, antisolar, firming, skin moisturizer
Syn®-Coll	Palmitoyl tripeptide-3/5	Synthetic	Signal peptide	Mimics thrombospondin I tripeptide sequence and promotes collagen formation	Improves stretch marks, antiwrinkle, skin moisturizer, improves skin's firmness and tone
Biopeptide-EL	Hydroglycolic solution of Pal-val-gly val-val-ala-pro-gly	Synthetic	Signal peptide	Upregulates transforming growth factor beta	Firming peptide and eye contour product, antiaging
Peptamide-6	FVAPFP or phe-val-ala-pro-phe-pro	Biotechnologic (*Saccharomyces* yeast fermentation)	Signal peptide	Increases collagen synthesis, upregulates growth factors, transmembrane, matrix, and cell shock proteins	Firming peptide ideal for all face/body/eye creams, antiaging
Acetyl Tetrapeptide-5	Eyeseryl®	Synthetic	Enzyme inhibitor peptide	Inhibits collagen glycation, increases dose-dependent vascular permeability, prevents liquid accumulation in eye bags and increases skin elasticity	Antiwrinkle, antipuffing, and reduces dark circles around eyes

(*continued*)

Table 3 (continued)

Peptides and proteins	Alternate/generic names	Source	Peptide type	Mechanism of action	Cosmeceutical uses
Acetyl tetrapeptide-9	AcTP1	Synthetic	Signal peptide	Increases collagen I synthesis, Stimulates lumican synthesis	Antiaging, antiwrinkle, firming peptide
Acetyl tetrapeptide-11	AcTP2	Synthetic	Signal peptide	Stimulates keratinocyte cell growth, Stimulates synthesis of syndecan-1	Antiaging, antiwrinkle, firming peptide
Acetyl hexapeptide-3	Argireline® or acetyl hexapeptide-8	Synthetic	Neurotransmitter-inhibitor peptide	Inhibits SNARE complex formation and catecholamine release	Antiwrinkle especially periorbital, skin moisturizer, improves skin's firmness and tone
Acetyl octapeptide-3	SNAP-8 or Acetyl glutamyl heptapeptide-1 or octapeptide	Synthetic	Neurotransmitter-inhibitor peptide	Mimics SNAP-25 N-terminal end which competes with it	Antiwrinkle especially periorbital, skin moisturizer, improves skin's firmness and tone
Pentapeptide-18	Leuphasyl®	Synthetic	Neurotransmitter-inhibitor peptide	Mimics the natural mechanism of enkephalins and inhibits neuronal activity and catecholamine release	Antiwrinkle (periorbital), skin moisturizer, improves skin's firmness and tone
Pentapeptide-3	Vialox®	Synthetic	Neurotransmitter-inhibitor peptide	Competitive antagonist at the acetylcholine receptors	Alternative to Botox®, Antiwrinkle (against expression wrinkles), antiaging
Pal-KTTKS	Palmitoyl pentapeptide-4 or palmitoyl pentapeptide-3 or palmitoyl oligopeptide or Matrixyl®	Synthetic (Pro-collagen I fragment)	Signal peptide	Stimulates collagen I, III, and VI, fibronectin, elastin, and glycosaminoglycans production	Antiaging, antiwrinkle
Pal-KT	Palmitoyl lysine-threonine	Synthetic (Pro-collagen I fragment)	Signal peptide	Stimulates collagen I, III, IV, fibronectin, elastin, and glycosaminoglycans production	Antiaging, antiwrinkle
Palmitoyl VGVAPG	Palmitoyl elastin-derived hexapeptide, Pal-val-gly-val-ala-pro-gly	Synthetic (elastin hexapeptide fragment)	Signal peptide	Stimulates angiogenesis, skin fibroblast proliferation and downregulates elastin expression. Induces DOPA-positive cell number and enhanced dendrite formation	Antiaging, skin moisturizer and smoother
Tripeptide-10 Citrulline	Decorin-like tetrapeptide (Decorinyl™)	Synthetic	Signal peptide	Regulates collagen fibrillogenesis and influences diameter and placement of collagen fibers	Antiaging, firming agent

Hexapeptide-11	–	Biotechnologic (yeast fermentation)	Signal peptide	Upregulates key genes responsible for collagen production and important extracellular matrix components	Antiaging, hair conditioner, hair growth promoter
Elaidyl -KFK	Lipospondin or elaidyl-lys-phe-lys	Synthetic	Signal peptide	Upregulates collagen and tissue inhibitor of metalloproteinase (TIMP)-1 production and downregulates MMP-1 in fibroblast cultures	Antiaging, antiwrinkle
SECMA 1®	Glu-Asp-Arg-Leu-Lys-Pro	Synthetic (green algae of *Ulva*)	Signal peptide	Modulates the production of proteoglycans and glycosaminoglycans in human fibroblasts	Antiaging, antiwrinkle
Human growth hormone	hGH	Biotechnologic (recombinant)	Signal peptide	Increased IGF-1 production, fibroblast and keratinocyte activity, and sebum production	Antiaging, antiwrinkle, after skin resurfacing
Transforming growth factors	TGF-α and TGF-β	Biotechnologic (recombinant)	Signal peptide	Reversibly inhibits keratinocytes and leukocytes growth, promotes keratinocyte migration, chemotactic for macrophages and fibroblasts	Anti-photoaging, antiwrinkle, post-laser uses
Interferon alpha	IFN-α	Biotechnologic (recombinant)	Signal peptide	Increases the concentration of dendritic cells and CD1a and HLA-DR positive cells	Antiaging, antiwrinkle
Melatonin	*N*-acetyl-5-methoxytryptamine OR MSH	Biotechnologic (recombinant)	Antioxidant and signal peptide	Reduces the oxidative damage and increases cell viability in fibroblasts	Antiaging, antisolar, hair growth promoter
Heat shock protein (70)	HSP70	Biotechnologic (recombinant)	Signal peptide	Protects the cells against apoptosis, aging, and UV damage	Antiaging, antiwrinkle
Syn®-Tacks	Palmitoyl dipeptide-5 diaminobutyloyl hydroxythreonine, palmitoyl dipeptide-6 diaminohydroxybutyrate	Synthetic	Signal peptide	Stimulates Laminin V, collagen type IV, VII, and XVII and integrin	Antiaging and antiwrinkle, firming product, sun-care products
Syn®-Ake	Tripeptide-3 or dipeptide diaminobutyroyl benzylamide diacetate	Synthetic	Neurotransmitter-inhibitor peptide	Mimics the effect of *Waglerin 1*, a peptide that is found in the venom of the Temple Viper, *Tropidolaemus wagleri*	Antiaging, intensive antiwrinkles
Soybean protein/amino acids	Glycine soja protein or Preregen®	Natural (soybean seed)	Enzyme inhibitor peptide	Inhibits the formation of proteinases, increases trichoblast and atrichoblast numbers without changing their localization pattern, increased the number and length of the root hairs	Antiaging, skin moisturizer, used in cleansing detergents, sensitive skin care, antisolar, regenerating effect. Hair-promoting agent

(*continued*)

Table 3 (continued)

Peptides and proteins	Alternate/generic names	Source	Peptide type	Mechanism of action	Cosmeceutical uses
Keratin proteins/amino acids	Keramino 25®	Natural (human hair and sheep's wool)	Structural peptide	Improves hydration and elasticity of the skin and hair	Skin and hair moisturizer, firming agent, hair shiner
Rice protein/ amino acids	Colhibin®	Natural (rice seed)	Enzyme inhibitor peptide	Inhibits MMP activity and induces expression of hyaluronan synthase 2 gene in keratinocytes	Antiaging, film-former, hair conditioner, skin moisturizer, antisolar
Kinetin	N6-furfuryladenine	Natural (plant-derived growth hormone)	Antioxidant and signal peptide	Delays the onset of aging characteristics in human fibroblasts. Inhibits keratinocyte growth	Antiwrinkle, antiaging, antisolar
Pyratine 6	N6-furfurylaminotetra-hydropyranyladenine	Synthesized from natural plants	Antioxidant and signal peptide	Has anti-ROS, and antisenescence effects on the growth of human skin cells	Antiwrinkle, antiaging, antisolar
Decorinyl™	Tripeptide-10 citrulline	Synthetic	Signal peptide	Mimics the sequences of decorin that bind to collagen fibrils. Regulates fibrillogenesis and control fibril growth and their uniformity	Antiwrinkle, increases skin suppleness and tone
Silk protein	Sericin	Natural (middle silk gland of the silkworm *Bombyx mori)*	Antioxidant, enzyme inhibitor protein, copper chelator protein	Chelates with copper, inhibits lipid peroxidation and tyrosinase activity and keratinocyte apoptosis	Antiaging, antiwrinkle, skin moisturizer
PEP-1-rpS3 fusion protein	–	Biotechnologic (Recombinant)	Signal protein	Increases epidermal cells viability and reduces DNA lesions in UV-exposed areas	Antiaging, antiwrinkle
Aquaporin	AQP	Natural (extracted from *Ajuga turkestanica*)	Signal protein	Increases epidermal proliferation and differentiation. Makes stratum corneum thicker	Antiaging, antiwrinkle, skin moisturizer

TIMP-1 tissue inhibitor of metalloproteinase 1, *MMP-1* matrix metalloproteinase 1, *IGF* Insulin growth factor, *ROS* reactive oxygen species, *rpS3* ribosomal protein S3, *SNARE* soluble *N*-ethylmaleimide-sensitive factor attachment protein receptors

significant improvement and best results were seen in texture, skin clarity, discrete and mottled pigmentation, fine wrinkling, and global appearance. No significant side effect was detected [70].

In a randomized double-blind 12-week trial [71], kinetin was compared to retinol-containing lotion. Both lotions made significant improvements for all outcomes. Kinetin produced better results in texture and clarity. Chiu et al. [72] – in another randomized double-blind study – compared topical kinetin plus niacinamide to niacinamide only and found significant reductions in spot, pore, wrinkle, and erythema index and evenness counts in kinetin group. Furthermore, significant increases in corneal hydration status were found in the same group.

In an unpublished data by Almay Research [70], nine kinetin-containing products were tested in 200 volunteers and no notable irritation was noted. Another unpublished study (Ivy Research laboratory, Philadelphia, PA) [70] did not find any significant adverse event.

Pyratine-6 has similar chemical structure to kinetin. It has modulatory, antireactive oxygen species (anti-ROS) and antisenescence effects on the growth of human skin cells [73]. Antiaging effects of Pyratine-6 was evaluated in an uncontrolled study. Fine wrinkles, roughness, mottled hyperpigmentation, TEWL, and moisture were all significantly improved at weeks 4 and 8. At week 12, everything improved except the number of wrinkles and mottled hyperpigmentation that were slightly higher than week 8 [73].

Melatonin, a peptide hormone that is secreted by pineal gland of mammals, has effects on day and night rhythm, seasonal rhythm, reproduction, hair growth, immunoregulation, and aging [74, 75]. It also has a highly lipophilic molecular structure facilitating penetration into cell membranes and serving as an extracellular and intracellular free radical scavenger. Melatonin seems to quench mainly hydroxyl radicals – the most damaging of all free radicals – and can protect cells against photoinduced oxidative stress [76, 77]. Melatonin diminishes the oxidative damage in the skin in disturbances of heme metabolism in porphyria [78]. It is able to increase cell viability in fibroblasts challenged by UVB irradiation and ionizing irradiation [79, 80]. Melatonin had a 17-fold more powerful antioxidant properties than control group [81]. It has the strongest radical suppressive potency when compared to vitamin C and trolox [82].

Topical melatonin in a noncolloid gel was applied on the back of healthy subjects. Melatonin suppressed UV erythema 24 h after exposure [83]. Melatonin has the potential to be applied as an active component of antiaging and antisolar products.

Interferon alpha increases the concentration of dendritic cells and CD1a and HLA-DR-positive cells [84, 85]. Ghersetich and Lotti [85] conducted a before-after study with three different inclusion protocols: five individuals aged 18–21 years, five aged 57–75 years, and five underwent cycles of PUVA therapy over a year and aged 30–45 years. Alpha-interferon cream (2,000,000 IU/day) in carboxymethylcellulose and glycerin was applied on periauricular area three times a day for 4 weeks. Counts for cells that expressed CD-1 and HLA-DR were significant compared to baseline only for aged and PUVA-exposed volunteers (5 ± 1.75 vs. 10 ± 4.47 and 6 ± 3.18 vs. 16 ± 2.15 for aged group and 4 ± 3.47 vs. 10 ± 3.53 and 3 ± 3.12 vs. 14 ± 1.75 for PUVA group, respectively).

Transforming growth factor α and β are recombinant growth factors that reversibly inhibit keratinocytes and leukocytes growth, promote keratinocyte migration, chemotactic for macrophages and fibroblasts [86–88]. Among major growth factors, tumor growth factor (TGF) α has the highest human keratinocyte pro-motility activity, reaching nearly 80 % of the activity in serum [87].

Several growth factors and cytokines have been applied to treat aging skin problems. Cell rejuvenation serum (CRS) contains liposome-encapsulated TGF-β1, ascorbic acid, and *Cimicifuga racemosa extract* in a silicone base. Rao et al. in an open-label uncontrolled pilot study [89] investigated the effects of 3-month CRS therapy on facial skin. Seven (58 %) participants saw improvement in their skin texture. This finding

Table 4 Efficacy data

Peptides	Study ID	Indication of topical use	Study design	Characteristics of subjects	Treatment arm(s)	Treatment protocol	Efficacy
Biotinyl-GHK	[38]	Skin conditioning (antiaging)	Ex vivo study	Ex vivo cell culture model containing dermal and epidermal cells	Biotinyl-GHK vs. control group	The solutions were applied to the cell culture	Biotinyl-GHK but not control solution stimulates collagen IV and laminin production and keratinocyte mitosis
GHK-Cu	[133]	Skin conditioning (antiaging)	Nonrandomized, active-controlled, clinical trial	Volunteer females	GHK-Cu-containing liquid foundation and GHK-Cu-containing cream concealer	Formulations were applied for 8 weeks	Sig. improvements in all evaluations of skin condition were found for both products
	[134]	Antiaging	Double-blind placebo-controlled clinical trial	71 Female volunteers with mild to advanced photodamage	GHK-Cu cream vs. placebo cream	The creams were applied on the faces twice daily for 12 weeks	Sig. improvements for GHK-Cu than placebo for all measurements by week 4
	[136]	Antiaging (periorbital)	Double-blind placebo-controlled clinical trial	41 Female volunteers with mild to advanced photodamage	GHK-Cu cream vs. Vitamin K cream	The creams were applied around the eyes twice daily for 12 weeks	Sig. improvements for GHK-Cu than placebo for all measurements by week 4
	[135]	Antiaging	Randomized, double-blind, parallel-group, placebo-controlled clinical trial	67 Female volunteers aged 50–59 with mild to advanced photodamage	GHK-Cu cream vs. placebo cream	Creams were applied on the face twice daily for 12 weeks	GHK-Cu improved skin laxity, clarity, and appearance, reduced fine lines, coarse wrinkles and mottled hyperpigmentation, and increased skin density and thickness
	[135]	Antiaging	Nonrandomized untreated-controlled clinical trial	5 Female volunteers aged 50–59 with mild to advanced photodamage	GHK-Cu cream vs. no treatment	GHK-Cu cream was applied on the face twice daily for 12 weeks	GHK-Cu strongly stimulated dermal keratinocyte proliferation

	[21]	Antiaging	Nonrandomized active-controlled parallel-group and within-patient clinical trial	20 Healthy volunteers	1. Topical tretinoin 2. Topical Vit C 3. Topical GHK-Cu 4. Topical melatonin	20 Subjects received creams to the extensor surface of thighs for 1 month	In terms of increase of procollagen synthesis, 4/10, 5/10, 5/10, and 7/10 of patients showed response for tretinoin, Vit C, melatonin, and GHK-Cu, respectively
Tripeptide-10	[42]	Antiaging	Single-blind placebo-controlled, parallel-group clinical trial	43 Female volunteers aged 40–58	0.01 % Liposomal Tripeptide-10 citrulline cream vs. placebo cream	The creams were applied on the face (temple) daily for 28 days	Tripeptide-10 induced a sig. increase in skin suppleness. No sig. increase in placebo group
Manganese tripeptide-1	[137]	Antiaging	Uncontrolled, evaluator-blind, clinical trial	15 Female volunteers aged 40–70 with moderate facial photodamage	Manganese peptide complex containing manganese tripeptide-1 serum base	The cream was applied to face and neck twice daily for 12 weeks	Best results in improving hyperpigmentation, but also seen in dryness, sallowness, mottled hyperpigmentation and actinic lentigo
Leuphasyl® vs. Argireline®	Centerchem fact sheet [127]	Antiaging	Active-controlled parallel-group clinical trial	43 Healthy female volunteers aged 39–64	Cream containing 5 % LEUPHASYL® solution (0.05 %) vs. cream containing 5 % ARGIRELINE® solution (0.05 %) vs. Combination	Each cream was applied twice daily around the eyes of 14 volunteers for 28 days	Mean wrinkle reductions were 11.64 % vs. 16.26 % vs. 24.62 % for Leuphasyl®, Argireline®, and combination, respectively

(*continued*)

Table 4 (continued)

Peptides	Study ID	Indication of topical use	Study design	Characteristics of subjects	Treatment arm(s)	Treatment protocol	Efficacy
Lipopentapeptide	[95]	Antiaging	Randomized active-controlled	Nine healthy photoaged volunteers (2 men and 7 women; aged 42–79)	6 % vs. 2 % Total active complex cream (lipopentapeptide, white lupin peptide, antioxidants); untreated sites have given Retin-A	Substances were patch tested separately to the extensor aspect of forearm on days 1, 4, and 8. Patch tests were removed on day 12	6 % Formula significantly increased fibrillin-1 and procollagen I deposition. Retin-A and 6 % complex were the best triggers for fibrillin-1 and procollagen I deposition, respectively
Peptamide®6	Arch personal care products technical sheet [44]	Antiaging (periorbital)	Placebo-controlled, within-patient clinical trial	25 Healthy volunteers	2.80 % Peptamide® 6 firming toner vs. control toner	Each cream was applied to half-face (periorbital and cheek) twice daily for 4 weeks	Initial skin elasticity and deformation response were improved at week 4
Pal-KTTKS	[20]	Antiaging	Randomized, double-blind, placebo-controlled, within-patient trial	93 Caucasian female volunteers aged 35–55	Pal-KTTKS oil-in-water moisturizer vs. placebo oil-in-water moisturizer	Each formulation was applied to the half-face skin twice daily for 12 weeks	Sig. better scores for expert grader assessment and subject self-assessment in age spots
	[22]	Antiaging	Randomized double-blind active-vehicle-controlled, within-patient round-robin clinical trial	180 Female volunteers aged 35–65	Pal-KTTKS facial moisturizer vs. Boswellia Serrata extract vs. moisturizer base (vehicle)	Each formulation was applied to the randomly selected half-face skin twice daily for 8 weeks	Pal-KTTKS made sig. reduction in bumpy texture and fine lines/wrinkles compared to other comparators and baseline
Acetyl tetrapeptide-9 (AcTP1)	[53]	Antiaging	Placebo-controlled clinical trial	17 Healthy female volunteers aged 45–55 with loss of elasticity on the forearms	3 % Cream containing AcTP1 vs. cream containing placebo	The creams were applied twice daily for 112 days	Sig. increase in skin thickness and firmness for active cream. AcTP1 was more effective than placebo too

Acetyl tetrapeptide-11 (AcTP2)	[53]	Antiaging	Placebo-controlled clinical trial	19 Healthy female volunteers aged 60–70 with loss of elasticity on the forearms	3 % Cream containing AcTP2 vs. Cream containing placebo	The creams were applied twice daily for 112 days	Sig. increase in biomechanical parameters of the superficial layers of epidermis was observed for active cream. AcTP2 had 5–10 % better effect than placebo
Acetyl tetrapeptide (Eyeseryl®)	[119]	Antiaging	Uncontrolled clinical trial	20 Female volunteers aged 18–65	10 % Eyeseryl® solution in cream base	The cream was applied under the eyes twice daily for 60 days	Puffy eye bag reduction in 14 days. 30 % increase in skin elasticity after 30 days
	[119]	Antiaging	Uncontrolled clinical trial	17 Female volunteers aged 34–54	1 % Eyeseryl® solution in cream base	The cream was applied under the eyes twice daily for 28 days	Eye bags were reduced in 70 % of volunteers. Sig. but clinically slight lightening effect
Acetyl hexapeptide-3 (Argireline)	[124]	Antiaging	Uncontrolled, open-label trial	14 Volunteers, aged 39–64	Cream containing 5 % Argireline® solution	The cream was applied twice daily around the eyes for 28 days	The depth of the furrow decreased a maximum value of 32 % in 28 days
	[23]	Antiaging	Vehicle-controlled, open-label, trial	10 Healthy women volunteers	O/W emulsion containing 10 % Argireline® solution	Solution was applied twice daily around the eyes during 30 days	Sig. more reduction in the depth of wrinkles for Argireline group
Elaidyl -KFK	[110]	Skin repair	Ex vivo study	Skin tissue section	Elaidyl-KFK solution	Different solutions were applied on skin tissue section	The inhibition of MMP-2 and MMP-9-mediated degradation of collagen fibers and elastin fibers, respectively, by elaidyl-KFK could be demonstrated
Acetyl octapeptide-3 (SNAP-8)	[128]	Antiaging	Uncontrolled open-label clinical trial	17 Healthy female volunteers	Cream containing 10 % of SNAP-8 solution	The cream was applied to periorbital area twice daily for 28 days	Sig. mean wrinkle reduction after 28 days

(*continued*)

Table 4 (continued)

Peptides	Study ID	Indication of topical use	Study design	Characteristics of subjects	Treatment arm(s)	Treatment protocol	Efficacy
Syn®- Ake Vs. Argireline		Antiaging	Placebo-controlled clinical trial	45 Healthy volunteers	4 % Syn®-Ake vs. 10 % acetyl hexapeptide-3 (Argireline®) vs. placebo	Each cream was applied to the skin of forehead twice daily for 28 days	Before-after measurements were sig. for Syn®-Ake only
Syn®-Tacks		Antiaging	Two case reports	2 Healthy volunteers aged 45 and 62.	1 % Syn®-Tacks	Cream was applied to their faces	Improved skin tonicity, skin anisotropy and cellular cohesion
Syn®-Coll	[40]	Antiaging	Active and placebo-controlled, clinical trial	60 Healthy volunteers	2.5 % Syn®-Coll cream vs. 10 % palmitoyl pentapeptide-3 cream vs. placebo cream	Creams were applied to facial skin twice daily for 84 days	Syn®-Coll significantly decrease average and maximum relief; when compared to pal-pentapeptide-3, it showed better sig. results for parameters
Fibronectin-like peptide	[114]	Antiaging	Randomized, double-blind, placebo-controlled, parallel-group trial	24 Healthy volunteers	1 % Fibronectin-like peptide cream vs. placebo cream	Creams were applied to lips once and evaluations occurred 1 and 3 h after application	Sig. improve in hydration, and smoothness in active group were seen
	[114]	Antiaging	Randomized, double-blind, placebo-controlled, within-patient trial	12 Healthy volunteers	1 % Fibronectin-like peptide cream vs. placebo cream	Each cream was applied to back of hands twice daily for 7 days	Increased smoothness and lightening effects, and skin appearance were noticed
Soy extract	[116]	Antiaging	Randomized, double-blind, placebo-controlled, within-patient trial	21 Healthy females (55 ± 6 years) with skin types of II and III	2 % Soy extract cream vs. placebo cream	Each cream was applied to volar forearm twice daily for 2 weeks	Papillae index was more increased by soy extract than placebo

	[117]	Antiaging	>Pseudo-randomized, volunteer-blind, within-patient trial	10 Healthy Caucasian females aged between 42 and 67	2 % *Soya biopeptide* emulsion vs. placebo emulsion	Control emulsion was applied to left side of the face and soya emulsion to right side twice daily for 4 weeks	Collagen and glycosaminoglycan contents were significantly stimulated by soya extract vs. placebo
Silk protein vs. Bovine serum albumin (BSA)	[122]	Antiaging and antitumor	Randomized active- and vehicle-controlled three-arm clinical trial	Thirty 4-week-old female Hos:HR-1 UVB-exposed hairless mice (three groups of five mice)	Single doses of 5-mg silk protein in 0.2 ml ethanol vs. 5-mg BSA in 0.2 ml ethanol vs. 0.2 ml ethanol	Each treatment group received its solution immediately after single application of 180 mJ/cm^2 UVB treatment	Silk protein significantly inhibited UVB-induced elevation and elevated expression of COX-2 protein more than BSA and vehicle
	[122]	Antiaging and antitumor	Randomized active- and vehicle-controlled three-arm clinical trial	Thirty 4-week-old female Hos:HR-1 UVB-exposed hairless mice (three groups of five mice)	5-mg silk protein in 0.2 ml ethanol vs. 5-mg BSA in 0.2 ml ethanol vs. 0.2 ml ethanol	Each treatment group received its solution immediately after 180 mJ/cm^2 of UVB treatment daily for 7 days	Silk protein significantly inhibited skin lesion formation and UVB-induced elevation and elevated expression of COX-2 protein more than BSA and vehicle
Silk protein	[120]	Skin moisturizer	Untreated-controlled within-patient clinical trial	6 Healthy human volunteers of both sexes (three men and three women) aged 22–25	0.2 g Sericin gel vs. no treatment	For hydroxyproline assay, Sericin gel (0.2 g) was applied on the dried skin of the forearm at the test site. For TEWL, the upper portion of forearm was used as the site for application of Sericin gel (0.2 g) and lower portion for control	No sig. difference in hydroxyproline content, skin impedance and TEWL content were seen; comparing silk peptides and untreated site
	[121]	Skin moisturizer	Active- and untreated-controlled	6 Healthy volunteers	1 % Fibrion vs. 3 % fibroin vs. 5 % fibroin vs. 5 % silk-Pro-100 solutions	1 ml of each solution was applied to inner upper portion of the forearm for 15 min	For TEWL, 5 % firoin solution-Silk-pro-100 > 1 % and 3 % fibroin solutions. Sig. drop in

(*continued*)

Table 4 (continued)

Peptides	Study ID	Indication of topical use	Study design	Characteristics of subjects	Treatment arm(s)	Treatment protocol	Efficacy
			within-patient clinical trial			and lower portion was left untreated as control (for impedance measurement, only 5 % solution were compared)	impedance was observed for both 5 % solutions within 1 h
Keratin peptide	[113]	Skin moisturizer	Randomized active- and placebo-controlled within-patient clinical trial	6 Healthy Caucasian female volunteers phototype III-IV, aged 24–36	Keratin peptide aqueous solution vs. keratin peptide liposome solution vs. IWL liposomes vs. water vs. 0.9 % NaCl solution	Each cream were applied onto marked areas of 9 cm^2 once a day for 4 days	Sig. differences of skin capacitance and elasticity parameters for keratin samples. Combination of keratin peptide with the IWL liposomes showed a sig. beneficial effect
	[112]	Skin moisturizer	Randomized placebo- and untreated-controlled, within-patient, clinical trial	16 Healthy female volunteers aged 24–50 with skin types of III-V	3 % Keratin peptide vs. 3 % deionized water in base cream vs. untreatment	Each cream was applied to a 9 cm^2 area of hand once a day for 12 days	Insignificant difference between topical therapies; although keratin was insignificantly effective for dry. Elasticity results were significantly better for it
	[112]	Skin moisturizer	Randomized placebo- and untreated-controlled, within-patient, clinical trial	9 Healthy female volunteers aged 24–50 with dry skin types of III-V	3 % Keratin peptide vs. 3 % deionized water in base cream vs. untreatment	The treated areas were exposed to 2 % sodium lauryl sulfate for 2 h to after 12-day daily application of each cream to a randomly assigned 9 cm^2 area of hand	There was a significantly smaller decrease in hydration for keratin peptide cream in terms of skin capacitance and TEWL

Aquaporins (protein)	[52]	Skin moisturizer	Untreated-controlled, within-patient, trial	15 Healthy female volunteers aged 22–56	*Ajuga turkestanica* extract formulated in a complex oil–water emulsion	The emulsion was applied to forearm skin twice daily for 21 days	Sig. TEWL decrease in treated site vs. untreated site (4.8 ± 0.4 vs. 5.4 ± 0.3)
PEP-1-rpS3 fusion protein	[111]	Antiaging, antitumor	In vivo study	Male ICR mice weighing about 30 g	Transductions of PEP-1-rpS3 fusion protein	50 μg PEP-1-rpS3 fusion proteins were topically applied to the shaved area of the animal skin for various time intervals	Transduced PEP-1-rpS3 fusion protein, time- and dose-dependently, efficiently protects against UV-induced DNA damage
Growth factors							
TNS	[91]	Antiaging (periorbital)	Uncontrolled, open-label trial	14 Individuals with at least Fitzpatrick class II facial photodamage	TNS cream	The cream was applied to the entire facial skin twice daily for 2 months	Best results in periorbital area, 30 % general average increase in epidermal thickness (especially Grenz zone), 8 (57 %) of patients accepted improvements in wrinkles
CRS	[89]	Antiaging	Uncontrolled, open-label, assessor-blind trial	12 Healthy females (mean age, 50 years) with facial wrinkling	CRS cream	The cream was applied to the entire facial skin twice daily for 3 months	Sig. patient-assessed and physician-assessed improvement
	[90]	Antiaging	Randomized, active-controlled, within-patient, assessor-blind, pilot	12 Healthy females with facial wrinkles (42–74 years of age)	CRS cream vs. same cream without TGF-β1 component (vitamin C base)	Each cream was applied twice daily for 3 months	Sig. improvement in wrinkle scores for CRS and nonsig. for Vit C
CRS Vs. TNS	[90]	Antiaging	Randomized, active-controlled, within-patient, assessor-blind, study	20 Healthy females with facial wrinkles (29–74 years of age)	CRS cream vs. TNS cream	Each cream was applied twice daily for 3 months	Sig. improvement in wrinkle score for CRS and nonsig. for Vit C

(*continued*)

Table 4 (continued)

Peptides	Study ID	Indication of topical use	Study design	Characteristics of subjects	Treatment arm(s)	Treatment protocol	Efficacy
PSP	[92]	Antiaging (periorbital)	Two-center, Uncontrolled, open-label study	20 Caucasian females with at least grade 2 Rao-Goldman's 5-point wrinkle scale (35–65 years of age)	PSP cream	The cream was applied to the randomly selected half-face skin twice daily for 2 months	17 %, 13 %, and 17 % wrinkle improvement in periorbital, perioral, and chin areas, respectively. Patients reported 9 % and 17 % decrease in periorbital and perioral wrinkles
	[94]	Antiaging	Two-center, randomized, double-blind, placebo-controlled, within-patient trial	20 Caucasian females with demonstrable facial wrinkles (35–65 years of age)	PSP cream vs. its physically identical placebo cream	Each cream was applied to the half-face skin twice daily for 2 months	Roughness parameters were significantly better in PSP group. No difference between two groups
	[93]	Antiaging (periorbital)	Four-center, Uncontrolled open-label trial	40 Female volunteers with demonstrable fine or deep wrinkles around both eyes (35–65 years of age)	PSP containing eye cream	The cream was applied to half-face twice daily for 6 weeks	PSP improved physician-assessed parameters. Subjects reported sig. improvement of all parameters except for infraorbital puffiness
Melatonin	[83]	Antiaging, antitumor	Randomized double-blind, placebo-controlled, within-patient, clinical trial	20 Healthy volunteers aged 22–33	50 µl Topical melatonin (0.6 mg/cm^2) vs. 50 µl topical vehicle	Creams were applied on 12 test sites; either 15 min before UV irradiation, or 240 min after irradiation	Best results for melatonin serum application before irradiation
Kinetin (cytokine)	[67]	Antiaging	Nonrandomized, open-label, vehicle-controlled, within-patient study	Three 10-year-old male hairless hybrid dogs	10, 100, 1,000, and 10,000 µM and 2 % kinetin solutions	Dorsum of each dog was divided into ten blocks: five of them for different kinetin concentrations and the other five as control for 50 days	All concentrations showed sig. improvement in skin color and decrease in the thickness of corneal layers and

							increase in epidermal thickness
	[69]	Antiaging	Uncontrolled open-label clinical trial	32 Healthy volunteers with mildly to moderately photodamaged facial skin	Kinetin (N6-furfuryladenine) 0.1 % lotion	The cream was applied onto the face twice daily for 24 weeks	Treatments lasting 12 and 24 weeks improved the appearance of skin texture, mottled hyperpigmentation, TEWL parameter, and fine wrinkles
	[68]	Antiaging	Uncontrolled open-label clinical trial	18 Patients with mild to moderate photodamaged skin aged 21–64	0.1 % Kinetin cream	The cream was applied to face and neck of patients twice daily for up to 24 weeks	At week 24, 55 % of subjects noted mild to moderate improvement. Average number of UV spots decreased from 69 to 43. Mean porphyrin count decreased from 262 to 101
	[71]	Antiaging	Randomized, double-blind, active-controlled, within-patient clinical trial	40 Female subjects aged 22–57	Kinetin-containing lotion vs. retinol-containing lotion	Creams were applied to the face twice daily for 12 weeks	Improvement in major parameters with both preparations at week 12
	Revlon research, unpublished data [70]	Antiaging	Uncontrolled clinical trial	98 Healthy volunteers	Kinetin-containing lotion and cream	The cream was applied to the face twice daily for 10 weeks	Best results in texture, skin clarity, pigmentation, fine wrinkling, and global appearance
Kinetin (cytokine) plus niacinamide	[72]	Antiaging	Randomized, double-blind, placebo-controlled, within-patient clinical trial	52 Healthy Taiwanese female and male subjects (age 30–60; 90 % female)	Aqueous serum containing kinetin 0.03 % plus niacinamide 4 % vs. aqueous serum containing only niacinamide 4 %	Each cream was applied to one side of the face daily for 12 weeks	Sig. reductions in spot, pore, wrinkle, erythema index and evenness counts and also sig. increase in corneal hydration status in Kinetin group

(*continued*)

Table 4 (continued)

Peptides	Study ID	Indication of topical use	Study design	Characteristics of subjects	Treatment arm(s)	Treatment protocol	Efficacy
Pyratine-6	[73]	Antiaging	Uncontrolled clinical trial	40 Healthy female volunteers aged 30–65 with skin type of I-III, and with mild to moderate signs of photodamaged facial skin	Pyratine 6 cream	The cream was applied onto the face of patients twice daily (early morning and 1 h before bedtime) for 12 consecutive weeks	All outcomes were significantly improved at weeks 4 and 8. At week 12, everything improved except number of wrinkles and mottled hyperpigmentation
Alpha-interferon	[85]	Antiaging	Before-after study with three inclusion protocols	15 Volunteers who experienced a periauricular area surgery (5 aged 18–21, 5 aged 57–75, and 5 underwent cycles of PUVA therapy over a year and aged 30–45)	Alpha-interferon cream (2,000,000 IU/day) in carboxymethylcellulose and glycerin	The cream was applied on periauricular area three times a day for 4 weeks	Expressed CD-1 and HLA-DR cell counts were sig. compared to baseline for aged and PUVA-exposed volunteers
Hsp70	[109]	Antiaging	Before-after studies with two inclusion protocols	10 Healthy volunteers aged 50–70	Artemia extract	Artemia extract was applied to half of subjects before UV exposure	Sig. effect of Artemia extract on Hsp70 expression of aged skin
				5 Healthy volunteers aged 31–40			

L: luminance, ITA: individual typological angle, CRS: cell rejuvenation serum, PSP: processed skin-cell proteins, Sig.: significant, RZmax: R3Z: RZISO, TNS: tissue nutrient solution recovery complex, Ra: average roughness, Rt: maximum difference between the highest peak and the deepest furrows, Rz: mean value of these different maxima

*In this study they provided a nontreatment control but did not mention the baseline and final results of that untreated half-face

was confirmed by four "blinded" dermatologists. In another trial [90], topical CRS was compared to placebo without TGF-β1 component to define the additive effect of TGF-β. TGF-β1 containing arm had 21.7 % significant mean improvement in physician-rated wrinkle score and the other arm had 6.2 % improvement ($p > 0.05$) compared to baseline. This trial [90] continued to compare topical CRS to another cream named TNS in 20 patients. TNS contains growth factors including VEGF, PDGF-A, G-CSF, HGF, IL-6, IL-8, and TGF-β1 without vitamin C. The results revealed that both creams produced significant improvement in wrinkle score.

Fitzpatrick and Rostan [91] conducted a pilot study on TNS cream and found best results in periorbital area (12.2 % improvement). They also reported 30 % general average increase in epidermal thickness, especially Grenz zone. Eight (57 %) patients accepted improvements in wrinkles.

Bio-restorative skin cream contains processed skin-cell proteins (PSP), a proprietary growth factor, and cytokine mixture extracted from cultured first trimester fetal human dermal fibroblasts in a moisturizing cream. Gold et al. [92] performed a study in two centers with open-label, uncontrolled design to evaluate antiaging effects of PSP cream. Periorbital and chin areas were reached to the best results (17 % physician-rated wrinkle improvement for each). Patients reported 9 % and 17 % decrease in periorbital and perioral wrinkles, respectively. In another uncontrolled study [93], 40 females with demonstrable fine or deep wrinkles around both eyes were given PSP containing eye cream to apply for 6 weeks. PSP cream improved periorbital wrinkles, dark circles, firmness, and texture significantly (14 %, 15 %, 26 %, and 28 %, respectively). Subjects reported significant improvement of all parameters except infraorbital puffiness. In a randomized placebo-controlled trial [94], Gold and colleagues concluded that some skin roughness parameters were significantly improved more in PSP group when compared to baseline, but no statistical difference between two groups was detected.

Lipopentapeptide, in combination with white lupin peptide and antioxidants, had significant effect on increasing fibrillin-1 and procollagen I deposition at a concentration of 6 %. It was also the best trigger for procollagen I deposition when compared to 2 % concentration of Retin-A and also untreated areas [95].

Heat shock proteins represent one of the principal mechanisms of cell defense and protection from stress. Among its family, Hsp70 has protective effects against UV, apoptosis, and ischemia and is recommended for wound healing and antiaging uses [96]. Hsp70 can effectively inhibit aggregation and assist in the refolding of denatured proteins. It can reduce cellular damage by retaining the damaged proteins in soluble form, as well as by binding to unfolded or misfolded proteins to assist in their proper refolding [96]. Hsp70 can be biotechnologically synthesized from yeasts [97]. Studies on both cultured human epidermal cells and ex vivo skin showed that induction or administration of Hsp70 prior to stress significantly diminished UV-related morphological changes and sunburn cell number [97–99]. It can also modulate inflammatory cytokine synthesis and reduce UV-induced inflammatory responses [100]. Hsp70 was proved to be able to block apoptosis by inhibiting signaling events upstream of SAPK/JNK activation [101, 102]. Aging alters the ability of cells to express Hsp70 in response to stress and any Hsp70 induction or application can reverse the process [102–108].

Generally, studies [103–109] showed that although aged skin exhibits a normal level of Hsp70 under nonstressful conditions, it fails to produce the typical protective Hsp70 increase, comparing to younger skin when exposed to UV. To sum up, Hsp70 can act against UV exposure especially in aged skin.

Lipospondin or elaidyl-KFK is a combination of elaidic acid and a tripeptide. It upregulates collagen and tissue inhibitor of metalloproteinase (TIMP)-1 production and downregulates matrix metalloproteinase 1 (MMP-1) production and activity in fibroblast cultures [110]. Different elaidyl-KFK solutions were applied on skin tissue section to evaluate its skin-repair abilities. Elaidyl-KFK inhibits degradation of collagen fibers and elastin fibers by MMP-2 and MMP-9, respectively [110].

PEP-1-rpS3 fusion protein is a recombinant protein, which is formed by conjugation of ribosomal protein S3 (rpS3) and PEP-1 carrier peptide. It increases epidermal cell viability and reduces DNA lesions in UV-exposed areas. Male mice were used to assess antiaging and antitumor properties of this protein. PEP-1-rpS3 protein was effective in protecting the skin against UV-induced damage and this protection was time-dependent and dose-dependent [111].

Keratin is a major protein in the structure of hair and skin that can be extracted from human hair or sheep's wool. Its topical application can improve hydration and elasticity of the skin and hair when applied topically. It is commonly used in skin and hair moisturizers, firming agents, and hair shiners. Barba et al. [112] conducted a randomized trial comparing 3 % keratin peptides to deionized water and untreated control in 16 healthy females. Keratin peptide was effective on disturbed but not undisturbed skin. In another recent trial [113], significant differences were achieved for skin capacitance (especially) and elasticity parameters with application of the keratin samples. Among all keratin-containing creams, a combination of keratin peptide with the internal wood lipid (IWL) liposomes had a significant beneficial effect compared to aqueous solution [113].

In two consecutive double-blind studies, dal Farra et al. [114] investigated the potential antiaging effects of a synthetic fibronectine-like peptide at a concentration of 0.5 % together with a booster molecule at 1 %. Twelve volunteers applied the cream formula containing the active ingredient twice a day on the back of one hand and the placebo on the other hand. Evaluations were performed after 1 h, 3 h, and 7 days. Increased smoothness of skin surface and also lightening effect on the skin were noticed by volunteers at all time points. Volunteers estimated a 40 % improvement on the peptide-treated side 1 h after application. A second study was performed on the lips and included two groups of 12 volunteers each. One group applied the cream formula with the active ingredient, and the other group applied the placebo. Evaluations were made at 1 and 3 h. Significant increase in smoothness, hydration, and repulping effect were mentioned.

Enzyme Inhibitor Peptides

Enzyme inhibitor peptides directly or indirectly inhibit an enzyme. Soybean protein (Soja protein) or peptides, enzyme inhibitor peptides naturally extracted from soybean seeds, inhibit the formation of proteinases, and increases trichoblast and atrichoblast numbers without changing their localization pattern [115]. It is frequently used as an antiaging, skin-moisturizing, antisolar, cleansing detergent, and hair-promoting agent. In a randomized, double-blind, placebo-controlled study [116], soy extract and placebo creams were applied to volar forearm of 21 healthy women. Papillae index was increased more by soy extract than placebo (3.76 vs. 4.56 in arbitrary units, $p < 0.05$). Another study with pseudo-randomized design in ten Caucasian females [117] concluded the superiority of 2 % soya biopeptide emulsion to placebo, in terms of collagen and glycosaminoglycan contents stimulation.

Rice protein/amino acids (Colhibin®) is another natural protein that inhibits MMP activity and induces expression of hyaluronan synthase-2 gene in keratinocytes. Antiaging, film-forming, and hair-conditioning products may contain this protein [118].

Acetyl Tetrapeptide-5 (Eyeseryl®) inhibits collagen glycation and increases dose-dependent vascular permeability and therefore prevents liquid accumulation in eye bags. It also increases skin elasticity. In two separate pharmaceutical-sponsored uncontrolled studies, 1 % and 10 % Eyeseryl® solution in cream base were administered under the eyes twice daily for 28 and 60 days, respectively. For 1 % Eyeseryl® solution, eye bags were reduced in 70 % of volunteers after 28 days, and significant increase in luminance (L*) and individual typological angle (ITA°) values showed slight lightening effect. For 10 % Eyeseryl® solution, puffy eye bag reduction in 14 days was noted in the majority and 30 % increase was reported in skin elasticity after 30 days [119].

Another enzyme inhibitor protein (silk protein, sericin), naturally extracted from middle silk gland of the silkworm *Bombyx mori*, has antioxidant properties with high affinity to chelate with copper. In addition, it inhibits lipid peroxidation and tyrosinase activity and keratinocyte apoptosis. In a within-patient untreated-controlled study [120], 0.2 g sericin gel was compared to untreated site with hydroxyproline assay and TEWL measurement to evaluate its hydrating effect. For hydroxyproline assay, Sericin gel was applied on the dried skin of the forearm at the test site. For TEWL, the upper portion of the forearm was used as the application site of sericin gel and lower portion of the forearm for control. Although hydroxyproline content was slightly promising in all related parameters for sericin, no significant differences in hydroxyproline content, skin impedance, and TEWL contents were seen when compared to no treatment. In another trial by Daithankar et al. [121], silk-protein-100 and different fibroin concentrations were tested. Five percent firoin solution had similar TEWL content to 5 % silk-protein-100 solution but more than 1 % and 3 % fibroin solutions. Significant drop in impedance was observed for both 5 % sericin and 5 % fibroin solutions within 1 h.

Silk protein was compared to bovine serum albumin and vehicle, and the results confirmed its superiority to both serum albumin and vehicle in reducing UVB-induced symptoms in short-term and long-term treatment courses [122].

Neurotransmitter Inhibitor Peptide

Neurotransmitter inhibitor peptides inhibit acetylcholine release at the neuromuscular junction and have curare-like effects. Seven types (A-G) of botulinum toxin target peripheral cholinergic neurons where they selectively proteolyze SNAP-25, syntaxin 1, and synaptobrevin, the soluble *N*-ethylmaleimide-sensitive factor attachment protein receptors (SNARE) responsible for transmitter release, to cause neuromuscular paralysis of different durations. Type A toxin proteolytically degrades SNAP-25, a type of SNARE protein. The SNAP-25 protein is required for the release of neurotransmitters from the axon endings. Botulinum toxin specifically cleaves these SNAREs, and so prevents neurosecretory vesicles from docking and or fusing with the nerve synapse plasma membrane and releasing their neurotransmitters. BXT-A paralysis lasts longest (4–6 months) in botulinum toxin subtypes, which makes it a good choice for antiwrinkle uses.

Researchers have found less invasive topical equivalents of these toxins [123]. Acetyl hexapeptide-3 (Argireline®) is a synthetic peptide that is especially marketed as a component of eye creams and patterned from the N-terminal end of the SNAP-25 protein that inhibits SNARE complex formation and catecholamine release. Inhibition of noradrenaline and adrenaline release was also demonstrated. This small peptide exhibits the great advantage of its insignificant acute toxicity (2,000 mg/kg) as compared to BTX-A (20 ng/kg) [23, 124]. Argireline® inhibits vesicle docking by preventing the ternary SNARE complex formation, which is involved in synaptic vesicle exocytosis [125, 126]. In one open-label trial, the cream containing 5 % Argireline® solution was examined around the eyes of 14 volunteers for 28 days. The depth of the furrow was reduced a maximum value of 32 % on day 28 [124].

Another open-label vehicle-controlled trial, 10 % acetyl hexapeptide-3, and placebo creams were applied twice daily on ten women and demonstrated nearly 30 % versus 10 % improvement in periorbital rhytids after 30 days as measured by silicone replica analysis, respectively [23].

Pentapeptide-18 (Leuphasyl®) mimics the natural mechanism of enkephalins and as a results inhibits neuronal activity and catecholamine release. An active-controlled trial compared the results of the use of a cream containing 5 % leuphasyl® solution (0.05 %), another containing 5 % Argireline® solution (0.05 %), and a combination of both. Mean wrinkle reductions were 11.64 % versus 16.26 % versus 24.62 % for Leuphasyl®, Argireline®, and combination, respectively. This study suggested a synergistic effects between leuphasyl® and Argireline® [127].

Acetyl octapeptide-3 (SNAP-8) is an elongated form of Argireline® with similar effect. It mimics SNAP-25 N-terminal end and competes with it. A cream containing 10 % SNAP-8 solution was applied to periorbital area twice daily for 4 weeks. Mean wrinkle reduction after 28 days was −34.98 % ($p < 0.05$) [128].

Pentapeptide-3 (Vialox®), a synthetic peptide that is a competitive antagonist at the acetylcholine receptors, safely blocks the sodium ion release at the synaptic membrane on muscles, so they cannot contract as frequently. In vitro tests showed muscle contractions reduced by 71 % within 1 min after treatment and 58 % 2 h later. Less frequent muscle contractions result in shallower lines. After 28 days of twice-daily use, wrinkle depth was reduced by 49 % [129].

Tripeptide-3 (Syn®-Ake) is used as an intensive antiwrinkle agent and mimics the effect of Waglerin 1, a peptide that is found in the venom of the temple viper, *Tropidolaemus wagleri*. SYN®-Ake (at a concentration of 0.5 mM) was able to reduce the frequency of innervated muscle cell contractions by 82 % ($p < 0.05$) after 2 h treatment.

In a study on 45 healthy subjects, Syn®-Ake, Argireline®, and placebo were compared. Syn®-Ake clearly showed a remarkable higher efficacy for all tested parameters. Before-after measurements were significant for Syn®-Ake only and not for Argireline®. Best results were seen on the forehead skin by up to 52 % (Parameter Rt) [128]. A high-quality randomized controlled trial is needed to confirm these robust results for Syn®-Ake.

Carrier Peptide

Carrier peptides belong to a general category that acts as a facilitator of an important substance transportation, but their major application is to deliver important trace elements (like copper and manganese) necessary for wound healing and enzymatic processes.

Recently, several peptides and proteins have been developed to accelerate and facilitate the delivery of bioactive molecules into the skin. These peptides and proteins are known as penetrating peptides or membrane transduction peptides and have basic transduction domains in their structure [130]. A study [131] demonstrated that short arginine-rich intracellular delivery peptides facilitate the transport of various proteins into living cells. Hou et al. [131] also investigate whether arginine-rich peptide could serve as carriers for topical and/or transdermal drug delivery and concluded that protein penetration can be stimulated by such peptides even without fusion between carrier peptide and protein. Another example of membrane transduction peptides is PEP-1 that has been mentioned earlier [132]. It facilitated the rpS3 protein's penetration [111].

Abdulghani and coworkers [21] conducted a nonrandomized, four-arm active-controlled trial on 20 participants to compare GHK-Cu to topical tretinoin, vitamin C, and melatonin. Ten subjects received tretinoin and vitamin C creams on the extensor surface of their right and left thighs, respectively, and the other ten subjects received GHK-Cu and melatonin creams to the extensor surface of their right and left thighs, respectively, for 1 month. Tretinoin, vitamin C, melatonin, and GHK-Cu increased procollagen synthesis in 4/10, 5/10, 5/10, and 7/10 of patients, respectively. Appa and colleagues [133] evaluated the efficacy of two cosmetic GHK-Cu-containing formulations for skin conditioning. The skin treatment benefits of a GHK-Cu-containing liquid foundation and cream concealer were evaluated over an 8-week period. Significant improvement in all visual evaluations of skin condition was found within first 2 weeks for both products. The skin's viscoelastic properties significantly improved.

GHK-Cu was tested in a 12-week placebo-controlled study [134] on facial skin of 71 women with mild to advanced photodamage. By week 1, the active cream delivered significant improvement in skin laxity, clarity, and overall appearance as compared with placebo. Significant improvement in fine lines was noted at week 2 and improvement in wrinkles was noted at week 4 over placebo. Significantly improved viscoelastic properties were consistent with ultrasound increase in overall skin density and thickness.

Subjects indicated strong performance acceptability of the cream. There were no adverse objective or subjective irritation findings.

In a randomized, double-blind, placebo-controlled study [135] that included 67 volunteers, GHK-Cu versus placebo were applied twice daily for 12 weeks on facial skin. GHK-Cu improved skin laxity, clarity, and appearance; reduced fine lines, coarse wrinkles, and mottled hyperpigmentation; and increased skin density and thickness. Five women participants also applied the cream to one forearm and leave the other forearm as untreated control. GHK-Cu strongly induced dermal keratinocyte proliferation.

GHK-Cu's efficacy and safety have been investigated on periorbital area of 41 females with mild to advanced photodamage. Within 4 weeks of this blind and controlled study with vitamin K-containing cream as the comparator, there was significant improvement in all parameters, including fine lines, wrinkles, and overall appearance of eyelids. The viscoelastic properties of periorbital skin – which was determined by a ballistometer – exhibited statistically significant improvement by week 1. Increase in overall skin density and thickness was demonstrated with ultrasound and digital images, which captured noticeable improvement in the appearance of periorbital skin [136].

Superoxide dismutase is important for defenses against oxidative damage in the body. Its manganese complex is also important to prevent or repair UV-induced photoaging. It also stimulates matrix protein growth [137–139]. Manganese tripeptide complex is another carrier and signal peptide and has been synthesized to act through this pathway [137]. In an uncontrolled assessor-blind study, Hussain and Goldberg [137] used GHK-Mn in serum base to treat 15 females – aged 40–70 years – with moderate facial photodamage and hyperpigmentation. The serum was applied to the face and neck twice a day for up to 12 weeks. Best results were seen for hyperpigmentation improvement, and also in dryness, sallowness, mottled hyperpigmentation, and actinic lentigo improvements. GHK-Mn was well tolerated and only one volunteer experienced mild erythema and the other experienced instance of tightness and drying associated with the treatment.

Conclusion

Taken together, some peptides have notable effects on chronologically aged and/or photodamaged skin. There is a large gap for permeability coefficient of major cosmeceutical peptides and proteins, and researchers should focus on this ambiguity to find more efficient substances with better permeability. Although topical peptides are frequently used in antiaging products, some do not have any well-designed in vivo studies with adequate sample size. High-quality randomized, double-blind, active-controlled large trials are needed to calculate their exact effect sizes in this regard.

Cross-References

▶ Aging and Antiaging Strategies
▶ Cosmetic Antiaging Ingredients
▶ Cosmetics and Aging Skin
▶ Topical Growth Factors for Skin Rejuvenation

References

1. Kosmadaki MG, Gilchrest BA. The demographics of aging in the United States: implications for dermatology. Arch Dermatol. 2002;138:1427–8.
2. Ranade VV. Drug delivery systems. 6. Transdermal drug delivery. J Clin Pharmacol. 1991;31:401–18.
3. Buri P, Puisieux F, Doelker E, et al. Formes pharmaceutiques nouvelles. Paris: Technique et Documentation; 1985.
4. Vecchia BE, Bunge AL. Evaluating the transdermal permeability of chemicals. In: Guy RH, Hadgraft J, editors. Transdermal drug delivery (electronic resource). New York: Dekker; 2003.
5. Guy RH. Current status and future prospects of transdermal drug delivery. Pharm Res. 1996;13:1765–9.
6. Roberts MS, Cross SE, Pellett MA. Skin transport. In: Walters AW, editor. Dermatological and transdermal formulations. New York: Dekker; 2002. p. 121.
7. Cullander C, Guy RH. Routes of delivery: case studies (6). Trasdermal delivery of peptides and proteins. Adv Drug Deliv Rev. 1992;8:291–329.

8. Nakamura RM, Einck L, Velmonte MA, Kawajiri K, Ang CF, Delasllagas CE, et al. Detection of active tuberculosis by an MPB-64 transdermal patch: a field study. Scand J Infect Dis. 2001;33:405–7.
9. Pai M, Kalantari S, Dheda K. New tools and emerging technologies for the diagnosis of tuberculosis: part II. Active tuberculosis and drug resistance. Expert Rev Mol Diagn. 2006;6:423–32.
10. Billich A, Aschauer H, Aszodi A, Stuetz A. Percutaneous absorption of drugs used in atopic eczema: pimecrolimus permeates less through skin than corticosteroids and tacrolimus. Int J Pharm. 2004;269:29–35.
11. Weiss M, Fresneau M, Monius T, Stutz A, Billich A. Binding of pimecrolimus and tacrolimus to skin and plasma proteins: implications for systemic exposure after topical application. Drug Metab Dispos. 2008;36:1812–18.
12. Frech SA, Dupont HL, Bourgeois AL, McKenzie R, Belkind-Gerson J, Figueroa JF, et al. Use of a patch containing heat-labile toxin from *Escherichia coli* against travellers' diarrhoea: a phase II, randomised, double-blind, placebo-controlled field trial. Lancet. 2008;371:2019–25.
13. Billich A, Vyplel H, Grassberger M, Schmook FP, Steck A, Stuetz A. Novel cyclosporin derivatives featuring enhanced skin penetration despite increased molecular weight. Bioorg Med Chem. 2005;13:3157–67.
14. Smith EW, Maibach HI. Percutaneous penetration enhancers. New York: Taylor & Francis; 2006.
15. Pillai O, Panchagnula R. Transdermal delivery of insulin from poloxamer gel: ex vivo and in vivo skin permeation studies in rat using iontophoresis and chemical enhancers. J Control Release. 2003;89:127–40.
16. Silva R, Little C, Ferreira H, Cavaco-Paulo A. Incorporation of peptides in phospholipid aggregates using ultrasound. Ultrason Sonochem. 2008;15:1026–32.
17. Goebel A, Neubert RH. Dermal peptide delivery using colloidal carrier systems. Skin Pharmacol Physiol. 2008;21:3–9.
18. Chen Y, Shen Y, Guo X, Zhang C, Yang W, Ma M, et al. Transdermal protein delivery by a coadministered peptide identified via phage display. Nat Biotechnol. 2006;24:455–60.
19. Foldvari M, Attah-Poku S, Hu J, Li Q, Hughes H, Babiuk LA, et al. Palmitoyl derivatives of interferon alpha: potential for cutaneous delivery. J Pharm Sci. 1998;87:1203–8.
20. Robinson LR, Fitzgerald NC, Doughty DG, Dawes NC, Berge CA, Bissett DL. Topical palmitoyl pentapeptide provides improvement in photoaged human facial skin. Int J Cosmet Sci. 2005;27:155–60.
21. Abdulghani AA, Sherr A, Shirin S, Solodkina G, Morales Tapia E, Wolf B, et al. Effects of topical creams containing vitamin C, a copper-binding peptide cream and melatonin compared with tretinoin on the ultrastructure of normal skin. Dis Manag Clin Outcomes. 1998;1:136–41.
22. Osborne R, Robinson LR, Mullins L, Raleigh P. Use of a facial moisturizer containing palmitoyl pentapeptide improves the appearance of aging skin. J Am Acad Dermatol. 2005;52:96.
23. Blanes-Mira C, Clemente J, Jodas G, Gil A, Fernandez-Ballester G, Ponsati B, et al. A synthetic hexapeptide (Argireline) with antiwrinkle activity. Int J Cosmet Sci. 2002;24:303–10.
24. Samuel M, Brooke RC, Hollis S, Griffiths CE. Interventions for photodamaged skin. Cochrane Database Syst Rev. 2005;CD001782.
25. Mazurowska L, Mojski M. Biological activities of selected peptides: skin penetration ability of copper complexes with peptides. J Cosmet Sci. 2008;59:59–69.
26. Ruland A, Kreuter J, Rytting JH. Transdermal delivery of the tetrapeptide hisetal (melanotropin (6-9)): II. Effect of various penetration enhancers. In vitro study across human skin. Int J Pharm. 1994;103:77–80.
27. Ruland A, Kreuter J, Rytting JH. Transdermal delivery of the tetrapeptide hisetal (melanotropin (6-9)). I. Effect of various penetration enhancers: in vitro study across hairless mouse skin. Int J Pharm. 1994;101:57–61.
28. Mazurowska L, Nowak-Buciak K, Mojski M. ESI-MS method for in vitro investigation of skin penetration by copper-amino acid complexes: from an emulsion through a model membrane. Anal Bioanal Chem. 2007;388:1157–63.
29. Ruland A, Kreuter J. Transdermal permeability and skin accumulation of amino acids. Int J Pharm. 1991;72:149–55.
30. Braun E, Wagner A, Furnschlief E, Katinger H, Vorauer-Uhl K. Experimental design for in vitro skin penetration study of liposomal superoxide dismutase. J Pharm Biomed Anal. 2006;40:1187–97.
31. Pickart L, Thaler MM. Tripeptide in human serum which prolongs survival of normal liver cells and stimulates growth in neoplastic liver. Nat New Biol. 1973;243:85–7.
32. Maquart FX, Siméon A, Pasco S, Monboisse JC. Regulation of cell activity by the extracellular matrix: the concept of matrikines. J Soc Biol. 1999;193:423–8.
33. Simeon A, Wegrowski Y, Bontemps Y, Maquart FX. Expression of glycosaminoglycans and small proteoglycans in wounds: modulation by the tripeptide-copper complex glycyl-L-histidyl-L-lysine-$Cu^{(2+)}$. J Invest Dermatol. 2000;115:962–8.
34. Simeon A, Emonard H, Hornebeck W, Maquart FX. The tripeptide-copper complex glycyl-L-histidyl-L-lysine-Cu^{2+} stimulates matrix metalloproteinase-2 expression by fibroblast cultures. Life Sci. 2000;67:2257–65.
35. Buffoni F, Pino R, Dal Pozzo A. Effect of tripeptide-copper complexes on the process of skin wound

healing and on cultured fibroblasts. Arch Int Pharmacodyn Ther. 1995;330:345–60.

36. Wegrowski Y, Maquart FX, Borel JP. Stimulation of sulfated glycosaminoglycan synthesis by the tripeptide-copper complex glycyl-L-histidyl-L-lysine-Cu^{2+}. Life Sci. 1992;51:1049–56.
37. Maquart FX, Pickart L, Laurent M, Gillery P, Monboisse JC, Borel JP. Stimulation of collagen synthesis in fibroblast cultures by the tripeptide-copper complex glycyl-L-histidyl-L-lysine-Cu^{2+}. FEBS Lett. 1988;238:343–6.
38. Lintner K. Promoting production in the extracellular matrix without compromising barrier. Cutis. 2002;70:13–6, discussion 21–3.
39. Croda, Croda USA – News and News Releases, Croda.
40. Pentapharm, Syn®-Coll, Basel.
41. Centerchem, Decorinyl™, Basel.
42. Puig A, Anton JMG, Mangues M. A new decorin-like tetrapeptide for optimal organization of collagen fibres. Int J Cosmet Sci. 2008;30:97–104.
43. Croda, Biopeptide EL™, Edison.
44. A.p.c. products, Peptamide™6, A firming hexapeptide. South Plainfield.
45. Osborne R, Mullins L, Jarrold B, Lintner K. In vitro skin structure benefits with a new antiaging peptide, Pal-KT. J Am Acad Dermatol. 2008;58:ab25 (Abstract).
46. Tajima S, Wachi H, Uemura Y, Okamoto K. Modulation by elastin peptide VGVAPG of cell proliferation and elastin expression in human skin fibroblasts. Arch Dermatol Res. 1997;289:489–92.
47. Wachi H, Seyama Y, Yamashita S, Suganami H, Uemura Y, Okamoto K, et al. Stimulation of cell proliferation and autoregulation of elastin expression by elastin peptide VPGVG in cultured chick vascular smooth muscle cells. FEBS Lett. 1995;368:215–19.
48. Fujimoto N, Tajima S, Ishibashi A. Elastin peptides induce migration and terminal differentiation of cultured keratinocytes via 67 kDa elastin receptor in vitro: 67 kDa elastin receptor is expressed in the keratinocytes eliminating elastic materials in elastosis perforans serpiginosa. J Invest Dermatol. 2000;115:633–9.
49. Chang CH, Kawa Y, Tsai RK, Shieh JH, Lee JW, et al. Melanocyte precursors express elastin binding protein and elastin-derived peptide (VGVAPG) stimulates their melanogenesis and dendrite formation. J Dermatol Sci. 2008;51:158–80.
50. Gruber JV, Bouldin L, Lou K. Can a topical scalp treatment reduce hair bulb extraction? J Cosmet Sci. 2007;58:369–74.
51. Ennamany R, Saboureau D, Mekideche N, Creppy EE. SECMA 1, a mitogenic hexapeptide from *Ulva* algae modulates the production of proteoglycans and glycosaminoglycans in human foreskin fibroblast. Hum Exp Toxicol. 1998;17:18–22.
52. Dumas M, Sadick NS, Noblesse E, Juan M, Lachmann-Weber N, Boury-Jamot M, et al. Hydrating skin by stimulating biosynthesis of aquaporins. J Drugs Dermatol. 2007;6:s20–4.
53. Pauly G, Contet-Audonneau J, Moussou P, Danoux L, Bardey V, Freis O, et al. Small proteoglycans in the skin: new targets in the fight against aging. IFSCC. 2008;11:21–9.
54. Marikovsky M, Breuing K, Liu PY, Eriksson E, Higashiyama S, Farber P, et al. Appearance of heparin-binding EGF-like growth factor in wound fluid as a response to injury. Proc Natl Acad Sci U S A. 1993;90:3889–93.
55. Deplewski D, Rosenfield RL. Growth hormone and insulin-like growth factors have different effects on sebaceous cell growth and differentiation. Endocrinology. 1999;140:4089–94.
56. Cohen IK, Crossland MC, Garrett A, Diegelmann RF. Topical application of epidermal growth factor onto partial-thickness wounds in human volunteers does not enhance reepithelialization. Plast Reconstr Surg. 1995;96:251–4.
57. Brown GL, Nanney LB, Griffen J, Cramer AB, Yancey JM, Curtsinger III LJ, et al. Enhancement of wound healing by topical treatment with epidermal growth factor. N Engl J Med. 1989;321:76–9.
58. Miller CO, Skong F, Von Saltza MH, Strong FM. Kinetin, a cell division factor from deoxyribonucleic acid. J Am Chem Soc. 1955;77:1392.
59. Miller CO, Skong F, Okumura FS, Von Saltza MH, Strong FM. Isolation, structure, and synthesis of kinetin, a substance promoting cell division. J Am Chem Soc. 1956;78:1375–80.
60. Berge U, Kristensen P, Rattan SI. Kinetin-induced differentiation of normal human keratinocytes undergoing aging in vitro. Ann N Y Acad Sci. 2006;1067:332–6.
61. Sharma SP, Kaur P, Rattan SIS. Plant growth hormone kinetin delays ageing, prolongs the lifespan and slows down development of the fruitfly *Zaprionus paravittiger*. Biochem Biophys Res Commun. 1995;216:1067–71.
62. Rattan SIS, Clark BFC. Kinetin delays the onset of ageing characteristics in human fibroblasts. Biochem Biophys Res Commun. 1994;201:665–72.
63. Barciszewski J, Rattan SI, Siboska G, Clark BFC. Kinetin- 45 years on. Plant Sci. 1999;148:37–45.
64. Olsen A, Siboska GE, Clark BFC, Rattan SIS. N6-furfuryladenine, kinetin, protects against Fenton reaction-mediated oxidative damage to DNA. Biochem Biophys Res Commun. 1999;265:499–502.
65. Verbeke P, Siboska GE, Clark BFC, Rattan SIS. Kinetin inhibits protein oxidation and glycoxidation in vitro. Biochem Biophys Res Commun. 2000;276:1265–70.
66. Hipkiss AR. On the "struggle between chemistry and biology during aging" – implications for DNA repair apoptosis and proteolysis, and a novel route of intervention. Biogerontology. 2001;2:173–8.

67. Kimura T, Doi K. Depigmentation and rejuvenation effects of kinetin on the aged skin of hairless descendants of Mexican hairless dogs. Rejuvenation Res. 2004;7:32–9.
68. Katz BE, Bruck MC. Efficacy and tolerability of kinetin 0.1% cream for improving the signs of photoaging in facial and neck skin. Cosmet Dermatol. 2006;19:736–41.
69. McCullough JL, Weinstein GD. Clinical study of safety and efficacy of using topical kinetin 0.1% (Kinerase(registered trademark)) to treat photodamaged skin. Cosmet Dermatol. 2002;15:29–32.
70. Levy SB. Kinetin. In: Elsner P, Maibach HI, editors. Cosmeceuticals and active cosmetics. New York: Marcel Dekker; 2005. p. 407–19.
71. Dickens MS, Levy SB, Helman MD, Nucci JE. Kinetin containing lotion compared with retinol containing lotion; comparable improvements in the signs of photoaging. In: American Academy of Dermatology 60th Annual Meeting, New Orleans; 2002. p. 28.
72. Chiu PC, Chan CC, Lin HM, Chiu HC. The clinical anti-aging effects of topical kinetin and niacinamide in Asians: a randomized, double-blind, placebo-controlled, split-face comparative trial. J Cosmet Dermatol. 2007;6:243–9.
73. McCullough JL, Garcia RL, Reece B. A clinical study of topical Pyratine 6 for improving the appearance of photodamaged skin. J Drugs Dermatol. 2008;7:131–5.
74. Arendt J. Melatonin. Clin Endocrinol (Oxf). 1988;29:205–29.
75. Fischer TW, Elsner P. The antioxidative potential of melatonin in the skin. Curr Probl Dermatol. 2001;29:165–74.
76. Halliwell B. Reactive oxygen species and the central nervous system. J Neurochem. 1992;59:1609–23.
77. Fischer T, Wigger-Alberti W, Elsner P. Melatonin in dermatology: experimental and clinical aspects. Hautarzt. 1999;50:5–11.
78. Karbownik M, Reiter RJ. Melatonin protects against oxidative stress caused by (delta)-aminolevulinic acid: implications for cancer reduction. Cancer Invest. 2002;20:276–86.
79. Chun Kim B, Sung Shon B, Wook Ryoo Y, Pyo Kim S, Suk Lee K. Melatonin reduces X-ray irradiation-induced oxidative damages in cultured human skin fibroblasts. J Dermatol Sci. 2001;26:194–200.
80. Young Wook R, Seong Il S, Kyo Cheol M, Byung Chun K, Kyu Suk L. The effects of the melatonin on ultraviolet-B irradiated cultured dermal fibroblasts. J Dermatol Sci. 2001;27:162–9.
81. Fischer TW, Scholz G, Knoll B, Hipler UC, Eisner P. Melatonin reduces UV-induced reactive oxygen species in a dose-dependent manner in IL-3-stimulated leukocytes. J Pineal Res. 2001;31:39–45.
82. Fischer TW, Scholz G, Knoll B, Hipler UC, Elsner P. Melatonin suppresses reactive oxygen species in UV-irradiated leukocytes more than vitamin C and trolox. Skin Pharmacol Appl Skin Physiol. 2002;15:367–73.
83. Fischer T, Bangha E, Elsner P, Kistler GS. Suppression of UV-induced erythema by topical treatment with melatonin. Influence of the application time point. Biol Signals Recept. 1999;8:132–5.
84. Ghersetich I, Comacchi C, Lotti T. Immunohistochemical and ultrastructural investigation of multiple common warts before and after therapy with alpha-interferon. G Ital Dermatol Venereol. 1992;127:207–10.
85. Ghersetich I, Lotti T. Alpha-interferon cream restores decreased levels of Langerhans/indeterminate (CD1a+) cells in aged and PUVA-treated skin. Skin Pharmacol. 1994;7:118–20.
86. Frank S, Madlener M, Werner S. Transforming growth factors beta1, beta2, and beta3 and their receptors are differentially regulated during normal and impaired wound healing. J Biol Chem. 1996;271:10188–93.
87. Li Y, Fan J, Chen M, Li W, Woodley DT. Transforming growth factor-alpha: a major human serum factor that promotes human keratinocyte migration. J Invest Dermatol. 2006;126:2096–105.
88. Govinden R, Bhoola KD. Genealogy, expression, and cellular function of transforming growth factor-beta. Pharmacol Ther. 2003;98:257–65.
89. Rao J, Ehrlich M, Goldman MP. Facial skin rejuvenation with a novel topical compound containing transforming growth factor (beta)1 and vitamin C. Cosmet Dermatol. 2004;17:705–10 + 13.
90. Ehrlich M, Rao J, Pabby A, Goldman MP. Improvement in the appearance of wrinkles with topical transforming growth factor beta(1) and l-ascorbic acid. Dermatol Surg. 2006;32:618–25.
91. Fitzpatrick RE, Rostan EF. Reversal of photodamage with topical growth factors: a pilot study. J Cosmet Laser Ther. 2003;5:25–34.
92. Gold MH, Goldman MP, Biron J. Efficacy of novel skin cream containing mixture of human growth factors and cytokines for skin rejuvenation. J Drugs Dermatol. 2007;6:197–201.
93. Lupo ML, Cohen JL, Rendon MI. Novel eye cream containing a mixture of human growth factors and cytokines for periorbital skin rejuvenation. J Drugs Dermatol. 2007;6:725–9.
94. Gold MH, Goldman MP, Biron J. Human growth factor and cytokine skin cream for facial skin rejuvenation as assessed by 3D in vivo optical skin imaging. J Drugs Dermatol. 2007;6:1018–23.
95. Watson RE, Long SP, Bowden JJ, Bastrilles JY, Barton SP, Griffiths CE. Repair of photoaged dermal matrix by topical application of a cosmetic "antiageing" product. Br J Dermatol. 2008;158:472–7.
96. Dal Farra C, Bauza E, Domloge N. Heat shock proteins for cosmeceuticals. In: Elsner P, Maibach HI,

editors. Cosmeceuticals and active cosmetics. New York: Marcel Dekker; 2005. p. 523–36.
97. Botto J, Cucumel K, Dal Farra C, Domloge N. Treatment of human cells with Hsp-70-rich yeast extract enhances cell thermotolerance and resistance to stress. J Invest Dermatol. 2001;117:452.
98. Cucumel K, Botto J, Bauza E, Dal Farra C, Roetto R, Domloge N. Artemia extract induces Hsp70 in human cells and enhances cell protection from stress. J Invest Dermatol. 2001;117:454.
99. Domloge N, Bauza E, Cucumel K, Peyronel D, Dal Farra C. Artemia extract toward more extensive sun protection. Cosmet Toiletries. 2002;2002:69–78.
100. Bauza E, Dal Farra C, Domloge N. Hsp70 induction by Artemia extract exhibits anti-inflammatory effect and down-regulates IL-1 and IL-8 synthesis in human hacat cells. J Invest Dermatol. 2001; 117:415.
101. Mosser DD, Caron AW, Bourget L, Denis-Larose C, Massie B. Role of the human heat shock protein hsp70 in protection against stress- induced apoptosis. Mol Cell Biol. 1997;17:5317–27.
102. Gabai VL, Meriin AB, Mosser DD, Caron AW, Rits S, Shifrin VI, et al. Hsp70 prevents activation of stress kinases: a novel pathway of cellular thermotolerance. J Biol Chem. 1997;272:18033–7.
103. Gutsmann-Conrad A, Heydari AR, You S, Richardson A. The expression of heat shock protein 70 decreases with cellular senescence in vitro and in cells derived from young and old human subjects. Exp Cell Res. 1998;241:404–13.
104. Wu B, Gu MJ, Heydari AR, Richardson A. The effect of age on the synthesis of two heat shock proteins in the HSP70 family. J Gerontol. 1993;48:B50–6.
105. Blake MJ, Fargnoli J, Gershon D, Holbrook NJ. Concomitant decline in heat-induced hyperthermia and HSP70 mRNA expression in aged rats. Am J Physiol Regul Integr Comp Physiol. 1991;260: R663–7.
106. Pardue S, Groshan K, Raese JD, Morrison-Bogorad M. Hsp70 mRNA induction is reduced in neurons of aged rat hippocampus after thermal stress. Neurobiol Aging. 1992;13:661–72.
107. Fargnoli J, Kunisada T, Fornace Jr AJ, Schneider EL, Holbrook NJ. Decreased expression of heat shock protein 70 mRNA and protein after heat treatment in cells of aged rats. Proc Natl Acad Sci U S A. 1990;87:846–50.
108. Muramatsu T, Hataoko M, Tada H, Shirai T, Ohnishi T. Age-related decrease in the inductability of heat shock protein 72 in normal human skin. Br J Dermatol. 1996;134:1035–8.
109. Cucumel K, Dal Farra C, Domloge N. Artemia extract "compensates" for age-related decrease of Hsp70 in skin. J Invest Dermatol. 2002;119:257.
110. Cauchard JH, Berton A, Godeau G, Hornebeck W, Bellon G. Activation of latent transforming growth factor beta 1 and inhibition of matrix metalloprotease activity by a thrombospondin-like tripeptide linked to elaidic acid. Biochem Pharmacol. 2004;67:2013–22.
111. Choi SH, Kim SY, An JJ, Lee SH, Kim DW, Ryu HJ, et al. Human PEP-1-ribosomal protein S3 protects against UV-induced skin cell death. FEBS Lett. 2006;580:6755–62.
112. Barba C, Mendez S, Roddick-Lanzilotta A, Kelly R, Parra JL, Coderch L. Wool peptide derivatives for hand care. J Cosmet Sci. 2007;58:99–107.
113. Barba C, Mendez S, Roddick-Lanzilotta A, Kelly R, Parra JL, Coderch L. Cosmetic effectiveness of topically applied hydrolysed keratin peptides and lipids derived from wool. Skin Res Technol. 2008;14:243–8.
114. dal Farra C, Oberto G, Berghi A, Domloge N. An anti-aging effect on the lips and skin observed in in vivo studies on a new fibronectin-like peptide. J Am Acad Dermatol. 2007;56:AB88.
115. Centerchem, Glycine soja (soybean) protein, Barcelona.
116. Sudel KM, Venzke K, Mielke H, Breitenbach U, Mundt C, Jaspers S, et al. Novel aspects of intrinsic and extrinsic aging of human skin: beneficial effects of soy extract. Photochem Photobiol. 2005;81: 581–7.
117. Andre-Frei V, Perrier E, Augustin C, Damour O, Bordat P, Schumann K, et al. A comparison of biological activities of a new soya biopeptide studied in an in vitro skin equivalent model and human volunteers. Int J Cosmet Sci. 1999;21:299–311.
118. Sim GS, Lee DH, Kim JH, An SK, Choe TB, Kwon TJ, et al. Black rice (*Oryza sativa* L. var. *japonica*) hydrolyzed peptides induce expression of hyaluronan synthase 2 gene in hacat keratinocytes. J Microbiol Biotechnol. 2007;17:271–9.
119. Centerchem, Eyeseryl®, Barcelona.
120. Padamwar MN, Pawar AP, Daithankar AV, Mahadik KR. Silk sericin as a moisturizer: an in vivo study. J Cosmet Dermatol. 2005;4:250–7.
121. Daithankar AV, Padamwar MN, Pisal SS, Paradkar AR, Mahadik KR. Moisturizing efficiency of silk protein hydrolysate: silk fibroin. Indian J Biotechnol. 2005;4:115–21.
122. Zhaorigetu S, Yanaka N, Sasaki M, Watanabe H, Kato N. Inhibitory effects of silk protein, sericin on UVB-induced acute damage and tumor promotion by reducing oxidative stress in the skin of hairless mouse. J Photochem Photobiol B Biol. 2003; 71:11–7.
123. Foran PG, Mohammed N, Lisk GO, Nagwaney S, Lawrence GW, Johnson E, et al. Evaluation of the therapeutic usefulness of botulinum neurotoxin B, C1, E, and F compared with the long lasting type A: basis for distinct durations of inhibition of exocytosis in central neurons. J Biol Chem. 2003;278:1363–71.
124. Centerchem, Argireline®, Barcelona.
125. Gutierrez LM, Viniegra S, Rueda J, Ferrer-Montiel AV, Canaves JM, Montal M. A peptide that mimics the C-terminal sequence of SNAP-25 inhibits

secretory vesicle docking in chromaffin cells. J Biol Chem. 1997;272:2634–9.

126. Gutierrez LM, Canaves JM, Ferrer-Montiel AV, Reig JA, Montal M, Viniegra S. A peptide that mimics the carboxy-terminal domain of SNAP-25 blocks Ca^{2+}-dependent exocytosis in chromaffin cells. FEBS Lett. 1995;372:39–43.
127. Centerchem, Leuphasyl®, Barcelona.
128. Lipotec, SNAP-8, Barcelona.
129. Centerchem, Vialox®, Basel.
130. Snyder EL, Dowdy SF. Recent advances in the use of protein transduction domains for the delivery of peptides, proteins and nucleic acids in vivo. Expert Opin Drug Deliv. 2005;2:43–51.
131. Hou YW, Chan MH, Hsu HR, Liu BR, Chen CP, Chen HH, et al. Transdermal delivery of proteins mediated by non-covalently associated arginine-rich intracellular delivery peptides. Exp Dermatol. 2007;16:999–1006.
132. Morris MC, Depollier J, Mery J, Heitz F, Divita G. A peptide carrier for the delivery of biologically active proteins into mammalian cells. Nat Biotechnol. 2001;19:1173–6.
133. Appa Y, Stephens T, Barkovic S, Finkey MB. A clinical evaluation of a copper-peptide-containing liquid foundation and cream concealer designed for improving skin condition. American Academy of Dermatology 60th Annual Meeting; 2002; New Orleans. p. 28.
134. Leyden JJ, Stevens T, Finkey MB, Barkovic S. Skin care benefits of copper-peptide containing facial cream. American Academy of Dermatology 60th Annual Meeting; 2002; New Orleans.
135. Finkey MB, Appa Y, Bhandarkar S. Copper peptide and skin. In: Elsner P, Maibach HI, editors. Cosmeceuticals and active cosmetics. New York: Marcel Dekker; 2005. p. 549–64.
136. Leyden JJ, Stevens T, Finkey MB, Barkovic S. Skin care benefits of copper peptide containing eye creams. American Academy of Dermatology 60th Annual Meeting; 2002; New Orleans.
137. Hussain M, Goldberg DJ. Topical manganese peptide in the treatment of photodamaged skin. J Cosmet Laser Ther. 2007;9:232–6.
138. Naderi-Hachtroudi L, Peters T, Brenneisen P, Meewes C, Hommel C, Razi-Wolf Z, et al. Induction of manganese superoxide dismutase in human dermal fibroblasts: a UV-B-mediated paracrine mechanism with the release of epidermal interleukin 1(alpha), interleukin 1(beta), and tumor necrosis factor (alpha). Arch Dermatol. 2002;138:1473–9.
139. Parat MO, Richard MJ, Leccia MT, Amblard P, Favier A, Beani JC. Does manganese protect cultured human skin fibroblasts against oxidative injury by UVA, dithranol and hydrogen peroxide? Free Radic Res. 1995;23:339–51.

138 Long-Term Estrogen Effects on Sun-Exposed Human Skin

Hyun Sun Yoon and Jin Ho Chung

Contents

Abstract
As human life expectancy has increased, the population of postmenopausal women increases, and interest in the effects of estrogen grows. Estrogen receptors are detected in the skin, so it is easily assumed that estrogens influence skin structure and function. For a long time, estrogen has been believed as an antiaging modality to improve the skin thickness, collagen, and wrinkles. This belief originated from a series of studies that investigated changes of collagen content and skin thickness in women receiving hormone replacement therapy in the 1980s. Despite different methodologies, the majority of studies have shown estrogen treatment in postmenopausal women to increase skin thickness and skin collagen content in sun-protected skin. However, estrogen effects on the skin are quite different between sun-protected and sun-exposed skin. The randomized placebo-controlled trials to investigate antiaging effect of estrogen supplementation in sun-exposed skin have shown inconsistent results. It seems that estrogen does not induce collagen in sun-exposed skin as much as in sun-protected skin. Taken together, estrogen could be beneficial to intrinsic aging but potentially harmful to photoaging in the skin. It is important to keep in mind the fact that estrogens might have differential effects on the skin in the presence of UV irradiation.

H.S. Yoon (✉)
Department of Dermatology, Seoul National University Boramae Hospital, Seoul, Korea
e-mail: hsyoon79@gmail.com

J.H. Chung
Department of Dermatology, Seoul National University College of Medicine, Seoul, Korea
e-mail: jhchung@snu.ac.kr

M.A. Farage et al. (eds.), *Textbook of Aging Skin*,
DOI 10.1007/978-3-662-47398-6_139

Introduction

Aging is a complex, multifactorial process resulting in several functional and esthetic changes in the skin. Aging is influenced at various extents by genetic, environmental, and hormonal factors [1]. All women experience menopause during their lifetime, and declining estrogen levels after menopause result to various physical and mood changes. As human life expectancy has increased, the population of postmenopausal women increases, and interest in the effects of estrogen grows [2].

The influence of estrogens on several body systems such as reproductive tissues, nervous and cardiovascular systems, and skeleton has been well documented [3]. Estrogen receptors are detected in the skin [4], so it is easily assumed that estrogens influence skin structure and function. Furthermore, estrogen has been believed as antiaging modality for a long time [5, 6].

However, skin aging is more complicated than any other organs, because of continuous exposure to external stimulus, ultraviolet (UV) radiation. Beyond the intrinsic aging process, sun-exposed areas such as the face, neck, and dorsum of hands and forearms encounter additional damages, largely due to exposure to UV [3].

Molecular Mechanisms of Estrogen Actions

There are several forms of estrogen that act within the body: estradiol, estrone, and estriol. Estradiol is synthesized in the ovary, estrone is a product of peripheral conversion by aromatase, and estriol is formed from the metabolism of estrone and estradiol. The most potent estrogen in human is 17-β-estradiol, whereas estriol is the least potent [6].

Estrogens regulate diverse cellular functions including proliferation, morphogenesis, differentiation, and apoptosis. The pathways by which estrogens influence cellular functions are complex [1]. The classical mechanism of estrogens is mediated through estrogen receptor (ER) α and β, which are members of a large superfamily of nuclear receptors [7]. After estrogens bind to estrogen receptors in the nucleus, the receptor-ligand complex binds to the specific DNA sequences located within the regulatory regions of the target genes, called estrogen response elements (EREs) [1, 7]. Steroid receptor complexes then interact with other cellular components to either activate or suppress transcription of the target gene in a promoter-specific and cell-specific manner [1, 8]. In addition, ERs can regulate gene expression without EREs by modulating the function of other transcription factors. The interaction of ERs with the activator protein 1 (AP-1) complex is a typical example of ERE-independent genomic actions [7]. The genomic effect of estrogen is characterized by its delayed onset of action and occurs within minutes to hours [1].

However, a number of estrogen effects are so rapid that they cannot depend on the activation of gene transcription and protein synthesis. These actions are known as nongenomic actions and are believed to be mediated through membrane-associated ERs or nonsteroid hormone receptors such as GPR30. The nonclassical pathways activate mitogen-activated protein (MAP) kinases that ultimately regulate transcription of specific genes. Via these nonclassical pathways, it appears that estrogens can also interact with other signaling pathways [9].

Cross talks between estrogen and other growth factors, such as insulin-like growth factor-1 and transforming growth factor-α (TGF-α), have been reported in several tissues [6].

In summary, estrogens have two different mechanisms of actions: (1) a genomic effect via nuclear estrogen receptors regulating the transcriptional expression of genes directly or indirectly and (2) a nongenomic effect that activates signaling pathways that affect cell survival and/or modulate other growth factor signaling [6].

Distribution of Estrogen Receptors in the Skin

Detection of ERs in human skin has yielded discordant results. ER-β is the predominant form of ERs in adult human skin. However, it is still uncertain whether ER-α is also expressed in the keratinocytes or fibroblasts of human skin in vivo.

Immunostaining-based studies reported that ER-α was not detected or was weakly detected, being restricted to sebocytes, whereas ER-β was strongly detected in the epidermis, eccrine glands, sebaceous glands, and hair follicles [10]. In contrast, mRNAs of ER-α, ER-β, and GPR30 are detected, and ER-α mRNA levels are even ten times greater than those of ER-β or GPR30 in human skin [11]. More studies are needed to precisely identify ER-expressing cells and the presence of functional ERs in human skin.

Meanwhile, estrogens and estrogen receptors are important modulators of the immune system. Due to the female predominance of autoimmune diseases, the role of gender and sex hormones in the immune system is of long-term interest [12].

Immune cells have been known to express ERs. Significant effects of estrogen and ERs on B cell function are well documented. Growing evidence indicates that ERs also impact dendritic cell development and function [12]. Mast cells and neutrophils are known to express ER-α not ER-β [13], whereas monocytes are known to express both ER-α and ER-β [14]. These immune cells exist in the skin and could be influenced by estrogens.

Estrogen and Skin Aging

Since estrogen receptors are detected in the skin, estrogen effects on skin structure and function are easily assumed. During peri- and postmenopausal period, women experience hot flushes, vaginal dryness, or dryness of the skin subsequent to significant decline of serum level of estrogen, especially estradiol. In addition, estrogen replacement may ameliorate some of these symptoms and stimulate collagen synthesis in restricted sites of the skin [6]. For a long time, estrogen has been believed as an antiaging modality to improve the skin thickness, collagen, and wrinkles [5, 6]. However, estrogen effects on the skin are quite different between sun-protected and sun-exposed skin.

Collagen Stimulating Effects Estrogen in Sun-Protected Skin

The belief in antiaging effects of estrogens originated from a series of studies that investigated changes of collagen content and skin thickness in hormone replacement therapy (HRT)-treated women in the 1980s. Despite different methodologies, the majority of studies have shown estrogen treatment in postmenopausal women to increase skin thickness and skin collagen content (Table 1). However, the studies reporting that estrogen treatment increased skin collagen content investigated the sun-protected skin such as the thigh [16, 20, 23], abdomen [17, 19, 21], or buttock [11, 15].

Clinical Trials to Investigate the Anti-wrinkle Effects of Estrogen in Photodamaged Skin

Collagen contents are decreased in intrinsically aged skin, and these decreases are accelerated in sun-exposed areas. In photoaged skin, collagen production is reduced, and collagen-degrading enzyme (MMP) is robustly upregulated [3].

Clinically, intrinsically aged skin shows thinning, loss of elasticity, and deepening of normal expression lines. In contrast, photoaged skin shows prominent wrinkles, dyspigmentation, laxity, telangiectasia, and cutaneous malignancies [24]. One of main histologic features of photoaging is loss of collagen and topical tretinoin; a well-established anti-photoaging modality improves wrinkles in photoaged skin [24]. Even though most previous studies to demonstrate collagen-stimulating effects of estrogen were obtained from sun-protected skin, people anticipated that estrogen could be used as a modality against photoaging.

Majority of clinical trials throughout the 1980s and 1990s to investigate whether estrogen treatment improve skin aging phenotypes especially wrinkles concluded that estrogen had anti-wrinkle effects in photoaged skin (Table 2) [25, 26, 29]. However, a lot of trials have major pitfalls:

Table 1 Review of studies evaluating collagen-stimulating effects (induction of collagen or reduction of MMPs) of estrogen in sun-protected skin[a]

References	Study design	N of subjects	Age, y (range)	Period	Treatment group	Biopsy site	Outcome
Topical estrogen treatment							
Son et al. [15]	Proof of concept, nonrandomized	16[b]	73.4[a] (62–79)	2 weeks	0.01 % estradiol three times per week, under occlusion	Buttock	Topical estradiol increased expressions of type I procollagen (mRNA, protein) and decreased MMP-1 (protein)
Rittie et al. [11]	Proof of concept, nonrandomized	17[c]	76 (66–94)	1 week	0.1–2.5 % estradiol three times every other day, under occlusion	Buttock	Topical estradiol increased procollagen I (mRNA, protein) and III (mRNA)
Systemic estrogen treatment							
Brincat et al. [16]	Open label, nonrandomized	118	50.4 (N.A.)	5.2 years (2–10 years)	Estradiol 50 mg + testosterone 100 mg implant ($n = 52$) Untreated control ($n = 66$)	Inner forearm, thigh	Skin thickness and collagen were increased by 30 % and 34 %, respectively, in HRT group than in untreated group
Brincat et al. [17]	Open label, single arm (no control)	16	48.9 (N.A.)	1 year	Estradiol gel, 1.5 mg daily	Abdomen, thigh	Increased collagen content only in the abdomen. No significant change in collagen content in the thigh at 1 year
		62	50.4 (N.A.)	6 months	Estradiol 50 mg implant ($n = 22$) Estradiol 50 mg + testosterone 100 mg implant ($n = 20$) Estradiol 100 mg implant ($n = 20$)	Thigh	Only 50 mg estradiol implant group showed significantly increased collagen content in the thigh at 6 months. Neither 50 mg estradiol + 100 mg testosterone implant group nor 100 mg estradiol implant group showed significant collagen induction at 6 months
Brincat et al. [18]	Open label, nonrandomized	41	52.7 (N.A.)	1 year	Estradiol subcutaneous implant 100 mg, every 6 months	Inner forearm	Skin thickness increased from 0.86 mm (baseline) to 0.97 mm at 6 months and to 1 mm at 1 year

Castelo-Branco et al. [19]	Open label, randomized	118	47.2 (N.A.)	1 year	Cyclic CEE group (n = 28) Transdermal group (n = 28, 50 μg/day estradiol for 24 days) Continuous CEE group (n = 30) Untreated control (n = 30)	Abdomen	The levels of collagen were significantly higher in transdermal (5.1 %) and continuous CEE (3.1 %) groups than in untreated group (−3.2 %) at 1 year
Maheux et al. [20]	Randomized, double blind, placebo controlled	60	61.0 (51–71)	1 year	Conjugated estrogen 0.625 mg (n = 30) Placebo control (n = 30)	Thigh, abdomen, neck	Skin thickness and dermal thickness were significantly increased in the thigh. However, there were no significant differences of skin thickness in the neck and lower abdomen
Haapassari [21]	Open label, nonrandomized	43	51 (46–58)	1 year	Estradiol 2 mg (n = 14) Estradiol 2 mg + norethisterone acetate 1 mg (n = 15) Untreated control (n = 14)	Abdomen	There were no changes of the de novo collagen synthesis or the total amount of collagen in the skin after 1-year HRT
Sauerbronn et al. [22]	Randomized, double blind, placebo controlled	41	N.A.	6 months	Estradiol 2 mg/day for 21 day + cyproterone acetate 1 mg/day for 10 days (n = 21) Placebo control (n = 20)	Upper arm	Collagen content of the upper arm increased after 6 months of treatment only in the hormonal group (+6.49 %)

[a] *CEE* conjugated equine estrogen, *HRT* hormone replacement therapy, *N.A.* not applicable
[b] Including eight male participants
[c] Even though this study included male participants, this table showed only data regarding female participants

Table 2 Review of studies evaluating clinical antiaging effects of estrogen treatment in the photoaged skin[a]

References	Study design	N of subjects	Age, y (range)	Period	Treatment group	Outcome
Topical estrogen treatment						
Creidi et al. [25]	Randomized, double blind, placebo controlled	54	N.A. (52–70)	6 months	Conjugated estrogen 0.625 mg per gram of cream ($n = 27$) Placebo control ($n = 27$)	Increased skin thickness No difference in wrinkle depth
Schmidt et al. [26]	Open label, single arm (no control)	28	54 (43–66)	6 months	0.01 % estradiol	Significant decrease in wrinkle depth Insignificant increase in hydration
		30	53 (41–67)	6 months	0.3 % estriol	Significant decrease in wrinkle depth Insignificant increase in hydration
Yoon et al. [27]	Randomized, double blind, placebo controlled	80	55.2 (51–60)	6 months	1 % estrone ($n = 40$) Placebo control ($n = 40$)	No improvement in wrinkle depth and skin elasticity
Systemic estrogen treatment						
Dunn et al. [28]	Cross sectional	3875[b]	61.6 (40–74)	N.A.	HRT ever ($n = 667$) HRT never ($n = 2736$)	Association between estrogen use and a significant decrease in the likelihood of senile dry skin and wrinkling
Pierard-Franchimont et al. [29]	Open label, nonrandomized	140	N.A. (40–52)	5 years	Conjugated estrogen 0.625 mg daily + medrogestone 5 mg for 12 days ($n = 90$) Untreated control ($n = 50$)	Control group showed a decrease in elasticity 1.5 % per year; HRT abated such impairments
Sumino et al. [30]	Open label, randomized	25	56.8 (49–71)	1 year	Conjugated estrogen 0.625 mg + MPA 2.5 mg daily ($n = 12$) Untreated control ($n = 13$)	No significant differences in skin elasticity between two groups
Wolff et al. [31]	Cross sectional	20	57.8 (N.A)	5 years	Longer-term HRT users ($n = 9$) Untreated control ($n = 11$)	Less severe wrinkling and more elastic skin in long-term HRT users
Sator et al. [32]	Randomized, double blind, placebo controlled	40	51.3 (44–55)	7 months	Estradiol 2 mg/ dydrogesterone 10 mg ($n = 20$) Placebo control ($n = 20$)	Increased skin elasticity at the mandible No differences in skin hydration at the forehead

(*continued*)

Table 2 (continued)

References	Study design	N of subjects	Age, y (range)	Period	Treatment group	Outcome
Kaatz et al. [33]	Open label, single arm (no control)	11	N.A. (38–58)	1 year	1 mg estradiol valerate and 2 mg dienogest	Decreased skin roughness (wrinkle depth) by 15 %
Phillips et al. [34]	Randomized, double blind, placebo controlled	485	53.6 (47–67)	48 weeks	NEA 1 mg/EE 5 μg ($n = 162$) NEA 1 mg/EE 10 μg ($n = 158$) Placebo control ($n = 165$)	No difference in facial wrinkling

[a]*EE* ethinyl estradiol, *HRT* hormone replacement therapy, *MPA* medroxyprogesterone acetate, *N.A.* not applicable, *NEA* norethindrone acetate
[b]Due to missing data, values do not always add up to 3875

lack of placebo-control group [26, 33, 35], small sample size [30, 35], no randomization [29], and no definite clinical end point [35].

To overcome the biased results, randomized, placebo-controlled trials are mandatory. There are three randomized, placebo-controlled trials in the 2000s to investigate the antiaging effects of estrogen in photoaged skin of postmenopausal women [27, 32, 34]. Two used systemic estrogen treatment [32, 34], and the other used topical estrogen [27].

Sator et al. evaluated the influence of estrogen on skin elasticity, skin surface lipids, skin hydration, and skin thickness in 40 postmenopausal women. They did not measure facial wrinkles. The dosage in the trial was a combination of 2 mg estradiol and 10 mg dydrogesterone. The results were different depending on the anatomic sites. Skin elasticity increased at the mandible, whereas there was no increase in skin elasticity at the upper arm where skin thickness was increased [32].

Phillips et al. assessed the effects of continuous combined norethindrone acetate (NA) and ethinyl estradiol (EE) in postmenopausal women. They enrolled 485 participants and randomly assigned the participants to one of three study arms: placebo group ($n = 165$), 1 mg NA/5 μg EE group ($n = 162$), or a 1 mg NA/10 μg EE group ($n = 158$). The primary endpoints were both investigator global assessment of coarse and fine facial wrinkling and subjective self-assessment changes in wrinkling at week 48. This is the largest randomized clinical trial to evaluate antiaging effects of estrogen treatment. However, they failed to find any statistical significant differences between the NA/EE groups and placebo and concluded that hormone therapy for 48 weeks in postmenopausal women did not significantly alter age-related facial skin changes [34].

Yoon et al. investigated the effects of topical estrogen treatment on photoaged facial skin in postmenopausal women. Eighty postmenopausal women are randomly assigned to receive the vehicle cream or estrone 1 % cream. All participants applied 1 g of the cream to the entire face every day for 24 weeks. They measured wrinkles using skin replicas and Visiometer and elasticity using Cutometer. After 24-week topical estrogen treatment, there were no improvements in wrinkles and skin elasticity in facial skin [27].

Therefore, the randomized placebo-controlled trials to investigate antiaging effect of estrogen supplementation in sun-exposed skin have shown inconsistent results despite estrogen's definite collagen induction ability in sun-protected skin (Table 2) [25, 26, 31, 35]. Contrary to the results in sun-protected skin, there has been only weak evidence to support antiaging properties of estrogen in sun-exposed skin.

Table 3 Review of studies evaluating collagen-stimulating effects (induction of collagen or reduction of MMPs) of estrogen in photoaged skin

References	Study design	N of subjects	Age, y (range)	Period	Treatment group	Outcome
Topical estrogen treatment						
Schmidt et al. [26][a]	Open label, single arm (no control)	46	54 (43–66)	6 months	0.01 % estradiol	No change in type I collagen (protein), increase in type III collagen (protein) after estrogen application
			53 (41–67)	6 months	0.3 % estriol	
Patriarca et al. [35]	Open label, single arm (no control)	15	51.3[b] (46–58)	16 weeks	0.01 % estradiol	Significant increases in epidermal thickness, dermal thickness, and collagen amount
Rittie et al. [11]	Proof of concept, nonrandomized	23[c]	75.2 (65–94)	1 week	0.1–2.5 % estradiol under occlusion, three times every other day on the forearm ($n = 18$)	No change of procollagen I (mRNA, protein) and III (mRNA) in estradiol-treated skin than in vehicle-treated skin
				2 weeks	0.2 % estradiol, twice a day on face ($n = 5$)	
Neder et al. [36]	Open label, single arm (no control)	40	53.3 (43–65)	30 days	0.05 % estradiol	No difference in MMP-1 expression in estradiol-treated skin compared to baseline values
Yoon et al. [27][a]	Randomized, double blind, placebo controlled	26	55.2 (51–60)	6 months	1 % estrone ($n = 13$) Placebo control ($n = 13$)	No change in type I procollagen (protein), and robust increase of MMP-1 (mRNA) were observed in estrone-treated skin

[a]In this table, the number of subjects indicates only the number of subjects who underwent skin biopsy, so the number is much smaller than overall study population

[b]All participants already received systemic estrogen therapy for at least 1 year (range 13–40 months)

[c]Even though this study included male participants, this table showed only data regarding female participants

Lack of Evidence of Collagen Stimulating Effects of Estrogen in Photodamaged Skin

Does estrogen induce collagen production in photoaged skin? There is a paucity of research on this subject (Table 3). Furthermore, no previous study measured the change of collagen content after systemic estrogen treatment. Because of small sample size, it is difficult to conclude the effect of estrogen on collagen synthesis in sun-exposed skin. However, it seems that estrogen does not induce collagen in sun-exposed skin as much as in sun-protected skin.

Rittie et al. reported a lack of effect of topical estradiol treatment on procollagen production in photoaged skin by a 2-week treatment. Even though they demonstrated 1-week topical estrogen treatment stimulates procollagen I and III expressions in sun-protected skin, no significant changes in production of procollagen types I and III were observed after 2-week estradiol treatment in the photoaged forearm or face skin [11]. The expression of estrogen receptors and the induction of estrogen responsive gene in the estrogen-treated sites were similar in both photoaged and sun-protected skin [11]. This is the first study that suggested the differential effects of estrogen between sun-exposed and sun-protected skin.

After 24 weeks of estrone 1 % treatment, mRNAs of procollagen type I and fibrillin type I were increased in face skin. However, MMP-1 mRNA was much more induced than procollagen or fibrillin mRNAs, and procollagen type I protein was not induced in the estrone-treated site than placebo treated [27].

One of the important signals to control collagen is activator protein 1 (AP-1). AP-1 consists of two subunits, c-Jun and c-Fos. Only c-Jun is UV inducible, whereas c-Fos expresses constitutively [37, 38]. The genes encoding the $\alpha1$ and $\alpha2$ chains of type I collagen do not contain an ERE [39]. Estradiol has been shown to regulate the transcription of many genes that lack an ERE but contain AP-1 binding site and suppressed collagen type I expression via AP-1 in murine mesangial cells [39]. Activation of AP-1 can be affected by pro-inflammatory cytokines such as IL-1β. IL-1β regulates the expression MMP-1 via AP-1 and NFκB [40]. Endogenous estrogen augmented the expression of pro-inflammatory cytokines including IL-1β and collagenase after UV irradiation in mice [41].

Potential Beneficial Effects of Estrogen on the Skin Other Than on Collagen

Few studies have investigated the effects of estrogen on the skin except on collagen. A few in vitro and animal studies have suggested that estrogen might stimulate keratinocyte proliferation [42, 43] and induce synthesis of glycosaminoglycan including hyaluronan and versican in the dermis [44]. However, these preclinical observations have not yet been proven in human skin in vivo. Even though some studies to evaluate antiaging effects of HRT or topical estrogen on skin measured epidermal hydration, the results were still conflicting [26, 32]. Further investigation is needed to understand the effects of estrogen on the epidermis or other dermal components such as glycosaminoglycan or elastic fiber.

Conclusion

Estrogen distinctly has many beneficial effects on various organs. However, under exogenous harmful stimuli, UV irradiation, estrogen may have a negative impact on the skin. Estrogen may be a double-edged sword in the skin, beneficial to intrinsic aging but potentially harmful to UV-induced skin responses. It is important to keep in mind the fact that estrogens have differential effects on the skin in the presence of UV irradiation.

References

1. Verdier-Sevrain S, Bonte F, Gilchrest B. Biology of estrogens in skin: implications for skin aging. Exp Dermatol. 2006;15:83–94.
2. Henry F, Pierard-Franchimont C, Cauwenbergh G, Pierard GE. Age-related changes in facial skin contours and rheology. J Am Geriatr Soc. 1997;45:220–2.
3. Rabe JH, Mamelak AJ, McElgunn PJ, Morison WL, Sauder DN. Photoaging: mechanisms and repair. J Am Acad Dermatol. 2006;55:1–19.
4. Hasselquist MB, Goldberg N, Schroeter A, Spelsberg TC. Isolation and characterization of the estrogen receptor in human skin. J Clin Endocrinol Metab. 1980;50:76–82.
5. Draelos ZD. Topical and oral estrogens revisited for antiaging purposes. Fertil Steril. 2005;84:291–2; discussion 295.
6. Hall G, Phillips TJ. Estrogen and skin: the effects of estrogen, menopause, and hormone replacement therapy on the skin. J Am Acad Dermatol. 2005;53:555–68; quiz 569–572.
7. Bjornstrom L, Sjoberg M. Mechanisms of estrogen receptor signaling: convergence of genomic and nongenomic actions on target genes. Mol Endocrinol. 2005;19:833–42.
8. Speroff L. A clinical understanding of the estrogen receptor. Ann N Y Acad Sci. 2000;900:26–39.
9. Lorenzo J. A new hypothesis for how sex steroid hormones regulate bone mass. J Clin Invest. 2003;111:1641–3.
10. Pelletier G, Ren L. Localization of sex steroid receptors in human skin. Histol Histopathol. 2004;19:629–36.
11. Rittie L, Kang S, Voorhees JJ, Fisher GJ. Induction of collagen by estradiol: difference between sun-protected and photodamaged human skin in vivo. Arch Dermatol. 2008;144:1129–40.
12. Cunningham M, Gilkeson G. Estrogen receptors in immunity and autoimmunity. Clin Rev Allergy Immunol. 2011;40:66–73.

13. Jensen F, Woudwyk M, Teles A, Woidacki K, Taran F, Costa S, et al. Estradiol and progesterone regulate the migration of mast cells from the periphery to the uterus and induce their maturation and degranulation. PLoS One. 2010;5:e14409.
14. Stefano GB, Cadet P, Breton C, Goumon Y, Prevot V, Dessaint JP, et al. Estradiol-stimulated nitric oxide release in human granulocytes is dependent on intracellular calcium transients: evidence of a cell surface estrogen receptor. Blood. 2000;95:3951–8.
15. Son ED, Lee JY, Lee S, Kim MS, Lee BG, Chang IS, et al. Topical application of 17beta-estradiol increases extracellular matrix protein synthesis by stimulating tgf-Beta signaling in aged human skin in vivo. J Invest Dermatol. 2005;124:1149–61.
16. Brincat M, Moniz CJ, Studd JW, Darby A, Magos A, Emburey G, et al. Long-term effects of the menopause and sex hormones on skin thickness. Br J Obstet Gynaecol. 1985;92:256–9.
17. Brincat M, Versi E, Moniz CF, Magos A, de Trafford J, Studd JW. Skin collagen changes in postmenopausal women receiving different regimens of estrogen therapy. Obstet Gynecol. 1987;70:123–7.
18. Brincat M, Yuen AW, Studd JW, Montgomery J, Magos AL, Savvas M. Response of skin thickness and metacarpal index to estradiol therapy in postmenopausal women. Obstet Gynecol. 1987;70:538–41.
19. Castelo-Branco C, Duran M, Gonzalez-Merlo J. Skin collagen changes related to age and hormone replacement therapy. Maturitas. 1992;15:113–9.
20. Maheux R, Naud F, Rioux M, Grenier R, Lemay A, Guy J, et al. A randomized, double-blind, placebo-controlled study on the effect of conjugated estrogens on skin thickness. Am J Obstet Gynecol. 1994;170:642–9.
21. Haapasaari K-M, Raudaskoski T, Kallioinen M, Suvanto-Luukkonen E, Kauppila A, Läärä E, et al. Systemic therapy with estrogen or estrogen with progestin has no effect on skin collagen in postmenopausal women. Maturitas. 1997;27:153–62.
22. Sauerbronn AV, Fonseca AM, Bagnoli VR, Saldiva PH, Pinotti JA. The effects of systemic hormonal replacement therapy on the skin of postmenopausal women. Int J Gynaecol Obstet. 2000;68:35–41.
23. Brincat M, Versi E, O'Dowd T, Moniz CF, Magos A, Kabalan S, et al. Skin collagen changes in postmenopausal women receiving oestradiol gel. Maturitas. 1987;9:1–5.
24. Weiss JS, Ellis CN, Headington JT, Tincoff T, Hamilton TA, Voorhees JJ. Topical tretinoin improves photoaged skin. A double-blind vehicle-controlled study. JAMA. 1988;259:527–32.
25. Creidi P, Faivre B, Agache P, Richard E, Haudiquet V, Sauvanet JP. Effect of a conjugated oestrogen (Premarin) cream on ageing facial skin. A comparative study with a placebo cream. Maturitas. 1994;19:211–23.
26. Schmidt JB, Binder M, Demschik G, Bieglmayer C, Reiner A. Treatment of skin aging with topical estrogens. Int J Dermatol. 1996;35:669–74.
27. Yoon HS, Lee SR, Chung JH. Long-term topical oestrogen treatment of Sun-exposed facial skin in post-menopausal women does not improve facial wrinkles or skin elasticity, but induces matrix metalloproteinase-1 expression. Acta Derm Venereol. 2014;94:4–8.
28. Dunn LB, Damesyn M, Moore AA, Reuben DB, Greendale GA. Does estrogen prevent skin aging? Results from the First National Health and Nutrition Examination Survey (NHANES I). Arch Dermatol. 1997;133:339–42.
29. Pierard-Franchimont C, Cornil F, Dehavay J, Deleixhe-Mauhin F, Letot B, Pierard GE. Climacteric skin ageing of the face – a prospective longitudinal comparative trial on the effect of oral hormone replacement therapy. Maturitas. 1999;32:87–93.
30. Sumino H, Ichikawa S, Abe M, Endo Y, Ishikawa O, Kurabayashi M. Effects of aging, menopause, and hormone replacement therapy on forearm skin elasticity in women. J Am Geriatr Soc. 2004;52:945–9.
31. Wolff EF, Narayan D, Taylor HS. Long-term effects of hormone therapy on skin rigidity and wrinkles. Fertil Steril. 2005;84:285–8.
32. Sator PG, Sator MO, Schmidt JB, Nahavandi H, Radakovic S, Huber JC, et al. A prospective, randomized, double-blind, placebo-controlled study on the influence of a hormone replacement therapy on skin aging in postmenopausal women. Climacteric. 2007;10:320–34.
33. Kaatz M, Elsner P, Koehler MJ. Changes in skin topography during hormone therapy. Menopause. 2008;15:1193–4.
34. Phillips TJ, Symons J, Menon S, HTS Group. Does hormone therapy improve age-related skin changes in postmenopausal women? A randomized, double-blind, double-dummy, placebo-controlled multicenter study assessing the effects of norethindrone acetate and ethinyl estradiol in the improvement of mild to moderate age-related skin changes in postmenopausal women. J Am Acad Dermatol. 2008;59:397–404; e393.
35. Patriarca MT, Goldman KZ, Dos Santos JM, Petri V, Simoes RS, Soares Jr JM, et al. Effects of topical estradiol on the facial skin collagen of postmenopausal women under oral hormone therapy: a pilot study. Eur J Obstet Gynecol Reprod Biol. 2007;130:202–5.
36. Neder L, Medeiros SF. Topical estradiol does not interfere with the expression of the metalloproteinase-1 enzyme in photo exposed skin cells. An Bras Dermatol. 2012;87:70–5.
37. Fisher GJ, Talwar HS, Lin J, Lin P, McPhillips F, Wang Z, et al. Retinoic acid inhibits induction of c-Jun protein by ultraviolet radiation that occurs subsequent to activation of mitogen-activated protein kinase pathways in human skin in vivo. J Clin Invest. 1998;101:1432–40.
38. Fisher GJ, Datta SC, Talwar HS, Wang ZQ, Varani J, Kang S, et al. Molecular basis of sun-induced premature skin ageing and retinoid antagonism. Nature. 1996;379:335–9.

39. Silbiger S, Lei J, Neugarten J. Estradiol suppresses type I collagen synthesis in mesangial cells via activation of activator protein-1. Kidney Int. 1999;55: 1268–76.
40. Vincenti MP, Coon CI, Brinckerhoff CE. Nuclear factor kappaB/p50 activates an element in the distal matrix metalloproteinase 1 promoter in interleukin-1beta-stimulated synovial fibroblasts. Arthritis Rheum. 1998;41:1987–94.
41. Yoon HS, Shin CY, Kim YK, Lee SR, Chung JH. Endogenous estrogen exacerbates UV-induced inflammation and photoaging in mice. J Invest Dermatol. 2014;134:2290–3.
42. Kanda N, Watanabe S. 17beta-estradiol enhances heparin-binding epidermal growth factor-like growth factor production in human keratinocytes. Am J Physiol Cell Physiol. 2005;288:C813–23.
43. Kanda N, Watanabe S. 17beta-estradiol stimulates the growth of human keratinocytes by inducing cyclin D2 expression. J Invest Dermatol. 2004;123: 319–28.
44. Rock K, Meusch M, Fuchs N, Tigges J, Zipper P, Fritsche E, et al. Estradiol protects dermal hyaluronan/versican matrix during photoaging by release of epidermal growth factor from keratinocytes. J Biol Chem. 2012;287:20056–69.

139 Solutions and Products for Managing Female Urinary Incontinence

Nancy Karapasha

Contents

N. Karapasha (✉)
The Procter & Gamble Company, Cincinnati, OH, USA
e-mail: nkarapasha@gmail.com

M.A. Farage et al. (eds.), *Textbook of Aging Skin*,
DOI 10.1007/978-3-662-47398-6_102

Abstract
Several options are available to women with urinary incontinence depending on key factors. Those key factors might include (1) type and severity of the problem, (2) level of acceptance or embarrassment of the incontinence problem, (3) available product options, (4) cost and affordability of disposable products, and (5) coverage and reimbursement by healthcare companies. These women deserve significant improvements in today's products as well as new product solutions.

Introduction

There are various solutions available to and chosen by women with urinary incontinence with the solution chosen dependent on a variety of factors. The key factors include: type and severity of the problem, level of acceptance and level of embarrassment of the problem, disposable income, product options available to her (choices vary by geography), and healthcare and reimbursement situation.

Types of Incontinence, Symptoms, and Impact of Symptoms on Solutions

The type of solutions an incontinent woman chooses is very dependent on the type of incontinence symptoms she experiences. Most women with bladder leakage have either stress urinary incontinence (SUI), urge urinary incontinence (UUI), or mixed (both stress and urge) urinary incontinence (MUI). SUI is the most common, with about 15 million women in the USA, followed by MUI, with about 11 million women in the USA, and UUI, with about five million women in the USA [1].

Stress incontinence is defined as involuntary urinary leakage on exertion, sneezing, or coughing and occurs when bladder pressure exceeds urethral resistance under conditions of increased abdominal pressure [2]. Generally, stress urinary incontinence occurs due to weakened pelvic muscles caused by childbirth, lack of estrogen, or from being overweight. Women with SUI typically have small amounts of urine loss described as urine drops or small spurts [3]. Urine loss episode from SUI can be up to 25 ml (approximately 1/10 of a cup) [3]. Therefore, many women with SUI use products designed for light incontinence because the amount of fluid is fairly slight.

Urge incontinence is defined as involuntary urinary leakage accompanied by or immediately preceded by urgency and is a function of uncontrolled detrusor contractions that overcome urethral resistance [2]. Women with UUI experience a strong, sudden need to urinate immediately followed by a bladder contraction, resulting in an involuntary loss of urine. Many women often have specific sounds that seem to trigger this sudden urge to urinate, such as the rattling of keys as they open the door to get home or the sound of running water. Urge incontinence is caused by a neurological issue in which signals are not properly sent to the bladder muscle. Women who have UUI often have urine loss of ¼ cup or more per episode [3]. Sometimes, a UUI episode could lead to a full bladder emptying, which is why many women with UUI tend to use products designed for moderate to heavy loss.

Women with MUI are dealing with both SUI and UUI symptoms, so they typically are using products designed for moderate to severe loss because they have to protect for the most severe condition, which is urge.

Another factor affecting her choice of solutions is the frequency she experiences urine loss. The data following shows that of the general population that experience incontinence, her incidence is approximately: 35 % experience urine loss one or more times daily, 25 % experience urine loss three or more times a week, 17 % experience urine loss about once a week, 13 % experience urine loss one to three times a month, and 10 % experience less than one time a month [4]. Obviously, the more frequent the urine loss, the more prepared she needs to be, and often the higher the level of protection she chooses.

The solutions chosen by women with incontinence are also dependent on her level of acceptance and level of embarrassment associated with the problem and general attitudes about how to manage problems. Some women are naturally proactive in managing solutions, while others tend to be more reactive. Some are early adopters who like to try new products, while others tend to find a solution that works for them and are slow to change to new options. Some have experienced a very embarrassing leak that has greatly impacted their solution system. In this case, she may overprotect in the future just to be on the safe side. All of these factors play a big role in how she approaches the problem and the solutions she chooses.

Where do women get information about products and solutions for incontinence? A recent study, in 2013, among those women experiencing bladder leakage, showed that about 45 % of incontinent women [5] had spoken to a doctor about their incontinence. Some women choose to confide in one or two close friends or family members to discuss the problem and possible solutions (see Table 1). There are several websites that provide

Table 1 Among adult incontinence sufferers: since experiencing bladder leakage, which of the following have you done? [5]

Consumers who experience AI and use a mix of AI and/or only feminine care products	$n =$ 785
Spoken to a doctor about my bladder leakage	46 %
Looked online for information about the condition or products to address it	30 %
Spoke about the issue with friends	27 %

information on how to manage the problem and different products and solutions available. Of course, manufacturers of various products reach consumers through television ads, print ads, websites, etc. Women's health magazines are also a source of information.

Behavior of Women with Incontinence

Before discussing details of the types of products used to manage bladder leakage, it is important to recognize the coping mechanisms and behavior modifications that are common among women with incontinence. These activities are common for women with slight urine loss as well as women with severe urine loss.

Controlling Fluid Intake

Many women simply choose to drink less liquids, in order to produce less urine. While the logic makes sense that less input equals less output, the issue is that this could lead to health issues, like dehydration.

Constantly Emptying the Bladder

Another way to reduce the risk of a bladder leak is to make frequent trips to the bathroom to urinate, leaving the bladder as empty as possible throughout the day. One very common practice is to always empty the bladder before leaving the house. A majority (56 %) of women claim to go to the bathroom before leaving the house [3]. This is extremely important if she is going to be away from the house for a significant period of time. In fact, if she will be gone from the house for a long time, she will often map out in advance exactly where the bathrooms are and when she will be able to go to the bathroom. She will sometimes avoid going to an unfamiliar place if she is not sure where a bathroom is. In addition, 18 % of women with incontinence claim to locate bathrooms when in a new place [3].

Avoiding Activities that Cause Leaks

Many women will consciously avoid activities that tend to cause leaks, particularly women with SUI, such as jogging, walking, lifting items, aerobics, running around with kids, or jumping on a trampoline. We have even heard women say that they will avoid going out with their "funny" friends to avoid laughter.

Changing Underwear/Clothing or Shower/Bathing More Often

Around 26 % of women claimed to change underwear or clothing more often as a way to help manage the problem, and 22 % claimed to shower or bathe more often [3].

Bracing Herself to Eliminate or Minimize the Amount of Leakage

Many women have talked about how they can sometimes prevent a leak by crossing their legs or by bracing herself (tightening the pelvic muscles) during a potential leak-causing situation. Women have told us they sometimes can fight their way through a leak by bracing herself or crossing her legs when she knows a sneeze is coming.

Bringing a Change of Clothes

Another common coping behavior is to bring a change of clothes when away from home, just in case of an accident. One clever trick is buying two pairs of the same pants, so that if a need arises to change pants when away from home due to a leaking accident, it can be done inconspicuously.

Exercise

Pelvic floor muscle exercises are a solution some women choose to manage their incontinence, particularly those with stress incontinence. Approximately 40 % of incontinent women claim they have done exercises designed to help reduce bladder leakage [5].

The pelvic muscles play a critical role in supporting the urethra and bladder neck. When the urethra and bladder neck are not supported properly, leaks can occur. Although recommendations regarding the number of repetitions necessary for treatment vary widely, efficacy has been shown with 30–50 daily contractions [6, 7].

If a woman has gone to her doctor, and if the symptoms appear to be those of stress urinary incontinence, the doctor will often advise the patient to try doing pelvic floor exercises on her own for the next 8–10 weeks. The doctor will often provide some general directions on how to do the Kegel exercises, encouraging her to do them while at a traffic light or when watching TV. Often, the doctor will ask the patient to come back for a visit in 2–3 months to discuss progress and options. Often, when she goes back to the doctor, she reports no progress because she has either not isolated the proper muscles (hard to do without any feedback system to confirm you have the right muscles) or she has not done the exercises frequent enough over several weeks. At this point, the doctor will often run urodynamic testing to confirm the type of incontinence. If stress incontinence is confirmed, the doctor may refer her to an incontinence clinic with programs which teach proper muscle isolation and can help ensure proper compliance.

There are also several pelvic floor exercise products available for home use. Some are available by prescription; others are available for purchase directly by consumers. While many of these devices have been proven effective clinically, compliance with routine usage of these devices is likely the biggest barrier to success. Vaginally inserted weighted "cones" are also available. These products are vaginally inserted and come in various sizes and weights. Vaginal cones are intended to provide internal pressure such that the pelvic muscles are contracted and exercised in order to keep the cones in the body.

Surgery is another option for some women with SUI. Very few women choose surgery as an option, due to perceived risks, recovery time, and costs. Two common procedures, the Burch colposuspension and fascial sling method, have shown success rates 2 years postsurgery to be 47 % and 38 %, respectively [8]. Both of these methods are designed to increase urethral support. The newer less invasive TVT (tension-free vaginal tape) surgery procedure has shown success rates of 81 % 7 years postsurgery [9].

Type of Products Used to Manage Urine Leakage

There are several types of absorbent products available for women to use (Table 2). First, it is important to note that 8 % of women choose to not treat their AI. Some choose to not use any products because the amount of fluid and frequency of leaks can be managed through different behaviors such as fluid intake management, frequent bathroom visits, underwear changes, etc. Some women choose to not use absorbent pads because they simply do not like the feeling of wearing an absorbent pad.

The most common type of absorbent product used for managing incontinence is a feminine care pantiliners. Pantiliners are inexpensive, thin, comfortable, and portable products that have enough absorbency to absorb small leaks. These are common among women with SUI because the amount of urine loss is small. Another reason many women choose pantiliners is because there is less embarrassment to buy these hygiene products than buying incontinent products. Recall this is a very private matter;; there are many women who do not talk to anyone about their condition, so keeping this condition a secret is very important. Being seen

Table 2 Among those that experience incontinence: what types of products used to treat incontinence? [4]

Products used to treat incontinence	*N* = 2433
Feminine care pads/pantiliners	56 %
Products designed especially for incontinence (pads/briefs)	10 %
Using both femcare and products especially for incontinence	27 %
Not using any products	8 %

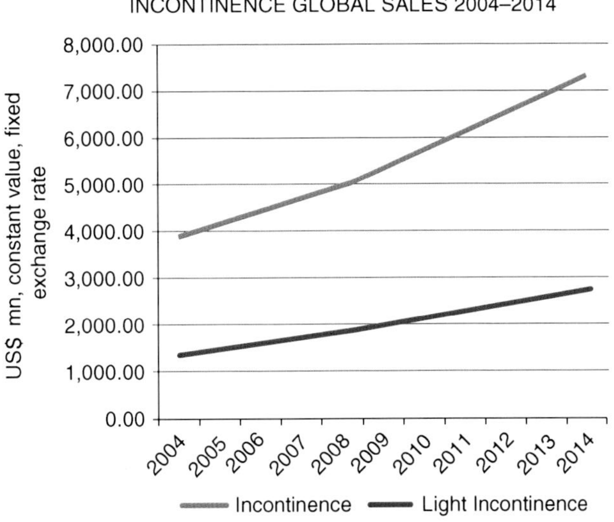

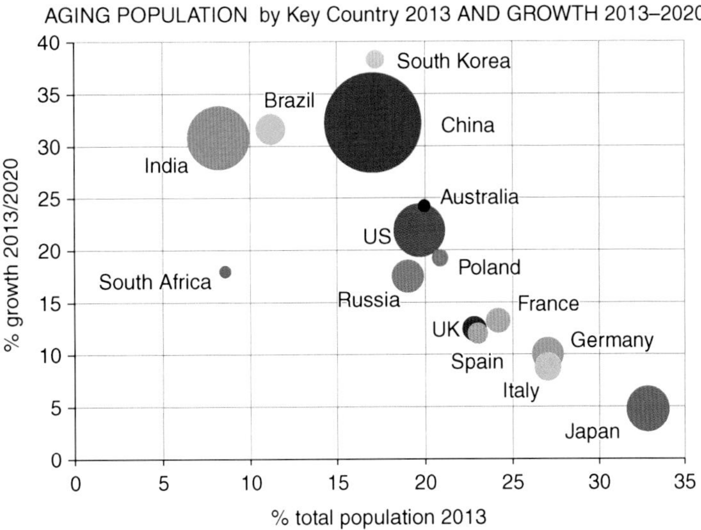

Fig. 1 Source: with kind permission from Euromonitor International [10, 12]

by a store clerk or someone she knows at a store checkout line purchasing a product designed for incontinence can be devastatingly embarrassing. Some women choose to use feminine care pads to manage incontinence. These offer more absorbency than a feminine care pantiliner and are often longer and thicker.

Some women choose pantiliners and pads designed specifically for incontinence. The key benefit of incontinence pads is they offer significantly more absorbency than menstrual products and, therefore, can often handle larger bladder leaks and help manage odor better. Some women choose to not buy these products because of the stigma associated with purchasing incontinent products, even if these products may work better than feminine care pantiliners and pads. These products come in various absorbencies. Depending on the absorbency a woman chooses, the median urine load while wearing an incontinent pad is between 7 g and 75 g, and the percentage of changes in which a woman says she "felt dry" ranges from 60 % to 85 % [3]. Obviously, the amount of urine loading and the level of dryness she feels are important in the design of these products.

Women with moderate to severe leakage often choose incontinent briefs and underwear. These products are designed to absorb full bladder leaks, often caused by UUI or MUI. They also are used by women who suffer from both urine and bowel incontinence.

Adult Incontinent Market

The adult incontinent market is growing and is driven by an aging population, developing markets with an increase of knowledge and awareness in incontinence, and the expanding retail market with multitiered approach to marketing has increased the affordability of incontinent products. Retail sales, in 2014, grew 8 % in volume and 6 % in value to exceed $7 billion. This growth is two times the global retail hygiene market in the past decade. It is projected that in 2014–2019, the sales will register a 7 % Compound Annual Growth Rate (CAGR) to $10 billion with a volume of 23 billion units (Fig. 1) [10, 12].

Table 3 Market size: incontinence total light, moderate/heavy (fixed 2014 exchange rate) (Source: Euromonitor International: Tissue and Hygiene [11])

Region	$ million
Asia Pacific	2328.7
Australasia	126.7
Eastern Europe	212.3
Latin America	1082.2
North America	1867.4
Western Europe	1660.5

In regard to volume and value share, the USA and Japan remain the world's largest markets for incontinence. The USA and Japan account for 53 % share of the global incontinent volume and 46 % of the global incontinent value [10]. In 2014, both markets showed upward trends that delivered an increase of 8 % in the USA and 6 % in Japan volume growth (Table 3).

Although the USA and Japan are developed and growing markets, developing markets such as Brazil and China are showing positive growth. The openness and growing understanding of incontinence, availability of a variety of products to meet the need, and rising incomes, with an increased affordability and availability, are igniting growth in these markets.

Brazil shows not only an increase in retail sales from 2013 to 2014 of 12 %, but with the Brazilian government subsidizing the purchase of incontinent products has allowed incontinent products to be offered to lower income consumers who previously would not have had the opportunity to purchase.

Emerging Markets: Retail Incontinence Sales Volume, 2004–2014

See Fig. 2.

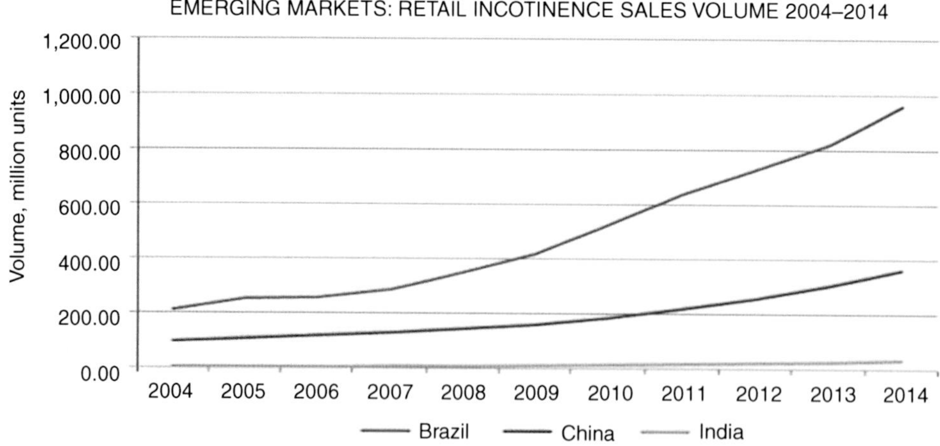

Fig. 2 Source: Euromonitor International [10]

Table 4 Additional products used among incontinent women (Source: Internal Procter & Gamble Study 2013)

	$n = 785$
Product used	% total use
Wipes (feminine, baby, etc.)	62 %
Intimate wash	22 %
Body wash	55 %
Powders	35 %
Diaper rash/cream/ ointment	17 %
Skin creams/lotions	31 %

Managing Incontinence

Skin irritation can be an issue with unintentional urine loss. Thirteen percent (13 %) of incontinent women claimed to experience skin irritation at least once a week, 16 % claimed at least once a month, and 72 % claimed once a month or less [3]. Given the long wear time of incontinent pads (6–10 h on average) and wetness from urine loss and perspiration, it is not surprising that skin irritation occurs. Also, given only 1/3 of loaded changes are changed immediately after urine loss [3], it is important that products acquire and store urine immediately to help the consumer feel dry and to reduce skin irritation.

Satisfaction of absorbent products tends to be fairly high, relative to other categories tested at P&G. One way to measure the biggest improvement opportunity is to compare several product attributes for both importance to the consumer and level of satisfaction. Those items with the greatest unmet needs are often those with high importance and low satisfaction. The greatest unmet needs for absorbent products among women with bladder leakage are daytime leak prevention, controlling urine odor, controlling skin irritation, and having products that stay in place [3].

Table 4 describes the use of a variety of products to help manage odor and skin health in addition to the absorbent products.

Conclusions

Overall, women use a wide variety of products and practices for managing unintentional urine loss. While satisfaction with these products individually is relatively high, as a whole, the fact that there are so many compensating behaviors (constant bladder emptying, fluid intake restrictions, activity avoidance, etc.) in addition to the products available to manage the problem indicates a need for a better experience for the incontinence sufferer. These women deserve significant improvements in today's products as well as new product solutions.

Cross-References

- ▶ Changes in Vulvar Physiology and Skin Disorders with Age and Benefits of Feminine Wipes in Postmenopausal Women
- ▶ Cutaneous Effects and Sensitive Skin with Incontinence in the Aged

References

External and Internal References

1. Mattson Jack Epidemiology Database.
2. Abrams P, Cardozo L, Fall M et al. Analysis of the standardisation of terminology of lower urinary tract dysfunction: report from the Standardisation Sub-Committee of the International Continence Society. Neurourol Urodyn. 2002;21:167–78.
3. Internal Procter & Gamble Study.
4. Internal Procter & Gamble Study 2014.
5. Internal Procter & Gamble Study 2013.
6. Burgio KL, Goode PS, Locher JL, et al. Behavioral training with and without biofeedback in the treatment of urge incontinence in older women: a randomized controlled trial. JAMA. 2002;288:2293–9.
7. Bo K. Pelvic floor muscle strength and response to pelvic floor muscle training for stress urinary incontinence. Neurourol Urodyn. 2003;22:654–8.
8. Albo ME, Richter HE, Brubaker L, et al. Burch colposuspension versus fascial sling to reduce urinary stress incontinence. N Engl J Med. 2007;356:2143–55.
9. Nilsson CG, Falconer C, Rezapour M. Seven-year follow-up of the tension-free vaginal tape procedure for treatment of urinary incontinence. Obstet Gynecol. 2004;104:1259–62.
10. Stevlana Uduslivaia, Euromonitor International. Tissue: from shame to fame: adult incontinence continues its global advance. 2015. www.euromonitor.com
11. Euromonitor International. Tissue and hygiene, market size, trade sources/national statistics. April 2015. www.euromonitor.com
12. Rob Walker, Euromonitor International. Procter & Gamble unlocks new sweet spot in incontinence finally. 2015. www.euromonitor.com

Therapeutic Alternatives for the Treatment of Epidermal Aging

140

Carla Abdo Brohem, Valéria Maria Di Mambro, and Márcio Lorencini

Contents

C.A. Brohem • V.M. Di Mambro • M. Lorencini (✉)
R&D Department, Grupo Boticário, São José dos Pinhais, PR, Brazil
e-mail: carla@grupoboticario.com.br; valeriamm@grupoboticario.com.br; marciolorencini@yahoo.com.br; marciolo@grupoboticario.com.br

M.A. Farage et al. (eds.), *Textbook of Aging Skin*,
DOI 10.1007/978-3-662-47398-6_140

Abstract

Over a lifetime, the epidermal layer of skin changes in structure and functionality, which contributes to the appearance of the clinical signs that characterize cutaneous aging, such as the appearance of wrinkles and pigmentation disorders, hydration dysfunction, and even cancer development. The search for effective treatments should consider the main biological functions of the epidermis affected by aging, including cell renewal and barrier integrity, antioxidant mechanisms and response to ultraviolet (UV) radiation, water-ion balance, and epidermal defense mechanisms. Several natural extracts and isolated compounds have been suggested in the literature as antiaging agents. However, a critical evaluation is essential to understand their mechanisms of action and how they could contribute to the development of promising therapeutic alternatives, in particular for the specific case of epidermal aging.

Introduction

Skin represents the largest and the most exposed organ of the human body and is indicative of an individual's health and well-being [1]. With time, the organism ages and the skin surface displays the cumulative effects of intrinsic (determined by genetic predisposition) and extrinsic (including but not limited to solar radiation, smoking, pollution, stress, and specific chemicals) factors [2, 3].

Despite several previous works describing the effects of aging on the skin, most of these works are focused on the dermis and the disorganization of its fiber-enriched extracellular matrix (ECM). The epidermis, the outer skin portion that is directly in contact with environmental factors, has largely not been discussed with respect to how aging affects its functional structure and how this could be prevented and/or treated. This chapter will focus on possible therapeutic approaches for the treatment of epidermal aging.

Epidermal Structure and the Effects of Aging

The structure of the epidermis represents an effective multilayered barrier that originates from the differentiation of keratinocytes, the most abundant epidermal cell type [4, 5]. The basal layer is the inner layer with highly proliferative keratinocytes, the spinous layer contains desmosome-enriched keratinocytes, the granular layer has keratinocytes abundant in lipid and protein granules, and the stratum corneum contains totally differentiated keratinocytes, also known as corneocytes [6–8]. The epidermis is a metabolically dynamic tissue that constantly undergoes renewal cycles [6, 9]. Keratinocyte differentiation involves the cross-linking of various proteins, and calcium is an important molecule in this process: lower concentrations stimulate cell renewal and division, while higher concentrations induce cell differentiation [10]. Additionally, other cell types are found in the epidermis, such as melanocytes, Langerhans cells (LC), Merkel cells, and stem cells [7, 11].

Over time, the epidermal primary functions may gradually fail, with signals that reveal skin aging becoming more apparent [12]. Some morphological and functional changes include a thinning of the epidermis, flattening of the dermal-epidermal junction (DEJ), decreased keratinocyte proliferation, and the appearance of senescent cells. Epidermal turnover takes 40–60 days in elderly people compared with 28 days in young people [13]. With age, an altered epidermal barrier permeability and epidermal homeostasis can induce the appearance of other skin disturbances, such as an increased susceptibility to irritants, development of contact dermatitis, and severe xerosis. Aged individuals show impaired epidermal repair capacity after tape stripping, evidenced by a more difficult recovery of transepidermal water loss (TEWL) and a slower gene expression activation [14]. Differential regulation of miRNAs in LC with age leads to immunosenescence, with an increased susceptibility to cutaneous viral and fungal infections as well as to skin cancer development [15]. UVB causes oxidative damages in keratinocytes and melanocytes through the genesis of reactive oxygen species (ROS), accelerating skin aging by the induction of epidermal hyperplasia, stratum corneum thickening, sunburn, synthesis of inflammatory cytokines, formation of pigmented spots and wrinkles, immunosuppression, and cancer [10, 16, 17].

A recent review published by Lorencini and colleagues [9] addressed the possible therapeutic alternatives for combating human epidermal aging based on the application of active ingredients. In addition to a review of the major topics of the epidermal functions affected by aging, current active ingredients for potential cosmetic and/or dermatological applications, specifically as regards their biological and biophysical effects on the regulation of age-impaired epidermal homeostasis, were discussed (Fig. 1).

Therapeutic Alternatives for Cell Renewal and Barrier Integrity

Cell renewal and barrier integrity are important characteristics for protection against mechanical and chemical insults, which are directly affected by differentiation and the proliferation rate of keratinocytes [18]. Age-affected skin shows a reduction in epidermal thickness as a consequence of decreased cell renewal [12, 19–21]. Physical treatments for epithelium renewal and keratinocyte proliferation have been suggested, such as photodynamic therapy [22, 23], high-energy pulsed CO_2 laser [24, 25], and a fractional CO_2 laser [26, 27]. However, the active ingredients in cosmetic and pharmacological formulas

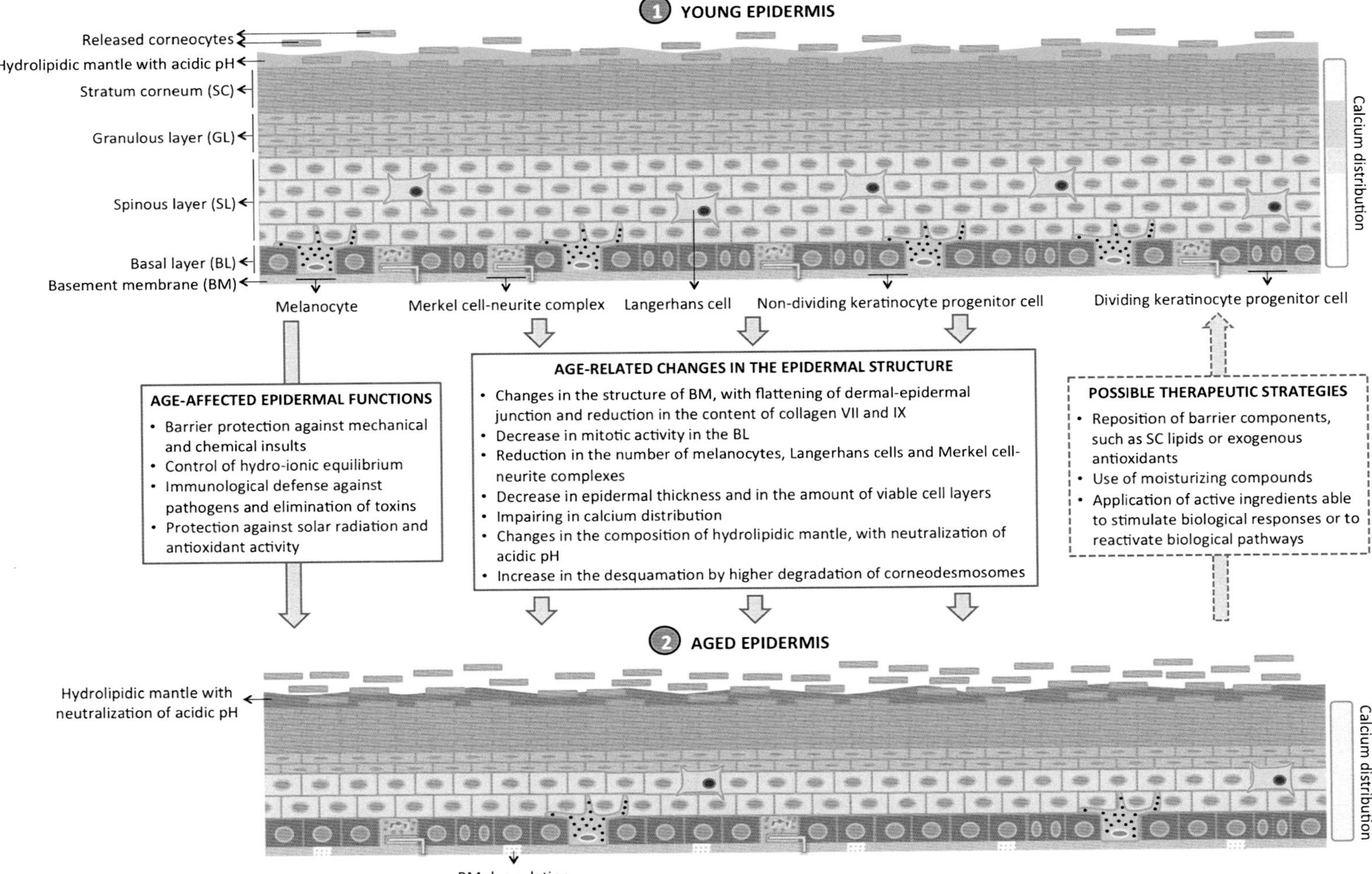

1 YOUNG EPIDERMIS
Released corneocytes
Hydrolipidic mantle with acidic pH
Stratum corneum (SC)
Granulous layer (GL)
Spinous layer (SL)
Basal layer (BL)
Basement membrane (BM)
Calcium distribution
Melanocyte
Merkel cell-neurite complex
Langerhans cell
Non-dividing keratinocyte progenitor cell
Dividing keratinocyte progenitor cell
AGE-AFFECTED EPIDERMAL FUNCTIONS
• Barrier protection against mechanical and chemical insults
• Control of hydro-ionic equilibrium
• Immunological defense against pathogens and elimination of toxins
• Protection against solar radiation and antioxidant activity
AGE-RELATED CHANGES IN THE EPIDERMAL STRUCTURE
• Changes in the structure of BM, with flattening of dermal-epidermal junction and reduction in the content of collagen VII and IX
• Decrease in mitotic activity in the BL
• Reduction in the number of melanocytes, Langerhans cells and Merkel cell-neurite complexes
• Decrease in epidermal thickness and in the amount of viable cell layers
• Impairing in calcium distribution
• Changes in the composition of hydrolipidic mantle, with neutralization of acidic pH
• Increase in the desquamation by higher degradation of corneodesmosomes
POSSIBLE THERAPEUTIC STRATEGIES
• Reposition of barrier components, such as SC lipids or exogenous antioxidants
• Use of moisturizing compounds
• Application of active ingredients able to stimulate biological responses or to reactivate biological pathways
2 AGED EPIDERMIS
Hydrolipidic mantle with neutralization of acidic pH
Calcium distribution
BM degradation

Fig. 1 (continued)

are used much more frequently for these purposes. Among these ingredients, many different types of molecules of different origins, including natural extracts and isolated compounds, retinoic acid and its derivatives, and alpha-hydroxy acids, can be found.

Achillea millefolium extract has been shown to help increase epidermal thickness in vitro and improve the appearance of wrinkles and pores in comparison with a placebo in vivo [28]. *Simarouba amara* extract has been shown to stimulate involucrin expression and activation of transglutaminase in skin fragments, which has an effect on improving barrier function and skin hydration ex vivo [29]. The compound hesperidin, isolated from natural orange rind extract, has been demonstrated to promote proliferation, differentiation, and secretion of lamellar bodies in mouse epidermis [30]. Green tea polyphenols and their well-described component epigallocatechin-3-gallate (EGCG) stimulated proliferation and differentiation of primary human keratinocytes, and induced higher levels of expression of keratin 1 and filaggrin and increased transglutaminase activity. In aged keratinocytes, green tea polyphenols stimulated DNA synthesis and succinate dehydrogenase activation, while EGCG modulated the expression of caspase 14, typically associated with keratinocyte differentiation and cornification [31, 32].

Vitamin A, also called retinoic acid, is a natural constituent of the epidermis, being the most widely used compound for epidermal renewal due to its ability to induce keratinocyte proliferation and differentiation, with a direct impact on wrinkle appearance and formation [16, 33, 34]. However, it is well known to be unstable in cosmetic formulations with typical collateral effects such as skin irritation [33, 34]. For this reason, vitamin A precursors and derivatives, such as retinaldehyde or retinol [34], retinyl retinoate [35, 36], and retinyl palmitate [37], are used as alternatives for cosmetic applications. Additionally, these molecules reduce skin hyperpigmentation caused by sunlight [38] and have inhibitory effects on metalloproteinase expression [39]. Lutein significantly increases the transcript activity of the retinoic acid responsive element, and its metabolites act as retinoic acid receptor ligands in keratinocytes, which makes this carotenoid a potential substitute for retinoids [40].

Alpha-hydroxy acids (AAA), such as glycolic acid and lactic acid, are used in cosmetic formulations due to their potential to stimulate epidermal renewal in photodamaged skin, to increase skin thickness and firmness, and to improve skin softness and the appearance of fine lines and wrinkles in clinical treatments [41–43]. Chemical peelings are also possible with AAA, once they reduce the amount of calcium ions in the epidermis, disrupting cell adhesions and resulting in desquamation [44].

Niacinamide, nicotinic acid, or vitamin B3 reduces TEWL, improves the moisture content of the cornified layer, and stabilizes the epidermal barrier function throughout by promoting keratin and ceramide synthesis, accelerating keratinocyte differentiation, and increasing intercellular nicotinamide adenine dinucleotide phosphate (NADP) levels. Topical application of niacinamide on aged skin has also been reported to improve the skin surface, softening wrinkles, and to inhibit photocarcinogenesis [45]. Myristyl nicotinate (MN), a nicotinic acid derivative, was developed for the treatment of photodamaged skin, which increases the content of nicotinamide adenine dinucleotide (NAD) in skin by 25 %, in addition

Fig. 1 Molecular, cell and morphological changes associated with epidermal aging. As the epidermis ages, it undergoes a series of structural modifications that directly impact its physiological functions, compromising the natural protective barrier of the organism. The diagram indicates calcium distribution points with a higher ion concentration in the granular layer (*GL*) and a darker colored region in the young epidermis (*1*). In older epidermis (*2*), the calcium gradient is lost and calcium is possibly distributed homogeneously among the skin layers. Possible therapeutic alternatives have different mechanisms of action, based on their active ingredients or compounds, which are capable of helping to recover age-affected physiological functions to an extent that will approximate those in the young epidermis as nearly as possible (This figure is reproduced from Lorencini and colleagues [9])

to increasing the thickness of the stratum corneum by 70 % and of the whole epidermis by 20 %. The epidermal renewal rate in skin treated with MN increases 6–11 %, and the TEWL rate decreases 20 % [46].

Therapeutic Alternatives for Antioxidant Mechanisms and UV Response

The generation of ROS has two main sources in the skin: the first is from endogenous metabolic processes, such as cell respiration, and the second is related to solar exposure, especially UV radiation [47, 48]. UVB can induce mutations in keratinocytes, which are usually prevented by the cellular machinery responsible for ROS elimination, cell cycle arrest, DNA repair, and, in the last instance, apoptosis induction [49]. These defense mechanisms are present in all body tissues but become vulnerable with age [50]. For example, in the epidermis of older individuals, the removal of DNA damage is slower and antioxidant ability is reduced, as there are lower concentrations of α-tocopherol, ascorbic acid, and glutathione [51, 52]. Consequently, epidermal aging is characterized by higher levels of oxidized and inactive proteins that accumulate inside of cells [53]. To reinforce ROS protection, exogenous antioxidant supplementation can be topical or orally administered. The most popular worldwide products are cosmetics formulated with antioxidants, usually obtained from natural plant extracts [54, 55]. Furthermore, sunscreens are also recommended to avoid the damaging effects of excessive solar radiation.

Regarding natural plant preparations, *Calluna vulgaris* extract, when topically applied on mouse skin, has been shown to protect skin from UV-induced DNA damage by diminishing tumor necrosis factor alpha (TNF-α) and interleukin 6 (IL-6) levels and inhibiting the formation of pyrimidine dimers and sunburn cells [56]. Green tea extract, rich in polyphenols, has an evident skin photoprotection potential by acting through anti-inflammatory, antioxidant, and DNA repair mechanisms, and when used as a topical treatment on human skin, it reduced UV-induced p53 expression – an important molecule in cell cycle regulation – and the number of apoptotic keratinocytes [57]. An extract from Jacquez grape wine was shown to maintain the epidermal redox state after exposure to UVB radiation when tested on reconstituted skin [58]. The polyphenol-rich pomegranate fruit extract also displayed an effect on photoaging prevention by inhibiting UVB effects, such as a reduction in cell viability and intracellular glutathione content and an increase in lipid peroxidation [59]. Red orange extract neutralized UVB-induced events associated with inflammation and apoptosis in the HaCaT human keratinocyte cell line [60]. Isoflavone-enriched soybean extract inhibited UVB-induced cell death in HaCaT cells in in vitro experiments, while the in vivo topical application prior to UV irradiation was able to reduce epidermal thickness and expression of cyclooxygenase 2 (COX-2) and proliferating cell nuclear antigen (PCNA), as well as to increase catalase concentration [61]. *Vitis vinifera* shoot extract showed antioxidant activity when applied to human keratinocytes, increasing the concentration of reduced glutathione and the activity of trans-plasma membrane oxidoreductase in a time- and dose-dependent manner [62, 63]. Flavonoid-enriched cocoa powder showed a reduction in erythemas, improved skin appearance and hydration, augmented skin layer thickness, and lowered the TEWL in female volunteers treated for 12 weeks [64].

Because the biological activity has been identified and well characterized for specific compounds, they can be isolated from plant extracts for potential therapeutic optimization. Astaxanthin was isolated from the microalga *Haematococcus pluvialis* and showed potential in suppressing oxidative melanocyte polymerization and epidermal inflammation and reducing aging spots [65]. β-carotene, a derivative from vegetables such as carrots, inhibited UVA-induced gene modulation in HaCaT cells and, in non-irradiated cells, significantly reduced the expression of genes related to oxidative stress and ECM degradation [66].

Catechins represent a class of chemicals – including epicatechin-3-gallate (ECG) and EGCG – isolated from green, white, and black teas with a significant antioxidant activity on skin. ECG has been shown to prevent keratinocyte death through inhibition of UVA-related hydrogen peroxide production and UVB-related membrane lipid peroxidation, while EGCG lowered UVB-induced cytotoxicity and inhibited mRNA expression for apoptosis-regulating genes and the enzyme inducible nitric oxide synthase (iNOS) in keratinocyte cultures. In a human in vivo study, the addition of EGCG to a broad-spectrum sunscreen decreased UV-induced damage compared with sunscreen alone [67–72].

Carotenoids can act in the recovery of epidermal antioxidants that are lost during UV exposure and protect skin from damage caused by UV. Lycopene can be used as a preventive agent for inhibiting the activity of epidermal ornithine decarboxylase, decreasing inflammation, maintaining an adequate cell proliferation rate, and avoiding DNA damage after UVB exposure [73, 74]. Moreover, carotenoids are also considered as excellent nutricosmetics, improving skin resilience and hydration [75].

Other molecules, such as ascorbic acid or vitamin C, have also been described for the treatment of skin aging, acting in deep and superficial wrinkles and promoting skin elasticity, firmness, roughness, and hydration [76, 77]. α-tocopherol, a form of vitamin E, has shown a high antioxidant potential by reducing the production of inflammation markers in UV-exposed human keratinocytes through an inhibition of NADPH oxidase activity [78].

Therapeutic Alternatives for Water-Ion Balance and Hydration

Homeostasis is represented by the exchange of substances with the environment, especially water and ions, and the epidermis plays a fundamental role in controlling that process [79]. To keep this functionality, different classes of lipids are essential in the epidermal structure, including ceramides, fatty acids, cholesterol, esters, triglycerides, and phospholipids [80]. The production of natural moisturizing factors (NMFs) and the presence of aquaporins (AQP) – channels that run along epidermal cell membranes – are also necessary to preserve adequate amounts of water and soluble ions [81]. However, age tends to modify the epidermal homeostatic control as a result of decreased lipid synthesis that leads to a more porous and less efficient ECM structure, reduced free amino acids in the NMF content of the stratum corneum, and a lower AQP3 expression [12, 82–84]. As alternatives for recovering the epidermal function of maintaining a water-ion balance in the skin, the list of possible active ingredients includes waxes, natural oils and their derivatives, and compounds that stimulate the endogenous synthesis of epidermal biomolecules.

Botryococcus braunii microalgae extract and hydroglycolic plant extracts increased the gene expression of AQP3 and cornified envelope proteins, such as filaggrin and involucrin in human keratinocytes in vitro [85, 86]. In the case of *P. colubrina*, a higher skin hydration was confirmed by increased corneometric indices and reduced TEWL in clinical studies after treatment with extract-containing formulations [85]. Treatment with glyceryl glucoside – an enhanced glycerol derivative – increased the levels of AQP3 mRNA and protein in cultured human keratinocytes, while in vivo studies on volunteer subjects demonstrated significantly increased AQP3 mRNA levels in the skin and reduced TEWL compared with vehicle-controlled areas [87]. Another compound that was shown to upregulate AQP mRNA expression was urea, which increased the gene expression of AQP3, AQP7, and AQP9 in cultivated normal human keratinocytes. The in vivo application of urea was also demonstrated to stimulate the production of lipids, enzymes related to lipid synthesis, such as transglutaminase-1, and proteins from the cornified envelope, such as filaggrin, loricrin, and involucrin [88].

The aqueous gromwell extract showed a potent effect on inducing keratinocyte migration and maintaining skin hydration through an increased synthesis of phospholipids, sphingolipids (ceramides and glucosylceramides), and neutral lipids [36]. The rice-derived glucosylceramide was shown to modify the ceramide profile in the stratum corneum when evaluated in a human skin-equivalent model, while its oral administration counterbalanced epidermal ceramide loss, resulting in TEWL reduction and barrier function improvement [89].

Many natural extracts able to mimic stratum corneum elements, due to their lipid composition or their ability to act as an adjuvant in skin hydration, have been described in the literature, including the following examples: amaranth oil, apricot oil, argan oil, candelilla wax, canola oil, carnauba wax, castor oil, coconut oil, corn oil, jojoba oil, jojoba wax, lanolin, lecithin, olive oil, palm oil, rice bran oil, safflower oil, sesame oil, shea butter, soybean oil, squalane, sunflower oil, sweet almond oil, wheat-germ oil, and yellow beeswax [90–92].

Therapeutic Alternatives for Epidermal Defense Mechanisms

The epidermis is an immunocompetent tissue able to create an immunological barrier against external aggressors. Epidermal cells are able to produce a high variety of cytokines, and the activation of the adaptive immune response is possible by the presence of LC, which can present antigens to T cells [93–95]. During the aging process, the epidermal immune defense also suffers some significant changes, including a reduction in the total number and functional capability of LC [15], a decreased secretion of IL-1 that impairs mitotic capacity and epidermal lipid synthesis [96], and a tendency to pH alkalinization in the stratum corneum [97]. Constant exposure to toxins and/or pollutants can accelerate skin aging, as demonstrated in a study by Vierkötter and Krutmann [98] that showed a significant correlation between air pollution and the signs of aging, such as dark spots and fine lines, in 400 Caucasian women. Cigarettes also present deleterious effects on the skin, such as impairing healing processes, inducing hair loss and deep wrinkle formation, and increasing the apoptosis frequency in keratinocytes [99, 100]. Alternative therapies to regulate epidermal immune defense functions should be able to modulate the inflammatory responses and/or stimulate the synthesis of natural defense compounds, but to date, few plant extracts and their derivatives have been identified that are efficient at this. At the moment, the most useful advice is to avoid excessive exposure to polluting or toxic substances and to follow a healthier lifestyle without smoking.

Leontopodium alpinum extract has shown anti-inflammatory and immunomodulation activities in human keratinocyte cell cultures exposed to UV radiation or LPS, through a dose-dependent inhibition of IL-8, interferon gamma-induced protein 10 (IP-10), monocyte chemoattractant protein-1 (MCP-1), and granulocyte-macrophage colony-stimulating factor (GM-CSF) [101]. Korean red ginseng extract was shown to control an LPS-stimulated inflammatory response with a dose-dependent decrease in TNF-α and IL-8 production in human keratinocytes [102]. Red orange (*Citrus sinensis* varieties) extract – enriched in anthocyanins, flavanones, hydroxycinnamic acids, and ascorbic acid – showed an anti-inflammatory activity in human keratinocytes exposed to IFN-γ and histamine [103]. In heat-stressed HaCaT cells, resveratrol or its natural precursor polydatin modulated the gene expression of IL-6, IL-8, and TNF-α and also stimulated the expression of heat shock protein 70B (Hsp70B), important for cytoprotection and cell repair, and human beta defensin (hBD2), a member of a class of antimicrobial peptides naturally produced in the epidermis [104].

Conclusion

Despite all of the complexity involved in skin aging, a great number of therapeutic treatments are continually being launched [105]. New approaches have been addressed in terms of differentiated ingredients that can be applied for cosmetics with effective results, which generally try to explore new mechanisms for antiaging claims. The development of natural plant extracts is a very promising alternative, but a lack of clinical evidence must be considered and critically analyzed before their use. Considering the focus of several studies on the dermis, a better understanding of the epidermis can certainly enrich discussions in the skin aging field.

References

1. Farage MA, et al. Psychological and social implications of aging skin: normal aging and the effects of cutaneous disease. In: Farage MA, Miller KW, Maibach HI, editors. Textbook of aging skin. 1st ed. Heidelberg: Springer; 2010. p. 949–57.
2. El-Domyati M, et al. Intrinsic aging vs. photoaging: a comparative histopathological, immunohistochemical, and ultrastructural study of skin. Exp Dermatol. 2002;11(5):398–405.
3. Nobile V, et al. Anti-aging and filling efficacy of six types hyaluronic acid based dermo-cosmetic treatment: double blind, randomized clinical trial of efficacy and safety. J Cosmet Dermatol. 2014;13 (4):277–87. doi:10.1111/jocd.12120.
4. Madison KC. Barrier function of the skin: "la raison d'être" of the epidermis. J Invest Dermatol. 2003;121 (2):231–41.
5. Baroni A, et al. Structure and function of the epidermis related to barrier properties. Clin Dermatol. 2012;30(3):257–62. doi:10.1016/j.clindermatol.2011.08.007.
6. Fuchs E, Raghavan S. Getting under the skin of epidermal morphogenesis. Nat Rev Genet. 2002;3 (3):199–209.
7. Brohem CA, et al. Artificial skin in perspective: concepts and applications. Pigment Cell Melanoma Res. 2011;24(1):35–50. doi:10.1111/j.1755-148X.2010.00786.x.
8. Eckhart L, et al. Cell death by cornification. Biochim Biophys Acta. 2013;1833(12):3471–80. doi:10.1016/j.bbamcr.2013.06.010.
9. Lorencini M, et al. Active ingredients against human epidermal aging. Ageing Res Rev. 2014;15:100–15. doi:10.1016/j.arr.2014.03.002.
10. Rinnerthaler M, et al. Oxidative stress in aging human skin. Biomolecules. 2015;5(2):545–89. doi:10.3390/biom5020545.
11. Choi HR, et al. Niche interactions in epidermal stem cells. World J Stem Cells. 2015;7(2):495–501. doi:10.4252/wjsc.v7.i2.495.
12. Elias PM, Ghadially R. The aged epidermal permeability barrier: basis for functional abnormalities. Clin Geriatr Med. 2002;18(1):103–20.
13. Dos Santos M, et al. In vitro 3-D model based on extending time of culture for studying chronological epidermis aging. Matrix Biol. 2015;47:85–97. doi:10.1016/j.matbio.2015.03.009.
14. Sextius P, et al. Analysis of gene expression dynamics revealed delayed and abnormal epidermal repair process in aged compared to young skin. Arch Dermatol Res. 2015;307(4):351–64. doi:10.1007/s00403-015-1551-5.
15. Xu YP, et al. Aging affects epidermal Langerhans cell development and function and alters their miRNA gene expression profile. Aging (Albany NY). 2012;4 (11):742–54.
16. Lee KO, Kim SN, Kim YC. Anti-wrinkle effects of water extracts of teas in hairless mouse. Toxicol Res. 2014;30(4):283–9. doi:10.5487/TR.2014.30.4.283.
17. Pérez-Sánchez A, et al. Protective effects of citrus and rosemary extracts on UV-induced damage in skin cell model and human volunteers. J Photochem Photobiol B. 2014;136:12–8. doi:10.1016/j.jphotobiol.2014.04.007.
18. Cangkrama M, Ting SB, Darido C. Stem cells behind the barrier. Int J Mol Sci. 2013;14(7):13670–86. doi:10.3390/ijms140713670.
19. Lock-Andersen J, et al. Epidermal thickness, skin pigmentation and constitutive photosensitivity. Photodermatol Photoimmunol Photomed. 1997;13 (4):153–8.
20. Crisan D, et al. Ultrasonographic assessment of skin structure according to age. Indian J Dermatol Venereol Leprol. 2012;78(4):519. doi:10.4103/0378-6323.98096.
21. Tsugita T, et al. Positional differences and aging changes in Japanese woman epidermal thickness and corneous thickness determined by OCT (optical coherence tomography). Skin Res Technol. 2013;19 (3):242–50. doi:10.1111/srt.12021.
22. Orringer JS, et al. Molecular effects of photodynamic therapy for photoaging. Arch Dermatol. 2008;144 (10):1296–302. doi:10.1001/archderm.144.10.1296.
23. Sjerobabski Masnec I, Situm M. Photorejuvenation – topical photodynamic therapy as therapeutic opportunity for skin rejuvenation. Coll Antropol. 2014;38 (4):1245–8.
24. Stuzin JM, et al. Histologic effects of the high-energy pulsed CO_2 laser on photoaged facial skin. Plast Reconstr Surg. 1997;99(7):2036–50.
25. Ratner D, et al. Pilot ultrastructural evaluation of human preauricular skin before and after high-energy pulsed carbon dioxide laser treatment. Arch Dermatol. 1998;134(5):582–7.
26. Sasaki GH, Travis HM, Tucker B. Fractional CO_2 laser resurfacing of photoaged facial and non-facial skin: histologic and clinical results and side effects. J Cosmet Laser Ther. 2009;11(4):190–201. doi:10.3109/14764170903356465.
27. Oram Y, Akkaya AD. Neck rejuvenation with fractional CO_2 laser: long-term results. J Clin Aesthet Dermatol. 2014;7(8):23–9.
28. Pain S, et al. Surface rejuvenating effect of Achillea millefolium extract. Int J Cosmet Sci. 2011;33 (6):535–42. doi:10.1111/j.1468-2494.2011.00667.x.
29. Bonté F, et al. Simarouba amara extract increases human skin keratinocyte differentiation. J Ethnopharmacol. 1996;53(2):65–74.

30. Hou M, et al. Topical hesperidin improves epidermal permeability barrier function and epidermal differentiation in normal murine skin. Exp Dermatol. 2012;21 (5):337–40. doi:10.1111/j.1600-0625.2012.01455.x.
31. Hsu S, et al. Green tea polyphenols induce differentiation and proliferation in epidermal keratinocytes. J Pharmacol Exp Ther. 2003;306(1):29–34.
32. Hsu S, et al. Green tea polyphenol-induced epidermal keratinocyte differentiation is associated with coordinated expression of p57/KIP2 and caspase 14. J Pharmacol Exp Ther. 2005;312(3):884–90.
33. Bellemère G, et al. Antiaging action of retinol: from molecular to clinical. Skin Pharmacol Physiol. 2009;22(4):200–9. doi:10.1159/000231525.
34. Sorg O, Saurat JH. Topical retinoids in skin ageing: a focused update with reference to sun-induced epidermal vitamin A deficiency. Dermatology. 2014;228 (4):314–25. doi:10.1159/000360527.
35. Kim H, et al. Retinyl retinoate, a novel hybrid vitamin derivative, improves photoaged skin: a double-blind, randomized-controlled trial. Skin Res Technol. 2011;17(3):380–5. doi:10.1111/j.1600-0846.2011.00512.x.
36. Kim H, et al. Water extract of gromwell (Lithospermum erythrorhizon) enhances migration of human keratinocytes and dermal fibroblasts with increased lipid synthesis in an in vitro wound scratch model. Skin Pharmacol Physiol. 2012;25(2):57–64. doi:10.1159/000330897.
37. Ro J, et al. Pectin micro- and nano-capsules of retinyl palmitate as cosmeceutical carriers for stabilized skin transport. Korean J Physiol Pharmacol. 2015;19 (1):59–64. doi:10.4196/kjpp.2015.19.1.59.
38. Gold MH, et al. Treatment of facial photodamage using a novel retinol formulation. J Drugs Dermatol. 2013;12(5):533–40.
39. Jurzak M, et al. Influence of retinoids on skin fibroblasts metabolism in vitro. Acta Pol Pharm. 2008;65 (1):85–91.
40. Sayo T, Sugiyama Y, Inoue S. Lutein, a nonprovitamin A, activates the retinoic acid receptor to induce HAS3-dependent hyaluronan synthesis in keratinocytes. Biosci Biotechnol Biochem. 2013;77 (6):1282–6.
41. Rendl M, et al. Topically applied lactic acid increases spontaneous secretion of vascular endothelial growth factor by human reconstructed epidermis. Br J Dermatol. 2001;145(1):3–9.
42. Yamamoto Y, et al. Effects of alpha-hydroxy acids on the human skin of Japanese subjects: the rationale for chemical peeling. J Dermatol. 2006;33(1):16–22.
43. Bhattacharyya TK, et al. Comparison of epidermal morphologic response to commercial antiwrinkle agents in the hairless mouse. Dermatol Surg. 2009;35(7):1109–18. doi:10.1111/j.1524-4725.2009.01196.x.
44. Wang X. A theory for the mechanism of action of the alpha-hydroxy acids applied to the skin. Med Hypotheses. 1999;53(5):380–2.
45. Gehring W. Nicotinic acid/niacinamide and the skin. J Cosmet Dermatol. 2004;3(2):88–93.
46. Jacobson EL, et al. A topical lipophilic niacin derivative increases NAD, epidermal differentiation and barrier function in photodamaged skin. Exp Dermatol. 2007;16(6):490–9.
47. Burke KE. Photoaging: the role of oxidative stress. G Ital Dermatol Venereol. 2010;145(4):445–59.
48. Rahimpour Y, Hamishehkar H. Liposomes in cosmeceutics. Expert Opin Drug Deliv. 2012;9 (4):443–55. doi:10.1517/17425247.2012.666968.
49. Schäfer M, et al. Nrf2: a central regulator of UV protection in the epidermis. Cell Cycle. 2010;9 (15):2917–8. doi:10.4161/cc.9.15.12701.
50. Keogh BP, et al. Expression of hydrogen peroxide and glutathione metabolizing enzymes in human skin fibroblasts derived from donors of different ages. J Cell Physiol. 1996;167(3):512–22.
51. Rhie G, et al. Aging- and photoaging-dependent changes of enzymic and nonenzymic antioxidants in the epidermis and dermis of human skin in vivo. J Invest Dermatol. 2001;117(5):1212–7.
52. Yamada M, et al. Aged human skin removes UVB-induced pyrimidine dimers from the epidermis more slowly than younger adult skin in vivo. Arch Dermatol Res. 2006;297(7):294–302.
53. Sander CS, et al. Photoaging is associated with protein oxidation in human skin in vivo. J Invest Dermatol. 2002;118(4):618–25.
54. Palmer DM, Kitchin JS. Oxidative damage, skin aging, antioxidants and a novel antioxidant rating system. J Drugs Dermatol. 2010;9(1):11–5.
55. Stamford NP. Stability, transdermal penetration, and cutaneous effects of ascorbic acid and its derivatives. J Cosmet Dermatol. 2012;11(4):310–7. doi:10.1111/jocd.12006.
56. Olteanu ED, et al. Photochemoprotective effect of Calluna vulgaris extract on skin exposed to multiple doses of ultraviolet B in SKH-1 hairless mice. J Environ Pathol Toxicol Oncol. 2012;31 (3):233–43.
57. Mnich CD, et al. Green tea extract reduces induction of p53 and apoptosis in UVB-irradiated human skin independent of transcriptional controls. Exp Dermatol. 2009;18(1):69–77. doi:10.1111/j.1600-0625.2008.00765.x.
58. Tomaino A, et al. In vitro protective effect of a Jacquez grapes wine extract on UVB-induced skin damage. Toxicol In Vitro. 2006;20(8):1395–402.
59. Zaid MA, et al. Inhibition of UVB-mediated oxidative stress and markers of photoaging in immortalized HaCaT keratinocytes by pomegranate polyphenol extract POMx. Photochem Photobiol. 2007;83 (4):882–8.
60. Cimino F, et al. Protective effects of a red orange extract on UVB-induced damage in human keratinocytes. Biofactors. 2007;30(2):129–38.
61. Chiu TM, et al. In vitro and in vivo anti-photoaging effects of an isoflavone extract from soybean cake.

J Ethnopharmacol. 2009;126(1):108–13. doi:10.1016/j.jep.2009.07.039.
62. Cornacchione S, et al. In vivo skin antioxidant effect of a new combination based on a specific Vitis vinifera shoot extract and a biotechnological extract. J Drugs Dermatol. 2007;6 Suppl 6:s8–13.
63. Fraternale D, et al. Aqueous extract from Vitis vinifera tendrils is able to enrich keratinocyte antioxidant defences. Nat Prod Commun. 2011;6(9):1315–9.
64. Heinrich U, et al. Long-term ingestion of high flavanol cocoa provides photoprotection against UV-induced erythema and improves skin condition in women. J Nutr. 2006;136(6):1565–9.
65. Tominaga K, et al. Cosmetic benefits of astaxanthin on humans subjects. Acta Biochim Pol. 2012;59 (1):43–7.
66. Wertz K, et al. Beta-Carotene interferes with ultraviolet light A-induced gene expression by multiple pathways. J Investig Dermatol. 2005;124(2):428–34.
67. Tobi SE, et al. The green tea polyphenol, epigallocatechin-3-gallate, protects against the oxidative cellular and genotoxic damage of UVA radiation. Int J Cancer. 2002;102(5):439–44.
68. Chung JH, et al. Dual mechanisms of green tea extract (EGCG)-induced cell survival in human epidermal keratinocytes. FASEB J. 2003;17(13):1913–5.
69. Luo D, et al. Effect of epigallocatechingallate on ultraviolet B-induced photo-damage in keratinocyte cell line. Am J Chin Med. 2006;34(5):911–22.
70. Song XZ, Bi ZG, Xu AE. Green tea polyphenol epigallocatechin-3-gallate inhibits the expression of nitric oxide synthase and generation of nitric oxide induced by ultraviolet B in HaCaT cells. Chin Med J (Engl). 2006;119(4):282–7.
71. Huang CC, et al. (−)-Epicatechin-3-gallate, a green tea polyphenol is a potent agent against UVB-induced damage in HaCaT keratinocytes. Molecules. 2007;12 (8):1845–58.
72. Nichols JA, Katiyar SK. Skin photoprotection by natural polyphenols: anti-inflammatory, antioxidant and DNA repair mechanisms. Arch Dermatol Res. 2010;302(2):71–83. doi:10.1007/s00403-009-1001-3.
73. Fazekas Z, et al. Protective effects of lycopene against ultraviolet B-induced photodamage. Nutr Cancer. 2003;47(2):181–7.
74. Andreassi M, et al. Antioxidant activity of topically applied lycopene. J Eur Acad Dermatol Venereol. 2004;18(1):52–5.
75. Lademann J, et al. Carotenoids in human skin. Exp Dermatol. 2011;20(5):377–82. doi:10.1111/j.1600-0625.2010.01189.x.
76. Yasuda S, et al. Suppressive effects of ascorbate derivatives on ultraviolet-B-induced injury in HaCaT human keratinocytes. In Vitro Cell Dev Biol Anim. 2004;40(3–4):71–3.
77. Haftek M, et al. Clinical, biometric and structural evaluation of the long-term effects of a topical treatment with ascorbic acid and madecassoside in photoaged human skin. Exp Dermatol. 2008;17 (11):946–52. doi:10.1111/j.1600-0625.2008.00732.x.
78. Wu S, et al. IL-8 production and AP-1 transactivation induced by UVA in human keratinocytes: roles of D-alpha-tocopherol. Mol Immunol. 2008;45 (8):2288–96. doi:10.1016/j.molimm.2007.11.019.
79. Tzaphlidou M. The role of collagen and elastin in aged skin: an image processing approach. Micron. 2004;35(3):173–7.
80. Lampe MA, Williams ML, Elias PM. Human epidermal lipids: characterization and modulations during differentiation. J Lipid Res. 1983;24(2):131–40.
81. Kezic S, et al. Natural moisturizing factor components in the stratum corneum as biomarkers of filaggrin genotype: evaluation of minimally invasive methods. Br J Dermatol. 2009;161(5):1098–104. doi:10.1111/j.1365-2133.2009.09342.x.
82. Jacobson TM, et al. Effects of aging and xerosis on the amino acid composition of human skin. J Invest Dermatol. 1990;95(3):296–300.
83. Ghadially R, et al. The aged epidermal permeability barrier. Structural, functional, and lipid biochemical abnormalities in humans and a senescent murine model. J Clin Invest. 1995;95(5):2281–90.
84. Li J, et al. Aquaporin-3 gene and protein expression in sun-protected human skin decreases with skin ageing. Australas J Dermatol. 2010;51(2):106–12. doi:10.1111/j.1440-0960.2010.00629.x.
85. del Pereda MC, et al. Expression of differential genes involved in the maintenance of water balance in human skin by Piptadenia colubrina extract. J Cosmet Dermatol. 2010;9(1):35–43. doi:10.1111/j.1473-2165.2009.00458.x.
86. Buono S, et al. Biological activities of dermatological interest by the water extract of the microalga *Botryococcus braunii*. Arch Dermatol Res. 2012;304(9):755–64. doi:10.1007/s00403-012-1250-4.
87. Schrader A, et al. Effects of glyceryl glucoside on AQP3 expression, barrier function and hydration of human skin. Skin Pharmacol Physiol. 2012;25 (4):192–9. doi:10.1159/000338190.
88. Grether-Beck S, et al. Urea uptake enhances barrier function and antimicrobial defense in humans by regulating epidermal gene expression. J Invest Dermatol. 2012;132(6):1561–72. doi:10.1038/jid.2012.42.
89. Shimoda H, et al. Changes in ceramides and glucosylceramides in mouse skin and human epidermal equivalents by rice-derived glucosylceramide. J Med Food. 2012;15(12):1064–72. doi:10.1089/jmf.2011.2137.
90. Huang ZR, Lin YK, Fang JY. Biological and pharmacological activities of squalene and related compounds: potential uses in cosmetic dermatology. Molecules. 2009;14(1):540–54. doi:10.3390/molecules14010540.
91. Budai L, et al. Natural oils and waxes: studies on stick bases. J Cosmet Sci. 2012;63(2):93–101.

92. de Waroux Yle P. The social and environmental context of argan oil production. Nat Prod Commun. 2013;8(1):1–4.
93. Corsini E, Galli CL. Epidermal cytokines in experimental contact dermatitis. Toxicology. 2000;142 (3):203–11.
94. Cumberbatch M, et al. Epidermal Langerhans cell migration and sensitisation to chemical allergens. APMIS. 2003;111(7–8):797–804.
95. Kupper TS, Fuhlbrigge RC. Immune surveillance in the skin: mechanisms and clinical consequences. Nat Rev Immunol. 2004;4(3):211–22.
96. Ye J, et al. Alterations in cytokine regulation in aged epidermis: implications for permeability barrier homeostasis and inflammation. I. IL-1 gene family. Exp Dermatol. 2002;11(3):209–16.
97. Choi EH, et al. Stratum corneum acidification is impaired in moderately aged human and murine skin. J Invest Dermatol. 2007;127(12):2847–56.
98. Vierkötter A, Krutmann J. Environmental influences on skin aging and ethnic-specific manifestations. Dermatoendocrinol. 2012;4(3):227–31. doi:10.4161/derm.19858.
99. Morita A, et al. Molecular basis of tobacco smoke-induced premature skin aging. J Investig Dermatol Symp Proc. 2009;14(1):53–5. doi:10.1038/jidsymp.2009.13.
100. Pedata P, et al. Interaction between combustion-generated organic nanoparticles and biological systems: in vitro study of cell toxicity and apoptosis in human keratinocytes. Nanotoxicology. 2012;6 (4):338–52. doi:10.3109/17435390.2011.579630.
101. Daniela L, et al. Anti-inflammatory effects of concentrated ethanol extracts of Edelweiss (*Leontopodium alpinum* Cass.) callus cultures towards human keratinocytes and endothelial cells. Mediators Inflamm. 2012;2012:498373. doi:10.1155/2012/498373.
102. Hong CE, Lyu SY. Anti-inflammatory and anti-oxidative effects of Korean red ginseng extract in human keratinocytes. Immune Netw. 2011;11 (1):42–9. doi:10.4110/in.2011.11.1.42.
103. Cardile V, et al. Antiinflammatory effects of a red orange extract in human keratinocytes treated with interferon-gamma and histamine. Phytother Res. 2010;24(3):414–8. doi:10.1002/ptr.2973.
104. Ravagnan G, et al. Polydatin, a natural precursor of resveratrol, induces β-defensin production and reduces inflammatory response. Inflammation. 2013;36(1):26–34. doi:10.1007/s10753-012-9516-8.
105. Lorencini M, Feferman IHS, Maibach HI. New perspectives in the control of the skin aging process. In: Barel AO, Paye M, Maibach HI, editors. Handbook of cosmetic science and technology. 4th ed. Boca Raton: CRC Press; 2014. p. 245–50.

Influence of Aging on Sensorial Perception of Skin Care Products

141

Valéria Maria Di Mambro, Carla Abdo Brohem, and Márcio Lorencini

Contents

Abstract

The process of sensory perception is composed of several steps including stimulation, sensation, perception, and response. Aging can affect the skin's ability to capture different stimuli from the environment; consequently, age represents an important variable affecting consumers' perceptions about skin care products. Considering the five human senses, touch is the most important for cosmetic evaluation because it is directly related to skin perception. With age, several sensorial and cognitive aspects are affected, such as impaired peripheral sensory function, a reduction of the number of mechanoreceptors in the skin, and a decrease in the conduction velocity of peripheral nerves. To improve the sensorial analysis of skin care products, this chapter will cover the main alterations in skin structure with aging, specifically those related to the sensory perceptions of cosmetic consumers.

Introduction

Sensory properties are perceived when the sensory organs interact with stimuli in the world surrounding the human body [1]. There are at least three steps in the process of sensory perception, as follows: (1) a stimulus hits a sense organ and is converted into a nerve signal that travels to the brain; (2) with previous experiences in memory, the brain interprets, organizes, and integrates

V.M. Di Mambro • C.A. Brohem • M. Lorencini (✉)
R&D Department, Grupo Boticário, São José dos Pinhais, PR, Brazil
e-mail: valeriamm@grupoboticario.com.br; carla@grupoboticario.com.br; marciolorencini@yahoo.com.br; marciolo@grupoboticario.com.br

M.A. Farage et al. (eds.), *Textbook of Aging Skin*,
DOI 10.1007/978-3-662-47398-6_141

the incoming sensations into perceptions; and (3) a response is formulated based on those particular perceptions [2]. Basically, sensory perceptions may differ from one person to another due to differences in their ability to capture stimuli or in their mental treatment of sensation.

It is already well known that higher cognitive functions decline over one's lifetime, as aging induces major reorganization and remodeling at all levels of brain structure and function [3–5]. Cognitive decline in aging theory suggests that generalized slowing of higher cognitive function can be explained by mechanisms involving poorer utilization of cognitive resources at an earlier sensory processing level [6, 7]. For generating perception, a minimum amount of stimulation (or a sensory threshold) is required, which can be classified into the following: (1) the absolute threshold is the lowest level of stimulus necessary for sensory detection, and (2) the differential threshold is the least noticeable difference or the smallest amount of change necessary to determine that a stimulus has become stronger [8]. As a person gets older, these sensory thresholds change, increasing the amount of stimulation needed for sensory awareness [9]. A study conducted by Heft and Robinson [10] with 178 healthy individuals aged 20–89 years suggests that sensory thresholds become elevated with age for multiple sensory somatosensory and taste modalities.

For the consumer goods industry, sensorial evaluation represents a method of evaluating the characteristics of products as perceived through the five senses, which include taste, hearing, vision, olfaction, and touch. Specifically for skin care products, significant perceived attributes usually include appearance, fragrance, consistency, texture, and skin sensation, and one's perception of most or all of them can overlap. Considering the importance of sensorial analysis as a powerful tool for accessing consumer preferences, the present chapter will address the impact of the different senses on the evaluation of skin care products and how aging may influence this process. Based on the intrinsic characteristics of skin care products, taste will not be discussed, whereas touch, as the most important sense for skin perception, will be covered in the most detail.

Hearing, Vision, and Olfaction

Hearing can contribute to one's understanding of a skin care product's attributes, such as the sound when opening or closing the package, and it represents the main channel for oral communication in advertising. The sense of hearing is based on the detection of sound-induced changes in air pressure, which are converted into electrical signals by hair cells in the inner ear that are then sent to the brain for analysis and interpretation [11]. With age, the ability to detect sounds might decrease, especially in the case of high-frequency sounds and with worse threshold deterioration in men than women [12]. Evidence for age-related deficits in central auditory processing has come from behavioral and electrophysiological studies. Older adults show impaired auditory sensory memory processing in the detection of changes in tone duration, interstimulus intervals, and short gaps in tones [13].

Vision is an important sense for the perceived quality of skin care products, as slight changes in color can lead to differences in consumer acceptance and pleasantness. Light waves reflected by an object enter the eye and reach the retina, in which receptor cells known as cones and rods convert light energy into neural impulses that travel via the optic nerve to the brain. The brain interprets these signals and constructs the appearance – color, shape, size, translucency, surface texture, etc. – of the object [1]. Over one's lifetime, visual acuity typically declines, the visual field becomes smaller, peripheral vision declines, and it is common to observe difficulty in focusing the eyes on close objects [14]. Regarding color appearance across the life span, it was observed that chromatic sensitivity improves in adolescence, reaches a maximum at approximately 30 years, and then undergoes a gradual decrease with marked acceleration after 60 years that is more pronounced for the blue-yellow system [15]. Based on this evidence, the use of materials with larger print and color contrast would be recommended when developing specific products for the elderly.

Olfaction is important not only for perceived quality but also for the emotions and olfactory memories that a smell brings to consumers when using a product. Considerable scientific evidence indicates that odors elicit emotion and are linked to emotional memories [16]. The binding of odor molecules to olfactory receptors in the nose generates neural impulses transmitted to the olfactory bulb in the brain, which are responsible for projecting information to the olfactory cortex and other cerebral areas. After some transmission steps, the captured information reaches the amygdala and hippocampus, which are involved with emotional response and memory, respectively [17]. A particular odor may be made up of several volatile compounds, but sometimes particular volatiles are associated with a particular smell. Individuals may perceive or describe single compounds differently, e.g., hexenol can be described as grass, green, or unripe. Similarly, a specific odor may be perceived or described in different compounds, e.g., minty is used to describe both menthol and carvone [1]. Studies report that age impairs the sense of smell, especially after 70 years, as a result of nerve ending loss and less mucus, which helps odors stay long enough to be detected and helps to clear odors from the nose [18–22]. In addition, there are changes in the temporal lobe, entorhinal cortex, hippocampus, and amygdala [21, 23]. Threshold loss, intensity loss, altered odor quality, and cognitive loss – characterized by loss of odor memory ability, including recall and recognition – may all play roles in handicapping an older person with respect to odor identification [23, 24]. Morgan and colleagues [25] showed that olfactory capacity is affected by age and gender, greater deficits being observed in older men than older women.

Touch

Touch is the detection of a mechanical stimulus impacting the skin and is very important for apprenticeship, social contacts, and sexuality [26]. Touch responses involve very precise coding of mechanical information, and the skin contains many different tactile receptors that can detect sensations related to contact and touch, e.g., force, particle size, stretch, vibration, and heat [1, 26, 27]. There are four major types of cutaneous mechanoreceptors distinguished by their distinctive structures and how their associated nervous fibers respond to stimulation: (1) Merkel receptors, with the function of sensing finely detailed surface patterns such as shapes and edges, are disk shaped and located near the border between the epidermis and dermis; (2) Meissner corpuscles are stacks of flattened disks in the dermis just below the epidermis that are particularly sensitive to touch and vibrations, controlling handgrip; (3) Ruffini cylinders are branched nervous fibers inside a cylindrical capsule located in the dermis, and their function is associated with perceiving stretching of the skin; and (4) Pacinian corpuscles are oval-cylindrical shaped, located deep in the skin and especially suited to feeling rough surfaces and detecting vibration [28] (Fig. 1).

Mechanoreceptors rely on the presence of ion channels that rapidly transform mechanical forces into electrical signals, thereby generating action potentials that propagate toward the central nervous system [26]. Nerve fibers from receptors in the skin are organized in bundles called peripheral nerves that enter the spinal cord and go to the brain through two major pathways: (1) the medial lemniscal pathway with large fibers that carry signals related to sensing the position of the limbs (proprioception) and perceiving touch and (2) the spinothalamic pathway with smaller fibers that transmit signals related to temperature and pain [26, 28]. In the brain, signals reach the thalamus and travel to the somatosensory cortex, which is organized into maps that correspond to

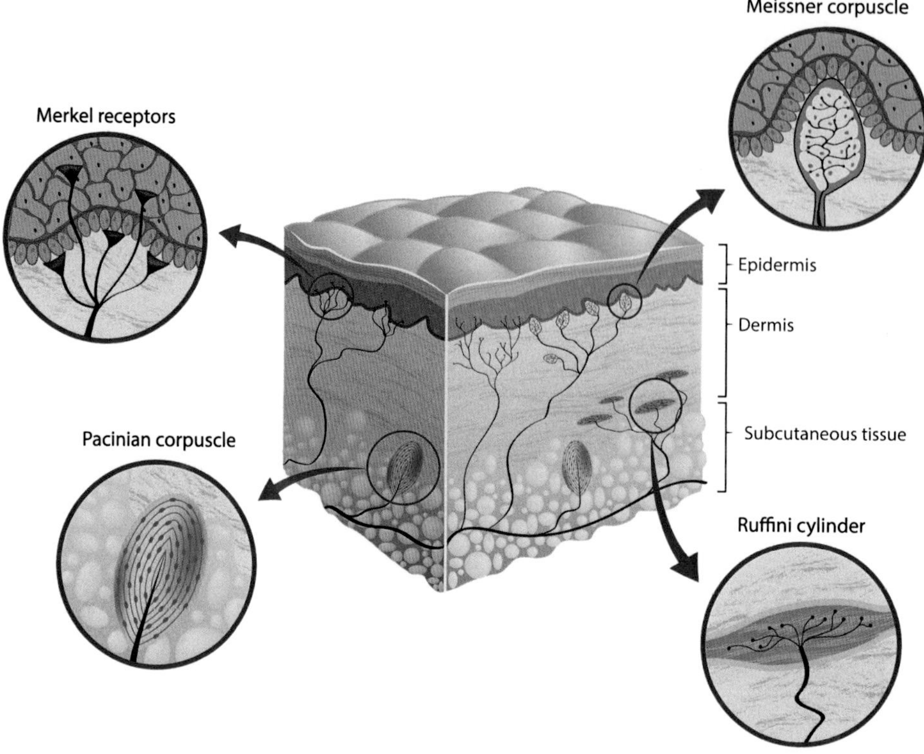

Fig. 1 Mechanoreceptors of the skin: Merkel receptors, Meissner corpuscles, Ruffini cylinders, and Pacinian corpuscles (Adapted from Goldstein [28])

specific locations on the body [28]. The brain interprets the type and magnitude of a touch sensation, considering the sensation as pleasant (such as being comfortably warm), unpleasant (such as being very hot), or neutral (such as being aware that you are touching something) [28, 29].

In addition to other structural changes that affect the skin over the years – leading to reductions of up to 50–60 % in principal cutaneous functions such as protection, excretion, secretion, absorption, thermoregulation, pigmentogenesis, immunological process regulation, and wound repair – aging is associated with a progressive decline in cutaneous sensory perception [30, 31] (Fig. 2). There is no clear consensus in the literature, but the sense of touch seems to become less acute, or sensations may change with age, impairing the detection of pain, temperature, and body position [9, 32]. Getting older is associated with impaired peripheral sensory function, a reduction of the number of mechanoreceptors in the skin, and a decrease in the conduction velocity of peripheral nerves [4, 33, 34]. Skin conformance is altered, although the mechanical properties of glabrous skin might only have a minor impact on the discriminative abilities of elderly subjects. Meissner and Pacinian corpuscles decrease in number and show structural deterioration with aging, while Merkel receptors appear to be less affected [31, 35]. A decline in the number of Ruffini corpuscles was reported in the ligaments of elderly subjects [31]. Nerve conduction velocity slows down, probably due to an age-related reduction in the number and density of myelinated peripheral nerve fibers and a decrease in myelin thickness on the remaining fibers [35]. Microneurography has shown a more pronounced activity-dependent slowing of mechanoresponsive C-fibers in aged subjects, which could, at least in part, explain the lower thresholds for mechanical stimuli with aging

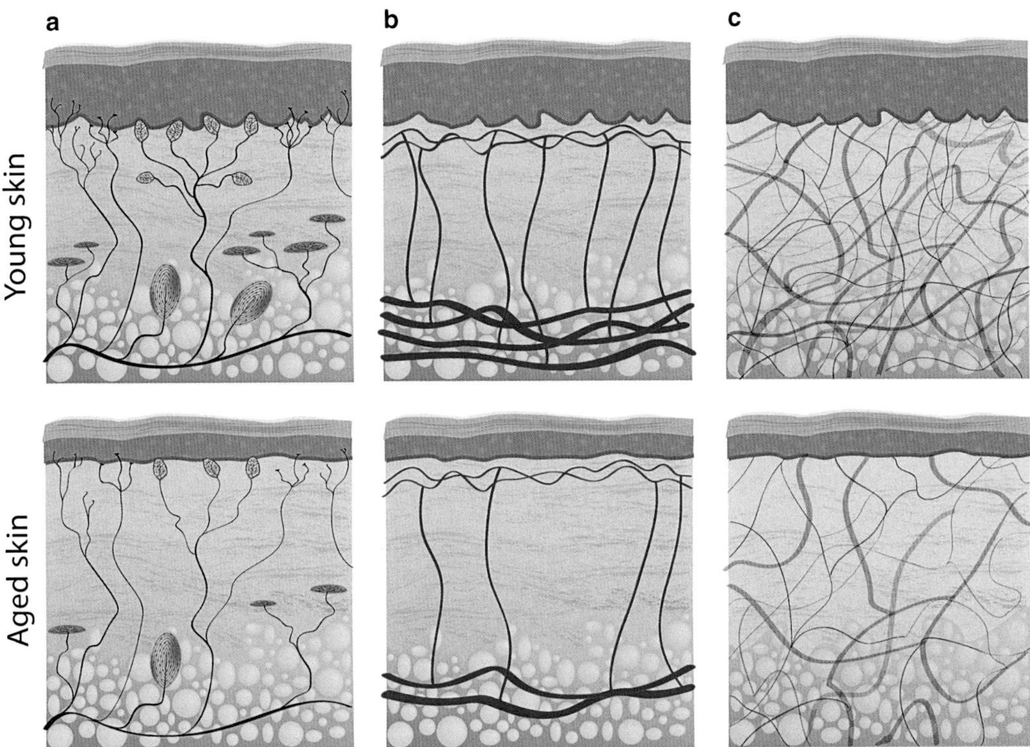

Fig. 2 Changes in skin structure with aging. (**a**) Modifications of cutaneous sensory perception system with reduction in the amount of mechanoreceptors in aged skin. (**b**) Vascular cutaneous system showing a decrease of capillary density and diameter with aging. (**c**) Extracellular matrix modification with age-related reduction in the content of cutaneous fibers, especially collagen and elastin

[31, 36]. The activation of mechanosensitive ion channels is at the origin of the electrical signals transmitted by sensory neurons, and although it was not described in the literature until now, the effects of aging on the structure and/or function of these channels could probably contribute to an age-related tactile defect [31]. Detection thresholds are generally independent of gender, whereas pain thresholds are significantly lower in women [37]. However, it seems that the changes in skin innervation with age are different according to the body site: decreased epidermal innervation in the face, trunk, and forearms has been reported, whereas it did not change in the abdomen and even increased in mammary skin [33, 38, 39]. In addition, loss of tactile acuity is particularly severe in the more distal extremities [40], which could have a major influence on how consumers perceive the application of topical skin care products.

Hydration also seems to play a role in the age-related decline of sensory perception. Dry skin is more common in older than in younger adults, and the skin has also been shown to become thinner with age [41]. Although cutaneous hydration does not affect vibrotactile detection thresholds, it does affect the perception of textured surfaces [31]. With aging, the skin is likely to become less hydrated, thereby increasing its resistance to electrical current, and this property, rather than sensorial/perceptual differences per se, may be the primary cause of differences between younger and older adults in somatosensorial perception when exposed to an electrical stimulus. Lowered skin hydration is also likely to result in increased thermal energy dispersion, and in this way it represents an impediment to the proper activation of sensory receptors [41].

Consumers' Perceptions

In 2014, our research group conducted several aesthetic and sensorial studies with skin care products to evaluate how the perceptions of Brazilian consumers could be influenced by age. An online survey was first carried with 477 women divided into four groups: 12 % aged 18–24 years, 55 % aged 25–34 years, 20 % aged 35–44 years, and 13 % aged 45–54 years. As expected, shopping and frequency of use for antiaging products were positively correlated with increasing age. Twenty-four percent of consumers aged 18–24 years affirmed to be antiaging users, while this number increased to 86 % after 35 years old. Regarding frequency of use, 69 % of consumers aged 18–24 years said they used a product once or twice a week, whereas 58 % of women aged 25–44 years said they used one every day, and 90 % of women older than 45 years said they used one every day. Regarding the moment of use, younger consumers usually apply the product only at night, whereas older consumers apply the product(s) at least twice a day.

Most attractiveness claims for antiaging products also varied according to age: claims such as "protection against free radicals" and "preservation of collagen and elastin fibers" were more important for younger people; "skin firmness" and "skin texture restoration" were the preferred claims for older women; and claims related to "skin firmer, tough and with fewer wrinkles and fine lines" and "UVA/UVB protection to prevent age marks" were considered important for all groups. Regarding the most attractive sensory attributes of an antiaging product, it was observed that attributes such as "rapid absorption," "leaves no sticky skin feeling," and "presence of sunscreen" were important for all consumers; "spreads easily" and "opaque" were more important for younger people, while consumers older than 45 years were more concerned about "leaves skin hydrated." When asked about preferences regarding formulation type, it was verified that oil-free formulas were the most preferred by younger women, while older consumers showed divided opinions between oil-free and serum formulas. This result is probably due to Brazil's weather. Formulas such as gels and creams showed very low preference among consumers.

The second phase of the study was focused on evaluating consumers' perceptions according to their age but also considered a Brazilian regional variable. The regions included were south (142 consumers), southeast (150 consumers), and northeast (150 consumers). The age groups included the following: 30–44, 45–59, and 60–70 years old. After 5 days of using an antiaging product, volunteers were asked about overall preference, texture, color, fragrance, and skin sensation. The results showed that Brazilian regions, rather than age, had a greater influence on consumers' perception concerning the attributes evaluated. Older consumers showed higher values of hedonic answers for skin sensation compared with younger consumers. When comparing the different regions, consumers from the southwest showed higher hedonic scores than the others, especially the south.

Conclusion

The techniques for evaluating cosmetic products have been evolving as a significant tool for achieving quality assurance, consumer satisfaction, and the acceptance of a product in the market. As cosmetics represent emotionally involved products, it is very important to consider that sensory characteristics can link them to consumer perceptions. The optimization of sensory characteristics leads to consumer satisfaction and a more successful development. However, specific characteristics such as the age of the target public are essential to greater effectiveness in the process of product evaluation. Aging represents a significant condition for skin care product evaluation as the skin changes drastically throughout life, and consequently, the application of products on the cutaneous surface can also represent a particular experience.

Of course aging is just one of several variables that must be considered when evaluating a skin care product or any other cosmetic. According to Jog and colleagues [42], sensory analysis is an invaluable set of methods for research and marketing, and any decision related to sensory evaluation begins with identifying what the researcher wants to accomplish. Access to consumer preferences in different parts of the world has been expanded through the exploration of Internet connectivity. In a future not so distant, sensory analysis will become increasingly accurate through the combination of well-defined methodologies with differentiated approaches such as the proposal of neuroscience. Then, it will be possible to access consumers' unconscious preferences for the development of products connected to their necessities, desires, and even their dreams.

References

1. Kemp SE, Hollowood T, Hort J. Sensory perception. In: Kemp SE, Hollowood T, Hort J, editors. Sensory evaluation, a practical handbook. 1st ed. Oxford: Wiley-Blackwell; 2009. p. 4–10.
2. Meilgaard M, Civille GV, Carr BT. Introduction to sensory techniques. In: Meilgaard M, Civille GV, Carr BT, editors. Sensory evaluation techniques. 4th ed. Boca Raton: CRC Press; 2006. p. 1–6.
3. Hedden T, et al. Insights into the ageing mind: a view from cognitive neuroscience. Nat Rev Neurosci. 2004;5(2):87–96.
4. Kalisch T, et al. Impaired tactile acuity in old age is accompanied by enlarged hand representations in somatosensory cortex. Cereb Cortex. 2009;19:1530–8. doi:10.1093/cercor/bhn190.
5. Lenz M, et al. Increased excitability of somatosensory cortex in aged humans is associated with impaired tactile acuity. J Neurosci. 2012;32(5):1811–6. doi:10.1523/JNEUROSCI.2722-11.2012.
6. Salthouse TA, et al. Interrelations of age, visual acuity, and cognitive functioning. J Gerontol B Psychol Sci Soc Sci. 1996;51(6):P317–30.
7. Cliff M, et al. Aging effects on functional auditory and visual processing using fMRI with variable sensory loading. Cortex. 2013;49:1304–13. doi:10.1016/j.cortex.2012.04.003.
8. Schultz M. Sensation and perception. In: Nicholas L, editor. Introduction to psychology. 2nd ed. Cape Town: UCT Press; 2008. p. 70–111.
9. Hills GA. The changing realm of the senses. In: Lewis CB, editor. Aging: the health-care challenge. 4th ed. Philadelphia: F. A. Davis Company; 2002. p. 83–103.
10. Heft MW, Robinson ME. Age differences in orofacial sensory thresholds. J Dent Res. 2010;89(10):1102–5. doi:10.1177/0022034510375287.
11. Schwander M, Kachar B, Müller U. Review series: the cell biology of hearing. J Cell Biol. 2010;190(12):9–20. doi:10.1083/jcb.201001138.
12. Ciorba A, et al. High frequency hearing loss in the elderly: effect of age and noise exposure in an Italian group. J Laryngol Otol. 2011;125(8):776–80. doi:10.1017/S0022215111001101.
13. Rimmele JM, Sussman E, Poeppel D. The role of temporal structure in the investigation of sensory memory, auditory scene analysis, and speech perception: a healthy-aging perspective. Int J Psychophysiol. 2015;95(2):175–83. doi:10.1016/j.ijpsycho.2014.06.010.
14. Sinfield M, Hatcher D, Jackson D. Ageing and health breakdown. In: Chang E, Daly J, Elliott D, editors. Pathophysiology applied to nursing practice. 1st ed. Marrickville: Mosby Elsevier; 2006. p. 404–24.
15. Paramei GV, Oakley B. Variation of color discrimination across the life span. J Opt Soc Am A Opt Image Sci Vis. 2014;31(4):A375–84. doi:10.1364/JOSAA.31.00A375.
16. Kadohisa M. Effects of odor on emotion, with implications. Front Syst Neurosci. 2013;7:66. doi:10.3389/fnsys.2013.00066.
17. Soudry Y, et al. Olfactory system and emotion: common substrates. Eur Ann Otorhinolaryngol Head Neck Dis. 2011;128(1):18–23. doi:10.1016/j.anorl.2010.09.007.
18. Doty RL, et al. Smell identification ability: changes with age. Science. 1984;226(4681):1441–3.
19. Stevens JC, Cain WS. Age-related deficiency in the perceived strength of six odorants. Chem Senses. 1985;10(4):517–29. doi:10.1093/chemse/10.4.517.
20. Cain WS, Gent JF. Olfactory sensitivity: reliability, generality, and association with aging. J Exp Psychol Hum Percept Perform. 1991;17(2):382–91.
21. Schiffman SS, Graham BG. Taste and smell perception affect appetite and immunity in the elderly. Eur J Clin Nutr. 2000;54 Suppl 3:S54–63.
22. Bitnes J, et al. Longitudinal study of taste identification of sensory panellists: effect of ageing, experience and exposure. Food Qual Prefer. 2007;18:230–41. doi:10.1016/j.foodqual.2005.11.003.
23. Murphy C, et al. Olfactory event-related potentials and aging: normative data. Int J Psychophysiol. 2000;36(2):133–45.
24. Stevens JC, Plantinga A, Cain WS. Reduction of odor and nasal pungency associated with aging. Neurobiol Aging. 1982;3(2):125–32.
25. Morgan CD, et al. Olfactory event-related potentials: older males demonstrate the greatest deficits. Electroencephalogr. Clin Neurophysiol. 1997;104(4):351–8.
26. Roudaut Y, et al. Touch sense: functional organization and molecular determinants of mechanosensitive receptors. Channels. 2012;6(4):234–45. doi:10.4161/chan.22213.
27. Fromy B, Sigaudo-Roussel D, Saumet JL. Cutaneous neurovascular interaction involved in tactile sensation.

Cardiovasc Hematol Agents Med Chem. 2008;6 (4):337–42.
28. Goldstein EB. The cutaneous senses. In: Goldstein EB, editor. Sensation and perception. 8th ed. Belmont: Wadsworth Cengage Learning; 2010. p. 329–52.
29. Hagen MC, et al. Somatosensory processing in the human inferior prefrontal cortex. J Neurophysiol. 2002;88(3):1400–6.
30. Farage MA, et al. Functional and physiological characteristics of the aging skin. Aging Clin Exp Res. 2008;20(3):195–200.
31. Decorps J, et al. Effect of ageing on tactile transduction processes. Ageing Res Rev. 2014;13:90–9. doi:10.1016/j.arr.2013.12.003.
32. Heft MW, Robinson ME. Age differences in suprathreshold sensory function. Age (Dordr). 2014;36(1):1–8. doi:10.1007/s11357-013-9536-9.
33. Besné I, Descombes C, Breton L. Effect of age and anatomical site on density of sensory innervation in human epidermis. Arch Dermatol. 2002;138(11): 1445–50.
34. Brodoehl S, et al. Age-related changes in the somatosensory processing of tactile stimulation–an fMRI study. Behav Brain Res. 2013;238:259–64. doi:10.1016/j.bbr.2012.10.038.
35. Kalisch T, Tegenthoff M, Dinse HR. Repetitive electric stimulation elicits enduring improvement of sensorimotor performance in seniors. Neural Plast. 2010;2010:690531. doi:10.1155/2010/690531.
36. Namer B, et al. Microneurographic assessment of C-fibre function in aged healthy subjects. J Physiol. 2009;587(Pt. 2):419–28. doi:10.1113/jphysiol.2008.162941.
37. Rolke R, et al. Quantitative sensory testing in the German research network on neuropathic pain (DFNS): standardized protocol and reference values. Pain. 2006;123(3):231–43.
38. Lauria G, et al. Epidermal innervation: changes with aging, topographic location, and in sensory neuropathy. J Neurol Sci. 1999;164(2):172–8.
39. Chang YC, Lin WM, Hsieh ST. Effects of aging on human skin innervation. Neuroreport. 2004;15 (1):149–53.
40. Stevens JC, Choo KK. Spatial acuity of the body surface over the life span. Somatosens Mot Res. 1996;13 (2):153–66.
41. Kemp J, et al. Age-related decrease in sensitivity to electrical stimulation is unrelated to skin conductance: an evoked potentials study. Clin Neurophysiol. 2014;125(3):602–7. doi:10.1016/j.clinph.2013.08.020.
42. Jog SV, et al. Sensorial analysis in cosmetics: an overview. Household Personal Care Today. 2012; 1:23–4.

The Role of Neuropeptides in Skin Wound Healing

142

Yun-Hee Choi, Sang Hyun Moh, and Ki Woo Kim

Contents

Y.-H. Choi
Anti-aging Research Institute of BIO-FD&C Co. Ltd, Incheon, Republic of Korea

Institute of Lifestyle Medicine and Nuclear Receptor Research Consortium, Wonju College of Medicine, Yonsei University, Wonju, Republic of Korea

S.H. Moh
Anti-aging Research Institute of BIO-FD&C Co. Ltd, Incheon, Republic of Korea
e-mail: shmoh@biofdnc.com; biofdnc@gmail.com

K.W. Kim (✉)
Departments of Pharmacology and Global Medical Science, Wonju College of Medicine, Yonsei University, Wonju, Republic of Korea

Institute of Lifestyle Medicine and Nuclear Receptor Research Consortium, Wonju College of Medicine, Yonsei University, Wonju, Republic of Korea
e-mail: kiwoo@yonsei.ac.kr

M.A. Farage et al. (eds.), *Textbook of Aging Skin*,
DOI 10.1007/978-3-662-47398-6_142

Abstract

The skin offers a well suited and clinically relevant model for studying communication between peripheral and central nervous system (CNS), due to its close connection with the brain. A variety of molecules such as neuropeptides, neurohormones, and neurotrophins and their specific receptors are expressed in both neuronal and skin cells, indicating a close functional interaction between the neurons and the skin. The skin acts as a protective barrier against mechanical and chemical damages; therefore, cutaneous innervation plays a critical role in modulating the wound healing process which functions in an orderly and timely manner to rebuild the skin's integrity and homeostasis. Furthermore, all these neuromediators are involved during all phases of the wound healing process. Neuropeptides circulate between the brain and peripheral tissues and functions as neurotransmitters, neuromodulators, and neurohormones. Neuropeptides have immunoregulatory roles and exhibit mitogenic property, which influence the function of various types of skin cells during the wound healing process.

Introduction

The skin is the largest organ in vertebrates and functions as a barrier against external environment, and it is also an important site for perception of multiple stimuli such as pain, temperature, and touch [1, 2]. The skin's ability to recognize, distinguish, and integrate various signals is very crucial for the immediate and appropriate response required to maintain skin homeostasis [1, 3]. The skin develops from neuroectoderm and this origin is reflected in its function as a sensory organ that is densely innervated by sensory and autonomic neurons [2]. Indeed, the skin is a major target and source of neuroendocrine signaling, indicating that the skin shares numerous neuromediators with the CNS and endocrine system [2, 4]. The communication between different cell types in the neuroendocrine and cutaneous systems is mediated by their specific receptors expressed in both neurons and skin [5]. Cutaneous injury initiates defense mechanisms to minimize damage and subsequently induce repair process to maintain homeostasis [6, 7]. Skin wound healing is a highly dynamic process made up of overlapping time-dependent phases including, homeostasis/coagulation, inflammation, migration/proliferation, and remodeling. For proper wound healing, the above processes in different phases require the interaction with multiple cell types, growth factors, chemokines, and cytokines [7, 8]. In a bid to understand skin homeostasis, previous studies sought to establish the various factors regulating the wound healing process. In the last three decades, numerous studies focused on neuropeptides in wound healing process because neuropeptides have been reported to play crucial roles in inflammation, proliferation, and migration, which are important for wound healing process [9]. Neuropeptides are released from peripheral terminals of primary afferent sensory neurons [10, 11] and different types of cells, including fibroblasts, mast cells, and keratinocytes, which are appropriately coupled to intracellular signaling pathways through their receptors [3]. Therefore, in this chapter, we will summarize the current understanding of the role of neuropeptides in skin wound healing.

Substance P (SP)

Substance P (SP) is an undecapeptide – an 11 amino acid (aa) peptide – member of the tachykinin neuropeptide family and acts as a neurotransmitter as well as a neuromodulator [12]. It is released from the central and peripheral endings of primary afferent neurons and also by C-nociceptive fibers in response to injury [12–14]. Immunoreactivity of SP is typically observed in blood vessel in the skin [15], however SP positive nerve fibers are found in the papillary layer near the epidermal basal membrane [16]. It has a higher affinity for the neurokinin 1 receptor (NK-1R) which is expressed in human keratinocytes, endothelial cells, and fibroblasts [17]. SP induces vasodilation action, alters vascular permeability, enhances delivery, and accumulates leukocytes to the tissues for local immune response through NK-1R [18–20]. In addition, SP stimulates endothelial cell differentiation, proliferation, and angiogenesis, which are important for inflammatory diseases and wound healing [21–23]. Exogenous injection of SP in the skin enhanced wound healing via neurite outgrowth as well as adhesion molecules [24]. In addition, NK-1R and SP promote the proliferation of human and murine-cultured keratinocytes directly or by releasing NGF [24–28]. Moreover, SP induces the remodeling of granulation tissue by stimulating proliferation and migration of dermal fibroblasts and increasing the expression of EGF/EGFR system [29–32]. EGF/EFGR system regulated by SP can modulate the synthesis and release of proinflammatory cytokines, such as interleukin-1 (IL-1), IL-6, and transforming growth factor (TGF)-α in different cell types of skin, which may play a crucial role in skin wound healing process [33, 34]. Furthermore, numerous studies have stressed the role of SP in impaired wound healing such as chronic wound in diabetic population since impaired wound healing in diabetic tissues is characterized by reduced number of nerve fibers and elevated neutral endopeptidase (NEP), an enzyme expressed in the skin and responsible for degradation of SP, activity [35–40]. In diabetic murine excisional wound model, duration of wound healing was longer compared to that in nondiabetic mice [20, 40, 41]. Moreover, topical application of SP or inhibition of NEP activity improved wound closure kinetics by increasing density of inflammatory cells in injured skin, implicating the crucial roles of SP in wound repair in the skin [20, 41–43].

Neurokinin-A (NKA)

Neurokinin-A, formerly known as substance K, is a neurologically active peptide encoded from preprotachykinin genes and closely related to substance P [44]. It has many excitatory effects on mammalian nervous system and influences inflammatory and pain response [44, 45]. NKA stimulates DNA synthesis in cultured human keratinocytes and fibroblasts suggesting that it might stimulate proliferation of connective tissue cells [29, 33]. It is mainly an inflammatory mediator and known to be less potent compared to SP. NKA upregulates mRNA expression of NGF both in human and mouse keratinocytes and promotes the release of NGF in the epidermis in mouse model [46].

Calcitonin Gene-Related Peptides (CGRP)

CGRP is a 37aa peptide produced majorly in neural body of dorsal root ganglion (DRG) and primarily localized to C and Aδ sensory fibers displaying a wide innervation throughout the body [47]. It belongs to the calcitonin peptide family and mediates biological effects through a heterodimeric receptor composed of the calcitonin receptor-like receptor (CALCRL, G protein-coupled receptor) and the receptor activity-modifying protein 1 (RAMP1). CGRP receptors are found throughout the body, indicating that CGRP may modulate physiological functions in all major systems including respiratory, endocrine, gastrointestinal, immune, and cardiovascular system [47–50]. Due to its numerous activities including vasodilatory effects on the skin, there is an increased interest in elucidating the role of CGRP in skin homeostasis [51, 52]. CGRP is released from sensory afferents and modulates cell proliferation, pigmentation, and wound healing in the skin [9, 53, 54]. Intravenous CGRP increased both blood flow and flap survival because normal wound healing is associated with early growth of new CGRP-containing sensory nerves, but depletion of CGRP using capsaicin led to decreased flap survival, highlighting the role of CGRP in tropic, regulatory, and repair process in wound healing [55, 56]. CGRP has also been shown to improve delayed wound contraction and prolonged time for wound healing in either capsaicin-treated or aged animal groups [57]. In addition, studies in CGRP KO mice or with CGRP antagonists which block CGRP receptors suggest beneficial effects of CGRP on skin wound healing [58, 59]. Toda et al. showed that defective wound healing in CGRP KO mice is likely due to impaired vasodilatory activity, in part, and also due to reduced expression of VEGF [59]. CGRP itself plays a role in the regeneration of skin through directly promoting proliferation of keratinocytes [60]. Together, CGRP enhanced human bronchial epithelial wound healing via PKA and MAPK signaling pathways [61]. Similarly, immunomodulatory effects of CGRP have also been suggested in Langerhans cells (LC) in esophageal mucosa and Merkel cells [62–66]. In human patients with thermal or soft tissue injuries, plasma levels of CGRP were increased significantly, indicating a crucial role of CGRP in pain, inflammation, and wound healing [67, 68].

Neuropeptide Y (NPY)

Neuropeptide Y (NPY) is a 36aa neuropeptide that is widely distributed in the brain and in the autonomic nervous system in humans where it acts as a neurotransmitter [69]. It serves as a strong vasoconstrictor and is thought to have various functions including food intake regulation, fat storage, and anxiety and stress reduction [70]. NPY also affects circadian rhythm, blood pressure, and epileptic seizures [70–74]. In the skin, NPY is found in sympathetic nerves in both the deeper layers and superficial dermal plexus near sweat glands and blood vessels, where it is stored either alone in small vesicles or in large vesicles in combination with catecholamines [39, 75, 76]. NPY stimulates proliferation and migration of human endothelial cells, which results in accelerating wound closure suggesting that NPY may act as an angiogenic factor through its receptors [77–79]. In addition, knockout mice lacking the Y2 receptor showed delayed skin wound healing, supporting the notion that NPY may have a crucial role in the regulation of angiogenesis and angiogenesis-related pathophysiological process [80]. It has been reported that the expression of NPY is closely correlated with impaired wound healing in diabetic patients [39]. Moreover, the levels of NPY were decreased in type 1 diabetic patients and in animal models of diabetes [81, 82]. Its reduced levels were observed at post-injury in diabetic wound compared to nondiabetic wound but no difference at the baseline [39]. Y2 receptor-deficient mice exhibit impaired skin wound healing, supporting important role of NPY as a proangiogenic factor in physiological conditions including wound healing [80].

Vasoactive Intestinal Peptide (VIP) and VIP-Related Peptides

Vasoactive Intestinal Peptide (VIP)

VIP is a 28aa neuropeptide belonging to the glucagon/secretin superfamily and works as a ligand for class II G protein-coupled receptor [83]. VIP is expressed in several organs including the heart, lung, eye, skin, ovary, and thyroid gland [84]. In the skin, its immunoreactivity is detected in nerve fibers around dermal arteries and capillaries, sweat and apocrine glands, and hair follicles [16]. VIP is more abundant in the dermis and subcutis as a potent vasoactive substance which regulates microcirculation [85]. It has been reported that VIP stimulates the proliferation and migration of human keratinocytes by an adenosine 3′,5′-cyclic monophosphate-dependent pathway [85, 86]. In addition, VIP stimulates angiogenesis in vitro and in vivo and the release of NGF or proinflammatory cytokines in human keratinocytes [87–89]. Studies on the rat sciatic nerve suggest the possible involvement of VIP in nerve regeneration after skin injury [90]. VIP immunoreactivity which is found in nerve fibers close to sites initiating epithelialization including hair follicles, sweat gland, and basal cell layer of epidermis supports the effect of VIP on skin wound healing [91].

Pituitary Adenylate Cyclase-Activating Peptide (PACAP)

PACAP is a 27aa (PACAP27) or 38aa (PACAP38) regulatory neuropeptide that is similar to VIP, 68 % homologous, and binds to VIP receptor 2 (VPAC2) and PACAP receptor [5, 92]. VPAC2 mRNA was found in the lung, CNS, and other peripheral organs including the skin [93]. In addition, the role of PACAP in the skin was studied in human keratinocyte, HaCaT cells, which express VPAC2 [93, 94]. The two forms of PACAP, PACAP27 and PACAP38, have similar biological functions and their expression varies in different tissues [95]. PACAP has been found in nerve fibers of various peripheral tissues, lymphoid tissues, and immunocompetent cells, co-localizing with SP and CGRP [96, 97]. PACAP is involved in pain, immunomodulation, and inflammatory process and induces vasodilatation, plasma extravasation, and increased blood flow in rodents [98, 99].

Bombesin-Like Peptide: Gastrin-Releasing Peptide (GRP)

GRP, a 27aa neuropeptide, is widely distributed in the CNS and peripheral nervous system, implicating a number of physiological and pathophysiological processes, and it also stimulates the release of gastrin from the stomach [100]. In the skin, GRP immunoreactivity was detected in primary afferent fibers and GRP-positive fibers [101]. GRP-positive nerve fibers are increased in the skin of mice with chronic dermatitis and in that of human dermatitis patients resulting in the increased secretion of GRP to the lesion of skin [101, 102]. Furthermore, recent studies indicate that GRP has mitogenic activity, and topical application of GRP on the skin accelerated epidermal regeneration and reepithelialization, showing improvement of cutaneous wound healing [103, 104].

Neurotensin (NT)

Neurotensin, a 13aa neuropeptide, is widely distributed throughout the brain, cardiovascular system, and gastrointestinal track and its action occurs via neurotensin receptors [105]. The role of NT in skin wound healing has been remotely suggested by its ability to downregulate proinflammatory cytokines and increase the expression of EGF in murine Langerhans cells and human skin fibroblasts [106, 107].

Galanin

Galanin, a neuropeptide encoded by GAL gene, is widely expressed in the brain, spinal cord, and gut in human [108]. There are four members of galanin peptides family including galanin (GAL), galanin message-associated protein (GMAP), galanin-like peptide (GALP), and alarnin [109]. They work through G protein-coupled GAL receptor (GALR) family, GALR1, 2, and 3 [109]. In human skin, GAL immunoreactivity was found in afferent sensory neurons, fibers of dermis, keratinocytes, and eccrine sweat glands [110]. GAL KO animal model and in vitro experiment demonstrate that the mitogenic and neurotrophic effects of GAL on axonal regeneration after neuronal injury [111–113]. Recent study showed that GAL induces proliferation and differentiation via GALR2 in human-cultured keratinocytes [114]. Moreover, the effects of GAL on skin wound healing have been suggested in a study using normal cultured human keratinocytes in which GAL induced proinflammatory cytokine production and increased neurotrophin, NGF, indicating that GAL plays a role in the modulation of cutaneous inflammation [115].

Opioids

Endogenous opioid system is one of the well-known pain-relieving systems, facilitated by the interaction between opioid receptors and their ligands. There are three distinct opioid systems, beta (β)-endorphin, methionine (met)- and leucine (leu)-enkephalin, and dynorphins, that are widely scattered in neurons [116]. These opioids act as neurotransmitters and neuromodulators with their receptors, μ-, delta (δ)-, and kappa (κ)-opioid receptors, and have analgesic effects [116, 117]. Recently, growing evidence shows the role of opioid receptors and endogenous ligands in different skin structures including peripheral nerve fibers, keratinocytes, melanocytes, hair follicles, and immune cells, implying that opioid-opioid receptor signaling may influence skin homeostasis [118]. Furthermore, several studies have examined the stimulating effect of agonists on granulation tissue formation, reepithelialization, and keratinocyte migration in the skin [118–121].

Beta (β)-Endorphin

β-endorphin is a 31aa endogenous opioid neuropeptide found in the neurons of both central and peripheral nervous system, produced by processing of the precursor pro-opiomelanocortin (POMC), and it acts as an agonist of the μ-opioid receptor (MOR) [118, 122]. In the skin, β-endorphin immunoreactivity was detected in keratinocytes of follicular matrix and in duct cells of sweat glands [123]. MOR and β-endorphin signal were also found in peripheral nerve endings [124, 125]. Human keratinocytes produce β-endorphin, and the serum concentration was found to be elevated in patients with severe atopic dermatitis [126]. In the skin, β-endorphin downregulates MOR and upregulates TGF-β receptor II and cytokeratin 16 which is not expressed in normal skin, but it was upregulated in the suprabasal and differentiating compartment of the epidermis during wound healing [127]. Recent study reported that β-endorphin stimulated the migration of human keratinocytes, while naltrexone, an opioid receptor antagonist, reduced the effect of β-endorphin on keratinocyte, implying that β-endorphin plays an essential role in the final reepithelialization and tissue regeneration during wound healing [128].

Enkephalin (ENK)

Enkephalin is a pentapeptide involved in regulation of nociception in the body [129]. Two forms of enkephalin have been identified, Met- and Leu-enkephalin, both of which are products of proenkephalin gene. Human skin and cultured skin cells express proenkephalin (PENK) gene, precursor form of Met- and Leu-ENK [130]. In addition, expression of Met- and Leu-ENK was observed in the epidermis with gradient pattern, the highest expression being in outer differentiated keratinocyte layers and along the basement membrane between nonvascular epidermis and vascularized dermis, suggesting the role of ENK to protect the skin [130]. ENK receptors include delta (δ)-opioid receptor (DOR) [131] which is expressed in murine and cultured human skin. Mice lacking DOR exhibit abnormal epidermal phenotypes and delayed wound healing, suggesting an essential role of DOR in skin proliferation, migration, and differentiation [132].

Dynorphins

Dynorphins are a class of opioid peptides that are cleaved from precursor protein prodynorphin. Cleaved peptides include dynorphin A, dynorphin B, and α-/β-neoendorphin [133]. All dynorphins exert their effects primarily through kappa (κ)-opioid receptor (KOR) [134]. Similar to other opioid peptides, dynorphins are analgesic, and KOR is involved in a natural addiction control mechanism, which suggests the effects of dynorphins and KOR system on perception of pain, consciousness, motor control, and mood [135, 136]. In addition, inducing dry skin dermatitis results in hypotrophic and thinner epidermis in mice lacking KOR compared to control mice, indicating a role of KOR system on epidermal homeostasis [137].

Conclusion

Increasing evidence suggests that the skin not only interacts with the immune system but also communicates with the nervous system [118, 138]. Although these interactions are not completely understood, clinical observations in patients with nervous system disorders indicate the role of cutaneous innervations in skin protection and repair [53, 139]. Cutaneous nerve fibers release neuromediators which play an important regulatory role in the skin under physiological and pathophysiological conditions including wound healing [140]. In recent years, experimental evidence shows that neuropeptides are implicated in various processes involved in skin wound healing such as induction of vasodilatation and angiogenesis, promotion of cell chemotaxis, modulation of immune response, and stimulation of migration and proliferation of keratinocytes and fibroblasts [125, 141, 142]. Therefore, a better understanding of skin homeostasis mediated by neuropeptides might be a possible option to intervene acute and chronic cutaneous wounds.

Acknowledgments We would like to thank Ann W. Kinyua (Yonsei University) for the critical reading of this manuscript. This work supported by Small and Medium Business Administration (Technological Innovation R&D Program S2178403) for S. H. M. and the National Research Foundation (NRF-2013R1A1A1007693 and 2014K1A3A1A19066980) for K.W.K.

References

1. Boulais N, Misery L. The epidermis: a sensory tissue. Eur J Dermatol. 2008;18:119–27.
2. Slominski A, Wortsman J, Luger T, Paus R, Solomon S. Corticotropin releasing hormone and proopiomelanocortin involvement in the cutaneous response to stress. Physiol Rev. 2000;80:979–1020.
3. Slominski AT, Zmijewski MA, Skobowiat C, Zbytek B, Slominski RM, Steketee JD. Sensing the environment: regulation of local and global homeostasis by the skin's neuroendocrine system. Adv Anat Embryol Cell Biol. 2012; 212: v, vii, 1–115.
4. Farber EM, Nickoloff BJ, Recht B, Fraki JE. Stress, symmetry, and psoriasis: possible role of neuropeptides. J Am Acad Dermatol. 1986;14:305–11.
5. Cheret J, Lebonvallet N, Carre JL, Misery L, Le Gall-Ianotto C. Role of neuropeptides, neurotrophins, and neurohormones in skin wound healing. Wound Repair Regen. 2013;21:772–88.
6. Theoret C. Tissue engineering in wound repair: the three "R"s–repair, replace, regenerate. Vet Surg. 2009;38:905–13.
7. Borena BM, Martens A, Broeckx SY, Meyer E, Chiers K, Duchateau L, Spaas JH. Regenerative skin wound healing in mammals: state-of-the-art on growth factor and stem cell based treatments. Cell Physiol Biochem. 2015;36:1–23.
8. Singer AJ, Clark RA. Cutaneous wound healing. N Engl J Med. 1999;341:738–46.
9. da Silva L, Carvalho E, Cruz MT. Role of neuropeptides in skin inflammation and its involvement in diabetic wound healing. Expert Opin Biol Ther. 2010;10:1427–39.
10. Yamaoka J, Di ZH, Sun W, Kawana S. Erratum to "changes in cutaneous sensory nerve fibers induced by skin-scratching in mice". J Dermatol Sci. 2007;47:172–82.
11. Joachim RA, Kuhlmei A, Dinh QT, Handjiski B, Fischer T, Peters EM, Klapp BF, Paus R, Arck PC. Neuronal plasticity of the "brain-skin connection": stress-triggered up-regulation of neuropeptides in dorsal root ganglia and skin via nerve growth factor-dependent pathways. J Mol Med. 2007;85:1369–78.
12. Datar P, Srivastava S, Coutinho E, Govil G. Substance P: structure, function, and therapeutics. Curr Top Med Chem. 2004;4:75–103.
13. Harrison S, Geppetti P. Substance p. Int J Biochem Cell Biol. 2001;33:555–76.
14. Otsuka M, Yoshioka K. Neurotransmitter functions of mammalian tachykinins. Physiol Rev. 1993;73:229–308.
15. Simone DA, Nolano M, Johnson T, Wendelschafer-Crabb G, Kennedy WR. Intradermal injection of capsaicin in humans produces degeneration and subsequent reinnervation of epidermal nerve fibers: correlation with sensory function. J Neurosci. 1998;18:8947–59.
16. Schulze E, Witt M, Fink T, Hofer A, Funk RH. Immunohistochemical detection of human skin nerve fibers. Acta Histochem. 1997;99:301–9.
17. Liu JY, Hu JH, Zhu QG, Li FQ, Sun HJ. Substance P receptor expression in human skin keratinocytes and fibroblasts. Br J Dermatol. 2006;155:657–62.
18. Pernow B. Substance P. Pharmacol Rev. 1983;35:85–141.
19. Baluk P. Neurogenic inflammation in skin and airways. J Investig Dermatol Symp Proc. 1997; 2: 76–81.
20. Scott JR, Tamura RN, Muangman P, Isik FF, Xie C, Gibran NS. Topical substance P increases inflammatory cell density in genetically diabetic murine wounds. Wound Repair Regen. 2008;16:529–33.
21. Jain M, LoGerfo FW, Guthrie P, Pradhan L. Effect of hyperglycemia and neuropeptides on interleukin-8-expression and angiogenesis in dermal microvascular endothelial cells. J Vasc Surg. 2011;53:1654–60. e2.
22. Walsh DA, Hu DE, Mapp PI, Polak JM, Blake DR, Fan TP. Innervation and neurokinin receptors during angiogenesis in the rat sponge granuloma. Histochem J. 1996;28:759–69.
23. Wiedermann CJ, Auer B, Sitte B, Reinisch N, Schratzberger P, Kahler CM. Induction of endothelial cell differentiation into capillary-like structures by substance P. Eur J Pharmacol. 1996;298:335–8.
24. Altun V, Hakvoort TE, van Zuijlen PP, van der Kwast TH, Prens EP. Nerve outgrowth and neuropeptide expression during the remodeling of human burn wound scars. A 7-month follow-up study of 22 patients. Burns. 2001;27:717–22.

25. Delgado AV, McManus AT, Chambers JP. Exogenous administration of Substance P enhances wound healing in a novel skin-injury model. Exp Biol Med. 2005;230:271–80.
26. Gibran NS, Tamura R, Tsou R, Isik FF. Human dermal microvascular endothelial cells produce nerve growth factor: implications for wound repair. Shock. 2003;19:127–30.
27. McGovern UB, Jones KT, Sharpe GR. Intracellular calcium as a second messenger following growth stimulation of human keratinocytes. Br J Dermatol. 1995;132:892–6.
28. Tanaka T, Danno K, Ikai K, Imamura S. Effects of substance P and substance K on the growth of cultured keratinocytes. J Invest Dermatol. 1988;90:399–401.
29. Nilsson J, von Euler AM, Dalsgaard CJ. Stimulation of connective tissue cell growth by substance P and substance K. Nature. 1985;315:61–3.
30. Parenti A, Amerini S, Ledda F, Maggi CA, Ziche M. The tachykinin NK1 receptor mediates the migration-promoting effect of substance P on human skin fibroblasts in culture. Naunyn Schmiedebergs Arch Pharmacol. 1996;353:475–81.
31. Ziche M, Morbidelli L, Pacini M, Dolara P, Maggi CA. NK1-receptors mediate the proliferative response of human fibroblasts to tachykinins. Br J Pharmacol. 1990;100:11–4.
32. Lai X, Wang Z, Wei L, Wang L. Effect of substance P released from peripheral nerve ending on endogenous expression of epidermal growth factor and its receptor in wound healing. Chin J Traumatol. 2002;5:176–9.
33. Luger TA, Lotti T. Neuropeptides: role in inflammatory skin diseases. J Eur Acad Dermatol Venereol. 1998;10:207–11.
34. Wei T, Guo TZ, Li WW, Hou S, Kingery WS, Clark JD. Keratinocyte expression of inflammatory mediators plays a crucial role in substance P-induced acute and chronic pain. J Neuroinflammation. 2012;9:181.
35. Olerud JE, Usui ML, Seckin D, Chiu DS, Haycox CL, Song IS, Ansel JC, Bunnett NW. Neutral endopeptidase expression and distribution in human skin and wounds. J Invest Dermatol. 1999;112:873–81.
36. Levy DM, Karanth SS, Springall DR, Polak JM. Depletion of cutaneous nerves and neuropeptides in diabetes mellitus: an immunocytochemical study. Diabetologia. 1989;32:427–33.
37. Scholzen TE, Luger TA. Neutral endopeptidase and angiotensin-converting enzyme – key enzymes terminating the action of neuroendocrine mediators. Exp Dermatol. 2004;13 Suppl 4:22–6.
38. Antezana M, Sullivan SR, Usui M, Gibran N, Spenny M, Larsen J, Ansel J, Bunnett N, Olerud J. Neutral endopeptidase activity is increased in the skin of subjects with diabetic ulcers. J Invest Dermatol. 2002;119:1400–4.
39. Pradhan L, Cai X, Wu S, Andersen ND, Martin M, Malek J, Guthrie P, Veves A, Logerfo FW. Gene expression of pro-inflammatory cytokines and neuropeptides in diabetic wound healing. J Surg Res. 2011;167:336–42.
40. Gibran NS, Jang YC, Isik FF, Greenhalgh DG, Muffley LA, Underwood RA, Usui ML, Larsen J, Smith DG, Bunnett N, Ansel JC, Olerud JE. Diminished neuropeptide levels contribute to the impaired cutaneous healing response associated with diabetes mellitus. J Surg Res. 2002;108:122–8.
41. Younan G, Ogawa R, Ramirez M, Helm D, Dastouri P, Orgill DP. Analysis of nerve and neuropeptide patterns in vacuum-assisted closure-treated diabetic murine wounds. Plast Reconstr Surg. 2010;126:87–96.
42. Kishimoto S. The regeneration of substance P-containing nerve fibers in the process of burn wound healing in the guinea pig skin. J Invest Dermatol. 1984;83:219–23.
43. Dunnick CA, Gibran NS, Heimbach DM. Substance P has a role in neurogenic mediation of human burn wound healing. J Burn Care Rehabil. 1996;17:390–6.
44. Nakanishi S. Molecular mechanisms of intercellular communication in the hormonal and neural systems. IUBMB Life. 2006;58:349–57.
45. Schaffer DA, Gabriel R. Two major tachykinins, substance P and substance K, are localized to distinct subsets of amacrine cells in the anuran retina. Neurosci Lett. 2005;386:194–8.
46. Burbach GJ, Kim KH, Zivony AS, Kim A, Aranda J, Wright S, Naik SM, Caughman SW, Ansel JC, Armstrong CA. The neurosensory tachykinins substance P and neurokinin A directly induce keratinocyte nerve growth factor. J Invest Dermatol. 2001;117:1075–82.
47. Russell FA, King R, Smillie SJ, Kodji X, Brain SD. Calcitonin gene-related peptide: physiology and pathophysiology. Physiol Rev. 2014;94:1099–142.
48. Caviedes-Bucheli J, Moreno GC, Lopez MP, Bermeo-Noguera AM, Pacheco-Rodriguez G, Cuellar A, Munoz HR. Calcitonin gene-related peptide receptor expression in alternatively activated monocytes/macrophages during irreversible pulpitis. J Endod. 2008;34:945–9.
49. Hagner S, Stahl U, Knoblauch B, McGregor GP, Lang RE. Calcitonin receptor-like receptor: identification and distribution in human peripheral tissues. Cell Tissue Res. 2002;310:41–50.
50. Hou Q, Barr T, Gee L, Vickers J, Wymer J, Borsani E, Rodella L, Getsios S, Burdo T, Eisenberg E, Guha U, Lavker R, Kessler J, Chittur S, Fiorino D, Rice F, Albrecht P. Keratinocyte expression of calcitonin gene-related peptide beta: implications for neuropathic and inflammatory pain mechanisms. Pain. 2011;152:2036–51.
51. Brain SD, Williams TJ, Tippins JR, Morris HR, MacIntyre I. Calcitonin gene-related peptide is a potent vasodilator. Nature. 1985;313:54–6.
52. Gibbins IL, Wattchow D, Coventry B. Two immunohistochemically identified populations of calcitonin gene-related peptide (CGRP)-

immunoreactive axons in human skin. Brain Res. 1987;414:143–8.
53. Roosterman D, Goerge T, Schneider SW, Bunnett NW, Steinhoff M. Neuronal control of skin function: the skin as a neuroimmunoendocrine organ. Physiol Rev. 2006;86:1309–79.
54. Cheret J, Lebonvallet N, Buhe V, Carre JL, Misery L, Le Gall-Ianotto C. Influence of sensory neuropeptides on human cutaneous wound healing process. J Dermatol Sci. 2014;74:193–203.
55. Kjartansson J, Dalsgaard CJ. Calcitonin gene-related peptide increases survival of a musculocutaneous critical flap in the rat. Eur J Pharmacol. 1987;142:355–8.
56. Karanth SS, Dhital S, Springall DR, Polak JM. Reinnervation and neuropeptides in mouse skin flaps. J Auton Nerv Syst. 1990;31:127–34.
57. Khalil Z, Helme R. Sensory peptides as neuromodulators of wound healing in aged rats. J Gerontol A Biol Sci Med Sci. 1996;51:B354–61.
58. Grant AD, Tam CW, Lazar Z, Shih MK, Brain SD. The calcitonin gene-related peptide (CGRP) receptor antagonist BIBN4096BS blocks CGRP and adrenomedullin vasoactive responses in the microvasculature. Br J Pharmacol. 2004;142:1091–8.
59. Toda M, Suzuki T, Hosono K, Kurihara Y, Kurihara H, Hayashi I, Kitasato H, Hoka S, Majima M. Roles of calcitonin gene-related peptide in facilitation of wound healing and angiogenesis. Biomed Pharmacother. 2008;62:352–9.
60. Roggenkamp D, Kopnick S, Stab F, Wenck H, Schmelz M, Neufang G. Epidermal nerve fibers modulate keratinocyte growth via neuropeptide signaling in an innervated skin model. J Invest Dermatol. 2013;133:1620–8.
61. Zhou Y, Zhang M, Sun GY, Liu YP, Ran WZ, Peng L, Guan CX. Calcitonin gene-related peptide promotes the wound healing of human bronchial epithelial cells via PKC and MAPK pathways. Regul Pept. 2013;184:22–9.
62. Singaram C, Sengupta A, Stevens C, Spechler SJ, Goyal RK. Localization of calcitonin gene-related peptide in human esophageal Langerhans cells. Gastroenterology. 1991;100:560–3.
63. Zaidi M, Moonga BS, Bevis PJ, Bascal ZA, Breimer LH. The calcitonin gene peptides: biology and clinical relevance. Crit Rev Clin Lab Sci. 1990;28:109–74.
64. Garcia-Caballero T, Gallego R, Roson E, Fraga M, Beiras A. Calcitonin gene-related peptide (CGRP) immunoreactivity in the neuroendocrine Merkel cells and nerve fibres of pig and human skin. Histochemistry. 1989;92:127–32.
65. Dalsgaard CJ, Jernbeck J, Stains W, Kjartansson J, Haegerstrand A, Hokfelt T, Brodin E, Cuello AC, Brown JC. Calcitonin gene-related peptide-like immunoreactivity in nerve fibers in the human skin. Relation to fibers containing substance P-, somatostatin- and vasocactive intestinalpolypeptide-like immunoreactivity. Histochemistry. 1989;91:35–8.
66. Hosoi J, Murphy GF, Egan CL, Lerner EA, Grabbe S, Asahina A, Granstein RD. Regulation of Langerhans cell function by nerves containing calcitonin gene-related peptide. Nature. 1993;363:159–63.
67. Onuoha GN, Alpar EK. Levels of vasodilators (SP, CGRP) and vasoconstrictor (NPY) peptides in early human burns. Eur J Clin Invest. 2001;31:253–7.
68. Onuoha GN, Alpar EK. Calcitonin gene-related peptide and other neuropeptides in the plasma of patients with soft tissue injury. Life Sci. 1999;65:1351–8.
69. Tatemoto K. Neuropeptide Y: complete amino acid sequence of the brain peptide. Proc Natl Acad Sci U S A. 1982;79:5485–9.
70. Decressac M, Barker RA. Neuropeptide Y and its role in CNS disease and repair. Exp Neurol. 2012;238:265–72.
71. Donoso MV, Miranda R, Irarrazaval MJ, Huidobro-Toro JP. Neuropeptide Y is released from human mammary and radial vascular biopsies and is a functional modulator of sympathetic cotransmission. J Vasc Res. 2004;41:387–99.
72. Donoso MV, Miranda R, Briones R, Irarrazaval MJ, Huidobro-Toro JP. Release and functional role of neuropeptide Y as a sympathetic modulator in human saphenous vein biopsies. Peptides. 2004;25:53–64.
73. Johnson MI, Tabasam G. A single-blind investigation into the hypoalgesic effects of different swing patterns of interferential currents on cold-induced pain in healthy volunteers. Arch Phys Med Rehabil. 2003;84:350–7.
74. Pedrazzini T, Pralong F, Grouzmann E. Neuropeptide Y: the universal soldier. Cell Mol Life Sci. 2003;60:350–77.
75. Polak JM, Bloom SR. Regulatory peptides–the distribution of two newly discovered peptides: PHI and NPY. Peptides. 1984;5 Suppl 1:79–89.
76. Tainio H, Vaalasti A, Rechardt L. The distribution of sympathetic adrenergic, tyrosine hydroxylase- and neuropeptide Y-immunoreactive nerves in human axillary sweat glands. Histochemistry. 1986;85:117–20.
77. Ghersi G, Chen W, Lee EW, Zukowska Z. Critical role of dipeptidyl peptidase IV in neuropeptide Y-mediated endothelial cell migration in response to wounding. Peptides. 2001;22:453–8.
78. Zukowska-Grojec Z, Karwatowska-Prokopczuk E, Rose W, Rone J, Movafagh S, Ji H, Yeh Y, Chen WT, Kleinman HK, Grouzmann E, Grant DS. Neuropeptide Y: a novel angiogenic factor from the sympathetic nerves and endothelium. Circ Res. 1998;83:187–95.
79. Marion-Audibert AM, Nejjari M, Pourreyron C, Anderson W, Gouysse G, Jacquier MF, Dumortier J, Scoazec JY. Effects of endocrine peptides on proliferation, migration and differentiation of human endothelial cells. Gastroenterol Clin Biol. 2000;24:644–8.
80. Ekstrand AJ, Cao R, Bjorndahl M, Nystrom S, Jonsson-Rylander AC, Hassani H, Hallberg B,

Nordlander M, Cao Y. Deletion of neuropeptide Y (NPY) 2 receptor in mice results in blockage of NPY-induced angiogenesis and delayed wound healing. Proc Natl Acad Sci U S A. 2003;100:6033–8.

81. Ahlborg G, Lundberg JM. Exercise-induced changes in neuropeptide Y, noradrenaline and endothelin-1 levels in young people with type I diabetes. Clin Physiol. 1996;16:645–55.
82. Kuncova J, Sviglerova J, Tonar Z, Slavikova J. Heterogenous changes in neuropeptide Y, norepinephrine and epinephrine concentrations in the hearts of diabetic rats. Auton Neurosci. 2005;121:7–15.
83. Umetsu Y, Tenno T, Goda N, Shirakawa M, Ikegami T, Hiroaki H. Structural difference of vasoactive intestinal peptide in two distinct membrane-mimicking environments. Biochim Biophys Acta. 1814;2011:724–30.
84. Zudenigo D, Lackovic Z. Vasoactive intestinal polypeptide: a potential neurotransmitter. Lijec Vjesn. 1989;111:354–9.
85. Granoth R, Fridkin M, Gozes I. VIP and the potent analog, stearyl-Nle(17)-VIP, induce proliferation of keratinocytes. FEBS Lett. 2000;475:78–83.
86. Kakurai M, Demitsu T, Umemoto N, Kobayashi Y, Inoue-Narita T, Fujita N, Ohtsuki M, Furukawa Y. Vasoactive intestinal peptide and inflammatory cytokines enhance vascular endothelial growth factor production from epidermal keratinocytes. Br J Dermatol. 2009;161:1232–8.
87. Dallos A, Kiss M, Polyanka H, Dobozy A, Kemeny L, Husz S. Effects of the neuropeptides substance P, calcitonin gene-related peptide, vasoactive intestinal polypeptide and galanin on the production of nerve growth factor and inflammatory cytokines in cultured human keratinocytes. Neuropeptides. 2006;40:251–63.
88. Yang J, Zong CH, Zhao ZH, Hu XD, Shi QD, Xiao XL, Liu Y. Vasoactive intestinal peptide in rats with focal cerebral ischemia enhances angiogenesis. Neuroscience. 2009;161:413–21.
89. Collado B, Carmena MJ, Clemente C, Prieto JC, Bajo AM. Vasoactive intestinal peptide enhances growth and angiogenesis of human experimental prostate cancer in a xenograft model. Peptides. 2007;28:1896–901.
90. Rayan GM, Johnson C, Pitha J, Cahill S, Said S. Vasoactive intestinal peptide and nerve growth factor effects on nerve regeneration. J Okla State Med Assoc. 1995;88:337–41.
91. Bjorklund H, Dalsgaard CJ, Jonsson CE, Hermansson A. Sensory and autonomic innervation of non-hairy and hairy human skin. An immunohistochemical study. Cell Tissue Res. 1986;243:51–7.
92. Conconi MT, Spinazzi R, Nussdorfer GG. Endogenous ligands of PACAP/VIP receptors in the autocrine-paracrine regulation of the adrenal gland. Int Rev Cytol. 2006;249:1–51.
93. Fischer TC, Hartmann P, Loser C, Springer J, Peiser C, Dinh QT, Fischer A, Groneberg DA. Abundant expression of vasoactive intestinal polypeptide receptor VPAC2 mRNA in human skin. J Invest Dermatol. 2001;117:754–6.
94. Granoth R, Fridkin M, Rubinraut S, Gozes I. VIP-derived sequences modified by N-terminal stearyl moiety induce cell death: the human keratinocyte as a model. FEBS Lett. 2000;475:71–7.
95. Vaudry D, Falluel-Morel A, Bourgault S, Basille M, Burel D, Wurtz O, Fournier A, Chow BK, Hashimoto H, Galas L, Vaudry H. Pituitary adenylate cyclase-activating polypeptide and its receptors: 20 years after the discovery. Pharmacol Rev. 2009;61:283–357.
96. Arimura A, Somogyvari-Vigh A, Miyata A, Mizuno K, Coy DH, Kitada C. Tissue distribution of PACAP as determined by RIA: highly abundant in the rat brain and testes. Endocrinology. 1991;129:2787–9.
97. Arimura A, Shioda S. Pituitary adenylate cyclase activating polypeptide (PACAP) and its receptors: neuroendocrine and endocrine interaction. Front Neuroendocrinol. 1995;16:53–88.
98. Odum L, Petersen LJ, Skov PS, Ebskov LB. Pituitary adenylate cyclase activating polypeptide (PACAP) is localized in human dermal neurons and causes histamine release from skin mast cells. Inflamm Res. 1998;47:488–92.
99. Cardell LO, Stjarne P, Wagstaff SJ, Agusti C, Nadel JA. PACAP-induced plasma extravasation in rat skin. Regul Pept. 1997;71:67–71.
100. Merali Z, McIntosh J, Anisman H. Role of bombesin-related peptides in the control of food intake. Neuropeptides. 1999;33:376–86.
101. Tominaga M, Ogawa H, Takamori K. Histological characterization of cutaneous nerve fibers containing gastrin-releasing peptide in NC/Nga mice: an atopic dermatitis model. J Invest Dermatol. 2009;129:2901–5.
102. Andoh T, Kuwazono T, Lee JB, Kuraishi Y. Gastrin-releasing peptide induces itch-related responses through mast cell degranulation in mice. Peptides. 2011;32:2098–103.
103. Regauer S, Compton CC. Cultured keratinocyte sheets enhance spontaneous re-epithelialization in a dermal explant model of partial-thickness wound healing. J Invest Dermatol. 1990;95:341–6.
104. Yamaguchi Y, Hosokawa K, Nakatani Y, Sano S, Yoshikawa K, Itami S. Gastrin-releasing peptide, a bombesin-like neuropeptide, promotes cutaneous wound healing. Dermatol Surg. 2002;28:314–9.
105. Vincent JP, Mazella J, Kitabgi P. Neurotensin and neurotensin receptors. Trends Pharmacol Sci. 1999;20:302–9.
106. da Silva L, Neves BM, Moura L, Cruz MT, Carvalho E. Neurotensin downregulates the pro-inflammatory properties of skin dendritic cells and increases epidermal growth factor expression. Biochim Biophys Acta. 1813;2011:1863–71.
107. Pereira da Silva L, Miguel Neves B, Moura L, Cruz MT, Carvalho E. Neurotensin decreases the

proinflammatory status of human skin fibroblasts and increases epidermal growth factor expression. Int J Inflam. 2014;2014:248240.

108. Mitsukawa K, Lu X, Bartfai T. Galanin, galanin receptors and drug targets. Cell Mol Life Sci. 2008;65:1796–805.

109. Bauer JW, Lang R, Jakab M, Kofler B. Galanin family of peptides in skin function. Cell Mol Life Sci. 2008;65:1820–5.

110. Kofler B, Berger A, Santic R, Moritz K, Almer D, Tuechler C, Lang R, Emberger M, Klausegger A, Sperl W, Bauer JW. Expression of neuropeptide galanin and galanin receptors in human skin. J Invest Dermatol. 2004;122:1050–3.

111. Hokfelt T, Wiesenfeld-Hallin Z, Villar M, Melander T. Increase of galanin-like immunoreactivity in rat dorsal root ganglion cells after peripheral axotomy. Neurosci Lett. 1987;83:217–20.

112. Hokfelt T, Zhang X, Wiesenfeld-Hallin Z. Messenger plasticity in primary sensory neurons following axotomy and its functional implications. Trends Neurosci. 1994;17:22–30.

113. Holmes FE, Mahoney SA, Wynick D. Use of genetically engineered transgenic mice to investigate the role of galanin in the peripheral nervous system after injury. Neuropeptides. 2005;39:191–9.

114. Dallos A, Kiss M, Polyanka H, Dobozy A, Kemeny L, Husz S. Galanin receptor expression in cultured human keratinocytes and in normal human skin. J Peripher Nerv Syst. 2006;11:156–64.

115. Jimenez-Andrade JM, Zhou S, Yamani A, Valencia de Ita S, Castaneda-Hernandez G, Carlton SM. Mechanism by which peripheral galanin increases acute inflammatory pain. Brain Res. 2005;1056:113–7.

116. Holden JE, Jeong Y, Forrest JM. The endogenous opioid system and clinical pain management. AACN Clin Issues. 2005;16:291–301.

117. Waldhoer M, Bartlett SE, Whistler JL. Opioid receptors. Annu Rev Biochem. 2004;73:953–90.

118. Bigliardi PL, Tobin DJ, Gaveriaux-Ruff C, Bigliardi-Qi M. Opioids and the skin–where do we stand? Exp Dermatol. 2009;18:424–30.

119. Charbaji N, Schafer-Korting M, Kuchler S. Morphine stimulates cell migration of oral epithelial cells by delta-opioid receptor activation. PLoS One. 2012;7, e42616.

120. Kuchler S, Radowski MR, Blaschke T, Dathe M, Plendl J, Haag R, Schafer-Korting M, Kramer KD. Nanoparticles for skin penetration enhancement–a comparison of a dendritic core-multishell-nanotransporter and solid lipid nanoparticles. Eur J Pharm Biopharm. 2009;71: 243–50.

121. Kuchler S, Wolf NB, Heilmann S, Weindl G, Helfmann J, Yahya MM, Stein C, Schafer-Korting M. 3D-wound healing model: influence of morphine and solid lipid nanoparticles. J Biotechnol. 2010;148:24–30.

122. Wintzen M, Gilchrest BA. Proopiomelanocortin, its derived peptides, and the skin. J Invest Dermatol. 1996;106:3–10.

123. Wintzen M, de Winter S, Out-Luiting JJ, van Duinen SG, Vermeer BJ. Presence of immunoreactive beta-endorphin in human skin. Exp Dermatol. 2001;10:305–11.

124. Stander S, Gunzer M, Metze D, Luger T, Steinhoff M. Localization of mu-opioid receptor 1A on sensory nerve fibers in human skin. Regul Pept. 2002;110:75–83.

125. Bigliardi-Qi M, Sumanovski LT, Buchner S, Rufli T, Bigliardi PL. Mu-opiate receptor and Beta-endorphin expression in nerve endings and keratinocytes in human skin. Dermatology. 2004;209:183–9.

126. Glinski W, Brodecka H, Glinska-Ferenz M, Kowalski D. Increased concentration of beta-endorphin in the sera of patients with severe atopic dermatitis. Acta Derm Venereol. 1995;75:9–11.

127. Bigliardi-Qi M, Bigliardi PL, Eberle AN, Buchner S, Rufli T. beta-endorphin stimulates cytokeratin 16 expression and downregulates mu-opiate receptor expression in human epidermis. J Invest Dermatol. 2000;114:527–32.

128. Bigliardi PL, Buchner S, Rufli T, Bigliardi-Qi M. Specific stimulation of migration of human keratinocytes by mu-opiate receptor agonists. J Recept Signal Transduct Res. 2002;22:191–9.

129. Noda M, Teranishi Y, Takahashi H, Toyosato M, Notake M, Nakanishi S, Numa S. Isolation and structural organization of the human preproenkephalin gene. Nature. 1982;297:431–4.

130. Slominski AT, Zmijewski MA, Zbytek B, Brozyna AA, Granese J, Pisarchik A, Szczesniewski A, Tobin DJ. Regulated proenkephalin expression in human skin and cultured skin cells. J Invest Dermatol. 2011;131:613–22.

131. Quock RM, Burkey TH, Varga E, Hosohata Y, Hosohata K, Cowell SM, Slate CA, Ehlert FJ, Roeske WR, Yamamura HI. The delta-opioid receptor: molecular pharmacology, signal transduction, and the determination of drug efficacy. Pharmacol Rev. 1999;51:503–32.

132. Bigliardi-Qi M, Gaveriaux-Ruff C, Zhou H, Hell C, Bady P, Rufli T, Kieffer B, Bigliardi P. Deletion of delta-opioid receptor in mice alters skin differentiation and delays wound healing. Differentiation. 2006;74:174–85.

133. Day R, Lazure C, Basak A, Boudreault A, Limperis P, Dong W, Lindberg I. Prodynorphin processing by proprotein convertase 2. Cleavage at single basic residues and enhanced processing in the presence of carboxypeptidase activity. J Biol Chem. 1998;273:829–36.

134. Shippenberg TS. The dynorphin/kappa opioid receptor system: a new target for the treatment of addiction and affective disorders? Neuropsychopharmacology. 2009;34:247.

135. Cahill CM, Taylor AM, Cook C, Ong E, Moron JA, Evans CJ. Does the kappa opioid receptor system contribute to pain aversion? Front Pharmacol. 2014;5:253.
136. Lalanne L, Ayranci G, Kieffer BL, Lutz PE. The kappa opioid receptor: from addiction to depression, and back. Front Psychiatr. 2014;5:170.
137. Bigliardi-Qi M, Gaveriaux-Ruff C, Pfaltz K, Bady P, Baumann T, Rufli T, Kieffer BL, Bigliardi PL. Deletion of mu- and kappa-opioid receptors in mice changes epidermal hypertrophy, density of peripheral nerve endings, and itch behavior. J Invest Dermatol. 2007;127:1479–88.
138. Bos JD, De Rie MA. The pathogenesis of psoriasis: immunological facts and speculations. Immunol Today. 1999;20:40–6.
139. Steinhoff M, Stander S, Seeliger S, Ansel JC, Schmelz M, Luger T. Modern aspects of cutaneous neurogenic inflammation. Arch Dermatol. 2003;139:1479–88.
140. Laverdet B, Danigo A, Girard D, Magy L, Demiot C, Desmouliere A. Skin innervation: important roles during normal and pathological cutaneous repair. Histol Histopathol. 2015;30(7):875–82.
141. Brain SD. Sensory neuropeptides: their role in inflammation and wound healing. Immunopharmacology. 1997;37:133–52.
142. Amadesi S, Reni C, Katare R, Meloni M, Oikawa A, Beltrami AP, Avolio E, Cesselli D, Fortunato O, Spinetti G, Ascione R, Cangiano E, Valgimigli M, Hunt SP, Emanueli C, Madeddu P. Role for substance p-based nociceptive signaling in progenitor cell activation and angiogenesis during ischemia in mice and in human subjects. Circulation. 2012;125:1774–86. S1-19.

143 Wound Healing as We Age

Jihane Abou Rahal and Dany Nassar

Contents

J. Abou Rahal
Department of Dermatology, American University of Beirut Medical Center, Beirut, Lebanon
e-mail: j.abourahal@gmail.com

D. Nassar (✉)
Department of Dermatology, American University of Beirut Medical Center, Beirut, Lebanon

Department of Anatomy, Cell Biology and Physiological Sciences, American University of Beirut Medical Center, Beirut, Lebanon
e-mail: dn18@aub.edu.lb

M.A. Farage et al. (eds.), *Textbook of Aging Skin*,
DOI 10.1007/978-3-662-47398-6_143

Abstract

The world population is aging and the prevalence of age-related diseases is increasing. Cutaneous ulcers are a major group of pathologies in the elderly that have high morbidity and economic burden. In this chapter, we review our current knowledge of age-related mechanisms underlying wound-healing alterations that occur with age.

Introduction

As the world population is aging, particularly in developed countries, there is a growing interest in the physiologic processes of aging, and age-related problems are being identified and studied. At the beginning of the twentieth century, the age expectancy varied between 30 years worldwide and 50 years in developed countries. Today, these numbers have risen to 67 and 78, respectively, and are expected to continue to rise [1]. Indeed, by 2030, one in five persons in the United States will be older than 65 years of age [2].

Understanding the processes of skin wound healing in this aging population, as well as defining the differences and characteristics of it, is essential for multiple reasons. For one, traumatic injuries are common in this age group. They even are the fifth leading cause of death of people over the age of 65 in the USA. [3]. In addition, over the last 20 years, the number of elderly people undergoing surgeries has increased, and these people are at risk of wound-healing complications [4]. Besides, chronic wounds affect an estimated seven million patients annually in the United States. Most common chronic wounds are pressure ulcers, venous leg ulcers, diabetic foot ulcers, and arterial ulcers [5]. All medical conditions associated with chronic wounds and ulcers are more frequent in the aging population including venous and arterial insufficiency, neuropathies, diabetes mellitus, and chronic pressure in long-term hospitalizations [5]. Direct and indirect medical costs of skin ulcers and wounds were estimated at nearly 12 billion USD in 2004, which makes them the most burdensome skin condition in the United States [6].

Aging is a complex process that is governed by both intrinsic and extrinsic factors. These factors combine to ultimately lead to a loss of structural and morphological functions. Intrinsic aging can usually be appreciated in sun-protected areas of the body. It is the result of the same aging conditions that affect other body organs and varies between different individuals and different body sites within the same individual [7]. On the other hand, extrinsic factors can play a major role in worsening or hastening the process of cutaneous aging. They are contributors that can be controlled to some degree and include sun exposure, pollution, smoking, and others. The most important of them is UV radiation that results from exposure to the sun, a process known as photoaging [8]. These factors will be discussed in further details at a later point.

As a result of both these intrinsic and extrinsic factors, many age-related changes develop in the normal skin of healthy older individuals. These include changes in practically all the components of the skin, leading to a progressive decline in morphologic and physiologic properties. Consequently, many of the skin functions are altered with age from skin permeability to angiogenesis, immune functions, and wound healing.

Skin wound healing is a complex and well-orchestrated process schematically divided into three consecutive phases of inflammation, proliferation, and remodeling [9]. It involves molecular and cellular processes like hemostasis, inflammation, angiogenesis, cell proliferation and migration, apoptosis, extracellular matrix deposition, and remodeling. Changes in any of these steps and processes can induce a delay of wound healing. Over the last century, studies have demonstrated that wounds of older individuals do not heal as well as those of their younger counterpart [10, 11]. Recent studies are shedding light on the mechanisms through which aging affects wound healing whether through changes that develop in the inflammatory response, the extracellular matrix, or angiogenesis [12].

Characteristics of the Aging Skin

Aging can be defined as what happens to an organism over time. Intrinsic aging, which is the normal or expected aging, is primarily driven by genetics and hormonal status [13, 14].

Genetic differences in aging are mostly seen in people from different ethnicities, with people having darker complexion being more protected from the cumulative effects of photoaging [15, 16]. This reflects in different signs of photoaging. While fairly colored people show atrophic skin changes with fine wrinkles, dark colored people show hypertrophic changes such as deep wrinkles, coarseness, and leathery appearance [16]. The other major intrinsic factor that contributes to skin aging is hormonal changes or changes in the endocrine environment [7]. The relative hypoestrogenism that occurs after menopause has a detrimental effect on skin aging. Indeed, estrogens increase collagen content and skin thickness and maintain skin moisture, thus influencing many skin functions and playing a role in cutaneous wound healing [17, 18]. Studies have shown that estrogen has the ability to improve wound healing in postmenopausal women [17, 18].

Alternatively, when it comes to extrinsic aging, UV radiation has, without contest, the biggest influence on skin senescence. Photoaging is defined as the superposition of solar damage on the intrinsic aging process. In fair skinned individuals, the majority of visible skin aging is a result of sun exposure. This is induced by several processes. For instance, UV radiation leads to the upregulation of metalloproteinases and the subsequent degradation of multiple components of the extracellular matrix such as collagen and elastin. Eventually, these changes become visible in the form of wrinkles and sagging skin [16]. Photoaging considerably accelerates the rate of intrinsic aging. As such, it is almost inevitable to find some degree of clinical skin damage in exposed areas in Caucasian Western individuals by 15 years of age, whereas these same changes will only become present in non-exposed areas in the early 30s. Other extrinsic factors that have been cited to affect aging include smoking and lifestyle influence. Cigarette smoking is strongly associated with elastolysis [19]. An obvious dose-response relationship between wrinkling and smoking had been observed [20].

Before dwelling into the different phases of wound healing and how they are altered in the elderly population, the age-related changes that occur in the skin must be examined. These changes are the culprit for the differences seen in wound healing between different age groups. The skin is a multilayered organ composed of the epidermis, dermis, and subcutaneous tissue from outermost to innermost. With age, morphological and functional changes can be seen in each of these compartments.

The epidermis is mostly composed of keratinocytes (squamous epithelial cells) maturing through stratified layers to ultimately ensure a barrier to water entry and preventing water loss. The keratinocytes are continuously replenished through actively dividing cells in the basal layer. With age, the thickness of the epidermis does not change significantly. However, flattening of the rete ridges at the dermal-epidermal junction is observed, which gives an atrophic appearance to this compartment. The flattening decreases the surface of contact between the epidermis and dermis and predisposes elderly people to a separation of the dermal-epidermal junction with latterly applied tension [21]. In addition, the progenitor cells of the basal layer show a decreased mitotic activity and increased duration of the cell cycle and migration time with age [22]. This delay in the migration of keratinocytes, a key process in skin healing, results in an expected delay of wound healing. Other cells such as melanocytes and Langerhans cells are present in the epidermis, albeit in a much lesser number than the epidermal squamous cells. A decrease in the number of melanocytes will cause graying of the hair. The Langerhans cells are antigen-presenting cells. They also display an age-related decline in their number and function with an ensuing diminished cutaneous immune function [12].

The second layer of the skin, or dermis, is composed of multiple types of cells and structures that are embedded in an extracellular matrix (ECM). It is subdivided into the upper papillary dermis and the deep reticular dermis. There is a decrease in the cellular components of the dermis with age, namely fibroblasts, mast cells, and macrophages. The extracellular matrix also shows several changes as visible by its generalized atrophy [21]. Consequently, the skin loses from its strength and resiliency. The most important components of the ECM are collagen, elastin, and fibronectin. As a result of decreased production and increased degradation, these proteins, and primarily collagen, are diminished with age [23]. Even the quality of the remaining collagen is altered, with the remaining collagen being less organized than that seen in younger dermis. Although there is also a decrease in the elastic fibers numbers and diameters in the upper layer of the dermis, the reticular dermis exhibits opposite findings [24]. The quantity of elastin, thus, remains relatively constant with age. However, similarly to collagen, it shows a distorted morphology that leads to decreased skin elasticity [24].

Another major age-related change that occurs in the skin is the reduction of the cutaneous vasculature that can reach up to a 40 % decrease by the age of 70 years [25]. The dermis loses with it some of its ability to adapt to injury. As dermal lymphatic drainage shows a parallel decrease, the skin is less capable of clearing pathogens and wound contraction diminishes [26].

Even dermal appendages are affected by the aging process. A decrease of hair follicles number, sweat glands, and sebaceous glands can be observed [27, 28].

Phases of Normal Cutaneous Wound Healing

Cutaneous healing has been traditionally divided into a series of four overlapping phases. Although the process by itself is a continuum, this division is useful to understand all the elements that come into play for a wound to properly heal. The first phase is hemostasis. It starts within seconds after an injury and represent the blood vessels attempt to stop bleeding. The vessels contract and the injury to the endothelial lining of a blood vessel will expose the normally hidden collagen and basement membrane. These molecules elicit the clotting cascade, leading to the formation of the thrombi clot. In parallel, exposed elements such as collagen and von Willebrand factor activate platelets, leading to their aggregation [29]. As the platelets adhere to the endothelial cells, they release many pro-inflammatory factors including platelet-derived growth factor (PDGF), vascular epidermal growth factors (VEGF), transforming growth factor (TGF)-β, and TGF-α. These chemokines will attract the cells of the inflammatory phase [30]. As such, the hemostasis phase serves not only in stopping any bleeding that incur from an injury but also has an important role in bringing forth the second step of healing. The inflammatory phase of healing is characterized by the sequential infiltration of the wound by neutrophils, macrophages, and lymphocytes. Neutrophils number peak at 24 h post injury. They function in cleaning the wound by phagocyting microbial agents that have infiltrated the injured site as well as damaged tissue debris. Although neutrophils are the first inflammatory cells to reach the site, it seems that the most important inflammatory cells in wound healing are the macrophages. Within 24–48 h after the trauma, monocytes will move into the wound and transform into macrophages. These cells carry many important functions. Firstly, they remove debris and apoptotic cells, leaving a clean wound bed where the proliferative cells can introduce a new matrix and angiogenesis can develop at a later stage. They are also important in controlling the inflammation and produce factors that recruit and activate other cells that are involved in the repair process [31]. Wound-associated macrophages stimulate keratinocytes, angiogenesis, and synthesis of extracellular matrix, thus promoting tissue regeneration [31]. The last cells to enter the wound, more than 3 days after the initiation of healing, are the lymphocytes. Although their role has not been fully elucidated yet, they might function through their secretion of cytokines or by interacting with other cells such as macrophages, keratinocytes, and fibroblasts [32]. Seventy two hours after the injury, the proliferation stage starts. It aims at replacing the tissue that has been destroyed and degraded, lasting for approximately 14 days. The fibrin matrix is replaced by granulation tissue and capillary growth occurs. Keratinocytes will proliferate and migrate to re-epithelialize the wound. Stem cells present in the basal cell layer of the epidermis and the hair follicle bulge aid in the re-epithelialization process [33]. Concomitantly, secreted cytokines such as PDGF, fibroblast growth factors, and TGF-β will induce proliferation of fibroblasts. In the dermis, a preliminary extracellular matrix is laid down by these cells that actively synthesize type I and type III collagen, proteoglycans, and glycosaminoglycans. As these events are taking place, new vessels develop in the response to the hypoxic milieu. A dense network of capillary is established and provides oxygen and nutrients to the cells in the wound bed. Eventually, some fibroblasts will differentiate into myofibroblasts, as the granulation tissue is formed. The myofibroblasts are very important for the subsequent wound contraction and remodeling of the newly formed matrix. The final stage of healing, remodeling, or resolution starts approximately at day 8 and is a long process that can persist for up to a year or longer. It is essential to restore tissue functionality and optimize the wound strength. In order to best acquire normal tissue architecture, the previously laid ECM is continuously broken down and synthesized. As the new collagen is deposited, less and less type III collagen is formed. Alternatively, the fraction of the stronger collagen type I increases. As these more resilient larger collagen bundles are formed, the wound acquires more tensile strength without regaining more than 80 % of its pre-injury strength. The dense blood vessel network regresses, leaving place to a normal capillary network [9, 30, 34]. The four stages described above have been shown to display multiple characteristic age-related changes. Although cutaneous healing is not defective, a definite delay has been reported in the healing process of people who are older than 65 years of age.

Age-Related Changes in Hemostasis and Inflammation

The first phase of healing culminates in the formation of a thrombi clot, a platelet plug, and the secretion of cytokines that attract inflammatory cells to the site of the injury. This phase seems to be boosted in the elderly as platelet adherence to the exposed collagen is enhanced. In addition, their release of PDGF, TGF-β, and TGF-α is increased [35]. In addition to the changes witnessed in the function of platelets, the clotting cascade shows age-related alterations. Studies have shown an elevated concentration of activated clotting factors such as d-dimers and inhibitors of clot-dissolving enzymes (plasminogen activator inhibitor-1). In addition, some coagulation inhibitors, namely, antithrombin III and activated protein C, show a decrease in their activity [36–39].

In contrast, there are conflicting conclusions regarding the age-related changes of the inflammatory phase. Some aspects of this phase are impaired, while others were shown to be enhanced in elderly. Inflammatory cells are recruited to the site of injury by the cytokines that have been secreted, starting with neutrophils within the first few hours and followed by monocytes/macrophages. As the inflammatory cells reach blood vessels adjacent to the injured area, they have to start by adhering to the endothelial cell lining before moving into the dermis. The process is governed by adhesion molecules on the immune cells as well as on the blood vessel lining. The expression of these molecules is altered in the elderly, probably affecting the early inflammatory response [40]. It has been shown that there is an increased early influx of neutrophils but a delay in the influx of monocytes with a relative increase in the number of mature macrophages in aged individuals as opposed to young controls. Lymphocytes infiltration into the wound seems also to be delayed as suggested by studies on middle-aged and elderly mice [40]. Moreover, studies showed that the function of neutrophils that were isolated from elderly people is defective in multiple areas, including their chemotactic ability, phagocytosis, and respiratory burst [41–43]. Indeed, in mouse models of wound infection, aged mice show decreased neutrophil chemotaxis and delayed infection clearance compared to young mice, thus affecting the dynamics of the inflammatory response in wound healing [44]. Macrophages play a key role in this process and changes in their function are thought to be crucial for age-related changes. Depletion of macrophage causes important defects in cutaneous healing. Indeed, delayed wound closure, decreased granulation tissue and angiogenesis, less collagen and cytokine production, and a lower number of myofibroblasts have been demonstrated upon selective depletion of macrophages in a study by Mirza et al. [45]. The pivotal role of macrophages was further demonstrated in an experiment on mice, where the healing of elderly mice was accelerated upon the injection of macrophages collected from young mice. The same was not noted after the injection of macrophages harvested from old mice [46]. Findings over the last few years suggest that there might be an age-related decline in the function of macrophages. Elderly macrophages have diminished chemotaxis and growth factors production abilities. In addition, a smaller percentage of these macrophages is able to phagocytose potential targets and still shows diminished functions of phagocytosis. Elderly macrophages were found to be able to ingest fewer particles than their counterpart isolated from younger animals [47, 48]. However, the mechanisms behind this functional deficit are not yet understood even though multiple defects were found in macrophages collected from elderly subjects. For instance, multiple transduction pathways in macrophages, such as MAP kinases ERK, p38, and JNK, were found to be negatively altered [49]. In addition, some macrophage receptors required for the cell's activation and recognition are less expressed with age [50]. Importantly, the Fcγ receptor, crucial for phagocytosis, is not affected by these changes [47, 51]. The effects of the alterations in the function of macrophages in the aged subject can be potentially detrimental even though many studies are still needed to further characterize and establish their role in changes seen with healing. This is because macrophages play a role that goes beyond the inflammatory phase of healing. Lucas et al. provided evidence to their different functions during different phases of repair [31]. During the inflammatory phase, the macrophages recruited to the site control major steps of the repair process from granulation tissue formation to re-epithelialization to angiogenesis. On the other hand, during the proliferative phase, an absence of macrophages causes hemorrhage and curbed tissue maturation.

Age-Related Changes in Proliferation

The proliferation phase is characterized by the restoration of the missing tissue in the epidermis through re-epithelialization and in the dermis via the formation of granulation tissue as well as through angiogenesis. Keratinocytes, fibroblasts, and endothelial cells are recruited, respectively, for each of these processes. All these cells show age-related changes, and subsequently, the above repair steps are disrupted and delayed in the elderly. As proliferation and migration are diminished and there is a reduced production of cytokines and response to growth factors, wound healing is delayed. Decreased angiogenesis as well as ECM deposition is also noted and contributes to this phenomenon [35]. The defects in wound re-epithelialization in elderly stem from multiple interlinked factors. Charruyer et al. have shown that although epidermal stem cell kinetics are maintained in aged epidermis, the kinetics of the transit-amplifying (TA) cells were altered [22]. They show that there is an increase in the numbers of TA cells due to a decrease in their proliferation rate and their differentiation, which might be needed to maintain the epidermal barrier functions in the elderly but, on the other hand, might explain the delay in cutaneous re-epithelialization [22]. Other studies have shown that keratinocytes exhibit a decreased proliferative ability with age [52, 53] and even a decreased turnover rate in normal, non-injured skin [54]. On top of their decreased proliferation, migration of keratinocytes is altered in aged skin. This may be due to an impaired responsiveness to hypoxia by the aged skin. Hypoxia develops in a wound as a result of disruption to the vasculature. In healthy young subjects, hypoxia induces the production of cytokines and growth factors that are important for repair and promote cell migration, proliferation, and angiogenesis. Older individuals show a reduced hypoxia inducible factor (HIF)-α signaling, resulting in a reduced stromal-derived factor-1 expression [55]. As hypoxia is an important stimulus for keratinocytes migration, the impaired response in the elderly was associated with a diminished migration [56]. Matrix metalloproteinase production is also disrupted when the response to hypoxia is abnormal. MMP-1 and MMP-9 are required for keratinocytes to be able to migrate without disruption. In elderly donors, these enzymes are not induced by hypoxia while it was found to be upregulated in cells of wound donors [56, 57].

Fibroblasts are the major proliferative cells in the dermis and are crucial for the production of a new matrix. In the dermis, fibroblasts decrease in number and size with age. Their life span has also been shown to decrease with age in some studies [58]. In addition, aged fibroblasts lose the ability to respond optimally to growth factors and to replicate efficiently [59, 60]. Senescent fibroblasts have a decreased responsiveness to a large number of cytokines and cell-signaling molecules and may become desensitized to many stimuli with age. Their mitogenic response to factors such as platelet-derived growth factors, epidermal growth factors, insulin, and other molecules is depressed [61]. Other studies have shown that fibroblasts of aged rats have decreased proliferation and migration deficits that are independent of chemotaxis. Fibronectin that is laid during previous phases of inflammation is a very important scaffold for the migration of fibroblasts. This type of migration is also depressed in aged fibroblasts [51, 62–64]. A possible explanation stems from the loss of responsiveness to hypoxia that leads to a depressed migratory activity. In parallel, obvious differences were found in the receptor expressions between dermal fibroblasts isolated from young adults as opposed to those isolated from old adults. Such findings involved epidermal growth factor receptors (EGFR) in regard to their number, affinity, and ratio of internalization, as well as insulin receptor numbers [65]. Other affected receptors include TGF- β type I and type II receptors which are decreased in hypoxic environments in aged fibroblasts, while still normal in a normoxic milieu [66].

On top of their decreased migration and proliferation rate, aged fibroblasts were shown to have decreased abilities to produce cytokines as well as some components of the extracellular matrix. Many fibroblast growth factors were found to be decreased in many studies [47, 67]. Measuring hydroxyproline content, it was shown that the rate of collagen production is also decreased with age [68]. The decreased production mainly expresses itself through a decreased deposit of type I collagen [57, 69]. However, even though the rate of collagen synthesis is delayed, the ultimate composition of collagen in the wound is similar in both young and old animals [48].

Age-Related Changes in Angiogenesis

Cutaneous vasculature displays age-related alteration with both types of aging. Both a decrease in the density of the cutaneous blood vessels as well as their size occurs, and a reduction in the surface area available for exchange has been described. Moreover, angiogenesis during wound healing is altered in older people [70]. Hypoxia is a well-known inducer of angiogenesis. Given that the response to hypoxia is altered in the elderly as described previously, it is expected to see an associated impairment in angiogenesis. The reduced levels of HIF-1α-dependent stromal-derived factor-1 expression were found to correlate with a depressed density of new vessels [55]. VEGF, one of the most important angiogenesis stimulators, was also found to be decreased with depressed HIF-1α signaling [48]. Furthermore, depression of this hypoxia pathway leads to an impaired mobilization and homing of bone marrow-derived angiogenic cells [71, 72].

Age-Related Changes in Remodeling

The last phase of wound healing aims at molding the new deposited tissue to become the closest possible to normal tissue architecture. Continuous collagen degradation and new synthesis occurs while the collagen structure matures. Unfortunately, few data are currently available on the age-associated changes of this phase. Studies have shown that collagen degradation appears to be increased in the older age group. Indeed, MMP-2 and MMP-9 were found to be upregulated in the wound of healthy older subjects, while the MMP inhibitors were downregulated, hence enhancing the breakdown of collagen [35]. As the balance between breakdown and synthesis tilts toward the degradation of collagen, a decreased collagen deposition is noted. This is further exacerbated because of the decreased levels of TGF- β1, which is known to promote the synthesis of collagen while suppressing its degradation. Finally, a study by Reed et al. suggested that there is an age-related defect in collagen remodeling and that old mice displayed less organized mature collagen [36].

As the ultimate result of remodeling is a durable dermis, many studies examine the final strength of a wound as a mean to evaluable the last step of repair. This will allow to indirectly assess collagen content and cross-linking of the new ECM, as the tensile strength of a tissue does not only correlate with the amount of collagen but also with the extent of cross-linking and the total architecture. Collagen cross-linking is carried through one of two methods. The first is through enzymatic posttranslational modifications via lysyl oxidase (LOX) that allows the formation of specific cross-linking [73]. The second mechanism is a nonspecific one that occurs secondary to chemical modifications [74]. Both of these mechanisms have been reported to be altered in aged tissue. A decrease in the activity of LOX was described in the skin of old monkeys [75]. Alternatively, and while specific cross-linking is depressed, the nonspecific chemical and glycosylation cross-links increase [73]. These changes possibly explain the stiffer extracellular matrix and coarser collagen found in elderly skin. Studies on abdominal and cutaneous wounds have shown that older patients and animals tend to gain strength slower and end up with less tensile strength than young counterparts [76, 77]. Similarly, in humans, patients older than 70 years displayed a lower tensile strength in their incisional wounds when compared to patients younger than 70 years [78]. Interestingly, and maybe in contradiction with previous available data, a recent observational study examining the maturation of human scars noted that the best maturation rate was seen in older subjects. This may point out that even though there is a delay in the early phases of healing in the elderly, the wound has the potential to mature faster and result in a better quality of scars if the healing is done under optimal conditions as was the case in the conducted study [79].

Conclusion

With the aging of the populations and the increasing prevalence of wound-associated morbidities, it becomes more and more important to understand the pathophysiological processes governing skin wound healing in the elderly. Several studies point out to defects in the cellular and molecular components intervening in the different phases of skin wound healing, including the kinetics of epidermal progenitor cells, the inflammatory cells, mainly macrophages, angiogenesis, and the fibroblasts. Nevertheless, our understanding of the mechanisms of age-related changes observed in these processes is still shallow and more cooperative and collaborative research is needed in the future to uncover the basics in order to prevent and treat wound-healing alterations in the elderly.

References

1. Cheung C. Older adults and ulcers: chronic wounds in the geriatric population. Adv Skin Wound Care. 2010;23(1):39–44. quiz 45–6.
2. Prevention C.f.D.C.a. The State of aging and health in America 2013. 2013.
3. McMahon DJ, Schwab CW, Kauder D. Comorbidity and the elderly trauma patient. World J Surg. 1996;20 (8):1113–9. discussion 1119–20.
4. Etzioni DA, et al. The aging population and its impact on the surgery workforce. Ann Surg. 2003;238(2):170–7.
5. Kirsner RS, Vivas AC. Lower-extremity ulcers: diagnosis and management. Br J Dermatol. 2015 Aug;173 (2):379–90.
6. Bickers DR, et al. The burden of skin diseases: 2004 a joint project of the American Academy of Dermatology Association and the Society for Investigative Dermatology. J Am Acad Dermatol. 2006;55(3):490–500.
7. Farage MA, et al. Intrinsic and extrinsic factors in skin ageing: a review. Int J Cosmet Sci. 2008;30(2):87–95.
8. Fisher GJ, et al. Pathophysiology of premature skin aging induced by ultraviolet light. N Engl J Med. 1997;337(20):1419–28.
9. Singer AJ, Clark RA. Cutaneous wound healing. N Engl J Med. 1999;341(10):738–46.
10. Du Nouy PL. Cicatrization of wounds: Iii. The relation between the age of the patient, the area of the wound, and the index of cicatrization. J Exp Med. 1916;24 (5):461–70.
11. Quirinia A, Viidik A. The influence of age on the healing of normal and ischemic incisional skin wounds. Mech Ageing Dev. 1991;58(2–3):221–32.
12. Gosain A, DiPietro LA. Aging and wound healing. World J Surg. 2004;28(3):321–6.
13. Kohl E, et al. Skin ageing. J Eur Acad Dermatol Venereol. 2011;25(8):873–84.
14. Farage MA, et al. Characteristics of the aging skin. Adv Wound Care (New Rochelle). 2013;2(1):5–10.
15. Rees JL. The genetics of sun sensitivity in humans. Am J Hum Genet. 2004;75(5):739–51.
16. Yaar M, Gilchrest BA. Photoaging: mechanism, prevention and therapy. Br J Dermatol. 2007;157 (5):874–87.
17. Gilliver SC, Ashworth JJ, Ashcroft GS. The hormonal regulation of cutaneous wound healing. Clin Dermatol. 2007;25(1):56–62.
18. Verdier-Sevrain S, Bonte F, Gilchrest B. Biology of estrogens in skin: implications for skin aging. Exp Dermatol. 2006;15(2):83–94.
19. Leow YH, Maibach HI. Cigarette smoking, cutaneous vasculature, and tissue oxygen. Clin Dermatol. 1998;16(5):579–84.

20. Kennedy C, et al. Effect of smoking and sun on the aging skin. J Invest Dermatol. 2003;120(4):548–54.
21. Kurban RS, Bhawan J. Histologic changes in skin associated with aging. J Dermatol Surg Oncol. 1990;16(10):908–14.
22. Charruyer A, et al. Transit-amplifying cell frequency and cell cycle kinetics are altered in aged epidermis. J Invest Dermatol. 2009;129(11):2574–83.
23. Bernstein EF, et al. Long-term sun exposure alters the collagen of the papillary dermis. Comparison of sun-protected and photoaged skin by northern analysis, immunohistochemical staining, and confocal laser scanning microscopy. J Am Acad Dermatol. 1996;34 (2 Pt 1):209–18.
24. Lavker RM, Zheng PS, Dong G. Aged skin: a study by light, transmission electron, and scanning electron microscopy. J Invest Dermatol. 1987;88 (3 Suppl):44s–51.
25. Tsuchida Y. The effect of aging and arteriosclerosis on human skin blood flow. J Dermatol Sci. 1993;5 (3):175–81.
26. Gniadecka M, Serup J, Sondergaard J. Age-related diurnal changes of dermal oedema: evaluation by high-frequency ultrasound. Br J Dermatol. 1994;131 (6):849–55.
27. Montagna W, Carlisle K. Structural changes in ageing skin. Br J Dermatol. 1990;122 Suppl 35:61–70.
28. Pochi PE, Strauss JS, Downing DT. Age-related changes in sebaceous gland activity. J Invest Dermatol. 1979;73(1):108–11.
29. Davi G, Patrono C. Platelet activation and atherothrombosis. N Engl J Med. 2007;357 (24):2482–94.
30. Shaw TJ, Martin P. Wound repair at a glance. J Cell Sci. 2009;122(Pt 18):3209–13.
31. Lucas T, et al. Differential roles of macrophages in diverse phases of skin repair. J Immunol. 2010;184 (7):3964–77.
32. Eming SA, Krieg T, Davidson JM. Inflammation in wound repair: molecular and cellular mechanisms. J Invest Dermatol. 2007;127(3):514–25.
33. Blanpain C, Fuchs E. Stem cell plasticity. Plasticity of epithelial stem cells in tissue regeneration. Science. 2014;344(6189):1242281.
34. Gurtner GC, et al. Wound repair and regeneration. Nature. 2008;453(7193):314–21.
35. Ashcroft GS, Mills SJ, Ashworth JJ. Ageing and wound healing. Biogerontology. 2002;3(6):337–45.
36. Reed MJ, et al. Age-related differences in repair of dermal wounds and myocardial infarcts attenuate during the later stages of healing. In Vivo. 2006;20(6B):801–6.
37. Bauer KA, et al. Aging-associated changes in indices of thrombin generation and protein C activation in humans. Normative aging study. J Clin Invest. 1987;80(6):1527–34.
38. Hager K, et al. Blood coagulation factors in the elderly. Arch Gerontol Geriatr. 1989;9(3):277–82.
39. Pieper CF, et al. Age, functional status, and racial differences in plasma D-dimer levels in community-dwelling elderly persons. J Gerontol A Biol Sci Med Sci. 2000;55(11):M649–57.
40. Ashcroft GS, Horan MA, Ferguson MW. Aging alters the inflammatory and endothelial cell adhesion molecule profiles during human cutaneous wound healing. Lab Invest. 1998;78(1):47–58.
41. Butcher SK, et al. Senescence in innate immune responses: reduced neutrophil phagocytic capacity and CD16 expression in elderly humans. J Leukoc Biol. 2001;70(6):881–6.
42. Di Lorenzo G, et al. Granulocyte and natural killer activity in the elderly. Mech Ageing Dev. 1999;108 (1):25–38.
43. Fortin CF, et al. Impairment of SHP-1 down-regulation in the lipid rafts of human neutrophils under GM-CSF stimulation contributes to their age-related, altered functions. J Leukoc Biol. 2006;79(5):1061–72.
44. Brubaker AL, et al. Reduced neutrophil chemotaxis and infiltration contributes to delayed resolution of cutaneous wound infection with advanced age. J Immunol. 2013;190(4):1746–57.
45. Mirza R, DiPietro LA, Koh TJ. Selective and specific macrophage ablation is detrimental to wound healing in mice. Am J Pathol. 2009;175(6):2454–62.
46. Danon D, Kowatch MA, Roth GS. Promotion of wound repair in old mice by local injection of macrophages. Proc Natl Acad Sci U S A. 1989;86 (6):2018–20.
47. Swift ME, et al. Age-related alterations in the inflammatory response to dermal injury. J Invest Dermatol. 2001;117(5):1027–35.
48. Swift ME, Kleinman HK, DiPietro LA. Impaired wound repair and delayed angiogenesis in aged mice. Lab Invest. 1999;79(12):1479–87.
49. Gomez CR, et al. Innate immunity and aging. Exp Gerontol. 2008;43(8):718–28.
50. Herrero C, et al. Immunosenescence of macrophages: reduced MHC class II gene expression. Exp Gerontol. 2002;37(2–3):389–94.
51. Ashcroft GS, Horan MA, Ferguson MW. The effects of ageing on cutaneous wound healing in mammals. J Anat. 1995;187(Pt 1):1–26.
52. Gilchrest BA. In vitro assessment of keratinocyte aging. J Invest Dermatol. 1983;81(1 Suppl):184s–9.
53. Rheinwald JG, Green H. Serial cultivation of strains of human epidermal keratinocytes: the formation of keratinizing colonies from single cells. Cell. 1975;6 (3):331–43.
54. Morris GM, Hamlet R, Hopewell JW. The cell kinetics of the epidermis and follicular epithelium of the rat: variations with age and body site. Cell Tissue Kinet. 1989;22(3):213–22.
55. Loh SA, et al. SDF-1 alpha expression during wound healing in the aged is HIF dependent. Plast Reconstr Surg. 2009;123(2 Suppl):65S–75.
56. Xia YP, et al. Differential activation of migration by hypoxia in keratinocytes isolated from donors of increasing age: implication for chronic wounds in the elderly. J Invest Dermatol. 2001;116(1):50–6.

57. Salo T, et al. Expression of matrix metalloproteinase-2 and -9 during early human wound healing. Lab Invest. 1994;70(2):176–82.
58. Schneider EL. Aging and cultured human skin fibroblasts. J Invest Dermatol. 1979;73(1):15–8.
59. Plisko A, Gilchrest BA. Growth factor responsiveness of cultured human fibroblasts declines with age. J Gerontol. 1983;38(5):513–8.
60. West MD. The cellular and molecular biology of skin aging. Arch Dermatol. 1994;130(1):87–95.
61. Phillips PD, Kaji K, Cristofalo VJ. Progressive loss of the proliferative response of senescing WI-38 cells to platelet-derived growth factor, epidermal growth factor, insulin, transferrin, and dexamethasone. J Gerontol. 1984;39(1):11–7.
62. Ashcroft GS, Horan MA, Ferguson MW. Aging is associated with reduced deposition of specific extracellular matrix components, an upregulation of angiogenesis, and an altered inflammatory response in a murine incisional wound healing model. J Invest Dermatol. 1997;108(4):430–7.
63. Albini A, et al. Decline of fibroblast chemotaxis with age of donor and cell passage number. Coll Relat Res. 1988;8(1):23–37.
64. Pienta KJ, Coffey DS. Characterization of the subtypes of cell motility in ageing human skin fibroblasts. Mech Ageing Dev. 1990;56(2):99–105.
65. Reenstra WR, Yaar M, Gilchrest BA. Effect of donor age on epidermal growth factor processing in man. Exp Cell Res. 1993;209(1):118–22.
66. Mogford JE, et al. Effect of age and hypoxia on TGFbeta1 receptor expression and signal transduction in human dermal fibroblasts: impact on cell migration. J Cell Physiol. 2002;190(2):259–65.
67. Komi-Kuramochi A, et al. Expression of fibroblast growth factors and their receptors during full-thickness skin wound healing in young and aged mice. J Endocrinol. 2005;186(2):273–89.
68. Viljanto J. A sponge implantation method for testing connective tissue regeneration in surgical patients. Acta Chir Scand. 1969;135(4):297–300.
69. Puolakkainen PA, et al. The enhancement in wound healing by transforming growth factor-beta 1 (TGF-beta 1) depends on the topical delivery system. J Surg Res. 1995;58(3):321–9.
70. Chung JH, et al. Differential effects of photoaging vs intrinsic aging on the vascularization of human skin. Arch Dermatol. 2002;138(11):1437–42.
71. Chang EI, et al. Age decreases endothelial progenitor cell recruitment through decreases in hypoxia-inducible factor 1alpha stabilization during ischemia. Circulation. 2007;116(24):2818–29.
72. Zhang X, et al. Aging impairs the mobilization and homing of bone marrow-derived angiogenic cells to burn wounds. J Mol Med (Berl). 2011;89(10):985–95.
73. Szauter KM, et al. Lysyl oxidase in development, aging and pathologies of the skin. Pathol Biol (Paris). 2005;53(7):448–56.
74. Au V, Madison SA. Effects of singlet oxygen on the extracellular matrix protein collagen: oxidation of the collagen crosslink histidinohydroxylysinonorleucine and histidine. Arch Biochem Biophys. 2000;384(1):133–42.
75. Reiser KM, Hennessy SM, Last JA. Analysis of age-associated changes in collagen crosslinking in the skin and lung in monkeys and rats. Biochim Biophys Acta. 1987;926(3):339–48.
76. Mendoza Jr CB, Postlethwait RW, Johnson WD. Veterans administration cooperative study of surgery for duodenal ulcer. II. Incidence of wound disruption following operation. Arch Surg. 1970;101(3):396–8.
77. Sussman MD. Aging of connective tissue: physical properties of healing wounds in young and old rats. Am J Physiol. 1973;224(5):1167–71.
78. Sandblom P, Petersen P, Muren A. Determination of the tensile strength of the healing wound as a clinical test. Acta Chir Scand. 1953;105(1–4):252–7.
79. Bond JS, et al. Maturation of the human scar: an observational study. Plast Reconstr Surg. 2008;121(5):1650–8.

Antiaging Effects of Algae-Derived Mycosporine-Like Amino Acids (MAAs) on Skin

144

Jeong Hun Lee, Hyeong-Sik Kim, Hyo Hyun Seo, Mi Young Song, Atul Kulkarni, Yun-Hee Choi, Ki Woo Kim, and Sang Hyun Moh

Contents

J.H. Lee • H.H. Seo • M.Y. Song • S.H. Moh (✉)
Anti-aging Research Institute of BIO-FD&C Co. Ltd., Incheon, Republic of Korea
e-mail: jhlee@biofdnc.com; hhseo@biofdnc.com; mysong@biofdnc.com; shmoh@biofdnc.com; biofdnc@gmail.com

H.-S. Kim
Department of Dermatology, Kangbuk Samsung Hospital, Sungkyunkwan University College of Medicine, Seoul, South Korea
e-mail: hskim@biofdnc.com

A. Kulkarni
Anti-aging Research Institute of BIO-FD&C Co. Ltd., Incheon, Republic of Korea

School of Mechanical Engineering, Sungkyunkwan University, Suwon, South Korea
e-mail: atulkin@gmail.com

Y.-H. Choi
Anti-aging Research Institute of BIO-FD&C Co. Ltd., Incheon, Republic of Korea

Departments of Pharmacology and Global Medical Science, Wonju College of Medicine, Yonsei University, Wonju, Republic of Korea
e-mail: imyunhee@gmail.com

K.W. Kim
Departments of Pharmacology and Global Medical Science, Wonju College of Medicine, Yonsei University, Wonju, Republic of Korea

Institute of Lifestyle Medicine and Nuclear Receptor Research Consortium, Wonju College of Medicine, Yonsei University, Wonju, Republic of Korea
e-mail: kiwoo@yonsei.ac.kr

M.A. Farage et al. (eds.), *Textbook of Aging Skin*,
DOI 10.1007/978-3-662-47398-6_144

Abstract

Skin aging is a complex biological process that is a consequence of both intrinsic and extrinsic aging. Intrinsic aging refers to genetically programmed aging with time. Extrinsic aging is mainly caused by environmental factors such as ultraviolet damage, pollution, harsh weather, and cigarette smoke. Chronic sun exposure is one of the main causes of extrinsic skin aging and is responsible for age-related changes such as wrinkles, roughness, mottled hyperpigmentation, dilated blood vessels, and loss of skin tone. The substantial loss in the stratospheric ozone layer and consequent increment in solar ultraviolet (UV) radiation on the earth's surface have augmented the interest in searching for natural photoprotective compounds. Several photosynthetic marine organisms have evolved defense mechanisms to counteract UV radiation by synthesizing UV-absorbing compounds, such as mycosporine-like amino acids (MAAs). MAAs have been reported in diverse organisms; they are a family of secondary metabolites that directly or indirectly absorb the energy of solar radiation and protect organisms from enhanced solar UV radiation. MAAs have maximum UV absorption between 310 and 362 nm and high molar extinction coefficients. In addition, they have a capability to dissipate absorbed radiation as heat efficiently without producing reactive oxygen species (ROS). And also MAAs increase the photostability and resistance to several abiotic stressors. Several MAAs are introduced in this chapter and their functional roles were suggested for antiaging. Among them, we will discuss three specific MAAs, porphyra-334, shinorine, and mycosporine-glycine (M-Gly), on their antiaging effects comprising antioxidant, anti-inflammation, and skin-firming properties.

Introduction

It is well understood that aging of the skin is a complex process and is mainly associated with morphological and chemical changes which are contributed to chronological aging. In general aging is divided into extrinsic and intrinsic aging. Extrinsic aging is mainly due to UV irradiation from the sun, called photoaging. Intrinsic aging is caused by radical oxygen species such as $O_2^{-\cdot}$ and $OH^{-\cdot}$. The term "photoaging" was first introduced in 1986 and describes the effects of chronic UV light exposure on skin [1]. Unlike other organs, the skin is in direct contact with the environment and therefore undergoes aging as a consequence of environmental damage (Fig. 1). The primary environmental factor that causes human skin aging is UV irradiation from the sun. This photoaging is a cumulative process and depends primarily on the degree of sun exposure and skin pigment distribution. Individuals who have outdoor lifestyles, live in sunny climates, and are lightly pigmented will experience the greatest degree of photoaging. The clinical signs associated with photoaging include dyspigmentation, wrinkles, and malignancies

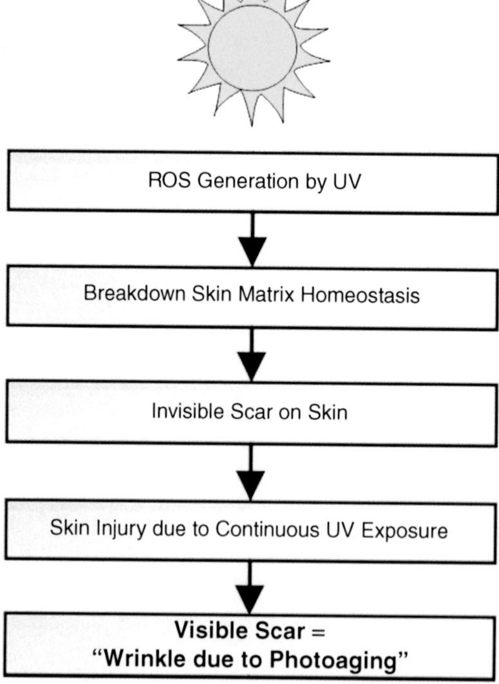

Fig. 1 Acute UV irradiation leads to generation of ROS. Repeated UV irradiation leads to accumulation of damage that results in visible solar scar or a wrinkle associated with photoaging

[2]. When skin is exposed to sunlight, UV radiation can generate harmful reactive oxygen species (ROS) in the skin, which then cause "oxidative damage" to cellular components like functional proteins, lipid membranes, RNA, and DNA. New insights regarding molecular mechanisms of photoaging might provide exciting opportunities for the development of new antiaging therapies, skin care products, and ingredients.

The ever-expanding market for skin care products and continual search for innovative ingredients have led to the development of a multitude of cosmetic products based on traditional marine sources, especially components derived from marine algae. Marine algae could be among the richest natural sources of known and novel bioactive compounds that can protect photoaging. Algal extracts can be used in cosmetics to decrease photodamage in two ways, as an excipient in the formulation (i.e., stabilizer or emulsifier) or as the therapeutic agent itself. There are growing interests in exploring bioactive materials that are beneficial for human life in marine organisms. Natural marine products have a variety of positive effects including anti-malaria, antituberculosis, anticancer, anti-inflammation, and antivirus, and diverse marine organisms such as cyanobacteria, macroalgae, and phytoplankton have been suggested for the effects [3]. In recent years, natural products from marine organisms have gained increasing research awareness, and a number of novel marine compounds of potential economic importance have been reported from different marine organisms [4–8].

During the past few decades, a substantial loss in the stratospheric ozone layer has been noticed that has aroused concern about the effects of increased solar ultraviolet radiation (UVR), particularly UV-B radiation (280–315 nm), on the earth's surface. Solar UV-B radiation is detrimental for most sun-exposed organisms, including humans [9, 10]. An increase in UV-B radiation has aroused interest in searching for the natural photoprotective compounds from various organisms such as microorganisms, plants, and animals of marine as well as freshwater ecosystems. A number of photoprotective compounds, such as melanins, mycosporines, mycosporine-like amino acids (MAAs), scytonemin, parietin, usnic acid, carotenoids, phycobiliproteins, phenylpropanoids, and flavonoids and several other UV-absorbing substances of unknown chemical structure, have been identified from different organisms [5, 11, 12].

Marine Photoprotective Compounds and MAAs

UVR is one of the most harmful exogenous agents and may affect a number of biological functions in all living organisms exposed to the sun. Solar radiation exposes the organisms to harmful doses of UV-B and UV-A (315–400 nm) in their natural habitats. In response to intense solar radiation, organisms have evolved certain mechanisms such as avoidance, repair, and protection by synthesizing or accumulating a series of photoprotective compounds, such as MAAs, scytonemin, carotenoids, and other compounds counteracting to the toxicity of UV (particularly UV-B) radiation [13, 14]. Among them, MAAs are known to be the most common compounds that have a potential role as UV sunscreens in marine organisms.

MAAs have been reported in diverse organisms; they are a family of secondary metabolites that directly or indirectly absorb the energy of solar radiation and protect organisms from enhanced solar UVR [7]. MAAs are intracellular, small (~400 Da), colorless, and water-soluble compounds that consist of cyclohexanone or cyclohexenimine chromophores conjugated with the nitrogen substituent of amino acids or its amino alcohol [14]. In general, MAAs have a glycine subunit at the third carbon atom, although some MAAs contain sulfate esters or glycosidic linkages through the imine substituents [15]. MAAs are favored as photoprotective compounds because they have maximum UV absorption between 310 and 362 nm, high molar extinction coefficients ($e = 28{,}100$–$50{,}000\ M^{-1}\ cm^{-1}$), the capability to dissipate absorbed radiation efficiently as heat without producing reactive oxygen species (ROS), and photostability and resistance to several abiotic stressors [16, 17].

High-performance liquid chromatography (HPLC) is the common method to detect the particular MAA using the distinctive nature of their retention times and absorption spectra. However, certain closely related unknown compounds have similar absorption maxima and retention times, which still cause difficulties in the identification process. Liquid chromatography coupled with electrospray ionization mass spectrometry (LC-ESI-MS) can be utilized to examine MAAs' structural diversity.

MAAs in Marine Cyanobacteria/Macroalgae/Microalgae

The accumulation of large amounts of MAAs in cyanobacteria was first reported by Shibata [18] from the Great Barrier Reef. Shinorine and porphyra-334 have been found to be the most dominant MAAs in several species of marine cyanobacteria [19]. MAA-producing cyanobacteria are abundant in hypersaline environments. Several species of macroalgae, belonging to Rhodophyceae (red), Phaeophyceae (brown), and Chlorophyceae (green), are commonly exposed to elevated solar radiation and synthesize and accumulate high concentrations of MAAs including porphyra-334, shinorine, and mycosporine-glycine (M-Gly). The structures of these MAAs with their absorption wavelength were depicted in Fig. 2. It has been reported that the imino-MAAs porphyra-334 and shinorine isolated from the red alga *Gracilaria cornea* were found to be highly stable against UV and heat stress. Zhaohui et al. in addition reported that the porphyra-334 from a marine alga was stable in water at a temperature of 60 °C [20]. MAAs have been reported to occur predominantly in members of the Dinophyceae, Bacillariophyceae, and Haptophyceae (or Prymnesiophyceae). Some species of dinoflagellates such as *Alexandrium excavatum* [21] and the prymnesiophyte *Phaeocystis pouchetii* are known to produce

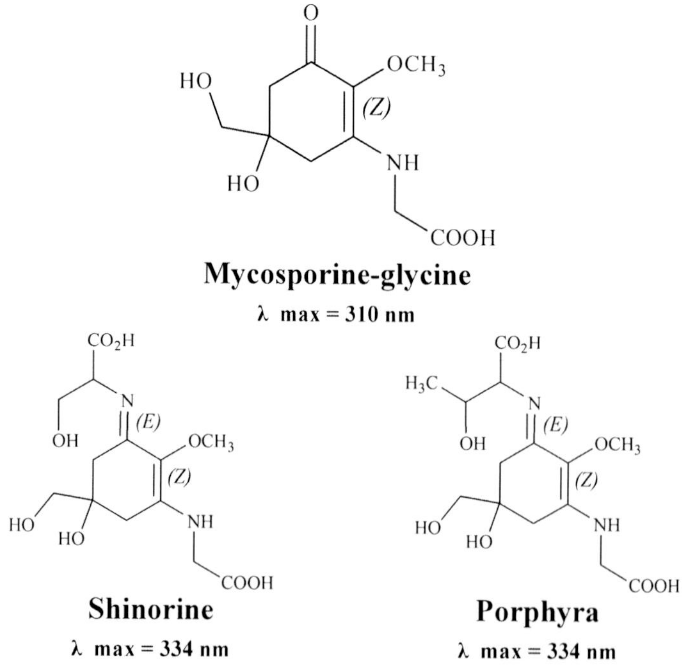

Fig. 2 Structures of MAAs; mycosporine-glycine, shinorine, and porphyra

MAAs in high concentrations. It has been suggested that accumulation of MAAs in marine organisms may be a result of alterations in amino acid synthesis induced by UV irradiation.

Antiaging Effects of MAAs

The observations of three MAAs (porphyra-334 (P334), shinorine (SH), and M-Gly) for their antiaging effects are described in Fig. 3 and described below.

Antioxidant Activity of MAAs

The 2,2-diphenyl-2-picrylhydrazyl (DPPH) is a stable radical source, and scavenging of DPPH is the basis of a common antioxidant assay [22]. Radical scavenging activity of M-Gly, a microalgae-derived MAA, was determined by DPPH assay. The radical scavenging activity of M-Gly was increased with proportion to its concentration up to 1.5 mM (Fig. 3a), suggesting that M-Gly may act as a strong antioxidant and prevent cellular damage by UV-induced free radicals. We in addition have examined antioxidant potentials for other MAAs including shinorine (SH) and P334, but there was no significant antioxidant activity of the MAAs in DPPH assay.

Anti-inflammation

We examined whether microalgae-derived MAAs had anti-inflammatory activity against UV irradiation. Immortalized human keratinocytes, HaCaT cells, were treated with MAAs plus UV irradiation. Real-time PCR was used to determine the mRNA levels of the COX-2 gene, a key player in the generation of inflammatory responses. The mRNA level of COX-2 was decreased by MAA treatment especially in M-Gly (Fig. 3b). However, P334 and SH had no effect on COX-2 expression at 0.3 mM concentration tested (Fig. 3b). It shows that M-Gly has inhibitory effect on UV-induced COX-2 expression and may blunt inflammatory responses caused by UV radiation.

Skin Firming

To evaluate the effects of MAAs on skin firming influenced by UV, we investigated the expression of procollagen C-endopeptidase enhancer (PCOLCE), elastin, and involucrin in cells with or without MAAs. Real-time PCR was used to determine the mRNA levels of PCOLCE, which binds to procollagen and enhances procollagen C-proteinase activity, and elastin, which is a major protein component of tissues that require elasticity in skin, and involucrin, which contributes to the formation of a cell envelope that protects corneocytes in the skin. The expression levels of PCOLCE and elastin mRNAs were strongly suppressed after UV irradiation (Fig. 3c, d), whereas that of involucrin was elevated (Fig. 3e). In the presence of three MAAs, decreased expression of PCOLCE and elastin by UV treatment was reverted and even increased compared with control (Fig. 3c, d). The involucrin mRNA level was significantly downregulated by pretreatment of MAAs, suggesting that MAAs might be an effective material for skin firming by modulation of procollagen, elastin, and involucrin expression (Fig. 3e).

Application of MAAs in Skin Care Cosmetic Products

Taking advantage of MAA properties, cosmetic companies in Korea are using them as an active ingredient in their cosmetic products such as (Fig. 4) Daily Defence Sun Cream and Complete Control Essence. In these cosmetic products, along with other standard ingredients, shinorine and porphyra were utilized, and the amount is decided by their efficacy studies carried out by the company. As per company claim, shinorine and porphyra complex prevents skin damage from UV exposure and contributes to skin matrix homeostasis. It is helpful for reducing skin aging process.

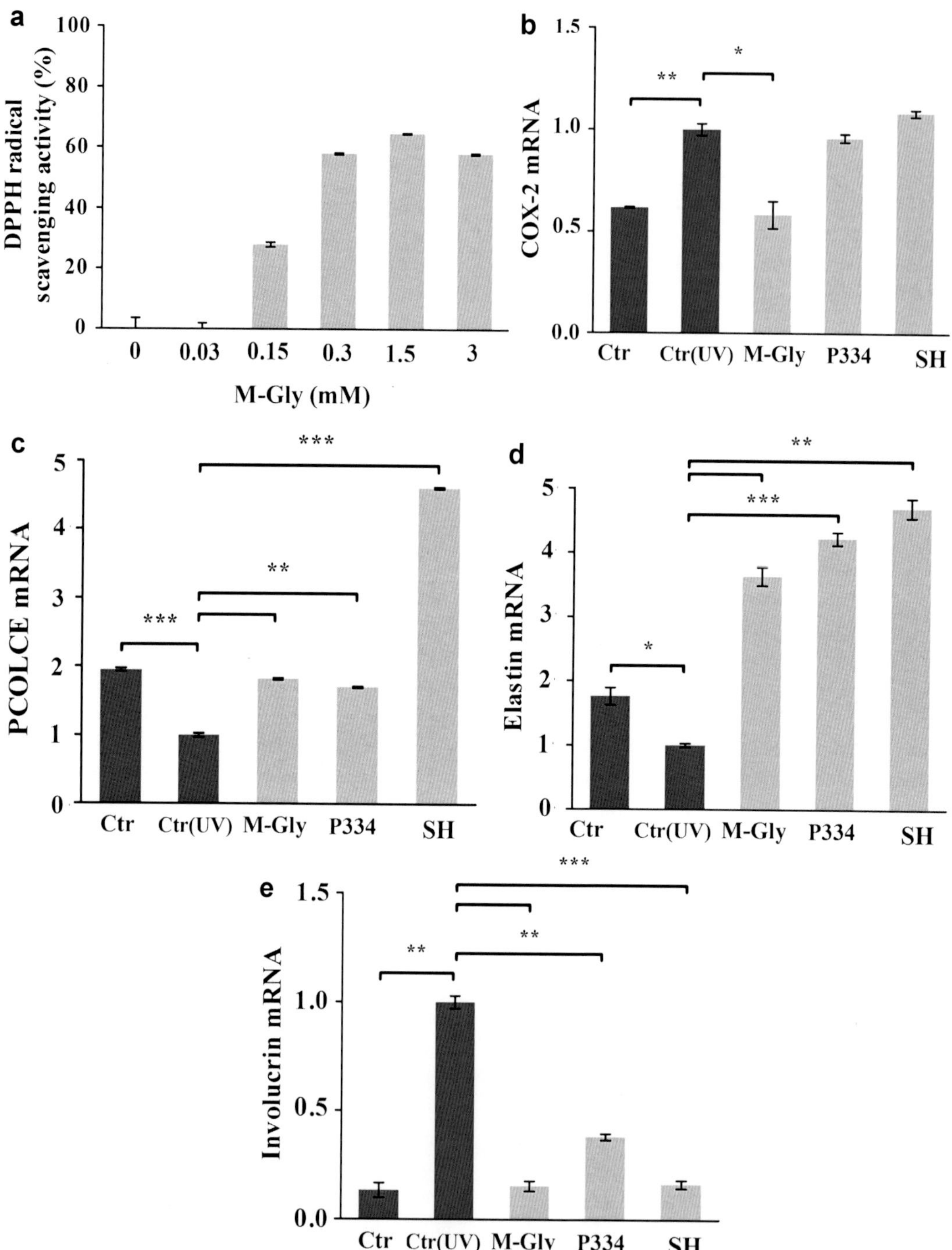

Fig. 3 (**a**) DPPH assay for radical scavenging activity of M-Gly. (**b**) Expression levels of COX-2 mRNAs in response to MAAs (0.3 mM) under UV radiation. Expression levels of PCOLCE (**c**), elastin (**d**), and involucrin (**e**) mRNAs in response to MAAs (0.15 mM) under UV radiation. Results are expressed as the mean ± s.e.m. of three independent experiments, $*p < 0.05$, $**p < 0.005$, and $***p < 0.0001$, versus control (UV) group. *Ctr* control, *M-Gly* mycosporine-glycine, *P334* porphyra-334, *SH* shinorine

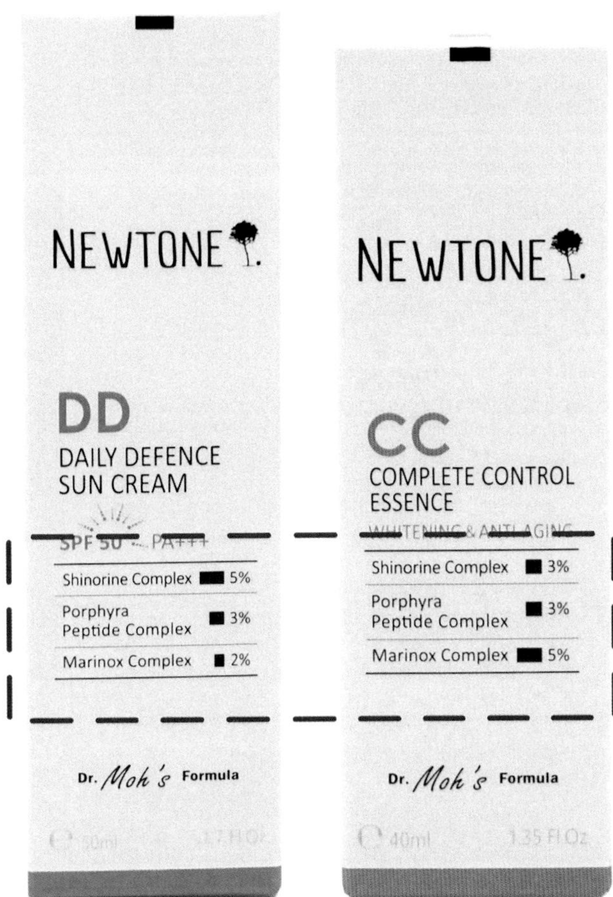

Fig. 4 Application of MAAs in cosmetic products

Conclusion

In conclusion, UV-absorbing MAAs may provide protection to the skin against the impact of UV radiation. In particular, MAAs act as UV-absorbing compounds, modulating the expression of genes associated with oxidative stress, inflammation, and skin aging caused by UV. Therefore, MAAs from marine organisms might be excellent biological substances for antiaging products.

Acknowledgments This work is supported by the Ministry of Ocean and Fisheries (20150071) for S. H. M. and the National Research Foundation (NRF-2013R1A1A1007693 and 2014K1A3A1A19066980) for K.W.K.

References

1. Kligman LH, Kligman AM. The nature of photoaging: its prevention and repair. Photodermatol. 1986;3 (4):215–27.
2. Leyden JJ. Clinical features of ageing skin. Br J Dermatol. 1990;122 Suppl 35:1–3.
3. Blunt JW, Copp BR, et al. Marine natural products. Nat Prod Rep. 2007;24(1):31–86.
4. Fenical W, Jensen PR. Developing a new resource for drug discovery: marine actinomycete bacteria. Nat Chem Biol. 2006;2(12):666–73.
5. Klisch M, Hader DP. Mycosporine-like amino acids and marine toxins – the common and the different. Mar Drugs. 2008;6(2):147–63.
6. Lebar MD, Heimbegner JL, et al. Cold-water marine natural products. Nat Prod Rep. 2007;24(4):774–97.
7. Usami Y. Recent synthetic studies leading to structural revisions of marine natural products. Mar Drugs. 2009;7(3):314–30.

8. Yuan YV, Westcott ND, et al. Mycosporine-like amino acid composition of the edible red alga, *Palmaria palmata* (dulse) harvested from the west and east coasts of Grand Manan Island, New Brunswick. Food Chem. 2009;112(2):321–8.
9. Hader DP, Kumar HD, et al. Effects of solar UV radiation on aquatic ecosystems and interactions with climate change. Photochem Photobiol Sci. 2007;6 (3):267–85.
10. Sinha RP, Rastogi RP, et al. Life of wetland cyanobacteria under enhancing solar UV-B radiation. Proc Natl Acad Sci Sect B. 2008;78:53–65.
11. Hylander S, Boeing WJ, et al. Complementary UV protective compounds in zooplankton. Limnol Oceanogr. 2009;54(6):1883–93.
12. Lee TM, Shiu CT. Implications of mycosporine-like amino acid and antioxidant defenses in UV-B radiation tolerance for the algae species *Ptercladiella capillacea* and *Gelidium amansii.* Mar Environ Res. 2009;67(1):8–16.
13. Fleming ED, Castenholz RW. Effects of periodic desiccation on the synthesis of the UV-screening compound, scytonemin, in cyanobacteria. Environ Microbiol. 2007;9(6):1448–55.
14. Singh SP, Kumari S, et al. Mycosporine-like amino acids (MAAS): chemical structure, biosynthesis and significance as UV-absorbing/screening compounds. Indian J Exp Biol. 2008;46(1):7–17.
15. Won JJW, Chalker BE, et al. Two new UV-absorbing compounds from *Stylophora pistillata*: sulfate esters of mycosporine-like amino acids. Tetrahedron Lett. 1997;38(14):2525–6.
16. Conde FR, Churio MS, et al. The photoprotector mechanism of mycosporine-like amino acids. Excited-state properties and photostability of porphyra-334 in aqueous solution. J Photochem Photobiol B. 2000;56 (2–3):139–44.
17. Whitehead K, Hedges JI. Photodegradation and photo sensitization of mycosporine-like amino acids. J Photochem Photobiol B. 2005;80(2):115–21.
18. Shibata K. Pigments and a UV-absorbing substance in coral and a blue-green alga living on the Great barrier reef. Plant Cell Physiol. 1969;10:325–35.
19. Sinha RP, Klisch M, et al. Induction of mycosporine-like amino acids (MAAS) in cyanobacteria by solar ultraviolet-B radiation. J Photochem Photobiol B. 2001;60(2–3):129–35.
20. Zhaohui Z, Xin G, Tashiro Y, Matsukawa S, Ogawa H. The isolation of prophyra-334 from marine algae and its UV-absorption behavior. Chinese J Oceanol Limnol. 2005;23:400–5.
21. Carreto JI, Carigan MO, Daleo G, DeMarco SG. Occurrence of mycosporine-like amino acids in the red tide dinoflagellate *Alexandrium* excavatum: UV-protective compounds? J Plankton Res. 1990;12:909–21.
22. Shimoji Y, Tamura Y, et al. Isolation and identification of DPPH radical scavenging compounds in Kurosu (Japanese unpolished rice vinegar). J Agric Food Chem. 2002;50(22):6501–3.

Innovative Nutraceutical Approaches to Counteract the Signs of Aging 145

Licia Genovese and Sara Sibilla

Contents

L. Genovese • S. Sibilla (✉)
Minerva Research Labs Ltd, London, UK
e-mail: lgenovese@minervalabs.com;
ssibilla@minervalabs.com

M.A. Farage et al. (eds.), *Textbook of Aging Skin*,
DOI 10.1007/978-3-662-47398-6_145

Abstract

The following chapter regards the benefits related to the daily consumption of nutraceutical liquid beauty supplements in the fight against skin aging. Aging is a complex biological phenomenon, caused by several factors which are genetically and environmentally determined. In the skin, aging induces a gradual decrease in the levels of collagen and elastin, which are the main proteins responsible for maintaining skin firmness and elasticity. As a consequence of aging, skin becomes more rigid and loses its ability to keep shape, and wrinkles and fine lines form. Following a healthy nutritional lifestyle can restore the homeostasis of macro- and micronutrients and support the physiology of cells and tissues in the skin. To this end, nutraceuticals offer formulations that increasingly represent a valid tool in the fight against skin aging. In this context, the consumption of hydrolyzed collagen-based beauty supplements can benefit the skin by restoring the natural production of collagen, hyaluronic acid and elastin. Blends of collagen peptides and multiple active ingredients can make them easily digestible, absorbed, and widely distributed in the human body. Importantly, they have been shown to restore skin hydration and elasticity and to reduce fine lines and wrinkles.

Introduction

Skin aging is characterized by a gradual structural deterioration due to intrinsic genetic factors, which may be accelerated by extrinsic aging factors such as chronic sun exposure (photoaging) [1, 2] or by lifestyle factors such as smoking, alcohol, stress, and lack of sleep [3, 4].

Skin constitutes an effective environmental interface providing protection for human body homeostasis, and as such it is also exposed to several environmental toxic insults (UV rays and chemical factors), which can lead to the production of reactive oxygen species (ROS). These molecules are known to be involved in the pathogenesis of a number of skin disorders and some types of cutaneous malignancy [5] and are also believed to lead to aging. In fact, in 1956, Denham Harman first proposed that the oxygen-free radicals, endogenously formed from normal metabolic processes, could cause aging [6, 7] (although this theory does not exclude other aging mechanisms such as cell senescence, telomere shortening, and genomic instability).

Skin is capable of counteracting the action of these molecules through efficient antioxidant defense mechanisms. Unfortunately, these processes weaken with time and can be overwhelmed by increased ROS production. One approach to prevent or treat these ROS-mediated disorders is based on the administration of different antioxidants [5].

There has been some controversy on the link between aging and ROS production. Several *in vivo* studies have in fact shown that inhibition of antioxidants expression leads on one side to increased oxidative damage, but on the other side does not lead to the expected signs of accelerated aging nor to a reduced lifespan. This suggests how the aging process may be triggered by many factors other than ROS production [8, 9].

Many functional foods (food containing additives which provide extra nutritional value), also known as nutraceuticals, which are able to counteract oxidative stress and ROS-mediated disorders, [5] have recently come into the market in many countries. For example, a study has shown that collagen peptides, as a dietary supplement, are beneficial in suppressing UVB-induced skin damage and photoaging [10]. Another study, conducted in hairless Sod1$^{-/-}$ double mutant mice, showed that co-treatment with collagen peptides and vitamin C corrected age-related skin thinning by attenuating oxidative damage [11]. Also, dietary intake of astaxanthin (a powerful antioxidant) combined with collagen hydrolysate can improve elasticity and barrier integrity in photo-aged human facial skin [12]. In addition, GOLD COLLAGEN® nutraceutical products have been shown to have beneficial effects on skin properties such as hydration, elasticity, and reduction of fine lines and wrinkles [13–15], making them a valid tool in the fight against skin aging.

Skin Structure and Function

Skin covers the whole human body and represents the principal barrier to the external environment [16]. Skin has many more roles other than guarding the underlying muscles, bones, ligaments, and internal organs. For example, skin plays a key role in immunity by protecting the body against pathogens (Langerhans cells in the skin are part of the adaptive immune system). Moreover, skin prevents excessive water loss, it has a role in insulation, temperature regulation, sensation, synthesis of vitamin D, excretion, and absorption.

The skin is composed of multiple layers: the epidermis, the dermis, and the subcutaneous tissues (Fig. 1). The epidermis itself is composed of several layers: the stratum corneum as the top layer, then proceeding deeper down, there are the *stratum lucidum* and *stratum granulosum*, followed by the *stratum spinosum*, and finally the *stratum basale* just above the dermis [17]. The *stratum corneum* is extremely difficult to penetrate, and it represents the first barrier to the external environment. Thus, the probability of external particles reaching the dermis through the epidermis is very limited. Below the epidermal layers lies the dermis, which is rich in proteins such as collagen, elastin, and glycosaminoglycans (such as hyaluronic acid). These proteins are the main components of the extracellular matrix (ECM) and are secreted by fibroblasts, cells of the

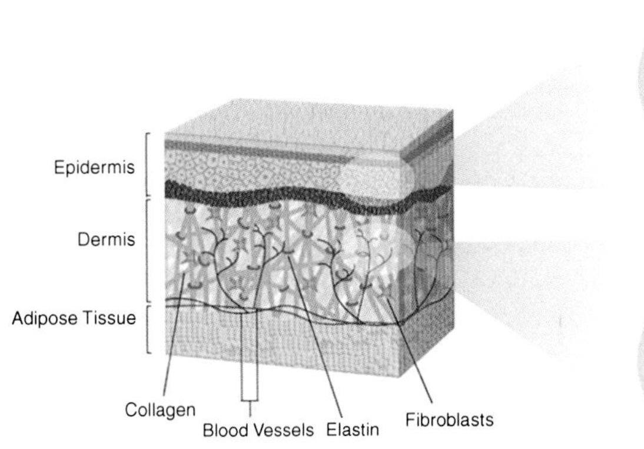

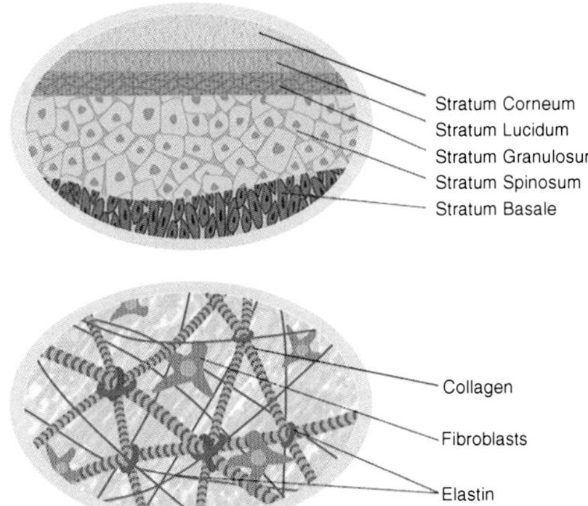

Fig. 1 Human skin structure

connective tissue. The subcutaneous tissue is the deepest layer of the skin, composed primarily of fat.

In the epidermis, melanocytes produce melanin and are responsible for skin pigmentation (skin color) and absorb some of the potentially dangerous UV rays present in sunlight. DNA repair enzymes help reverse UV damage in the skin, such that people lacking the genes coding for these enzymes suffer higher rates of skin cancer.

Skin is directly exposed to periodical changes in light and temperature, as it forms an interface between the external environment and the body. Many physiological processes are characterized by periodic daily fluctuations such as changes in skin temperature, sebum production, pH, and transepidermal water loss [18]. Also cell division is associated with specific times of the day and exhibits a circadian periodicity [19]. Epidermal cell proliferation is in fact regulated by a circadian clock, and this could serve as a mechanism for protecting against UV-induced DNA damage by minimizing DNA replication during exposure to the sun UV rays [20].

Collagen

The extracellular matrix of connective tissues is formed by different protein families involved in providing structural integrity and several other physiological functions. In the dermis, one of the principal proteins of the ECM is collagen, an insoluble fibrous protein which, together with elastin and hyaluronic acid, is the main component of skin and has a key role in providing integrity and elasticity to this organ.

Collagen is mostly found in fibrous tissues, such as tendons and ligaments, and it is also abundant in the cornea, cartilage, bones, blood vessels, the gut, and intervertebral disks.

Collagen protein is composed of three polypeptide chains named α-chains, which form a triple helix [21]. Based on their structure and three-dimensional organization, they can be grouped into fibril-forming collagens, fibril-associated collagens (FACIT), network-forming collagens, anchoring fibrils, transmembrane collagens (MACIT), basement membrane collagens, and others with unique functions. 28 triple helical proteins have been named as collagens [22, 23].

The five most common types of collagen are:

- ***Type* I**: dermis, tendon, ligaments, and bone
- ***Type II***: cartilage, vitreous body, and nucleus pulposus
- ***Type III***: skin, vessel wall, and reticular fibers of most tissues (lungs, liver, spleen)
- ***Type IV***: forms the basal lamina and the epithelium-secreted layer of the basement membranes
- ***Type V***: lung, cornea, hair, and fetal membranes

A collagen fibril is composed of multiple triple helices and multiple fibrils form a collagen fiber. Collagen fibrils are made of different collagen types: collagen I and III in the skin and collagen II and III in cartilage [21]. Type I collagen is the most abundant in the human body: it forms more than 90 % of bone organic mass, and it is the major collagen present in tendons, ligaments, cornea, and many interstitial connective tissues. It is also the main component of human skin (80 %) with collagen type III making up the remainder of skin collagen (15 %) [23, 24].

Together collagen fibers form a dense network throughout the dermis that confers structural integrity to the skin and also provides structural support to the epidermis.

In the connective tissues, collagen is mainly produced by fibroblasts [22]. In the dermis, fibroblasts are the main cells responsible for producing and organizing the collagen matrix. The activation of fibroblasts results in an increase in the production of collagen. Also myofibroblasts [25] and numerous epithelial cells make certain types of collagens in other tissues [26].

Studies have shown that collagen synthesis varies at different stages of life. The relative proportion of the types of collagen in skin also changes with age. Young skin is composed of 80 % type I collagen and about 15 % collagen type III. With age, the ability to replenish collagen naturally decreases by about 1 % per year [27].

Elastin

The elasticity of many tissues depends on the presence of elastic fibers which are composed by elastin and microfibrils. Elastin is a very important protein for arteries and helps in the pressure wave propagation for blood flow. Elastin is also very important for the lungs, elastic ligaments, and skin. The principal characteristic of elastic fibers is that they stretch rapidly under a load and return quickly to their original form once the load is removed.

Elastin contains many cross-linking sites [28]. Thus, elastic fibers are freely mobile with respect to one another, except at points of cross-linking. The major cross-links in elastin are two polyfunctional amino acids, desmosine and isodesmosine, which account for both the elasticity and insolubility of elastic fibers. These fibers are mainly composed of an amorphous component, which is extensively cross-linked elastin, and a fibrillar component, which are primarily the microfibrils, such as fibrillin. Fibroblasts produce multiple tropoelastin molecules, which covalently bind together with cross-links to form the final elastin protein.

Hyaluronic Acid

Another essential ECM protein is hyaluronic acid (HA). This molecule is found mainly in soft connective tissues, in particular skin and joints. HA is formed by alternating units of glucuronic acid and *N*-acetylglucosamine.

In the skin HA is synthesized by fibroblasts, keratinocytes, and other cells [29]. HA is found not only in the dermis but also in the epidermal intercellular spaces. HA has a high molecular weight (10–104 KDa), and this represents a key factor in influencing its physical-chemical properties, such as viscosity, elasticity, and the ability to retain water. In fact, HA is essential for tissue hydration, lubrication, and the production of collagen in the dermis.

Though HA is known to play a structural role in connective tissue, its overall turnover rate appears to be surprisingly quick. Studies have shown that HA has a turnover rate of 0.5 to a few (2–3) days [29, 30].

It has been shown that HA is absorbed and distributed to organs and joints after a single oral administration [31]. *In vitro* studies have shown that collagen peptides can stimulate not only dermal fibroblasts proliferation but also synthesis of hyaluronic acid [32].

HA has been widely used as an antiaging cosmetic ingredient. Its beneficial effects on skin are controlled by varying its molecular size. For example, lower-molecular-weight HA was shown not only to lead to a significant reduction of wrinkle depth [33] but also to penetrate the skin better and to influence the expression of many genes involved in keratinocyte differentiation and in the formation of intercellular tight junction complexes, which are reduced in aged skin [34].

Skin Aging

Aging is the process of becoming older and in humans it refers to a psychological and physical processes. In particular, aging of the skin is a complex biological phenomenon which affects several of its constituents and hence its appearance, and for this reason it can have a big social impact.

There are two primary skin-aging mechanisms, intrinsic and extrinsic [3, 4]. Both intrinsic and extrinsic aging (discussed later on) act simultaneously and are associated with phenotypic changes such as wrinkle formation.

In aged skin, collagen fibers become thicker and much shorter, resulting in a loss of collagen type I, which alters the ratio of collagen types [35]. The density of collagen and elastin in the dermis declines, and as a consequence, skin support and elasticity degrade and skin becomes thinner and more rigid. Reduced collagen can reflect two different underlying mechanisms: cellular fibroblast aging and a lower level of fibroblast cell stimulation. Hence, there is a destruction of existing collagen and a failure to replace damaged collagen with newly synthesized material [36]. Moreover, it has been shown that in the presence of damaged collagen fibers, fibroblasts have a reduced proliferative capacity and synthesize less collagen [37–39].

The aging process results also in the loss of hyaluronic acid. This reduces the moisture, suppleness, and elasticity of the skin. The diminished elasticity of the skin reduces its ability to retain its shape, and therefore, it will not conform as closely to the contours of the face. The skin appears looser and sags, lines and furrows emerge to enable movement. Gravity then pulls on the skin, all leading to sagging eyelids and bags under the eyes and jowls.

Intrinsic Aging

Intrinsic aging depends on time, it is genetically determined and the changes that occur are a result of different factors:

- Cumulative endogenous damage due to the formation of ROS which affects cellular constituents such as membranes, enzymes, and DNA.
- Decreased sex hormone levels (estrogen, testosterone, dehydroepiandrosterone) and other hormones (i.e., melatonin, insulin).
- Shortening of telomere length. It has been reported, for example, that in fibroblasts of quiescent skin, more than 30 % of telomere length is lost during adulthood [40].
- Decreased levels of cytokines and their receptors with consequent loss of several skin functions.

Several changes occur in skin layers: there is a decreased number of melanocytes and Langerhans cells in the epidermis, alteration in the epidermal-dermal junction (with a consequent reduction of exchange of nutrients between the two), loss of dermal volume, decrease in blood supply, and reduced tyrosinase activity (which is linked to melanin production) [41].

Deep inside in the dermis, fibrillar collagens, elastin fibers, and hyaluronic acid undergo different structural and functional changes. Collagen and elastin are long-life proteins and are predisposed to intrinsic molecular aging and have a half-life measured in years [3]. For this characteristic, these fibers accumulate damage over time, and this reduces their ability to function correctly. As a consequence, intrinsically aged skin is generally characterized by dermal atrophy with reduced density of collagen fibers, elastin, and hyaluronic acid (Fig. 2).

All these changes lead to the formation of wrinkles and fine lines, which are exacerbated by gravitational forces and the loss of subcutaneous fat.

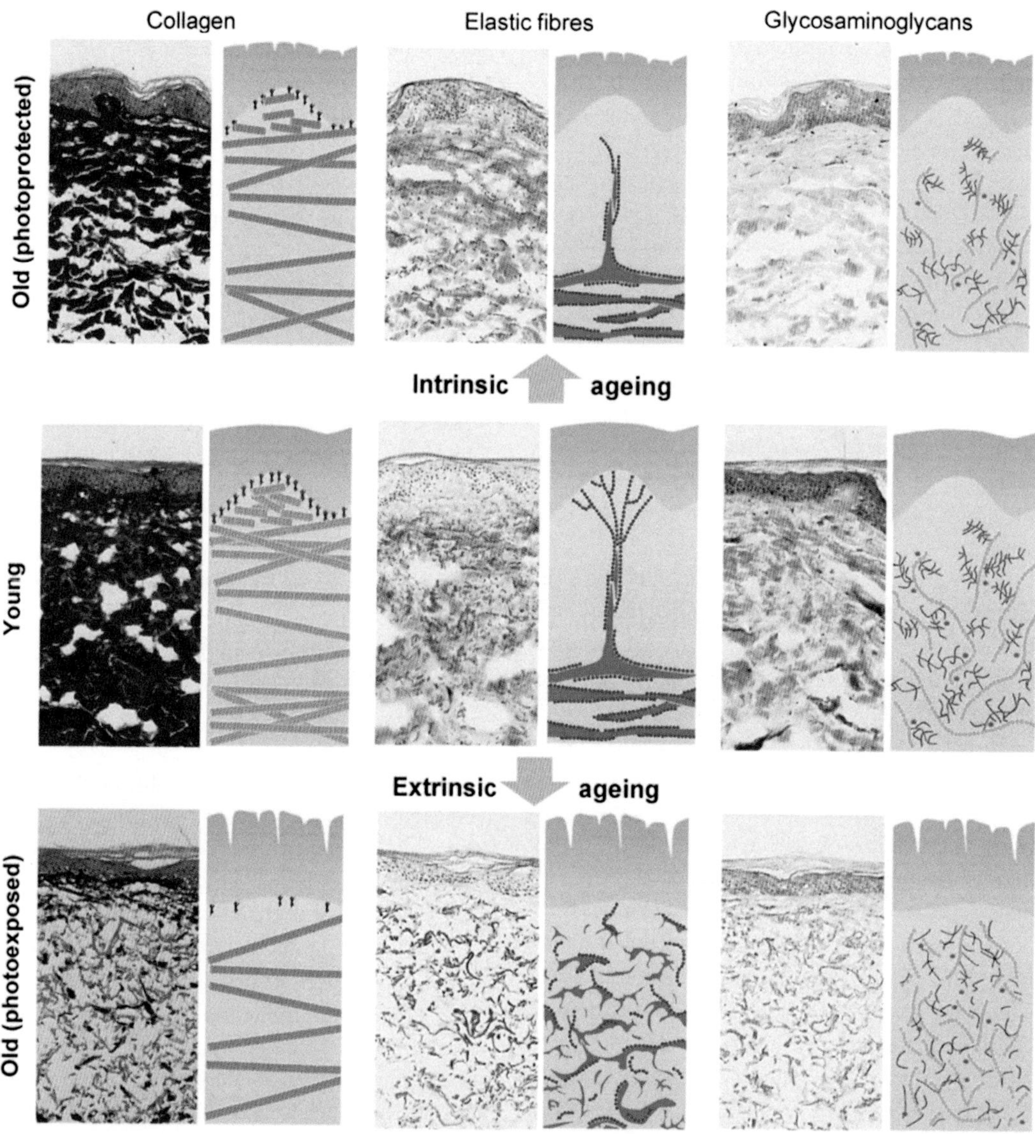

Fig. 2 Extracellular matrix remodeling in intrinsically and extrinsically aged skin. Dermal collagens, elastic fibers, and glycosaminoglycans undergo significant changes in both photo-protected and photo-exposed aged skin. When comparing with young skin, intrinsically aged skin (photo-protected) is characterized by atrophy of dermal collagens and of the elastic fiber system. Extrinsically aged skin (photo-exposed) is characterized both by a marked reduction in fibrillar collagen and by an accumulation of disorganized elastic fiber proteins throughout the dermis, a process termed solar elastosis [3].

Extrinsic Aging

Extrinsic aging is caused by several factors:

- Chronic sun exposure (UV radiation is the most important factor for skin aging). It damages DNA in keratinocytes and melanocytes and induces the production of proteolytic enzymes, such as collagen-degrading enzymes. It is also responsible for the formation of thymidine dimers ("UV fingerprints"), which lead to an accumulation of DNA mutations. Clinically UV radiation leads to the formation of actinic keratosis, solar elastosis, lentigines, and carcinomas [41].

- High alcohol intake
- Smoking
- Poor nutrition
- Overeating
- Environmental pollution
- Stress

Extrinsically aged skin is characterized by the degradation and the alteration of collagen fibers and the accumulation of disorganized elastin proteins throughout the dermis, a process known as elastosis (Fig. 2). Metalloproteinases can be induced by UVA and UVB [42], and their proteolytic activity results in the degradation of collagen and elastin fibers. For example, metalloproteinases were found to be induced in cells obtained from old versus young subjects [43], and many other studies show their upregulation in photodamaged skin [44–47]. As a consequence, the collagen density decreases each year with a faster rate in photo-exposed skin [4]. In fact, aged fibroblasts synthesize lower levels of collagen, both *in vitro* and *in vivo*, compared to young adult fibroblasts [36], and photo-aged dermis contains disorganized collagen fibers and accumulated abnormal elastin [46, 48].

Another important aging phenomenon that takes place, especially in tissues very rich in proteins, is the production of advanced glycation end products (AGEs). These molecules form because of a chemical reaction between glucose and the free amino groups in proteins, and they remain in the tissue as they cannot be degraded normally by enzymes [49].

Clinical manifestations of extrinsic aging include leathery appearance, increased wrinkle formation, reduced recoil capacity, increased fragility of the skin, and altered color pigmentation (age spots).

The skin has two photo-protective mechanisms: the melanin in the lower layer of the epidermis and the urocanic barrier of the *stratum corneum* which absorbs a good amount of UV rays.

In addition, a very important role is played by antioxidants, which help counteract ROS damage. Antioxidants are naturally occurring in the skin and include superoxide dismutase, catalase, alpha-tocopherol, ascorbic acid, ubiquinone, and glutathione. A proper diet, rich in vitamins and antioxidants (e.g., coenzyme Q10 and alpha-lipoic acid), can help protect from oxidative damage [50].

Interestingly, alteration in diet can change the way skin functions as evidenced by the effects of dietary deprivation on skin health. For example, essential fatty acid deficiency [51] or the accumulation of abnormal fatty acids [52] results in the so-called skin scaling and poor barrier function.

Thus, it is important to have a correct nutritional approach, maintaining a balanced diet and a good supply of food supplements to restore the homeostasis of cells and tissues in the human body.

The Use of Hydrolyzed Collagen as a Nutraceutical

Hydrolyzed collagen is becoming an increasingly popular nutraceutical. It is produced from native collagen, and it consists of small collagen peptides with low molecular weight (0.3–8 KDa). It is formed through a process of hydrolysis which involves breaking down the molecular bonds between individual collagen strands using a combination of heat, acids, alkalis, or enzymes. Hydrolyzed collagen is widely used in cosmetics as a moisturizer, for example, in creams. The main advantage of using small collagen peptides, compared to native collagen, is that they are highly digestible, easily absorbed, and distributed in the human body. In literature there are numerous clinical trials that have been performed showing the efficacy and benefits of collagen peptides on skin properties (such as hydration, elasticity, and reduction of wrinkles). A reduction in skin collagen levels, which comes with age, can lead to a reduced mechanical tension on fibroblasts with a consequent loss in matrix production and stimulation instead of matrix-degrading enzymes [53]. In this context, hydrolyzed collagen supplementation has a dual mechanism: (1) collagen peptides and free amino acids are used as building blocks for the formation of new collagen and elastin fibers; (2) the collagen peptides bind to fibroblasts receptors and stimulate the production of new collagen, elastin, and hyaluronic acid.

When administered orally, hydrolyzed collagen reaches the small intestine and then it is absorbed into the bloodstream. The collagen peptides are distributed in the human body and to the dermis through the circulatory system.

The **bioavailability** of hydrolyzed collagen was demonstrated first in mice by a study published in 1999. In this study the authors showed that when orally administered ^{14}C-labeled hydrolyzed collagen was digested, more than 90 % was absorbed within the first 12 h from the intake. In fact, radioactivity in skin peaked 12 h after the administration of ^{14}C-labeled hydrolyzed collagen, and in contrast to plasma, the radioactivity levels remained high up to 96 h [54]. In a more recent study (published in 2005), the authors found that hydrolyzed collagen from porcine skin, chicken feet, and cartilage, ingested by healthy human volunteers after 12 h of fasting, was absorbed in the blood as small peptides. In fact, hydroxyproline-containing peptides were found to be increased in the plasma, reaching a peak level after 2 h and then decreasing to half of the maximum level after 4 h from the oral ingestion. The authors also identified a small peptide proline-hydroxyproline (Pro-Hyp) in the blood, which was present only after intake of hydrolyzed collagen [55].

The safety of collagen peptides and gelatin (from which hydrolyzed collagen is prepared) is widely recognized. The Food and Drug Administration (FDA) has classified gelatin as a safe substance. In addition, based on international research results, both the World Health Organization (WHO) and the European Commission for Health and Consumer Protection have confirmed that hydrolyzed collagen is safe. There may be only rarely minor side effects, such as nausea, flatulence, or dyspepsia.

The **distribution** of collagen peptides to the skin was demonstrated in a study in which ^{14}C-labeled proline or ^{14}C-labeled collagen peptides were administered to Wistar rats. After ingestion of the collagen peptides, radioactivity was measured in the different tissues until 14 days. The results showed that the radioactivity remained at high levels in the skin up to 14 days. This indicates the ability of collagen peptides to reach the dermis in the skin and stay there for prolonged periods [56].

Several *in vitro* and *in vivo* studies have demonstrated the efficacy of collagen peptides on skin health.

An *in vitro* study example is given by the work of Chen and coworkers [57]. These authors studied the effect of different concentrations of hydrolyzed collagen from fish on fibroblasts and keratinocytes. In particular, they investigated cell proliferation, collagen production, and mRNA type I collagen expression. The authors found that an optimal concentration of collagen ranging between 48 and 97 μg/mL resulted in 191% increase in the percentage of fibroblast cell proliferation. Also the highest keratinocytes proliferation was achieved with a collagen concentration between 0.76 and 1.53 μg/mL, and this induced an increase of 242% in proliferation percentage. They also reported an increase in the expression of collagen I mRNA in fibroblasts.

In addition to these studies, Ohara et al. [32] further demonstrated that collagen peptides can stimulate not only the proliferation of dermal fibroblasts but also the synthesis of hyaluronic acid. In this study eight different collagen-derived peptides containing Hyp were analyzed, and a positive effect on proliferation was observed for Ala-Hyp, Ala-Hyp-Gly, and Pro-Hyp. The same eight peptides were also used to evaluate their effect on hyaluronic acid synthesis, and the results were consistent with the proliferation study. In both studies, Pro-Hyp showed highest efficacy in proliferation and hyaluronic acid synthesis.

Examples of *in vivo* studies are those by Matsumoto et al. [58]. This research group carried out a preclinical trial in which they showed that daily ingestion of collagen peptides improved skin hydration in female volunteers after supplementation with fish collagen peptides for 6 weeks. This study was followed by a double-blind placebo-controlled study by the same research group [59]. Healthy female volunteers aged 25–45 ingested 2.5, 5, and 10 g of fish collagen peptide, and the results were compared to a placebo group. *Stratum corneum* hydration was measured at baseline and after 4 weeks. When all subjects were included in the analysis no significant difference between the treated groups (2.5/5/10 g) and the placebo was observed. However, when only subjects older than 30 years were considered, there was a significant difference between the treated group (5 and 10 g) and the placebo.

Koyama et al. [60] demonstrated that women ingesting 5 or 10 g of pig skin collagen had an improvement of their skin condition already after 3 weeks and at the end of the treatment after 7 weeks. Furthermore, in a double-blind, placebo-controlled study, Proksch and colleagues investigated the effects of collagen hydrolysate on skin biophysical parameters such as skin elasticity, skin moisture, transepidermal water loss, and skin roughness. Sixty-nine women (35–55 years old) were randomized to receive collagen hydrolysate (2.5 g or 5.0 g) or placebo once daily for 8 weeks. At the end of the study, skin elasticity in both collagen hydrolysate dosage groups showed a statistically significant improvement in comparison to placebo [61]. Results from several clinical trials, showing the efficacy of liquid hydrolyzed collagen-based dietary supplements, such as PURE GOLD COLLAGEN®, in reducing wrinkles and nasolabial fold depth and increasing skin hydration and elasticity, have been published recently [13–15].

A study involving 265 volunteers was carried out independently by 40 dermatologists across 5 different countries: USA, UAE, Greece, Czech Republic, and Spain. The subjects were given a standardized daily dose of PURE GOLD COLLAGEN® for 20 days before and 40 days after a cosmetic procedure. The outcome of the study showed that there was a significant increase in collagen density and skin firmness along with a significant reduction in skin dryness, wrinkles, and depth of nasolabial folds [13].

A double-blind, randomized, placebo-controlled study including 108 healthy volunteer subjects was performed by an independent Clinical Research Organization to assess the efficacy of PURE GOLD COLLAGEN® on skin condition. Volunteers consumed the products daily for 12 weeks. The effect on the skin was investigated and a significant improvement in wrinkles (19 % reduction compared to placebo) was achieved, primarily a decrease in the surface area and the mean length of wrinkles [14].

Another recent 12 weeks double-blind, randomized, placebo-controlled clinical trial was conducted on 18 female healthy subjects (between the ages of 45 and 64) to assess whether the oral consumption of PURE GOLD COLLAGEN® could improve certain specific skin properties of postmenopausal women such as depth of facial wrinkles, skin elasticity, and hydration. The results showed that the combination of specific ingredients such as hydrolyzed collagen, hyaluronic acid, and essential vitamins and minerals present in the nutritional drink acts to significantly reduce the depth of facial wrinkles within 9 weeks and increase skin elasticity (between week 9 and week 12) as well as skin hydration (after 6 weeks) [15].

Thus, on the basis of the significant amount of data now present in the literature, hydrolyzed collagen can be considered an important nutraceutical weapon in the everyday fight against skin aging.

GOLD COLLAGEN® Products: An Overview

Nutraceuticals containing collagen peptides together with vitamins and minerals are innovative liquid, nutritional food supplements. These dietary supplements help promote healthy skin, fight the early signs of aging, such as fine lines and wrinkles and promote healthy looking hair and nails. Examples of these innovative nutricosmeceuticals are the GOLD COLLAGEN® products, conceived and created by MINERVA Research Labs (http://www.gold-collagen.com).

Collaborative studies which are analyzing the mechanisms of action, safety, and efficacy of hydrolyzed collagen-based supplements, such as GOLD COLLAGEN® products, involving research and academic institutes in the UK, Europe, and USA, are currently ongoing.

Non-collagen Anti-aging Ingredients (Table 1)

Summary of Results Obtained with PURE GOLD COLLAGEN®

Numerous clinical trials on PURE GOLD COLLAGEN® (patented formula) have been carried out since 2012, and as mentioned above, three clinical studies have been successfully completed and published to date [13–15].

One of these studies [13] was an open-label multicenter study conducted by 40 dermatologists who worked independently in different countries (namely, the UK, USA, UAE, Greece, and the Czech Republic). The study involved 265 healthy volunteer subjects, ingesting one bottle (50 ml) of the dietary supplement daily for 60 days. Subjects had a skin assessment before, during, and at the end of the treatment.

In summary this study showed:

1. **Significant reduction in wrinkles and depth of nasolabial folds** (Fig. 3)
2. **Twelve and nineteen percent increase in collagen density after 12 weeks of treatment both in the forearm and Crow's feet area** (Fig. 4)
3. **Significant increase in skin firmness after 80 and 130 days of treatment** (Fig. 5)

Preliminary Results Obtained with GOLD COLLAGEN® FORTE

An independent double-blind, randomized, placebo-controlled clinical trial was performed to investigate the effects of GOLD COLLAGEN® FORTE on skin elasticity in subjects who underwent a cosmetic treatment (fillers and Botox in the face) and subjects who did not while using this nutraceutical supplement.

Subjects participating in the trial were divided into two groups: 30 volunteer subjects (28 females and 2 males, between 40 and 60 years old) who consumed GOLD COLLAGEN® FORTE daily and other 30 volunteer subjects (27 females and 3 males, between 40 and 60 years old) who consumed placebo. Subjects drank one bottle (50 ml) of product daily over a period of 90 days.

DermaLab SkinLab USB elasticity module was used to measure skin elasticity on each subject forearm at baseline (day 0) and at the end of the treatment at day 90.

A self-assessment questionnaire including questions related to skin, hair, nails, joints, mood, and photoaging conditions and questions regarding the subjects' opinion about the product was filled by each subject. The questionnaire comprised of two parts: the first section was completed by the subjects at baseline (day 0), while the second section was completed at the end of the trial (day 90).

To evaluate the efficacy of the product on skin, histological examination was performed in two subjects who took the product for 90 consecutive days. Histological exam was performed staining the sections with hematoxylin and eosin (E-E) for the assessment of skin structures and, in particular, of collagen and elastin fibers.

In summary this study showed:

1. **Increase in skin elasticity after 90 days of treatment**, Fig. 6.

   Interestingly, the overall increase in skin elasticity in the subjects taking GOLD COLLAGEN® FORTE (from 8.42 to 9.17 mm) was statistically significant ($p < 0.05$, *T*-test), and an increase in skin elasticity was observed singularly both in subjects who underwent a cosmetic treatment and subjects who did not. Moreover, no significant change in skin elasticity was observed in the placebo group, both in subjects who underwent or did not undergo a cosmetic treatment. The increase in skin elasticity suggests that this functional food supplement, containing collagen peptides among other active ingredients, has an effect in restoring the correct levels of extracellular matrix proteins such as elastin. In fact, hydrolyzed collagen has a dual action mechanism in the dermis: (1) collagen peptides and free amino acids provide building blocks for the formation of collagen and elastin fibers; (2) hydrolyzed

Table 1 Ingredients present in nutraceutical supplements: properties, benefits, and approved claims

PROPERTIES	BENEFITS/APPROVED CLAIMS
Borage oil	
Borage oil is the richest known source (24 %) of gamma-linolenic acid (GLA), an essential fatty acid. GLA is converted, via a sequence of biochemical steps, into prostaglandin 1 (PG1), a key molecule for maintaining healthy skin. PG1 exhibits a potent anti-inflammatory effect on the skin and is very effective in regulating water loss and protecting the skin from injury and damage [62]	Borage oil, both taken orally and used topically, has been used for soothing disorders such as atypical dermatitis, psoriasis, eczema, and other inflammatory skin conditions [63, 64]
Borage oil/evening primrose oil	
Evening primrose oil is often used in combination with borage oil for skin benefit. It contains very high levels of GLA	The combination of borage oil and evening primrose oil is often used for the treatment of eczema [65, 66]
N-acetylglucosamine	
Both glucosamine and its derivative *N*-acetylglucosamine are substrate precursors for the biosynthesis of polymers such as glycosaminoglycans (e.g., hyaluronic acid) and for the production of proteoglycans	Because of its ability to stimulate hyaluronic acid synthesis, *N*-acetylglucosamine has been shown to accelerate wound healing, improve skin hydration, and decrease wrinkles [67]
Vitamin A	*Approved claim*:
Vitamin A consists of a group of unsaturated nutritional organic compounds that includes retinol, retinal, retinoic acid, and several provitamin A carotenoids, among which beta-carotene is the most important. Vitamin A has multiple functions such as vision, gene transcription, immune function, embryonic development and reproduction, bone metabolism, hematopoiesis, skin and cellular health, and antioxidant activity. This vitamin can be obtained from foods of animal origin such as organ meats, fish oil, and dairy products and from plant-origin foods. Aging may reduce the efficiency of the conversion of provitamin A carotenoids to their active form [68]. Retinoids are well known as antiaging agents. For many years this vitamin has been used for the prevention and treatment of photoaging. Retinyl palmitate (vitamin A ester) has been used in skin creams, where it is broken down to retinol and metabolized to retinoic acid, which has potent biological activity. Retinoic acid, in fact, appears to maintain normal skin health by switching on genes and differentiating keratinocytes (immature skin cells) into mature epidermal cells [69]. This suggests that retinoids also play a role in the prevention of aging, because of their inhibitory effects on metalloproteinases expression (which degrade collagen) [70].	Vitamin A contributes to the maintenance of normal skin and vision and to normal iron metabolism
Vitamin B3	*Approved claim*:
Vitamin B3, also known as niacin, is a hydrophilic endogenous substance which can have antipruritic, antimicrobial, vasoactive, photo-protective, sebostatic, and lightening effect depending on its concentration. Niacin deficiency was described some centuries ago as it was responsible for *pellagra* (one of the most devastating nutritional diseases) characterized by extreme weakness and crusty skin. Vitamin B3 can be found in meats, cereals and grain products, and vegetables. Vitamin B3 is a well-tolerated and safe substance often used in cosmetics. It has been shown to protect from inflammatory dermatoses and photoaging [71]	Vitamin B3 contributes to the maintenance of normal skin and to the reduction of tiredness and fatigue

(*continued*)

Table 1 (continued)

PROPERTIES	BENEFITS/APPROVED CLAIMS
Vitamin B6	*Approved claim*:
Vitamin B6 is a water-soluble vitamin that is naturally present in many foods, and it is a cofactor in many cell reactions (primarily in the metabolism of amino acids but also carbohydrates and lipids). Vitamin B6 plays a role in cognitive development through the biosynthesis of neurotransmitters and in maintaining normal levels of homocysteine, an amino acid in the blood. Vitamin B6 affects all aspects of metabolic function and cellular homeostasis, and it is a vitamin widely distributed in foods of plant and animal origin	Vitamin B6 contributes to normal energy-yielding metabolism and to the reduction of tiredness and fatigue
Vitamin B12	*Approved claim*:
Vitamin B12 is involved in: Nervous system maintenance Formation of blood Cell metabolism (DNA synthesis and regulation, fatty acid metabolism and amino acid metabolism). Humans obtain vitamin B12 from products of animal origin including meats, fish, shellfish, dairy products, and eggs. Altered vitamin B12 levels are associated with dermatological manifestations such as hyperpigmentation, hair and nail changes, vitiligo, atopic dermatitis, and acne [72].	Vitamin B12 contributes to a normal function of the immune system
Vitamin C	*Approved claim*:
Vitamin C (L-ascorbic acid) is a powerful antioxidant and a common enzymatic cofactor in mammals used in the synthesis of collagen. It is a powerful reducing agent capable of rapidly scavenging a number of reactive oxygen species (ROS). It is therefore involved into the development and maintenance of several biological systems: immune system, blood vessels, bones, gums and teeth, cell metabolism, nervous system, and skin condition. Low intakes of fresh fruits and vegetables increase the risk of scurvy (characterized by fatigue, skin spots, and bloody gums). Dietary vitamin C can aid with iron absorption. Vitamin C is widely used in cosmetic products to improve several skin parameters such as wrinkles [73–75]	Vitamin C contributes to normal collagen formation and the normal function of bones, cartilage, and skin
Vitamin D	*Approved claim*:
Vitamin D is responsible for enhancing intestinal absorption of calcium, iron, magnesium, phosphate, and zinc. The intake of Vitamin D can be through the diet, but mainly the body can synthesize it in the skin, from cholesterol, and with sun exposure. Sunlight exposure is the primary source of vitamin D for the majority of people. In the skin, vitamin D is produced in the two innermost layers, the *stratum basale* and *stratum spinosum* of the epidermis. One of the most important roles of vitamin D is to maintain skeletal calcium balance by promoting calcium absorption in the intestine, promoting bone resorption by increasing osteoclast number, maintaining calcium and phosphate levels for bone formation, and allowing proper functioning of parathyroid hormone to maintain serum calcium levels. Also other physiological systems respond to vitamin D such as the cardiovascular system, the immune system, muscle, pancreas, metabolic homeostasis, and the brain. Vitamin D reduces DNA damage, inflammation, and photo-carcinogenesis caused by UV rays, and it is very often recommended as a supplement, especially during childhood and pregnancy [76, 77]	Vitamin D contributes to normal absorption of calcium and phosphorous and maintenance of normal bones, normal muscle function, teeth, and the immune system

(*continued*)

Table 1 (continued)

PROPERTIES	BENEFITS/APPROVED CLAIMS
Vitamin E	*Approved claim*:
Vitamin E (or tocopherol) is a fat-soluble compound and has many biological functions: enzymatic activity, gene expression, neurological function and antioxidant function (which is the most important). It neutralizes reactive oxygen species, and as such, it protects cells and tissues from free radical damage; this is the reason why it is often used in antiaging skin creams. Vitamin E often works together with vitamin C, as the latter can help to activate vitamin E. Vitamin E works in lipid environment and halts lipid peroxidation in lipoproteins and membranes. The richest sources of vitamin E are plant oils, such as soya, corn, and olive oil. This vitamin works as a soothing and anti-inflammatory agent. In fact, vitamin E has been shown to protect the skin from chemical-induced irritation [78] and has been shown to have photo-protective effects against skin UV photodamage [79]	Vitamin E contributes to the protection of cell constituents from oxidative damage
Zinc	*Approved claim*:
Zinc is a trace element which has a role in catalytic, structural, and regulatory reactions. It serves as structural ions in transcription factors, and it stabilizes the tertiary structure of many proteins. Zinc is stored and transferred in metallothioneins. It is important in helping the body to make new cells, process food, and heal wounds. It also has antioxidant effects and is pivotal for the body's resistance to infection and for tissue repair. Classic signs of zinc deficiency include reduced growth, diarrhea, skin and eye lesions, neuropsychiatric changes, and alopecia [80]. The food plants that contain the most zinc are wheat (germ and bran) and various seeds (sesame, poppy, alfalfa, celery, mustard). Zinc is also found in beans, nuts, almonds, whole grains, pumpkin seeds, sunflower seeds, and blackcurrant	Zinc contributes to the maintenance of normal skin, hair, and nails
Copper	*Approved claim*:
Copper is a transition metal that is vital for all eukaryotic organisms. It is involved in important biochemical reactions including cellular respiration, antioxidant defense, detoxification, blood clotting, melanin production, and connective tissue formation. Copper is part of several enzymes and proteins that are essential for an adequate use of iron by the body. Copper is required for the formation of hemoglobin, red blood cells, and bones. It also helps with the formation of collagen and elastin, making them available for wound healing. Copper is useful to maintain joint and nerve health. Copper deficiency may lead to anemia, neutropenia, hypopigmentation, and abnormalities in the skeletal, cardiovascular, and immune system. Copper is present in many common foods, including legumes (beans), grains, and nuts	Copper contributes to normal skin and hair pigmentation and protects cell constituents from oxidative damage
Biotin	*Approved claim*:
Biotin, also known as vitamin H, is a water-soluble B vitamin. It is an essential coenzyme for several important enzymes, and it is necessary for cell growth, energy production, and maintenance of adequate blood sugar levels. Biotin helps in the production of fatty acids and the metabolism of amino acids. It is sometimes used as part of weight reduction efforts. Proper fat production is critical for the health of the skin because fatty acids protect skin cells against damage and water loss. Biotin is often recommended as a dietary supplement for strengthening hair and	Biotin contributes to the maintenance of normal skin and hair

(*continued*)

Table 1 (continued)

PROPERTIES	BENEFITS/APPROVED CLAIMS
nails, and it is found in many cosmetic and health products for hair and skin. Biotin deficiency may lead to developmental delay in children and to skin and hair disorders. Food rich in biotin include egg yolk, liver, and some vegetables	
Bioperine®	
Bioperine® is an extract derived from black pepper, *Piper nigrum*. Piperine is what gives peppers their spicy taste. This extract is marketed as a nutritional supplement, and it is believed to enhance cell bioavailability and so to increase the absorption of a variety of nutrients [81, 82]	Black pepper extract is clinically proven to increase bioavailability by 60 %
Glucosamine hydrochloride	
Glucosamine is a derivative of cellular glucose metabolism. It is also a component of glycosaminoglycans and proteoglycans of the cartilage matrix, covering the ends of bones, and hyaluronic acid which is a part of the synovial fluid within the joints. The primary source of exogenous glucosamine is the exoskeleton of shellfish. It exists in primarily two formulations, glucosamine hydrochloride and glucosamine sulfate. Glucosamine hydrochloride lacks the sulfate group and has 99 % purity. Glucosamine is readily absorbed from the gastrointestinal tract with oral administration, rapidly undergoes metabolism via the liver, and is eliminated through feces and urine. Because glucosamine is a part of the cartilage matrix in joint tissues, it has been theorized for many years that its administration could affect symptomatic relief for osteoarthritis	Glucosamine and chondroitin sulfate are often used together in the treatment of osteoarthritis [83–85]
L-Carnitine	
L-Carnitine is a naturally occurring compound, synthesized in the body from the essential amino acids lysine and methionine. L-carnitine is mainly found in the skeletal muscle, where it is required for the transport of fatty acids from the cytosol into the mitochondria for the beta-oxidation process. For its properties in increasing oxidative metabolism of fatty acids and muscle glycogen, supplementation of carnitine could have a potential role in muscular performance enhancement, in mental function increase and may be considered as a fat burner in weight loss diets (although all these properties need further scientific investigation)	Although the results present in literature related to the role of L-carnitine to improve energy performance are controversial, some studies have shown that this compound can positively impact the muscle recovery process after exercise, therefore allowing a more active lifestyle [86, 87]
Chondroitin sulfate	
Chondroitin sulfate is a sulfated glycosaminoglycan. It is usually found attached to proteins as part of a proteoglycan. Chondroitin sulfate is an important structural component of cartilage and provides much of its resistance to compression. Along with glucosamine, chondroitin sulfate has become a widely used dietary supplement for the treatment of osteoarthritis	Chondroitin sulfate and glucosamine sulfate have been shown to exert beneficial effects on the metabolism of *in vitro* models of cells derived from synovial joints: chondrocytes, synoviocytes, and cells from subchondral bone, all of which are involved in osteoarthritis. They increase type II collagen and proteoglycan synthesis in human articular chondrocytes and are also able to reduce the production of some pro-inflammatory mediators and proteases, to reduce cellular death process, and to improve the anabolic/catabolic balance of the extracellular cartilage matrix [88]. *See glucosamine hydrochloride above for other references*

(*continued*)

Table 1 (continued)

PROPERTIES	BENEFITS/APPROVED CLAIMS
Resveratrol	
Resveratrol is an antioxidant polyphenol found in the skin of red grapes and in other fruits. It has several benefits: cardiovascular system (via increased nitric oxide production, downregulation of vasoactive peptides, lowered levels of oxidized low-density lipoprotein, and cyclooxygenase inhibition), Alzheimer's disease (by breakdown of beta-amyloid and direct effects on neural tissues), phytohormonal actions, anticancer properties (via modulation of signal transduction, which translates into anti-initiation, anti-promotion, and anti-progression effects), and antimicrobial effects [89]	A study showed that resveratrol helped to increase the rate of skin fibroblast proliferation and inhibited collagenase activity [90]. In fact, resveratrol is used also for skin care formulations against a wide range of cutaneous disorders including skin aging and skin cancers [91]. Also, resveratrol is responsible for epidermal homeostasis and has therefore potential cosmetic and/or dermatological applications [74]
Acai berry	
The fruit of *Euterpe oleracea*, commonly known as acai berry, has been shown to exhibit significantly high antioxidant activity *in vitro*, especially as a scavenger for superoxide and peroxyl radicals, and it has therefore health benefits	Together with licorice, green tea, arbutin, soy, turmeric, and pomegranate, acai berry exhibits strong antioxidant properties, and it is among those plants and compounds found to be most beneficial to treat skin hyperpigmentation [92] It is a natural compound often used in cosmetic dermatology [93]
Coenzyme Q10	
Coenzyme Q10 (CoQ10) is an antioxidant, and it is a vitamin-like substance found throughout the body, especially in the heart, liver, kidney, and pancreas. It is present in most eukaryotic cells, primarily in the mitochondria. This molecule can exist in a completely oxidized form and a completely reduced form, and this enables it to perform its functions as an antioxidant [94]. Besides endogenous synthesis, CoQ10 is also supplied to the organism by various foods (present in small amounts in meat and seafood)	CoQ10 positively influences the age-affected cellular metabolism and helps to counteract signs of aging at the cellular level. As a consequence to topical application, CoQ10 is beneficial for human skin as it rapidly improves mitochondrial function in skin *in vivo* [95]. Moreover, CoQ10 has been shown to promote proliferation of fibroblasts, increase collagen expression, and reduce UVR-induced matrix metalloproteinases. It also increased elastin production, and it was shown to have depigmentation properties [96]
Pomegranate	
Pomegranate is rich of polyphenols and has therefore antioxidant properties which have been shown to have health-promoting effects [97]. In fact, the oil of pomegranate contains ellagic acid, which is a natural phenol antioxidant and it is found in many fruits and is believed to have anticancer properties	Pomegranate is considered part of the botanic ingredients used in the prevention of skin aging [98]. Moreover, it was shown that ellagic acid, of which pomegranate is rich, prevented collagen destruction and inflammatory responses caused by UVB. Therefore, its dietary supplementation may be a promising treatment strategy to reduce skin wrinkling and inflammation (which come with photoaging) [99]
Lycopene	
Lycopene is known to be one of the most effective antioxidants in the carotenoids family, with excellent stability and bioavailability. Its powerful antioxidant activity is effective in maintaining the strength, thickness, and fluidity of cellular membranes which form the cell external layer. Strong and healthy cellular membranes are of pivotal importance in the prevention from many diseases. Moreover, lycopene acts as an antioxidant preventing free radicals from disrupting the balance of new bone formation and bone loss that naturally occurs with age [100]	Carotenoids are widely used in the cosmetic industry as skin care products [101]. Moreover, it has been shown that β-carotene and lycopene are able to modulate skin properties when ingested as supplements or as dietary products. While they cannot be compared with sunscreen, there is evidence that they protect the skin against sunburn (solar erythema) by increasing the basal defense against UV light-mediated damage [102]

(continued)

Table 1 (continued)

PROPERTIES	BENEFITS/APPROVED CLAIMS
L-Carnosine	
Carnosine is an endogenous free radical scavenger. It is concentrated in muscles when they are working, and it is also found in the heart, brain, and many other parts of the body. Carnosine is used to prevent aging and to prevent or treat complications of diabetes such as nerve damage, eye disorders (cataracts), and kidney problems	The latest research has indicated that apart from the function of protecting cells from oxidation-induced stress damage, carnosine is able to extend the lifespan of cultured cells, rejuvenate senescent cells, and maintain cellular homeostasis [103]. Thus, carnosine-containing products can be used in preparations to reduce skin wrinkles [104, 105]

collagen binds to receptors present on the membrane of fibroblasts and stimulates the production of new collagen, elastin, and hyaluronic acid.

2. **Reduction in solar elastosis and in hyperkeratosis**, Fig. 7.

   Histological sections of healthy skin (by hematoxylin-eosin staining) relative to two female subjects before and after 90 days of treatment with GOLD COLLAGEN® FORTE revealed a reduction in epidermal hyperkeratosis and of solar elastosis in the dermis.
3. **Self-assessment questionnaire outcome**.

   The subjects' perception of GOLD COLLAGEN® FORTE versus placebo on skin, hair, nails, joints, and mood and their feedback about the product were further investigated. Results from the self-assessment questionnaires showed that the perception of the overall skin, hair, nails, and joints condition was dramatically improved after 90 days of treatment. Importantly, these improvements were not observed in the subjects taking placebo.

   Together with other cosmetic treatments or taken alone, daily consumption of a liquid hydrolyzed collagen-based nutritional supplement, such as GOLD COLLAGEN® FORTE, led to significant benefits in terms of efficacy and patient compliance, suggesting that hydrolyzed collagen can help counteract signs of aging and boost the effect of cosmetic treatments (Fig.6 and Fig.7).

Preliminary Results Obtained with ACTIVE GOLD COLLAGEN®

An in-house clinical trial has been carried out to evaluate the effect of the systemic treatment with a hydrolyzed collagen-based nutraceutical supplement, such as ACTIVE GOLD COLLAGEN®, on collagen density, skin elasticity, and body composition in healthy and active volunteer subjects.

The study was conducted in 20 male volunteer subjects aged 20–60 years. Each subject was administered 1 × 50 ml daily dosage for a maximum of 14 weeks.

In summary this study showed:

1. **Increase in skin elasticity**, Fig. 8.

   An increase in skin elasticity was observed at 7 and 14 weeks in the subjects who were taking ACTIVE GOLD COLLAGEN® with a statistically significant improvement detected at week 14 (65% increase).
2. **Increase in collagen density**, Fig. 9.

   The same subjects were also measured for collagen density in the ventral forearm. In 55% of the subjects, a constant statistically significant increase was observed in the collagen density over 14 weeks.

   This study supports published literature demonstrating increased collagen production in the skin as a result of an oral treatment with collagen peptides [106].
3. **Improvement in body composition and fitness level**, Fig. 10.

   Body fat, muscle mass, bone density, and hydration were measured in the 20 subjects

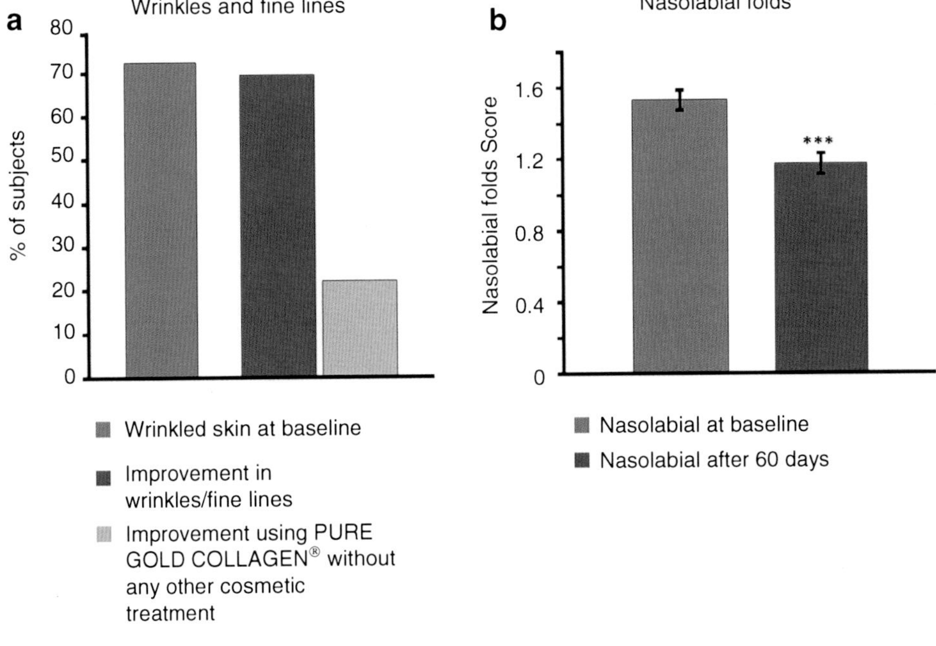

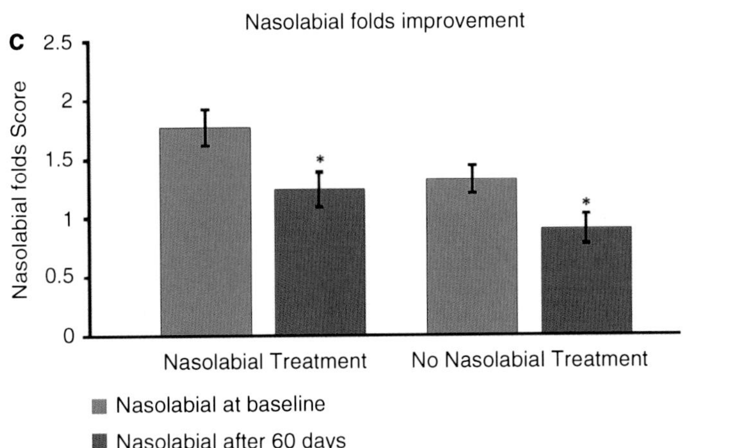

Fig. 3 Percentage of subjects showing an improvement in wrinkles (**a**) and an improvement in the average score of nasolabial folds (**b**) after 60 days of treatment with PURE GOLD COLLAGEN®. (**c**) Significant and comparable decrease of nasolabial folds, after 60 days, both in subjects who underwent a specific treatment for nasolabial folds or not.

who took part in this study using Ozeri Touch II Digital Scale, a multifunction scale that provides profile-driven measurements for these parameters. A decrease in weight and body fat was detected over the 14-week treatment with ACTIVE GOLD COLLAGEN®, together with an improvement in hydration, muscle mass, and bone density (Fig. 10).

As shown in Table 2, the resting heart rate can vary according to the fitness level and with age: the fitter a person is, generally the lower the resting heart rate. This is due to the heart getting bigger and stronger with exercise and getting more efficient at pumping blood around the body – so at rest more blood can be pumped around with each beat, and therefore, less beats per minute are required. In 55 % of the

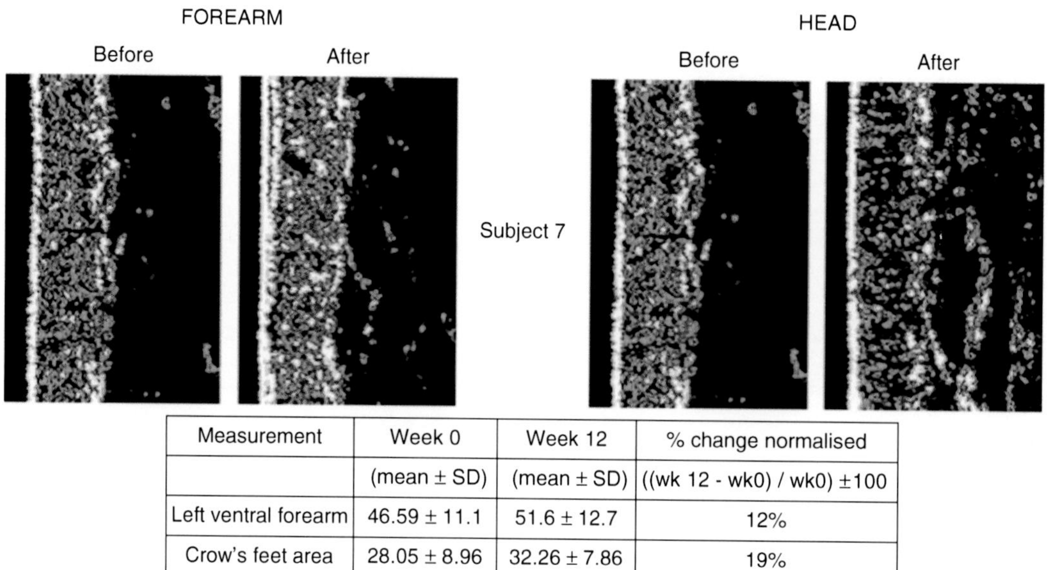

Measurement	Week 0	Week 12	% change normalised
	(mean ± SD)	(mean ± SD)	((wk 12 - wk0) / wk0) ±100
Left ventral forearm	46.59 ± 11.1	51.6 ± 12.7	12%
Crow's feet area	28.05 ± 8.96	32.26 ± 7.86	19%

Fig. 4 Collagen density measurements in the left ventral forearm and in the crow's feet area around the left eye. An increase in collagen density (12 % increase in forearm and 19 % in the crow's feet area) is clearly visible after 12 weeks in the both areas measured.

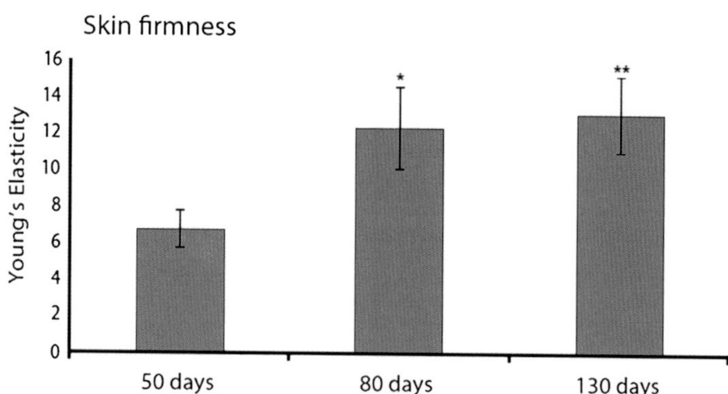

Fig. 5 Increase in skin firmness after 80 and 130 days.

subjects, a 9 % reduction in the resting heart rate (from 71 to 64 on average) was noticed after 5 weeks (Fig. 10). According to Table 2, this means that those subjects moved from an average level (highlighted in yellow) to a good level (highlighted in cyan) of fitness, improving their performances.

These results suggest that daily oral consumption of a dietary supplement containing collagen peptides, vitamins, and minerals, in this case ACTIVE GOLD COLLAGEN®, does lead to a detectable improvement in skin properties, such as elasticity and collagen density. Moreover, the active ingredients present in this liquid supplement have a positive effect on the level of fitness, muscle mass, bone density and decrease body fat and resting heart rate (Fig. 8, Fig. 9, Fig. 10 and Table 2).

Conclusions

Innovation in Liquid Hydrolyzed Collagen-Based Supplementation

The novelty of nutraceutical supplements (sometimes referred to as *nutricosmeceuticals*) for skin care, such as GOLD COLLAGEN® products, is

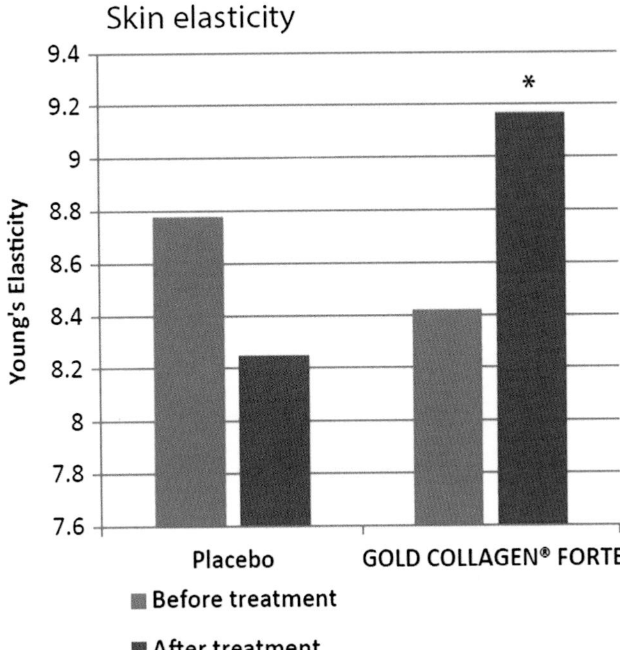

Fig. 6 Overall increase in skin elasticity in subjects consuming GOLD COLLAGEN® FORTE versus placebo for 90 days.

based on their orally ingestible formulation and the use of the highest-quality hydrolyzed collagen together with a specific blend of active ingredients that can be easily absorbed and distributed, by the bloodstream, throughout the whole body.

Many topical collagen-containing products such as creams, lotions, and serums are unable to reach the dermis to boost the production of skin collagen. This is because collagen has a large molecular size and cannot penetrate the skin surface (epidermis). A daily oral intake of a product containing hydrolyzed collagen is therefore more effective, as collagen peptides are able to reach the dermis from the inside, with no need to penetrate the epidermis. Liquid nutritional supplements are easier to swallow than a pill and work from within, in the dermis, to nourish and rejuvenate your skin.

Proven Benefits of GOLD COLLAGEN® Products

Several independent clinical trials have shown visible and significant benefits on skin, hair, and nails after daily intake of GOLD COLLAGEN® nutricosmeceutical supplements. The subjects taking these hydrolyzed collagen-based drinks also perceived an improvement in their mood and energy levels. Additional clinical trials and explorative research projects are currently in progress to further investigate the benefits and mechanisms of action of these supplements.

Nutricosmeceutical products represent an innovative and powerful tool in the fight against skin aging. It is important to underline how the interaction between the ensemble of all the ingredients present in these liquid supplements, such as GOLD COLLAGEN® products, gives these nutricosmeceuticals the ability to have a multipurpose action so to benefit not only the skin but also other structures of the connective tissue such as hair and nails, to boost the body's energy and to contribute to the person's general well-being. Although aging is in fact an irreversible biological process, which is mostly visible on skin, it involves the whole body leading to a slow and progressive deterioration of all human tissues, particularly cartilage in the joints. In this context, nutricosmeceutical supplements containing collagen peptides and other active ingredients, such as vitamins, minerals, and antioxidants, might appear to represent a powerful tool to slow down the aging process.

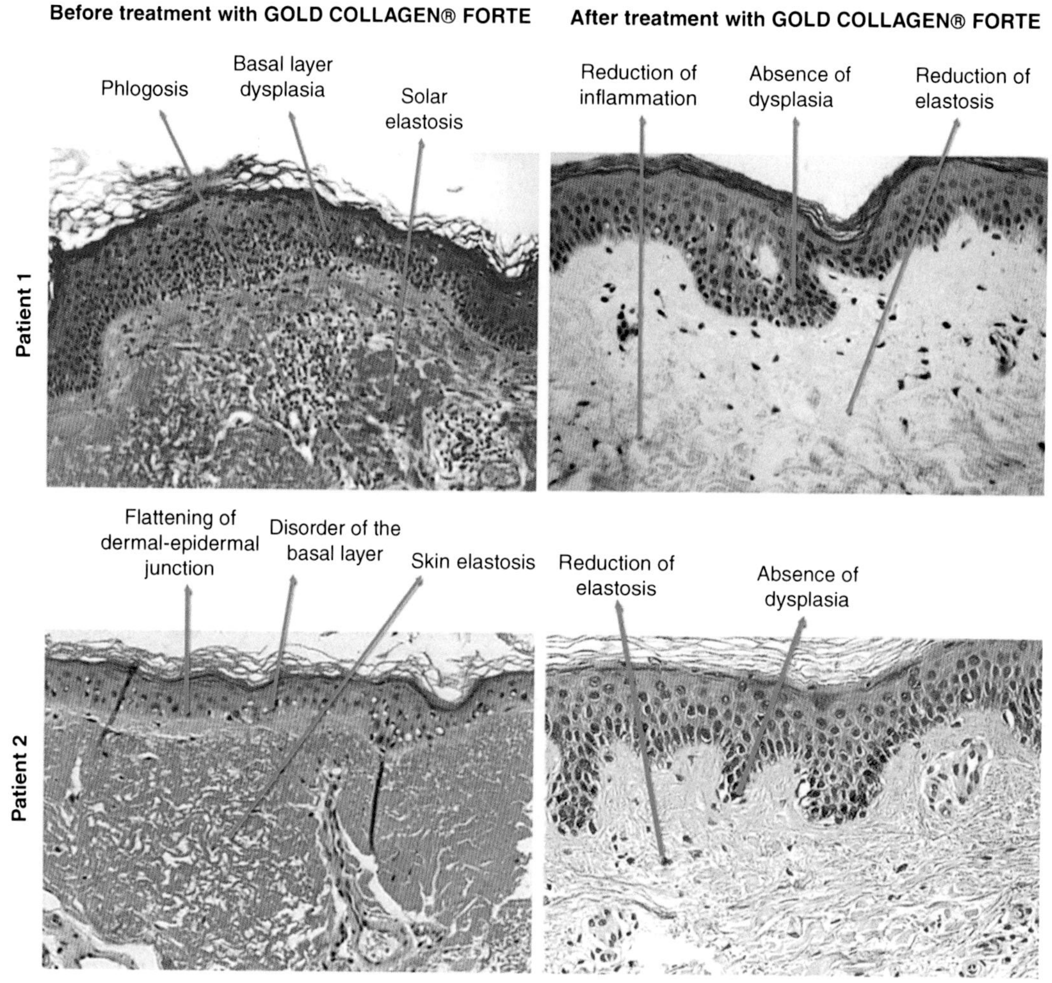

Before treatment with GOLD COLLAGEN® FORTE
After treatment with GOLD COLLAGEN® FORTE
Phlogosis
Basal layer dysplasia
Solar elastosis
Reduction of inflammation
Absence of dysplasia
Reduction of elastosis
Patient 1
Flattening of dermal-epidermal junction
Disorder of the basal layer
Skin elastosis
Reduction of elastosis
Absence of dysplasia
Patient 2

Fig. 7 Skin histological sections from two patients before and after treatment with GOLD COLLAGEN® FORTE.

Skin elasticity
Skin Elasticity (VE)
% OF CHANGE FROM WEEK 0
70
60
50
40
30
20
10
0
*
0
7
14
WEEKS

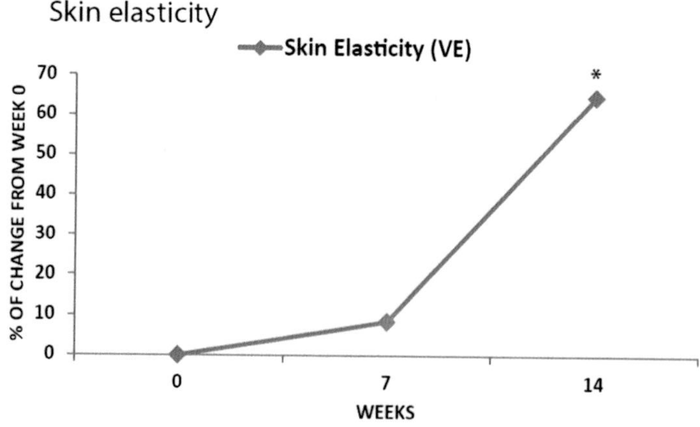

Fig. 8 Increase in skin elasticity (*blue line*) at 7 and 14 weeks of treatment ($* = p \leq 0.05$).

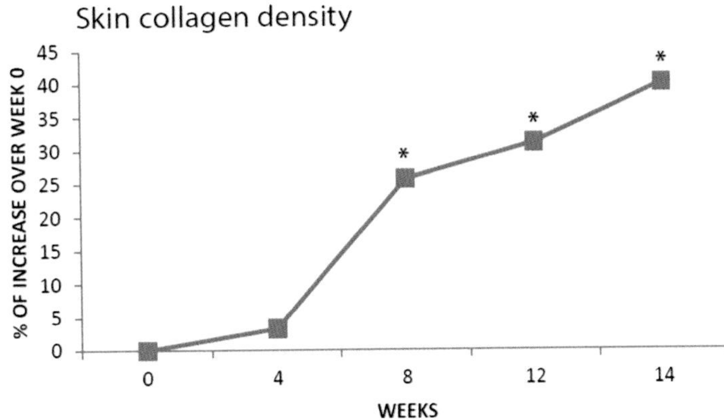

Fig. 9 Increase in collagen density in 55 % of the subjects after 4, 8, 12, and 14 weeks of treatment.

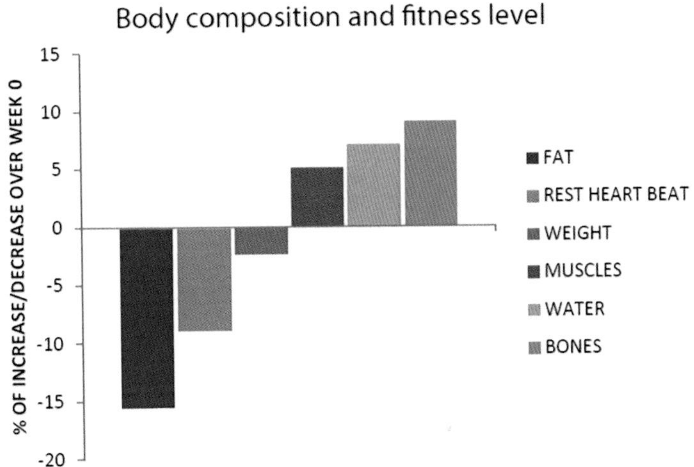

Fig. 10 Effects of ACTIVE GOLD COLLAGEN® on body fat, muscle mass, bone density, hydration, and heart beat at rest.

Table 2 Chart relating resting heart rate and fitness level.

Resting heart rate for men						
Age	**18–25**	**26–35**	**36–45**	**46–55**	**56–65**	65+
Athlete	49–55	49–54	50–56	50–57	51–56	50–55
Excellent	56–61	55–61	57–62	58–63	57–61	56–61
Good	62–65	62–65	63–66	64–67	62–67	62–65
Above average	66–69	66–70	67–70	68–71	68–71	66–69
Average	70–73	71–74	71–75	72–76	72–75	70–73
Below average	74–81	75–81	76–82	77–83	76–81	74–79
Poor	82+	82+	83+	84+	82+	80+

Acknowledgments We would like to thank Dr. Martin Godfrey for his time and expertise in critically reviewing the manuscript. We would also like to thank all the dermatologists who collected the data, in particular Professor Andrea Corbo.

References

1. Kligman LH. Photoaging. Manifestations, prevention, and treatment. Clin Geriatr Med. 1989;5:235–51.
2. Guercio-Hauer C, Macfarlane DF, Deleo VA. Photodamage, photoaging and photoprotection of the skin. Am Fam Physician. 1994;50:327–32. 34.
3. Naylor EC, Watson RE, Sherratt MJ. Molecular aspects of skin ageing. Maturitas. 2011;69:249–56.
4. Baumann L. Skin ageing and its treatment. J Pathol. 2007;211:241–51.
5. Bickers DR, Athar M. Oxidative stress in the pathogenesis of skin disease. J Invest Dermatol. 2006;126:2565–75.
6. Harman D. Free radical theory of aging: an update: increasing the functional life span. Ann N Y Acad Sci. 2006;1067:10–21.
7. Benz CC, Yau C. Ageing, oxidative stress and cancer: paradigms in parallax. Nat Rev Cancer. 2008;8:875–9.
8. Van Raamsdonk JM, Hekimi S. Deletion of the mitochondrial superoxide dismutase sod-2 extends lifespan in *Caenorhabditis elegans*. PLoS Genet. 2009;5:e1000361.
9. Speakman JR, Selman C. The free-radical damage theory: accumulating evidence against a simple link of oxidative stress to ageing and lifespan. Bioessays. 2011;33:255–9.
10. Tanaka M, Koyama Y, Nomura Y. Effects of collagen peptide ingestion on UV-B-induced skin damage. Biosci Biotechnol Biochem. 2009;73:930–2.
11. Shibuya S, Ozawa Y, Toda T, Watanabe K, Tometsuka C, Ogura T, Koyama Y, Shimizu T. Collagen peptide and vitamin C additively attenuate age-related skin atrophy in Sod1-deficient mice. Biosci Biotechnol Biochem. 2014;78:1212–20.
12. Yoon HS, Cho HH, Cho S, Lee SR, Shin MH, Chung JH. Supplementating with dietary astaxanthin combined with collagen hydrolysate improves facial elasticity and decreases matrix metalloproteinase-1 and -12 expression: a comparative study with placebo. J Med Food. 2014;17:810–6.
13. Borumand M, Sibilla S. Daily consumption of the collagen supplement Pure Gold Collagen(R) reduces visible signs of aging. Clin Interv Aging. 2014;9:1747–58.
14. Borumand M, Sibilla S. A study to assess the effect on wrinkles of a nutritional supplement containing high dosage of hydrolysed collagen. Cosmeceuticals 2014;2014:93–96.
15. Borumand M, Sibilla S. Effects of a nutritional supplement containing collagen peptides on skin elasticity, hydration and wrinkles. J Med Nutr Nutraceuticals 2015;4:47–53.
16. Freinkel RK, Woodley DT. The biology of the skin. Pantheon Publishing, USA (New York) and UK (London), 2001.
17. Wickett RR, Visscher MO. Structure and function of the epidermal barrier. Am J Infect Control. 2006;34:98–110.
18. Le Fur I, Reinberg A, Lopez S, Morizot F, Mechkouri M, Tschachler E. Analysis of circadian and ultradian rhythms of skin surface properties of face and forearm of healthy women. J Invest Dermatol. 2001;117:718–24.
19. Matsuo T, Yamaguchi S, Mitsui S, Emi A, Shimoda F, Okamura H. Control mechanism of the circadian clock for timing of cell division in vivo. Science. 2003;302:255–9.
20. Geyfman M, Kumar V, Liu Q, Ruiz R, Gordon W, Espitia F, Cam E, Millar SE, Smyth P, Ihler A, Takahashi JS, Andersen B. Brain and muscle Arnt-like protein-1 (BMAL1) controls circadian cell proliferation and susceptibility to UVB-induced DNA damage in the epidermis. Proc Natl Acad Sci U S A. 2012;109:11758–63.
21. Ricard-Blum S. The collagen family. Cold Spring Harb Perspect Biol. 2011;3:a004978.
22. Matsuda N, Koyama Y, Hosaka Y, Ueda H, Watanabe T, Araya T, Irie S, Takehana K. Effects of ingestion of collagen peptide on collagen fibrils and glycosaminoglycans in the dermis. J Nutr Sci Vitaminol (Tokyo). 2006;52:211–5.
23. Gelse K, Poschl E, Aigner T. Collagens – structure, function, and biosynthesis. Adv Drug Deliv Rev. 2003;55:1531–46.
24. Fleischmajer R, MacDonald ED, Perlish JS, Burgeson RE, Fisher LW. Dermal collagen fibrils are hybrids of type I and type III collagen molecules. J Struct Biol. 1990;105:162–9.
25. Hinz B. Formation and function of the myofibroblast during tissue repair. J Invest Dermatol. 2007;127:526–37.
26. Langness U, Udenfriend S. Collagen biosynthesis in nonfibroblastic cell lines. Proc Natl Acad Sci U S A. 1974;71:50–1.
27. Shuster S, Black MM, McVitie E. The influence of age and sex on skin thickness, skin collagen and density. Br J Dermatol. 1975;93:639–43.
28. Wagenseil JE, Mecham RP. New insights into elastic fiber assembly. Birth Defects Res C Embryo Today. 2007;81:229–40.
29. Laurent TC, Fraser JR. Hyaluronan. FASEB J. 1992;6:2397–404.
30. Fraser JR, Laurent TC, Laurent UB. Hyaluronan: its nature, distribution, functions and turnover. J Intern Med. 1997;242:27–33.
31. Balogh L, Polyak A, Mathe D, Kiraly R, Thuroczy J, Terez M, Janoki G, Ting Y, Bucci LR, Schauss AG. Absorption, uptake and tissue affinity of high-molecular-weight hyaluronan after oral administration in rats and dogs. J Agric Food Chem. 2008;56:10582–93.
32. Ohara H, Ichikawa S, Matsumoto H, Akiyama M, Fujimoto N, Kobayashi T, Tajima S. Collagen-derived dipeptide, proline-hydroxyproline, stimulates

cell proliferation and hyaluronic acid synthesis in cultured human dermal fibroblasts. J Dermatol. 2010;37:330–8.

33. Pavicic T, Gauglitz GG, Lersch P, Schwach-Abdellaoui K, Malle B, Korting HC, Farwick M. Efficacy of cream-based novel formulations of hyaluronic acid of different molecular weights in anti-wrinkle treatment. J Drugs Dermatol. 2011;10:990–1000.
34. Farwick M, Gauglitz G, Pavicic T, Kohler T, Wegmann M, Schwach-Abdellaoui K, Malle B, Tarabin V, Schmitz G, Korting HC. Fifty-kDa hyaluronic acid upregulates some epidermal genes without changing TNF-alpha expression in reconstituted epidermis. Skin Pharmacol Physiol. 2011;24:210–7.
35. Oikarinen A. The aging of skin: chronoaging versus photoaging. Photodermatol Photoimmunol Photomed. 1990;7:3–4.
36. Varani J, Dame MK, Rittie L, Fligiel SE, Kang S, Fisher GJ, Voorhees JJ. Decreased collagen production in chronologically aged skin: roles of age-dependent alteration in fibroblast function and defective mechanical stimulation. Am J Pathol. 2006;168:1861–8.
37. Varani J, Spearman D, Perone P, Fligiel SE, Datta SC, Wang ZQ, Shao Y, Kang S, Fisher GJ, Voorhees JJ. Inhibition of type I procollagen synthesis by damaged collagen in photoaged skin and by collagenase-degraded collagen in vitro. Am J Pathol. 2001;158:931–42.
38. Varani J, Perone P, Fligiel SE, Fisher GJ, Voorhees JJ. Inhibition of type I procollagen production in photodamage: correlation between presence of high molecular weight collagen fragments and reduced procollagen synthesis. J Invest Dermatol. 2002;119:122–9.
39. Varani J, Schuger L, Dame MK, Leonard C, Fligiel SE, Kang S, Fisher GJ, Voorhees JJ. Reduced fibroblast interaction with intact collagen as a mechanism for depressed collagen synthesis in photodamaged skin. J Invest Dermatol. 2004;122:1471–9.
40. Allsopp RC, Vaziri H, Patterson C, Goldstein S, Younglai EV, Futcher AB, Greider CW, Harley CB. Telomere length predicts replicative capacity of human fibroblasts. Proc Natl Acad Sci U S A. 1992;89:10114–8.
41. Puizina-Ivic N. Skin aging. Acta Dermatovenerol Alp Pannonica Adriat. 2008;17:47–54.
42. Berneburg M, Plettenberg H, Krutmann J. Photoaging of human skin. Photodermatol Photoimmunol Photomed. 2000;16:239–44.
43. Millis AJ, Sottile J, Hoyle M, Mann DM, Diemer V. Collagenase production by early and late passage cultures of human fibroblasts. Exp Gerontol. 1989;24:559–75.
44. Quan T, Little E, Quan H, Qin Z, Voorhees JJ, Fisher GJ. Elevated matrix metalloproteinases and collagen fragmentation in photodamaged human skin: impact of altered extracellular matrix microenvironment on dermal fibroblast function. J Invest Dermatol. 2013;133:1362–6.
45. Quan T, Qin Z, Xia W, Shao Y, Voorhees JJ, Fisher GJ. Matrix-degrading metalloproteinases in photoaging. J Investig Dermatol Symp Proc. 2009;14:20–4.
46. Fisher GJ, Wang ZQ, Datta SC, Varani J, Kang S, Voorhees JJ. Pathophysiology of premature skin aging induced by ultraviolet light. N Engl J Med. 1997;337:1419–28.
47. Vayalil PK, Mittal A, Hara Y, Elmets CA, Katiyar SK. Green tea polyphenols prevent ultraviolet light-induced oxidative damage and matrix metalloproteinases expression in mouse skin. J Invest Dermatol. 2004;122:1480–7.
48. El-Domyati M, Attia S, Saleh F, Brown D, Birk DE, Gasparro F, Ahmad H, Uitto J. Intrinsic aging vs. photoaging: a comparative histopathological, immunohistochemical, and ultrastructural study of skin. Exp Dermatol. 2002;11:398–405.
49. Tanaka H, Ono Y, Nakata S, Shintani Y, Sakakibara N, Morita A. Tobacco smoke extract induces premature skin aging in mouse. J Dermatol Sci. 2007;46:69–71.
50. Perricone N. The wrinkle cure: unlock the power of cosmeceuticals for supple, youthful skin. New York: Warner books; 2001.
51. Prottey C. Essential fatty acids and the skin. Br J Dermatol. 1976;94:579–85.
52. Dykes PJ, Marks R, Davies MG, Reynolds DJ. Epidermal metabolism in heredopathia atactica polyneuritiformis (Refsum's disease). J Invest Dermatol. 1978;70:126–9.
53. Lambert CA, Soudant EP, Nusgens BV, Lapiere CM. Pretranslational regulation of extracellular matrix macromolecules and collagenase expression in fibroblasts by mechanical forces. Lab Invest. 1992;66:444–51.
54. Oesser S, Adam M, Babel W, Seifert J. Oral administration of(14)C labeled gelatin hydrolysate leads to an accumulation of radioactivity in cartilage of mice (C57/BL). J Nutr. 1999;129:1891–5.
55. Iwai K, Hasegawa T, Taguchi Y, Morimatsu F, Sato K, Nakamura Y, Higashi A, Kido Y, Nakabo Y, Ohtsuki K. Identification of food-derived collagen peptides in human blood after oral ingestion of gelatin hydrolysates. J Agric Food Chem. 2005;53:6531–6.
56. Watanabe-Kamiyama M, Shimizu M, Kamiyama S, Taguchi Y, Sone H, Morimatsu F, Shirakawa H, Furukawa Y, Komai M. Absorption and effectiveness of orally administered low molecular weight collagen hydrolysate in rats. J Agric Food Chem. 2010;58:835–41.
57. Chen RH, Hsu C, Chung MY, Tsai WL, Liu CH. Effect of different concentrations of collagen, ceramides, *n*-acetyl glucosamine, or their mixture on enhancing the proliferation of keratinocytes, fibroblasts and the secretion of collagen and/or the

expression of mRNA of type i collagen. J Food Drug Anal. 2008;16:66–74.

58. Matsumoto H, Ohara H, Ito K, Nakamura Y, Takahashi S. Clinical effect of fish type I collagen hydrolysate on skin properties. ITE Lett. 2006;7:386–390.
59. Ohara H, Ito K, Iida H, Matsumoto H. Improvement in the moisture content of the stratum corneum following 4 weeks of collagen hydrolysate ingestion. Nippon Shokuhin Kogaku Kaishi. 2009;56:137–145.
60. Koyama Y. Effect of collagen peptide on the skin. Shokuhinto Kaihatsu. 2009;44:10–12.
61. Proksch E, Segger D, Degwert J, Schunck M, Zague V, Oesser S. Oral supplementation of specific collagen peptides has beneficial effects on human skin physiology: a double-blind, placebo-controlled study. Skin Pharmacol Physiol. 2014;27:47–55.
62. Ziboh VA, Miller CC. Essential fatty acids and polyunsaturated fatty acids: significance in cutaneous biology. Annu Rev Nutr. 1990;10:433–50.
63. De Spirt S, Stahl W, Tronnier H, Sies H, Bejot M, Maurette JM, Heinrich U. Intervention with flaxseed and borage oil supplements modulates skin condition in women. Br J Nutr. 2009;101:440–5.
64. Foster RH, Hardy G, Alany RG. Borage oil in the treatment of atopic dermatitis. Nutrition. 2010;26:708–18.
65. Bamford JT, Ray S, Musekiwa A, van Gool C, Humphreys R, Ernst E. Oral evening primrose oil and borage oil for eczema. Cochrane Database Syst Rev. 2013;4:CD004416.
66. Bath-Hextall FJ, Jenkinson C, Humphreys R, Williams HC. Dietary supplements for established atopic eczema. Cochrane Database Syst Rev. 2012;2: CD005205.
67. Murad H, Tabibian MP. The effect of an oral supplement containing glucosamine, amino acids, minerals, and antioxidants on cutaneous aging: a preliminary study. J Dermatolog Treat. 2001;12:47–51.
68. Wang Z, Yin S, Zhao X, Russell RM. Tang G: beta-Carotene-vitamin A equivalence in Chinese adults assessed by an isotope dilution technique. Br J Nutr. 2004;91:121–31.
69. Fuchs E, Green H. Regulation of terminal differentiation of cultured human keratinocytes by vitamin A. Cell. 1981;25:617–25.
70. Fisher GJ, Talwar HS, Lin J, Voorhees JJ. Molecular mechanisms of photoaging in human skin in vivo and their prevention by all-trans retinoic acid. Photochem Photobiol. 1999;69:154–7.
71. Surjana D, Damian DL. Nicotinamide in dermatology and photoprotection. Skinmed. 2011;9:360–5.
72. Brescoll J, Daveluy S. A review of vitamin B12 in dermatology. Am J Clin Dermatol. 2015;16:27–33.
73. Tran D, Townley JP, Barnes TM, Greive KA. An antiaging skin care system containing alpha hydroxy acids and vitamins improves the biomechanical parameters of facial skin. Clin Cosmet Investig Dermatol. 2015;8:9–17.
74. Lorencini M, Brohem CA, Dieamant GC, Zanchin NI, Maibach HI. Active ingredients against human epidermal aging. Ageing Res Rev. 2014;15:100–15.
75. Fitzpatrick RE, Rostan EF. Double-blind, half-face study comparing topical vitamin C and vehicle for rejuvenation of photodamage. Dermatol Surg. 2002;28:231–6.
76. Gordon-Thomson C, Tongkao-on W, Song EJ, Carter SE, Dixon KM, Mason RS. Protection from ultraviolet damage and photocarcinogenesis by vitamin D compounds. Adv Exp Med Biol. 2014;810:303–28.
77. Leccia MT. Skin, sun exposure and vitamin D: facts and controversies. Ann Dermatol Venereol. 2013;140:176–82.
78. Schempp CM, Meinke MC, Lademann J, Ferrari Y, Brecht T, Gehring W. Topical antioxidants protect the skin from chemical-induced irritation in the repetitive washing test: a placebo-controlled, double-blind study. Contact Dermatitis. 2012;67:234–7.
79. Wu Y, Zheng X, Xu XG, Li YH, Wang B, Gao XH, Chen HD, Yatskayer M, Oresajo C. Protective effects of a topical antioxidant complex containing vitamins C and E and ferulic acid against ultraviolet irradiation-induced photodamage in Chinese women. J Drugs Dermatol. 2013;12:464–8.
80. Aggett PJ. Severe zinc deficiency. In: Colin F. Mills (ed.) Zinc in human biology. International Life Sciences Institute, Springer, London, 1989:259–79.
81. Umesh K Patil, Amrit Singh, Anup K Chakraborty. Role of piperine as a bioavailability enhancer. Int J Recent Adv Pharm Res. 2011;4:16–23.
82. Johnson JJ, Nihal M, Siddiqui IA, Scarlett CO, Bailey HH, Mukhtar H, Ahmad N. Enhancing the bioavailability of resveratrol by combining it with piperine. Mol Nutr Food Res. 2011;55:1169–76.
83. Henrotin Y, Lambert C. Chondroitin and glucosamine in the management of osteoarthritis: an update. Curr Rheumatol Rep. 2013;15:361.
84. Sawitzke AD, Shi H, Finco MF, Dunlop DD, Bingham 3rd CO, Harris CL, Singer NG, Bradley JD, Silver D, Jackson CG, Lane NE, Oddis CV, Wolfe F, Lisse J, Furst DE, Reda DJ, Moskowitz RW, Williams HJ, Clegg DO. The effect of glucosamine and/or chondroitin sulfate on the progression of knee osteoarthritis: a report from the glucosamine/chondroitin arthritis intervention trial. Arthritis Rheum. 2008;58:3183–91.
85. Clegg DO, Reda DJ, Harris CL, Klein MA, O'Dell JR, Hooper MM, Bradley JD, Bingham 3rd CO, Weisman MH, Jackson CG, Lane NE, Cush JJ, Moreland LW, Schumacher Jr HR, Oddis CV, Wolfe F, Molitor JA, Yocum DE, Schnitzer TJ, Furst DE, Sawitzke AD, Shi H, Brandt KD, Moskowitz RW, Williams HJ. Glucosamine, chondroitin sulfate, and the two in combination for painful knee osteoarthritis. N Engl J Med. 2006;354:795–808.

86. Wachter S, Vogt M, Kreis R, Boesch C, Bigler P, Hoppeler H, Krahenbuhl S. Long-term administration of L-carnitine to humans: effect on skeletal muscle carnitine content and physical performance. Clin Chim Acta. 2002;318:51–61.
87. Huang A, Owen K. Role of supplementary L-carnitine in exercise and exercise recovery. Med Sport Sci. 2012;59:135–42.
88. Henrotin Y, Marty M, Mobasheri A. What is the current status of chondroitin sulfate and glucosamine for the treatment of knee osteoarthritis? Maturitas. 2014;78:184–7.
89. Baxter RA. Anti-aging properties of resveratrol: review and report of a potent new antioxidant skin care formulation. J Cosmet Dermatol. 2008;7:2–7.
90. Giardina S, Michelotti A, Zavattini G, Finzi S, Ghisalberti C, Marzatico F. [Efficacy study in vitro: assessment of the properties of resveratrol and resveratrol + *N*-acetyl-cysteine on proliferation and inhibition of collagen activity]. Minerva Ginecol. 2010;62:195–201.
91. Ndiaye M, Philippe C, Mukhtar H, Ahmad N. The grape antioxidant resveratrol for skin disorders: promise, prospects, and challenges. Arch Biochem Biophys. 2011;508:164–70.
92. Fowler Jr JF, Woolery-Lloyd H, Waldorf H, Saini R. Innovations in natural ingredients and their use in skin care. J Drugs Dermatol. 2010;9:S72–81; quiz s2-3.
93. Baumann L, Woolery-Lloyd H, Friedman A. "Natural" ingredients in cosmetic dermatology. J Drugs Dermatol. 2009;8:s5–9.
94. Littarru GP, Tiano L. Bioenergetic and antioxidant properties of coenzyme Q10: recent developments. Mol Biotechnol. 2007;37:31–7.
95. Prahl S, Kueper T, Biernoth T, Wohrmann Y, Munster A, Furstenau M, Schmidt M, Schulze C, Wittern KP, Wenck H, Muhr GM, Blatt T. Aging skin is functionally anaerobic: importance of coenzyme Q10 for anti aging skin care. Biofactors. 2008;32:245–55.
96. Zhang M, Dang L, Guo F, Wang X, Zhao W, Zhao R. Coenzyme Q(10) enhances dermal elastin expression, inhibits IL-1alpha production and melanin synthesis in vitro. Int J Cosmet Sci. 2012;34:273–9.
97. Mertens-Talcott SU, Jilma-Stohlawetz P, Rios J, Hingorani L, Derendorf H. Absorption, metabolism, and antioxidant effects of pomegranate (Punica granatum l.) polyphenols after ingestion of a standardized extract in healthy human volunteers. J Agric Food Chem. 2006;54:8956–61.
98. Suggs A, Oyetakin-White P, Baron ED. Effect of botanicals on inflammation and skin aging: analyzing the evidence. Inflamm Allergy Drug Targets. 2014;13:168–76.
99. Bae JY, Choi JS, Kang SW, Lee YJ, Park J, Kang YH. Dietary compound ellagic acid alleviates skin wrinkle and inflammation induced by UV-B irradiation. Exp Dermatol. 2010;19:e182–90.
100. Rao LG, Krishnadev N, Banasikowska K, Rao AV. Lycopene I – effect on osteoclasts: lycopene inhibits basal and parathyroid hormone-stimulated osteoclast formation and mineral resorption mediated by reactive oxygen species in rat bone marrow cultures. J Med Food. 2003;6:69–78.
101. Schagen SK, Zampeli VA, Makrantonaki E, Zouboulis CC. Discovering the link between nutrition and skin aging. Dermatoendocrinology. 2012;4:298–307.
102. Stahl W, Heinrich U, Aust O, Tronnier H, Sies H. Lycopene-rich products and dietary photoprotection. Photochem Photobiol Sci. 2006;5:238–42.
103. Wang AM, Ma C, Xie ZH, Shen F. Use of carnosine as a natural anti-senescence drug for human beings. Biochemistry (Mosc). 2000;65:869–71.
104. Babizhayev MA, Deyev AI, Savel'yeva EL, Lankin VZ, Yegorov YE. Skin beautification with oral non-hydrolized versions of carnosine and carcinine: effective therapeutic management and cosmetic skincare solutions against oxidative glycation and free-radical production as a causal mechanism of diabetic complications and skin aging. J Dermatolog Treat. 2012;23:345–84.
105. Kaczvinsky JR, Griffiths CE, Schnicker MS, Li J. Efficacy of anti-aging products for periorbital wrinkles as measured by 3-D imaging. J Cosmet Dermatol. 2009;8:228–33.
106. Schwartz SR, Park J. Ingestion of BioCell Collagen ((R)), a novel hydrolyzed chicken sternal cartilage extract; enhanced blood microcirculation and reduced facial aging signs. Clin Interv Aging. 2012;7:267–73.

Neck Rejuvenation with Fractional CO_2 Laser

146

A. Deniz Akkaya and Yasemin Oram

Contents

Abstract

Treatment of the aging neck remains to be one of the most challenging aspects of the rejuvenative procedures, because of the unique aging pathogenesis and the limited healing capacities of this area. Although there are several surgical or nonsurgical techniques available for the treatment of the aging neck, successful results can only be achieved after establishing the main pathologic process and selecting the procedure accordingly for each individual patient. Consecutive to the advances in technology and the demand for noninvasive procedures, nonsurgical treatment modalities have gained popularity among the treatment options for aging neck. Ablative CO_2 laser rejuvenation has been considered the gold standard of resurfacing, resulting in impressive clinical improvements. However, the high incidence of side effects and long recovery period was an impetus for the development of the term "fractional photothermolysis." Ablative fractional resurfacing results in clinical improvements comparable or even superior to traditional ablative resurfacing, with a shorter down time and fewer side effects. Collagen remodeling that has been shown to continue for several months after the procedure is reflected as significant clinical improvements on skin tightening and texture. For a patient with an aging neck with prominent skin laxity, jowling, and pigmentary changes, fractional CO_2 laser resurfacing is a safe and effective

A.D. Akkaya (✉)
Department of Dermatology, Koç University Hospital, Istanbul, Turkey

Department of Dermatology, V.K. Foundation, American Hospital of Istanbul, Istanbul, Turkey
e-mail: drdenizakkaya@yahoo.com

Y. Oram
Department of Dermatology, V.K. Foundation, American Hospital of Istanbul, Istanbul, Turkey
e-mail: dryaseminoram@mynet.com

M.A. Farage et al. (eds.), *Textbook of Aging Skin*,
DOI 10.1007/978-3-662-47398-6_146

treatment alternative. However, procedure should be done with caution, with a thorough understanding of the laser-tissue interactions at various laser parameters used in different anatomic units, in order to achieve successful clinical results without side effects. Post-procedure frequent follow-up is also necessary for the early recognition of the signs of side effects that could result in scarring.

Introduction

Neck is an important part of the overall perception of a youthful appearance and is one of the first areas to reveal the signs of aging. When viewing an aging face, anterior neck is often captured first. Patients may lay a stress on the neck contour, even at the initial visit for facial rejuvenation [1]. Although facial rejuvenation is performed frequently, neck rejuvenation is often overlooked. Patients, who have gone under facial rejuvenation procedures, can be left with a demarcation line, between the face and the untreated neck [2]. On the other hand, patients may be interested in neck surgery alone [3].

In recent years, minimally invasive and noninvasive facial rejuvenation options have grown tremendously, consecutive to the advances in technology and the demand for noninvasive procedures, lacking downtime. Many of these options can be applied to the neck, including peelings, fillers and botulinum toxin injections, radiofrequency tissue tightening, phototherapy with lasers and light sources, and minimally invasive surgical rejuvenation techniques, either alone or in combination. However, improvement of the aging neck remains one of the most challenging aspects of rejuvenation procedures [4]. In order to achieve successful results and patient satisfaction, preoperative evaluation should address the individual patient's characteristics and include an appropriate patient-technique matching. Also, vigilant utilization of the selected procedure is crucial. Either alone or combined with other surgical or nonsurgical procedures, neck rejuvenation should be executed with significant caution, as the neck is very prone to scarring due to fewer pilosebaceous units and the limited healing properties.

Neck Aging

Neck is one of the first areas to show telltale signs of aging. The majority of changes associated with senescent appearance are related to photoaging, while chronological aging also plays a role. Photoaging is most prominent in people with fair skin complexions and is seen mostly on the frequently sun-exposed areas, including the neck [5]. Chronic sun damage is mainly responsible for pigmentary alterations, formation of benign and malignant growths, deep furrows, rhytides, and laxity of the skin, while the deleterious effects of solar radiation is on dermal connective tissue [6]. With aging, due to chronic sun damage, the mass of dermal collagen is reduced and elastic fibers lose their regular arrangement. Histologically, readily diminished dermal collagen is replaced by these rearranged elastic fibers and solar elastotic material, which is known as solar elastosis. Surface vascular changes can cause poikiloderma of Civatte. The skin develops laxity because of these alterations in connective tissue matrix, which is accentuated with the downward vector effect of the gravity. Submandibular glands may become ptotic. Dynamic changes in time cause hypertrophy of the platysma, leading to formation of platysmal bands. Fat accumulation or fat repositioning in the subcutaneous and subplatysmal planes results in localized adiposity, mainly provoked by changes in weight [4]. Bone resorption at the level of mentum and mandibular body results in loss of contours of the neck, a recessed chin, and changes at the cervicomandibular angle that contributes to the appearance of an aging neck [5]. Moreover, position of the hyoid bone, natural height of the cervical spine, and presence of arthritic changes on the cervical spine that modifies its height and curvature also affects the aesthetics of the neck [7].

Table 1 Brant and Bellman's classification of age-related neck degeneration [12, 13]

Category	Horizontal neck rhytides	Platysmal bands	Skin laxity	Jowls
I	Subtle	Only detectible with neck contraction	–	–
II	Mild	Thin	Mild	Minimal
III	Moderate	Moderate	Moderate	Moderate
IV	Deep	Severe hypertrophy at rest	Severe	Prominent

In summary, the related characteristics of an aging neck are the decreased skin quality and wrinkles, skin laxity, submental and subplatysmal lipodystrophy, prominent submandibular glands, platysmal bands and redundancy, with an increase at the cervicomandibular angle, loss of the definitive mandibular contours, and nasolabial jowls extending into to the neck [1, 8]. Hence, the skin represents the most conspicuous marker of the aging neck [9].

On the other hand, a youthful neck is described as follows: (1) a distinct inferior mandibular border from mentum to angle, with no jowl overhang; (2) subhyoid depression; (3) visible thyroid cartilage; (4) visible anterior border or the sternocleidomastoid muscle, distinct in its entire course from mastoid to sternum; and (5) a cervicomental angle between 105° and 120°, with a good skin quality [10].

With realistic expectations, to obtain the best results from neck rejuvenation techniques, establishing the main pathologic process and selecting the procedure accordingly is critical.

Evaluation of the Neck

Preoperative evaluation of the neck is critical for establishing the proper procedure addressing the pathologies contributing to the aging neck to obtain desirable results [2]. In fact, matching the technique chosen to a particular patient's needs is one of the most important determinants of a successful outcome [11]. The first step in evaluation of the neck is visual inspection. The neck is observed during normal conversation at the initial visit for dynamic changes, horizontal rhytides, and jowling, and adiposity of the neck. The patient is then asked to contract the anterior neck for evaluation of the lateral and medial platysmal banding. The cervicomental angle is assessed from the lateral view. An additional view with the patient's neck flexed is helpful in evaluating the platysmal laxity and redundancy [1]. Adiposity of the neck, ptotic glands, elasticity of the skin, and the degree of skin laxity should be evaluated with palpation. Skin texture and quality, with vascular changes, and benign and malignant growths should be considered and noted during the physical examination.

A standard facial photographic series, including anterior, lateral, and oblique views, should be obtained before performing any treatment. There are several classification systems that describe and categorize the changes seen in the lower face and neck. Brant and Bellman's classification on age-related neck degeneration establishes the grade of platysmal deformity and was initially developed for determining dosage requirements and prediction of degree of success after botulinum toxin injections [12, 13] (Table 1). Baker's classification for neck aging was originally developed for designating the good candidates for minimal incision rhytidectomy [14] (Table 2). However, both of these classifications can be adapted to different treatment modalities, for an objective and quantitative assessment of the results.

Proper patient selection is likely the most important determinant of successful results with the selected neck rejuvenation technique. Among the several available surgical and nonsurgical techniques, due to the complexity of the aging process of the neck, there is no one single treatment option that can address all of the pathologies contributing to neck aging. Realistic patient expectations should be established, and patients should be informed about the benefits, risks, and limitations of different treatment modalities regarding their main pathology.

Table 2 Baker classification for neck aging [14]

Type I	Aged early to late 40s Slight cervical skin laxity, early jowls, submental/submandibular fat
Type II	Aged late 40s to late 50s Moderate cervical skin laxity, moderate jowls, submental/submandibular fat
Type III	Aged late 50s, 60s, early 70s Moderate cervical skin laxity, significant jowls, submental/submandibular fat, active platysma bands
Type IV	Aged late 60s and 70s Loose redundant cervical skin and skin folds below the cricoid, significant jowls, submental/submandibular fat, active platysma bands, deep cervical creases

Laser Rejuvenation

Phototherapy with lasers and light sources is the most effective way to address photoaged skin [2]. Patients' desire for avoiding an operated look and resistance to invasive treatments have resulted in the popularity of laser resurfacing to improve skin laxity and induce tissue tightening, as an alternative to surgery [15]. There are a number of different ablative and nonablative lasers that can be used to resurface the skin of the neck [2].

Since the introduction of CO_2 laser resurfacing in 1980s, it has been accepted as the gold standard among skin rejuvenation modalities [16]. With the concept of selective photothermolysis, ablative lasers, mainly CO_2 and Er:YAG, target dermal water as the chromophore. Laser energy absorbed by intercellular water is converted to heat, leading to tissue ablation at the epidermis and residual thermal damage at the superficial dermis, with consequent wound-healing process and initiation of an inflammatory response. The extent of residual thermal damage can be controlled by a choice of laser wavelength, irradiance, and exposure duration. The CO_2 laser energy penetrates down to 20–30 μm into tissue, and residual thermal damage is seen at 200–250 μm or deeper around the ablated tissue [17]. The residual thermal injury to the upper dermis stimulates neocollagenesis, collagen remodeling, and neoelastogenesis, resulting with dramatic and long-lasting clinical changes reflected as reduction in rhytides, skin tightening, and removal of photodamaged skin. The clinical results are obtained after an intense postoperative wound care until complete reepithelialization is seen, in order to prevent the complications such as pigmentary alterations and scarring. Patients experience a social downtime for several weeks. With the modified devices, including high-energy pulsed CO_2 lasers and flash scanner CO_2 laser systems, scarring continued to remain a concern [18]. Despite the impressive clinical improvements, high risk for scarring and permanent delayed hypopigmentation, related with nonspecific thermal damage, and the trend towards no downtime procedures has diminished the popularity of fully ablative laser resurfacing [15].

In order to overcome the problems of ablative laser resurfacing, nonablative dermal remodeling techniques emerged next, which selectively heat dermal tissue, to induce a wound repair response and consequent neocollagenesis, while protecting the epidermis by cooling. However, the degree of dermal coagulation generated with these devices is not sufficient to result in satisfactory clinical results [19, 20].

In 2004, the introduction of the concept of "fractional photothermolysis" revolutionized laser surgery. By creation of a pixilated pattern of multiple microscopic vertical columns of thermal injury, known as microthermal treatment zones, surrounded by unlasered viable tissue, rapid healing is achieved, due to small wounds and short migratory paths for keratinocytes from the adjacent viable tissue [20, 21]. Fractional laser technology became increasingly popular, providing minimal downtime, rapid recovery, and satisfying cosmetic results [22]. The first devices employing fractional photothermolysis were the nonablative lasers *(1550 nm erbium-doped laser)*; however the results were still inferior to ablative strategies [18]. Shortly after the introduction of nonablative fractionated lasers, ablative lasers in a fractional mode were developed [23, 24]. With these devices, controlled tissue vaporization and dermal coagulation extending to greater depths (up to 1.5 mm) than those of traditional ablative and nonablative devices is achieved, without significant risk of complications [15, 23–25]. It is known that deeper zones of thermal damage result in greater clinical efficacy, inducing a long-lasting wound-healing process [26]. Moreover, tissue tightening effects may even be superior than ablative lasers because of this ability to ablate deeper into the reticular dermis. Another major advantage of ablative fractional resurfacing is the lower risk of delayed-onset hypopigmentation, since epidermal melanocytes are spared in the viable unlasered tissue [15]. Histological and ultrastructural studies after ablative fractional resurfacing treatment have revealed changes consistent with a wound repair mechanism and confirmed evidence of new collagen deposition [27].

Ablative fractional resurfacing treatment results in significant improvements in moderate to severe rhytides; skin laxity; and dyschromia on the face, neck, and chest [25, 26, 28]. Several fractional CO_2 devices, from different manufacturers, are now available on the market. Major differences between devices pertain to the depth of ablation and coagulation and to variations in treatment handpieces. Handpieces vary in spot sizes, shapes, and mode of application (rolling or stamping) [25]. Rolling handpieces work in a continuous motion with an optical tracking system and adjust the scanning system according to the operator's hand speed. Stamping handpieces need operator's devotion to avoid leaving untreated areas or overlapping. However, clinical results and downtime of different devices have been shown to be similar [29].

In the neck skin, pilosebaceous units are low in density, epidermis and dermis are thin, vasculature is poor, and the platysma runs superficially underneath. These tissue characteristics of the neck, especially on the lower part, may result in prolonged times for reepithelialization and deeper penetration of the laser energy, leading to greater tissue contraction and scarring after fractional ablative laser rejuvenation [26, 30] Therefore, utilization of fractional ablative lasers to neck should be done with great caution [2].

Fractional CO_2 Laser Resurfacing of the Neck: Contraindications

The optimal candidate for neck rejuvenation with fractional CO_2 laser is a patient with Fitzpatrick skin types I to IV with photodamage, especially with skin laxity, jowling, and dyschromia and with moderate postoperative expectations [4, 31]. Contraindications to treatment include active cutaneous infection, history of keloid formation, connective tissue diseases, dermatologic conditions that result in a reduced adnexal structures, and inhibited healing. History of radiation therapy or surgery at the treatment siteand a history of skin diseases that Koebnerize such as vitiligo and psoriasis can serve as relative contraindications [31, 32].

Previous isotretinoin therapy has been associated with atypical scarring after resurfacing procedures. It is generally recommended to perform the ablative fractional laser treatment, 6–12 months after isotretinoin therapy [31]. However, patients receiving isotretinoin treatment or who have completed the treatment 1–3 months prior to fractional ablative laser surgery revealed normal reepithelialization with no associated hypertrophic scarring or keloid formation [33].

Fractional CO_2 Laser Resurfacing of the Neck: Pre-procedural Strategies

Patients should be evaluated in a similar fashion to fully ablative resurfacing; however, fractional laser treatments offer flexibility in patients of all skin types and ages [18]. After fully informing the patients about necessary pretreatment prophylaxis, post-procedure skin care, possible side effects and outcomes of the procedure, written consent forms should be obtained. Patients are instructed to avoid sun exposure and to apply sunscreens before the procedure. Topical retinoid acid products, started several weeks beforehand, can be used to help speed reepithelialization after fractional ablative resurfacing, although it may promote post-procedure erythema [32]. On the other hand, topical bleaching agents are not usually recommended, since they have not been shown to reduce the risk of postinflammatory hyperpigmentation [31].

Since ablative fractional resurfacing may be complicated with infections, resulting in scarring, appropriate antimicrobial prophylaxis must be given. In order to prevent herpetic infections, which can be widespread and persistent after resurfacing, herpetic infections should be covered with prophylactic systemic antivirals (valacyclovir, 500 mg, twice daily), starting 1 day before the procedure, for 10 days or until full epithelialization is achieved. Prophylactic antivirals are given to patients with a history of recurrent herpetic infections; however, because of the considerable rates of unknown underlying HSV infection and the relative innocuous nature of the antiviral medications, some advocate that it should be given to all patients undergoing fractional ablative resurfacing, regardless of HSV history [22, 31]. Oral antibiotics are not routinely recommended, and should be decided upon individual patient characteristics. If recommended, broad-spectrum antibiotics should be chosen, considering that antibiotics covering for Gram (+) organisms can promote Gram (−) infections. Chlorhexidine washes and intranasal mupirocin ointment applications before the procedure may be recommended to decrease the risk of infection. Likewise, systemic antifungals (fluconazole, 200 mg) can be given on the day of procedure. To reduce the post-procedure edema, systemic corticosteroids (oral prednisone, 30 mg) can be recommended, started on the procedure day, continued for 2–3 days [18].

Fractional CO_2 Laser Resurfacing of the Neck: Procedure

Ablative fractional laser rejuvenation of the neck is generally performed in an outpatient office setting under topical anesthesia. Oral or intramuscular analgesics and sedatives may be administered, 30 min prior to the procedure. Additionally, appropriate nerve blocks, local or tumescent anesthetic infiltrations, intravenous sedation, or general anesthesia may be preferred to lessen patient discomfort [32, 34]. A topical anesthetic cream, consisting of mixtures of lidocaine, prilocaine, or tetracaine, either commercial or compounded (i.e., 2.5 % lidocaine/2.5 % prilocaine or 7 % lidocaine/7 % tetracaine), is liberally applied to the neck under occlusion for 1 h before the laser treatment. Eye protection with plain glasses is provided. Forced cold air cooling can be applied during the procedure. Prior to the procedure, the skin is cleansed.

Treatment techniques and parameters vary between different devices. Besides, one set of parameters of a particular device cannot be used for all patients to achieve the same outcome. It is essential to fully understand the laser-tissue interactions and the depth and width of tissue injury resulted at various laser settings used for the treatment of the neck. With smaller spot sizes, the laser energy would penetrate deeper. With increasing energy levels or density (distance between microthermal treatment zones), the width of the microthermal treatment zones and the percentage of the treated area would increase, resulting in larger zones of ablation and coagulation and longer time needed for recovery. Similarly, with longer pulse durations, the collateral heating and, thus, the width of microthermal treatment zones would increase. Hence, a safe treatment, avoiding a delayed recovery period and scarring can be obtained by selecting large spot sizes (shallower depth), lower energy and density settings at shorter pulse durations. For a more effective skin tightening, higher settings of density, energy, coverage, and pulse durations can be selected with caution [26]. However, treatment densities should not be greater than 35 % for the upper neck, and 20 % for the lower neck [30]. Overlapping will result in bulk heating, similar to fully ablative laser surfacing. User's instructions of each device can be referred for appropriate treatment parameters for different devices from different manufacturers. With most devices, one single pass laser treatment, avoiding to overlap or to leave untreated areas is performed [4, 32]. Devices with rolling handpieces require parallel, overlapping treatment passes in the horizontal and vertical directions [34].

After treating the area, without wiping the skin, cold saline compresses or cold packs are applied. This is effective in reducing the edema. Afterward, a single application of topical steroids can be used to help reduce both the edema and erythema. Patients may experience a burning sensation for the following hours. A bland moisturizer, such as pure petroleum jelly, is applied in order to alleviate patient discomfort and provide hydration for wound healing. Patients are strictly instructed to use the recommended skin care and to avoid sun exposure.

Fractional CO_2 Laser Resurfacing of the Neck: Post-procedural Strategies

Fractionally ablated skin should be cared in a similar fashion to fully ablative resurfacing. Although less extensive and limited to the ablated percentage of skin, there is an open wound for several days, followed by edema and erythema. Prudent wound care is essential to fasten epithelialization and for the prevention of complications. Both occluded and open wound care can be employed. Occlusive dressings may help speed healing and reduce inflammation.

Cold soaks with saline, dilute white vinegar (5 ml vinegar in 250 ml water), or aluminum acetate applied several times a day, help to reduce edema and erythema and provide antisepsis [32]. This is followed by the application of pure petrolatum jelly for enhancing epithelialization. Other topical products should be avoided, because of the disrupted barrier function of the skin and the related risk of irritant or allergic contact dermatitis.

Erythema, edema, oozing, and petechial bleeding are seen immediately after the procedure and can continue for 24 h [35]. Post-procedure erythema is most prominent in the first 2 of days of the treatment, which gradually decreases and fades in several weeks. A thin layer of dark brown crusting is seen as a result of oozing. Patients should be strictly instructed not to pick the desquamated areas or crusts. Epithelialization after neck rejuvenation with fractional CO_2 is usually seen after 3–6 days, and the expected downtime is up to 7 days. After reepithelialization, switching to a water-based cream and application of sunscreens is recommended for the prevention of acneiform eruptions and postinflammatory hyperpigmentation. To further decrease the risk of hyperpigmentation, a mid-potency topical corticosteroid cream can also be recommended on the third day for reducing the inflammation. Patients should be closely followed up in the first weeks of the procedure for monitoring postoperative wound care and the signs of complications.

Fractional CO_2 Laser Resurfacing of the Neck: Complications

Fractional ablative laser resurfacing of the neck is a safe procedure when performed by experienced laser surgeons, with appropriate laser settings. Reepithelialization is faster, infections are less frequent, duration of posttreatment skin care is shorter, fewer acneiform eruptions occur, and the duration of postoperative erythema is shorter when compared to traditional resurfacing [36]. The overall complication rate for fractional CO_2 resurfacing is low, ranging from 0 % to 5.5 % and totaling 13.9 % [22]. However, the complications are mainly related to improper technique, aggressive energy and density settings, and postoperative infections [37]. Hence, neck should always be treated with conservative parameters, with meticulous post-procedure care.

Acneiform eruption and infections (bacterial, viral, yeast) are the most common complications, followed by hyperpigmentation, prolonged erythema, contact dermatitis, scarring, and hypopigmentation [22, 38]. The majority of these complications are mild, short-lived, and easily managed [22].

Premature removal of the crust or desquamated skin, like any kind of trauma can result with prolonged erythema and postinflammatory hyperpigmentation. In patients with darker skin types, postinflammatory hyperpigmentation is a common complication. Broad-spectrum sunscreens and topical depigmenting agents are used for management. In refractory cases, low-dose, high-frequency Q-switched Nd:YAG laser treatments can be an effective treatment option.

Although the risk of hypertrophic scarring after fractional CO_2 resurfacing is low, especially the lower portion of the neck is prone to develop scarring. Any elevated lesion after the first weeks at the treatment area should be immediately treated to minimize scarring. Potent topical or intralesional corticosteroids should be started promptly. Additionally, if reepithelialization is complete, pulse dye laser treatment can be performed [4].

Postoperative infections may also result in scar formations [30]. Any area that fails to heal, or becomes painful, swollen, and ulcerates after healing, should be assumed to have developed an infection, until proven otherwise. Bacterial and fungal cultures should be taken to identify the causative organisms, and appropriate topical and systemic antimicrobial treatment should be started immediately. HSV activation can be seen in patients that did not receive antiviral prophylaxis.

Fractional CO_2 Laser Resurfacing of the Neck: Outcomes

Significant improvements in skin texture, skin tightening, and skin rhytides, similar to that of ablative CO_2 laser treatment has been reported with fractional CO_2 rejuvenation of the neck [39]. Skin laxity, jowling, and surface pigmentation are significantly improved, even after one session of treatment. Although fat deposition is not affected from fractional CO_2 rejuvenation, effects in skin tightening provide a better appearance of fat tissue [4].

Conclusions

The unique aging pathogenesis and limited healing properties of the neck leave the treatment of the aging neck as one of the most challenging aspects of rejuvenation procedures. Development and utilization of fractional ablative laser resurfacing revolutionized laser surgery, with improved safety profile and clinical efficacy, when compared to traditional laser resurfacing. For a patient with an aging neck with prominent skin laxity, jowling, and pigmentary changes, fractional CO_2 laser resurfacing is a safe and effective treatment alternative. However, procedure should be done with caution, since the excessive ablation and thermal damage can result in scarring. Post-procedure frequent follow-up is necessary, to recognize the signs of infection which may result in scarring as well if left untreated.

References

1. Rohrich RJ, Rios JL, Smith PD, Gutowski KA. Neck rejuvenation revisited. Plast Reconstr Surg. 2006;118 (5):1251–63.
2. Roy D. Neck rejuvenation. Dermatol Clin. 2005;23 (3):469–74.
3. Matarasso A. Managing the components of the aging neck: from liposuction to submentalplasty, to neck lift. Clin Plast Surg. 2014;41(1):85–98. doi:10.1016/j.cps.2013.09.013.
4. Oram Y, Akkaya AD. Neck rejuvenation with fractional CO_2 laser: long-term results. Clin Aesthet Dermatol. 2014;7(8):23–9.
5. Shadfar S, Perkins SW. Anatomy and physiology of the aging neck. Facial Plast Surg Clin North Am. 2014;22 (2):161–70. doi:10.1016/j.fsc.2014.01.009.
6. Kligman LH. Photoaging. Manifestations, prevention, and treatment. Dermatol Clin. 1986;4(3):517–28.
7. Ramirez OM. Multidimensional evaluation and surgical approaches to neck rejuvenation. Clin Plast Surg. 2014;41(1):99–107. doi:10.1016/j.cps.2013.09.011.
8. Stebbins WG, Hanke CW. Rejuvenation of the neck with liposuction and ancillary techniques. Dermatol Ther. 2011;24(1):28–40. doi:10.1111/j.1529-8019.2010.01376.x.
9. Fedok FG, Sedgh J. Managing the neck in the era of the short scar face-lift. Facial Plast Surg. 2012;28 (1):60–75. doi:10.1055/s-0032-1305791.
10. Ellenbogen R, Karlin JV. Visual criteria for success in restoring the youthful neck. Plast Reconstr Surg. 1980;66(6):826–37.
11. Beaty MM. A progressive approach to neck rejuvenation. Facial Plast Surg Clin North Am. 2014;22 (2):177–90. doi:10.1016/j.fsc.2014.01.001.
12. Brandt FS, Bellman B. Cosmetic use of botulinum A exotoxin for the aging neck. Dermatol Surg. 1998;24 (11):1232–4.

13. Matarasso A, Matarasso SL, Brandt FS, Bellman B. Botulinum A exotoxin for the management of platysma bands. Plast Reconstr Surg. 1999;103 (2):645–52.
14. Baker DC. Minimal incision rhytidectomy (short scar face lift) with lateral SMASectomy: evolution and application. Aesthet Surg J. 2001;21(1):14–26. doi:10.1067/maj.2001.113557.
15. Ortiz AE, Goldman MP, Fitzpatrick RE. Ablative CO_2 lasers for skin tightening: traditional versus fractional. Dermatol Surg. 2014;40 Suppl 12:S147–51. doi:10.1097/DSS.0000000000000230.
16. Fitzpatrick RE, Goldman MP, Satur NM, Tope WD. Pulsed carbon dioxide laser resurfacing of photo-aged facial skin. Arch Dermatol. 1996;132 (4):395–402.
17. Walsh Jr JT, Flotte TJ, Anderson RR, Deutsch TF. Pulsed CO_2 laser tissue ablation: effect of tissue type and pulse duration on thermal damage. Lasers Surg Med. 1988;8(2):108–18.
18. Brightman LA, Brauer JA, Anolik R, Weiss E, Karen J, Chapas A, Hale E, Bernstein L, Geronemus RG. Ablative and fractional ablative lasers. Dermatol Clin. 2009;27(4):479–89. doi:10.1016/j.det.2009.08.009.
19. Goldberg DJ, Whitworth J. Laser skin resurfacing with the Q-switched Nd:YAG laser. Dermatol Surg. 1997;23 (10):903–6.
20. Manstein D, Herron GS, Sink RK, Tanner H, Anderson RR. Fractional photothermolysis: a new concept for cutaneous remodeling using microscopic patterns of thermal injury. Lasers Surg Med. 2004;34(5):426–38.
21. Huzaira M, Anderson RR, Sink K, Manstein D. Intradermal focusing of near-infrared optical pulses: a new approach for non-ablative laser therapy. Lasers Surg Med. 2003;S15:21. doi:10.1002/lsm.1151.
22. Shamsaldeen O, Peterson JD, Goldman MP. The adverse events of deep fractional CO[2]: a retrospective study of 490 treatments in 374 patients. Lasers Surg Med. 2011;43(6):453–6. doi:10.1002/lsm.21079.
23. Hantash BM, Bedi VP, Chan KF, Zachary CB. Ex vivo histological characterization of a novel fractional resurfacing device. Lasers Surg Med. 2007;39 (2):87–95.
24. Hantash BM, Bedi VP, Kapadia B, Rahman Z, Jiang K, Tanner H, Chan KF, Zachary CB. In vivo histological characterization of a novel fractional resurfacing device. Lasers Surg Med. 2007;39(2):96–107.
25. Hunzeker CM, Weiss ET, Geronemus RG. Fractionated CO_2 laser resurfacing: our experience with more than 2000 treatments. Aesthet Surg J. 2009;29(4):317–22. doi:10.1016/j.asj.2009.05.004.
26. Tierney EP, Hanke CW, Petersen J. Ablative fractionated CO_2 laser treatment of photoaging: a clinical and histologic study. Dermatol Surg. 2012;38(11):1777–89. doi:10.1111/j.1524-4725.2012.02572.x.
27. Berlin AL, Hussain M, Phelps R, Goldberg DJ. A prospective study of fractional scanned nonsequential carbon dioxide laser resurfacing: a clinical and histopathologic evaluation. Dermatol Surg. 2009;35 (2):222–8. doi:10.1111/j.1524-4725.2008.34413.x.
28. Chapas AM, Brightman L, Sukal S, Hale E, Daniel D, Bernstein LJ, Geronemus RG. Successful treatment of acneiform scarring with CO_2 ablative fractional resurfacing. Lasers Surg Med. 2008;40(6):381–6. doi:10.1002/lsm.20659.
29. Carniol PJ, Hamilton MM, Carniol ET. Current status of fractional laser resurfacing. JAMA Facial Plast Surg. 2015;17(5):360–6. doi:10.1001/jamafacial.2015.0693.
30. Fife DJ, Fitzpatrick RE, Zachary CB. Complications of fractional CO_2 laser resurfacing: four cases. Lasers Surg Med. 2009;41(3):179–84. doi:10.1002/lsm.20753.
31. Alexiades-Armenakas MR, Dover JS, Arndt KA. The spectrum of laser skin resurfacing: nonablative, fractional, and ablative laser resurfacing. J Am Acad Dermatol. 2008;58(5):719–37. doi:10.1016/j.jaad.2008.01.003.
32. Ramsdell WM. Fractional carbon dioxide laser resurfacing. Semin Plast Surg. 2012;26(3):125–30. doi:10.1055/s-0032-1329414.
33. Kim HW, Chang SE, Kim JE, Ko JY, Ro YS. The safe delivery of fractional ablative carbon dioxide laser treatment for acne scars in Asian patients receiving oral isotretinoin. Dermatol Surg. 2014;40 (12):1361–6. doi:10.1097/DSS.0000000000000185.
34. Woodward JA, Fabi SG, Alster T, Colón-Acevedo B. Safety and efficacy of combining microfocused ultrasound with fractional CO_2 laser resurfacing for lifting and tightening the face and neck. Dermatol Surg. 2014;40 Suppl 12:S190–3. doi:10.1097/DSS.0000000000000228.
35. Rahman Z, MacFalls H, Jiang K, Chan KF, Kelly K, Tournas J, Stumpp OF, Bedi V, Zachary C. Fractional deep dermal ablation induces tissue tightening. Lasers Surg Med. 2009;41(2):78–86. doi:10.1002/lsm.20715.
36. Duplechain JK. Fractional CO_2 resurfacing: has it replaced ablative resurfacing techniques? Facial Plast Surg Clin North Am. 2013;21(2):213–27. doi:10.1016/j.fsc.2013.02.006.
37. Avram MM, Tope WD, Yu T, Szachowicz E, Nelson JS. Hypertrophic scarring of the neck following ablative fractional carbon dioxide laser resurfacing. Lasers Surg Med. 2009;41(3):185–8. doi:10.1002/lsm.20755.
38. Campbell T, Goldman P. Adverse events of fractional CO_2 lasers, a review of 373 treatments. Dermatol Surg. 2010;36(11):1645–50. doi:10.1111/j.1524-4725.2010.01712.x.
39. Tierney EP, Hanke CW. Ablative fractionated CO_2 laser resurfacing for the neck: prospective study and review of the literature. J Drugs Dermatol. 2009;8 (8):723–31.

147 Changes in Vulvar Physiology and Skin Disorders with Age and Benefits of Feminine Wipes in Postmenopausal Women

Miranda A. Farage, Kenneth W. Miller, and William J. Ledger

Contents

M.A. Farage (✉)
Winton Hill Business Center, The Procter & Gamble Company, Cincinnati, OH, USA
e-mail: farage.m@pg.com

K.W. Miller
Margoshes-Miller Consulting, LLC, Cincinnati, OH, USA

W.J. Ledger
Department of Obstetrics and Gynecology, The New York-Presbyterian Hospital, Weill Medical College of Cornell University, New York, NY, USA
e-mail: wjledger@med.cornell.edu

M.A. Farage et al. (eds.), *Textbook of Aging Skin*,
DOI 10.1007/978-3-662-47398-6_103

Abstract

Postmenopausal estrogen deficiency may lead to vulvar atrophy and irritation. This chapter reviews the morphology and physiology of the vulva over a woman's lifetime, discusses vulvar irritation associated with the menopause, and reports the benefits of feminine wet wipes' use by postmenopausal women. As women age, the skin of the vulva becomes less elastic and the underlying fat and connective tissues can break down. These changes can lead to a variety of disorders and symptoms which result in vulvar irritation, such as atrophic vaginitis, incontinence dermatitis, vulvar intertrigo, fungal infections secondary to urinary incontinence, bacterial infections, pruritis ani and perianal inflammation, and decubitus ulcers. A 28-day, examiner-blind, randomized, prospective trial compared skin effects of a prototype wet wipe to dry toilet tissue. The treatment group used individual sheets of tissue moistened with a lotion that contained skin cleansers and moisturizing agents. The comparison group used a commercially available dry toilet tissue. Skin condition was assessed at two time points, and the participants also reported subjective symptoms and product preferences. In general, mild to barely discernible irritation was present at study inception. Erythema, when present, improved over the course of the study in both groups. Genital moisture significantly increased in wet wipe users ($p = 0.01$) compared to dry tissue users. Most postmenopausal women in the study favored wet wipes over dry toilet tissue, which may suggest improved comfort of atrophied vulvar skin and amelioration of dryness associated with postmenopausal estrogen depletion.

Introduction

Vulvar skin changes over time. The most significant changes, which are hormonally mediated, are linked to the onset of puberty, the menstrual cycle, pregnancy, and menopause. Postmenopausal estrogen deficiency can lead to vulvar atrophy and irritation. This chapter reviews the morphology and physiology of the vulva over a woman's lifetime, vulvar irritation associated with the menopause, and studies on the benefits of feminine wet wipes in postmenopausal women.

Effects of Aging on Vulvar Morphology, Physiology, and Susceptibility to Irritation

The female lower urogenital tract is unique in that it is derived from all three embryonic germ cell layers: the ectoderm, the endoderm, and the mesoderm [1, 2]. Like the skin at other anatomical sites, the cutaneous epithelia of the mons pubis, labia, clitoris, and perineum originate from the embryonic ectoderm and exhibit a keratinized, stratified squamous structure with sweat glands, sebaceous glands, and hair follicles [3, 4]. The degree of keratinization is greatest on the mons pubis and labia majora; it decreases over the clitoris and the outer surface and inner two-thirds of the labia minora, the epidermis of the labia minora being thinner than that of the labia majora. From the inner third of the surface of the labia minora through the vestibule, the vulvar epithelium is nonkeratinized and is comprised of mucosal tissue originating from the embryonic endoderm [2, 5]. The vagina originates from the embryonic mesoderm and bears a nonkeratinized squamous epithelium that is responsive to estrogen cycling [1].

Table 1 summarized changes in the morphology and physiology of the vulva over a woman's lifetime. The most significant changes are hormonally mediated and linked to the onset of puberty, the menstrual cycle, pregnancy, and menopause.

From birth until about 4–6 weeks of age, the effects of residual maternal estrogens on the vulva are evidenced by swollen labia majora, well-developed labia minora, and a relatively large clitoris [3, 11]. During early childhood, the female genitalia receive little estrogen stimulation, resulting in flattened labia majora and thin labia minora and hymen [11]. Although vulvar hair follicles and sebaceous glands are present at birth, these structures do not mature until the adrenal glands are activated at puberty. Prior to puberty, the labia minora have barely discernible vellus hair follicles; these disappear when the follicles of the labia majora and mons pubis terminally differentiate at puberty [12].

At puberty, adrenal and gonadal maturation induce further changes in vulvar skin. Follicular development causes estrogen production to rise: as estrogen stimulation increases, the vulvar epithelium thickens, the labial skin becomes rugose, and the clitoris becomes more prominent [4].

During the reproductive years, vulvar changes are linked to the menstrual cycle and pregnancy. The vulvar epidermis and dermis reach their fullest thickness during the reproductive years [3, 4] (see Fig. 1). While vulvar epithelial thickness remains constant throughout the menstrual cycle, cytologic changes associated with sex hormone cycling have been observed [14]: orthokeratosis predominates at the beginning of the menstrual cycle, parakeratosis increases at mid-cycle, then orthokeratosis rises once again by the end of the cycle.

During pregnancy, an increase in total blood volume heightens the coloration of the vulva and the vagina. Saphenous, vulvar, and hemorrhoidal swelling also occur due to increased blood volume and venous pressure in femoral and pelvic vessels from the enlarging uterus [9]. Increases in progesterone levels also elevate venous distensibility; this may lead to vulvar varices that typically regress postpartum [3, 9, 10].

Following menopause, circulating estrogen levels (primarily estradiol) are dramatically reduced (from >120 pg per mL to around 18 pg

Table 1 Vulvar physiology and characteristics from birth to postmenopause

Life stage	Pertinent physiology	Vulvar characteristics
Newborn	Effects of residual, transplacental maternal estrogens	Plump labia majora
		Well-developed labia minora
		Immature hair follicles and sebaceous glands
Early childhood	Lack of stimulation by adrenal or gonadal steroid hormones	Mons pubis and labia major lose fat
		Benign labial adhesions, if present, normalize without treatment [6]
Puberty	Adrenal and gonadal maturation ensues. Secondary sex characteristics are acquired and menstruation begins [7]	Subcutaneous fat is deposited in the mons pubis and labia majora
		Vulvar epithelium thickens
		The labia minora and clitoris become more prominent
		Pubic hair emerges
Reproductive years	Menstruation	The morphology of the vulva is mature
		Vulvar skin thickness remains constant throughout the menstrual cycle [1]
		Parakeratosis of the vulvar stratum conreum rises at mid-cycle [1, 8]
	Pregnancy: blood volume increases; menstrual cycle ceases during gestation	Hair may darken along the midline of the abdomen
		Increased blood flow heightens vulvar coloration
		Susceptibility to vulvar varicose veins increases [9, 10]
		Flattening of the fourchette and perineal trauma may occur during delivery
Menopause	Follicular function and menstrual cycle cease. The prevalence of urinary and fecal incontinence rises. Physical health, immune function, tissue regeneration capacity, and cognition may be compromised with increasing age	Pubic hair becomes sparse
		Subcutaneous fat is lost
		Vulvar tissue atrophies
		Risk of perineal dermatitis rises in older women with incontinence

Adapted from Farage and Maibach [3]. Adapted and reprinted with permission from Springer Science and Business Media

per mL) [15]. Concurrent with this change, levels of gonadotropins increase: follicle-stimulating hormone (FSH) rises earlier and to a greater extent than luteinizing hormone (LH). Sex hormone levels pre- and postmenopause are shown in Fig. 2.

Postmenopausal estrogen depletion induces further changes. At a cytological level, estrogen-linked parakeratosis decreases during menopause and is essentially nonexistent by the eight decade [18]. On the morphological level, connective tissue proliferates, elastin fragmentation rises, and hyalinization of collagen occurs. The endometrium becomes thinner, the labia majora lose subcutaneous fat, and the labia minora, vulvar vestibule, and vaginal epithelium progressively atrophy [4, 19]. Vaginal secretions diminish, and vaginal pH rises. These effects make the vulvovaginal epithelium more susceptible to inflammatory changes such as atrophic vaginitis [3, 13, 20].

Characteristics of Aging Vulvar Skin

Vulvar skin differs from exposed (forearm) skin in several characteristics: skin hydration, skin friction, permeability, and visually discernible

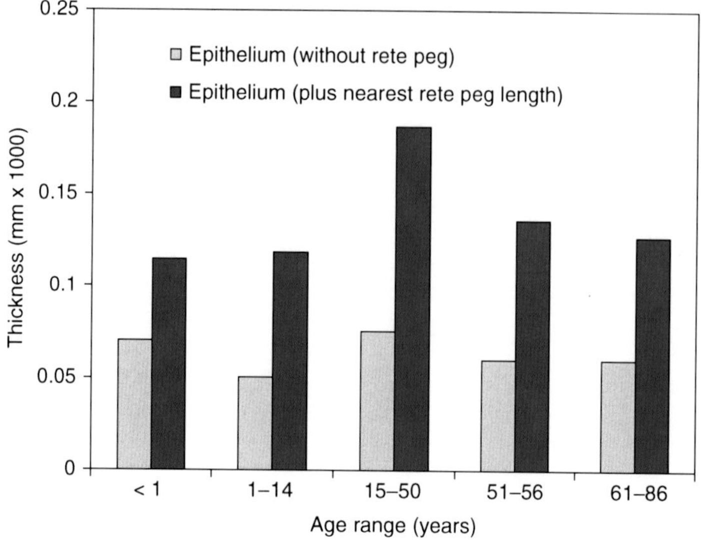

Fig. 1 Changes in epithelial thickness of the labia majora with age [13] (Reprinted with permission from Informa Healthcare, New York)

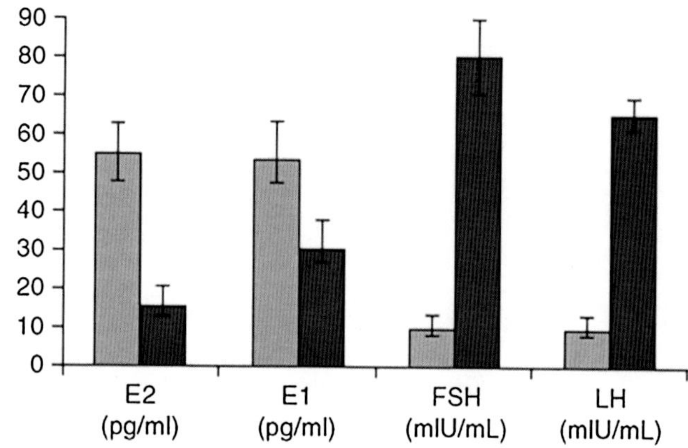

Fig. 2 Differences in hormone concentration premenopause (*shaded lighter Color bar*) and postmenopause (*solid bar*). E_2 estradiol, E_1 estrone, *FSH* follicle-stimulating hormone, *LH* luteinizing hormone (From Yen [16], Phillips et al. [17]. Reprinted with permission from Elsevier)

irritation [3, 13, 21]. However, aging does not appear to induce significant changes in the vulvar skin, as evidenced by studies of pre- and postmenopausal women (Table 2).

For example, vulvar skin is more hydrated than forearm skin (as measured by transepidermal water loss [TEWL]) [22, 25] and has a higher friction coefficient ($p < 0.001$) [22]. Small age-related differences in these two parameters were observed in forearm skin but not in vulvar skin.

Effects on skin permeability depend on the nature of the penetrant. For example, vulvar skin was more permeable to hydrocortisone than forearm skin, but both regions exhibited comparable permeability to testosterone [23]. Age-related changes depended on the penetrant. Hydrocortisone absorption from the vulva was significantly higher ($p < 0.01$) in premenopausal women compared to postmenopausal women; a trend was also observed without significance for forearm skin. However, no significant differences ($p > 0.05$) in percutaneous testosterone absorption from vulvar or forearm skin were observed in pre- or postmenopausal women.

Studies with a model irritant (1 % aqueous sodium lauryl sulfate [SLS]) suggest a lower erythematous response on the vulva than on the

Table 2 Physiologic skin parameters in pre- and postmenopausal women

Parameter	Site	Age group	N	Measured value	Significance[a]	References
Water barrier function (TEWL, g/m^2 h)	Forearm	Premenopausal	34	3.7 ± 0.4	$p < 0.05$	[22]
		Postmenopausal	10	2.6 ± 0.3		
	Vulva	Premenopausal	34	14.8 ± 1.5	n.s	
		Postmenopausal	10	13.5 ± 1.8		
Skin hydration (capacitance, AU)	Forearm	Premenopausal	34	93.3 ± 2.3	n.s	[22]
		Postmenopausal	10	91.9 ± 2.8		
	Vulva	Premenopausal	34	116.8 ± 4.1	n.s	
		Postmenopausal	10	118.0 ± 8.2		
Friction coefficient (μ)	Forearm	Premenopausal	34	0.49 ± 0.02	$p < 0.05$	[22]
		Postmenopausal	10	0.45 ± 0.01		
	Vulva	Premenopausal	34	0.60 ± 0.04	n.s	
		Postmenopausal	10	0.60 ± 0.06		
Hydrocortisone penetration (% dose absorbed)	Forearm	Premenopausal	9	2.8 ± 2.4	n.s	[23]
		Postmenopausal	9	1.5 ± 1.1		
	Vulva	Premenopausal	9	8.1 ± 4.1	$p < 0.01$	
		Postmenopausal	9	4.4 ± 2.8		
Testosterone penetration (% dose absorbed)	Forearm	Premenopausal	9	20.2 ± 8.1	n.s	[23]
		Postmenopausal	9	14.7 ± 4.2		
	Vulva	Premenopausal	9	26.7 ± 8.0	n.s	
		Postmenopausal	9	24.6 ± 5.5		
Visual erythema scores (scored on day 2 after 24 h exposure to 1 % sodium lauryl sulfate [SLS])	Forearm	Premenopausal	10	9	$p = 0.03$	[24]
		Postmenopausal	10	5		
	Vulva	Premenopausal	10	0	n.s.	
		Postmenopausal	10	0		

Source: Farage and Maibach [3]. Reprinted with permission from Springer Science and Business Media
n.s. not significant, *TEWL* transepidermal water loss
[a]Level of statistical significance of age-group differences

forearm [24]. Following patch testing with SLS, more intense erythema was observed on the forearms of premenopausal women compared to postmenopausal women; however, no visually discernable erythema was observed in the vulvar region of either pre- or postmenopausal women.

Vulvar Irritation in Older Women

As women age, the skin of the vulva becomes less elastic and the underlying fat and connective tissues can break down, leading to a variety of disorders and symptoms which result in vulvar irritation [26, 27]. A summary of the most common inflammatory vulvar disorders in older women follows.

Atrophic Vaginitis

Up to 40 % of postmenopausal women have symptoms of atrophic vaginitis, an inflammatory condition of the vulva and vagina linked to estrogen depletion [28–30]. Estrogen receptors of the vagina, vulva, urethra, and bladder trigone atrophy as postmenopausal estrogen levels diminish. Concurrently, the vaginal epithelium thins, vaginal secretions decline, and vaginal pH rises. In total, such changes weaken the lining of the vagina and urinary tract and increase susceptibility to inflammation and urinary tract infections [28, 29, 31–33].

Even at the moment, there is no consensus on the definition and assessment of vaginal atrophy. Weber et al. propose to define vaginal atrophy as a

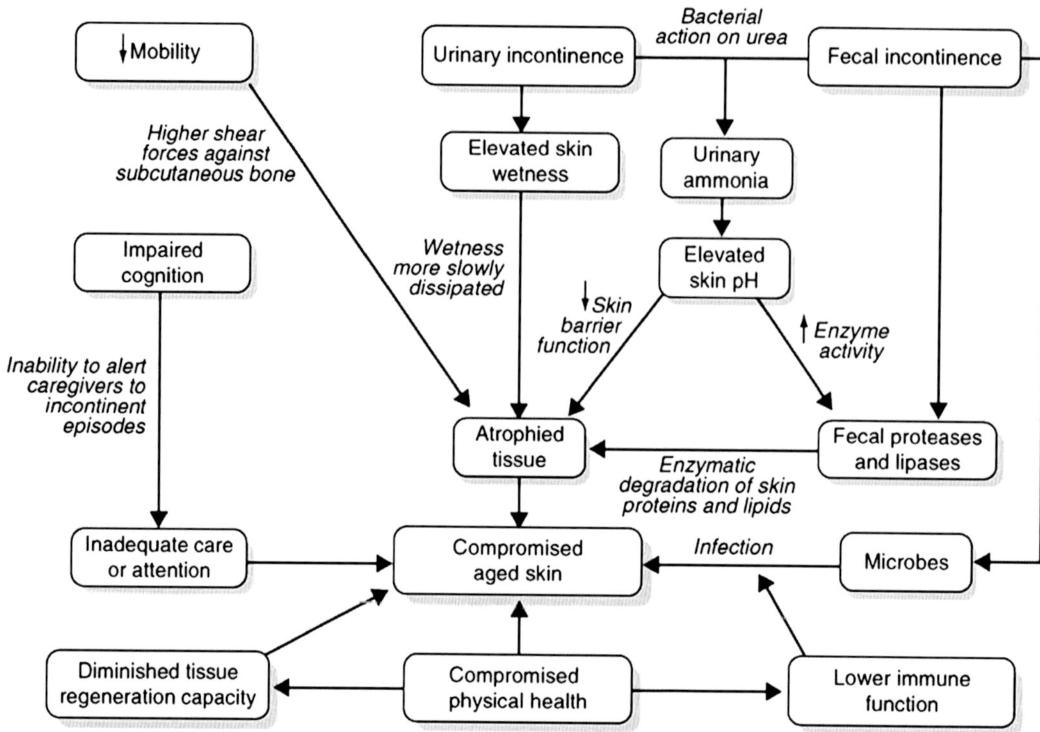

Fig. 3 Factors contributing to the morbidity of incontinence dermatitis in the elderly population (From Reference [41]. Reprinted with permission from Informa Healthcare, New York)

common manifestation of estrogen decline associated with specific symptoms of which the most common are vaginal dryness, itching or irritation, and dyspareunia [34]. Symptoms of atrophic vaginitis include vaginal and vulvar discomfort, dryness, burning, itching, and dyspareunia (painful intercourse). Inflammation of the vaginal epithelium also can contribute to urinary symptoms, including increased frequency, urgency, dysuria, stress incontinence, and/or recurrent infection [29].

Atrophic vaginitis is usually treated with low-dose, hormone replacement therapy (HRT). Studies have compared a variety of treatment regimens including creams, tablets, suppositories, pessaries, and rings with no treatment being demonstrated as superior to another [29]. Due to the nature of the atrophic epithelia, initial systemic absorption is low; however, as vascularity improves, absorption increases [35]. In addition, it has been demonstrated through cytology that low doses of estrogen are needed to maintain vaginal elasticity [36]. It is therefore recommended that initial estrogen treatment consists of low doses [29, 37, 38].

Incontinence Dermatitis

Women often experience greater urinary urgency as they age; bladder capacity and voiding efficiency also may decline [39]. When accompanied by illness, obstetrical injury, changes in nutrition or hormonal status, side effects of medication, and/or decreased cognitive function, such changes can contribute to urinary incontinence [39, 40]. While prevalence rates vary, urinary incontinence rises among older people and is relatively common after the age of 50 [41, 42].

Although research studies found no significant age-related decrease in the barrier function and hydration of vulvar skin nor any significant difference in susceptibility to model irritants, older women with incontinence nevertheless are at increased risk for developing incontinence dermatitis. This risk results from a combination of factors, including tissue atrophy, delayed dissipation of excess skin moisture, shear forces of bone against skin due to limited mobility, and lower tissue regeneration capacity. In addition, skin occlusion associated with incontinence garments can have an irritating effect on the skin [43]. Skin occluded by incontinence garments or pads is wetter and with a higher pH, bacterial count, and susceptibility to erosion [44]. Barrier permeability and molecular and cellular homeostasis are also affected [45]. Factors contributing to the morbidity of incontinence dermatitis in the elderly are displayed in Fig. 3.

Incontinence dermatitis begins with mild skin erythema, which, if untreated, may intensify and be accompanied by blisters and erosions in severe cases [41, 46]. In women, urinary dermatitis first appears between the labial folds; signs of fecal dermatitis begin in the perianal area and progress to the posterior aspect of the upper thighs [47]. Secondary infections can occur (see below).

Treatment of urinary and fecal incontinence dermatitis must take into account the fragility of the older skin as well as concurrent cutaneous damage due to secondary infections or cleansing. Limited systematic research exists on specific cleansing regimens and their impact on the prevention or treatment of incontinence dermatitis. One prospective trial of the impact of preventative care was a preliminary examination of structured intervention in 15 institutionalized patients with dementia [48]. In this study, the number of patients who developed dermatitis was unchanged regardless of whether or not preventative treatments were used. Dermatitis developed only in patients with urofecal incontinence with more than four episodes in a 24-h period. None of the patients were able to inform caregivers of incontinent episodes. While the small number of subjects and their poor mental health limit the conclusions that can be drawn from this study, the results suggest that patient incapable of reporting incontinent episodes should be monitored closely.

Vulvar Intertrigo

Vulvar intertrigo is an inflammation of the genitocrural folds, the labia, and the perineum caused by skin-on-skin friction. It is characterized initially by mild erythema that may progress to more intense inflammation. While most commonly seen in morbidly obese women, the condition can also ensue from urinary and fecal incontinence that traps moisture in folds of the skin [41, 49, 50].

Fungal Infections Secondary to Urinary Incontinence

Fungal infections of vulvar and perineal skin related to urinary incontinence generally involve two species: *Candida albicans* and *Tinea cruris*. *C. albicans* infections of the vagina often manifest as an itchy erythema with a creamy white discharge. Infections that involve the vulva or perineum create erythematous patches with satellite pustules. *Candida* intertrigo can develop in moist skin folds [43, 51, 52]. Because the gastrointestinal tract is a primary reservoir for *C. albicans*, fecal incontinence increases the risk of secondary infection [53]. Routine antibiotic use may also increase the risk for secondary infections of the vulva with *Candida* [43]. Treatment of candidiasis consists of keeping the skin dry and use of topical antifungal treatments containing nystatin or clotrimazole [40, 51] or combination of isoconazole nitrate and diflucortolone valerate [54]. *Tinea cruris* is a fungal infection of the inguinal folds, perineum, and buttocks [51]. Although rare and more commonly seen in men, its prevalence increases in older women due to the diminished cellular immune response [55]. *T. cruris* usually presents as a ring-shaped eruption with an actively advancing border and a scaly, healing center. It often occurs in patients with *Tinea pedis* and onychomycosis and is thought to spread to the groin from contaminated clothing. Most patients with *T. cruris* can be treated easily with topical antifungal agents; maintaining dry skin helps prevent this condition.

Bacterial Infections

Aging skin that has been compromised by incontinence dermatitis may facilitate the proliferation and invasion of microbials such as *Staphylococcus* in elderly subjects [53]. Vulvar folliculitis, characterized by red, tender pus-filled papules surrounding the hair follicles, often involves infection by *Staphylococci* and *Streptococci* species [43, 56]. Some surgical incontinence therapies, such as transobturator and tension-free vaginal tape (TVT), have resulted in serious subdermal infections by these organisms, progressing to cellulitis and potentially fatal, necrotizing fasciitis, which are rare but serious [57, 58].

Pruritis Ani and Perianal Inflammation

Anogenital pruritus, characterized by perianal itching, erythema, and/or lesions, can stem from incontinence but also may result from cleansing with harsh soaps. Chronic scratching exacerbates perianal inflammation and may compromise the skin. This condition is more common among with people with impaired mental function or dementia [59].

Decubitus Ulcers

Pressure or decubitus ulcers, commonly known as bedsores, occur when soft tissues become compressed between bony protuberances and contact surfaces. Under these conditions, friction or shearing forces contribute to tissue ischemia, infarction, and tissue erosion [60, 61]. Pressure ulcers occur most often in patients with cognitive impairment, immobility, or both. Over 60 % of decubitus ulcers occur in patients over 70 years old; the prevalence rate in nursing homes is estimated to be 20–40 % [60]. Excessive skin hydration associated with urinary incontinence increases the susceptibility to pressure ulcers: the frequency of pad changes for incontinent patients correlates directly to the risk of stage II pressure ulcers (defined as partial thickness skin loss involving the epidermis, dermis, or both) [43, 62].

Benefits of Feminine Wet Wipes in Postmenopausal Women

Clinical studies suggest a potential benefit of feminine wet wipes to vulvar skin of postmenopausal women. A 28-day, examiner-blind, randomized, prospective trial compared skin effects of a prototype wet wipe to dry toilet tissue in 120 premenopausal and 60 postmenopausal women [63]. Results in the postmenopausal group are discussed here. These participants were women aged 55–80 years, free of vulvovaginal infection (e.g., candidiasis, genital herpes, chlamydia, *Trichomonas vaginalis*, and bacterial vaginosis), who were not on hormone replacement therapy (HRT). Women with stress or urge urinary incontinence were included; approximately 30 % of the participants reported a history of stress incontinence.

Thirty-one (31) women were randomly assigned to the treatment group and 29 to the comparison group. The treatment group used individual sheets of tissue moistened with a lotion that contained skin cleansers and moisturizing agents (>90 % water with low levels of humectants, surfactants, emulsifiers, fragrance, and preservatives). This product was used in lieu of toilet tissue to clean the vulva, perineum, and/or anal area after every episode of urination or defecation during the 28-day study period. The comparison group (controls) used a commercially available dry toilet tissue. Skin condition was assessed after 14 ± 2 and 28 ± 2 consecutive days. Participants also reported subjective symptoms and product preferences.

In general, mild to barely discernible irritation was present at study inception. Erythema of the mons pubis, labia majora, labia minor, vestibule, perineum, buttocks, or upper thighs, when present, improved over the course of the study in both groups.

Genital moisture on the labia majora and the perineum significantly increased in wet wipe users ($p = 0.01$) compared to dry tissue users.

Subjective reports from participants were instructive (Table 3). Wet wipes were significantly preferred to dry toilet tissue by postmenopausal

Table 3 Subjective product ratings following 28 days use of wet wipes of dry toilet tissue by postmenopausal women

	Treatment	
	Wet wipes	Dry toilet tissue
	$N = 31$	$N = 29$
Assessment	N (%)	N (%)
Comfort ratings		
Excellent	10 (32)	8 (28)
Very good	16 (52)	11 (40)
Good	3 (10)	8 (28)
Fair	2 (6)	1 (3)
Poor	0 (0)	1 (3)
Severity of subjective comments about sensory effects		
Dryness	1 (3.2) Slight	3 (10) Slight
Sticky sensation	3 (9.7) Slight	0 (0) None
Burning	4 (12.9) Slight	1 (3.4) Slight
Itching	1 (3.2) Slight	0 (0) None
Stinging	3 (9.7) Slight	1 (3.4) Slight

The first evaluation occurred at day 14 (±2) of product use
Source of data: Farage et al. [63]. Reprinted with permission from Science Printers and Publishers

women: 26 of 31 (84 %) of wet wipe users rated their assigned product *excellent* to *very good* for skin comfort compared to 19 of 29 (66 %) of dry tissue users. However, 4 of 31 (13 %) of women using wet wipes reported more burning and 3 of 31 (10 %) experienced more stinging compared to the product they typically used. In addition, 3 of 31 (10 %) reported a more of a "sticky" sensation with the wet product. Overall, 3 of the 31 (10 %) postmenopausal participants considered the wipes to be too wet [63]. Hence, a significant majority of postmenopausal users favored wet wipes over conventional products, although some did not care for the associated sensations of wetness. However, postmenopausal wipes users were less likely to be bothered by skin wetness than premenopausal women (see original report) and were more likely to favor wet wipes over dry tissue for genital cleaning. Taken together, the results suggest that the hydrating effect of the wet wipes on genital skin was perceived to be beneficial by most postmenopausal women in the study, a group more likely to experience vulvar atrophy and skin dryness.

Conclusion

The vulva undergoes morphological and physiological changes over the course of a woman's lifetime. Many of these changes are mediated by sex hormones. Estrogen depletion alters the structure of vulvovaginal tissues, making them more susceptible to inflammation. Vulvovaginal skin disorders associated with aging include atrophic vaginitis, incontinence dermatitis, fungal and bacterial infections secondary to incontinence, anogenital pruritus, perianal inflammation, and decubitus ulcers. Clinical trials indicate that feminine hygiene wet wipes may improve skin comfort in postmenopausal women. Four weeks of exclusive use of wet wipes in lieu of dry toilet tissue caused negligible effects on vulvar skin irritation but a clinically observable increase in genital skin moisture. Most postmenopausal women in the study favored wet wipes over dry toilet tissue, which may suggest improved comfort of atrophied vulvar skin and amelioration of dryness associated with postmenopausal estrogen depletion.

Cross-References

- ▶ Aging Genital Skin and Hormone Replacement Therapy Benefits
- ▶ Solutions and Products for Managing Female Urinary Incontinence
- ▶ Unique Skin Immunology of the Lower Female Genital Tract with Age
- ▶ Vaginal Secretions with Age

References

1. Nauth H. Anatomy and physiology of the vulva. In: Elsner P, Martius J, editors. Vulvovaginitis. New York: Marcel Dekker; 1993.
2. Sargeant P, Moate R, Harris JE, et al. Ultrastructural study of the epithelium of the normal human vulva. J Submicrosc Cytol Pathol. 1996;28:161–70.
3. Farage MA, Maibach H. Lifetime changes in the vulva and vagina. Arch Gynecol Obstet. 2006;273:195–202.
4. Jones IS. A histological assessment of normal vulval skin. Clin Exp Dermatol. 1983;8:513–21.
5. Woodruff JD, Friedrich EGJ. The vestibule. Clin Obstet Gynecol. 1985;28:134–41.
6. Williams TS, Callen JP, Owen LG. Vulvar disorders in the prepubertal female. Pediatr Ann. 1986;15:588–9. 592–601, 604–5.
7. Marshall W, Tanner J. Puberty. In: Davis J, Dobbing J, editors. Scientific foundations of paediatrics. London: Heinemann; 1981.
8. Nauth HF, Haas M. Cytologic and histologic observations on the sex hormone dependence of the vulva. J Reprod Med. 1985;30:667–74.
9. Torgerson RR, Marnach ML, Bruce AJ, et al. Oral and vulvar changes in pregnancy. Clin Dermatol. 2006;24:122–32.
10. Wong RC, Ellis CN. Physiologic skin changes in pregnancy. J Am Acad Dermatol. 1984;10:929–40.
11. Chang L, Muram D. Pediatric & adolescent gynecology. In: DeCherney AH, Nathan L, editors. Current diagnosis & treatment obstetrics and gynecology. New York: McGraw-Hill; 2002.
12. Harper WF, McNicol EM. A histological study of normal vulval skin from infancy to old age. Br J Dermatol. 1977;96:249–53.
13. Farage MA, Maibach HI, Deliveliotou A, et al. Changes in the vulva and vagina throughout life. In: Farage MA, Maibach HI, editors. The vulva: anatomy, physiology, and pathology. New York: Informa Healthcare; 2006.
14. Nauth HF, Schilke E. Cytology of the exfoliative layer in normal and diseased vulvar skin: correlation with histology. Acta Cytol. 1982;26:269–83.
15. Pandit L, Ouslander JG. Postmenopausal vaginal atrophy and atrophic vaginitis. Am J Med Sci. 1997;314:228–31.
16. Yen SS. The biology of menopause. J Reprod Med. 1977;18:287–96.
17. Phillips TJ, Demircay Z, Sahu M. Hormonal effects on skin aging. Clin Geriatr Med. 2001;17:661–72.
18. Nauth HF, Böger A. New aspects of vulvar cytology. Acta Cytol. 1982;26:1–6.
19. Erickson KL, Montagna W. New observations on the anatomical features of the female genitalia. J Am Med Womens Assoc. 1972;27:573–81.
20. Farage MA, Miller KW, Elsner P, et al. Intrinsic and extrinsic factors in skin ageing: a review. Int J Cosmet Sci. 2008;30:87–95.
21. Oriba HA, Elsner P, Maibach HI. Vulvar physiology. Semin Dermatol. 1989;8:2–6.
22. Elsner P, Maibach HI. The effect of prolonged drying on transepidermal water loss, capacitance and pH of human vulvar and forearm skin. Acta Derm Venereol. 1990;70:105–9.
23. Oriba HA, Bucks DA, Maibach HI. Percutaneous absorption of hydrocortisone and testosterone on the vulva and forearm: effect of the menopause and site. Br J Dermatol. 1996;134:229–33.
24. Elsner P, Wilhelm D, Maibach HI. Effect of low-concentration sodium lauryl sulfate on human vulvar and forearm skin. Age-related differences. J Reprod Med. 1991;36:77–81.
25. Elsner P, Wilhelm D, Maibach HI. Frictional properties of human forearm and vulvar skin: influence of age and correlation with transepidermal water loss and capacitance. Dermatologica. 1990;181:88–91.
26. Stiles M, Redmer J, Paddock E, et al. Gynecologic issues in geriatric women. J Womens Health (Larchmt). 2012;21:4–9.
27. Seyfarth F, Schliemann S, Antonov D, et al. Dry skin, barrier function, and irritant contact dermatitis in the elderly. Clin Dermatol. 2011;29:31–6.
28. Bachmann GA, Nevadunsky NS. Diagnosis and treatment of atrophic vaginitis. Am Fam Physician. 2000;61:3090–6.
29. Castelo-Branco C, Cancelo MJ, Villero J, et al. Management of post-menopausal vaginal atrophy and atrophic vaginitis. Maturitas. 2005;52 Suppl 1: S46–52.
30. Nyirjesy P, Leigh RD, Mathew L, et al. Chronic vulvovaginitis in women older than 50 years: analysis of a prospective database. J Low Genit Tract Dis. 2012;16:24–9.
31. Parish SJ, Nappi RE, Krychman ML, et al. Impact of vulvovaginal health on postmenopausal women: a review of surveys on symptoms of vulvovaginal atrophy. Int J Womens Health. 2013;5:437–47.
32. Reimer A, Johnson L. Atrophic vaginitis: signs, symptoms, and better outcomes. Nurse Pract. 2011;36:22–8; quiz 29.

33. Pearson T. Atrophic vaginitis. J Nurse Pract. 2011;7:502–5.
34. Weber MA, Limpens J, Roovers JP. Assessment of vaginal atrophy: a review. Int Urogynecol J. 2015;26:15–28.
35. Heimer GM, Englund DE. Effects of vaginally-administered oestriol on post-menopausal urogenital disorders: a cytohormonal study. Maturitas. 1992;14:171–9.
36. Fraser IS, Ayton R, Farrell E, et al. A multicentre Australian trial of low dose estradiol therapy for symptoms of vaginal atrophy using a vaginal ring as delivery system. Maturitas. 1995;22(Suppl):S41.
37. Santen RJ, Pinkerton JV, Conaway M, et al. Treatment of urogenital atrophy with low-dose estradiol: preliminary results. Menopause. 2002;9:179–87.
38. Cano A, Estévez J, Usandizaga R, et al. The therapeutic effect of a new ultra low concentration estriol gel formulation (0.005% estriol vaginal gel) on symptoms and signs of postmenopausal vaginal atrophy: results from a pivotal phase III study. Menopause. 2012;19:1130–9.
39. Millard RJ, Moore KH. Urinary incontinence: the Cinderella subject. Med J Aust. 1996;165:124–5.
40. Resnick NM. Geratric medicine. In: Tierney L, McPhee S, Papdakis M, editors. Current medical diagnosis and treatment. New York: McGraw Hill; 2000.
41. Farage MA, Bowtell P, Katsarou A. The relationship among objectively assessed vulvar erythema, skin sensitivity, genital sensitivity, and self-reported facial skin redness. J Appl Res. 2006;6:272.
42. Farage MA, Maibach HI. Morphology and physiological changes of genital skin and mucosa. Curr Probl Dermatol. 2011;40:9–19.
43. Farage MA, Miller KW, Berardesca E, et al. Incontinence in the aged: contact dermatitis and other cutaneous consequences. Contact Dermatitis. 2007;57:211–7.
44. Aly R, Shirley C, Cunico B, et al. Effect of prolonged occlusion on the microbial flora, pH, carbon dioxide and transepidermal water loss on human skin. J Invest Dermatol. 1978;71:378–81.
45. Zhai H, Maibach HI. Skin occlusion and irritant and allergic contact dermatitis: an overview. Contact Dermatitis. 2001;44:201–6.
46. Gray M, Beeckman D, Bliss DZ, et al. Incontinence-associated dermatitis: a comprehensive review and update. J Wound Ostomy Continence Nurs. 2012;39:61–74.
47. Gray M. Preventing and managing perineal dermatitis: a shared goal for wound and continence care. J Wound Ostomy Continence Nurs. 2004;31:S2–9; quiz S10-2.
48. Lyder CH, Clemes-Lowrance C, Davis A, et al. Structured skin care regimen to prevent perineal dermatitis in the elderly. J ET Nurs. 1992;19:12–6.
49. Mistiaen P, Poot E, Hickox S, et al. Preventing and treating intertrigo in the large skin folds of adults: a literature overview. Dermatol Nurs. 2004;16:43–6.
50. Norman RA, Young EM. Intertrigo. In: Atlas of geriatric dermatology. London: Springer; 2014.
51. Martin ES, Elewski BE. Cutaneous fungal infections in the elderly. Clin Geriatr Med. 2002;18:59–75.
52. Black JM, Gray M, Bliss DZ, et al. MASD part 2: incontinence-associated dermatitis and intertriginous dermatitis: a consensus. J Wound Ostomy Continence Nurs. 2011;38:359–70; quiz 371-2.
53. LeLievre S. Skin care for older people with incontinence. Elder Care. 2000;11:36–8.
54. Veraldi S. Rapid relief of intertrigo-associated pruritus due to Candida albicans with isoconazole nitrate and diflucortolone valerate combination therapy. Mycoses. 2013;56 Suppl 1:41–3.
55. Shenefelt PD, Fenske NA. Aging and the skin: recognizing and managing common disorders. Geriatrics. 1990;45:57–9.
56. Kumar N, Behera B, Sagiri SS, et al. Bacterial vaginosis: etiology and modalities of treatment-A brief note. J Pharm Bioallied Sci. 2011;3:496–503.
57. Caquant F, Collinet P, Deruelle P, et al. Perineal cellulitis following trans-obturator sub-urethral tape Uratape. Eur Urol. 2005;47:108–10.
58. Connolly TP. Necrotizing surgical site infection after tension-free vaginal tape. Obstet Gynecol. 2004;104:1275–6.
59. Fiers S, Thayer D. Management of intractable incontinence. In: Doughty D, editor. Urinary and fecal incontinence: nursing management. St. Louis: Mosby; 2000.
60. Harold C, ed. Professional guide to diseases. 9th Edition. Ambler, PA: Lippincott, Williams and Wilkins. pp 775–781. 2009.
61. Edlich RF, Winters KL, Woodard CR, et al. Pressure ulcer prevention. J Long Term Eff Med Implants. 2004;14:285–304.
62. Fader M, Clarke-O'Neill S, Cook D, et al. Management of night-time urinary incontinence in residential settings for older people: an investigation into the effects of different pad changing regimes on skin health. J Clin Nurs. 2003;12:374–86.
63. Farage MA, Stadler A, Chassard D, et al. A randomized prospective trial of the cutaneous and sensory effects of feminine hygiene wet wipes. J Reprod Med. 2008;53:765–73.

Part XV

Cosmetic Surgeries

A New Paradigm for the Aging Face 148

Samuel M. Lam

Contents

S.M. Lam (✉)
Willow Bend Wellness Center, Lam Facial Plastic Surgery Center and Hair Restoration Institute, Plano, TX, USA
e-mail: drlam@lamfacialplastics.com

M.A. Farage et al. (eds.), *Textbook of Aging Skin*,
DOI 10.1007/978-3-662-47398-6_104

Abstract

This chapter encapsulates the process of facial aging as primarily a result of volumetric involution. In particular, the important concept of framing the eye rather than elevating and excavating is discussed as a principal method of facial rejuvenation. Other concepts like reducing facial transitions and improving facial shape are explored as adjunctive measures to improve the youthfulness of the face. The pros, cons, and limitations of facial fat grafting as a method of facial volumization are detailed, and a hair transplant model of graft take is also used to illustrate longevity of fat grafting. Today, fat grafting and facial fillers are the two principal methods for facial volumization, and restoring volume to the face should be a vital component to an overall strategy for facial rejuvenation.

Introduction

This textbook is dedicated to a thorough understanding of the aging skin that encompasses both basic science and clinical topics. However, the effects of skin aging extend well beyond the inherent microarchitecture of the cutis itself. Concomitant aging processes have a remarkable impact on the appearance of the skin as well, which will be covered in this chapter. An outdated perspective of the aging process for the human face is that the only two components of facial aging include manifest skin changes, e.g., rhytids, textural worsening, solar elastosis, and dyschromias, and gravitational effects, e.g., brow, periorbital, midface, jawline, and neck descent. However, the concept of volume deflation via loss of both soft tissue and bone has increasingly been recognized not only as an ancillary part of the aging process but also as a core facet of aging [1]. Although various components of the aging process will be discussed in this chapter, the central role of volume loss will be elucidated in great detail and the effect that volume loss and volume repletion have on the appearance of the skin will be explored.

Although some fundamental scientific ideas will be evaluated, this chapter is almost entirely of a clinical nature. It discusses how the facial aging process is seen as well as how surgical and nonsurgical interventions are made to ameliorate this condition. Autologous facial fat transfer is the mainstay of therapy for facial rejuvenation followed by other adjunctive measures including rhytidectomy, hair restoration, and skin therapies. Regarding facial fat transfer, some new theories about the observed stem-cell changes to the skin in which scarring, dyschromias, and rhytids diminish over a period of 1–2 years following a fat transfer will also be discussed.

From a surgeon's perspective, this textbook is principally focused on educating the students and researchers on aging skin, and in this case, the overall aging process related to cutaneous aging. Accordingly, very little will be addressed as far as elaborate technical execution of surgical methods is concerned. Instead, the primary focus will be in alignment with the objectives of this textbook, which are to provide current and comprehensive understandings of the aging process, i.e., to teach the reader to see more than to do.

Understanding the Facial Aging Process Using a Volume-Centric Model

As alluded to earlier, the effect of gravity on the facial aging process has been greatly overestimated. What was once thought to be distinctly gravitational has been reconsidered as representing volume deflation. Lambros studied the aging process by superimposing the face of a mature individual over the exact pose of that same individual at 20 years of age [2]. He then evaluated the effects that accounted for periorbital, midface, and jawline aging. His results are nothing short of remarkable: the brow was seen on occasion to descend approximately 1 mm but no further, the lower eyelid-cheek interface did not fall at all, the cheek and nasolabial groove did not descend at all, and the jawline actually went up with aging. This latter observation can be quite confusing without further explanation. The jowl that appears with aging has been thought in the past to represent descent of that part of the jawline. What Lambros discovered was that the entire jawline that was once volumetrically full (by virtue of replete fat, soft tissue, and bone) was actually, at one point, situated below the jowl along its entire length. In other words, the entire jawline recedes superiorly to expose the jowl. In addition, by examining the relative position of nevi to the surrounding anatomic landmarks, he found that nevi do not fall downward, but either do not change position at all or migrate horizontally along muscle pull directions, indicating a volumetric deflation rather than a descent.

With this almost unassailable empiric study, it is hard to argue that gravity is the principal mechanism by which facial aging occurs. Further, simply having patients bring in their own photographs during their youth will help educate both the patient and the surgeon regarding what techniques would be ideal to rejuvenate that patient so that the result will approximate their own youthful mien and avoid the unnatural alteration of identity that can occur through overzealous, traditional, excisional techniques. Lambros states: "The brows do not fall as much as we pick them up" [3]. Accordingly, using old photographs can be an instructive guide to plan surgical intervention.

Interestingly, traditional textbooks on plastic surgery are perhaps the worst source of information to understand the aging process and what is required to rejuvenate the face. Brows are arbitrarily lifted upward and upper eyelid skin aggressively removed along with upper eyelid fat. Lower eyelids have fat extracted and skin

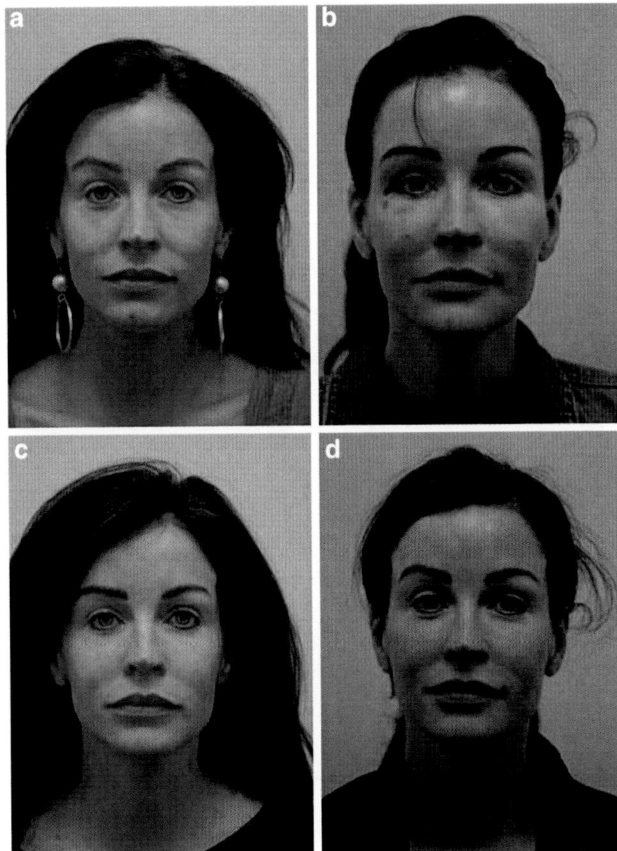

Fig. 1 This 45-year-old woman is shown (**a**) before fat transfer but after eyelid and browlift surgery (done elsewhere) that have in combination left her looking different and not more youthful. She is shown (**b**) 1 week following full facial fat transfer, (**c**) 3 months after the procedure with a slight dip in appearance, and (**d**) 1 year after a single session of fat transfer

tightened leaving the area hollower and the canthal position unnaturally changed. Instead, the "textbooks" that have the most accurate information on what defines youth are entitled *Glamour*, *Allure*, and *Vogue* and can be purchased at any newsstand. The reader is encouraged to review these exemplars of youthful beauty to understand facial shape, proportion, and what exactly defines youth. In many instances, the very low brows that are robustly full will perhaps shock a complacent surgeon/physician into rethinking the aging process entirely.

Framing the Eye

Traditional reductive surgery, especially in the periorbital region, oftentimes leads to an acceleration of the aging process in which the hollower eyelid and brow are manifestly more so after the procedure (Fig. 1). *In* short, traditional eyelid and brow surgery can actually render an individual even older in appearance than the desired rejuvenation. A model to understand what in fact happens with the brow is to think of a balloon that deflates, in which the goal is not to excise the hanging and deflated skin but to refill the lost volume (Fig. 2). Now, in selected individuals, a very small degree of skin (1–3 mm) is removed but almost always in conjunction with fat transfer to the brow and upper eyelid for the aforementioned reasons. Performing browlifts was stopped several years ago realizing today that a browlift is rarely, if ever, indicated and can be counterproductive in the ultimate goal of framing the eye with fat. The lower eyelid "eyebag" that appears most oftentimes does not need to be removed, but additional fat is added along the exposed periorbital bony rim. This again represents the opposite strategy of traditional surgery in which

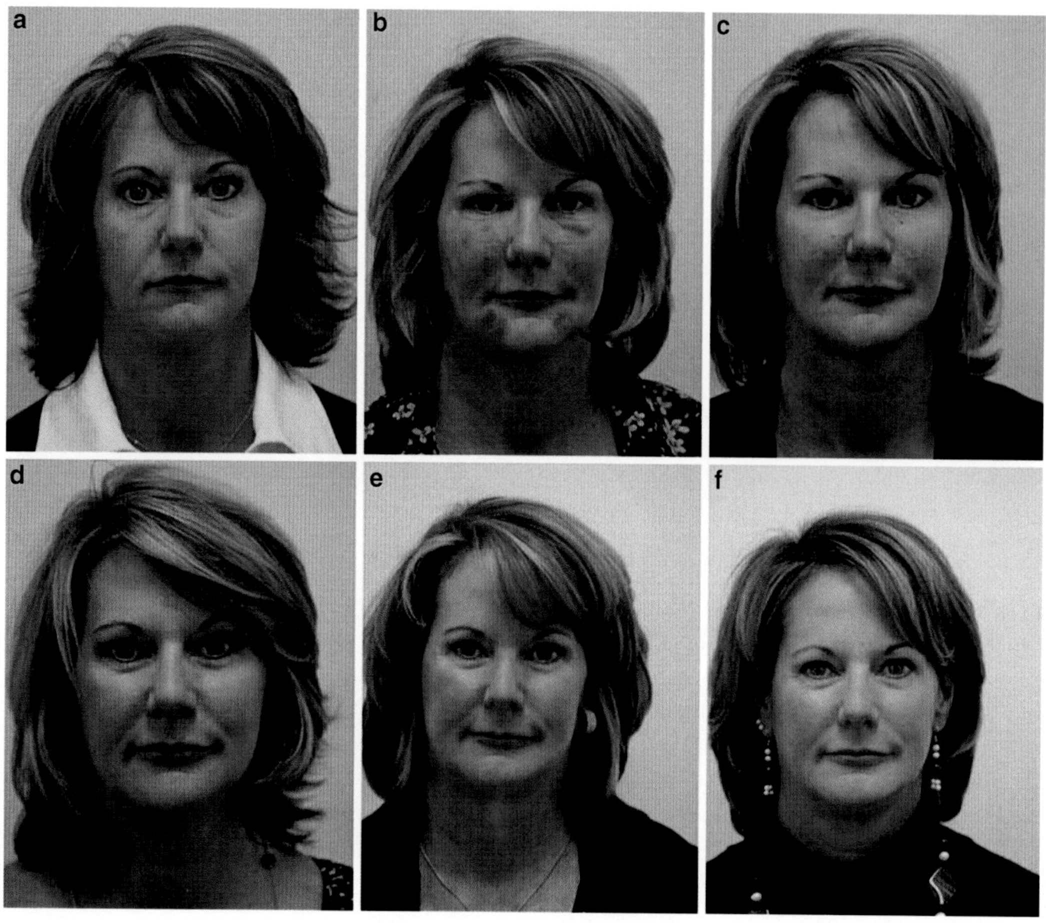

Fig. 2 This 46-year-old woman appears to require traditional eyelid surgery. However, with closer inspection she exhibits a hollow eye deformity due to volume loss that also involves the entire face. She is shown (**a**) before fat transfer, (**b**) 1 week after fat transfer, (**c**) 1 month after, (**d**) 3 months after, (**e**) 1 year after, and (**f**) 1.5 years following a single session of fat grafting

the eyebag is removed and the skin is tightened. A model for the lower eyelid may be informative to understand this concept better: the rocks (eyebag) are covered by high tide (fat along the orbital rim), but when the shoreline recedes (panfacial fat loss), the rocks that were once covered become evident. In a lecture, William Little explained it this way, and his analogy makes quite a bit of sense. In other words, the exposed orbital fat may be thought of as being camouflaged in youth with the presence of fat surrounding it along the orbital rim. A transconjunctival blepharoplasty is performed to remove excessive orbital fat only in about 5 % of operative cases but almost always in conjunction with adding fat along the bony orbital rim. Skin resurfacing and botulinum toxin are used to address the cutaneous changes in the lower periorbital region, and no skin is almost ever removed along the lower half of the periorbital frame for fear of changing the lower eyelid and/or canthal position in an unfavorable way.

Another finding that Lambros discovered in his seminal study was that the eyelid shape is more almond configured in youth no matter the race and that in turn becomes increasingly smaller and rounder in shape with age. This narrower eyelid shape of aging is more accentuated via traditional browlifting techniques and aggressive reductive eyelid blepharoplasty, which has been facetiously termed blepharectomy (Fig. 1). Although there is no known method to safely re-enlarge the lateral canthus to resemble the almond shape of youth without risking unpredictable scleral show, fat transfer to the lateral brow can help draw one's attention to the illusory widening of the eye shape rather than a further narrowing of it. These concepts are very difficult to explain with superlative clarity, and the reader is advised to study young and old (unoperated) eyes in the quest to understand what takes place in nature rather than what happens in the preconceived brain or biased surgical training history that can taint perceptions of the aging process.

Recalibrating Perceptions and Redefining Aging

Most individuals, specifically women, seek microchanges to their face, namely, improvement in the appearance of small folds and creases around their mouth, reduction of the "crepiness" of their upper eyelid, etc. The reason for this desire in change is that women in particular apply makeup at close range so that the small facial flaws take center stage and appear to be the focus for aesthetic improvement. The first goal of the aesthetic surgeon/physician is to recalibrate what may be more important for the patient when evaluating the face for aging and related cosmetic enhancement. Gladwell's [4] brilliant thesis, *Blink*, argues that we judge another individual in a blink of an eye. When evaluating the face for aging, it should be understood what programs us to make an almost immediate, visceral response to another person's attractiveness and aging. It is certainly not the micro skin effects in the perioral region in most cases, but a larger gestalt that is quickly apparent upon first glance.

Before wrinkles and small flaws can be appreciated, the gut response of a bystander judging another individual regarding age and attractiveness at even a relatively far social distance of 10–20 f. should be the measure of how aging is understood. What is the fundamental element, then, if it is not the prescribed traditional vocabulary of wrinkles, folds, and other minor flaws? In a word – geometry. The facial shape of another as being older or younger is recognized almost instantaneously. This concept is further refined in this chapter.

The shape of the face of a baby, a young child, a teenager, and an individual in his/her early 20s is round owing to the abundance of so-called baby fat despite overall body weight or habitus. The ongoing volume loss of the face is a continuous process that begins from infancy forward. An individual in his/her early 20s has proportionately less fat in the face than a child or a baby. Accordingly, this process continues for the remainder of one's life. Most women in fact who are dreadfully afraid of looking fat oftentimes when they pass 35 years of age look retrospectively at their youth and in the majority of cases prefer the look of their face in their early 30s than in their 20s due to the slimming effect that further soft-tissue loss affords them. However, passing through the early 30s into the mid to late 30s, a slight fatigue and aging become more apparent as they mature passing through the narrow window of full-framed youth to thinner 30-something youth to now slight aging with further volume loss.

These volume changes can be redefined more precisely with geometric terminology in broad strokes. From infancy to early 20s, the predominant facial shape is round. With a slight slimming effect that occurs in the early 30s and loss of fat in the buccal area among other areas, the face transforms into a triangle with the apices in the anterior cheek and chin. In the intervening mid to late 20s, a hybrid shape is observed somewhere between a circle and a triangle, i.e., a less circular circle or a slightly widened triangle. Keep in mind that these geometric assumptions are not meant to describe each and every individual person, as variances occur owing to gender, race, genetics, weight, and environmental insults like sun exposure, smoking, etc.

As volume loss progresses from mid 30s into the early 40s, the face assumes a more masculine appearance whether the individual is a man or a woman. The eyes and the cheeks flatten, and the padding of the anterior chin starts to dissipate exposing the underlying malar and chin bone protuberances. With volume loss across the expanse of the jawline minus the jowl region, the apices of a new geometry shift toward the appearance of a square: the malar bone and the jowl become the new apices of this square. The flattening effect of the face further accentuates the masculine contour along with the exposed bone, which is a masculinizing attribute. Many male models are chosen for their flatter anterior cheek profile, as they look more chiseled and attractive for these masculine hallmarks. It has been noticed that even very young male models are chosen for this attribute of greater bone exposure than their female counterparts.

As metabolism slows in the late 30s and beyond, weight gain is oftentimes more prevalent at this juncture. The mid to late 40s and thereafter exposes the curious mixture of weight gain and soft-tissue volume loss further unbalancing the face. The soft tissue of the periorbital region, upper anterior cheek, and anterior chin continues to dissipate in the face of weight gain that becomes more pronounced in the lower anterior cheek and the jowl region along with neck adiposity. The dominance of the lower face and ongoing recession of the upper face with marked depressions running superomedially down inferolaterally in the anterior cheek transform the face into the shape of an upside triangle. These progressive changes become even more apparent with further aging of the 50s and beyond as the lower face dominates with concurrent volume loss of the periorbital region and midface.

Beyond Geometry: Understanding Transitions and Highlights

Is gross geometry then the only perception of aging? Obviously not, as the neck does suffer from gravitational forces with the exposure of loosening platysma. There are also readily apparent signs of cutaneous damage with the onset of rhytids, dyschromias, etc. However, what can be more important than both neck descent and skin changes is what could be termed microgeometry. The aforementioned geometry in the previous section can be smoothly presented with minimal transitions or with multiple abrupt demarcations. Take for example an overweight child or young adult versus an overweight 50 years something. If they are both replete with fat, how does the brain determine their aging even before a wrinkle or a hanging neck is perceived? The answer lies in the fact that an overweight youth is uniformly convex and uniformly round. An overweight person past 35 years of age or so will exhibit areas of marked hollowness that become even more pronounced alongside pockets of excessive weight gain in the lower cheek, jowl, and neck area. These abruptions in gross geometry further accentuate perception of aging. That is how it is possible to tell if someone is young and simply full with their natural baby fat, someone overweight and young, and someone overweight and older.

The young person even when very thin will still maintain a soft-tissue padding that is relatively uniform unless they are so thin that they look emaciated. An older individual will show abrupt transition points as the underlying bone is exposed and retaining ligaments exacerbate transition points. In short, a young face exhibits relative uniformity, whereas an older face displays signs of obvious transitions between various facial regions despite weight, neck descent, and signs of skin aging.

With that respect, another word to introduce in perception is convexity. The reader is reminded that in daily life, most situations involve the play of overhead lighting. Indoors, top-down lighting is the norm, and even outdoors, the sun shines from a relatively high vantage point. Flash photography, on the other hand, tends to wash out facial features that can improve one's appearance. Daily life is not so kind. With overhead lighting, everyone can look a bit worse. The more pointed the light source from above, the worse that facial features can appear. The well-known "mug shot" look of celebrities caught after a bad night of partying reflects as much their torrid state as the harsh overcast lighting. With all of that in mind, two attributes of the aging process become sharply defined in relief with standard overhead lighting: the appearance of unwelcome facial transition zones (previously discussed) and the presence/absence of light convexity. The flatter the face with aging, the less is the light bounce that the face transmits back to the viewer. Relative convexity of the lateral brow, upper cheek, and chin with reflected light bounce back to the viewer is the hallmark of a youthful face. Softening abrupt transitions and creating facial convexity are two major objectives of facial fat transfer. Interestingly, when it comes to the appearance of skin, more light on the skin will make it look brighter and thereby more youthful. Other effects of fat transfer on the skin will be discussed next.

Stem-Cell Changes and Other Cutaneous Manifestations Following Fat Transfer

Although skin resurfacing techniques and botulinum toxin remain the gold standards for addressing the signs of aging skin, there has been a consensus among fat-transfer surgeons that favorable skin changes can occur down the road following fat transfer [5]. Wrinkles, scars, pores, texture, and other pathologies have been noted to diminish in areas overlying transplanted fat. These cutaneous effects, if they manifest, require months if not a year or more to start to show up. Personal findings noted the reduction of acne scarring after a year or more as well as scar reductions in areas that failed to be corrected with conventional scar revision surgery. Reports have claimed improvement in conditions such as radiation damage, chronic ulceration, breast capsular contracture, and damaged vocal cords. Thoughts include that transplanted fat cells may contain adipocyte-derived stem cells or preadipocytes that can repair surrounding tissues and perhaps even transform into bone, cartilage, muscle, blood vessels, nerves, and skin [6]. Thinking and research on these purported claims are still in their nascent phase, but the clinical evidence is difficult to deny.

Long-Term Outcomes Using a Hair Transplant Model

A major drawback that has been expressed regarding transplanted fat is its equivocal longevity. Simply put, this problem was not observed. With proper hand harvesting using gentle negative pressure, centrifugation to purify the fat cells, and atraumatic cannula injection techniques using microdroplet technique, transplanted fat holds remarkably well. It is with rare exception that an additional session is required to attain the optimal results. However, to understand the nature of this longevity, the evolution of fat grafting results over the first 2 years and beyond must be understood.

A critical study [7] documents the evolution of a fat grafting result over the first 18 months using three-dimensional computer VECTRA modeling. Using this method, the author quantified the volume a fat-transfer result would have preoperatively and at points measured at 3 months and every 3 months thereafter for the first year and a half. What they found was that the fat-transfer results at 3 months in many cases had the same volume as preoperatively, i.e., there was no appreciable volumetric gain. However, at 6 months the result started to increase in volume and steadily did so in each recorded interval, i.e., every 3 months. The obvious question then is: why should this happen? Why would the result apparently evaporate at 3 months and then steadily increase thereafter. Hair transplant surgery using follicular-based grafts is very similar to a fat transfer for the following reasons. First, they both rely on free grafts, i.e., no direct microvascular attachment, just freely transplanted with surrounding blood supply creeping in over time. Second, both types of grafts are relatively small and numerous (tiny parcels of fat the size of 1/50th of a cubic centimeter compared with tiny hair grafts containing one to four hairs). Third, they are both transplanted into the same general body region, i.e., the head. Finally, albeit least importantly, they are both performed for cosmetic purposes.

Walter Unger's book, *Hair Transplantation* [8], explains how transplanted hair grafts attain their blood supply over time. During the first few days, nutrients from the surrounding tissue enter the graft through a process known as plasmatic imbibition. Thereafter, a tenuous blood supply maintains graft viability through a process known as primary and secondary inosculation. It is not until 6 months following a hair transplant that formal neovascularization is fully attained. This time period also correlates with clinical onset of substantive hair growth. From experience, except for occasional examples of significant hair growth at 3–4 months, in most cases pronounced clinical growth is generally evident starting approximately 6 months following hair transplant surgery. Hair grafts then continue to grow at variable rates for the first 18 months.

Not surprisingly, a similar progress in the evolution of a fat grafting result was clinically observed. The only difference would be that hair grafts typically fall out after the first few weeks, whereas a fat grafting result can persist for the first 6 weeks or so owing to the presence of edema since fat grafting is contingent upon soft-tissue volume, whereas a hair transplant result obviously is not. Like a hair transplant, a process of vascular inosculation maintains the fat graft alive, which does not become clinically apparent until typically 6 months following the procedure at which time neovascularization has been established with ongoing growth of a result in the majority of cases for the first 18 months or so just like a hair transplant.

The longevity of a hair transplant and fat grafting result is also correlative. An individual who undergoes a hair transplant will retain the transplanted grafts but suffer ongoing hair loss in susceptible hairs that have not been transplanted. Similarly, once the fat grafting attains a mature blood supply, the grafts survive but ongoing volume loss of nontransplanted fat occurs with ineluctable aging. Generally, a fat transfer may require a minor touch-up procedure 3–4 years later in someone with a genetic predisposition toward more accelerated aging but will not require anything further for 5–10 years in most individuals.

It has been speculated that fat grafting has been so roundly condemned in the past with regard to longevity due to several reasons. First, poor technique can compromise longevity with speculated errors including traumatic donor harvesting, inadequate or excessive processing, and improper infiltration techniques. Second, physicians may not sufficiently follow clinical results over time or understand the nature of a transplant result. More specifically, the 3-month interval that often presents a clinical situation that is quite unimpressive and may discourage surgeons from continuing, since the result appears to have dissipated. Conversely, filling a patient repeatedly during these time intervals of volume descent may lead to an uncorrectable overfilling when the fat grafting result attains maturity 2 years later.

Some of the stem-cell changes that have been proposed for fat transfer have also been observed clinically when hair transplanted into regions of scarring alopecia can actually heal the damaged and cicatricial skin. Obviously, the effect that a transplanted hair graft has on surrounding tissues may arise through a recognized stem-cell process. The pilosebaceous unit is considered the source for skin regeneration with stem cells understood to reside in the bulge region of the hair shaft. In addition, the long-standing premise of modern hair transplant surgery that transplanted hairs fully retain the native characteristics of their donor region is being recently challenged [9]. For example, hairs grafted from the occiput into the eyebrow region have shown a retardation of hair growth rate to match that of native eyebrow hairs. In addition, hairs transplanted from the body to the scalp in individuals who have depleted their occipital donor hair have been shown to start growing more rapidly and become finer in caliber over time. These profound clinical observations reveal how little is known about the nature of a transplanted graft and skin and hair changes in general.

Conclusion

The landscape of understanding facial aging is constantly a shifting terrain. Most of the traditional thinking that dominated perception of aging (i.e., gravity and wrinkles) this past century has been recently upended by distilling the concept of aging through the primary mechanism of soft-tissue (and bony) volume depletion. The juncture between dermatologic and surgical worlds to restore the aging face has become more apparent than ever. The novel concepts of stem-cell changes that can manifest following fat transfer push this idea to an even greater measure. Ongoing clinical and basic science research will ensure that more natural results are attained for facial rejuvenation that also more closely parallel the true nature of facial aging with possible derivative benefits to the understanding and treatment of the aging skin.

Cross-References

▶ Cosmetic Surgery in the Elderly
▶ Facial Rejuvenation: A Chronology of Procedures

References

1. Lam S, Glasgold M, Glasgold R. Complementary fat grafting. Philadelphia: Lippincott; 2007.
2. Lambros V. Observations on periorbital and midface aging. Plast Reconstr Surg. 2007;120(5):1367–76.
3. Lambros V. Lecture at Cedars-Sinai Medical Center. Los Angeles, October 26, 2008.
4. Gladwell M. Blink: the power of thinking without thinking. Boston: Little, Brown; 2005.
5. Having spoken to well-respected and experienced fat transfer surgeons over the years, the consensus is that these surgeons have clinically observed cutaneous benefits that have been thought to be related to fat transplant beyond what would have been observed through any other more direct skin therapy.
6. Coleman S. Structural fat grafting: more than a permanent filler. Plast Reconstr Surg. 2006;118:108S–20.
7. Meier JD, Glasgold RA, Glasgold MJ. Autologous fat grafting: long-term evidence of its efficacy in midfacial rejuvenation. Arch Facial Plast Surg. 2009;11(1):24–8.
8. Unger W, Shapiro R, editors. Hair transplantation. 4th ed. London: Informa Healthcare; 2004.
9. Lee S, Kim D, Jun J, et al. The changes in hair growth pattern after autologous hair transplantation. Dermatol Surg. 1999;25:605–9.

Cosmetic Surgery in the Elderly

149

Richard Scarborough, Dwight Scarborough, Kimberly M. Eickhorst, and Emil Bisaccia

Contents

R. Scarborough (✉)
University Hospitals Case Medical Center, Cleveland, OH, USA
e-mail: Richard.scarborough@uhhospitals.org

D. Scarborough
Clinical Assistant Professor of Medicine, Division of Dermatology, The Ohio State University Wexner Medical Center, Columbus, OH, USA
e-mail: Scarbor@ccf.org

K.M. Eickhorst
Dermatology Associates Of W CT, Danbury, CT, USA
e-mail: kimuva21@hotmail.com

E. Bisaccia
Columbia University College of Physicians and Surgeons, New York, NY, USA
e-mail: ebisaccia@gmail.com

M.A. Farage et al. (eds.), *Textbook of Aging Skin*,
DOI 10.1007/978-3-662-47398-6_105

Abstract
Cosmetic surgery in the elderly is an increasingly sought-after means to augment the "aging gracefully" process. It has been long known that looking better supports feeling better, and through thoughtful and careful discussion with older patients, the surgeon may be able to preserve and bolster self-confidence. By maintaining who they have been appearance wise, seniors are motivated to get more life out of their years. In this chapter, we have provided a review of common surgical interventions to counter the effects of aging.

Introduction

Aging is a dynamic, biological process of tissue involution and evolution. In the skin, these physiologic and morphologic changes occur throughout many tissue layers. With time, both the epidermis and the dermis become thin. However, in the facial region, changes in the dermis, supporting tissues, adipose, and superficial muscular aponeurotic system (SMAS) are the most marked ones. It is specifically the alterations in the reticular cutis, the structures that lie between the skin and the SMAS (unique to the facial and neck regions), that most significantly contribute to the clinical signs of facial aging.

From an etiologic perspective, there are two categories of aging: extrinsic and intrinsic. Extrinsic changes result in pigmentary and textural differences that tend to leave the skin with blotchy discoloration. These types of skin changes are environmentally linked to ultraviolet radiation, oxidative damage, exposure to the elements, and smoking. In contrast, intrinsic changes are secondary to dermal, bone, and fat remodeling and are inevitable. Intrinsic changes are dependent on genetic and hormonal influences and are apparent in the sagging skin, rhytids, and subdermal atrophy seen in the elderly.

Changes in the reticular cutis of the face exemplify intrinsic aging. Many fibrous septa tightly connect the SMAS to the dermis and serve as a scaffold for the overlying skin. However, with time, intrinsic alterations in collagen, elastin, and ground substance cause the reticular cutis to become more compact, and the integrity of these connections is lost. As a consequence, the dermis is more lax and simply drapes the facial musculature rather than closely adhering and enveloping the underlying facial structures. These changes, in addition to the reduction in bony skeletal mass, lost facial muscular tone, and protrusion of fat pads, result in less structural support for the skin. Thus, the skin tends to hang off the face creating signs of gauntness, laxity, and rhytids.

Clinically, aging skin often appears "tarnished" with dyspigmentation, laxity, yellow hue, wrinkles, telangiectasias, and leathery appearance, as well as potential cutaneous malignancies and scars from their removal. But, on a microscopic level, aging skin begins to lose the orderly maturation of keratinocytes and melanocytes, Langerhans cells decrease in number, the dermis thins as it loses glycosaminoglycans and type I and III collagens, and disorganized, abnormal collagen and elastin replace their predecessors [1].

Regardless of the exact etiologic mechanism of aging, it is complex and variable. This wide range of complexities and variabilities is echoed in the potential dermatologic interventions that can be employed to correct or reverse the signs of aging. Dermatologic options for such revitalization range from nonsurgical modalities (Botox, filler substances, and nonablative lasers) to more aggressive resurfacing procedures (chemical peels, dermabrasion, and ablative lasers) and to more traditional, surgical procedures (liposuction, blepharoplasty, and various types of face- and neck lifting). The application of these revitalizing tools, along with their associated risks and expected outcomes, is explored over the course of this chapter.

Botox

Surgical options for rejuvenation continue to improve with increased numbers of minimally invasive procedures that are becoming available. However, many patients, either due to preexisting medical conditions or pure concern over associated surgical risks, desire esthetic correction from a nonsurgical approach. Aging of the upper face can be defined by varying degrees of forehead laxity, brow ptosis, horizontal creases in the mid forehead, and deepening glabellar furrows. For these patients, cosmetic injectables are simple modalities that can safely and efficaciously improve one's appearance.

Most wrinkles and undesirable facial lines are worsened by continued muscle movement. The hypertonic condition of the underlying muscular structure can render a harsh look to the face. Botox, a neurotoxin, can inhibit muscular contraction and diminish the excess, undesirable lines that communicate fatigue and/or negative expressions. Approved by the Food and Drug Administration (FDA) in 2002 for cosmetic treatment of glabellar lines, botulinum toxin type A (BTX-A), Botox, has become widely available for facial rejuvenation. By inhibiting muscular contraction, Botox helps to reduce the evidence of dynamic lines and correct facial asymmetry. Its appeal is largely due to its impressive safety profile in the appropriate trained professional's hands, lack of downtime, and relatively quick onset of action.

Botulinum toxin A is a naturally occurring exotoxin produced by *Clostridium botulinum*, which ultimately inhibits acetylcholine release and prevents local neuromuscular transmission. Botox is also used "off-label," or without the official approval of the FDA, for several other cosmetic indications. For example, horizontal forehead lines, "crow's feet," "bunny lines," chin dimpling, and platysmal bands are safely corrected by Botox [2]. The toxin binds to the receptor sites on motor nerve terminals and blocks neuromuscular conduction by inhibiting the release of acetylcholine. More specifically, BTX-A facilitates the cleavage of synaptosomal-associated membrane protein (SNAP-25), which is required for exocytosis of acetylcholine.

BTX-A has not been without competition. There are seven subtypes of botulinum neurotoxin (BTX-A through BTX-G). Type A is currently the most effective for human use, although BTX-B has also become available. Dysport (BTX-A), currently used only outside the United States, and Myobloc (BTX-B), approved by the FDA in 2000 only for the treatment of cervical dystonia, are not currently FDA approved for cosmetic use. It should be noted that all three of these toxins have completely different profiles in relation to manufacturing, action at the muscular junction, and potency and therefore should not be used interchangeably. For example, Dysport is known to diffuse farther away from injection sites, whereas Myobloc is much more painful on injection, compared to BTX-A toxins, due to its higher acidity. Myobloc also has a shorter duration of effectiveness [3].

Each vacuum-dried vial of Botox contains 100 U of (mouse) toxin, 0.5 mg of "human" albumin, and 0.9 mg of sodium chloride in sterile form, without preservative. Different physicians choose to dilute the Botox to different concentrations. Preserved saline dilution tends to be less painful upon administration. Once the Botox product is reconstituted, it should be stored at 28 °C. The degree of dilution can alter the manner in which the physician chooses to deliver the Botox. While higher doses of BTX-A delivered in smaller volumes (50 or 100 units/mL) keep the effects more localized and enable precise delivery of the toxin with little diffusion, smaller doses in larger volumes (5–10 units/mL) may generate more widespread effects [4, 5]. The effects of BTX-A at the neuromuscular junction are evidenced in about 1–2 weeks and last for about 3–4 months. Clinically, however, patients may reap the benefit of relaxed skin tension lines for up to 6 months, depending on the patient and treated location [6].

Botox injection is ideal in the upper face (Figs. 1 and 2). Men, in comparison to women, usually require a greater amount of the toxin to achieve the same result. Most commonly used on the forehead, crow's feet area, and glabella, Botox paralyzes the dynamic facial muscles and helps to decrease brow furrows, while widening the eyes. When used on the lower face, it can be especially helpful in correcting facial asymmetry. Other areas, such as the "bunny lines" and platysmal bands of the lower face, have also been treated with success; however, even the well-trained and experienced physicians with a thorough understanding of facial anatomy should proceed with

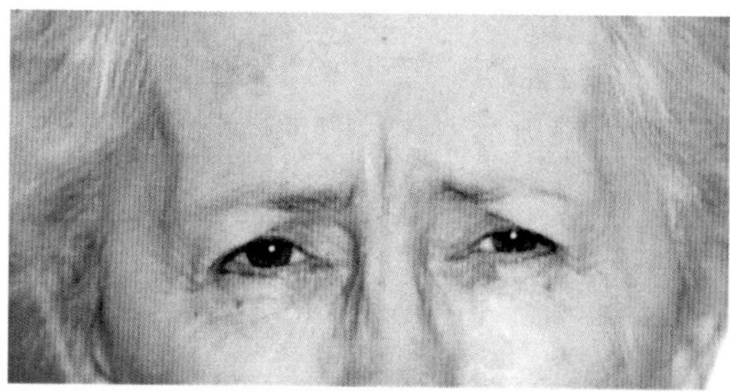

Fig. 1 Pre-Botox

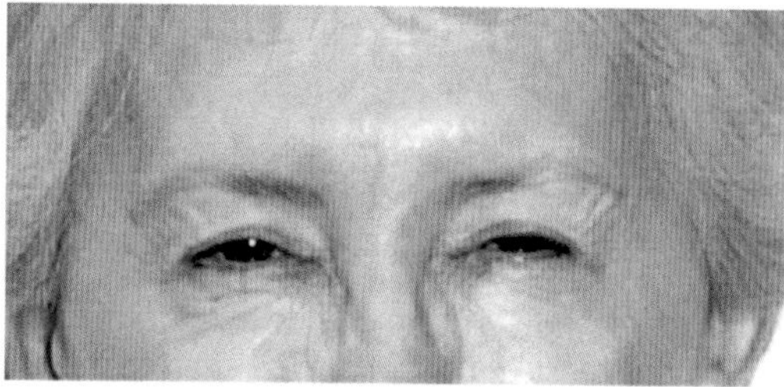

Fig. 2 Post-Botox

caution in these areas. Dysphagia is a much-feared complication of platysmal band treatment.

As a category C drug, Botox is not recommended for pregnant or breastfeeding women. Other contraindications include therapy with aminoglycosides or acetylsalicylic acid prior to treatment, as well as certain neuromuscular conditions (i.e., Eaton-Lambert syndrome, myasthenia gravis, amyotrophic lateral sclerosis, etc.). These conditions may potentiate the effects of Botox. Temporary side effects include bruising, headache, pain at injection site, asymmetry, muscle twitching, numbness, eyebrow or eyelid ptosis, and double vision. The most commonly encountered complications from Botox include an overtreated frontalis, dropped brow, asymmetry, and bruising, particularly in the lateral canthus [3]. These complications are best avoided by injecting 1 cm or more from the bony orbital rim and injecting at or above the middlebrow. Request that the patient remain upright for about 2 h after the procedure, and avoid any manipulation to the treated areas. These tips will help minimize unwanted side effects.

Newer trends with Botox emphasize the need for decreased number of toxin units in the forehead and greater amounts in the crow's feet region. These new recommendations are based on a finding that 20 or more units of Botox in the forehead are more likely to lead to suboptimal outcomes [3]. There has also been an increased desire to couple Botox with other nonsurgical fillers to achieve not only a more relaxed look but also a smoother, fuller, and more youthful appearance.

Fillers

BoNTA remains the cornerstone of treatment in the rejuvenation of the upper face. But its effects are only two-dimensional. By "volumizing" the face with injectable fillers, a more three-dimensional outcome can augment results achieved from Botox and maximize cosmesis. Studies have shown that BoNTA and hyaluronic acid filler, in combination, synergistically improve the appearance of the lower face, in comparison to the use of either injectable alone [3]. Fillers are therefore central to the midface revitalization, due to their ability to restore lost volume throughout the aging process. As another nonsurgical modality, fillers are also very attractive to the aging population. Instantly gratifying results and minimal downtime after administration make these products a win-win among patients. The "ideal" filler that maximizes longevity and ease of delivery and minimizes downtime and side effects has yet to be developed. But the discussion that follows highlights some of the more commonly used fillers and their associated indications and challenges.

Fillers are either biodegradable (12–18 months), slowly biodegradable (2–5 years), or permanent. Some of the more commonly used injectables can be broadly categorized into three main groups based on their duration: (1) temporary biodegradables (autologous fat, human collagen, bovine collagen, and hyaluronic acid), (2) long-lasting biodegradables (calcium hydroxylapatite, poly-L-lactic acid), and (3) permanent (polymethyl methacrylate). While dermal fillers tend to correct fine lines, more permanent injectables are placed in the subdermis and reserved for deeper furrows and longer-lasting volume restoration. Some fillers also have a secondary effect on volume enhancement, in that they additionally stimulate collagen neogenesis.

Unfortunately, the advantage of longer-lasting fillers is often offset by their tendency to create tissue reactions, such as granulomas and extrusion. The permanency of these products may also not adequately address changes in the dynamically aging face, resulting in an unnatural look with the progression of time. In choosing the appropriate filler for a given individual, there are many considerations. These include antigenicity of the injectable material and need for prior skin testing, duration of action, ease of delivery, number of sessions required to achieve the desired degree of correction, product longevity, and overall side effect profile. In choosing the appropriate filler, the patient's skin quality and age must also be taken into account; older patients may require a greater amount of a particular injectable product to attain results similar to those of a younger patient.

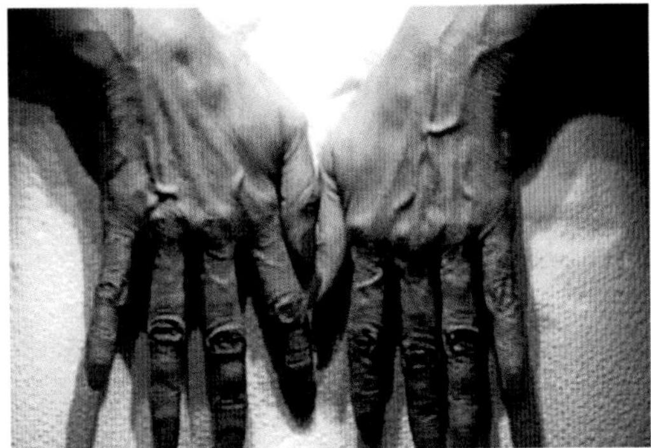

Fig. 3 Pre-fat transfer

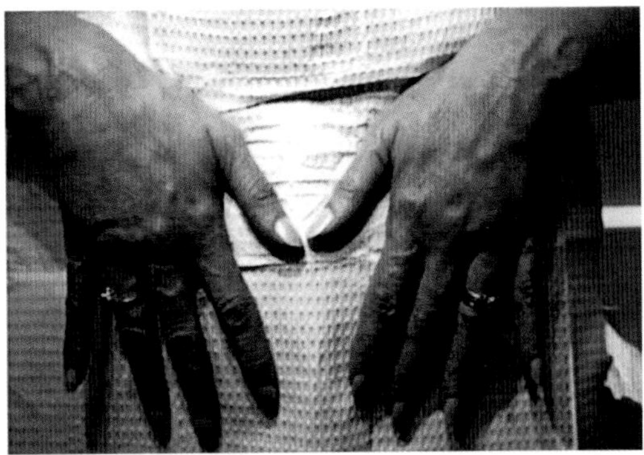

Fig. 4 Post-fat transfer

Temporary Biodegradable Fillers

Historically, autologous fat has provided safe, inexpensive volume replacement. Cosmetic areas that lend themselves to treatment with fat transplantation included deepened nasolabial folds, the fallen and receding upper lip with radial perioral lines, sunken cheeks, and transverse forehead creases. The dorsal hands also are an ideal location for the use of autologous fat (Figs. 3, 4, 5, and 6). However, due to the multistep nature of tissue harvest and implantation, as well as the controversy over the effective, longevity of fat transplantation, this filler has become a less ideal option for controlled volume replacement.

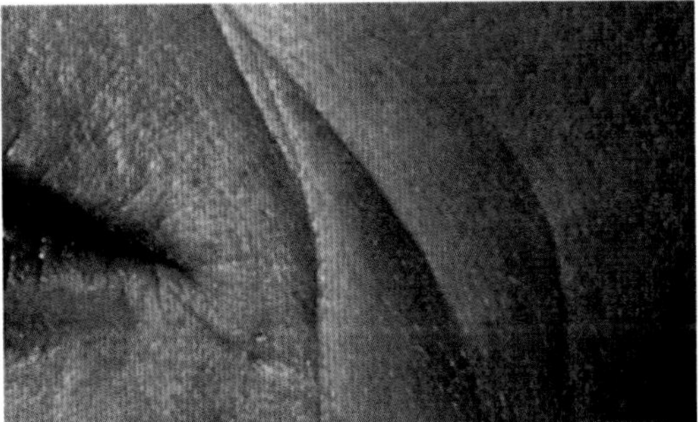

Fig. 5 Pre-collagen

Historic trends in temporary biodegradable fillers once included the use of either collagen derivatives (human or bovine) or hyaluronic acid. These products were injected into the superficial and mid-dermis to treat finer rhytids. Bovine-derived injectables (Zyderm® and Zyplast®) require two pretreatment allergy tests to screen for hypersensitivity reactions, whereas human-derived collagens (CosmoDerm® and CosmoPlast®) required none. The reported rate of bovine collagen sensitivity reactions ranges from 1 % to 2 %, and injection-related events include swelling, redness, itching, nodule formation, granulomas, and abscesses [7]. Therefore,

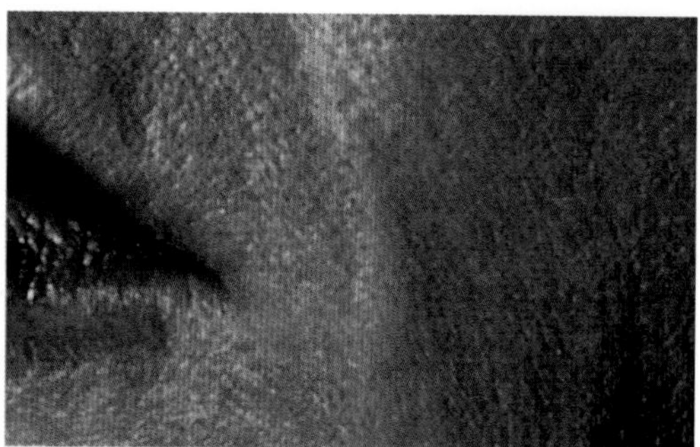

Fig. 6 Post-collagen

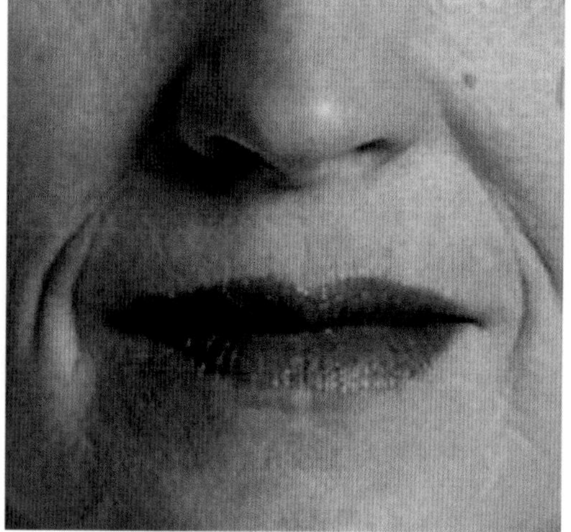

Fig. 7 Pre-Restylane

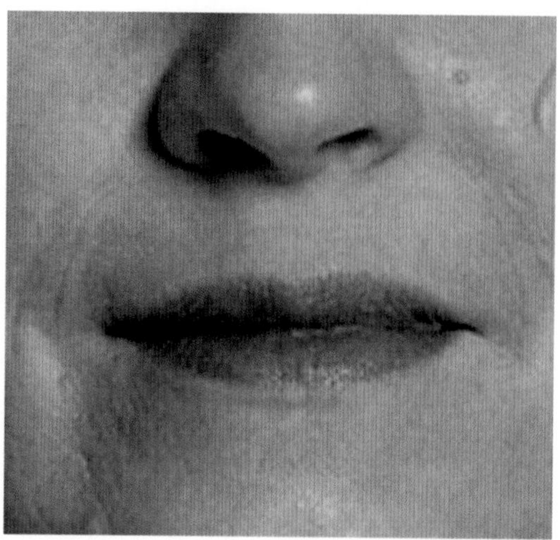

Fig. 8 Post-Restylane

the type III and I collagens that compose CosmoDerm and CosmoPlast, approved by the FDA in 2003, clearly offer a safety benefit over bovine collagens. All of these products also contained some amount of local anesthetic as part of their suspension but are no longer available.

Cross-linked or stabilized hyaluronic acid (HA) is currently the most used resorbable filler [8]. In 2008, there were eight HA dermal fillers approved for commercialization by the FDA [9]. HA fillers are so appealing due to their low immunogenicity and rare, limited side effects (i.e., bruising). This is largely due to HA's biocompatibility across species. It can be produced from animal origin and rooster combs. However, it is mostly extracted from a nonpathogenic bacterium, *Streptococcus equi*, as in Restylane® [8] (Figs. 7 and 8).This product must be correctly placed intradermally. If placed too high above the dermis, bumpy bluish nodules may be seen. If placed too deep into the dermis, durability is sacrificed. The most feared complication is the vascular injection leading to vascular occlusion and necrosis [7]. Retrograde injection helps to minimize this risk. Although the different HA products vary in longevity, one of the newer HAs to market, Juvederm®, was shown to have treatment efficacy for up to 12 months [3] (Figs. 9 and 10).

Long-Lasting Biodegradable Fillers

Calcium hydroxylapatite (Radiesse®) and poly-L-lactic acid (Sculptra®) represent devises injected below the dermis, which are more appropriate for moderate to severe rhytids. These products offer the advantage of new collagen production, in addition to the increased volume created by the injectable itself. Radiesse® promises improvement of deeper furrows and creases for about 1 year, whereas the response to Sculptra® can last for more than 2 years [7]. A crosshatched threading technique is unique to the delivery of Sculptra®. Caveats regarding Radiesse® include not placing the product in the lips due to higher

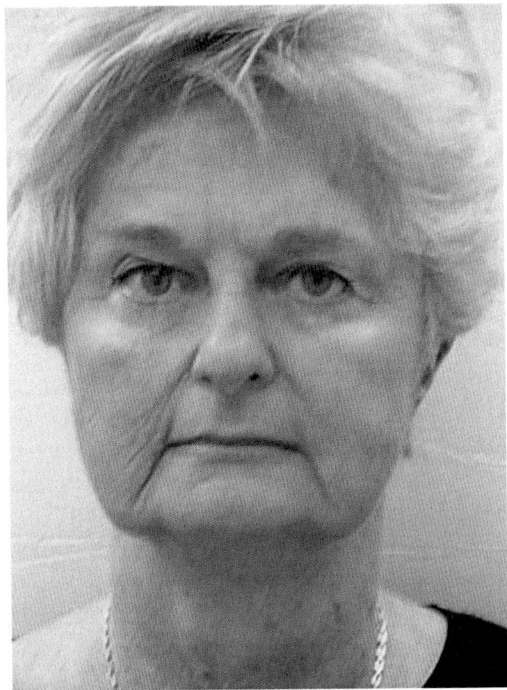

Fig. 9 Pre-Juvederm

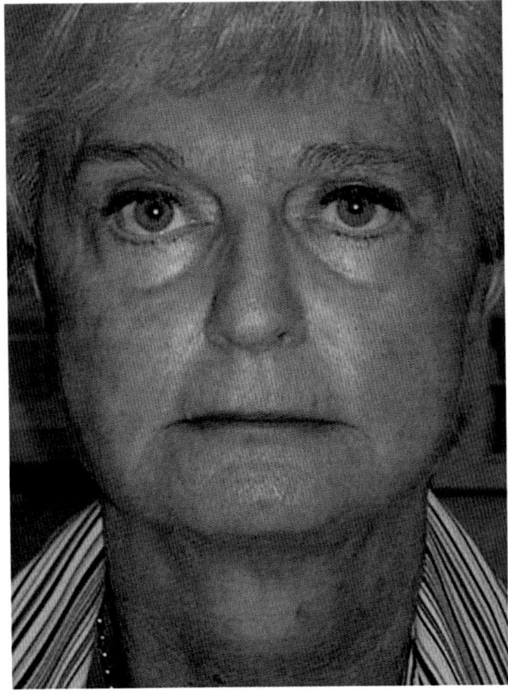

Fig. 10 Post-Juvederm

reports of granuloma formation. Similarly, caution is advised with Sculptra®, which usually requires subsequent, touch-up injections. Once Sculptra® is initially placed, the dermal thickness gradually increases over a period of about 1 month. Therefore, care should be taken not to overcorrect for volume during initial administration of poly-L-lactic acid. Posttreatment massage is recommended for both products to ensure even distribution.

Permanent Fillers

It should be noted that no filler will yield truly permanent correction of wrinkles, due to the ongoing forces of gravity and senescence at work in the skin. However, this class of fillers is composed of materials that are more permanent and maintained within the skin for prolonged periods. Artefill® is a dual-acting injectable filler. Composed of 20 % polymethyl methacrylate (PMMA) microspheres and 80 % purified bovine collagen with lidocaine, this suspension is injected into the sub- or deep dermis to treat deep facial rhytids. Unlike Sculptra®, which is a more optimal global volume filler, Artefill® is reserved for treatment of defined lines or scars. Due to its bovine collagen component, allergy testing is required by the FDA.

In addition to the pure volume of the injected suspension, the PMMA microspheres within the Artefill® induce a delayed foreign body response, which results in the deposition of new collagen. So, although the initial correction of the product slowly decreases as the bovine collagen is resorbed over a 1–3-month time period [10], 50–75 % of the correction is maintained long term, due to the permanence of the PMMA microspheres. Two to four treatments at intervals of about 3–4 months are often needed for complete correction [7]. Disadvantages associated with Artefill's® PMMA predecessors included granuloma formation thought to be primarily due to material impurities. But Artefill's® improved purification and reconstitution process has lowered granuloma formation [11]. The relative advantages of Artefill are (1) unique microsphere technology providing a complete smooth surface of the microspheres, (2) indications similar to those of collagen and hyaluronic acid, (3) ease of injection despite higher viscosity than collagen alone, (4) permanent stimulation of the connective tissue and collagen deposition, (5) long-lasting esthetic effect over many years, and (6) a low rate of granuloma formation similar to collagen and hyaluronic acid injections [11]. However, since the consequence of granuloma formation can be severely disfiguring, caution must be exercised.

So, whether the physician's aim is to correct fine or deep wrinkles or replace lost volume in certain cosmetic units of the face, there are a variety of nonsurgical options to rejuvenate the aging face. The "art" in choosing the most appropriate injectable "media" for the composition at hand is what separates a nonsurgical outcome from an esthetically pleasing cosmetic result. Fillers can be utilized alone or in combination with one another, as well as with other rejuvenating techniques, to achieve impressive changes in appearance.

Chemical Peels

Decreasing the visibility of dynamic rhytids with Botox and replenishing facial areas of lost volume with fillers only partially correct the many signs of photodamaged skin. Textural and pigmentary changes also contribute to an aged look and need to be addressed. On a histologic level, these changes are characterized by decreased microcirculation, elastosis, epidermal atrophy, cellular atypia, and preneoplastic dysplasia [12]. Chemical peels, classified by their depth of skin penetration (superficial, medium, and deep), have long been used to address these changes.

Depending on the chemical agent's depth of penetration, a skin wound is created during the peeling process. Superficial peels penetrate to the epidermis. Medium-depth peels create both epidermal and dermal injuries. And deep peels wound the skin to the area of the deep papillary or reticular dermis. Reepithelialization is then driven by the remaining, uninjured adnexal structures, which generate cellular division and differentiation. Within 24 h of a chemical peel, these epidermal appendages, located primarily in the remaining dermis, begin the production of the "new skin," and the entire process is usually completed in 7–10 days [13]. Overall, chemical peels create a thinner, more compact stratum corneum, a thicker acanthotic epidermis without atypia, and a uniform dispersion of melanin [13]. Additionally, as the skin regrows after injury, new collagen and glycosaminoglycans are produced. Although these added components are most pronounced in deeper peels, they result in increased skin elasticity and volume, leading to tighter and firmer skin, which minimizes the appearance of wrinkles [13].

Depending on the histologic depth of the photodamaged change, the appropriate level of peel is chosen to reverse those changes; the peel must penetrate to the histologic depth of the skin abnormality. For example, superficial peels treat textural skin changes, active acne, actinic keratoses, and superficial dyschromias confined to the epidermis. Medium-depth peels are reserved for solar lentigines, multiple solar keratoses, fine wrinkles, or acne scars. In addition, although the deep peel has largely fallen out of favor due to its side effect profile, deep peels are primarily indicated for coarse wrinkles and premalignant skin tumors [14]. Of note is that nevi, dermal and mixed melasma, dermal and mixed postinflammatory hyperpigmentation, and seborrheic keratoses respond poorly to superficial and medium-depth peels [13].

The pretreatment of the areas to be peeled with agents that "defat" the skin (e.g., scrubbing with alcohol or acetone) will significantly alter the depth of the peel. Also, patients who use topical retinoid products generally have less stratum corneum (the barrier layer) and thus tend to have a stronger reaction to peeling agents. Older patients have a flattened epidermis with less rete ridges as well as less dermal vascularity, diminishing their regenerative potential; thus, a certain degree of caution is warranted when using peeling agents.

Superficial Peels

Superficial peels exfoliate the skin and are primarily used to treat acne and its associated hyperpigmentation, as well as photodamaged (actinic keratoses, poor skin texture, superficial dyschromia) skin. Due to the minimal depth of penetration, a serial number of sessions is usually needed to accomplish the desired goal. Superficial peels include alpha hydroxy acid peels such as glycolic acid (up to 70 %), Jessners solution (resorcinol, lactic acid, and salicyclic acid in ethanol), trichloroacetic acid (TCA) (10–30 %), salicylic acid, and Retin-A peels [13, 14]. In contrast to the many superficial peels, which self-neutralize, the alpha hydroxy acid peels (i.e., glycolic acid) require an alkaline neutralizing agent, such as sodium bicarbonate, to terminate the peel's destructive action.

Medium-Depth Peels

Various strengths of trichloroacetic acid (TCA) peels exist, ranging from 25 % to 100 %. However, TCA (35 %) is considered a medium-depth peel. Other medium-depth agents include glycolic acid (70 %) applied for a more prolonged duration, TCA (35–50 %), carbon dioxide plus TCA, Jessners solution plus TCA (35 %), and glycolic acid (70 %) plus TCA (35 %). Due to the associated dermal penetration, these peels help improve mild to moderate mobile rhytids around the eyes and on the cheeks. Deeper, fixed, perioral, and nasolabial rhytids will not respond well. Melasma and more severe postinflammatory hyperpigmentation may improve, but results are very variable.

Deep Peels

Historically, phenol-based peels were reserved for patients with dyschromia, fine and coarse wrinkles, premalignant skin tumors, and severe acne scars. Phenol-based agents not only penetrate to the midreticular dermis but also create significant production of new collagen [14]. Unfortunately, phenol is directly toxic to the myocardium. Cardiac arrhythmias have been recorded in up to 23 % of patients who underwent full-face peel in less than 30 min [15]. Additional side effects include prolonged or permanent erythema, hypopigmentation, and porcelain scarring. Therefore, due to its toxicity, need for full cardiopulmonary monitoring with intravenous hydration throughout the procedure, and prolonged recovery period with variable outcome, deep peeling has fallen out of favor. In instances in which deep peeling is required, it is the author's preference to turn to the carbon dioxide (CO_2) laser. The CO_2 laser allows for less risk and more controlled results.

Overall, the risks associated with chemical peeling increase proportionately to the increased depth of the peel. Broadly categorized, postpeel complications include infection, altered pigmentation, and scarring. Bacterial, viral, and candidal infections are also possible, especially if the skin peels prematurely and exposes non-reepithelialized skin. Acneiform eruptions and milia may also follow a peel. Prior to the peel, patients should always be asked about a history of herpes simplex. Luckily, all of these infections can be easily treated with the appropriate topical and oral regimens.

Postinflammatory pigmentation, most common in darker skin types, can occur immediately or months following a peel. Pigmentation changes are often precipitated by premature sun exposure. Bleaching agents such as hydroquinone and retinoids may aid in improving unwanted pigmentary alterations. However, prolonged postpeel erythema (>3 months) is a rare complication that can occur with any depth of peel.

Associated scarring can be either hypertrophic or atrophic. The most common area of scarring is the lower face [14], especially the mandible. But the periorbital region is also at risk. To avoid this complication, it is best to inquire pre-procedure as to whether the patient has a history of scar formation or isotretinoin use in the last 18 months. Regardless, should scarring result after a peel, it is imperative to quickly intervene with high-potency topical or intralesional steroids. Q-switched pulse dye laser treatments may also serve as a necessary adjunct.

Chemical peels are an economical, readily available, and safe alternative to many other types of resurfacing modalities. The choice of peel is customized based on the desired treatment skin "target" and offers the advantage of minimal downtime. If used alone or in combination with other resurfacing and rejuvenating technique, peels are another great option in helping to refresh the skin's appearance.

Microdermabrasion

An alternative to chemical resurfacing of the skin is microdermabrasion. On par with a superficial chemical peel, this revitalizing tool enables chemical-free, partial skin ablation or "skin polishing" with a negative pressure device, which delivers debrading particles. A compressor and an aspirator are the essential components of the system. Aluminum oxide crystals or sodium chloride salt are projected from a reservoir via a tubing system and handpiece onto the patient's skin. These crystals and loosened skin debris are evacuated from the treatment surface into a second tubing system and finally deposited in another closed container, thereby preventing contamination.

In comparison to the open microdermabrasion techniques of the past, today's dermabrasion is a closed loop vacuum-assisted abrasive procedure, harnessing the physical action of inert crystals to exfoliate the skin. The closed loop system helps to ensure operator safety from possible viral released particles like herpes simplex virus and HIV. The operator can also adjust the device settings including vacuum pressure, speed of crystals, particle size, angle of impaction, number of passes, and speed of movement of the probe. These adjustments allow for ablation of different depths, as needed to accomplish the cosmetic goal.

Because microdermabrasion creates partial skin ablation, the skin responds to this injury by stimulating epidermal turnover and producing new collagen. Various studies reviewing the resultant histologic changes have reported stratum corneum thinning and homogenization immediately following microdermabrasion. More chronic changes demonstrate an increase in epidermal thickness, flattening of the rete pegs, improvement in loss of polarity, liquefaction of basal cells, and hyalinization of the papillary dermis [16].

Indications for microdermabrasion run the gamut: fine rhytids, photoaging, active acne, mild acne scarring, comedones, dyschromia, correction of enlarged pores, stretch marks, tattoo removal, and scar revision. Microdermabrasion has also become particularly useful in blending cosmetic transition zones in areas previously treated with laser. Treating the photoaged neck in patients who have previously undergone facial laser resurfacing helps diminish the often pronounced contrast between the rejuvenated facial skin and the untreated neck without adverse sequela. It may take five to seven monthly microdermabrasion treatments to blend an area on the lower two-thirds of the neck with an area already treated by CO_2 laser [17].

The overall effect of the procedure is a subtle, smoothing of the skin. Advantages of microdermabrasion include that it is chemical-free, and in contrast to peels, lasers, and dermabrasion, it can be used on any skin type with few complications or morbidity. Additionally, the technique is relatively bloodless, does not require anesthesia, requires very little downtime, and can be customized to individual patients due to its high degree of operator control. On the other hand, microdermabrasion should be avoided in those with active skin infection or rosacea. Microdermabrasion can trigger a rosacea flare, which may result in permanent, unfavorable change to the skin. Furthermore, the procedure is not without risk of pigment streaking and hyperpigmentation, persistent erythema, herpes simplex activation, or ocular complications due to the entrance of crystals into the cornea.

Prior to the procedure, it is important to specifically ask the patient about his/her use of antioxidants like vitamin E and ginkgo biloba, as well as anticoagulants or any other antiplatelet agent (including aspirin). These medications can increase posttreatment edema and erythema and even lead to petechiae. Patients should also be advised to discontinue any alpha hydroxy acid or retinoid-containing products about 2 days prior to the procedure. Continued use of these topical regimens can lead to a brisk and more unpredictable response to treatment.

During microdermabrasion, a patient can expect to experience mild and limited discomfort.

If too great, the level of discomfort can easily be decreased by adjusting the apparatus settings. Mild erythema, the usual procedure endpoint, and tingling may be experienced after the procedure. In general, most patients feel their skin to be smoother and less mottled after microdermabrasion [16]. However, deep rhytids, melasma, deep scars, telangiectasias, and actinic keratoses will not disappear.

Microdermabrasion is an effective and nonsurgical solution for the older patient population. Although its results may not be as dramatic as other resurfacing techniques, it has the advantages of little to no discomfort, no required anesthesia, few complications, and minimal to no recuperation time. It is a simplistic resurfacing tool, whether used alone or in conjunction with other resurfacing techniques, which can grant facial rejuvenation to the patient.

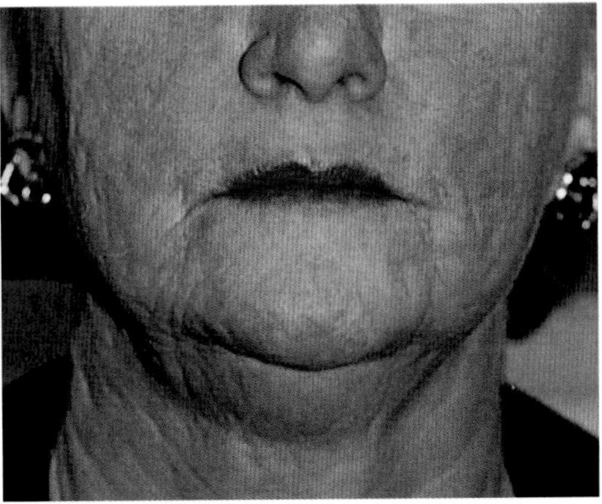

Fig. 11 Pre-dermabrasion

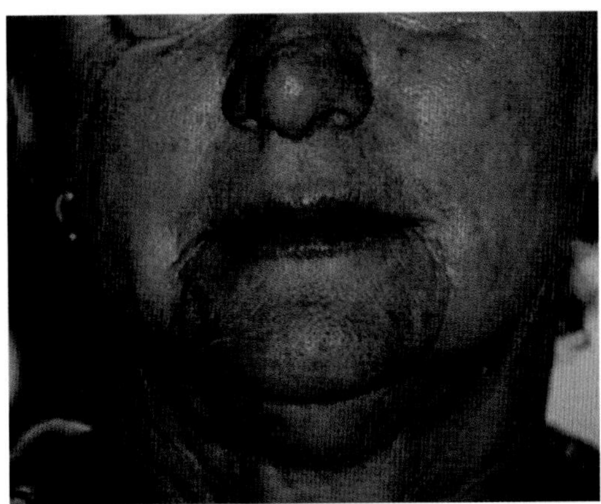

Fig. 12 Post-dermabrasion

Dermabrasion

Prior to the development of lash technology, dermabrasion was the mainstay in treatment for deep rhytids and significant acne scarring. The aerosolization of blood products is its main limiting factor, but if used for focal areas, it remains a viable treatment option.

Dermabrasion differs from microdermabrasion in that a wire brush or diamond fraise creates a wound that penetrates more deeply into the papillary dermis. Subsequently, reepithelialization occurs via the still vital underlying adnexal structures. Thus, dermabrasion supersedes microdermabrasion, when attempting to treat deeper, facial defects. Due to decreased vascular supply and decreased numbers of adnexal structures on nonfacial areas, dermabrasion has an increased tendency to leave a scar if used in areas other than the face.

Dermabrasion alters the primary scar formation by creating a repair zone of new, more organized collagen within the papillary dermis. New collagen exhibits an increase in collagen bundle density and size, with unidirectional orientation of collagen fibers that tend to be more parallel to the epidermal surface. Histologically, there appears to be an upregulation of tenascin expression throughout the papillary dermis and the expression of alpha-6/beta-4 integrin subunit on the keratinocytes throughout the stratum spinosum [18]. Clinically, these changes result in more evenly contoured skin (Figs. 11 and 12).

In contrast to lasers that thermally ablate the skin, dermabrasion is a "cold" form of ablation that minimizes vascular stimulation throughout the healing phase, allowing for less intense, postoperative erythema that is quicker to resolve in some cases [19]. Although there are numerous uses for this resurfacing technique (Table 1), actinically photodamaged skin, wrinkles, superficial scarring (acne and varioliform), and surgical

Table 1 Indications for dermabrasion

Indications for dermabrasion
Scarring
Acne scarring
Surgical scars/posttraumatic scars
Pigmentary lesions
Congenital pigmented nevi
Lentigines
Tattoo
Epithelial-derived growths
Actinic keratoses
Seborrheic keratoses
Growths with dermal components
Angiofibromas
Neurofibromas
Syringomas
Trichoepitheliomas
Xanthelasma
Others
Photoaging-solar elastosis-rhytids
Resistant acne
Rhinophyma

scar revision are the more common indications. Of note is that burn scars do not respond to dermabrasion, as they lack the necessary revitalizing adnexal structures. Additionally, patients with pigmentary conditions such as melasma encounter problems with recurrence, just as with many other resurfacing procedures. Interestingly, despite major resurfacing advances in the realm of lasers, many still find dermabrasion to be an excellent option for treating acne scars. However, others will argue that the CO_2 ablative laser, which is operated in a bloodless field, is superior. Regardless, assessing the depth of acne scarring is critical as to whether the technique will result in substantial improvement. Pigmentary irregularities, tattoos, and actinic keratoses may also improve with dermabrasion. But more efficacious lasers and topical treatments have largely replaced the use of dermabrasion in treating these entities.

Clearly, dermabrasion (as with aggressive laser resurfacing discussed in the next section) should be contraindicated for any patients with decreased dermal appendageal structures, such as those who have recently taken isotretinoin, or with a history of radiation to the treatment area. These predisposing conditions significantly increase the potential for scarring. With specific regard to isotretinoin, the recommended delay before undergoing dermabrasion is 6–18 months. However, poor wound healing has occurred in isotretinoin patients even 38 months post-drug. Therefore, it is recommended to delay dermabrasion after isotretinoin for as long as possible (normally not a concern in the aging patient population). Other concerns regarding the treatment are activation of herpes simplex, spread of existing verruca vulgaris and keloidal or hypertrophic scarring, and post-procedure solar-induced pigmentary change. Prior to the procedure, it is also important to document the bleeding time and platelet counts, as well as HIV and hepatitis status. Regardless, universal precautions should always be taken for every dermabrasion procedure with all persons present in the operating suite wearing protective gears including face masks, face shields, surgical gowns, and gloves.

Dermabrasion is a valuable tool in the surgeon's resurfacing armamentarium, when a skilled operator is paired with an optimal candidate. Although the list of resurfacing options continues to lengthen with the development of newer laser technology, dermabrasion remains particularly effective for the treatment of facial acne scarring, rhytids, and scar revision.

Lasers

Laser technology dates back to Einstein's study of quantum mechanics in the early twentieth century. But light amplification by stimulated by emission of radiation (LASER) has drastically evolved since its inception. Today, the theory of selective photothermolysis is utilized by cosmetic lasers to directly treat specific targets in the skin, resulting in a more rejuvenated appearance. By selecting a laser with the appropriate wavelength, pulse duration, and fluence, certain unwanted skin changes (i.e., increased melanin and telangiectasias) can be targeted and "erased," while other favorable skin components, such as collagen, can be induced.

A vast array of cosmetic lasers is currently available. However, before profiling different types of lasers, it is important to understand some key laser principles. The physical properties of laser light include the following: monochromaticity, coherence, and collimation. Monochromaticity refers to the ability of laser light to selectively target chromophores with a corresponding *single* wavelength. Melanin, hemoglobin, and water are the three intrinsic skin chromophores or laser "targets." Coherence defines the relationship of individual laser light waves as they travel next to one another with respect to both time and space. Collimation is described as the ability of lasers to transmit parallel rays of light without divergence and loss of intensity, despite increasing distance.

As described by Parrish and Anderson, the theory of selective photothermolysis states that a specific chromophore can be selectively targeted (with a specific wavelength) and destroyed with minimal damage to surrounding tissues. This is usually best accomplished with the delivery of energy using a pulse duration that is less than or equal to the thermal relaxation time of the chosen target tissue. Thermal relaxation time is defined as the amount of time needed for the target tissue to lose 50 % of its incident heat, by diffusion to the surrounding tissue.

The first lasers that came to the cosmetic market in the 1980s and 1990s were ablative lasers, namely, the carbon dioxide (10,640 nm) and erbium-doped yttrium aluminum garnet (Er: YAG) (2,940 nm) lasers. This class of lasers, through superficial destruction of the tissue, clinically enabled resurfacing of unwanted solar damage and scarring by targeting intra- and extracellular water. By vaporizing the epidermis with continued destruction to the papillary dermis, extrinsic skin changes could be removed allowing for the reepithelialization of the skin. Most patients with wrinkles were able to attain a 50–90 % improvement after treatment with this subset of lasers [20] (Figs. 13 and 14). But, despite impressive postoperative results, the procedure is painful and requires sedation. In addition, facial bandaging and 2–6 weeks of downtime with sun avoidance can be a barrier to treatment for many patients. A CO_2 laser peel remains the gold standard for those looking to attain a more dramatic youthful appearance. One must be aware of the

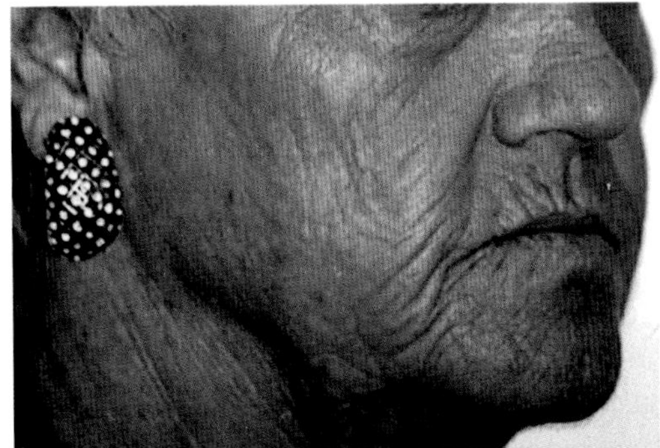

Fig. 13 Pre-CO_2 laser

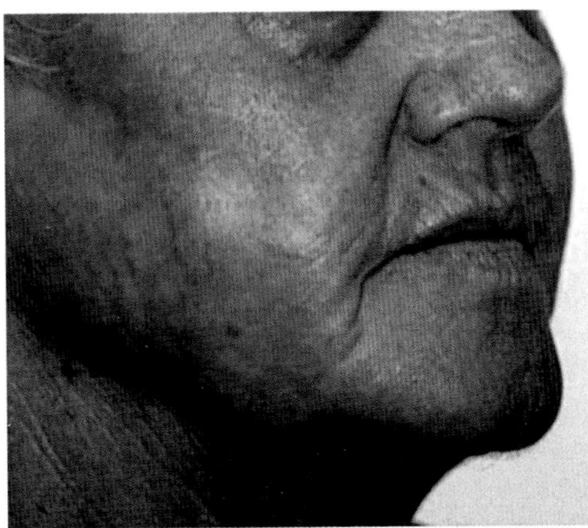

Fig. 14 Post-CO_2 laser

associated but uncommon risks such as erythema, dyspigmentation, acne eruptions, infections, and scarring. These ablative laser disadvantages then drove the demand for a laser system with less risk and less downtime. Hence, a supply of nonablative lasers began to populate the marketplace. These nonablative lasers produced thermal energy, which reduced rhytids and extrinsic changes while preserving the epidermis.

This recent subset of rejuvenating lasers promised decreased pain upon delivery, little or no healing time, and additional advantage of collagen stimulation. To deliver this promise, increasingly longer-wavelength lasers were employed to target not only hemoglobin and melanin but collagen structures too. In general, the nonablative lasers can be subdivided into three main types of lasers or light systems: (1) visible light lasers, (2) infrared lasers, and (3) intense pulsed light systems. Overall, visible light lasers somewhat improve texture but greatly reduce redness and telangiectasias. The infrared lasers improve texture. Intense pulsed light devices improve both vascular imperfections and brown discoloration, as well as skin texture [21]. Regardless of these advancements, discontent arose over the lack of drastic improvement attained by the nonablative lasers and the requirement of a series of treatments prior to any noticeable skin enhancement.

Thus, a new technology was embraced: fractional resurfacing. This laser system is a "compromise" between the dichotomous poles of ablative and nonablative lasers. Fractional resurfacing entails thermally ablating about 15–25 % of a skin surface during a treatment while sparing the remaining skin surface. The thermally ablated, vertical columns of the skin, which are about 70–150 μm in width, are evenly distributed over the treatment area [20]. As these microthermal zones repair and heal after ablation, they can draw upon the neighboring spared tissue for fibroblasts and epidermal stem cells to increase the speed and ease of healing. Overall outcomes are associated with decreased morbidity and healing time and increased improvement in skin changes as compared to a nonablative approach.

Classification of Lasers

Ablative

The carbon dioxide (CO_2, 10,640 nm) and erbium-doped yttrium aluminum garnet (Er: YAG, 2,940 nm) lasers classically define ablative lasers. These lasers work independent of melanin or hemoglobin because they primarily target the water chromophore. Because water makes up 80 % of the skin, the wavelengths produced by these lasers are absorbed by the tissue that is then vaporized. The erbium wavelength is 12–18 times more efficiently absorbed by water than the CO_2 wavelength. Thus, the erbium laser's tissue penetration is not as deep, but the laser is able to vaporize the tissue with more precision and control. Conversely, due to the CO_2 laser's ability to penetrate deeper into the tissue, it offers the advantage of blood vessel coagulation. This decreases the intraoperative bleeding and postoperative ecchymosis and edema. A debate once existed as to which of these lasers is the gold standard in ablation. The verdict often rested in the opinion of the operating surgeon. The "trade-off" exists in that although the erbium may provide more precision and control, it also usually requires multiple passes. Up to ten passes can be required. The erbium has also been associated with less tissue contraction in comparison to the CO_2 laser, and in the author's opinion, the CO_2 laser gave routinely superior results.

Patient Selection

The two most common indications for ablative lasers are photoaging (rhytids, dyspigmentation, vascularity, elastosis, actinic keratoses) and scarring [20]. While fine lines and wrinkles tend to respond quite well to ablative laser, deeper rhytids may improve slightly but are difficult to eradicate. The glabella and nasolabial folds are areas particularly resistant to laser resurfacing secondary to their dynamic movement [20]. Treating areas of scarring should also be approached with caution, as ablative results are highly dependent on the type of scar undergoing treatment. Elevated or minimally deep, distensible acne scars are much more amenable to treatment, as compared to ice-picked or bound-down scarring. The latter usually requires concomitant treatment with microexcision and/or punch grafting to see worthwhile improvement. Although improvement in acne scarring is usually seen about 3 months postoperatively, it can take up to 1 year to realize the final healed outcome of the procedure. Of note is that more drastic improvement in scarring is seen if resurfacing is undertaken within 6–10 weeks from the inciting event [20].

Anesthesia

Ablative lasers as a class are painful, though the CO_2 laser is known to be more painful than the erbium. Nonetheless, the choice of anesthesia is based on the location and overall surface area undergoing treatment. For localized treatment of individualized cosmetic units such as the periorbital or perioral regions, local anesthesia with topical creams or nerve blocks can be employed. For more extensive or full-face laser resurfacing intravenous, conscious sedation is recommended.

Technique

CO_2 lasers usually require one to two passes to the resurfaced area. Feathering of edge borders can soften lines of demarcation. Treatment areas are not overlapped. Usually, it is preferred that an entire cosmetic unit or the entire face be resurfaced rather than "a scar," as this helps to avoid obvious lines between treated and nontreated areas. Any vaporized tissue should be removed from the surface of the treatment area between subsequent passes. Any sign of yellow or brown discoloration after wiping should cease treatment. Ideally, the treatment endpoint is improvement of prior area of concern. With the erbium laser, the desired endpoint is removal of rhytids or pinpoint bleeding. Postoperative care includes application of ointments such as petroleum jelly and an "open" or "closed" technique of wound dressing. The closed technique consists of a totally occlusive or semiocclusive dressing that promotes a moist healing environment and protects against postoperative scratches or abrasion. The potential drawback to this approach is increased rate of infection. The compromise is the application of a semiocclusive dressing for the first 24–48 h after surgery, and thereafter using a bland emollient seems to be the ideal approach.

Side Effects

Recovery period for both laser types are characterized by serous discharge, crusting, and burning sensation. Patients treated with the erbium laser generally experience faster reepithelialization and shorter duration of erythema than is seen with the CO_2. However, these differences are dependent on the energy level settings. Accordingly, edema and pruritus are of notably shorter duration with erbium laser resurfacing. A history of keloid formation, connective tissue disease, koebnerizing conditions (psoriasis, vitiligo, etc.), ongoing sun exposure, undermining of treatment area in the last 6 months, or use of isotretinoin in the last year should preclude treatment. Complications include erythema, dyspigmentation, milia, acne, eczematous dermatitis, infections, and scarring. The most feared complications of laser resurfacing are hypertrophic scarring and ectropion.

After the procedure, the patient can expect to see reepithelialization between 3 and 10 days. By this time, epithelial oozing should have ceased. Pruritus, which may be present for the first few postoperative weeks, can be treated with antihistamines, cold packs, and topical corticosteroid creams. It is recommended that prophylactic antivirals (continued until reepithelialization is complete), antibiotics, and potentially anti-candidal agents be given to all patients. It is important to set the patient's expectation with regard to postoperative healing. Postoperative erythema is particularly variable. From 1 to 4 months of postoperative erythema is considered "normal," but rarely erythema, especially associated with emotional or exertional flushing, may persist for up to 1 year.

Nonablative

In general, nonablative lasers can be subdivided into three main categories: (1) visible light lasers, such as the vascular, pulsed dye lasers at 585–595 nm; (2) infrared lasers, such as Nd: YAG laser at 1,320 nm (CoolTouch) or diode lasers at 1,450 nm (Smoothbeam) or the erbium: glass laser at 1,540 nm; and (3) intense pulsed light (IPL) systems. The Q-switched Nd:YAG laser is unique among the above grouping in that it can emit either an invisible, near infrared light beam with a wavelength of 1,064 nm or a green light with a wavelength of 532 nm when a frequency-doubling crystal is used. This Q-switching technique allows for a large amount of energy to build up prior to its sudden, powerful release. It is this distinctive laser capability that makes the Q-switched 532 nm Nd:YAG a favorite for targeting the superficial melanin chromophore in lentigos (Figs. 15 and 16).

Overall, nonablative lasers spare the epidermis of injury, many with adjunct epidermal cooling modalities, as they target skin chromophores. Additionally, this subset of lasers stimulates collagen remodeling, which is the key to the improvement in fine lines and wrinkles, as well as acne scarring. As there are many different lasers within the nonablative class of lasers, many different mechanisms are used to stimulate collagen. Regardless, the end result is usually a softening, rather than an eradication, of fine lines.

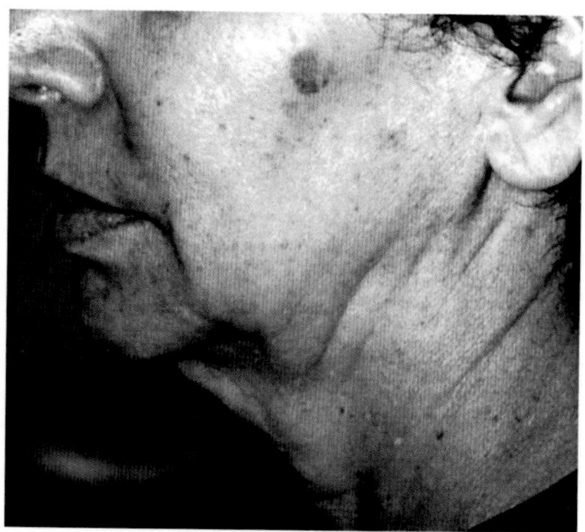

Fig. 15 Pre-frequency-doubled 532 nm Nd:YAG

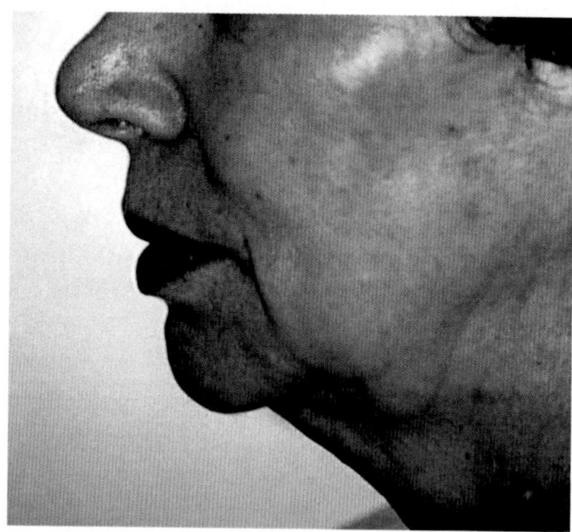

Fig. 16 Post-frequency-doubled 532 nm Nd:YAG

Visible Lasers

The pulsed dye laser (585 nm) employs low fluences at short enough pulse durations to selectively target a specific chromophore in the dermis – namely, the vessels of the upper dermal plexus, at a subpurpuric level of energy (Figs. 17 and 18). With one pass, the tissue response of these vessels includes the creation of low-grade inflammation and a growth response. Inflammatory mediators are released from endothelial cells, subsequently stimulating fibroblast activity and collagen neogenesis. Pulse dye laser studies have shown histological changes in collagen [20]; however, clinical outcomes have been disappointing even after about five treatments at monthly intervals. Despite the US FDA approval for treating photodamage with the long-pulsed PDL, only modest results have been observed with these short wavelengths, presumably because of predominantly vascular targeting and superficial penetration to the papillary dermis [20]. Due to lack of more drastic improvement for the aging skin, the vascular lasers have been largely replaced by the ablative and nonablative lasers. Instead, the pulsed dye laser has found its strength in the treatment of vascular birthmarks, facial telangiectasias, and certain forms of rosacea [20].

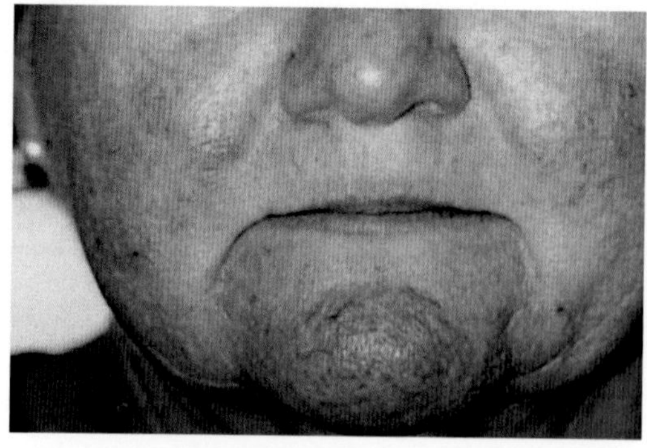

Fig. 17 Pre-pulsed dye laser

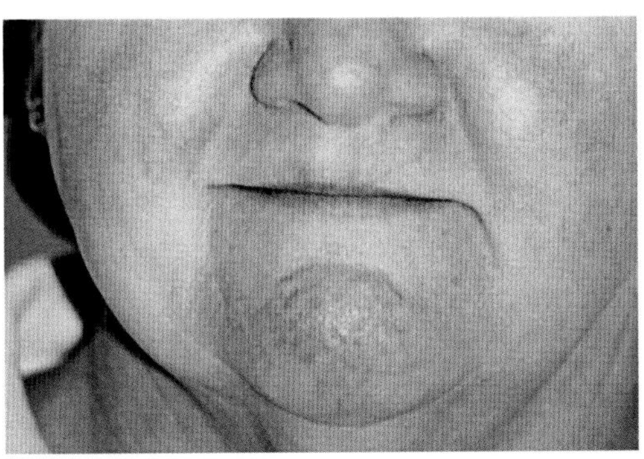

Fig. 18 Post-pulsed dye laser

Infrared Lasers

With longer wavelengths the infrared (IR) lasers offer deeper penetration creating a more promising collagen-tissue interaction. However, these lasers lack the benefit of improvement in epidermal changes such as dyschromia and vascular photoaging. The goal of nonablative IR laser treatments is to induce selective dermal injury while keeping the overlying epidermis intact. Clinically, the epidermis is not visibly disrupted. After thermal injury to the dermis, there is new production of type I collagen. This collagen is then deposited and reorganized into parallel arrays. Because of these collagen effects, rhytids, pore size, and acne scarring may improve during treatment. With all IR sources, epidermal protection is provided with a variety of cooling techniques. The ideal epidermal surface temperature is 40–48 °C, which correlates with a dermal temperature of 70 °C, the temperature required for collagen denaturation [21]. Unfortunately, these laser systems have delivered suboptimal results for the majority of patients hoping for more.

Patient Selection

Patients with mild to moderate rhytid formation and possibly mild atrophic acne scarring, particularly when present in isolated cosmetic units, are ideal. Good candidates are young with minimal facial sagging. Nonablative laser systems may also serve as a supplement to augment and/or maintain the rejuvenating effect of ablative laser treatments.

Anesthesia

The higher the fluence used (without blistering), the greater the degree of improvement, but the greater the discomfort of treatment. Some tolerate the procedure well with no anesthesia, but application of topical anesthesia for about 1 h before the treatment makes the procedure quite well tolerated by almost all individuals.

Technique

Usually, five to six treatments are needed at 2–4-week intervals, using about one to three passes per each treatment session.

Intense Pulsed Light

Intense pulsed light instruments (IPLs) emit nonmonochromatic and noncoherent light: specific filters allow to select wavelengths (ranging from 515 to 1,200 nm) to be emitted by a single light source. The use of IPL has led to modest clinical improvement in wrinkles, with concomitant significant improvement in pigment and vascular abnormalities of photodamaged skin.

Patient Selection

While the infrared lasers are a more optimal choice for patients with textural changes, IPL is a better choice for those who have varying degrees of photodamage with telangiectasias and unevenly distributed pigment. The great advantage to this modality is that a large surface area can be treated simultaneously for vascular and pigmentary changes with practically no downtime. Small improvements in texture may also be achieved.

Anesthesia

A topical anesthetic cream may be applied and then removed prior to the laser treatment. However, many patients are able to tolerate the procedure without anesthesia.

Technique

All IPLs require application of a cold aqueous gel, as one to multiple passes of the handpiece are delivered. A series of five or six sessions at 4–6-week intervals is usually required to visualize clinical improvement.

All of the nonablative laser choices discussed require little to no postoperative care. Although blistering, transient hyperpigmentation, and pinpoint scarring have been reported with some devices [20], overall risks of the procedure are minimal. Most patients experience slight erythema and edema for a few hours following the treatment session but return to baseline shortly thereafter. Contraindications to the use of nonablative lasers include oral retinoid use within the past year, intake of drugs that increase light sensitivity, tanned skin, and pregnancy.

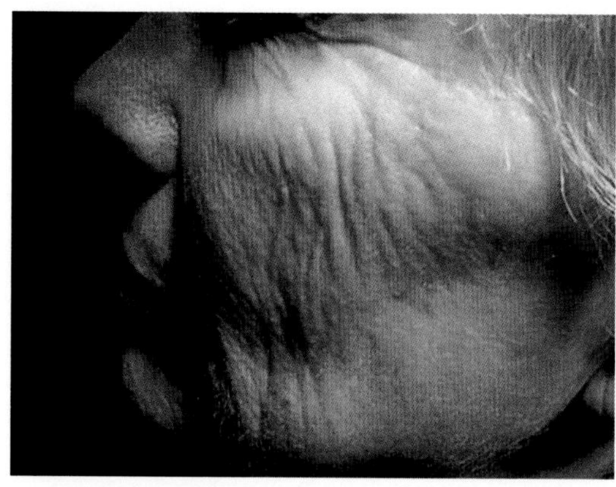

Fig. 19 Pre-fractional laser

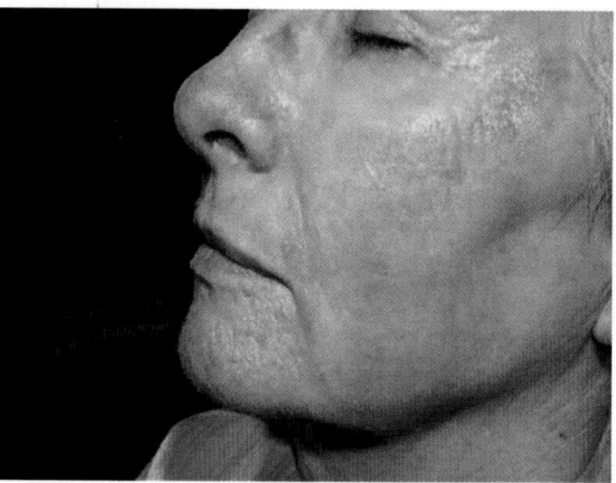

Fig. 20 Post-fractional laser

Fractional

Fractional lasers provide a minimally invasive method for laser intervention, using fractional, nonablative thermal energy for creation of microthermal zones of necrosis paired with induction of dermal remodeling. This clinically results in more impressive changes in overall skin appearance at a decreased cost of downtime for the patient (Figs. 19 and 20).

Patient Selection

These patients must be willing to sacrifice more postoperative downtime for more drastic improvements in skin texture and pigmentation. Patients with extrinsic photoaging and dyschromia usually require about two to three treatments, in comparison to those patients with significant rhytids who require at least five treatments.

Anesthesia

Topical anesthesia is usually recommended, though some patients are able to tolerate the discomfort associated with the treatment without any prior numbing. A topical numbing cream such as LMX [previously named Elamax, contains 4% or 5% Lidocaine in a liposomal delivery system] may be applied about an hour prior to the procedure. But many of the newer fractional laser models have been developed to provide decreased pain on delivery [20]. Forced cool air, which additionally can help to decrease discomfort, is also delivered during the procedure.

Technique

After the anesthetic cream is removed with a dry gauze, a gel is applied and multiple passes are made over the treatment area. Upon completion of the treatment session, cold compresses are applied to soothe the treatment area and a moisturizer is applied.

Side Effects

The epidermis is primarily intact, with most patients experiencing only transient erythema, edema, and mild pruritus for about 2–5 days following the treatment. Scarring, dyspigmentation, or other adverse effects are rare if ever present [22]. Depending on the area to be treated, a course of prophylactic antivirals should be considered, whereas prophylactic antibiotics are generally unnecessary.

Today, the options available for laser treatment seem almost boundless, with new laser technologies coming to the marketplace each day. Chronologically, laser applications have moved from strictly ablative devices, to nonablative systems, to a more fractionalized approach. But the field of cosmetic laser treatment will continue to evolve with the development of the "magic wand" that instantly erases both the extrinsic and intrinsic changes of aging, while minimizing associated risks and downtime.

Liposuction

The previously discussed cosmetic interventions have primarily concentrated on efforts to improve and rejuvenate the face and sun-exposed skin. However, body habitus also significantly contributes to the overall "youthfulness" of an individual's appearance. As the body ages, there is a tendency for fat to collect in certain, localized areas. Common sites of excessive fat collection, which can be corrected by liposuction, are the hips, flank, buttocks, abdomen, male breasts, outer and inner thighs, knees, calves, and arms (Figs. 21 and 22). With minimal scarring, liposuction can remove these unwanted body bulges and collections of excess fat, helping to improve body contour (Figs. 23, 24, 25, and 26). Areas of localized fat hypertrophy on the face and neck can also be liposuctioned to improve appearance (Figs. 27 and 28). When considering liposuction in the elderly, the degree of skin laxity must be taken into account, as well as the underlying health status of the patient. Therefore, patient selection is critical to a successful outcome. It should be clearly understood that the goal is for them to look better in their clothes.

Although, dry and wet techniques were historically used to perform the procedure, the current standard of care is tumescent liposuction. Tumescent liposuction involves subcutaneous infiltration of high volumes of crystalloid fluid containing low concentrations of lidocaine and epinephrine followed by suction-assisted aspiration of fat with small aspiration cannulas. There is a higher proportion of pure fat aspirated during tumescent liposuction, with a very small component of blood compared with the aspirate obtained by other techniques of liposuction [23]. This method of liposuction can be performed while the patient is only under local anesthesia, thus, obviating the risk associated with general anesthesia. Additionally, the tumescent technique helps to reduce blood loss and postoperative pain, while maximizing fat harvest. Tumescent anesthesia for liposuction with dilute lidocaine has been well documented to result in peak serum levels 4–14 h after infiltration [24]. Traditional tumescent liposuction requires completed infusion time plus about 20 min for the desired vasoconstrictive effects of epinephrine. In order to decrease systemic absorption of lidocaine, it is the author's preference to adjunctly use intravenous conscious sedation when liposuctioning. This approach decreases the total procedure time, thereby lowering systemic absorption of lidocaine, while still reaping the vasoconstrictive, anesthetic, and tissue-expanding benefits of the

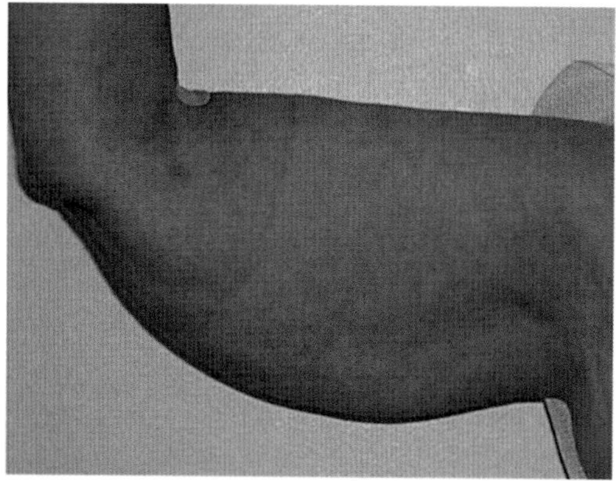

Fig. 21 Pre-liposuction of the arm

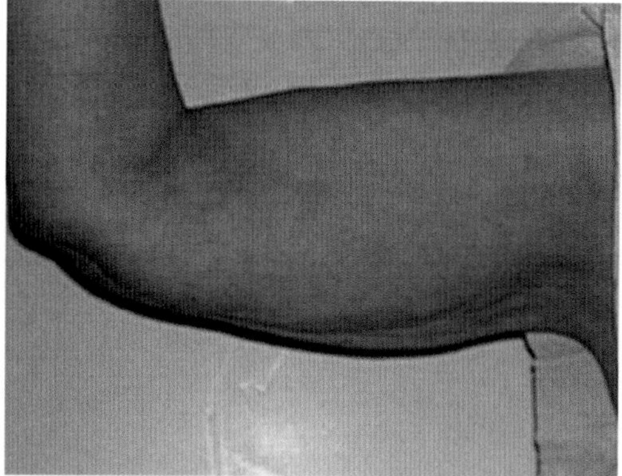

Fig. 22 Post-liposuction of the arm

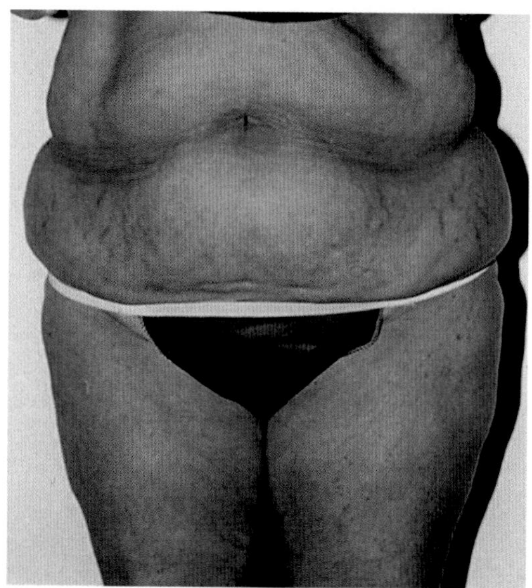

Fig. 23 Pre-lower abdomen, high hips, and waist

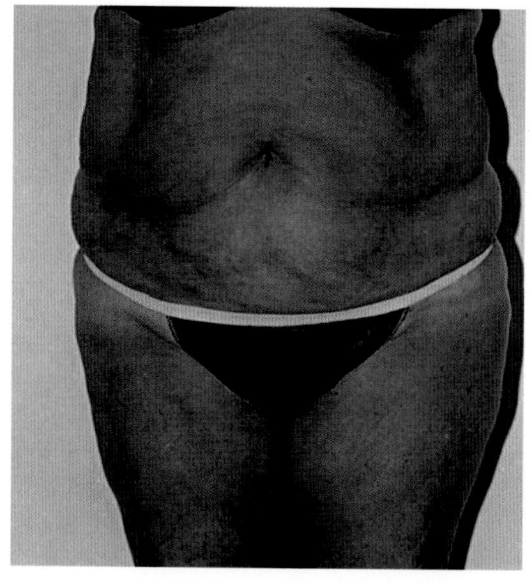

Fig. 24 Post-lower abdomen, high hips, and waist

infused tumescent fluid. Although the recommended maximal dose of lidocaine is 55 mg/kg, it is usually unnecessary to infuse dosages beyond 35 mg/kg [25].

Prior to liposuction, all patients should have a thorough consultation, including preoperative photos and discussion of realistic expectations. In addition to obtaining medical clearance, physical exam with the patient in the standing position should be performed. The skin is examined for fat distribution, skin elasticity, tone, and redundancy. Facial and neck liposuction are especially dependent on accurate assessment of not only fat distribution but also skin tone and facial contour. Good skin and muscular tone in body liposuction patients will also help optimize surgical results.

Contraindications to liposuction include, but are not limited to, clotting disorders that risk thromboembolism, bleeding diatheses, severe cardiovascular disease, pregnancy, and recent abdominal surgery. Any liver disease or current medications that might interfere with the metabolism of lidocaine should also be considered. It is imperative that all patients are informed that

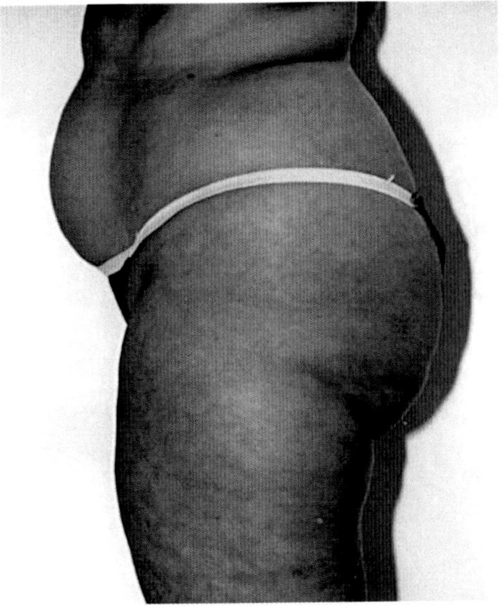

Fig. 25 Pre-liposuction

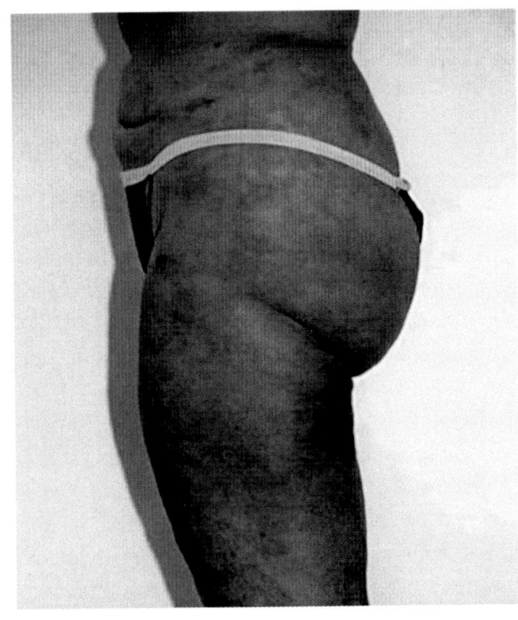

Fig. 26 Post-liposuction

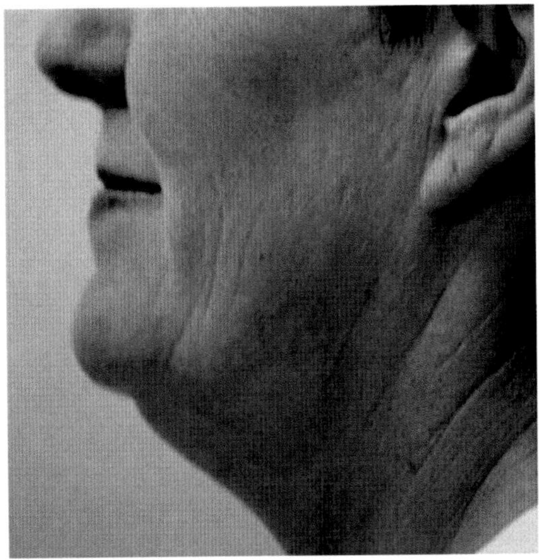

Fig. 27 Pre-neck jawline liposuction

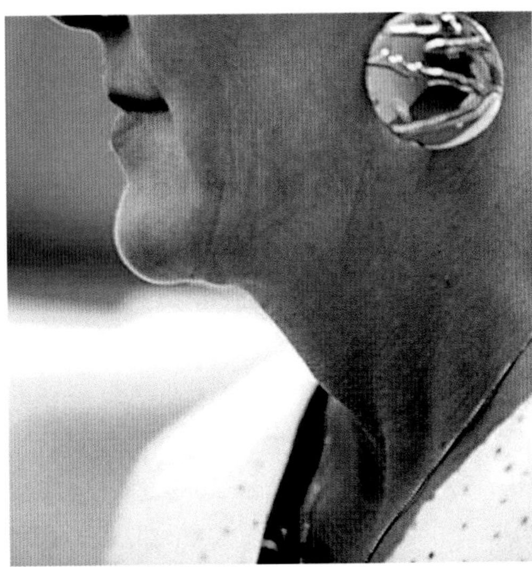

Fig. 28 Post-neck jawline liposuction

liposuction is not a weight loss procedure; it may remove inches from one's waistline, but one's weight will predominantly remain unchanged. The ideal candidate for liposuction has a lifestyle focused on maintenance of weight and muscular tone. If weight gain occurs following the procedure, it is common for weight to preferentially localize to the breast and buttocks. Similarly, it should be emphasized that liposuction is not a treatment for cellulite, striae, poor muscular tone, or inelastic skin tissue.

Liposuction can be safely performed in an office or ambulatory surgical setting. The patient first undergoes intravenous conscious sedation. Next, the tumescent anesthesia is infused into the localized fatty deposits through cannulas, hydrodissecting the tissue plane. Subsequently, suction-assisted cannulas are introduced through the same incisions used for tumescent anesthesia delivery. The syringe-assisted cannulas tunnel through the fat and remove excess fat from the treatment area. Cannulas come in many different sizes, diameters, lengths, and tip shapes. Treatment location, as well as fat density and thickness or the presence of any fibrosis, dictates the choice of cannula employed (Figs. 29 and 30). Currently, it is recommended that not more than 4 L of supranatant fat should be removed during one operative session [23].

After the procedure, patients are required to wear special surgical garments that help support the skin over the treatment area. These binders, girdles, or elastic tapes worn for about 1–4 weeks postoperatively deliver compression and minimize fluid shifts, bruising, and discomfort. There may be some drainage from the incision sites for several days, but overall the recovery period is remarkably rapid. Pain is minimal and is usually controlled by nonnarcotic analgesic agents. Although some pain and bruising are normal, they are usually minimal and well tolerated. On occasion, there is temporary fluid or blood accumulation under the skin. However, this is easily treated and resolved with no long-term adverse effects. The skin overlying the treatment area may be numb during the healing process, but generally numbness resolves over 3–6 months.

Many recent studies have documented the safety of tumescent liposuction [23, 25, 26]. In 2002 in a national survey of over 66,000 liposuction cases performed using the tumescent local anesthesia technique, no deaths were reported, and the rate of serious adverse events was 0.68 per 1,000 cases [24]. When complications do occur secondary to liposuction, they can be either systemic or localized. Systemic complications include fat and pulmonary emboli, infection, perforations, excessive blood loss, lidocaine toxicity, or death. Local complications include contour irregularities, paradoxical weight gain, hematoma or seroma, paresthesias, scarring, pigment irregularities localized to incision sites, and superficial skin necrosis.

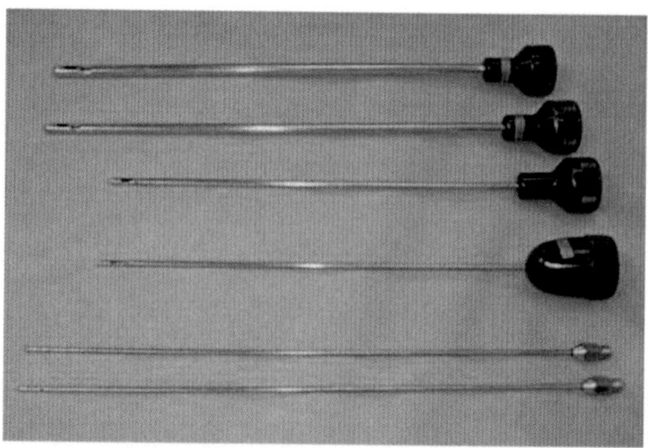

Fig. 29 Cannulas used for body liposuction

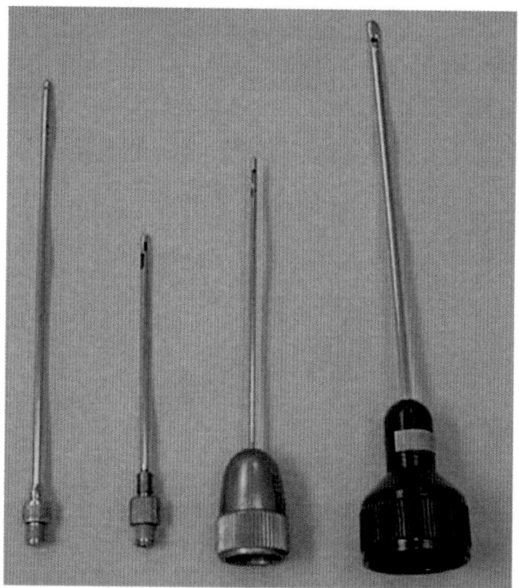

Fig. 30 Cannulas used for facial liposuction

In the first few days after liposuction, patients may be both sore and weak, but most are able to return to work within a week's time. Red-tinged drainage from incision sites, dependent swelling, and temporary numbness in overlying skin can all be encountered postoperatively. Pain and bruising can be controlled with oral narcotics. The incisional drainage should not persist more than

3 days. The tight-fitted binder garments help to prevent any collection of this fluid. However, regardless of garment wear after abdominal liposuction, fluid/edema will often collect in the groin and genital region. This swelling can persist for about 6–8 weeks. Any numbness in the skin overlying the treatment area usually improves by 6 months. Patients are also often frustrated by lack of immediate change in body contour following the procedure. It may take anywhere from 6 weeks to 6 months to appreciate the new, altered post-liposuction silhouette. Patients are advised to avoid alcohol, hot tubs, smoking, and any blood-thinning medication such as aspirin for about 2 weeks after the procedure. Nonvigorous daily walking is also strongly encouraged, as it helps to speed recovery.

Liposuction, in essence, is a tool used to sculpt the body by removing localized fat deposits. It is clearly not a form of weight loss and is ideally suited for younger patients who maintain good skin elasticity and muscular tone, although good results can be achieved in the older population. Whether large or small volumes of fat are removed, in the appropriate candidate, the results can be drastic. Clothes fit better. A facial profile appears more youthful. Therefore, liposuction can remove not only fat but years off one's appearance. Perhaps, this is why it has become one of the most popular cosmetic procedures currently performed by dermatologic and plastic surgeons [26].

Blepharoplasty

As Ralph Waldo Emerson once said, "The eyes indicate the antiquity of the soul." With the eyes being such an age-defining feature, there exists a natural tendency for patients to desire correction of periorbital signs of aging to rejuvenate facial appearance as a whole. Blepharoplasty is a pivotal procedure in "turning back the years" with regard to aging changes in the upper third of the face. When considering blepharoplasty in the elderly population, it is important to also note the brow position. A sagging brow will significantly add to upper eyelid skin redundancy, as well as contribute to an overall tired appearance. It is therefore advised that significant brow ptosis be corrected prior to undergoing blepharoplasty or concomitantly. Although contributory, brow ptosis is a distinct phenomenon from the periocular bags, sags, and folds, which develop over time secondary to loss of skin strength and supporting structures. It is specifically these unwanted periocular changes that blepharoplasty, alone, can "repair."

Although differences in opinion exist across cultures, the Western world has a fairly clear definition of "beautiful" eye architecture. For males, a flat eyebrow that rests upon the orbital rim is considered attractive, whereas for females, a brow that medially is positioned at or slightly above the orbital rim and ascends gently in the lateral aspect to reach a peak at the lateral limbus is preferred. Male and female differences also exist regarding the esthetic position of the eyelid crease. Generally, the male eyelid crease is positioned at approximately 10 mm above the eyelid margin at the superior border of the tarsus. The female eyelid crease is positioned slightly higher than the male, creating a more open appearance with greater depth. It is the attachment of the levator aponeurosis to the orbicularis muscle and subdermal skin that contributes to the eyelid crease structure.

In the upper eyelids, there are two fat pads: a small medial pad and a larger central one. There is no lateral fat pad. The anatomic caveat here is not to mistake a prolapsed lacrimal gland in the lateral position for a fat pad; if a prolapsed lacrimal gland is accidentally removed, chronic dry eye is likely to result. The lower eyelid has three fat pads: medial (nasal), central, and lateral (temporal). The inferior oblique muscle separates the medial and central fat collections and must not be injured, as trauma to this muscle can result in permanent diplopia on upward gaze. Additionally, the preaponeurotic fat pads are highly vascular, and great care must be taken when excising them so as to control bleeding and prevent retrobulbar hematoma. Eyelid surgery can treat loose or sagging skin that creates folds or disturbs the natural contour of the upper eyelid, sometimes impairing vision, excess fatty deposits that appear as puffiness in the upper eyelids, bags under the eyes, droopiness of the lower eyelids causing scleral show, or excess skin and fine wrinkles of the lower eyelid. Unfortunately, some of these ocular findings may have hereditary associations, and neither diet nor exercise will change these unwanted periocular characteristics.

As discussed previously, all cosmetic procedures require a thorough consultation outlining realistic expectations. Preoperative condition is documented with a series of photos, and the eyelids are evaluated for excess skin texture, herniated fat, level of supratarsal crease, ptosis, lacrimal gland position, and lower eyelid laxity. Special attention is directed to any evidence of contributory brow ptosis, a consequence of aging that can give the illusion of excess skin (pseudoblepharochalasis). It is critical to first surgically correct significant brow ptosis before proceeding with blepharoplasty. General medical clearance, with specific screening for a history of Graves' disease, connective tissue diseases associated with a clinical or subclinical sicca syndrome, or a history of a bleeding disorder, is recommended. Additionally, an ophthalmology consult should provide baseline visual acuity testing, visual filed mapping, fundoscopic examination, and Schirmer test to determine tear secretion. Specific ophthalmologic history pertaining to laser-assisted in situ keratomileusis and other refractive surgery should be documented, as they predispose the patient to postblepharoplasty dry eye exposure and visual changes [27].

The generic term blepharoplasty can be further divided into procedures specific to the upper and lower lid. Upper blepharoplasty can be employed to correct cosmetic and functional facial imperfections like drooping eyelids with skin redundancy (Figs. 31, 32, 33, 34, 35, and 36). In comparison, lower blepharoplasty, which helps correct the "bags" created from anteriorly, herniated retro-orbital fat, is employed primarily for cosmesis (Figs. 37 and 38). Depending upon the location and degree of necessary correction, patients may require excision of excess skin alone, skin and fat, or skin, fat, and muscle.

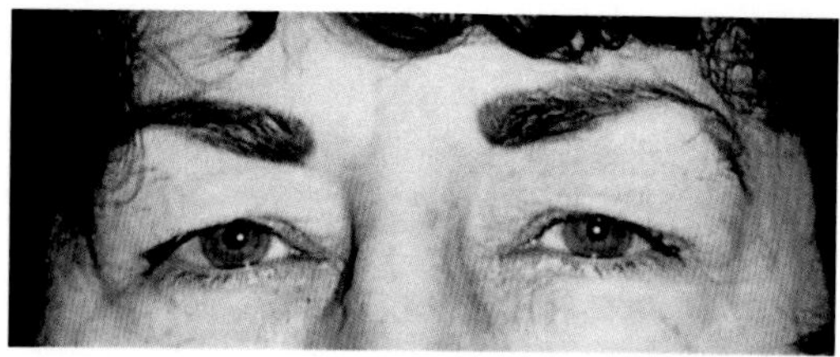

Fig. 31 Pre-upper blepharoplasty

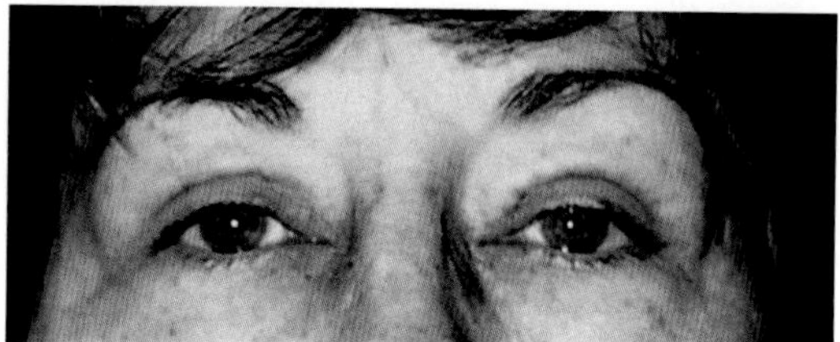

Fig. 32 Post-upper blepharoplasty

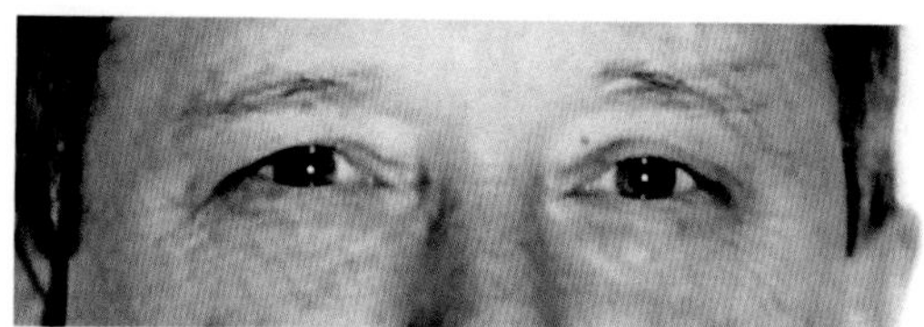

Fig. 33 Pre-upper blepharoplasty

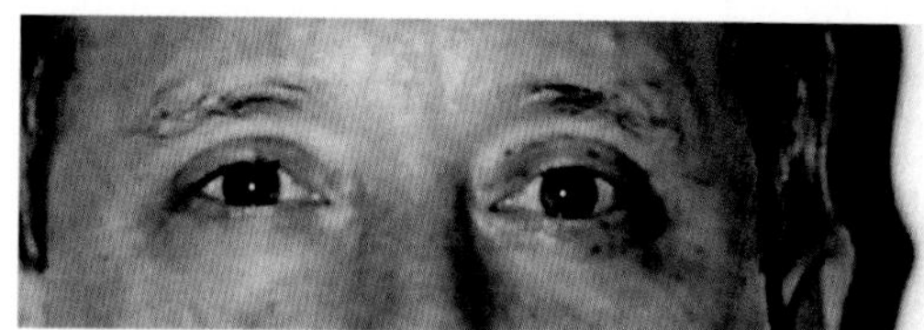

Fig. 34 Post-upper blepharoplasty

Most patients seek upper lid blepharoplasty for correction of redundant upper lid skin. This can either be a cosmetic concern secondary to unfavorable signs of aging or a functional concern in which the excess skin impedes vision or activities of daily living. The upper eyelid skin flap technique is exercised in instances where it is necessary to only excise excess skin and/or fat, as the orbicularis musculature is left intact. The skin is first appropriately marked with the patient in an

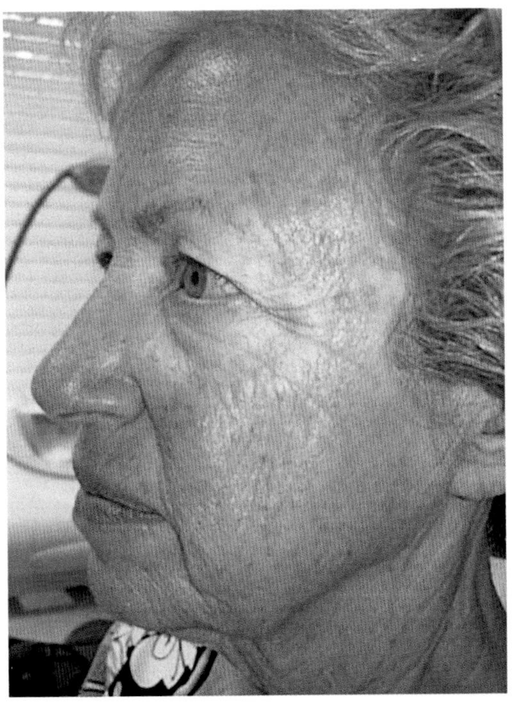

Fig. 35 Pre-upper blepharoplasty, side view

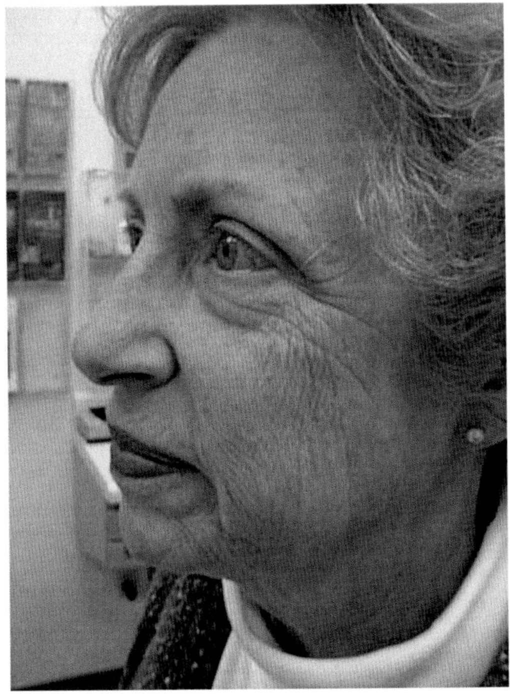

Fig. 36 Post-upper blepharoplasty, side view

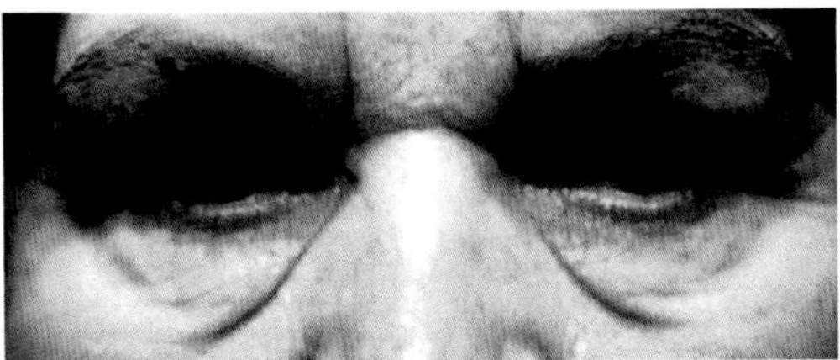

Fig. 37 Pre-lower blepharoplasty

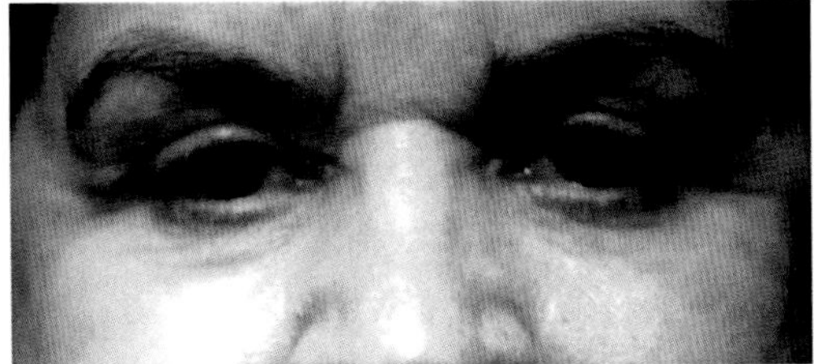

Fig. 38 Post-lower blepharoplasty

upright position, followed by eyelid excision, undermining, exposure of the orbicularis, dissection and removal of any unwanted fat, and finally a sutured closure. The myocutaneous upper blepharoplasty is exceedingly similar, with one exception. After the orbicularis muscle is dissected and visualized, a 5–6-mm strip of orbicularis muscle is excised just above the interior wound margin, exposing the orbital septum and levator aponeurosis. Subsequently, excess fat is also removed and the area closed with suture. This myocutaneous technique is primarily reserved for patients who have not only redundant skin and fat but also a component of hypertrophic musculature. If there also exists the need to recreate the supratarsal crease, nylon sutures are then placed with deep fixation to the underlying levator aponeurosis.

In contrast to upper lid blepharoplasty, lower lid procedures are usually performed for cosmetic reasons. If the desired goal is to simply remove the lower eyelid skin or fat "bags," a skin flap that allows for concomitant fat removal is all that is needed. An alternative method, in which the conjunctiva, rather than the skin, is incised, is the transconjunctival approach. The transconjunctival approach places the incision line approximately 4–6 mm inferior to the eyelid margin. This technique is preferred over transcutaneous incision, as it touts two major advantages. The risk of ectropion is decreased, and cosmesis is superior due to lack of visible scar. Unfortunately, if there is also a need for lower lid tightening, or if there exist excess fat and minimal excess skin (common in younger patients), a transcutaneous approach is necessary to address the needed myocutaneous abnormalities. It is recommended that the blepharoplasty procedure be performed under a combination of local (injectable and topical [eyeball]) anesthetic and conscious sedation.

Blepharoplasty-associated risks include corneal irritation, milia, cyst formation, allergic reactions, chemosis, dehiscence, loss of eyelashes, lagophthalmos (inability to close eyelids), overresection of fat, ectropion, ptosis, lacrimal gland injuries, diplopia, hematoma, asymmetry, persistent edema, and, rarely, retrobulbar hemorrhages with associated loss of vision. Penetration of the orbital septum introduces increased risk for retrobulbar hemorrhages. The overall incidence of blindness resulting from a retrobulbar hematoma following blepharoplasty is estimated to be only 0.04 % [28]. Signs of retrobulbar bleeding include pain, ecchymosis, proptosis (bulging eye), and visual loss.

Postoperatively, patients should be instructed regarding aggressive corneal lubrication with eye protection, eyedrops, and ointment [27]. Most patients do very well, but many may need reassurance that any swelling or bruising will resolve by the end of 2 weeks. Most patients resume normal activities within 2–3 days and return to work within a week. Contact lens wearers may return to contact eyewear 7–10 days after surgery. And women may return to eye makeup wear 10–24 days postoperatively. The quick healing and immediate results seen in association with blepharoplasty make it quite appealing to patients. But even more attractive are the procedure's long-lasting results. Depending on the age and inherent skin properties of an individual, the procedure's effects may endure from 5 to 15 years.

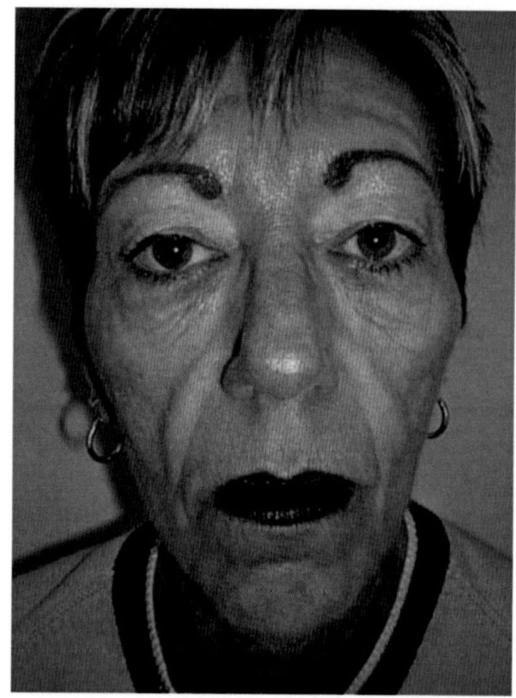

Fig. 39 Pre-upper and lower blepharoplasty

Blepharoplasty, though, namely, targeting aging in the periocular region, can drastically change overall appearance (Figs. 39 and 40). Caution is advised not to remove too much fat and underlying tissue from the periocular region, as a hollowed appearance will threaten cosmesis. In skilled hands, blepharoplasty will open up the eye and leave expressions of tiredness behind. By coupling blepharoplasty with browpexy and other cosmetic procedures (Figs. 41 and 42), the look of even younger years can be achieved. Laser resurfacing is commonly combined with eyelid surgery, to further improve skin tone and pigment irregularities. It is also the standard practice to combine the blepharoplasty procedure with CO_2 laser resurfacing. The tissue contraction associated with the CO_2 laser can further enhance blepharoplasty outcome, especially when treating lid laxity.

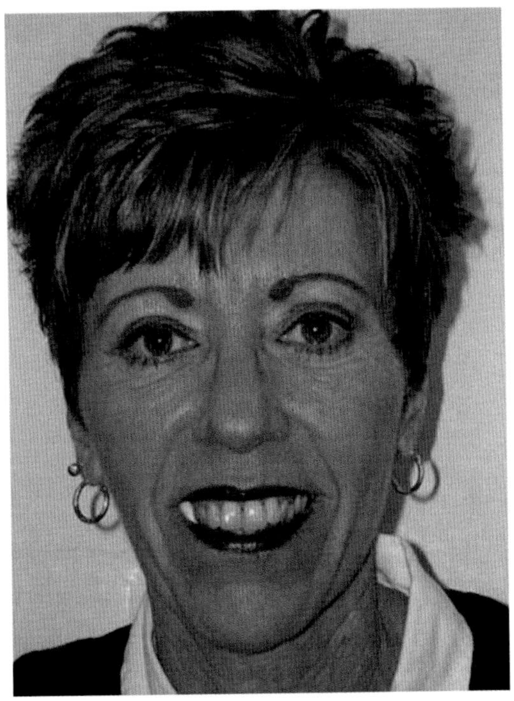

Fig. 40 Post-upper and lower blepharoplasty

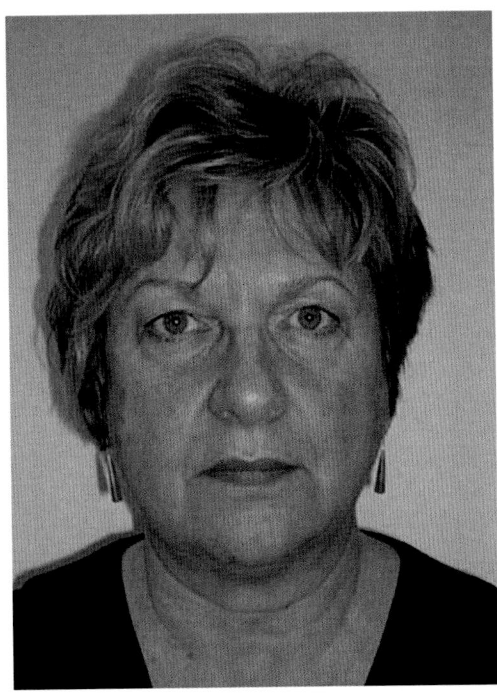

Fig. 41 Pre-combination upper and lower blepharoplasty, jawline tuck, neck jawline liposuction, and fractional laser to lower eye area

Face-Lift

The ultimate technique in surgical management of facial restoration has traditionally been considered the face-lift. However, with ongoing advancements in laser technology, this dogma may change in the future. Regardless, the primary means of manipulating both skin and underlying structures to restructure facial appearance in one surgical procedure remains the face-lift. The degree of necessary alteration varies with each patient and is dependent on inherent facial structure, the presence of intrinsic and extrinsic aging change, as well as the patient's expectation for dramatic improvement. Clearly, risks and morbidity are directly proportional to the invasiveness of a face-lift. Therefore, it has been the authors' goal to employ an individualized face-lift technique for each patient; the technique is minimally invasive but delivers equivalent if not superior results, in comparison to the traditional face- and neck lifting.

Using a limited undermining technique and superficial muscular aponeurotic system (SMAS) plication, the SMAS can be tightened and the skin carefully removed, restoring an oval jawline and well-defined chin-neck angle. Although early intervention is not uncommon for younger patient (aged 38–45 years), this technique can also be modified to treat an elderly population (65–80 years of age). In more mature patients, it is necessary to not only tighten the SMAS but also actually resuspend it. Due to limited undermining and lack of compromise to the facial vascular supply, this method may be safely used for face-lifts in certain cases where the patient's underlying health may be partially compromised.

As with most cosmetic, surgical procedures, there is a trade-off of invasiveness, risk, recuperation, and expense, with the degree of improvement in appearance. Thus, there is a range of different techniques, which vary in aggressiveness and should be tailored to the patient's present

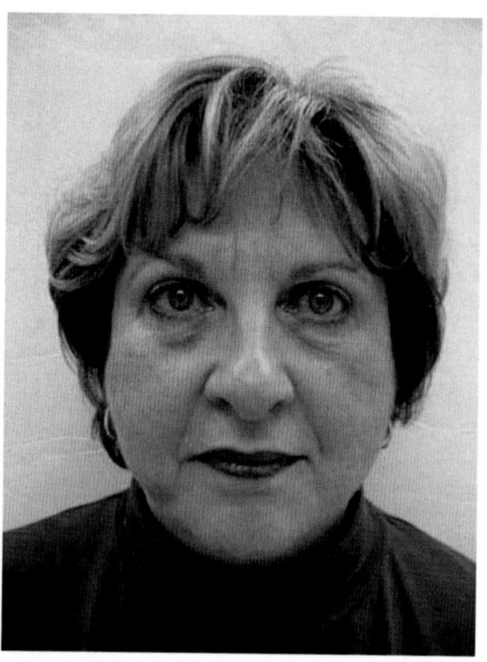

Fig. 42 Post-combination upper and lower blepharoplasty, jawline tuck, neck jawline liposuction, and fractional laser to lower eye area

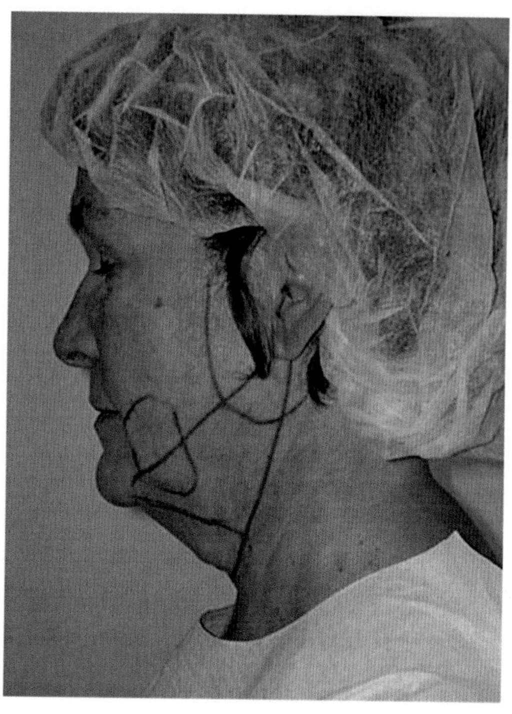

Fig. 43 Presurgical markings for jawline tuck procedure

appearance and the cosmetic state they hope to achieve. Patient selection criteria include general health, age, asymmetry, dysmorphic fat, weight gain or loss, muscle tone, bony structure, skin tone, skin thickness, and patient expectations. Of note is that age is not as important as the integrity of the facial skin and its underlying structures. Early tissue sagging and mild rhytids, depending on the skin's elasticity, can be substantially helped by limited skin procedures, whereas severe photodamage, prior trauma, scarring, and radiation changes may require more involved techniques.

The optimal candidate for a sutureless face-lift technique includes a patient with early mandibular angle blurring and potentially subtle neck droop with minimal fatty deposit. Conversely, a patient who presents with similar but more severe changes, as well as mild to moderate skin laxity, is a better candidate for a modified face-lift. And on the most severe end of the spectrum, those patients that have a large degree of tissue laxity and sag and/or platysmal banding are better suited for the conventional face-lift.

After a thorough patient consultation including an exam and preoperative photographs, informed consent with appropriately set patient expectations, and medical clearance, a patient is ready to undergo the face-lift procedure. All the authors' patients undergo cervicofacial rhytidectomy in an outpatient ambulatory surgical setting. Intravenous conscious is employed to ensure a comfortable patient experience. Patients are marked while seated in an upright position and then prepped and draped for sterility.

The procedure to which the authors subscribe involves incision, dissection, plication, skin removal, redraping, and closure. First, small skin incisions are placed bilaterally in the preauricular fold inferior to the tragus, at the base of the earlobe, postauricularly in the auricular sulcus to the level of the tragus, and in the midline under the mentum (Figs. 43, 44, and 45). Through these minute incisions, tumescent anesthesia is infused, and hydrodissection, along with undermining, ensues to create a cervical neck flap. As more invasive technique is

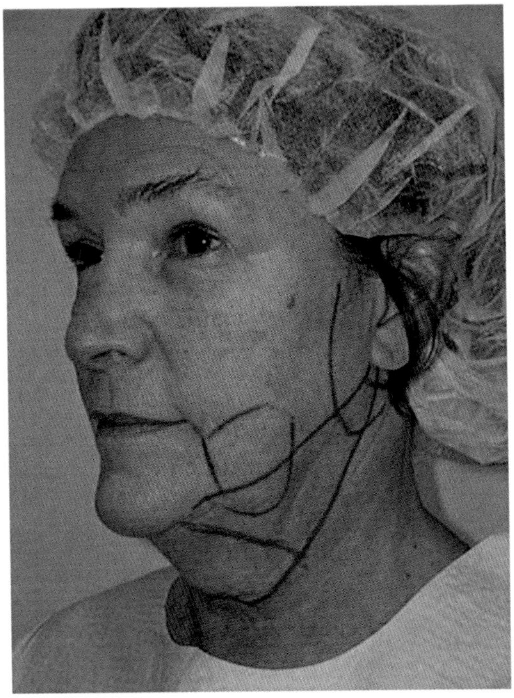

Fig. 44 Presurgical markings for jawline tuck procedure

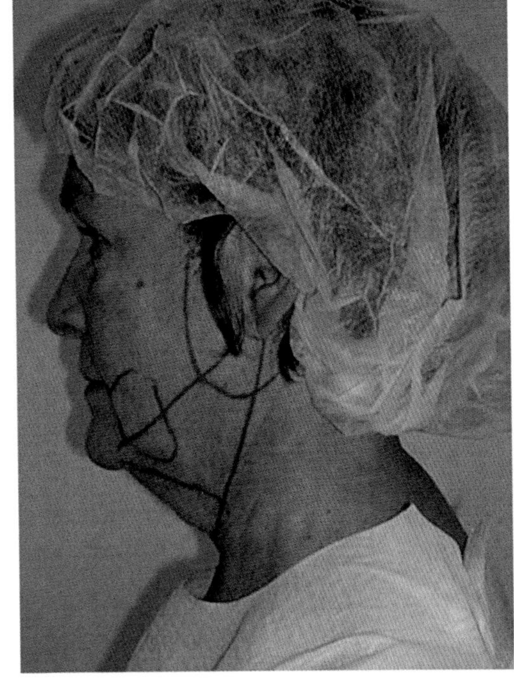

Fig. 45 Presurgical markings for jawline tuck procedure

required to accomplish the esthetic goal, the incisions can be lengthened, allowing for better access and further alteration of underlying tissue structures and creation of a larger flap (Fig. 46). The degree of undermining and extent of flap creation, as well as the degree of restructuring the SMAS, is what distinguishes a lunchtime lift, from a modified "minilift," from a traditional face-lift. Facial liposuction may also be employed at this time to remove any excess fat from the area. Subsequently, the SMA tissue is plicated by being folded over itself and pulled up with the use of nonabsorbable suture. Redundant skin is trimmed, redraped, and sutured, depending on the extent of the lift. The Webster variation lift is defined by sutures limited to the natural anterior and posterior cosmetic units of the ear, whereas in the traditional lift the incision/closure rises above the ear and into the temporal hairline.

The postoperative course involves typical wound care with twice a day topical antibiotic ointment and any necessary suture removal in about 7–10 days. Patients with more involved procedures may be fitted with a facial elastic garment. All patients are advised to avoid bending and lifting and are instructed to sleep in a 30–45° upright position so as to minimize swelling. While any swelling and bruising usually resolves by about postoperative day 10, the face may feel numb, especially along the neck, in the mandibular line, and in the periauricular area, for about 6–12 weeks after the procedure. Sun exposure also should be avoided. Overall, complications are few, and the major complications (large hematomas, skin loss, hair loss, and nerve loss) more commonly associated with the traditional face-lift are avoided. The patients' high level of satisfaction with their outcomes is a testament to the safety and efficacy of the Webster-style face-lift.

Although there are countless different approaches to rejuvenating the face within the realm of cervicofacial rhytidectomy, none has

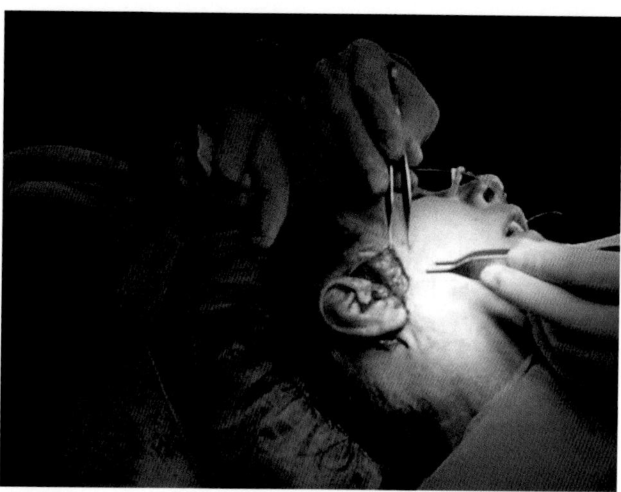

Fig. 46 Intraoperative face-lift flap dissection

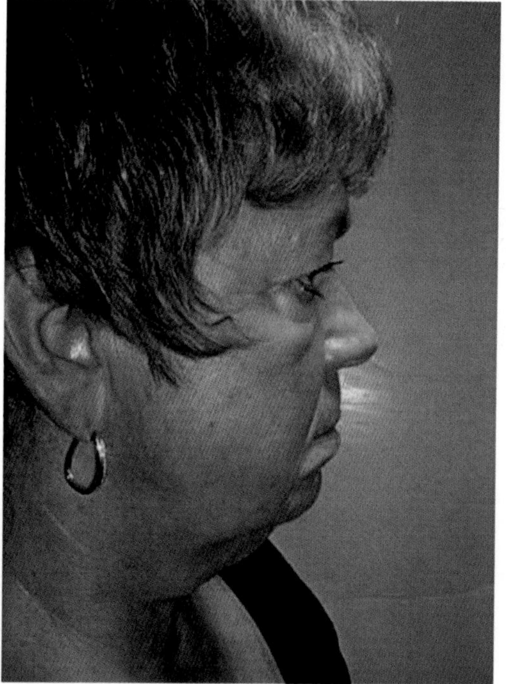

Fig. 47 Pre-jawline tuck; female

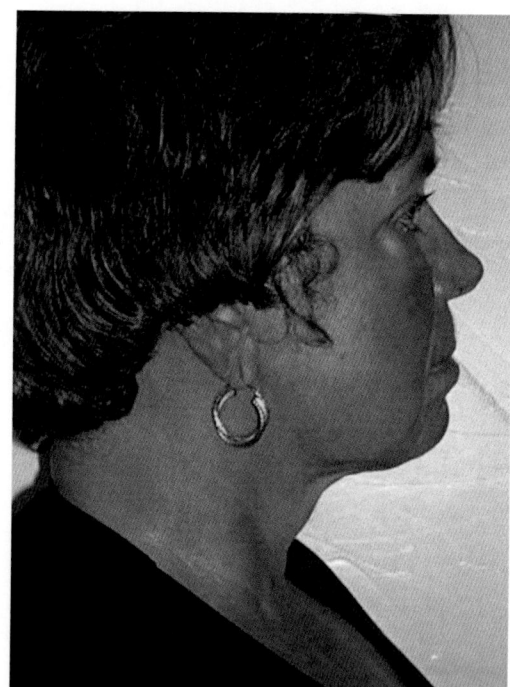

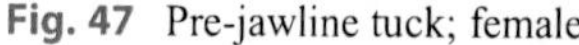

Fig. 48 Post-jawline tuck; female

been shown to produce consistently better or longer-lasting results. Many of the more aggressive techniques extend operating time, heighten the potential morbidity of the operation, and prolong the duration of convalescence. The Webster-type lift, to which the authors subscribe, has proven time and again, that a less invasive approach often gives the best and longest-lasting result, while limiting risk and avoiding serious complications (Figs. 47, 48, 49, and 50).

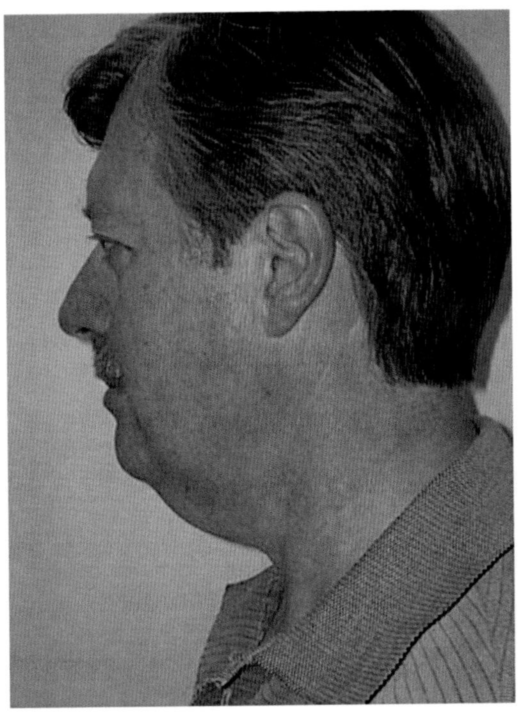

Fig. 49 Pre-jawline tuck; male

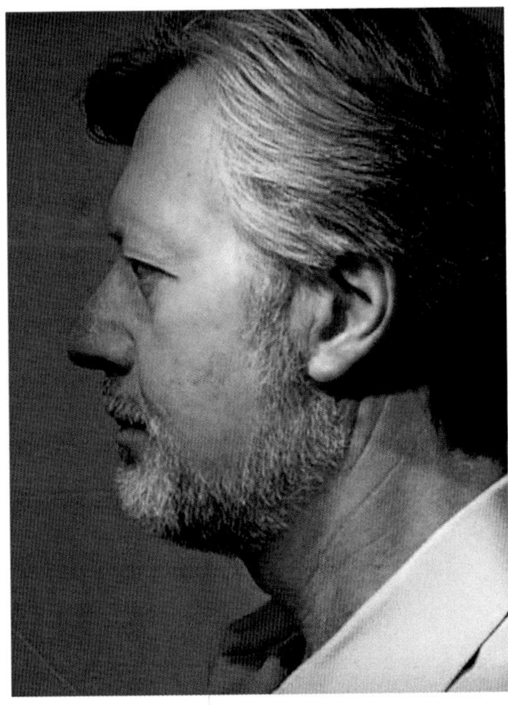

Fig. 50 Post-jawline tuck; male

Conclusion

With baby boomers reaching a critical mass, the pursuit of "aging gracefully" is particularly coveted in the elderly and can provide significant health benefits. It has been long known that looking better supports feeling better, and through thoughtful and careful discussion with older patients, the surgeon may be able to preserve and bolster self-confidence. By maintaining who they have been appearance wise, seniors are motivated to get more life out of their years.

Cross-References

- ▶ A New Paradigm for the Aging Face
- ▶ Facial Rejuvenation: A Chronology of Procedures

References

1. Rabe J, et al. Photoaging: mechanisms and repair. J Am Acad Dermatol. 2006;55(1):1–19.
2. Carruthers J, Botox Consensus Group, et al. Consensus recommendations on the use of botulinum toxin type a in facial aesthetics. Plast Reconstr Surg. 2004;114 (6):1S–22.
3. Carruthers J, Facial Aesthetics Consensus Group Faculty, et al. Advances in facial rejuvenation: botulinum toxin type a, hyaluronic acid dermal fillers, and combination therapies – consensus recommendations. Plast Reconstr Surg. 2008;121(5):5S–30.
4. Carruthers A, Carruthers J. Botulinum toxin type A: history and current cosmetic use in the upper face. Semin Cutan Med Surg. 2001;20:71–84.
5. Carruthers A, Carruthers J. Dose dilution and duration of effect of botulinum toxin type A (BTX-A) for the treatment of glabellar rhytids. Presented at the American Academy of Dermatology Winter Meeting, 22–27 Feb 2002, New Orleans, 2002.
6. Wise JB, Greco T. Injectable treatments for the aging face. Facial Plast Surg. 2006;22(2):140–6.
7. Lupo MP. Natural look in volume restoration. J Drugs Dermatol. 2008;7(9):833–9.
8. Romagnoli M, Belmontesi M. Hyaluronic acid-based fillers: theory and practice. Clin Dermatol. 2008;26:123–59.
9. Brandt FS, Cazzaniga A. Hyaluronic acid gel fillers in the management of facial aging. Clin Interv Aging. 2008;3(1):153–9.

10. Thioly-Bensoussan D. Non-hyaluronic acid fillers. Clin Dermatol. 2008;7(9):833–9.
11. Lemperle G, et al. Soft tissue augmentation with Artecoll: 10-year history, indications, techniques, and complications. Dermatol Surg. 2003;29:573–87.
12. Ortonne JP, Marks R. Photodamaged skin. London: Martin Dunitz; 1999. p. 11–28.
13. Clark E, Lawrence S. Superficial and medium-depth chemical peels. Clin Dermatol. 2008;26:209–18.
14. Landau M. Chemical peels. Clin Dermatol. 2008;26:200–8.
15. Truppman F, Ellenbery J. The major electrocardiographic changes during chemical face peeling. Plast Reconstr Surg. 1979;63:44.
16. Bhalla M, Thami GP. Microdermabrasion: reappraisal and brief review of literature. Dermatol Surg. 2006;32 (6):809–14.
17. Sadick NS, Finn NA. New applications for microdermabrasion technology. Int J Cosmet Surg Aesth Dermatol. 2002;4(63):44.
18. Campbell RM, Harmon CB. Dermabrasion in our practice. J Drugs Dermatol. 2008;7(2):124–8.
19. Lawrence N. History of dermabrasion. Dermatol Surg. 2000;26:95–101.
20. Alexiades-Armenakas MR, et al. The spectrum of laser skin resurfacing: nonablative, fractional, and ablative laser resurfacing. J Am Acad Dermatol. 2008;58 (5):719–37.
21. DeHoratius D. Nonablative tissue remodeling and photorejuvenation. Clin Dermatol. 2007;25:474–9.
22. Stewart N, Lim AC, Lowe PM, Goodman G. Laser and laser-like devices: part one. Australas J Dermatol. 2013;54(3):173–83.
23. Coldiron B, et al. Liposuction council bulletin: ASDS guidelines of care for tumescent liposuction. Dermatol Surg. 2006;32:709–16.
24. Butterwick KJ, Goldman MP, Sriprachya-Anunt S. Lidocaine levels during the first two hours of infiltration of dilute anesthetic solution for tumescent liposuction: rapid versus slow delivery. Dermatol Surg. 1999;25(9):681–5.
25. Coleman W, American Academy of Dermatology Guidelines/Outcomes Committee, et al. Guidelines of care for liposuction. J Am Acad Dermatol. 2001;45 (3):438–47.
26. Housman T, et al. The safety of liposuction: results of a national survey. Dermatol Surg. 2002;28(11):971–8.
27. Trussler A, Rohrich R. Blepharoplasty. Plast Reconstr Surg. 2008;121(1):1–10.
28. DeMere M, et al. Eye complications with blepharoplasty or other eyelid surgery: a national survey. Plast Reconstr Surg. 1974;53:634–7.

Facial Rejuvenation: A Chronology of Procedures

150

Alexander S. Donath

Contents

Abstract

The past two decades have borne witness to a remarkable increase in the demand for facial rejuvenation, with recent advances in minimally invasive procedures driving substantial growth in such procedures. This chapter aims to outline the procedures which are appropriate for the various decades of adult life, beginning when the earliest signs of aging typically present themselves – in the thirties. It should be emphasized that the following are general guidelines for the respective decades and that major factors such as ultraviolet light exposure and tobacco smoking, along with lesser factors such as diet and exercise, can accelerate the natural aging process. Additionally, one's genetic construct also certainly influences the period in which the various stigmata outlined below become evident. The utility of nonsurgical procedures such as injection of botulinum toxin A and synthetic soft tissue fillers, chemical peels, and laser resurfacing is outlined for the decades in which their use commonly begins. Surgical rejuvenation procedures are detailed as well, including fat transfer, blepharoplasty, facelifting (rhytidectomy), necklifting, and browlifting, in the chronological order in which they are typically employed. Newer technologies such as radiofrequency- and ultrasound-based tightening devices are discussed. Finally, future applications and techniques are proposed, including

A.S. Donath
Cincinnati Facial Plastic Surgery, Cincinnati, OH, USA
e-mail: drdonath@cincyfacialplastics.com

M.A. Farage et al. (eds.), *Textbook of Aging Skin*,
DOI 10.1007/978-3-662-47398-6_106

current evidence for the potential for platelet-rich plasma and adipose-derived stem cells.

Introduction

The past two decades have borne witness to a remarkable increase in the demand for facial rejuvenation [1], with recent advances in minimally invasive procedures driving substantial growth in such procedures [2]. Fueled in part by reality television programming and the associated increase in public familiarity with, and acceptance of, the available procedures, this trend is also a reflection of increasing life expectancies and the entrance of baby boomers into their fifth through seventh decade (40s through 60s) – a period of heightened manifestation of aging face stigmata. Indeed, this cohort, born between 1946 and 1964 [3], is characterized as having been the healthiest and wealthiest generation to that time and among the first to grow up genuinely expecting the world to improve with time [4]. It logically follows that with such optimism comes the desire to maintain a youthful countenance during the expected period of global progress.

While the estimated 80 million boomers are certainly a major driving force in the economy, the marketing dollars spent in pursuit of their spending power have yielded messages that have also piqued the interest of other generations. This chapter aims to outline the procedures which are appropriate for the various decades of adult life, beginning when the earliest signs of aging typically present themselves – in the thirties. It should be emphasized that the following are general guidelines for the respective decades and that major factors such as ultraviolet light exposure and tobacco smoking, along with lesser factors such as diet and exercise, can accelerate the natural aging process. Thus, a heavy smoker who also sunbathes excessively and without UV protection will perhaps be a candidate for many procedures described below in his/her early forties, in contrast to his/her healthier counterparts in the expected decades outlined herein. Additionally, one's genetic construct also certainly influences the period in which the various stigmata outlined below become evident.

Thirties

Most adults begin to show mild rhytides at rest (without animation) in the glabellar, forehead, and periorbital regions in the early to mid-30s. Some patients wish to prevent formation of these dynamic lines prior to their presentation at rest, as they note their appearance in animation in their late twenties and are frequently fearful of permanence, but the majority of patients tend to delay intervention until the persistence of rhytides at rest. The primary treatment modality for these rhytides is neurotoxin, specifically botulinum toxin type A. Botulinum toxin causes a temporary paralysis of the targeted muscle(s) by preventing acetylcholine release from motor nerve endings. The paralysis typically lasts for 3–4 months, with increased durability of effect realized by patients after multiple treatments at regular intervals; some patients are able to extend their treatment intervals to 6 months or more. Muscles most frequently treated in this fashion include the *procerus* and *corrugator supercilii* muscles, for horizontal and vertical glabellar rhytides, respectively; the *frontalis* muscle for horizontal forehead rhytides; and the *orbicularis oculi* muscles for lateral periorbital rhytides, commonly called "crow's feet." Additional sites for the use of neurotoxins in the later decades are outlined below. The specific US FDA approval for botulinum toxin A for cosmetic purposes is for glabellar lines and crow's feet, and as such it has shown an excellent safety profile since its approval in 2002 [5].

In addition to neuromodulators, synthetic fillers have seen a surge in utility for lines and folds of the aging face, and hyaluronic acid (HA) fillers are the most commonly employed. While the primary goal of such fillers is overall improvement in wrinkles and folds, recent studies have shown stimulation of collagen production by HA fillers, which may lead to further applications in treatment of aging skin [6].

For patients who do not wish to receive neurotoxin injections or fillers, or for whom they are contraindicated, facial resurfacing procedures are also effective in reducing fine rhytides. A variety of modalities are available for this aim, including medium strength chemical peels (e.g., 35 %

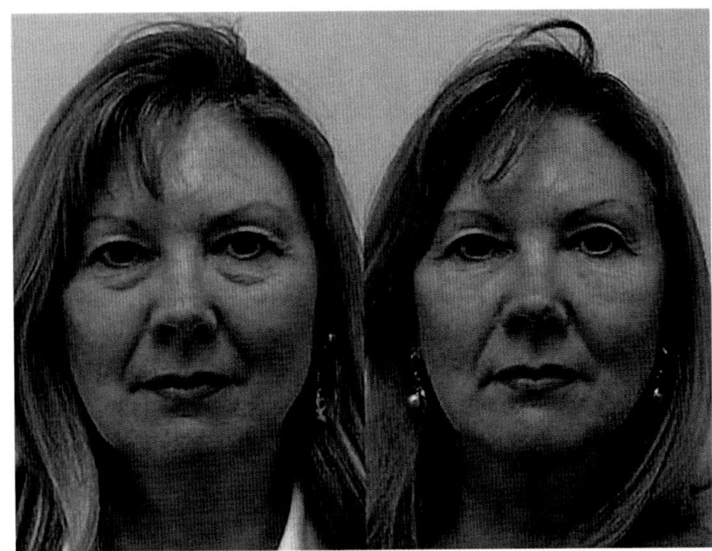

Fig. 1 A 56-year-old patient who requested improvement in the infraorbital region. Patient shown before (*left*) and after (*right*) hyaluronic acid filler augmentation of the tear trough region, using <1.0 cc total for both sides. Patients have been treated in a similar fashion in the author's practice as early as the late twenties, when genetically predisposed to early tear trough deformity

trichloroacetic acid [TCA]) and light-based therapies such as the erbium laser; a full discussion of the available chemical and light-based resurfacing modalities is beyond the scope of this chapter.

In addition to the role of rhytides in portending age, there has been a dramatic increase in appreciation for the role of *volume loss* in the aging face [7]. This volume loss is exhibited in diminishment of skin thickness, subcutaneous adipose volume, and bony volume, as well as in muscular atrophy. The earliest site to yield evidence of this volume loss is the infraorbital region, beginning in the late twenties or early thirties. Here, patients begin to show the "tear trough deformity" or "dark circles" beneath the eyes. While commonly attributed to allergic, fatigue, or vascular etiologies, the elimination of these "circles" is most effectively achieved by volume augmentation of the tear trough region [8], rather than by reversal of the other proposed etiologies. Indeed, many patients who have previously used numerous under-eye "concealers" unsuccessfully in hopes of camouflaging what is perceived as darkly pigmented skin are relieved when volume augmentation is quickly effective. This is because volume loss results in a depression, or concavity, between the convexities of the bony inferior orbital rim and/or lower lid fat pads above and the cheek mass below. The appropriateness of a patient for volume augmentation here may be determined by shining light directly into the "dark circle," perpendicular to the skin – this will fill the shadow in the tear trough created by overhead light, such as that in a typical examination room. If the resulting appearance is desired by the patient, they are excellent candidates for this procedure; any pigmentary issues are thus excluded as causative. Volume replacement can be performed with either synthetic materials, such as hyaluronic acid (HA) fillers, or the patient's own fat cells (Fig. 1). The specific FDA approval for most HA fillers is for "correction of moderate to severe facial wrinkles and folds, such as the nasolabial folds," and volume restoration in the infraorbital area and others is therefore categorized as "off-label," though well-accepted in the medical community [9–13].

The next most common site of use for filling materials in our practice in this decade is the lips. Rejuvenation or augmentation of genetically suboptimal fullness in the vermillion of the lips is easily accomplished with synthetic fillers, such as the HA fillers. Certain anatomic norms must be respected, however, if the physician is to achieve a natural result: the upper lip vermillion show should not exceed one half of the lower lip vermillion in vertical height; the upper lip vermillion should be viewed as three separate aesthetic units, central (tubercle), left, and right, with the lateral units comprising the majority of the horizontal length; and the lower lip vermillion is comprised of two aesthetic units – left and right – with a central sulcus between them. Rarely is more than 1 cc of HA filler required to achieve the desired results in this age group.

Forties

With the progressive thinning of skin comes increased visibility of rhytides at rest. In addition to the periorbital and glabellar regions, lines become more evident in the forehead and perioral regions, as well as the sidewalls of the nose. While neurotoxin is commonly used in the frontalis muscle for horizontal forehead rhytides, less commonly treated muscles include the *orbicularis oris*, for vertical rhytides of the white portions of the lips, and the transverse portion of the *nasalis*, for vertical lines on the sidewalls of the nose ("bunny lines") [14]. Treatment of the *orbicularis oris* muscle in this fashion is done conservatively, so as not to affect animation, oral intake, or oral competency.

Synthetic fillers may also be used to eliminate fine lines in the skin. In contradistinction to neurotoxins, which are injected into the muscles that cause the rhytides, fillers are placed in the dermis directly beneath the line of depression and typically last from 6 months to 1 year or more. Hyaluronic acid fillers are exceedingly well tolerated in this manner and may also be used in conjunction with neurotoxins for particularly deep rhytides, such as commonly develop in the glabellar region. A significant advancement of the past 5 years has been the introduction of cannulas for synthetic filler injection. As opposed to traditional needles for infiltration, cannulas have blunt tips which seem to cause less vascular injury and therefore decreased posttreatment bruising, with a corresponding reduction in social downtime. Additionally, the blunt tip, as well as the location of the injection port on the side of the cannula, would be expected to provide improved safety from intravascular injection, though no studies could be identified to document this.

In the areas of fine rhytides at rest not amenable to neurotoxin treatment, or in patients apprehensive about such treatments or otherwise not candidates, chemical peels and laser resurfacing are excellent options. Both types of modalities can be customized to the depth of the patient's rhytides and the available downtime; those with predominantly fine rhytides or with limited capacity for skin erythema beyond 1-week posttreatment are best treated with a medium-depth peel, such as 35 % trichloroacetic acid (TCA) or a medium strength croton oil/phenol peel (e.g., Hetter's medium-light peel) [15, 16], or an erbium laser set to medium penetration depth [17]. For patients with deeper rhytides at rest and greater capacity for downtime, a deeper chemical peel (e.g., Hetter's medium–heavy or heavy croton oil/phenol peel) or erbium laser set to deeper penetration will be more effective. Fractionated carbon dioxide lasers have also been utilized in this fashion, with promising results and significantly diminished downtime and unwanted effects such as scarring and pigmentary changes [18], although detracting effects are possible [19].

In addition to fine lines noted above, the face begins to show deepening of the nasolabial folds (from the sides of the nose to the corners of the mouth) and labiomandibular folds (from the oral commissures toward the jawline, commonly called "marionette lines") in this decade. Synthetic fillers are excellent remedies for such folds, and these areas are among the most commonly treated with HA fillers. Indeed, it was the augmentation of nasolabial folds which served as the basis for FDA approval of the initial HA fillers [12]. Calcium hydroxylapetite and poly-L-lactic acid fillers are also used frequently for temporary improvement in folds as well as facial volume restoration, while polymethylmethacrylate is used for permanent enhancement of folds and volume loss.

In the periorbital region, volume loss becomes evident in the medial infrabrow region, where the convex highlight of youth gives way to a relative concavity and associated shadow. Accompanying this shadow, particularly toward the end of the fifth decade, is the accumulation of folds of skin in the upper eyelids, termed dermatochalasis. While traditional aging theory attributes this skin

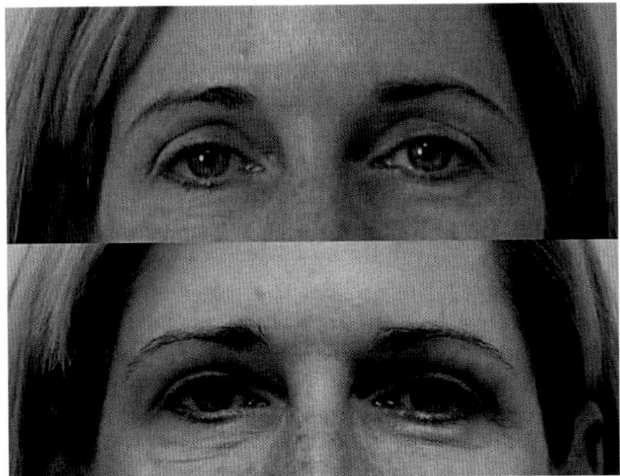

Fig. 2 Patient at 50 years of age before (*above*) and after (*below*) soft tissue augmentation in the superior orbital rim/infrabrow area using an HA filler. Note the age-associated atrophy in medial infrabrow soft tissue creating concavity with resultant shadowing as well as skin redundancy prior to treatment (*above*), the latter seen best on patient's left side. Note improvement of atrophy and skin redundancy in posttreatment image (*below*) resulting in reduction of upper eyelid show to a more youthful amount of vertical height

excess purely to loss of skin elasticity and descent of the brow, current understanding of this presentation recognizes the important role of volume loss, both in the soft tissue (adipose) and the bony orbital rim. Thus, refilling of the infrabrow region restores the youthful convexity and associated highlight to the medial infrabrow area and elevates a finite portion of the infrabrow skin from the lashline (Fig. 2). This reinflation of the infrabrow area can create an appearance of brow elevation, as elegantly demonstrated by Coleman [20]. As described below, when infrabrow skin excess exceeds the capacity for elevation by soft tissue augmentation, upper lid blepharoplasty, with excision of redundant skin, may be entertained as an adjunctive procedure or in isolation.

Fifties

One of the most important events contributing to the aging face stigmata in women is menopause, for which the average age is 51. The associated decline in circulating body estrogen has been linked to multiple facial cutaneous aging phenomena, including wrinkling, dryness, laxity, and atrophy; it has been demonstrated that some 30 % of skin collagen is lost in the first 5 years after menopause and that the average annual decline over 20 years following menopause is 2.1 % [21, 22]. Estrogen replacement, particularly in the form of topical application of *estriol*, a weak estrogen, may ameliorate some of these effects and could be considered as part of a comprehensive skin care regimen in postmenopausal women [23, 24].

In the periocular region, the infrabrow shadow noted above and resulting from volume loss, progresses laterally across the infrabrow region, creating an appearance of darkness across the upper eyelid region. In this sixth decade, the deflation of the infrabrow area also results in greater accumulation of folds of skin near the eyelashes, which prompt visits to the facial cosmetic surgeon for blepharoplasty consultation to a larger extent than during the fifth decade. At this relatively early age, however, the degree of skin laxity may be best treated not by skin excision but by volume restoration in the infrabrow area; refilling the subcutaneous volume in this area results in radial expansion of the skin, restoring a youthful convexity and highlight to this area (Figs. 2, 3, and 4) and frequently elevating the overlying brow hair.

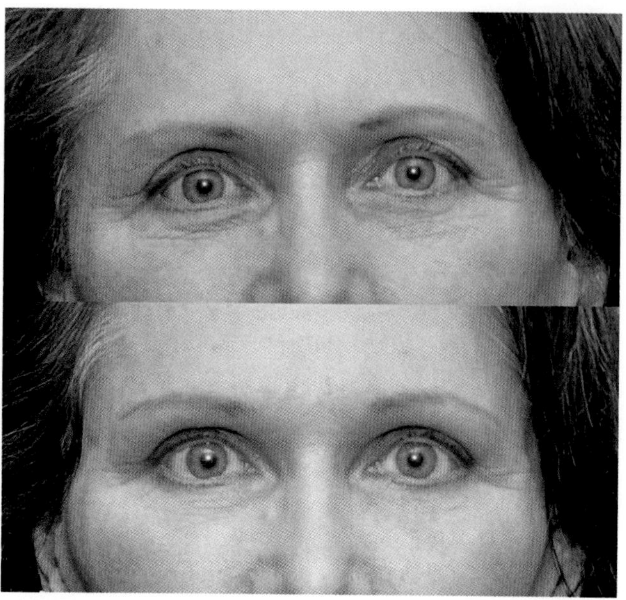

Fig. 3 Patient at 59 years of age before (*above*) and 1 month after (*below*) fat transfer to the superior orbital rim/infrabrow and infraorbital areas. Note the age-associated atrophy in medial infrabrow soft tissue creating concavity with resultant shadowing and upper eyelid show as well as skin redundancy prior to treatment (*above*). Note also improvement of atrophy and skin redundancy in posttreatment image (*below*) resulting in reduction of upper eyelid show to a more youthful amount of vertical height. The infraorbital hollowing is improved as well

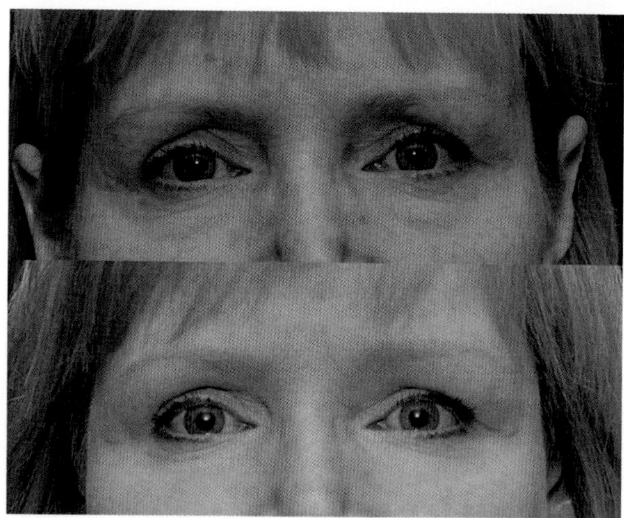

Fig. 4 Sixty-year-old female preoperative (*above*) and 5 months postoperative (*below*) from fat transfer to periocular regions. Note improvement in periorbital hollowing with reduction in supra- and infraorbital concavity and associated shadowing, creating more natural, youthful convexity, and associated highlights. Note also the modest reduction in upper eyelid show

Along with the *infraorbital* filling, which is begun in the thirties and forties, such *infrabrow* filling aids in restoring highlights around the eyes, a technique frequently termed "framing the eye" [25]. The reader is encouraged to review covers of beauty and fashion magazines for depictions of society's "ideal" periorbital constructs: a relatively low eyebrow, full infrabrow soft tissue with associated highlight, and a full lower eyelid–cheek interface. It is this anatomy that draws the viewer's eye toward the iris and pupil. Careful study of these anatomic relationships allows more natural restoration of the youthful visage, as eloquently demonstrated by Coleman [20]. Indeed without such examination, one may be beguiled by the optical illusion that a hollowed infrabrow region represents a *descended* brow and thereafter undertake to surgically elevate the brow, all too often creating an unnatural, surprised look [25, 26]. Additionally, the lateral brow descends earlier and to a greater extent than the central or medial brow, and therefore in early brow rejuvenation, greater emphasis should be placed on lateral browlifting than the more traditional lift, which incorporates all brow components. In addition to surgical brow lifting, some have shown benefit of focused ultrasound in achieving nonsurgical brow elevation [27].

In the lower periorbital region, the tear trough deformity described above becomes more prominent, while the lower lid fat pads become more protuberant as well. Although the latter is partially due to weakening of the lower eyelid retaining structures, it is the same atrophy that causes the tear trough deformity to manifest that also results in uncovering of the infraorbital fat pads. Pseudoherniation of the lower eyelid fat pads may necessitate surgical removal, via lower eyelid blepharoplasty, particularly if they are too large to be concealed by volume restoration in the tear trough and inferior orbital rim regions. Techniques for addressing lower eyelid fat pseudoherniation include *transconjunctival* and *transcutaneous* blepharoplasty. Our practice employs predominantly the transconjunctival approach, so as to limit the possibility of weakening the lower eyelid support mechanisms, which may result in lid retraction and scleral show [28]. Regardless of the chosen approach, it is recommended that blepharoplasty be done in conjunction with infraorbital volume restoration, either by formal lipotransfer, synthetic filler injection, or by lower lid fat *transposition* [29], to both increase the longevity of the result and to create a more youthful eyelid–cheek interface.

Another anatomic site of volume loss is the lips. Frequently overtreated at the patient's unwitting request, a conservative, natural restoration of more youthful volume in the lip vermillion is an important aspect of facial rejuvenation. Here again, both synthetic fillers and autologous fat are excellent options. As noted above for patients in their thirties, the aesthetic norms should be respected in order to prevent an unnatural appearance. In addition to restoration of vermillion volume, however, patients in their fifties frequently begin to benefit from restoration of the philtral ridges, vermillion borders, and the white rolls, including the central "cupid's bow" of the upper lip and vertical lip lines. To this end, a newly FDA-approved small-particle HA filler (Restylane Silk®, Galderma, Fort Worth, TX) has shown promise in addressing such fine details of the lips.

Many patients begin to note an interruption of their jawline with "jowls" in their late forties or early fifties. While frequently attributed entirely to gravity-induced descent of the cheek and loss of cutaneous elasticity, jowling is also partially a function of subcutaneous atrophy in the cheek, with resultant hanging of the deflated, less elastic tissue inferiorly under the influence of gravity. Thus, gravity is not primarily causative, but rather simply determines the direction in which the deflated, elastotic cheek tissue hangs. Reinflation of the cheek with fat, synthetic fillers, or implants aids in the reduction of jowling along the mandibular border. However, the primary benefit of volume augmentation in the anterior and lateral cheek is in restoring the convexities of youth, which have typically become replaced by concavities in this decade (Fig. 5). It would not be advisable to rely *solely* on cheek augmentation to elevate any more than subtle amounts (a few millimeters of vertical height) of jowling.

Bony loss is also thought to contribute to jowling: atrophy of the mandible anterior to the jowl leads to the formation of the *prejowl sulcus*, creating a superomedial indentation in the overlying soft tissue, which exacerbates the appearance of jowling [30, 31]. Bony loss also occurs in the lateral/posterior mandibular region, and thus, when combined with augmentation of the prejowl sulcus, volume restoration of this postjowl region may effectively postpone surgical elevation of the jowl (Fig. 6).

Once accumulation of jowls has progressed to a point unwelcome to the patient and if deemed too pronounced to be addressed by volume restoration alone, or if this is otherwise not necessary or desired, facelifting becomes a viable remedy (Fig. 7). There are many variations of this procedure, and a complete review of the techniques is beyond the scope of this chapter [32]. Most methods, however, rely on elevation of a skin flap, suture suspension of the underlying superficial musculoaponeurotic system (SMAS) in a superoposterior direction, redraping and trimming

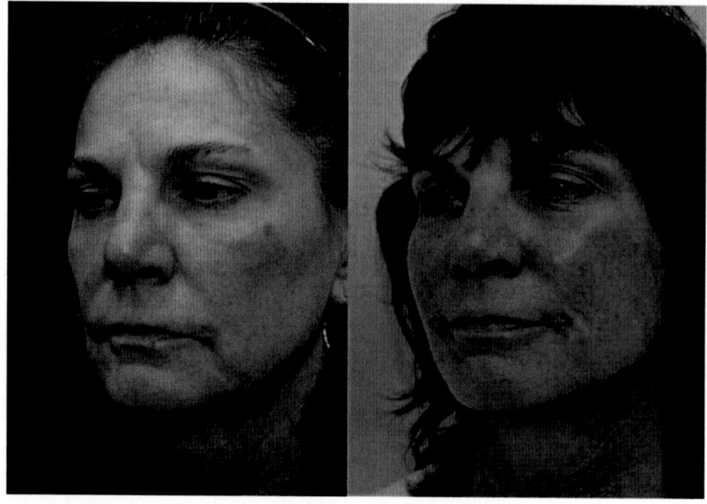

Fig. 5 A 51-year-old woman who underwent fat transfer to the midface to complement facelifting, shown before (*left*) and 2 months postoperatively (*right*). Notable is the improvement in the cheek fullness seen in both the near and far cheek and the associated improvement in continuity of the lid–cheek interface; neither benefit is likely with facelifting alone

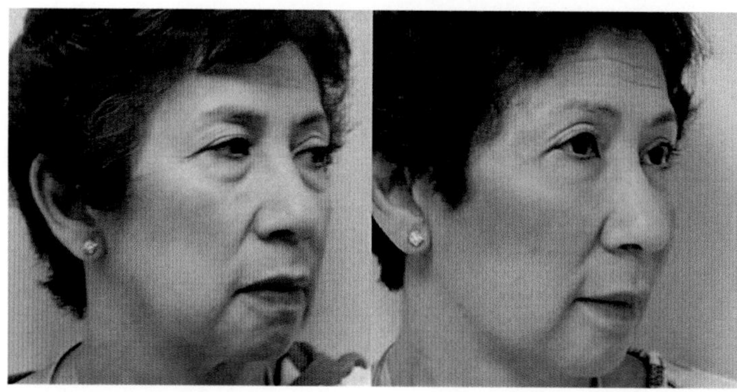

Fig. 6 A 64-year-old woman who requested fat transfer for facial rejuvenation, which was performed in the pre- and postjowl regions, as well as the midface and superior orbital rim/infrabrow area; lower lid transconjunctival blepharoplasty was also performed. Note the atrophic pre- and postjowl regions prior to treatment (*left*), as well as upper eyelid dermatochalasis and lower eyelid pseudoherniation. Significant improvement was evident along the jawline at the 1-month postoperative visit (*right*), with a straightening effect without the employment of facelifting. Also notable is improvement in upper eyelid skin redundancy via volume restoration alone and improvement in midfacial contour achieved with combination of blepharoplasty and lipoaugmentation; the mentum was augmented as well

of excess skin, and suturing the cut skin edges. Facelifting addresses primarily the lower third of the face, from the nasal ala to the jawline and jowl, in addition to the neck; improvement is expected in the labiomandibular fold and jowl, as well as modest platysmal banding, particularly when coupled with a submentoplasty, as noted below. Importantly, however, facelifting does *not* appreciably efface the majority of the nasolabial fold, although some improvement can be seen in the inferior aspect. Liposuction of the jowls, while unlikely to independently give a satisfactory result, is a useful adjunct to the above mentioned techniques and is frequently performed in conjunction with cervical liposuction. Neck liposuction may also be indicated as an isolated procedure, though more frequently in younger age groups, and a recently approved treatment with deoxycholic acid (Kybella®, Kythera Biopharmaceuticals, Westlake Village, CA) provides a nonsurgical alternative for preplatysmal fat deposits.

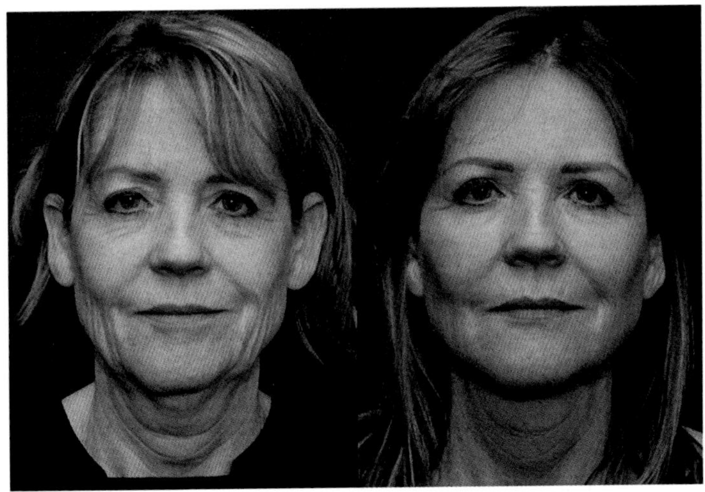

Fig. 7 Fifty-nine-year-old woman preoperative (*left*) and 1½ years postoperative (*right*) from facelift, necklift, and fat transfer, along with upper blepharoplasty. Note improvement in the lower face and neck achieved with face- and necklifting and the improvement in the periorbital and cheek volumes attributable to fat transfer

For patients with more advanced platysmal banding and interplatysmal (midline neck) fat accumulation, directly addressing the neck through a submental incision – *submentoplasty* – is beneficial. In this procedure the neck skin is elevated in the subcutaneous plane, the interplatysmal and subplatysmal neck fat – which is poorly responsive to liposuction – is excised sharply with scissors, and the medial platysmal edges are sutured together at the midline, from the immediate submental region to the level of the hyoid bone. A notch is then frequently created in the platysmal edges just inferior to this level to further define the cervicomental angle. Excess skin may also be conservatively removed by advancing the skin flap anteriorly and excising the redundant skin prior to closure of the submental incision.

In addition to the surgical solutions above, an increasing number of patients are seeking nonsurgical tightening of the facial and neck soft tissue. Options in this category include intense focused ultrasound (US) [33], radiofrequency (RF), and microneedling. A commonly used US device delivers microfocused ultrasound energy to the mid-dermis and subcutaneous tissue to effect tightening of these layers and resultant refinement of appearance, with moderately good success in appropriately selected patients [34]. Multiple RF devices are currently available for the same goal of collagen denaturing and tightening through thermal injury, including a newer minimally invasive device which delivers the energy via a probe insinuated in the dermal–subdermal junction; each device has shown modest clinical improvement with the advantage of minimal downtime [35]. Microneedling, also known as collagen induction therapy, has shown improvement in tightening of aged skin and is cost-effective despite the need for multiple treatments to realize a substantial benefit [36].

Finally, an often overlooked feature of the aging face is that of ptosis of the nasal tip. Typically manifesting first in the late fifties and sixties, this presentation results from weakening of the fibrocartilaginous support of the nasal tip, allowing the lower lateral nasal cartilages to become more inferiorly directed. This is effectively corrected by placement of a cartilaginous graft termed a *columellar strut graft*, usually harvested from the nasal septum and placed in the columella. Rhinoplasty surgeons often also employ this grafting technique in the younger rhinoplasty patient as a preventive measure.

Sixties

In addition to the regions of volume loss in earlier decades noted above, patients in their seventh decade show more advanced volume loss in the temporal regions, with a resultant step-off lateral to the lateral orbital rim. Likewise, atrophy on the inferior aspect of the zygomatic arch, in the submalar region, becomes more evident, along with that of the buccal region. Left uncorrected, these areas represent subtle cues of aging, which are often overlooked by cosmetic specialists unfamiliar with volume restoration. Periorbital, labial/perioral, and mandibular atrophy also become more pronounced in this decade and can be restored in conjunction with the perizygomatic and buccal areas.

Facelifting is beneficial for most patients in their seventh decade, and progression of neck laxity is such that necklifting (submentoplasty) is performed in conjunction with the majority of facelifts in this age group or can be performed in isolation for those patients who have previously undergone facelifting alone and have maintained their mandibular line.

If the patient has not sought a facial resurfacing procedure in earlier decades, they will usually be candidates by their sixties, with most patients having progressed to a Glogau classification of III–IV (advanced to severe) [37]. Resurfacing at these stages frequently requires a deeper chemical peel, such as a croton oil/phenol peel, or a deeper laser resurfacing procedure [16, 38–40].

Blepharoptosis, or descent of the upper eyelid margin over the iris and even the pupil of the eye, may become apparent in this decade and is addressed by a variety of suspensory procedures [41]. Dermatochalasis, or laxity of the upper eyelid skin, may begin as early as the fourth decade, but may progress to the point of obscuring the patient's visual fields by their sixties, thus becoming of greater functional concern than of cosmetic significance alone, and is addressed by upper lid blepharoplasty. As noted above, volume loss in the infrabrow region, as well as loss of bony orbital rim, contributes to the deflation of the infrabrow skin, exacerbating the accumulation of the skin resulting from loss of elasticity, or *elastosis*; volume restoration to the infrabrow region to complement upper eyelid blepharoplasty is therefore routinely recommended. Correction of lower eyelid skin redundancy may also become warranted during this decade and can be addressed with either a resurfacing procedure such as a chemical peel or laser resurfacing or with surgical excision via lower eyelid transcutaneous blepharoplasty or skin pinch; caution and conservatism must be exercised in lower lid skin excision, however, so as not to cause lower lid retraction and scleral show, lid eversion with epiphora, or even lagophthalmos and possible exposure keratitis [42].

The brow of the seventh decade is more likely to show modest descent in the middle and medial portions in addition to the lateral descent noted above during the fifties. Thus, while many patients at this point benefit from lateral browlifting in conjunction with lipotransfer to the infrabrow region, patients in their sixties may also require conservative elevation of the more medial components, as in endoscopic, coronal, trichophytic, direct, or trans-blepharoplasty browlifting; the emphasis nonetheless remains on lateral brow elevation.

Seventies and Beyond

The eighth decade and beyond are manifested by a continuation of the processes noted in the above sections: gradual progression of subcutaneous volume loss, depletion of skin thickness with associated progression of facial rhytides, and elastosis with resultant increase in skin laxity. Patients who have undergone facelifting or browlifting in their fifties or sixties may wish to undergo a repeat procedure to restraighten the jawline and resuspend their brows, respectively; blepharoplasty may be successfully repeated as well. The typical facelift should be expected to provide a youthful jawline and neck for approximately 7–10 years, although the associated skin removal is permanent, the fibrosis that occurs between the elevated SMAS and the redraped skin flap is long-lasting, and some surgeons use permanent sutures for elevation of the SMAS. Patients are informed that the aging process continues following surgical rejuvenation, with associated continued decline in skin thickness and elasticity, but that they will always display a more youthful countenance following such endeavors than if no such procedure had been undergone. Similar longevity is to be generally expected with other surgical results, including those of volume replacement with lipotransfer.

Future Directions

Much excitement surrounds the seemingly limitless potential for stem cells in the rejuvenative efforts for the aging face. Adipose tissue has been shown to provide the richest source of stem cells in the body, by mass, and such fat-derived stem cells have been successfully encouraged in vitro to develop into adipose tissue, nerves, blood vessels, and other tissues [43, 44]. It is hoped that, provided the proper biochemical milieu, adipose-derived stem cells will develop into these and other tissues in vivo. With associated improvement in nutrient supply to the skin, fat, muscle, and bone of the face, it may be possible to achieve more durable maintenance of the youthful facial glow. Anecdotally, this has been noted in our practice and others in the months and years following autologous fat transfer to the face as a general improvement in the texture of the facial skin [45, 46], and support for this has now been shown in animal models, in which increased dermal thickness has occurred through new collagen synthesis [47]. A skin analysis system (such as Visia®, Canfield Imaging Systems, Fairfield, NJ) may provide important documentation of this effect, which might ultimately allow physicians to offer volume restoration and modest cutaneous rejuvenation with a single procedure, particularly as efforts to improve the durability of fat grafts continue to yield positive returns [48]. Significant work remains in the elucidation of best harvest methods and specific mechanisms whereby stem cells may be beneficial, but recent research has begun to show microscopic structural changes suggestive of rejuvenation following both stem cells alone and fat plus stromal vascular fraction [49–52].

Additional optimism surrounds the burgeoning use of platelet-rich plasma (PRP) applications for facial rejuvenation, either alone or coupled with fat transfer [53–59]. A recent review of the available data on PRP concluded that the vast majority of studies to date indicate an effect from both topical and injectable PRP on facial aesthetics, although there has been an inability to show dramatic results with quantifiable evidence to support those results, and this may explain the lack of widespread adoption of its use in plastic surgery. Large, robust random-controlled trials are needed to further define the potential benefits [60].

Conclusion

Appreciation for the causative factors in the phenotype of the aging face is rapidly evolving. Along with this enhanced understanding come novel techniques for rejuvenation in each decade of age, each potentially more natural and durable than its predecessors, but balanced by the public's yearning for limited downtime and maximum safety. Such procedures are unlikely to wane in widespread societal acceptance, though modest fluctuations in adoption can occur with cyclical economic phenomena, such as the increase in nonsurgical procedures relative to surgical methods during the recent recession of 2007–2009 [2]. While the specific procedures sought will undoubtedly also undergo transformation, what seems constant is the quest for improved self-esteem that accompanies what the public regards as quick and effortless solutions provided by cosmetic procedures [61]. Also constant is the duty of the physician to ensure that motivating factors are healthy and recommended remedies are appropriate for the patient's state of facial aging, whatever the chronologic age.

Cross-References

▶ A New Paradigm for the Aging Face
▶ Cosmetic Surgery in the Elderly

References

1. Liu TS, Miller TA. Economic analysis of the future growth of cosmetic surgery procedures. Plast Reconstr Surg. 2008;121:404e–12.
2. Wilson SC, Soares MA, Reavey PL, et al. Trends and drivers of the aesthetic market during a turbulent economy. Plast Reconstr Surg. 2014;133:783e–9.

3. http://www.census.gov/Press-Release/www/releases/archives/facts_for_features_special_editions/006105.html. Accessed 03 Jan 2006.
4. Jones L. Great expectations: America and the baby boom generation. New York: Coward, McCann and Geoghegan; 1980.
5. US FDA. http://www.fda.gov/newsevents/newsroom/pressannouncements/ucm367662.htm. Accessed 06 oct 2015.
6. Carruthers JDA, Carruthers JA, Humphrey S. Fillers and neocollagenesis. Dermatol Surg. 2014;40:S134–6.
7. Donath AS, Glasgold RA, Glasgold MJ. Volume loss versus gravity: new concepts in facial aging. Curr Opin Otolaryngol Head Neck Surg. 2007;15(4):238–43.
8. Donath AS, Glasgold RA, Meier J, Glasgold MJ. Quantitative evaluation of volume augmentation in the tear trough with a hyaluronic acid-based filler: a three-dimensional analysis. Plast Reconstr Surg. 2010;125(5):1515–22.
9. US FDA. http://www.fda.gov/cdrh/pdf2/p020023a.pdf. Accessed 29 jun 2009.
10. Kane MA. Treatment of tear trough deformity and lower lid bowing with injectable hyaluronic acid. Aesthetic Plast Surg. 2005;29:363–7.
11. Airan LE, Born TM. Nonsurgical lower eyelid lift. Plast Reconstr Surg. 2005;116(6):1785–92.
12. Goldberg RA, Fiaschetti D. Filling the periorbital hollows with hyaluronic acid gel: initial experience with 244 injections. Ophthalmic Plast Reconstr Surg. 2006;22(5):335–41.
13. Carruthers JDA, Glogau RG, Blitzer A, et al. Advances in facial rejuvenation: Botulinum toxin type A, hyaluronic acid dermal fillers, and combination therapies – consensus recommendations. Plast Reconstr Surg. 2008;121(Suppl):5S–30.
14. Carruthers J, Fagien S, Matarasso SL, et al. Consensus recommendations on the use of botulinum toxin type A in facial aesthetics. Plast Reconstr Surg. 2004;114 (Suppl):1S–22.
15. Monheit GD. Medium-depth chemical peels. Dermatol Clin. 2001;19(3):413–25, vii.
16. Hetter GP. An examination of the phenol-croton oil peel: part IV. Face peel results with different concentrations of phenol and croton oil. Plast Reconstr Surg. 2000;105(3):1061–83.
17. Alster TS, Lupton JR. Erbium: YAG cutaneous laser resurfacing. Dermatol Clin. 2001;19(3):453–66.
18. Berlin AL, Hussain M, Phelps R, Goldberg DJ. A prospective study of fractional scanned nonsequential carbon dioxide laser resurfacing: a clinical and histopathologic evaluation. Dermatol Surg. 2009;35:222–8.
19. Fife DJ, Fitzpatrick RE, Zachary CB. Complications of fractional CO_2 laser resurfacing: four cases. Lasers Surg Med. 2009;41:179–84.
20. Coleman SR. Facial augmentation with structural fat grafting. Clin Plast Surg. 2006;33:567–77.
21. Brincat M, Moniz CF, Studd JWW, et al. Sex hormones and skin collagen content in postmenopausal women. Br Med J. 1983;287:1337.
22. Schuster S, Black MM, McVitie E. The influence of age and sex on skin thickness, skin collagen and density. Br J Dermatol. 1975;93:639–43.
23. Hall G, Phillips TJ. Estrogen and skin: the effects of estrogen, menopause, and hormone replacement therapy on the skin. J Am Acad Dermatol. 2005;53:555–68.
24. Baumann L. Hormones and aging skin. In: Bauman L, Weisberg E, editors. Cosmetic dermatology: principles and practice. New York: McGraw-Hill; 2002. p. 25–8.
25. Lam SM, Glasgold MJ, Glasgold RA. Complementary fat grafting. Philadelphia: Lippincott Williams & Wilkins; 2006. p. 10–1.
26. Chiu ES, Baker DC. Endoscopic brow lift: a retrospective review of 628 consecutive cases over 5 years. Plast Reconstr Surg. 2003;112:628–33.
27. Alam M, White LE, Martin N, et al. Ultrasound tightening of facial and neck skin: a rater-blinded prospective cohort study. J Am Acad Dermatol. 2010;62 (2):262–9.
28. Palmer FR, Rice DH, Churukia MM. Transconjunctival blepharoplasty. Complications and their avoidance: a retrospective analysis and review of the literature. Arch Otolaryngol Head Neck Surg. 1993;119:993–9.
29. Goldberg RA, Edelstein C, Shorr N. Fat repositioning in lower blepharoplasty to maintain infraorbital rim contour. Facial Plast Surg. 1999;15(3):225–9.
30. Mittleman H. The anatomy of the aging mandible and its importance to facelift surgery. Facial Plast Surg Clin North Am. 1994;2:301–9.
31. Romo T, Yalamanchili H, Sclafani A. Chin and prejowl augmentation in the management of the aging jawline. Facial Plast Surg. 2005;21(1):38–46.
32. Perkins SW, Naderi S. Rhytidectomy. In: Papel ID et al., editors. Facial plastic and reconstructive surgery. 3rd ed. New York: Thieme; 2011. p. 207–26.
33. Lee HS, Jang WS, Cha YJ, et al. Multiple pass ultrasound tightening of skin laxity of the lower face and neck. Dermatol Surg. 2012;38:20–7.
34. Fabi SG. Noninvasive skin tightening: focus on new ultrasound techniques. Clin Cosmet Investig Dermatol. 2015;8:47–52.
35. Carruthers J, Fabi S, Weiss R. Monopolar radiofrequency for skin tightening: our experience and a review of the literature. Dermatol Surg. 2014;40:S168–73.
36. El-Domyati M, Barakat M, Awad S, et al. Multiple microneedling sessions for minimally invasive facial rejuvenation: an objective assessment. Int J Dermatol. 2015;1–9.
37. Glogau RG. Aesthetic and anatomic analysis of the aging skin. Semin Cutan Med Surg. 1996;15(3):134–8.
38. Rinaldi F. Laser: a review. Clin Dermatol. 2008;26:590–601.
39. Fulton JE, Porumb S. Chemical peels – their place within the range of resurfacing techniques. Am J Clin Dermatol. 2004;5(3):179–87.

40. Carniol PJ, Harmon CB, Hamilton MM. Ablative laser facial skin rejuvenation. In: Papel ID et al., editors. Facial plastic and reconstructive surgery. 3rd ed. - New York: Thieme; 2009. p. 321–30.
41. Baroody M, Holds JB, Vick VL. Advances in the diagnosis and treatment of ptosis. Curr Opin Ophthalmol. 2005;16:351–5.
42. Morax S, Touitou V. Complications of blepharoplasty. Orbit. 2006;25(4):303–18.
43. Zuk PA, Zhu M, Mizuno H, et al. Multilineage cells from human adipose tissue: implications for cell-based therapies. Tissue Eng. 2001;7:211–28.
44. Urbich C, Dimmeler S. Endothelial progenitor cells functional characterization. Trends Cardiovasc Med. 2004;14:318–22.
45. Coleman SR. Structural fat grafting: more than a permanent filler. Plast Reconstr Surg. 2006;118 (3 Suppl):108S–120.
46. Lam SM. A new paradigm for the aging face. In: Farage MA, Miller KW, Maibach HI, editors. Textbook of aging skin. New York: Springer; 2009.
47. Mojallal A, Lequeux C, Shipkov C, et al. Improvement of skin quality after fat grafting: clinical observation and an animal study. Plast Reconstr Surg. 2009;124:765–74.
48. Gerth DJ, King B, Rabach L, et al. Long-term volumetric retention of autologous fat grafting processed with closed-membrane filtration. Aesthet Surg J. 2014;34(7):985–94.
49. Conde-Green A, de Amorim NF, Pitanguy I. Influence of decantation, washing and centrifugation on adipocyte and mesenchymal stem cell content of aspirated adipose tissue: a comparative study. J Plast Reconstr Aesthet Surg. 2010;63:1375–81.
50. McArdle A, Senarath-Yapa K, Walmsley GG, et al. The role of stem cells in aesthetic surgery: fact or fiction? Plast Reconstr Surg. 2014;134:193–200.
51. Charles-de-Sa L, Gontijo-de-Amorim NF, Takiya CM, et al. Antiaging treatment of the facial skin by fat graft and adipose-derived stem cells. Plast Reconstr Surg. 2015;135:999–1009.
52. Kim D-Y, Ji Y-H, Kim D-W. Effects of platelet-rich plasma, adipose-derived stem cells, and stromal vascular fraction on the survival of human transplanted adipose tissue. J Korean Med Sci. 2014;29:S193–200.
53. Park KY, Kim IS, Kim BJ, et al. Letter: autologous fat grafting and platelet-rich plasma for treatment of facial contour defects. Dermatol Surg. 2012;38:1572–4.
54. Modarressi A. Platelet rich plasma (PRP) improves fat grafting outcomes. World J Plast Surg. 2013;2(1):6–13.
55. Willemsen JC, Lindenblatt N, Stevens HP. Results and long-term patient satisfaction after gluteal augmentation with platelet-rich plasma-enriched autologous fat. Eur J Plast Surg. 2013;36:777–82.
56. Gentile P, De Angelis B, Pasin M, et al. Adipose-derived stromal vascular fraction cells and platelet-rich plasma: basic and clinical evaluation for cell-based therapies in patients with scars on the face. J Craniofac Surg. 2014;25(1):267–72.
57. Willemsen JC, van der Lei B, Vermeulen KM, Stevens HP. The effects of platelet-rich plasma on recovery time and aesthetic outcome in facial rejuvenation: preliminary retrospective observations. Aesthetic Plast Surg. 2014;38(5):1057–63.
58. Cervelli V, Bocchini I, Di Pasquali C. PRL platelet rich lipotransfer: our experience and state of art in the combined use of fat and PRP. BioMed Res Int. 2013;434191:1–9.
59. Leo MS, Kumar AS, Kirit R, et al. Systematic review of the use of platelet-rich plasma in aesthetic dermatology. J Cosmet Dermatol. 2015;0:1–9.
60. Sclafani AP, Azzi J. Platelet preparations for use in facial rejuvenation and wound healing: a critical review of current literature. Aesthetic Plast Surg. 2015;39:495–505.
61. Haas CF, Champion A, Secor D. Motivating factors for seeking cosmetic surgery. A synthesis of the literature. Plast Surg Nurs. 2008;28(4):177–82.

Elderly Face No Added Risk from Cosmetic Surgery

151

Julian Winocour, Varun Gupta, K. Kye Higdon, James C. Grotting, and Max Yeslev

Contents

J. Winocour • V. Gupta • K.K. Higdon • M. Yeslev (✉)
Department of Plastic Surgery, Vanderbilt University, Nashville, TN, USA
e-mail: julian.winocour@vanderbilt.edu; varun.gupta@vanderbilt.edu; kent.higdon@vanderbilt.edu; max.yeslev@kp.org

J.C. Grotting
Department of Plastic Surgery, University of Alabama, Birmingham, AL, USA
e-mail: jcgrotting@gmail.com

M.A. Farage et al. (eds.), *Textbook of Aging Skin*,
DOI 10.1007/978-3-662-47398-6_148

Abstract

The proportion of elderly patients in North America is increasing. As aesthetic procedures become less invasive and more available to the general public, more elderly patients are undergoing cosmetic surgery. With this increase in the number of elderly patients undergoing cosmetic surgery, there is a pressing need for a detailed evaluation of safety of aesthetic surgery in this population. Current chapter provides comprehensive review of available surgical literature on safety of cosmetic procedures in patients of advanced age. Specifically, the role of elderly person in contemporary society, the demand for aesthetic surgery among older individuals, factors associated with safety of cosmetic procedures, and review of major adverse outcomes among elderly cosmetic patients are discussed in details.

Elderly Individual in Contemporary Society

Definition of Elderlies and "Generians"

The World Health Organization (WHO) defines an "elderly person" as an individual 65 years of age and older [1]. This is largely an arbitrary chronological age and is viewed by many as primarily applying to developed countries. It often coincides with the age a person becomes eligible for statutory and occupational retirement pensions [2]. This definition is often not generalizable to many other countries and continents, including Africa where great differences in healthcare access and life expectance exist. Factors such as gain or loss of societal roles based on physical decline have more importance and meaning toward "old age" rather than chronological age. Equally, placing a chronological age on the state when a person becomes "old" assumes a relationship with biological age, which is not always the case [2]. A United Nations standard criterion for defining an "elderly person" does not currently exist; however, the terminology of the older population is generally accepted to apply to a population of age greater than 60 years.

Elderly Persons as Part of World Population

The United States of America (USA) is seeing a growth in the proportion of elderly persons that is unprecedented in history [3]. According to the US Census Bureau, the proportion of the population aged ≥65 is projected to increase from 12.4 % in 2000 to 19.6 % in 2030. This represents a more than doubling of the absolute number of elderly persons from 35 to 71 million [4]. The expected growth of the proportion of elderly population in North America is only surmounted by Europe, where the proportion is projected to increase from 15.5 % to 24.3 % during that same time frame [5]. North America and Europe mirror the overall global trend, where during the same years the proportion of elderly persons has been projected to increase from 6.9 % to 12.0 % worldwide [5]. This is equally being seen universally in Asia, Latin America, and the Caribbean.

In North America, this population change has been attributed mainly to an increased fertility seen in the two decades following World War II (the "baby boom" phenomenon), combined with a decline in fertility and increase in life expectancy during the second half of the twentieth century [6]. The leading edge of the baby boomers reached age 65 in 2011 with the tail end expected to be in 2030. However, in addition to the increasing elderly population equally is the increasing racial and ethnic diversity among this population. The demographic transition in the non-Western world is equally being attributed to a decreased fertility rate with delayed mortality. Equally, there has been an epidemiologic transition in the leading causes of death over the last half century from infectious diseases and acute ailments to more chronic and degenerative diseases. This is especially true in developed countries where the leading causes of death are currently cardiovascular disease and cancer, compared to developing countries where infectious diseases and parasites are often the leading cause [6]. This growing global trend has placed a greater burden on national healthcare systems, with new challenges and increasing costs. This has included a greater number of chronic illnesses, injuries, and disabilities as well as concerns about future caregiving [6]. The cost of healthcare per capita in persons aged ≥65 is three to five times that of persons <65.

Cosmetic Surgery Among Elderlies

The Elderly Patient

In general, there are many negative stereotypes in North America about elderly persons, mostly related to their transitional role in society. The impression exists that this age group no longer serves a productive role to society, but rather simply imposes a burden on younger persons [7]. In fact, for the mass majority, elderly persons as a whole are living longer but equally more productive lives with improved "well-being." There are many aspects to "well-being" in the daily lives of people that include domains such as material/economic well-being, physical well-being, social engagement, and emotional well-being. The Index of Well-Being in Older Populations (IWOP), developed by the Stanford Center on Longevity and the Population Reference Bureau, incorporates all of these domains into a global score which can be used to compare countries [8]. The USA ranks in the top four countries in the world for the well-being for adults greater than 65 years of age. Also, many studies, including Feinson et al., have demonstrated that older adults do not report more distress or depressive symptoms than other age groups when race, gender, and income are controlled [9].

It is important to appreciate that there can be a discrepancy between a person's chronological age and their perceived age. Gerontology literature has demonstrated that people that maintain a "middle-age" identity despite having an older chronological age are better adjusted and satisfied in life [7, 10, 11]. Altering the perception of social cues, most notably physical appearance that would otherwise label someone as "elderly," would maintain this "middle-age" identity. Cosmetic surgery thus can be a mechanism to resolve the discord between an internal youthful state and an elderly physical appearance [7]. Napoleon et al. describe a second general category of elderly patients seeking cosmetic surgery that have poor social functioning in society and do not have a younger perceived age. These patients often have expectations that are unrealistic because they anticipate that they will gain a more positive internal state through changing their physical appearance [7]. It is important to appreciate these different motivations and expectations of patients, in order to best understand the psychology of the elderly patient.

Increasing Demand for Aesthetic Surgery: Noninvasive and Invasive

The increase in medical utilization seen in the elderly population is not limited to disease states, but equally in terms of aesthetic procedures. Currently, aesthetic surgery encompasses a much wider audience with respect to gender, ethnicity, socioeconomic means, and particularly, in regard to age. As aesthetic procedures become less invasive and more available to the general public, more elderly patients are undergoing cosmetic surgery. According to the American Society for Aesthetic Plastic Surgery (ASAPS) statistics report (2014), patients over age 65 underwent 10.9 % of the total number of nonsurgical procedures (967,814) and 7.9 % of the surgical procedures (138,612). This has more than doubled since 2000, where patients above age 65 underwent a total of 407,339 procedures (both surgical and nonsurgical combined). This also represents a 3.3 % overall increase in the proportion of cosmetic surgery being performed in patients above age 65 [12].

As mentioned previously, there are multiple reasons for the increased demand for aesthetic surgery in the elderly population. Often in elderly patients, the goals of aesthetic surgery are to restore or rejuvenate features to their youthful appearance, rather than refine or transform features. There are multiple motivations that elderly patients have to seek a more youthful look. Elderly persons are living longer more productive lives and many people are equally retiring later in life. Beauty and youth in many fields are a determinant of economic security as well as there are strong negative stereotypes with aging, especially in North America. In women, many stipulate that signs of aging are perceived as a loss of femininity, sexual identity, social power, and social visibility [13, 14]. Males are equally seeing a dramatic increase in aesthetic procedures, with a 273 % increase from 1997 to 2014. These procedures are mostly related to the face and body from the belief that it will enhance their job prospects or public image [13]. This was described by Figueroa et al. who emphasized the relationship between body image and self-image and self-esteem in both males and females [15].

From a societal standpoint, there has been a major influence in the last couple decades from the beauty industry. The push for antiaging products and social stigma against aging has led to a surge in aesthetic surgery procedures. This has been combined with more minimally invasive procedures and safer anesthesia. There has equally been more literature emerging demonstrating the safety of aesthetic surgical procedures in elderly patients, even in the octogenarian population [15, 16].

Specifics of Cosmetic Procedures in Elderly Patients

Surgical Cosmetic Procedures in Elderly

The American Society for Aesthetic Plastic Surgery maintains a national data (the Cosmetic Surgery National Data Bank) for surgical and nonsurgical cosmetic procedures performed since 1997. This includes data from over 900 board-certified plastic surgeons, dermatologists, and otolaryngologists, which is projected to reflect nationwide statistics.

Since 1997, there has been an 82 % increase in surgical cosmetic procedures, with nearly 1.8 million performed in the USA in 2014. Surgical procedures accounted for 60 % of the total expenditures on aesthetic procedures at a cost of 7.5 billion dollars. The top five cosmetic surgical procedures in 2014 were liposuction (342,494 procedures), breast augmentation (286,694 procedures), eyelid surgery (165,714 procedures), abdominoplasty (164,021 procedures), and rhinoplasty (145,909 procedures). People age 35–50 years of age were the largest consumers of cosmetic surgery with 39 % of all surgical procedures performed on this group. People aged 65 years and older underwent 138,612 surgical procedures, 8 % of total, representing a 61 % increase since 2002. There is a unique pattern of aesthetic procedures that is specific for elderly patients. In contrast to younger patients, who more commonly choose to have aesthetic surgery focused on breast and body areas, older individuals more frequently undergo procedures focused on the face. The most common procedures in this population were facelift, blepharoplasty, rhinoplasty, and neck lift followed by liposuction. Among all cosmetic patients in the ASAPS database, 30 % of all facelifts, 24 % of neck lifts, 22 % of eyelid surgeries, and 20 % of brow lifts were performed on elderly patients. A similar trend of increasing popularity of cosmetic surgery among older patients is evident in the CosmetAssure™ database (Birmingham, Alabama, USA). CosmetAssure™ is an insurance program that covers the cost of unexpected major complications from covered cosmetic surgical procedures and tracks outcomes of aesthetic procedures [16, 17].

The percentage of elderly patients undergoing cosmetic surgery recorded in CosmetAssure™ database has increased yearly, from 3.9 % in 2008 to 6.4 % in 2012 (Fig. 1). Equally, similar to ASAPS data, elderly patients undergo more facial procedures and less breast and body procedures compared to younger population of patients (Table 1).

Nonsurgical Cosmetic Procedures in Elderly

Nonsurgical cosmetic procedures encompass injectables (botulinum toxin, hyaluronic acid,

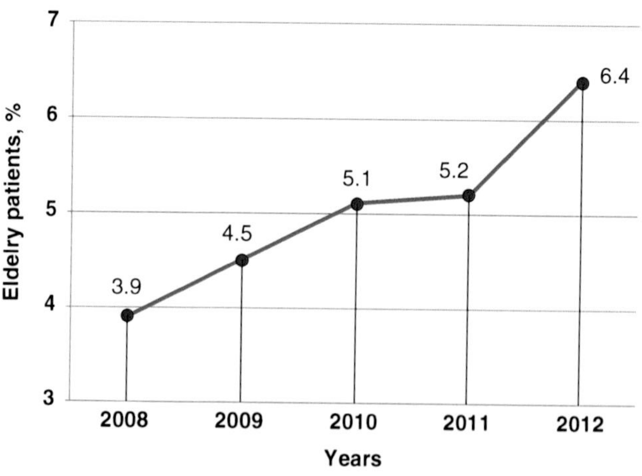

Fig. 1 Proportion of elderly individuals among patients undergoing aesthetic surgical procedures over 5 years (according to CosmetAssure™ database)

Table 1 Incidence of cosmetic procedures and major complications in elderly and young patients

Body area	Procedures, %		Major complications, %	
	<65	>65	<65	>65
Face	36.8	63.2	1.3	1.4
Breast	81.1	18.9	1.9	1.8
Body	73.4	26.6	2.9	3

etc.), skin rejuvenation (chemical peel, dermabrasion, laser resurfacing, etc.), and other procedures such as hair removal, nonsurgical fat reduction, and sclerotherapy. Since 1997, there has been a five times increase in nonsurgical procedures, with almost nine million procedures performed in the USA in 2014. The top five nonsurgical procedures were injection of botulinum toxin and hyaluronic acid, nonsurgical hair removal, and skin treatment with chemical peels and microdermabrasion. According to the ASAPS database, people age 65 and over underwent 967,814 nonsurgical procedures, which comprise 11 % of total number of the procedures performed among all cosmetic patients, representing a 95 % increase since 2002. The most common nonsurgical cosmetic treatments among elderly patients were botulinum toxin injection, hyaluronic acid fillers, laser skin resurfacing, chemical peel, and photo rejuvenation. Additionally, a significant proportion of dermabrasions (26 %) and laser skin resurfacing (17 %) were performed on elderly patients.

Safety of Cosmetic Surgery in Elderly Patients

Complications in Cosmetic Surgery

The essential goal of cosmetic surgery is to perform improvement of patient's aesthetic appearance by the means of a safely performed surgical procedure. This may involve restoration or rejuvenation of features to their youthful appearance or a transformation or refinement of specific features. Therefore, given that this is purely elective surgery, safety remains an essential factor. Traditionally, perioperative morbidity and mortality serve as indicators of safety associated with a surgical procedure. Because mortality after aesthetic procedures is extremely low, it is incidence of postoperative complications that serves as a surrogate for safety in contemporary cosmetic surgery. These can be further categorized into minor and major complications. Minor complications are usually small deviations from the ideal postoperative course that are not inherent in the procedure and do not signify a failure of treatment. Such complications traditionally require minor additional postoperative care such as localized wound infections requiring oral antibiotic therapy, nonsignificant tissue necrosis requiring local debridement, and topical wound care. These complications of aesthetic surgery traditionally can be managed in the office setting and generally do not require hospital admission or operating room treatment. In contrast, major postoperative complications are serious medical conditions occurring as a result of surgical procedures, which can be immediately or consequentially life-threatening to a patient or result in significant physical disability. Examples of such dramatic conditions are pulmonary embolism, major uncontrolled bleeding, myocardial infarction, stroke. Such complications require prompt diagnoses and medical attention and generally hospitalization of the patient with initiation of complex therapeutic measures. Although, minimizing risks of both major and minor complications after surgical intervention is an ultimate goal of any surgical specialty, avoiding major complications is essential for the safe practice of aesthetic plastic surgery.

The Role of Homeostenosis and Comorbid Conditions

The influence of advanced age on the safety of surgical procedures has recently gained more attention. The number of manuscripts evaluating surgical outcomes of patients with advanced age has significantly increased over the last years (Fig. 2). Recently, the concept of homeostenosis of aging human organism has been intensively studied and can be applied to elderly surgical

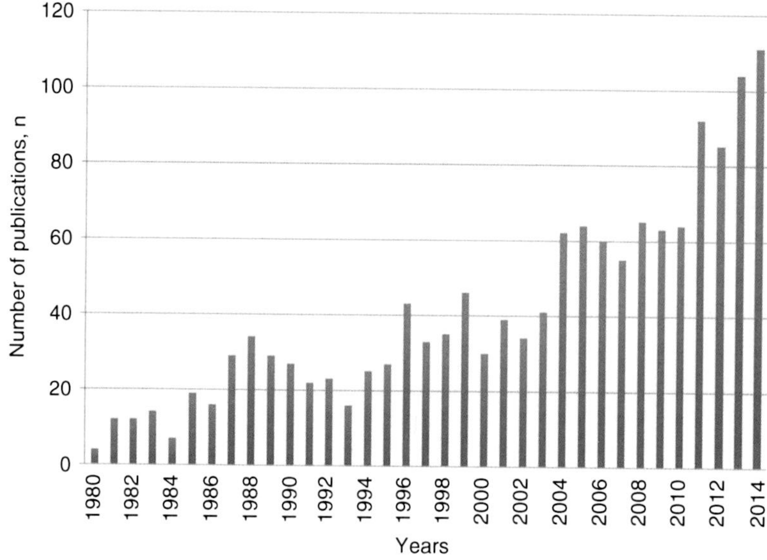

Fig. 2 Number of scientific publications per year on surgery in elderly patients

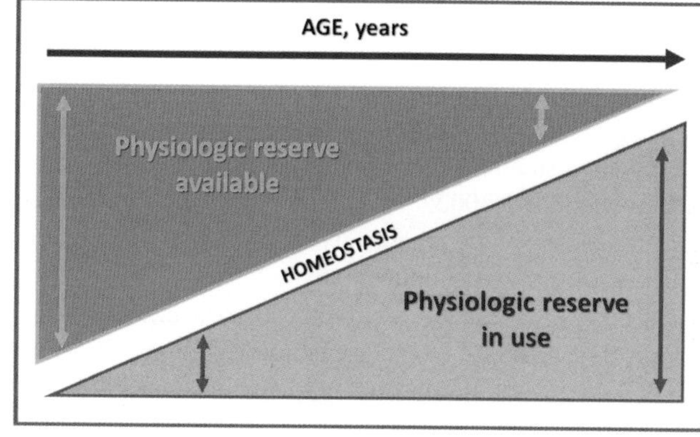

Fig. 3 Concept of homeostenosis. As an individual ages, more physiologic reserve is recruited to maintain homeostasis, leaving less physiological reserve to resist and recover from stress stimuli such as surgery

patients [17, 18]. Homeostenosis represents a process of characteristic, progressive constriction of homeostatic reserve on organ systems that occurs with aging. Additionally, homeostenosis is believed to be responsible for the accumulation of chronic pathological conditions throughout a lifetime. Younger individuals possess a larger physiological reserve to deal with physiological stress. As a patients age, maintaining homeostasis utilizes more of one's physiological reserve, which leaves less reserve to adequately react to stressful stimuli (Fig. 3). Surgical procedures represent such a disturbance of physiological balance, and, therefore, postoperative recovery can be negatively impacted in the elderly patient.

Elderly patients presenting for surgery have a higher incidence of comorbid conditions (such as diabetes mellitus, cardiac atherosclerotic disease, etc.) compared to younger patients. As a person ages, there is commonly a steady increase in the number of pathological comorbid conditions. Therefore, advanced age and pre-existing comorbidities traditionally have been seen as risk factors for postoperative complications. The impact of comorbid conditions on surgical outcomes and safety has been intensively studied in various surgical specialties (nonaesthetic surgical

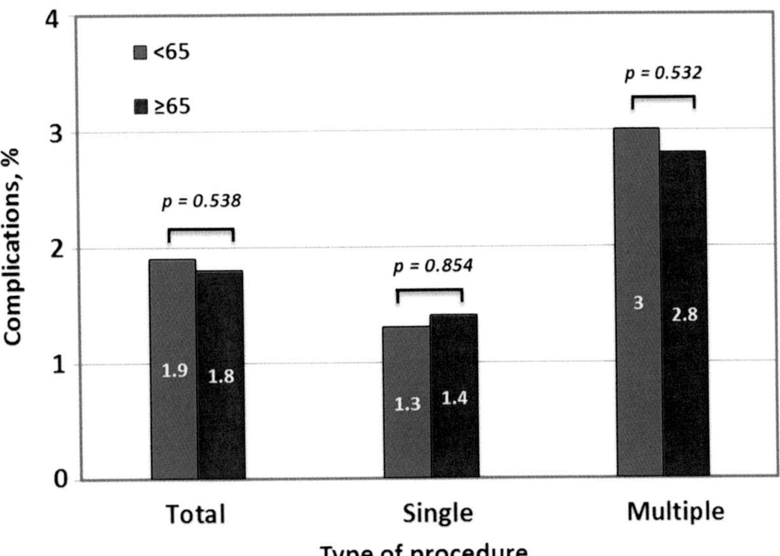

Fig. 4 Incidence of major postoperative complications in elderly and younger patients (Yeslev M, et al. Safety of Cosmetic Procedures in Elderly and Octogenarian Patients. Aesthetic Surgery Journal, published online April, 2015. Reprinted with permission from Oxford University Press)

procedures). Multiple clinical studies have demonstrated direct correlation between number of preoperative comorbidities and increased risk of postoperative complications in various surgical disciplines. In aesthetic surgery, however, the effect of advanced age and comorbid conditions on adverse outcomes remains more controversial, with a paucity of literature.

Incidence of Major Complications After Cosmetic Procedures in Elderly Patients

The frequency of major postoperative complications after aesthetic procedures is poorly reported in surgical literature. To present, studies based on individual surgeons' experience and single institution studies rarely provided sufficient statistical power to draw conclusions regarding the true incidence of such dramatic and rare events after aesthetic procedures. However, recently several initiatives on tracking patient outcomes after cosmetic and reconstructive surgery have led to the development the number of multi-institutional prospectively followed databases. Such mega-scale databases, such as NSQIP, TOPS, and CosmetAssure^{TM}, are nationally based and contain clinical information on hundreds of thousands of plastic surgery procedures. Data from such databases allow accurate tracking of the incidence of even very rare occurring major postoperative complications such as death, pulmonary embolism and severe bleeding. Although each database has its own advantages and drawbacks, CosmetAssure^{TM} is a unique database system that exclusively follows outcomes of aesthetic procedures. Outcomes of cosmetic procedures, including complications among elderly patients, have been thoroughly studied using the CosmetAssure^{TM} database and have resulted in a number of publications and recent media attention.

Yeslev et al. performed a thorough analysis of postoperative complications in elderly patients compared to younger patients using the CosmetAssure^{TM} database [16]. This study revealed that the overall postoperative complication rate was not significantly different between the elderly and younger patients (1.8 % vs. 1.9 %, $p = 0.54$, Fig. 4). Among patients who underwent single cosmetic procedures, postoperative complications developed in 55 elderly (1.3 %) and 1,198 younger (1.4 %) patients ($p = 0.85$). Both groups demonstrated a significant increase in the incidence

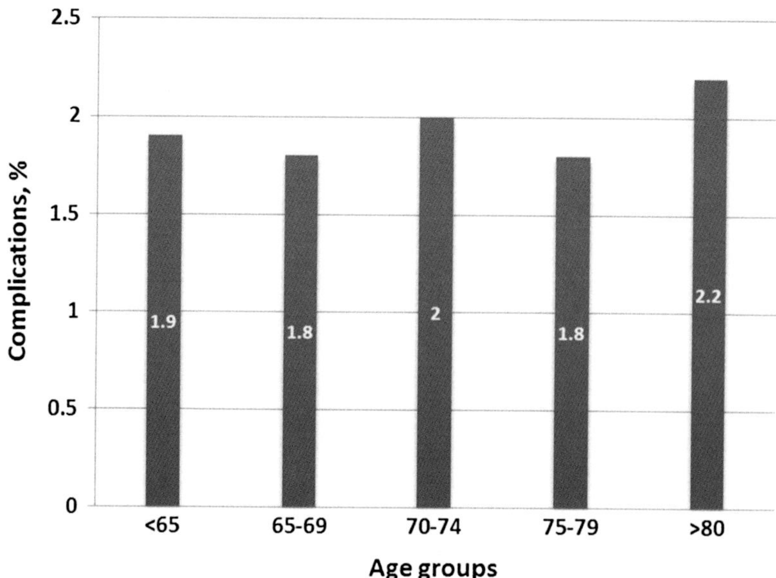

Fig. 5 Major complications after aesthetic procedures in elderly patients stratified by age group

of complications with additional cosmetic procedures (combined procedures). In young patients, the overall complication rate in combined procedures was 3.0 % (n = 1,183) compared to 1.3 % with single procedures (n = 1,198, $p < 0.01$). Similarly, the incidence of postoperative complications among elderly patients almost doubled in the combined procedure group (2.8 % vs. 1.4 %, $p < 0.01$). However, no statistically significant difference in the complication rate was detected between elderly and young patients when the two groups were compared. Analysis of complications within the elderly patient population stratified by age group failed to demonstrate statistically significant difference in the incidence of major postoperative complications among the different age groups (Fig. 5, p = NS).

Frequency of complications varied based on body area on which aesthetic procedure was performed. The highest major complication rate was among elderly patients undergoing aesthetic procedures on the torso and extremities, followed by breast procedures, and finally face procedure (Table 1). However, when stratified by type of cosmetic procedure, only abdominoplasty was associated with a higher postoperative complication rate in elderly compared to younger patients (5.4 % vs. 3.9 %, p = 0.03). The most common postoperative complications in elderly patients after aesthetic surgery were hematoma and infection (Fig. 6).

Equally, a specific analysis was performed of complications after aesthetic surgical procedures in the subset of octogenarians (patients 80 years old and older). Interestingly, octogenarians demonstrated acceptably low incidence of major complications after aesthetic procedures, which was not statistically significantly different from younger patients (Fig. 7).

Despite these encouraging findings, several critical points regarding specifics of aesthetic procedures in elderly patients require mentioning. The CosmetAssure^{TM} database collects data from aesthetic procedures performed by board-certified or board-eligible plastic surgeons. Elderly patients almost universally undergo thorough preoperative clinical evaluation and selection of appropriate surgical candidates by their plastic surgeon. Therefore, existing selection bias of surgical candidates is an explanation for the low incidence of postoperative complications in patients of older age. Nevertheless, cosmetic procedures in

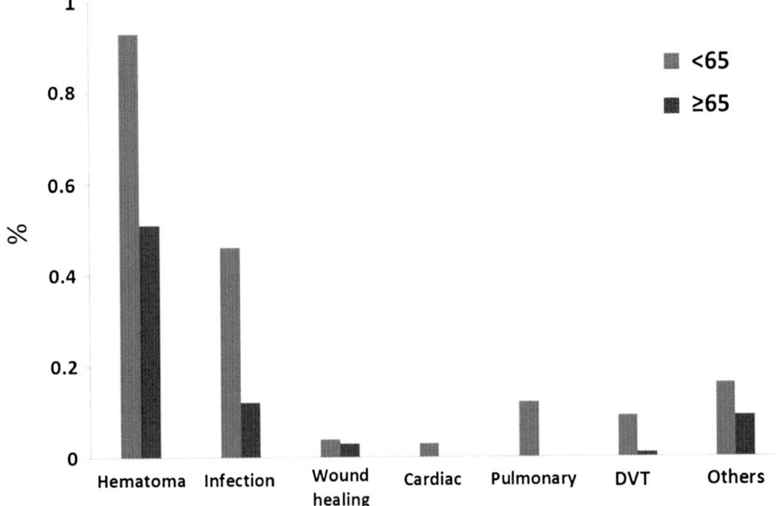

Fig. 6 Incidence of major complications in elderly patients compared to younger group

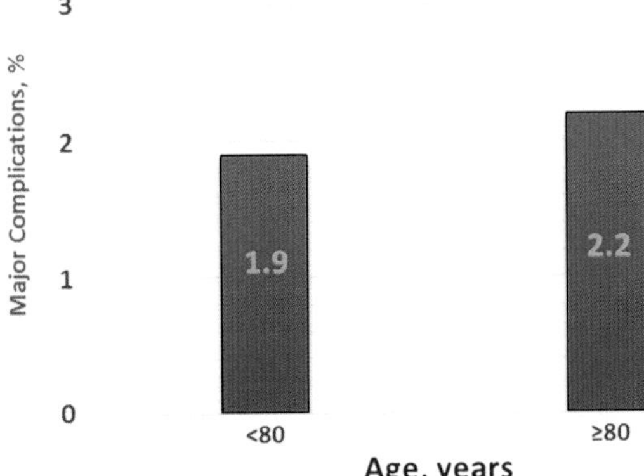

Fig. 7 Incidence of major complication after aesthetic procedures in octogenarians compared to younger patients (Yeslev M, et al. Safety of Cosmetic Procedures in Elderly and Octogenarian Patients. Aesthetic Surgery Journal, published online April, 2015. Reprinted and modified with permission from Oxford University Press)

carefully selected elderly patients (including octogenarians) remain safe with a low major complication rate that is comparable to that of younger patients.

Perioperative Safety Measures in Aesthetic Surgery

Recently, significant advances have been made in aesthetic surgery with the aim of providing safer surgery and increasing the quality of medical care. Recommendations for surgical and perioperative measures to minimize perioperative risk of complications and increase patients' safety have been proposed by several institutions and organizations. These include VTE prophylaxis, prevention of hypothermia during surgery, and patient risk stratification to name a few (Table 2). Although the efficacy of some of these measures remains debatable in the literature, it is without a doubt that implementation of entire complexes of safety measures can significantly decrease incidence of both minor and major complications. This will result in safer aesthetic surgery not only for elderly but equally younger patients.

Table 2 Risk factor for complications and risk-reducing measures aimed to increase safety of aesthetic procedures

Risk factor/ complication	Risk-reducing measures
Patient risk stratification	Standard pre-evaluation questionnaire Thorough physical examination Preoperative medical clearance by appropriate specialist
Anesthesia risk	Using ASA classification Airway evaluation Selection an appropriate location of the procedure (office- vs. hospital-based OR)
Hypothermia	Avoiding intraoperative body temperature below 36°C: prewarming patient preoperatively, continuous body temperature monitoring, increasing room temperature, covering patient, limiting exposure, using warm irrigation and injection fluids, using warming blankets
Length of surgery	Avoiding procedures >6 h Staging surgical procedure
Venous thromboembolism	Screening high-risk patients, appropriate mechanical and/or chemoprophylaxis
Surgical site infection	Perioperative antibiotic therapy, thorough aseptic, antiseptic, and surgical techniques
Hypertension	Thorough preoperative screening, accurate perioperative blood pressure monitoring and control
Lidocaine toxicity	Appropriate weight-based administration of local anesthetic, prompt recognition of toxicity

Conclusion

The number of aesthetic surgical procedures among elderly patients continues to increase in North America. Facial and breast surgery are among most commonly performed procedures among elderly patients. Based on the analysis of the CosmetAssure^{TM} database, elderly patients demonstrate similar incidence of major postoperative complications compared to younger patients. Aesthetic surgical procedures, therefore, remain safe in carefully selected patients of older age and even octogenarians. Proper selection of surgical candidates and implication of perioperative safety measures aimed to reduce the postoperative complication rate are essential for safe aesthetic surgery on the elderly patient.

References

1. World Health Organization website. http://www.who.int. Accessed 12 Mar 2015.
2. "Definition of an older or elderly person." World Health Organization. http://www.who.int/healthinfo/survey/ageingdefnolder/en/. Accessed 12 Mar 2015.
3. US Department of Health and Human Services. Aging statistics. http://www.aoa.acl.gov/Aging_Statistics/index.aspx. Accessed 12 Mar 2015.
4. U.S. Census Bureau. International database. http://www.census.gov/population/www/projections/natdet-D1A.html. Accessed 12 Mar 2015.
5. Kinsella K, Velkoff V. U.S. Census Bureau. An Aging World: 2001. Washington, DC: U.S. Government Printing Office, 2001; series P95/01-1.
6. "Public health and aging: trends in aging – United States and Worldwide." Centers for Disease Control and Prevention. http://www.cdc.gov/mmwr/preview/mmwrhtml/mm5206a2.htm. Accessed 12 Mar 2015.
7. Napoleon A, Carson ML. Psychological considerations in the elderly cosmetic surgery candidate. Ann Plast Surg. 1990;24:165–9.
8. Jacobsen L, Kent M, Lee M, Mather M. America's aging population, vol. 66. 1st ed. Washington, DC: Population Reference Bureau; 2011.
9. Feinsom MC. Aging and mental health: distinguishing myth from reality. Res Aging. 1985;7:155.
10. Havighurst RJ, Albrecht R. Older people. New York: Longmans Green and Company; 1953.
11. Riley M, Foner A. Aging and society, An inventory of research findings, vol. 1. New York: Russell Sage Foundate; 1968.
12. 2014 National totals for cosmetic Procedures. American Society for Aesthetic Plastic Surgery (ASAPS). www.surgery.org Accessed 12 Mar 2015.
13. Honigman R, Castle D. Aging and cosmetic enhancement. Clin Interv Aging. 2006;1:115–9.
14. Featherstone M. The body of the consumer culture. Theory Cult Society. 1982;1:18–33.
15. Figueroa C. Self-esteem and cosmetic surgery: is there a relationship between the two? Plast Surg Nurs. 2003;23:21–5.
16. Yeslev M, Gupta V, Winocour J, Shack RB, Grotting JC, Higdon KK (2015) Safety of cosmetic procedures in elderly and octogenarian patients. Aesthet Surg J. Published online April 2015
17. www.cosmetassure.com. Accessed 12 Mar 2015.
18. Karp JF, Shega JW, Morone NE, Weiner DK. Advances in understanding the mechanisms and management of persistent pain in older adults. Br J Anaesth. 2008;101:111–20.

Punctural Face Rejuvenation

152

Igor Roganin

Contents

I. Roganin (✉)
DAO Clinic, Moscow, Russia
e-mail: a5109144@yandex.ru; dr.roganin@gmail.com

M.A. Farage et al. (eds.), *Textbook of Aging Skin*,
DOI 10.1007/978-3-662-47398-6_149

Abstract

Punctural Face Rejuvenation (PFR) is an exclusive technique for those, seeking for solutions to preserve the natural beauty and individuality with no botox or fillers. Serving to prevent the visible signs of aging and to intesify the regeneration of all layers of skin. The technique smoothes skin, boosts cellular metabolism, enhances the production of collagen, hialuronic acid and elastine, prevents fold formation. It has been popular with clients for more than 10 years.

It would seem what else new could be done in the field of rejuvenation technologies with such an abundance of modern techniques, and whether it is worth it, when almost all problems are solved effectively today. Nevertheless, there is always a small percentage of women looking for alternative, safe, and more effective ways to maintain a youthful skin. It is for them that the author has been developing punctural face rejuvenation (PFR) for more than 10 years.

The History of Cosmetic Acupuncture

In China, the birthplace of the acupuncture method, a needle as a beauty tool has been known for a long time. The acupuncture is first introduced in 960–1280 AC, the time of Song Dynasty. One important work was written in *Zhen Ju Zhi Shen Jing* by Wang Zhi-zhong [1] about the single point acupuncture and moxibustion.

Chinese medicine doctors sought to restore an overall balance of the body, through which people could not only look young but keep the young state inside. Based on the traditional Chinese medicine (TCM), it is not only the hormones and the state of the intestine and liver that affect the skin, as commonly believed in Western medicine, but also separate organs, interconnected by meridians (pathways), where qi energy circulates. Each organ is related to certain elements (water, wood, fire, metal, earth), continuously interacting with each other conforming to the rule of the five elements in accordance with the principle of u-sin – the principle of mutual stimulation and oppression, as everything should be in a state of dynamic equilibrium.

To determine the disbalance through inspection, survey, measuring of pulse, and physical configuration of the language, a Chinese doctor looks for a "deficiency of yang-qi" or "liver qi stagnation" or "cold of the stomach, spleen deficiency, and accumulation of phlegm." It is a set of unknown words and terms for European doctors, and for the Chinese ones, it's a clear understanding of the processes going on in the body and a guide to action. For the face, for example, the predominance of yin means the tendency to stagnation and succulence, while for yang, dryness, inflammation, and excessive bleeding. Disorders associated with the stomach certainly have an impact on the area under the eyes (gray circles, succulence), as it is where stomach meridian starts. Disorders in the gall and urinary bladders affect the eyelids, as the first points of the meridian of these organs start in the inner and outer corners of the eyes (Fig. 1).

In general, the skin condition depends a lot on the condition of the lungs. If the qi of the lungs is weakened, then the skin will be dull and faded. The lungs are also connected to the large intestine with outer-inner connections. It is more clear to us that disbacteriosis is often the cause of skin inflammation. Thus, it is a complex system of interconnections that is impossible to understand without a good understanding of the fundamentals of TCM. The main principle of TCM says: "To restore the balance of yin and yang necessary to fill the missing, redistribute the excess."

This universal, at first glance, very simple and well-known formula requires a doctor to have a deep understanding of the theory of TCM and more experiences. As a result, four main processes of good health are performed well, digestion, excretion, circulation, and relaxation, provided with the methods of traditional Chinese medicine such as the use of herbal medicine, acupuncture (tuina and qigong exercises), and proper nutrition. Moreover, eastern practices affect remarkably epigenetic regulation, that is, the activity of our genes.

Thanks to modern scientific discoveries, regulatory mechanisms used by TCM and the benefits

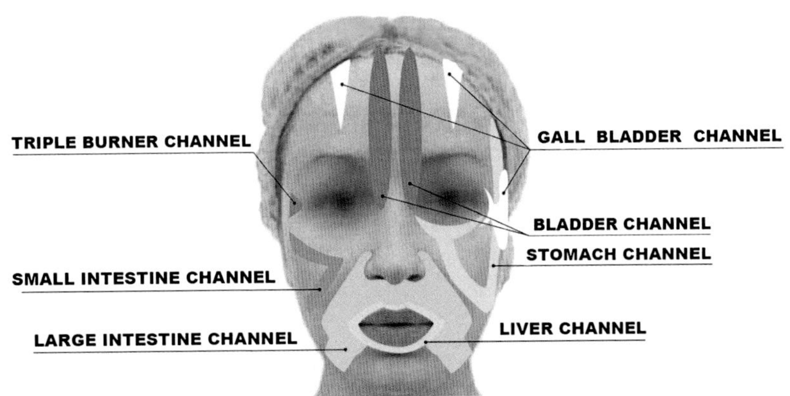

Fig. 1 Points of meridians of the internal organs on the face

we can extract from it for cosmetic purposes are becoming more clear.

It is important to remember that beauty does not only mean a good condition of the skin and lack of wrinkles, it is also a sparkle in the eyes, a zest for life, and an overall vitality, or, in other words, a never-give-up attitude. Thus, it is not only about health, sparing energy that must be generated, consumed, and restored in a correct way, but also about the psychology and philosophy of life, restoring peace of mind and balance. And eastern practices, e.g., qigong, meditation, and acupuncture, help us in that.

The Aim of the Method of Punctural Face Rejuvenation (PFR)

The aim of punctural face rejuvenation is to activate the regeneration of different skin elements of subcutaneous fat, initiated by multiple microdamages. General regulatory effects arising in the tissues due to the Chinese approach can be identified in the methodology, as well as local effects due to highly specific techniques developed by the author of this article. So, we have a combined technology, where the Chinese method is just based on the foundation of which copyrights techniques are realized quickly and efficiently. It is these techniques, being at the crossroads of several modern medical disciplines (physiology, dermatology, cosmetology, surgery, reflexology), that ultimately lead to the corresponding results.

The author used the knowledge of regeneration, degeneration, and atrophy from physiology; the information about the skin structure and functions and various factors affecting the skin condition from dermatology; the percutaneous method of inducing the synthesis of collagen, modern technologies of care, revitalization, the principles of replenishment, and the impact of botulinum toxin on our facial expressions from cosmetology; the features of wound healing and surgical rejuvenation procedures from surgery; and the basic TCM theory and acupuncture from reflexology.

The Procedure Technique

The PFR technique differs from acupuncture in a fundamental way. As the name implies, puncture is a prick, perforation; acupuncture is a shot in a biologically active point, which is not so much on the face (about 50). As a well-known American beautician said: "In order to obtain the effects from acupuncture, not less than 200–300 punctures should be made." This idea was realized while creating dermarollers (mezorollers), through which it is possible to get pronounced activation of collagen and elastin synthesis (PCI – percutaneous collagen induction).

Histological examination of the thigh skin before and after 6 months after PCI showed an increase of these important components of youthful skin which was almost 400 % [2]. Without dwelling on the advantages and disadvantages of this method, we can say that with all the indications and contraindications, it gives good visible results. However, not everyone will bear such results. Moreover, the hope that the PCI-toned skin will take on all the "carcass" load is not always justified, especially if we are dealing with gravity (strain) type of facial aging.

Punctural facial rejuvenation works not only with the epidermal and dermal layers of the skin but, more importantly, with subcutaneous fat and muscles, where, as is known, age-related changes of the trophics, tone, density, and mass redistribution occur. Therefore many patients during and after treatment experience pleasant feelings of the activation not only on the skin surface but also deep in the facial tissues. Needle works on the entire thickness of the superficial musculoaponeurotic layer, thereby achieving good lifting effect.

Thus, the differences between acupuncture and PFR are significant. In PFR sometimes up to 100 needles are used, especially when the patient needs a faster result. So, thanks to PFR, you can see the changes after the first procedure already, which is impossible for the acupuncture. In cosmetic acupuncture (commonly referred to as acupuncture facelift), the number of procedures reaches 50 and the duration of each of them is 30–60 min. This is popular with Hollywood stars. Moreover, we just do not get the same results with the help of a simple acupuncture on facial points that Chinese doctors usually do, due to the difference in technologies.

Mode of Action of the PFR

Modes of action of the punctural face rejuvenation can be divided into several groups: one for the wrinkles, to make the facial outlines distinct, another for the ptosis, and so on. To receive visible results, we should clearly understand how and what to do. So, to reduce the wrinkles, we should understand what this most unpleasant sign of aging represents at the histological level. The most complete study of the wrinkle structures is discussed in the article, by J. L. Content-Audonneau, C. Jeanmaire, and G. Pauly, "A histological study of human wrinkle structures" [3].

A wrinkle is the thinning of the epidermal, dermal, and hypodermal layers, due to the dystrophic and even atrophic processes in the tissues. And this is nothing but substitution of high-specific skin cells for fibrosis (in rough and deep wrinkles). On the analogy of laser nanoperforation, these changed layers are penetrated by the needles, but in a rougher, more active, and more directional manner (in fact, we can affect the different skin layers with the needle). This starts a cascade of wound healing and in series all stages of regeneration. As a result of this, over repeatedly iterative sessions, reduction (elimination) of the wrinkles occurs, and through the phases of revascularization and reepithelialization, a normal skin appears (Fig. 2).

Certainly, facial mobility, age, and other factors stand against this reparative process. That's why this procedure is good only in the case of moderate facial mobility; otherwise botulinum toxin therapy is needed. The PFR can be associated with botulinum toxin (conducted in 3–4 weeks after injections). Thus, due to the PFR, we can apply two times less botulinum toxin therapy. This is especially indicated for women who can't tolerate injections of botulinum toxin, or those who seek to minimize any adverse effects of this procedure. The combination of the PFR and botulinum toxin therapy can be justified when the wrinkles are quite deep, and due to the accumulated dystrophic changes in the skin of the wrinkle after injections of botulinum toxin, they become less noticeable, but don't disappear completely. Then the combination of the PFR and botulinum toxin therapy can give the best results.

How Is the Procedure Conducted?

The skin is disinfected and anesthetized with cream "EMLA" most commonly. The needles are inserted in the wrinkles at small distances with different angles, depths, and lengths.

Contour Remodeling of the Face (e.g., lower contour, ptosis of the cheeks, "marionette folds," double chin): The PFR is effective in the case of wrinkled and mixed (tired face) type of aging. In case of gravitative (deformational) type of aging, the PFR may be effective only under the following conditions: age up to 37 years, no smoking, no

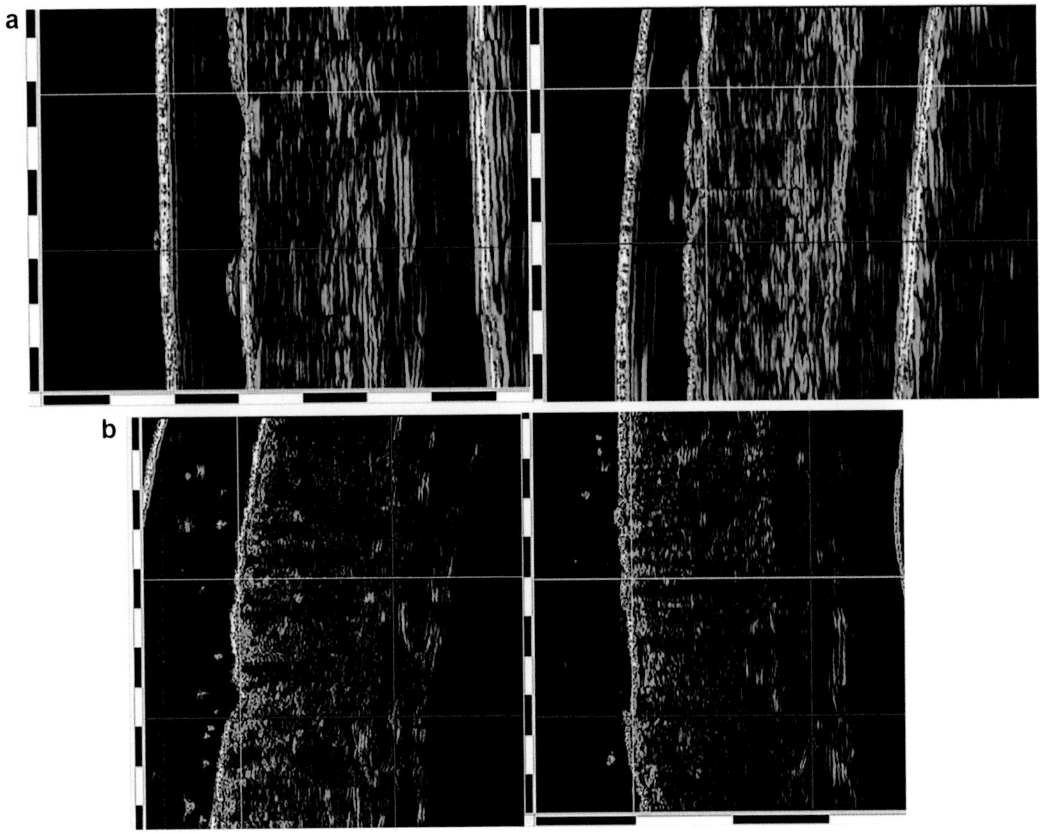

Fig. 2 (**a**, **b**) Example of the PFR effect on the transversal forehead wrinkle (male of 47 years old). Photo of an ultrasound skin examination with the equipment DUB SkinScanner before and after PFR (15 min since the procedure). Alignment surface of skin is noted. (**a**) DUB SkinScanner 22 MHz. (**b**) DUB SkinScanner 75 MHz

hormonal dysregulations, and with normal diet and sleep. Surgical technologies propose facelifting of the middle and lower third of the face in many ways, which is certainly justified in the case of expressed changes. Threads and fillers in the zygomatic region are also mostly good at skin tightening. But these methods are not always sufficient for good effect. And then the PFR may be a good addition to the above procedures. How? If insertion of fillers in the "in short supply" areas can be called "plus technology," the effect of the PFR can be called "minus technology." Due to the good lipolytic effect of the needles on the adipose tissue, we can reduce the volume and doughiness of the adipose tissue of the face very selectively, sensitively, and manageably. Then the fat in the "jowl" area will be reduced, as well as in the double chin and "marionette folds," plus the SMAS lifting effect results in smoother lower facial contour and more gentle line of chin and lower jaw.

This method makes an absolutely unique opportunity for the facial rejuvenation in the nasolacrimal area! It is the practice to correct by means of fillers a prominent fold, beginning at the wing of the nose and proceeding in nasolabial fold. But by no means always good result can be achieved. What to do? To use lipolytics is risky. To lift the middle part of face using threads is ineffective. In this case, the PFR can sensationally solve the problem! Reduction of the prominent fold occurs due to the lipolytic effect of needles and incremental recovery of normal density of the subcutaneous fat. The fold is flattening, the tissue is firming and becomes more compact, and visual profit is evident. This effect required studying and scientific evidence.

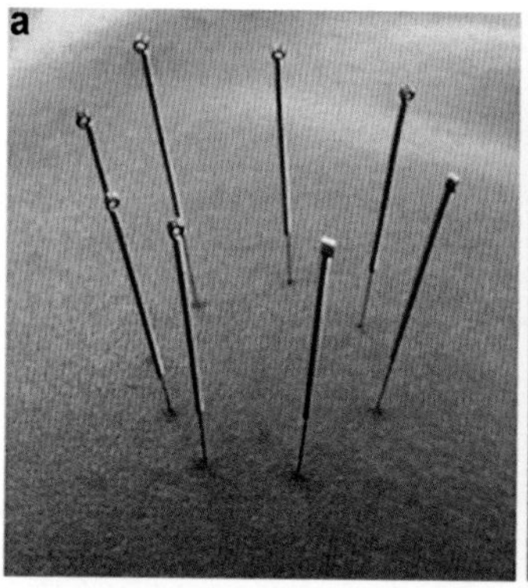

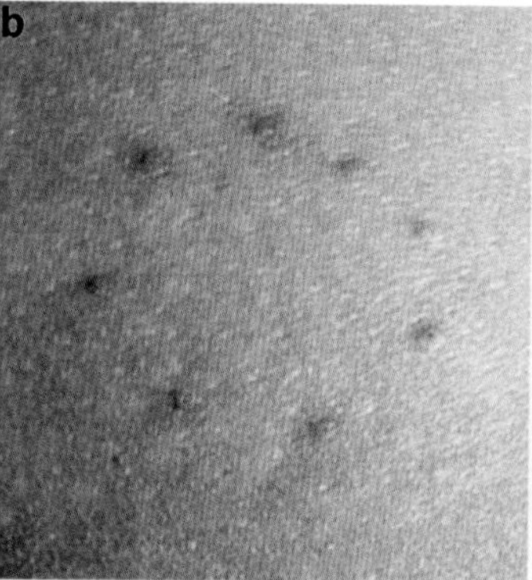

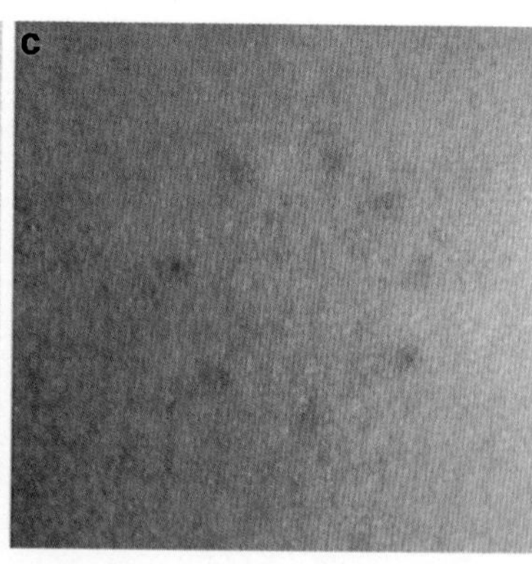

Fig. 3 (**a**) This is the view of positioning needles using the "dragon fence" method. Eight needles, thickness 0.25 mm, are installed with a radius of 2.5 cm, in depth up to 2 cm. (**b**) Traces of needles 15 min after extraction from the skin. (**c**) Traces of needles 6 h after extraction from the skin. The traces of microdamages, which activate all the subsequent stages of an aseptic inflammation, proliferation, and remodeling of the skin, are visible

Local Effect on the Tropism of the Facial Tissues

The needle, inserted in the tissue to a depth of 1 cm, causes around itself an "injury" within a radius of up to 2.5 cm. As a result, in this area the circulation of blood and plasma is enhanced, and the local metabolism and fibroblasts with all relevant subsequent reactions are activated.

In terms of physiology of the key cells and tissues involved in the local reactions after active acupuncture, the following phases could be estimated in analogy with wound healing process:

1. Hemostasis with the involvement of platelets and fibrin
2. Inflammation with the involvement of neutrophils, lymphocytes, and macrophages
3. Proliferation with the involvement of fibroblasts, collagen, and epithelium and endothelium cells
4. Remodeling with the involvement of astringent collagen fibers and maturing scar [4]

The process includes a variety of physiologic paths with a number of involved biochemical substances, which can be divided into several groups:

- Cytokines (IL-1,4,6,3, tumor-necrotizing factor-α(TNF- α), and others).
- Growth factors, proliferation inducers, and inhibitors of apoptosis. They include KGF (keratinocyte growth factor), EGF (epidermal growth factor), TrGF (transforming growth factor), granulocyte-macrophage colony-stimulating factor (GM-CSF), AP-1 (activating protein-1), ILGF-1,2 (insulin-like growth factor-1,2), and PDGF (platelet-derived growth factor).
- Glycoproteins of intercellular space: fibronectin, collagen, and metalloproteinase.
- Chalones and antichalones.
- Cell adhesion molecule [5].

It should be noted that physicians of ancient China with no awareness of such complicated biochemical processes in the skin used to stimulate wound healing by active pricking all around the site of the injury. This method was referred to as "dragon fence" [6] (Fig. 3).

Additionally, the needle causes microdamages in tissues, causing a cascade of healing, and this in turn leads to an increase in tone, elasticity, and moisture of the skin, which are the major factors in its rejuvenation.

Segmental Effect on Tissues

As it was mentioned above, the needle does not only affect the skin but also the subcutaneous fat and muscles. Afferent pathway signals move to the rear horns of the spinal cord, partially "switch" on the "path" of the autonomic innervation, and return to the place of impact, thus activating local metabolism. This effect is important for neck rejuvenation. In other words, to the local influence segmental influence is added, more common in area and more stable in the duration. On these effects metameric reflexotherapy technique mainly works [7].

Total Effect of Acupuncture on the Central Nervous System

It was proven long before that acupuncture stimulates the production of serotonin, the "hormone of joy," and endogenous opioids – endorphins. Therefore, patients receive during the procedure further portion of positive emotions, relaxation, and comfort that are not superfluous in the modern life in big cities. Especially in patients who are in significant chronic stress, protracted treatment reduces the level of the hormone cortisol, which is by our foreign colleagues called the "silent killer"; they observed a decrease in inflammatory activity in the tissues, including the skin, resulting in improved regeneration and therefore skin rejuvenation. It should be noted that reflexotherapy does not only affect the CNS and ANS but also cardiovascular, endocrine, and immune systems of the body [8].

Cosmetic Effects Obtained Using PFR

Cosmetic effects of punctural rejuvenation are different. We can say that the technique is particularly successful in solving major cosmetic problems of women from 35 to 45 years old. But this does not mean that it is ineffective in older patients, and it should not be used by younger patients. Just each time interval is characterized by its changes, and, perhaps, the main in the technique efficiency is not even your age but lifestyle – the right way of life, that is, balanced food, nutraceutical reception, yoga, tai chi, the regulation of body functions using Chinese medicine, and good skin care using high-quality natural cosmetics.

The most effective procedure is the removal of wrinkles, and where they are located is not so important. The needle is a wonderful tool in that it can help reduce almost any wrinkles in the face. Of course, the effect of the PFR remains durable enough in the case of moderate or weak mimic activity. Otherwise we can't do it without botulinum toxin. Wrinkles on the nose, "crow's feet," "purse-string lines," and "marionette folds" yield particularly well to the reduction. Much more difficult to cope with is ptosis of facial tissues, especially in the case of gravitational (deformation) type of aging. But even in these cases, we can achieve certain lifting; however, it will have to be maintained by certain repetitive procedures with individually prescribed intervals (at least once or twice a month).

With the method of punctural rejuvenation, you can treat the following anatomic face areas:

Transversal forehead wrinkles	Lineae frontales transversae
Vertical wrinkles of glabella	Lineae verticales glabellares
Vertical wrinkles of nose	Lineae nasales transversae
The fold under the lower eyelid	Lineae palpebrales inferiores (sulcus infraorbitalis)
Lateral eye wrinkles	Lineae orbitales laterales
Orbitozygomatic wrinkles	Linea orbitozygomatica
Nasolabial fold	Sulcus nasolabialis
Buccomandibular fold	Sulcus buccomandibularis
Oromentalis fold	Sulcus oromentalis
Circumoral folds	Striae circumoralis
Mentolabial fold	Sulcus mentolabialis

Factors Affecting the Efficiency of the Method

There are a lot of factors affecting the effectiveness of the method. First is the patient's health. The skin is a separate organ, and it is not healthy when illnesses are present. Unhealthy skin is difficult to correct using PFR. It must be said that you can achieve visible results almost always using special methods, but how long it will last and how much will be emphasized depends on "internal resources" of the skin and the whole body. Such factors as hormones, sleep, the state of the function of detoxification, nutrition, relaxation, and so on are very important. For the author's opinion, the most pernicious to the skin is smoking as it reduced detoxifying activity of the body. A special term "cigarette skin" is used abroad. In this case, special programs of "protection" of the vessels, liver, and intestines are required, in which the methods of TCM are also quite effective.

Nothing can be done by PFR if there is a significant excess of tissue. It is impossible to "pack" a large area on a smaller area without losing tone and folds. Patients with such problems should be treated by plastic surgeons.

PFR Painfulness and Consequences

A sense of pain during PFR is moderate. Approximately every fifth patient can bear the procedure without anesthesia. In patients with low bias of pain sensitivity, surface anesthesia is used by applying on face skin the cream, "EMLA," with lidocaine. In 1 % of cases ultrahigh pain sensitivity is observed. In such cases PFR is not carried out.

It should be said that besides the innate level of pain sensitivity, there are different factors that can influence the acceptability of the procedure.

For example, the author noticed that pain sensation increases with:

- Menses
- Disturbed sleep (insomnia) before the procedure
- Distress
- Any pain syndrome

That is why the patients are recommended to get enough sleep before the procedure, not to be nervous, and to pass sessions if with menses and different pain syndromes. These recommendations may be general for all intrusive cosmetic procedures.

Certainly, the acceptability of PFR is also influenced by:

- The quality, thickness, and number of needles
- Intensity of manipulations with needles
- Influenced area

For example, double chin and cheeks are less sensible, while orbital and nasolabial zones are more sensible. The anesthesia may be local in view of individual sensibility.

In any case, PFR may be classified as well-accepted procedures for most patients. Moreover, every patient adapts his or her own combination of techniques, taking into consideration the set problem and the level of pain sense.

PFR Stages

The first stage is maximum result achievement. Sessions are performed once a week on one face zone. It's allowed to perform the sessions with less intensity but greater frequency, e.g., once every 2 or 3 days. After the desired result is achieved, you may go to supportive scheme.

The second stage is sustaining and support. Procedure frequency may vary a lot, from once in a month to short courses of two to three sessions half a year or a year. The most suitable schemes are defined individually in each particular case.

Indications for PFR

Punctural face rejuvenation primarily is recommended to those:

- Who would like to avoid or less frequently use injections of botulinum toxin and fillers
- Who are susceptible to allergic reactions to various cosmetic products and procedures
- Who have lower sensitivity to Botox
- Who would like to use as long as possible "natural technologies of beauty"
- Who were not satisfied by the results of conventional cosmetic procedures completely
- Who are focused on maintenance of appearance as a healthy state mark

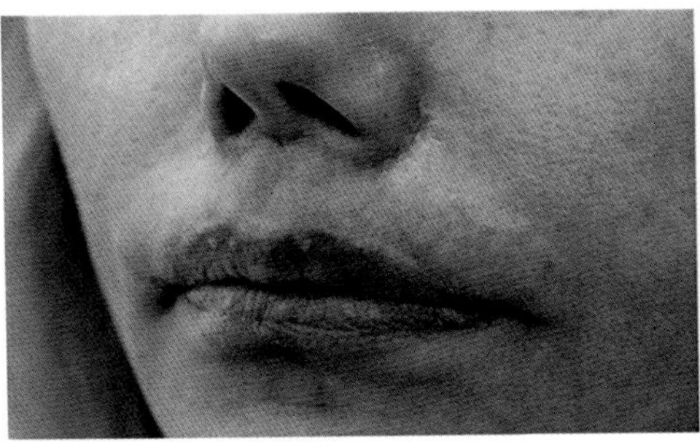
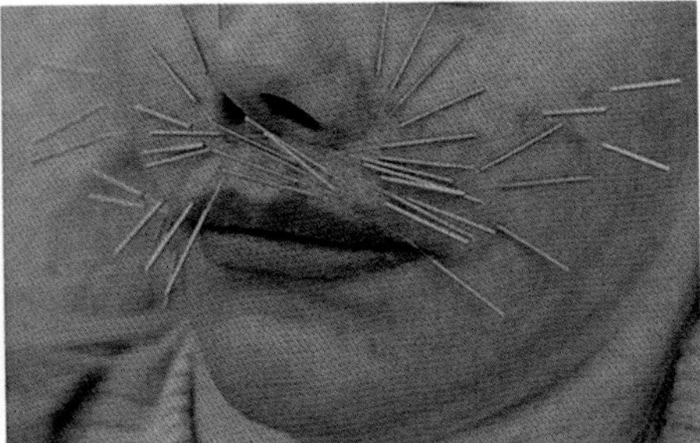

Fig. 4 Scars treatment

Contraindications for PFR

Absolute

- Infectious, allergic, hormonal skin diseases (acne, dermatitis, herpes (herpes labialis), warts, vitiligo, etc.)
- Skin tendency to expressed cicatricial keloids formation
- Hemophilia
- Infectious diseases (ARVI, flu, conjunctivitis, sinusitis, otitis, increased temperature)
- Oncological diseases
- Epilepsy
- Anticoagulants intake (warfarin, heparin)

Relative

- Skin tendency to bruises, hematomas, cicatricial keloids formation
- Hypertensive illness (existence of hypertensive crises)
- Insulin-dependent diabetes
- Vibrating arrhythmia
- Pregnancy

Combination with Other Cosmetic Procedures

PFR can be conducted 3–4 weeks after botulinum toxin and fillers injections. PFR can be combined with fillers injections, for example, eliminating remaining wrinkles in nasolabial zone, nose bridge, after contour correction procedures.

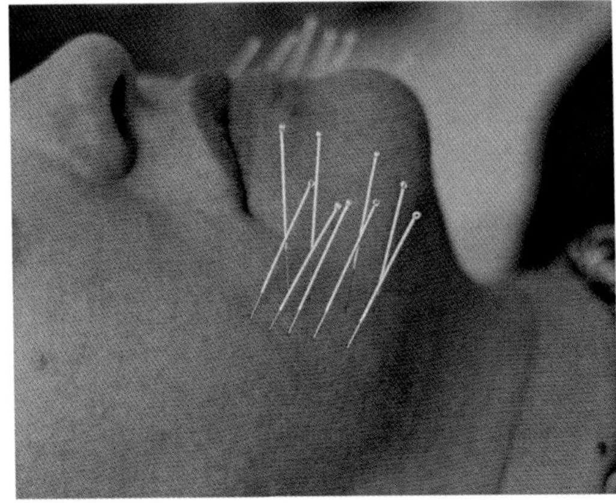

Fig. 5 Treating of the cheeks area

PFR can be conducted a week after superficial peeling, 1–2 months after median peeling, and 6 months after deep peeling.

It is not recommended to combine PFR with laser. At least 6 months have to pass after a laser course before PFR is performed. The more traumatic the procedure was, the more time has to pass (on the average from 3 to 6 months).

PFR is well combined with a mesotherapy and a revitalization. It is possible to combine procedures with an interval in a week. PFR and revitalization perfectly supplement each other, strengthening final effect.

After plastic surgery with the help of PFR, it is possible to remove the scar (Fig. 4).

By analogy with wrinkles the "needling" of most cicatricial tissue itself is carried out with various intensities and depths. Frequency is once in 1–2 weeks, and duration depends on the extent of facial expressions and is about 6–7 months. The process is slow.

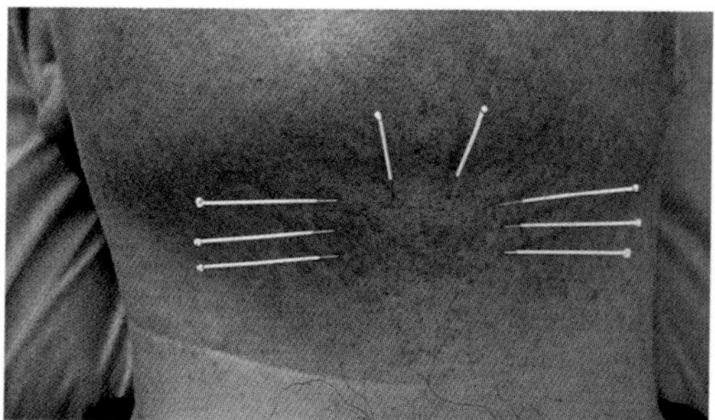

Fig. 6 Treating of the double chin area

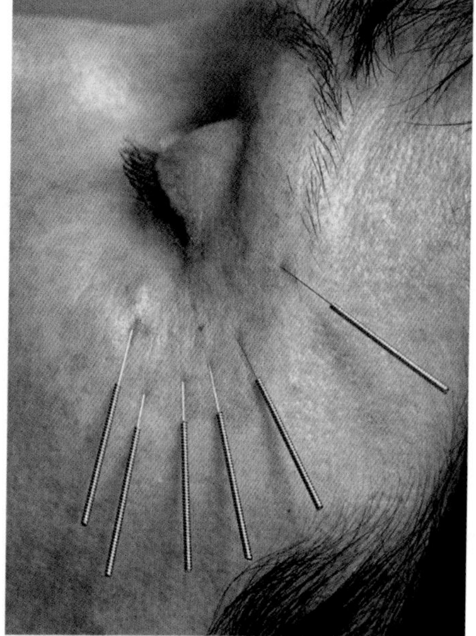

Fig. 7 Treating of the crow's feet area

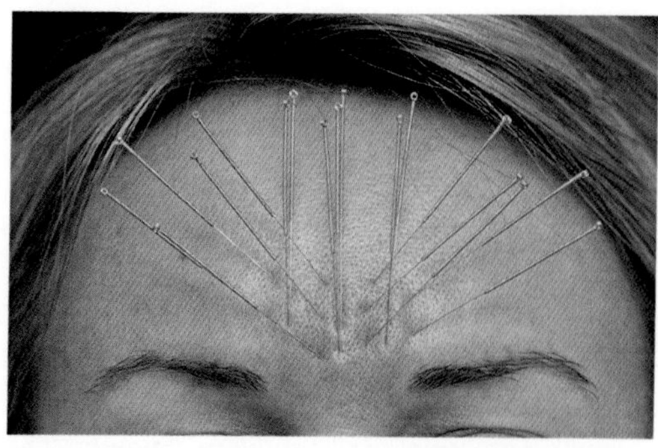

Fig. 8 Treating of the area between the eyebrows

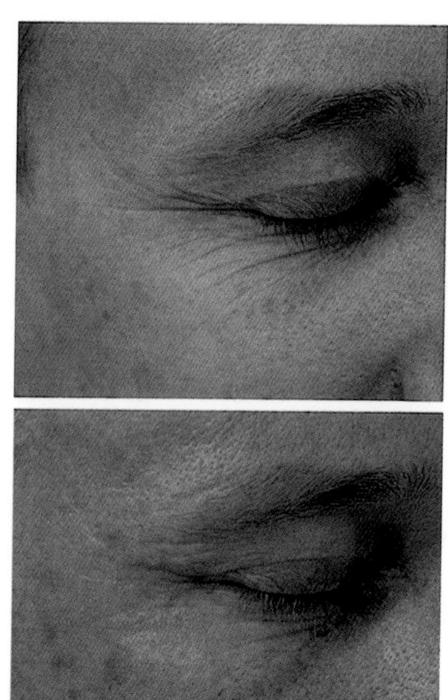

Fig. 9 Treating of the crow's feet area 5 sessions, 6 weeks

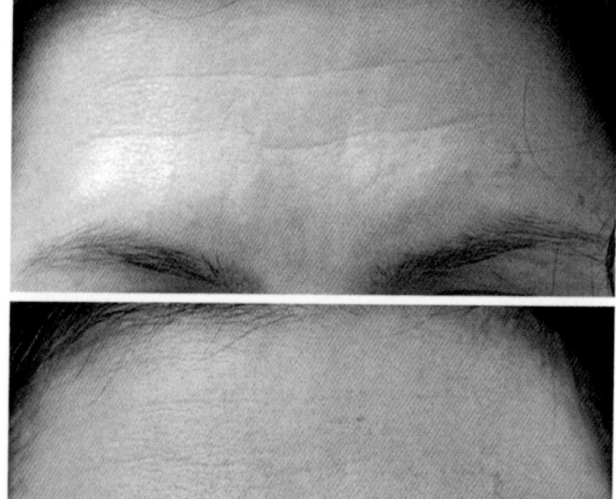

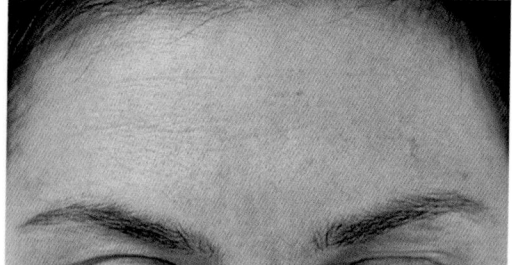

Fig. 10 Treating of the forehead 5 sessions, 8 weeks

Additional Opportunities of PFR

With the help of PFR, side effects after fillers injections can be eliminated. Similar to scars, in case fillers are exposed asymmetrically, multiple

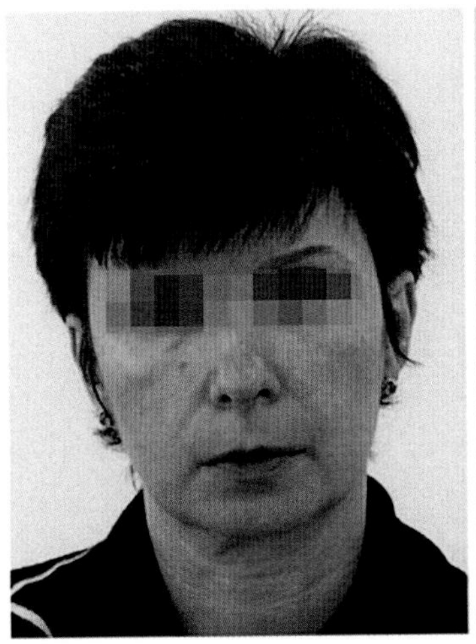
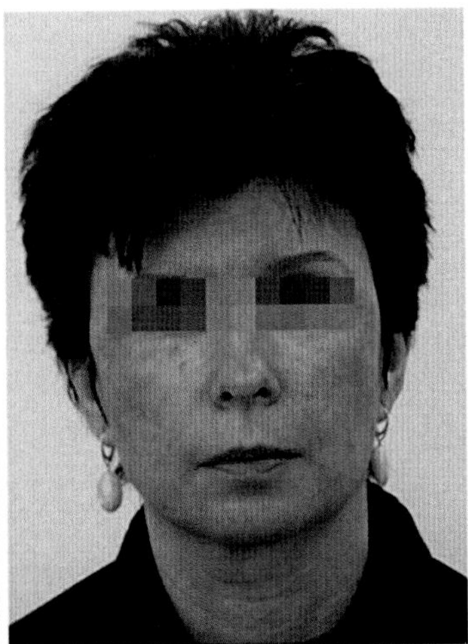

Fig. 11 Punctural face rejuvenation 7 sessions, 8 weeks

punctures of fillers can be done with the necessary intensity. Gradually symmetry is restored. Frequency is once in 1–2 weeks, and duration is from 1 to 2 months.

Unfortunately there are no panaceas in rejuvenation, reasonable combination of various cosmetic technologies.

Photo Examples of PFR

With cheeks, the needles are put in the subcutaneous fat of the cheeks at the length up to 4–5 cm. They stimulate splitting of fatty tissues (lipolysis) in this zone, gradual volume reduction, and skin lifting.

The same principle, as in Fig. 5, is used. As a result of repetition of procedures, the reduction of volume of subcutaneous fat and lifting of double chin are achieved (Fig. 6).

With crow's feet area, thinner needles (thickness of 0.20 mm) with a superficial passage at an acute angle to an extent of 1 cm are used (Fig. 7).

With the area between the eyebrows, the techniques are directed on the stimulation of skin regeneration and relaxation of the muscles (Fig. 8).

Conclusion

PFR is not a technique of external impact on the person; it is rather natural rejuvenation technology which activates the organism's own resources. PFR can easily be combined with the majority of cosmetic techniques, and also it can be used as an independent method for face age-specific changes prevention. Thanks to it, it is possible to carefully and efficiently support your potential, considerably suppressing age-specific changes and preventing radical interventions.

Photo of the Results

See Figs. 9, 10, and 11.

References

1. Zhang P. A comprehensive handbook for traditional Chinese medicine facial rejuvenation. Port Washington: A Nefeli Corporation Publication; 2006. p. 6–7.
2. Under the editorship of Joseph Riatmu 3, Richard H. Hog. Minimum invasive cosmetic surgery. «Medpress-inform», 2007:77.
3. Farage MA, et al. Textbook of aging skin. Berlin/Heidelberg: Springer; 2010. p. 364.
4. Falabella AF, Kirsner RS. In: Chin GA, Diegelmann RF, editors. Wound healing. p. 18.
5. Myadelets OD, Adskevich VP. Morphofunctional dermatology. – M.: Medical literature. 2006. p. 688.
6. White A, Cummings M, Filshie J. An introduction to western medical acupuncture. Edinburgh: Churchill Livingstone/Elsevier; 2008. p. 20.
7. Prihodko E. Candidate of Medical Science inaugural dissertation "The correction of age-specific involutional changes in cervico-facial region tissues through metameric acupuncture". Tver, 2004.
8. Ma Y-T, Ma M, Cho ZH. Biomedical acupuncture for pain management. St. Louis: Churchill Livingstone/Elsevier; 2005. p. 24.

Bridging Science and Beauty

153

Christine C. Kim and Paul S. Yamauchi

Contents

Abstract

The pursuit of beauty can be traced back to ancient times. The history of human beautification spans the realms of religion, medicine, and philosophy, and the means by which humans have attempted to enhance their appearance evolved from a practice of rituals based on empirical knowledge to a legitimate medical specialty. Humans first used natural resources from their environment – plants, animals, and minerals – for beautification. Unfortunately, at times this experimentation led to deleterious results. Modern-day aesthetic medical techniques are subjected to rigorous scientific testing, although some discoveries were made by pure serendipity. This chapter highlights the past, present, and future of the closely intertwined relationship between science and beauty.

Introduction

What constitutes beauty is a question that artists, philosophers, and scientists have debated over millennia. What is beauty? A simple answer is elusive. Is there an objective beauty ideal, or does beauty, according to Plato, lie in the eyes of the beholder? Is beauty a constant that transcends geographical and chronological borders, or does it change with place and time? Is our sense of beauty innate or learned? Can beauty be quantified? In *Survival of the Prettiest*, Nancy Etcoff takes a

C.C. Kim (✉)
Dermatology Institute and Skin Care Center, Santa Monica, CA, USA
e-mail: drkim@discc.com

P.S. Yamauchi
Dermatology Institute and Skin Care Center, Santa Monica, CA, USA

David Geffen School of School of Medicine at UCLA, Los Angeles, CA, USA
e-mail: paulyamauchi@yahoo.com

M.A. Farage et al. (eds.), *Textbook of Aging Skin*,
DOI 10.1007/978-3-662-47398-6_151

Darwinian stance and theorizes that the human pursuit of beauty is a struggle to ensure the survival of one's genes [1]. Phi, or the golden ratio, is used to mathematically define the ideal human face and body shape [2]. A complete discourse on the meaning of beauty is beyond the scope of this chapter, but interested readers will find a plethora of opinions on the matter.

Historical Methods of Beautification

Dating back to prehistoric times, humans have experimented with botanical ingredients, animal products, and minerals to enhance their appearance. Tattooing, or placing tints under the skin to make them permanent, was among the first cosmetic procedures [3]. Since the ancient Egyptians, beautification rituals were important for religious purposes or to attract members of the opposite sex. The *Ebers Papyrus* devoted a chapter to hair care that recommended ointments made of animal fat or blood to facilitate hair growth [3]. *Mesdemet*, the "black paste" for the eyes, was composed of plumbic sulfate or antimony sulfide, while green-colored cosmetics were produced with copper salts [4]. Henna, a vegetable dye derived from *Lawsonia inermis* or *Lawsonia alba*, was used to paint the skin, hair, and nails a dark red color [4]. It is said that Cleopatra bathed in goat's milk, almond, and honey [5]. Unrefrigerated milk sours to produce lactic acid, an alpha-hydroxy acid, which acts as a chemoexfoliant [6] while honey is a natural humectant. The Egyptians also used clay and herbal masks to draw out toxins from the skin, flower and tree oils for aromatherapy, and fruit acids of sugar cane, mangos, and apples to smoothen the skin [5].

The history of beautification methods is also fraught with examples of risky and potentially harmful practices. The ancient Greeks used lead-based makeup to lighten the skin, a technique that persisted through the European Elizabethan era to modern nineteenth-century America. Elizabethan women painted their faces with ceruse, a mixture of white lead and vinegar, which unfortunately slowly poisoned its users [3]. Both women and men took great measures to acquire pallor, going so far as to apply leeches for bloodletting [3]. Women of Renaissance Italy used eye drops prepared from the berries of the deadly nightshade plant, *Atropa belladonna*, to dilate their pupils, an effect considered to enhance their beauty [7]. In the 1800s, Victorian women swallowed the cysts of tapeworms in a quest to stay slim, a dangerous practice that continues to resurface in modern times among diet faddists [8].

Beautification in Modern Times

Aesthetic surgery gained momentum in the nineteenth century, aided by the widespread knowledge of antiseptic technique pioneered by the British surgeon Josef Lister as well as the advent of general anesthesia. Rhinoplasty, blepharoplasty, and facelifts were introduced at this time. In the latter half of the twentieth century, mammoplasty, hair transplantation, and liposuction became commonplace procedures [9].

A revolutionary discovery that truly bridged science and beauty was that of selective photothermolysis which succeeded in harnessing lasers and light sources to enhance the skin's appearance. Rox Anderson and John Parrish theorized that specific wavelengths of light emitted in suitably brief pulses could precisely target different structures in the skin while allowing the surrounding area to remain relatively undisturbed [10]. Lasers and light sources are now used to treat pigmentation, vascular lesions, and aid in tattoo removal, hair removal, and collagen remodeling. An important milestone in laser technology was introduced in 2004 by Dieter Manstein and called fractional photothermolysis [11]. By treating only a fraction of the skin's surface, the remaining undamaged surrounding tissue could promote rapid repair, thus reducing downtime and side effects. Radiofrequency, microwave, and high-frequency ultrasound energy sources are currently used in devices for skin tightening, axillary hyperhidrosis, and noninvasive fat removal, respectively. Cryolipolysis is another method of noninvasive fat reduction.

The latter part of the twentieth century and the beginning of the twenty-first century saw the serendipitous discovery of cosmetic benefits from medications already in use for non-cosmetic indications. Researchers discovered that minoxidil, a vasodilator that reduces blood pressure, could also grow hair. Topical minoxidil was approved by the Food and Drug Administration (FDA) in 1988 for male pattern baldness and is available today over the counter for both men and women. In 1992, Alastair and Jean Carruthers published their discovery that injecting *Clostridium* botulinum-A exotoxin, previously used for blepharospasm, could also treat glabellar frown lines [12]. Botulinum toxin was approved for cosmetic use in 2002 and in 2004 acquired the FDA indication for treating severe axillary hyperhidrosis. In 2001, the FDA approved bimatoprost, a prostaglandin analog for the reduction of high intraocular pressure in open-angle glaucoma or ocular hypertension. One of the "side effects" reported was longer, fuller, and darker eyelashes [13]. This accidental discovery led to the FDA approval of bimatoprost in 2008 for eyelash hypotrichosis.

The use of dermal and subcutaneous fillers for nonsurgical facial rejuvenation evolved from early bovine collagen in the 1980s to hyaluronic acid, poly-L-lactic acid, and calcium hydroxylapatite in the early 2000s. Fillers are used to correct fine lines, wrinkles, folds, and loss of volume. Injectables are also used to remove unwanted volume. In 2015, deoxycholic acid was FDA approved for the treatment of moderate-to-severe submental fat.

The Future of Science and Beauty

According to the American Society for Aesthetic Plastic Surgery (ASAPS), in 2013 more than 11 million cosmetic surgical and nonsurgical procedures were performed by board-certified plastic surgeons, dermatologists, and otolaryngologists in the United States, totaling more than 12 billion dollars [14]. The pursuit of beauty has reached insatiable levels and in turn has driven the scientific community to focus on developing less invasive, more effective, and more accessible techniques to enhance the human form. What does the future hold?

Nanotechnology is the rapidly developing discipline that uses particles 1,000 nm in size and smaller. It allows the potential to deliver molecules into the skin, which ordinarily do not penetrate the stratum corneum. In the dermatologic setting nanotechnology is most commonly used for sunscreens containing zinc oxide, rendering more elegant sun protection [15]. Topical botulinum toxin which is being studied for treatment of facial rhytides and hyperhidrosis has the potential to revolutionize the landscape of aesthetic medicine [16].

The personalization of aesthetic treatments is a fast-growing movement. The possibility of harvesting one's own blood to extract precious substances such as growth factors and anti- inflammatory cytokines is the basis of an autologous antiaging serum [17]. An injectable suspension of autologous fibroblasts was FDA approved in 2011. In a multicenter, double-blind, placebo-controlled study, it was shown to be a safe and effective way to improve the appearance of moderate-to-severe nasolabial fold wrinkles with the added benefit of being a natural, biological treatment modality [18]. In the near future the application of genomics technologies will offer insights into skin cell biology that can be harnessed for the development of new products [19].

Also forecasted is the increasing market for home-use laser and light devices for self-administered beauty treatments. Although not as powerful as office versions, the currently available devices for hair removal, photoaging, and acne have a wide margin of safety and are less costly [20].

In an interesting arc, the use of natural botanical ingredients has gained increasing popularity in recent years. Perhaps as the pendulum swings toward scientific breakthroughs, there is a counterbalancing desire to use simple remedies for beautification. The discovery of antioxidants in various botanical ingredients, such as feverfew, green tea, licorice, soy, and coffee berry, has led to an expanding cosmeceutical market targeting the effects of photoaging [21]. The burgeoning natural beauty market will likely continue to grow as topical vehicles improve the delivery of active ingredients to their targets in the skin.

Conclusion

Science and technology have influenced the quest for human beautification in unforeseen ways. Due to the efficiency of international travel and the Internet, the exchange of ideas occurs at a rapid pace. Cosmetic companies are capitalizing on this move toward globalization. Korean beauty trends have made their way onto American shores, with BB creams and sleeping masks becoming mainstream [22]. The Internet has produced a generation of bloggers whose influence eclipses traditional mass marketing [23]. Meanwhile, photo-perfecting smartphone applications and Madison Avenue airbrushed images promote an unattainable ideal of beauty for humans to try and emulate. As novel methods of beautification arise from scientific advances, the eternal pursuit of beauty will continue.

References

1. Etcoff N. Survival of the prettiest. 1st ed. New York: Anchor; 1999.
2. Atiyeh BS, Hayek SN. Numeric expression of aesthetics and beauty. Aesthet Plast Surg. 2008;32:209–16. doi:10.1007/s00266-007-9074-x.
3. Blanco-Davila F. Beauty and the body: the origins of cosmetics. Plast Reconstr Surg. 2000;105 (3):1196–204.
4. Murube J. Ocular cosmetics in ancient times. Ocul Surf. 2013;111(1):2–7. doi:10.1016/j.jtos.2012.09.003.
5. Oumeish OY. The cultural and philosophical concepts of cosmetics in beauty and art through the medical history of mankind. Clin Dermatol. 2001;19:375–86.
6. Hoenig LJ. Beauty tips from ancient queens. Arch Dermatol. 2012;148(10):1164. doi:10.1001/archdermatol.2012.2407.
7. http://www.nlm.nih.gov/medlineplus/druginfo/natural/531.html
8. http://www.bbc.com/news/science-environment-25968755
9. Kreuger N, et al. The history of aesthetic medicine and surgery. J Drugs Dermatol. 2013;12 (7):737–42.
10. Anderson RR, Parrish JA. Selective photothermolysis: precise microsurgery by selective absorption of pulsed radiation. Science. 1983;220:524–7.
11. Manstein D, et al. Fractional photothermolysis: a new concept for cutaneous remodeling using microscopic patterns of thermal injury. Lasers Surg Med. 2004;34:426–38.
12. Carruthers JD, Carruthers JA. Treatment of glabellar frown lines with C. botulinum-A exotoxin. J Dermatol Surg Oncol. 1992;18(1):17–21.
13. Cohen JL. Commentary: from serendipity to pilot study and then pivotal trial: bimatoprost topical for eyelash growth. Dermatol Surg. 2010;36(5):650–1. doi:10.1111/j.1524-4725.2010.01532.x.
14. http://www.surgery.org/media/news-releases/the-american-society-for-aesthetic-plastic-surgery-reports-americans-spent-largest-amount-on-cosmetic-surger
15. Nasir A, Friedman A. Nanotechnology and the nanodermatology society. J Drugs Dermatol. 2010;9 (7):879–82.
16. Collins A, Nasir A. Topical botulinum toxin. J Clin Aesthet Dermatol. 2010;3(3):35–9.
17. Pinto H, Garrido LG. Study to evaluate the aesthetic clinical impact of an autologous antiaging serum. J Drugs Dermatol. 2013;12(3):322–6.
18. Smith SR, et al. A multicenter, double- blind, placebo-controlled trial of autologous fibroblast therapy for the treatment of nasolabial fold wrinkles. Dermatol Surg. 2012;38(7pt2):1234–43. doi:10.1111/j.1524-4725.2012.02349.x.
19. Tiesman JP. From bench to beauty counter: using genomics to drive technology development for skin care. J Drugs Dermatol. 2009;8(7 Suppl):12–4.
20. Chapas A, Bergstrom KG. Home laser treatments: acne, aging, and unwanted hair. J Drugs Dermatol. 2012;11(5):666.
21. Bowe WP, Pugliese S. Cosmetic benefits of natural ingredients. J Drugs Dermatol. 2014;13 (9):1021–5.
22. http://www.fastcompany.com/3038283/why-korean-skincare-is-booming
23. http://www.corporate-eye.com/main/the-influence-of-blogs-on-purchase-decisions/

154 Botulinum Toxin Type A and Laser Resurfacing Provide Adjunctive Benefit to Skin Aging

Paul S. Yamauchi and Christine C. Kim

Contents

Abstract

The combination of intrinsic skin aging, chronic exposure to ultraviolet light, and the repetitive motion of the dynamic muscles in the face leads to wrinkles in the forehead, glabella, and the periorbital area. Combination treatment that addresses various contributing factors can enhance outcomes to rejuvenate these areas. Studies conducted in the past have demonstrated that combination of botulinum toxin and laser resurfacing improves the textural changes as well as pigmentation in the treated areas compared to either treatment performed alone. This chapter illustrates the benefits of an adjunctive approach to treating aging skin in the dynamic areas of the face.

Introduction

There are numerous cosmetic procedures designed to treat facial lines and solar elastosis such as soft tissue fillers, neurotoxin injections, chemical peels, microdermabrasion, and ablative and non-ablative laser treatments. The understanding that hyperkinetic or dynamic musculature contributes to the etiology of facial rhytides [1, 2] has broadened the treatment options for these facial cosmetic blemishes. However, one single procedure may not adequately address all the issues that contribute to photoaging. For example, while neurotoxins may alleviate hyperkinetic facial lines such as crow's feet, horizontal forehead lines,

P.S. Yamauchi (✉)
Dermatology Institute and Skin Care Center, Santa Monica, CA, USA

David Geffen School of School of Medicine at UCLA, Los Angeles, CA, USA
e-mail: paulyamauchi@yahoo.com

C.C. Kim
Dermatology Institute and Skin Care Center, Santa Monica, CA, USA
e-mail: paulyamauchi@yahoo.com

M.A. Farage et al. (eds.), *Textbook of Aging Skin*,
DOI 10.1007/978-3-662-47398-6_152

and glabellar furrows, they do not address pigmentation and solar elastosis. Conversely, while laser resurfacing can correct lentigines and textural irregularities of the skin, the underlying cause of dynamic rhytides due to functional muscular contraction is not addressed. Frequently, combination therapy and not just one single therapy is necessary to achieve the desired results.

Various commercial type A botulinum toxins (BTX-A) are potent neurotoxins that irreversibly block presynaptic acetylcholine release and have been successfully utilized to correct facial spastic conditions such as blepharospasm, strabismus, focal dystonias, spasmodic dysphonia, and achalasia [3–5]. Consequently, many clinicians have noted improvement of facial rhytides in patients who received BTX-A for these spastic disorders. Indeed, Carruthers and Carruthers first noted improvement of glabellar frown lines while treating patients with blepharospasm [6].

Ablative skin resurfacing lasers provide significant improvement, rapid healing, and minimum complications in patients with mild to moderate facial wrinkling and scarring. They produce laser energy in a wavelength that gently penetrates the skin and scatters the heat effects of the laser light. There are several case reports and studies that examine of the effect of combination therapy with ablative laser resurfacing and the administration of BTX-A and the additive benefits derived from each type of treatment.

Combination Therapy with BTX-A and Laser Resurfacing

One objective of a single-center, prospective, randomized, placebo-controlled, paired comparison study was to compare the safety and efficacy of combining intramuscular injections of BTX-A with ablative laser resurfacing versus ablative laser resurfacing without BTX-A by substituting placebo intramuscular injections of saline in subjects with bilateral crow's feet [7].

Thirty-three patients with bilateral, symmetrical periorbital rhytides characterized by a minimum measurement of +2 during maximum attempted contraction were selected for the study. Female subjects who were pregnant, breastfeeding, or of childbearing potential and not practicing reliable method of birth control, patients with disorders or on agents that interfere with neuromuscular function, or subjects with profound atrophy or excessive weakness of the muscles in the target areas of injection were excluded from the study.

Study patients were randomized to receive placebo saline injections on one side of their face and 18 units of BTX-A on the contralateral side of their face. Two to six weeks postinjection, all study subjects received erbium:YAG laser resurfacing to both sides of crow's feet areas. Follow-up visits were scheduled at days 1 and 3 and weeks 1, 2, 4, 8, 12, 16, 20, and 24 post-laser resurfacing. At week 12, study subjects received a second injection of BTX-A (18 units) and placebo according to their random allocation at baseline. At the end of the 24 weeks, study subjects were given BTX-A (18 units) to both sides of their face.

Resurfacing was performed with the erbium: YAG laser at standardized laser settings of 4 Hz, 6 mm spot size, and 700 mJ. Three passes were performed periorbitally except for the upper eyelids where only one pass was done. A final pass at 500 mJ was performed at the outer edges of crow's feet for feathering.

A total of 33 female patients were enrolled in the study. Figure 1 demonstrates that at rest following laser resurfacing in both treatment groups, there was an increase in the percentage of patients with none to mild rhytides over the next 12 weeks. While laser resurfacing alone resulted in improvement of the rhytides in the placebo group, this trend was more evident in the BTX-A-treated group indicating that the combined therapy was more efficacious in reducing the rhytides at rest.

The results were more evident when rhytides were assessed during maximum contraction. Figure 2 shows that severe wrinkles were greatly reduced with BTX-A compared to the placebo group for up to 12 weeks.

Adjunctive therapy with BTX-A and laser resurfacing demonstrated a greater reduction in rhytides. Figure 3 shows photographs from one female patient who exhibited a greater improvement of crow's feet at rest with BTX-A versus the

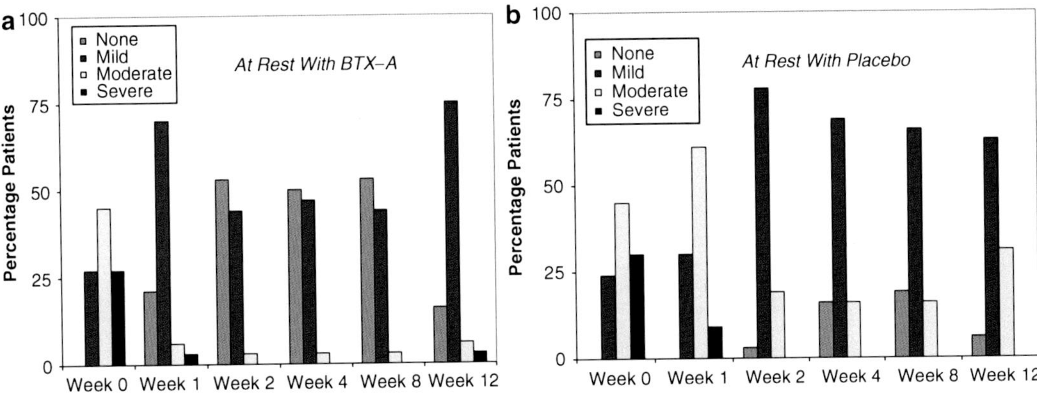

Fig. 1 Percentage of patients exhibiting none, mild, moderate, or severe rhytides at (**a**) rest during a 12-week interval treated with BTX-A (**b**) or placebo in conjunction with erbium:YAG laser resurfacing

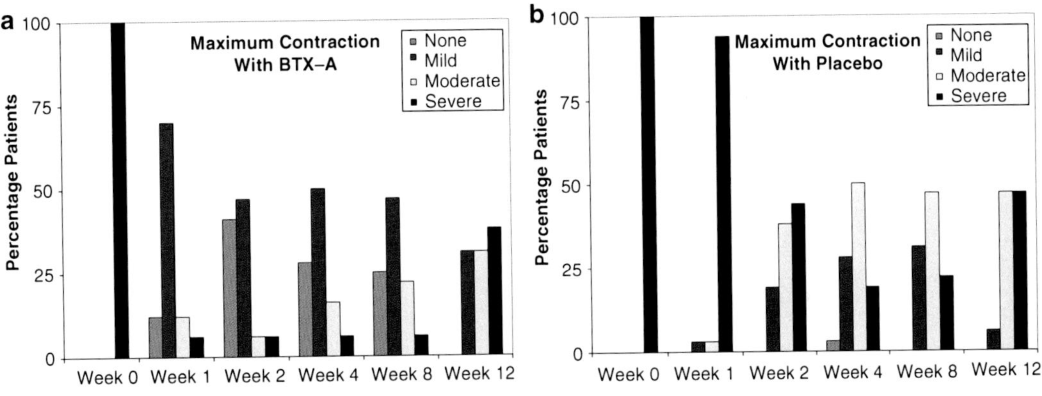

Fig. 2 Percentage of patients exhibiting none, mild, moderate, or severe rhytides at (**a**) maximal contraction during a 12-week interval treated with BTX-A or (**b**) placebo in conjunction with erbium:YAG laser resurfacing

placebo side in conjunction with erbium:YAG laser. Upon maximal contraction, the BTX-A-treated side had a clearer diminution of wrinkles. In addition, there was overall reversal of photodamage with a reduction of lentigines and improvement in skin texture. In combination with BOTOX®, there was greater enhancement of rejuvenation.

57.5 % (19/33) of patients reported at least one adverse event and the most common adverse events seen were pain on injection and bruising. There was no scarring, hyper- or hypopigmentation, blistering, or infections from the treatment. No serious adverse events occurred during this study.

This study demonstrated that erbium:YAG laser produces some reduction of periorbital rhytides both at rest and at maximum contraction at 12 weeks. In addition, erbium:YAG laser with Botox® produces higher reduction of periorbital rhytides at rest and at maximum contraction at 12 weeks. Combination therapy yields better reduction of dynamic wrinkles and also improves the texture of photodamaged skin.

In another study, 10 female subjects had one side of their face injected for their crow's feet, horizontal forehead furrows, and glabellar frown lines with BTX-A 1 week before undergoing laser treatment on both sides of the face with either a carbon dioxide or an erbium dual-mode laser [8].

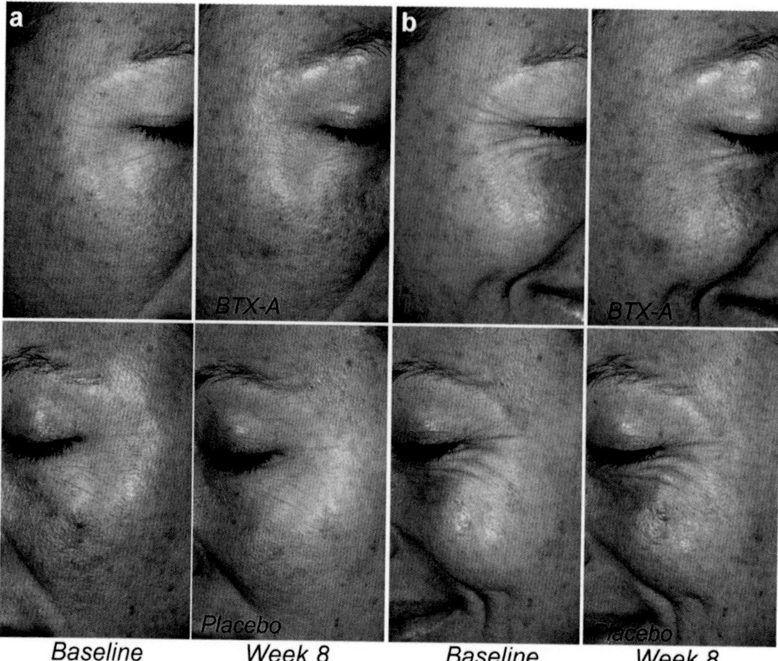

Fig. 3 Photograph of a female patient at baseline and 8 week at (**a**) rest and with (**b**) maximum contraction after treatment with BTX-A on the *right* face and placebo on the *left* face following erbium:YAG laser resurfacing

The target sites that were pretreated with BTX-A showed statistically significant visual improvement over the nontreated side, with crow's feet region showing the greatest improvement. The outcomes between the carbon dioxide and erbium lasers did not result in any statistically significant differences.

The purpose of another study was to evaluate the effect of BTX-A injections on movement-associated rhytides following cutaneous laser resurfacing [9]. Several patients who undergo CO2 laser resurfacing for correction of rhytides experience recurrence of movement-associated wrinkles within 6–12 months following the laser procedure. Forty patients who had received full-face CO2 laser resurfacing for the treatment of facial rhytides were randomized to receive BTX-A injections to the glabella, forehead, or lateral canthal regions or to receive no additional treatment. There was enhanced and more prolonged correction of forehead, glabellar, and/or lateral canthal rhytides observed in patients treated with BTX-A injections postoperatively compared to non-BTX-A-treated control patients. The use of BTX-A following CO2 laser resurfacing results in prolonged correction of movement-associated rhytides. It is advised that patients receive information regarding the benefits of maintenance therapy with botulinum toxin as part of their routine preoperative education.

A case report described the use of fractional resurfacing and fractionally ablative CO2 resurfacing in combination with BTX-A injections for the cheek area [10]. Injections of BTX-A were performed 1 day prior to the first fractional resurfacing session. Each cheek was treated with four injections that utilized approximately one unit of BTX-A in each injection. The distance between each BTX-A injection was approximately 1 cm. Significant improvement of the radiating rhytides was noted after the first laser treatment. This improvement increased after the second fractional resurfacing treatment and was enhanced slightly by a third treatment.

Discussion

The aforementioned case studies and reports have demonstrated that the combination utilization of BTX-A injections and laser resurfacing provides an added benefit than either one alone. BTX-A provides stability to the hyperkinetic facial lines by inhibiting the contraction of muscle groups in the areas treated that is not addressed by laser resurfacing. Conversely, laser resurfacing improves the texture and dyspigmentation of the skin caused by prolonged sun exposure that BTX-A injections do not correct. The recommendations from these studies are to pretreat the desired areas with BTX-A injections prior to laser resurfacing to improve outcomes. In addition, maintenance therapy with BTX-A injections is recommended to enhance and maintain the durability of the results attained by laser resurfacing.

References

1. Fagien S. BOTOX for the treatment of dynamic and hyperkinetic facial lines and furrows: adjunctive use in facial aesthetic surgery. Plast Reconstr Surg. 1999;103:701–13.
2. Pierard GE, Lapier CM. The microanatomical basis of facial frown lines. Arch Dermatol. 1989;125:1090–2.
3. Jankovic J, Brin MF. Therapeutic uses of botulinum toxin. N Engl J Med. 1991;324:1186–94.
4. Ward AB, Molenaers G, Colosimo C, Berardelli A. Clinical value of botulinum toxin in neurological indications. Eur J Neurol. 2006;4:20–6.
5. Simpson LL. Botulinum toxin: a deadly poison sheds its negative images. Ann Intern Med. 1996;125:616–7.
6. Carruthers JDA, Carruther JA. Treatment of glabellar frown lines with C. botulinum A exotoxin. J Dermatol Surg Oncol. 1991;18:17–21.
7. Yamauchi PS, Lask G, Lowe NJ. Botulinum toxin type A gives adjunctive benefit to periorbital laser resurfacing. J Cosmet Laser Ther. 2004;3:145–8.
8. Beer K, Waibel J. Botulinum toxin type A enhances the outcome of fractional resurfacing of the cheek. J Drugs Dermatol. 2007;11:1151–2.
9. Zimbler MS, Holds JB, Kokoska MS, Glaser DA, Prendiville S, Hollenbeak CS, Thomas JR. Effect of botulinum toxin pretreatment on laser resurfacing results: a prospective, randomized, blinded trial. Arch Facial Plast Surg. 2001;3:165–9.
10. West TB, Alster TS. Effect of botulinum toxin type A on movement-associated rhytides following CO2 laser resurfacing. Dermatol Surg. 1999;4:259–61.

Update on Asian Eyelid Anatomy and Periocular Aging Change

155

Preamjit Saonanon and Katherine M. Whipple

Contents

P. Saonanon (✉)
Department of Ophthalmology, King Chulalongkorn Memorial Hospital, The Thai Red Cross Society, Chulalongkorn University, Bangkok, Thailand
e-mail: drpreamjit@gmail.com

K.M. Whipple
Envision Eye and Aesthetics, Fairport, NY, USA
e-mail: whipplekatherine@yahoo.com

M.A. Farage et al. (eds.), *Textbook of Aging Skin*,
DOI 10.1007/978-3-662-47398-6_157

Abstract

This chapter discusses East and Southeast Asian eyelids and highlights the differences between Asian and Caucasian eyelids. Recent research focused on the Asian eyelid has led to improved understanding of its unique anatomy and notable precautions when performing surgery. The Asian eyelid can be categorized broadly into three types: single eyelid, low/partial eyelid crease, and double eyelid. Multiple factors such as dermal extension of levator aponeurosis and thickness of orbicularis oculi muscle are involved in eyelid crease formation. The presence of an epicanthal fold, the medial skin fold covering the inner corner of the eye, in Asian eye is extremely common. Redundant preseptal orbicularis oculi muscle causes the epicanthal fold. If removal of the epicanthal fold is desired, removing this portion of the orbicularis is necessary during epicanthoplasty. Unique periocular aging changes also occur in the Asian eyelid. Although rhytid formation is less common in Asian skin due to darker pigment and a thicker dermis, the eyelid is subjected to a greater amount of gravitational force due to increased weight of the soft tissue.

Introduction

The eyes are among the most important and recognizable areas of the face. Communication and expression is enhanced greatly with our eyelids and periocular area. Humans are able to be identified promptly by acquaintances from seeing his or her eyes and periocular area. Ethnicity is usually guessable by only seeing the eye area. Eyeball morphology is quite universal in all ethnicities with the exception of iris color. However, the eyelid varies greatly. A different external eyelid appearance is created by variations in each tissue layer, from skin composition to the orbital bones. As Asians are the nation's fastest growing ethnic group in the USA as of 2012, understanding of the differences between Asian and Caucasian eyelid is very important.

The eyelid is the key distinctive feature of the Asian eye. The most obvious characteristic of Asian eyelid is the absent or very low lid crease and fuller upper eyelid. When examining an Asian patient, the external appearance of Asian eyelid should be appreciated. In particular, three distinct portions of the eyelid should be noted. First, the medial part, whether the epicanthal fold is present and how severe the epicanthal fold is. Second, the central part, whether the eyelid crease is present. The central portion can be subcategorized into three types: single eyelid; low eyelid crease; and double eyelid. Third, the lateral part, where the lateral canthal tendon inserts to the orbital rim. Understanding these differences is the key to achieving optimal and reproducible surgical results while maintaining ethnic characteristics.

External Asian Eyelid Appearance

The average Asian male and female adult palpebral fissure is 27.0 ± 1.8 mm and 26.8 ± 1.7 mm in width, respectively, and 8.0 ± 1.0 mm and 8.2 ± 1.1 mm in height, respectively [1]. The stereotypical Asian eye has been described as seen in a famous Disney's character "Mulan," a single eyelid with an up-slant lateral angle and prominent epicanthal fold [2]. Ironically, only a minority of Asians possess this appearance. Previous articles in English and Chinese attempted to categorize the Asian eye, but none are universally accepted as all variations of Asian eye are not included. Asian eyes can be any shape (e.g., round, narrow, almond, triangular, slant, prominent, or deep set), but the absent or very low lid crease and fuller upper eyelid are almost always present. Narrower nasal lid contour is also common in Asian eye, in contrast to a medially or central lid peak in Caucasian [3]. The average Caucasian and Asian periorbital measurements and anatomical differences are summarized in Table 1.

The external appearance of Asian eyelid should be appreciated in three distinct parts:

1. Medial part: epicanthal fold
2. Central part: eyelid crease
3. Lateral part: lateral canthal angle

Medial Part: The Epicanthal Fold

Medial canthus is the inner corner of the eye. In Caucasians, a rounded medial canthal angle with total visualization of caruncle and plica semilunaris is ubiquitous. In Asians, the inner skin fold called the "epicanthal fold" covers the medial part of the eye, giving the illusion of a wider distance between eyes and causing the eye to look shorter horizontally [6]. Epicanthal fold also lowers the nasal lid contour compared to the temporal one [3]. In severe cases, epicanthal fold causes a decrease in overall palpebral fissure height. Prevalence of epicanthal fold in the general population has not been reported. However, single eyelid subjects almost always possess epicanthal fold, and around 50–90 % of general population in East and Southeast Asians possess a single eyelid. Therefore, prevalence of an epicanthal fold would likely be similar. Causative theories of epicanthal fold include:

- A low nasal bridge with less tenting effect.
- The oblique intermuscular fiber of the preseptal orbicularis oculi muscle attached to the skin [7].
- The preseptal orbicularis oculi arises more lateral than Caucasian counterparts and is not angled high enough to avoid overriding the pretarsal portion and the medial canthus [8].

Table 1 Differences between East/Southeast Asian and Caucasian eyelid character

	Asian	Caucasian
External appearance		
Medial part: epicanthal fold	Usually present	Usually none
Central part: eyelid crease Average height	None, partial, double 4–6 mm (male) 6–8 mm (female)	Double 6–8 mm (male) 8–10 mm (female)
Lateral part: lateral canthal angle	9.4° [4]	4.6° [4]
Horizontal palpebral fissure	27.2 ± 1.2 mm [1]	27–30 mm
Vertical palpebral fissure	8.5 ± 0.9 mm [1]	8–10 mm
Internal variation		
Skin	More melanin and thicker dermis	Less melanin
Orbicularis oculi	Thicker, form epicanthal fold and lower eyelid love band	Thinner
Superficial fat layer (SMFAT)	Well-formed	Less identifiable, often none
Orbital septum	Same	Same
Orbital fat	Descended preaponeurotic fat when eye open	Preaponeurotic fat retract when eye open
Eyelid retractor	Same	Same
Upper tarsal height	9.2 ± 0.8 mm	11.3 ± 1.7 mm [5]

Epicanthal fold is categorized into four types [9] (see Fig. 1):

1. Epicanthus tarsalis: epicanthal fold rising from the upper lid and merging into the skin near the medial canthus.
2. Epicanthus palpebralis: epicanthal fold covers the upper and lower lids equally across the medial canthus.
3. Epicanthus supraciliaris: epicanthal fold rises near the eyebrow and runs toward the tear trough area (not shown).
4. Epicanthus inversus: epicanthal fold rises from the lower lid and ascends into the upper lid over the medial canthus.

Epicanthus tarsalis and palpebralis are typical but not exclusive feature in Asians. Epicanthus supraciliaris and inversus are signs of congenital anomaly and not found in general population.

Severity of epicanthal fold can be graded as mild, moderate, and severe by degree of caruncular obliteration. Mild epicanthal fold means less than half of caruncle is covered and the width of the epicanthal fold is <2 mm. Moderate means more than half but not whole of caruncle is covered and the width of the epicanthal fold is 2–4 mm. Severe means no caruncle is visible and the width of epicanthal fold is >4 mm (see Fig. 2) [10].

Central Part: Eyelid Crease

The central part of the eyelid is categorized into three types (see Fig. 3): single eyelid, low/incomplete/partial eyelid crease, and double eyelid [1]. Double eyelid type then can be subcategorized based on eyelid crease morphology [10]. In the past, the single eyelid has been perceived as dull, tired, and less attractive. Therefore, the double eyelid crease procedure is among the most common cosmetic procedures performed in Asia.

An average eyelid crease height in Caucasian is 8–10 mm in female and 6–8 mm in male. An average Asian eyelid crease is 2 mm lower than Caucasian: 6–8 mm in females and 4–6 mm in

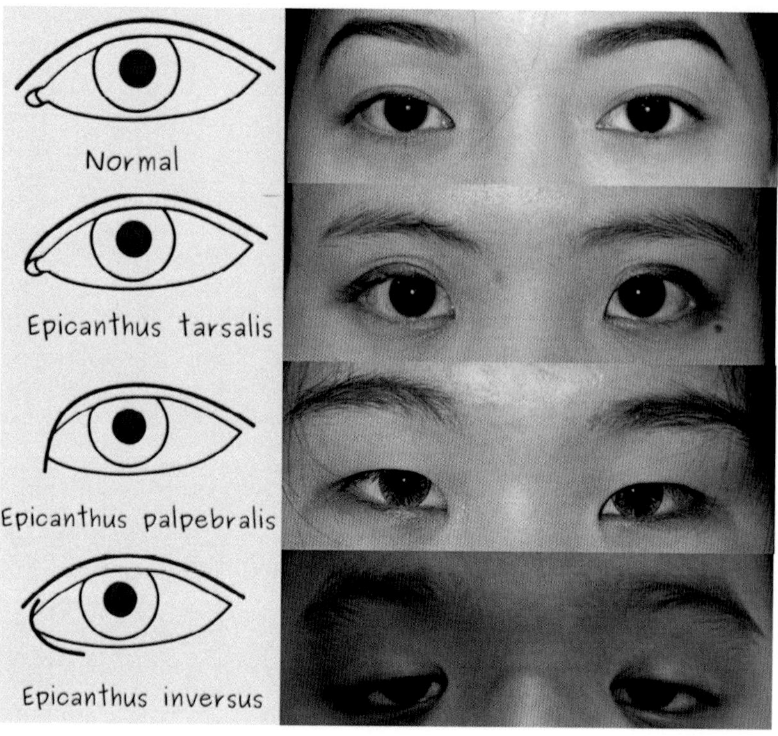

Fig. 1 Types of epicanthal fold

males [1]. Many theories in eyelid crease formation have been postulated but none scientifically proved. Studies in single and double eyelid fail to demonstrate significant differences between the two. Current evidence suggests multiple factors are responsible for eyelid crease formation [8]. Factors involved in eyelid crease formation include:

- The levator expansion theory: the levator aponeurosis penetrating orbital septum and orbicularis oculi muscle giving rise to the dermal extension [11]. When the eye opens, the levator palpebrae superioris contracts and transmits force through the levator aponeurosis. Then, the dermal extension of levator aponeurosis pulls the eyelid skin and creates the eyelid crease. It may also play a role in the everted position of the eye lashes [12, 13]. This theory is among the most popular; however, a later study found the dermal extension fiber in single eyelid subject as well [14].
- The width and tightness of the skin-orbicularis-tarsus complex: a single tight unit is needed. At the lid margin, the tarsus serves as the structural support of the eyelid. In double eyelid, strong attachment of all tissue layers to the tarsus is evidenced. When the eye open, all tissue layers are pulled up together as a single unit and the eyelid crease is created above the tarsus. In single eyelid, the skin and orbicularis muscle slip down along the rising tarsal plate and no eyelid crease is created [15].
- The thickness of orbicularis oculi muscle: thinner orbicularis oculi is found in double eyelid group [14]. Increased thickness of orbicularis oculi muscle is proposed to bar eyelid crease formation.
- Decreased lifting force from levator aponeurosis: less lifting force due to descended preaponeurotic fat or the existence of the lower-positioned transverse ligament is evidenced in single eyelid. Descended preaponeurotic fat during eye open was present

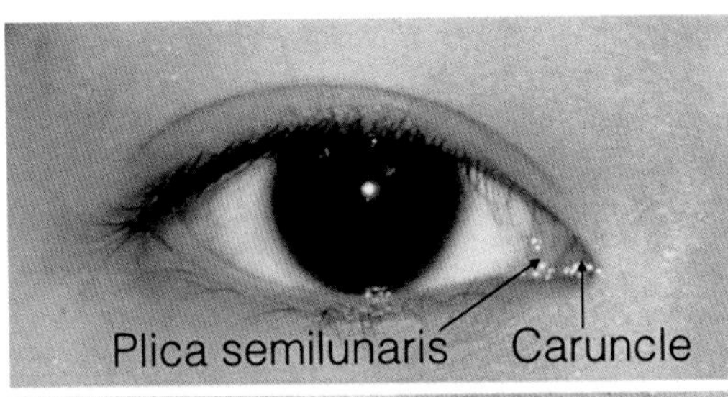

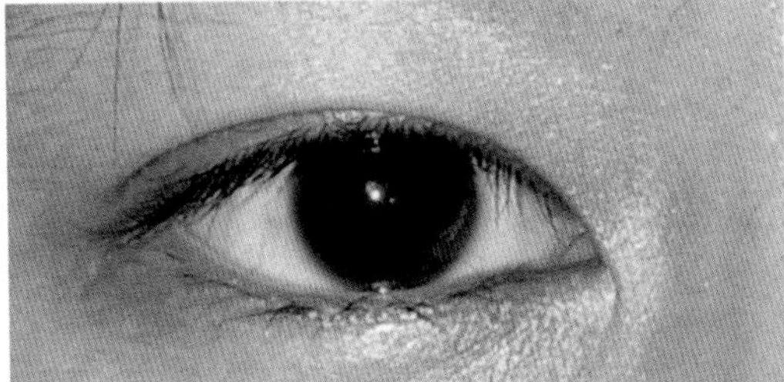

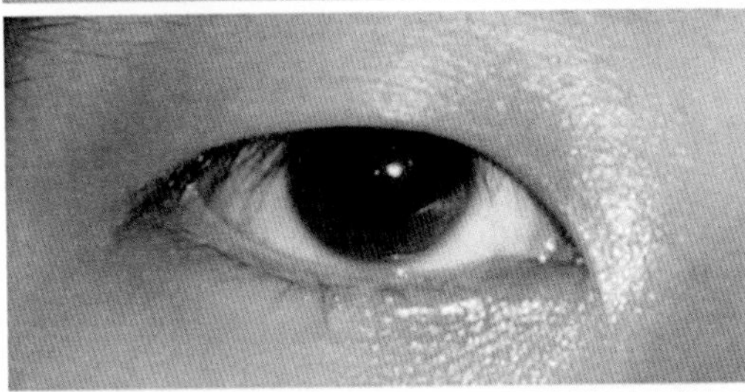

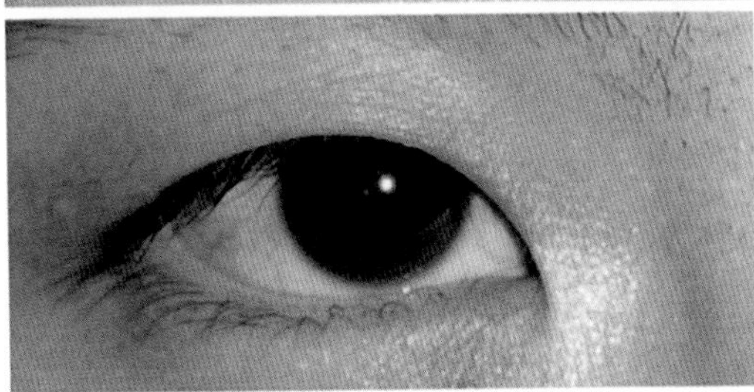

Fig. 2 Severity of epicanthal fold. Mild epicanthal fold means less than half of caruncle is covered (*top*). Moderate means more than half of caruncle is covered (*middle*). Severe means no caruncle is visible (*bottom*)

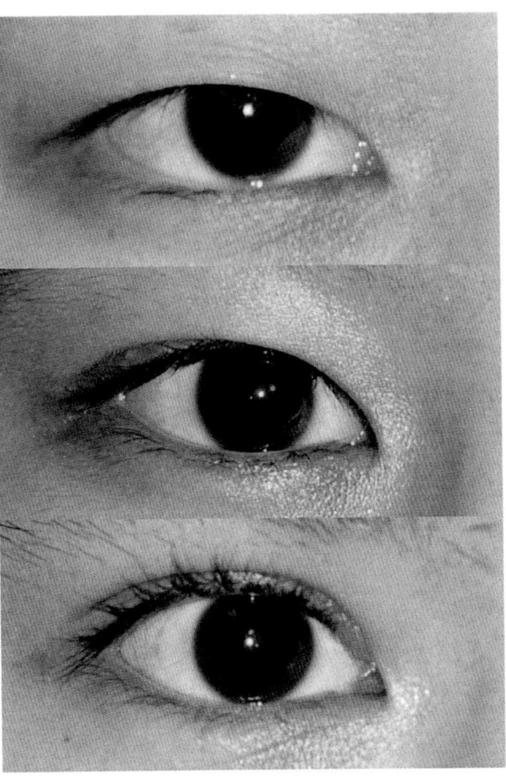

Fig. 3 Types of Asian eyelid. Asian eyelid was categorized into three types: single eyelid (*top*), low eyelid crease (*middle*), and double eyelid (*bottom*)

in the single eyelid as opposed to its deeper position in the orbit of a double eyelid. This herniated fat interferes with levator lifting force and crease formation [16]. Another factor contributing to the decreased lifting force of the levator aponeurosis is the lower-positioned transverse ligament, a structure above the line of fusion of the orbital septum and the levator aponeurosis [17]. This ligament is well-developed exclusively in the single eyelid and is believed to antagonize levator function. Severing of this ligament is recommended when performing blepharoplasty to allow further excursion of the upper eyelid [18].

Lateral Part: Lateral Canthal Angle

The lateral canthal tendon attaches upper and lower tarsus to the inner aspect of the lateral orbital rim. The lateral canthal angle is usually appreciated by comparing its height with the medial canthus. By comparing, the lateral canthal angle can be categorized into three types: up-slant, parallel, and down-slant eye. Majority of Asians possess an up-slant eye with an average of 9.4°

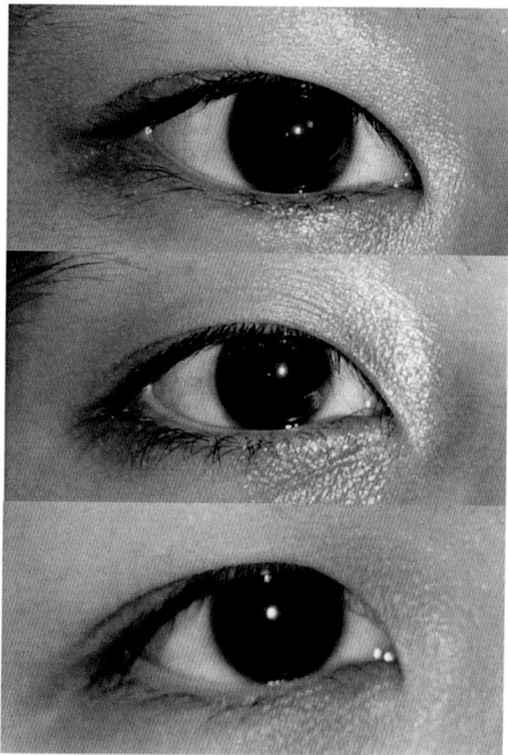

Fig. 4 Type of lateral canthal angle. Lateral canthal angle can be categorized by comparing its height with the medial canthus: up-slant (*top*), parallel (*middle*), and down-slant eye (*bottom*)

upward lateral canthus [4]. The Caucasians tend to be more parallel with an average of 4.6° upward [4]. Excessive up-slant is known as "mongoloid slant," found in a number of syndrome, e.g., Down's syndrome. Down-slant or anti-mongoloid slant can be found periodically in general Asian population (see Fig. 4).

Layer by Layer Anatomical Variation

Bony Orbit

Mean orbital volume was 26.0 and 23.3 mL in Asian male and female subjects, respectively, and was 25.6 mL in Caucasians [19, 20]. When comparing entrance height and width, the shape of Asian and Caucasian orbits was similar [20, 21]. Nevertheless, the shape of the orbit has a role in ethnic identity in forensic anthropology. In a front view, Asians tend to have a taller, more circular shape, whereas Caucasians tend to have a square shape orbit. In a lateral view, Caucasians possess more prominent superior rim and deeper lateral rim [22]. The relationship between the globe and the orbital rim makes the Caucasian eye more dimensional with a higher and deeper eyelid crease.

Eyelid

The eyelid is a complex structure and can be divided into the following eight structural layers. Figure 5 shows diagram of Asian upper eyelid:

- Skin and subcutaneous tissue
- Orbicularis oculi muscle
- Superficial fat layer
- Orbital septum
- Orbital fat
- Eyelid retractor
- Tarsus
- Conjunctiva

Skin

The eyelid skin is the thinnest skin in the body with range of thickness of 0.3–1 mm from the thinnest part at eyelid margin to the thickest part just below eyebrow [23]. The thickness remains constant with age. The eyelid aging process was evident as solar elastosis.

The Orbicularis Oculi

The orbicularis oculi, innervated by CN VII, is divided into palpebral (subdivided into pretarsal and preseptal) and orbital parts. The palpebral part functions in involuntary blinking. The orbital portion is responsible for forceful eyelid closure. The orbicularis oculi originates and inserts mainly from medial canthal tendon. When comparing with Caucasians, Asian orbicularis oculi tends to be thicker. This leads to two noteworthy external appearances:

1. The hypertrophy of the pretarsal orbicularis oculi in the lower eyelid creates dynamic under-eye bulges, sometimes referred to

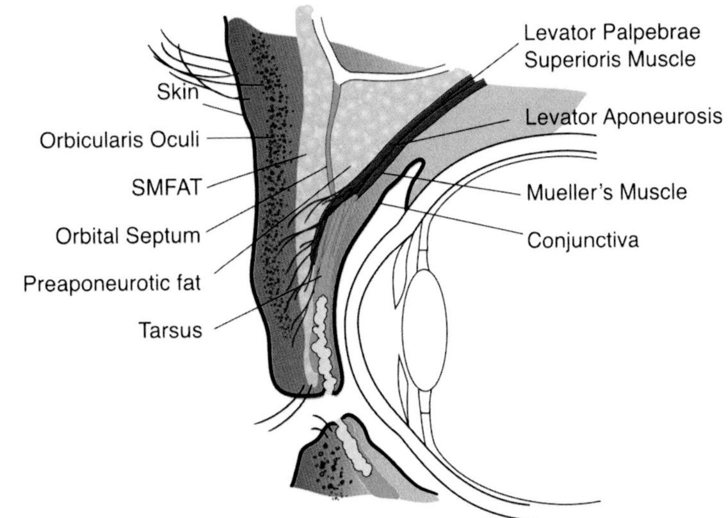

Fig. 5 Diagram of Asian upper eyelid. The submuscularis fibroadipose tissue (SMFAT) extends down to pretarsal area. The levator muscle divides into superior and inferior division before transitions into levator aponeurosis and Mueller's muscle

anecdotally as the love band, charming eye, or smiley eye. This muscle hypertrophy becomes more prominent when one smiles and creates a cuter, younger look [24].

2. The epicanthal fold, as discuss earlier [7].

Orbicularis muscle volume does not change with age but dynamic wrinkles are created. Crow's feet or rhytids at the lateral canthus are often seen during the smile but become static with age and photodamage to the skin.

The Superficial Fat Layer

Submuscular fibroadipose tissue (SMFAT) lies between the orbicularis oculi and orbital septum as shown in Fig. 6. This fat layer is well formed exclusively in Asian and causes a puffier look of the eyelid [25, 26]. The SMFAT continues beyond arcus marginalis as retro-orbicularis oculi fat (ROOF) in the upper eyelid and sub-orbicularis oculi fat (SOOF) in the lower eyelid. The ROOF extends beneath the frontalis muscle as part of the galeal fat pad, causing lateral hooding of the upper eyelid in aging as the lid descends secondary to gravity. Excision of this tissue layer is almost always recommended during Asian blepharoplasty and double eyelid procedure.

The Orbital Septum

A sheet of fibrous tissue arises from the orbital periosteum, i.e., the periorbita. The orbital septum fuses with levator aponeurosis approximately 5 mm above superior tarsal border [27]. This fibrous layer serves as a barrier preventing orbital contents from bulging and infections from spreading, among others. Weakening and stretching of orbital septum, as occurs in the aging process, allows preaponeurotic fat to bulge anteriorly, causing medial fat protrusion in the upper eyelid and the dreaded "under-eye bags" in the lower lid.

Preaponeurotic Fat/Extraconal Orbital Fat

There are two fat pads in the upper eyelid, the central and the medial fat pads. These fat pads are found posterior to the orbital septum and anterior to the levator aponeurosis, leading to its name, the "preaponeurotic fat." The preaponeurotic fat is the important surgical landmark in blepharoptosis repair to identify the levator aponeurosis. With aging, the medial fat pad becomes prominent whereas the central fat pad atrophies. Trimming of the medial fat while preserving the central one is recommended in modern upper blepharoplasty [28].

In the lower eyelid, there are three fat pads: the medial, central, and lateral. These lower fat pads' volume increased until the 60 years of age and then decreased in both male and female groups [29]. Protrusion of the lower fat pads and descent of the malar fat pads create the appearance of a baggy eyelid. Repositioning and occasionally

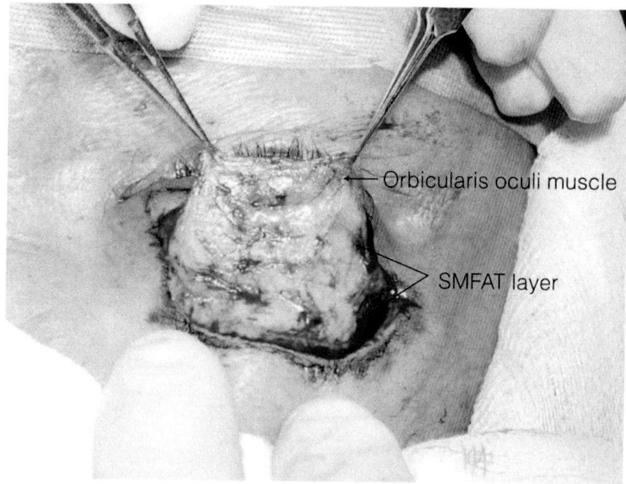

Fig. 6 Submuscularis fibroadipose tissue (SMFAT). Preseptal orbicularis oculi was dissected and reflexed down to show SMFAT layer

minor excision of the lower fat pads are the main step of the lower eyelid blepharoplasty.

Eyelid Retractors

There are four retractor muscles in the eyelid: the levator palpebrae superioris and Mueller's muscle in the upper eyelid and the capsulopalpebral fascia and the inferior tarsal muscle in the lower eyelid.

The Upper Lid Retractor

1. The levator palpebrae superioris: Innervated by superior division of CN III. Originates from orbital apex and distally gives rise to two lamellas below Whitnall's ligament: the anterior lamella which becomes the levator aponeurosis and the posterior lamella which becomes Mueller's muscle [30]. Medially and laterally, the aponeurosis expands transversely and forms the weaker medial and the stronger lateral horn, respectively [31].
2. Mueller's muscle: Innervated by sympathetic nervous system. Originates from levator palpebrae superioris at Whitnall's ligament and extends inferiorly to insert along the superior tarsal margin via its tendon and functions to aid in lifting the tarsus.

The Lower Lid Retractor

3. Capsulopalpebral fascia: The analog of levator aponeurosis in the lower eyelid. Arises from inferior rectus and inferior oblique muscle.
4. Inferior tarsal muscle: The analog of Mueller's muscle in the lower eyelid.

The upper lid retractors were thought to be thinner and smaller in Asian eye but studies proved similar shape and thickness comparing to previous studies in Caucasians [32]. Smaller vertical palpebral fissure in the Asian eye is not due to smaller upper lid retractors but caused by surrounding soft tissue that weakens the levator force (discuss earlier). To open the eye, the double eyelid structure with eyelid crease is also more labor saving than single eyelid [14].

The Tarsus

The tarsus is a dense trapezoid plate of connective tissue that serves as the structural support of the eyelid. The tarsus attaches to the periosteum through the medial and lateral canthal tendons. In Caucasian, the upper and lower eyelid tarsus height is 10–12 mm and 4–5 mm, respectively. An average upper tarsus height was significantly shorter in Asians (11.3 ± 1.7 mm in Caucasian vs. 9.2 ± 0.8 mm in Asians; $p < 0.05$) [5]. However, the lower eyelid tarsus heights were not significantly different.

There are three distinct morphological categories of upper eyelid tarsus in Asians: the sickle (55.6 %), round upper margin and short height; the triangular (29.6 %), the narrow upper margin with longer height; and the trapezoid (16.7 %), the flat upper margin with long height [33].

Conjunctiva

The conjunctiva is a nonkeratinizing squamous epithelium layer that covers the eyeball. It is divided into bulbar part which covers the eyeball and palpebral part which forms the most posterior layer of the eyelid.

Aging Changes Around the Eye

The aging process in the eye area is among the most prominent and frustrated areas. Contemporary words to describe facial aging include "descent and deflation." Loss of facial volume, especially the subcutaneous and superficial fat layers, combined with tissue laxity causes the typical involutional changes of the face. Periocular aging changes include rhytid formation, droopiness of the eyelid, and protrusion of inferior eyelid fat. Although Asian skin ages more gracefully due to darker pigment and thicker dermis, the eyelid contour is subjected to a greater amount of gravitational force due to heavier soft tissue. Puffiness and bulginess of the eyelid, both upper and lower, are present earlier and become more prominent with age [34].

Periocular area includes the eyebrow superiorly and the midface inferiorly. Upper eyelid-eyebrow complex and lower eyelid-midface complex should always be evaluated and managed concurrently as a single confluent unit [35].

There are three main factors of environmentally induced periocular aging change: photoaging, gravitational force, and facial expression.

1. Photoaging

   Photoaging causes skin texture and color change. Most Asians become bothered by this by their fifth decade and the predominant complaint is with skin pigmentation. Less wrinkles are noted as Asian skin has stronger natural defense mechanisms against UV exposure account to more melanin pigment and thicker dermis. In addition, most Asians habitually avoid sun exposure as they prefer light rather than tan skin color.

2. Gravitational force and tissue laxity

   Periocular soft tissue sags down from a combination of gravity and degenerative changes. On the upper eyelid, it may evidence as brow ptosis, dermatochalasis, and blepharoptosis [36]. Decrease in marginal reflex distance and palpebral fissure height especially in temporal sector is evident as aging occur in Asians [3]. This change seems to affect women more than men.

   - Brow ptosis, or drooping of the forehead and eyebrow, is caused by stretching and degenerative changes of the forehead area. In most females, the brow is arch shape and located above the superior orbital rim. In males, the brow is more straight and lower, usually positioned at the superior orbital rim. The brow is considered ptotic when it falls below the superior orbital rim. Temporal brow ptosis is common in elders as frontalis muscle thins laterally. Asymmetrical brow ptosis should be noted and causes for asymmetry, especially CN VII palsy, should be investigated.

   Surgical correction: Brow ptosis surgery can be performed by various approaches but can be broadly categorized into external and endoscopic approaches (see Fig. 7). External approaches include direct brow lift and midforehead, pretrichial, and coronal brow lift. Due to visible surgical scar, most external approaches are preferred only in functional brow ptosis.

   - Dermatochalasis refers to redundancy of eyelid skin. Dermatochalasis may become severe and block superior vision. Upper blepharoplasty can be performed for functional purposes when more than 30° of superior visual field is blocked or skin is redundant enough to compress the eyelashes [37]. Bulging of orbital fat is usually present concurrently and can be excised during corrective procedure.

   Surgical correction: Dermatochalasis can be managed by upper blepharoplasty to remove excessive skin. In Asian eye, double eyelid can be created simultaneously by performing eyelid crease fixation procedure [38] (see Fig. 8).

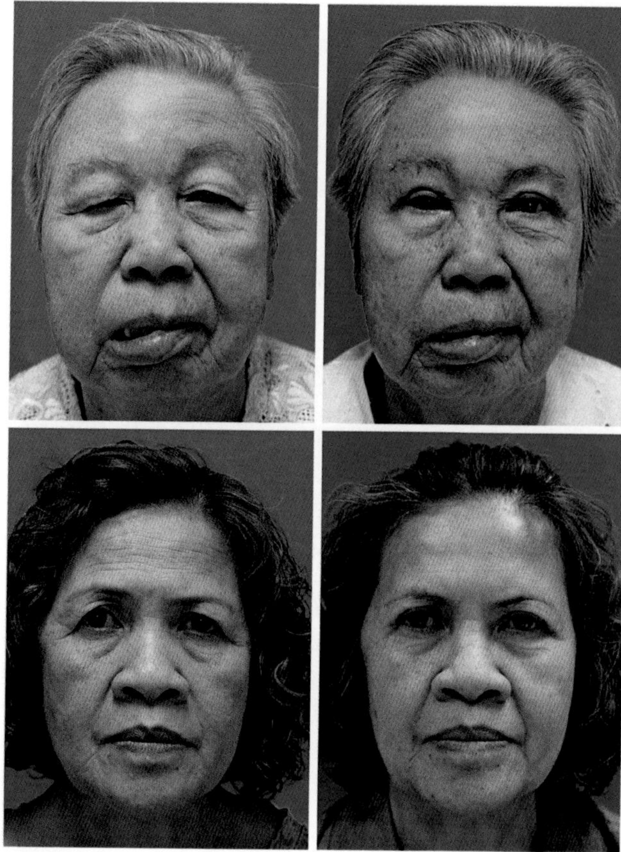

Fig. 7 Direct and endoscopic brow lift. Patient with severe brow ptosis from long standing CN VII palsy pre-operation (*upper left*) and post direct brow lift of the right eye and bilateral upper blepharoplasty (*upper right*). Patient with brow ptosis and dermatochalasis pre-operation (*lower left*) and post endoscopic brow lift and bilateral upper blepharoplasty (*lower right*)

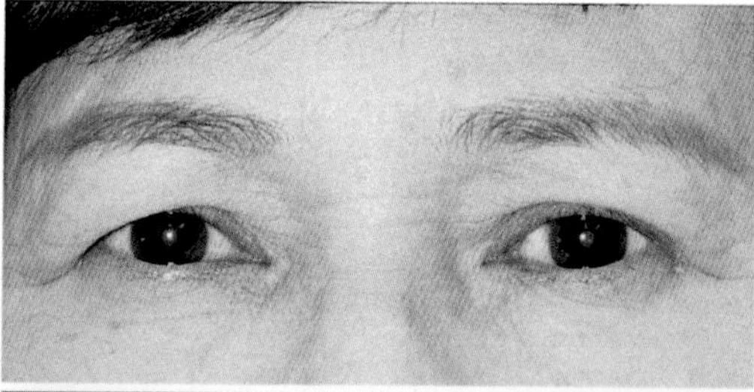

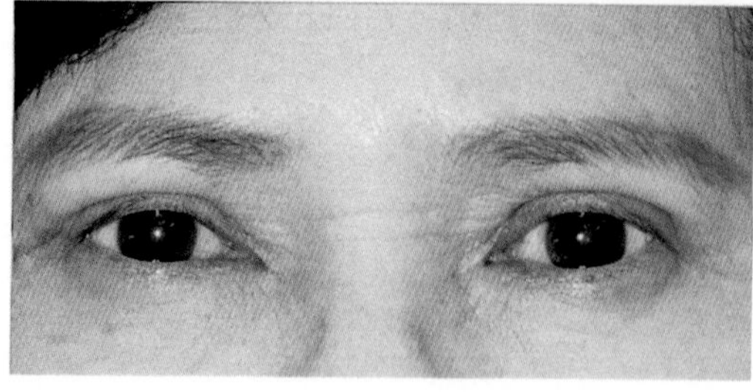

Fig. 8 Dermatochalasis, excessive skin of the upper eyelid. Pre and post upper blepharoplasty. Noted that the distance from the upper eyelid margin to the corneal light reflex in primary position is normal

- Blepharoptosis or ptosis is drooping of the eyelid. Levator palpebrae superioris opens the eye by transmitting its force through levator aponeurosis. Stretching or disinsertion of levator aponeurosis causes aponeurotic ptosis, the most common form of ptosis. Blepharoptosis is diagnosed when the distance from the upper eyelid margin to the corneal light reflex in primary position is less than normal. Normal range varies depending on ethnic: 4–5 mm in Caucasian and 3–4 mm in Asian. Blepharoptosis is usually diagnosed when the number is less than 2.0–2.5 mm [36].

Surgical correction: Blepharoptosis has to be managed by eyelid retractor muscle strengthening procedure. For aponeurotic ptosis, most common procedures are levator

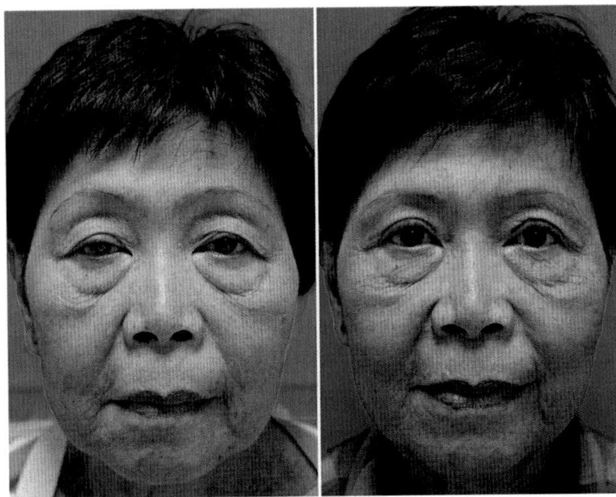

Fig. 9 Aponeurotic blepharoptosis, drooping of the eyelid. Noted that the distance from the right upper eyelid margin to the corneal light reflex in primary position is lower than normal. Pre and post external levator advancement of the right eye and bilateral upper blepharoplasty

advancement and conjunctivo-mullerectomy. In levator advancement, part of levator aponeurosis is resected and shortened aponeurosis is reattached to the tarsus [39] (see Fig. 9). Conjunctivo-mullerectomy removes part of Mueller's muscle to strengthen its force [40]. Managing blepharoptosis patient with blepharoplasty will result in unnatural high eyelid crease and more senile appearance.

On the lower eyelid, changes can be evidenced as baggy eyelid and double convexity deformity.

- Baggy eyelids are caused by prolapse of orbital fat pad. With aging, the orbital septum stretches, bulges, or dehisces, allowing fat to prolapse anteriorly. Lower eyelid orbital fat pad volume also increases with age, making baggy eyelid more prominent [29].

Surgical correction: Baggy eyelid can be managed by lower blepharoplasty. Repositioning and occasional excision of bulging fat are the main steps of the lower eyelid blepharoplasty. Transcutaneous approach was traditionally used but the transconjunctival approach is now preferred by most cosmetic surgeons. In the transconjunctival approach, there is less likely to have complications, such as eyelid retraction. Additionally, no skin scarring is another advantage of the transconjunctival approach [41].

- Double convexity deformity is the combination of baggy eyelid and descending midface. Drooping malar fat pad produces the skeletonization of the inferior orbital rim. Hollowness of the inferior orbital rim between prominence baggy eyelid fat and bulge of descending malar fat develops deep orbital sulcus called double convexity deformity.

Surgical correction: Lysis of orbitomalar ligament and midface lift can be performed concurrently with lower blepharoplasty. Orbital fat transposition or liposuction with fat injection procedure will alleviate deep orbital sulcus and smoothen lower lid-cheek junction area [42] (see Fig. 10).

3. Facial expression

Movement of facial muscle expression may cause overlying skin rhytids with time. Rhytids only noticed during facial movement are called dynamic wrinkles. Creases and lines that are present without facial expression are termed static wrinkles. Static wrinkles occur with photodamage and as collagen and elastin fiber of the dermis break down. Asians tend to have rhytid formation later in life and to a milder degree than Caucasians.

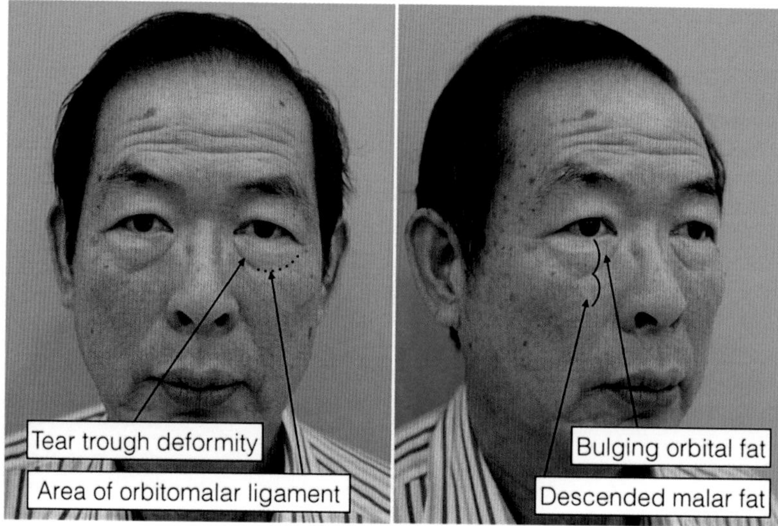

Fig. 10 Double convexity deformity. Hollowness of the inferior orbital rim between prominence baggy eyelid fat and bulge of descending malar fat develops deep orbital sulcus

Conclusion

The East and Southeast Asian population presents exciting and interesting eyelid and periocular variations that are unique. Intimate understanding of its anatomy is imperative for surgeons operating on this population. The most obvious characteristic of Asian eye is the absent or very low lid crease and fuller upper eyelid. Upper eyelid morphology should be appreciated separately into three parts: medial, central, and lateral. The submuscular fibroadipose tissue is well formed exclusively in Asian eyelid and causes fuller eyelid. More than one factor is responsible for eyelid crease formation; familiarity with all components is critical to the success of Asian eyelid surgery.

References

1. Liu D, Hsu WM. Oriental eyelids. Anatomic difference and surgical consideration. Ophthal Plast Reconstr Surg. 1986;2:59–64.
2. Chen WP. Asian blepharoplasty. Ophthal Plast Reconstr Surg. 1987;3:135–40.
3. Lee H, Lee JS, Chang M, et al. Analysis of lid contour change with aging in Asians by measuring midpupil lid distance. Plast Reconstr Surg. 2014;134:521.
4. Hanada AL, de Souza Jr EN, Moribe I, et al. Comparison of palpebral fissure obliquity in three different racial groups. Ophthal Plast Reconstr Surg. 2001;17:423–6.
5. Kakisaki H, Goold LA, Casson RJ, et al. Tarsal height. Ophthalmology. 2009;116:1831.
6. Wu XS, Jian XC, He ZJ, et al. Investigation of anthropometric measurements of anatomic structures of orbital soft tissue in 102 young Han Chinese adults. Ophthal Plast Reconstr Surg. 2010;26:339–43.
7. Kakizaki H, Ichinose A, Nakano T, et al. Anatomy of the epicanthal fold. Plast Reconstr Surg. 2012;130:494e–5.
8. Saonanon P. Update on Asian eyelid anatomy and clinical relevance. Curr Opin Ophthalmol. 2014;25:436–42.
9. Johnson CC. Epicanthus. Am J Ophthalmol. 1968;66:939e46.
10. Wang S, Shi F, Luo X, et al. Epicanthal fold correction: our experience and comparison among three kinds of epicanthoplasties. J Plast Reconstr Aesthet Surg. 2013;66:682–7.
11. Sayoc BT. Absence of superior palpebral fold in slit eyes; an anatomic and physiologic explanation. Am J Ophthalmol. 1956;42:298–300.
12. Malik KJ, Lee MS, Park DJ, et al. Lash ptosis in congenital and acquired blepharoptosis. Arch Ophthalmol. 2007;125:1613–5.
13. Lee TE, Lee JM, Lee H, et al. Lash ptosis and associated factors in Asians. Ann Plast Surg. 2010;65:407–10.
14. Kakizaki H, Takahashi Y, Nakano T, et al. The causative factors or characteristics of the Asian double eyelid: an anatomic study. Ophthal Plast Reconstr Surg. 2012;28:376–81.
15. Zhu L, Chen X. Mechanical analysis of eyelid morphology. Acta Biomater. 2013;9:7968–76.
16. Miyake I, Tange I, Hiraga Y. MRI findings of the upper eyelid and their relationship with single- and double-eyelid formation. Aesthetic Plast Surg. 1994;18:183–7.
17. Yuzuriha S, Matsuo K, Kushima H. An anatomical structure which results in puffiness of the upper eyelid

and a narrow palpebral fissure in the Mongoloid eye. Br J Plast Surg. 2000;53:466–72.
18. Ban M, Matsuo K, Ban R, et al. Developed lower-positioned transverse ligament restricts eyelid opening and folding and determines Japanese as being with or without visible superior palpebral crease. Eplasty. 2013;13:289–98.
19. Kwon J, Barrera JE, Most SP. Comparative computation of orbital volume from axial and coronal CT using three-dimensional image analysis. Ophthal Plast Reconstr Surg. 2010;26:26–9.
20. Ji Y, Qian Z, Dong Y, et al. Quantitative morphometry of the orbit in Chinese adults based on a three-dimensional reconstruction method. J Anat. 2010;217:501–6.
21. Weaver AA, Loftis KL, Tan JC, et al. CT based three-dimensional measurement of orbit and eye anthropometry. Invest Ophthalmol Vis Sci. 2010;51:4892–7.
22. Xing S, Gibbon V, Clarke R, et al. Geometric morphometric analyses of orbit shape in Asian, African, and European human populations. Anthropol Sci. 2013;121:1–11.
23. Hwang K, Kim DJ, Hwang SH. Thickness of Korean upper eyelid skin at different levels. J Craniofac Surg. 2006;17:54–6.
24. Chen MC, Ma H, Liao WC. Anthropometry of pretarsal fullness and eyelids in oriental women. Aesthetic Plast Surg. 2013;37:617–24.
25. Ichinose A, Tahara S. Extended preseptal fat resection in Asian blepharoplasty. Ann Plast Surg. 2008;60:121–6.
26. Chen WP. Concept of triangular, trapezoidal, and rectangular debulking of eyelid tissues: application in Asian blepharoplasty. Plast Reconstr Surg. 1996;97:212–8.
27. Kakizaki H, Leibovitch I, Selva D, et al. Orbital septum attachment on the levator aponeurosis in Asians: in vivo and cadaver study. Ophthalmology. 2009;116:2031–5.
28. Oh SR, Chokthaweesak W, Annunziata CC, et al. Analysis of eyelid fat pad changes with aging. Ophthal Plast Reconstr Surg. 2011;27:348–51.
29. Lee JM, Lee H, Park M, et al. The volumetric change of orbital fat with age in Asians. Ann Plast Surg. 2011;66:192–5.
30. Kakizaki H, Prabhakaran V, Pradeep T, et al. Peripheral branching of levator superioris muscle and Müller muscle origin. Am J Ophthalmol. 2009;148:800–3.
31. Kakizaki H, Zako M, Ide A, et al. Causes of undercorrection of medial palpebral fissures in blepharoptosis surgery. Ophthal Plast Reconstr Surg. 2004;20:198–201.
32. Hwang K, Huan F, Kim DJ, et al. Size of the superior palpebral involuntary muscle (Müller muscle). J Craniofac Surg. 2010;21:1626–9.
33. Nagasao T, Shimizu Y, Ding W, et al. Morphological analysis of the upper eyelid tarsus in Asians. Ann Plast Surg. 2011;66:196–201.
34. Shirakabe Y, Suzuki Y, Lam SM. A new paradigm for the aging Asian face. Aesthetic Plast Surg. 2003;27:397–402.
35. Lam SM, Chang EW, Rhee JS, et al. Perspective: rejuvenation of the periocular region: a unified approach to the eyebrow, midface, and eyelid complex. Ophthal Plast Reconstr Surg. 2004;20:1–9.
36. John BH, editor. Basic and clinical science course section 7: orbit, eyelid and lacrimal system. San Francisco: American Academy of Ophthalmology; 2013.
37. Bajric J, Levin JJ, Bartley GB, et al. Patient and physician perceptions of medicare reimbursement policy for blepharoplasty and blepharoptosis surgery. Ophthalmology. 2014;121:1475–9.
38. Chen WP, Park JD. Asian upper lid blepharoplasty: an update on indications and technique. Facial Plast Surg. 2013;29:26–31.
39. Ben Simon GJ, Lee S, Schwarcz RM, et al. External levator advancement vs. Muller's muscle-conjunctival resection for correction of upper eyelid involutional ptosis. Am J Ophthalmol. 2005;140:426–32.
40. Putterman AM, Fett DR. Muller's muscle in the treatment of upper eyelid ptosis: a ten-year study. Ophthalmic Surg. 1986;17:354–60.
41. Fagien S, Putterman AM. Putterman's cosmetic oculoplastic surgery. In: Putterman AM, editor. Transconjunctival approach to resection of lower eyelid herniated orbital fat. 4th ed. Philadelphia: Saunders; 2008.
42. Korn BS, Kikkawa DO, Cohen SR. Transcutaneous lower eyelid blepharoplasty with orbitomalar suspension: retrospective review of 212 consecutive cases. Plast Reconstr Surg. 2010;125:315–23.

Part XVI

Mind/Skin/Body Interaction

Unified Mind/Body for a Healthy Aging Skin

156

Miranda A. Farage, Kenneth W. Miller, Gabe Tzeghai, and Howard I. Maibach

Contents

Gabe Tzeghai has retired.

M.A. Farage (✉)
Winton Hill Business Center, The Procter & Gamble Company, Cincinnati, OH, USA
e-mail: farage.m@pg.com

K.W. Miller
Margoshes-Miller Consulting, LLC, Cincinnati, OH, USA
e-mail: miller.kw.1@pg.com; bbbns2@fuse.net

G. Tzeghai
Wyoming, OH, USA
e-mail: gtzeghai@cinci.rr.com

H.I. Maibach
Department of Dermatology, University of California, San Francisco, CA, USA

M.A. Farage et al. (eds.), *Textbook of Aging Skin*,
DOI 10.1007/978-3-662-47398-6_110

Abstract
One of the most troublesome organ systems in old age, causing both physical and psychosocial discomfort, is the skin. The elderly usually have at least one skin disease if not several. This review focuses on mind–body interactions and interventions in skin disease in old age. Aging is affected by many factors, including the individual's genetic foundation, environmental insult, nutrition, exercise, disease, and injury, as well as psychosocial factors that create stress. Mind–body interactions are an integral part of the aging process. The mind/body connection, once mysterious, is increasingly recognized as a complex web of neurological, immunological, and endocrine actions which modulate the function of a more basic web of effectors that provide a communication network among body systems. Recognition of the effects of psychosocial stress in the development of skin complaints of the elderly but also in all other medical complaints can only lay the foundation for better treatments.

Introduction

Western medicine has historically been conceptualized as a series of silos, i.e., a whole consisting of individual disparate body systems with well-defined boundaries and little relevant interaction. This model, however, ignores the myriad interactive functions that each system requires and hinders understanding of syndromes for which etiology is not confined to one organ system, particularly those with a strong psychosocial component. In addition, this model is increasingly shown to be antiquated. Evidence is rapidly accumulating that the human body is a sophisticated, inalienable whole, a complex web of neurological, immunologic, and endocrine interactions that in turn modulate a fluid epigenetic base, namely, evidence of Pavlovian conditioning of physiological processes (i.e., placebo and nocebo effects) [1], immune system conditioning [1], physiological distinctions between multiple personalities [1], and inexplicable clustering of seemingly unrelated diseases, with each increasing risk for onset of the others. For example, psoriasis – a skin disease – increases risk for a host of comorbidities related to metabolic syndrome, including chronic pulmonary disease, diabetes, liver disease, cardiovascular disease, peptic ulcer, kidney disease, and squamous cell carcinoma [2]. Emergence of one autoimmune disease has also been observed to increase the risk of various others such as rheumatoid arthritis (RA), systemic lupus erythematosus (SLE), Type I diabetes, ankylosing spondylitis (AS), Crohn's disease, celiac disease, and ulcerative colitis, which all may show familiar clustering.

Moreover, as the destructive and pervasive effects of psychosocial stress are progressively demonstrated in every body system (down to the level of the genome), it has become clear that the traditional paradigm must be revised [1]. Firmly planted in the rationalistic viewpoint that is the foundation of Western medicine, but inclusive of the more holistic (mind and body) view inherent to Eastern medicine, a nexus model which views the body as a series of multi-connected, continually interacting physiological webs, is essential to continued progress in medicine.

Mind/Body Medicine and Aging Skin

It is hypothesized that the integration of mind and body processes may contribute more significantly to disease in the elderly than in other populations, due to the onset of chronic disease(s), an overall increase in the risk of injury, dwindling sensory input as the function of both eyes and ears becomes increasingly compromised, and the individual becoming increasingly isolated. Chronic pain and isolation produces depression and fatigue, which further isolates the individual and in turn causes stress with its many injurious effects on physiological function [3].

One of the most troublesome organ systems in old age, causing both physical and psychosocial discomfort, is the skin; more than 90 % of the elderly, in fact, have at least one skin disease and many have several [4]. This review will focus on mind–body interactions and interventions in skin disease in old age.

Influences on Aging Skin

Aging is affected by many factors, including the individual's genetic foundation, environmental insult, nutrition, exercise, disease, and injury, as well as psychosocial factors that create stress. The effects of psychosocial stress on the physical body were recognized even in ancient texts, for example, "A merry heart doeth good like a medicine" (King James Bible "Authorized Version," Cambridge Edition, Prov 17:22). Only recently, however, have the numerous physiological changes that stress can induce come to light. Stress associated with major life events (e.g., bereavement, caregiving), as well as seemingly more trivial sources of stress (e.g., school exams), has been demonstrated to have consistent and clinically consequential effects on multiple immune parameters such as changes in the production of cytokines, cortisol, specific lymphocytes, and other immune effectors and changes in susceptibility to both infectious and noninfectious diseases. Detailed information on the specific physiological effects of stress are shown in Table 1.

Hormones: Estrogen and Progesterone

Physiological effects of estrogen, with cyclical variations of estrogen levels during a woman's reproductive years (as well as various forms with similarly varying levels over the female lifespan),

Table 1 Physiological responses to psychosocial stressors

Psychosocial factor	Physiological effect	Reference
Self-report (women) with induced skin blisters	Decreased IL-1α, IL-9 at wound sites	Glaser et al. [52]
Depression	Delayed wound healing	Gouin and Kiecolt-Glaser [53]
Caregivers (Alzheimer's disease)	Poorer response to influenza vaccine as compared to matched controls	Glaser et al. [54]
Caregivers (dementia)	Decreased immunoglobulin production	Black et al. [55]
	Increased proinflammatory NF-κB production	Black et al. [55]
Loneliness	Reduction in natural killer cell activity	Kiecolt-Glaser et al. [56]
Lack of social support	Poorer response to hepatitis B vaccine	Glaser et al. [54]
	Decrease T-cell respond to HBsAg	Glaser et al. [54]

HBsAg surface antigen of the hepatitis B virus, *IL* interleukin, *NF-κB* nuclear factor kappa-light-chain-enhancer of activated B cells

are recognized as a physiological mediator throughout the female body. Estrogen receptors exist in nearly every body tissue of the human female, with numerous effects on cognitive and emotional function, immune function, the skin, and various other physiological processes. The skin has highly sensitive receptors for both estrogen and progesterone, affecting many skin disorders, including autoimmune disorders known as estrogen dermatitis and autoimmune progesterone dermatitis, believed to be cutaneous reactions to the female endogenous sex hormones themselves.

Estrogen is also a modulator of the immune system; high estrogen levels inhibit many autoimmune processes, with high estrogen levels acting to inhibit allergic response. Peak estrogen levels at the time of ovulation are associated with mast cell degranulation, as well as decreases in T-cell numbers, leading to a depression of cellular immune response. However B-cell numbers increase in coincidence with ovulation [5]. Cyclically fluctuating levels of estrogen and progesterone influence numerous characteristics of the epidermis, including skin-surface lipid secretion and sebum production, skin thickness, fat deposition, skin hydration, and barrier function. Dermal collagen content, which contributes to skin elasticity and resistance to wrinkling, is also influenced. Interestingly, estrogen levels also influence skin pigmentation and ultraviolet (UV) susceptibility, as well as resident microflora on both vaginal and keratinized skin [6, 7].

In addition, changing hormone levels across the menstrual cycle produce measurable variations in immune function and disease susceptibility. An understanding of the profound influence that fluctuating estrogen and progesterone levels have on the biological responses of the premenopausal adult woman is critical to optimizing the efficiency of medical therapies in this population [7].

Although the web of physiological effects induced by the complex, interdependent fluctuation of estrogen and progesterone over the course of the female human lifespan has long been recognized as a dominant influence on the female body, the substantial influence that these hormones have on neurological and psychosocial development has only more recently come to light. Estrogen and progesterone impact brain function, cognition, emotional status, sensory processing, appetite, and more [7–10]. The ability of reproductive hormones to impact neuropsychological processes involves the interplay of several body systems, lending credibility to the view of premenstrual syndrome (PMS) as a disorder founded in real biochemical disturbances [11].

Autoimmune diseases show a clear predominance in women, implying a central role for estrogen in their development. A thorough elucidation of that role, however, has been challenged by the observation of undeniable contributions to autoimmune disease by genetics, immunosenescence, and environmental triggers as well. The global

Table 2 Changes in psychosocial function associated with hormone levels in women

Life stage	Psychosocial effects	Reference
Menopause	Rapid deterioration of overall mental function	Halbreich et al. [57]
	Deterioration of memory	Sherwin [58]
	Decrease in abstract reasoning capability	Sherwin [58]
	Decreased reaction times	Sherwin [58]
	Decline in brain volume	Murphy et al. [59]
	Decreased verbalization acuity	Ashman et al. [60]
	Decreased attention	Stankov [61]
	Decreased processing speed	Halbreich et al. [57]
	Increased anxiety	Palmer et al. [62]
	Increased mood disturbance	Palmer et al. [62]
	Increased motivation	Palmer et al. [62]
Estrogen replacement therapy	Better performance on memory testing	Sherwin [58]
	Better performance on abstract reasoning tests	Jacobs et al. [63]
	Better performance on general cognitive tests	Kimura [64]
	Better performance in name recall	Robinson et al. [65]

incidence of autoimmune disease has risen steadily in recent years, worldwide and in all ages, in parallel with steadily increasing global lifespans [12].

Interestingly however, some evidence exists which suggests that PMS, a disorder characterized by depressed mood, anxiety, affective lability, irritability, decreased interest in usual activities, difficulty concentrating, low energy, changes in appetite, sleep disturbances, a sense of being overwhelmed or out of control, headaches, joint or muscle pain, breast tenderness, and abdominal bloating, may in fact be an autoimmune disease [13]. PMS impacts the majority of adult women on some level, with millions of women affected severely enough to disrupt daily life; nevertheless, it is an under-investigated disorder still lacking a definitive etiology. The pronounced gender discrepancy in the prevalence of autoimmune diseases strongly implicates estrogen and/or progesterone as a culprit. Again, hormonal fluctuations of the menstrual cycle are known to cause exacerbation of the many autoimmune diseases, particularly those with cutaneous manifestations. The demonstration of a dramatic comorbidity of premenstrual exacerbations of cutaneous allergic and autoimmune disorders with PMS, the documentation of hypersensitivity reactions to estrogen and progesterone in PMS patients but not in normal controls, and the ability of desensitization therapy to improve symptoms in PMS patients suggest that autoimmunity may play a role in the origin of PMS symptoms [11]. A substantial list of both physiological and psychological effects on the woman's body is in Table 2.

Neurological Interactions Among the Endocrine System, the Skin, and the Immune System

The nervous system interacts with every body system through signals conveyed by sensory nerves and motor nerves; the brain–skin connection particularly is made up of a vast neurosensory web perfused with, in the woman, estrogen and progesterone as well as other hormones. Brain neurotransmitters as well as receptors are also known to exist in the immune system, with interferon and interleukin (IL)-1 effects on the brain [14]. Blalock, a neuroimmunologist, in fact called the immune system a "sixth sense" (in that sense, a branch of the neurological system) that enables us to respond to not only "the universe of things we can see, hear, taste, touch and smell but also the other universe of things we cannot" [15]. The immune system affects regulation in response to stress signals from the nervous and endocrine systems through the production of cytokines; these cytokines, as well, feed back to the central nervous system (CNS) and regulate further neurochemical response. This provides an intrinsic system of regulation, through cytokine production that links physiological response to psychosocial and environmental events [16]. Cytokines and the autoinflammatory reactions they can create are implicated in the pathology of numerous chronic pain diseases with still dubious etiologies, for example, psoriasis, irritable bowel syndrome (IBS), vulvodynia, and autoimmunity. Even a mild stress such as sleep deprivation, for example, is known to activate inflammatory processes (in a gender-specific manner), with cellular markers of inflammation associated with cardiovascular disease, autoimmune diseases, diabetes mellitus, and arthritis. Females evidence more cellular immune activation than males, with a functional alteration of monocyte-specific inflammatory cytokine responses [17].

Contributors to Skin Aging

UV exposure accounts for about 80 % of external aging [18]. Intrinsic aging, in contrast, occurs primarily because of cumulative damage due to oxygen-containing highly reactive by-products of cellular metabolism in the mitochondria called reactive oxygen species (ROS). While ROS at moderate concentrations act as intercellular messengers, when under stress individuals produce these reactive oxygen species at much higher levels (called oxidative stress) and the abundance of ROS act to degrade other biological molecules through free-radical reactions.

Aging consists of a progressive decline in maintenance of homeostasis throughout all body tissues, a decline which has remained somewhat unexplained but which is considered to result from both genetically determined and external environmentally induced factors. Because ROS inflict oxidative damage to protein and lipids as well as deoxyribonucleic acid (DNA), ROS are considered an important component of the aging process [19], with the ability of the individual to ameliorate ROS-induced cellular damaging contributing significantly to life expectancy [20]. Numerous studies have linked cellular damage caused by ROS with aging [21].

ROS interact with DNA to oxidize nucleotide bases in the DNA, excise bases, and create strand breaks, thus creating genomic aberrations that contribute to aging, cancer, abasic sites, and DNA strand breaks, which ultimately lead to genomic instability [22], ROS have also been implicated in cellular proliferation [23], cellular senescence [24], and cell death [25]. As cellular metabolism proceeds primarily in the mitochondria, mitochondrial DNA is particularly vulnerable to oxidative damage. Oxidative damage of mitochondrial DNA also has been associated with cancer, neurodegenerative diseases, and other disease of the aged [21]. Mitochondria also help to regulate apoptosis; degeneration of mitochondrial DNA may also deregulate apoptosis and further contribute to aging by promoting premature cell death [26]. Neurodegenerative diseases common to the aged, such as Alzheimer's, Huntington disease, and Parkinson's disease, have particularly been attributed to mitochondrial defects related to oxidative stress [27, 28].

Oxidative stress is also an important contributor to skin aging. ROS have been shown to downregulate collagen production, accelerating the thinning of the dermis and diminished tensile strength (caused by loss of collagen in the dermis), that is, characteristic of aging skin [29]. Mice lacking *Sod2*, a mitochondrial antioxidant enzyme, were characterized by increased nuclear DNA damage and cellular senescence as well as a decreased thickness of and number of cells in the epidermis. Mice lacking *Sod2* also evidenced an increased rate of terminal differentiation [30]. Prolonged exposure to ROS has been show to accelerate skin aging, wrinkle formation, and the onset of melanoma [31].

A second significant contributor to aging, only recently identified, is the inexorable shortening of the DNA's telomeres, protein caps at each end of every chromatid which are truncated slightly with each cell division. Telomerase is an enzyme that has the ability to rebuild shortened telomeres with telomeric DNA, thereby preventing premature cell death or senescence. Although shortening of the telomeres is an inherent contributor to aging, psychosocial stress has also shown to both accelerate telomere loss and induce cell senescence.

Patients with obvious sources of stress (e.g., long-term caregivers, mothers of handicapped children, difficult financial situations) were found to be associated with shorter telomere lengths [32, 33] as have those with major depression [34]. Telomere length, in turn, is considered closely related to aging body-wide, with shorter telomere length associated with heart disease, vascular dementia, osteoarthritis, osteoporosis, diabetes, Alzheimer's, stroke, and even mortality [35].

Epigenetics

Ultimately, the foundation of all body structures and systems in the foundation encoded in the DNA and that genetic sequence is the determinate factor in body structure as well as many physiological functions; for example, ethnicity influences numerous characteristics of skin structure and function [36], and many diseases (including autoimmune and skin diseases) have familial affiliations, including psychological function. Nocebo and placebo effects have a genetic basis, and dissociative identity disorder (DID) appears to have genetic basis as well. The genetic sequence which provides the blueprint for the developing child is essentially set in stone; only recently however, has medical science begun to understand that structural changes occur with dramatic effects on health, structural changes that can be influenced by psychosocial events. In addition, it was recently reported that stress acts to shorten telomeres (the protein cap on every chromosome which influences cellular senescence by inducing apoptosis) which in turn accelerates cellular aging in every organ system [37].

Modification of physiological function by non-genomic changes in DNA which act to regulate gene transcription (a regulatory process known as *epigenetics*) is a biological phenomenon which has come to light only over the last couple of decades. Epigenetic actions are cell-specific and stable changes to DNA that act to regulate gene expression but which do not cause mutation. Epigenetic changes do not alter DNA sequence, but instead control gene expression [38]. These epigenetic changes affect real-time control of homeostasis in the body, maintaining normal function of virtually every single body cell and cellular metabolism.

Epigenetic mechanisms confer "phenotypic plasticity" upon the genotypic platform by giving the body, at the cellular level, ability to respond to both internal and external environmental cues [39]. Cells, for example, monitor inventories of necessary compounds and are able to modulate transcription of appropriate genes through epigenetic mechanisms [40]. Epigenetic modifications of DNA are abundant in every cell, changes which are stable because they are heritable during cell division [39].

Epigenetic changes are involved in normal development as well as in disease. Epigenetic variation over time depends on genotype, environment, sex hormone interactions, and undoubtedly other undetermined stochastic factors [41]. Such epigenetic changes in fact provide a ready explanation for discordance in monozygotic (MZ) twins with regard to epigenetic diseases that clearly have strong genetic foundation [38], literally serving as the physiological link between the nervous, endocrine, and immunological systems; the genome; and the genesis of disease.

Epigenetics provides a mechanism (transcriptional control of cytokines, immune factors, or any gene product) through which psychosocial events can cause physiological distress and disease. The effects of this transcription control can be devastating. Childhood neglect and other early life social adversity cause transcriptional modulation of the developing immune system with patterns of enhanced inflammatory gene expression and inhibited antiviral gene expression; for example, social distress perceived by the CNS influences transcription decision-making in leukocytes [16]. Alterations to immune processing can alter immune function irrevocably, with disturbation of physical function through adulthood [42].

Monkey data, moreover, shows that social adversity can play a role in activating conserved transcriptional response to adversity (CTRA) dynamics during the earliest stages of postnatal immune system development.

Body functions, in conclusion, with input from estrogen levels and environmental impacts, act on the genetic foundation of the individual at both genomic and extra-genomic levels to influence pathways of gene regulation and intra-system communication, with often synergistic effects on disparate organ systems, to influence health and disease.

Mind–Body Interventions for Aging Skin

A wide variety of natural compounds are now believed to have antioxidant capabilities, including vitamins (e.g., vitamin E, vitamin C, carotene, and selenium), enzymes (e.g., superoxide dismutase [SOD], catalase [CAT] and glutathione peroxidase), and other molecules (e.g., coenzyme Q, uric acid, isoflavones, anthocyanins, catechins, phenols, and a variety of molecules produced in plants called phytochemicals), are now known to exist in a wide variety of natural sources and are increasingly being associated with antiaging benefits [43, 44]. In one recent study, extracts were prepared from a variety of fruits and medicinal herbs cultivated in the Gyeongnam area of Korea and the antioxidant capacity of each extract analyzed through an oxygen radical absorbance activity assay. Phenolic content of each extract was also determined. All of the juices exerted a protective effect on ROS-induced oxidative stress; phenolic content, higher in the extracts of medicinal herbs than in those of the fruits studied, was associated with greater reduction of oxidative stress [45]. A systematic review including 70 independent articles, furthermore, found that cinnamon (*Cinnamomum zeylanicum*, called "true cinnamon," also containing phenols) had antiaging effects as well, including antioxidant and free-radical scavenging and inhibition of inflammatory processes [46].

Interestingly, mind–body interactions have demonstrated capacity to act as antiaging therapies as well. Stress-reduction techniques such as meditation, yoga, and prayer in multiple randomized trials have been shown to decrease stress arousal, reduce urinary free cortisol and epinephrine, reduce hypothalamic–pituitary–adrenal (HPA) axis, enhance coping skills [35], and improve mood [47].

Mind–body researchers, furthermore, have very recently demonstrated that meditation may, in fact, increase telomerase activity as well as telomerase length [48].

Conclusion

The mind/body connection, once mysterious, is increasingly recognized as a complex web of neurological, immunological, and endocrine actions which modulate the function of a more basic web of effectors that provide a communication network among body systems. In that respect, the interest in mind/body medicine is not an assault on the traditional Western medical model, but an appeal to take both a wider view (one which encompasses psychological and social functioning into the disease process and looks at all body systems as integrated whole [49, 50]) and a deeper one (one which seeks fundamental causes until the responsible physiological mechanisms are understood). This view recognizes that all body systems (brain and body), together with psychosocial factors (and environmental exposures), act in concert to determine health.

Mind–body interactions are an integral part of the aging process. Skin aging, the most visible and pervasive form of aging (90 % of elderly individuals have skin disease), is no exception. As the population of people over 60 years of age is expected to double by 2050 [51], the diseases common to aging skin will only increase in importance. Recognition of the effects of psychosocial stress, in the development of skin complaints of the elderly but also in all other medical complaints, can only lay the foundation for better treatments, particularly those which may harness mind–body physiology for healing.

References

1. Farage MA, Miller KW, Tzeghai G, et al. A body divided: toward reunification of the paradigm. Br J Med Med Res. 2014;4:3339–65.
2. Yeung H, Takeshita J, Mehta NN, et al. Psoriasis severity and the prevalence of major medical comorbidity: a

population-based study. JAMA Dermatol. 2013;149:1173–9.

3. Rejeski WJ, Gauvin L. The embodied and relational nature of the mind: implications for clinical interventions in aging individuals and populations. Clin Interv Aging. 2013;8:657–65.
4. Dugdale DI. Aging changes in skin. http://www.nlm.nih.gov/medlineplus/ency/article/004014.htm. Accessed 27 Mar 2015.
5. Farage MA, Berardesca E, Maibach HI. The effect of sex hormones on irritant and allergic response: possible relevance for skin testing. Br J Dermatol. 2009;160:450–1.
6. Muizzuddin N, Marenus KD, Schnittger SF, et al. Effect of systemic hormonal cyclicity on skin. J Cosmet Sci. 2005;56:311–21.
7. Farage MA, Neill S, MacLean AB. Physiological changes associated with the menstrual cycle: a review. Obstet Gynecol Surv. 2009;64:58–72.
8. Farage MA, Miller KW. Effects of estrogen decline of aging on the mental health of women. Int J Med Biol Front. 2011;17:1–23.
9. Farage MA, Osborn TW, MacLean AB. Estrogen and the female brain. Mental notes. Spring; 2009. p.12–13.
10. Farage MA, Osborn TW, MacLean AB. Cognitive, sensory, and emotional changes associated with the menstrual cycle: a review. Arch Gynecol Obstet. 2008;278:299–307.
11. Farage MA, Miller KW, Ajayi F, et al. Premenstrual syndrome: a disease with an autoimmune component? In: Petrov ME, editor. Autoimmune disorders: symptoms, diagnosis and treatment. Hauppauge: Nova Science Publishers; 2010.
12. Farage MA, Miller KW, Maibach HI. Effect of menopause on autoimmune diseases. Expert Rev Obstet Gynecol. 2012;7:557–71.
13. American Psychiatric Association. Diagnostic and statistical manual of mental disorders. Washington, DC: American Psychiatric Association; 2000.
14. Bedford FL. A perception theory in mind-body medicine: guided imagery and mindful meditation as cross-modal adaptation. Psychon Bull Rev. 2012;19:24–45.
15. Blalock JE. The immune system as the sixth sense. J Intern Med. 2005;257:126–38.
16. Irwin MR, Cole SW. Reciprocal regulation of the neural and innate immune systems. Nat Rev Immunol. 2011;11:625–32.
17. Irwin MR, Carrillo C, Olmstead R. Sleep loss activates cellular markers of inflammation: sex differences. Brain Behav Immun. 2010;24:54–7.
18. Park JS. Walnut husk ethanol extract possess antioxidant activity and inhibitory effect of matrix metalloproteinase-1 expression induced by tumor necrosis factor alpha in human keratinocyte. Kor J Aesthet Cosmetol. 2013;11:715–9.
19. Halliwell B. Reactive oxygen species in living systems: source, biochemistry, and role in human disease. Am J Med. 1991;91:14S–22.
20. Harman D. Aging: a theory based on free radical and radiation chemistry. J Gerontol. 1956;11:298–300.
21. Cui H, Kong Y, Zhang H. Oxidative stress, mitochondrial dysfunction, and aging. J Signal Transduct. 2012;2012:646354.
22. Krokan HE, Standal R, Slupphaug G. DNA glycosylases in the base excision repair of DNA. Biochem J. 1997;325(Pt 1):1–16.
23. Clément MV, Pervaiz S. Reactive oxygen intermediates regulate cellular response to apoptotic stimuli: a hypothesis. Free Radic Res. 1999;30:247–52.
24. Burdon RH. Control of cell proliferation by reactive oxygen species. Biochem Soc Trans. 1996;24:1028–32.
25. Burdon RH. Superoxide and hydrogen peroxide in relation to mammalian cell proliferation. Free Radic Biol Med. 1995;18:775–94.
26. Mather M, Rottenberg H. Aging enhances the activation of the permeability transition pore in mitochondria. Biochem Biophys Res Commun. 2000;273:603–8.
27. DiMauro S, Andreu AL. Mutations in mtDNA: are we scraping the bottom of the barrel? Brain Pathol. 2000;10:431–41.
28. Wallace DC. Mouse models for mitochondrial disease. Am J Med Genet. 2001;106:71–93.
29. Qin Z, Robichaud P, He T, et al. Oxidant exposure induces cysteine-rich protein 61 (CCN1) via c-Jun/AP-1 to reduce collagen expression in human dermal fibroblasts. PLoS One. 2014;9:e115402.
30. Velarde MC, Flynn JM, Day NU, et al. Mitochondrial oxidative stress caused by Sod2 deficiency promotes cellular senescence and aging phenotypes in the skin. Aging (Albany NY). 2012;4:3–12.
31. Decker EA. Phenolics: prooxidants or antioxidants? Nutr Rev. 1997;55:396–8.
32. Epel ES, Blackburn EH, Lin J, et al. Accelerated telomere shortening in response to life stress. Proc Natl Acad Sci U S A. 2004;101:17312–5.
33. Cherkas LF, Aviv A, Valdes AM, et al. The effects of social status on biological aging as measured by white-blood-cell telomere length. Aging Cell. 2006;5:361–5.
34. Simon NM, Smoller JW, McNamara KL, et al. Telomere shortening and mood disorders: preliminary support for a chronic stress model of accelerated aging. Biol Psychiatry. 2006;60:432–5.
35. Epel E, Daubenmier J, Moskowitz JT, et al. Can meditation slow rate of cellular aging? Cognitive stress, mindfulness, and telomeres. Ann N Y Acad Sci. 2009;1172:34–53.
36. Farage MA, Maibach HI. Sensitive skin: closing in on a physiological cause. Contact Dermatitis. 2010;62:137–49.
37. Choi J, Fauce SR, Effros RB. Reduced telomerase activity in human T lymphocytes exposed to cortisol. Brain Behav Immun. 2008;22:600–5.
38. Meda F, Folci M, Baccarelli A, et al. The epigenetics of autoimmunity. Cell Mol Immunol. 2011;8:226–36.

39. Feinberg AP. Phenotypic plasticity and the epigenetics of human disease. Nature. 2007;447:433–40.
40. Luo J, Kuo M. Linking nutrient metabolism to epigenetics. Cell Sci Rev. 2009;6:49–54.
41. Aguilera O, Fernández AF, Muñoz A, et al. Epigenetics and environment: a complex relationship. J Appl Physiol (1985). 2010;109:243–51.
42. McGowan PO, Sasaki A, D'Alessio AC, et al. Epigenetic regulation of the glucocorticoid receptor in human brain associates with childhood abuse. Nat Neurosci. 2009;12:342–8.
43. Cai Y, Luo Q, Sun M, et al. Antioxidant activity and phenolic compounds of 112 traditional Chinese medicinal plants associated with anticancer. Life Sci. 2004;74:2157–84.
44. Kaur C, Kapoor HC. Anti-oxidant activity and total phenolic content of some Asian vegetables. Int J Food Sci Technol. 2002;37:153–61.
45. Shon M, Lee Y, Song J, et al. Anti-aging potential of extracts prepared from fruits and medicinal herbs cultivated in the Gyeongnam area of Korea. Prev Nutr Food Sci. 2014;19:178–86.
46. Ranasinghe P, Pigera S, Premakumara GAS, et al. Medicinal properties of 'true' cinnamon (*Cinnamomum zeylanicum*): a systematic review. BMC Complement Altern Med. 2013;13:275.
47. Bormann JE, Carrico AW. Increases in positive reappraisal coping during a group-based mantram intervention mediate sustained reductions in anger in HIV-positive persons. Int J Behav Med. 2009;16:74–80.
48. Hoge EA, Chen MM, Orr E, et al. Loving-kindness meditation practice associated with longer telomeres in women. Brain Behav Immun. 2013;32:159–63.
49. Engel GL. The need for a new medical model: a challenge for biomedicine. Science. 1977;196:129–36.
50. Engel GL. The clinical application of the biopsychosocial model. Am J Psychiatry. 1980;137:535–44.
51. Facts about ageing. http://www.who.int/ageing/about/facts/en/. Accessed 27 Mar 2015.
52. Glaser R, Kiecolt-Glaser JK, Marucha PT, et al. Stress-related changes in proinflammatory cytokine production in wounds. Arch Gen Psychiatry. 1999;56:450–6.
53. Gouin J, Kiecolt-Glaser JK. The impact of psychological stress on wound healing: methods and mechanisms. Crit Care Nurs Clin North Am. 2012;24:201–13.
54. Glaser R, Kiecolt-Glaser JK, Malarkey WB, et al. The influence of psychological stress on the immune response to vaccines. Ann N Y Acad Sci. 1998;840:649–55.
55. Black DS, Cole SW, Irwin MR, et al. Yogic meditation reverses NF-κB and IRF-related transcriptome dynamics in leukocytes of family dementia caregivers in a randomized controlled trial. Psychoneuroendocrinology. 2013;38:348–55.
56. Kiecolt-Glaser JK, Garner W, Speicher C, et al. Psychosocial modifiers of immunocompetence in medical students. Psychosom Med. 1984;46:7–14.
57. Halbreich U, Lumley LA, Palter S, et al. Possible acceleration of age effects on cognition following menopause. J Psychiatr Res. 1995;29:153–63.
58. Sherwin BB. Estrogen and cognitive functioning in women. Endocr Rev. 2003;24:133–51.
59. Murphy DG, DeCarli C, McIntosh AR, et al. Sex differences in human brain morphometry and metabolism: an in vivo quantitative magnetic resonance imaging and positron emission tomography study on the effect of aging. Arch Gen Psychiatry. 1996;53:585–94.
60. Ashman T, Mohs R, Harvey P. Cognition and aging. In: Hazzard W, Blass J, Ettinger S, Hatter J, Ouslander J, editors. Principles of geriatric medicine and gerontology. New York: McGraw Hill; 1999.
61. Stankov L. Aging, attention, and intelligence. Psychol Aging. 1988;3:59–74.
62. Palmer K, Berger AK, Monastero R, et al. Predictors of progression from mild cognitive impairment to Alzheimer disease. Neurology. 2007;68:1596–602.
63. Jacobs DM, Tang MX, Stern Y, et al. Cognitive function in nondemented older women who took estrogen after menopause. Neurology. 1998;50:368–73.
64. Kimura D. Estrogen replacement therapy may protect against intellectual decline in postmenopausal women. Horm Behav. 1995;29:312–21.
65. Robinson D, Friedman L, Marcus R, et al. Estrogen replacement therapy and memory in older women. J Am Geriatr Soc. 1994;42:919–22.

Brain-Skin Connection: Impact of Psychological Stress on Skin

157

Ying Chen, Robert Maidof, and John Lyga

Contents

Abstract

The intricate relationship between stress and skin conditions has been documented since ancient times. Recent clinical observations also link psychological stress to the onset or aggravation of multiple skin diseases. However, the exact underlying mechanisms have only been studied and partially revealed in the past 20 years or so, involving both the central and peripheral pathways. Psychological stress can play important roles in skin's inflammation responses, barrier function, and wound healing. Long-term chronic stress can also lead to premature skin aging. In this chapter, the authors will discuss the recent discoveries in the field of "brain-skin connection," summarizing findings from the overlapping fields of psychology, endocrinology, skin neurobiology, skin inflammation, immunology, and pharmacology.

Introduction

Psychological stress arises when people are under mental, physical, or emotional pressure and when an individual perceives that the pressure exceeds his adaptive power. Stress can vary in both intensity and duration. Acute stress usually lasts minutes to hours, while repeated exposure to stressful situations can lead to chronic stress that lasts for days, months, or even longer [1]. Stress is perceived by the brain and causes hormones such

Conflict of Interest: None

Y. Chen (✉)
Global R&D, Equity and Claims, Reckitt Benckiser, Montvale, NJ, USA
e-mail: azureling@gmail.com

R. Maidof • J. Lyga
Avon Global R&D, Suffern, NY, USA

M.A. Farage et al. (eds.), *Textbook of Aging Skin*,
DOI 10.1007/978-3-662-47398-6_153

as corticotropin-releasing hormone (CRH), glucocorticoids, and epinephrine to be released. This triggers a wide range of physiological and behavioral responses that adapt the body to the stress [2]. However, if the stress responses are inadequate or excessive, they may trigger adverse physiological events [3]. It has been shown that stress can trigger and/or exacerbate multiple conditions, including cardiovascular disease [4, 5], migraine [6], multiple sclerosis [7], epileptic seizures [8], and neurodegeneration [9].

Recent research has confirmed that skin is both an immediate stress perceiver and a target of stress responses. As the largest organ of the body, skin plays important barrier and immune functions, maintaining homeostasis between the external environment and internal tissues. Skin is composed of two major layers: the epidermis and dermis. The epidermis is constantly under renewal and regeneration where basal proliferating keratinocytes gradually differentiate, are pushed upward, and eventually slough off the surface. The primary role of the epidermis is to provide a barrier and the first-line defense system against the external environment. The outermost layer of the epidermis is called the stratum corneum (SC) and is composed of dead and flattened corneocytes embedded in a matrix of lipids. Corneocytes contain numerous keratin filaments bound to a peripheral cornified envelope composed of cross-linked proteins. In the epidermis, secreted lipid vesicles flatten to form intercellular lamellar disks, which then disperse and join together to form multiple, continuous membrane sheets in the SC [10, 11]. The dermis is composed of fibroblasts and extracellular matrix proteins including collagen, elastin, and hyaluronic acid which provide elasticity and tensile strength. It is composed of the upper papillary dermis and lower reticular dermis. It also contains hair follicles, blood vessels, nerve endings, sweat glands, and sebaceous glands [12].

In this chapter, we will summarize the recent findings on how the brain and skin communicate with each other, how the skin reacts to the stress by activating the endocrine and immune systems, and the negative impact of chronic stress on skin health.

Stress Mediators and Effector Cells

Skin is the primary sensing organ for external stressors, including heat, cold, pain, and mechanical forces. Three classes of nerve receptors are responsible for transmitting the outside signals to the spinal cord and then to the brain: thermoreceptors for heat and cold, nociceptor for pain, and mechanoreceptors for mechanical signals [13]. The cutaneous sensory fibers also convey changes in temperature, pH, and inflammatory mediators to the central nervous system (CNS). The nerve terminals are often associated with receptors indicating close interactions between the two [14]. The brain responds to these signals, which in turn influence the stress responses in the skin (Table 1).

Skin and its appendages are not only targets of key stress mediators, but they are also a local source for these factors which induce various immune and inflammation responses. In this section, we will discuss key players in mediating the stress response from both the central nervous system and the resident skin cells (Fig. 1).

Central HPA Axis and SAM Axis

Stress conditions exert their effects to skin mainly through the hypothalamic-pituitary-adrenal (HPA) axis. Upon sensing stress, neurons in the hypothalamus secrete corticotropin-releasing hormone (CRH), which is transported to the pituitary gland, where it binds to the CRH receptor type-1 (CRH-R1) and stimulates the secretion of proopiomelanocortin (POMC)-derived neuropeptides, including α-melanocyte-stimulating hormone (α-MSH), β-endorphin, and adrenocorticotropin (ACTH). In turn, ACTH travels to the outer layer of adrenal cortex through the bloodstream, binds to the MC2 receptors (MC2-R), and stimulates production of glucocorticoids (GC) including cortisol and corticosterone. Cortisol is the primary stress hormone in humans that regulates a wide range of stress responses [15]. Cortisol works by binding to the glucocorticoids receptor (GR), which undergoes conformational change, dissociates from the heat shock

Table 1 Major stress mediators in skin

Stress mediator	Source	Effector cell	Functions in skin
CRH	Hypothalamus	CRH-R1 is expressed in epidermis, dermis, and subcutis layer; CRH-R2 is expressed in hair follicle keratinocytes and papilla fibroblasts	Stimulation of downstream ACTH and cortisol production
	Skin keratinocytes, sebocytes, and mast cells		Proliferation, differentiation, apoptosis, inflammation, and angiogenesis
ACTH	Pituitary gland	MC2-R is expressed in skin melanocytes, hair follicles, epidermal keratinocytes, sebaceous and eccrine glands, as well as dermal fibroblasts, sebaceous and eccrine glands, and muscle and dermal blood vessels	Stimulation of cortisol and corticosterone production
	Skin melanocytes, epidermal and hair follicle keratinocytes, and dermal fibroblasts; Langerhans cells, monocytes, and macrophages		Melanogenesis, cytokine production, cell proliferation, dendritic formation, hair growth, and immune and inflammation regulation
Cortisol	Adrenal cortex	Glucocorticoids receptor (GR) is ubiquitously expressed in all skin cells	Major impact on the immune and inflammation system
	Skin hair follicles, melanocytes, and fibroblasts		Cell proliferation and survival via the PI3K/Akt pathway
			Hair follicle proliferation and differentiation; Epidermal barrier formation
Neurotrophins	Central nervous system	Two receptors TrK and p75 are expressed in mast cells, immune cells, keratinocytes, fibroblasts, and melanocytes	Promote skin innervations
	Skin sympathetic neurons, mast cells, T cells and B cells, keratinocytes, fibroblasts, and melanocytes		Promote survival and differentiation of mast cells and modify inflammatory cytokine expressions
			Promote proliferation of keratinocytes; important for melanocytes migration, viability, and differentiation and protect them from oxidative stress and apoptosis
			Promote fibroblast differentiation and migration and possibly contraction and MMP secretion
Substance P	Sensory nerve fibers	Mast cells, macrophages, T cells	Cytokine release to induce inflammation, activate mast cells, and induce lymphocyte proliferation
			Induce vascular permeability
Prolactin	Pituitary gland	Prolactin receptor (PRLR) is ubiquitously expressed except in fibroblasts	Autocrine hair growth modulator by promoting catagen (hair regression)
	Skin hair follicle and epidermal keratinocytes, fibroblasts, adipocytes, sweat glands, and sebaceous glands		Stimulate keratinocytes growth and keratin production in keratinocytes
			Sebum production in sebaceous glands
			Immunomodulation

(*continued*)

Table 1 (continued)

Stress mediator	Source	Effector cell	Functions in skin
Catecholamines (epinephrine and norepinephrine)	Adrenal medulla	Adrenergic receptors are expressed by natural killer cells, monocytes, T cells, keratinocytes, and melanocytes	Regulate keratinocyte proliferation, differentiation, and migration
	Skin nerve fibers, keratinocytes		Promote melanogenesis in melanocytes
			Decrease fibroblast migration and collagen secretion and impair wound healing
			Suppress IL-12 in dendritic cells leading to blunted Th1 and increased Th2 differentiation
			Important for lymphocyte trafficking, circulation, proliferation, and cytokine production

protein-binding complex, translocates to the nucleus, and affects gene expression through glucocorticoid response elements (GREs) on gene promoter regions or direct interactions with transcription factors like activating protein-1 (AP-1) and nuclear factor-κB (NF-κB) [16, 17].

Normally cortisol levels undergo daily oscillation regulated by the internal circadian clock system, with peak level at early morning and lowest point around midnight [18, 19]. Stress can significantly disrupt cortisol level and the oscillation curve. It was shown that in mice under restraint stress, there is diurnal dysregulation of HPA axis activation resulting in a fourfold increase in plasma corticosterone [20]. Under stress conditions, significantly upregulated cortisol can have a major impact on the immune system (mainly being immunosuppressive), including antigen presentation, lymphocyte proliferation and traffic, secretion of cytokines and antibodies, and shift of the T helper (Th1 toward Th2) responses [21].

Stress also induces the release of catecholamines through the sympathetic-adrenal medullary (SAM) axes. The inner layer of the adrenal medulla releases epinephrine (adrenaline) and norepinephrine (noradrenaline) upon activation by stress. They are the critical components of the "fight or flight response": acceleration of heart rate and respiration, constriction of blood vessels except in the muscles, increased perspiration, and dilation of pupils. Epinephrine acts by binding to a variety of adrenergic receptors, leading to decreased skin blood flow and altered immune and inflammation functions, including lymphocyte trafficking, circulation, proliferation, and cytokine production [22–24]. In monocytes and dendritic cells, adrenergic signaling can inhibit IL-12 production via increased cAMP, thus blunting TH1 response and promoting TH2 differentiation [25]. It also impacts various cytokines' production in dendritic cells [26].

Skin Peripheral HPA and SAM Axis

The skin also develops a fully functional peripheral HPA system where CRH, ACTH, and their receptors are produced in skin cells [27, 28]. CRH is produced by epidermal and hair follicle keratinocytes, melanocytes, sebocytes, and mast cells upon stress, including immune cytokines, UV irradiation, and cutaneous pathology [29, 30]. In humans, CRH receptor (CRH-R) 1 is expressed in all major cellular populations of epidermis, dermis, and subcutis layers, while CRH-R2 is only expressed in hair follicle

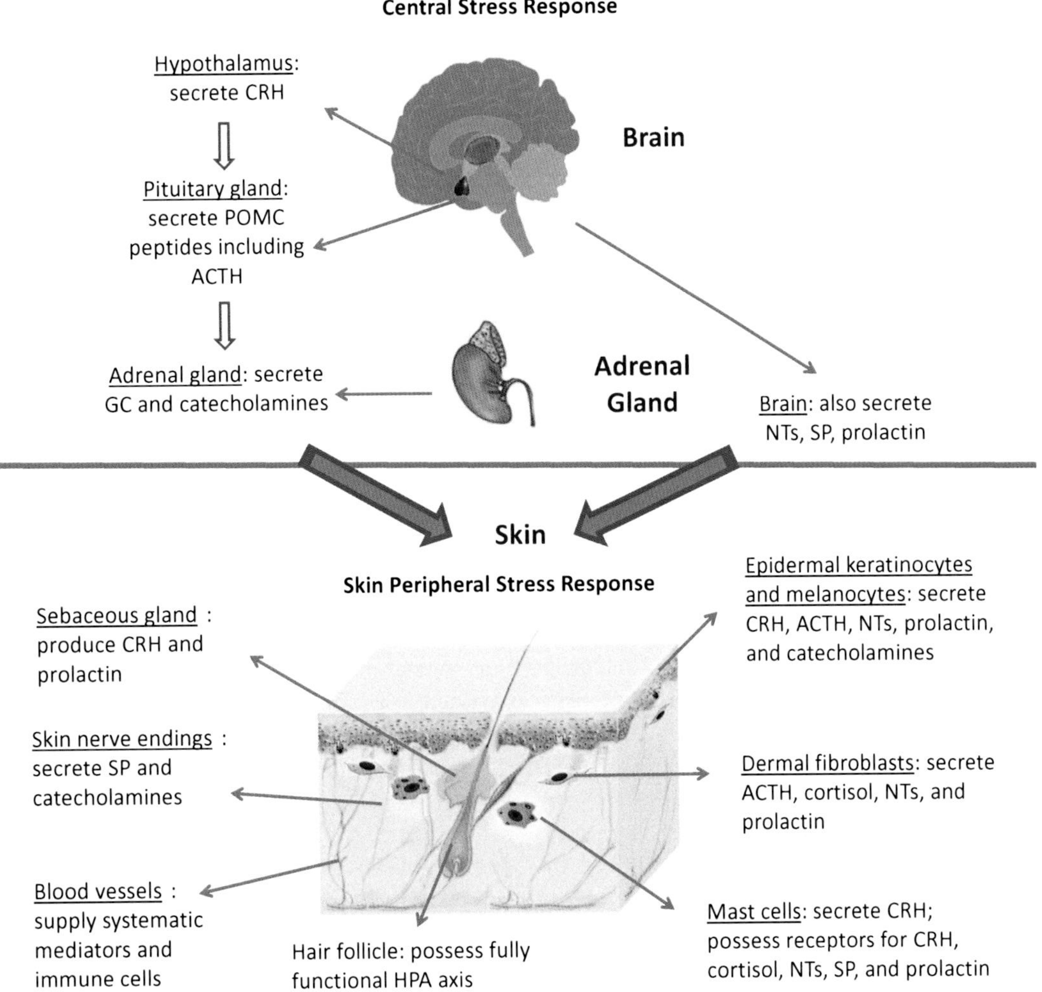

Fig. 1 Central stress response and skin peripheral stress response. This figure illustrates how brain or the central stress response system secrete CRH, ACTH, and GC to adapt to stress. The skin also possesses peripheral stress response system with participation from skin cells, glands, nerve endings, and blood vessels

keratinocytes and papillary fibroblasts [31, 32]. Human melanocytes and dermal fibroblasts respond to CRH signaling via the cAMP pathway and lead to ACTH and corticosterone production [33, 34]. ACTH has also been detected in keratinocytes, Langerhans cells, monocytes, and macrophages [35].

The function of CRH in the skin is very diverse and cell-type specific. In epidermal keratinocytes, CRH inhibits proliferation by arresting cells at the G0/1 cycle and induces differentiation by calcium influx via the AP-1 transcription pathway [36, 37]. The MAPK pathway and VEGF downregulation were also proposed to be a possible mechanism [38]. In melanocytes and dermal fibroblasts, CRH acts as growth factor that stimulates proliferation. It also inhibits apoptosis in the same cells by starvation stress [39]. In mast cells, CRH induces degranulation and increases vascular permeability, demonstrating a pro-inflammatory function [40]. It also leads to selective secretion of vascular endothelial growth factor (VEGF) to promote angiogenesis [41]. In keratinocytes, CRH stimulates the pro-inflammatory IL6 production [42]. However, in melanocytes, CRH inhibits

NF-κB signaling, possibly to self-inhibit the inflammation response [43]. In a human sebocyte model, CRH stimulated lipid production through upregulation of key lipogenesis enzymes [44].

ACTH stimulates IL-18 production in skin keratinocytes. IL-18 is a pro-inflammatory cytokine that enhances T-cell activity and promotes T helper type 2 (Th2) cytokine production [45]. Since CRH downregulates IL-18 in keratinocytes [46], IL-18 may participate in the negative feedback loop to regulate HPA axis activity. In melanocytes, ACTH stimulates proliferation and melanogenesis with a similar effect of α-MSH [47, 48]. Endogenous ACTH can stimulate hair growth in a mouse model [49]. In sebocytes, ACTH works through the MC5R receptor and induces sebocyte differentiation [50].

The skin also holds a peripheral catecholamine system where epinephrine is synthesized in keratinocytes while the adrenergic receptors are present in both epidermal keratinocytes and melanocytes [51]. In keratinocytes, after epinephrine activates the β2-adrenoceptor, it induces a major increase in cAMP, which in turn increases calcium concentration through protein kinase C (PKC) activation [52, 53]. Since calcium level can regulate both epidermal proliferation and differentiation, it is possible that epinephrine can affect epidermal health. In melanocytes, the epinephrine produced by surrounding keratinocytes can promote melanogenesis [54]. Fibroblast functions are also impacted by epinephrine, including migration and collagen production, both being important steps in wound healing [55]. For a detailed review of epinephrine's effect on wound healing, please refer to the wound healing section.

Neurotrophins, Substance P, and Prolactin

The skin is highly innervated, and peripheral nerves also impact skin health through secreted factors such as neuropeptides (e.g., substance P or SP) and neurotrophins (NT). They serve as local stress responders that mediate neurogenic inflammation [56]. NGF contributes to stress-induced cutaneous hyperinnervation and affects all hallmarks of allergic inflammation and cutaneous stress responsiveness upstream of SP [57].

Nerve growth factor (NGF) is one of four NT family members. It binds to the high affinity tyrosine kinase receptor (TrkA, TrkB, and TrkC) and low affinity p75 NT receptor and promotes neurogenic inflammation by stimulating cytokine releases from skin mast cells [58]. In keratinocytes, NGF promotes proliferation and protects cells from UV-induced apoptosis [59–61]. In fibroblasts, NGF induces proliferation, migration, and differentiation into myofibroblasts, which may play a vital role in cutaneous wound healing [62]. In melanocytes, NGF receptors are induced by UV irradiation and can induce migration and dendricity [63, 64]. In a stress-induced hair loss mouse model, sonic stress induced rapid increases of NGF and p75 NTR, which in turn significantly increased the number of substance P-positive sensory neurons and eventually caused premature hair growth termination [65].

Substance P (SP) is a stress-related pro-inflammatory neuropeptide which is released from cutaneous peripheral nerve terminals. During repeated sonic stress, SP+ nerve fibers are significantly increased [65]. It is the key mediator in connecting the brain to the hair follicle by stimulating mast cell degranulation and increasing macrophage infiltration. SP receptor antagonist can indeed normalize stress-induced phenotypes [66]. Antioxidant enzyme levels, autophagy pathway, and hair cycle are normalized by both SP receptor antagonist and antioxidant treatment [67]. Substance P participates in the effect of CRH on mast cell degranulation during stress, an important process in neuroinflammation [68]. It also induces neutrophil and inflammatory cell infiltrates [69]. SP can induce a variety of cytokines to be released from monocytes and T cells, including IL-1, IL-6, and IL-12, leading to T-cell proliferation and inflammation [70, 71]. Very interestingly, SP can increase the virulence of multiple skin microflora by increasing caspase and altering the actin cytoskeleton. This could be another mechanism contributing to its role in neurogenic inflammation [72].

Prolactin is the hormone best known for its function in lactation and reproduction. It also has a global effect on body weight and adipose tissue [73, 74] and is immediately induced by psychological stress [75]. Recent research has revealed its function and implication in the brain-skin connection [76]. Prolactin stimulates proliferation and regulates keratin expression in keratinocytes [77, 78]. It stimulates sebum production in sebaceous glands [79]. In human monocytes/macrophages, prolactin stimulates heme oxygenase-1 production and VEGF production, contributing to angiogenesis [80]. Prolactin was proposed to have immunoprotection functions during stress because it can antagonize glucocorticoid function and maintain survival and function of T lymphocytes and macrophages [81, 82].

Mast Cells

Skin mast cells have emerged as a central player of the skin stress responses. It was proposed as the "central switchboard" of neurogenic inflammation [83]. In skin they are located near SP+ nerve endings and blood vessels, where they are the first-line defense of the innate immune system. All the major stress pathways discussed above can impact various aspects of mast cell functions, including survival, activation, and downstream effectors' secretion (see above for details). These include various vasodilatory and pro-inflammatory mediators such as histamine, VEGF, cytokines, nitric oxide (NO), and proteases. In turn, they serve as central players in the skin neurogenic immune response activated by stress.

Stress-Induced Immune Dysfunction

The interdisciplinary field of psychoneuroimmunology (PNI) has revealed key mechanistic evidence on how the immune system responds and communicates with the nervous and endocrine system under stress conditions and how these interactions can affect skin health. Almost all immune cells express receptors for one or more stress hormones. Alternatively, stress can also indirectly affect immune cells by regulating the production of cytokines, such as interleukins, tumor necrosis factor (TNF), and interferon-γ (IFN-γ) [84].

It has been widely accepted that very brief stress can be immune-enhancing, while chronic stress is generally immune-repressing. Mice under acute restraint stress for 2 h exhibit higher numbers of activated macrophages and enhanced recruitment of surveillance T cells in the skin [85]. In humans, interview stress briefly increases natural killer cell number and activity [86]. On the other hand, chronic stress-induced immune dysfunction can increase susceptibility and severity of infection, increase inflammation, slow wound healing, and lead to various skin health risks [87].

Skin Neurogenic Inflammation Plays a Central Role in Stress-Triggered or Exacerbated Skin Diseases

Stress is known to affect various diseases and conditions, for example, asthma, arthritis, migraines, and multiple sclerosis [88–91]. Specifically in skin multiple neuroinflammatory conditions can be triggered or aggravated by stress, such as psoriasis, atopic dermatitis, acne, contact dermatitis [92, 93], alopecia areata [94–97], itch or pruritus [98], and erythema. This section will focus on several skin conditions.

Psoriasis

Psoriasis is a chronic skin inflammatory disease, affecting about 2 % of the population worldwide. It is characterized by over-proliferation of keratinocytes and inflammation, which lead to epidermal hyperplasia, a hallmark of lesional psoriatic skin. The psoriatic plaques are most commonly seen over the elbows, knees, and scalp. Other pathological signatures include dysregulated angiogenesis, skin infiltrating T lymphocytes, and expression of pro-inflammatory T helper (Th) 1 cytokines

[99–101]. Although recent research has revealed parts of the pathogenesis and the intricate cross talk between nerves, immune system, endocrine system, and skin cells, there is still no cure for psoriasis.

Stress is both a consequence of living with psoriasis and a cause for psoriasis exacerbation [102, 103]. The pro-inflammatory cytokines that are highly expressed in psoriasis are potent activators of the HPA axis. This could lead to a vicious cycle and amplify the negative effects [104]. Stress leads to a hyporesponsive central HPA axis with blunted cortisol response and upregulation of inflammatory cytokines [105, 106]. In psoriasis stress also has an impact on the skin peripheral HPA axis and the SAM axis. However, the exact role and mechanism still need to be elucidated due to conflicting data from different research groups [107].

The role of NGF and substance P in psoriasis has been extensively studied. It was discovered that psoriatic tissue expresses high levels of NGF [108, 109]. NGF can contribute to keratinocyte proliferation [59, 60] and mast cell activation [58, 110], both being early events of psoriatic lesion formation. NGF also contributes to inflammation, by activating T lymphocytes [111] and inducing chemokine expression from keratinocytes [112]. The critical role of NGF in psoriasis development is further confirmed when blocker of TrkA, the high affinity NGF receptor, significantly improved transplanted psoriatic plaques in a mouse model [113]. Substance P and SP+ cutaneous sensory nerves are both increased in psoriasis skin [114, 115]. This could be downstream of NGF signaling since NGF and its receptors play a crucial role in regulating innervation and upregulating neuropeptides [116]. In fact, cutaneous denervation can improve inflammation and reduce T-cell numbers, which is prevented by restoration of SP signaling [117].

It was recently discovered that in keratinocytes, prolactin enhances interferon-gamma-induced production of (C-X-C motif) ligand 9 (CXCL9), CXCL10, and CXCL11. Thus, prolactin may promote type 1 T-cell infiltration into psoriatic lesions via these chemokines [118]. It can also stimulate keratinocyte proliferation [77], potentially promoting the development of psoriatic plaques.

Acne

Acne vulgaris (or simply acne) is a very common skin disease affecting a majority percentage of the population at some point in their life. It affects skin with the densest population of sebaceous follicles, including the face, the upper part of the chest, and the back. Acne pathogenesis is characterized by increased colonization of P. acne anaerobic bacteria, increased sebum production from the sebaceous glands, inflammation, and hyperkeratinization [119].

Stress has long been suspected to induce acne flares by clinical experiences and anecdotal observations [120, 121], but it was only confirmed 10 years ago by a well-controlled study. In a student examination stress study, increased acne severity is significantly associated with stress levels [122].

The role of skin peripheral HPA axis has been studied in the pathogenesis of acne. CRH and its receptors have been detected on sebocytes [29, 44]. It was shown that CRH promotes lipogenesis in sebocytes through upregulation of a key enzyme [44]. In addition, it induces cytokine (IL-6 and IL-11) production in keratinocytes [42], contributing to inflammation. ACTH and α-MSH also contribute to sebum production and possibly worsen the acne phenotype [123, 124]. The role of neuropeptide, specifically SP, in acne has been studied extensively [125]. Facial skin from acne patients shows marked increase of SP+ nerve fibers around the sebaceous glands and around acne lesions [126]. SP can promote both proliferation and differentiation of sebaceous glands [127]. SP induces gene expression of PPAR-γ, which plays a unique role in stimulating sebocyte lipogenesis. It also stimulates various pro-inflammatory cytokine release from sebocytes, including IL-1, IL-6, and TNF-α [128]. In addition, SP can activate mast cells, adding another important player to the neurogenic inflammation [68].

Atopic Dermatitis

Atopic dermatitis (AD) is a chronic and relapsing inflammatory skin disease often associated with eczema and itch [129]. A complex interaction of genetic, environmental, and immunological factors is manifested in AD. Skin barrier function defect is a key feature of AD because null mutations in the filaggrin gene are an important predisposing factor for AD. Filaggrin protein is essential for the final cell compacting process to form the terminally differentiated stratum corneum [130–132]. Environmental factors such as allergens or microbial organisms are critical triggers or complications in the disease [133]. Toll-like receptor 2 (TLR-2) has emerged as another important player. It recognizes cell wall components of bacteria, and its gene polymorphism has been associated with AD [134]. AD is also characterized by an acute phase with predominant TH2 response (IL-4, IL-13, and IL-31) and a chronic phase toward a TH1 (IL-5, IL-12, and IFN-γ) feature [135].

Similar to psoriasis, AD symptoms and psychological stress seem to form a vicious cycle. AD patients have been reported to have anxiety and depression, while psychological stress in turn can exacerbate AD pathology [136–138].

Stress can impact AD symptoms through different mechanisms. Stress can negatively affect skin's permeability barrier function and homeostasis. In AD patients, barrier dysfunction can lead to increased sensitization to allergens and microbial organisms, increased transepidermal water loss, and lowered threshold for itch [139]. For a detailed review of how stress impacts barrier function, please refer to the next section.

Stress also contributes to the immune and inflammation dysfunction in AD patients. HPA response after stress was found to be impaired in AD patients. This hyporesponsiveness was linked to severity of inflammation [136]. The blunted HPA response was proposed to lead to immune function dysregulation, allergic inflammation, and exacerbation of disease [140]. On the other hand, the SAM axis is over-reactive. Both basal and stress-induced levels of catecholamines are higher in AD patients compared to control [136]. However, the adrenergic receptor mutation or polymorphisms have been discovered in AD. A point mutation in the β2-adrenoceptor gene could alter the structure and function of the receptor, thereby leading to a low density of receptors on both keratinocytes and peripheral blood lymphocytes [141]. Receptor mutation or polymorphism is also associated with AD [14, 141]. Therefore, the catecholamine signaling is probably still dysfunctional even with upregulated ligand. It was discovered that adrenoceptor signaling defect with TLR activation can shift the recall memory response to the Th1 type, releasing multiple cytokines. This could be a mechanism where the SAM axis can contribute to chronic AD pathogenesis [142]. Further research is warranted to elucidate the role of the SAM axis in AD pathogenesis.

In a mouse model for atopic dermatitis, it was discovered that stress increased cutaneous but not serum or hypothalamic NGF. Treatment with NGF-neutralizing antibody can partially recover the skin inflammation phenotype by reducing epidermal thickening, decreasing pro-inflammatory cytokine induction, and attenuating allergy-characteristic cellular infiltration [143]. However, there are conflicting data on NGF expression in AD patients. Some research showed increased NGF [138, 144–146], while others demonstrated no significant difference or even decreased NGF level [84, 147]. Further research is needed in this area to elucidate the differences. In a pilot study where AD patients were subjected to Trier social stress test (TSST), it was shown that AD patients had more NGF+ nerve fibers, and after acute stress, nonneuronal cholinergic system (NNCS) markers are decreased in healthy skin but increased in inflamed AD skin suggesting a role in the fine tuning of proliferative and inflammatory responses in the skin's response to stress [135]. SP was also involved in the neurogenic inflammation that worsens dermatitis because the exacerbation was not seen in mice lacking the SP receptor [148]. It was shown that SP receptor expression is much higher in AD patients' peripheral blood mononuclear cells (PBMCs) than in healthy control. SP can increase PBMCs proliferation rate and TNF-α and IL-10 production

[13]. However, in an atopic mouse model, the SP+ nerve fibers in skin are decreased in stressed animals [149]. The exact role of SP in AD remains to be clarified. Mast cells also play a role in AD neurogenic inflammation. Mast cell numbers are increased in lesional AD skin, as well as mast cell-nerve contacts [150, 151]. Recently, it was discovered that oxytocin (OXT), a neuropeptide playing a major role in behavior regulation, is downregulated in lesional AD skin. Both oxytocin and its receptor are detected in keratinocytes and fibroblasts, and it affects cell proliferation, inflammatory cytokine release, and oxidative stress responses [152].

Impact of Stress on Skin Barrier Function and Wound Healing

The stratum corneum (SC) plays important barrier functions by regulating epidermal permeability and homeostasis. This protein/lipid barrier creates a surface seal essential for maintenance of hydration and protection against microbial infection. Disruption of the skin barrier function can lead to flaky or dry skin [133]. Alternation of the lipids composition has also been linked to skin diseases like atopic dermatitis and psoriasis [153, 154].

Stress can cause detrimental physiological and functional consequences in the skin. Overcrowding stress in mice caused higher transepidermal water loss, lower water retention, and impaired barrier function, leading to moderate exfoliation and slight wrinkle formation. The exact mechanism is still unclear, but a decrease in ceramide and pyrrolidone carboxylic acid was observed [155, 156]. Other studies have corroborated the result and further confirmed the involvement of stress by demonstrating that treatment of glucocorticoid receptor antagonist or CRH receptor antagonist can block the adverse events [157, 158]. A study using topical glucocorticoid-treated mice proposed that lipid synthesis inhibition is key for the stress-induced abnormalities [159]. In a later insomnia study, the authors discovered that stress can significantly impair epidermal proliferation and differentiation, decrease size and density of corneodesmosomes, and decrease lipid synthesis and lamellar body production. It also confirmed the critical role of lipids because topical application of physiological lipids including ceramides and free fatty acids can restore barrier homeostasis and stratum corneum integrity [160].

Similar effects were also observed in human subjects. For example, final exam stress on students caused a decline in permeability barrier recovery kinetics [161]. Interview stress caused barrier function recovery delay, increased plasma cortisol level, and activated several inflammation and immune players, including interleukin-1β, interleukin-10, tumor necrosis factor α, and circulating natural killer cells [86]. Stress due to marital disruption significantly delayed skin barrier recovery after tape stripping [162]. Students who are under stress due to final exam or returning from vacation showed significant decline in barrier function and deterioration in barrier disruption and recovery [163]. Interestingly, relaxation intervention before or after tape stripping can significantly improve skin barrier recovery compared to control [139].

One of skin's major functions is physical protection and wound repair upon injury. Wound healing is an intricate process that involves both resident skin cells, skin extracellular matrix, and systemic factors. Mechanosensing and mechanotransduction also play vital roles in wound closure [164]. It is divided into three major yet overlapping phases: inflammation, proliferation, and remodeling. During inflammation, cytokines and chemokines including IL-1α,IL-1β, IL8, transforming growth factor-β, vascular endothelial growth factor (VEGF), and tumor necrosis factor alpha (TNF-α) play important roles. They protect against infection, attract phagocytes, and recruit fibroblasts. In proliferation, new granulation tissue is rebuilt with collagen, blood vessel, and other ECM proteins. Finally, in remodeling, collagen is remodeled and realigned, and apoptosis removes unnecessary cells, which may take weeks or months [165].

An extensive literature search has revealed that chronic systemic corticosteroids have a negative impact on all three phases of wound healing

[166]. A meta-analysis also concluded that stress was associated with impaired healing or dysregulation of healing biomarkers [167].

The negative impact of stress on wound healing was first observed clinically in humans when caregivers of demented relatives needed 20 % more time for complete dermal wound healing [168]. Anxiety and depression is also associated with delayed healing in chronic wounds [169]. It was found that perceived stress and elevated cortisol level are two contributing factors [170].

Subsequent mouse and human studies have revealed some important molecular mechanisms. The HPA axis plays a vital role because glucocorticoid receptor antagonist treatment can restore proper healing rate [20]. Inflammatory marker (including IL1α and IL1β) kinetics are disrupted [171]. Two key cytokines (IL-1α and IL8) were found to be significantly lower at the wound site in stressed patients [172]. MMP2 expression in blister wound was found to be negatively correlated with plasma cortisol level [173]. Rotational stress in mice can delay wound closure by delaying immune cell infiltration, lowering TNF-α level at wound site, and reducing MMP activity [174]. Bacterial infections during early stages of wound healing are also more prominent due to compromised skin immune function [175]. Antimicrobial peptide expression was also decreased by stress leading to increased severity of infection at the wound site [176]. Furthermore, myofibroblast differentiation is delayed, leading to severely impaired wound contraction [177]. TGF-β signaling could also be involved since it was shown that endogenous glucocorticoids play an important part in wound healing by altering TGF-β expression which affects fibroblast proliferation, migration, and differentiation [178, 179].

Alternatively, stress can also work through the SAM-epinephrine pathway to negatively impact keratinocyte motility and wound reepithelialization. Epinephrine can be induced by stress systematically and can also be produced locally at the wound site. Epinephrine binds to the β2-adrenergic receptor (β2AR) in keratinocytes and decreases downstream PI3K/AKT signaling. This leads to stabilization of actin cytoskeleton and increased focal adhesion formation, both inhibiting migration and proper wound healing. β2AR antagonist was shown to be effective at reversing this impairment [180]. Antagonist can also accelerate skin barrier recovery and reduce epidermal hyperplasia [181]. Epinephrine was found to decrease fibroblast migration and MMP2 secretion in vitro [174]. It can also reduce collagen deposition by fibroblasts [55]. Recent research discovered that neutrophil trafficking alternation and IL-6 upregulation were induced by epinephrine and inflammatory responses are impaired in wound healing [182]. Stress-activated SAM pathway can alter blood flow. Peripheral vasoconstriction can limit the blood and oxygen supply at the wounding site, which limits the rate of healing by increasing the production of nitric oxide (NO). Hyperbaric oxygen therapy was shown to effectively correct stress-impaired wound healing in a mouse model [183]. In humans, emotional disclosure intervention was shown to significantly improve wound healing after skin biopsy [184]. Recently it was discovered that higher stress levels are associated with fewer macrophages and less immune cell activation, both of which can contribute to slow wound healing [185].

Long-Term Skin Damage of Chronic Stress

Under short-term acute stress, the HPA axis is tightly regulated through feedback mechanisms. Increased cortisol levels can keep the HPA activity in check through both a slow genomic and a fast non-genomic negative feedback mechanism [186]. Acute stress can induce a significant redistribution of lymphocytes from the blood to the skin, leading to enhanced skin immunity and successful stress adaptation [187]. In a mouse restraint stress study, both innate and adaptive immunities are involved: dendritic cells mature and traffic from skin to the lymph nodes, macrophages are activated, and surveillance T cells are recruited to the skin [85]. Acute stress also suppresses ROS production [188].

In contrast to acute stress, which may augment innate and adaptive immune responses, chronic stress usually suppresses immunoprotection, increases susceptibility to infections, and exacerbates some allergic and inflammatory diseases [189]. This is due to altered stress responses after repeated or prolonged stress termed stress habituation, which reduces HPA axis activation but also sensitizes reactivity to new stimuli [190]. Aging also has a negative effect on the feedback system, as shown in both rats and humans [191, 192].

In a mouse study, chronic stress induced by fox urine can significantly accelerate UV-induced skin neoplasma development. The stressed group starts to develop skin tumors much earlier than the control group, and the survival rate is significantly lower [193]. It was later discovered that chronic stress caused a significant decrease in T-cell infiltration in the skin and cell-mediated immunity was greatly compromised. Several important skin immune markers are decreased by stress, including IL12 (Th-1 response promotion and cellular immunity mediator), IFN-γ (tumor recognition and elimination), and CCL27 (skin homing T-cell attraction) [194].

Skin aging is characterized by formation of lines and wrinkles, increased pigmentation, loss of elasticity and firmness, and dull skin. It is a consequence of both intrinsic factors and extrinsic factors. There are two major theories for aging: the programmatic theory which focuses on reduced cellular life span, decreased responsiveness and functionality, and dysfunctional immune responses and the stochastic theory which points toward environmental damages, focusing on DNA damage, inflammation, and free radical formation [195–197].

The exact mechanism of how stress impacts skin aging is still quite elusive. However, recent research has provided evidence of possible pathways that might contribute to skin aging [198]. UV irradiation is one of the major extrinsic stressors responsible for premature skin aging, thus the term "photoaging." UV irradiation is one of the major stimulants of the skin HPA axis. It induces expression of CRH, POMC peptides, ACTH, cortisol, and β-endorphin [199]. Considering that skin is under daily UV stress, the repeated activation of the HPA axis can have detrimental effects on skin. Long-term glucocorticoid (GC) therapy for treating skin inflammatory disease has a severe skin atrophy side effect, including decreased epidermal thickness, flat dermal-epidermal junction, reduced number of fibroblasts, and disruption of the dermal fibrous network, which are also hallmarks of skin aging. Several extracellular matrix proteins are negatively impacted by GC, including collagen I, collagen III, proteoglycans, and elastin [200].

Epinephrine, norepinephrine, and cortisol were found to increase DNA damage, interfere with DNA repair, and alter transcriptional regulation of the cell cycle [201]. It has been demonstrated that stress can induce DNA damage through the β2-adrenoreceptor (β2AR) pathway. Chronic catecholamine stimulation leads to p53 degradation and accumulation of DNA damage [202]. Furthermore, blockage of the β2AR pathway can prevent DNA damage accumulation [203]. Thus, stress-induced SAM axis can also contribute to skin aging by compromising genome integrity.

Reactive oxygen species (ROS) was recently discovered to play a role in the stress-SP-mast cell pathway. In chronic restraint stress mice, oxidative stress pathway has a two-way cross talk with the SP pathway, and antioxidant Tempol was shown to also be effective for normalizing hair growth [204]. Repeated short-term stress can induce ROS production by upregulation of NF-κB in the skin induced by toxicant and UVB. Stress augments depletion of cellular antioxidant machinery, shown by significant loss of GSH (glutathione- and GSH-dependant enzymes), superoxide dismutase, and catalase activity [205]. It was also discovered that in the brain, stress leads to increased oxidative stress and mitochondria dysfunction [206, 207]. Considering that ROS production in the mitochondria is the major determinant of aging and life span [208], stress can have a major impact on skin aging through the ROS pathway.

Smoking and air pollution have been confirmed as critical chronic stressors that impact skin aging significantly. In photoprotected skin, years of smoking and packs smoked per day are strong indicators of premature skin aging [209]. In an identical twin study, it was observed that a 5-year difference in smoking history led to noticeable changes in skin aging [136]. A significant increase in temperature and decrease in oxygen content were observed in skin after smoking [71]. ROS production and aryl hydrocarbon receptor (AhR) signaling pathway lead to dermal matrix breakdown and wrinkle formation [210]. Airborne particle exposure from traffic was associated with a significant increase in pigment spots and facial wrinkles [211]. ROS production is the major underlying mechanism. It can induce vitamin E depletion and lipid peroxidation, as well as MMP induction [116, 212]. Direct mitochondria damage and the AhR pathway have also been proposed as possible mechanisms [213–215].

Recently, telomere shortening has emerged as another possible cellular mechanism linking chronic psychological stress and aging. Telomeres are DNA repeats at the ends of chromosomes and shorten with each cell division, eventually leading to replicative senescence and premature cellular aging. Various chronic stress situations have been associated with shorter telomere length, including caregiving for sick child with chronic conditions or elderly dementia patients, major depression, childhood adversity, and exposure to intimate partner violence [126, 128, 145, 216]. Although the exact mechanism of how stress induces telomere shortening is still under debate, cortisol and epigenetic modulation have been proposed as possible routes [125, 217]. Telomere shortening can lead to the downregulation of mitochondria biogenesis and ROS production [119, 218]. This could constitute a vicious cycle where stress from lifestyle or habits further exacerbates the skin damage and signs of aging.

A recent study established the negative effect of sleep deprivation on skin aging [127]. It was found that poor quality sleepers showed increased signs of intrinsic skin aging including fine lines, uneven pigmentation, and reduced elasticity. They also recover much slower after skin barrier disruption. Sleep-deprived subjects also showed higher skin conductance level after completing a difficult perceptual task with false feedback. This indicated that sleep deprivation augments allostatic responses to increasing psychosocial stress [219]. Hypoxia stress induced during wound healing can also impact skin aging by disrupting basement membrane involving laminin and integrins [220].

Conclusions and Future Perspectives

In recent years, emerging research has demonstrated that skin is not only a target of psychological stress signaling modulation, but it also actively participates in the stress response by a local HPA axis, peripheral nerve endings, and local skin cells including keratinocytes, mast cells, and immune cells. There are also feedback mechanisms and cross talk between the brain and the skin, and pro-inflammatory cytokines and neurogenic inflammatory pathways play huge roles in mediating such responses. In this chapter, we summarized findings that shed light on how the "brain-skin connection" actually works: what are the major pathways and effector cells, how do they negatively impact skin functions and diseases, and how chronic stress can have a detrimental effect on skin aging.

As of today, there is no proven medical treatment that can either prevent or treat stress-induced or exacerbated skin conditions or skin aging. Several key players have been proposed which might give rise to potential therapeutics. Skin mast cells are activated by stress, and in turn they also produce stress hormones and inflammatory factors. This could lead to a vicious cycle of stress-induced inflammatory events. Indeed mast cells have been implicated in numerous skin diseases including acne, atopic dermatitis, psoriasis, and pruritus [221]. Several compounds have been found to be effective in inhibiting cytokine release from mast cells [134]. Dietary supplements combining active flavonoids with proteoglycans could also be helpful in atopic and inflammatory conditions [150]. Specific receptor antagonists against CRH receptors, NGF receptors, or SP receptors could also prove to be effective in relieving stress-induced neurogenic inflammation [222].

In the future, researchers should further investigate the HPA axis, pro-inflammatory hormones and cytokines, and their downstream effectors that mediate the brain-skin connection. Future researchers can look into ways to modulate this connection and discover novel therapeutics for skin diseases and antiaging treatments.

References

1. Dhabhar FS. Psychological stress and immunoprotection versus immunopathology in the skin. Clin Dermatol. 2013;31(1):18–30.
2. Papadimitriou A, Priftis KN. Regulation of the hypothalamic-pituitary-adrenal axis. Neuroimmunomodulation. 2009;16(5):265–71.
3. Cohen S, Janicki-Deverts D, Miller GE. Psychological stress and disease. JAMA: J Am Med Assoc. 2007;298(14):1685–7.
4. Schwartz BG, French WJ, Mayeda GS, Burstein S, Economides C, Bhandari AK, Cannom DS, Kloner RA. Emotional stressors trigger cardiovascular events. Int J Clin Pract. 2012;66(7):631–9.
5. Steptoe A, Kivimäki M. Stress and cardiovascular disease. Nat Rev Cardiol. 2012;9(6):360–70.
6. Haque B, Rahman KM, Hoque A, Hasan AT, Chowdhury RN, Khan SU, Alam MB, Habib M, Mohammad QD. Precipitating and relieving factors of migraine versus tension type headache. BMC Neurol. 2012;12:82.
7. Schumann R, Adamaszek M, Sommer N, Kirkby KC. Stress, depression and antidepressant treatment options in patients suffering from multiple sclerosis. Curr Pharm Des. 2012;18(36):5837–45.
8. Novakova B, Harris PR, Ponnusamy A, Reuber M. The role of stress as a trigger for epileptic seizures: a narrative review of evidence from human and animal studies. Epilepsia. 2013;54(11):1866–76.
9. Hemmerle AM, Herman JP, Seroogy KB. Stress, depression and Parkinson's disease. Exp Neurol. 2012;233(1):79–86.
10. Downing DT. Lipid and protein structures in the permeability barrier of mammalian epidermis. J Lipid Res. 1992;33(3):301–13.
11. Madison KC. Barrier function of the skin: "la raison d'etre" of the epidermis. J Invest Dermatol. 2003; 121(2):231–41.
12. Haake A, Scott GA, Holbrook KA. Structure and function of the skin: overview of the epidermis and dermis. Biol Skin. 2001;2001:19–45.
13. Schmelz M. Neuronal sensitivity of the skin. Eur J Dermatol. 2011;21 Suppl 2:43–7.
14. Slominski AT, Zmijewski MA, Skobowiat C, Zbytek B, Slominski RM, Steketee JD. Sensing the environment: regulation of local and global homeostasis by the skin's neuroendocrine system. Adv Anat Embryol Cell Biol. 2012;212:v. vii, 1–115.
15. Smith SM, Vale WW. The role of the hypothalamic-pituitary-adrenal axis in neuroendocrine responses to stress. Dialogues Clin Neurosci. 2006;8(4):383–95.
16. Pratt WB. The role of heat shock proteins in regulating the function, folding, and trafficking of the glucocorticoid receptor. J Biol Chem. 1993;268(29): 21455–8.
17. Ray A, Prefontaine KE. Physical association and functional antagonism between the p65 subunit of transcription factor NF-kappa B and the glucocorticoid receptor. Proc Natl Acad Sci U S A. 1994; 91(2):752–6.
18. Weitzman ED, Fukushima D, Nogeire C, Roffwarg H, Gallagher TF, Hellman L. Twenty-four hour pattern of the episodic secretion of cortisol in normal subjects. J Clin Endocrinol Metab. 1971;33(1):14–22.
19. Debono M, Ghobadi C, Rostami-Hodjegan A, Huatan H, Campbell MJ, Newell-Price J, Darzy K, Merke DP, Arlt W, Ross RJ. Modified-release hydrocortisone to provide circadian cortisol profiles. J Clin Endocrinol Metab. 2009;94(5):1548–54.
20. Padgett DA, Marucha PT, Sheridan JF. Restraint stress slows cutaneous wound healing in mice. Brain Behav Immun. 1998;12(1):64–73.
21. Elenkov IJ, Webster EL, Torpy DJ, Chrousos GP. Stress, corticotropin-releasing hormone, glucocorticoids, and the immune/inflammatory response: acute and chronic effects. Ann N Y Acad Sci. 1999;876:1–11. discussion 11-3.
22. McCarty R, Horwatt K, Konarska M. Chronic stress and sympathetic-adrenal medullary responsiveness. Soc Sci Med. 1988;26(3):333–41.
23. Sanders VM, Baker RA, Ramer-Quinn DS, Kasprowicz DJ, Fuchs BA, Street NE. Differential expression of the beta2-adrenergic receptor by Th1 and Th2 clones: implications for cytokine production and B cell help. J Immunol. 1997;158(9):4200–10.
24. Marino F, Cosentino M. Adrenergic modulation of immune cells: an update. Amino Acids. 2013;45(1): 55–71.
25. Panina-Bordignon P, Mazzeo D, Lucia PD, D'Ambrosio D, Lang R, Fabbri L, Self C, Sinigaglia F. Beta2-agonists prevent Th1 development by selective inhibition of interleukin 12. J Clin Invest. 1997;100(6):1513–19.
26. Goyarts E, Matsui M, Mammone T, Bender AM, Wagner JA, Maes D, Granstein RD. Norepinephrine modulates human dendritic cell activation by altering cytokine release. Exp Dermatol. 2008;17(3):188–96.
27. Kim JE, Cho BK, Cho DH, Park HJ. Expression of hypothalamic-pituitary-adrenal axis in common skin diseases: evidence of its association with stress-related disease activity. Acta Derm Venereol. 2013;93(4):387–93.
28. Slominski A, Zbytek B, Nikolakis G, Manna PR, Skobowiat C, Zmijewski M, Li W, Janjetovic Z, Postlethwaite A, Zouboulis CC, Tuckey RC. Steroidogenesis in the skin: implications for

local immune functions. J Steroid Biochem Mol Biol. 2013;137:107–23.

29. Kono M, Nagata H, Umemura S, Kawana S, Osamura RY. In situ expression of corticotropin-releasing hormone (CRH) and proopiomelanocortin (POMC) genes in human skin. FASEB J. 2001;15(12):2297–9.
30. Slominski A, Wortsman J, Pisarchik A, Zbytek B, Linton EA, Mazurkiewicz JE, Wei ET. Cutaneous expression of corticotropin-releasing hormone (CRH), urocortin, and CRH receptors. FASEB J. 2001;15(10):1678–93.
31. Pisarchik A, Slominski A. Molecular and functional characterization of novel CRFR1 isoforms from the skin. Eur J Biochem. 2004;271(13):2821–30.
32. Slominski A, Pisarchik A, Tobin DJ, Mazurkiewicz JE, Wortsman J. Differential expression of a cutaneous corticotropin-releasing hormone system. Endocrinology. 2004;145(2):941–50.
33. Slominski A, Zbytek B, Semak I, Sweatman T, Wortsman J. CRH stimulates POMC activity and corticosterone production in dermal fibroblasts. J Neuroimmunol. 2005;162(1–2):97–102.
34. Slominski A, Zbytek B, Szczesniewski A, Semak I, Kaminski J, Sweatman T, Wortsman J. CRH stimulation of corticosteroids production in melanocytes is mediated by ACTH. Am J Physiol Endocrinol Metab. 2005;288(4):E701–6.
35. Slominski A, Wortsman J, Luger T, Paus R, Solomon S. Corticotropin releasing hormone and proopiomelanocortin involvement in the cutaneous response to stress. Physiol Rev. 2000;80(3):979–1020.
36. Zbytek B, Pikula M, Slominski RM, Mysliwski A, Wei E, Wortsman J, Slominski AT. Corticotropin-releasing hormone triggers differentiation in HaCaT keratinocytes. Br J Dermatol. 2005;152(3):474–80.
37. Zbytek B, Slominski AT. Corticotropin-releasing hormone induces keratinocyte differentiation in the adult human epidermis. J Cell Physiol. 2005;203(1): 118–26.
38. Zhou CL, Yu XJ, Chen LM, Jiang H, Li CY. Corticotropin-releasing hormone attenuates vascular endothelial growth factor release from human HaCaT keratinocytes. Regul Pept. 2010;160(1–3): 115–20.
39. Slominski A, Zbytek B, Pisarchik A, Slominski RM, Zmijewski MA, Wortsman J. CRH functions as a growth factor/cytokine in the skin. J Cell Physiol. 2006;206(3):780–91.
40. Theoharides TC, Singh LK, Boucher W, Pang X, Letourneau R, Webster E, Chrousos G. Corticotropin-releasing hormone induces skin mast cell degranulation and increased vascular permeability, a possible explanation for its proinflammatory effects. Endocrinology. 1998; 139(1):403–13.
41. Cao J, Papadopoulou N, Kempuraj D, Boucher WS, Sugimoto K, Cetrulo CL, Theoharides TC. Human mast cells express corticotropin-releasing hormone (CRH) receptors and CRH leads to selective secretion of vascular endothelial growth factor. J Immunol. 2005;174(12):7665–75.
42. Zbytek B, Mysliwski A, Slominski A, Wortsman J, Wei ET, Mysliwska J. Corticotropin-releasing hormone affects cytokine production in human HaCaT keratinocytes. Life Sci. 2002;70(9):1013–21.
43. Zbytek B, Pfeffer LM, Slominski AT. CRH inhibits NF-kappa B signaling in human melanocytes. Peptides. 2006;27(12):3276–83.
44. Zouboulis CC, Seltmann H, Hiroi N, Chen W, Young M, Oeff M, Scherbaum WA, Orfanos CE, McCann SM, Bornstein SR. Corticotropin-releasing hormone: an autocrine hormone that promotes lipogenesis in human sebocytes. Proc Natl Acad Sci U S A. 2002;99(10):7148–53.
45. Park HJ, Kim HJ, Lee JY, Cho BK, Gallo RL, Cho DH. Adrenocorticotropin hormone stimulates interleukin-18 expression in human HaCaT keratinocytes. J Invest Dermatol. 2007;127(5):1210–16.
46. Park HJ, Kim HJ, Lee JH, Lee JY, Cho BK, Kang JS, Kang H, Yang Y, Cho DH. Corticotropin-releasing hormone (CRH) downregulates interleukin-18 expression in human HaCaT keratinocytes by activation of p38 mitogen-activated protein kinase (MAPK) pathway. J Invest Dermatol. 2005;124(4):751–5.
47. Suzuki I, Cone RD, Im S, Nordlund J, Abdel-Malek ZA. Binding of melanotropic hormones to the melanocortin receptor MC1R on human melanocytes stimulates proliferation and melanogenesis. Endocrinology. 1996;137(5):1627–33.
48. Dissanayake NS, Mason RS. Modulation of skin cell functions by transforming growth factor-beta1 and ACTH after ultraviolet irradiation. J Endocrinol. 1998;159(1):153–63.
49. Paus R, Maurer M, Slominski A, Czarnetzki BM. Mast cell involvement in murine hair growth. Dev Biol. 1994;163(1):230–40.
50. Zhang L, Li WH, Anthonavage M, Eisinger M. Melanocortin-5 receptor: a marker of human sebocyte differentiation. Peptides. 2006;27(2): 413–20.
51. Grando SA, Pittelkow MR, Schallreuter KU. Adrenergic and cholinergic control in the biology of epidermis: physiological and clinical significance. J Invest Dermatol. 2006;126(9):1948–65.
52. Schallreuter KU, Wood JM, Lemke R, LePoole C, Das P, Westerhof W, Pittelkow MR, Thody AJ. Production of catecholamines in the human epidermis. Biochem Biophys Res Commun. 1992; 189(1):72–8.
53. Koizumi H, Tanaka H, Ohkawara A. beta-Adrenergic stimulation induces activation of protein kinase C and inositol 1,4,5-trisphosphate increase in epidermis. Exp Dermatol. 1997;6(3):128–32.
54. Gillbro JM, Marles LK, Hibberts NA, Schallreuter KU. Autocrine catecholamine biosynthesis and the beta-adrenoceptor signal promote pigmentation in human epidermal melanocytes. J Invest Dermatol. 2004;123(2):346–53.

55. Romana-Souza B, Otranto M, Almeida TF, Porto LC, Monte-Alto-Costa A. Stress-induced epinephrine levels compromise murine dermal fibroblast activity through beta-adrenoceptors. Exp Dermatol. 2011;20 (5):413–19.
56. Botchkarev VA, Yaar M, Peters EM, Raychaudhuri SP, Botchkareva NV, Marconi A, Raychaudhuri SK, Paus R, Pincelli C. Neurotrophins in skin biology and pathology. J Invest Dermatol. 2006;126(8):1719–27.
57. Babizhayev MA, Savel'yeva EL, Moskvina SN, Yegorov YE. Telomere length is a biomarker of cumulative oxidative stress, biologic age, and an independent predictor of survival and therapeutic treatment requirement associated with smoking behavior. Am J Ther. 2011;18(6):e209–26.
58. Marshall JS, Gomi K, Blennerhassett MG, Bienenstock J. Nerve growth factor modifies the expression of inflammatory cytokines by mast cells via a prostanoid-dependent mechanism. J Immunol. 1999;162(7):4271–6.
59. Wilkinson DI, Theeuwes MJ, Farber EM. Nerve growth factor increases the mitogenicity of certain growth factors for cultured human keratinocytes: a comparison with epidermal growth factor. Exp Dermatol. 1994;3(5):239–45.
60. Pincelli C, Haake AR, Benassi L, Grassilli E, Magnoni C, Ottani D, Polakowska R, Franceschi C, Giannetti A. Autocrine nerve growth factor protects human keratinocytes from apoptosis through its high affinity receptor (TRK): a role for BCL-2. J Invest Dermatol. 1997;109(6):757–64.
61. Marconi A, Terracina M, Fila C, Franchi J, Bonte F, Romagnoli G, Maurelli R, Failla CM, Dumas M, Pincelli C. Expression and function of neurotrophins and their receptors in cultured human keratinocytes. J Invest Dermatol. 2003;121(6):1515–21.
62. Palazzo E, Marconi A, Truzzi F, Dallaglio K, Petrachi T, Humbert P, Schnebert S, Perrier E, Dumas M, Pincelli C. Role of neurotrophins on dermal fibroblast survival and differentiation. J Cell Physiol. 2012;227(3):1017–25.
63. Peacocke M, Yaar M, Mansur CP, Chao MV, Gilchrest BA. Induction of nerve growth factor receptors on cultured human melanocytes. Proc Natl Acad Sci U S A. 1988;85(14):5282–6.
64. Yaar M, Grossman K, Eller M, Gilchrest BA. Evidence for nerve growth factor-mediated paracrine effects in human epidermis. J Cell Biol. 1991;115(3):821–8.
65. Peters EM, Handjiski B, Kuhlmei A, Hagen E, Bielas H, Braun A, Klapp BF, Paus R, Arck PC. Neurogenic inflammation in stress-induced termination of murine hair growth is promoted by nerve growth factor. Am J Pathol. 2004;165 (1):259–71.
66. Arck PC, Handjiski B, Hagen E, Joachim R, Klapp BF, Paus R. Indications for a 'brain-hair follicle axis (BHA)': inhibition of keratinocyte proliferation and up-regulation of keratinocyte apoptosis in telogen hair follicles by stress and substance P. FASEB J. 2001;15(13):2536–8.
67. Wang L, Guo LL, Wang LH, Zhang GX, Shang J, Murao K, Chen DF, Fan XH, Fu WQ. Oxidative stress and substance P mediate psychological stress-induced autophagy and delay of hair growth in mice. Arch Dermatol Res. 2015;307(2):171–81.
68. Singh LK, Pang X, Alexacos N, Letourneau R, Theoharides TC. Acute immobilization stress triggers skin mast cell degranulation via corticotropin releasing hormone, neurotensin, and substance P: a link to neurogenic skin disorders. Brain Behav Immun. 1999;13(3):225–39.
69. Smith CH, Barker JN, Morris RW, MacDonald DM, Lee TH. Neuropeptides induce rapid expression of endothelial cell adhesion molecules and elicit granulocytic infiltration in human skin. J Immunol. 1993;151(6):3274–82.
70. Lotz M, Vaughan JH, Carson DA. Effect of neuropeptides on production of inflammatory cytokines by human monocytes. Science (New York, NY). 1988;241(4870):1218–21.
71. Fan GB, Wu PL, Wang XM. Changes of oxygen content in facial skin before and after cigarette smoking. Skin Res Technol. 2012;18(4):511–15.
72. Mijouin L, Hillion M, Ramdani Y, Jaouen T, Duclairoir-Poc C, Follet-Gueye ML, Lati E, Yvergnaux F, Driouich A, Lefeuvre L, Farmer C, Misery L, Feuilloley MG. Effects of a skin neuropeptide (substance p) on cutaneous microflora. PLoS One. 2013;8(11):e78773.
73. Ben-Jonathan N, Hugo ER, Brandebourg TD, LaPensee CR. Focus on prolactin as a metabolic hormone. Trends Endocrinol Metab. 2006;17 (3):110–16.
74. Langan EA, Foitzik-Lau K, Goffin V, Ramot Y, Paus R. Prolactin: an emerging force along the cutaneous-endocrine axis. Trends Endocrinol Metab. 2010; 21(9):569–77.
75. Rossier J, French E, Rivier C, Shibasaki T, Guillemin R, Bloom FE. Stress-induced release of prolactin: blockade by dexamethasone and naloxone may indicate beta-endorphin mediation. Proc Natl Acad Sci U S A. 1980;77(1):666–9.
76. Foitzik K, Langan EA, Paus R. Prolactin and the skin: a dermatological perspective on an ancient pleiotropic peptide hormone. J Invest Dermatol. 2009;129(5): 1071–87.
77. Girolomoni G, Phillips JT, Bergstresser PR. Prolactin stimulates proliferation of cultured human keratinocytes. J Invest Dermatol. 1993;101 (3):275–9.
78. Ramot Y, Biro T, Tiede S, Toth BI, Langan EA, Sugawara K, Foitzik K, Ingber A, Goffin V, Langbein L, Paus R. Prolactin – a novel neuroendocrine regulator of human keratin expression in situ. FASEB J. 2010;24(6):1768–79.
79. Gosain A, DiPietro LA. Aging and wound healing. World J Surg. 2004;28(3):321–6.

80. Malaguarnera L, Imbesi R, Di Rosa M, Scuto A, Castrogiovanni P, Messina A, Sanfilippo S. Action of prolactin, IFN-gamma, TNF-alpha and LPS on heme oxygenase-1 expression and VEGF release in human monocytes/macrophages. Int Immunopharmacol. 2005;5(9):1458–69.
81. Bernton EW, Meltzer MS, Holaday JW. Suppression of macrophage activation and T-lymphocyte function in hypoprolactinemic mice. Science. 1988;239 (4838):401–4.
82. Krishnan N, Thellin O, Buckley DJ, Horseman ND, Buckley AR. Prolactin suppresses glucocorticoid-induced thymocyte apoptosis in vivo. Endocrinology. 2003;144(5):2102–10.
83. Paus R, Theoharides TC, Arck PC. Neuroimmunoendocrine circuitry of the 'brain-skin connection'. Trends Immunol. 2006;27(1):32–9.
84. Padgett DA, Glaser R. How stress influences the immune response. Trends Immunol. 2003;24(8):444–8.
85. Viswanathan K, Daugherty C, Dhabhar FS. Stress as an endogenous adjuvant: augmentation of the immunization phase of cell-mediated immunity. Int Immunol. 2005;17(8):1059–69.
86. Altemus M, Rao B, Dhabhar FS, Ding W, Granstein RD. Stress-induced changes in skin barrier function in healthy women. J Invest Dermatol. 2001;117(2): 309–17.
87. Segerstrom SC, Miller GE. Psychological stress and the human immune system: a meta-analytic study of 30 years of inquiry. Psychol Bull. 2004;130(4):601–30.
88. Trueba AF, Ritz T. Stress, asthma, and respiratory infections: pathways involving airway immunology and microbial endocrinology. Brain Behav Immun. 2013;29:11–27.
89. Harris ML, Loxton D, Sibbritt DW, Byles JE. The influence of perceived stress on the onset of arthritis in women: findings from the Australian Longitudinal Study on women's health. Ann Behav Med. 2013;46 (1):9–18.
90. Theoharides TC, Donelan J, Kandere-Grzybowska K, Konstantinidou A. The role of mast cells in migraine pathophysiology. Brain Res Brain Res Rev. 2005;49 (1):65–76.
91. Mohr DC, Hart SL, Julian L, Cox D, Pelletier D. Association between stressful life events and exacerbation in multiple sclerosis: a meta-analysis. BMJ. 2004;328(7442):731.
92. Flint MS, Valosen JM, Johnson EA, Miller DB, Tinkle SS. Restraint stress applied prior to chemical sensitization modulates the development of allergic contact dermatitis differently than restraint prior to challenge. J Neuroimmunol. 2001;113(1):72–80.
93. Kaneko K, Kawana S, Arai K, Shibasaki T. Corticotropin-releasing factor receptor type 1 is involved in the stress-induced exacerbation of chronic contact dermatitis in rats. Exp Dermatol. 2003; 12(1):47–52.
94. Picardi A, Pasquini P, Cattaruzza MS, Gaetano P, Baliva G, Melchi CF, Papi M, Camaioni D, Tiago A, Gobello T, Biondi M. Psychosomatic factors in first-onset alopecia areata. Psychosomatics. 2003;44 (5):374–81.
95. Brajac I, Tkalcic M, Dragojevic DM, Gruber F. Roles of stress, stress perception and trait-anxiety in the onset and course of alopecia areata. J Dermatol. 2003;30(12):871–8.
96. Willemsen R, Vanderlinden J, Roseeuw D, Haentjens P. Increased history of childhood and lifetime traumatic events among adults with alopecia areata. J Am Acad Dermatol. 2009;60(3):388–93.
97. Paus R, Arck P. Neuroendocrine perspectives in alopecia areata: does stress play a role? J Invest Dermatol. 2009;129(6):1324–6.
98. Steinhoff M, Bienenstock J, Schmelz M, Maurer M, Wei E, Biro T. Neurophysiological, neuroimmunological, and neuroendocrine basis of pruritus. J Invest Dermatol. 2006;126(8):1705–18.
99. Bjerke JR, Krogh HK, Matre R. Characterization of mononuclear cell infiltrates in psoriatic lesions. J Invest Dermatol. 1978;71(5):340–3.
100. Bata-Csorgo Z, Hammerberg C, Voorhees JJ, Cooper KD. Flow cytometric identification of proliferative subpopulations within normal human epidermis and the localization of the primary hyperproliferative population in psoriasis. J Exp Med. 1993;178(4): 1271–81.
101. Bata-Csorgo Z, Hammerberg C, Voorhees JJ, Cooper KD. Intralesional T-lymphocyte activation as a mediator of psoriatic epidermal hyperplasia. J Invest Dermatol. 1995;105(1 Suppl):89s–94.
102. O'Leary CJ, Creamer D, Higgins E, Weinman J. Perceived stress, stress attributions and psychological distress in psoriasis. J Psychosom Res. 2004; 57(5):465–71.
103. Verhoeven EW, Kraaimaat FW, Jong EM, Schalkwijk J, van de Kerkhof PC, Evers AW. Effect of daily stressors on psoriasis: a prospective study. J Invest Dermatol. 2009;129(8):2075–7.
104. Turnbull AV, Rivier CL. Regulation of the hypothalamic-pituitary-adrenal axis by cytokines: actions and mechanisms of action. Physiol Rev. 1999;79(1):1–71.
105. Evers AW, Verhoeven EW, Kraaimaat FW, de Jong EM, de Brouwer SJ, Schalkwijk J, Sweep FC, van de Kerkhof PC. How stress gets under the skin: cortisol and stress reactivity in psoriasis. Br J Dermatol. 2010;163(5):986–91.
106. Kunz-Ebrecht SR, Mohamed-Ali V, Feldman PJ, Kirschbaum C, Steptoe A. Cortisol responses to mild psychological stress are inversely associated with proinflammatory cytokines. Brain Behav Immun. 2003;17(5):373–83.
107. Hunter HJ, Griffiths CE, Kleyn CE. Does psychosocial stress play a role in the exacerbation of psoriasis? Br J Dermatol. 2013;169(5):965–74.
108. Fantini F, Magnoni C, Bracci-Laudiero L, Pincelli CT. Nerve growth factor is increased in psoriatic skin. J Invest Dermatol. 1995;105(6):854–5.

109. Raychaudhuri SP, Jiang WY, Farber EM. Psoriatic keratinocytes express high levels of nerve growth factor. Acta Derm Venereol. 1998;78(2):84–6.
110. Aloe L, Bracci-Laudiero L, Bonini S, Manni L. The expanding role of nerve growth factor: from neurotrophic activity to immunologic diseases. Allergy. 1997;52(9):883–94.
111. Lambiase A, Bracci-Laudiero L, Bonini S, Bonini S, Starace G, D'Elios MM, De Carli M, Aloe L. Human CD4+ T cell clones produce and release nerve growth factor and express high-affinity nerve growth factor receptors. J Allergy Clin Immunol. 1997;100(3):408–14.
112. Raychaudhuri SP, Farber EM, Raychaudhuri SK. Role of nerve growth factor in RANTES expression by keratinocytes. Acta Derm Venereol. 2000;80(4):247–50.
113. Raychaudhuri SP, Raychaudhuri SK. Role of NGF and neurogenic inflammation in the pathogenesis of psoriasis. Prog Brain Res. 2004;146:433–7.
114. Naukkarinen A, Nickoloff BJ, Farber EM. Quantification of cutaneous sensory nerves and their substance P content in psoriasis. J Invest Dermatol. 1989;92(1):126–9.
115. Eedy DJ, Johnston CF, Shaw C, Buchanan KD. Neuropeptides in psoriasis: an immunocytochemical and radioimmunoassay study. J Invest Dermatol. 1991;96(4):434–8.
116. Thiele JJ, Traber MG, Polefka TG, Cross CE, Packer L. Ozone-exposure depletes vitamin E and induces lipid peroxidation in murine stratum corneum. J Invest Dermatol. 1997;108(5):753–7.
117. Ostrowski SM, Belkadi A, Loyd CM, Diaconu D, Ward NL. Cutaneous denervation of psoriasiform mouse skin improves acanthosis and inflammation in a sensory neuropeptide-dependent manner. J Invest Dermatol. 2011;131(7):1530–8.
118. Kanda N, Watanabe S. Prolactin enhances interferon-gamma-induced production of CXC ligand 9 (CXCL9), CXCL10, and CXCL11 in human keratinocytes. Endocrinology. 2007;148(5):2317–25.
119. Sahin E, Depinho RA. Linking functional decline of telomeres, mitochondria and stem cells during ageing. Nature. 2010;464(7288):520–8.
120. Perry JC, Guindalini C, Bittencourt L, Garbuio S, Mazzotti DR, Tufik S. Whole blood hypoxia-related gene expression reveals novel pathways to obstructive sleep apnea in humans. Respir Physiol Neurobiol. 2013;189(3):649–54.
121. Georgin-Lavialle S, Moura DS, Bruneau J, Chauvet-Gelinier JC, Damaj G, Soucie E, Barete S, Gacon AL, Grandpeix-Guyodo C, Suarez F, Launay JM, Durieu I, Esparcieux A, Guichard I, Sparsa A, Nicolini F, Gennes C, Trojak B, Haffen E, Vandel P, Lortholary O, Dubreuil P, Bonin B, Sultan S, Teyssier JR, Hermine O. Leukocyte telomere length in mastocytosis: correlations with depression and perceived stress. Brain Behav Immun. 2014;35:51–7.
122. Chiu A, Chon SY, Kimball AB. The response of skin disease to stress: changes in the severity of acne vulgaris as affected by examination stress. Arch Dermatol. 2003;139(7):897–900.
123. Zhang X, Lin S, Funk WE, Hou L. Environmental and occupational exposure to chemicals and telomere length in human studies. Occup Environ Med. 2013;70(10):743–9.
124. Boesten DM, de Vos-Houben JM, Timmermans L, den Hartog GJ, Bast A, Hageman GJ. Accelerated aging during chronic oxidative stress: a role for PARP-1. Oxid Med Cell Longev. 2013;2013:680414.
125. Tyrka AR, Price LH, Marsit C, Walters OC, Carpenter LL. Childhood adversity and epigenetic modulation of the leukocyte glucocorticoid receptor: preliminary findings in healthy adults. PLoS One. 2012;7(1):e30148.
126. Tyrka AR, Price LH, Kao HT, Porton B, Marsella SA, Carpenter LL. Childhood maltreatment and telomere shortening: preliminary support for an effect of early stress on cellular aging. Biol Psychiatry. 2010;67(6):531–4.
127. Oyetakin-White P, Koo B, Matsui M, Yarosh D, Fthenakis C, Cooper K, Baron E. In: Effects of sleep quality on skin aging and function. J Invest Dermatol Nature Publishing Group. 2013. p. S126.
128. Epel ES, Blackburn EH, Lin J, Dhabhar FS, Adler NE, Morrow JD, Cawthon RM. Accelerated telomere shortening in response to life stress. Proc Natl Acad Sci U S A. 2004;101(49):17312–15.
129. Bieber T. Atopic dermatitis. Ann Dermatol. 2010;22(2):125–37.
130. Dhabhar FS. Stress, leukocyte trafficking, and the augmentation of skin immune function. Ann N Y Acad Sci. 2003;992:205–17.
131. Barker JN, Palmer CN, Zhao Y, Liao H, Hull PR, Lee SP, Allen MH, Meggitt SJ, Reynolds NJ, Trembath RC, McLean WH. Null mutations in the filaggrin gene (FLG) determine major susceptibility to early-onset atopic dermatitis that persists into adulthood. J Invest Dermatol. 2007;127(3):564–7.
132. Brown SJ, Kroboth K, Sandilands A, Campbell LE, Pohler E, Kezic S, Cordell HJ, McLean WH, Irvine AD. Intragenic copy number variation within filaggrin contributes to the risk of atopic dermatitis with a dose-dependent effect. J Invest Dermatol. 2012;132(1):98–104.
133. Elias P, Man MQ, Williams ML, Feingold KR, Magin T. Barrier function in K-10 heterozygote knockout mice. J Invest Dermatol. 2000;114(2):396–7.
134. Kempuraj D, Huang M, Kandere K, Boucher W, Letourneau R, Jeudy S, Fitzgerald K, Spear K, Athanasiou A, Theoharides TC. Azelastine is more potent than olopatadine n inhibiting interleukin-6 and tryptase release from human umbilical cord blood-derived cultured mast cells. Ann Allergy Asthma Immunol. 2002;88(5):501–6.
135. Peters EM, Michenko A, Kupfer J, Kummer W, Wiegand S, Niemeier V, Potekaev N, Lvov A, Gieler U. Mental stress in atopic dermatitis – neuronal

plasticity and the cholinergic system are affected in atopic dermatitis and in response to acute experimental mental stress in a randomized controlled pilot study. PLoS One. 2014;9(12):e113552.
136. Okada HC, Alleyne B, Varghai K, Kinder K, Guyuron B. Facial changes caused by smoking: a comparison between smoking and nonsmoking identical twins. Plast Reconstr Surg. 2013;132(5):1085–92.
137. Everson CA. Functional consequences of sustained sleep deprivation in the rat. Behav Brain Res. 1995;69 (1–2):43–54.
138. Oh SH, Bae BG, Park CO, Noh JY, Park IH, Wu WH, Lee KH. Association of stress with symptoms of atopic dermatitis. Acta Derm Venereol. 2010;90(6):582–8.
139. Robinson H, Jarrett P, Broadbent E. The effects of relaxation before or after skin damage on skin barrier recovery: a preliminary study. Psychosom Med. 2015;77(8):844–52.
140. Buske-Kirschbaum A, Ebrecht M, Hellhammer DH. Blunted HPA axis responsiveness to stress in atopic patients is associated with the acuity and severeness of allergic inflammation. Brain Behav Immun. 2010;24(8):1347–53.
141. Barcelo A, Pierola J, Lopez-Escribano H, de la Pena M, Soriano JB, Alonso-Fernandez A, Ladaria A, Agusti A. Telomere shortening in sleep apnea syndrome. Respir Med. 2010;104(8):1225–9.
142. Manni M, Maestroni GJ. Sympathetic nervous modulation of the skin innate and adaptive immune response to peptidoglycan but not lipopolysaccharide: involvement of beta-adrenoceptors and relevance in inflammatory diseases. Brain Behav Immun. 2008;22(1):80–8.
143. Peters EM, Liezmann C, Spatz K, Daniltchenko M, Joachim R, Gimenez-Rivera A, Hendrix S, Botchkarev VA, Brandner JM, Klapp BF. Nerve growth factor partially recovers inflamed skin from stress-induced worsening in allergic inflammation. J Invest Dermatol. 2011;131(3):735–43.
144. Vedhara K, Cox NK, Wilcock GK, Perks P, Hunt M, Anderson S, Lightman SL, Shanks NM. Chronic stress in elderly carers of dementia patients and antibody response to influenza vaccination. Lancet. 1999;353(9153):627–31.
145. Damjanovic AK, Yang Y, Glaser R, Kiecolt-Glaser JK, Nguyen H, Laskowski B, Zou Y, Beversdorf DQ, Weng NP. Accelerated telomere erosion is associated with a declining immune function of caregivers of Alzheimer's disease patients. J Immunol. 2007;179 (6):4249–54.
146. Teresiak-Mikolajczak E, Czarnecka-Operacz M, Jenerowicz D, Silny W. Neurogenic markers of the inflammatory process in atopic dermatitis: relation to the severity and pruritus. Postepy Dermatol Alergol. 2013;30(5):286–92.
147. Papoiu AD, Wang H, Nattkemper L, Tey HL, Ishiuji Y, Chan YH, Schmelz M, Yosipovitch G. A study of serum concentrations and dermal levels of NGF in atopic dermatitis and healthy subjects. Neuropeptides. 2011;45(6):417–22.
148. Pavlovic S, Daniltchenko M, Tobin DJ, Hagen E, Hunt SP, Klapp BF, Arck PC, Peters EM. Further exploring the brain-skin connection: stress worsens dermatitis via substance P-dependent neurogenic inflammation in mice. J Invest Dermatol. 2008;128 (2):434–46.
149. Glaser R, Sheridan J, Malarkey WB, MacCallum RC, Kiecolt-Glaser JK. Chronic stress modulates the immune response to a pneumococcal pneumonia vaccine. Psychosom Med. 2000;62(6):804–7.
150. Theoharides TC, Bielory L. Mast cells and mast cell mediators as targets of dietary supplements. Ann Allergy Asthma Immunol. 2004;93(2 Suppl 1):S24–34.
151. Jarvikallio A, Harvima IT, Naukkarinen A. Mast cells, nerves and neuropeptides in atopic dermatitis and nummular eczema. Arch Dermatol Res. 2003; 295(1):2–7.
152. Deing V, Roggenkamp D, Kuhnl J, Gruschka A, Stab F, Wenck H, Burkle A, Neufang G. Oxytocin modulates proliferation and stress responses of human skin cells: implications for atopic dermatitis. Exp Dermatol. 2013;22(6):399–405.
153. Hara J, Higuchi K, Okamoto R, Kawashima M, Imokawa G. High-expression of sphingomyelin deacylase is an important determinant of ceramide deficiency leading to barrier disruption in atopic dermatitis. J Invest Dermatol. 2000;115(3):406–13.
154. Ghadially R, Reed JT, Elias PM. Stratum corneum structure and function correlates with phenotype in psoriasis. J Invest Dermatol. 1996;107(4):558–64.
155. Denda M, Tsuchiya T, Hosoi J, Koyama J. Immobilization-induced and crowded environment-induced stress delay barrier recovery in murine skin. Br J Dermatol. 1998;138(5):780–5.
156. Aioi A, Okuda M, Matsui M, Tonogaito H, Hamada K. Effect of high population density environment on skin barrier function in mice. J Dermatol Sci. 2001;25 (3):189–97.
157. Denda M, Tsuchiya T, Elias PM, Feingold KR. Stress alters cutaneous permeability barrier homeostasis. Am J Physiol Regul Integr Comp Physiol. 2000;278 (2):R367–72.
158. Choi EH, Demerjian M, Crumrine D, Brown BE, Mauro T, Elias PM, Feingold KR. Glucocorticoid blockade reverses psychological stress-induced abnormalities in epidermal structure and function. Am J Physiol Regul Integr Comp Physiol. 2006;291 (6):R1657–62.
159. Kao JS, Fluhr JW, Man MQ, Fowler AJ, Hachem JP, Crumrine D, Ahn SK, Brown BE, Elias PM, Feingold KR. Short-term glucocorticoid treatment compromises both permeability barrier homeostasis and stratum corneum integrity: inhibition of epidermal lipid synthesis accounts for functional abnormalities. J Invest Dermatol. 2003;120 (3):456–64.
160. Choi EH, Brown BE, Crumrine D, Chang S, Man MQ, Elias PM, Feingold KR. Mechanisms by which psychologic stress alters cutaneous permeability

barrier homeostasis and stratum corneum integrity. J Invest Dermatol. 2005;124(3):587–95.

161. Garg A, Chren MM, Sands LP, Matsui MS, Marenus KD, Feingold KR, Elias PM. Psychological stress perturbs epidermal permeability barrier homeostasis: implications for the pathogenesis of stress-associated skin disorders. Arch Dermatol. 2001;137(1):53–9.
162. Muizzuddin N, Matsui MS, Marenus KD, Maes DH. Impact of stress of marital dissolution on skin barrier recovery: tape stripping and measurement of trans-epidermal water loss (TEWL). Skin Res Technol. 2003;9(1):34–8.
163. Fukuda S, Baba S, Akasaka T. Psychological stress has the potential to cause a decline in the epidermal permeability barrier function of the horny layer. Int J Cosmet Sci. 2015;37(1):63–9.
164. Wong VW, Gurtner GC, Longaker MT. Wound healing: a paradigm for regeneration. Mayo Clin Proc. 2013;88(9):1022–31.
165. Reinke J, Sorg H. Wound repair and regeneration. Eur Surg Res. 2012;49(1):35–43.
166. Wang AS, Armstrong EJ, Armstrong AW. Corticosteroids and wound healing: clinical considerations in the perioperative period. Am J Surg. 2013;206(3):410–17.
167. Walburn J, Vedhara K, Hankins M, Rixon L, Weinman J. Psychological stress and wound healing in humans: a systematic review and meta-analysis. J Psychosom Res. 2009;67(3):253–71.
168. Kiecolt-Glaser JK, Marucha PT, Malarkey WB, Mercado AM, Glaser R. Slowing of wound healing by psychological stress. Lancet. 1995;346(8984):1194–6.
169. Cole-King A, Harding KG. Psychological factors and delayed healing in chronic wounds. Psychosom Med. 2001;63(2):216–20.
170. Ebrecht M, Hextall J, Kirtley LG, Taylor A, Dyson M, Weinman J. Perceived stress and cortisol levels predict speed of wound healing in healthy male adults. Psychoneuroendocrinology. 2004;29(6):798–809.
171. Mercado AM, Padgett DA, Sheridan JF, Marucha PT. Altered kinetics of IL-1 alpha, IL-1 beta, and KGF-1 gene expression in early wounds of restrained mice. Brain Behav Immun. 2002;16(2):150–62.
172. Glaser R, Kiecolt-Glaser JK, Marucha PT, MacCallum RC, Laskowski BF, Malarkey WB. Stress-related changes in proinflammatory cytokine production in wounds. Arch Gen Psychiatry. 1999;56(5):450–6.
173. Yang EV, Bane CM, MacCallum RC, Kiecolt-Glaser JK, Malarkey WB, Glaser R. Stress-related modulation of matrix metalloproteinase expression. J Neuroimmunol. 2002;133(1–2):144–50.
174. Romana-Souza B, Otranto M, Vieira AM, Filgueiras CC, Fierro IM, Monte-Alto-Costa A. Rotational stress-induced increase in epinephrine levels delays cutaneous wound healing in mice. Brain Behav Immun. 2010;24(3):427–37.
175. Rojas IG, Padgett DA, Sheridan JF, Marucha PT. Stress-induced susceptibility to bacterial infection during cutaneous wound healing. Brain Behav Immun. 2002;16(1):74–84.
176. Aberg KM, Radek KA, Choi EH, Kim DK, Demerjian M, Hupe M, Kerbleski J, Gallo RL, Ganz T, Mauro T, Feingold KR, Elias PM. Psychological stress downregulates epidermal antimicrobial peptide expression and increases severity of cutaneous infections in mice. J Clin Invest. 2007;117(11):3339–49.
177. Horan MP, Quan N, Subramanian SV, Strauch AR, Gajendrareddy PK, Marucha PT. Impaired wound contraction and delayed myofibroblast differentiation in restraint-stressed mice. Brain Behav Immun. 2005;19(3):207–16.
178. Grose R, Werner S, Kessler D, Tuckermann J, Huggel K, Durka S, Reichardt HM, Werner S. A role for endogenous glucocorticoids in wound repair. EMBO Rep. 2002;3(6):575–82.
179. Kondo T, Ishida Y. Molecular pathology of wound healing. Forensic Sci Int. 2010;203(1):93–8.
180. Sivamani RK, Pullar CE, Manabat-Hidalgo CG, Rocke DM, Carlsen RC, Greenhalgh DG, Isseroff RR. Stress-mediated increases in systemic and local epinephrine impair skin wound healing: potential new indication for beta blockers. PLoS Med. 2009;6(1):e12.
181. Denda M, Fuziwara S, Inoue K. Beta2-adrenergic receptor antagonist accelerates skin barrier recovery and reduces epidermal hyperplasia induced by barrier disruption. J Invest Dermatol. 2003;121(1):142–8.
182. Kim MH, Gorouhi F, Ramirez S, Granick JL, Byrne BA, Soulika AM, Simon SI, Isseroff RR. Catecholamine stress alters neutrophil trafficking and impairs wound healing by beta-adrenergic receptor-mediated upregulation of IL-6. J Invest Dermatol. 2013;314:809.
183. Gajendrareddy PK, Sen CK, Horan MP, Marucha PT. Hyperbaric oxygen therapy ameliorates stress-impaired dermal wound healing. Brain Behav Immun. 2005;19(3):217–22.
184. Weinman J, Ebrecht M, Scott S, Walburn J, Dyson M. Enhanced wound healing after emotional disclosure intervention. Br J Health Psychol. 2008;13(Pt 1):95–102.
185. Koschwanez H, Vurnek M, Weinman J, Tarlton J, Whiting C, Amirapu S, Colgan S, Long D, Jarrett P, Broadbent E. Stress-related changes to immune cells in the skin prior to wounding may impair subsequent healing. Brain Behav Immun. 2015.
186. Zarzer CA, Puchinger MG, Kohler G, Kugler P. Differentiation between genomic and non-genomic feedback controls yields an HPA axis model featuring hypercortisolism as an irreversible bistable switch. Theor Biol Med Model. 2013;10:65.
187. Dhabhar FS, McEwen BS. Acute stress enhances while chronic stress suppresses cell-mediated immunity in vivo: a potential role for leukocyte trafficking. Brain Behav Immun. 1997;11(4):286–306.

188. Atanackovic D, Brunner-Weinzierl MC, Kroger H, Serke S, Deter HC. Acute psychological stress simultaneously alters hormone levels, recruitment of lymphocyte subsets, and production of reactive oxygen species. Immunol Invest. 2002;31(2):73–91.
189. Dhabhar FS. Enhancing versus suppressive effects of stress on immune function: implications for immunoprotection versus immunopathology. Allergy Asthma Clin Immunol. 2008;4(1):2–11.
190. Herman JP. Neural control of chronic stress adaptation. Front Behav Neurosci. 2013;7:61.
191. Mizoguchi K, Ikeda R, Shoji H, Tanaka Y, Maruyama W, Tabira T. Aging attenuates glucocorticoid negative feedback in rat brain. Neuroscience. 2009;159(1):259–70.
192. Born J, Ditschuneit I, Schreiber M, Dodt C, Fehm HL. Effects of age and gender on pituitary-adrenocortical responsiveness in humans. Eur J Endocrinol. 1995;132(6):705–11.
193. Parker J, Klein SL, McClintock MK, Morison WL, Ye X, Conti CJ, Peterson N, Nousari CH, Tausk FA. Chronic stress accelerates ultraviolet-induced cutaneous carcinogenesis. J Am Acad Dermatol. 2004;51(6):919–22.
194. Saul AN, Oberyszyn TM, Daugherty C, Kusewitt D, Jones S, Jewell S, Malarkey WB, Lehman A, Lemeshow S, Dhabhar FS. Chronic stress and susceptibility to skin cancer. J Natl Cancer Inst. 2005; 97(23):1760–7.
195. Yaar M, Gilchrest BA. Cellular and molecular mechanisms of cutaneous aging. J Dermatol Surg Oncol. 1990;16(10):915–22.
196. Goto M. Inflammaging (inflammation + aging): a driving force for human aging based on an evolutionarily antagonistic pleiotropy theory? Biosci Trends. 2008;2(6):218–30.
197. Poljsak B, Dahmane R. Free radicals and extrinsic skin aging. Dermatol Res Pract. 2012;2012:135206.
198. Dunn JH, Koo J. Psychological stress and skin aging: a review of possible mechanisms and potential therapies. Dermatol Online J. 2013;19(6):18561.
199. Skobowiat C, Dowdy JC, Sayre RM, Tuckey RC, Slominski A. Cutaneous hypothalamic-pituitary-adrenal axis homolog: regulation by ultraviolet radiation. Am J Physiol Endocrinol Metab. 2011;301(3):E484–93.
200. Schoepe S, Schacke H, May E, Asadullah K. Glucocorticoid therapy-induced skin atrophy. Exp Dermatol. 2006;15(6):406–20.
201. Flint MS, Baum A, Chambers WH, Jenkins FJ. Induction of DNA damage, alteration of DNA repair and transcriptional activation by stress hormones. Psychoneuroendocrinology. 2007;32(5):470–9.
202. Hara MR, Kovacs JJ, Whalen EJ, Rajagopal S, Strachan RT, Grant W, Towers AJ, Williams B, Lam CM, Xiao K, Shenoy SK, Gregory SG, Ahn S, Duckett DR, Lefkowitz RJ. A stress response pathway regulates DNA damage through beta2-adrenoreceptors and beta-arrestin-1. Nature. 2011; 477(7364):349–53.
203. Hara MR, Sachs BD, Caron MG, Lefkowitz RJ. Pharmacological blockade of a beta(2)AR-beta-arrestin-1 signaling cascade prevents the accumulation of DNA damage in a behavioral stress model. Cell Cycle. 2013;12(2):219–24.
204. Liu N, Wang LH, Guo LL, Wang GQ, Zhou XP, Jiang Y, Shang J, Murao K, Chen JW, Fu WQ, Zhang GX. Chronic restraint stress inhibits hair growth via substance P mediated by reactive oxygen species in mice. PLoS One. 2013;8(4):e61574.
205. Ali F, Sultana S. Repeated short-term stress synergizes the ROS signalling through up regulation of NFkB and iNOS expression induced due to combined exposure of trichloroethylene and UVB rays. Mol Cell Biochem. 2012;360(1–2):133–45.
206. Lucca G, Comim CM, Valvassori SS, Reus GZ, Vuolo F, Petronilho F, Gavioli EC, Dal-Pizzol F, Quevedo J. Increased oxidative stress in submitochondrial particles into the brain of rats submitted to the chronic mild stress paradigm. J Psychiatr Res. 2009;43(9):864–9.
207. Seo JS, Lee KW, Kim TK, Baek IS, Im JY, Han PL. Behavioral stress causes mitochondrial dysfunction via ABAD up-regulation and aggravates plaque pathology in the brain of a mouse model of Alzheimer disease. Free Radic Biol Med. 2011;50(11):1526–35.
208. Treiber N, Maity P, Singh K, Kohn M, Keist AF, Ferchiu F, Sante L, Frese S, Bloch W, Kreppel F, Kochanek S, Sindrilaru A, Iben S, Hogel J, Ohnmacht M, Claes LE, Ignatius A, Chung JH, Lee MJ, Kamenisch Y, Berneburg M, Nikolaus T, Braunstein K, Sperfeld AD, Ludolph AC, Briviba K, Wlaschek M, Florin L, Angel P, Scharffetter-Kochanek K. Accelerated aging phenotype in mice with conditional deficiency for mitochondrial superoxide dismutase in the connective tissue. Aging Cell. 2011;10(2):239–54.
209. Helfrich YR, Yu L, Ofori A, Hamilton TA, Lambert J, King A, Voorhees JJ, Kang S. Effect of smoking on aging of photoprotected skin: evidence gathered using a new photonumeric scale. Arch Dermatol. 2007; 143(3):397–402.
210. Morita A, Torii K, Maeda A, Yamaguchi Y. Molecular basis of tobacco smoke-induced premature skin aging. J Investig Dermatol Symp Proc. 2009;14(1):53–5.
211. Vierkotter A, Schikowski T, Ranft U, Sugiri D, Matsui M, Kramer U, Krutmann J. Airborne particle exposure and extrinsic skin aging. J Invest Dermatol. 2010;130(12):2719–26.
212. Valacchi G, Pagnin E, Okamoto T, Corbacho AM, Olano E, Davis PA, van der Vliet A, Packer L, Cross CE. Induction of stress proteins and MMP-9 by 0.8 ppm of ozone in murine skin. Biochem Biophys Res Commun. 2003;305(3):741–6.
213. Donaldson K, Tran L, Jimenez LA, Duffin R, Newby DE, Mills N, MacNee W, Stone V. Combustion-derived nanoparticles: a review of their toxicology following inhalation exposure. Part Fibre Toxicol. 2005;2:10.

214. Li N, Sioutas C, Cho A, Schmitz D, Misra C, Sempf J, Wang M, Oberley T, Froines J, Nel A. Ultrafine particulate pollutants induce oxidative stress and mitochondrial damage. Environ Health Perspect. 2003;111(4):455–60.
215. Morhenn VB. Langerhans cells may trigger the psoriatic disease process via production of nitric oxide. Immunol Today. 1997;18(9):433–6.
216. Simon NM, Smoller JW, McNamara KL, Maser RS, Zalta AK, Pollack MH, Nierenberg AA, Fava M, Wong KK. Telomere shortening and mood disorders: preliminary support for a chronic stress model of accelerated aging. Biol Psychiatry. 2006;60(5):432–5.
217. Choi J, Fauce SR, Effros RB. Reduced telomerase activity in human T lymphocytes exposed to cortisol. Brain Behav Immun. 2008;22(4):600–5.
218. Sahin E, DePinho RA. Axis of ageing: telomeres, p53 and mitochondria. Nat Rev Mol Cell Biol. 2012; 13(6):397–404.
219. Liu JC, Verhulst S, Massar SA, Chee MW. Sleep deprived and sweating it out: the effects of total sleep deprivation on skin conductance reactivity to psychosocial stress. Sleep. 2015;38(1):155–9.
220. Rezvani HR, Ali N, Serrano-Sanchez M, Dubus P, Varon C, Ged C, Pain C, Cario-Andre M, Seneschal J, Taieb A, de Verneuil H, Mazurier F. Loss of epidermal hypoxia-inducible factor-1alpha accelerates epidermal aging and affects re-epithelialization in human and mouse. J Cell Sci. 2011;124(Pt 24):4172–83.
221. Arck PC, Slominski A, Theoharides TC, Peters EM, Paus R. Neuroimmunology of stress: skin takes center stage. J Invest Dermatol. 2006;126(8): 1697–704.
222. Arck PC, Handjiski B, Peters EM, Hagen E, Klapp BF, Paus R. Topical minoxidil counteracts stress-induced hair growth inhibition in mice. Exp Dermatol. 2003;12(5):580–90.

Place Your Bets, the Die Is Cast: The Skin at the Retiring Age Today and Tomorrow

158

Claudine Piérard-Franchimont, Gérald E. Piérard, Marianne Lesuisse, and Trinh Hermanns-Lê

Contents

C. Piérard-Franchimont
Laboratory of Skin Bioengineering and Imaging, Department of Dermatopathology, University Hospital of Liège, Liège, Belgium

Department of Dermatology, Regional Hospital of Huy, Huy, Belgium
e-mail: claudine.franchimont@ulg.ac.be

G.E. Piérard (✉)
Laboratory of Skin Bioengineering and Imaging, Department of Dermatopathology, University Hospital of Liège, Liège, Belgium
e-mail: gerald.pierard@ulg.ac.be

M. Lesuisse
Department of Dermatology, Unilab Lg, Regional Hospital Citadelle, Liège, Belgium

Department of Dermatology, Regional Hospital of Huy, Huy, Belgium
e-mail: marianne.lesuisse@chrcitadelle.be

T. Hermanns-Lê
Laboratory of Skin Bioengineering and Imaging, Department of Dermatopathology, University Hospital of Liège, Liège, Belgium

Electron Microscopy Unit, Department of Dermatopathology, Unilab Lg, University Hospital of Liège, Liège, Belgium
e-mail: trinh.hermanns@chu.ulg.ac.be

M.A. Farage et al. (eds.), *Textbook of Aging Skin*,
DOI 10.1007/978-3-662-47398-6_154

Abstract
The skin, similarly to any other organ, is aging in particular ways. Over the past century, the time effects on the skin have been expressed differently. The skin of any individual presently engaged in the Third Age looks different from that of his/her line ancestral. What is the expected future? The Third Age population is expanding, and skin problems call for a variety of management procedures. Prevention of the diverse types of skin aging has made tremendous progresses particularly in the field of preventive and corrective dermocosmetology. The future should further speed up such trends.

Introduction

Senescence of people represents the global expression of obsolescence of their various organs, tissues, cells, and constitutive molecules. The skin, similarly to any other organ, is aging in various ways. Over the past century, the time effects on the skin have been expressed differently. The skin of any individual getting on in age looks different from that of his/her line ancestral. What is the expected future? The aged population is expanding, and skin problems call for a variety of management procedures. Prevention of the diverse types of skin aging has made tremendous progresses particularly in the field of preventive and corrective dermocosmetology. The future should further speed up such trends.

Inescapably, skin aging progresses in any individual over the passing time. Diverse intrinsic and extrinsic factors including peculiar social compartments alter the regular common aging evolution. The impact of these factors has changed over the past century. Thus, at a given legal age, the skin at the present time does not exactly fit with the regular aspect of the skin of individuals at the same age a century ago. Taking into account the prominent increase in life expectancy of about 10 years over the past half of century in developed countries, the aging population has considerably progressed. What is the future? Should further aging progression or improvement in the aging quality be expected?

The skin is aging over time. Some intrinsic and extrinsic factors, as well as peculiar social behaviors, concur to modulate the aging process. The impact of these factors has probably changed over the past century. At similar legal ages, the skin at the retiring age nowadays has not the same look as most subjects a century ago. In certain respect of the large increase in the life expectancy, about 10 years during the past 50 years in developed countries, the aging part of the life covers an increasing part of the life.

The noticeable modifications of the skin aging signs are not similar in all individuals. In addition, in a given subject, the modalities and time of apparition of the signs, as well as their extent, vary according to the nature of cell types, tissues, and organs [1, 2]. Aging is usually a slow and insidious process. Most of the effects become perceptible only when clinical lesions become spontaneously irreversible. In addition, the adaptation potential of any physiological system declines with the aging progression. The decrease in performance related to aging corresponds to a decline in the adaptation potential of diverse biological and physical stresses. The intra- and interindividual heterogeneity of the skin quality requires the assessment of the biological age before rating the efficacy of any procedure aiming at reducing the visible signs of skin aging [3].

Our purpose is not to comment problems linked to demographic shift in the population. Everybody acknowledges the numerical growth of the aged population and of its important social impact. We are rather looking at the clinical aspect of aged skin at different time periods of the last century and inside different ethnic groups.

Legal Versus Biological Age?

Some differences exist between the actual skin aspect of aging people and their legal age. When things are on the road to ruin, the legal age only reflects in part the global aging. It is therefore appropriate to be more discriminative for better appreciating the actual organic state by considering a reference other than the legal age. Indeed, the biological age refers to the physiological and functional status of the subject. It occasionally corresponds to the legal age, but it is not rare to meet people who are not looking their ages. They appear either younger or older than their contemporary people. In general, people looking younger share healthy biological parameters.

A Century Ago

At the onset of the past century, the average life expectancy in developed countries reached about 50 years, and people older than 65 only represented a minute proportion of the population. At that time, most acknowledged observations in dermatology were confined to Europe. The archetype of older skin was that of the sailor or farmer exposed without any protection to the environment. The working conditions at that time accentuated the effects of chronic sun exposures.

At Present

At present, native populations in Western countries are diversified and different ethnic groups are mixed. Retired people are progressively more numerous and the global socioeconomic status has improved. The distinct aspects of skin aging are better identified [4]. The prevention of skin alterations at the retiring age has also made prominent advances, in particular, in the field of dermocosmetology, camouflaging, and wrinkle obliteration. By contrast, the problematics of skin cancers have grown in scale [5, 6]. The factors influencing the overall aging, and in particular skin aging, are better perceived and considered, allowing to better appreciate preventive measures.

In the past century, fatalism prevailed in the field of aging as the expression of the ravages of time. The quest of endless youth appeared mythical and out of reach. Aging appeared as the major factor invalidating efforts aiming at increasing life expectancy. Hopefully, factual studies performed by scientists were detrimental of medical charlatans.

Numerous scientific developments are still needed to understand the involved processes of aging [7–11]. Many facets of the knowledge about aging are currently available, and a fastened spreading of expansion was burning during the past decade [7] distinguishing two possible theories, namely, the clock (cell/DNA programming) and the accumulation of successive mistakes created by stresses generated by different origins. Among them, the oxidative stress following the intervention of oxygen species appears as a major biological mechanism involved as a supplier of aging [7].

Skin Aging Modalities

The problematic of skin aging cannot be dissociated from the global events in the organism. A particularity of aging is the variable multimorbidity in the organs, their respective tissues, and their diverse cell lines. However, the skin often reveals the initial visible signs of aging. The subject becomes aware of changes in color, texture, and tonicity of the skin, as well as the installation of the initial wrinkles followed by more obvious signs such as couperosis, a progressive laxity, and increased skin fragility, as well as the occurrence of benign and malignant tumors. Such an evolution is neither stereotyped nor inescapable. The skin alterations are more or less early and severe according to each individual and the different parts of the body.

According to a common axiom, two major types of skin aging are distinguished. One type corresponds to chronologic aging. Its typical manifestations develop on photoprotected areas. It is opposed to aging induced by environmental factors, particularly actinic radiations or selected ultraviolet light irradiations (sunbeds). This latter type of aging develops on photoexposed areas.

Another more diversified classification of skin aging has been proposed considering seven groups of mechanisms (Table 1). Each of these factors acts at different levels in the global skin aging, and they explain in part some differences between temporal influence and the biological age (Table 2). Aging and its signs represent the outcome of the autobiography of the subject.

Arbitrarily, some people consider that any individual begins aging (young-old) about mid-60s. The next step (medium-old) at the gate of geriatry takes place at about 75 years old. The last step (old-old) initiates at the age of 85. For each individual, the reality is frequently different and more complex. As another concept, human aging commonly begins in early adulthood. It presents diverse aspects according to the physiological systems, and it progresses distinctly according to the organs, the genetic inheritance, the past medical history, the environment, and the way of life. The diversity of the physiological stage according to the cutaneous area represents one of the most salient aspects in the aged population. This concept implies that aging must be addressed from distinctive perspectives. The medical approach of skin aging cannot dismiss the dermocosmetic management.

Table 1 Modalities of skin aging

Modality	Main factor
Temporal	Evolving time
Genetic	Phototype, abnormal DNA repair, premature aging syndromes
Actinic	Ultraviolet light and infrared irradiations
Behavioral	Tobacco, alcohol, starvation, drug abuses
Catabolic	Debilitating diseases (chronic infections, cancer)
Endocrine	Aging and dysfunctions of hormonal glands (perimenopause, thyroid dysfunction, etc.)
Mechanical	Earth gravitation, platysma muscles

Diversity in Aging Modalities

There exists a time-related aging, probably related to the progressive shortening of telomere in cell nuclei [12, 13]. Such an aging aspect is independent from environmental influences and from any acquired physiopathological alterations. Within this context, legal age is primordial. The elapsed time exerts an impact on all modalities of getting older. In other respects, there exists a pathological genetic aging involving specific DNA mutations responsible for premature aging (Werner syndrome, progeria, xeroderma pigmentosum, etc.).

Photoaging is the result of cumulative effects of ultraviolet light and at a lesser extent of infrared light on the functions of nuclei in cells of the skin. The epidermis becomes atrophic showing alterations in the relationship between melanocytes

Table 2 Clinical signs of skin aging

	Skin aging						
Clinical signs	Temporal	Genetic	Actinic	Behavioral	Catabolic	Endocrine	Mechanical
Alopecia	+	+		+	+	+	
Dermal atrophy	+	+		+	+	+	
Canitia	+	+			+	+	
Stellate scar		+	+		+	+	+
Cutis variegata	+	+	+				
Actinic elastosis		+	+				
Sebaceous hypertrophy		+	+				
Onychopathy	+				+	+	+
Bateman purpura	+				+	+	+
Wrinkles and expression	+			+	+		+
Wrinkles and laxity	+	+			+		+
Wrinkles and elastosis			+				
Gray complexion	+			+	+	+	
Sallow complexion		+	+				
Xerosis	+		+		+	+	

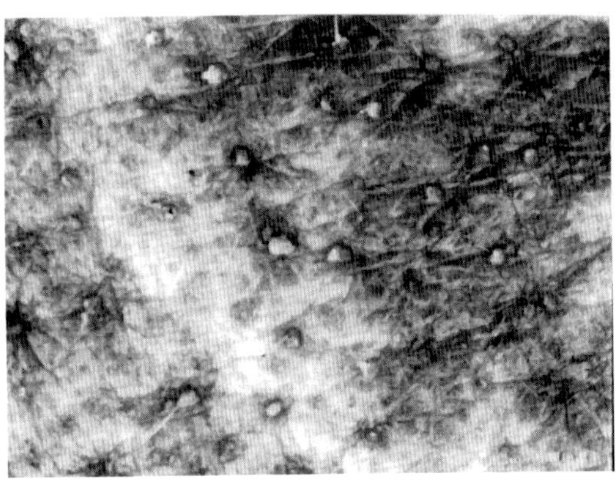

Fig. 1 Faint mosaic melanoderma on the facial skin of an older woman

and keratinocytes [14]. Clinically, the faint mosaic melanoderma progressively develops. The face is particularly involved since early adulthood [15], and the abnormal pattern of subtle melanin variegation increases with skin aging (Fig. 1). Such a skin condition is possibly involved in the initiation of skin malignancies [15, 16].

In addition to a remodeling of the dermal structure, a dermal atrophy takes place in some skin areas, and, at other sites, actinic elastosis develops. Field cancerogenesis is frequently induced on the face and hairless scalp [11]. Photoaging is under ethnic influences [17] and on the individual behavior regarding sun exposures.

Some behaviors induce a premature aging aspect. For instance, chronic alcoholism, nicotine abuse, and various drug addictions lead to wrinkle deepening on the face [18].

The aging process of the skin depends in its greater part on an increased degradation of the dermal extracellular matrix. The atrophy of the issue is occasionally severe and called "transparent skin," atrophodermia, or dermatoporosis [19]. Some chronic infections (AIDS, tuberculosis, etc.), cancers, and nutritional deficiencies are responsible for such a process.

A series of endocrine dysfunctions are responsible for worsening the aspect of skin aging, particularly by reducing synthesis of the extracellular matrix [20, 21].

A diversity of mechanical factors related to the repetitive action of facial muscles exerts a prominent influence. Gravity represents the earth attraction on the skin. It is responsible for a series of skin folds and for ptosis at specific body sites.

The overall aspect of skin aging results from the conjunction of the abovementioned modalities and of any interference with various treatments [22–24]. Each of the single aging modalities is possibly countered by specific preventive, corrective, or adequately fitted therapeutic modalities. Some correlations possibly exist between some signs of skin aging and a series of internal degradations including age-related osteoporosis [25].

To curb skin aging and to plan youthfulness have progressively evolved from inactive procedures to more realistic concepts. Active cosmetology has progressively evolved [26, 27]. It allows to wipe out and cover up some manifestations of skin aging. Another skin care management requires fillers for wrinkle or agents such as botulinum toxin responsible for facial muscle paralysis. Beyond such procedures, plastic surgery (lifting) remodels and advisedly stretches again the skin.

Prevention particularly targets photoaging following the use of topical photoprotectors [28, 29] and adequate clothing. Some supplementary foodstuffs have been also offered [30].

The correction of hormonal aging is attempted using drugs [31, 32]. Postmenopausal hormonotherapy correcting specific effects of hypoestrogenemia has been extensively studied [20, 31–38].

Tomorrow

Tomorrow should generate new preventive modalities against skin aging. Some corrective innovative procedures and improvements in various therapies, in particular, those oriented toward molecular biology are expected. Scientifically supported facts will prevail over publicity campaigns and artificial unsubstantiated claims.

Some of the main lines of progress are expected in the prevention and treatment of field cancerogenesis and in the control of the dermal texture as well. Cosmeceutical products are expected by an increasing proportion of the population. Some improvements are further expected in the field of laser therapies. All those expected evolutions will require refined formation of physicians devoted to the future methods for controlling skin aging.

Objective measurements of the biological age of the skin represent a priority in dermometrology in order to support specialized physicians in skin aging. This discipline should bring adequate means of objective evaluations of the skin effects at short, medium, and long term.

Conclusion

Skin aging is multifactorial and protean in the population. Dermoscosmetic treatments help concealing or reducing some clinical signs. "Evidence-based dermocosmetology" in the field of efficacy relies on objective evaluations of the skin presentation using biometeorological methods. The field of claimed product efficacy is variable, going from imperceptibility to convincing. The future in this field is promising. When we will get old, the younger generation will probably be testing with objectivity any real antiaging strategy.

References

1. Piérard GE. The quandary of climacteric skin ageing. Dermatology. 1996;193:273–4.
2. Piérard GE. Ageing across the life span: time to think again. J Cosmet Dermatol. 2004;3:50–3.
3. Tamburic S, et al. Exploring the effects of non-medical versus medical approaches to the management of skin aging in women over sixty. Int J Cosmet Sci. 2012;34:481–8.
4. Piérard GE, Piérard-Franchimont C. From cellular senescence to seven ways of skin aging. Rev Med Liege. 1997;52:285–8.
5. Farage MA, et al. Neoplastic skin lesions in the elderly patient. Cutan Ocul Toxicol. 2008;27:213–29.
6. Piérard GE, et al. The thousand and one facets of actinic keratosis. Hauppauge: Nova Science Publishers; 2013. p. 1–129.
7. Toussaint O, et al. Experimental gerontology in Belgium: from model organisms to age-related pathologies. Exp Gerontol. 2000;35:901–16.
8. Petit L, et al. Regional variability in mottled subclinical melanoderma in the elderly. Exp Gerontol. 2003;38:327–31.
9. Henry F, et al. Towards obsolete senescence. Everything wanes ... old age no longer exists! Rev Med Liege. 2000;55:110–3.
10. Hermanns-Lê T, et al. Skin tensile properties revisited during ageing. Where now, where next? J Cosmet Dermatol. 2004;3:35–40.
11. Piérard GE, et al. Field melanin mapping of the hairless scalp. Skin Res Technol. 2012;18:431–5.
12. Kim Sh SH, et al. Telomeres, aging and cancer: in search of a happy ending. Oncogene. 2002;21:503–11.
13. Imbert I, et al. Modulation of telomere binding proteins: a future area of research for skin protection and anti-aging target. J Cosmet Dermatol. 2012;11:162–6.
14. Schiller M, et al. Solar-simulated ultraviolet radiation-induced upregulation of the melanocortin-1 receptor, proopiomelanocortin, and alpha-melanocyte-stimulating hormone in human epidermis in vivo. J Invest Dermatol. 2004;122:468–76.
15. Hermanns-Lê T, et al. Scrutinizing skinfield melanin patterns in young Caucasian women. Expert Opin Med Diagn. 2013;7:455–62.
16. Piérard GE, et al. In vivo skin fluorescence imaging in young Caucasian adults with early malignant melanomas. Clin Cosmet Investig Dermatol. 2014;7:225–30.
17. de Rigal J, et al. The effect of age on skin color and color heterogeneity in four ethnic groups. Skin Res Technol. 2010;16:168–78.
18. Piérard GE, et al. Update on the histological presentation of facial wrinkles. Eur J Dermatol. 2002;12: XIII–IV.
19. Piérard-Franchimont C, et al. Dermatoporosis, a vintage for atrophoderma and transparent skin. Rev Med Liege. 2014;69:210–3.
20. Wines N, Willsteed E. Menopause and the skin. Australas J Dermatol. 2001;42:149–58. quiz 159.
21. Piérard-Franchimont C, Piérard GE. Postmenopausal aging of the sebaceous follicle: a comparison between women receiving hormone replacement therapy or not. Dermatology. 2002;204:17–22.
22. Calvo E, et al. Pangenomic changes induced by DHEA in the skin of postmenopausal women. J Steroid Biochem Mol Biol. 2008;112:186–93.
23. Farage MA, et al. Gender differences in skin aging and the changing profile of the sex hormones with age. J Steroid Horm Sci. 2012;3:1000109.
24. Castelo-Branco C, et al. Facial wrinkling in postmenopausal women. Effects of smoking status and hormone replacement therapy. Maturitas. 1998;29:75–86.
25. Piérard GE, et al. Relationship between bone mass density and tensile strength of the skin in women. Eur J Clin Invest. 2001;31:731–5.
26. Saint-Léger D. 'Cosmeceuticals'. Of men, science and laws. Int J Cosmet Sci. 2012;34:396–401.
27. Krause M, et al. Sunscreens: are they beneficial for health? An overview of endocrine disrupting properties of UV-filters. Int J Androl. 2012;35:424–36.
28. L'Alloret F, et al. New combination of ultraviolet absorbers in an oily emollient increases sunscreen

efficacy and photostability. Dermatol Ther (Heidelb). 2012;2:4.
29. Bouilly-Gauthier D, et al. Clinical evidence of benefits of a dietary supplement containing probiotic and carotenoids on ultraviolet-induced skin damage. Br J Dermatol. 2010;163:536–43.
30. Braverman ER. Ageprint for anti-ageing medicine. J Eur Anti-Ageing Med. 2005;1:7–8.
31. Zouboulis CC, Makrantonaki E. Hormonal therapy of intrinsic aging. Rejuvenation Res. 2012;15:302–12.
32. Piérard-Franchimont C, et al. Climacteric skin ageing of the face – a prospective longitudinal comparative trial on the effect of oral hormone replacement therapy. Maturitas. 1999;32:87–93.
33. Sauerbronn AV, et al. The effects of systemic hormonal replacement therapy on the skin of postmenopausal women. Int J Gynaecol Obstet. 2000;68:35–41.
34. Raine-Fenning NJ, et al. Skin aging and menopause: implications for treatment. Am J Clin Dermatol. 2003;4:371–8.
35. Guinot C, et al. Effect of hormonal replacement therapy on skin biophysical properties of menopausal women. Skin Res Technol. 2005;11:201–4.
36. Piérard GE, et al. Place your bets, the die is cast . . . the skin at the retiring age today and tomorrow. Rev Med Liege. 2014;69:366–71.
37. Piérard GE, et al. La cosméceutique, oxymoron de la quête d'une efficacité cosmétique? Dermatol Actual. 2009;113:16–9.
38. Piérard GE, et al. Women's skin throughout lifetime. Biomed Res Int. 2014;2014, 328981.

159 Sleep and Aging Skin

Linna Guan, Reena Mehra, and Elma Baron

Contents

L. Guan (✉) • E. Baron
Department of Dermatology, Case Western Reserve University, Cleveland, OH, USA
e-mail: Linna.Guan@case.edu; Elma.Baron@UHhospitals.org

R. Mehra
Sleep Medicine Center, The Cleveland Clinic, Cleveland, OH, USA
e-mail: Mehrar@ccf.org

M.A. Farage et al. (eds.), *Textbook of Aging Skin*,
DOI 10.1007/978-3-662-47398-6_155

Abstract

Aging is a process that is universal and commonly outwardly manifested on the skin and often most significantly noticed on the skin. The prevention of skin aging is currently a multibillion dollar industry with progressive rapid expansion and continues to expand. Intact sleep and circadian rhythm regulation is known to have protective effects against systemic inflammation, oxidative stress, hormone dysregulation, DNA damage, and other variables that contribute to aging. This chapter is focused upon the examination of factors that relate sleep to skin aging. To dissect this relationship, it is necessary to recognize the definitions of adequate sleep quality and how it is assessed. Sleep occurs in alternating cycles of NREM sleep and REM sleep and disruption can decrease sleep quality. In fact, here are over 90 sleep disorders characterized by the International Classification of Sleep Disorders. Various tools in our armamentarium can assess sleep quality and identify sleep disorders including subjective measures collected from questionnaires and objective sleep measures gleaned from polysomnography. Sleep helps regulate physiological hormone levels and metabolism. When quality sleep is disrupted, these hormone levels become abnormal and cause aberrant metabolism and increased stress on the body. Some of the major hormones regulated by sleep are cortisol, glucose, and melatonin. Furthermore, sleep deprivation enhances inflammation, increased DNA damage, and decreased DNA repair; oxidative stress and emerging data implicate sleep disruption in carcinogenic risk. These adverse pathophysiologic consequences may contribute to signs of aging such as wrinkling and alterations in pigmentation. Biologic plausibility of these underlying mechanisms and available data identifying sleep disruption as a factor compromising skin health suggest that it is important to consider methods of improving sleep quality as part of maintaining a healthy skin, in order to minimize or delay such effects.

Introduction

Every night an individual goes through a period of rest during which the body is subjected to reduced activity and decreased sensitivity to external stimuli. Such experience is loosely defined as sleep [1]. During sleep the body's temperature, blood pressure, and physiological demands drop. Sleep is a vital part of life and plays an important role in information retention and processing, hormone and metabolism regulation, cellular repair, immune response, and aging, including skin aging [2]. To better understand the effect of sleep on skin aging, we must understand sleep's complexity and its effects.

Defining Sleep

Although people experience sleep slightly differently, there are common patterns found in normal sleep. Sleep is an easily reversible process characterized by cycles of NREM (non-rapid eye movement) and REM (rapid eye movement) sleep [2]. During NREM sleep, the body experiences decreased physiological activity with decreased heart rate, decreased blood pressure, and prolonged brain waves with greater amplitudes, the latter specific to slow-wave sleep [2]. NREM sleep consists of four stages. Each progressive stage represents a deeper and more restful state. Stage 1 is defined as the transition from wakefulness to sleep characterized by slow rolling eye movements. It is often during this stage that people experience the feeling of falling followed by sudden muscle jerks (so-called myoclonic or hypnic jerks) [2]. During stage 2, the body begins to relax as brain waves become slower and the heart rate and body temperature decrease. Sporadic surges of rapid waves called sleep spindles (fast alpha waves, 12–14 Hz) are observed on encephalography reflective of thalamocortical oscillations. Stages 3 and 4 (slow-wave sleep) are defined by profound relaxation of the body. The blood pressure, breathing rate, heart rate, and body temperature further decrease while brain waves are characterized by slow delta waves at times mixed with smaller and faster waves [2]. The body becomes immobile and it is often difficult to awake during these two stages. REM sleep differs from NREM sleep in that REM sleep is characterized by fast and chaotic brain waves with rapid and shallow breathing, increased heart rate and blood pressure, and paralyzed limbs – a tumultuous state of sleep. Dream recall often occurs during REM sleep. Healthy sleep contains alternating NREM and REM sleeps in cycles of approximately 90–110 min, repeated four to six times with progressive lengthening of REM periods such that the predominance of REM sleep occurs during the latter part of the sleep cycle [2].

Measuring Sleep Quality

It is important clinically to be able to define sleep quality because of the immense role sleep plays in various aspects of aging. There are tools that have been used in sleep-related research and/or clinical care to evaluate sleep quality, which can also be used to determine the effect of sleep on skin aging.

Sleep Quality Questionnaires

The evaluation of sleep quality accounts for not only sleep duration but also other factors. One tool for measuring sleep quality is the Pittsburgh Sleep Quality Index (PSQI). The PSQI utilizes several parameters including subjective sleep quality, sleep latency, sleep duration, habitual sleep efficiency, sleep disturbances, use of sleep medication, and daytime dysfunction over the last month [3]. The PSQI, developed in 1989, is a survey taken by an individual or clinical study subject that yields a number of points that then translate into a quantitative score. The maximum number of points on the survey is 21 and the minimum number of points is 0. The higher the number of points, the poorer the sleep. A score greater than 5 is associated with poor sleep quality [3]. It is one of the simple but effective tools for determining patient sleep quality and often used for research studies with large sample sizes. Other sleep-focused questionnaires that may assist with understanding subjective sleep quality include the Sleep Quality Questionnaire, Epworth Sleepiness Scale (assesses dozing propensity), Functional Outcomes of Sleep Questionnaire, and questionnaires focused on screening for sleep-disordered breathing such as the Berlin and STOP-BANG questionnaires. Furthermore, questionnaires targeted toward other sleep disorders such as insomnia and restless legs syndrome are also available.

Polysomnography

The gold standard tool for evaluating sleep disorders such as sleep-disordered breathing and disruption of sleep architecture is polysomnography. It requires the patient to sleep overnight in a sleep laboratory while his brain activity and vitals are monitored using sensors attached to the scalp and the body [4]. Some of the commonly monitored physiologic parameters measured include brain electrical activity using an electroencephalogram (EEG), eye movements using an electrooculogram (EOG), and heart rate using an electrocardiogram (EKG). Other vitals such as respirations (airflow and nasal transducer), thoracoabdominal effort (typically via inductance plethysmography), and oxygen saturation are also often monitored. Polysomnography is a clinical diagnostic tool that can be used to detect sleep disorders such as narcolepsy, idiopathic hypersomnia, parasomnias, and sleep apnea. The main drawback of polysomnography, particularly in research, is that it is expensive and time consuming to perform in large scale.

Actigraphy

An increasingly common tool for assessing outpatient sleep quality is wrist actigraphy [5]. The actigraph estimates a patient's activity using the frequency of movement in the patient's arm. Usually the actigraph is a small, watch-like device that the patient wears on the nondominant wrist. Since muscle movements are more limited during sleep, the actigraph can measure sleep-wake cycles by monitoring the patient's movements. Actigraphy is an excellent tool for sleep studies that involve longer periods of time and unlike polysomnography can characterize sleep quality measures and patterns over multiple days/nights. Usually the actigraph is used to monitor patients for 1–2 weeks at a time [5]. It is relatively inexpensive. However, it lacks some details of sleep quality that the sleep questionnaires and polysomnography can provide.

The Effect of Sleep on Hormone Regulation and Skin Aging

Skin aging is classified into two types, intrinsic and extrinsic. Extrinsic skin aging is attributed to external factors such as UV radiation. Intrinsic aging of the skin is defined by structural changes due to genetics and normal physiology [6]. Unlike extrinsic aging that is accounted for by UV and toxin exposure, hormone changes and dysregulation are responsible for the majority of intrinsic aging of the skin [6]. Hormone dysregulation not only leads to aberrant metabolism which is ultimately responsible for the generation of reactive oxygen species (ROS) but also prevents the production of important antioxidants responsible for counteracting ROS and the damage they cause [7]. Sleep is one of the main regulators of hormone balance and rate of metabolism.

Cortisol

It has long been known that cortisol levels cycle in a circadian rhythm [8]. Cortisol is released in a pulsatile manner following adrenocorticotropic hormone (ACTH) release. The level of cortisol typically falls during the night, shortly after falling asleep, and reaches its lowest around midnight [9]. It then slowly reaches its peak in the morning around 3–9 a.m. [10]. Many diseases are associated with the dysfunction of this cyclical process including Cushing's syndrome, Alzheimer's disease, metabolic syndrome, and various mood disorders [11].

Studies have shown that short-term sleep deprivation of only one night corresponded with a 45 % elevation of cortisol levels the following night [9]. Long-term sleep deprivation showed similar results with elevated levels of glucocorticoids [12]. In the skin, elevated levels of glucocorticoids translate to lower permeability barrier homeostasis, less stratum corneum cohesion, decreased wound healing, and depressed innate immunity in the epidermis [13], all of which in turn could lead to intrinsic aging of the skin. Furthermore, sleep deprivation can cause physiological stress which induces excess glucocorticoid secretion and thus enhance skin aging. Insomniac psychologic stress, also known as IPS, is known to decrease epidermal cell proliferation, impair epidermal differentiation, and decrease the density and size of corneodesmosomes which hold keratinocytes together [14]. This can disrupt the skin's barrier against exogenous insults. The excess glucocorticoids also inhibit the synthesis of lipids, causing lower production and secretion of lamellar bodies which can lead to further damage to the epidermal barrier [15].

Glucose

During restful sleep, metabolic rate is reduced by approximately 15 % [16]. During the day when metabolic demand and glucose utilization are high, there is an increase in oxidative stress leading to increase in the production of radical oxygen species. During parts of non-REM sleep, there is a decrease in metabolic rate and brain temperature. This decrease helps the repair of damage from metabolically active periods.

When sleep deprivation occurs, glucose clearance is reduced by 40 % and the response of insulin to glucose is also reduced, leading to an elevated level of serum glucose [17]. The reduction of glucose tolerance after sleep deprivation is partially attributed to the increased levels of glucocorticoids. However, there also seem to be other mechanisms involved [7]. Studies have shown that slow-wave sleep (SWS) plays an important role in regulating insulin and maintaining glucose homeostasis [8].

The elevation of glucose concentration negatively impacts the proliferation of keratinocytes as well as fibroblasts of the skin [18, 19]. Impairment of proliferation of skin fibroblasts leads to delayed wound healing [19], similar to the delay in wound healing observed in the skin of the elderly [20]. There is also evidence that an increase in glucose concentration leads to the terminal differentiation and change in morphology of these keratinocytes [18]. These terminally differentiated cells lose their ability to generate new cells and are arrested in a terminal state through the upregulation of cyclin-dependent kinase inhibitors and downregulation of positive mediators of the cell cycle [21]. This parallels the phenomenon of cellular senescence in that these keratinocytes treated with high-glucose levels show characteristics similar to senescent cells [21]. At high concentrations of glucose, the keratinocytes are larger and flatter and did not exhibit orientation toward each other which can negatively impact the function and integrity of the keratinocytes [18].

Melatonin

Melatonin is another hormone that has been extensively studied in relationship to sleep. Its release from the pineal gland via stimulation from the suprachiasmatic nuclei (SCN) of the anterobasal hypothalamus displays circadian rhythm [8]. Its levels are higher in the biological night and lower in the biological day [8]. Melatonin can also be produced in extrapineal organs such as cutaneous cells, but the level of secretion is variable and usually displays no circadian rhythm [22]. The release of melatonin can help reduce sleep latency, increase total sleep time, and improve sleep maintenance [8]. Furthermore, the therapeutic effects of melatonin on the skin are extensive. Skin cells express both membrane-bound and nuclear melatonin receptors which allow melatonin to play a role in multiple vital functions such as hair growth cycling, hair pigmentation, melanoma control, antioxidant activity, and suppression of ultraviolet-induced damage to skin cells [23]. Melatonin has been shown to decrease aging-related skin changes from oxidative stress and prevent extrinsic aging of the skin through protection against UV-induced skin aging [24, 25], both of which will be discussed later in more detail.

The induction of melatonin expression from the SCN is dependent primarily on the light/dark cycling within the day [26]. Because light is the most effective suppressor, the introduction of artificial light in modern-day life alters the induction of melatonin secretion through the SCN [26]. Studies have shown that the intensity of light used directly correlates to the amount of suppression of melatonin levels [27]. The common practice of using artificial light at night to increase productivity has a negative impact on the circadian rhythm of melatonin. Dysregulation of melatonin ultimately has an adverse effect on the integrity of the skin and prevents melatonin's natural antiaging benefits on the skin. This leads to both increases in extrinsic aging of the skin from UV damage as well as intrinsic aging of the skin from oxidative stress.

The interplay among various hormones involved in the maintenance of skin health and integrity is extensive and complex. While significant research efforts are still ongoing on how sleep can impact these hormones, it is agreed that sleep deprivation negatively impacts changes in these hormone levels that ultimately result in damage and accelerated aging of the skin.

Cellular Repair and Sleep

Sleep is a process indispensable for cellular repair. During sleep, the body undergoes cellular repair and renewal and protects against other harmful exposures. This process is vital to the maintenance of the integrity and structure of the skin and recovery of the skin from UV damage [28]. Dysregulation of sleep is linked with an increase in inflammatory activity [29], increase in cellular injury [30], increase in DNA damage [31], increase in radical oxygen species production [32], and change in transcription levels of various genes [33], all of which may contribute to both intrinsic and extrinsic aging of the skin.

Inflammation

Inflammation is a process mediated by various cytokines, notably IL-6 and TNF-α [34]. IL-6 has many functions including elevating body temperature through activation of C-reactive protein, activating other inflammatory cytokine pathways, stimulating the production of neutrophils in the bone marrow, and attracting neutrophils to the site of inflammation [35]. TNF-α also plays many roles in the body from coordination of organ development to mediation of acute adaptive immune response and apoptosis [36]. Elevated levels of both IL-6 and TNF-α are observed in modest sleep restriction [29]. These cytokines have been linked to the loss of facial subcutaneous fat through the inhibition of preadipocyte differentiation [37]. Adipocytes are the fat-storing cells of the dermis and loss of adipocyte differentiation can ultimately cause increased wrinkling and sagging, resulting in the appearance of an aged face [38].

DNA Damage and Repair

A vital process for the retardation of aging is DNA repair. Repairing DNA helps maintain cellular function and regulation and prevents apoptosis of the cell. Sleep deprivation not only causes cell damage but also predisposes the cells to replication errors. Significantly increased DNA damage has been found in murine models that suffer total sleep deprivation over the control [30]. Diseases that disrupt sleep and cause poor sleep quality in humans such as sleep apnea can cause increased stress on the DNA. Sleep apnea patients are found to have a significant increase in susceptibility to DNA damage and reduction in DNA repair [39]. Although total sleep deprivation studies on humans cannot be fully replicated due to ethical concerns, it can be inferred that similar results can be obtained.

Furthermore, DNA repair has been shown to be regulated by factors that display a circadian pattern [31]. Numerous proteins, including several that regulate DNA repair, are controlled by the biological clock. Timeless, Tipin, and human CLK-2 are all factors that regulate the biological clock that also have been shown to directly affect ATR/Chk1-controlled DNA damage checkpoints during S-phase progression [31]. ATR and its downstream effects, Chk1, are responsible for the regulation of replication checkpoints where ssDNA have stalled which can result in deleterious conformations or collapsed replication forks [40].

NPAS2, neuronal PAS domain protein 2, is a core circadian gene and a transcriptional regulator, which has been linked to DNA repair [41]. NPAS2 protein forms a heterodimer with BMAL1 protein as a part of the positive circadian feedback loop to activate circadian genes and regulate circadian rhythm [41]. Silencing the NPAS2 gene has been shown to decrease cell viability, increase susceptibility to DNA damage, and decrease DNA damage repair capacity [41]. Dysregulation of sleep and circadian rhythm can impair the DNA repair mechanisms. Skin aging and carcinogenesis are closely linked with DNA damage and inhibition of DNA repair [42]. Poor sleep quality can result in elevated levels of DNA damage and reduced levels of DNA repair.

Oxidative Stress

Along with increased DNA damage, sleep deprivation and sleep-disordered breathing also have been associated with elevated levels of reactive oxygen species (ROS) [30]. ROS refers to free radicals such as hydroxyl (OH•), superoxide ($O2^{-}$), nitric oxide (NO•), thyl (RS•), and peroxyl (RO_2•) and non-free radicals such as peroxynitrite ($ONOO^{-}$), hypochlorous acid (HOCl), hydrogen peroxide (H_2O_2), singlet oxygen ($^1O_2$), and ozone (O_3) [43]. Even normal metabolism naturally generates ROS. The electron transport system in the mitochondria of many cells uses electron carriers such as nicotinamide dinucleotide (NAD+) and flavin adenine dinucleotide (FAD) which are later reoxidized in the mitochondria to generate ATP [43]. During this process of ATP production, significant ROS by-products are generated. It is estimated that approximately 1–2 % of all consumed oxygen is used for superoxide production [44]. In most cells, ROS is generated mainly in the mitochondria, although it is important to note that cells like hepatocytes can produce more ROS in the peroxisomes and endoplasmic reticulum than in the mitochondria [43].

ROS is also produced by various other pathways such as inflammation and UV damage. ROS plays important functions in normal physiology from destroying microbes in macrophages to regulating apoptosis [43]. However, superfluous levels of ROS can be produced during sleep deprivation. Being awake requires high levels of neuronal metabolism to retain electric potentials of the neurons [32]. As mentioned previously, sleep decreases levels of metabolism which can reduce ROS generation and provide for a state of increased antioxidant action to protect against free radicals [32]. Increased oxidative stress from sleep deprivation causes unwarranted apoptosis and cellular dysfunction through DNA damage and modification of proteins and lipids [43].

Oxidative damage is the major cause of skin aging. In the dermis, ROS imbalance leads to the destruction of collagen or impairment of collagen synthesis [44]. Breakdown of the dermal matrix causes wrinkling, a major sign of skin aging. ROS also increases destruction or impairment of differentiation of melanocytes, leaving the skin hypopigmented and vitiligo-like, which is another manifestation of skin aging [45].

Role of Antioxidants

Antioxidants can prevent and even reverse damage done by ROS. There are both enzymatic antioxidants and nonenzymatic antioxidants. Nonenzymatic antioxidants include compounds such as vitamin C, vitamin E, beta-carotene, and CoQ10 [45]. Most of these compounds such as vitamin C and vitamin E exert their antioxidant effects through the donation of an electron to a dangerous free radical. After donation of an electron, both vitamin C and vitamin E form radicals. However, they are relatively unreactive compared with the ROS and may be reduced back to its original state or donate its other electron [45]. Beta-carotene takes the free radical from the ROS to form an epoxide that can be later degraded while CoQ10 blocks lipids from forming peroxides. Enzymatic antioxidants function to "dismutate" superoxides to hydrogen peroxide through various mechanisms [45]. Some of these enzymes include superoxide dismutases, catalases, glutathione peroxidases, ferritin, and peroxiredoxins [45].

Melatonin functions as both a nonenzymatic antioxidant and an activator of enzymatic antioxidants. It scavenges ROS through single electron transfer, hydrogen transfer, and radical adduct formation [46]. It also activates antioxidant enzymes, inhibits prooxidant enzymes, and improves mitochondrial function to reduce radical formation [46]. Skin aging is marked by decrease in skin thickness, flattening of the dermoepidermal junction, and decrease in hair follicles and dermal papillae [24]. Interestingly, melatonin has also been proved to be able to reverse the process of skin aging through increasing the thickness of the epidermis and dermis, hair follicles, and papillae in murine models [24]. This further lends support to the role of melatonin as an important antioxidant that can relieve oxidative stress to hinder the skin aging process.

Carcinogenesis

As the skin ages, it becomes more susceptible to carcinogenesis. The effects of UV light accumulate over time and contribute to photoaging of the skin. Some of the mechanisms involved in the increase in susceptibility to carcinogenesis include increase in ROS production leading to damage of DNA, reduction in DNA repair ability, and decline in immune surveillance. These are all processes that may be associated with sleep deprivation. Sleep deprivation also causes increase in ROS production, decrease in RNA repair ability, and attenuation in immune function [43]. Various cohort studies have shown that "long sleepers" of greater than 9 h have been shown to have decreased risk of breast cancer compared with those who sleep less [47]. Sleep is a time when the body can undergo repair and renewal, which likely explains the association between sleep deprivation, skin aging, and cancer development.

Sleep and Skin Aging

Sleep Quality and Skin Aging

The effectiveness of sleep is dependent on more than just the duration of sleep. Other factors such as sleep latency and sleep disturbances are also critical measurements of sleep quality. Sleep quality has a significant impact on the aging of the skin. It has been reported that chronic poor sleep quality, evaluated using the PSQI score, is associated with lower skin function, integrity, and perception [28]. Those with scores less than 5 on the PSQI and an average sleep duration of 7–9 h are considered good sleeper, while those with scores greater than 5 on the PSQI and an average sleep duration of less than 5 h were considered poor sleepers. The good sleepers were shown to have significantly lower intrinsic aging than the poor sleepers, determined using SCINEXA [28].

SCINEXA is an index used to evaluate intrinsic versus extrinsic skin aging based on 5 noninvasive parameters of intrinsic aging and 18 noninvasive parameters of extrinsic aging [48]. Major intrinsic aging parameters are reduced fat tissue and uneven pigmentation. Major extrinsic aging parameters include carcinomas and permanent erythema [48].

Good sleepers have better recovery from erythema 24 h after UV radiation compared with poor sleepers. Good sleepers also have better skin barrier recovery [28]. To test skin barrier recovery, both good sleepers and poor sleepers were tape stripped to the same transepidermal water loss (TEWL). After 3 days, good sleepers showed markedly greater barrier recovery (30 %) than poor sleepers [28]. The good sleepers also had better satisfaction with their overall appearance than the poor sleepers did [28].

Chronic poor sleep quality affects intrinsic aging of the skin, recovery from UV erythema, and skin barrier recovery. Poor sleep quality not only affects the integrity and function of the skin but also negatively impacts self-perception.

Sleep and Facial Appearance

In a separate study, subjects' facial appearances were evaluated post good sleep and post sleep deprivation [49]. The study used pictures of subjects following 8 h of sleep and subjects following 5 h of sleep and then 31 h of sleep deprivation. Random evaluators were asked to rate the pictures on various signs of fatigue. The factors include perceived fatigue, hanging eyelids, swollen eyes, glazed eyes, dark circles under eyes, pale skin, wrinkles/lines around the eyes, rash/eczema, sadness, tense lips, and droopy corners of the mouth. It was noted that those with 5 h of sleep followed by 31 h of sleep deprivation had more hanging eyelids, redder eyes, more swollen eyes, darker circles under the eyes, paler skin, more wrinkles and fine lines around the eyes, and droopier corners of the mouth [49]. They were also noted to look more fatigued and sad [49]. Items that did not seem to differ between the two groups were level of glazed eyes, rash/eczema, and tense lips [49].

The idea that sleep has a significant impact on facial appearance is not a new one. However, with consumers spending billions of dollars on cosmetic products to enhance facial appearance, it is important to remember that just having a good sleep can significantly improve facial appearance.

Diurnal Cycle of Skin Wrinkling

One of the major signs of skin aging that can be visualized is wrinkling. A study published in 2004 found that wrinkle formation on the face differed in the morning versus the afternoon [50]. It was revealed that measurements of skin wrinkling were significantly higher in the afternoon versus in the morning on the forehead, corner of the eye, and nasolabial groove. Skin thickness and skin elasticity were also measured and were both found to be significantly less in the afternoon than in the morning. It is speculated that this phenomenon is caused by a shift of fluid from the skin of the face into the limbs from the morning to the afternoon [50]. Sleep would have a significant impact on this diurnal cycle since the horizontal position of sleeping would bring the shift in fluid back to the face. Therefore, it can be inferred that sleep deprivation would prevent the shift of fluid back to the face and promote wrinkle formation.

Sleep Lines and Facial Wrinkles

Sleep position can also affect the formation of facial wrinkles. Wrinkles or sleep lines are caused by continuous and repetitive pressure placed on the face from sleeping in the same position [51]. This constant force can eventually lead to elongation of the facial muscles and compression of wrinkles that persists even throughout the day. Since on average a person sleeps for one-third of his life, sleeping causes deepening of the wrinkles that worsens with aging [51]. Sleep lines are generally found as 2–3 parallel lines within a general area of the face [52]. Common areas of these lines are found in the lateral orbital, temporal, frontal, and buccal regions. People who sleep in prone positions are more likely to develop sleep lines than those who sleep in supine positions [52]. Furthermore, those who sleep on their left side are more likely to develop sleep lines than those who sleep on their right side [53]. Certain pillows can relieve the pressure on certain areas of the face and redistribute the gravitational force [51], but ultimately the only way to eliminate any pressure on the face is to sleep supine.

Independent of sleep position, individuals who have a mutation in the melanocortin-1 receptor (MC1R) gene also demonstrate an increased likelihood to form sleep lines [54]. The MC1R protein binds to melanocortin hormones such as ACTH (adrenocorticotropic hormone) and MSH (melanocyte-stimulating hormone) to regulate skin and hair color. It was also shown to have a role in photoaging of the skin. Certain mutations of this gene have been linked to significantly increased risk for photoaging when compared with wild type [54]. The same mutations of MC1R that are linked with photoaging have been implicated in increase in development of sleep lines.

The Role of Gender

Gender differences affect many aspects of the brain, most notably cognition and sleep. Some cognitive differences between the genders include that women perform better on verbal and memory tasks, while men performed better in spatial tasks [55]. Studies have also shown that women display less age-associated cognitive decline than men and that men show age-related neurocognitive decline at a younger age than women [55–57].

Differences in the sleep quality between the two genders have been well documented in previous literature [58]. Sleep differences that have been reported include: females experience longer sleep latency than males, women younger than 55 years of age report more sleepiness than men, older women sleep on average 20 min less than men, and women have more SWS and less NREM stage 1 than men [59]. As women age, they are 40 % more likely to develop insomnia and two times more likely to develop restless legs syndrome than men [60]. Mouse models have shown that some of these differences are due to the different sex hormones' involvement with each gender [59]. Murine models have shown that gonadectomy in female and male rates eliminated gender differences in the sleep-wake cycle, but hormone replacement of physiological levels restored these differences [61]. Furthermore, ovarian steroids were shown to inhibit NREM and REM sleep with greater suppression in female rats than in male rats [61].

On a different note, a study found that aging affected gender categorization of male and female adult faces differently. Compared to images of younger females, aging female faces took progressively longer amount of time to categorize. On the other hand, images of aging male faces took progressively shorter time to categorize [62]. The study suggests that female faces are progressively more difficult to categorize as female, while male faces are more easily identifiable as male as they age.

These findings suggest that although women display less cognitive decline as they age, their sleep quality is lower when compared to men. This puts the females at elevated risk for skin aging compared to the males. Furthermore, a large part of societal beauty standards comes from the distinction between the two genders. Since female faces seem to lose its "feminine" characteristics as they age, the desire to prevent facial aging is even more pronounced in aging females.

Recommendations for Good Sleep

Knowing the benefits of sleep and the detrimental effects of sleep deprivation on the skin, it is natural to want to know what it takes to achieve good quality sleep. There are different approaches to improving sleep quality. Two approaches are discussed here, sleep hygiene and lavender.

Sleep Hygiene

Sleep hygiene is a term coined by Dr. Peter Hauri to define various ways for patients to deal with their insomnia [63]. It recommends incorporation of various behaviors and environmental conditions that are conducive to good quality sleep and avoidance of behaviors and environmental conditions that result in poor quality sleep [64]. It is often used to treat or prevent sleep disorders and is a major component of cognitive behavioral therapy or multimodal therapy for treating insomnia [65]. Although there has been mixed findings on the effectiveness of incorporating sleep hygiene to improve sleep quality in the experimental setting, the components of sleep hygiene can still provide useful information to aid individuals with finding good quality sleep solutions.

Up to date, there has not been a consensus on what elements to include in a sleep hygiene treatment. However, some of the factors often associated with sleep hygiene include consistency of sleep and wake times, avoidance of daytime naps, avoidance of alcohol particularly close to bedtime, and exercise (preferably in the morning) before bedtime [64]. Having a regular bedtime helps align the circadian rhythm for the promotion of sleep [64]. It has been demonstrated that sleeping at approximately the same time every night and aligning light exposure around the same time increase the propensity for sleep. Daytime naps reduce nocturnal sleep pressure and are associated with decrease in depth of nighttime sleep and increased latency before sleep onset. Avoidance of daytime naps is associated with good sleep hygiene. Alcohol is well documented as a suppressant of nocturnal REM sleep and reduces upper airway muscle tone, hence resulting in worsening of sleep-disordered breathing [64]. It interferes with good quality sleep and should be avoided before bedtime. Studies have shown that exercise has a mixed effect on sleep. Exercising later in the day can help promote sleep depth. However, exercising prior to bedtime can delay sleep onset [64]. Increasing body temperature before bedtime has been shown to increase the depth of sleep. Activities such as taking a hot bath before bedtime have been proven conducive to good quality rest. It is suggested that a rapid decline in core body temperature before sleep can decrease sleep latency [64]. It is also recommended that the average adult obtain 7–8 h of sleep as in particular reduced sleep duration has been associated with long-term adverse health consequences such as weight gain and increased cardiovascular risk as well as compromise of alertness and vigilance.

Improving sleep hygiene can positively impact sleep quality. However, each individual is different and may be affected by different factors. An effective way to find out what constitutes good sleep hygiene is to experiment with different routines and environments.

Lavender and Sleep

Various studies have noted that there is a positive effect of lavender on sleep quality. A study on healthy Japanese students reported that nighttime exposure to lavender helps prevent sleepiness upon awakening [66]. In postpartum women, a similar effect was observed. Postpartum women using lavender aromatherapy at night were shown to have a significant increase in sleep quality at 8 weeks follow-up evaluated using PSQI [67]. Lavender has also been indicated in attenuation of depression [68].

For those with mild sleep disturbances and those who would like to improve sleep quality, lavender aromatherapy at night can be suggested. There are no negative side effects of this inhaled essential oil when used appropriately [69].

Conclusion

One of the obvious signs of aging occurs where everyone can see it – on the skin. The market's demand to prevent and slow skin aging drives a multibillion dollar industry today. However, sound approaches to improve skin function and protect skin against aging do not come from expensive creams or gels. One of the effective ways to protect the skin is through adequate quantity and quality of sleep. Good quality sleep can attenuate sleep aging through many mechanisms highlighted in this chapter.

On the other hand, skin plays an integral role in regulating sleep from thermoregulation during sleep-to-sleep onset and sleep latency. All of which can in return augment the quality of sleep. Since the discovery of the relationship between sleep and skin aging, there is a stronger focus on improvement of sleep quality from a dermatological standpoint. We expect more studies in the future that are aimed at understanding this dynamic field.

References

1. WGBH Educational Foundation. Division of sleep medicine at Harvard Medical School: the characteristics of sleep. 2007. http://healthysleep.med.harvard.edu/healthy/science/what/characteristics
2. National Sleep Foundation. National Sleep Foundation: sleep-wake cycle: its physiology and impact on health. 2006. http://sleepfoundation.org/sites/default/files/SleepWakeCycle.pdf
3. Buysse D, Reynolds C, Monk T, Berman S, Kupfer D. The Pittsburgh Sleep Quality Index (PSQI): a new instrument for psychiatric research and practice. Psychiatry Res. 1989;28(2):193–213.
4. Kushida C, Littner M, Morgenthaler T, et al. Practice parameters for the indications for polysomnography and related procedures: an update for 2005. Sleep. 2005;28:499–521.
5. Sadeh A, Sharkey K, Carskadon M. Activity-based sleep-wake identification: an empirical test of methodological issues. Sleep. 1994;17:201–7.
6. Poljšak B, Dahmane R, Godić A. Intrinsic skin aging: the role of oxidative stress. Acta Dermatovenerol Alp Pannonica Adriat. 2012;21:33–6. doi:10.2478/v10162-012-0009-0.
7. Sharma S, Kavuru M. Sleep and metabolism: an overview. Int J Endocrinol. 2010. doi:10.1155/2010/270832.
8. Kim TW, Jeong J, Hong S. The impact of sleep and circadian disturbance on hormones and metabolism. Int J Endocrinol. 2015. doi:10.1155/2015/591729.
9. Leproult R, Copinschi G, Buxton O, Van Cauter E. Sleep loss results in an elevation of cortisol levels the next evening. Sleep. 1997;20(10):865–70.
10. Kreiger DT. Rhythms of acth and corticosteroid secretion in health and disease, and their experimental modification. J Steroid Biochem. 1975;6(5):785–91.
11. Chung S, Son GH, Kim K. Circadian rhythm of adrenal glucocorticoid: its regulation and clinical implications. Biochim Biophys Acta. 2011;1812(5):581–91. doi:10.1016/j.bbadis.2011.02.003.
12. Mirescu C, Peters JD, Noiman L, Gould E. Sleep deprivation inhibits adult neurogenesis in the hippocampus by elevating glucocorticoids. Proc Natl Acad Sci. 2006;103(50):19170–5.
13. Lin TK, et al. Paradoxical benefits of psychological stress in inflammatory dermatoses models are glucocorticoid mediated. J Invest Dermatol. 2014;134(12):2890–7. doi:10.1038/jid.2014.265.
14. Choi EH, et al. Mechanisms by which psychologic stress alters cutaneous permeability barrier homeostasis and stratum corneum integrity. J Invest Dermatol. 2005;124(3):587–95.
15. Kahan V, Andersen ML, Tomimori J, Tufik S. Can poor sleep affect skin integrity? Med Hypotheses. 2010;75(6):535–7. doi:10.1016/j.mehy.2010.07.018.
16. Goldberg GR, Prentice AM, Davies HL, Murgatroyd PR. Overnight and basal metabolic rates in men and women. Eur J Clin Nutr. 1988;42(2):137–44.
17. Spiegel K, Leproult R, Van Cauter E. Impact of sleep debt on metabolic and endocrine function. Lancet. 1999;354(9188):1435–9.
18. Spravchikov N, et al. Glucose effects on skin keratinocytes: implications for diabetes skin complications. Diabetes. 2001;50(7):1627–35.
19. Hehenberger K, Heilborn JD, Brismar K, Hansson A. Inhibited proliferation of fibroblasts derived from chronic diabetic wounds and normal dermal fibroblasts treated with high glucose is associated with increased formation of L-lactate. Wound Repair Regen. 1998;6:135–41.

20. Gerstein A, et al. Wound healing and aging. Dermatol Clin. 1993;11(4):749–57.
21. Gandarillas A. Epidermal differentiation, apoptosis, and senescence: common pathways? Exp Gerontol. 2000;35(1):53–62.
22. Slominski A, et al. Melatonin in the skin: synthesis, metabolism and functions. Trends Endocrinol Metab. 2008;19(1):17–24.
23. Slominski A, et al. On the role of melatonin in skin physiology and pathology. Endocrine. 2005;27(2):137–48.
24. Eşrefoğlu M, et al. Potent therapeutic effect of melatonin on aging skin in pinealectomized rats. J Pineal Res. 2005;39(3):231–7.
25. Kleszczynski K, Fischer TW. Melatonin and human skin aging. Dermatoendocrinology. 2012;4(3):245–52. doi:10.4161/derm.22344.
26. Reiter RJ, et al. Obesity and metabolic syndrome: association with chronodisruption, sleep deprivation, and melatonin suppression. Ann Med. 2012;44(6):564–77. doi:10.3109/07853890.2011.586365.
27. McIntyre IM, et al. Human melatonin suppression by light is intensity dependent. J Pineal Res. 1989;6(2):149–56.
28. Oyetakin-White P, et al. Does poor sleep quality affect skin ageing? Clin Exp Dermatol. 2015;40(1):17–22. doi:10.1111/ced.12455.
29. Vgontzas AN, et al. Adverse effects of modest sleep restriction on sleepiness, performance, and inflammatory cytokines. J Clin Endocrinol Metab. 2004;89(5):2119–26.
30. Everson CA, et al. Cell injury and repair resulting from sleep loss and sleep recovery in laboratory rats. Sleep. 2014;37(12):1929–40. doi:10.5665/sleep.4244.
31. Collis SJ, Boulton SJ. Emerging links between the biological clock and the DNA damage response. Chromosoma. 2007;116(4):331–9.
32. Villafuerte G, et al. Sleep deprivation and oxidative stress in animal models: a systematic review. Oxid Med Cell Longevity. 2015. doi:10.1155/2015/234952.
33. Anafi RC, et al. Sleep is not just for the brain: transcriptional responses to sleep in peripheral tissues. BMC Genomics. 2013;14:362. doi:10.1186/1471-2164-14-362.
34. Irwin MR, Carrillo C, Olmstead R. Sleep loss activates cellular markers of inflammation: sex differences. Brain Behav Immun. 2010;24(1):54–7. doi:10.1016/j.bbi.2009.06.001.
35. Ataie-Kachoie P, et al. Gene of the month: interleukin 6 (IL-6). J Clin Pathol. 2014;67(11):932–7. doi:10.1136/jclinpath-2014-202493.
36. Bradshaw RA, Dennis EA. Handbook of cell signaling. 2nd ed. Oxford: Academic; 2009. p. 265–75.
37. Li WH, et al. IL-11, IL-1α, IL-6, and TNF-α are induced by solar radiation in vitro and may be involved in facial subcutaneous fat loss in vivo. J Dermatol Sci. 2013;71(1):58–66. doi:10.1016/j.jdermsci.2013.03.009.
38. Pessa JE, et al. The anatomical basis for wrinkles. Aesthet Surg J. 2014;34(2):227–34. doi:10.1177/1090820X13517896.
39. Kontogianni K, et al. DNA damage and repair capacity in lymphocytes from obstructive sleep apnea patients. Environ Mol Mutagen. 2007;48(9):722–7.
40. Paulsen RD, Cimprich KA. The ATR pathway: fine-tuning the fork. DNA Repair. 2007;6(7):953–66.
41. Hoffman AE, et al. The circadian gene NPAS2, a putative tumor suppressor, is involved in DNA damage response. Mol Cancer Res. 2008;6(9):1461–8. doi:10.1158/1541-7786.MCR-07-2094.
42. Hadshiew IM, Eller MS, Gilchrest BA. Skin aging and photoaging: the role of DNA damage and repair. Am J Contact Dermat. 2000;11(1):19–25.
43. Noguti J, et al. Oxidative stress, cancer, and sleep deprivation: is there a logical link in this association? Sleep Breath. 2013;17(3):905–10. doi:10.1007/s11325-012-0797-9.
44. Masaki H. Role of antioxidants in the skin: anti-aging effects. J Dermatol Sci. 2010;58(2):85–90. doi:10.1016/j.jdermsci.2010.03.003.
45. Rinnerthaler M, et al. Oxidative stress in aging human skin. Biomolecules. 2015;5(2):545–89. doi:10.3390/biom5020545.
46. Zhang HM, Zhang Y. Melatonin: a well-documented antioxidant with conditional pro-oxidant actions. J Pineal Res. 2014;57(2):131–46. doi:10.1111/jpi.12162.
47. Blask DE. Melatonin, sleep disturbance and cancer risk. Sleep Med Rev. 2009;13(4):257–64. doi:10.1016/j.smrv.2008.07.007.
48. Vierkötter A, et al. The SCINEXA: a novel, validated score to simultaneously assess and differentiate between intrinsic and extrinsic skin ageing. J Dermatol Sci. 2009;53(3):207–11. doi:10.1016/j.jdermsci.2008.10.001.
49. Sundelin T, et al. Cues of fatigue: effects of sleep deprivation on facial appearance. Sleep. 2013;36(9):1355–60. doi:10.5665/sleep.2964.
50. Tsukahara K, et al. A study of diurnal variation in wrinkles on the human face. Arch Dermatol Res. 2004;296(4):169–74.
51. Poljsak B, et al. The influence of the sleeping on the formation of facial wrinkles. J Cosmet Laser Ther. 2012;14(3):133–8. doi:10.3109/14764172.2012.685563.
52. Sarifakioğlu N, et al. A new phenomenon: “sleep lines” on the face. Scand J Plast Reconstr Surg Hand Surg. 2004;38(4):244–7.
53. Kotlus BS. Effect of sleep position on perceived facial aging. Dermatol Surg. 2013;39(9):1360–2. doi:10.1111/dsu.12266.
54. Jdid R, et al. MC1R major variants are a risk factor of sleep lines in Caucasian women. J Eur Acad Dermatol Venereol. 2014;28(6):805–9. doi:10.1111/jdv.12119.
55. Gur RE, Gur RC. Gender differences in aging: cognition, emotions, and neuroimaging studies. Dialogues Clin Neurosci. 2002;4(2):197–210.

56. Gur RC, Moberg PJ, Gur RE. Aging and cognitive functioning. Geriatric secrets. Philadelphia: Hanley & Belfus; 1996. p. 126–9.
57. Saykin AJ, et al. Normative neuropsychological test performance: effects of performance: effects of age, education, gender and ethnicity. Appl Neuropsychol. 1995;2:79–88.
58. Ohayon MM, Reynolds CF, Dauvilliers Y. Excessive sleep duration and quality of life. Ann Neurol. 2013;73:785–94.
59. Mallampalli MP, Carter CL. Exploring sex and gender differences in sleep health: a Society for Women's Health Research Report. J Womens Health. 2014;23(7):553–62.
60. Guidozzi F. Gender differences in sleep in older men and women. Climacteric. 2015;5:1–7.
61. Cusmano DM, Hadjimarkou MM, Mong JA. Gonadal steroid modulation of sleep and wakefulness in male and female rats is sexually differentiated and neonatally organized by steroid exposure. Endocrinology. 2014;155:204–14.
62. Kloth N, et al. Aging affects sex categorization of male and female faces in opposite ways. Acta Psychol. 2015;158:78–86.
63. Hauri P. Current concepts: the sleep disorders. Kalamazoo: The Upjohn Company; 1977.
64. Stepanski EJ, Wyatt JK. Use of sleep hygiene in the treatment of insomnia. Sleep Med Rev. 2003;7 (3):215–25.
65. Voinescu BI, Szentagotai-Tatar A. Sleep hygiene awareness: its relation to sleep quality and diurnal preference. J Mol Psychiatry. 2015;3(1):1.
66. Hirokawa K, Nishimoto T, Taniguchi T. Effects of lavender aroma on sleep quality in healthy Japanese students. Percept Mot Skills. 2012;114 (1):111–22.
67. Keshavarz AM, et al. Lavender fragrance essential oil and the quality of sleep in postpartum women. Iran Red Crescent Med J. 2015;17:4. doi:10.5812/ircmj.17(4) 2015.25880.
68. Szafrański T. Herbal remedies in depression – state of the art. Psychiatr Pol. 2014;48(1):59–73.
69. Lillehei AS, Halcon LL. A systematic review of the effect of inhaled essential oils on sleep. J Altern Complement Med. 2014;20(6):441–51. doi:10.1089/acm. 2013.0311.

Part XVII

Global Market Place, Social and Emotional Aspects for the Aged

Marketing and Product Design of Antiaging Skin Care Products

160

Nancy C. Dawes

Contents

N.C. Dawes (✉)
The Procter and Gamble Company, Cincinnati, OH, USA
e-mail: dawes.nc@pg.com

M.A. Farage et al. (eds.), *Textbook of Aging Skin*,
DOI 10.1007/978-3-662-47398-6_107

Abstract

Designing and marketing of antiaging skin care products for consumers is a huge global business. Often, the principles for successful design and marketing of antiaging skin care products have not been well articulated to guide product developers or researchers. This chapter seeks to fill that void.

Introduction

Designing and marketing of antiaging skin care products for consumers is a huge global business. Often, the principles for successful design and marketing of antiaging skin care products have not been well articulated to guide product developers or researchers. This chapter seeks to fill that void.

According to Euromonitor International's 2008 cosmetics and toiletries database, skin care is the largest category of beauty care products, larger than hair care products, bath and shower products, color cosmetics, men's grooming products, fragrances, and deodorants. Skin care products represent over 25 % of market sales in the beauty care product category. Of all the major segments in the category excluding men's skin care, antiaging facial care products now exhibit the fastest market growth (11 % annually), and this segment represents over 20 % of the market for skin care products. In 2007, consumers in North America, Western Europe, and Australia spent a combined US$7.7 billion on wrinkle-reducing facial creams. In Asia, unlike in the West, antiaging is considered less important than skin whitening or skin cleansing, toning, and moisturizing. For example, in Japan, the largest skin care market in the world (US$13.1 billion), spending on antiaging products accounts for less than 10 % of overall spending on skin care, whereas in the USA and UK, the figure is closer to 30 %. In 2007, the top five beauty companies based on market share were L'Oreal Group (10.6 %), Beiersdorf AG (7.2 %), Shiseido Co LTd (5.7 %), Procter & Gamble (4.8 %), and Avon Products, Inc (4.8 %). The top five brand leaders were Avon (4.8 %), Olay (3.8 %), Nivea Visage/Vital (3.3 %), L'Oreal Dermo-Expertise (3.2 %), and Nivea Body (2.3 %) [1].

The Social and Psychosociological Importance of Facial Appearance

While overall body shape and body size are the dominant attributes that affect a woman's perception of her attractiveness, her facial skin is central to her social presentation and hence is the focus of this chapter. The scientific discipline of evolutionary psychology has identified the face as particularly important to human social communication and to body image [2, 3] and even minor imperfections often can disproportionately impact a person's state of mind and quality of life. Evolutionary and socialization theories suggest that human facial appearance influences the development of social behavior (e.g., social skills, dating, and sexual experience) and personal traits (e.g., mental and physical health) [4, 5]. However uncomfortable the implications may be, several studies have shown that there is a tendency to assign more positive qualities to facially attractive adults and children than to unattractive ones [4, 6]. Moreover, facial attractiveness correlates positively with success in finding a partner; this supports the hypothesis that in humans, facial attractiveness is an important criterion for selecting a mate [7]. Only very recently researchers have started to correlate facial skin biology with the psychology of perception; indeed, this is now the leading way to define how companies are approaching technology development [8–11].

From the viewpoint of the consumer, the importance of the face is captured in everyday sayings, such as "face the day" or "don't lose face." Women recognize that their face communicates who they are, as captured in the following quotes from personal interviews (Internal data):

> "The face is the first thing I notice about someone." (Becky age 26)
>
> "A face portrays emotions." (Laura age 26)
>
> "The face is the most visible part of body." (Carol age 56)
>
> "What women do with their face represents how they perceive themselves and how they want society to see them." (Sandy age 36)
>
> "The face reflects the true person." (Harriet age 41)

The insights in the chapter derive from interviews with consumers worldwide, from quantitative market research studies across multiple geographies, and from the development of several major brands of skin care products sold globally, some of which have ranked among the top-10, best-selling-facial skin care products sold in mass market retail channels in the past decade.

Seven Principles for Designing and Marketing for Antiaging Skin Care products

Principle 1: Don't Spend Marketing Money All At Once

Antiaging facial skin care is a business that grows relatively slowly over time, driven in large part by certain fundamental dynamics in the product category. The annual purchase frequency for facial moisturizers is about 3/year, compared to about 4.5/per year for body wash, 6/per year for laundry detergent, and about 9/per year for toilet paper. Team sport provides a useful analogy to describe the fundamental impact of purchase frequency on revenue: purchase frequency is analogous to an individual team member's "play time" on a sports team. A team player whom the coach places in play more frequently will gain more points in a season than a player with equal skill, who is placed in play less frequently. Toilet paper is "played by the coach" about three times as often as a facial moisturizer – in effect, consumers will shop in the toilet paper aisle about three times as often as they shop the facial moisturizer aisle. If, in a concept test, the same percentage of consumers claim that they "definitely would buy" toilet paper and facial moisturizer, then toilet paper trial will be predicted to be three times the frequency of moisturizer trial in the first base year of analysis (this is an example of category purchase frequency dynamics.)

Because the consumer purchases only a small number of antiaging facial care products in a given year, it is critical that a skin care company reaches her at the right time – i.e., when she is ready to buy. Thus, media or marketing spending must be spread out over a long period of time, because although slower buyers may like the product offering as much as faster buyers – they need to hear the marketing message at the point at which they have a need for the product.

Within the facial skin care category, a marketer can influence several business elements to increase revenue. These functions control the size of revenue:

- The overall size of a business's *Revenue* in year one is a function of the dollar amount of sales from *Triers* (i.e., those consumers purchasing a product for the first time), known as *Trial Revenue*, and the amount of sales from *Repeaters* (i.e., consumers purchasing a product for a second or more time) known as *Repeat Revenue*. Because facial skin care is both a low purchase and a slow purchase category, most of Year One revenue comes from *Triers*; this also means that trial will continue for more than 1 year, and hence marketing dollars should be spread over time.
- *Trial Revenue* is a function of *Population Size*, the *Year-One-Trial-Rate*, and the relevant *Currency Amount* for each purchase. Although higher-priced skin care products can deliver more trial revenue, a higher price will likely mean that fewer women will be willing to purchase it. Thus, pricing strategy will optimize revenue.
- To further dissect *Trial Revenue*, the *Year-One-Trial-Rate* is a function of *Year-One-Base-Trial*, the level of *Awareness*, and product *Distribution*. *Year-One-Base-Trial* is a level of *Trial* that assumes 100 % *Awareness* and 100 % *Distribution* and is driven by concept or copy appeal and category purchase frequency. Advertising is a key marketing variable that drives awareness. Because facial skin care products are sold in multiple retail outlets (ranging from drug stores to mass market retailers to department stores and specialty stores) and also through other channels such as the Internet, catalogs, and direct marketers, it is critical to consider product distribution. Moreover, the target consumers should shop via the distribution outlets selected.
- *Out-Year Volume* depends on how many *Triers* repeat their purchase again and again, as well as on the generation of new trial. Product performance, product improvements, and new advertising claims and messages can impact out-year volume. Consequently, product design and performance are critical components of great marketing.

Although a company can influence consumers' product purchases by spending more money on advertising, increasing the number of outlets that sell the target products, and optimizing pricing, the crux of this first principle is to pace marketing spending in such a way that women are reached when and where they are receptive to buying the antiaging skin care product.

Principle 2: Innovate! Innovate! Innovate!

The market for antiaging skin care products thrives on innovation. Women are keenly aware that science and technology advance rapidly – women over age 50 have seen a man walk on the moon, have observed the Internet change how they communicate and get information, and know that the genome has been decoded. Consumer research in 2006 showed that 38 % of the US facial moisturizer buyers agreed with the statement that "I'm always on the lookout for new facial skin care products even if I like what I'm currently using." Technological changes that the consumer has experienced in her life convince her that new and more effective antiaging solutions are always on the horizon.

Overall, the strength and sustainability of product innovation in this product category is a function of (a) the number of women who want the benefit(s) that the product delivers, (b) the magnitude of the antiaging benefit that the product delivers, (c) the importance of the benefit (and thus, the trade-offs the consumer is willing to make), and (d) other enhancements that accompany the product.

When designing an antiaging facial skin care product, the product technology must be linked to "solving" a woman's skin concern (e.g., fine lines, age spots). The ultimate size of the market opportunity depends on the number of potential Triers. This is controlled by the number of women who want the product benefit – which, in turn, is derived from the types of age-related issues that women actually experience. In the USA and Europe, about 60–70 % of women are concerned with fine lines and/or wrinkles; fewer (about 30 %) are concerned with uneven facial skin color, age or brown spots, or loss of firmness/sagging. In Japan and China, however, a large proportion of women are interested in improving overall fairness or "whitening," which is perceived to be a combination of overall skin color and "translucency." In Japan, many women (70 %) are concerned about pigmented (melanized) spots. The importance of these attributes varies by hereditary, ethnicity, and age; consequently, these affect how many women will be interested in the product.

Historically, facial skin care products delivered "hope in a bottle" and the magnitude of change was difficult to measure. However, over the past 10 years, modern techniques that capture and measure "before-and-after" changes (such as standardized high-resolution digital facial imaging and analysis) lead women to expect perceptible changes in their facial skin in response to treatment with the product.

The importance of the benefit can also be dimensionalized as follows:

- Bigger skin care benefits are better than smaller benefits: eliminating a wrinkle is better than reducing the size of a wrinkle.
- Multiple benefits are better than single benefits: a single product that both fades spots and reduces wrinkles is better than a product that elicits only one of these benefits.
- Benefits that are noticeable sooner are better than those that take longer to notice – this is precisely why products such as Botox® have created new markets within a very short period of time.
- Benefits that are permanent are better than those that are temporary.

However, the benefits that the product delivers can be offset by "trade-offs." Hence, one must consider: What is the cost to the consumer for the benefits the product delivers? The classic cost is currency, but in the antiaging skin care category, trade-offs also can include irritation, healing time, inconvenience, and poor aesthetics. The professional skin treatment market illustrates the importance of trade-offs. Over the past 10 years, this market has grown as new procedures are created that improve appearance with limited healing time. For instance, in 2000, a typical superficial laser treatment required at least a week of recovery (and associated patient downtime), due to the extent of the controlled injury inflicted upon the epidermis; however, in 2008, many professional procedures, such as Fraxel laser treatments, incur minimal downtime (less than a day). With topical products, the primary side effect that minimizes consumer acceptance of a product is irritation – especially if the product creates visible changes such as redness, peeling, or flaking.

Finally, skin care products can provide additional lifestyle enhancements. Data show that women enjoy their skin care routine and look forward to this part of their day. Skin care products can deliver emotional benefits such as relaxation, refreshment, or perceived rejuvenation; they can deliver in use experiences via warming or cooling sensations. On a more rational side, they can deliver convenience if multiple skin care steps are achieved by applying a single product.

However, even with the most advanced antiaging treatments, women's skin continues to change as they age; interviews with women who have undergone professional treatments (such as microdermabrasion, chemical peels, or Botox® injections) show that they nonetheless continue to use topical skin care products to further improve their skin appearance. Thus, there are ongoing opportunities for newer and better technologies for women to experience, which require continual product innovation.

Principle 3: Link "Kitchen Logic" to Product Design

Women have ingrained beliefs about how products work, and if products are designed and tailored to fit intuitively with their "kitchen logic," such products will be more successful than products that try to convince them of a "new truth."

For example, consumers implicitly expect antiaging products to be moisturizing, because they surmise that "when things dry out, wrinkles form and sagging happens"; this logic is gleaned not only by observing older skin but also by observing that fruit or vegetables in the refrigerator dry out and get limp and wrinkled. Women intuitively know that moisturization is the foundation of firm, smooth skin: they connect this "kitchen logic" to their skin care products and believe that moisturizers must penetrate the skin to work. Thus, if a product feels sticky after it is applied to the face, it "signals" that the product remains on the surface. This not only creates an uncomfortable sensation but also implies that the product "can't be moisturizing."

Some successful brands of moisturizers have been built on consumers' beliefs about how brown or age spots are created. For example, a high proportion of 40-year-old women have noticed "brown spots that used to fade in the autumn, when we were out of sun, are now lasting through the winter." A woman intuitively believes that brown or age spots reside deep within the skin, because she has tried scrubbing them off, and they do not disappear. She has also heard that brown spots are caused by sun damage. Also, she draws an analogy to acne breakouts or pimples from her teenage days: she believes that pimples break out unexpectedly due to something happening inside her skin (e.g., dirt and oil buildup inside a pore). Thus, the general logic is developed: "The sun causes damage to cells inside my skin; this causes the cells to create something that becomes a brown spot; a brown spot has roots deep inside my skin. Therefore, if a product is going to fade a brown spot, it will work best if it penetrates deep inside my skin."

Intuitively, in the consumer's mind, this penetration belief is more strongly connected to a foaming facial care product than to a serum or lotion because foams are lighter in consistency. Lighter products are perceived to be absorbed faster and more deeply. Thus, women believe and expect that a light, airy, foaming product will be more effective in preventing brown or age spots than a lotion.

Concept testing confirms this. Women were presented with a written concept describing a facial skin care product that improved appearance by reducing brown or age spots. In one version of the concept, the product was presented as a "foaming moisturizer" while, in the other, the product was presented as a "serum." Based on the written concept alone, they rated the foaming moisturizer significantly higher ($p < 0.10$) than the serum for "preventing future brown or age spots," "improving skin's health" and "making skin more radiant."

Consumers' kitchen logic-based beliefs about ingredients can reinforce the perception of product benefits. Indeed, certain ingredients enhance women's perceptions and awareness of core product attributes. For example, women shown a packaged product labeled either "WrinkLift Treatment

Cream" or "WrinkleLift Treatment Cream with Vitamins E and A" were asked their level of agreement with various statements. Significantly more women ($p < 0.10$) agreed that the cream with Vitamin E/A would "moisturize my facial skin," "help my skin to heal itself," and "make my skin smooth" compared to the same cream that did not reference these ingredients.

Leveraging "kitchen logic" is a powerful tool for marketers because less marketing money is spent to communicate messages if the form or description of the product intuitively communicates either a benefit or a mechanism of action.

Principle 4: Attitude Drives Action

As mentioned earlier, the ultimate market size for an antiaging product is controlled by the number of women who desires the benefit offered by the product. Women are more apt to alter their behavior – in this case, by using a facial skin care product – if they want to improve or change something. Thus, people who have visible signs of aging on their face are more prone to "do something about them" than people who have perfect skin. However, not all people who have "signs of aging" are bothered enough to do something about them.

Although all women eventually develop facial signs of aging, they show various degrees of concern and involvement. Women around the globe can be divided into three broad groups: those who want to enhance their skin's condition to appear younger looking; those who want to maintain the feel and/or appearance of their skin; and those who want to fix their skin's problem areas. These groups will be referred to as "Enhancers," "Maintainers," and "Fixers."

Enhancers are the consumers with the highest potential for antiaging marketers, as they are actively involved in category purchases and are seeking new products and solutions. They are willing to pay more for facial skin care products and are more discerning about how they work. In 2001, they were estimated to represent approximately 35 % of women in the USA, 30 % in the UK, and 50 % in large cities in China. In the USA and the UK, 60–70 % of Enhancers strongly agree with the statement: "I want to reduce the signs of aging so my skin looks the best it can for my age." Across all three countries, 25–35 % of Enhancers claimed to have used a facial moisturizer containing antiaging ingredients (as opposed to a regular facial moisturizer) in the past 3 months. In the USA, it appears that this percentage is increasing over time.

Maintainers are women who are either satisfied with how their skin is aging or who do not have signs of aging – this group represents approximately 35 % of US women, 50 % of UK women, and 40 % of Chinese women. In 2001, 12–16 % of Maintainers in the USA, the UK, and China claimed to have used a facial moisturizer containing antiaging ingredients in the past 3 months, significantly fewer ($p < 0.10$) than the percentage of Enhancers that did so in each country.

Fixers, for the most part, are women who are dealing with oily skin or pimples and breakouts: in the USA, Germany, and China, respectively, 65 %, 56 %, and 25 % of these women indicated that they had pimples/breakouts in the past 3 months. Within each country, these women tend to be younger than their Enhancer or Maintainer counterparts. *Fixers* represent approximately 30 % of US women, 20 % of UK women, and 10 % of Chinese women. In 2001, fewer than 15 % of these women used any type of facial moisturizer three or more times a week, a lower percentage than among either Enhancers or Maintainers in each country.

Women's attitudes toward aging affect their receptivity to products and to marketing messages. Enhancers, who comprise most of the market of antiaging products, are more likely than Maintainers or Fixers to try leading-edge products, are more open to trying new forms (serums vs. creams, for instance), and are more responsive to semi-technical language that communicates antiaging benefits ("regenerates skin" vs. "renews skin"). While designing skin care products or developing advertising copy, it is important to know which type of consumer among these three broad classes is providing input or feedback on the message or product.

Principle 5: Reframe Relative to an Aspirational Standard of Excellence

In recent years, the most successful facial skin care brands have redefined the mass market for such products through an unprecedented strategy – positioning the product's performance relative to the standards of expensive department store brands. The importance of consumer aspirations is highlighted by a case study on the launch of Olay Total Effects®, currently one of the top-selling facial skin care items in US mass market retailers.

Prior to 2000, the most expensive facial skin care products sold in US mass market retailers cost about US$12, the bulk of facial creams sold in the US$5–8 range. By contrast, in department stores, facial moisturizer prices began at about US$30. A dramatic change in the market occurred when Olay Total Effects® launched at a US$19.99 price point in US mass market retailers, accompanied by prestige claims but at an unprecedented price for this retail channel.

Several critical insights influenced the success of the product launch. Women aspired to buy prestige brands that were sold in department stores. However, market research indicated that about one third of women shopped for facial skin care only in mass retailers, about one third shopped only in department stores (with beauty counters), and one third shopped in both types of stores. Department store prestige brands were perceived as luxurious: these brands were the first to market new antiaging ingredients and they often had innovative, upscale packaging. Women believed that department store brands were better than mass brands but that the higher price was largely due to in-store consultation and attractive presentation. Hence, women also believed that, with enough research, they could find lower cost skin care products that would deliver similar performance to the department store brands.

Olay Total Effects®, a product that delivered meaningful and visible benefits, met this need. In a global consumer use study involving thousands of women, the product was tested against seven leading prestige antiaging skin care products (with brand names concealed). Results demonstrated that more "real women" saw improvements in their skin using this product than when using prestige products. These data were leveraged strongly by briefing beauty magazine editors and thought leaders as well as in direct marketing to women in TV and press copy.

By understanding both the perceptions and the realities of mass market and department store products, the launch of Olay Total Effects® shifted the entire US skin care market. In 2007, Olay Total Effects was sold in 50 countries and was a top-10 best-selling item in US mass retail skin care, having propelled the Olay® brand as a whole to market leadership.

As another case study, Olay Regenerist® launched in 2003 using marketing copy that positioned the product not against prestige brands but against "professional treatments." In the early 2000s, Botox®, an injectable botulinum toxin treatment for wrinkles, had not received FDA approval in the USA; consumers were just becoming aware of professional treatments such as chemical peels. Women were not knowledgeable about the details of these treatments; however, these professional treatments were perceived to be more effective than typical topical products.

These consumer perceptions were incorporated into the Olay Regenerist® design theme and in the language used to describe its benefits. When Botox® received FDA approval in the spring of 2002, print advertising for the Regenerist® product evoked this professional treatment as a standard of excellence: the statement "Dramatically improved skin need not require drastic measures" was coupled with visuals of a syringe (Fig. 1). Subsequent product offerings were positioned relative to other well-known professional treatments such as eyelifts and light chemical peels. In 2007, this product also held a position among the top-10 best-selling US mass retail skin care products.

In summary, in-market results over the past 10 years demonstrate that reframing a skin care product relative to a standard of excellence builds businesses in the antiaging skin care market. Inspecting web site and print advertising from several manufacturers in 2007 revealed a

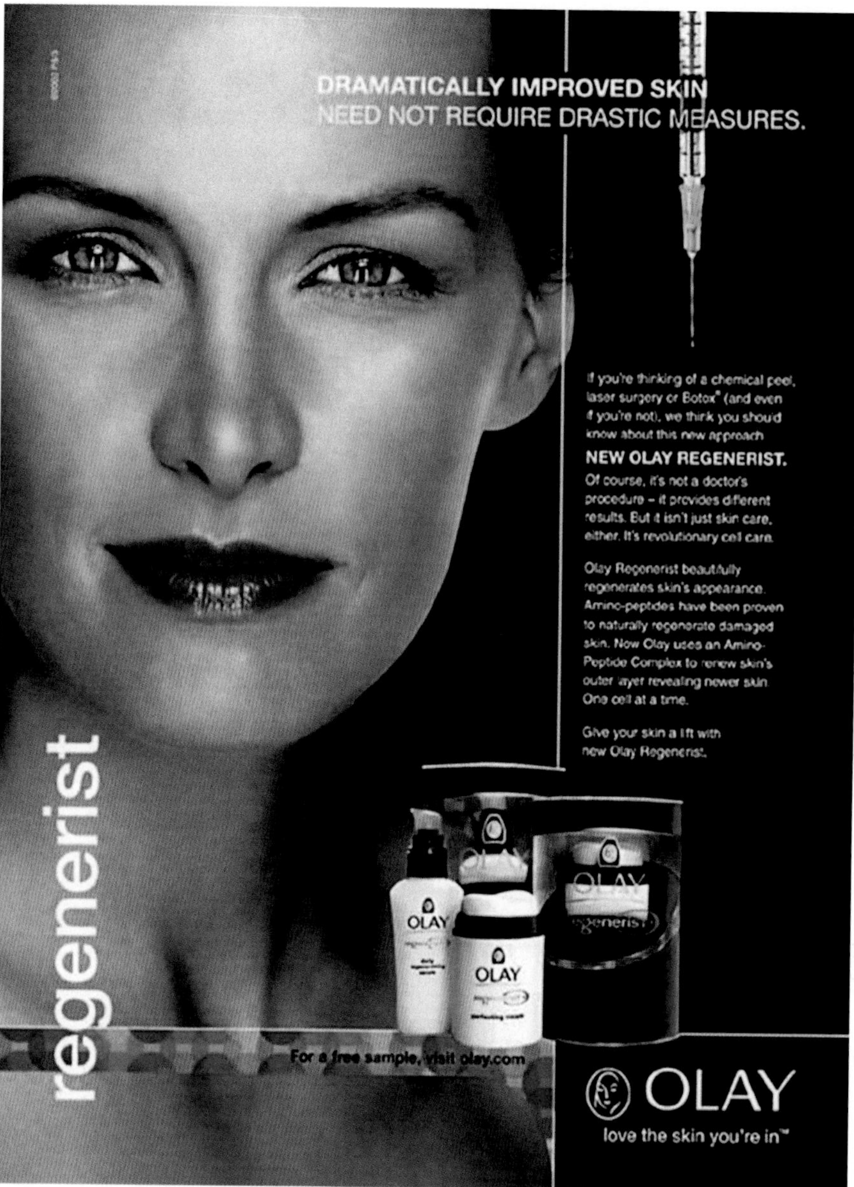

Fig. 1 Example how consumer perceptions and visual benefits were incorporated into Olay Regenerist® design theme

multitude of product descriptions leveraging doctor endorsements, physician-developed formulas, and comparison to Botox®. The ability to identify relevant or emerging standards of excellence, coupled with opportunities to reframe skin care products toward these aspirational standards, is needed to remain competitive in the antiaging skin care market.

Principle 6: Tell Her a Story

Beauty care is an emotionally driven category. For most women, the facial skin care regimen is a process that women look forward to and enjoy as a start or an end to their day. Although daily skin care is a repetitive process, it is a "ritual" and "me-time" – not a chore, like doing the laundry or washing the dishes. Thus, engaging the consumer in a holistic story that builds on the technical credentials of the product – an experience encompassing the product, the package, the name, the credentials, and the ingredients – will evoke both a "right brain" (emotional) and "left brain" (analytical) response.

Here are some approaches to this principle:

Use positive language: The consumer of antiaging skin care products is typically an intelligent, aware woman who wants to *look* younger, though not necessarily *be* younger. Language should give her hope that she can, once again, look the way she used to. Benefit language that captures this utilizes words that begin with "re-," because this prefix communicates the idea of "regaining what she once had." Thus, benefit language of "renewing," "restoring," "reactivating," "regenerating," "replenishing" resound with her better than "fixing" or "antiaging."

Recognize that she is intelligent: Today's consumer is more informed and educated than women were 20 years ago. Appeal to her wisdom without making her feel guilty for her mistakes. Today's consumer of antiaging products looks for information from multiple sources. One 2006 market research study showed that 29 % of female purchasers of facial moisturizers always or frequently "search for additional information regarding my facial skin care products online"; 38 % of them "look for in-store materials such as brochures or pamphlets to provide additional information about a skin care line and its products," and 66 % of them "will read a product's ingredient list before I purchase it for the first time." Therefore, use various forms of media to communicate the product story.

Provide ways to let her be in control: Although women know that they cannot stop aging, they believe they have the power to slow it down. Consequently, do not treat aging like a disease – they do not want to hear that a new product "cures aging" – instead, they want the product to provide them with tools to manage their destiny. A 2007 market research study showed that 83 % of buyers of facial moisturizer agreed with the statement: "How I take care of my skin now will affect how it looks later in life." Do not assume that antiaging products are for the aged – younger and younger people want to deal with aging proactively.

The tone of the story is one aspect of the overall marketing message, and today's woman is open to positive, empowering messages. The 50-year-old of today knows that she looks better than 50-year-old women did 20 years ago. To her, facial skin care products are empowering – but they are also fun, relaxing, self-indulgent, and enjoyable. Thus, positive messages that recognize her intelligence and provide ways to let her be in control resound better than negative, authoritative messages.

Principle 7: Write Chapters in Her Journey

Once the overall proposition is designed for a consumer, assembling them into a coherent marketing communication plan that "tells the story" is essential. Considering the consumer journey with the intended Brand as chapters in a story provides a framework for designing and leveraging a holistic marketing experience.

Hearing there's a Good Book: Hearing a credible source that recommends a new antiaging product is a critical source of awareness that leads to product trial. In one market research study, 24 % of purchasers of facial moisturizer indicated that magazines/editors/books influenced their decision. Thus, beauty awards or articles influence purchase more than advertisements. Hearing that independent agencies (such as the Good Housekeeping Institute or Consumer Reports) have tested specific skin care products is a proven model for building business. However, TV and/or print advertisements are still the mainstay of how women hear about new products. Whatever format is used, a marketer wants to create the response: "I'd like to learn more about this product."

The introduction: In the actual introduction, women get firsthand experience with a product.

For beauty care products, the type of introduction varies by shopping outlet. For instance, when products are sold at a counter, the introduction is often enabled by a trained beauty consultant who provides information, helps the woman understand why this product is right for her, and provides product samples. In a self-serve (mass retailer) environment, women often read packages and compare on-pack claims, benefits, and pricing to determine "is this the right product for me?" Simple product names and clear benefit descriptions help women make this decision. In-store testers (where women can actually try the product) enable a more interactive and engaging introduction.

The purchase: Purchasing is the moment when product design and marketing efforts "close the deal" and deliver the critical "revenue-producing trial." Given the complexity of the facial skin care category, having a distinctive package and product name that the consumer can easily identify is important. Purchase can be hindered if a retailer is concerned about pilferage of costly, easily shoplifted products and decides to store the product behind a counter or in a locked cabinet.

Usage: For an antiaging product, the usage experience is critical. In the antiaging category, longer-term benefits often are delivered after use of more than one package of product. Delivering immediate and short-term benefits, therefore, encourages the consumer to continue using the product so that she will experience the longer-term skin improvement. However, within a week a woman will decide if she does not like the product – sometimes, in as little as a day! Her first filter is product aesthetics (e.g., fragrance, skin feel). If a woman finds the product greasy or does not like its fragrance, she will not continue using it. The next stopping-point is if a woman decides that the product is "not right for her skin" – and these signs are typically sensitivity (itching, burning) or pimples/breakouts. However, with ongoing use of a product, a woman will begin to look for positive skin changes in about 3 weeks – thus, palpable improvement in critical short-term measures of skin condition and health (e.g., those technically assessed as improved stratum corneum [SC] barrier function or optimized SC turnover) is crucial.

Buying again!: Repurchase is critical for establishing the longevity of a product or brand. Making repurchase simply enhances business. In a mass retail environment with hundreds of products, a well-differentiated package that is easily identified is a simple way to strengthen repurchase; coupons and in-store advertisements also remind women to repurchase; transparent primary packages where women can see the amount of remaining product remind them to repurchase. Department store counter brands and direct sales brands employ beauty consultants who form a personal relationship with the client and provide reminder phone calls or mailed cards to remind them to repurchase. Product regimens sold in retail or mail-order channels often use automatic replenishment as a way to ensure that their consumers remain committed. When a product enters a woman's selected set of skin care products, she often skips browsing and simply goes directly to the store or counter to make a repeat purchase; other times, she will repurchase but also "browse" to see what new products are available.

Telling others: Word of mouth is a great way to spread the story about a product. In a 2006 market research study, 43 % of those who purchased facial moisturizer indicated friends and family as "sources of skin care information that influenced the decision to purchase a new facial skin care product." Hence, having a message that can be communicated by others, a distinctive brand name, and a unique yet identifiable package, all are attributes that will maximize the benefits of informal, word-of-mouth communication.

A coherent marketing communication plan should consider the multiple ways in which women hear (and tell) a product story. Often, different agencies are used to develop package copy, in-store copy, magazine copy, and TV copy; this makes it critical for the marketer to coordinate the overall story line and design theme. A marketer should consider (a) what messages are best communicated via different media (i.e., magazine copy vs. in-store messages);

(b) whether color and design themes are consistent in print ads, TV copy, package artwork, and in-store display to coherently communicate the brand's message; and (c) through what channels compelling claims are best communicated to the target consumer. Consistent messaging through multiple media is a key opportunity for engaging the consumer in the product or brand.

Conclusion

Intensive marketing of antiaging, facial skin care products is anticipated in the next 10 years, as the average age of the world's population increases and as younger consumers take a more proactive view in minimizing the effects of age. Advances in medicine and science present opportunities for companies to continue to deliver products that improve how a woman's skin ages. Linking these technological breakthroughs with strong product platforms, and communicating these ideas in compelling ways to increasingly knowledgeable global consumers, will provide marketing challenges and opportunities for the next decade and beyond.

The seven principles discussed in this chapter will enable the product developers and technologists to create great products that enable great marketing. Knowing the seven principles – (1) Don't spend marketing money all at once; (2) Innovate, innovate, innovate; (3) Link kitchen logic to product design; (4) Attitude drives action; (5) Reframe relative to an aspirational standard of excellence; (6) Tell her a story; and (7) Write chapters in her journey – will guide stronger technology, product design, and marketing strategy. Product designers and technologists should understand these principles, as, ultimately, product performance and design are the foundations of competitive marketing.

Cross-References

▶ Key Trends Driving Antiaging Skin Care in 2009 and Beyond

References

1. Euromonitor International. Category Watch: cosmeceuticals lead the anti-ageing market, Alexander Kirillov. Other material used: all data sourced from Euromonitor International Passport: cosmetics and toiletries 2008 edition. 2008.
2. Haxby JV, Hoffman EA, Gobbini MI. The distributed human neural system for face perception. Trends Cogn Sci. 2000;4:223–33.
3. Haxby JV, Hoffman EA, Gobbini MI. Human neural systems for face recognition and social communication. Biol Psychiatry. 2002;51:59–67.
4. Langlois JH, Kalakanis L, Rubenstein AJ, Larson A, Hallam M, Smoot M. Maxims and myths of beauty? A meta-analytic and theoretical review. Psychol Bull. 2000;126:390–423.
5. Hoss RA, Ramsey JL, Griffin AM, Langlois JH. The role of facial attractiveness and facial masculinity/femininity in sex classification of faces. Perception. 2005;34:1459–74.
6. Mobius MM, Rosenblat TS. Why beauty matters. J Econ. 2006;93:267–91.
7. Rhodes G, Simmons LW. Peters attractiveness and sexual behavior: does attractiveness enhance mating success? Evol Hum Behav. 2005;26:186–201.
8. Fink B, Grammer K, Matts PJ. Visible skin colour distribution plays a major role in the perception of age, attractiveness and health in female faces. Evol Hum Behav. 2006;27(6):433–42.
9. Fink B, Matts PJ, Klingenberg H, Kuntze S, Weege B, Grammer K. Visual attention to variation in female facial skin colour distribution. J Cosmet Dermatol. 2008;7(2):155–61.
10. Fink B, Matts PJ. The effects of skin colour distribution and topography cues on the perception of female facial age and health. J Eur Dermatol Venereol. 2008;22(4):493–8.
11. Matts PJ, Fink B, Grammer K, Burquest M. Colour homogeneity and visual perception of age, health and attractiveness of female facial skin. J Am Acad Dermatol. 2007;57(6):977–84.

161 Key Trends Driving Antiaging Skin Care in 2009 and Beyond

Mary Carmen Gasco-Buisson

Contents

Abstract

Antiaging products are expected to be key drivers of the global skin care market. This chapter aims at overviewing the key trends which impact the industry to better recognize and prepare for the future.

Introduction

Antiaging skin care is a large and dynamic business, accounting for 22 % of the global skin care market worth US$ 66 billion and growing at 11 % compound annual growth rate (CAGR) between 2001 and 2007 according to data from Euromonitor International. Euromonitor predicts skin care to grow by 24 % to US$82 billion by 2012, a very impressive increase for a mature market. Antiaging products are expected to be key drivers of that growth [1–3]. While none of us possess crystal balls, understanding the key trends which impact the industry will help to better recognize and prepare for the future.

This chapter focuses on seven of the trends considered most influential in driving the antiaging skin care business, based on extensive consumer, market, technology, and regulatory reviews either conducted or studied over 7 + years by Procter & Gamble's beauty business.

M.C. Gasco-Buisson (✉)
P&G Brand Creation & Innovation, Procter & Gamble, Cincinnati, OH, USA
e-mail: gascobuisson.mc@pg.com

M.A. Farage et al. (eds.), *Textbook of Aging Skin*,
DOI 10.1007/978-3-662-47398-6_108

Some of the trends discussed are driving the skin care business as a whole, while others are more specifically impacting the antiaging segment. Some provide background on the business opportunities the category presents; some others outline the spaces most promising for new innovation, and the rest focus on important market and regulatory changes. This chapter aims to provide a foundational overview of these trends and hopes to inspire further study, as a solid understanding of these dynamics is critical for anyone who wants to successfully enter or lead in this fascinating business.

Key Trend 1: Shifting Perceptions Regarding Health, Beauty, and Aging

Advances in medicine, better nutrition, and improved standards of living have been driving life expectancy and mean age increases for years. According to the CIA's World Factbook 2008 estimate, most countries in Western Europe have life expectancies of about 79–81 years, and the USA has a life expectancy of 78.1 years [4]. This reflects a steady increase over the years, with the USA seeing an increase of about 8 years since the early 1960s, according to data from the US Center for Disease Control and Prevention. These increases are projected to continue at least for the next few years [5].

The expectations of living longer and of having years of healthy, active living ahead have contributed to significant shifts in attitudes about health, beauty, and aging in the last decade. Phrases like "60 is the new 40" capture the spirit of a generation of the US and European "Baby Boomers" (people born between 1946 and 1964) who have seen extraordinary technological and medical advances as well as life expectancy increases in their lifetime. Retirement is becoming an outdated idea, as many Boomers seek second careers and look to continue working as long as possible. This desire to be in the work force longer increases Boomers' interest in health and beauty, to ensure they remain at the top of their game and respected by their younger peers.

Boomers not just expect to live longer; they also expect to look as good as they feel. According to Procter & Gamble research, 44 % of US Boomers say they are bothered by the signs of aging and want to do something about them. This incredibly influential group, 78 million strong in the USA and spending more than US$2 trillion each year according to the same P&G research, has set in motion some of the key movements experienced today – including the health and wellness revolution, the social responsibility movement, and the growth of industries like antiaging skin care and cosmetic procedures [6].

Another group significantly influencing attitudes regarding health, beauty, and aging are the LOHAS consumers. LOHAS is an acronym for Lifestyles of Health and Sustainability. LOHAS consumers account for 19 % of US adults, according to the LOHAS online website, and are the driving force behind movements like natural/organic food and personal care, planet sustainability, integrative health, and ecotourism. The typical LOHAS consumer is a well-educated middle-aged woman who is very active intellectually and physically. LOHAS consumers are particularly influential because they are involved in their communities, tend to be "in the know" information seekers and sharers, and are among the first to try health and wellness and natural/organic products [7].

LOHAS consumers believe in the body-mind-spirit connection and are driving the growth in acceptance and popularity of yoga, meditation, ayurvedic treatments, acupuncture, holistic spa retreats, and other alternative modalities. These practices are beginning to influence beauty, as evidenced by the growth of Eastern-inspired brands like Aveda, Avon Anew Alternative, and Sundari. In-depth understanding of the LOHAS consumer and market is available through the LOHAS online website (www.lohas.com) and the Natural Marketing Institute website (www.nmisolutions.com).

The importance of this trend lies in its direct impact to both the growth of antiaging solutions, including antiaging skin care, and the degree of consumers' expectations. While one can revel in the promise of a growing industry, to succeed in antiaging, one must also remember that consumers are multidimensional beings and that they are coming to expect no physical or emotional trade-offs for themselves, their communities, or the planet.

Key Trend 2: Developing Markets as Key Drivers of Growth

Skin care is truly a global business, with the biggest regions, according to Euromonitor data, being Asia Pacific (40 %) and Western Europe (29 %). North America is about 14 % of the total market. While developed Asian markets are the largest for skin care as a whole (Japan and South Korea rank #1 and #3 in skin care sales globally), antiaging significantly lags behind in importance there versus whitening products. In Japan, for example, antiaging only accounts for about 10 % of sales, while it exceeds 30 % in the USA and the UK, according to Euromonitor International [8]. Other large developed markets where antiaging is of great importance are France, Australia, Italy, Germany, and Spain.

Now, while all regions have been growing by at least 4 % CAGR from 2001 to 2007, the fastest growth is occurring in developing regions like Latin America and Eastern Europe, both growing at 15–16 % CAGR. At a country level, the BRIC economies (Brazil, Russia, India, and China) are expected to be key drivers of growth for cosmetic products, including antiaging skin care. The growth in Latin America, Eastern Europe, and the BRIC markets is linked to their fast developing economies, where consumer's access to discretionary income and to products (via strengthened retail channels) is rapidly increasing. While these economies are undoubtedly affected by the 2008–2009 recession, growth is expected to slow down but not stop.

China and India are considered the markets with the most potential, driven by their fast growth and large populations. Increased wealth for the prosperous, middle class expansion and exposure to western values are driving significant increases in demand for luxury and lifestyle goods. Antiaging is expected to grow exponentially in these markets, given that their standards of beauty are being significantly influenced by western values. According to Euromonitor, skin care sales in China increased by 132 % from 2002 to 2007, reaching US$5.3 billion. India's growth lags behind China due to foreign investment restrictions, price sensitivity, and lack of modernized infrastructure. In both markets, skin care per capita consumption is still very low, as the affluence and ability to purchase discretionary products is concentrated in the young, urban, educated population.

In Brazil, economic growth is translating into middle class expansion, driving retail sale increases and more access to technology. Importantly, Brazilians are very "beauty involved" and closely associate outer appearance with identity, status, and well-being. All of this bodes very well for skin care products, which grew by 128 % from 2002 to 2007 to reach US$2.6 billion. Similarly, in Russia, economic prosperity is translating into increases in average income and discretionary spending. But unlike in Brazil, where premium skin care sales are very small, urban Russian consumers are willing to splurge in premium brands. Between 2002 and 2007, Russia's skin care sales increased by 106 % to reach US$1.6 billion [9, 10].

There are many other emerging and transition markets – like Ukraine and Vietnam – where skin care is expected to grow significantly in the years ahead, fueled by some of the same dynamics observed in the BRIC countries. Comprehensive reports for these markets are available from business intelligence companies like Euromonitor International.

The key message here is that while the skin care category promises significant growth globally, much of that growth is driven by countries where consumer income and access to products are increasing rapidly – like the BRIC economies. Companies that seek to win globally in the long run must not only play in the big, developed markets but also establish a strong presence in key developing markets.

Key Trend 3: Explosion of New Technologies to Slow or Reverse Aging

Antiaging is among the most dynamic of all cosmetic and toiletry categories when it comes to pace and breadth of innovation. As discussed previously, consumer demand for new and better ways to reverse, delay, and prevent signs of skin aging is high and increasing. This, coupled with significant scientific advances and relentless competitive pressures, ensures that there is never a lull in the category's innovation pipeline. Not all innovation spaces are equal, though. Some meaningfully shift consumers' expectations at large, while others result in specialized niches with fewer but highly committed followers. This section provides an overview of some of the technologies considered most influential.

Ingredients

Most innovations in antiaging skin care are new ingredients, often touted as the next "fountain of youth." While no one has discovered how to stop or reverse aging yet, there are some ingredients that have truly transformed what is possible in antiaging skin care. Some of the most effective ingredients (like retinoids, peptides, and antioxidants) have become the leading skin aging fighters in the industry. Hydroxy acids, vitamins (like B, C, and E), hyaluronic acid, coenzyme Q10, alpha-lipoic acid, and green tea are also among the industry's staples. However, in this ever-changing landscape, there are always new additions. Some recent ones include growth factors, sirtuins, resveratrol, hydroquinone, argireline, dimethylaminoethanol (DMAE), and açai berry.

Providing definitions and benefits for the myriad of antiaging ingredients is beyond the scope of this chapter, but there are resources where this information is readily available. One of the most comprehensive is Paula Begoun's Cosmetic Ingredient Dictionary, accessible via her Cosmetics Cop website (www.cosmeticscop.com). Another good reference is her widely consulted book *Don't Go to the Cosmetics Counter Without Me*.

Beauty Hybrids

While incorporating new ingredients helps manufacturers deliver better skin benefits and build credibility with consumers, companies cannot derive lasting differentiation from them due to low barriers to entry in the industry. In their relentless effort to differentiate their products from competitors and deliver bigger benefits faster, antiaging skin care developers have expanded their reach to ingredients once reserved for professional use only. Similarly, propelled by the desire to partake in the profitable and growing antiaging skin care market, some pharmaceutical companies have begun to develop cosmetic improvement lines. In this process, the once obvious division line between cosmetics and drugs has increasingly become unclear, even to the savviest of consumers.

More recently, a plethora of nutritional supplement and food manufacturers have joined the skin improvement bandwagon. Product descriptors trying to capture the myriad of hybrid possibilities – like cosmeceuticals, nutricosmetics, and nutraceuticals – have become part of the complex category lexicon and offering. The 2006 report "Beauty Drugs: Consumer Perceptions and Blurring Boundaries in the Global Cosmetics and Toiletries Market" by Euromonitor International examines this complex and evolving panorama in depth. The authors depict the landscape in a very simple way, recreated in Fig. 1 [11].

Among these hybrid categories, cosmeceuticals are the best established in most markets, represented by success stories like

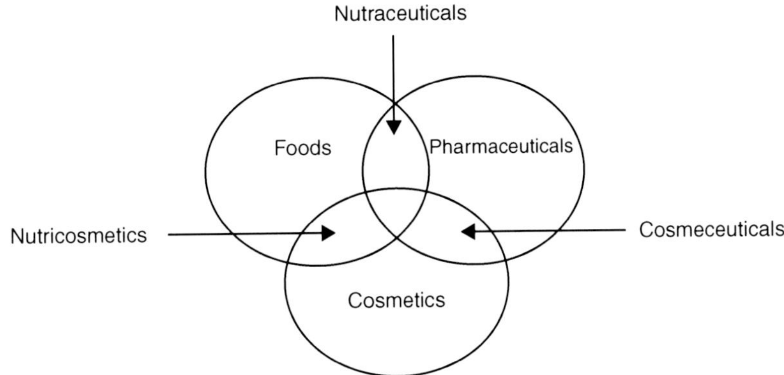

Fig. 1 The evolving landscape in antiaging skin care

StriVectin SD® wrinkle reducer (originally a pharmaceutical product to combat stretch marks) and the myriad of "doctor" or "professional" skin care brands like Murad®, PerriconeMD Cosmeceuticals®, and DDF®. According to a May 2008 online article from Cosmetics Design, citing Kline & Company research, professional skin care is a US$5.9 billion global business, and its growth is outpacing the general market both in the USA and Europe. The report describes the segment as an "explosive opportunity" with strong potential in both developed and developing markets [12].

Nutraceuticals, like foods and drinks including omega-3s and probiotics (live bacteria that offer health benefits), long prevalent in Japan, are increasing in acceptance and popularity. Some examples are the trendy Borba® beauty waters and Danone's highly successful Activia® yogurt line, which according to the Food Industry Report soared past the US$100 million mark in its first year in the USA [13]. Nutricosmetics are also increasing in popularity, fueled by the entry of some big cosmetics and food players like L'Oréal and Nestlé, partners in the creation of Inneov®, a skin and hair care supplement.

From a consumer point of view, the merging of categories, while exciting, causes significant confusion as there is no industry-wide agreement on definitions and players use the same terms in different ways. Aggravating the confusion is the fact that these evolutions do not reflect corresponding changes in legislation, which still regulates drugs, cosmetics, and nutritional supplements separately. For example, the US FDA does not recognize nor has established regulations for "cosmeceuticals." Some of the implications of this lack of regulation will be discussed later in the chapter.

Alternatives to Cosmetic Procedures

According to the American Society of Plastic Surgeons (ASPS), almost 12 million surgery procedures were performed for cosmetic purposes in the USA in 2007, representing a 7 % increase from 2006. This excludes the 5.1 million surgery procedures conducted for reconstructive (non-cosmetic) purposes. The growth was driven by "minimally invasive" procedures, which approached 10 million. The report lists the most popular as Botox® injections (4.6 million, up 13 % from 2006), hyaluronic acid fillers (1.1 million, up 35 %), chemical peels (1 million, down 4 %), laser hair removal (906,000 procedures, up 2 %), and microdermabrasion (897,000 procedures, up 10 %). Almost half (46 %) of these "minimally invasive" procedures were conducted on patients 40–54 years old, 26 % on patients 55 and over, and 91 % of all treated were women [14]. While these are all US statistics, this is certainly not a US-only phenomenon, with cosmetic procedures growing in the double digits across many European, Asian, and Latin American countries.

This dramatic increase in cosmetic procedures has been accompanied by a corresponding rise in topical innovations aimed at mimicking or extending their benefits. Some brands have developed lines that provide topical alternatives for women who are not willing to undergo cosmetic procedures, but want significant skin improvement. Olay's Regenerist™ line, for example, has derived global success behind its "dramatic results without drastic measure" positioning. Other innovations in this area include at-home procedure alternatives like L'Oréal's Dermo Expertise ReFinish™ Micro Dermabrasion Kit and at-home cosmetic devices like Safetox®, which claims to relax forehead wrinkles without injections and retails for 265 €. Another device example is Perricone MD LIGHT Renewal™, which promises to improve skin's texture, tone, and firmness and retails for US$270 on the brand's website.

Development of these kinds of products, as well as versions to help extend benefits after surgery, is expected to continue, mirroring the increased interest in cosmetic procedure benefits. Partnerships between beauty companies and device technology companies are key enablers of these types of developments. For example, Johnson & Johnson (manufacturer of skin care brands like Neutrogena® and Aveeno®) has partnered with Palomar Medical Technologies to develop light-based devices to treat concerns like aging, acne, and cellulite. Procter & Gamble (manufacturer of brands like Olay® and Gillette®) also has an agreement with Palomar to develop light-based hair-removal devices for women and another one with Syneron to develop a noninvasive energy-based device to treat signs of aging. Other big beauty players, like L'Oréal and Estée Lauder, have similar agreements of their own.

Bio-rejuvenation and Customization

Another significant development in antiaging skin care is the emergence of advanced biological treatments beyond the growing use of youth-promoting nanotechnologies, growth factors, and hormone replacement therapies. While many of these advances – like the use of stem cells to regenerate damaged skin, DNA-customized formulas, mitochondria- and enzyme-boosting treatments, neural rejuvenation, and plasma therapies – are still in their infancy and are highly controversial, they are expected to eventually change the way the fight against aging is approached. With advances in longevity science and the use of genomics becoming mainstream among the big beauty companies, it is a matter of time before antiaging products begin to address aging at the most basic biological levels.

Diagnostic tools are also becoming more sophisticated and portable, allowing researchers to customize products and treatments to an individual's skin and even genotype. In response, consumer expectations are increasing, and they are beginning to look for effective, customized treatments and solutions with minimal or no trade-offs in timeliness, affordability, and ease of use. These advances are further accelerating the blurring between cosmetics and pharmaceuticals, and some of them challenge the conceptions of what is going "too far" in the quest for beauty and agelessness.

Advances in ingredient technologies, new approaches, devices, and skin understanding are creating many opportunities for new products and segments that are more profitable. The breadth and depth of these advances can be intimidating. The key is to understand which are most promising and which can be best synergized with one's existing capabilities to deliver better results and breakthrough news in this category where promises abound.

Key Trend 4: Naturals/Organics Go Mainstream

Along with the growth in the use of advance scientific and pharmaceutical ingredients in skin care, there is an opposing trend that rejects synthetic chemicals in beauty products. This trend is reflected in the steady growth of natural/organic personal care products, which often avoid ingredients like parabens and other synthetic preservatives, phthalates (solvents often used in fragrances), silicones, petrochemical derivatives (like mineral oil), sulfates (like sodium lauryl/laureth sulfate), and chemical sunscreens.

According to the UK-based business research and consulting company Organic Monitor, global sales of natural and organic cosmetics approached US$7 billion in 2007, with North America and Western Europe making up for most of the recent double-digit growth [15]. Some of the key drivers of this growth are increasing concerns about chemicals in relationship to health issues like cancer and allergy, growing interest in the environment and social responsibility, increased awareness of the benefits of natural ingredients, and growing natural/organic retailers like The Body Shop, The Organic Pharmacy, and Whole Foods Market.

According to "The Age of Naturals," a 2008 report by The Benchmarking Company, 70 % of US women who buy natural beauty products and 31 % of those who buy traditional beauty products claim to read labels carefully before buying beauty products. The same report also states that 45 % of all US women said that the main reason why they buy natural/organic beauty products is their fear of chemicals. This is particularly true for skin care products, which account for over 40 % of natural/organic personal care product sales [16].

All this has led to a huge proliferation of natural and organic brands, increased investment and innovation by large beauty companies, acceleration in distribution of existing brands in traditional stores like Wal-Mart and Tesco, and explosive growth of cosmetic sales at natural or "green" retailers like Whole Foods and The Body Shop. Globally, some of the leading brands in this highly fragmented segment are Weleda, Burt's Bees, The Body Shop, L'Occitane, and Aveda. One of the beauty giants capitalizing on the segment's growth is L'Oréal, which acquired The Body Shop and Sanoflore, a French organic cosmetic brand, in 2006. In recent years, Estée Lauder has expanded its investment in natural-positioned brands like Origins and Aveda. In addition, even bleach giant Clorox entered this growing market with the acquisition of Burt's Bees natural cosmetics in 2007. Acquisitions like these are expected to continue, as the segment continues to grow and mature.

Two of the key challenges this segment faces are similar to the challenges faced by the hybrid products discussed earlier – lack of clear regulation and consumer confusion. In fact, most products sold as "natural" or "organic" are not purely natural or organic. Many are what some industry insiders call "natural inspired" or "pseudo-natural," meaning a significant portion of their ingredients is synthetic. Truly natural products and "pseudo-natural" products compete side to side, making similar claims, which causes confusion and loss of credibility. Some government standards like the USDA Organic seal in the USA, which requires products to be made with at least 95 % organic ingredients, exist but are not yet commonly adopted. The industry has resorted to self-regulation, evidenced by the growing influence of standards like the ones by France-based EcoCert, UK-based Soil Association, Germany-based BDIH, and US-based OASIS. The industry recognizes the need for a global, cohesive standard, and many talks toward that goal have taken place in recent years.

As noted earlier, environmental sustainability and social responsibility are key motivators for consumers of natural and organic products. This has led to natural/organic and "green" becoming somewhat synonymous in many consumers' minds, even though they are in reality quite distinct. Natural/organic refers to the origin of the ingredients, while "green" refers to the product's reduced impact on the environment. Most natural/organic companies also adopt "green" practices, leading to some of the interchangeability in the use of the terms in the industry. One of the leaders in "green beauty" is Aveda, owned by Estée Lauder. It claims to be the first beauty company to use 100 % wind energy and showcases its ongoing commitment to using organic and sustainable materials behind its "Beauty is as beauty does" campaign. The lack of regulation and clear standards for what is truly "green" is another issue for this industry segment. The industry needs to find a way to manage "greenwashing" (or misrepresentation of a product's environmental friendliness and level of social responsibility) and the resulting tendency of many consumers to distrust or ignore such claims.

One final challenge the natural/organic segment faces is continuing to innovate and deliver bigger and better benefits. While ingredient suppliers constantly improve their ability to extract, formulate, and process natural ingredients for maximum efficacy and reliability, avoiding synthetic ingredients can be limiting. Formulators of natural/organic products are not able to leverage many of the new ingredients and technologies being developed, which is problematic in an industry where having "news" is key to winning.

Despite all the challenges mentioned above, most industry experts agree that natural and organic products are just in their infancy and will continue to grow in popularity. Consumer-led movements like health and wellness and planet sustainability are sure to keep fueling their growth. The key will be for natural/organic manufacturers, as well as conventional manufacturers, to find ways to deliver products that require no compromises – in performance, safety, environmental and social responsibility, and value.

Key Trend 5: Blurring Distribution Channels

Skin care retails in several channels are very distinct from each other. The biggest channel is food/drug/mass (F/D/M), which includes retailers like Kroger and Tesco (food/grocery), Walgreens and Boots (drug stores), and Wal-Mart and Carrefour (mass/hypermarkets). Food/drug/mass stores accounted for 33 % of skin care sales in 2007, according to Euromonitor data. Other large channels are department stores (like Saks and Harrods), direct to consumer (sold through independent representatives like "Avon ladies"), and specialty/perfumery outlets like Sephora. Globally, only F/D/M and the still small E-Commerce channel are growing, as shown in Table 1.

The retail landscape varies dramatically across markets. In some regions, like Latin America and Eastern Europe, the direct model is predominant, while specialty/perfumery retailers are particularly strong in Europe, and F/D/M brands generate the most sales in the USA. However, as with other areas in this highly competitive business, the lines between channels are beginning to become blurry [17], as demonstrated by the examples below:

Table 1 Share of global skin care market by channel

Channel	2001 (%)	2007 (%)
Food/drug/mass (F/D/M)	31	33
Department stores	17	17
Direct to consumer	18	17
Specialty/perfumery	16	14
Pharmacy	7	7
E-Commerce	2	3
Others	10	9

Source: Internal Procter & Gamble Skin Care report citing Euromonitor International data

- Some brands like Olay® play in F/D/M only in the USA but in both F/D/M and department stores in China and in some European countries.
- Some brands, like Origins, previously only sold in department and specialty stores, are now available at mass retailers like Target in the USA.
- Other brands, like La Roche-Posay® and Vichy®, are sold in dermatologist's offices in some countries, in pharmacies in others, and now in some drug stores in the USA.
- Avon® entered China as a direct business, given the government's lift of its direct-selling ban in 2006, but is also offering their products in new Avon Specialty Stores.
- Some F/D/M retailers are establishing their own beauty specialty stores (like Shoppers Drug Mart's Murale in Canada and CVS's Beauty 360 in the USA), offering a wide selection of premium products, expert advice, and skin diagnosis.
- Some specialty chains, like Ulta in the USA, compete by purposely crossing the boundaries between channels and offering what its website calls "one-stop shopping for prestige, mass and salon products, and salon services."

While department stores' share of the market remained stable between 2001 and 2007 at 17 %, there is a growing concern among department store-only companies, as consumers continue to look for the best value for their money. The biggest players in that channel (brands like Shiseido® and Estée Lauder®) are losing share to F/D/M brands like Olay® and direct brands like Avon®.

At the same time, there is a growing presence of high-end brands in the Internet and in TV home-shopping channels (like QVC), which diverts traffic from brick-and-mortar department stores.

However, some department store chains are also innovating and contributing to the blurring of channels, as evidenced by the recently announced partnership between the US upscale department store chain Bloomingdales and the UK-based specialty store chain Space NK. Consumers looking for the luxurious apothecary experience and unbiased expert advice of Space NK will soon find it inside select Bloomingdales stores in the USA. In another interesting twist in this increasingly blurred panorama, the Sonia Kashuk brand, previously only sold at mass merchandiser Target, will now be offered at some of the Space NK sites, including the one at Bloomingdales' 59th street flagship store in Manhattan. The line between mass and luxury has never been less clear.

The expected growth of E-Commerce is likely to add interest to all these dynamics, as brands from all channels are strengthening their online selling efforts. Internet sales are particularly important for natural/organic brands and for small niche brands, which choose to not participate in traditional channels or do not have enough scale to secure distribution at brick-and-mortar retailers.

No one knows where the division lines between channels will stop moving – or if there will be any solid lines at all. But one thing is for sure: this industry will never be the same again. Any company trying to win in or enter this business needs to embrace that and evolve its business, retail, and innovation models accordingly.

Key Trend 6: Simultaneous Globalization and Regionalization

Globalization, the process by which regional or local norms and behaviors become global, has become a major buzzword in the business world. It is evident that the world is becoming more connected and multicultural. Nations geographically "worlds apart" can have tremendous financial and cultural influence on each other. However, in some ways globalization may be an overstatement, as regional and local differences remain critically important. In the world of beauty, a piece of evidence for globalization and multiculturalism is the ethnic and nationality diversity of some of today's most celebrated beauties, including Halle Berry, Penelope Cruz, Zhang Ziyi, Nicole Kidman, and Freida Pinto. However, at the same time, it is undeniable that ethnic and cultural norms continue to play a key role in standards of beauty, as evidenced by the importance of skin-whitening products in Asia and the preference for natural ingredients in Latin America.

Globalization is also evident in the growth of many multinational beauty brands, like L'Oréal, which often successfully market the same products and use the same spokeswomen and models across regions. However, these companies also hire people from the key regions where they compete, to ensure that local customs and needs are properly accounted for. Many of them have regional brands that cater to specific regions, and all customize their communications to ensure they speak to the mind-set of the specific consumers they serve. Not doing so would result in sure failure eventually, as consumers expect products and messages to speak to them and their circumstances, not to an "averaged out" global prime prospect or foreign version of themselves.

Another important aspect of globalization is consumer's ability to influence one another across the Internet, even if they are physically "worlds apart." A satisfied consumer in China, blogging in English, can influence the skin care-purchasing decisions of thousands of consumers across the world. This, however, does not deny the importance of local endorsement from trusted people and organizations in each consumer's home country. Furthermore, changes in industry governance and legislation in one key region or country influence other regions, but they are ultimately managed at the country level. Failure to properly account for these simultaneous dynamics can be devastating for a brand or business.

None of this is to imply that global success cannot be achieved with one cohesive initiative. Some propositions manage to find the important "sweet spot" of global appeal and regional relevance. As an example, Olay® was able to capitalize on the universal consumer desire for better value with the launch of Olay Regenerist® Micro-Sculpting Cream, which promised better results than US$350 creams for under US$30 and backed the claim via an independent study by the reputable Good Housekeeping Institute. The product quickly rose to the #1 position in skin care sales across the USA, followed by highly successful regional adaptations for diverse countries like China, the UK, Spain, Germany, and Australia.

The key takeaway from this trend is that to win in antiaging skin care, at a multinational level, one must think globally but act locally. Thinking globally enables understanding of key consumer trends, development of economies of scale, and reapplication of learning from one market to another. Acting locally ensures that products and messages are customized enough to meet the unique needs of each market that regional opportunities are best leveraged and that local regulations and constraints are properly managed. It is indeed both a global and a regional world.

Key Trend 7: Evolving Regulations and Industry Governance

As discussed earlier, the skin care industry has evolved and innovated beyond the scope of most current regulatory systems. Hybrid products that challenge the boundaries between cosmetics, pharmaceuticals, and nutritional supplements and the growing number of claims for natural/organic products demand further regulation. Globalization and the Internet create the need for common standards across regions. Global brands can significantly benefit from cohesive standards that can enable product development and marketing, and the Internet makes products available globally – crossing regulatory lines – almost instantly.

Given that foods and drugs are regulated by government agencies, like the FDA in the USA, regulations involving these categories are managed via complex processes and often take a long time. However, consumer and public concerns with the safety and environmental friendliness of chemicals used in cosmetics are prompting changes expected to result in regulatory reform over the next 10 years. The European Union is implementing new chemical regulations under its REACH program. According to the website of the European Chemical Agency (www.echa.europa.eu), which manages the program, "REACH places greater responsibility on industry to manage the risks that chemicals may pose to the health and the environment [18]." Other countries are also increasing regulation of chemicals in cosmetic products based on their potential environmental effect, as seen with Canada's recent call out of siloxanes as concerning.

In the USA, California has been a leader in state-level regulation, with the approval of its Safe Cosmetics Act that banned potentially carcinogenic ingredients several years ago and a 2008 bill that regulates "non-green" chemicals. Other states like Massachusetts, New Jersey, and Minnesota are following suit with bills of their own. Nationwide, the FDA is looking to increase oversight of cosmetics through provisions in the proposed FDA Globalization Act. Nongovernmental organizations like the Environmental Working Group (EWG) and the Campaign for Safe Cosmetics are also very influential through efforts like EWG's Skin Deep ingredient database, which rates the potential dangers of substances in cosmetic products. Advertising boards, like the National Advertising Division (NAD) in the USA, also play a key governance role, as they ensure advertising claims are valid, not exaggerated, and not misleading to consumers. Because they are not bound to a certain type of product or standard, the governance efforts of these boards reach across product lines and include cosmetics, nutritional supplements, drugs, and all the hybrids in between.

In the case of natural/organic products, government involvement is still relatively limited. In the European Union, several industry-led standards coexist, including the UK-based Soil Association, Germany-based BDIH, Brussels-based NaTrue, and France-based EcoCert. In the USA, some companies have adopted the government-led

USDA's standard for organic products, which is very stringent and not specific to personal care. The Natural Products Association has created its own standard for natural products and, more recently, NSF International, a not-for-profit public health and safety-certifying organization, introduced another one. The NSF standard is the first one approved by the American National Standards Institute for personal care products made with organic ingredients [19].

At the same time, a group of key industry players – including L'Oréal, Estée Lauder, and other smaller companies like Juice Beauty – collaborated to create the Organic and Sustainability Industry Standards (OASIS) organic seal. Other groups – like Toronto-based Certech Registration, personal care brand Burt's Bees, and even retailer Whole Foods – have also developed their own standards. The degree of stringency varies widely across these standards, with some like the USDA being very strict, while others are considered lax by many in the industry. The Organic Consumers Association offers a comparison of these standards, for anyone interested in understanding them in a bit more detail. The article entitled "Comparing USDA & EU 'Organic,' 'Made with Organic' & 'Natural' Standards on Body Care Products" was written by David Bronner (president of the all-natural, organic soap brand Dr. Bronner's Soaps) and is available at www.organicconsumers.org [20].

In terms of harmonization of standards, there has been much effort toward that goal in recent years. Some of the European agencies have been working for several years to agree to one EU-wide standard, and some groups are collaborating for harmonization across the Atlantic. Unfortunately, a common standard has not yet been established. To help ease consumer concern and confusion in this environment, some personal care industry trade organizations, like the Personal Care Products Council (PCPC), are making safety and regulatory information available to consumers through their websites.

There are two potential outcomes of this situation. The less desirable scenario is that the proliferation causes enough confusion that it invalidates some of the benefits of all standards. If, in the worst case of this scenario, the different standards are carried into regulations, global trade and economies of scale will be significantly hindered. The more desirable, and arguable more likely, outcome is that a multi-region standard is agreed upon. This would simplify innovation and accreditation for manufacturers and certifying agencies, reduce consumer confusion and skepticism, and limit the ability of imitators to make the same claims as legitimate products. Consumers, manufacturers, and governments would all benefit.

It is evident that evolutions in the governance and regulatory environment can have a huge impact in the skin care business, its consumers, and its members. Changes could be very positive for some and very negative for others, depending on what course governance and regulations take and how equally and consistently they are applied. On one hand, unambiguous standards can result in clearer criteria for researchers and manufacturers, simplifying their processes and mitigating their risks. Consumer concern and confusion would also be significantly reduced. On the other hand, increased regulations can mean stricter controls, more complex testing requirements, technology limitations, longer development times, and higher costs for all. Staying current and, where possible, actively participating in these discussions are critical for any skin care company that wants to win in this changing environment.

Conclusion

Diving into the trends driving antiaging skin care globally is a complex undertaking, and trying to forecast the industry's future can be a bit daunting. However, a good understanding of the seven trends discussed in this chapter should provide a good foundation and hopefully help inspire further studies. And some things are fairly certain. The exciting antiaging skin care category is only going to get more interesting and rewarding, as people continue to live longer and lead more active lives, different approaches in health and antiaging gain momentum, competition sparks imagination and better solutions, new retail models emerge, new technologies break the limitations of current paradigms, and consumers throughout the world prosper and reach for higher standards in beauty and in life. The role of regulators will be to continue to safeguard consumer's safety and interests, without delaying progress in the quest to look and feel our best.

Cross-References

▶ Marketing and Product Design of Antiaging Skin Care Products

References

1. All data not otherwise credited sourced from Euromonitor International Passport: Cosmetics & Toiletries. Euromonitor International. 2001–2008.
2. Category watch: naturals and cosmeceuticals point to the future of skin care. Euromonitor International. 19 Sep 2008.
3. Global cosmetics and toiletries: facing tougher times ahead. Euromonitor International. Nov 2008.
4. Rank order – life expectancy at birth. Central Intelligence Agency. The World Factbook. Accessed 8 Feb 2009. www.cia.gov/library/publications/the-world-factbook/index.html
5. QuickStats: life expectancy at birth, by race and sex – United States, 1970–2005. US Center for Disease Control. MMWR Weekly. 2008. Accessed 8 Feb 2009. www.cdc.gov/mmwr/preview/mmwrhtml/mm5651a7.htm
6. Boomers, the generation that could and will. Procter & Gamble Healthcare Consumer Institute, 2008.
7. LOHAS Background. LOHAS Online. Accessed 22 Feb 2009. www.lohas.com/about.html
8. Kirillov A. Category watch: cosmeceuticals lead the anti-ageing market. Euromonitor International. 18 Apr 2008.
9. Lee V. Category watch: five trends driving the global skin care market. Euromonitor International. 3 Sep 2008.
10. 25 global consumer trends 2008: back to basics – it's still the old economy in a cool climate. Euromonitor International. June 2008.
11. Beauty drugs: consumer perceptions and blurring boundaries in the global cosmetics and toiletries market. Euromonitor International. Dec 2007.
12. Montague-Jones G. Professional skin care market booms. Cosmetics Design.Com. 16 May 2008. Accessed 28 Feb 2009. www.cosmeticsdesign.com/content/view/print/64205
13. In the Year since the Dannon Company Introduced Activia, Sales in U.S. Stores Soared Well Past the $100 Million Mark. The Food Industry Report excerpt in Goliath. 29 Jan 2007. Accessed 25 Jan 2009. http://goliath.ecnext.com/coms2/gi_0199-6262827/In-the-year-since-the.html.
14. 2008 Report of the 2007 Statistics. American Society of Plastic Surgeons. Procedural Statistics Press Kit. Accessed 8 Feb 2009. www.plasticsurgery.org/Media/Press_Kits/Procedural_Statistics.html
15. Global Natural Cosmetic Sales Approaching US$7 Billion. Organic Monitor. Research News. 17 Sep 2007. Accessed 7 Feb 2009. www.organicmonitor.com/r1709.htm
16. The Age of Naturals. The Benchmarking Company. Online Report Overview. 2007. Accessed 8 Feb 2009. www.benchmarkingco.com/pinkreports.html
17. Lee V. Category watch: competition is heating in global anti-ageing. Euromonitor International. 27 May 2008.
18. About REACH. European Chemicals Agency. REACH Guidance. Accessed 15 Mar 2009. http://guidance.echa.europa.eu/about_reach_en.htm
19. Montague-Jones G. NSF's "Made with Organic" Standard becomes an American National Standard. Cosmetics Design.Com. 19 Feb 2009. Accessed 15 Mar 2009. www.cosmeticsdesign.com/content/view/print/237118
20. Bronner D. Comparing USDA & EU "Organic," "Made with Organic" & "Natural" Standards on body care products. Organic Consumers Association. 2008. Accessed 9 Mar 2009. www.organicconsumers.org/articles/article_15106.cfm

Index

M.A. Farage et al. (eds.), *Textbook of Aging Skin*,
DOI 10.1007/978-3-662-47398-6

B

I

J

K

L

O

P

W

X